W9-DIE-729

Textbook of SMALL ANIMAL SURGERY

Second Edition

Douglas Slatter, B.V.Sc., M.S., Ph.D., F.R.C.V.S.
Diplomate, American College of Veterinary Surgeons
Diplomate, American College of Veterinary Ophthalmologists

Volume II

W.B. SAUNDERS COMPANY
A Division of Harcourt Brace & Company
Philadelphia London Toronto Montreal Sydney Tokyo

W.B. SAUNDERS COMPANY
A Division of
Harcourt Brace & Company

The Curtis Center
Independence Square West
Philadelphia, Pennsylvania 19106

Library of Congress Cataloging-in-Publication Data

Textbook of small animal surgery / edited by Douglas Slatter.
— 2nd ed.

p. cm.

Includes bibliographical references and index.

ISBN 0-7216-8330-4 (set)

1. Veterinary surgery. I. Slatter, Douglas II. Title: Small animal surgery.

SF911.T49 1993

636.089'7—dc20 92-21883

Textbook of Small Animal Surgery, Second Edition

ISBN Volume I 0-7216-8328-2
Volume II 0-7216-8329-0
Two Volume set 0-7216-8330-4

Printed in the United States of America.

Last digit is the print number: 9 8 7 6 5 4 3

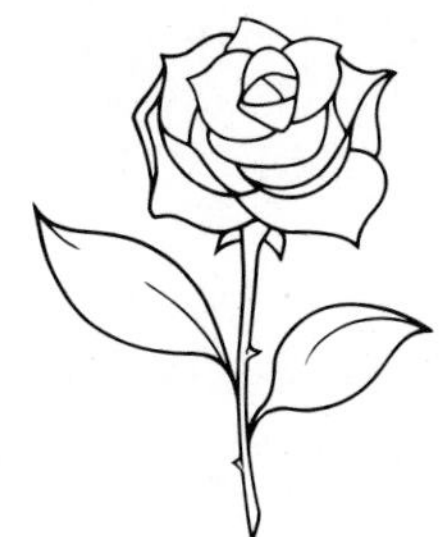

To:
Edith and Horton, my parents
Elizabeth, my wife and colleague
Christine and Diane, my daughters

Section Editors

SECTION	SECTION EDITORS
Surgical Biology	Eberhard Rosin
Surgical Methods	David Holmberg
Skin and Adnexa	Michael M. Pavletic
Body Cavities & Hernias	Christopher Bellenger
Gastrointestinal System	David T. Matthiesen
Respiratory System	A. Wendell Nelson
Cardiovascular System	George E. Eyster
Hemolymphatic System	Gary W. Ellison
Nervous System	Howard B. Seim III
Eye and Adnexa	Douglas Slatter
Reproductive System	Elizabeth Arnold Stone
Urinary System	Dale E. Bjorling
Endocrine System	Thomas D. Scavelli
Ear	Howard B. Seim III
Musculoskeletal System	Philip B. Vasseur and Douglas Slatter
Oncology	Dennis D. Caywood
Anesthesia	Richard M. Bednarski and William W. Muir III
Dentistry	Albert S. Dorn

Contributors

Sarah K. Abood, D.V.M.
Clinical Instructor and Resident, Clinical Nutrition of Large and Small Animals, Veterinary Teaching Hospital, Ohio State University, Columbus, Ohio.
Nutritional Support of Hospitalized Patients

Lorel K. Anderson, D.V.M.
Associate Professor, Department of Small Animal Clinical Sciences, College of Veterinary Medicine, and Clinical Veterinarian, Department of Cardiology, Veterinary Teaching Hospital, Michigan State University, East Lansing, Michigan.
Surgical Anatomy; Diagnostic Methods

Lawrence W. Anson, D.V.M.
Diplomate, American College of Veterinary Surgeons. Staff Surgeon, Veterinary Referral Clinic, Cleveland, Ohio
Emergency Management of Fractures

Michael Aronsohn, V.M.D.
Diplomate, American College of Veterinary Surgeons. Director of Surgery, Angell Memorial Animal Hospital, Boston, Massachusetts.
Large Intestine

Rodney S. Bagley, D.V.M.
Resident, Department of Neurology, School of Veterinary Medicine, North Carolina State University, Raleigh, North Carolina, and Assistant Professor, Department of Veterinary Clinical Medicine and Surgery, College of Veterinary Medicine, Washington State University, Pullman, Washington.
Central Nervous System

Claudia J. Baldwin, D.V.M., M.S.
Diplomate, American College of Veterinary Internal Medicine. Assistant Professor, Department of Veterinary Clinical Sciences, College of Veterinary Medicine, Iowa State University, Ames, Iowa.
Hemostasis: Physiology, Diagnosis, and Treatment of Bleeding Disorders in Surgical Patients

R. Randy Basinger, D.V.M.
Diplomate, American College of Veterinary Surgeons. South Carolina Surgical Referral Service, Columbia, South Carolina.
The Prostate

Michael S. Bauer, D.V.M.
Diplomate, American College of Veterinary Surgeons. Assistant Professor of Small Animal Surgery, Department of Veterinary Clinical Sciences, School of Veterinary Medicine, Purdue University, West Lafayette, Indiana.
Basic Operative Techniques; Intervertebral Disc Disease

Gary B. Beard, D.V.M.
Diplomate, American Veterinary Dental College. Assistant Dean for Continuing Education, College of Veterinary Medicine, Auburn University, Auburn, Alabama.
Occlusion and Orthodontics

Richard M. Bednarski, D.V.M., M.S.
Diplomate, American College of Veterinary Anesthesiologists. Associate Professor, Department of Veterinary Clinical Sciences, College of Veterinary Medicine, Ohio State University, Columbus, Ohio.
Equipment and Techniques for Inhalation Anesthesia; Section Editor: Section 17, Anesthetic Considerations in Surgery

Jamie R. Bellah, D.V.M.
Diplomate, American College of Veterinary Surgeons. Associate Professor of Surgery, College of Veterinary Medicine, and Chief, Small Animal Surgery Service, Department of Small Animal Clinical Sciences, Veterinary Medical Teaching Hospital, University of Florida, Gainesville, Florida.
Surgical Management of Specific Skin Disorders; The Thymus

Christopher R. Bellenger, B.V.Sc., Ph.D., F.A.C.V.Sc.
Associate Professor of Veterinary Surgery, and Head, Department of Veterinary Clinical Sciences, University of Sydney, Sydney, New South Wales, Australia.
Abdominal Wall; Hernias; Perineal Hernia; Section Editor: Section 4, Body Cavities and Hernias

John Berg, D.V.M., M.S.
Diplomate, American College of Veterinary Surgeons. Associate Professor of Surgery, Tufts University School of Veterinary Medicine, North Grafton, Massachusetts.
Sterilization

C. W. Betts, D.V.M.
Diplomate, American College of Veterinary Surgeons. Professor of Surgery, College of Veterinary Medicine, and Surgery Service Chief, Veterinary Teaching Hospital, North Carolina State University, Raleigh, North Carolina.
Pelvic Fractures

Stephen J. Birchard, D.V.M., M.S.
Diplomate, American College of Veterinary Surgeons. Associate Professor, Department of Veterinary Clinical Sciences, Ohio State University, Columbus, Ohio.
Adrenalectomy

Stephen I. Bistner, D.V.M.
Diplomate, American College of Veterinary Ophthalmologists. Professor, Comparative Ophthalmology, School of Veterinary Medicine, University of Minnesota, St. Paul, Minnesota.
Ocular Emergencies and Trauma; Eye and Orbit

Dale E. Bjorling, D.V.M., M.S.
Diplomate, American College of Veterinary Surgeons. Associate Professor and Chair, Department of Surgical Sciences, School of Veterinary Medicine, University of Wisconsin, Madison, Wisconsin.
Peritoneum and Peritoneal Cavity; Pathophysiology and Therapeutics of Urinary Tract Disorders; Principles of Urinary Tract Surgery; Kidneys; Ureters; Section Editor: Section 12, Urinary System

Mark Bloomberg, D.V.M., M.S.
Diplomate, American College of Veterinary Surgeons. Professor and Chairman, Department of Small Animal Clinical Sciences, College of Veterinary Medicine; Chief of Staff, Small Animal Surgery, Veterinary Medical Teaching Hospital; and Director, Center for Veterinary Sports Medicine, University of Florida, Gainesville, Florida.
Muscles and Tendons

Julia Blue, D.V.M., Ph.D.
Associate Professor of Clinical Pathology, College of Veterinary Medicine, Cornell University, Ithaca, New York.
Spleen

E. G. Boone, D.V.M.
Adjunct Professor, Department of Veterinary Clinical Medicine, College of Veterinary Medicine, University of Illinois, Urbana, Illinois, and Staff Surgeon, Animal Surgical Services, Lisle, Illinois.
Fractures of the Tibia and Fibula

Harry W. Boothe, D.V.M., M.S.
Diplomate, American College of Veterinary Surgeons. Professor of Surgery, Department of Small Animal Medicine and Surgery, College of Veterinary Medicine, and Professor of Surgery, Veterinary Teaching Hospital, Small Animal Clinic, Texas A&M University, College Station, Texas.
Suture Materials, Tissue Adhesives, Staplers and Ligating Clips; Testes and Epididymides; Penis, Prepuce, and Scrotum

Adele L. Boskey, Ph.D.
Professor, Biochemistry, Cornell University Medical College, and Director, Laboratory for Ultrastructural Biochemistry, The Hospital for Special Surgery, New York, New York.
Connective Tissues of the Musculoskeletal System

Kenneth C. Bovèe, D.V.M., M.Med.Sc.
Professor of Medicine, School of Veterinary Medicine, University of Pennsylvania, Philadelphia, Pennsylvania.
Pathophysiology and Therapeutics of Urinary Tract Disorders

Kyle G. Braund, B.V.Sc., Ph.D., F.R.C.V.S.
Diplomate, American College of Veterinary Internal Medicine (Neurology). Professor and Director of Neuromuscular Laboratory, Scott-Ritchey Research Center, College of Veterinary Medicine, Auburn University, Auburn, Alabama.
Neurologic Examination and Localization

William R. Brawner, Jr., D.V.M., Ph.D.
Diplomate, American College of Veterinary Radiology. Assistant Professor, Department of Radiology, College of Veterinary Medicine, Auburn University, Auburn, Alabama.
Neuroradiology

William G. Brewer, Jr., D.V.M.
Diplomate, American College of Veterinary Internal Medicine (Oncology). Assistant Professor, Internal Medicine, College of Veterinary Medicine, Auburn University, Auburn, Alabama.
Skin and Subcutis

Alan H. Brightman II, D.V.M., M.S.
Diplomate, American College of Veterinary Ophthalmologists. Professor, Department of Clinical Sciences, College of Veterinary Medicine, Kansas State University, Manhattan, Kansas.
Eyelids

Scott A. Brown, V.M.D., Ph.D.
Assistant Professor, Department of Physiology, College of Veterinary Medicine, University of Georgia, Athens, Georgia.
Physiology of the Urinary Tract

Kenneth A. Bruecker, D.V.M., M.S.
Diplomate, American College of Veterinary Surgeons. Staff Surgeon, Veterinary Medical and Surgical Group, Ventura, California.
Caudal Cervical Spondylomyelopathy; Spinal Fractures and Luxations

C. A. Tony Buffington, D.V.M., Ph.D.
Diplomate, American College of Veterinary Internal Medicine (Neurology). Assistant Professor, College of Veterinary Medicine, Ohio State University, Columbus, Ohio.
Nutritional Support of Hospitalized Patients; Feline Urological Syndrome

Rhondda B. Canfield, B.V.Sc., Ph.D.
Professional Officer, Department of Veterinary Anatomy, University of Sydney, Sydney, New South Wales, Australia.
Perineal Hernia

Charles G. Cantrell, V.M.D.
Practitioner, Malvern, Pennsylvania.
Ovary and Uterus

Dennis D. Caywood, D.V.M., M.S.
Diplomate, American College of Veterinary Surgeons. Professor, Small Animal Surgery, College of Veterinary Medicine, University of Minnesota, St. Paul, Minnesota.
Urinary System; Section Editor: Section 16, Oncology

Irshad H. Chaudry, Ph.D.
Professor of Surgery and Physiology, Director of Surgical Research, Department of Surgery, College of Medicine, Michigan State University, East Lansing, Michigan.
Shock; Pathophysiology and Management of Hypovolemia and Sepsis

Bruce A. Christie, B.V.Sc., M.V.Sc.
Diplomate, American College of Veterinary Surgeons. Senior Associate, School of Veterinary Science, and Senior Registrar (part time), Veterinary Clinic and Hospital, University of Melbourne, Werribee, Victoria, Australia.
Anatomy of the Urinary Tract; Principles of Urinary Tract Surgery; Kidneys; Ureters

Cynthia S. Cook, D.V.M., Ph.D.
Diplomate, American College of Veterinary Ophthalmologists. Research Assistant Professor, Department of Growth and Development, School of Veterinary Medicine, University of California, San Francisco, California, and Ophthalmologist, Veterinary Vision, San Mateo, California.
Iris and Ciliary Body

James R. Cook, Jr., D.V.M., Ph.D.
Diplomate, American College of Veterinary Internal Medicine (Neurology). Staff Neurologist, Animal Emergency and Referral Center, Fort Pierce, Florida
Electrodiagnosis

Susan M. Cotter, D.V.M.
Diplomate, American College of Veterinary Internal Medicine. Professor, Medicine, School of Veterinary Medicine, Tufts University, North Grafton, Massachusetts.
The Hematopoietic System

Rick L. Cowell, D.V.M., M.S.
Diplomate, American College of Veterinary Pathologists. Associate Professor, Clinical Pathology, College of Veterinary Medicine, and Director of Clinical Pathology, Boren Veterinary Medical Teaching Hospital, Oklahoma State University, Stillwater, Oklahoma.
The Hematopoietic System; Hemostasis: Physiology, Diagnosis, and Treatment of Bleeding Disorders in Surgical Patients

Stephen W. Crane, D.V.M.
Diplomate, American College of Veterinary Surgeons. Adjunct Professor of Surgery, College of Veterinary Medicine, North Carolina State University, Raleigh, North Carolina.
Surgical Lasers

Dennis T. Crowe, Jr., D.V.M.
Diplomate, American College of Veterinary Surgeons. Director, Surgery and Nutritional Support Services, Animal Emergency Center, and Director of Research, Veterinary Institute of Trauma, Emergency, and Critical Care, Milwaukee, Wisconsin.
Peritoneum and Peritoneal Cavity

Michael B. Curtis, D.V.M., Ph.D.
Diplomate, American College of Veterinary Anesthesiologists. Assistant Professor, Department of Companion Animals, and Section Chief, Department of Anesthesiology, Atlantic Veterinary College, University of Prince Edward Island, Charlottetown, Prince Edward Island, Canada
Anesthesia for Gastrointestinal Surgery

William R. Daly, D.V.M.
Diplomate, American College of Veterinary Surgeons. Surgeon, Houston Veterinary Referral Surgery Service, Houston, Texas.
Surgical Wound Infection and Use of Antibiotics

Thomas K. Day, D.V.M., M.S.
Assistant Professor, Department of Anesthesiology, College of Veterinary Medicine, Mississippi State University, Mississippi State, Mississippi.
Anesthesia for Elective Soft-Tissue and Orthopedic Procedures

Charles E. DeCamp, D.V.M., M.S.
Associate Professor, Department of Small Animal Clinical Sciences, College of Veterinary Medicine, and Chief, Small Animal Surgery, Veterinary Medical Center, Michigan State University, East Lansing, Michigan.
External Coaptation

Jon F. Dee, D.V.M., M.S.
Diplomate, American College of Veterinary Surgeons. Partner and Staff Surgeon, Hollywood Animal Hospital, Hollywood, Florida.
Tarsus and Metatarsus

David J. DeYoung, D.V.M.
Diplomate, American College of Veterinary Surgeons, and Diplomate, American College of Veterinary Anesthesiologists. Associate Professor of Surgery, Department of Companion Animal and Special Species Medicine, College of Veterinary Medicine, and Orthopedic Surgeon, Veterinary Teaching Hospital, North Carolina State University, Raleigh, North Carolina.
Methods of Internal Fracture Fixation

S. P. DiBartola, D.V.M.
Professor of Medicine, Department of Veterinary Clinical Sciences, College of Veterinary Medicine, and Internist, Veterinary Teaching Hospital, Ohio State University, Columbus, Ohio.
Feline Urological Syndrome

Albert S. Dorn, D.V.M., M.S.
Diplomate, American College of Veterinary Surgeons. Professor of Surgery, Department of Urban Practice, College of Veterinary Medicine, University of Tennessee, Knoxville, Tennessee.
Dental Extractions and Complications; Introduction to Veterinary Dentistry; Section Editor: Section 18, Dentistry

Steven W. Dow, D.V.M., M.S.
Special Assistant Professor, Department of Pathology, College of Veterinary Medicine and Biomedical Sciences, Colorado State University, Fort Collins, Colorado.
Surgical Wound Infection and Use of Antibiotics

Mary L. Dulisch, D.V.M., M.S.
Diplomate, American College of Veterinary Surgeons. Staff Surgeon, Angell Memorial Animal Hospital, Boston, Massachusetts.
Lymphatics, Lymph Nodes, and Tonsils

Erick L. Egger, D.V.M.
Diplomate, American College of Veterinary Surgeons. Associate Professor of Surgery, College of Veterinary Medicine and Biomedical Sciences, and Orthopedic Surgeon, Veterinary Teaching Hospital, Colorado State University, Collins, Colorado.
External Skeletal Fixation; Fractures of the Radius and Ulna; Skull and Mandibular Fractures

A. D. Elkins, D.V.M., M.S.
Assistant Professor, School of Veterinary Medicine, Louisiana State University, Baton Rouge, Louisiana, and Surgeon and Owner, Indiana Surgical Referral Service, Indianapolis, Indiana.
External Skeletal Fixation

Gary W. Ellison, D.V.M., M.S.
Diplomate, American College of Veterinary Surgeons. Associate Professor, Department of Small Animal Clinical Sciences, College of Veterinary Medicine, University of Florida, Gainesville, Florida.
Section Editor: Section 8, Hemolymphatic System

A. Thomas Evans, D.V.M., M.S.
Diplomate, American College of Veterinary Anesthesiologists. Associate Professor of Anesthesia, College of Veterinary Medicine, and Section Chief, Anesthesia Veterinary Medical Center, Michigan State University, East Lansing, Michigan.
Common Complications and Anesthetic Emergencies

George E. Eyster, V.M.D., M.S.
Diplomate, American College of Veterinary Surgeons. Professor, College of Veterinary Medicine, and Staff Surgeon, Veterinary Clinical Center, Michigan State University, East Lansing, Michigan.
Cardiac Disorders; Basic Cardiac Surgical Procedures; Section Editor: Section 7, Cardiovascular System

Daniel A. Feeney, D.V.M., M.S.
Diplomate, American College of Veterinary Radiology. Professor of Comparative Radiology, College of Veterinary Medicine, and Radiologist, Veterinary Teaching Hospital, University of Minnesota, St. Paul, Minnesota.
Radiation Therapy

James M. Fingeroth, D.V.M., B.S.
Diplomate, American College of Veterinary Surgeons. Chief of Surgery, Veterinary Specialists of Rochester, Pittsford Animal Hospital, Rochester, New York.
The Esophagus

Roger B. Fingland, D.V.M., M.S.
Diplomate, College of Veterinary Surgeons. Assistant Professor, College of Veterinary Medicine, Kansas State University, Manhattan, Kansas.
Surgical Diseases of the Endocrine Pancreas

James A. Flanders, D.V.M.
Diplomate, American College of Veterinary Surgeons. Associate Professor, Department of Clinical Sciences, Section of Surgery, New York State College of Veterinary Medicine, Cornell University, Ithaca, New York.
Parathyroid Gland

Theresa W. Fossum, D.V.M., M.S.
Diplomate, American College of Veterinary Surgeons. Assistant Professor, Department of Small Animal Medicine and Surgery, Texas A&M University, College Station, Texas.
Lymphatics, Lymph Nodes, and Tonsils; Respiratory System

C. L. Fries, D.V.M., D.V.Sc.
Diplomate, American College of Veterinary Surgeons. Associate Professor, Department of Veterinary Anesthesiology, Radiology and Surgery, Western College of Veterinary Medicine, University of Saskatchewan, Saskatoon, Saskatchewan, Canada.
Assessment and Preparation of the Surgical Patient

Cathy E. Gaber, D.V.M., M.S.
Private Practitioner, Bath, Michigan
Cardiac Disorders

James S. Gaynor, D.V.M., M.S.
Assistant Professor, Department of Anesthesiology, College of Veterinary Medicine and Biomedical Sciences, Colorado State University, Fort Collins, Colorado.
Anesthesia for Elective Soft-Tissue and Orthopedic Procedures

Stephen D. Gilson, D.V.M.
Diplomate, American College of Veterinary Surgeons. Staff Surgeon, Sōnōra Veterinary Surgery and Oncology, Scottsdale, Arizona.
Cesarean Section

Ira M. Gourley, D.V.M., Ph.D.
Professor (retired), Department of Surgery, School of Veterinary Medicine, University of California, Davis, California.
Organ Transplantation in Clinical Veterinary Practice

John Grandage, B.Vet.Med., D.V.R.
Associate Professor of Anatomy, School of Veterinary Studies, Murdoch University, Perth, Western Australia.
Functional Anatomy of the Digestive System; Functional Anatomy

Gregory F. Grauer, D.V.M., M.S.
Diplomate, American College of Veterinary Internal Medicine. Associate Professor, Department of Clinical Sciences, College of Veterinary Medicine and Biomedical Sciences, and Staff Internist, Veterinary Teaching Hospital, Colorado State University, Fort Collins, Colorado.
Medical Treatment of Canine Uroliths

Raymond T. Greer, Ph.D.
Professor of Aerospace Engineering and Engineering Mechanics, Iowa State University, Ames, Iowa.
Biomaterials

Clare R. Gregory, D.V.M.
Diplomate, American College of Veterinary Surgeons. Associate Professor, Department of Surgery, School of Veterinary Medicine, University of California, Davis, California.
Organ Transplantation in Clinical Veterinary Practice

T. Keith Grove, D.D.S., M.S., V.M.D.
Diplomate, American Veterinary Dental College. Clinician and Director, Florida Veterinary Dental Clinic, Vero Beach, Florida.
Periodontal Disease; Endodontics and Root Canal Therapy

Kevin A. Hahn, D.V.M., Ph.D.
Assistant Professor of Oncology, Department of Environmental Practice, College of Veterinary Medicine, University of Tennessee, Knoxville, Tennessee.
Diagnosis of Neoplasia

Nils Håkanson, M.V.S.
Diplomate, American College of Veterinary Ophthalmologists. Clinician, The Animal Hospital in Strānsholm, Kolbāck, Sweden.
Cornea and Sclera

Terrance A. Hamilton, D.V.M.
Resident in Comparative Oncology, School of Veterinary Medicine, Purdue University, West Lafayette, Indiana.
Diagnosis of Neoplasia

Joseph Harari, D.V.M., M.S.
Assistant Professor of Veterinary Clinical Medicine and Surgery, College of Veterinary Medicine, Washington State University, Pullman, Washington.
Surgery of the Exocrine Pancreas

Elizabeth M. Hardie, D.V.M., Ph.D.
Department of Companion Animal and Special Species Medicine, College of Veterinary Medicine, North Carolina State University, Raleigh, North Carolina.
The Prostate

R. M. Hardy, D.V.M., M.S.
Professor, Department of Small Animal Clinical Sciences, College of Veterinary Medicine, University of Minnesota, St. Paul, Minnesota.
Alimentary Tract, Liver, and Pancreas

Benjamin L. Hart, D.V.M., Ph.D.
Professor of Physiology and Behavior, School of Veterinary Medicine, and Director, Animal Behavior Services, University of California Veterinary Medical Teaching Hospital, Davis, California.
Pathophysiology and Therapeutics of Urinary Tract Disorders

Colin E. Harvey, B.V.Sc., F.R.C.V.S.
Diplomate, American College of Veterinary Surgeons. Professor of Surgery and Dentistry, Department of Clinical Studies, School of Veterinary Medicine, and Department of Periodontics, School of Dental Medicine, University of Pennsylvania, Philadelphia, Pennsylvania.
Oral Cavity

Ralph C. Harvey, D.V.M., M.S.
Diplomate, American College of Veterinary Anesthesiologists. Associate Professor, Department of Urban Practice, and Associate Professor of Anesthesiology, College of Veterinary Medicine, University of Tennessee, Knoxville, Tennessee.
Anesthesia for Central Nervous System and Ophthalmic Surgery

Steven C. Haskins, D.V.M., M.S.
Diplomate, American College of Veterinary Anesthesiologists. Associate Professor, Department of Veterinary Surgery, School of Veterinary Medicine, and Section of Anesthesiology and Intensive Care, Veterinary Medical Teaching Hospital, University of California, Davis, California.
Operating Room Emergencies

Joseph Hauptman, D.V.M., M.S.
Diplomate, American College of Veterinary Surgeons. Professor of Surgery, Department of Small Animal Clinical Services, College of Veterinary Medicine, Michigan State University, East Lansing, Michigan.
Shock; Pathophysiology and Management of Hypovolemia and Sepsis

B. Jean Hawkins, D.V.M., M.S.
Fellow, Academy of Veterinary Dentistry, and Diplomate, American Veterinary Dental College. Associate Veterinarian, Orchard Animal Clinic, Boise, Idaho.
Restorative Dentistry

Stuart C. Helfand, D.V.M.
Diplomate, American College of Internal Medicine (Oncology). Assistant Professor of Internal Medicine and Oncology, Department of Medical Sciences, School of Veterinary Medicine, University of Wisconsin, Madison, Wisconsin.
Hematopoietic System

Peter W. Hellyer, D.V.M., M.S.
Diplomate, American College of Veterinary Anesthesiologists. Assistant Professor of Anesthesiology, College of Veterinary Medicine, North Carolina State University, Raleigh, North Carolina.
Anesthesia for Cesarean Section

Ralph A. Henderson, D.V.M., M.S.
Diplomate, American College of Veterinary Surgeons and American College of Veterinary Internal Medicine (Oncology). Professor, Department of Small Animal Surgery and Medicine, School of Veterinary Medicine, Auburn University, Auburn, Alabama.
The Pinna; Skin and Subcutis

H. Philip Hobson, B.S., D.V.M., M.S.
Diplomate, American College of Veterinary Surgeons. Professor, Department of Small Animal Surgery, College of Veterinary Medicine, Texas A&M University, College Station, Texas.
Surgical Facilities and Equipment

David L. Holmberg, D.V.M., M.V.Sc.
Diplomate, American College of Veterinary Surgeons. Professor of Small Animal Surgery, Department of Clinical Studies, Ontario Veterinary College, and Chief, Small Animal Surgery, Veterinary Teaching Hospital, University of Guelph, Guelph, Ontario, Canada.
Cryosurgery; Extracorporeal Circulatory Support; Section Editor: Section 2: Surgical Methods

Patrick E. Hopper, D.V.M.
Diplomate, American College of Veterinary Internal Medicine. Internist, Center for Veterinary Care, New York, New York.
Immune-Mediated Joint Diseases

R. D. Horne, D.V.M., M.S.
Diplomate, American College of Veterinary Surgeons. Professor, Department of Small Animal Surgery and Medicine, School of Veterinary Medicine, Auburn University, Auburn, Alabama.
The Pinna

Don Hulse, D.V.M.
Diplomate, American College of Veterinary Surgeons. Professor of Surgery, College of Veterinary Medicine, Texas A&M University, College Station, Texas.
Fracture Biology and Biomechanics

Bill Hyman, S.c.D.
Professor of Surgery, College of Veterinary Medicine, Texas A&M University, College Station, Texas.
Fracture Biology and Biomechanics

Wolfgang Janas
Research Assistant, Biomedical Engineering, Purdue University, West Lafayette, Indiana.
Diagnosis of Neoplasia

Ann L. Johnson, D.V.M., M.S.
Diplomate, American College of Veterinary Surgeons. Associate Professor, Department of Veterinary Clinical Medicine, College of Veterinary Medicine, University of Illinois, Urbana, Illinois.
Fractures of the Tibia and Fibula

Kenneth A. Johnson, M.V.Sc., Ph.D.
Diplomate, American College of Veterinary Surgeons. Associate Professor of Surgery, Department of Surgical Sciences, School of Veterinary Medicine, and Associate Professor of Surgery, Veterinary Medical Teaching Hospital, University of Wisconsin, Madison, Wisconsin.
Diaphragmatic, Pericardial, and Hiatal Hernia

Gary R. Johnston, D.V.M., M.S.
Diplomate, American College of Veterinary Radiology. Professor of Comparative Radiology, College of Veterinary Medicine, University of Minnesota, St. Paul, Minnesota.
Radiation Therapy

Shirley D. Johnston, D.V.M., Ph.D.
Diplomate, American College of Theriogenologists. Professor, Department of Small Animal Clinical Sciences, College of Veterinary Medicine, University of Minnesota, St. Paul, Minnesota.
Reproductive Systems

Spencer A. Johnston, V.M.D.
Assistant Professor, Virginia-Maryland Regional College of Veterinary Medicine, Virginia Polytechnic Institute and State University, Blacksburg, Virginia.
Other Orthopedic Diseases

Robert L. Jones, D.V.M., Ph.D.
Diplomate, American College of Veterinary Microbiologists. Professor, Department of Microbiology, College of Veterinary Medicine and Biomedical Sciences, Colorado State University, Fort Collins, Colorado.
Principles of Surgical Asepsis

Robert E. Kaderly, D.V.M., Ph.D.
Diplomate, American College of Veterinary Surgeons. Professor of Surgery, Department of Companion Animals, Atlantic Veterinary College, University of Prince Edward Island, Charlottetown, Prince Edward Island, Canada.
Delayed Union, Nonunion, and Malunion

David B. Kestenman, D.V.M.
Staff Surgeon, Bloomington Cat Hospital, Bloomington, Indiana.
Radiation Therapy

Jeffrey S. Klausner, D.V.M., M.S.
Diplomate, American College of Veterinary Internal Medicine (Internal Medicine and Oncology). Professor, Department of Small Animal Clinical Sciences, College of Veterinary Medicine, University of Minnesota, St. Paul, Minnesota.
Alimentary Tract, Liver, and Pancreas; Urinary System

Ronald J. Kolata, D.V.M., M.S.
Diplomate, American College of Veterinary Surgeons. Principal Scientist, Ethicon-Endosurgery, Cincinnati, Ohio.
Trauma: Epidemiology and Mechanisms; Monitoring the Surgical Patient

J. Komtebedde, D.V.M.
Staff Surgeon, Solano Veterinary Consultants, Cordelia, California.
Elbow Luxation

Joe N. Kornegay, D.V.M., Ph.D.
Professor of Neurology, College of Veterinary Medicine, and Neurologist and Neurosurgeon, Veterinary Teaching Hospital, North Carolina State University, Raleigh, North Carolina.
Pathogenesis of Diseases of the Central Nervous System; Discospondylitis; Central Nervous System

Marilyn Kostolich, D.V.M.
Diplomate, American College of Veterinary Surgeons. Associate Professor, Department of Medicine and Surgery, College of Veterinary Medicine, Oklahoma State University, Stillwater, Oklahoma.
Hemostasis: Physiology, Diagnosis, and Treatment of Bleeding Disorders in Surgical Patients

D. J. Krahwinkel, D.V.M., M.S.
Diplomate, American College of Veterinary Surgeons, American College of Veterinary Anesthesiologists, and *American College of Veterinary Emergency and Critical Care.* Professor of Surgery, Department of Urban Practice, College of Veterinary Medicine, University of Tennessee, Knoxville, Tennessee.
External Ear Canal

J. D. Lavach, D.V.M., M.S.
Diplomate, American College of Veterinary Ophthalmologists. Staff Surgeon, Eye Clinic for Animals, Garden Grove, California.
The Lacrimal System

Arnold S. Lesser, V.M.D.
Diplomate, American College of Veterinary Surgeons. Private Practitioner, Veterinary Surgical Referral Service, Centerport, New York.
Arthrodesis

Stephen H. Levine, D.V.M., M.S.
Diplomate, American College of Veterinary Surgeons. Staff Surgeon, Crossroads Animal Hospital, Burnsville, Minnesota.
Surgical Therapy

James Lincoln, D.V.M., M.S.
Associate Professor of Veterinary Clinical Medicine and Surgery, College of Veterinary Medicine, Washington State University, Pullman, Washington.
Surgery of the Exocrine Pancreas

Alan J. Lipowitz, D.V.M., M.S.
Diplomate, American College of Veterinary Surgeons. Professor of Surgery, Department of Small Animal Clinical Sciences, College of Veterinary Medicine, University of Minnesota, St. Paul, Minnesota.
Spleen; Degenerative Joint Disease

Philip Litwak, D.V.M., Ph.D.
Diplomate, American College of Veterinary Surgeons. Vice President, Thoratec Laboratories Corporation, Berkeley, California.
Principles of Vascular Surgery; Peripheral Vascular Procedures and Disorders

John W. Ludders, D.V.M.
Diplomate, American College of Veterinary Anesthesiologists. Associate Professor, Section of Anesthesiology, Department of Clinical Sciences, College of Veterinary Medicine, Cornell University, Ithaca, New York.
Anesthesia for Central Nervous System and Ophthalmic Surgery

George Lust, Ph.D.
Professor of Physiological Chemistry, New York State College of Veterinary Medicine, Cornell University, Ithaca, New York
Other Orthopedic Diseases

Paul A. Manley, D.V.M., M.Sc.
Diplomate, American College of Veterinary Surgeons. Associate Professor, School of Veterinary Medicine, University of Wisconsin, Madison, Wisconsin.
The Hip Joint; Other Orthopedic Diseases

Sandra Manfra Marretta, D.V.M.
Diplomate, American College of Veterinary Surgeons. Assistant Professor, Small Animal Surgery and Dentistry, Department of Veterinary Clinical Medicine, University of Illinois, Urbana, Illinois.
Diseases of the Anus and Rectum

Charles L. Martin, D.V.M., M.S.
Diplomate, American College of Veterinary Ophthalmologists. Professor, Department of Small Animal Medicine, College of Veterinary Medicine, and Director, Veterinary Teaching Hospital, University of Georgia, Athens, Georgia.
Glaucoma

Robert A. Martin, D.V.M.
Diplomate, American College of Veterinary Surgeons. Associate Professor, Virginia-Maryland Regional College of Veterinary Medicine, and Section Chief, Small Animal Surgery and Anesthesiology, Veterinary Teaching Hospital, Virginia Polytechnic Institute and State University, Blacksburg, Virginia.
Liver and Biliary System

Diane E. Mason, D.V.M., M.S.
Diplomate, American College of Veterinary Anesthesiologists. Assistant Professor, Department of Veterinary Clinical Sciences, College of Veterinary Medicine, Ohio State University, Columbus, Ohio.
Anesthesia and the Urinary System

David T. Matthiesen, D.V.M.
Diplomate, American College of Veterinary Surgeons. Senior Staff Surgeon, The Animal Medical Center, New York, New York, and Surgeon, Veterinary Surgical Specialists, Tinton Falls, New Jersey.
Stomach; Diseases of the Anus and Rectum; Section Editor: Section 5, Gastrointestinal System

John V. Mauterer, D.V.M.
Clinical Instructor and Resident in Small Animal Surgery, College of Veterinary Medicine, Ohio State University, Columbus, Ohio.
Nutritional Support of Hospitalized Patients

Dennis M. McCurnin, D.V.M.
Diplomate, American College of Veterinary Surgeons. Professor of Clinical Sciences, School of Veterinary Medicine, and Associate Dean and Hospital Director, Veterinary Teaching Hospital and Clinics, Louisiana State University, Baton Rouge, Louisiana.
Principles of Surgical Asepsis

Mary A. McLoughlin, D.V.M., M.S.
Assistant Professor of Small Animal Surgery, Department of Veterinary Clinical Sciences, College of Veterinary Medicine, Ohio State University, Columbus, Ohio.
Nutritional Support of Hospitalized Patients

David F. Merkley, D.V.M., M.S.
Diplomate, American College of Veterinary Surgeons. Professor of Veterinary Surgery, College of Veterinary Medicine, and Staff Surgeon, Veterinary Teaching Hospital, Iowa State University, Ames, Iowa.
Surgical Instruments

Craig W. Miller, D.V.M., M.V.Sc.
Diplomate, American College of Veterinary Surgeons. Associate Professor of Small Animal Surgery, Department of Clinical Studies, Ontario Veterinary College, University of Guelph, Guelph, Ontario, Canada.
Bandages and Drains

Darryl L. Millis, D.V.M., M.S.
Assistant Professor, College of Veterinary Medicine, Mississippi State University, Starkville, Mississippi.
Carpus and Digits

J. L. Milton, D.V.M., M.S.
Diplomate, American College of Veterinary Surgeons. Professor of Surgery, Department of Small Animal Surgery and Medicine, School of Veterinary Medicine, Auburn University, Auburn, Alabama.
Fractures of the Femur

Cecil P. Moore, D.V.M., M.S.
Diplomate, American College of Veterinary Ophthalmologists. Associate Professor, Department of Veterinary Medicine and Surgery, College of Veterinary Medicine, and Section Leader, Ophthalmology Section, Veterinary Teaching Hospital, University of Missouri, Columbia, Missouri.
Conjunctiva; Third Eyelid

M. Morandi, M.D.
Aiuto Orthopedico, Divisioné di Orthopedia, Bologna, Italy.
External Skeletal Fixation

Wallace B. Morrison, D.V.M., M.S.
Associate Professor, School of Veterinary Medicine, Purdue University, West Lafayette, Indiana.
Biology of Neoplastic Disease; Diagnosis of Neoplasia

William W. Muir III, D.V.M., PhD.
Professor, Department of Veterinary Clinical Sciences, College of Veterinary Medicine, Ohio State University, Columbus, Ohio.
Anesthetics and Techniques; Section Editor: Section 17, Anesthetic Considerations in Surgery

A. Wendell Nelson, D.V.M., M.S., Ph.D.
Diplomate, American College of Veterinary Surgeons. Professor of Clinical Sciences, College of Veterinary Medicine and Biomedical Sciences, and Director, Veterinary Teaching Hospital, Colorado State University, Fort Collins, Colorado.
Upper Respiratory System; Lower Respiratory System; Section Editor: Section 6, Respiratory System

Gert W. Niebauer, D.V.M., M.S., Dr. Med. Vet. Habil.
Assistant Professor of Surgery, School of Veterinary Medicine, University of Pennsylvania, Philadelphia, Pennsylvania.
Hypophysectomy

Mary Ann Nieves, D.V.M.
Assistant Professor, Department of Clinical Sciences, College of Veterinary Medicine, and Orthopedic Surgeon, Veterinary Teaching Hospital, Iowa State University, Ames, Iowa.
Surgical Instruments

Phillip N. Ogburn, D.V.M., Ph.D.
Associate Professor of Cardiology, Department of Small Animal Clinical Sciences, College of Veterinary Medicine, University of Minnesota, St. Paul, Minnesota.
Cardiovascular System

N. Bari Olivier, D.V.M., Ph.D.
Assistant Professor of Medicine, Department of Small Animal Clinical Sciences and Department of Physiology, College of Veterinary Medicine, Michigan State University, East Lansing, Michigan.
Pathophysiology of Cardiac Failure

Marvin L. Olmstead, D.V.M., M.S.
Diplomate, American College of Veterinary Surgeons. Professor, College of Veterinary Medicine, Ohio State University, Columbus, Ohio.
Fractures of the Humerus

Patricia N. Olson, D.V.M.
Diplomate, American College of Theriogenologists. Clinical Associate Professor of Small Animal Clinical Sciences, College of Veterinary Medicine, University of Minnesota, St. Paul, Minnesota.
Vagina, Vestibule, and Vulva; Normal and Abnormal Parturition

Robert J. Orsher, V.M.D.
Diplomate, American College of Veterinary Surgeons. Adjunct Assistant Professor of Surgery, Department of Clinical Studies, School of Veterinary Medicine, University of Pennsylvania, Philadelphia, Pennsylvania, and Staff Surgeon and Owner, Veterinary Surgical Center, Oakford, Pennsylvania.
Small Intestine

E. Christopher Orton, D.V.M., Ph.D.
Diplomate, American College of Veterinary Surgeons. Associate Professor, Department of Clinical Sciences, College of Veterinary Medicine and Biomedical Sciences, and Staff Surgeon, Veterinary Teaching Hospital, Colorado State University, Fort Collins, Colorado.
Thoracic Wall; Pleura and Pleural Space; Evaluation of the Surgical Respiratory Patient

Robert R. Paddleford, D.V.M.
Diplomate, American College of Veterinary Anesthesiologists and *American College of Veterinary Emergency and Critical Care.* Associate Professor, Department of Urban Practice, College of Veterinary Medicine, University of Tennessee, Knoxville, Tennessee.
Anesthesia for Central Nervous System and Ophthalmic Surgery

Rodney L. Page, D.V.M., M.S.
Associate Professor, College of Veterinary Medicine, North Carolina State University, Raleigh, North Carolina.
Central Nervous System

Anthony D. Pardo, D.V.M., M.D.
Diplomate, American College of Veterinary Surgeons. Assistant Professor of Surgery, Department of Urban Practice, College of Veterinary Medicine, University of Tennessee, Knoxville, Tennessee.
Methods of Internal Fracture Fixation

Richard D. Park, D.V.M., Ph.D.
Diplomate, American College of Veterinary Radiology. Professor, Department of Radiological Health Sciences, College of Veterinary Medicine and Biomedical Sciences, and Radiologist, Veterinary Teaching Hospital, Colorado State University, Fort Collins, Colorado.
Evaluation of the Surgical Respiratory Patient

Robert B. Parker, D.V.M.
Diplomate, American College of Veterinary Surgeons. Associate Professor and Chief, Small Animal Surgery, College of Veterinary Medicine, University of Florida, Gainesville, Florida.
Scapula

Peter J. Pascoe, B.V.Sc.
Assistant Professor, Department of Surgery, School of Veterinary Medicine, and Small Animal Anesthesiologist, Veterinary Medical Teaching Hospital, University of California, Davis, California.
Patient Aftercare

Michael A. Pass, B.V.Sc., M.Sc., Ph.D.
Reader in Physiology, Department of Physiology and Pharmacology, University of Queensland, St. Lucia, Queensland, Australia.
Physiology of the Digestive System

Michael M. Pavletic, D.V.M.
Diplomate, American College of Veterinary Surgeons. Professor of Surgery, School of Veterinary Medicine, Tufts University, North Grafton, Massachusetts, and Head of Small Animal Surgery.
The Integument; Pedicle Grafts; Section Editor: Section 3, Skin and Adnexa

Phillip T. Pearson, D.V.M., Ph.D.
Diplomate, American College of Veterinary Surgeons. Professor of Veterinary Clinical Sciences, College of Veterinary Medicine, and Small Animal Orthopedic Surgeon, Veterinary Teaching Hospital, Iowa State University, Ames, Iowa.
Biomaterials

Robert L. Peiffer, Jr., D.V.M., Ph.D.
Diplomate, American College of Veterinary Ophthalmologists. Professor and Director of Laboratories, Department of Ophthalmology, School of Medicine, University of North Carolina, Chapel Hill, North Carolina.
Iris and Ciliary Body; The Lens; Surgery of the Vitreous and Retina

Roger C. Penwick, V.M.D.
Diplomate, American College of Veterinary Surgeons. President and Surgeon, Tucson Veterinary Surgical Service, P.C., Tucson, Arizona.
Surgical Wound Infection and Use of Antibiotics

Mark E. Peterson, D.V.M.
Diplomate, American College of Veterinary Internal Medicine. Head, Division of Endocrinology, Department of Medicine, The Animal Medical Center, New York, New York.
The Thyroid

Steven W. Petersen, D.V.M.
Surgeon, Alameda East Veterinary Hospital, Denver, Colorado.
Surgical Wound Infection and Use of Antibiotics

Steven L. Peterson, D.V.M.
Fourth-Year Veterinary Student, Cardiac Electrophysiology, School of Medicine, Health Science Center, University of Colorado, Denver, Colorado.
Liver and Biliary System

Eric R. Pope, D.V.M., M.D.
Diplomate, American College of Veterinary Surgeons. Associate Professor of Surgery, College of Veterinary Medicine, University of Missouri, Columbia, Missouri.
Burns: Thermal, Electrical, Chemical, and Cold Injuries

Raymond G. Prata, D.V.M.
Diplomate, American College of Veterinary Surgeons. Staff Surgeon, Oradell Animal Hospital, Inc., Oradell, New Jersey.
Cauda Equina Syndrome

Curtis W. Probst, D.V.M.
Diplomate, American College of Veterinary Surgeons. Associate Professor, Department of Small Animal Clinical Sciences, Veterinary Medical Center, Michigan State University, East Lansing, Michigan.
Wound Healing and Specific Tissue Regeneration; Methods of Internal Fracture Fixation; Carpus and Digits; Hip Dysplasia in Dogs

Maralyn Probst, A.H.T.
Research Assistant, College of Veterinary Medicine, Michigan State University, East Lansing, Michigan.
Cardiac Disorders

Jane E. Quandt, D.V.M., M.S.
Assistant Professor, Small Animal Medicine, College of Veterinary Medicine, University of Georgia, Athens, Georgia.
Anesthesia for Upper Airway and Thoracic Surgery

Marc R. Raffe, D.V.M., M.S.
Diplomate, American College of Veterinary Anesthesiologists and American College of Veterinary Emergency and Critical Care. Professor of Veterinary Medicine, Department of Small Animal Clinical Sciences, College of Veterinary Medicine, University of Minnesota, St. Paul, Minnesota.

Fluid, Electrolyte, and Acid-Base Therapy in the Surgical Patient; Anesthesia for Upper Airway and Thoracic Surgery

Rose E. Raskin, D.V.M., Ph.D.
Diplomate, American College of Veterinary Pathologists. Assistant Professor of Clinical Pathology, Department of Physiological Sciences, College of Veterinary Medicine, University of Florida, Gainesville, Florida.
Bone Marrow

Richard A. Read, B.V.Sc., Ph.D.
Senior Lecturer, Small Animal Surgery, School of Veterinary Studies, Murdoch University, Murdoch, Western Australia.
Hernias

Virginia T. Rentko, V.M.D., M.S.
Staff Surgeon, School of Veterinary Medicine and Foster Hospital for Small Animals, Tufts University, North Grafton, Massachusetts.
The Hematopoietic System

Ken Richardson, B.Sc., B.V.Sc., Ph.D.
Senior Lecturer, School of Veterinary Studies, Murdoch University, Murdoch, Western Australia.
Functional Anatomy

Ralph C. Richardson, D.V.M.
Professor of Internal Medicine and Oncology, School of Veterinary Medicine, Purdue University, West Lafayette, Indiana.
Biology of Neoplastic Disease; Diagnosis of Neoplasia

C. Lee Robinette, D.V.M., Ph.D.
Department of Anatomy, Physiological Sciences, and Radiology, College of Veterinary Medicine, North Carolina State University, Raleigh, North Carolina.
The Prostate

Elaine P. Robinson, B.Vet.Med.
Diplomate, American College of Veterinary Anesthesiologists. Associate Professor, College of Veterinary Medicine, University of Minnesota, St. Paul, Minnesota.
Pediatric and Geriatric Anesthetic Technique

William G. Rodkey, D.V.M.
Diplomate, American College of Veterinary Surgeons. Director, Research and Education, Steadman Sports Medicine Foundation, Vail, Colorado, and (formerly) Chief, Division of Military Trauma Research, Letterman Army Institute of Research, San Francisco, California.
Peripheral Nerve Surgery

Kenita S. Rogers, D.V.M., M.S.
Diplomate, American College of Veterinary Internal Medicine (Oncology). Associate Professor, Department of Small Animal Medicine and Surgery, Texas A&M University, College Station, Texas.
Lymphatics, Lymph Nodes, and Tonsils; Respiratory System

Janet Amundson Romich, D.V.M., M.S.
Instructor, Madison Area Technical College, Madison, Wisconsin
Other Orthopedic Diseases

Robert C. Rosenthal, D.V.M., Ph.D.
Chief of Medicine, Veterinary Specialists of Rochester, Rochester, New York.
Chemotherapy

Anne E. Rosin, D.V.M., M.S.
Student, School of Medicine, University of Wisconsin, Madison, Wisconsin.
Pathophysiology and Therapeutics of Urinary Tract Disorders

Eberhard Rosin, D.V.M., Ph.D.
Diplomate, American College of Veterinary Surgeons. Professor of Surgery, School of Veterinary Medicine, University of Wisconsin, Madison, Wisconsin.
Surgical Wound Infection and Use of Antibiotics; Small Intestine; Section Editor: Section 1, Surgical Biology

E. Kathleen Salisbury, D.V.M.
Diplomate, American College of Veterinary Surgeons. Associate Professor of Surgery, School of Veterinary Medicine, Purdue University, West Lafayette, Indiana.
Oral Cavity

Thomas D. Scavelli, D.V.M.
Diplomate, American College of Veterinary Surgeons. Director, Veterinary Surgical Specialists, Tinton Falls, New Jersey.
The Thyroid; Section Editor: Section 13, Endocrine System

Kay L. Schwink, D.V.M.
Diplomate, American College of Veterinary Ophthalmology. Resident in Ophthalmology, College of Veterinary Medicine, Iowa State University, Ames, Iowa
Surgical Approaches to the Spine

Howard B. Seim, III, D.V.M.
Diplomate, American College of Veterinary Surgeons. Associate Professor and Section Chief, Small Animal Surgery, College of Veterinary Medicine and Biomedical Sciences, Colorado State University, Fort Collins, Colorado.
Caudal Cervical Spondylomyelopathy; Spinal Fractures and Luxations; Middle Ear; Section Editor: Section 9, Nervous System; Section 14, Ear

Douglas C. Sempere, D.V.M.
Visiting Instructor, Department of Medicine and Surgery, College of Veterinary Medicine, Oklahoma State University, Stillwater, Oklahoma.
Hemostasis: Physiology, Diagnosis, and Treatment of Bleeding Disorders in Surgical Patients

Nicholaus J. H. Sharp, M.R.C.V.S., Ph.D.
Diplomate, American College of Veterinary Surgeons. Clinical Instructor, College of Veterinary Medicine, North Carolina State University, Raleigh, North Carolina.
Ovary and Uterus

G. Diane Shelton, D.V.M., Ph.D.
Associate Clinical Professor, Department of Pathology, School of Medicine, and Director, Comparative Neuromuscular Laboratory, University of California at San Diego, La Jolla, California.
The Esophagus

Peter K. Shires, B.V.Sc., M.S.
Diplomate, American College of Veterinary Surgeons. Professor, Small Animal Surgery, Virginia-Maryland Regional College of Veterinary Medicine, and Staff Surgeon, Veterinary Medical Teaching Hospital, Virginia Polytechnic Institute and State University, Blacksburg, Virginia.
Atlantoaxial Instability

Andy Shores, D.V.M., M.S., Ph.D.
Associate Professor, Neurology/Neurosurgery, Department of Small Animal Clinical Sciences, Veterinary Teaching Hospital, Michigan State University, East Lansing, Michigan.
Neurological Examination and Localization; Intracranial Surgery

Douglas Slatter, B.V.Sc., M.S., Ph.D., F.R.C.V.S.
Diplomate, American College of Veterinary Surgeons and American College of Veterinary Ophthalmologists. Adjunct Professor, Southern California College of Optometry, Fullerton, California, and Veterinary Ophthalmologist and Surgeon, Animal Eye Clinics of Nevada and California, Reno, Nevada.
Principles of Ophthalmic Surgery; Cornea and Sclera; Orbit; Section Editor: Section 10, Eye and Adnexa; Section 15, Musculoskeletal System

Barclay Slocum, D.V.M.
Slocum Clinic Animal Foundation, Eugene, Oregon.
Cauda Equina Syndrome

Theresa D. Slocum, M.S.
Slocum Animal Foundation, Eugene, Oregon.
Cauda Equina Syndrome

Daniel D. Smeak, D.V.M.
Diplomate, American College of Veterinary Surgeons. Associate Professor, Small Animal Surgery, Department of Veterinary Clinical Sciences, College of Veterinary Medicine, Ohio State University, Columbus, Ohio.
Abdominal Hernias

C. W. Smith, D.V.M., M.S.
Diplomate, American College of Veterinary Surgeons. Professor, Department of Veterinary Clinical Medicine, College of Veterinary Medicine, and Chief, Small Animal Surgery, Veterinary Medical Teaching Hospital, University of Illinois, Urbana, Illinois.
Surgical Diseases of the Urethra

Mark M. Smith, V.M.D.
Diplomate, American College of Veterinary Surgeons. Assistant Professor, Department of Small Animal Clinical Sciences, Virginia-Maryland Regional College of Veterinary Medicine, Virginia Polytechnic Institute and State University, Blacksburg, Virginia.
Orthopedic Infections; Other Orthopedic Diseases

Kathy A. Spaulding, D.V.M.
Department of Anatomy, Physiological Sciences, and Radiology, College of Veterinary Medicine, North Carolina State University, Raleigh, North Carolina.
The Prostate

Sharon Stevenson, D.V.M., Ph.D.
Diplomate, American College of Veterinary Surgeons. Assistant Professor, Department of Orthopaedics, Case Western Reserve University, Cleveland, Ohio; Adjunct Clinical Assistant Professor, Department of Veterinary Clinical Sciences, College of Veterinary Medicine, Ohio State University, Columbus, Ohio, and Staff Surgeon, Akron Veterinary Surgical Associates, Metropolitan Veterinary Hospital, Akron, Ohio
Bone Grafting

Elizabeth Arnold Stone, D.V.M., M.S.
Diplomate, American College of Veterinary Surgeons. Professor of Surgery, College of Veterinary Medicine, and Surgeon, Veterinary Teaching Hospital, North Carolina State University, Raleigh, North Carolina.
Ovary and Uterus; Section Editor: Section 11, Reproductive System

G. Sumner-Smith, B.V.Sc., M.Sc., D.V.Sc., F.R.C.V.S.
Professor, Ontario Veterinary College, University of Guelph, Guelph, Ontario, Canada.
Gait Analysis and Orthopedic Examination

Rodney C. Straw, B.V.Sc.
Diplomate, American College of Veterinary Surgeons. Associate Professor, College of Veterinary Medicine and Biomedical Sciences, and Associate Professor of Oncology and Surgeon, Veterinary Teaching Hospital, Colorado State University, Fort Collins, Colorado.
Limb-Sparing Surgery for Dogs with Bone Neoplasia

Steven F. Swaim, D.V.M., M.S.
Professor, Small Animal Surgery, College of Veterinary Medicine, and Staff Surgeon, Scott-Ritchey Research Center and Department of Small Animal Surgery and Medicine, Auburn University, Auburn, Alabama.
Principles of Plastic and Reconstructive Surgery; Skin Grafts

Robert A. Taylor, D.V.M., M.S.
Diplomate, American College of Veterinary Surgeons. Alameda East Veterinary Hospital, Denver, Colorado.
Tarsus and Metatarsus

Christopher Thacher, D.V.M.
Diplomate, American College of Veterinary Surgeons. Chairman, Department of Surgery, The Animal Medical Center, New York, New York.
Other Orthopedic Diseases

Donald E. Thrall, D.V.M., Ph.D.
Professor of Radiology, College of Veterinary Medicine, North Carolina State University, Raleigh, North Carolina.
Central Nervous System

James Tomlinson, D.V.M., M.V.Sc.
Diplomate, American College of Veterinary Surgeons. Associate Professor of Surgery, Department of Veterinary Medicine and Surgery, College of Veterinary Medicine, and Head of Surgery and Small Animal Hospital Coordinator, Veterinary Teaching Hospital, University of Missouri, Columbia, Missouri.
Surgical Approaches to the Spine

James P. Toombs, D.V.M., M.S.
Diplomate, American College of Veterinary Surgeons. Associate Professor of Small Animal Orthopedics and Neurosurgery, Department of Veterinary Clinical Sciences, School of Veterinary Medicine, Purdue University, West Lafayette, Indiana.
Basic Operative Techniques; Intervertebral Disc Disease

William J. Tranquilli, D.V.M., M.S.
Diplomate, American College of Veterinary Anesthesiologists. Professor of Anesthesiology, Veterinary Medical Teaching Hospital, University of Illinois, Urbana, Illinois.
Anesthesia for the Trauma or Shock Patient

Peter B. Trevor, B.V.Sc., M.S., M.R.C.V.S.
Chief Resident, Small Animal Surgery, Virginia-Maryland Regional College of Veterinary Medicine, Virginia Polytechnic Institute and State University, Blacksburg, Virginia.
Management of Superficial Skin Wounds

Cynthia Trim, B.V.Sc.
Professor, College of Veterinary Medicine, University of Georgia, Athens, Georgia.
Anesthesia and the Endocrine System

Alan Tucker, Ph.D.
Professor of Physiology and Assistant Dean for Graduate and Undergraduate Education, College of Veterinary Medicine and Biomedical Sciences, Colorado State University, Fort Collins, Colorado.
Pathophysiology of the Respiratory System

Ronald D. Tyler, D.V.M., Ph.D.
Diplomate, American College of Veterinary Pathologists. Adjunct Professor, Department of Pathology, College of Veterinary Medicine, Oklahoma State University, Stillwater, Oklahoma, and Senior Research Pathologist, Schering-Plough Research Institute, Lafayette, New Jersey.
Hemostasis: Physiology, Diagnosis, and Treatment of Bleeding Disorders in Surgical Patients; The Hematopoietic System

David M. Vail, D.V.M., M.S.
Diplomate, American College of Veterinary Internal Medicine (Oncology). Assistant Professor of Internal Medicine and Oncology, Department of Medical Sciences, School of Veterinary Medicine, University of Wisconsin, Madison, Wisconsin.
Hematopoietic System

Frederik J. Van Sluys, D.V.M.
Lecturer in Small Animal Surgery, Faculty of Veterinary Medicine, State University of Utrecht, The Netherlands.
Stomach

Philip B. Vasseur, D.V.M.
Diplomate, American College of Veterinary Surgeons. Professor, Department of Veterinary Surgery, School of Veterinary Medicine, and Chief, Small Animal Surgery Service, Veterinary Medical Teaching Hospital, University of California, Davis, California.
Luxation of the Scapulohumeral Joint; Elbow Luxation; Stifle Joint; Section Editor: Section 15, Musculoskeletal System

Frank J. M. Verstraete, Dr.Med.Vet., M.Med.Vet.(Chir.)
Associate Professor of Surgery, Faculty of Veterinary Science, University of Pretoria, Onderstepoort, South Africa.
Dental Pathology and Microbiology

Mary Ann Vonderhaar, D.V.M.
Resident in Comparative Oncology, School of Veterinary Medicine, Purdue University, West Lafayette, Indiana.
Biology of Neoplastic Disease

Stanley D. Wagner, D.V.M.
Assistant Professor, College of Veterinary Medicine, and Orthopaedic Section, Veterinary Teaching Hospital, Iowa State University, Ames, Iowa.
Preparation of the Surgical Team; Surgical Instruments

Don R. Waldron, B.S., D.V.M.
Diplomate, American College of Veterinary Surgeons. Associate Professor of Surgery, Virginia-Maryland Regional College of Veterinary Medicine, and Staff Surgeon, Veterinary Medical Teaching Hospital, Virginia Polytechnic Instutute and State University, Blacksburg, Virginia.
Management of Superficial Skin Wounds; Urinary Bladder

Patricia A. Walters, D.V.M., M.S.
Diplomate, American College of Veterinary Radiology. Associate Professor of Comparative Radiology, College of Veterinary Medicine, University of Minnesota, St. Paul, Minnesota.
Urinary System

David J. Waters, D.V.M., Ph.D.
Diplomate, American College of Veterinary Surgeons. Assistant Professor of Small Animal Surgery, Purdue University, West Lafayette, Indiana.
Musculoskeletal System

Joseph P. Weigel, D.V.M.
Diplomate, American College of Veterinary Surgeons. Associate Professor of Surgery, College of Veterinary Medicine, University of Tennessee, Knoxville, Tennessee.
Amputations

Steven L. Wheeler, D.V.M., M.S.
Diplomate, American College of Veterinary Internal Medicine. Staff Internist, Animal Medical Specialists of Colorado, Denver, Colorado.
Care of Respiratory Patients

Marcia B. Whiteley, D.V.M.
Diplomate, American College of Veterinary Radiology. Tri-State Veterinary Imaging, Cincinnati, Ohio.
Radiation Therapy

Pamela G. Whiting, D.V.M.
Post-Doctoral Fellow–Research, University of California, Davis, California.
Liver and Biliary System

Alida P. Wind, D.V.M.
Senior Lecturer, Department of Surgery, School of Veterinary Medicine, and Staff Surgeon, Veterinary Medical Teaching Hospital, University of California, Davis, California.
Other Orthopedic Diseases

Stephen J. Withrow, D.V.M.
Diplomate, American College of Veterinary Surgeons. Professor, College of Veterinary Medicine and Biomedical Sciences, and Section Chief, Clinical Oncology, Veterinary Teaching Hospital, Colorado State University, Fort Collins, Colorado.
Limb-Sparing Surgery for Dogs with Bone Neoplasia

E. Dan Wolf, D.V.M.
Diplomate, American College of Veterinary Ophthalmologists. Adjunct Clinical Assistant Professor, Department of Small Animal Clinical Sciences, College of Veterinary Medicine, University of Florida, Gainesville, Florida, and Staff Surgeon, Animal Eye Clinic, Tampa, Florida.
Orbit

Peggy M. Wykes, D.V.M.
Diplomate, American College of Veterinary Surgeons. Staff Surgeon, Reference Surgery Practice, Englewood, California.
Vagina, Vestibule, and Vulva; Normal and Abnormal Parturition

Preface

Since publication of the first edition, the *Textbook of Small Animal Surgery* has been widely accepted by the veterinary profession as a definitive clinical, reference, and teaching work in veterinary surgery in many countries. The enormous task of translation of the book into several foreign languages has been completed. As with the first edition, it is the aim of this edition to provide the current, scientifically accepted facts of veterinary surgery.

We are faced with an ever-expanding literature of inconsistent quality, increasingly complex procedures, the difficulty of separating true advances from the spurious, and the challenge of limiting the size and cost of the text. I have deliberately avoided the shortsighted current trend to omit vital material, because this denies access to important concepts by the reader. Veterinary medicine has matured considerably in recent decades, and our major scholarly works must remain comparable with those of other professions.

As the volume of material in our specialty grows, the difficulty in using the information becomes apparent. In this edition, all authors have been requested to include decision-making algorithms and illustrations of procedures for clinical use.

The section editors and authors have labored with persistence and diligence in identifying new material and organizing it in a useful fashion. On every page we are reminded of the remarkable depth of talent of the contributing authors, both as authors and veterinarians.

I am indebted to the many colleagues who have made helpful suggestions for this edition, and to the staff of the W.B. Saunders Company including Ray Kersey, Larry McGrew, Linda Mills, and Darlene Pedersen. It is a pleasure to acknowledge Dr. James Archibald's *Canine Surgery*, the watershed in veterinary surgical publishing that originally inspired this textbook; the professional examples of Drs. Ralph Vierheller and Bill Lumb and many fellow Diplomates of the American College of Veterinary Surgeons; and the formative influence of Dr. Ghery Pettit, professor, editor, and friend.

DOUGLAS SLATTER

Contents

Volume I

Textbook of
SMALL ANIMAL SURGERY

SECTION 10

Eye and Adnexa

Douglas Slatter ■ *Section Editor*

CHAPTER 81

Principles of Ophthalmic Surgery

Douglas Slatter

Meticulous attention to detail is essential to success in ophthalmic surgery. Failure to attend to seemingly minute pharmacological preoperative, procedural, or postoperative details may cause unnecessary complications with intraocular or corneal surgery. Consequently, considerable discussion of apparently similar surgical techniques that differ in small details is encountered in the literature. The authors of the ophthalmic surgery section have compared techniques when sufficient information exists and have described the most appropriate techniques in their experience when information is limited. Despite its rigors, ophthalmic surgery offers great potential for relief of distress and improvement of quality of life and cosmetic appearance.

ANESTHESIA

General anesthesia is used for all but the most minor ophthalmic procedures (e.g., suture removal and superficial foreign body removal). A useful regimen follows. The simplest method that achieves anesthesia is recommended, without unnecessary use of complicated drug cocktails.

1. Minimum data base, including a preoperative physical examination and a complete blood count, serum chemistry profile, and thoracic radiographs for all patients over 6 years of age.
2. Preoperative medication with atropine[19] or glycopyrrolate. In ophthalmic surgery, the presence of the oculocardiac reflex probably indicates that atropine should be used.
3. Induction of anesthesia with sodium thiamylal, thiopental, or alfaxalone (in cats) and immediate intubation. Muscle relaxants may be used but are unnecessary in properly anesthetized patients. Aged or high-risk patients may be anesthetized by inhalation with isoflurane.
4. Maintenance with methoxyflurane, halothane, or isoflurane.

Compared with halothane, methoxyflurane provides the advantages of postoperative analgesia and tranquilization and reduced dangers of inducing cardiac arrhythmias or ventricular fibrillation with intraocular epinephrine ("epinephrine syncope") during the surgical procedure. Epinephrine is a common constituent of intraocular irrigating solutions for veterinary ophthalmic surgery. Reports of pulmonary edema associated with concurrent use of methoxyflurane and mannitol have not been confirmed by subsequent research or decades of clinical use. Methoxyflurane should be used with caution in patients with established kidney disease if extended anesthesia (> 2 hours) is contemplated. Most general anesthetics decrease intraocular pressure and tear production. For methods of monitoring physiological parameters during anesthesia, see Chapter 175.

PREOPERATIVE PREPARATION

Pharmacological Preparation

Anti-Inflammatory Agents

The canine eye (and to a lesser degree the feline eye) rapidly becomes inflamed during or after ocular surgical procedures. Corticosteroids are frequently used both systemically and topically for several days before ophthalmic procedures or cyclocryotherapy to reduce miosis and release of protein into the aqueous when the anterior chamber is opened, and to limit postoperative inflammation. Corticosteroids reduce release of prostaglandins, which mediate some of the protein release through vascular walls, and diminish the direct action of prostaglandins on the smooth muscle of the iris sphincter, the cause of miosis during intraocular surgery. In addition to preoperative topical and systemic administration of corticosteroids, an intravenous bolus may be given about 30 minutes before surgery.

Complications with the use of steroids include slower wound healing and decreased resistance to bacterial and fungal infections.[12] To reduce these complications, use of preoperative antibiotics and disinfecting solutions to reduce conjunctival bacterial numbers is recommended. Topical corticosteroids reduce serum cortisol, suppress adrenocorticotropic hormone response, and cause accumulation of hepatic glycogen.[9, 11, 23] Long-term use in healthy dogs produces few effects, but caution is necessary in patients with pre-existing hepatic dysfunction. These effects are reversible in 7 to 14 days.

Prophylactic antibiotics are bactericidal and are changed regularly during the pre- and postoperative periods.

Prostaglandins are important mediators of ocular inflammation, including protein release during intraocular surgery.[30] Inhibitors of prostaglandin synthetase reduce vascular permeability when administered preoperatively.[11, 27] In dogs, acetylsalicylic acid (30 mEq/kg PO every 8 hours for 40 hours before surgery) reduces aqueous protein concentrations.[4] Unfortunately, platelet numbers are depressed by acetylsalicylic acid, with consequent effects on clotting time, a particularly undesirable complication in intraocular surgery.[15] Indomethacin also inhibits prostaglandin synthetase in the eye[20] but must be administered carefully and with food because of systemic toxicity in dogs. Topical indomethacin (1 per cent) [26, 32] and flurbiprofen[1, 2, 10, 17, 18] are particularly useful preoperatively to reduce protein release during surgery. Although not approved for use in dogs, flunixin meglumine (0.5 mg/kg) is widely and effectively used[14, 17, 18, 22] systemically as a preoperative prostaglandin inhibitor and analgesic. Antihistamines are used by some ophthalmic surgeons 30 to 60 minutes before the eye is opened to reduce protein release.

Osmotic Agents

Mannitol decreases intraocular pressure and vitreous body volume[13] and is widely used to reduce loss of vitreous during intraocular surgery. Although its need has been questioned,[20] it is beneficial and without complications if the patient is normally hydrated and normotensive before surgery. A potential interaction between mannitol and methoxyflurane resulting in pulmonary edema has been reported[6] but was not reproducible experimentally and has not been confirmed by clinical reports. The frequency of simultaneous use of mannitol and methoxyflurane makes a significant association unlikely.

Antibacterials

Because of the normal bacterial flora of the conjunctival sac (Tables 81–1 and 81–2) and tarsal glands and the frequent use of immunosuppressive drugs, preoperative preparation for several days with a broad-spectrum bactericidal antibiotic and povidone-iodine solution (diluted 1:25 with saline)[2] immediately before surgery during preparation is advised for elective procedures. Before intraocular procedures, solutions are preferable to ointments to prevent entry of oily bases into the eye, with subsequent chronic inflammation.

After induction of anesthesia, the periocular area is carefully clipped and cilia on the upper lid are removed. "Clipper burn," or traumatic dermatitis, is avoided to minimize postoperative scratching. Special care is taken, if the globe has been penetrated, to prevent hair from entering the conjunctival sac during clipping and to avoid placing pressure on the eye. K-Y jelly may be placed in the sac before clipping and removed with the adherent hair after clipping.

1. Gross contamination is removed with gauze sponges soaked in sterile saline.
2. The periocular area is carefully scrubbed with povidone-iodine solution diluted with saline. (Note: Povidone scrub solution contains detergents harmful to the cornea).
3. The corneal and conjunctival surfaces are irrigated with balanced salt solution or saline, and a drop of broad-spectrum antibiotic solution may be instilled before surgery.
4. A final preparation of ethyl alcohol followed by povidone-iodine may be used. The alcohol must not enter the conjunctival sac.

TABLE 81–1. NORMAL FLORA OF THE CANINE CONJUNCTIVAL SAC

	Percentage of Cases with Positive Cultures		Percentage of Cases with Positive Cultures
Western United States[3]		Eastern Australia[16]	
Staphylococcus epidermidis	46	*Staphylococcus epidermidis*	16
Staphylococcus aureus	24	*Staphylococcus aureus*	39
Streptococcus spp. (β-hemolytic)	2	*Bacillus* spp.	29
Streptococcus spp. (α-hemolytic)	4	*Corynebacterium* spp.	19
Bacillus spp.	12	*Streptococcus* spp. (β-hemolytic)	1
Gram-negative organisms *(Mima [Acinetobacter]* spp., *Neisseria* spp., *Moraxella* spp., *Pseudomonas* spp.*)*	7	*Streptococcus* spp. (α-hemolytic)	3
		Streptococcus spp. (nonhemolytic)	3
		Yeasts	5
Diphtheroids	75	*Micrococcus* spp.	3
Midwestern United States[28]		*Neisseria* spp.	2
Staphylococcus epidermidis	55	*Pseudomonas* spp.	1
Staphylococcus aureus	45	*Nocardia* spp.	1
Streptococcus spp. (β-hemolytic)	7.3	*Escherichia coli*	1
Streptococcus spp. (α-hemolytic)	34	*Clostridium* spp.	1
Neisseria spp.	26	*Enterobacter* spp.	1
Pseudomonas spp.	14	*Flavobacterium* spp.	1
Diphtheroids	30	*Branhamella catarrhalis*	1

TABLE 81–2. NORMAL FLORA OF THE FELINE CONJUNCTIVAL SAC IN THE WESTERN UNITED STATES

Organism	Percentage of Cases with Positive Cultures	
	Conjunctiva	*Lids*
Staphylococcus aureus	10.4	8.8
Staphylococcus epidermidis	16.3	13.3
Mycoplasma spp.	5	—
Bacillus spp.	2.9	1.7
Streptococcus spp. (α-hemolytic)	2.5	1.7
Corynebacterium spp.	1.3	—
Escherichia coli	—	0.4

From Campbell L: Ocular bacteria and mycoplasma of the clinically normal cat. *Feline Pract 3*:10, 1973.

Positioning of Patient and Surgeon

Ophthalmic surgery is performed with the surgeon seated. An arm rest is used to steady both wrists for fine movements. An adjustable stool and arm rest are commonly combined (Fig. 81–1). The patient's head is placed on an elevated conforming rest (e.g., evacuated bag filled with polystyrene beads) so that the eye can be positioned exactly as required (Fig. 81–2).

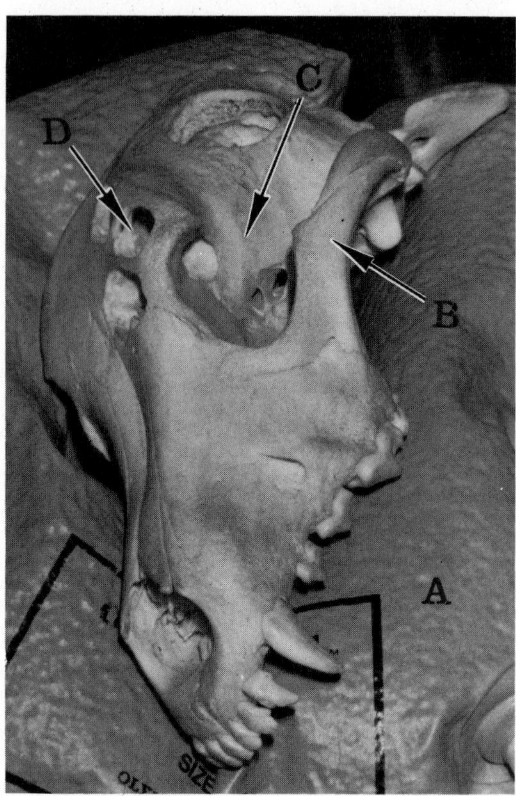

FIGURE 81–2. A canine skull positioned in a vacuum-evacuated bag (A). Note the relationship of the orbit (C), zygomatic arch (B), and frontal sinus (D). The eye can be positioned as required.

Draping

Three field drapes are placed around the eye and fastened with small towel clamps (Fig. 81–3). A fenestrated drape with a 3-cm eccentrically placed hole is positioned over the eye. An adhesive drape may be used to prevent penetration by moisture and bacteria. This drape should be large enough to cover the remainder of the patient. Full aseptic precautions are used for intraocular surgery, although some requirements may be relaxed for simple external procedures involving the lids and third eyelid. For intraocular procedures, starch powder, which may cause postoperative endophthalmitis, is removed from surgical gloves with sterile saline. Similarly, cellulose sponges are preferable to cotton-tipped applicators, which may shed fibers.

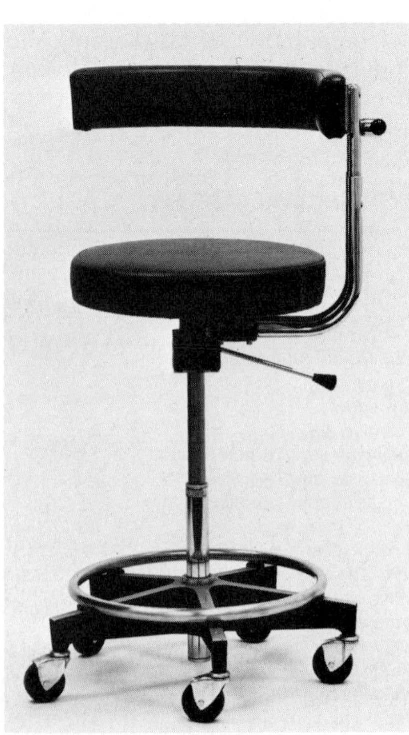

FIGURE 81–1. An ophthalmic operating stool with arm rest.

SURGICAL EQUIPMENT AND SUPPLIES

Illumination and Magnification

Ophthalmic surgery is performed in a semidarkened room with a focal light to reduce reflections in the transparent ocular media that make inner structures difficult to see. For adnexal surgery, a standard operating light is suitable, but for finer procedures, a focal or head-mounted light source (Fig. 81–4) that generates little heat is desirable to limit drying and heating of delicate structures.

Surgical procedures involving cilia, lacrimal puncta, or globe usually require magnification. A loupe as used in ocular examination (Fig. 81–5) (2.5 to 4.0 ×), and focal length of 20 to 30 cm is recommended. For more intricate procedures (e.g., correction of distichiasis or intraocular surgery), an operating microscope is essential. Available microscopes vary from simple table-mounted models (Fig. 81–6) with fixed magnification and illumination for one surgeon, to elaborate and expensive instruments with power focusing, variable

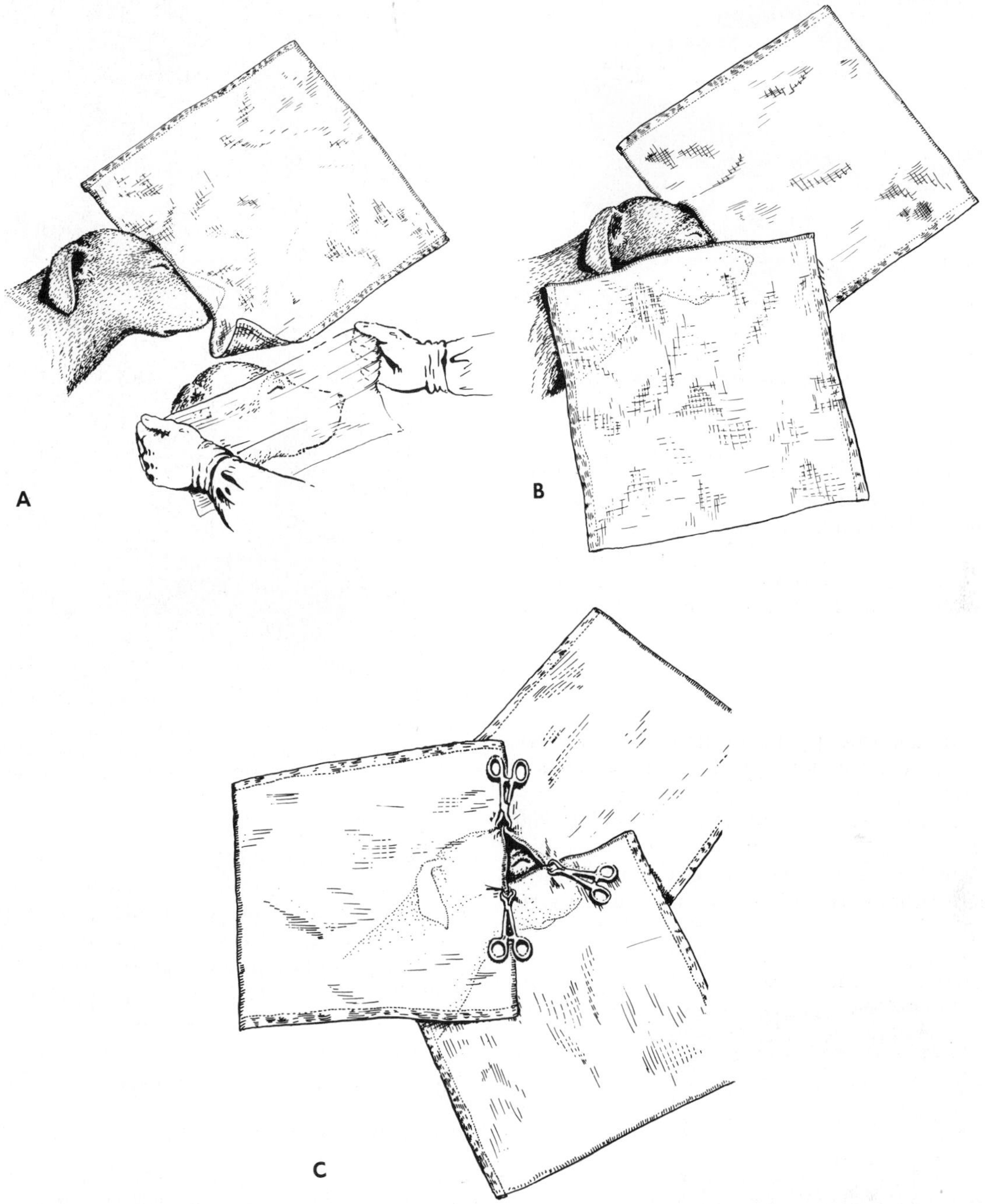

FIGURE 81–3. Draping for ocular surgery. *A,* The first field drape in position. *B,* The second field drape in position. *C,* The third field drape and Backhaus towel clamps in position.

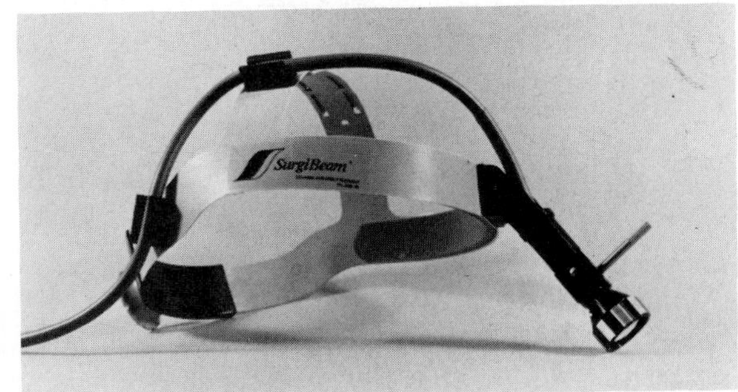

FIGURE 81–4. Head-mounted fiber-optic light source.

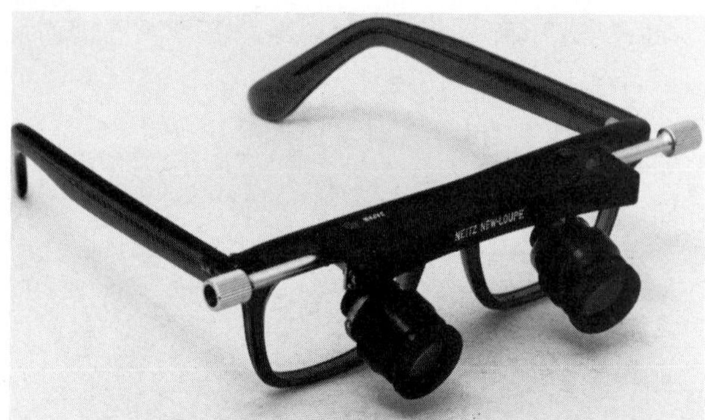

FIGURE 81–5. A simple magnifying loupe with interchangeable lenses of different magnification suitable for basic ophthalmic surgery. Such an instrument can be worn with the light source shown in Figure 81–4.

magnification, photographic outlets, assistant's eyepieces, multiple light sources, and provision for video recording (Fig. 81–7). Successful microsurgery requires training and practice. Microsurgical instruments are small and delicate and have matte surfaces to prevent reflection.

Hemostasis

Methods of hemostasis used in ophthalmic surgery include pressure with a cotton-tipped applicator; ligation of vessels, especially in lid and orbital surgery; electrocautery; electrohemostasis; and the use of 1:10,000 epinephrine solution. Electrocautery may be applied by small hand-held disposable battery-driven units (Fig. 81–8). Electrohemostasis with alternating current supplied by larger units (Fig. 81–9) capable of supplying cutting or blended currents is particularly useful if profuse hemorrhage is expected (e.g., in tumor excision, blepharoplastic procedures, and procedures involving the iris and choroid). These latter units are not to be used for epilation (Fig. 81–10). Smaller direct-current units are available, although microcryoepilation is a less destructive and more effective technique.

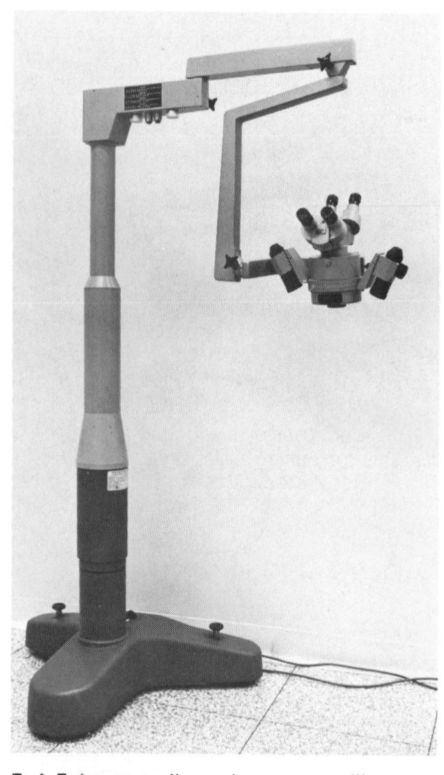

FIGURE 81–7. A Zeiss operating microscope with power-operated focus and zoom, multiple light sources, and an assistant's eyepiece.

Cryotherapy

In veterinary ophthalmic surgery, cryotherapy is used for selective destruction of neoplasms, removal of luxated lenses, treatment of distichiasis and trichiasis (microcryoepilation) (Fig. 81–11), and destruction of parts of the ciliary body in control of glaucoma[5] (cyclocryotherapy) (Fig. 81–12). Microcryoepilation and cyclocryotherapy are major advances in veterinary ophthalmic surgery. General cryosurgical equipment (Fig. 81–12) may be used for periocular tumors, but for small lesions or for use on the globe, ophthalmic cryosurgical units with a probe diameter of approximately 3 mm are necessary (see Fig. 81–11). These units are

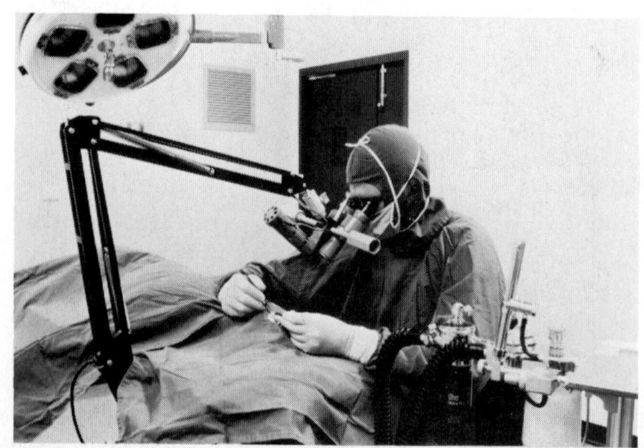

FIGURE 81–6. A basic operating microscope with a magnification of 10× and sterile handles to allow manipulation by the surgeon.

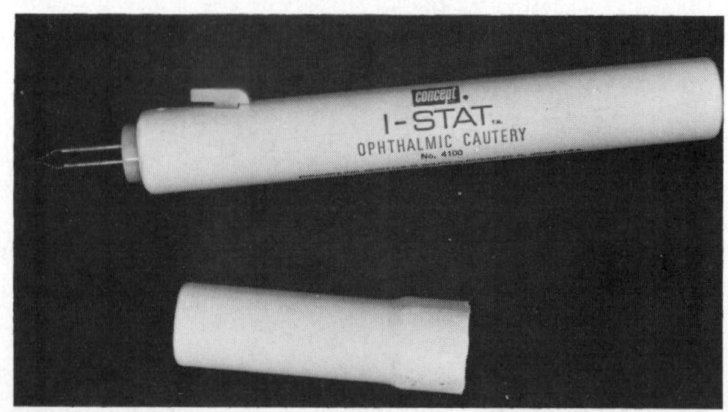

FIGURE 81–8. A disposable battery-driven hand-held electrocautery unit. The unit has a continuous operating time of 20 to 30 minutes and, although disposable, may be resterilized with ethylene oxide for repeated use.

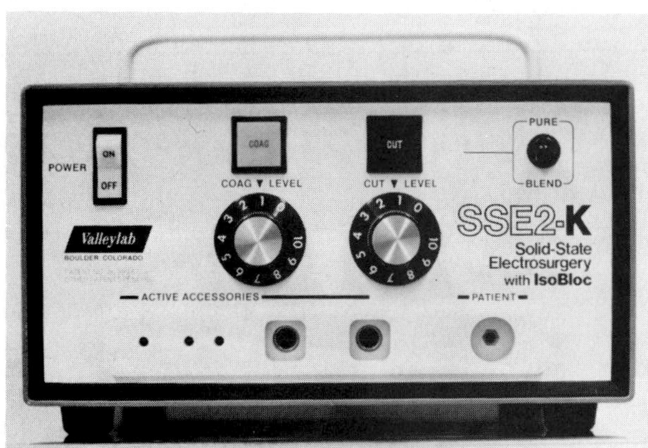

FIGURE 81–9. An electrosurgical unit capable of supplying pure or blended currents for cutting or coagulation or both. These units should not be used for electroepilation.

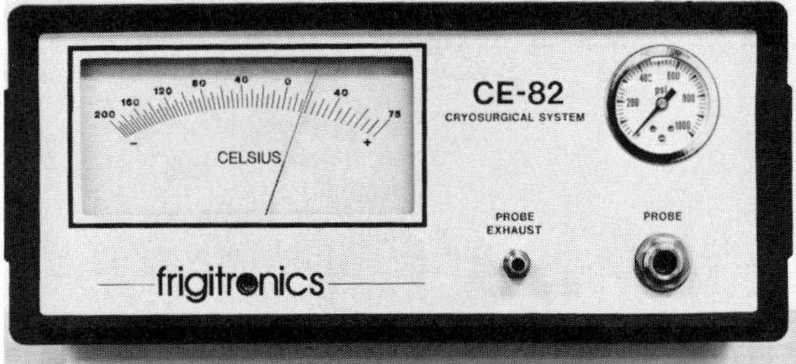

FIGURE 81–11. Frigitronics N20 cryosurgical unit for direct ocular use. A temperature of −89°C is reached with this equipment. A large variety of probes is available, but the glaucoma and lens probes are most suited to veterinary use.

cooled by nitrous oxide and have a minimum temperature of approximately −89°C.

Suture Materials and Needles (Table 81–3)

The principles of selection of ophthalmic suture material are as follows:

1. The suture should be as fine as possible, consistent with the surgeon's ability and training, and the patient's temperament.
2. Suture materials that touch the cornea are soft and pliable.
3. Chromic gut is not used in the cornea because of local tissue reactions. For buried sutures (e.g., beneath the conjunctiva), in subcutaneous sites, and in the cornea, polyglycolic acid (Dexon), polyglactin 910 (Vicryl), modified polyglycolic acid (Maxon), and polydioxanone (PDS) sutures have many advantages (see Chapter 19). Modified polyglycolic acid and polydioxanone are monofilaments that retain strength longer but may irritate the cornea.
4. Absorbable materials should be used with caution as the sole suture in a major corneal or scleral wound when nonabsorbable materials are available. A mixture of suture types may be used. The tendency for difficult infections to occur with these sutures has been recorded in other tissues.[29]

Fine, nonirritant suture materials limit postoperative inflammation. Fine nylon may be left in the cornea much longer than silk. Recommended suture materials for different situations are listed in Table 81–3. Nylon also results in less inflammation around the suture in the upper lid when used for third-eyelid flaps.

Surgical Needles

For corneal suturing, a micropoint spatula GS-9 (Ethicon) or cutting micropoint G-1 needle is recommended. For eyelids and the third eyelid, a cutting PS-2 needle is recommended. Swaged needles cause much less trauma on passage through tissue than needles with eyes, and are recommended.

Scalpel Blades

Three systems are commonly used:

1. Beaver handle with number 64 or 65 blade (Fig.

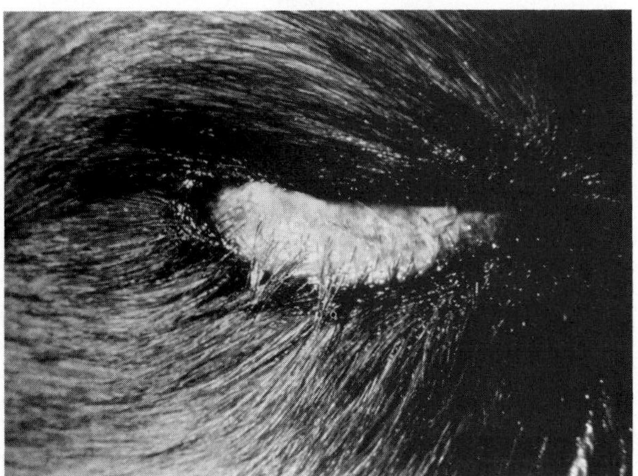

FIGURE 81–10. Severe necrosis of the lower lid resulting from use of an electrosurgical unit for epilation. (Courtesy of Dr. G. Severin.)

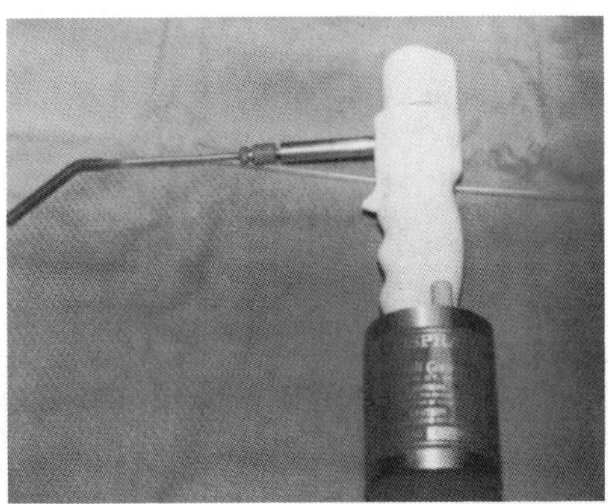

FIGURE 81–12. A cryosurgical unit cooled by liquid nitrogen, with specific probes for cyclocryotherapy. (From Slatter DH: *Fundamentals of Veterinary Ophthalmology.* 2nd ed. W.B. Saunders, Philadelphia, 1990.)

TABLE 81–3. SUTURE MATERIAL SELECTION

Tissue	Recommended Sutures	Size
Lids	Silk—soft and pliable	6-0, 4-0
	Nylon—nonirritating, but short sutures may be traumatic	6-0, 4-0, 3-0
Conjunctiva	Polydioxanone (PDS)	7-0, 6-0, 5-0
	Polyglactic acid (PGL)	
	Polyglycolic acid (PGA)	
	Chromic gut	6-0
Third eyelid	Silk	4-0
	Nylon	3-0, 4-0
Cornea	Nylon (preferred)	10-0, 9-0, 8-0, 7-0, 6-0 (10-0, 9-0—operating microscope)
	Silk	8-0, 7-0, 6-0
	PDS, PGA, PGL	9-0, 8-0, 7-0, 6-0

From Slatter D: *Fundamentals of Veterinary Ophthalmology*. 2nd ed. W. B. Saunders, Philadelphia, 1990.

81–13) or their generic equivalents. Numerous other Beaver blades are available for special purposes in ophthalmic surgery (Fig. 81–21*E*), but the number 64 and 65 are generally most useful.

2. Standard number 3 handle with number 11 and 15 blades (Fig. 81–14).

3. Special-purpose blades (e.g., 3-mm keratome for anterior chamber entry, corneal diamond knives). These have generally replaced the broken edge of razor blades once used.

MISCELLANEOUS SUPPLIES

Irrigating Solutions

Balanced salt solution* is preferable to saline for ocular irrigation because it causes less osmotic damage to the corneal endothelium.[8] For continuous intraocular irrigation, heparin and epinephrine are often added. For preoperative preparation, saline may be used. Solutions containing glutathione cause even less endothelial damage but are expensive. Sterile water is never used near the eye, because intraocular use causes severe osmotic damage to the endothelium.

*Alcon Laboratories, Fort Worth, TX.

Viscoelastic Substances

Viscoelastic substances such as hyaluronic acid and methycellulose are placed in the anterior chamber to retain its shape during intraocular surgery and to prevent contact between intraocular objects and the corneal endothelium. Methylcellulose is safe and sterile when correctly prepared and has few if any demonstrated disadvantages over much more expensive hyaluronic acid.

Sponges

Cellulose sponge wedges* (Fig. 81–15) are recommended for penetrating ocular wounds. Sterile cotton-tipped applicators are useful for controlling conjunctival hemorrhage but should not be placed inside the eye or near a penetrating wound because of the danger of cotton strands entering the eye. Standard cotton surgical sponges are treated similarly.

*Weck-cel, Edward Weck Surgical Co., Long Island, NY.

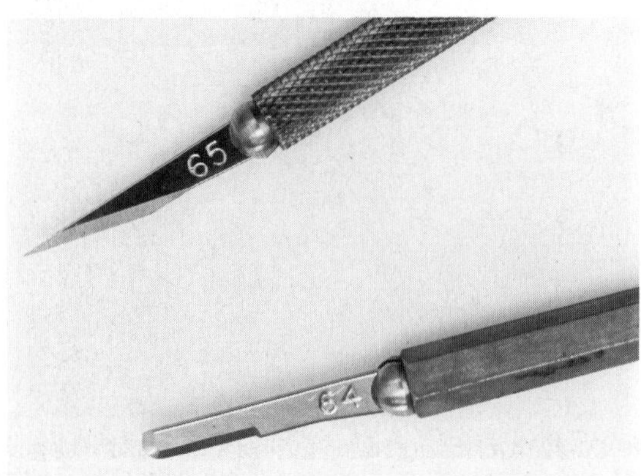

FIGURE 81–13. Hexagonal and circular milled Beaver handles with number 64 and number 65 blades, respectively.

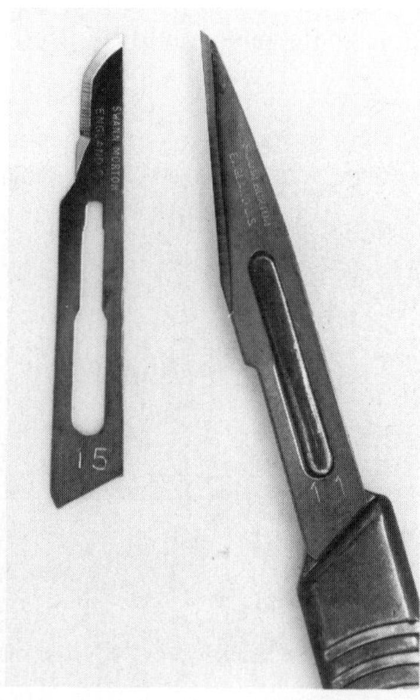

FIGURE 81–14. Standard number 3 handle with number 15 and number 11 blades.

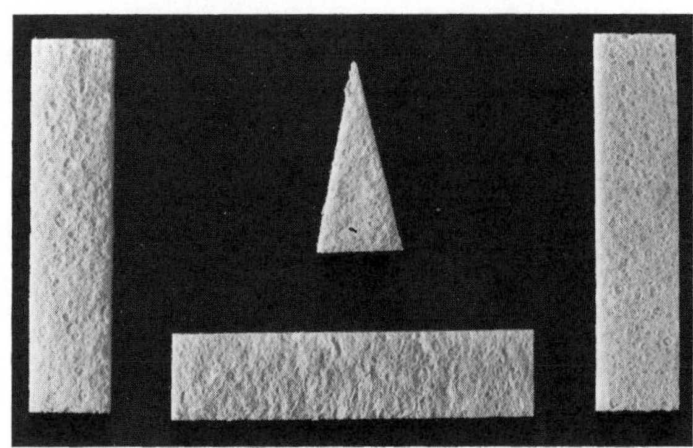

FIGURE 81–15. Cellulose surgical sponges for ophthalmic use.

CARE AND STERILIZATION OF OPHTHALMIC INSTRUMENTS

Ophthalmic instruments require special care because they are delicate, fragile, and expensive. Instruments are individually cleaned and dried to preserve teeth, points, and cutting edges. They must not be placed in groups for washing, because damage occurs. Ultrasonic cleaning is useful and limits damage to delicate surfaces by handling. Instruments are inspected regularly by the surgeon and repaired early. Tubular silicone cuffs may be placed over the ends of instruments to protect them during autoclaving (plastics may melt). Instruments may be protected during autoclaving or storage by placing them on racks or boards or, ideally, in a perforated instrument case (Fig. 81–16).

Three methods of sterilization are commonly used: autoclaving, ethylene oxide, and dry heat (see also Chapter 11). Ethylene oxide sterilization is least damaging to instruments but is very toxic to tissues, and instrument packs must be aired for 48 hours before use. Special precautions are required to prevent exposure of personnel to ethylene oxide. Steam sterilization is commonly used, although over a long period, fine cutting edges are subject to corrosion and damage, especially with poor-quality equipment. The dry heat sterilizer is useful for fine instruments but has the disadvantage of requiring sterilization at 302°F (150°C) for 1½ hours (320°F [160°C] damages fine edges). Dry heat ovens contain a fan and thermostatic switch.

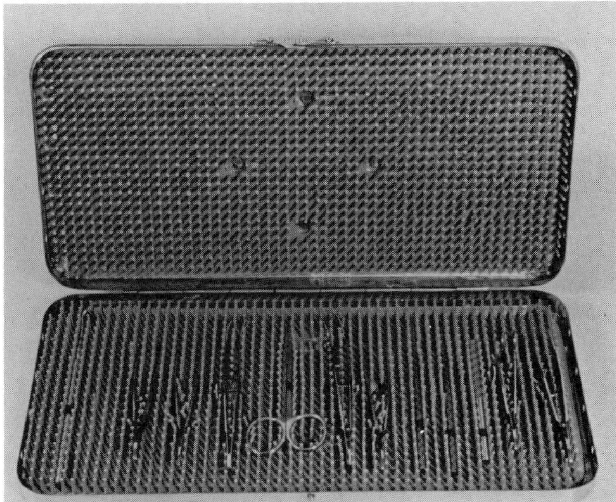

FIGURE 81–16. A perforated instrument case with flexible rubber fingers suitable for autoclaving or storing instruments.

PREVENTION OF SELF-TRAUMA

Prevention of self-trauma after ophthalmic surgical procedures is important, especially when a cycle of scratching has been established before surgery and when fine sutures are used. Various methods are available, either singly or in combination:

1. An Elizabethan collar or plastic bucket (Fig. 81–17). These are recommended for all external ophthalmic surgical procedures (e.g., entropion) but are usually not indicated for intraocular surgery and may be detrimental if the animal attempts to remove it vigorously.
2. Bandaging dewclaws on the forelegs.
3. Bandaging the eye. This method is rarely necessary; the bandage is difficult to keep on and limits the frequency of observation and medication.
4. Painful anterior segment lesions can be rendered less painful with appropriate cycloplegics for ciliary spasm (e.g., in uveitis) or with third-eyelid flaps for corneal lesions. Topical anesthetics are not used because they are toxic to the cornea with repeated application.
5. Tranquilization in severe cases (e.g., diazepam or acetylpromazine as necessary). Analgesics such as morphine, meperidine hydrochloride, and butorphanol may occasionally be necessary.

It is often useful to leave a collar or bucket in place for several days after suture removal until all irritation has

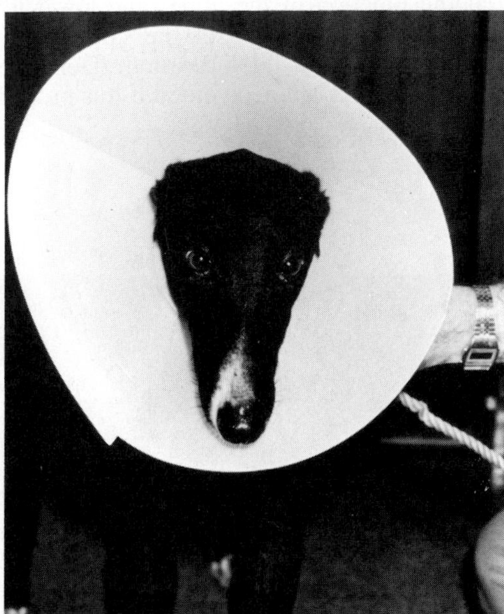

FIGURE 81–17. An Elizabethan collar to protect the eye from being rubbed or scratched. A plastic bucket with the bottom removed may be used similarly, attached to the animal's collar.

subsided, because some patients commence rubbing or scratching soon after leaving the clinic.

EXPOSURE AND FIXATION OF THE GLOBE

Good exposure and control of the globe are prerequisites for successful ophthalmic surgery. The effort required to achieve exposure in animal patients differs markedly from the simpler methods necessary in humans, primarily because the eye deviates in an inferomedial direction under general anesthesia (reversed Bell phenomenon) in animals. The third eyelid also restricts exposure.

Exposure

Numerous designs of lid retractors and specula are available. For short procedures, especially when an animal is conscious, a lid speculum is useful (Fig. 81–18). For major ophthalmic procedures, the Castroviejo and Maumenee-Park specula are recommended (Fig. 81–19).

Canthotomy

A lateral canthotomy greatly improves exposure of the eye (Fig. 81–20). The lateral canthus is incised with straight Mayo scissors up to but not including the orbital ligament. The area should *not* be crushed with hemostats before incision, or healing is retarded. Infiltration with dilute epinephrine solution reduces hemorrhage. After the ophthalmic procedure is completed, the incision is closed in two layers. The first layer of simple interrupted sutures of 6-0 polyglactin 910 or polyglycolic acid apposes the conjunctiva underlying the incision. The second layer of simple interrupted sutures of 4-0 or 6-0 silk closes the skin. In the second layer, the first suture is placed at the junction of the upper and lower lids and emerges from the lid margin in the same way as the suture used to close a lid laceration. Dehiscence of canthotomy incisions can be avoided if this procedure is followed.

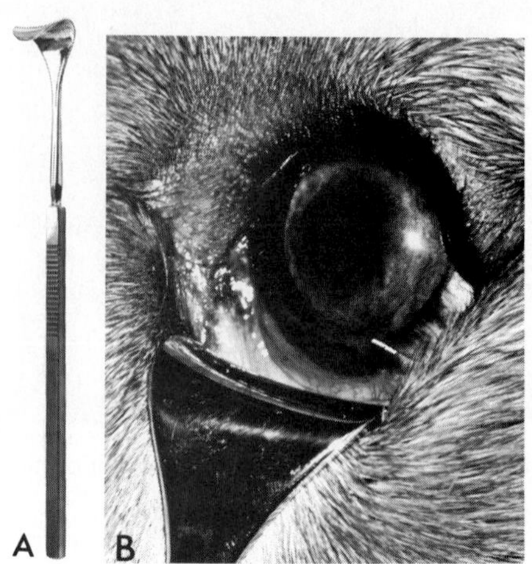

FIGURE 81–18. *A*, A lid retractor. A number of different sizes are available. *B*, Lid retractor in place.

Fixation

Scleral Fixation Sutures

Scleral fixation sutures are invaluable but must be placed partially through the sclera (unlike the human eye). Passing the suture beneath the insertion of the dorsal rectus muscle is usually inadequate in animals because the muscle either cannot be identified or is too thin and flat for secure anchorage. A suture of 3-0 or 4-0 silk with a swaged cutting needle is placed 1 to 2 mm from the limbus and is tagged lightly with either a small hemostat or serrefines. Care is taken not to penetrate the sclera with the suture. Additional sutures may be placed inferiorly, nasally, or temporally as required. When the suture is removed, one arm is cut close to the conjunctiva to reduce trauma rather than drawing the whole suture through the tissue. Subconjunctival hemorrhage is frequent with scleral fixation sutures.

Oschner forceps (mosquito hemostats with a small tooth near the tip) are useful for fixing the globe when attached to the conjunctiva near the limbus.

Text continued on page 1156

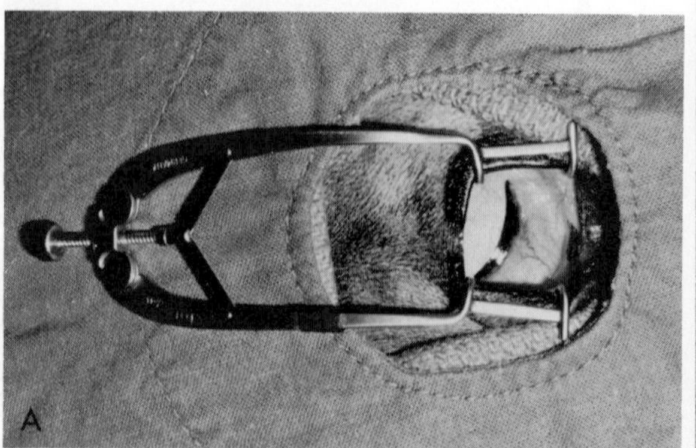

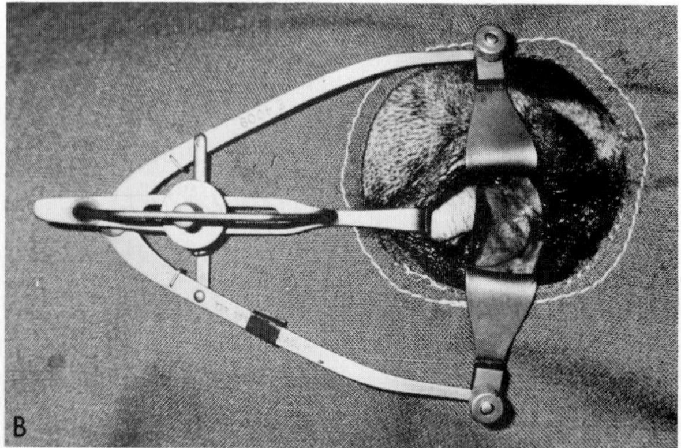

FIGURE 81–19. *A*, A self-retaining Castroviejo lid speculum in place. If additional exposure is needed, a lateral canthotomy may be performed. *B*, A self-retaining Maumenee-Park lid speculum in place. This speculum has the advantage of being able to retract in three directions.

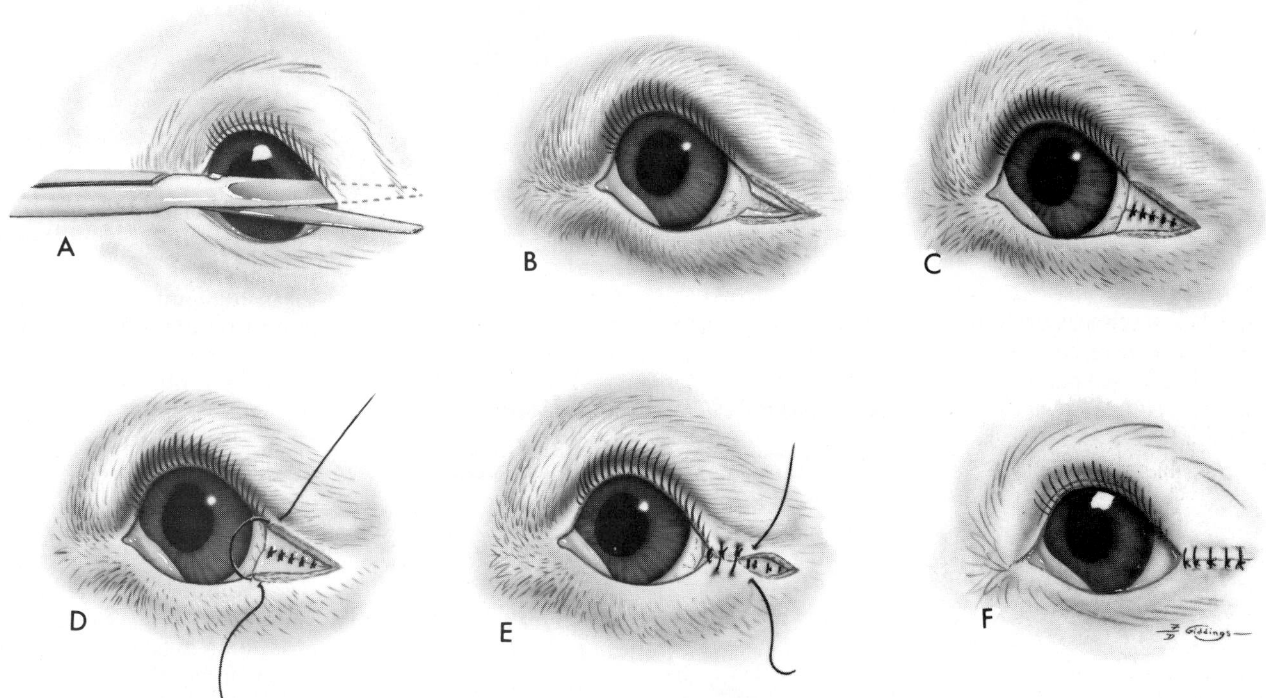

FIGURE 81–20. Lateral canthotomy. *A*, Position of the scissors. *B*, The canthotomy performed. *C*, Closure of the conjunctiva with simple interrupted sutures of 6–0 Vicryl or Dexon. *D*, The first suture of the second layer is placed at the lateral canthus and emerges at the lid margin. *E*, The incision is closed with simple interrupted sutures of 4–0 silk or Ethibond. *F*, The incision accurately sutured.

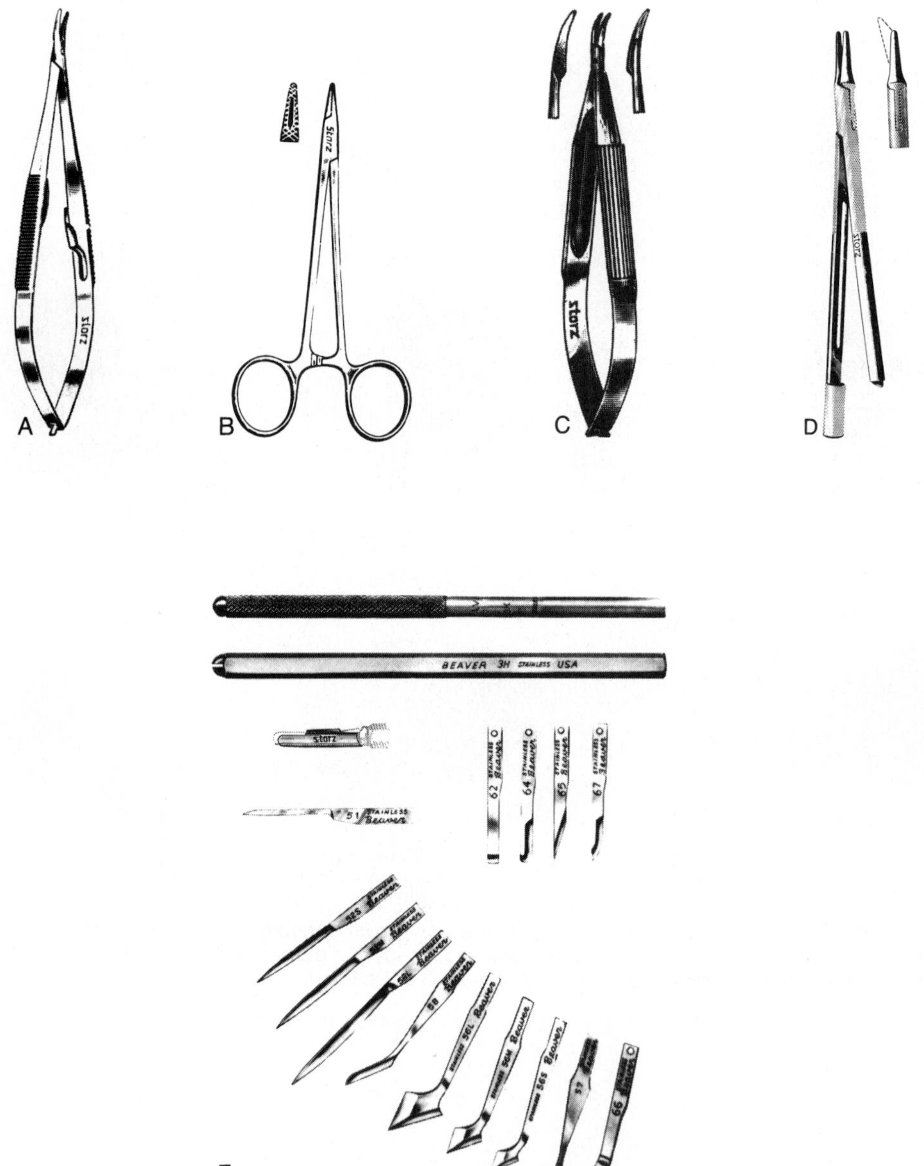

FIGURE 81–21. Common ophthalmic instruments. *A*, Castroviejo curved needle holders. *B*, Derf needle holders. *C*, Troutman needle holders (microsurgery). *D*, Swiss blade breaker. *E*, Selection of Beaver blades and handles.

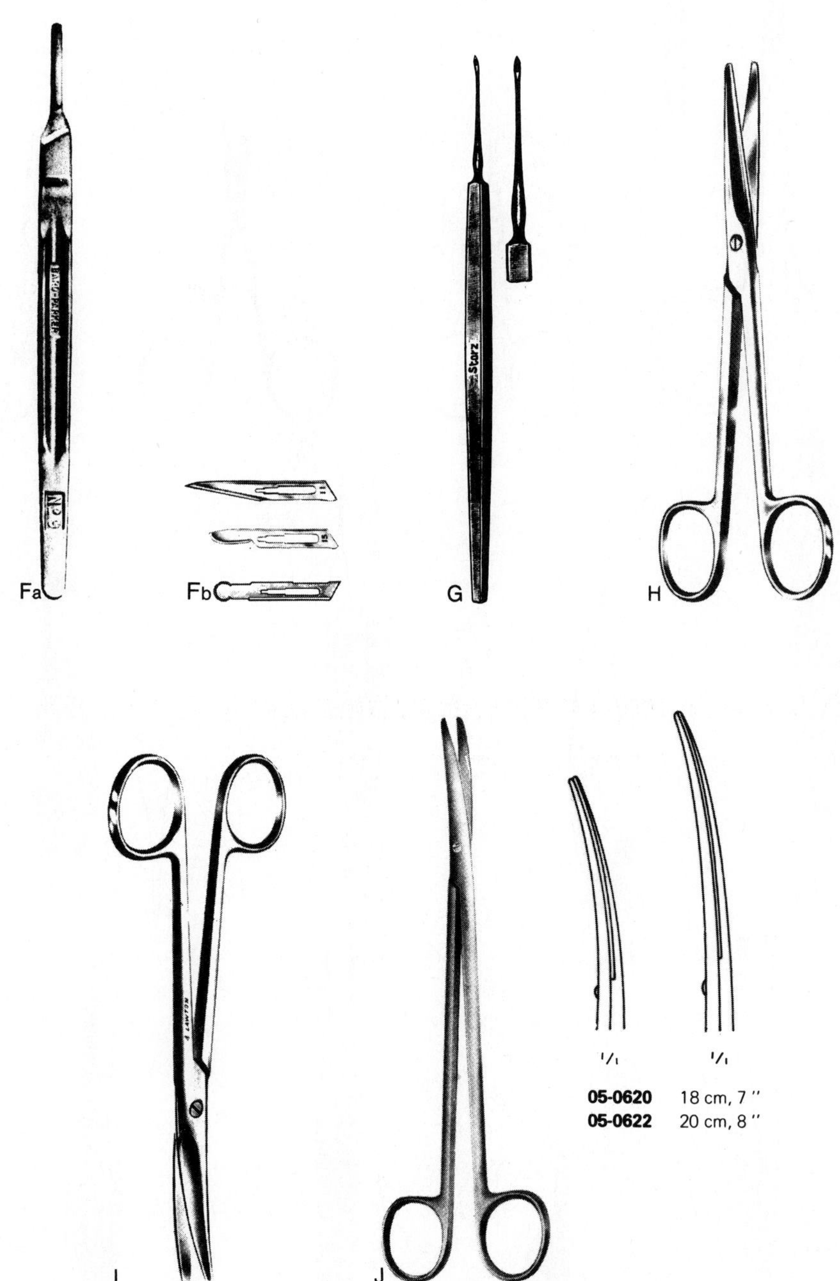

FIGURE 81–21 *Continued Fa* and *Fb*, Bard-Parker blades. *G*, Foreign body spud. *H*, Straight Mayo scissors. *I*, Curved Mayo scissors. *J*, Curved Metzenbaum scissors.

Illustration continued on following page

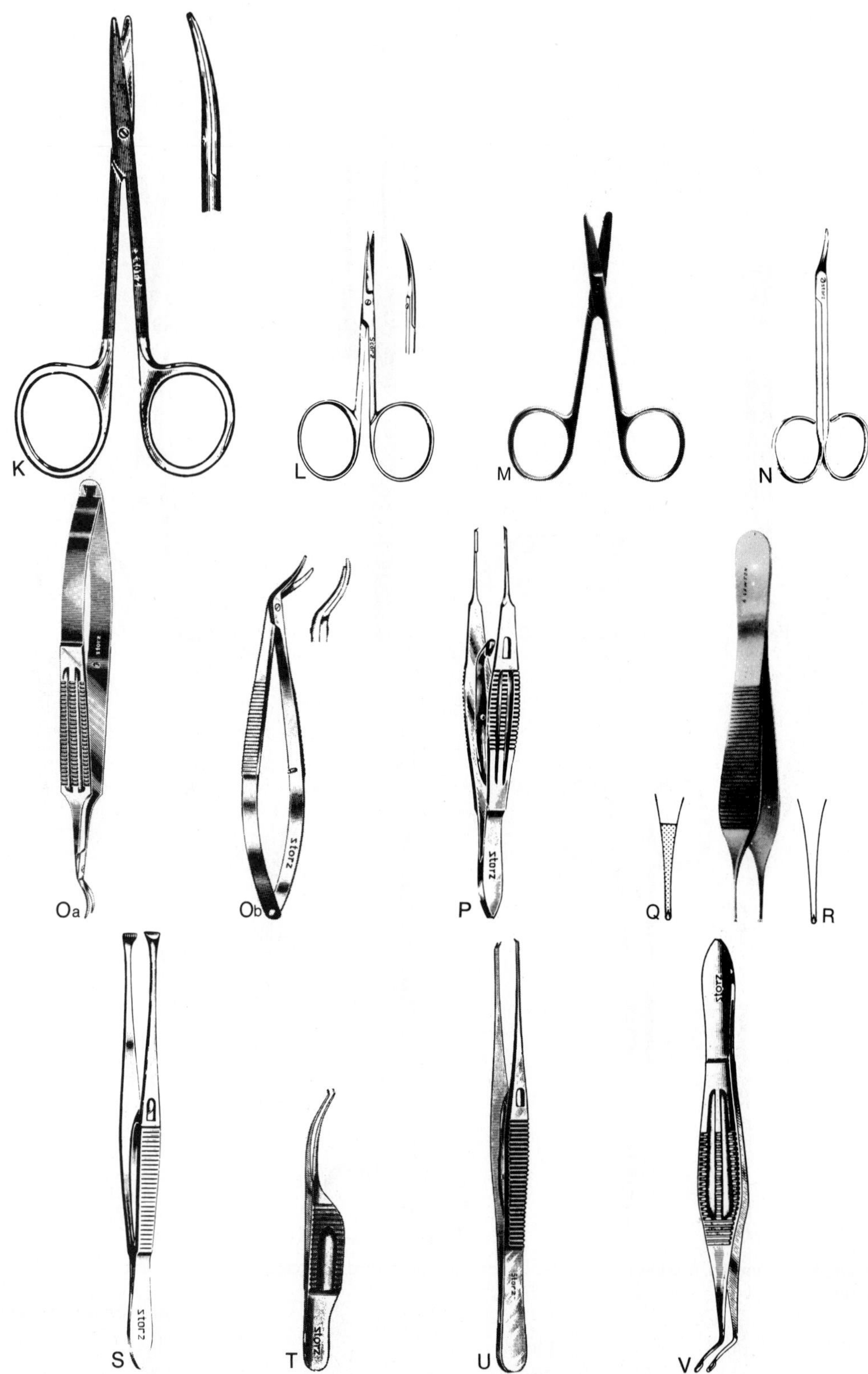

FIGURE 81–21 *Continued K*, Strabismus scissors. *L*, Iris scissors. *M*, Spencer suture scissors. *N*, McGuire corneal scissors. *Oa* and *Ob*, Castroviejo corneal scissors (left- and right-handed). *P*, Castroviejo forceps with tying platforms. *Q*, Adson tissue forceps. *R*, Adson tissue forceps (toothed). *S*, Von Grafe fixation forceps. *T*, Colibri forceps. *U*, Elschnig-O'Brien forceps. *V*, Arruga capsule forceps.

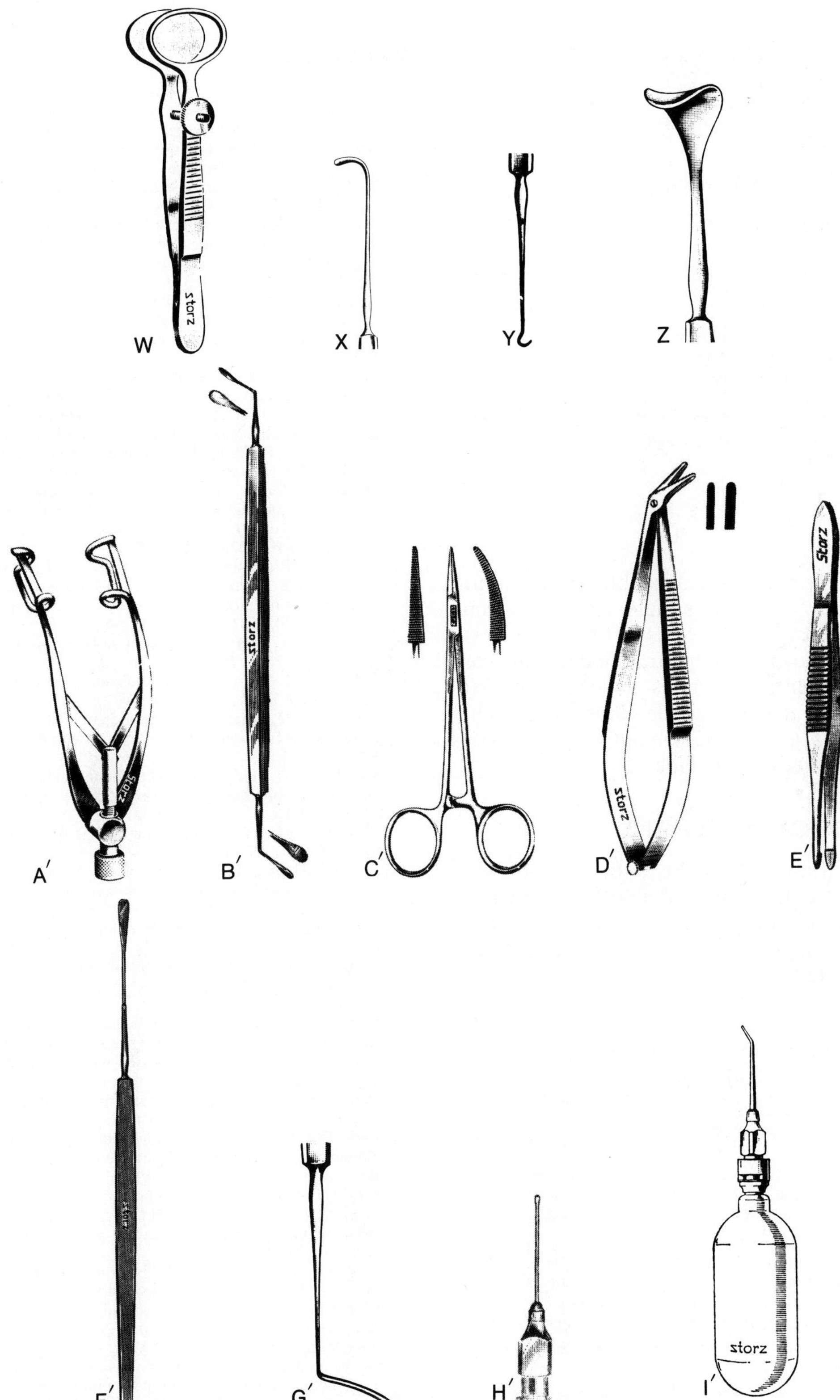

FIGURE 81–21 *Continued W,* Chalazion forceps. *X,* Muscle hook. *Y,* Iris hook. *Z,* Lid retractor. *A′,* Castroviejo lid speculum. *B′,* Martinez corneal knife dissector. *C′,* Halsted curved hemostats. *D′,* Scleral punch. *E′,* Cilia forceps. *F′,* Kimura spatula. *G′,* Cyclodialysis spatula. *H′,* Lacrimal cannula. *I′,* Silicone irrigating bulb and anterior chamber needles.

TABLE 81–4. BASIC OPHTHALMIC INSTRUMENT SET

Instrument tray (35 × 25 cm)
Saline bowl (10-cm diameter)
Sponges (7 cm)
Cellulose sponges
Scalpel handle (number 3), blades (number 11, 15)
Castroviejo lid speculum
Castroviejo conjunctival forceps
Adson toothed (1 × 2) tissue forceps
Colibri corneal forceps
Castroviejo corneal forceps
Elschnig-O'Brien fixation forceps
Derf needle holders
Strabismus scissors
Straight Mayo scissors
Spencer suture scissors
McGuire corneal scissors
Silicone irrigating bulb
Curved Halsted mosquito hemostats
Curved Metzenbaum scissors
Curved mosquito hemostats
Irrigating cannula

From Slatter D: *Fundamentals of Veterinary Ophthalmology*. 2nd ed. W. B. Saunders, Philadelphia, 1990.

Instruments

A number of instruments are available for fixation to restrict movement, but each suffers from the same disadvantage: When placed securely enough to grasp the sclera firmly, the instrument traumatizes the conjunctiva. If the conjunctiva alone is grasped, poor fixation results because it is so mobile. Fine Halsted hemostats (Fig. 81–21*C′* and Elschnig-O'Brien forceps (Fig. 81–21*U*) are used for the globe.

OPHTHALMIC SURGICAL INSTRUMENTS

Ophthalmic instruments are illustrated in Figure 81–21. A basic list of instruments suitable for procedures commonly performed in general practice is given in Table 81–4. More sophisticated extra- and intraocular instruments are listed in Table 81–5. Eponyms applied to instruments denote the designer. Many different designs of similar instruments often can do the same job.

TABLE 81–5. ADVANCED OPHTHALMIC INSTRUMENT SET

Extraocular	Intraocular
Distichiasis clamps	Iris scissors
Castroviejo needle holders	Lens loupe
Troutman needle holders	Arruga lens capsule forceps
Beaver scalpel handle (blades number 64, 65)	McGannon lens capsule forceps
	Scleral punch
Cystitome	Cystitome
Foreign body spud	Iris hook (sharp, dull)
Desmarres chalazion clamp	O'Gawa irrigation cannula
Chalazion spoon	Cyclodialysis spatula
Muscle hook	Flieringa fixation righs
Martinez corneal elevator	Jamieson calipers
Maumenee-Park lid speculum	
Tying forceps	

References

1. Anderson JA, Chen CC: Multiple dosing increases bioavailability of topically administered flurbiprofen. *Arch Ophthalmol 106:*1107, 1988.
2. Anderson JA, et al: Disposition of topical flurbiprofen in normal and aphakic rabbit eyes. *Arch Ophthalmol 100*:642, 1982.
3. Bistner SI, et al: Conjunctival bacteria: Clinical appearances can be deceiving. *Mod Vet Pract 50*:45, 1969.
4. Brightman AH, et al: Effect of aspirin on aqueous protein values in the dog. *J Am Vet Med Assoc 178*:572, 1981.
5. Brightman AH, et al: Cryosurgery for the treatment of canine glaucoma. *J Am Anim Hosp Assoc 18*:319, 1982.
6. Brock KA, Thurmon JC: Pulmonary edema associated with mannitol administration. *Canine Pract 6*:31, 1979.
7. Campbell L: Ocular bacteria and mycoplasma of the clinically normal cat. *Feline Pract 3*:10, 1973.
8. Edelhauser HF, et al: Comparative toxicity of intraocular irrigating solutions on the corneal endothelium. *Am J Ophthalmol 81*:473, 1976.
9. Eichenbaum JD, et al: Effect in large dogs of ophthalmic prednisolone acetate on adrenal gland and hepatic function. *Am J Vet Res 24*:705, 1988.
10. Feinstein NC, Rubin B: Toxicity of flurbiprofen sodium. *Arch Ophthalmol 106*:311, 1988.
11. Floman N, Zor U: Mechanism of steroid action in ocular inflammation. Inhibition of prostaglandin production. *Invest Ophthalmol 16*:69, 1977.
12. Gelatt KN, Rubin LF: Delayed postoperative staphylomas in dogs. *J Am Vet Med Assoc 154*:283, 1969.
13. Havener WH: *Ocular Pharmacology*. 4th ed. C.V. Mosby, St. Louis, 1983.
14. Krohne SDG, Vestre WA: Effects of flunixin meglumine and dexamethasone on aqueous protein values after intraocular surgery in the dog. *Am J Vet Res 48*:420, 1987.
15. Magrane WG: Cataract extraction: A follow-up study (429 cases). *J Small Anim Pract 10*:545, 1969.
16. McDonald PJ, Watson ADJ: Microbial flora of normal canine conjunctivae. *J Small Anim Pract 17*:809, 1976.
17. Millichamp NJ, Dziezyc J: Comparison of flunixin meglumine and flurbiprofen for control of ocular irritative response in dogs. *Am J Vet Res 52*:1452, 1991.
18. Millichamp NJ, et al: Acute effects of anti-inflammatory drugs on neodymium:yttrium aluminum garnet laser-induced uveitis is dogs. *Am J Vet Res 52*:1279, 1991.
19. Muir WW: Effects of atropine on cardiac rate and rhythm in dogs. *J Am Vet Med Assoc 172*:917, 1978.
20. Nuefeld AH, et al: Degeneration release of norepinephrine causes transient ocular hyperemia mediated by prostaglandins. *Invest Ophthalmol 12*:167, 1973.
21. Peiffer RL: Current concepts in ophthalmic surgery. *Vet Clin North Am 10*:455, 1980.
22. Regnier A, et al: Effect of flunixine meglumine breakdown of the blood aqueous barrier following paracentesis in the canine eye. *J Ophthalmol Pharmacol 2*:165, 1986.
23. Roberts SM, et al: Effect of ophthalmic prednisolone on the canine adrenal gland and hepatic function. *Am J Vet Res 45*:1711, 1984.
24. Roberts SM, et al: Antibacterial activity of dilute povidone-iodine solutions used for ocular surface disinfection in dogs. *Am J Vet Res 47*:1207, 1986.
25. Slatter D: *Fundamentals of Veterinary Ophthalmology*. 2nd ed. W.B. Saunders, Philadelphia, 1990.
26. Spiess BM, et al: Kinetics of uptake and effects of topical indomethacin on protein concentration in the aqueous humor of dogs. *Am J Vet Res 52*:1159, 1991.
27. Stark WJ, et al: Reduction of pupillary constriction during cataract surgery using suprofen. *Arch Ophthalmol 104*:364, 1986.
28. Urban M, et al: Conjunctival flora of clinically normal dogs. *J Am Vet Med Assoc 161*:201, 1972.
29. Varma S, et al: Further studies with polyglycolic acid (Dexon) and other sutures in infected experimental wounds. *Am J Vet Res 42*:571, 1981.
30. Waitzman MB, King CD: Prostaglandin influences on intraocular pressure and pupil size. *Am J Physiol (Lond) 212*:329, 1967.
31. Whitelocke RAF, Eakins KC: Vascular changes in the anterior uvea of rabbits produced by prostaglandins. *Arch Ophthalmol 89*:495, 1973.
32. Yoshimoto T, Ito Y: Effects of indomethacin and prostaglandins on the dog iris sphincter and dilator muscles. *Invest Ophthalmol Vis Sci 29*:127, 1988.

CHAPTER

82 Eyelids

Alan H. Brightman II

ANATOMY

The eyelids are thin, mobile folds of skin that normally cover the eyes. In cross section, the lids are composed of the external epidermal surface, the orbicular muscle of the eye, the tarsal plate, the meibomian glands, and the palpebral conjunctiva (Fig. 82–1).[18] The lid margins are demarcated from the skin by a mucocutaneous border 2 to 3 mm from the lid margin. The openings of the tarsal glands (20 to 40 per lid) can be seen on the surface of the lid margins. On everting the lids, these glands can be seen under the conjunctiva as white cords extending ventrally 5 to 7 mm from the lid margin. The tarsal glands secrete a phospholipid-rich sebaceous material that forms the superficial lipid layer of the tear film.

The tarsal plate is a poorly defined fibrous sheet that supports the lids and is continuous with the orbital septum, which is attached to the orbital periosteum.

The cilia (eyelashes) in dogs are found on the outer surface of the upper lid margin. Dogs have no cilia on the lower lid, and cats have no cilia at all.[8] At the base of these cilia, sweat glands (glands of Moll) and sebaceous glands (glands of Zeis) open near or into the adjacent hair follicle.[18]

Muscles of the Eyelids

The orbicular muscle of the eye lies anterior to the tarsal plate and encircles the palpebral fissure (Fig. 82–2). It is innervated by the palpebral nerve, a branch of the facial nerve (cranial nerve VII).[8]

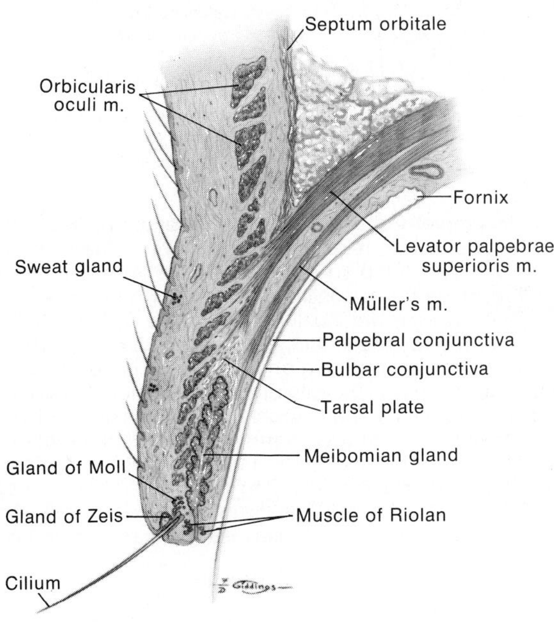

FIGURE 82–1. Anatomy of the normal eyelid.

The orbicular muscle of the eye functions as a sphincter to close the lids. In most species, the muscle is anchored medially to the orbit by fascia and laterally by the retractor muscle of the lateral angle of the eye. These attachments of the orbicular muscle of the eye preserve the elliptical shape of the palpebral fissure. The muscle that elevates the upper lid is the superior palpebral levator. It is innervated by the oculomotor nerve (cranial nerve III). The Müller muscle, which is indistinguishable from the superior palpebral levator, provides sympathetic tone to keep the upper lid elevated without conscious effort. The sensory nerve to the lids is the ophthalmic branch of the trigeminal nerve (cranial nerve V).[8]

DIFFERENTIAL DIAGNOSIS OF EYELID DISEASE

A concise review of differential diagnosis of primary and secondary eyelid diseases can be found in Table 82–1.

CONGENITAL ABNORMALITIES OF THE EYELIDS REQUIRING SURGICAL CORRECTION

Ophthalmia Neonatorum

The lids in newborn puppies normally separate at 10 to 15 days. In some puppies but rarely in other species, an acute purulent conjunctivitis occurs before lid separation. The lids are swollen, and a purulent exudate is

TABLE 82–1. DIFFERENTIAL DIAGNOSIS OF EYELID DISEASE

Eyelid mass	Distichiasis
Chalazion/hordeolom	Nasal fold
Neoplasia	Chalazion
Staphylococcal granuloma	Staphylococcal blepharitis
Parasitic—*Cuterebra*	*Blepharospasm*
Scar—dermatomycosis	Ectopic cilia
Eyelid dermatitis	Distichiasis
Autoimmune	Entropion
Allergic	Staphylococcal infection
Toxic	Tumor
Parasitic	Laceration
Infectious	Trichiasis
Staphylococcal dermatitis	*Keratitis*
Tear excoriation	Entropion
Dermatomycosis	Ectopic cilia
Tearing	Facial folds
Entropion	Lid tumor
Ectopic cilia	Agenesis
Ectropion	Foreign body
Nasolacrimal blockage	

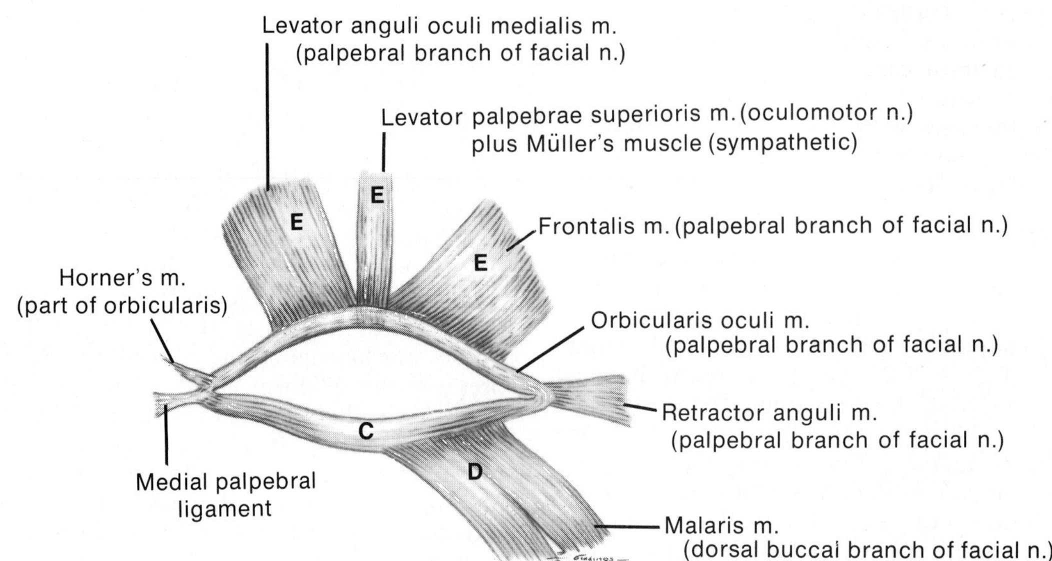

FIGURE 82–2. Actions and innervations of the muscles of the eyelid. (E, elevate upper eyelid; D, depress lower lid; C, constrict palpebral fissure.)

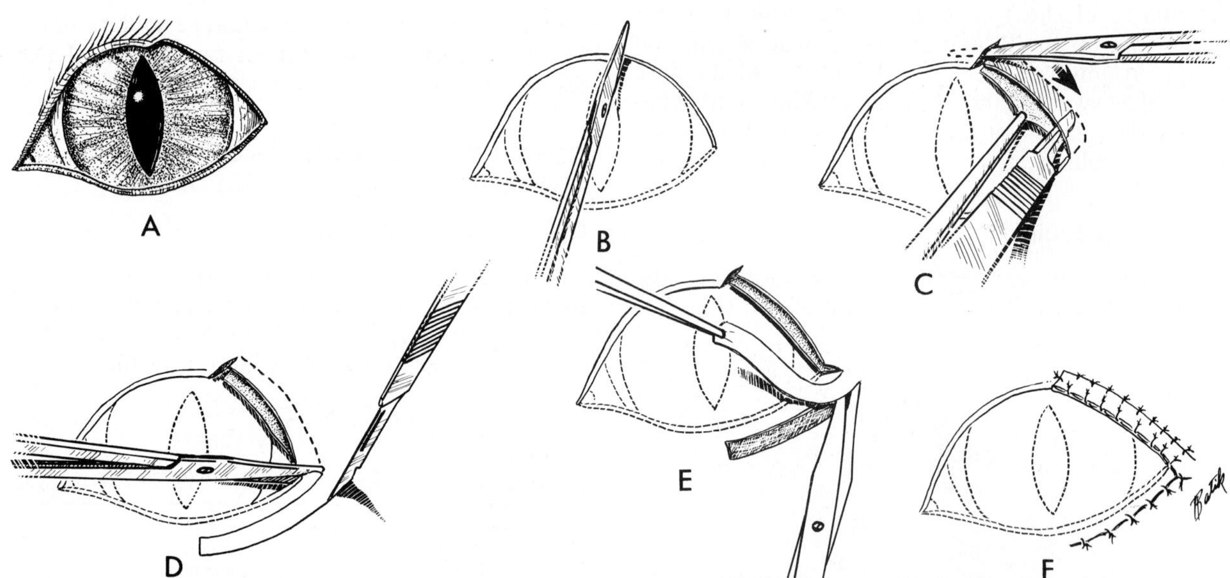

FIGURE 82–3. Horizontal pedicle graft for correction of eyelid coloboma. *A,* Incomplete development of the temporal aspect of the upper eyelid can result in chronic keratitis. *B,* A recipient bed is prepared in the upper lid to receive the pedicle graft. The nasal end of the lid defect is made square by trimming the defect with Stevens tenotomy scissors. *C,* The lid is split along the length of the upper defect, separating the skin-orbicularis layer from the underlying conjunctiva. The lid splitting is continued nasally for a distance of 3 mm into the normal lid. *D,* The horizontal pedicle flap to be transposed is prepared by making two incisions through the skin and orbicularis of the lower lid. The first incision is made parallel to and 2 mm from the lid margin; the second incision is made 5 mm from the lid edge, providing a 3-mm horizontal flap. The length of the pedicle flap depends on the size of the defect to be filled. The incisions into the lower lid are parallel but diverge slightly to form a broader base as they reach the lateral canthus. The lateral canthus is cut to the uppermost edge of the pedicle, permitting the pedicle to be rotated to its new position in the upper lid. The horizontal skin-orbicularis oculi pedicle flap is bluntly dissected free. *E,* A thin strip of skin-orbicularis muscle in the recipient bed is removed from the upper lid to create a fresh wound to receive the pedicle graft. The pedicle graft is moved to its new position. *F,* The pedicle flap is sutured in place with interrupted 6-0 silk, nylon, or polyglycolic acid. The conjunctiva is sutured to the edge of the pedicle flap, creating a new lid margin. All sutures should be placed to avoid corneal irritation. Hair does not grow on the new lid margin, which consists of tarsus that becomes epithelialized and heals with a smooth border. The lower lid defect is closed with simple interrupted sutures. (Reprinted with permission from Bistner S, et al: *Atlas of Veterinary Ophthalmic Surgery.* W.B. Saunders, Philadelphia, 1977.)

observed from the medial canthus or nares. In these cases, it is imperative to open the lids surgically as soon as possible to prevent corneal damage.[14] A muscle hook or tenotomy scissors are inserted medially or laterally at the canthus. In most cases, the lids separate when gentle upward pressure is applied with the instrument. Flushing the cul-de-sacs with a sterile eye wash and applying an appropriate antibiotic four to six times a day for several days usually result in rapid recovery.[14]

Colobomas

A coloboma, or agenesis of the eyelid, is a defect in the lid margin. The disease rarely occurs in dogs but has been reported in cats.[2, 8, 20] In cats, the defect usually involves the lateral portion of the upper lid. Depending on the severity of the defect, the condition can result in entropion, trichiasis, blepharospasm, or secondary keratitis.

Surgical correction of the defect using a horizontal pedicle graft (Fig. 82–3) is usually required if the lesion is causing clinical signs of disease.[1] The procedure involves preparing a graft site by splitting the skin and conjunctiva. A pedicle graft is harvested from the lower lid and is sutured into the defect. Care must be taken to suture the conjunctiva to the pedicle so that hair from the skin does not rub on the cornea. The conjunctiva-to-pedicle sutures are 6-0 or 7-0 polyglactin 910, and 5-0 or 6-0 silk is used for the skin sutures.

Narrow Palpebral Fissure (Blepharophimosis, Micropalpebral Fissure)

A narrow palpebral fissure is congenital in the chow chow, Kerry blue terrier, collie, Shetland sheepdog, and bull terrier.[2, 14, 20] If the condition is associated with concomitant microphthalmia, surgical correction may not be necessary. In a dog with a normal-sized globe, however, this condition may result in entropion (inversion of the lid margins). Enlargement of the palpebral fissure by performing a canthotomy and canthoplasty usually corrects the entropion (Fig. 82–4).[1]

The canthotomy is performed by drawing the lateral canthus laterally with the thumb and forefinger. The canthus is cut with blunt scissors to the desired length. After the canthotomy has been performed, permanent lengthening of the palpebral fissure can be achieved with a canthoplasty.[1]

Large Palpebral Fissure (Macropalpebral Fissure)

Too large a palpebral fissure, in the presence of a normal-sized globe, can result in ectropion (eversion of the lid margins). Although the condition rarely causes ocular disease, certain breeds, such as the English bulldog, spaniel, and hounds, may require shortening of the fissure.[14, 20] The procedure may also be indicated in cases of phthisis bulbi or endophthalmos secondary to loss of orbital fat. Also, brachycephalic breeds with corneal

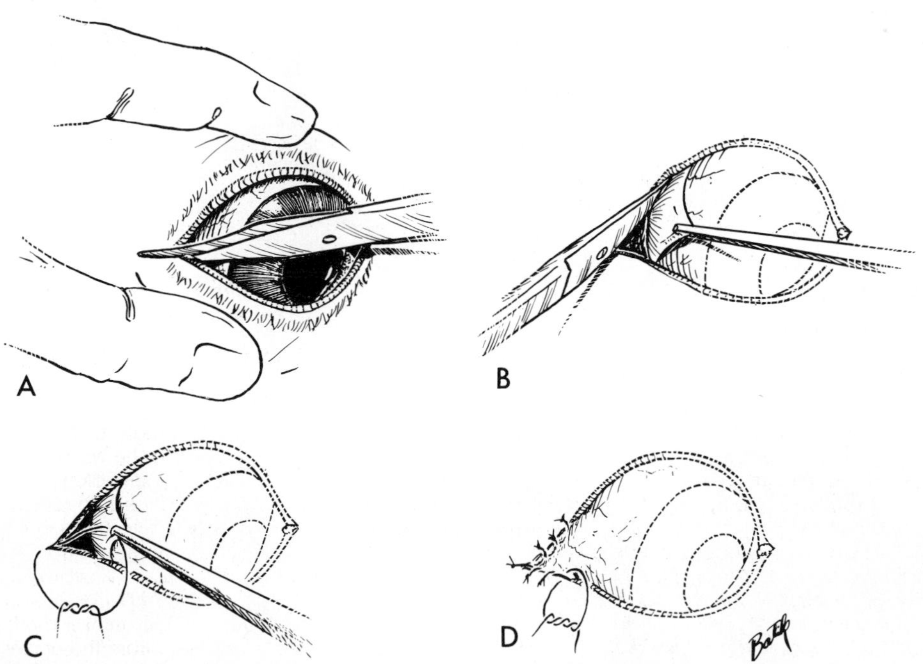

FIGURE 82–4. Lengthening palpebral fissure by lateral canthoplasty. *A,* A lateral canthotomy is performed. The size of the canthotomy is equivalent to the desired size of palpebral fissure. Hemorrhage is minimal and is controlled by pinpoint electrocautery. *B,* After performing the canthotomy, the palpebral conjunctiva is undermined by blunt dissection using Stevens tenotomy scissors. The blunt dissection, involving the conjunctiva of both the upper and lower temporal lids, is carried to the fornix. *C,* The conjunctiva is sutured to the new lateral canthus with simple interrupted 6-0 silk sutures, and the knots are tied on the outside of the lid. The canthotomy incision must be lined by conjunctiva to prevent the development of adhesions between raw lid surfaces. *D,* The palpebral fissure is lenghtened. The sutures are removed in 14 to 21 days. (Reprinted with permission from Bistner S, et al: *Atlas of Veterinary Ophthalmic Surgery.* W.B. Saunders, Philadelphia, 1977.)

exposure or melanosis benefit from a medial tarsorrhaphy.

The procedure performed to shorten the palpebral fissure is a permanent tarsorrhaphy. The lateral lid margins are removed to the canthus. The amount of tissue to be removed varies with each individual. Between one-quarter and one-third of the margins can usually be closed without causing an unacceptable cosmetic appearance. A strip of tissue 2 to 3 mm wide and parallel to to the margins is removed (Fig. 82–5). In performing a medial tarsorrhaphy, care must be taken not to remove or occlude the puncta of the nasolacrimal system. The cut margins are sutured with 5-0 silk in an interrupted pattern. The sutures are be left in place for about 14 days.

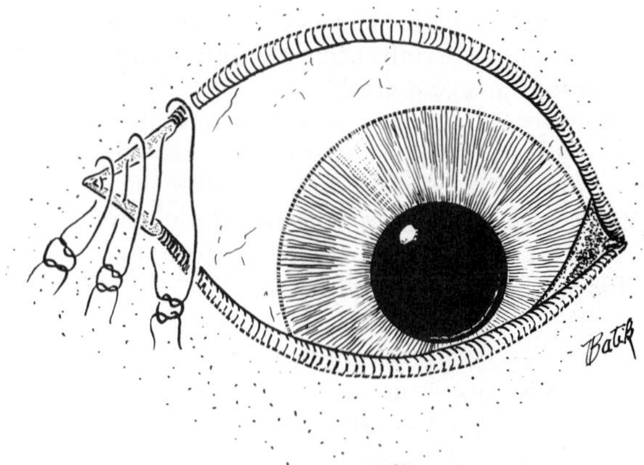

FIGURE 82–5. Permanent shortening of palpebral fissure.

CONGENITAL AND ACQUIRED EYELID DISEASES

Entropion

Entropion is defined as an inversion of the eyelid margin in which the eyelashes rub the cornea. This condition often results in a superficial irritation of the conjunctiva and cornea. Chronic ocular discharge and blepharospasm are commonly seen (Fig. 82–6). If not surgically treated, the condition can lead to vasculariza-

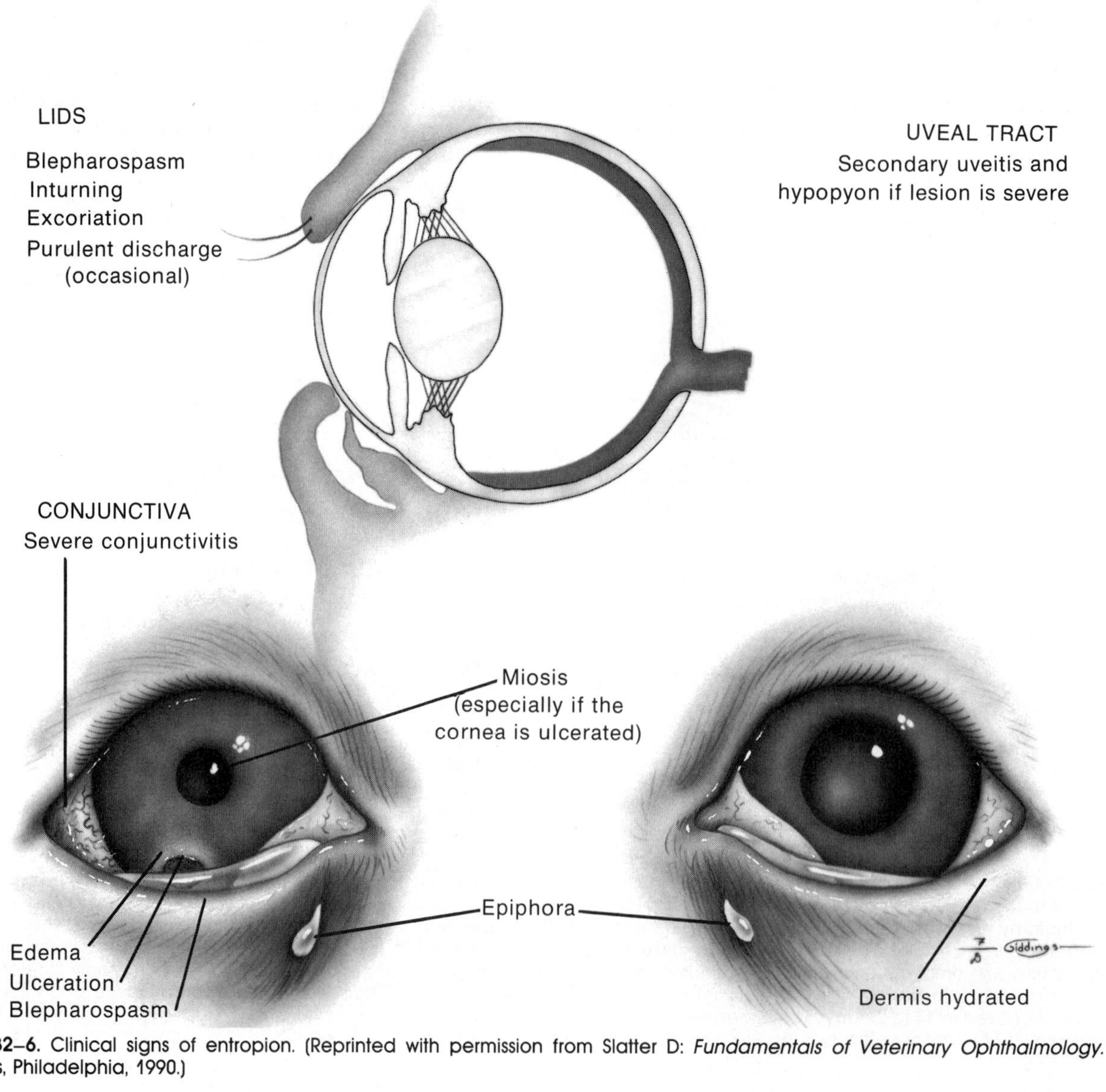

FIGURE 82–6. Clinical signs of entropion. (Reprinted with permission from Slatter D: *Fundamentals of Veterinary Ophthalmology.* W.B. Saunders, Philadelphia, 1990.)

tion, pigmentation, and possible ulceration of the cornea. Three commonly accepted etiologies are congenital, spastic, and acquired.

Congenital Entropion

Congenital entropion is usually a bilateral condition that is commonly noted in dogs. The lower lateral lid is most frequently affected, followed by the upper lid and, infrequently, the medial lower lid. The chow chow, bloodhound, Labrador retriever, English bulldog, Doberman pinscher, Chesapeake Bay retriever, Saint Bernard, rottweiler, poodle, Irish setter, and Sharpei are predisposed to entropion.[14, 20]

Diagnosis of this disease is usually easy. Surgical correction is satisfactory in most cases. Whenever possible, it is wise to postpone entropion correction until the dog is 4 to 6 months of age and its facial features have matured. Application of a topical antibiotic ointment three to four times a day coats the eyelashes and hairs rubbing on the cornea and is used until surgery is performed. Sharpei puppies as young as 3 weeks of age often may require surgical intervention to prevent severe corneal disease. The preferred method is "lid tacking." This procedure is performed with 3-0 nylon in a vertical matress pattern (Fig. 82–7).[11] The sutures are removed in 14 to 20 days. Permanent correction of entropion is often necessary at a later date.

Surgical Correction

Many techniques have been suggested for correcting simple entropion. The technique that provides the most consistent result is a modified Holtz-Celsus procedure (Fig. 82–8)[8, 20] involving excision of a half-moon-shaped flap of skin 2 to 3 mm from the lid margin. The skin excision is 3 to 4 mm wider than the affected area of lid. The area of skin to be removed is crushed with Halsted or Crile forceps by grasping the fold of skin with the edge of the instrument. After the forceps are initially placed on the skinfold, fine adjustments in the size of the fold can be made by releasing skin or pulling more skin into the jaws of the forceps before crushing. The hemostats are clamped tightly and left in place for about 30 seconds before being removed. The fold of skin is removed with blunt scissors. Some surgeons prefer to make a freehand incision with a scalpel to reduce most operative scarring. This method has the advantage of causing slightly less tissue trauma, but more hemorrhage is encountered. In severe cases of entropion, a small strip of orbicular muscle may be removed in an effort to create greater internal scarring and reduce the amount of postoperative skin stretching. This is accomplished by grasping the exposed muscle with small Bishop-Harmon forceps and cutting a strip of muscle with tenotomy scissors. Care is taken not to cut through the palpebral conjunctiva. The skin is closed with 5-0 or 6-0 silk sutures placed about 2 mm apart in a simple interrupted pattern. Subcutaneous suturing is not necessary.

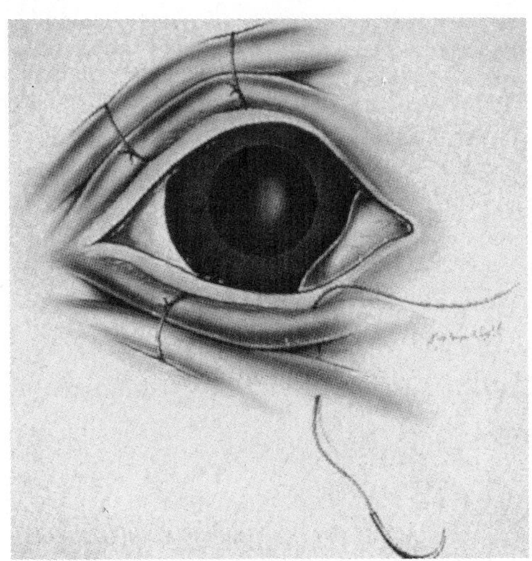

FIGURE 82–7. Placement of the sutures in the tacking procedure.

Immediately postoperatively, the lids should be in a normal position. During the first few days of recovery, the lids appear to be slightly overcorrected, but as the swelling subsides, they return to normal. When in doubt, it is better to slightly undercorrect than to overcorrect and create an ectropion. Postoperative treatment consists of placing an antibiotic ointment in the eye and on the wound twice a day. A plastic Elizabethan collar is placed on the animal to prevent self-injury. Sutures are removed 10 to 14 days postoperatively.

The two major reasons for failure to achieve a good cosmetic result are (1) not making the incision close enough to the lid margin and (2) placing the sutures too far apart.

Spastic Entropion

Spastic entropion is usually unilateral and can occur at any age. The cause of the lid inversion is spasm of the orbicular muscle of the eye secondary to ocular irritation. The etiology includes conjunctivitis, foreign bodies, keratoconjunctivitis sicca, trichiasis, distichiasis, ectopic cilia, and corneal ulceration. A detailed ocular examination should be performed to determine the underlying cause. Initial therapy is directed at correcting the original problem. Many cases of spastic entropion resolve after the inciting irritant is removed. One diagnostic method to help differentiate spastic from congenital or acquired entropion is to place several drops of topical anesthetic on the eye. If the entropion resolves spontaneously, it was most likely spastic in character.

If the entropion persists once the underlying cause has been corrected, one can use a soft contact lens or a temporary tarsorrhaphy (Fig. 82–9) to reduce further irritation. Sutures for both of these procedures are removed in 2 to 3 weeks. If all else fails, a standard entropion correction cures the condition.

Acquired Entropion

Entropion is a common sequela of endophthalmos from loss of orbital fat or temporal muscle atrophy. Endophthalmos caused by contraction of the retractor

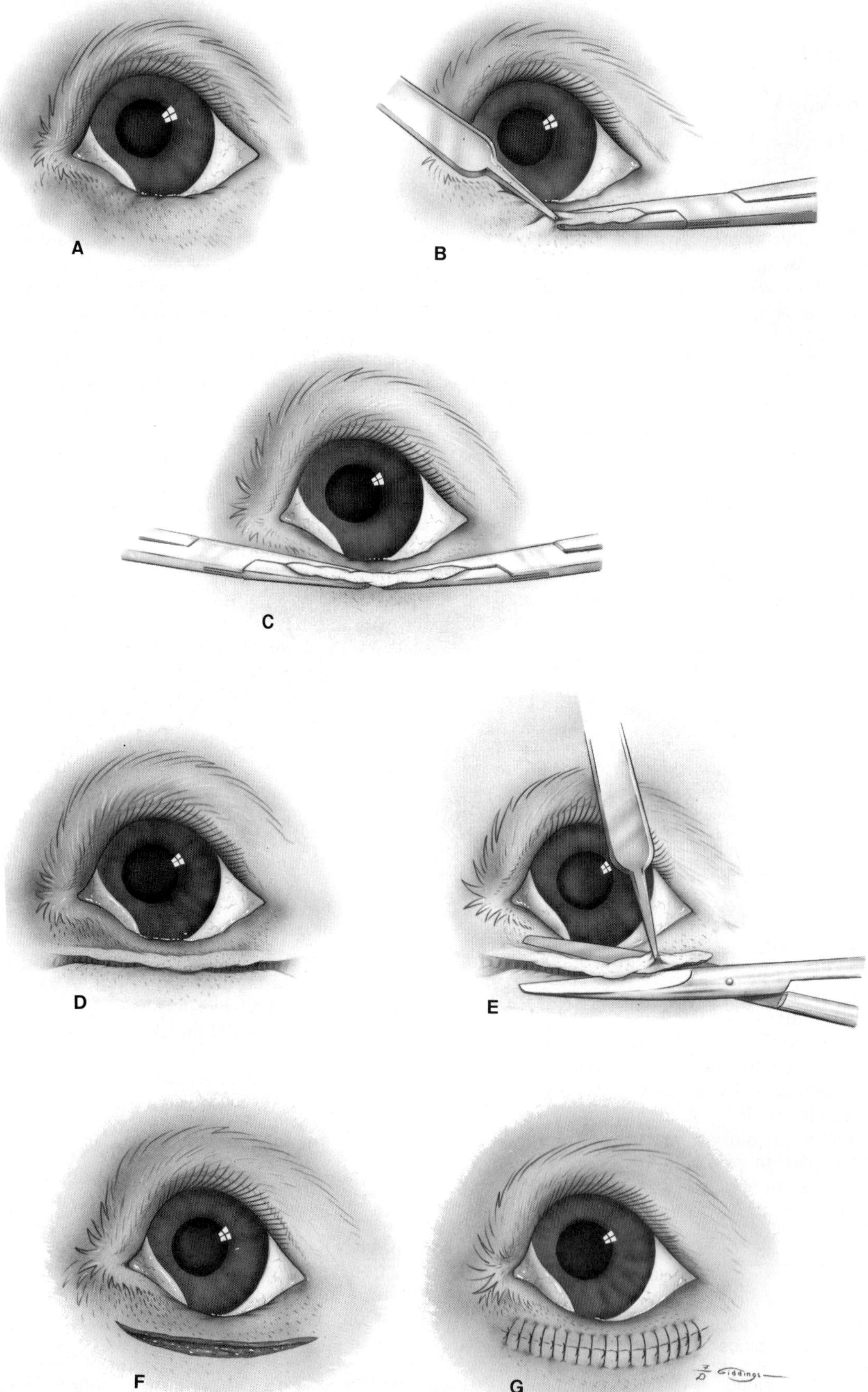

FIGURE 82–8 *See legend on opposite page*

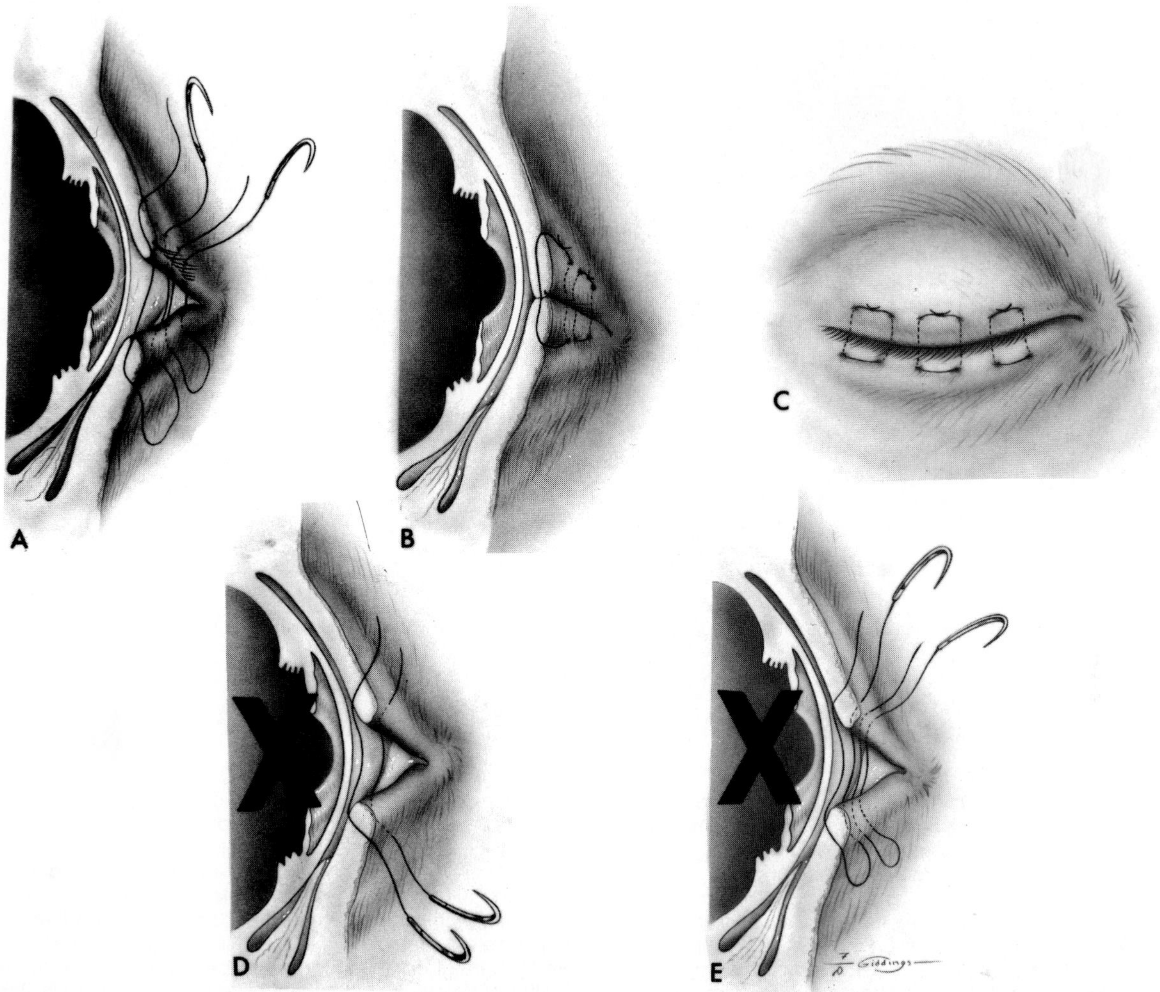

FIGURE 82–9. *A, B,* and *C,* Placement of interrupted intermarginal horizontal mattress sutures in temporary tarsorrhaphy. *D* and *E,* Incorrect suture placement, which results in corneal abrasions from the sutures. (After Severin GA: *Veterinary Ophthalmology Notes.* Fort Collins, CO, 1976. Reprinted with permission from Slatter D: *Fundamentals of Veterinary Ophthalmology.* W.B. Saunders, Philadelphia, 1990.)

muscles of the globe, secondary to ocular pain, generally does not cause entropion. An abnormally small globe with normal lids, as seen with phthisis bulbi or microphthalmos, can also result in entropion. Surgical correction of this type of entropion is performed by a lateral canthoplasty to shorten the palpebral fissure (Fig. 82–10). This is accomplished by separating the skin from the orbicular muscle of the eye at the lateral canthus with a small scalpel (number 64 Beaver blade). A triangular flap of skin, in proportion to the amount of closure required, is removed from the upper lid. A flap from the lower lid is sutured into the defect in the upper lid. Suturing is completed with 6-0 silk in an interrupted pattern. This procedure has the advantage of providing a palpebral fissure proportionate to the globe size while correcting the acquired entropion.

Medial Entropion and Facial Folds

In poodles, Pekingeses, and pugs, the lid margins at the medial canthus may be slightly inverted. This condition is occasionally seen in Persian cats. The lacrimal puncta are slightly compressed, and epiphora may be the only presenting sign. Cats and dogs having only

FIGURE 82–8. Pinch technique for entropion. *A,* Preoperative appearance of the entropion. *B,* The "rolled-in" area is everted, and the necessary amount of skin is placed between the forceps. *C,* The second pair of forceps is applied, and final adjustments are made before clamping. *D,* The forceps are removed. *E,* The strip of skin is excised, starting at the temporal canthus, including *all* of the clamped area. The strip is kept taut throughout the excision. *F,* The excised area with orbicularis oculi *undisturbed. G,* The incision sutured with simple interrupted sutures of 6-0 silk, 1.5 to 2.0 mm apart. A generous bite of tissue should be taken to prevent premature pulling out as the wound heals, but the sutures should not be tied tight, because postoperative edema may cause tearing of the surrounding tissue. (After Severin GA: *Veterinary Ophthalmology Notes.* Fort Collins, CO, 1976. Reprinted with permission from Slatter D: *Fundamentals of Veterinary Ophthalmology.* W.B. Saunders, Philadelphia, 1990.)

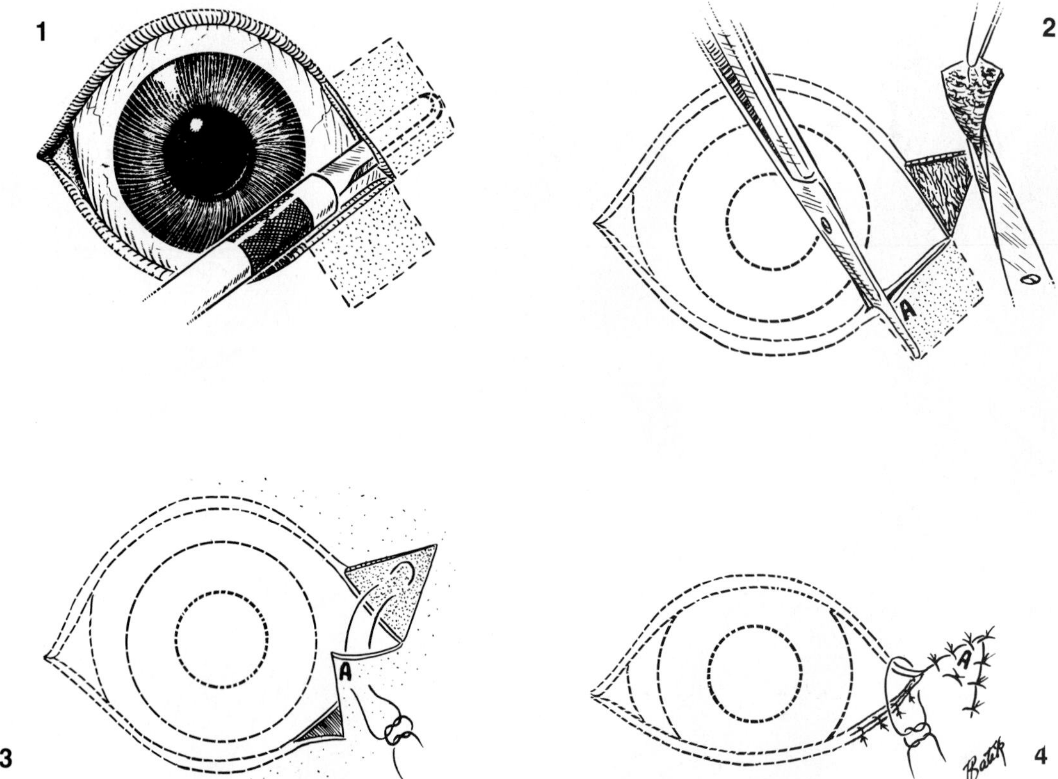

FIGURE 82–10. *1,* The amount of palpebral fissure to be closed is estimated by pinching the lids closed at the lateral canthus. The upper and lower lids are then split over an area that encompasses the amount of closure desired. The lid-splitting technique separates skin-orbicularis muscle from the underlying conjunctiva. *2,* A cut *(A)* is made at the nasal end of the lid split in the lower lid, and the tarsal (ciliary) margin of this undermined lower lid flap is removed. A similar cut at the nasal end of the upper lid split is made, and the incision is extended outward and downward to end at the lateral canthus. This triangular piece of skin-orbicularis muscle is removed from the upper lid. *3,* A double-armed 4-0 silk suture is used to place a mattress suture in the upper eyelid tarsoconjunctiva and then through the lower lid skin-muscle flap. The lower lid is then drawn upward to fit into the defect created in the upper lid, and the mattress suture is tied. *4,* Additional 6-0 silk sutures are used to secure the flap and recreate the lateral canthus. Care must be taken to close the lid-splitting defect in the lower lid. (Reprinted with permission from Bistner SI, et al: *Atlas of Veterinary Ophthalmic Surgery.* W.B. Saunders, Philadelphia, 1977.)

minor epiphora may not benefit from surgical intervention because the defect may be so slight that the problems associated with overcorrection outweigh the potential benefit of surgery. Medical therapy using 25 mg of oral tetracycline once a day often eliminates the staining of the tears on the facial fur of these patients and obviates surgical intervention. The brachycephalic breeds such as the Pekingese and pug often have a combination of medial entropion and prominent facial folds.[8, 14, 20] One or both of these conditions can cause keratitis and eventually pigment infiltration of the cornea from the medial limbus. Once this pigmentary keratitis is diagnosed, it is necessary to determine if surgery is necessary and what kind. In older dogs (7 to 8 years and older) in which the pigment has infiltrated only one-fourth or less of the cornea and no visual loss is observed, surgery is generally not necessary. In younger dogs with progressive pigmentary keratitis, close examination usually reveals the cause of the irritation, which may require surgical intervention.

Medial entropion is repaired by the same technique as for congenital entropion (see Fig. 82–8). Care is taken not to cut or suture the lacrimal puncta. Removal or reduction of the nasal folds is indicated when the hairs on the folds rub on the cornea. This can be accomplished by crushing the tissue to be removed with forceps and excising it with blunt scissors (Fig. 82–11). A better cosmetic result is obtained if the incision is made on the posterior aspect of the folds. The nasal folds must usually be reduced to at least half their original height. Sutures are placed in an interrupted pattern with 6-0 or 5-0 silk and are removed 10 to 14 days postoperatively. Concurrent superficial keratectomy for pigmentary keratitis is unnecessary, because correction of the medial entropion or nasal folds stops the physical irritation to the cornea. Pigmentation decreases with time and *judicious* use of corticosteroids.

Combined Entropion-Ectropion

Certain breeds, such as the Saint Bernard, Doberman pinscher, English bulldog, and cocker spaniel, may exhibit a lid deformity that involves both an inversion and eversion of one or both lids.[2, 20] These dogs typically have lateral entropion and central ectropion of both the upper and lower lids. They are usually present with a profound mucopurulent discharge and severe keratoconjunctivitis.

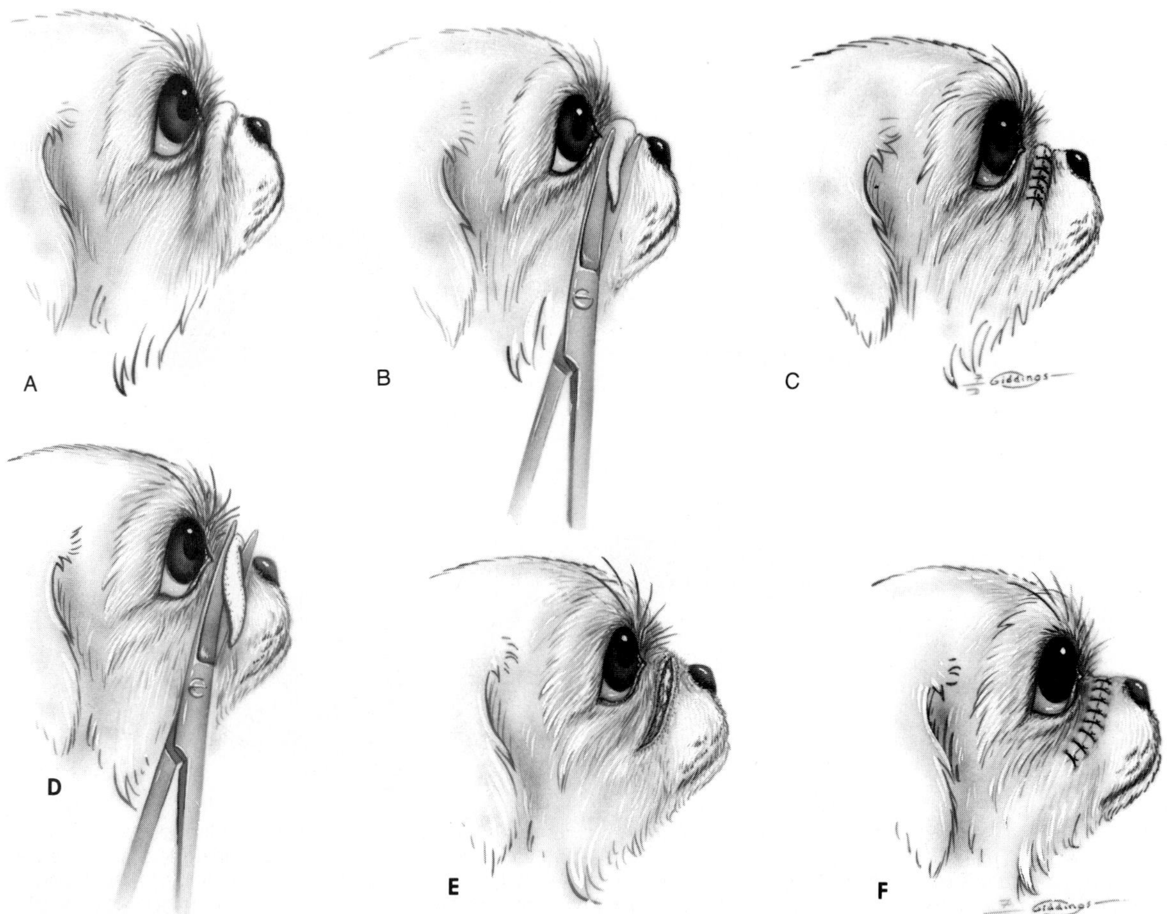

FIGURE 82–11. *A–C*, Partial removal of the nasal fold. *A*, Lateral view of nasal fold. *B*, Removal of nasal portion with curved scissors. Note that the anterior portion of the fold is removed. *C*, The sutured wound with a small remaining fold that is more prominent laterally. The knots are placed on the anterior side of the incision to limit corneal contact. *D–F*, Total removal of the nasal fold. *D*, Removal of the fold starting laterally. *E*, The fold removed. *F*, The fold sutured. The knots are placed on the anterior side of the incision to reduce the chance of corneal contact. (After Severin GA: *Veterinary Ophthalmology Notes*. Fort Collins, CO, 1976. Reprinted with permission from Slatter D: *Fundamentals of Veterinary Ophthalmology*. W.B. Saunders, Philadelphia, 1990.)

There are several theories regarding the cause of this disease. It has been proposed that an absent or poorly functioning retractor muscle of the angle of the eye may be responsible for providing lateral tension on the lid.[22] This muscle may perform the function of the lateral canthal ligament in humans. The possibility that the underlying cause is simply excessive facial skin in breeds such as the Saint Bernard must also be considered.

The condition requires a surgical procedure that not only corrects the entropion but also provides lateral traction on the canthus to correct the ectropion. Wyman originally outlined a lateral canthoplasty procedure for this lid abnormality.[22] A simpler technique can currently be used (Fig. 82–12).[17] The procedure involves making a crush-and-cut incision extending half the length of both the upper and lower lids. It continues around the lateral canthus. The incision should be 3 mm from the lid margins and the lateral canthus. A second incision is made from the area of the lateral canthus to the orbital ligament. A 3-0 polyglycolic acid suture is passed through the lateral canthus margin and then the orbital ligament. As it is tightened, the lid margins are straightened, correcting the ectropion. The skin is closed with 5-0 silk, which corrects the entropion.

Most cases show more postoperative swelling than is encountered with a standard entropion correction. Hot packing twice a day for 2 or 3 days while the animal is still hospitalized is recommended. An Elizabethan collar is placed on the animal, and sutures are removed after 14 days.

Ectropion

Ectropion, or eversion of the lid margin, is a common finding in many breeds of dogs. It is particularly common in the Saint Bernard, bloodhound, American cocker spaniel, basset hound, and bulldog.[8, 14, 20] The condition is usually congenital and generally involves the lower eyelids but can result from scarring.

Most dogs with congenital ectropion do not require surgical correction. Only those animals experiencing chronic keratitis or conjunctivitis that is unresponsive to medical therapy are considered for surgery (Fig. 82–13).

Of the numerous techniques available for correcting both congenital and acquired ectropion, the Wharton-Jones blepharoplasty (V-Y technique) is the simplest and most commonly used (Fig. 82–14).[20] In this procedure,

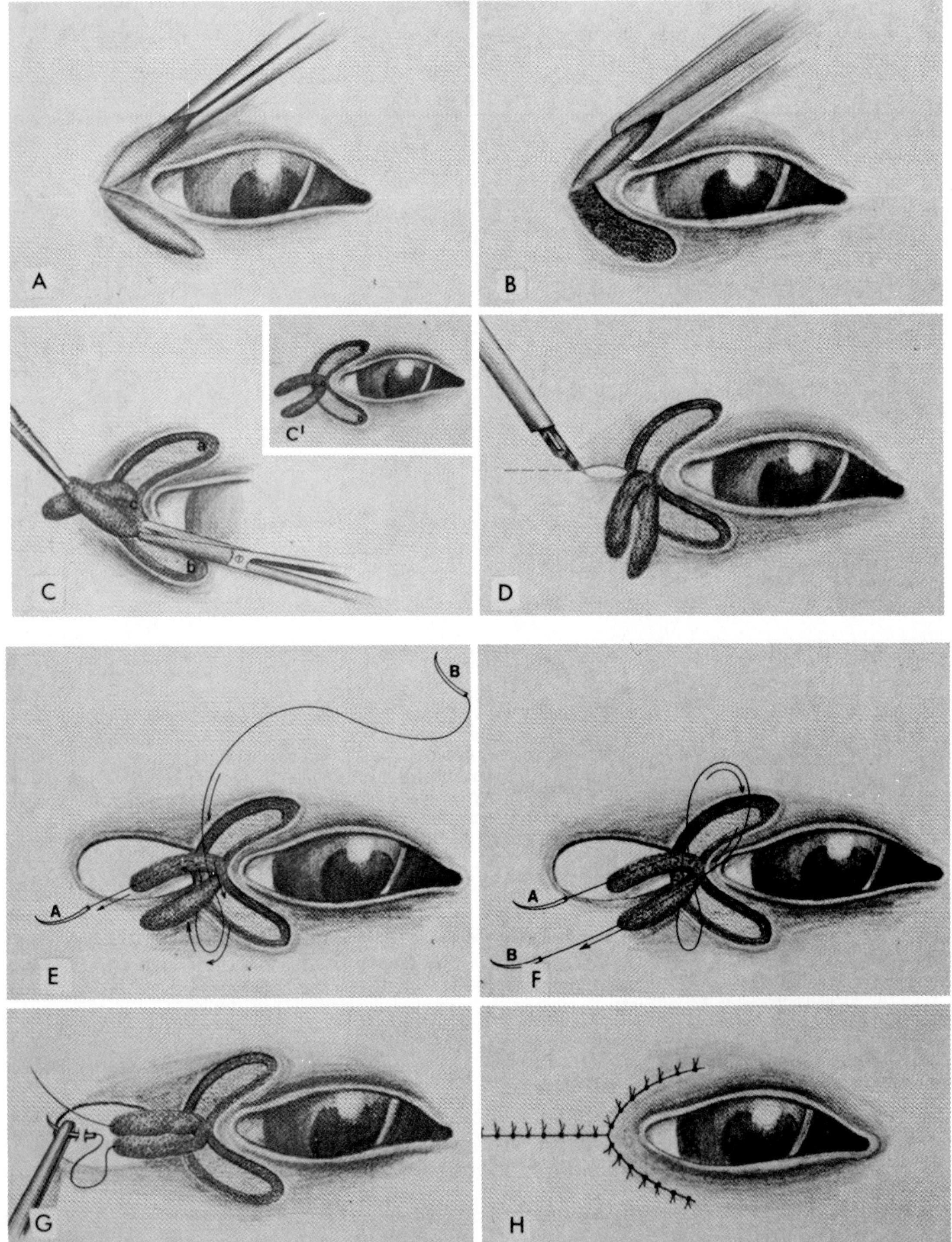

FIGURE 82–12. Wyman lateral canthoplasty (modified) for correction of combined entropion-ectropion. *A*, Folds of upper and lower lids are made to meet opposite the lateral canthus. *B*, Excision of folds. *C*, Commencing at a and b, tongues of orbicularis muscle are dissected to terminate in a single bundle base. *C'*, Step completed. *D*, Skin incision is made from the base of the muscle bundle to an area over the temporal bone. *E*, Tongues are brought together at the base. One needle (A) traverses the base, is turned and brought up through the opposite tongue. F, The second needle (B) is brought up the length of the other tongue. *G*, The bundle is "tacked" to the periosteum over the zygomatic arch of the temporal bone. *H*, Skin closure.

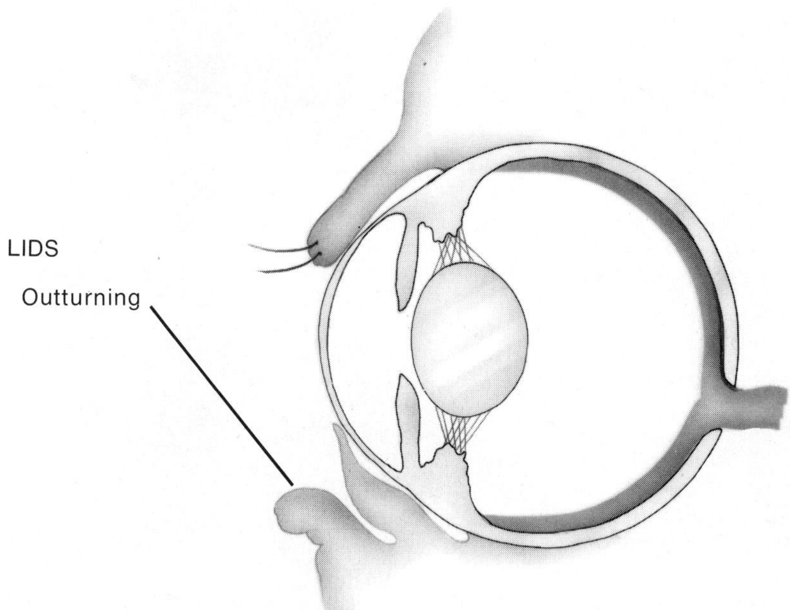

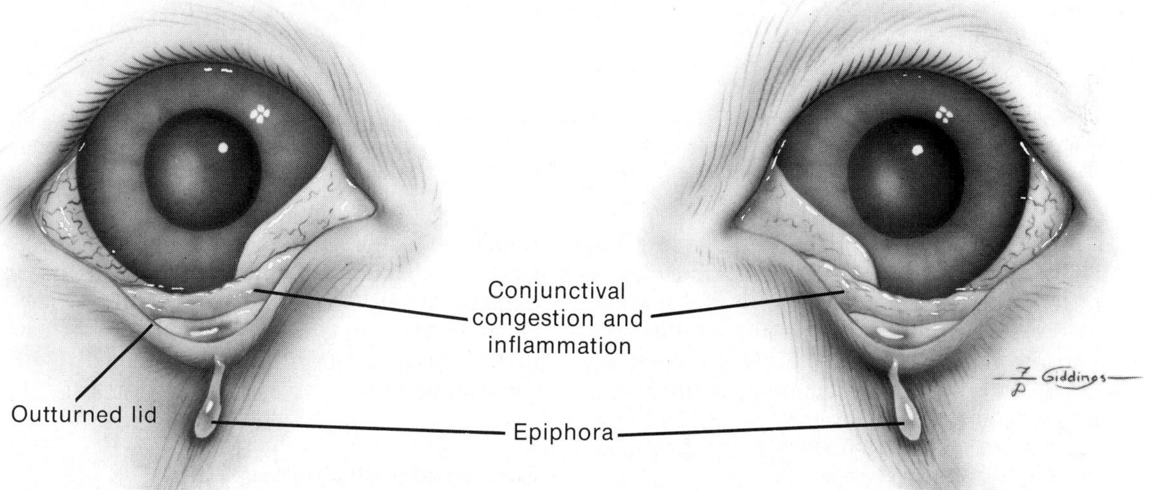

FIGURE 82–13. Clinical signs of ectropion. (Reprinted with permission from Slatter D: *Fundamentals of Veterinary Ophthalmology.* W.B. Saunders, Philadelphia, 1990.)

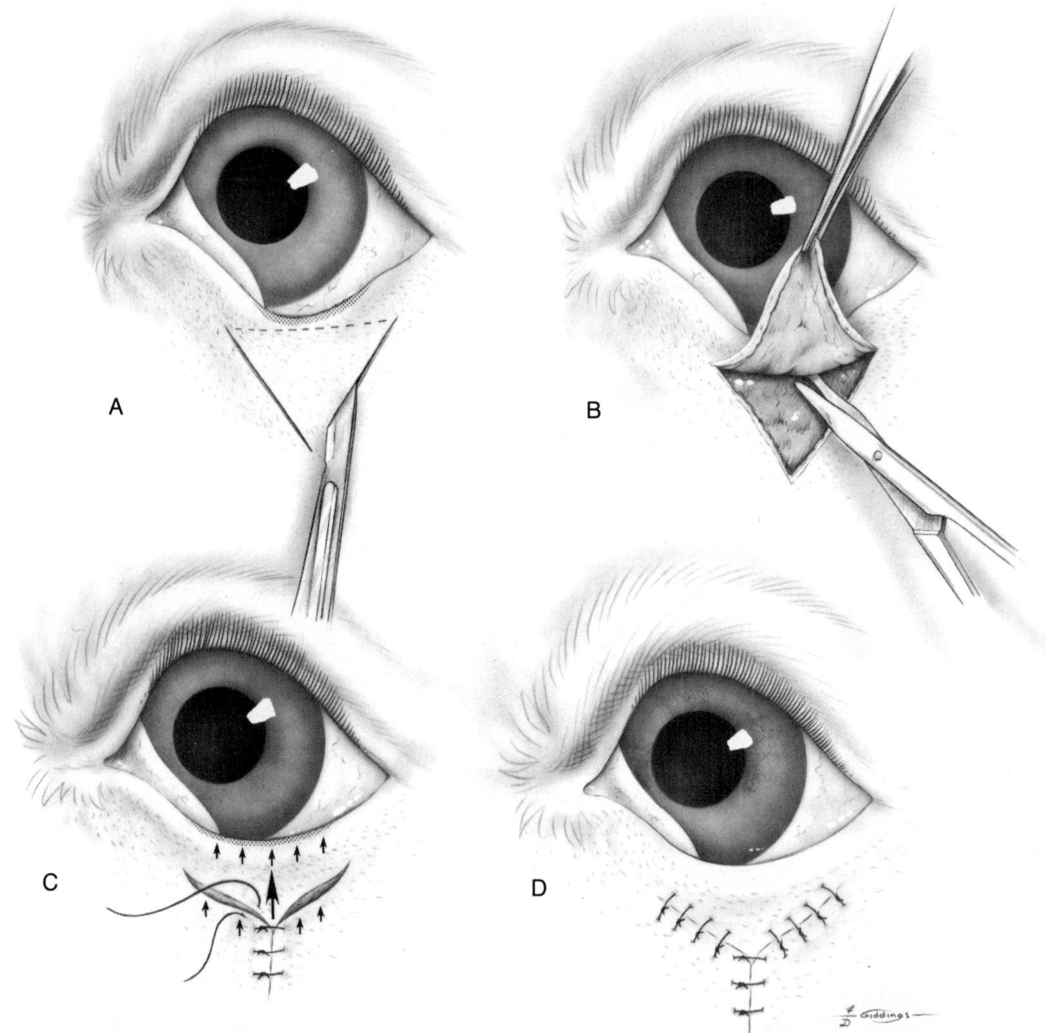

FIGURE 82–14. Wharton-Jones blepharoplasty. *A*, Skin triangle outlined and incisions made. *B*, Skin flap elevated and dissected beneath. *C*, Vertical portion formed (defect + 3 mm). *D*, Completed Y incision sutured with 6-0 or 4-0 silk. (Reprinted with permission from Slatter D: *Fundamentals of Veterinary Ophthalmology.* W.B. Saunders, Philadelphia, 1990.)

a V-shaped incision is made through the skin ventral to and slightly wider than the everted area. The flap is undermined to within 2 to 3 mm of the eyelid margin. The incision is closed from the base to the margin. The amount of closure can be gauged by moving the flap up until the eversion is corrected. Subcutaneous suturing is neither indicated nor needed in this procedure. The incision is closed with 5-0 or 6-0 silk in an interrupted pattern.

In severe cases in which the V-Y technique will not correct the ectropion, a modification of the Kuhnt-Szymanowski technique can be used (Fig. 82–15).[8, 20] This procedure involves removing a wedge of lid margin of appropriate width to shorten the margin adequately. The crush-and-cut technique can be used to outline the area to be excised. Once the tissue is removed, the conjunctiva and tarsal tissues are closed in a continuous pattern to ensure accurate apposition. The skin is closed with 5-0 or 6-0 silk in an interrupted pattern.

EYELID TUMORS

Eyelid tumors are common in dogs. Tarsal gland adenomas are the most frequently diagnosed eyelid tumors in dogs.[12] Less commonly found are adenocarcinomas, melanomas, and papillomas. Tarsal gland adenoma, as with most tumors of the canine eyelid, is clinically benign, and surgical excision is usually curative. Cryosurgery using liquid nitrogen at −4°F (−20°C) can also be used to treat these tumors (discussed later).

Excision of Eyelid Tumors

A full-thickness eyelid resection is the simplest procedure for removing tarsal gland adenomas in dogs (Fig. 82–16).[3] This procedure can be used in lesions that involve up to one-third of the lid margin on either the upper or lower lid. Immobilizing the lesion with a Desmarres chalazion clamp or using hemostats to crush along the proposed incisions decreases bleeding. A V incision is made with blunt scissors, including a 2- to 3-mm strip of normal tissue on each side of the tumor. If a chalazion clamp is used, the tissue edges can be moved closer together and the clamp retightened before suturing. The wound is closed by suturing only the conjunctiva and skin, allowing the lid to stretch and return to a nearly normal appearance postoperatively. The con-

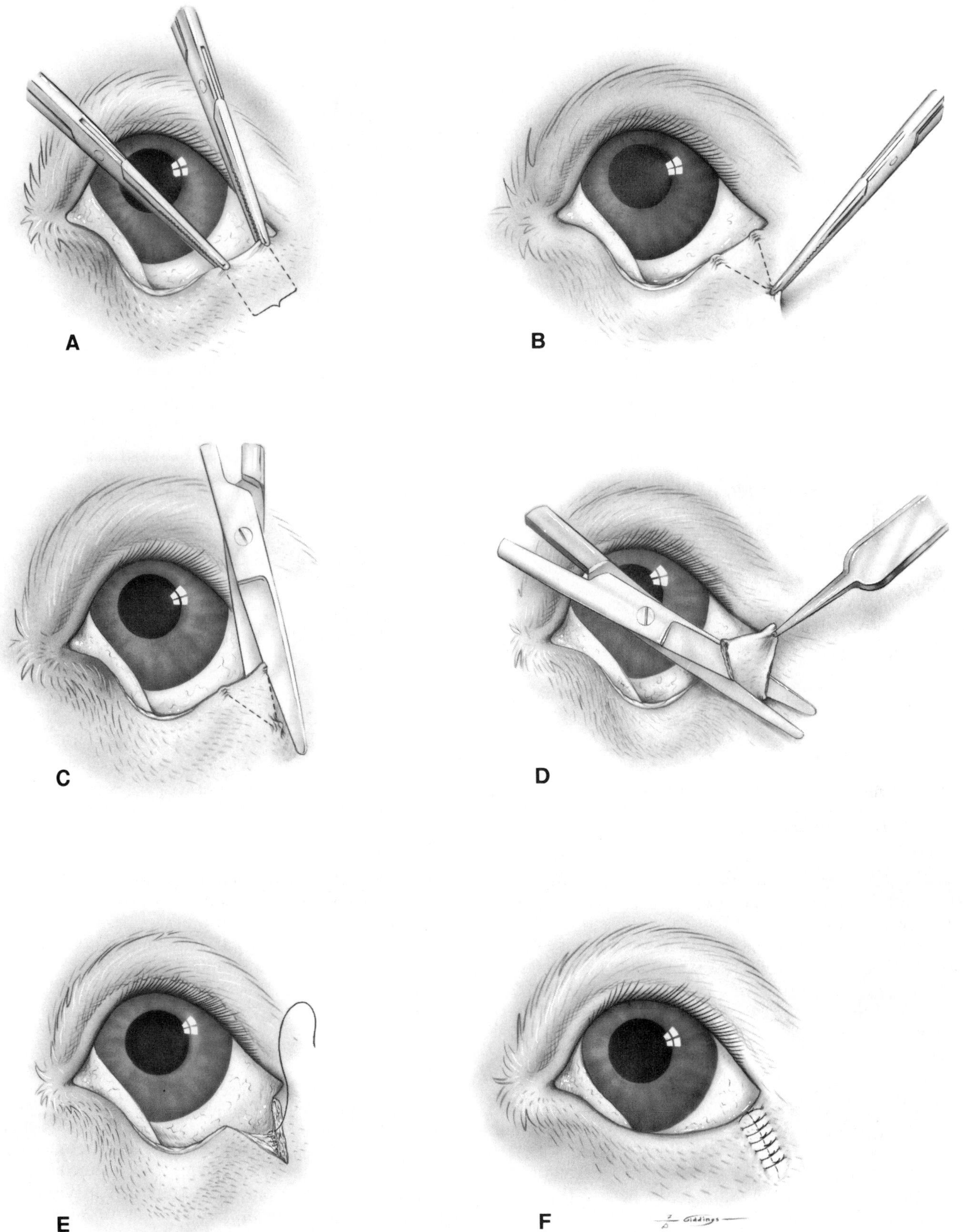

FIGURE 82–15. Modified Kuhnt-Szymanowski procedure. *A,* The lid margin is marked laterally. *B,* An estimate of the amount of margin to be removed is made, and the lid is marked. The ventral end of the triangle is marked 10 to 14 mm below. *C,* The first incision is made with straight Mayo scissors. *D,* The second incision is made. *E,* The triangular piece removed. Note that the conjunctival defect is smaller, justifying one layer of sutures in the skin in some cases. *F,* The wound sutured with 6-0 silk.

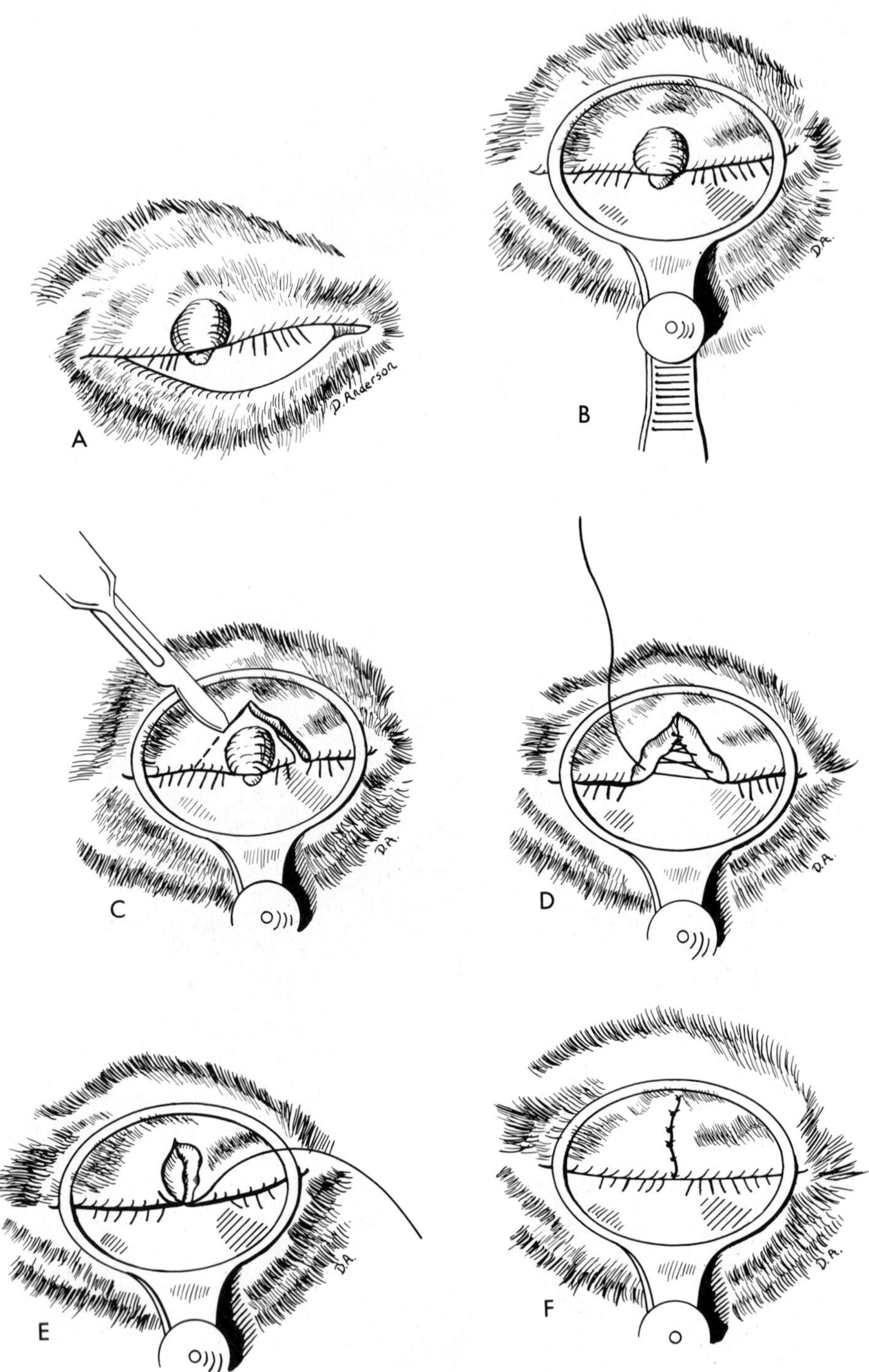

FIGURE 82–16. Full-thickness resection of the eyelid. *A*, Typical appearance of a meibomian gland adenoma in a dog. *B*, Chalazion forceps in place over the neoplasm. *C*, Full-thickness incision of the lid. The plate of the chalazion forceps protects the globe. *D*, Continuous 6-0 gut suture is used to close the conjunctiva; the knots are buried, and the orbicularis muscle is not sutured. *E*, The skin incision is closed with silk suture starting 1 mm from the lid margin. *F*, Simple interrupted pattern is used to close the skin. (Reprinted with permission from Brightman A, Helper L: Full thickness resection of the eyelid. *J Am Anim Hosp Assoc 14*:483, 1978.)

junctiva is closed using 5-0 or 6-0 chromic gut in a continuous pattern, starting at the bottom of the V and working toward the margin. The skin is closed with 5-0 or 6-0 silk in an interrupted pattern starting at the lid margin.

Tumors that require excision of one-third or more of the eyelid require more extensive restoration techniques. For lesions that do not involve the full thickness of the eyelid, partial-thickness tissue advancement may be used (Fig. 82–17).[2, 20] This technique preserves the palpebral conjunctiva. If, however, the majority of the lower lid is removed, a mucocutaneous flap from the lower lip can be used for restoring the lid.[15] The use of a mucocutaneous subdermal plexus flap has several advantages over other procedures. It can replace extensive areas of eyelid and provides a new mucous membrane to replace the palpebral conjunctiva. Good cosmetic results have been obtained in dogs with this procedure.

Alternative methods for removing small tumors of the eyelid include electrocautery and cryosurgery. A loop attached to a surgical electrocautery unit aids in removal of papillomas, melanomas, and small basal cell carcinomas. The cornea must be protected, because heat

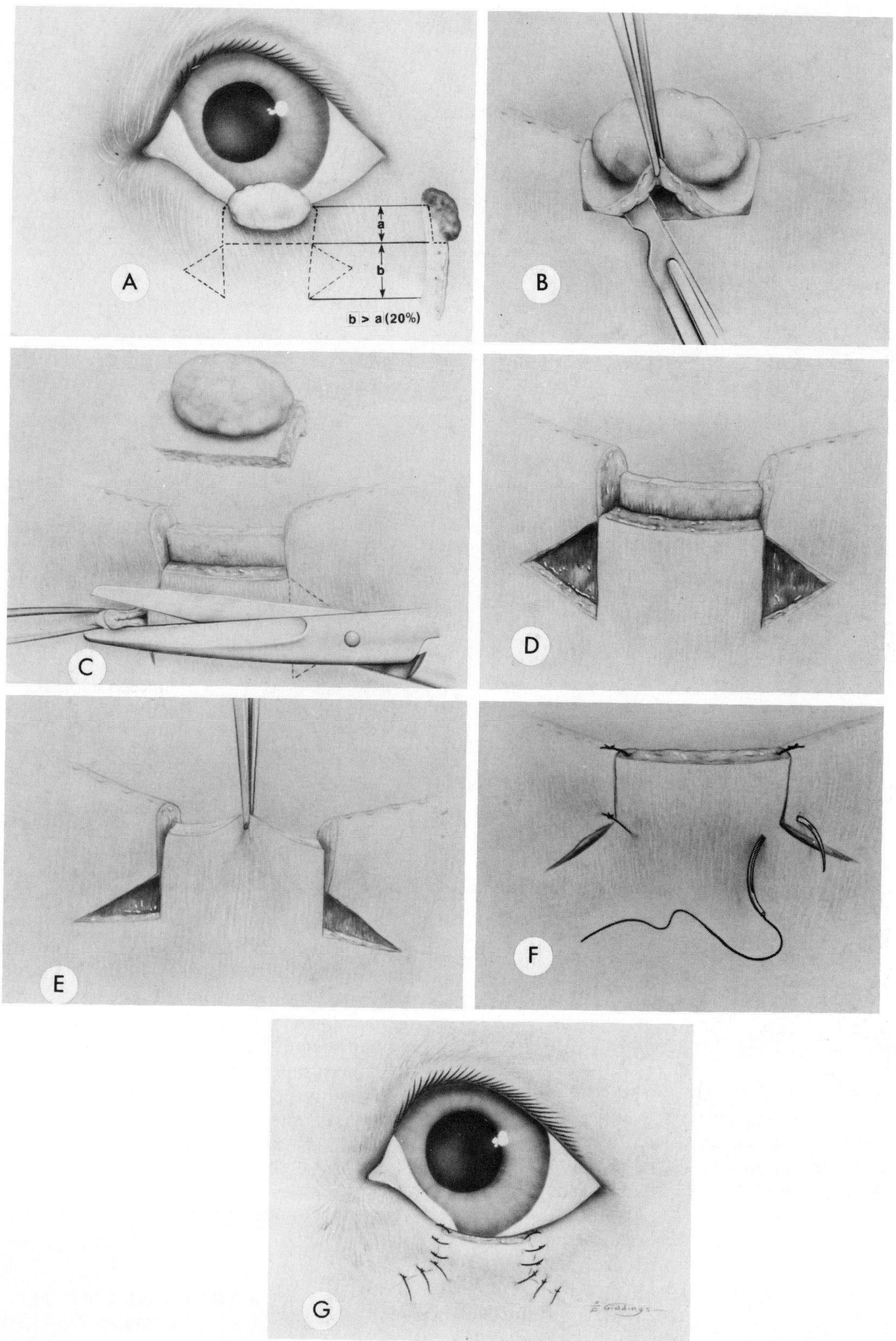

FIGURE 82–17. Advancement flap for partial-thickness lesions. *A,* The tumor (or defect) before excision. Because the conjunctiva is not involved, it is not removed. Incisions are outlined by broken lines. The incisions are marked on the patient with a plastic surgery marking pen. The vertical sides of the triangles are 20 per cent longer than the vertical incisions adjacent to the tumor to allow for wound contraction. *B,* A square or rectangular incision is made around the tumor. The tumor is dissected off from the base toward the lid margin. *C,* The tumor is removed and placed in fixative. The tumor is pinned to a piece of cardboard to allow the ophthalmic pathologist to examine the margins for evidence of tumor. Note: If tumor is present in any margin, excision has been incomplete. The previously marked triangle is elevated and excised. *D,* The triangles have been removed and all incisions completed. *E,* To prevent tension on the wound, the tissues surrounding the triangles and the flap are undermined. The flap is advanced to the margin with no tension on it. *F,* Simple marginal sutures of 6-0 silk are placed. Sutures are placed at the corners of the incision to assist in accurate placement of subsequent sutures. *G,* Remaining sutures in place 2 mm apart. If the conjunctiva is mobile, it is sutured to the skin edge, filling the defect with a simple continuous suture. This helps prevent retraction of the advancement flap. (Reprinted with permission from Slatter D: *Fundamentals of Veterinary Ophthalmology.* W.B. Saunders, Philadelphia, 1990.)

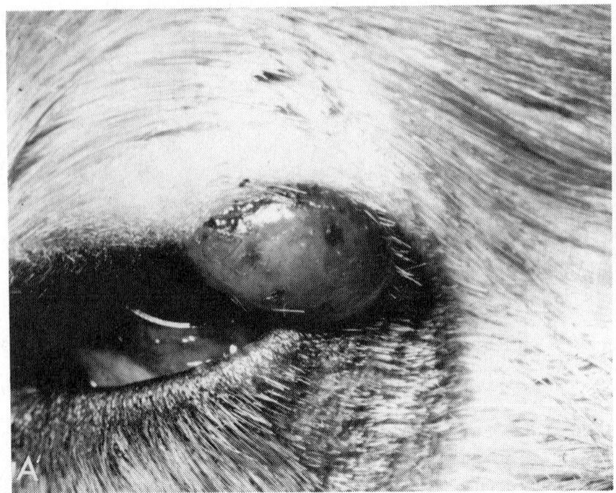

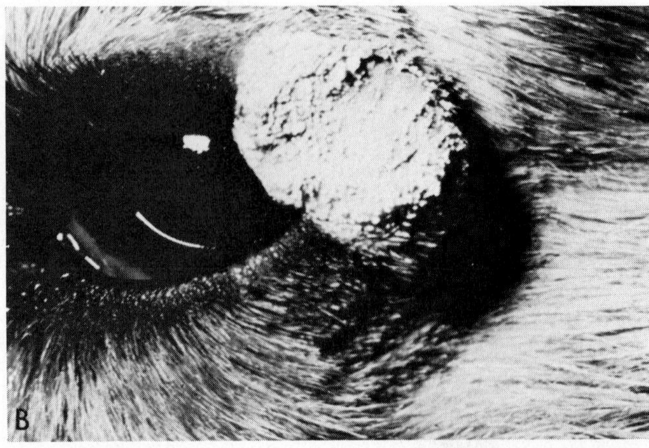

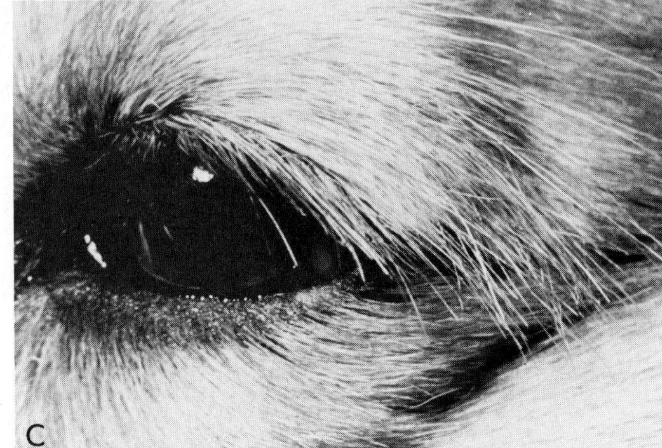

FIGURE 82–18. *A*, A palpebral neoplasm. *B*, Frozen. *C*, Sixty days after cryosurgery. (Courtesy of S. J. Withrow.)

cautery wounds of the cornea are very slow to heal. Also, electrocautery may be contraindicated if microscopic examination of the excised tissue is desired, because it coagulates small tumors and alters their histological architecture.

Cryosurgery (see also Chapter 173)

Cryosurgery is an alternative to excision of eyelid tumors.[6] Only liquid nitrogen is used as the cooling agent because other substances, such as nitrous oxide, may not yield temperatures low enough to destroy neoplastic tissues (Fig. 82–18). General anesthesia is recommended for cryosurgery.

The most commonly used cryosurgical technique for removing eyelid tumors is the freeze-thaw-refreeze method.[6] Thermocouples should be placed under and at the edges of the lesion before freezing. Liquid nitrogen is sprayed (Fig. 82–19) on the center of the mass until thermocouples indicate −4°F (−20°C). The tissue is allowed to thaw to 32°F (0°C) and is then refrozen to −4°F (−20°C). Lesions can be expected to slough in 5 to 7 days. Bleeding and postoperative infections are uncommon complications. One drawback to the use of cryosurgery in dogs is that hair that grows into the previously frozen area is depigmented, and the resulting white spot may be objectionable in black or dark-colored animals.

EYELASH-RELATED DISEASES

Distichiasis, districhiasis, trichiasis, and ectopic cilia all result in corneal irritation or ulceration (Fig. 82–20). These cilia-related diseases are most frequently encountered in dogs. In some breeds, such as the cocker spaniel, distichiasis (cilia emerging from the tarsal [meibomian] gland openings) and districhiasis (more than one cilium emerging from the gland opening) are common findings.[12] Many of these dogs have few or no adverse effects from the presence of these cilia and therefore do not require surgical treatment. In other

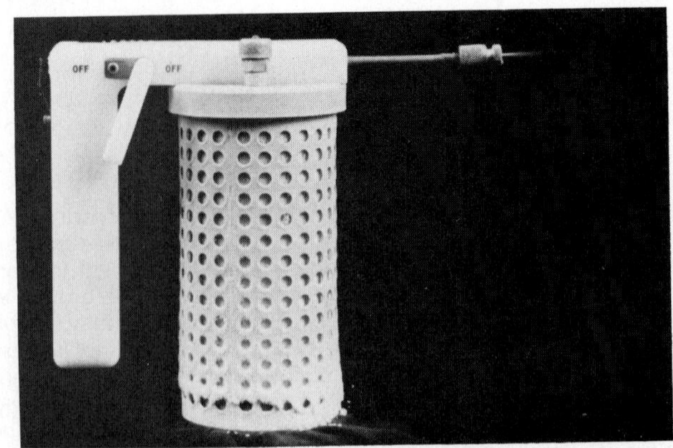

FIGURE 82–19. Liquid nitrogen applicator.

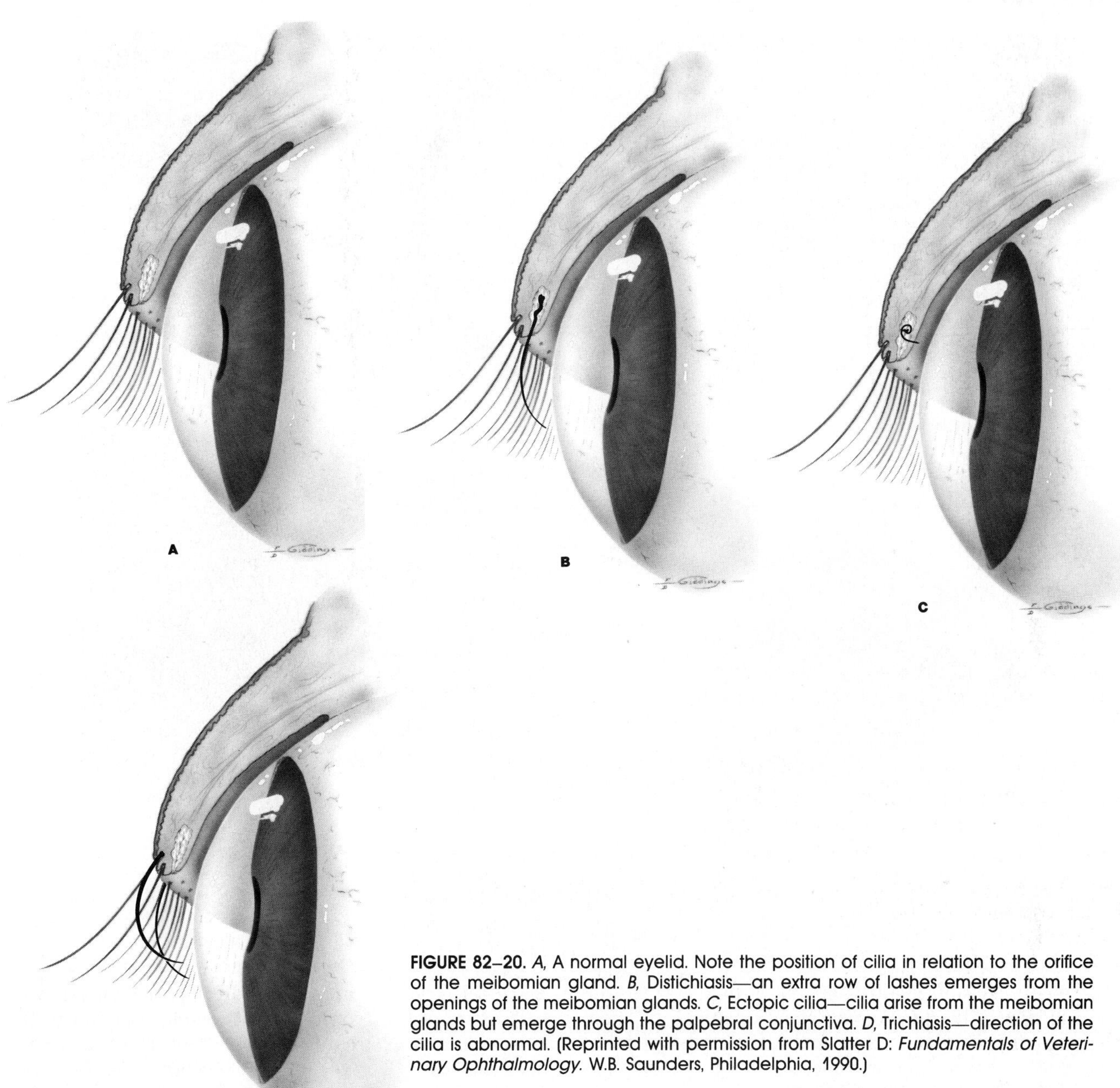

FIGURE 82–20. *A*, A normal eyelid. Note the position of cilia in relation to the orifice of the meibomian gland. *B*, Distichiasis—an extra row of lashes emerges from the openings of the meibomian glands. *C*, Ectopic cilia—cilia arise from the meibomian glands but emerge through the palpebral conjunctiva. *D*, Trichiasis—direction of the cilia is abnormal. (Reprinted with permission from Slatter D: *Fundamentals of Veterinary Ophthalmology.* W.B. Saunders, Philadelphia, 1990.)

dogs, however, chronic keratitis or ulceration may result and surgery is indicated (Fig. 82–21).

Surgical Correction

Several methods have been described to treat distichiasis or districhiasis. Manual epilation can be accomplished using either cilia forceps or jeweler's forceps. This method may be useful when a corneal ulcer has developed in a dog that has had distichiasis without complications for years. Once the cornea becomes ulcerated, the distichiasis may prevent healing by mechanically rubbing the loosely adhered, healing epithelium. Manual epilation yields only temporary results but often relieves the irritation long enough for the cornea to heal before the cilia grow back.

Electroepilation can be used to treat distichiasis permanently when only five or six cilia are present on each lid. To permanently destroy the hair follicle in the tarsal gland, a thin wire (25 gauge or less) is passed down the hair shaft and current is applied until the cilia can be removed with little tension. Caution should be taken not to use excessive power, which can coagulate surrounding tissues (Fig. 82–22). The failure rate is fairly high because it is difficult to accurately know if the cilia have been destroyed.

When the cilia on each eyelid are too numerous to be easily removed with electroepilation, other procedures are indicated. Various techniques have been described for resecting the cilia at the lid margin.[7, 9, 16] These include partial tarsal plate excision, transconjunctival *en bloc* resection, and electrocautery.[8, 10, 19, 20, 21] Partial

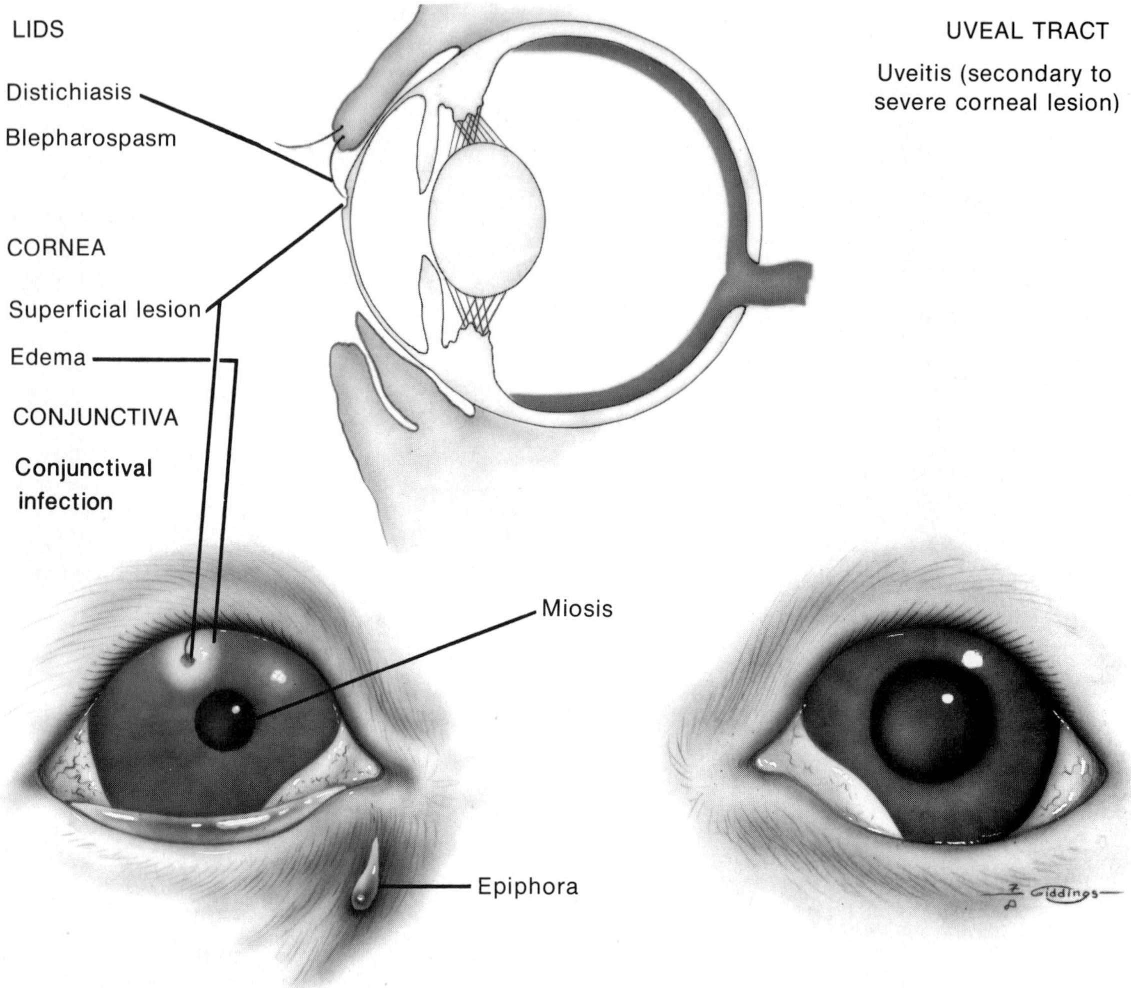

LIDS

Distichiasis

Blepharospasm

CORNEA

Superficial lesion

Edema

CONJUNCTIVA

Conjunctival infection

UVEAL TRACT

Uveitis (secondary to severe corneal lesion)

Miosis

Epiphora

FIGURE 82–21. Clinical signs of distichiasis. (Reprinted with permission from Slatter D: *Fundamentals of Veterinary Ophthalmology.* W.B. Saunders, Philadelphia, 1990.)

tarsal plate excision involves making a parallel incision on each side of the meibomian gland opening and then removing the glandular tissue and associated hair follicles. This technique and modifications of it are difficult to perform in smaller dogs with thin eyelids and often create cicatricial entropion. Entering the eyelids and performing a transconjunctival *en bloc* resection of the hair follicles or destroying them with electrocautery have been used in selected cases.[4, 19, 21] Care must be taken not to cut through the entire eyelid.

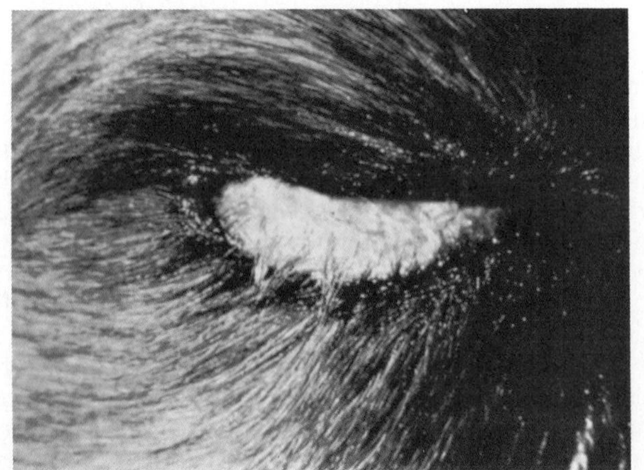

FIGURE 82–22. Severe necrosis of the lower lid resulting from use of an electrosurgical unit for epilation. (Courtesy of Dr. G. Severin.)

Microcryoepilation

Microcryoepilation has recently been reported to be the most effective and efficient therapy for distichiasis removal.[5, 7] A 4-mm nitrous oxide cryoprobe and an operating microscope are required. A freeze-thaw-freeze cycle is used. The probe is placed 4 to 6 mm from the lid margin or over the hair follicle if visible. The ice ball is allowed to progress until it reaches the center of the lid margin. The tarsal gland is not permanently damaged, and if done with precision, the procedure yields excellent results. The only complications are temporary and include conjunctivitis and occasional depigmentation of the eyelid margin.

Ectopic Cilia

Ectopic cilia originate from the tarsal gland and penetrate the conjunctiva (see Fig. 82–20). Superficial cor-

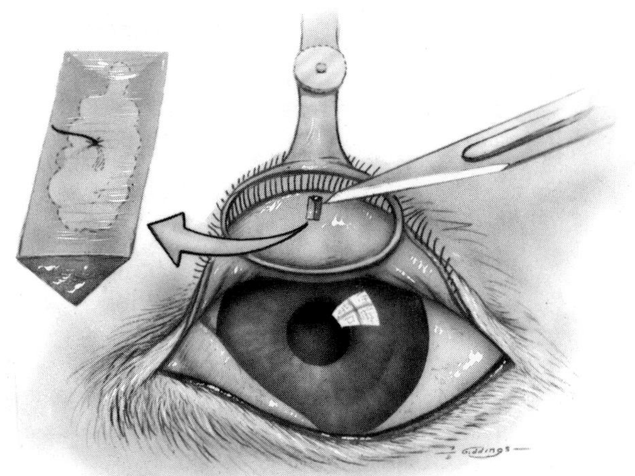

FIGURE 82–23. Ectopic cilium resection. The offending area of the lid is clamped with a Desmarres chalazion clamp for hemostasis, and the lid is everted. The wedge for resection is outlined. (Reprinted with permission from Slatter D: *Fundamentals of Veterinary Ophthalmology.* W.B. Saunders, Philadelphia, 1990.)

neal ulceration is a common finding associated with ectopic cilia, and the condition should be suspected when any small ulcer fails to heal with medical therapy, especially in a young dog.[10] Most ectopic cilia develop at the base of the tarsal glands in the center of the upper lid. Unlike distichiasis, ectopic cilia usually involve one individual cilium rather than a row. They may be very difficult to locate, and careful examination under anesthesia with high magnification may occasionally be necessary to make the diagnosis. Simple *en bloc* excision is the preferred treatment (Fig. 82–23). Suturing the defect in the conjunctiva is not necessary.

CHALAZION

A chalazion is an accumulation of secretory products in a blocked tarsal gland. It is a relatively common disease in dogs but rare in other species and is usually recognized as a painless swelling 4 to 6 mm from the lid margin. It appears as a thickened yellow-white swelling

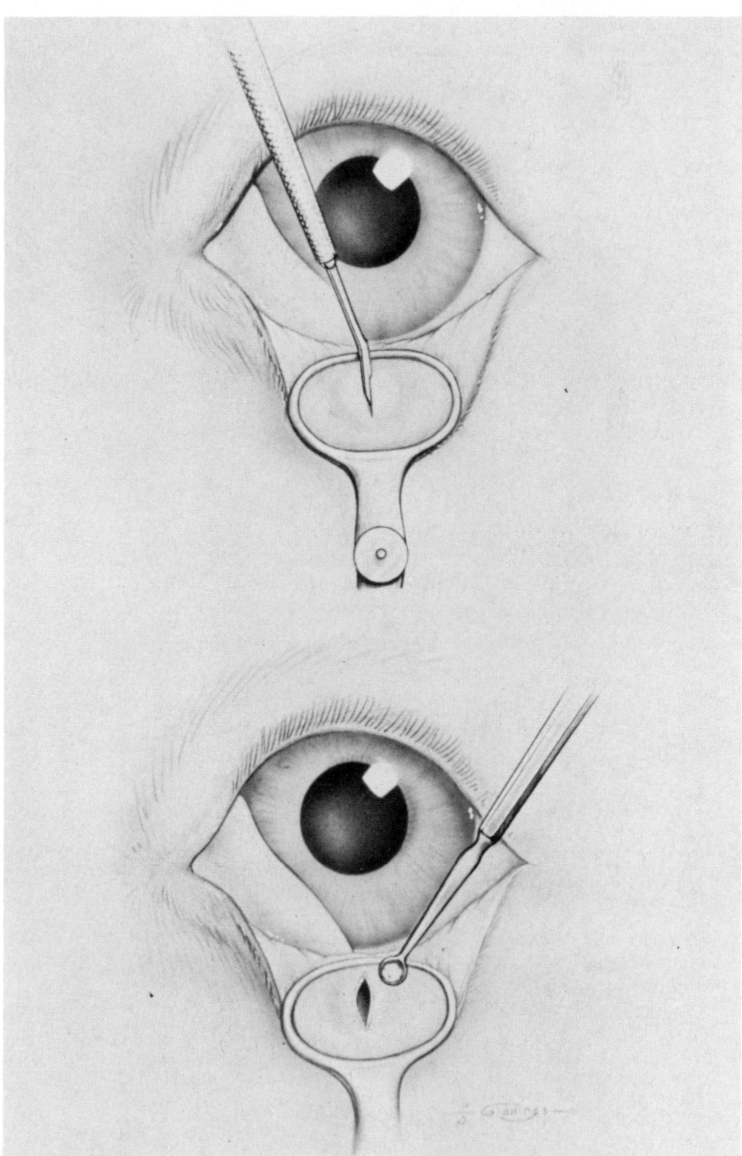

FIGURE 82–24. Treatment of chalazion. *A,* A chalazion clamp has been applied, and the lesion is incised through the palpebral conjunctiva with a number 11 blade. *B,* Removal of granulomatous material and secretion with a chalazion spoon or curette. (Reprinted with permission from Slatter D: *Fundamentals of Veterinary Ophthalmology.* W.B. Saunders, Philadelphia, 1990.)

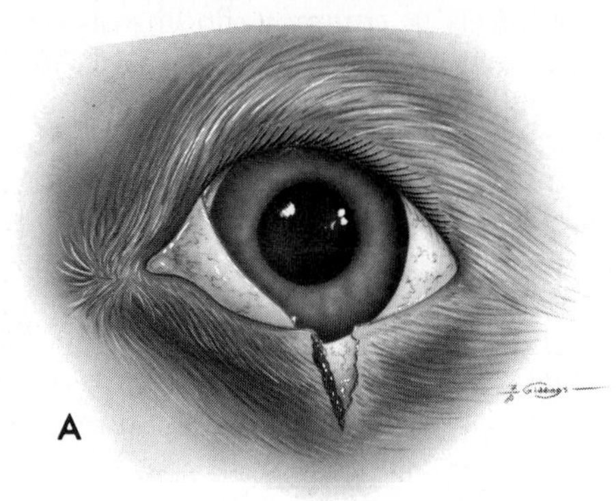

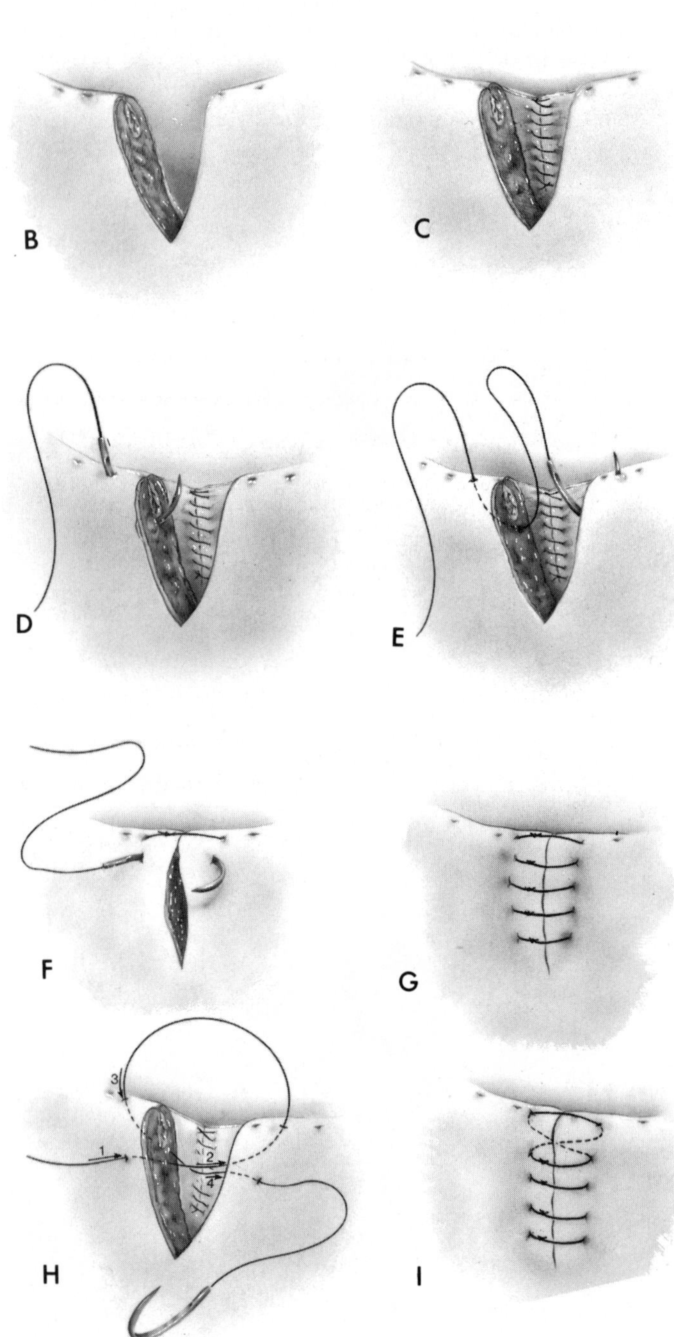

FIGURE 82–25. Simple two-layer repair. *A,* Initial injury before débridement. *B,* Wound after débridement and ready for suturing. *C,* The conjunctiva is sutured with 6-0 polyglactin 910 in a simple continuous pattern. *D,* The marginal suture is placed first, in two separate bites. *E,* The second bite. *F,* The marginal suture is carefully tied to ensure apposition of the margins. The knot lies along the margin. The wound is sutured with simple interrupted suture of 6-0 silk 2 mm apart. The first suture beneath the margin relieves tension on the marginal suture. *G,* The wound sutured. *H,* A figure-eight suture pattern may be used in place of the first two sutures. *I,* The wound sutured using a figure-eight technique. (After Severin GA: *Veterinary Ophthalmology Notes.* Fort Collins, CO, 1976. Reprinted with permission from Slatter D: *Fundamentals of Veterinary Ophthalmology.* W.B. Saunders, Philadelphia, 1990.)

seen through the palpebral conjunctiva when the eyelid is everted. A chalazion must be differentiated from a tarsal gland adenoma, which becomes more invasive, and a hordeolum, which contains purulent material. The treatment of choice for chalazion is incision and curettage of the lesion (Fig. 82–24). This may be done under either manual restraint or general anesthesia, depending on the patient. With general anesthesia, a chalazion clamp can be used to stabilize the lid. Attempts to express a chalazion manually should be avoided, because rupture of the gland may lead to lipid granulomas in the surrounding tissue as a result of the release of inspissated material.

HORDEOLUM

A hordeolum is a bacterial (usually *Staphylococcus aureus*) infection of either the lash follicle and associated gland of Zeis (external hordeolum) or the tarsal gland (internal hordeolum). Unlike a chalazion or a lid tumor, a hordeolum is characterized by marked inflammation of the surrounding tissue. External hordeolums are usually raised, painful pustules on the external lid margin. Internal hordeolums are not raised as much as the external lesions. They appear as small white pustules along the base of the tarsal glands. Treatment consists of incising the lesions with the tip of a scalpel or the point of an 18-gauge needle. The purulent material is expressed from the lids. Hot packing and topical and systemic antibiotics may also be used, depending on the severity of the disease.

LACERATIONS

A full-thickness laceration of the eyelid is best repaired using a simple two-layer technique. If the wound is near the medial canthus, the nasolacrimal puncta and canaliculi are examined to ensure they are not involved in the wound. If the nasolacrimal system is involved, the canaliculi are cannulated with a large monofilament suture or polyethylene tube to maintain patency during healing.

Two-layer closure is accomplished after débridement of the wound edges. The conjunctiva is sutured in a simple continuous pattern with 6-0 polyglactin 910 or gut. The lid margins are carefully apposed using the suture pattern shown in Figure 82–25. No subcutaneous sutures are used in this technique. This has the advantage of allowing the natural elasticity of the skin and conjunctiva to stretch back to a nearly normal eyelid shape. If the tarsal plate is sutured, the resultant scarring may prevent the eyelid from healing with the excellent cosmetic result obtained by the two-layer closure.

References

1. Bistner SI, et al: *Atlas of Veterinary Ophthalmic Surgery*. W.B. Saunders, Philadelphia, 1980.
2. Blogg JR: *The Eye in Veterinary Practice*. W.B. Saunders, Philadelphia, 1980.
3. Brightman AH, Helper LC: Full thickness resection of the eyelid. *J Am Animal Hosp Assoc 14*:483, 1978.
4. Campbell LH, McCree AV: Conjunctival resection for the surgical management of canine distichiasis. *J Am Vet Med Assoc 171*:275, 1977.
5. Chambers ED, Slatter DH: Cryotherapy (N_2O) of canine distichiasis and trichiasis: An experimental and clinical report. *J Small Anim Pract 25*:647, 1984.
6. Farris HE, Fraunfelder FT: Cryosurgical treatment of ocular squamous cell carcinoma of cattle. *J Am Vet Med Assoc 168*:213, 1976.
7. Frueh BR: Treatment of distichiasis with cryotherapy. *Ophthalmic Surg 12*:100, 1981.
8. Gelatt KN: *Textbook of Veterinary Ophthalmology*. Lea & Febiger, Philadelphia, 1981.
9. Grier RL, et al: Treatment of bovine and equine ocular squamous cell carcinoma by radiofrequency hyperthermia. *J Am Vet Med Assoc 177*:55, 1980.
10. Helper LC, Magrane WG: Ectopic cilia of the canine eyelid. *J Small Anim Pract 11*:185, 1970.
11. Johnson BW, et al: Nonsurgical correction of entropion in Shar Pei puppies. *Vet Med 83*:482, 1988.
12. Krehbiel JD, Langham RF: Eyelid neoplasms of dogs. *Am J Vet Res 36*:115, 1975.
13. Lavach JD, Severin GA: Neoplasia of the equine eye, adnexa and orbit—a review of 68 cases. *J Am Vet Med Assoc 170*:202, 1977.
14. Magrane WG: *Canine Ophthalmology*. 3rd ed. Lea & Febiger, Philadelphia, 1977.
15. Pavletic MM, et al: Mucocutaneous subdermal plexus flap from the lip for lower eyelid restoration in the dog. *J Am Vet Med Assoc 180*:921, 1982.
16. Peiffer RL, et al: Surgery of the canine and feline orbit, adnexa and globe Part 2. *Companion Animal Practice 1*:27, 1986.
17. Peiffer RL, et al: Surgery of the canine and feline orbit, adnexa and globe Part 3. *Companion Animal Practice 1*:20, 1987.
18. Prince JH, et al: *Anatomy and Histology of the Eye and Orbit in Domestic Animals*. Charles C Thomas, Springfield, IL, 1960.
19. Riis R: Basal meibomian gland cautery, a surgical technique for distichiasis. *Proc Am Soc Vet Ophthalmol 1*:88, 1982.
20. Slatter D: *Fundamentals of Veterinary Ophthalmology*. 2nd Ed. W.B. Saunders, Philadelphia, 1990.
21. White JH: Correction of distichiasis by tarsal resection and mucous membrane grafting. *Am J Ophthalamol 80*:507, 1975.
22. Wyman M: Lateral canthoplasty. *J Am Anim Hosp Assoc 7*:196, 1971.

CHAPTER

83 Conjunctiva

Cecil P. Moore

APPLIED ANATOMY AND PHYSIOLOGY

The conjunctiva is the richly vascularized ocular mucous membrane that covers the inner aspects of the upper and lower eyelids, both sides of the third eyelid, and the anterior portion of the globe with the exception of the cornea. The conjunctiva is divided into bulbar, fornix, palpebral (tarsal), and third-eyelid portions (Fig. 83–1).

The conjunctiva is supplied by blood vessels originating from the anterior ciliary arteries. Conjunctival vessels are distinguished from episcleral vessels because they are superficial, branch extensively, and are movable within the conjunctiva. Episcleral vessels are deeper, radiate from the limbus with little branching, and do not move with shifting of the conjunctiva. Sensory innervation of the conjunctiva is provided by branches of the ophthalmic and maxillary nerves, which initiate reflexes that are important preservation mechanisms for the eye in response to frictional irritants, foreign bodies, or noxious stimuli.

The conjunctival mucosa allows smooth, friction-free movements between the globe, the third eyelid, and the eyelids. The conjunctiva is a protective physical and immunological barrier. The epithelium is covered by a layer of mucus, produced by epithelial goblet cells, that contributes to the preocular tear film by serving as an interface between the aqueous tear and the hydrophobic epithelial cell membranes. This mucus also traps particulate material and debris and contains immunoglobulin A. Aggregates of lymphoid cells are prevalent in the substantia propria of the conjunctiva.

SURGICAL CONSIDERATIONS

Conjunctival Healing

Because of the high density of vessels and lymphatics within the conjunctiva, edema (chemosis) occurs quickly after conjunctival insult. Neutrophils and lymphocytes enter the injured area directly from blood vessels and lymphatics. Primary healing of mucosal lesions results as epithelial cells divide and slide rapidly (i.e., in 24 to 36 hours) to cover small defects occurring from punctures, abrasions, chemical irritation, or surgical wounds. Histiocytic macrophages and fibrocytes transform to fibroblasts to allow healing of subepithelial defects. Large denuded areas heal by granulation in 4 to 7 days.

Surgical Manipulation of Conjunctiva

The conjunctiva is securely attached at the limbus, the upper and lower tarsal plates, the leading edge of the third eyelid, and the lateral and medial canthi. Its movability and elasticity make the conjunctiva a challenging tissue to manipulate surgically.

When performing conjunctival surgery, a surgeon must take into account the forces exerted on the tissues by their normal attachments and, when necessary, exert localized traction on movable areas to accomplish the desired surgical procedure.[7] Strategic placement of traction by fine forceps counters or complements tissue attachments and stabilizes the conjunctiva, thus allowing precise incisions and dissection. Stabilization and manipulation of the globe by placement of one or more limbal fixation sutures may be quite helpful, minimizing common errors such as deviation of incisions and perforation or "buttonholing" of the membrane.[20]

Superficial dissection of the conjunctiva (e.g., when preparing conjunctival flaps) is generally more difficult than performing procedures necessitating deep dissection and entry into the episcleral space. Successful superficial dissection requires a balance of tension created by normal conjunctival attachments and skillful application of tension and countertension on the mobile conjunctiva and globe to achieve sharp dissection.[7, 20] By contrast, access to the episcleral space may be accomplished relatively easily by epibulbar dissection.

CONGENITAL DISORDERS

Dermoid

Dermoids are congenital ocular tumors that are easily identified because of the characteristic growth of hair from the lesion. Ocular dermoids commonly occur on the epibulbar surface and conjunctiva between the limbus and the lateral canthus. Although ocular dermoids may occur in any breed, dachshunds and Saint Bernards have higher incidences.[2, 17] In cats, Burmese are more commonly affected than other breeds.[10]

Clinically significant dermoids are removed surgically. Conjunctivectomy, keratectomy, or eyelid reconstruction may be needed to restore anatomy and normal ocular function.

Lacrimal Caruncle Trichiasis

Hairs growing from the lacrimal caruncle may cause epiphora, mild conjunctivitis, or superficial medial keratitis. In brachycephalic dogs, medial pigmentary keratitis has also been noted and is often complicated by conformational lagophthalmos. The term *aberrant dermis* has been used to describe the more prominent forms of lacrimal caruncle trichiasis in brachycephalic dogs.[4]

Clinical signs are resolved by removing caruncle tissue containing the follicles of offending cilia. Because the nasolacrimal puncta and canaliculi lie dorsal and ventral

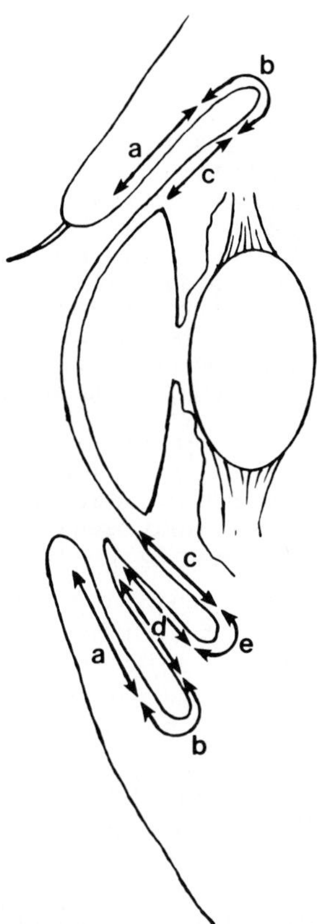

FIGURE 83–1. Cross-sectional view of conjunctiva illustrating anatomical areas. (a, palpebral [tarsal]; b, dorsal fornix and anterior ventral fornix; c, bulbar; d, anterior and posterior third eyelid; e, posterior ventral fornix conjunctivae.)

to the lacrimal caruncle, care must be taken to avoid these excretory structures. Cannulation of each canaliculus with monofilament material (2-0 or 3-0 nylon) is recommended before surgery. The conjunctival defect resulting from caruncle excision is repaired by undermining adjacent conjunctiva and closing the wound as illustrated (Fig. 83–2) with 5-0 absorbable suture. In brachycephalic dogs, removal of lacrimal caruncle hairs may be combined with a permanent medial tarsorrhaphy.[23]

Conjunctival Hypoplasia/Eyelid Colobomas

Maldevelopment of the eyelid may result in congenital absence of all normal eyelid components including the palpebral conjunctiva. Therefore, when surgical reconstruction of the eyelid is performed, particularly when defects are extensive, conjunctival grafting is indicated to line skin grafts.[6] A strip of conjunctiva may be freed from the palpebral surface of the third eyelid or from the epibulbar area. In either case, the pedicle is based laterally and formed long enough to allow graft rotation up to 180° (Fig. 83–3).

As the conjunctival portion of the reconstruction is completed, the conjunctival pedicle is sutured at the limbus and to the leading edge of the skin graft with 7-0 braided absorbable suture (polyglycolic acid [Dexon] or polyglactin 910 [Vicryl]). The donor site may be sutured or be left to heal by granulation. Topical broad-spectrum antibiotics are administered for 10 to 14 days. Trichiasis is the most common postoperative problem following eyelid and conjunctival reconstruction and may require hair removal by cryoepilation or a modified Holtz-Celsus procedure to evert the skin margin.

INFLAMMATORY DISORDERS

Symblepharon

As conjunctival ulcerations heal after infections, chemical injuries, or trauma, fibrosis of two apposing ulcerated areas may cause permanent adhesions (symblepharon). Severe neonatal conjunctivitis in kittens, usually caused by feline herpesvirus, is the most common cause of extensive conjunctival adhesions in small animals.

Adhesions of palpebral and bulbar conjunctiva may reduce or obliterate the conjunctival fornices, and scarring of the lacrimal puncta may cause persistent epiphora. When the initial ulcerative process involved the cornea, extensive symblepharon may occur between the cornea and the palpebral or third eyelid bulbar conjunctiva, resulting in considerable corneal scarring. In such instances, symblepharon may also result in reduced ocular mobility, including immobility of the third eyelid, and various degrees of enophthalmos.

Prevention of adhesions by regular use of a blunt instrument, such as a glass rod or blunt spatula, has been advocated to maintain separation of healing surfaces while the eye is treated with topical lubricant antibiotics.[16] Once symblepharon has occurred, treatment involves surgical dissection of the adhered surfaces. In the absence of epiphora, impaired mobility of the globe, or significant corneal opacity, focal symbleph-

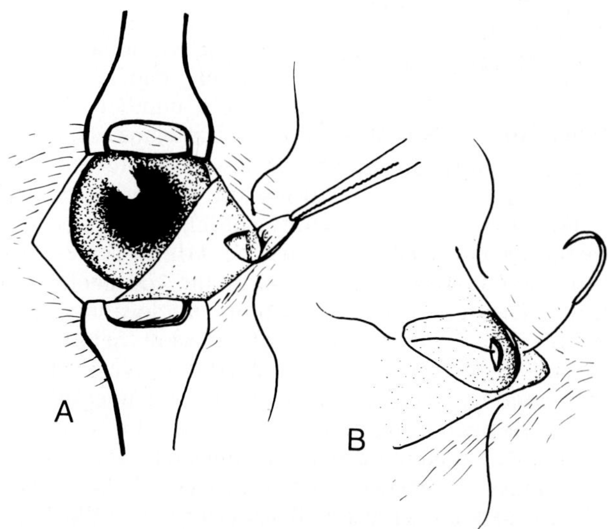

FIGURE 83–2. Removal of lacrimal caruncle tissue for treatment of medial canthal trichiasis (aberrant dermis). After dissection of the dermis, adjacent conjunctiva is undermined and the wound is closed by suturing conjunctiva to the medial canthal ligament with interrupted sutures of 6-0 polyglactin 910. (Redrawn from Carter JD: Medial conjunctivoplasty for aberrant dermis of the Lhasa Apso. *J Am Anim Hosp Assoc* 9:242, 1979.)

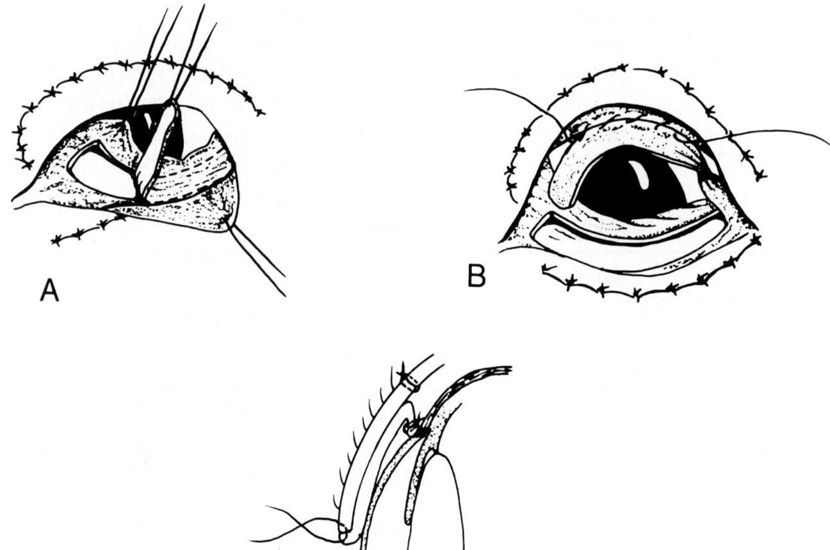

FIGURE 83–3. Placement of a conjunctival pedicle to line a cutaneous graft in repair of a full-thickness eyelid defect. *A*, A strip of conjunctiva is dissected from either the ventral bulbar conjunctiva or the anterior third eyelid conjunctiva. *B*, The conjunctival pedicle is rotated and positioned into the defect under the cutaneous graft; the ventral edge of the conjunctival flap is sutured to the limbal conjunctiva. *C*, Side view illustrating placement of suture through the reconstructed eyelid margin. Note the slight evertion of conjunctiva at the lid margin to minimize postoperative trichiasis. (Redrawn from Dziezyc J, Millichamp NJ: Surgical correction of eyelid agenesis in a cat. *J Am Anim Hosp Assoc 25*:513, 1989.)

aron may not merit repair. Minor adhesions that interfere with ocular mobility may be incised and separated by sharp dissection. After surgery, topical treatment with antibiotic ophthalmic ointment several times daily for 14 days and regular separation of affected surfaces is recommended to discourage additional adhesions.

In more severe cases of symblepharon, conjunctivectomy and superficial keratectomy, combined with grafting of adjacent healthy conjunctiva or application of overlays to prevent adhesions, provide means of restoring or improving ocular function. When the cornea is extensively opacified, a lamellar keratectomy may be needed to remove superficial corneal scar tissue (see Chapter 86). Because affected cornea may be thinner than normal, removal of only the most superficial corneal layers is indicated.

When possible, extensive conjunctival adhesions are undermined and freed as a mobile flap. The initial perilimbal incision is made using a number 15 Bard-Parker or number 64 Beaver surgical blade. Dissection is completed with conjunctival scissors or Stevens tenotomy scissors. Subconjunctival scar tissue is dissected and removed. If sufficient healthy conjunctiva is preserved to allow reconstruction, either the Arlt or Teale-Knapp technique may be used to repair the conjunctival defect.[16] Depending on the extent and location of the symblepharon, mobilization of adjacent healthy conjunctiva with reconstruction of the fornices may be attempted using either technique. Buccal mucosal grafts have also been suggested.[11]

The Arlt technique may be indicated when corneal adhesions are extensive but somewhat localized. Focal superficial keratectomy is first performed, followed by dissection of the fornix and palpebral conjunctiva to near the eyelid margin (Fig. 83–4). A free flap is created and is secured in the fornix by placing 6-0 suture into the tip of the flap, then into the fornix and through the skin, where the suture is tied and anchored over stent material. The epibulbar defects are closed by undermining, sliding, and suturing adjacent bulbar conjunctiva. The Teale-Knapp technique may be used for extensive scarring of the ventral or dorsal fornix and involves constructing and rotating conjunctival pedicle flaps from bulbar conjunctiva on both nasal and lateral aspects of the globe.[16] However, extensive scarring of the bulbar conjunctiva may preclude this form of conjunctival grafting.

In extensive generalized symblepharon, I prefer the application of a corneal-scleral overlay to prevent readhesions after keratoconjunctivectomy.[14] With this procedure, after dissecting adhesions and removing scar tissue, a bandage soft contact lens* is placed over the corneal surface and a broad-spectrum antibiotic ophthalmic ointment is applied into the conjunctival cul-de-sac. A corneal-scleral shield is then placed over the ocular surface, inserted under the eyelids, and secured by three temporary tarsorrhaphy mattress sutures (Fig. 83–5).

A commercially available plastic corneal protector may be used as the corneal-scleral shield and fornix conformer. Because the corneal protector is only available in one size, it may be reduced by trimming the perimeter with utility scissors (Fig. 83–5), smoothing the cut margins with a file or fine sandpaper, and rinsing the plastic of sanded particles. A number of different sizes may be prepared in this manner and then gas sterilized before surgery. The temporary tarsorrhaphy sutures are removed in 10 to 14 days. Systemic antibiotics are indicated because the presence of temporary tarsorrhaphy sutures over the conformer precludes effective topical treatments. To prevent self-trauma, an Elizabethan collar is placed on the animal until sutures are removed. Mild sedation or systemic analgesics may be indicated during the immediate postoperative period. The conformer allows conjunctival re-epithelialization while minimizing further adhesions and allowing re-

*Plano-T, Bausch & Lomb, Rochester, NY.

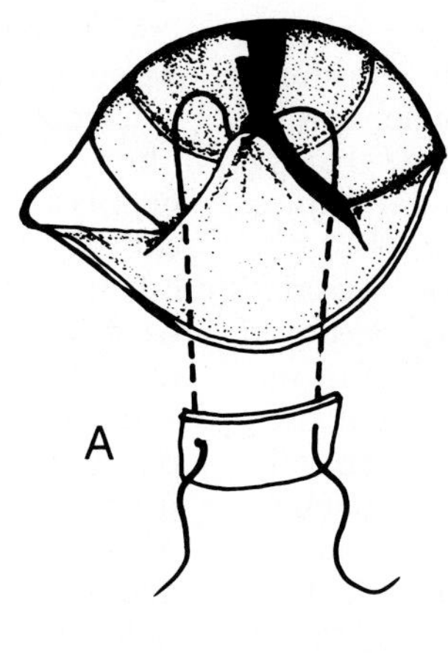

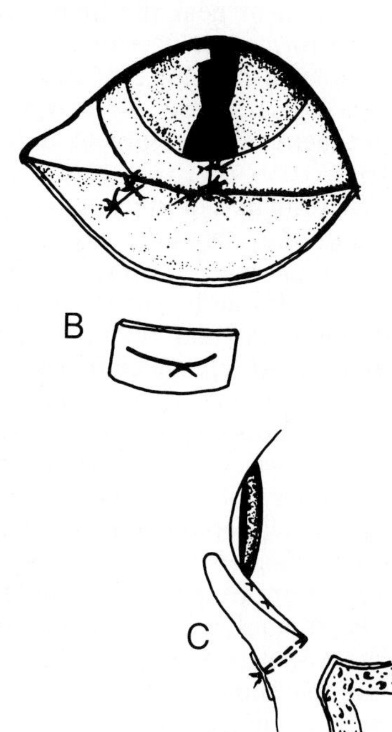

FIGURE 83–4. Arlt technique with forniceal anchor suture for repair of focal symblepharon. *A*, Adherent conjunctiva is dissected from the cornea; the incision is continued on each side of the adhesion onto the palpebral surface. *B, C*, The resultant flap is undermined and then engaged with double-armed nonabsorbable braided 5-0 suture and sutured over a stent to the skin. The bulbar conjunctiva is undermined and advanced to cover the sclera. The conjunctival incisions are closed with 7-0 absorbable suture. (Redrawn from Munger RJ: The conjunctiva. *In* Slatter DH [ed]: *Textbook of Small Animal Surgery.* W.B. Saunders, Philadelphia, 1985.)

establishment of relatively normal depth to the conjunctival fornices.

Readhesions and additional corneal scarring may occur after attempts to correct symblepharon. In severe cases, the goal of surgical correction is improvement of ocular function rather than total correction of all associated abnormalities.

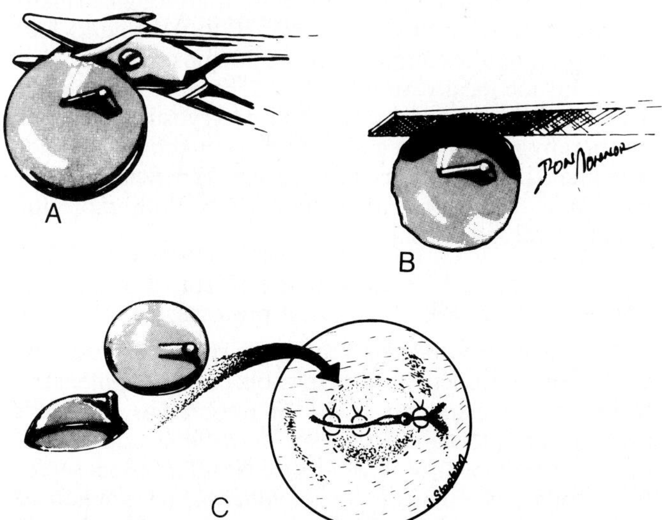

FIGURE 83–5. Use of a Crouch corneal protector (Storz, St. Louis, MO) as a corneal-scleral conformer to prevent readhesions after dissection to correct extensive symblepharon. *A*, The corneal protector is reduced to the appropriate size by trimming with utility scissors. *B*, The margins are smoothed with a file or fine sandpaper; the protector is rinsed thoroughly, dried, and gas sterilized. *C*, After surgery to remove adhesions, the protector is inserted under the eyelids and seated into the conjunctival fornices. Temporary tarsorrhaphy sutures secure the protector in position (right eye). (Redrawn from Moore CP: Surgery of the conjunctiva. *In* Bojrab MJ [ed]: *Current Techniques in Veterinary Surgery.* 3rd ed. Lea & Febiger, Philadelphia, 1990.)

Follicular Conjunctivitis (Follicle Abrasion)

Abnormal conjunctival lymphoid follicles, or *follicular conjunctivitis,* occur as a nonspecific immunological response to ocular surface antigens. In dogs, this condition usually occurs in animals younger than 18 months and is characterized by a mildly inflamed conjunctiva and mucoid ocular discharge. The discharge may be partially due to frictional rubbing of follicles on apposing conjunctival surfaces. Treatment of follicular conjunctivitis in dogs consists of topical or intralesional (subconjunctival) corticosteroids. In cats, follicular conjunctivitis is most often associated with subacute or chronic stages of chlamydial infections, and affected eyes are treated with topical tetracycline.

When lymphoid follicles are associated with conjunctival infections in dogs, the discharge is mucopurulent, and antibiotic-corticosteroid solutions or ointments are administered topically. A solution is instilled four times daily, or an ointment is applied three times daily for 2 weeks or slightly longer until follicles regress. In resistant cases, physical abrasion of the affected surface with gauze may induce an acute inflammatory response to stimulate resolution of the follicles.

CONJUNCTIVAL TUMORS

Neoplasia

Types of Conjunctival Neoplasia

The conjunctiva is an uncommon site for primary tumors; however, neoplasms arising from adjacent tissues are relatively common and may secondarily involve the conjunctiva. When a conjunctival mass is identified, a complete examination of the periocular area and globe is essential and should include biomicroscopy and ophthalmoscopy. A proliferative conjunctival lesion occurring at or near the limbus requires that gonioscopy be performed as part of the examination to determine possible involvement of the iridocorneal angle. Histopathological study of incisional or excisional biopsy specimens is necessary to differentiate possible tumor types.

Of primary conjunctival neoplasms in dogs, vascular tumors (i.e., hemangiomas and hemangiosarcomas) are among the more common.[16] The anterior surface of the third eyelid and bulbar conjunctiva are the usual sites for these vascular tumors. Hemangiomas are typically small raised telangiectatic lesions. Conjunctival hemangiosarcomas may appear similar but are larger, broader-based tumors characterized by aggressive behavior (i.e., rapid growth, local invasion, and metastatic tendency). Squamous cell carcinomas originate from nonpigmented conjunctival epithelium. Ocular squamous cell tumors, which often involve both the eyelids and conjunctiva, occur more frequently in cats than dogs.[22]

Papillomas, presumably of viral origin, may arise from the conjunctiva of dogs[1] but rarely cats.[22] Other less common tumors originating from the conjunctiva include angiokeratomas and mastocytomas.[3, 8] Primary conjunctival melanocytic tumors are rare in animals.[5] Limbal melanocytomas are more common than primary conjunctival melanomas but originate from scleral melanocytes and only secondarily involve the conjunctiva. Limbal melanocytomas are typically noted as elevated pigmented lesions at the dorsolateral limbus and are static or grow slowly. A breed predisposition occurs in German shepherds.[12]

Secondary tumors may have various appearances depending on the site of origin and the tumor type. Adenomas and adenocarcinomas most commonly arise from the tarsal glands; however, these tumors may also arise from the gland of the third eyelid. Conjunctival involvement is by direct extension, and the location of the mass suggests the tissue of origin. Periocular and orbital fibrosarcomas and neurofibrosarcomas are uncommon but when present are locally invasive and may infiltrate the conjunctiva. Systemic neoplasms (e.g., lymphosarcoma) may infiltrate around the eye as fleshy conjunctival or subconjunctival masses.

Therapeutic Procedures for Conjunctival Neoplasia

Local Excision. Masses localized to the bulbar conjunctiva are readily removed by grasping the mass with forceps and excising the tumor with conjunctival or tenotomy scissors. Small conjunctival wounds from local tumor excision generally do not require suturing and heal in 2 to 4 days. Conjunctival wounds 5 mm in diameter or larger are sutured with 7-0 braided absorbable suture in a continuous suture pattern. Palpebral tumors may require full-thickness eyelid resection.

Conjunctival Reconstruction. Undermining and sliding of adjacent conjunctiva usually facilitates closure of wounds greater than 5 mm in diameter. Primary closure of large defects may be accomplished by constructing pedicle grafts of adjacent healthy conjunctiva. Similar to their use for symblepharon repair or to line eyelid grafts, conjunctival grafts may also be used to replace tissue excised with neoplastic lesions.

Cryosurgery. Although cryosurgery has been most often used to treat eyelid neoplasia, freezing of non-neoplastic proliferative conjunctival lesions with a probe cooled with nitrous oxide or liquid nitrogen is also effective.[21] Liquid nitrogen spray is not recommended because imprecise freezing may result in inadvertent damage to the cornea or other ocular tissues.

Radiation Therapy. After surgical excision of a neoplastic lesion, beta radiation (5,000 to 10,000 cGy/site) from a strontium 90 applicator may be used at the base of the tumor. Beta particles have a relatively shallow depth of penetration (i.e., 2 to 3 mm); therefore, beta radiation application is unsuitable as the sole treatment for most ocular surface neoplasms.

Hyperthermia. Low-current radiofrequency hyperthermia provides an alternative to surgical removal of localized conjunctival masses. When a tumor is heated to 122°F (50°C) for 30 seconds, the radiofrequency current penetrates about 4 mm.

Therapy for Specific Conjunctival Neoplasms

A single treatment or combined modalities may be appropriate depending on the location, extent, and type of tumor. With papillomas, adenomas, and mastocytomas, surgical excision alone is usually curative. With squamous cell carcinomas or adenocarcinomas, excision plus ancillary treatment with local radiation therapy (i.e., beta application) is recommended. Hyperthermia has been an effective treatment for small epibulbar carcinomas in large animals.[9] Excision and beta radiation are used for treating vascular tumors, although hemangiosarcomas are generally refractory to treatment. Despite treatment, conjunctival hemangiosarcomas may recur, invade locally, or metastasize. Surface melanomas are generally treated by excision or cryosurgery. Chemotherapy results in regression of conjunctival lymphosarcoma. Topical corticosteroids are beneficial as supplemental treatment to systemic chemotherapy for conjunctival lymphosarcoma.

Conjunctival Cysts

The location and causes of cystic periocular lesions vary.[13] Subconjunctival cysts may occur developmentally from ectopic glandular tissue or anomalous duct formation, or alternatively, cysts may be acquired and occur secondary to periocular diseases that affect secretory structures. Invagination of mucosa, obstruction of glandular ducts, and disruption and sequestration of secretory cells are possible mechanisms for acquired cyst formation.

With subconjunctival cysts, the conjunctiva typically bulges over a fluctuating translucent mass. The overlying conjunctiva may be minimally inflamed. Cysts are usually readily differentiated from foreign bodies, neoplasia, or dacryoadenitis by aspirates that yield serous or seromucoid fluid. Treatment consists of surgical exploration and excision of the cyst and associated secretory tissue.

Pseudotumor

Non-neoplastic proliferative lesions of the conjunctiva occur as smooth, pink, focal, multifocal, or diffuse lesions that progress and enlarge until tissue protrudes through the eyelid fissure. One form of proliferative inflammatory ocular surface disease occurs with high frequency in collies.[19] Several terms have been used to describe these lesions, including *collie granulomas, fibrous histiocytomas, inflammatory pseudotumors, proliferative keratoconjunctivitis,* and *nodular episclerokeratoconjunctivitis.* Although the conjunctiva and subconjunctival tissues are commonly involved, the cornea and third eyelid are also frequent sites.

Treatment consists of surgical reduction and administration of corticosteroids topically, intralesionally, or systemically. In refractory or recurring cases, immunosuppressive chemotherapeutic agents (e.g., azathioprine or chlorambucil) may be administered orally. Cryosurgery has also been advocated as an effective method of treating these proliferative lesions.[21]

TRAUMA

Punctures/Lacerations

Because the conjunctiva repairs rapidly, many lacerations and punctures heal spontaneously without suturing. Conjunctival lacerations or puncture wounds are explored for foreign bodies and irrigated liberally with 1:50 betadine:saline solution.[18] After exploration and irrigation of the wound, large lacerations (i.e., 6 mm or greater in length) are sutured in a continuous pattern with 6-0 to 7-0 polyglactin 910. Whether or not the conjunctiva is sutured, broad-spectrum antibiotics are applied topically three to four times daily and systemic antibiotics are administered for 1 week to prevent opportunistic infections.

In conjunctival trauma, other ocular structures are carefully examined for evidence of trauma because the orbit, eyelids, or globe may be involved. In addition, the orbit is palpated for fractures and a thorough examination is performed for foreign bodies. Radiography allows detection of radiopaque foreign bodies.

Traumatically induced subconjunctival hemorrhage resorbs spontaneously in 7 to 14 days depending on the amount of blood present and the area involved. When conjunctival or subconjunctival hemorrhage is present, antibiotics are applied topically to prevent secondary infections of damaged tissues. Corticosteroids are of equivocal value in ocular surface hemorrhage, because the process of spontaneous resorption is not hastened by steroid application. When conjunctival hemorrhage occurs with no evidence of puncture or without a history of trauma, a systemic clotting disorder is considered.

Avulsion

Facial trauma may result in abrasion of the ocular surface with loss of conjunctival tissue. Conjunctival avulsion usually accompanies lacerated or avulsed eyelids and corneal ulcerations. Small conjunctival defects generally heal spontaneously and uneventfully with empirical topical therapy. Because of the elasticity of the conjunctiva, defects up to 5 mm in width can usually be sutured directly without placing excessive tension on the tissues or distorting ocular position. A 6-0 or 7-0 absorbable (e.g., polyglactin 910) suture is used in a continuous pattern to close the defect. When large areas of conjunctiva are lost (e.g., with concurrent eyelid avulsion), conjunctival grafting may be indicated as part of the blepharoplastic repair.

MISCELLANEOUS SURGICAL PROCEDURES

Conjunctival Biopsy

Biopsy of the conjunctiva is indicated for differentiating inflammatory from neoplastic diseases and in suspected cases of preocular goblet cell (mucin) deficiency.[15] In tractable animals, conjunctival biopsy is performed under local anesthesia. Topical anesthesia is generally sufficient for biopsy of the fornix conjunctiva, whereas subconjunctivally administered local anesthetic may be needed for biopsy of perilimbal or third-eyelid conjunctival lesions.

After four instillations of 0.5 per cent proparacaine on the ocular surface (at 30-second intervals over a 2-minute period), a fornix biopsy sample may be harvested by grasping and tenting the conjunctiva with 0.3-mm rat-tooth forceps and snipping a 3- × 4-mm specimen with conjunctival scissors. A small amount of hemorrhage is anticipated but is usually minimal because fibrin formation quickly seals the wound. The biopsy specimen is gently spread out on a flat surface, such as a small styrofoam pad or a section of wooden tongue depressor. The specimen is then immediately fixed in 10 per cent buffered formalin.

In animals that resist grasping and tenting of the conjunctiva after only topical anesthetic, administration of a tranquilizer/analgesic combination and infiltration of the biopsy site with lidocaine 2 per cent (0.25 ml) may be needed. Defects resulting from conjunctival biopsy that are less than 4 × 4 mm heal uneventfully with topical antibiotic treatment. Larger iatrogenic wounds are sutured, and general anesthesia may be necessary.

References

1. Bonney CH, et al: Papillomatosis of the conjunctiva and adnexa in dogs. *J Am Vet Med Assoc 176*:48, 1980.
2. Brandsch H, Schmidt V: Erbanalytische Untersuchungen zum Dermoid des Auges Beim Hund [Analysis of heredity of dermoid in dog eye]. *Mh Vet-Med 37*:305, 1982.
3. Buyukmihci N, Stannard AA: Canine conjunctival angiokeratomas (two cases). *J Am Vet Med Assoc 178*:1279, 1981.
4. Carter JD: Medial conjunctivoplasty for aberrant dermis of the Lhasa Apso. *J Am Anim Hosp Assoc 9*:242, 1979.
5. Cook CS, et al: Malignant melanoma of the conjunctiva in a cat. *J Am Vet Med Assoc 186*:505, 1985.
6. Dziezyc J, Millichamp NJ: Surgical correction of eyelid agenesis in a cat. *J Am Anim Hosp Assoc 25*:513, 1989.
7. Eisner G: *Eye Surgery—An Introduction to Operative Techniques*. Springer-Verlag, New York, 1980.
8. Johnson BW, et al: Conjunctival mast cell tumor in two dogs. *J Am Anim Hosp Assoc 24*:439, 1988.

9. Kainer RA, et al: Hyperthermia for treatment of ocular squamous cell tumors in cattle. *J Am Vet Med Assoc 176*:356, 1980.
10. Koch SA: Congenital ophthalmic abnormalities in the Burmese cat. *J Am Vet Med Assoc 174*:90, 1979.
11. Magrane WG: *Canine Ophthalmology*. 3rd ed. Lea & Febiger, Philadelphia, 1977, pp 101–102.
12. Martin CL: Canine epibulbar melanomas and their management. *J Am Anim Hosp Assoc 17*:83, 1981.
13. Martin CL, et al: Cystic lesions of the periorbital region. *Comp Cont Educ Pract Vet 9*:1022, 1987.
14. Moore CP: Surgery of the conjunctiva. *In* Bojrab MJ (ed): *Current Techniques in Veterinary Surgery*. 3rd ed. Lea & Febiger, Philadelphia, 1990, pp 76–82.
15. Moore CP, et al: Selection of biopsy site for quantitation of canine conjunctival goblet cells. Transactions of the American College of Veterinary Ophthalmology, New Orleans, LA, Nov. 1986, pp 272–300.
16. Munger RJ: The conjunctiva. *In* Slatter DH (ed): *Textbook of Small Animal Surgery*. W.B. Saunders, Philadelphia, 1985.
17. Priester WA: Congenital ocular defects in cattle, horses, cats and dogs. *J Am Vet Med Assoc 160*:1504, 1972.
18. Roberts SM, et al: Antibacterial activity of dilute povidone-iodine solutions used for ocular surface disinfection in dogs. *Am J Vet Res 47*:1207, 1986.
19. Smith JS, et al: Infiltrative corneal lesions resembling fibrous histiocytoma: Clinical and pathological findings. *J Am Vet Med Assoc 169*:722, 1976.
20. Troutman RC: *Microsurgery of the Anterior Segment of the Eye*. Vol I. *Introduction and Basic Techniques*. C.V. Mosby, St. Louis, 1974.
21. Wheeler CA, et al: Cryosurgery for treatment of recurrent proliferative keratoconjunctivitis in five dogs. *J Am Vet Med Assoc 195*:354, 1989.
22. Williams LW, et al: Ophthalmic neoplasms in the cat. *J Am Anim Hosp Assoc 15*:999, 1981.
23. Wyman M: Permanent medial tarsorrhaphy. *Vet Clin North Am 2*:322, 1979.

CHAPTER 84 The Lacrimal System

J. D. Lavach

The lacrimal system produces and removes tears. In normal animals, there is a coordinated secretion of glandular products that combine to form the precorneal tear film. This film is distributed across the cornea and performs several important functions. A substantial portion of tear volume is lost through evaporation, and the remainder is removed through drainage channels (Fig. 84–1).

ANATOMY OF THE LACRIMAL SYSTEM*

The lacrimal glands are responsible for producing most of the tears.[10] Histologically, they are similar to the serosalivary glands.[19, 39] They are modified skin glands with a tubuloalveolar arrangement, containing both serous and mucous acini.[39] Lacrimal glands are located in the region of the orbit between the globe nasally and orbital ligament and zygomatic process of the frontal bone temporally.[12] They are enclosed within a fold of periorbita but are isolated from the rectus muscles by a fascial plane. The size varies, with the following dimensions reported in dogs: 0.5 to 2.0 cm long, 1.5 to 3.0 cm wide, and 0.7 to 1.5 cm thick.[12] The emptying ducts are continuous from the deeper lobe through the superficial lobe; hence damage to the superficial portions of the ducts or their openings renders the glands nonfunctional. The ducts in dogs (3 to 20) are not visible but open through the conjunctiva in the superior temporal fornix.[12, 48]

The gland of the third eyelid is an accessory lacrimal gland. The gland encompasses the stem of the cartilaginous shaft in the third eyelid. The secretions are mixed and seromucoid in dogs and serous in cats.[33, 39] In dogs, 29 to 57 per cent of the serous tear component may be produced by this gland.[10, 26] The secretions pass through two to four invisible ducts[12] that open into the inferior cul-de-sac between the globe and third eyelid.

The tarsal glands are grossly visible through the thin palpebral conjunctiva, perpendicular to the margin of the eyelid (Fig. 84–2). In dogs, approximately 40 openings are found in the upper eyelid and fewer (usually 28 to 34) in the lower eyelid. Each opening is about 80 μm (0.08 mm) in diameter.[39] The secretion is a lipid-laden sebaceous material, which can be manually expressed on the margin of the eyelid as a cream-colored exudate.

The intraepithelial goblet cells are the primary source of the mucoid layer of the tears. The cells are scattered throughout the palpebral conjunctiva, including the reflections on the third eyelid, but are most prevalent in the fornices. Goblet cells are not normally found on the bulbar conjunctiva.

The upper and lower eyelids each have a small opening, the lacrimal punctum—the beginning of the lacrimal drainage system. The puncta are 2 to 5 mm from the nasal canthus.

After entering a punctum, the tears pass into the upper or lower canaliculus. The total length of each canaliculus is between 4 and 7 mm, and the diameter varies in dogs from 0.5 to 1.0 mm.[12, 17, 19]

The lacrimal sac at the confluence of the canaliculi is not always a distinct structure in animals, as it is humans. It occupies the fossa in the lacrimal and frontal bones posterior to the lacrimal crest.

The nasolacrimal duct begins at the lacrimal sac. The duct continues rostrally through the bony channel of the lacrimal bone and into the lacrimal sulcus of the maxilla. This section is the narrowest portion of the nasolacrimal duct. The duct emerges from the bony capsule at the level of the conchal crest, which is adjacent to the

*For a more detailed discussion consult standard ophthalmology texts.

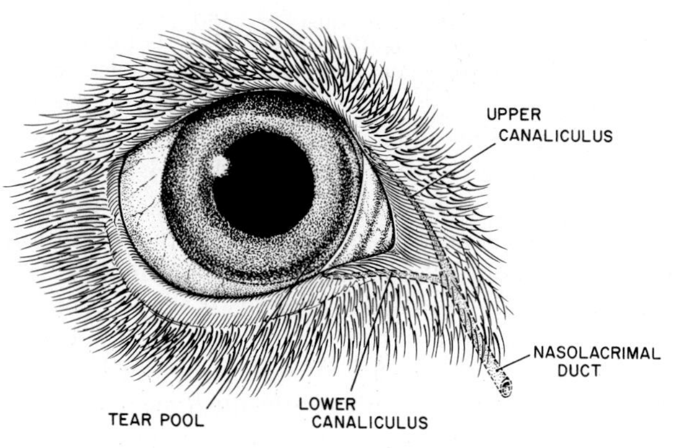

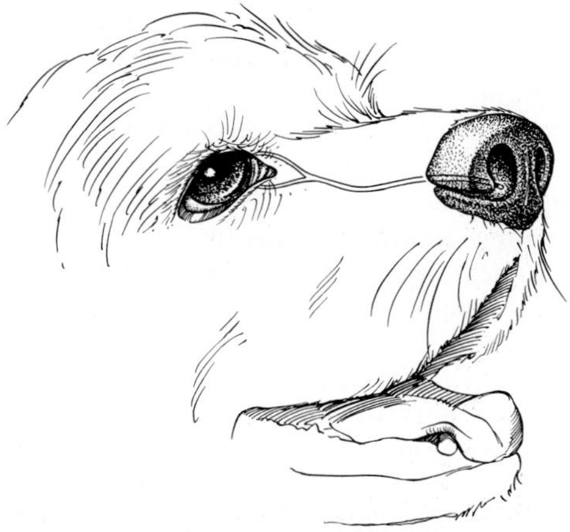

FIGURE 84–1. The nasolacrimal system.

second premolar tooth, or at the infraorbital canal.[12, 19] After leaving the bony canal, the duct continues in the medial wall of the maxilla, deep to the nasal mucosa. An accessory opening is present at the root of the upper canine tooth in approximately 50 per cent of dogs.[35] The duct makes an abrupt 90° turn 2 mm from the orifice and opens onto the floor of the nasal cavity at the junction of the ventral and lateral walls, approximately 1 cm inside the opening of the external nares. A nasal speculum or forceps must be used to retract the alar cartilage laterally to see the opening in the nasal vestibule. The feline nasolacrimal system is similar to the canine; however, a communication with the oral cavity is noted, and the opening is located on the small papillae just behind the upper incisor teeth.

TEAR MOVEMENT

The flow of tears begins in the lacrimal gland, passes across the cornea, blends with other secretory components, and pools in the lacrimal lake. The pool is not always evident owing to eyelid and globe relations but exists interiorly in the nasal canthus. The heavy, oily secretions from the tarsal glands help to prevent spillage of tears onto the face and direct the tears toward the lacrimal lake. Several theories have evolved to explain the passage of tears from the palpebral fissure to the lacrimal lake and down into the nose.[36, 48, 51, 52] A combination of contraction of the orbicularis muscle, gravity, capillary action, and a syphoning effect from the lacrimal sac may be required to propel the tears. Consequently, a patent outflow apparatus does not ensure removal of tears unless physiological function is present. Little tear secretion occurs during sleep in humans, and approximately half of the total tear volume is lost through evaporation.[51] A discussion of the composition and function of tears and mucous threads is beyond the scope of this chapter, and the reader is referred to other sources.[27, 34]

Principles of Diagnosis

Readers are referred to standard ophthalmology texts for principles of diagnosis.[18, 46]

EPIPHORA AND LACRIMATION

Epiphora is an overflow or spillage of tears onto the face as a result of impaired outflow apparatus. Lacrimation is increased production of tears that may result in tear overflow when the production exceeds the capacity for drainage and evaporation.[14] Lacrimation caused by psychic stimulation is not recognized as a phenomenon in lower animals, but lacrimation may be provoked by various external stimuli including pain (Table 84–1).

CONGENITAL ANOMALIES OF DRAINAGE

Congenital anomalies of the drainage apparatus are occasionally encountered in small animals. Some anomalies are insignificant, and epiphora is not present. In

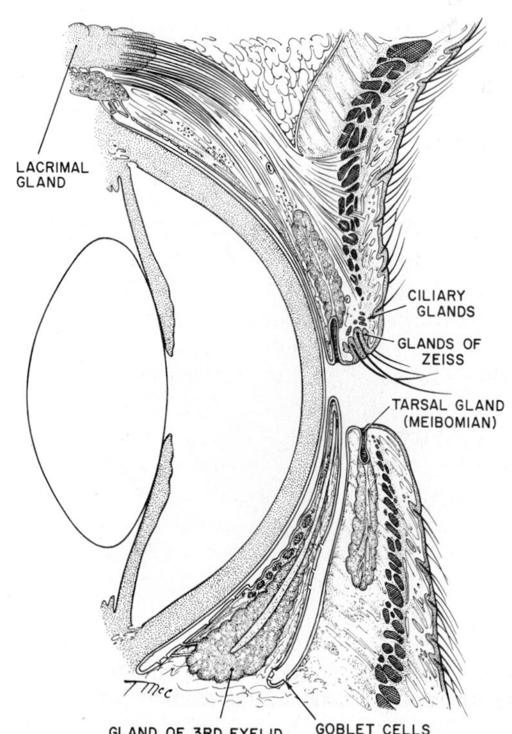

FIGURE 84–2. A cross section of the globe and eyelids showing sources of the precorneal tear film.

TABLE 84–1. ETIOLOGY OF OVERFLOW OF TEARS

I. Lacrimation
  A. Parasympathetic stimulation
    1. Cholinergic drugs (pilocarpine)
    2. Anticholinesterase drugs (demecarium bromide)
  B. Lacrimal gland inflammation
    1. Traumatic lesions
    2. Infectious process
  C. Trigeminal irritation
    1. Lesions of the eyelids, conjunctiva, cornea, and iris
    2. Glaucoma
  D. Retinal stimulation by glare and excessive light
II. Epiphora
  A. Eyelid abnormalities
  B. Congenital anomalies of the nasolacrimal system
    1. Atresia
    2. Hypoplasia
  C. Acquired anomalies
    1. Trauma
    2. Infection
  D. Foreign bodies
  E. Neoplasia
III. Tear staining syndrome

others, a constant state of increased moisture is noticed during the first 3 to 4 months of life. The discharge is clear and free of copious amounts of mucoid or purulent material. The chief complaint is altered appearance and not discomfort or disability. In a few patients, copious moisture causes scalding of the skin and secondary dermatitis.

Absence of the Punctum

Several dog breeds,[2, 18] including cocker spaniels, golden retrievers, Samoyeds, toy poodles, miniature poodles, and Bedlington terriers, as well as Persian cats, may lack one or more puncta.

If either the upper or lower punctum is present, epiphora may not exist. If only the lower is absent, epiphora is more likely than if only the upper is absent, because the lower punctum is more important in removing tears. A thorough examination with magnification is necessary to establish the absence of a punctum. If the upper and lower puncta are absent, a slight depression in the conjunctiva may be identified where the opening would normally be located. If one punctum is present, it may be cannulated, and gentle flushing may cause a tenting up or slight ballooning of the conjunctiva at the site of the atretic punctum (Fig. 84–3). Retrograde catheterization from the nasal orifice may allow the catheter to push up against the conjunctiva as a landmark for incision.

A conjunctival excision is performed parallel to the lid margin at the anticipated site of the punctum. A 2- × 3-mm piece of conjunctiva is excised with scissors. Minimal bleeding occurs with this technique.

After the punctal opening is established, the nasolacrimal system is flushed to expel any debris and confirm patency. Postoperative treatment consists of the use of a topical antibiotic-corticosteroid solution four times daily for 7 days. Tears should continue to flow through the new punctum, and patency should be maintained without further surgery. In a small number of patients, two complications may occur: First, the punctal opening may close with granulation tissue or cicatrix, necessitating reoperation; this event is more likely in the presence of concurrent infectious conjunctivitis or infection in the canaliculus. Second, epiphora may still be present when the drainage system does not have adequate functional

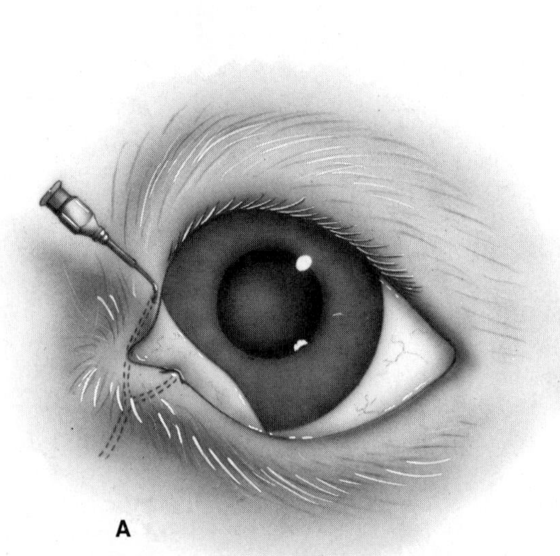

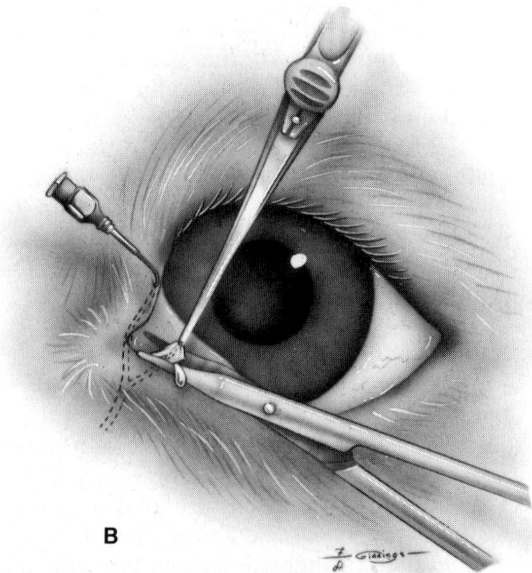

FIGURE 84–3. Repair of imperforate punctum using pressurized fluid. *A,* The opposing punctum is cannulated, and pressure is applied via a saline-filled syringe to elevate the obstructing conjunctiva over the other punctum. The use of methylene blue solution aids in locating the bleb. Some loss of saline occurs down the nasolacrimal duct. *B,* The tissue is grasped with fine forceps and incised with strabismus scissors. Antibiotic and corticosteroid preparations are applied for 7 to 10 days to prevent scarring and obstruction. Daily dilation may be necessary for a few days to prevent closure. (Reprinted with permission from Slatter D: *Fundamentals of Veterinary Ophthalmology,* 2nd ed. W.B. Saunders, Philadelphia, 1990.)

capacity, even though the punctum is open and patency is established.[14]

If a new punctal opening is established and is not satisfactory, a monofilament nylon suture may be passed as previously described. A larger polyethylene catheter is threaded over the monofilament nylon and pulled through the nasolacrimal system.[43, 46] The nylon guide is removed, and the tubing is sutured in place at the nasal canthus and on the hair-bearing skin just posterior to the planum nasale (Fig. 84–4). This drainage tube remains in place for 4 weeks until the wounds have epithelialized and postsurgical inflammation has subsided.

Congenital Membrane

A condition similar to congenital absence of the punctum occurs when a conjunctival membrane or flap is present over the punctum, providing partial or complete obstruction. The treatment is similar to that for establishing a punctal opening.

Stenotic Punctum

Stenotic puncta are occasionally found in Manx and Persian cats. Small, apparently hypoplastic or incomplete openings are seen in some dogs.[2] They may represent incomplete atresia of punctal openings. A lacrimal dilator, a blunt, taper-point instrument, may be introduced through the small punctum and gradually advanced into the canaliculus. Additionally, the punctum may be enlarged by excision. A one-, two-, or three-snip technique may be used immediately after dilation.[2, 37, 48] A canaliculus knife or scissors are gently inserted into the punctum while the eyelid is stretched medially. The blade edge is parallel to the lid margin, and the incision is made horizontally through the posterior portion of the canaliculus for 1 to 2 mm (one snip). The second and third snips, if made, are performed with scissors and result in the removal of a triangular flap of conjunctiva (Fig. 84–5). Failures are attributed to reclosure of the punctum.[15] Tension sutures can be placed through the eyelid skin to pucker the punctum and keep it dilated during the first 5 days after surgery.[13]

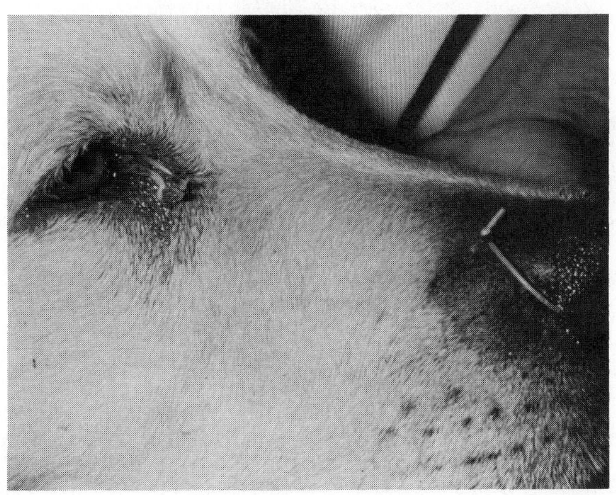

FIGURE 84–4. Polyethylene tubing sutured in place for treatment of dacryocystitis.

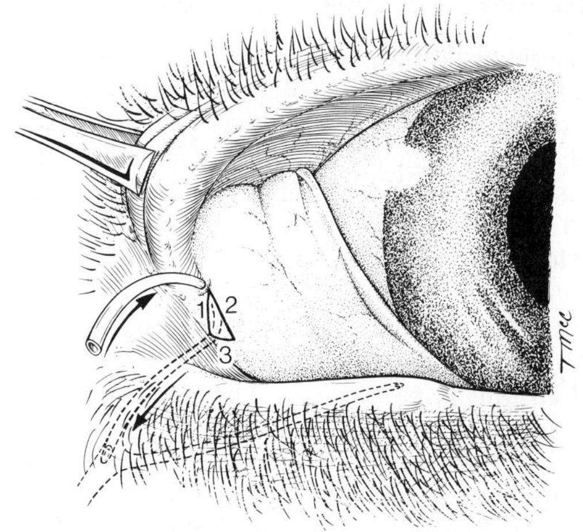

FIGURE 84–5. 1,2,3-snip procedure.

Atresia of Canaliculi or Lacrimal Duct

The canaliculi or nasolacrimal duct may be obstructed by a membrane owing to failure of the facial fissure to close properly. This anomaly is usually associated with lethal defects. Rarely a dog is presented with a normal punctum and canaliculus but an obstruction of the bony canal. This condition requires surgery to establish communication between the nasolacrimal sac and the nasal cavity to provide relief of the epiphora.

Tear Staining Syndrome

The tear staining syndrome is a poorly defined clinical entity of chronic facial moisture and secondary staining of facial hairs. The nasolacrimal system is patent when flushed, but a functional blockage exists. The absence of obvious abnormalities or obstructions to drainage makes this condition a diagnostic enigma. Previous treatments of epiphora have included medical and surgical techniques.[3, 7, 8, 16, 21–28, 29, 41, 50]

Medical Treatment of Tear Staining

Palliative management with topical creams and pastes is an attempt to protect the facial hair and skin but has been uniformly unsuccessful. One medical approach is based on a theory that tetracyclines may bind with circulating porphyrins[21, 45] or lactoferrin-like pigments[46] and prevent hair staining. The face remains wet, but the hair is not stained; therefore, the tear staining is less noticeable. Another medical treatment is based on the concept that affected dogs have a chronic low-grade inflammation of the nasal or pharyngeal area and tonsils.[7, 8] This inflammation could produce edema of the nasolacrimal system and lead to functional blockage. Systemic and topical treatment with antibiotics and corticosteroids for 2 weeks is required to improve most cases.

Surgical Treatment of Tear Staining

A histological study of 91 glands of the third eyelid was performed on glands obtained from 47 dogs with epiphora.[32] The results could not be correlated with clinical signs, suggesting that the gland of the third eyelid is not responsible for epiphora and that the benefit derived by removing the gland is a reduction of the total tear volume. Surgical removal of the gland of the third eyelid effectively reduces the tear volume by up to 50 per cent. This relatively simple procedure *should not be attempted* unless the Schirmer test values are known to exceed 20 mm in 60 seconds. The potential for keratoconjunctivitis sicca and its consequences should be thoroughly discussed and explained before using this approach to control epiphora.

Hair may be observed growing from the nasal canthal conjunctiva and third eyelid. The hairs can cause corneal irritation and serve as wicks for the tears. If this condition leads to facial staining and constant moisture on the face, the offending tissue may be excised or removed by cryoepilation. Sutures are placed with care to avoid excessive tension that would alter the position or function of the punctum and canaliculi. In a similar procedure described by Carter,[9] the dermal tissue is dissected from the conjunctiva and the margins are bluntly undermined, exposing the medial palpebral ligament (Fig. 84–6). A 6–0 absorbable suture attaches the cut edge of the conjunctiva to the margin of the medial palpebral ligament.

ACQUIRED ANOMALIES OF TEAR OUTFLOW

Spastic Entropion

Proper eyelid position and function are essential for even distribution and removal of excessive tears. Orbicularis muscle spasm produces a spastic entropion, which, if not treated early by reducing the source of pain, remains as a permanent entropion. Surgical correction of the entropion is necessary to restore eyelid function and normal tear outflow.

Cicatricial Entropion

Old wounds or infected tissues around the eyelid may lead to cicatrix formation and may inhibit eyelid movement. The scar tissue must be freed and the eyelid function restored to regain normal function of the lacrimal system.

Blepharitis

Swelling of the eyelids may result from systemic or localized disease processes. Insect bites and local injury may produce enough hemorrhage and edema to alter eyelid and lacrimal function.

Conjunctivitis

Acquired occlusion of the punctum may follow several disease processes and may result in epiphora. Conjunctival infections or inflammatory processes may cause enough edema and catarrhal thickening to occlude the puncta. In cats with upper respiratory diseases (e.g., herpesvirus infection), the symblepharon may be extensive. This altered anatomical relationship often results in epiphora even though patency can be established. The adhesions may be incised, but there is a propensity for postoperative re-formation.

Folliculosis

Extensive follicle or papule formation may inhibit tear flow and occlude the punctum. Increased lacrimation or epiphora may be associated with folliculosis in young dogs. The cause is unknown, but the condition is presumed to be an allergic phenomenon. Appropriate treatment of the follicles eliminates the tearing.

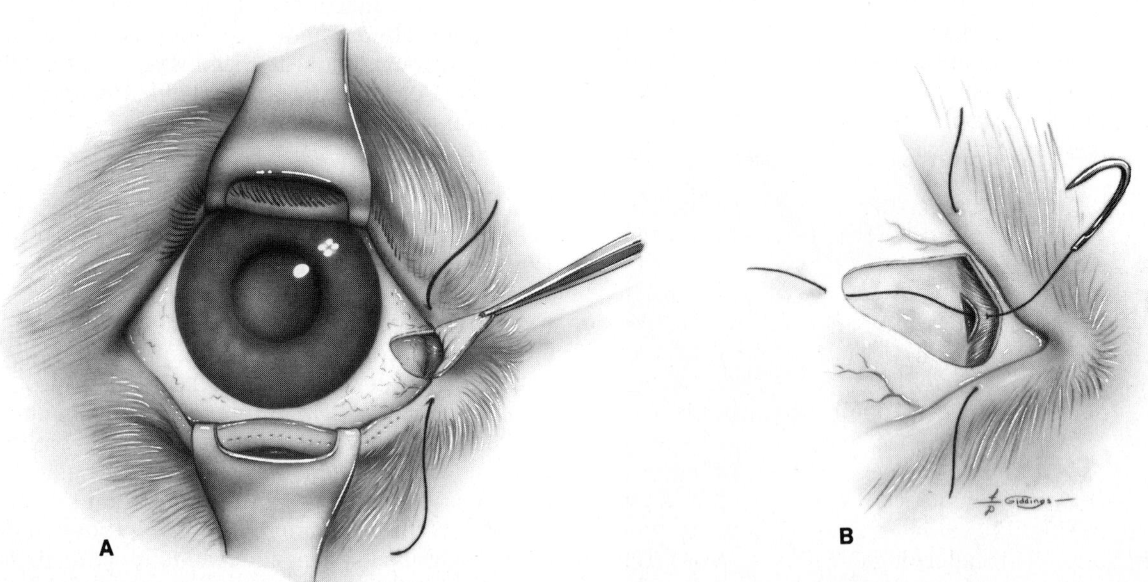

FIGURE 84–6. Sliding conjunctival flap for treatment of dermoid. *A*, The dermis is dissected off, and a conjunctival flap is created. *B*, The sliding flap is sutured to the edge of the medial palpebral ligament with one or two simple interrupted sutures of 5-0 Vicryl. (Reprinted with permission from Slatter D: *Fundamentals of Veterinary Ophthalmology*, 2nd ed. W.B. Saunders, Philadelphia, 1980.)

Autoimmune Disease

Autoimmune erosions of the mucocutaneous junction, as in the pemphigoid diseases, may be associated with closure of the punctum and epiphora. Each condition must be correctly diagnosed and treated specifically. Once the condition is under control, the patency of the nasolacrimal system may be established with stents and tubing. The creation of a new drainage pathway may be considered if patency cannot be established.

Neoplasia

Neoplastic tissue involving the eyelids may interfere with normal eyelid function or may obstruct the punctum and create epiphora.

ACQUIRED OCCLUSION OF THE CANALICULI, SAC, OR NASOLACRIMAL DUCT

Upper Respiratory Infections

In small animals, occlusion of the canaliculi, sac, or nasolacrimal duct may follow any of several disease processes. Upper respiratory infections in cats and chronic bacterial infections can extend into the canaliculus and sac. The primary disease often responds to appropriate treatment, but the infectious organisms remain in the isolated sac, and reinfection is possible. Repeated flushing with antibiotic-steroid combinations is indicated.

Dacryocystitis

Dacryocystitis is inflammation of the nasolacrimal sac. Chronic low-grade dacryocystitis is characterized by epiphora and persistent conjunctivitis. In humans, this has been described as a "silent dacryocystitis."[49] Typical infections in small animals result in epiphora with a mucoid to mucopurulent discharge from the lower punctum. The discharge has a stringy consistency and often contains bubbles. Digital pressure over the nasal canthus may result in extrusion of material from the upper and lower puncta. Chronic infections have an associated canaliculitis, and the punctum may be elevated and hyperemic. The most obvious signs involve the lower punctum and canaliculus. Pain may be evident over the sac, but only in a few patients can a detectable swelling of the sac be seen.

The treatment for dacryocystitis is the establishment of patency of the outflow system by mechanical flushing and removal of any foreign material and debris.[38] Chronic cases are difficult to catheterize, and a complete evaluation, including culturing of the exudate and dacryocystorhinography, is necessary. Localized bony involvement of the sac may be encountered. Periosteal reaction may narrow or occlude the lumen and prevent catheterization. If a catheter cannot be passed, repeated efforts using a smaller-diameter monofilament nylon suture are indicated. Once the catheter is in place, a larger polyethylene tube is threaded and passed. As the polyethylene tube is passed over the suture, resistance may be encountered at the sac, and considerable effort may be required to force a channel through obstructing fibrous tissue. Follow-up care consists of appropriate topical and systemic antibiotic therapy. If the stent tube cannot be passed or if the tube is passed but the infections persists, the patient is a candidate for surgical exploration of the lacrimal sac.

Laing and colleagues described a technique for a dacryocystotomy.[30] It begins as a skin incision at the level of the ventromedial orbital rim. The incision is 2 to 3 cm long and parallel to the lower eyelid. A catheter is inserted into the upper or lower canaliculus and palpated where it enters the lacrimal fossa. The lacrimal sac is 5 mm on the ventral side of the orbital rim from this site. A drill is used to penetrate the lacrimal bone and enter the lacrimal sac. Hemorrhage is controlled by gauze packing. The sac can be flushed with saline to remove any debris. The stent tube or catheter can be passed through the system to the nares as previously described. The periosteum and deep tissues are closed with 4-0 absorbable suture. The skin wound is closed with nonabsorbable material. Follow-up care consists of topical and systemic antibiotics.

Mucocele

Mucocele of the lacrimal sac is rare but may be either congenital or acquired. Facial swelling by a fluctuating mass over the lacrimal sac with minimal pain and an absence of signs of infection suggests a mucocele. Radiographs may assist in the diagnosis.

Neoplasia

Primary neoplasia of the canaliculus, sac, or duct is rare (Fig. 84–7).

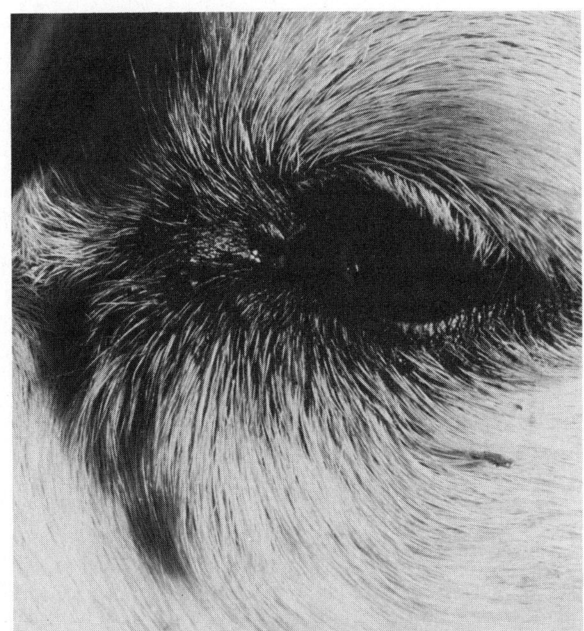

FIGURE 84–7. Metastatic adenocarcinoma of the lacrimal sac.

Lacerations

Superficial lacerations of the conjunctiva may involve the punctum or canaliculus. If only the punctum is damaged, it is unlikely that sufficient scarring will occur to produce epiphora. If the canaliculus is lacerated, however, surgical repair is indicated. Passage of a monofilament nylon suture from the punctum into the lacerated end is possible by visual inspection. The distal portion is not visible until nasal (retrograde) passage is accomplished. Because about 50 per cent of affected dogs have an accessory opening, it may be impossible for the suture to follow the nasolacrimal duct out through the cut end. If the suture does pass, it is usually easy to thread the previously identified proximal end carefully out through the punctum. If it cannot be catheterized, retrograde flushing may permit a stream of fluid to identify the cut end. Pigtail probes (Worst) are available with hook ends or eye holes and may assist in identifying the cut ends of the canaliculus and in passing catheters (Fig. 84–8).[6, 46] Once the canaliculus is catheterized, a single simple interrupted suture of a 7-0 absorbable material is placed through the deep tissue below the canaliculus (Fig. 84–9). A second suture is placed above the canaliculus in a similar fashion, and a 4-0 suture is placed full thickness from skin to conjunctiva and back out to skin to complete the closures. Sutures are not placed directly through the canaliculus.[40] The tube is left in place for 12 weeks in dogs to ensure healing without stricture.[47]

SURGICAL CREATION OF A NEW DRAINAGE APPARATUS

Dacryocystorhinostomy

Dacryocystorhinostomy may be used in patients with a patent canaliculus but an obstruction of the sac or

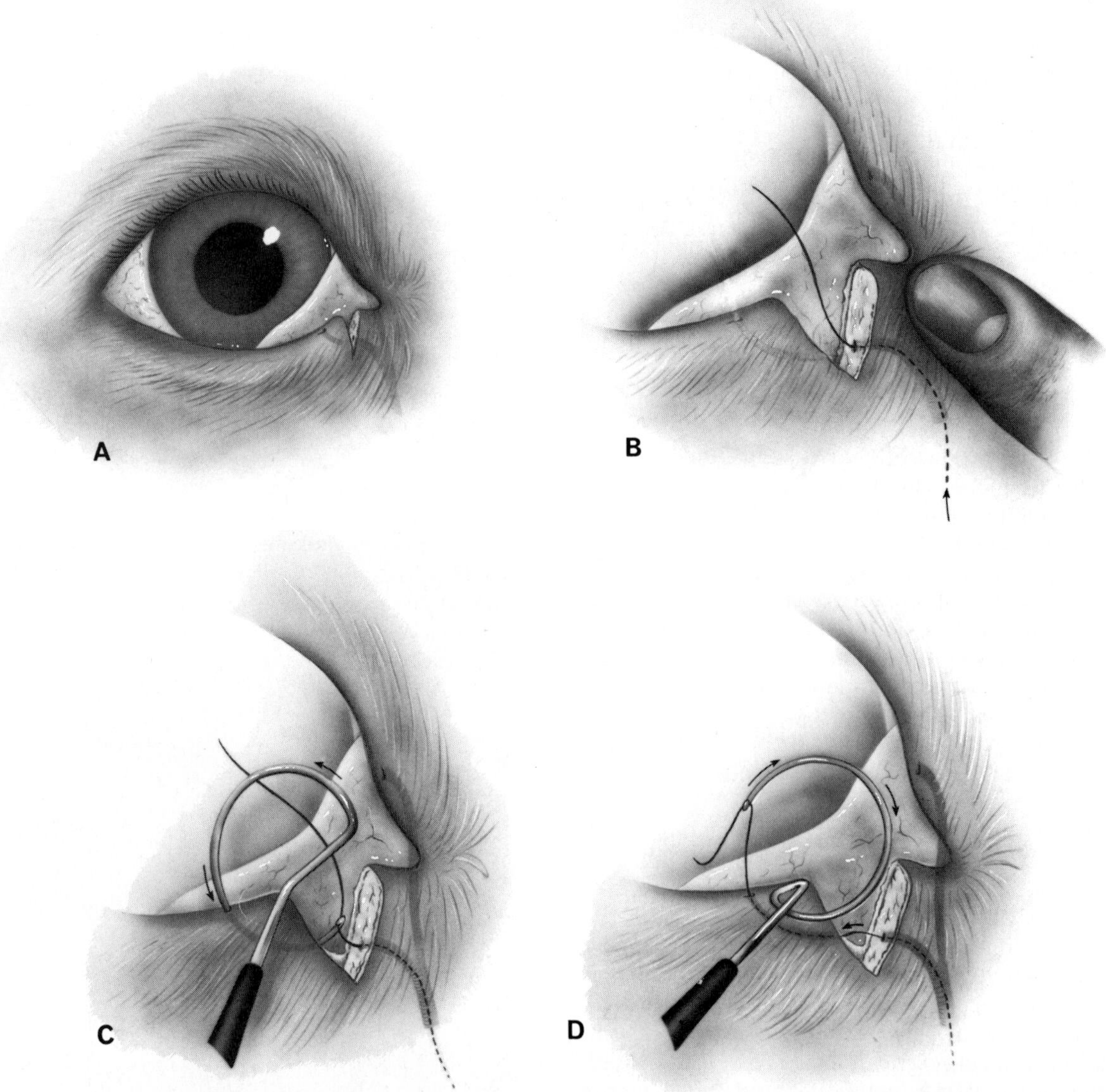

FIGURE 84–8. Nasolacrimal catheterization for canalicular laceration. *A,* Laceration of lid margin and canaliculus. *B,* A fine nylon (e.g., 2-0) thread is passed up the nasolacrimal duct from the nose. The superior punctum from which it normally emerges is occluded by finger pressure, and the thread is manipulated to emerge from the severed inferior canaliculus. *C,* A Worst probe is passed, and the suture is tied to it and pulled through the punctum *(D).* (Reprinted with permission from Slatter D: *Fundamentals of Veterinary Ophthalmology,* 2nd ed.. W.B. Saunders, Philadelphia, 1990.)

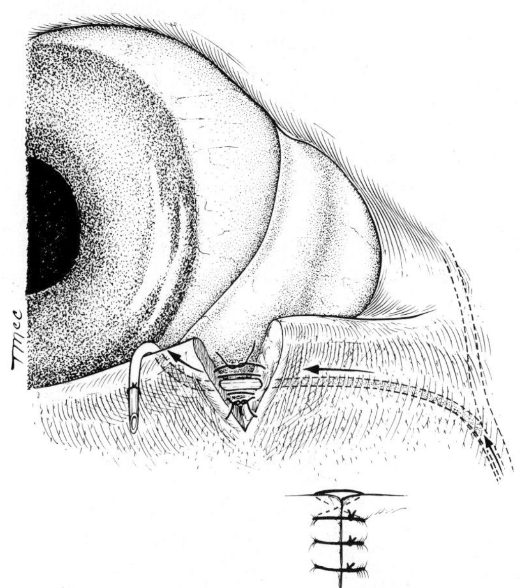

FIGURE 84–9. Closure of canalicular laceration.

canal. A skin incision is made parallel to the nose and 2 to 3 mm medial to the nasal canthus. The incision continues ventrally 2 cm over the sac. The exact position of the sac is determined by palpating the inferior rim of the orbit. The incision should be full thickness through the skin but not deep enough to injure the large vessels. The skin and vessels are retracted, and the sac is identified. If the sac is redundant and not readily visible, palpation of the maxillary bone and lacrimal bones may reveal the lacrimal crest and fossa; catheterization of the canaliculi may "point" to the junction of the upper and lower canaliculi. A bone drill or trephine is used to enter the bone at the level of the sac.

In dogs and cats, the largest polyethylene tubing that can pass through the punctum and canaliculus is threaded through the new bony canal and sutured in place as described for dacryocystitis. The catheter is left in place for at least 4 months to ensure continued patency. Continued evaluation of the tubing is necessary. In the event of loss, it is replaced immediately. This procedure has not been previously described for use in small animals; however, a similar approach, dacryocystotomy, has been used in the treatment of chronic dacryocystitis in three dogs.

Conjunctivorhinostomy

In the technique described by Covitz and colleagues, a small Steinmann pin is directed ventromedially into the orbital rim toward the nasal cavity (Fig. 84–10).[11] The pin is aimed at the ipsilateral external nares, with the shaft of the pin. A series of larger pins is used until one larger than the outside diameter of the catheter to be placed is used. The tract is flushed with saline before catheterization. Hemorrhage can be considerable. Either polyethylene or Silastic tubing may be used in lengths of 2.5 to 3.8 cm. A flanged end or rim is applied to the tubing and is used to suture the tubing in place at the mucocutaneous junction of the nasal canthus. If the tubing does not slide easily into place, nasal mucosal folds are most likely obstructing the bony opening and need to be flushed out of the way.

A topical antibiotic-steroid ointment is applied three times daily for 3 to 4 days and then once daily until the tubing is removed. The tube is flushed at least once weekly. The sutures are removed 2 weeks after surgery; however, the tubing is left in place for at least 8 weeks. Premature removal results in overgrowth of the canal with granulation tissue. If the tube is accidentally lost, it is replaced immediately. The actual relief of epiphora is usually not noticed until after the final tube is removed. If tubing with a flange or collar is not available, the surgeon may suture polyethylene tubing to the skin of the face and at the exit of the nares as described previously for other conditions.

The previously described surgical techniques are rarely used in veterinary practice. Only an experienced ophthalmic surgeon should attempt any of these procedures.

DEFICIENCY OF PRECORNEAL TEAR FILM

Diseases resulting in reduced or absent precorneal tear film are commonly encountered in small animals. Readers are referred to standard ophthalmology texts for details and medical therapy.[73]

Surgical Treatment

Punctal Occlusion

This technique is of no proven value in small animals.

Permanent Partial Tarsorrhaphy (see Chapter 82)

Parotid Duct Transposition

Parotid duct transposition is recommended for dogs and cats without measurable tear volume and for chronic keratoconjunctivitis sicca that has not responded to medical treatments.[4, 20, 31, 43, 44] Before surgery, medical treatment is necessary to ascertain complete loss of

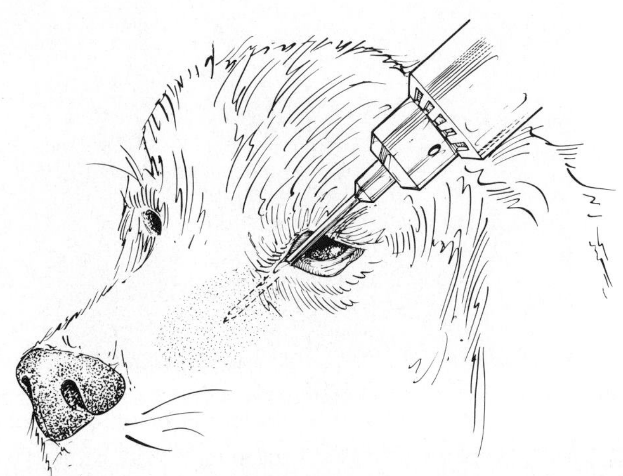

FIGURE 84–10. Position of pin and chuck to create a new outflow channel.

lacrimal function. The function of the parotid salivary gland is evaluated by stimulating salivation and observing saliva flowing from the duct opening. The client must be well informed of the disease process, the alternative use of topical therapy instead of surgery, and what to expect after surgery. Only an experienced surgeon should perform this procedure.

Surgical Technique[20, 31, 44] (Fig. 84–11). After catheterization, the duct is palpated through the skin over the masseter muscles. A skin incision is made directly over the duct for 2 to 5 cm, depending on the size of the dog. The incision is carefully continued down to the level of the duct, and the duct is isolated and retracted by applying a loop of moist umbilical tape around it. The loop allows manipulation of the duct without forceps, reducing iatrogenic damage to the duct. The duct is freed from the tissues posterior to the level of the parotid gland. The overlying tissues are carefully and patiently dissected from the duct. The surgeon should avoid transecting the branches of the buccal nerves when

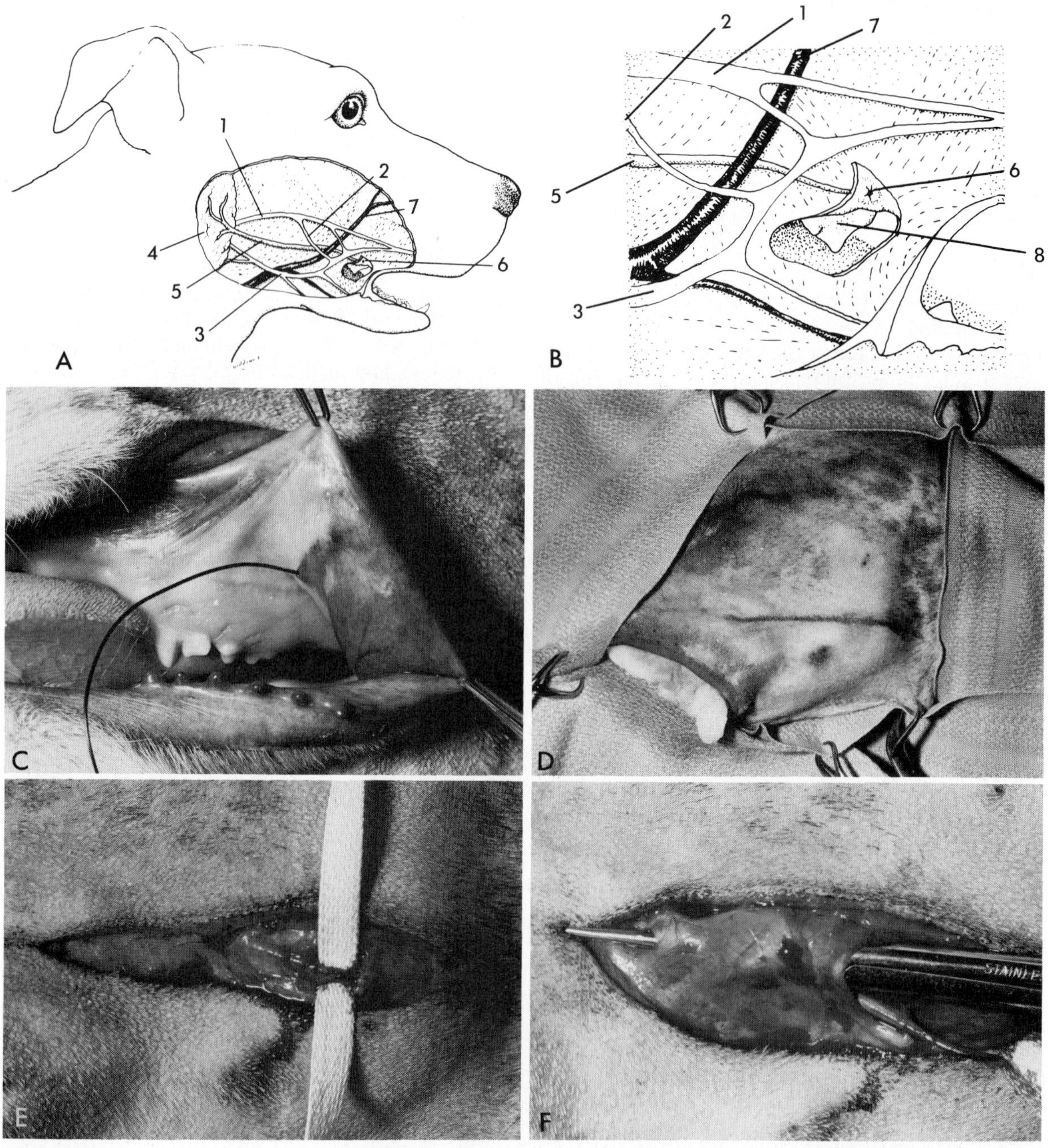

FIGURE 84–11. Parotid duct transposition. *A* and *B*, Cutaway diagram of the face *(A)* and enlargement of area where duct enters mouth *(B)*. (1, Dorsal buccal nerve; 2, anastomosis of dorsal and ventral buccal nerves; 3, ventral buccal nerve; 4, parotid salivary gland; 5, parotid duct; 6, papilla of parotid duct; 7, facial vein; 8, upper carnassial tooth.) *C*, Monofilament nylon suture marker in place in the parotid duct. *D*, Pledget of cotton soaked with 1:750 aqueous benzalkonium chloride placed over the parotid duct papilla. The course of the duct is marked on the skin. *E*, Umbilical tape passed beneath parotid duct so that the duct can be manipulated without damaging it with forceps. *F*, Completed dissection beneath the facial vein and branches of buccal nerve with blunt scissors.

possible. The duct passes beneath the superficial facial vein, which is also avoided. An accidental incision into the vein produces hemorrhage and necessitates ligation of the vein. The deep side of the duct is not freed from its attachments at this point. Careful dissection is continued until the duct enters the oral mucosa. The last centimeter before the duct's entrance into the oral cavity is difficult to dissect, because the duct is tightly adherent to the oral mucosa. The lip is retracted, and a 6-mm Keyes skin biopsy punch is used to outline the oral mucosa around the papilla. The punch is rotated gently, with its greatest pressure anteriorly because the duct lies just under the mucosa posteriorly. Too much pressure will transect the duct. The papilla is cut free from the remaining mucosal attachments with small scissors. Once the papilla is completely freed, it is passed back through the canal under the superficial facial vein and into the skin incision. Some additional dissecting may be performed from the deeper side of the duct to free it from muscular fascia. Scissors are directed from the skin incision to the lower conjunctival cul-de-sac, and the conjunctiva is entered between the lateral margin of the third and lower eyelids. This pathway lies on the fascia of the masseter muscle and should not be placed at other levels. The papilla and free duct are carried through the canal, and the papilla is sutured in place with six to eight 7-0 absorbable sutures. The skin and oral wounds are closed in a routine fashion.

Immediate postoperative care consists of systemic and topical antibiotic therapy for 5 days. Several small meals during each day stimulate the parotid flow (a small blood clot can be milked from the duct through the skin on the first postoperative day). Proper flow must be ascertained immediately to correct any complications.

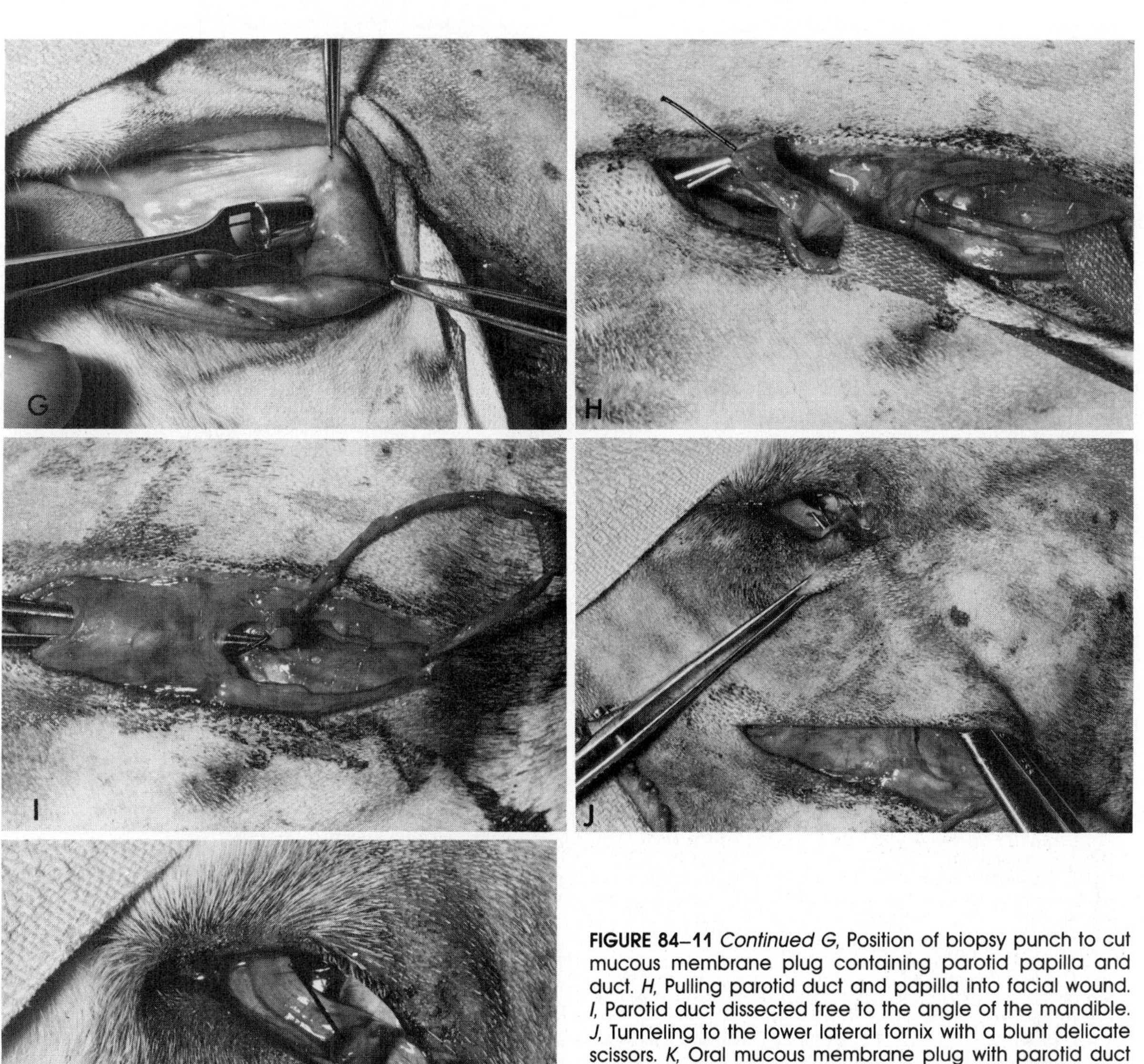

FIGURE 84–11 *Continued G,* Position of biopsy punch to cut mucous membrane plug containing parotid papilla and duct. *H,* Pulling parotid duct and papilla into facial wound. *I,* Parotid duct dissected free to the angle of the mandible. *J,* Tunneling to the lower lateral fornix with a blunt delicate scissors. *K,* Oral mucous membrane plug with parotid duct papilla positioned for suturing to the conjunctiva. (Reprinted with permission from Severin GA: Keratoconjunctivitis sicca. *Vet Clin North Am* 3:407, 1973.)

The major postoperative complication is failure of the duct to function.[1, 5, 22, 42] This usually results from twisting the duct during surgery. Preoperative catheterization and careful placement of the transposed duct reduce the likelihood of this complication. Postsurgical stricture formation may impede the flow of saliva at any time after the surgery has been performed. Strictures probably result from poor dissection of the duct or rough handling of the tissues, which stimulates more fibrosis. Uncontrolled conjunctival infections may also lead to fibrosis and closure of the duct.[42] If a duct fails to function, it should be catheterized and evaluated for patency. If a stricture is found, the duct is surgically exposed and examined. When a stricture is near the papilla, the duct may be transected below the stricture and the cut end of the duct sutured into the conjunctival sac. If a stricture occurs farther from the papilla, the duct may not be of sufficient length to reach the conjunctival sac, and a surgical solution may have to be abandoned.

Complications of Parotid Duct Transposition. Immediate complications of parotid duct transposition include a nonfunctioning parotid gland, twisting or kinking of the duct, bending around a vessel or nerve, and suturing through the duct. Delayed complications include slippage of papilla into subcutaneous tissues, stricture formation, skin maceration, and solid deposits on the cornea and eyelids.

Skin infections resulting from maceration by saliva are a potential problem, and it may be necessary to apply petrolatum or other ointment around the eyelids to protect the skin. When maceration occurs, it is usually transient, because the volume of saliva seems to diminish with time. The hair should be kept short around the eyelids to reduce the amount of retained moisture. A few dogs have a continuous large volume of saliva accumulation on the eyelids and face. Another potential complication is the appearance of chalklike deposits on the eyelid margins and on and in the cornea.[44] The material in the deposits may be irritating and may require superficial corneal abrasion and the use of EDTA to remove them. Periodic use of mucolytic agents (acetylcysteine) or 1 per cent EDTA solution slows the accumulation of these deposits.

References

1. Baker GJ, Formston C: An evaluation of transplantation of the parotid duct in the treatment of keratoconjunctivitis sicca in the dog. *J Small Anim Pract 9*:261, 1968.
2. Barnett KC: Imperforate and microlachrymal puncta in the dog. *J Small Anim Pract 20*:481, 1979.
3. Barrows GT: Canine tearing operation. *Norden News Spring:* 26, 1968.
4. Bennett JE: The management of total xerophthalmia. *Trans Am Ophthalmol Soc 66*:503, 1968.
5. Betts DM, Helper LC: The surgical correction of parotid duct transposition failures. *J Am Anim Hosp Assoc 13*:695, 1977.
6. Billson FA, et al: Trauma to the lacrimal system in children. *Am J Ophthalmol 86*:828, 1978.
7. Bryan GM: Diseases of the nasolacrimal system. *In* Kirk RW (ed): *Current Veterinary Therapy VI.* W.B. Saunders, Philadelphia, 1977, pp 618–624.
8. Bryan GM, Michelson E: Epiphora in the poodle. *West Vet 16*:13, 1978.
9. Carter JD: Reconstructive surgery for juxtapunctal neoplasms of the lower eyelid. *J Am Vet Med Assoc 157*:199, 1970.
10. Chang SH, Lin AC: Effects of main lacrimal gland and third eyelid gland removal on the eye of dogs *J Chin Soc Vet Sci 6*:13, 1970.
11. Covitz D, et al: Conjunctivorhinostomy: A surgical method for the control of epiphora in the dog and cat. *J Am Vet Med Assoc 171*:251, 1977.
12. Diesem C: Organ of vision. *In* Getty R (ed): *Sisson and Grossman's The Anatomy of Domestic Animals.* 5th ed. W.B. Saunders, Philadelphia, 1975.
13. Dolin SL, Hecht SD: The punctum pucker procedure for stenosis of the lacrimal punctum. *Arch Ophthalmol 104*:1086, 1986.
14. Duke-Elder S, MacFaul PA: *The System of Ophthalmology.* Vol 13. C.V. Mosby, St. Louis, 1974.
15. Fein W: Cautery applications to relieve punctal stenosis. *Arch Ophthalmol 95*:145, 1977.
16. Filipek ME, Rubin LF: Effect of metronidazole on lacrimation in the dog: A negative report. *J Am Anim Hosp Assoc 13*:339, 1977.
17. Gelatt KN, et al: Dacryocystorhinography in the dog and cat. *J Small Anim Pract 13*:381, 1972.
18. Gelatt KN, Gwin RM: Canine lacrimal and nasolacrimal systems. *In* Gelatt KN (ed): *Veterinary Ophthalmology.* Lea & Febiger, Philadelphia, 1981, 309–329.
19. Getty R: The eye, orbit, and adnexa. *In* Miller ME, et al (eds): *Anatomy of the Dog.* W.B. Saunders, Philadelphia, 1964.
20. Gwin RM, et al: Parotid duct transposition in a cat with keratoconjunctivitis sicca. *J Am Anim Hosp Assoc 13*:42, 1977.
21. Harrison VA: Letter to the editor. *Vet Rec 76*:437, 1964.
22. Harvey CE, Koch SA: Surgical complication of parotid transposition in the dog. *J Am Anim Hosp Assoc 7*:122, 1971.
23. Harvey CE, et al: Orbital cyst with conjunctival fistula in a dog. *J Am Vet Med Assoc 153*:1432, 1968.
24. Hayes KC: Vitamin A. *In Nutritional Management of Dogs and Cats.* Ralston-Purina Company, St. Louis, 1975.
25. Helper LC: The effect of lacrimal gland removal on the conjunctiva and cornea of the dog. *J Am Vet Med Assoc 157*:72, 1970.
26. Helper LC, et al: Surgical induction of keratoconjunctivitis sicca in the dog. *J Am Vet Med Assoc 165*:172, 1974.
27. Holly FJ, Lemp MA: Tear physiology and dry eyes *Surv Opthalmol 22*:69, 1977.
28. Howard DR: The surgical correction of epiphora. *Vet Med Small Anim Clin* 64:683, 1969.
29. Kerpsack RW, Kerpsack WR: The orbital gland and tear staining in the dog. *Vet Med Small Anim Clin 61*:121, 1966.
30. Laing EJ, et al: Dacryocystotomy: A Treatment for chronic dacaryocystitis in the dog. *J Am Anim Hosp Assoc 24*:223, 1988.
31. Lavignette AM: Keratoconjunctivitis sicca in a dog treated by transposition of a parotid salivary duct. *J Am Vet Med Assoc 148*:778, 1966.
32. Leoffler VK, et al: Histologische unterscuchungen an nickhautdrusen von hunden mit vermehrtem tranenflub. *Kleintierprazis 23*:215, 1978.
33. Martin CL, Anderson PG: Ocular anatomy. *In* Gelatt KN (ed): *Veterinary Ophthalmology.* Lea & Febiger, Philadelphia, 1981, pp 12–121.
34. McDonald JE: Surface phenomena of tear films. *Trans Am Ophthalmol Soc 66*:905, 1968.
35. Michel G: Anatomy of the lachrymal glands and ducts in the dog and cat. *DTW Dtsch Tierarztl Wochenschr 62*:347, 1955.
36. Milder B: The lacrimal apparatus. *In* Moses RA (ed): *Adler's Physiology of the Eye.* 7th ed. C.V. Mosby, St. Louis, 1981.
37. Miller SJH: Diseases of the lacrimal apparatus. *In Parson's Diseases of the Eye.* 16th ed. Churchill Livingstone, New York, 1978.
38. Murphy JM, et al: Nasolacrimal catheterization for treating chronic dacryocystitis. *Vet Med Small Anim Clin 72*:883, 1977.
39. Prince JH, et al: *Anatomy and Histology of the Eye and Orbit in Domestic Animals.* Charles C Thomas, Springfield, IL, 1960.
40. Putterman AM: *In* Peyman GA, et al (eds): *Principles and Practice of Ophthalmology.* Vol 3. W.B. Saunders, Philadelphia, 1980.
41. Roberts SR: Abnormal tear secretion in the dog. *Mod Vet Pract 43*:37, 1962.
42. Schmidt G, et al: Parotid duct transposition: A followup study of 60 eyes. *J Am Anim Hosp Assoc 6*:235, 1970.
43. Severin GA: Nasolacrimal duct catheterization in the dog. *J Am Anim Hosp Assoc 8*:13, 1972.
44. Severin GA: Keratoconjunctivitis sicca. *Vet Clin North Am 3*:407, 1973.
45. Severin GA: *Veterinary Ophthalmology Notes.* 2nd ed. Colorado State University, Ft Collins, 1976.
46. Slatter DH: *Fundamentals of Veterinary Ophthalmology.* 2nd ed. W.B. Saunders, Philadelphia, 1990.
47. Snead JW, et al: The effects of silicone tube on the canaliculus: An animal experiment. *Ophthalmology 87*:1031, 1980.
48. Startup FG: *Diseases of the Canine Eye.* William & Wilkins, Baltimore, 1969.
49. Theodore FK: Silent dacryocystitis. *Arch Ophthalmol 40*:157, 1948.
50. Thun R, et al: Effect of tetracycline on tear production in the dog. *J Am Anim Hosp Assoc 11*:802, 1975.
51. Veirs ER (ed): *The Lacrimal System, Clinical Application.* Grune & Stratton, New York, 1955.
52. Yamaguchi M (ed): Recent advances on the lacrimal system. Proceedings of the 3rd International Lacrimal Symposium, Kyoto, 1978.

CHAPTER

85 Third Eyelid

Cecil P. Moore, DVM, MS

ANATOMY AND PHYSIOLOGY

The third eyelid is a triangular structure that arises from the anterior ventromedial aspect of the orbit. A T-shaped hyaline cartilage supports the third-eyelid gland, connective tissue stroma, and conjunctiva that covers the anterior (palpebral) and posterior (bulbar) surfaces (Fig. 85–1). A seromucous gland surrounds the base of the cartilage and provides a significant portion of the basal tear secretion in dogs.[8] A fascial retinaculum secures the base of the gland and cartilage to the ventromedial orbit.[6] The position of the third eyelid depends on normal size and position of the globe and sympathetic tone of smooth-muscle fibers within the orbital fascia.

The third eyelid protects the globe and secretes and distributes tears. When the retractor bulbi muscle retracts the globe, the third eyelid passively covers the eye and serves as a protective barrier. Movements of the third eyelid aid in expulsion of particulate matter from the eye. The tapered leading margin (free border) spreads the tear and sweeps across the ocular surface, serving as a "windshield wiper" for the cornea. Because the free border of the third eyelid is usually pigmented and blends in with the eyelids and iris, the anterior surface is generally inconspicuous. In an animal with a nonpigmented third eyelid, the free border and anterior surface appear pink and therefore are more noticeable.

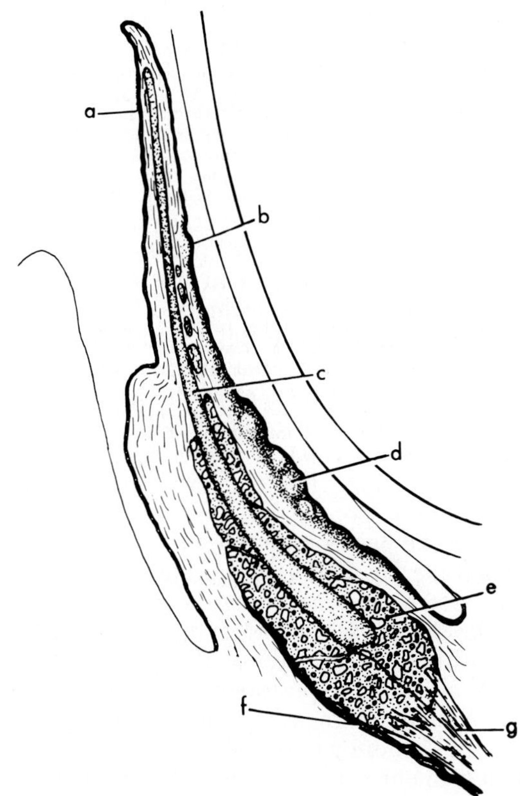

FIGURE 85–1. Cross section of third eyelid. a, anterior conjunctiva; b, posterior conjunctiva; c, stem of cartilage; d, lymphoid follicles; e, gland of third eyelid; f, branch of ventral palpebral artery; g, orbital fascia (muscular fasciae of endorbit). (From Moore CP: Diseases of the eyelids, conjunctiva, and third eyelid. *In* Bojrab MJ [ed]: *Disease Mechanisms in Small Animal Surgery.* Lea & Febiger, Philadelphia, in press.)

PATHOPHYSIOLOGY—SURGICAL IMPLICATIONS

Because of the contribution of the third eyelid to production and distribution of preocular tear fluid, every effort *must* be made to preserve its integrity. The rigid, tapered margin of the third eyelid provides a unique mechanism for effectively removing debris from the cornea. Furthermore, because the third eyelid occupies a substantial space between the ventromedial aspect of the globe and the medial canthal tissues, removal of the third eyelid in small animals creates a space that may harbor debris and microorganisms and predispose the eye to severe surface disease. For these reasons, if the third eyelid is removed, chronic keratoconjunctivitis with or without keratoconjunctivitis sicca often results. Careful repair and preservation of the third eyelid are important.

CONGENITAL/DEVELOPMENTAL DISORDERS

Cartilage Eversion

In animals with cartilage eversion, defective cartilage allows the third eyelid to roll toward or, more commonly, away from the globe. A predisposition is noted in large canine breeds (e.g., Great Danes, Saint Bernards, Newfoundlands, and German shorthaired pointers).[14, 20] Clinical problems are associated with chronic irritation of exposed tissue, poor third-eyelid function, and a cosmetically unacceptable appearance.

Treatment is removal of the scrolled portion of the cartilage from the posterior side while the anterior conjunctival surface, the leading margin, and the gland are left intact. Using mosquito forceps to stabilize the third eyelid margin, the posterior surface is exposed and a number 15 blade is used to incise the conjunctiva along one side of the everted cartilage. Small tissue scissors are used to tunnel under the conjunctiva to free

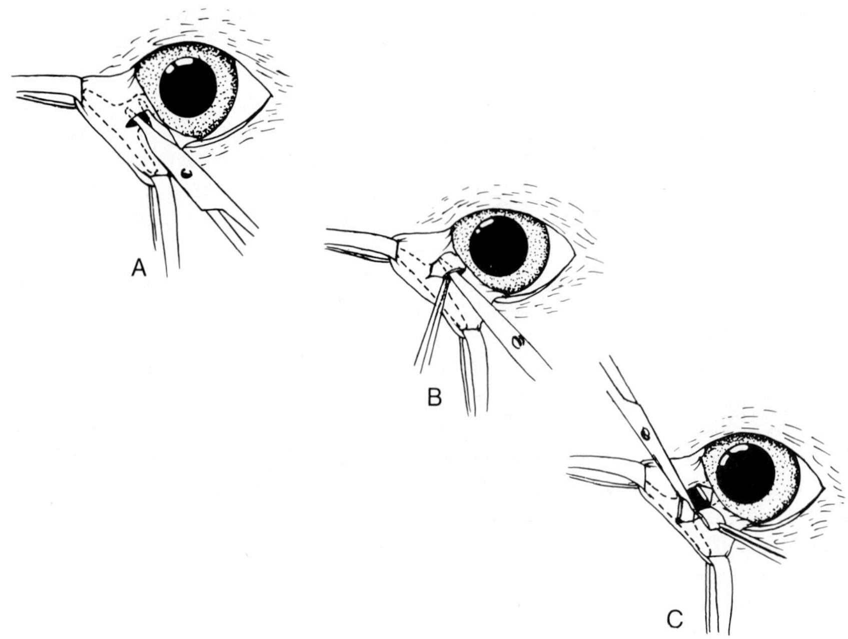

FIGURE 85–2. Cartilage eversion surgery. *A*, After the third eyelid is retracted, the posterior third eyelid conjunctiva is incised with a scalpel blade and the posterior conjunctiva is dissected free from the cartilage with small tissue scissors (e.g., conjunctival scissors or Stevens tenotomy scissors). *B*, Scissors are used to bluntly dissect between the cartilage and the anterior conjunctiva. *C*, The cartilage is cut with scissors at two locations: under the scrolled portion near its base (without removing glandular tissue) and at the junction of the stem and wings. (Redrawn from Bromberg N: Lacrimal apparatus and nictitating membrane. *In* Bojrab MJ [ed]: *Current Techniques in Veterinary Surgery*. 2nd ed. Lea & Febiger, Philadelphia, 1983.)

it from the cartilage and to expose its posterior surface (Fig. 85–2). The affected cartilage is bluntly dissected from the anterior third-eyelid conjunctiva.

The scissors are retracted and reinserted with one blade under the cartilage while the other blade is left on the posterior side of the cartilage. The cartilage is incised with scissors near its base, and the cut stem is grasped with thumb forceps and reflected. The scissors are placed at the junction of the stem and the wings of the cartilage, and the defective portion is cut and removed. Care is taken to remove only the defective portion of the cartilage. After surgery, an immediate resolution of the eversion is achieved. No suturing is needed, and topical antibiotics are administered postoperatively to prevent secondary bacterial infection.

Protrusion (Prolapse) of the Third-Eyelid Gland

Third-eyelid gland protrusion or prolapse (also referred to as "haws" or "cherry eye") is seen in puppies and dogs usually less than 1 year of age. Because a breed predisposition is noted in beagles, American cocker spaniels, Boston terriers, poodles, and brachycephalic breeds,[20] a genetic anatomical defect is suspected. However, a specific abnormality has not been demonstrated.

The third-eyelid gland, which is normally hidden from view, protrudes above the free border of the membrane and typically becomes swollen and inflamed. Clinical problems associated with gland prolapse include ocular discharge, conjunctivitis, and the cosmetic concern of a pink mass being visible in the medial canthus. Definitive treatment of third-eyelid gland prolapses is surgical. Manual replacement of a prolapsed gland followed by medical therapy, consisting of topical antibiotic-corticosteroid, may be attempted in puppies. However, this usually produces a temporary response only. Replacement is the definitive treatment.

Replacement Techniques

A number of replacement techniques have been described.[1, 2, 7, 10, 15, 16] Most involve inverting the gland and using suture to anchor the gland to adjacent fibrous tissue.[1, 2, 7, 10] Other techniques stimulate conjunctival fibrosis to maintain the gland in its proper position.[15, 16] Less invasive techniques are generally simpler to perform but may be less likely to accomplish permanent replacement, particularly in cases of chronic gland prolapses.

Techniques for correction of third-eyelid gland prolapse have been described by several authors. The Blogg technique was the first described and involves dissecting the gland free and suturing it to the ventral epibulbar fascia.[2] Gross modified the technique by anchoring the gland to the ventral equatorial sclera.[7] Albert used a similar technique in cats but further modified it by anchoring the gland to the ventral oblique muscle.[1] Each of these procedures involves dissection on the posterior aspect of the third eyelid, which is believed to be the area where excretory ducts of the glands are located. The most serious potential complication of these procedures is globe penetration.

To avoid the possibility of altering the gland's excretory duct system or penetrating the globe, Kaswan and Martin developed a technique that is primarily performed on the anterior side of the third eyelid.[10] This technique also avoids postoperative contact of suture material with the cornea. An incision is made in the ventral fornix anterior to the base of the third eyelid. A 3-0 monofilament suture is placed through the periosteum of the orbital rim and passed through the base of the third eyelid into the gland. The needle leaves the dorsal surface of the prolapsed gland and is redirected horizontally through the same exit hole. It is passed through to the opposite side of the exposed gland and is then redirected ventrally through the second exit hole. The needle is directed through the base of the third eyelid and is pulled out the initial incision (Fig. 85–3). The 3-0 suture is tied and buried, and the conjunctival incision is closed with 6-0 absorbable suture.

Slatter recommends modifying Kaswan's technique by extending dissection ventrally to expose the zygomatic periosteum after making the initial incision.[22] This more extensive exposure allows precise placement of the nylon anchor suture into the periosteum. Precise suturing in this procedure produces a highly reliable method of gland prolapse repair.[22]

Because previously described techniques are moderately invasive and may result in immobility of the third eyelid, I have developed two imbrication techniques that are minimally invasive to replace prolapsed third-eyelid gland.[15, 16] The first technique is a modified purse-string suture technique used for repair of acute third-eyelid gland prolapses in puppies.[16] A 7-0 absorbable braided suture (polyglactin 910 or polyglycolic acid) with a small cutting needle is used. After the third eyelid is extended to expose the bulbar side and the prolapsed gland, a number 15 Bard-Parker blade is used to mildly scarify the conjunctiva overlying the prolapsed gland. After the repair, this stimulates symblepharon and thereby fixes the gland in position.

The needle with swaged-on suture is passed into the ventral fornix conjunctiva below the center of the gland (Fig. 85–4). After a 4-mm bite is taken, the needle is pulled through the conjunctiva, reversed, and reinserted into the conjunctiva just under the leading edge of the third eyelid. The second bite is taken parallel the margin of the third eyelid and incorporates 6 mm of conjunctiva. The needle is pulled through, reversed again, and reinserted into the ventral fornix. It is directed into the conjunctiva for 4 mm toward the original point of entry. The initial entry point and the final exit point of the suture allow the knot to be tied so that it rests in the ventral fornix. To replace the prolapsed gland, a cotton-tipped applicator is used to apply gentle downward pressure, and the suture is drawn together.

When the prolapse has been subacute or chronic or is a recurring problem, conjunctivectomy with Lembert imbrication may be performed to stimulate more extensive fibrosis over the gland.[15] Similar to the purse-string imbrication technique, this procedure is performed on the bulbar side of the third eyelid. Over the central portion of the gland prolapse, an elliptical section of conjunctiva (3 mm wide at its widest point) is removed. The remaining conjunctiva overlying the gland is freed by bluntly undermining in both directions (i.e., toward the free margin of the third eyelid and toward the ventral fornix). Two or three subconjunctival Lembert sutures are preplaced, gentle pressure is placed on the exposed gland to replace it to its normal position, and the sutures are tied (Fig. 85–5). If the sutures are strategically placed, the knots lie just under the conjunctiva.

With either of these inverting techniques, an external anchor suture may be placed through the base of the third eyelid to hold the third eyelid in normal position while the postoperative inflammation resolves and the conjunctiva heals (Fig. 85–6). After surgery with any of the techniques described here, topical antibiotics are applied for 7 to 10 days to prevent secondary bacterial infection. Fluorescein stain application to the operated eye is recommended on postoperative day 1 and at any time during the immediate postoperative period if ocular pain becomes evident.

Encircling Third Eyelid

Dorsal remnants of the third eyelid may be noted as curvilinear pigmented lesions on the upper bulbar con-

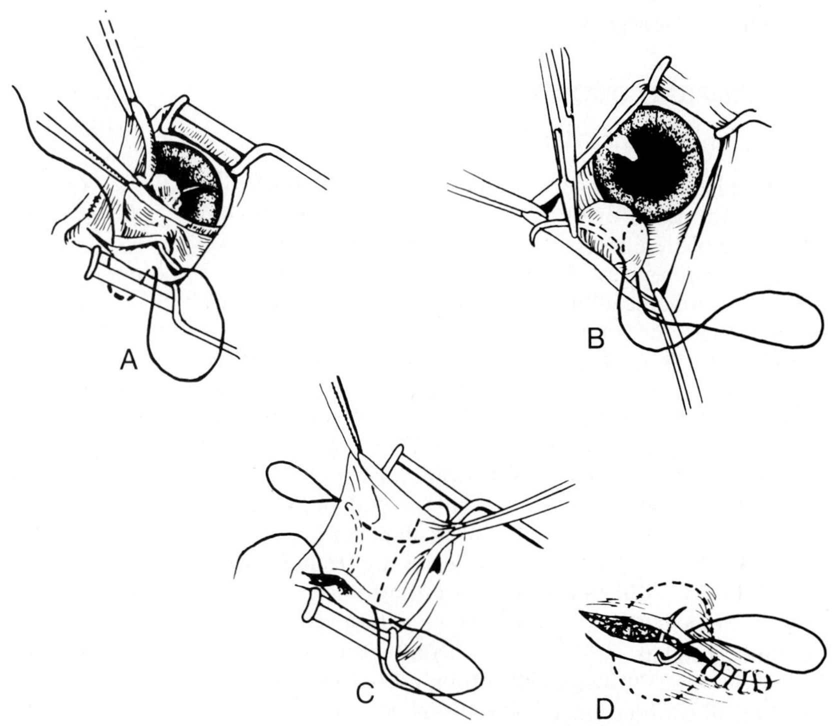

FIGURE 85–3. Kaswan technique of repair of third-eyelid gland prolapse. *A,* After incision of the anterior fornix conjunctiva and blunt dissection exposing the rim of the orbit, a 3-0 monofilament suture is placed through fascia attached to the periosteal rim of the orbit then passed through the third eyelid, exiting through the prolapsed gland. *B,* A horizontal bite is taken through the most prominent portion of the prolapsed gland. *C,* The suture is passed back ventrally through the gland and exits through the conjunctival incision. *D,* The 3-0 suture is tied, and the conjunctival incision is sutured with 6-0 absorbable suture. (Redrawn from Kaswan RL, Martin CL: Surgical correction of third eyelid prolapse in dogs. *J Am Vet Med Assoc 186*:83, 1985.)

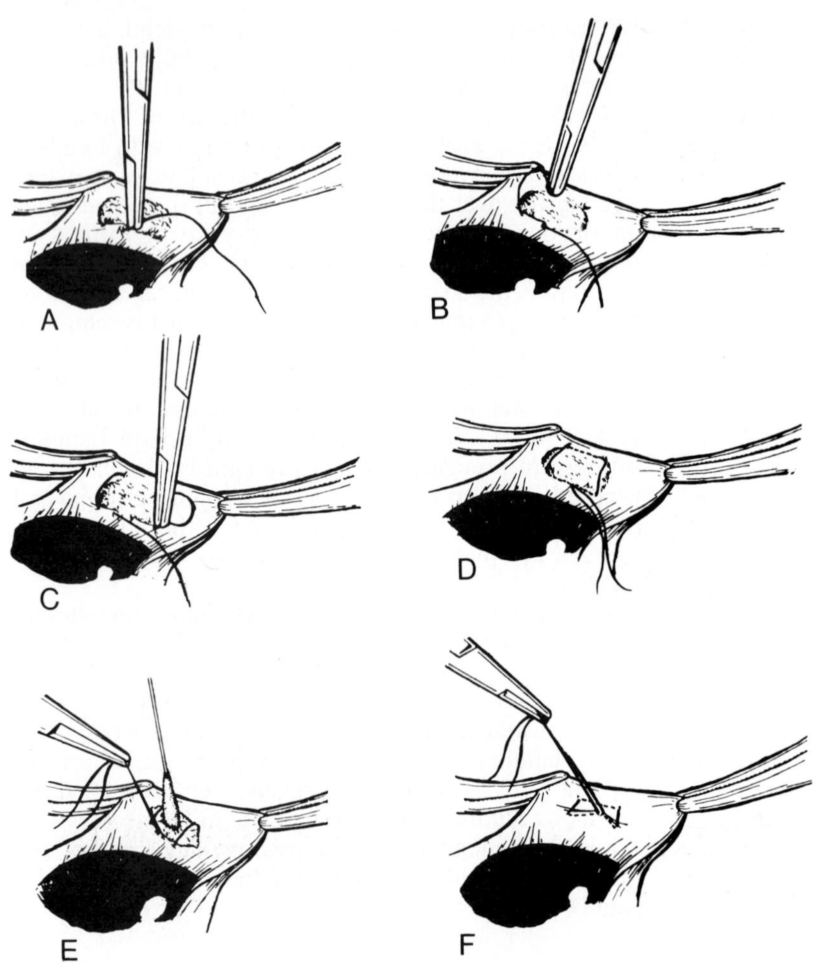

FIGURE 85–4. Moore purse-string technique. *A*, Conjunctiva over the surface of the prolapsed gland is scarified. A microcutting suture needle (attached to 7-0 braided absorbable material) is passed into the conjunctiva below the center of the gland. *B*, The needle is pulled through as illustrated and placed into the conjunctiva dorsal to the gland. This second bite should encompass approximately 6 mm of conjunctiva as it is passed parallel to the third-eyelid margin. *C*, A third bite of conjunctiva is taken in a reverse manner from the initial bite. The needle is passed ventral to the gland and is directed toward the original point of entry. *D*, Proper placement of suture will allow it to be drawn together easily and the knot to be tied so that it rests in the ventral fornix. *E*, Before tying the suture, a cotton-tipped applicator is used to replace the prolapsed gland. *F*, As the suture is tightened, the cotton-tipped applicator is withdrawn. (Redrawn from Moore CP: Imbrication technique for replacement of third eyelid gland. *In* Bojrab MJ [ed]: *Current Techniques in Veterinary Surgery*. 3rd ed. Lea & Febiger, Philadelphia, 1989.)

junctiva. These often occur as incidental findings in dogs, particularly in American cocker spaniels, and do not require treatment.

INFLAMMATORY DISORDERS

Follicular Conjunctivitis

Lymphoid follicles are normally present on the bulbar side of the third eyelid. The presence and hypertrophy of lymphoid elements on the anterior side of the third eyelid occur as a nonspecific ocular surface response to chronic antigenic stimulation. In cats, follicular conjunctivitis occurs with chronic chlamydial infections.[4]

Mucoid discharge, mild epiphora, and a red cobblestone appearance of the anterior surface of the third eyelid are characteristic findings. Treatment is aimed at removing stimulating antigens—for example, by eliminating chronic bacterial infections, environmental irritants (e.g., dust, pollen), or chlamydial organisms (in cats). Because nonspecific follicular conjunctivitis is often present in dogs, corticosteroids are frequently used to shrink the follicles. Removing the follicles by physically abrading the affected surface with gauze or with a chemical agent (i.e., an astringent such as iodine or copper sulfate) has been previously recommended.[13] Chemical cautery apparently stimulates an acute inflammation that results in regression of the follicles. Because cauterizing agents cause severe, acute chemical conjunctivitis, they are *not* recommended.

Plasmacytic Infiltrates

In German shepherds, thickened, hyperemic third eyelids with bilateral third-eyelid protrusions occur as a result of diffuse plasmacytic infiltration of the conjunctiva (plasmacytoma). The cytological features of this disease are identical to those of cases of chronic immune-mediated keratoconjunctivitis syndrome. Therefore, plasmacytic infiltration of the third eyelid is considered a variant form of this disease.

Plasmacytic infiltrates of the third eyelid is a particularly challenging disease to treat. Variable responses result from local and systemic corticosteroids used either separately or in combination. Systemic chemotherapeutic agents may reduce clinical severity but pose a potential for systemic toxicity.[5] Preliminary indications are that topical 1 to 2 per cent cyclosporine in oil is promising as a safe and effective treatment.[9]

Pseudotumors

Proliferative granulomatous lesions of the third eyelids in dogs may accompany similar lesions of the eyelids, conjunctiva, or cornea or appear as isolated lesions involving only the third eyelid. These appear as smooth,

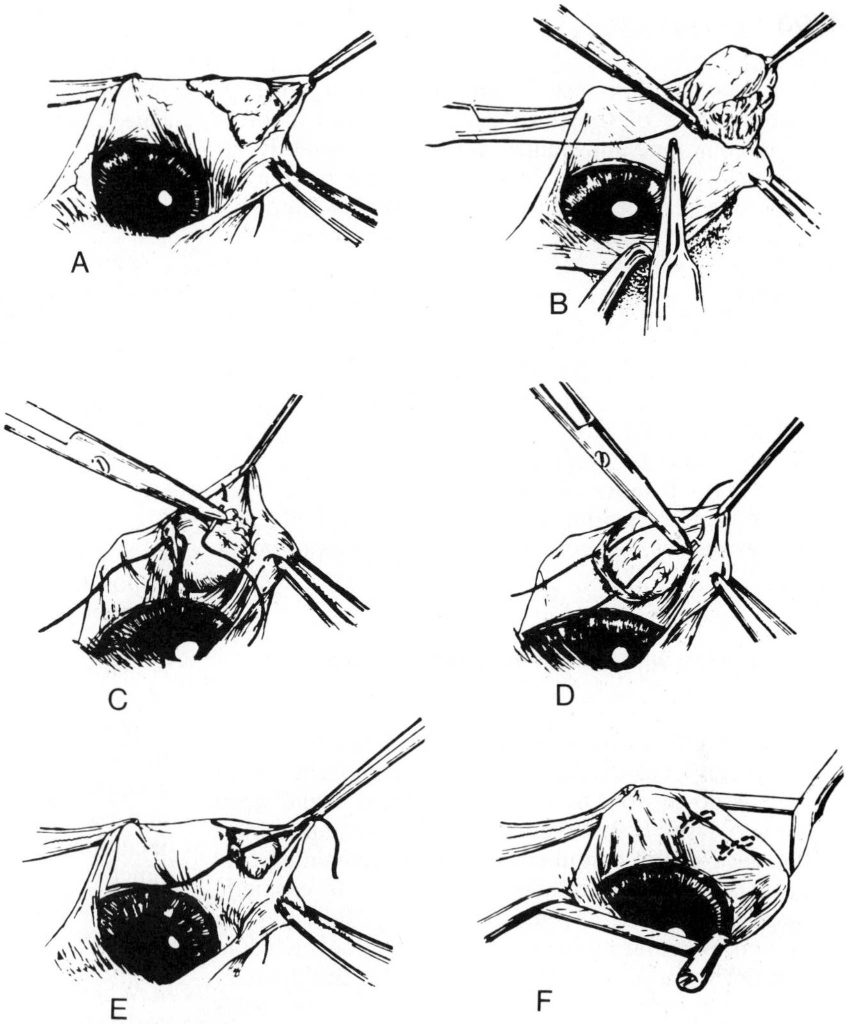

A B C D E F

FIGURE 85–5. Moore-Lembert suture technique. *A,* An elliptical incision is made in the conjunctiva over the prolapsed gland, and a segment of conjunctiva (3 mm at widest point) is removed. The conjunctiva is bluntly dissected, exposing subconjunctival connective tissues dorsal and ventral to the gland. *B,* A needle with attached 7-0 braided absorbable suture is passed deep to the gland and is anchored into the epibulbar connective tissue. *C,* The suture is then passed over the gland, and the needle is placed into the subconjunctival tissue between the gland and the free margin of the third eyelid. *D,* The initial suture is left untied, and a second suture is placed alongside but on the opposite side of the gland. *E,* As each suture is drawn down and tied, the underlying gland should be divided approximately into thirds by the overlying sutures. Gentle downward pressure is exerted on the gland as the sutures are tied. *F,* The knots are trimmed closely and should lie under the conjunctiva. (Redrawn from Moore CP: Alternative technique for prolapsed gland of the third eyelid. *In* Bojrab MJ [ed]: *Current Techniques in Veterinary Surgery.* 2nd ed. Lea & Febiger, Philadelphia, 1983.)

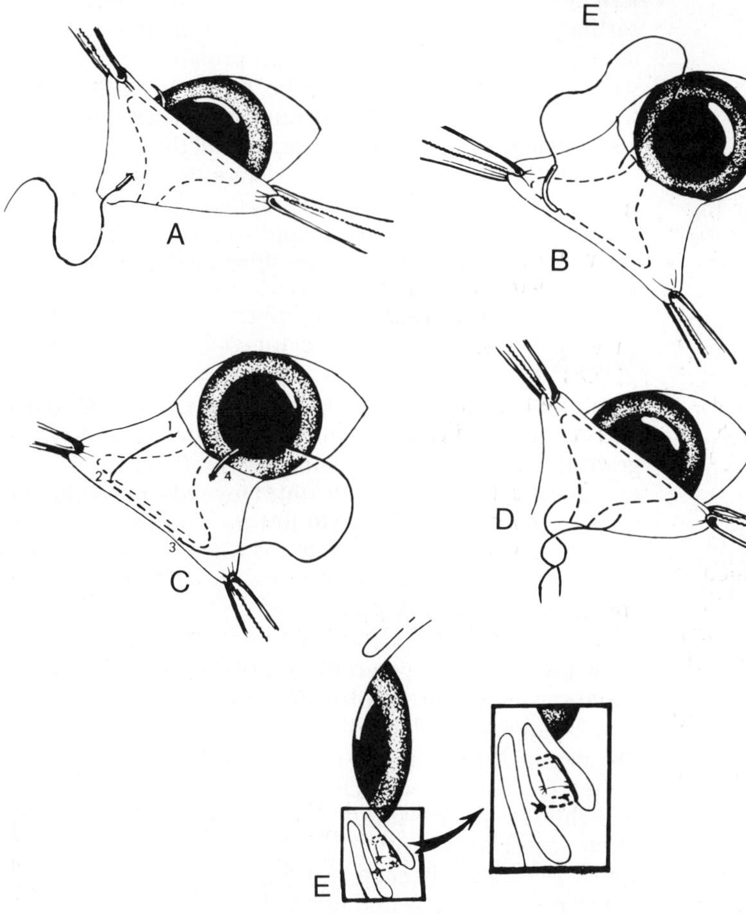

A B 1 2 3 4 C D E

FIGURE 85–6. Anchor suture for third-eyelid stabilization. *A,* The needle is passed through the base of the third eyelid and retrieved from the posterior side. *B,* The needle is inserted horizontally into the posterior conjunctiva dorsal to the repaired prolapse. *C,* The needle is then removed and redirected through the base of the third eyelid as shown. *D,* The suture is secured and tied in the anterior ventral fornix. This anchor suture may be used to reinforce either the purse-string (see Fig. 85–4) or the Lembert suture (see Fig. 85–5) techniques. *E,* Cross-sectional view of the third eyelid after placement of anchor suture over the purse-string repair.

raised, usually pink lesions on the leading edge or anterior surface of the third eyelid. Bilateral involvement is common, and collies are more frequently affected than other canine breeds. (See the section on proliferative keratoconjunctivitis in Chapters 83 and 86.)

NEOPLASIA

Ocular squamous cell carcinoma is the most common tumor of the third eyelid. Most third-eyelid neoplasms, including squamous cell tumors, arise from the conjunctiva. The clinical features and approaches to therapy are similar to those of other conjunctival neoplasms (see Chapter 83). Tumors of the third eyelid that do not originate from the conjunctiva include third-eyelid gland adenocarcinomas, fibrosarcomas, and lymphosarcomas.[3, 17, 23]

Local Excision with Partial Removal of Third Eyelid

If the neoplasm involves only the leading edge of the third eyelid, local excision may be accomplished with curved tissue scissors by incising the third eyelid deep to the neoplastic tissue. Removal of the mass and repair of the third eyelid conjunctiva over the remaining cartilage and gland usually allow functional and cosmetic healing of the third eyelid. If necessary, this may be facilitated by undermining the conjunctiva on each side of the third eyelid and then suturing the conjunctival margins in a continuous pattern with 6-0 or 7-0 polyglactin 910.

Total Excision with Reconstruction of Third Eyelid

Extensive neoplastic invasion constitutes one of the rare indications for complete surgical removal of the third eyelid. The neoplasm is exteriorized, curved scissors are placed at the base of the third eyelid, and the tissue is excised. To replace lost tissue, a buccal mucosal graft may be constructed.[12] This procedure involves placing a chalazion clamp on the labial mucosa of the upper lip, removing a mucosal strip (approximately 20 × 5 mm), and suturing the graft to the conjunctiva with 7-0 absorbable suture at the base of the amputated third eyelid.[12] A similar technique may also be used for traumatic avulsions or iatrogenic causes (prior removal) of the third eyelid.[11] Kuhns reported a case in which bilateral buccal mucosal grafts simulated true third eyelids and remained functional (i.e., protecting the ventral cornea and conserving the preocular tear film) for 2 years after surgery.[11] Slatter reports a survival rate of approximately 65 per cent using the mucosal grafting technique.[22]

Ancillary Therapy

Ancillary oncotherapy (e.g., radiation, cryosurgery, or chemotherapy) is an adjunct to partial or total removal of the third eyelid in cases of extensive neoplasia (see Chapters 83 and 158).

TRAUMA

Punctures and Lacerations

Third-eyelid lacerations are most commonly encountered as a result of claw punctures due to cat-scratch injuries. Small superficial punctures or partial-thickness lacerations involving only mucosa do not require suturing. With such lesions, irrigation with saline or 1:50 betadine:saline solution[19] and topical antibiotic application are usually sufficient.

Linear lacerations, particularly those involving the third-eyelid margin, are sutured. Repair of marginal tears or lost tissue from the anterior surface of the third eyelid may be performed by first undermining then apposing the anterior conjunctiva with 6-0 or 7-0 absorbable suture. The knot is tied on the anterior side of the third eyelid. A conjunctival pedicle graft may be constructed when extensive avulsion of the third-eyelid mucosa has occurred.

If the cartilage is torn, it is generally not trimmed unless jagged edges are present. Repairing lacerated conjunctiva over torn cartilage usually allows functional and cosmetic healing of the third eyelid. This may be facilitated by undermining the external (palpebral) conjunctiva and apposing the conjunctival margins. The conjunctival margins are minimally débrided and sutured on the anterior side in a continuous pattern with 6-0 polyglactin 910.

When linear lacerations involving the third-eyelid cartilage occur parallel to the free margin and very near it, a primary repair may not be possible and a small strip of marginal tissue may be removed with curved tissue scissors. With surgical removal of lacerated marginal tissue, it is extremely important that the leading edge of the third eyelid be left smooth. After surgical repair of injured third eyelids, systemic antibiotics are administered for 5 to 7 days and topical antibiotics are applied for 10 to 14 days. In third-eyelid trauma, removal of the third eyelid is avoided.

Avulsion

In unusual trauma (e.g., avulsion or irreparable damage to third eyelid), removal may be necessary. A grafting procedure (e.g., mucosal graft as used after amputation of a neoplastic third eyelid) may also be used to replace a third eyelid lost as a result of trauma.

PROMINENT THIRD EYELID

Congenital and acquired diseases or conformational variations may cause protruding, conspicuous third eyelids. Prominence of the third eyelid due to extension of the membrane over the globe without concurrent lesions, e.g., a prolapsed mass, gland, or cartilage eversion is identified as *protrusion.* Protruding third eyelids are often associated with breed-related enophthalmos, which is frequently seen in larger canine breeds (e.g., Doberman pinschers and Great Danes).

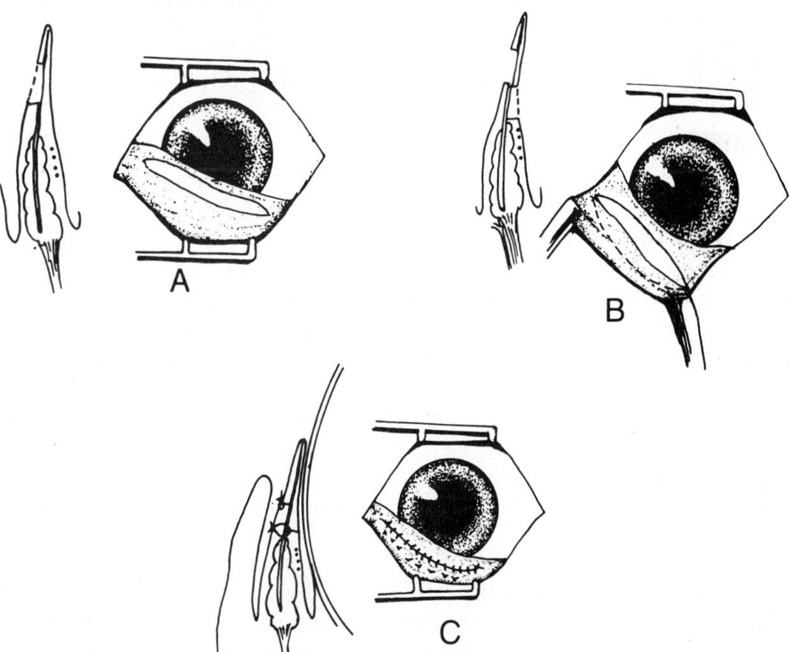

FIGURE 85–7. Third-eyelid shortening procedure. An elliptical incision is made on the anterior surface of the third eyelid. *A,* Anterior conjunctiva and a portion of the cartilage are removed. *B,* On the posterior side of the third eyelid, just ventral to the level of the initial (anterior) incision, a second elliptical segment of conjunctiva without cartilage is incised and removed. *C,* The resulting wounds are repaired at two different levels with interrupted sutures. For each row of sutures, note that the knots are tied on the anterior side of the third eyelid. (Redrawn from Peruccio C: Surgical correction of prominent third eyelid in the dog. *Calif Vet 35*:24, 1981.)

Changes in orbital volume can have a profound effect on third-eyelid position. Because a normal globe-orbit relationship is necessary for normal third-eyelid position, an anterior shift in globe position from an increase in orbital contents (e.g., neoplasms, abscesses, or hematomas) or, conversely, a posterior shift from reduction of orbital contents (e.g., atrophy of orbital fat, microphthalmia, phthisis bulbi) causes third-eyelid protrusion.

Systemic diseases that cause dehydration or emaciation with subsequent loss of retrobulbar tissue volume may cause third-eyelid protrusion. Animals with malaise or lethargy associated with generalized illnesses often exhibit prominent third eyelids. Tetanus causes contraction of extraocular muscles with retraction of the globe and third-eyelid protrusion. Ocular pain may also stimulate retraction of the eye with third-eyelid prominence.

Sympathetic denervation of periocular tissues is associated with prominence of the third eyelid(s). Horner's syndrome may be caused by a number of diseases involving the head, neck, or anterior thorax.[21] Loss of sympathetic innervation to the orbit also results in miosis, ptosis (upper eyelid drooping), and enophthalmos on the affected side. In cats, a syndrome of bilateral third-eyelid protrusion (haws syndrome) is associated with loss of sympathetic tone in both third eyelids.[21]

In breeds with prominent or nonpigmented third eyelids, owners may find the appearance aesthetically displeasing and request correction. A technique that can be used to remedy this cosmetic problem involves excision of two linear strips from the third eyelid, from each of the anterior and posterior surfaces.[18] Incisions are sutured as illustrated in Figure 85–7. This procedure results in a staggered but full-thickness resection of the third eyelid. The third eyelid retains its function, but the ventral-dorsal dimension of the third eyelid is reduced and thus the free margin becomes less visible.

References

1. Albert RA, et al: Surgical correction of everted third eyelid in two cats. *J Am Vet Med Assoc 180*:763, 1982.
2. Blogg JR: Surgical replacement of a prolapsed gland of the third eyelid ("cherry eye"), a new technique. *Aust Vet J 9*:75, 1979.
3. Buyukmihci N: Fibrosarcoma of the nictitating membrane in a cat. *J Am Vet Med Assoc 167*:934, 1975.
4. Cello RM: Clues to differential diagnosis of feline respiratory infections. *J Am Vet Med Assoc 158*:968, 1971.
5. Collins BK: Systemic toxicity of azathioprine therapy for the eyes. Resident's Forum. 17th Annual Scientific Program of the American College of Veterinary Ophthalmology, New Orleans, LA, Nov, 1986.
6. Constantinescu GM, McClure RC: Anatomy of the orbital fasciae and the third eyelid in the dog. *Am J Vet Res 51*:260, 1990.
7. Gross S: Effectiveness of a modification of the Blogg technique for replacing the prolapsed gland of the canine third eyelid. *Trans Am Coll Vet Ophthalmol 14*:28, 1983.
8. Helper LC, et al: Surgical induction of keratoconjunctivitis sicca in the dog. *J Am Vet Med Assoc 165*:172, 1974.
9. Kaswan RL: Personal communication, 1990.
10. Kaswan RL, Martin CL: Surgical correction of third eyelid prolapse in dogs. *J Am Vet Med Assoc 186*:83, 1985.
11. Kuhns EL: Oral mucosal grafts for membrana nictitans replacement. *Mod Vet Pract 58*:768, 1977.
12. Kuhns EL: Replacement of canine membrana nictitans with a lip graft. *Mod Vet Pract 62*:773, 1981.
13. Magrane WG: *Canine Ophthalmology*. 3rd ed. Lea & Febiger, Philadelphia, 1977.
14. Martin CL, Leach R: Everted membrana nictitans in German shorthaired pointers. *J Am Vet Med Assoc 157*:1229, 1970.
15. Moore CP: Alternative technique for prolapsed gland of the third eyelid. *In* Bojrab MJ (ed): *Current Techniques in Veterinary Surgery*. 2nd ed. Lea & Febiger, Philadelphia, 1983, pp 52–53.
16. Moore CP: Imbrication technique for replacement of prolapsed third eyelid gland. *In* Bojrab MJ (ed): *Current Techniques in Veterinary Surgery*. 3rd ed. Lea & Febiger, Philadelphia, 1989, pp 126–128.
17. Moore CP: Diseases of the eyelids, conjunctiva, and third eyelid. *In* Bojrab MJ (ed): *Disease Mechanisms in Small Animal Surgery*. Lea & Febiger, Philadelphia, in press.
18. Peruccio C: Surgical correction of prominent third eyelid in the dog. *Calif Vet 35*:24, 1981.
19. Roberts SM, et al: Antibacterial activity of dilute povidone-iodine solutions used for ocular surface disinfection in dogs. *Am J Vet Res 47*:1207, 1986.
20. Rubin LF: *Inherited Eye Diseases in Purebred Dogs*. Williams & Wilkins, Baltimore, 1989.
21. Slatter D: *Fundamentals of Veterinary Ophthalmology*. 2nd Ed. W.B. Saunders, Philadelphia, 1990.
22. Slatter D: Personal communication, 1990.
23. Wilcock B, Peiffer R: Adenocarcinoma of the gland of the third eyelid in seven dogs. *J Am Vet Med Assoc* 193:1549–1550, 1988.

CHAPTER

86

Cornea and Sclera

Douglas Slatter and Nils Håkanson

Corneal structure and function are uniquely specialized. Knowledge of these features and normal corneal reactions to disease is necessary for acceptable surgical results. For a detailed discussion, the reader is referred to standard texts.[1, 4, 25, 49]

ANATOMY[36, 37, 42]

The cornea is the transparent anterior window in the fibrous coat of the eye, the sclera is the posterior opaque part, and the limbus is the transition zone between. The canine cornea is 0.61±0.01 mm thick centrally and 0.67±0.01 mm peripherally. In older dogs, corneal thickness may increase to 0.9 mm owing to failing endothelial cell function.[20] The feline cornea is 0.57 ±0.04 mm thick in the center.[9]

The canine sclera is 1 mm thick in the ciliary region, 0.3 mm at the equator, and 0.55 mm near the optic disc. The feline sclera is 1.6 mm thick at the scleral venous plexus and otherwise similar to canine sclera.[43] The prominent intrascleral venous plexus is located 2 mm behind the limbus in dogs.[3]

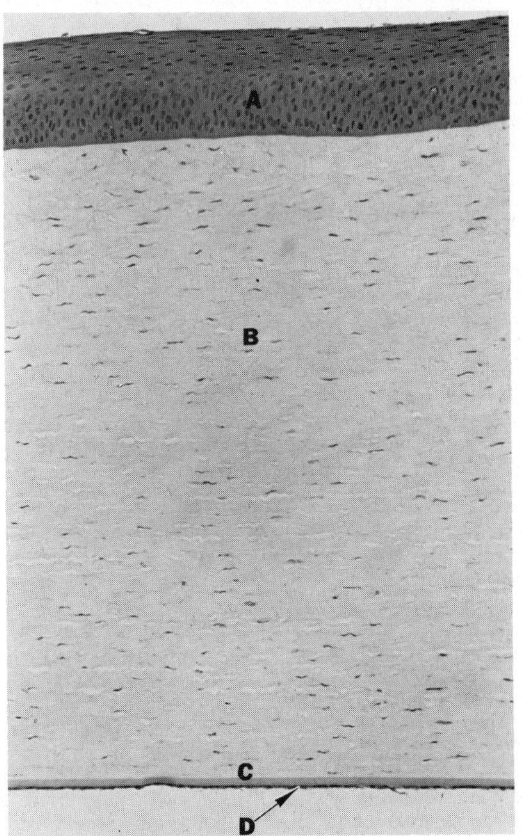

FIGURE 86–1. Microscopic structure of the cornea. (A, Epithelium; B, stroma; C, Descemet membrane; D, endothelium.)

The cornea has five layers (Fig. 86–1): the precorneal tear film, epithelium and basement membrane, stroma, Descemet membrane (basement membrane of the endothelium), and endothelium. The precorneal tear film covers the cornea and conjunctiva to a depth of 7 μm. Its three layers differ in composition and function (Fig. 86–2). The outer superficial layer is composed of oily materials and phospholipids from the tarsal glands and serves two functions: (1) to increase surface tension and bind the precorneal tear film to the corneal surface and (2) to limit evaporation of the aqueous layer beneath. The middle, or aqueous, layer is mostly water, derived from the lacrimal and nictitans glands. It has the following functions:

1. It flushes foreign material from the conjunctival sac.
2. It lubricates passage of the lids and third eyelid over the epithelium.
3. It serves as a medium for passage of oxygen, inflammatory cells, and immunoglobulins A and G to the cornea.
4. It provides a smooth corneal surface for greatest optical efficiency.

The inner, or mucoid, layer consists of mucoproteins derived from conjunctival goblet cells, which bind the hydrophilic, lipophobic aqueous layer to the hydrophobic, lipophilic corneal epithelium with bipolar mucoprotein molecules.

The corneal epithelium is composed of simple stratified squamous and nonkeratinized cells, attached to its basement membrane by hemidesmosomes. As the basal cells near the basement membrane undergo mitosis, daughter cells are forced toward the surface and lose their organelles. Fibrocytes, keratocytes, collagen, and ground substance account for about 90 per cent of the corneal stromal substance.[24] Collagen fibrils in it are arranged in parallel, forming interlacing sheets or lamellae. The regular spacing of stromal collagen fibrils maintains corneal transparency and distinguishes the stroma from collagen in scar tissue and sclera (Figs. 86–3 and 86–4). Stromal keratocytes can synthesize collagen, glycosaminoglycans, and mucoprotein of the ground substance.

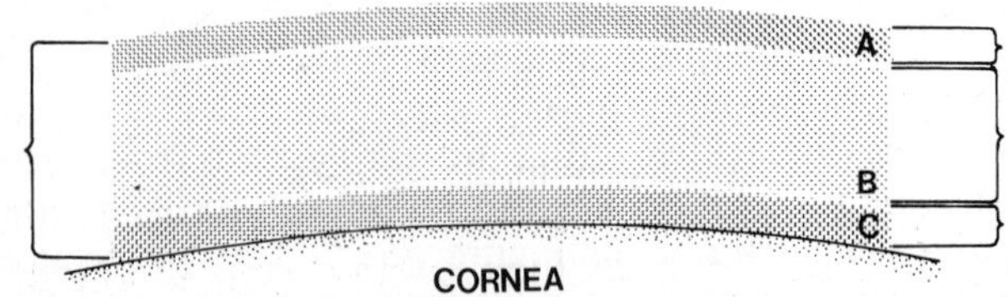

FIGURE 86–2. Precorneal tear film. (A, Superficial lipid layer; B aqueous layer; C, inner mucoid layer.)

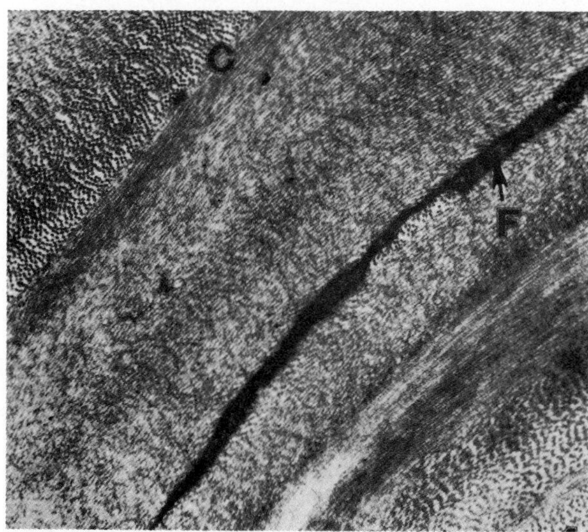

FIGURE 86–3. Interlacing lamellae cross at right angles in a dog's cornea. The lamellae consist of regularly spaced collagen fibrils (C) separated by ground substance. A process of a keratocyte (F) is present between lamellae. (Reprinted with permission from Shively JN, Epling GP: Fine structure of the canine eye: Cornea. *Am J Vet Res 31*:713, 1970.)

The Descemet membrane (see Fig. 86–1) is the basement membrane of the endothelium and is continuously laid down by the endothelium throughout life. It is composed of fine collagen fibrils and is elastic; if it is ruptured, the ends curl (Fig. 86–5). In a descemetocele in which the overlying stroma has been destroyed, the Descemet membrane often protrudes dramatically because of this elasticity. After rupture, the endothelium secretes a new membrane to fill small defects. The Descemet membrane does not stain with fluorescein, and its presence as a dark, transparent bulge in the center of a corneal ulcer or wound signals impending rupture.

The endothelium is one cell thick and posterior and adjacent to the Descemet membrane (see Fig. 86–1). It has a limited ability to replicate depending on age and species,[20] and when endothelium is lost, the defect is replaced by migration of existing adjacent cells. With advancing age, the number of endothelial cells decreases.[20] The endothelium is important to a surgeon; it is extremely susceptible to osmotic and traumatic damage during surgery.[1] Loss of corneal endothelium beyond the ability of adjacent cells to compensate or replicate causes permanent corneal edema and opacity.[1]

The sclera consists of an outer episclera, the sclera proper, and the lamina fusca adjacent to the choroid (Fig. 86–6). The episclera is a dense, highly vascular connective tissue that binds the Tenon capsule to the sclera. Near the limbus, the episclera blends with the Tenon capsule and subconjunctival connective tissue. The sclera is composed of collagen fibers and fibroblasts. The collagen fibers vary in diameter and orientation in different parts of the globe. Scleral collagen fibrils differ from corneal fibrils in their considerable variation in diameter and absence of regular fixed spacing between them.

The sclera is perforated posteriorly by the optic nerve. The short posterior ciliary nerves and arteries pierce the sclera around the optic nerve and enter the choroid. The long posterior ciliary nerves and arteries also enter near the optic nerve and extend forward horizontally within the sclera to the ciliary body. In dogs, these arteries carry most of the blood supply to the anterior

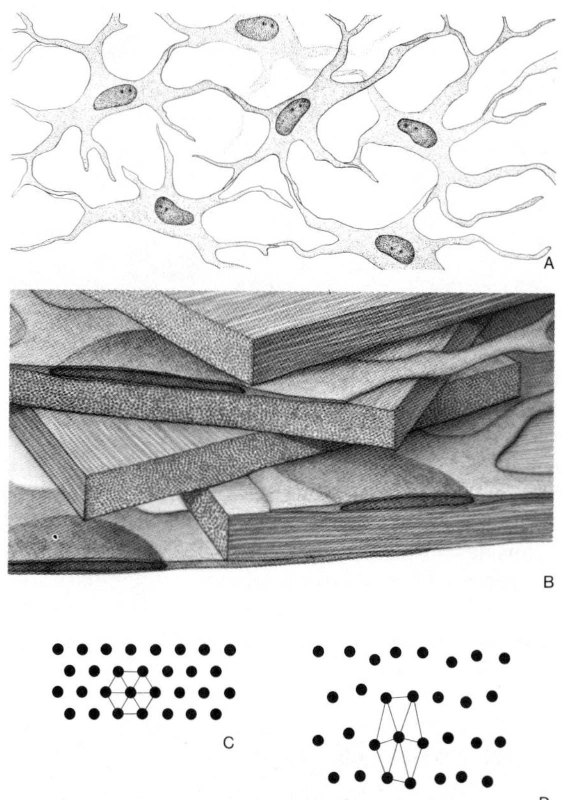

FIGURE 86–4. Summary diagram of the corneal stroma. *A,* Fibroblasts. This diagram shows six fibroblasts lying between the stromal lamellae. The cells are thin and flat, with long processes that contact fibroblast processes of other cells lying in the same plane. These cells were once believed to form a true syncytium, but electron microscopy has disproved this idea. There is almost always a 200-nm-wide intercellular space separating the cells. Unlike fibroblasts elsewhere, these cells occasionally join each other at a macula occludens.

B, Lamellae. The cornea is composed of a very orderly, dense fibrous connective tissue. Its collagen, which is a very stable protein having a half-life estimated at 100 days, forms many lamellae. The collagen fibrils within a lamella are parallel to each other and extend the full length of the cornea. Successive lamellae pass across the cornea at an angle to each other. Three fibroblasts are seen between the lamellae.

C, Diagram to show the theoretical orientation of the corneal collagen fibrils. Each of the fibrils is separated from its fellows by an equal distance. Maurice has explained the transparency of the cornea on the basis of this very exact equidistant separation. As a result of this arrangement, the stromal lamellae form a three-dimensional array of diffraction gratings. Scattered rays of light passing through such a system interact with each other in an organized way. resulting in the elimination of scattered light by destructive ir rference. The mucoproteins, glycoproteins, and other components of the ground substance are responsible for maintaining the proper position of the fibrils.

D, Orientation of the collagen fibrils in an opaque cornea. The diagram shows the orderly positions of the fibrils to have been disturbed. Because of this disarrangement, scattered light is not eliminated by destructive interference and the cornea becomes hazy. Edema fluid in the ground substance also produces clouding of the cornea by disturbing the interfibrillar distance.

(Reprinted with permission from Hogan MJ, et al: *Histology of the Human Eye.* W. B. Saunders, Philadelphia, 1971.)

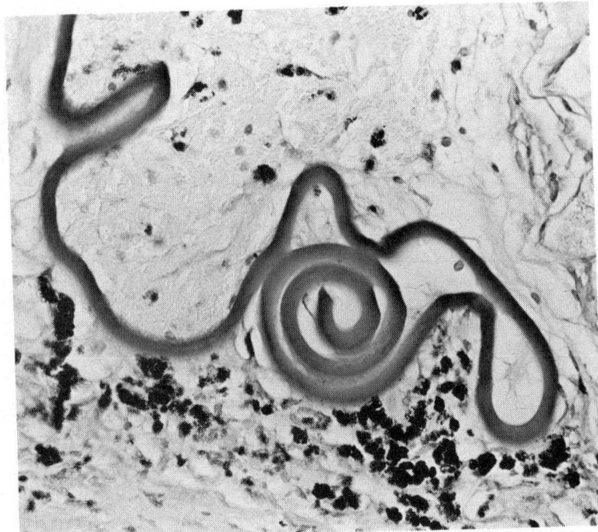

FIGURE 86–5. Retraction of Descemet's membrane after rupture. PAS stain.

segment,[25] a feature of considerable importance in prognosis after ocular prolapse when the anterior ciliary arteries are torn from their insertions with the extraocular muscles. The anterior ciliary arteries and vortex veins enter and leave the sclera over the ciliary body.

PHYSIOLOGY

The cornea is the most powerful refractive component of the eye. The cornea but not the sclera is transparent owing to the following features:

1. Lack of blood vessels and few stromal cells
2. Lack of pigment
3. Control of water content
4. A smooth optical surface provided by precorneal tear film
5. A high mucopolysaccharide content
6. Orderly arrangement of collagen fibrils of uniform diameter and spacing, which eliminates light scattering by destructive interference

Glucose metabolism is the most important source of energy. Two-thirds of the glucose is metabolized via the Embden-Meyerhof pathway and the Kreb cycle, and one-third via the hexose-monophosphate shunt.[37] The endothelium receives most of its oxygen from aqueous, whereas the rest of the avascular cornea receives oxygen mainly from the atmosphere via the precorneal tear film and from limbal and conjunctival capillaries (Fig. 86–7). The endothelium receives most of its oxygen from the aqueous, but atmospheric oxygen is the major source for the remainder of the cornea.

Water enters the cornea under the influence of intraocular pressure and the hydrophilic character of stromal collagen and mucopolysaccharides. Endothelial and epithelial barriers limit entry of water into the cornea. Water leaves by evaporation from the anterior corneal surface. The endothelium functions as an active energy-dependent pump, removing electrolytes and water from the corneal stroma.[33] The corneal state of relative dehydration is important to transparency.

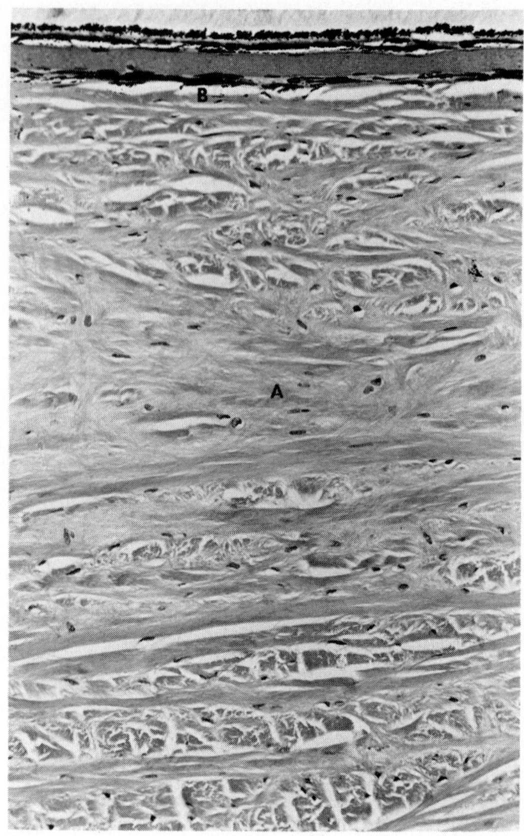

FIGURE 86–6. Layers of the canine sclera. *A*, Scleral stroma; *B*, lamina fusca.

Corneal transparency is affected by changes in the properties just described. Increased water content separates the corneal collagen lattice, causing opacity by scattering light. In glaucoma, elevated intraocular pressure and endothelial damage cause corneal edema and opacity. Digital pressure on the globe distorts the lattice mechanically, causing immediate opacification. In scars,

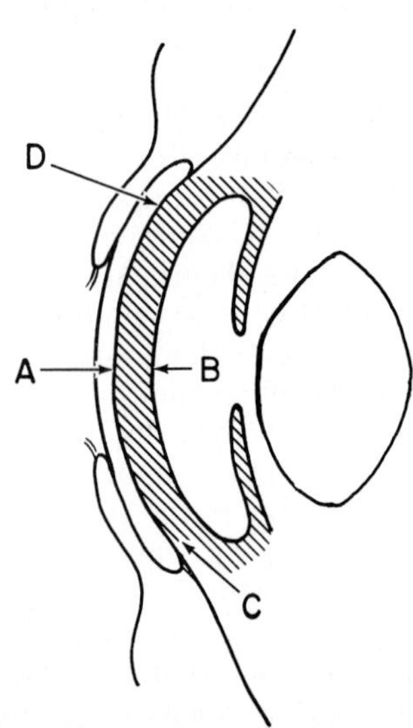

FIGURE 86–7. Sources of oxygen available to cornea. A, Precorneal film; B, aqueous humor; C, limbal capillaries; D, palpebral conjunctival capillaries. (Reprinted with permission from Scheie HG, Albert DM: *Textbook of Ophthalmology.* 9th ed. W.B. Saunders, Philadelphia, 1977.)

irregular size and arrangement of collagen fibrils cause opacity.

Interference with oxygen supply (e.g., by an impermeable contact lens) increases anaerobic glycolysis and causes corneal edema due to accumulation of lactic acid and water. Removal of epithelium allows entry of water from tears into the stroma and causes gross corneal swelling. This is seen after superficial keratectomy. Destruction of the endothelial barrier causes even worse corneal swelling.

PATHOLOGICAL RESPONSES[49]

The normal cornea is avascular. Penetration of new vessels and immunoglobulins into the cornea is impeded by the compact stromal tissue. These features make corneal pathological reactions sluggish, chronic, and intractable. The precarious state of transparency depends on unstable factors like fluid balance and degree of hydration. Changes that would be mild in other tissues (e.g. edema, minor scars, or tissue tension changes) may greatly alter transparency and are more significant in the cornea. The corneal epithelium forms an effective barrier against exogenous influences (e.g., bacteria and their toxins). Bacteria rarely cause primary keratitis in dogs and cats, but once the epithelial barrier has been broken, microorganisms may establish themselves within the avascular stroma. Extension of disease processes from other ocular tissues is a common cause of corneal disease. Examples include entry of infectious canine hepatitis virus into the cornea from the aqueous, effects of uveitis on the cornea including corneal edema, and trauma due to misplaced cilia in distichiasis. Endogenous conditions arising within the cornea include lipid deposition in hyperlipoproteinemia, endothelial dystrophy in dogs, and corneal bullae formation in corneal dystrophy in Manx cats.

NORMAL CORNEAL HEALING

Epithelium

The regenerative capacity of the epithelium is great. Within a short time, cells around a lesion slide over the defect (Fig. 86–8). An entirely denuded cornea can be re-epithelialized in 4 to 7 days.[41] Once cells have covered the defect, mitosis occurs and a multilayered epithelium is reconstituted. During cell migration, melanocytes from the limbus may be carried into formerly transparent areas. Small defects in the stroma may be filled with thickened epithelium, forming an epithelial facet (Fig. 86–9).

Stroma

Superficial stromal defects are filled by epithelial facets. Deeper defects are covered initially by epithelium, with regeneration of stroma from beneath. Regeneration often is incomplete, causing reduced corneal thickness. Uncomplicated stromal wounds heal without vascularization, but infected or destructive lesions heal with vascularization.

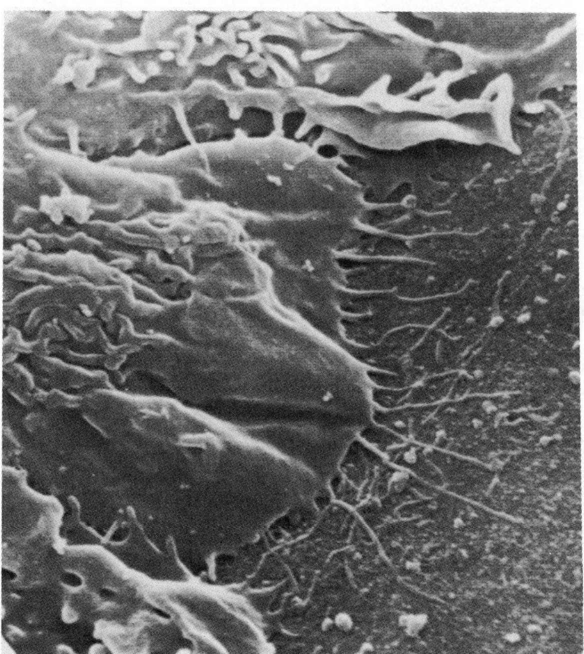

FIGURE 86–8. Filopodia extending from an epithelial cell over bare basement membrane at the edge of an epithelial defect. (Reprinted with permission from Pfister RR: The healing of corneal epithelial abrasions in the rabbit: A scanning electron microscope study. *Invest Ophthalmol 14*:648, 1975.)

Avascular Stromal Healing

Edema formation begins immediately after stromal injury. Within 1 to 2 days, neutrophils from tears and limbal blood vessels infiltrate the wound under chemotactic influences. Keratocytes adjacent to the wound die. In surrounding areas, keratocytes transform into fibroblasts, migrate to the damaged area, and produce collagen and mucopolysaccharides of corneal ground substance. From about 48 hours after injury, macrophages invade the lesion, remove cellular debris, and subse-

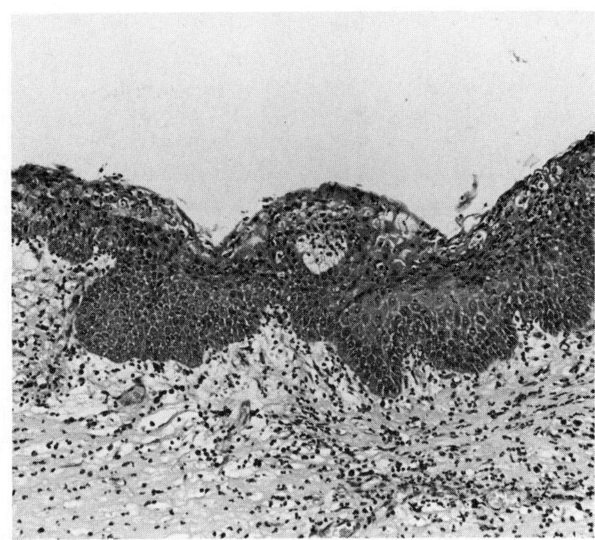

FIGURE 86–9. Epithelial facet and associated subepithelial inflammatory cell infiltration after a superficial corneal injury in a canine cornea.

quently transform into keratocytes. The collagen fibrils of regenerated stroma are irregular, causing opacity. Within weeks to months, the density of the scar decreases, although it does not disappear totally. Scar resolution is more complete in cats than in dogs. A sutured full-thickness corneal wound depends on mechanical support by sutures for 16 days when using polyglactin 910 (Vicryl) or nylon sutures.[51]

Vascular Stromal Healing

In vascular healing of destructive lesions, cellular infiltration is more extensive than in avascular healing. Blood vessels originating from the limbal vascular plexus invade the area (Fig. 86–10). Granulation tissue is laid down and forms a denser scar than in avascular healing. Blood vessels eventually collapse but do not disappear. They remain as "ghost vessels," visible with a slit-lamp biomicroscope. As damaged corneal nerves regenerate, sensation slowly returns.

Endothelium and Descemet Membrane

The Descemet membrane is elastic and retracts and curls when damaged, exposing corneal stroma. Neighboring endothelial cells slide in to cover the area, and a new Descemet membrane is laid down. In extensive lesions, endothelium may not cover the defect, causing a persisting area of swollen, edematous stroma. The endothelium is very delicate; if widely damaged, permanent opacity results. Endothelial regeneration occurs in dogs and rabbits[3, 53] but to a lesser extent in cats,[53] primates, and humans.[52]

CORTICOSTEROIDS AND CORNEAL HEALING[24]

Corticosteroids inhibit epithelial and endothelial regeneration, infiltration with inflammatory cells, and fibroblastic activity.[5, 12, 48] The tensile strength of the healing wound is lessened, collagenases are potentiated many times,[8] and the risk of infection is greatly increased (Fig. 86–11). Corticosteroids are useful after an epithelial cover has been achieved, to reduce scar formation.

The effects of corticosteroids on wound healing are dose dependent. Also, if topical corticosteroid therapy can be delayed for 7 days after wounding, fibroblastic activity will be well under way and wound healing will be much less impeded. This may not be possible in the presence of uveitis. The nonsteroidal anti-inflammatory drug flurbiprofen when given topically inhibits corneal stromal healing similarly to topical prednisolone.[35]

INTERPRETATION OF CORNEAL PATHOLOGICAL REACTIONS

The majority of clinically important corneal disorders exhibit one or more of the following: edema, vascularization, scar formation, pigmentation, and accumulation of abnormal substances in the cornea.

Edema

Corneal edema results from excess fluid in the stroma. It distorts the collagen lattice, causing opacity, and

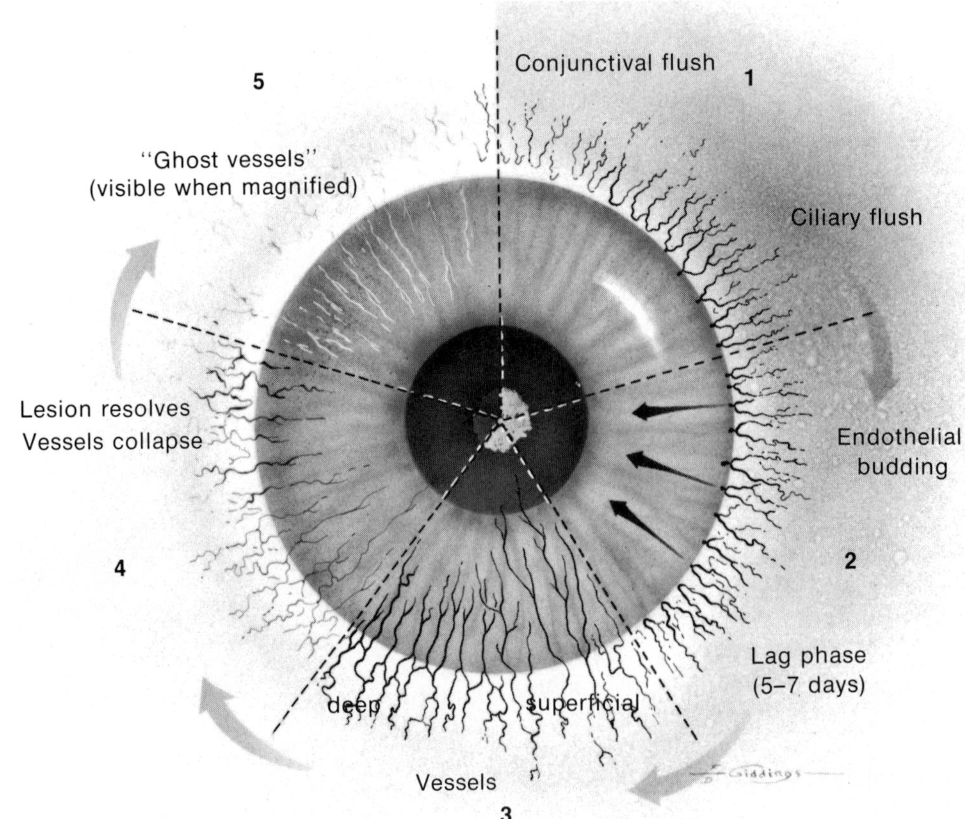

FIGURE 86–10. Diagrammatic sequence of corneal vascularization in a simple injury.

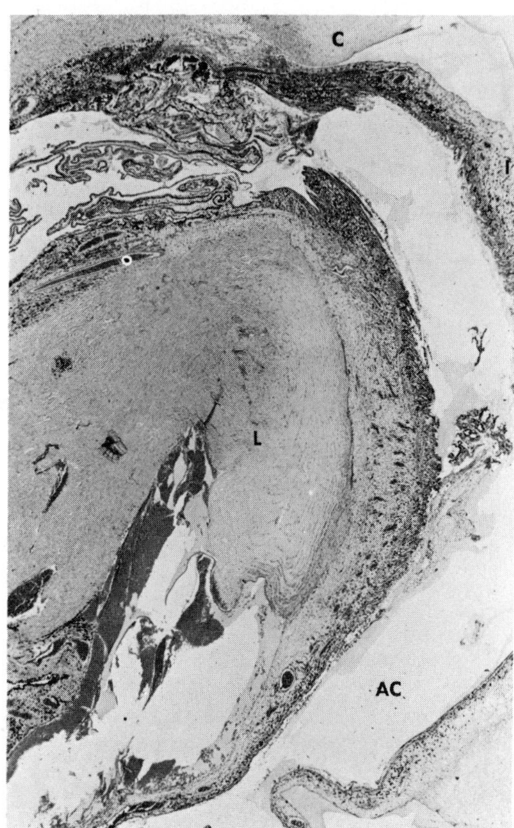

FIGURE 86–11. Ruptured descemetocele, endophthalmitis, and disorganization due to infection by *Pseudomonas* spp. after treatment of a minor corneal wound with subconjunctival corticosteroids in a dog. (C, cornea; I, iris; L, lens; AC, anterior chamber.)

occurs when regulating functions of epithelium or endothelium are lost, either by removal or functional alteration. Edematous cornea is hazy gray to blue, either in localized areas around injuries or throughout as in glaucoma and endothelial disorders. Edema is usually reversible if the underlying cause is removed and fluid balance is re-established. Chronic edema may cause corneal vascularization or, less commonly, bullous keratopathy,[45] in which fluid-containing vesicles form in or beneath the epithelium. Corneal edema may be cleared temporarily for examination by topical application of hypertonic solutions (e.g., 5 per cent sodium chloride, 40 per cent glucose, or 50 per cent glycerin).

Vascularization

There are no blood vessels in normal cornea. Vessels invade corneal stroma in response to various pathological processes and during vascularized stromal healing. Vascularization may be induced by different stimuli, including stimulated lymphocytes or their elaborated lymphokines.[14]

Corneal vascularization may be superficial or deep. Superficial vessels occur in the anterior third of the stroma and are continuous with the conjunctival circulation at the limbus. These superficial vessels branch (arborize) more than deep vessels and are brighter red than deep vessels. The latter branch less and are often short, straight, and darker red. Deep vessels are continuous with the ciliary circulation and disappear from view at the limbus. The depth of invading vessels gives some indication about the depth of the inciting lesion. Knowledge of the timing sequence of corneal vascularization is important both for diagnostic evaluation of corneal lesions and during postoperative assessment (see Fig. 86–10).

In complicated stromal lesions, especially when the stimulus in the cornea remains, vessels may not collapse and further vascularization and granulation occur. In general, vascularization is a beneficial response (e.g., during stromal repair after prolapse of the globe in dogs), but vessels result in decreased transparency, ingrowth of pigment, and occasionally transport of antibodies and inflammatory cells that decrease corneal transparency. Control of vascularization is often attempted with topical corticosteroids or beta radiation (e.g., when re-epithelialization has occurred after superficial keratectomy for superficial erosion). Beta radiation can be used before re-epithelialization.

Scar Formation

Corneal stromal repair results in disorganized collagen fibrils of uneven diameter, causing loss of transparency. Scars increase in transparency with time, but in dogs, pigmentation and lipid deposition may occur. The deeper the initial injury, the more dense and permanent the resulting scar and the less the tendency for clearing. Very superficial stromal defects are filled with epithelial facets, without scarring. Corneal opacities are termed *nebula, macula,* and *leukoma,* in increasing order of size and density (Fig. 86–12). Extensive loss of stroma with subsequent cicatrization may cause a thin cornea that bulges (corneal ectasia or kerectasis). If the stroma is destroyed full thickness and a bare Descemet membrane bulges forward, the lesion is called a *descemetocele* (Fig. 86–13). Descemetoceles frequently form after unremitting ulceration, and if untreated, the membrane either ruptures, with loss of aqueous and collapse of the anterior chamber, or becomes surrounded by scar tissue. Descemetoceles do not stain with fluorescein (Fig. 86–14). In corneal perforation, escaping aqueous carries the iris forward into the defect. If the iris is incorporated into the healing wound, an anterior synechia is formed. If the iris is carried out through the wound, an iris prolapse exists (Fig. 86–15).

Opacity due to uncomplicated corneal stromal wounds may be limited by judicious use of corticosteroids, provided that (1) infection has been controlled, (2) an epithelial covering can be demonstrated with fluorescein, and (3) the structural integrity of the cornea is not compromised. Under such circumstances, topically applied corticosteroids (e.g., 1 per cent prednisolone acetate or 0.1 per cent dexamethasone drops three to four times a day) decrease vascularization, reduce scarring and pigmentation, and improve final transparency.

Pigmentation

Corneal pigmentation (pigmentary keratitis) is a nonspecific response to corneal inflammation, either severe

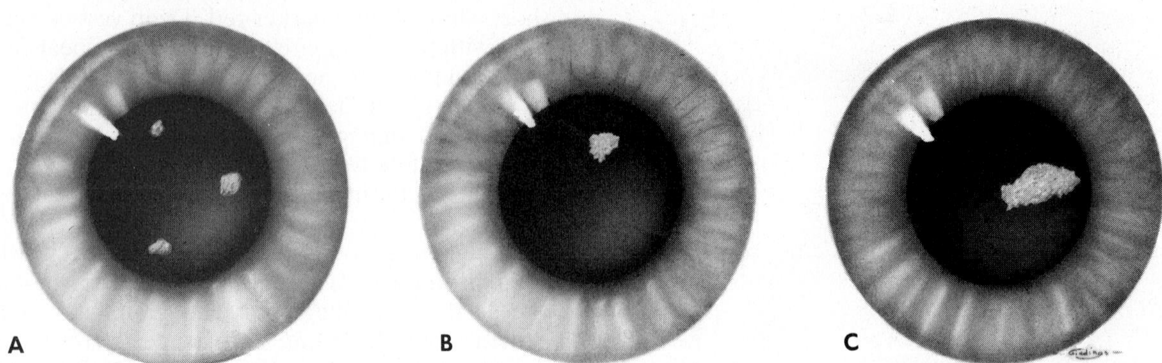

FIGURE 86–12. Types of corneal scars. *A*, Nebula. *B*, Macula. *C*, Leukoma. If the iris attaches to the leukoma, it is called an *adherent leukoma.*

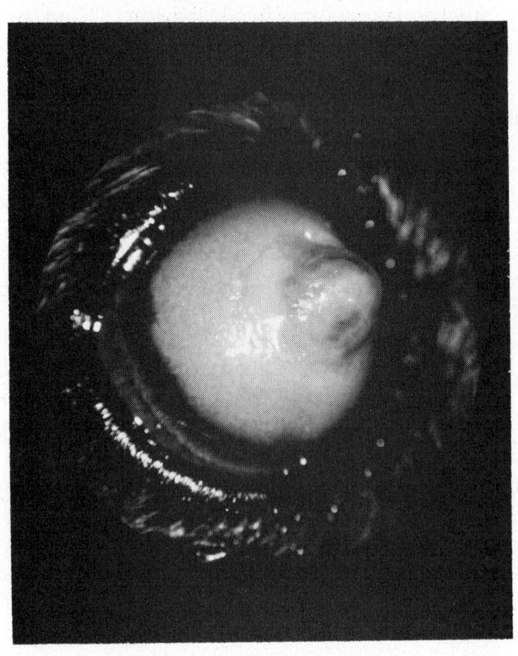

FIGURE 86–13. A descemetocele with corneal edema and vascularization in a Pekingese.

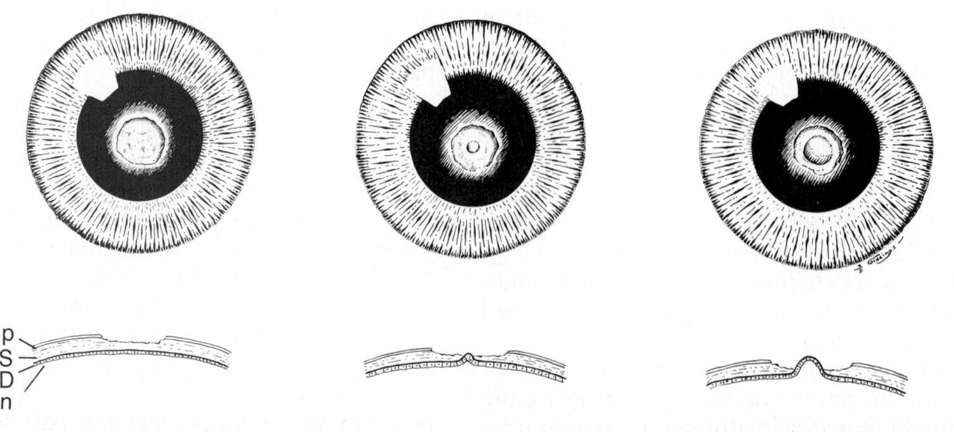

FIGURE 86–14. Staining characteristics of corneal lesions. (Ep, epithelium; S, stroma; D, Descemet membrane; En, endothelium.)

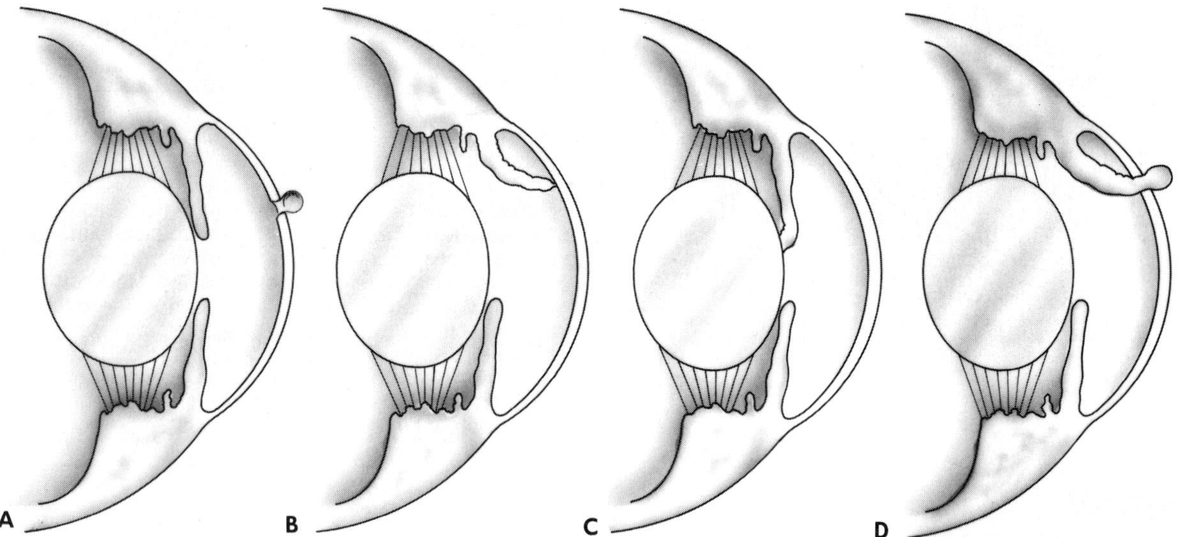

FIGURE 86–15. Corneal lesions. *A,* Descemetocele. *B,* Anterior synechia. *C,* Posterior synechia. *D,* Iris prolapse.

or mild, and not a primary disease. Stromal melanin originates from proliferation of normal limbal melanoblasts that migrate into the cornea along with blood vessels. Pigment in the corneal epithelium arises from the basal layer, which is of the same embryological origin as the layer containing pigment in the conjunctiva. Epithelial pigmentation is more common in chronic corneal diseases, especially when continuous exposure or irritation is present (e.g., distichiasis, nasal fold trichiasis, corneal exposure). Removal of the stimulus usually prevents progression of pigmentation. Stromal pigmentation usually is associated with more severe corneal disease and vascularization. With chronic corneal exposure or lack of precorneal tear film, the corneal epithelium may revert to a simple skin pattern with thickening, rete peg formation, keratinization, and pigmentation. In cats, melanin pigmentation must be distinguished from focal corneal necrosis in which the color may be due to necrotic tissue and keratin.[15] Pigmentation itself is not normally treated unless vision is threatened. The underlying cause is removed whenever possible (e.g., removal of nasal folds in trichiasis, reduction of the eyelid aperture in brachycephalic dogs with corneal exposure, or control of inflammation in chronic immune-mediated keratitis syndrome).[48] Methods used to control pigmentation include superficial keratectomy,[40, 48] beta irradiation,[48] and control of inflammation with topical corticosteroids.

GENERAL PRINCIPLES OF SURGICAL MANIPULATION OF CORNEA

The cornea has unique features of practical surgical importance. Handling the multilayered solid stroma requires knowledge of such features.[13, 50]

Grasping the cornea often requires toothed forceps that allow wound edges to be held (e.g., when suturing corneal lacerations). Corneal endothelium must not be included in such a grip (Fig. 86–16).

In *cutting corneal stroma,* regulation of tissue sectility becomes important. Sectility refers to the ability of the tissue to be cut. The higher the sectility of a tissue, the more easily it can be divided by a cutting edge. This regulation of sectility is used in superficial corneal dissections to increase sectility of the fibers between two corneal lamellae by increasing tissue tension focally (Fig. 86–17). Corneal sectility also depends on intraocular pressure. Increased intraocular pressure increases tissue tension and sectility.

The corneal stroma causes *lamellar deflection* of incisions: An incision is deflected to become more parallel to the lamellae (Fig. 86–18). If the intention is to cut through lamellae, incisions are easier to make at a high tissue tension and sectility. If the intention is lamellar dissection of the cornea, lamellar deflection is increased by working at a low intraocular pressure. Tissue tension is increased focally as described earlier.

When corneal stroma is cut *with scissors,* the resulting cut has an S-shaped profile (Fig. 86–19).

This distortion of incision shape can be minimized by preliminary reduction of the tissue thickness to be cut (e.g., by making a groove incision with a knife before cutting with scissors).

Corneal suturing requires precise placement and guid-

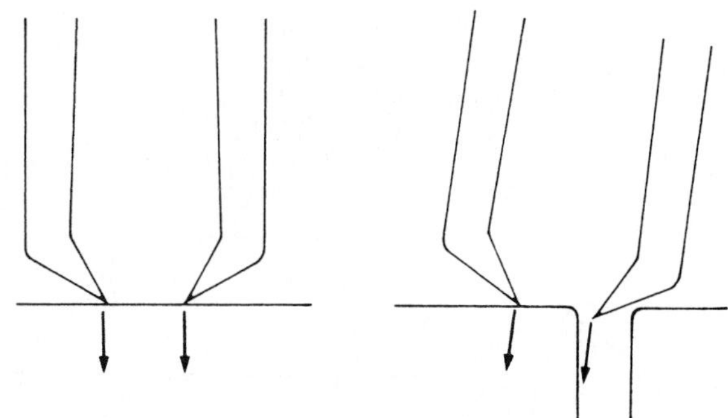

FIGURE 86–16. Possible points of attack of the thrust vector. Owing to the forward-directed vector, mouse tooth forceps can grab into flat surfaces *(left)* or penetrate into the space between wound edges *(right).* (From Eisner G.: *Eye Surgery: An Introduction to Operative Technique.* Springer-Verlag, Berlin, 1980.)

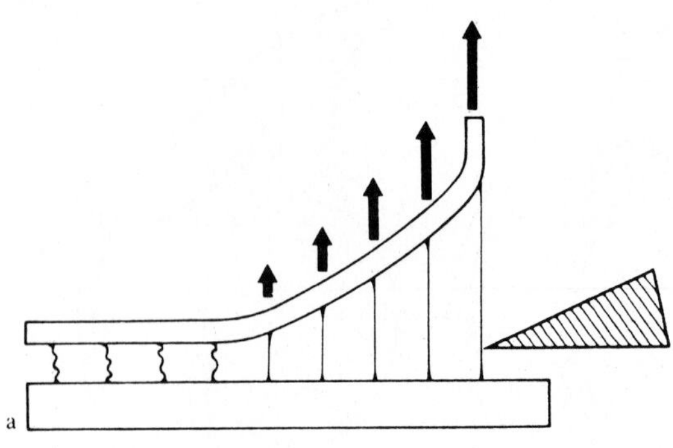

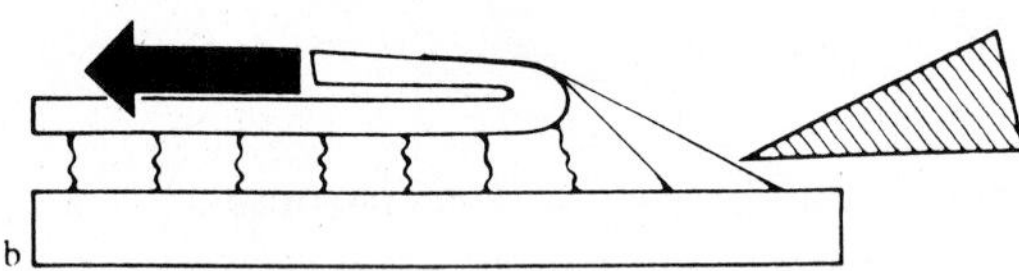

FIGURE 86–17. Regulation of tissue sectility. *A,* Diffuse tissue tension. The tissue layer that transmits forceps traction to the target fibers is lifted vertically away from the underlying layer so that tension is exerted on a great number of fibers. This produces good sectility over a large area. *B,* Selective tissue tension. The layer that transmits the traction is drawn back so that tension is exerted only on the most peripheral fibers. The remaining fibers and the overlying layer have poor sectility and, thus, are protected from inadvertent lesions. (From Eisner G: *Eye Surgery: An Introduction to Operative Technique.* Springer-Verlag, Berlin, 1980.)

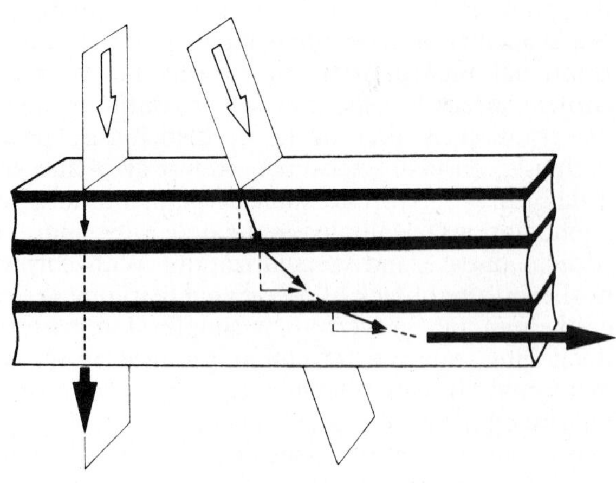

FIGURE 86–18. Lamellar deflection. Lamellar tissues consist of a regular arrangement of layers with varying resistances. If a blade is applied to the lamellae at right angles *(left),* it encounters a symmetrical lateral resistance and can advance in the direction intended. If the blade is applied obliquely *(right),* the lateral resistance becomes asymmetrical. The incision deviates until it terminates in loose interlamellar tissue, where the lateral resistance is again symmetrical. (From Eisner G: *Eye Surgery: An Introduction to Operative Technique.* Springer-Verlag, Berlin, 1980.)

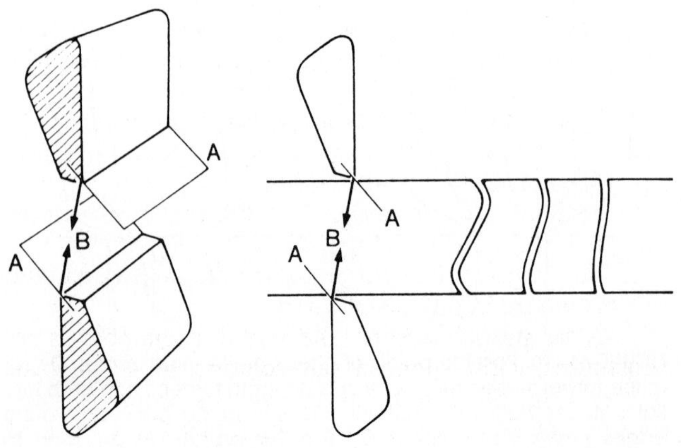

FIGURE 86–19. The profile of a scissors cut. In thick tissue layers, not only the point cutting edge but also the cutting properties of the blades play a role. By their nature, scissors always create an angle between the guidance direction, *B,* and the preferential path of the edge, *A*. This results in an S-shaped cut profile whose curvature depends on the resistance, displaceability, and thickness of the tissue. Note: The obliquity of the guidance path *B* is due to the camber of the blades. (From Eisner G: *Eye Surgery: An Introduction to Operative Technique.* Springer-Verlag, Berlin, 1980.)

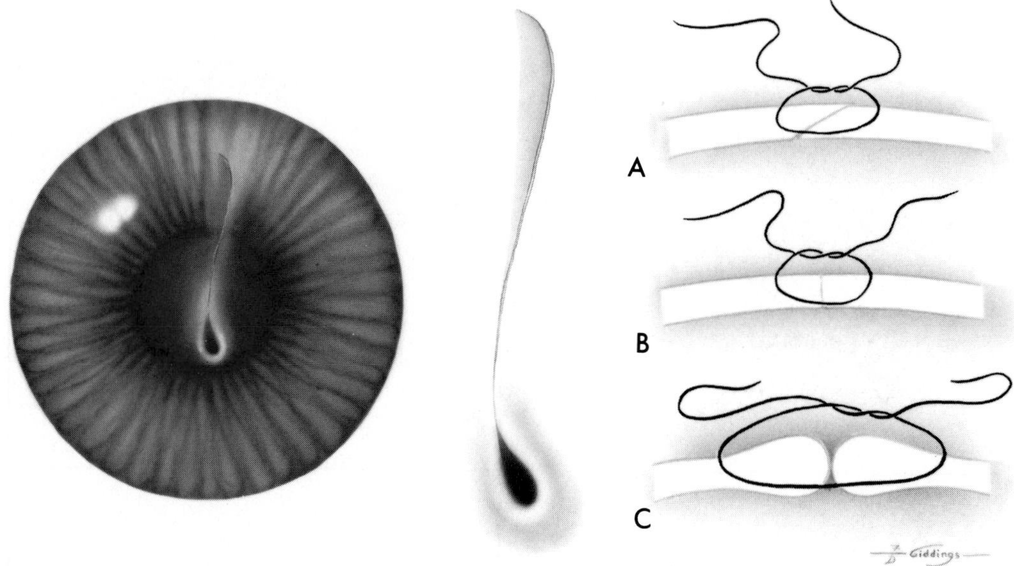

FIGURE 86–20. Repair of corneal laceration. The diagram illustrates suggested placement of nylon suture material for shelved laceration *(A)*, vertical laceration *(B)*, and laceration with edematous margins *(C)*. (Redrawn after Paton D, Goldberg MF: *Management of Ocular Injuries.* W.B. Saunders, Philadelphia, 1976.)

ance of the needle. In full-thickness wounds, sutures are placed deeply but not totally through the stroma (Fig. 86–20). The radius of curvature of the needle and the angle of initial penetration into the stroma are important. The smaller the radius of curvature, the deeper the preferential path of the needle. The initial penetration into stroma is made perpendicular to the surface to facilitate deep needle passage. Sutures distort tissue when tightened. Simple interrupted sutures form a circle when tightened, whereas a continuous suture tends to form a straight line. Both suture types shift tissue so that the suture lies in one plane. These distortions must be controlled when suturing delicate ocular tissues.[13]

SURGICAL PROCEDURES

Treatment of Corneal Injuries

With a penetrating wound of the globe, pressure may cause further intraocular damage. A third-eyelid flap is initially placed over the eye to prevent further damage until skilled assistance is available. A careful examination is required to evaluate intraocular injuries. One of the most common causes of severe endophthalmitis and secondary glaucoma leading to enucleation in dogs is unsuspected damage to the lens and its capsule after a perforating injury. If no other intraocular damage is evident, the wound is sutured after routine exposure and fixation of the globe.

Equipment

Magnifying loupe (× 2 to × 4) or operating microscope
Lid retractors
Ophthalmic needle holders
Corneal scissors
Iris scissors
Corneal forceps
Cyclodialysis spatula
Anterior chamber irrigating bulb and needle
Fine suture (7-0 or 8-0 silk or 8-0 to 10-0 nylon with a swaged-on needle)
Cellulose sponge
Balanced salt solution for irrigation (epinephrine [1:10,000] and dilute heparin may be added to control hemorrhage and fibrin, respectively)

Closure of a Corneal Wound

1. The corneal endothelium is exquisitely sensitive to trauma. It must not be touched with instruments or flushed vigorously with irrigating solutions. When the edges of a corneal wound are held, only stroma and epithelium are touched with forceps.
2. The edges of corneal wounds are not débrided; as much tissue as possible is left in place to complete closure.
3. If the wound is fresh, an attempt is made to replace protruding iris with an iris repositor. This may be facilitated if the anterior chamber is reconstituted with methylcellulose, air, or sodium hyaluronate. If the tissue is damaged, protruding iris is excised with iris scissors. Hemorrhage may be severe if the excision is near the major arterial circle of the iris. Electrocautery is advised.
4. Blood and fibrin clots in the anterior chamber are carefully removed with a cyclodialysis spatula or blunt iris hook before the wound is closed.
5. Partial-thickness rather than full-thickness sutures are used in the cornea (Figs. 86–20 and 86–21).
6. The cornea is sutured with simple interrupted sutures placed about 1 mm apart.
7. After partial closure, the anterior chamber is reconstituted with balanced salt solution or a small air bubble (Fig. 86–22). In uncomplicated wounds, some sutures may be removed after 7 days. Generally, corneal wounds depend on sutures for tensile strength for 16 days.[51]

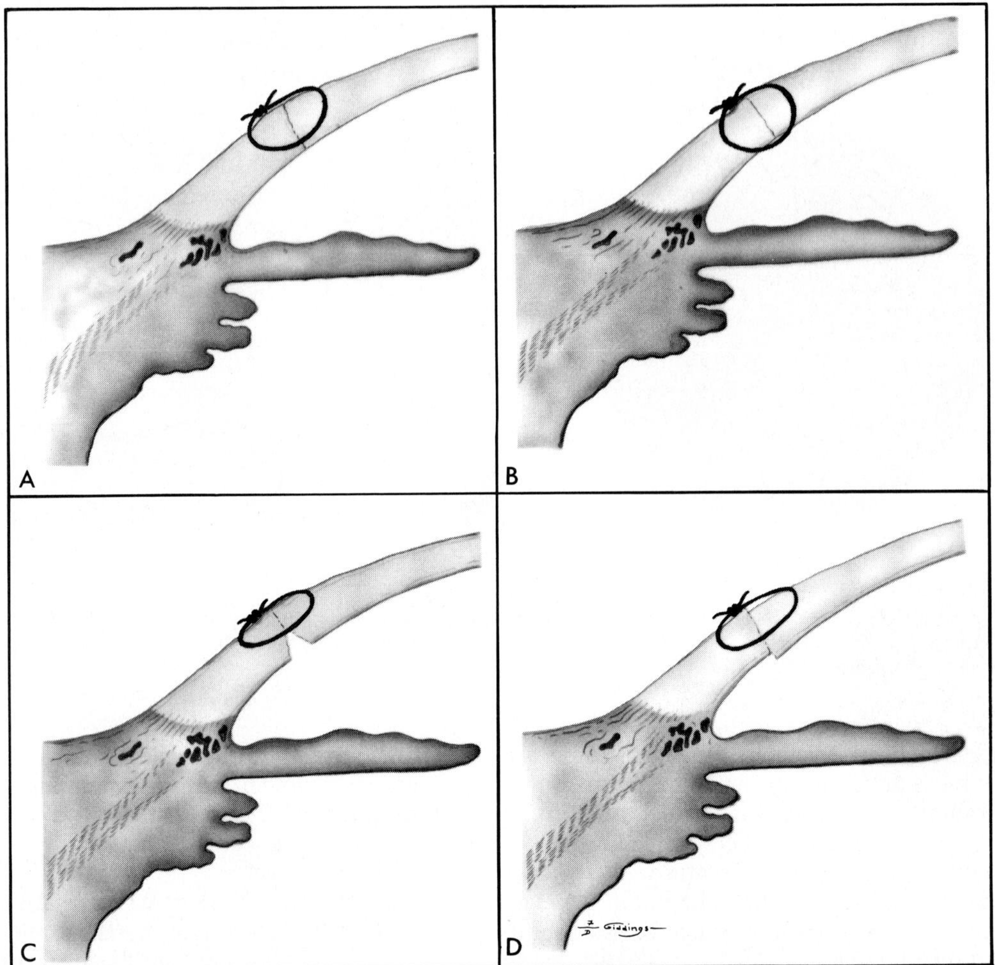

FIGURE 86–21. *A,* A correctly placed corneal suture. *B,* Suture incorrectly penetrates the anterior chamber. *C,* Suture is too superficial, resulting in poor endothelial closure and persistent edema. *D,* Bites of the suture are uneven, resulting in poor apposition of the wound edges. (Redrawn after Severin G: *Veterinary Ophthalmology Notes.* 2nd ed. Colorado State University Bookstore, Ft. Collins, CO, 1976.)

The prognosis for a corneal wound depends on its initial depth and severity. Lacerations usually have a favorable prognosis, as do wounds that do not perforate the cornea. Perforating wounds heal with more vascularization, scarring, and opacity. Corneal ruptures due to blunt trauma have a poorer prognosis owing to disruption of tissue at the wound edges.

Removal of Corneal Foreign Bodies

Corneal foreign bodies are removed to limit pain, reduce infection, and prevent vascularization and scarring. Many corneal foreign bodies can be flushed off with a jet of physiological saline through a 23- to 27-gauge needle. Small embedded foreign bodies are removed with an instrument called a *foreign body spud* (see Fig. 81–21*G*). In an emergency, the tip of a 25- or 27-gauge needle may be used with magnification. Deeply embedded foreign bodies may require an incision in the overlying epithelium and stroma over the long axis of the object. Adherent foreign bodies (e.g., flakes of paint) frequently lie in a depression in the corneal epithelium, with the lids passing over them. Such objects may be removed by lifting the edge with an instrument. Thorns from bushes and cacti that penetrate the anterior chamber may be difficult to pull out because of barbs on the surface. Extraction via the anterior chamber and a limbal corneal incision may be necessary. Foreign body extractions are performed with the utmost care. Inappropriate attempts at removal may result in penetration into the anterior chamber or corneal damage with more severe vascularization and scarring.

After suture removal, a topical broad-spectrum antibiotic (applied four times a day) and atropine are administered to control infection and ciliary spasm due to secondary uveitis, respectively. In cats, atropine ointment is preferred over drops to reduce salivation because of the bitter taste of atropine drops. Corneal epithelial healing normally is rapid. Topical anesthetics inhibit epithelialization and are both unnecessary and contraindicated postoperatively.

Superficial Keratectomy

Keratectomy is removal of the corneal epithelium or stroma. Because the stroma does not regenerate, the number of successive keratectomies that can be performed on the same site is limited to two or three,

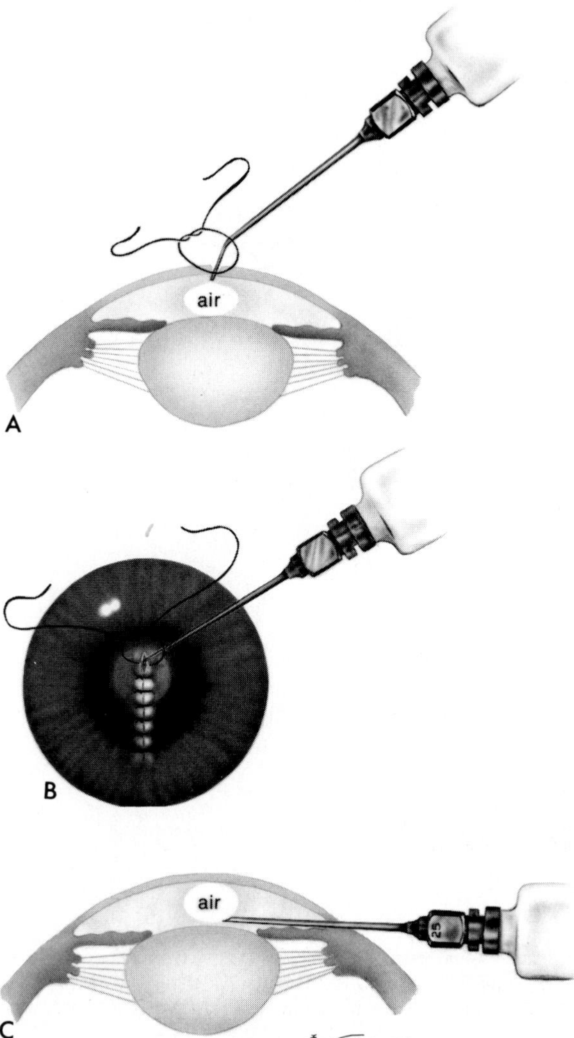

FIGURE 86–22. Reconstruction of the anterior chamber with a sterile air bubble or balanced salt solution. *A* and *B*, A cannula may be placed between the wound edges or *(C)* via a 25-gauge needle from the limbus. With the sterile air bubble method, care must be taken to use as little air as possible, because if air gets behind the iris, "air block" glaucoma can occur. Balanced salt solution is preferable to air.

depending on the depth of each excision. Therefore, keratectomy is of limited value in a pathological process that is likely to continue postoperatively. The safety of performing a successive keratectomy can be determined by measuring the corneal thickness by ultrasonic pachymetry. Use of an operating microscope greatly improves the safety and results of this procedure. Superficial keratectomy is indicated in several situations:

1. Removal of neoplasms encroaching on the cornea from the limbus
2. Treatment of specific keratopathies (e.g., chronic superficial erosion syndrome in boxers and corgis and focal corneal necrosis [mummification, sequestration] in cats)
3. Débridement of any superficial epithelial corneal wound

Procedure

Superficial keratectomy is either complete or partial. In complete keratectomy, the area to be removed may be outlined with a corneal trephine set to a predetermined depth (e.g., 0.3 to 0.4 mm) or by dividing the cornea into segments (Fig. 86–23). The initial incision is made under magnification with a number 64 Beaver blade. Dissection is continued with a Martinez corneal dissector (see Fig. 81–21*B′*). The stroma is removed in sheets to the limbus, where it is cut. Postoperatively, the cornea is stained as necessary with fluorescein to evaluate epithelialization. Topical antibiotic and atropine drops are applied. A third-eyelid flap may be constructed after keratectomy and removed after 7 to 10 days. Although it precludes daily evaluation of the cornea, it provides support for the growing epithelium. When the cornea is moderately vascularized before keratectomy (e.g., in boxers with chronic superficial erosions), indicating possible progression of vascularization postoperatively, dexamethasone drops may be given once daily from the fourth postoperative day and twice daily from the seventh postoperative day, as well as cyclosporine drops once daily after surgery. Although this therapy may delay re-epithelialization, it does reduce vascularization and scarring.[48]

Keratoplasty[2]

Corneal transplantation (keratoplasty) is not widely used in veterinary ophthalmic surgery but may be useful in selected cases. It is the only specific treatment for chronic corneal edema due to canine endothelial dystrophy[21] (Fig. 86–24). Corneal transplants should be considered only in animals with a severe bilateral visual handicap. The cornea should be free of vascularization, a condition that often is not met. The surgeon should be trained in the use of an operating microscope[50] and keratoplasty techniques.

Reports of long-term success in clinical cases are few owing to graft rejection. Microsurgical technique and immunosuppression are important for success.[11, 31, 34] Generally, indications for keratoplasty are fewer in cats, but the long-term prognosis is better. The two main types of corneal grafts are penetrating and lamellar (Fig. 86–25).

Penetrating Keratoplasty

Penetrating keratoplasty is used to replace scarred or diseased cornea. Affected tissue is removed full thickness and replaced with a donor button lined with viable endothelium. Major problems encountered with penetrating keratoplasty in dogs are formation of protein-rich ("plasmoid") aqueous, shrinkage of the donor button, and postoperative vascularization.

Formation of plasmoid aqueous may be minimized by pretreatment with

1. Systemic corticosteroids (oral prednisolone, 1 to 2 mg/kg daily for 3 days)
2. Topical corticosteroids (dexamethasone, 0.1 per cent QID for several days before surgery)

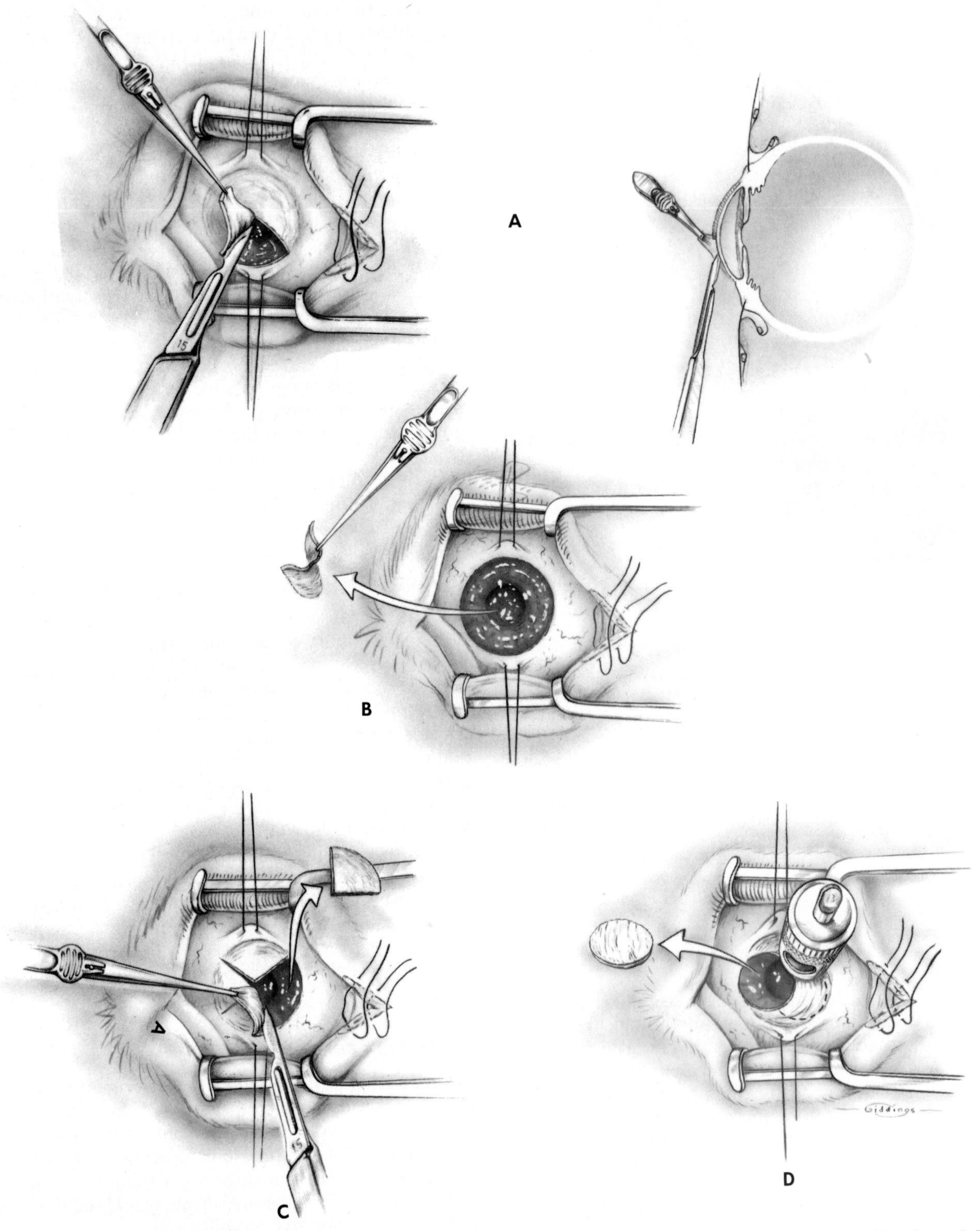

FIGURE 86–23. *A* and *B*, Removal of a large lesion *en bloc*. Although clear at this stage, the cornea soon becomes edematous. *C*, Division of the cornea into quadrants. *D*, Outline of the area to be removed with a corneal trephine. The canthotomy is closed.

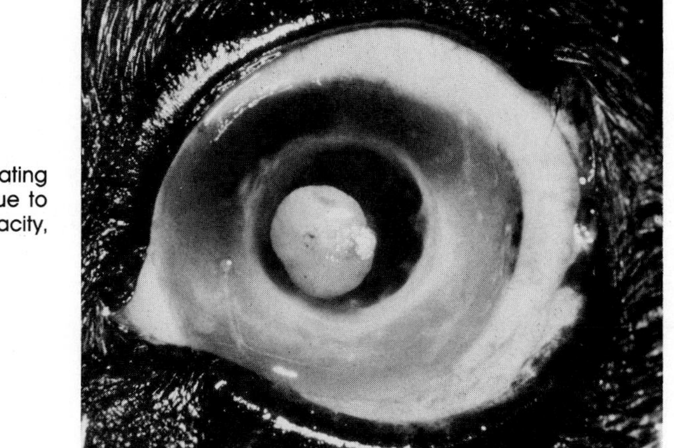

FIGURE 86–24. Postoperative appearance 16 months after a penetrating corneal graft in a 12-year-old Boston terrier with corneal edema due to corneal dystrophy. The clear donor button contains an area of opacity, probably calcification. (Courtesy of Dr. G. L. Gwin.)

3. Topical antiprostaglandins (e.g., topical flurbiprofen or indomethacin) (see Chapter 81)

4. Systemic antiprostaglandins (flunixin meglumine, 1 mg/kg IV at induction; acetylsalicylic acid, 25 mg/kg PO daily for 1 to 2 days before surgery)

5. Heparin and epinephrine in the intraocular flushing solution used

Technique

1. The lesion is removed with the trephine set at 1 mm depth (Fig. 86–26*A*). The trephine is withdrawn immediately on entering the anterior chamber (Fig. 86–26*B*).

2. Corneal scissors may be needed to complete the incision (Fig. 86–26*C* and *D*).

3. Any bevel or tissue tags are trimmed from the incision edges with corneal scissors and fine forceps (Fig. 86–26*E* and *F*).

4. The donor button surface is washed with bacitracin-neomycin-polymyxin solution, and the button is removed from the donor eye (Fig. 86–26*G* and *H*). Alter-

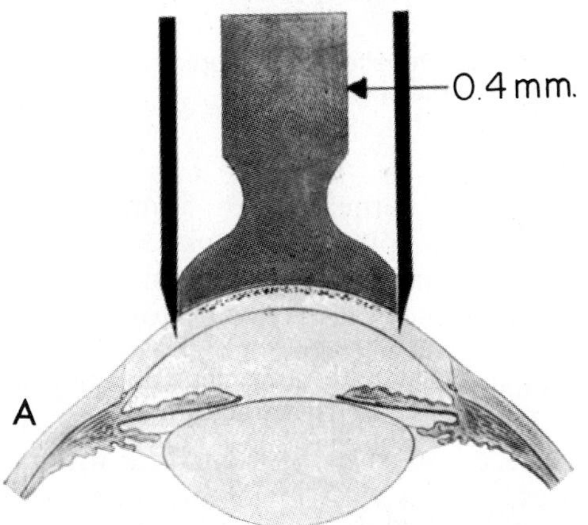

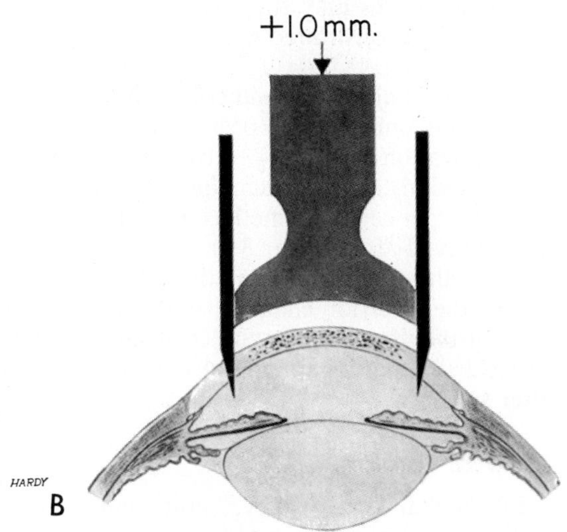

FIGURE 86–25. Lamellar *(A)* and penetrating *(B)* keratoplasty with a corneal trephine. (Reprinted with permission from Castroviejo R: *Atlas of Keratectomy and Keratoplasty.* W.B. Saunders, Philadelphia, 1966.)

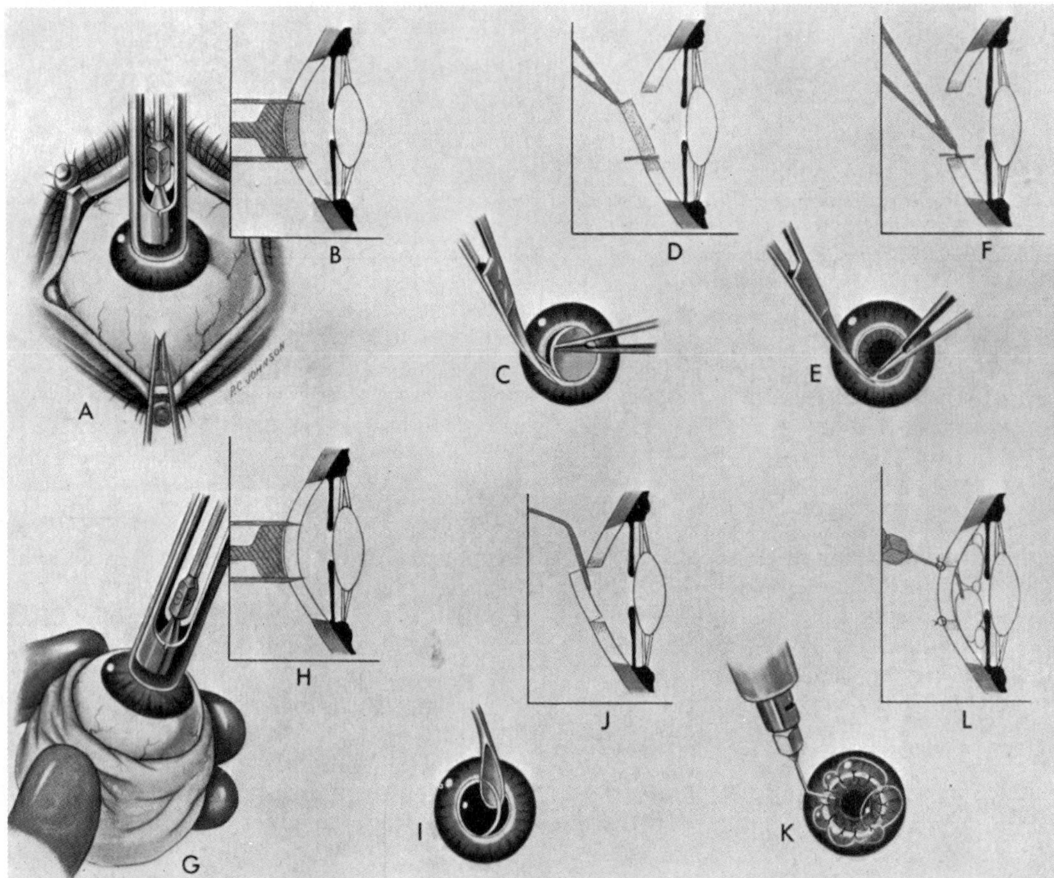

FIGURE 86–26. Penetrating keratoplasty. (Reprinted with permission from Castroviejo R: *Atlas of Keratectomy and Keratoplasty.* W.B. Saunders, Philadelphia, 1966.)

natively, the cornea and a 5-mm rim of sclera are removed, the epithelium is placed on a Teflon block, and the donor button is cut from the endothelial side with a trephine. The donor button is 0.5 mm larger in diameter than the recipient bed to allow for shrinkage.[34] Endothelium must not be touched during any procedure.

5. The donor button is removed (Fig. 86–26*I* and *J*) and placed in the recipient bed with four cardinal sutures, one in each quadrant. Suturing is completed with either multiple interrupted or a continuous suture. Cardinal sutures may then be removed.[50] The anterior chamber is reconstituted with balanced salt solution and an air bubble.

6. Topical antibiotic and corticosteroids are administered (four times a day) postoperatively. Postoperative vascularization is minimized by use of fine sutures (8-0 to 10-0 nylon), careful technique, and topical corticosteroids (0.1 per cent dexamethasone TID to QID). Sutures are removed after 12 to 18 days.

7. Hyaluronic acid or methylcellulose (see Chapter 81) in the anterior chamber and on the edges of the corneal incision protects the corneal endothelium from surgical trauma. The material is irrigated from the eye after suturing.

Lamellar Keratoplasty

In lamellar keratoplasty,[26] epithelium and superficial stroma are dissected free and replaced with donor tissue, usually for structural support during healing of a wound (e.g., in a descemetocele or after removal of a scar or an opacity).

Technique

1. The area to be removed is outlined with a trephine set at 0.3 mm (Fig. 86–27*A* and *C*).

2. The lesion is removed with a corneal dissector, a number 64 Beaver blade, or scissors (Fig. 86–27*B*).

3. The donor eye is washed with bacitracin-neomycin-polymyxin solution. The lamellar graft is removed from the donor eye with an electrokeratome or a Martinez corneal dissector (Fig. 86–27*D*). The graft is made 0.5 mm larger than the recipient bed.

4. The graft is sutured into the recipient bed with either a continuous suture with a buried knot[50] or multiple interrupted sutures (Fig. 86–27*E*).

5. Postoperatively, topical antibiotic and corticosteroids are applied four times daily.

Autogenous lamellar corneal transplantation in the treatment of corneal ulcers and descemetoceles has been described, and good success rates are reported.[7] A square block of tissue is excised at the ulcer site for débridement and graft site preparation. A slightly larger graft is harvested by superficial keratectomy elsewhere on the same cornea or on the contralateral cornea. The graft is sutured into the recipient bed at the ulcer. The use of autogenous tissue prevents graft rejection, but vascularization of the site often occurs.

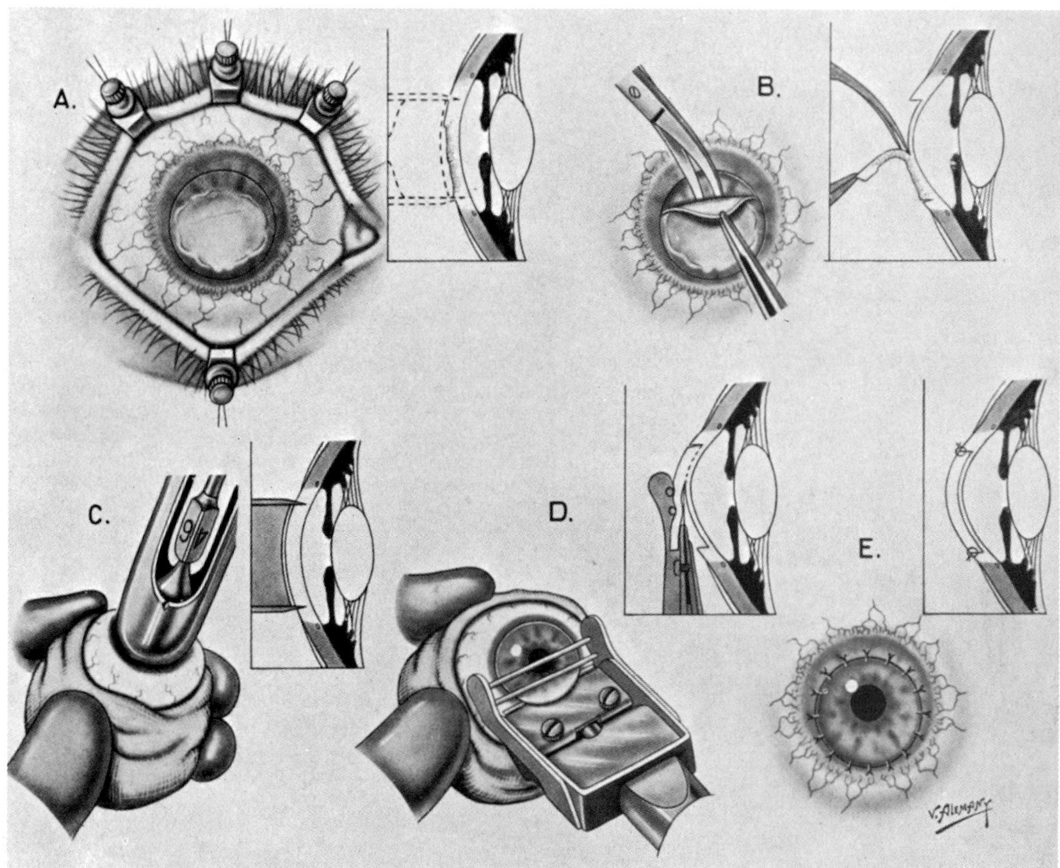

FIGURE 86–27. The technique of lamellar keratoplasty. *D,* A Martinez corneal dissector may be used in place of an electrokeratome. (Reprinted with permission from Castroviejo R: *Atlas of Keratectomy and Keratoplasty.* W.B. Saunders, Philadelphia, 1966.)

Corneal Preservation

Corneas can be preserved by various techniques for subsequent keratoplasty. Shortage of donor tissue has not stimulated their use in veterinary surgery.

Penetrating Corneoscleral Allograft

Replacement of continuous cornea and sclera from a donor of the same species is the treatment of choice for canine epibulbar melanomas when the tumor infiltrates the cornea or sclera. Canine epibulbar melanoma (Fig. 86–28) is a distinct tumor entity[32] and must be distinguished from melanosis of the conjunctiva and extension of intraocular melanoma[16] through the cornea and sclera. In intraocular melanoma, the intraocular mass or its sequelae are visible in the anterior chamber. Melanosis of the conjunctiva has the potential for malignant transformation in dogs; local resection with beta irradiation is the treatment of choice.[48]

Corneoscleral donor tissue is collected aseptically as soon as possible before resection of the lesion and is kept on a sterile gauze pad moistened with balanced salt solution. All traces of uveal tissue are removed from the graft to reduce the severity of postoperative immune reactions. The technique for resection and placement of the graft is illustrated in Figure 86–29. The graft is sutured with 8-0 to 10-0 monofilament nylon. The eye is treated topically with broad-spectrum antibiotics and corticosteroids four to six times daily for 7 to 10 days. The graft slowly vascularizes around its margins, sutures are removed, and therapy is gradually discontinued.

Corneoscleral Transposition

Corneoscleral transposition[39] is partial replacement of the cornea by the adjacent sclera to fill a defect resulting from removal of a lesion (Fig. 86–30). It is indicated

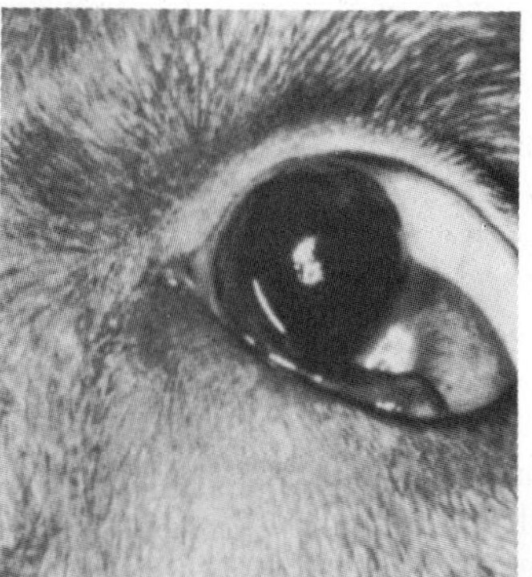

FIGURE 86–28. An epibulbar melanoma in a dog. Note penetration of the cornea by the neoplasm. (Courtesy of Dr. G. A. Severin. Slatter DH: Fundamentals of Veterinary Ophthalmology. 2nd ed. Philadelphia, W.B. Saunders, 1990.)

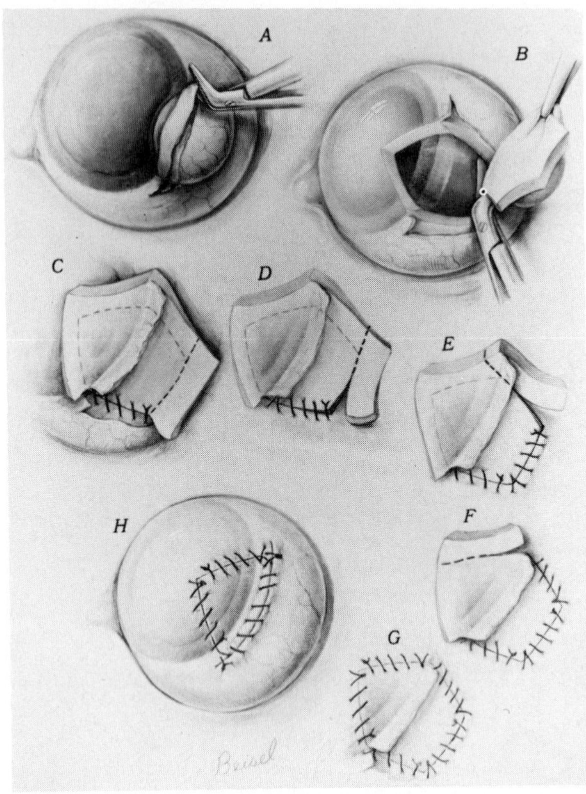

FIGURE 86–29. Penetrating corneoscleral allograft. *A*, The conjunctiva is incised and retracted. *B*, The affected cornea and sclera are excised full thickness with scissors or scalpel after initial use of an electroscalpel to reduce hemorrhage. *C*, Oversized donor tissue is sutured along one scleral edge. *D–G*, Remaining edges of the graft are trimmed and sutured. *H*, Adjacent conjunctiva is mobilized and sutured to the graft. (Reprinted with permission from Martin CL: Canine epibulbar melanomas and their management. *J Am Anim Hosp Assoc 17*:83, 1981.)

when insufficient tissue remains to fill a defect after lesion removal. Alternatives to this technique include penetrating keratoplasty, autogenous lamellar corneal transplantation, and penetrating corneoscleral allograft.

CORNEAL DISORDERS OF SURGICAL IMPORTANCE

Superficial Corneal Erosion

Superficial corneal erosion is most common in boxers[44] and corgis,[48] although other breeds are affected. Affected dogs usually have a history of blepharospasm and epiphora resistant to treatment with topical antibiotics for weeks to months.

Clinical Signs

Unilateral chronic blepharospasm, epiphora, and photophobia are common. In boxers and corgis, the lesions are due to separation of the epithelium from the basement membrane secondary to a defect in hemidesmosomes[18, 46, 48] or in the layers of the basement membrane.[27, 28] Abnormalities in basal epithelial cells and anterior stroma have also been noted.

In other breeds, some cases may have similar causes, whereas some may be due to mild endothelial dysfunction with diffuse, persistent corneal edema. Affected areas are usually 3 to 4 mm in diameter, have a ragged outline, cause pain, and stain with fluorescein. Epithelium does not adhere to underlying stroma but often accumulates at the periphery of the ulcer, causing a rolled-up appearance.

Treatment

If the lesion is discovered early, débridement and placement of a dissolving collagen shield, followed by topical antibiotics and hyperosmotic solutions, constitute the first treatment. About 30 per cent heal with this method. For refractory cases, superficial keratectomy is the treatment of choice.[40, 48] The lesion and a margin of 2 mm of normal surrounding tissue are removed superficially, preferably using an operating microscope. The cornea is covered with a third-eyelid flap and treated as for a superficial ulcer (see Table 86–2) until re-epithelialization is complete. Thereafter, topical corticosteroid therapy is used to reduce scar formation. The third-eyelid flap is removed 7 days (10 days in aged animals) postoperatively.

The use of vitamin A, estrogens, or chemical cautery (phenol, iodine) is not recommended for superficial corneal erosions.

Epithelial Inclusion Cysts

An epithelial inclusion cyst[30] is a rare fluid-filled sac lined with epithelium in the corneal stroma. The cyst appears as an elevation 3 to 4 mm in diameter on the corneal surface. It may be caused by traumatic inclusion of epithelium into the stroma. The cyst is removed by superficial keratectomy.

Superficial Pigmentary Keratitis

Superficial pigmentary keratitis occurs frequently in Pekingeses, pugs, and similar breeds. It is a nonspecific,

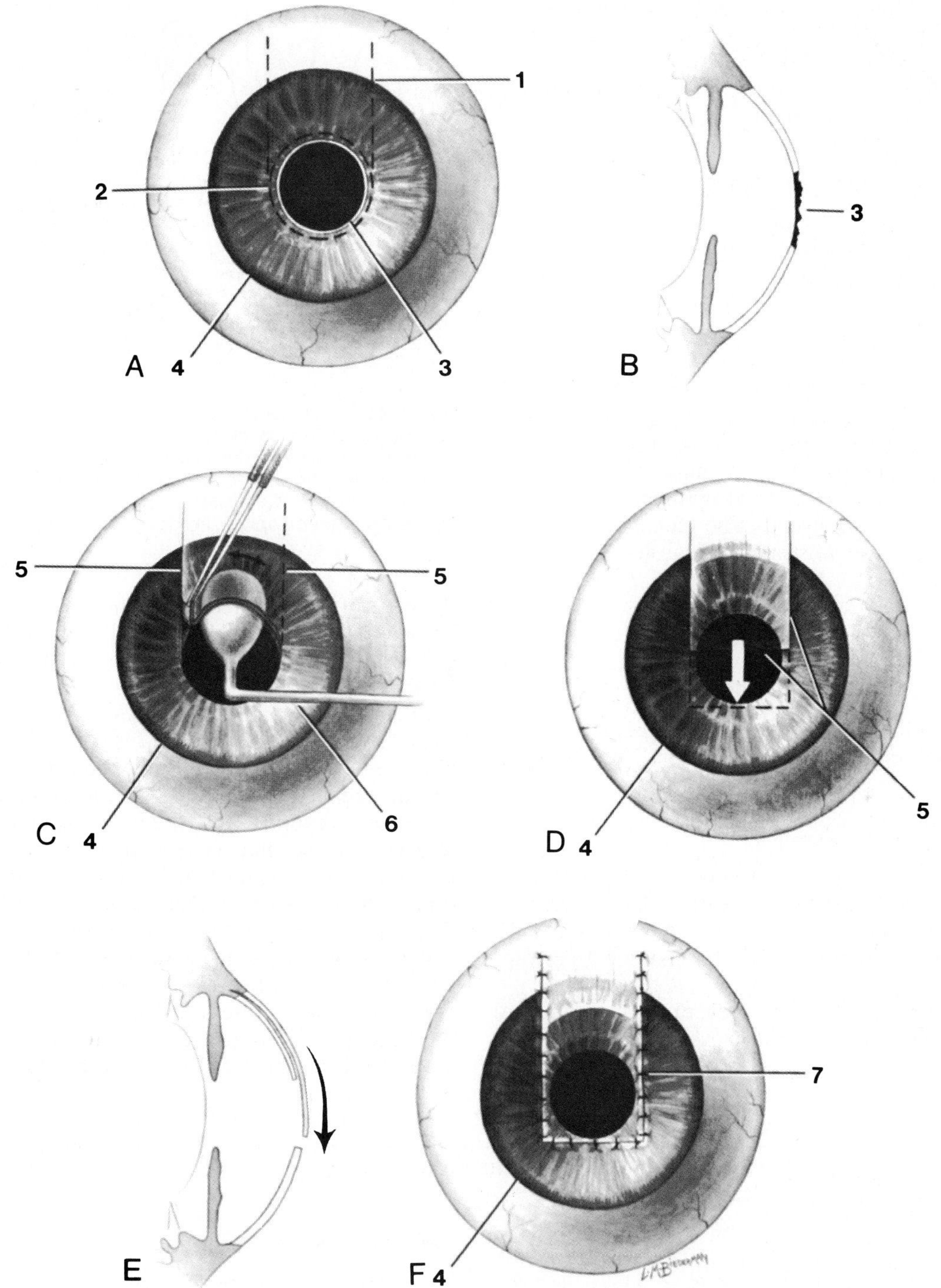

FIGURE 86–30. Corneoscleral transposition (method of Parshall). *A,* Line of graft excision (1); borders of surgically excised lesion (2); limits of necrotic tissue (3); limbus (4). *B,* Necrotic tissue (3). *C,* Limbus (4); edge of graft (5); corneal elevator (6). *D,* Limbus (4); end of graft (5). *E,* Graft is moved ventrally to cover defect. *F,* Limbus (4); placement of sutures (7). (Slatter DH: Fundamentals of Veterinary Ophthalmology. 2nd ed. Philadelphia, W.B. Saunders, 1990.)

chronic low-grade keratitis with pigmentation of the superficial stroma and epithelium[48] due to prominent exposed globes and a large palpebral fissure (euryblepharon) with chronic exposure of the cornea, distichiasis, and nasal fold trichiasis. Pigmentation frequently advances to interfere with vision before the owner is aware of its presence. Therapy aims at correction of causative factors to prevent progression of pigmentation, rather than removal of pigment.

Pseudopterygium and Symblepharon

Pseudopterygium is an adhesion of the conjunctiva to the cornea. When palpebral conjunctiva adheres, the condition is termed *symblepharon.* It bears a superficial resemblance to the human condition called *pterygium,* which does not occur in animals. Its most common cause is feline herpesvirus infection in young cats. In severe cases, the whole cornea may be affected. The conjunctival adhesion may be removed by superficial keratectomy, but regrowth may occur. With more extensive adhesions, reconstructive surgery may be needed to achieve a continuous conjunctival epithelial cover over the sclera or inside the eyelid. The techniques of Arlt and Teale-Knapp are illustrated (Figs. 86–31 through 86–33).

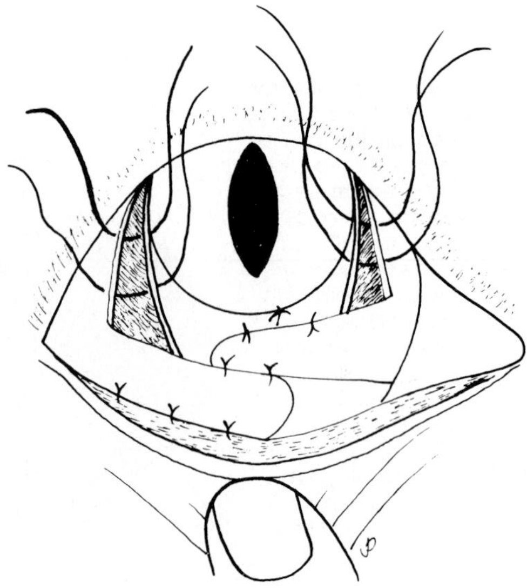

FIGURE 86–31. Teale-Knapp technique of symblepharon repair. Following mobilization of the symblepharon, the fornix is reconstructed using rotating conjunctival pedicle flaps from each side of the cornea. (Reprinted with permission from Peiffer RL: Feline ophthalmology. *In* Gelatt KN, [ed]: *Textbook of Veterinary Ophthalmology.* Lea & Febiger, Philadelphia, 1981.)

Ulcerative Keratitis[48]

A corneal ulcer is present when corneal epithelium and a variable amount of stroma are missing. Small acute ulcers heal rapidly, but chronic lesions may heal slowly if at all.

Progression

Corneal ulcers may progress to involve deeper layers, as shown in the box below. In treating corneal ulceration, the most important steps are to determine and remove the causes, to prevent progression, and to create an ideal environment for healing.

Surgical treatment is used to prevent or treat rupture of the cornea. Regardless of the cause, all corneal ulcers have the potential to evolve to perforation and endophthalmitis if not treated. The most common causes of corneal ulceration are listed in Table 86–1. The pathogenesis and progression of corneal ulcers have been reviewed.[38]

In simple traumatic injuries with small epithelial defects, healing is rapid. If the ulcer becomes infected or if the epithelium is unable to attach to the underlying stroma, healing is delayed and progression to a deep ulcer and beyond may occur. In chronic or infected ulcers, proteases may speed progression ("melting") of a simple ulcer to perforation and iris prolapse, sometimes within 24 hours. Proteases are produced by epithelium, bacteria (*Pseudomonas* spp. especially), neutrophils, and possibly stroma.[4, 19, 47] Their action is potentiated by corticosteroids. Proteases are not important in the pathogenesis of all ulcers. Those in which they are active have a gelatinous, bluish appearance around the margin, which must be distinguished from

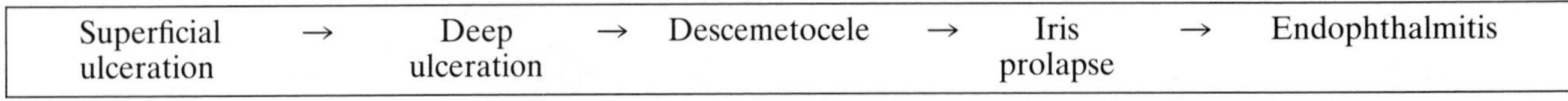

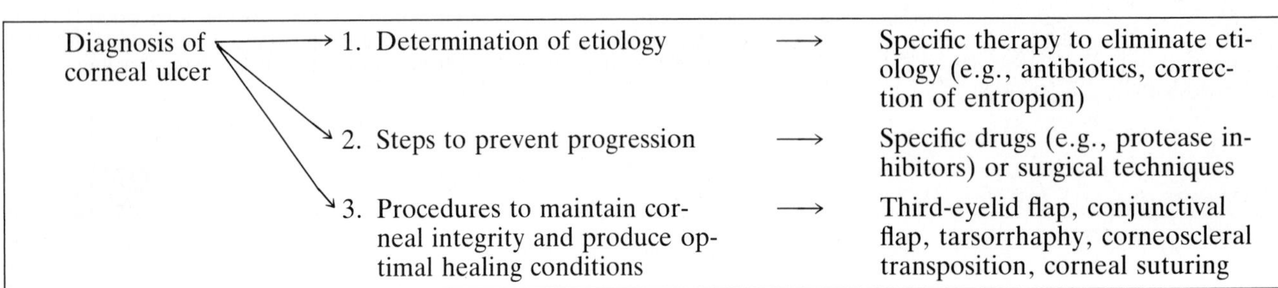

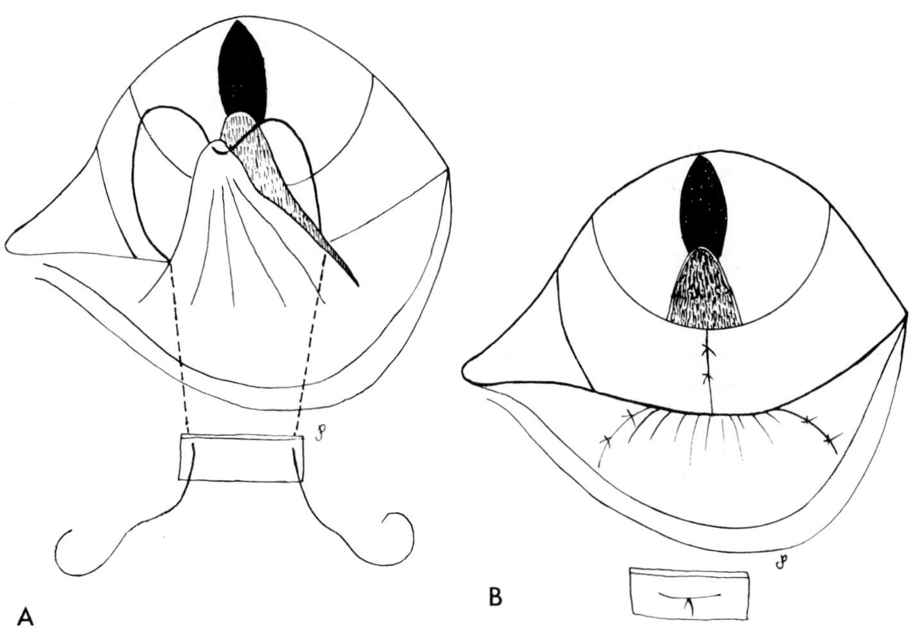

FIGURE 86–32. Arlt technique for symblepharon repair. *A,* The adherent conjunctiva is shaved off the cornea, and the incision continued onto the palpebral surface. A double-armed 4-0 (or 5-0) silk suture is passed through the mobilized flap and the eyelid to emerge at the edge of the lower orbital rim. *B,* The bulbar conjunctiva is mobilized by blunt dissection and sutured with 6-0 absorbable material. The flap of conjunctiva is sutured to the fornix with similar material. The knots may be buried. The skin sutures are tightened and tied over a tension device. (Reprinted with permission from Peiffer RL: Feline ophthalmology. *In* Gelatt KN: *Textbook of Veterinary Ophthalmology.* Lea & Febiger, Philadelphia, 1981.)

uncomplicated corneal edema found around most corneal wounds.

Diagnosis (Fig. 86–34)

Corneal ulcers are frequently invisible even with good lighting. Therefore, all red and painful eyes must be stained with fluorescein and the intraocular pressure measured. Ancillary diagnostic tests like bacterial culture and corneal scrapings for Gram and Giemsa staining are also useful.

The clinical handling of a corneal ulcer is summarized in Table 86–2. Occasionally, it is necessary to institute treatment phases 1 and 2 without knowing the cause of the ulcer, either because it is obscure or because the structural integrity of the eye must be preserved while awaiting laboratory results. The stage reached by the ulcer determines which methods are chosen in phases 2 and 3. In addition to the measures outlined, topical atropine (1 per cent TID) is applied to relieve pain due to ciliary spasm and secondary uveitis and to decrease formation of synechiae between a miotic pupil and the lens or central cornea.

No attempt is made to inhibit secondary uveitis or to

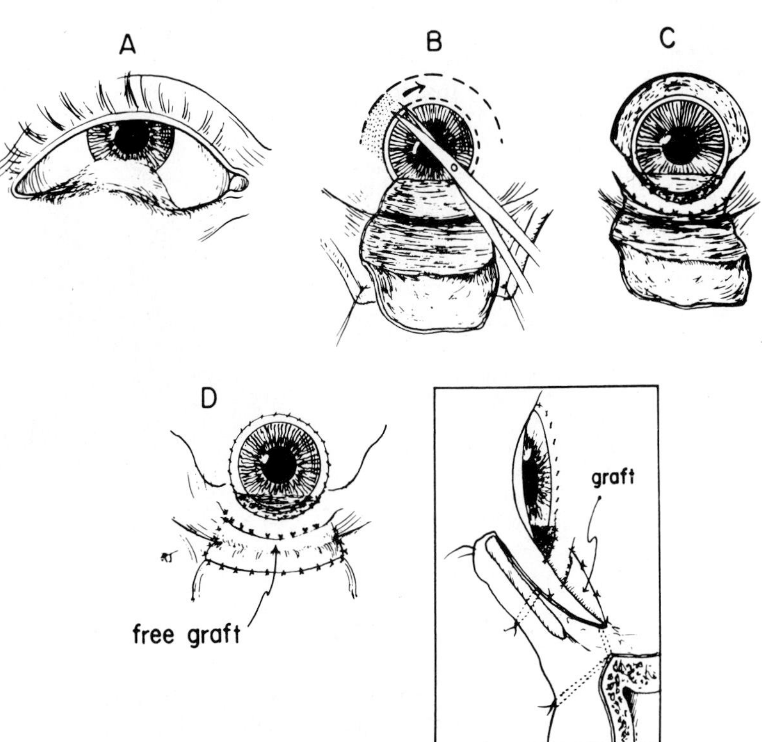

FIGURE 86–33. Variation of the Arlt technique for repair of symblepharon involving the cornea. *A, B,* and *C,* After freeing the conjunctiva from the cornea and sclera, a strip of bulbar conjunctiva is dissected 180° from the defect and mobilized across the cornea as a bridge flap to cover the sclera adjacent to the limbus. *D,* The conjunctiva dissected from the cornea is used to reline the palpebral surface, and a free graft has been used to reconstruct the fornix. Note deep sutures anchoring the forniceal portion of the graft to the orbital rim and passing through the skin. (Reprinted with permission from Tenzel RR: Statement of the problem and treatment of chemical injuries. *In* Guibor P, Gougleman H [eds]: *Problems and Treatments of Contracted Sockets, Exenterated Orbits and Alkali Burns.* Intercontinental Medical Book Co., New York, 1973.)

TABLE 86–1. ETIOLOGY OF CORNEAL ULCERATION

Dog	Cat
Trauma	Trauma
Foreign body	Foreign body
Distichiasis	Herpetic keratitis
Keratitis sicca	Entropion
Entropion	
Superficial corneal erosion	
Chronic corneal edema	
Tumors of lid margin	

remove purulent exudate from the anterior chamber. Chemical cautery (phenol, iodine) of corneal ulcers is not recommended. Careful débridement, use of antibiotics, and physical coverage of the lesion are more consistent with the principles of corneal wound healing. The following combination of antibiotics, atropine, antiprotease agents, and base is commonly and effectively used[48]:

Acetylcysteine 20 per cent 6 ml
Atropine ophthalmic solution 1 per cent 6 ml
Gentamicin 1.5 ml
Artificial tear solution daily to 25 ml

Acetylcysteine retains its potency at room temperature,[10] reducing the need for refrigeration. For details on other antiprotease agents, see standard veterinary ophthalmology texts.[17, 48]

In deep ulceration, descemetoceles, and perforated ulcers, systemic antibiotic therapy is used (e.g., amoxicillin *per os*). In perforated ulcers, systemic anti-inflammatory agents (acetylsalicylic acid) also are warranted.

Surgical Therapy

Mechanical support for ulcers often is warranted. Tarsorrhaphy, third-eyelid flaps, direct suturing of descemetoceles, and conjunctival flaps have been used successfully.

In uncomplicated ulcers, coverage with a third-eyelid flap should be maintained for 7 to 10 days. During this time, medications are placed on top of the flap. If any of the following signs appear, the flap is removed and the cornea examined:

1. Purulent discharge
2. Sudden voluminous watery discharge
3. Hemorrhagic discharge
4. Sudden, painful blepharospasm

Flaps usually relieve much of the discomfort of painful corneal lesions. A small amount of discharge from an eye with a third-eyelid flap is to be expected. The use of tissue adhesive has been described in humans[43] and anecdotally in animals, but its use has not become widespread, nor has it been confirmed by controlled studies.[29]

Deep ulcers may be treated with third-eyelid flaps or conjunctival grafts. With descemetoceles, third-eyelid flaps are insufficient to prevent rupture. Direct suturing of descemetoceles followed by a 360° conjunctival flap[48] or a conjunctival graft is preferred. Autogenous lamellar corneal transplantation or corneoscleral transposition also may be used (discussed earlier). Temporary partial lateral tarsorrhaphy may be used for additional support.

During the healing of any ulcer, corneal vascularization and scar formation may occur. Scar formation may

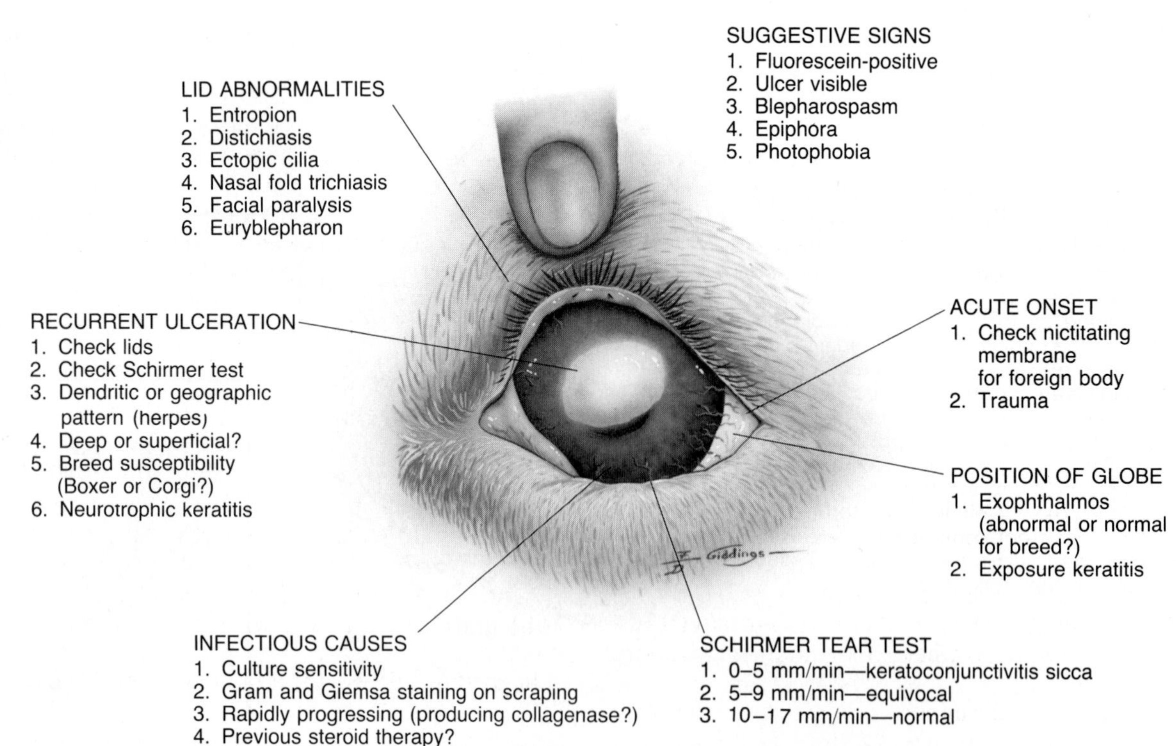

FIGURE 86–34. Clinical signs of corneal ulceration.

TABLE 86–2. TREATMENT OF CORNEAL ULCERATION

Type of Ulcer	Phase 1	Phase 2	Phase 3
Simple superficial ulcer	Topical antibiotics Correction of lid defects (e.g., entropion, cilia) Topical atropine	Rarely necessary	Rarely necessary
Uncomplicated deep ulcer	Topical antibiotics Topical atropine	Antiprotease agents Débridement	Third-eyelid flap Tear replacement
Complicated deep ulcer	Topical, subconjunctival, and systemic antibiotics (subpalpebral lavage) Topical atropine	Antiprotease agents Débridement (surgical, chemical)	Conjunctival or third-eyelid flap, conjunctival pedicle graft Tear replacement
Descemetocele	Topical, subconjunctival, and systemic antibiotics (subpalpebral lavage) Topical atropine	Antiprotease agents	Conjunctival or third-eyelid flap Tear replacement or corneoscleral transposition, conjunctival pedicle graft
Iris prolapse	Topical, subconjunctival, and systemic antibiotics (subpalpebral lavage) Topical atropine	Antiprotease agents	Resection or replacement of prolapsed iris Conjunctival or third-eyelid flap, conjunctival pedicle graft Suture lacerations Reconstitution of anterior chamber

be reduced by judicious topical use of corticosteroids after re-epithelialization is complete.

Conjunctival Pedicle Grafting

Conjunctival pedicle grafting is effective in saving the integrity of the eye in severe ulceration, with or without perforation.[22, 23] In the majority of cases, functional vision is also preserved. Conjunctival grafts are effective against enzymatic corneal melting, infection, and pain. They support the cornea well and supply vessels and fibroblasts to aid corneal healing.

Conjunctival pedicle grafts are prepared under general anesthesia with the eye positioned with the direction of gaze perpendicularly upward. Magnification with loupes or an operating microscope is necessary. Fixation sutures of 5-0 to 6-0 silk or nylon or microhemostats are attached at the limbus to stabilize the globe. Lateral canthotomy may be needed for exposure.

A recipient bed on the cornea is prepared by débriding the ulcer. Epithelium is scraped off the ulcer and off a 0.5- to 1-mm-wide zone around it with a number 64 Beaver blade. Loose, devitalized tissue and debris in the ulcer also are removed, if this can be done without risking perforation.

The pedicle is prepared from dorsolateral or dorsomedial bulbar conjunctiva. Dissection begins with a small conjunctival cut perpendicular to the limbus. This starting point is as far from the 12 o'clock position as the desired length of pedicle. Conjunctiva is undermined toward the 12 o'clock position with Stevens tenotomy scissors or smaller McPherson conjunctival scissors. Only the thin, transparent conjunctiva is freed. This is easier to accomplish when dissection is not begun immediately at the limbus, where the conjunctiva is more firmly attached.

The edge of the undermined conjunctiva is lifted with fine, toothed corneal forceps, and two parallel cuts are made with scissors to free a strip of conjunctiva along the limbus. The strip is made as wide as the width of the de-epithelialized zone around the ulcer, though not less than 3 to 4 mm. At the 12 o'clock position, the incision closest to the limbus is carried slightly farther than the more peripheral incision.

The conjunctival wound is closed by a continuous suture of 7-0 polyglactin 910, beginning at the pedicle base to appose this to the limbus.

The pedicle graft is spread flat on the cornea. Its end may be trimmed slightly to roughly fit the contour of the ulcer. Precise fitting is aided by the inherent elasticity of the conjunctiva. The graft must reach and cover the recipient bed on the cornea without tension. If additional length is needed, the two parallel conjunctival incisions are extended.

The graft is sutured to firm corneal stroma around the recipient bed with simple isolated sutures of 7-0 polyglactin 910, beginning ventrally and proceeding laterally and medially around the ulcer. The last sutures are placed dorsomedially and dorsolaterally to the ulcer. In large grafts and perforated, leaking ulcers, one suture is placed through the middle of the pedicle into the dorsal rim of the ulcer, taking care not to strangulate vessels in the pedicle. If pedicle width makes exposure difficult for placement of this suture, it can be placed as the first suture.

After completion of suturing, the de-epithelialized recipient bed is covered by a flatly spread graft end. Care is taken not to stretch the graft across the ulcer, causing graft ischemia, which is seen as immediate graft paleness on suture tightening.

Excessive slackness of the pedicle is also avoided. This can be adjusted by placing one suture at each side of the pedicle base to the limbus at completion of surgery.

In melting ulcers, the graft edges must cover all of the devitalized stroma and are sutured into viable stroma around the lesion. For medially and laterally located ulcers, the graft can be prepared more medially and laterally, respectively. The graft need not be vertical, but an angle of more than 45° from the vertical should be avoided. Otherwise, eyelid movements tend to dislodge the graft.

Canthotomies are closed in two layers. A partial temporary lateral tarsorrhaphy is performed with 4-0 to 3-0 nylon to close the lateral one-third to two-thirds of the eyelid opening. Elizabethan collars are not needed routinely.

Aftercare includes daily cleaning of the eye with warm, wet compresses. Medications include topical antibiotic solution (three to four times daily), topical atropine solution (three times daily), and possibly systemic antibiotics and anti-inflammatory drugs.

Patients are re-evaluated 2 to 4 days after surgery and then weekly or as indicated. After 1 to 3 weeks, when the graft has adhered securely and the cornea is fluorescein negative, topical corticosteroid therapy is added to the regimen to decrease corneal neovascularization and scarring. This begins with one application daily and is increased to twice daily after another week. Antibiotics are given topically as long as the cornea is fluorescein positive or as long as signs of infection are present. Systemic antibiotics are given for 7 to 10 days with corneal perforation. Systemic anti-inflammatory therapy is tapered off slowly in accordance with clinical progress. Low-dose anti-inflammatory therapy is often continued for several weeks. The graft is left in place for several months to allow for corticosteroid treatment of keratitis under protection of the vascularized graft. In recurrent deep ulceration (e.g., in brachycephalic dogs), the pedicle graft is left intact permanently. The pedicle may be removed under topical anesthesia using small scissors. Pretreatment with one drop of epinephrine (1 per cent) decreases hemorrhage. A scar and graft remnants remain at the ulcer site but thin with time.

Conjunctival flaps covering parts or all of the cornea (360° flaps) are prepared by undermining the conjunctiva from the limbus peripherally and suturing it to the cornea or to conjunctiva from across the eye.

Corneal Neoplasia

Corneal neoplasms are uncommon in dogs and cats. Squamous cell carcinomas are the most common, especially in lightly pigmented animals. These tumors may involve conjunctiva, lids, and cornea. Depending on the extent of invasion, they are treated by surgical excision, beta irradiation, or cryotherapy. Surgical methods include superficial keratectomy, corneoscleral transposition, and corneoscleral allografting. Chemotherapy and immunotherapy for squamous cell carcinomas have not been described extensively in small animals.

Dermoids (Dermolipoma)

Dermoids usually afflict both conjunctiva and cornea. Those involving the cornea are removed by superficial keratectomy with local conjunctivectomy. Dermoids may extend into deep corneal layers. Even after uneventful keratectomy, corneal scarring may occur.

Feline Focal Corneal Necrosis[15]

Focal corneal necrosis (corneal mummification,[54] sequestration[6, 48]) occurs most commonly in Persian and Siamese cats. The cause is unknown, but the disease usually occurs after previous ulceration or keratitis (e.g., herpesvirus felis keratitis). It consists of brown to black areas of necrotic stroma tightly attached to the cornea. The lesion may extend down to the Descemet membrane.

Clinical Signs

Clinical signs include (1) a slowly progressive, focal, brownish-black corneal lesion, often of several months duration; (2) corneal vascularization; (3) epiphora; and (4) pain and blepharospasm. Very mild lesions appear like a superficial ulcer with an amber hue in the stroma.

Treatment

Before treatment is attempted, the lesion should have ceased to enlarge, because a nonprogressive lesion is less likely to recur postoperatively. If herpetic keratitis is present, the lesion must be quiescent. The necrotic material is removed by superficial keratectomy before healing occurs. The use of an operating microscope is recommended because the lesion often is deep. Extreme care must be used not to perforate the cornea during surgery. Postoperatively, the eye is covered with a third-eyelid flap and treated with topical antibiotics and atropine as for an ulcer (see Table 86–2). Topical corticosteroids should not be used at any stage because of the frequency of herpesvirus as the cause. The condition tends to recur. After excision of very deep or large lesions, a conjunctival pedicle graft may be placed. Recurrence seems to be less likely in the presence of vascularization, as with a pedicle in place.

ADVANCES IN CORNEAL SURGERY AND THERAPEUTICS

Viscoelastic Substances

Sodium hyaluronate is a viscous disaccharide polymer that is widely used during intraocular procedures in humans. It is instilled into the anterior chamber during surgery to facilitate dissection, protect the corneal endothelium, and prevent adhesions between tissues. Sterile methycellulose is more economical for use in animals and has equivalent properties.

Hydrophilic Contact Lenses

Hydrophilic contact lenses may be used to cover corneas with severe bullous keratopathy or persistent epithelial erosions. They can also be used to deliver drugs to the cornea in high concentrations.[50] A lens that fits the eye properly is soaked in an antibiotic solution until saturated with the drug and then is applied to the eye. Antibiotic diffuses from the lens and enters the cornea in high concentrations. The lens must be recharged with drug several times daily, the frequency depending on the properties of the drug and the composition of the lens. A dissolving collagen lens is available for similar coverage and application of drugs. This lens or shield is never used to cover deep ulcers or in the presence of uncontrolled infection.

References

1. Bahn CF, et al: Complications associated with bovine corneal endothelial cell-lined homografts in the cat. *Invest Ophthalmol Vis Sci 22*:73, 1982.
2. Barraquer JI: Corneoplastic surgery. Proceedings of the International Corneoplastic Conference, London, England, 1967.
3. Barrie KP, et al: Quantitation of uveoscleral outflow in normotensive and glaucomatous beagles by 3H-labeled dextran. *Am J Vet Res 46*:84, 1985.
4. Befanis PJ, et al: Endothelial repair of the canine cornea. *Am J Vet Res 21*:113, 1981.
5. Berman MB, et al: Characterization of collagenolytic activity in the ulcerating cornea. *Exp Eye Res 11*:225, 1971.
6. Blogg JR: *The Eye in Veterinary Practice.* W.B. Saunders, Philadelphia, 1980.
7. Brightman AH, et al: Autogenous lamellar corneal grafting in dogs. *J Am Vet Med Assoc 195*:469, 1989.
8. Brown SI: Collagenase and corneal ulcers. *Invest Ophthalmol 10*:203, 1971.
9. Chan-Ling T, et al: Diurnal variation of corneal thickness in the cat. *Invest Ophthalmol Vis Sci 26*:102, 1985.
10. Costa ND, Slatter DH: The potency of acetylcysteine in pharmaceutical preparations—effects of temperature and storage. *Aust Vet J 60*:195, 1983.
11. Dice PF, et al: Experimental autogenous and homologous corneal transplantation in the dog. *J Am Anim Hosp Assoc 9*:245, 1973.
12. Duke-Elder S, Leigh AG: *System of Ophthalmology.* Vol VIII. *Diseases of the Outer Eye, Part 2.* Henry Kimpton, London, 1965.
13. Eisner G: *Eye surgery: An Introduction to Operative Technique.* Springer-Verlag, Berlin, 1980.
14. Epstein RJ, Stunting ROD: Corneal neovascularization induced by stimulated lymphocytes in inbred mice. *Invest Ophthalmol Vis Sci 28*:1505, 1987.
15. Formston C, et al: Corneal necrosis in the cat. *J Small Anim Pract 15*:19, 1974.
16. Gelatt KN: Excision of adenocarcinoma of iris and ciliary body. *J Am Anim Hosp Assoc 6*:59, 1970.
17. Gelatt KN: *Veterinary Ophthalmology.* Lea & Febiger, Philadelphia, 1981.
18. Gelatt KN, Samuelson DA: Recurrent corneal erosions and epithelial dystrophy in the boxer dog. *J Am Anim Hosp Assoc 18*:453, 1982.
19. Gordon JM, et al: Collagenase in human cornea immunologic localization. *Arch Ophthalmol 98*:341, 1980.
20. Gwin RL, et al: Decrease in canine corneal endothelial cell density and increase in corneal thickness as functions of age. *Invest Ophthalmol Vis Sci 22*:267, 1982.
21. Gwin RL, et al: Primary canine corneal endothelial cell dystrophy: Specular microscopic evaluation and therapy. *J Am Anim Hosp Assoc 18*:471, 1982.
22. Håkanson NE, Merideth RE: Conjunctival pedicle grafting in the treatment of corneal ulcers in the dog and cat. *J Am Anim Hosp Assoc 23*:641, 1987.
23. Håkanson NE, et al: Further comments on conjunctival pedicle grafting in the treatment of corneal ulcers in the dog and cat. *J Am Anim Hosp Assoc 24*:602, 1988.
24. Havener WH: *Ocular Pharmacology.* 3rd ed. C.V. Mosby, St. Louis, 1983.
25. Hogan MJ, et al: *Histology of the Human Eye.* W.B. Saunders, Philadelphia, 1962.
26. Khodadoust AA: Lamellar corneal transplantation in the rabbit. *Am J Ophthalmol 66*:1111, 1968.
27. Kirschner SE, et al: Ultrastructural morphology of persistent corneal erosions in dogs: A preliminary report. Proceedings of the American College of Veterinary Ophthalmologists, New Orleans, LA, Nov, 1986, p 492.
28. Kirschner SE, et al: Idiopathic persistent corneal erosions: Clinical and pathological findings in 18 dogs. *J Am Anim Hosp Assoc 25*:84, 1989.
29. Koch SA: Presented at the American College of Veterinary Ophthalmologists 12th Annual Scientific Meeting, Incline Village, NV, Oct–Nov, 1982.
30. Koch SA, et al: Corneal epithelial inclusion cysts in four dogs. *J Small Anim Pract 164*:1192, 1974.
31. Kuhns EL, et al: The treatment of pannus in dogs by use of a corneal scleral graft. *J Am Vet Med Assoc 162*:950, 1973.
32. Martin CL: Canine epibulbar melanomas and their management. *J Am Anim Hosp Assoc 17*:83, 1981.
33. Maurice DM: The location of the fluid pump in the cornea. *J Physiol (Lond) 221*:43, 1972.
34. McIntyre J: Experimental penetrating keratoplasty in the dog. *Arch Ophthalmol 80*:372, 1968.
35. Miller D, et al: Topical flurbiprofen or prednisolone: Effect on corneal wound healing in rabbits. *Arch Ophthalmol 99*:681, 1981.
36. Morrin LA, et al: Oval lipid opacities in beagles: Ultrastructure of normal beagle cornea. *Am J Vet Res 43*:443, 1982.
37. Moses RA: *Adler's Physiology of the Eye.* 6th ed. C.V. Mosby, St. Louis, 1975.
38. Nassise, MY: Canine ulcerative keratitis. *Comp Cont Educ Pract Vet 7*:686, 1985.
39. Parshall CJ: Lamellar corneal-scleral transposition. *J Am Anim Hosp Assoc 9*:270, 1973.
40. Peiffer RL, et al: Superficial keratectomy in the management of indolent ulcers of the boxer cornea. *Canine Pract 3*:31, 1976.
41. Pfister RR: The healing of corneal epithelial abrasions in the rabbit: A scanning electron microscope study. *Invest Ophthalmol 14*:648, 1968.
42. Prince JH, et al: *Anatomy and Histology of the Eye and Orbit in Domestic Animals.* Charles C Thomas, Springfield, IL, 1960, pp 73, 107.
43. Refojo MF, et al: Evaluation of adhesives for corneal surgery. *Arch Ophthalmol 80*:645, 1968.
44. Roberts SR: Superficial indolent ulcer of the cornea in boxer dogs. *J Small Anim Pract 6*:111, 1966.
45. Rosenthal JJ: Bullous keratopathy: A latent complication of chronic corneal diseases. *Vet Med Small Anim Clin 69*:181, 1974.
46. Shively JN, Epling GP: Fine structure of the canine eye: Cornea. *Am J Vet Res 31*:713, 1970.
47. Slansky HH, Dohlman CH: Collagenase and the cornea. *Surv Ophthalmol 14*:402, 1970.
48. Slatter D: *Fundamentals of Veterinary Ophthalmology.* 2nd ed. W.B. Saunders, Philadelphia, 1990.
49. Spencer WH (ed): *Ophthalmic Pathology—An Atlas and Textbook.* W.B. Saunders, Philadelphia, 1985.
50. Troutman RC: *Microsurgery of the Anterior Segment of the Eye.* C.V. Mosby, St. Louis, 1974.
51. van Ee RT, et al: The effects of nylon and polyglactin 910 suture material on corneal wound healing in the canine. Proceedings of the American College of Veterinary Ophthalmologists, Atlanta, GA, Nov, 1984, pp 144–145.
52. Van Horn DL, Hyndiuk RA: Endothelial wound repair in primate cornea. *Exp Eye Res 21*:113, 1975.
53. Van Horn DL, et al: Regenerative capacity of the corneal endothelium in the rabbit. *Invest Ophthalmol 16*:597, 1977.
54. Verger MA: Partial mummification of the cornea in cats—the corneal sequestrum. Proceedings of the 32nd annual meeting of the American Animal Hospital Association, Apr, 1965, p 112.

CHAPTER

87 Iris and Ciliary Body

Cynthia S. Cook and Robert L. Peiffer, Jr.

Indications for surgical manipulation of the iris and ciliary body are infrequent in veterinary ophthalmology, with the exception of treatment of glaucoma (see Chapter 92). This chapter examines iridotomy as a means of controlling pupillary aperture, pupillary membranectomy to manage common complications of cataract surgery, iridectomy and iridocyclectomy for removing localized anterior segment neoplasms, and aspiration of iris and ciliary body epithelial cysts.

SURGICAL ANATOMY AND PHYSIOLOGY

The iris and ciliary body consist of connective tissue stroma of neural crest origin, lined posteriorly by a two-layered epithelium of neuroectodermal origin. The iris epithelium is heavily pigmented with melanin in both layers; the basilar portion of the anterior layer is made up of smooth muscle, which forms the dilator muscle of the iris, an alpha-adrenergic smooth muscle. This layer continues posteriorly over the ciliary body as a densely pigmented sheet of cuboidal cells continuous with the retinal pigmented epithelium. The posterior pigmented iris epithelium lines the pupil as the "pupillary ruff" and continues as a nonpigmented epithelial layer over the surface of the ciliary body, continuous with the neural retina. The bilayered posterior iris epithelium is pigmented even in blue-eyed individuals; only in true albinos is it devoid of melanin granules. The stromal melanin gives the iris its characteristic color. The iris is grossly divided by the collarette into a peripheral ciliary zone and a thinner central pupillary zone.

The pupillary zone contains the sphincter muscle, formed by a 1.5-mm ring of smooth muscle encircling the pupil within the posterior stroma. The pupillary sphincter is a cholinergic smooth muscle that constricts to produce miosis. The phenomenon can be induced with parasympathomimetic drugs and also occurs in response to the release of prostaglandins and other mediators of inflammation.[11]

Ciliary body landmarks include the ora ciliaris retinae, or junction between the pars plana of the ciliary body and the peripheral retina; this area in dogs is located 8 mm posterior to the limbus superiorly and temporally but only 4 mm inferiorly and nasally.[3] Iridocyclectomy extending posterior to the ora may cause peripheral retinal dialysis and detachment. The ciliary epithelium produces aqueous humor; although it is not clear to what extent this tissue can be excised without impairing aqueous humor dynamics, it is probably less than 25 per cent. The zonules arise from both the pars plana and the pars plicata of the ciliary body. Manipulations that cause extensive zonular disruption may lead to lens dislocation or ciliary body hemorrhage.

The iris and ciliary body receive a vascular supply from the long posterior ciliary arteries, which originate from the ophthalmic artery near the posterior pole and follow a trans-scleral and intrachoroidal route to the anterior segment. The anterior ciliary arteries, which are continuations of the muscular branches of the ophthalmic artery, enter the globe at the insertions of the extraocular muscles. They contribute less significantly to anterior uveal perfusion in dogs than in primates. Each long posterior ciliary artery terminates as a medial and lateral branch entering the iris at the 9 and 3 o'clock positions. They branch dorsally and ventrally along the peripheral half of the ciliary zone to form the major arterial circle, which is incomplete at the 12 and 6 o'clock positions. Radial vessels emanate from this circle, traveling toward the pupil as well as retrograde into the ciliary body, where they anastomose with the short posterior ciliary arteries. The vessels lack perivascular connective tissue sheaths, which minimize surgical hemorrhage in primates.[10] Significant bleeding is usually avoided, however, if the major arterial circle is not transected. Fibrinous exudation from the iris vasculature and miosis are frequent surgical complications that can be minimized by preoperative treatment with systemic and topical antiprostaglandins (aspirin, 32.5 mg/kg; flunixin, 1.1 mg/kg; flurbiprofen or indomethacin drops) and topical mydriatics and corticosteroids. Intracameral application of agents such as epinephrine (1:100,000) and heparin (2 units/ml) can be helpful in maintaining mydriasis and inhibiting fibrin clot formation. Topical, subconjunctival, and systemic corticosteroids and topical mydriatics are used postoperatively to reduce surgically induced inflammation, thereby decreasing the incidence of complications.

SPHINCTER IRIDOTOMY

The most common indication for sphincter iridotomy is enlargement of the pupillary aperture during cataract surgery. If the pupil constricts before lens extraction or is less than 3 mm after extraction, a one- to four-quadrant sphincterotomy is performed as necessary to enhance exposure or achieve at least a 5-mm pupil. The technique is described and illustrated in Figure 87–1. Incision with scissors is preferable to grasping and tearing because it is less traumatic and more readily controlled. Significant hemorrhage can usually be avoided if the major arterial circle in the base of the ciliary zone is avoided; an incision can safely be made to a depth of 2 to 3 mm. Incisions at the 12 or 6 o'clock positions, where the major arterial circle is incomplete, are preferred. If hemorrhage does occur, closing the eye and re-establishing the anterior chamber and intraocular pressure may be helpful to hasten clot formation. After

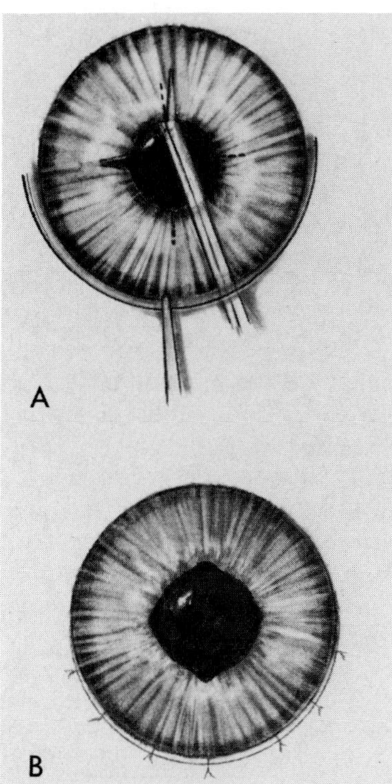

FIGURE 87–1. Iridotomy. *A,* Enlargement of the pupillary aperture may be achieved by incising the sphincter muscle of the iris. The procedure is best performed with sharp scissors and a formed anterior chamber in the superior and lateral quadrants; gentle retraction of the cornea and an "open sky" technique are necessary to incise the iris at the 12 o'clock position. Minimizing the incision to a depth of 2 mm prevents significant hemorrhage. *B,* The resultant pupil appears diamond shaped rather than round if four-quadrant sphincterotomy is performed.

several minutes, blood and clots may be gently irrigated or extracted from the anterior chamber.

The neodymium:yttrium-aluminum-garnet (Nd:YAG) laser at low energy levels (1.0 to 1.7 mJ) has also been used to perform iridotomies in primates.[13] Elevation in aqueous humor prostaglandin levels and a transient increase in intraocular pressure were observed after this procedure,[7, 9] although the lens was not damaged.[6] As with any surgical manipulation of the iris and ciliary body, the differences in the structure of the uveal vasculature of the canine eye may predispose to a more exaggerated inflammatory response.[10]

As in all intraocular surgery, care is taken to avoid corneal endothelial damage; gentle irrigation is minimal and directed away from the endothelium, and instruments must not contact the endothelial surface.

PUPILLARY MEMBRANECTOMY

The formation of opaque pupillary iridocapsular membranes is one of the more common complications of extracapsular cataract extraction in dogs and may also occur after anterior uveitis, especially lens-induced uveitis. If extensive, these membranes may impair vision or block the flow of aqueous, precipitating secondary glaucoma. When the lens is present, a sector iridectomy may be indicated in a combined procedure to increase aqueous humor outflow. However, in an aphakic animal, membranectomy is a simple and effective secondary procedure that frequently allows the patient to see, salvaging an otherwise unsuccessful cataract surgery. When available, a Nd:YAG laser is ideally suited to the incision of such membranes. The technique for needle capsulotomy is illustrated in Figure 87–2. One needle is used for infusion to maintain the anterior chamber, and another for transection of the membrane.

EXCISIONAL PROCEDURES FOR TREATMENT OF ANTERIOR UVEAL NEOPLASIA

The therapeutic approach required for management of an anterior uveal mass is based on an accurate diagnosis (Fig. 87–3). Proliferative ocular lesions may be either neoplastic or inflammatory in origin. In cats, iritis may mimic neoplasia, with a nodular appearance unassociated with classic signs of flare and miosis. In such cases, a positive response to systemic and topical corticosteroids is usually diagnostic. For masses that are clearly neoplastic, a thorough systemic evaluation is necessary to differentiate primary ocular neoplasia from neoplasia that has metastasized from a distant site. The

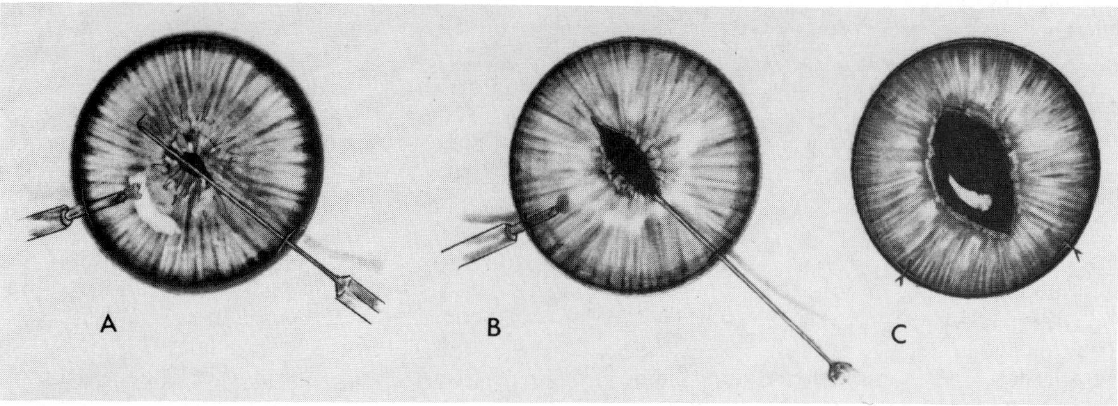

FIGURE 87–2. Pupillary membranectomy. *A,* Two 2- to 3-mm limbal incisions are made at the 4 and 8 o'clock positions. An infusion port or needle is placed through one incision, and a 27-gauge needle with its tip bent 90° is placed through the other. *B,* The needle is rotated and its tip manipulated to engage the iris. The needle is gently depressed and drawn across the membrane. *C,* The instruments are withdrawn, and the incisions are closed with interrupted sutures of 7-0 polyglactin 910 (Vicryl).

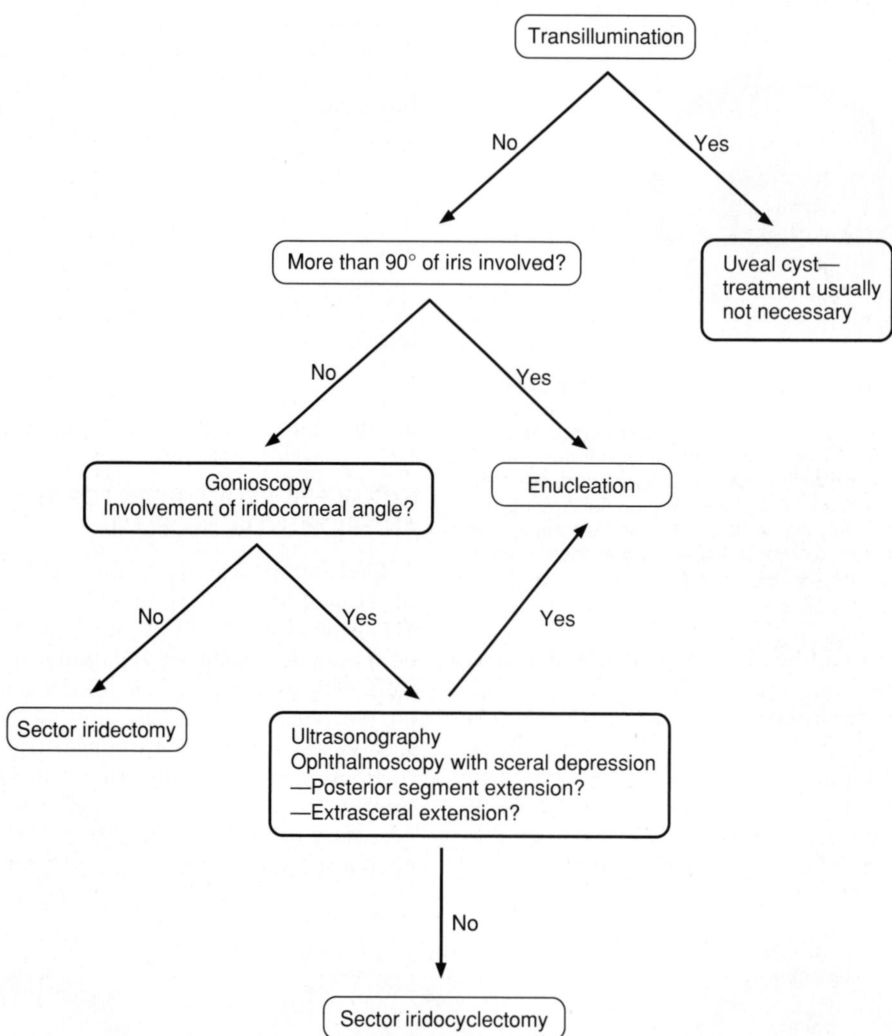

FIGURE 87–3. Diagnosis and management of an anterior uveal mass. Visual globe with no evidence of metastatic disease or inflammatory etiology.

excisional surgical procedures described here are applicable only to primary tumors with limited ocular involvement. The risks of a surgical procedure on an eye with a potentially malignant tumor must be weighed against the advantages of preserving a cosmetic, visual globe. Ocular melanomas in cats are often highly malignant, with widespread and fatal metastases.[2, 8] In one retrospective evaluation of ocular melanomas in dogs, 16 of 91 were histologically malignant, with metastasis confirmed in 3 cases.[12] In contrast, limbal melanomas are consistently benign, although they may be locally invasive. The preferred treatment for limbal melanomas is partial excision and cryotherapy; iridocyclectomy is indicated only if the base of the iris is involved to a depth of more than 3 mm.

IRIDECTOMY

Sector iridectomy (Fig. 87–4) is indicated for excisional biopsy of iris neoplasia. The iris may be incised to a depth of 2 to 3 mm without significant hemorrhage; deeper incisions should be made using wet-field cautery. In addition to the usual care taken to prevent trauma to the corneal endothelium, contact with the anterior lens capsule is avoided because the underlying epithelium may be damaged, resulting in cataract formation.

Iridocryothermy has been applied experimentally in dogs[1] and might be clinically useful in the management of localized benign iris neoplasms.

IRIDOCYCLECTOMY

Partial excision of the iris and ciliary body is used infrequently for anterior uveal tumors. This technique may be used to remove cilary adenomas, which usually involve only the ciliary processes. Anterior uveal malignant melanomas and ciliary body adenocarcinomas are usually diagnosed only when they have been present for some time and have extended into the aqueous outflow pathways or posteriorly into the choroid, retina, or deep sclera. The ideal surgical candidate has an uninvolved iridocorneal angle on gonioscopic examination, a discrete, well-defined lesion confined to the iris or ciliary body, and no secondary uveitis or glaucoma. A thorough clinical examination, including indirect ophthalmoscopy with scleral depression under general anesthesia, critical transillumination, and ultrasonography,[4] facilitates this challenging clinical diagnosis (see Fig. 87–3). In most

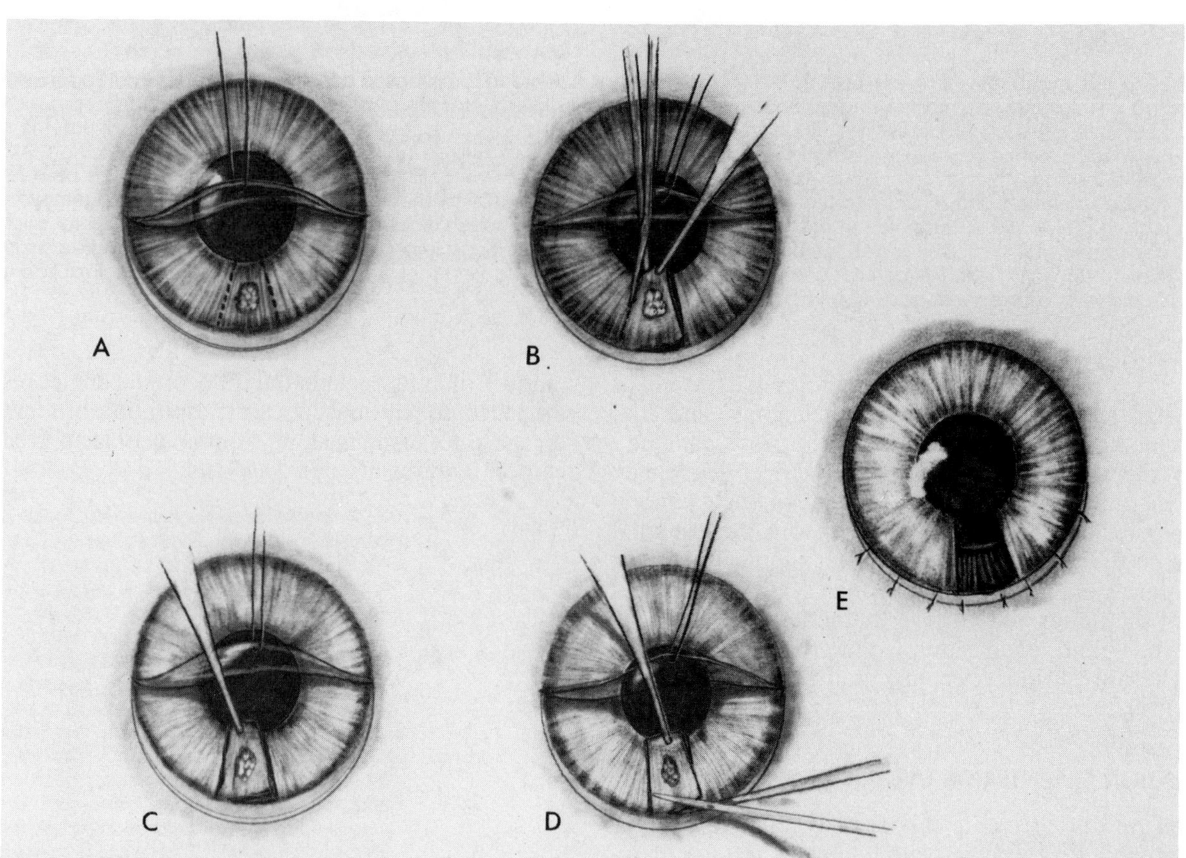

FIGURE 87–4. Sector iridectomy for excisional biopsy of an inferior iris lesion. *A*, After an inferior 180° corneoscleral incision, the cornea is gently retracted. Lesions in the superior quadrants are excised with a similar incision and a formed anterior chamber. Broken lines indicate area of planned excision. Note that liberal margins of grossly normal tissue are allowed. *B*, While exerting gentle traction on the pupillary margin, the lateral iris margins are incised with scissors or cautery. If hemorrhage does occur, the corneal flap is replaced, the anterior chamber is formed, and the bleeding vessels are allowed to clot before irrigating the anterior chamber and proceeding. *C* and *D*, The base of the iris can be transected by tearing *(C)* or by incision *(D)*. *E*, Postoperative appearance. The corneoscleral incision is closed with interrupted sutures of 7-0 polyglactin 910 (Vicryl), and the anterior chamber is reformed with lactated Ringer or a similar solution. The lens equator, zonules, and ciliary processes will be seen through the keyhole pupil.

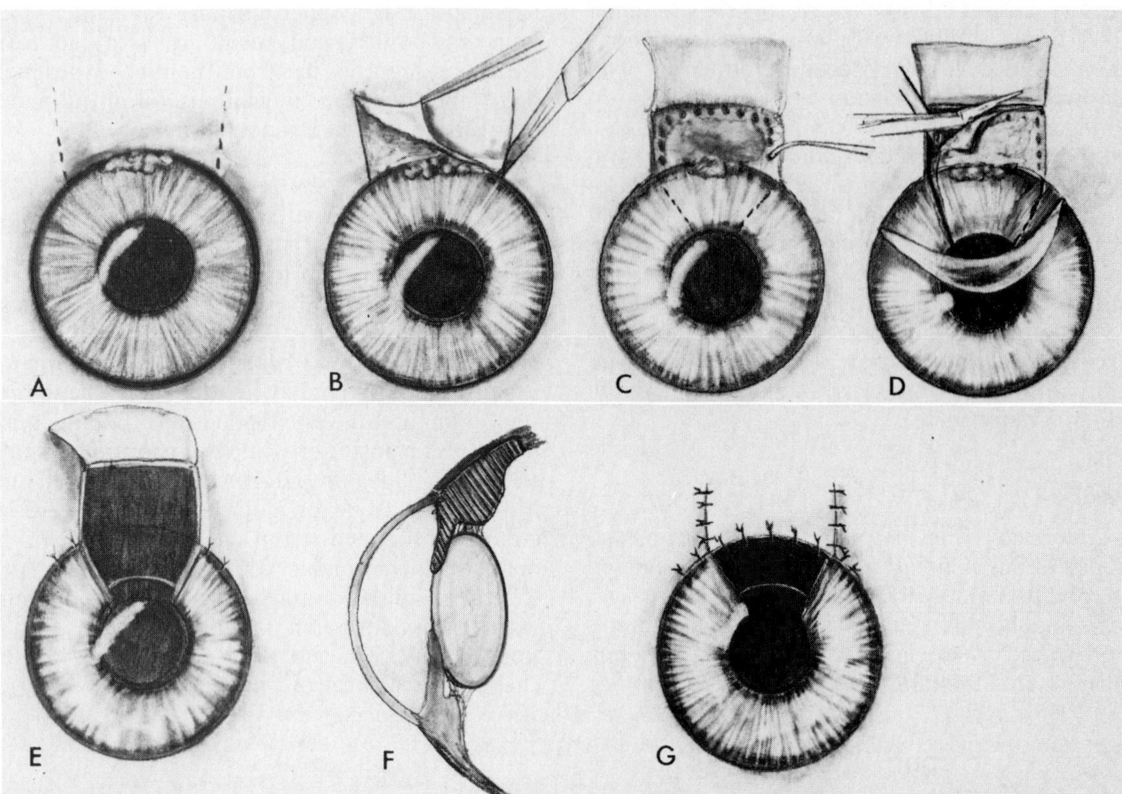

FIGURE 87–5. Iridocyclectomy for excision of an anterior uveal tumor. *A*, A broad fornix-based conjunctival flap is prepared and retracted; conjunctiva is not shown to simplify the drawings. Broken lines indicate lateral margins of planned scleral flap and deeper excision. *B*, With sharp dissection, a half-thickness posterior-based scleral flap is prepared. *C*, Cautery is applied around the margins of the excised flap to minimize hemorrhage when the underlying ciliary body is excised. Broken lines indicate extent of planned iris excision. *D* and *E*, A corneoscleral incision is made beyond the extent of planned excision to allow mobility of the corneal flap. Scissors are used to excise the iris, the deep cornea and sclera, and the ciliary body along the area made by the flap. A suction cutter is used to remove vitreous if it appears in the wound. *F*, The hatched area indicates the tissues excised, which include the deep sclera and peripheral cornea, the iridocorneal angle structures, the iris, and the ciliary body. *G*, The flap and corneoscleral incision are closed with interrupted sutures of 7-0 polyglactin 910 (Vicryl), and the anterior chamber is reformed with lactated Ringer or a similar solution. The conjunctival flap may be sutured in place or allowed to reposition and heal without sutures.

cases, 45° to 60° is the maximum tolerable extent of uveal excision. Although invasive melanomas and adenocarcinomas may be removed with this technique,[5] involvement of the angle structures and deep sclera may makes it difficult to define the extent of such tumors. The possibility of residual neoplasm with the potential for metastasis is high. In addition, manipulation during the surgical procedure may enhance seeding or metastasis of the tumor. We believe that unless the contralateral eye is blind, enucleation is the procedure of choice in such cases. Iridocyclectomy is illustrated in Figure 87–5.

ASPIRATION OF ANTERIOR UVEAL CYSTS

Cysts of the iris and ciliary body epithelium may develop spontaneously or subsequent to trauma or inflammation. They may be attached to the ciliary processes or pupillary margin or may be observed floating free in the anterior chamber. These are distinguished clinically by their regular margins and transparency when transilluminated. Although benign, they may be aspirated if they become excessively large, if they contact the corneal endothelium, or rarely, when a large number of cysts occlude the iridocorneal angle, resulting in glaucoma. In unusual cases, aspiration of a cyst may be used to distinguish it from a neoplasm when the clinical features are not diagnostic.

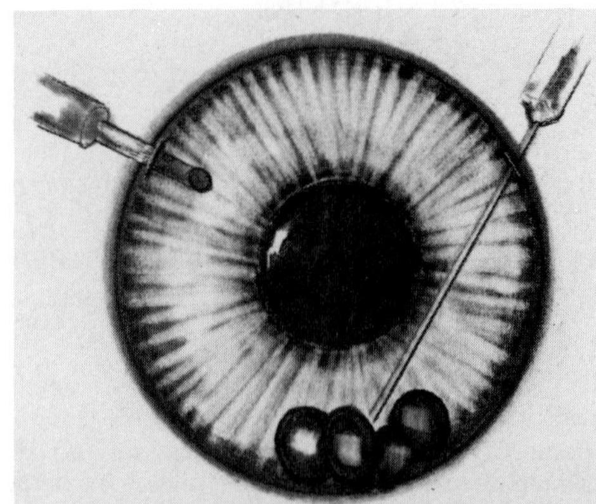

FIGURE 87–6. Aspiration of pupillary cysts. Incisions identical to those described for membranectomy are made at the 10 and 2 o'clock positions, and the infusion port is inserted. A straight 25-gauge needle is used to aspirate the cysts.

If available, a Nd:YAG laser is ideally suited to the disruption of this avascular uveal tissue. An alternative surgical technique uses two needles as described for a membranectomy; a straight 25-gauge needle is used for aspiration (Fig. 87–6). As the cyst is aspirated, the bevel of the needle is used to transect the base of the cyst if it is attached to uveal tissue. Aspirated tissue is submitted for histopathological examination.

References

1. Barrie K, et al: Effects of iridocryothermy in the normal dog. *Am J Vet Res 41*:51, 1980.
2. Bertoy RW, et al: Intraocular melanoma with multiple metastases in a cat. *J Am Vet Med Assoc 192*:87, 1988.
3. Donovan RJ, et al: Histology of the normal collie eye. II. Uvea. *Ophthalmology 6*:1175, 1974.
4. Dziezyc J, et al: Two-dimensional real-time ocular ultrasonography in the diagnosis of ocular lesions in dogs. *J Am Anim Hosp Assoc 23*:501, 1987.
5. Gelatt K, et al: Excision of an adenocarcinoma of the iris and ciliary body in a dog. *J Am Anim Hosp Assoc 6*:59, 1970.
6. Higginbotham EJ, Ogura Y: Lens clarity after argon and neodymium-YAG laser iridotomy in the rabbit. *Arch Ophthalmol 105*:540, 1987.
7. Liu SJ, et al: Study of prostaglandins and intraocular pressure in rabbits after Nd:YAG laser anterior segment procedure. *Ophthalmic Surg 19*:112, 1988.
8. Patnaik AK, Mooney S: Feline melanoma: A comparative study of ocular, oral, and dermal neoplasms. *Vet Pathol 25*:105, 1988.
9. Tawara A, Inomata H: Histological study on transient ocular hypertension after laser iridotomy in rabbits. *Graefes Arch Clin Exp Ophthalmol 225*:114, 1987.
10. Van Buskirk EM: The canine eye: The vessels of aqueous drainage. *Invest Ophthalmol Vis Sci 18*:223, 1979.
11. Van Buskirk EM: The ciliary vasculature and its perturbation with drugs and surgery. *Trans Am Ophthalmol Soc 86*:794, 1989.
12. Wilcock BP, Peiffer RL Jr: Morphology and behavior of primary ocular melanomas in 91 dogs. *Vet Pathol 23*:418, 1986.
13. Wise JB: Large iridotomies by the linear incision technique using the neodymium:YAG laser at low energy levels. A study using cynomologus monkeys. *Ophthalmology 94*:82, 1987.

CHAPTER 88 The Lens

Robert L. Peiffer, Jr.

Surgery of the lens is limited to extraction, which is indicated when visual impairment is due to opacification, when the lens is dislocated, and when lens-induced uveitis does not respond to medical therapy.

EMBRYOLOGY

The lens forms from the lens placode, which develops from surface ectoderm by induction by the underlying optic vesicle between days 15 and 17 of gestation in dogs. The placode invaginates and separates from the surface to form the spherical lens vesicle by the 19th gestational day. The cells lining the posterior of the sphere elongate anteriorly, resulting in a solid structure totally enclosed by epithelial cell basement membrane (lens capsule) and lined anteriorly by cuboidal epithelial cells. Obliteration of the lens vesicle cavity is completed by 30 days of gestation. These fibers remain at the central core of the lens as the embryonic nucleus.

The cells along the equator elongate in an anterior and posterior direction between the capsule, with its anterior monolayer of epithelium, and the embryonic nucleus by the 25th day of gestation. As fibers from the opposite side meet, they are sealed together by an amorphous cement substance. These terminal junctions collectively form a Y pattern called the *anterior and posterior suture lines;* the posterior Y is inverted, compared with the upright anterior Y. The fibers formed before birth make up the fetal nucleus. Cell division and elongation continue after birth and throughout life, resulting in compaction of central lens fibers and forming the adult nucleus. The zone of "young" lens fibers between capsule and nucleus is the cortex.

Although the lens is an avascular tissue in adults, *in utero* it is enveloped posteriorly by the tunica vasculosa lentis and anteriorly by the developing anterior uveal vasculature and pupillary membrane. Both are fully developed in dogs by 30 days of gestation and may persist in a neonate. Persistent tunica vasculosa lentis can be associated with posterior lenticonus and posterior axial capsular cataracts, and adherent persistent pupillary membranes may cause anterior capsular cataract.

Development of the zonular fibers, which suspend the lens, is the result of secretion of the tertiary vitreous by the ciliary neuroepithelium. These fibers extend from the equatorial lens capsule to the pars plicata and pars plana of the ciliary body.[1]

ANATOMY

A fully developed lens is composed of anterior and posterior capsules, anterior epithelium, and elongated cells (fibers). It is an optically transparent structure located between the iris and vitreous and suspended by the zonular fibers, which join the lens to the ciliary body. The lens is bounded by the anterior and posterior chambers and iris anteriorly and the vitreous posteriorly. Firm vitreolenticular adhesions, the hyaloid-capsular ligament, are present.

The anterior lens capsule is thicker (about 50 μm) than the posterior capsule (about 4 μm), which is formed by the posterior lens epithelium during lens development. The capsule is composed of a collagen framework with interstices of mucopolysaccharide and has elastic properties that permit alteration in lens shape owing to the effect of the ciliary muscle, which exerts traction on the lens capsule via the zonular fibers during accommodation. The ciliary muscle is generally poorly developed in subprimates, and accommodation is not as active nor as important in subprimates. The lens capsule also acts as a semipermeable membrane between the ocular fluids and the lens.

The anterior lens epithelium is a monolayer of cuboidal cells, which divide equatorially, elongate, and migrate centrally.

The cortex is the zone of developing lens fibers, the nuclei of which are arranged at the lens bow. As the cells elongate, they extend anteriorly and posteriorly as lens fibers and take a more central position, increasing in length with loss of the nucleus. Opposing fibers meet to form the suture lines. The cortex is less dense than the nucleus.

The center of the lens consists of the innermost embryonic nucleus, the fetal nucleus, and the adult nucleus. The embryonic nucleus has no Y sutures, because the fibers are formed by the anterior elongation of the posterior lens epithelium. The fetal nucleus is the next layer of the lens to form and surrounds the embryonic nucleus. The adult nucleus is continuously formed throughout life. As the cortical fibers are compressed concentrically, they become relatively dehydrated; in older animals, this process commonly results in nuclear sclerosis.

PHYSIOLOGY AND BIOCHEMISTRY

The lens refracts light, controlled to some extent by the process of accommodation. The ability of a medium to refract light requires (1) optical clarity for the transmission of light and (2) an interface between tissues of different optical density and thus a difference in velocity of the light passing through the medium (refractive index). The greatest degree of refraction in the eye takes place at the cornea and, to a lesser degree, at the lens, to result in images focused on the retina.

The lens in humans and some animals has the ability to change shape, thus allowing focus adjustments for objects at various distances. This process, called *accommodation,* requires a pliable lens and capsule, intact zonular fibers, and a functional ciliary muscle. The process involves a complex, poorly defined reflex pathway; to accommodate for near vision, the ciliary muscle contracts, releasing tension on the zonular fibers, allowing the lens capsule to relax and the lens to assume a more spherical shape. As the lens ages, it loses its elasticity owing to compaction and dehydration of lens fibers, with an associated decrease in ability to accommodate.

Maintaining lens transparency is a primary function of the anterior lens epithelium and intact lens capsule. The anterior lens epithelium has a high metabolic rate and actively transports carbohydrates, electrolytes, and amino acids into the lens. Glucose is the primary energy source for lens epithelial metabolism, and abnormal glucose metabolism may result in lens opacification, as in diabetic and galactose cataracts.

The lens substance is composed primarily of intercellular protein (60 per cent) and water (40 per cent). Potassium is sequestered intracellularly, and sodium is extruded.

IMMUNOLOGY

The lens is immunologically unique. If lens protein is exposed to the immune system, it is recognized as a foreign substance. Lens protein is sequestered and potentially antigenic for the following reasons: (1) The lens capsule is formed before the immune system develops; lens protein is thus never recognized as "self." (2) The lens is avascular. (3) The lens is enclosed by a capsule that is impermeable to cells and large molecules.

An animal immunized by injection of lens protein develops serum antibodies against lens protein regardless of the animal species from which it came, demonstrating that lens protein is organ specific rather than species specific.

Lens protein may be exposed to the body as a result of leakage through the lens capsule during liquefaction and resorption of a cataract, traumatic lens rupture, or extracapsular lens extraction. The characteristics of the antigen, including potency, quantity, and duration of exposure, govern the severity of the inflammatory reaction. Leakage of soluble lens protein from a hypermature cataract may result in mild to moderate anterior uveitis, which may be either granulomatous or nongranulomatous and which usually responds to topical corticosteroid therapy. Acute traumatic lens rupture may result in severe intraocular inflammation. Planned extracapsular lens extraction exposes residual lens material to the immune system; if most of the lens material is successfully removed, the resultant inflammation is mild and responsive to anti-inflammatory therapy. Intracapsular lens extraction results in minimal inflammation relative to the other manipulations of the globe.

ROLE OF THE LENS IN AN ANIMAL'S VISION

Accommodation is poorly developed in domestic animals: Dogs and cats possess one to two diopters of accommodative power compared with ten diopters in humans. Although mature cataracts may permit light and dark perception, they result in functional blindness. Although many dogs and cats adjust remarkably well to vision loss, successful cataract extraction allows restoration of functional vision—the ability to recognize people and objects.

CATARACTS

Cataracts are a nonspecific disease that results in opacification of the lens fibers or capsule. Cataracts may be characterized clinically according to stage of development, location within the lens, age of the animal at the time of development, and etiology.

Stages of Development

The stages of development are incipient, immature, mature, and hypermature.[12]

Incipient. Focal opacification of the lens or its capsule characterizes an incipient cataract. An affected animal can still see well, and the fundus is readily observed with an ophthalmoscope.

Immature. In an immature cataract, opacity is more or less diffuse, although there may be areas of variable density. The fundic reflex is present, and the animal may experience some visual impairment.

Mature. A mature cataract shows total dense opacification of the lens with absence of the fundic reflex. Visual function is significantly impaired. Cataract surgery is recommended at this stage.

If a cataract becomes hydrated, the lens swells and increases in size (intumescence). Resultant shallowing of the anterior chamber or pupillary block may cause secondary glaucoma.

Hypermature. Lens protein liquefies and may leak through the capsule. If leakage is extensive with significant resorption of protein, the lens capsule becomes wrinkled, initially at the equator. The nucleus, which is insoluble albuminoid protein, may migrate inferiorly within the lens capsule to form a morgagnian cataract. Uveitis may result from leakage of lens protein. The fundic reflex may be present peripherally, and the animal may see if resorption is extensive.

Location

Location is an aid in defining etiology, and cataracts may be capsular, subcapsular, cortical, or nuclear. These are further described as axial or equatorial and anterior or posterior.

Age of the Animal

Age of the animal when the cataract first appears may be used to classify the cataract as congenital, developmental, or senile.

Congenital. A congenital cataract is present at birth. Congenital cataracts may be inherited or noninherited; inherited congenital cataracts are most commonly encountered in miniature schnauzers.

Developmental. A developmental cataract is an inherited bilateral cataract that occurs after birth, usually in young animals, but in such breeds as the American cocker spaniel, miniature poodle, and Boston terrier, may not appear until later in life.

Senile. Occurring in aged animals, senile cataracts are preceded or accompanied by nuclear sclerosis.

Etiology

Etiology may be difficult to determine; cataracts may occur secondary to ocular diseases, including uveitis, retinal degeneration, lens dislocation, and glaucoma. They may occur in association with systemic metabolic disease, including diabetes mellitus and Cushing's disease, or may be secondary to blunt or penetrating trauma. They may also represent a congenital developmental disorder. The majority of canine cataracts are inherited; cataracts occur less commonly in cats and when encountered are likely to be secondary.

CATARACT SURGERY

Cataracts are a surgical disease; there is no reliable topical, systemic, or intraocular medication that prevents progression or induces resorption of cataracts.

Extracapsular lens extraction is routinely performed for the majority of cataract extractions owing to the strong hyaloideocapsular ligament; intracapsular extraction almost invariably results in disruption of the hyaloid membrane, with vitreous presentation and associated complications, including corneal edema, glaucoma, and retinal detachment. With the extracapsular technique, the posterior lens capsule and vitreous face are not disturbed. In addition, enzymatic dissolution of the zonules is unreliable in dogs, and intracapsular extraction results in excessive traction on the ciliary processes.

Although not all patients presented with cataracts are candidates for surgery, cataract extraction is a most successful and rewarding procedure.

Selection of Patients

The objective of cataract surgery is to restore functional vision. Because of the ability of dogs and cats to adjust and compensate for incomplete lens opacity or monocular blindness, functional vision is not significantly impaired until bilateral cataracts approach maturity. The owner of the pet is the best judge of when surgery should be contemplated. When the animal is constantly bumping into objects and is unable to maintain its normal life-style and personality, cataract extraction should be considered.

Of prime importance is the establishment of integrity of the retina and the central visual pathways. It is discouraging to both client and surgeon to have a technically successful procedure fail to restore vision because of disease of the retina or optic nerve. To evaluate the neural visual components, history, ophthalmoscopy, visual function tests, and electrophysiology should be used in combination.

Inherited retinal degenerations are the primary cause of failure in technically successful cataract surgery. Probably because of soluble lens photosensitizing substances released by degenerating retinal tissue, animals with inherited or inflammatory retinal degeneration are likely to develop associated cataracts. The problem is complicated by the fact that breeds with a high incidence of inherited retinal degeneration, such as the miniature and toy poodle and the Irish setter, also have primary genetic cataracts unassociated with retinal disease.

Pupillary responses are unreliable as the sole method of assessing peripheral and central vision potential. The majority of cataract patients should demonstrate complete, brisk direct and consensual responses to a bright focal light source in a darkened room in the presence of even the densest cataract. These responses may persist in the presence of well-advanced retinal degeneration. The ganglion cell fibers that mediate this reflex are distinct from the visual fibers that extend to the lateral geniculate body and thus provide no information about the status of the optic radiation and visual cortex. Iris atrophy is frequently observed in miniature poodles, and lesions involving the third cranial nerve may also result in absence of pupillary reflexes in the presence of intact visual components. Although it is always reassuring to observe normal pupillary reflexes, they provide minimal information.

History is helpful in relation to the owner's observation of changes in the animal's appearance and behavior. Without exception, visual and ophthalmoscopic changes in inherited retinal degeneration precede associated cataract development. Thus, a reliable history of visual impairment accompanied or followed by noticeable cataract development rather than preceded by it suggests an intact visual system. If inherited retinal degeneration is present, a history of initial nyctalopia (night blindness) may be elicited. Critical ophthalmoscopy performed while the cataracts are still immature, rather than waiting until the fundus cannot be critically examined, is beneficial. Rare dogs with genetic tendencies to develop both retinal degeneration and primary cataracts cause occasional disappointment if the retinal degeneration develops subsequent to the primary cataract.

The ability to negotiate an obstacle course under photopic and scotopic (a red filtered light works well) conditions may be of value in those cases in which the fundus reflex can be obtained although lens changes prohibit a critical fundic examination. Generally, if a fundic reflex can be obtained, some vision should be present and should change minimally with alterations in ambient light if the retina is healthy.

Electrophysiology provides the most reliable criterion for critical evaluation. Electroretinography should be performed on all patients with cataracts and unobservable fundi; in those breeds with predisposition to inherited retinal degeneration, electroretinography is a prerequisite to cataract surgery. If history, pupillary responses, or neurological findings suggest the possibility of a defect in the central visual system, evaluation of visually evoked responses may be considered in addition to electroretinography. Ultrasonography may be of value in detecting retinal detachment.

Young dogs (between 1 and 3 years of age) with inherited developmental cataracts (most frequently encountered in the Afghan hound, American cocker spaniel, Irish setter, and miniature and toy poodle) may undergo spontaneous resorption of their cataracts. Active resorption, demonstrated by mild lens-induced uveitis and an irregular lens capsule, is a reason to delay surgery. Although these liquefied cataracts may be aspirated, many resorb so that cataract surgery is unnecessary. We prefer to manage these animals with topical application of 1.0 per cent atropine sulfate to enhance peripheral vision and corticosteroids to temper the uveitis. The animal should be examined monthly, and cataract surgery is recommended only when active resorption has subsided without restoration of visual function. Success rates in animals with previous uveitis are somewhat lower than in uncomplicated cataracts.[7]

Cataract surgery is an elective procedure; thorough multisystem evaluation should be performed before surgery. Concurrent related diseases (such as diabetes mellitus or Cushing's disease) or unrelated diseases (such as renal decompensation or heartworm disease) should be identified and controlled. In older patients that have systemic disease and have adjusted reasonably well to their visual impairment, the complications of anesthesia should be weighed against the benefits of improved vision.

Philosophies of Cataract Surgery

With few exceptions, I perform cataract surgery on one eye only because of the ability of an animal to function well with monocular vision, lower cost to the owner, and the reduced insult to the patient in terms of anesthesia time and postoperative discomfort. Also, it is reassuring to know that in case of failure, one can offer the client an alternative operation on the contralateral eye. Both cataracts may be removed at one or two sittings at the owner's request or if acute visual function is desirable or necessary, as in active young hunting dogs or obedience dogs.

The procedure for cataract removal, when performed with appropriate preoperative treatment and instrumentation, is not difficult. However, the incidence of intraoperative or postoperative complications is high compared with other procedures, and these complications frequently have disastrous effects on the visual outcome. An experienced cataract surgeon, using an operating microscope and having the instrumentation necessary to perform vitrectomy, should anticipate success rates of 90 to 95 per cent.

Routine Procedures and Techniques

Adequate preoperative preparation minimizes intraoperative and postoperative complications. Canine eyes respond to even meticulous surgery with intraoperative constriction of the pupil, which hampers exposure and necessitates increased intraocular manipulation, with resultant intensified postoperative inflammation. Pretreatment with antiprostaglandins and topical antibiotic-corticosteroids and mydriatics minimizes these problems.[15] Prostaglandins have a role in both pupillary constriction and inflammation, and systemic aspirin or topical flurbiprofen, which inhibits synthesis of prostaglandin, provides results superior to those of corticosteroids alone. In addition, flunixin meglumine is administered intravenously immediately before surgery.

Two general approaches are available for the extraction of cataractous lenses: manual extracapsular extraction[3, 4, 9, 13, 16] and phacoemulsification.[1, 5] Principles common to both include controlled intraocular manipulations, maintenance of a formed anterior chamber, and total removal of lens nucleus and cortex.

Stable deep anesthesia and smooth recovery are important. Under light anesthesia, the animal may move when the iris is touched and intraocular pressure may increase owing to extraocular muscle contraction. Quiet recovery minimizes the likelihood of self-inflicted trauma; these patients should be closely observed to prevent problems.

The positioning of the patient is crucial to the success of the procedure. The muzzle is elevated to enable the surgeon to see the iris and lens surface in a horizontal plane. Lateral canthotomy is routinely performed. A traction suture of 4-0 silk placed through the conjunctiva and episclera superiorly may be necessary; a similar suture is placed through the third eyelid and is used to retract it if required. The incision in extracapsular procedures should be a minimum of 180°; it is difficult to accurately predict lens size before surgery, and attempting to deliver an intumescent lens through a small incision results in undue trauma to corneal endothelium and residual lens material in the anterior chamber.

A beveled corneoscleral incision under a limbus-based conjunctival flap heals more rapidly than a clear corneal incision. Corneal scarring at the incision site is minimized, and accurate apposition of the surgical wound margin is facilitated. If corneal dehiscence occurs, the intraocular contents are not exposed to the environment. Absorbable suture knots may be covered by the flap so that postoperative irritation does not occur. These advantages offset the additional 3 to 5 minutes needed to dissect the flap and control the minimal hemorrhage associated with a corneoscleral incision. A clear corneal incision is more efficient in terms of time and provides slightly better exposure, without obstruction by the flap. Preplaced sutures hinder exposure and maneuverability, and I prefer to have unobstructed access to the anterior segment should complications arise.

Capsulectomy may be performed with a bent needle, scissors, cryoprobe, or capsule forceps. Needle capsulectomy is carried out in a formed chamber with a bent 27- or 30-gauge needle. After the initial half to three-quarter thickness perpendicular grooved incision, a 2- to 3-mm penetrating stab incision is made at 12 o'clock, the chamber formed with viscoelastic material or an infusion of commercial balanced salt solution, and the needle used to incise and tear (capsulorhexis) and remove the anterior capsule. Various techniques and patterns may be used to remove the capsule. Although a good equatorial capsular tear can be made with a cryoprobe, the incidence of posterior capsule disruption is high and the remaining capsule is not conducive to implant insertion. The instrument is placed somewhat superiorly on a thoroughly dry anterior capsule, and the capsule torn by simultaneous elevating and rotating movements while the cornea is reflected. If forceps are used, the capsule is grasped as superficially and as widely as the dilated pupil allows without obstructing the view of the forceps teeth. The forceps are closed, elevated minutely, and gently rotated.

The lens cortex and nucleus are mobilized using intracapsular irrigation (hydrodissection) with saline solution and expressed by applying inferior traction on the scleral wound lip and posterior pressure inferiorly. Liquefied or residual cortex may be gently irrigated and aspirated after partial wound closure.

If a pupil of less than 3 mm results (a rare occurrence), sphincter iridotomy may be performed. To enhance exposure, scissors are used to incise 2 to 3 mm into the sphincter in three or four quadrants. Blood and fibrin clots are extracted with an iris hook. Closure is with 7-0 to 9-0 absorbable suture or 9-0 or 10-0 nylon. I prefer 7-0 polyglactin 910 in an interrupted or continuous X pattern with the knots buried (Figs. 88–1 and 88–2).

Phacoemulsification or phacofragmentation uses ultrasonic energy to disrupt and liquefy the cataract, which is simultaneously aspirated; although the instrumentation is expensive, this technique represents the optimum in formed chamber surgery and greatly facilitates total cortical removal. The technique involves a smaller incision, formed chamber needle capsulectomy or capsulotomy, and disruption and aspiration of the cataract. Phacoemulsification can be performed entirely within the capsular bag (endocapsular phacoemulsification).

Postoperative care is critical and is aimed at reducing inflammation and maintaining pupil size. Corticosteroids may be administered subconjunctivally, and oral corticosteroids are continued for 7 days except in diabetic patients. Topical 1.0 per cent atropine sulfate, 2.5 per cent phenylephrine, and antibiotic-corticosteroid solutions are applied as required to control pupillary size and to temper inflammation. Bandages, Elizabethan collars, sedation, and analgesics are not routinely used because the surgery is tolerated remarkably well. Mydriatics and topical corticosteroids are continued until the inflammation has subsided, usually by 4 to 6 weeks. Patients should be re-examined frequently after surgery.

Complications

Operative complications include miosis, which can be largely prevented by adequate premedication and minimal intraocular manipulations; hemorrhage from the ciliary processes while performing the capsulectomy or from the sphincterotomy incision if one is necessary; posterior capsular tears with vitreous presentation; and posterior capsular opacity. A small pupil is managed intraoperatively by use of intracameral epinephrine or sphincterotomy and postoperative medication. Ciliary process hemorrhage is uncommon; iris hemorrhage may occur in animals subjected to three- or four-quadrant sphincterotomy. In both instances, bleeding is minimal and self-limited. The vessels are encouraged to clot by re-forming the anterior chamber and delaying manipulations for 3 to 5 minutes. Blood can be irrigated or gently teased from the anterior chamber. A small amount of residual hyphema, although undesirable, is resorbed over 2 to 3 weeks without consequences.

Vitreous presentation occurs when the posterior capsule or zonules are unintentionally disrupted or in the presence of lens subluxation; the incidence is higher in animals with incomplete cataract resorption or microphthalmia. Vitreous presentation is managed with an anterior chamber air bubble if the hyaloid membrane is intact. Unfortunately, the hyaloid membrane usually ruptures, and the vitreous must be removed from the anterior chamber to reduce the likelihood of disastrous sequelae, including corneal edema associated with vitreous touch, pupillary block glaucoma, and retinal detachment. Anterior vitrectomy may be performed with cellulose sponges, excising the vitreous as close to the plane of the iris as possible, or ideally with a vitrectomy instrument. A vitreophage is preferred because it mini-

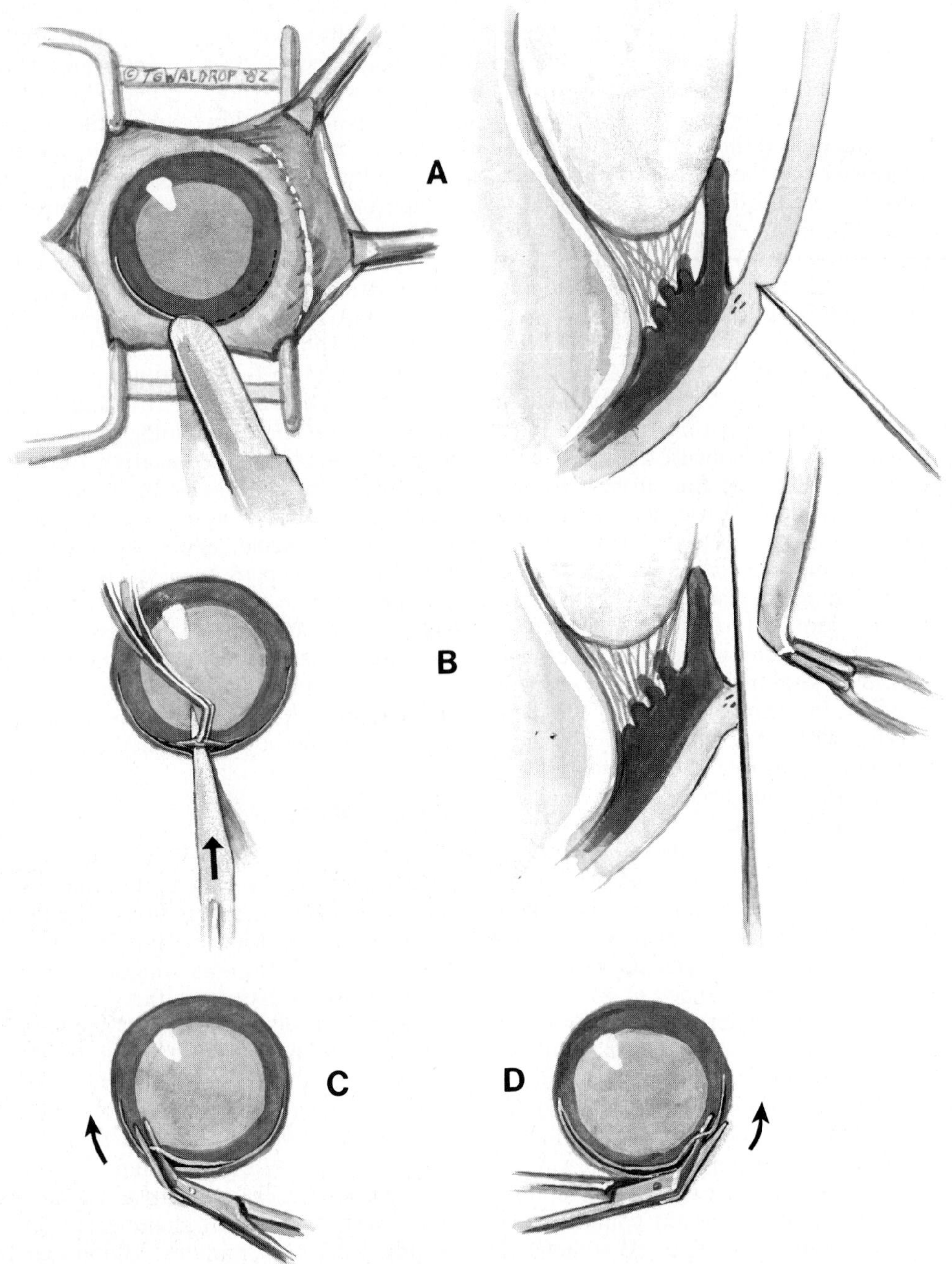

FIGURE 88–1. Extracapsular cataract extraction via a clear corneal incision. *A,* Using a number 64 Beaver blade 1 mm anterior to the limbus, a 180° ¾-depth corneal incision is made. *B,* The anterior chamber is entered with a number 65 Beaver blade at the 12 o'clock position. *C* and *D,* The cornea incision is completed with left- and right-handed corneoscleral scissors, following the previously made corneal groove.

mizes intraocular manipulation and traction to the retina. Vitrectomy is performed until the anterior chamber is completely free of vitreous and the iris plane assumes a concave appearance. A spatula is used to sweep any vitreous from the wound after closure.

If the cataract has been present for some time, the posterior capsule may be translucent or opaque at the time of surgery. If the fundus cannot be readily observed at surgery, the capsule is incised or removed. Except for a 3-mm superior opening, the corneal incision is closed and the anterior chamber re-formed with saline or viscoelastic material; the posterior capsule is then incised with a bent 25-gauge needle. The linear incision usually widens to prevent unimpaired observation of the posterior pole. If it does not, the incision is opened and the incised margins are grasped and the capsule teased away from the hyaloid membrane and excised with scissors. Vitrectomy is performed if necessary. Alternatively, capsular opacities of significance may be managed postoperatively by laser capsulotomy.

Postoperative complications include (1) pupillary membrane with or without pupillary occlusion and secondary glaucoma, (2) corneal edema, (3) glaucoma without pupillary obstruction, and (4) retinal detach-

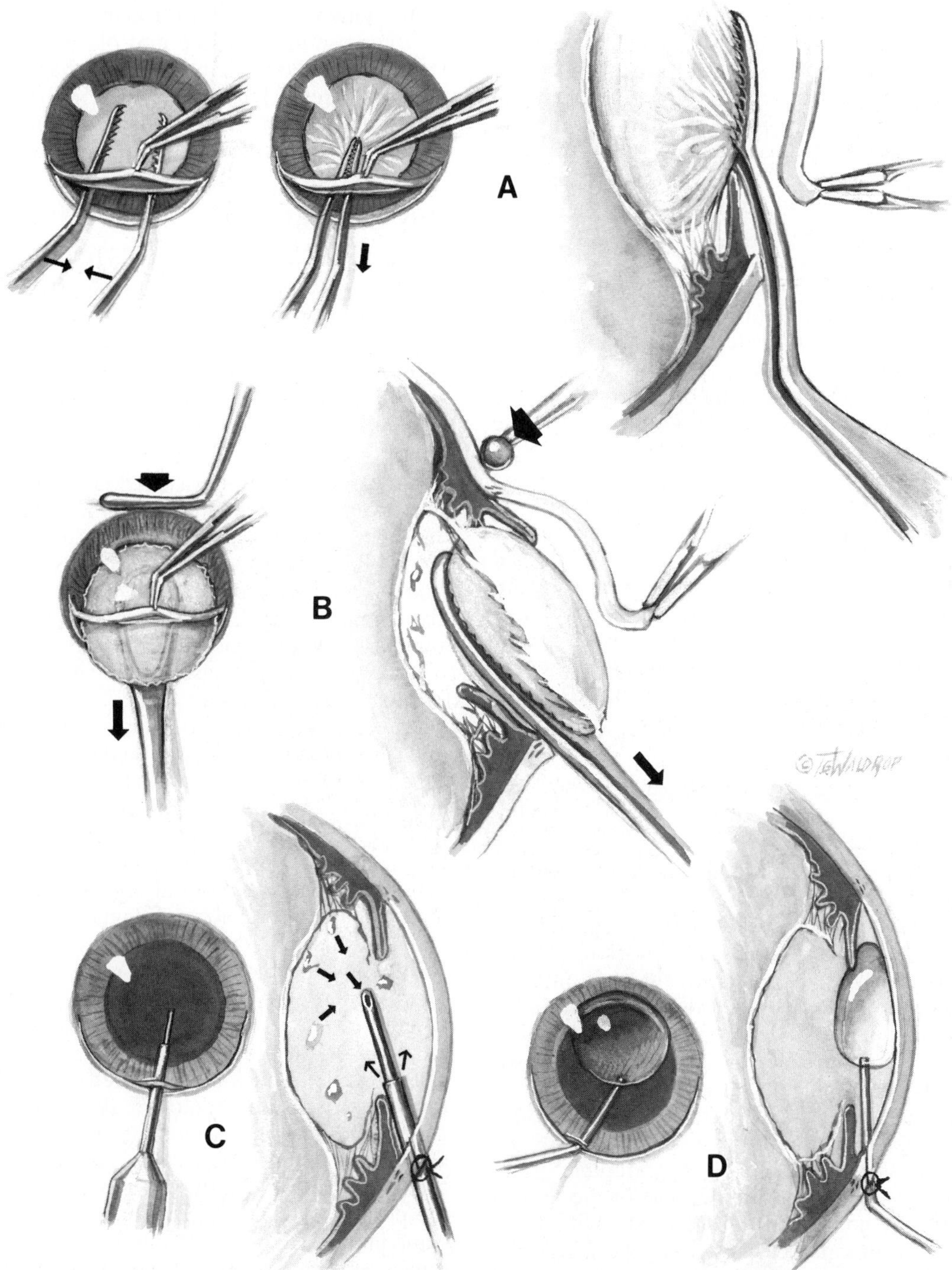

FIGURE 88–2. Extracapsular cataract extraction (continued). *A,* The corneal flap is grasped with fine-toothed forceps and gently elevated to allow entrance of the toothed capsulotomy forceps. The capsulotomy forceps are inserted into the anterior chamber with closed jaws. As the forceps are positioned over the anterior lens capsule, the jaws are opened, gently depressed, and closed to grasp the anterior lens capsule. With gentle elevation and rotation of the capsulotomy forceps, the anterior lens capsule tears at the equator. *B,* A lens loop is positioned to gently depress the superior iris. An extraocular muscle hook is placed opposite the lens loop on the outside of the globe 2 mm posterior to the limbus; gentle pressure is exerted to deliver the lens. *C,* After anterior chamber irrigation, the corneal incision is closed with simple interrupted sutures; the anterior chamber is re-established with saline solution. Residual lens debris may be aspirated. *D,* An air bubble one-third the volume of the anterior chamber reconstitutes the anterior chamber, and closure is completed. Balanced salt solution may be used instead of air.

ment.[4, 6, 7] The first complication is almost invariably associated with intense postoperative inflammation related to residual lens material or excessive intraocular manipulation, and the last to unplanned intracapsular extraction and anterior vitrectomy. Although focal opacification of the posterior capsule and synechiae of the iris to the posterior capsule are common, functional vision persists around the secondary cataract if a pupil is maintained. Scarring of the limbal cornea in the area of incision is expected and is of no consequence even if associated with peripheral anterior synechiae.

Coreoplasty may be performed as a salvage procedure in dogs with pupillary membrane with or without iris bombé. Using a spatula in a viscoelastic-formed chamber, it may be possible to bluntly free iris-to-iris or iris-to-capsule adhesions. Sector iridectomy may likewise be considered. Currently available suction cutting machines manipulated through the pars plana offer promise in the management of this common complication, and the use of ophthalmic lasers may be considered if the instrumentation is available.

Mild transient corneal edema is a common postoperative feature that occurs in proportion to (1) mechanical trauma due to intraocular irrigation or lens endothelial contact during extraction and (2) postoperative inflammation. Severe persistent corneal edema is associated with excessive trauma, glaucoma, or vitreous touch. Because the canine endothelium possesses some regenerative capabilities, especially in younger animals, some recovery may occur over time.

INTRAOCULAR LENSES IN CANINE CATARACT SURGERY*

Although aphakic canine patients function reasonably well, postoperative vision can be improved by inserting an artificial intraocular lens after cataract removal.[11, 14] Because of the sensitivity of the canine uvea to contact with intraocular lenses, a posterior chamber implant inserted within the capsular bag is the best location. A broad, modified C-loop polymethyl methacrylate implant provides optimum stability and centration.[10] Although there is some individual variability in refractive need, an implant of about 40 diopters brings the majority of canine patients acceptably close to emmotropia.[2]

Needle or scissor capsulotomy is preferable if an intraocular lens is to be inserted because of the desirability of having a controlled capsular tear with large anterior flaps. After cataract extraction, the incision is closed, with the exception of an 8-mm superior wound (or extended to 8 mm, if phacoemulsification is used). The anterior chamber and capsular bag are re-formed with viscoelastic solution (hyaluronic acid, methylcellulose, chondroitin sulfate, or collagen alone or in combination all have been used, with little significant difference), and the implant is inserted into the capsular bag. The lower haptic is inserted directly, and the superior haptic either "dialed" with a hooked 30-gauge needle or otherwise manipulated into place. Dialing, however, ensures capsular placement of both haptics with minimal capsular stress. Intraocular lens insertion presents an additional variable and as such poses another potential chance for operative and postoperative complications.

*Editor's note: Intraocular lens placement is ***controversial*** among veterinary ophthalmologists and ophthalmic surgeons. Some experienced practitioners believe that dogs do not function better in the long term and that the complications (which include uveitis, lens decentering, and capsule opacification) are significant. These practitioners believe that intraocular lenses are contraindicated at their current state of development.

LENS DISLOCATION

Lens dislocation can be complete (luxation) or partial (subluxation, with some intact zonules remaining). The lens may dislocate into the anterior chamber (anterior luxation) or the vitreous (posterior luxation) or may remain within the retropupillary space (subluxation). The condition may occur after blunt trauma but most frequently is a spontaneous bilateral problem in the terrier breeds, most likely related to inherited zonular weakness. Obstruction of aqueous flow from the posterior to anterior chamber by the dislocated lens or displaced vitreous frequently causes secondary glaucoma. Primary lens dislocation must be distinguished from secondary displacement associated with chronic glaucoma, in which megaloglobus (buphthalmos) and zonular stretching lead to this condition. Lens extraction is rarely indicated in cases of lens dislocation associated with chronic glaucoma.

Prevention or effective management of glaucoma secondary to primary lens luxation demands lens extraction, which is recommended in all cases of anterior lens luxation and subluxation associated with clinical disease (glaucoma or anterior uveitis). Asymptomatic subluxations and posterior luxations may be managed by observation and pharmacological miosis, but sooner or later they are likely to cause problems. Extraction is usually indicated as well.

Intracapsular cryoextraction is the technique of choice for a primary dislocated lens.[3, 8] Although the zonular attachments are damaged, the hyaloidocapsular ligament is usually intact, and a surgeon who operates on a dislocated lens must be prepared to perform a vitrectomy before or after removing the lens.

Preoperative preparation of the eye varies with the location of the dislocated lens. Anterior lens luxation is considered a nonelective surgical procedure owing to the potential for damage to the corneal endothelium or glaucoma as a result of pupillary block. Preoperative topical pilocarpine may maintain a small pupil, which traps the lens in the anterior chamber and facilitates extraction; however, miosis may precipitate vitreous pupillary block, and topical pilocarpine is used immediately before surgery only. If the intraocular pressure is significantly elevated (greater than 40 mm Hg), intravenous mannitol is given at 1 mg/kg 1 hour before surgery to minimize vitreous presentation and spontaneous choroidal hemorrhage.

Exposure of the anterior chamber and approach to it are identical to those used during extracapsular lens extraction. An *ab externo* incision may be used to avoid puncture of the lens capsule if the lens is luxated anteriorly. If vitreous protrudes during the corneoscleral incision, it is ignored until the incision is complete. Once the anterior chamber is exposed, the technique for intracapsular extraction varies with the position of the lens.

With anterior luxation or subluxation of the lens, the cornea is retracted and vitrectomy performed, if necessary, to allow direct access to the lens. Posterior lens luxation involves a more extensive vitrectomy to remove the vitreous between the surgeon and the lens. The lens capsule is dried with a cellulose sponge, and the tip of the cryoprobe is applied to the lens capsule superiorly. Once the cryoprobe is firmly adherent, the lens is carefully extracted as the surgeon separates the posterior vitreal attachments with a cyclodialysis spatula in a gentle sweeping movement or transects the vitreous with scissors in the plane of the iris. Anterior vitrectomy is performed if vitreous is present within the anterior chamber after extraction. Closure is identical to that for extracapsular lens extraction. When completed, an air bubble one-third the size of the anterior chamber is injected, and routine closure of the canthotomy is performed (Fig. 88–3). Postoperative therapy is similar to that after extracapsular lens extraction. Intraocular inflammation is less than after extracapsular extraction, because lens protein is not released and is completely removed.

Postoperative complications include corneal edema,

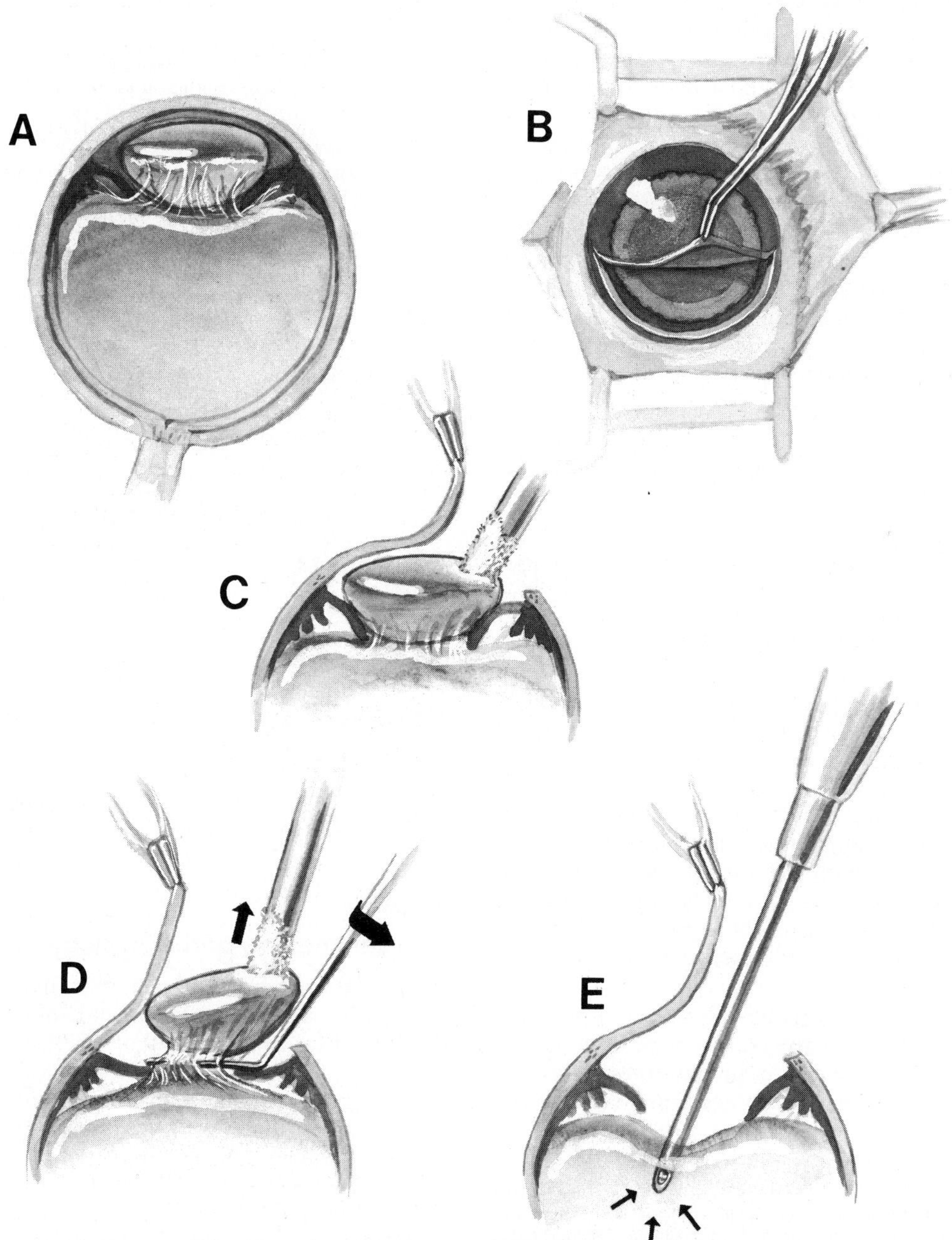

FIGURE 88–3. Intracapsular cryoextraction of dislocated lenses. *A*, Anterior dislocation of the lens with the vitreal attachments to the posterior lens capsule intact. *B*, The approach to the anterior chamber is the same as in Figure 88–1. *C*, The corneal flap is retracted with corneal forceps, and a cryoprobe is applied to the lens. *D*, Once the cryopexy to the lens is achieved, the lens is removed while relieving vitreal attachment with a spatula. *E*, Intracapsular lens extraction is followed by an anterior vitrectomy as demonstrated with a Kaufman vitrector.

pupillary membrane, persistent glaucoma, and retinal detachment. Significant corneal edema may be associated with preoperative mechanical trauma due to an anteriorly luxated lens or postoperative vitreous in the anterior chamber in direct contact with the endothelium. The former complication may be managed by thin conjunctival flaps or corneal transplantation if time and topical hyperosmotic agents fail to restore vision.

Pupillary membranes are uncommon with extracapsular cataract extraction and are usually associated with intraocular hemorrhage during or after surgery; if significant, surgical management as discussed previously may be considered. Such membranes are rare after phacoemulsification.

Postoperative intraocular pressure should be monitored closely and regularly. Continued elevation uncontrollable by medication is an indication for further surgical intervention. Such circumstances are unusual, because removal of the dislocated lens generally cures glaucoma.

Retinal detachment is the most common and perhaps most discouraging of complications. The majority of detachments occur 2 to 4 weeks postoperatively and are associated with peripheral tears of the retina. Surgical correction may be attempted, with drainage of the subretinal fluid and cryopexy followed by scleral buckling or intraocular gas injection. Reports of such treatment of retinal detachments after cataract surgery in dogs are lacking.

References

1. Aguirre GD, et al: Development of the canine eye. *Am J Vet Res 33*:2399, 1972.
2. Gaiddon J, et al: Use of biometry and keratometry for determining optimal power for intraocular lens implants in dogs. *Am J Vet Res 52*:781, 1991.
3. Knight GC: The extraction of dislocations and the cataractous crystalline lens of the dog with the objective of preserving some useful vision. *Vet Rec 68*:318, 1957.
4. Magrane WG: Cataract extraction: A follow-up study (429 cases). *J Small Anim Pract 10*:545, 1969.
5. Miller TR, et al: Phacofragmentation and aspiration for cataract extraction in dogs: 56 cases (1980–1984). *J Am Vet Med Assoc 190*:1577, 1987.
6. Murphy JM, et al: Sequelae of extracapsular lens extraction in the normal dog. *J Am Anim Hosp Assoc 16*:47, 1980.
7. Paulsen ME, et al: The effect of lens-induced uveitis on the success of extracapsular cataract extraction: A retrospective study of 65 lens removals in the dog. *J Am Anim Hosp Assoc 22*:49, 1986.
8. Peiffer RL Jr: Surgical management of dislocated lenses with vitrectomy using a disposable vitreophage. *Vet Med Small Anim Clin 75*:1299, 1980.
9. Peiffer RL Jr: Current concepts in ophthalmic surgery. *Vet Clin North Am 10*:455, 1980.
10. Peiffer RL Jr, et al: Personal communication (unpublished data), 1992.
11. Peiffer RL Jr, Gaiddon J: Posterior chamber intraocular lens implantation in dogs: Results of 65 implants in 61 patients. *J Am Anim Hosp Assoc, 27*:453, 1991.
12. Playter RF: The development and maturation of a cataract. *J Am Anim Hosp Assoc 13*:317, 1977.
13. Rooks RL, et al: Extracapsular cataract extraction: An analysis of 240 cases. *J Am Vet Med Assoc 287*:1013, 1985.
14. Simpson HD: Intraocular plastic lens implantation in canine cataract surgery. *North Am Vet 37*:573, 1956.
15. Szymanski CM, et al: Effective mydriasis for cataract surgery in the dog. *J Am Vet Med Assoc 163*:260, 1973.
16. Vierheller RC: Canine cataract surgery: Suggested technique for the occasional operator. *Vet Med 52*:487, 1957.

CHAPTER 89 Surgery of the Vitreous and Retina

Robert L. Peiffer, Jr.

"Open sky" anterior vitrectomy is a commonly performed, essential technique in the treatment of anterior vitreous presentation with rupture of the anterior hyaloid membrane that may occur during removal of dislocated or cataractous lenses. Otherwise, vitreoretinal surgery is undeveloped in veterinary ophthalmic surgery for two reasons.

First, the number of animals with posterior segment disease that would benefit by manipulative intervention is low; removal of posterior segment foreign bodies, vitreous hemorrhage and membranes, and opaque vitreous due to anterior hyalosis are infrequent. Fortunately, animal species do not experience the florid vitreoretinal fibrovascular proliferations with associated vitreous hemorrhage and tractional retinal detachments that devastate human eyes. Rhegmatogenous retinal detachments occur both spontaneously and as a complication after lens extraction.

Second, surgery in the posterior segment (i.e., pars plana vitrectomy) requires instrumentation not readily available and skills not highly developed by most veterinary ophthalmic surgeons.

VITREOUS

Surgical Anatomy and Physiology

The vitreous is a transparent hydrated connective tissue consisting of collagen and mucopolysaccharides, primarily hyaluronic acid, that fills the posterior segment of the globe. The definitive (secondary) vitreous is of neuroectodermal origin and is formed around the fetal hyaloid artery system (primary vitreous) by gestational day 45 in dogs.[1] The volume of this tissue is approximately 3 ml in dogs and cats.[7] In adults, the vitreous is avascular, atrophy of the hyaloid artery occurring during the first 2 postnatal months. The zonular fibers attaching the lens to the ciliary body constitute the tertiary vitreous, but this classification is academic rather than practical.

Collagen fibrils within the vitreous are continuous

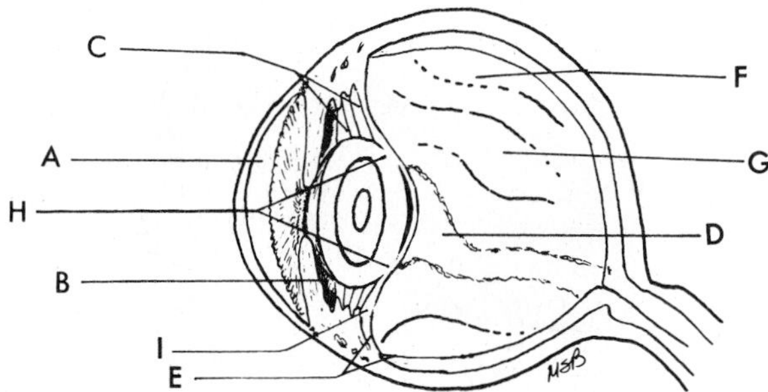

FIGURE 89–1. Zones within the vitreous. A, Anterior chamber; B, posterior chamber; C, zonules (tertiary vitreous); D, Cloquet's canal (remnant of primary vitreous); E, vitreous base; F, cortical vitreous; G, intermediate zone of vitreous; H, hyaloideocapsular ligament; I, anterior hyaloid membrane.

with Müller cell processes, which form the internal limiting membrane of the retina.[9] Firm areas of attachment to adjacent structures occur at three locations: the peripheral posterior lens capsule (hyaloideocapsular ligament), the ora ciliaris retinae (vitreous base), and the margin of the optic nerve. Vitreal attachments are likely stronger along retinal blood vessels. The main body of the vitreous is divided into a peripheral cortical portion; an intermediate zone; and the central primary vitreal remnant, Cloquet's canal (Fig. 89–1). The cortical vitreous is loosely attached to the retina and, unlike that of humans, is less dense than the central zone.[20] Cellular components of the vitreous are scarce, consisting primarily of macrophages called *hyalocytes.* These cells are most numerous near the vitreal base. At its boundaries, the vitreous condenses to form the hyaloid membrane.

Development of Vitrectomy

Removal of opaque vitreous was first performed in humans in 1890 using an approach through the pars plana.[10] Modifications of this technique have been used extensively to clear vitreal opacities (hemorrhage, amyloidosis), to treat retinal detachment by reducing traction and removing vitreous sequestered behind the detachment, to remove posterior segment foreign bodies, and to prevent anterior vitreal prolapse in aphakic eyes.* An anterior approach to vitrectomy through a limbal incision was introduced in the late 1960s and was subsequently applied to treatment of persistent hyperplastic vitreous, vitreociliary block (malignant glaucoma), vitreous opacities, and vitreal incarceration in corneal wounds.†

Techniques of vitreous removal have involved use of cellulose sponges, which readily adhere to and absorb liquefied vitreous, with transection of fibrils using scissors.[2, 13, 14] Mechanized suction cutters, either rotating or oscillating, minimize retinal traction.[3, 6, 7, 19, 22]

Early in development of vitrectomy, controversy existed over proper replacement of vitreous with a substance of similar properties to maintain normal anatomical relationships, tamponade the retina against the pigmented epithelium, and reduce traction. Absorbable and nonabsorbable materials that have been used include saline, gases (air, oxygen, nitrogen, nitrous oxide, sulfur hexafluoride), body fluids (cerebrospinal fluid, aqueous humor, vitreous grafts), hyaluronic acid, and silicone oil.[23] No substance is completely satisfactory, and a balanced salt solution, which is replaced by aqueous humor, currently is most practical for use in veterinary ophthalmology.[14, 15]

*See references 4, 11, 15, 17–19, 21, and 25.

†See references 3, 4, 12, 14, 16, 21, 24, and 26.

Pathophysiology and Indications

Owing to intimate anatomical relationships between the vitreous and the retina, any process altering the volume or structure of the vitreous may cause retinal detachment. Syneresis, or liquefaction, of the vitreous can occur as a result of senile changes or inflammation. Postinflammatory scarring, or cicatrization, can result in the formation of traction bands that separate the inner retina from the underlying pigmented epithelium.

Lack of vascular supply to the vitreous results in delayed clearing of hemorrhage and response to infection. Abnormal vascularization can occur by ingrowth of retinal blood vessels (neovascularization) and is a challenging problem in persons with diabetic retinopathy. These neovascular proliferations are fragile and can bleed into the vitreous; this is rare in animals.

Vitreal surgery in animals is rarely a primary or elective procedure. Asteroid hyalosis, even in extreme cases, is unlikely to significantly affect functional vision. Vitreous or subretinal aspiration may be performed as a diagnostic tool in posterior segment inflammatory disease for vitreous culture and cytological study. Vitrectomy may be used to remove posterior segment foreign bodies and vascular membranes associated with persistent hyperplastic primary vitreous. The most frequent indication for vitrectomy occurs during intracapsular extraction of a dislocated lens in which some degree of vitreal prolapse is expected owing to the firm attachment of the posterior lens capsule to the anterior hyaloid membrane. Inadvertent tearing of the posterior lens capsule or partial rupture of zonules during extracapsular cataract extraction may also result in appearance of vitreous through the pupil.

The surgeon may observe signs of imminent rupture of the hyaloid face, such as iris prolapse through the initial limbal incision, ballooning forward of the iris and narrowing of the anterior chamber, and the actual appearance of the vitreous face. In such cases, it may be possible to sweep the anterior hyaloid behind the iris with a cyclodialysis spatula or prevent anterior vitreal prolapse by aspiration of liquefied vitreous through the pupil or by a pars plana approach. Rupture of the anterior hyaloid with vitreous presentation into the anterior chamber is an indication for anterior vitrectomy.

Vitreous in the anterior chamber is removed because (1) it can physically obstruct circulation of aqueous through the pupil and iridocorneal angle; (2) it provides a scaffolding for growth of membranes and adhesions; and (3) when in contact with corneal endothelium, it causes endothelium dysfunction and corneal edema.

Techniques

Vitreous Aspiration

Aspiration of liquefied vitreous can be performed through the pars plana with a 1-inch 22-gauge needle or through the aphakic pupil to alleviate vitreous pressure and prevent prolapse; success depends unpredictably on finding vitreous liquefied adequately to allow aspiration without creating undue traction on the retina; these techniques are not recommended unless a suction cutting machine is not available. With the pars plana technique, the needle is advanced through the sclera 6 mm posterior to the limbus at 12 o'clock and directed toward the optic nerve to avoid the lens.

Pars Plana Vitrectomy

Pars plana vitrectomy may be performed in either phakic or aphakic globes and is uncommonly used. It allows for removal of vitreous and intravitreal membranes or cells in a closed eye (the lens may be removed piecemeal with this technique as well). Control and exposure, especially near the posterior pole, are optimal compared with anterior vitrectomy. The globe is entered over the pars plana ciliaris, 6 to 8 mm behind the limbus. Anatomical relationships are critical (Fig. 89–2); an anterior approach may result in ciliary trauma and hemorrhage or damage to the lens. If the retina is penetrated by the needle posterior to the pars plana, the retinal hole may lead to detachment. The technique involves use of a vitreous suction cutter, with infusion, in combination with an operating microscope, a corneal contact lens, and fiber-optic illumination.

Anterior Vitrectomy

Once formed vitreous is present in the anterior chamber, anterior vitrectomy is necessary. A technique that requires minimal instrumentation uses cellulose sponges to absorb the liquid components and adhere to formed vitreous, facilitating gentle elevation (Fig. 89–3). Vitreous is excised, a little at a time, at the level of the iris to minimize traction on the retina until the anterior chamber deepens, the iris face is concave, and no further vitreous appears. Great care is taken to avoid contact with the corneal endothelium and iris as the cellulose swells; a broad, 180° corneoscleral incision and corneal retraction facilitate the procedure. Small particles of cellulose left within the eye may cause granulomas and chronic inflammation.[14]

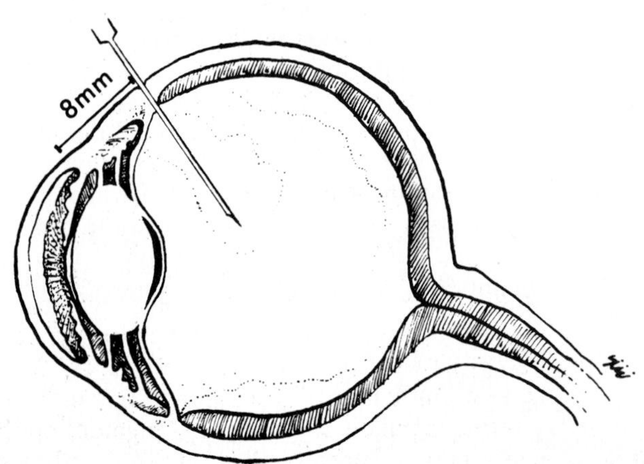

FIGURE 89–2. Anatomical relationships in a pars plana vitrectomy. Similar techniques are used to aspirate vitreous for diagnostic purposes.

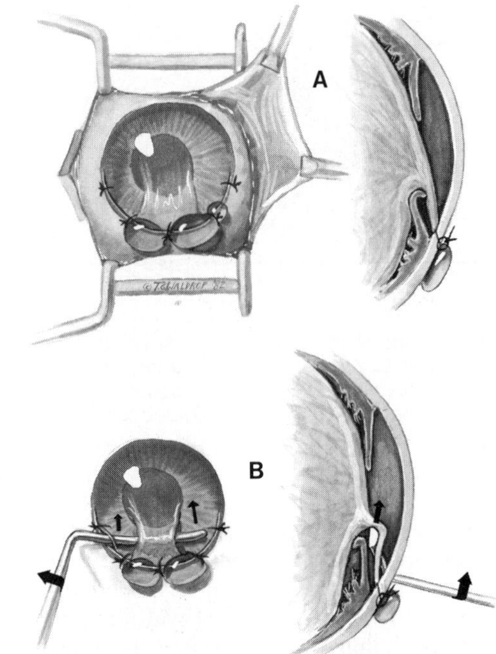

FIGURE 89–3. *A*, Vitreous incarcerated in a corneoscleral wound. *B*, Sweeping vitreous from incision using a cyclodialysis spatula, with replacement of vitreous behind the iris.

If vitreous is incarcerated into a corneoscleral wound (as suggested by a peaked or irregular pupil), it may be swept behind the iris with a cyclodialysis spatula[5] (Fig. 89–4).

Vitreophages combine controlled suction with atraumatic tissue resection via a rotating or guillotine-like blade within an aspirating needle (Fig. 89–5). These instruments markedly reduce the time required for vitrectomy, minimize traction on the retina, and are particularly applicable when more than a small amount of vitreous must be removed. The excised vitreous is replaced with saline, and an air bubble is used to reform the anterior chamber. This technique is most frequently used in cryoextraction of a dislocated lens. If vitreous appears as the globe is entered, the incision is extended and vitreous is excised until the cryoprobe can be applied directly to the lens capsule; the cryoprobe is used to elevate the lens through the incision. Vitreous attachments are separated from the posterior lens capsule in the plane of the iris with a lens loop or cyclodialysis spatula. Vitreous is removed until the anterior chamber is empty and the iris is concave. Limitations of this technique are as its name implies—the open sky anterior vitrectomy does not allow observation or control much beyond the equator.

Complications

Complications of vitrectomy may occur at surgery or in the postoperative period. In humans, these include

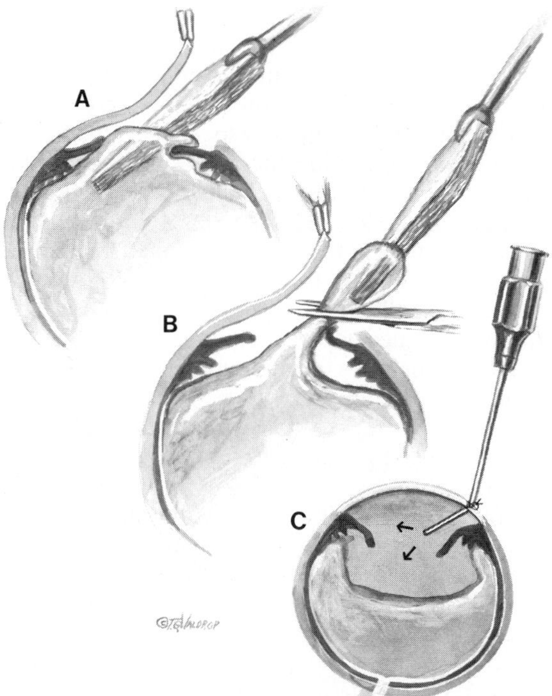

FIGURE 89–4. Anterior vitrectomy using a cellulose sponge. *A*, Vitreous is allowed to adhere to the sponge. *B*, The sponge is gently retracted, and vitreous fibrils are transected at the level of the iris. *C*, After closure of the corneal incision, an infusion of balanced salt solution is used to reform the anterior chamber and re-establish normal anatomical relationships.

cystic macular edema, persistent uveitis, retinal detachment, vitreous hemorrhage, keratopathy, peaked pupil, and glaucoma.[6, 12]

Complications of anterior vitrectomy associated with canine lens removal include corneal edema, retinal detachment, and glaucoma. Incomplete removal of vitreous from the anterior chamber can lead to glaucoma due to blockage of outflow pathways, pupillary and cyclitic membranes, and endothelial damage due to vitreocorneal contact. Excessive manipulation and traction on the vitreous can lead to the most serious complication of vitrectomy—retinal detachment. During pars plana vitrectomy, failure to cut cleanly through the vitreous base may push the vitreous ahead of the needle, the resulting traction producing retinal dialysis and detachment. Hemorrhage may result from cutting fibrovascular membranes.

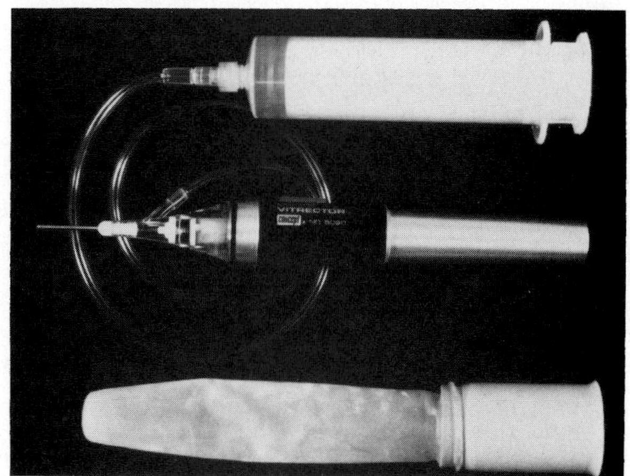

FIGURE 89–5. The disposable vitreophage consists of a battery-powered motor, an assistant-operated syringe to provide suction, and a rotary cutting blade. The power source is enclosed in a sterile latex sleeve and coupled to the cutting unit during the procedure.

RETINA

Repair of retinal detachments requires an understanding of the pathophysiology of the posterior segment as well as an appreciation of the anatomy of the globe, its relationships to the extraocular muscles and other surrounding tissue, its vascular supply, and the relationships of the intraocular tissues to one another. Species differences exist, notably in regard to the insertion of the extraocular muscles, the location of the ora ciliaris retinae in relation to the limbus, and retinal vascular patterns that are critical.

Historical Perspectives

At the International Congress of Ophthalmology in 1929, Jules Gonin, a Swiss, presented the principles on which contemporary retinal detachment surgery is based. His contributions were preceded in 1851 by Helmholz's invention of the ophthalmoscope, which allowed identification of retinal breaks and tears, and followed by the invention of the binocular indirect ophthalmoscope by Schepens in 1947 and, more recently, posterior segment biomicroscopy.

Gonin's principles included (1) drainage of subretinal fluid and (2) identification of retinal breaks and tears, sealing them with cautery. Evolution of technique has included the development of various methods to create chorioretinal adhesions, notably trans-scleral diathermy, cryosurgery, and photocoagulation, and methods to appose the retina to the choroid, including intraocular gas tamponade, scleral shortening or imbricating techniques, and the use of exogenous implants to indent or buckle the sclera. Appreciation of the relationships between the vitreous and retina and the development of closed-eye vitrectomy surgery by Machemer in the early 1970s, followed by the invention of numerous devices to facilitate intraocular manipulations, have set the stage for veterinary ophthalmic surgeons who attempt retinal detachment repair.

Pathophysiology and Indications

Retinal detachments can be classified by cause into those that are (1) rhegmatogenous—that is, associated with a retinal tear or hole through which, when combined with vitreous traction and liquefication, vitreous enters and dissects the neurosensory retina off of the retinal pigment epithelium; (2) tractional, in which neurosensory retina is pulled off the retinal pigment epithelium by contraction of preretinal or vitreal membranes; and (3) exudative/hemorrhagic, in which the primary disease involves the choroidal vasculature or retinal pigment epithelium to allow plasma transudate, exudate, or hemorrhage to accumulate between the photoreceptors and retinal pigment epithelium. Regardless of cause, separation of photoreceptors from their source of nutrition (the choriocapillaris) and their photopigment recycling factories (the retinal pigment epithelium) initiates photoreceptor degeneration that is progressive and largely irreversible. Thus prognosis for vision depends on duration; although specifics have not been determined for animals' eyes, it is not likely that reattachments will result in vision if the detachment is prolonged.

Indications for surgical reattachment include a rhegmatogenous detachment, ideally where the tear or hole can be identified, or a tractional detachment, either of relatively short duration. The smaller the tear or hole in a rhegmatogenous detachment, the better the chance of reattachment. Focal serous detachments associated with optic disc colobomas in collies have been treated with xenon photocoagulation with good results; however, the natural history of this process has not been defined, and thus treatment recommendations and critical evaluation of treatment efficacy are not known.

Techniques

Tractional detachments require pars plana vitrectomy as well as appositional techniques. Rhegmatogenous detachments are repaired by the drainage of subretinal fluid, apposition of neurosensory retina to retinal pigment epithelium at the hole or tear, and creation of chorioretinal adhesions adjacent to the defect.

Drainage of subretinal fluid is performed by a 360° peritomy and posterior dissection over the area of detachment; the sclera, choroid, and retinal pigment epithelium are perforated with a 25-gauge needle, and gentle compression on adjacent sclera is used to facilitate fluid escape. Depending on the extent of the detachment, multiple drainage sites may be necessary.

Trans-scleral cryosurgery is a safe, effective way to create a chorioretinal adhesion; nitrous oxide is the preferred refrigerant. Freezing retina creates an adhesion stronger than treating only the retinal pigment epithelium. Adhesion effect is time dependent and increases linear to maximum after 10 to 12 days. Freezing is performed with observation provided by indirect ophthalmoscopy, and the area over the tear or hole and adjacent to it is treated. Adhesions can also be generated with photocoagulation.

Apposition of neurosensory retina and retinal pigment epithelium is acheived using either scleral buckles or pneumatic retinopexy. Silicone buckling elements are available in a wide assortment of designs selected on the basis of the location and size of the tear or hole; encircling bands are placed posterior to the insertion of the rectus muscles and secured with intrascleral mattress sutures of 5-0 nonabsorbable material in each quadrant. A spatulated needle is essential for intrascleral suture placement. Silicone "tires" or sponges are used beneath the band to enhance the indentation effect.

Intraocular gases can be used alone or in conjunction with scleral buckles to tamponade the retina against retinal pigment epithelium. Pneumatic retinopexy relies on the effects of an expanding intravitreal gas bubble to reappose the retina. Air is the most common gas used; expanding gases include sulfur hexafluoride and perfluoropropane, which via diffusion can expand to 2.5 and 4 times their original volumes respectively, in the first 24 hours after injection. Half-life values are 1 to 5 days for air, 2 to 2.5 days for sulfur hexafluoride, and 4 to 6 days for perfluoropropane. Because gas bubbles rise, they are most effective if the tear or hole is located in the superior quadrants (as the detachments following cataract surgery usually are).

Other techniques used to repair severe human retinal detachments include intravitreal silicone oil, sodium hyaluronate, heavier-than-water perfluorocarbon liquids, and retinal tacks and cyanoacrylate glues, all of which may have application to retinal detachment repair in animals.

Common complications of cryotherapy include hemorrhage (4 per cent in humans) and choroidal effusion (18 per cent); scleral buckling, infection, or extrusion (up to 15 per cent); and intravitreal gas injection, elevation of intraocular pressure, and corneal endothelial toxicity. Complications of vitrectomy include proliferative vitreoretinopathy, which, as the name implies, is a relentless process that prevents reattachment. Of course, the most common complication regardless of technique is failure to reattach the retina. Although scant data are available to determine success rates in animals, repair was successful in three of four dogs treated with scleral buckles for postcataract extraction retinal detachments.[8]

References

1. Aguirre GD, et al: Development of the canine eye. *Am J Vet Res 33*:2399, 1972.
2. Barraquer F: Surgery of the dislocated lens. *Trans Am Acad Ophthalmol Otolaryngol 76*:44, 1972.
3. Binder PS: Anterior vitrectomy in cataract surgery, aphakic keratoplasty, and patients with vitreous pathology using a simple vitreophage. *Ann Ophthalmol 6*:947, 1974.
4. Binder PS: Present surgical approaches to vitrectomy. *Ann Ophthalmol 7*:1377, 1975.
5. Castroviejo R: Handling of eyes with vitreous prolapse. *Am J Ophthalmol 48*:397, 1959.
6. Cerasoli JR, Kasner D: A follow-up study of vitreous loss during cataract surgery managed by anterior vitrectomy. *Am J Ophthalmol 71*:1040, 1971.
7. Cole DF: Comparative aspects of the intraocular fluids. *In* Dawson H, Graham LT (eds): *Comparative Physiology*. Vol 1, Academic Press, New York, 1974.
8. Dziezyc J, et al: Surgical repair of rhegmatogenous retinal detachments in dogs. *J Am Vet Med Assoc 189*:902, 1986.
9. Foos RY: Vitreoretinal juncture, topographical variations. *Invest Ophthalmol 12*:801, 1972.
10. Ford V: Proposed surgical treatment of opaque vitreous. *Lancet 1*:462, 1890.
11. Freeman H: Recent advances in vitreous surgery. *Invest Ophthalmol 12*:549, 1973.
12. Gardner RC: Anterior vitrectomy. *Ann Ophthalmol 7*:723, 1975.
13. Iliff CE: Management of vitreous loss after cataract extraction. *Arch Ophthalmol 83*:319, 1970.
14. Kasner D: Vitrectomy: A new approach to the management of vitreous. *Highlights Ophthalmol 11*:304, 1969.
15. Kasner D, et al: Surgical treatment of amyloidosis of the vitreous. *Trans Am Acad Ophthalmol Otolaryngol 72*:410, 1968.
16. Kaufman HE: Vitrectomy from the anterior approach. Vitrectomy for the anterior segment surgeon. *Ophthalmic Surg 6*:58, 1975.
17. Machemer R: A new concept for vitreous surgery. 2. Surgical technique and complication. *Am J Ophthalmol 74*:1022, 1972.
18. Machemer R, Norton E: A new concept for vitreous surgery. 3. Indications and results. *Am J Ophthalmol 74*:1034, 1972.

19. Machemer R, et al: A new concept for vitreous surgery. 1. Instrumentation. *Am J Ophthalmol 73*:1, 1972.
20. Martin CL, Anderson BG: Ocular anatomy. *In* Gelatt K (ed): *Veterinary Ophthalmology*. Lea & Febiger, Philadelphia, 1981, pp 80–84.
21. Michaels RG, et al: Vitreous surgery: History and concepts. *Ophthalmic Surg 5*:13, 1974.
22. Peiffer RL Jr: Removal of a luxated lens and anterior vitrectomy using a disposable vitreophage. *Vet Med Small Anim Clin 75*:1249, 1980.
23. Peyman GA, et al: A review of substances and techniques of vitreous replacement. *Surv Ophthalmol 17*:41, 1972.
24. Peyman GA, et al: Techniques of vitreous removal. *Surv Ophthalmol 17*:29, 1972.
25. Tolentino FI, et al: Biomicroscopy of the vitreous in collie dogs with fundus abnormalities. *Arch Ophthalmol 73*:700, 1965.
26. Turtz AI: Anterior vitrectomy. *Ophthalmic Surg 1*:14, 1970.

CHAPTER 90

Orbit

Douglas Slatter and E. Dan Wolf

The orbit is the bony cavity surrounding the eye. Many orbital disorders are treated surgically, and manipulative procedures are frequently used in the diagnosis of orbital disease. In this chapter, major features of orbital anatomy and pathophysiology are discussed before the diseases themselves. For discussion of nonsurgical orbital disease, readers are referred to veterinary ophthalmology texts.[10, 25] Orbital surgery should not be attempted without a thorough understanding of orbital anatomy. Close observation of a skull of the same species before and during surgery is suggested.

The orbit of the dog and cat[7] surrounds and protects the eye and separates the eye from the cranial cavity. Blood vessels and nerves serving orbital structures pass through numerous foramina in the bony orbital walls (Figs. 90–1 through 90–7). The length of the optic nerve is greater than the distance from the eye to the optic foramen (Fig. 90–8).

The dorsolateral wall of the orbit is not composed of bone but is formed by the dense collagenous orbital ligament between the zygomatic process of the frontal bone and the frontal process of the zygomatic bone (see

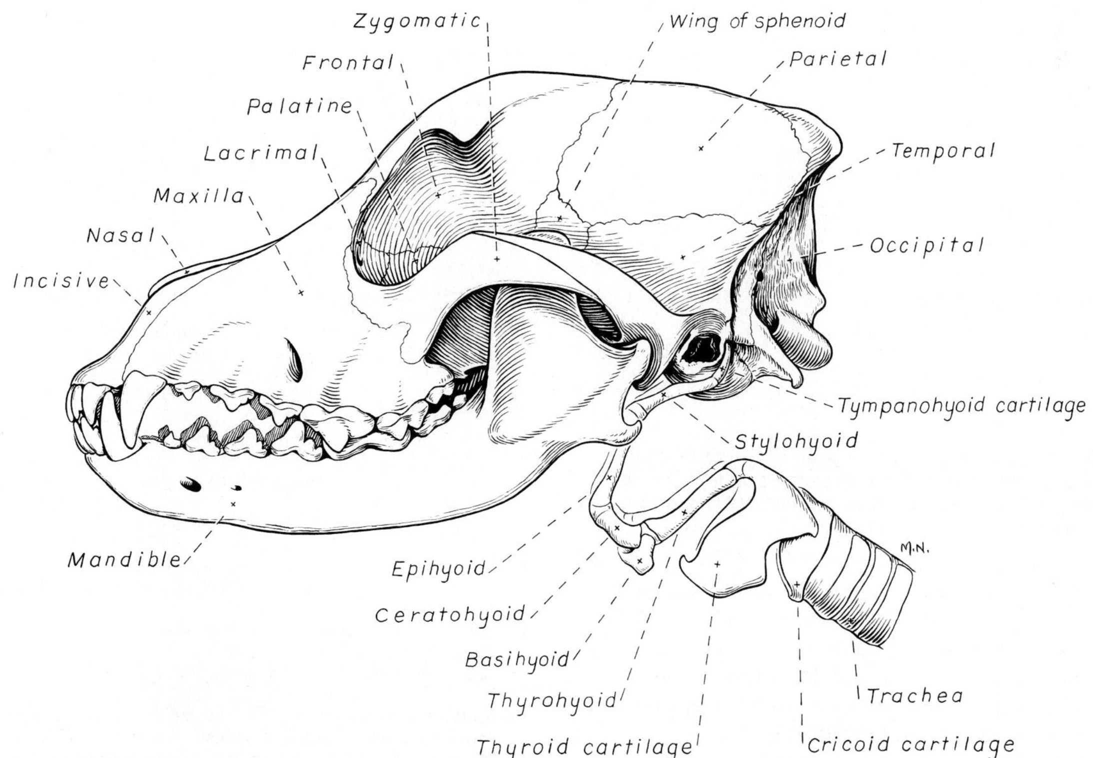

FIGURE 90–1. Bones of the skull, hyoid apparatus, and laryngeal cartilages. (Reprinted with permission from Evans HE (ed): *Miller's Anatomy of the Dog.* 3rd ed. W.B. Saunders, Philadelphia, 1993.)

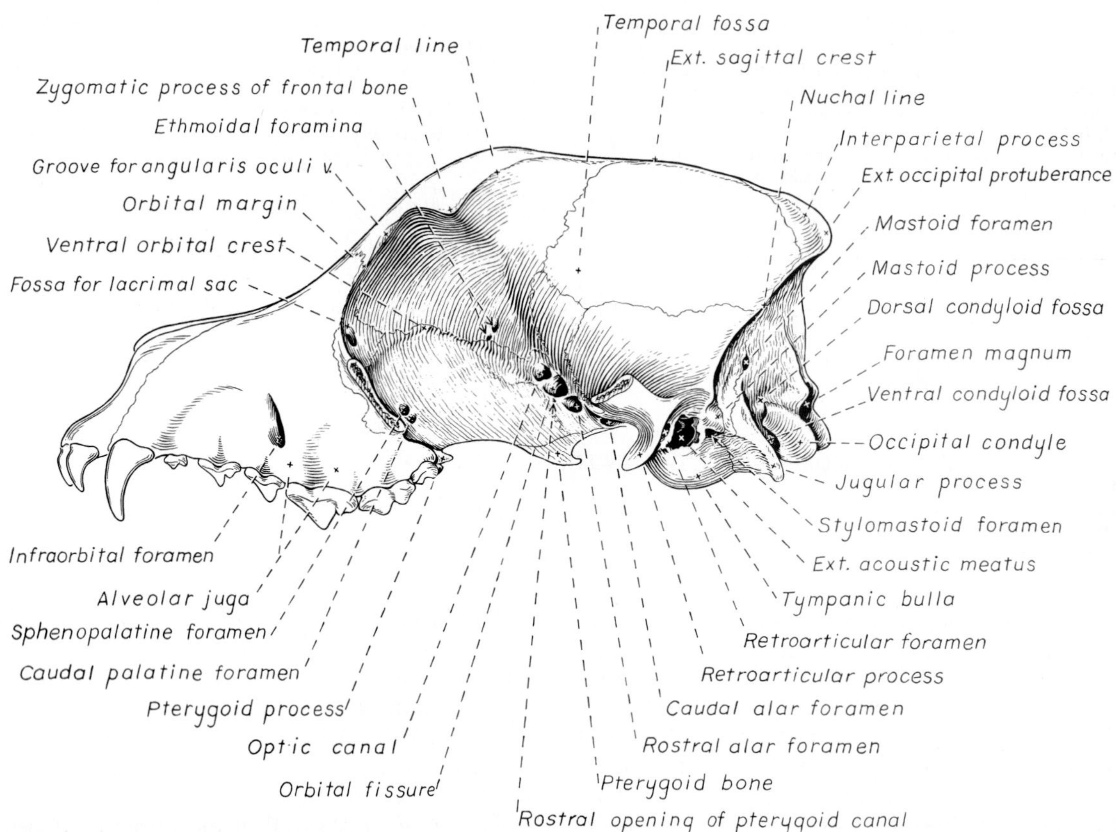

FIGURE 90–2. Skull, lateral aspect (zygomatic arch removed). (Reprinted with permission from Evans HE (ed): *Miller's Anatomy of the Dog.* 3rd ed. W.B. Saunders, Philadelphia, 1993.)

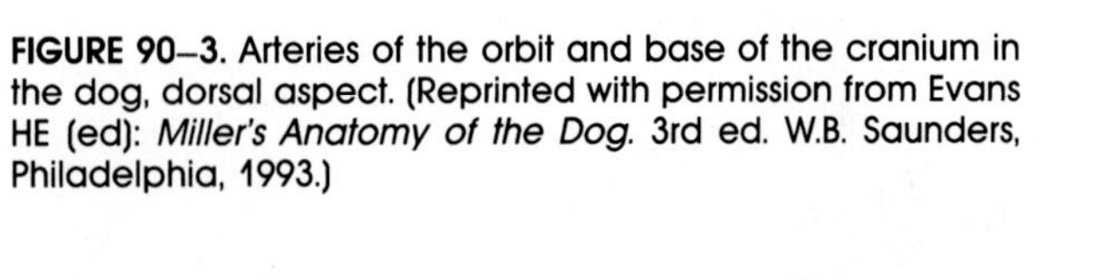

FIGURE 90–3. Arteries of the orbit and base of the cranium in the dog, dorsal aspect. (Reprinted with permission from Evans HE (ed): *Miller's Anatomy of the Dog.* 3rd ed. W.B. Saunders, Philadelphia, 1993.)

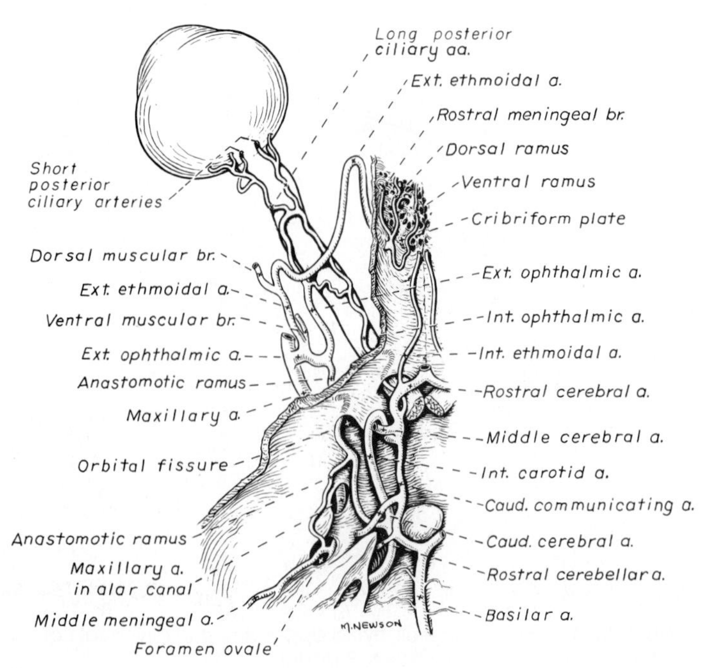

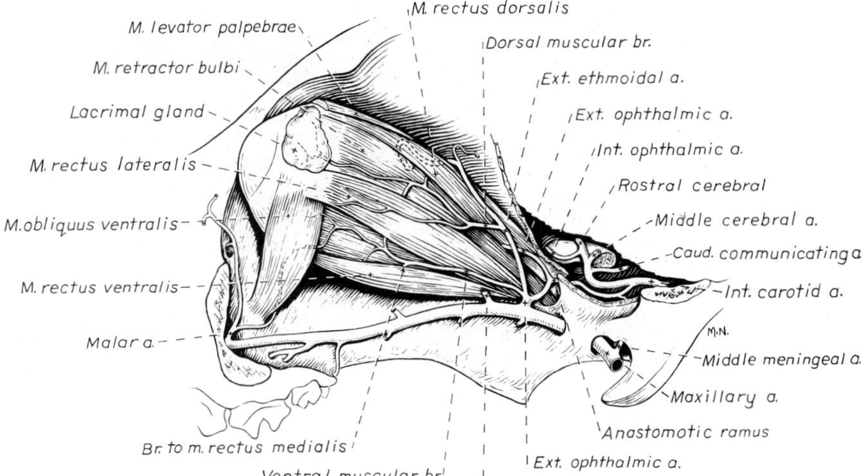

FIGURE 90–4. Arteries of the orbit and extrinsic ocular muscles in the dog, lateral aspect. (Reprinted with permission from Evans HE (ed): *Miller's Anatomy of the Dog.* 3rd ed. W.B. Saunders, Philadelphia, 1993.)

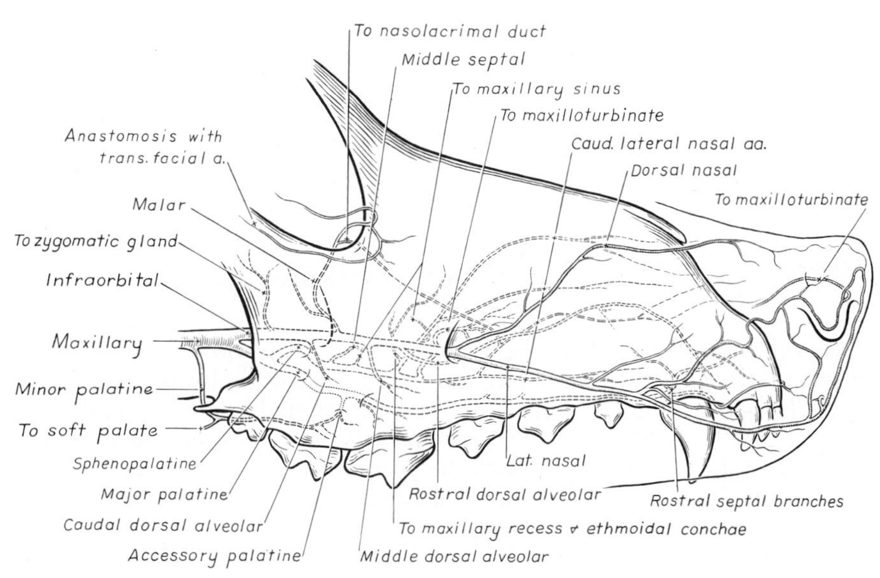

FIGURE 90–5. Scheme of the terminal branches of the maxillary artery in the dog, lateral aspect. (Reprinted with permission from Evans HE (ed): *Miller's Anatomy of the Dog.* 3rd ed. W.B. Saunders, Philadelphia, 1993.)

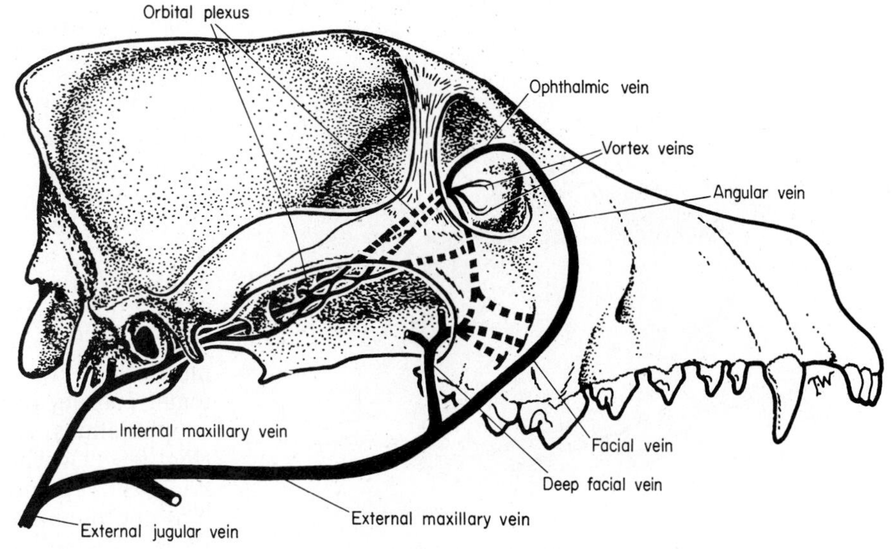

FIGURE 90–6. The venous drainage of the eye and orbit. (Reprinted with permission from Startup FG: *Diseases of the Canine Eye.* Williams & Wilkins, Baltimore, 1969.)

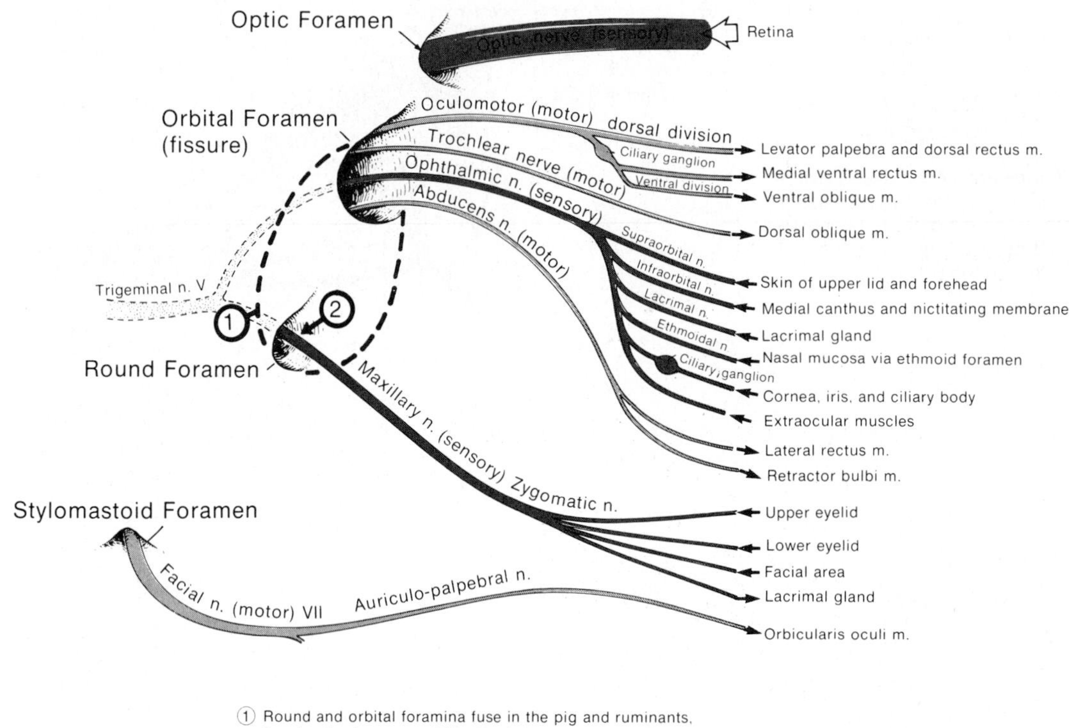

FIGURE 90–7. Nerve supply to the eye.

Fig. 90–1).[9] The soft-tissue contents of the orbit are enclosed by the periorbita, connective tissue that lies next to the bony walls and is thickened laterally as the orbital ligament (see Fig. 90–8).

The periorbita also surrounds the extraocular muscles and forms the Tenon capsule, which blends with the sclera and conjunctiva near the limbus. Incorporated in the retrobulbar portion of the periorbita is smooth muscle innervated by sympathetic nerve fibers. Normal sympathetic tone helps maintain the typical position of the eye within the orbit. The periorbita is continuous with the periosteum of the facial bones around the orbital rim, the orbital septum, and the dura of the optic nerve at the optic foramen. The orbital fat pad lies between the periorbita and the orbital wall posteriorly. Extraocular muscles arise from the fibrous annulus of Zinn, which surrounds the posterior orbital foramina and blends with the periosteum (Figs. 90–9 and 90–10). Innervation and function of the extraocular muscles are listed in Table 90–1.

The lacrimal gland lies beneath the orbital ligament on the dorsolateral surface of the globe and is surrounded by the periorbita (see Fig. 90–8).

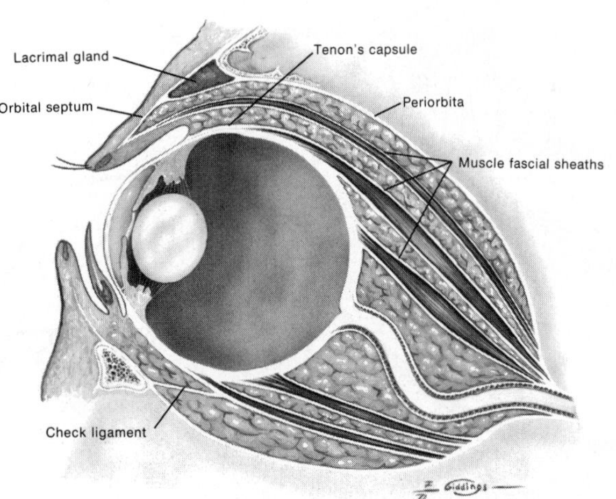

FIGURE 90–8. Division of the periorbita.

PATHOLOGICAL MECHANISMS

The orbit is a confined space. Changes in the volume and contents of the orbit affect the position of the globe in relation to the orbital rim, the face, and the other eye. The position of the margin of the third eyelid is usually affected also. The periorbita and extraocular muscles provide three possible compartments for disease processes (see Fig. 90–8): (1) within the muscle cone, (2) outside the muscle cone but within the periorbita, or (3) within the bony walls of the orbit but outside the periorbita (i.e., beneath the periosteum [periorbita] or behind the periorbita laterally).

Space-occupying lesions (e.g., tumors,[4, 22] zygomatic mucocele,[24] and abscesses) displace normal orbital contents, causing protrusion of the third eyelid rostrally, exophthalmos, and swelling behind the last upper molar (Fig. 90–11), where the periorbita is unrestrained by a bony wall. Accurate differentiation between exophthalmos and buphthalmos is essential and is discussed elsewhere. Reduction in volume of orbital contents or loss

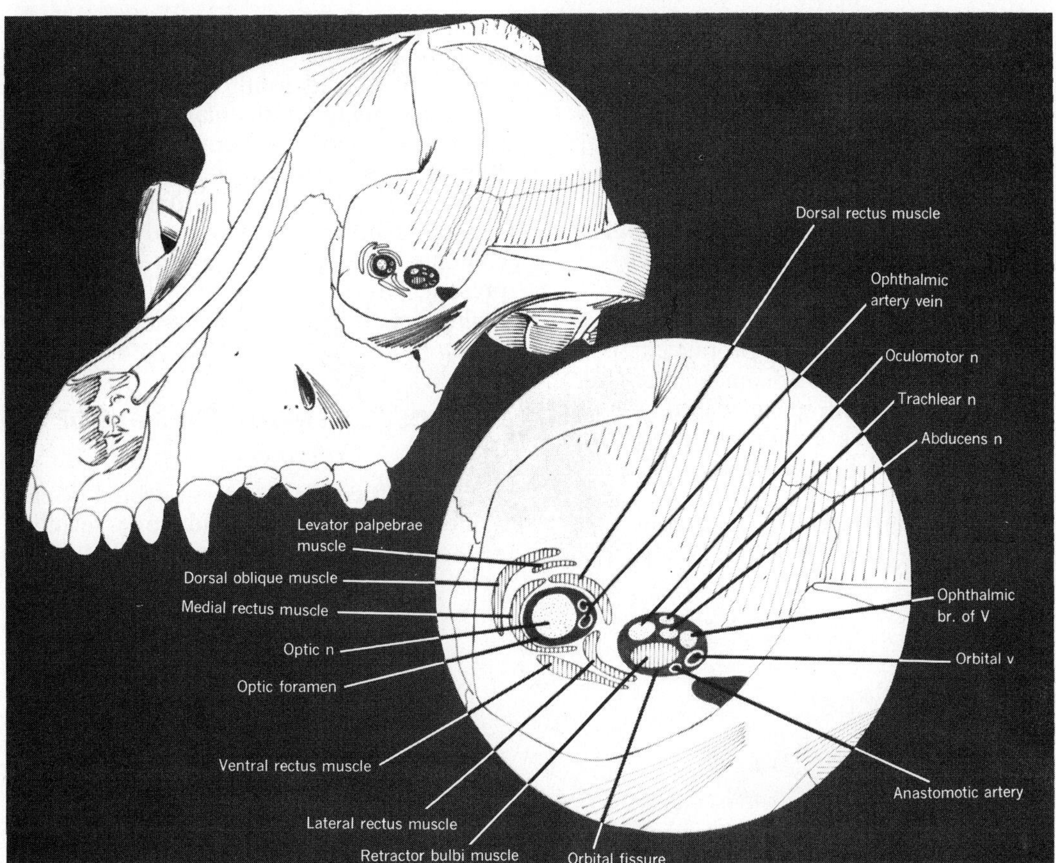

FIGURE 90–9. Orbital apex of dog illustrating structures passing through the optic foramen and orbital fissure as well as extraocular muscle attachments. (Reprinted with permission from Gelatt KN: *Textbook of Veterinary Ophthalmology.* Lea & Febiger, Philadelphia, 1981.)

of sympathetic innervation (Horner's syndrome) causes the eye to recede into the orbit (enophthalmos) and the third eyelid to protrude. With the exception of displaced orbital fractures, enophthalmos usually does not require surgery unless it causes severe entropion and chronic infection with dermatitis and pain. Periorbital epidermoid cysts may cause swelling in the medial canthal area.[5]

The position of space-occupying lesions alters the direction in which the globe is displaced and is useful in localizing a mass for fine-needle aspiration, biopsy, or excision (Fig. 90–12). Exophthalmos leads to increased evaporation of the precorneal tear film with exposure keratitis, ulceration, and conjunctivitis. Orbital edema typically extends anteriorly to cause chemosis, and obstruction of retrobulbar venous drainage exacerbates the condition.

The proximity of the paranasal sinuses (Fig. 90–13), teeth, zygomatic gland, and vertical ramus of the mandible to the orbit influences the extension of disease processes in these structures by affecting the orbital tissues. Infections and neoplasms in the sinuses or nasal cavity may invade the orbit, usually through the thin medial wall[9] of the orbit where the frontal, lacrimal, and palatine bones join. Orbital emphysema may result from fracture of an adjacent sinus wall, an osteolytic

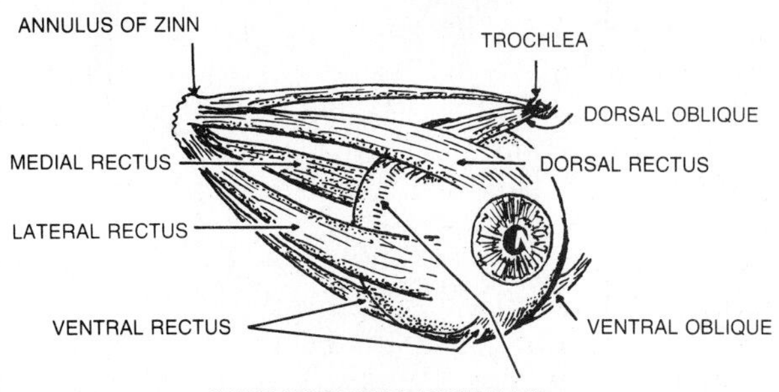

FIGURE 90–10. General arrangement of the orbital muscles. (After Prince JH, et al: *Anatomy and Histology of the Eye and Orbit in Domestic Animals.* Charles C Thomas, Springfield, 1960. Courtesy of Charles C Thomas, Publisher, Springfield, Illinois.)

TABLE 90–1. INNERVATION OF THE EXTRAOCULAR MUSCLES

Muscle	Innervation	Action
Dorsal rectus	Oculomotor III	Elevates globe
Ventral rectus	Oculomotor III	Depresses globe
Medial rectus	Oculomotor III	Turns globe nasally (medially)
Lateral rectus	Abducens VI	Turns globe temporally (laterally)
Dorsal oblique	Trochlear IV	Intorts globe (rotates 12 o'clock position nasally)
Ventral oblique	Oculomotor III	Extorts globe (rotates 12 o'clock position temporally)
Retractor of the globe	Abducens VI	Retracts globe
Superior levator	Oculomotor III	Elevates upper lid

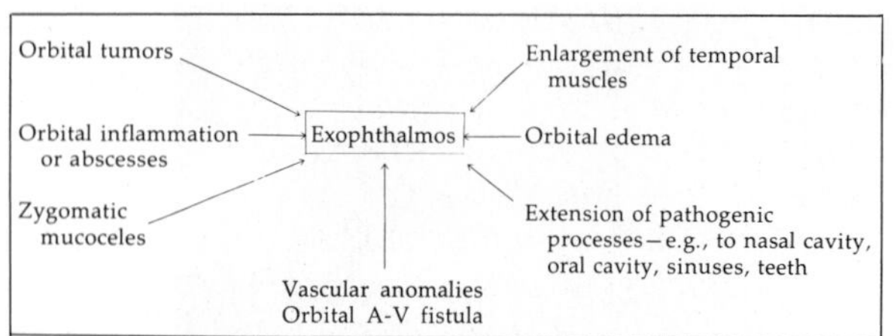

FIGURE 90–11. Mechanisms of exophthalmos.

process of the sinus wall, or enucleation (air enters via the nasolacrimal duct).[1, 16] Although uncommon, such passage of air may be caused by increased pressure within the nasal cavity during expiration in brachycephalic dogs with collapsed external nares and elevated intranasal pressure.

Orbital infection or cellulitis can be caused by infections of the roots of the molar teeth or foreign body penetration of the ventral orbit via the oral cavity. A discharging fistula beneath the eye is also a common sign of abscessed tooth roots. Sialocele of the canine zygomatic gland[18] with enlargement can cause the gland to protrude into the ventral orbit and appear in the ventral conjunctival fornix or behind the last upper molar. When the mouth is opened, the vertical ramus of the mandible moves forward, pressing on the orbital contents and causing pain if cellulitis or abscess is present. Dislocation of the mandible may cause exophthalmos if the vertical ramus impinges on orbital contents.

DIAGNOSTIC METHODS AND SIGNS OF ORBITAL DISEASE

The most common sign of orbital disease is displacement of the third eyelid and globe, resulting from either an increase or decrease in orbital soft-tissue mass. Other

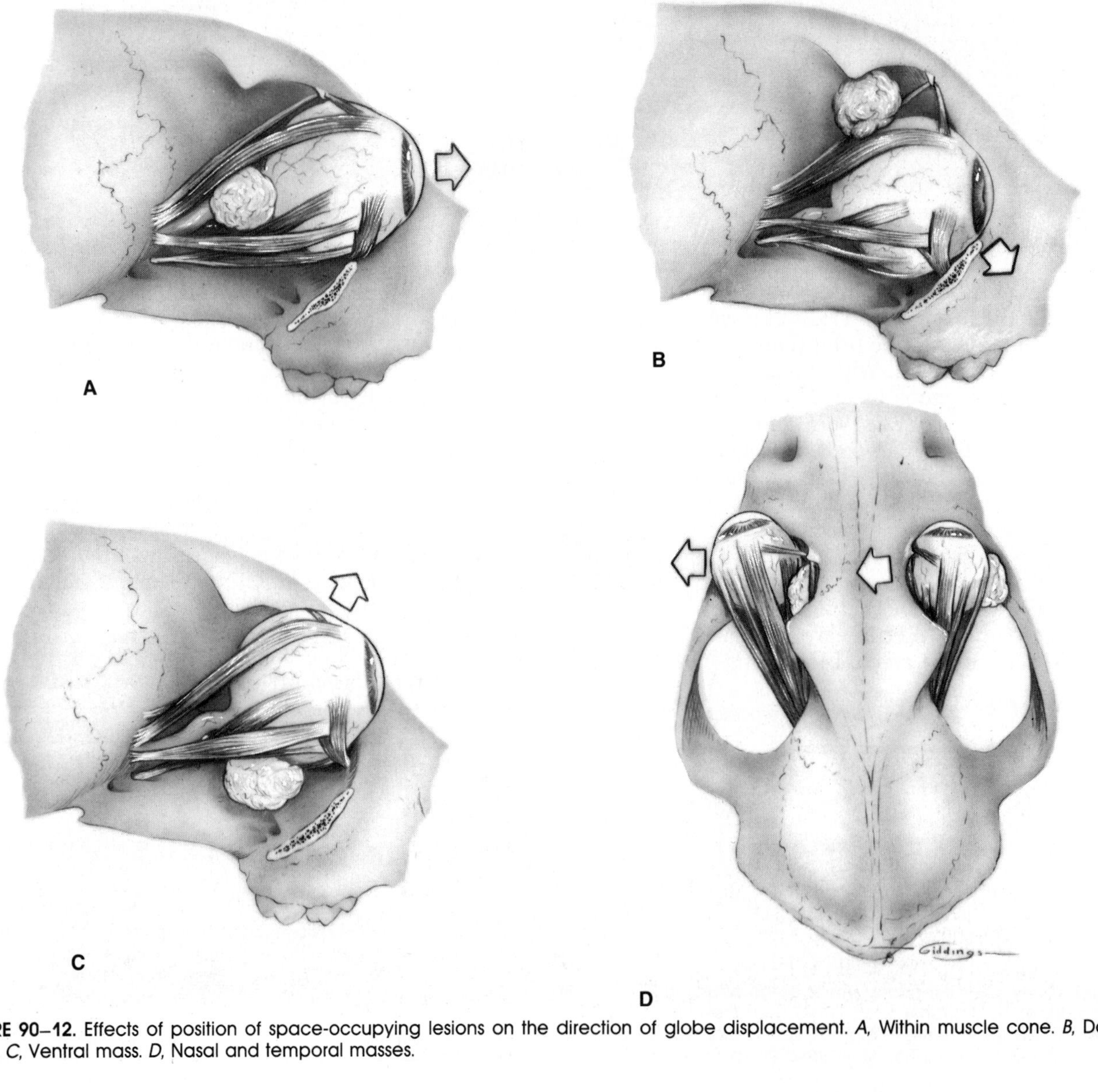

FIGURE 90–12. Effects of position of space-occupying lesions on the direction of globe displacement. *A*, Within muscle cone. *B*, Dorsal mass. *C*, Ventral mass. *D*, Nasal and temporal masses.

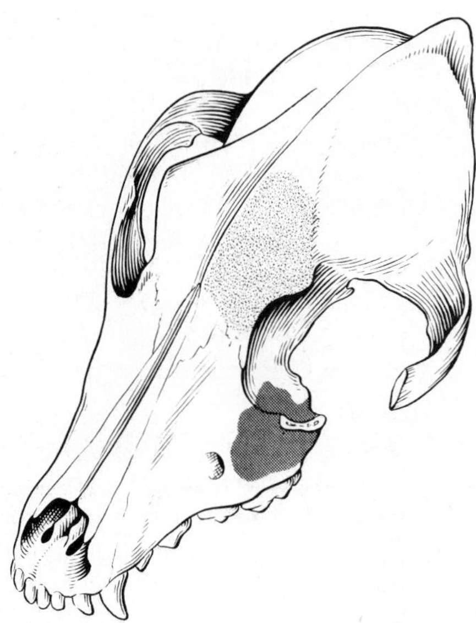

FIGURE 90–13. Relationship of the paranasal sinuses to the orbital walls in the dog. (Reprinted with permission from Evans HE (ed): *Miller's Anatomy of the Dog.* 3rd ed. W.B. Saunders, Philadelphia, 1993.)

signs include chemosis, conjunctival erythema, periorbital swelling, pain on opening the mouth if inflammation is present, neurological deficits including blindness, and posterior indentation of the globe. Because extension of neoplasia from the nasal sinuses into the orbit is common, nasal discharge and incomplete passage of air through the nose may be present.

Although an aggressive diagnostic and therapeutic approach to orbital disease is recommended, thorough diagnostic evaluation can help differentiate surgical disease from nonsurgical disease and permit more directed surgical approaches.

Thorough palpation, complete cranial nerve evaluation, ocular examination (including the fundus), and examination of the oral cavity and nasal passages represent a preliminary evaluation of the orbit, orbital contents, and contiguous structures. Other evaluations and special tests may be necessary, including serum chemistry and hematological studies, fine-needle aspiration and cytological study, biopsy, and special radiographic and alternative imaging techniques (e.g., orbital venography [Fig. 90–14],[6] arteriography,[28] sialography,[4] thecography,[15] contrast orbitography,[20] ultrasonography,[8] computed tomography scanning,[14] and magnetic resonance imaging).

Palpation of the orbit is essential; the bony orbital rim and ventral orbit (via the oral cavity) may be palpated directly. The posterior orbit may be palpated by using the globe as an extension of the palpating finger (ballotement). The globe under gentle pressure normally retropulses posteromedially to various degrees depending on species and breed. Inability to retropulse the globe or retropulsion in an abnormal direction may suggest the location and extent of retrobulbar lesions.

If fundus examination demonstrates indentation of the posterior wall of the globe, the extent and location of the indentation define the adjacent aspects of the lesion. If the indentation is "fixed in the fundus," it moves within the extraocular muscle cone. If it "rolls" across the fundus as the eye moves, the lesion usually is outside the cone. Exophthalmos that resists retropulsion, as well as loss of ocular movement, is usually associated with diffuse orbital disease.

Elevation and palpation of the base of the third eyelid may localize the lesion to the third eyelid. Ultrasonography of orbital lesions[5, 8] helps differentiate localized from diffuse involvement and solid from cystic lesions. Fine-needle aspiration of the localized lesion or of a medial retrobulbar space with a diffuse lesion often results in a specific diagnosis. These relatively inexpensive and noninvasive procedures decrease the indications for exploratory orbitotomy, which should be reserved for therapeutic purposes if possible.

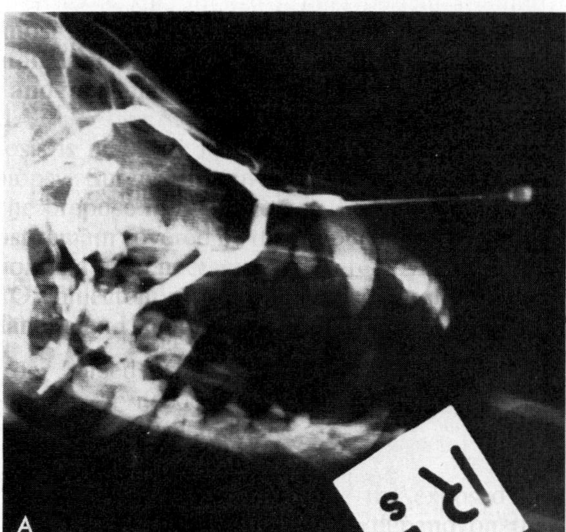

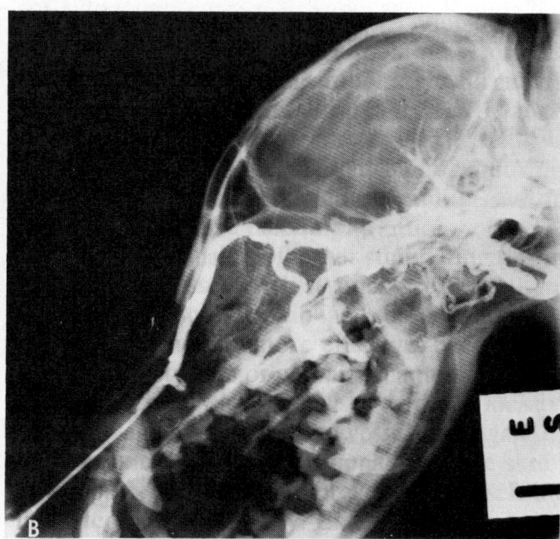

FIGURE 90–14. *A,* Lateral orbital venogram (right eye). *B,* Venogram of left orbit in a 5-year-old poodle with a lymphoid pseudotumor in the inferonasal orbit. The inferior ophthalmic vein has been obliterated. (Courtesy of Dr. R. Dixon.)

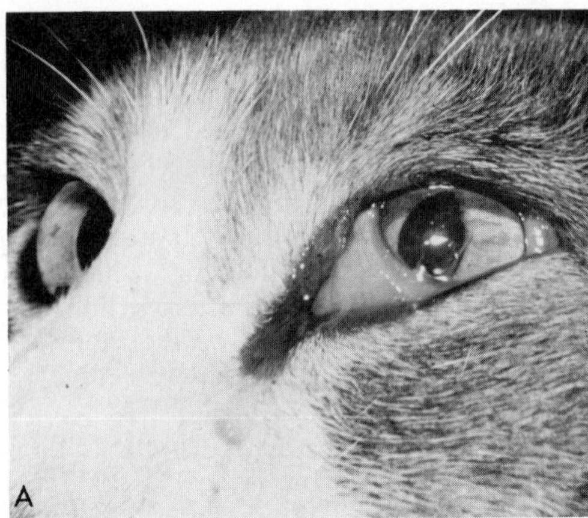

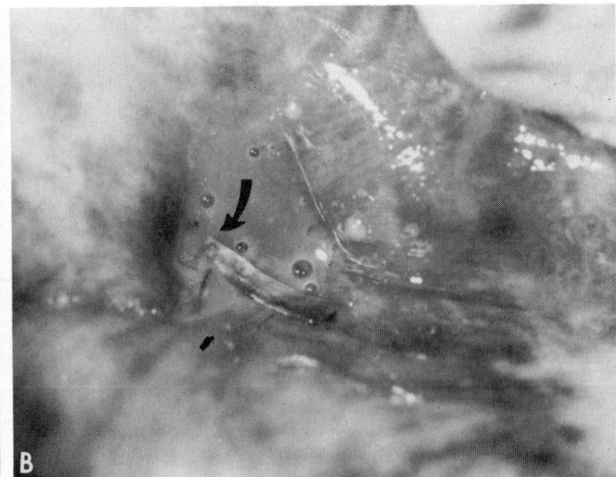

FIGURE 90–15. *A*, Acute retrobulbar abscess in a cat with exophthalmos, protrusion of the third eyelid, chemosis, and pain on opening the mouth. *B*, Foreign body behind the last molar tooth of a dog with acute retrobulbar abscess. The foreign body was 6 cm in length. (Courtesy of Dr. Stephen Bistner.)

ORBITAL DISORDERS

Orbital Inflammation

Orbital inflammation occurs in both dogs and cats and may be diffuse, with or without abscessation, or may be localized involving masticatory muscles, extraocular muscles, or other specific orbital structures (e.g., adenitis). Diffuse cellulitis, which can progress to a retrobulbar abscess (Fig. 90–15), is often associated with a foreign body or infection introduced locally or by hematogenous spread. Mycotic and other opportunistic organisms can also invade the retrobulbar space.

Clinical signs of orbital inflammation include pyrexia, chemosis, protrusion of the third eyelid, conjunctival congestion, decreased or painful retropulsion of the globe, pain on opening the mouth, variable exophthalmos, fluctuating red swelling in the oral mucous membrane behind the last upper molar tooth (Fig. 90–16), periorbital swelling, and anorexia. The clinical signs are usually subacute to acute but may be intermittent initially. Immune-mediated myositis generally causes fever and systemic effects and is usually bilateral.

Based on clinical signs alone, it is often impossible to distinguish orbital cellulitis from abscess. In cellulitis, pain, pyrexia, and anorexia are less severe. The two can usually be differentiated by the lack of discharge when the orbit is drained to the oral cavity. Orbital inflammation is distinguished from other causes of exophthalmos by its acute onset, pain, pyrexia, and the frequent occurrence of leukocytosis with neutrophilia. Diagnosis of orbital inflammation is based on clinical signs, hematological and serum chemistry evaluations, ultrasonography, fine-needle aspiration and cytological study, and possibly exploratory biopsy. Accurate diagnosis should be pursued vigorously, because major differential diagnoses include aggressive neoplasia and systemic mycoses, which require early and specific treatment.

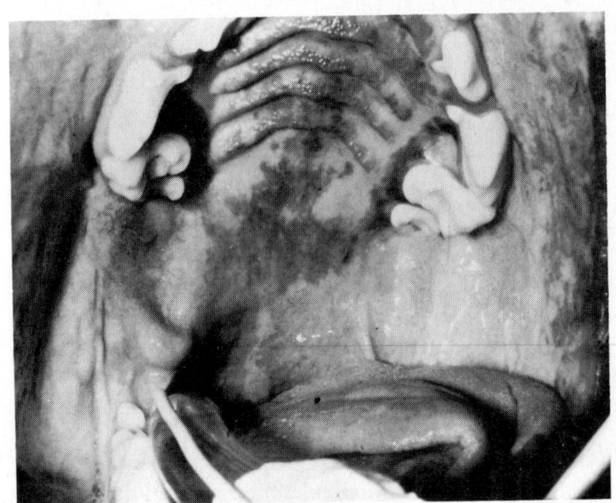

FIGURE 90–16. Fluctuant reddened mucous membrane behind the last upper molar.

Treatment

Cellulitis and abscesses are treated by ventral drainage to the oral cavity and systemic and local antibiotics. If immune-mediated myositis is present, corticosteroids are indicated. Drainage is through an incision behind the last upper molar (Fig. 90–17). The mucous membrane is incised, and a pair of curved Crile hemostats or a blunt probe is inserted (Fig. 90–18) and gradually advanced and opened in small steps until the orbit is reached. Dependent drainage to the orbit is established, and small pockets of exudate (sometimes under pressure) may be released.

The orbit is flushed with sterile saline or crystalline penicillin solution via the oral incision with a blunt needle or lacrimal cannula. Systemic antibiotics are administered for 5 to 7 days, and soft foods are fed during the recovery period, which is usually short (1 to 2 days). Topical antibiotics and tear replacement solutions may be used if severe conjunctivitis was present before drainage. Exploratory orbitotomy may occasionally be required if response to therapy is poor or to locate foreign bodies.

Zygomatic Mucocele[17, 24]

A mucocele is a leakage of saliva from a gland or duct with inflammation and fibrosis. Mucocele of the zygomatic salivary gland beneath the eye occurs spon-

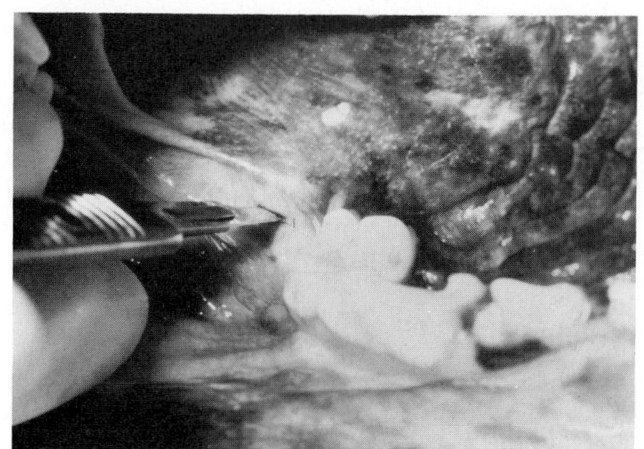

FIGURE 90–17. Site of incision for drainage of retrobulbar abscess.

taneously in dogs, as well as after trauma to the head. Although not common, it must be considered in the differential diagnosis of exophthalmos, space-occupying orbital lesions, and posterior oropharyngeal masses.

The clinical signs include protrusion of the oral mucous membrane behind the last upper molar, the presence of a mass in the ventral conjunctival fornix, protrusion of the third eyelid, exophthalmos, and painless orbital swelling. The clinical signs vary with the position of the mucocele in the orbit. Aspiration of fluid from within the mucocele reveals tenacious straw-colored fluid. A zygomatic sialogram may be useful in outlining the mucocele for therapy.

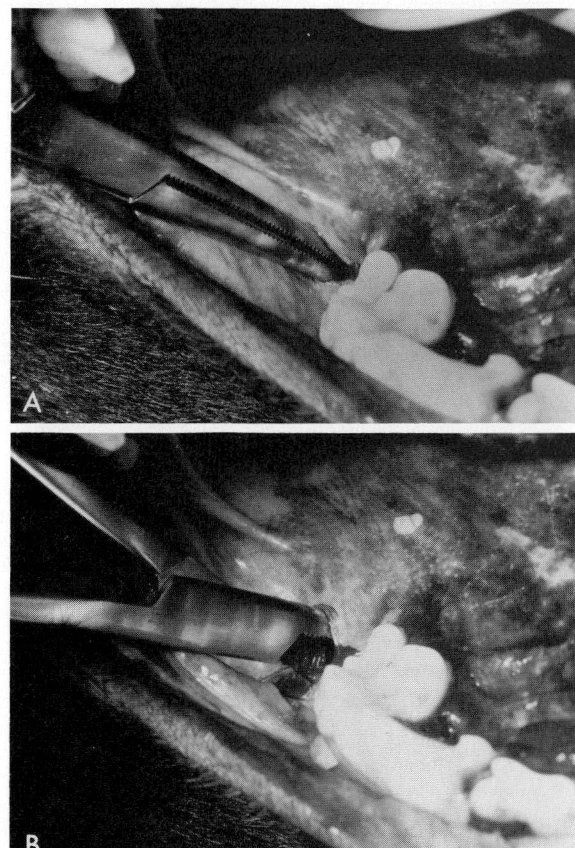

FIGURE 90–18. Gradual insertion of hemostats to establish drainage from the orbit to the oral cavity.

Treatment is resection of the gland and mucocele via local orbitotomy. Any of the following approaches may be used: (1) posterior to the orbital ligament, (2) dorsal to the zygomatic arch, (3) through the ventral conjunctival fornix, or (4) behind the last upper molar for orally visible lesions.

Orbital Emphysema[1, 16]

Air may enter the orbit from the paranasal sinuses after trauma (Fig. 90–19), from the nasolacrimal duct after enucleation (Fig. 90–20), or from an erosion of the wall of an adjacent sinus. The air is palpable as crepitus beneath the conjunctiva or periocular skin.

If emphysema is present, a radiographic study may demonstrate the source. Systemic antibiotics are used to prevent infection of the orbit from the sinuses. In the few cases reported, spontaneous resolution has occurred. If emphysema occurs after enucleation, the nasolacrimal duct may be cannulated from the nasal end, exposed at its upper end at its emergence from the lacrimal bone, and ligated.

Orbital emphysema after enucleation is more common in brachycephalic breeds, possibly because of the higher pressure in the nasal cavity near the exit of the nasolacrimal duct during expiration, collapsed nares, or a narrowed airway. Ligation of the dorsal end of the duct during enucleation in these breeds should prevent emphysema.

Orbital Cyst[11, 18]

Cystic structures of the orbit or periorbital tissue develop in glandular structures (lacrimal, salivary), cys-

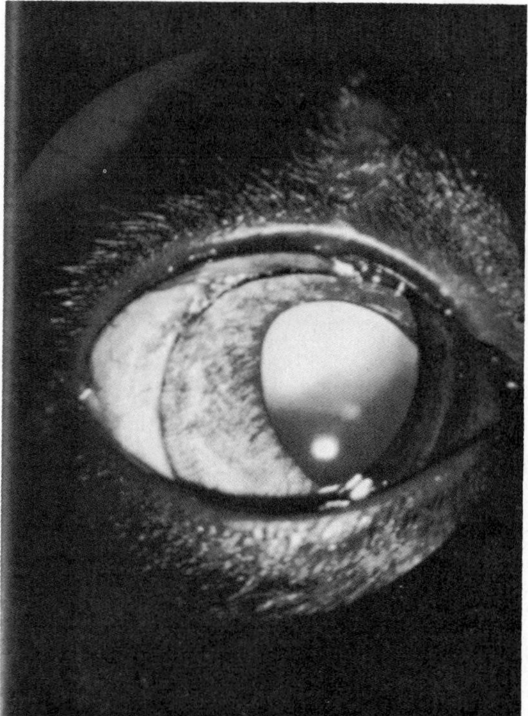

FIGURE 90–19. Subconjunctival emphysema following orbital trauma in a cat. (Reprinted with permission from Bryan G: Subconjunctival emphysema in a cat. *Vet Med Small Anim Clin 72*:1087, 1977.)

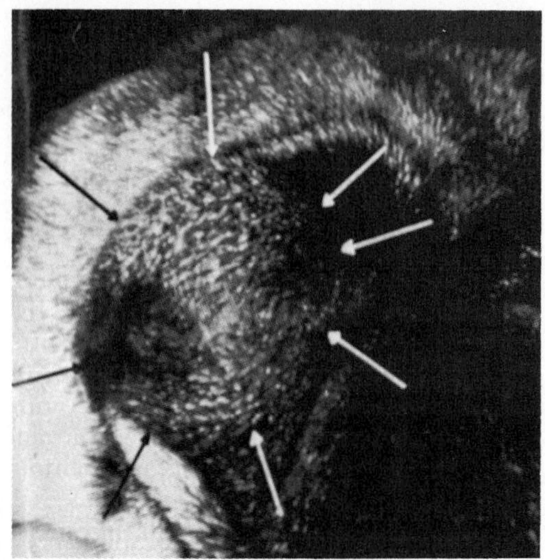

FIGURE 90–20. Orbital emphysema following enucleation in a pug. (Reprinted with permission from Martin CL: Orbital mucocele in a dog. *Vet Med Small Anim Clin 66*:986, 1971.)

tic neoplasia, or congenital lesions.[5] Cysts usually progress gradually, are unilateral, and are not painful causes of exophthalmos. Diagnosis is by clinical signs, ultrasonography, and fine-needle aspiration. Treatment is surgical removal of the cyst and associated glandular tissue.

Orbital cysts rarely occur because either the lacrimal gland or the gland of the third eyelid has been left in the orbit during enucleation. Care must be taken to remove these glands. If the cyst ruptures, a fistula may form. Because of its position within the periorbita, the cyst is often difficult to see and remove. If a cyst has formed, the orbit is opened, and the tissue is located and removed.

Vascular Abnormalities[13, 19, 22, 23]

Orbital arteriovenous fistulas and varices have been reported. Both conditions are rare but require an accurate diagnosis and specific therapy. Experience with vascular surgical techniques is necessary before treating such lesions.

Other Orbital Disorders[7, 27]

The differential diagnoses of other orbital conditions are considered in Table 90–2.

SURGICAL PROCEDURES

Orbital Drainage

Ventral orbital drainage to the oral cavity was discussed previously.

TABLE 90–2. SUMMARY OF ORBITAL DISEASES*

Type of Disorder	Condition	Clinical Signs
Developmental abnormalities	1. Shallow orbit (brachycephalic breeds)	1. Exophthalmos, exposure keratitis, corneal ulceration, pigmentation
	2. Microphthalmos, anophthalmos	2. Small or absent globe, narrow palpebral fissure, prominent third eyelid, epiphora, blindness
	3. Hydrocephalus with orbital malformation	3. Exotropia, hypotropia, poor vision
	4. Euryblepharon	4. Long palpebral fissure resulting in apparent exophthalmos
	5. Orbital arteriovenous fistula	5. Exophthalmos, fremitus, pulse detectable ("exophthalmos pulsans")
Trauma	1. Hemorrhages	1. Subconjunctival and episcleral hemorrhages; retrobulbar hemorrhage with exophthalmos or proptosis
	2. Penetrating foreign bodies (grass awns, needles, etc., from mouth)	2. Discharging sinus fluid through the conjunctiva, periocular skin, buccal mucosa; pain on opening mouth
	3. Orbital fractures	3. Pain, crepitus; skin abrasions, displacement of globe
Infections	1. Bacterial, fungal	1. Ocular discharge usually secondary to penetrating foreign bodies from conjunctiva or oral cavity; sinusitis, rhinitis, or infections of roots of teeth
	2. Parasites (*Dirofilaria immitis; Pneumonyssus caninum*)	2. Granulomatous lesions due to wandering larvae, e.g., *Dirofilaria* (rare), or extension of infection from nasal cavity (*Pneumonyssus*)
Neoplasia	1. Primary orbital neoplasms—sarcoma, meningioma, adenocarcinoma from nasal cavity, lymphosarcoma in cattle	1. Exophthalmos, exposure keratitis, strabismus, displacement of globe
	2. As for (1), plus nasal or neurological signs	
Miscellaneous conditions	1. Zygomatic mucocele	1. Exophthalmos, strabismus, swelling in any part of orbit or behind upper last molar tooth
	2. Infections of roots of teeth (especially carnassial)	2. Discharging fistula beneath eye in dogs
	3. Dehydration	3. Enophthalmos, protrusion of third eyelid
	4. Eosinophilic myositis	4. Exophthalmos, pain with dysphagia in acute stage; enophthalmos potentiated by opening mouth in chronic stage when temporal muscles have atrophied
	5. Horner's syndrome	5. Enophthalmos, miosis, ptosis, protrusion of nictitating membrane, ipsilateral sweating in horses, dermal vasodilation, and hypothermia

*Reprinted with permission from Slatter D: *Fundamentals of Veterinary Ophthalmology*. W.B. Saunders, Philadelphia, 1990.
Modified from Smith JS: Diseases of the orbit. *In* Kirk RW (ed): *Current Veterinary Therapy* VI. W.B. Saunders, Philadelphia, 1977.

Enucleation

Enucleation is removal of the globe and the third eyelid (Fig. 90–21). It is indicated for intraocular neoplasia, severe perforating ocular trauma, uncontrollable endophthalmitis or panophthalmitis, and intractable glaucoma when other treatment methods have failed. The use of cryotherapy, intrascleral prostheses, and intraocular drainage implants has almost eliminated the need for enucleation in glaucoma therapy. In dogs and cats, the lateral subconjunctival technique gives excellent results and leaves more orbital tissue than the transpalpebral method.

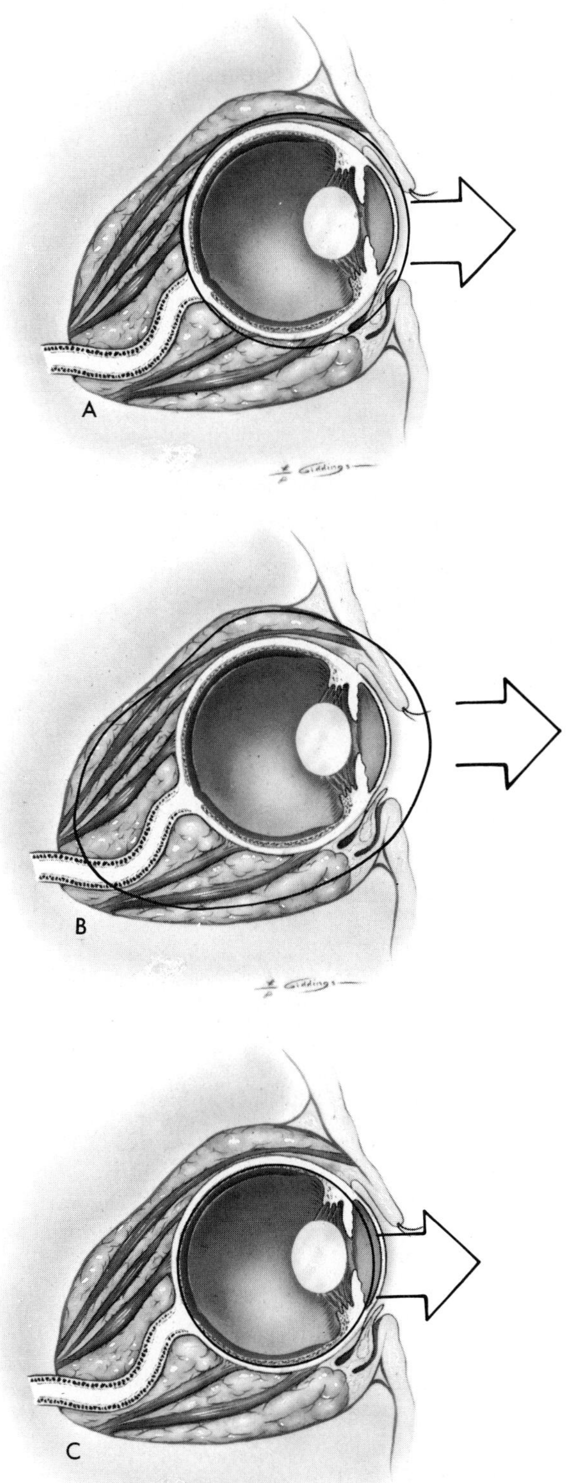

FIGURE 90–21. Diagram of *(A)* enucleation, *(B)* exenteration, and *(C)* evisceration.

Lateral Subconjunctival Enucleation[2]

A lateral canthotomy is performed for 1 to 2 cm to improve exposure. The conjunctiva is grasped near the limbus with toothed forceps, and a 360° perilimbal incision is made (Fig. 90–22*A*). The conjunctiva, fascia, and extraocular muscles are elevated from the sclera with curved Metzenbaum or Mayo scissors to the optic nerve (Fig. 90–22*B*). If possible, the lacrimal gland, which is found dorsolaterally over the globe, should be left attached to it.

The optic nerve is severed with either scissors or an electrosurgical tonsil snare (Fig. 90–22*C*). Excess traction on the optic nerve, especially in cats, may damage the optic chiasm and impair vision in the contralateral eye. A ligature may be placed around the optic nerve and nearby long and short posterior ciliary vessels. Hemorrhage in the orbit is controlled by either ligation or pressure from surgical sponges. The third eyelid is grasped and removed (Fig. 90–22*D*), and the orbit is temporarily packed with sponges. The eyelids are removed entirely (Fig. 90–22*E*) at this later stage to prevent blood from obscuring the earlier dissection during removal of the globe.

Surgical sponges are removed, and the conjunctiva and Tenon capsule are closed with simple interrupted sutures of 4-0 absorbable material. Any further hemorrhage is contained by the sutured conjunctiva (Fig. 90–22*F*). The lid incisions are closed with simple interrupted sutures of 4-0 silk, nylon, or polyglactin 910 (Fig. 90–22*G*).

Postoperative swelling is common, especially if hemorrhage has continued, but usually resolves in 3 to 4 days. The owner may observe a drop of red fluid on the nose from the nasal end of the nasolacrimal duct during the postoperative period as clots within the orbit break down. With enucleation, orbital fat and extraocular muscles are retained, making the defect after healing more cosmetic than after exenteration. A number of techniques have been used to reduce the orbital defect. Silicone prostheses are the latest to gain acceptance.

The size of the orbital implant (16 to 22 mm) is determined by the depth and diameter of the orbital defect (see Fig. 90–29). The silicone sphere is prepared by removing one-third of the circumference with a clean horizontal slice and contouring the cut edges using a number 10 scalpel blade (Fig. 90–23). The prosthesis is inserted into the orbit with the flat surface uppermost. It is secured by suturing the periorbital fascia with a simple continuous suture of 4-0 polyglactin 910. Crystalline sodium penicillin (1 million units) is instilled into the orbital space before closure of the conjunctiva and also before the skin incision is closed.

All enucleated globes should be examined histologically, because the clinical reason for enucleation is

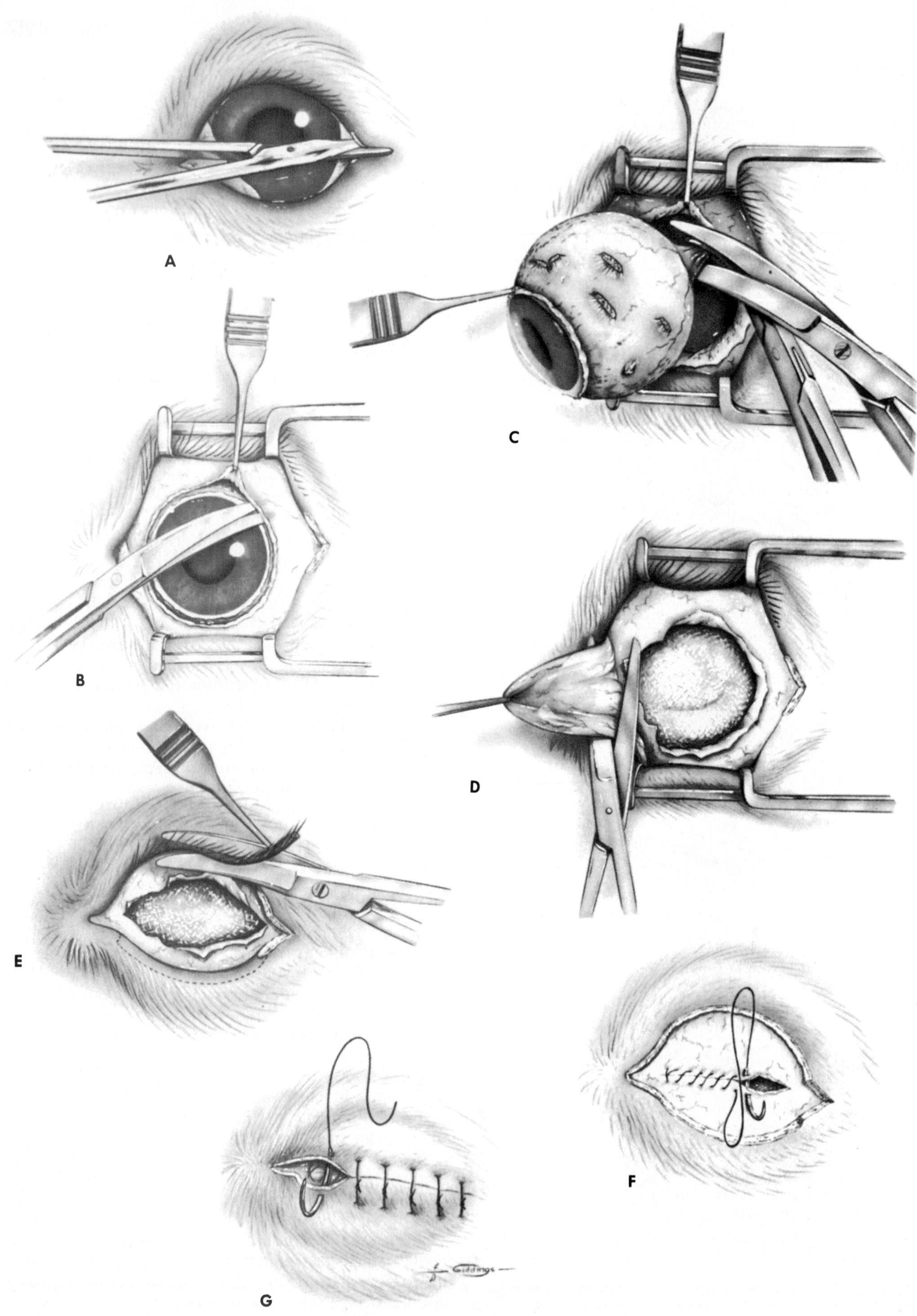

FIGURE 90–22 *See legend on opposite page*

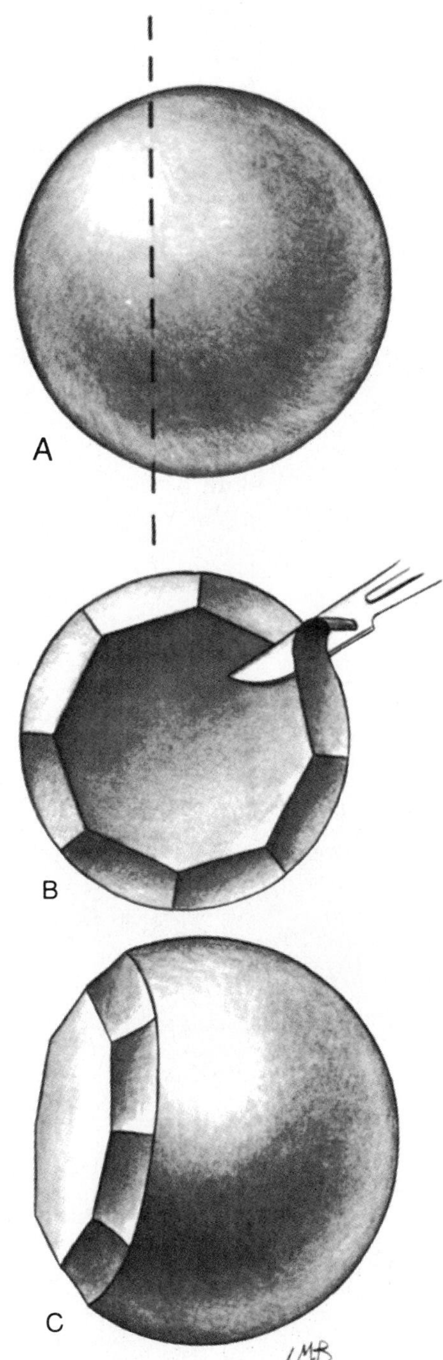

FIGURE 90–23. Preparation of the orbital prosthesis. *A,* One-third of the silicone sphere is removed. *B* and *C,* The cut edge is contoured. (From Slatter DH [ed]: Fundamentals of Veterinary Ophthalmology. 2nd ed. W.B. Saunders, Philadelphia, 1990.)

frequently inaccurate (e.g., intraocular neoplasia may masquerade as endophthalmitis or glaucoma).[25] Foreign materials (e.g., antibiotic powders, setons, or irritating antiseptic solutions) should not be placed in the orbit before closure.

Exenteration

Exenteration is removal of the globe, adnexa, and orbital contents (see Fig. 90–21). It is performed to stop a noxious disease process (e.g., neoplasia or fulminating, uncontrollable infection). The technique of transpalpebral exenteration is illustrated in Figure 90–24. The technique differs from enucleation in that the lids are incised initially and the plane of dissection is outside the extraocular muscles rather than adjacent to the sclera. Because more of the orbital contents are removed with this method than with enucleation, the postoperative defect is greater. Orbital implants are contraindicated after this procedure because of the removal of orbital contents and the possibility of recurrence of the disease process.

Evisceration

Evisceration is removal of the contents of the globe (see Fig. 90–21) but not of the sclera and cornea. It is performed before insertion of an intrascleral prosthesis in the treatment of advanced glaucoma.

Orbitotomy

There are a number of approaches to the orbit, depending on the site and degree of desired exposure.

1. Dorsal, nasal, and temporal transconjunctival approach, for lesions anterior to the equator of the globe
2. Limited orbitotomy with transection of the orbital ligament for lesions posterior to the globe
3. Dorsal orbitotomy for exposure of the dorsal and medial orbit
4. Complete orbitotomy with zygomatic arch resection for extensive orbital exposure

Preliminary examination and diagnostic techniques should suggest which is the most appropriate approach for the lesion being treated. Any approach to the ventral orbit or exenteration must carefully avoid the maxillary artery. If this artery is severed accidentally or is involved in the pathological process, it must be ligated. If it cannot be identified, temporary occlusion of the ipsilateral carotid artery may be necessary to obtain a bloodless field.

Dorsal Conjunctival Approach

The dorsal conjunctival approach is used for lesions either inside or outside the muscle cone. A perilimbal incision is made through the conjunctiva, and dissection is continued either above or beneath the insertions of the dorsal rectus and dorsal oblique muscles, depending on the site of the lesion in relation to the muscle cone (Fig. 90–25*A*). The use of electrocautery aids hemostasis. Dorsally, a vortex vein may be encountered 4 to 6

FIGURE 90–22. Enucleation. *A,* A lateral canthotomy is performed. *B,* The globe is dissected free from the conjunctiva via a perilimbal incision. Extraocular muscle insertions and periorbita are dissected from the globe back to the optic nerve. *C,* The optic nerve is transected, and the eye removed. *D,* The cavity is packed with sponges for *temporary* hemostasis, and the third eyelid is removed completely. *E,* The lid margins are removed. *F,* The sponges are removed, and the conjunctiva is sutured with 3-0 polyglactin 910 or chromic gut. *G,* The entire lid incision is sutured with 3-0 silk.

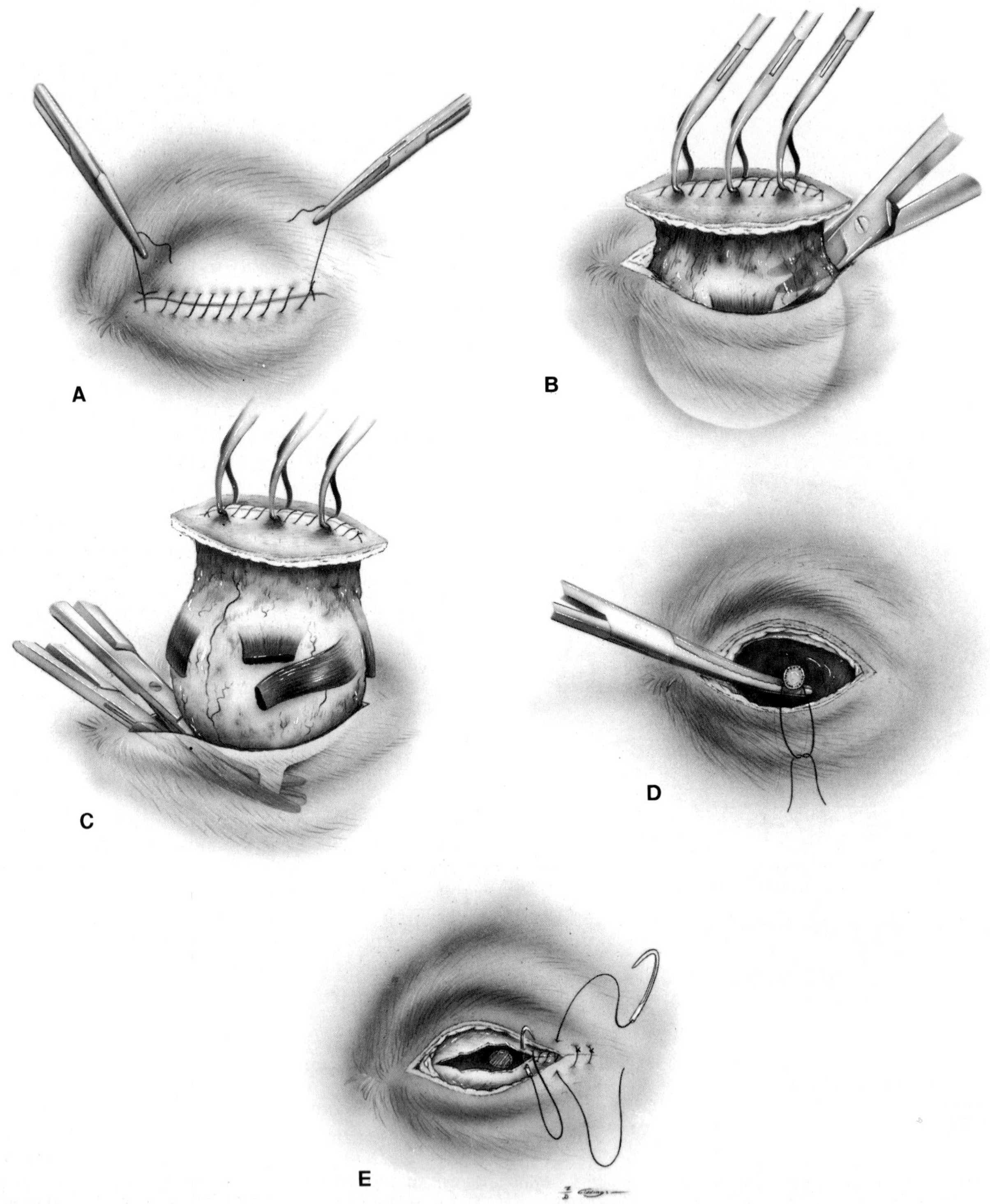

FIGURE 90–24. Transpalpebral exenteration. *A,* The eyelids are sutured with a simple continuous suture tied at either end and are held with hemostats. *B,* A periocular incision is made and dissection carried down to, but not perforating the conjunctiva. Posterior dissection separates fascia and muscles from the sclera to expose the optic nerve. *C* and *D,* The optic nerve and associated vessels are clamped, ligated, and transected. *E,* Muscles, fascia, and Tenon capsule are sutured with 3-0 chromic gut or polyglactin 910, and the skin is closed with simple interrupted sutures of a nonabsorbable material appropriate for the size and environment of the patient (e.g., 4-0 silk or nylon for cats and dogs).

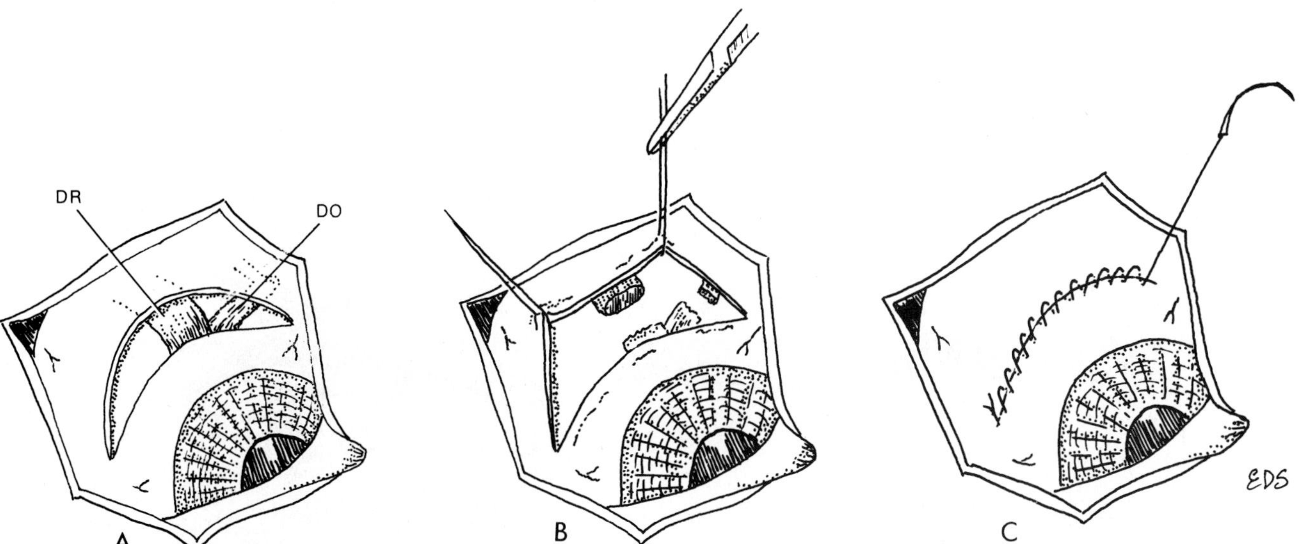

FIGURE 90–25. Dorsal conjunctival approach to the orbit. *A*, The dorsal rectus (DR) and dorsal oblique (DO) muscles are exposed. *B*, The muscles are transected to increase surgical exposure. *C*, The conjunctiva is closed with a simple continuous suture of 4-0 polyglactin 910 or silk.

mm posterior to the limbus. If the lesion is inside the muscle cone, dorsal rectus and dorsal oblique muscles may be transected 3 to 4 mm from their scleral insertions to aid exposure (Fig. 90–25*B*). In closing, these muscles are sutured with mattress sutures of 4-0 to 6-0 polyglactin 910 or chromic gut and the conjunctiva closed with a simple 6-0 continuous suture of the same material (Fig. 90–25*C*).

Nasal and Temporal Transconjunctival Approaches

Nasal and temporal transconjunctival approaches may be used for lesions located nasally or temporally and anterior to the equator. They are performed in a manner similar to the dorsal approach (Fig. 90–26). An infero-nasal approach is useful for periorbital epidermoid cysts, masses, or foreign bodies involving the base of the third eyelid. Complete hemostasis is required.

Partial Orbitotomy with Orbital Ligament Transection

Partial orbitotomy with orbital ligament transection is useful for removal of zygomatic mucoceles and lesions in the lateral orbit of a dog. Transecting the short ligament in cats seldom improves exposure (Fig. 90–27). The dense collagenous orbital ligament may be transected above or slightly below the lateral canthus. It should be resutured with nonabsorbable monofilament nylon (e.g., 2-0) to prevent disruption during the slow healing process.

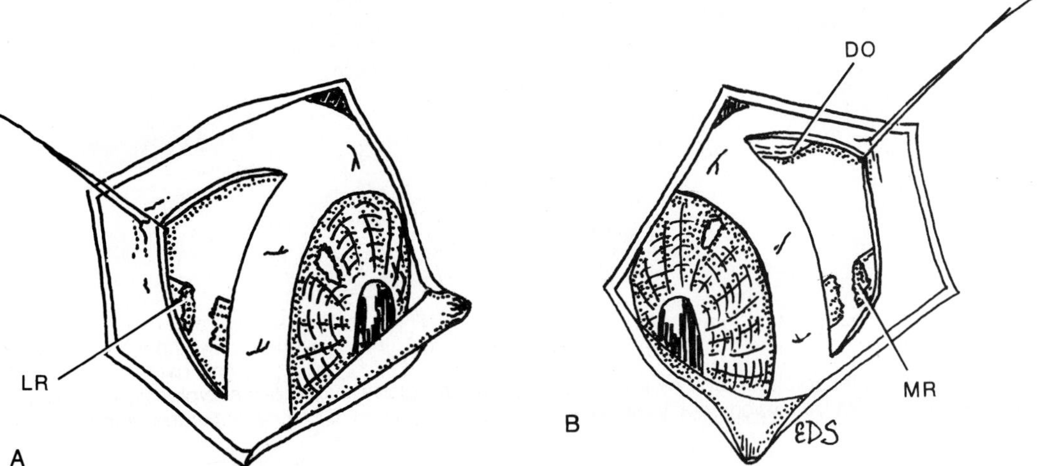

FIGURE 90–26. *A*, Temporal (lateral) conjunctival approach to the right eye with exposure and transection of the lateral rectus (LR) muscle. *B*, Nasal (medial) conjunctival approach to the right eye with exposure of the medial rectus (MR) and dorsal oblique (DO) muscles and transection of the medial rectus muscle.

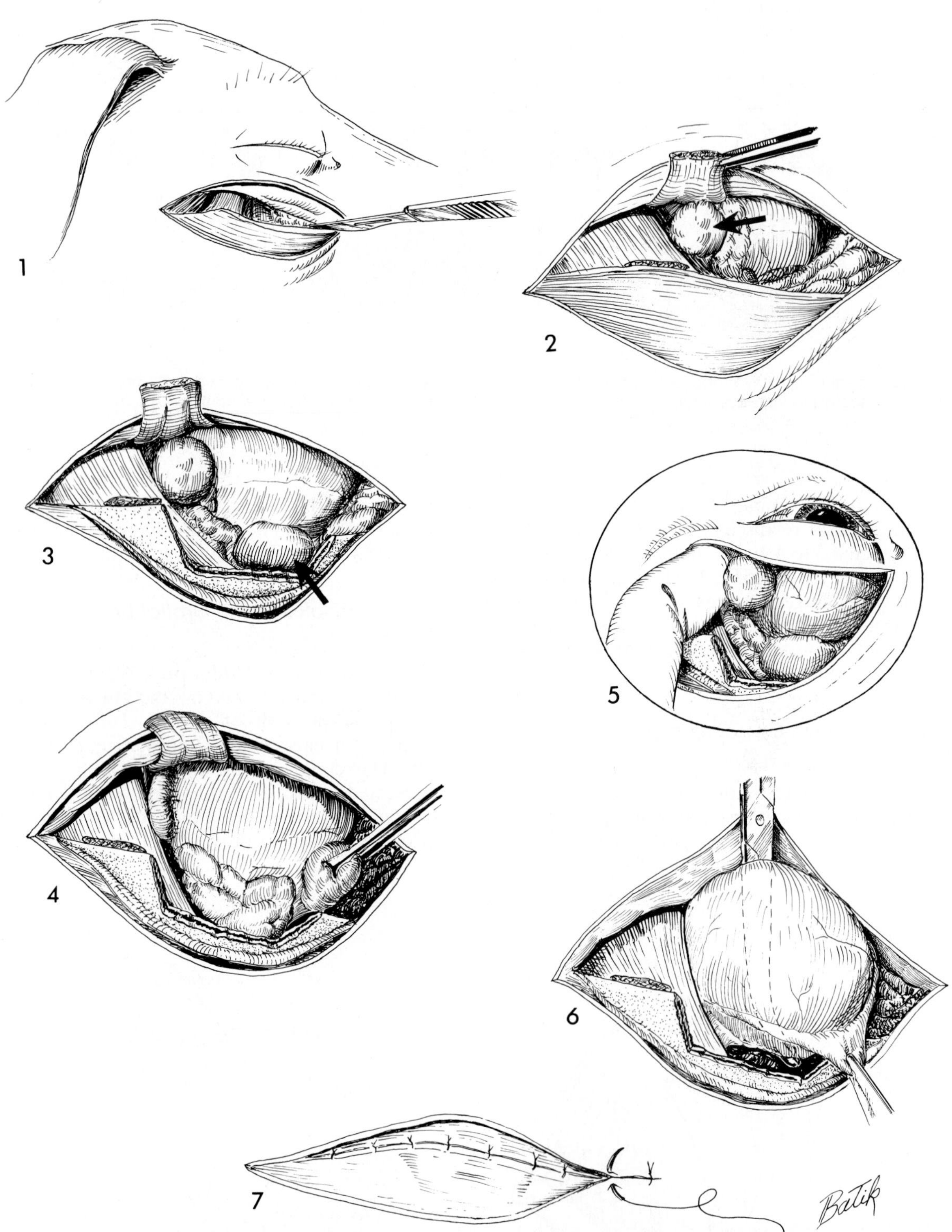

FIGURE 90–27. Exposure of the inferior lateral orbit by limited orbitotomy. The globe, zygomatic salivary gland, and transected orbital ligament are visible. (Reprinted with permission from Bistner SI, et al: *Atlas of Veterinary Ophthalmic Surgery.* W.B. Saunders, Philadelphia. 1977.)

Lateral Orbitotomy with Zygomatic Arch Resection[26]

Lateral orbitomy with zygomatic arch resection is an extensive and time-consuming approach. It affords excellent exposure of deeper orbital structures and is indicated for removal of neoplasms and foreign bodies and for diagnostic and experimental procedures. The technique is illustrated in Figure 90–28, and further details have been published.[26]

Dorsal Orbitotomy[29]

The superior and superonasal orbit may be approached through a curved incision from the midpoint of the parietal bone, extending rostrally to the frontal process of the zygomatic bone and laterally along the posterior margin of the orbital ligament (Fig. 90–29). The skin and frontal muscle flap are reflected laterally and posteroventrally, and the periosteum along the external sagittal crest is incised. The temporal muscle is

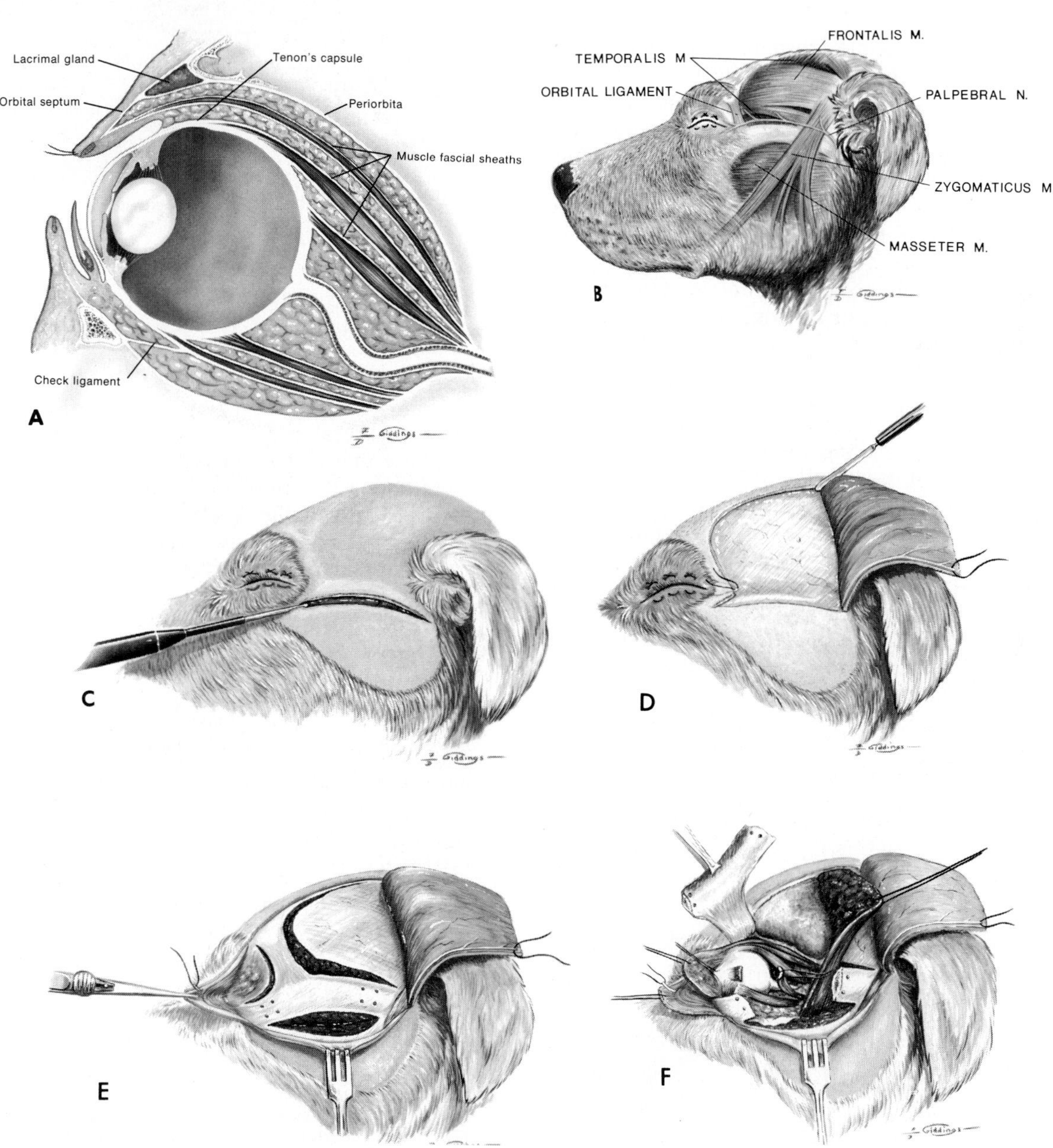

FIGURE 90–28. Lateral orbitotomy with zygomatic arch resection. *A,* Diagram of the three divisions of the orbital fascia: Tenon capsule, periorbita, and fascial sheaths of extraocular muscles. *B,* Major anatomical structures in the operative field. *C,* Initial horizontal skin incision over the zygomatic arch. *D,* Outline of skin incisions, with reference to palpable surface landmarks. The initial skin flap with adherent frontal muscle is reflected posteriorly. *E,* Incision of the aponeurosis of the temporal muscle along the external frontal and sagittal crests and the dorsal margin of the zygomatic arch. Temporal muscle attachment to periosteum of parietal and temporal bones is broken down, and the muscle is reflected posteriorly. *F,* Zygomatic arch is reflected dorsally. (Reprinted with permission from Slatter DH, Abdelbaki Y: Lateral orbitotomy by zygomatic arch resection in the dog. *J Am Vet Med Assoc 175:*1179, 1979.)

dissected from the parietal and frontal bones to the orbital ligament to create a temporal muscle flap, exposing the superior compartment of the orbit, orbital fat, and muscle cone. Closure requires careful replacement and resuturing of these structures.

OCULAR PROSTHESES

Prostheses for ocular use in animals are of three types: intraorbital, intrascleral, and extrascleral.

Orbital Prosthesis

Implantation of a silicone prosthesis after enucleation or exenteration reduces the facial distortion caused by removal of orbital contents. The major complication is dislodgment of the prosthesis and rotation within the orbit; this can be minimized by making incisions into the posterior part of the prosthesis to allow ingrowth of tissue. Preoperative bacterial invasion is minimized by prophylactic use of bactericidal antibiotics. Extrusion of the prosthesis is rare. Although methyl methacrylate prostheses have been used,[21] silicone prostheses are preferred because they can be contoured for a better cosmetic appearance.

Intrascleral Prosthesis

An intrascleral silicone prosthesis is used in dogs and cats in the treatment of chronic intractable glaucoma in blind, painful eyes. It provides the clinician and the owner with an acceptable alternative to enucleation. The prosthesis (Fig. 90–30) is inserted in the eye with a prosthesis inserter after evisceration. In buphthalmic eyes, the sclera and cornea shrink to conform to the size of the prosthesis. Complications of the technique are minimal when careful tissue handling and strict aseptic technique are used. A complication rate of about 10 per cent[12] has not been confirmed by other reports[3] or our observations.

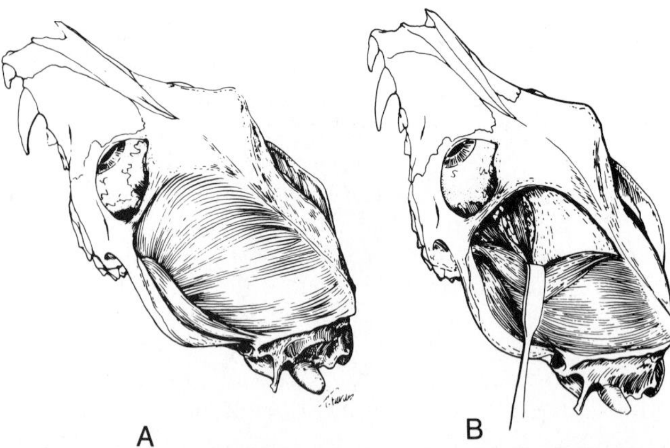

FIGURE 90–29. Dorsal exposure of the orbit is achieved by incising the skin to expose the dorsolateral area of the head *(A)*. The temporalis muscle is incised along the posterior boundary of the orbital ligament and is extended posteriorly along the external sagittal crest. Posterolateral reflection of the temporal muscle exposes the dorsal orbit *(B)*. (From Wolf ED, Wilkes DA: Exploratory surgery of the orbit. *In* Bojrab MJ [ed]: *Current Techniques in Small Animal Surgery*. 3rd ed. Lea & Febiger, Philadelphia, 1990, p 128.)

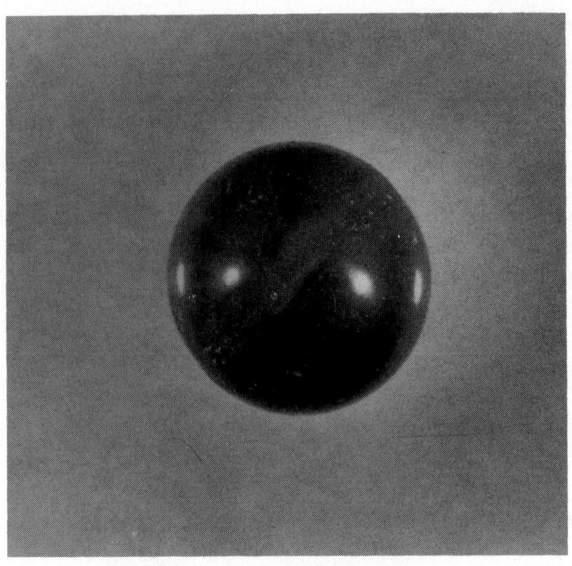

FIGURE 90–30. Silicone prosthesis.

Extrascleral Prosthesis

An extrascleral prosthesis is a porcelain or acrylic hemisphere that is manufactured to fit over the surface of a phthitic or deformed eye. An eye is painted on the surface of the prosthesis after it has been accurately fitted. These prostheses are rarely used in small animals but are more commonly fitted to horses.

References

1. Bedford PGC: Orbital pneumatosis as an unusual complication to enucleation. *J Small Anim Pract 20*:551, 1979.
2. Bellhorn RW: Enucleation technique. A lateral approach. *J Am Anim Hosp Assoc 8*:59, 1972.
3. Brightman AH et al: Intraocular prosthesis in the dog. *J Am Anim Hosp Assoc 13*:481, 1977.
4. Cottril NB, et al: Bilateral orbital parosteal osteoma in a cat. *J Am Anim Hosp Assoc 23*:405, 1987.
5. Davidson HJ, Blanchard GL: Periorbital epidermoid cyst in the medial canthus of three dogs. *J Am Vet Med Assoc 198*:271, 1991.
6. Dixon RT, Carter JD: Canine orbital venography. *J Am Vet Radiol Soc 13*:43, 1973.
7. Duke-Elder S: *System of Ophthalmology*. Vol 1. *The Eye in Evolution*. H. Kimpton, London, 1958.
8. Dziezyc J, Hager DA: Ocular ultrasonography in veterinary ophthalmology. *Semin Vet Med Surg 3*:1, 1988.
9. Evans HE, Christensen GC: *Miller's Anatomy of the Dog* 2nd ed. W.B. Saunders, Philadelphia, 1981.
10. Gelatt KN (ed): *Veterinary Ophthalmology*. 2nd ed. Lea & Febiger, Philadelphia, 1991.
11. Harvey CE, et al: Orbital cyst with conjunctival fistula in a dog. *J Am Vet Med Assoc 153*:1432, 1968.
12. Koch SA: Intraocular prosthesis in the dog and cat—the failures. *J Am Vet Med Assoc 179*:883, 1981.
13. Komar G, Schuster A: Exophthalmos pulsans in a dog. *Munch Tierarztl Wochenschr 80*:359, 1967.
14. Le Couteur RA et al: Computed tomography of orbital tumors in the dog. *J Am Vet Med Assoc 180*:910, 1982.
15. Le Couteur RA et al: Indirect imaging of the canine optic nerve using metrizamide (optic thecography). *J Am Vet Med Assoc 43*:1424, 1982.
16. Martin CL: Orbital emphysema. *Vet Med Small Anim Clin 66*:986, 1971.
17. Martin CL: Orbital mucocele in a dog. *Vet Med Small Anim Clin 66*:36, 1971.

18. Martin CL, et al: Cystic lesions of the periorbital region. *Comp Cont Educ Pract Vet 19*:1022, 1987.
19. Millichamp N, Spencer CP: Orbital varix in a dog. *J Am Anim Hosp Assoc 27*:56, 1991.
20. Munger RT, Ackerman N: Retroorbital injections in the dog: A comparison of three techniques. *J Am Anim Hosp Assoc 14*:490, 1978.
21. Nasisse MP, et al: Use of methylmethacrylate orbital prostheses in dogs and cats (1980–1986). *J Am Anim Hosp Assoc 14*:490.
22. Olivier NB: Pathophysiology of arteriovenous fistulae. *In* Slatter D (ed:) *Textbook of Small Animal Surgery*. W.B. Saunders, Philadelphia, 1985.
23. Rubin LF, Patterson DF: Arteriovenous fistula of the orbit in a dog. *Cornell Vet 55*:471, 19
24. Schmidt GM, Betts CW: Zygomatic salivary mucoceles in the dog. *J Am Vet Med Assoc 172*:940, 1978.
25. Slatter D: *Fundamentals of Veterinary Ophthalmology*. 2nd ed. W.B. Saunders, Philadelphia, 1990.
26. Slatter DH, Abdelbaki Y: Lateral orbitotomy by zygomatic arch resection in the dog. *J Am Vet Med Assoc 175*:1179, 1979.
27. Smith JS: Diseases of the orbit. *In* Kirk RW (ed): *Current Veterinary Therapy* VI. W.B. Saunders, Philadelphia, 1977.
28. Ticer JW: *Radiographic Technique in Small Animal Practice*. W.B. Saunders, Philadelphia, 1975.
29. Wolf D, Wilkes DA: Exploratory surgery of the orbit. *In* Bojrab MJ (ed): *Current Techniques in Small Animal Surgery*. Lea & Febiger, Philadelphia, 1990, pp 128–132.

CHAPTER 91

Glaucoma

Charles L. Martin

Glaucoma is an important therapeutic enigma in dogs because of its relatively high incidence in certain breeds (Table 91–1) and in cats because the subtle signs usually result in presentation late in the disease. Glaucoma is a syndrome, and many causes may result in the "final common pathway" leading to increased intraocular pressure (IOP). Because various conditions may precipitate glaucoma, a thorough examination should be performed on the normal and the affected eye. Therapy may be specific for the cause.

Glaucoma is defined as an elevation in IOP that is accompanied by impaired ocular function. In humans, 50 per cent of optic nerve fibers are lost before the milder visual field disturbances are detected, and 90 per cent of the fibers are lost in patients with severe glaucomatous field losses.[67, 69] In view of the advanced state of nerve fiber loss that is present in animals before visual signs are manifested, it is obvious why it is difficult to keep animals seeing when presented with this complaint.

The reported upper limit of normal IOP is 27 to 30 mm Hg, as measured with a Schiøtz tonometer and using the human conversion tables.[13, 34, 43] Two separate conversion tables for the Schiøtz tonometer have been calculated for dogs and one for cats. Comparable scale readings result in higher IOP readings than in the human conversion tables.[62, 65] The earliest table did not receive widespread acceptance because the upper limits of normal IOP would presumably have been increased to 38 mm Hg.[62] The most recent canine table does not have this spurious high pressure at scale readings considered normal and correlates more closely with applanation tonometry readings (Tables 91–2 and 91–3).[65] The IOP should not vary more than 5 mm Hg between eyes of the same dog.[34]

TABLE 91–1. BREED PREDISPOSITION AND USUAL FORMS OF GLAUCOMA

Breed	Form
American cocker spaniel	Closed angle
Bouvier des Flandres	Closed angle
Basset hound	Closed angle
Chow chow	Closed angle
Samoyed	Closed angle
Siberian husky	Closed angle
Norwegian elkhound	Closed and open angle
Brittany spaniel	Closed angle
Beagle	Open angle
Miniature toy poodle	Open and closed angle
Welsh springer spaniel	Closed angle
Wire- and smooth-haired fox terrier	Lens displacement ± closed angle
Sealyham terrier	Lens displacement

ANATOMY AND PHYSIOLOGY

Aqueous humor is produced continuously by the ciliary processes and leaves the eye mainly via the iridocorneal angle.[60] Alterations in production, outflow, or both may be responsible for variations in IOP. Aqueous is produced by a combination of passive ultrafiltration and active secretion. Secretion is usually given the dominant role (65 to 70 per cent).[16, 77]

The ciliary body is divided into the anterior pars plicata (ciliary processes) and the posterior pars plana. Grossly, the ciliary processes are 60 to 70 triangular blades separated by deep valleys (Fig. 91–1).[56, 82] In relation to external landmarks, the ciliary processes are 5 mm posterior to the limbus dorsally and 3 mm in the remaining regions.

Aqueous produced in the posterior chamber flows through the pupil and leaves mainly through the iridocorneal angle. The iridocorneal angle is that region where the base of the iris attaches to the peripheral cornea and sclera (Figs. 91–2 and 91–3; see Fig. 91–1). In viewing the angle from the anterior chamber, the

TABLE 91–2. CALIBRATION TABLE FOR SCHIØTZ TONOMETRY IN DOGS*

Schiøtz Scale Reading	IOP (mm Hg) 5.5 g wt.	IOP (mm Hg) 7.5 g wt.	IOP (mm Hg) 10.0 g wt.
0.5	46	61	75
1.0	44	59	73
1.5	43	56	70
2.0	40	53	66
2.5	33	47	61
3.0	26	40	55
3.5	23	35	49
4.0	21	32	44
4.5	20	29	41
5.0	19	27	38
5.5	18	26	36
6.0	17	24	33
6.5	16	23	31
7.0	15	22	30
7.5		20	28
8.0	14	19	27
8.5	13		25
9.0		18	24
9.5	12	17	23
10.0		16	22
10.5	11	15	21
11.0			20
11.5	10	14	19
12.0		13	18
12.5			17
13.0		12	16
13.5	8	11	15
14.0			
14.5		10	14
15.0	7		13
15.5		9	12
16.0			
16.5	6	8	11
17.0			10
17.5		7	
18.0	5		9
18.5		6	
19.0			8
19.5			7
20.0		5	

IOP, intraocular pressure.
*From Pickett P, et al: Calibration of the Schiøtz tonometer for the canine and feline eye. Transactions of the 19th Annual Scientific Program of the American College of Veterinary Ophthalmologists *19*:47, 1988.

main structure observed is the pectinate ligament, which originates from the anterior extremity of the iris base and inserts in the peripheral cornea. The pectinate ligament consists of numerous strands that, in general, are single strands with relatively wide spaces between them. An accessory row of strands arises slightly deeper in the angle. On gonioscopy, a bluish-white zone denotes the uveal trabeculae that loosely fill the ciliary cleft between the base of the ciliary body and iris and the sclera (see Figs. 91–2 and 91–3). The pectinate ligament has the same pigmentation as the adjacent iris. The insertion of the pectinate ligament strands may have a dark, narrow zone of pigmentation (deep zone) that usually continues obliquely and superficially onto the scleral shelf and is visible as a grayer, wider zone of pigmentation that extends beyond the deep zone.[4, 39, 51, 52, 54, 84]

In addition to the previously described angle structures, compact corneoscleral trabeculae (cribriform ligament)—meridional ciliary muscles that extend anteriorly to insert near the termination of the Descemet membrane—are found on sagittal section. Numerous small vascular channels, the angular plexus, drain aqueous from the corneoscleral trabeculae into larger collecting veins and then into the large channels of the scleral venous plexus in the midsclera. The scleral venous plexus consists of two to four large interwoven channels that communicate posteriorly with the vortex venous system and anteriorly with the episcleral and conjunctival veins (see Fig. 91–1).[8, 52, 54, 83, 86]

In addition to vascular uptake in the trabecular meshwork, aqueous drainage via a posterior uveoscleral route has been demonstrated.[18, 27] Uveoscleral flow is through the iridocorneal angle into the ciliary muscle interstitium and to the suprachoroidal space, where aqueous is probably absorbed by choroidal vessels and transsclerally into orbital lymphatics (see Fig. 91–1).

TABLE 91–3. CALIBRATION TABLE FOR SCHIØTZ TONOMETRY IN CATS*

Schiøtz Scale Reading	IOP (mm Hg) 5.5 g wt.	IOP (mm Hg) 7.5 g wt.	IOP (mm Hg) 10.0 g wt.
0.5	44	73	
1.0	42	71	
1.5	40	68	
2.0	37	65	80
2.5	33	61	76
3.0	30	56	71
3.5	27	48	66
4.0	25	42	61
4.5	24	37	56
5.0	22	34	51
5.5	21	31	47
6.0	20	29	44
6.5	18	27	40
7.0		25	37
7.5	17	24	35
8.0	16	22	33
8.5	15	21	31
9.0	14	20	29
9.5	13	19	27
10.0		18	25
10.5		17	23
11.0	12	16	22
11.5	11	15	20
12.0		14	19
12.5	10	13	18
13.0		12	17
13.5	9		15
14.0		11	14
14.5	8	10	13
15.0			12
15.5		9	11
16.0	7	8	10
16.5			9
17.0	6	7	8
17.5		6	7
18.0			6
18.5	5	5	5
19.0			
20.0			

IOP, intraocular pressure
*From Pickett P, et al: Calibration of the Schiøtz tonometer for the canine and feline eye. Transactions of the 19th Annual Scientific Program of the American College of Veterinary Ophthalmologists *19*:47, 1988.

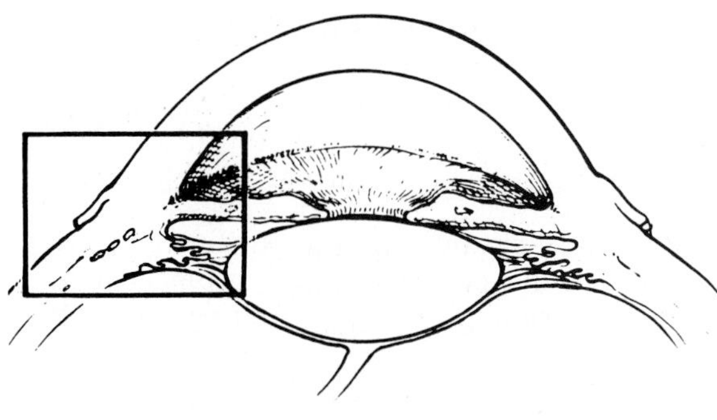

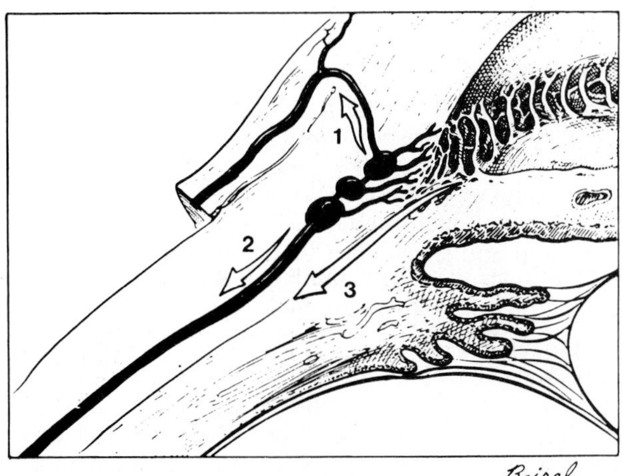

FIGURE 91–1. The routes of aqueous drainage from the canine iridocorneal angle. Aqueous taken up by the venous system in the angle may drain anteriorly to the episceral and conjunctival veins (1), posteriorly into the vortex venous system (2), or through the ciliary muscle interstitium to the suprachoroid and diffuse through the sclera (uveoscleral flow, 3).

CLINICAL SIGNS AND DIAGNOSTIC TECHNIQUES

The signs of glaucoma are generally pressure dependent. IOP in the 30s to low 40 mm Hg range is occult. It is not until the IOP reaches the mid-40s and 50 mm Hg that typical external signs of vascular injection, pupillary dilation, and corneal edema appear.

Increased Intraocular Pressure

All signs of glaucoma are nonspecific, necessitating an objective means of measurement of IOP. Although an accurate objective measurement may not be necessary in patients with very high IOP for the initial diagnosis, it is required when monitoring the response to therapy when an obvious hypotony does not develop.

Tonometry is the measurement of intraocular tension. Digital tonometry, using two fingers (not thumbs) to palpate the firmness of the eye through the closed upper lid, is a crude technique and differentiates only soft, medium, and hard eyes. The most practical instrument for tonometry in dogs is the Schiøtz tonometer, which measures the amount of corneal indentation that a plunger with a given weight produces (Fig. 91–4). The higher the IOP, the less the indentation. The amount of indentation is measured on a scale, with each scale reading representing 0.1 mm of indentation. The scale reading is usually converted to millimeters of mercury on a table. The tonometer must be vertical to avoid plunger friction, the plunger should be freely movable, and the instrument should be near the central cornea to conform to the curved footplate. After applying a topical anesthetic, the entire weight of the instrument is rested on the globe for 1 to 2 seconds, and two to four readings are taken to determine consistency. The lids are held open by distant pressure near the orbital rim to avoid

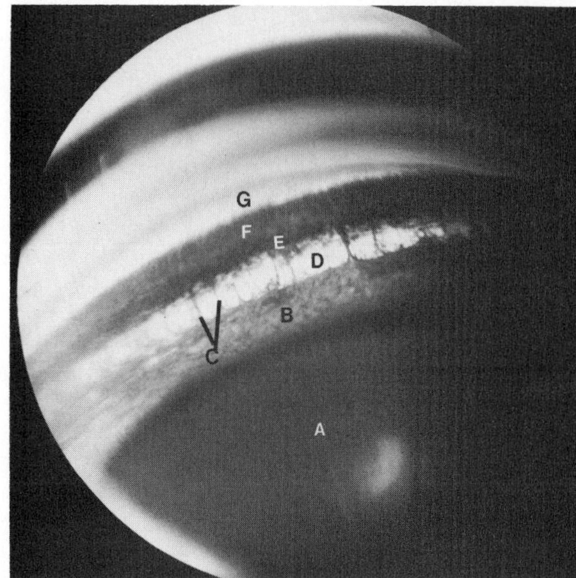

FIGURE 91–2. Goniophotograph of a normal dog. (A, Pupil; B, iris; C, pectinate ligament strands; D, bluish-white zone of the uveal trabeculae; E, deep pigmented zone; F, superficial pigmented zone; G, cornea.)

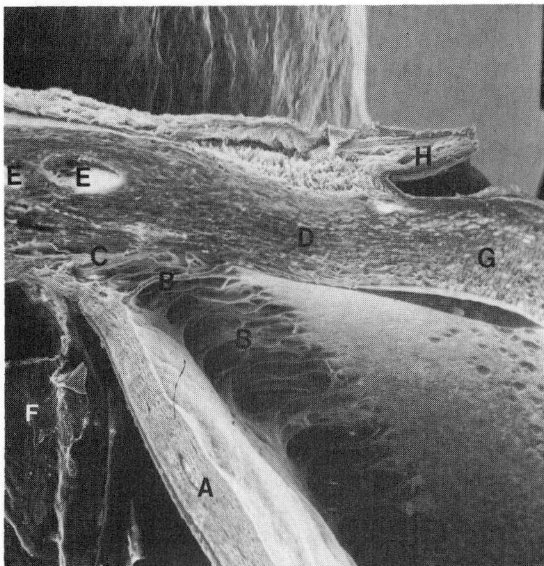

FIGURE 91–3. Combined frontal and sagittal scanning electron micrograph of the canine iridocorneal angle (× 32). (A, iris; B, primary row of pectinate ligament fibers; C, uveal trabeculae; D, limbus; E, scleral venous plexus; F, ciliary process; G, corner; H, conjunctiva.)

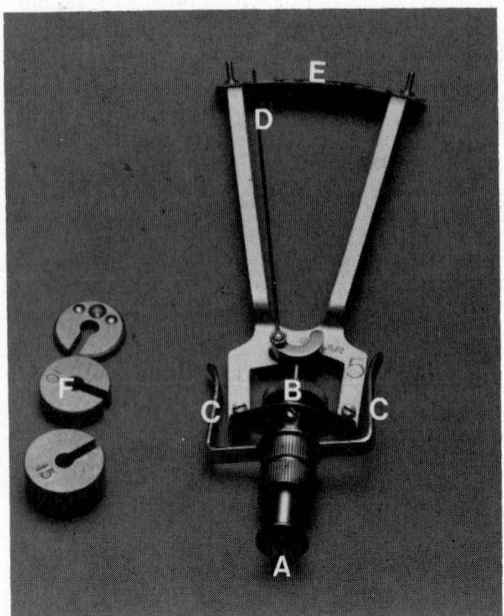

FIGURE 91–4. Schiøtz tonometer with additional weights. (A, Footplate with protruding plunger; B, weight on proximal portion of plunger; C, tabs used to hold tonometer; D, pointer that plunger pushes, indicating scale reading; E, scale of tonometer (out of view); F, additional weights used on glaucomatous eyes.)

transferring pressure to the globe. Additional sources of error with Schiøtz tonometry are deviations in corneal curvature (buphthalmos or microphthalmos), corneal scars and irregularities, and severe corneal edema. Applanation tonometry measures the force necessary to flatten or applanate the cornea over a given surface area of a plunger. In general, this technique is more accurate and subject to fewer errors, but the new electronic instruments* that make this adaptable to veterinary medicine are expensive (Fig. 91–5).

Dilated Pupil

In uncomplicated glaucoma without iris adhesions, the pupil dilates at about 45 to 50 mm Hg. Thus, although it is a frequent sign, mydriasis is neither a sensitive nor specific sign of glaucoma. The pathogenesis of pupillary dilation with increased IOP is associated with a lack of vascular perfusion of the iris.[14, 75, 76] Direct and consensual reflexes are absent, and miotics are ineffective until IOP is lowered.

Conjunctival and Episcleral Vascular Injection

Various degrees of vascular injection are present in most cases of canine glaucoma, depending on cause, chronicity, abruptness of onset, and degree of pressure elevation. Vascular injection occurs before pupil dilation and is similar to that in intraocular inflammation. Large conjunctival veins that bend near the limbus and drain the episcleral and scleral plexus are selectively injected. With acute high IOP, capillary engorgement as well as large-vessel engorgement may be present. The presumed cause of conjunctival injection is collapse of the posterior intrascleral veins in the thin equatorial sclera, resulting in increased venous drainage via the anterior routes (see Fig. 91–1).[47]

*Tonopen, Oculab, Glendale, CA.

Corneal Pathology

Corneal opacification occurs with increased IOP by disruption of the normal corneal stromal lamellar arrangement, resulting in light scattering, and from corneal edema.[90] Corneal edema may be mild or severe enough to hamper evaluation of intraocular structures. Although corneal edema is pressure dependent, considerable individual susceptibility exists. Chronic edema usually results in corneal vascularization. Epithelial edema combined with the cellular toxicity of topical anesthetics and perhaps mechanical trauma of tonometry or lagophthalmos may result in epithelial erosions and ulcer complications. Severe edema may interfere with accurate tonometry.

Stretching of the globe frequently results in breaks in the Descemet membrane (Descemet streaks) that are permanent and specific for glaucoma. Descemet streaks appear as double curvilinear lines that may branch and can be localized with the slit-lamp to the posterior cornea (Fig. 91–6).

Chronic corneal edema combined with lagophthalmos and decreased corneal sensation usually results in a degenerative pannus or a superficially scarred cornea. In those individuals or breeds with marked limbal pigmentation, corneal pigmentation accompanies the scarring. Corneal scarring may significantly alter Schiøtz tonometer readings.

Fundus Abnormalities

The fundus may appear normal in acute, modest pressure elevations, but with higher pressure, retinal vascular attenuation, optic disc hemorrhages, and papilledema may be visible. Papilledema is due to the interference in axoplasmic flow from a pinching of axons in the lamina cribrosa. In chronic IOP elevations, peripapillary or diffuse hyper-reflectivity of the tapetum and attenuation of the retinal vessels may be seen. The optic nerve usually develops cupping, loss of myelin, and

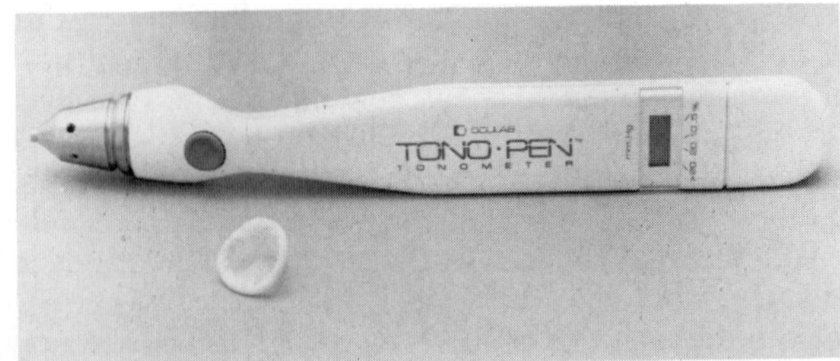

FIGURE 91–5. Tonopen applanation tonometer. Latex cover protects plunger from tears and transmission of infectious agents between patients. The tonometer is activated by pushing the button behind the head, and the plunger is lightly and quickly pressed on the cornea until four good contacts are made. At this time, a beep is produced and a digital readout in millimeters of mercury is seen in the window, with a mark indicating percentage of variance between recorded readings.

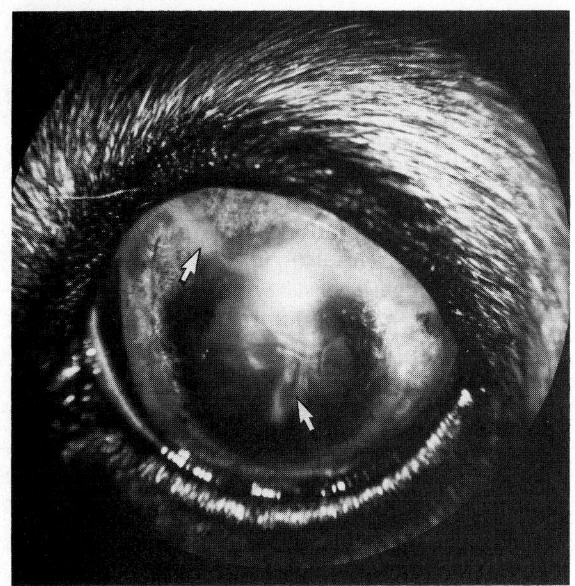

FIGURE 91–6. Breaks in the Descemet membrane *(arrows)* associated with glaucoma.

change in color to grayish white in chronic cases (Fig. 91–7). Advanced changes may appear similar to those in progressive retinal degeneration, with attenuated retinal vessels, hyper-reflectivity of the tapetum, and atrophy of the optic disc.[47] Glaucomatous posterior segment changes may be differentiated from progressive retinal degeneration by lack of bilateral symmetry, presence of optic disc cupping, and other ocular lesions associated with glaucoma.

Ocular Pain

Most animals with primary glaucoma have epiphora but lack blepharospasm or ocular pain that is recognized by the owner. Once the IOP is reduced to normal, it is common for owners to comment on how playful the animal appears. Pain with glaucoma is usually manifested as sleepiness, depression, irritability, and reduced playfulness. Relief of ocular pain is one of the main goals in the therapy of chronic glaucoma. Pain should be considered present even if it is not a complaint.

Decreased Vision or Blindness

Increased IOP for 2 to 4 hours to a few days may cause loss of vision in acute high-pressure glaucoma,[33, 68, 71] or an insidious loss may occur with modest elevations of IOP or pressure that has gradually increased. One of the frustrations of treating glaucoma is late presentation for therapy. Client education and experience usually result in earlier presentation of the second eye in patients with primary glaucoma.

There are two main theories of glaucoma-induced optic nerve and retinal damage: vascular and mechanical.[59] The vascular theory states that tissue damage results from ischemia when IOP interferes with tissue perfusion.[32] The retina can sustain only 100 minutes of complete anoxia before irreversible damage occurs.[33] A cat's retina suffers complete ischemia at an IOP of 100 mm Hg.[95] In the mechanical theory, increased IOP causes the lamina cribrosa to bow outward, distorting and disregistering its pores or passages. The resulting distortion pinches the axon bundles, thus interfering with axoplasmic flow and causing axonal death.[21, 40, 59, 70] Interference in axoplasmic flow has been demonstrated in beagles with glaucoma.[12, 94] Both of these mechanisms are probably involved in the usual case of acute canine glaucoma with high IOP.[11]

Buphthalmos

Enlargement of the globe is a typical and specific but not sensitive sign of canine glaucoma. Once significantly stretched, the globe remains large even after the IOP returns to normal. Young eyes are most susceptible to stretching, and extreme buphthalmos may cause lagophthalmos and a grotesque appearance. In buphthalmic eyes, accurate Schiøtz tonometer readings may be unobtainable because the corneal curvature does not fit the tonometer footplate or because of corneal scarring and altered scleral rigidity.

Luxated Lens

Various degrees of lens luxation are commonly associated with glaucoma, and it is often difficult to determine cause and effect. Buphthalmos frequently results in rupture of part of the zonular circumference, with consequent subluxation that usually does not progress to complete luxation. The signs of subluxation are an aphakic crescent, iridodonesis, and alterations in depth of the anterior chamber and vitreous strands. How a subluxated lens induces glaucoma is unclear, and the

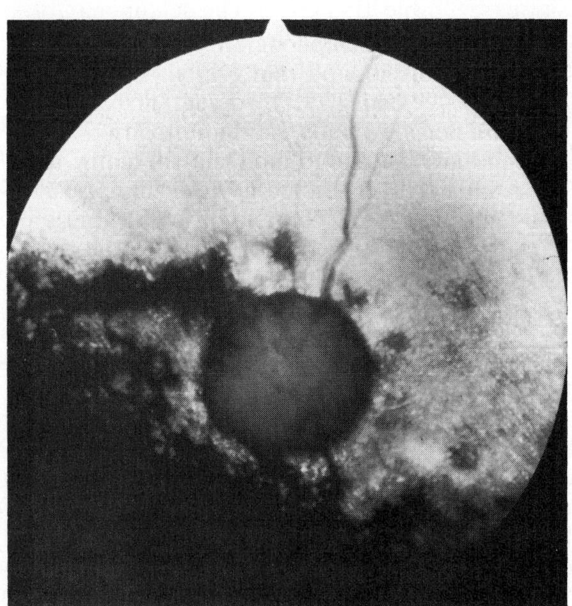

FIGURE 91–7. Optic disc atrophy with mild cupping, retinal vascular attenuation, loss of vessels, and diffuse tapetal hyper-reflectivity from chronic glaucoma.

usual theories of pupil block and angle closure are often unconfirmed clinically.

Lens luxation into the anterior chamber may precipitate glaucoma or may turn chronic glaucoma into an acute syndrome. Anterior lens luxation with a normal iridocorneal angle may not precipitate pressure elevations or may do so intermittently. The lens may be clear or cataractous. Anterior lens displacements are usually obvious but may be hidden by corneal edema. Posterior luxations may be overlooked if the pupil is not dilated or if the lens is transparent. A deep anterior chamber, iridodonesis, and vitreous herniation through the pupil suggest possible lens displacement.

Aqueous Flare

Increased aqueous protein and pigment clumps may be observed in many forms of glaucoma. Increased protein in the aqueous is caused by increased vascular permeability (i.e., with anterior uveitis). The protein content is often as high as 4.5 to 5.0 g/100 ml, and it is suspected that the protein may precipitate pressure elevations by obstructing trabecular spaces.

CLASSIFICATION AND PATHOGENESIS OF GLAUCOMA (Table 91–4)

The classification of glaucoma in animals is similar to that in humans, although there are species differences in the relative incidence of types.[91] Glaucoma is divided into two broad categories, primary and secondary, and these in turn are each subdivided according to the gonioscopic findings of an open, narrow, or closed angle.

Primary glaucoma is glaucoma not caused solely by acquired intraocular lesions. Primary glaucoma is potentially bilateral, although the onset is usually asynchronous (often by years), and a genetic inheritance is suspected in most cases as reflected in the breed predisposition (see Table 91–1).[2, 44, 48] The definition of primary glaucoma is not clear-cut; detailed examinations reveal that in many instances of apparent "secondary" glaucoma the acquired lesion may have been an initiating event in an eye predisposed by an abnormal angle or anterior chamber conformation. When two or more conditions produce ocular decompensation, it is difficult to determine the relative importance of each condition. The genetics of most types of glaucoma have proved elusive, possibly indicating the influence of environmental or compound factors.[1, 45, 96]

Congenital glaucoma is rare, and classification by age of onset overlaps other methods of classification, serving little purpose.

Most cases of primary glaucoma in dogs are associated with bilateral closed angles (Fig. 91–8).[5, 25, 44, 57] The cause of closure cannot be determined in many cases, but it is present in the absence of inflammation, is often tolerated for years without decompensation, and can be encountered at any age.[58] In many of these eyes, a severe form of goniodysgenesis or an arrest in angle development is present, but in aged dogs, one may question the likelihood of a congenital lesion.[53] In the severe manifestations of goniodysgenesis, a sheet of iris-like tissue replaces the pectinate ligament. On close inspection of closed angles in normotensive eyes, flow holes can be observed near the corneal insertion of the obstructing sheet (Fig. 91–9).[55, 58] These holes are presumably more prone to obstruction than the normal open spaces between the pectinate ligament, and if obstruction occurs suddenly, an acute syndrome may develop. If slowly progressive closure occurs, an insidious onset of glaucoma results. Acquired intraocular lesions may obstruct these pores and be overinterpreted, or normal covert intraocular changes may precipitate obstruction (i.e., lens growth, pupil size, and endothelial proliferation). Obstruction of the sheet creates a pressure differential, pushing it outward to collapse the ciliary cleft and causing it to adhere to the inner sclera (Fig. 91–10). The latter finding is usually interpreted histopathologically as a peripheral anterior synechia.[44, 58]

TABLE 91–4. CLASSIFICATION OF CANINE GLAUCOMA

- I. Open-angle glaucoma: normal, wide angle on gonioscopy
  - A. Primary: no observable predisposing factors, angle normal on gonioscopy, bilateral, breed predisposition (see Fig. 91–2)
  - B. Secondary: normal angle obstructed by aqueous contents or elevated episcleral venous pressure interferes with aqueous drainage
    1. Inflammation—leukocytes and fibrin obstruct outflow
    2. Hyphema—erythrocytes and fibrin obstruct outflow
    3. Pigment—deposition or proliferation obstructs outflow
    4. Lipids in anterior chamber obstruct outflow
    5. Anterior luxated lens—may obstruct angle or create pupil block
    6. Elevated episcleral venous pressure—arteriovenous fistula, orbital lesion, or increased blood pressure (rare)
- II. Closed-angle glaucoma: angle is collapsed or covered with peripheral iris or connective tissue
  - A. Primary
    1. Congenital: goniodysgenesis—maldeveloped angle covered with mesodermal tissue; usually bilateral; age of glaucoma onset varies (see Figs. 91–8 to 91–10)
    2. Acquired: closure associated with abnormal anterior chamber conformation
       - a. Forward displacement of lens presumably due to slack zonules; creates a relative pupillary blockage from increased adhesive forces between lens and iris (see Fig. 91–11)
       - b. Shallow anterior chamber with small anterior segment; pupillary block may occur, resulting in peripheral anterior synechia
       - c. Plateau iris—iris plane is flat, but peripheral iris has a recess adjacent to angle, which is susceptible to angle closure with pupillary blockage
  - B. Secondary closed angle: acquired lesions precipitate closure of previously normal angle; also, angle conformations under IIA have an increased susceptibility to pupillary blockage
    1. Associated with pupillary block
       - a. Intumescent lens
       - b. Posterior synechia, iris bombé
       - c. Subluxated lens, luxated lens
       - d. Aphakic vitreous herniation
       - e. Increased volume in vitreous compartment (i.e., accumulation of aqueous, swelling of vitreous)
    2. No pupillary block
       - a. Neoplasia with invasion of angle and/or pushing iris forward or thickening of iris
       - b. Inflammation with peripheral anterior synechia
       - c. Subluxated lens pushing iris base forward
       - d. Epithelial downgrowth—perforating corneal wound with epithelium proliferating over angle

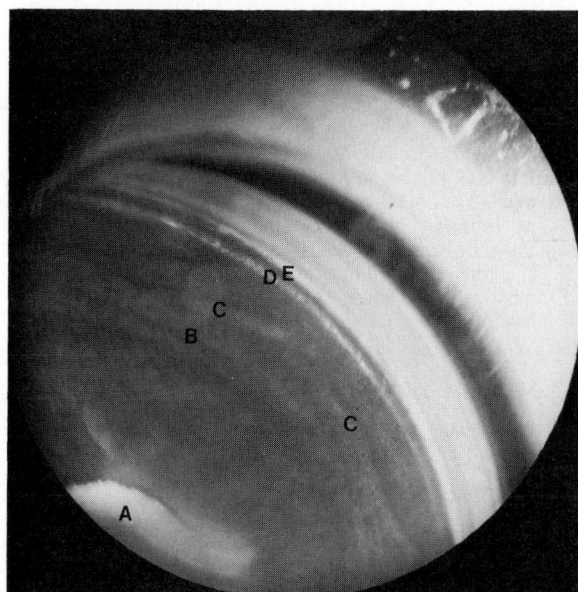

FIGURE 91–8. Goniophotograph of a basset hound's angle with severe goniodysgenesis. The opposite eye had glaucoma and a similar-appearing angle, but IOP in this eye was normal. Note the absence of an obvious pectinate ligament. (A, Pupil; B, iris in a deep anterior chamber; C, major arterial circle of the iris; D, angle covered with lightly pigmented mesoderm; E, deep pigmented zone.) The thin white zone with pigment streaks simulates a narrow angle with a short pectinate ligament at low magnification but with high magnification can be identified as a sheet continuous with the iris.

A closed angle is usually seen gonioscopically as a thin, lighter circumferential zone that may have some radial pigment streaks but no distinct pectinate ligament.[4, 57, 58] The latter appearance may be misinterpreted as a narrowed filtering cleft and is often erroneously called a *narrow angle* (see Fig. 91–8).

Primary open-angle glaucoma is relatively rare in dogs but has been studied in detail in beagles, in which it is a simple recessive trait.[24] Many beagles with open-angle glaucoma later develop a closed angle, but this differs from the primary closed angle glaucoma in the sequence of events (i.e., in the latter instance, closed angles present before pressure elevation).[29, 61]

Feline glaucoma is typically more subtle in its presentation and consequently is presented in the late stages. Primary forms of glaucoma are observed, although secondary glaucoma associated with inflammation is the most common form. In a review of 87 enucleated feline eyes with glaucoma, 50 per cent did not have obstructive pathology at the pupil or angle, but 44 per cent of the latter had plasmacytic-lymphocytic uveitis.[93]

Secondary glaucoma is caused by acquired intraocular abnormalities and, depending on the etiology, may be unilateral or bilateral. Secondary glaucoma is associated with acquired diseases that alter fluid dynamics at the pupil or angle and may vary from inflammation to neoplasia.[49]

EMERGENCY THERAPY

All recently functional eyes should be treated with emergency medical therapy to reduce IOP whether surgery is planned or not. A delay of several hours may be critical, considering the high IOPs that are often present. Surgical patients should have normal pressures, if possible, to minimize the internal shock to homeostasis that occurs when decompressing the eye from a high IOP to zero.

Systemic Therapy

The first line of emergency therapy is osmotic diuretics. The osmotic diuretics create a hyperosmolar vascular space, which withdraws extravascular fluid into the vessels. The ocular effect is to withdraw fluid from the vitreous as well as the aqueous.[72, 89] Osmotic agents that remain in the vascular system without leaking into the eye produce longer hypotony with less rebound of water into the eye. The effect is dependent on dose and rate. Thirst is stimulated; therefore, water is restricted for 2 to 3 hours so that the drug effect is not neutralized. Mannitol also increases ocular perfusion and retinal oxygen tension, benefiting the glaucomatous eye.[19]

Many agents, such as mannitol, glycerol, urea, sorbitol, lactate, ascorbate, ethyl alcohol, dextrose, sucrose, and isosorbide, have potential as osmotic agents, but in veterinary practice, mannitol and glycerol are routinely used. Mannitol, 1 to 2 g/kg, is given by slow push intravenous injection over 5 minutes or by slow intravenous drip. The hypotensive effect occurs in about 15 to 30 minutes and usually lasts for 4 to 6 hours, although some patients have a prolonged response for up to 48 hours after emergency therapy before the pressure rises again.[22, 42] Repeat injections of mannitol can be given, but dehydration of the patient may reach critical levels,

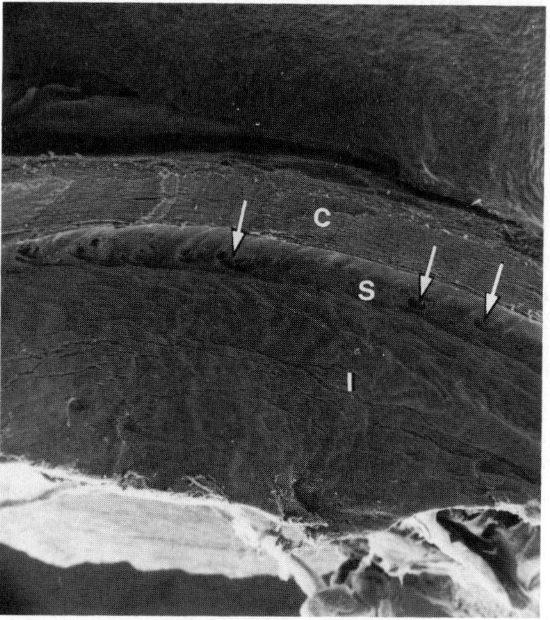

FIGURE 91–9. Frontal scanning electron micrograph of an American cocker spaniel with moderate goniodysgenesis (× 21). Arrows indicate holes in sheet that allows aqueous passage. (I, Iris; S, sheet covering angle; C, cut cornea.) (Reprinted with permission from Martin CL, Wyman M: Primary glaucoma in the dog. *Vet Clin North Am* 8:257, 1978.)

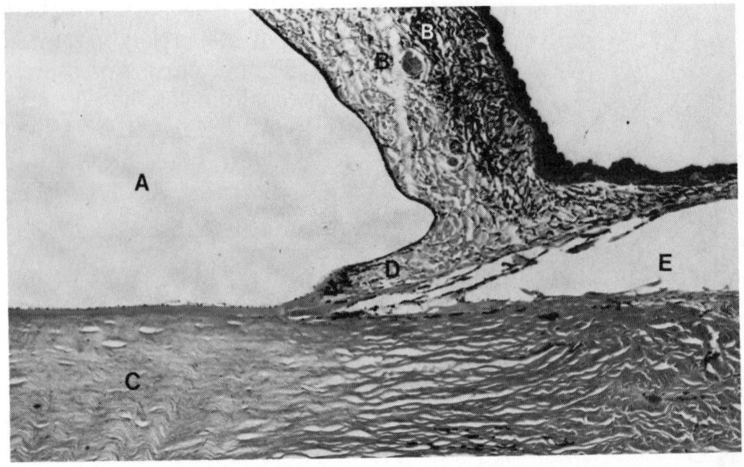

FIGURE 91–10. Sagittal histological section of the angle of a basset hound with goniodysgenesis. The pressure in this eye was normal, but the opposite eye was glaucomatous. (A, anterior chamber; B, iris; C, cornea; D, mesodermal sheet covering the angle and pulling the iris base forward; E, ciliary cleft.) If the sheet becomes occluded, obstructing aqueous flow, the sheet and iris base are pushed against the inner sclera, obliterating the ciliary cleft.

and the response to subsequent injections is greatly diminished after the second dose. Caution should be used in animals with cardiac disease, because rapid infusion of mannitol may overload the circulatory system and create pulmonary edema.

Orally administered glycerol (glycerin), although not as effective as mannitol, lowers the IOP within 15 to 30 minutes.[22, 42] A dose of 1 to 2 g/kg PO may cause gastric irritation and vomiting, but it is nontoxic and does not induce the diuresis that mannitol does.

Carbonic anhydrase inhibitors (CAIs) are the second type of drug used. The hypotensive effect of CAIs is independent of the diuretic effect, because the ocular effect occurs in nephrectomized patients and other potent non-CAI diuretics have minimal ocular effect.[20] Although the exact ocular mechanism is unknown, CAIs decrease aqueous secretion by about 40 to 50 per cent and have a minimal effect on the facility of outflow.[32, 46, 50] The IOP was decreased with a single administration of CAI by 24 per cent in normal and 29 per cent in glaucomatous beagles.[28] In general, the decrease in pressure begins within 1 hour and lasts for about 8 hours, with minor variations with drug and dosage. An intravenous form of acetazolamide is available and may produce a recognizable reduction in pressure after 10 minutes.

Four CAI preparations are available, and the recommended dosages are given (Table 91–5). Acetazolamide (Diamox, Vetamox) is the best known and most available of the group. Side effects are similar with all the preparations, but individual tolerance to side effects and to individual products is quite variable. Some patients do not tolerate any of the products at therapeutic doses, but intolerance to one does not imply intolerance to all. The primary side effects noted are panting, vomiting, anorexia, and acidosis.[30] Vestibular signs of nystagmus and circling and apparent paresthesias have also been noted on several occasions.

TABLE 91–5. CARBONIC ANHYDRASE INHIBITORS FOR GLAUCOMA THERAPY

Drug	Dose (mg/kg)	Frequency of Administration
Acetazolamide	10–30	BID to TID
Dichlorphenamide	2–4	BID to TID
Methazolamide	2–4	BID to TID

Topical Therapy

Epinephrine decreases aqueous formation and increases outflow facility.[35, 81] Decreased aqueous formation with epinephrine is independent of the effect of the CAI decrease, and together they have an additive effect. As epinephrine dilates the pupil, it may create or aggravate angle closure. The main indication for use of epinephrine is open-angle glaucoma. Epinephrine is available as hydrochloride, borate, and bitartrate in concentrations of 0.5 to 2.0 per cent.

The use of miotics in emergency therapy is restricted to direct-acting agents such as pilocarpine. The more potent cholinesterase inhibitors are avoided because of their systemic toxicity if used frequently, as well as their potentiation of bleeding and inflammation if surgery is performed.[31] The mydriasis of glaucoma is not overcome with miotics until the pressure is lowered.

Pilocarpine solution is available in concentrations of 0.25 to 10.0 per cent, but 2.0 per cent was the most efficient concentration in a study in beagles, with no additional benefits resulting from the higher concentrations.[92] Pilocarpine 4 per cent gel (Pilopine HS) allows twice-a-day therapy. Although minimal ocular effects are noted while the IOP is elevated, pilocarpine is given to be present when the pressure is lowered. Administration at 30-minute intervals for two treatments and then at 6-hour intervals delivers adequate drug concentration without complicating systemic side effects. Some individuals are very sensitive to pilocarpine-induced ciliary spasms, and if a tolerance does not develop, therapy may have to be discontinued. Miotic therapy is contraindicated with secondary glaucomas due to inflammation.

Timolol maleate (Timoptic), betaxolol (Betoptic), and levobunolol (Betagan) are beta-adrenergic blockers that decrease aqueous production up to 48 per cent in humans and have little effect on the pupil.[15] Although laboratory evidence in cats demonstrates some effect with the commercial concentrations of 0.25 and 0.5 per cent of timolol, a significant lowering of IOP has not been noted in normal dogs given commercial concentrations.[41, 64]

In summary, emergency medical therapy consists of an osmotic diuretic, a CAI (oral or intravenous), and topical pilocarpine. Once the IOP is lowered, maintenance therapy with a CAI and pilocarpine is continued to determine the chronic response to therapy. Most acute high-pressure glaucomas are associated with closed angles or mechanical obstructive phenomena and respond poorly to chronic medical therapy. Persistence with medical therapy simply prolongs the inevitable surgical procedure, allowing more ocular damage to occur from erratic control. Owners should be forewarned so that the decision for surgery can be made early in the course of therapy.

SURGICAL THERAPY

Before surgical procedures are attempted on a glaucomatous eye, a thorough ophthalmic examination must be performed to determine the cause of the glaucoma and select the most rational therapy and prognosis. Retinal and optic nerve damage must be accurately defined, because the selection of therapy may depend on restoration of vision as opposed to cosmetic appearance and pain relief alone. If CAIs have been administered, blood gas determinations may be important, because acidosis may persist for up to 36 hours after their withdrawal.[30] Acid-base and electrolyte imbalances are corrected before induction of general anesthesia.

Surgical therapy is categorized into those procedures that increase aqueous outflow (e.g., filtering procedures), those that decrease aqueous production (e.g., cyclocryosurgery), and salvage procedures used to relieve pain and provide a cosmetically acceptable eye (i.e., intraocular prosthesis or chemical induction of hypotony). Salvage procedures destroy the retina and are not acceptable for a potentially functional eye.

Surgical procedures such as iridencleisis, corneoscleral trephination, cyclodialysis, sclerectomy, anterior chamber implantation of aqueous shunts, and combinations of these procedures have been used to overcome the angle obstruction. The success rate has been reported to be 30 to 50 per cent—an optimistic estimate in my experience—and few surgeons persist with these procedures.[6, 23, 63] Silicone aqueous shunts of various designs are not a recent concept but are the subject of new interest.* The cause of failure of most filtering procedures and shunts has been fibroplasia of the sclera and conjunctival filtering bleb.[78] Revised designs of the shunt devices, perhaps in conjunction with drugs that counteract fibroplasia, offer the possibility of bypassing the angle obstruction. A series of 21 eyes with aqueous shunts had a success rate of 80 per cent in controlling IOP, although 50 per cent also needed medical glaucoma therapy.[3] Silicone shunts may block up with fibrin in the small-diameter anterior chamber tubing or have the distal subconjunctival or orbital filtering bleb develop fibroplasia with subsequent retention of fluid.[26] Modifications of the distal end of the shunt by attaching to an encircling silicone strap or band to allow fluid absorption over a large surface area have apparently increased the success rate.

Aqueous shunts are placed by dissecting a limbus-based conjunctival flap and partial-thickness scleral flap and inserting the tubing into the anterior chamber through a small limbal stab incision or needle centesis. The tubing is secured with sutures to the sclera to prevent migration. The distal end of the tubing may end near the limbus, extend into the orbit, or attach to a Silastic band that partially or completely encircles the globe near the equator (Fig. 91–11). Topical anti-inflammatory agents and antibiotics are administered postoperatively. Loss of function of the implant is initially due to obstruction of the tube by inflammatory debris or later to fibrosis of the filtering bleb.

Focused high-frequency ultrasound has been applied transconjunctivally to produce necrosis of the sclera and the ciliary processes. Damage to the ciliary body may decrease aqueous production, or a scleral hole can be formed to produce a filtering conjunctival bleb.[17]

Luxated Lens Removal

The role of lens displacement and lens luxation in canine glaucoma is not understood. Lens displacement may produce glaucoma, may be the result of glaucoma, or may be an exciting event in precipitating glaucoma. Removal of a displaced lens may simplify or eliminate the need for medical management if the drainage angle remains partially open. In some breeds in which zonular defects are often the primary disease (e.g., terriers), removal of a luxated lens may control glaucoma without long-term medical management.

Anteriorly luxated lenses should be removed from eyes that are still functional, but in chronically blind glaucomatous eyes, they may pose a therapeutic dilemma. Removal of the lens in the latter case may not control the pressure, and a more pragmatic and less expensive mode of therapy is usually preferred (i.e., salvage surgical procedure). The pathogenesis of glaucoma associated with subluxated or partially luxated lenses is often not obvious even when subjected to detailed clinical examinations. A posteriorly luxated lens without pressure elevation is usually not removed. Lens extraction is discussed elsewhere, but several points are crucial in the removal of the anterior luxated lens. Preoperative treatment consists of medically controlling the IOP and inducing miosis to trap the lens in the anterior chamber. In anticipation of vitreous loss, intravenous mannitol and complete muscle relaxation with pancuronium are valuable adjuncts. Prostaglandin inhibitors are routinely given before intraocular surgery.

Removal of a luxated lens is an intracapsular procedure, and the vitreous must be gently teased away from the posterior capsule as the lens is elevated. Vitreous that remains herniated through the pupil is excised using scissors and cellulose sponges until all solid vitreous is well behind the pupil. Postoperative management is similar to routine cataract extraction. The IOP is gently monitored in the immediate postoperative period as well

*See references 3, 7, 25, 37, 38, 66, and 80.

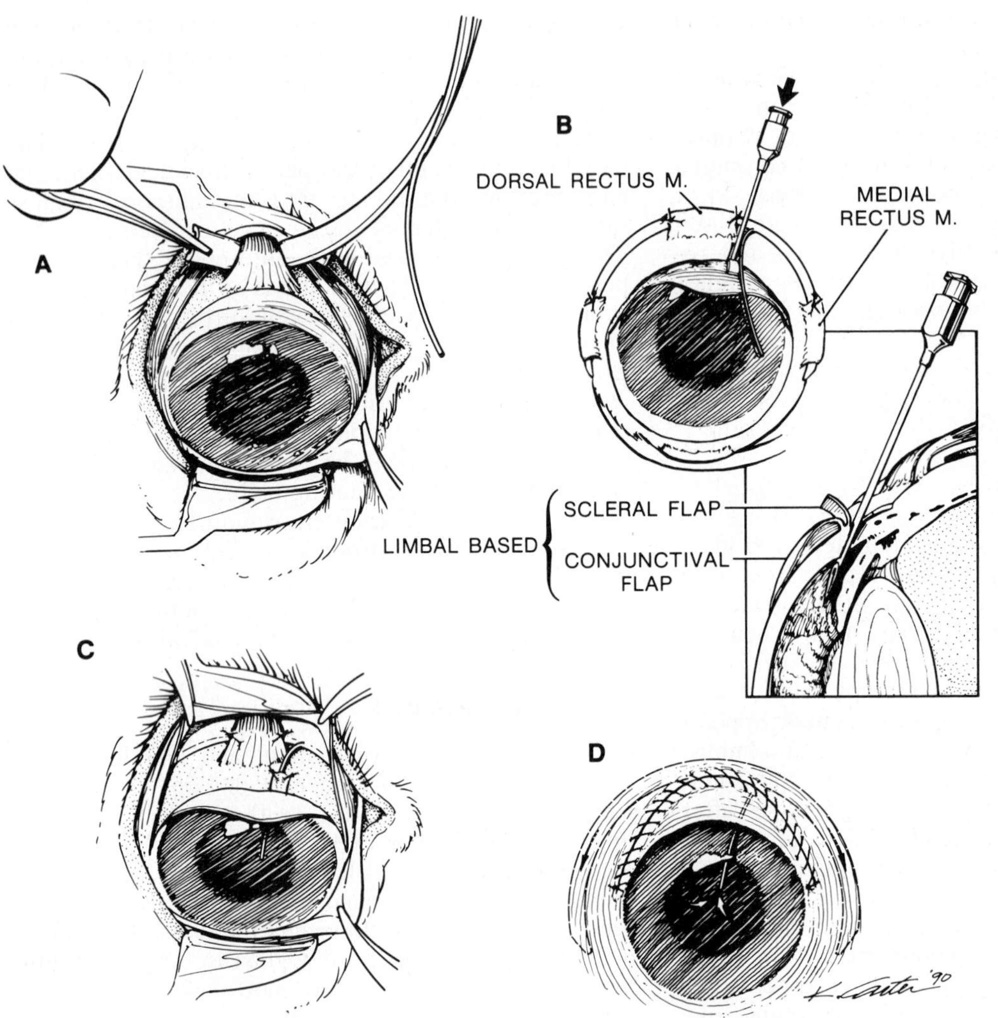

FIGURE 91–11. Placement of aqueous shunt. A grooved scleral buckling silicone strip is modified by notching and gluing a silicone tube of 0.02 inches internal diameter into the groove and leaving the proximal end long. *A,* A limbus-based conjunctival flap has been fashioned, the Tenon capsule removed, and the dorsal rectus exposed. The silicone band is being placed under the dorsal rectus muscle. *B,* The silicone band has been cut to encircle 180° to 270° of the circumference of the globe, placed under the medial and lateral rectus muscle, and fixed with 8-0 nylon sutures to their tendons. The anterior chamber component lies beside the dorsal rectus. A small partial-thickness limbus-based scleral flap is dissected using electrocautery for hemostasis, and a 20-gauge needle is used to enter the anterior chamber. *C,* The silicone tube is cut so that the end will extend near the pupillary axis, and it is then placed into the anterior chamber through the needle tract after heparin flushing. The scleral flap is reappositioned with two 8-0 nylon sutures to fixate the tubing. *D,* The conjunctival flap is sutured with a 7-0 absorbable suture.

as in the follow-up period of 1 to 2 years. Retinal detachments are relatively common after intracapsular extractions with vitreous loss.

Procedures That Decrease Aqueous Production

Decreasing aqueous production by ciliary body destruction to balance the decreased outflow is a relatively crude method to normalize IOP. Methods of damaging the ciliary body are cyclodiathermy, cyclocryotherapy, laser ablation, focused ultrasound, and chemical ablation.

Cyclodiathermy is the application of intense heat within the ciliary body, usually by inserting a diathermy needle through the sclera 5 to 6 mm posterior to the limbus. This technique produces severe postoperative inflammation and is unpredictable, frequently resulting in phthisis bulbi. The technique is rarely used. Transscleral application of a nonpulsed neodymium:yttrium-aluminum-garnet (Nd:YAG) laser at 8 joules per site has been used to produce necrosis of the ciliary body. The most important complication was vitreal hemorrhage.[60] The expense of this form of Nd:YAG laser precludes its wide availability.

Cyclocryotherapy or cold applications to the ciliary body also destroy the ciliary epithelium and decrease aqueous production. A wide range of cryotherapy techniques may produce the desired decrease in IOP.[88] The cryogen used for freezing the ciliary epithelium can be liquid nitrogen or nitrous oxide.* A cryoprobe with a thermocouple incorporated to monitor tip temperature is preferred. When the nitrous oxide cryoprobe tip is −60° to −80°C, a predictable cooling curve in the ciliary body is obtained. Freezing of the ciliary processes to 14°F (−10°C) is reached in 135 seconds using a 2.5-mm-diameter nitrous oxide cryoprobe. The ciliary epithelium appears to be sensitive to cold, and a temperature of 14°F (−10°C) is adequate to cause hypotony in dogs.[87]

Cyclocryotherapy is performed under general anesthesia. The cryoprobe tip is placed firmly on the conjunctiva 5 mm posterior to the limbus, and each site is frozen for 2 minutes (Fig. 91–12). The process is repeated at six to eight (nitrous oxide) or two to three (liquid nitrogen) approximately equally spaced locations around the globe. In cats and in dogs with a small palpebral fissure, it is more difficult to place the cry-

*Editors note: Some investigators report that liquid nitrogen equipment produces a much more reliable effect.

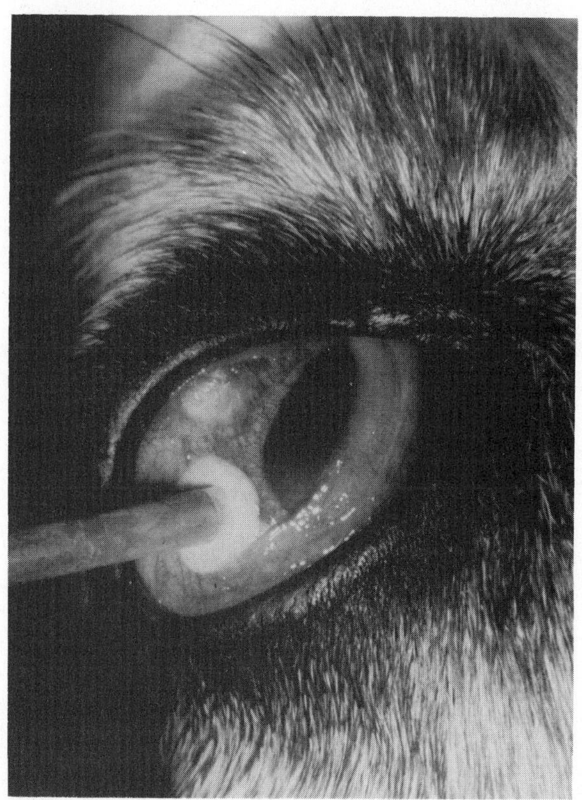

FIGURE 91–12. Cyclocryotherapy with formation of ice ball at cryoprobe tip placed 5 mm posterior to limbus. A previously frozen area is thawing, and the conjunctiva is chemotic and inflamed.

oprobe over the 360° without contacting excess adjacent tissue. The freezing site under the third eyelid is exposed by rolling the globe upward with forceps placed adjacent to the limbus near the freezing site, not by pulling on the third eyelid, which shortens the cul-de-sac so that the probe cannot be positioned. Once freezing has begun, cryoadhesion allows easy manipulation of the globe. Repeat freeze-thaw cycles in a given location are no more effective than single freezes and result in more severe postoperative chemosis. Overzealous cryotherapy may occasionally result in phthisis bulbi. Liquid nitrogen as a cryogen allows more profound freezing. The probe is placed similarly to the nitrous oxide probe, but freezing is discontinued when the ice ball reaches the cornea. Freezing occurs more rapidly, and because of a larger probe and ice ball, fewer individual freezes are necessary. The need for repeat freezes is questionable.[73]

After cryotherapy, marked conjunctivitis, chemosis, and uveitis occur. A subconjunctival injection of 0.5 to 1.0 mg of dexamethasone is administered at the end of the cryotherapy, and topical antibiotic-steroids are administered for 10 to 14 days. CAIs are continued until the IOP is normal. After cryotherapy, about one-fourth to one-third of eyes have a transient increase in IOP that may be difficult to control and may destroy the last vestiges of vision in advanced cases or require several days to recover the lost vision. Once the IOP has returned to normal, patients are challenged by withdrawal of the glaucoma medications.

Patients are re-evaluated at 2 to 3 weeks and 2 months postoperatively and then at 3-month intervals. The IOP may gradually increase as ciliary epithelium regenerates. If IOP increases, medical management may control the pressure, or in about 30 per cent of patients, cyclocryotherapy must be repeated. Cyclocryotherapy with liquid nitrogen was more successful than nitrous oxide in controlling IOP in patients requiring repeat freezing.[74]

Cyclocryotherapy is advantageous over filtering procedures because it is noninvasive, easily repeatable, less expensive, technically easier, and more successful. Success rates as high as 90 per cent have been reported, but cats do not respond as well as dogs to cyclocryotherapy.[10]

Complications of cyclocryotherapy include phthisis bulbi, hyphema, and choroidal and retinal detachments. Owing to a high incidence of retinal detachments produced by cryotherapy in normal eyes, prophylactic cryotherapy on an eye with ocular hypertension but no clinical signs of glaucoma is not recommended.[88]

Cyclocryotherapy is useful for narrow-, closed-, and open-angle glaucoma. Glaucoma secondary to uveal inflammation responds but with a lower success rate than primary glaucoma. The procedure was originally designed for pain relief in blind eyes but has been used on glaucomatous globes, with preservation of vision in 25 to 73 per cent of cases.[79, 85]

Salvage Surgical Procedures for Glaucoma

Ocular Prosthesis

Ocular evisceration and insertion of a prosthesis is indicated in chronically blind, painful eyes that do not have an ocular tumor, infection, or deep corneal ulcer. Preservation of a nearly normal eye is very desirable to most owners, who invariably elect the prosthesis over enucleation.

A prosthesis 1 to 2 mm larger than the horizontal corneal diameter is selected. If the globe is greatly enlarged, the contralateral normal eye is measured for the size of implant. Most canine eyes accept a sphere of 17 to 22 mm in diameter.[9]

The limbus-based conjunctival and Tenon flap is made beginning 5 mm posterior to the limbus and extending approximately 150°. The sclera may be incised by various methods, but using an electroscalpel to incise 2 to 3 mm posterior and parallel to the limbus for 150° to 160° helps control hemorrhage. The uvea is separated from the sclera by traction and blunt dissection using instruments such as a cyclodialysis spatula, a lens loop, or a cotton-tipped applicator. Hemorrhage is profuse, and suction is useful to keep the field free of blood. The uvea, retina, lens, and vitreous are removed, leaving only the fibrous tunic. The corneal endothelium is avoided during the intraocular manipulations. Once all intraocular contents are removed, the black sphere* is positioned with a sphere introducer (Fig. 91–13). The scleral incision is closed with simple interrupted absorbable sutures. A small amount of air or balanced salt solution is injected between the implant and cornea,

*Jardon Plastic Research, Southfield, MI.

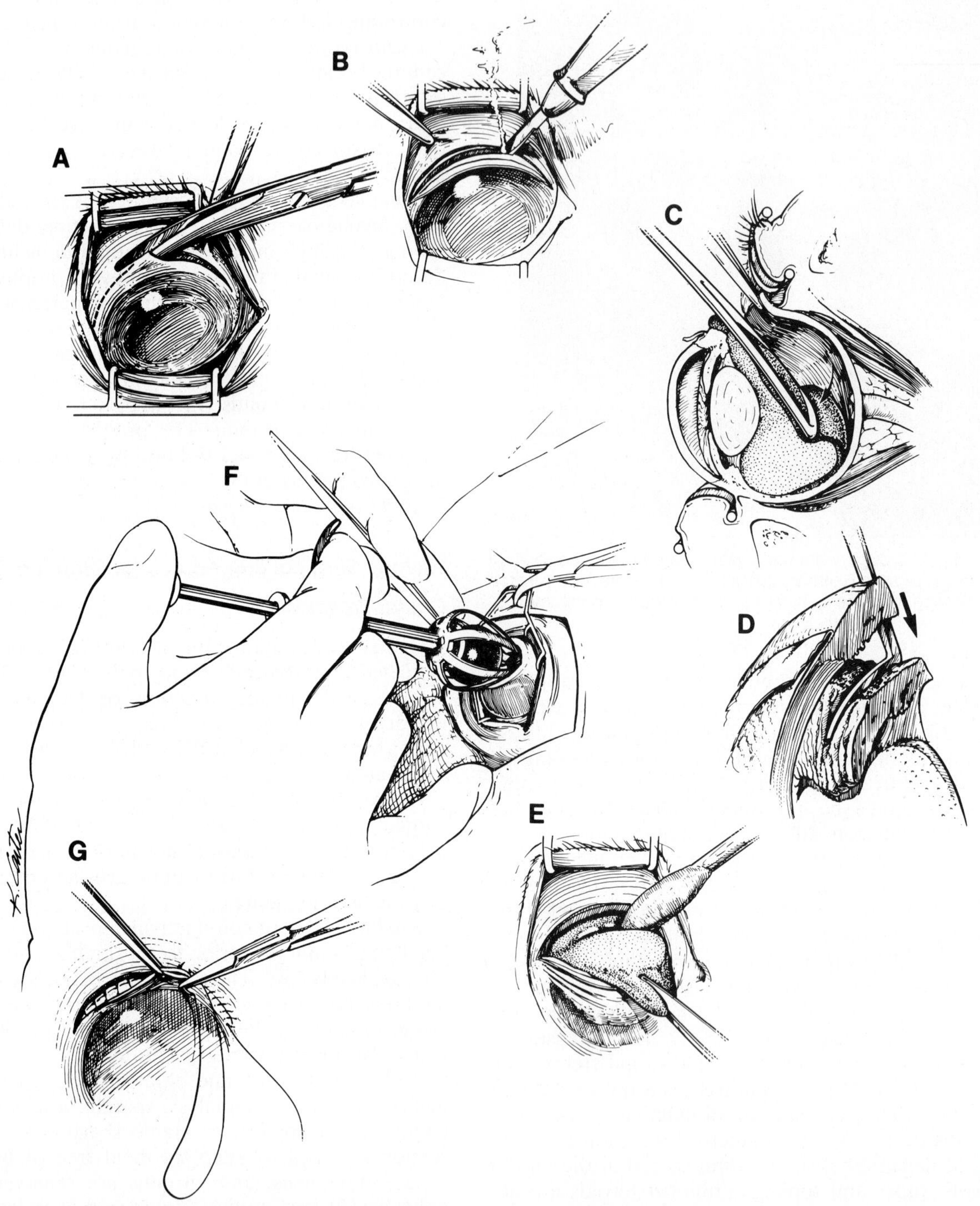

FIGURE 91–13. Ocular implant insertion. *A*, Limbus-based conjunctival flap dissection. *B*, Incision into globe with electrosurgery. *C*, Blunt separation of posterior uvea from the sclera. *D*, Separation of the base of the iris with a cyclodialysis spatula. *E*, Removal of ocular contents using a cotton-tipped applicator for hemostasis. *F*, Insertion of black silicone sphere with a sphere inserter. *G*, Continuous suture in conjunctiva after a series of interrupted sutures in the sclera.

and the conjunctiva is closed with a simple continuous suture. In buphthalmic eyes, a temporary tarsorrhaphy may be performed to protect the cornea during postoperative swelling. The ocular contents should be submitted for histopathological examination in patients that have not had clear media (i.e., the genesis of the glaucoma is unknown). In feline eyes enucleated for glaucoma, 33 per cent were associated with ocular melanoma, and in many instances, the tumor was not suspected on clinical examination.[93]

Postoperative complications include extrusion of the implant through a central corneal ulceration, recurrence of an unsuspected ocular tumor around the implant, and extrusion due to intraocular infection.[36] Despite occasional failures, the prosthesis is a viable alternative to enucleation for a painful glaucomatous globe.

Enucleation (see Chapter 109)

Although once considered standard surgical therapy for chronic canine glaucoma, enucleation is indicated mainly in glaucoma associated with an intraocular tumor or overwhelming infection. Pragmatic pet owners may select this option. The low cost and high efficacy of cyclocryosurgery and intraocular implants make enucleation the last choice of all the surgical procedures available in treating canine glaucoma. An orbital prosthesis* (see Chapter 90) may be used to improve the postoperative cosmetic appearance.

SUMMARY

Most cases of glaucoma cannot be adequately or consistently controlled with medical therapy and require surgery. The type of surgical procedure selected depends on the equipment available, whether return of vision is a goal, the cause of glaucoma, and the surgeon's preference. Cyclocryotherapy is the procedure of choice.

References

1. Alsbirk PH: Anterior chamber depth and primary angle closure glaucoma II. A genetic study. *Acta Ophthalmol 53*:436, 1975.
2. Barnett KC: Glaucoma in the dog. *J Small Anim Pract 11*:113, 1970.
3. Bedford PG: A clinical evaluation of a one-piece drainage system in the treatment of canine glaucoma. *J Small Anim Pract 30*:68, 1989.
4. Bedford PG: Gonioscopy in the dog. *J Small Anim Pract 18*:615, 1977.
5. Bedford PG: A gonioscopic study of the iridocorneal angle in the English and American breeds of cocker spaniel and the basset hound. *J Small Anim Pract 12*:631, 1977.
6. Bedford PG: The surgical treatment of canine glaucoma. *J Small Anim Pract 18*:713, 1977.
7. Bedford PG: Use of a one-piece drainage system in the treatment of a closed angle glaucoma in a dog. *J Small Anim Pract 29*:231, 1988.
8. Bedford PG: Aqueous drainage in the dog. *Res Vet Sci 41*:172, 1986.
9. Brightman AH, et al: Intraocular prosthesis in the dog. *J Am Anim Hosp Assoc 13*:481, 1977.
10. Brightman AH, et al: Cryosurgery for the treatment of canine glaucoma. *J Am Anim Hosp Assoc 18*:319, 1982.
11. Brooks DE, et al: Ultrastructural changes in laminar optic nerve capillaries of beagles with primary open-angle glaucoma. *Am J Vet Res 50*:929, 1989.
12. Brooks DE, et al: Morphologic changes in the lamina cribrosa of beagles with primary open-angle glaucoma. *Am J Vet Res 50*:936, 1989.
13. Bryan G: Tonometry in the dog and cat. *J Small Anim Pract 6*:117, 1965.

*Storz Instrument Co., St. Louis, MO.

14. Charles ST, Hamasaki DI: The effect of intraocular pressure on the pupil size. *Arch Ophthalmol 83*:729, 1970.
15. Coakes RL, Brubaker RF: The mechanism of timolol in lowering intraocular pressure. *Arch Ophthalmol 96*:2045, 1978.
16. Cole DF: Aqueous humour formation. *Doc Ophthalmol 21*:116, 1966.
17. Coleman DJ, et al: Therapeutic ultrasound in the treatment of glaucoma. II. Clinical applications. *Ophthalmology 92*:347, 1985.
18. Cruise L, McClure R: Posterior pathway for aqueous humor drainage in the dog. *Am J Vet Res 42*:992, 1981.
19. Ernest JT, et al: The effect of mannitol infusion on retinal function and oxygen tension. *Invest Ophthalmol Vis Sci 16*:670, 1977.
20. Friedman Z, et al: Ocular and systemic effects of acetazolamide in nephrectomized rabbits. *Invest Ophthalmol Vis Sci 23*:209, 1982.
21. Gaasterland D, et al: Axoplasmic flow during chronic experimental glaucoma. *Invest Ophthalmol Vis Sci 17*:838, 1978.
22. Galin MA, et al: Ophthalmological use of osmotic therapy. *Am J Ophthalmol 62*:629, 1966.
23. Gelatt KN: The canine glaucomas. *In* Gelatt KN (ed): *Veterinary Ophthalmology*. Lea & Febiger, Philadelphia, 1981, pp 390–434.
24. Gelatt KN, Gum GG: Inheritance of primary glaucoma in the beagle. *Am J Vet Res 42*:1691, 1981.
25. Gelatt KN, Ladds PW: Gonioscopy in dogs and cats with glaucoma and ocular tumors. *J Small Anim Pract 12*:105, 1971.
26. Gelatt KN, et al: Evaluation of the Krupin-Denver valve implant in normotensive and glaucomatous Beagles. *J Am Vet Med Assoc 191*:1404, 1987.
27. Gelatt KN, et al: Uveoscleral flow of aqueous humor in the normal dog. *Am J Vet Res 40*:845, 1979.
28. Gelatt KN, et al: Ocular hypotensive effects of carbonic anhydrase inhibitors in normotensive and glaucomatous beagles. *Am J Vet Res 40*:334, 1979.
29. Gelatt KN, et al: Clinical manifestations of inherited glaucoma in the Beagle. *Invest Ophthalmol Vis Sci 16*:1135, 1977.
30. Haskins SC, et al: Effect of acetazolamide on blood acid-base and electrolyte values in dogs. *J Am Vet Med Assoc 179*:792, 1981.
31. Havener W: *Ocular Pharmacology*. 4th ed. C.V. Mosby, St. Louis, 1978.
32. Hayreh SS: Pathogenesis of cupping of the optic disc. *Br J Ophthalmol 58*:863, 1974.
33. Hayreh SS, Weingeist TA: Experimental occlusion of the central artery of the retina IV: Retinal tolerance time to acute ischemia. *Br J Ophthalmol 64*:818, 1980.
34. Heywood R: Intraocular pressures in the beagle dog. *J Small Anim Pract 12*:119, 1971.
35. Kaufman PL, Barany EH: Adrenergic drug effects on aqueous outflow facility following ciliary muscle retrodisplacement in the cynomolgus monkey. *Invest Ophthalmol Vis Sci 20*:644, 1981.
36. Koch SA: Intraocular prosthesis in the dog and cat: The failures. *J Am Vet Med Assoc 179*:883, 1981.
37. Krupin T, et al: Valve implants in filtering surgery. *Am J Ophthalmol 81*:232, 1976.
38. Krupin T, et al: A long Krupin-Denver valve implant attached to a 180° scleral explant for glaucoma surgery. *Ophthalmology 95*:1174, 1988.
39. Lescure G: L'angle camerulaire du chien etude goniophotographique. *Proc World Vet Cong 17*:1001, 1963.
40. Levy ND: The effect of elevated intraocular pressure on axoplasmic transport in the optic nerve of the rhesus monkey. *Doc Ophthalmol 43*:181, 1977.
41. Liu HK, Chiou CY: Ocular hypotensive effects of timolol in cat eyes. *Arch Ophthalmol 98*:1467, 1980.
42. Lorimar DW, et al: The effect of intravenous mannitol or oral glycerol on intraocular pressure in dogs. *Cornell Vet 79*:249, 1989.
43. Lovekin L: Primary glaucoma in dogs. *J Am Vet Med Assoc 145*:1081, 1964.
44. Lovekin L, Bellhorn RW: Clinicopathologic changes in primary glaucoma in the cocker spaniel. *Am J Vet Res 29*:379, 1968.
45. Lowe RF: Primary angle-closure glaucoma inheritance and environment. *Br J Ophthalmol 56*:13, 1972.
46. Macri FJ, Cevario SJ: A possible vascular mechanism for the inhibition of aqueous humor formation of ouabain and acetazolamide. *Exp Eye Res 20*:563, 1975.
47. Magrane WG: Canine glaucoma. I. Method of diagnosis. *J Am Vet Med Assoc 131*:311, 1957.
48. Magrane WG: Canine glaucoma. II. Primary classification. *J Am Vet Med Assoc 131*:372, 1957.
49. Magrane WG: Canine glaucoma. III. Secondary classification. *J Am Vet Med Assoc 131*:374, 1957.
50. Maren TH: The rates of movement on Na^+, Cl^-, and HCO^- from plasma to posterior chamber: Effect of acetazolamide and relation to the treatment of glaucoma. *Invest Ophthalmol Vis Sci 15*:356, 1976.
51. Martin CL: Biomicroscopic examination of the normal canine anterior segment. Master's thesis, Ohio State University, 1968.
52. Martin CL: Gonioscopy and anatomical correlations of the drainage angle of the dog. *J Small Anim Pract 10*:171, 1969.
53. Martin CL: Development of pectinate ligament structure of the dog: Study by scanning electron microscopy. *Am J Vet Res 35*:1433, 1974.
54. Martin CL: The normal canine iridocorneal angle as viewed with the scanning electron microscope. *J Am Anim Hosp Assoc 11*:180, 1975.

55. Martin CL: Scanning electron microscopic examination of selected canine iridocorneal angle abnormalities. *J Am Anim Hosp Assoc 11*:301, 1975.
56. Martin CL, Anderson BG: Ocular antomy. *In* Gelatt KN (ed): *Veterinary Ophthalmology*. Lea & Febiger, Philadelphia, 1981, pp 12–121.
57. Martin CL, Wyman M: Glaucoma in the basset hound. *J Am Vet Med Assoc 53*:1320, 1968.
58. Martin CL, Wyman M: Primary glaucoma in the dog. *Vet Clin North Am 8*:257, 1978.
59. Minckler DS, Spaeth GL: Optic nerve damage in glaucoma. *Surv Ophthalmol 26*:128, 1981.
60. Nasisse MP, et al: Neodymium:yttrium, aluminum, and garnet laser energy delivered transsclerally to the ciliary body of dogs. *Am J Vet Res 59*:1972, 1988.
61. Peiffer RL, Gelatt KN: Aqueous humor outflow in Beagles with inherited glaucoma: Gross and light microscopic observations of the iridocorneal angle. *Am J Vet Res 41*:861, 1980.
62. Peiffer RL, et al: Calibration of the Schiotz tonometer for the normal canine eye. *Am J Vet Res 38*:1881, 1977.
63. Peiffer RL, et al: Combined posterior sclerectomy, cyclodialysis and transscleral iridencleisis in the management of primary glaucoma. *Canine Pract 4*:54, 1977.
64. Pickett P, Majors L: Short-term and long-term effects of topical timolol maleate and betaxolol on intraocular pressure, heart rate, and blood pressure in normal dogs. Transactions of the 20th Annual Scientific Program of the American College of Veterinary Ophthalmology *20*:115, 1989.
65. Pickett P, et al: Calibration of the Schiotz tonometer for the canine and feline eye. Transactions of the 19th Annual Scientific Program of the American College of Veterinary Ophthalmology *19*:47, 1988.
66. Pritchard DL, Hamlet MP: A Silastic-darcon implant for the treatment of glaucoma. *Vet Med Small Anim Clin 65*:1191, 1970.
67. Quigley HA: Glaucoma's optic nerve damage: Changing clinical perspectives. *Ann Ophthalmol 14*:611, 1982.
68. Quigley HA, Addicks EM: Chronic experimental glaucoma in primates. II. Effect of extended intraocular pressure elevation on optic nerve head and axonal transport. *Invest Ophthalmol Vis Sci 19*:137, 1980.
69. Quigley HA, et al: Optic nerve damage in human glaucoma. III. Quantitative correlation of nerve fiber loss and visual field defect in glaucoma, ischemic neuropathy, papilledema, and toxic nephropathy. *Arch Ophthalmol 100*:135, 1982.
70. Quigley HA, et al: The mechanism of optic nerve damage in experimental acute intraocular pressure elevation. *Invest Ophthalmol Vis Sci 19*:505, 1980.
71. Radius RL, Anderson DF: Reversibility of optic nerve damage in primate eyes subjected to intraocular pressure above systolic blood pressure. *Br J Ophthalmol 65*:661, 1981.
72. Robbins R, Galin MA: Effect of osmotic agents on the vitreous body. *Arch Ophthalmol 82*:694, 1969.
73. Roberts S, et al: Cyclocryotherapy—part I evaluation of a liquid nitrogen system. *J Am Anim Hosp Assoc 20*:823, 1984.
74. Roberts S, et al: Cyclocryotherapy—part II clinical comparison of liquid nitrogen and nitrous oxide cryotherapy on glaucomatous eyes. *J Am Anim Hosp Assoc 20*:282, 1984.
75. Rutkowski PC, Thompson HS: Mydriasis and increased intraocular pressure. I. Pupillographic studies. *Arch Ophthalmol 87*:21, 1972.
76. Rutkowski PC, Thompson HS: Mydriasis and increased intraocular pressure. II. Iris fluorescein studies. *Arch Ophthalmol 87*:25, 1972.
77. Sears ML: The aqueous. *In* Moses RA (ed): *Adler's Physiology of the Eye*. 7th ed. C.V. Mosby, St. Louis, 1981, pp 204–226.
78. Skuta GL, Parish RK II: Wound healing in glaucoma filtering surgery. *Surv Ophthalmol 32*:149, 1987.
79. Stades F, Boeve M: Methods, techniques and results of glaucoma therapy in dog and cat. Transactions of the 17th Annual Scientific Program of the American College of Veterinary Ophthalmology and International Society of Veterinary Ophthalmology *17*:813, 1986.
80. Stanley SS, et al: Anterior chamber tube shunt to an encircling band in the treatment of neovascular glaucoma. *Ophthalmology 89*:1188, 1982.
81. Townsend DJ, Brubaker RF: Immediate effect of epinephrine on aqueous formation in the normal human eye as measured by fluorophotometry. *Invest Ophthalmol Vis Sci 19*:256, 1980.
82. Troncoso MU: Microanatomy of the eye with the slitlamp microscope. II. Comparative anatomy of the ciliary body, zonula and related structures in mammallia. *Am J Ophthalmol 25*:1, 1942.
83. Troncoso MU: The intrascleral vascular plexus and its relations to the aqueous outflow. *Am J Opthalmol 25*:1153, 1942.
84. Troncoso MU, Castroveijo R: Microanatomy of the eye with the slitlamp microscope. I. Comparative anatomy of the angle of the anterior chamber in living and sectioned eyes of mammalia. *Am J Ophthalmol 19*:481, 1936.
85. Vainisi S, Schmidt G: Retrospective survey of cyclocryosurgery for the control of canine glaucoma. Transactions of the Scientific Program of the American College of Veterinary Ophthalmology and International Society of Veterinary Ophthalmology *17*:194, 1986.
86. VanBuskirk ME: The canine eye: The vessels of aqueous drainage. *Invest Ophthalmol Vis Sci 18*:223, 1979.
87. Vestre WA, Brightman AH: Ciliary body temperatures during cyclocryotherapy in the clinically normal dog. *Am J Vet Res 44*:135, 1983.
88. Vestre WA, Brightman AH: The effects of cyclocryotherapy on the clinically normal canine eye. *Am J Vet Res 44*:187, 1983.
89. Vucicevic ZM, et al: Echographic studies of osmotic agents. *Ann Ophthalmol 11*:1331, 1979.
90. Waltman SR: The cornea. *In* Moses RA (ed): *Adler's Physiology of the Eye*. 7th ed. C.V. Mosby, St. Louis, 1981, pp 38–62.
91. Watson P: Comparative aspects of glaucoma. *J Small Anim Pract 11*:129, 1970.
92. Whitley RD, et al: Dose response of topical pilocarpine in the normotensive and glaucomatous beagle. *Am J Vet Res 41*:417, 1980.
93. Wilcock B, Peiffer R: The causes of glaucoma in cats. Transactions of the American College of Veterinary Ophthalmology *19*:97, 1988.
94. Williams LW, et al: Orthograde rapid axoplasmic transport and ultrastructural changes of the optic nerve of normotensive, acute ocular hypertensives and glaucomatous beagles. Transactions of the 11th Annual Scientific Program of the American College of Veterinary Ophthalmology *11*:172, 1980.
95. Wundsch L: Experimentall-kritische Studie zum Problem der retinalen Ischamie. *Albrecht von Graefes Arch Klin Exp Ophthalmol 197*:241, 1975.
96. Wyman M, Ketring K: Congenital glaucoma in the basset hound: A biologic model. *Trans Am Acad Ophthalmol Otolaryngol 81*:645, 1976.

CHAPTER 92 Ocular Emergencies and Trauma

Stephen I. Bistner

EVALUATION OF THE TRAUMATIZED EYE

Ocular emergencies include corneal abrasion or chemical irritation, lid laceration, corneal foreign body, acute infectious keratitis, corneal or scleral laceration, contusion and penetrating intraocular injury, proptosis of the globe, endophthalmitis, and acute glaucoma. When an animal is presented with an ocular emergency, the following procedures are performed to obtain a diagnosis and institute effective therapy:[23]

1. Obtain an adequate history from the owner. This may reveal previous ocular disease, the instillation of some chemical irritant, or trauma. Determine when the injury occurred and if any medication or eye wash was used.

2. Examine the eye for any discharge, blepharospasm, or photophobia. Note the type of any discharge present. If the animal is in extreme discomfort and the eye is completely closed, *do not* try to force open the

lids—intraocular contents may be extruded if a corneal laceration is present. If a severe corneal ulcer, laceration, or penetrating wound is present, the animal is anesthetized and preparations are made for surgery before examination.

3. Note the position of the globe within the orbit and the presence of exophthalmos or proptosis. Exophthalmos is frequently attended by strabismus and protrusion of the third eyelid, exposure keratitis, and, with retrobulbar or zygomatic salivary gland inflammation, pain on opening the mouth. Note displacement of the globe medially or temporally.

4. Note swelling, contusions, or lacerations of the lids and whether the lids cover the cornea. Determine the depth of any lid lacerations. Penetrating lid lacerations may be associated with secondary injury to the globe.

5. Palpate the orbital margins for fractures, crepitus, air, and cellulitis.

6. Examine the conjunctiva for hemorrhage, chemosis, lacerations, or foreign bodies and the superior and inferior conjunctival cul-de-sacs for foreign bodies. With the animal under topical anesthesia, a sterile cotton swab can be used to "sweep" the conjunctival fornix free of foreign bodies. Elevate the third eyelid with small, fine-toothed forceps and examine its bulbar aspect for foreign bodies.

7. Examine the cornea for opacities, ulcers, foreign bodies, abrasions, or lacerations. A loupe and a focal source of bright illumination are important. A Finoff transilluminator with halogen illumination (3.5 V) is an excellent source of focal illumination.

8. Record pupil size; shape; and response to light, both direct and consensual; and the presence of anisocoria.

9. Examine the anterior chamber and note its depth and the presence of hyphema, iridodonesis, or iridodialysis.

10. If indicated and if the cornea is undamaged, measure intraocular pressure.

11. Dilate the eye with 1 per cent tropicamide drops and examine the fundus with a direct or indirect ophthalmoscope, noting intraocular or retinal hemorrhage, edema, or retinal detachment.

OCULAR EMERGENCIES

Differential Diagnosis

Acute Vision Loss

Sudden loss of vision or marked visual impairment may involve one or both eyes. The differential diagnosis includes the following:

1. Massive vitreous or retinal hemorrhage from any cause (no pain)
2. Bilateral optic neuritis or retrobulbar optic neuritis (painful)
3. Retinal detachment (no pain)
4. Severe anterior or posterior uveitis (painful)
5. Severe keratitis with blepharospasm (painful)
6. Acute congestive glaucoma (painful)

Asymmetry of Pupils

Pupillary asymmetry may be caused by any of the following:

1. Traumatic uveitis with miosis of the pupil
2. Horner's syndrome—miosis of the ipsilateral side
3. Intraorbital trauma to ciliary nerves or ganglia—mydriasis.
4. Optic neuritis or optic nerve avulsion—mydriasis with acute vision loss
5. Iridodialysis and rupture of iris sphincter—mydriasis
6. Unilateral use of topical mydriatic or miotic drugs
7. Diffuse central neurological disease—increased cerebrospinal fluid pressure

Chemical Burns

Chemical irritation of the eye may result from accidental contact with a noxious agent, such as a cleaning solution containing soap or sodium hydroxide, or from intentional discharge of chemical agents, such as mace, lye, or other noxious gases, into the face of an animal.[23, 24, 32]

Immediate first aid is aimed at removing the offending chemical from the eye with irrigation using large amounts of water or saline. Particles of solid material that adhere to the cornea or remain in the conjunctival cul-de-sacs are removed.

In general, acidic compounds are less dangerous than basic compounds.[24] Acidic compounds denature surface proteins and stop their penetration, whereas basic compounds destroy protein and penetrate deeper ocular structures.[32]

A classification of chemical ocular irritation indicates the extent of ocular injury following chemical irritation:

1. Mild
   a. Erosion of corneal epithelium
   b. Faint haziness of cornea
   c. No ischemic necrosis of conjunctiva and sclera
2. Moderately severe
   a. Corneal opacity blurs iris details
   b. Minimal ischemic necrosis of conjunctiva and sclera
3. Very severe
   a. Blurring of pupillary outline
   b. Blanching of conjunctiva and sclera

With mild chemical irritation, epithelial tags and remnants are carefully removed under topical anesthesia using a fine cotton swab. The pupil is dilated with atropine and, if necessary, 10 per cent phenylephrine. A synergistic effect is obtained when indirect-acting atropine and the direct-acting phenylephrine are combined. Infection, especially with gram-negative organisms, may be prevented by topical application of gentamicin ointment or drops five times daily.

An Elizabethan collar prevents the animal from rubbing its eye. If pain is severe, hospitalization and systemic administration of pethidine (Demerol), 3 to 6 mg/kg every 6 to 8 hours, may be indicated. Once reepithelization has taken place and if interstitial keratitis, vascularization, or granulation tissue remains, topical corticosteroids such as 0.1 per cent dexamethasone can be used topically.

If stromal necrosis of the cornea accompanies moderately severe anterior ocular segment injury, additional steps may be necessary. Antiprotease agents,[7] such as acetylcysteine 10 per cent, may be administered, using two drops five to seven times daily topically. Thin conjunctival flaps in combination with topical acetylcysteine 10 per cent, antibiotics, and atropine aid in controlling secondary uveitis.

Lid Injuries

Lid contusions and lacerations are most commonly associated with bite wounds or vehicular trauma. Surgical treatment of lid lacerations is similar to that of other areas of the body, except that careful primary repair is undertaken to ensure adequate physiological and cosmetic results. An accurate understanding of lid anatomy is necessary before attempting lid surgery (see Chapter 82).[5]

The lids are a two-layered structure; the anterior layer is composed of skin and orbicular muscle, and the posterior layer is composed of tarsal glands, connective tissue, and conjunctiva. Meticulous repair of lid lacerations is important if good cosmetic and physiological results are to be obtained. The age and type of injury are important considerations. Lacerations of the lid margin *without* lid avulsion that are presented 24 to 48 hours after injury and are grossly contaminated should not be immediately operated on but carefully cleaned, the eye evaluated for further injury, the lids treated with topical antibiotics, and systemic infections controlled. The animal can undergo surgical repair of the lid in 5 to 7 days.

When the lid is torn away from its lateral or medial attachments, blood supply to the lid may be compromised and atrophy of the damaged piece of lid may occur (Fig. 92–1). Although avulsions may be grossly contaminated and 24 to 48 hours old, they are carefully cleaned, minimally débrided, and resutured to restore adequate circulation.[5]

Treatment

The lid laceration is lavaged with sterile saline, and any foreign material removed aseptically. All hair is carefully clipped and irrigated from the wound, and a 1 per cent povidone-iodine solution is applied around the wound margins but not in the wound itself. The surgical field is draped aseptically.

A full-thickness lid wound laceration involves the conjunctiva, muscle-fascial layer, and skin. A minimum of two suture layers gives well-approximated lid closure. Ragged wound margins are trimmed, and necrotic tissue is débrided. However, *as much tissue as possible* is saved to minimize wound contracture and lid deformity. When a ragged lid margin is corrected, the tarsus is trimmed in a slightly curved fashion, permitting slight overcorrection and "pouting" of the suture incision when the lid is sutured vertically. This helps ensure tight lid closure and reduces scarring.[15]

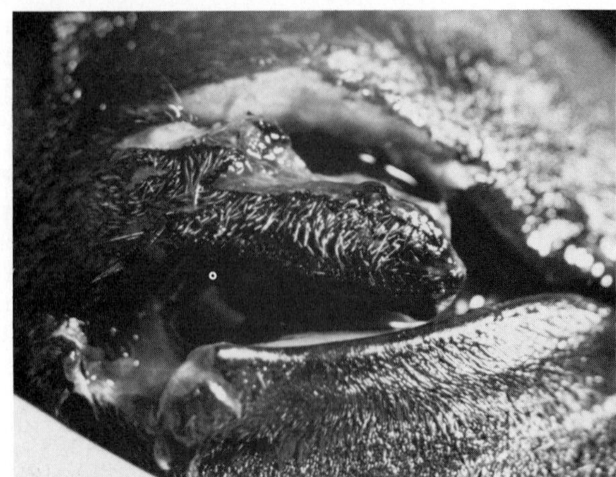

FIGURE 92–1. Severe lacerations of the lid with avulsion of the lid from the lateral canthus. Very careful débridement, cleaning, and reapposition of lid were required using a two-layer closure.

The conjunctiva is closed with interrupted absorbable sutures (5-0 to 7-0) of collagen, chromic gut, or polyglycolic or polyglactic acid. All knots are buried beneath the conjunctiva to prevent corneal abrasion. The lid margins must be parallel. The skin is closed with nylon, silk, or polyglycolic or polyglactic acid, and small sutures (5-0 to 7-0) are used. An everting effect is achieved at the skin closure line. It is especially important to close the marginal lid defect to prevent notching of the lid margin.

Closure of lid margin defects not involving more than one-fourth to one-third of the lid margin can usually be accomplished without placing abnormal tension on the lid margin. If more than one-fourth of the lid margin has been lost, blepharoplasty must be performed to close the defect while preserving normal lid structure. Numerous blepharoplastic techniques can be used.[5, 15, 16, 24, 30, 31]

The two-layer technique to close extensive lid lacerations is shown in Figures 92–2 and 92–3. Splitting the lid separates the skin-muscle layer from the tarsoconjunctival layer, permitting mobilization of the skin. Interrupted 6-0 chromic gut sutures are used to close the tarsoconjunctival layer, with the knots buried on the anterior surface of the conjunctiva (see Fig. 92–2*D*). The skin-muscle layer is closed with interrupted 6-0 silk sutures (see Fig. 92–2*F–I*). Thus, the conjunctival and skin-muscle sutures are in two different planes.

Lacerations of the lids near the medial canthus can present difficult problems if a canalicular laceration is also present. For repair of canalicular defects, see Chapter 84.

Corneal Foreign Bodies

Foreign bodies are frequently encountered in dogs and occasionally in cats. In working dogs, awns, grass seeds, and oat hulls may enter the anterior segment of the eye and become embedded in the conjunctival

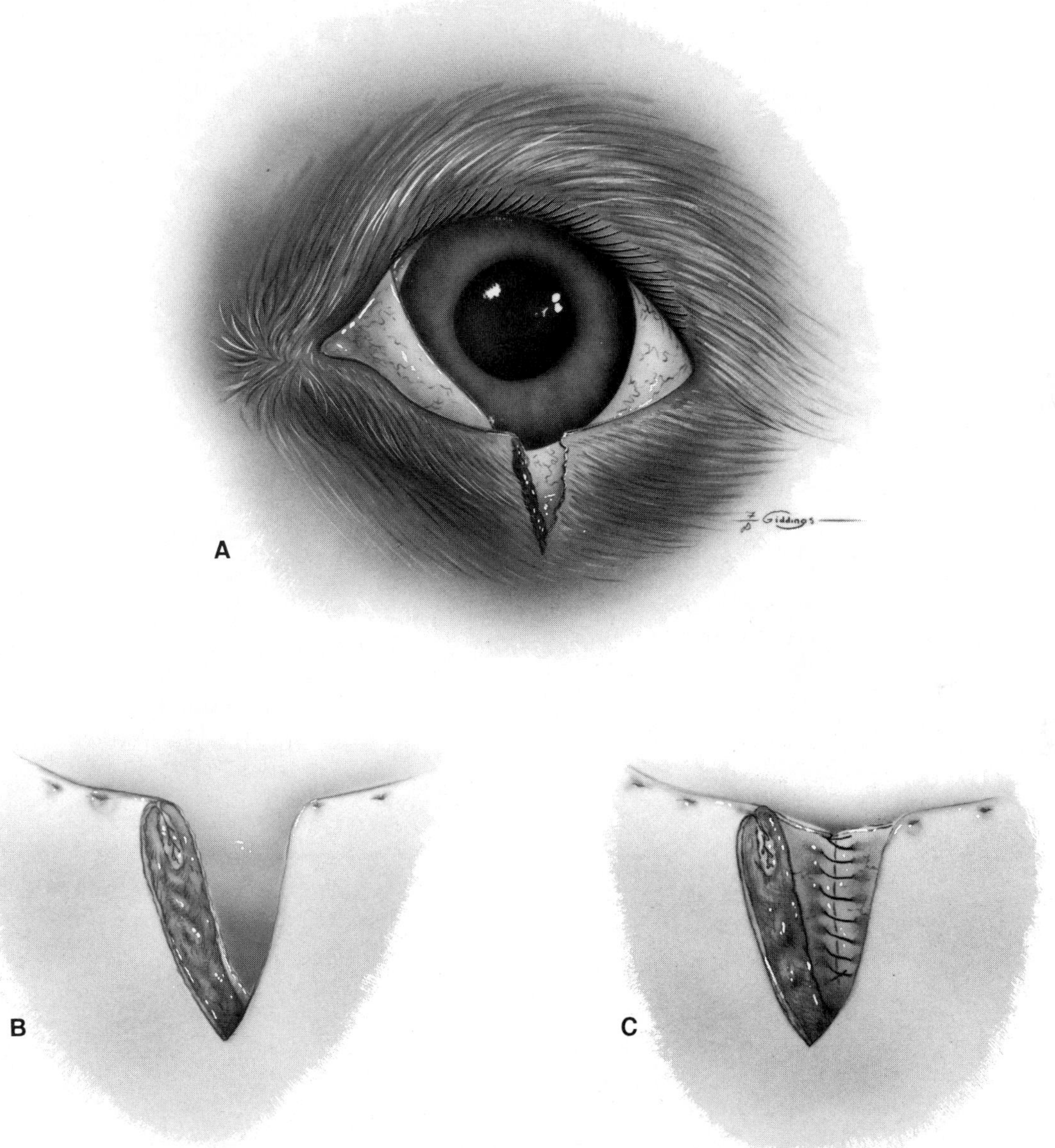

FIGURE 92–2. Simple two-layer repair. *A*, Initial injury before débridement. *B*, Wound after débridement and ready for suturing. *C*, The conjunctiva is sutured with 6-0 polyglactin 910 in a simple continuous pattern.

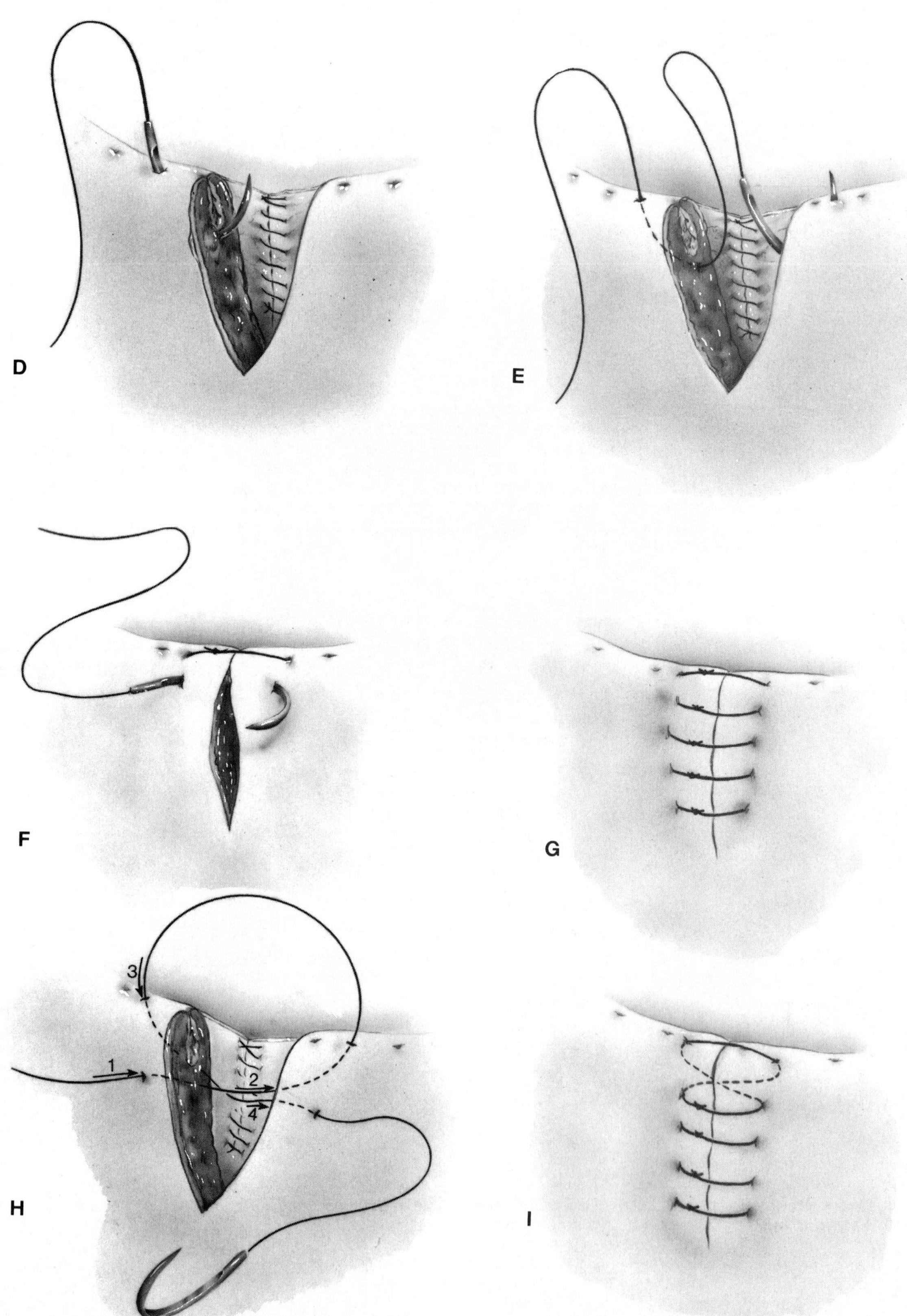

FIGURE 92–2 *Continued D*, The marginal suture is placed first, in two separate bites. *E*, The second bite. *F*, The marginal suture is carefully tied to ensure apposition of the margins. The knot lies along the margin. The wound is sutured with simple interrupted suture of 6-0 silk, 2 mm apart. The first suture beneath the margin relieves tension on the marginal suture. *G*, The wound sutured. *H*, A figure-eight suture pattern may be used in place of the first two sutures. *I*, The wound sutured using a figure-eight technique. (Reprinted with permission from Slatter DH: *Fundamentals of Veterinary Ophthalmology*. 2nd ed. W.B. Saunders, Philadelphia, 1990.)

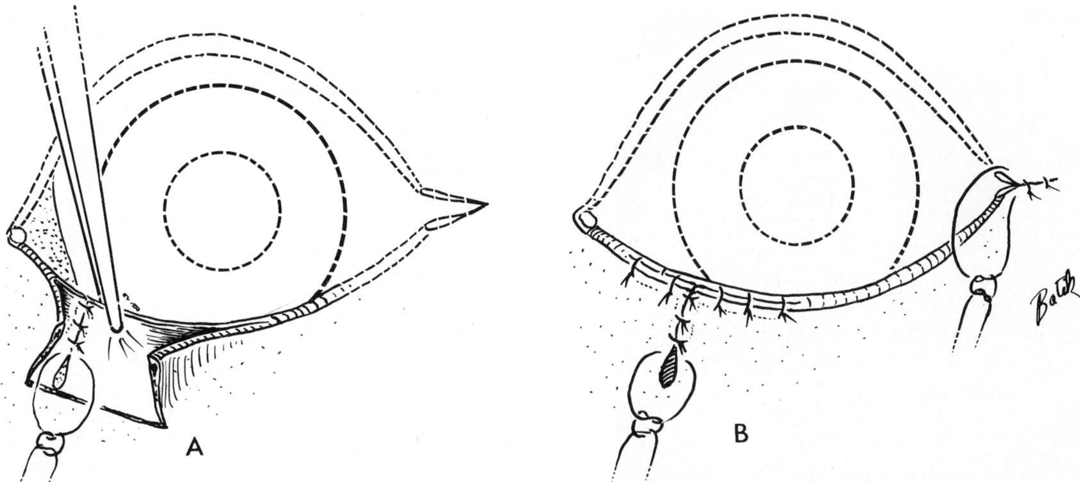

FIGURE 92–3. Marginal lid wound repair by lid splitting and conjunctival resection. *A,* The lower lid in the area of the lower punctum has been split into skin-orbicular muscle and conjunctiva. The punctum is not incised. The tumor-containing portions of the epidermal and conjunctival tissues have been removed as wedge resections. The edges of the skin-orbicular portion are undermined. If mobilization of the skin is difficult, a lateral canthotomy should be performed. The conjunctiva is closed with 6-0 chromic gut, tied with the knots lying between the conjunctiva and the skin. *B,* The undermined skin-orbicular area is closed with simple interrupted 6-0 silk sutures. The lateral canthotomy permits the lid to be moved nasally to facilitate closure. The split lid margin is closed with 6-0 silk sutures, with the knots tied on the outside of the lid margin. Sutures are removed in 10 to 14 days. (Reprinted with permission from Bistner SI, et al: *Atlas of Veterinary Ophthalmic Surgery.* W.B. Saunders, Philadelphia, 1977.)

fornices or cornea (Figs. 92–4 and 92–5). Blepharospasm, photophobia, pain, keratitis, and secondary uveitis may develop. The foreign body may penetrate the corneal stroma and enter the anterior chamber.

Dogs may have paint chips fall on their corneas when they are in the area while their owner is removing paint from a wall. Animals are presented with active keratitis caused by this foreign body.

In all cases of corneal foreign bodies, removal of the foreign body is the most effective treatment. Removal usually requires topical or general anesthesia. If a foreign body is embedded in the cornea, the epithelium may have to be carefully incised to remove it. After removal, the active keratitis is treated with topical antibiotics and atropine, and interstitial keratitis and granulation tissue are controlled with topical corticosteroids (e.g., 0.1 per cent dexamethasone ointment or drops).

Acute Infectious Keratitis

(Tables 92–1 and 92–3)

Infectious keratitis is an ocular emergency because of the rapidity with which certain forms of infection spread, destroy the corneal stroma, and result in corneal perforation, endophthalmitis, and loss of the affected eye.

Clinical Diagnosis

The following may signal active keratitis associated with microbial infection: (1) rapidly developing keratitis

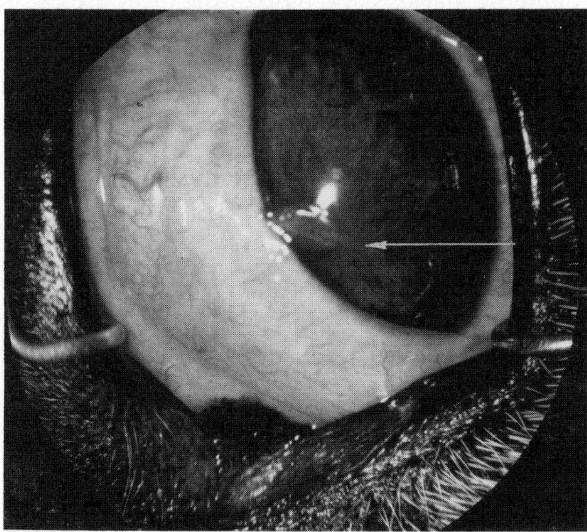

FIGURE 92–4. Corneal foreign body. A grass awn, partially hidden by the prolapsed third eyelid, is embedded in the corneal stroma. Note the miotic pupil resulting from secondary uveitis.

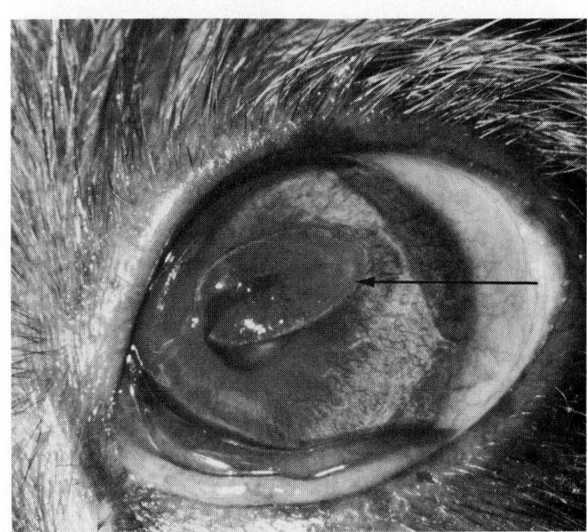

FIGURE 92–5. An oat hull *(arrow)* is attached to the cornea and must be surgically removed.

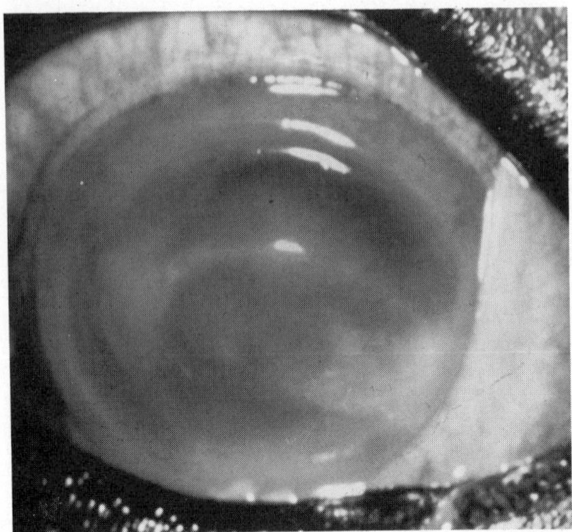

FIGURE 92–6. Acute infectious keratitis with rapid development of corneal edema, corneal stromal cellular infiltrates, mucopurulent stromal necrosis, and secondary anterior uveitis with possible hypopyon formation. The infectious organism was a *Pseudomonas* spp.

TABLE 92–1. SUBCONJUNCTIVAL ANTIBIOTIC DOSES FOR TREATMENT OF KERATITIS

Antibiotic	Dose
Ampicillin	50 to 250 mg
Bacitracin	10,000 U
Carbenicillin	100 mg
Cephaloridine	100 mg
Cephalothin	100 mg
Chloramphenicol, sodium succinate suspension	50 to 100 mg
Colistin	15 to 30 mg
Erythromycin (lactobionate or gluceptate)	50 to 100 mg
Gentamicin	10 to 20 mg
Kanamycin	10 to 20 mg
Lincomycin	50 to 150 mg
Methicillin	100 to 200 mg
Neomycin	100 to 500 mg
Penicillin G	300,000 to 1,000,000 U
Polymyxin B	10 mg
Streptomycin	50 to 100 mg
Tobramycin	40 mg
Vancomycin	25 mg

Reprinted with permission from Bistner SI: Clinical diagnosis and treatment of infectious keratitis. *Comp Cont Educ* 3:1056, 1981.

in a previously normal eye (signs appear and within 24 to 48 hours become much more severe); (2) loss of corneal epithelium accompanied by stromal cellular infiltrates and stromal edema; (3) mucopurulent stromal necrosis; and (4) secondary anterior uveitis with possible hypopyon (Figs. 92–6 and 92–7).

Confirmation of Infectious Keratitis

Corneal and conjunctival cultures are easy to perform and can quickly confirm a diagnosis of infectious keratitis. The following materials are needed to perform a corneal or conjunctival culture: (1) sterile cotton-tipped applicators or calcium alginate swabs; (2) bacterial culture media including blood agar plate, thioglycollate broth, and Sabouraud dextrose agar plates; (3) a Kimura platinum spatula or other spatula that can be sterilized in the heat of an open flame; (4) an alcohol lamp; (5) glass slides with etched ends; (6) Gram stain; and (7) Giemsa stain.

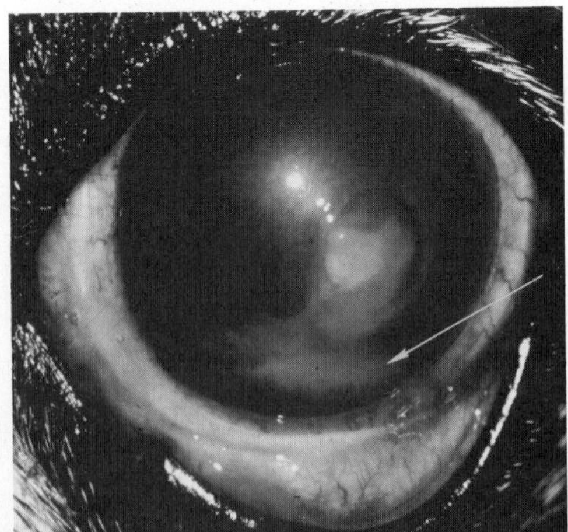

FIGURE 92–7. Intrastromal corneal abscess in a Boston terrier. There is secondary uveitis with hypopyon formation *(arrow)*. Care must be taken in handling these dogs, because the stromal abscesses are often very deep and descemetoceles are present (see the section on complicated corneal lacerations).

To obtain viable corneal cultures, a wet swab is used. Topical anesthetics are not placed in the eye before obtaining a sample because anesthetics contain antiseptics that may alter bacterial growth. A sterile swab is moistened in thioglycollate broth, the excess fluid is wiped off, and the moistened swab is gently wiped over the cornea. The swab is immediately plated onto culture media.

Corneal scrapings are made with the Kimura platinum spatula. A topical anesthetic (e.g., 0.5 per cent proparacaine hydrochloride*) is used on the cornea. The glass slides are dipped in 95 per cent methanol and wiped clean, and the margins and base of the ulcer are carefully scraped. Mucus or mucopurulent discharge is disregarded; corneal cellular infiltrate is spread onto the surface of two slides. The slides are stained with Gram and Giemsa stains. New methylene blue stain can be used for immediate evaluation of cytological detail.[4, 21]

Treatment

The initial selection of antibiotics is based on the results of Gram staining. Until culture results prove otherwise, it can generally be assumed that gram-positive infections are caused by penicillin-resistant *Staphylococcus* spp. and gram-negative rod infections are caused by *Pseudomonas* spp.[3, 21]

The treatment for gram-positive infections includes subconjunctival therapy with cefamandole, 75 mg, or cefazolin, 100 mg. (Tables 92–1 and 92–2); topical

*Ophthaine, E. R. Squibb & Sons Inc., Princeton, NJ.

TABLE 92–2. PREPARATION OF ANTIBIOTICS FOR SUBCONJUNCTIVAL INJECTION

	Cefamandole	Cefazolin	Clindamycin	Gentamycin	Tobramycin
Concentration in commercially prepared vial	1 g	1g	150 mg/ml	80 mg/2.0 ml	40 mg/ml
Antibiotic dose in injejction volume	75 mg	100 mg	30 mg	20 mg	20 mg

treatment with a concentrated solution of gentamicin and cefazolin (Table 92–3), if it can be applied frequently (requires hospitalization). In severe cases, systemic therapy with intravenous methicillin or ampicillin.

Infection with gram-negative rods can be treated subconjunctivally with gentamicin, 20 mg, tobramycin, 20 mg, and topically with fortified gentamicin drops or gentamicin ointment. In many cases, topical fluoroquinolone (ciprofloxacin) drops (see later) have replaced the previously discussed antibiotics in the treatment of infectious keratitis.

Pseudomonas Infections

Keratitis produced by *Pseudomonas aeruginosa* is a rapidly spreading and destructive corneal disease. In *Pseudomonas*-induced keratitis, the cornea becomes

TABLE 92–3. PREPARATION OF FORTIFIED ANTIBIOTIC EYE DROPS

Penicillin G

1. Remove 5 ml "tears" from 15-ml tear substitute squeeze bottle.
2. Add 5 ml "tears" to one vial penicillin G (5 million units).
3. Replace 5 ml reconstituted penicillin into tear squeeze bottle (10 ml + 5 ml = 15 ml).
4. Final concentration of penicillin = 333,000 U/ml.

Oxacillin

1. Remove 7 ml "tears" from a 15-ml tear substitute squeeze bottle.
2. Add 7 ml "tears" to ampule oxacillin (1 g).
3. Replace 7.2 ml reconstituted oxacillin into tear squeeze bottle (8 ml + 7.2 ml = 15.2 ml).
4. Final concentration of oxacillin = 66 mg/ml.

Carbenicillin

1. Reconstitute one vial carbenicillin (1 g) with 9.5 ml sterile water.
2. Add 1 ml reconstituted carbenicillin into 16-ml tear substitute squeeze bottle (15 ml + 1 ml = 16 ml).
3. Final concentration of carbenicillin = 6.2 mg/ml.

Ticarcillin

1. Reconstitute one vial ticarcillin (1 g) with 10 ml sterile water.
2. Add 1 ml reconstituted ticarcillin into 15-ml tear substitute squeeze bottle.
3. Final concentration of ticarcillin = 6.3 mg/ml.

Cephaloridine

1. Remove 2 ml "tears" from a 15-ml tear substitute squeeze bottle and discard.
2. Add 2 ml sterile saline to 1 ampule cephaloridine (500 mg).
3. Replace 2.4 ml reconstituted cephaloridine into tear squeeze bottle (13 ml + 2.4 ml = 15.4 ml).
4. Final concentration of cephaloridine = 32 mg/ml.

Cefazolin

1. Remove 2 ml "tears" from a 15-ml tear substitute squeeze bottle and discard.
2. Add 2 ml sterile saline to one ampule cefazolin (500 mg).
3. Replace 2.2 ml reconstituted cefazolin into tear squeeze bottle (13 ml + 2.2 ml = 15.2 ml).
4. Final concentration of cefazolin = 33 mg/ml.

Vancomyin

1. Remove 9 ml "tears" from a 15-ml tear substitute squeeze bottle and discard.
2. Add 10 ml sterile water to one vial vancomycin (500 mg).
3. Replace 10.2 ml reconstituted vancomycin into tear substitute squeeze bottle.
4. Final concentration of vancomycin = 31 mg/ml.

Gentamicin

1. Add 2 ml parenteral gentamicin to the 5-ml dropper bottle of commercial ophthalmic gentamicin.
2. Final concentration of gentamicin = 14 mg/ml.

Tobramycin

1. Remove 2 ml "tears" from a 15-ml tear substitute squeeze bottle and discard.
2. Add 2 ml parenteral tobramycin (80 mg) to tear substitute squeeze bottle (13 ml + 2 ml = 15 ml).
3. Final concentration of tobramycin = 5 mg/ml.

Amikacin

1. Remove 2 ml "tears" from a 15-ml tear substitute squeeze bottle and discard.
2. Add 2 ml parenteral amikacin (100 mg) to tear substitute squeeze bottle (13 ml + 2 ml = 15 ml).
3. Final concentration of amikacin = 6.7 mg/ml.

Bacitracin

1. Remove 9 ml "tears" from a 15-ml tear substitute squeeze bottle.
2. Add 3 ml "tears" to each of three commercial vials of bacitracin (50,000 U each).
3. Replace 9.6 ml reconstituted bacitracin into tear squeeze bottle (9.6 ml + 6 ml = 15.6 ml).
4. Final concentration of bacitracin = 9,600 U/ml.

Neomycin

1. Remove 2 ml "tears" from a 15-ml tear substitute squeeze bottle.
2. Add 2 ml "tears" to one vial neomycin (500 mg).
3. Replace 2 ml reconstituted neomycin into tear squeeze bottle (13 ml + 2 ml = 15 ml).
4. Final concentration of neomycin = 33 mg/ml.

Adapted from Baum I: Antibiotic use in ophthalmology. *In* Tasman W, Jaeger EJ (eds): *Clinical Ophthalmology*. Vol 4. J.B. Lippincott, Philadelphia, 1980.

edematous and necrotic, and uveitis with hypopyon is frequently associated (see Fig. 92–6). *Pseudomonas* produces proteolytic enzymes[4, 7, 20, 21] and additionally may stimulate collagenase production,[4, 7] which causes the rapid spread of infection and the destruction of corneal stroma with perforation.

Gentamicin can be used for *Pseudomonas* infections. Additionally, tobramycin, polymyxin B, and colistin have been effective in treating *Pseudomonas* ulcers.

Additionally, disodium EDTA* is used to inhibit the proteoglycan enzyme produced by *Pseudomonas.* A solution is made by adding 0.4 ml of EDTA (150 mg/ml) to a 15-ml bottle of Adapt† drops. Two drops are administered five times daily.

A new fluoroquinolone ophthalmic antibiotic appears to offer an excellent therapeutic option in the management of anterior ocular segment infections. Studies of this new fluoroquinolone Ciprofloxacin‡ shows that this agent is highly effective against a broad spectrum of gram-positive and gram-negative organisms. *In vitro* studies showed that Ciprofloxacin 0.3 per cent solution killed bacteria when used at one to four times the minimal inhibitory concentration. Findings involving animal models confirm that Ciprofloxacin is highly active against ocular pathogens including *P. aeruginosa*. Ciprofloxacin does not have to be enhanced by the addition of another antibiotic. It is stable at room temperature at the 0.3 per cent concentration.

Additional Treatment

Additional treatment measures include the following:

1. The animal is hospitalized whenever possible to provide intensive treatment.
2. Pain associated with secondary uveal inflammation is controlled with a mydriatic-cycloplegic agent such as atropine (1 to 4 per cent).
3. If the cornea appears soft, collagenase may be present and an antiprotease agent such as 10 per cent acetylcysteine drops§ may be used (two drops every 2 hours for the first 24 to 48 hours).
4. Careful cleaning to remove necrotic corneal tissue may be helpful. A sterile swab and a small amount of 2 per cent iodine solution may be used to remove necrotic tissue. The eye is washed carefully with a sterile collyrium.¶
5. Self-multilation is prevented by an Elizabethan collar.
6. Pain is relieved with systemic agents.‖
7. When extensive loss of corneal stroma may result in imminent perforation, a conjunctival or third-eyelid flap may be placed over the cornea. In severe corneal infections, I prefer not to cover the cornea; however, good results have been obtained with covered corneas and the previously mentioned treatment.

*Endrate, Abbott Laboratories, North Chicago, IL.
†Burton, Parsons & Co., Inc., Washington, DC.
‡Ciprofloxacin 0.3% (Ciloxan, Alcon Laboratories, Ft. Worth, TX).
§Mucomyst, Mead Johnson Pharmaceuticals, Evansville, IN.
¶Dacriose, CooperVision Pharmaceuticals, Inc., San German, PR.
‖Demerol, Winthrop Laboratories, New York, NY.

Corneal Lacerations

Corneal lacerations may be penetrating or perforating (passing through the cornea). Perforating corneal lacerations may cause prolapse of intraocular contents. Pieces of uveal tissue or fibrin often effectively but temporarily seal the wound and permit the anterior chamber to re-form. Manipulation of these wounds is avoided until the animal has been anesthetized. If the examiner cannot determine if an injury has perforated the cornea, a Seidel test may be useful. A small amount of concentrated fluorescein is applied to the cornea, and the cornea is examined for any evidence of aqueous leakage from the perforation site.

In the initial management of corneal perforations and lacerations, the wound site is cultured using blood agar, chocolate agar, thioglycollate broth, and Sabouraud agar.

Care is used in anesthetizing an animal with a corneal laceration, because struggling or excitement during administration of anesthetic may result in loss of the temporary seal in the corneal laceration and extrusion of intraocular contents. In addition, an intraocular foreign body may be present concurrently with a perforating corneal laceration. The globe should be examined carefully, and radiographs of the globe and orbit taken if necessary.[1, 5, 16, 18, 22, 23]

Management of Small Corneal Lacerations

Tissue adhesive in the form of a cyanoacrylate monomer can be used for closure of corneal perforations measuring less than 2 mm. Tissue adhesives are especially useful in management of irregular small wounds that may not hold sutures well.

Before adhesive application, loose necrotic tissue around the corneal wound is completely débrided. A flat anterior chamber is not a contraindication to the application of a tissue adhesive. The corneal surface must be meticulously cleaned of any debris before adhesive is applied. The corneal epithelium adjacent to the wound margin for 2 mm must be removed with a number 64 Beaver blade. The corneal surface is carefully dried using cellulose sponges. Cyanoacrylate monomer is placed in a tuberculin syringe with a 27-gauge needle on the end. Tissue glue is then carefully applied to the wound, sealing the wound without allowing excess glue to cover the cornea. Check the wound for leakage with a cellulose sponge or by a Seidel test. If the anterior chamber is shallow, re-form the anterior chamber with sterile saline.

Corneal lacerations or perforations greater than 2 to 3 mm in diameter are best managed by surgical intervention.[18, 23]

Complicated Corneal Lacerations

Complicated corneal lacerations are accompanied by one or a combination of the following: iris prolapse, hyphema, cataract formation, luxation of the lens, or loss of vitreous (Figs. 92–8 and 92–9).

If examination of the eye reveals a damaged lens with

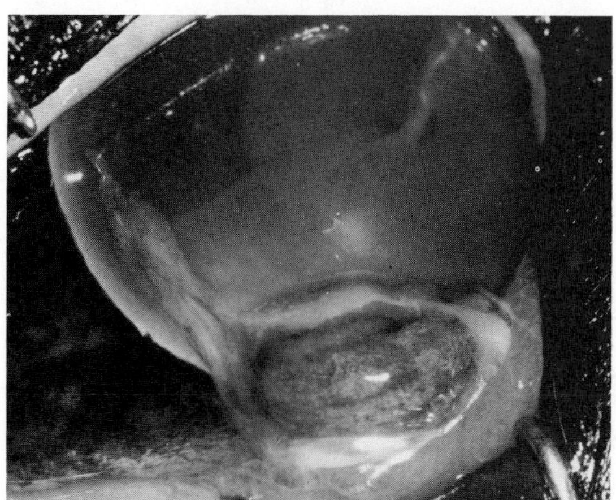

FIGURE 92–8. Corneal laceration with incarcerated uveal tissue in the wound and severe secondary uveitis.

rupture of the anterior lens capsule, extraction of the lens via an extracapsular approach may be indicated. If the corneal wound is small, the wound is first closed and a limbal or corneal section made to extract the lens. Damage to the lens is a frequent problem with cat-scratch injuries of the eyes of dogs or cats. The claws are long and penetrate the cornea and anterior chamber, lacerating the anterior lens capsule. The lens becomes intumescent (swollen), and cataractous changes occur. The anterior chamber narrows as the lens swells. These lenses have been removed by phacofragmentation and suction as well as with a standard planned extracapsular approach following repair of the corneal laceration. If the lens is not removed, phacolytic uveitis and secondary glaucoma develop.

Incarceration or prolapse of uveal tissue in corneal wounds presents a difficult surgical problem. The tendency for iris prolapse depends on the size of the wound. If the wound is small and the iris prolapse is small and of short duration, the iris may be repositioned with an iris spatula. The spatula is introduced into the anterior chamber through the corneal wound to sweep free possible anterior synechiae. If hyphema is present, the anterior chamber is irrigated with BSS* and the blood clots are removed. The wound is closed with 7-0 or 8-0 silk, nylon, or 7-0 polyglactin 910 sutures, and the anterior chamber is re-formed (Fig. 92–10). Mydriatics are used postoperatively to correct the associated traumatic uveitis and to prevent anterior synechia formation if the wound is in the central cornea.

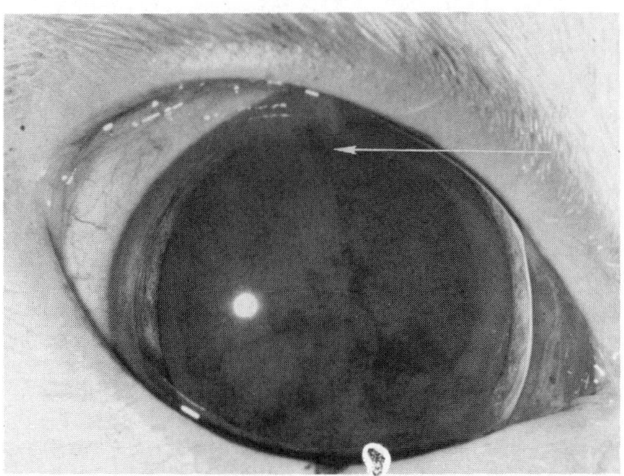

FIGURE 92–9. Corneal laceration *(arrow)* in a cat caused by a cat's claw. Note that the aqueous is plasmoid and that hyphema is present. Immediate treatment for traumatic uveitis is indicated, and the corneal laceration must be sutured. The pupil is widely dilated because the cat had already been given topical atropine as part of the uveitis treatment.

At the time of surgical repair, if the surgeon cannot effectively replace a prolapsed iris or if the iris is excessively contaminated and necrotic, it is excised.

The uveal tissue can be trimmed from the corneal wound using an electroscalpel or scissors, and the wound swept with a blunt cyclodialysis spatula to free additional adhesions. An electroscalpel is preferred, because it minimizes the profuse hemorrhage that accompanies iridectomies in domestic animals. The corneal wound is repaired as previously described.

When a corneal laceration is attended by prolapse of the iris, lens, vitreous, and ciliary processes, a decision must be made whether, under these circumstances, it is better to perform immediate enucleation. If the eye is soft and extensively damaged, enucleation is the procedure of choice once the animal has been medically stabilized. On the other hand, if there is any chance of saving the eye, repair can be attempted and enucleation performed if necessary in 10 days to 2 weeks.

In suturing the cornea, attempt to use a corneal spatula needle with suture bites approximately 75 to 90 per cent of the corneal depth and perpendicular to the laceration. Equal bites of corneal tissue with the needle on either side of the wound are made usually about 1 to 2 mm long. If the wound edges are edematous, longer sutures are required and must extend deeper into healthy tissue.

The use of a conjunctival flap as a primary wound closure procedure in the cornea is not recommended because the wound can seldom be effectively sealed with only a conjunctival flap. Optical results after conjunctival flaps as primary closure techniques are also poor. We have used conjunctival flaps as additional protection over a cornea that has been sutured, especially when adjacent corneal epithelial erosive disease is present.[1, 5, 18, 22, 24]

Contusion and Penetrating Injury

Severe ocular contusions are caused by injury resulting from sudden acceleration or deceleration imparted by a blunt force.[19] In animals, contusions commonly result from being hit by a car, kicked, hit with a blunt object, or kicked by a larger animal (e.g., a horse). A number of factors determine the effect of this form of trauma on the eye: (1) impact of the force on the globe at the point of injury, (2) contrecoup impact in direct line with the force but on the opposite side of the globe, and (3) indirect force when the globe is pushed or "hurled" against the orbital contents.[9, 16, 24, 28, 33]

Ocular damage can result from disturbance of func-

*Balanced Salt Solution, Alcon Laboratories, Fort Worth, TX.

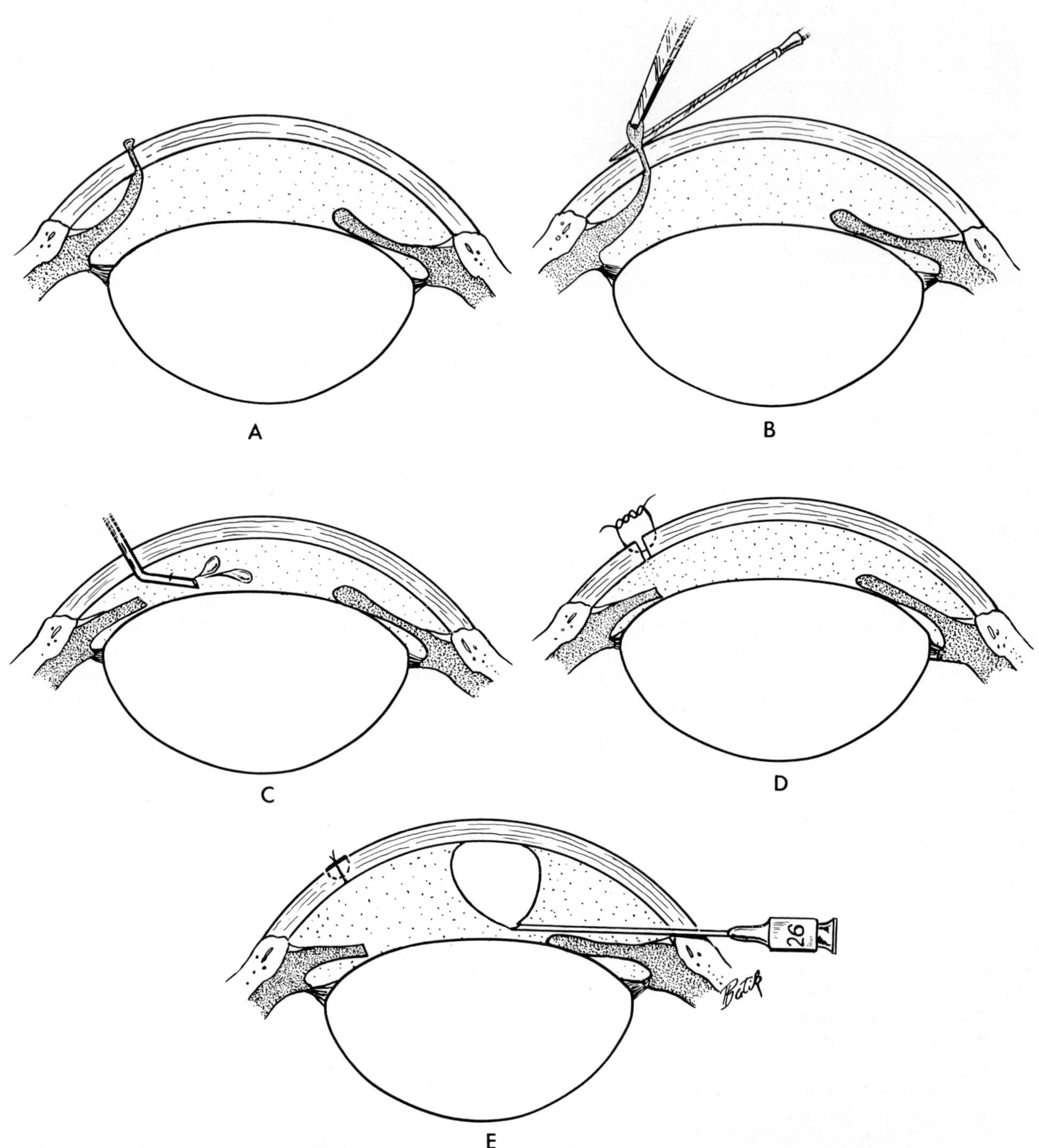

FIGURE 92–10. Primary reconstruction of corneal laceration. *A*, Corneal laceration with incarcerated iris and secondary hyphema and uveitis. *B*, Incarcerated viable iris should be repositioned whenever possible. The corneal wound may have to be enlarged to replace the iris with either a cyclodialysis spatula or an iris spatula. If extensive anterior synechiae have already occurred, incarcerated iris may be removed using an electroscalpel or scissors. *C*, If possible, the iris is swept free from its adhesion to the cornea with an anterior chamber irrigating needle or iris spatula. If the lens capsule appears ruptured or the lens dislocated, a limbal incision is made and the lens extracted. *D*, In repairing corneal wounds, a 4.5-mm atraumatic needle is used if adequate magnification is available. I prefer 8-0 silk or nylon or 7-0 collagen. The sutures are placed in the deeper two-thirds of the cornea to ensure coaptation of the Descemet membrane and to prevent posterior gaping of the wound. If possible, the needle bite is approximately 1 mm on either side of the wound margin. *E*, Once the anterior chamber has been closed, it is reformed with balanced salt solution via a limbal injection using a 26-gauge needle. (Reprinted with permission from Bistner SI, et al: *Atlas of Veterinary Ophthalmic Surgery.* W.B. Saunders, Philadelphia, 1977.)

tional integrity of tissues, hemorrhage or ischemia due to vascular damage, or mechanical tearing of tissue.

The orbits of dogs and cats are not completely enclosed in bone; therefore, these animals do not suffer from fractures of the orbital floor, as in humans. However, fractures of the zygomatic arch or maxillary, frontal, or lacrimal bones can occur. Therefore, animals with concussive ocular injuries are radiographed to evaluate damage. Attention is paid to the maxillary and mandibular bones for evidence of mandibular fracture or luxation of the temporomandibular joint.

Hyphema is blood in the anterior chamber of the eye. Blood within the eye may come from the anterior uveal tract, posterior uveal tract, or both. Trauma may result in tearing of the iris at its root (iridodialysis), permitting excessive bleeding from the iris and ciliary body.[33]

Simple hyphema usually resolves spontaneously in 7 to 10 days and does not cause vision loss.[17, 25] Loss of vision following hyphema is associated with secondary ocular injuries, including glaucoma, traumatic iritis, cataract, retinal detachment, endophthalmitis, and corneal scarring.

Severe trauma to the globe or a direct blow to the head can result in retinal or vitreous hemorrhage, with a distinctive ophthalmoscopic appearance.[30] Retinal and vitreous hemorrhage associated with trauma usually resorbs spontaneously over a 2- to 3-week period.[28] Unfortunately, vitreous hemorrhage can produce vitreous traction bands as it organizes, eventually leading to retinal detachment. Extensive retinal hemorrhage may be associated with scarring and glial proliferation as the blood resorbs. Expulsive choroidal hemorrhage can occur at the time of injury and usually leads to retinal detachment, severe visual impairment, and total vision loss.

Several basic principles are significant in the management of traumatic hyphemas in animals. Because of the vascular anatomy of the uveal tract, traumatic uveitis is also present after concussive or penetrating intraocular injury with hyphema. Bleeding usually stops spontaneously unless a traumatic iridodialysis or retinal detachment and posterior choroidal rupture have occurred. Very little can be done to control intraocular bleeding. Animals are confined and kept as quiet as possible. Rebleeding may occur within the first 5 days after injury.

Secondary uveal inflammation is controlled. Topical prednisolone acetate 1 per cent drops, seven to nine times daily, and atropine drops 1 to 2 per cent, three to four times daily, may be used.

Intraocular pressure is monitored. Hyphema and secondary uveitis can lead to secondary pupillary block or angle-closure glaucoma. If pressure increases, an oral carbonic anhydrase inhibitor is administered (e.g., dichlorphenamide, 125 mg TID for a 15-kg dog).

The animal is repeatedly observed for the initial 5 to 10 days during resorption of blood. If intraocular complications such as lens subluxation or luxation occur, surgery is indicated to remove the lens if pupillary block exists.

After 5 to 7 days, blood in the anterior chamber changes from bright red to a bluish black ("eight-ball hemorrhage"). If total hyphema persists and elevated pressure is evident despite medical therapy, surgical intervention is indicated. Surgical therapy varies, depending on the hyphema and the availability of instrumentation and skilled surgical assistance.*

Surgical Intervention

If the blood has formed a firm, well-organized clot, it can be removed by entering the anterior chamber through a limbus-based corneal incision in the same manner as for cataract surgery.† The anterior chamber may be gently irrigated with a balanced salt solution,‡ the incision closed, and the eye treated for traumatic uveitis.

If the hyphema is still partially liquefied, anterior chamber irrigation and suction can be carefully carried out. Many techniques are available to do this, but in general (unless very sophisticated automatic irrigators with handpieces are available), two surgeons are needed, one to irrigate and the other to aspirate, even when a double-walled needle is used.

Sophisticated anterior chamber irrigating and vitreous cutting units using microsurgical handles and needles are available. They work well in hyphemas of both the anterior and posterior chamber. The only unit that might be economically feasible is the Concept Portable Vitreophage Unit (Kaufman Vitrector II§ vitreous suction cutter with reciprocating cutting action).

The use of vitamin C, vitamin K, calcium, rutin, or estrogenic substances does not accelerate normal clotting. There is some evidence that aminocaproic acid¶ may minimize rebleeding by inhibiting fibrinolysis in the damaged blood vessels.[12]

Surgical intervention and blind probing of the anterior chamber in an attempt to remove blood or blood clots may cause *serious* surgical complications, such as rebleeding, luxated lens, extensive iris damage, and damage to the corneal endothelium.

Ocular Foreign Bodies

Periorbital, scleral, or corneal punctures or lacerations may be due to penetrating foreign bodies. The most common foreign bodies associated with ocular injuries in small animals are birdshot, air gun pellets, and glass. The site of intraocular penetration may be obscured by the eyelids (Figs. 92–11 and 92–12).

A foreign body entering the eye may follow one of several trajectories, depending on its velocity and angle of entry. It may penetrate the cornea and fall into the anterior chamber or become lodged in the iris, or it may penetrate the anterior capsule of the lens, producing a cataract. Some metallic high-speed foreign bodies may perforate the cornea, iris, and lens to lodge in the posterior wall of the eye or in the vitreous or may pass entirely through the eye and remain within the orbit.[23]

---

*See references 5, 8, 11, 19, 24, 25, 27, 28, and 29.
†See references 5, 8, 10, 24, 25, 29, and 30.
‡Balanced Salt Solution, Alcon Laboratories, Fort Worth, TX.
§Concept Inc., Clearwater, FL.
¶Amicar, Lederle Laboratories, Pearl River, NY.

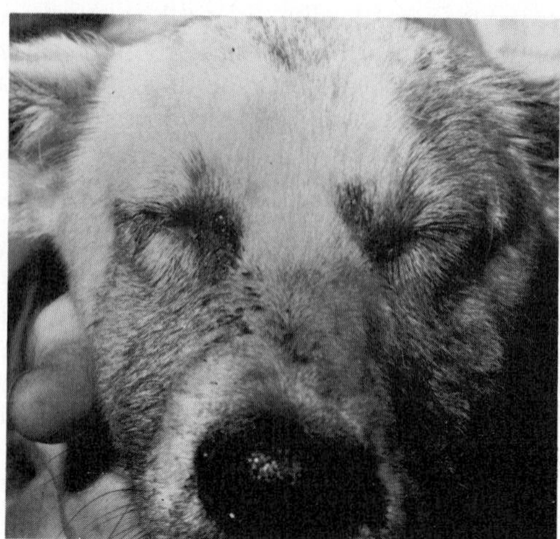

FIGURE 92–11. This dog was shot in the head with a shotgun. Severe blepharospasm is evident because of traumatic uveitis from the wounds in and around the eye.

Numerous techniques are available to determine the presence and location of ocular foreign bodies.[6, 11, 13, 15, 16] Direct observation is the best means of locating a foreign body. Examination with a biomicroscope or indirect ophthalmoscope may prove invaluable in locating foreign bodies. The anterior chamber and anterior drainage angle can be directly viewed with a gonioprism. Careful ocular examination is performed as early as possible before secondary ocular inflammation or cataract formation opacifies the ocular media. Indirect demonstration of an intraocular foreign body may be achieved by radiography or ultrasonography.[11, 16, 17]

In addition to radiography, the more refined technique of ultrasonography may be used to locate foreign bodies. This technique is most valuable in evaluating the extent of intraocular damage in the presence of extensive corneal edema or secondary cataract formation. Ultrasonic evaluation of the traumatized globe may be helpful in evaluating the presence of hyphema, lens luxation, lens rupture, vitreous hemorrhage, retinal detachment, and foreign bodies.

Intraocular penetration by a foreign body always warrants a guarded prognosis, and the outcome depends on the foreign body's chemical nature and its position within the eye. Foreign bodies made of iron or copper can produce extensive ocular inflammation.[13, 16, 26]

Chalcosis is produced by retention of copper or its alloys of bronze or brass and results in rapid inflammation, hypopyon, and localized abscess formation. Slow release of copper results in deposition of copper on limiting membranes within the eye, especially the Descemet membrane and the anterior lens capsule.

Retained foreign bodies of iron and steel may lead to repeated episodes of ocular inflammation and siderosis.[13] In siderosis, iron pigments are deposited in the cornea, iris, and lens, and degenerative changes occur in these areas as well as in the retina.

Other metals besides copper and iron may produce ocular inflammatory reactions.[13] Precious metals, stone, carbon, glass, building plaster, and rubber are usually inert in the eye; however, the mechanical trauma produced by these objects may lead to serious sequelae.

When considering removing any foreign body from an eye, the dangers of leaving the foreign body in the eye must be weighed against the dangers of surgical removal. Foreign objects in the anterior chamber are much easier to remove than objects at the posterior pole. Removal of foreign bodies from the vitreous has consistently produced poor results.

Proptosis of the Globe

Proptosis of the globe secondary to trauma is common in brachycephalic animals. A greater degree of initiating contusion is required in doliocephalic than brachycephalic dogs. Therefore, secondary damage to the eye and central nervous system associated with proptosis of the globe may be far greater in a collie than in a Pekingese.

One should not disregard the general physical condition of an animal presented with a proptosed globe, despite the urgency of globe replacement. Careful evaluation of the cardiovascular system for evidence of shock and examination of the respiratory and nervous systems should be carried out. Treatment to establish an adequate airway and control shock and overt bleeding is carried out before any attempt is made to replace the eye. While this initial examination and treatment are being carried out, the proptosed globe must be protected against further exposure and drying. This can be accomplished by using sponges soaked in cold hypertonic 10 per cent dextrose to reduce edema and prevent corneal drying.

Proptosis of the globe results in several pathological phenomena that must be considered in establishing treatment and prognosis. (1) Occlusion of the vortex and ciliary veins of the eye by the lids produces venous

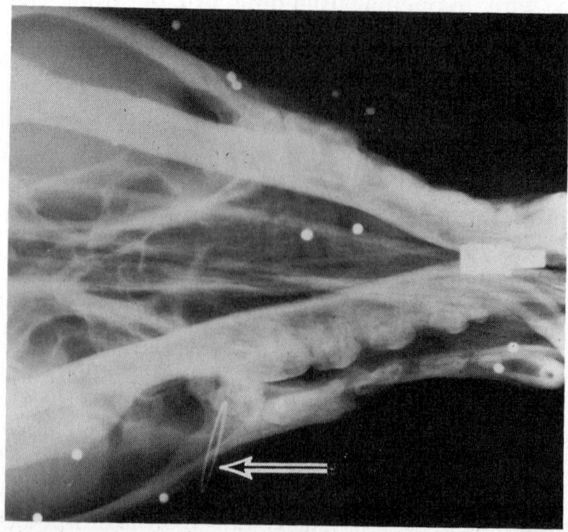

FIGURE 92–12. Radiographs were taken of the skull of the dog in Figure 92–11, and a Flieringa metallic ring was placed under the lids *(arrow)* to help outline the location of the orbit. Penetrating wounds of the globe such as this must be sutured, and the eyes treated for traumatic uveitis. Pieces of "shot" should not be recovered from the eye unless they are easily retrievable.

stasis and a form of congestive glaucoma. The resulting venous stasis also limits accessibility of intravenous medication to the eye. Venous stasis is relieved once the eye is replaced in the orbit. (2) Proptosis results in marked exposure keratitis and corneal necrosis. Initial protection of the eye with moist gauze soaked in a hypertonic solution prevents excessive drying. (3) Proptosis of the globe can be associated with iritis, chorioretinitis, retinal detachment, luxation of the lens, and avulsion of the optic nerve.

An attempt is made to replace most proptosed globes. Exceptions are eyes in which the intraocular contents have been extruded or in which massive destruction of the intraocular contents has taken place. The owner may wish to have the eye removed because of cosmetic or economic considerations.

*Treatment**

1. Anesthetize the patient.
2. Replace the globe as soon as possible to prevent severe corneal damage. If first aid is to be administered by a client in a distant location prior to transport, advise keeping the eye moist with wet cotton or whatever is available and to avoid additional trauma from movement.
3. Flush the conjunctival sac free of extraneous debris with sterile saline solution and lubricate the cornea with tear replacement solution and antibiotic drops.
4. Using fine Vetafil or 4/0 nylon, place three or four simple, interrupted sutures as shown in Figure 92–13*A* and *B*. If possible, sutures should emerge on the lid margin rather than on the conjuctival surface to prevent corneal abrasion after replacement of the globe.
5. Apply a suitable antibiotic ointment (e.g., chloramphenicol) to the eye.
6. Place a scalpel handle across the cornea, beneath the sutures, and draw up on each of the sutures simultaneously, as shown in Figure 92–13*C* and *D*. This pulls the lids forward to protect the cornea and replaces the globe within the orbit.
7. The sutures are tied (Fig. 92–13*E*). If necessary, that is, if pressure is extensive, additional intermarginal lid sutures may be placed between the original traction sutures.
8. Using the dorsal rim of the orbit as a landmark, inject 10 to 20 mg of triamcinolone 2 to 3 cm by retrobulbar injection.
9. Apply atropine ointment (1 per cent) and chloromycetin ointment to the conjuctival sac between the sutures.
10. Give an intravenous injection of dexamethasone (10 to 15 mg), and flunixin meglumine (1 mg/kg) to limit and control secondary uveitis. (For maintenance therapy, see further on.)

Postoperative treatment is designed to control traumatic iritis and the extensive corneal damage that is associated with proptosis and exposure. Systemic broad-spectrum antibiotics are indicated. Atropine ointment (1 per cent) is used topically, and topical steroids* and antiobiotics are used five to six times daily. Although steroids are a "two-edged sword," the extensive vascularization, inflammation, and scar tissue that can form after ocular injury make them a valuable aid in treating traumatic proptosis. Topical medication can be delivered as either an ointment or drops (in the case of prednisolone acetate, 1 per cent placed through the eyelid margins directly on the cornea). If trauma to an eye has been extensive, topical steroids are supplemented with systemic steroids for 1 week.

Sutures are left in place until intraorbital swelling is markedly reduced, usually 10 days to 3 weeks. The sutures are removed, and the globe is inspected. If proptosis recurs, the sutures are replaced and removed after an additional 2 weeks.

Extraocular muscle injury and the resultant strabismus are common after proptosis. The most frequent deviation observed is upward and outward, suggesting possible paralysis or rupture of the medial rectus, dorsal oblique, and ventral rectus muscles or an overaction of the lateral or dorsal rectus muscle. Strabismus is most noticeable immediately after removal of the lid sutures. In most cases, a relatively normal visual axis returns in 3 to 4 months after the initial injury. Keratitis sicca and optic nerve atrophy are common sequelae to proptosis of the globe.

Endophthalmitis

Endophthalmitis (inflammation of the eye and its contents) is more severe than uveitis, and an infectious agent is often associated with this inflammatory reaction. In dogs and cats, endophthalmitis is most associated with penetrating intraocular wounds, postsurgical infections, and ruptured corneal wounds with secondary infections.

Signs of endophthalmitis are more severe than those of uveitis and include extreme pain, very deep scleral vascular engorgement, corneal edema with large numbers of cells and proteins in the anterior chamber, large amounts of vitreous exudate, systemic signs (e.g., anorexia and pyrexia), and neutrophilia.

Treatment

If very severe structural damage is not evident and the cornea has not been ruptured with intraocular tissue loss, treatment may be attempted.

An anterior or vitreous chamber aspiration for culture and cytological examination is performed. This requires either a short-acting anesthetic or sedation of the patient. Endophthalmitis in animals produces a plasmoid aqueous, and although small-gauge needles (25- or 26-gauge) are less traumatic, they frequently become plugged with fibrin. A 20-gauge needle is used to enter the anterior chamber at the limbus, and the aspirate is examined by culture and cytological study.[2, 5, 14] Large

*Modified from Severin GA: Veterinary Ophthalmology Notes, 2nd ed. Fort Collins, CO, 1976.

*Editor's note: The use of *topical* steroids in the control of corneal vascularization after proptosis is controversial and is regarded as contraindicated by some veterinary ophthalmologists.

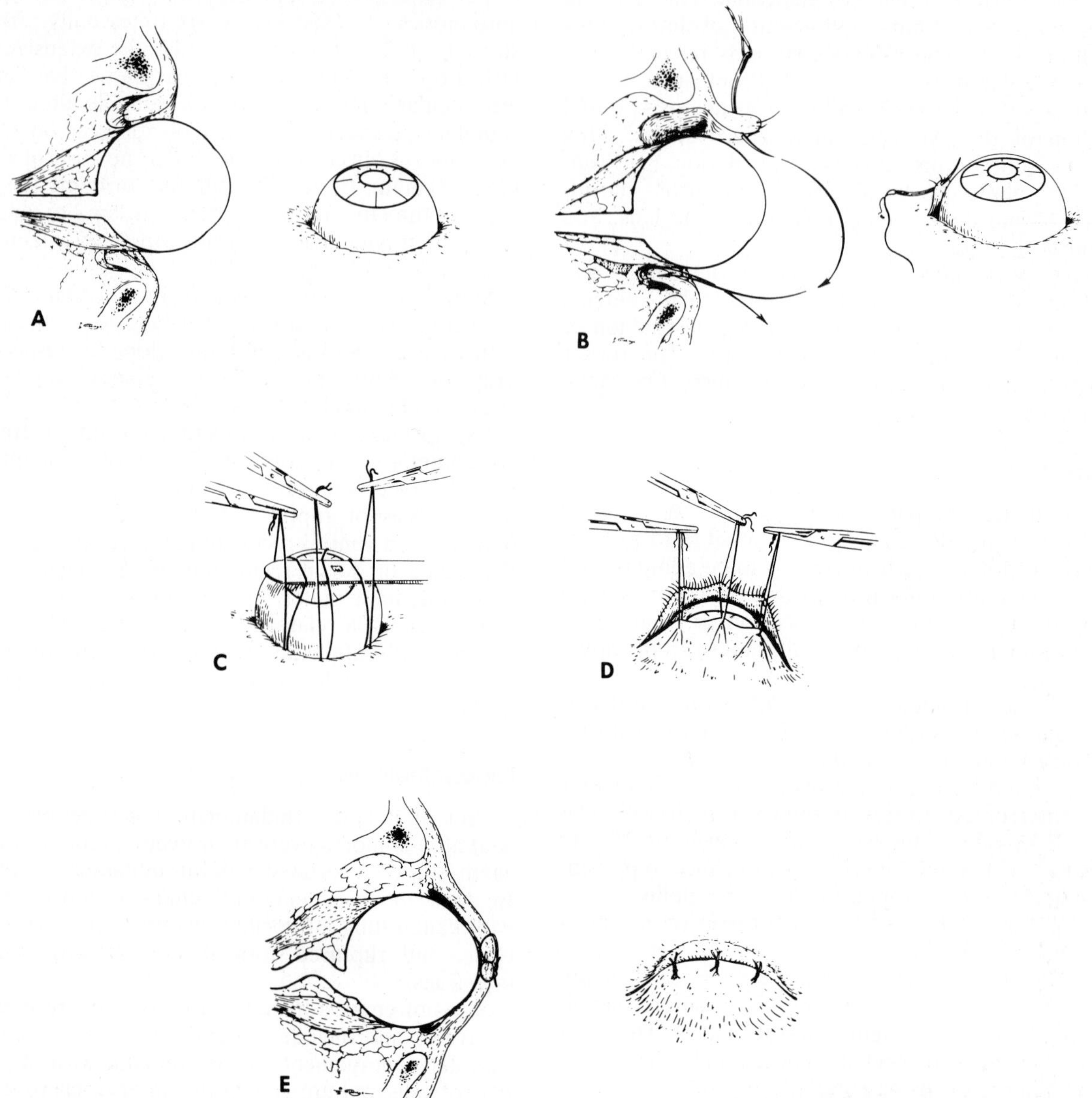

FIGURE 92–13. Procedure for replacement of prolapsed globe. *A*, Prolapsed globe. *B*, Placement of simple interrupted traction sutures of 4/0 nylon or fine Vetafil. *C*, Placement of scalpel handle. *D*, Traction on the sutures and replacement of the globe. *E*, Completion of the sutures. (Courtesy of Dr. G. A. Severin.)

numbers of polymorphonuclear leukocytes and gram-negative or gram-positive bacteria signal active infection, and treatment should begin immediately without awaiting culture results.

Rapid determination of glucose content in the vitreous may aid in distinguishing infectious from noninfectious endophthalmitis.[34] Material is applied to a Dextrostix from a vitreous tap. In bacterial infections, bacteria use glucose in the vitreous and glucose is reduced or absent. In noninfectious endophthalmitis, the vitreous glucose content is normal (greater than 10 mg/100 ml).

Antibiotics and anti-inflammatory agents at prescribed doses are placed in the aqueous and vitreous cavity.[2] Additionally, in vitreal disease, a vitrectomy may be performed (see Chapter 89).

Initial Therapy. The intraocular antibiotic regimen for the treatment of endophthalmitis is as follows:

1. Intraocular gentamicin, 0.1 mg, and cephaloridine, 0.25 mg
2. Subconjunctival gentamicin, 25 mg, and cephaloridine, 1 mg, or methicillin, 100 mg
3. Topical gentamicin ophthalmic ointment
4. Systemic cephaloridine intravenously

Intraocular aspiration is repeated at 48 hours, and if bacteria are still evident and culture positive, the intraocular antibiotic regimen is repeated.

Because infections associated with endophthalmitis can spread via the optic nerve and meninges to the central nervous system, resulting in meningitis, it is important either to treat endophthalmitis or, if treatment is not successful, to enucleate the diseased globe.

Preparation of Gentamicin and Cephaloridine for Intraocular Injection

Intraocular Gentamicin, 0.1 mg

1. Withdraw 0.1 ml (4 mg) from the vial (40 mg/100 ml gentamicin).
2. Add to 9.9 ml of nonbacteriostatic saline if final volume of 0.25 ml for injection is desired *or* to 3.9 ml of nonbacteriostatic saline if 0.1 ml volume is desired.
3. Ten milliliters contains 4 mg of gentamicin; 1 ml contains 0.4 mg; 0.25 ml contains 0.1 mg; *or* 4 ml contains 4 mg; 1 ml contains 1 mg; 0.1 ml contains 0.1 mg.
4. Inject either 0.25 ml containing 0.1 mg gentamicin *or* 0.1 ml containing 0.1 mg gentamicin.

Cephaloridine

1. Reconstitute powder with 10 ml sterile sodium chloride (1,000 mg in 10 ml).
2. Add 0.1 (10 mg) of suspension to 3.9 ml nonbacteriostatic saline; 10 mg in 4 ml contains 1 mg cephaloridine in 0.4 ml.
3. Inject 0.1 ml, containing 0.25 mg cephaloridine.

ACUTE ELEVATION IN INTRAOCULAR PRESSURE—GLAUCOMA (see also Chapter 91)

Glaucoma is an ocular emergency because uncontrolled elevated intraocular pressure causes irreversible damage to the ganglion cells of the retina and optic nerve, resulting in irreversible vision loss. This damage can take place within 24 to 48 hours of the onset of acute pressure elevation. For the pathogenesis of glaucoma see Chapter 91.

In dogs and cats, acute rises in pressure are associated with preceding intraocular disease (secondary glaucoma) that severly compromises the anterior drainage angle. In the initial treatment of acute congestive glaucoma, it is important to consider the differential diagnosis of the major problems producing secondary narrow-angle glaucoma.

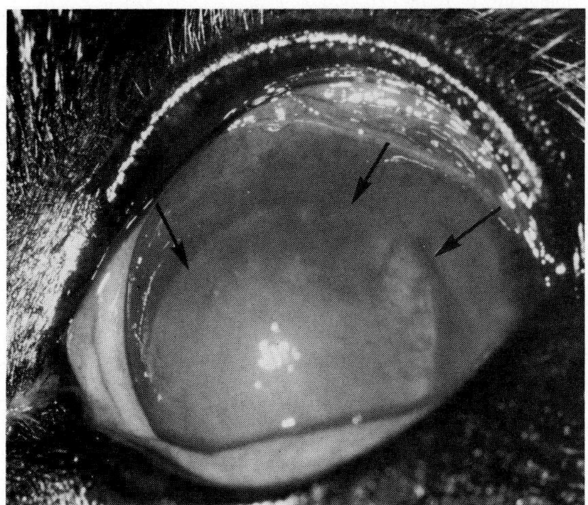

FIGURE 92–14. Acute congestive glaucoma and a subluxated lens in a dog with cyclitis (inflammation of the ciliary body). The zonular ligaments ruptured secondary to inflammation, and the lens moved forward, becoming trapped in the pupillary space. The outline of the lens is marked by the arrows. Severe uveitis as well as elevated intraocular pressure is evident. Treatment involved treating the uveitis and surgically removing the subluxated lens.

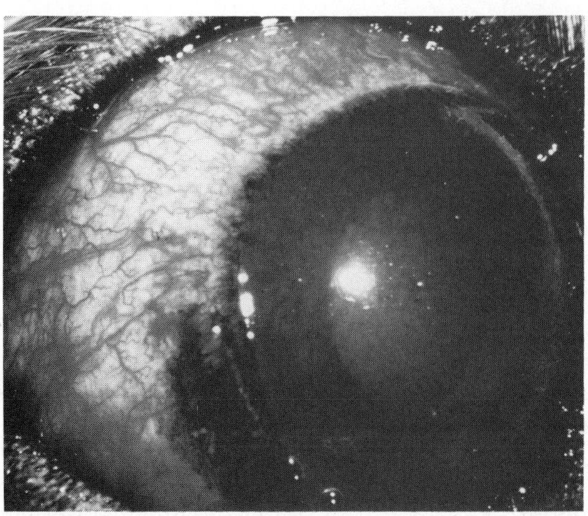

FIGURE 92–15. Acute glaucoma with episcleral engorgement and corneal edema.

Anterior Uveitis

Uveitis is one of the most common causes of glaucoma. It rapidly produces a plasmoid aqueous, which can lead to blockage of the trabecular meshwork with fibrin and cells, secondary broad-based anterior synechia, and elevations in intraocular pressure. Cyclytis is a diagnosis that often remains undetected until the zonular ligaments supporting the lens are broken and the lens subluxates or luxates through the pupil or into the anterior chamber (Fig. 92–14). Careful examination with a biomicroscope in many early lens luxation cases has shown protein in the anterior chamber and vitreous; inflammatory cells, especially in the vitreous; and active cyclytis. Cyclytis and lens luxations are primarily encountered in terriers and small breeds of dogs.

Basset hounds with acute congestive unilateral glaucoma (Fig. 92–15) have active severe uveitis that has caused decompensation of a poorly formed anterior drainage angle and secondary glaucoma. When the normal eye is gonioscopically evaluated, the angle is usually poorly developed and narrowed and appears as if it too could develop increased pressure if anything caused "decompensation."

Animals with acute lens subluxation or luxation into the anterior chamber and secondary anterior uveitis and cyclytis can be helped by surgical removal of the lens and control of underlying intraocular inflammation. Early diagnosis of pupillary block glaucoma *is essential* for a favorable prognosis.

Lens Intumescence

Intumescence means enlargement or swelling of the lens.[30] It leads to pupillary block and narrowing of the anterior drainage angle because fluid in the posterior chamber pushes the iris forward, with resultant peripheral anterior synechia.

Treatment (see also Chapter 91)

Initial treatment in acute elevations of intraocular pressure is directed at the reduction of pressure using osmotic agents such as mannitol, 1 g/kg IV given slowly. The effect of the drug develops during a 30- to 60-minute period and lasts 3 to 4 hours. Oral osmotic agents (glycerin 50 to 75 per cent) can also be given (8 to 12 ml to a 15-kg dog every 8 hours).

Carbonic anhydrase inhibitors can be used to decrease the production of aqueous fluid. Numerous drugs are available. However, an initial loading dose can be achieved with acetazolamide, 250 to 500 mg by intravenous bolus to a 15- to 20-kg dog. The initial loading dose can be followed with oral dichlorphenamide, 50 mg/20 kg every 8 hours. Dichlorphenamide produces fewer serious side effects, including vomiting, diarrhea, panting, and weakness, than other carbonic anhydrase inhibitors.

Once the initial acutely elevated intraocular pressure is controlled, careful examination may indicate the underlying cause of the glaucoma, and further appropriate therapy, such as treatment for uveitis, lens removal, cyclocryotherapy, or intraocular implant can be undertaken.[2]

References

1. Arentensen H, et al: Management of corneal descemetoceles and perforations. *Ophthalmic Surg 16*:29, 1985.
2. Baum JL: Bacterial endophthalmitis. *In* Fraunfelder FT, Roy TH (eds): *Current Ocular Therapy*. W.B. Saunders, Philadelphia, 1980, pp 439–440.
3. Baum JL: Antibiotic use in ophthalmology. *In* Duane TD (ed): *Clinical Ophthalmology*. Vol 4. Harper & Row, New York, 1980.
4. Bistner SI: Clinical diagnosis and treatment of infectious keratitis. *Comp Cont Educ 3*:1056, 1981.
5. Bistner SI, et al: *Atlas of Veterinary Ophthalmic Surgery*. W.B. Saunders, Philadelphia, 1977.
6. Bronson NR II: Management of magnetic foreign bodies. *In* Freeman HM (ed): *Ocular Trauma*. Appleton-Century-Crofts, New York, 1979, pp 179–186.
7. Brown SI, Weller CA: The pathogenesis and treatment of collagenase induced disease of the cornea. *Trans Am Acad Ophthalmol Otolaryngol 74*:375, 1970.
8. Byron HM: The contused globe: Management of traumatic hyphema and secondary glaucoma. Instruction course, American Academy of Ophthalmology, Rochester, MN, 1975.
9. Cherry PMH: Indirect traumatic rupture of the globe. *Arch Ophthalmol 96*:252, 1978.
10. Coleman JD: Surgical management of traumatic lens injuries. *In* Freeman HM (ed): *Ocular Trauma*. Appleton-Century-Crofts, New York, 1979, pp 205–214.
11. Coleman JD, Smith ME: Ultrasound in the preoperative evaluation of trauma. *In* Freeman HM: *Ocular Trauma*. Appleton-Century-Crofts, New York, 1979, pp 23–30.
12. Crouch ER Jr, Frenkel M: Aminocaproic acid in the treatment of traumatic hyphema. *Am J Ophthalmol 81*:355, 1976.
13. Ellis PP: Intraocular foreign body—steel or iron. *In* Fraunfelder FT, Hampton R (eds): *Current Ocular Therapy*. W.B. Saunders. Philadelphia, 1980, pp 286–288.
14. Forster RK: Endophthalmitis. *In* Duane TD (ed): *Clinical Ophthalmology*. Vol 4. Harper & Row, New York, 1980.
15. Fox SA: *Ophthalmic Plastic Surgery*. 4th ed. Grune & Stratton, New York, 1970.
16. Freeman HM (ed): *Ocular Trauma*. Appleton-Century-Crofts, New York, 1979.
17. Hanafee WN (ed): Symposium on radiology of the orbit. *Radiol Clin North Am 10*:1, 1972.
18. Hersh PS, Renyon KK: Anterior segment reconstruction following ocular trauma. *Int Ophthalmol Clin 28*:57, 1988.
19. Hoondeph BC: Blunt ocular trauma. *Emerg Med Clin North Am 6*:147, 1988.
20. Jones DB: Initial therapy of suspected microbial corneal ulcers. II. Specific antibiotic therapy based on the corneal smears. *Surv Ophthalmol 24*:97, 1979.
21. Jones DB, et al: *Laboratory Diagnosis of Ocular Infections*. Cumitech 13. American Society for Microbiology, Washington, DC, 1981.
22. Lin DT, et al: Repair of corneal lacerations and perforations: *Int Ophthalmol Clin 28*:69, 1988.
23. Mattews J, Zun LS (eds): Ophthalmologic emergencies and ocular trauma. *Emerg Med Clin North Am 6*:1988.
24. Paton D, Goldberg MF: *Management of Ocular Injuries*. W.B. Saunders, Philadelphia, 1976.
25. Read JE: Trauma: Ruptures and bleeding. *In* Duane TD (ed): *Clinical Ophthalmology, External Diseases*. Vol 4. Harper & Row, New York, 1980, pp 5–12.
26. Rosenthal AR, et al: Intraocular copper foreign bodies. *Am J Ophthalmol 78*:671, 1974.
27. Rynne MV, Romano P: Systemic corticosteroids in the treatment of traumatic hyphema. *J Pediatr Ophthalmol 17*:141, 1980.
28. Sarin LK, Reinert G: Retinopathy in ocular trauma. *In* Duane TD (ed): *Clinical Ophthalmology*. Vol 3. Harper & Row, Hagerstown, MD, 1976.
29. Sholiton DB, Soloman OD: Surgical management of black ball hyphema with sodium hyaluronate. *Ophthalmic Surg 12*:820, 1981.
30. Slatter D: *Fundamentals of Veterinary Ophthalmology*. 2nd ed. W.B. Saunders, Philadelphia, 1990.
31. Smith B: Eyelid reconstruction. *In* Soll DB, Asbell RL (eds): *Management of Complications in Ophthalmic Plastic Surgery*. Aesculapius Publishing Co., Birmingham, 1976, pp 221–243.
32. Thoft RA, Dohlman CH: Chemical and thermal burns of the eye. *In* Freeman HM (ed): *Ocular Trauma*. Appleton-Century-Crofts, New York, 1979.
33. Wilson FM II: Traumatic hyphema, pathogenesis and management. *Ophthalmology 87*:910, 1980.
34. Wong R: Endophthalmitis. An exhibit at the American Academy of Ophthalmology, Atlanta, GA, Nov. 1981.

SECTION 11

Reproductive System

Elizabeth Arnold Stone ■ *Section Editor*

CHAPTER 93

Ovary and Uterus

Elizabeth Arnold Stone, Charles G. Cantrell, and Nicholaus J. H. Sharp

ANATOMY

Ovary

Canine ovaries are oval, flattened, and about 1.5 cm in length in a 20-kg dog.[54] The feline ovary is about 1 cm in diameter.[63] The ovaries are located close to both the abdominal wall and the caudal poles of the kidneys. In multiparous animals, the ovaries are located more caudally and ventrally.[54] Canine ovaries are completely concealed within a peritoneal pouch, the *ovarian bursa,* which contains fat and is closed except for a narrow slitlike opening ventrally.[63] The feline ovarian bursa is much smaller, contains no fat, and covers only the lateral surface of the ovary.[115]

The ovary is attached to the dorsolateral region of the abdominal wall by the mesovarium, in which the ovarian blood vessels course. The mesovarium is continuous cranially with the suspensory ligament and caudally with the mesometrium (Fig. 93–1). The *suspensory ligament* of the ovary extends to the last rib.[115] The *proper ligament* of the ovary is a continuation of the suspensory ligament.[53] It connects the caudal end of the ovary to the cranial end of the uterine horn.[54]

The ovary is divided into a medulla and a cortex. The ovarian follicles are embedded in the cortex. Each follicle is made up of an oocyte and its surrounding granulosa cells encompassed by a basement membrane. A connective tissue capsule, the *tunica albuginea,* envelops the ovary.[54]

The ovarian artery is a branch of the aorta. Branches of the uterine artery may also supply the ovary.[115] The right ovarian vein drains into the caudal vena cava. The left ovarian vein enters the left renal vein.[54]

Uterine Tube

The uterine tube, or oviduct, of a bitch is 6 to 10 mm long.[115] The funnel-shaped infundibulum forms the cranial end of the uterine tube and opens into the ovarian bursa at the abdominal ostium. Multiple fimbriae project

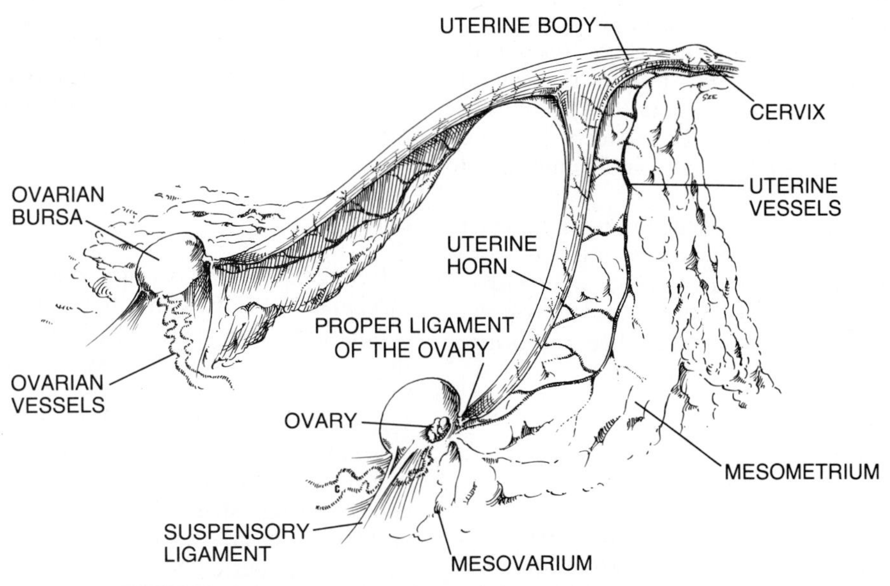

FIGURE 93–1. Anatomy of ovaries and uterus (dorsal recumbency).

from the end of the infundibulum. The uterine tube opens into the uterine horn at the uterine ostium.[54] The ovarian and uterine arteries supply the uterine tube, and drainage is via satellite veins.

Uterus

The uterus consists of the cervix, body, and two uterine horns. The uterine horns in a 10-kg dog average 10 to 14 cm in length and 0.5 to 1 cm in diameter.[54] In cats, they are about 9 to 10 cm long.[115] They lie completely within the abdominal cavity and extend from the uterine tubes to the uterine body.

The uterine body is about 1.5 cm long and 1 cm wide in dogs and 2 cm long in cats.[54, 115] It is located partly in the pelvic cavity but in multiparous animals may be entirely within the abdominal cavity.[54] It lies between the descending colon and the urinary bladder. An internal musculomembranous projection, not visible externally, extends 1 cm into the body of the uterus, dividing the uterine lumen longitudinally.[54] The cervix in dogs is about 1 cm long. The internal orifice of the cervix faces almost dorsally; the external orifice is directed ventrally toward the vaginal floor.[63] The feline cervix feels like a hard oval knot at the uterovaginal junction.[115]

The *mesometrium* is part of the broad ligament and attaches the uterus to the dorsolateral body wall. The *round ligament* of the uterus extends from the tip of the uterine horn, through the inguinal canal, to end between the groin and the vulva.[53, 115]

The peritoneal outer covering of the uterus is termed the *tunica serosa.* The tunica muscularis or myometrium consists of a thin outer longitudinal layer and a thick inner circular layer of smooth muscle, between which lies a network of blood vessels. The innermost layer of the uterus is the tunica mucosa or endometrium. It has a lamina propria with simple branched tubular uterine glands that open into the uterine lumen. Low columnar epithelium, which is temporarily ciliated, faces the uterine lumen.[54, 115]

The ovarian and uterine arteries supply blood to the uterus. The uterine branch of the ovarian artery supplies the cranial uterine horns. The uterine artery arises from the internal pudendal artery[117] and supplies the caudal uterus, cervix, and parts of the vagina.[115] The uterine veins follow the course of the arteries, except that the left ovarian vein enters the left renal vein as mentioned earlier.[54, 115]

Parasympathetic innervation reaches the genital tract via the pelvic nerves. Sympathetic innervation is from the caudal mesenteric ganglion via the hypogastric nerves and pelvic plexus. Lymphatic drainage of the ovary and uterus passes to the medial iliac and aortic lumbar nodes.[115, 117]

PHYSIOLOGY OF THE OVARIAN CYCLE

Ovarian Cycle in the Bitch

The ovarian cycle in a bitch is monestrous, with considerable individual variation in the extent and timing of hormonal changes.

The interval between cycles varies among breeds, ranging from 4 to 13 months, and averaging 7 months. Generally, smaller breeds have shorter cycle lengths than larger breeds. Some breeds have only one ovarian cycle a year (e.g., Basenjis and Tibetan mastiffs). Environmental factors (e.g., photoperiod and pheromone-induced and olfactory-dependent responses) can also affect the interval length.[34]

Puberty begins in most dogs at 6 to 9 months of age. Larger dogs may have their first ovarian cycle as late as 2 years of age. Endometrial infection, ovarian cysts, or genetic aberrations such as XO syndrome in a female with normal female phenotype should be considered in bitches that have not cycled by 24 months of age.[135] The follicular and luteal phases of the ovarian cycle have corresponding changes in estrogen, luteinizing hormone (LH), and progesterone concentrations. The ovarian cycle is divided into four stages: proestrus, estrus, diestrus, and anestrus.

Proestrus

Proestrus averages 5 to 9 days, ranging from 2 to 22 days. Ovarian follicles produce estradiol as they develop. Increased estrogen causes the external signs of proestrus, including vaginal discharge of uterine blood by diapedesis; enlargement, edema, and hyperemia of the vulva and perineum; and hypertrophy of the flow of the caudal vagina. Vulvar tumescence reaches maximal size in late proestrus, with peak estrogen concentrations. Increased estrogen concentrations also promote secretion of sex pheromones.

Hormonal changes from proestrus to estrus reflect the transition from the follicular phase to the luteal phase of the cycle. The follicle begins to luteinize during midproestrus, before peak estrogen levels, then undergoes more rapid luteinization during the preovulatory LH surge. LH released from the anterior pituitary acts as a trigger for ovulation, which occurs 36 to 50 hours after the LH surge. LH is luteotropic, and basal LH levels are required for progesterone secretion during the luteal phase of the cycle. Release of LH is suppressed by ovarian estrogen through a negative-feedback inhibition mechanism.[58] After ovulation, the follicles form corpora lutea, which secrete progesterone.

Estrus

Behavioral estrus occurs when a bitch stands firmly for a male, usually with reflex tail deviation, and permits copulation. The change from refusal to acceptance of the male usually occurs synchronously with the LH surge. It may begin as early as 5 days before the LH surge or as late as 6 days after the LH surge.[34] Estrogen concentrations decline from the peak at 1 to 2 days before the LH surge, whereas progesterone levels increase during estrus. Behavioral estrus last 6 to 12 days, varying from 2 days to more than 3 weeks.[34] The period of fertility is better assessed by vaginal cytological study, vaginoscopy, and hormonal assay than by behavior.

Metestrus

The period after estrus is described by loss of estrus behavior and vaginal cornification, vaginal crenulation, and reappearance of leukocytes in the vaginal smear.[34] The duration of metestrus varies, depending on criteria used.

The increase in progesterone during the first part of the luteal phase promotes growth and development of uterine mucosa and mammary epithelium.[34] Rising progesterone levels also cause elongation and coiling of the uterine horns. By day 20 to 25, the endometrium becomes secretory for 1 month or more, during which time cystic endometrial hyperplasia may develop. The endometrium returns to the anestrus state between day 120 and 130 of the ovarian cycle.[34, 58]

The term diestrus has been substituted for *metestrus.*[79, 48] Diestrus is the period during which the reproductive organs are mainly under the influence of progesterone.[79] In this classification, the term *metestrus* is restricted to the 3- to 5-day period when the corpora lutea are becoming functional and progesterone concentrations are increasing.

Anestrus

Anestrus is the transition from one cycle to the next and is characterized by low progesterone levels. The termination of metestrus (diestrus) and the beginning of anestrus are not obvious. Anestrus may last from 1 to 6 months.

Pseudopregnancy

Mammary gland development occurs during the external luteal phase of all nonfertile ovarian cycles. Overt pseudopregnancy, or pseudocyesis, occurs when mammary development and behavior are indistinguishable from that of late pregnancy or lactation. Many of the clinical signs of pseudopregnancy are due to excessive prolactin caused by abrupt decline in progesterone.[34]

Ovarian Cycle in the Queen

Cats usually reach sexual maturity by 6 to 9 months of age. An adult queen is seasonally polyestrous. Multiple periods of estrus behavior in a given season are caused by sequential waves of follicle development, maturation, and degeneration.[58, 98] The photoperiod has a major impact on the onset and duration of ovarian activity. A queen does not ovulate spontaneously; ovulation usually occurs 24 to 30 hours after copulation. A queen may remain receptive to a male for several days after ovulation. In queens mated daily, the average length of estrus was 6.5 days.[58, 98]

The ovarian cycle is divided into proestrus, estrus, anestrus, and frequently a nonestrus or interestrus interval phase. The terms *diestrus* and *metestrus* are not used as commonly to describe phases of the ovarian cycle in cats as in dogs.

Proestrus is not routinely observed in queens. A queen may cry and posture as if in estrus but will not accept the male. Proestrus usually lasts 12 to 48 hours.[58, 98]

Estrus begins when a queen allows a male to mount and ends when this behavior ceases. The plasma estrogen concentrations rapidly rise, remain increased for 3 to 4 days, and abruptly decrease. Estrogen effects are characterized by a queen's crouching, treading her feet, elevating her pelvis, holding her tail to one side, rubbing, and vocalizing. LH levels peak after vaginal stimulation.[98]

A queen must have coital contact or similar vaginal stimulation to induce ovulation. Diestrus begins 24 to 48 hours after ovulation, with the development of functioning corpora lutea. Peak progesterone levels are reached about 21 days after ovulation.[58, 98]

Anestrus is the period of ovarian inactivity after estrus when ovulation has not occurred. These periods of inactivity are periods of quiescence or interestrus intervals. The follicles regress to a nondetectable state within 1 week after estrus.[58, 98]

DISORDERS OF THE OVARY AND UTERUS

Diagnostic Techniques

Abdominal Palpation

Palpation of the ovaries is not possible unless they are grossly enlarged. The tubular uterus is palpated ventral to the descending colon. It may be difficult to feel the anestral or early estral uterus in a dog. Generally, it is easier to feel a cat's uterus.

Pregnancy Determination. Abdominal palpation is frequently used to diagnosis pregnancy in dogs and cats. In a dog at 17 to 18 days of gestation, the uterus is about the same size as in a pseudopregnant bitch. Round swellings, approximately 1.25 cm in diameter, may be palpable in the uterine horns at 18 to 21 days of gestation. From 24 to 32 days, the readily palpable, spherical swellings are about 2.5 to 4.0 cm in diameter. From 35 to 45 days of gestation, the swellings increase in size, elongate, become flaccid, and lie in the ventral abdomen. By day 50, it is no longer possible to palpate individual swellings. After 55 days of gestation, the fetuses are easily palpable.[54, 109, 135]

In cats, pea-sized swellings are felt at 21 days of gestation. By 28 days, the swellings are firm and are about 2.0 to 2.5 cm in diameter. The uterus is evenly distended during days 35 to 50 and may be difficult to differentiate from pyometra.[135]

Radiography is useful in diagnosing pregnancy after fetal skeletal ossification during the last 15 days of gestation. Radiographs taken after pneumoperitoneum may delineate uterine swellings as early as 30 to 35 days of pregnancy.[135] Using ultrasonography, pregnancy can be diagnosed in dogs as early as 28 days after breeding.[29, 161] Exact litter size cannot be determined. In cats, a gestational sac is visible at days 11 to 14, with fetal cardiac activity present at day 14.[36] Ultrasonography is also useful for identifying the origin of soft-tissue masses on caudal abdominal radiographs (e.g., enlarged uterus or uterine stump).[132]

Exploratory Laparotomy

The diagnosis of some ovarian or uterine diseases may require exploratory laparotomy and biopsy. If the ovaries are not grossly enlarged, the ovarian bursa is first incised to expose the ovaries. The presence of follicles, cysts, and corpora lutea is noted. The bursal incision is closed with synthetic absorbable suture material. The uterine tubes can be examined, but patency cannot be determined because of the uterotubal valve.[146]

Uterine biopsy and culture samples can be taken. A 2- to 3-mm skin biopsy punch instrument is used for punch biopsy. A sterile swab is inserted into the uterine lumen through the biopsy hole to obtain a sample of uterine contents for culture. The small hole in the uterus is closed with 3-0 absorbable suture.

Congenital Anomalies of the Ovary

Agenesis of one or both ovaries occurs in dogs.[88, 101, 135] If both ovaries are absent, the uterus may also be absent or hypoplastic. Hypoplastic, supernumerary, or accessory ovaries are rarely reported.[135] A supernumerary ovary is a third ovary separate from the normally positioned ovary. An accessory ovary is located near the normally positioned ovary, usually connected to it, and appears to develop after splitting of the embryonic gonad.[88] Congenital ovarian anomalies are usually found incidentally during elective ovariohysterectomy or during a laparotomy to determine a cause of sterility.

Acquired Ovarian Lesions

Ovarian Cysts

Follicular cysts develop from graafian follicles. Smaller cysts are lined by several layers of granulosa cells within a capsule composed of regressing theca and compressed ovarian stroma.[47] Solitary follicular cysts range from 1 to 5 cm in diameter. Multiple follicular cysts can form masses up to 10 cm in diameter. The component cysts are small and monolocular with no communication between individual cysts. Both ovaries may have follicular cysts.[47]

Follicular cysts were found in 16 per cent of 400 canine ovaries examined during a random postmortem study. They were more prevalent in nulliparous bitches and in bitches older than 5 years. No histological evidence of estrogenic activity was noted in the endometrium or vagina of any of the dogs studied.[47] However, clinical signs associated with follicular cysts have been reported as prolonged estrus with bloody vaginal discharge, cystic mammary hyperplasia, and genital fibroleiomyomas.[88, 138, 164] Follicular cysts can develop after incomplete removal of the ovary during ovariohysterectomy. Viable remnants of ovarian tissue develop follicles that become cystic.[88, 108]

In cats, cysts from atretic follicles can be functional. Excessive estrogen can cause prolonged estrus, nymphomania, and behavior changes such as aggressiveness and viciousness. Pathogenesis of these cysts is unknown. Cats may be predisposed to follicular cysts because ovulation and subsequent LH release are not spontaneous.[135]

Lutein cysts form from the corpus luteum after ovulation. In the postmortem study previously mentioned, 2 per cent of the ovaries had lutein cysts 1.5 to 3.0 cm in diameter. They were thicker and more opaque than follicular cysts. The ovaries in all dogs contained normal corpora lutea. Histological examination of the uterus and vagina revealed changes consistent with the progesterone phase of the ovarian cycle.[47] They may also be associated with cystic endometrial hyperplasia or pyometra. They are found incidentally during routine ovariohysterectomy or during laparotomy for pyometra.

Parovarian cysts originate from the remnants of either mesonephric (wolffian) or paramesonephric tubules and ducts. They are more frequently encountered in dogs than cats[135] and are located between the ovary and uterine horn. They are found incidentally during ovariohysterectomy.

Inflammatory Disease of the Ovary

Inflammatory disease of the ovary and oviduct is not a distinct disease. Ovaritis or pyosalpinx may occur secondary to pyometra.

Ovarian Tumors (see Chapter 159)

Ovarian tumors are uncommon in dogs and cats, accounting for only 1.2 per cent of 4,187 canine neoplasms in one survey.[35] They occur more frequently in older, nulliparous bitches.[78] Ovarian tumors may stimulate the luteinization of theca cells, with concomitant production of progesterone and associated cystic endometrial hyperplasia and pyometra. Larger tumors may be palpable in the cranial right or left abdominal quadrant.[82, 83] Signs may be consistent with a cranial abdominal space-occupying mass (e.g., vomiting, dyspnea). Radiographic evaluation may reveal a soft-tissue-density mass in the same area.[5, 56]

Sex cord-stromal tumors of the ovary are divided into two main groups, granulosa-theca cell tumors, which are the most common canine ovarian tumors,[47, 88, 135] and Sertoli-Leydig cell tumors. Granulosa cell tumors are composed of cells that differentiate to female-type cells. Bitches with granulosa cell tumors may show signs of elevated levels of estrogen (e.g., hyperplasia and cornification of the vaginal epithelium).[47]

Sertoli-Leydig cell tumors are composed of cells that differentiate into male-type cells. Of 71 dogs with primary ovarian neoplasms, 12 (17 per cent) had Sertoli-Leydig cell tumors. Cystic endometrial hyperplasia was common, suggesting active hormonal effects.[127]

Surgical therapy is ovariohysterectomy. If tumor has invaded the body wall, it may be necessary to excise part of the wall with the tumor. Unilateral nephrectomy may also be required to successfully remove a large, invasive tumor. Chemotherapy has been described for granulosa cell tumor.[106]

Papillary cystadenomas and cystadenocarcinomas occur only in bitches. Cystadenomas are either unilocular, varying in size from 0.8 to 1.5 cm, or multilocular, varying in size from 6 to 8 cm. They are thin walled and usually cause no derangement of the estrous cycle.[47, 88] Bitches with cystadenocarcinomas may have irregular estrous cycles, cystic endometrial hyperplasia, or ascites.[47, 135] Papillary adenocarcinoma is always considered in the differential diagnosis of ascites in adult intact bitches. The ascites develops from obstruction of diaphragmatic lymphatic vessels by tumor fragments and fluid secretion by tumor epithelium. The tumors vary from microscopic to 10 cm or larger. When the tumor is confined within the ovarian bursa, the papillae are compressed and have a cauliflower appearance. Once the papillae outgrow the bursa, their papillary nature becomes apparent, and peritoneal implantation occurs readily. The presence of papillae signals malignancy. Cysts of various sizes are usually scattered throughout the neoplastic mass.[88]

Surgical treatment of a confined papillary cystadenocarcinoma is ovariohysterectomy. Because even a confined papillary cystadenocarcinoma frequently is marked by peritoneal implantation and lung metastasis, prognosis is poor.

Germ cell tumors, including teratomas and dysgerminomas, originate from primordial germ cells of the gonads. Teratomas are composed of derivatives of more than one germ layer and may contain skin, muscle, fat, bone, and nervous tissue. They are diagnosed more often in young bitches.[62, 177] Teratomas containing anaplastic or undifferentiated elements can be malignant and metastatic.[82, 83] A dysgerminoma does not undergo further differentiation and has the same histological appearance as a testicular seminoma.[81] In some instances, it is possible to excise only the affected ovary, permitting future pregnancies.[177]

Congenital Anomalies of the Uterus

Congenital anomalies of the uterus are rare in cats and dogs. The incidence of uterus unicornis is 1:5,000 to 1:10,000 necropsies.[135] Uterus unicornis complicates routine ovariohysterectomy, because the absence of one uterine horn is unexpected. The ovary on the side of the undeveloped uterus may be small but is removed.[43, 73, 150] Agenesis of one uterine horn may be accompanied by unilateral renal agenesis.[136] Other congenital abnormalities of the uterus include hypoplasia, agenesis, atresia, segmental aplasia, septate uterine body, double cervix, and cornual fusion.[17, 101, 110, 150] Most anomalies are found incidentally during elective ovariohysterectomy, but some may cause infertility or dystocia.

Acquired Diseases of the Uterus

Pyometra

The term *pyometra* describes a pus-filled uterus and associated ovarian changes and extragenital disorders. Pyometra is one stage of the *cystic hyperplasia-pyometra complex.* As described by Dow, type I is cystic endometrial hyperplasia, which occurs in middle-aged dogs and is not related to the ovarian cycle. The thickened endometrium is lined by numerous thin-walled translucent cysts. Type II occurs only during diestrus when the cervix is relaxed and patent. A diffuse plasma cell infiltrate is noted in addition to cystic endometrial hyperplasia. In type III, cystic endometrial hyperplasia is accompanied by an acute inflammatory reaction of the endometrium. Bitches found to have pyometra usually have type III uterine changes. Uterine size is proportional to the patency of the cervix. Affected dogs usually present within 8 weeks of their last estrus.[48–50, 154] In chronic endometritis, type IV, the cervix can be either open or closed. If the cervix is open, chronic vaginal discharge occurs. (Fig. 93–2). The horns are not greatly enlarged, the walls are thickened, and there is little pus. Myometrial hypertrophy and fibrosis are noted. If the cervix is closed, the uterus is greatly distended and the uterine walls may be thin. The endometrium is atrophied and infiltrated with lymphocytes and plasma cells.[48–50]

In cats, focal areas of polypoid proliferation are more common than diffuse cystic endometrial hyperplasia. Localized cysts are interspersed with normal endometrial tissue. Larger cysts attached by slender pedicles can be found. These are usually asymptomatic, unless torsion of a pedunculated cyst causes hemorrhage.[88]

Pyometra is a disease of the diestrous phase of the ovarian cycle, when the corpus luteum is actively secreting progesterone, which increases secretions of the uterine glands, inhibits myometrial contraction, and maintains closure of the cervix.[76] Ovarian or exogenous progesterone must be present for maintenance of pyometra.[50] Estrogen alone given to ovariectomized dogs causes a mild, chronic endometrial hyperplasia and decreases the amount of progesterone required to produce pyometra.[157]

Long-acting progestational compounds administered to intact bitches cause endometrial hyperplasia with progression to pyometra in some animals.[25, 66, 92, 131, 149, 178] Biological activity of medroxyprogesterone in dogs is about 24 to 48 times the activity of naturally occurring progesterone.[5] Short-term progestational compounds, administered when endogenous estrogen concentrations are high, may also cause pyometra.[149]

In bitches with naturally occurring pyometra, endogenous progesterone and estrogen concentrations are similar to concentrations in diestrual or pregnant bitches.[13, 33, 70, 71] However, endometrial cell receptors in bitches with pyometra may have an increased affinity for progesterone, or the receptors may maintain a prolonged influence on uterine endometrium.[149] Even when the pyometra persists, luteolysis may occur at the normal time about 60 days after ovulation.[30]

Because cats do not ovulate spontaneously, a progesterone-dependent disease like pyometra should occur only after sterile matings. However, pyometra is encountered in unbred cats. A queen may respond to mild stimulation that is sufficient to cause ovulation and production of a corpus luteum.[46, 51] Pyometra is diagnosed in fewer cats in the latter part of the year, which corresponds to anestrus from September to December in most cats.

Even though infection is not the primary cause of pyometra, it is usually present. The progesterone-primed uterus is more susceptible to infection,[116] possibly because of an inhibition of leukocyte response[77] and greater binding of *Escherichia coli* antigens by the early diestrual uterus.[142]

The most common bacterium cultured from the uterine contents of dogs with pyometra is *E. coli.*[21, 32, 67, 134, 154]

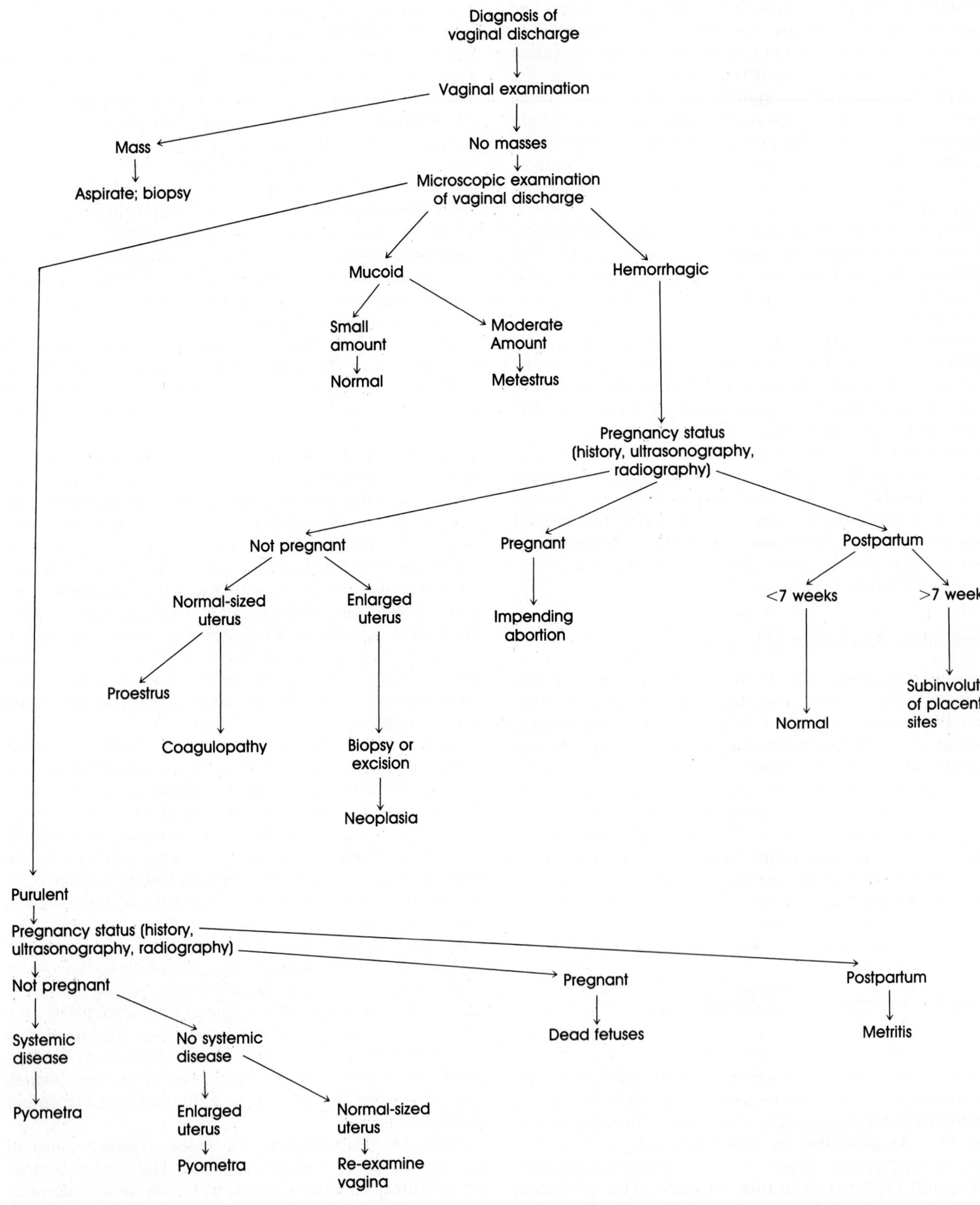

FIGURE 93–2. Algorithm for the diagnosis of vaginal discharge.

Other bacteria cultured include *Streptococcus, Staphylococcus,* enterococci, *Klebsiella, Proteus, Pseudomonas, Aerobacter, Hemophilus,* and *Serratia marcescens.*[32, 91, 154, 171] Rarely, the uterus is sterile, as determined by aerobic bacterial culture,[21, 170] but anaerobic infections may be present. *Bacteroides, Clostridium,* and other anaerobes have been cultured.[14, 123] Endotoxemia was documented in 15 bitches with pyometra.[170]

Bacteria have been isolated from 68 to 85 per cent of uteri of cats with pyometra.[51, 90] Organisms cultured include *E. coli, Staphylococcus, Streptococcus, Pasteurella* spp., *Klebsiella* spp., and *Moraxella* spp.[32, 90] Fifteen to 31 per cent of cats with pyometra had negative results of aerobic bacterial cultures.[51, 90] Attempts to produce pyometra in cats by intrauterine injection of bacteria, with or without simultaneous estrogen administration, have been unsuccessful. Simultaneous injection of progesterone and intrauterine bacteria produced signs of pyometra in 25 per cent of cats.[46]

Pyometra is a polysystemic disease. Leukocytosis, anemia, hypoalbuminemia, hyperglobulinemia, increased alkaline phosphatase levels, azotemia, and acidosis all can occur to various degrees.* Leukocytosis and hyperglobulinemia correlate with the inflammatory condition of the uterus. Hypoalbuminemia is not caused by a loss of protein in the urine[170] but could be caused by decreased hepatic production, reduced protein intake, and loss into the uterus. The nonregenerative anemia is associated with diapedesis of erythrocytes into the uterine lumen and by toxic depression of erythropoiesis.[74]

Twenty to 25 per cent of dogs and 12 per cent of cats with pyometra are azotemic.† In the majority, serum creatinine values return to within reference range after fluid therapy and ovariohysterectomy because prerenal factors are important in the azotemia. Glomerular filtration rate is often reduced even in dogs that are not azotemic.[10, 12, 154] Diminished glomerular filtration rate suggests some factor associated with pyometra decreases renal perfusion with and without azotemia.

Nonazotemic dogs with pyometra are not proteinuric by quantitative evaluation of 24-hour urine collection[154] Increased quantitative urine protein concentrations are noted using single urine samples collected by catheter.[41] Analysis of a voided urine sample may demonstrate protein because of contamination by uterine discharge. If a cystocentesis sample reveals proteinuria, the dog is re-evaluated after resolution of the pyometra to determine the cause and appropriate management.

Dogs with pyometra have decreased urine-concentrating ability, although diluting ability may be retained.[9, 75, 154] The cause of the low urine specific gravity values is multifaceted. In some dogs, it may be caused by the effect of *E. coli* endotoxin on renal tubules.[11] Other bacterial toxins, obligatory solute load from glomerular filtration rate reduction, and unknown factors contribute.

The reduction in glomerular filtration rate is a functional abnormality not correlated with structural damage in the glomerulus.[154] Pyometra is an immune complex disease based on studies of 12 dogs without evaluation of morphological or functional changes. Immunofluorescent evaluation of the glomeruli from dogs with pyometra did not support this conclusion.[154] Glomerular lesions described previously[16, 119] may have been caused by intercurrent disease and age-related changes.

The rate of urinary tract infection is at least 22 per cent[154] and may be as high as 69 per cent.[147] Cystocentesis at the time of surgery is routinely performed, and the urine submitted for bacterial culture and antibiotic sensitivity.

Alkaline phosphatase concentrations may be increased.[147, 154, 171] The liver isoenzyme and perhaps the steroid-induced bile canaliculi isoenzyme have been identified.[147] Primary hepatic disease in older dogs, steroid administration, and toxemia may contribute to increased alkaline phosphatase levels. Serum alanine transaminase concentrations are usually within normal limits.

Some dogs with pyometra may have respiratory alkalosis, but the most important acid-base disturbance associated with pyometra is metabolic acidosis.[18, 154] Dogs with severe acidosis are most likely hypovolemic and septic.

Death rates of 16 to 17 per cent[55] were reported in the 1960s and 1970s. Earlier diagnosis and better monitoring and management probably contributed to the improved survival (death rates of 0 to 5 per cent) reported in the 1980s.[154, 171] Rupture of the uterus produces peritonitis and sepsis, with accompanying hypoglycemia and leukopenia.[126] Dogs that are septic are treated as described in Chapter 99 for dogs with prostatic abscesses. An 8 per cent incidence of death or euthanasia after surgery for pyometra in cats was reported, with causes including sepsis and bacterial peritonitis secondary to rupture of the uterus, liver disease, and nonregenerative anemia and anorexia.[90]

Diagnosis. The diagnosis of pyometra can usually be made from the clinical history, physical examination, and laboratory values. Pyometra is considered in any ill diestrual bitch or queen. Vaginal discharge may not be present if the cervix is not patent. Pyometra occurs at any age after the first estrus (age ranges from 6 months to 16 years in dogs[147, 154] and 1 to 20 years in cats).[90] It occurs more frequently in bitches over 6 years of age within 8 weeks of the last estrus.[19, 48, 74, 154, 155] The incidence of pyometra is no greater in dogs with a history of irregular estrous cycles, abnormal estrus, or pregnancies. The occurrence is less frequent in dogs with a history of pseudopregnancy.[59] Estrogen and progesterone administration increases the risk of pyometra.

In cats, pyometra occurs most frequently within 4 weeks of estrus.[90] It also occurs in spayed cats after treatment with megestrol acetate for dermatological disease.[86, 99]

The type and severity of clinical signs depend on patency of the cervix, duration of the illness, and associated extragenital disease. In dogs, the most frequently reported signs include anorexia, polydipsia, depression, vaginal discharge, vomiting, and diarrhea.* Digital ex-

*See references 20, 38, 39, 69, 91, 147, and 170.
†See references 20, 38, 39, 41, 69, 75, 90, 124, 144, and 170.

*See references 19, 38, 39, 40, 50, 68, 69, 74, 75, 118, 134, 144, 154, 155, 167, and 171.

amination of the vagina differentiates vaginal tumors as a cause of vaginal discharge. If necessary, a vaginoscopic examination may be performed to identify vaginitis. The majority of dogs and cats with pyometra have normal body temperatures, 20 to 30 per cent are febrile, and a few may have subnormal temperatures because of sepsis.[90, 154]

Signs of pyometra in cats are more subtle than in dogs. Cats may show mild anorexia and depression until the disease is well advanced. Primary signs detected by owners are vaginal discharge, anorexia, and lethargy. Less commonly reported are vomiting, weight loss, abdominal distension, and polydipsia/polyuria.[90] Copious vaginal discharge is not seen because of the grooming habits of cats. Physical examination may disclose soiling of the perineal hair.[151]

An enlarged uterus may be felt during abdominal palpation. Care must be taken to avoid rupturing a distended uterus. Many dogs with pyometra are also obese, making them difficult to palpate.

Laboratory findings are not pathognomonic for pyometra. Total leukocyte count is usually greater than 15,000, although some animals have a normal count[90, 147, 154] and even leukopenia.[90] A left shift that may be degenerative is common.[15] The hematocrit may be decreased, but the severity of the anemia can be masked by dehydration.

Renal function is carefully evaluated. A midstream urine sample is collected for evaluation of specific gravity. If a dehydrated or azotemic dog has a urine specific gravity value suggesting lack of concentrating ability (< 1.030), primary renal dysfunction is present. Serum creatinine and urea nitrogen concentrations may reflect both primary renal disease and prerenal dehydration and hypovolemia. The chronicity and severity of renal disease may be difficult to determine until after pyometra is corrected. The owners are forewarned that chronic renal failure may be present.

Urine for bacterial culture and urinalysis is obtained by cystocentesis during surgery. If medical therapy is planned, cystocentesis is not performed until after the uterus has returned to normal size. Because 30 per cent of dogs with pyometra have urinary tract infection, follow-up diagnosis and treatment are important.

When radiographic examination is necessary for confirmation, abdominal preparation such as enemas or withholding food is not recommended. On survey abdominal radiographs, homologous tubular structures of fluid density may be seen in the caudal abdomen. The uterus has a similar appearance during early pregnancy and immediately postpartum.[74, 134] Some dogs with pyometra, even with a closed cervix, may have no visible uterine silhouette on abdominal radiography.[165] Abdominal compression with a belly band or spoon to push the intestines cranially may help outline the uterus in the caudal abdomen. It should be applied selectively to avoid rupturing a distended uterus. Ultrasonography is useful for determining uterine size, thickness of the uterine wall, and presence of fluid within the uterus.

Treatment. The usual treatment for pyometra is ovariohysterectomy. Broad-spectrum antibiotics are administered intravenously at the time of anesthetic induction and continued for 7 to 10 days after surgery. Corrective therapy for fluid deficits, acidosis, and sepsis is started before surgery and continued as needed during and after surgery (see Chapter 99 for treatment of sepsis). In a sick animal, surgery is not postponed for more than a few hours because the diseased uterus continues to contribute to bacteremia and septicemia.

If renal function is impaired before surgery, 20 per cent mannitol (0.25 to 0.5 g/kg IV) is administered. Urine output is usually monitored by observing the bladder size during surgery and the frequency of voiding afterward. Insertion of a urinary catheter is avoided to prevent introducing bacteria into the bladder. However, if the animal is hypotensive or urine output is questionable, a urinary catheter must be placed so that response to volume expansion and diuretics can be measured.

The surgical procedure for ovariohysterectomy, as described in this chapter, needs little modification for the removal of an enlarged uterus in dogs and cats. Special precaution is taken to avoid lacerating an enlarged, friable uterus. The recommended method for handling the uterine body is the classic triple-clamp method with individual ligation of the uterine arteries. The ligatures are placed on the cranial cervix to avoid leaving any uterine body. The uterus is isolated from the abdomen with laparotomy sponges before it is severed, to prevent abdominal contamination. The small amount of exposed uterus is lavaged and suctioned to remove residual pus. A Parker-Kerr oversew is not necessary, unless the cervix is greatly distended. The disadvantages of oversewing the uterine stump are that (1) the cavity between the oversewn area and the cervix may continue as an abscess; (2) the oversewn stump contains more tissue and suture material, which contributes to a stump granuloma; and (3) the oversew technique increases operative time.

If the uterus has ruptured or is torn during surgery, the abdomen is copiously washed with warm multiple-electrolyte solution (50 ml/kg). Intensive therapy for peritonitis and sepsis is initiated.

Postoperative complications for pyometra include those described for ovariohysterectomy later in this chapter, plus those related to generalized septicemia. Splenic infarcts, vascular thrombosis caused by endocarditis, or myocarditis with thromboemboli to the brain and musculoskeletal system occurs.[171]

Medical therapy for pyometra is directed at lowering the progesterone concentrations, eliminating bacteria, and opening the cervix.[112] Several investigators have reported the use of prostaglandin F_2 in dogs and cats.* A precise dosing regimen should be followed.[112, 113] At this time, the drug has not been approved for use in dogs or cats. Clinical improvement is not observed for at least 48 hours after prostaglandin therapy. Thus, the clinician must weigh the relative risks of anesthesia and surgery versus the delay in response with medical therapy. Bitches and queens with open-cervix pyometra often have complete resolution of their infection and whelp normal litters.[107, 112, 113] Recurrence of pyometra is

*See references 4, 7, 8, 28, 37, 76, 85, 107, 112, 125, and 174.

quite likely, thus breeding at the first estrus after treatment is recommended.[107, 113]

Bitches with closed-cervix pyometra may be so ill that immediate ovariohysterectomy is performed. Ovariohysterectomy may be also be necessary for animals that do not respond to prostaglandins.[112, 113]

Some bitches have required repeated treatments with prostaglandins.[57] Uterine drainage was performed in three bitches with pyometra treated unsuccessfully with prostaglandins. Drains were inserted through the cervix under fluoroscopic control. Catheters allowed better drainage by keeping the walls of the cervical canal apart and may also have caused mechanical stimulation of the uterine wall.[93]

Hydrometra and Mucometra

Hydrometra and mucometra are sterile accumulations of fluid within the uterus from endometrial gland secretions under progesterone stimulation. The type of accumulation is determined by the amount of mucin present. Drainage is impeded by a closed cervix or a polypoid cyst from cystic endometrial hyperplasia. The fluid may extend into the oviducts, causing hydrosalpinx or mucosalpinx. Hydrometra and mucometra are uncommon and are usually found incidentally during elective ovariohysterectomy.[88, 103, 104] Chronic abdominal distension secondary to hydrometra was reported in two cats that had a congenital absence of an internal cervical os with accumulation of uterine secretions.[111]

Subinvolution of Placental Sites

Normal involution of the uterus is complete by 12 weeks after parturition. During the first week, the uterine horns are dilated and edematous. Decidual cells are found throughout the lamina propria. The placental sites are 1.5 to 3 cm in width and are rough, granular, and covered with mucus and a few blood clots. By the fourth week, the dilated uterine glands are degenerating and the placental sites are thick and nodular. The uterine horns are contracted, and the placental sites are narrow with few nodules by the seventh week. The endometrial glands have a normal shape. By 9 weeks after parturition, the uterine horns are uniform in shape and have a narrow lumen. The placental sites are a narrow brown band.[2]

With subinvolution of placental sites, a disturbance in the normal postparturient placental degeneration and endometrial reconstruction takes place. During pregnancy, fetal trophoblastic cells invade the myometrium. These cells should die promptly and spontaneously after an abortion or full-term pregnancy. If they do not regress or degenerate, they can continue to invade the deep glandular layer and the myometrium. Retention of these cells for a prolonged time after parturition interferes with normal involution.[1]

Subinvolution of placental sites causes persistent serosanguineous vaginal discharge 7 to 12 weeks after parturition. It usually occurs in bitches less than 2½ years of age after the first or second whelping. Severe anemia may develop. Abdominal palpation may reveal discrete, firm, spherical enlargements of the uterine horns.[64, 143] Subinvolution of placental sites must be differentiated from cystitis, urinary bladder tumors, metritis, and vaginitis. Coagulopathies such as von Willebrand's disease and factor VII deficiency are also considered.[72, 172] The cause of the hemorrhage in dogs with subinvolution of placental sites may be failure of the vessels of the exposed placental bed to occlude, failure of endometrial blood vessels to thrombose, or damage to vessels by trophoblast-like cells.[1]

Spontaneous remission usually occurs, and bitches with subinvolution of placental sites rarely require medical or surgical therapy.[173] If bleeding continues and anemia is worsening, ovariohysterectomy is recommended.

Metritis

Acute metritis occurs most commonly in the immediate postpartum period and is usually associated with dystocia, obstetrical manipulations, or retained placentas or fetuses. Acute metritis may also develop after a normal whelping or following contaminated artificial insemination.[97]

Clinical signs begin within a few days of parturition, including a malodorous, mucopurulent vaginal discharge and signs of systemic illness, such as fever, anorexia, and vomiting. The enlarged uterus may be palpable. Mastitis may also be present.[97, 151]

A complete blood count may reveal neutrophilia and a degenerative left shift. If the animal is dehydrated, the hematocrit and total proteins are increased. Anemia may be masked by the increased hematocrit. Vaginal cytological evaluation reveals degenerative neutrophils and bacteria.

Ovariohysterectomy is recommended. Supportive therapy may be necessary before surgery. The puppies or kittens are weaned and hand-fed. Medical treatment can be attempted for a breeding animal that is not too sick. A soft rubber catheter with a stylet is manipulated through the external opening of the cervix. Care is taken to avoid contacting the uterine wall. The uterus is evacuated, and an antibiotic solution instilled. Broad-spectrum antibiotics are used until antibiotic sensitivity of uterine bacteria is known. Antibiotics are instilled into the uterus daily until there is no uterine discharge, white blood cell count is normal, and temperature is normal.[97]

In animals that do not respond to this treatment or in which an intrauterine catheter cannot be placed through the cervix, a laparotomy can be performed. If the uterus is discolored, swollen, or eroded, ovariohysterectomy is performed. If the uterine wall looks healthy, a hysterotomy incision is made at the uterine bifurcation to remove the uterine contents. Gentle massage of the uterus may help break down adhesions and debris. A catheter is passed from the uterus through the cervix. Antibiotics are placed into the uterus, and the uterine incision is closed. The abdominal incision is closed routinely. The catheter can be used to instill antibiotics after surgery.[52, 97]

Uterine Torsion

Uterine torsion is an uncommon condition in dogs and cats. One or both uterine horns can twist along the long axis or around the opposite horn, or the entire uterine body can rotate. The gravid or nongravid uterus can twist clockwise or counterclockwise from 90° to more than 200° of rotation.* Reported uterine torsions in cats have been in one horn of a gravid uterus.[61, 166, 179] The following causes of uterine torsion have been suggested: (1) jumping or running late in pregnancy, (2) active fetal movement, (3) premature uterine contraction, (4) partial abortion, (5) variations in length and mobility of the proper ovarian ligament, and (6) abnormalities of the uterus.[151]

Signs of uterine torsion are not specific and usually reflect abdominal pain. The onset is often acute. The bitch or queen may crouch and strain as if in labor and may attempt to defecate. Prior delivery of a healthy or dead puppy or kitten may have occurred. Vaginal discharge may be noted. The abdomen can be tense and distended. On vaginal examination, the caudal aspect of the rotated uterus may occasionally be felt. Radiographic examination often discloses a large air- or fluid-filled tubular structure.[133, 151]

The treatment of choice is ovariohysterectomy. If viable fetuses remain in the normal horn, a cesarean section can be performed. Because massive sequestration of fluid within the uterus and vascular obstruction are possible, preoperative supportive therapy may be necessary.

Uterine Prolapse

Prolapse of the uterus is infrequent in dogs and cats. Primiparous queens and queens and bitches that have had several normal litters without complication have developed uterine prolapse.[6, 102, 105, 114] One horn or the entire uterus can prolapse during prolonged labor or up to 48 hours after parturition, when the cervix is extremely dilated.[6, 150] Fetuses may be expelled from one horn, which subsequently prolapses while the other horn is still gravid. Both horns have usually emptied before the prolapse.[151]

Possible mechanisms include (1) excessive relaxation and stretching of pelvic musculature, (2) uterine atony due to metritis, (3) incomplete separation of placental membranes, (4) severe tenesmus, and (5) postpartum contractions intensified by oxytocin release during lactation.[105, 151]

An animal with a prolapsed uterus has one or two tubular masses protruding from the vulva. If a mass is not visible at the time of presentation, digital examination reveals a uterine horn in the vagina. The uterus may be hemorrhagic, ulcerated, and encrusted with litter, hair, feces, or placental membranes. Tenesmus may continue.[151]

If the animal is in good physical condition and the uterus is healthy, manual reduction can be attempted.[168] Sterile gauze sponges are soaked in warm sterile saline and placed around the uterus. General anesthesia or epidural anesthesia is usually necessary. The uterus is cleaned with warm saline followed by an antibiotic wash and lubricated with a water-soluble jelly. Gentle manipulation with gloved fingers, a sterile smooth syringe plunger, or a long glass tube may assist reduction. After reduction, the uterus can be palpated abdominally to determine its position. If partial reduction is achieved, further reduction and positioning can be done via laparotomy. Uterine prolapse seldom recurs after replacement.[135] A successful pregnancy in a queen 6 months after reduction of a uterine prolapse has been reported.[105]

Extensive uterine devitalization necessitates ovariohysterectomy after reduction of the prolapse. If reduction of the uterus is impossible, the uterus is amputated and the stump is reduced.[6, 114, 151, 176] It may be necessary to stabilize a shocked, toxic animal before anesthesia and surgery. To amputate the prolapsed uterus, an incision is made into the cranial part of the uterine body near the vulva. The cranial ends of the uterine horns are visible. Gentle traction on the uterine horns may expose the ovaries. If possible, the ovarian artery is ligated proximal to the ovary. If the ovary cannot be seen, the uterine horn is divided between two ligatures. The uterine arteries are ligated and severed; the uterus is severed and closed with simple interrupted absorbable sutures. The uterine stump is reduced through the vagina. Remaining ovaries are removed through an abdominal incision.[102, 150, 151]

Uterine Rupture

Rupture of a gravid uterus is a rare occurrence during parturition or after severe trauma.[3, 31, 140, 169] Fetuses expelled into the peritoneal cavity may die immediately and resorb or remain intact, causing peritonitis. If the fetal circulation remains intact, the fetuses may live to term. The extrauterine location may not be recognized until whelping, when the fetus is not delivered. Routine palpation of the abdomen may reveal extrauterine masses.[160] An exploratory laparotomy reveals one or more fetuses within the peritoneal cavity, surrounded by adhesions. In some instances, the fetus may be easily removed by dissecting the adhesions from their attachments.[160] If removal of the fetuses and fetal membranes is impossible, the prognosis is poor.

Acute rupture of the uterus is usually treated by ovariohysterectomy. A unilateral ovariohysterectomy may preserve fertility. A small laceration can be sutured, but a repaired area is more likely to rupture during subsequent pregnancies. Fibrotic and constricted areas predispose to infertility.[151]

A uterus that is enlarged from pyometra may rupture before or during surgery. Extensive peritoneal contamination can result. Copious lavage and careful suctioning during laparotomy minimize contamination and the potential for peritonitis.

Uterine Intussusception

Uterine intussusception has been reported in a chow chow with vaginal discharge for 4 weeks. At laparotomy,

*See references 23, 27, 80, 133, 141, 151, 162, 166, and 179.

the left uterine horn was telescoped into itself near its junction with the uterine tube. Ovariohysterectomy was successfully performed.[65]

Uterine Neoplasia (see also Chapter 159)

The incidence of uterine tumors in dogs is 0.3 to 0.4 per cent of canine tumors.[158] Comparable data are not available for cats. In dogs, leiomyoma is the most frequent tumor; leiomyosarcomas occur much less frequently.[78, 158] In cats, endometrial carcinoma is the most frequently reported malignant uterine tumor.[152]

The clinical signs may be abdominal enlargement or a palpable abdominal mass. If the tumor obstructs the lumen, a hydrometra or mucometra may develop.[78] Tumors of the uterine body may cause dysuria, hematuria, and vaginal discharge.[128] The tumor may be found incidentally during ovariohysterectomy or during exploratory laparotomy. Surgical treatment is ovariohysterectomy.

OVARIOHYSTERECTOMY

Indications

Elective sterilization is the most common indication for ovariohysterectomy. Removal of the ovaries and uterus is the usual treatment for many of the ovarian and uterine diseases discussed previously (e.g., ovarian cysts, pyometra, uterine torsion, uterine prolapse, and uterine rupture). Ovariohysterectomy is also indicated to prevent recurrence of vaginal hyperplasia. Animals with diabetes or epilepsy may be spayed to prevent hormonal changes that can interfere with medication.

The customary age for spaying dogs and cats is around 6 months, either just before or after their first estrus. Ovariohysterectomy before the first ovarian cycle decreases the incidence of mammary gland tumors to less than 0.5 per cent. If ovariohysterectomy is performed after the first ovarian cycle, risk of mammary gland tumors increases to 8 per cent; after two ovarian cycles, risk increases to 26 per cent. After 2½ years, ovariohysterectomy has no preventive effect on mammary gland tumor development.[145] Intact female cats have a sevenfold higher risk of mammary cancer than ovariectomized females.[45]

At some humane society shelters, pups and kittens are neutered at 8 to 12 weeks of age, with no reported adverse effects.[95, 96] Advocates for neutering animals at 2 months of age suggest that the procedure is less stressful on the animal and requires less operative time. It also ensures that an adopted animal will not reproduce.

After very early ovariohysterectomy, there may be a greater potential for hypoplasia of the vagina and vulva, leading to perivulvar dermatitis. In addition, juvenile behavior may persist. However, controlled studies examining these possibilities have not been carried out. We do not recommend very early neutering because of the risk of distemper and other infectious diseases for puppies and kittens that may not be protected by maternal antibodies or vaccinations.

Procedure[153]

The length of the midline abdominal incision is based on the size of the animal and whether it is a dog or cat. The distance between the umbilicus and the pubis is divided into thirds. In a dog, the incision is made in the cranial third because the ovaries are more difficult to exteriorize than the uterine body. In a cat, the incision is made in the middle third because the uterine body is more difficult to exteriorize than the ovaries. If the uterus is distended or enlarged, the incision is lengthened. We do not use a flank incision in dogs or cats because the entire uterine body is difficult to remove using this approach.

The right uterine horn is located by means of an ovariohysterectomy hook or the index finger. The spleen is avoided. A clamp is placed on the proper ligament of the ovary (Fig. 93–3*A*) and is used to retract the ovary, while the suspensory ligament is stretched or broken with the index finger (Fig. 93–3*B*). A window is made in the mesovarium caudal to the ovarian vessels. The ovarian pedicle is triple clamped, and the pedicle is severed between the clamp closest to the ovary and the middle clamp (Fig. 93–3*C*). The clamp most distant from the ovary is removed so that the pedicle ligature can be placed in its groove (Fig. 93–3*D*).

Absorbable suture material is used for ligatures. The pedicle is grasped with small hemostats, the remaining clamp is removed, and the pedicle is inspected for bleeding. The pedicle is gently replaced into the abdomen, and the hemostat is released. The procedure is repeated on the opposite ovarian pedicle. In young dogs or cats, two clamps can be used because it is not necessary to groove the pedicle. The broad ligament is severed or torn. If the broad ligament is vascular, it is ligated with one or two sutures before it is cut (Fig. 93–3*E*).

Three clamps are placed on the uterine body just cranial to the cervix. The uterine body is severed between the proximal and middle clamps (Fig. 93–3*F*). The uterine arteries are individually ligated caudal to the most caudal clamp. The caudal clamp is removed, and the uterus is ligated in the groove that remains (Fig. 93–3*G*). The uterine pedicle is grasped with a small hemostat above the clamp, the clamp is removed, and the pedicle is inspected for bleeding. The pedicle is gently replaced into the abdomen, and the hemostat is removed.

Complications

Ovariohysterectomy can have the same complications as any abdominal procedure (e.g., anesthesia complications, delayed wound healing, suture abscesses and infection, and self-inflicted trauma to the wound).[44, 87, 150]

Hemorrhage is reported as the most common cause of death after ovariohysterectomy.[129] Operative hemorrhage may be caused by rupture of the ovarian vessels when the suspensory ligament is stretched or by tearing the vessels in the broad ligament. The uterine vessels may be torn by excessive traction on the uterine body. This can be avoided by lengthening the abdominal

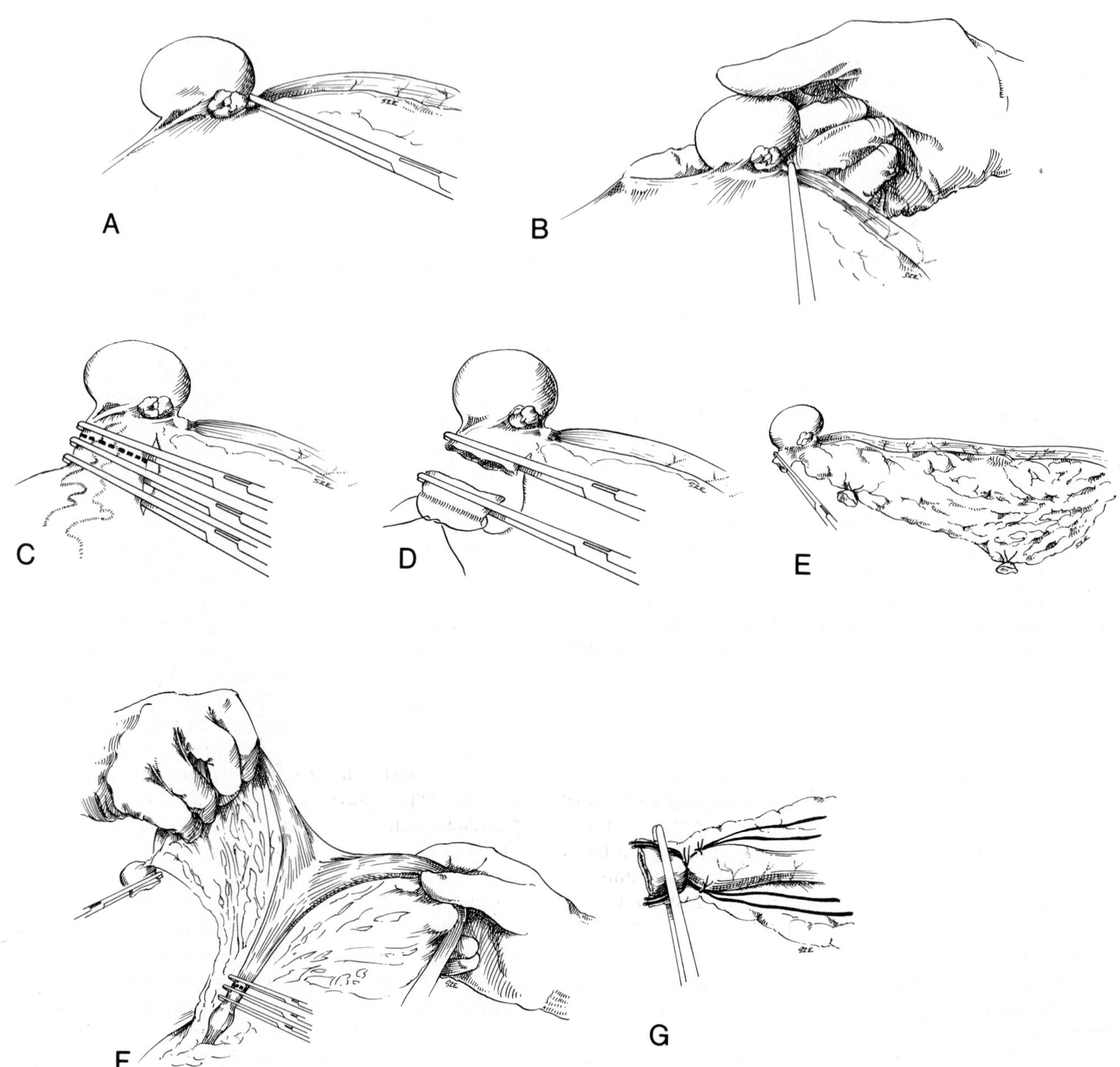

FIGURE 93–3. *A*, Ovariohysterectomy. After a uterine horn is located with a hook or the surgeon's finger, a clamp is placed on proper ligament of ovary. *B*, The clamp is used to retract the ovary while the suspensory ligament is stretched or broken with the index finger. *C*, A window is made in the mesovarium caudal to the ovarian vessels. The ovarian pedicle is triple clamped, and the pedicle is severed between the clamp closest to the ovary and the middle clamp. *D*, The clamp most distant from the ovary is removed so that the ligature can be placed in its groove. *E*, After the opposite ovarian pedicle is ligated and severed, the broad ligament is examined. If it is vascular, it should be ligated with one or two ligatures before is cut or torn. *F*, Three clamps are placed on the uterine body just cranial to the cervix. The uterine body is severed between the proximal and middle clamps. *G*, The uterine arteries are individually ligated caudal to the most caudal clamp. The caudal clamp is removed, and the uterus is ligated in the groove that remains.

incision so the uterine body can be easily exposed. Improperly placed ligatures or defective suture material may result in hemorrhage during or after surgery. Transfixation sutures around the ovarian pedicle or the uterine arteries keep the ligature from dislodging but do not prevent bleeding if the ligature loosens. Coagulopathies may also cause hemorrhage.[129, 150]

To determine the source of bleeding, each ligature is inspected. To do this efficiently, the abdominal incision is lengthened. The right ovarian pedicle is found by using the mesoduodenum to retract the jejunum and expose the right paravertebral space. The left ovarian pedicle ligature is located by using the descending colon and its mesentery to retract the jejunum and expose the left paravertebral space. The ovarian pedicles are found just caudal to the kidneys. The bladder is retracted ventrally and caudally to reveal the uterine pedicle between its neck and the rectum. The broad ligament is also examined for bleeding vessels.

Erosion of the uterine vessels or infection around the uterine vessel ligatures can cause intermittent bleeding from the vagina 4 to 16 days after ovariohysterectomy.[129] Erosion of the uterine vessels occurs most frequently when a single ligature is placed around the uterine body and the uterine vessels. Localized infection can occur when a transfixation suture is passed through the lumen of the uterus. An exploratory laparotomy is indicated because the bleeding may quickly become severe. The vessels may not be bleeding into the peritoneal cavity. The uterine vessels are individually ligated at the cranial cervix. The cervix is also ligated.[129]

Recurrent estrus following ovariohysterectomy is caused by residual ovarian tissue.[26, 120, 129, 150] Ovarian tissue remaining after an incomplete ovariohysterectomy often becomes cystic and may be the cause of recurrent estrus.[108] The right ovary is incompletely removed more often than the left.[120, 129] Ovarian remnants may be more common in cats that have been spayed through a flank incision.[151] Vulval swelling, proestral bleeding, and behavioral changes may occur. Serum progesterone concentrations are usually greater than the basal concentrations measured in ovariectomized dogs.[120] Uterine stump pyometra can develop if a uterine horn or the uterine body is also present.* *Brucella canis* has been reported in a uterine stump abscess in a bitch that had both ovaries.[42]

The diagnosis and treatment of recurrent estrus require an exploratory laparotomy through a midline incision and removal of all remaining tissue. It may be easier to find residual ovarian tissue if the operation is performed during estrus. Even if the ovarian remnant cannot be seen because it is hidden in fat, the ovarian vessels may be enlarged on the functional side. The pedicle is clamped, ligated, and severed closer to the aorta. The excised tissue is submitted for histopathological examination.

Active ovarian tissue that is separate from the ovarian blood supply has not been documented after routine ovariohysterectomy. In an experimental study in cats, the ovarian cortex was severed from its vascular supply and sutured to the lateral abdominal wall. Estrus occurred in two of four cats. The other two cats had cystic follicles. Collateral circulation revascularized the ovarian remnants several months after ligation of the ovarian vessels.[148]

Uterine stump pyometra can occur in dogs and cats after incomplete ovariohysterectomy. The source of progesterone may be from residual ovarian tissue or from exogenous progestational compounds.[99, 122, 156, 175] Uterine stump pyometra is prevented by complete removal of uterine horns and body. The uterine ligature is placed just cranial to the cervix. In cats, it may be necessary to extend the abdominal incision caudally to reach the cervix. *Uterine stump inflammation and granuloma* can be caused by ligatures of nonabsorbable suture material,[89, 120] poor aseptic technique, or excessive remaining devitalized uterine body. Proper materials and technique and wrapping the uterine stump with omentum minimize this complication.

Fistulous tracts can develop from inflammatory response to ligature material.[129] The tract extends from the ligature around the ovarian pedicle or uterine body through the muscle planes to the skin. A soft, painful swelling forms beneath the skin in the flank (ovarian ligature) or *precrual* fold, medial thigh, or inguinal region (uterine ligature). Blood-tinged fluid or pus may intermittently drain. Antibiotic administration may stop the drainage, but the drainage recurs after cessation of the antibiotics. In one report of 20 cases of ovariohysterectomy-related fistulous tracts, the tract originated unilaterally from an ovarian ligature in 12 animals and from the uterine ligature in 4 animals. Braided nonabsorbable suture material (silk, nylon, linen) was used for ligatures.[129]

Dissection of the fistulous tracts is of little value. A midline exploratory laparotomy is performed, and all pedicles examined. If the ligature is deeply embedded in reactive tissue, the entire mass is removed. When the inflammatory tissue around the ovarian pedicle is adhered to the kidney, a nephrectomy may be necessary. Obstruction of the ureter by adhesions causes hydronephrosis, which may also necessitate a nephrectomy. Uterine stump fistulous tracts can produce extensive adhesions to the bladder, ureters, mesentery, omentum, and intestines. The ureters must be protected during dissection to prevent further damage.[22]

Accidental *ligation of a ureter,* causing hydronephrosis or atrophy of the kidney,[87, 121, 150, 163] is prevented by careful identification of uterine horns and body before ligating the uterine body. Inclusion of the ureter in the ligature is more likely with a distended bladder, which moves the trigone and ureterovesical junction cranially and slackens the ureters.

Urinary incontinence following ovariohysterectomy can be caused by adhesions or granulomas of the uterine stump that interfere with urinary bladder sphincter function.[120, 139] A common ligature around the vagina and ureter may produce vaginoureteral fistulation and urinary incontinence.[100, 130]

Estrogen-responsive incontinence can occur in older spayed bitches.[124, 137, 159] The recommended therapy is either oral administration of diethylstilbestrol (0.1 to 1.0 mg/day for 3 to 5 days, followed by a maintenance dose

*See references 60, 87, 99, 122, 129, 156, and 175.

of 1.0 mg/week) or parenteral administration of estradiol cypionate (0.1 to 1.0 mg at intervals of weeks to months, as needed).[137]

Body weight gains of 26 to 38 per cent have been reported after ovariohysterectomy.[24, 44] Inactivity and increased food intake contribute to weight gain.

Ovariectomy may produce a *eunuchoid syndrome* in working dogs (i.e., decreased aggression, interest in working, and stamina).[94] To prevent this syndrome, ovarian tissue is transferred after ovariohysterectomy to an area of the stomach that is drained exclusively by the portal vein. The graft continues to produce estradiol and progesterone, which are partially metabolized by the liver. Estrus is avoided, but occasional brief periods of proestrus occur. Concentrations of estradiol in the systemic circulation are sufficient to prevent the eunuchoid state.[94] Because the prevalence and significance of the eunuchoid syndrome are uncertain, routine use of ovarian grafts is not recommended.

References

1. Al-Bassam MA, et al: Involution abnormalities in the postpartum uterus of the bitch. *Vet Pathol 18*:208, 1981.
2. Al-Bassam MA, et al: Normal postpartum involution of the uterus in the dog. *Can J Comp Med 45*:217, 1981.
3. Allcock J, Penhale BM: Rupture of the uterus in a bitch. *Vet Rec 64*:353, 1952.
4. Amano T, Koi Y: Treatment of feline pyometra with prostaglandin F2α. *J Jpn Vet Assoc 33*:115, 1980.
5. Andersen GL: Granulosa cell tumor in a dog. *Comp Cont Educ Pract Vet 8*:158, 1986.
6. Arnall L: Prolapse of the uterus. *Vet Rec 73*:750, 1961.
7. Arnbjerg J, Flagstad A: Prostaglandin F2α treatment of feline open pyometra. *Nord Vet Med 37*:286, 1985.
8. Arnold S, et al: Use of low dose prostaglandin for the treatment of canine pyometra. *J Small Anim Pract 29*:303, 1988.
9. Asheim A: Renal function in dogs with pyometra. 2. Concentrating and diluting ability. *Acta Vet Scand 4*:293, 1963.
10. Asheim A: Renal function in dogs with pyometra. 3. Glomerular filtration rate, effective renal plasma flow, and the relation between solute excretion rate and maximum urine osmolarity during dehydration. *Acta Vet Scand 5*:26, 1964.
11. Asheim A: Renal function in dogs with pyometra. 8. Uterine infection and the pathogenesis of the renal dysfunction. *Acta Pathol Microbiol Scand 60*:119, 1964.
12. Asheim A: Renal function in dogs with pyometra. 9. Comparative pathophysiological aspects of the glomerulonephritis associated with pyometra in dogs. *Acta Vet Scand 5*:125, 1964.
13. Austad R, et al: Pyometra in the dog—pathophysiological investigation. III. Plasma progesterone levels and ovarian morphology. *Nord Vet Med 31*:258, 1979.
14. Berg JN, et al: Occurrence of anaerobic bacteria in diseases of the dog and cat. *J Am Vet Med Assoc 40*:876, 1979.
15. Bloom F: The blood and bone marrow in pyometra. *North Am Vet 25*:483, 1944.
16. Bloom F: The extragenital lesions of canine pyometra. *Cornell Vet 36*:324, 1946.
17. Bloom F: *Pathology of the Dog and Cat.* American Veterinary Publications, Santa Barbara, CA, 1954.
18. Borresen B: Pyometra in the dog—a pathophysiological investigation. VI. Acid-base status and serum electrolytes. *Nord Vet Med 36*:1, 1984.
19. Borresen B: Pyometra in the dog—a pathophysiological investigation. II. Anamnestic, clinical and reproductive aspects. *Nord Vet Med 31*:251, 1979.
20. Borresen B: Pyometra in the dog—a pathophysiological investigation. IV. Functional derangement of extragenital organs. *Nord Vet Med 32*:255, 1980.
21. Borresen B, Naess B: Microbial, immunological and toxicological aspects of canine pyometra. *Acta Vet Scand 18*:569, 1977.
22. Borthwick R: Unilateral hydronephrosis in a spayed bitch. *Vet Rec 90*:244, 1972.
23. Brear N: Torsion of the uterus with tubal gestation in the bitch. *Vet Rec 51*:422, 1939.
24. British Small Animal Vet Assoc Congress Report: Sequelae to bitch sterilization: Regional survey. *Vet Rec 96*:371, 1975.
25. Brodey RS, Fidler IJ: Clinical and pathologic findings in bitches treated with progestational compounds. *J Am Vet Med Assoc 149*:1406, 1966.
26. Brodey RS, Harvey CE: Letter to the editor: Excision of ovarian remnant for post ovariohysterectomy estrus *J Small Anim Pract 12*:699, 1971.
27. Brown AJ: Torsion of the gravid uterus in a bitch. *Vet Rec 94*:202, 1974.
28. Burke TJ: Prostaglandin F2 alpha in the treatment of pyometra-metritis. *Vet Clin North Am Small Anim Pract 12*:107, 1982.
29. Cartee RE, Rowles T: Preliminary study of the ultrasonographic diagnosis of pregnancy and fetal development in the dog. *Am J Vet Res 45*:1259, 1984.
30. Chaffaux S, Thibier M: Peripheral plasma concentrations of progesterone in the bitch with pyometra. *Ann Rech Vet 9*:587, 1978.
31. Chivers AW: Letter to the editor: An unusual finding in a cat. *Vet Rec 88*:560, 1971.
32. Choi W-P, Kawata K: O group of *Escherichia coli* from canine and feline pyometra. *Jpn J Vet Res 23*:141, 1975.
33. Christie DW, et al: Plasma progesterone levels in canine uterine disease. *Vet Rec 90*:704, 1972.
34. Concannon PW, Lein DH: Hormonal and clinical correlates of ovarian cycles, ovulation, pseudopregnancy, and pregnancy in dogs. *In* Kirk RW (ed): *Current Veterinary Therapy X.* W.B. Saunders, Philadelphia, 1989, pp 1269–1282.
35. Cotchin E: Canine ovarian neoplasms. *Res Vet Sci 2*:133, 1961.
36. Davidson AP, et al: Pregnancy diagnosis with ultrasound in the domestic cat. *Vet Radiol 27*:109, 1986.
37. Delverdier M, et al: Traitement du pyometre de la chienne par les prostaglandines. *Rev Med Vet 135*:155, 1984.
38. De Schepper J, et al: The morphological and chemical blood profile in 62 dogs with a typical endometritis post oestrum (pyometra) with or without renal failure. Proceedings of the 4th International Symposium of Veterinary Laboratory Diagnosis 1986, pp 117–120.
39. De Schepper J, et al: The morphological chemical blood profile in 96 dogs with endometritis post oestrum (pyometra). *Vlaams Diergeneeskd Tijdschr 54*:455, 1985.
40. De Schepper J, et al: Renal injury in dogs with pyometra. *Tijdschr Diergeneeskd (suppl) 112*:124, 1987.
41. De Schepper J, et al: Urinary γ glutamyl transferase and the degree of renal dysfunction in 75 bitches with pyometra. *Res Vet Sci 46*:396, 1989.
42. Dillon AR, Henderson RA: *Brucella canis* in a uterine stump abscess in a bitch. *J Am Vet Med Assoc 178*:987, 1981.
43. Doley PB: Instances of reproduction with uterus unicornis and uterus didelphys. *Vet Med 46*:60, 1951.
44. Dorn AS, Swist RA: Complications of canine ovariohysterectomy. *J Am Anim Hosp Assoc 13*:720, 1977.
45. Dorn CR, et al: Survey of animal neoplasms in Alameda and Contra Costa Counties, Calif. II. Cancer morbidity in dogs and cats from Alameda County. *J Natl Cancer Ints 40*:307, 1968.
46. Dow C: Experimental uterine infection in the domestic cat. *J Comp Pathol 72*:303, 1962.
47. Dow C: Ovarian abnormalities in the bitch. *J Comp Pathol 70*:59, 1960.
48. Dow C: The cystic hyperplasia-pyometra complex in the bitch. *J Comp Pathol 69*:237, 1959.
49. Dow C: The cystic hyperplasia-pyometra complex in the bitch. *Vet Rec 69*:1409, 1957.
50. Dow C: The cystic hyperplasia-pyometra complex in the bitch. *Vet Rec 70*:1102, 1958.
51. Dow C: The cystic hyperplasia-pyometra complex in the cat. *Vet Rec 74*:141, 1962.
52. Durfee PT: Surgical treatment of postparturient metritis in the bitch. *J Am Vet Med Assoc 153*:40, 1968.
53. Dyce KM, et al: *Textbook of Veterinary Anatomy.* W.B. Saunders, Philadelphia, 1987, p 432.
54. Evans HE, Christensen GC: *Miller's Anatomy of the Dog.* W.B. Saunders, Philadelphia, 1979.
55. Ewald BH: A survey of the cystic hyperplasia-pyometra complex in the bitch. *Small Anim Clin 1*:383, 1961.
56. Faulkner RT: Removal of a thecoma in a poodle. *Vet Med Small Anim Clin 73*:451, 1978.
57. Feldman EC, Nelson RW: Diagnosis and treatment alternatives for pyometra in dogs and cats. *In* Kirk RW (ed): *Current Veterinary Therapy X.* W.B. Saunders, Philadelphia, 1989, p 1305.
58. Feldman EC, Nelson RW: *Canine and Feline Endocrinology and Reproduction.* W.B. Saunders, Philadelphia, 1987, pp 399–480, 525–548.
59. Fidler IJ, et al: Relationship of estrous irregularity, pseudopregnancy and pregnancy to canine pyometra. *J Am Vet Med Assoc 149*:1043, 1966.
60. Fitts RH: Pyometra following incomplete oophorectomy in a bitch. *J Am Vet Med Assoc 128*:449, 1956.
61. Freeman LJ: Feline uterine torsion. *Comp Cont Educ Pract Vet 10*:1078, 1988.
62. Frye FL: Canine ovarian teratoma. *Vet Med Small Anim Clin Dec 78*:1863, 1983.
63. Getty R: *Sisson and Grossman's The Anatomy of the Domestic Animals.* W.B. Saunders, Philadelphia, 1975.
64. Glenn BL: Subinvolution of placental sites in the bitch. 18th Gaines Veterinary Symposium, 1968, pp 7–10.

65. Gorham MF, Spink RR: Uterine intussusception in a chow chow. *Mod Vet Pract 56*:35, 1975.
66. Goyings LS, et al: Clinical, morphologic, and clinicopathologic findings in beagles treated for two years with melengestrol acetate. *Am J Vet Res 38*:1923, 1977.
67. Grindlay M, et al: O-groups of *Escherichia coli* associated with canine pyometra. *Res Vet Sci 14*:75, 1973.
68. Gyula H, et al: Observations on the pathophysiology and clinical signs of chronic pyometra in dogs. I. Histories, clinical signs and examination of ovarian function. *Magy Allatorv Lapja 40*:229, 1985.
69. Gyula H, et al: Observations on the pathophysiology and clinical signs of pyometra in dogs. II. Laboratory investigations of extrauterinal changes. *Magy Allatorv Lapja 40*:236, 1985.
70. Hadley JC: Unconjugated oestrogen and progesterone concentrations in the blood of bitches with false pregnancy and pyometra. *Vet Rec 96*:545, 1975.
71. Hadley JC: Variations in peripheral blood concentrations of progesterone and total free oestrogens in the nonpregnant bitch. *Vet Rec 93:*77, 1973.
72. Hamilton H, et al: Von Willebrand's disease manifested by hemorrhage from the reproductive tract: Two case reports. *J Am Anim Hosp Assoc 21*:637, 1985.
73. Hansen JS: Ectopic pregnancy in a queen with one uterine horn and a urachal remnant. *Vet Med Small Anim Clin 69*:1135, 1974.
74. Hardy RM, Osborne CA: Canine pyometra—a polystemic disorder. *In* Kirk RW (ed): *Current Veterinary Therapy VI.* W.B. Saunders, Philadelphia, 1977, pp 1229–1233.
75. Hardy RM, Osborne CA: Canine pyometra: Pathophysiology, diagnosis and treatment of uterine and extra-uterine lesions. *J Am Anim Hosp Assoc 10*:245, 1974.
76. Hardy RM, Senior DF: Canine pyometra. *In* Kirk RW (ed): *Current Veterinary Therapy VII.* W.B. Saunders, Philadelphia, 1980, pp 1216–1219.
77. Hawk HW, et al: The effect of ovarian hormones on the uterine defense mechanism during the early stages of induced infection. *Am J Vet Res 21*:644, 1960.
78. Herron MA: Tumors of the canine genital system. *J Am Anim Hosp Assoc 19*:981, 1983.
79. Holst PA, Phemister RD: Onset of diestrus in the beagle bitch: Definition and significance. *Am J Vet Res 135*: 401, 1974.
80. Homer BL, et al: Left horn uterine torsion in a nongravid nulliparous bitch. *J Am Vet Med Assoc 176*:634, 1980.
81. Jackson ML, et al: Ovarian dysgerminoma in a bitch. *Can Vet J 26*:285, 1985.
82. Jergens AE, Shaw DP: Tumors of the canine ovary. *Comp Cont Educ Pract Vet 9*:489, 1987.
83. Jergens AE, et al: Ovarian teratoma in a bitch. *J Am Vet Med Assoc 191*:81, 1987.
84. Jochle W, Andersen AC: The estrous cycle in the dog: A review. *Theriogenology 7*:113, 1977.
85. Johnson CA, Wasserfall JL: Prostaglandin therapy in feline pyometra. *J Am Anim Hosp Assoc 20*:247, 1984.
86. Jones AK: Letter to the editor: Pyometra in the cat. *Vet Rec 97*:100, 1975.
87. Joshua JO: The spaying of bitches. *Vet Rec 77*:462, 1965.
88. Jubb KVF, Kennedy PC: *Pathology of Domestic Animals.* Academic Press, New York, 1970.
89. Kassem MM, et al: Studies on some modifications of ovariohysterectomy in bitches and its complications. *Assiut Vet Med J 15*:197, 1985.
90. Kenney KJ, et al: Pyometra in cats: 183 cases (1979–1984). *J Am Vet Med Assoc 191*:1130, 1987.
91. Kivisto A-K, et al: Laboratory diagnosis of canine pyometra. *Acta Vet Scand 18*:308, 1977.
92. Knecht CD: A brief survey of progestogen involvement in utero-ovarian disorders. *Ill Vet 9*:3, 1966.
93. Lagerstedt A-S, et al: Uterine drainage in the bitch for treatment of pyometra refractory to prostaglandin F2α. *J Am Anim Pract 28*:215, 1987.
94. LeRoux PH, Van Der Walt LA: Ovarian autograft as an alternative to ovariectomy in bitches. *J South Afr Vet Assoc 48*:117, 1977.
95. Lieberman LL: A case for neutering pups and kittens at two months of age. *J Am Vet Med Assoc 191*:518, 1987.
96. Lieberman LL: Advantages of early spaying and neutering. *J Am Vet Med Assoc 181*:420, 1982.
97. Lipowitz AJ, Larsen RE: Acute metritis. *In* Kirk RW (ed): *Current Veterinary Therapy VII.* W.B. Saunders, Philadelphia, 1980, pp 1214–1215.
98. Lofstedt RM: The estrous cycle of the domestic cat. *Comp Cont Educ Pract Vet 4*:52, 1982.
99. Long RD: Letter to the editor: Pyometritis in spayed cats. *Vet Rec 91*:105, 1972.
100. MacCoy DM, et al: Postovariohysterectomy ureterovaginal fistula in a dog. *J Am Anim Hosp Assoc 24*:469, 1988.
101. Marcella KL, et al: Segmental aplasia of the uterine horn in a cat. *J Am Vet Med Assoc 186*:179, 1985.
102. Maxson FB, Krausnick KE: Dystocia with uterine prolapse in a Siamese cat. *Vet Med Small Anim Clin 64*:1065, 1969.
103. McAfee LT: Hydrouterus and hydrovarium in a beagle bitch. *Can Pract Aug 4*:46, 1977.
104. McAfee LT, McAfee JT: Hydrometra in a bitch. *Mod Vet Pract 57*:829, 1976.
105. McCaig J: Prolapse of the uterus in the bitch. *Vet Rec 73*:628, 1961.
106. McKee WM: Granulosa cell tumour and attempted chemotherapy in a 17-month-old bitch. *Vet Rec 117*:501, 1985.
107. Meyers-Wallen VN, et al: Prostaglandin F2α treatment of canine pyometra. *J Am Vet Med Assoc 189*:1557, 1986.
108. Miller DM, et al: Polycystic ovarian tissue in a spayed bitch. *Mod Vet Pract 64*:749, 1983.
109. Morrow DA: *Current Therapy in Theriogenology.* W.B. Saunders, Philadelphia, 1980.
110. Morrow LL, Howard DR: Genital tract anomaly. *Vet Med Small Anim Clin 67*:1313, 1972.
111. Nash AS, et al: Hydrometra in cats. *J Small Anim Pract 27*:265, 1986.
112. Nelson RW, Feldman EC: Treatment of canine pyometra with prostaglandin F2 alpha. 31st Gaines Veterinary Symposium, 1981, pp 10–16.
113. Nelson RW, et al: Treatment of canine pyometra and endometritis with prostaglandin F2α. *J Am Vet Med Assoc 181*:899, 1982.
114. Newman MAH: Letter to the editor: Prolapse of the uterus in the bitch and the cat. *Vet Rec 73*:680, 1961.
115. Nickel R, et al: *The Viscera of the Domestic Mammals.* Verlag, Paul Parey, New York, 1973.
116. Nishikawa Y, et al: Effect of the estrous cycle on uterine infection induced by *Escherichia coli. Infect Immun 43*:678, 1984.
117. *Nomina Anatomica Veterinaria and Nomina Histologica.* International Committee on Veterinary Gross Anatomical Nomenclature, Ithaca, NY, 1983.
118. Nomura K: Clinical signs, intrauterine bacteria and plasma progesterone levels in bitches with pyometra. *J Jpn Vet Med Assoc 37*:83, 1984.
119. Obel AL, et al: Light and electron microscopical studies of the renal lesions in dogs with pyometra. *Acta Vet Scand 5*:93, 1964.
120. Okkens AC, et al: Gynaecological complications following ovariohysterectomy in dogs, due to (1) partial removal of the ovaries, (2) inflammation of the uterocervical stump. *Tijdschr Diergeneeskd 106*:1142, 1981.
121. Okkens AC, et al: Urologic complications following ovariohysterectomy in dogs. *Tijdschr Diergeneeskd 106*:1189, 1981.
122. Orhan UA: Letter to the editor: Pyometritis in spayed cats. *Vet Rec 90*:77, 1972.
123. Osbaldiston GW: Bacteriological studies of reproductive disorders of bitches. *J Am Anim Hosp Assoc 14*:363, 1978.
124. Osborne CA, Polzin DJ: Canine estrogen-responsive incontinence: An enigma. DVM *10*:42, 1979.
125. Ott RS, Gustafsson BK: Therapeutic application of prostaglandins for postpartum infections. *Acta Vet Scand 77*:363, 1981.
126. Pages JP, Trouillet JL: Hypoglycemie grave par choc septique lors de pyometres perfores chez deux chiennes. *Pratique Med Chir Anim Compagnie 20*:597, 1985.
127. Patnaik AK, et al: Morphology of canine ovarian Sertoli-Leydig cell neoplasms. *Cancer 62*:577, 1988.
128. Payne-Johnson CE, et al: Endometrial carcinoma in a young dog. *J Comp Pathol 96*:463, 1986.
129. Pearson H: The complications of ovariohysterectomy in the bitch. *J Small Anim Pract 14*:257, 1973.
130. Pearson H, Gibbs C: Urinary incontinence in the dog due to accidental vagino-ureteral fistulation during hysterectomy. *J Small Anim Pract 21*:287, 1980.
131. Petit GD: Progesterone-induced pyometra in the bitch. *Anim Hosp 1*:151, 1968.
132. Poffenbarger EM, Feeney DA: Use of gray-scale ultrasonography in the diagnosis of reproductive disease in the bitch: 18 cases (1981–1984). *J Am Vet Med Assoc 189*:90, 1986.
133. Rendano VT, et al: Hematometra associated with pseudocyesis and uterine torsion in a dog. *J Am Anim Hosp Assoc 10*:577, 1974.
134. Renton JP, et al: Pyometra in the bitch. *J Small Anim Pract 12*:249, 1971.
135. Roberts SJ: *Obstetrics and Genital Diseases (Theriogenology).* Published by the author, Ithaca, NY, 1971.
136. Robinson G: Uterus unicornis and unilateral renal agenesis in a cat. *J Am Vet Med Assoc 147*:516, 1965.
137. Rosin AH, Ross L: Diagnosis and pharmacological management of disorders of urinary continence in the dog. *Comp Cont Educ Pract Vet 3*:601, 1981.
138. Rowley J: Cystic ovary. *Vet Med Small Anim Clin 75*:1888, 1980.
139. Ruckstuhl B: Urinary incontinence in the bitch as a complication of spaying. *Schweiz Arch Tierheilkd 120*:143, 1978.
140. Rudolph L: Clinical rupture of the uterus in a dog. *North Am Vet 12*:46, 1931.
141. Salzmann GB: Torsion of the canine uterus. *Mod Vet Pract 55*:250, 1974.
142. Sandholm SM, et al: Pathogenesis of canine pyometra. *J Am Vet Med Assoc 167*:1006, 1975.
143. Schall WD, et al: Spontaneous recovery after subinvolution of placental sites in a bitch. *J Am Vet Med Assoc 159*:1780, 1971.
144. Schalm OW: Pyometra in the dog. *Calif Vet 27*:18, 1973.
145. Schneider R, et al: Factors influencing canine mammary cancer development and postsurgical survival. *J Natl Cancer Inst 43*:1249, 1969.
146. Senior DF: Infertility in the cycling bitch. *Comp Cont Educ Pract Vet 1*:17, 1979.

147. Sevelius E, et al: Pyometra in the dog. *J Am Anim Hosp Assoc 26*:33, 1990.
148. Shemwell RE, Weed JC: Ovarian remnant syndrome. *Obstet Gynecol 36*:299, 1970.
149. Shille VM: Canine pyometra. *Vet Med Newsletter* (Univ Florida), *Aug* 9:6, 1980.
150. Smith KW: Female genital system. *In* Archibald J (ed): *Canine Surgery*. American Veterinary Publications, Santa Barbara, 1974, pp 762–782.
151. Stein BS: The genital system. *In* Catcott EJ (ed): *Feline Medicine and Surgery*. American Veterinary Publications, Santa Barbara, 1975, pp 303–354.
152. Stein BS: Tumors of the feline genital tract. *J Am Anim Hosp Assoc 17*:1022, 1981.
153. Stone EA: Uterus. *In* Slatter D (ed): *Textbook of Small Animal Surgery*. W.B. Saunders, Philadelphia, 1985.
154. Stone EA, et al: Renal dysfunction in dogs with pyometra. *J Am Vet Med Assoc 193*:457, 1988.
155. Sumner-Smith G: The diagnosis of "open" and "closed" pyometra in the dog and cat—I. Clinical aspects and differential diagnosis. *J Small Anim Pract 6*:429, 1965.
156. Teale ML: Letter to the editor: Pyometritis in spayed cats. *Vet Rec 90*:129, 1972.
157. Teunissen GHB: The development of endometritis in the dog and the effect of oestradiol and progesterone on the uterus. *Acta Endocrinol* 9:407, 1952.
158. Theilen GH, Madewell BR: *Veterinary Cancer Medicine*. Lea & Febiger, Philadelphia, 1979.
159. Thrusfield MV: Association between urinary incontinence and spaying in bitches. *Vet Rec 116*:695, 1985.
160. Tirgari M: Secondary ectopic pregnancy in a cat: A case report. *J Small Anim Pract 27*:383, 1986.
161. Toal RL, et al: A comparison of real-time ultrasound, palpation and radiography in pregnancy detection and litter size determination in the bitch. *Vet Radiol 27*:102, 1986.
162. Tompsett JW, Bezner GA: Torsion of the dog's uterine horn. *Mod Vet Pract 52*:52, 1971.
163. Turner T: An unusual case of hydronephrosis in a spayed Alsatian bitch. *Vet Rec 91*:588, 1972.
164. Vaden P: Surgical treatment of cystic ovaries in the dog (a case report). *Vet Med Small Anim Clin 73*:1160, 1978.
165. Van Bree H, et al: The significance of radiology in the diagnosis of pyometra (endometritis postoestrum) in dogs: An evaluation of the correlation between radiographic and laboratory findings in 131 cases. *J Am Vet Med Assoc 35*:200, 1988.
166. Vlcek Z, Kozumplik J: Uterine torsion. *Veterinarstvi 12*:334, 1962.
167. Walker RG: The diagnosis of "open" and closed" pyometra in the dog and cat—II. Diagnosis and clinical assessment of closed pyometritis in the bitch. *J Small Anim Pract 6*:437, 1965.
168. Wallace LJ, et al: Manual reduction of uterine prolapse in a domestic cat. *Vet Med Small Anim Clin 65*:595, 1970.
169. Webb AI: Ventral hernia and ruptured uterus in a cat. *Aust Vet J 48*:212, 1972.
170. Wessels BC, Wells MT: Antiendotoxin immunotherapy for canine pyometra endotoxemia. *J Am Anim Hosp Assoc 25*:455, 1989.
171. Wheaton LG, et al: Results and complications of surgical treatment of pyometra. *J Am Anim Hosp Assoc 25*:563, 1989.
172. Wheeler SL, et al: Persistent uterine and vaginal hemorrhage in a beagle with factor VII deficiency. *J Am Vet Med Assoc 185*:447, 1984.
173. Wheeler SL, et al: Postpartum disorders in the bitch: A review. *Comp Cont Educ Pract Vet June 6*:493, 1984.
174. Wildt DE, et al: Effect of prostaglandin F2 on endocrine-ovarian function in the domestic cat. *Prostaglandins 18*:883, 1979.
175. Wilkins DB: Pyometritis in spayed cats. *Vet Rec 90*:24, 1972.
176. Wilkinson GT: Prolapse of the uterus in the bitch. *Vet Rec 73*:679, 1961.
177. Wilson RB, et al: Ovarian teratoma in two dogs. *J Am Anim Hosp Assoc 21*:249, 1985.
178. Withers AR, Whitney JC: The response of the bitch to treatment with medroxyprogesterone acetate. *J Small Anim Pract 8*:265, 1967.
179. Young RC, Hiscock R: Torsion of the uterus in the cat. *Vet Rec 75*:872, 1963.

CHAPTER 94

Vagina, Vestibule, and Vulva

Peggy M. Wykes and Patricia N. Olson

VAGINA AND VESTIBULE

Congenital Anomalies

Congenital abnormalities of the vagina probably occur commonly in bitches but are only occasionally associated with clinical disease. They result from abnormal development of the paramesonephric ducts (müllerian ducts) or urogenital sinus. Congenital abnormalities of a dog's reproductive tract are caused by either developmental inhibition of portions of the paramesonephric ducts or aberrations in the pattern of fusion to each other or to the urogenital sinus.

Segmental Vaginal Aplasia; Hypoplasia

Segmental aplasia of the paramesonephric duct system is commonly reported in humans and cattle but is uncommonly found in dogs.[6, 15] The defect can occur anywhere along the vaginal wall. The occlusion may be partial (hypoplasia) and interfere with breeding or parturition, or it may be complete (aplasia) and cause retention of uterine fluids during estrus. The latter can appear similar to a closed pyometra radiographically.

The method of treatment for complete or partial vaginal occlusion depends on its location within the vagina, the degree of obstruction, and the breeding potential of the dog. In breeding bitches, caudal and midvaginal strictures have been successfully resected and the vaginal segments anastomosed.[6] No treatment may be necessary for nonbreeding asymptomatic female dogs with partial obstruction. Nonbreeding symptomatic animals may require ovariohysterectomy or vaginectomy.

Whether some of the asymptomatic developmental defects should be surgically corrected in breeding animals is ethically debatable. The cause of segmental aplasia of the paramesonephric ducts system in cattle may be a sex-linked trait, but a genetic etiology has not been established in dogs.[6]

Persistent Hymen

Various forms of persistent hymen occur as the paramesonephric ducts fail to unite with each other or fail to fuse or cannulate with the urogenital sinus. Incomplete perforation of the hymen, taking the form of a

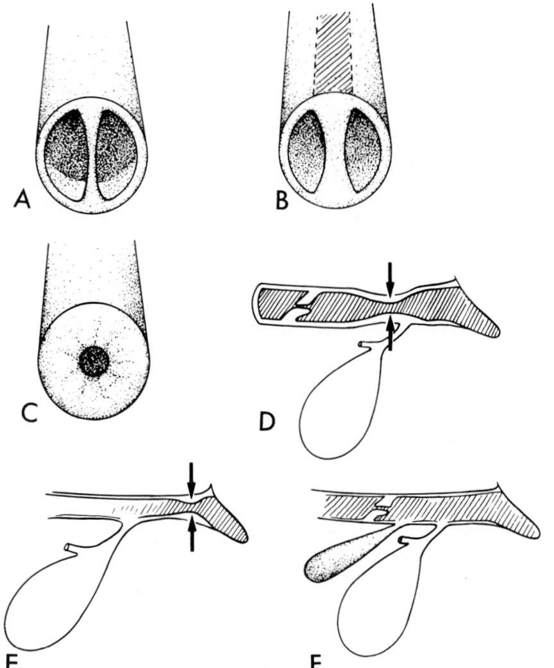

FIGURE 94–1. Congenital anomalies of the vagina and vulva. *A*, Vertical septum at vaginovestibular junction. *B*, Incomplete fusion of the paramesonephric ducts resulting in incomplete partitioning of the vagina. *C*, Annular stricture at the vaginovestibular orifice. *D*, Hypoplasia of the vaginovestibular junction. *E*, Stenosis at the vestibulovulvar junction. *F*, Secondary vaginal pouch (double vagina).

vertical septum or annular fibrous stricture, results in stenosis at the vaginovestibular junction (Fig. 94–1*A* and *C*).[7, 16] The latter may be confused with hypoplasia of the genital canal at the vaginal entrance, which also has a reduced lumen but lacks a fibrous ring as seen with hymen remnants (Fig. 94–1*D*). Normal contraction of the constrictor vestibular muscle during vaginal palpation of a nervous animal may falsely represent stenosis at the vaginovestibular junction.

Incomplete fusion of the caudal paramesonephric ducts, with retention of a medial partition, results in an elongated vertical vaginal band or, rarely, a double (bifid) vagina with one segment ending as a blind pouch[5, 18, 19] (Fig. 94–1*B* and *F*).

Clinical Signs

Annular fibrous strictures or vertical septa in dogs may contribute to breeding or whelping difficulties, chronic vaginitis, and urine pooling. Affected female dogs have normal cycles and exhibit normal mating behavior by flagging and allowing the male to mount, but they experience pain on intromission by the male and are unable to complete the "tie." If the male is allowed to penetrate to the level of the obstruction, he may experience pain and dismount or may refuse further attempts to breed.

A history of intermittent vaginal discharge with intense licking at the vulva also has been reported in females with vaginitis associated with vaginal obstruction.[16] The persistent vaginitis results from inadequate drainage of the cranial portion of the vagina and uterus. Abnormal sloping of the vagina in a cranioventral direction ("up-and-over" vagina) due to pelvic angulation may also contribute to retention of fluids or signs of apparent urinary incontinence.[7, 8] In the latter case, urine collects in the vagina cranial to the vaginovestibular stenosis and overflows intermittently as the dog changes position.

Diagnosis

A digital vaginal examination is the most informative and least expensive method of diagnosing vaginal anomalities. A vaginal band, elongated vaginal septa, or a double vagina is considered when a small stoma is palpated on either side of a central partition, just cranial to the urethral tubercle. Bitches with annular strictures and hypoplastic lesions have a single small vaginal opening that prevents digital penetration of the ostium vaginum. In questionable cases, the patient is examined under sedation or general anesthesia or during estrus when the diameter of the vaginovestibular junction is greatest, to rule out a false stricture due to contraction of the vestibular muscle.[19] These defects are often missed during vaginal examination with vaginal specula or otoscopic cones that bypass the anomaly. Likewise, vaginal bands and strictures are not readily appreciated with fiber-optic equipment, although it is helpful for examination and biopsy of the vaginal mucosa.

A vaginogram may demonstrate the location and expandability of a vaginal or vaginovestibular stricture or may delineate double vaginas. [2, 16]

Treatment

Surgical correction of vertical vaginal bands or stenotic defects at the vaginovestibular junction is indicated when persistent urogenital signs (e.g., vaginitis) fail to respond to medical therapy and when no other cause can be found (allergies, foreign bodies) or if the anomaly interferes with natural breeding or parturition. Some bands can be digitally resected through the vagina by speculum. Large or thick vaginal bands that resist digital breakdown or the presence of annular strictures requires surgical correction using an episiotomy to permit exposure of the defect.

An episiotomy extends from the dorsal vulvar commissure toward the anus, along the median raphe. Fascia and constrictor vestibular and vulvar muscles are incised, followed by separation of the deeper vestibular bulb tissue and vaginal mucosa. The incisional edges are retracted laterally to expose the vaginovestibular junction. A urethral catheter is placed before resection of ring strictures or septa to avoid incising the urethral tubercle. A curved instrument placed cranial to the band assists exposure and resection at the dorsal and ventral attachment (Fig. 94–2). Closure of the vaginal mucosa with an absorbable suture may be necessary for hemostatis if broad-based bands are removed (Fig. 94–3).

Some animals possess both types of perforate hymen (annular stricture and vertical bands). Consequently, the diameter of the vaginal opening is carefully evaluated after septum removal. In some cases, a short, intact

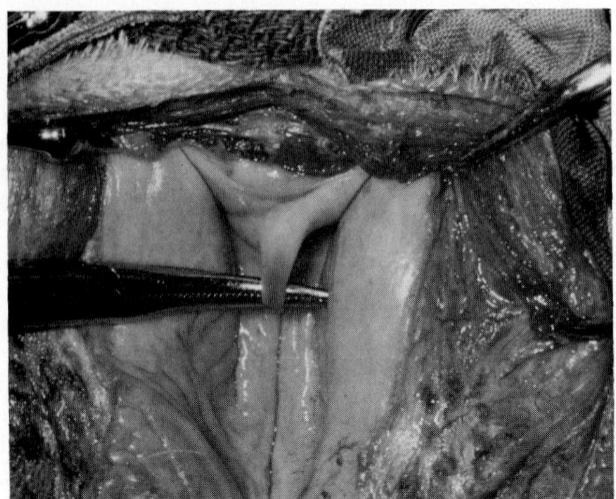

FIGURE 94–2. Episiotomy to expose the vaginovestibular junction. A curved hemostat is used to isolate a vertical band before resection at its dorsal and ventral attachments.

vertical band may flatten the vaginal entrance to suggest an associated stricture, but the vaginal opening expands normally after band excision.

Annular strictures located at the vaginovestibular junction require resection of submucosal fibrous tissue through an incision in the mucosa. Only the ventral 180° of the stricture is removed in mild cases to allow adequate drainage of vaginal fluids in spayed bitches. Expansion of these strictures by digital dilation alone is usually unsuccessful.

When considering surgery for segmental vaginal hypoplasia, a vaginogram is performed to evaluate the extent and location of a hypoplastic region and to determine the feasibility of surgery. For short segmental hypoplastic areas (less than 1.5 cm in length) located near the ostium vaginum, a vaginovestibuloplasty can be attempted. The episiotomy incision is extended through the dorsal vaginal wall beyond the stenotic region. The vaginal wall is closed in a T fashion using a single layer of 3-0 polyglactin 910 in an interrupted pattern[7] (Fig. 94–4) to increase the diameter of the vaginal lumen. A more viable option is rotation of a vestibular mucosal flap, with the base located at the vaginovestibular junction. The flap is sutured into the vaginal defect created after extending the dorsal episiotomy.

After correction of the previously mentioned abnormalities, the episiotomy is closed in three layers, consisting of interrupted absorbable sutures in the vaginal mucosa, a continuous layer in the submucosa, and a subcuticular row in the skin. Permanent relief of signs can be expected after septum removal if no other genital abnormalities exist. If a ring stricture requires intermittent digital dilation after surgery to prevent cicatricial narrowing of the vaginal canal, the prognosis is guarded.

Strictures that are located more than 2 cm cranial to the vaginal opening cannot be adequately exposed with a standard episiotomy. An abdominal approach and possible pubic osteotomy may be necessary to surgically correct such strictures. When the vagina is to be preserved, an *en bloc* resection of the stricture can be performed, followed by anastomosis of the vaginal components.

Abdominal exposure of the vagina is necessary when treatment by vaginectomy is considered.[7] Vaginectomy is indicated for cranial vaginal strictures, if urine pooling persists after septum removal, or when surgical removal of the occlusive tissue at the vaginovestibular junction is unsuccessful. In intact females, an ovariohysterectomy is performed, in addition to removal of the entire vagina. For vaginectomy, the vagina is isolated from its perito-

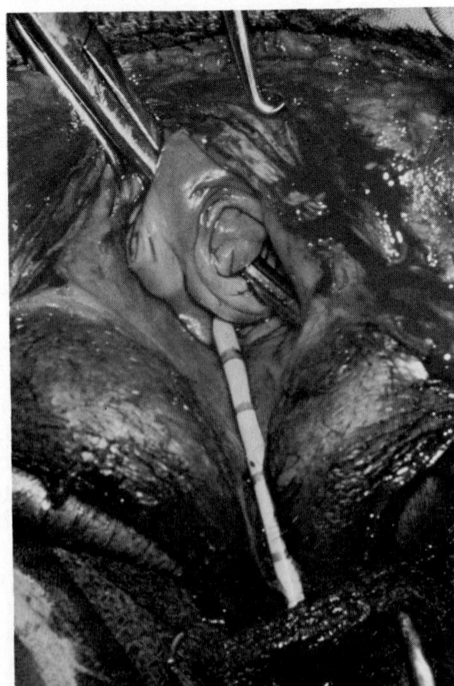

FIGURE 94–3. Episiotomy exposure of a broad and lengthy vaginal band that partially partitions the caudal vagina.

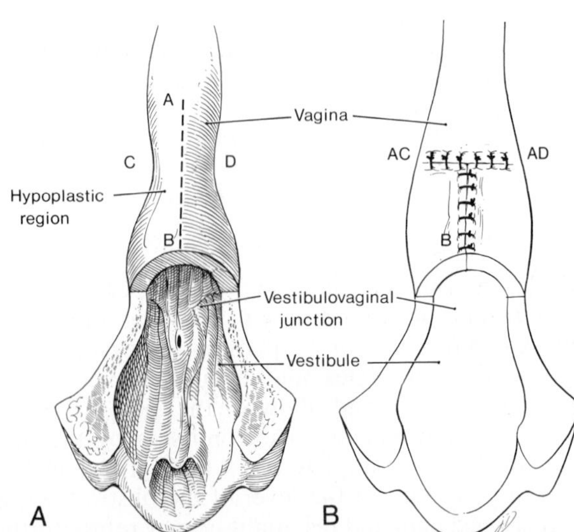

FIGURE 94–4. Vaginoplasty. *A*, Dorsal view of the vestibule and vagina, demonstrating a hypoplastic region (C–D). A longitudinal incision is made beyond the limits of the stenotic area (A–B). *B*, The vaginal incision is closed in a T fashion to increase the diameter of the vaginal lumen.

neal support, followed by ligation of the vaginal branches of the urogenital arteries and veins. The vagina is transfixed just cranial to the urethral tubercle. Extreme care is taken to avoid interruption of the nerve and blood supply to the urethra and bladder, as well as to avoid compression or distortion of the urethral opening.

The incidence of vaginal abnormalities in animals without clinical signs is unknown. Many of these animals are spayed early in life, making hereditary predisposition difficult to evaluate.[19]

Rectovaginal/Vestibular Fistula

In rectovaginal/vestibular fistula, the rectum forms an abnormal communication with either the vagina or the vestibule, and the vulva functions as a common orifice for both the urogenital and gastrointestinal tracts (Fig. 94–5). This congenital condition is often associated with imperforate anus. A barium sulfate enema can be given to demonstrate the fistula, and if atresia ani is present, the barium is given via the vagina.

The severity of clinical signs varies with the size of the fistula and the dog's diet. An animal that has a large fistula and is on a liquid diet evacuates enough soft feces through the fistula to decompress the colon. Megacolon is a complicating factor when excessive feces collect in the colon after the diet is changed to solid food, especially if atresia ani is also present.[12]

Vaginal cytological study demonstrates large amounts of debris and a mixed population of bacteria with rectogenital fistula. Mature dogs with a recessed vulva and associated vaginal fecal contamination occasionally may simulate females with acquired rectovaginal fistulas because of similar vaginal cytological findings. Large populations of vaginal anaerobic bacteria have also been noted with this condition and may be associated with bacterial overgrowth.

Treatment. The objective of surgery is to restore the lumen of both the rectum and the vagina or vestibule. A linear incision is made along the median raphe from just ventral to the anal sphincter, extending to the vulva. The fistula is located and isolated by blunt dissection. The dorsal communication with the rectum is ligated with absorbable sutures placed around the fistula, and the fistula is incised. Oversewing the rectal ligature ensures a tight seal. If the tract is very short and wide and ligation is not feasible, the stoma must be oversewn primarily. The tract is also divided where it joins the vaginal or vestibular wall, and the resulting vaginal defect is closed with a double line of absorbable sutures.

Cellulitis is a complicating factor if the operative site is contaminated with feces or if the rectal incision leaks. Use of regional rotational muscle flaps to patch the rectal closure site and insertion of drains may be appropriate. Fecal incontinence often persists when this condition occurs with imperforate anus. These animals frequently lack an anal sphincter and remain incontinent even after surgical reconstruction of the anal opening.[12]

Acquired Abnormalities

Vaginal Edema (Formerly "Vaginal Hyperplasia")

During the follicular phase of the estrous cycle, the vaginal and vestibular mucosa normally becomes edematous and thickened. Exaggeration of this estrogenic response occasionally results in excessive mucosal folding of the vaginal floor cranial to the urethral tubercle.[16] This redundant mucosa begins to protrude through the vulvar labia as a fleshy red mass (Fig. 94–6*A*). The exposed tissue is subject to trauma, inflammation, and ulceration. The urethra does not become exteriorized and can usually be catheterized. Vaginal edema is most frequently seen during the first estrous period and usually regresses spontaneously during the luteal phase. Recurrence is common during succeeding estrous peri-

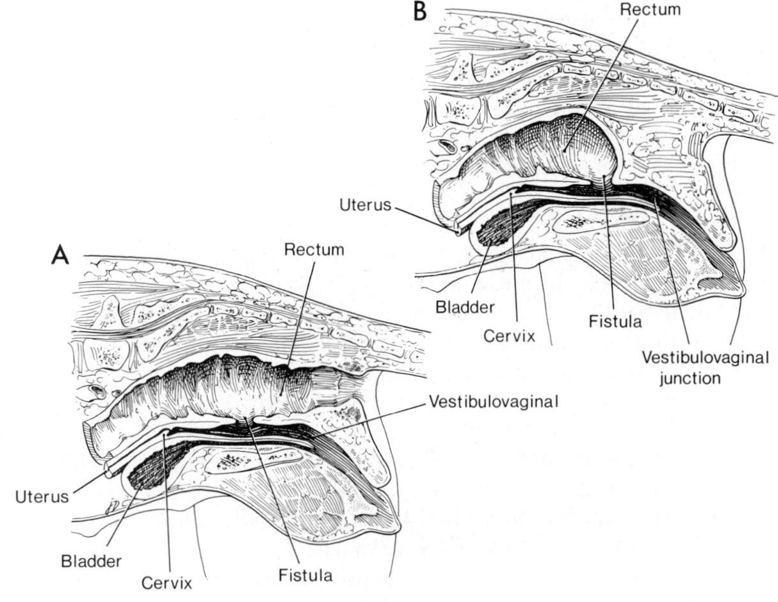

FIGURE 94–5. Rectovaginal fistula. *A*, Rectum communicates directly with the vagina but terminates in a normal anus. *B*, Rectum terminates at the vagina. Atresia ani is present.

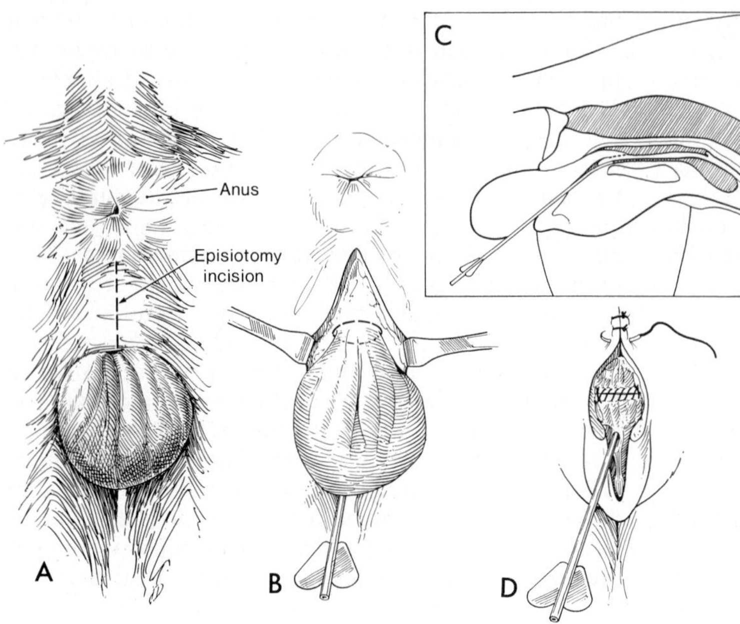

FIGURE 94–6. Vaginal edema. *A*, Protrusion of edematous tissue through the vulvar labia. An episiotomy is necessary for better exposure. *B*, The mass is lifted off the vestibular floor to catheterize the urethra. Note that the mass originates from the vaginal floor just cranial to the urethral tubercle. *C*, A transverse elliptical incision is made at the base of the mass, avoiding the urethral tubercle. *D*, Vaginal wall defect is closed with a continuous suture followed by closure of the episiotomy.

ods. The edematous tissue may prevent natural breeding, and affected bitches may be artificially inseminated. Owners should be cautioned that the edematous tissue occasionally recurs at parturition and may result in dystocia. A secondary vaginal prolapse has been encountered in association with this condition.

Because English bulldogs, boxers, and other brachycephalic breeds are most commonly afflicted, owners should be informed that the condition may be hereditary.[3]

Megestrol acetate (2 mg/kg PO daily for 7 days) can be given in early proestrus in an attempt to prevent the development of vaginal edema in bitches with a predisposition. Megestrol acetate is a synthetic progestogen and may be antagonistic to estrogens in the target tissue. Owners wishing to breed their bitches during the current cycle should be advised that this treatment prevents ovulation.

Gonadotropin-releasing hormone (GnRH) has also been used to treat vaginal edema in bitches (50 μg GnRH IV once). Administration of GnRH in early proestrus or when ovarian follicles are still immature and not capable of ovulating could result in preovulatory luteinization of follicles or the development of ovarian cysts.

Temporary relief can be provided by application of K-Y Jelly or normal saline to minimize drying of the exposed mucosa. In addition to interfering with coitus, the edematous tissue is aesthetically displeasing to many owners, and surgical resection becomes the treatment of choice. After surgical correction, vaginal edema occasionally recurs during subsequent estrous periods. Only ovariohysterectomy prevents further recurrence.

Surgical Treatment. The patient is placed in sternal recumbency and positioned and prepared for episiotomy, which exposes the caudal vaginal floor and allows delineation of the prolapsed tissue margins. The mass is lifted off the vestibular floor to identify the urethra for catheterization (Fig. 94–6*B*). Redundant vaginal tissue is amputated by making a transverse elliptical incision around its base (Fig. 94–6*C*). Closure of the vaginal defect is with a simple continuous pattern of an absorbable suture, avoiding the urethral orifice (Fig. 94–6*D*).

Vaginal Prolapse

Vaginal prolapse is less common than vaginal edema in dogs and can be either partial or complete. In contrast to partial vaginal prolapse, the cervix is exteriorized with complete prolapses. In either case, a doughnut-shaped eversion of the complete vaginal circumference (including the urethral tubercle) protrudes through the vulvar labia (Fig. 94–7). This must be differentiated from vaginal edema, in which redundant mucosa arises primarily from the vaginal floor. The everted tissue often becomes discolored from venous congestion, ulcerates, and is easily traumatized. Displacement of abdominal or pelvic organs into the prolapse is rare, although vaginal prolapse may precede prolapse of the uterus.[14]

Brachycephalic breeds such as boxers and Boston terriers appear predisposed to vaginal prolapse. The cause of this condition is complex, but hereditary weakness of the perivaginal tissue is a predisposing factor.[14] Constipation, forced separation during coitus, and size discrepancy between breeding partners may also have a role in vaginal prolapse.[1] This condition occurs in normal estrus when estrogen production is increased and with pathological hyperestrogenism (e.g., cystic ovaries). Vaginal displacement during pregnancy is rare in bitches but has been reported in late gestation.[14]

Both vaginal prolapse and vaginal edema must be differentiated from tumors arising from the vaginal and vestibular wall (leiomyomas, fibromas, polyps). The presenting signs are similar, and careful vaginal examination and biopsy are performed if a neoplasm is suspected (see Chapter 159).

Treatment. With mild prolapse, no treatment may be

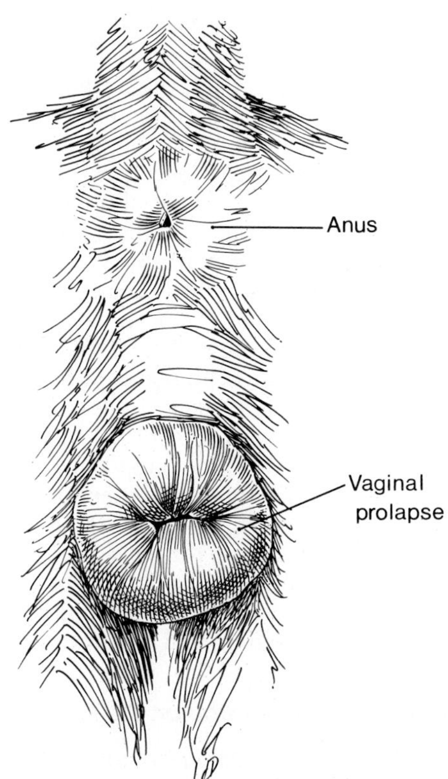

FIGURE 94–7. Vaginal prolapse. Eversion of the complete vaginal circumference through the vulvar labia, demonstrating the typical doughnut-shaped appearance.

necessary, because spontaneous regression occurs during diestrus. More severe prolapses require protection of exposed tissues until estrus passes. Attempts to replace the vaginal mucosa usually require general anesthesia. The everted tissue is first cleaned with saline or a dilute antiseptic solution (povidone-iodine). Tissue edema can be reduced by manual compression or by application of 50 per cent dextrose to the mucosal surface. The solution is later rinsed off to minimize mucosal irritation. A lubricated plastic syringe case can be used to push the everted tissue back into place. Episiotomy provides additional exposure for easier reduction. Once the vagina is repositioned, a urinary catheter is placed until the swelling resolves, and the reduction is maintained by placing nonabsorbable sutures across the labia. If repositioning is unsuccessful with the vulvar approach, reduction can be assisted by traction on the uterus through a ventral abdominal incision. After vaginal repositioning, recurrent prolapse can be minimized by suturing the uterine body or the broad ligaments to the abdominal wall.[1]

Severe acute or long-standing vaginal prolapse may be attended by hemorrhage, infection, or necrosis of the prolapsed tissue. Affected animals may become hypotensive or septic and are treated accordingly. Surgical resection of the devitalized tissue is necessary to prevent further sepsis and self-mutilation and to restore the vaginal lumen. Repair is often preceded by an episiotomy for better exposure, and a urinary catheter is inserted to identify and protect the urethra (Fig. 94–8*A*). A circumferential incision is carried out in relays through the vaginal wall. One to 2 cm of the outer mucosal layer is incised, followed by resection of the inner noninverted mucosal layer (Fig. 94–8*B*).[1] Hemorrhage is controlled by electrocautery and ligation and closure of the incision edges with a series of horizontal mattress sutures. The ring-shaped incision is extended, and the next section is sutured until the entire circumference of the prolapsed vaginal tissue is resected.

A bitch with a vaginal prolapse during late pregnancy will probably have difficulty with parturition.[14] Therefore, surgical resection of the prolapsed tissue at the time it occurs is perferred to waiting until parturition is evident. Future breeding is seldom impaired after surgical resection. Breeding is undesirable for bitches that have a tendency to prolapse, because the condition may be hereditary. Ovariohysterectomy causes permanent regression of vaginal prolapse and is recommended for patients with a tendency to prolapse.[14] In long-standing prolapse, ovariohysterectomy may not cause complete regression of the prolapsed vaginal tissue, and subse-

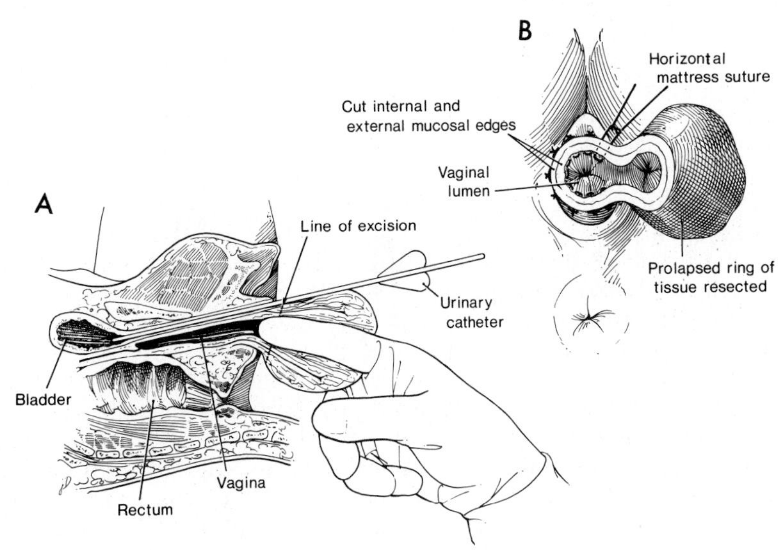

FIGURE 94–8. Surgical correction of vaginal prolapse. *A*, The dog is placed in dorsal recumbency. A urethral catheter is placed to identify urethral tubercle; a finger can be inserted into the center of the prolapsed tissue. Note the intended line of resection. *B*, A stepwise full-thickness circumferential incision is made in the vaginal wall. Horizontal mattress sutures are placed to close the incisional edges.

quent surgical removal of the remaining prolapsed tissue is necessary.

Vaginal Trauma

Injury of the vagina most often occurs with the use of obstetrical equipment during assisted parturition. Other causes include forceful separation of dogs during mating, traumatic insult, and malicious injuries.[13] Hemorrhage may be profuse in these cases. Spontaneous vaginal hemorrhage due to factor VII or VIII deficiency or warfarin poisoning must be considered as an alternative diagnosis.[11] Vaginal douching is used commonly by practitioners as a form of treatment for vaginitis. This therapy, especially if performed frequently by inexperienced people, can often severely traumatize the vaginal and vestibular region and perpetuate the underlying condition. This therapy for treatment of vaginal disease is discouraged.

THE VULVA

Congenital Abnormalities

Congenital abnormalities of the canine vulva are uncommon; they may contribute to the development of vestibulitis, clitoritis, cystitis, and difficulty with natural breeding. Some of these anomalies include vulvar stenosis, anovulvar cleft, vulvar atresia, and clitoral hypertrophy. Double vulvar formation and total vulvar agenesis are uncommon.

Vulvar Stenosis

Stenosis may occur within the body of the vestibule or, more commonly, in the vulvar region (see Fig. 94–1*E*). The vulva consists of the labia, the commissures of the labia, and the rima vulvae between the labia. The cranial boundary of the vulva is the cranial portion of the clitoral fossa.[13] Vulvar strictures may be caused by imperfect joining of the genital folds or genital swellings.

Affected female dogs experience pain when coitus is attempted and often require artificial insemination. The condition is most common in collies and shelties. A partial episiotomy can be performed to permanently enlarge the vulvar opening to prevent dyspareunia (difficult mating) and potential dystocia. This procedure is performed as for episiotomy; the ventral third of the incision is closed in a mucocutaneous fashion, resulting in an elongated vulvar cleft.[9] As a result of the increased vestibular exposure to microorganisms in the environment, the flora of the vestibule and vagina may change and predispose to urinary tract infection.[16] Another surgical option to treat vulvar strictures is to rotate a vestibular mucosal flap into the episiotomy closure at the level of the stricture. Incorporation of the graft in the episiotomy closure can adequately enlarge the vulvar opening for normal breeding and parturition.

Anovulvar Cleft (Vulvovestibular Cleft)

Anovulvar cleft results from incomplete closure of the skin between the dorsal vulvar commissure and the anus (Fig. 94–9*A*).[4, 17] Failure of the urogenital folds to fuse dorsally allows the vestibular floor and clitoris to be directly observed. Clitoritis and hyperemia of the vestibular mucosa frequently occur subsequent to environmental exposure and fecal contamination. This anomaly may occur in sexually normal female dogs or with intersex disorders. The rarity of this defect suggests it is not hereditary.[4]

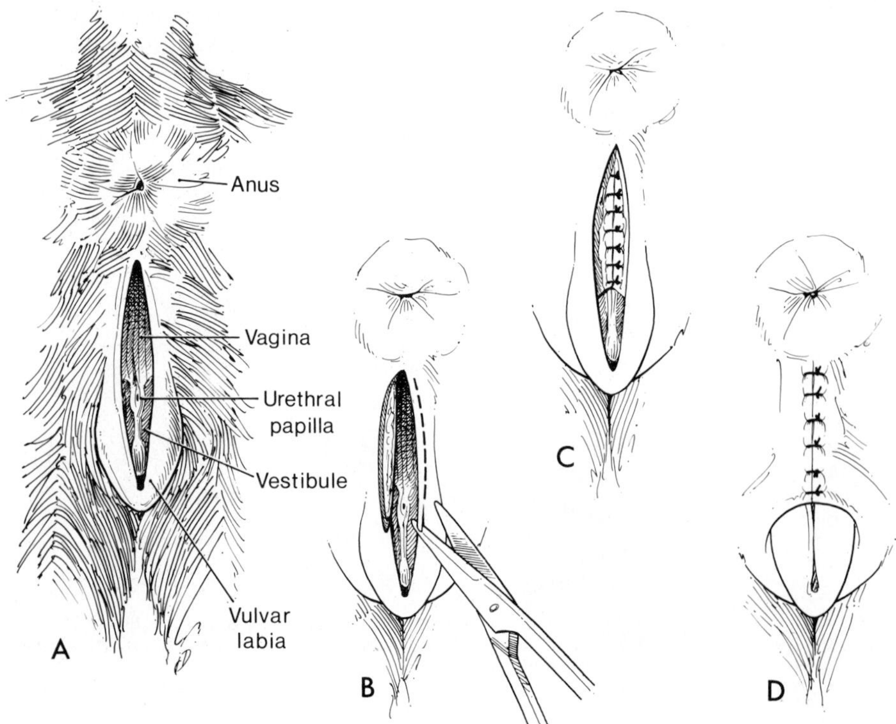

FIGURE 94–9. Anovulvar cleft. *A*, Incomplete closure of skin from the anus to the dorsal vulvar commissure. *B*, A V-shaped incision is made along the mucocutaneous junction between the anus and vulvar labia. *C*, Simple interrupted sutures are used to close the vestibular wall. *D*, Skin closure with simple interrupted sutures.

Treatment. Surgical repair is performed to reduce infection and abrasion of exposed mucous membranes and to provide a more cosmetic appearance of the perineal region. The cleft is repaired by making an inverted V perineoplasty incision along the mucocutaneous junction between the anus and vulva (Fig. 94–9*B*).[4] Enough tissue is removed to create a gap between the vestibular mucosal margin and skin edge of about 1 cm. Interrupted absorbable sutures are used in the vestibular mucosa and submucosa to close the dorsal defect, followed by placement of interrupted nonabsorbable sutures in the skin (Fig. 94–9*C* and *D*).

Atresia of the Vulva

Vulvar hypoplasia or atrophy is most frequently recognized in spayed female dogs.[10] The vulva appears small (infantile) and is often retracted into the perineal skin folds. This results in a moist dermatitis that may be accentuated by retention of urine or feces within the folds of skin. Recurrent vestibulitis, clitoritis, and cystitis may be encountered in many of these animals and may be due to continual reinfection caused by bacteria retained in the perivulvar folds. Surgical removal of the perivulvar folds, in conjunction with antibiotic treatment, may be necessary to alleviate signs of cystitis or vestibulitis.

Estrogens should not be used to treat this condition. Continual administration of estrogens is necessary for retained vulvar size, and prolonged use of estrogens can result in fatal bone marrow suppression. Episioplasty improves exteriorization of the vulva by removing excessive perivulvar skin folds and the underlying subcutaneous fat and is the preferred treatment.

Clitoral Hypertrophy

A dog with an enlarged clitoris is often presented by an owner for aesthetic reasons rather than for health reasons. These animals may have disorders of sexual differentiation, may be receiving anabolic steroids, or may be suffering from hyperadrenocorticism. The condition is occasionally found in normal females.[10] The clitoris may protrude through the vulvar cleft if hypertrophy is severe and may result in clitoritis (Fig. 94–10). The clitoris sometimes resembles a small penis and may even possess an os clitidoris. The mechanical irritation of an enlarged clitoris can result in secondary inflammation of the vestibule. In contrast, primary inflammation of the vestibule can contribute to secondary enlargement of the clitoris. When an os is present, clitoral enlargement may persist even after removal of the gonads; consequently, the os is surgically removed by simple dissection. Large "phalluses" in dogs with intersex disorders bleed profusely when removed, and an episiotomy may be needed for improved surgical exposure and to assist with hemostatis.

Acquired Vulvar Abnormalities

Vulvar Hypertrophy

The vulva normally becomes swollen and edematous during the follicular stages of the estrous cycle in response to estrogen stimulation. This vulvar enlargement occasionally becomes excessive, but the swelling should dissipate with the conclusion of normal estrus. In animals experiencing prolonged estrogen stimulation due to cystic ovaries or granulosa cell tumor, vulvar hypertrophy may persist. In chronic cases, the labia become thickened, pigmented, and hairless.[10] Ovariohysterectomy is an effective treatment.

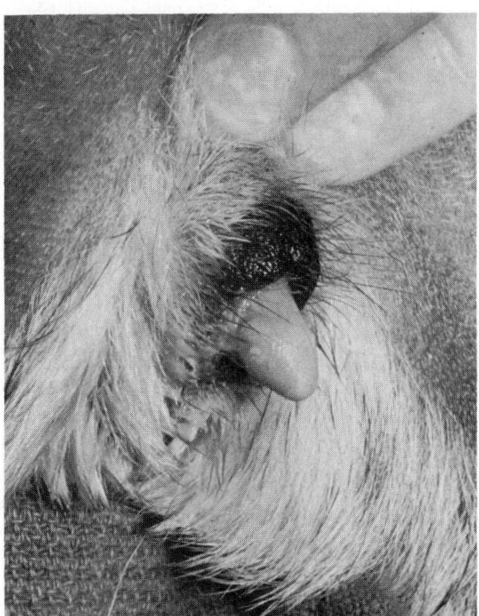

FIGURE 94–10. Hypertrophied clitoris protruding through the vulvar cleft.

Vulvar Trauma

Vulvar trauma is uncommon but usually results from dog fights, sadistic acts, injury during breeding, attempts to disrupt mating during a tie, or difficult parturition. The injuries are usually lacerations, contusions, or puncture wounds.[16] Determination of the extent of the injury and subsequent treatment may require vaginoscopy or episiotomy. Lacerations and large puncture wounds are débrided and sutured. Penrose drains are placed if needed. Bitches in estrus are separated from other dogs to prevent mating and reinjury. Large vulvar hematomas are allowed to organize 1 to 2 days before resection. Failure to remove these may result in vulvovestibular obstruction. Vaginal and vestibular douching is not recommended in trauma patients because it is traumatic. To minimize infection, systemic antibiotics are suggested rather than douching.

References

1. Alexander JE, Lennok WJ: Vaginal prolapse in the bitch. *Can Vet J 2*:428, 1961.
2. Allen WE, France C: A contrast radiographic study of the vagina and uterus of the normal bitch. *J Small Anim Pract 26*:153, 1986.
3. Burke TJ, Reynald HA: The female genital system. *In* Bojrab MJ (ed): *Pathophysiology in Small Animal Surgery*. Lea & Febiger, Philadelphia, 1981, p 425.
4. Burt TJ, Smith CW: Vulvovaginal cleft in a dog. *J Am Anim Hosp Assoc 11*:774, 1975.
5. Capel-Edwards K: Double vagina with perineal agenesis in a bitch. *Vet Rec 101*:57, 1977.

6. Gee, BR, et al: Segmental aplasia of the mullerian duct system in the dog. *Can Vet J 18*:281, 1977.
7. Holt PE, Salye B: Congenital vestibulovaginal stenosis in the bitch. *J Small Anim Pract 22*:67, 1981.
8. Jones DE, Joshua JO: *Reproductive Clinical Problems in the Dog*. Boston, Wright P.S.G., 1982, p 42.
9. McConnell DA: Correction of vaginovestibular strictures in the bitch. *J Am Anim Hosp Assoc 13*:92, 1977.
10. Olson PN: Accepted terms for theriogenology. *Soc Theriogenol Newsletter 12*:1, 1989.
11. Olson PN, Wheeler SL: Persistent uterine and vaginal hemorrhage in a beagle with factor VII defeciency. *J Am Vet Med Assoc 185*:447, 1984.
12. Rawlings CA, Capps WF: Rectovaginal fistula and imperforate anus in the dog. *J Am Vet Med Assoc 159*:320, 1971.
13. Smith KW: Female genital system. *In* Archibald J (ed): *Canine Surgery*. American Veterinary Publications, Santa Barbara, 1974, p 751.
14. Troger CP: Vaginal prolapse in the bitch. *Mod Vet Pract 53*:73, 1972.
15. Wadsworth PF, et al: Segmental aplasia of the vagina in a beagle bitch. *Lab Anim 12*:65, 1978.
16. Welser JR: The vagina and vulva. *In* Bojrab MJ (ed): *Current Techniques in Small Animal Surgery*. Lea & Febiger, Philadelphia, 1981, p 249.
17. Wilson CF, Clifford DH: Perineoplasty for anovaginal cleft in the dog. *J Am Vet Med Assoc 159*:871, 1971.
18. Wykes PM, Olson PN: The vagina. *In* Slatter DH (ed): *Textbook of Small Animal Surgery*. W.B. Saunders, Philadelphia, 1985, p 1672.
19. Wykes PM, Soderberg SF: Congenital abnormalities of the canine vagina and vulva. *J Am Anim Hosp Assoc 19*:995, 1983.

CHAPTER 95 Normal and Abnormal Parturition

Peggy M. Wykes and Patricia N. Olson

An understanding of the physiology and endocrinology of normal parturition (eutocia) is necessary for diagnosing and treating abnormal parturition (dystocia). Although the exact mechanisms that allow parturition to begin and proceed normally in a bitch are still unknown, studies of canine parturition and extrapolations from other species provide information on the physiological and endocrinological changes important for normal parturition.

PHYSIOLOGY OF PARTURITION

Changes in the concentrations of the various hormones in a dam's serum (progesterone, prolactin, estradiol) preceding and following whelping have been discussed.[1, 8–10, 27]

Fetal Factors Contributing to Parturition

The fetus is important in initiating parturition; normal fetal adrenal-pituitary-hypothalamic axis is necessary for eutocia in many animals. Normal fetal stress near parturition results in increased release of fetal corticotropin-releasing hormone, which stimulates release of adrenocorticotropic hormone (ACTH) and subsequently of cortisol[24] (Fig. 95–1). Although other tropic agents produced by the pituitary or placenta may stimulate fetal adrenals in some species, no such tropic agent has been identified for bitches.

The increase in corticoids produced by the fetal adrenal gland is believed to stimulate the release of uterine prostaglandins, which can directly stimulate uterine contractions or enter the maternal circulation to stimulate release of oxytocin from the pituitary gland (see Fig. 95–1). Mean concentrations of 13,14-dihydro-15-keto-prostaglandins $F_{2\ alpha}$ in plasma of pregnant bitches increase at the time of parturition.[7] Because fetal factors are important in initiating parturition, gestational length is often increased in a bitch with a single fetus. Similarly, puppies born with head defects may also have prolonged gestation periods, possibly owing to an abnormality of the adrenal-pituitary-hypothalamic axis that interferes with fetal steroid production.[3]

Maternal Factors Contributing to Parturition

A decrease in the progesterone/estrogen ratio at the myometrium is accepted as important for initiating normal parturition. The decrease can occur as a result of increasing concentrations of estradiol, decreasing concentrations of progesterone, or both. Because progesterone inhibits myometrial cell contractility, parturition does not occur in many species until concentrations of progesterone in the serum or placenta decline.[10] As progesterone declines (or estradiol increases) in the serum, oxytocin initiates and maintains uterine contractions. As a fetus enters the birth canal and causes mechanical distension, nerve impulses pass to the hy-

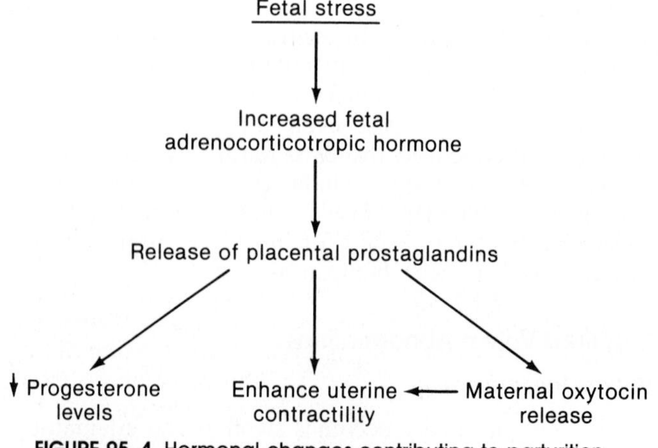

FIGURE 95–1. Hormonal changes contributing to parturition.

pothalamus and cause release of more oxytocin into the systemic circulation. Mechanical distension of the birth canal also stimulates the sensory part of a spinal reflex arc, resulting in efferent contractions of the abdominal muscles.

Relaxin, a polypeptide hormone and homologue of insulin, has an important role in remodeling the reproductive tract for parturition. Plasma relaxin levels in pregnant, lactating, and pseudopregnant bitches have been reported.[24] Immunoreactive relaxin was not detectable in plasma of pseudopregnant bitches but increased by the third or forth week of diestrus in pregnant retrievers and beagles. Peak levels were reached 2 to 3 weeks before whelping.[23]

Corticoids are elevated in the serum before whelping, but their contribution to lowering concentrations of serum progesterone and initiating labor is unclear. It is also uncertain whether the corticoids are of fetal or maternal origin. Dexamethasone (5 mg BID for 10 days) reportedly results in intrauterine death followed by fetal resorption when medication is initiated at day 30 of pregnancy or abortion when initiated at day 45 of pregnancy.[1] Because the exact role of corticoids in inducing parturition in bitches is still unknown, it seems prudent to avoid treating pregnant dogs with glucocorticoids.

HEMATOLOGICAL CHANGES DURING PREGNANCY

The packed cell volume declines in pregnant bitches, with an observed anemia (PCV < 40 per cent) reportedly occurring between 7 and 9 weeks after estrus. Smaller decreases occur in nonpregnant bitches during diestrus. Serum cholesterol and protein levels increase during diestrus in pregnant and nonpregnant bitches.[24] Increases in circulating activity of coagulation factors VII, VIII, IX, and XI occur in pregnant but not in nonpregnant diestrous bitches.[15] Various reproductive states affect the relative proportions of T_3 and T_4 secreted by the thyroid gland, peripheral conversion of T_4 to T_3, protein binding of thyroid hormones, or metabolic clearance rates of these hormones.[20] Basal concentrations of cortisol in dogs did not differ among reproductive states. Concentrations of cortisol after ACTH administration are different, with anestrus = diestrus > lactation = pregnancy = male > proestrus.[20] Therefore, the reproductive state of a dam should be considered when evaluating function of the thyroid and adrenal or pituitary glands.

SIGNS OF IMPENDING PARTURITION

Physical examination reveals signs of impending parturition. The rectal temperature drops to less than 99°F (37.22°C) approximately 8 to 24 hours before parturition and 10 to 14 hours after concentrations of progesterone in the serum decline to less than 2 ng/ml.[8] The hypothermia is transient, with the temperature rising during or immediately after parturition and remaining slightly elevated for several days. Transient hypothermia has also been observed for 1 to 2 days after ovariohysterectomy in bitches with pyometra, presumably because of the rapid decrease in concentrations of progesterone after removal of the ovaries.[5] If parturition does not occur after the decline in progesterone (i.e., dystocia), a bitch soon becomes euthermic as the thermoregulatory mechanisms readjust. Therefore, the return of a normal rectal temperature does not preclude the possibility of dystocia.

For several days before parturition, a bitch becomes restless, seeks seclusion, and may not eat. In one study, the most consistent indicator of impending parturition was relaxation of the pelvic and abdominal musculature.[13] Mammary turgidity and secretion of milk may be seen 1 to 2 weeks and nesting behavior 12 to 24 hours before parturition.[13, 14]

STAGES OF NORMAL PARTURITION

Stage 1

The first stage of labor is characterized by subclinical uterine contractions and dilation of the cervix. Although the uterine contractions are not usually externally visible a bitch may appear restless and may pant and tremble. Occasionally she vomits, and respiratory and heart rates may be elevated. She may seek seclusion and establish a nest. This first stage of labor usually lasts 6 to 12 hours, but it may persist for 36 hours in primiparous animals.

Stage 2

During the second stage of labor, each fetus passes through the birth canal and is expelled. Although the average duration of this stage is 6 to 12 hours, it may continue for 24 hours. Abdominal straining is apparent and coincides with uterine contractions. As a fetus enters the birth canal, the neuroendocrine reflex (Ferguson reflex) results in oxytocin release, which enhances uterine contractions. A bitch usually lies down during the second stage of labor. Stage 2 can be inhibited if she is disturbed or distressed. The allantois usually ruptures as a fetus enters the birth canal, and a clear, water-like fluid may pass from the vulva. The allantoic membranes occasionally may cover a newborn, but a fetus is more likely covered by only amniotic membranes at birth. A bitch frequently removes and consumes the surrounding amnion. This cleaning action aids in stimulating cardiovascular and respiratory function in the puppies. Vomiting is not uncommonly associated with consumption of the placental membranes by the dam, particularly if the entire placenta is consumed. Aspiration pneumonia due to placental vomitus can be life threatening, therefore she is discouraged from eating the placentas if possible.

Approximately 60 per cent of puppies are born in a cranial presentation, the remaining presenting in the caudal position. A caudal presentation (rear limbs first) does not predispose to dystocia like the breech presentation (complete retention or extension of the rear limbs beneath the body). Although puppies are usually delivered every one-half to 1 hour until whelping is finished, the interval between puppies can be variable, with up to 4 hours between eutocic births.

Stage 3

The third stage of parturition involves expulsion of the fetal membranes and involution of the uterus. Fetal membranes usually pass 5 to 15 minutes after birth of each pup. Because fetuses may be alternately delivered from each uterine horn, 2 puppies may be delivered consecutively before passage of their placentas. In this case, two placentas must be passed before another pup is delivered. In one study in which puppies were marked, after the birth of one pup, the next pup came from the contralateral horn in 78.2 per cent of the births.[25]

A thick greenish discharge (lochia) accompanies normal placental separation and may be observed in all three stages of labor. It may even precede the first puppy by several hours. The pigment in this discharge is uteroverdin, the product of erythrocyte breakdown in the placenta. Because expulsion of fetal membranes occurs during labor in polytocous species (producing many young at birth), stage 3 actually begins in stage 2 for dogs.

Uterine Involution

Uterine involution may continue for a period of several weeks after whelping, with complete endometrial recovery occurring by 3 months postpartum. Lochia, produced by the breakdown of hemoglobin at the placental borders, may be observed passing from the vulva of normal females for up to 3 weeks postpartum and must be differentiated from abnormal uterine discharges. Degenerative neutrophils with engulfed bacteria are frequently present on vaginal smears from animals with metritis, in contrast to healthy neutrophils frequently observed in vaginal smears from normal females after whelping. A bright red, bloody discharge may be observed postpartum with coagulopathies, trauma, or subinvolution of placental sites. Animals with subinvolution of placental sites are frequently less than 3 years of age and primiparous. These females are not systemically ill unless the retained placental tags of tissue, characteristic of the condition, become secondarily infected. Generally, the hemorrhagic discharge resolves by the next estrus and no therapy is required. Rarely, the hemorrhage is so severe that ovariohysterectomy is necessary. Although subinvolution of placental sites is fairly common in young females, retention of the whole placenta is unusual at any age. Individuals retaining entire placentas are often systemically ill, with metritis occurring as a sequel.

ABNORMAL PARTURITION

Taking a thorough history is important in establishing whether dystocia is present. Although breeding dates are helpful in determining whether gestation is prolonged, they may be of limited value because a normal female may be in estrus (and hence be mated) for up to 21 days. Gestation lengths, when based on single breeding dates, can range from 59 to 71 days.[6, 17] Nevertheless, a pregnancy longer than 68 days is considered suspect for dystocia and is evaluated; some normal pregnant bitches may be examined. The owner is questioned about past whelping and previous dystocias, because some causes of dystocia (e.g., uterine inertia, vaginal anomalies, pelvic fractures) may result in subsequent whelping difficulties.

A complete physical examination assists in determining the stage of gestation. The animals general health status must be established, and a thorough evaluation of the genital system performed. A digital examination of the vestible and vagina is carried out to determine whether (1) a fetus is lodged in the birth canal, (2) vaginal anomalies exist that might result in dystocia, or (3) firm pressure placed on the ventral or dorsal vaginal wall results in abdominal straining (Ferguson reflex). Absence of the Ferguson reflex suggests that the bitch is premature for delivery, that uterine inertia is present and she is incapable of responding to vaginal pressure, or that she is severely stressed and preventing a normal response. A vaginal examination helps characterize the presence and nature of uterine discharges. The presence of lochia suggests that placental separation has begun for at least one puppy and whelping should ensue within 2 hours.

Rectal palpation is beneficial in evaluating pelvic diameter and identifying old pelvic fractures that may cause obstructive dystocia. Abdominal palpation is routinely performed to determine whether fetuses are present. A bitch that is not pregnant or that has already completed delivery may occasionally be presented for dystocia.

Fetal heartbeats are difficult to hear through the abdominal wall in most females. Therefore, the absence of fetal heartbeats does not always correlate with fetal death, nor does the presence of fetal heartbeats guarantee viability of each puppy. Real-time ultrasonographic equipment can accurately evaluate the heart rate and viability of individual fetuses. If fetal heart rates are absent or decreased (normal rate 142 to 162 beats per minute in anesthetized dams) or if fetal motion is absent on real-time ultrasonographic evulation, dystocia is likely and the owner must be cautioned that it is unlikely that all puppies will survive.[19]

Survey radiographs of the abdomen can also be used to evaluate fetal viability; radiographic changes denoting fetal death usually do not occur until puppies have been dead for several hours (Fig. 95–2). Intravascular fetal gas, usually found in the heart, is not apparent radiographically until 6 hours after death. Overlap of the cranial bones is a less reliable sign and results from calvarial collapse around the shrunken brain about 2 days postmortem. Another sign of fetal death is an alteration of the spatial relationships between the bones of the fetal skeleton. This is especially seen in the vertebral column as a collapse of the spine following loss of axial muscle tone. The fetus may appear radiographically like a bag of bones.[11]

Survey radiographs are probably most valuable in determining the number of fetuses yet to be delivered. However, radiographic evaluation of progressive uterine enlargement and fetal mineralization has been reported and can be used as a guideline for estimation of the time until delivery.[21] The stage of fetal development can be more accurately predicted when times to luteinizing

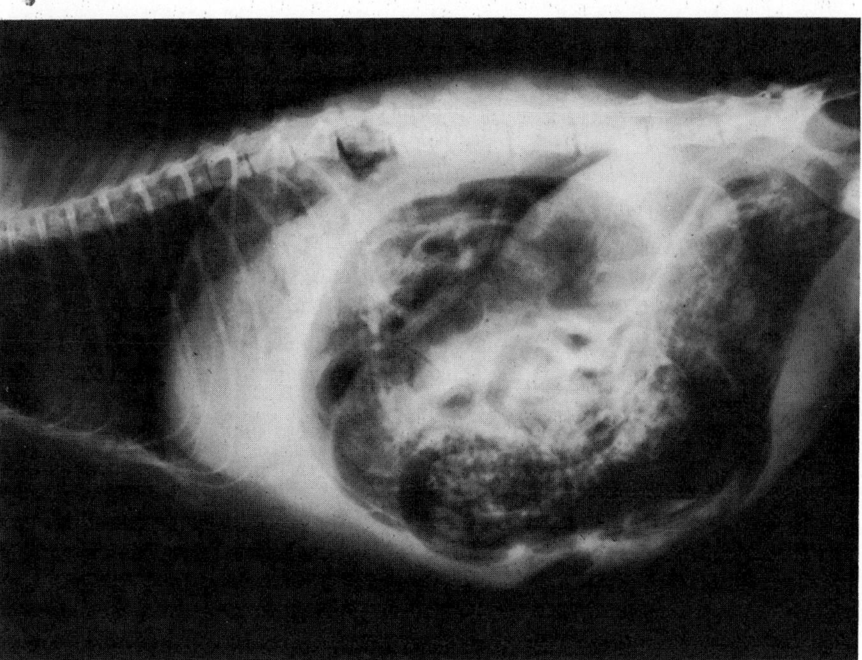

FIGURE 95–2. Free intrauterine gas or fetal gas is evidence of fetal death.

hormone peak or parturition are used rather than breeding dates. Fetal skeletal development was first detectable 45 days after luteinizing hormone peak (20 to 22 days prepartum), with uterine enlargement and fetal mineralization being detected earlier on lateral radiographs versus the dorsoventral view. At 45 days, portions of the fetal spine, skull, and ribs were seen, followed by the long bones by 48 days after luteinizing hormone peak (17 days before parturition). Mineralization of the teeth occurs by 61 days after luteinizing hormone peak. The fetuses are delivered within 8 days of radiographic appearance of teeth.

There have been no reports of fetal harm associated with late term diagnostic irradiation,[13, 14] although one study did suggest an increased risk of neoplasia after perinatal (late fetal or neonatal period) irradiation in dogs, but doses and exposure times exceeded those used diagnostically.[2]

By clinical monitoring of fetal heart rate, transcutaneous oxygen and carbon dioxide pressures, and tissue pH, investigators were able to record changes in these parameters during periods of induced fetal hypoxia. Late decelerations of the fetal heart rate are an early sign of fetal hypoxia, and a decline in fetal blood pH is a late and advanced sign of fetal distress due to hypoxia. In a toxic dam, evaluation of these parameters may be of value in identifying abnormal fetal states.[19]

Criteria for Dystocia

The following criteria for determining the presence of dystocia are guidelines and are not absolute.

Signs of Toxicity in a Pregnant Bitch. Any toxic bitch in late pregnancy should be critically evaluated for dystocia. If lochia is present in the caudal reproductive tract of a term bitch, placental separation has begun for at least on one fetus. The entire litter of puppies may die within 24 hours after the onset of dystocia that continues unrelieved. Signs of toxemia are evident in a bitch by 48 to 72 hours after intrauterine fetal death.

Prepartum pregnancy toxemia (ketosis) may occur when energy demands are high for developing fetuses and nutrient demands cannot be met by the dam. Ketonuria without glucosuria occurs in prepartum pregnancy toxemia. Hepatic lipidosis frequently accompanies this disorder.

Strong and Frequent Abdominal Straining with Failure to Produce a Puppy Within 30 Minutes. This usually suggests that a puppy is present in the birth canal but cannot pass. A puppy lodged in the birth canal can become asphyxiated if complete placental separation occurs before birth. Prolonged straining eventually results in secondary uterine inertia and cessation of labor.

Weak Straining That Fails to Produce a Puppy Within 2 Hours. Weak abdominal straining without delivery of a puppy suggests that uterine contractions are incapable of advancing the fetus into the birth canal.

More Than 4 Hours Since the Birth of the Last Puppy. If more than 4 hours has lapsed since the birth of the last puppy, parturition may be completed. If not, uterine inertia is considered, especially if the delivery has been prolonged and the myometrium is fatigued. Although some dams can deliver a live puppy after 4 hours or more, the incidence of stillbirths rises as the time interval between delivered puppies increases. If inertia develops, she will require an assisted delivery by caesarean section.

Prolonged Gestation. The average length of estrus ranges from 3 days to 3 weeks. Therefore, giving a due date for whelping based on 63 to 65 days from breeding can be erroneous. Although whelping usually occurs 57 days from the onset of diestrus as determined by vaginal cytological study, the date of onset of cytological diestrus is usually not available for an animal presented for prolonged gestation.[19] Because breeding dates frequently are an owner's only guidelines, a dam is evaluated for dystocia if 68 days or more has elapsed since the last mating. With this parameter, some normal bitches may be included, but dogs with uterine inertia may also be identified (see the later section on uterine inertia). Because a nonpregnant diestrous bitch develops mammary gland tissue and occasionally lactates, owners may occasionally present a nonpregnant animal for prolonged gestation. Radiographic evaluation can be performed to determine whether fetuses are present (fetal skeletons are usually visible between day 45 and 50 of gestation), to evaluate fetal maturity, to measure fetal size and maternal pelvic diameter, and to detect signs of fetal death. Ultrasonography is invaluable in detecting fetal motion and determining heart rates to evaluate fetal viability.

Retained Puppy Visible at Vulva. An owner may observe a puppy that cannot pass between the vulvar lips.

The Presence of Normal and Abnormal Discharge at the Vulva. The presence of lochia (a greenish discharge) indicates that placental separation has occurred and is a reliable sign that whelping should occur within a few hours for the puppies for the puppies to survive. Rarely, a single fetus may die *in utero* several days before term and lochia is passed, with the remaining puppies being born normally at term. Because this occurrence is rare, any bitch that is near term and passes a greenish discharge should be critically evaluated for dystocia.

A copious amount of a clear water-like discharge suggests that the allantoic or amniotic fluids have passed. A bloody discharge seen near term may be due to a traumatic birth or uterine torsion. Severe hemorrhage occurs at whelping in animals that have inadequate or dysfunctional clotting factors.[16, 17] Hemorrhagic discharges observed earlier in gestation are frequently associated with abortion.

TYPES OF DYSTOCIA AND BREED INCIDENCE[3, 4, 12–14, 22]

Both maternal and fetal factors can contribute to abnormal parturition, with most episodes of dystocia rarely being caused by a single morphological or physiological problem. Some of the factors have been categorized (Fig. 95–3). Maternal factors most frequently resulting in dystocia include decreased pelvic canal size (from immaturity, fractures, breed predisposition); ab-

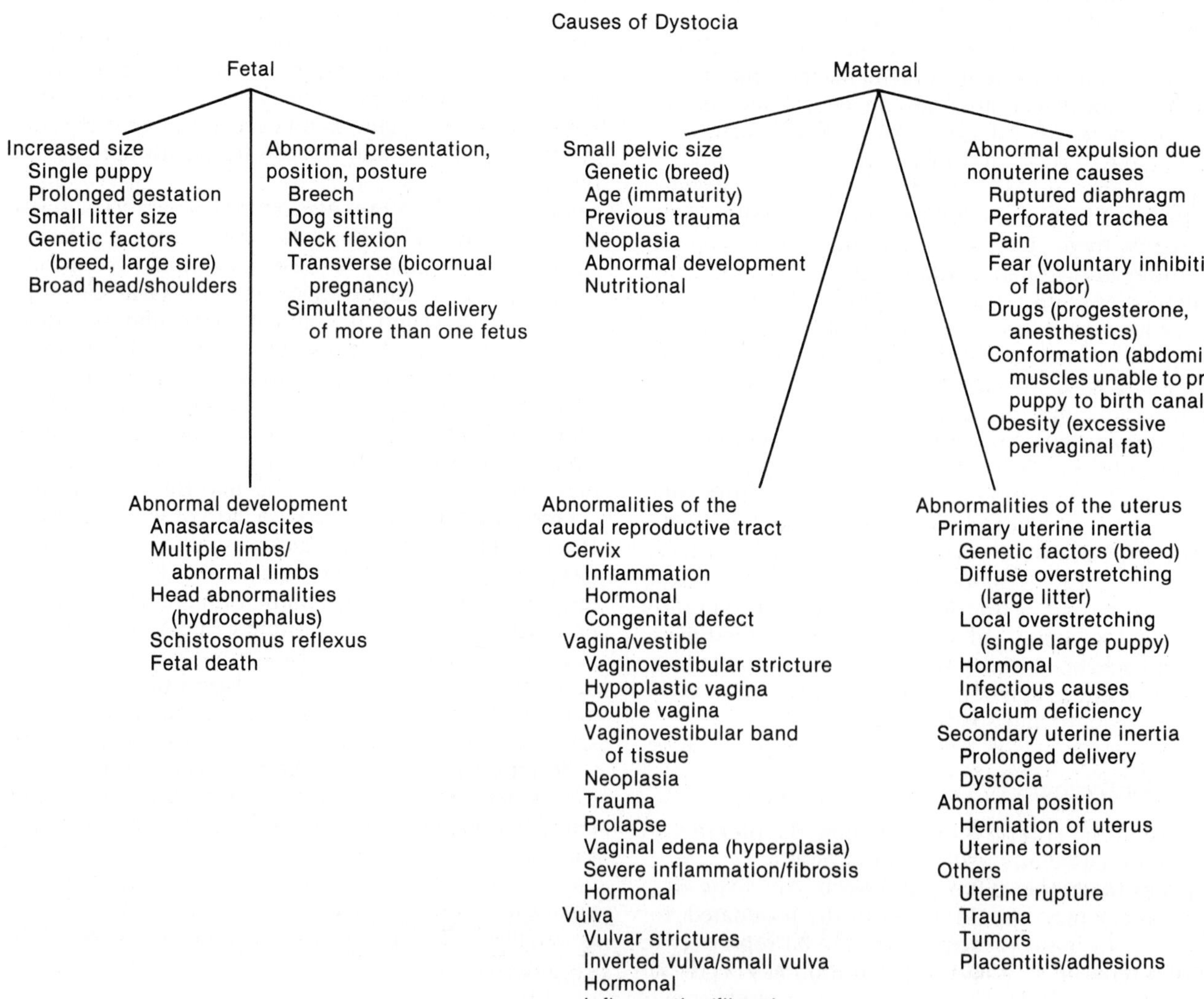

FIGURE 95–3. Causes of canine dystocia.

normalities of the vagina or vestibule (vaginal bands, vaginovestibular strictures, vaginal hypoplasia, vaginal tumors); abnormalities of the vulva (vulvar stricture); and uterine malfunction (uterine inertia, uterine rupture, uterine malposition through a hernia, or uterine torsion). Fibrosis of the cervix may prevent adequate cervical dilation and contribute to dystocia.[14]

The most common factors leading to dystocia are an oversize fetus (single puppy or puppy of a breed predisposed to large head or shoulder widths); developmental defects (fetal monsters, ascites, anasarca, hydrocephalus or hydropic conditions, hypothalamic-pituitary-adrenal axis abnormalities); and faulty presentations, positions, or postures at birth. Inadequate fetal fluids can result in fetal death due to inadequate lubrication of the birth canal.

The brachycephalic breeds frequently have obstructive dystocias owing to large fetal head sizes relative to small maternal pelvic diameters. Bulldogs may experience inadequate abdominal contractions, resulting in inconsistent advancement of a fetus into the pelvic canal. Dachshunds and Scottish terriers have a higher incidence of primary uterine inertia, whereas Saint Bernards frequently develop secondary uterine inertia as a sequel to large litter size. Greyhounds have a relatively high incidence of arrested fetal development during pregnancy and fetal death resulting in dystocia.[3, 4, 12] In one study of 118 cases of dystocia, Chihuahuas and miniature poodles had the highest incidence of dystocia.[13]

UTERINE INERTIA

Uterine inertia is failure of the uterus to expel a fetus normally and is a common cause of canine dystocia. Uterine inertia is either primary or secondary. The primary form is characterized by inability of the uterus to contract sufficiently to expel a normal-sized fetus through an unobstructed birth canal.[13] It can be due to an inherited breed predisposition, overstretching of the uterus (large litter), inadequate uterine stimulation (small litter), systemic disease (hypocalcemia, obesity, septicemia), age-related changes, or psychogenic influences.

Primary inertia is complete if no signs of second-stage labor occur. With any gestation lasting longer than 68 days, primary inertia should be suspected. Lochia is frequently observed in the vagina with complete uterine inertia, suggesting that parturition should be occurring but cannot. Partial primary inertia occurs if parturition begins normally, but uterine contractions soon fail, with insufficient activity to expel the remaining puppies. Because calcium is necessary for normal myometrial function, serum calcium should be evaluated.

In secondary uterine inertia, the uterine muscles become exhausted after prolonged contraction against an obstructing fetus or following efforts to expel a large litter or an oversized puppy. In both types of inertia, the uterine musculature fails to respond to the administration of oxytocin and the bitch fails to strain when pressure is applied *per vaginam* to the pelvic canal (lack of the Ferguson reflex).

Normal animals not yet ready to whelp may be confused with those with uterine inertia in that they may fail to demonstrate the Ferguson reflex, lack evidence of lochia, or demonstrate other signs of dystocia.

NONSURGICAL TREATMENT OF DYSTOCIA

Whether to use medical or surgical treatment to alleviate dystocia depends on the duration and cause of the dystocia. A physical examination should identify signs of toxemia, and a history might indicate the stage of labor. Pelvic obstruction of a fetus is ruled out by vaginal examination and abdominal radiographs. The number and viability of fetuses may be determined by radiographs or ultrasonography.

Ecbolics are administered only with *nonobstructive* dystocias and when uterine inertia is not complete (pups produced but not for 2 to 3 hours). The most commonly used ecbolic is oxytocin, which can be given intramuscularly or subcutaneously at 0.2 U/5 kg every 30 minutes. Although higher doses of oxytocin relieve dystocia, 0.05 U/kg IV increased uterine motility in 100 per cent.[26] Because higher doses of oxytocin may be associated with fetal hypoxemia, conservative doses are given initially. Oxtyocin stimulates uterine contraction, reduces uterine hemorrhage, promotes uterine involution, and decreases the incidence of fetal membrane retention.[13] It has the advantage of a short duration of action and is not as likely to cause uterine rupture if dystocia is present. Premature placental separation occurs with oxytocin. If a bitch fails to respond to therapy during the first hour or delivers only a single puppy every 2 or 3 hours, surgical intervention should be considered.

Ergot drugs are also ecbolics but have a much longer duration of action than oxytocin. They are more likely to cause uterine rupture and also interfere with lactation by inhibiting prolactin release from the pituitary gland.

When oxytocin fails to improve uterine contraction, calcium gluconate solution 10 per cent (1 ml/3 kg) or glucose (5 to 10 ml of 20 per cent glucose solution) may be given intraveneously.[18] Calcium solutions are frequently given with dystocias, because calcium is required for myometrial contractions. However, because most bitches presented for dystocia have normal concentrations of calcium in the serum, it is probably safer to use a balanced electrolyte solution (lactated Ringer solution) without additional calcium unless she is showing clinical signs of hypocalcemia (prepartum eclampsia).

Although some researchers have suggested tranquilizing apprehensive bitches to promote a normal delivery, many sedatives cross the placenta and affect the fetus. Barbiturates and promazine derivatives traverse the placenta, resulting in fetal depression, and are poorly metabolized by the fetal liver. If a dam is toxic, surgical intervention is beneficial to remove necrotic debris as well as the diseased uterus. On the other hand, a toxic patient is a greater anesthetic risk, and certain precautions must be taken (Section 17).

OBSTETRICAL MANAGEMENT OF DYSTOCIA: VAGINAL DELIVERY BY DIGITAL AND FORCEPS MANIPULATION

Delivery *per vaginam* by digital or forceps manipulation can be attempted for a fetus lodged within the birth canal. The indications for assisted deliver *per vaginam* are (1) to correct abnormal fetal positions (breast-head, lateral head deviation); (2) to relieve obstruction due to slight fetal oversize (assuming secondary uterine inertia has not occurred); (3) to extract the last remaining fetus in secondary uterine inertia; or (4) to relieve obstruction by extracting a dead fetus. Manipulation of a fetus within the vagina is done carefully to avoid trauma to the fetus and the vaginal wall. Vaginal infection and injury can be avoided if aseptic technique is maintained and if sufficient lubrication (K-Y Jelly)* is used during fetal extraction. With a dam standing, simple digital manipulation is attempted before extraction with obstetrical instruments. Correction of abnormal fetal disposition is often necessary to allow fetal extraction. If the obstructed fetus is beyond digital reach, vaginal delivery of the fetus is discouraged.

Several types of instruments are available for fetal extraction. Among these are Rampley sponge-holding forceps and Hobday forceps.[3, 27] Extreme care must be taken when traction is applied to the fetus with these instruments to avoid disarticulation or amputation of tails or limbs. Vaginal mucosal entrapment in obstetrical forceps is also of concern. Some people discourage use of instrumentation for fetal extraction because of the increased potential for trauma.

In some cases, fetal membranes can also be removed *per vaginam*. A pair of obstetrical forceps padded with gauze are inserted into the uterus and then twisted to "wind up" the membranes before withdrawal.[3]

---

*K-Y Jelly, Johnson & Johnson, New Brunswick, NJ.

References

1. Austad R, et al: Peripheral plasma levels of estradiol 17B and progesterone in the bitch during the estsrous cycle, in normal pregnancy, and after dexamethasone treatment. *J Reprod Fertil 46*:129, 1976.
2. Benjamin J: Neoplasms in young dogs after perinatal irradiation. *J Nat Cancer Inst 77*:563, 1989.
3. Bennett D: Normal and abnormal parturition. *In* Morrow DA (ed): *Current Therapy in Theriogenology*. W. B. Saunders, Philadelphia, 1980, p 595.
4. Bennett D: Canine dystocia—a review of the literature. *J Small Anim Pract 15*:101, 1974.
5. Blevins M: Personal communication, 1982.
6. Concannon PW: Radiographic diagnosis of canine pregnancy: Onset of fetal skeletal radiopacity in relation to times of breeding, preovulatory luteinizing hormone release, and parturition. *Am J Vet Res 44*:1506, 1983.
7. Concannon PW: Ovulation, pregnancy and parturition in the dog. *Jo Reprod Fertil 39* (Suppl):3, 1989.
8. Concannon PW, et al: The ovarian cycle of the bitch: Plasma estrogen, LH and progesterone. *Biol Reprod 13*:112, 1975.
9. Concannon PW, et al: Parturition and lactation in the bitch: Serum progestrone, cortisol and prolactin. *Biol Reprod 19*:1113, 1978.
10. Edquist LE, et al: Blood plasma levels of progesterone and estradiol in the dog during the estrous cycle and pregnancy. *Acta Endocrinol 78*:544, 1975.
11. Farrow CW, et al: Late term fetal death in the dog: Early radiographic diagnosis. *J Am Vet Radiol 17*:11, 1976.
12. Freak MJ: Practitioners'-breeders' approach to canine parturition. *Vet Rec 96*:303, 1975.
13. Gaudet DA: Retrospective study of 118 cases of canine dystocia. *J Am Anim Hosp Assoc 21*:813, 1985.
14. Gaudet DA, Kitchell BE: Canine dystocia *Comp Cont Educ 7*:406, 1985.
15. Gentry PA, Fiptrap RM: Plasma levels of specific coagulation factors and estrogens in the bitch during pregnancy. *J Small Animal Pract 18*:267, 1977.
16. Hamilton H, et al: Von Willibrands disease manifested by hemorrhage from the reproductive tract: Two case reports. *J Am Anim Hosp Assoc 21*:637, 1985.
17. Holst PA, Phemister RD: Onset of diestrus in the beagle bitch: Definition and significance. *Am J Vet Res 35*:401, 1974.
18. Irvine CHG: Hypoglycemia in the bitch. *N Z Vet J 13*:140, 1964.
19. Monheit AG, et al: Fetal heart rate and transcutaneous monitoring during experimentally induced hypoxia in the fetal dog. *Pediatr Res 23*:548, 1988.
20. Reimers TJ, et al: Effects of reproductive state on concentrations of thyroxine, 3,5,3′-triidothyronine and cortisol in serum of dogs. *Biol Reprod 31*:148, 1984.
21. Rendano VT, et al: Radiographic evaluation of prenatal development in the beagle. Correlation with time of breeding, LH release and parturition. *Vet Radiol 25*:132, 1984.
22. Soderberg SF: Vaginal disorders. *Vet Clin North Am Small Anim Pract 16*:534, 1986.
23. Steinetz BG, et al: Plasma relaxin levels in pregnant and lactating dogs. *Biol Reprod 37*:719, 1987.
24. Tietz WJ, et al: Anemia and cholesterolemia during estrus and pregnancy in the beagle. *Am J Physiol 212*:693, 1967.
25. Vander Weyden GC, et al: Intrauterine position of canine fetuses and their sequence of expulsion at birth. *J Small Anim Pract 22*:503, 1981.
26. Wheaton LG: Recording uterine motility in the nonanesthetized bitch. *Am J Vet Res 47*:1220, 1986.
27. Wykes PM, Olson PN: *In* Slatter DH (ed): *Textbook of Small Animal Surgery*. W. B. Saunders, Philadelphia, 1985, p 1681.

CHAPTER 96 Cesarean Section

Stephen D. Gilson

Although dystocia is a relatively uncommon problem in companion animals, delivery of puppies or kittens by hysterotomy (cesarean section) is a procedure most veterinarians perform many times during their careers. The decision to perform surgery for the treatment of dystocia is often made subjectively and requires consideration of the best interests of the dam, neonates, and owner (Table 96–1).[1, 6, 14] In a 10-year single-institution review of dystocia, 59 per cent of dogs required surgery.[4] The remaining 41 per cent were successfully managed by various combinations of medical therapy and manipulation.

TREATMENT OF DYSTOCIA

Perhaps the most important step in successful completion of cesarean section is appropriate treatment of the dam, including physiological stabilization, efficient surgical preparation, and safe and effective anesthesia. When the decision for surgery is made, the dam has

TABLE 96–1. GUIDELINES FOR THE USE OF CESAREAN SECTION IN TREATMENT OF DYSTOCIA

Complete primary uterine inertia (gestation > 70 days)
Incomplete primary uterine inertia refractory to medical management
Secondary uterine inertia
Relative or absolute fetal oversize
Anatomical abnormality of maternal pelvic canal
Fetal monstrosities
Uncorrectable fetal malpresentation
Fetal death with putrefaction
Previous cesarean section?

often endured hours of intensive labor. Abnormalities can include physical exhaustion, dehydration, acid-base disorders, hypotension, hypocalcemia, or hypoglycemia. Recommended laboratory tests before surgery include determination of hematocrit, total plasma protein concentration, urine specific gravity, and blood urea nitrogen and glucose concentrations. Other useful tests, which may be indicated by clinical signs, are complete blood count, blood calcium determination, or blood gas analysis. Before anesthetic induction, physiological abnormalities are stabilized or corrected to minimize risks to the dam and fetuses. Intravenous fluids (balanced electrolyte solution with dextrose if indicated, given at minimum of 10 ml/kg/hour), corticosteroids, antibiotics, and calcium gluconate are administered as needed.

Preparation for surgery should be quickly, efficiently, and quietly performed before anesthetic induction. The abdomen is clipped from xyphoid to pubis and antiseptically scrubbed. Anesthetic induction and final surgical scrubbing are performed in the operating room.

ANESTHESIA (see Chapter 173)

Various anesthetic protocols have been recommended for pregnant animals.[5, 7, 9, 13] No single protocol is best. A surgeon must consider the physiological condition of the dam and fetuses (Table 96–2) and the advantages and disadvantages of each protocol. The regimen selected should meet the needs of the patient and be familiar to the surgeon. Regional or general anesthetic techniques can be used.

TABLE 96–2. PHYSIOLOGICAL CHANGES IN THE DAM AND FETUSES DURING PREGNANCY AND PARTURITION

Dam
Increased cardiac work and decreased reserve from
Increased cardiac output
Increased blood volume, decreased erythrocyte count
Decreased pulmonary reserve and safety from hypoxia and increased anesthetic gas exchange from
Decreased lung volume and functional residual capacity
Increased oxygen consumption
Increased minute volume and alveolar ventilation
Fetuses
Inefficient drug metabolism, minimal cardiopulmonary reserve, and risk of hypothermia from
Immature hepatic and renal metabolic pathways
Immature cardiovascular-pulmonary system
Immature thermoregulatory system

TABLE 96–3. GENERAL ANESTHETIC PROTOCOLS FOR CESAREAN SECTION

Protocol 1
Atropine (0.04 mg/kg IM)
Induction with diazepam (0.2 mg/kg) and thiopental (8–12 mg/kg IV)
Maintain anesthesia with isoflurane or halothane
Protocol 2
Induction with ketamine (5–10 mg/kg) and diazepam (0.2 mg/kg IV)
Maintain anesthesia with isoflurane or halothane
Protocol 3
Atropine (0.04 mg/kg IM)
Induction with diazepam (0.2 mg/kg IV) and oxymorphone (0.05–1.0 mg/kg IV)
Maintain anesthesia with isoflurane or halothane

Regional anesthesia is induced by epidural administration of bupivacaine (1 ml/3.5 kg) or a similar drug.[13] Most patients require concurrent narcotization (oxymorphone, 0.1 mg/kg IV) for immobilization.[13] Intravenous fluid administration (20 ml/kg/hour) is essential to counteract induced vasodilation and hypotension. Advantages include minimal depression of the fetuses and dam, immobilization of the hindquarters, and reasonable visceral analgesia. Disadvantages are regional vasodilation, often resulting in hypotension, fetal hypoxia, and exacerbation of surgical bleeding. Local anesthesia (abdominal and uterine wall infiltration with lidocaine) can be used with epidural anesthesia.

General anesthesia can be provided by various combinations of drugs. Advantages are complete analgesia and immobilization. Disadvantages are depression of the fetuses and dam. Premedications are generally omitted to lessen fetal depression, and the dam is preoxygenated by face mask to prevent fetal hypoxia. Intravenous fluids are administered, and anesthetic depth is maintained at the minimum required for analgesia and immobilization. After delivery of the fetuses, routine anesthetic techniques can be used. Table 96–3 presents three examples of general anesthesia protocols.[5, 7, 9, 13]

SURGICAL TECHNIQUE

The animal is moved to the operating room, rapidly anesthetized, and placed in dorsal recumbency for final preparation. For very large animals, it may be advantageous to tilt the patient 10° to 15° to the side to remove the weight of the gravid uterus from the caudal vena cava, preventing supine hypotension syndrome.[12] In most animals (< 30 kg) this is unnecessary.[10, 11] During induction, the surgeon scrubs, gowns, and prepares the instrument table.

The animal is surgically draped, and a ventral midline incision is made from umbilicus to pubis. The linea alba is often stretched thin and the abdomen distended, so care is taken not to incise underlying organs. The uterus is exteriorized and isolated from the abdomen with moistened laparotomy sponges. A ventral midline incision is made in the uterine body (Fig. 96–1). Care is taken not to lacerate a fetus. The incision should be long enough to allow easy, rapid removal of fetuses. The fetus in the uterine body is removed first, followed in order by those in the horns. Each fetus is moved to

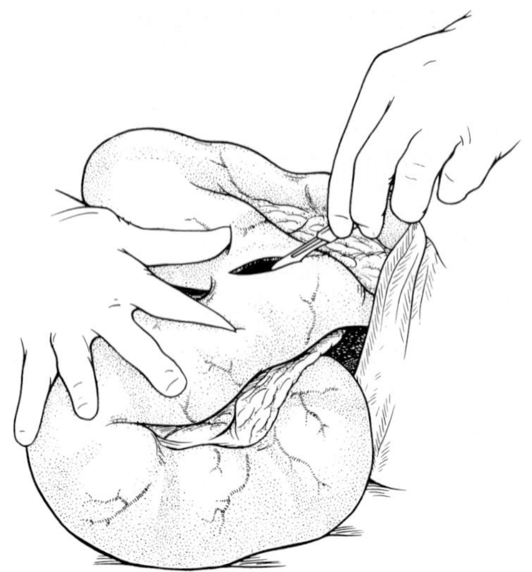

FIGURE 96–1. The uterus is exteriorized and isolated with moistened laparatomy sponges. A ventral midline incision is made in the body.

the incision site by gentle peristaltic motion on the uterine horn with the nondominant hand. The surgeon concurrently grasps the fetus intraluminally with the dominant hand and exerts gentle traction (Fig. 96–2). Once exteriorized, the amniotic sac is broken and the fetal fluids wiped or suctioned from the neonate and surgical site. If the placenta readily separates from the uterus, it is removed with the neonate, both placed in a sterile towel, and handed to an attendant. After a few minutes, the umbilicus is clamped 2 to 3 cm from the body wall and the placenta severed free. If the placenta is difficult to separate or bleeds excessively, it is left in place until all fetuses are removed. The umbilicus is clamped and cut as described, and the fetus removed.

After removal of all apparent fetuses, thorough palpation of the uterus is performed from ovaries to cervix to ensure that no fetuses remain. The uterine serosa and incision are wiped clean in preparation for closure.

The hysterotomy is closed with fine (3-0 or 4-0) absorbable suture material on a taper-point needle. Single- and double-layer closures have been recommended using various suture patterns.[1, 9, 14] A simple continuous suture pattern in the first layer (avoid penetrating the lumen), followed by a continuous Cushing pattern oversew, is generally adequate (Fig. 96–3). If sutures are carefully placed and knots buried, adhesion formation will be minimal. If the uterus does not begin involuting during closure or hemorrhage is excessive, oxytocin (5 to 20 IU IM) is given. If the abdomen is contaminated with fetal fluids, it is lavaged with 100 to 200 ml/kg of warm saline or balanced electrolyte solution. The abdomen and skin are closed routinely.

CARE OF NEONATES AND DAM

Neonatal resuscitation is instituted immediately by attendants. The amniotic membranes are vigorously wiped away to clean the neonate and stimulate respiration. The oral cavity and nostrils are cleared of fluid with suction or cotton swabs or by gently swinging the neonate in a downward arc, removing fluid by centrifugal force. If spontaneous respiration is still not evident, artificial respiration by catheter intubation or mouth-to-mouth resuscitation is instituted or respiration stimulated pharmacologically (doxapram, 1 to 2 drops PO). If narcotics were used as part of the dam's anesthetic regimen, naloxone can be given to the neonates (1 to 2 drops PO). Oxygen is administered if cyanosis or respiratory depression is present. After several minutes, the clamps are removed from the umbilicus and the stump dipped in povidone-iodine solution. If hemor-

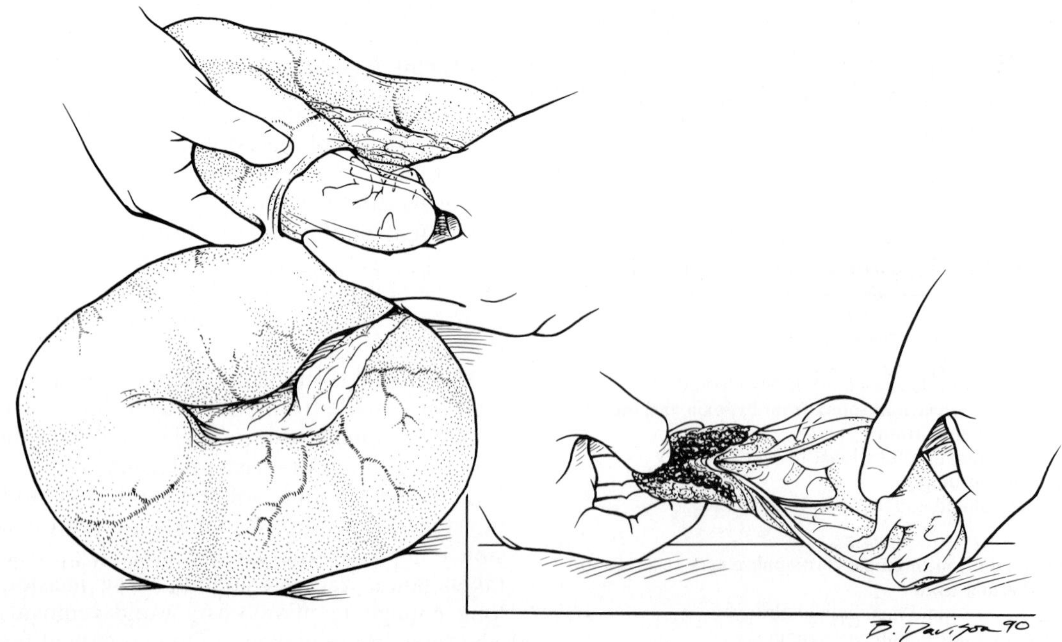

FIGURE 96–2. A fetus is gently brought to the incision site and removed with the placenta. The amniotic sac is broken and removed from the fetus.

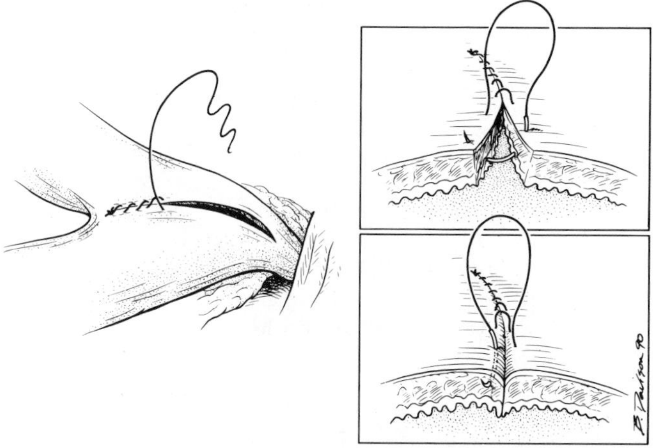

FIGURE 96–3. Fetal fluids are cleaned from the surgical field. *Upper right,* the hysterotomy incision is closed with a simple continuous suture pattern (avoid penetrating the uterine lumen). *Lower right,* A Cushing's pattern oversew follows.

rhage persists, the umbilicus is ligated. The neonate is quickly inspected for obvious birth defects (e.g., cleft palate, atresia ani, limb deformities) and placed in a warm container (91.4°F [33°C]).

Neonates are introduced to the dam after both have completely recovered from the effects of anesthesia. If the dam rejects the neonates, vaginal placental fluids rubbed onto their fur may facilitate acceptance. A few bitches require a muzzle or tranquilization in the early postpartum period. The dam is checked for the presence of colostrum and monitored for hemorrhage.

COMPLICATIONS

Potential postoperative complications include hemorrhage, hypovolemia and hypotension, and peritonitis due to exposure to uterine fluids. In animals in which uterine viability is questionable, ovariohysterectomy (with prior owner approval) is performed concurrently with cesarean section. This does not adversely affect the dam's milk production because prolactin and cortisol maintain lactation.[14]

Once an animal has undergone a cesarean section, it is not known whether subsequent litters should be delivered by cesarean section. For women, the addage has been "once a cesarean, always a cesarean. . . ."[2] This remains true for hysterotomies made along the anterior uterine body midline (similar to that described here) in women but is no longer held true for the more often performed low transverse hysterotomy incision.[3, 8] Based on experience in women and until further information is available, it is probably advisable to deliver subsequent litters surgically. Further studies are needed to evaluate the use of low transverse hysterotomy incisions and subsequent trials of labor in animals.

References

1. Bennett D: Canine dystocia—a review of the literature. *J Small Anim Pract 15*:101, 1974.
2. Craigin EB: Conservatism in obstetrics. *NY State J Med 104*:1, 1916.
3. Duff P, et al: Outcome of trial of labor in patients with a single previous low transverse cesarean section for dystocia. *Obstet Gynecol 71*:380, 1988.
4. Gaudet DA: Retrospective study of 128 cases of canine dystocia. *J Am Anim Hosp Assoc 21*:813, 1985.
5. Gilroy Ba, De Young DJ: Cesarean section. Anesthetic management and surgical technique. *Vet Clin North Am Small Anim Pract 16*:483, 1986.
6. Jones DE, et al: *Reproductive Clinical Problems in the Dog*. Wright, London, 1988, pp 87–112.
7. Marcella KL, Short CE: Anesthetic management of the pregnant animal. *Comp Cont Educ Pract Vet 6*:942, 1984.
8. Martin JN Jr, et al: Vaginal birth after cesarean section: The demise of routine repeat abdominal delivery. *Obstet Gynecol Clin North Am 15*:719, 1988.
9. Probst CW, Webb AI: Cesarean section in the dog and cat: Anesthetic and surgical techniques. *In* Bojrab MJ (ed): *Current Techniques in Small Animal Surgery*. Lea & Febiger, Philadelphia, 1983, pp 346–351.
10. Probst CW, Webb AI: Postural influence on systemic blood pressure, gas exchange, and acid/base status in the term-pregnant bitch during general anesthesia. *Am J Vet Res 44*:1963, 1983.
11. Probst CW, et al: Postural influence on systemic blood pressure in large full-term pregnant bitches during general anesthesia. *Vet Surg 16*:471, 1987.
12. Scott DB: Inferior vena caval occlusion in late pregnancy and its importance in anesthesia. *Br J Anaesth 40*:120, 1968.
13. Wright M: Anesthesia for the pregnant bitch. *In* Morrow DA (ed): *Current Therapy in Theriogenology*. 2nd ed. W. B. Saunders, Philadelphia, 1986, pp 502–504.
14. Wykes PM, Olson PN: Surgical management of dystocia. *In* Slatter D (ed): *Textbook of Small Animal Surgery*. W. B. Saunders, Philadelphia, 1985, pp 1689–1691.

CHAPTER **97**

Testes and Epididymides

Harry W. Boothe

ANATOMY

Testes

The testes are positioned obliquely within the scrotum, with their long axis directed dorsocaudally. Average testicular dimensions for a 12-kg dog are a length of 3 cm, a width of 2 cm, and thickness of 2 cm.[12]

The testes, epididymides, and spermatic cords are covered by peritoneum originating from within the abdomen (Figs. 97–1 through 97–3). The parietal vaginal tunic is the outer layer, whereas the visceral vaginal tunic is continuous with the parietal peritoneum of the abdominal cavity.[12] Deep to the vaginal tunic is the tunica albuginea, a dense white fibrous capsule.[12] Su-

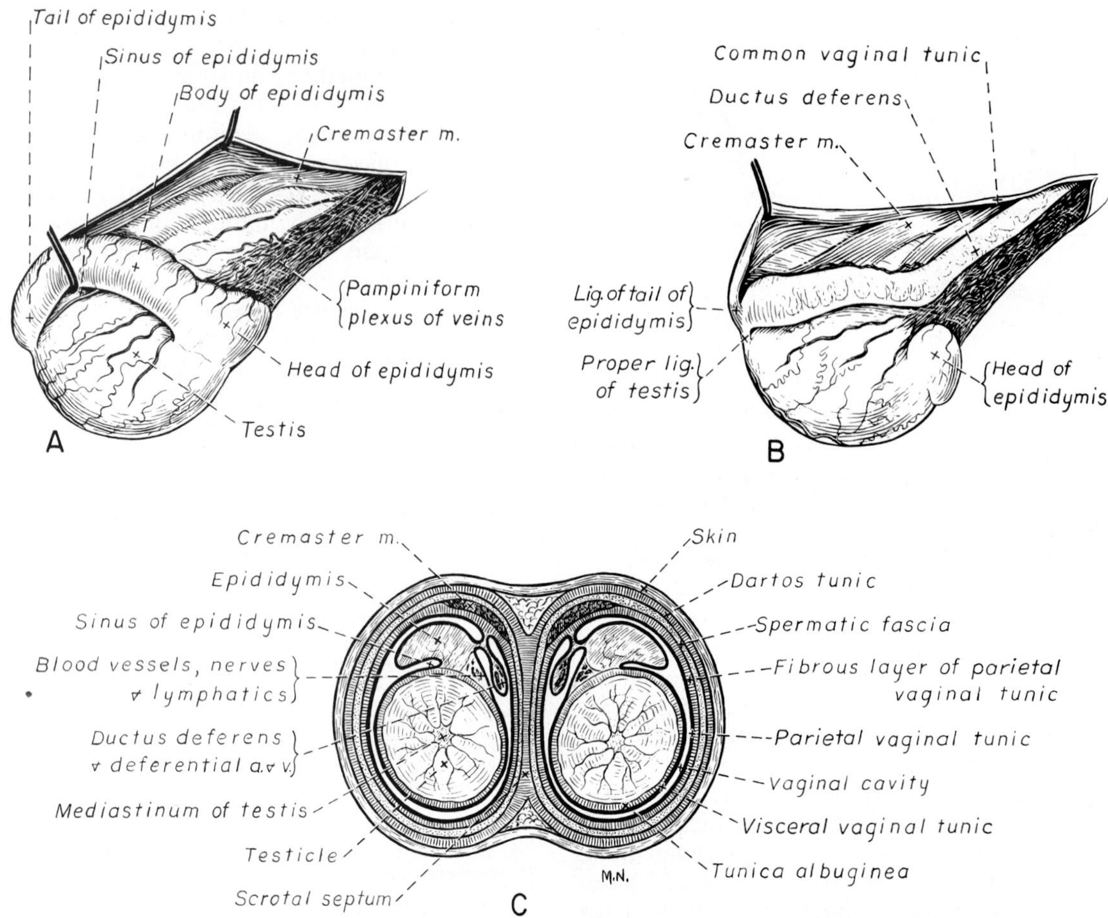

FIGURE 97–1. Structures of testes and scrotum. *A*, Right testis, lateral aspect. *B*, Left testis, medial aspect. *C*, Schematic cross section through scrotum and testes. (Reprinted with permission from Evans HE, Christensen GC (eds): *Miller's Anatomy of the Dog.* 2nd ed. W. B. Saunders, Philadelphia, 1979.)

perficial branches of the testicular artery and vein are contained in this inelastic covering. The testes are divided into lobules by connective tissue septa (septula testis), which contain blood vessels, lymphatics, and nerves.[30] These connective tissue lamellae connect the deep surface of the tunica albuginea to the centrally located mediastinum testis.

The testes and epididymides are connected to the parietal vaginal tunic at the caudal extremity of the epididymides by the caudal ligaments of the epididymides, which stabilize the testes. The testes are also indirectly stabilized by the spermatic cords and their reflected vaginal tunics (see Fig. 97–3).

The testicular arteries are tortuous and arise from the aorta at the level of the fourth lumbar vertebra.[12] The right testicular artery originates cranial to the left. The testicular veins follow the arterial pattern but form an extensive pampiniform plexus in the spermatic cord. The right testicular vein empties into the caudal vena cava, and the left terminates in the left renal vein.

Testicular lymphatics anastomose into a variable number of trunks that drain into the iliac lymph nodes. The testicular nerve supply is autonomic and contains postganglionic sympathetic fibers arising from the third to fifth lumbar sympathetic ganglia.[13]

Epididymides

The epididymides are relatively large in dogs. They lie along the dorsolateral border of the testes in both dogs and cats, being attached to the testes by the visceral vaginal tunic. The three parts of the epididymis are head, body, and tail.[31] The head communicates with the testis, beginning on its medial surface, but immediately twists around the cranial extremity to reach the lateral side.[12] The body is the middle part, being slightly smaller than the head. The tail is attached by the tough proper ligament of the testis to the caudal testicular extremity and is continuous with the ductus deferens.

The artery of the ductus deferens, a branch of the prostatic artery, supplies the epididymis and anastomoses with the testicular artery.[12] Epididymal lymphatics drain into the iliac lymph nodes. The ductus deferentes extend along the dorsomedial border of the testes, ascend in the spermatic cords, and connect the epididymides with the pelvic urethra.

PHYSIOLOGY

Testes

The testes release spermatozoa and fluid into the seminiferous tubules and elaborate male sex hormones.[17]

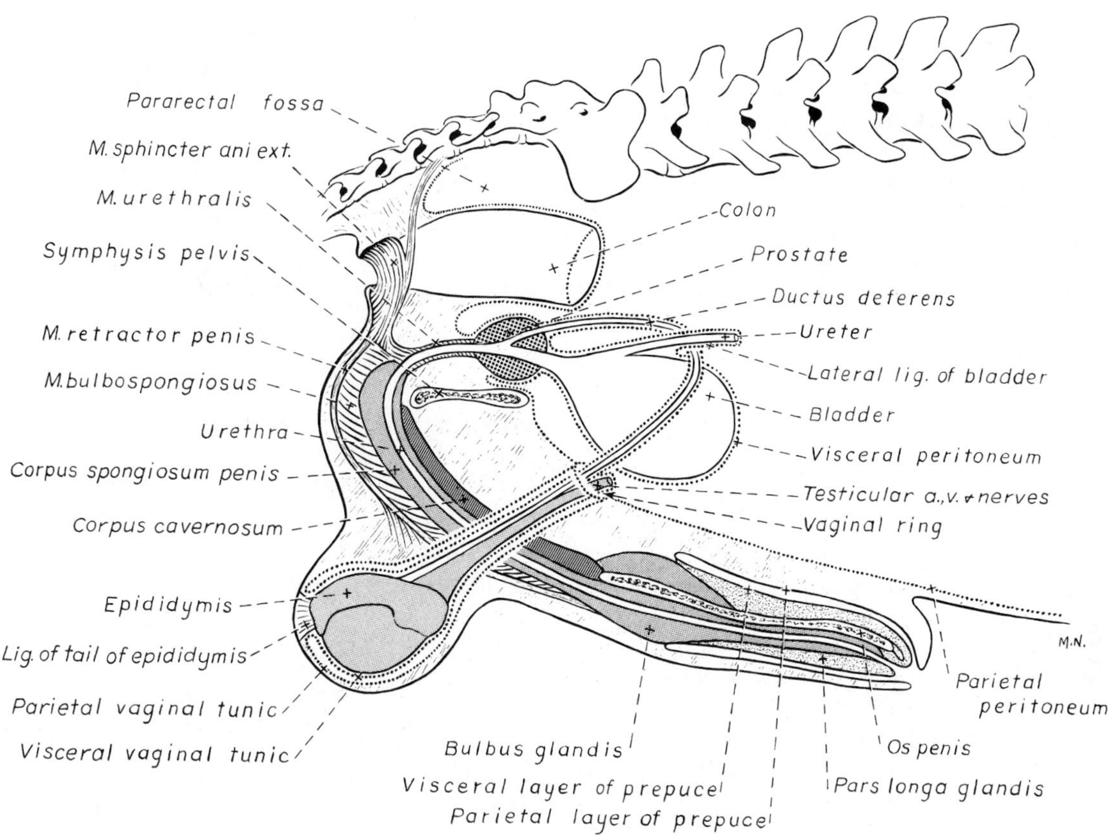

FIGURE 97–2. Peritoneal reflections and the male genitalia. (Reprinted with permission from Evans HE, Christensen GC (eds): *Miller's Anatomy of the Dog.* 2nd ed. W. B. Saunders, Philadelphia, 1979.)

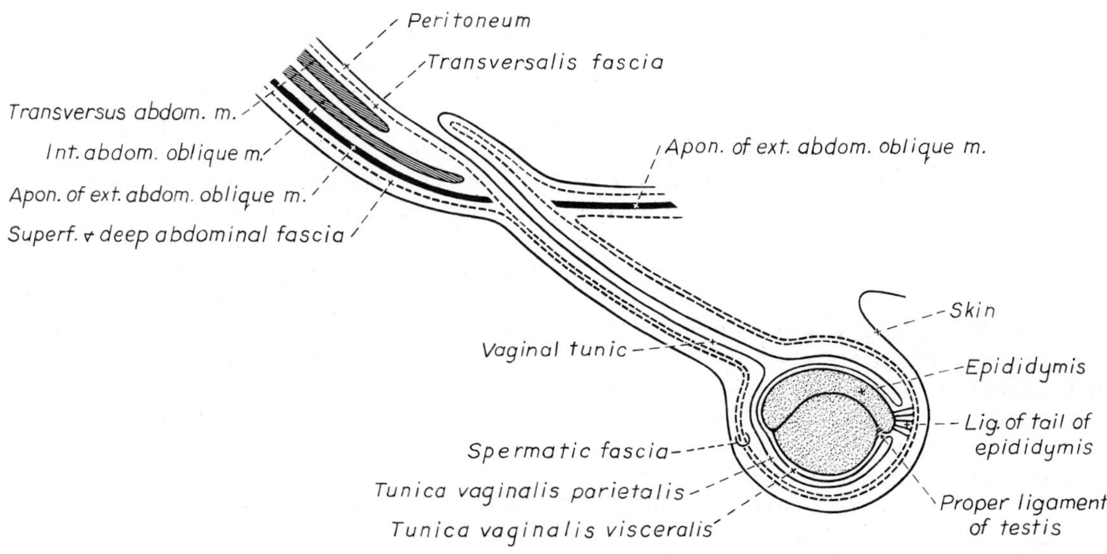

FIGURE 97–3. Sagittal section of the inguinal canal and vaginal process of the male. (Reprinted with permission from Evans HE, Christensen GC (eds): *Miller's Anatomy of the Dog.* 2nd ed. W. B. Saunders, Philadelphia, 1979.)

Both testicular functions are regulated by gonadotropins and depend on precise thermoregulation. Spermatic cord vascular architecture, cremaster muscle function, and scrotal structure and function all help maintain the scrotal temperature below general body temperature.

The exocrine portion of the testes is the seminiferous tubules. They are composed of supporting cells and spermatogenic cells.[4] Sertoli cells provide support and are involved in the release of spermatozoa (spermiation). Sertoli cells are more resistant to many noxious agents than other testicular cells.[36]

Spermatogenesis is the sequence of events by which spermatogonia are transformed into spermatozoa.[4] This process consists of mitotic and meiotic activity, as well as a maturation phase.[36] Spermatogenesis is a continuous process that is controlled by gonadotropins from the pituitary. It is decreased by elevated testicular temperatures, nutritive deficiencies, and many noxious agents.

The principal constituent of the endocrine portion of the testes is the interstitial cells (Leydig cells); however, Sertoli cells also have a role. Leydig cells produce androgens in response to interstitial cell-stimulating hormone in synergy with follicle-stimulating hormone and probably prolactin.[36] Androgens are involved with spermatogenesis, maintenance of the accessory glands and secondary sex characteristics, and changes associated with sexual maturity. Interstitial cell function is not severely reduced in ectopic testes, in contrast to the severely damaging effect that the intra-abdominal or other ectopic position of the testes has on the germinal epithelium.[36] Sertoli cells are the most probable source of testicular estrogens, which have been isolated from the testes of dogs and other species.[36]

A blood-testis barrier comparable to the blood-brain barrier has been described; however, its significance is not fully understood.[17] The barrier may be responsible for the gradient between androgen levels in the blood and in the seminiferous tubules. The antigenic properties of spermatozoa are also, in part, associated with the blood-testis barrier. Gonadotropins and temperature influence this barrier.[17]

Epididymides

The epididymides function in the storage, maturation, and transport of spermatozoa.[17] Functional regions of the epididymides (head, body, and tail) do not necessarily correspond to anatomical regions.

Spermatozoa are stored primarily in the tail of the epididymis, which is capable of preserving them for fairly long periods. Ejaculated spermatozoa in dogs and cats originate mainly from the epididymides. The epididymal tail is located in the coolest part of the scrotum, which may be related to its storage function. Sperm maturation also occurs in the epididymides. Maturation is characterized by changes in both structure and function. Spermatozoa acquire the progressive forward motility of mature sperm, develop the capacity for fertility, and become less resistant to thermal stress. Epididymal spermatozoa also have a different metabolic pattern from testicular spermatozoa.[36]

Maintenance of epididymal functions and cellular integrity depends on androgenic hormones.[43] Androgen receptors have been demonstrated in the canine epididymides.[43, 44] Circulating androgen as well as testicular fluid androgen probably regulate epididymal function (e.g., the effect of androgen on epididymal contractile activity).[17]

DISORDERS

Testes

Anorchism and Monorchism

Congenital absence of both testes in small animals is rare.[1, 10] Monorchism is reported, with the left testis usually being absent.[21] Diagnosis of these conditions is made after careful palpation of the scrotum and inguinal region and exploratory celiotomy. A thorough search of the abdomen is performed to establish the lack of one or both testes, epididymides, and ductus deferentes.

Testicular Hypoplasia

Testicular hypoplasia may be present unilaterally or bilaterally. Hypoplastic testes are usually freely movable within the scrotum and may be difficult to palpate, particularly in obese patients. Hypoplastic testes are usually of normal or soft consistency. When accompanied by excessive connective tissue, however, a hypoplastic testis is firmer than normal.[23] Hypoplastic testes usually are incapable of spermatogenesis; however, interstitial (Leydig) cell function may be present. Some dogs with testicular hypoplasia exhibit signs of feminization. Treatment is orchidectomy.

Cryptorchidism

Cryptorchidism, the most common congenital testicular defect, is a failure of one or both testes to descend into the scrotum at the usual time.[9] The usual time of testicular descent is at birth, although descent may occur normally at any time up to 6 months of age.[9] Cryptorchidism may be unilateral or bilateral, and the position of an ectopic testis may be prescrotal, inguinal, or abdominal.[9] Unilateral cryptorchidism is more common, with the right testis being more commonly undescended.[9, 38] Ectopic testes are probably more commonly located in the abdomen than in the inguinal region.[8, 37] Reported incidences of canine cryptorchidism vary widely, from 0.8 per cent for a large study involving dogs of all ages, to 10 per cent for a smaller study involving dogs at least 6 months of age.[8]

Cryptorchidism may be a hereditary condition involving a single recessive autosomal gene.[6] Because of its atypical environment, an ectopic testis is exposed to normal body temperatures. Long-term exposure to normal body temperatures results in degeneration of the germinal epithelium and loss of exocrine function. Because the interstitial cells and Sertoli cells continue to function, endocrine function of the ectopic testis is nearly normal. Secondary characteristics develop normally, even in a bilaterally cryptorchid animal. Unilateral cryptorchidism results in disturbed function of the scrotal testis.[22]

Ectopic testes, particularly intra-abdominal testes, are more susceptible to torsion and neoplasia than descended testes.* Presumably, the ectopic position allows greater movement of the testes than is possible in the scrotum.[32] The abnormal environment of an ectopic testis may partially explain why neoplasia, particularly Sertoli cell tumor and seminoma, is more commonly observed in an ectopic testis.[37] Cryptorchid dogs have a risk of testicular tumors 13.6 times that of normal dogs.[19] Approximately 50 per cent of Sertoli cell tumors and 33 per cent of seminomas occurred in cryptorchid testes in one study of canine testicular neoplasia, compared with 10.2 and 11.8 per cent, respectively, in breed-matched noncryptorchid control dogs.[8] Signs of feminization have also been more commonly observed with Sertoli cell tumors of cryptorchid testes than scrotal testes.[8, 27] Neoplasms of ectopic testes are also observed at a younger age than neoplasms of descended testes.

Diagnosis of cryptorchidism, particularly in a young pup, may be difficult. Testes may be located in the scrotum but be difficult to palpate because of their small size, especially in an obese pup. Testes may also be freely movable between the scrotum and inguinal canal. A final diagnosis of cryptorchidism should not be made until the dog is approximately 6 months of age.[2, 9] Ectopic testes, unless tumorous or diseased, are uniformly smaller than descended testes. Locating an extra-abdominal ectopic testis by palpation is usually possible, although often difficult. Intra-abdominal ectopic testes are usually palpable only when enlarged (Fig. 97–4).

Cryptorchidism is more common in the Chihuahua, miniature schnauzer, Pomeranian, poodle, Shetland sheepdog, Siberian husky, and Yorkshire terrier.[33] Small breeds have a 2.7 times greater risk of cryptorchidism than other breeds.[33] Although the specific genetic basis of canine cryptorchidism is unclear, the hereditary nature of this problem in miniature schnauzers has been discussed.[8]

Medical and surgical attempts to move ectopic testes into the scrotum have been largely unsuccessful in dogs.[42] Orchiopexy is not condoned in veterinary medicine because of the heritable nature of cryptorchidism.[6] Although the incidence of testicular neoplasia in dogs is unknown, the higher risk of neoplasia in cryptorchid testes may justify prophylactic removal of undescended testes. The high incidence of multiple tumors of more than one histological type in the same or opposite testis justifies bilateral orchidectomy.[6] Another advantage of early bilateral orchidectomy in a unilaterally cryptorchid dog is that it decreases the possibility of perpetuating the defect.

The surgical technique for removal of a cryptorchid testis varies with its location. An extra-abdominal ectopic testis is removed by the usual technique, except that the skin incision is usually made directly over the testis. Abdominal testes are generally approached from a ventral median and parapreputial abdominal incision. An ectopic testis can be located by tracing (1) the ductus deferens from its prostatic termination to the testis, (2) the testicular artery from its aortic origin to the testis, (3) the testicular vein from its termination in the caudal vena cava (or left renal vein) to the testis, or (4) the gubernaculum testis to the testis. I prefer tracing the ductus deferens from its prostatic termination to the testis. Once located, the vessels and ductus deferens are doubly ligated and divided. Histological evaluation of the testes is performed.

The prognosis for a cryptorchid dog after castration is generally favorable, even with testicular neoplasia. Testicular neoplasms are generally benign, and the incidence of observed metastasis is low (Chapter 159).

*See references 8, 11, 20, 28, 32, 39, and 41.

Orchitis

Infection of the testis in a dog is not uncommon and is frequently accompanied by epididymitis. Clinical signs of acute orchitis include testicular pain, tenseness, and scrotal edema. Acute orchitis is usually suppurative, with the formation of one or more abscesses in the testis and epididymis. Systemic signs of infection, including leukocytosis, pyrexia, and listlessness, may be present. Involvement of the parietal vaginal tunic in the inflammatory process may result in formation of a fistula through the scrotal skin to the exterior.[23] Signs of chronic orchitis are usually limited to the finding of a small, firm, irregular testis with an enlarged epididymis.[23] The scrotal contents usually adhere to the tunics and cannot be moved freely.[38] Diagnosis is made by physical examination, cytological and bacteriological examination of the semen, and possibly serological examination.

Infection may be acute or chronic and unilateral or bilateral. Infection reaches the testis most commonly by reflux along the ductus deferens from the urinary bladder, urethra, or prostate, although the hematogenous route or local extension from penetrating wounds of the scrotum are also possible.[21, 23] Bacterial organisms frequently found are *Escherichia coli, Proteus* spp., *Staphylococcus* spp., and *Streptococcus* spp.[40] Although not a common feature, orchitis may be encountered in *Brucella canis* infection.[15] Because of accompanying inflammation and autoimmune reactions, testicular infection relatively rapidly results in reduced fertility or infertility.[14, 21, 40] Atrophy and fibrosis of the testes as well as fibrotic stenosis of the epididymis are possible sequelae of infection.[6]

Treatment of orchitis depends on the extent of involvement and breeding usefulness of the dog (see Fig. 97–4). Severely traumatized or abscessed testes are surgically removed. Removal of chronically inflamed testes is justified to prevent continuing episodes of acute inflammation.[6] Antibacterial drugs, local hypothermia, and possibly anti-inflammatory drugs are used to treat less severe orchitis.[14] Primary foci of infection elsewhere in the urogenital tract are eliminated. Local treatment of sinus tracts in the parietal tunic and scrotum consists of excision, drainage, and flushing with an appropriate antibiotic. The prognosis for maintaining fertility is guarded, because orchitis is quite resistant to antibiotic or chemotherapeutic treatment. Orchidectomy is usually

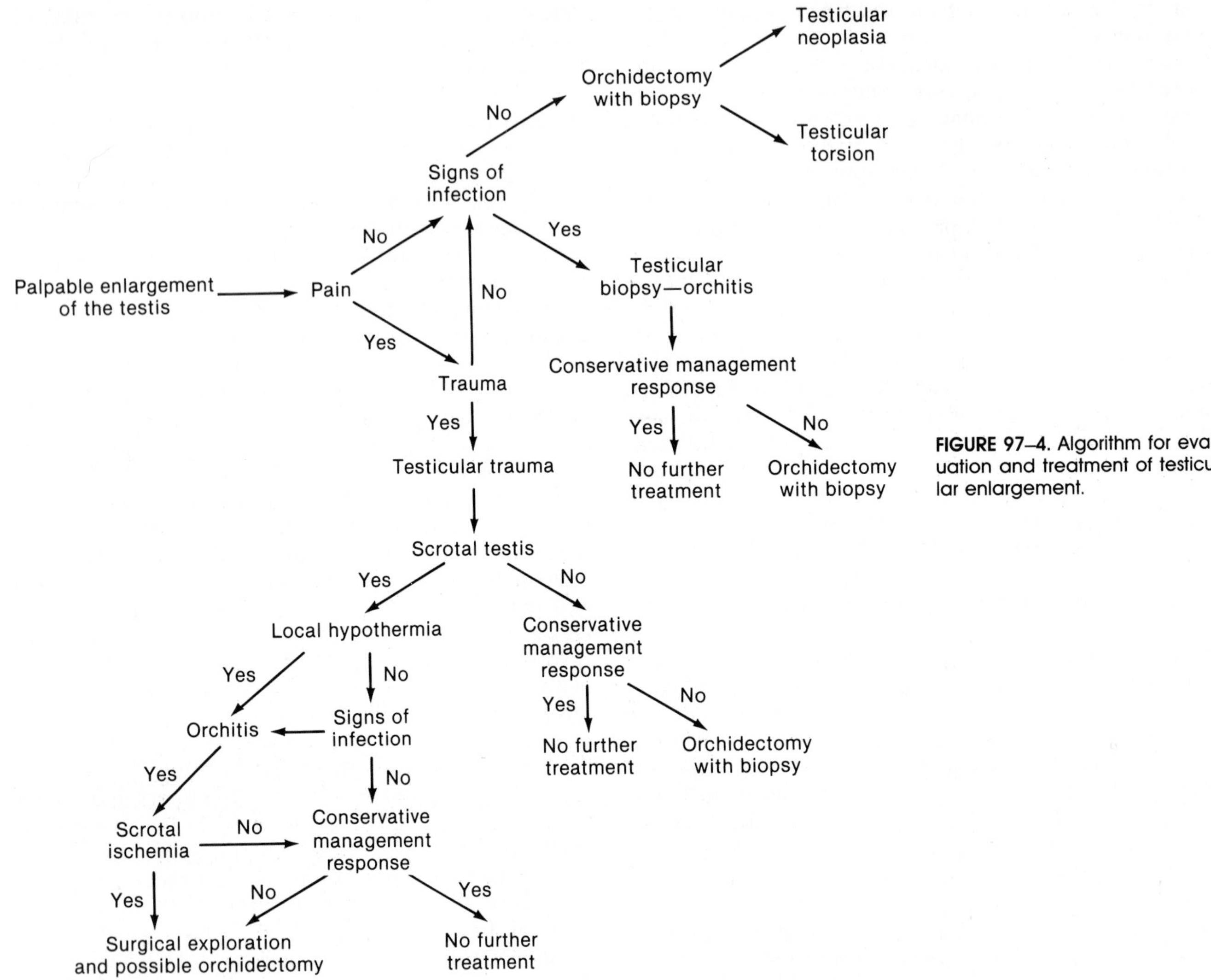

FIGURE 97–4. Algorithm for evaluation and treatment of testicular enlargement.

the treatment of choice, particularly if the patient is not a valuable breeding dog.[26]

Testicular Trauma

Despite their exposed location, testes are not commonly traumatized in dogs and cats. Clinical signs usually include local pain and swelling of the testis with possible hindlimb lameness. Scrotal swelling and bruising may be seen in more severe testicular lesions. Local hemorrhage and rupture of the tunica albuginea with resulting massive scrotal hematoma may accompany severe blunt testicular trauma.[6] Penetrating wounds frequently cause hemorrhage and may lead to local infection.

Testes may be injured by either blunt trauma or penetrating wounds. Any trauma to the testis, epididymis, or spermatic cord is potentially dangerous because it is frequently accompanied by hemorrhage. The expansile nature of the scrotum permits development of large hematomas after rupture of even small blood vessels.[6] Damage to testicular tissue can lead to leakage of sperm into the interstitial tissue and eventually the formation of spermatic granulomas, which develop because of the antigenic properties of sperm. Immune-mediated orchitis may develop, with reduction of spermatogenesis throughout both testes.[24] Local testicular hyperthermia following trauma can result in temporarily or permanently reduced fertility. A traumatized testis is predisposed to infectious orchiepididymitis because of accompanying edema and congestion.[24] The original injury can be aggravated if the animal persists in licking the traumatized scrotum and testes.

Diagnosis of testicular trauma is established by physical examination. Careful palpation often reveals an abnormal testicular contour.[16] Rupture of the tunica albuginea may be difficult to detect because of swelling of the scrotum and testis. Swelling, local hypothermia, loss of sensation, and blue discoloration of the scrotum are grave signs indicating irreversible damage due to ischemia.[6]

Medical treatment is indicated for minor testicular trauma. Local hypothermia, possibly supportive bandaging, and antibiotics and corticosteroids are often used. Analgesics and diuretics may also be indicated. Fluid accumulations are aseptically aspirated. If blood refills the scrotum, surgical exploration is considered for hemostasis.[6]

Surgical exploration of the scrotum is performed by longitudinally incising the cranial aspect of the scrotum. After the fluid accumulations are removed, a systematic search of the scrotum and testes is performed. The parietal vaginal tunic may be incised to repair wounds of the tunica albuginea. Bleeding vessels are ligated with fine synthetic absorbable sutures. Tears in the tunica albuginea are sutured with fine synthetic absorbable sutures after excision of protruding testicular tissue and thorough lavage with physiological saline. Fine sutures are used to close the parietal vaginal tunic and scrotum separately. Appropriate antibiotics are continued postoperatively.

Severe testicular trauma often requires unilateral or bilateral orchidectomy, possibly with scrotal ablation. Orchidectomy is delayed until the injury can be assessed.[21] Indications for orchidectomy following trauma include persistent pain, swelling, or local hyperthermia (see Fig. 97–4).[6]

Testicular Tumors

Testicular tumors occur commonly in dogs, particularly older dogs (Chapter 159). Clinical signs may include increased firmness or nodular enlargement of the scrotal or ectopic testis. Signs of pain or feminization may be noted.[3]

Testicular tumors are the second most frequently reported tumors in male dogs.[19] The three common neoplasms are seminoma, interstitial cell tumor, and Sertoli cell tumor, each with about equal frequency.[19] They can occur individually, although a combination of two or more tumors in a testis is common.[19] The differential diagnosis includes torsion of the spermatic cord, testicular and spermatic cord trauma, orchitis, epididymitis, spermatocele, scrotal hernia, and scrotal neoplasia (see Fig. 97–4).

Definitive diagnosis of testicular neoplasia is by biopsy of the involved testis. An excisional wedge biopsy of the testis away from the epididymis is preferred to percutaneous needle techniques.[5] Hemorrhage is controlled with digital pressure and closure of the tunica albuginea. The chance of adhesions may be reduced by offsetting incisions in the parietal vaginal tunic and the tunica albuginea.[25]

Orchidectomy

Orchidectomy in Dogs

Canine orchidectomy can be performed by either open or closed methods. Both methods use a midline prescrotal skin incision (Fig. 97–5*A*). The testis is pushed cranially to the skin incision, and the subcutaneous tissue and spermatic fascia are incised over the testis to expose the parietal vaginal tunic (Fig. 97–5*B*).[35] The testis is exteriorized and freed from its scrotal attachment by incising the spermatic fascia and scrotal ligament close to the testis (Fig. 97–5*C*). Fat and fascia surrounding the parietal vaginal tunic are reflected using a gauze sponge (Fig. 97–5*D*), enabling greatest exteriorization of the testis and spermatic cord (Fig. 97–5*E*).

In the open method, an incision is made through the parietal vaginal tunic covering the spermatic cord at the point where ligatures are to be placed. The components of the spermatic cord are double ligated using a transfixation ligation. The parietal vaginal tunic and cremaster muscle are ligated in an encircling ligature distal to the spermatic cord ligation. Alternatively, the parietal vaginal tunic can be incised just before exteriorization of the testis. The tunics are separated from the remainder of the spermatic cord (Fig. 97–6*A*), and these two structures are double ligated separately (Fig. 97–6*B*).

In the closed method, the intact spermatic cord and vaginal tunics are double ligated using two transfixation ligatures. The needle can be safely inserted through the spermatic cord between the cremaster muscle and the ductus deferens (Fig. 97–7*A* and *B*). The spermatic cord is transected distal to the ligature and returned to the inguinal region (Fig. 97–7*C* and *D*).

The other testis is removed in the same manner and through the same skin incision, if indicated. The subcutaneous tissues are closed with 3-0 absorbable suture material. The skin may be closed with nonabsorbable interrupted sutures or by a subcuticular pattern of 3-0 absorbable suture material.

Orchidectomy in Cats

Feline orchidectomy is usually performed by making a separate longitudinal scrotal incision over each testis (Fig. 97–8*A*). The testis is pushed caudally to the skin incision, and the subcutaneous tissue and parietal vaginal tunic are incised. The parietal vaginal tunic is grasped with hemostats, separated from the testis, and excised (Fig. 97–8*B* and *C*). Occlusion of the components of the spermatic cord can be accomplished by ligation, overhand or figure-eight knot in the spermatic cord, or square knot of the ductus deferens to the testicular vessels.[34] The latter technique involves transection (using scissors or traction) of the ductus deferens near the testis (Fig 97–8*D*). Two square knots are placed in the spermatic cord using the ductus deferens and spermatic vessels (Fig. 97–8*E*). The spermatic cord is transected distal to these square knots (Fig. 97–8*F*), and the scrotal incision is left unsutured.

Complications

Complications following orchidectomy include scrotal bruising and swelling, hemorrhage, and infection. Bruising and swelling of the scrotum are common after canine orchidectomy; however, the closed technique of canine orchidectomy has a lower incidence of scrotal swelling.[35] Hemorrhage after orchidectomy may be serious, particularly if it occurs within the abdomen. Serious hemorrhage mandates ligation of the bleeding spermatic cord, intravenous fluid therapy, and possibly a blood transfusion. A ventral median abdominal approach is often necessary to locate and ligate the spermatic cord. Infection following orchidectomy usually requires both local (irrigation and drainage) and parenteral antibiotic treatment.

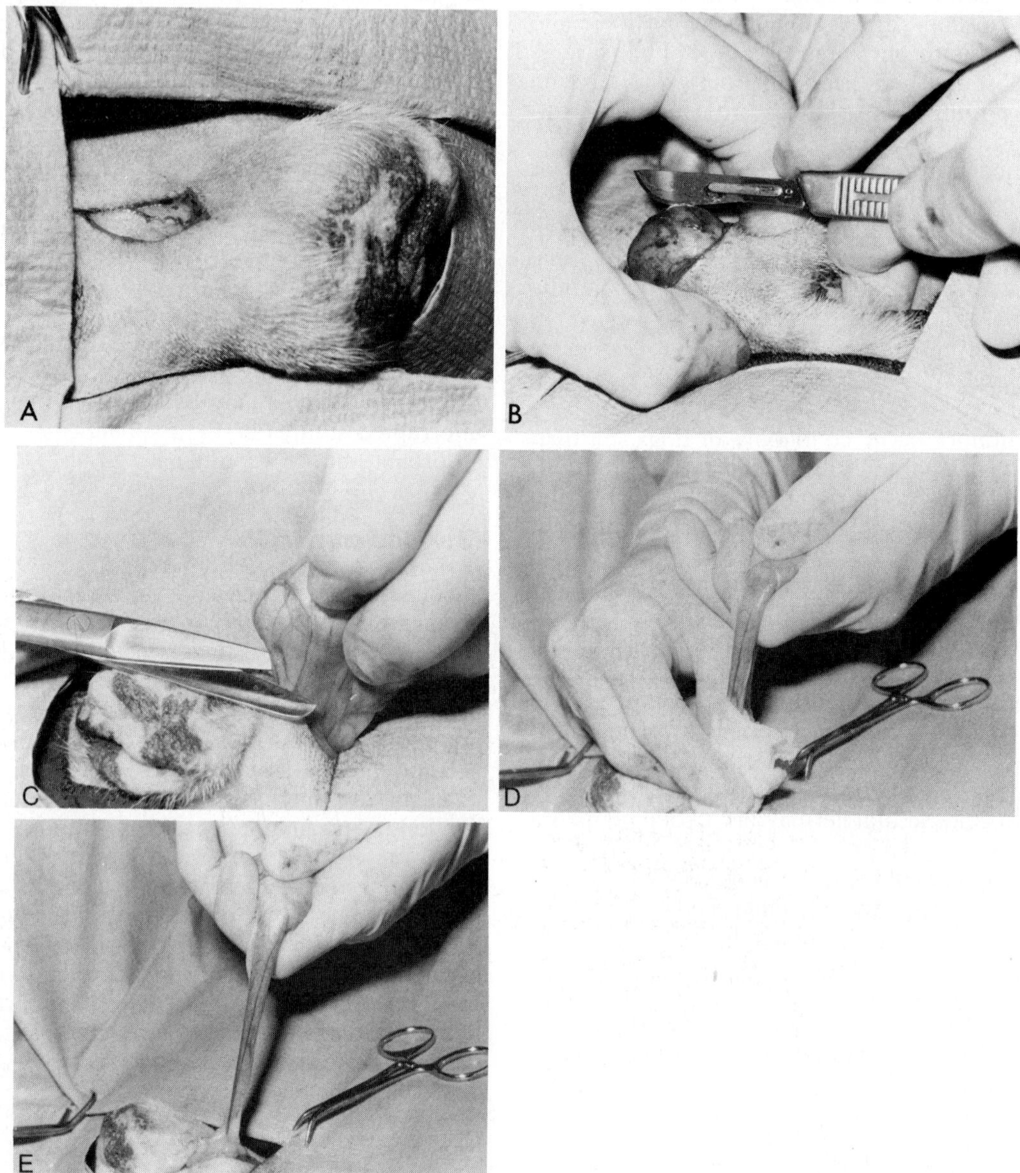

FIGURE 97–5. Canine orchidectomy. *A,* A prescrotal skin incision is made. *B,* The testis is pushed cranially to the skin incision. The subcutaneous tissue and spermatic fascia are incised over the testis, exposing the parietal vaginal tunic. *C,* After exteriorization of the testis, the spermatic fascia and scrotal ligament are incised close to the testis with scissors. *D,* The fat and fascia that surround the spermatic cord are reflected proximally with a gauze sponge. *E,* The spermatic cord has been maximally exteriorized and is ready for ligation.

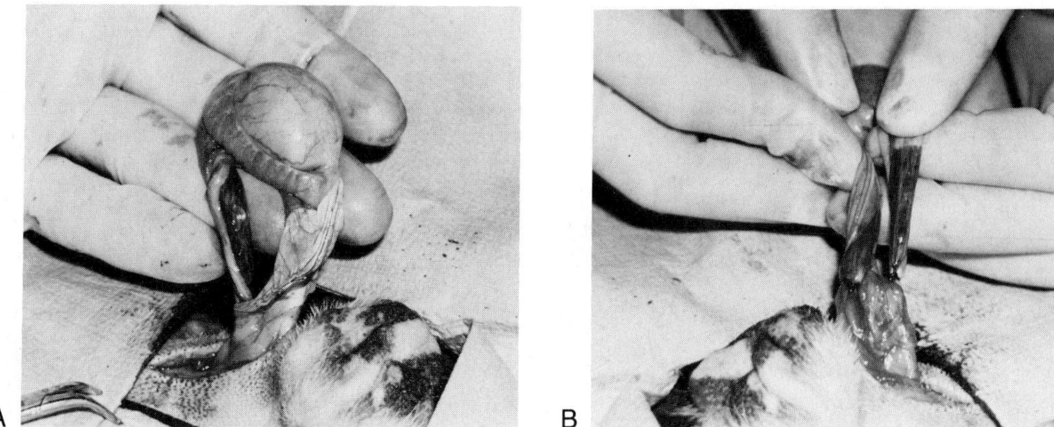

FIGURE 97–6. Canine orchidectomy—alternative open technique. *A*, The tunics and associated cremaster muscle are separated from the rest of the spermatic cord. *B*, Transfixation sutures have been placed in the tunics and the rest of the spermatic cord.

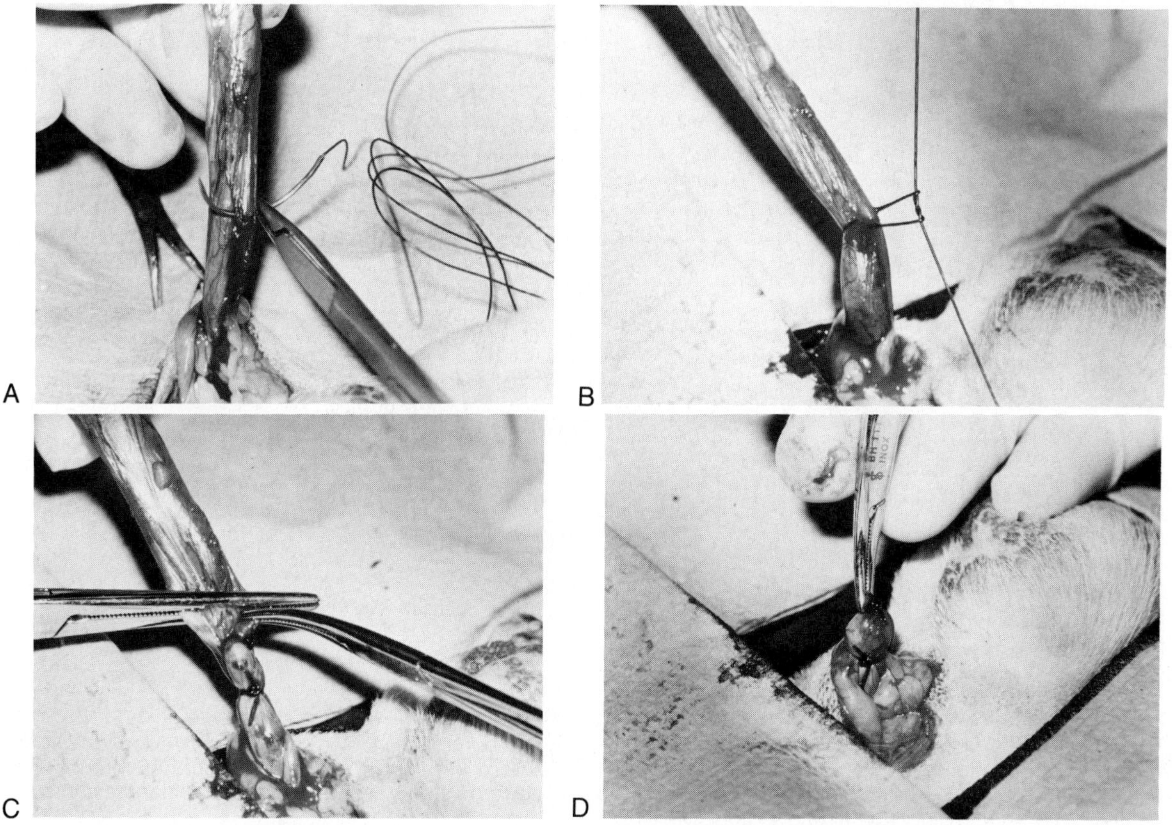

FIGURE 97–7. Canine orchidectomy—closed technqiue. *A*, The suture needle is inserted between the cremaster muscle (right) and the ductus deferens in preparation for transfixation ligation. *B*, A figure-eight transfixation ligature is being tied. The entire spermatic cord is enclosed in the ligature. *C*, Two transfixation ligatures have been placed. The spermatic cord will be transected between the two hemostats. *D*, The ligated spermatic cord is returned to the inguinal region.

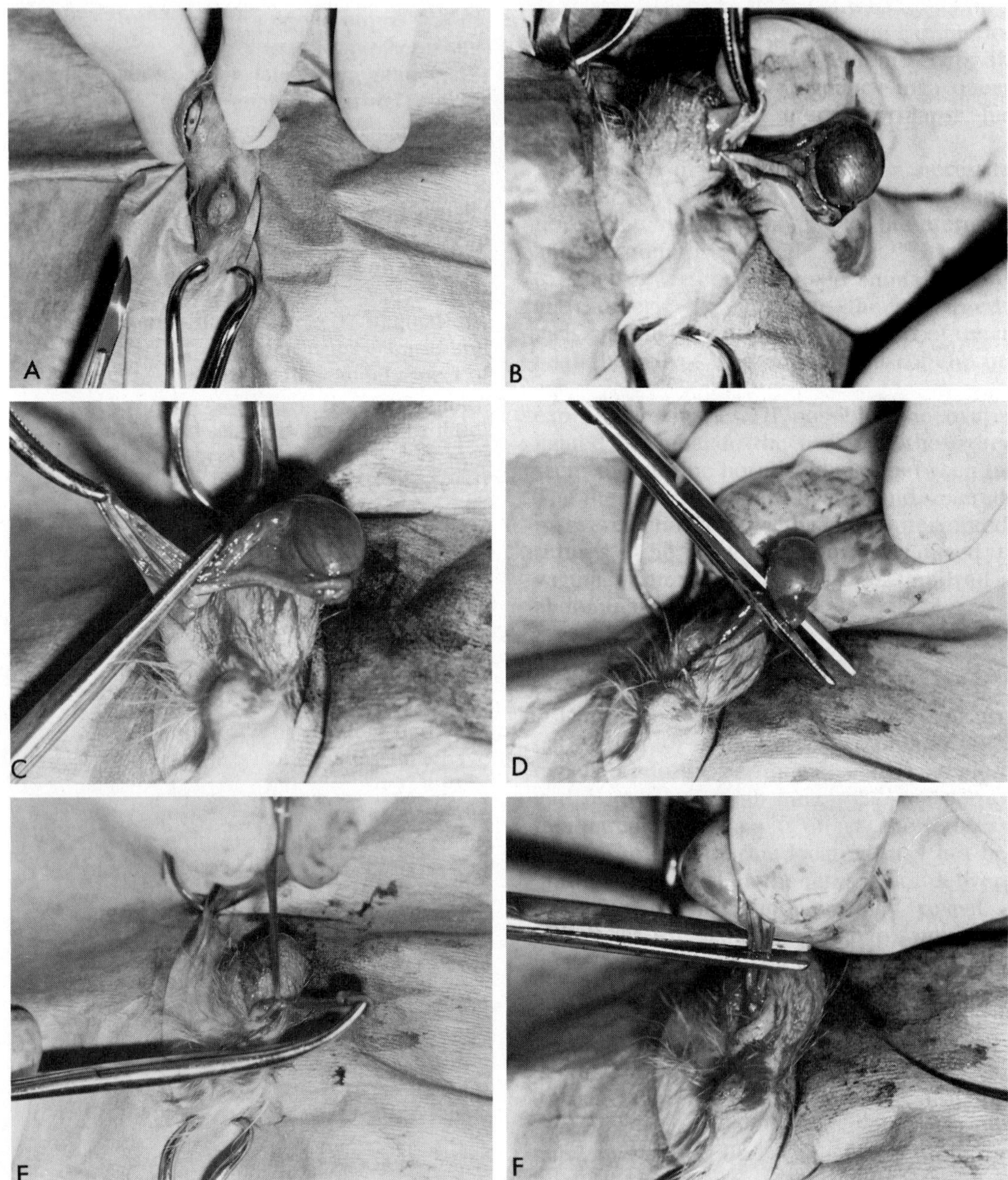

FIGURE 97–8. Feline orchidectomy—open technique. *A*, A separate longitudinal scrotal incision is made over each testis. *B*, The parietal vaginal tunic is grasped with hemostats, separated from the testis, and excised with scissors *(C)*. *D*, The ductus deferens is transected with scissors near the testis. *E*, The ductus deferens and spermatic vessels are used to tie two square knots in the spermatic cord. *F*, The spermatic cord is transected distal to the square knots.

Scrotal Ablation

Scrotal ablation is recommended at the time of orchidectomy whenever trauma to the scrotum is severe and suggests ischemia. Ablation of the scrotum may be preferred at orchidectomy in old dogs with pendulous scrotums to avoid postoperative problems such as scrotal irritation and edema.[18] Curvilinear incisions are made on both sides of the scrotum at its base. The incisions curve toward the scrotum to provide adequate skin for closure (Fig. 97–9).[18] Bleeders are controlled by ligation, and both testes are removed. Care is taken to avoid damage to the urethra or penis during dissection. After transection of the scrotal septum, the skin is closed in the usual manner.

Epididymides

Aplasia and Occlusion of the Epididymis

Segmental aplasia of the epididymis, due to failure of development of a portion of the mesonephric duct, has been reported in dogs.[7, 23, 29] Bilateral epididymal aplasia results in obstruction to flow of spermatozoa and infertility. Spermatoceles and spermatic granulomas develop immediately proximal to the obstructed segment.[23]

Biopsy is necessary to establish a diagnosis; however, careful palpation of the scrotal contents assists in the diagnosis of aplasia of the epididymis.[7] Repair of epididymal aplasia and occlusion is usually not attempted in dogs and cats; orchidectomy is generally performed.

Epididymitis

Epididymitis usually accompanies orchitis. Epididymitis may produce only clinical signs of slight pain associated with epididymal enlargement.[15] More severe inflammation results in fluid accumulations between the parietal and visceral vaginal tunics, epididymal fibrosis, spermatocele, spermatic granuloma, and possibly abscess formation. Pyrexia and anorexia can accompany acute epididymitis.

Epididymitis can result from an ascending infection of the genital tract, canine distemper virus, or a hematogenous infection. Canine distemper virus produces cytoplasmic and intranuclear inclusions in the epididymal epithelial cells.[23] Hematogenous infection, particularly *B. canis*, can result in epididymitis without orchitis.[16] Diagnosis of the causative organism often requires microbiological testing of fluid within the vaginal tunics, semen, urine, and possibly blood. Diagnosis of canine brucellosis involves both serological and bacteriological testing.[5] Canine distemper-induced epididymitis is diagnosed by histopathology.

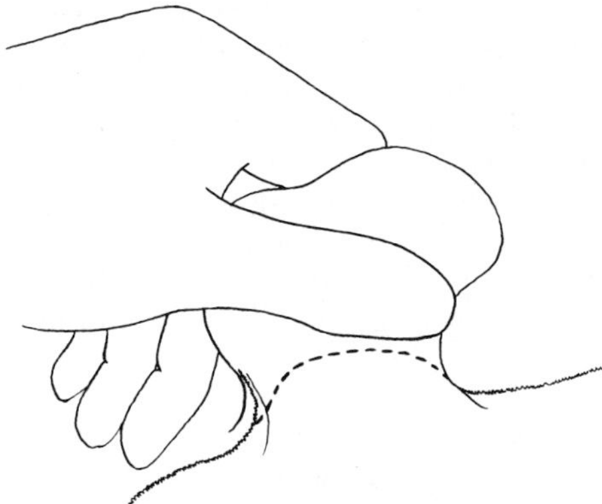

FIGURE 97–9. Ablation of the scrotum in a dog. The scrotum is retracted ventrally. The curved scrotal skin incision is shown as a broken line. (Reprinted with permission from Harvey CE: Scrotal ablation and castration in the dog. *J Am Anim Hosp Assoc 9*:170, 1973.)

Treatment of acute suppurative epididymitis is orchidectomy. The cavity of the vaginal tunics is drained and allowed to heal by second intention.[21] Antibacterial drugs are used to control infection. There is no uniformly successful treatment for canine brucellosis.[5] The prognosis for maintaining fertility after epididymitis is guarded. Testicular atrophy and chronic epididymitis are common sequelae of *B. canis* infections.[5, 15]

Epididymal Tumors

Primary epididymal tumors are rarely reported in dogs and cats. Local invasion of the epididymis by testicular tumors can occur.[23] Fibromas of the epididymis have been observed.[3, 21] Orchidectomy with excision of as much of the spermatic cord and vaginal tunics as necessary is the method of diagnosis and treatment.

References

1. Arey LB: *Developmental Anatomy*. W. B. Saunders, Philadelphia, 1965, pp 315–341.
2. Ashdown RR: The diagnosis of cryptorchidism in young dogs: A review of the problem. *J Small Anim Pract 4*:261, 1963.
3. Barrett RE, Theilen GH: Neoplasms of the canine and feline reproductive tracts. *In* Kirk RW (ed): *Current Veterinary Therapy VI*. W. B. Saunders, Philadelphia, 1977, pp 1263–1267.
4. Bloom W, and Fawcett DW (eds): *A Textbook of Histology*. 10th ed. W. B. Saunders, Philadelphia, 1975, pp 805–857.
5. Burke TJ: Reproductive disorders. *In* Ettinger SJ (ed): *Textbook of Veterinary Internal Medicine*. 2nd ed. W. B. Saunders, Philadelphia, 1983, pp 1711–1725.
6. Burke TJ, Reynolds HA: The testis. *In* Bojrab MJ (ed): *Pathophysiology in Small Animal Surgery*. Lea & Febiger, Philadelphia, 1983, pp 454–459.
7. Copeland MD, MacLachlan NJ: Aplasia of the epididymis and vas deferens in the dog. *J Small Anim Pract 17*:443, 1976.
8. Cox VS, et al: An anatomic and genetic study of canine cryptorchidism. *Teratology 18*:233, 1978.
9. Dunn ML, et al: Cryptorchidism in dogs: A clinical study. *J Am Anim Hosp Assoc 4*:180, 1968.
10. England GCW, et al: Evaluation of the testosterone response to hCG and the identification of a presumed anorchid dog. *J Small Anim Pract 30*:441, 1989.
11. Eskew NE, Kuhn EF: Abdominal pain due to torsion of a retained testicle. *Vet Med 56*:212, 1961.
12. Evans HE, Christensen GC (eds): *Miller's Anatomy of the Dog*. 2nd ed. W. B. Saunders, Philadelphia, 1979, pp 554–565.
13. Evans HE, deLahunta A (eds): *Miller's Guide to the Dissection of the Dog*. 3rd ed. W. B. Saunders, Philadelphia, 1988, p 182.
14. Feldman EC: Infertility. *In* Ettinger SJ (ed): *Textbook of Veterinary Internal Medicine*. 3rd ed. W. B. Saunders, Philadelphia, 1989, pp 1851–1858.
15. George LW, et al: Semen examination in dogs with canine brucellosis. *Am J Vet Res 40*:1589, 1979.
16. Glenn JF, Weinerth JL: The male genital system. *In* Sabiston DC Jr (ed): *Davis-Christopher Textbook of Surgery: The Biological Basis of Modern Surgical Practice*. 12th ed. W. B. Saunders, Philadelphia, 1981, pp 1761–1786.
17. Glover TD: Recent progress in the study of male reproductive physiology: Testis stimulation; sperm formation, transport and maturation (epididymal physiology); semen analysis, storage and artificial insemination. *In* Greep RO (ed): *International Review of Physiology: Reproductive Physiology I*. University Park Press, Baltimore, 1975.

18. Harvey CE: Scrotal ablation and castration in the dog. *J Am Anim Hosp Assoc 9*:170, 1973.
19. Hayes HM Jr, Pendergrass TW: Canine testicular tumors: Epidemiologic features of 410 dogs. *Int J Cancer 18*:482, 1976.
20. Jarlov N, Blixenkrone-Moller M: Two cases of torsio testis in the dog. *Nord Vet Med 38*:244, 1986.
21. Johnston DE, Archibald J: Male genital system. *In* Archibald J (ed): *Canine and Feline Surgery*. Vol I. American Veterinary Publications, Santa Barbara, 1984, pp 293–356.
22. Kawakami E, et al: Testicular function of scrotal testes after the cryptorchidectomy in dogs with unilateral cryptorchidism. *Jpn J Vet Sci 50*:1239, 1988.
23. Ladds PW: The male genital system. *In* Jubb KUF, Kennedy PC (eds): *Pathology of Domestic Animals*. 3rd ed. Academic Press, New York, 1985, pp 409–459.
24. Larsen RE: Evaluation of fertility problems in the male dog. *Vet Clin North Am Small Anim Pract 7*: 735, 1977.
25. Larsen RE: Testicular biopsy in the dog. *Vet Clin North Am Small Anim Pract* 7:747, 1977.
26. Lein DH: Canine orchitis. *In* Kirk RW (ed): *Current Veterinary Therapy VI*. W. B. Saunders, Philadelphia, 1977, pp 1255–1259.
27. Lipowitz AJ, et al: Testicular neoplasms and concomitant clinical changes in the dog. *J Am Vet Med Assoc 163*:1364, 1973.
28. MacDonald DS, et al: Torsion of an ectopic testicle simulating a foreign body in the intestine. *Can Vet J 2*:117, 1961.
29. Majeed ZZ: Segmental aplasia of the Wolffian duct; report of a case in a poodle. *J Small Anim Pract 15*:263, 1974.
30. Nickel R, et al (eds): *The Viscera of Domestic Mammals*. 2nd ed. Springer-Verlag, New York, 1979, pp 304–350.
31. Orsi AM: Regional histology of the epididymis of the dog. A light microscope study. *Anat Anz 153*:441, 1983.
32. Pearson H, Kelly DF: Testicular torsion in the dog: A review of 13 cases. *Vet Rec 97*:200, 1975.
33. Pendergrass TW, Hayes HM Jr: Cryptorchidism and related defects in dogs: Epidemiologic comparisons with man. *Teratology 12*:51, 1975.
34. Pettit GD: There's more than one way to castrate a cat. *Mod Vet Pract 62*:713, 1981.
35. Phillips JT, Leeds EB: A closed technique for canine orchidectomy. *Canine Pract 3*:23, 1976.
36. Pineda MH, Faulkner LC: Male reproduction. *In* McDonald LE (ed): *Veterinary Endocrinology and Reproduction*. 3rd ed. Lea & Febiger, Philadelphia, 1980, pp 235–273.
37. Reif JS, Brodey RS: The relationship between cryptorchidism and canine testicular neoplasia. *J Am Vet Med Assoc 155*:2005, 1969.
38. Reif JS, et al: A cohort study of canine testicular neoplasia. *J Am Vet Med Assoc 175*:719, 1979.
39. Saypol DC, et al: Influence of surgically induced varicocele on testicular blood-flow, temperature, and histology in adult rats and dogs. *J Clin Invest 68*:39, 1981.
40. Smith F, Larsen RE: The infertile stud dog. *In* Kirk RW (ed): *Current Veterinary Therapy VIII*. W. B. Saunders, Philadelphia, 1983, pp 962–964.
41. White PT, Johnson P Jr: Strangulated testicle of a cryptorchid (dog). *J Am Vet Med Assoc 126*:312, 1955.
42. Wilson GP: Surgery of the male reproductive tract. *Vet Clin North Am Small Anim Pract 5*:537, 1975.
43. Younes MA, Pierrepoint CG: Androgen steroid-receptor binding in the canine epididymis. *Prostate 2*:133, 1981.
44. Younes M, et al: Steroid receptors in the canine epididymis. *J Reprod Fertil 56*:45, 1979.

CHAPTER 98

Penis, Prepuce, and Scrotum

Harry W. Boothe

ANATOMY

Penis

The penis is composed of three principal divisions: root, body, and distal portion (Fig. 98–1). The root is attached to the tuber ischii by the left and right crura. Each crus is composed of the proximal part of the corpus cavernosum and the ischiocavernous muscle covering it (Figs. 98–2 through 98–5).[18] The corpus spongiosum contains the penile urethra and is situated ventrally within the penile root. The bulb of the penis is a bilobed expansion of the corpus spongiosum, located between the crura at the ischial arch.

The body of the penis begins at the blending of the crura and extends just beyond the proximal end of the os penis. The body is directly continuous with the root. The corpus cavernosum and the corpus spongiosum constitute the main substance of the penile body.

The distal portion, the glans, is subdivided in dogs into a smaller proximal portion, the bulbus glandis, and a larger distal portion, the pars longa glandis (see Fig. 98–2). The distal half of the bulbus glandis is overlapped by the caudal third of the pars longa glandis.

The corpora of the penis contain enlarged venous spaces. The corpora cavernosa arise from the ischial tuberosity and continue distally in the dorsolateral part of the body of the penis as far as the os penis. The right and left cavernous bodies are separated by a fibrous median septum. Each corpus cavernosum is covered by a thick layer of collagenous and elastic fibers, the tunica albuginea. The corpus spongiosum originates within the pelvic cavity and surrounds the penile urethra throughout its course. It is located in a groove on the urethral side of the penis. The corpus spongiosum narrows in diameter until it enters the glans penis, where it gives off numerous shunts that supply the bulbus glandis with blood. The corpus spongiosum continues in the pars longa glandis to the external urethral orifice.

The bulbus glandis surrounds the proximal part of the os penis. Its thickest dimension and greatest potential for expansion are located dorsally. The bulbus glandis is separated from the pars longa glandis by a fibrous septum. The pars longa glandis is structurally similar to the bulbus glandis, but it has erectile tissue dorsally and laterally only. The pars longa glandis is not capable of expansion comparable to that of the bulbus glandis.

The os penis begins caudal to the bulbus glandis and extends almost to the tip of the glans. The distal end is extended by a slightly curved fibrocartilaginous projection. The proximal two-thirds of the os penis is indented ventrally by a distinct groove, which is occupied by the penile urethra and surrounding corpus spongiosum. The

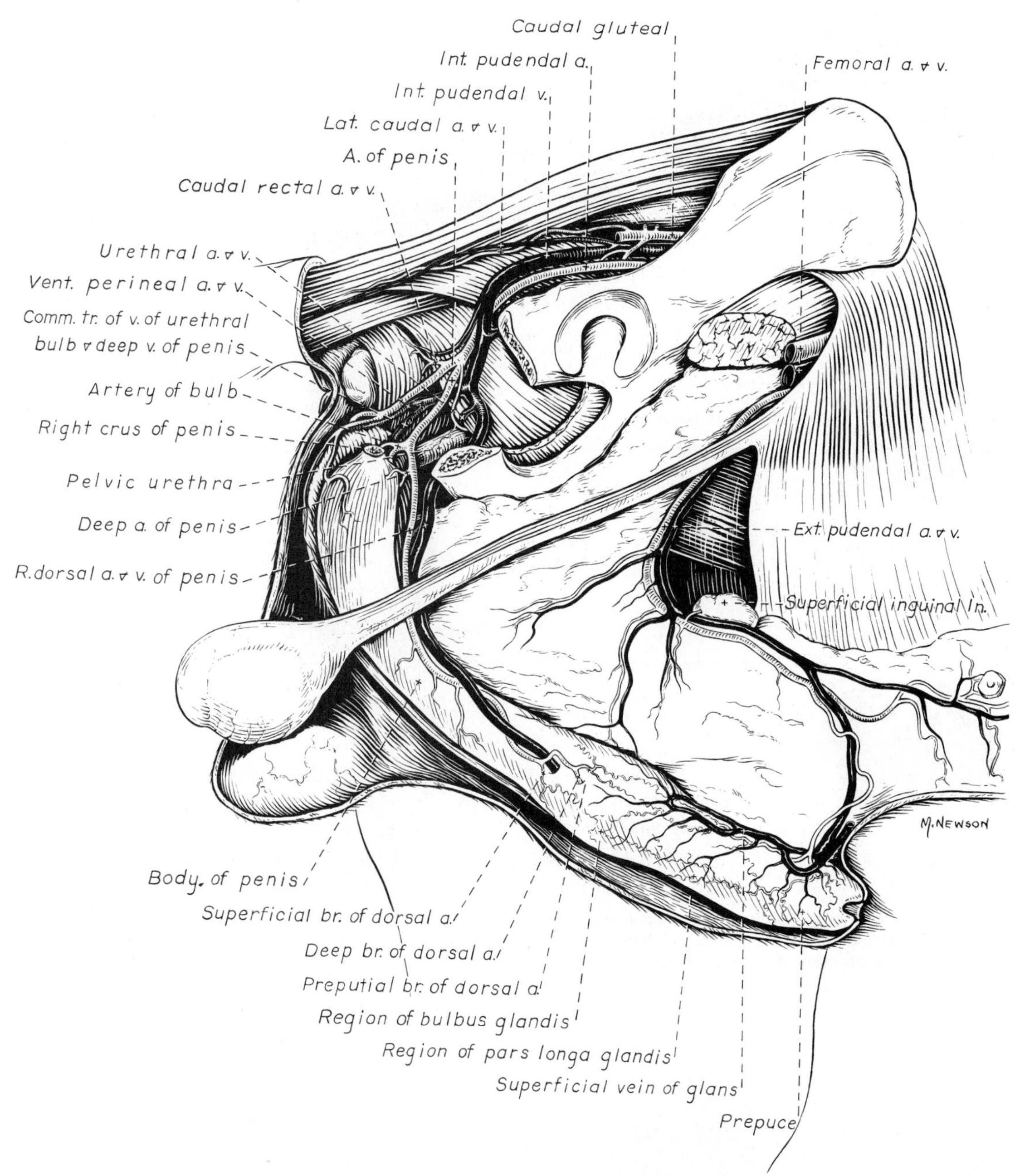

FIGURE 98–1. Topographic relations of the penis and other pelvis structures. (The right ischium is removed.) (Reprinted with permission from Christensen GC: Angioarchitecture of the canine penis and the process of erection. *Am J Anat 95*:230, 1954.)

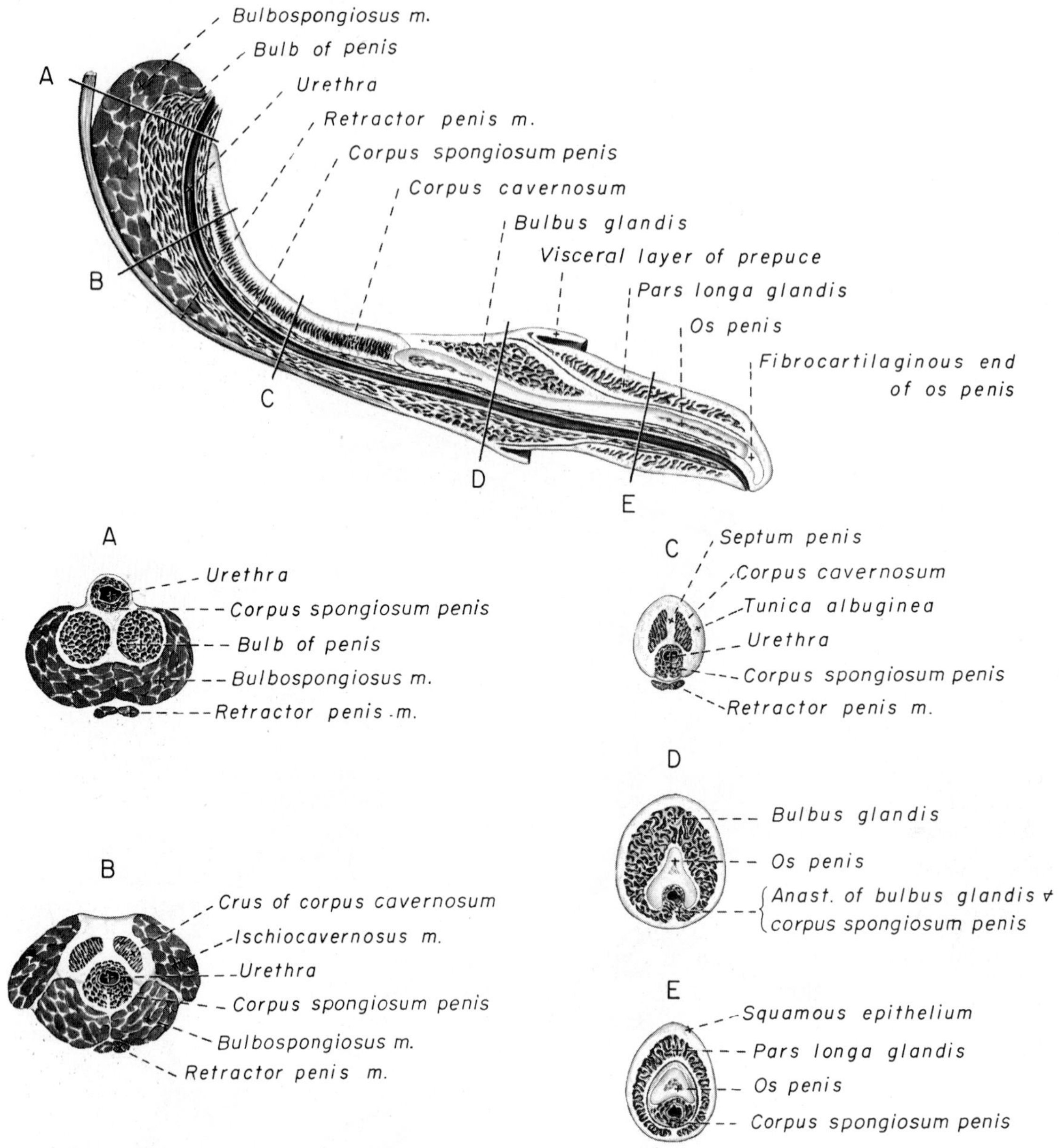

Bulbospongiosus m.
Bulb of penis
Urethra
Retractor penis m.
Corpus spongiosum penis
Corpus cavernosum
Bulbus glandis
Visceral layer of prepuce
Pars longa glandis
Os penis
Fibrocartilaginous end of os penis
A
B
C
D
E
A
Urethra
Corpus spongiosum penis
Bulb of penis
Bulbospongiosus m.
Retractor penis m.
B
Crus of corpus cavernosum
Ischiocavernosus m.
Urethra
Corpus spongiosum penis
Bulbospongiosus m.
Retractor penis m.
C
Septum penis
Corpus cavernosum
Tunica albuginea
Urethra
Corpus spongiosum penis
Retractor penis m.
D
Bulbus glandis
Os penis
Anast. of bulbus glandis & corpus spongiosum penis
E
Squamous epithelium
Pars longa glandis
Os penis
Corpus spongiosum penis

FIGURE 98–2. Internal morphology of the penis. *Upper drawing*, A parasagittal section. *Lower drawing*, Cross sections made at five levels indicated by corresponding letters on upper drawing. (Reprinted with permission from Christensen GC: Angioarchitecture of the canine penis and the process of erection. *Am J Anat 95*:233, 1954.)

M. bulbospongiosus
M. ischiocavernosus
M. ischiourethralis
Tuber ischii
Sacrotuberous lig.
M. obturator int.
M. coccygeus
M. levator ani
M. retractor penis
Cut bulb of urethra
Urethra
Fibrous ring
Common trunk of dorsal vv. of penis
Int. pudendal a. & v.
M.N.
Urethra
Prostate

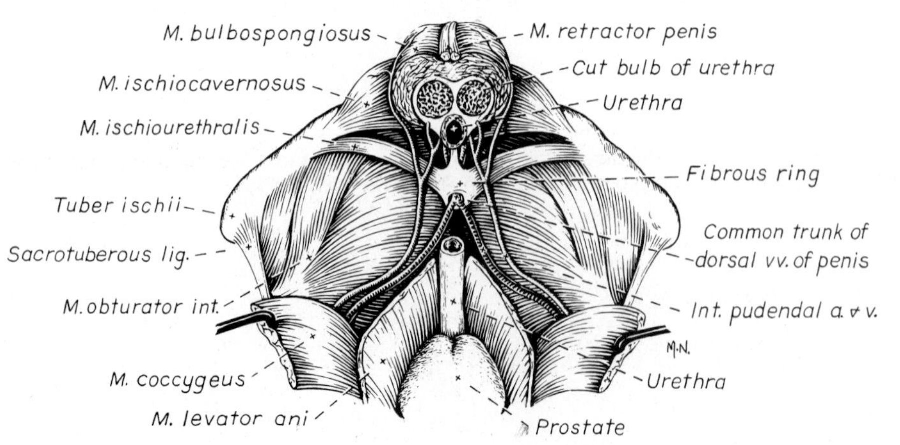

FIGURE 98–3. Dorsal view of ischiourethral muscles. (The pelvic urethra is cut off at the urethral bulb and removed.) (Reprinted with permission from Evans, H. E., and Christensen, G. C. (eds.): *Miller's Anatomy of the Dog.* 2nd ed. W. B. Saunders, Philadelphia, 1979.)

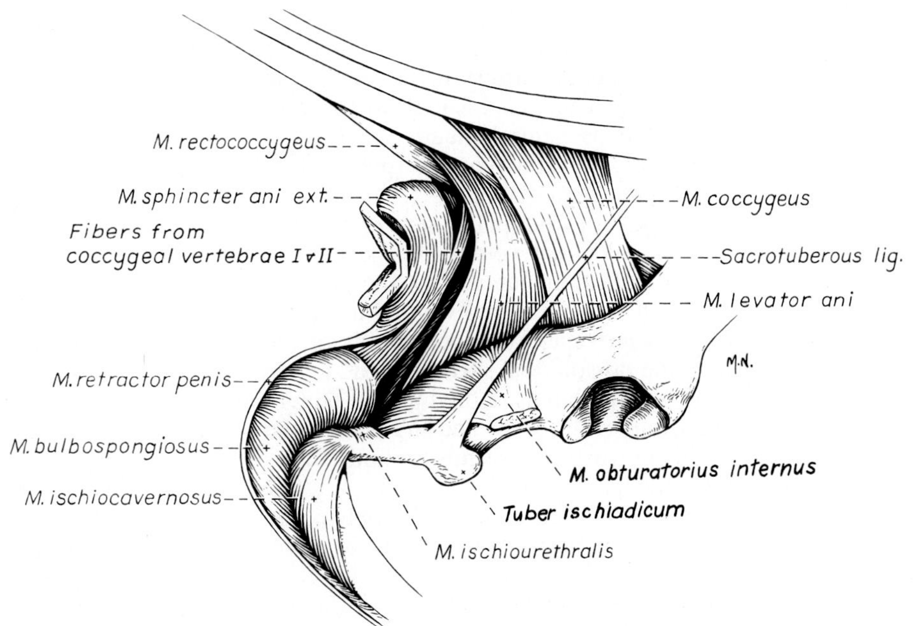

FIGURE 98–4. Root of the penis with superficial muscles, lateral aspect. (Reprinted with permission from Evans HE, Christensen GC (eds): *Miller's Anatomy of the Dog.* 2nd ed. W. B. Saunders, Philadelphia, 1979.)

os penis is attached to the bulbus glandis, pars longa glandis, and tunica albuginea.

Dogs have four paired extrinsic penile muscles: retractor penis, ischiocavernous, bulbocavernous, and ischiourethral muscles (see Figs. 98–3 to 98–5). The retractor penis muscles are composed principally of smooth muscle fibers. They arise from the first two caudal vertebrae, blend with the external anal sphincter, extend along the ventral surface of the penis, and insert on the penis at the level of the preputial fornix. The ischiocavernous muscles originate from the ischial tuberosity and insert on the corpus cavernosum. The bulbocavernous muscles arise from the external anal sphincter, cover the superficial surface of the bulb of the penis, and fuse with the retractor penis muscles at the proximal third of the penile body. The ischiourethral muscles originate from the dorsal aspect of the ischial tuberosity and insert into a fibrous ring at the urethral bulb.

The principal source of blood to the penis is derived from three branches of the artery of the penis, the continuation of the internal pudendal artery (see Fig. 98–1).[18] All three branches—artery of the bulb, deep artery of the penis, and dorsal artery of the penis—anastomose with one another. The paired arteries of the bulb enter and supply the corpus spongiosum, penile

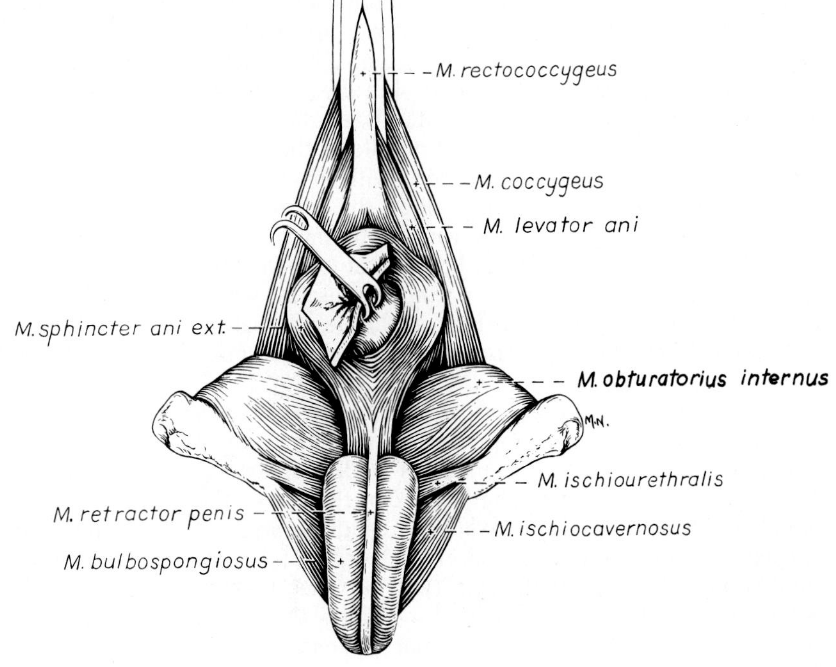

FIGURE 98–5. Superficial muscles of male perineum, caudal aspect. (Reprinted with permission from Evans HE, Christensen GC (eds): *Miller's Anatomy of the Dog.* 2nd ed. W. B. Saunders, Philadelphia, 1979.)

urethra, and pars longa glandis. The deep artery of the penis passes through the tunica albuginea to enter the corpus cavernosum. The dorsal artery of the penis, the continuation of the main trunk, is located on the dorsolateral surface of the os penis beneath the erectile tissue. This branch supplies the corpus spongiosum, bulbus glandis, and pars longa glandis.

The venous drainage of the penis occurs via the internal and external pudendal veins. The pars longa glandis is drained by both the deep vein of the glans to the bulbus glandis and the superficial vein of the glans to the external pudendal vein. The dorsal veins of the penis extend along the dorsolateral surface of the penile body and drain the bulbus glandis to the internal pudendal vein. The deep vein of the penis and the vein of the urethral bulb drain the corpus cavernosum and corpus spongiosum, respectively.

The penis is supplied by nerves from the pelvic and sacral plexuses. The dorsal nerve of the penis passes on the dorsolateral surface of the penis and is the chief sensory nerve to the penis. Penile lymphatics drain into the superficial inguinal lymph nodes.

A cat's penis is shorter and directed caudally. Its urethral surface faces caudodorsally, and its dorsal aspect cranioventrally.[32] Like a dog's penis, a cat's penis consists of a proximal cavernous and a distal osseous part. The free part of the penis of a sexually mature cat is studded with small cornified papillae, called *penile spines*.[2, 32]

Prepuce

The *canine* prepuce is a complete tubular sheath that covers the pars longa glandis and part of the bulbus glandis in a nonerect penis. It is firmly attached and continuous with the skin of the ventral abdominal wall.[18] The dorsal prepuce is composed of two layers of integument. On its ventral and lateral surfaces and cranial aspects of its dorsal surface, the prepuce is composed of three layers of integument. The outer layer is skin, and the inner layers, parietal and visceral, are made up of thin, stratified squamous epithelium. The parietal layer is a continuation of the outer skin layer onto the wall of the preputial cavity. It extends to the fornix, which is located at the level of the middle of the bulbus glandis. The parietal layer is stippled with many lymph nodules and nodes, particularly along the fornix. The visceral, or inner, layer extends from the preputial fornix to the external urethral orifice. It is continuous with the cavernous urethra. The paired preputial muscles, which extend from the xiphoid cartilage to the dorsal wall of the prepuce, are derived from the cutaneus trunci muscle.[18]

The blood supply to the visceral and parietal layers of the prepuce is derived primarily from the dorsal artery of the penis and the external pudendal artery. The artery of the bulb of the penis contributes to the blood supply of the visceral layer. The caudal superficial epigastric artery supplies the preputial skin. The principal venous drainage of the visceral and parietal layers is the superficial and deep veins of the glans, the dorsal vein of the penis, and the external pudendal veins. Preputial lymphatics drain to the superficial inguinal lymph nodes.

Scrotum

The *canine* scrotum is a membranous pouch located approximately two-thirds of the distance from the preputial orifice to the anus. It is spherical, divided into two cavities by a median septum, and located between the thighs. The scrotal wall consists of two layers, skin and dartos. The outer skin is thin and pigmented and covered with fine scattered hairs. The dartos is composed of smooth muscle mixed with collagenous and elastic fibers. The dartos forms a common lining for both halves of the scrotum and contributes to the scrotal septum. The septum is continuous with the abdominal fascia dorsally. The scrotum contains the testes, the epididymides, the distal part of the spermatic cord with its associated spermatic fascia and vaginal tunics, and the distal cremaster muscle. The external spermatic fascia attaches to the caudal aspect of the scrotum as the scrotal ligament. The external pudendal artery is the principal blood vessel to the scrotum. The draining veins parallel the arteries. Lymphatic drainage is to the superficial inguinal lymph nodes.

The *feline* scrotum is located just ventral to the anus. It is densely covered with hair.

PHYSIOLOGY

Penis

Erection is essential for the penis to function during copulation in all species except dogs.[33] The canine os penis facilitates vaginal entry without full erection. The basis for erection of the penis is a profound increase in blood supply. Parasympathetic stimulation increases blood flow through the internal pudendal artery, the principal source of blood to the penis.[15] Erection is accomplished by synergy of two mechanisms. First, engorgement of the cavernous bodies of the penis occurs through expansion of the arteries and contraction of the veins.[12] Second, the dorsal penile vein is compressed against the ischial arch by contraction of the ischiocavernous and bulbocavernous muscles.[13, 33] The extent to which the cavernous spaces expand during erection depends on development and composition of the connective tissue tunics of the penis. Erection involves primarily the glans penis in dogs and cats.[33] Enlargement of the bulbus glandis in dogs is an important part of the "tie" that occurs during copulation. The cornified spines of a cat's penis are proposed to stimulate ovulation.[2]

Prepuce

At birth, the epithelial surfaces of the prepuce and penis adhere. Separation of the prepuce from the penis is under androgenic influence and usually occurs at puberty. The preputial muscles keep the prepuce over the penis. They are classified as "slow" muscles and are similar to the cremaster muscle in their contraction properties.[40]

Scrotum

The scrotum functions in thermoregulation of the testes.[21] The scrotal skin is thin, sparsely covered with hair, and richly supplied with sweat glands. This structure favors the dissipation of heat from the testes. The dartos also regulates the distance of the testes from the body. Contraction of the dartos helps bring the testes closer to the abdomen, whereas relaxation does the opposite.

DISORDERS

Penis

Hypospadias

Hypospadias, the most common developmental anomaly of the male external genitalia, is most frequently encountered in Boston terriers (Fig. 98–6).[26] Clinical signs may be absent if the prepuce is normal and the external urethral orifice is near the end of the penis. The skin and hair around the urethral orifice occasionally are urine soaked and irritated.[39] Failure of fusion of the urogenital folds and incomplete formation of the penile urethra are noted.[1] The external urethral orifice can be located anywhere on the ventral aspect of the penis from the normal opening to the perineal region, with glandular, penile, scrotal, and perineal hypospadias occurring (Fig. 98–7).[1] Hypospadias is usually associated with failure of fusion of the prepuce and underdevelopment of the penis (see the later section on abnormalities of the prepuce). Diagnosis of hypospadias is made by close inspection of the penis.

Surgical correction is not usually attempted in dogs, because the urethra cranial to the abnormal orifice is deficient.[26] Excision of the remnants of the prepuce and penis as well as bilateral orchidectomy may be indicated in severe cases. The urethral orifice is maintained in the perineal region.[39]

Deformity of the Os Penis

The os penis may rarely develop with a pronounced curvature.[26] Because of the curvature, the dog may not be able to retract the distal part of the penis into the prepuce. The exposed part becomes dry and fissured, resulting in infection and necrosis.[8, 26]

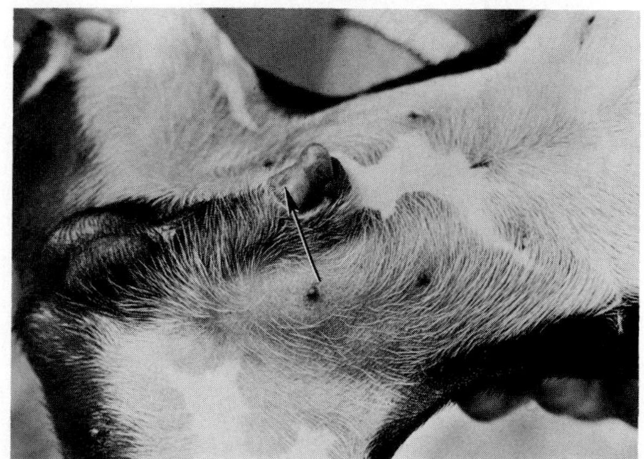

FIGURE 98–6. Hypospadias. The urethral orifice is located on the ventral aspect of the penis (*arrow*). The prepuce is not fully developed.

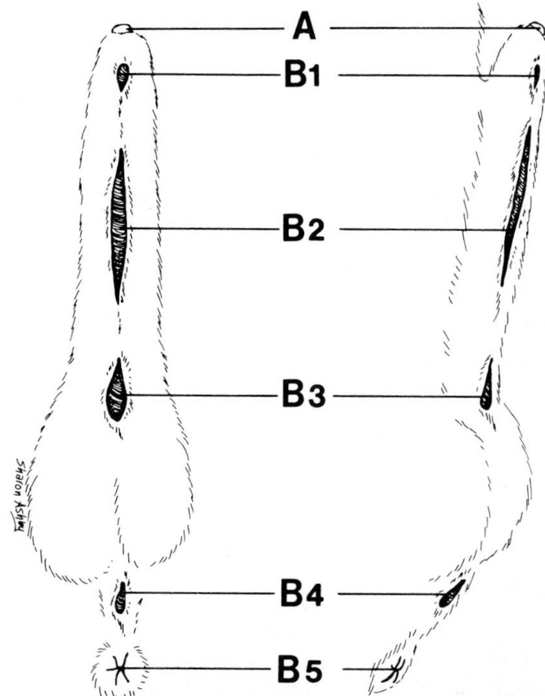

FIGURE 98–7. Normal urethral meatus (A) and types of hypospadias: glandular (B1); penile (B2); scrotal (B3); perineal (B4); and anal (B5). (Reprinted with permission from Ader PL, Hobson HP: Hypospadias: A review of the veterinary literature and a report of three cases in the dog. *J Am Anim Hosp Assoc 14*:722, 1978.)

Treatment depends on the condition of the penis. Local treatment of the exposed penis is usually not effective without treatment of the bony curvature. It may be possible to fracture and straighten the os penis, if infection and necrosis are not present.[8] Partial penile amputation may be necessary in severe cases (see the later section on strangulation of the penis).

Penile Wounds

The most common clinical sign of penile wounds is hemorrhage. Hemorrhage is frequently intermittent but often profuse. Repeated hemorrhage is associated with penile erection, which in turn is caused by irritation due to injury. Rupture of the penile urethra is usually accompanied by fluctuating subcutaneous swelling associated with urine extravasation.

Because of its exposed location, the penis is relatively accessible to injury. Penile wounds may occur during mating, dog fights, and fence jumping or from automobile or gunshot accidents.[22, 26, 31] Penile lacerations and gunshot wounds may involve the urethra. Severe penile trauma may produce a fracture of the os penis (see the later section on fracture of the os penis).

Minor injuries of the penis can be cleaned and treated with a topical antibiotic ointment. These wounds are usually allowed to heal by second intention. If significant hemorrhage occurs, the wound is debrided and sutured.

Arterial bleeding is controlled by ligation, and cavernous bleeding is controlled by suturing the tunica albuginea with fine absorbable material. The penile mucosa is closed with fine absorbable material. Parenteral and local antibiotics are used postoperatively. Erection of the penis is prevented by sedating the animal.[26]

Wounds of the penile urethra are usually treated by catheterization, provided that the urethra has not been transected. A transected urethra is sutured with fine absorbable material and catheterized. Catheters remain in place, using a closed collection system, for 5 to 7 days with minor penile urethral tears and up to 10 days after urethral anastomosis. Severe wounds may require partial penile amputation (see the later section on strangulation of the penis) and a scrotal urethrostomy.

The prognosis for penile wounds is generally favorable if the urethra has not been transected. Urethral stricture is possible, especially after transection and anastomosis.

Fracture of the Os Penis

Fracture of the os penis occurs rarely. Clinical signs depend on the degree of soft-tissue damage and fracture displacement. Dysuria and hematuria are often present. Crepitus is apparent, and urethral obstruction may be present. Urethral obstruction may also be observed with callus formation.[41]

Fractures usually are transverse, with limited soft-tissue damage, although they may be comminuted.[26] Radiography determines the amount of damage to the os penis.

Conservative management of this fracture is often successful.[26, 31, 41] Minimally displaced simple fractures do not require immobilization.[26] More severe fractures can be adequately immobilized with a urethral catheter. The end of the catheter is positioned beyond the fracture site. The catheter is maintained as a closed system for 7 days. If a catheter cannot be passed because of urethral damage, or if the fracture is unstable after urethral catheterization, open reduction and fixation with a finger plate has been successful.[41] Fractures accompanied by severe penile trauma may necessitate partial penile amputation (see the later section on strangulation of the penis). If urethral obstruction occurs because of callus formation, a prescrotal urethrostomy can be performed.

Balanoposthitis

Infections of the penis and prepuce are fairly common, constituting 20 per cent of canine penile and preputial lesions in one study.[31] A copious yellow or blood-tinged preputial discharge suggests balanoposthitis or prostatic disease. A slight purulent preputial discharge is normal in mature dogs, because it is not associated with inflammation of the penile or preputial mucosa. The affected dog frequently licks the prepuce. Examination of a dog with balanoposthitis reveals an inflamed, thickened mucosa of the penis and prepuce. Enlarged lymphoid nodules are noted, particularly near the fornix of the preputial cavity. The significance of these nodules is unknown, because they have been observed in both symptomatic and nonsymptomatic dogs.[4] Adhesions may develop between the prepuce and penis in severe cases. Balanoposthitis may be seen after penile injury or accompanying phimosis, preputial foreign bodies, or neoplasia. Treatment is elimination of the primary cause. Patients are usually anesthetized to allow complete examination. Thorough irrigation of the penis and preputial cavity is performed with warm saline solution. Superficial curettage of the lymphoid nodules with a gauze sponge is often necessary. Adhesions between the penis and prepuce are severed. Local instillation of povidone-iodine or chlorhexidine solution is also helpful. An antibiotic ointment is instilled into the preputial cavity for a few days after curettage. The prognosis following treatment is guarded, because balanoposthitis tends to recur.

Strangulation of the Penis

Malicious application of a rubber band around the penis or constriction by a ring of preputial hairs can cause strangulation of the penis. The dog usually seems to be in pain and may frequently lick the prepuce. Dysuria can also be noted. The penile mucosa becomes swollen with a necrotic circle, or the entire penis distal to the constriction may be necrotic (Fig. 98–8).[26]

This condition must be distinguished from paraphimosis because the treatment differs (see the later section

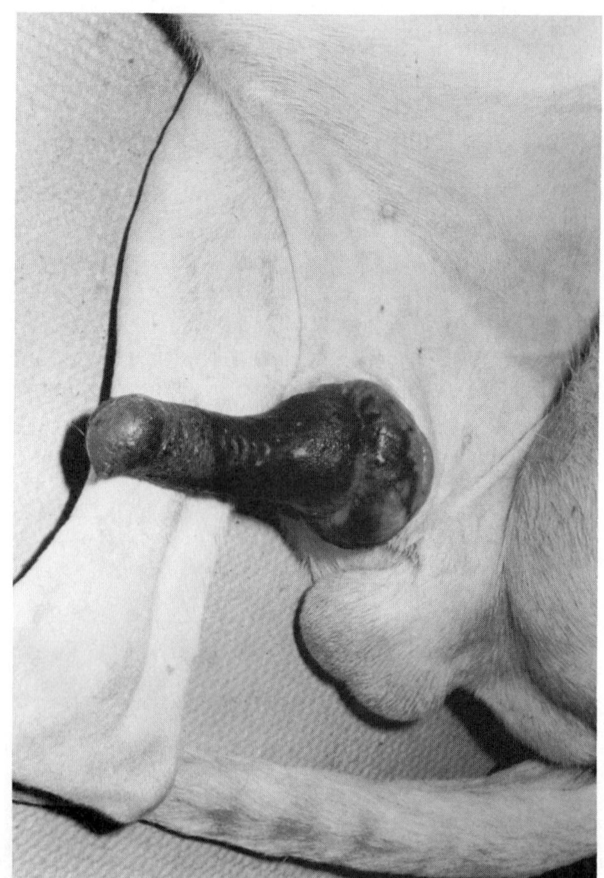

FIGURE 98–8. Strangulation of the penis. This lesion necessitated penile amputation, orchidectomy, scrotal ablation, and perineal urethrostomy.

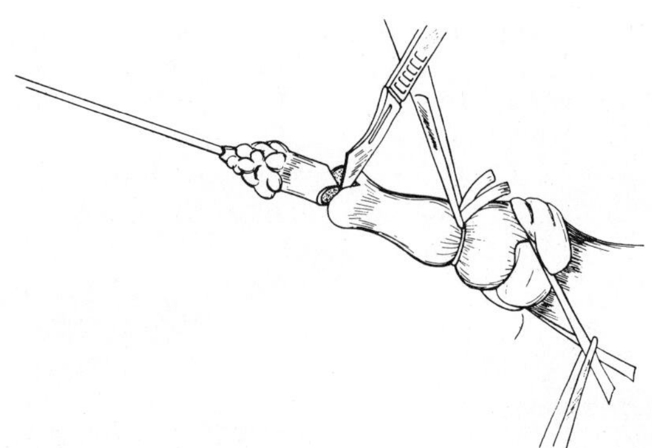

FIGURE 98–9. Partial penile amputation: creation of bilateral flaps in the pars longa glandis. The penis is extruded, and the prepuce is retracted with umbilical tape. After urethral catheterization, a tourniquet is placed around the penis. The pars longa glandis is incised to create two flaps. (Reprinted with permission from Bojrab MJ (ed): *Current Techniques in Small Animal Surgery I.* Lea & Febiger, Philadelphia, 1975.)

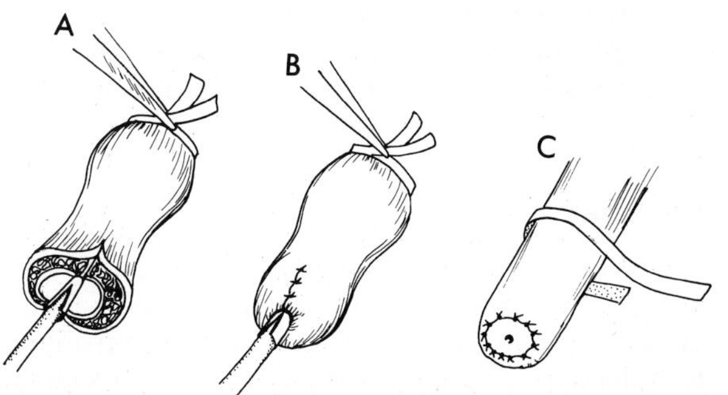

FIGURE 98–11. Partial penile amputation: closure of the distal end of the penis. *A,* The distal urethra is incised longitudinally on its dorsal surface. *B,* The cavernous tissue is closed on the dorsal aspect of the penis with fine absorbable sutures placed in the tunica albuginea. *C,* The urethral margin is sutured to the epithelium of the penis with simple interrupted absorbable sutures. (Reprinted with permission from Bojrab MJ (ed): *Current Techniques in Small Animal Surgery I.* Lea & Febiger, Philadelphia, 1975.)

on paraphimosis). When damage to the penis is minor, removal of the cause and topical application of an antibiotic ointment result in prompt healing. Licking is controlled. More severe cases accompanied by urethral swelling and constriction require an indwelling urethral catheter as well as local antibiotics.

Partial amputation of the penis is indicated when the distal portion is gangrenous or when the urethra is severely damaged. The surgical area, including the preputial cavity, is prepared in the usual manner after induction of general anesthesia. The urethra is catheterized. The penis is withdrawn from the prepuce and kept exteriorized with a rubber tourniquet placed around the penis as far caudally as possible. The prepuce may also be retracted caudally with umbilical tape. If the penis cannot be adequately exteriorized, the prepuce is incised on the ventral midline. Bilateral flaps are created proximal to the os penis while leaving the urethra intact (Fig. 98–9). The urethra is dissected from the groove in the os penis. The catheter is removed, and the urethra is transected just distal to the proposed amputation site. The os penis is transected with bone-cutting forceps at the base of the flap (Fig. 98–10). The tourniquet is loosened to identify and ligate blood vessels in the erectile tissue. The flaps of erectile tissue and tunica albuginea are apposed with simple interrupted sutures of 4-0 absorbable material. The urethra is incised along its dorsal midline. Urethral edges are sutured to penile mucosa over the ventral portion of the end of the penile stump. Penile mucosa is sutured to penile mucosa on the dorsal portion of the penile stump (Fig. 98–11) to prevent too large a urethral orifice.

Shortening the prepuce may be necessary when a large part of the glans penis has been removed.[23] A rectangular full-thickness segment of the ventral wall of the prepuce is excised (Fig. 98–12). The preputial mucous membrane is sutured with fine absorbable material

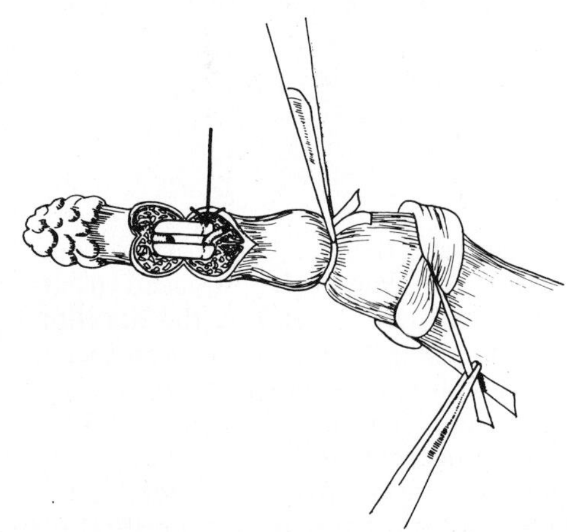

FIGURE 98–10. Partial penile amputation: transection site in the os penis after dissection of the urethra. The urethra is transected distal to the proposed ostectomy site (arrow) and dissected from the groove of the os penis. (Reprinted with permission from Bojrab MJ (ed): *Current Techniques in Small Animal Surgery I.* Lea & Febiger, Philadelphia, 1975.)

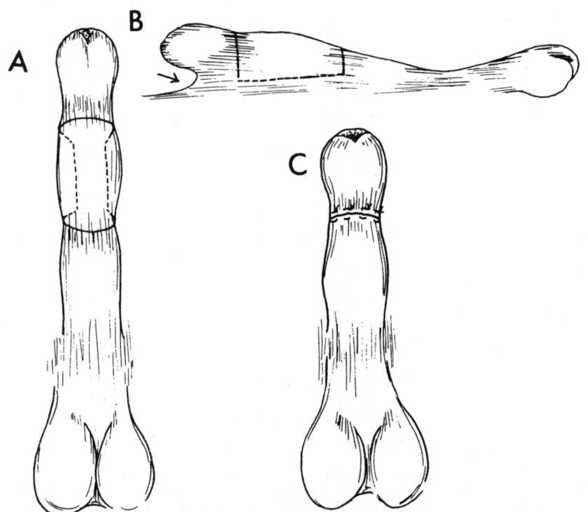

FIGURE 98–12. Technique for shortening the prepuce in conjunction with partial penile amputation. *A,* A rectangular portion of prepuce is excised. *B,* A sliding skin flap will facilitate retraction of the cranial prepuce (*arrow*). *C,* The segments are apposed with three layers of suture. (Reprinted with permission from Bojrab MJ (ed): *Current Techniques in Small Animal Surgery I.* Lea & Febiger, Philadelphia, 1975.)

in an everting pattern. The subcutaneous tissue is closed with simple interrupted absorbable sutures. The skin is apposed with simple interrupted or horizontal mattress sutures.

Penile Tumors

Tumors of the canine penis are not uncommon. There are almost no reports of genital neoplasia in male cats. Tumors of the penis in dogs include transmissible venereal tumor, papilloma, and squamous cell carcinoma.[4] Licking and a serosanguineous preputial discharge are common clinical signs of penile transmissible venereal tumors.[11] Diagnosis is frequently made by cytological evaluation of fine-needle aspirates or impression smears from the mass. Transmissible venereal tumors respond to many modes of treatment, including radiation therapy, chemotherapy, and surgery.[36] Tumors of the distal portion may require partial penile amputation (see the earlier section on strangulation of the penis).

Tumors involving most of the penis may require more extensive penile amputation and perineal urethrostomy. Bilateral orchidectomy and scrotal ablation may also be necessary. An elliptical incision is made along each side of the prepuce to an appropriate level on the perineal midline (Fig. 98–13). Branches from the caudal superficial epigastric vessels are ligated in the subcutaneous tissue. The testes and scrotum are removed in a standard fashion (see Chapter 97). The penis is isolated cranially to the scrotum and is temporarily encircled with a heavy ligature proximal to the site of initial transection. The penis is transected and removed. The proximal portion of the penis is exteriorized through a separate midline perineal incision. The ventral abdominal incision is closed in a routine manner.

The temporary ligature is removed, and the penis is cut at a 45° angle dorsoventrally in preparation for perineal urethrostomy. Severed arteries are ligated with 4-0 absorbable material, and the tunica albuginea is apposed over the end of the penis. The urethra is incised along its dorsal midline and sutured to the skin with simple interrupted sutures of nonabsorbable material.[23]

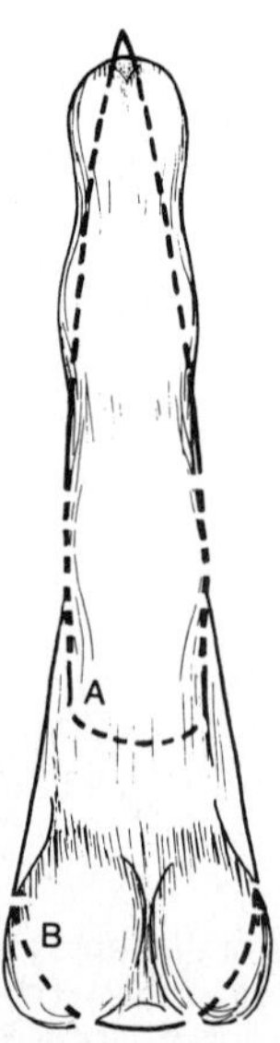

FIGURE 98–13. Incision sites for amputation of the prepuce (A) and combined amputation of the prepuce and scrotum (B) are shown. (Reprinted with permission from Bojrab MJ (ed): *Current Techniques in Small Animal Surgery I.* Lea & Febiger, Philadelphia, 1975.)

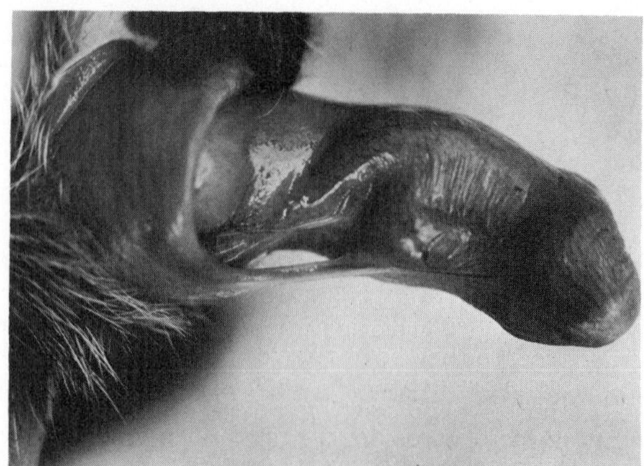

FIGURE 98–14. The persistent penile frenulum is evident, connecting the ventral aspect of the penis and the prepuce.

Persistent Penile Frenulum

Persistence of the penile frenulum occurs in cocker spaniels, miniature poodles, mixed-breed dogs, and Pekingeses (Fig. 98–14).* Pain may be evident during sexual excitement or when an attempt is made to retract the prepuce. The patient may also continually lick the area. Ventral deviation of the glans is usually noted when retraction is attempted. Balanoposthitis may also be seen.

In most domestic animals, the epithelial surfaces of the penis and prepuce are fused at birth and remain so until the onset of puberty.[9, 29] In immature dogs, the penis and prepuce are joined ventrally by a fine band of connective tissue, the frenulum. The frenulum normally ruptures by puberty, under androgenic influences.[3, 14]

Surgical severing of the minimally vascular connective tissue is readily performed after administration of a short-acting anesthetic. The prognosis is favorable after surgery.

Paraphimosis

In paraphimosis, the penis protrudes from the preputial sheath and cannot be replaced to its normal position. Clinical signs depend on the duration of paraphimosis. The exteriorized glans penis becomes congested and discolored owing to the constricting band of retracted prepuce. The dog frequently licks at the exposed penis, exacerbating the inflammation. Severe penile damage can result from prolonged paraphimosis. Necrosis of the exposed penis and urethral obstruction can occur quickly.

Inability to retract the penis completely into the prepuce has both congenital and acquired causes. Con-

*See references 3, 6, 7, 25, 28, 35, and 37.

genital causes include a narrowed preputial orifice and an abnormally shortened prepuce. Acquired causes include trauma, infection, and priapism.[14, 26] Paraphimosis is usually seen after coitus, trauma, or masturbation, particularly in young male dogs.[26]

Treatment is directed at retracting the penis into the prepuce. Lubricants, hyperosmolar solutions, and local heat or cold may be adequate to reduce the size of the penis and permit replacement. The penis is pushed caudally as the prepuce is drawn cranially. If replacement cannot be accomplished within a few hours, an indwelling urethral catheter is sutured in place. Temporary or permanent surgical enlargement of the preputial orifice may be necessary (see the later section on phimosis). Long-standing paraphimosis accompanied by necrosis can require partial penile amputation (see the earlier section on strangulation of the penis).

The prognosis after repair is guarded. Recurrence is common.[14] Paraphimosis accompanied by a deficient prepuce usually requires partial penile amputation to be effective.

Priapism

Priapism—persistent erection not associated with sexual excitement—is uncommon in small animals. It is usually secondary to spinal cord injury, although it may accompany constipation or genitourinary infection.[26] Priapism is distinguished from paraphimosis because the penis can be manually replaced into the prepuce. With additional penile congestion and swelling because of drying and licking, this distinguishing feature is lost.

Treatment is elimination of the primary cause. Some cases subside spontaneously.[26] The exposed penis is kept clean and moist by applying a soothing ointment. Licking is also controlled.

Prolapse of the Urethra

Prolapse of the urethra occurs uncommonly in male dogs. Intermittent hemorrhage from the penis unassociated with urination is often noted. Affected dogs frequently lick the preputial orifice. This condition is mainly encountered in young English bulldogs, although it has been reported in a Boston terrier.[16, 19, 24, 38] Prolapse may follow genitourinary infection or excessive sexual excitement.[24] Swelling, hemorrhage, and drying of the prolapsed tissue occur relatively early, and self-inflicted trauma perpetuates the inflammation.

Diagnosis is made by finding a small red pea-shaped mass at the end of the penis (Fig. 98–15). Treatment is surgical, because spontaneous recovery does not occur.[38] The primary cause is identified and treated. The prolapse can be reduced by inserting a lubricated catheter in the urethra or by gentle manipulation with a moistened gauze sponge. A purse-string suture of fine nonreactive nonabsorbable material is inserted around the exterior of the urethral orifice and tied sufficiently tightly to prevent recurrence. The suture is removed in 5 days. Amputation of the prolapse and anastomosis of urethral and penile mucosa are performed when the prolapse is irreducible, necrotic, or recurrent after the purse-string

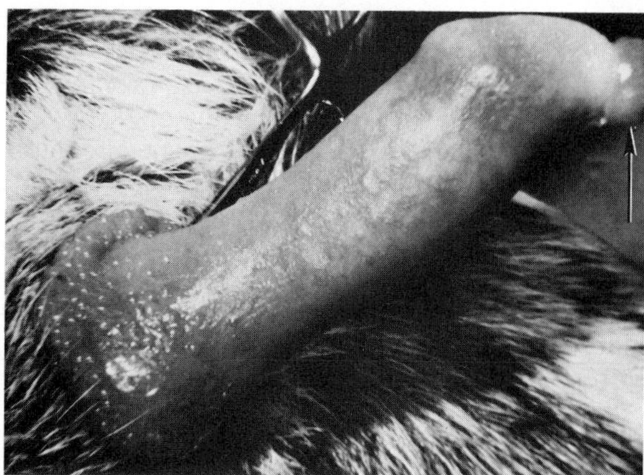

FIGURE 98–15. Prolapsed urethra in a dog. The exposed hemorrhagic urethral mucosa is evident at the end of the penis (*arrow*).

suture has been removed. An incision is made on the ventral surface of the penis through both penile and urethral mucosa, extending halfway around its circumference.[38] Urethral mucosa is sutured to penile mucosa with simple interrupted sutures of 4-0 absorbable material to prevent retraction of the urethral mucosa and to eliminate the need for stay sutures. The dorsal surface of the urethral mucosa is incised and sutured (Fig. 98–16).

The dog is prevented from licking the area postoperatively. Smooth-muscle relaxants and tranquilizers may be helpful in controlling postoperative hemorrhage, which frequently persists for at least 7 to 10 days. The prognosis after surgical repair is favorable, and prolapse usually does not recur.

Prepuce

Phimosis

Phimosis is the inability to protrude the penis beyond the preputial orifice. Clinical signs depend on the cause (congenital or acquired) and the size of the preputial orifice. Congenital phimosis is usually accompanied by

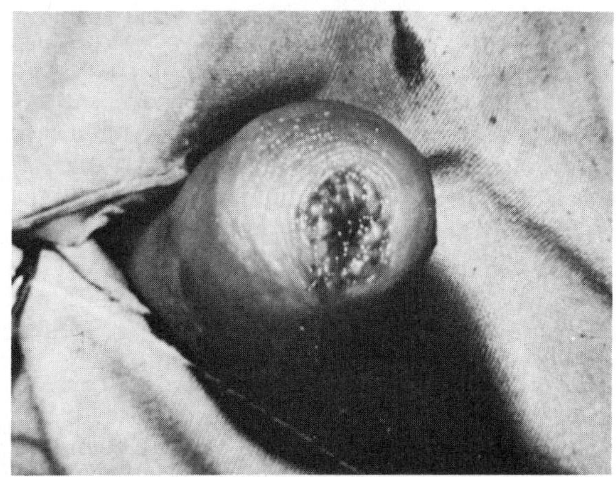

FIGURE 98–16. Amputation of prolapsed urethra. The urethra is sutured to the epithelium of the penis after amputation of the prolapsed portion.

a distended prepuce and inability to urinate normally. Urine can often be passed only in drops or a thin stream.[26] Despite these signs, affected pups are rarely distressed. Urinary outflow obstruction and early death have been reported in one case of congenital phimosis.[27] Preputial retention of urine results in balanoposthitis, and the infected area may ulcerate.[34] Acquired phimosis results from scarring after preputial trauma or neoplasia. Inflammation and edema of the prepuce and associated licking of the area are common. A neoplasm or healing wound can also be present. Retention of urine within the prepuce can occur in severe cases.

Surgical enlargement of the preputial orifice and correction of the primary condition result in successful treatment. A triangular incision is made over the preputial orifice after induction of general anesthesia and appropriate preparation of the site. The skin, subcutaneous tissue, and preputial mucosa are excised, usually on the dorsal surface of the prepuce. As much tissue as possible is removed, although one ensures that the penis remains covered by prepuce. Neoplasms are excised or treated appropriately, and stenosis of the preputial orifice is avoided (see the later section on preputial tumors). Bleeding vessels are ligated or cauterized, and the preputial mucosa is sutured to the skin. Simple interrupted fine nonabsorbable sutures are used.

The prognosis after repair of congenital phimosis is generally favorable. Another operation may be necessary to enlarge the preputial orifice further after the patient is fully grown. Acquired phimosis caused by neoplasia may be complicated by recurrence of the tumor. A larger than normal preputial orifice is created, because postoperative fibrosis can be significant. If too much tissue is removed, particularly from the ventral surface, paraphimosis may result.

Abnormalities of the Prepuce

The prepuce may be hypoplastic or absent or may fail to fuse normally (Fig. 98–17). Clinical signs of congenital preputial abnormalities usually are due to exposure of the distal part of the penis. Affected dogs frequently lick at the penis, causing inflammation. Trauma results in hemorrhage. Normal embryological closure of the genital folds over the penis does not occur, resulting in a deficient prepuce. Failure of preputial fusion usually accompanies hypospadias and underdevelopment or absence of the penis.[17, 39] A deficiency in the length of the prepuce is occasionally seen in dogs. The end of the penis is exposed, subjecting it to trauma and drying. This condition may also be a source of annoyance to the owner.[30]

Surgical management of congenital preputial abnormalities other than phimosis is difficult. Failure of preputial fusion is usually treated by removal of the open prepuce, partial penile amputation, and scrotal or perineal urethrostomy.[17, 39] An elliptical incision is made along each side of the exposed preputial mucosa. The mucosa is dissected to the level of the glans penis. Hemorrhage is controlled with fine absorbable material. Partial penile amputation is performed to excise the exposed distal penis. The preputial mucosa and distal

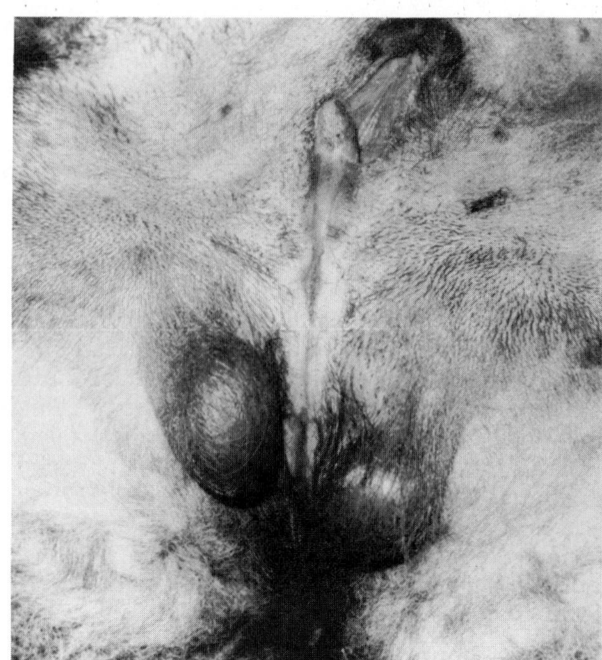

FIGURE 98–17. Failure of preputial fusion, resulting in exposure of the distal penis and abnormal scrotal development.

penis are excised, and the urethra is sutured to the ventral abdominal skin with fine nonabsorbable material. Orchidectomy, scrotal ablation, and perineal urethrostomy may be necessary if the preputial defect is severe.

A deficiency in the length of the prepuce is corrected by advancing the prepuce cranially along the abdominal wall or by partial penile amputation. Simple cranial advancement of the prepuce is often unsuccessful if much of the distal portion of the penis is exposed. After routine preparation of the area, a U-shaped incision is made in the abdominal skin immediately cranial to the prepuce. This part of the prepuce is freed from the abdominal skin and advanced cranially until the penis is covered. This point is marked. A second U-shaped skin incision is made at this level. The skin between the two incisions is excised. The prepuce is sutured in its new position using fine absorbable material in the subcutaneous tissue and fine nonabsorbable material in the skin.[26, 30]

The prognosis after repair of congenital preputial defects is guarded. Even if adequate coverage of the penis has been achieved after cranial preputial advancement with the dog anesthetized, the distal part of the penis may remain exposed postoperatively. Partial penile amputation usually corrects this problem. Urethral stricture may follow partial penile amputation if healing is complicated.

Preputial Foreign Bodies

Foreign bodies such as grass awns, plant seeds, pieces of straw, and urinary calculi can lodge in the preputial cavity. Clinical signs are often mild and may be overlooked. A purulent, blood-tinged preputial discharge may be present, and the animal frequently licks the prepuce. Migration of the foreign body through the preputial mucosa at the fornix results in swelling and abscess of the tissues surrounding the penis. The animal usually is in pain, listless, and mildly pyrectic and walks stiffly. A draining tract may be present ventral or lateral to the penis.

Removal of the foreign body from the preputial cavity usually corrects the associated balanoposthitis. Irrigation of the preputial cavity may be necessary. Draining tracts are opened and explored for foreign bodies. After removal of the foreign body, the tract is flushed with antiseptic solution and drained. Systemic antibiotics may be indicated. The prognosis is usually favorable if the foreign body is removed.

Preputial Wounds

Preputial wounds are not uncommon in dogs. Superficial lacerations and abrasions usually cause mild clinical signs, including local swelling, edema, and irritation. Wounds may be inflicted during mating or by trauma caused by barbed wire, motor accidents, and gun pellets.[31] Wounds that penetrate into the preputial cavity or are near the preputial orifice are most likely to require surgical management.

Management of superficial wounds often involves avoiding self-inflicted trauma by preventing the patient's licking the wound. Initial cleaning of the wound followed by topical application of antiseptics or antibiotics may also be indicated. Surgical management of preputial wounds involves suturing the preputial mucosa and skin separately after thorough cleaning of the wound and preputial cavity and possibly wound débridement. Some wounds are allowed to heal by second intention.

Preputial Tumors

The prepuce is affected by the same tumors as the skin.[4, 26] Clinical signs are often minimal, unless the tumor ulcerates or involves the preputial orifice. Phimosis and balanoposthitis can result. Mast cell tumors are the most frequently reported tumors of the external genitalia.[4] Transmissible venereal tumors, melanomas, and perianal gland tumors have also been reported.[4, 29, 39]

Diagnosis is made by incisional, excisional, or cytological biopsy. Surgical removal of the tumor with closure of the prepuce in two layers is the treatment. The penis must remain covered by the prepuce. Partial penile amputation may be necessary after removal of large tumors. Orchidectomy is recommended after removal of a perianal gland tumor.

Scrotum

Scrotal Injury

Scrotal injury is uncommon despite the exposed location of the scrotum.[26] Clinical signs depend on the severity of the injury. Minor abrasions and lacerations may be initially undetected because of the paucity of clinical signs. Inflammation with or without signs of infection is seen, and the scrotum is sensitive to palpation. An affected animal frequently licks at scrotal wounds, causing further inflammation and possible infection. A stiff gait may be noted, and the dog prefers to sit. Significant wounds are likely to become infected if treatment is delayed. Trauma to the parietal vaginal tunic of the testis can result in infection within the cavity of the vaginal tunic and even orchitis.

Minor abrasions and lacerations are treated by gently cleaning the wound with saline, applying topical antibiotics, and preventing self-inflicted trauma. Antiseptics are usually not used on the scrotum because of the irritation they produce. More extensive wounds require suturing with fine nonreactive skin sutures after cleaning, débridement, and local antibiotic irrigation. Severely contaminated wounds may require orchidectomy with scrotal ablation (see Chapter 97).

The prognosis after scrotal injury is favorable if contamination has been minimal and the parietal vaginal tunic has not been traumatized. Prevention of self-mutilation of the scrotum is the usual aftercare. Systemic antibiotics may be indicated in extensive scrotal wounds.

Infection of the Scrotal Skin

The exposed location and delicacy of the scrotal skin make it relatively susceptible to irritants. A disinfectant such as iodine is frequently the cause of scrotal irritation and subsequent infection, particularly in surgical procedures and in kennels. Scrotal dermatitis is a prominent feature of *Brucella canis* infection of male dogs.[20] Infection can also be secondary to scrotal laceration. The scrotal skin is inflamed, edematous, exudative, and sensitive to palpation. Culture and susceptibility testing of the exudate determine appropriate antibiotic therapy. Treatment is avoidance of further scrotal irritation and local treatment with emollients and antibiotics. Systemic antibiotics are indicated in severe cases. The prognosis is generally favorable; severe cases may require orchidectomy and scrotal ablation (see Chapter 97).

Varicosities of the Scrotal Blood Vessels

Varicose dilation of scrotal veins occurs in older dogs.[29, 42] The varicosities are seen as flattened and irregular thickenings of the scrotal skin.[29] They are subepithelial, with the overlying epithelium normal or ulcerated. Trauma leads to ulceration and repeated episodes of profuse bleeding.

Treatment consists of either stimulating thrombosis of the varicose vessels with styptics or surgically removing the involved scrotal skin and blood vessels. Surgical removal is generally more effective, because recurrence after use of styptics or chemical cautery is common. All involved scrotal skin is excised without incision of the parietal vaginal tunic. Blood vessels are ligated, and the incision is closed with fine nonabsorbable skin sutures. A support bandage and prevention of self-injury are indicated postoperatively. Extensive lesions may require excision of the majority of the scrotum. The testes can be transposed to the subcutaneous tissues lateral to the penis; however, orchidectomy is generally indicated. The prognosis depends on the severity of the lesion.

Chronic Hyperplasia of the Scrotum

Hyperplasia of the scrotum is common in older dogs.[26] The ventral part of the scrotum is thickened, wrinkled, and usually heavily pigmented. This condition presumably results from chronic irritation of the scrotum. Because of the insulating effect of the thickened scrotum, fertility may be reduced. Scrotal hyperplasia usually is not clinically significant unless secondary infection occurs. Simple cases of scrotal hyperplasia usually are not treated. Resistant infections are treated by excision of the involved tissue and closure of the scrotum with fine sutures. It is important to avoid incising the parietal vaginal tunic. Extensive hyperplasia with infection may require orchidectomy and scrotal ablation (see Chapter 97).

Scrotal Neoplasms

Many cutaneous neoplasms involve the scrotum.[5, 10, 26] Mastocytomas are commonly reported. Because of their accessible location, scrotal neoplasms can often be differentiated by fine-needle aspiration or impression smears (see Section 17). Wide excision of a scrotal neoplasm may necessitate orchidectomy and scrotal ablation. Closure of scrotal skin after removal of a neoplasm is performed with fine nonabsorbable sutures.

References

1. Ader PL, Hobson HP: Hypospadias: A review of the veterinary literature and a report of three cases in the dog. *J Am Anim Hosp Assoc 14*:721, 1978.
2. Aronson LR, Cooper ML: Penile spines of the domestic cat: Their endocrine-behavior relations. *Anat Rec 157*:71, 1967.
3. Balke J: Persistent penile frenulum in a Cocker Spaniel. *Vet Med Small Anim Clin 76*:988, 1981.
4. Barrett RE, Theilen GH: Neoplasms of the canine and feline reproductive tracts. *In* Kirk RW (ed): *Current Veterinary Therapy VI*. W. B. Saunders, Philadelphia, 1977, pp 1263–1267.
5. Barron CN: Scrotal neoplasms—a report of two cases in the dog. *J Am Vet Med Assoc 115*:13, 1949.
6. Begg TB: Persistent penile frenulum in the dog. *Vet Rec 75*:930, 1963.
7. Belkin PB: Persistence of penile frenulum in a dog. *Mod Vet Pract 50*:80, 1969.
8. Bennett D, et al: Wedge osteotomy of the os penis to correct penile deviation. *J Small Anim Pract 27*:379, 1986.
9. Bharadwaj MB, Calhoun ML: Mode of formation of the preputial cavity in domesticated animals. *Am J Vet Res 22*:764, 1961.
10. Brodey RS: Multiple genital neoplasia (mast cell sarcoma, seminoma, and sertoli cell tumor) in a dog. *J Am Vet Med Assoc 128*:450, 1956.
11. Brown NO, et al: Chemotherapeutic management of transmissible venereal tumors in 30 dogs. *J Am Vet Med Assoc 176*:983, 1980.
12. Carati CJ, et al: Vascular changes during penile erection in the dog. *J Physiol 400*:75, 1988.
13. Christensen GC: Angioarchitecture of the canine penis and the process of erection. *Am J Anat 95*:227, 1954.
14. Christie TR: Phimosis and paraphimosis. *In* Bojrab MJ (ed): *Pathophysiology in Small Animal Surgery*. Lea & Febiger, Philadelphia, 1981, pp 442–443.
15. Colleen S, et al: An angiographic study of erection in the dog. *Urol Res 9*:297, 1981.
16. Copland MD: Prolapse of the penile urethra in a dog. *NZ Vet J 23*:180, 1975.
17. Croshaw JE Jr, Brodey RS: Failure of preputial closure in a dog. *J Am Vet Med Assoc 136*:450, 1960.
18. Evans HE, Christensen GC (eds): *Miller's Anatomy of the Dog*. 2nd ed. W. B. Saunders, Philadelphia, 1979, pp 554–565.
19. Firestone WM: Prolapse of the male urethra. *J Am Vet Med Assoc 99*:135, 1941.
20. George LW, et al: Semen examination in dogs with canine brucellosis. *Am J Vet Res 40*:1589, 1979.
21. Glover TD: Recent progress in the study of male reproductive physiology: Testis stimulation; sperm formation, transport and maturation (epididymal physiology); semen analysis, storage and artificial insemination. *In* Greep RO (ed): *International Review of Physiology: Reproductive Physiology I*. University Park Press, Baltimore, 1975.
22. Hall MA, Swenberg LN: Genital emergencies. *In* Kirk RW (ed): *Current Veterinary Therapy VI*. W. B. Saunders, Philadelphia, 1977, pp 1216–1227.
23. Hobson HP: Surgical procedures of the penis. *In* Bojrab MJ (ed): *Current Techniques in Small Animal Surgery*. 3rd ed. Lea & Febiger, Philadelphia, 1990, pp 423–430.
24. Hobson HP, Heller RA: Surgical correction of prolapse of the male urethra. *Vet Med Small Anim Clin 66*:1177, 1971.
25. Hutchison, JA: Persistence of the penile frenulum in dogs. *Can Vet J 14*:71, 1973.
26. Johnston DE, Archibald J: Male genital system. *In* Archibald J (ed): *Canine and Feline Surgery*. Vol. 1. American Veterinary Publications, Santa Barbara, 1984, pp 293–356.
27. Johnston SD: Disorders of the external genitalia of the male. *In* Ettinger SJ (ed): *Textbook of Veterinary Internal Medicine*. 3rd ed. W. B. Saunders, Philadelphia, 1989, pp 1881–1889.
28. Joshua JO: Persistence of the penile frenulum in a dog. *Vet Rec 74*:1550, 1962.
29. Ladds PW: The male genital system. *In* Jubb KUF, Kennedy PC (eds): *Pathology of Domestic Animals*. 3rd ed. Academic Press, New York, 1985, pp 409–459.
30. Leighton RL: A simple surgical correction for chronic penile protrusion. *J Am Anim Hosp Assoc 12*:667, 1976.
31. Ndiritu CG: Lesions of the canine penis and prepuce. *Mod Vet Pract 60*:712, 1979.
32. Nickel R, et al (eds): *The Viscera of Domestic Mammals*. 2nd ed. Springer-Verlag, New York, 1979, pp 304–350.
33. Pineda MH, Faulkner LC: Male reproduction. *In* McDonald LE (ed): *Veterinary Endocrinology and Reproduction*. 3rd ed. Lea & Febiger, Philadelphia, 1980, pp 235–273.
34. Proescholdt TA, et al: Preputial reconstruction for phimosis and infantile penis. *J Am Anim Hosp Assoc 13*:725, 1977.
35. Pugh DG, et al: A persistent penile frenulum in a dog. *Canine Pract 14*:38, 1987.
36. Richardson RC: Canine transmissible venereal tumor. *Comp Cont Educ Pract Vet 3*:951, 1981.
37. Ryer KA: Persistent penile frenulum in a cocker spaniel. *Vet Med Small Anim Clin 74*:688, 1979.
38. Sinibaldi KR, Green RW: Surgical correction of prolapse of the male urethra in three English bulldogs. *J Am Anim Hosp Assoc 9*:450, 1973.
39. Smith CW: Developmental anomalies. *In* Bojrab MJ (ed): *Pathophysiology in Small Animal Surgery*. Lea & Febiger, Philadelphia, 1981, pp 445–447.
40. Spurgeon TL, et al: Physiologic properties of contraction of the canine cremaster and cranial preputial muscles. *Am J Vet Res 39*:1884, 1978.
41. Stead AC: Fracture of the os penis in the dog—two case reports. *J Small Anim Pract 13*:19, 1972.
42. Weipers WL, Jarrett WFH: Haemangioma of the scrotum of dogs. *Vet Rec 66*:106, 1954.

CHAPTER

99 The Prostate

R. Randy Basinger, C. Lee Robinette,
E. M. Hardie, and Kathy A. Spaulding

ANATOMY AND PHYSIOLOGY

Anatomy

The prostate gland is the only accessory sex organ in male dogs.[77] Although cats have a prostate gland, prostatic disease is rare. Embryologically, the prostate is formed by buds arising from the pelvic urethra at about the sixth week of gestation.[18] The gland lies within the abdomen after birth until degeneration of the urachal remnant occurs around 2 months of age, after which it assumes a position in the pelvic cavity.[18] The prepubertal prostate is a small nodular enlargement around the proximal urethra. It is generally no more than 1 cm in diameter in dogs of beagle size.[77] At puberty, it grows to normal mature proportions, being bounded dorsally by the rectum and ventrally by the symphysis pubis and abdominal wall.[18, 77] A normal mature prostate weighs 0.64 to 0.96 g/kg of body weight in beagle-sized dogs.[77] The weight of the prostate of adult Scottish terriers, when expressed relative to body weight, was described as unusually large compared with other breeds. Because this observation was based on measurements of seven Scottish terriers that were older than the other breeds in the study, its validity is unknown and further confirmation is needed.[66] With advancing age, the prostate continues to increase in size by hyperplasia,[11] and it moves cranially.[18] By 4 years of age, approximately half of the gland is located in the abdomen, and by 10 years, it may be completely abdominal.[18]

A normal mature prostate is ovoid to spherical on transverse section and possesses a dorsal and ventral sulcus. The dorsal portion of the gland encircles the urethra close to the neck of the bladder.[18, 77] The vasa deferentia enter each side of the craniodorsal prostate, pass caudoventrally through the gland, and empty into the urethra.[18] A fibromuscular capsule surrounds the gland.[77]

Histology

The prostate has epithelial and stromal (smooth muscle, fibroblasts, and collagen) components. The epithelial cells predominate, with the stroma occupying 10 per cent of the organ. The architecture of the prostate is characterized by compound tubuloalveoli that drain into the urethra.[77] Irregular smooth-muscle septa, which extend from the prostatic capsule to the periurethral connective tissue, divide the organ into well-defined lobules.[11]

Although a large proportion (90 to 95 per cent) of the epithelial cells produce secretions, the secretory material is generally stored within the cellular cytoplasm rather than in alveoli.[77] The secretory cells are columnar to cuboidal in shape, show an intensely eosinophilic cytoplasm, and often form characteristic alveolar infoldings.[11, 77] Undifferentiated basal cells, located along the basement membrane, constitute the remainder of the epithelial cells, which are identified by their nuclei when routine histological methods are used.[77]

Vessels and Nerves

The blood supply of the gland is provided by branches of the prostatic artery that penetrate the prostatic capsule on the dorsolateral surface. The prostatic artery arises from the internal pudendal or the umbilical artery. Anastomoses can be found between the prostatic vessels and the urethral artery and the cranial and caudal rectal arteries. Venous return is provided by the prostatic and urethral veins that connect to the internal iliac vein. Lymph drains into the iliac lymph nodes.[18]

The gland is innervated by the hypogastric and pelvic nerves. The hypogastric nerve follows the artery of the ductus deferens to the prostate. The pelvic nerve follows the prostatic artery to the pelvic plexus before projecting fibers to the gland.[18] Neurons from the hypogastric nerve, part of the sympathetic nervous system, stimulate the secretory epithelium, as well as the contractile smooth muscle.[74] The postganglionic hypogastric neurons innervating the secretory epithelium are short and cholinergic,[74] compared with the long, adrenergic fibers characteristic of most postganglionic sympathetic nerves.[86a] The postganglionic motor fibers from the hypogastric nerve are short and adrenergic. The pelvic nerve provides parasympathetic cholinergic innervation to the smooth muscle, with little influence on the secretory epithelium.[74]

Based on anatomical determinants and experimental nerve stimulation studies, the active secretory process of the epithelium is under cholinergic regulation by postganglionic fibers of the hypogastric nerve.[74] Muscle contractions that expel the prostatic fluid are primarily controlled by the adrenergic postganglionic neurons of the hypogastric nerve, but cholinergic pelvic nerve fibers may contribute.[74, 84]

In addition to these neural pathways, evidence now suggests that the canine prostate also contains opioidergic nerves and ganglia. The opioids produced by these structures may regulate prostatic stromal tone and local vascular perfusion.[3]

Physiology

Secretions

Despite the large numbers of studies that have focused on canine prostate structure, the physiological functions of the gland remain poorly understood. Although prostatic secretions provide a vehicle for spermatozoa, they may not be essential for fertility.[47] Prostatic contribution to seminal plasma varies from dog to dog and from time to time in the same animal. Quantitative studies during ejaculation have shown that a volume of prostatic fluid varying from 2 to 30 ml can be secreted during a period of 3 to 35 minutes. This fluid becomes part of the semen during the third phase of ejaculation, after the contributions of the urethral mucous glands and the testes have been expressed. The secretions provided by the prostate during this process consist of components that are newly synthesized, as well as preformed.[74]

Experimental studies have shown that resting secretion of 0.1 to 2.0 ml/hour occurs independently of neural stimulation and that fluids produced by this process are hypotonic and slightly acidic.[74, 84] Sodium, potassium, and chloride, the major electrolytes found in these fluids, are less concentrated than in plasma, and the protein concentration is low. Active secretion induced by ejaculation produces a product that is high in protein, slightly acidic, and isotonic. In these secretions, the sodium concentration is equivalent to plasma, and the potassium and chloride concentrations are higher than in plasma.[74]

Zinc is also secreted by the prostate in relatively high concentrations. Although the functions of zinc are incompletely understood, it may be important for normal sperm function and antibacterial activity.[13]

A prostate-derived enzyme, arginine esterase, is found in high concentrations (10 mg/ml) in seminal plasma and constitutes more than 90 per cent of the total protein in the ejaculate.[16, 50] Maintenance of the normal quantity and quality of prostatic secretion requires adequate stimulation by androgenic hormones,[49, 51] and the androgen-dependent level of arginine esterase in prostatic secretions reflects the hormonal status of the dog.[17, 51] Acid phosphatase, a common marker of human prostatic function, is also present in canine prostatic secretions but in smaller quantities.[23] The functions of these enzymes are unknown.[23, 50]

Benign Prostatic Hyperplasia

As a dog ages, the prostate undergoes spontaneous enlargement, commonly referred to as *benign prostatic hyperplasia*.[14] Clinically, it can sufficiently enlarge the prostate to cause obstruction of the colon and rectum, and under severe conditions, urethral obstruction can also occur.[77] Hyperplasia begins as early as 1 to 2 years of age, and its prevalence increases with age. More than 80 per cent of 6-year-old dogs show histological evidence of benign prostatic hyperplasia. By 9 years of age, a 95 per cent prevalence rate has been documented. In the 8.1 to 10-year-old range, the prostate in some dogs with pre-existing benign prostatic hyperplasia undergoes additional accelerated growth that can greatly enhance the already enlarged gland.[11] Despite these changes in size, prostatic secretory capacity per gram of tissue decreases as benign prostatic hyperplasia develops.[9, 14, 87]

Various factors associated with the disease process have been characterized in beagles.[11, 14] Two distinct histotypes, glandular hyperplasia and complex hyperplasia, have been described.[77] The glandular form may be an antecedent of the complex form.[11, 14, 77] Glandular hyperplasia begins at 1 to 2 years of age and its prevalence peaks at 5.1 to 6 years. During this time, the prostate develops a proliferation of secretory structures that are distributed uniformly throughout the organ. The histological appearance of this growth reveals an increase in the number and size of the epithelial cells, accompanied by a smaller but significant proliferation of stromal fibroblasts and smooth muscles.[11, 77] These changes are reflected in a more elaborate branching of the glandular structures and in enlarged alveoli that have more pronounced papillary infoldings.[11] Although the wet weight of the gland increases from a normal of approximately 12 g to 20 g in benign prostatic hyperplasia, its overall consistency remains relatively normal.[11, 77]

The second histotype, complex hyperplasia, generally develops later, with the first evidence of complex benign prostatic hyperplasia appearing at 2 to 3 years of age.[11, 77] This histotype increases with age and affects 70 per cent of dogs between 8 and 9 years old.[11] Light microscopic analysis shows a diverse morphological pattern compared with glandular benign prostatic hyperplasia. Cystic, dilated alveoli filled with eosinophilic material are a characteristic feature and can give the surface of the prostate an irregular contour. The epithelial lining of these cysts varies from a columnar appearance with eosinophilic cytoplasm to cuboidal cells with no evidence of secretory capacity. Although distributed throughout the prostate, the cysts are more numerous in periurethral areas. Inflammation consisting of lymphocytes and plasma cells is common, appearing as clusters or nodules of cells in the stroma.[11, 77] The inflammatory reactions have raised the possibility of concurrent infectious or autoimmune processes.[77] Frequent epithelial atrophy and occasional epithelial squamous metaplasia are associated with these areas of inflammation. Other portions of the same gland may look normal or have characteristics more representative of glandular hyperplasia. In general, the stroma of cystic hyperplasia is more prominent than in glandular hyperplasia.[11, 77] Prostatic weight with this type of hyperplasia (average approximately 23 g) is similar to the glandular form.[11]

That hormones may be involved in the induction or maintenance of benign prostatic hyperplasia has long been recognized, because dogs castrated early in life do not develop the problem.[48] If dogs with pre-existing benign prostatic hyperplasia are castrated, the hyperplasia regresses but is restored if exogenous testosterone is administered.[10]

Glandular hyperplasia can be induced when young, intact dogs are injected with the active intracellular androgen dihydrotestosterone or with 3α-androstane3α, 17β-diol, which can be converted to dihydrotestosterone. To induce hyperplasia in castrated dogs, estradiol-17β had to be coadministered with dihydrotestosterone or androstanediol.[14] These studies have been interpreted as demonstrating that hormonal manipulation can induce benign prostatic hyperplasia but that some testicular factor such as an estrogen in addition to androgens may be required.[14, 24] The estrogenic stimulation may enhance the sensitivity of the prostate to intracellular dihydrotestosterone.[83]

In addition to endogenous estrogens, phytoestrogens

were detected in the urine of dogs fed commercial diets that naturally contained these substances.[53]

Although glandular benign prostatic hyperplasia has been induced experimentally, complex benign prostatic hyperplasia has not.[14] Additional studies are required to gain more insight into the factors influencing this particular expression of the disease process. Because benign prostatic hyperplasia in men is primarily a stromal disease, further evaluation of the stromal proliferation of canine complex benign prostatic hyperplasia may provide insights into the pathogenesis of the disorder in humans.[77]

RADIOGRAPHY AND ULTRASONOGRAPHY

Radiography and ultrasonography are used to characterize architectural abnormalities of the canine prostate gland. A complete sonographic and radiographic examination of the male reproductive tract includes evaluation of the prostate gland, testes, entire urinary tract, periprostatic tissue, lumbar spine, pelvis, and regional lymph nodes. Contributing to a presumptive diagnosis of prostatic disease are changes in the size, topography, location, and opacity of the prostate gland; iliac lymph node enlargement; and proliferative or invasive changes in the lumbar vertebrae or pelvis.

Prostatic Radiography[26, 28, 34, 76, 79]

The position of the prostate depends on bladder distension and the age and conformation of the dog, as well as pathological prostatic enlargement. An immature or involuted prostate in a castrated dog may be too small to be apparent on radiographs. A normal mature prostate appears as an ovoid homogeneous soft-tissue opacity caudal to the bladder and primarily within the pelvic canal. The cranial margin is often apparent on a lateral recumbent radiograph, cranial to the brim of the pelvis, especially with an enlarged prostate (Fig. 99–1). A triangular area of fat lies between the caudoventral border of the bladder and the cranioventral margin of the prostate gland. The peripheral border is smooth. When the bladder is distended, in obese animals, or with prostatomegaly, the entire prostate gland may lie within the abdominal cavity. A normal prostate occupies less than 50 per cent of the pelvic canal, as measured from the sacrum to the promontory of the pubis. Soft-tissue opacities, including feces in the intestinal tract, pelvic limb skinfolds, and quadriceps muscles, when superimposed over the prostate may mimic prostatic disease. The pelvic limbs are extended caudally to avoid superimposition over the prostate. On a ventrodorsal view, the prostate frequently appears, reduced in size because of feces in the colon and the superimposed pubic bones. In some instances, administration of contrast material is necessary to identify the bladder and to outline the border of the prostatic urethra. Spread or extension of disease to the skeleton, regional organs, and lungs necessitates radiographic evaluation of these areas.

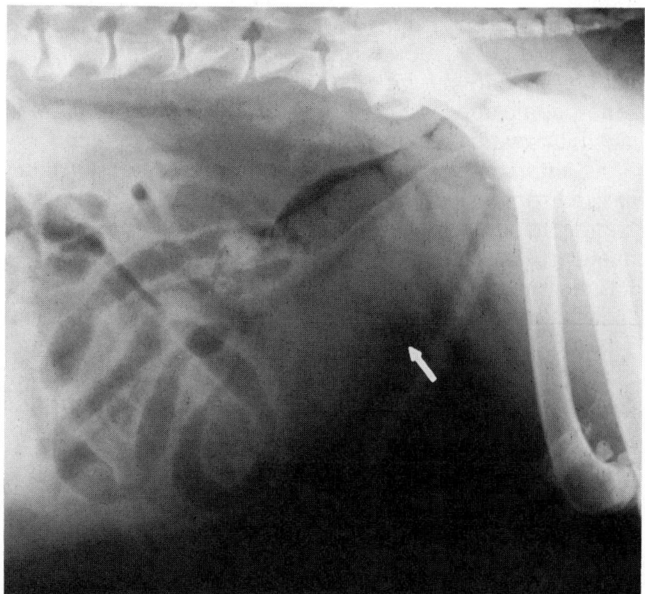

FIGURE 99–1. Lateral radiograph of a dog with an enlarged prostate. A triangular area of fat (*arrow*) lies between the caudoventral border of the bladder and the cranioventral margin of the prostate.

Prostatic Ultrasonography*

The clinical usefulness and safety of ultrasonography makes it an integral part of the assessment and management of prostatic disease. Ultrasonography is more informative and sensitive than radiology for detecting intraparenchymal prostatic disease, but neither is specific for investigating the underlying cause. Ultrasonography is useful in guiding a biopsy needle into diseased areas to help establish a final diagnosis.

A 10- or a 7.5-MHz transducer or both are recommended for most dogs because they provide clear resolution of the prostatic parenchyma. A 5- or 3-MHz transducer may provide useful information about the prostate's size, location, and architecture but does not show detail. Use the most powerful transducer available to penetrate to the needed depth. Either a sector or linear type of probe may be used. Large linear probes cannot completely access the prostate because of interference by the bony pelvic canal.

The entire prostate is evaluated. Sagittal, dorsal, or and transverse planes are recommended. Because the caudal border of the prostate gland may be obscured by overlying pelvic bone and the penis and os penis are on the abdominal midline, oblique or angled planes of the prostate may be necessary. If the caudal border is still difficult to see, the gland can be pushed cranially by an assistant with rectal manipulation. The urethra is traced through the prostate gland in both sagittal and transverse planes. The urinary tract, testicles, periprostatic tissue, and medial iliac lymph nodes are also examined.

The prostate is evaluated for size, shape, symmetry, echogenicity, and cavitational areas. The parenchyma is described as normal, focally involved, or diffusely af-

*See references 1, 8, 15, 25, 27, 42, 68, and 82.

fected. Ultrasonography may differentiate prostatomegaly attributable to cysts, abscesses, cystic hyperplasia, neoplasm, and paraprostatic cysts and abscesses. The sonographic appearance of these disease processes overlaps. (Disorders of the prostate are discussed later.)

An immature prostate encircles the urethra, is small, has indistinguishable or faintly distinct lobes, and has a homogeneous hypoechoic appearance. A fully developed prostate has a uniform homogeneous echoic pattern throughout both lobes. Prostatic echogenicity is slightly hyperechoic, relative to splenic parenchyma. This quality may be influenced by the transducer and other factors such as the sexual maturity of the dog. The urethra may be traced from the trigone of the urinary bladder through the prostate gland. The mucosal surface of the urethra resembles a doughnut; a hypoechoic center appears within the echoic prostate. A distended urethra has an anechoic lumen. The cranial prostatic urethra may appear wider than the caudal prostatic urethra when the bladder is distended. It narrows in the middle part of the prostate where the ductus deferens enters the dorsal urethral wall. The periurethral region is frequently hypoechoic relative to the remainder of the prostate. This quality may reflect the smooth muscle normally located in the periurethral area. Shadowing in the periurethral area, seen in some dogs, may be attributed to absorption of the ultrasound beam by the periurethral tissues.

The prostate gland becomes diffusely enlarged with benign prostatic hyperplasia. Early benign prostatic hyperplasia does not cause appreciable change in size or echo. With more advanced hyperplasia, the prostate gland may be more hyperechoic. Age changes or chronic hyperplasia may lead to a heterogeneous echoic pattern. Focal scarring causes focal hyperechoic regions, whereas other areas appear relatively hypoechoic.

Cystic hyperplasia, which frequently accompanies benign prostatic hyperplasia, is recognized by small hypoechoic to anechoic areas in the parenchyma. The cysts are usually of millimeter size but may reach centimeter size. Clinical history, physical examination, and laboratory findings are important in differentiating cystic hyperplasia from prostatitis or small abscesses because they have a similar ultrasonographic appearance. Large cavitary areas (> 1 cm) are more likely abscesses, cysts, or hemacysts (Fig. 99–2). Abscesses frequently have irregular borders, and the surrounding parenchyma shows decreased echogenicity. The remainder of the prostate may have normal echogenicity or may exhibit a patchy hyperechoic appearance. Periprostatic cysts are present as cystic structures usually extending from the prostate gland. Concomitant cavitary intraprostatic involvement may be present. A parenchymal cyst may communicate with the urethra.

Acute prostatitis has a varying sonographic pattern. No change may be apparent in mild or early prostatitis, or it may resemble benign prostatic hyperplasia. Diffusely hypoechoic or a patchy, complex hyperechoic and hypoechoic pattern may be seen with chronic or more severe inflammatory process (Fig. 99–3). Chronic disease may also have nonspecific focal hyperechoic areas indicating fibrosis, stromal proliferation, or glandular aging. Areas of fibrosis may occasionally attenuate the beam sufficiently to cause a bright echo and shadowing. Gas within the prostate creates a bright echo and usually a reverberation artifact. Gas occasionally mimics mineralization. Extensive gas or mineralization interferes with complete evaluation of the gland.

After castration, the involuted prostate is small and hypoechoic and the lobes less distinct. Residual disease may persist within the diseased prostate after castration,

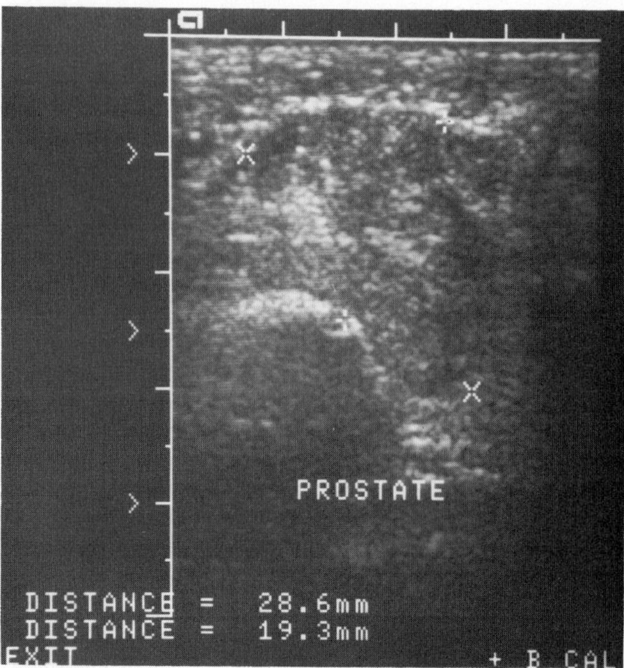

FIGURE 99–2. Sonogram of a canine prostate with complex echo pattern with focal areas of hyperechogenicity and hypoechogenicity (transverse plane).

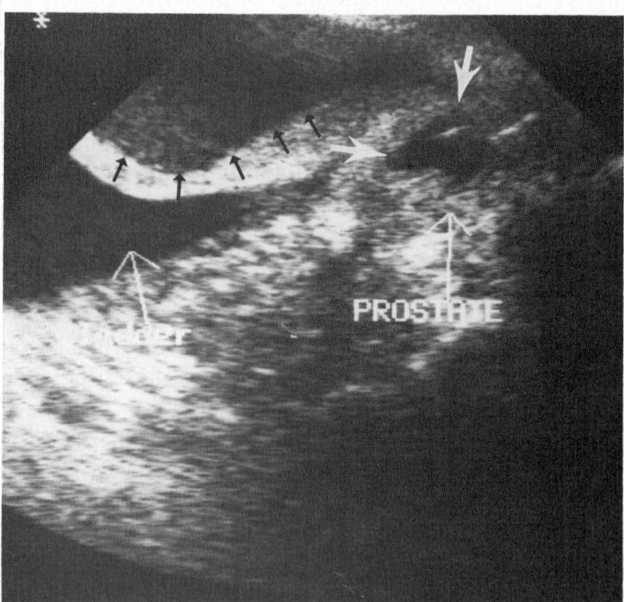

FIGURE 99–3. Sonogram of an enlarged prostate with large cavitary area (*white arrows*) that could be an abscess or cyst. A large paraprostatic cyst (*black arrows*) extends ventral to the bladder (sagittal plane).

surgery, or antibiotic therapy. Repeated sonographic evaluation is important for monitoring progression or regression of disease.

Tumors of the prostate are often hyperechoic and contain mineralization (Fig. 99–4). Early tumors may have a hypoechoic appearance. Concurrent prostatic abscesses or other significant disease may obscure a tumor. If the continuity of the urethra is disrupted and an abscess is not apparent, a urethral or prostatic tumor should be considered. Focal hyperechoic areas with or without shadowing arouse suspicion of tumor. Disruption of the prostatic capsule may occur with tumor, cyst, periprostatic cyst, or abscess.

The lymph nodes in the sublumbar area are evaluated for enlargement. The medial iliac lymph nodes are located adjacent to the bifurcation of the aorta and caudal vena cava. Normal lymph nodes cannot be identified by ultrasonographic examination. Enlarged lymph nodes are typically hypoechoic and elliptical. They may become hyperechoic or contain hyperechoic shadowing areas of mineralization.

PROSTATE DISORDERS

Clinical Disorders

Diseases of the prostate can produce clinical signs from weight loss and lethargy to septic shock with cardiovascular collapse. Male dogs that demonstrate tenesmus, penile discharge, hematuria, pyuria, stranguria, urinary incontinence, caudal abdominal pain, an acute abdomen, or ambulatory difficulty due to pelvic cavity discomfort are evaluated for prostatic disease.

Complete agreement has not been reached about classification of prostatic disease with respect to pathophysiological origin. The system presented here correlates with clinical presentation and takes into account two concerns of other investigators: (1) Multiple disease processes are often present microscopically, and (2) suppurative prostatitis may be an early stage of a disease continuum leading to prostatic abscessation.

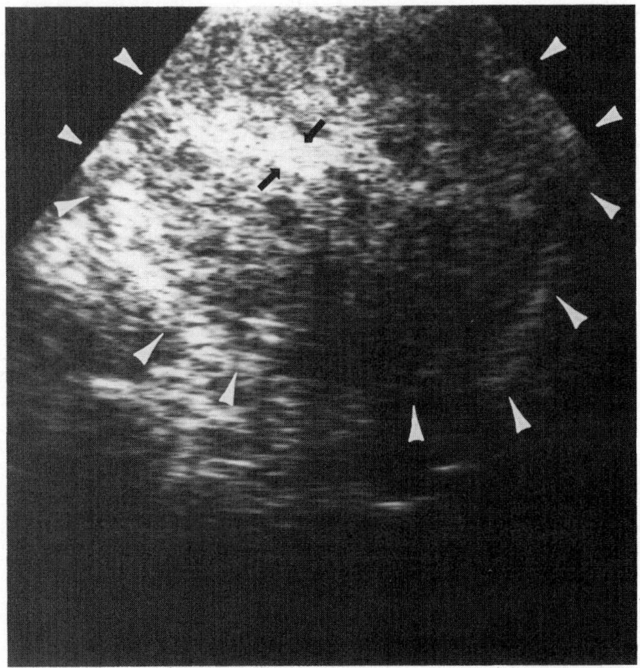

FIGURE 99–4. Sonogram of an enlarged prostate with focal hyperechoic shadowing areas (*black arrows*) containing mineralization (transverse plane). Prostatic adenocarcinoma was confirmed by microscopic examination.

Diagnostic Techniques

A complete anamnesis should be obtained. Reproductive, urinary, and gastrointestinal system questions are emphasized. It is important to determine if any nearby female dogs are in estrus.

Hematuria and penile discharge at the end of urination are often reported. If the prostate is greatly enlarged, urine retention and constipation are noted. Dogs with bacterial prostatic infections are frequently ill with fever, lethargy, anorexia, dehydration, vomiting, or weight loss. Caudal abdominal, lumbar, or pelvic pain suggests prostatitis, peritonitis, or neoplasia. Cachexia may accompany neoplasia.

Physical examination includes careful abdominal and rectal palpation. In larger dogs, elevating the forequarters or lifting the caudal abdominal contents while the examiner's finger is within the rectum facilitates digital examination of the prostate. The position, sensitivity, contour, texture, mobility, symmetry, and size of the prostate are noted. In some dogs, it is possible to palpate enlarged iliac lymph nodes. Both testicles are palpated for tumors. If urinary retention or obstruction is suspected, catheterizing the urethra allows determination of urethral lumen patency and measurement of residual urine volume.

Minimum data base includes a complete blood count, biochemistry profile, *Brucella canis* titer, urinalysis, and caudal abdominal radiographs.[72]

Many dogs with prostatic disease have disorders of urine storage or voiding.[5] Urodynamic abnormalities may be exacerbated by surgery or biopsy. Early identification and characterization of these abnormalities allow for appropriate treatment and avoids clients' misunderstanding.

Prostatic fluid may be obtained for cytological study and culture by ejaculation, prostatic wash, or fine-needle aspiration. Cytological criteria obtained by prostatic wash and fine-needle aspiration for diagnosis of prostatic disease have been reviewed.[80] Prostatic tissue may be obtained for histopathological examination and culture by percutaneous techniques or during laparotomy.

Collection of ejaculate and interpretation of results have been described.[57] Disadvantages of ejaculate samples are the difficulty in obtaining samples in dogs with prostatic disease and the inaccuracy in localizing lesions to the prostate because of testicular, epididymal, or urethral contamination of the sample.

Prostatic wash has been advocated for collecting cytological and bacterial specimens for evaluating prostatic disease. Prostatic fluid is not always obtained with this technique in normal dogs.[4] Comparison of premassage and postmassage samples is critical for appropriate interpretation of results. Disadvantages of prostatic wash are increased laboratory costs and failure to define localized disease processes that do not communicate with the prostatic urethra and, hence, the sample pool. Advantages of this technique are the ease of obtaining samples and the increased specificity compared with ejaculate samples.

Fine-needle aspiration of the prostate can be performed percutaneously via a perineal or prepubic approach.[4, 72] The location of the prostate, as determined by palpation or radiographic examination, determines the approach. Prepubic aspiration minimizes potential complications including hemorrhage and peritonitis by avoiding the rectum and paired neurovascular supply to the bladder, prostate gland, and urethra. Disadvantages of this technique are potential failure to diagnose localized disease and seeding infection or tumor along the needle tract. Advantages are ease of obtaining samples and specificity. Cytological diagnosis correlated with eventual definitive diagnosis in 96 per cent of 23 dogs.[80]

Percutaneous biopsy is performed with an actuated biopsy cutting needle* via an abdominal or perineal approach.[6] An assistant may be required to immobilize the prostate to aid the surgeon performing the biopsy. Alternatively, a keyhole incision enables the surgeon to immobilize the prostate against the ventral abdominal wall for prepubic biopsy.[19] The prostate is aspirated first to rule out abscessation. If prostatic abscessation is suspected, percutaneous biopsy is not performed. Disadvantages of percutaneous biopsy are the potential failure to diagnose localized disease, the possibility of rupturing a cyst or abscess, and the risk of hemorrhage. Advantages are low patient morbidity and avoidance of laparotomy and general anesthesia.

Whenever possible, a laparotomy for biopsy is preferred.[6, 19] Inspection of the prostate before biopsy increases the chance of diagnosing localized disease. Multiple biopsy samples may be collected if more than one disease process is suspected. A wedge-shaped incisional specimen is collected, avoiding the centrally located urethra. Hemorrhage is controlled by placing 2-0 or 3-0 monofilament absorbable horizontal mattress sutures across the defect. An actuated cutting needle may also be used to collect the material. Disadvantages of open abdomen biopsy are increased anesthetic time, increased patient morbidity, and a possible need for a second laparotomy to treat the condition after diagnosis.

Caudal abdominal plain radiographs and positive-contrast cystourethrography are helpful in diagnosing and localizing pathology of the prostate or surrounding structures. Ultrasonography is excellent for detecting cavitary changes within the prostatic parenchyma (see the preceding section on radiography and ultrasonography).

Benign Prostatic Hyperplasia and Cystic Hyperplasia

Benign prostatic hyperplasia is arguably a normal aging change, and physical findings of an enlarged prostate must be interpreted cautiously (see the preceding section on physiology of the prostate). Clinical signs of constipation, tenesmus, hemorrhagic urethral discharge, or urine retention may be noted. As an enlarging prostate obstructs the pelvic canal, defecation becomes more difficult. Dyschezia is much more common than dysuria. The resultant straining may lead to breakdown of the pelvic diaphragm, resulting in perineal hernia.

Rectal palpation reveals a symmetrically enlarged, nonpainful prostate of normal spongy consistency. Hemogram and blood chemistry findings are normal. Urinalysis or prostatic fluid analysis may show hemorrhage, especially with cystic hyperplasia. Bacterial cultures are negative. Biopsy is necessary for definitive diagnosis but is seldom indicated unless response to treatment is unsatisfactory.

Treatment objectives are to decrease the size of the prostate and to alleviate signs of pelvic canal obstruction. The recommended treatment is castration. Permanent involution of the prostate and relief of clinical signs occur[5] in 2 or 3 weeks. If no response is noted after 3 weeks, further diagnostic procedures are indicated.

Estrogen administration reduces the size of the prostate temporarily but can lead to bone marrow suppression and squamous metaplasia of the prostate, causing ductal obstruction with retention cyst formation. Its use is restricted to valuable breeding dogs. The dose is 0.2 to 1.0 mg of diethylstilbestrol orally every 2 to 3 days for 3 to 4 weeks.[52]

Medical therapy for constipation and urine retention may be indicated until the prostate shrinks. Constipation may be alleviated with a low-residue diet supplemented with a bulk laxative. Enemas or glycerin suppositories* may occasionally be needed. Urine retention may require placement of an indwelling urinary catheter and closed collection system if the bladder has become atonic. Manual expression of the bladder for several days is usually sufficient.

Suppurative Prostatitis and Prostatic Abscessation

The proximity of the prostate to the urethra, with its normal bacterial flora, predisposes the prostate to infection. Additionally, *B. canis* or other bacterial infection can ascend from the testicles during orchitis. Normal defense mechanisms of the urethra include mechanical flushing during urination, the urethral high-pressure zone, surface characteristics of the urethral mucosa, and urethral peristalsis.[54] Prostatic fluid has a zinc-associated antibacterial factor that serves as a natural defense mechanism. Despite these protective barriers, the prostatic parenchyma can be colonized by various bacteria. *Escherichia coli, Proteus* spp., staphylococci, streptococci, and *Pseudomonas* are commonly cultured.

Suppurative prostatitis occurs when bacteria colonize the prostatic parenchyma. If the infection is not quickly eliminated, microabscessation can result. As multiple

*Tru-Cut disposable biopsy needle, Travenol Laboratories, Deerfield, IL.

*Glycerin suppositories, C. B. Fleet Co., Lynchburg, VA.

foci of purulent material coalesce, large abscesses form, even as the prostate attempts to contain or localize the infection. Prostatic abscesses can rupture into the peritoneal cavity or retroperitoneal space, causing acute deterioration of physiological status.

Clinical Signs and Diagnosis. Acute prostatitis typically causes lethargy, anorexia, and fever. Urine retention and constipation may occur. A purulent or bloody urethral discharge is frequently noted. Caudal abdominal or pelvic pain may cause abnormal posture or gait. Physical examination findings often suggest low-grade sepsis. Injected mucous membranes and dehydration may be detected. Caudal abdominal or rectal palpation elicits a painful response. The prostate is enlarged and usually asymmetrical, and it often has fluctuating areas of purulent material. Firm areas and adhesions may be palpated. Chronic suppurative prostatitis is likely to cause abscesses extending into the caudal abdomen or pelvic canal. Hindlimb edema may result from interference with venous and lymphatic drainage and the altered vascular permeability that accompanies sepsis. If an abscess ruptures, acute peritonitis causes overt septic shock with cardiovascular collapse.

Diagnosis of suppurative prostatitis or prostatic abscess is confirmed by recovering a septic, suppurative exudate from urethral discharge, prostatic wash, ejaculate, or fine-needle aspirate. Urinalysis usually shows hematuria and pyuria. A neutrophilic leukocytosis with left shift is often present with low-grade sepsis. With septic shock, leukopenia or degenerative left shift may be detected. Caudal abdominal radiographs may show an enlarged prostate, and a decrease in detail may be noted if peritonitis is present.

Treatment. Treatment of suppurative prostatitis requires vigorous antibiotic supportive follow-up therapy. If the infection is not eliminated, chronic recurrent urinary and prostatic infection with resistant bacteria is likely.

Antibiotic therapy is based on culture and sensitivity testing of prostatic fluid. Many antibiotics do not readily cross the intact epithelium of the prostate acinus to reach therapeutic concentrations.[54] Whether this is true in an infected prostate is unknown. Trimethoprim-sulfadiazine or chloramphenicol is recommended initially until the sensitivity is determined.

With chronic infection, aminoglycosides may be indicated for resistant bacteria. Quinolone antibiotics are effective against resistant bacteria. Oral enrofloxacin is the drug of choice for resistant genitourinary infections. Antibiotic therapy is continued for 3 weeks. Urinalysis and urine or prostatic fluid culture are performed several days after discontinuing antibiotics to document response to therapy.

Castration is indicated for suppurative prostatitis to decrease the size and activity of the prostate and the chance of recurrence. Castration is not performed when a patient is ill.

Prostatic abscessation complicates medical management of prostatic infection. When available, ultrasonography can determine the degree of cavitation within the prostate. Dogs with extensive cavitary lesions and known prostatic infection are less likely to respond to medical therapy. Surgery is indicated to drain or excise large prostatic abscesses. Surgical techniques include drainage of parenchymal abscesses with gravity or suction drains and prostatectomy. Large prostatic abscesses may be marsupialized or resected during prostatectomy.

Prostatic Cysts and Paraprostatic Cysts

The pathophysiology of prostatic cysts is uncertain. Ductal occlusion from squamous metaplasia may result in progressive secretory stasis. Oversecretion by glandular tissue with functional obstruction of the ducts causes fluid retention with cyst formation. The cysts may occur as multiple cavitary areas within the gland or as large fluid-filled structures extending into the abdominal cavity or pelvic canal.

Cysts typically cause signs from compression of adjacent intestinal or urinary structures. A significant inflammatory component may be associated with prostatic cysts, manifested by localized adhesions, pain, and hematological changes. Prostatic cysts may become secondarily infected, causing signs of prostatic abscessation.

Paraprostatic cysts may originate from the blind-ended uterus masculinus, an embryonic structure formed from the müllerian duct system.[55] These cysts have no direct communication with the prostatic parenchyma and can become quite large. The source of these cysts is unclear; the müllerian duct attaches to the dorsal side of the prostate at the seminal hillock. No paraprostatic cyst has been reported to originate from this area.[88] They typically are large oval structures that extend in a cranial-caudal direction from the caudal part of the abdomen to the perineal fossa.[55] A large amount of pale yellow to orange fluid is contained within the cyst. The interior of the cyst is lined by a smooth, shiny surface and may have a trabecular supporting structure; cartilage and calcified areas may be present. They are less likely to become secondarily infected because they have no communication with the urogenital tract.

Clinical Signs and Diagnosis. Patients with prostatic or paraprostatic cysts may have vague clinical signs related to the large caudal abdominal mass. Inappetance, dysuria, constipation, and tenesmus are common. Incontinence, dysuria, or retention may be more common with cysts than with other prostatic diseases[88]; pelvic pain may result in ambulatory difficulties. Results of urinalysis are frequently normal, but hematuria may be present. Hematological studies cannot diagnose this problem; azotemia, neutrophilic leukocytosis, and an increase in alkaline phosphatase may occur.[84] Radiographs document a caudal abdominal mass, which is usually fluid dense but may have calcified areas. Positive-contrast cystourethrography is particularly helpful in guiding a surgical approach. Fine-needle aspiration yields a modified transudate with erythrocytes and occasional epithelial and inflammatory cells. Results of bacterial culture are negative, unless secondary infection is encountered.

Treatment. Therapy is restricted to treatment of urine retention or constipation. Estrogen therapy is contraindicated.

The goal of surgical therapy is to remove, reduce, or

drain the cyst. Castration decreases the secretory activity of the prostate. Cyst resection may be coupled with partial or complete prostatectomy. Semipermanent drainage is achieved by marsupialization or temporarily by Penrose or suction drainage. It is unknown if secretory activity by the lining of the cyst is affected by castration.

Prostatic Neoplasia (see also Chapter 159)

Adenocarcinoma and transitional cell carcinoma are the most common types of prostatic neoplasia in dogs; the cause is unknown. Older dogs typically are affected. A direct androgenic hormonal influence from the testes is not necessary, because castration does not prevent prostatic carcinoma. In two studies, more intact dogs than castrated dogs developed prostatic carcinoma[56, 66, 85]; in another, castrated dogs were as likely to develop prostatic carcinoma as intact dogs.[41]

Clinical Signs and Diagnosis. Prostatic carcinoma may be focal or disseminated throughout the gland; metastasis is common. Metastasis occurs via the vertebral venous sinuses and lymphatics, with the iliac lymph nodes most frequently involved. Local metastasis to the bladder, rectum, pelvis, lumbar vertebrae, and pelvic musculature is observed. Distant metastasis is less common.

Clinical signs include rear limb weakness, edema, stranguria, tenesmus, polyuria, polydipsia, and emaciation. Hematuria, urethral bleeding, and incontinence may also occur. Rectal or caudal abdominal palpation reveals a painful, firm, irregular, and nodular prostate. Prostatic carcinoma can cause severe clinical signs before reaching a large size. The prostate may be fixed to surrounding pelvic structures. Iliac lymphadenopathy is palpable.

Differentiating prostatic carcinoma from suppurative prostatitis may be difficult without biopsy. Percutaneous biopsy may be used after the suspicious area is localized by palpation or ultrasonography. If doubt exists, open abdomen biopsy is preferred. As with other malignant tumors, complete staging is indicated before treatment.

Treatment. Successful treatment of prostatic carcinoma is difficult because of its aggressive biological behavior. Estrogen administration or castration may temporarily decrease clinical signs. Chemotherapy and immunotherapy have been discussed, but no reports of their clinical usefulness are available. If the diagnosis is made before detectable metastasis, prostatectomy is recommended.

Prostatic Trauma

The prostate is susceptible to trauma from displaced pelvic fractures or penetrating injury to the caudal abdomen. Patients with major caudal abdominal wall defects due to blunt trauma are at risk for prostatic injury (Fig. 99–5). Focal tears of the prostatic urethra, avulsion of the prostate and bladder from the postprostatic membranous urethra, and crush injuries with complete disruption of the prostate may be seen. Evaluation of prostate trauma is similar to lower urinary tract

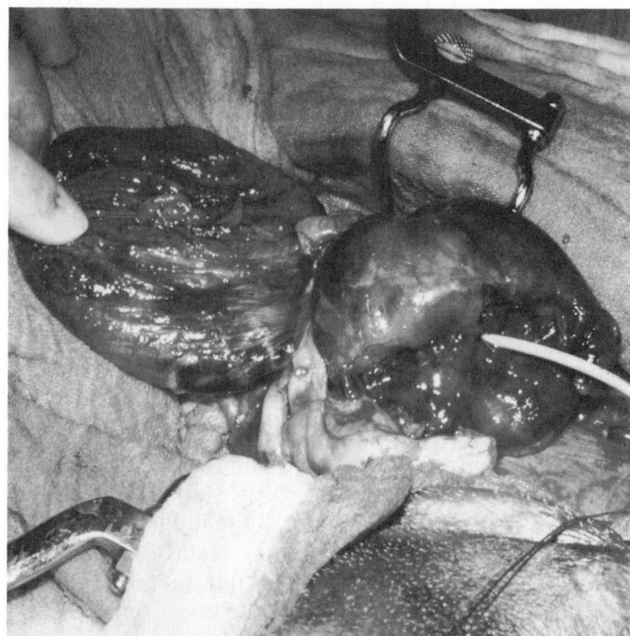

FIGURE 99–5. Traumatic avulsion of the bladder and prostate (avascular).

trauma. Initial evaluation and stabilization focus on the integrity of the urethra (Fig. 99–6). Urethral catheterization can establish gross urethral patency. Positive-contrast urethrocystography localizes leakage to a specific area of the urethra. Short-term management requires maintaining urine outflow via catheterization and a closed collection system. For small tears, several days of catheterization may allow complete healing. Gross leakage or inability to pass the urethral catheter into the bladder warrants exploratory laparotomy. Subtotal or complete prostatectomy may be required. Prognosis for long-term maintenance of normal voiding and storage and preservation of fertility in breeding dogs is guarded. Crush and avulsion injuries often cause extensive damage to the neurovascular supply to the bladder and prostate, necessitating permanent urinary diversion.

Prostatic Calculi

Prostatic calculi are rare in dogs, and their significance is unknown. If calculi cause obstruction, cystic prostatic disease may result. If secondary infection occurs, signs of suppurative prostatitis and sepsis may be encountered. No information suggests that prostatic calculi should be treated as a primary disease entity.

Surgical Procedures and Complications

General Considerations and Surgical Approach

The prostate gland is usually approached by caudal laparotomy. It may also be approached from the perineum, usually as part of surgical repair of perineal hernia. As for any operation on the urogenital tract,

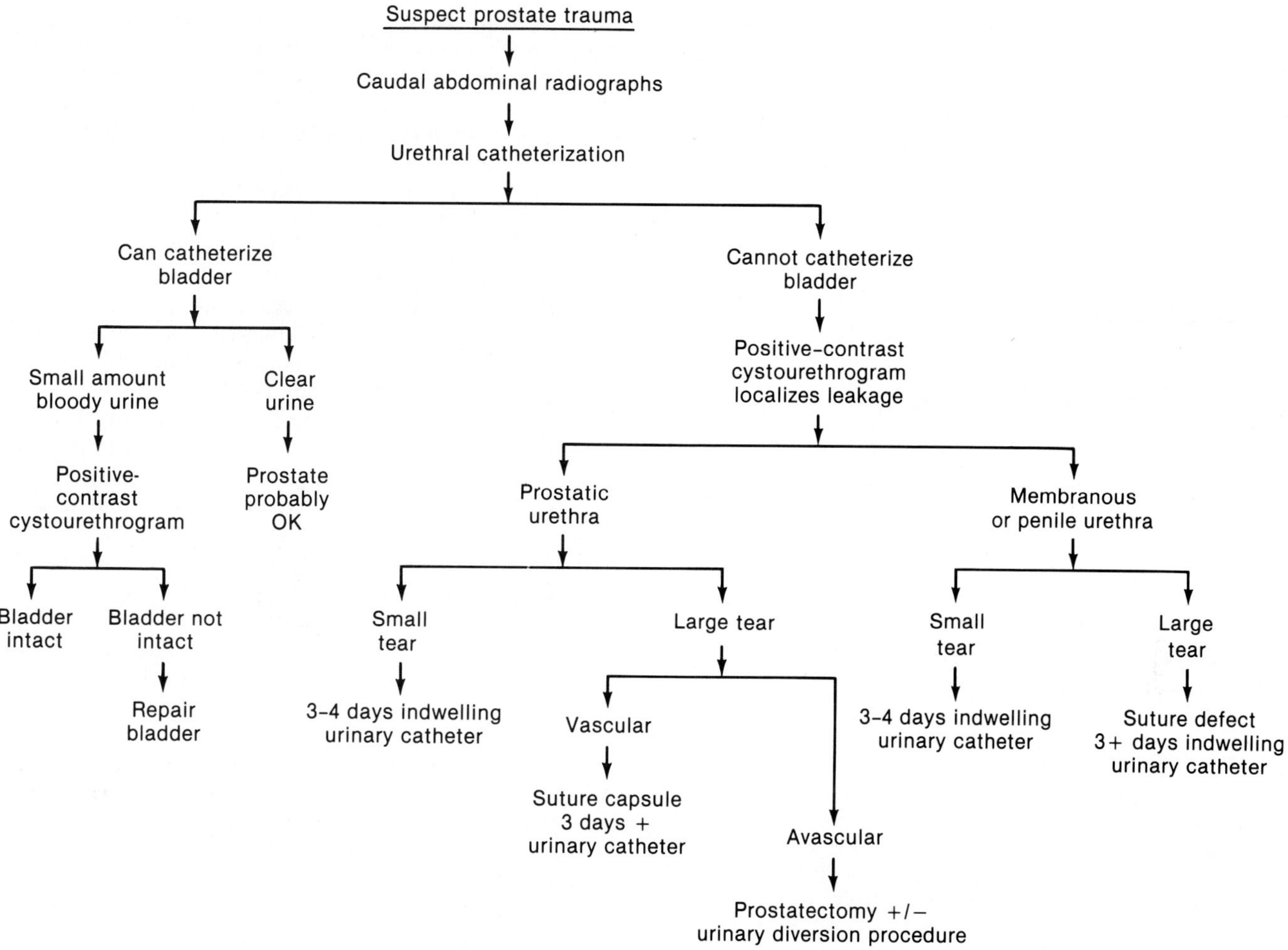

FIGURE 99–6. Algorithm for management of prostatic trauma.

preparations are made for aseptic urethral catheterization at any point in the procedure. With the patient in dorsal recumbency, the prepuce is flushed repeatedly with either 0.1 per cent povidone-iodine or a 1:40 dilution of 2 per cent chlorhexidine diacetate before preparing the abdomen. The prepuce is left in the surgical field.

During caudal laparotomy, the skin incision deviates from the midline lateral to the prepuce and extends to the cranial pubis. If lateral pathology of the prostate is suspected, the skin incision is on the side of the prepuce where maximum exposure is desired. Moistened laparotomy pads and a Balfour retractor are placed. A Gelpi retractor directed cranially facilitates retraction of the prepuce and caudal abdominal wall. Separating the middle umbilical ligament from the ventral abdominal wall and placing retention sutures for cranial retraction of the bladder increase exposure. The prostate can be further mobilized by cutting the connective tissue band between the pubic floor and the ventral surface of the pelvic urethra.

If further caudal exposure is necessary, pubic osteotomy is indicated.[46] Pubic osteotomy exposes the cranial portion of the pelvic canal. Three osteotomies are made, two connecting the craniomedial third of each obturator foramen to the pubic brim and one connecting the medial border of each obturator foramen to the other (Fig. 99–7). Care is taken to avoid the obturator nerve, traversing the lateral foramen. The pubis is reflected caudoventrally. After the prostate procedure is completed, the pubis is attached with four orthopedic wires placed through drilled holes.

Drainage Techniques. When fluid accumulates within the prostatic parenchyma, drainage is indicated. Gravity or suction drains can be quickly placed in septic patients that cannot withstand more time-consuming resection techniques.

In most drainage techniques, a stab incision is made into one prostate lobe, and suction is used to remove any purulent material. Bacterial cultures are collected. Digital breakdown of individual accumulations of pus results in one large abscess cavity. The procedure is repeated on the other lobe. Alternately, by passing a hemostat or a finger dorsal to the urethra, the other lobe is similarly broken down. Both lobes are thoroughly irrigated with an antibacterial solution. Careful isolation of the infected prostate with laparotomy pads and minimal dissection of periprostatic fat help localize contamination. After the drainage procedure is completed, the caudal abdominal portion is lavaged and suctioned. Elevating the cranial portion of the dog's abdomen by 15° limits the cranial extension of leakage. If leakage is

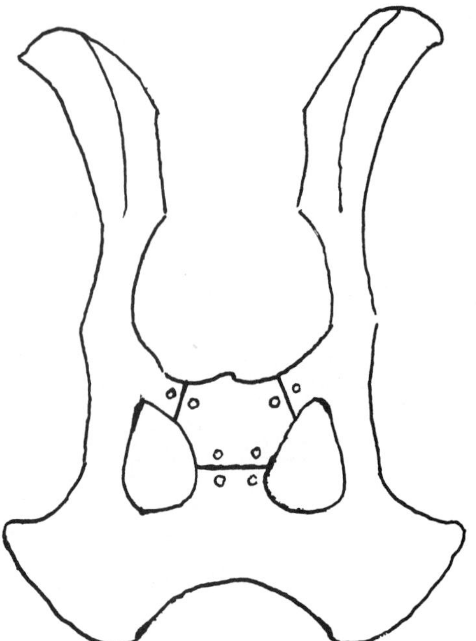

FIGURE 99–7. Pubic osteotomy—osteotomy and wire hole locations.

severe, abdominal drains or open abdomen drainage after surgery is considered.

Gravity drainage with various configurations of Penrose drains has been described[6] (Fig. 99–8). In the first technique, a stab incision is created in the dorsal limit of each abscess cavity.[89] Two to four 1-cm Penrose drains are placed in each side and secured dorsally with a single 4-0 gut suture. The drains exit together through an abdominal stab incision on their respective sides of the prepuce and are secured to the skin. Multiple periprostatic drains are placed to exit through separate abdominal stab incisions (Fig. 99–8*A*).

In a second technique,[52] a hemostat is used to create a blunt opening into the abscess cavity, and purulent material is aspirated. The surgeon's finger is inserted to cross the midline of the prostate dorsal to the urethra. A second blunt opening is created on the side opposite the first opening. A single 5-mm Penrose drain is passed through the abscess cavity, allowing the ends to be exteriorized lateral to the prepuce (Fig. 99–8*B*). Care is taken to ensure that the drain is loosely placed as it passes over the urethra to prevent obstruction. No periprostatic drains are used. The drain is left in place for 3 weeks.

In a third technique,[40] two abscess cavities are created as in the first technique. A single 5-mm Penrose drain is passed ventrally to dorsally on both sides of the urethra. As the drains exit the dorsal surface of the prostate, they are retrieved and passed lateral to the gland to exit through the same stab incision in the abdominal wall (Fig. 99–8*C*). No internal tacking sutures are used. The drains are secured to the skin and left in place 2 to 4 weeks.

When gravity drains are used, preventing ascending infection by covering drain exit sites with a sterile dressing is a difficult but important postoperative goal. The use of an Elizabethan collar or side brace helps to maintain bandages and drains. Duration of drainage is based on the amount and character of the drainage. Drains are removed as soon as possible to decrease the risk of nosocomial infections and urethrocutaneous fistula.

Because of the difficulty in maintaining clean drain exit sites and the inability to accurately quantitate discharge from gravity drains, I use closed-system suction drains. In this technique, a single large abscess cavity is created from a ventral stab incision in one prostate lobe. The cavity is cultured and lavaged. Several new side holes are cut in a feeding tube. The catheter is inserted through a stab incision in the abdominal wall, advanced into the prostate, and passed dorsal to the urethra into the abscess cavity of the other lobe. It is secured with a single 3-0 gut suture as it leaves the prostate and to the skin with 3-0 nylon as it leaves the abdominal wall. A closed-system suction reservoir is connected to the suction catheter. The site of the reservoir is based on the size of the patient and anticipated drainage, a small suction reservoir* for smaller patients and a larger suction reservoir† for larger patients. The suction reservoir is attached to a fitted side brace. The gross and cytological appearance of the exudate changes from purulent or hemorrhagic to serous or serohemorrhagic as the infection resolves.

Regardless of the technique chosen for drainage of the infected prostate, aggressive antibiotic, fluid, electrolyte, and supportive therapy is indicated. If infection recurs after surgical drainage, castration, and proper antibiotic therapy, partial or complete prostatectomy is indicated.

Cyst Resection. Discrete paraprostatic cysts or true prostatic cysts that have a narrow attachment to the prostate gland may be amenable to local resection. Most cysts have some adhesions to caudal abdominal or pelvic structures. Aggressive dissection must not be performed dorsolateral to the bladder neck, prostate, or proximal pelvic urethra unless the lateral umbilical ligaments are clearly separated from the cyst.[6] Incomplete cyst resection is preferable to producing incontinence or detrusor atony. It has not been determined if prostatic or paraprostatic cysts continue to enlarge after castration. Reduction and suction drainage of these cysts often alleviate clinical signs.

When paraprostatic cysts adhere to the prostate or when prostatic cysts narrow to a manageable stalk at the prostate, partial prostatectomy may be possible. The prostatic capsule is sutured with a monofilament absorbable suture.

Perineal prostatic or paraprostatic cysts associated with perineal hernia are difficult to resect because of limited surgical exposure. Surgical reduction and suction drainage of the cysts during herniorrhaphy are performed. An indwelling suction drainage system may be established for postoperative drainage. Although perineal gravity drainage has been described,[61] inability to

*Axiom, Adler Co., Norcross, GA.

†Snyder Hemovac, Snyder Laboratories, Dover, OH.

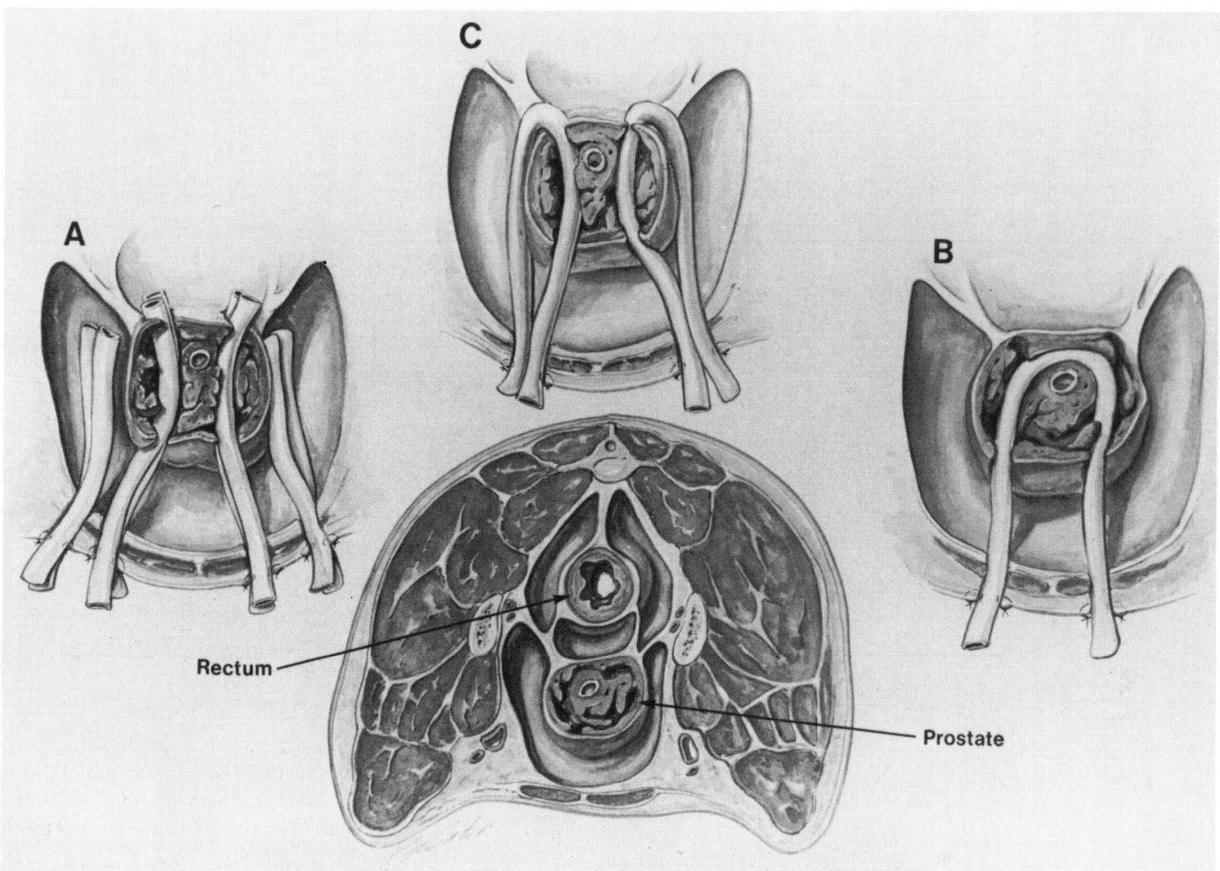

FIGURE 99–8. Techniques for Penrose drainage of multiple prostatic abscesses. Note that all loculations are broken down to form a single cavity that is subsequently drained. *A*, Multiple ½-inch Penrose drains secured dorsally with a single 4-0 surgical gut suture. Multiple ½-inch Penrose periprostatic drains are present. *B*, Single 5-mm Penrose drain looping over the prostatic urethra with both ends exiting the abdominal wall. *C*, Two 5-mm Penrose drains draining both the prostate and the periprostatic areas.

achieve ventral drainage and drain contamination are major problems.

Marsupialization. Marsupialization is used for prostatic or paraprostatic cysts.[35, 44, 62] Abscesses within the parenchyma cannot be treated with this technique. A permanent stoma is created into the cyst for drainage. For marsupialization, the cyst must be mobilized to the ventral abdominal wall, and the capsule of the cyst must be strong enough to hold sutures without tearing. An oval stoma is created by sharp dissection in the skin, subcutaneous tissue, and fascia, lateral to the prepuce (Fig. 99–9*A*). The cyst is freed of adhesions and mobilized to the body wall. Blunt dissection is used to create a muscular stoma (Fig. 99–9*B*). The cyst wall is sutured to the external rectus sheath with a simple continuous pattern of 3-0 monofilament absorbable suture. The cyst is incised, cultured, and flushed. Simple interrupted sutures appose the incised cyst wall to the skin (Fig. 99–9*C–E*). The cyst interior may be flushed with antibacterial solutions postoperatively. Drainage decreases over several weeks, and the stoma contracts and closes. Persistent drainage and infection for 3 to 4 months have been reported.[35, 44] It is not known if the drainage is from continued fluid production by the cyst, failure to eliminate the primary cause, or ascending infection at the marsupialization site.

Reported advantages of marsupialization are that continuous drainage is established, the interior of the cyst may be treated postoperatively, morbidity is less than with prostatectomy, and more aggressive surgical treatment involving removal of prostatic parenchyma is still possible.

Marsupialization may have major postoperative complications. Urinary tract infection, abscessation, urinary incontinence, and chronic drainage have been reported. Persistence of the stoma may necessitate reoperation and excision of the shrunken cyst. Some of these complications may have been caused by inappropriate use of marsupialization to treat parenchymal abscesses.

When cysts or abscesses are large enough to extend caudodorsally into the perineum, creating a permanent stoma in a contaminated perineum is risky. Perineal hernia is frequently a concurrent problem with large perineal cysts. Herniorrhaphy, castration, and surgical reduction and suction drainage of the cyst are performed.

Prostatectomy. The incidence of chronic recurrent urinary tract infection and reabscessation is lowest with prostatectomy. Unfortunately, prostatectomy may have unacceptable complications. Complete or total prostatectomy removes the entire prostate. Partial prostatectomy (prostatic fillet) eliminates substantial portions of

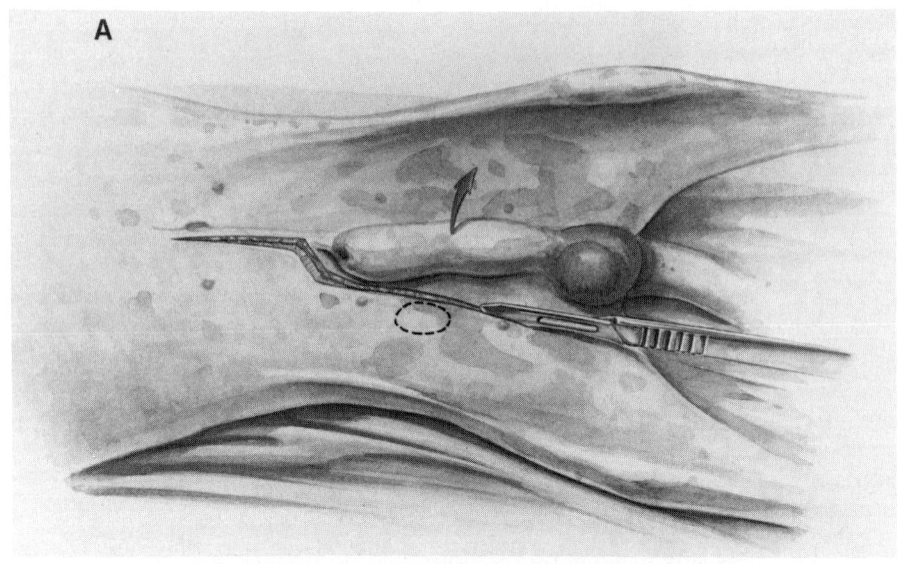

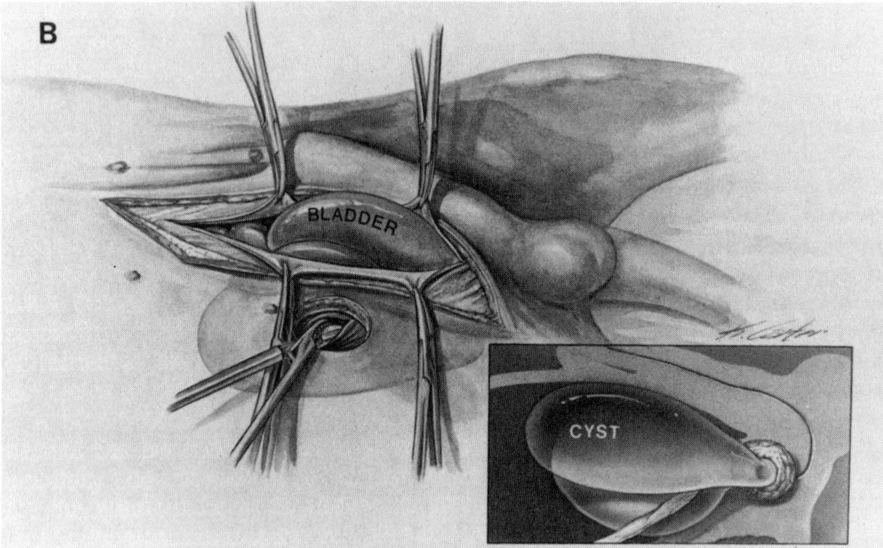

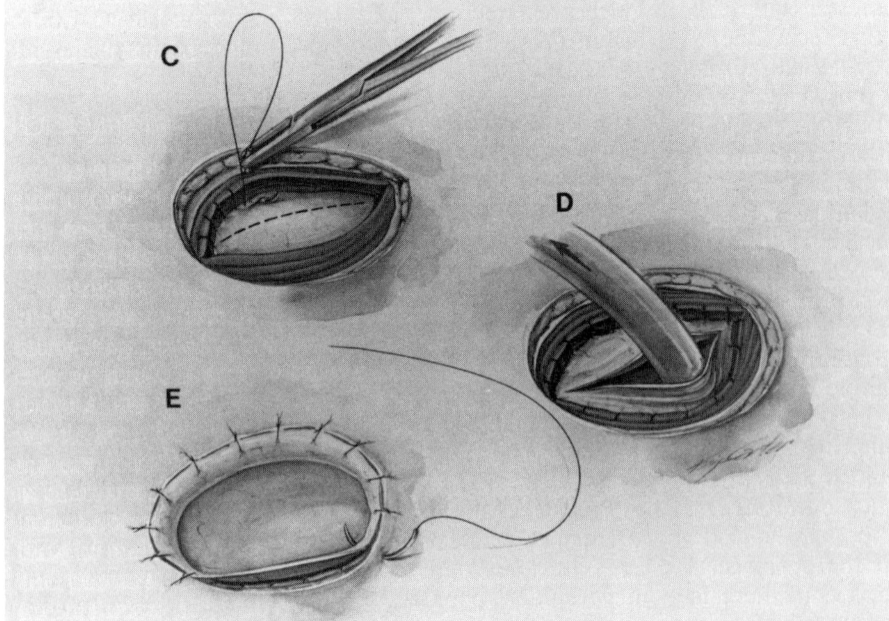

FIGURE 99–9. Technique for marsupialization of a large prostatic cyst or abscess. *A*, After parapreputial incision, an oval stoma is created in the skin lateral to the prepuce. *B*, A caudal abdominal laparotomy is performed. The cyst or abscess is mobilized to the abdominal wall, and a muscular stoma is created. *C*, The cyst or abscess wall is sutured to the abdominal wall with a simple continuous pattern of monofilament suture. *D*, The cyst or abscess is incised, cultured, and flushed. *E*, Simple interrupted sutures appose the cyst or abscess wall to the skin.

diseased tissue. The term *transurethral prostatectomy* is not used because it implies that the procedure is performed from within the prostate, using an endoscope as performed in men.

Complete prostatectomy is performed during laparotomy. A pubic osteotomy is occasionally necessary for better exposure. The periprostatic fat is reflected laterally from the ventral midline until the lateral umbilical ligaments are encountered on the dorsolateral surfaces of the gland. Blood vessels and nerve branches supplying the bladder and urethra are identified dorsal to the prostate and preserved. Short vessels supplying the prostate are individually ligated or cauterized and transected close to the gland. The vasa deferentia are ligated and divided. A dissection plane is established between the prostate gland and bladder neck cranially, reflecting as much prostatic tissue caudally as possible. Similar manipulation reflects prostatic tissue cranially off the membranous urethra. After the dissection is completed, the urethra is transected cranially, leaving as much of the bladder neck as possible. Retention sutures are placed in the outer fibrous coat of the membranous urethra, and the urethra is transected at the caudal margin of the prostate. The prostate is removed and saved for bacterial culture and microscopic examination. A urethral catheter is placed to facilitate approximation of the urethra. An end-to-end anastomosis of the bladder neck to the membranous urethra is performed using simple interrupted or interrupted mattress sutures of 4-0 or 5-0 monofilament absorbable material (Fig. 99–10*A–D*). These sutures are placed into the lumen of the urethra, but the amount of suture material exposed to the urethral lumen is minimized. Eight to 12 sutures are usually necessary. A urethral catheter is placed to keep the bladder decompressed and limit tension on the anastomosis. If delayed healing or suture line tension is anticipated, a cystostomy catheter is placed. The abdomen is lavaged before routine closure. If contamination is severe, caudal abdominal drains or open abdominal drainage may be used. A side brace is placed to prevent catheter and drain dislodgment. The cystostomy catheter is removed after 6 to 7 days, and the urethral catheter the following day.

In the first 2 days after surgery for prostatic infection, shock and oliguria were the most common complications.[38] Postoperative monitoring of vital signs, fluid and electrolyte balance, urine production, biochemical values, and nutritional status allows early identification and treatment of complications.

Dogs that have undergone prostatectomy for prostatic disease are usually incontinent.[5] Incontinence does not occur after prostatectomy in normal dogs[7] and is a rare complication of prostatectomy in men. Unfortunately, postprostatectomy incontinence in dogs responds poorly to medical therapy. Until this complication can be avoided or treated effectively, prostatectomy is reserved for severe prostatic trauma or prostatic neoplasia or is used in dogs in which minimizing recurrence of prostatic disease is more important than urinary continence.

Partial prostatectomy reduces glandular parenchyma without causing permanent incontinence. An intracapsular technique that removes 80 per cent of the parenchyma has been described in normal dogs.[70] In this technique, successive longitudinal half-moon incisions are created into the prostate and prostatic urethra with an electroscalpel. Glandular parenchyma is removed except for 2 to 3 mm inside the capsule and a dorsal roof of prostatic urethra and parenchyma (Fig. 99–11*A*). The capsule of the prostate is closed with a double inverting suture pattern. Normal dogs were not incontinent, but results in dogs with diseased prostates have not been reported.

In a different partial prostatectomy technique, all tissue is removed by electroscalpel, except for the prostatic urethra surrounded by a thin rim of glandular tissue around the urethra[33] (Fig. 99–11*B*). The prostate is completely isolated from its neurovascular attachments and ductus deferens as for complete prostatectomy. No attempt is made to suture any defects into the urethral lumen. No urethral catheter is used. Several periprostatic drains are placed to exit on either side of the prepuce and are removed when drainage ceases and the dog urinates entirely through the penile urethra. Clinical observations suggest that postoperative incontinence may not be a problem in dogs with a diseased prostate.[32]

The results of a similar technique using the neodymium:yttrium-aluminum-garnet laser for cutting and hemostasis have been reported.[40] The laser was helpful for controlling parenchymal bleeding but not capsular vein bleeding. The technique could be performed as well with the electroscalpel. Two configurations of partial prostatectomy were used, depending on the location of the prostatic disease as determined by ultrasonography and visual observation (Fig. 99–11*C–D*). When compared with prostatic drainage in a randomized group of dogs, subtotal prostatectomy resulted in more complete resolution of prostate and bladder infection with a shorter hospital stay. Urinary incontinence was noted but was less severe than with complete prostatectomy. Operative mortality was higher, and surgical time was longer with partial prostatectomy than with drainage.[40]

The role of partial prostatectomy in the treatment of prostatic abscessation will become better defined as more data accumulate. At present, it is reserved for stable patients with prostatic abscessation and dogs with localized prostatic disease. A surgical drainage procedure is performed on septic patients to help stabilize them. Prostatectomy can be performed later if needed.

TREATMENT OF CANINE PROSTATIC ABSCESSATION

Complications of surgical treatment of prostatic abscessation are common. Sepsis and shock occurred in 32 to 64 per cent of dogs undergoing surgery.[38, 60] Hypoproteinemia occurred in 59 per cent of dogs, hypokalemia in 59 per cent, hypoglycemia in 59 per cent, anemia in 46 per cent, and peripheral edema in 43 to 69 per cent.[71] Less frequent complications included polyuria/polydipsia, diarrhea, wound infection, ventricular arrhythmias, and hemorrhage.[38, 60]

Mortality rates for dogs with prostatic abscessation are high. An overall mortality rate of 51 per cent for 23 dogs with abscessation was reported in 1978,[45] whereas

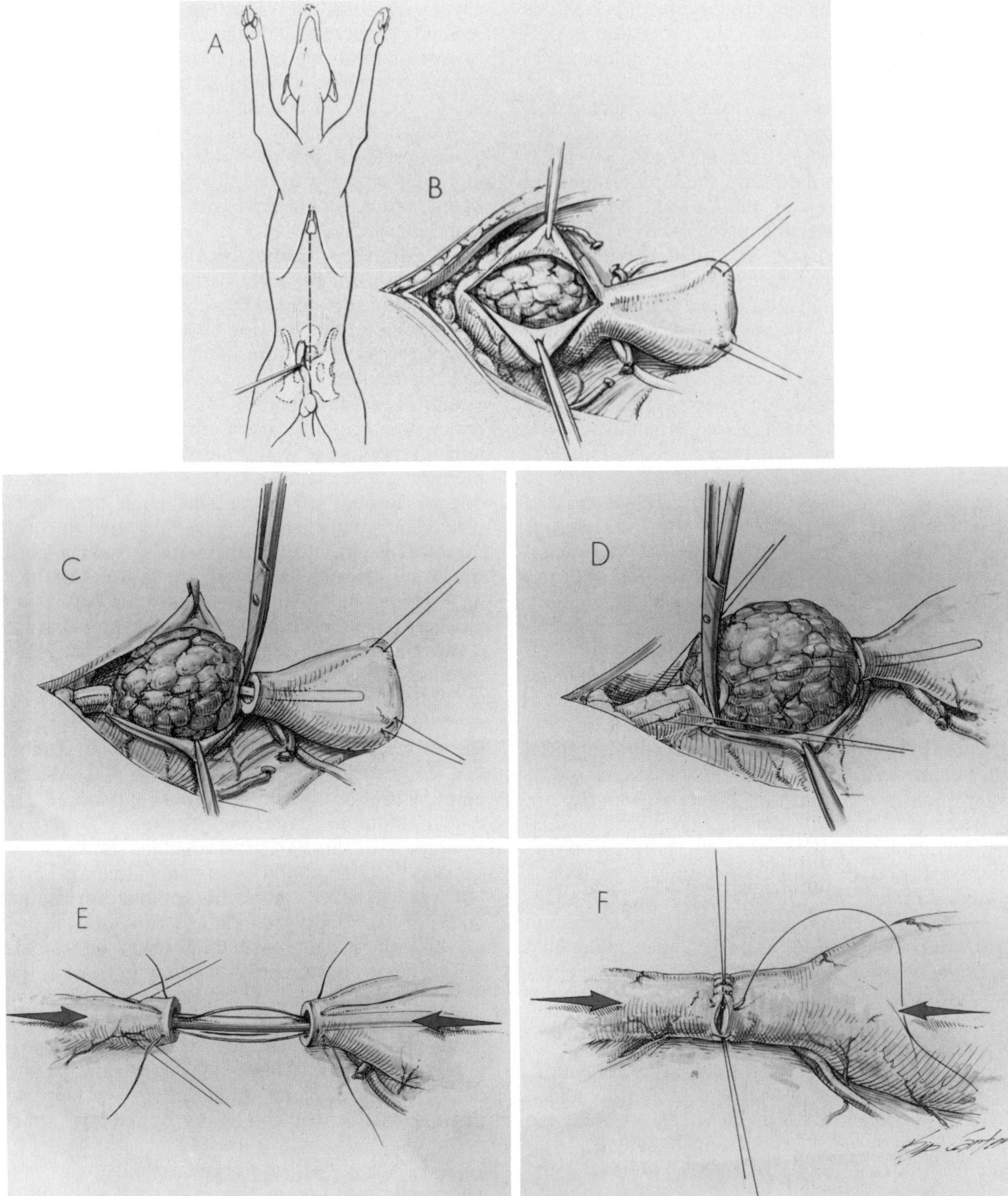

FIGURE 99–10. Technique for total prostatectomy. *A*, The prostate is approached by caudal laparotomy. *B*, The periprostatic fat is dissected off the prostate gland. *C*, The urethra is transected at the caudal border of the prostate. *D*, The urethra is transected at the caudal border of the prostate. *E*, The prostate is removed, and the catheter is reinserted into the bladder. *F*, An end-to-end anastomosis is performed, between the bladder neck and membranous urethra.

21 per cent of 89 dogs that survived surgical drainage for an abscessed prostate died within 1 week of surgery.[63] Sepsis and associated shock were the most common causes of death. All the listed complications, including death, should be anticipated in a dog with a life-threatening septic process. A plan for recognizing and treating sepsis is necessary.

History and physical examination findings suggesting sepsis can be vague.[39] Depression, anorexia, vomiting, or diarrhea in association with other signs of prostatic disease suggests possible sepsis. Fever is a fairly reliable indicator of bacteremia.[20] but often is not present during shock or when infection is localized within an abscess.[39] Increased heart rate or respiratory rate may also signal

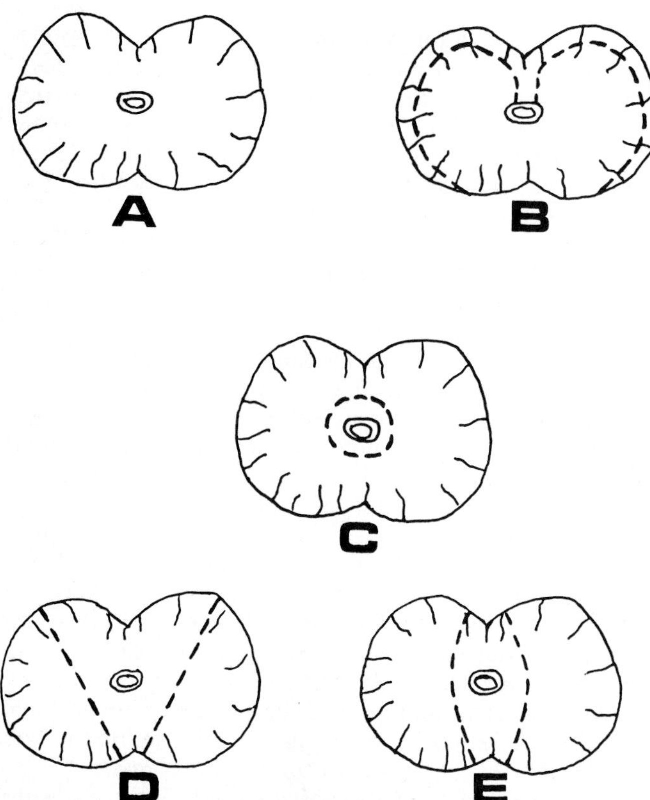

FIGURE 99–11. Subtotal prostatectomy techniques. *A*, Transverse section through the center of the prostate gland and prostatic urethra. *B*, Subtotal intracapsular. *C*, Fillet subtotal prostatectomy. *D* and *E*, Modified fillet with preservation of dorsal innervation.

sepsis. Shock in sepsis can be hyperdynamic (high cardiac output, normal or low blood pressure, low peripheral resistance, brick-red mucous membranes) or hypodynamic (low cardiac output, low blood pressure, high peripheral resistance, cold extremities, pale mucous membranes). Overt hypodynamic shock is usually associated with disseminated gram-negative infection or peritonitis secondary to a ruptured abscess.

A complete blood count, serum biochemical panel, and urinalysis are obtained before surgery. If available, a platelet count, arterial blood gas analysis, and assessment of clotting function are performed (Table 99–1). Multiple abnormal serum biochemical values have been associated with advanced sepsis and a poor prognosis.[39] The blood is crossmatched with blood from available donors because transfusion is often necessary during or after surgery.

In a septic patient, several intravenous lines (including one central line) are placed to supply fluids, administer drugs, and withdraw blood samples. An indwelling urinary catheter is placed to monitor urine output. To assess the progress of treatment and watch for the development of multiple organ failure, numerous variables (Table 99–2) must be monitored. Pretreatment values for these variables are determined.

Systemic antibiotic therapy is initiated, not to treat the abscess but to avert potential dissemination of infection. Intravenous antibiotics are usually required because of shock and gastrointestinal failure. *E. coli* is most often cultured from prostatic abscesses, but other gram-negative organisms are often present. Staphylococcal and streptococcal organisms are occasionally cultured.[38, 45] Antibiotic therapy includes coverage for anaerobes, which are often present in suppurative infections.[21]

A combination of amikacin (7 to 10 mg/kg IV every 8 hours) and ampicillin (20 to 40 mg/kg IV every 8 hours) is recommended if renal function is normal. If renal function is compromised, cefoxitin (20 mg/kg IV every 8 hours) is safe and usually effective.[37] Rapid identification of organism antibiotic sensitivities is necessary if cefoxitin is used, because bacteria are more likely to be resistant to a cephalosporin than to an aminoglycoside-antianaerobe drug combination. If oral antibiotics can be used, enrofloxacin (5 to 8 mg/kg PO every 12 hours) is recommended.

The choice of cardiovascular support therapy (Table 99–3) before surgery depends on the presence of shock. If hypodynamic shock is present, resuscitation using hypertonic solutions (see Table 99–3) may be initiated. The two major hypertonic solutions in use are hypertonic saline[62, 64, 71] and glucose-insulin-potassium.[59] Administration of one dose of hypertonic saline may result in beneficial cardiovascular effects and reduce the amounts of crystalloids needed for hours.[71] Glucose-insulin-potassium helps treat hypoglycemia and has cardiovascular effects that are similar to hypertonic saline.[12, 58, 59] This solution must be continuously infused, and the cardiovascular effects diminish with prolonged administration.[12] Because no studies have examined the effects of combining hypertonic saline and glucose-insulin-potassium, clinicians should choose between the two solutions.

Once fluid administration has been initiated, the need for metabolic therapy is assessed (see Table 99–3). Glucose and potassium levels are often decreased,[60] and replacement therapy with a glucose-insulin-potassium solution or routine supplementation of crystalloid solutions may be needed. Metabolic acidosis is often present, and bicarbonate therapy may be indicated.

Antiendotoxin therapy (see Table 99–3) is chosen carefully. Corticosteroids are effective when used before shock or within the first hour of onset.[43] One shock dose of corticosteroids is given before surgery if shock is not yet present. If corticosteroids are given, the dog is

TABLE 99–1. LABORATORY RESULTS COMPATIBLE WITH SEPSIS

Complete Blood Count	Serum Biochemistry
Neutrophilia or neutropenia	Hyper- or hypoglycemia
Increased band neutrophils	Increased alkaline phosphatase
Degenerative left shift	Hypoalbuminemia
Toxic changes in neutrophils	Increased alanine aminotransferase
Monocytosis	Bilirubinemia
Decreased platelet count	
Clotting Tests	**Acid-Base**
Prolonged prothrombin and activated partial thromboplastin times	Metabolic acidosis with respiratory compensation
Increased fibrin degradation products	

TABLE 99–2. MONITORING VARIABLES FOR DOGS WITH PROSTATIC ABSCESS

Parameter (Frequency of Monitoring)	Possible Interpretation
Core temperature (every 6 hours)	<100.4°F (38°C): hypodynamic shock >104°F (40°C): bacteremia
Toe web temperature (every 6 hours)	>10°F (5.5°C) lower than core: hypodynamic shock
Pulse rate (hourly, if critical)	>160–200 beats per minute based on body size: shock
Respiratory rate (hourly)	Steady increase: metabolic acidosis, pulmonary thromboembolism, lung failure
Capillary refill time (hourly)	>2 seconds: shock
Mucous membrane color (hourly)	Pale: anemia, hypodynamic shock
Blood pressure (hourly, if critical)	<60 mm Hg or undetectable: shock
Central venous pressure (every 6 hours)	<5 cm H_2O: hypovolemia >10 cm H_2O: fluid overload, heart failure
Urine output (hourly)	<2 ml/kg/hour: shock, renal failure
Glucose (every 6–8 hours)	<70 mEq/100 ml: sepsis, replacement therapy needed
Packed cell volume (every 6–8 hours)	<20%: hemorrhage, volume overload dilution, replacement therapy needed
Total solids (every 6–8 hours)	<5 g/100 ml: third-space loss, volume overload dilution
Albumin (if total solids <5 g/100 ml)	<1 g/100 ml: replacement therapy needed
Serum electrolytes (every 24 hours)	Potassium <3.5 mEq/L: replacement therapy needed Calcium decreasing: sepsis, continued albumin loss
Blood urea nitrogen (every 24 hours)	>30 mg/100 ml: hypovolemia or renal failure
Serum bilirubin, alkaline phosphatase, alanine aminotransferase (every 48 hours)	Increasing values: sepsis
Arterial blood gases (as needed)	Metabolic acidosis: shock or sepsis Hypoxemia: lung failure, pulmonary thromboembolism, pneumonia

monitored for secondary infections, which occur at an increased rate in human patients after shock doses of corticosteroids.[75] If shock has been present for longer than 2 hours, corticosteroids have no proven value. Potent nonsteroidal anti-inflammatory drugs such as flunixin meglumine are useful after the onset of shock.[31] One dose of flunixin meglumine is recommended before surgery if shock is already present. Side effects associated with use of nonsteroidal anti-inflammatory drugs in endotoxic shock include exacerbation of renal failure[30] and hemorrhagic gastroenteritis.[22] They should not be combined with corticosteroids because of additive toxicity.[21, 22]

The clotting status of septic dogs can range from hypercoagulable to disseminated intravascular coagulation.[29] If clotting times and platelet counts are normal, low-dose heparin (see Table 99–3) is probably indicated to prevent activation of clotting cascades.[67, 73] If platelet counts are low and clotting times are prolonged, replacement therapy with heparin-activated platelet-rich plasma[73] (see Table 99–3) can be used to treat disseminated intravascular coagulation. Heparin therapy is not combined with dextran administration because both therapies decrease clotting function.

During surgery, anesthetic management of patients with prostatic abscess is similar to that of any patient in critical condition. Anesthetic regimens that can be quickly adjusted and that require minimal hepatic metabolism should be used. Dopamine or dobutamine (see Table 99–3) may be needed to support cardiac function. Dobutamine provides maximal increases in cardiac performance and oxygen delivery but results in increased fluid needs owing to vasodilation.[80] Dopamine increases cardiac performance and renal perfusion without altering fluid needs but does not improve cardiovascular function in septic shock to the same degree as the combination of dobutamine plus fluids.[81] Packed cell volume, total solids, and glucose levels are monitored frequently during surgery, because they may decrease rapidly as a result of ongoing hemorrhage, release of endotoxin, and rapid fluid administration. If hypertonic solutions have not been given recently, mannitol (see Table 99–3) is administered for renal protection.

If samples of prostatic abscess fluid and urine were not collected previously, they are collected at surgery. Prostate fluid samples are submitted for Gram staining, cytological evaluation, aerobic and anaerobic cultures, and sensitivity testing. Urine is submitted for aerobic culture and sensitivity studies. Gram stain results are used to guide antibiotic therapy, particularly when unsuspected organisms are found.

After surgery, patients are closely monitored for expected complications (i.e., anemia, hypoglycemia, hypoproteinemia, hypokalemia, and shock—see Table 99–2). Therapy (see Table 99–3) is instituted as soon as a downward trend is noted rather than waiting until minimally acceptable values are reached.

Patients that are in obvious septic shock at the onset of surgery or that develop shock after surgery are carefully monitored for multiple organ failure. The order of organ failure in dogs is usually gastrointestinal tract, liver, kidneys, lungs, and heart.[78] Signs of gastrointestinal tract failure include bloody vomitus, melena, anorexia, and ileus. Liver failure can be detected by the development of icterus, increasing liver enzyme and bilirubin values, and worsening hypoalbuminemia. Renal failure can be detected by monitoring urine output, blood urea nitrogen, and serum creatinine levels. Creatinine clearance is easily measured in a dog with an indwelling urinary catheter. Sepsis-associated respiratory failure is a rare event in dogs[78] and usually requires other contributing factors (such as fluid overload or pulmonary thromboembolism) to become clinically evident. Subclinical heart failure is present early in sepsis,[36] but overt failure usually occurs as a terminal event.

Gastrointestinal tract failure and ulceration are treated with H_2-receptor antagonists, metoclopramide, and gastrointestinal coating agents (see Table 99–3).

TABLE 99–3. DOSES FOR SEPTIC DOGS WITH PROSTATIC ABSCESS

Category	Dose	Frequency
Fluid Therapy		
Hypertonic crystalloids		
7.5% sodium chloride (NaCl) solution (70 ml 23.4% NaCl in 180 ml 0.9% NaCl)	4 ml/kg IV	Once, for resuscitation from shock
GIK solution (3 g glucose, 1–2 U insulin; potassium, 0.5 mEq/kg in 250 ml lactated Ringer)	IV, 10% volume bolus, rest infused over 4–5 hours	Once, for resuscitation from shock
Colloids		
Plasma	Maximum: 30 ml/kg/24 hours IV	Based on albumin value
Dextran 40 (10%) Dextran 70 (6%)	Maximum: 30 ml/kg/24 hours IV	Slow infusion
3% albumin (12 ml 25% human albumin in 488 ml lactated Ringer)	20 ml/kg IV	Once, for resuscitation from shock
Isotonic crystalloids		
Lactated Ringer	20–80 ml/kg IV 10–20 ml/kg/hour IV	Resuscitation Ongoing needs in sepsis
Metabolic Therapy		
Potassium chloride	0.125–0.25 mEq/kg/hour IV, not to exceed 0.5 mEq/kg/hour	Based on serum potassium concentration
Glucose	50–500 mg/kg/hour IV	Infuse to maintain normal blood glucose concentration
Antiendotoxin Therapy		
Corticosteroids		
Methylprednisolone Sodium succinate	30 mg/kg IV	Once, early in shock or before surgery
Nonsteroidal anti-inflammatory drugs		
Flunixin meglumine	0.25–1.0 mg/kg IV	Once; may repeat once in 6–12 hours
Drugs for Altered Clotting Function		
Heparin (low dose)	75–100 units/kg SC	Every 6–8 hours
Heparin-activated plasma (incubate 5–10 units/kg heparin with 1 unit fresh plasma for 30 minutes)	10 mg/kg	Every 3 hours, based on clotting function
Cardiovascular Support Drugs		
Dopamine	5–10 μg/kg/minute IV	Continuous, until cardiovascular status stable
Dobutamine	5–20 μg/kg/minute IV	Continuous, until cardiovascular status stable
Drugs for Gastrointestinal Tract Failure		
Cimetidine	5–10 mg/kg IV, IM, or PO	Every 6–8 hours, stagger 2 hours from sucralfate
Ranitidine	2–4 mg/kg PO	Every 12 hours, stagger 2 hours from sucralfate
Sucralfate	<20 kg: 500 mg PO >20 kg: 1 g PO	Every 6–8 hours
Kaolin/pectin	1–2 ml/kg PO	Every 6–8 hours
Metoclopramide	0.2–0.5 mg/kg SC or 1–2 mg/kg/24 hours IV	Every 6–8 hours or 24-hour infusion
Drugs for Acute Renal Failure		
Mannitol	0.25–1 g/kg IV	Once, slow bolus
Furosemide	1–2 mg/kg IV	Once, if no effect, repeat in 2 hours, increase dose 1 mg/kg
Dopamine	1–3 μg/kg/minute IV	Until urine production consistently >2 ml/kg/hour

Liver failure usually resolves without specific therapy. Lack of urine production is often noted immediately after surgery. If fluid therapy is adequate and blood pressure is normal, low-dose dopamine or furosemide (see Table 99–3) is given. If hypertonic solutions have not previously been administered, mannitol is also given. Once urine flow is established, fluid balance is carefully monitored because polyuria often ensues. The development of either respiratory or heart failure is a poor prognostic sign.

As soon as a dog is alert enough to eat, a diet including high-quality protein is fed. The energy requirements of septic patients are 1.5 to 1.8 higher than the resting energy requirement.[69] These dogs are weighed daily. Continued weight loss and inappetence may indicate supplemental feeding, using a palatable liquid or tube feeding through a nasogastric or percutaneously placed gastrostomy tube.[2] Appetite usually returns once gastrointestinal tract and liver failure begin to resolve.

Antibiotic sensitivity patterns for organisms cultured from the prostatic abscess are used to guide postoperative antibiotic therapy as soon as possible. Intravenous therapy is continued as long as sepsis is obvious. When sepsis resolves and the gastrointestinal tract is functioning, oral antibiotic therapy is used for prolonged therapy.

References

1. Abu-Yousef MM: Benign prostatic hyperplasia: Tissue characterization using suprapubic ultrasound. *Radiology 156*:169, 1985.
2. Armstrong PJ, Hardie EM: Percutaneous endoscopic gastrostomy. *Vet Med Rep 1*:404, 1989.
3. Aumuller G, et al: Regional distribution of opioidergic nerves in human and canine prostates. *Prostate 14*:279, 1989.
4. Barsanti JA, et al: Evaluation of diagnostic techniques for canine prostatic diseases. *J Am Vet Med Assoc 177*:160, 1980.
5. Basinger RR, Barsanti JA: Urodynamic abnormalities associated with canine prostatic diseases and therapeutic intervention. *In* Kirk RW (ed): *Current Veterinary Therapy X*. W. B. Saunders, Philadelphia, 1989, p 115.
6. Basinger RR, Rawlings CA: Surgical management of prostatic diseases. *Comp Cont Educ Pract Vet 9*:993, 1987.
7. Basinger RR, et al: Urodynamic alterations after prostatectomy in dogs without clinical prostatic disease. *Vet Surg 16*:405, 1987.
8. Berry SJ, et al: Methods for monitoring canine prostate size: Internal and external caliper measurements. *Prostate 6*:303, 1985.
9. Berry SJ, et al: Effects of aging on prostate growth in beagles. *Am J Physiol 250*:R1039, 1986.
10. Berry SJ, et al: Effect of age, castration, and testosterone replacement on the development and restoration of canine benign prostatic hyperplasia. *Prostate 9*:295, 1986.
11. Berry SJ, et al: Development of canine benign prostatic hyperplasia with age. *Prostate 9*:363, 1986.
12. Bornsveld W, et al: Ventricular function, hemodynamics, and oxygen consumption during infusions of blood, and glucose-insulin-potassium (GIK) in canine endotoxin shock. *Circ Shock 9*:145, 1982.
13. Branam JE, et al: Selected physical and chemical characteristics of prostatic fluid collected by ejaculation from healthy dogs and from dogs with bacterial prostatitis. *Am J Vet Res 45*:825, 1984.
14. Brendler CB, et al: Spontaneous benign prostatic hyperplasia in the beagle—age-associated changes in serum hormone levels, and the morphology and secretory function of the canine prostate. *J Clin Invest 71*:1114, 1983.
15. Cartee RE, Rowles T: Transabdominal sonographic evaluation of the canine prostate. *Vet Radiol 24*:156, 1983.
16. Chapdelaine P, et al: Identification of arginine esterase as the major androgen-dependent protein secreted by dog prostate and preliminary molecular characterization in seminal plasma. *J Androl 5*:206, 1984.
17. Chapdelaine P, et al: Androgen regulation of canine prostatic arginine esterase mRNA using cloned cDNA. *Mol Cell Endocrinol 56*:63, 1988.
18. Christensen GC: The urogenital apparatus. *In* Evans HE, Christensen GC (eds): *Miller's Anatomy of the Dog* 2nd ed. W. B. Saunders, Philadelphia, 1979.
19. Christie TR: Prostate gland and testes. *In* Bojrab MJ (ed): *Current Techniques in Small Animal Surgery*. Lea & Febiger, Philadelphia, 1983, pp 360–369.
20. Dow SW, et al: Bacterial culture of blood from critically ill dogs and cats: 100 cases (1985–1987). *J Am Vet Med Assoc 195*:113, 1989.
21. Dow SW, et al: Anaerobic bacterial infections and response to treatment in dogs and cats: 36 cases (1983–1985). *J Am Vet Med Assoc 189*:930, 1986.
22. Dow SW, et al: Adverse effects of flunixin meglumine administered with and without prednisone, on the gastrointestinal tract of dogs. *Proceedings of the 7th Annual ACVIM Forum*, Chicago, IL, Oct. 1989, p 1045.
23. Dubé JY, et al: Biochemical characteristics of the proteins secreted by dog prostate, a review, *Exp Biol 43*:149, 1985.
24. Ewing LL, et al: Testicular androgen and estrogen secretion and benign prostatic hyperplasia in the beagle. *Endocrinology 114*:1308, 1984.
25. Feeney DA, et al: Two-dimensional, gray-scale ultrasonography: Application in canine prostatic disease. *Vet Clin North Am Small Anim Pract 15*:1159, 1985.
26. Feeney DA, et al: Canine prostatic disease—comparison of radiographic appearance with morphologic and microbiologic findings; 30 cases (1981–1985). *J Am Vet Med Assoc 190*:1018, 1987.
27. Feeney DA, et al: Canine prostatic disease—comparison of ultrasonographic appearance with morphologic and microbiologic findings: 30 cases (1981–1985). *J Am Vet Med Assoc 8*:1027, 1987.
28. Feeney DA, et al: Dimensions of the prostatic and membranous urethra in normal male dogs during maximum distension in retrograde urethrocystography. *Vet Radiol 25*:249, 1984.
29. Feldman BF: Disseminated intravascular coagulation. *Comp Cont Educ Pract Vet 3*:46, 1981.
30. Fink MP, et al: Effects of nonsteroidal anti-inflammatory drugs on renal function in septic dogs. *J Surg Res 36*:516, 1984.
31. Fink MP, et al: Inhibition of prostaglandin synthesis restores normal hemodynamics in canine hyperdynamic sepsis. *Ann Surg 200*:619, 1984.
32. Gahring DR: Personal communication, San Diego, 1989.
33. Gahring DR: Surgical management of prostatic diseases. Proceedings of the 6th Annual *ACVS Forum*, Chicago, IL, Oct. 1978.
34. Gordon N: The position of the canine prostate gland. *Am J Vet Res 22*:142, 1961.
35. Gourley IMG, Osborne CA: Marsupialization—a treatment for prostatic abscess in the dog. *Anim Hosp 2*:100, 1966.
36. Guntheroth WG, et al: Left ventricular performance in endotoxin shock in dogs. *Am J Physiol 242*:H172, 1982.
37. Hardie EM: Peritonitis from urogenital conditions. *Probl Vet Med 1*:36, 1989.
38. Hardie EM, et al: Complications of prostatic surgery. *J Am Anim Hosp Assoc 20*:50, 1984.
39. Hardie EM, et al: Severe sepsis in selected surgical patients. *J Am Anim Hosp Assoc 22*:33, 1986.
40. Hardie EM, et al: Subtotal prostatectomy using the neodymium:yttrium aluminum garnet laser in the dog. *Vet Surg, 19*:349, 1990.
41. Hargiss AM, Miller LM: Prostatic carcinoma in the dog. *Comp Cont Educ Pract Vet 5*:647, 1983.
42. Hasegawa Y, Kumazawa J: Relationship between echogram and histology of benign prostatic hyperplasia. *Eur Urol 13*:378, 1987.
43. Hinshaw LB, et al: Current management of the septic shock patient: Experimental basis for treatment. *Circ Shock 9*:543, 1982.
44. Hoffer RE, et al: Marsupialization as a treatment for prostatic disease. *J Am Anim Hosp Assoc 13*:98, 1977.
45. Hornbuckle WE, et al: Prostatic disease in the dog. *Cornell Vet 68*:284, 1978.
46. Howard DR: Surgical approach to the canine prostate. *J Am Vet Med Assoc 155*:2026, 1969.
47. Huggins C: The physiology of the prostate gland. *Physiol Rev 25*:281, 1945.
48. Huggins C, Clark PJ: Quantitative studies of the prostatic secretion, 2. The effect of castration and of estrogen injection on the normal and on the hyperplastic prostate glands of dogs. *J Exp Med 72*:747, 1940.
49. Isaacs JT, et al: Differential effects of estrogen treatment on canine seminal plasma components. *Invest Urol 17*:495, 1980.
50. Isaacs WB, Coffey DS: The predominant protein of canine seminal plasma is an enzyme. *J Biol Chem 259*:11520, 1984.
51. Isaacs WB, Shaper JH: Isolation and characterization of the major androgen-dependent glycoprotein of canine prostatic fluid. *J Biol Chem 258*:6610, 1983.
52. Johnston DE: Prostate. *In* Slatter (ed): *Textbook of Small Animal Surgery*. W. B. Saunders, Philadelphia, 1985, pp 1635–1650.
53. Juniewicz PE, et al: Identification of phytoestrogens in the urine of male dogs. *J Steroid Biochem 31*:987, 1988.
54. Klausner JS, Osborne CA: Management of canine bacterial prostatitis. *J Am Vet Med Assoc 182*:292, 1983.
55. Knecht CD: Diseases of the canine prostate gland (part I). *Comp Cont Educ Pract Vet 1*:385, 1979.
56. Leav I, Ling GV: Adenocarcinoma of the canine prostate. *Cancer 22*:1329, 1968.
57. Ling GV, et al: Canine prostatic fluid: Techniques of collection, quantitative bacterial culture, and interpretation of results. *J Am Vet Med Assoc 183*:201, 1983.
58. Luypaert P, et al: Fluid resuscitation with hypertonic saline in endotoxic shock. *Circ Shock 20*:311, 1986.
59. Manny J, et al: Effect of glucose-insulin-potassium on survival in experimental endotoxic shock. *Surg Gynecol Obstet 147*:405, 1978.
60. Matthiesen DT, Manfra Marretta S: Complications associated with the surgical treatment of prostatic abscessation. *Probl Vet Med 1*:63, 1989.
61. McLain DL: Surgical treatment of perineal prostatic abscesses. *J Am Anim Hosp Assoc 19*:794, 1982.
62. Muir WW, et al: Small-volume resuscitation with hypertonic saline solution in hypovolemic cats. *Am J Vet Res 50*:1883, 1989.
63. Mullen HS, et al: Abstract: Abscessation of the prostate gland treated with a multiple drain technique: An evaluation of postoperative complications and results in 92 dogs. *Vet Surg 18*:70, 1989.
64. Mullins RJ, Hudgens RW: Hypertonic saline resuscitates dogs in endotoxic shock. *J Surg Res 43*:37, 1985.
65. Obradovich J, et al: The influence of castration on the development of prostatic carcinoma in the dog. *J Vet Intern Med 1*:183, 1987.
66. O'Shea JD: Studies on the canine prostate gland I. Factors influencing its size and weight. *J Comp Pathol 72*:321, 1962.
67. Perry MO: Anticoagulation: A surgical perspective. *Am J Surg 155*:268, 1988.
68. Pontes JE, et al: Transrectal ultrasonography of the prostate. *Cancer 53*:1369, 1984.
69. Remillard RL, Thatcher CD: Parenteral nutritional support in the small animal patient. *Vet Clin North Am Small Anim Pract 19*:1287, 1989.
70. Robertson JJ, Bojrab MJ: Subtotal prostatectomy results in normal dogs. *Vet Surg 13*:6, 1984.
71. Rocha-e-Silva M, et al: Hypertonic resuscitation from severe hemorrhagic shock: patterns of regional circulation. *Circ Shock 19*:165, 1986.
72. Rogers KS, et al: Diagnostic evaluation of the canine prostate. *Comp Cont Educ Pract Vet 8*:11, 1988.
73. Ruehl W, et al: Rational therapy in disseminated intravascular coagulation. *J Am Vet Med Assoc 181*:76, 1982.

74. Smith ER: The canine prostate and its secretion. *Adv Sex Horm Res 1*:168, 1975.
75. Sprung CL, et al: The effects of high dose corticosteroids in patients with septic shock. *N Engl J Med 311*:1137, 1984.
76. Stone EA, et al: Radiographic interpretation of prostatic disease in the dog. *J Am Anim Hosp Assoc 14*:115, 1978.
77. Strandberg JD, Berry SJ: The pathology of prostatic hyperplasia in the dog. *In* Rodgers CH, et al (eds): *Benign Prostatic Hyperplasia*. Volume II. NIH Publication 87–2881. National Institutes of Health, Bethesda, MD, 1985.
78. Sugarman HJ, et al: Hemodynamics, oxygen consumption and serum catecholamine changes in progressive, lethal peritonitis in the dog. *Surg Gynecol Obstet 154*:8, 1982.
79. Thrall DE: Radiographic aspects of prostatic disease in the dog. *Comp Cont Educ Pract Vet 3*:718, 1981.
80. Thrall MA, et al: Cytologic diagnosis of canine prostatic disease. *J Am Anim Hosp Assoc 21*:95, 1984.
81. Vincent JL, et al: Dopamine compared with dobutamine in experimental septic shock: Relevance to fluid administration. *Anesth Analg 66*:565, 1987.
82. Wade DR, et al: A noninvasive technique for monitoring changes in canine prostatic size in vivo. *Invest Urol 18*:266, 1981.
83. Walsh PC: Benign prostatic hyperplasia. *In* Walsh PC, et al (eds): *Campbell's Urology*. 5th ed. W. B. Saunders, Philadelphia, 1986.
84. Watanabe H, et al: Dynamic study of nervous control on prostatic contraction and fluid excretion in the dog. *J Urol 140*:1567, 1988.
85. Weaver AD: Discrete prostatic (paraprostatic) cysts in the dog. *Vet Rec 102*:435, 1978.
86. Weaver AD: Fifteen cases of prostatic carcinoma in the dog. *Vet Rec 109*:71, 1981.
86a. Weiner N, Taylor P: Neurohumoral transmission: The autonomic and somatic nervous systems. *In* Gilman AG, Goodman LS, Rall TW, et al. (eds.): *Goodman and Gilman's The Pharmacological Basis of Therapeutics*. 7th ed. Macmillan Publishing Co., New York, 1985.
87. Wheaton LG, et al: Relationship of seminal volume to size and disease of the prostate in the beagle. *Am J Vet Res 40*:1325, 1978.
88. White RAS, et al: The diagnosis and management of paraprostatic and prostatic retention cysts in the dog. *J Small Anim Pract 28*:551, 1987.
89. Zolton GM, Greiner TP: Prostatic abscesses—a surgical approach. *J Am Anim Hosp Assoc 14*:698, 1978.

SECTION 12

Urinary System

Dale E. Bjorling ■ *Section Editor*

CHAPTER 100

Anatomy of the Urinary Tract

Bruce A. Christie

DEVELOPMENT OF THE URINARY SYSTEM

The urinary and genital systems share a common mesodermal origin and pursue an integrated development. Much of this chapter's content is drawn from several textbooks.[1, 19, 37]

Normal Development

Kidneys and Ureters

Kidneys are compound tubular glands composed of uriniferous tubules. They arise in the embryo in a mesodermal plate called the *nephrotome*, which lies between the somatic and splanchnic mesoderm (Fig. 100–1*A*). From the nephrotome, three classes of organs develop sequentially (Fig. 100–1*B* and *C*). The first to form is the pronephros. This is the functional kidney of primitive vertebrates such as cyclostomes and the provisional kidney of larval fishes and amphibians. Pronephric tubules arise as buds from the nephrotome plate. The growing extremities of the buds unite to produce a pronephric duct. The caudal blind end of the duct grows toward the cloaca and penetrates it. Pronephric tubules degenerate, but the duct is retained and used by tubules of the mesonephros, the second nephrogenic organ to develop. The duct is now known as the *mesonephric* or *wolffian* duct. The mesonephros is the permanent kidney of fishes and amphibians. In mammals, some portions of the mesonephric duct and some tubules are salvaged for use in the genital system of the male. The metanephric kidney, the third class in the sequence, is the functional kidney of reptiles, birds, and mammals. It has a dual origin. Secretory units, or nephrons, consist of the Bowman capsule, proximal and distal convoluted tubules, and the loop of Henle. These units arise in the caudalmost portion of the nephrogenic cord, the metanephros.

The drainage duct system of the metanephros is derived from a bud growing off the mesonephric duct close to the cloaca. This bud pushes into the metanephrogenic mesoderm and, by a process of repeated dichotomous branching and absorption, differentiates into ureter, pelvis, calyces, papillary ducts, and straight collecting tubules (Fig. 100–2).

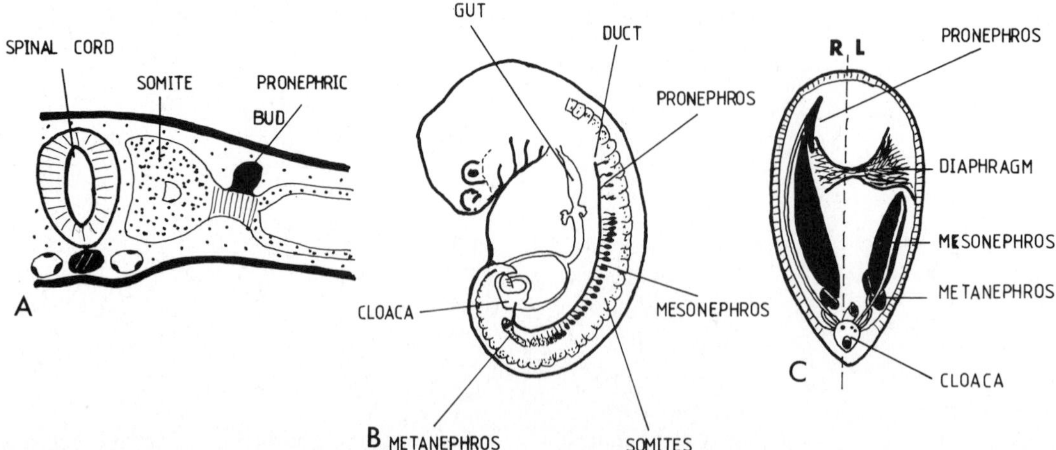

FIGURE 100–1. Development of the kidney and ureter. *A*, Transverse section. *B*, Sequential development of the three kidney types in mammals. *C*, Ventral dissection. The left side is drawn at a later stage than the right. (Reproduced with permission from Arey LB: *Developmental Anatomy*. W. B. Saunders, Philadelphia, 1965.)

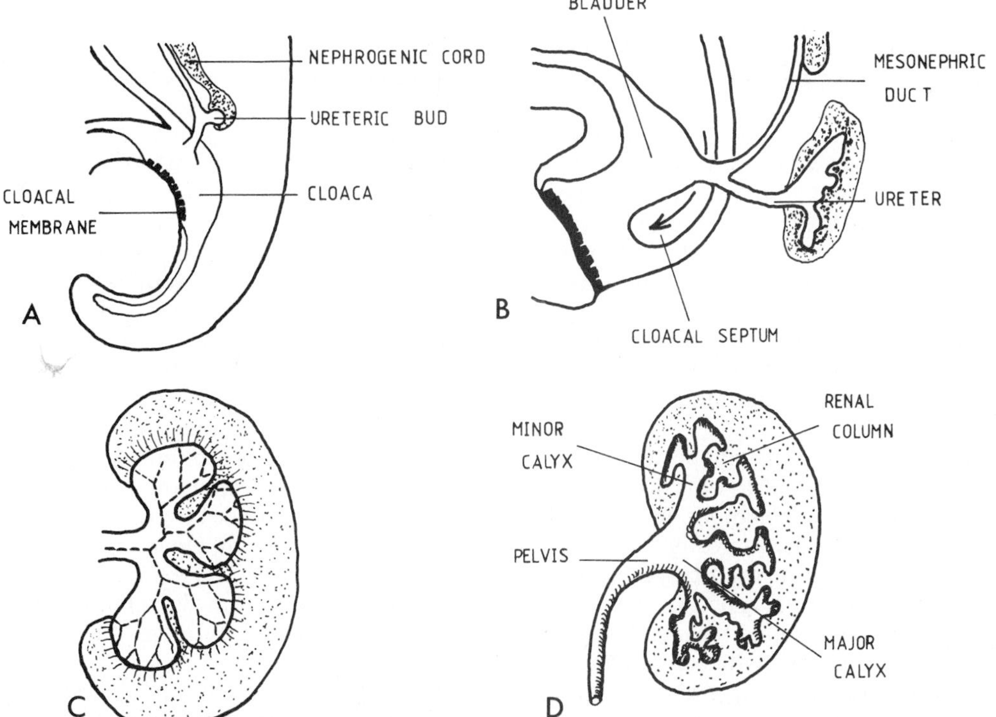

FIGURE 100–2. Development of the metanephros and drainage duct system. *A*, Ureteric bud from the mesonephric duct pushing into metanephrogenic cord. The cloacal membrane is the fused ectodermal/endodermal plate. *B*, A septum divides the cloaca into dorsal rectum and ventral urogenital sinus. *C* and *D*, The duct system is formed from repeated dichotomous branching. Absorption of the first 15 generations forms the pelvis and calyces. (*A*, *B*, and *D* reproduced with permission from Arey LB: *Developmental Anatomy*. W. B. Saunders, Philadelphia, 1965.)

Microdissection studies have shown that human kidneys contain 25 to 30 generations of buds.[27] The renal pelvis is formed from the first 5 generations, major calyces generations 10 through 15, and collecting tubules from succeeding generations. Each bud consists of an interstitial or tubular segment and the advancing end or ampulla. Up to 25 papillary ducts, or ducts of Bellini, open into each minor calyx via the fenestrated papillary tip known as the *area cribrosa*. All papillary ducts that drain into the same minor calyx form the medullary pyramid. Straight collecting tubules are abundant in the medulla and project into the cortex as medullary rays (Fig. 100–3). The metanephrogenic mesoderm, which caps the medullary pyramid, is the cortex. This tissue also divides and increases in volume as the collecting tubules divide. Renal columns are regions where the cortex extends between individual pyramids. The terminal ampulla of the last generation of buds induces nephron formation. The tiny masses of metanephrogenic tissue around each terminal collecting tubule hollow into

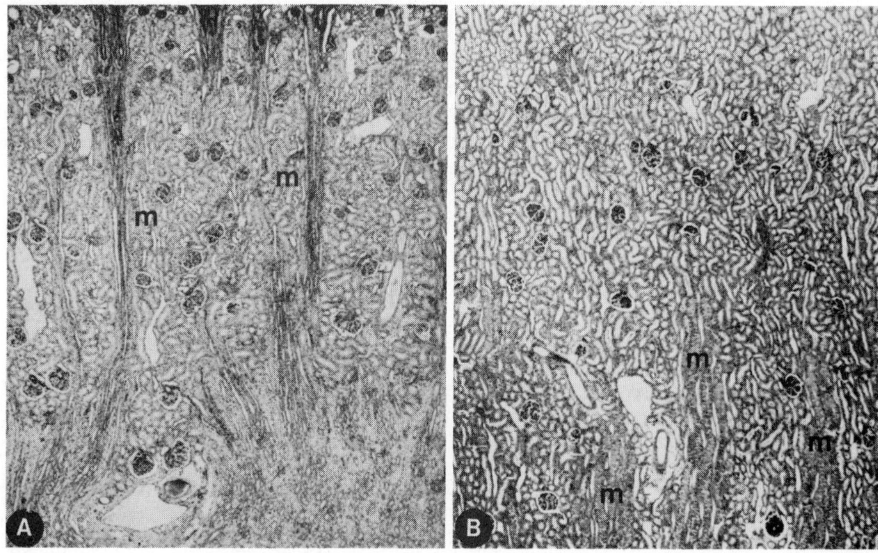

FIGURE 100–3. Photomicrograph of a dog's kidney to show the underdevelopment of the outer cortex in a 1-week-old pup *(A)* compared with a mature dog *(B)*. The medullary rays (m) are prominent. (H and E, × 10.)

vesicles, elongate, and become tortuous. A Bowman capsule and glomerulus differentiate at one end, whereas the other end becomes continuous with a nearby collecting duct.

Newer generations of nephrons develop centrifugally as the terminal ampulla grows toward the kidney capsule. From 12 to 15 nephrons ultimately attach to each of the terminal branches. It follows, therefore, that the subcapsular glomeruli are youngest. Nephron formation in each human kidney is finished at birth. Each kidney contains approximately 1,000,000 nephrons. Enlargement of the kidney after birth is due to maturation of nephrons already present. In dogs[2] and presumably cats, induction of more nephrons continues into the postnatal period.

Ascent of the Kidneys. The metanephros originates near the bifurcation of the aorta, but its definitive position is closer to the thoracolumbar junction. The cranial movement is brought about mostly by growth of the lumbosacral region as the marked curvature of the body of the embryo straightens out. As the kidneys ascend out of the pelvis, they rotate through 90° so that the hilus faces medially rather than dorsally. In addition, the blood supply to the kidneys sequentially shifts from iliac arteries to the final point of origin off the aorta level with lumbar vertebral segments 2 and 3.

Lobation, Pyramids, and Lobules. As the cortex organizes over a primary pyramid, the boundary of the cortical cap is established by a deep groove on the surface of the kidney. Each primary pyramid, but not its papilla, subsequently divides into two or more secondary pyramids. The site of the secondary pyramids is also demonstrated on the surface of the kidney, giving it a lobed appearance. Fetal lobation in human kidneys progressively disappears in infancy and childhood as kidney growth causes the cortical cap on the pyramids to fuse. In dogs, the cortex and medullary pyramids fuse completely. The composite broad-based papilla is called the *renal crest*. Such kidneys are known as *unipyramidal* or *unilobar* kidneys even though they consist of several fused lobes. A cat's kidney is a true unilobar kidney, because it contains only one lobe.

Within the lobes are found lobules. These are the functional units of a kidney, containing all the uriniferous tubules whose collecting ducts course in a particular medullary (cortical) ray.

Cloacal Differentiation. The cloaca is the common endodermal chamber into which fecal, urinary, and reproductive products pass. Reptiles, birds, and nonplacental mammals retain this organ. In placental mammals, the cloaca is further subdivided into dorsal rectum, ventral bladder, and urogenital sinus by the growth of a wedge-shaped mesenchymal mass called the cloacal septum (see Fig. 100–2*B*). When this reaches the cloacal membrane (the fused ectodermal/endodermal plate), the membrane ruptures, exposing the projecting wedge, which is now called the *perineal body*. The perineal body merges with the lateral folds flanking the fissure that was left when the cloacal membrane was resorbed. This area becomes covered by advancing ectoderm and fuses at the median raphe. When the bladder is first formed, it still receives on either side the common stem of a mesonephric duct and ureter (Fig. 100–4*A*). Growth now occurs with absorption of these stems so that the four ducts acquire individual openings (Fig. 100–4*B*). The mesonephric ducts are displaced caudally and open close together on an elevation in the future urethra known as the *Müller tubercle*, or *seminal colliculus*. The triangular area on the dorsal wall of the bladder and urethra demarcated by these ducts is the trigone (Fig. 100–4*C*).

With further growth, the bladder expands into an elongated sac. It has a tapering cranial extremity leading to the urachus, which is continuous at the umbilicus with the allantois. The caudal extremity, the neck, is continuous with the urethra.

The urogenital sinus (Fig. 100–5*A*) has pelvic and phallic portions. In females, the short neck connecting the bladder and urogenital sinus elongates into the permanent urethra (Fig. 100–5*B*), and the pelvic and phallic portions of the sinus merge to create the slitlike vestibule. A female's urethra does not extend into the clitoris. In males, the prostatic urethra between the bladder neck and Müller tubercle is equivalent to the entire female urethra. The pelvic portion of the urogenital sinus completes the prostatic and all the membranous urethra (Fig. 100–5*C*). The phallic portion of the sinus contributes the penile urethra, which extends through the penis to the exterior.

Abnormal Development

Renal Agenesis. This can occur if the mesonephric ducts fail to develop or if no ureteric bud forms. It is primarily the branching ureteric bud penetrating into the metanephrogenic tissue that stimulates the devel-

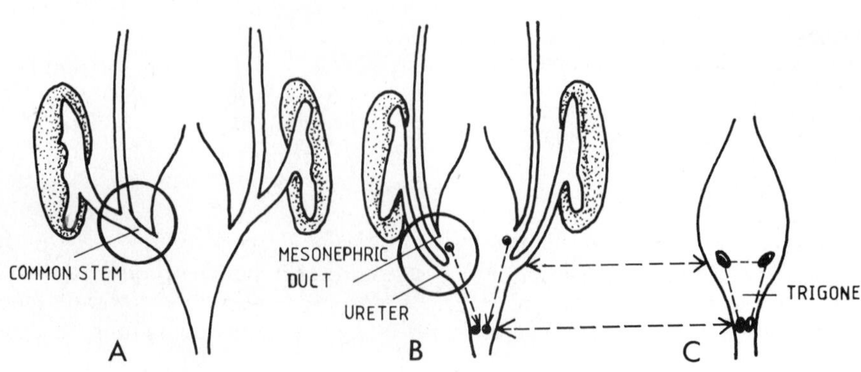

FIGURE 100–4. Differentiation of the cloaca. *A* and *B*, Growth and absorption of the ureter and mesonephric duct so that they acquire separate openings. These openings outline the bladder trigone *(C)*.

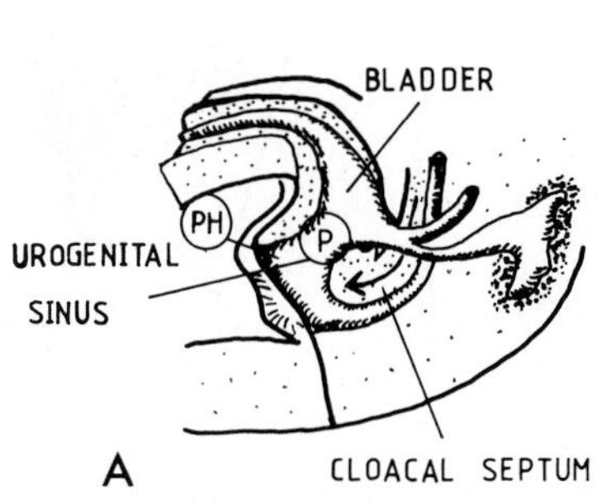

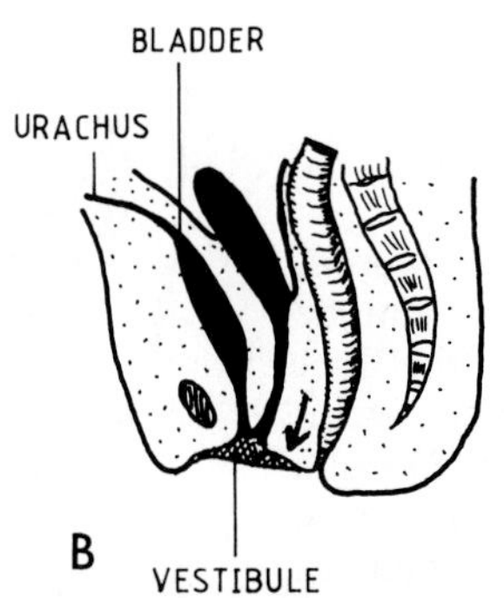

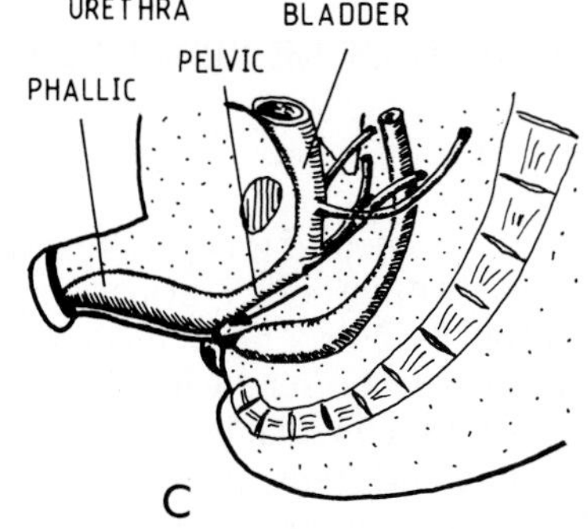

FIGURE 100–5. *A,* Development of the urogenital sinus with its pelvic (P) and phallic (PH) portions. *B,* In the female, the pelvic and phallic portions merge to create the vestibule. *C,* In the male, the phallic portion of the sinus forms the penile urethra. (Reproduced with permission from Arey LB: *Developmental Anatomy.* W. B. Saunders, Philadelphia, 1965.)

opment of nephrons. That is, in true renal agenesis, there is no ureter.

Supernumerary Kidneys. If two ureteric buds grow from the same mesonephric duct, supernumerary kidneys will result. Separate renal development is induced around each duct system. In this situation, the upper metanephric duct drains the upper (cranial) part of the kidney and the lower drains the caudal region. The upper duct is usually ectopic because it migrates with the mesonephric duct into the urethra.[7]

Renal Hypoplasia. This is a deficiency in the total nephron population. A defect in the "inducer capability" of the ureteric bud or in the nephrogenic cord can produce renal abnormalities.[31] With extreme sites of ureteral ectopia, the abnormally placed bud unites with defective involuting nephrogenic or stromagenic mesenchymal tissue, leading to hypoplasia and dysplasia. *Dysplasia* refers to the presence of abnormal nephrons. Normal renal parenchymal development is also impaired by complete obstruction of the urinary tract but not by incomplete obstruction.[31]

Nonascent of the Kidneys. This can affect one or both kidneys. The kidney remains in its primary pelvic position.

High Renal Ectopia. This can result in an intrathoracic kidney.[24] The diaphragm does not form completely until about 8 weeks of gestation in human beings. Continued ascent of the kidney exerts pressure on the incompletely formed diaphragm, displacing it anteriorly and producing a thin membrane covering the cranial pole of the kidney.

Fused Kidneys. If the ureteric buds take a converging course during development, fused kidneys may result. The fused kidneys might or might not ascend properly.

Renal Polycystic Disease. The traditional anatomical explanation attributes renal cysts to nonunion of secretory and collecting tubules.[18] The blind secretory tubules dilate and become cysts. It is now known as a result of microdissection studies that polycystic disease can be due to dilatation and hyperplasia of collecting ducts, inhibited ampullary activity with failure to induce nephrons, or multiple abnormalities in the ureteric bud derivatives and the nephrons.[28] The developing cysts apply pressure to surrounding normal tubules and compromise their function.

Ureteral Ectopia. In males, the bladder neck, prostatic urethra, seminal vesicles, and vasa deferentia all develop from the mesonephric duct and urogenital sinus. If the ureter buds off the mesonephric duct too far cranially, then with growth and absorption the metanephric duct (ureter) might not open separately into the bladder. It can be carried caudally to open into the vas deferens, seminal vesicles, or urethra.[30] The same explanation accounts for ureters that open into the bladder neck or urethra in females and also accounts for the upper (cranial) ureter being ectopic when the ureters are duplicated, as the lower (caudal) metanephric duct is absorbed normally into the bladder wall. It is less certain how ureters can open into the vagina, cervix, or uterus, because these structures are müllerian duct derivatives. One explanation is that part of the vagina is derived from the mesonephric system and urogenital sinus.[5] However, embryological connection through the Gartner duct, a wolffian derivative that normally atrophies and disappears, is the most common explanation of an ectopic opening into the cervix and uterus.[14] In humans, rare cases of an ectopic ureteral opening into the rectum have been reported.[23] Such an abnormality could be accounted for by faulty division of the cloaca by the cloacal septum.

Ureterocele. A ureterocele is a cystic dilatation of the intravesicular portion of the ureter. It may be related to a congenitally small ("pinpoint") ureteral meatus due to faulty mesonephric duct development. Urine pressure builds up, and the bladder mucosa over the region of the submucosal ureter bulges. Ureteroceles can also occur when the ureteral orifice or meatus is large. This usually occurs in an ectopic ureter. The distal portion of the ureter expands in response to the same stimulus that causes the fetal bladder to expand.[33]

Faulty Differentiation of the Cloaca. This can result in incomplete separation of the rectum and urogenital sinus. The outcome is a rectovestibular fistula in a female or a rectovesicular or rectourethral fistula in a male (Fig. 100–6). If invasion by somatic mesoderm fails to reduce the extensive cranial extent of the early cloacal membrane (see Fig. 100–2), subsequent rupture of the membrane exposes the lining of the bladder. This condition is known as *exstrophy* of the bladder.

GROSS ANATOMY OF THE URINARY SYSTEM

Overview[9, 15, 36]

When the abdomen of a dog is opened and explored, most of the "within-body" urinary apparatus can be seen (Fig. 100–7). For a more complete view, the floor of the pelvis has to be removed. The renal artery, vein, and ureter enter the medial border of the kidney through a fissure called the *hilus*. The hilus leads to a central recess, the renal sinus, which is lined by a continuation of the kidney capsule and contains much fat. Lymph vessels and renal nerves are closely related to the renal vein and artery, respectively. Because the aorta and vena cava lie side by side with the aorta to the left of the cava, the left kidney has a relatively long renal vein and the right kidney a relatively long renal artery.

The ureters, like the kidneys, are retroperitoneal structures. They extend caudomedially along the sublumbar muscles toward the bladder. As they approach the pelvic inlet, they leave the sublumbar position and gain access to the bladder between the two layers of peritoneum that form the lateral ligaments of the bladder. The spermatic or ovarian vessels cross the cranial ureter ventrally, but the deep circumflex iliac vessels cross the caudal ureter dorsally.

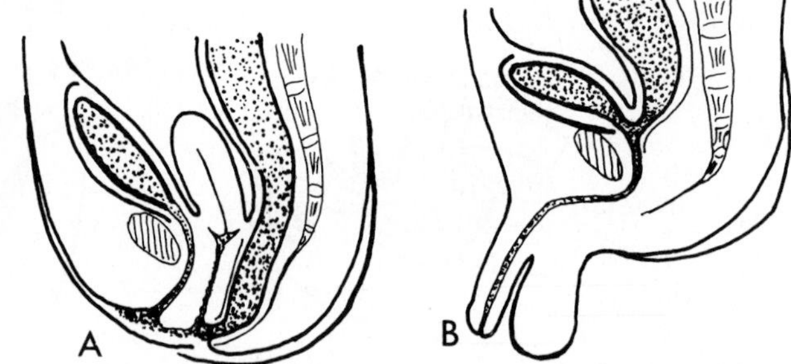

FIGURE 100–6. Faulty separation of the rectum and urogenital sinus can lead to rectovestibular fistula in a female *(A)* and rectourethral fistula in a male *(B)*. (Reproduced with permission from Arey LB: *Developmental Anatomy*. W. B. Saunders, Philadelphia, 1965.)

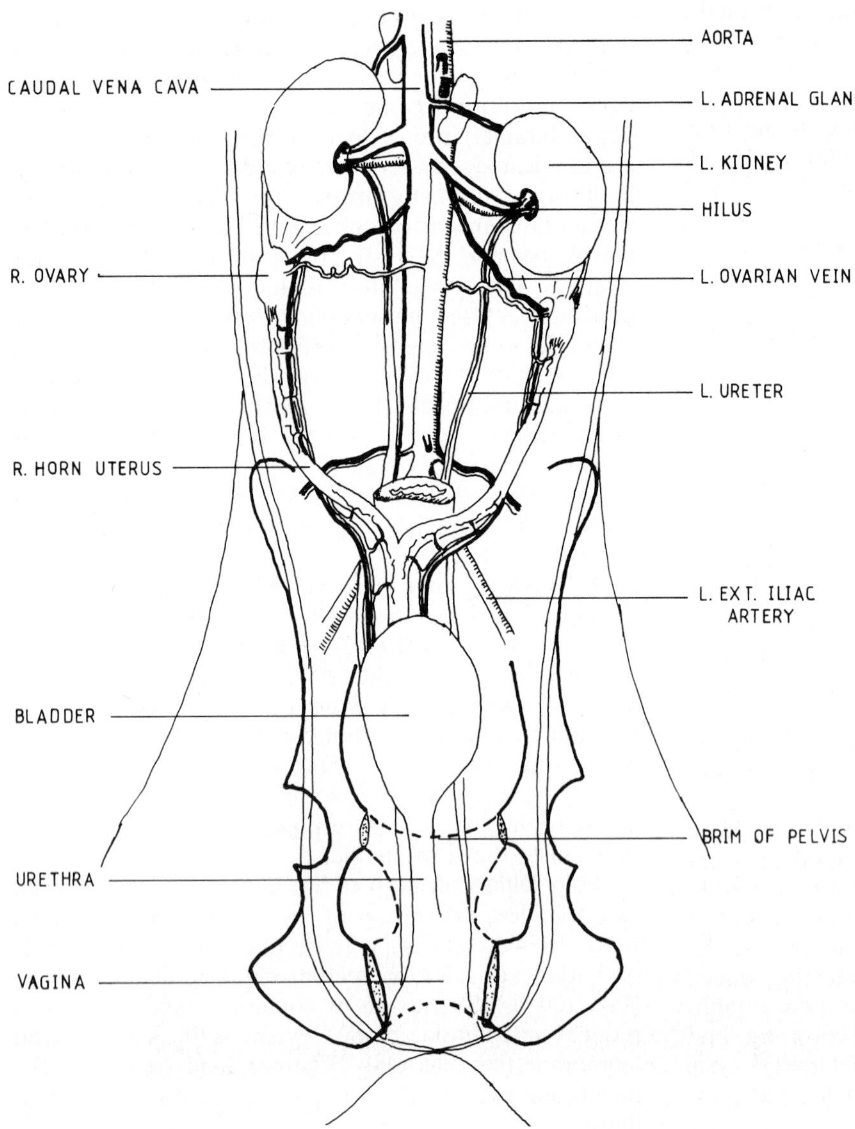

FIGURE 100–7. The relationships of the urinary genital apparatus to each other and to the bony pelvis in a female dog.

Radiographic Anatomy

Contrast agents infused into the lower urinary tract or excreted into the upper urinary tract outline the urinary apparatus (Fig. 100–8). An intravenous pyelogram opacifies the entire kidney parenchyma, renal pelvis, and ureters. A pneumocystogram highlights the thin-walled bladder and provides negative contrast against which the ureterovesical junction can be seen. A retrograde pyelogram outlines the renal pelvis and ureters. Finally, a positive-contrast voiding cystogram illustrates bladder volume and shape and also the capacity of the bladder neck and proximal urethra to dilate.

Kidneys

Topography

The topographical anatomy of the kidneys is well illustrated in canine whole-body longitudinal, horizontal, and transverse sections (Fig. 100–9). The kidneys are retroperitoneal. The cranial pole of each kidney is covered by peritoneum on both dorsal and ventral surfaces, but only the ventral surface of the caudal pole is covered. The kidneys are embedded in adipose tissue and are held in the sublumbar position by subperitoneal fibroareolar tissue or renal fascia. Ventrally, this renal fascia is continuous with the connective tissue around the aorta and caudal vena cava. Medially and dorsally, it is attached to the thoracolumbar fascia. The fixation is not rigid. Both kidneys are displaced by movement of the diaphragm during respiration. The right kidney is related to the liver and is firmly attached. The left kidney is less firmly attached and can be displaced caudally by a full stomach. In cats, both kidneys are equally mobile.

Characteristics

The characteristic features of the kidneys of dogs and cats are summarized in Table 100–1. Both cats and dogs have bean-shaped, unipyramidal or unilobar kidneys. A feline kidney has only one lobe, but a canine kidney contains a number of fused lobes.[12] Canine kidneys are brownish red to brownish blue, depending on the degree of oxygenation of the blood they contain. Feline kidneys are red to yellowish red because of a large amount of intracellular fat stored in the proximal convoluted tubules.[16] Lipid content is greatest in mature cats, castrated males, and pregnant females. Feline kidneys are comparatively large, representing 0.6 to 1.0 per cent of body weight, compared with 0.6 per cent of body weight for dogs.[29] Many investigators have measured the size of normal kidneys of dogs and cats from raidographs.[11, 22, 34] The most recent study[22] recorded measurements from lateral radiographs of 167 dogs and 33 cats. Length varied between 2.5 and 3.2 lumbar vertebrae in dogs and 2.5 to 3.0 in cats. Width ranged from 1.4 to 1.8 for dogs and 1.6 to 1.9 for cats. That is, feline kidneys are shorter and broader than canine kidneys. This study

TABLE 100–1. CHARACTERISTIC FEATURES OF THE KIDNEYS

Feature	Dog	Cat
Type	Unipyramidal (fused pyramids)	Unipyramidal (single pyramid)
Weight per kidney (g)	50 to 60	7.5 to 15
Color	Brownish red to reddish blue	Red to yellowish red
Kidney mass as a percentage of body weight	0.6	0.6 to 1.0
Total nephrons per kidney	415,000	190,000
Kidney length in proportion to length of lumbar vertebra (L2)	2.9	2.7
Kidney width in proportion to length of L2	1.6	1.7
Ventral displacement in proportion to length of L2	L 0.7 R 0.3	0.7 0.7

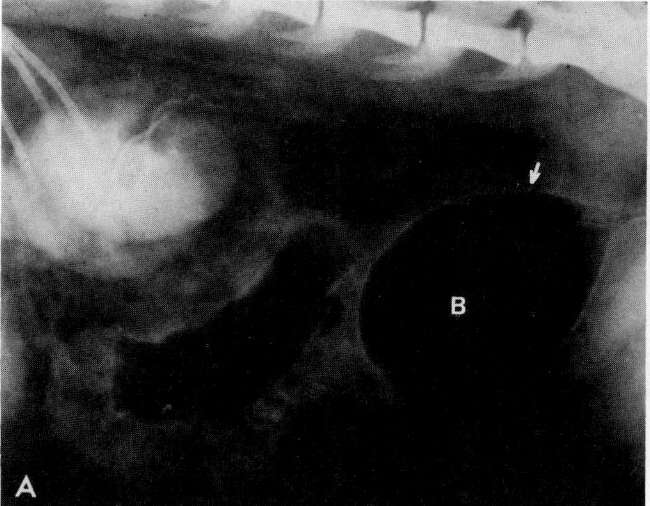

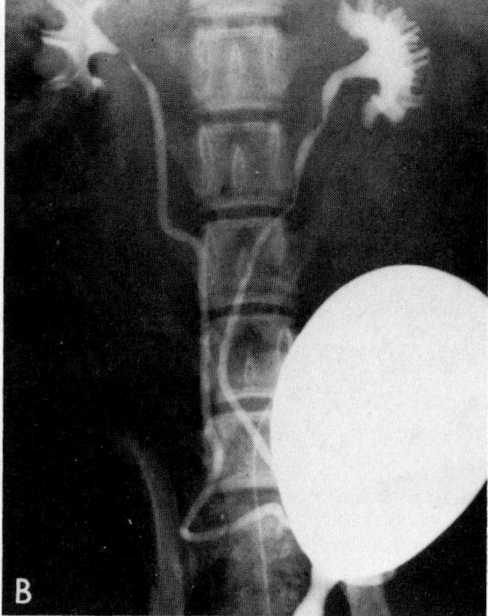

FIGURE 100–8. *A*, Intravenous urogram in a cat to show the point of entry of the ureters (*arrow*) into the bladder (B). *B*, Cystogram and retrograde pyelogram outlining the urinary apparatus in a young male dog.

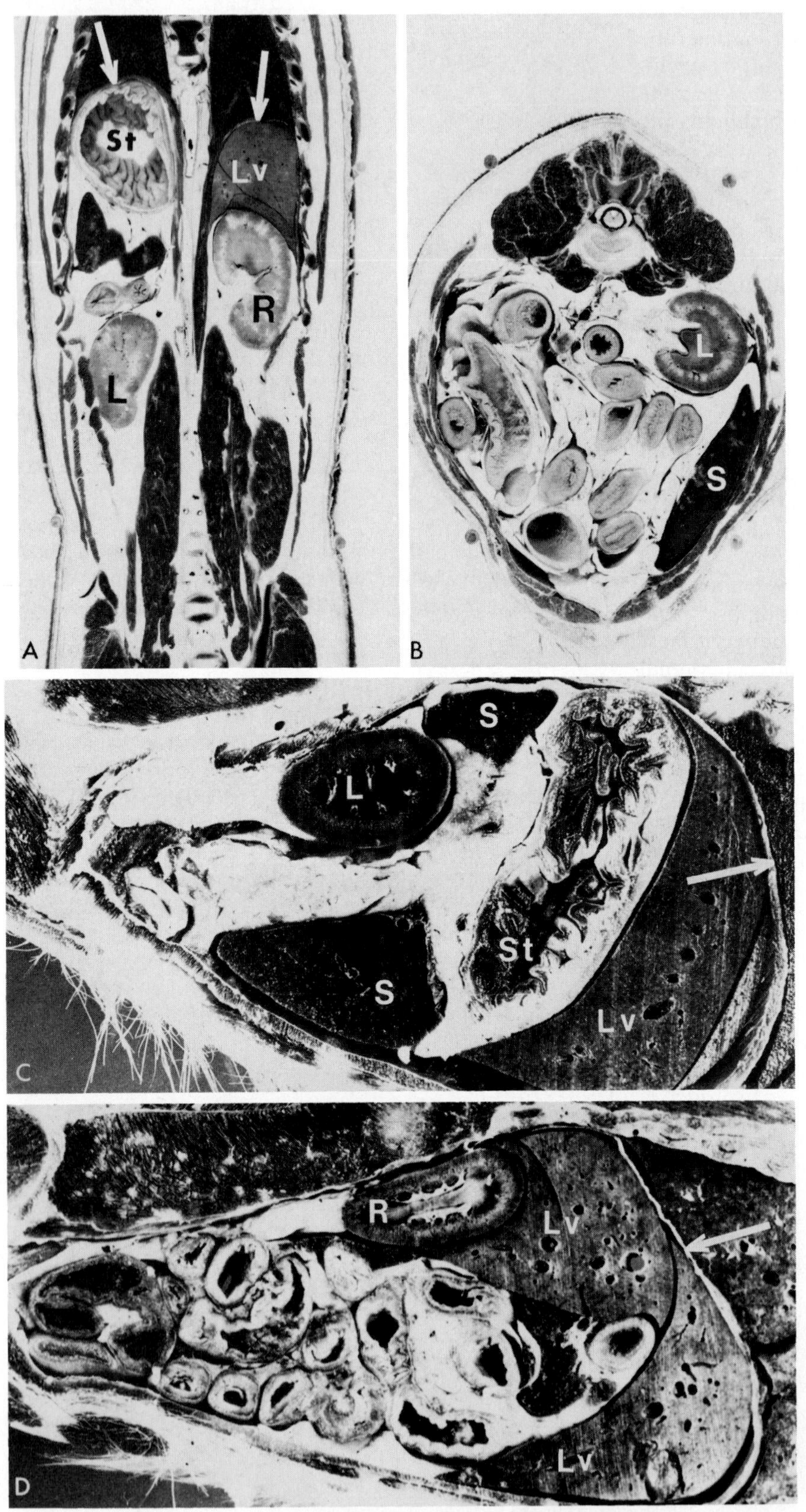

FIGURE 100–9. Frozen whole-body sections of dogs to show the topography of the kidneys. *A*, Horizontal section. *B*, Transverse section. *C*, Left longitudinal section. *D*, Right longitudinal section. (St, stomach; S, spleen; L, left kidney; R, right kidney; Lv, liver; *arrows*, line of the diaphragm.)

also showed that kidneys from male dogs were proportionally larger than those from female dogs and that the kidneys from immature dogs were proportionally larger than those from mature dogs.

The measured ventral displacement of the kidney from the line of the lumbar vertebrae indicates that the right kidney of a dog is less likely to be displaced than the left, whereas both kidneys of a cat are equally mobile.

Structure

The adipose capsule that envelops the kidney (see Fig. 100–9) varies in thickness with the nutritional state of the animal. The surface of a canine kidney is smooth, but that of a cat is grooved owing to the presence of large subcapsular veins that join the renal vein at the hilus (Fig. 100–10*A* and *B*).

Longitudinal midsagittal sections of canine and feline kidneys demonstrate their gross internal structure (Fig. 100–10*C*). The outer region, the cortex, is granular owing to the presence of glomeruli. The cortex also contains many radially directed striations of medullary substance called *medullary rays*. The inner region, the medulla, is paler than the cortex and divides into outer and inner zones at the point where the ascending thin loop of Henle gives way to the thick loop of Henle. The inner zone, the papilla in a cat or renal crest in a dog, projects into the renal pelvis. This region contains only thin loops of Henle, collecting ducts, and blood vessels. The renal crest is wedge shaped with a long craniocaudal axis. Clay models of the renal crest of a dog show transversely oriented finger-like ridges that project from each side of the renal crest into the pelvic cavity.[5]

Kidney sections dorsal or ventral to the longitudinal axis of the crest (Fig. 100–10*D*) cut the transverse ridges and expose the recesses (diverticulae) of the renal pelvis, simulating a multipyramidal kidney with calyces. A feline kidney also has recesses in its medullary pyramid. These recesses are related more to the presence of "interlobar" blood vessels than to well-developed medullary transverse ridges. The renal pelvis is shaped like an everted umbrella and is adapted to the configuration of the ridged renal crest. The perimeter of attachment of the pelvis to the medulla courses over each ridge, thus creating a scalloped configuration and simulating a calyceal pattern on pyelography (see Fig. 100–8).

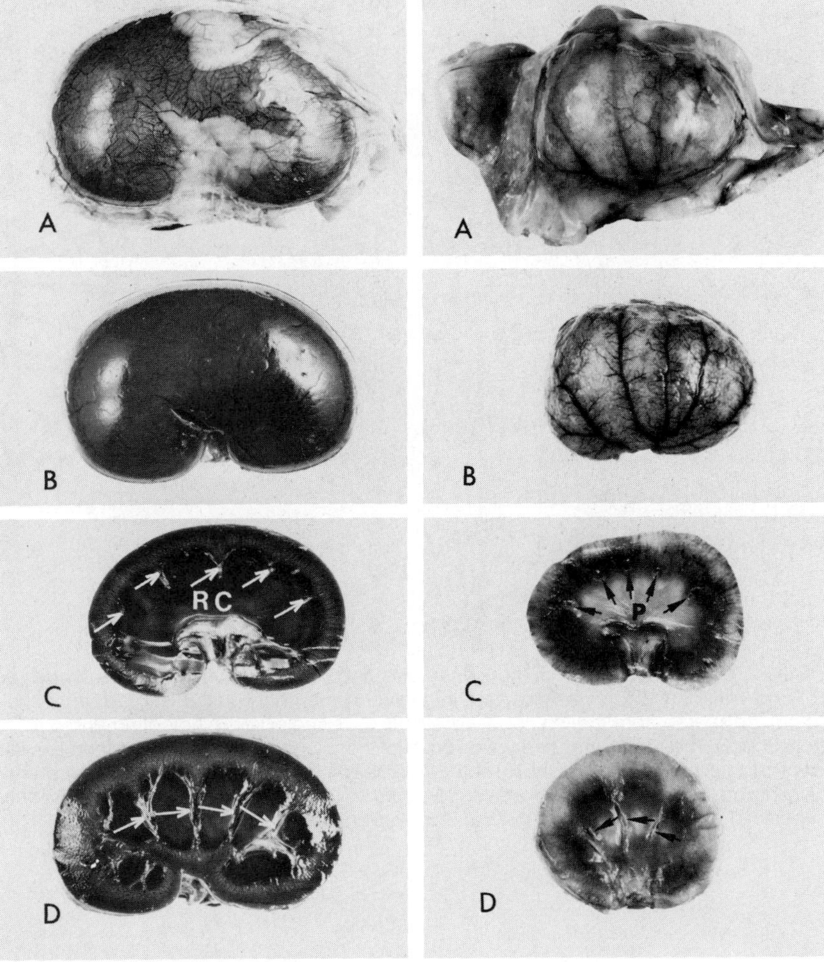

FIGURE 100–10. Dog and cat kidneys. *A*, With capsule in place. Capsular vessels and capsular fat are prominent features. *B*, With capsule removed, the surface of a dog's kidney is smooth, whereas a cat's shows prominent subcapsular veins. *C*, Midsagittal sections illustrate the renal crest (RC) in a dog and papilla (P) in a cat. The arrows point to the arcuate vessels. *D*, Sagittal sections to one side of the midline cut through the transverse ridges on the renal crest of a dog, simulating a multipyramidal kidney. The arrows point to the interlobar arteries, which in a cat also groove the medulla and simulate a multipyramidal kidney.

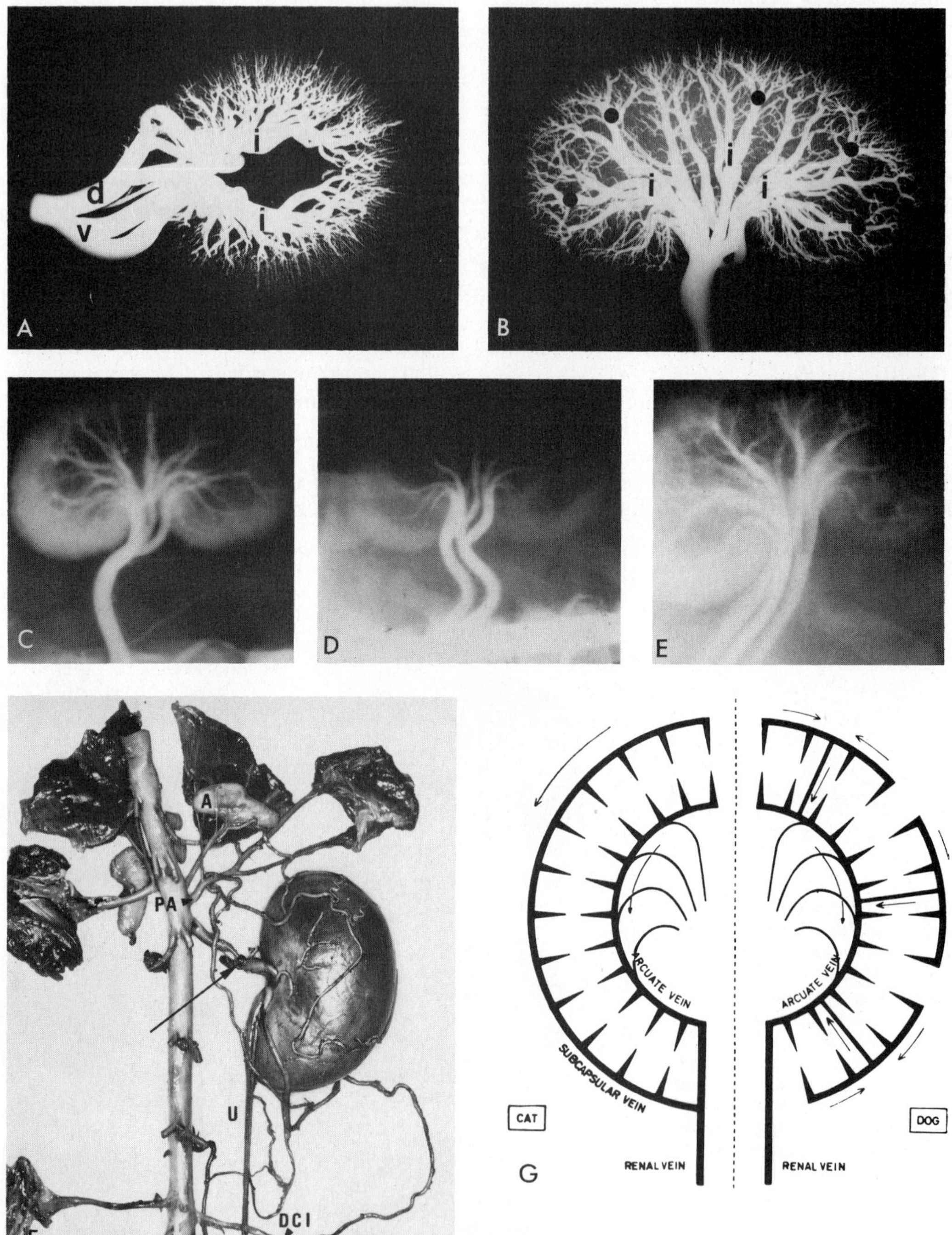

FIGURE 100–11. Vasculature of the kidney of a dog. *A*, Angiogram in the transverse plane showing the renal artery branching into dorsal (d) and ventral (v) branches and then into interlobar branches (i). *B*, Angiogram in the lateral plane indicating where the arcuate vessels (*black dots*) arise from the interlobar vessels (i). *C–E*, Angiograms indicating single *(C)*, double *(D)*, and triple *(E)* renal arteries. *F*, Specimen from a dog. The right renal artery was gradually occluded, and the left kidney excised. (A, Adrenal gland; PA, phrenicoabdominal trunk; *arrow*, ligated right renal artery; U, ureter; DCI, deep circumflex iliac artery.) Note prominent collateral vessels on the surface of the kidney. *G*, Diagram showing the different vein systems of dog and cat kidneys. (*G* reproduced with permission from Nissen OI: The function of superficial and deep areas of the cat kidney. *Danish Med Bull 16*:Suppl III, 1969.)

Vasculature

Arterial Circulation. After the renal artery leaves the aorta, it bifurcates into dorsal and ventral branches (Fig. 100–11*A* and *B*). Each branch gives rise to five to seven interlobar arteries. These travel between the medullary ridges outside the pelvic diverticulae and branch into arcuate arteries at the corticomedullary junction. The arcuate arteries radiate toward the periphery of the cortex, giving rise to radially directed interlobular arteries, the smallest arteries that can be readily identified by renal angiography. These arteries supply the afferent arterioles of the glomerulus.

Multiple renal arteries (Fig. 100–11*D*) have been observed in the left kidney in 13 per cent of dogs[29, 32] but are uncommon in cats. Most dogs have a single renal artery to the right kidney.

Although the renal arteries are usually described as "end arteries," a significant number of interlobar and arcuate arteries in dogs perforate the renal substance and make vascular connections with the adrenal gland, phrenicoabdominal trunk, deep circumflex iliac artery, caudal mesenteric artery, spermatic artery, and ureteral artery.[9] These vessels form an arterial circle around the kidney. They can hypertrophy (Fig. 100–11*F*) and provide an alternative blood supply if renal artery flow is gradually obstructed.

Venous Drainage. Venous drainage of the kidneys has deep and superficial components.[26] Capillary beds in the outer cortex drain toward the surface by superficial cortical veins, which join stellate veins beneath and within the capsule in dogs and cats. Interlobular veins drain the stellate veins into the arcuate and major renal veins in dogs, but in cats they converge and drain via a second route into the renal vein at the hilus (Fig. 100–11*G*). The deeper cortical capillaries drain into deep cortical veins and from there to the renal vein. In dogs, the left renal vein also receives the left ovarian vein.[15]

Lymphatics. Renal capsular and parenchymal lymphatics are connected to interlobular plexes, which converge and leave the kidney at the hilus to terminate in the lumbar lymph nodes.[15, 35]

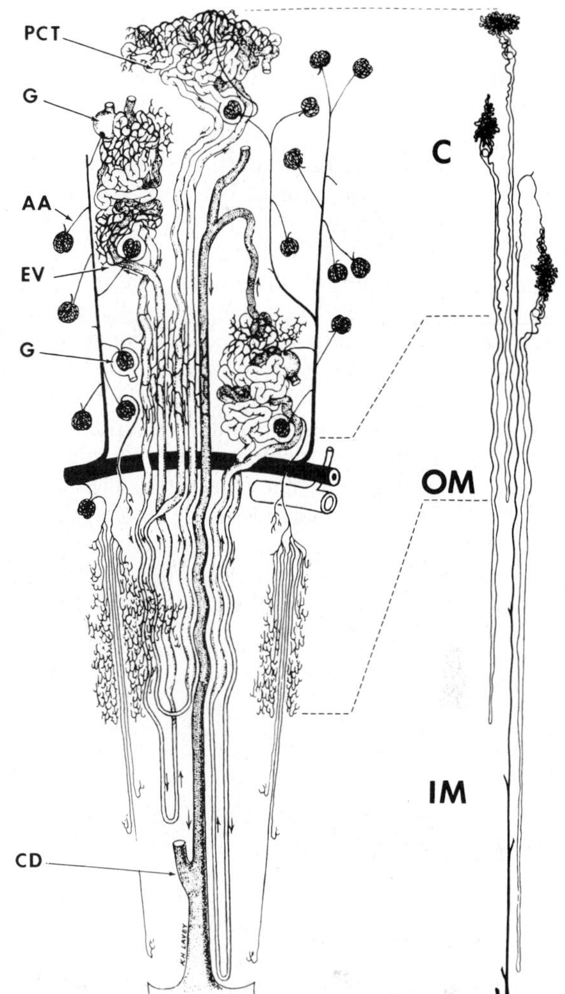

FIGURE 100–12. Arrangement of nephrons and collecting ducts in the kidney. (C, cortex; OM, outer medulla; IM, inner medulla; PCT, proximal convoluted tubules; G, glomeruli; AA, afferent arteriole; EV, efferent vessel; CD, collecting duct.) (Reproduction with permission from Beeuwkes R III: The vascular organization of the kidney. *Ann Rev Physiol 42*:531, 1980.)

Innervation

Autonomic sympathetic innervation to the kidneys comes from ganglia in the region of the celiac and phrenicoabdominal arteries and lumbar splanchnic nerves to form a plexus around the renal arteries. Branches of the dorsal vagal trunk (parasympathetic) also join the renal plexus.[15]

Microstructure

Medullary rays (see Fig. 100–3) form the core of the kidney lobule.[17] The core of the medullary ray is the branched collecting tubule, which receives filtrate from the many nephrons that surround it (Fig. 100–12). The medullary ray also contains descending and ascending limbs of the *loops of Henle*. Mammals have long and short loops of Henle named according to whether the U-bend occurs in the outer or inner medulla, respectively. The relative proportion of each loop depends on the species (see Chapter 101). The loops of Henle in dogs and cats all are long loops.[26] After the *efferent arteriole* leaves the vascular pole of the Bowman capsule, it forms a peritubular plexus around the uriniferous tubules of the cortex. The efferent network has many anastomotic links. Single nephron perfusion depends on the efferents of many glomeruli. The efferent arterioles of the juxtamedullary glomeruli descend into the medulla along straight paths to form a network around the medullary uriniferous tubules. Venules from this capillary network return blood to the interlobular veins and arcuate veins and from there to the renal vein.[3] When a glomerular tuft invaginates into the expanded proximal end of the nephron, a *renal corpuscle* is formed. A renal corpuscle consists of the glomerular capillaries plus the parietal and visceral layers of the Bowman capsule.

The glomerular capillary is lined by fenestrated endothelial cells that lie on a basement membrane. The visceral layer of the Bowman capsule consists of highly specialized epithelial cells called *podocytes*. Foot processes on the podocytes interdigitate with each other and are separated by filtration slits, or pores. The site where the afferent and efferent arterioles enter and leave glomeruli is the vascular pole. At this site, the ascending limb of the loop of Henle of each nephron returns to the glomerulus of that nephron before it continues on as the distal convoluted tubule. There is a concentration of nuclei where the tubule touches the root of the glomerulus and the afferent arteriole. This group of cells is the macula densa. Between it and the glomerulus is an aggregation of smaller cells termed the *polar cushion*, or laser cells. In some parts of the glomerulus, the basement membrane derived from epithelial cells does not completely surround each capillary. Support is provided by mesangial cells, which also have phagocytic and contractile properties. The cells of the media of the afferent arteriole in the region of the glomerular root have rounded nuclei and contain granules. They are called juxtaglomerular cells and, together with the cells of the macula densa, form the juxtaglomerular complex.

Ureters

The ureters are retroperitoneal urine conduits that pursue a relatively tortuous route to the bladder (see Fig. 100–8).

The Ureteropelvic Junction

The ureter expands within the renal sinus in dogs and cats to form the renal pelvis. The periphery of the renal pelvis is adapted to the configuration of the ridged renal crest, giving it a scalloped appearance on pyelography (see Fig. 100–8). The pelvic diverticula simulates calyces radiographically, but because the kidneys of dogs and cats are unipyramidal, calyces are not found.

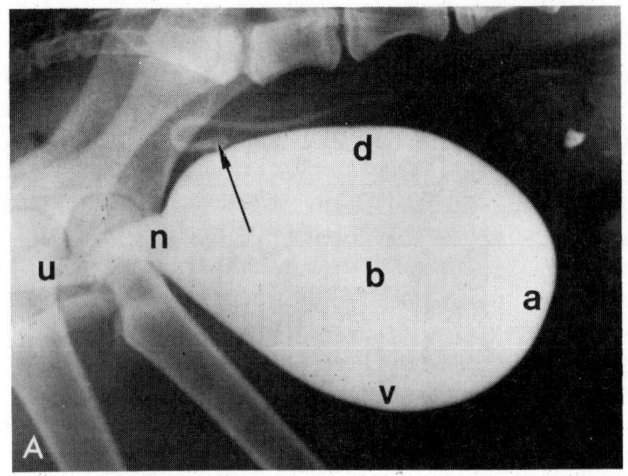

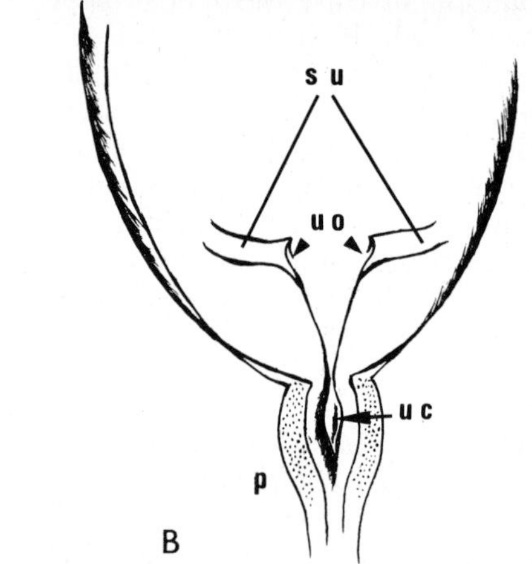

FIGURE 100–13. Ureterovesicular junction. *A*, Cystogram and ureterogram showing the ureter entering the bladder on its dorsal surface (d), near the bladder neck (n). Other regions of the bladder are identified as body (b), apex (a), ventral surface (v), and proximal urethra (u). *B*, Mucosal view of the dorsal half of the bladder of a young male dog, showing submucosal ureters (su), ureteral orifices (uo), urethral colliculus (uc), and prostate gland (p).

Ureterovesical Junction

Ureters must be long enough to reach their point of attachment to an empty bladder retracted within the bony pelvis. As the bladder fills with urine, it becomes an intra-abdominal organ. The angle of approach of the ureter to the bladder must pass beyond 90° and may even strongly recurve (Fig. 100–13). When the ureter pierces the bladder wall, it loses its outer layer of circular muscle and is surrounded by a connective tissue sheath into which detrusor muscle fasicles insert. This is the principal means by which the ureter is connected to the bladder.[8] The ureter reaches a submucosal position and extends obliquely toward the bladder neck.

The ureteral orifices are characteristically horseshoe shaped and form the base limits of the bladder trigone. The long, narrow submucosal ureter acts as a flap valve to prevent vesicoureteral reflux as bladder hydrostatic pressure is raised above ureteral peristaltic pressure.

Vessels and Nerves

The ureter has a cranial blood supply from the renal artery and a caudal blood supply from the prostatic or vaginal arteries. Cranial and caudal ureteral arteries anastomose on the ureter in the outer layers of adventitia.[25] Additional supply from surrounding vessels frequently joins the ureteral artery.[9]

Autonomic nerves supply the ureter, but their function is not clear, because ureteral peristalsis is not propagated by nervous impulses as it is in the gut but is myogenic in origin.[20]

Bladder

The bladder is a urine reservoir that varies in form, size, and position, depending on the volume of urine it contains. The bladder (Fig. 100–13*A*) has a neck (vesicourethral junction), a body, and a vertex (apex). The body has dorsal (roof) and ventral (floor) surfaces. The *fundus* (base), used as a descriptive term in human anatomy, is equivalent to the dorso-caudal region of the body of the bladder of a dog. This term is appropriate for humans because it relates to an erect posture, but it is an inappropriate term for quadrupeds. The distended bladder lies on the floor of the abdomen and occupies a considerable volume of the abdominal cavity (Fig. 100–14*A*). The bladder of dogs and cats has a peritoneal covering over the entire bladder and bladder neck (Fig. 100–14*B* and *C*). Peritoneal reflections (lateral ligaments) attach the bladder to the lateral abdominal wall and ventral abdominal wall (median ligament). Obliquely oriented detrusor muscle fascicles are continuous with urethral smooth muscle at the bladder neck.[21, 38] When the detrusor muscle is relaxed, deployment of fibers at the vesicourethral junction constricts the bladder neck. This action is assisted by a concentration of submucosal elastic tissue in the region. Thus, the internal urinary sphincter is formed. It should be noted, however, that although a constriction is present at the bladder neck, the region is not an anatomical sphincter. Alpha-adrenergic receptors are found in the bladder neck and proximal urethra. These receptors are active during the late phase of bladder filling, indicating that sympathetic stimulation of the smooth muscle of this region contributes to urine continence. (Refer to Chapters 101 and 102 for physiology and pathophysiology of bladder function.)

Electrical conduction within the bladder is along each smooth-muscle fiber.[4] There are few neuromuscular

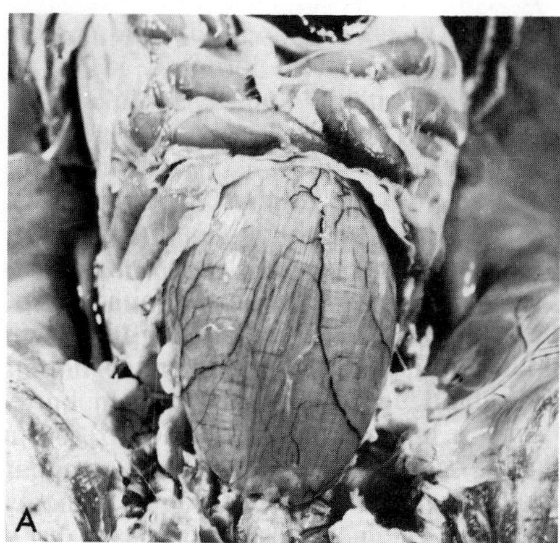

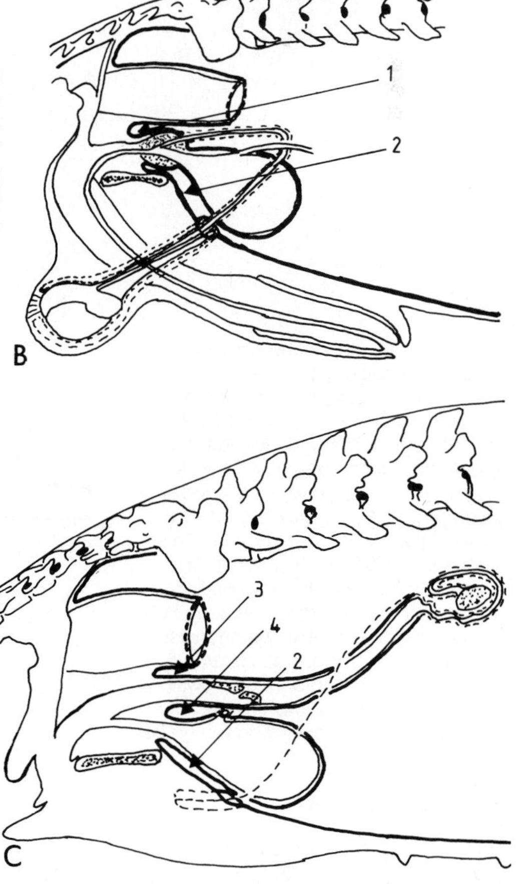

FIGURE 100–14. Location of the bladder in a dog. *A*, The ventral body wall has been removed to show the position of a full bladder. *B* and *C*, Longitudinal sections of male *(B)* and female *(C)* dogs showing the peritoneal covering of the bladder. Peritoneal reflections form the rectovesicular pouch (1) and the pubovesicular pouch (2). In a female, the presence of the uterus divides the rectovesicular pouch into the rectogenital pouch (3) and vesicogenital pouch (4). (*B* and *C* modified from Evans HE (ed): *Miller's Anatomy of the Dog.* 3rd ed. W. B. Saunders, Philadelphia, 1993.)

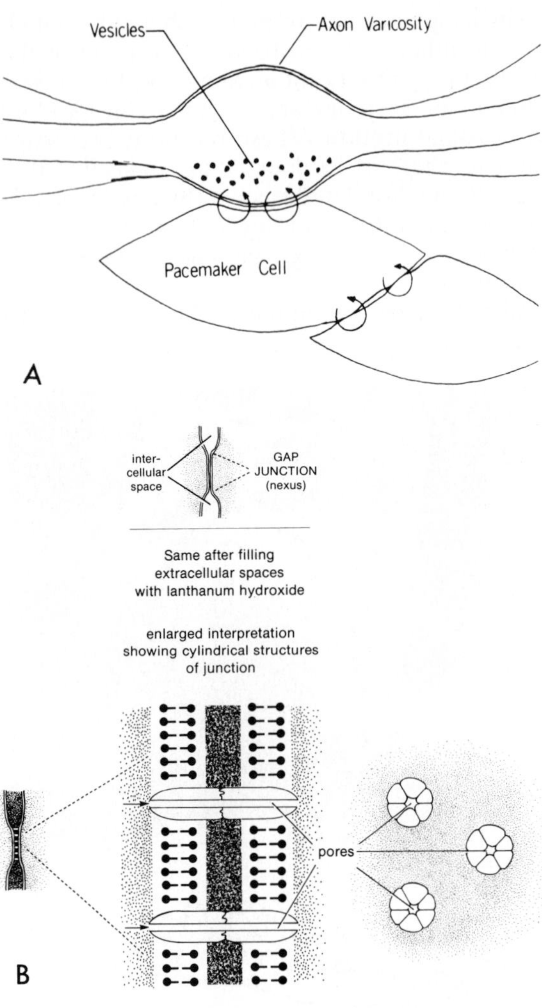

FIGURE 100–15. Electrical conduction in the bladder. *A,* Electrical impulses are generated at axon varicosities. *B,* The pacemaker cell depolarizes, and impulses pass to adjacent smooth-muscle cells through areas of close contact called *gap junctions.* (*A* reproduced with permission from Bradley WE, et al: Innervation of the detrusor muscle and urethra. *Urol Clin North Am* *1*:3, 1974. *B* reproduced with permission from Ham AW, Cormack DH: *Histology.* 8th ed. J. B. Lippincott, Philadelphia, 1979.)

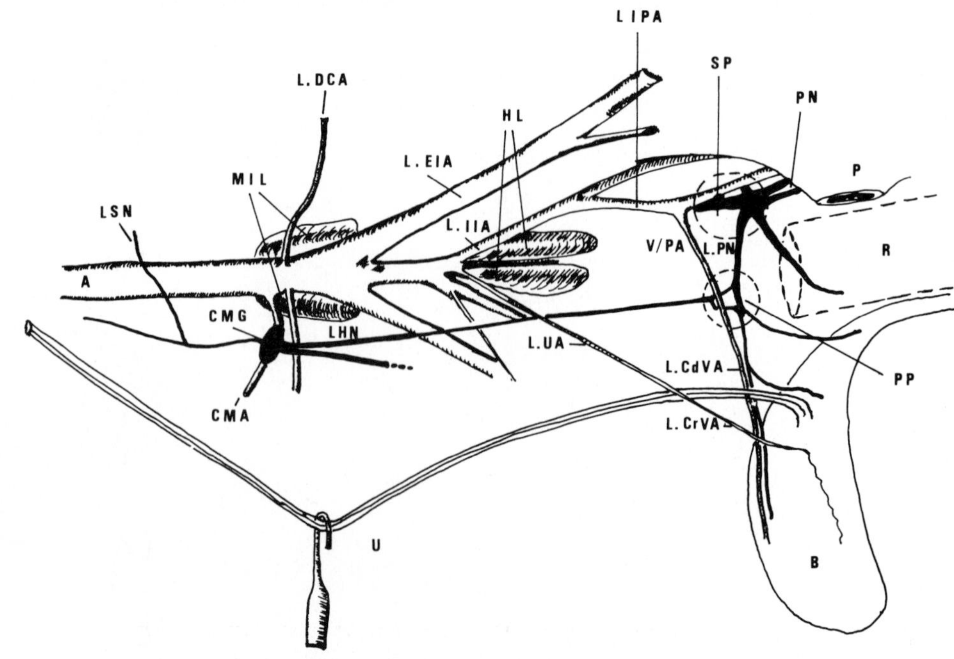

FIGURE 100–16. Blood and nerve supply to the bladder of a dog, viewed from the ventral surface with the bladder and left ureter displaced to the right. The prefix L stands for left, the suffix A stands for artery, and N for nerve. (*Arteries:* A, aorta; CM, caudal mesenteric; CdV, caudal vesical; CrV, cranial vesical; DC, deep circumflex iliac; EI, external iliac; II, internal iliac; IP, internal pudendal; UA, umbilical; V/P, vaginal or prostatic. *Nerves:* H, hypogastric; SN, lumbar splanchnic; LPN, pelvic; PN, pudendal. *Plexus:* PP, pelvic; SP, sacral. *Ganglion:* CMG, caudal mesenteric. *Lymph nodes:* HL, hypogastric; MIL, middle iliac.)

junctions in visceral smooth muscle. Those that are present are of the axon varicosity type rather than the motor end-plate of skeletal muscle. When depolarization occurs in a "pacemaker" cell, impulses cross from one fiber to the next at areas of close apposition of their cell membranes (Fig. 100–15). These junctions (nexuses) are areas of low electrical resistance and are probably of the "gap junction type"[17] rather than the "tight junction type," as stated by others.[4]

Vessels and Nerves

The blood supply and innervation to the bladder of a female dog are shown in Figure 100–16. Close to its origin, the internal iliac artery gives rise to the umbilical artery. The lumen of this artery is obliterated in 50 per cent of adult dogs, forming the lateral umbilical ligament. In the remaining 50 per cent of adult dogs, the artery continues patent and supplies the cranial end of

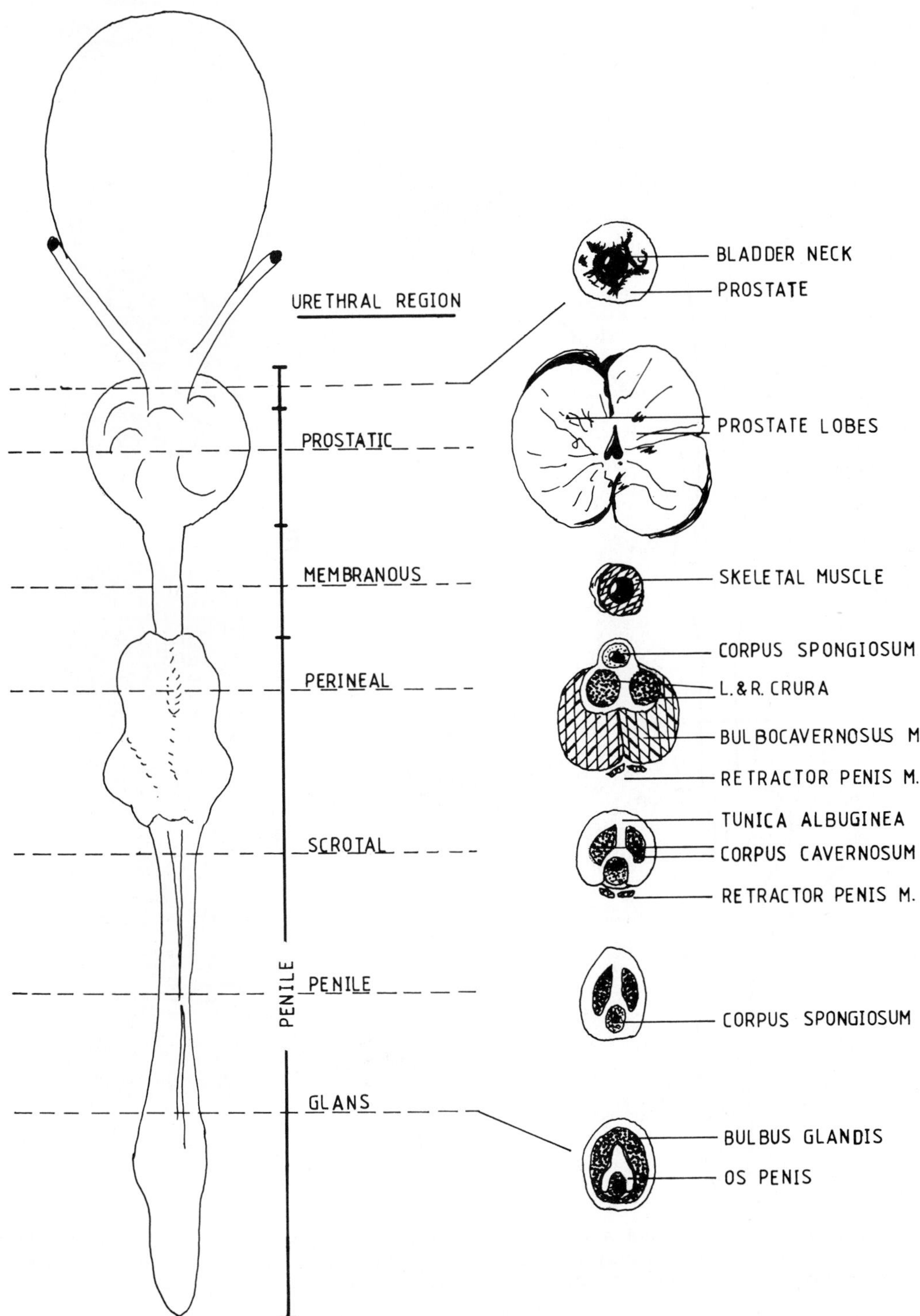

FIGURE 100–17. Structure of the urethra in a male dog. Transverse sections are drawn from the levels indicated in the diagram. Note that the membranous urethra has a large, transversely oriented skeletal muscle component.

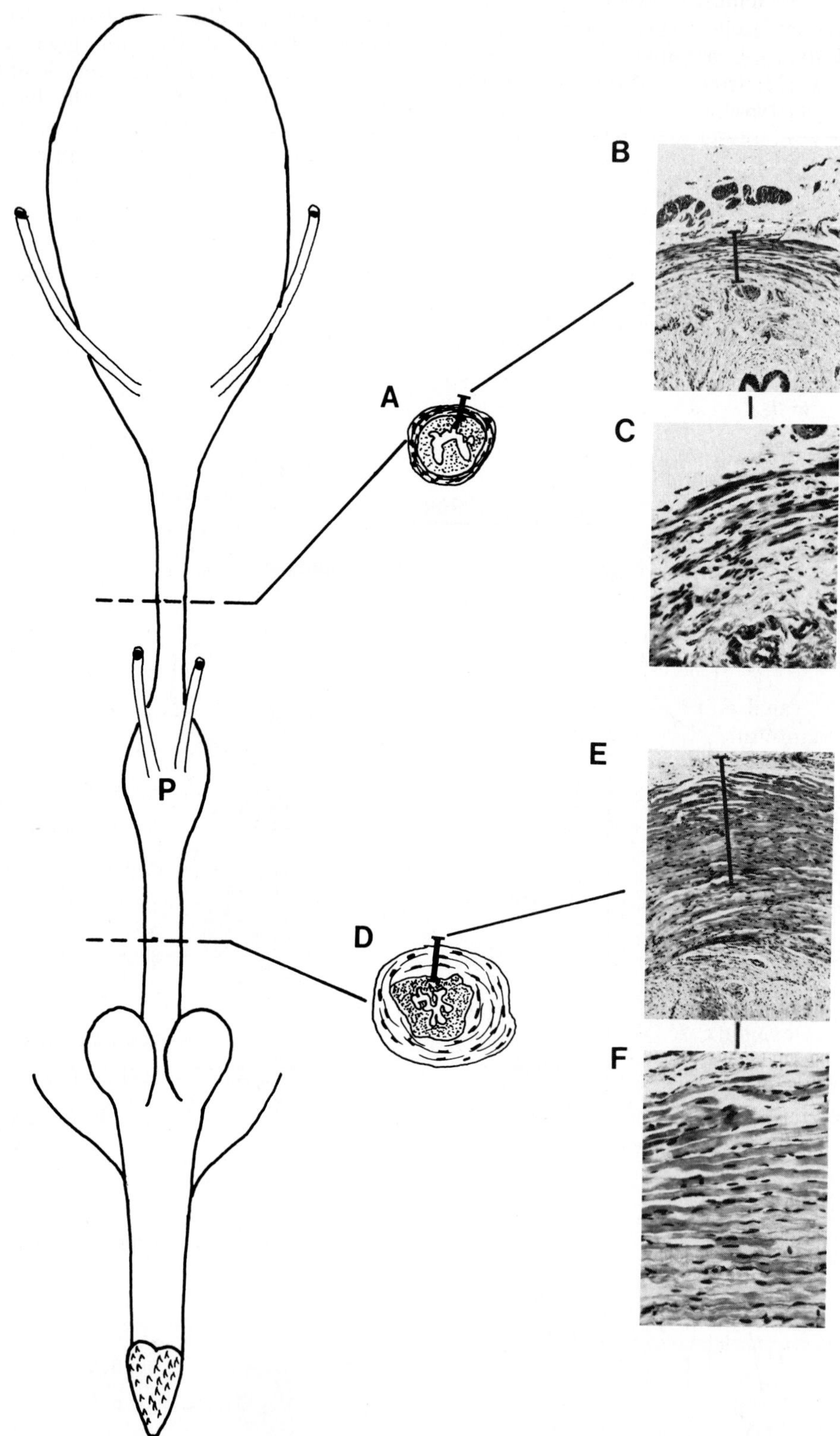

FIGURE 100–18. Urinary apparatus of a male cat. *A*, Transverse section of the elongated bladder neck. *B* and *C*, Photomicrographs indicate that the major component of the wall is smooth muscle. (*B*, H and E × 40; *C*, H and E × 100.) *D*, Transverse section of the membranous urethra shows a dense outer skeletal muscle layer. *E* and *F*, Photomicrographs. (*E*, H and E × 40; *F*, H and E × 100.)

the bladder as the cranial vesical artery. The internal iliac artery branches into caudal gluteal and internal pudendal arteries. The vaginal (or prostatic) branch of the internal pudendal artery lies in the pelvic fascia with the pelvic plexus of nerves approximately level with the brim of the pelvis. Arising from this vessel is the major supply to the bladder, the caudal vesical artery, which also gives rise to the caudal ureteral artery.

The plexus of veins drain into the vaginal (or prostatic) vein, a satellite of the artery, and then into the internal iliac vein.

The bladder lymphatics drain into the hypogastric nodes, which lie in the angle between the internal iliac and median sacral arteries, and the lumbar lymph nodes, which are variably located along the aorta and caudal vena cava.[15]

The nerve supply of the urinary bladder[4] is via the pelvic parasympathetic nerves, which stimulate contraction of the detrusor muscle, and the hypogastric sympathetic nerves, which help maintain bladder neck tone. Nerve trunks from the pelvic plexus pass into the bladder adventitia near the ureters. They follow a tortuous course, pass into smooth muscle fascicles, and terminate as free nerve endings. Pudendal somatic innervation is to the striated muscle of the external urethral sphincter.

Urethra

The urethra is the canal that extends from the neck of the bladder to the urethral meatus. It conveys urine from the bladder to the external environment. In males, the urethra also carries seminal secretions.

The male urethra is shown for a dog (Fig. 100–17) and cat (Fig. 100–18). The bladder neck is short in a dog, and the urethra is divisible into prostatic, membranous, and cavernous or penile segments. In a cat, however, the prostate gland is located 3 or 4 cm from what appears to be the bladder neck. This preprostatic region has been variably called an *elongated bladder neck*[13] or a *preprostatic portion of the membranous urethra*.[10] Histological examination of these two regions shows no striated muscle surrounding the preprostatic membranous urethra, but striated muscle is present around the true membranous urethra. Anatomically, therefore, the region is bladder neck, and the term *elongated bladder neck* is quite appropriate.

References

1. Arey LB: *Developmental Anatomy*. 7th ed. W. B. Saunders, Philadelphia, 1965, p 295.
2. Banks WJ: *Applied Veterinary Histology*. Williams & Wilkins, Baltimore, 1981, p 424.
3. Beeuwkes R III: The vascular organization of the kidney. *Ann Rev Physiol 42*:531, 1980.
4. Bradley WE, et al: Innervation of the detrusor muscle and urethra. *Urol Clin North Am 1*:3, 1974.
5. Brodsky SL, et al: Gross and radiological anatomy of the canine kidney. *Invest Urol 14*:356, 1977.
6. Bulmer D: The development of the human vagina. *J Anat 91*:490, 1957.
7. Campbell MF: Anomalies of the ureter. *In* Campbell MF, Harrison JH (eds): *Urology*. Vol 2, 3rd ed. W. B. Saunders, Philadelphia, 1970, p 1493.
8. Christie BA: The ureterovesical junction in dogs. *Invest Urol 9*:10, 1971.
9. Christie BA: Collateral arterial blood supply to the normal and ischemic canine kidney. *Am J Vet Res 41*:519, 1980.
10. Crouch JE: *Text-Atlas of Cat Anatomy*. Lea & Febiger, Philadelphia, 1969, p 167.
11. Douglas SW, Williamson HD: *Principles of Veterinary Radiography*. 2nd ed. Williams & Wilkins, Baltimore, 1972.
12. Ellenport CR: Carnivore urogenital apparatus. *In* Getty R (ed): *Sisson and Grossman's The Anatomy of the Domestic Animals*. Vol. 2. W. B. Saunders, Philadelphia, 1975, p 1576.
13. Elliot R: *Reighard and Jennings Anatomy of the Cat*. 3rd ed. Holt, Rinehart & Winston, New York, 1935.
14. Emmett JL: *Clinical Urography*. 2nd ed. W. B. Saunders, Philadelphia, 1964.
15. Evans HE, Christensen GC: *Miller's Anatomy of the Dog*. 2nd ed. W. B. Saunders, Philadelphia, 1979, pp 544, 551, 554.
16. Finco DR, et al: Diseases of the urinary system. *In* Catcott EJ (ed): *Feline Medicine and Surgery*. 2nd ed. American Veterinary Publications, Santa Barbara, 1975, p 251.
17. Ham AW, Cormack DH: *Histology*. 8th ed. J. B. Lippincott, Philadelphia, 1979, pp 200, 757.
18. Hildebrant A: Weiterer Beitrag zur pathologischen Anatomie der Nierengeschwülste. *Arch Klin Chir 48*:343, 1894.
19. Hilderbrand M: Analysis of vertebrate structure. John Wiley & Sons, New York, 1974, p 303.
20. Kiil F: Physiology of the renal pelvis and ureter. *In* Campbell MF, Harrison JH (eds): *Urology*. Vol 1. 3rd ed. W. B. Saunders, Philadelphia, 1970, p 72.
21. Kirulata HG, et al: The continence mechanisms. The effect of bladder filling on the urethra. *Invest Urol 18*:460, 1981.
22. Lee R, Leowijuk C: Normal parameters in abdominal radiology of the dog and cat. *J Small Anim Pract 23*:251, 1982.
23. Lepoutre MC: Sur un cas d'absence congenitale de la vessie. *J Urol Med Chir 48*:334, 1939.
24. Malter IJ, Stanley RJ: The intrathoracic kidney. *J Urol 107*:538, 1972.
25. Mingledorff WE, et al: Experimental study of the blood supply of the distal ureter with reference to cutaneous ureterostomy. *J Urol 92*:424, 1964.
26. Nissen OI: The function of superficial and deep areas of the cat kidney. *Danish Med Bull 16*:Suppl III, 1969.
27. Osathanondh V, Potter EL: Development of human kidney as shown by microdissection. *Arch Pathol 76*: 271, 1963.
28. Osathanondh V, Potter EL: Pathogenesis of polycystic kidneys. *Arch Pathol 77*:459, 1964.
29. Osborne CA, et al: *Canine and Feline Urology*. W. B. Saunders, Philadelphia, 1972, p 3.
30. Owen RR: Canine ureteral ectopia—a review. 1. Embryology and aetiology. *J Small Anim Pract 14*:407, 1973.
31. Schwartz RD, et al: The pathogenesis of renal dysplasia, II and III. Invest. *Urology 19*:97, 1981.
32. Shively MJ: Origin and branching of renal arteries in the dog. *J Am Vet Med Assoc 173*:986, 1978.
33. Stephens FD: Caecoureterocele and concepts on the embryology and aetiology of ureteroceles. *Aust NZ J Surg 40*:239, 1971.
34. Suter PF: Portal vein anomalies in the dog. Their angiographic diagnosis. *J Am Vet Radio Soc 16*:84, 1975.
35. Trautmann A, Fiebiger J: *Fundamentals of the Histology of Domestic Animals* (translated and revised from the 8th and 9th German editions, 1949, by Habel RE, Biberstein EL). Comstock, Ithaca, 1952.
36. Warwick R, Williams PL: *Gray's Anatomy*. 35th ed. Longman Group, Edinburgh, 1973.
37. Webster D, Webster M: *Comparative Vertebrate Morphology*. Academic Press, New York, 1974, p 427.
38. Woodburne RT: Anatomy of the bladder and bladder outlet. *J Urol 100*:474, 1968.

CHAPTER

101

Physiology of the Urinary Tract

Scott A. Brown*

OVERVIEW OF RENAL FUNCTION

The primary function of the kidneys is regulation of the composition of extracellular fluid. Thus the kidneys indirectly control the composition of intracellular fluid as well. These functions are accomplished through filtration, reabsorption, secretion, and hormone production. A partial list of systemic parameters wholly or partially regulated by the kidneys includes

1. Blood volume, extracellular fluid volume, and systemic arterial pressure
2. Concentration of a wide variety of waste products in the blood (some known and others unknown)
3. Concentration of electrolytes (sodium, potassium, chloride, phosphate, magnesium, and calcium) in plasma
4. Plasma pH
5. Hematocrit

STRUCTURAL ORGANIZATION OF THE KIDNEYS

Renal function is the sum of the function of individual nephrons, approximately 190,000 per kidney in cats and 430,000 to 580,000 per kidney in dogs.[74, 87] A nephron consists of several anatomical divisions, each with characteristic functions. Ultrafiltrate forms across the glomerular filtration barrier, entering the urinary space within the Bowman capsule. The fluid then enters the proximal tubule, whose role is to reabsorb most of the glomerular ultrafiltrate without regard for body needs. At its termination, the proximal tubule descends and thins to form the beginning of the loop of Henle, responsible for the generation of medullary hypertonicity, a prerequisite for the formation of concentrated urine. The loop of Henle forms a hairpin turn in the medulla and ascends into the cortex to reach the glomerulus from which the tubule originated. Here the tubule lies between the afferent and efferent arterioles (vascular pole of the glomerulus), with this portion of the tubule being referred to as the *macula densa* segment. This area of the nephron—where the arterioles, macula densa, and glomerulus are immediately adjacent, referred to as the *juxtaglomerular apparatus*—is responsible for the release of renin and participates in the tubuloglomerular feedback mechanism (see the later section on mechanisms controlling renal blood flow and glomerular filtration). The portion of the tubule from the macula densa to the collecting ducts is the distal tubule. This portion of the tubule is responsible for reabsorption of filtered water and solutes in accordance with body needs.

RENAL CIRCULATION

The kidneys receive approximately 20 to 25 per cent of cardiac output, despite the fact that they account for less than 1 per cent of total body weight. Normal renal blood flow in dogs is approximately 4 ml/minute/g of kidney weight (Table 101–1).[16, 57, 58] This high flow rate exceeds that of the brain, liver, and heart. Although formation of urine represents a high metabolic energy requirement, the renal arteriovenous oxygen gradient is small, demonstrating that oxygen demand is not the determining factor for this high perfusion rate.

Blood flow is determined by perfusion pressure divided by renal vascular resistance. Renal perfusion pressure is equal to mean arterial pressure. Although the interlobular arteries (and perhaps larger arteries) contribute to renal vascular resistance, the combined resistance of these arteries is very small or negligible.[18] It is afferent and efferent arteriolar tone that provides the bulk of renal vascular resistance and hence exerts the predominant control over renal blood flow. When assessed by micropuncture techniques, pre- and postglomerular resistances are approximately equal in normal dogs.[16, 57, 58]

Cortical blood flow is considerably greater than medullary. Inert gas washout studies in anesthetized dogs demonstrated that blood flow in the cortex averaged 4.59 ml/minute/g of wet kidney tissue, 0.7 ml/minute/g in the outer medulla, and 0.1 ml/minute/g in the inner medulla.[7] Approximately 90 per cent of renal blood flow traverses the cortex, 10 per cent perfuses the outer medulla, and 1 to 2 per cent reaches the inner medulla and papilla.[61]

The microcirculation of the kidneys is composed of several separate units (glomerular, peritubular, and vasa recta), each with a distinct anatomy and function. The glomerular microcirculation consists of an afferent arteriole, immediately branching into numerous glomerular capillaries, which coalesce to form the efferent arteriole. Glomerular filtration, the process of formation of glomerular ultrafiltrate, occurs across these glomerular capillary walls.

Efferent arterioles of cortical nephrons give rise to peritubular capillaries, a dense network of vessels surrounding cortical convoluted tubules. These vessels facilitate the important function of solute and water reabsorption in proximal tubules.

Efferent arterioles of the juxtamedullary nephrons give rise to the vasa recta, long unbranched capillary loops that extend into the medulla. The slow blood flow within these loops has a critical role in the maintenance of medullary hypertonicity in the urine-concentrating mechanism.

*The author acknowledges the assistance of Dr. D. Finco in the preparation of this chapter.

TABLE 101–1. REPRESENTATIVE VALUES FOR PARAMETERS OF RENAL FUNCTION IN DOGS AND CATS

	Dog	Cat
Renal blood flow		
(ml/minute/g kidney)	4	2
(ml/minute/kg body weight)	20	15
(ml/minute/nephron)	400	200
Glomerular filtration rate		
(ml/minute/g kidney)	0.7	0.4
(ml/minute/kg body wt)	4.0	3.0
(ml/minute/nephron)	60	30
Hydrostatic pressures (mm Hg)		
Mean renal arterial	100	100
Glomerular capillary	55	59
Peritubular capillary	12	10
Proximal tubule	20	18

GLOMERULAR FILTRATION

Formation of glomerular filtrate, which is the central function of the kidneys, occurs as a result of Starling forces in the glomerular capillary bed. The filtrate formed is most accurately termed *glomerular ultrafiltrate*. The determinants of glomerular ultrafiltration have been evaluated in dogs (Fig. 101–1). The Starling forces under consideration are the colloid (protein) osmotic and hydrostatic pressure gradients. The glomerular filtration rate of individual single nephrons (SNGFR) can be expressed as follows (see Fig. 101–1):

$$SNGFR = Kf\,[(\pi GC - \pi T) - (PGC - PT)]$$

where πGC and πT are the colloid (protein) osmotic pressure within the glomerular capillary and proximal tubule, respectively, PGC and PT represent the hydrostatic pressure within the glomerular capillary and proximal tubule, and Kf is the glomerular ultrafiltration coefficient.

The force driving the filtration process, referred to as *net effective filtration pressure* (EFP), is defined as follows:

$$EFP = (\Delta P - \Delta\pi)$$

where $\Delta P = PGC - PT$ and $\Delta\pi = \pi GC - \pi T$. The magnitude of this force (approximately 10 to 15 mm Hg) has been well defined in dogs (see Fig. 101–1).

Although plasma protein concentration averages 6 to 8 g/100 ml, the protein content of filtrate rarely exceeds 10 mg/100 ml, and the colloid osmotic pressure within the early proximal tubule (πT) is so small that its contribution to the filtration process is negligible. Consequently, the process of glomerular filtration is driven only by glomerular capillary pressure and is opposed by plasma colloid osmotic pressure and proximal tubule hydrostatic pressure (see Fig. 101–1).

The magnitude of the pressure decrease along the vascular tree up to the afferent arteriole in a dog is comparatively small, and proximal afferent arteriolar hydrostatic pressure is only 10 to 15 mm Hg less than that of the systemic arteries.[58] Most (70 per cent) of the preglomerular reduction in hydrostatic pressure occurs along the length of the afferent arteriole. This decline is considerably less than in systemic arterioles, and the resultant hydrostatic pressure in glomerular capillaries is high (see Table 101–1). Micropuncture techniques in dogs have yielded values for glomerular capillary pressure of 53 to 63 mm Hg.[16, 57, 58] Because of the abundance of parallel glomerular capillaries and the relatively large cross-sectional area of the glomerular capillaries relative to the afferent and efferent arterioles, the overall pressure decrease along the glomerular capillary path is negligible.

The hydrostatic pressure opposing the formation of glomerular filtrate is that of the Bowman space. Because there are no flow restrictions at the urinary pole of the glomerulus, proximal tubule pressure is the same as in the capsule and can be directly measured by micropuncture techniques. Direct measurements of proximal tubule pressure demonstrate values of 18 to 22 mm Hg in dogs.[16, 57, 58]

Single-nephron glomerular filtration rate can be expressed as the product of effective filtration pressure and the ultrafiltration coefficient. The ultrafiltration coefficient can be further expressed as the product of

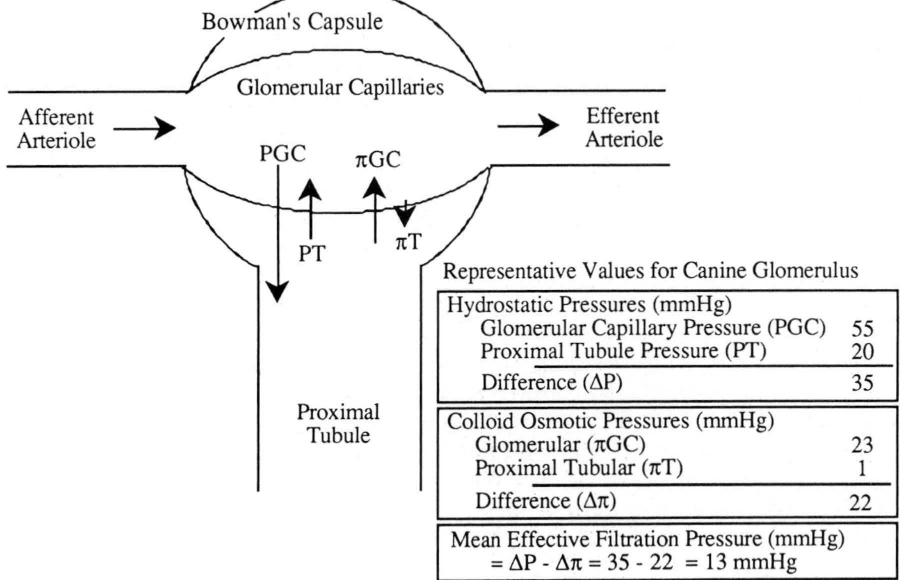

FIGURE 101–1. The primary driving force for formation of glomerular ultrafiltrate is glomerular capillary pressure (PGC), which is opposed by proximal tubule hydrostatic pressure (PT) and glomerular capillary colloid osmotic pressure (πGC).

glomerular capillary hydraulic conductivity and total glomerular surface area. Alterations of either of these factors greatly affect filtration. Conceptually, hydraulic conductivity can be considered as the permeability of the glomerular capillary wall to fluid (water). Although the glomerular capillary wall is poorly permeable to large protein molecules, such as albumin, its permeability to plasma fluid exceeds that of other capillaries.

The relative amount of plasma traversing the capillary wall is referred to as the *filtration fraction*. On a whole-organ basis, filtration fraction is equal to glomerular filtration rate divided by renal plasma flow. The relative tone of the afferent and efferent arterioles determines the filtration fraction. For example, an increase in efferent arteriolar resistance produces a proportionately greater decrease in renal plasma than glomerular filtration rate, with a resultant increase in filtration fraction. However, the relationship between arteriolar tone and filtration fraction is complex.[19]

As protein-free ultrafiltrate leaves glomerular capillary plasma and enters the urinary space, plasma colloid osmotic pressure rises, leading to a decline in net filtration pressure along the length of the glomerular capillaries. In certain strains of rats, the increment in colloid osmotic pressure along the glomerular capillary leads to an equality of $\Delta\pi$ and ΔP. Hence, effective filtration pressure reaches zero, and there is no further formation of filtrate along the rest of the length of the glomerular capillary. This phenomenon is referred to as *filtration pressure equilibrium*. In rats that reach filtration pressure equilibrium, an increase in glomerular plasma flow delays the onset of filtration pressure equilibrium and results in an increase in single-nephron glomerular filtration rate. This causes "plasma flow dependence" of the filtration process. In normal dogs, unless the arterial plasma oncotic pressure is greatly elevated, filtration pressure equilibrium does not occur.[58] Glomerular capillary pressure and the ultrafiltration quotient are important determinants of the filtration process in dogs.

MECHANISMS CONTROLLING RENAL BLOOD FLOW AND GLOMERULAR FILTRATION

The driving force for glomerular filtration rate, glomerular capillary hydrostatic pressure, is controlled through the relative resistance of the afferent and efferent arterioles. Most vasoactive compounds affecting renal blood flow and glomerular filtration rate act by altering the relative or absolute tone of these arterioles.

A central concept of renal hemodynamics is that renal blood flow and glomerular filtration rate tend to remain constant despite variations in systemic arterial pressure between 75 and 160 mm Hg. This capacity is referred to as *autoregulation*, and because it occurs in a denervated, isolated-perfused kidney, it is an intrinsic property of the kidney. In dogs, both cortical[16] and medullary[20, 55] blood flow are autoregulated. Whole-kidney and single-nephron glomerular filtration rate are also autoregulated. Because the tone of preglomerular vessels controls glomerular perfusion pressure, the vascular site responsible for autoregulatory adjustments of renal blood flow and glomerular filtration rate is the afferent arteriole.[76]

In some tissues, such as the brain, blood flow is autoregulated to allow perfusion to match metabolic demands. This is unlikely to be the case in the kidneys, where only 10 to 15 per cent of available oxygen is extracted. In addition, if renal blood flow (and consequently glomerular filtration rate) decreases, a parallel decrease occurs in sodium reabsorption in the proximal tubule. Because a decrease in sodium reabsorption results in a decrease in energy demand, energy needs of the kidneys are determined by renal blood flow, not vice versa as in most other tissues.

This autoregulatory property of the kidneys has generally been attributed to one of two basic mechanisms.[55] The *myogenic theory* argues that alterations in preglomerular vascular wall tension or diameter are opposed by active vasoconstriction so that increases in perfusion pressure are met with an increase in vascular resistance. The alternate hypothesis, referred to as the *tubuloglomerular feedback hypothesis*, argues that the macula densa region of the distal tubule controls afferent arteriolar resistance. Proponents of this hypothesis suggest that the macula densa cells sense some component of distal tubular fluid character and act to adjust afferent arteriolar tone in response to changes in the tubular fluid composition. Micropuncture experiments have clearly demonstrated that perfusion of the macula densa with fluids of various osmolality or chloride concentrations results in appropriate adjustments in vascular resistance.[58] Thus, an increase in renal perfusion pressure results in a transient (few seconds) increase in tubular fluid flow. The cells of the macula densa detect this change and produce afferent arteriolar vasoconstriction. Studies have supported a preglomerular effector site for the tubuloglomerular feedback mechanism.[55]

Atrial natriuretic factor, a peptide released from atrial myocytes in response to distension, causes an increase in renal blood flow, glomerular filtration rate, and urinary sodium excretion.[35, 66] The vasodilatory effects of atrial natriuretic factor apparently occur at the afferent arteriole.[82] Prostanoids (prostaglandins, thromboxanes, and leukotrienes) have dramatic effects on renal vasculature.[12] Vasodilatory prostanoids (prostaglandins E_2 and I_2) are opposed by the vasoconstrictive effects of thromboxane A_2 and several of the leukotrienes. Although apparently having insignificant effects on renal function in normal animals, vasodilatory prostanoids are particularly critical for the maintenance of renal blood flow and glomerular filtration rate when renal hemodynamics are compromised (e.g., dehydration, anesthesia, renal failure, urinary tract obstruction). Two compounds, endothelin and endothelium-derived relaxing factor, are released by vascular endothelial cells and produce either marked, prolonged contraction (endothelin) or relaxation (endothelium-derived relaxing factor) of vascular smooth muscle, with important effects on the renal arterioles.[10]

Renin is released from the granular cells of the juxtaglomerular apparatus in response to various stimuli, including a decline in systemic arterial pressure and direct sympathetic stimulation. Renin cleaves angiotensin I from a plasma protein of hepatic source (angiotensinogen or renin substrate). Converting enzyme, present in the vasculature of the lungs and elsewhere, cleaves a terminal 2 amino acid fragment from angiotensin I, converting it to angiotensin II. The latter two compounds (angiotensin I and II) have short half-lives, generally less than 1 minute.

$$\text{Angiotensinogen} \xrightarrow{\text{renin}} \text{angiotensin I} \xrightarrow{\text{converting enzyme}} \text{angiotensin II}$$

Angiotensin II is a potent systemic vasoconstrictor and increases renal vascular resistance in both afferent and efferent arterioles.[18] It may preferentially constrict the efferent arteriole.[39] Angiotensin II also stimulates proximal tubular reabsorption of sodium[59] and stimulates release of aldosterone from the adrenal cortex, which subsequently enhances distal tubular sodium reabsorption. The result of these effects of angiotensin II is to increase systemic arterial pressure and decrease renal blood flow. Angiotensin II may either decrease, increase, or have little effect on glomerular filtration rate, depending on the physiological state of the animal.[39, 56, 59]

Beyond the effects of changes in arteriolar tone, additional local control of the filtration process is provided by glomerular mesangial cells, which possess actin and myosin contractile filaments. The main effect of mesangial contraction is to reduce glomerular capillary surface area or capillary wall permeability to water.[11] Mesangial cells contract in response to several hormones and other vasoactive substances.

Both nonmyelinated and myelinated nerve fibers are found in the kidneys. These are predominantly alpha adrenergic (sympathetic), and enter the renal parenchyma with the renal artery and its branches. These fibers innervate the afferent arteriole, efferent arteriole, vasa recta, veins, tubular epithelium, and juxtaglomerular apparatus. In a normal dog at rest, the renal nerves have little influence on glomerular filtration rate or renal blood flow. During exercise or such pathophysiological states as congestive heart failure or cardiac arrhythmias, increased sympathetic nerve activity may be responsible for a decrease in renal blood flow and glomerular filtration rate.[4, 43]

RENAL SOLUTE HANDLING

Although in excess of 100 L of glomerular filtrate is formed daily in the average dog, less than 1 per cent of this ultimately remains in the urine. Because of the large quantity of electrolytes, water, amino acids, and glucose in the filtrate, tubular modification is essential for the maintenance of homeostasis. The reabsorptive process is arranged axially along the nephron, with most reabsorption occurring in an isosmotic manner without regard to body needs via high-capacity, low-affinity transport systems in the early portions of the tubule. As fluid progresses along the length of the tubule, reabsorption occurs in accordance with body needs through low-capacity, high-affinity transport processes. For some solutes, such as glucose and amino acids, this entire process occurs within the proximal tubule, and all filtered solute is normally removed from the tubular fluid. For other solutes, such as sodium and potassium, the bulk of filtered solute is reabsorbed in a poorly regulated fashion in the proximal tubule, and the amount of solute finally to appear in the urine is adjusted according to body needs in the distal tubule and collecting duct.

Transport of solutes occurs by the action of carrier molecules, which are generally glycoproteins. Reabsorption of two solutes occurring in the same direction in concert is referred to as *cotransport* or *symport.* An antiporter exchanges solutes (e.g., reabsorption of Na^+ and secretion of H^+ via the Na^+-H^+ antiporter). The primary active membrane transport in the kidneys, Na^+-K^+ antiport activity in the basolateral membrane of tubular epithelia, is used to generate an electrochemical gradient for sodium reabsorption.

Sodium is a classic example of the complexity of reabsorptive function. Sodium is the main extracellular cation and a principal determinant of extracellular fluid volume and systemic arterial pressure. Thus, sodium reabsorption would theoretically be closely regulated. However, reabsorption of most other solutes and water is linked secondarily to the sodium-potassium adenosine triphosphatase (Na^+-K^+ATPase) activity in the basolateral membrane. The apparent contradiction between the need for tight control of sodium reabsorption and the use of the sodium gradient to secondarily drive other solute handling is met by the spatial arrangement of transport processes along the length of the nephron. Most of the reabsorptive process that is coupled to sodium transport occurs in the proximal portions of the nephron, without regard for body needs. This accounts for 50 to 75 per cent of filtered water and solutes. Fluid remaining in the tubular lumen at the end of the proximal tubule is isosmotic with plasma (approximately 300 mOsm/kg). In the loop of Henle, an additional, smaller amount of solute and water is reabsorbed. As a result of the reabsorptive processes of the proximal tubule and loop of Henle, nearly 85 per cent of glomerular filtrate is reclaimed, in a poorly regulated fashion. In the more distal portions of the nephron, tubular modification of fluid occurs in accordance with body needs.

Secretion of protons, potassium, and organic acids and bases from tubular cells into the tubular lumen is an important regulatory function of the kidneys. Secretory processes occur at various tubular sites, depending on the solute (e.g., proximal nephron secretion of organic ions and distal nephron potassium secretion). The secretion of a wide variety of exogenous drugs and chemicals occurs via organic ion transport in the proximal tubule.

The saturability of transport proteins is reflected in the presence of a characteristic maximal rate of reabsorption or excretion for some solutes (e.g., glucose reabsorption). This is defined on a whole-kidney basis as the tubular maxima for reabsorption. Tubular maxima is generally expressed as milligrams of solute excreted or reabsorbed per unit of time or per 100 ml of glomerular filtration rate.[15, 72]

The fraction of filtered solute that ultimately appears in the urine is termed the *fractional excretion:*

$$\text{Fractional excretion (\%)} = 100 \times \frac{\text{urine volume} \times [\text{solute}]_u}{\text{GFR} \times [\text{solute}]_p}$$

where $[\text{solute}]_u$ and $[\text{solute}]_p$ represent the concentrations of solute in the urine and plasma, respectively, and GFR is the glomerular filtration rate. For glucose and amino acids, the fractional excretion is normally less than 1 per cent. Normal fractional excretion values for other solutes depend on body needs for maintenance of homeostasis. For example, if a dog's ration were switched from a low-salt (0.1 per cent sodium) to a normal-salt (0.3 per cent sodium) diet, urinary fractional excretion for sodium would be expected to increase threefold. This would be a normal homeostatic response, not a defect in tubular reabsorption of sodium. Hence, interpretation of values for fractional excretion rates for balanced solutes (i.e., sodium, chloride, potassium, calcium, phosphate, magnesium, and bicarbonate) requires some knowledge of the animal's solute balance. Conserved solutes (i.e., amino acids and glucose) normally are completely reabsorbed, and fractional excretion rates greater than 1 per cent are not expected, with the notable exception of felinine (see the later section on amino acids). Glucosuria or aminoaciduria may be attributed to increased plasma concentrations or reduced renal reabsorption.

Some clinical utility may be obtained from calculation of fractional excretion from a single urine sample, according to the following formula:

$$\text{Fractional excretion (\%)} = 100 \times \frac{[\text{creatinine}]_p \times [\text{solute}]_u}{[\text{creatinine}]_u \times [\text{solute}]_p}$$

However, there are several limitations to this single sample or spot determination of fractional excretion. Because of tubular secretion of creatinine and noncreatinine chromogens present in plasma, creatinine is not a valid marker of glomerular filtration rate. Fluctuations in urinary excretion of solute related to food intake or circadian rhythms are not time averaged by single sample determinations.

Glucose

At normal plasma concentrations, reabsorption of glucose is complete as the filtrate passes through the first 20 per cent of the proximal tubule.[83] Reabsorption of glucose at the luminal membrane is via cotransport with sodium, driven by the electrochemical gradient for sodium reabsorption created by the Na^+-K^+ ATPase activity in the basolateral membrane. This mechanism of solute reabsorption is referred to as *secondary active transport*. The transport protein is stereospecific for D-glucose, and it has been isolated and characterized.[53] Completion of the reabsorptive process for glucose involves a second transport step, with exit of glucose from the proximal tubule cell occurring via a different transporter at the basolateral membrane.

As plasma glucose concentration increases, the filtered load of glucose and glucose reabsorption initially increase in unison. Eventually, as plasma glucose continues to increase, a maximal rate of glucose reabsorption is reached—the transport maximum for glucose (TmG).[15, 72] Filtered loads of glucose that exceed this value result in glucosuria. The plasma glucose concentration at which glucosuria first occurs is referred to as the *renal threshold for glucosuria*, which is approximately 180 to 200 mg/100 ml in dogs[64, 74] and 290 mg/100 ml in cats.[49] Glucosuria may occur at normal plasma glucose concentrations if the transport maximum of individual nephrons is reduced. This may occur as a defect for only glucose (renal glucosuria) or in concert with other proximal tubular reabsorptive defects (Fanconi's syndrome).[8, 13, 14, 26, 29]

Amino Acids

Amino acid reabsorption is nearly complete (> 99 per cent) in the proximal tubule. One exception is felinine, which is normally present in the urine of cats.[38, 85] The functional significance of this sulfur-containing amino acid is unknown.

The transport system for individual amino acids depends on the chemical nature of the amino acid. Carrier systems for basic (lysine, arginine, and ornithine), acidic (glutamic and aspartic acids), and neutral (e.g., glycine, alanine, phenylalanine) alpha amino acids have been described.[17] Transport systems exist for beta amino acids (e.g., taurine) as well. Some of the amino acid transporters are driven by secondary active transport through linkage with sodium, whereas others are driven by potassium transport. Conversely, amino acid reabsorption may also secondarily stimulate proximal tubular sodium reabsorption.[88] As with glucose, a second transport step in amino acid reabsorption occurs at the basolateral membrane. This step is not sodium dependent. One unusual exception is the glutamic acid transport system in the basolateral membrane, which is sodium linked, transporting glutamic acid into the cell to serve as a substrate for renal ammoniagenesis.

Sodium

Sodium is the principal extracellular cation, and its concentration and total body content are important determinants of extracellular fluid composition. Total body sodium content and plasma sodium concentration are not equivalent, and changes in one do not necessarily imply changes in the other. The concentration of sodium in plasma is a main determinant of plasma osmolality. Body sodium content determines extracellular fluid volume and influences systemic arterial pressure.

Although sodium reabsorption occurs along the length of the tubule, most filtered sodium is reabsorbed in the proximal tubule. Sodium movement from the lumen into the epithelial cell is driven by Na^+-K^+ ATPase activity in the basolateral membrane.[17] Sodium transport in the ascending limb of the loop of Henle is passive in the thin portion and active in the thick portion. Sodium reabsorption in the thick portion of the loop occurs in concert with other ions, in the ratio of $1Na^+{:}1K^+{:}2Cl^-$, commonly referred to as *Na^+-K^+-$2Cl^-$ cotransport*. Some diuretic agents (e.g., ethacrynic acid or furosemide) are referred to as *loop diuretics* because they block sodium transport (Na^+-K^+-$2Cl^-$ cotransport) in the loops of Henle.

In both the proximal tubule and the loop of Henle, sodium reabsorption occurs without regard to body needs. In the distal tubule and collecting duct, aldosterone enhances sodium reabsorption in accordance with needs. This is a low-capacity system, and marked reductions in sodium reabsorption in either upstream site (proximal tubule or loop of Henle) can result in the delivery of a quantity of sodium ions that exceeds the capacity of this distal site for sodium reabsorption.

Chloride

Chloride transport in the proximal tubules occurs by secondary active transport and passive transport through intercellular spaces.[17] Similar to the glucose and amino acid transport system, chloride reabsorption is a two-step process. In the proximal tubular luminal membrane, a Na^+-H^+ antiporter transports H^+ into the lumen and Na^+ into the tubular epithelial cell. This antiporter is driven by the sodium gradient created by Na^+-K^+ ATPase in the basolateral membrane. As a consequence, chloride transport across the luminal membrane can be coupled to a cation (e.g., HCl) or can occur via an anion antiporter (e.g., Cl^-/HCO_3^-). Both are driven by the cell-to-lumen pH/bicarbonate gradient, which is maintained by the Na^+-/H^+ antiporter.

Potassium

Potassium is predominantly an intracellular ion. A high intracellular potassium concentration is required for optimal cellular functions and for maintenance of the transmembrane potential. Maintenance of extracellular potassium concentration within a narrow range is a result of two separate, equally important potassium balances: (1) external balance, which occurs between intake (gastrointestinal) and excretion (predominantly renal and colonic), and (2) internal balance, which occurs between the intracellular and extracellular fluid compartments. Because we generally assess potassium status by measuring its concentration in the plasma (a component of extracellular fluid), a shift in either of these two balances affects the measured parameter.[36] Plasma potassium concentration does not provide a reliable method to assess whole-body potassium homeostasis.

Like glucose, amino acids, and sodium, potassium is freely filtered across the glomerular filtration barrier. Approximately 75 per cent of the filtered load of potassium is reabsorbed in the proximal tubule. Further reabsorption occurs in the loop of Henle (Na^+-K^+-$2Cl^+$ cotransport). Potassium secretion in the distal tubule and collecting duct adjusts the potassium content of the urine in accordance with needs. This secretion is passive and under the influence of aldosterone. Aldosterone stimulates the activity of existing basolateral Na^+-K^+ ATPase carriers and the production of new ones. Other important factors influencing distal potassium secretion include tubular flow rate and the concentration of anions in the luminal fluid. A large concentration of anions (e.g., bicarbonaturia) or rapid flow rates (e.g., diuresis) in the distal nephron enhance potassium secretion and may cause body depletion of potassium, if prolonged. Other factors promoting potassium secretion include low concentration of protons in luminal fluid, glucocorticoids, antidiuretic hormone, and catecholamines.[34]

Normal kidneys adapt urinary excretion of potassium to dietary intake. A high potassium intake enhances potassium excretion.[67] Hence, fractional excretion of potassium varies widely in normal animals. On "normal diets," fractional excretion of potassium may be 5 to 15 per cent, whereas an increase in potassium intake or a decrease in glomerular filtration rate may cause fractional excretion that exceeds 100 per cent of filtered load.

Cats with normal or diseased kidneys are predisposed to urinary losses of potassium and subsequent development of a polymyopathy secondary to potassium depletion.[25] The relative contributions of inadequate dietary potassium intake versus enhanced urinary potassium losses have not been determined.

Phosphate

The kidneys are the main organs responsible for phosphate homeostasis.[44] Phosphate is freely filtered and reabsorbed in the proximal tubule by a sodium-dependent mechanism, which is inhibited by parathyroid hormone. Although parathyroid hormone has a prominent role in the control of phosphate reabsorption in the kidneys of normal animals, plasma phosphate concentration can be grossly regulated in the absence of parathyroid hormone, suggesting important contributions to control of renal phosphate reabsorption from parathyroid hormone-independent mechanisms.

Calcium

The most important mechanism for maintenance of homeostasis of calcium is gastrointestinal absorption, which is influenced by vitamin D. Although only ionized calcium is physiologically active, calcium exists in plasma in protein-bound, chelated, or ionized forms. Only chelated and ionized forms are freely filtered by the kidneys and account for approximately 50 per cent of total calcium in normal animals. The relationship between filterable and total plasma calcium is not fixed. For example, acidemia preferentially reduces the two freely filtered fractions. Reabsorption of filtered calcium parallels that of sodium, and manipulations that affect sodium excretion often have the same effect on calcium reabsorption.[27, 79] An exception is thiazide diuretics, which often enhance renal calcium reabsorption.

Magnesium

Plasma magnesium concentration is regulated by the kidneys. Most magnesium in plasma is freely filtered, and about 25 per cent of this is reabsorbed in the proximal tubules. The major site of magnesium reabsorption and regulatory control is the loops of Henle.[84]

ACID-BASE BALANCE

Acid-base homeostasis is controlled by the kidneys and lungs. The CO_2/HCO_3^- buffer system has an integral role in maintenance of acid-base balance by both kidneys and lungs via the following reactions:

$$H_2O + CO_2 \underset{}{\overset{\text{carbonic anhydrase}}{\rightleftharpoons}} H_2CO_3 \rightleftharpoons HCO_3^- + H^+$$

This relationship demonstrates the ready interconversion of carbon dioxide and bicarbonate in the presence of carbonic anhydrase. Although the lungs can bring about an acute change in body acid-base status by altering carbon dioxide pressure, the kidneys provide long-term control of body acid-base status through the related processes of bicarbonate reabsorption and proton excretion.

Bicarbonate Reabsorption

Bicarbonate freely passes the glomerular filtration barrier and must normally be reabsorbed to maintain acid-base homeostasis. Bicarbonate is reabsorbed by proton secretion into the proximal tubular lumen (Fig. 101–2). The predominant carrier protein is the sodium-hydrogen antiporter, which transports protons into the luminal fluid and is driven by the transmembrane sodium gradient (generated by the basolateral Na^+-K^+ ATPase). Filtered bicarbonate is converted to carbon dioxide and water by carbonic anhydrase. The carbon dioxide passively diffuses into the epithelial cells and is reconverted to bicarbonate, which subsequently enters the blood. Bicarbonate leaves the tubular cells via a transporter in the basolateral membrane, which may cotransport sodium.[6] This process is cyclical, because the proton is regenerated within the cell to be used for reabsorption of another bicarbonate ion. Unlike most electrolytes, bicarbonate has several mechanisms contributing to control of its reabsorption in the proximal tubules. Bicarbonate reabsorption in the proximal tubules is normally complete (99 per cent), but bicarbonate reabsorption in the proximal tubules can be inhibited by volume expansion, alkalemia, elevated plasma concentrations of parathyroid hormone, and heightened carbon dioxide pressure. It is stimulated by potassium depletion, elevated luminal pH, and increased glomerular filtration rate. The mechanism of these effects on bicarbonate transport in the proximal nephron is unknown, although parathyroid hormone inhibits the Na^+-H^+ antiporter.[68] If needed, new bicarbonate ions can be synthesized from metabolically generated carbon dioxide in the tubular cells. These bicarbonate ions are transported to the interstitium and diffuse into a peritubular capillary.

Proton Excretion

Although the addition of alkalinizing agents (e.g., sodium bicarbonate, potassium citrate, or calcium carbonate) or the ingestion of a cereal-based diet may have a net alkalinizing effect, cats and dogs ingesting a meat-based diet must usually generate acidic urine to maintain acid-base balance. Proton secretion by the distal tubules and collecting ducts is responsible for the final adjustment of urine pH and the maintenance of total-body acid-base balance.

The process of proton secretion by the distal tubules (Fig. 101–3) is similar to that in the proximal nephron.[45] While secreted protons in the proximal tubules combine with bicarbonate and are reabsorbed as carbon dioxide and water (see Fig. 101–2), protons secreted into the distal tubular lumen combine with ammonia and phosphate, resulting in the production of ammonium (NH_4^+) and titratable acid ($H_2PO_4^-$), two nonreabsorbable ions (see Fig. 101–3). Ammonia passively diffuses into the luminal fluid, having been derived from glutamine by tubular epithelial cells. Phosphate in the distal tubular fluid represents filtered solute that has not been reabsorbed. The final urine pH is thus a product of distal tubular proton excretion and the net secretion of hydrogen ions and can be quantitated as the sum of urinary content of ammonium and titratable acid.

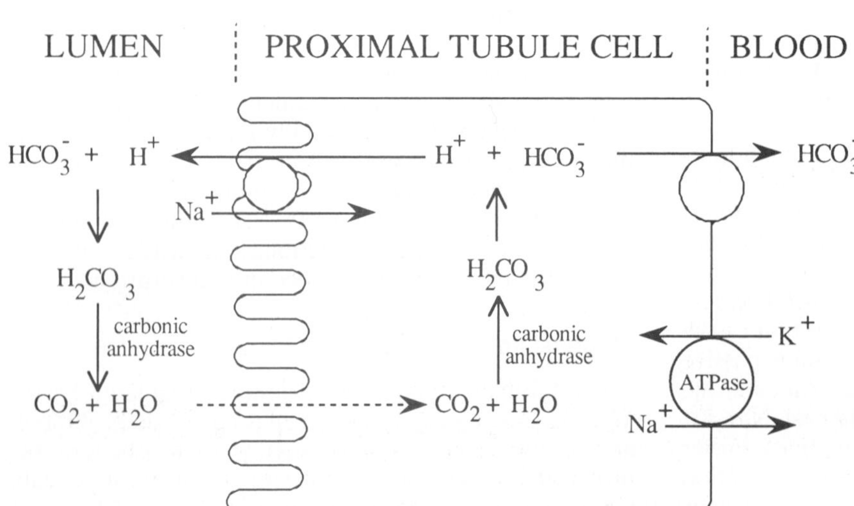

FIGURE 101–2. In the proximal tubule epithelial cell, the basolateral Na^+-K^+ ATPase produces a gradient favoring sodium reabsorption and hydrogen ion secretion by the Na^+-H^+ antiporter in the luminal membrane. This proton then combines with a bicarbonate ion, producing carbonic acid, which in turn is converted to carbon dioxide and water in a reaction aided by the enzyme carbonic anhydrase. The process is cyclical, resulting in regeneration of the hydrogen ion within the epithelial cell.

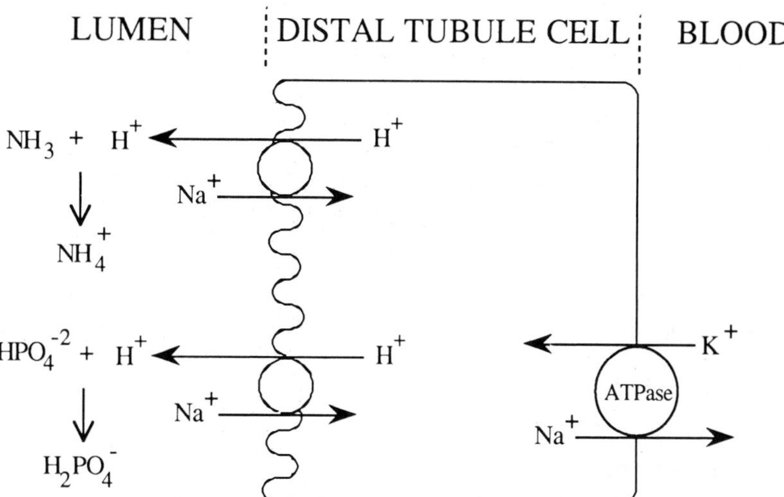

FIGURE 101–3. As a result of proximal reabsorption, bicarbonate ions are not normally present in the distal tubular fluid. At this site, secreted hydrogen ions combine with ammonia or phosphate, producing nonreabsorbable anions. These urinary buffers increase the tubular fluid content of hydrogen ions, and the final urine pH is determined by hydrogen ion secretion in the distal tubule.

Factors Affecting Tubular Reabsorption

The influx of fluid into the peritubular capillary lumen can be described as follows (Fig. 101–4):

$$\text{Fluid influx (Jv)} = K\,[(\pi c - \pi i) - (Pc - Pi)]$$

where πc and πi are the colloid (protein) osmotic pressure within the peritubular capillary and interstitium, respectively, Pc and Pi represent the hydrostatic pressure within the proximal tubule and interstitium, and K is the effective hydraulic permeability of the capillary wall (also referred to as the *reflection coefficient*). K is a constant that is a characteristic of the vessel itself. Because of the large decrease in hydrostatic pressure along the length of the efferent arteriole, peritubular capillary pressures average 10 to 14 mm Hg in a dog's kidneys (see Table 101–1). The formation of protein-free filtrate in the glomeruli leads to an elevation of oncotic pressure at the origination of canine peritubular capillaries to values (πc) of approximately 30 to 40 mm Hg. The interstitial hydrostatic and oncotic pressures are unknown but are estimated to be approximately equal and less than 5 mm Hg.[11] Consequently, the high oncotic pressure within the peritubular capillary, which exceeds the intracapillary hydrostatic pressure (Pc), results in a net force of approximately 20 to 25 mm Hg, forcing fluid movement into the capillary.

The hydraulic conductivity, K, of a capillary is the product of the vessel surface area times the hydraulic permeability to fluid. Compared with other capillary beds in the body, the K value for a peritubular capillary is high, exceeded only by that of a glomerulus. Both capillary types are several times more permeable to water than are capillaries of skeletal muscle.

Although the uptake of solutes and water from the lumen depends on cellular transport mechanisms, the transit of solutes and water from the interstitium into the peritubular capillaries depends on these Starling forces (see Fig. 101–4). Hence, peritubular physical forces—specifically interstitial colloid osmotic and hydrostatic pressures—greatly affect renal handling of solutes and water. Consequently, any process that causes fluid to accumulate in the interstitium lowers interstitial colloid osmotic pressure and raises interstitial hydrostatic pressure, both changes that hinder fluid movement out of the tubule. An example of these forces at work occurs during extracellular volume expansion when a decrease in interstitial colloid osmotic pressure and an increase in interstitial hydrostatic pressure inhibit tubular solute and water reabsorption. The resultant diuresis and natriuresis return extracellular fluid volume to normal. Conversely, volume contraction has the opposite effects, appropriately enhancing renal reabsorption of solute and water.

An important property of the kidneys is the presence of glomerulotubular balance, which allows that for most solutes, the rate of transport reflects the rate of

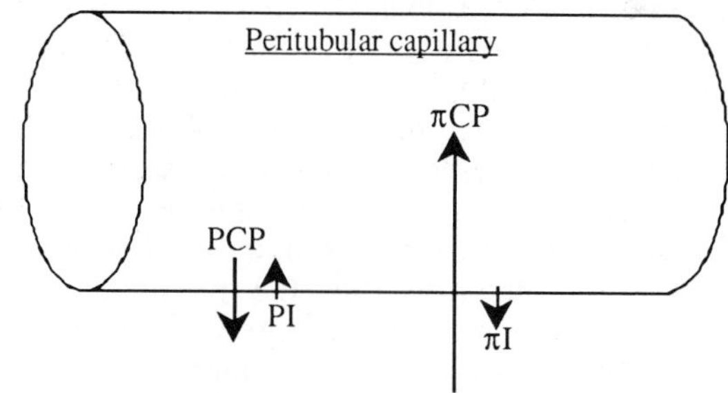

Representative Values - Canine

Hydrostatic Pressures (mmHg)	
Peritubular Capillary (PCP)	12
Interstitial (PI)	5
Difference (ΔP)	7
Colloid Osmotic Pressures (mmHg)	
Peritubular capillary (πCP)	35
Interstitial (πI)	5
Difference (Δπ)	30
Mean Effective Reabsorptive Pressure (mmHg)	
$= \Delta\pi - \Delta P = 30 - 7 = 23$ mmHg	

FIGURE 101–4. The primary driving force for reabsorption of solute and water into the peritubular capillaries is peritubular capillary colloid osmotic pressure (πCP), which is opposed by peritubular capillary hydrostatic pressure (PCP). The opposing interstitial pressures, colloid osmotic (πI) and hydrostatic pressures (PI), are small and of approximately equal magnitude (5 mm Hg).

filtration.[47] Thus, elevations of glomerular filtration rate lead to increases in filtered load, which are met with increases in absolute reabsorption. As a consequence, transient changes in glomerular filtration rate do not cause wide fluctuations in urinary content of solutes or in concentrations of solutes within the extracellular fluid. Glomerulotubular balance thus represents an important homeostatic mechanism. Because more distal portions of a nephron do not possess a large reabsorptive reserve and their regulatory functions can be readily overcome, much of the explanation for glomerulotubular balance lies within the proximal tubules. Here, increased flow rate (increased glomerular filtration rate) prevents development of a concentration gradient between epithelial cells and luminal fluid, favoring continued isosmotic reabsorption. In addition, at a normal filtration rate for most solutes (e.g., glucose or amino acids), reabsorption is nearly complete in the initial portion of the proximal tubules. As the filtered load of solute increases, this process of reabsorption extends axially along a proximal tubule, exceeding reabsorptive capacity of this tubular segment only at very high filtered loads.

Many hormones have direct effects on tubular reabsorptive processes. Some important examples include stimulation of Na^+ reabsorption by angiotensin II, aldosterone, and vasopressin; inhibition of sodium reabsorption by atrial natriuretic factor; inhibition of phosphorus and bicarbonate reabsorption by parathyroid hormone; and stimulation of calcium reabsorption by parathyroid hormone. Renal nerves, via innervation of tubular epithelia, can modify tubular transport processes directly.

WATER REABSORPTION: THE URINE-CONCENTRATING MECHANISM

The kidneys are responsible for maintaining water homeostasis. This includes the ability to conserve or excrete water, depending on body needs. In a normal 20-kg dog, the daily glomerular filtration rate exceeds 100 L, and even polyuric animals must reclaim the majority of filtrate. As with most filtered substances, water reabsorption occurs primarily in the proximal portions of the nephrons. In the proximal tubules, because of the massive surface area of the proximal tubular brush border and the high water permeability of this epithelium, water reabsorption occurs at a high rate with solute reabsorption, and luminal fluid remains isosmotic. Consequently, luminal fluid tonicity is approximately 300 mOsm/kg (isosmotic) at the beginning of the descending limb of Henle. As a consequence of water reabsorption in the proximal tubules and the loops of Henle, approximately 10 per cent of the filtered load of water reaches the final portion of distal tubules, regardless of body needs.

Although many issues pertaining to urine-concentrating mechanisms remain unanswered, the function of the loops of Henle in water homeostasis is generally accepted.[37] In contrast to the proximal tubules, solute reabsorption in the ascending limb of the loops of Henle is not followed by water reabsorption, because this portion of a nephron is not permeable to water. Solute reabsorbed by the ascending limb of a loop of Henle remains concentrated in the medullary interstitium (Fig. 101–5).

In contrast, the descending limb of a loop of Henle is permeable to water. Because of medullary hypertonicity, water passively leaves the tubular lumen and tubular fluid becomes progressively more hypertonic. At the hairpin turn of a loop of Henle and in the initial portion of the ascending limb of a loop of Henle, tubular fluid is hypertonic. In the thin portion of the ascending limb, sodium and chloride passively exit the tubular fluid. The thick portion of the ascending limb actively reabsorbs solute (Na^+-K^+-$2Cl^-$ cotransport), causing a progressive decrease in tubular fluid tonicity and eventually leading to tubular fluid hypotonicity in the latter portions of the ascending limb and the distal tubules. This solute reabsorption contributes to medullary hypertonicity. In cats, tubular fluid may not become hypotonic but remains isotonic in the final segments of the ascending limb.[40, 80]

As the tubular fluid reaches the terminal portion of the distal tubules and the collecting ducts, water could be passively reabsorbed along the osmotic gradient provided by medullary hypertonicity. Antidiuretic hormone, released from the posterior hypothalamus in response to an increase in plasma tonicity, has a central role in maintenance of water permeability of this portion of the tubule. Antidiuretic hormone bound to receptors on the basolateral membrane of collecting duct cells stimulates membrane-bound adenyl cyclase enzyme activity, resulting in increased intracellular levels of cyclic adenosite monophosphate, which enhances water

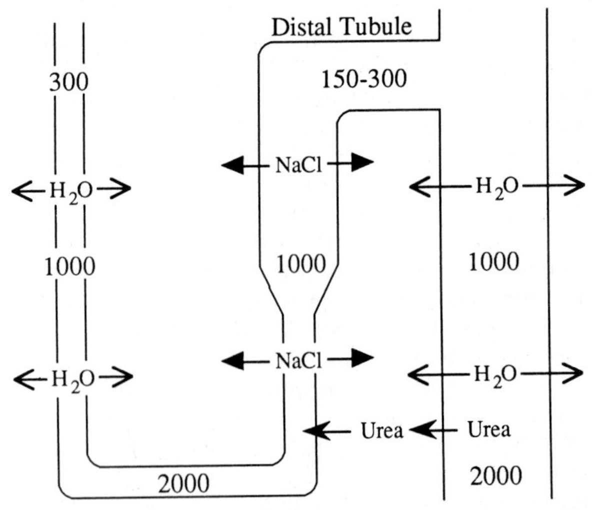

FIGURE 101–5. The countercurrent theory of the urine-concentrating mechanism suggests that sodium chloride movement out of the water-impermeable ascending limb of the loop of Henle (passive movement in the thin, active in the thick portion) combined with the water permeability of the descending limb is responsible for the generation of medullary hypertonicity. Antidiuretic hormone causes the collecting duct to be permeable to water, which is passively reabsorbed along its osmotic gradient, and concentrated urine is produced. Urea, through passive recycling in the collecting duct and ascending limb, further contributes to medullary hypertonicity. (Values in mOsm/kg.)

permeability. In the absence of antidiuretic hormone, the collecting duct epithelium is impermeable to water, resulting in formation of dilute urine. Water movement from collecting duct to interstitium is promoted by antidiuretic hormone, resulting in the production of concentrated urine.

As a solute, urea also contributes to the urine-concentrating mechanism.[37] In the tubules, filtered urea is concentrated as water is passively reabsorbed. Under the influence of antidiuretic hormone, water is reabsorbed across the collecting duct epithelium, and as a consequence, urea is highly concentrated in the medullary portion of the collecting ducts. Urea permeability is enhanced by antidiuretic hormone binding to the ductal epithelium, and urea passively diffuses into the interstitium along its concentration gradient. This leads to high concentrations of urea in the medullary interstitium, favoring movement of urea into the ascending limb of the loops of Henle, along the concentration gradient. The addition of urea to the medullary interstitium and the recycling of reabsorbed urea in the collecting ducts and ascending limb of the loops of Henle contribute to medullary hypertonicity.

The anatomy and slow flow of the vasa recta prevent removal of solute, further contributing to maintenance of medullary hypertonicity.

ASSESSMENT OF RENAL FUNCTION

Renal function is assessed by analysis of urine, measurement of serum concentrations of creatinine (SCr) and blood urea nitrogen (BUN), or specialized tests to assess glomerular filtration rate, renal blood flow, or renal solute handling.

Urinalysis includes dipstick methods for qualitative urine chemistry analysis, measurement of urinary enzymes to assess renal damage, urine sediment examination, and determination of the urine protein/creatinine ratio. The urine protein/creatinine ratio is calculated as urine [protein]/urine [creatinine], with both values expressed as milligrams per 100 milliliters. Although the urine protein/creatinine ratio is a useful method for qualitative assessment of urinary protein excretion, accurate evaluation of proteinuria is best obtained by timed collection of urine.[86] Values for the urine protein/creatinine ratio, which depend on analytical methods, are less than 1.0 for normal dogs and cats.

Serum Creatinine and Blood Urea Nitrogen

Urea is the product of the combination of two ammonia molecules by enzymes of the hepatic urea cycle. Urea is passively filtered through the renal glomeruli. Because some segments of the tubular epithelium are permeable to urea, urea may exit or enter tubular fluid and undergo recycling in the urine-concentrating process.

Creatine produced by the liver is taken up by muscle cells, where it eventually undergoes an irreversible decomposition to creatinine. Creatinine is excreted by the kidneys through filtration in dogs and cats and also by proximal tubular secretion in dogs.

Because of wide interanimal variability and the effects of nonrenal factors (Table 101–2), measurement of SCr and BUN is generally worthwhile only for clinical detection of marked impairment of renal function (glomerular filtration rate). Normal BUN and SCr values may be noted in dogs and cats with as little as 25 per cent of normal glomerular filtration rate. Any mechanism that reduces glomerular filtration rate (i.e., prerenal, renal, or postrenal) may lead to increases in SCr and BUN. The use of BUN/SCr ratios has been advocated in humans to distinguish these causes of azotemia. These ratios have little use in dogs.[32]

The ratio 1/SCr has been used to assess the temporal pattern of renal function in animals with chronic renal failure.[1] The limitations of SCr remain, and although some dogs have a linear relationship,[1] others do not,[5] and the utility of this ratio has been questioned because of increasing extrarenal creatinine catabolism in end-stage renal disease and poor correlation between rates of change of glomerular filtration rate and reciprocal SCr.[52]

Measurement of Renal Clearance

The standard measure of renal function is the clearance procedure in which a timed, total collection of urine is used with the standard clearance formula:

$$C = UvUc/Pc$$

where C = clearance (milliliters per minute), Uv = urine flow rate (milliliters per minute), Uc = concentration of solute in urine, and Pc = concentration of solute in plasma.

Inulin, a fructose polymer that is freely filtered, not metabolized, and neither reabsorbed nor secreted, is the standard compound for measurement of glomerular fil-

TABLE 101–2. CONDITIONS THAT MAY AFFECT BLOOD CONCENTRATIONS OF CREATININE AND UREA

	Increase	Decrease
Creatinine	Reduced GFR	Tubular secretion (male dog)
	Noncreatinine chromogens*	Intestinal degradation
	Protein ingestion	
	Strenuous exercise	
	Muscle injury	
Urea	Reduced GFR	
	Slow urine flow rates	Rapid urine flow rates
	Protein ingestion	Anabolic steroid administration
	Protein catabolism	Hepatic insufficiency
	Tetracycline administration	Urea cycle defects
	Steroid administration	Intestinal degradation
	Gastrointestinal hemorrhage	
	Fever	
	Burns	
	Infection	

*Falsely elevates measured serum creatinine value in many commercial assays but does not affect true plasma concentration of creatinine.
GFR, glomerular filtration rate.

tration rate (inulin clearance). At low plasma concentrations, all *p*-aminohippuric acid is removed from renal plasma in one passage, and clearance of *p*-aminohippuric acid is used to measure renal plasma flow.

A timed collection of urine in a metabolism cage (24 hours) is used to measure endogenous creatinine clearance. This method is useful clinically. Many laboratory assays for creatinine measure both noncreatinine chromogens and creatinine,[3] and SCr values may thus be falsely increased. Because noncreatinine chromogens are not present in urine, the urine creatinine value reflects only creatinine, and the calculated clearance is often less than inulin clearance. Tubular secretion of creatinine in dogs,[60, 81] but not cats,[30] may modestly increase the clearance value. As a consequence of variable tubular secretion and differences in analytical assays, it is difficult to predict normal values for this clearance measurement, and normal values for endogenous creatinine clearance are established for each veterinary facility.

Exogenous infusion/injection of creatinine for short-term measurement of clearance (20 to 60 minutes) minimizes the contribution of noncreatinine chromogens, providing a reliable method for measuring glomerular filtration rate in dogs.[33]

Quantitative renal scintigraphy, using the compound ^{99m}Tc-diethylenetriaminopentaacetic acid (DTPA), can be used to measure glomerular filtration rate.[21, 48] This method has the advantages of being noninvasive and rapid, allowing separate evaluation of individual kidney glomerular filtration rate and kidney size. However, the procedure requires specialized equipment and methods for handling radioisotopes.

MICTURITION

The urinary tract provides a means for delivery of urine (ureteral peristalsis) from the renal pelvis to a storage reservoir (bladder) and a route (bladder and urethra) for voiding urine to the exterior. The entire process of urine storage and voiding is referred to as *micturition*. During the storage phase, detrusor (bladder muscle) relaxation allows urine to accumulate at an intravesicular pressure that is below the outlet resistance. Detrusor relaxation occurs through both passive and neural (sympathetic inhibition) mechanisms.[22, 23] Bladder distension activates receptors within the wall, leading to the detrusor reflex. The neural pathway involves transmission from bladder wall tension receptors to the sacral spinal cord and to the pontine micturition center.[62] Parasympathetic fibers originating at the pontine level descend to innervate postganglionic fibers, which in turn terminate on the detrusor muscle, stimulating a coordinated contraction. During the voiding phase, detrusor contraction is coupled with urethral relaxation to allow bladder emptying. Urethral resistance is the result of a combination of passive and active resistance. The active component of resistance is attributable to both smooth muscle fibers ("internal sphincter") innervated by the sympathetic nervous system and striated muscle fibers ("external sphincter") innervated by the pudendal (somatic) nerve. Although they function as sphincters, these two components of active resistance of the urethra are not organized into anatomically recognizable sphincters. During the voiding phase, both components of the urethral musculature are inhibited. There is cerebrocortical (voluntary) input into the micturition process, including direct cortical innervation of the micturition center and somatic innervation of the striated muscle of the urethra. The cerebellum inhibits the pontine micturition center.[9] A lesion of the bladder, urethra, or any component of the neural pathway may lead to a disorder of the storage or voiding phase of micturition.[62, 63, 65]

References

1. Allen TA, et al: A technique for estimating progression of chronic renal failure in the dog. *J Am Vet Med Assoc 190*:866, 1987.
2. Amiel C, et al: Evidence for a parathyroid hormone-independent calcium modulation of phosphate transport along the nephron. *J Clin Invest 57*:256, 1976.
3. Balint P, Visy M: "True creatinine" and "pseudocreatinine" in blood plasma of the dog. *Acta Physiol Acad Sci Hung 28*:265, 1965.
4. Barger AC, et al: Role of the kidney in the pathogenesis of congestive heart failure. *Circulation 20*:273, 1959.
5. Barsanti JA, Finco DR: Dietary management of chronic renal failure in dogs. *J Am Anim Hosp Assoc 21*:371, 1985.
6. Boron WF, Boulpaep EL: Intracellular pH regulation in the renal proximal tubule of the salamander: Basolateral bicarbonate transport. *J Gen Physiol 81*:53, 1983.
7. Bovee KC, Webster GD: Values for intrarenal distribution of blood flow using xenon 133 in the anesthetized dog. *Am J Vet Res 33*:501, 1972.
8. Bovee KC, et al: Characterization of renal defects in dogs with a syndrome similar to Fanconi syndrome in man. *J Am Vet Med Assoc 174*:1094, 1979.
9. Bradley WE, Teague CT: Cerebellar influence on the micturition reflex. *Exp Neurol 23*:399, 1969.
10. Brenner BM: Endothelium-dependent vascular responses. *J Clin Invest 84*:1373, 1989.
11. Brenner BM, et al: The renal circulations. *In* Brenner BM, Rector FC (eds): *The Kidney*. W. B. Saunders, Philadelphia, 1986, pp 93–124.
12. Brown SA: Renal effects of nonsteroidal antiinflammatory drugs. *In* Kirk RW (ed): *Current Veterinary Therapy X*. W. B. Saunders, Philadelphia, 1989, pp 1158–1161.
13. Brown SA: Fanconi's syndrome: Inherited and acquired. *In* Kirk RW (ed): *Current Veterinary Therapy X*. W. B. Saunders, Philadelphia, 1989, pp 1163–1165.
14. Brown SA, et al: Fanconi syndrome and acute renal failure associated with gentamicin therapy in a dog. *J Am Anim Hosp Assoc 22*:635, 1986.
15. Brown SA, et al: Glucose conservation by the kidney and effect of systemic glucose infusion on inulin clearance in female goats. *Am J Vet Res 51*:587, 1990.
16. Brown SA, et al: Single nephron adaptations to partial renal ablation in the dog. *Am J Physiol 258*:F495, 1990.
17. Burg MB: Renal handling of sodium, chloride, water, amino acids, and glucose. *In* Brenner BM, Rector FC (eds): *The Kidney*. W. B. Saunders, Philadelphia, 1986, pp 145–176.
18. Carmines PK, et al: Angiotensin II effects on microvascular diameters of *in vitro* blood-perfused juxtamedullary nephrons. *Am J Physiol 251*:F610, 1986.
19. Carmines PK, et al: Effects of preglomerular and postglomerular vascular resistance alterations on filtration fraction. *Kidney Int 31*:S229, 1987.
20. Cohen HJ, et al: Autoregulation in vasa recta of the rat kidney. *Am J Physiol 245*:F32, 1983.
21. Cowgill L, Hornof W: Assessment of individual kidney function by quantitative renal scintigraphy. *In* Kirk RW (ed): *Current Veterinary Therapy IX*. W. B. Saunders, Philadelphia, 1986, pp 1108–1110.
22. DeGroat WC: Nervous control of the urinary bladder of the cat. *Brain Res 87*:201, 1975.
23. DeGroat WC, Saum WE: Sympathetic inhibition of the urinary bladder and of pelvic ganglionic transmission in the cat. *J Physiol 220*:297, 1972.
24. Dossetor JB: The relative significance of blood urea nitrogen and serum creatinine concentrations in azotemia. *Ann Intern Med 65*:1287, 1966.
25. Dow SW, LeCouteur RA: Hypokalemic polymyopathy of cats. *In* Kirk RW (ed): *Current Veterinary Therapy X*. W. B. Saunders, Philadelphia, 1989, pp 1158–1161.
26. Easley JR, Breitschwerdt EG: Glucosuria associated with renal tubular dysfunction in three Basenji dogs. *J Am Vet Med Assoc 168*:938, 1976.
27. Edwards BR, et al: Micropuncture study of diuretic effects on sodium and calcium reabsorption in the dog nephron. *J Clin Invest 52*:2418, 1973.

28. Feinstein EI, Massry SG: Nutritional therapy in acute renal failure. *In* Mitch WE, Klahr S (eds): *Nutrition and the Kidney*. Little, Brown, Co, Boston, 1988, pp 80–103.
29. Finco DR: Familial renal disease in Norwegian elkhounds: Physiologic and biochemical examinations. *Am J Vet Res 37*:87, 1976.
30. Finco DR, Barsanti JA: Mechanism of urinary excretion of creatinine by the cat. *Am J Vet Res 43*:2207, 1982.
31. Finco DR, Duncan JR: Relationship of glomerular number and diameter to body size of the dog. *Am J Vet Res 33*:2447, 1972.
32. Finco DR, Duncan JR: Evaluation of blood urea nitrogen and serum creatinine as indicators of renal dysfunction. *J Am Vet Med Assoc 168*:593, 1976.
33. Finco DR, et al: Simple, accurate method for clinical estimation of glomerular filltration rate in the dog. *Am J Vet Res 42*:1874, 1981.
34. Fried TA, Stein JH: Glomerular dynamics. *Arch Intern Med 143*:787, 1983.
35. Gellai M, et al: Contrasting views on the action of atrial peptides: Lessons from studies of conscious animals. *Fed Proc 45*:2387, 1986.
36. Giebisch G, et al: Renal transport and control of potassium excretion. *In* Brenner BM, Rector FC (eds): *The Kidney*. W. B. Saunders, Philadelphia, 1986, pp 177–205.
37. Gottschalk CW, et al: Neural control of renal function in health and disease. *In* Seldin DW, Giebisch G (eds): *The Kidney: Physiology and Pathophysiology*. Raven Press, New York, 1985, pp 581–611.
38. Greaves JP, Scott PP: Urinary amino-acid pattern of cats on diets of varying protein content. *Nature 187*:242, 1960.
39. Hall JE, et al: Control of glomerular filtration rate by renin-angiotensin system. *Am J Physiol 233*:F366, 1977.
40. Jamison RL: The urinary concentrating mechanism. *In* Brenner BM, Rector FC (eds): *The Kidney*. W. B. Saunders, Philadelphia, 1976, pp 391–441.
41. Jones JD, Burnett PC: Creatinine metabolism in humans with decreased renal function: Creatinine deficit. *Clin Chem 20*:1204, 1974.
42. Jones SM, et al: Regional renin release by the cat kidney *in vitro* and *in vivo*. *Am J Physiol 237*:F188, 1979.
43. Katholi RE: Renal nerves in the pathogenesis of hypertension in experimental animals and humans. *Am J Physiol 245*:F1, 1983.
44. Knochel JP, Jacobson HR: Renal handling of phosphorus, clinical hypophosphatemia, and phosphorus deficiency. *In* Brenner BM, Rector FC (eds): *The Kidney*. W. B. Saunders, Philadelphia, 1986, pp 619–662.
45. Koeppen B, et al: Mechanism and regulation of renal tubular acidification. *In* Seldin DW, Giebisch G (eds): *The Kidney: Physiology and Pathophysiology*. Raven Press, New York, 1985, pp 1491–1526.
46. Kopple JD, Coburn JW: Importance of serum urea nitrogen, serum creatinine, and their ratio. *JAMA 227*:41, 1974.
47. Kramp RA, et al: A study by microdissection and micropuncture of the structure and function of the kidneys and the nephrons of rats with chronic renal damage. *Kidney Int 5*:147, 1974.
48. Krawiec DR, et al: Evaluation of^{99m} Tc-diethylenetriaminepentaacetic acid nuclear imaging for quantitative determination of the glomerular filtration of dogs. *Am J Vet Res 47*:2175, 1986.
49. Kruth SA, Cowgill LD: Abstract: Renal glucose transport in the cat. Proceedings of the American College of Veterinary Internal Medicine Scientific Forum, San Diego, May 1982, p 78.
50. Kumar R, et al: Chronic renal failure or simple starvation? A case report. *Lancet 2*:1005, 1972.
51. Kuntziger H, et al: Localization of parathyroid-hormone-independent sodium bicarbonate inhibition of tubular phosphate reabsorption. *Kidney Int 17*:749, 1980.
52. Levey AS, et al: Abstract: Poor correlation of rates of change of creatinine clearance, reciprocal serum creatinine, and GFR. *Kidney Int 35*:197, 1989.
53. Malathi P, Preiser H: Isolation of the sodium-dependent D-glucose transport protein from brush border membranes. *Biochim Biophys Acta 735*:314, 1983.
54. Mitch WE: Nutritional therapy and progression of renal disease. *In* Mitch WE, Klahr S (eds): *Nutrition and the Kidney*. Little, Brown, Co, Boston, 1988, pp 154–179.
55. Moore LC, Casellas D: Tubuloglomerular feedback dependence of autoregulation in rat juxtamedullary afferent arterioles. *Kidney Int 37*:1402, 1990.
56. Navar LG, Rosivall L: Contribution of the renin-angiotensin system to the control of intrarenal hemodynamics. *Kidney Int 25*:857, 1984.
57. Navar LG, et al: Evaluation of the single nephron glomerular filtration coefficient in the dog. *Kidney Int 12*:137, 1977.
58. Navar LG, et al: The regulation of glomerular filtration rate in mammalian kidneys. *In* Andreoli TE, et al (eds): *Physiology of Membrane Disorders*. Plenum, New York, 1986, pp 637–667.
59. Navar LG, et al: The tubular effects of angiotensin II. *Kidney Int 31*:S81, 1987.
60. O'Connell JM, et al: Renal tubular secretion of creatinine in the dog. *Am J Physiol 203*:985, 1962.
61. Ofstad J, Aukland K: Renal circulation. *In* Seldin DW, Giegisch G (eds): *The Kidney: Physiology and Pathophysiology*. Raven Press, New York, 1985, pp 471–496.
62. Oliver JE: Disorders of micturition. *In* Oliver JE, et al (eds): *Veterinary Neurology*. W. B. Saunders, Philadelphia, 1987, pp 342–352.
63. Oliver JE, Osborne CA: Neurogenic urinary incontinence. *In* Kirk RW (ed): *Current Veterinary Therapy VII*. W. B. Saunders, Philadelphia, 1980, pp 1159–1164.
64. Osborne CA, et al: *Canine and Feline Urology*. Philadelphia, W. B. Saunders, 1972, pp 39–61.
65. Osborne CA, et al: Nonneurogenic urinary incontinence. *In* Kirk RW: *Current Veterinary Therapy VI*. W. B. Saunders, Philadelphia, 1980, pp 1165–1172.
66. Paul RV, et al: Renal autoregulation and pressure natriuresis during ANF-induced diuresis. *Am J Physiol 253*:F424, 1987.
67. Pickering EC: The role of the kidney in sodium and potassium balance. *Proc Nutr Soc 24*:73, 1965.
68. Pollack AS, et al: Parathyroid hormone induced decrease in Na/H antiporter activity in a cultured opossum kidney cell line. Proceedings of the 9th International Congress of Nephrology 387A, Helsinki, June 1984, p 387 A.
69. Refsum HE, Stromme SB: Urea and creatinine production and excretion in urine during and after prolonged heavy exercise. *Scand J Lab Invest 33*:247, 1974.
70. Ross LA, Finco DR: Relationship of selected clinical renal function tests to glomerular filtration rate and renal blood flow in cats. *Am J Vet Res 42*:1704, 1990.
71. Shannon JA: Glomerular filtration and urea excretion in relation to urine flow in the dog. *Am J Physiol 117*:206, 1936.
72. Shannon JA, et al: The measurement of glucose Tm in the normal dog. *Am J Physiol 133*:752, 1941.
73. Shils ME: Renal disease and the metabolic effects of tetracycline. *Ann Intern Med 58*:389, 1963.
74. Smith HW: *The Kidney: Structure and Function in Health and disease*. Oxford University Press, London, 1951.
75. Spielman WS, Osswald H: Characterization of the postocclusive response of renal blood flow in the cat. *Am J Physiol 235*:F286, 1978.
76. Steinhausen M, et al: Visualization of renal autoregulation in the split hydronephrotic kidney of rats. *Kidney Int 35*:1151, 1989.
77. Street AE, et al: Prolonged blood urea elevation observed in the beagle after feeding. *Toxicol Appl Pharmacol 13*:363, 1968.
78. Strombeck DR, et al: Hyperammonemia due to a urea cycle enzyme deficiency in two dogs. *J Am Vet Med Assoc 166*:1109, 1975.
79. Sutton RAL, Dirks JH: Calcium and magnesium: Renal handling and disorders of metabolism. *In* Brenner BM, Rector FC (eds): *The Kidney*. W. B. Saunders, Philadelphia, 1986, pp 551–618.
80. Suzuki A: Micropuncture study of distal tubular function of cat kidney. *Jpn J Pharmacol 21*:75, 1971.
81. Swanson RE, Hakim AA: Stop-flow analysis of creatinine secretion in the dog. *Am J Physiol 203*:9880, 1962.
82. Veldkamp PJ, et al: Direct evaluation of the microvascular actions of ANP in juxtamedullary nephrons. *Am J Physiol 254*:F440, 1988.
83. Von Baeyer H, et al: Determination of transport constants for glucose in proximal tubules of the rat kidney. *Pfluegers Arch 343*:273, 1973.
84. Wen SF, et al: Micropuncture study of magnesium transport in proximal and distal tubule of the dog. *Am J Physiol 219*:570, 1970.
85. Westall RG: The amino acid and other ampholytes of urine. 2. Isolation of a new sulfur-containing amino acid from cat urine. *Biochem J 55*:244, 1953.
86. White JV: Diagnostic approach to proteinuria. *In* Kirk RW (ed): *Current Veterinary Therapy X*. W. B. Saunders, Philadelphia, 1989, pp 1139–1141.
87. Williams RH, et al: Autoregulation of nephron filtration rate in the dog assessed by indicator-dilution technique. *Am J Physiol 233*:F282, 1977.
88. Woods LL, et al: Mechanisms controlling renal hemodynamic and electrolyte excretion during amino acids. *Am J Physiol 251*:F303, 1986.

CHAPTER

102 Pathophysiology and Therapeutics of Urinary Tract Disorders

Kenneth C. Bovée, Anne E. Rosin, and Benjamin L. Hart
Revised by Dale E. Bjorling

RENAL INSUFFICIENCY AND RENAL FAILURE

This section deals with reduced renal function in three characterized syndromes: urinary tract obstruction, acute renal failure, and chronic renal failure. Detection of these syndromes requires clinical and laboratory data from a routine examination. After confirmation, the syndrome should be analyzed to determine severity, causal factors, and therapeutic approaches. A surgeon's most common questions concerning an animal with renal failure are, Is the animal safe for surgery? What is the rationale for surgery? Is renal failure reversible? What are the relative benefits and risks of surgery?

The three syndromes have significant pragmatic value, because each is easily recognized and requires different medical and surgical treatment. Each syndrome is caused by a large number of abnormalities that affect renal function. After the diagnosis is confirmed, natural distinctive characteristics, categories of pathophysiology, and specific etiologies become apparent.

Renal insufficiency is defined as reduction in renal function in the absence of dramatic clinical signs. Renal insufficiency may be transient or permanent and may occur in any of these three syndromes. Overt clinical signs or significant azotemia may not be recognized until renal function has been reduced by 70 per cent of normal. The term *renal failure* refers to more significant loss of renal function with dramatic clinical signs. Failure usually implies the loss of a major portion of renal tissue on a permanent basis. Renal failure is associated with a group of metabolic abnormalities termed *uremia*.

Urinary Tract Obstruction

Obstruction of urine outflow is a common and potentially reversible cause of renal failure. Urinary tract obstruction is generally divided into two forms, acute and chronic. When acute obstruction is complete and bilateral, it threatens life. Death results within 65 to 70 hours if the obstruction is not relieved. After relief of the obstruction, renal function may return to normal in several days. Acute incomplete or acute unilateral obstruction might not be clinically obvious. Overdistension of the bladder and subsequent loss of detrusor function are most often encountered after acute, complete urethral obstruction of 3 to 5 days duration but can be observed after long-standing partial urethral obstruction.

Chronic urinary tract obstruction is commonly unilateral or incomplete and may remain unrecognized for long periods. If obstruction persists, the kidney may be irreversibly damaged. The presence of chronic obstruction may be obvious or silent. It may be recognized readily with anuria, dysuria, or abdominal pain or may be undetected for long periods with manifestations of pyuria, fever, or vague abdominal pain. Urinary tract obstruction is secondary to other diseases of the urinary tract, abdomen, or pelvis.

Causes

The incidence of acute obstruction is generally thought to be higher than that of chronic obstruction, but many cases of chronic obstruction are undetected. Males have a higher incidence than females owing to different anatomy of the urethra. A combination of factors, including diameter of the urethra, predisposition to metabolic urinary calculi in males, and obstruction due to prostatic disease, contributes to the higher incidence in males. Obstruction may be mechanical or functional. The most common mechanical cause of obstruction is urinary calculi (Chapters 108 and 110). The most common cause of functional obstruction is neurogenic or atonic bladder (see the later section on urine incontinence). Acute obstruction is usually not associated with anatomical defects of the urinary tract. In contrast, chronic obstruction is commonly associated with neoplasia, strictures, urolithiasis, atonic bladder, and prostatic diseases.

Clinical Signs and Laboratory Findings

The clinical signs of acute complete obstruction are straining on urination, increased frequency of attempts to urinate, dysuria with oliguria or anuria, and abdominal pain. Table 102–1 outlines the clinical and laboratory data commonly used to identify urinary tract obstruction and distinguish it from acute or chronic renal failure. Pain due to urinary tract obstruction is secondary to stretching of the collecting system or renal capsule. The severity of pain appears to correlate with the rate of distension rather than the degree of dilation. Pain is usually associated with anorexia, restlessness, and stranguria.

Clinical signs of chronic obstruction may include moderate polydipsia and polyuria, which might not be associated with azotemia. It should be emphasized that large volumes of urine suggest rather than rule against chronic obstructive disease. Animals with chronic obstruction may not show symptoms of uremia until renal failure is far advanced.

Animals with acute obstruction have a tense and

TABLE 102–1. CLINICAL AND LABORATORY DATA BASE

Finding	Urinary Tract Obstruction	Acute Renal Failure	Chronic Renal Failure
Azotemia	X	X	X
Uremic symptoms		X	X
Urinary retention	X		
Edema/ascites		X	X
Anuria/oliguria	X	X	
Tender bladder	X		
Distended bladder after voiding	X		
Gross polyuria			X
Blood chemistry			
↑ Urea nitrogen/ creatinine	X	X	X
↑ or ↓ sodium			
↑ potassium	X	X	
↑ chloride or ↓ carbon dioxide		X	X
↑ phosphorus	X	X	X
↑ or ↓ calcium			X
Blood count anemia			X
Urinalysis			
proteinuria		X	X
glycosuria	X	X	
casts		X	X

painful abdomen, distended urinary bladder, engorged external genitalia, and enlarged and sensitive kidneys. Azotemia will ultimately result in vomiting, "uremia breath," dehydration, and hypothermia. Labored respiration may be observed owing to metabolic acidosis. A sterile catheter should be passed into the urethra to determine its patency. Careful rectal examination and abdominal palpation are essential to evaluate pelvic or abdominal masses.

Physical findings associated with chronic obstruction are more discrete, and affected animals may require special diagnostic tests including radiography. Abdominal palpation may reveal an enlarged kidney or bladder or other abdominal masses such as a tumor or cystic calculus. Observation of the voiding pattern and force of the urine stream may suggest bladder atony. Hematuria is commonly noted by owners. This finding suggests calculi, infection, inflammatory disease, or neoplasia.

Laboratory evaluation should include a urinalysis, urine culture, complete blood count, plasma creatinine concentration, and sodium, potassium, calcium, chloride, and phosphorus measurements if azotemia is present. Obstruction is usually associated with microscopic and gross hematuria. Careful examination of urine sediment is particularly important during chronic obstruction to determine the presence of inflammatory or infectious disease.

Urine is commonly dilute in all forms of obstruction. Glycosuria occurs transiently during and after acute obstruction. Azotemia due to acute obstruction is marked by elevated plasma creatinine and urea nitrogen levels, hyperphosphatemia, hyperkalemia, and metabolic acidosis.

Animals with chronic obstruction may be azotemic after a variable period of time associated with chronic renal failure. There are no specific blood chemistry tests to distinguish urinary tract obstruction from other causes of chronic failure.

Pathophysiology

The effects of urinary tract obstruction on renal function must be considered during and after relief of obstruction. Dramatic changes in renal function occur during the first 24 hours of complete bilateral obstruction. After relief of obstruction, sodium and water excretion in the urine markedly increases despite a severe reduction in glomerular filtration rate (GFR), a natriuretic state referred to as postobstructive diuresis. After relief of unilateral obstruction or incomplete obstruction, there may be no dramatic increase in sodium and water excretion, even though fractional excretion of these substances is increased from the previously obstructed kidney. During unilateral obstruction, the nonobstructed kidney undergoes changes that may mask the presence of obstruction in the opposite kidney. Relief of chronic obstruction usually leads to less dramatic changes in renal function.

Urine-concentrating capacity is the first function lost after any form of urinary tract obstruction.[110] GFR and renal plasma flow are decreased during acute obstruction.[15, 39] Loss of the ability to excrete acid occurs when urine is not excreted.

After 24 hours of complete ureteral obstruction in dogs, renal blood flow decreases to approximately 50 per cent of normal.[108] This reduction occurs in both unilateral and bilateral complete obstruction. During chronic unilateral obstruction, renal blood flow progressively decreases and, after 2 months, flow is about 10 per cent of normal.[102]

After relief of complete obstruction of 24 hours duration, renal blood flow returns to approximately 60 per cent of normal in dogs.[108] It appears that renal blood flow gradually returns to normal over a period of days after relief of obstruction.

During acute bilateral urinary tract obstruction, GFR is markedly reduced and is approximately 20 per cent of normal immediately after relief of 24 hours of obstruction.[109] Although GFR returns toward normal, as does renal blood flow, after relief of obstruction, it remains reduced for several days. During chronic obstruction, GFR is variably decreased from 20 to 70 per cent of normal.[107] After relief of unilateral obstruction, recovery of GFR to between 50 and 75 per cent occurs within 6 weeks in dogs.[76] These results suggest that a return of renal function may be seen after relief of chronic obstruction and may be greater if the more severely obstructed kidney is released first.

Postobstructive diuresis that occurs immediately after relief of obstruction is an important phenomenon related to renal function. This diuresis is marked by a transient increase in urine volume and excessive loss of solutes in the urine. Urine is usually dilute and contains large quantities of sodium, leading to inappropriate losses after the relief of bilateral obstruction. The phenomenon of postobstructive diuresis has been described in cats with complete urethral obstruction.[22] Excessive urinary loss of sodium may lead to negative sodium balance persisting for 2 days after the relief of obstruction. A concomitant loss of excessive water in the urine may persist for 3 to 4 days. Although an animal may have dramatic polyuria and may suffer from dehydration, serum sodium concentration remains normal during the diuresis.

During acute bilateral obstruction, plasma potassium concentration increases. After relief of obstruction, potassium loss in the urine increases.[15] Excessive urinary potassium loss during the postobstructive diuresis may lead to a negative potassium balance 3 to 5 days after relief of the obstruction. Although the functional defect is self-limiting, it may lead to significant hypokalemia during the diuretic phase.

Reduced ability to concentrate the urine is a feature of almost all types of obstruction. After relief of bilateral obstruction, many factors may influence urine concentration, including decreased reabsorption of filtrate resulting in increased delivery in collecting ducts, increased osmotic load per nephron due to azotemia, and a direct effect of sustained increase in intrapelvic hydrostatic pressure on collecting duct transport. The clinical significance of the concentrating defect is potential dehydration that may occur for several days after relief of obstruction.

During acute obstruction, metabolic acidosis occurs in both cats and dogs.[22, 104] After relief of 24 hours of unilateral obstruction, urine pH and plasma bicarbonate are decreased, which may lead to acidosis for a short interval.

Urethral obstruction (complete or partial) can cause overdistension of the bladder, resulting in loss of tight junctions within the bladder wall. Impaired detrusor function may improve in response to drug therapy, but the owner should be informed that this may be permanent.

Treatment

Animals with acute complete obstruction have a potentially lethal disease that must be treated immediately. The site of blockage must be determined and the obstruction removed as soon as possible. The most direct measure is to bypass the obstruction with a catheter that decompresses the fluid column behind the obstruction. Surgical correction of the primary disease is advisable as soon as the patient is stabilized. Severe acidosis, hyperkalemia, and azotemia may preclude immediate surgery. Animals with azotemia, hypothermia, and dehydration should be hospitalized for intensive treatment.

An intravenous catheter should be placed in a peripheral vein for administration of warmed fluids (2.5 per cent dextrose in 0.5 per cent saline) to replace the estimated fluid deficit, which ranges between 5 and 15 per cent. Rate of administration should be 5 to 15 ml/kg/hour. Expansion of the extracellular fluid volume may partially correct the reduced GFR associated with obstruction.[26] The urinary obstruction should be mechanically relieved or the bladder decompressed per urethra or by cystocentesis with a urinary catheter that can be maintained in the bladder (cystostomy catheter). Based on the severity of clinical signs or on specific measurement of the severity of acidosis, sodium bicarbonate should be administered intravenously. The rate varies between 3 and 9 mEq/kg, depending on the severity of clinical signs. Half of the calculated dose is given as a slow intravenous bolus and the rest administered intravenously with the rehydrating fluids during the next few hours. When the fluid deficit has been replaced, administration of fluid is slowed to the maintenance rate of 60 to 80 ml/kg/day. When serum potassium is normal, a balanced electrolyte solution is substituted for the dextrose/saline solution. Although potassium-containing solutions are contraindicated initially because of hyperkalemia, reduced potassium intake combined with increased urinary potassium loss tends to cause hypokalemia during recovery, possibly resulting in anorexia, muscle weakness, ileus, and bladder atony. This may be corrected by adding 10 to 20 mEq of potassium to each liter of maintenance fluids or by giving oral potassium supplementation.

Using these measures, azotemia should be corrected within 24 to 48 hours after initiation of treatment. In some animals, fluid administration must be dramatically increased to match urinary output. Potassium supplementation is usually not necessary once animals begin to eat voluntarily. Permanent surgical correction of the mechanical obstruction may take place as soon as hyperkalemia, acidosis, and severe azotemia are corrected. The timing of surgery is highly variable, depending on the severity of these metabolic abnormalities; it may require 6 to 48 hours to make the patient stable for surgery.

Chronic incomplete obstruction usually requires extensive radiographic studies to confirm the diagnosis. Complications of obstruction, such as renal failure, anemia, calculi, and infection, require specific management before or after surgery. Surgical correction need not be hastily entered into in the majority of cases.

Finally, all animals that have had recurrent obstruction with or without infection require careful long-term surveillance. Periodic evaluation should include complete physical examination, urinalysis, urine culture, and renal function tests, as well as a radiographic examination.

Acute Renal Failure

Acute renal failure is defined as recent loss of renal function owing to potentially reversible damage of the renal parenchyma. It may be difficult to distinguish from chronic renal failure. Anuria or oliguria may be present during the early stages of the disease but may change to polyuria, which may be confusing. Additional evidence is the occurrence of renal failure without anemia, a finding that is less common in chronic renal failure. Rapid increases in blood urea nitrogen (BUN), serum creatinine, potassium, and phosphate concentrations and metabolic acidosis are consistent findings. It is particularly helpful to know if the serum creatinine concentration and GFR were normal within a reasonable time before the illness. Hence, these measurements should be part of the data base in all "at risk" patients.

Causes

Reduced renal hemodynamics represent a major predisposing factor to acute renal failure.[32] Reduced renal perfusion, hypotension, hypovolemia, and sudden circulatory collapse are the most common initiating factors. These may result from a large number of disease processes, including hemorrhage, trauma, prolonged anesthesia, extensive surgery, and reduced cardiovascular function.

Various nephrotoxins may also cause acute renal failure, including heavy metals, organic compounds, antimicrobial agents, pigments, acute infectious agents, and hypercalcemia. Antimicrobials are important nephrotoxins, particularly the aminoglycosides and amphotericin B. The aminoglycoside gentamicin disrupts renal tubular cell function and causes ultrastructural changes in the glomeruli.[4, 13] The onset of acute renal failure due to aminoglycosides ranges from a few days to 2 weeks. Therefore, the onset of clinical signs is much later than with primary reduction of renal hemodynamics. Hypercalcemic nephropathy as a result of malignancy may also cause acute renal failure. Serum calcium concentrations in excess of 13 mg/100 ml may result in a renal concentrating defect, tubular necrosis, and calcification of the kidney.[27] Hypervitaminosis D may cause a similar nephropathy.[93]

Clinical Signs and Laboratory Findings

Animals with acute renal failure are generally depressed, hypovolemic, and hypothermic and have acute and severe gastrointestinal signs. Kidneys are usually normal in size or enlarged. Oliguria with concentrated urine suggests acute rather than chronic renal failure. Laboratory studies should include a complete blood count; BUN, serum creatinine, sodium, potassium, phosphorus, and calcium determinations; acid-base evaluation; and urinalysis (see Table 102–1). The complete blood count is usually nonspecific unless there is an infectious cause. Animals with acute renal failure usually have a normal hematocrit, whereas those with chronic renal failure tend to have anemia. Moderate to severe azotemia is usually present. Serum inorganic phosphorus is elevated, as in chronic failure. Hyperkalemia and acidosis are commonly present in acute failure but would not be expected until the terminal stages of chronic failure. Serum potassium concentration may range from 6 to 10 mEq/L. Acidosis is commonly accompanied by deep and labored respiratory motions. Bicarbonate deficits are frequently 5 to 15 mEq/L.

Urinalysis may be helpful in differentiating acute failure from other forms of renal failure. Urinary concentrating capacity is lost in the early stages of this disease, but urine specific gravity in the absence of fluid deprivation is highly variable. Proteinuria and glycosuria are commonly present. Glycosuria is usually transient and is due to reduced tubular reabsorption of glucose. A urine sediment examination is helpful to confirm acute failure, because the sediment may contain many casts that suggest an acute inflammatory or ischemic process. Increased activity of urine enzymes as an early indicator of aminoglycoside nephrotoxicosis has been investigated in sheep.[37, 38] Concentrations of specific enzymes increased in the urine several days before overt evidence of functional damage.

Radiographic studies to confirm acute failure are of limited practical value. Normal or enlarged kidneys suggest acute failure, in contrast to small, shrunken kidneys, which suggest chronic disease. Conventional intravenous urograms are seldom helpful in differentiating the two forms of disease, because reduced blood flow to the kidneys occurs in both. A renal arteriogram may confirm the presence of the normal vascular pattern and suggest acute failure. However, this procedure is not practical and may not be safe in many cases of acute failure during the early stages of the disease. Whether contrast radiography further decreases renal function in this situation is controversial.

The diagnosis may be confirmed by renal biopsy. A biopsy may be helpful to rule out chronic renal disease, but it seldom provides a specific etiology or prognosis in acute failure. A wedge biopsy or even a percutaneous needle biopsy may be contraindicated owing to the dangers of anesthesia and bleeding tendencies associated with renal failure.

Pathophysiology

Acute renal failure occurs in four stages: (1) onset, (2) oliguric or maintenance stage, (3) diuretic stage, and (4) recovery. During the initial stage, the renal insult occurs followed by reduction in glomerular filtration and urine volume. The time period varies from 1 to a few days. The oliguric or maintenance stage may persist for several days or weeks, with continued reduction in GFR and oliguria. During this time, the initiating factors of failure persist or trigger additional factors that maintain the disease. The diuretic phase is recognized by a progressive increase in urine output that may or may not be associated with improved renal function. Urine volume may increase dramatically for 1 to 2 weeks while healing and repair continue or while the disease process is maintained. If azotemia subsides during the diuretic phase, a recovery phase begins and may last for days or weeks. Complete stabilization of renal function may require 1 to 2 months, and the animal may be left with subclinical chronic renal failure.

Four major mechanisms participate in the production and maintenance of acute failure. No single event or sequence of events uniformly represents the pathophysiological sequence.[29] After an ischemic or nephrotoxic insult, alterations in renal hemodynamics, cellular injury to the glomerulus, arteriolar vasoconstriction, tubular ischemia, tubular leakage, intratubular obstruction, and decreased glomerular permeability occur. The exact sequence of these events is unclear. If nephrotoxins are the initial insult, it is presumed that altered function and structure of tubules and glomeruli are primary, with hemodynamic changes occurring as a secondary event. When ischemia is the initial insult, vasoconstriction appears to initiate reduced renal blood flow, filtration formation, and urine output. In the maintenance stages, many of these factors appear to be interrelated to maintain vasoconstriction, tubular back-leak, and altered glomerular permeability.

Treatment

Surgery is seldom indicated in the treatment of acute renal failure. In fact, surgery is likely to be contraindicated in most animals because of hyperkalemia, acidosis, and prolonged bleeding time. Treatment is divided into conservative measures and dialysis. Conservative measures are directed at correcting major metabolic disturbances such as reduced extracellular fluid volume, hyperkalemia, acidosis, and azotemia. The first priority is correction of renal hemodynamic disorders and alleviation of biochemical abnormalities until renal repair can take place.

Conservative measures can be pursued only when an indwelling intravenous catheter is maintained for repeated sampling of blood and administration of fluid and electrolytes. A catheter that will remain secure and sterile for several days should be implanted. The animal should be given a reduced dose of antibiotics (owing to renal failure) to prevent vascular infection. A urinary catheter attached to a closed sterile drainage system is placed in the urinary bladder for continuous measurement of urine volume.

Diuretic agents have been advocated in the treatment of oliguric acute renal failure when volume replacement alone fails to initiate urine production. The protective effects of diuretics are related to reduced vascular resistance, increased renal blood flow, and increased solute excretion.[31] These agents are of little benefit during the maintenance stage and later than 12 to 24 hours after initiation of acute failure. Mannitol has been extensively used and reported to improve renal function and survival secondary to traumatic injury, surgery, and shock. In dogs, mannitol increases GFR, renal blood flow, urine output, and survival when administered before or shortly after the induction of several models of acute renal failure.[11, 21, 77, 90]

After surgery, trauma, or nephrotoxic exposure resulting in oliguria, mannitol administration may be of considerable benefit in protecting renal function. Infusion of 0.25 to 0.5 g/kg given with fluid replacement to dogs is beneficial. If diuresis results, a maintenance infusion of 5 to 10 per cent mannitol in normal saline or a balanced electrolyte solution can be continued to promote diuresis for 12 to 24 hours. If diuresis does not occur within 1 hour of the first dose, additional doses should not be given.

Expansion of extracellular fluid volume using isotonic saline or hypertonic saline is of little benefit compared with mannitol.[77] Although hypertonic glucose has been suggested in place of mannitol, there are no clinical or experimental studies to support its efficacy in acute failure. If osmolar excretion is the major factor in protecting renal function in acute renal failure, mannitol is likely to be more effective than glucose owing to its limited volume of distribution and specific influence on renal hemodynamics and tubular reabsorption.

Diuretics that work on the loop of Henle have been recommended for treatment of acute failure. These agents have been inconsistently effective compared with mannitol in improving renal function experimentally. The efficacy of these agents in clinical medicine remains controversial. The use of dopamine or dobutamine in conjunction with mannitol enhances renal blood flow in dogs with acute renal failure.[69]

Metabolic acidosis is treated in a manner similar to that described for urinary obstruction. Repeated bicarbonate administration every 6 to 12 hours may be necessary for several days to combat acidosis.

The management of persistent hyperkalemia and severe azotemia requires more aggressive therapy during the second and third days of acute failure if conservative management is not adequate. Peritoneal dialysis and hemodialysis may be considered and applied for 3 to 14 days until it is clear whether renal function will return and be adequate to support the animal. Peritoneal dialysis and hemodialysis are discussed elsewhere (Chapter 103).[84, 99]

Chronic Renal Failure

In chronic renal failure, GFR has been reduced for a long interval, and there is little likelihood of rapid deterioration or hope of significant improvement. This diagnosis includes all degrees of azotemia including renal insufficiency, which may be detected before the uremic symptoms appear. The duration is months to years.

Causes

The causes of chronic failure are multiple, varied, and commonly unknown. The causes are not detailed here. The causes of chronic failure are usually not surgical diseases and cannot be corrected by surgical intervention. The exceptions include diseases resulting in chronic urinary tract obstruction and pyelonephritis. When animals are presented with clinical signs of chronic renal failure, the cause cannot be determined with certainty at the end-stage. A renal biopsy with tissue diagnosis of chronic interstitial nephritis reveals little about the pathogenesis or time course of the disease.

A prospective study of 111 dogs with chronic renal disease found that in dogs for which histological diagnosis was available (76), glomerular (52 per cent) and nonglomerular (48 per cent) disease each accounted for nearly half of the cases. This study concluded that although interstitial nephritis occurs frequently in dogs, glomerular disease is a common cause of chronic renal failure in dogs.[70, 74]

Clinical Signs and Laboratory Findings

The common clinical and laboratory findings seen with chronic failure are outlined in Table 102–1. Evidence of chronicity includes stable azotemia and stable reduced GFR for more than 3 months and a gradual decline of function over years. Most animals have some degree of polyuria, anorexia, or osteodystrophy or small kidneys observed on routine x-ray films. In conjunction with signs of renal disease, nonresponsive anemia suggests chronic rather than acute failure.

Chronic renal failure in dogs and cats can also result in systemic hypertension.[18, 65] When more than 70 per cent of the total functional renal mass is lost, sodium and water are retained. Increased extracellular fluid has a direct effect on blood pressure, and systemic pressure also rises in an attempt to be more effective than sodium restriction alone in the regulation of blood pressure in these animals.[18]

Hyperphosphatemia or abnormalities in serum calcium concentration are indicators of chronicity but are seldom helpful, because serum phosphorus alterations may also be present in acute failure. Chronic failure may also include the coexistence of acute renal failure, which may obscure the duration of disease. Chronic failure includes irreversible nephron loss with permanent reduction in renal function, whereas acute failure includes reductions in GFR resulting from reversible causes such as volume depletion, heart failure, and urinary tract obstruction. Although these factors are generally minor and their correction usually does not return GFR to an improved state, they should be recognized and corrected. The value of the search for reversible factors contributing to chronic failure is often determined by judgment of the severity and duration of azotemia.

Metabolic Abnormalities in Uremia

As chronic failure progresses, a number of complex alterations in renal function occur to maintain metabolic balance until the later stages of renal failure. These functional responses to nephron loss have been described for dogs.[16] Three basic patterns of adaptation occur during progressive renal failure in regard to specific types of solutes. For example, one group of solutes has a pattern of no regulation by surviving nephrons. These solutes, including urea and creatinine, are characterized by a rise in plasma concentration as GFR is reduced. A second group of solutes has limited regulation during renal failure (e.g., phosphate ion). Phosphate is excreted in higher quantities into the urine during the early stages of renal failure, resulting in normal plasma phosphate concentrations. However, adaptive ability fails when GFR falls below 25 per cent of normal, and plasma concentration progressively rises as GFR falls. A third pattern of solutes is associated with complete regulation (sodium and potassium). These solutes are regulated by renal tubular mechanisms that maintain normal plasma concentrations throughout the course of renal disease and failure.

The pattern of metabolic abnormalities in uremia is irregular. In some animals, regulatory failure may occur first for sodium and water. This may lead to inability to regulate extracellular fluid volume. Alternatively, inadequate production of erythropoietin may result in anemia as the first sign. Certain endocrinopathies may result in, for example, excess production of parathyroid hormone associated with malabsorption of calcium and impaired release of calcium ions from bone, or a group of vague gastrointestinal symptoms, malnutrition, anorexia, poor energy utilization, and abnormal metabolism of carbohydrates may lead to clinical signs. Therefore, during the early course of chronic failure, the presenting signs may be highly variable and confusing.

The rate of progression of chronic renal failure in 11 dogs was investigated. It was found that a plot of the reciprocal of the serum creatinine concentration versus age provided a regression line that accurately predicted the dog's age at the time of death due to chronic renal failure.[3] This technique should be validated in a larger study, but it may prove useful.

A typical animal with progressive chronic failure may pass through four stages.

Stage 1. During this stage there is only a reduction in renal reserve. Until at least 50 per cent of normal nephrons have been lost, there is no evidence of chemical abnormalities or azotemia. The excretory and regulatory functions of the kidneys are preserved in this stage, and clinical signs are absent. This stage is commonly missed in clinical evaluation unless renal clearance studies are performed

Stage 2. This stage may be termed *renal insufficiency*. Manifestations include mild azotemia, impaired ability to concentrate urine, nocturia, and polyuria. Anorexia may occur intermittently, but body weight and physical appearance are relatively normal. A mild anemia may be present. The animal is in a precarious state, which may be revealed by reduced fluid intake, vomiting, or diarrhea leading to more pronounced azotemia.

Stage 3. This stage is associated with persistent and frank renal failure with anemia, hyperphosphatemia, isosthenuria, and marked polyuria. Intermittent anorexia, weakness, listlessness, and intermittent vomiting with debilitation occur.

Stage 4. The final stage is uremia, when all the consequences of metabolic abnormalities become obvious. Clinical signs are more advanced than in stage 3 and include severe gastrointestinal disturbances, nervous signs, and severe anemia.

Consideration of these four stages is helpful to determine if animals are safe candidates for surgery. Those in stages 1 and 2 are generally considered safe for mandatory surgery but should be carefully evaluated for elective procedures, particularly if prolonged general anesthesia is required. Animals in stage 3 are poor candidates for general surgery. If surgery is necessary, renal function and the degree of metabolic abnormalities must be evaluated. During and after surgery, special care must be given to maintain extracellular fluid volume, renal blood flow, hematopoietic function, and electrolyte and acid-base balance.

The major metabolic abnormalities of uremia are listed in Table 102–2. All these abnormalities have been reviewed.[17] Three important and newly elucidated disturbances (endocrine disturbances, anemia, and renal osteodystrophy) are discussed here.

Uremia is associated with various endocrine abnormalities, including excessive production of hormones, inadequate production of hormones, reduced metabolic or renal clearance of hormones, and abnormal metabolism of hormones. In some cases, as with parathyroid hormone, clinical disturbances have been identified, and the role of the hormone has been clarified. The important polypeptide hormones that are not removed from

TABLE 102–2. METABOLIC DISTURBANCES OF UREMIA

Uremic toxins
Cellular function and composition
Biochemical disturbances
Nitrogen metabolism
Fat metabolism
Endocrine alterations
Gastrointestinal changes
Fluid, electrolyte, and acid-base changes
Hematological abnormalities
Renal osteodystrophy
Neurological changes
Cardiovascular abnormalities

the circulation in adequate quantities during renal failure include parathyroid hormone, glucagon, insulin, and pituitary hormones. Therefore, increased plasma concentrations of these hormones occur during renal failure (Table 102–3). Parathyroid hormone is a key element in renal osteodystrophy and is discussed later.

The significance of increases in plasma concentration of other polypeptide hormones such as growth hormone, prolactin, calcitonin, gastrin, and the sex hormone precursors is unclear. Increased plasma insulin concentration is associated with peripheral insensitivity to the action of insulin caused by a uremic toxin and reduced renal clearance of insulin during renal failure. Increased glucagon concentrations are related to carbohydrate metabolism but may also have a role in the regulation of blood flow to specific tissues during renal failure. Decreased production of hormones such as erythropoietin and thyroid hormone may have a role in the uremic syndrome.

It is clear that reduced erythropoietin production during renal failure leads to reduced production of red blood cells. Reduced thyroid function may be partly due to a defect in the peripheral conversion of thyroxin to T_3 (triiodothyronine). Although some uremic subjects have reduced plasma thyroid hormone concentrations, it is not clear whether this reflects the metabolic state of subjects with renal failure. A reduced thyroid hormone concentration may be appropriate for subjects with reduced metabolism due to renal failure. The side effects of these multiple endocrinopathies and their interrelationships may explain many of the mechanisms of metabolic disturbances in uremia.

The anemia of chronic renal failure may be a major limiting factor in survival of these animals. Fatigue, listlessness, weakness, and anorexia are clinical signs contributed to by the presence of anemia. The pathogenesis of anemia includes deficiency of erythropoietin. Experiments in animals suggest that reduction in the availability of this hormone is the central factor in reduced erythropoiesis, and replacement of the hormone increases bone marrow production.[101] In an experimental model of chronic renal disease in dogs, it was shown that increased concentrations of parathyroid hormone had a negative effect on erythropoietin concentrations, but this effect did not completely explain anemia associated with chronic renal disease.[85] Reduced erythrocyte life span may also be a factor contributing to anemia. The hemostatic mechanism is abnormal during uremia, leading to insidious loss of erythrocytes. The major hemostatic defect in uremia appears to be related to abnormal platelet function. The result may be prolonged bleeding time although the number of circulating platelets is normal. This qualitative platelet defect has been described in dogs with acute renal failure.[68] It is likely that the most significant blood loss during uremia is through insidious gastrointestinal bleeding.

Renal osteodystrophy is a major metabolic abnormality with widespread secondary effects. Although the bony changes may be associated with rubber jaw, a fractured mandible, or bowed long bones, the most devastating lesions may occur in soft tissues and may lead to progression of renal failure. The pathogenesis of renal osteodystrophy involves three main abnormalities: malabsorption of calcium, altered vitamin D metabolism, and hyperparathyroidism. Their interrelationships are shown in a simplified schematic fashion in Figure 102–1. Chronic failure is characterized by marked impairment in the intestinal absorption of calcium. This intestinal defect appears restricted to the vitamin D–dependent active or carrier-mediated calcium transport sites in the duodenum and jejunum. The defect appears to be a derangement of vitamin D metabolism. Because $1,25\text{-}(OH)_2D_3$ functions principally to regulate calcium absorption, acquired alterations in its production by

TABLE 102–3. ALTERATIONS IN PLASMA CONCENTRATION OF SOME HORMONES IN UREMIA

Increased	Decreased
Parathyroid hormone	Somatomedin
Growth hormone	Erythropoietin
Prolactin	Triiodothyronine
Insulin	Testosterone
Glucagon	
Calcitonin	
Gastrin	
Follicle-stimulating hormone	
Luteinizing hormone	

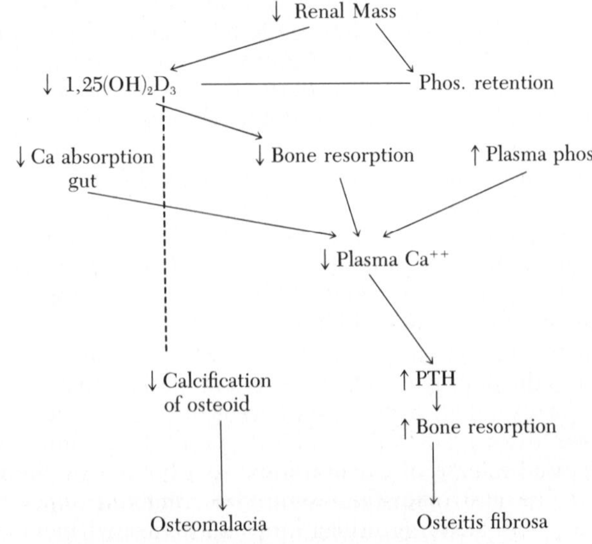

FIGURE 102–1. Pathogenesis of renal osteodystrophy.

renal disease could have a major role in altering the intestinal absorption of calcium.

Secondary hyperparathyroidism in uremic patients represents the cellular and biochemical adaptations of the parathyroid gland to sustained reduction in calcium intake or slight hypocalcemia. As a result of excessive parathyroid hormone release, serum calcium concentration remains normal during renal failure owing to a release of calcium from bone stores. In this situation, the parathyroid gland enters an autonomous secretory state. Control of phosphate balance is achieved primarily by renal excretion of filtered phosphate, with parathyroid hormone having a significant role. The subsequent rise in circulating parathyroid hormone promotes a greater degree of phosphaturia by the remaining nephrons and normalizes circulating phosphate concentration. Hyperphosphatemia was initially caused by reduced GFR but is now corrected by altered tubular excretion of phosphate due to parathyroid hormone. The importance of phosphate balance in the control of hyperparathyroidism has been confirmed in studies using uremic dogs, in which it was found that dietary phosphate restriction controls hyperparathyroidism.[60] The long-standing increases in circulating parathyroid hormone have several effects in addition to remodeling bone.

Several toxic effects have been attributed to excessive parathyroid hormone, and this substance may now be considered a uremic toxin. As previously mentioned, increased parathyroid concentrations may contribute to the development of anemia. The possible relationship of excessive parathyroid hormone, calcium, and phosphorus abnormalities in uremia includes soft-tissue calcification, bone pain, fractures, retarded growth, neuropathy, altered mental state, and sodium and bicarbonate renal reabsorption. The most significant of these is probably soft-tissue calcification. Both metastatic and dystrophic calcification occur during chronic failure. Metastatic calcification is a reflection of abnormal chemical balance resulting in mineral deposition in normal tissues. Hyperphosphatemia or an increased [calcium] × [phosphate] product probably is an important component in this complication. It is generally believed that when the [calcium] × [phosphate] product is greater than 60, soft-tissue calcification occurs. Although the tissue sites of calcification have not been carefully quantitated in uremic animals, mineralization is common in the lungs, kidneys, arteries, stomach, and myocardium. The significance of soft-tissue calcification is that it may cause serious injury to renal tissues and further advance renal failure. This observation leads to the therapeutic approach of dietary phosphate restriction or other medical management of phosphate concentration.

METABOLIC CONSEQUENCES AND ALTERED RENAL FUNCTION AFTER URINARY DIVERSION

Urinary diversion procedures include ureteroileostomy, ureterosigmoidostomy, trigonal-colonic anastomosis, transureteroureterostomy, and cutaneous end ureterostomy. Experience with these procedures is primarily in dogs. The objectives of urinary diversion are to provide for adequate urinary drainage, to preserve renal function, and to minimize secondary effects of diversion. Untoward consequences are not expected when a technically competent transureteroureterostomy is performed.[30] Problems associated with the use of bowel as a urinary conduit include ascending infection resulting in pyelonephritis and reduced renal function, electrolyte imbalances secondary to absorption of urinary solutes, and stenosis at the site of intestinal anastomosis causing impaired ureteral function, leakage of urine, or progressive hydronephrosis. The problems of cutaneous end ureterostomy in domestic animals have not been studied because this procedure is considered impractical in domestic animals.

Infection of the upper urinary tract is a major concern when using any urinary diversion technique.[111] Infections include pyelonephritis, pyelitis, and ureteritis. Pyelonephritis is the most serious infection, because it may lead to reduced renal function or permanent loss of renal mass. Ureteritis may also be important in that it leads to altered function of the submucosal ureter, which may allow vesicoureteral reflux and renal infection.[29] Vesicoureteral reflux in the presence of chronic partial urethral obstruction can result in loss of normal peristaltic contraction of the ureter.[58] Bacterial cultures from the ureters, renal pelvis, and renal parenchyma usually contain the same organisms as those found in the gastrointestinal contents (i.e., *Escherichia coli, Proteus* spp., and *Klebsiella*). The incidence of pyelonephritis in dogs with trigonal-colonic anastomosis was 30 per cent regardless of duration of anastomosis.[19] Similar results were found with trigonal-ileal anastomosis and ureterocolonic anastomosis in dogs.[86, 96] The rate of pyelonephritis in ureteroileostomy varied from 25 to 80 per cent.[87, 92] In similar studies, the incidence of pyelonephritis ranged from 7 to 67 per cent for ureterosigmoidostomy.[89, 92] The lower incidence of pyelonephritis after diversion to the large bowel seemed to be related to the preservation of a normal ureterovesicular junction, as in trigonal-colonic anastomosis, or to the creation of a long submucosal tunnel, as in ureterocolonic anastomosis. The valvelike function of these structures is thought to protect against ascending infection.[75] This so-called antireflux anastomosis prevents pressure waves within the lumen of the bowel from ascending the ureter to the renal pelvis, whereas end-to-side, mucosa-to-mucosa anastomosis allows transmission of pressure from the lumen of the bowel to the ureter.[59] Pyelonephritis was also found in 50 per cent of dogs with an ileal conduit to the skin.[94] Pyelonephritis may lead to rapid deterioration of renal function or it may persist as a minor infection that smolders for years without causing major renal insufficiency.

Abnormal levels of plasma electrolytes and other solutes are less likely with urine diversion into the colon compared with diversion into the small intestine.[59, 72] Electrolytes are more readily absorbed from the small intestine than from the colon. However, ureterocolonic anastomosis in dogs has been accompanied by uremia due to dehydration, ureteral obstruction, renal dysfunction or absorption of urea, and metabolic acidosis and hyperchloremia.[96, 97] In studies using isolated intestinal loops, it was found that chloride, urea, and phosphate are absorbed more readily than sodium or potassium. Bicarbonate is readily lost in an intestinal loop.[72] Serum inorganic phosphorus and blood urea are the most frequently increased constituents in the plasma as a result of absorption from the colon.[19] The increases in concentration may be minor, and values may remain in the high-normal range. It should be understood that these changes may have no relation to renal function in this situation.

Changes in glomerular filtration rate have been studied in dogs after trigonal-colonic anastomosis.[19] In dogs from which bacteria were not cultured from the kidneys, the mean reduction in GFR was only 12 per cent. In dogs from which bacteria were cultured from the kidneys, the mean decrease was 40 per cent. Although renal function as measured by filtration rate was reduced after the surgical procedure, serum creatinine values remained within normal limits. The decrease in GFR in dogs that did not have a kidney infection suggests that mild pyelitis or perhaps increased ureteral pressure may have been responsible for reduced renal hemodynamics.

Problems associated with urinary diversion are usually obvious within a few days of surgery. Their presence must be investigated along with other postsurgical problems such as stenosis at the site of anastomosis, hydronephrosis, abnormal gastrointestinal motility, and urinary obstruction. The metabolic complications mentioned previously must be distinguished from deterioration of renal function, which is monitored by long-term surveillance. Once the postsurgical period is passed without complications, serum creatinine measurements, intravenous urogram, or radioisotope imaging should be used to monitor renal function.

PATHOPHYSIOLOGY AND PHARMACOLOGICAL MANAGEMENT OF URINARY INCONTINENCE

Urinary incontinence is the failure of voluntary control of the urinary bladder and urethral sphincters, resulting in inability to control urination. Dysfunction of any of the various components that control micturition or the storage and voiding of urine can result in incontinence. This disorder is more common in dogs than in cats and in females than in males. An understanding of the anatomy of the lower urinary tract and of the physiology of normal urination and continence is essential if one is to establish the cause of urinary incontinence or institute proper drug therapy for the specific disorder (see Chapters 100 and 101).

Pathophysiology of Urinary Incontinence

Urinary incontinence and urinary outflow obstruction are frequently encountered in small animal practice. These problems can occur secondary to neurological lesions, hormonal imbalances, congenital abnormalities, and diseases of the bladder, urethra, or prostate gland.

Neurological Causes of Urinary Incontinence

Neurological lesions that affect micturition can usually be divided into upper motor neuron lesions and lower motor neuron lesions. Abnormalities of the cerebral cortex, brain stem, cerebellum, or spinal cord above the L7 spinal cord segment (L5 vertebral body) may result in incontinence and are considered upper motor neuron lesions with respect to micturition. Abnormalities of the sacral spinal cord segments or sacral nerve roots or branches may result in lower motor neuron incontinence.

Upper Motor Neuron Lesions

Lesions from the pons L7 spinal cord segments may result in detrusor areflexia, with hyperreflexia and increased tone of the external urethral sphincter. Thus, there is loss of voluntary control of urination, and manual expression of the bladder is difficult. One to two weeks following the injury, spinal reflexes usually initiate a sequence of bladder filling, contraction, and emptying, which is incomplete and involuntary. The bladder is referred to as spastic, hyperreflexic, or automatic. The external urethral sphincter remains hypertonic. The combination of incomplete bladder emptying and increased urethral resistance to urine flow results in residual urine.

Abnormalities of the cerebellum or partial long tract lesions may result in detrusor hyperreflexia with little or no residual urine. In these cases, urination is frequent and inappropriate. Partial long tract lesions may also result in detrusor urethral dyssynergia or reflex dyssynergia, a condition in which bladder contraction and urethral relaxation are not synchronous.[36] Interruption of the reflex pathways from the pelvic and pudendal nerve origin in the caudal spinal cord to the sympathetic origin in the thoracolumbar spinal cord may result in increased smooth-muscle tone of the urethra. Additionally, decreased inhibition of the skeletal muscle of the external urethral sphincter may contribute to increased outflow resistance. Reflex dyssynergia creates functional urethral obstruction, characterized by sudden cessation of voiding with continued straining to urinate and a residual urine volume. This condition mimics mechanical urethral obstruction.

Lower Motor Neuron Lesions

Injuries of the sacral spinal cord or nerve roots or branches may result in detrusor areflexia with or without sphincter areflexia. Atony of the detrusor muscle results in overdistension, which, if prolonged, may cause separation of the tight junctions and increased bladder capacity with large amounts of residual urine. If the pudendal nerve is damaged, the external urethral sphincter is incompetent. As the bladder fills and intravesical pressure increases, the sphincter is no longer able to maintain continence, and urine leakage occurs.

Non-Neurological Causes of Urinary Incontinence

Congenital Abnormalities

The most common congenital abnormality resulting in urinary incontinence is ectopic ureter (see Chapter 106). Although ectopic ureters may be found in both male and female dogs and cats, the abnormality is primarily associated with incontinence in female dogs.[82] If the ectopic ureters empty distal to the external urethral sphincter, involuntary dribbling of urine occurs. Surgery may correct the urinary incontinence, depending on the location of the ectopic ureters. Although dogs with vaginal ectopic ureters often become continent after surgery, there is a high incidence (50 to 60 per cent) of persistent urinary incontinence in female dogs whose ureters terminated in the urethra before surgery.[59, 101] This observation suggests inherent urethral incompetence, and treatment with phenylpropanolamine or diethylstilbestrol may improve continence after surgery.[89, 95]

Other congenital abnormalities that may result in urinary incontinence include patent urachus, urethrorectal fistulas, and urethrovaginal fistulas. In patients with patent urachus, urine is voided through the umbilicus, and surgical correction is warranted. Urethrorectal and urethrovaginal fistulas also require surgery for correction of incontinence.

Hormone-Responsive Urinary Incontinence

Estrogen-responsive incontinence in female dogs is an uncommon and poorly understood sequela to ovariohysterectomy. It develops in dogs after a variable period of time following surgery. The reported mean age of dogs in which this type of incontinence has been recognized is 8.3 years. The incidence of urinary incontinence in spayed female dogs has been reported to be 5 to 20 per cent, whereas the incidence of urinary incontinence in intact female dogs was less than 1 per cent.[5, 100] The pathogenesis of this syndrome is unclear; it appears that the proper maintenance and function of urethral mucosa and musculature are dependent on estrogen, and the removal of an important source of this hormone results in incontinence in some female dogs.[85] Estrogen therapy in ovariectomized female baboons was found to significantly increase urethral length, the length of the zone of increased pressure within the urethra corresponding to the sphincter mechanism, and maximal urethral closing pressure.[20]

Hormone-responsive incontinence has also been reported in a castrated male dog. The time of onset after castration and response to testosterone therapy supported an endocrine etiology. This syndrome is apparently similar to estrogen-responsive incontinence in neutered bitches.

Incontinence Due to Cystitis, Urethritis, or Prostatic Disease

The urinary bladder, urethra, and prostate gland are subject to non-neurogenic diseases that may result in incontinence of varying magnitude. An inflamed or irritated bladder may become hyperactive or unstable, resulting in a syndrome called *urge incontinence*, which is characterized by detrusor contractions that cannot be voluntarily inhibited. Loss of urine by uncontrolled detrusor contraction occurs immediately after a sensation of bladder fullness. Urge incontinence is often accompanied by increased frequency of urination and nocturia.[24, 82] Urge incontinence in humans is commonly associated with neurological or psychological abnormalities,[24] but in dogs it is recognized most frequently as a sequela to cystitis. Urinary incontinence due to detrusor instability and hyperactivity in the absence of bacterial cystitis and evidence of urge has been reported in dogs and cats.[67] It is also known as *small bladder syndrome* because the bladder is abnormally small and incapable of storing a normal volume of urine.

Chronic cystitis, urethritis, or prostatic disease can also cause urethral incompetence resulting in urinary incontinence. In these cases, as the bladder fills with urine and intravesical pressure increases, the diseased or damaged urethra is unable to prevent the flow of urine through its lumen. Dogs with urethral incompetence secondary to chronic prostatic disease may have a history of urethral obstruction during the acute phase of the disease.

Paradoxical Incontinence Due to Mechanical Obstruction of the Urethra

Mechanical obstruction of the urethra by calculi, foreign bodies, neoplasms, or strictures can result in paradoxical urinary incontinence. Resistance to urine flow through the urethra is increased by the obstruction, and normal micturition is hampered or cannot occur. As the bladder distends with urine, intravesical pressure exceeds the increased urethral resistance, and urinary incontinence results. Treatment of these disorders generally requires invasive techniques such as surgery or hydropropulsion of calculi.

Bladder Position and Urethral Length

Caudal displacement of the bladder (pelvic bladder) in female dogs has been variously reported to be a cause of urinary incontinence[1, 53] or an incidental finding.[57, 73] It is clear that not all female dogs with pelvic bladder suffer urinary incontinence, but the incidence of pelvic bladder may be higher in incontinent female dogs.[53] Caudal displacement of the bladder shortens urethral length, which may contribute to decreased pressure within the urethral sphincter and, subsequently, incontinence.[53] This concept is supported by the observation of improved urinary continence in female dogs with caudal displacement of the bladder treated by cranial displacement and fixation of the vagina.[54]

Idiopathic Urinary Incontinence

The specific cause of urinary incontinence occasionally cannot be determined. The urinary incontinence frequently is due to urethral incompetence, but a neurological, hormonal, or inflammatory basis for the urethral weakness cannot be proved. These cases can be considered idiopathic, and therapy should be attempted because results are often positive.

Diagnosis

An accurate history, recorded chronologically, is important in the diagnosis of the cause of urinary incontinence. The owner should be asked to describe the present problem and how the animal's urination habits have changed. Whether the onset of the micturition disorder paralleled or followed another disease or procedure should also be established. Knowledge of recent ovariohysterectomy, abdominal or neurological surgery, prostatic or urinary tract disease, or trauma could be important to the diagnosis.

Observation of the animal's urination, attempted urination, or lack of urination can provide important clues to the dysfunction. Measuring residual urine may provide additional information. Normally, residual urine volume should be less than 10 ml.[80]

The presence of voluntary control of urination is important in the diagnosis of urinary incontinence. If an animal initiates and maintains urination until the bladder is emptied, it can be assumed that a detrusor reflex is present and that functional urethral obstruction does not exist. If the animal dribbles urine, has a distended bladder, and does not voluntarily initiate urination, a denervated bladder is likely, and neurological examination will help localize the lesion. Dribbling of urine in an animal that can voluntarily urinate suggests urethral sphincter incompetence; normal initiation of urination followed by sudden interruption of urine flow and continued staining implies functional urethral obstruction or detrusor urethral dyssynergia. Increased frequency of urination, inappropriate urination, and urge incontinence may occur with inflammatory diseases of the bladder and urethra such as cystitis and urethritis with certain neurological diseases, or with idiopathic detrusor instability.

In addition to observation of urination, a complete physical and neurological examination is essential to the correct diagnosis of disorders of continence. Palpation and careful manual expression of the bladder provide information about bladder and urethral tone. Expression of the bladder in a male dog is more difficult than in a female dog, but in either sex if the bladder can be easily expressed with only slight pressure, the intrinsic tone of the urethra is probably decreased.

If the physical examination reveals dribbling of urine and an easily expressed bladder, the urethral sphincter mechanism is inefficient. A neurological examination should be carried out to assess concurrent deficits and localize the lesion. Diseases of the sacral spinal cord, sacral roots, or pudendal nerves can cause these clinical signs, and examination of the animal's perineal region for intact sensation and anal sphincter tone and reflexes should support such a diagnosis.

If neurological disease cannot be documented, other causes of urethral incompetence should be considered, including ectopic ureter syndrome, hormone-responsive urinary incontinence in neutered animals, and inefficiency of the urethra following prostatic or urethral disease.

Difficulty in expressing the bladder in a dog with signs of bladder-urethral incoordination is further evidence that dyssynergia exists. It is difficult on the basis of physical examination to determine whether the dyssynergia is somatic, with urethral striated muscle contraction, or sympathetic, with urethral smooth-muscle contraction. Response to therapy may provide the diagnosis. Strictly somatic dyssynergia is uncommon in human patients, and in those dyssynergics with somatic and sympathetic components, the major urethral resistance is due to sympathetic overdischarge.[8]

Increased urethral tone due to sympathetic discharge can occur in animals with cauda equina lesions such as intervertebral disc protrusion, lumbosacral instability, or cauda equina tumors. Interruption of the reflex pathway from the pelvic and pudendal nerve centers in the sacral spinal cord to the sympathetic center in the thoracolumbar cord can result in overdischarge of sympathetic impulses when the animal attempts to urinate or when manual expression of the bladder is attempted.[2, 10] Sympathetic tone in the urethra can increase rapidly and can be strong enough to cause functional obstruction to urination. This obstruction is largely due to smooth-muscle contraction, but striated urethral muscle via its sympathetic innervation will contribute to obstruction as well.

In all continence disorders, thorough examination must be performed for urinary tract infection or mechanical obstruction to urination. Urinalysis and urine culture may provide important information. Although urinary tract infection alone infrequently causes incontinence, it often exists concurrently, may exacerbate the signs, and should be treated definitively.

If functional obstruction is suspected but mechanical obstruction cannot be ruled out on the basis of physical and neurological examination, further examination of the urethra and bladder should be initiated. Catheterization of the bladder with no obstruction to passage of the catheter implies absence of mechanical obstruction of the urethra. Infrequently, urethral polyps or mucosal flaps can cause intermittent mechanical obstruction to urine flow but not to catheter passage, and these possibilities should be ruled out before a diagnosis of functional obstruction is made. Plain and contrast radiography can provide valuable information about the bladder and urethra and the patency of the urethral lumen.

Other diagnostic tests that are usually available through referral centers and that may be necessary in making a definitive diagnosis include the electromyogram (EMG), the cystometrogram (CMG), and the urethral pressure profile (UPP). EMG of the anal sphincter provides indirect information on the innervation of the urethral sphincter, because branches of the pudendal nerve innervate both structures. EMG of limb and paraspinal muscles may also aid in localizing a neurological lesion.

CMG measures intravesical pressure during a detrusor reflex, and, besides documenting the presence or absence of a detrusor reflex, provides information on threshold volume and pressure capacity, elasticity, and function of the bladder.[80]

UPP measures intraluminal urethral pressure and allows the effective closure pressure of the urethra at rest to be determined.[90] It can be a valuable tool in the diagnosis and management of certain types of urinary incontinence in dogs and may help identify the site and extent of urethral incompetence or obstruction. UPP was performed in 50 continent and 50 incontinent female dogs.[62, 58] Significant differences were identified between the two groups, but there was considerable overlap of data.[50] Only the resting urethral pressure is measured by UPP, and conditions that are not problems during rest, such as functional urethral obstruction, may not be diagnosed by UPP alone. However, clinical signs and the exclusion of mechanical obstruction by radiology and UPP allow a presumptive diagnosis of functional obstruction.

Treatment

Once the cause of urinary incontinence or obstruction has been identified, a therapeutic plan can be established. Micturition disorders that are responsive to specific drug therapy are listed in Table 102–4. These pharmacological agents have been tested in dogs either clinically or experimentally and have demonstrated effectiveness in alleviating the disorders for which they are advocated. However, pharmacological manipulation of the lower urinary tract is a palliative measure.

Clinical effectiveness of the drugs depends greatly on accurate assessment of the voiding disorder and the patient's response to the dose of drug used. It should be emphasized that the drug dosages and maintenance intervals used are empirical: They were established on the basis of uncontrolled clinical observations or were extrapolated from recommended children's dosages. Doses should begin at the low end of the range given and are increased gradually until the desired response is seen or the maximum dose is reached. The duration of the therapeutic trial at maximum dose depends on the individual drug but in general should be 1 to 2 weeks. If no response to the chosen drug is noted within this time period, the drug can be considered ineffective and discontinued.

Each drug mentioned has certain side effects related to its mode of action, and although the majority of adverse effects are inconsequential, they must be understood before therapy is implemented (see Table 102–4). Consulting a pharmacology text before using an unfamiliar drug is axiomatic.

Hormone-Responsive Urinary Incontinence

See Table 102–4 for recommended drugs and dosages, mode of action, and potential side effects. In female dogs with urinary incontinence presumed due to low circulating concentrations of hormones, the response to estrogen therapy is variable, and some dogs that fail to improve may show a favorable response to alpha stimulants.[78] The dose and route of administration of testosterone to control incontinence in castrated male dogs are not well established. Oral testosterone is less effective than parenteral because of hepatic degradation.[12] Testosterone esters, such as testosterone cypionate, that are absorbed more slowly than testosterone itself are recommended.

Urethral Incompetence

Phenylpropanolamine is an alpha stimulant that is effective in increasing urethral pressure and resistance to urine leakage when given orally.[10, 88, 106] It is preferable to use products that contain phenylpropanolamine alone rather than those that contain antihistamines or caffeine. Ephedrine is another alpha stimulant that can be used for incontinence due to urethral incompetence.[10, 78]

Urge Incontinence

Propantheline, an anticholinergic drug, is commonly the drug of choice in cases of detrusor hyperactivity. It is effective in dogs.[64] Unfortunately, the therapeutic and toxic doses are similar, and side effects may occur at therapeutically effective doses. Therefore, direct-acting smooth-muscle relaxants may be more rewarding.

Oxybutynin and flavoxate are antispasmodic drugs with little or no anticholinergic action and fewer potential side effects than propantheline. They may require several weeks of therapy before maximum response is achieved.[10] Oxybutynin has been used successfully to treat incontinence due to detrusor instability in a dog and a cat.[67] The prototypical anticholinergic drug, atropine, is relatively ineffective in alleviating uninhibited detrusor contractions.[10]

Imipramine pamoate is a tricyclic antidepressant that has been used successfully in humans to treat detrusor instability and facilitate urine storage.[25, 98] Imipramine has systemic anticholinergic effects, but the direct inhibitory effect on the detrusor appears to be neither anticholinergic nor adrenergic.[14, 83] Clinically, the drug appears to decrease bladder contractility and increase resistance to urine outflow.[74]

Empronium bromide is an anticholinergic drug with antimuscarinic and antinicotinic actions. It has been used to decrease intravesicular pressure in humans with detrusor instability.[50] In one study, only 7 of 21 female dogs with urinary incontinence responded favorably to treatment with empronium bromide (10 mg/kg/day divided TID or QID).[52] Lack of response to empronium bromide may be a sign that incontinence is not due to detrusor instability. This drug has not been approved for use in the United States.

Functional Urethral Obstruction

Sympathetically induced urethral obstruction can be treated effectively with the alpha-adrenergic blocking agents phenoxybenzamine or prazosin hydrochloride.[9, 63, 71] Phenoxybenzamine has also been useful in alleviating functional urethral obstruction in human patients with prostatic disease.[38] Phenoxybenzamine is long acting, but therapeutic blood levels are attained slowly;

TABLE 102–4. DISORDERS OF MICTURITION AND DRUGS USED IN THEIR MANAGEMENT

Disorder	Drug	Brand Name and Manufacturer*	Dosage†	Mode of Action	Potential Side Effects‡
Estrogen-responsive incontinence	Estrogens: diethylstilbestrol	Stilbestrol, North American Pharmacol.	Initially 0.1 to 1.0 mg/day for 3 to 5 days Maintenance 1 mg/week	Unknown, thought to enhance alpha receptor response to sympathomimetics[16]	Bone marrow toxicity
Testosterone-responsive incontinence	Testosterone cypionate	Depo-Testosterone Cypionate, The Upjohn Co.	200 mg/month IM	Unknown	None noted in dogs
Urethral incompetence due to postprostatic or posturethral disease, ectopic ureter syndrome (see text), neurogenic disorders	Phenyl-propanolamine OR	Dexatrim Capsules, Thompson Medical Co., Inc.	12.5 to 50.0 mg TID, titrate to effect	Sympathomimetic alpha receptor stimulation and increased urethral resistance	Minimal; restlessness may be noted
	Ephedrine	Ephedrine Sulfate, Eli Lilly & Co.	20 to 50.0 mg BID	Same as that of phenylpropanolamine	Same as those of phenyl-propanolamine; may cause urine retention
Urge incontinence	Propantheline	Pro-Banthine, Searle & Co.	7.5 to 30.0 mg TID to QID	Anticholinergic: decreased uninhibited bladder contractions	Urine retention
	Oxybutynin	Ditropan, Marion Laboratories, Inc.	5 mg BID to TID	Direct antispasmodic effect on smooth muscle to allow increased bladder capacity	Urine retention
	Flavoxate	Urispas, Smith Kline & French Laboratories	100 mg TID to QID		
	Imipramine pamoate	Tofranil, Geigy Pharmaceuticals	0.5 to 1.0 mg/kg TID	Decreased bladder contractions and increased urethral resistance	Depression; myocardial depression; gastrointestinal upset
Functional urethral obstruction Sympathetic	Phenoxybenzamine	Dibenzyline, Smith Kline & French Laboratories	2.5 to 30.0 mg once daily or in divided doses	Sympatholytic: alpha receptor blockage and decreased urethral resistance	Postural hypotension, tachycardia
	Prazosin HCl	Minipress, Pfizer Inc.	1.0–5.0 mg once daily or in divided doses	Same as phenoxybenzamine	Same as phenoxybenzamine
Somatic	Diazepam	Valium, Roche Laboratories	2 to 10 mg TID	Skeletal muscle relaxation and decreased external sphincter resistance	Sedation
	Dantrolene	Dantrium, Norwich-Eaton Pharmaceuticals	3 to 15 mg/kg daily in divided doses		Generalized muscle weakness, hepatotoxicity (long-term use)
Detrusor atony	Bethanechol	Urecholine, Merck Sharp & Dohme	5 to 15 mg TID	Cholinergic: stimulation of detrusor contractions	Abdominal discomfort due to increased intestinal peristalsis
Detrusor atony with urethral resistance	Bethanechol and phenoxybenzamine	See above	As listed above	Stimulation of detrusor contraction and decreased urethral resistance	As listed above

*Products may be available from other manufacturers or as generic drugs.
†Dosage is for dogs and administered orally unless otherwise indicated.
‡Consult a pharmacopeia for a complete description of each drug and its mode of action, contraindications, and adverse reactions before use.

several days to 2 weeks may be required for noticeable effect.

Somatically induced urethral obstruction can be treated with diazepam or dantrolene.[10, 6] Diazepam is a centrally acting muscle relaxant and provides nonspecific action in the treatment of somatic dyssynergia. Dantrolene is a more specific skeletal muscle relaxant, but it can cause generalized muscle weakness. It is effective in decreasing intraurethral pressure in dogs.[61]

Detrusor Atony and Detrusor Atony with Functional Urethral Obstruction

Bethanechol is a cholinergic agent that has been used successfully to stimulate detrusor contraction in neurogenic and non-neurogenic hypotonic bladder dysfunction.[10, 62] It is indicated in atony of the bladder with urine retention. Bethanechol is a potent drug that stimulates contractions of the detrusor muscle as well as contractions of the smooth muscle of the gastrointestinal tract. High parenteral doses can cause increased gastric motility, diarrhea, and abdominal discomfort. Atropine is the antidote. Although oral therapy is less successful in low doses, up to 50 mg is clinically effective while avoiding undue systemic effects in humans.[91]

Because bethanechol stimulates the parasympathetic receptors of smooth muscle, it may cause increased urethral resistance, and its efficacy in improving bladder emptying depends on its effect on the detrusor exceeding its effect on the urethra.[92, 105] In cases of suspected outlet resistance or dyssynergia, phenoxybenzamine should be used concurrently with bethanechol. Combined administration allows increased intravesical pressure with lowered urethral resistance.[62, 105]

Bethanechol should not be used in patients with a mechanical obstruction to urination or defecation or if the integrity of the patient's urinary bladder or gastrointestinal wall is in question.

Surgical Treatment of Urinary Incontinence

Various surgical procedures have been performed to increase resistance to urine outflow, including urethroplasty using bladder flaps,[23] cranial displacement of the vagina (colosuspension),[54] periurethral injection of Teflon,[6] and implantation of artificial sphincters. Although all these techniques have been reported to improve urinary incontinence, they have not gained widespread acceptance in veterinary medicine.

URINE SPRAYING AND MARKING IN CATS

Even though male cats are castrated to prevent urine spraying and female cats spray urine infrequently, this behavior remains a clinical problem in feline practice. Alternative therapeutic approaches include behavioral control, administration of progestins and, as a last resort, neurosurgical bilateral ischiocavernosus myectomy techniques. Urine spraying is a serious behavioral problem. If therapy is not successful, often the only other solution is euthanasia. A number of hormonal preparations, including estrogen, testosterone, and progestins, have been advocated. Attempts to alter an animal's ability to spray by performing a perineal urethrostomy have not been successful because the animal eventually regains the ability to direct a jet of urine in a spray (unpublished observations). None of the therapeutic approaches currently used are 100 per cent effective. Progestin therapy is much more effective in males than females, but satisfactory results are obtained with olfactory tractotomy in virtually all females and 50 per cent of males.

Normal Urine Spraying and Urine Marking Behavior

Territorial Marking

Urine spraying is usually initiated when a cat smells a vertical target and then turns around and directs a stream of urine toward the investigated target. Males and females spray using basically the same posture. The squatting posture is used in urine marking, but the urination is in places that would not be normal toilet areas, such as specific places on a carpet, the shoes or clothes of a family member, or an owner's bed.

Cats have a tendency to spray particular objects in their environment, and this seems to be associated with an attempt to make their environment familiar.[34, 43, 103] By creating a recognizable olfactory field in the home environment, it is believed that the cat may feel more self-assured and confident, especially in regard to agonistic encounters with other cats.[34]

Sexually Dimorphic Aspects

Spraying is a behavior normally associated with tomcats, and the onset is related to sexual maturation. Like sexual activity, spraying occurs most frequently during the breeding season,[103] presumably as a function of an increase in seasonal secretion of testosterone and also because of increased agonistic interactions with other male cats. Urine marks are undoubtedly useful in attracting sexually receptive females to a male's territory.

Like fighting, roaming, and sexual behavior, urine spraying is sexually dimorphic behavior that occurs less frequently in females than males. Under natural conditions, one would expect females to spray at estrus when the deposition of urine on prominent vertical objects would "advertise" their sexual condition.[35, 103]

Differential Diagnosis of Problem Spraying

To treat urine spraying effectively it is imperative to distinguish urine spraying from other types of urination problems, namely, inappropriate urination and urinary disorders. When urine is found 1 to 2 feet above the ground on vertical objects, it is a result of spraying. In both urine spraying and marking, certain objects are usually selected and repeatedly hit. Usually the cat is still using a litter box or the outdoors for most urination and all defecation.

Inappropriate Urination

If a cat has an aversion to the litter box or the outdoors, it often ceases using a litter box or going outdoors entirely. Defecation as well as urination will occur in inappropriate areas. The treatment of inappropriate elimination involves some conditioning principles to induce the cat to use the litter box or the outdoors again.[40]

Urinary Disorders

The presence of a urinary disorder is usually evident from the medical history. Problem urination stemming from a urinary infection should be indiscriminate in terms of target areas, and the pattern of urination is consistent with the behavior of an animal unable to make it to the litter box or the outdoors. Straining at the time of urination and frequent urination may also be noted. A urinalysis may be conducted to differentiate spraying from a disease of the urinary tract.

It is not uncommon for a cat to start urine spraying after one or more bouts with urinary cystitis with possible blockage. Perhaps some discomfort in the urinary tract is one of the factors that predisposes the cat to spraying.

Androgenic Steroids

An occasional cause of spraying may be administration of androgenic steroids to stimulate metabolism, increase muscle tone, or treat certain skin conditions. The steroids may have sufficient androgenic activity to activate the neural circuitry for spraying, similar to the activation that occurs as male cats go through puberty.

Incidence of Urine Spraying

Effects of Postpubertal Castration

Castration of tomcats after puberty, even after spraying has begun, is quite effective in eliminating or markedly reducing spraying. We found that about 80 per cent of adult males castrated because of problem spraying underwent a rapid decline in the behavior, with an additional 10 per cent experiencing a more gradual decline.[47] One could expect from these data that approximately 10 per cent of male cats castrated because of problem spraying persist indefinitely in the behavior.

The persistence in spraying after castration is not due to residual amounts of testosterone, because within 8 to 16 hours after castration the concentration of testosterone in the blood is reduced to castrate levels and is behaviorally insignificant.[42]

Effects of Prepubertal Castration

It is common for male cats to be castrated before puberty, and there is an assumption among veterinarians and cat owners that prepubertal castration is more effective in preventing objectionable urine spraying, fighting, and roaming than postpubertal castration is in eliminating these behaviors once they have begun. However, urine spraying is common enough in prepubertally castrated males and spayed females that the administration of progestins in an attempt to control this behavior has become routine in feline practice.[42, 44] It is not unusual to find male or female cats, neutered at 6 months of age, begin spraying as late as 3 or 4 years of age. The onset of spraying is often related to the introduction of new cats into a household with other cats, changing households, or altering a major aspect of the cat's life-style, such as making an outdoor cat an indoor cat.

A survey including 136 male and 124 female cats gonadectomized between 6 and 10 months of age found no relationship between age of male cats at the time of castration and the likelihood of spraying; there was also no relationship between age at ovariohysterectomy in female cats and the incidence of spraying.[40] Furthermore, there was no greater spraying tendency in females coming from litters in which all the other littermates were male and in which androgenization was likely than in females coming from all-female litters. In this survey, the incidence of frequent urine spraying by prepubertally castrated male cats was very close to 10 per cent, and the incidence of frequent spraying by prepubertally spayed females was 5 per cent. Because only 10 per cent of male cats castrated in adulthood for spraying continue to spray, this survey revealed that prepubertal castration is not likely to be more effective in preventing objectionable spraying than postpubertal castration is in eliminating the behavior once it has started.

Therapy for Problem Spraying

Predisposing and Causal Factors

When treating urine spraying and marking, it is a good idea to determine why the cat started spraying and continues to spray. Some of the factors provoking spraying may be transient, such as the breeding season or a move to a new house, and therefore the problem may resolve itself. Other causal factors may be more permanent and may continue to maintain spraying activity. Therapy is more difficult for these problems.

Therapeutic approaches at three levels are discussed here: behavioral and management approaches, use of synthetic progestins, and neurosurgical procedures. Of course, a combination of approaches may be attempted. For example, a cat for which progestin treatment did not satisfactorily suppress the behavior may be subjected to an olfactory tractotomy. If the operation is not completely effective, the additional use of a progestin may control the behavior.

Behavioral Approaches and Management

Before seeking the services of a veterinarian, cat owners have often tried punishment such as yelling or throwing something at the cat when it is caught in the act of spraying. In some instances, this has been effective for a time. Most cat owners understand the futility of bringing the cat to the urine-soiled spot and either pointing it out or rubbing the cat's nose in it. This usually just makes the cat wary of the owner.

A remote punishment, such as upside-down mouse traps near the soiled areas, may be effective. Ambushing a cat with a squirt gun or water sprayer when it is beginning to spray is another technique. It is important that remote punishment be delivered without the cat knowing that the owner is involved in the punishment process. In this way the animal makes the association between the target areas and the punishment rather than between the owner and the punishment. Remote punishment is useful only if a cat is spraying very few objects. Obviously, one cannot have an entire house booby-trapped with upside-down mouse traps. A comprehensive discussion of the use of remote punishment is available.[41, 43]

Another technique for dealing with spraying in just one or two spots in the house is to feed the animal at these spots during its regular mealtime. Cats are unlikely to eliminate in the same spot in which they eat.

Progestin Therapy

Synthetic progestins are related to the hormone progesterone; the progestins suppress malelike behavior, such as spraying, even when the behavior occurs in females. The long-acting progestins effective in correcting spraying include the commercially available medroxyprogesterone (MPA; Depo-Provera) and megestrol acetate (MA; Ovaban). MPA is given as an injection and MA orally. One injection or an oral treatment series may permanently eliminate the behavior, especially if transient environmental factors evoked the behavior. If the cat is continuously anxious or nervous or if other factors are continuously stimulating the behavior, only repeated injections or continuous oral therapy may be effective. In these instances, the potential side effects of the progestin therapy must be noted. Given the objectionable nature of urine spraying, there may be no option but to continue progestin therapy despite the potential for adverse side effects.

Our clinical survey of the overall effectiveness of progestin therapy in gonadectomized cats revealed that problem spraying or urine marking was resolved for a month or longer in about 30 per cent of cats.[44] However, the sex of the cat and the number of cats in the household were important considerations. Of males, 50 per cent responded favorably, compared with less than 20 per cent of spayed females. About 50 per cent of cats (both sexes) from single-cat households responded favorably, compared with only 18 per cent of cats from multicat households. Thus, the prognosis for progestin therapy is highly dependent on the sex of the cat and its home environment. Females from multicat environments appear to warrant the poorest prognosis, and males from single-cat homes the most favorable prognosis.

Both MPA and MA were about equally effective in the initial treatment of spraying. However, as many as one-half of the cats not responding to MPA treatment were found to respond favorably to subsequent MA treatment.

Common side effects included an increase in appetite and signs of behavioral depression. These side effects, which developed shortly after initial administration of the drug, were more common with MA than with MPA, occurring in up to 30 per cent of patients after MA treatment. Mammary gland hyperplasia[33, 34] and tumors[44] have been reported after both MA and MPA treatment. The hyperplasia regresses after treatment is terminated. Other side effects have been reported in the literature, including precipitation of diabetes mellitus in prediabetic patients, depression of corticosteroid output, and corticosteroid-like effects.[44] One would expect these more serious side effects to follow rather long-term therapy.

Because MPA and MA seem to be about equally effective in the initial treatment of spraying but MA results in more depression and appetite stimulation than MPA, it is recommended that injectable MPA be used in most cases for initial treatment. The use of an injectable drug also eliminates the need for a client to follow a complex dosage regimen. A dose of 10 to 20 mg/kg of MPA is recommended. Because of occasional loss of hair or change in hair pigmentation immediately over the site of injection, a subcutaneous injection into the inguinal region is recommended. For treatment with MA alone or following unsuccessful MPA treatment, the recommended initial oral dosage is 5 mg/kg/day. If the treatment is effective, the dose should be gradually reduced over intervals of 2 weeks to a dosage of 5 mg once a week. This treatment should then be terminated in about 2 to 6 months, depending on the severity of the problem. If the initial MA treatment is not effective in 1 week, no additional MA should be given.

Bilateral Ischiocavernosus Myectomy

Bilateral ischiocavernosus myectomy has been reported to significantly decrease chronic urine spraying in castrated male cats that did not respond to hormonal therapy.[66, 70] The exact cause of the beneficial effect is unknown, but it is postulated that the surgery prevents the cat from holding the penis at the preferred position to spray urine. Bilateral skin incisions are made lateral to the scrotum and prepuce and medial to the tuber ischii. The ischiocavernosus muscles are isolated at their attachment to the ischium. The ischiocavernosus muscles and the associated penile crura are sharply dissected from the ischium. Hemorrhage is controlled with ligatures or electrocautery. The wound is closed routinely.

Olfactory Tractotomy

When progestin therapy is not effective, many cat owners wish to consider more extreme measures to resolve the spraying or marking problem. Olfactory tractotomy has been successfully used to eliminate spraying in cats that do not respond to progestin treatment.[45, 46] The operation is a simple neurosurgical procedure, carrying little surgical and recovery risk, and requires little in the way of specialized instruments and neuroanatomical background. The rationale for the operation is that spraying is usually initiated by a cat's smelling the target area. The cat then usually turns

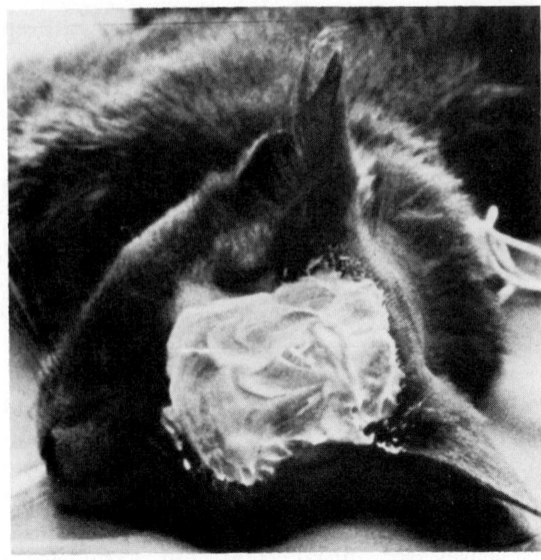

FIGURE 102–2. Depilatory cream used for hair removal, which is necessary for adhesion of a plastic drape. The cream, which is applied after the hair is clipped, should remain on the skin for 5 to 10 minutes.

around and directs a stream of urine toward the investigated target. The operation is a modification of that used by other investigators in their study of the sensory control of sexual behavior.[3] The olfactory tracts and caudal parts of the olfactory bulbs are approached dorsally through the frontal sinus. No adverse behavioral changes have been noted.

The complications that have been reported include transient anorexia and occasional and transient subcutaneous emphysema over the incision site. Subcutaneous emphysema, if it does occur, is due to passage of air from the frontal sinus to the wound site and usually disappears within a day or two.

Transient anorexia occurs in about half of the patients, but one can usually stimulate a cat to start eating by placing chicken or turkey baby food in its mouth or smearing the food on its lips. After it has eaten baby food, a cat will usually accept its regular semimoist or dry food, but it may be necessary to mix the normal food with baby food for a period of time. To verify complete anosmia, cat owners can be asked to conduct a "hidden food" test by placing food (tuna) under paper towels and determining if the cat can find the hidden food.

Individual responses to the operation vary. Spraying in some cats is markedly reduced or eliminated on a permanent basis. In others it is reduced to an occasional level that is tolerable to the owner. One might find that a cat sprays inside the house while under postoperative confinement, but after it is allowed access to the outdoors, no further spraying is noted. A number of cats show an increase in affection toward the owner. Other cats have an increase in appetite or at least seem willing to consume a greater variety of food than preoperatively. Occasional cats become more finicky eaters.

Our clinical evaluation of the effectiveness of this operation is 50 per cent for male cats and 80 to 90 per cent for female cats.

Another neurosurgical operation, the creation of bilateral hypothalamic lesions,[49] was found to be 100 per cent effective in eliminating spraying in male cats but completely ineffective in female cats. This operation is lengthy and requires equipment for stereotaxic brain surgery and is not reviewed here.

Surgical Procedure. Perhaps the greatest concern in performing this surgery is that one can miss completely severing the olfactory tracts bilaterally, thus leaving the animal with a sense of smell. It is suggested that the surgeon practice on a cadaver with subsequent dissection of the surgical area. The technique might also be performed at least once on a practice cat.

An inhalant anesthetic for general anesthesia is appropriate. The hair over the incision site should be clipped, and a depilatory cream can be used for additional hair removal, especially if the area is to be draped

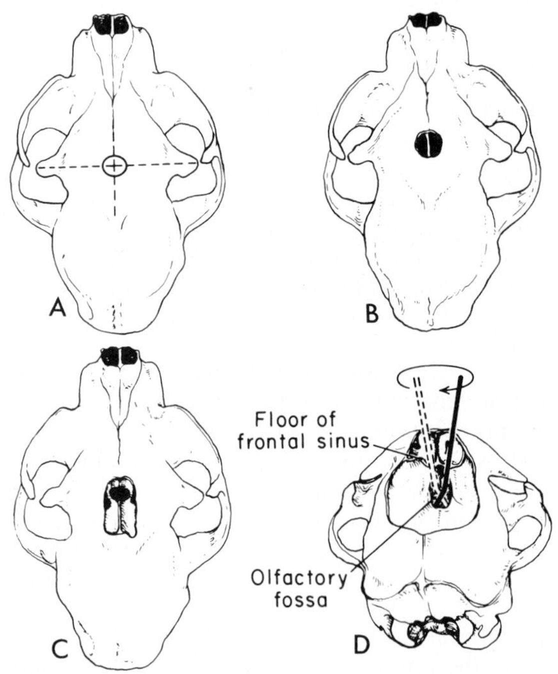

FIGURE 102–3. Surgical approach to olfactory tractotomy. *A*, A hole 6 to 8 mm in diameter is made in the roof of the frontal sinus at the intersection of the sagittal suture and a line passing through the tips of the zygomatic processes of the frontal bones. Dorsal view. *B*, The opening to the frontal sinus reveals a midsagittal septum, which must be removed. Dorsal view. *C*, A hole 6 mm (transversely) by 3 mm (longitudinally) is made in the floor of the sinus to expose the olfactory fossa and to allow lateral movement of the aspiration tube. In this illustration, the hole in the roof of the frontal sinus is enlarged to show the opening in the floor of the frontal sinus, which lies about 12 mm below the roof. Part of the septum of the sinus is evident. Dorsal view. *D*, In this caudal view, the relationship of the roof and floor of the frontal sinus to the olfactory fossa is shown. At the rostral end of the olfactory fossa is the cribriform plate, through which pass olfactory nerves to terminate in the olfactory bulb, which occupies the olfactory fossa. The range of movement of the aspiration tube (with the angled tip directed caudally) is illustrated. In this operation, the olfactory bulb cannot be completely removed, but the olfactory tracts passing along the floor of the olfactory fossa are completely severed. (Reprinted with permission from Hart BL: Olfactory tractotomy for control of objectionable urine spraying and urine marking in cats. *J Am Vet Med Assoc 179*:231, 1981.)

with an adhesive plastic drape such as one designed for eye surgery (Fig. 102–2).

An opening into the frontal sinus, 6 to 8 mm in diameter, is made after making a midline incision through the skin (Fig. 102–3). Removal of the bone is best accomplished with a pneumatic drill. Care is taken to avoid cutting into the ethmoturbinates, which project into the frontal sinus. The midsagittal septum is removed to completely expose the floor of the frontal sinus, which overlies the olfactory (ethmoidal) fossa enclosing the olfactory bulbs and tracts (Fig. 102–4). A hole about 6 × 3 mm is made in the floor of the frontal sinus to allow access to the olfactory bulbs.

The caudal parts of the olfactory bulbs and the olfactory tracts can be removed by aspiration through a metal suction tube number (8 French). Although not necessary, it is best to modify the tube by bending the last 10 mm to about a 30° angle (see Fig. 102–4). The olfactory tracts are located on the ventral side of the olfactory fossa, and the tractotomy is accomplished by rubbing the aspiration tube across the floor and sides of the olfactory fossa. Visual inspection of the area is usually not possible because of seepage of blood into the fossa. To be sure that the tracts are completely severed, the bent part of the cannula should be directed caudally.

Minor hemorrhage can be controlled by packing the olfactory fossa with absorbable hemostatic material such as gelatin foam. Subcutaneous fascia and skin are closed separately. The surgery itself should take about 30 minutes. Minor bleeding from the nose may occur in some cats. Because the frontal sinus communicates with the nasal cavity, it is recommended that 1 day before surgery cats be placed on a prophylactic (5-day) regimen of a broad-spectrum antibiotic, such as ampicillin.

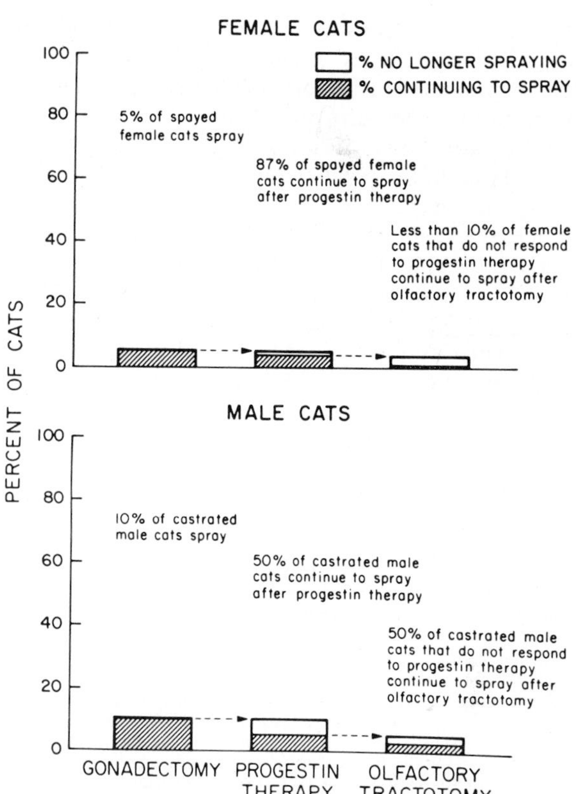

FIGURE 102–5. Clinical results of successive approaches to treatment of urine spraying in neutered female and male cats.

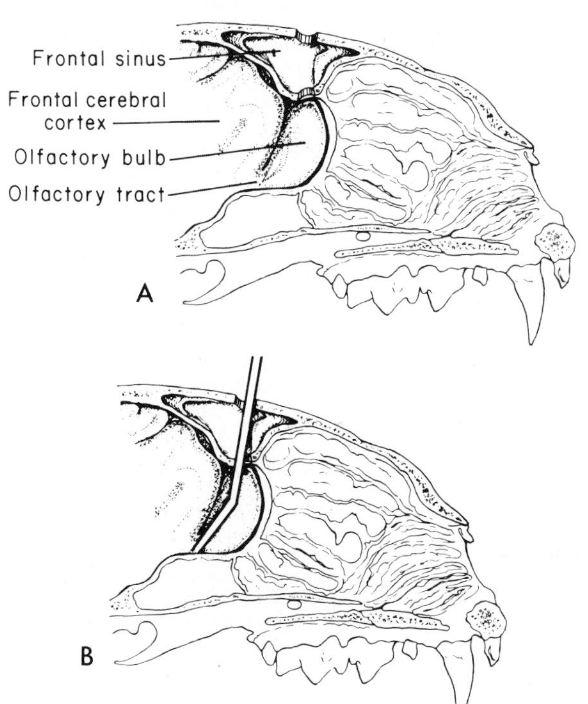

FIGURE 102–4. Parasagittal view of olfactory bulb lying in the olfactory fossa. *A,* Anatomical relationships of cerebral cortex, olfactory bulb, and olfactory tract. *B,* View of insertion of aspiration tube to perform the olfactory tractotomy. (Reprinted with permission from Hart BL: Olfactory tractotomy for control of objectionable urine spraying and urine marking in cats. *J Am Vet Med Assoc* *179*:231, 1981.)

Graphic representation to highlight successive approaches to the treatment of urine spraying in gonadectomized female and male cats is shown (Fig. 102–5). Gonadectomy, which refers to prepubertal[48] and postpubertal[47] castration of male cats or spaying of female cats,[48] is tried first. For those that do not respond, progestin therapy with either MPA or MA[44] is used. Neurosurgery is tried last, not first. Data on olfactory tractotomy include previously published clinical trials[45, 46] substantiated by more recent unpublished clinical results.

SUMMARY

Urine spraying is an innate behavior that is difficult to control by training, punishment, and management procedures. Even when causative factors in the environment can be identified, clients are often unable or unwilling to alter their own or their pet's habits that led to the problem urination. The simplest measures are management and punishment techniques, but these are often only temporarily effective, if at all. Progestin treatment is effective in some cats, depending on sex and number of cats in the home. The results of bilateral ischiocavernosus myectomy for urine spraying in male cats have been reported in only 10 cats. The reliability of this technique needs to be confirmed in a larger study. Surgical placement of bilateral hypothalamic lesions reliably eliminates urine spraying in male cats. However, this operation is lengthy and requires specialized equipment for stereotaxic brain surgery. Olfactory tractotomy, a much more practical operation requiring little in the way of specialized equipment, is rapid and carries minimal surgical risk. Viewed in the light of an alternative to euthanasia, elimination of a cat's sense of smell cannot be considered inhumane. It should be emphasized, however, that the neurosurgical approach described here represents the end of a continuum of therapeutic measures aimed at treating the problem behavior.

References

1. Adams WM, DiBartola SP: Radiographic and clinical features of pelvic bladder in the dog. *J Am Vet Med Assoc 182*:1212, 1983.
2. Albert NE, et al: Effect of pelvic and retroperitoneal surgery on the urethral pressure profile and perineal floor electromyogram in dogs. *Invest Urol 15*:140, 1977.
3. Allen TA, et al: A technique for estimating progression of chronic renal failure in the dog. *J Am Vet Med Assoc 190*:866, 1987.
4. Appel GB, New HC: Gentamicin in 1978. *Ann Intern Med 89*:528, 1978.
5. Arnold S, et al: Urinary incontinence in spayed female dogs: Frequency and breed disposition. *Schweiz Arch Tierheilkd 131*:259, 1989.
6. Arnold S, et al: Treatment of urinary incontinence in dogs by endoscopic injection of Teflon. *J Am Vet Med Assoc 195*:1369, 1989.
7. Aronson LR, Cooper ML: Olfactory deprivation and mating behavior in sexually experienced male cats. *Behav Biol 11*:459, 1974.
8. Awad SA, Downie JW: Sympathetic dyssynergia in the region of the external sphincter: A possible source of lower urinary tract obstruction. *J Urol 118*:636, 1977.
9. Awad SA, et al: Alpha adrenergic agents in urinary disorders of the proximal urethra. Part II. Urethral obstruction due to sympathetic dyssynergia. *Br J Urol 50*:336, 1978.
10. Awad SA, et al: Pharmacologic treatment of disorders of bladder and urethra: A review. *Can J Surg 22*:515, 1979.
11. Balint P, et al: Renal haemodynamics in dogs with dehydration azotemia. *Acta Med Acad Sci Hung 32*:193, 1975.
12. Barsanti JA, et al: Testosterone responsive urinary incontinence in a castrated male dog. *J Am Anim Hosp Assoc 17*:117, 1981.
13. Baylis C, et al: Mechanisms of the defect in glomerular ultrafiltration associated with gentamicin administration. *Kidney Int 12*:344, 1977.
14. Benson GS, et al: Comparative effects and mechanisms of action of atropine, propantheline, flavoxate, and imipramine on bladder muscle contractility. *Urology 9*:31, 1977.
15. Bercovitch DD, et al: The postobstructive kidney. Observations on nephron function after the relief of 24 hours of ureteral ligation in the dog. *J Clin Invest 50*:1154, 1971.
16. Bovee KC: Functional responses to nephron loss. *In* Bovée KC (ed): *Canine Nephrology*. Harwal, Media, PA, 1983.
17. Bovee KC: Metabolic disturbances of uremia. *In* Bovée KC (ed): *Canine Nephrology*. Harwal, Media, PA, 1983.
18. Bovee KC, Littman MP: Hypertension and renal dysfunction. *Tijdschr Diergeneeskd 112*(Suppl 1):1215, 1987.
19. Bovee KC, et al: Trigonal-colonic anastomosis: A urinary diversion procedure in dogs. *J Am Vet Med Assoc 174*:184, 1979.
20. Bump RC, Friedman CI: Intraluminal urethral pressure measurements in the female baboon: Effects of hormonal manipulation. *J Urol 136*:508, 1986.
21. Burke TJ, et al: Ischemic and tubule obstruction during acute renal failure in dogs: Mannitol in protection. *Am J Physiol 238*:F305, 1980.
22. Burrows CF, Bovee KC: Characterization and treatment of acid-base and renal defects due to urethral obstruction in cats. *J Am Vet Med Assoc 172*:801, 1978.
23. Bushby PA, Hankes GH: Sling urethroplasty for the correction of urethral dilation and urinary incontinence. *J Am Anim Hosp Assoc 16*:115, 1980.
24. Cardozo LD, Stanton SL: An objective comparison of the effects of parenterally administered drugs in patients suffering from detrusor instability. *J Urol 122*:58, 1979.
25. Castleden C, et al: Imipramine—A possible alternative to current therapy for urinary incontinence in the elderly. *J Urol 125*:318, 1981.
26. Chander M, et al: The influence of extracellular fluid volume expansion on postobstructive diuresis in the dog. *Invest Urol 11*:114, 1973.
27. Chew DJ, Capen CC: Hypercalcemia nephropathy and associated disorders. *In* Kirk RW (ed): *Current Veterinary Therapy VII*. W. B. Saunders, Philadelphia, 1980.
28. Christie BA: Vesicoureteral reflux in dogs. *J Am Vet Med Assoc 162*:772, 1973.
29. Cowgill L: Acute renal failure. *In* Bovee KC (ed): *Canine Nephrology*. Harwal, Media, PA, 1983.
30. Crane SW, Waldron DR: Ureteral function and healing following microsurgical transureteroureterostomy in the dog. *Vet Surg 9*:108, 1980.
31. Cronin RE, et al: Pathogenic mechanisms in early norepinephrine-induced acute renal failure: Functional and histological correlates of protection. *Kidney Int 14*:115, 1978.
32. Divers TJ, et al: Acute renal failure in six horses resulting from haemodynamic causes. *Equine Vet J 19*:178, 1987.
33. Dorn AS, et al: Mammary hyperplasia in a male cat receiving progesterone. *J Am Vet Med Assoc 182*:621, 1983.
34. Eisenberg JF, Kleiman DG: Olfactory communication in mammals. *Ann Rev Ecol Syst 3*:1, 1972.
35. Ewer RF: *The Carnivores*. Cornell University Press, Ithaca, 1973.
36. Fletcher TE, Bradley WE: Neuroanatomy of the bladder-urethra. *J Urol 119*:153, 1978.
37. Garry F, et al: Enzymuria as an index of renal damage in sheep with induced aminoglycoside nephrotoxicosis. *Am J Vet Res 51*:428, 1990.
38. Gerstenberg T, et al: Phenoxybenzamine reduces bladder outlet obstruction in benign prostatic hyperplasia. *Invest Urol 18*:29, 1980.
39. Gillenwater JY, et al: Renal function one week after release of chronic unilateral hydronephrosis in man. *Kidney Int 7*:179, 1975.
40. Hart BL: Inappropriate urination and defecation. *Feline Pract 6*:6, 1976.
41. Hart BL: Water sprayer therapy. *Feline Pract 8*:13, 1978.
42. Hart BL: Problems with objectionable sociosexual behavior of dogs and cats: Therapeutic use of castration and progestins. *Comp Cont Ed 1*:461, 1979.
43. Hart BL: Behavioral therapy with mousetraps. *Feline Pract 9*:10, 1979.
44. Hart BL: Objectionable urine spraying and urine marking in cats: Evaluation of progestin treatment in gonadectomized males and females. *J Am Vet Med Assoc 177*:529, 1980.
45. Hart BL: Olfactory tractotomy for control of objectionable urine spraying and urine marking in cats. *J Am Vet Med Assoc 17*:231, 1981.
46. Hart BL: Neurosurgery for behavioral problems. A curiosity or the new wave? *Vet Clin North Am 12*:707, 1982.
47. Hart BL, Barrett RE: Effects of castration on fighting, roaming, and urine spraying in adult male cats. *J Am Vet Med Assoc 163*:290, 1973.
48. Hart BL, Cooper L: Factors relating to urine spraying and fighting in prepubertally gonadectomized male and female cats. *J Am Vet Med Assoc 184*:1255, 1984.
49. Hart BL, Voith VL: Changes in urine spraying, feeding and sleep behavior of cats following medial preoptic-anterior thalamic lesions. *Brain Res 145*:406, 1978.
50. Hebjorn S, Walter S: Treatment of female incontinence with empronium bromide. *Urol Int 33*:120, 1978.
51. Hinton M, Gaskell CJ: Non-neoplastic mammary hypertrophy in the cat associated with pregnancy or with oral progestational therapy. *Vet Rec 100*:277, 1977.
52. Holt PE: Efficacy of empronium bromide in the treatment of physiological incontinence in the bitch. *Vet Rec 114*:355, 1984.
53. Holt PE: Importance of urethral length, bladder neck position, and vestibulovaginal stenosis in sphincter mechanism imcompetence in the incontinent bitch. *Res Vet Sci 39*:364, 1985.
54. Holt PE: Urinary incontinence in the bitch due to sphincter mechanism incompetence: Surgical treatment. *J Small Anim Pract 26*:237, 1985.
55. Holt PE: 'Simultaneous' urethral pressure profilometry: Comparisons between continent and incontinent bitches. *J Small Anim Pract 29*:761, 1988.
56. Holt PE, et al: Canine ectopic ureter—a review of twenty-nine cases. *J Small Anim Pract 23*:195, 1982.
57. Johnston GR, et al: Effects of urinary bladder distention on location of the urinary bladder and urethra of healthy dogs and cats. *Am J Vet Res 47*:405, 1986.
58. Jorgensen TM: Dynamics of the urinary tract in long-term vesico-ureteral reflux and intravesical obstruction and infection in pigs. IV. *Scand J Urol Nephrol 19*:193, 1985.
59. Kamizaki H, Cass AS: Conduit and renal pelvic pressures after ileal and colonic urinary diversion in dogs. *Invest Urol 16*:27, 1978.
60. Kaplan MA, et al: Interrelations between phosphorus, calcium, parathyroid hormone, and renal phosphate excretion in response to an oral phosphorus load in normal and uremic dogs. *Kidney Int 14*:207, 1978.
61. Khalaf IM, et al: The effect of Dantrium on the canine urethral pressure profile. *Invest Urol 17*:188, 1979.
62. Khanna OP: Disorders of micturition. Neuropharmacologic basis and results of drug therapy. *Urology 8*:316, 1976.
63. Khanna OP, Gonick P: Effects of phenoxybenzamine hydrochloride on canine lower urinary tract: Clinical implications. *Urology 6*:323, 1975.
64. Khanna OP, et al: Cholinergic and adrenergic neuroreceptors in urinary tract of female dogs: Evaluation of function with pharmacodynamics. *Urology 5*:616, 1975.
65. Kobayashi DL, et al: Hypertension in cats with chronic renal failure or hyperthyroidism. *J Vet Intern Med 4*:58, 1990.

66. Komtebedde J, Hauptman J: Bilateral ischiocavernosus myectomy for chronic urine spraying in castrated male cats. *Vet Surg 19*:293, 1990.
67. Lappin MR, Barsanti JA: Urinary incontinence secondary to idiopathic detrusor instability: Cystometrographic diagnosis and pharmacologic management in two dogs and a cat. *J Am Vet Med Assoc 19*:1439, 1987.
68. Larrain C, Langdell RD: The hemostatic defect of uremia. II. Investigation of dogs with experimentally produced acute urinary retention. *Blood 11*:1067, 1956.
69. Lindner A, et al: Synergism of dopamine plus furosemide in preventing acute renal failure in the dog. *Kidney Int 16*:158, 1979.
70. Macdougall DF, et al: Caninechronic renal disease: Prevalence and types of glomerulonephritis in the dog. *Kidney Int* 29:1144, 1986.
71. MacGregor R, Diokno A: The α-adrenergic blocking action of prazosin hydrochloride on the canine urethra. *Invest Urol 18*:426, 1981.
72. Madsen PO: The etiology of hyperchloremic acidosis following intestinal anastomosis: An experimental study. *J Urol 92*:448, 1964.
73. Mahaffey MB, et al: Pelvic bladder in dogs without urinary incontinence. *J Am Vet Med Assoc 184*:1477, 1984.
74. Mahony DT, et al: Observations on sphincter augmenting effect of imipramine in children with urinary incontinence. *Urology 1*:317, 1973.
75. Maydl I: Neue Beobachtungen von Ureterenimplantation die Flexura Romana bei Ectopia Vesicae. *Wien Med Wochenschr 46*:1241, 1896.
76. Miller JB, et al: Patterns of recovery of renal function after surgical relief of chronic bilateral partial ureteral obstruction. *Invest Urol 17*:69, 1979.
77. Morris CR, et al: Restoration and maintenance of glomerular filtration by mannitol during hypoperfusion of the kidney. *J Clin Invest 51*:1555, 1972.
78. Nendick PA, Clark WT: Medical therapy of urinary incontinence in ovariectomized bitches: A comparison of the effectiveness of diethylstilboestrol and pseudoephedrine. *Aust Vet J 64*:117, 1987.
79. Oliver JE: Diseases of micturition. *In* Hoerlein BF (ed): *Canine Neurology: Diagnosis and Treatment*. W. B. Saunders, Philadelphia, 1978, p 461.
80. Oliver JE, Young WO: Air cystometry in dogs under xylazine induced restraint. *Am J Vet Res 34*:1433, 1973.
81. Osborne CA, Polzin DJ: Canine estrogen responsive incontinence: An enigma. *DVM Newsmag 10*:42, 1979.
82. Osborne CA, et al: Non-neurogenic urinary incontinence, *In* Kirk RW (ed): *Current Veterinary Therapy VII*. W. B. Saunders, Philadelphia, 1980, p 1128.
83. Olubadewo J: The effect of imipramine on rat detrusor muscle contractility. *Arch Int Pharmacodynam 245*:84, 1980.
84. Parker HR: Peritoneal dialysis and hemoperfusion. *In* Bovee KC (ed): *Canine Nephrology*. Harwal, Media, PA, 1983.
85. Petrites-Murphy MB, et al: Role of parathyroid hormone in the anemia of chronic terminal renal dysfunction in dogs. *Am J Vet Res 50*:1898, 1989.
86. Pond HS, Texter JH: Trigonal-ileal anastomosis: Experimental studies. *J Urol 103*:746, 1970.
87. Richie JP, et al: The effect of reflux on the development of pyelonephritis in urinary diversion: An experimental study. *J Surg Res 16*:256, 1974.
88. Richter KP, Ling GB: Clinical response and urethral pressure profile changes after phenylpropanolamine in dogs with primary sphincter incompetence. *J Am Vet Med Assoc 187*:605, 1985.
89. Rigg DL, et al: Neoureterostomy and phenylpropanolamine therapy for incontinence due to ectopic ureter in a dog. *J Am Anim Hosp Assoc 19*:237, 1983.
90. Selkurt EE: Changes in renal clearance following complete ischemia of the kidney. *Am J Physiol 144*:395, 1945.
91. Sondal LP, et al: Further observations on the cystometric and uroflowmetric effects of bethanechol chloride on the human bladder. *J Urol 122*:775, 1980.
92. Spence B, et al: Bacteriuria in intestinal conduit urinary diversion in dogs. *Invest Urol 10*:290, 1973.
93. Sprangler WI, et al: Vitamin D intoxication and the pathogenesis of vitamin D nephropathy in the dog. *Am J Vet Res 40*:73, 1979.
94. Starr A, et al: Antireflux ureteroileal anastomosis: Two experimental techniques. *Invest Urol 12*:165, 1974.
95. Stone EA, Mason LK: Surgery of ectopic ureters: Types, methods of correction and postoperative results. *J Am Anim Hosp Assoc 3*:627, 1990.
96. Stone EA, et al: Ureterocolonic anastomosis in clinically normal dogs. *Am J Vet Res 49*:1147, 1988.
97. Stone EA, et al.: Ureterocolonic anastomosis in ten dogs with transitional cell carcinoma. *Vet Surg 17*:147, 1988.
98. Sundin T, et al: The sympathetic innervation and adrenoreceptor function of the human lower urinary tract in the normal state and after parasympathetic denervation. *Invest Urol 14*:322, 1977.
99. Thornhill JA: Hemodialysis. *In* Bovee KC (ed): *Canine Nephrology*. Harwal, Media, PA, 1983.
100. Thrusfield MV: Association between urinary incontinence and spaying in bitches. *Vet Rec 116*:695, 1985.
101. Van Stone JC, Max P: Effect of erythropoietin on anemia of peritoneally dialyzed anephric rats. *Kidney Int 15*:370, 1979.
102. Vaughan ED Jr, et al: The renal hemodynamic response to chronic unilateral complete ureteral occlusion. *Invest Urol 8*:78, 1970.
103. Verberne G, Leyhausen P: Marking behavior of some viverridae and felidae. Time-interval analysis of marking pattern. *Behaviour 58*:192, 1976.
104. Walls J, et al: Nature of the acidifying defect after the relief of ureteral obstruction. *Kidney Int 7*:304, 1975.
105. Westmore DD: Urinary incontinence: Which drugs to use. *Drugs 17*:418, 1979.
106. White RAS, Pomeroy CJ: Phenylpropanolamine: An α-adrenergic agent for the management of urinary incontinence in the bitch associated with urethral sphincter mechanism incompetence. *Vet Rec 125*:478, 1989.
107. Wilson DR: Micropuncture study of chronic obstructive nephropathy before and after release of obstruction. *Kidney Int 2*:119, 1972.
108. Yarger WE, Griffith LD: Intrarenal hemodynamics following chronic unilateral ureteral obstruction in the dog. *Am J Physiol 227*:816, 1974.
109. Yarger WE, et al: A micropuncture study of postobstructive diuresis in the rat. *J Clin Invest 51*:625, 1972.
110. Zetterstrom R, et al: Separate renal function studies in predominantly unilateral hydronephrosis. *Acta Paediatr Scand 47*:540, 1958.
111. Zincke H, Seruga JW: Ureterosigmoidostomy: Critical review of 173 cases. *J Urol 113*:324, 1975.

CHAPTER 103 Principles of Urinary Tract Surgery

Bruce A. Christie and Dale E. Bjorling

PATIENT EVALUATION

The aim of evaluation of patients is to determine the location and extent of disease and to recommend a definitive treatment. A method of proceeding diagnostically is outlined in Figure 103–1. The physical examination narrows the examiner's focus and, with the history, supplies most of the information needed to make a diagnosis. Laboratory evaluation of blood and urine samples helps confirm or rule out urinary tract bleeding or urinary tract infection and demonstrates the degree of reduction of renal function.

Radiography

The presence of urinary tract disease or injury may be suggested by plain radiographs. The observation of

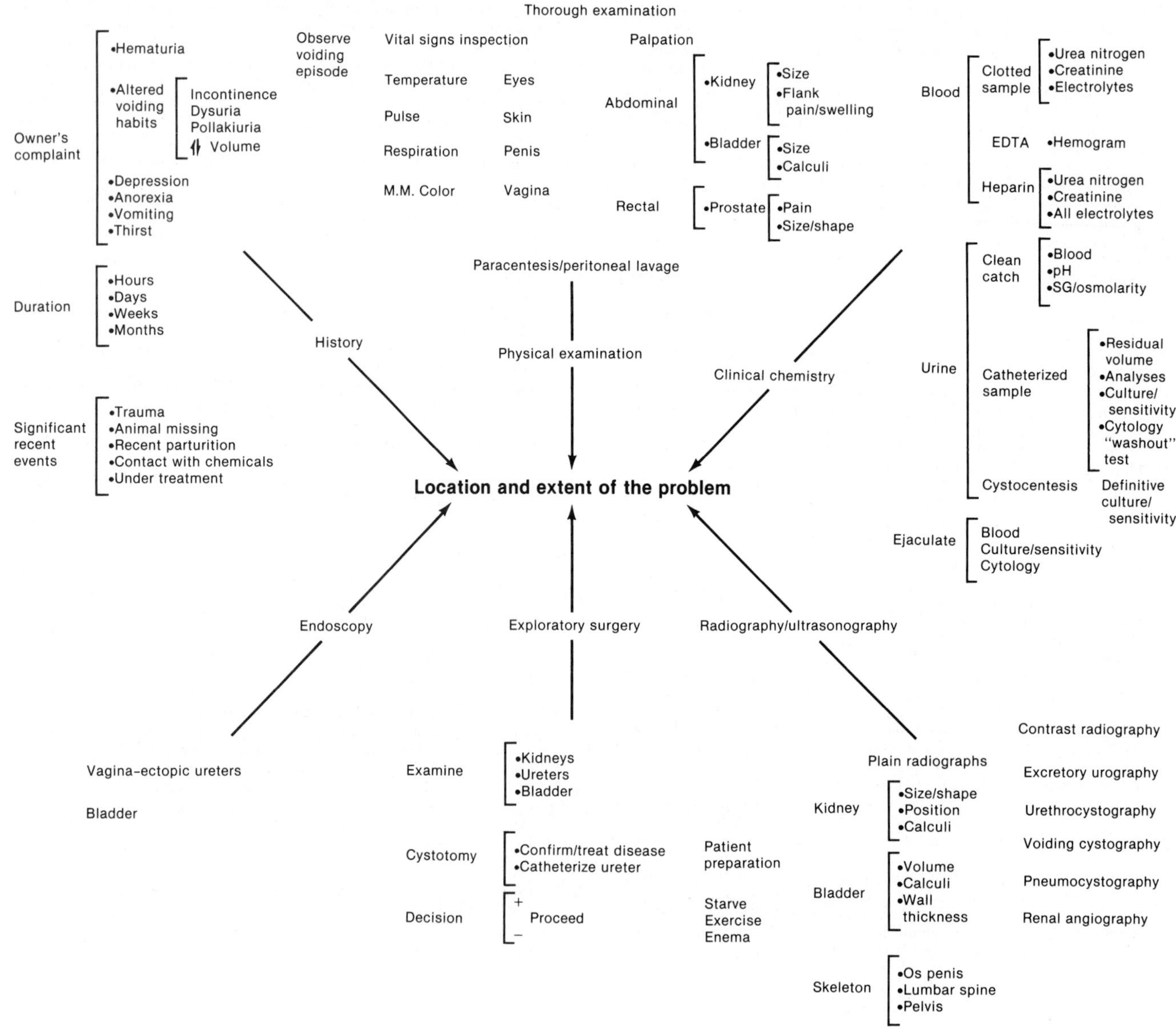

FIGURE 103–1. Method of diagnosing urinary tract abnormalities.

calculi is diagnostic, but contrast studies are frequently required to confirm the presence, location, and extent of urinary tract disease.[100, 120] Displacement or asymmetry of the kidneys, loss of the renal shadow, and reduction in size or absence of the bladder are indications for contrast studies.[69, 98, 123] In one survey of urinary tract injuries in animals with a fractured pelvis, the most consistent finding on plain radiographs was enlargement with increased density, streaking, or mottling of the retroperitoneal space due to perirenal hemorrhage or disruption of the ureters, bladder, or urethra.[111]

Excretory Urography

If the renal blood supply is intact and the kidneys are capable of concentrating and excreting contrast material, excretory urography (intravenous pyelography) outlines the kidneys and ureters and provides information about the junction of the ureters and the trigone of the bladder. The location of injury to the kidneys or ureters can often be identified precisely.[83, 98] The ability of the kidneys to extract contrast material from the blood is an imprecise indicator of renal function. Intravenous injection of contrast material can cause hypotension and bradycardia. Also, renal blood flow may be decreased in hypovolemic patients. These prerenal factors may confound evaluation of renal function. Excretory urography should not be performed when cardiovascular function is impaired.[51, 123]

Rapid intravenous administration of aqueous organic iodide (880 mg/kg) is recommended.[50] A wide variety of contrast media can be used (Table 103–1). Sodium salts give better definition than methylglucamine (meglumine) at the same concentration but can stimulate vomiting in unanesthetized animals. If sodium retention is a problem (i.e., in heart failure), meglumine is the

TABLE 103–1. RADIOGRAPHIC CONTRAST AGENTS FOR UROGRAPHY AND RENAL ANGIOGRAPHY

Contrast Medium				
Generic Name	*Trade Name*	Manufacturer	Iodide Content (mg/ml)	Viscosity at 37° C (Centipoises)
Sodium iothalamate	Conray 420	May & Baker, Australia Pty. Ltd.	420	5.2
	Conray 400	Mallinckrodt, Inc., St. Louis, MO	400	4.7
Methylglucamine iothalamate	Conray 280	May & Baker, Australia Pty. Ltd.	280	4.0
	Conray 60	Mallinckrodt, Inc., St. Louis, MO	282	3.8
Methylglucamine (66%) and sodium (10%) diatrizoate combination	Renografin-76	E.R. Squibb & Sons, Inc., Princeton, NJ	370	8.4
	Urografin-76	Schering Corp., Kenilworth, NJ	370	9.0
	Hypaque-76	Winthrop Aust., Ermington, NSW	370	9.0

alternative cation. Meglumine salts are more viscous than sodium salts; therefore, larger intravenous catheters are used, and the solution is warmed to body temperature to make injection easier and faster.

The first exposure is made 10 seconds after the injection, and a second is made as soon as possible after the first (Fig. 103–2). The 10-second exposure usually shows the bolus of contrast agent as an intravenous aortogram, which should reveal any abnormality of the renal vascular pedicle. The renal outline is visible in the second radiograph during the nephrogram phase. If the kidney is functioning normally, the ureters are best evaluated after 5 minutes. Opacification of the renal pelvis is optimum 10 to 20 minutes after the contrast agent has been injected. If excretory urography does not outline the urinary tract, renal angiography is used.

Renal Angiography

Renal angiography is infrequently done. Options include selective or nonselective renal angiography. Nonselective renal angiography is performed by passing an arterial cather into the aorta and advancing the tip to a position in the abdominal aorta immediately cranial to the renal arteries. A 5- to 10-ml bolus of contrast agent is injected as rapidly as possible. One radiograph is exposed ½ to 1 second after the start of the injection to outline the renal artery and its branches, and a second is exposed approximately 5 to 10 seconds later, when the contrast agent is in the renal vein.[16] Selective angiography requires specialized catheters that may be inserted into the renal arteries, providing greater opacification of the kidneys and allowing the kidneys to be studied separately.[7] Both techniques require some mechanism for rapidly exposing several radiographs.

Retrograde Urethrocystography

The integrity of the urethra and bladder is best assessed by retrograde positive-contrast urethrocystography. In traumatized patients, the bladder should be distended with contrast material in case small leaks are present (Fig. 103–3). Negative-contrast or double-contrast studies may identify intraluminal calculi, masses, or blood clots. Negative-contrast cystography adds little to the evaluation of the urinary tract in traumatized patients and may be dangerous. Fatal air embolism has been reported after negative-contrast cystography in animals, and carbon dioxide or nitrogen should be used if this procedure is performed.[1, 122, 139]

Ultrasonography

The equipment and expertise needed to perform ultrasonographic evaluation of the urinary tract are becoming more prevalent in veterinary medicine. Ultrasonography is useful in evaluating the internal structure of the kidneys, and although low renal blood flow or diminished renal function may severely limit the use of contrast radiographic studies, ultrasonography accurately evaluates the position and structure of the kidney with these physiological alterations.[71, 73, 132–134] The contour and size of the kidneys are easily determined, and mass or cystic lesions of the kidneys are readily detected and biopsy performed using ultrasonography.[59, 72, 73, 133, 134] It may be difficult to evaluate normal ureters in dogs and cats, but when these structures are dilated, they are easily observed. Ultrasonography is efficacious in evaluating the bladder (Fig. 103–4).[17]

Abdominoparacentesis

If fluid is present in the abdomen or if intra-abdominal urinary tract trauma is suspected, abdominoparacentesis and diagnostic peritoneal lavage (if necessary) should be performed.[41, 71] Diagnostic peritoneal lavage is only performed if abdominoparacentesis does not yield a sample of fluid. The concentration of creatinine or urea in the fluid retrieved from the abdomen is compared with that in peripheral blood when samples are collected. The urea and creatinine concentrations in abdominal fluid contaminated with urine are initially greater than in peripheral blood; however, within 4 days, the urea concentration in abdominal fluid is similar but the intra-abdominal creatinine concentration remains higher.[24, 113] This is because the creatinine molecule is larger than the urea molecule and less readily absorbed.[118] If urine is detected within the abdominal cavity, the source is identified by contrast radiography. Diagnostic peritoneal lavage is not performed before plain abdominal radiographs because it introduces air and fluid and complicates interpretation of subsequent radiographic studies.

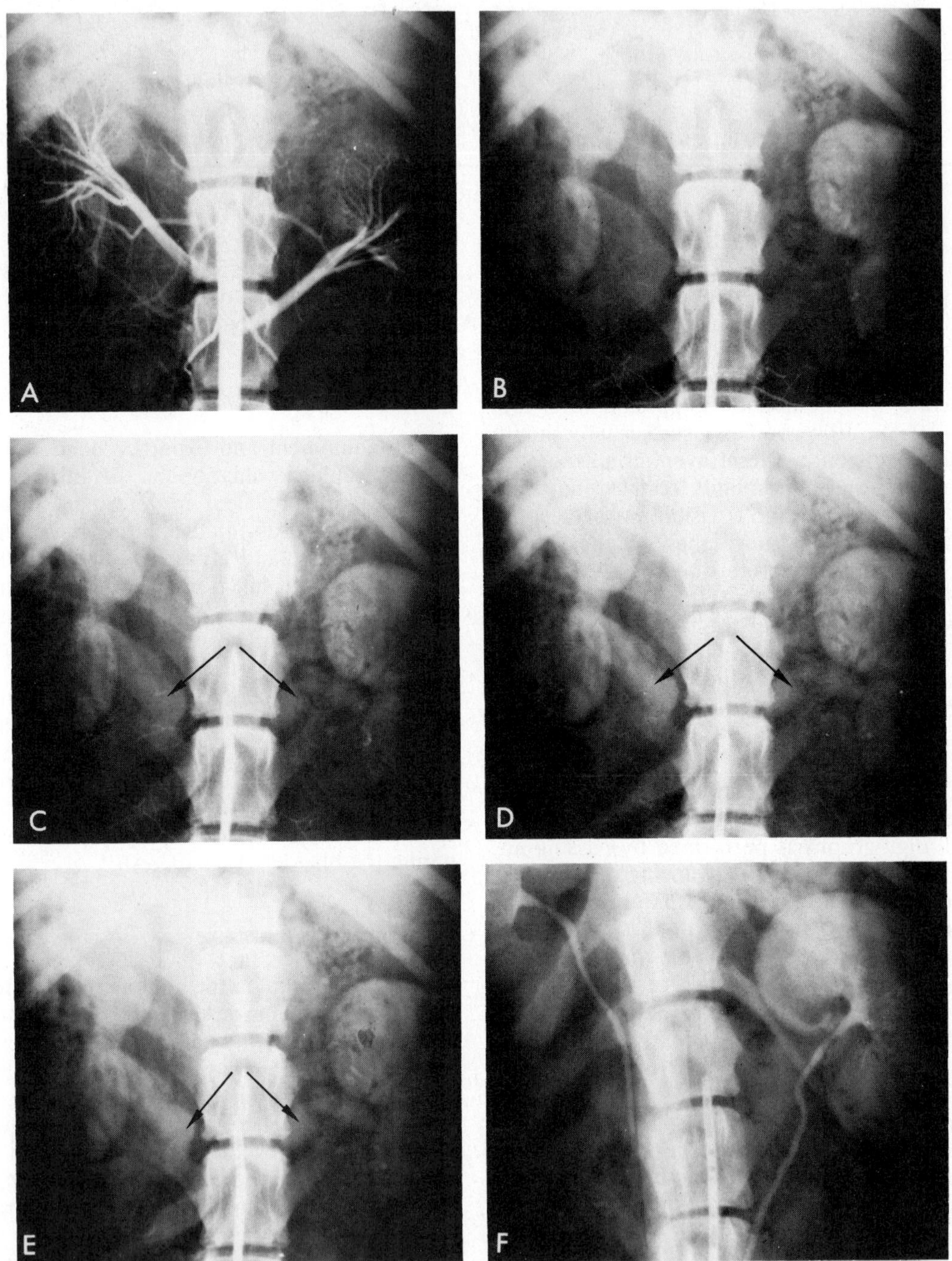

FIGURE 103–2. Nonselective renal angiography in a 15-kg dog. Individual 5-ml boluses of contrast agent were given and radiographs exposed 1.5 (*A*), (*B*), 6 (*C*), 8 (*D*), and 10 seconds (*E*) after commencing each injection. The five exposures were all taken within 1 minute. Features visible include renal artery and major branches (*A*), renal veins (arrows in *C* through *E*), and, after 3 minutes, the origin of the ureter (excretory urogram) (*F*).

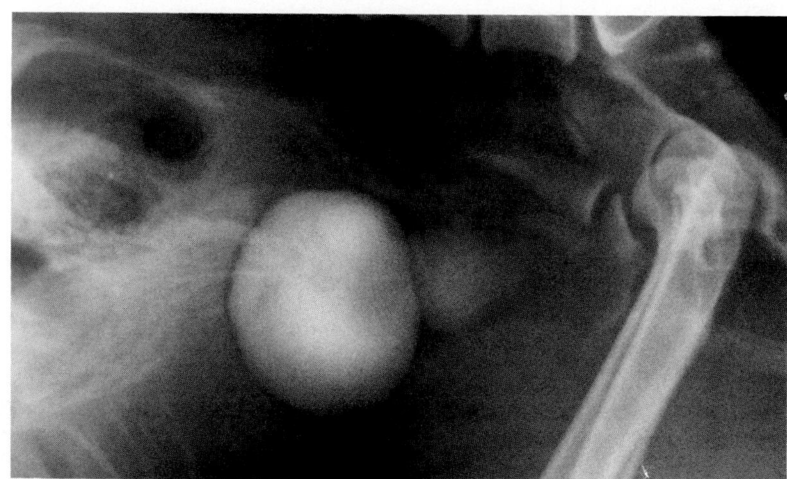

FIGURE 103–3. Positive-contrast cystogram demonstrating leakage of dye from the bladder after traumatic injury.

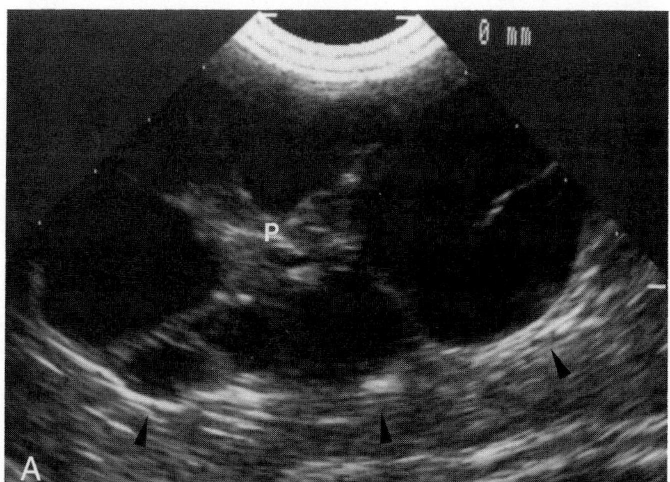

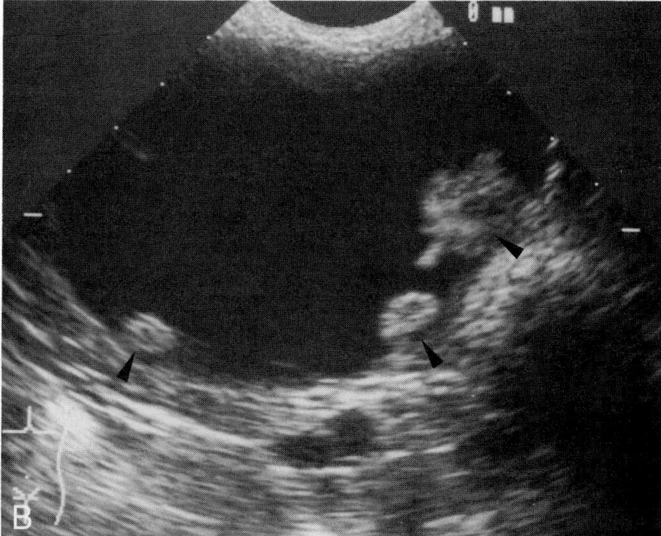

FIGURE 103–4. Ultrasonographic image of a bladder mass (*arrow*).

Endoscopy

Endoscopes small enough to be inserted into the renal pelvis can be used to evaluate unilateral hematuria.[57] Endoscopes can be used to search for an ectopic ureteral orifice in the vagina. Most operations on the urinary tract are elective, but if the urinary tract is obstructed or ruptured or if bleeding is severe, emergency surgery is justified.

SURGICAL PRINCIPLES

Surgical Instruments

A gentle touch with delicate, high-quality equipment and minimal handling of the tissues minimizes edema. A scalpel cut causes minimal tissue trauma. A scalpel can be used to make an incision in any part of the urinary tract. The jaws of scissors twist past each other, cutting and crushing tissue; however, high-quality scissors can be useful for making incisions in the ureters or urethra.

An electroscalpel is a useful tool for incising the bladder and urethra and for hemostasis by coagulation of small vessels. When an electric radiofrequency current is applied to tissues, it produces heat proportional to the frequency of oscillation and inversely proportional to the contact area of the electrode used.[14] Needle electrodes can be used, and tips should be kept clean of carbonized biological material. The tissues are parted by generation of steam bubbles, which rupture cells near the tip of the electrode.[62] Healing of skin wounds is delayed 48 to 72 hours when compared with scalpel incisions.[70] This disadvantage is offset by the precision and ease with which the tissue can be cut, as well as rapid hemostasis.

Grasping instruments with strong jaws and large teeth are not required for operating on delicate urinary tract tissues. Smooth-tipped dissecting forceps can be used to manipulate tissue gently without crushing. Mosquito forceps are sometimes needed to control hemorrhage but are also useful for grasping stay sutures for tissue retraction. Needle holders must have fine jaws when small needles are used to maximize effective needle length and minimize the straightening stress as the needle holder is applied (Fig. 103–5). The most gentle way to stabilize and retract the kidneys and the bladder often is to use the fingers and thumb. The renal vascular pedicle can also be gently occluded by digital pressure.

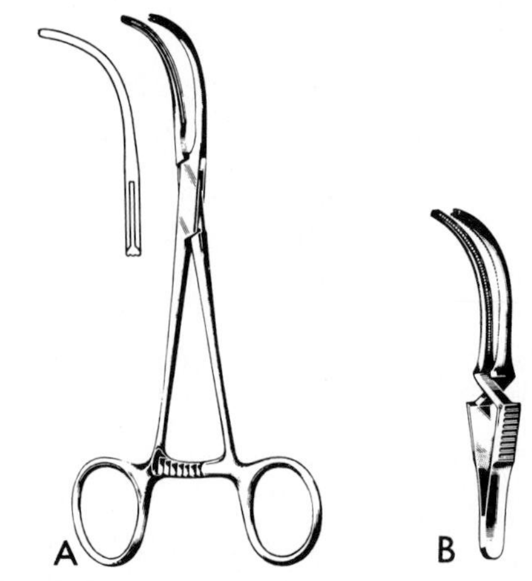

FIGURE 103–6. Peripheral vascular clamps. *A*, Adjustable pressure forceps. When the ratchet is engaged in the first notch, the jaws are still open. Enough pressure is applied just to occlude the blood vessel. *B*, Bulldog clamp. These clamps can be purchased with a specific pressure rating.

Hemostats are never used for temporary vascular occlusion because they crush vessels and promote clotting and stricture. Bulldog clamps (serrefines) or, preferably, vascular forceps (Fig. 103–6) can be used when adjustable closing pressure is needed. Alternatively, the renal vasculature can be occluded by using a snare-type (Rommel) tourniquet, which can be constructed by placing umbilical tape around the vessels and passing both ends through a short length of tubing.

Polypropylene catheters with rounded, sealed ends and a side hole in a range of sizes from 3 to 8 French can be used for catheterizing the urethra or ureters of cats and dogs. Open-ended number 3.5 French catheters are also available for catheterizing the urethra in male cats. Catheters can be used to test patency, to flush the urinary tract, to act as a landmark to help locate the urethra when performing urethrotomy, and to serve as a splint or stent during urethral and ureteral surgery. For irrigating the renal pelvis during nephrotomy, a lacrimal needle or a modified disposable hypodermic needle can be used (Fig. 103–7). Some type of suction apparatus is useful to aspirate urine and flushing solutions. For fine work on ureters, operating loupes with 2 to 4 × magnification are helpful.

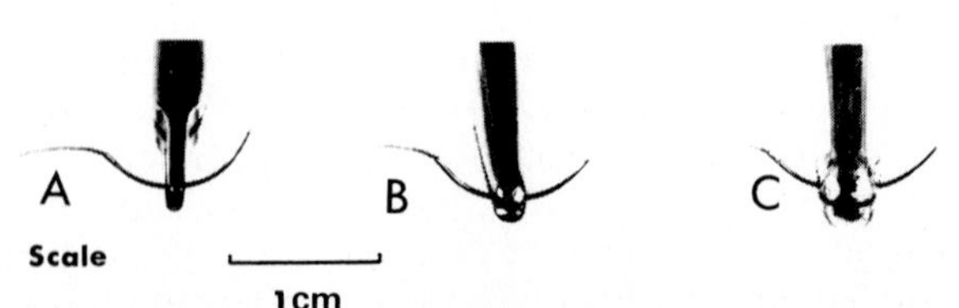

FIGURE 103–5. Three different sizes of needle holders are applied to the same size needle. The effective working length of the needle from the needle tip to the needle holder decreases from *A* to *C*. As the largest needle holder (*C*) is applied, the curved needle is stressed as it straightens out.

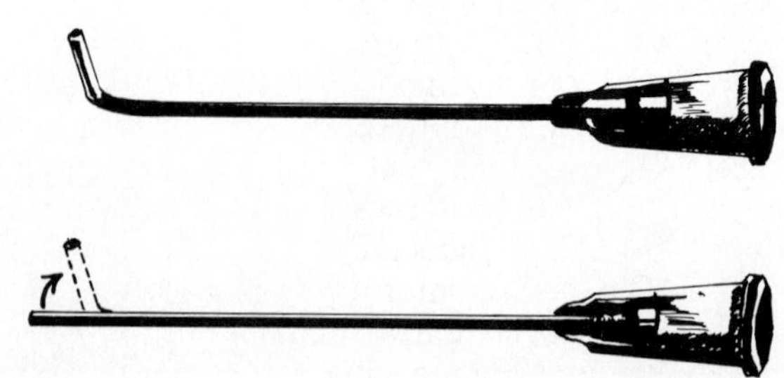

FIGURE 103–7. A disposable hypodermic needle modified to irrigate the diverticula of the renal pelvis. The sharp tip has been ground off, and the distal 5 mm bent approximately 70°.

Suture Materials

The choice of suture material depends on the normal strength of the tissues, the rate at which the wound recovers strength, the strength of the suture material, the rate at which the suture material loses strength in tissues, and interactions that occur between sutures and tissues.[126] The bladder, along with the proximal colon, is one of the weakest organs in the body;[126] however, tissues regain nearly 100 per cent of prewounded strength in 14 to 21 days.[103] Sutures should be at least as strong as the tissue through which they are placed. Nonabsorbable sutures are not used in the urinary tract, because they provide a nidus for formation of urinary calculi. The following remarks concern absorbable suture materials only.

When 6-0 (0.7 μ) plain surgical gut and 7-0 (0.3 μ) chromic gut were used to close the incised bladder of rats, all three suture materials retained tensile strength long enough for satisfactory healing.[2] During bursting tests, pressures as great as 550 mm Hg were reached, and although some bladders burst, sutures cutting through tissues were the cause, not sutures breaking.[2] Because a "desire to void" reflex is triggered at approximately 17 mm Hg and voiding pressures are usually about 20 to 40 mm Hg in normal dogs,[28] there is little justification for using suture materials much outside this size range. Polyglycolic acid (Dexon) sutures have a greater tensile strength than surgical gut of the same diameter,[126] but when placed in tissues, this material loses tensile strength more rapidly than surgical gut.[126] It is reasonable to equate 5-0 polyglycolic acid with 7-0 surgical gut.

Most suture materials in contact with urine for any length of time can act as a nidus for calculus formation,[66, 138] but when concretions occurred on polyglycolic acid suture material used to close cystotomy incisions in rabbits, the cause was the specific type of suture material used.[12] This conclusion prompted work in rabbits,[66] rats,[87] dogs,[20, 26, 66] and cats.[105] The results substantiated the previous findings in rabbits, but it was found that polyglycolic acid was less likely than surgical gut to stimulate the formation of calculi in rats, dogs, and cats.[20]

Two braided synthetic absorbable suture materials are commonly used in surgery of the urinary tract: polyglycolic acid and polyglactin 910 (Vicryl). Both sutures are degraded by hydrolysis and absorbed by the body with minimal tissue reaction. Size 4-0 polyglactin 910 is significantly thicker than 4-0 polyglycolic acid, and the strength is correspondingly greater.[105] When diameters are normalized, the strength of the two materials is approximately equal. Knotting reduces the strength of polyglactin 910 by 40 per cent and polyglycolic acid by 32 per cent.[105] These materials have a high coefficient of friction, and square knots are secure. From a practical point of view, a granny knot with a double first throw should be tied first to allow the knot to be set and advanced until snug; then a square knot can be tied on top to ensure knot security.

Both sutures lose all their strength after 28 days of tissue implantation.[36] Polyglycolic acid decays more slowly than polyglactin 910,[37] but polyglycolic acid sutures placed in dog bladders sloughed by 3 to 6 weeks.[89] Both suture materials retain adequate strength to make them satisfactory for use in the urinary tract.

Some investigators have observed accelerated hydrolysis of polyglycolic acid sutures in the presence of bacteria in urine and high urine pH,[110] but another study failed to confirm this.[63] The reasons for the discrepancies between studies are unclear, but it may be safer to assume that polyglactin 910 maintains its strength characteristics over a wider range of pH than does polyglycolic acid.

Two monofilament synthetic absorbable suture materials are now widely available, polydioxanone (PDS)[104] and modified polyglycolic acid (Maxon).[68] These suture materials have less drag, are approximately 20 per cent stronger than synthetic braided absorbable sutures of similar size, and have satisfactory knot security.[106] Modified polyglycolic acid suture is 60 per cent stiffer than polydioxanone.[106] Both monofilament sutures decay slowly in tissues and retain their strength far in excess of the time required for healing of the urinary tract.[119] Significantly less bacterial adhesion was observed on the surface of polydioxanone than on the surface of polyglycolic acid, polygalactin 910, or chromic gut.[30] This finding, reduced tissue drag, and relative greater strength at smaller sizes are the primary advantages of the monofilament synthetic absorbable suture materials over the braided synthetic absorbable suture materials. Prolonged decay may make these sutures less useful in the urinary tract.

Splinting (Stenting) in Urethral and Ureteral Surgery

Urinary epithelium is damaged by indwelling urethral catheters.[47] Stomal stricture after perineal urethrostomy in cats has been attributed to early use of catheters postoperatively.[55] If primary intention healing is sought, splinting catheters are avoided because of (1) interference with healing and (2) risk of ascending infection.[67, 76, 124] Urine leakage at the urethral anastomosis can delay healing; if this is considered a possibility, urine can be diverted during healing by placing a Foley catheter in the bladder and exteriorizing it in the antepubic position.[44, 107]

When the urethra has been damaged but a segment of intact urethral mucosa bridges the defect, a splinting catheter can be placed to allow the wall of the urethra to heal and mucosa to regenerate over the site of injury.[135] Placement of a catheter across a urethral defect when the mucosa has been completely disrupted does not result in satisfactory healing. The defect is filled with scar tissue not covered by epithelium, and a stricture forms. Ureteral epithelium has the capacity to regenerate over a splint.[88] Although ureteral splints are not invariably necessary in uncomplicated ureteroneocystostomy, they are routinely used in human patients and thought to do little or no harm.[125] The duration of splinting can range from 4 to 5 days for ureteral reimplantation to 10 to 15 days for ureteral anastomosis and as long as 45 days for ureteral regeneration. In animals, lack of cooperation by patients makes management of indwelling catheters difficult. If sound microsurgical techniques are used for ureteral anastomosis in dogs, splinting catheters are not required.[39, 64]

ALTERED RENAL FUNCTION DUE TO ANESTHESIA, SURGERY, AND DRUGS

Ether anesthesia causes urine flow to decrease from 50 ml/hour to 1.2 ml/hour during surgery, but urine flow returns to normal postoperatively, usually within a few hours.[34, 102] After extensive surgery and prolonged anesthesia, direct and indirect secondary effects were noted.

Indirect Effects of Anesthesia

Circulation. Renal blood flow is decreased owing to renal vasoconstriction and systemic hypotension. Catecholamine release and subsequent renal vasoconstriction are pronounced with cyclopropane or ether anesthesia.[101] Thiopentone and halothane do not provoke a catecholamine response but cause myocardial depression and peripheral vasodilation. The result is hypotension, which causes some renal vasoconstriction.[43]

Sympathetic Nervous System. Renal blood vessels are innervated by the celiac and renal plexes with sympathetic constrictor fibers. In response to moderate stress, efferent arteriolar constriction occurs. Thus, although renal blood flow has decreased, glomerular filtration rate remains constant. With further stress, afferent arteriolar constriction occurs and glomerular filtration rate decreases (see Chapter 101). When the kidneys are denervated, anesthetic exposure does not affect renal function.[13]

Endocrine Effects. These are significant and are closely related to circulatory changes. Signals from baroreceptors in the right atrium mediate antidiuretic hormone release and antidiuresis. Angiotensin II, a potent vasoconstrictor, is produced by the action of renin on renin substrate (angiotensinogen). Control of renin release is multifactorial, and these factors (sodium content of tubular fluid, catecholamine levels, sympathetic nervous system impulses, and pressure within the afferent arterioles[56]) all are influenced by anesthesia.

Direct Effects of Anesthesia

Immediate effects are masked by the indirect effects outlined previously. Delayed effects are related to direct nephrotoxicity as a result of anesthetic agents containing fluorinated hydrocarbons, principally methoxyflurane.[38] Affected patients are unable to concentrate urine, resulting in high-output renal insufficiency. The effect is usually transient but occasionally can lead to renal failure. Two metabolites of methoxyflurane are inorganic fluoride and oxalate. Inorganic fluoride has been suggested as the toxic agent,[91, 120] but oxalic acid might also be a factor in patients that develop permanent renal insufficiency.[55, 85, 86] If methoxyflurane anesthesia is limited to less than 2 hours, nephrotoxicity is unlikely. If anesthesia must continue beyond 2 hours, the concentration of methoxyflurane is reduced, and the use of narcotics, nitrous oxide, and muscle relaxants is recommended.[34] Fluorinated anesthetics with the potential to cause direct renal toxicity, in decreasing order of toxicity, include methoxyflurane, enflurane, isoflurane, and halothane. Isoflurane and halothane are metabolized to fluoride to a negligible extent.[35, 82, 116] Acute renal failure was not observed in dogs with decreased renal mass after 4 hours of halothane anesthesia during which an exploratory laparotomy was performed and dogs were maintained in a hypotensive state (arterial blood pressure < 75 mm Hg).[117] Light anesthesia and an adequate fluid regimen with a balanced electrolyte solution ensure that patients have only minimal and transient depression of renal function.[34, 117] Premedication with drugs with mild alpha-blocking properties, such as the neuroleptics acepromazine and droperidol, helps prevent catecholamine-induced vasoconstriction and depressed renal function during anesthesia.[34]

Certain antimicrobial agents, analgesics, and contrast agents are potentially nephrotoxic.

Antimicrobial Agents

The kidneys are a major excretory pathway for many antibiotics. Nephrons are exposed to high concentrations by glomerular filtration, tubular reabsorption, and secretion. The relative nephrotoxicity of various antimicrobials[3] is listed (Table 103–2). Of the cephalosporins, cephaloridine is much less protein bound than cephalothin or cephazolin. It achieves a higher serum concentration and is more nephrotoxic than cephalothin or cephazolin. There is considerable species variation in renal handling of cephalosporins, and with the exception of cephaloridine, they are not considered nephrotoxic.[100]

Degradation products from outdated tetracycline may cause reversible Fanconi's syndrome, and demethylchlortetracycline produces reversible nephrogenic diabetes insipidus.[3] These drugs also have an antianabolic effect and can lead to progressive azotemia. Anabolic steroids prevent these effects,[46] whereas concurrent use of diuretics exacerbates them.[121] Tetracyclines potentiate the nephrotoxicity of methoxyflurane in humans,[25] but when this combination of drugs was administered to ten healthy dogs, nephrotoxicity was not observed.[90] Nephrotoxicity is a well-recognized side effect of treatment with polymyxins B and E.[127] These drugs are only used if less toxic antibiotics are not available.

The sulfonamides had a reputation for crystallization within renal parenchyma.[3, 45] When it was found that a mixture of sulfonamides could be dissolved to the limits of their individual solubilities and that the combination had antibacterial effectiveness, crystallization was no longer a problem. The availability of short-acting, highly soluble sulfonamides such as sulfisoxazole and sulfamethizole has eliminated crystallization problems. In burn therapy, topical silver sulfadiazine produces the nephrotic syndrome in humans by inducing immune-complex glomerulonephritis.[97] When combined with trimethoprim, which has no nephrotoxicity associated with its use, the renal disposition of the sulfa drugs is the same. However, azotemia has been reported with this

TABLE 103–2. NEPHROTOXICITY OF ANTIBIOTICS

Agent	Frequency of Nephrotoxicity*
Amikacin	S
Amoxicillin	N
Ampicillin	R
Carbenicillin	R
Cefazolin	N
Cephalexin	R
Cephaloridine	S
Cephalothin	R
Chloramphenicol	N
Chlortetracycline	R
Ciprofloxacin	N
Cloxacillin	N
Colistin	S
Enrofloxacin	N
Erythromycin	N
Gentamicin	S
Kanamycin	S
Lincomycin	N
Methenamine mandelate	N
Methicillin	R
Nalidixic acid	N
Neomycin	S
Nitrofurantoin	N
Norfloxacin	N
Oxacillin	R
Oxytetracycline	R
Penicillin G	R
Polymyxin	S
Streptomycin	S
Sulfadiazine	R
Sulfamethoxazole	R
Sulfisoxazole	R
Tetracycline hydrochloride	R
Ticarcillin	N
Trimethoprim	R
Tobramycin	S

Modified from Appel GB, Neu HC: The nephrotoxicity of antimicrobial agents (first of three parts). *N Engl J Med 296:*663, 1977.
*N, none reported; R, rare; S, substantial.

combination,[65] possibly owing to altered renal function, which does not affect glomerular filtration rate.

Aminoglycoside antibiotics are not absorbed orally but, after parenteral administration, disperse within the extracellular space. The aminoglycosides are excreted 99 per cent by the kidneys and 1 per cent in the bile. They are filtered and have a predilection for uptake by the proximal tubules and retention within the renal cortex.[136] The proximal tubule is the specific site for nephrotoxicity. In addition to the kidneys, the inner ear and neuromuscular junctions are target sites for toxicity. Streptomycin is the least[3, 49] and neomycin the most nephrotoxic.[27] The toxicities of other aminoglycosides—kanamycin,[49] gentamicin,[129] tobramycin,[42] and amikacin[3]—are within these limits. If any of the more toxic antibiotics has to be used during treatment, monitoring of renal function is essential. Although serial laboratory testing does not always detect aminoglycoside-induced nephrotoxicity early enough to prevent its progression, the earliest signs of nephrotoxicity are detected by urinalysis; urine is evaluated for proteinuria, glucosuria, hematuria, cylindruria, or reduction in specific gravity in the absence of fluid therapy.[21, 40] If changes are detected, administration is stopped.

Analgesic Nephropathy

In humans, nephropathy after administration of nonsteroidal anti-inflammatory drugs has been recognized since 1953. Inhibition of prostaglandin synthesis by nonsteroidal anti-inflammatory agents has little effect on renal blood flow or glomerular filtration rates in normal animals but profoundly diminishes these indices in animals subjected to hemorrhage, salt depletion, general anesthesia, biliary cirrhosis, or heart failure.[32] Paracetamol (acetaminophen), a metabolite of phenacetin, in massive doses can cause papillary necrosis and toxicity in cats.[19] Aspirin in high doses causes papillary necrosis in rats.[92] It has a long half-life in cats (36 hours) and can cause cumulative toxicity.[19] Phenylbutazone and indomethacin can also have toxic renal effects.[4] The vasodilatory effects of renal prostaglandins, which offset ischemic vasoconstriction resulting from sympathetic stimuli associated with anesthesia, surgery, and other stresses, are lost with *prolonged* antiprostaglandin therapy.[6, 32*]

Radiographic Contrast Agents

Acute renal failure lasting 3 to 5 days has been reported in humans after contrast studies of the kidneys, heart, and brain.[128] If an iodinated contrast agent is injected through a catheter that is obstructing arterial blood flow, organ damage results.[18] Damage is demonstrated by prolonged and intense accumulation of contrast agent within the perfused organ, called *contrast staining*. Such a result might be unintentional or can be used for therapeutic nephrectomy.[18] Renal atrophy occurs because of diffuse infarction of the renal arteries.

URINARY TRACT INFECTION

Most urinary tract pathogens originate in the gut or on the skin. Organisms ascend from the urethral orifice,[90, 96] and most are mechanically cleared by normal voiding.[36] The long urethra of males provides protection against ascending infection. Urinary tract infection is potentiated by impairment of normal voiding and retention of urine after voiding. The bladder does have an intrinsic defense mechanism. The bladder mucosa resists the binding of microorganisms, and if organisms do become established in the bladder wall, they are engulfed by phagocytes and are acted on by humoral defense mechanisms.[95, 99] Although urine has been described as an excellent culture medium,[36] bacterial multiplication in rabbit urine is inhibited when the pH is less than 5 or greater than 8 or by urine osmolality in excess of 800 mOsm.[91, 109] A 4 per cent urea concentration is bacteriostatic for most urinary tract pathogens, and this concentration is reached in the renal medulla unless diuresis is ongoing.[109] Cat urine has enhanced bactericidal properties.[75]

Urine may be collected by free catch, catheterization, or cystocentesis for analysis and microbial culturing.

*Editor's note: Experimental reports of nephrotoxicity after flunixin administration in dogs anesthetized with methoxyflurane are unsubstantiated by clinical reports and widespread use.

Quantitative urine cultures may be performed to determine if an infection is present. The number of organisms present depends on the method[25] and time[115] of urine collection, whether or not the patient is undergoing diuresis, and whether or not the patient is on antibacterial therapy. Samples of urine obtained from dogs by catheterization suggest urinary tract infection when bacteria exceed 10,000/ml in males and 100,000/ml in females.[8, 9, 25] Manual compression of the bladder with sufficient force to initiate voiding induces vesicoureteral reflux[52] and is therefore not recommended for patients suspected of having cystitis for fear of producing pyelonephritis.[29] Contamination of the urine can occur from the urethra, prepuce, or vagina when a clean-catch or catheterized specimen is obtained. In 50 normal dogs (25 females and 25 males), urine specimens were obtained for microbial culturing from all animals by cystocentesis and from 30 dogs by catheterization and 20 dogs by free catch. No growth was observed from any of the samples obtained by cystocentesis, whereas bacteria were cultured from 26 per cent of the samples obtained by catheterization and 85 per cent of voided samples.[33] These findings reinforce the importance of performing quantitative cultures to distinguish contamination from infection. Care should be taken to avoid introducing bacteria into the bladder during catheterization. Contamination can be minimized by first cleaning the external genitalia or flushing the preputial cavity or vagina with sterile water or saline. Cleaning the external genitalia with antiseptics such as 0.05 per cent aqueous chlorhexidine is recommended before catheterization as long as a urine culture is not contemplated. Even very small traces of antiseptic interfere with colony counts.[115] The risk of mechanically seeding the bladder with organisms from the preputial cavity or perineum is greater in females than in males.[15, 33] If contamination occurs and catheterization was rough, the mucosal injury provides an opportunity for contaminating organisms to become established within the bladder wall and to produce an infection. For this reason, a bladder rinse with 0.2 per cent neomycin before removing the catheter significantly decreases the incidence of postcatheterization bacteriuria.[31]

Open indwelling urethral catheters are frequently used for temporary urine diversion in animals and humans. Their use has to be weighed against the known risk of infection. Organisms can enter around or through the lumen of the catheter,[9, 124] and most patients with previously sterile urine have bacteriuria within 24 hours of catheter placement.[67, 76] Closed catheter drainage systems with nonreturn valves prevent catheter-associated urinary tract infection for short periods.[124] EDTA-tris-lysozyme lavage has been advocated to treat *Pseudomonas* spp. infections and coliform cystitis associated with indwelling catheters.[58, 138] However, neither flushing catheter systems with antiseptics nor administering systemic antibiotics prevents catheter-related infections with prolonged catheterization.[9] Prophylactic antibiotic therapy is not recommended during catheterization, because although the initial rate of infection may decrease slightly, infection with antibiotic-resistant strains of bacteria occurs much more frequently.[9] It is preferable to culture the urine after the catheter has been removed and use appropriate antibiotics to treat urinary tract infection.

TABLE 103–3. ORGANISMS COMMONLY ISOLATED FROM DOGS AND CATS WITH URINARY TRACT INFECTION

Dogs	Cats
Escherichia coli	*Escherichia coli*
Proteus spp.	Enterococci
Staphylococcus aureus	*Proteus* spp.
Enterococci	*Pasteurella*
Klebsiella	β-hemolytic streptococci
Enterobacter	
Pseudomonas spp.	

There should be no delay in processing urine once it has been collected, because bacterial numbers can double at room temperature in 45 minutes.[5] If the specimen is refrigerated at 39.2°F (4°C), it can be stored for 24 hours and meaningful results can still be obtained from the cultures.[27] The test to confirm renal infection is culture of the renal pelvis or ureteric urine. In animals, this is usually done by catheterizing the ureteric orifices during cystotomy. However, it is possible to sample urine from the renal pelvis by percutaneous nephropyelocentesis.[80] An indirect method used in humans is the bladder washout test.[48] Serial quantitative urine cultures are performed, first on a catheterized urine sample. The bladder is sterilized by infusing enzymes and antibiotics, which are then washed out with sterile saline. Urine is sampled at regular intervals and cultured. If successive cultures remain sterile, the infection arose from the bladder. If colony counts increase with successive cultures, the infection is seated in the kidneys. This test is simple but time-consuming and costly and in animals might be unreliable.[53, 54] Organisms that commonly infect the urinary tract of dogs and cats are listed in Table 103–3. *Escherichia coli, Proteus* spp., and *Staphylococcus aureus* account for 80 per cent of isolates in dogs.[137] The prevalence of urinary tract infections in cats is less than in dogs,[27] possibly because of superior antibacterial qualities of cat urine.[75]

Antibiotic, Antibacterial, and Analgesic Therapy (Table 103–4)

Antibiotics

Penicillins. These drugs are bactericidal and, except for cloxacillin and oxacillin, are destroyed by bacterial penicillinase. As a group, the penicillins are generally active against gram-positive organisms. Penicillin G and ampicillin, when given orally, reach urine concentrations 100 times greater than serum concentrations and can be effective against gram-negative as well as gram-positive organisms.[79] Food in the stomach interferes with penicillin absorption; therefore, food should be withheld for 20 minutes after administration to aid absorption.

Voiding opportunities should be limited to 15 to 20 minutes before the next dose to maintain high urine

TABLE 103–4. ANTIBIOTIC, ANTIBACTERIAL, AND ANALGESIC THERAPY FOR URINARY TRACT INFECTION

Therapy	Dose Rate (mg/kg) Oral	Dose Rate (mg/kg) Intramuscular	Dose Frequency/Day
Antibiotic			
Penicillin G	12*	12	6
Penicillin V	8		3
Ampicillin	10	7	3
Amoxicillin	10	7	3
Amoxicillin with clavulanic acid	15		3
Streptomycin		20	1
Gentamicin		2	3
Neomycin	0.2% solution for bladder infusion		
Cephalexin	10		2
Cephaloridine		11	2
Tetracycline	20		3
Oxytetracycline	27		2
		10	1
Chloramphenicol	40		3 (dog) 2 (cat)
Ciprofloxacin	10–15		2
Enrofloxacin	5–10		2
Norfloxacin	22		2
Antibacterial			
Sulfamethizole	50		4
Sulfisoxazole	50		4
Trimethoprim/ sulfadiazine (1:5)	15 30		2 (dog) 1 (cat)
Nitrofurantoin	4		3
Methenamine	25		2
Methenamine mandelate or hippurate	25		2
Analgesic			
Phenazopyridine	5		2

*Penicillin G, 1,595 units/mg.

levels of the drug. Amoxicillin is an analogue of ampicillin and has the same antibacterial spectrum but is better absorbed in the presence of food.[19] The combination of clavulanic acid and amoxicillin has greater activity against gram-negative bacteria than other penicillins. Carbenicillin and ticarcillin are semisynthetic penicillins with activity against *Pseudomonas* spp. and are synergistic with gentamicin.[19]

Aminoglycosides. Streptomycin at the recommended dose is bactericidal against many gram-negative organisms, including *Proteus* spp. and *Pseudomonas* spp. Penicillin-streptomycin mixtures are compatible and have a broad spectrum of activity. Streptomycin resistance can develop as rapidly as within a week.[19] Neomycin is bactericidal and has a broad spectrum of activity. It is not recommended for parenteral use because of the risk of nephrotoxicity and ototoxicity. It is useful for local instillation into the bladder after catheterization. Gentamicin is bactericidal and has a broad spectrum of activity. It is particularly effective against *Pseudomonas* spp. Resistance occurs in proportion to usage, so as a rule, this drug should not be used as a first-line antibiotic. Ototoxicity, renal toxicity, and neuromuscular blockade with the risk of respiratory paralysis can occur with this drug. Nephrotoxicity is potentiated by dehydration and concomitant administration of diuretics.[21] Cats are most at risk.[19] Because of its mechanism of action, gentamicin can be given less frequently at higher doses, resulting in similar efficacy with less toxicity. Gentamicin enters bacteria and binds to the ribosomal subunits, interfering with RNA function and protein synthesis. The effects of gentamicin depend less on maintaining serum concentrations above minimum inhibitory concentrations and depend more on the amount of drug that enters the bacteria.[23, 84, 94] Tobramycin is like gentamicin and is active against *Pseudomonas* spp.

Cephalosporins. These antibiotics are bactericidal with a spectrum of activity similar to ampicillin. The second- and third-generation cephalosporins have a greater spectrum of activity against gram-negative organisms than do the penicillins or first-generation cephalosporins. Cephadroxil and cephalexin are effective in the treatment of urinary tract infection due to *E. coli* and *Klebsiella pneumoniae,* respectively.[10, 78] The cephalosporins occasionally cause nephrotoxicity in humans but are not nephrotoxic (with the exception of cephaloridine) in dogs and cats.[100]

Tetracyclines. These antibiotics have a broad spectrum of activity and are bacteriostatic at usual concentrations. They are absorbed in the gut and undergo enterohepatic circulation but are not metabolized and are mainly excreted in urine. Oxytetracycline is more freely excreted in the urine than chlortetracycline. Tetracycline, from which chlor- and oxytetracycline are derived, is absorbed well from the gastrointestinal tract. Blood levels are higher and are maintained longer than with the other tetracyclines. This drug is inexpensive and has a high cure rate against *Pseudomonas* spp. urinary tract infections in dogs.[81] Nephrotoxicity has been reported when degraded, out-of-date tetracycline was used in conjunction with methoxyflurane anesthesia in a stressed patient.[74]

Chloramphenicol. This antibiotic is bacteriostatic with a broad spectrum of activity and is rapidly absorbed after oral dosing. As much as 45 per cent of the drug binds to serum proteins.[19] It is effective in treating urinary tract infections in dogs, including *Proteus* spp. and *Pseudomonas* spp. infections. Chloramphenicol may suppress bone marrow function and interfere with hematopoiesis, particularly in cats. It also depresses liver mitochondrial activity; therefore, treated animals may have greatly delayed recovery after barbiturate anesthesia.[19]

Fluoroquinolones. The fluoroquinolones are bactericidal and are effective against many gram-positive and gram-negative bacteria. They are structurally related to nalidixic acid[93] and have a broader spectrum of activity against gram-negative bacteria than most other orally administered antibiotics. Enrofloxacin is approved for veterinary use; norfloxacin and ciprofloxacin are approved for use in humans, but their administration in dogs has not been evaluated.[22, 130, 131] Norfloxacin in particular appears to be concentrated in the urine.[11]

Renal toxicity has not been observed with fluoroquinolones.

Polymyxins. These antibiotics have a gram-negative spectrum and are synergistic with oxytetracycline. Therefore, the doses of each in combination can be cut by 1/2 to 1/16.[19] These drugs are decidedly nephrotoxic and are only used if other, less toxic drugs are unavailable.[127]

Antibacterials

Sulfonamides. These drugs are bacteriostatic, with a gram-positive spectrum of activity. Sulfacrystalluria can occur in acid urine and at low urine flows but is not likely with the more soluble sulfonamides such as sulfisoxazole and sulfamethizole. Resistant strains may develop following sulfa drugs.

Enhanced Sulfonamides. When a sulfonamide is combined with trimethoprim, another bacteriostatic drug, the combination is bactericidal and has a broad spectrum of activity.[19, 114] Antibacterial effects are enhanced because each drug inhibits a different step in the synthesis of folic acid, which is needed by microorganisms.[77]

Nitrofurans. These agents are bactericidal and have a broad spectrum of activity in acid urine. In patients with oliguria or anuria, toxic levels can be reached. Many urinary tract pathogens are resistant to nitrofurans.[112]

Methenamine and Its Salts. Methenamine is excreted in the urine, where, in the pH range of 5 to 6, it breaks down to form ammonia and formaldehyde. To provide the acid medium, methenamine has been coupled with the organic acids mandelamine and hippuric acid. Methenamine mandelate and hippurate are absorbed as individual components, and *in vitro* tests suggest that if the pH is maintained between 5 and 6, methenamine by itself is not inferior to the combination with acid salts.[60] Bacterial resistance to methenamine has not been demonstrated; therefore, it can be used with its acid salts for long-term therapy. If necessary, urine pH can be adjusted to between 5 and 6 with ammonium chloride or sodium acid phosphate.

Some urinary antiseptics contain methylene blue. These agents should not be used in cats, because severe hemolytic anemia can result.[108]

Urinary Tract Analgesia

Phenazopyridine is an azo dye that, when excreted in the urine, has a topical analgesic effect. It also turns urine bright orange. This drug is therapeutically hazardous in cats, because it can cause methemoglobinemia and Heinz body hemolytic anemia.[61] It should never be used in dogs, because it produces acute keratoconjunctivitis sicca owing to lacrimal gland damage. This drug is not recommended for use in animals with renal or hepatic insufficiency.

References

1. Ackerman N, et al: Fatal air embolism associated with pneumourethrography and pneumocystography in a dog. *J Am Vet Med Assoc 160*:1616, 1972.
2. Adams H, et al: Sutures and bladder wound healing in the experimental animal. *Invest Urol 12*:267, 1975.
3. Appel GB, Neu HC: The nephrotoxicity of antimicrobial agents. Parts 1, 2, and 3. *N Engl J Med 296*:663, 1977.
4. Arnold L, et al: Further studies of the acute effects of phenylbutazone, oxyphenbutazone and indomethacin on the rat kidney. *Pathology 8*:135, 1976.
5. Asscher AW, et al: Urine as a medium for bacterial growth. *Lancet 2*:1037, 1966.
6. Attallah AA, Lee JB: Prostaglandins, renal function and blood pressure regulation. *In* Lee JB (ed): *Prostaglandins*. Elsevier, New Holland, New York, 1982.
7. Barber DL: Renal angiography in veterinary medicine. *Vet Radiol 16*:187, 1975.
8. Barsanti JA, Finco DR: Laboratory findings in urinary tract infection. *Vet Clin North Am 9*:729, 1979.
9. Barsanti JA, et al: Urinary tract infection due to indwelling bladder catheters in dogs and cats. *J Am Vet Med Assoc 187*:384, 1985.
10. Barsanti JA, et al: Efficacy of cephadroxil in experimental canine cystitis. *J Am Anim Hosp Assoc 21*:89, 1985.
11. Bergeron MG, et al: Norfloxacin penetration into human renal and prostatic tissues. *Antimicrob Agents Chemother 28*:349, 1985.
12. Bergman FO, et al: Synthetic absorbable suture material (P.G.A.). *Acta. Chir Scand. 137*:193, 1971.
13. Berne RM: Hemodynamics and sodium excretion of denervated kidney in anesthetized and unanesthetized dog. *Am J Physiol 171*:148, 1952.
14. Bierman W: Electrosurgery. *Am J Surg 50*:768, 1951.
15. Bierteumpel PH, et al: Urinary tract infection resulting from catheterization in healthy adult dogs. *J Am Vet Med Assoc 178*:989, 1981.
16. Biery DN: Upper urinary tract. *In* O'Brien TR (ed): *Radiographic Diagnosis of Abdominal Disorders in the Dog and Cat.* W.B. Saunders, Philadelphia, 1978.
17. Biller DS, et al: Diagnostic ultrasound of the urinary bladder. *J Am Anim Hosp Assoc 26*:397, 1990.
18. Brady TM, et al: Angiographic nephrectomy using iodinated contrast agent. *Invest Radiol 17*:479, 1982.
19. Brander GC, et al: *Veterinary Applied Pharmacology and Therapeutics.* 4th ed. Balliere Tindall, London, 1982, pp 228, 383, 392.
20. Brannan W, et al: Laboratory and clinical experience with polyglycolic acid suture in urogenital surgery. *J Urol 110*:571, 1973.
21. Brown SA, et al: Gentamicin-associated acute renal failure in the dog. *J Am Vet Med Assoc 186*:686, 1985.
22. Budsberg SC, et al: Norfloxacin therapy in infections of the canine urogenital tract caused by multiresistant bacteria. *J Am Anim Hosp Assoc 25*:713, 1989.
23. Bundtzen RW, et al: Postantibiotic suppression of bacterial growth. *Rev Infect Dis 3*:28, 1981.
24. Burrows CF, Bovee KC: Metabolic changes due to experimentally induced rupture of the canine urinary bladder. *Am J Vet Res 35*:1083, 1974.
25. Carter JM, et al: Comparison of collection techniques for qualitative urine collection in dogs. *J Am Vet Med Assoc 173*:296, 1978.
26. Case GD, et al: Comparison of absorbable sutures in urinary bladder. *Urology 7*:165, 1976.
27. Chew DJ, Kowalski JP: Urinary tract infection. *In* Bojrab MJ (ed): *Pathophysiology in Small Animal Surgery*. Lea & Febiger, Philadelphia, 1981.
28. Christie BA: Incidence and etiology of vesico-ureteral reflux in apparently normal dogs. *Invest Urol 9*:184, 1971.
29. Christie, BA: The occurrence of vesicoureteral reflux and pyelonephritis in apparently normal dogs. Invest Neurol *10*:359, 1973.
30. Chu C-C, Williams DF: Effects of physical configuration and chemical structure of suture materials on bacterial adhesion. *Am J Surg 147*:197, 1984.
31. Clark LW: Neomycin in the prevention of postcatheterization bacteriuria. *Med J Aust 1*:1034, 1973.
32. Clive DM, Stoff JS: Renal syndromes associated with nonsteroidal antiinflammatory drugs. *N Engl J Med 310*:563, 1984.
33. Comer KM, Ling GV: Results of urinalysis and bacterial culture of canine urine obtained by antepubic cystocentesis, catheterization, and the midstream voided methods. *J Am Vet Med Assoc 179*:891, 1981.
34. Cousins MJ, Mazze RI: Anesthesia surgery and renal function. *Anaesth Intensive Care 1*:355, 1973.
35. Cousins MJ, et al: A comparison of the renal effects of isoflurane and methoxyflurane in Fischer 344 rats. *Anesthesiology 38*:556, 1973.
36. Cox CE, Hinman F Jr: Experiments with induced bacteriuria, vesical emptying and bacterial growth on the mechanism of bladder defense to infection. *J Urol 86*:739, 1961.
37. Craig PH, et al: A biological comparison of polyglactin 910 and polyglycolic acid synthetic absorbable sutures. *Surg Gynecol Obstet 141*:1, 1975.
38. Crandell WB, et al: Nephrotoxicity associated with methoxyflurane anaesthesia. *Anaesthesiology 27*:591, 1966.
39. Crane S: Transureteroureterostomy in the dog. *Vet Surg 9*:108, 1980.
40. Cronin RE, et al: Natural history of aminoglycoside nephrotoxicity in the dog. *J Lab Clin Med 95*:463, 1980.
41. Crowe DT Jr, Crane SW: Diagnostic paracentesis and lavage in the evaluation of abdominal injuries in dogs and cats: Clinical and experimental investigations. *J Am Vet Med Assoc 168*:700, 1976.

42. DeRosa F, et al: Tobramycin: Toxicological and pharmacological studies in animals and pharmacokinetic research in patients with varying degrees of renal impairment. *J Int Med Res 2*:100, 1974.
43. Deutsch S, et al: Effects of anaesthesia with thiopental, nitrous oxide, and neuromuscular blockers on renal function in normal man. *Anesthesiology 20*:184, 1968.
44. Dhein CR, et al: Prepubic (suprapubic) catheterization of the dog. *J Am Anim Hosp Assoc 25*:261, 1989.
45. Dowling HF, Lepper MH: Toxic reactions following therapy with sulfapyridine, sulfathiozole, and sulfadiazine. *JAMA 121*:1190, 1943.
46. Editorial: The danger of giving tetracyclines to patients with kidney disease. *NZ Med J 77*:397, 1973.
47. Edwards L, Trot PA: Catheter-induced urethral inflammation. *J Urol 100*:678, 1973.
48. Fairley KF, et al: Simple test to determine the site of urinary tract infection. *Lancet 2*:427, 1967.
49. Falco FG, et al: Nephrotoxicity of the aminoglycosides. *J Infect Dis 119*:406, 1969.
50. Feeney DA, et al: Normal canine excretory urogram: Effects of dose, time, and individual dog variation. *Am J Vet Res 40*:1596, 1979.
51. Feeney DA, et al: The excretory urogram; Parts I and II. *Comp Cont Educ Pract Vet 4*:233, 1982.
52. Feeney DA, et al: Vesicoureteral reflux induced by manual compression of the urinary bladder of dogs and cats. *J Am Vet Med Assoc 182*:795, 1983.
53. Finco DR, Kern A: Pyelonephritis. *In* Kirk RW (ed): *Current Veterinary Therapy VI*. W.B. Saunders, Philadelphia, 1977.
54. Finco DR, et al: Evaluation of methods for localization of urinary tract infection in the female dog. *Am J Vet Res 40*:707, 1979.
55. Franscino JA, et al: Renal oxalosis and azotaemia after methoxyflurane anaesthesia. *N Engl J Med 283*:676, 1970.
56. Ganong WF: *Review of Medical Physiology*. 8th ed. Lange Medical Publications, Los Altos, 1977, p 346.
57. Gittes RF, Varady S: Nephroscopy in chronic unilateral hematuria. *J Urol 126*:297, 1981.
58. Goldschmidt MC, et al: EDTA and lysozyme lavage in the treatment of pseudomonas and coliform bladder infections. *J Urol 197*:969, 1972.
59. Hager DA, et al: Ultrasound-guided biopsy of the canine liver, kidney, and prostate. *Vet Radiol 26*:82, 1985.
60. Hamilton-Miller JMT, Brumfitt W: Methenamine and its salts as urinary tract antiseptics. *Invest Urol 14*:287, 1977.
61. Harvey JW, Kronick HP: Phenazopyridine toxicosis in the cat. *J Am Vet Med Assoc 169*:327, 1976.
62. Honig WM: The mechanisms of cutting in electrosurgery. *IEEE Trans Biomed Eng 22*:58, 1975.
63. Hovendal CP, Schwartz W: Polyglycolic acid (Dexon) sutures in *Escherichia coli* infected urine. *Scand J Urol Nephrol 13*:105, 1979.
64. Jonas D, et al: Splintless microsurgical anastomosis of the ureter in the dog. *Urol Res 9*:271, 1981.
65. Kalowsky S, et al: Deterioration of renal function in association with co-trimoxazole therapy. *Lancet 1*:394, 1973.
66. Kaminski JM, et al: Urinary bladder calculus formation on sutures in rabbits, cats, and dogs. *Surg Gynecol Obstet 146*:353, 1978.
67. Kass EH, Sossen HS: Prevention of infection of urinary tract in the presence of indwelling catheters. *JAMA 169*:1181, 1959.
68. Katz AR, et al: A new synthetic monofilament absorbable suture made from polytrimethylene carbonate. *Surg Gynecol Obstet 161*:213, 1985.
69. Kleine LJ, Thornton GW: Radiographic diagnosis of urinary tract trauma. *J Am Anim Hosp Assoc 7*:318, 1971.
70. Knecht CD, et al: Healing of sharp incisions and electroincisions in dogs. *J Am Vet Med Assoc 159*:1447, 1971.
71. Kolata RJ: Diagnostic abdominal paracentesis and lavage: Experimental and clinical evaluation in the dog. *J Am Vet Med Assoc 168*:697, 1976.
72. Konde LJ, et al: Ultrasonographic anatomy of the normal canine kidney. *Vet Radiol 25*:173, 1984.
73. Konde LJ, et al: Sonographic appearance of renal neoplasia in the dog. *Vet Radiol 26*:74, 1985.
74. Konde LJ, et al: Comparison of radiography and ultrasonography in the evaluation of renal lesions in the dog. *J Am Vet Med Assoc 188*:1420, 1986.
75. Lees GE, Osborne CA: Antibacterial properties of urine: A comparative review. *J Am Anim Hosp Assoc 15*:125, 1979.
76. Lees GE, et al: Adverse effects of indwelling urethral catheterization in clinically normal male cats. *Am J Vet Res 42*:825, 1981.
77. Ling GV, Ruby AL: Chloramphenicol for oral treatment of canine urinary tract infections. *J Am Vet Med Assoc 172*:914, 1978.
78. Ling GV, Ruby AL: Cephalexin for oral treatment of canine urinary tract infection caused by *Klebsiella pneumoniae*. *J Am Vet Med Assoc 182*:1346, 1983.
79. Ling GV, Gillmore CJ: Penicillin G or ampicillin for oral treatment of canine urinary tract infections. *J Am Vet Med Assoc 171*:358, 1977.
80. Ling GV, et al: Percutaneous nephropyelocentesis and nephropyelostomy in the dog: A description of the technique. *Am J Vet Res 40*:1605, 1979.
81. Ling GV, et al: Tetracycline for oral treatment of canine urinary tract infections caused by *Pseudomonas aeruginosa*. *J Am Vet Med Assoc 179*:578, 1981.
82. Loew G, et al: Quantum chemical studies of the metabolism of the inhalation anesthetics methoxyflurane, enflurane and isoflurane. *Mol Pharmacol 10*:406, 1974.
83. Lord PF, et al: Intravenous urography for evaluation of renal diseases in small animals. *J Am Anim Hosp Assoc 10*:139, 1974.
84. Mattie H, et al: Determinants of efficacy and toxicity of aminoglycosides. *J Antimicrob Chemother 24*:281, 1989.
85. Mazze RI, et al: Strain differences in metabolism and susceptibility to the nephrotoxic effects of methoxyflurane in rats. *J Pharmacol Exp Ther 184*:481, 1973.
86. Mazze RI, et al: Methoxyflurane metabolism and renal dysfunction: Clinical correlation in man. *Anesthesiology 35*:247, 1971.
87. Milroy E: An experimental study of the calcification and absorption of polyglycolic acid and catgut sutures within the urinary tract. *Invest Urol 14*:151, 1976.
88. Mobley DF: Studies in ureteral regeneration. *Invest Urol 14*:269, 1976.
89. Morrow FA, et al: *In vivo* comparison of polyglycolic acid, chromic catgut and silk in tissue of the genitourinary tract: An experimental study of tissue retrieval and calculogenesis. *J Urol 112*:655, 1974.
90. Mulholland SG: Lower urinary tract antibacterial defense mechanisms. *Invest Urol 17*:93, 1979.
91. Mulholland SG, et al: The antibacterial effects of urine. *Invest Urol 6*:569, 1969.
92. Nanra RS, Kincaid-Smith P: Papillary necrosis in rats caused by aspirin and aspirin containing mixtures. *Br Med J 3*:559, 1970.
93. Neer TM: Clinical pharmacologic features of fluoroquinolone antimicrobial drugs. *J Am Vet Med Assoc 193*:577, 1988.
94. Nordstrom L, et al: Does administration of an aminoglycoside in a single daily dose affect its efficacy and toxicity? *J Antimicrob Chemother 25*:159, 1990.
95. Orikase S, Hinman F Jr: Reaction of the vesical wall of bacterial penetration. *Invest Urol 15*:185, 1977.
96. Osborne CA, et al: *Canine and Feline Urology*. W.B. Saunders, Philadelphia, 1972.
97. Owens JC, et al: Nephrotic syndrome following topically applied sulfadiazine silver therapy. *Arch Intern Med 134*:332, 1974.
98. Pechman RD: Urinary trauma in dogs and cats: A review. *J Am Anim Hosp Assoc 18*:33, 1982.
99. Perez JR, et al: Evidence for bladder bactericidal factor. *Invest Urol 11*:489, 1974.
100. Perkins RL, et al: Cephaloridine and cephalothin: Comparative studies of potential nephrotoxicity. *J Lab Clin Med 71*:75, 1968.
101. Price HL, et al: Sympathoadrenal responses to general anesthesia in man and their relation to hemodynamics. *Anesthesiology 20*:563, 1959.
102. Pringle H, et al: Clinical effects of ether anesthesia on renal activity. *Br Med J 2*:542, 1905.
103. Rasmussen F: Biochemical analysis of wound healing in the urinary bladder. *Surg Gynecol Obstet 124*:553, 1967.
104. Ray JA, et al: Polydiozanone (PDS): A novel monofilament synthetic absorbable suture. *Surg Gynecol Obstet 153*:497, 1981.
105. Rodeheaver GT, et al: Mechanical performance of polyglycolic acid and polyglactin 910 synthetic absorbable sutures. *Surg Gynecol Obstet 153*:835, 1981.
106. Rodeheaver GT, et al: Mechanical performance of monofilament synthetic absorbable sutures. *Am J Surg 154*:544, 1987.
107. Rosenberg M: Experience with extended use of Foley catheter following repair of the bladder. *Surg Gynecol Obstet 141*:734, 1975.
108. Schechter RD, et al: Heinz body hemolytic anemia associated with the use of urinary antiseptics containing methylene blue in the cat. *J Am Vet Med Assoc 162*:37, 1973.
109. Schlegel JU, et al: Bactericidal effect of urea. *J Urol 86*:819, 1961.
110. Sebeseri O, et al: The physical properties of polyglycolic acid sutures (Dexon) in sterile and infected urine. *Invest Urol 12*:490, 1975.
111. Selcer BA: Urinary tract trauma associated with pelvic trauma. *J Am Anim Hosp Assoc 18*:785, 1982.
112. Seneca H, et al: Efficacy of drugs in Gram negative urinary pathogens. *J Urol 99*:337, 1968.
113. Shah PM, et al: Elevated blood urea nitrogen: An aid to the diagnosis of intraperitoneal rupture of the bladder. *J Urol 122*:741, 1979.
114. Siegel CW, et al: Pharmacokinetics of trimethoprim and sulfadiazine in the dog. Urine concentrations after oral administration. *Am J Vet Res 42*:996, 1981.
115. Stamey TA, Pfau A: Urinary infections. A selective review and some observations. *Calif Med 113*:16, 1970.
116. Stevens WC, et al: Comparative toxicities of halothane, isoflurane and diethylether at subanesthetic concentrations in laboratory animals. *Anesthesiology 42*:408, 1975.
117. Stone EA, et al: Renal function after prolonged hypotensive anesthesia and surgery in dogs with reduced renal mass. *Am J Vet Res 42*:1675, 1981.
118. Sullivan MJ, et al: Intraperitoneal extravasation of urine. *JAMA 221*:491, 1972.
119. *Summary of Laboratory and Clinical Assessment of Maxon*. Davis & Geck, American Cyanamid Company, Danbury, CT, June, 1987.
120. Taves DR, et al: Toxicity following methoxyflurane anesthesia. *JAMA 214*:91, 1970.
121. Tetracycline and drug attributed rises in blood urea nitrogen. A report

from the Boston Collaborative drug surveillance program. *JAMA 220*:377, 1972.

122. Thayer GW, et al: Fatal venous air embolism associated with pneumocystography in a cat. *J Am Vet Med Assoc 176*:643, 1980.
123. Thornhill JA, Cechner PE: Traumatic injuries to the kidneys, ureter, bladder and urethra. *Vet Clin North Am 11*:157, 1981.
124. Thornton GF, Andriode VT: Bacteriuria during indwelling catheter drainage. *JAMA 214*:339, 1970.
125. Turner MD, et al: Ureteral splints: Results of a survey. *J Urol 127*:654, 1982.
126. Van Winkle W, Hastings JC: Considerations in the choice of suture material for various tissues. *Surg Gynecol Obstet 135*:113, 1972.
127. Vinnicombe J, Stamey TA: The relative nephrotoxicity of polymyxin B sulfate, sodium sulfomethyl-polymyxin B, sodium sulfamethyl-colistin (Colymycin) and neomycin sulfate. *Invest Urol 6*:505, 1969.
128. Wagoner RD: Acute renal failure associated with contrast agents. *Arch Intern Med 138*:353, 1978.
129. Waitz JA, et al: Aspects of chronic toxicity of gentamycin sulphate in cats. *J Infect Dis 124*(Suppl):125, 1971.
130. Walker RD, et al: Serum and tissue fluid norfloxacin concentrations after oral administration of the drug to healthy dogs. *Am J Vet Res 50*:154, 1989.
131. Walker RD, et al: Serum and tissue cage fluid concentrations of ciprofloxacin after oral administration of the drug to healthy dogs. *Am J Vet Res 51*:896, 1990.
132. Walter PA, et al: Renal ultrasonography in healthy cats. *Am J Vet Res 48*:600, 1987.
133. Walter PA, et al: Ultrasonographic evaluation of renal parenchymal diseases in dogs: 32 cases (1981–1986). *J Am Vet Med Assoc 191*:999, 1987.
134. Walter PA, et al: Applications of ultrasonography in the diagnosis of parenchymal kidney disease in cats: 24 cases (1981–1986). *J Am Vet Med Assoc 192*:92, 1988.
135. Weaver RG, Schulte JW: Experimental and clinical studies of urethral regeneration. *Surg Gynecol Obstet 115*:729, 1962.
136. Whelton A, Solez K: Aminoglycoside nephrotoxicity. *J Lab Clin Med 99*:148, 1982.
137. Wooley RE, BLle JL: Quantitative bacteriological studies of urine specimens from canine and feline urinary tract infections. *J Clin Microbiol 4*:326, 1976.
138. Wooley RE, et al: Efficacy of EDTA-tris-lysozyme lavage in the treatment of experimentally induced Pseudomonas aeruginosa cystitis in the dog. *Am J Vet Res 35*:27, 1974.
139. Zontine WJ, Andrews LK: Fatal air embolism as a complication of pneumocystography in two cats. *Vet Radiol 29*:8, 1978.

CHAPTER 104

Kidneys

Bruce A. Christie and Dale E. Bjorling

CONGENITAL ABNORMALITIES

The embryological basis for development of congenital abnormalities of the urinary tract is discussed in Chapter 100.

Number

If the metanephrogenic blastema fails to produce nephrons, renal aplasia or agenesis results. Bilateral agenesis is incompatible with life. Unilateral agenesis (Fig. 104–1) occurs infrequently in dogs and cats[25, 41, 75] and is often associated with ipsilateral abnormalities of the genitalia (Fig. 104–2). The remaining kidney is usually hypertrophied and is capable of maintaining normal function throughout life. If renal surgery, particularly nephrectomy, is contemplated, it is vital to know that a second kidney is present and functioning. Removal of a solitary kidney is indefensible. Supernumerary kidneys can develop as a consequence of ureteric bud malformation (see Chapter 105).

Volume

Hypoplasia or dysgenesis means arrested development or maldevelopment and results in a small kidney. Histological examination is necessary to confirm the diagnosis, because renal disease can cause a previously normal kidney to become scarred and shrunken. The glomeruli and tubules in a hypoplastic kidney have normal architecture with no interstitial scar tissue. Hypoplasia is more common than aplasia. In dogs, hypoplasia may be unilateral (Fig. 104–3), but it more often affects both kidneys.[41] Cocker spaniels are most frequently affected, but this disease also occurs in German shepherds, Doberman pinschers, Norwegian elkhounds, and malamutes.[37, 42, 46] The prognosis is poor. Affected dogs usually die of renal failure before 2 years of age. The clinical signs are those of chronic renal failure. In cats, the condition is usually asymmetrical, affecting the left kidney, and is accompanied by compensatory hypertrophy of the right kidney. Hypertrophy of the kidney occurs in response to the loss or nonfunction of renal tissue. Increase in mass is mainly due to increase in cell size. No new nephrons are formed, but tubular cell multiplication (hyperplasia) does occur.[40] Renal hypertrophy can be induced in many ways, including partial or complete nephrectomy, ureteral ligation, high-protein diet, high-sodium diet, and exposure to cold and certain hormones.[29] The stimuli that trigger hypertrophy are humoral;[96] so-called renotrophins are produced by the kidneys and inactivated by the liver.[7]

Position

Renal ectopia has been described in dogs[99] and cats.[39] The kidney is found in its embryonic position near the

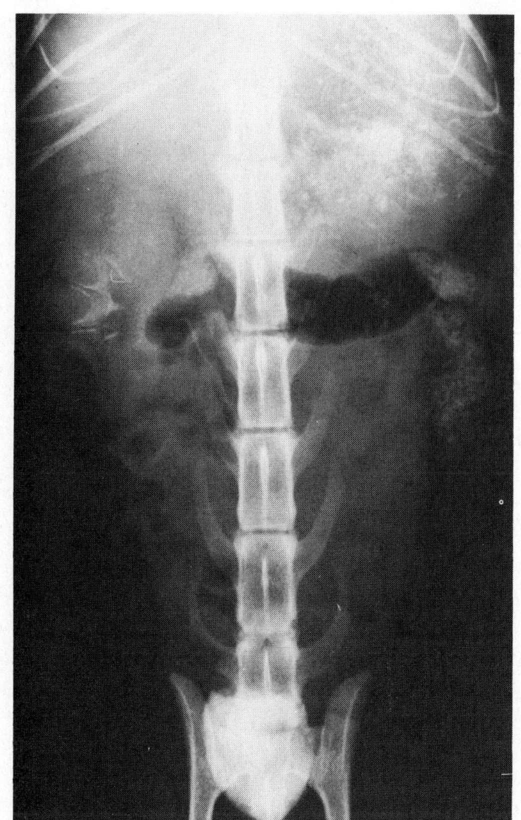

FIGURE 104–1. Unilateral renal agenesis in a dog. An excretory urogram outlines the right kidney, but there is no evidence of a left kidney.

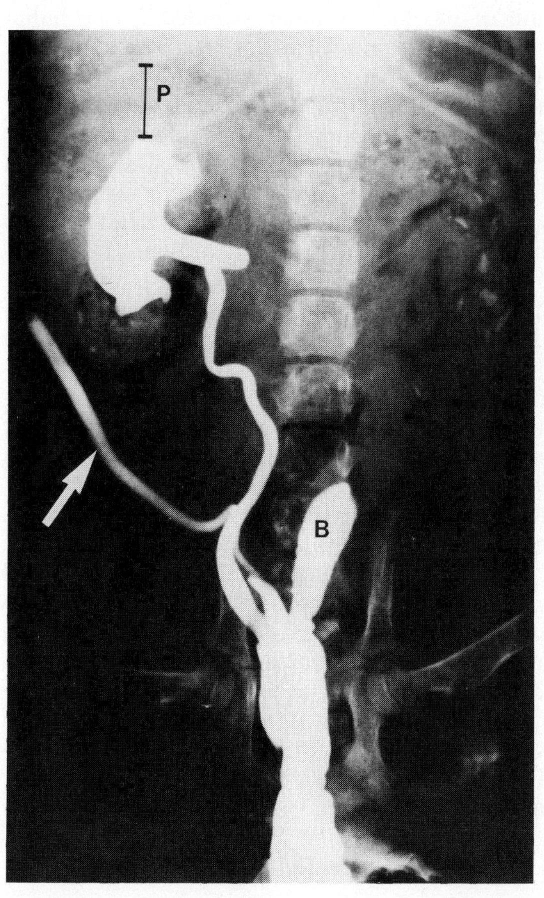

FIGURE 104–2. Unilateral renal agenesis and ipsilateral absence of the uterus in a dog demonstrated by vaginography. The right ureter has an ectopic opening into the uterus. The bladder (B) is infantile, and the ureter and renal pelvis of the right kidney are outlined by retrograde flow of contrast agent. The right uterine horn is visible *(arrow).* The kidney is enlarged. There is mild hydronephrosis, but the thickness of the renal parenchyma (P) demonstrates hypertrophy of the kidney.

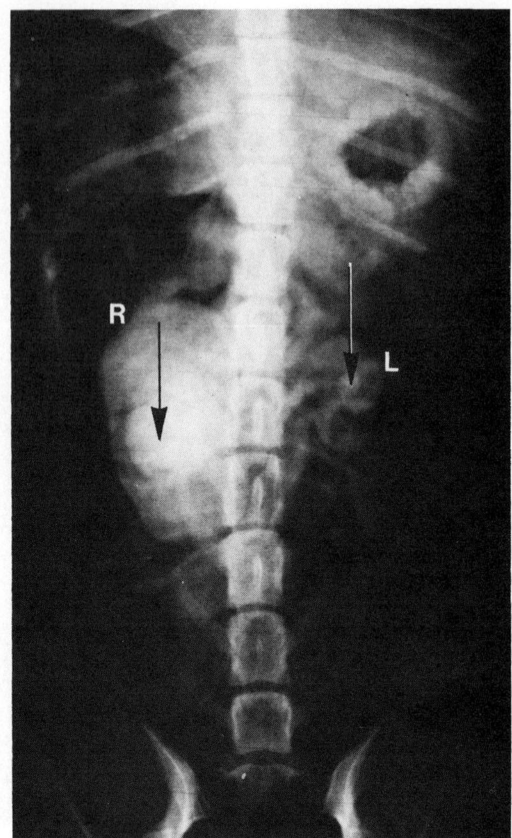

FIGURE 104–3. Unilateral renal hypoplasia in a dog. The left kidney (L) is much smaller than the right (R), and both kidneys contain calculi *(arrows)*.

pelvis and fails to ascend. The diagnosis of ectopic kidney is usually made radiographically, during investigation of a caudal abdominal mass. The condition is occasionally noted as an incidental finding during abdominal surgery. Kidney function is not usually compromised, but pressure exerted by the kidney could compress the colon or uterus, producing constipation or dystocia. The incidental finding of an ectopic kidney is no cause for concern unless the malposition is causing a problem.

Fusion

During early development, the kidneys lie close to each other near the origin of the iliac arteries. Fusion anomalies can occur in all species.[41] The most common abnormality is horseshoe kidney with fusion at the caudal pole.[25] The fusion may involve only a portion of the capsule or parenchyma[66] or may be so extensive that a common pelvis is formed. When fusion is extensive, the renal mass cannot ascend normally and remains in the pelvic cavity.[78] Fusion is unlikely to be clinically significant.

Cysts

Cysts can develop in any part of the nephron and collecting duct system. Some cystic lesions are heritable and arise during organogenesis. Others develop in normal renal tissue after the kidneys are fully formed. Cysts may be few and large or multiple and small. Solitary cysts are infrequently reported and are rarely pathological.[88] Large isolated cysts or multiple cysts can be identified in the renal parenchyma by intravenous pyelography or ultrasonography.[4, 52] Polycystic disease affecting the kidneys and liver occurs in Cairn terriers[56] and long-haired cats.[19] Polycystic kidney disease displaying an autosomal dominant pattern of heritability occurs in Persian cats.[4] It has been observed in cats from less than a year to 10 years of age.* Clinical signs include abdominal distension due to renal enlargement or depression, anorexia, emesis, polydipsia, polyuria, and weight loss due to renal failure.[4, 62] Polycystic disease can be unilateral, and removal of the affected kidney may be advisable because it is predisposed to infection.[3]

ACQUIRED ABNORMALITIES

Trauma

Automobiles inflict most injuries to the urinary tracts of dogs and cats. The most common injury is rupture of the urinary bladder, followed by rupture of the kidney, urethra, and ureter. A laceration of the kidney or renal vasculature causes a perirenal hematoma.[72] Rupture of the abdominal musculature or diaphragm may allow the kidney to be displaced into a subcutaneous position[16, 100] and still function normally. Reports of foreign body penetration of the kidney have included a rifle bullet lodged in the renal pelvis of a dog,[51] an air gun pellet in the renal parenchyma of a cat,[5] and a 5-cm-long sewing needle that penetrated the duodenum of a dog and entered the right kidney.[21]

Renal parenchymal damage as a result of blunt trauma can vary from minor subcapsular bleeding with hematuria to a shattered kidney from which death due to exsanguination, hemorrhagic shock, or acute renal failure may occur. If the peritoneum remains intact, the expanding perirenal hematoma may produce flank swelling with local pain. If the peritoneum is ruptured, blood accumulates in the abdominal cavity. Perirenal extravasation of blood and urine can occur if the renal parenchymal injury communicates with the collecting duct system or if the ureter has been avulsed. Those lesions are called *pararenal* or *perinephric pseudocysts.*[36]

The diagnosis of renal trauma is based on history, clinical examination, laboratory findings, radiographic findings, and exploratory surgery (Chapter 103). Renal injury is confirmed by observation of extravasated contrast agent on excretory urography.[72] Rapid administration of an organic iodine contrast agent (880 mg/kg) is recommended.[72] If the animal is in shock, renal perfusion may be decreased, and study results are poor.[90] Rapid administration of contrast material to a hypovolemic animal may also cause profound bradycardia or cardiac arrest.[23] If an animal is not hypovolemic or in

*See references 3, 4, 11, 19, 54, 62, and 74.

shock and the kidney is not excreting the contrast agent within 20 minutes, the renal blood supply is evaluated by renal arteriography.[17] Renal angiography is frequently used in human medicine to detect traumatic lesions such as aneurysms, infarcts, and arteriovenous fistulas.[48]

The therapeutic objectives of treatment of renal trauma are to control hemorrhage, excise devitalized tissue, and repair injured structures. Most renal lesions respond to rest and osmotic or volume diuresis. If major renal damage is suspected, shock is stabilized by appropriate fluid therapy and exploratory surgery is undertaken. Parenchymal tears can be packed with a topical hemostatic agent such as gelatin sponge* or polymerized methyl cellulose.† If the damage is confined to one pole, partial nephrectomy may be considered. If the kidney is shattered, it is removed, provided the other kidney is present and functioning satisfactorily.

Nephrectomy

The kidneys are surrounded in the sublumbar region by peritoneum, renal fascia, and various amounts of perirenal fat. The renal artery of dogs, particularly the left renal artery, is often paired, whereas multiple renal veins are frequently found in cats.

The kidney can be exposed through a retroperitoneal flank or ventral midline approach. The abdominal approach is favored because both kidneys and the abdomen can be thoroughly examined. The incision starts in the cranial abdomen and extends as far caudally as necessary. The left kidney is exposed by packing abdominal viscera behind the mesentery of the descending colon (Fig. 104–4*A*). The right kidney is exposed by using the mesoduodenum in a similar fashion (Fig. 104–4*B*) and retracting the viscera. The kidney is freed from its sublumbar attachment by a combination of sharp dissection with scissors and blunt dissection with a finger or gauze sponge (Fig. 104–5). Minor hemorrhage may be encountered from hypertrophied capsular vessels,[15] but it soon stops or is easily controlled by cautery or ligation. The arterial supply is isolated close to the aorta proximal to any interlobar branches. In dogs, the left ovarian vein is identified because it does not drain into the posterior vena cava but into the renal vein. The ureter is isolated by dissection as far as the bladder. Mass ligation of the renal artery and vein is convenient but is not recommended because of the possibility of displacement of the ligature or the development of an arteriovenous fistula.[14] Cardiovascular silk (2-0 to 1 for cats and 0 to 1 for dogs) is an excellent material for ligating blood vessels. Ligatures can be placed and tied directly around the blood vessels or tied around previously placed forceps. The ureter is ligated and divided close to the bladder to prevent retention of urine in the ureteral remnant, which could promote infection, and to decrease the risk of spread of a renal tumor. Unless a patient is uremic or in shock, no special care is required after unilateral nephrectomy.

*Gelfoam, Upjohn Company, Kalamazoo, MI.
†Oxycel, Parke-Davis, Morris Plains, NJ.

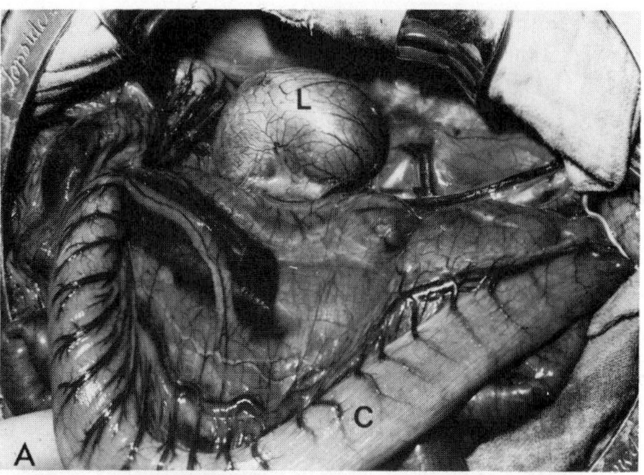

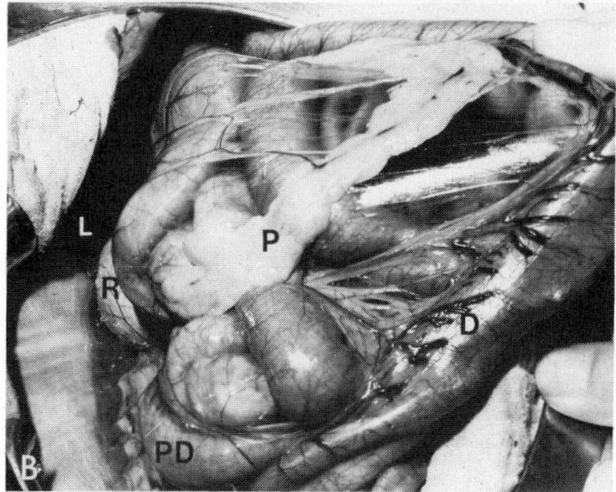

FIGURE 104–4. Transperitoneal approach to the kidney. *A,* The left kidney (L) is exposed by retracting the colon (C) to the right and packing the abdominal viscera behind the mesocolon. *B,* The cranial part of the right kidney (R) is embedded in the caudate lobe of the liver (L). The duodenum (D) has been retracted to the left. The pancreas (P) is visible, and viscera have been packed behind the mesoduodenum. The kidney is exposed completely by retracting the proximal duodenum (PD) to the left.

Partial Nephrectomy

Czerny performed the first partial nephrectomy in a human in 1887.[28] Wedge resection and transverse resection have been used since that time.[58] Partial nephrectomy was unpopular because postoperative hemorrhage, infection, and urine fistulas were common complications. Nevertheless, the operation became a necessity as a treatment for renal tuberculosis. Newer techniques for partial nephrectomy use either a single[102] or triple[45] thread to cut through the renal parenchyma and simultaneously control hemorrhage. The multiple-suture method is preferred because there is less chance of ligatures slipping (Fig. 104–6).

The renal capsule is stripped back from the area to be resected, and two long, straight needles threaded with number 1 chromic gut are inserted into the kidney at the proposed site of resection. The needles and thread are passed through the kidney. The thread is cut to make three separate nooses, which are tied. Renal tissue is excised distal to these ligatures. Bleeding points are ligated, and open diverticula are closed with suture ligatures of 3-0 or 4-0 synthetic absorbable suture material. The capsule is approximated over the exposed

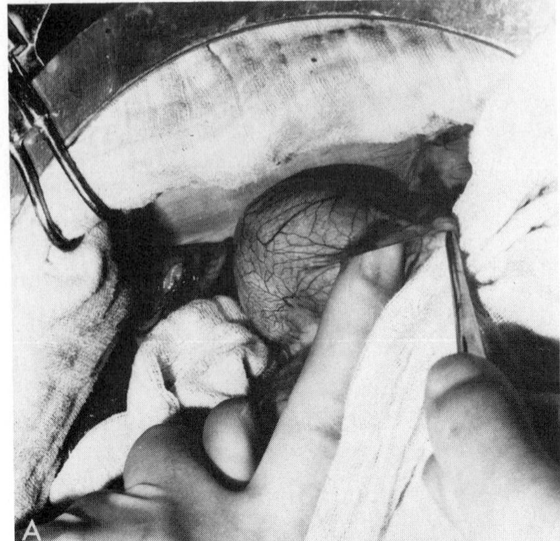

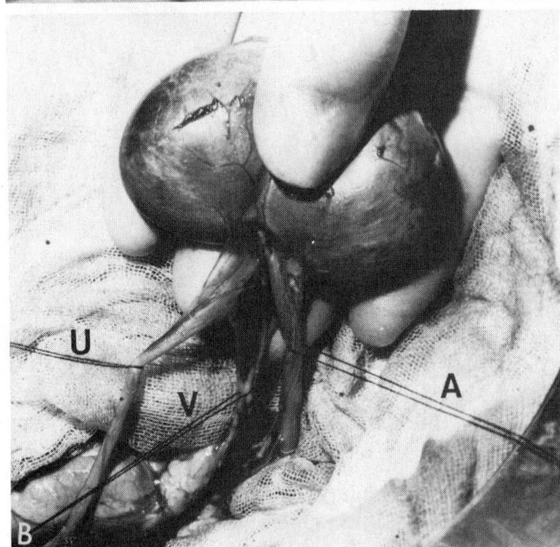

FIGURE 104–5. Mobilization of the left kidney of a dog. *A*, The peritoneum and caudal renal fascia have been elevated with forceps and cut with scissors. They are peeled from the kidney with a finger and gauze sponge. *B*, When mobilized, the kidney can be elevated from its sublumbar position to expose the renal artery (A), vein (V), and ureter (U).

parenchyma, and some additional sutures are placed to anchor the capsule to the abdominal wall to prevent accidental rotation.

Alternatively, a tourniquet or vascular forceps may be applied to the renal vasculature, and the diseased portion of the kidney removed by excision. The renal pelvis and calyces are closed with 3-0 or 4-0 absorbable suture, and the vessels are ligated. Vascular flow is restored, and the exposed renal parenchyma is covered with the remaining renal capsule, peritoneum, or omentum.[47]

Idiopathic Hematuria

Hematuria is expected with accidental or iatrogenic renal trauma or renal infection. It can also occur as a consequence of discrete renal hemangioma.[10, 50] Spontaneous hemorrhage of no apparent cause has been reported in five dogs.[35, 86] In four, hemorrhage was potentially fatal if left untreated. Histologically, two of the kidneys removed appeared normal, one had evidence of chronic pyelitis, and infarcts were observed in the renal cortical vessels of the other.[35, 86]

Selective embolization of intrarenal vessels with a suspension of gelatin sponge or placement of a steel coil has been used to treat hematuria of renal origin in humans.[2, 8, 98] Unilateral nephrectomy of the affected kidney (identified during surgery by ureteral catheterization) has successfully resolved idiopathic hematuria of renal origin in dogs.[35, 86]

Nephrolithiasis

Calculi may form anywhere along a dog's urinary tract, but the kidneys are involved in only 4 per cent.[9] Calculi are occasionally found in the kidneys of cats.[79] (For a detailed account of canine and feline urolithiasis, including medical management, see Chapters 108 and 109.) Clinical signs of nephrolithiasis are often lacking, but depression, anorexia, hematuria, and flank pain may be noted. Bilateral renal calculi can reduce renal function to such a degree that signs of uremia may occur. The diagnosis is confirmed by radiography or ultrasonography. If the affected kidney still has adequate function, medical dissolution may be attempted (see Chapter 109). If renal function is already depressed, surgical removal of the calculi may prevent further deterioration of the kidney and may be lifesaving.

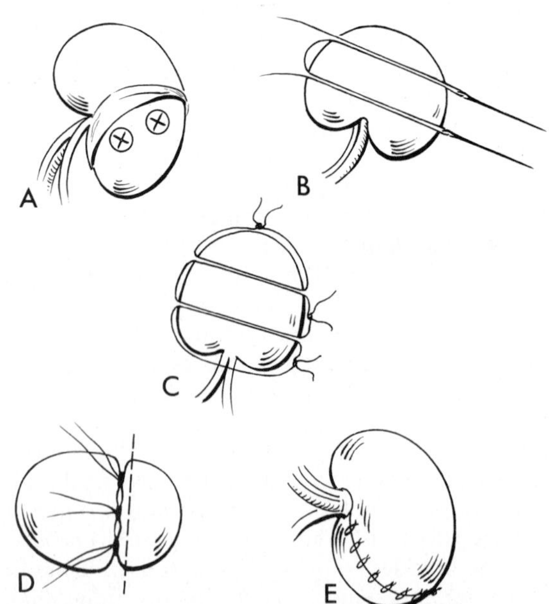

FIGURE 104–6. Partial nephrectomy. *A*, The kidney capsule is peeled back, and the points of insertion of the needles are denoted by crosses. *B*, The needles are drawn through the kidney parenchyma. *C*, The thread is cut to make three separate nooses. *D*, The nooses are tightened and tied, and guillotine amputation *(broken line)* is performed. *E*, The capsule is reapproximated.

Nephrotomy

Nephrotomy temporarily decreases renal function by 20 to 50 per cent.[26, 27] If calculi are present in both kidneys, a choice of one operation or two operations spaced a few weeks apart must be made. Bilateral nephrotomy can be performed during one operation; if a patient is severely azotemic or surgical trauma during the first nephrotomy is excessive, the operations should be staged.

The best access to the kidney is via a long ventral midline abdominal incision. The renal artery and vein can be temporarily occluded with vascular forceps or a tourniquet (see Chapter 103). Both kidneys usually are sufficiently mobile to be held between thumb and fingers to expose their convex lateral surfaces. This avoids dissection of the kidney from its sublumbar attachments, minimizing damage to functional collateral vessels and surgical trauma. When bisection nephrotomy is performed, a longitudinal sagittal incision is made with a scalpel through the convex lateral surface of the kidney (Fig. 104–7). The length of the incision is limited to the dimensions of the renal pelvis. Less damage is done to the renal parenchyma if an incision is made with a scalpel through the renal capsule and the renal parenchyma is bluntly separated with forceps to expose the calculus within the pelvis and calyces.[84] Alternatively, an intersegmental nephrotomy can be performed by dividing the kidney along an avascular plane between the terminal branches of the renal artery identified by intra-arterial injection of dye.[34] Because the intraparenchymal vessels are spared, intersegmental nephrotomy does not depress postoperative renal function to the same degree as bisection nephrotomy; no differences were observed postoperatively in the function of kidneys randomly subjected to either nephrotomy technique.[87] After nephrotomy, passive blood flow is removed to expose the calculus, which is removed. Mineral aggregates can be flushed from each diverticulum with saline, using a modified hypodermic needle. The ureter is catheterized with a 3.5 French catheter, and saline is gently flushed through the ureter to confirm patency. The nephrotomy is closed by apposing the two renal parenchymal flaps with gentle digital pressure while renal blood flow is restored. Hemorrhage usually ceases within 5 minutes, and the clotted blood has virtually glued the two halves of the kidney together (Fig. 104–8). Although this method is called the *sutureless nephrotomy closure,* the incision in the renal capsule is closed with 3-0 or 4-0 absorbable suture placed through the capsule and superficial parenchyma in a simple continuous pattern (see Fig. 104–8). This technique is used in humans[69] and dogs.[27]

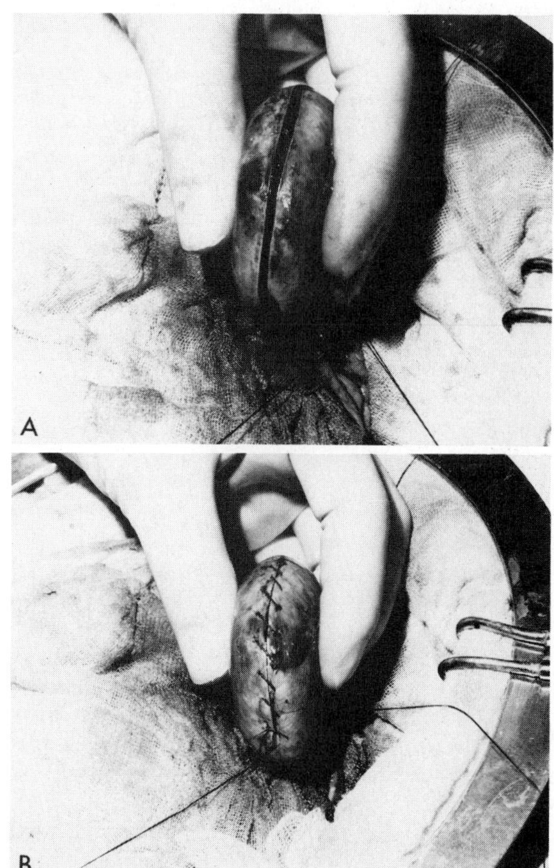

FIGURE 104–8. Sutureless nephrotomy closure. *A,* The renal parenchymal flaps are united by a fibrin bond. *B,* The capsule is apposed with a continuous suture.

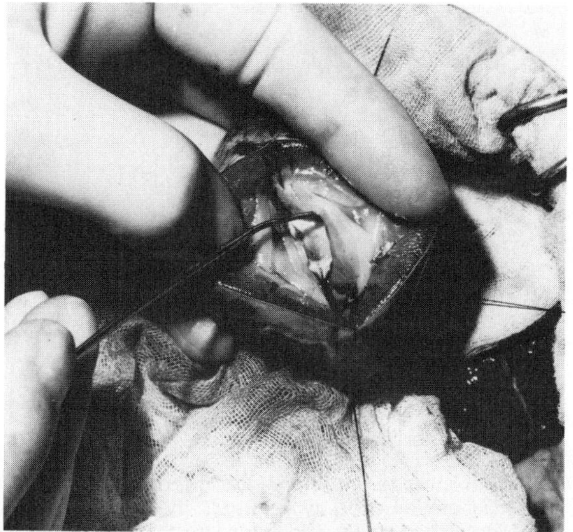

FIGURE 104–7. Sagittal nephrotomy exposing the renal pelvis of a dog. The renal crest has been elevated with a probe.

After nephrotomy, minor hematuria may continue for a few days. Intravenous fluids are given during surgery and postoperatively to establish diuresis and flush blood clots from the urinary tract. If hematuria persists after a few days, treatment with a hemostatic agent such as aminocaproic acid (Amicar) can be tried.[83] This drug promotes clotting by inhibiting urokinase, which is an activator of plasminogen and plasmin (fibrinolysin) in urine. Tranexamic acid (Vasolamin) has the same action and applications as aminocaproic acid, but it is 10 minutes more potent and is less toxic. It is given at an

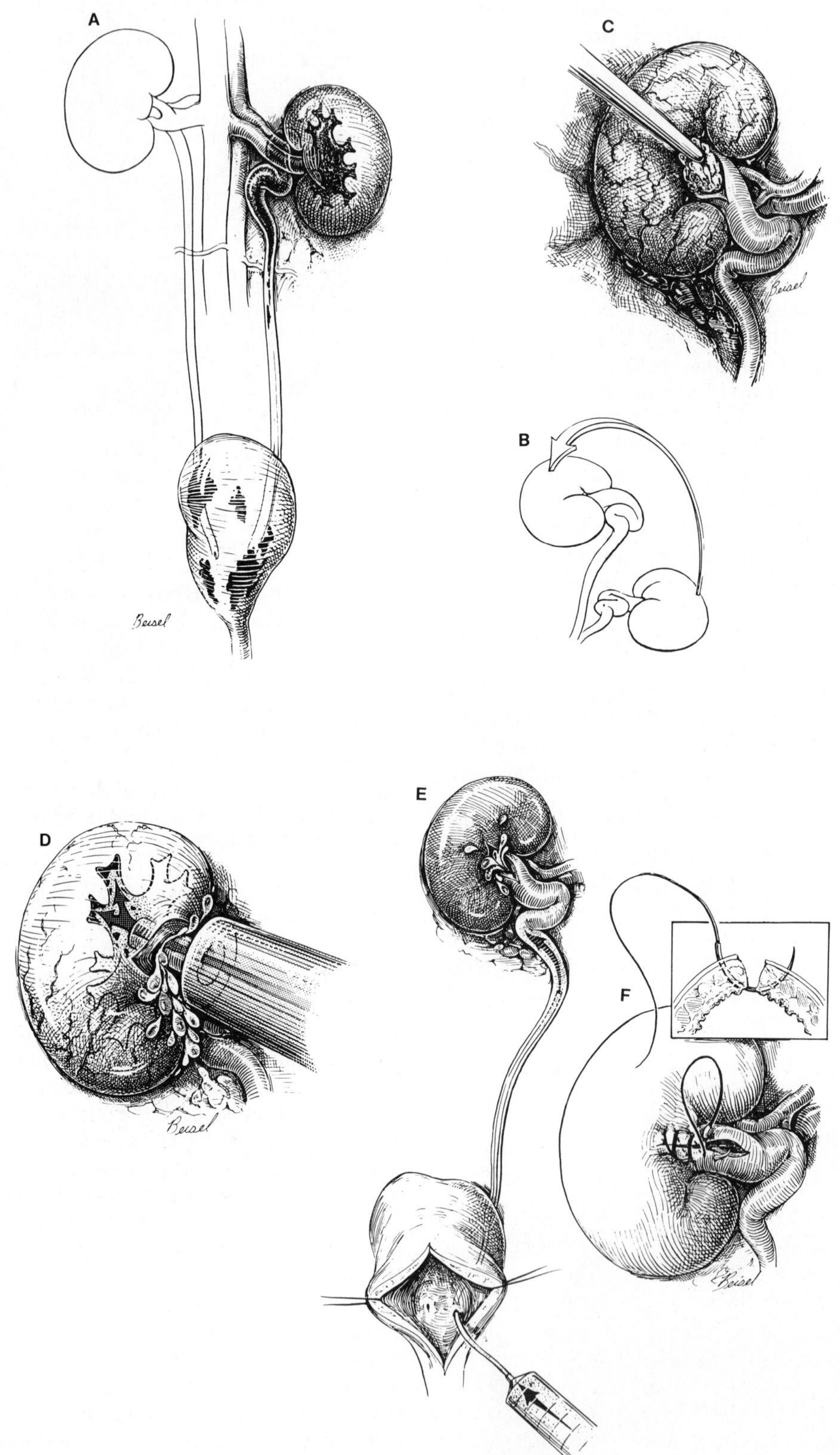

FIGURE 104–9. Pyelolithotomy. *A,* The ventral surface of the proximal ureter and renal pelvis is obscured from view by the renal artery and vein. *B,* The kidney is freed of its attachments and rotated medially. *C,* An incision is made into the dilated renal pelvis and proximal ureter, and the calculi are removed. *D,* Small calculi that remain within the diverticuli are removed by flushing. *E,* The ureter is catheterized to ensure patency. *F,* The incision in the renal pelvis and proximal ureter is closed with a simple continuous pattern. (From Greenwood KM, Rawlings CA: Removal of canine renal calculi by pyelolithotomy. *Vet Surg 10*:12, 1981.)

initial dose of 25 mg/kg, followed by 10 mg/kg every 6 hours.

Pyelolithotomy

If renal calculi have resulted in dilation of the proximal ureter and renal pelvis, they may be removed through an incision made into these structures (pyelolithotomy).[31] This approach to remove renal calculi does not require occlusion of the renal vasculature and avoids trauma to the renal parenchyma, thereby minimizing the deleterious effects of removal of the calculi on postoperative renal function.

As the kidney is viewed in its normal position when a ventral midline approach is made to the abdominal cavity, the renal pelvis and proximal ureter are hidden by the renal vessels. The kidney is dissected free of its peritoneal attachments and rotated medially, exposing the renal pelvis and proximal ureter (Fig. 104–9). An incision is made over the pelvis and proximal ureter, and the calculi are removed. The renal pelvis and calyces are flushed with saline to remove small calculi that may remain. A 3.5 French catheter is passed into the bladder through the ureter to ensure patency. The incision in the renal pelvis and ureter is closed with 4-0 or 5-0 continuous absorbable suture.[31]

If the renal pelvis and proximal ureter are not dilated, this technique is not attempted. Use of this technique in cats has not been reported.

Alternative Methods for Removing Renoliths

An experimental evaluation of percutaneous nephrolithotomy in dogs has been reported.[20] Although this method appeared successful, it requires sophisticated percutaneous placement of specialized instruments under fluoroscopic guidance, making its application limited. In humans, percutaneous nephrolithotomy and fragmentation of renal calculi by extracorporeal shock-wave lithotripsy have generally replaced other techniques.[71] The equipment required to perform extracorporeal shock-wave lithotripsy is not readily available for veterinary use.

Hydronephrosis

Hydronephrosis is progressive dilation of the renal pelvis and progressive atrophy of the renal parenchyma, most often due to ureteral obstruction.[65] Dogs are more often affected than cats.[33, 61] When urine outflow obstruction affects both kidneys, the animal dies before pressure atrophy can cause much reduction in renal mass. When the obstruction is unilateral, the degree of hydronephrosis can reach such proportions that the renal parenchyma is only a shell (Fig. 104–10). Urine production continues after the lower urinary tract is obstructed, because the obstruction is not complete. Urine is reabsorbed through the renal vein and the renal hilar lymphatics.[59] If the obstruction is relieved within 1 week, the renal damage is totally reversible. Although up to

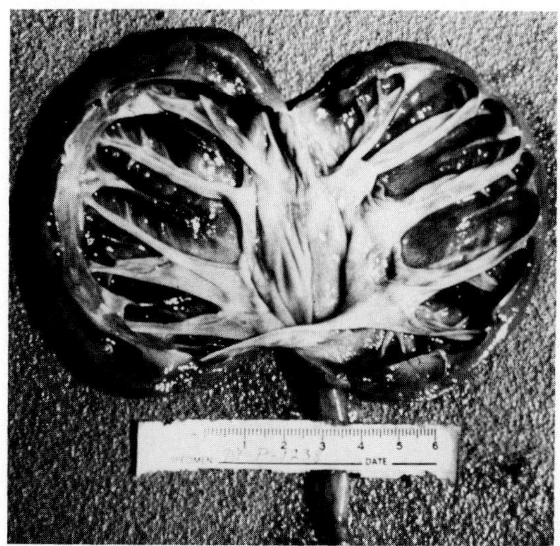

FIGURE 104–10. Hydronephrosis in a dog. The renal pelvis is dilated, and the parenchyma remains as a thin shell. (Courtesy of R. Mitten.)

25 per cent of normal renal function can return after 4 weeks of total obstruction, ureteral obstruction of this duration may result in complete loss of renal function.[97, 103] Relief of chronic partial ureteral obstruction can result in an improvement in the radiographic appearance of the ureters and associated kidneys.[77]

Urine outflow obstruction can be congenital. Torsion, kinking, stenosis, and atresia of the ureters or urethra or aberrant renal vessels that constrict the ureters have been reported.[65] Hydronephrosis may also be acquired as a result of compression of the ureters or urethra by neoplasia or other masses, such as hematomas, cysts, or abscesses. Urinary obstruction may also be the result of urinary calculi or accidental ligation of the ureter during ovariohysterectomy.[92]

The clinical signs and pathophysiology of urinary tract obstruction are discussed in Chapter 102. The usual clinical sign of uncomplicated unilateral hydronephrosis is an enlarged abdomen, and abdominal radiographs show an enlarged renal shadow (Fig. 104–11). The degree of dilation can be seen with excretory urography as long as sufficient functioning nephrons are present within the kidney (Fig. 104–12). If the kidney is not excreting contrast agent, renal angiography may demonstrate hydronephrosis by the appearance of an attenuated vascular pattern and an enlarged renal shadow (Fig. 104–13). Palpation of an enlarged kidney and lack of renal opacification on an excretory urogram are sufficient justification to explore the abdomen to confirm the diagnosis and to effect a treatment. In acute ureteral obstruction, the affected kidney is tense and the renal hilar lymphatics are prominent.

A condition called *capsular hydronephrosis* has been described in cats, in which the kidney capsule is separated from the renal parenchyma by a large collection of fluid.[1, 13, 76, 93] Capsular hydronephrosis is possibly related to lymphatic obstruction and is effectively treated by excising the wall of the pseudocyst.[1, 13, 65] If hydronephrosis is advanced and the kidney is only a

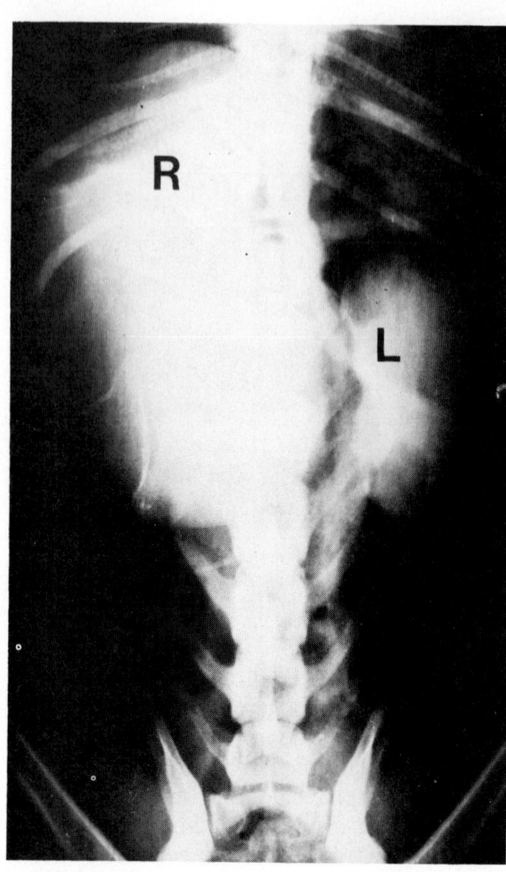

FIGURE 104–11. Unilateral hydronephrosis in a dog demonstrated radiographically against the contrast of a pneumoperitoneum. The dimensions of the left kidney (L) are normal, but the right kidney (R) is enlarged.

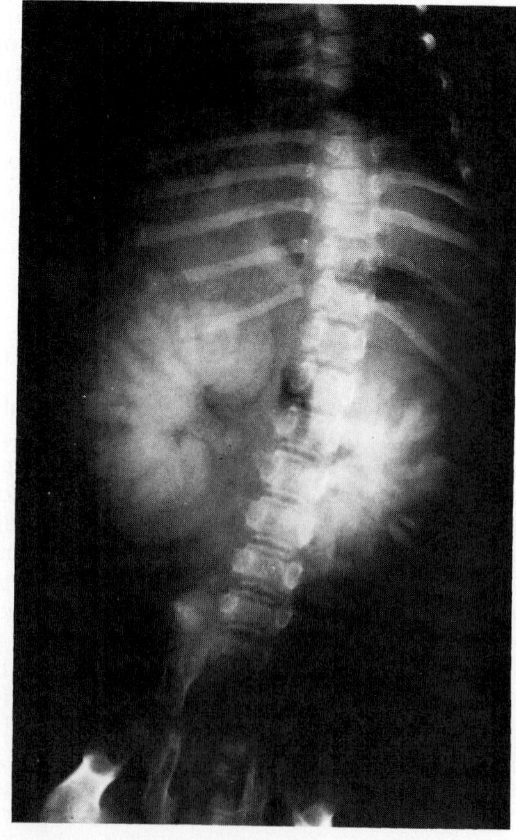

FIGURE 104–12. Bilateral hydronephrosis in a 1-week-old pup with urethral obstruction. Excretory urography shows that both renal pelves are dilated.

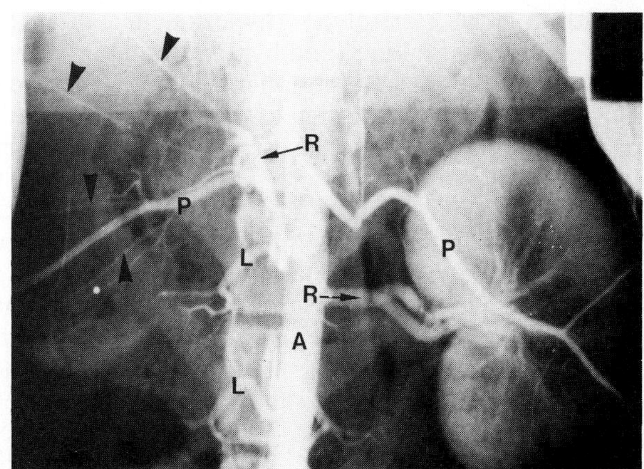

FIGURE 104–13. Unilateral hydronephrosis seen as an incidental finding during arteriography of the infrarenal aorta. Contrast agent has passed into both renal arteries. The left kidney shows a normal vascular pattern. The interlobar vessels of the right kidney *(arrows)* are regular but attenuated, and the right renal shadow is enlarged. Vessels opacified are the aorta (A), renal artery (R), phrenicoabdominal artery (P), and lumbar arteries (L).

fluid-filled sac, the prognosis is hopeless, and the remains of the kidney are removed. If some kidney function is evident on excretory urography and if the cause of the urine obstruction can be identified and corrected, it is vital to try to save that kidney, particularly if the other kidney is also damaged.

Nephrostomy drainage of urine immediately relieves intrarenal pressure. The kidney is mobilized, and a length of fenestrated latex or silicone rubber tubing 5 or 6 mm in diameter is positioned in the dilated renal pelvis (Fig. 104–14). The catheter is exteriorized through the abdominal wall, and the urine diverted into a closed container. Drainage can be maintained until the cause of the obstruction has been corrected. The kidney is anchored to the abdominal wall with a few capsular sutures. If necessary, this type of nephrostomy tube can be replaced, because when the tube is removed, a urine fistula will remain for a short while.[105] If distal obstruction still exists, the fistula persists.

Purulent Nephritis

If a cat's ureter is obstructed and a systemic bacterial infection is established, the kidney with the obstructed ureter becomes infected.[44] Clinical experience has shown that bacterial infection by the hematogenous route is a common complication of obstructive uropathy.[18, 24] Renal injury also predisposes the kidney to blood-borne infection.[24] Purulent nephritis also can occur as an ascending infection from the lower urinary tract, particularly in the presence of vesicoureteral reflux.[24]

When both kidneys are infected, the relative contribution of each kidney to total renal function is important. Their relative contributions can be determined by renal scans after injection of radioactively labeled substances that are excreted by the kidneys.[43] Selective catheterization of the ureters and determination of the function of the individual kidneys by clearance of various indicators may also be performed. In bilateral renal infection, it is feasible to remove foreign bodies or excise focal abscesses. If an abscess is unilateral, partial or total nephrectomy, with systemic antibiotic therapy, is an effective treatment.

Kidney Worm

Dioctophyma renale, the giant kidney worm, is found sporadically in dogs and wild fish-eating carnivores, particularly mink. Cats are resistant to this parasite.[67] Dogs become infected by eating fish or frogs that contain infective larvae. The larvae penetrate the gut wall of the host and mature into adults, usually within the peritoneal cavity. However, they often penetrate the

FIGURE 104–14. Nephrostomy. *A,* Increased resistance in urine outflow *(arrow)* results in dilation of the renal pelvis (P). *B,* A fenestrated tube (T) is drawn into the renal pelvis with narrow, long forceps passed through the renal parenchyma and pelvis in a sagittal plane. *C,* Each end of the tube is exteriorized through the abdominal wall. One end is sealed, and the other end is connected to a closed urine collection system. The kidney is anchored to the abdominal wall with a few capsular sutures, and the nephrostomy tube is secured to the skin.

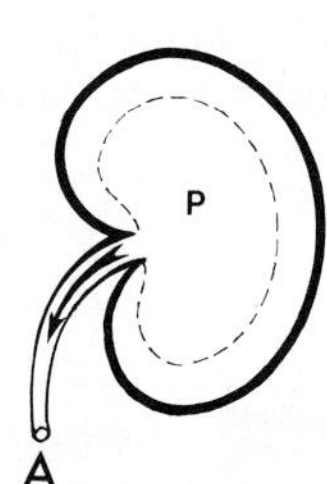

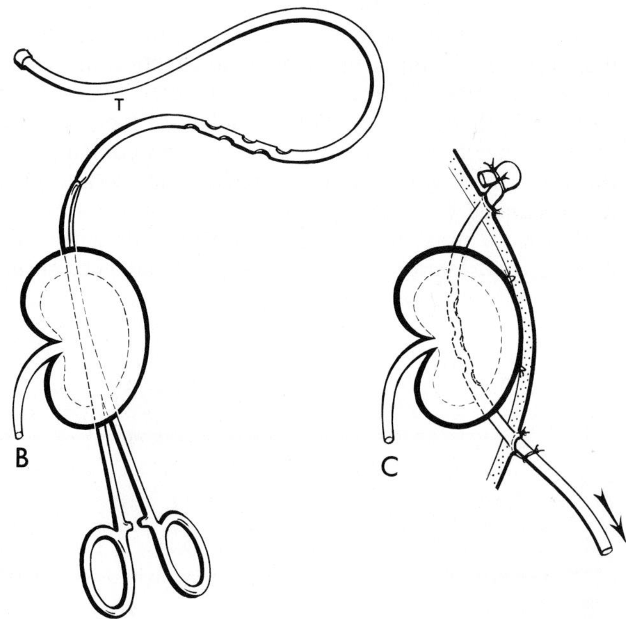

kidney and may completely destroy the renal parenchyma. Giant kidney worms are usually discovered incidentally after ova are found in urine. Alternatively, adult worms are found in the peritoneal cavity during abdominal surgery. The treatment is nephrectomy or nephrotomy, depending on the degree of renal damage and whether one or both kidneys are harboring parasites. Prevention depends on blocking access to raw fish, particularly the North American catfish.

Acute Renal Failure

Acute renal failure is characterized by the rapid onset of oliguria or anuria, reduced renal blood flow, reduced glomerular filtration rate, and sudden azotemia. Acute renal failure is potentially reversible, but some renal tubular damage has invariably occurred. Recovery depends on the extent of renal injury and the capacity of the remaining nephrons to regain normal function.

Two major predisposing factors that contribute to acute renal failure are decreased renal blood flow and exposure of the kidneys to nephrotoxic agents such as heavy metals, organic compounds, and antimicrobial drugs. Decreased renal perfusion can be the result of hemorrhage, trauma, prolonged anesthesia, extensive surgery, or impaired cardiac function. Any of these inciting factors may be present in various proportions in all surgery. However, prolonged hemorrhagic shock in dogs resulted in death before the onset of acute renal failure.[73] The effects of hypotension, anesthesia, and surgery on renal function have been investigated experimentally in dogs in which functional renal mass was reduced by unilateral nephrectomy followed by ligation of four of the six terminal branches of the renal artery of the remaining kidney.[85] Anesthesia was induced and maintained with halothane, the plane of anesthesia was adjusted to maintain mean systemic arterial pressure less than 75 mm Hg for 4 hours, and a 1-hour exploratory laparotomy was performed while the dogs were anesthetized. One week after the hypotensive episode, the glomerular filtration rate was significantly (15 per cent) lower than before surgery, but acute renal failure was not observed.[85] Impairment of renal function may have a multifactorial etiology, and during elective surgery on patients with no preoperative renal disorders, infusion of a balanced salt solution such as lactated Ringer at the rate of 11 ml/kg/hour diminishes the likelihood of renal damage.

If surgery must be performed on animals with renal disease, consideration is given to fluid balance, serum concentrations of electrolytes (hyperkalemia often occurs in acute renal failure, and hyponatremia in chronic failure), and the pH of peripheral blood (metabolic acidosis accompanies the impaired ability to excrete hydrogen ions). Acidosis causes myocardial irritability and also results in decreased barbiturate binding to plasma protein, increasing the potency of the barbiturate. If proteinuria has been present for any length of time, hypoproteinemia develops. Fluid replacement in hypoproteinemic animals is given as colloid (plasma) rather than crystalloid. As protein is lost from the plasma, more barbiturate and narcotic remain unbound, increasing the concentration and thus the potency of these drugs.

Patients with chronic renal failure are anemic as a result of decreased erythropoietin production. If the blood oxygen saturation is less than 70 g/L, adequate oxygenation during anesthesia is impossible. Patients require a blood transfusion with crossmatched blood, because even minor transfusion reactions cannot be tolerated by animals with renal disease.

Because it is possible for animals with compensated chronic renal failure to decompensate and experience a uremic crisis, it is important for therapeutic and prognostic reasons first to distinguish between acute and chronic renal failure (see Chapter 102). One of the best ways of doing this is by renal biopsy.[68] Even in kidneys with diffuse lesions, histological examination does not always predict reversibility and functional compensation. In focal lesions, chance sampling errors obviously can lead to diagnostic and prognostic mistakes. Sampling errors are minimized if a wedge biopsy, partial nephrectomy, or nephrectomy is performed.

Needle Biopsy

It is possible to obtain a sample of kidney tissue without having to open the abdomen using the blind percutaneous, keyhole, or percutaneous approach guided by ultrasonography.[68] A great deal of information can be gained by exposing the two kidneys and sampling from one or both under direct observation. The kidneys can also be sampled under direct observation during laparoscopy.[31] Before biopsy, the benefits must be weighed against the risks. Absolute contraindications to needle biopsy are hemorrhagic tendencies, inexperienced diagnosticians, and damaged equipment.[63] Complications observed after keyhole kidney biopsy in dogs and cats have included gross and microscopic hematuria, fatal hemorrhage, and hydronephrosis.[38] Arteriovenous

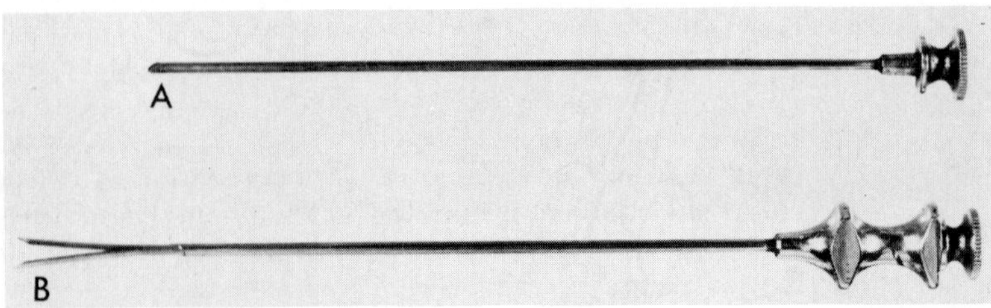

FIGURE 104–15. The Franklin modified Vim-Silverman biopsy needle. *A*, Obturator. *B*, the obturator has been removed from the sheath and replaced by cutting prongs, which are thrust into the tissue to be sampled. When the sheath is advanced over the cutting prongs, the specimen is retained, and the needle can be withdrawn.

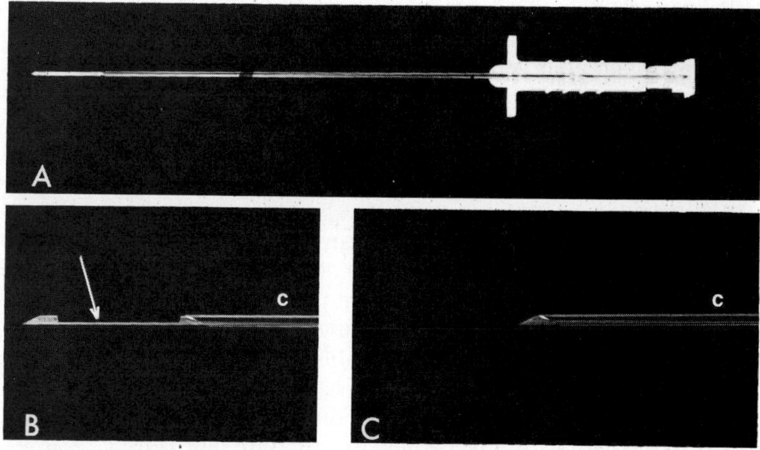

FIGURE 104–16. *A,* Vim Tru-Cut biopsy needle. *B,* When the obturator specimen rod is advanced, tissue fills the specimen notch *(arrow).* *C,* When the sheath (C) is advanced, its sharp cutting tip severs a sample of tissue, which is retained in the specimen notch as the needle is withdrawn.

fistulas have developed after renal biopsy in humans[22, 95] but have not been encountered in dogs and cats.[64] We have observed severe, uncontrollable hemorrhage that necessitated nephrectomy after performing needle biopsy of a kidney.

Two types of needles are currently in use, the modified pediatric Franklin-Silverman biopsy needle* (Fig. 104–15) and the Vim Tru-Cut biopsy needle† (Fig. 104–16). The Franklin needle is reusable and can be resharpened but is less widely used than the Vim Tru-Cut needle. If this needle is not cared for, much damage is done to the kidney, and the sample is often unsatisfactory. The Tru-Cut needle is disposable, sharp, and easy to use. It can be cleaned and resterilized with ethylene oxide.[63]

The components of the Vim Tru-Cut needle are shown in the retracted and fully advanced positions (see Fig. 104–16). With the obturator specimen rod fully retracted within the outer cannula, the tip of the instrument is placed on the surface of the lesion, and the specimen rod is thrust into the lesion by advancing the plastic handle. The outer sheath of the needle is advanced into the tissue to sever the biopsy sample from its attachment. The material is retained within the specimen notch. As the needle is withdrawn, hemorrhage is often profuse for a short while. It is controlled by finger pressure and soon stops. If gross hematuria persists after 24 hours, the animal can be treated with a hemostatic agent such as tranexamic acid (see the earlier section on nephrotomy).

The keyhole approach is performed by making an incision that bisects the angle formed by the 13th rib and the sublumbar musculature. The internal abdominal oblique and transverse abdominal muscles are bluntly separated, and the kidney is identified in its retroperitoneal position by inserting a finger into the opening created. A stab incision is made through the 12th or 13th intercostal space to insert the biopsy needle. The needle must be directed toward one of the poles of the kidney and not at the hilus to avoid damaging the renal vessels, pelvis, or ureter. The kidney is immobilized against the body wall by digital pressure applied by the finger inserted through the incision caudal to the ribs, and the biopsy sample is obtained. At least two specimens are taken, and digital pressure is maintained for at least 5 minutes after completion of the biopsy procedure to control hemorrhage. The wound is closed in a routine fashion. Although inadequate material may be obtained, the necropsy diagnosis was identical to the biopsy diagnosis in 97 of 101 dogs and cats reviewed in one study.[38]

*Mueller Company, Chicago, IL.
†Travenol Laboratories, Deerfield, IL.

Wedge Biopsy

A larger sample of renal tissue can be obtained during nephrotomy. A wedge of tissue 2 to 5 mm thick can be removed from the exposed parenchyma by making a scalpel incision parallel to the nephrotomy incision. This provides an excellent sample for histological evaluation or mineral analysis. The effects of removal of this amount of tissue on renal function after surgery depend on the function of remaining tissue. If at least one-third of the nephrons are functioning normally, renal function is normal.[32]

Dialysis

The metabolic waste products that accumulate during acute renal failure and contribute to the signs of uremia can be eliminated by dialysis. Two techniques of dialysis are available, hemodialysis and peritoneal dialysis. Fluid and solute in the extracellular fluid are exchanged across a semipermeable membrane. This membrane is cellulose in hemodialysis and the peritoneum in peritoneal dialysis. Hemodialysis is more efficient, but it requires special equipment and trained staff because the blood has to be removed from the body, circulated through an artificial kidney, and returned to the body. For chronic hemodialysis, an arteriovenous fistula or vascular shunt must be created to allow chronic vascular access in the patient. A disadvantage of hemodialysis is the need for anticoagulation therapy to be given for the life of the shunt. A patient also has to face the risks of hemorrhage resulting from the reduction of platelets during extracorporeal circulation, hypotension and hemolysis during each episode of dialysis, and infection at the site of vascular access.[89]

Peritoneal dialysis is quite feasible in dogs and cats,[70] and a dog has been maintained without kidneys for 54 days using ambulatory peritoneal dialysis.[91] The dialysate contains at least 1.5 per cent glucose* to prevent rapid water absorption from the peritoneum due to the hyperosmotic state of uremic plasma. Hyperosmotic dialysis solutions with 4.25 and 7 per cent glucose are also available, and their use effectively reduces plasma volume in edematous patients. In an emergency, lactated Ringer solution can be used by adding 30 ml of 50 per cent dextrose per liter of fluid to make a 1.5 per cent solution. A disadvantage of Ringer solution is its low sodium content. It also contains potassium and phosphate, two of the electrolytes already present in excess in renal failure. Warming the dialysate to 104° to 107.6°F (40° to 42°C) promotes vasodilation and enhances blood flow to the peritoneum. Intraperitoneal vasodilators such as isoproterenol increase urea clearance by approximately 25 per cent[60] but are not commonly used.

The major difficulty with peritoneal dialysis has been removing the bulk of the fluid instilled. This problem has largely been overcome by the development of two efficient silicone rubber peritoneal dialysis cannulas.[70, 89] These catheters are flexible and are designed to be attached to the abdominal wall. Removing the omentum at the time of catheter placement significantly decreases the incidence of obstruction of the dialysis catheters.[12, 80] The peritoneal catheters can be maintained for a number of weeks during the period of chronic intermittent dialysis. The expected drainage rate by gravity alone from these catheters is about 100 ml/minute, with a recovery rate of 90 to 100 per cent.[6] Dialysis has also been performed by instilling dialysate into the pleural space.[82] The pleura was a satisfactory surface for exchange, and the absence of the omentum or a similar structure within the pleural space decreased obstruction of the dialysis catheter.

The recommended volume of dialysis fluid to infuse is 30 to 40 ml/kg.[12, 89] It remains in the abdominal cavity (dwell) for 30 minutes. A cycle of infusion, dwell, and recovery takes about 1 hour. During the first exchange, as much as 20 per cent of the dialysate may be taken up by the intestines and other organs. The first few exchanges may be blood tinged as a result of hemorrhage that may have occurred during insertion of the cannula. Six to eight exchanges can be completed in 24 hours. After each session, the cannula is flushed with heparinized saline, and an appropriate antibiotic is instilled into the peritoneal cavity.[12] Fluid balance and plasma chemistry values are recorded before treatment and after every 12 to 24 hours. Patients are weighed daily.

Complications of peritoneal dialysis include peritonitis, hypoproteinemia, malnutrition, hydrothorax, and signs associated with renal failure. Peritonitis is a frequent complication of peritoneal dialysis and is best prevented. Strict attention is paid to asepsis, and antibiotics are used judiciously.[12, 89] Hypoproteinemia and malnutrition are the result of protein loss in the dialysate and vomiting and anorexia due to failure. Various forms of alimentation are considered, and vomiting is controlled pharmacologically if necessary. Hydrothorax is the result of passage of dialysate across the diaphragm, possibly via the lymphatics; direct communication between the abdominal and thoracic cavities has not been demonstrated.[12] Hydrothorax associated with peritoneal dialysis has resolved after cessation of dialysis, thoracentesis, pleurodesis, or modification of the dialysate volume, dwell time, or a patient's posture during dwell.[12, 57, 81, 94]

*Dianeal, Travenol Laboratories, Deerfield, IL.

Chronic Renal Failure

Chronic renal failure is the result of progressive nephron loss, regardless of etiology, eventually leading to uremia when the process has reached its end-stage. Dialysis is considered in treating chronic renal disease only when acute decompensation that can be reversed has occurred. There is no justification for dialysis of an animal in terminal renal failure unless renal transplantation is being contemplated.

Renal Transplantation

Renal transplantation is described in Chapter 7. This procedure is technically feasible in dogs and cats, but its use in clinical practice is limited by the cost of immunosuppressive therapy and postoperative care and by the incidence of complications.

Renal Autotransplantation

In renal autotransplantation, the kidney is removed from its orthotopic position and transferred to a heterotopic position, such as the iliac fossa. This procedure could be an alternative to nephrectomy if a damaged distal ureter were too short to be reimplanted into the bladder. The kidney is implanted in the iliac fossa of the recipient with the renal artery anastomosed end to end with the external iliac artery and the renal vein anastomosed end to side to the common iliac vein. The ureter is implanted into the bladder using techniques outlined in Chapter 106. As an adjunct to autotransplantation, extracorporeal or "workbench" surgery has become established as a technique to treat certain renal vascular lesions in humans.[49] The kidney is excised and cooled, the lesion is dealt with on the bench top, and then the kidney is reimplanted, usually in a heterotopic site. This technique has also been used in selected cases of renal tumor and urinary calculi.[49] An experimental study in dogs comparing bench surgery with *in situ* repair of induced renal trauma showed that both methods were equally effective.[55] Hilar injuries with segmental artery involvement benefit most from bench microsurgery and bench angiography.

Renal Neoplasia

A wide range of tumors occur in the kidneys of dogs and cats. Their diagnosis, biological behavior, and de-

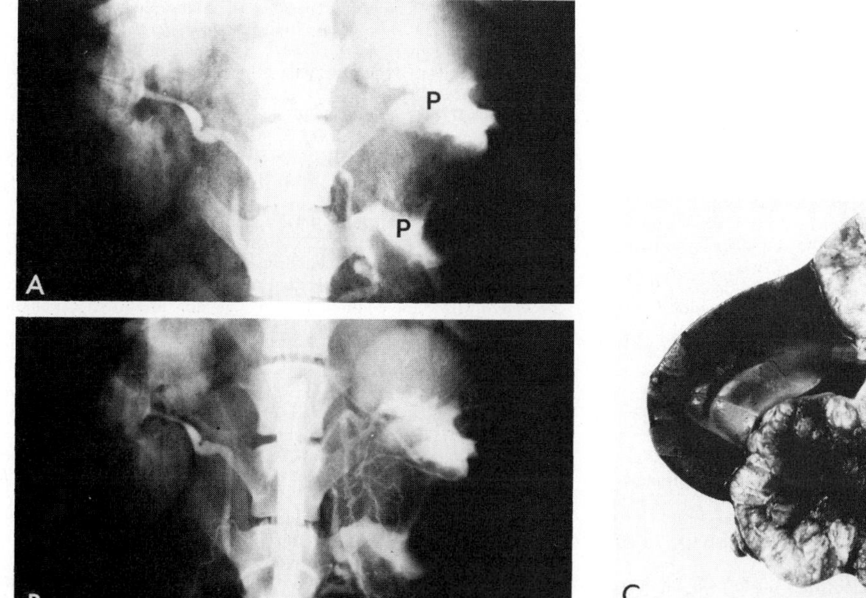

FIGURE 104–17. Renal carcinoma in a dog. *A*, An excretory urogram shows contrast agent being excreted by both kidneys. The left kidney is enlarged, and its pelvis (P) is misshapen and contains a large filling defect. *B*, A renal angiogram shows increased vascularity of the caudal pole. *C*, The kidney and tumor after excision.

tails of treatment are covered in Section 17. It is important not to be too pessimistic when a space-occupying lesion is detected in a kidney. It may be benign, in which case the prognosis is excellent with partial or total nephrectomy. Even if carcinoma is diagnosed (Fig. 104–17), nephrectomy is tried, provided thoracic radiographs show clear lung fields and exploratory surgery does not reveal enlarged regional lymph nodes. Survival for 4 years after excision of a renal carcinoma has been observed in dogs.[53]

References

1. Abdinoor DJ: Perinephric pseudocysts in a cat. *J Am Vet Med Assoc 16*:763, 1980.
2. Ankenman GJ, Murray JB: Control of postoperative renal hemorrhage by embolization with a Gianturco coil. *Can J Surg 25*:269, 1982.
3. Battershell D, Garcia JP: Polycystic kidney in a cat. *J Am Vet Med Assoc 154*:665, 1969.
4. Biller DS, et al: Polycystic kidney disease in a family of Persian cats. *J Am Vet Med Assoc 196*:1288, 1990.
5. Borthwick R: Foreign body in a cat's kidney. *J Small Anim Pract 12*:623, 1971.
6. Bovee KC: Peritoneal dialysis, hemodialysis and prospects of renal transplantation. *Nephrology, Urology and Diseases of the Urinary Tract.* No. 61. Proceedings of the University of Sydney Postgraduate Committee in Veterinary Science. Sydney, August 1982, p 299.
7. Brickner NS, Fine LG: The renal response to progressive nephron loss. *In* Brenner BM, Rector FC (eds): *The Kidney.* Vol 1. 2nd ed. W.B. Saunders, Philadelphia, 1981.
8. Brooker WJ, et al: Renal bleeding due to congenital vascular malformation: Control by arterial embolization. *J Urol 119*:261, 1978.
9. Brown NO, et al: Canine urolithiasis: Retrospective analysis of 438 cases. *J Am Vet Med Assoc 170*:414, 1977.
10. Cadwallader JA, et al: Renal haemangioma in a dog. *NZ Vet J 21*:48, 1973.
11. Caputo CA: Polycystic kidney disease in a cat. *Feline Pract 10*:36, 1980.
12. Carter LJ, et al: Clinical experience with peritoneal dialysis in small animals. *Comp Cont Educ Pract Vet 11*:1335, 1989.
13. Chastain CB, Grier RL: Bilateral retroperitoneal perirenal cysts in a cat. *Feline Pract 5*:41, 1975.
14. Chew QT, Madayag MA: Post nephrectomy arteriovenous fistula. *J Urol 109*:546, 1973.
15. Christie BA: Collateral arterial blood supply to the normal and ischemic canine kidney. *Am J Vet Res 41*:1519, 1980.
16. Churchward RE: Subcutaneous herniation of a kidney of a dog. *Aust Vet J 47*:178, 1971.
17. Cowgill LD: Diseases of the kidney. *In* Ettinger SJ (ed): *Textbook of Veterinary Internal Medicine.* Vol 2. 2nd ed. W.B. Saunders, Philadelphia, 1983, p 1812.
18. Crow SW, et al: Pyonephrosis associated with *Salmonella* infection in a dog. *J Am Vet Med Assoc 169*:1324, 1976.
19. Crowell WA, et al: Polycystic renal disease in related cats. *J Am Vet Med Assoc 175*:386, 1979.
20. Donner GS, et al: Percutaneous nephrotomy in the dog. An experimental study. *Vet Surg 16*:411, 1987.
21. Dorn AS, Stoloff D: Renal foreign body in a dog. *J Am Vet Med Assoc 167*:755, 1975.
22. Ekelund L, et al: Arteriovenous fistulae following renal biopsy with hypertension and hemodynamic changes. *J Urol 108*:373, 1972.
23. Feeney DA, et al: The excretory urogram: Parts I and II. *Comp Cont Educ Pract Vet 4*:233, 1982.
24. Finco DR, Barsanti JA: Bacterial pyelonephritis. *Vet Clin North Am 9*:645, 1979.
25. Finco DR, et al: Diseases of the urinary system. *In* Catcott EJ (ed): *Feline Medicine and Surgery.* 2nd ed. American Veterinary Publications, Santa Barbara, 1975, p 263.
26. Fitzpatrick JM, et al: Intrarenal access: Effects on renal function and morphology. *Br J Urol 52*:409, 1980.
27. Gahring DR, et al: Comparative renal function studies of nephrotomy closure with and without sutures in dogs. *J Am Vet Med Assoc 171*:537, 1977.
28. Goldstein AE, Abeshuse BS: Partial resection of the kidney. *J Urol 38*:15, 1937.
29. Goss RJ, Dittmer JE: Compensatory renal hypertrophy: Problems and prospects. *In* Nowinski WW, Goss RI (eds): *Compensatory Renal Hypertrophy.* Academic Press, New York, 1969, p 299.
30. Grauer GF, et al: Evaluation of laparoscopy for obtaining renal biopsy specimens from dogs and cats. *J Am Vet Med Assoc 183*:677, 1983.
31. Greenwood KM, Rawlings CA: Removal of canine renal calculi by pyelolithotomy. *Vet Surg 10*:12, 1981.
32. Guyton AC: Renal disease, diuresis, and micturition. *In Textbook of Medical Physiology.* 6th ed. W.B. Saunders, Philadelphia, 1981, p 463.
33. Hall MA, et al: Hydronephrosis with heteroplastic bone formation in a cat. *J Am Vet Med Assoc 160*:857, 1972.
34. Harrison LH: Anatrophic nephrolithotomy: Update 1978. *AUA Courses in Urology 1*:1, 1979.
35. Hitt ME, et al: Idiopathic hematuria of unilateral renal origin in a dog. *J Am Vet Med Assoc 187*:1371, 1985.

36. Hurwitz SP, Weisenthal CL: Pararenal pseudocysts. *J Urol 97*:8, 1967.
37. Iliff WJ, Galdabini JJ: Massive intratubular hemorrhage with herniations into renal veins requiring nephrectomy. *J Urol 108*:44, 1972.
38. Jeraj K, et al: Evaluation of renal biopsy in 197 dogs and cats. *J Am Vet Med Assoc 181*:367, 1982.
39. Johnson CA: Renal ectopia in a cat. *J Am Anim Hosp Assoc 15*:599, 1979.
40. Johnson HA: Cytoplasmic response to overwork. *In* Nowinski WW, Goss RI (eds): *Compensatory Renal Hypertrophy*. Academic Press, New York, 1969, p 14.
41. Jubb KVF, Kennedy PC: *Pathology of Domestic Animals*. Vol 1. 2nd ed. Academic Press, New York, 1970, p 288.
42. Kaufman CF, et al: Renal cortical hypoplasia with secondary hyperparathyroidism in the dog. *J Am Vet Med Assoc 155*:167, 1969.
43. Kawamura J, et al: Preoperative and postoperative cortical function of the kidney with staghorn calculi assessed by ^{99m}technetium-dimercaptosuccinic acid renal scintigraphy. *J Urol 130*:430, 1983.
44. Kelly DF, et al: Experimental pyelonephritis in the cat. *J Comp Pathol 89*:125, 1979.
45. Kim SK: New techniques of partial nephrectomy. *J Urol 102*:165, 1969.
46. Klopfer U, et al: A nephropathy similar to renal cortical hypoplasia in a Yorkshire terrier. *Vet Med Small Anim Clin 73*:327, 1978.
47. Kolata RJ: Abdominal trauma. *Comp Cont Educ Pract Vet 1*:445, 1979.
48. Lang EK, et al: Renal arteriography in the assessment of renal trauma. *Radiology 98*:103, 1971.
49. Lawson R: Extracorporeal renal surgery. *J Urol 123*:301, 1980.
50. Lee R, et al: Persistent haematuria in a dog due to discrete renal haemangioma. *J Small Anim Pract 15*:621, 1974.
51. Lipson MP, et al: Bullet lodged in the kidney of a dog. *J Am Vet Med Assoc 161*:293, 1972.
52. Lord PF, et al: Intravenous urography for evaluation of renal disease in small animals. *J Am Anim Hosp Assoc 10*:139, 1974.
53. Lucke VM, Kelly DF: Renal carcinoma in the dog. *Vet Pathol 13*:264, 1976.
54. Lulich JP, et al: Feline idiopathic polycystic kidney disease. *Comp Cont Educ Pract Vet 10*:1030, 1988.
55. McAninch JW, et al: Experimental penetrating renal trauma: A comparison of bench and in situ repair. *Invest Urol 17*:33, 1979.
56. McKenna SC, Carpenter JL: Polycystic disease of the kidney and liver in the Cairn terrier. *Vet Pathol 17*:436, 1980.
57. Milutinovic J, et al: Acute massive unilateral hydrothorax: A rare complication of chronic peritoneal dialysis. *South Med J 73*:827, 1980.
58. Murphy JJ, Best R: The healing of renal wounds. 1. Partial nephrectomy. *J Urol 78*:504, 1957.
59. Nabar KG, Madson PO: Renal function during acute total ureteral occlusion and the role for the lymphatics. An experimental study in dogs. *J Urol 109*:330, 1973.
60. Nolph KD, et al: The effects of intraperitoneal vasodilator on peritoneal clearances. *Trans Am Soc Artif Intern Organs 22*:586, 1976.
61. North DC: Hydronephrosis and hydroureter in a kitten. *J Small Anim Pract 19*:237, 1978.
62. Northington JW, Juliana MM: Polycystic kidney disease in a cat. *J Small Anim Pract 18*:663, 1977.
63. Osborne CA: General principles of biopsy. *Vet Clin North Am 4*:213, 1974.
64. Osborne CA, et al: *Canine and Feline Urology*. W.B. Saunders, Philadelphia, 1972, p 114.
65. Osborne CA, et al: *Canine and Feline Urology*. W.B. Saunders, Philadelphia, 1972, p 198.
66. Osborne CA, et al: Congenital fusion of kidney in a dog. *Vet Med Small Anim Clin 67*:39, 1972.
67. Osborne CA, et al: Dioctophyma renale in the dog. *J Am Vet Med Assoc 155*:605, 1969.
68. Osborne CA, et al: Kidney biopsy. *Vet Clin North Am 4*:351, 1974.
69. Paramo PG, et al: Sutureless nephrotomy. *J Urol 98*:456, 1967.
70. Parker HR: Current status of peritoneal dialysis. *In* Kirk RW (ed): *Current Veterinary Therapy VIII*. W.B. Saunders, Philadelphia, 1980.
71. Payne SR, Webb DR: The role of endourology in combination with extracorporeal shockwave lithotripsy. *In Percutaneous Renal Surgery*. Churchill Livingstone, New York, 1988, p 123.
72. Pechman RD: Urinary trauma in dogs and cats: A review. *J Am Anim Hosp Assoc 18*:33, 1982.
73. Phillips RA, et al: Effects of acute hemorrhagic and traumatic shock on renal function of dogs. *Am J Physiol 145*:314, 1946.
74. Rendano VT, Parker RB: Polycystic kidneys and peritoneopericardial diaphragmatic hernia in the cat: A case report. *J Small Anim Pract 17*:479, 1976.
75. Robbins GR: Unilateral renal agenesis in the beagle. *Vet Rec 77*:1345, 1965.
76. Robotham GR: Unilateral hydronephrosis in a cat. *Feline Pract 8*:23, 1978.
77. Ross LA, Lamb CR: Reduction of hydronephrosis and hydroureter associated with ectopic ureters in two dogs after ureterovesical anastomosis. *J Am Vet Med Assoc 196*:1497, 1990.
78. Ryan CP: Fused pelvic kidney. *Feline Pract 9*:32, 1979.
79. Ryan CP, Smith RA: Bilateral nephrolithiasis in a cat. *J Am Vet Med Assoc 158*:1946, 1971.
80. Salusky IB, et al: Continuous ambulatory peritoneal dialysis in pediatric patients: A 20-month experience. *Kidney Int 24*:101, 1983.
81. Scheldewaert R, et al: Management of a massive hydrothorax in a CAPD patient: A case report and a review of the literature. *Peritoneal Dialysis Bulletin 2*:69, 1982.
82. Shahar R, Holmberg DL: Pleural dialysis in the management of acute renal failure in two dogs. *J Am Vet Med Assoc 187*:952, 1985.
83. Silverberg DS, et al: Arteriovenous fistula and prolonged hematuria after renal biopsy: Treatment with epsilon amino caproic acid. *Can Med Assoc J 110*:671, 1974.
84. Stone EA: Canine nephrotomy. *Comp Cont Educ Pract Vet 9*:883, 1987.
85. Stone EA, et al: Renal function after prolonged hypotensive anesthesia and surgery in dogs with reduced renal mass. *Am J Vet Res 42*:1675, 1981.
86. Stone EA, et al: Massive hematuria of nontraumatic origin in dogs. *J Am Vet Med Assoc 183*:868, 1983.
87. Stone EA, et al: Glomerular filtration rate after nephrotomy: A comparison of intersegmental and bisection nephrotomy. *Vet Surg 19*:76, 1990.
88. Stowater JL: Congenital solitary renal cyst in a dog. *J Am Anim Hosp Assoc 11*:199, 1975.
89. Thornhill JA: Peritoneal dialysis in the dog and cat: An update. *Comp Cont Educ 3*:20, 1981.
90. Thornhill JA, Cechner PE: Traumatic injuries to the kidneys, ureter, bladder and urethra. *Vet Clin North Am 11*:157, 1981.
91. Thornhill JA, et al: Support of an anephric dog for 54 days with ambulatory peritoneal dialysis and a newly designed peritoneal catheter. *Am J Vet Res 45*:1156, 1984.
92. Thun R, et al: Iatrogenic hydronephrosis in a bitch. *J Am Vet Med Assoc 167*:388, 1975.
93. Ticer JW: Capsulogenic renal cyst in a cat. *J Am Vet Med Assoc 143*:613, 1963.
94. Townsend R, Fragola JA: Hydrothorax in a patient receiving continuous ambulatory peritoneal dialysis. *Arch Intern Med 142*:1571, 1982.
95. Tynes WV, et al: Surgical treatment of renal arteriovenous fistulas. *J Urol 103*:692, 1970.
96. Van Vroonhoven TJ, et al: Humoral regulation of renal mass. *Surgery 72*:300, 1972.
97. Vaughan ED Jr, et al: Unilateral ureteral occlusions: Pattern of nephron repair and compensatory response. *J Urol 109*:979, 1973.
98. Wallace S, et al: Therapeutic vascular occlusion utilizing steel coil technique: Clinical applications. *Am J Roentgenol 127*:381, 1976.
99. Webb AI: Renal ectopia in a dog. *Aust Vet J 50*:519, 1974.
100. Wells MJ, et al: Ectopic kidney in a cat. *Mod Vet Pract 61*:693, 1980.
101. Weyrauch HM, Rous SN: U-tube nephrostomy. *J Urol 97*:225, 1967.
102. Williams DF, et al: A new technique of partial nephrectomy. *J Urol 97*:955, 1967.
103. Wilson DR: Renal function during and following obstruction. *Annu Rev Med 28*:329, 1977.

CHAPTER

105 Ureters

Dale E. Bjorling and Bruce A. Christie

CONGENITAL ABNORMALITIES

Ectopic Ureters

Failure of the ureters to open into the bladder in the normal location has been reported in dogs,[3, 35, 57, 75, 80] cats,* horses,[14, 67, 82] cattle,[19] poultry,[83] and humans.[10, 21] Ureteral ectopia is due to abnormal differentiation of the mesonephric and metanephric ducts. The ureters open into the uterus, neck of the bladder, urethra, or vagina rather than the normal location in the trigone of the bladder. Although the condition has been reported in both male and female dogs and cats, it is more common in dogs than cats and occurs more frequently in females of both species. The majority of reported cases in dogs are bilateral, whereas in cats, bilateral and unilateral ectopic ureters occur with equal frequency.

The most commonly described location of ectopic ureters in relation to the bladder is intramural, within the wall of the bladder, usually between the muscularis and submucosa.[80] The ectopic ureter may have a single opening in an abnormal location or it may have an elongated opening into the bladder (ureteral trough), a double opening, or a blind end.[18, 31, 75, 80] Excretory urography alone may not identify the ectopic ureters. Combined use of excretory urography and negative-contrast cystography may improve the accuracy.[51] Partial obstruction of the ectopic ureter may occur, and hydronephrosis and hydroureter have been observed in dogs in association with ectopic ureters.[28, 68] This condition may improve after neoureterocystostomy of affected ureters.[68] Ectopic ureters that have a blind end may not be diagnosed on plain or contrast radiography owing to loss of functional tissue of the associated kidney.[5, 80] Ureters lacking a distal opening have also been identified as a cause of unilateral renal enlargement. Ectopic ureters that completely bypass the bladder (extramural) are observed less commonly, and it has been suggested that not all the ectopic ureters considered to be extramural when evaluated by contrast radiography actually are in this position.[51, 80] In one study of dogs with ectopic ureters, other abnormalities of the urogenital tract were identified before surgery by special radiographic studies in 17 of 18 dogs.[51]

The heritability of this condition has not been established, and the majority of cases have been reported in mixed-breed dogs.[33, 35, 57, 75] A familial predisposition occurs in Siberian huskies, Newfoundland retrievers, poodles, Labrador retrievers, and golden retrievers,[33, 34, 80] but the mode of inheritance is unknown.

The most common complaint of owners of animals with ectopic ureter(s) is urinary incontinence. Many of these animals void a small to nearly normal quantity of urine at appropriate intervals. The perineal area (females) or tip of the prepuce (males) is constantly damp from the uncontrolled flow of urine.[7, 55, 80] Incontinence associated with this condition may be intermittent or positional or may be observed at rest.[18, 35, 80] Incontinence is primarily attributed to discharge of urine into the uterus, vagina, or urethra, but abnormal function of the urethral sphincter may accompany ectopic ureter in dogs and cats.[66] Incontinence may occur less frequently in male dogs with ectopic ureter because the ureter opens into the urethra between the urethral sphincter and the bladder.[55] Surgical treatment (see Chapter 106) frequently corrects incontinence associated with ectopic ureter in cats, but as many as 50 to 60 per cent of dogs treated surgically for ectopic ureter may have some degree of incontinence (positional, exertional, nocturnal, or other) after surgery.[18, 35, 80] Treatment with phenylpropanolamine (an alpha-adrenergic receptor agonist that may increase urethral sphincter tone) or diethylstilbestrol may improve incontinence observed after surgery.[66, 80] Urinary tract infection may also accompany ectopic ureter.[80] The reasons for this are not clear, although infection is probably due to migration of bacteria through the ectopic ureter or failure of competence of the urethral sphincter.

Ureterocele

A ureterocele is a cystic dilation of the intravesicular, submucosal segment of the distal ureter (Fig. 105–1). This disorder is rare in dogs[52, 58, 72, 73, 81] and has not been described in cats. In humans, although the distal orifice of a ureter affected by a ureterocele may be tiny,

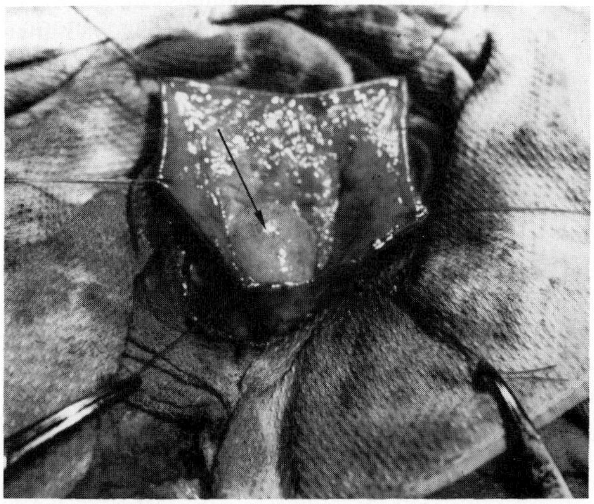

FIGURE 105–1. Ureterocele (*arrow*) in a dog, exposed by a ventral cystotomy. (Courtesy of Dr. D. E. Johnston.)

*See references 4, 6, 24, 27, 45, 64, and 74.

ureteroceles have been observed in the presence of a normal ureterovesicular orifice.[78] This observation discredits one theory of the development of ureteroceles that suggests that they are the result of at least partial obstruction of the distal ureter.[52] The exact embryological causes of the development of ureteroceles are unknown. Ureters affected by ureteroceles are frequently ectopic, and incontinence may be observed if the affected ureter is ectopic.[52]

Ureteroceles may cause pain, stranguria, pollakiuria, or hematuria. Stranguria is the result of the physical presence of the dilated distal ureter, which applies pressure on the neck of the bladder.[26] Ureteral obstruction may predispose the animal to the development of infection and calculi.[72] Obstruction of the flow of urine from the ureter into the bladder may also cause hydronephrosis and loss of functional renal tissue of the associated kidney.[52]

Preoperatively, the diagnosis of ureterocele is most often made by excretory urography. If the kidney associated with the ureterocele is nonfunctional, the bladder is filled with urine containing contrast material, excreted by the contralateral kidney, and the ureterocele appears as a filling defect in the neck of the bladder.[52, 81] If the kidney is functional, a dilation of the distal intravesicular portion of the ureter is observed as the ureterocele fills with contrast material. A filling defect may then be observed in the neck of the bladder as the ureterocele empties.

If the associated kidney is still functional, the affected ureter can be severed and reimplanted into the bladder (see Chapter 106). The ureterocele is dissected from the wall of the bladder and removed. Damage to the urethral sphincter is avoided. The ureterocele can be approached via a ventral cystotomy, and the resulting mucosal defect is closed.[52] If the kidney is severely affected and has lost function, the kidney, ureter, and ureterocele are removed.

Absence or Duplication of Ureters

During embryonic development, penetration by the growing ureteric bud into the metanephrogenic tissue stimulates development of nephrons. If the ureteric bud fails to form, the consequence is renal agenesis. If two ureteric buds grow out of the same mesonephric duct or if division of the ureteric bud is faulty, separate renal development is induced around each duct system. Each moiety fuses to form a duplex kidney. The ureter associated with the more cranial part of the duplicated kidney usually migrates with the mesonephric duct to the urethra—that is, it is ectopic and is usually associated with urinary incontinence.[10]

Ureteral and renal agenesis is more common in dogs than renal or ureteral duplication. It is difficult to diagnose duplex kidneys at postmortem examination, because there is probably a common capsule, a common renal artery, and a common peritoneal fold around the two ureters.[54] The prevalence of this disorder may therefore be greater than suspected. In the only case of renal and ureteral duplication reported in a dog, incontinence was observed, and pyelonephritis due to gram-negative bacteria was present in both normal and duplex kidneys.[54]

Ureteral Valves

Ureteral valves are rare in humans[10] and animals.[62] They have been reported in a dog; however, the diagnosis was made by observing transverse filling defects on excretory urography and was not confirmed by surgery or necropsy.[62] This dog was presented for evaluation of incontinence. The radiographic appearance made the presence of ectopic ureter(s) unlikely, but the cause of incontinence was not determined, and it is unclear how ureteral valves could contribute to incontinence. In humans, ureteral valves are seldom the cause of a urological problem.[10]

VESICOURETERAL REFLUX

Retrograde flow of urine from the bladder into the ureter and renal pelves is prevented by the valvelike effect of the bladder wall on the intravesicular portion of the ureter (Fig. 105–2). However, vesicoureteral reflux of urine may be common in younger dogs, but the prevalence may decline with age.[14] The incidence of vesicoureteral reflux in dogs and cats during manual compression of the bladder and distension of the bladder with radiographic contrast material has been evaluated.[22, 23] In these studies, in sedated or lightly anesthetized animals, vesicoureteral reflux was a relatively common occurrence (50 per cent of dogs and 40 per cent of cats). This finding may have been due to the ages of the animals (although age of the animals was difficult to absolutely determine in these reports) or the effects of drugs administered for sedation. In addition to its rela-

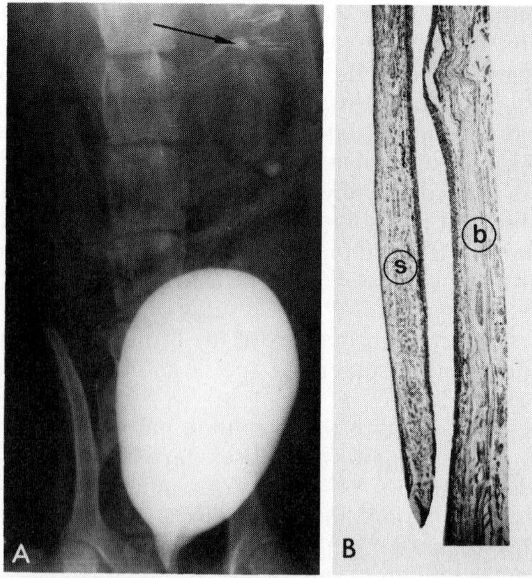

FIGURE 105–2. *A*, Unilateral vesicoureteral reflux in a dog, demonstrated by voiding cystourethrography. Contrast agent, which had run back to the renal pelvis (*arrow*), is being cleared by ureteral peristaltic action. *B*, A normal ureterovesical junction showing the submucosal ureter (s), which is compressed against the bladder wall (b) as pressure in the bladder rises. (H&E, × 10.)

tionship to manual compression of the bladder, vesicoureteral reflux may also occur in association with cystitis, obstruction of the bladder neck or urethra, or neurogenic bladder disease. Vesicoureteral reflux has been observed in a cat with urological disease, but the prevalence in normal cats is probably low.[42]

The prevalence of vesicoureteral reflux in normal, unsedated dogs is not clear, but the previously cited studies suggest that it may be fairly common. Chronic retrograde flow of urine in humans may result in deterioration of renal function, regardless of the presence or absence of infection.[38, 70] Certainly, reflux of urine containing bacteria leads to pyelonephritis and loss of renal function.[14] Short-term reflux of sterile urine has no apparent effect on renal function in dogs.[87] If chronic vesicoureteral reflux occurs in dogs and cats, it may not have a significant effect on renal function because of the relatively low incidence of urinary tract infection in the total population and the short life span of these species. Numerous surgical procedures have been described for the prevention and treatment of vesicoureteral reflux in humans, but surgical treatment specifically to prevent vesicoureteral reflux in dogs and cats is not recommended.

ACQUIRED ABNORMALITIES

Ureteral Injury—Accidental

Ureteral disruption may be the result of accidental or iatrogenic injury or it may be a sequel to ureteral obstruction.[9, 30, 43, 46] Because of their position ventral to the lumbar musculature, the ureters are injured much less frequently than other abdominal organs as a result of blunt trauma.[44] The presence of ureteral injury due to penetrating trauma may be suggested by the location of the entry and exit wounds. The presence of calculi lodged within the ureter can cause necrosis and subsequent disruption of the ureteral wall.[9] Crushing injuries may result in transient or permanent ureteral obstruction or disruption. Compressive injuries often cause spasm of the ureter, which resolves if compression and inflammation are relieved as the injury resolves.[20] Prolonged compression may disrupt the ureteral blood supply, resulting in necrosis of a segment of the ureter. Permanent obstruction of the ureter due to the presence of blood clots and subsequent fibrosis is rare in the absence of extensive injuries to the mucosa or wall of the ureter.

Ureteral Injury—Iatrogenic

Iatrogenic injuries of the ureter occur most commonly during ovariohysterectomy. Although this injury has been reported more frequently in dogs, cats may be at greater risk because of the proximity of the ureters to the body of the uterus as the ureters pass from their association with the broad ligament of the uterus into the lateral ligaments of the bladder. The ureters may also be inadvertently cut, crushed, or devascularized during exploratory laparotomy, as in human patients.[13, 53, 69]

If a ligature or clamp has been applied to the ureter, the ultimate degree of injury may be difficult to assess initially. Obviously, the constricting appliance is removed. Experimental studies have shown that the duration (from 1 to 60 minutes) of application of a crushing instrument to the ureters of dogs does not influence the degree of injury.[7] Although contrast radiography consistently demonstrated localized narrowing at the site of injury and increased tortuosity along the length of the ureter during the first week, by the 12th week after injury, 90 per cent of the strictures had resolved and 41 per cent had formed aneurysmal dilations. It has been recommended that crush injuries not be treated immediately but instead be evaluated at regular intervals by excretory urography and treated if abnormalities persist.[7] If a ligature is removed from the ureter within 1 week of application, normal function of the ureter and kidney may be regained. Obstruction of the ureter for 4 weeks or longer results in total loss of function of the associated kidney.[90, 91] Chronic partial obstruction of the ureter causes a variable loss of function of the kidney and ureter as a result of prolonged distension.

Experimental devascularizing trauma in dogs was achieved by removing 2 or 3 cm of adventitia from the ureter.[7] The effects of this injury were more serious than those of experimentally induced crush injury. Forty per cent of the damaged ureters developed early strictures, and 50 per cent of the strictures persisted, leading to hydronephrosis, calculus, and urine fistula formation. For these reasons, prompt resection of the damaged segment and anastomosis are recommended.

Diagnosis of Ureteral Trauma

Radiography. The presence of ureteral rupture may be suggested on plain abdominal radiographs by an increase in the size of the retroperitoneal space due to accumulation of urine. This possibility is pursued by performing excretory urography.

Excretory Urography. Excretory urography usually allows the presence and location of ureteral disruption to be precisely determined (Fig. 105–3). If the vascular supply of the kidney is intact and the kidney is functioning normally, contrast material is excreted by the kidney, outlines the urinary tract on radiographs made at appropriate time intervals, and conclusively demonstrates the location of injury to the urinary tract (see Chapter 103).[50, 59]

Renal Angiography. Renal angiography is described in Chapter 103. Specialized catheters of appropriate size and shape, as well as the ability to rapidly expose radiographic film or continuously record a fluoroscopic image, are required to perform this technique. Nonselective angiography may be performed by injecting contrast material into the abdominal aorta cranial to the origin of the renal arteries.[15] This technique may not have significant advantages over excretory urography.

Exposures made within seconds of dye injection allow identification of the vascular structures of the kidney. The dye, which is concentrated and excreted, begins to opacify the proximal ureter within 3 to 5 minutes of injection. A prolonged delay in dye excretion suggests that an inadequate volume was given, renal function may be poor, or the dye was injected in an inappropriate location.

Antegrade Ureterography. The technique of percu-

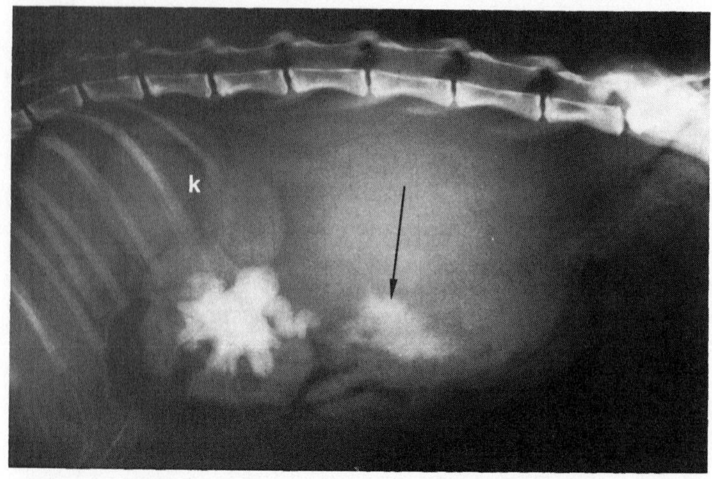

FIGURE 105–3. Ruptured ureter in a dog (*arrow*) demonstrated by excretory urography. Note that the ureter is dilated proximal to the site of rupture; this is a common finding. There is retroperitoneal accumulation of fluid in the sublumbar region. The right kidney (k) is nonfunctional.

taneous nephropyelocentesis has been described in dogs[48] and may be used to obtain samples of urine from the renal pelves and perform antegrade ureterography.[1] A catheter is passed through the renal parenchyma into the pelvis or ureter, and contrast material is injected. This method of examination of the ureters reveals more anatomical detail than excretory urography and does little damage to the kidney.[48] To monitor the position of the catheter, fluoroscopy, ultrasonography, or computed tomography is required.

Management of Ureteral Trauma

When the ureters have been injured, four treatment options exist: ureteronephrectomy, placement of a ureteral catheter, ureteral anastomosis, or reimplantation of the ureter into the bladder (neoureterocystostomy—see Chapter 106). A common solution to ureteral trauma in veterinary medicine is to perform ureteronephrectomy. In humans, the surgical approach to trauma of the urinary tract has become more conservative.[53] Extravasation of sterile urine is relatively harmless for 24 to 36 hours.[53] Extravasation of infected urine, however, results in rapidly spreading cellulitis. Therefore, animals with suspected ureteral or renal injury and urinary tract infections are treated with broad-spectrum antibiotics (see Chapter 103). Small ureteral tears ultimately heal completely, so extravasation of urine is not an absolute indication for immediate surgery.[53] In humans, percutaneous nephrostomy allows diversion of urine for the management of ureteral injury.[60] When feasible, early exploratory surgery and definitive therapy are preferred to protracted conservative management in animals for economic as well as humane reasons.

Reimplantation of a ureter after it has avulsed from the renal pelvis is technically difficult. A catheter is placed as a stent across the site of reimplantation to promote healing (Fig. 105–4). In small patients, ureteronephrectomy may be the only recourse unless some form of magnification is available.

Ureteral anastomosis is difficult in small patients[13] and is associated with an extremely high rate of postoperative obstruction in cats. Magnification of the operative field using magnifying loupes or an operating microscope can be helpful in performing a precise, atraumatic ureteral anastomosis. In most dogs, no more than 3 to 5

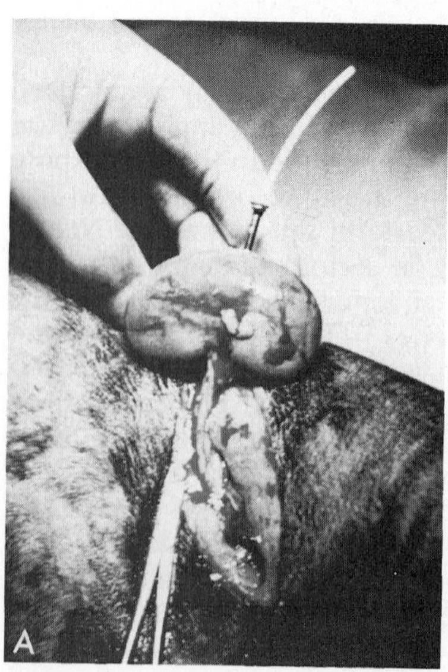

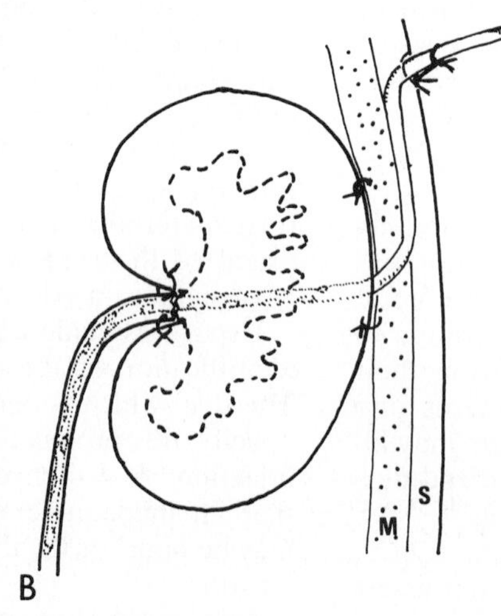

FIGURE 105–4. Splinting an avulsed ureter. *A*, A trocar and cannula are passed into the renal pelvis through the parenchyma. The trocar is withdrawn, and a number 5 French fenestrated flexible catheter is inserted into the renal pelvis. The cannula is then withdrawn. The catheter is advanced into the distal ureter. The ureter is anchored to the kidney adjacent to the site of avulsion. The catheter is exteriorized through a subcutaneous tunnel and anchored to the skin (S). Nephropexy is performed with a few capsular sutures to anchor the kidney to the abdominal wall muscles (M).

cm of ureter can be resected without creating tension on the anastomosis. However, some investigators have suggested that the amount of tension on the anastomosis does not correlate with scar tissue and stricture formation, and as much as 10 cm of ureter has been removed in dogs weighing 22 to 34 kg without subsequent stricture formation at the site of anastomosis.[61] These researchers suggested that the limits of the amount of tension that can safely be placed on the anastomosis are unknown. A tension-free anastomosis is preferred.[11, 40, 61]

To increase the circumference of the ureteral anastomosis, the ends of the ureter are spatulated by making longitudinal incisions 3 to 5 mm in length in each end (Fig. 105–5). The spatulating incisions are placed on opposite sides of the ends of the ureter. Interrupted sutures of 5-0 to 7-0 polyglycolic acid or polyglactin 910 are placed in the apex of the spatulating incisions, and the remainder of the anastomosis is completed in an interrupted or continuous pattern.[12, 76] Care is taken to avoid twisting the ureter during the anastomosis, because this may result in obstruction of the longitudinal blood supply. It is impossible to place the sutures in a

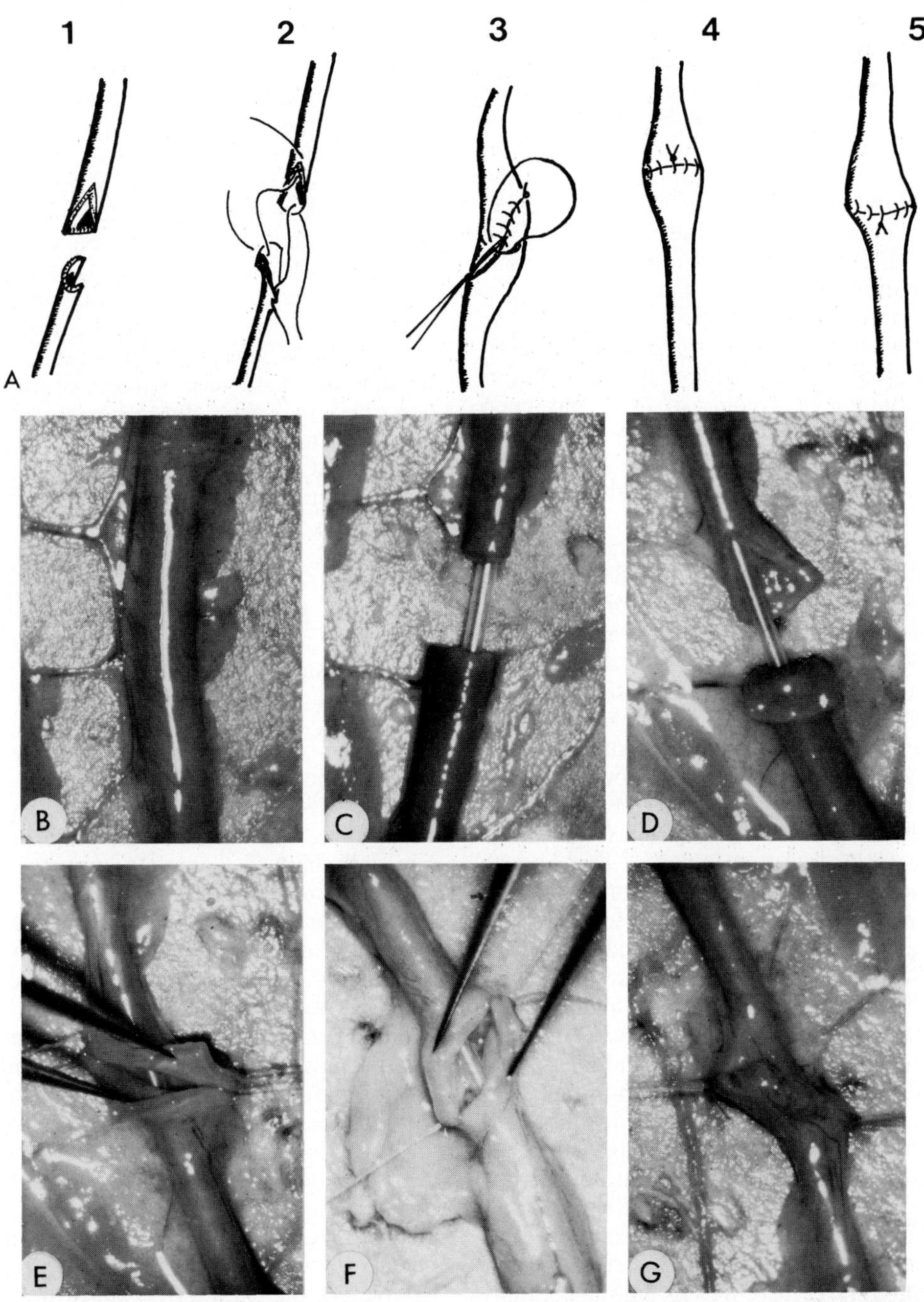

FIGURE 105–5 *A*, Continuous suture pattern for ureteral anastomosis. 1, Spatulate ureter; 2, place stay sutures; 3, insert running stitch; 4 and 5, finished anastomosis viewed from opposite sides. *B*, Normal ureter of a dog viewed through an operating microscope using ×6 magnification. Longitudinally oriented blood vessels in the adventitia supply regular transversely oriented blood vessels to the wall of the ureter. *C*, Ureter cut and splinted with vinyl tubing. *D*, Ends of ureter spatulated. *E*, Stay sutures placed. *F*, First row of stitches completed and ureter rolled through 180°. *G*, Anastomosis completed.

partial-thickness (submucosal) manner without magnification, and sutures are usually placed through the full thickness of the ureteral wall. Calculi formation usually does not occur in the absence of infection. Although leakage across the suture line is an infrequent occurrence, the line of anastomosis may be sealed with a thin film of the tissue adhesive fluoralkyl cyanoacrylate.[86] This tissue adhesive is less toxic than other cyanoacrylates, invokes only a mild inflammatory reaction, and does not interfere with normal ureteral healing.

Compensation for Loss of Ureteral Length

If a segment of ureter is permanently damaged, the surgeon can reduce the distance between the kidney and the bladder to facilitate reimplantation of the ureter or attempt to replace the ureter. The kidney can be freed of its retroperitoneal attachments and displaced caudally.[63] The capsule of the kidney can be tacked to the fascia of the sublumbar musculature using absorbable or nonabsorbable sutures. The kidney should not be displaced such a distance that renal arterial or venous blood flow is impaired. The bladder may also be drawn cranially and sutured to the fascia of the sublumbar musculature (psoas hitch).[65] The ureter is then reimplanted into a segment of the bladder that is immobilized. Normal spontaneous voiding of urine has been observed after this procedure. Obviously, if one is attempting to overcome loss of ureteral length, the ureter is reimplanted into the most cranial portion of the bladder.

The most successful techniques for replacing the ureter have used autogenous tissues. Bladder flaps, pedicle grafts of the intestine or bladder mucosa, or free grafts of buccal mucosa all have been used successfully, clinically in humans or experimentally in animals.[32, 37, 39, 77, 85, 87] If the mucosa is left intact in intestinal pedicle grafts, a significant amount of mucus is produced. The mucosa regenerates if removed, and if the submucosa is removed, the graft becomes lined with urothelium but consistently produces extensive osteoid.[74] Free autologous bladder mucosal grafts 5 to 20 cm in length have functioned satisfactorily as ureters in dogs.[37] These grafts regenerate a smooth-muscle coat, presumably from submucosal cellular elements in the graft. It is unlikely that these grafts develop the ability to form and propagate peristaltic contractions similar to normal ureters. However, tubular grafts of buccal mucosa used to replace 3-cm defects in the ureters of baboons proved quite successful, despite a complete lack of peristalsis.[77] Other biological materials including skin, fallopian tubes, vermiform appendix, and vessels have proved less successful as replacements for the ureter.[3, 32] Collagen film has been used to buttress the repair of ureteral defects but is not an effective substitute for the ureter.[71]

Various synthetic ureteral prostheses composed of glass, metals, plastics, Dacron, silicone rubber, and polytetrafluoroethylene (Gore-Tex), among others, have been investigated and found to be uniformly unsatisfactory.[3, 15, 36, 84] These implants have been associated with a high incidence of infection, obstruction, excessive scar formation, calculi formation, leakage, and migration of the implant. A 3-year study of the implantation of a silicone rubber prosthesis reinforced with metal spirals and secured to the ureter and bladder with Dacron cuffs suggested that this particular design was more successful than others.[36] However, significant scar tissue formation was observed, and concern was expressed about the long-term patency of the prosthesis.

Ureteral Obstruction

Ureteral obstruction may be the result of trauma, intraluminal objects or structures, intramural mass lesions, or extramural compression. Intraluminal obstruction of the ureters by calculi in cats and dogs is rare.[8, 9, 92] Bilateral hydronephrosis due to ureteral fibrosis has been reported in a cat.[47] Histological evaluation of the ureters and kidneys demonstrated the presence of infiltration of these structures by fibrous tissue and thickening of the ureteral mucosa, but the cause of these changes was undetermined. When ureteral passage of artificial calculi was investigated in dogs, it was observed that solid spheres with diameters of 2.3 mm were freely passed and those of 2.8 mm became firmly impacted. When the diameter was 3.9 mm or greater, the calculi could not even be introduced into the ureter.[41] Intramural lesions causing obstruction are also rare, but benign[49] and malignant[5] tumors of the ureter have been described in dogs, and a malignant transitional cell tumor of the renal pelvis of a cat has been reported.[56] Extramural causes of compression, apart from tumors, include intrapelvic cysts,[89] which are developmental abnormalities, and uterine stump granulomas, which occur as sequelae of ovariohysterectomy.[2]

Ureteral obstruction invariably results in dilation of the ureter proximal to the site of obstruction due to dilation of the lumen and some hyperplasia and hypertrophy of smooth muscle in the ureteral wall.[17]

Treatment

Experimental studies in dogs have shown that if ureteral obstruction is relieved within 10 weeks of its occurrence, the dilated segment returns to its normal size and shape.[88] Complete ureteral obstruction for 4 weeks or longer results in permanent loss of function of the associated kidney.[90, 91] If the ureter does not regain its normal diameter or if the dilation is not related to obstruction, ureteral plication can be tried.[78] Ureteral plication was developed in dogs to reduce the caliber of a dilated ureter, thereby restoring normal coaptation and propulsion of urine into the bladder without disrupting the ureteral blood supply. The plication is performed over a number 10 to 12 French catheter by inserting interrupted Lembert stitches of 4-0 to 5-0 absorbable suture through the medial and lateral walls of the ureter. The sutures are placed about 1 cm apart and are reinforced with simple interrupted stitches placed between them. When the plication has been completed, the catheter is removed.

Ureterotomy. In humans, ureteral calculi are initially treated by administering antispasmodics and oral or intravenous fluids. Ureteral calculi are identified so infrequently in dogs and cats[9] that the efficacy of this form of treatment is unclear. Because of the nonspecific

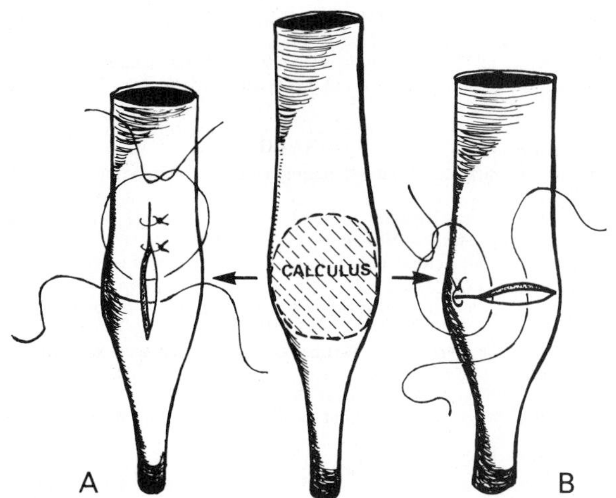

FIGURE 105–6. Longitudinal (*A*) or transverse (*B*) ureterotomy over a calculus. Closure may be by interrupted (illustrated) or continuous sutures to bring the edges of the ureteral wall into loose apposition.

signs associated with ureteral calculi in dogs and cats, the diagnosis may be delayed. The prolonged presence of calculi within the ureter may result in necrosis of the ureteral wall. Ureteral transit time for solid artificial calculi varies from 1 to 24 hours.[41] If there is no radiographic evidence within this time that the stone has moved, ureterotomy is indicated. Before surgery, the kidneys, bladder, and urethra are carefully evaluated radiographically for the presence of other calculi. Either a longitudinal[29] or transverse[79] incision may be made over the calculus (Fig. 105–6); however, sutures may tear out of longitudinal incisions more easily. Transverse incisions heal well if one-third to one-half of the ureteral circumference is left intact.[25] The ureter is flushed proximally and distally with sterile saline, and a number 3 to 5 French catheter passed in both directions to ensure that no calculi remain within the ureter. The incision is closed with 5-0 to 7-0 absorbable suture in an interrupted or continuous pattern. Sutures are placed through the entire thickness of the wall of the ureter and are tied with the tissues in loose apposition. If a segment of the ureter has been damaged by the presence of the calculus, the damaged portion is resected and an anastomosis performed. If a portion of the ureteral mucosa and wall bridging the damaged area is intact, a catheter can be left in place for 2 to 4 weeks to allow the ureter to heal (see Chapter 103).

References

1. Ackerman N, et al: Percutaneous nephropyelocentesis and antegrade ureterography. A fluoroscopically assisted diagnostic technique in canine urology. *Vet Radiol 1*:117, 1980.
2. Bartells JE: Radiology of the genital tract. *In* O'Brien TR (ed): *Radiographic Diagnosis of Abdominal Disorders in the Dog and Cat.* W.B. Saunders, Philadelphia, 1978.
3. Baum N, et al: Ureteral replacements. *Urology 5*:165, 1975.
4. Bebko RL, et al: Ectopic ureters in a male cat. *J Am Vet Med Assoc 171*:738, 1977.
5. Berzon JL: Primary leiomyosarcoma of the ureter in a dog. *J Am Vet Med Assoc 175*:374, 1979.
6. Biewenga WJ, et al: Ectopic ureters in a cat—a report of two cases. *J Small Anim Pract 19*:531, 1978.
7. Brodsky SL, et al: Effects of crush and devascularizing injuries to the proximal ureter. An experimental study. *Invest Urol 14*:361, 1977.
8. Brown NO, et al: Canine urolithiasis: Retrospective analysis of 438 cases. *J Am Vet Med Assoc 70*:414, 1977.
9. Campbell KL: Ureteral rupture associated with struvite nephrolithiasis and ureterolithiasis. *Canine Pract 8*:41, 1981.
10. Campbell MF: Anomalies of the ureter. *In* Campbell MF, Harrison JH (eds): *Urology*. 3rd ed. Vol 2. W.B. Saunders, Philadelphia, 1970.
11. Carlton CE, et al: The initial management of ureteral injuries: A report of 78 cases. *J Urol 105*:335, 1971.
12. Cass AS, et al: Ureteral anastomosis in the dog comparing continuous sutures with interrupted sutures. *Invest Urol 6*:94, 1968.
13. Chomchark C, Eckert C: Repair of the ureter severed at operation. *Ann Surg 177*:748, 1973.
14. Christie BA: Vesicoureteral reflux in dogs. *J Am Vet Med Assoc 162*:772, 1973.
15. Christie BA, Wood AKW: Renal angiography in dogs. Proceedings of the 5th International Veterinary Radiology Congress, Munich, September, 1979.
16. Christie B, et al: Surgical correction of bilateral ureteral ectopia in a male Appaloosa foal. *Aust Vet J 57*:336, 1981.
17. Cussen LJ: The effect of incomplete chronic obstruction on the ureteric muscle of a dog. *Invest Urol 10*:208, 1972.
18. Dean PW, et al: Canine ectopic ureter. *Comp Cont Educ Pract Vet 10*:146, 1988.
19. Devlin A: Surgical correction of congenital ectopic ureter in a calf. *Irish Vet News 10*:22, 1988.
20. Docimo SG, DeWolf WC: High failure rate of indwelling ureteral stents in patients with extrinsic obstruction: Experience at 2 institutions. *J Urol 142*:277, 1989.
21. Emmett JL: *Clinical Urography*. 2nd ed. W.B. Saunders, Philadelphia, 1964.
22. Feeney DA, et al: Maximum-distention retrograde urethrocystography in healthy male dogs: Occurrence of vesicoureteral reflux. *Am J Vet Res 45*:953, 1984.
23. Feeney DA, et al: Normal canine excretory urogram: Effects of dose, time, and individual dog variation. *Am J Vet Res 40*:1596, 1979.
24. Filippich LJ, et al: Ectopic ureter in a cat—a case report. *Aust Vet Pract 15*:7, 1985.
25. Gil-Vernat JM: Transverse ureterotomy. *J Urol 111*:755, 1974.
26. Gingell JC, et al: Acute obstructive uropathy due to prolapsed ectopic ureterocele: Case report. *Br J Urol 43*:305, 1971.
27. Grauer GF, et al: Urinary incontinence associated with an ectopic ureter in a female cat. *J Am Vet Med Assoc 182*:707, 1983.
28. Greene JA, et al: Hydronephrosis and hydroureter associated with a unilateral ectopic ureter in a spayed bitch. *J Am Anim Hosp Assoc 14*:708, 1978.
29. Greene RW, Greiner TP: The ureter. *In* Bojrab MJ (ed): *Current Techniques in Small Animal Surgery*. Lea & Febiger, Philadelphia, 1975.
30. Gumbrell RC, McLeavey BJ: Traumatic atresia of a ureteral orifice in a dog. *NZ Vet J 20*:59, 1972.
31. Hager DA, Blevins WE: Ectopic ureter in a dog: Extension from the kidney to the urinary bladder and to the urethra. *J Am Vet Med Assoc 189*:309, 1986.
32. Hatch CS: Intestinal seromuscular pedicle graft to defects of the ureteropelvic junction. *J Urol 95*:764, 1966.
33. Hayes HH: Breed associations of canine ectopic ureter: A study of 217 female cases. *J Small Anim Pract 25*:501, 1984.
34. Hayes HM Jr: Ectopic ureter in dogs: Epidemiological features. *Teratology 10*:129, 1974.
35. Holt PE, et al: Canine ectopic ureter—a review of twenty-nine cases. *J Small Anim Pract 23*:195, 1982.
36. Homann W, et al: Long-term results of prosthetic ureteral replacement in minipigs. *Urol Int 39*:95, 1984.
37. Hovnanian AP, Kingsley IA: Reconstruction of the ureter by free autologous bladder mucosa graft. *J Urol 96*:167, 1966.
38. Itatani H, Sonoda T: New techniques of ureteroileal anasotomosis and its clinical experience. *J Urol 119*:735, 1978.
39. Ivancevic LD, et al: Total replacement of the ureter using a bladder flap and cinematographic studies on the newly constructed ureter. *J Urol 107*:576, 1972.
40. Jonas D, et al: Splintless microsurgical anastomosis of the ureter in the dog. *Urol Res 9*:271, 1981.
41. Kim HL, et al: An experimental model of ureteric colic. *J Urol 104*:390, 1970.
42. Kipnis RM: Vesicoureteral reflux in a cat. *J Am Vet Med Assoc 167*:288, 1975.
43. Kleine LJ, Thornton GW: Radiographic diagnosis of urinary tract trauma. *J Am Anim Hosp Assoc 7*:318, 1971.
44. Kolata RJ, et al: Patterns of trauma in urban dogs and cats: A study of 1000 cases. *J Am Vet Med Assoc 164*:499, 1974.
45. Kuzma AB, Holmberg DL: Ectopic ureter in a cat. *Can Vet J 29*:59, 1988.
46. Leeds EB: The diagnosis and treatment of ruptured ureters in the dog. *Arch Am Coll Vet Surg 3*:45, 1973.
47. Lieb MS, et al: Bilateral hydronephrosis attributable to bilateral ureteral fibrosis in a cat. *J Am Vet Med Assoc 192*:795, 1988.

48. Ling GV, et al: Percutaneous nephropyelocentesis and nephropyelostomy in the dog: A description of the technique. *Am J Vet Res 40*:1605, 1979.
49. Liska WD, Patnaik AK: Leiomyoma of the ureter of a dog. *J Am Anim Hosp Assoc 13*:83, 1977.
50. Lord PF, et al: Intravenous urography for evaluation of renal diseases in small animals. *J Am Anim Hosp Assoc 10*:139, 1974.
51. Mason LK, et al: Surgery of ectopic ureters: Pre- and postoperative radiography morphology. *J Am Anim Hosp Assoc 26*:73, 1990.
52. McLoughlin MA, et al: Canine ureteroceles: A case report and literature review. *J Am Anim Hosp Assoc 25*:699, 1989.
53. Mitchell JP: Trauma to the urinary tract. *N Engl J Med 288*:90, 1973.
54. O'Handley P, et al: Renal and ureteral duplication in a dog. *J Am Vet Med Assoc 174*:484, 1979.
55. Osborne CA, Perman V: Ectopic ureter in a male dog. *J Am Vet Med Assoc 154*:273, 1969.
56. Osborne CA, et al: Renal pelvic carcinoma in a cat. *J Am Vet Med Assoc 159*:1238, 1971.
57. Owen R, ap R: Canine ureteral ectopia—a review. 1: Embryology and aetiology. *J Small Anim Pract 14*:407, 1973.
58. Pearson H, Gibbs C: Urinary tract abnormalities in the dog. *J Small Anim Pract 12*:67, 1971.
59. Pechman RD Jr: Urinary trauma in dogs and cats: A review. *J Am Anim Hosp Assoc 18*:33, 1982.
60. Persky L, et al: Percutaneous nephrostomy and ureteral injury. *J Urol 125*:298, 1981.
61. Pohl J, et al: On the importance of resection length and tension for ureter end-to-end anastomoses. *Urol Int 40*:107, 1985.
62. Pollock S, Schoen SS: Urinary incontinence associated with congenital ureteral valves in a bitch. *J Am Vet Med Assoc 59*:332, 1971.
63. Popesco C: Replacement of the pelvic ureter by lowering the kidney. *Presse Med 77*:2061, 1969.
64. Reis RH: Renal aplasia, ectopic ureter and vascular anomalies in a domestic cat. *Anat Rec 135*:105, 1959.
65. Riedmiller H, et al: Psoas-hitch ureteroneocystostomy: Experience with 181 cases. *Eur Urol 10*:145, 1984.
66. Rigg DL, et al: Neoureterostomy and phenylpropanolamine therapy for incontinence due to ectopic ureter in a dog. *J Am Anim Hosp Assoc 19*:237, 1983.
67. Robertson JT, et al: Repair of ureteral defect in a foal. *J Am Vet Med Assoc 183*:799, 1983.
68. Ross LA, Lamb CR: Reduction of hydronephrosis and hydroureter associated with ectopic ureters in two dogs after ureterovesical anastomosis. *J Am Vet Med Assoc 196*:1497, 1990.
69. Schapira HE, et al: Ureteral injury during vascular surgery. *J Urol 125*:293, 1981.
70. Schellhammer PF, Texter JH: An experimental ureteroileal anastomosis to prevent reflux. *Invest Urol 11*:319, 1974.
71. Scott R, et al: The evolution of a biodegradable membrane for use in urological surgery. A summary of 109 *in vivo* experiments. *Fr J Urol 62*:26, 1988.
72. Scott RC, et al: Unilateral ureterocele associated with hydronephrosis in a dog. *J Am Anim Hosp Assoc 10*:126, 1974.
73. Smith CW, Park RD: Bilateral ectopic ureteroceles in a dog. *Canine Pract 10*:28, 1974.
74. Smith CW, et al: Bilateral ureteral ectopia in a male cat with urinary incontinence. *J Am Vet Med Assoc 182*:172, 1983.
75. Smith CW, et al: Ectopic ureter in the dog—a review of cases. *J Am Anim Hosp Assoc 17*:245, 1981.
76. Smith MW, et al: Ureteral reaction to suture material. *Invest Urol 21*:279, 1983.
77. Somerville JJF, Naude JH: Segmental ureteric replacement: An animal study using a free non-pedicled graft. *Urol Res 12*:115, 1984.
78. Starr A: Ureteral plication. *Invest Urol 17*:153, 1979.
79. Stone EA: Surgical management of urolithiasis. *Comp Cont Educ 3*:627, 1981.
80. Stone EA, Mason LK: Surgery of ectopic ureters: Types, method of correction, and postoperative results. *J Am Anim Hosp Assoc 26*:81, 1990.
81. Stowater JL, Springer AL: Ureterocele in a dog. *Vet Med Small Anim Clin 74*:1753, 1979.
82. Sullins KE, et al: Ectopic ureter managed by unilateral nephrectomy in two female horses. *Equine Vet J 20*:463, 1988.
83. Tudor DC: Congenital defects of poultry. *World's Poultry Science Journal 35*:20, 1979.
84. Varady S, et al: Ureteral replacement with a new synthetic material: Gore-Tex. *J Urol 128*:171, 1982.
85. Vargas AS, Silva EI: Mobilization of the ureter by a posterior vesical flap in dogs: Preliminary report of a new technique. *J Urol 107*:742, 972.
86. Vargas AD, et al: Experimental use of fluoroalkyl cyanoacrilate in ureteral anastomosis. *Invest Urol 5*:416, 1982.
87. Vatandaslar F, et al: Ileal segment replacement of ureter. I. Effects on kidney of refluxing vs. nonrefluxing anastomosis. *Urology 23*:549, 1984.
88. Wan SP, et al: A second look at ureteral plication. *J Urol 127*:803, 1982.
89. Weaver AD: Intrapelvic cyst as a urinary obstruction in a bitch. *J Am Vet Med Assoc 169*:798, 1976.
90. Wilson DR: Renal function during and following obstruction. *Annu Rev Med 28*:329, 1977.
91. Wilson DR: Nephron functional heterogeneity in the postobstructive kidney. *Kidney Int 7*:19, 1975.
92. Wolf AM, et al: Uric acid ureteral calculus and pararenal cyst in a cat. *J Am Anim Hosp Assoc 5*:767, 1979.

CHAPTER 106 Urinary Bladder

Don R. Waldron

ANATOMY

The bladder is a hollow muscular organ that receives urine from the kidneys via both ureters and stores the urine until expulsion through the urethra. The bladder musculature (detrusor muscle) is smooth muscle. In dogs and cats, the bladder is partially covered by peritoneum and loosely supported by peritoneal reflections that form bilateral lateral ligaments and a single midventral ligament.[14] The lateral ligaments connect the bladder to the lateral walls of the pelvic canal, and the ventral ligament connects the ventral surface of the bladder to the pelvic symphysis and ventral abdominal midline. The bladder's size and location in the caudal abdomen depend on the volume of urine. In dogs, the bladder usually lies within the pelvic canal when empty but moves cranially and ventrally as it distends. In cats, the bladder is almost always located within the caudal abdomen.

The bladder in both dogs and cats may be divided into the fundus (cranial portion), body (midportion), and neck (caudal portion).[9] Internally, the neck area is considered the trigone. The base of this triangular area is formed by the two ureteral orifices and the apex by the urethral orifice. The mucosa of the bladder is made up of transitional epithelium. The ureters are retroperitoneal in location on the ventral border of the psoas muscle before entering the peritoneal space and coursing through the lateral ligaments of the bladder. The ureters enter the bladder serosal surface on its dorsolateral aspect and travel obliquely through the muscular wall a short distance before opening into the bladder through two small slitlike orifices.

The dorsal surface of the bladder wall is in contact with the small intestine and descending colon. In intact females, the uterine body and cervix are just dorsal to the bladder. In males, the vaso deferentia are dorsal to the neck of the bladder. A short expanse of urethra lies between the bladder neck and the prostate in males. Diseases of surrounding structures in close proximity to the bladder may cause clinical signs of bladder dysfunction.

The bladder receives its blood supply through the cranial vesical artery, a branch of the umbilical artery, and the caudal vesical artery, a branch of the urogenital artery.[13]

Innervation of the bladder is complex, with both autonomic and somatic input. The hypogastric nerve provides sympathetic innervation of the bladder. Its preganglionic branches originate from the thoracolumbar spinal cord. Parasympathetic innervation is via the pelvic nerve, which originates in the sacral spinal cord (S1–S3). There are numerous synapses between sympathetic and parasympathetic nerves.[26]

Somatic innervation originates in fibers from the sacral spinal cord (S1–S3) that form the pudendal nerve. One branch of the pudendal nerve supplies the external urethral sphincter, and others supply the perineal area.

PHYSIOLOGY

The bladder is responsible for storage and intermittent expulsion of urine. In the storage phase of micturition, the bladder acts as a flaccid, low-pressure reservoir for urine and the urethra acts as a high-pressure valve preventing passage of urine. Urethral smooth muscle provides the major resistance to urine flow in the resting state. Sympathetic innervation via the hypogastric nerve dominates this phase of micturition while parasympathetic activity is inhibited.

During bladder filling, sensory endings of the pelvic nerve detect stretching of the bladder wall. When a threshold bladder capacity is reached, afferent impulses travel to the spinal cord and brain. After brain-stem integration, efferent impulses descend the spinal cord and stimulate parasympathetic nuclei, interrupting the sympathetic storage phase of micturition. Parasympathetic input begins to dominate the emptying phase, which is initiated by smooth-muscle (detrusor) depolarization and contraction. As the detrusor muscle contracts, the bladder neck opens. Simultaneously, the sympathetically innervated urethral smooth muscle and the somatically innervated urethral striated muscle relax, resulting in normal micturition.[26, 27]

After bladder emptying, impulses in the parasympathetic fibers stop and the detrusor muscle relaxes. The pudendal and hypogastric nerve effects predominate, and the internal and external urethral sphincters return to the normal tone maintained during bladder filling.

Disorders of micturition, including urinary incontinence, are not uncommon in small animal medicine. These disorders are classified as neurogenic or non-neurogenic. Non-neurogenic causes of urinary incontinence include ovariohysterectomy, ectopic ureters, and chronic disease of the bladder, urethra, or prostate. Central or peripheral lesions anywhere in the normal neural pathway of micturition may cause dysuria or incontinence.

Chronic bladder or urethral disease can cause incontinence. An inflamed bladder becomes hyperactive, resulting in "urge incontinence." Dogs with ectopic ureter may have a bladder that is abnormally small and incapable of storing a normal volume of urine. Partial cystectomy necessitated by neoplasia may result in inability to store urine normally until the volume of the remaining bladder increases. Surgical invasion of the bladder without interruption of its innervation does not usually cause urinary storage problems or incontinence, although temporary hematuria is common after bladder surgery.

DIAGNOSIS OF BLADDER DISEASE

Physical Examination

When empty, the bladder is relatively difficult to palpate because of its pelvic location and small size. As it fills, it becomes more accessible to palpation. Findings noted on palpation include size, pain, wall thickness, calculi, and intraluminal or intramural masses.

Complete palpation of the caudal abdomen, perineum, and rectum allows the examiner to evaluate the urethra and prostate, which may be involved. Simultaneous digital rectal examination and caudal abdominal palpation facilitate palpation of the trigone region, prostate, and pelvic urethra.

Urinalysis/Microbiology

Examination and interpretation of a urine sample that has been properly collected may yield valuable information. It is recommended that all nonelective surgical patients have a urinalysis performed as part of a preoperative data base. Urinalysis is of most benefit when performed before drug or fluid therapy is begun.

Urine may be obtained by voiding ("catch" sample), manual expression of the bladder, catheterization, or cystocentesis. In general, urine obtained by cystocentesis is most easily interpreted because contamination with cells and bacteria from the distal urethra is avoided. Cystocentesis is easily and safely performed in small animals using a 22-gauge or smaller needle and syringe. Urinalysis includes examination of the physical and chemical properties of the urine and microscopic examination of the urine sediment.[12]

Specific components of the urinalysis that may assist in diagnosis of bladder disease include microscopic examination of urine sediment and urine culture. Microscopic examination may reveal transitional epithelial cells or bacteria. The presence of transitional epithelial cells is normal.[12] Results of microscopic examination of urine should be correlated with other diagnostic techniques including physical examination, radiology, and microbiology. Cytological evaluation of urine sediment is especially important if bladder neoplasia is suspected. A bladder wash technique using saline to flush and obtain mucosal cells after the bladder has been emptied may assist in diagnosis of neoplastic diseases;[9, 23] however, false-negative findings are common.

Bacteria are not present in the urine of normal dogs or cats; however, both false-positive and false-negative findings are common, depending on the method of urine collection. Samples obtained by cystocentesis are sterile in normal dogs and cats. Urinary tract infections are common in dogs and may be the cause of specific types of urinary calculi. Culture and antimicrobial susceptibility testing aid in identifying specific bacterial pathogens.

Radiology/Ultrasonography

Radiographic examination of the bladder is begun with survey radiographs, but contrast radiographs are often required to demonstrate most diseases. Before radiography of the abdomen, patients are fasted for 12 hours and given a cleaning enema. If neoplasia of the bladder is part of the differential diagnosis, survey radiographs (right and left lateral and dorsoventral) of the thorax are taken to rule out radiographically detectable metastasis.

Positive-, negative-, and double-contrast cystography may assist in identifying mucosal irregularities, thickening of the bladder wall, diverticula, leakage, and space-occupying masses. Excretory urography is valuable when assessing diseases of the trigonal area.

Ultrasonography is a useful aid to radiography in evaluating the bladder, especially when space-occupying masses are present. It may help delineate the extent of neoplasia or perivesicular masses without invasive techniques.

Cystoscopy

Cystoscopy as a diagnostic technique was previously limited to the use of rigid endoscopes in females. With the advent of flexible fiber-optic instruments, the bladders of large male dogs can be examined without the need for surgical intervention.

Two studies described cystoscopy for diagnosis and biopsy of the canine bladder.[7, 16] A flexible 3.6-mm-diameter fiber-optic pediatric bronchoscope was successfully used in 13 of 21 male dogs weighing 20 to 55 pounds. The os penis, even in large dogs, may limit passage of the scope. Twenty-five of 27 female dogs were examined or successfully underwent biopsy using a 13 to 21 French rigid pediatric cystoscope.

Cystoscopy using a 5-mm rigid laparoscope and a 2.7-mm rigid arthroscope inserted through a prepubic percutaneous approach has been described.[25] A disadvantage of this procedure is the need to maintain bladder drainage via a urethral catheter for 48 to 72 hours after the procedure. Cystoscopy may also be valuable for postoperative examination and surgical follow-up when repeated cystotomy is undesirable.

Cystometrogram/Urethral Pressure Profile

Urinary incontinence is the lack of voluntary control over the flow of urine from the body.[27] Neurological dysfunction is a common cause of urinary incontinence in dogs and cats. Neurological disease may disrupt the upper motor neuron or lower motor neuron segment of the micturition reflex.

Non-neurogenic disease may also cause urinary incontinence. Both congenital (ectopic ureter and urethral fistula) and acquired disease (neoplasia, prostatic disease) may cause signs of urinary incontinence.

Clinical evaluation of patients with urinary incontinence includes a hemogram, biochemical profile, and urinalysis/culture. Radiography and ultrasonography may be valuable in detecting causes of urinary incontinence.

Urodynamic studies provide functional data that may give a diagnosis and prognosis and aid in treatment of a micturition disorder. Urodynamic studies measure pressure, volume, and flow relationships within the bladder and urethra during various phases of micturition. Cystometry and urethral pressure profilometry evaluate bladder and urethral function in incontinent dogs.[26, 27, 34, 35]

Cystometry or cystometrograms can provide objective data about bladder tone, bladder capacity, detrusor reflex, threshold volume and pressure, and maximum contraction pressure.[26, 35] If sedation is required for cystometry, intravenous or subcutaneous xylazine is recommended as the drug of choice.[33] Narcotics may also be used without adversely affecting collected data.[26]

The urethral pressure profile assesses nonvoiding urethral pressure measured from the bladder to the external urethral meatus and is plotted against that distance. Urethral musculature and connective tissue response to distension by water is measured. The urethral pressure profile may localize areas of increased urethral resistance (obstruction) or decreased urethral resistance (incompetence).[34] The test has proved valuable in dogs for diagnosis of incontinence related to prostatic disease, urethral masses, cauda equina syndrome, and reflex dyssynergia of unknown origin.[26] Both normal and abnormal urethral pressure profiles have been described.[33, 34]

CONGENITAL SURGICAL DISEASES

Ectopic Ureters (see also Chapter 105)

Ectopic ureter is a congenital anomaly in which one or both ureters terminate and drain at a site other than the bladder. Normally, the ureters enter the dorsolateral caudal surface of the bladder and open into the trigone after a short intramural course. In dogs, approximately 70 to 80 per cent are unilateral, whereas cats more frequently have bilateral involvement.[18, 37] Most ectopic ureters contact and enter the bladder wall normally but lack a normal orifice at the trigonal area of the bladder (intramural ectopic ureter). In some cases, the ureter remains completely extramural and totally bypasses the bladder before terminating in the urethra, vagina, or uterus.

Most animals with ectopic ureters are females, and they exhibit some urinary incontinence at the time of birth or weaning. In a review of 17 cases, all dogs had urinary incontinence and 15 were able to urinate normally, reflecting the predominance of unilateral ectopia.[38] In those rare cases in males in which the ureter opens into the urethra, distal urethral pressure and resistance are high enough to cause retrograde flow of urine into the bladder; thus, males may not show urinary incontinence. Physical findings in animals with ectopic ureter are usually normal; however, urine dribbling may cause wetness of perivulvar hair or of the preputial opening and irritation of surrounding skin.

A tentative diagnosis of ectopic ureter may be confirmed by radiography, vaginoscopy, or exploratory laparotomy. The method of choice for confirming the diagnosis of ectopic ureter is excretory urography, which provides information about the renal pelvis and ureter size and may identify the site of termination of the ureters. The site of termination of ectopic ureters is often difficult to determine owing to accumulation of contrast material within the bladder. Intramural ectopic ureters are more difficult to observe than extramural ureters. In its normal course, the ureter has a J-shaped ureterovesicular junction[24]; alteration of this angle to a straight line suggests ectopia. Hydroureter in a young, incontinent bitch suggests ectopic ureter.

Several radiographic techniques are useful in improving observation of the ureters. Radiographs are made both early and late after administration of contrast media. Extramural ectopic ureters may be best observed early in the study before the bladder becomes distended with radiopaque contrast media.[2] A pneumocystogram performed concurrently with the excretory urogram may help outline the ureters and be the most useful technique for assessing ureteral morphology. A patient is placed in ventral recumbency to allow the gas to rise adjacent to the ureters.[24] Some ectopic ureters can best be seen on oblique lateral radiographs rather than lateral or ventrodorsal views, especially if the ureter is totally extramural (Fig. 106–1).

Vaginoscopy may reveal the orifice of an ectopic ureter. Direct examination is difficult because of patients' small size. Before surgery, patients with ectopic ureters are placed on appropriate antibiotic therapy for urinary tract infection as indicated by urine culture and sensitivity tests. Urinary tract infection is found in many animals with ectopic ureters and may cause pyelonephritis in both the affected and contralateral kidneys if not properly treated.

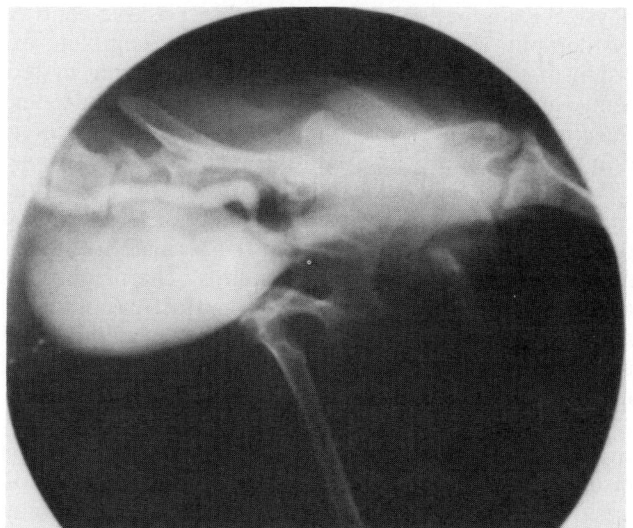

FIGURE 106–1. Ventrodorsal oblique radiograph during excretory urography of a dog with an extramural ectopic ureter. The ureter terminates in the vagina.

Before surgery, the prognosis is discussed with the owner. The prognosis for health in most cases is favorable if renal function is normal. The prognosis for urinary continence after surgery is guarded and depends on several factors. Bilateral ectopia is accompanied by cystic hypoplasia, thereby reducing bladder storage volume postoperatively. The bladder may be evaluated by cystometrograms, and urethral pressure profiles may help assess urethral sphincter integrity. These studies are difficult to perform in small patients. The incidence of ectopic ureter and concurrent urethral sphincter incompetence is unknown. Similarly, the cause of continued incontinence after correction of ectopic ureter in some animals is unknown. In two series, approximately 40 per cent of patients continued to show some degree of incontinence after surgical correction of the ectopic ureter.[18, 38] It is unclear whether this incontinence is permanent or transient.

The choice of surgical technique for correcting ectopic ureter depends on whether the condition is unilateral or bilateral, the type of ectopic ureter, and functional status of the kidneys. Nephrectomy-ureterectomy is selected only when severe hydronephrosis or pyelonephritis and unilateral ectopic ureter are present. Ectopic ureter can be difficult to demonstrate radiographically; therefore, a surgeon should be cautious in performing nephrectomy for unilateral ectopia until bilateral ectopia has been ruled out.[2]

Ectopic ureters may be intramural or extramural. In either case, a thorough exploration of the urinary tract precedes a ventral cystotomy. The bladder incision is generous, extending into the proximal urethra. Stay sutures are placed through the bladder wall to facilitate atraumatic tissue handling and retraction. The trigonal area is inspected for ureteral openings. In most cases, only one orifice is observed. Digital occlusion of the urethra causes enlargement of an intramural ureter, which appears as a submucosal swelling or ridge within the bladder wall. A number 15 scalpel blade is used to make a 5-mm longitudinal incision through the bladder mucosa into the ureteral lumen. The ureteral mucosa is sutured to the bladder mucosa with 5-0 or 6-0 coated polyglactin 910 (Vicryl) or polydioxanone (PDS) (Fig. 106–2). A number 3 French urinary catheter is passed distally through the ureter, and the distal portion of the ureter is ligated with 3-0 absorbable suture caudal to the new ureteral stoma. The suture is passed from the serosal surface of the bladder and tied as the catheter is withdrawn. Failure to adequately ligate the distal ureter results in continued urinary incontinence postoperatively.

If an ectopic ureter is extramural, it is ligated and transected, preserving the maximum length of ureter available, and ureteroneocystostomy is performed. The goal of implantation is to salvage the affected ureter and

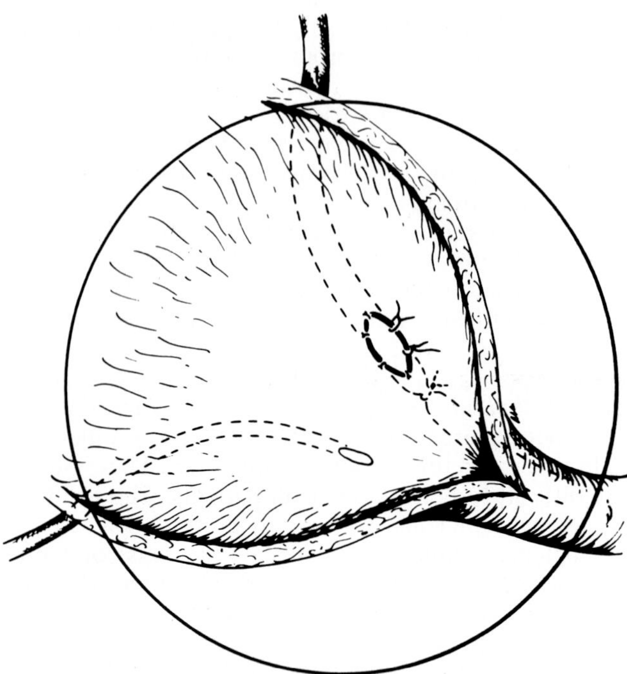

FIGURE 106–2. Creation of a new stoma for an intramural ectopic ureter. An incision is made into the lumen of the ectopic ureter, and the bladder and ureteral mucosa are apposed with 5-0 or 6-0 absorbable suture.

kidney and prevent vesicoureteral reflux of urine into the operated ureter. The importance of preventing vesicoureteral reflux in animals is unknown, and the creation of long submucosal tunnels may promote resistance to urine flow and contribute to hydroureter and hydronephrosis. I prefer the intravesical technique of implantation (Fig. 106–3). After a ventral cystotomy and excision of an ellipse of bladder mucosa, a short oblique submucosal tunnel is created in the bladder wall, through which the previously ligated ureter is drawn. The terminal ureter is excised, spatulated, and sutured to the bladder mucosa with 5-0 or 6-0 coated polyglactin 910 or polydioxanone on a tapered needle. The tunnel and ureteral orifice are situated so that closure of the cystotomy incision does not impinge on the ureter. It is important to minimize trauma to the ureter and bladder, and care is taken to avoid twisting the ureter and occluding its vascular supply. The use of stay sutures, pediatric surgical instruments, and 2.5 × optical loupes for magnification assists in decreasing tissue trauma. After the ureter is implanted, urine is observed flowing from the newly created ureteral orifice. Because of small bladder size, a one-layer continuous Lembert or appositional continuous suture pattern is used to close the cystotomy incision.

Complications of all methods of implantation or neoureterostomy include hydroureter and hydronephrosis and continued incontinence. Normal ureteral peristaltic activity is disturbed by transection of the ureter and tissue trauma to the ureter and bladder. The duration and severity of postoperative hydroureter and hydronephrosis are related to the degree of tissue trauma and swelling, which usually resolves in 2 to 6 weeks if there are no other contributing factors. A more serious cause of hydroureter and hydronephrosis is partial or complete ureteral stomal stenosis. Stomal stenosis may be secondary to poor surgical technique, ureteral trauma, or bladder wall edema.

Urachal Anomalies

The urachus is an embryonic conduit providing communication between the bladder and the allantoic sac. During later fetal development, the urachus is no longer needed as a conduit for urine, and urethral function increases. Normally, the urachus is nonfunctional at birth, and urine is evacuated completely through the urethra.

Four types of congenital urachal anomalies have been classified in humans and animals (Fig. 106–4).[29] A persistent urachus exists if the entire urachal tube remains patent between the bladder and umbilicus. Urine evacuation occurs through both the umbilicus and the urethra. Omphalitis and urinary tract infection are often present with patent urachus.

A vesicourachal diverticulum occurs when the external opening of the urachus closes but the bladder attachment of the urachus remains patent, creating a blind diverticulum at the bladder apex (Fig. 106–5). Vesicourachal diverticula are clinically significant in dogs because they predispose to recurrent urinary tract infections.[41] In cats, vesicourachal diverticula are usually detected in animals with lower urinary tract dysfunction, especially urethral obstruction.[29, 30] A cause-and-effect relationship has not been demonstrated between obstruction and diverticula.

A urachal cyst exists when secreting urachal epithelium persists in isolated segments of a persistent urachus. It is rare in dogs and is unreported in cats.[29] A urachal sinus develops when the distal urachus remains patent and is open at the umbilicus. This anomaly is asymptomatic and rarely diagnosed.

Patent urachus is diagnosed on clinical signs and physical examination and confirmed by positive-contrast cystography. Surgical therapy consists of complete excision of the urachal tube, necessitating partial cystectomy, and excision of the umbilicus. Urine culture and sensitivity tests are performed, and urinary tract infection treated appropriately.

Vesicourachal diverticulum is considered a potential cause of recurrent urinary tract infection in dogs and therefore may also contribute to the formation of magnesium ammonium phosphate uroliths. The diagnosis is confirmed by positive- or double-contrast cystography, and treatment consists of partial cystectomy/diverticulectomy, urolith removal (if present), and treatment of urinary tract infection.

In cats, diverticula of the bladder may spontaneously regress after proper treatment of bladder or urethral disease; therefore, diverticulectomy may not be indicated initially. It is recommended that cats be re-evaluated by urinalysis and radiography 4 weeks after initial detection of diverticula to assess whether the problem is responsive to therapy and is self-limiting.[30] The pres-

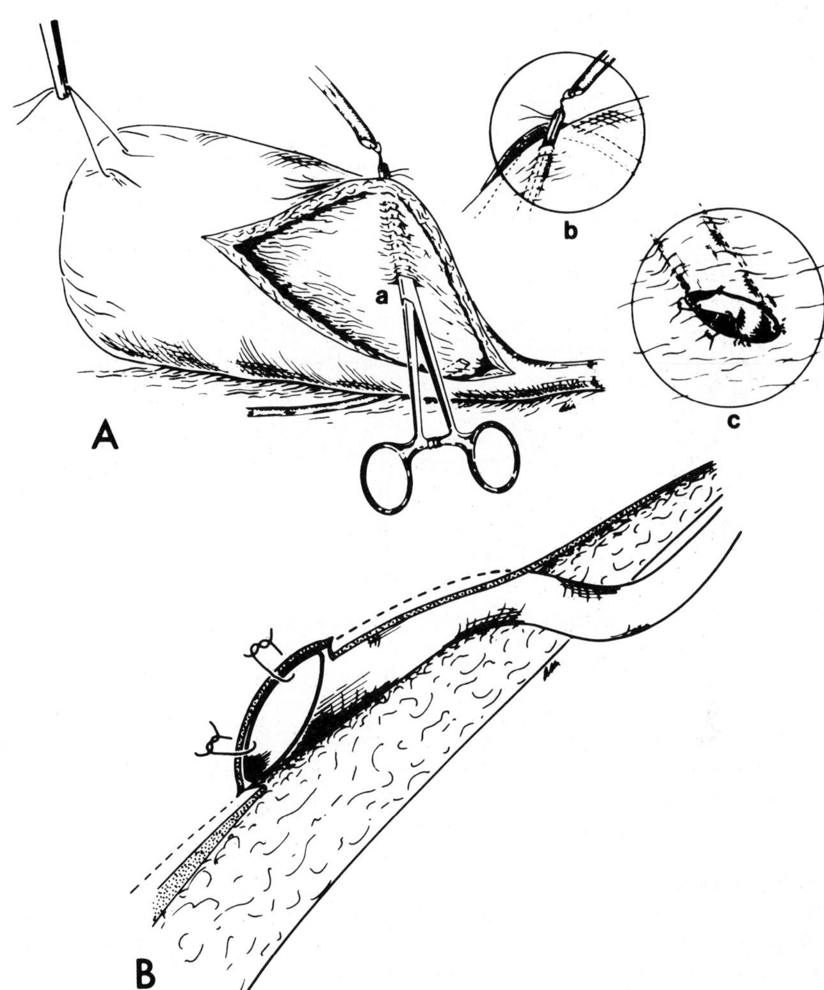

FIGURE 106–3. Implantation of an extramural ectopic ureter into the bladder wall. *A,* A submucosal tunnel is formed by undermining the bladder mucosa and penetrating the bladder musculature with forceps (a). A stay suture in the end of the ureter is grasped with forceps (b), and the ureter is gently delivered through the tunnel. The spatulated tip of the ureter is sutured to the bladder mucosa (c). *B,* The ureter passes beneath the mucosa and out through the muscular wall of the bladder.

ence of diverticula and continued urinary tract infection is an indication for diverticulectomy.

ACQUIRED SURGICAL DISEASE

Bladder Rupture

Bladder rupture may be caused by blunt or penetrating abdominal trauma or improper catheterization.

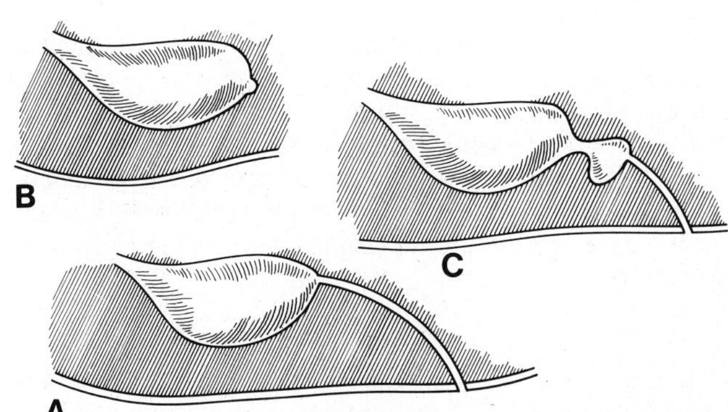

FIGURE 106–4. Congenital urachal anomalies. *A,* Persistent urachus. *B,* Vesicourachal diverticulum. *C,* Urachal cyst. Urachal sinus is not shown.

Spontaneous rupture is uncommon but may occur secondary to prolonged urethral obstruction or necrosis. Urine leakage into the peritoneal cavity results in uremia, dehydration, hypovolemia, and death if undiagnosed or untreated. Injury to the urinary system and bladder is most often encountered after motor vehicle trauma. Many animals have concurrent orthopedic injury, especially pelvic fractures. Dogs and cats presented for evaluation after vehicular trauma should be suspected of having injury to the cardiovascular, respiratory, nervous, and urinary systems. A high index of suspicion and complete physical examination result in more rapid diagnosis and decreased morbidity and mortality.

Clinical signs of urinary tract trauma can be vague. Hematuria, dysuria, abdominal pain, lack of a palpable bladder, fluid accumulation within the abdomen, and abdominal and perineal bruising are early signs. Progressive depression, vomiting, and metabolic changes associated with worsening uremia occur later. The ability of a patient to urinate or the retrieval of urine on bladder catheterization does not rule out bladder rupture.

Radiographic examination of the abdomen is indicated if urinary tract trauma is suspected. Radiographic signs that suggest urinary tract injury include nonvisual-

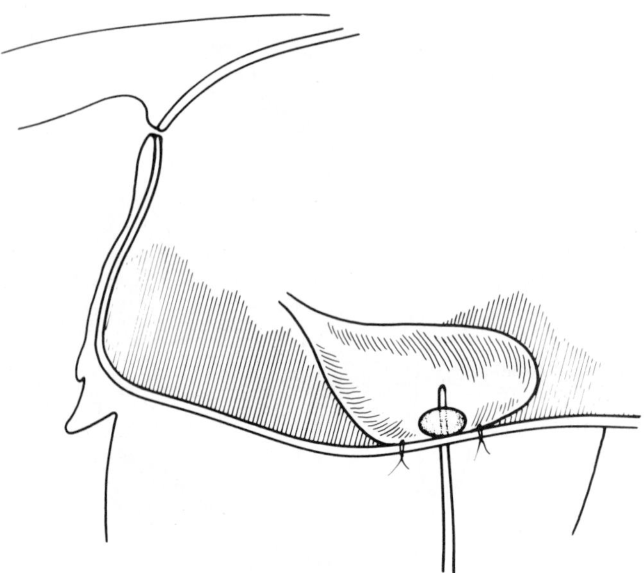

FIGURE 106–5. Vesicourachal diverticulum in a cat examined for urethral obstruction.

ization or asymmetry of the kidneys, enlargement of the retroperitoneal space, loss of normal intra-abdominal contrast, and reduced size or absence of the bladder.[32]

Contrast examination of the urinary system is the most reliable noninvasive method of establishing the site and extent of urinary tract injury. Positive-contrast cystography is the method of choice to evaluate bladder integrity. If the bladder has ruptured, contrast medium is free within the abdominal cavity and outlines other intra-abdominal organs (Fig. 106–6). The site of contrast leakage from the bladder may be seen if there is a small tear in the bladder wall and contrast material is injected while radiographs are made.

Surgical repair is the definitive treatment for most rents in the bladder. The timing of surgical intervention is important. If the diagnosis is made early (less than 12 hours after rupture), surgery is performed after hypovolemia has been corrected with intravenous fluids.[10] If a patient is metabolically unstable and hypothermic, supportive therapy is instituted before anesthesia and surgery. Fluid and electrolyte imbalances are corrected with intravenous fluid therapy.

In the preoperative period, urinary diversion can be accomplished by inserting an indwelling urinary catheter into the bladder and connecting the catheter to a closed collection system. A peritoneal dialysis catheter may be placed directly into the abdomen to divert urine that has accumulated within the peritoneal cavity. The latter technique is especially useful if urethral trauma makes catheterization difficult. Temporary cystostomy is another alternative for temporary urinary diversion (see the next section on cystostomy).

A caudal ventral midline approach is used for surgical repair. Most bladder ruptures occur near the apex. The bladder rent is débrided of devitalized tissue, and the bladder is closed with polydioxanone in a double-layer continuous inverting suture pattern using a Cushing pattern oversewn with a Cushing or Cushing oversewn with a Lembert. The bladder is tested by injecting saline to ensure a watertight seal. In some cases, leakage may occur because of friable or bruised tissue. Serosal patching is a useful technique to buttress the leaking suture line. The antimesenteric border of a jejunal segment of intestine is sutured to healthy tissue surrounding the bladder defect. The serosal patch provides an early mechanical and physiological barrier to urine leakage. Indwelling urinary catheters are avoided. An exception is bladder rupture secondary to urethral obstruction, when continued bladder decompression after repair is indicated because of poor tissue quality and bruising. Indwelling catheters may also assist in treating bladder atony secondary to obstructive disease.

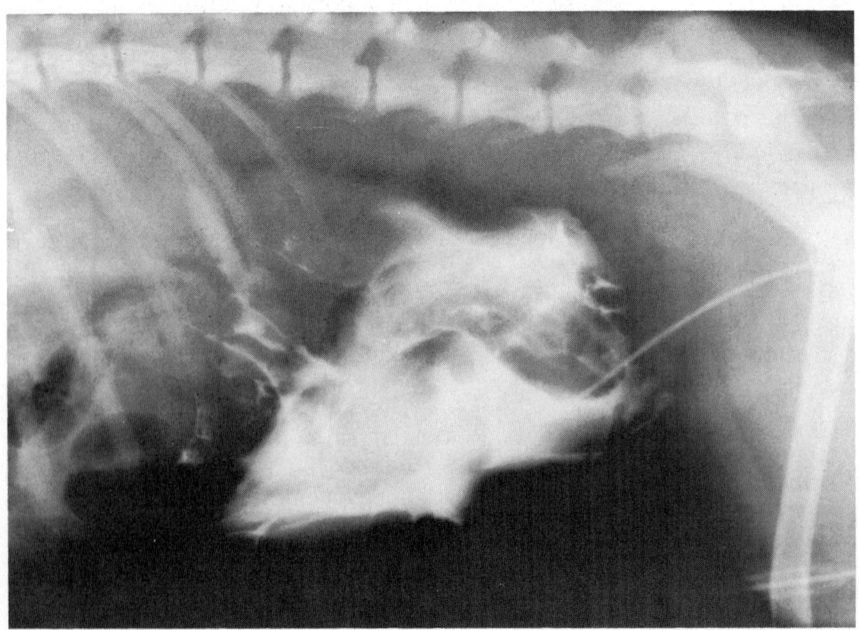

FIGURE 106–6. Positive-contrast cystogram of ruptured urinary bladder in a dog. Contrast material is free within the abdomen.

Cystostomy

Antepubic urinary diversion by temporary cystostomy provides urinary drainage that may allow stabilization of an ill patient before definitive urological surgery. It may also serve to divert urine from a urethra that has been traumatized or surgically repaired.

Either of two methods of cystostomy that have been previously described provide satisfactory urine diversion.[3, 4, 6] The first method requires a 6 to 12 French Foley catheter (Fig. 106–7).[4] Local abdominal analgesia augmented by sedation or mask general anesthesia is adequate for patients that are metabolically unstable. A minilaparotomy incision is made on the caudal ventral midline in a female or the peripreputial position in a male. The bladder is located, and a purse-string suture is placed using 3-0 absorbable material, which is left untied. A stab incision is made into the bladder in the middle of the purse-string suture, and the Foley catheter is placed into the bladder lumen. The balloon is inflated with saline, and the purse-string suture tied, securing the catheter within the bladder lumen. A second small abdominal incision is made lateral to the first incision through which the Foley catheter is passed. Traction is placed on the Foley catheter to bring bladder into apposition with the abdominal wall. Several absorbable sutures are used to tack the bladder to the abdominal wall. The catheter is connected to a sterile closed urinary collection system. When removal of the urinary catheter is desired, the balloon is deflated, the catheter removed, and the wound allowed to heal by second intention. Generally, the catheter remains 5 to 7 days to diminish the probability of urine leakage on removal.

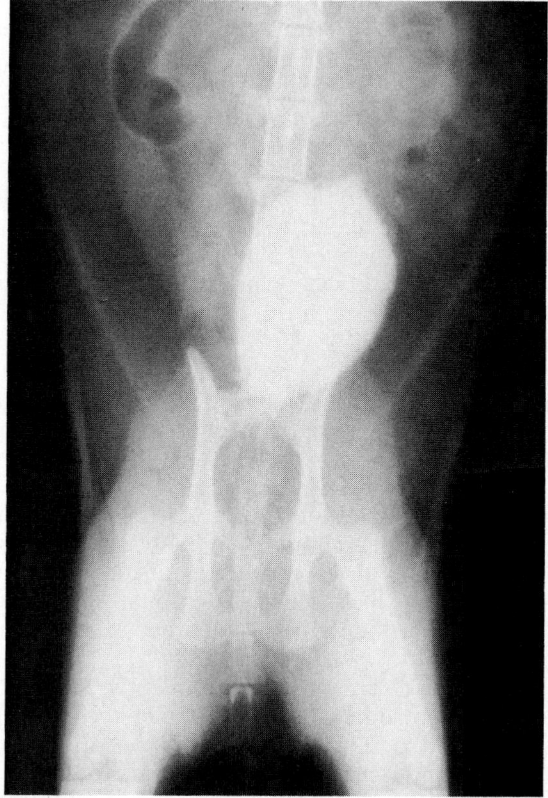

FIGURE 106–7. Urinary diversion accomplished by cystotomy using a Foley catheter. The catheter is connected to a closed urinary collection system.

A second method of urine diversion is by percutaneous placement of a Stamey catheter.[3, 6] The catheter may be placed using local anesthesia. A palpable bladder is a prerequisite for catheter placement. The patient is placed in right or left lateral recumbency, and the lateral caudal abdominal wall is surgically prepared. A small stab incision is made through the skin, and the catheter is advanced through the incision and abdominal wall. The bladder is palpated and is steadied against the body wall, and the catheter is thrust into the bladder lumen. The catheter, after placement, is secured to the skin by sutures and tape and connected to a closed urinary system. An abdominal bandage is applied to cover the catheter and prevent premature removal by the patient. Removal of the catheter is by gentle traction as early as 3 days after placement.

Cystic Calculi

The most common surgical procedure performed on the bladder in companion animals is cystotomy for removal of uroliths. Calculi develop most often in middle-aged animals but may also be found in puppies and kittens. Magnesium ammonium phosphate (struvite) is the main component of approximately 60 to 70 per cent of all calculi in dogs.[8, 28] These stones are commonly associated with urinary tract infection but may also form in sterile urine. In decreasing incidence, the other types of calculi found in dogs are calcium oxalate, urate, cystine, silicate, and calcium phosphate.[28] The composition of calculi may be reasonably determined without surgery based on urinalysis and identification of crystals within the urine and bacterial culture and sensitivity tests. If the calculi are magnesium ammonium phosphate, dietary and appropriate antibiotic therapy may result in stone dissolution. Disadvantages of dietary therapy include cost, low protein content of the diet, and questionable owner compliance. Patients treated medically or surgically are closely monitored for response to therapy with repeated urine cultures and radiographs. Preoperative identification of other types of uroliths by urinalysis may also be worthwhile—urate stones in a young dog of any breed should alert the clinician to the possibility of a metabolic or anatomical defect such as a portosystemic shunt.

Diagnostic radiographs are indicated in the clinical evolution of any patient with cystic calculi. Survey radiographs may reveal the presence of calculi elsewhere in the urinary tract, including the kidneys or urethra. Contrast studies are indicated, especially in patients with recurrent disease. An excretory urogram may reveal underlying disease such as pyelonephritis. Contrast cystography may reveal radiolucent calculi or anatomical defects such as a urachal diverticulum.

Surgical removal of cystic calculi is indicated for stones other than magnesium ammonium phosphate or stones that are causing or may cause urinary tract obstruction. The bladder is approached through a caudal ventral midline incision. In male dogs, the incision begins at the umbilicus and curves peripreputially. Branches of the caudal superficial epigastric vessels are encountered and ligated. The abdomen is entered on the ventral midline.

The bladder is located, and a stay suture is placed in the apex. The bladder is elevated and isolated from surrounding viscera with saline-moistened laparotomy pads to minimize abdominal contamination. A second stay suture is placed at the caudal aspect of the proposed incision site. The incision site for cystotomy and removal of uroliths is made in the most avascular and convenient area of the bladder. A second consideration is avoidance of the trigonal area and the ureteral orifices. Dorsal cystotomy incisions have been recommended to decrease the occurrence of urine leakage, avoid adhesions of the bladder to the abdominal wall, and reduce the incidence of calculi formation from sediment accumulation on exposed sutures.[22, 42] There are no data supporting these recommendations. In a study using normal dogs, ventral cystotomy incisions closed with polydioxanone did not result in abdominal wall adhesions.[20]

A stab incision is made between the previously placed stay sutures, and residual urine is removed by suction. Alternatively, the bladder may be emptied before incision by inserting a butterfly catheter and applying suction with a three-way valve and syringe. The incision between stay sutures is lengthened to permit access to the entire bladder. Calculi may be removed with curettes, forceps, or other instruments designed for stone removal. Palpation of the bladder neck and passage of a catheter through the urethra are indicated to ensure that the bladder neck or urethra is not blocked by calculi. Repeated flushing and aspiration are indicated to remove all discrete calculi and small particles of sand. Samples may be obtained from the bladder wall or the center of calculi, or whole calculi may be used for microbial culturing. The stones are submitted for quantitative analysis of their mineral content. Watertight closure of the bladder wall is ensured by a double-layer inverting suture pattern. Contact of suture with urine is avoided by use of simple continuous Cushing or Lembert suture patterns using 3-0 or 4-0 synthetic absorbable suture placed no deeper than the submucosa. Polydioxanone is an ideal choice because its monofilament structure does not damage or saw through tissue as braided suture may. If the bladder wall is thickened as a result of chronic cystitis or previous surgery, a double layer of simple continuous sutures is used. A study of normal dogs showed no difference in bursting strengths of cystotomy incisions closed with single-layer appositional or two-layer inverting patterns. The bladder closure is tested for security by injection and distension of the bladder with saline.

Thorough medical management by dietary therapy, induced diuresis, or appropriate antimicrobial therapy is indicated to minimize the incidence of calculi recurrence, which ranges from 12 to 25 per cent.[8, 21]

Neoplasia

Bladder neoplasia accounts for less than 1 per cent of all canine neoplasia, and the prevalence is even lower in cats.[36] Malignant neoplasms are more common than benign tumors in both dogs and cats. Transitional cell carcinoma is the most commonly diagnosed tumor in dogs and cats, followed by squamous cell carcinoma and adenocarcinoma. Fibromas, leiomyomas, and papillomas are the most common benign tumors of the bladder.[40]

Patients with bladder neoplasia usually show clinical signs of hematuria, stranguria, and pollakiuria. Most animals are not systemically ill unless the ureters are obstructed, resulting in progressive renal disease. Physical examination and blood values are often normal. Urinalysis and urine sediment cytological tests performed on urine collected by cystocentesis may reveal neoplastic cells in addition to white and red blood cells. The appearance of transitional cells is variable; therefore, caution is used in making a diagnosis by cytological study alone.[17]

Radiography is of significant value in evaluating patients with bladder neoplasia. Survey abdominal radiographs may show sublumbar lymph node enlargement and may reveal other causes of hematuria such as prostatic disease or cystic calculi. Thoracic radiographs should be made to rule out metastatic disease.

Contrast radiography is often necessary to detect bladder masses as well as to assess the remainder of the urinary tract. Positive- and double-contrast cystography are the most useful procedures for outlining bladder masses. Excretory urograms are performed if surgery is considered, because obstructive uropathy, as evidenced by hydroureter or hydronephrosis, may influence the surgical plan and prognosis (Fig. 106–8).

Confirmation of the diagnosis of bladder tumor usually requires biopsy. Specimens may be obtained by percutaneous fine-needle aspiration if the mass is palpable. Urethral catheterization with a large-bore catheter may help exfoliate cells and confirm the diagnosis. Cystoscopy may be useful in confirming tumor type and determining the extent of disease.

Surgical therapy for bladder neoplasia consists of partial cystectomy if the location of the mass allows complete excision of the tumor while sparing the urethral and ureteral orifices (trigone). A margin of at least 1 cm of normal tissue removed with the tumor is desirable to minimize local tumor recurrence. If the trigone is preserved, 75 per cent of the bladder may be resected, with return to near normal function over a period of weeks.[31, 36] An indwelling bladder catheter is placed if a large portion of bladder is excised. Closure of the bladder after partial cystectomy may be with inverting or appositional suture patterns. A simple continuous appositional pattern is used if a large portion of bladder has been excised. Before abdominal closure, the regional lymph nodes are examined. If the nodes are enlarged, an incisional or excisional biopsy should be performed to determine accurate staging of the disease.

Transitional cell carcinoma frequently involves the trigone of the bladder, making partial cystectomy a poor treatment option. Urinary diversion consisting of total cystectomy and ureteral transplantation into the gastrointestinal tract may be considered as a treatment option. The ideal goals of treatment are cure or palliation of the disease and maintenance of urinary conti-

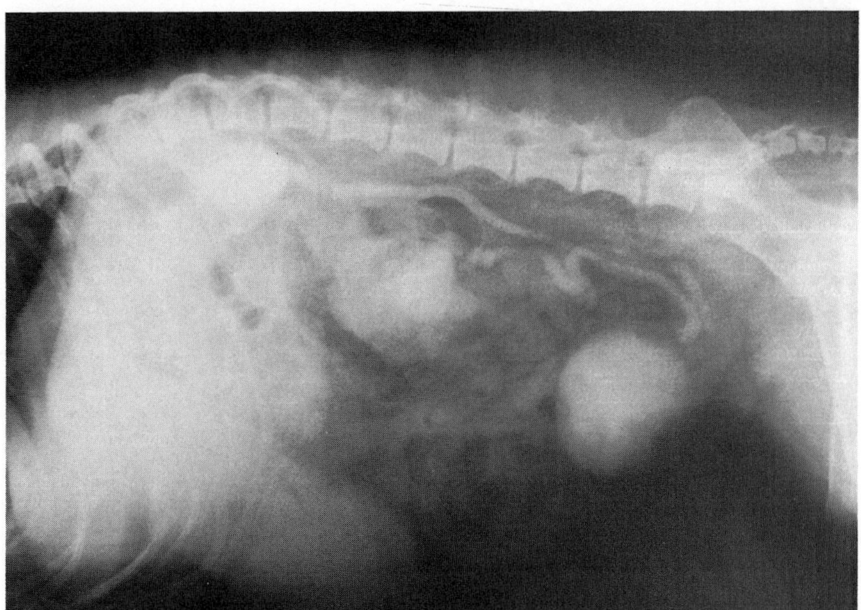

FIGURE 106–8. Excretory urogram demonstrating a trigonal mass. Bilateral hydroureter is noted. Biopsy confirmed the presence of a transitional cell carcinoma.

nence. In human surgery, an isolated bowel loop is commonly used as a conduit for urine. A portion of small intestine, usually ileum, is isolated along with its vascular supply. The isolated loop of bowel is used as a conduit (as is) or fashioned into a reservoir to allow urine accumulation. As a conduit, the loop is sutured to the skin surface, and an appliance is fixed to the stoma. As a reservoir, the loop is refashioned to allow intermittent catheterization and drainage of urine. Successful use of continent urinary reservoirs has not been reported clinically in veterinary medicine.

Ureterocolonic anastomosis and trigonal colonic anastomosis have been used successfully in animals to maintain urinary continence after cystectomy. Because transitional cell carcinomas frequently involve the trigonal area, ureterocolonic anastomosis is the surgical procedure of choice.[5]

Preoperative preparation of patients undergoing ureterocolonic anastomosis begins with a 24-hour fast and saline enemas the night before. Morning surgery is planned. Systemic antibiotic therapy is indicated. Gentamicin combined with cephalosporins provides efficacy against gram-negative, gram-positive, and anaerobic bacteria. Metronidazole and trimethoprim-sulfonamide offer the advantage of oral administration and are also effective against these bacteria. Long-term antibiotic therapy (8 weeks) is continued after surgery because of the risk of pyelonephritis.

A caudal ventral midline incision is made into the abdomen. The bladder and proximal urethra are excised, and the ureters are ligated and transected. The ureters are dissected free from their retroperitoneal attachments and the psoas musculature. Fecal material, if present, is expressed away from the site of proposed ureterocolonic anastomosis. Doyen forceps are used to isolate this segment of the colon. Two separate seromuscular flaps of the colon are prepared to accept the right and left ureters (Fig. 106–9). The right ureter is usually anastomosed to the colon 1 to 2 cm proximal to the left. The three-sided serosal-muscular flaps are created so that the ureter lies in a 3- to 4-cm submucosal tunnel. A 3- to 5-mm defect is created in the colonic mucosa, and the ureter is spatulated and sutured to the mucosa with 5-0 or 6-0 absorbable suture using a single interrupted pattern. The flap is loosely apposed to its bed, taking care not to compress the ureter. The opposite ureter is anastomosed, and the abdomen is thoroughly flushed with warm saline before closure.

Metabolic abnormalities including hyperchloremic metabolic acidosis, hyperammonemia, and elevated creatinine levels are common after urinary diversion into the colon; therefore, careful monitoring of electrolytes, acid-base status, and renal serum chemistry values is mandatory. Pyelonephritis is also common, and renal function is monitored with serum chemistry determinations and excretory urograms postoperatively.

Aggressive surgical therapy has not resulted in significantly increased survival times in dogs. In a study of ten cases of bladder transitional cell carcinoma treated by ureterocolonic diversion, nine of the dogs survived 1 to 5 months after surgery.[39] Six dogs had confirmed metastatic disease at death. The development of effective adjunctive therapy may make ureterocolonic anastomosis more effective in the future.

One report suggests that the ureters may be successfully diverted into the uterus.[1] The metabolic consequences of diversion may be decreased, but incontinence remains a problem.

Radiation during surgery has been used in conjunction with surgical reduction of bladder neoplasms. After irradiation, the ureters and bladder became fibrotic, resulting in secondary hydronephrosis and urinary incontinence in 12 dogs.[36, 43]

URINARY INCONTINENCE

Urinary incontinence is a complex problem with multiple causes. A complete medical and neurological eval-

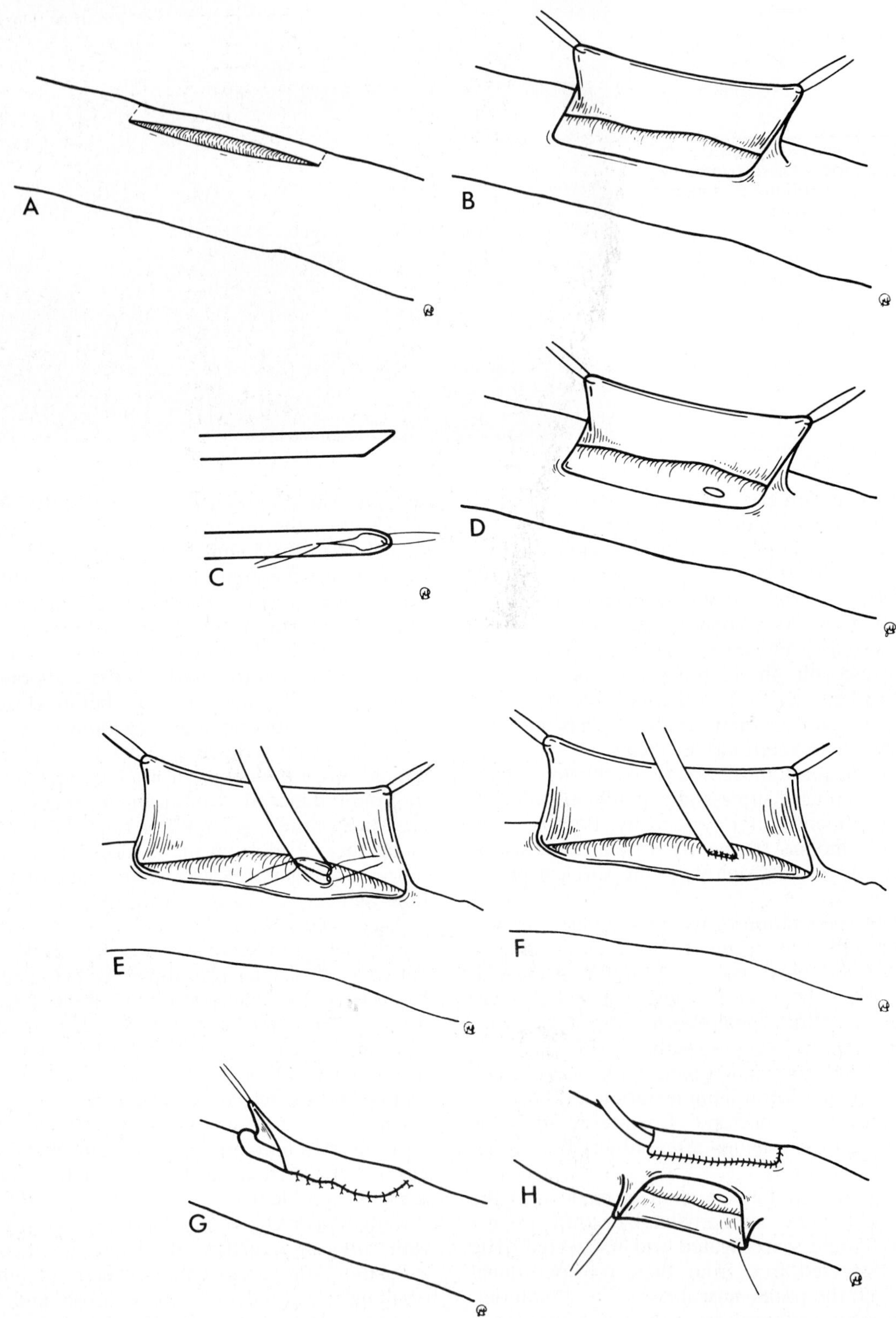

FIGURE 106–9. Ureterocolonic anastomosis. A three-sided seromuscular flap is created, and the ureter is sutured to the colonic mucosa. A separate flap is prepared for the contralateral ureter. (From Stone EA, et al: Urinary diversion. *Vet Clin North Am 14*:123, 1984.)

uation is necessary before considering surgical treatment of urinary incontinence. Urethral pressure profiles and cystometrograms may assist in localizing the cause of incontinence. Determination of a specific cause may allow successful medical management of urinary incontinence. Several surgical techniques have been described for managing incontinence caused by bladder neck and proximal urethral dysfunction. All of the procedures described provide a mechanical means of increasing urethral resistance to urine flow. There are insufficient data on clinical cases to document the success of any procedure. Patients treated medically or surgically for urinary incontinence are monitored periodically for urinary tract infection.

Cystourethroplasty

The creation of a bladder neck sling using autogenous fascia has been described.[15] A fascial strip is harvested from the fascia lata or rectus abdominus muscle sheath. After mobilization of the bladder neck, the strip of fascia is passed dorsally over the neck and proximal urethra. The ends of the fascial strip are passed through bilateral stab incisions made 2 cm off the midline in the abdominal wall.[15, 23] Tension is placed on the ends of the fascial strip, and the bladder neck is pulled in a cranioventral direction, resulting in compression of the neck and urethra against the abdominal wall. The amount of compression applied to the bladder neck and urethra is important and has been crudely estimated. More accurate determination of compression may be made by performing a urethral pressure profile during surgery. An increase in absolute urethral pressure to 50 to 60 mm Hg has been suggested as a satisfactory endpoint.[19]

A sling urethroplasty technique using seromuscular urethral flaps has also been described.[11] An extremely dilated proximal urethra, as observed on contrast radiography, is required. Two seromuscular flaps are created from the dorsal urethral wall. The flaps are reflected laterally to join on the ventral urethra and are apposed with suture. The dilated urethra is reduced in size by one-third of its circumference.

Three female dogs with sphincter incontinence were treated using Dacron-impregnated Silastic strips to increase pressure on the proximal urethra while allowing the bladder to maintain its normal position.[19] A 0.5- to 1.0-cm-wide Silastic strip is passed around the urethra in a circular fashion and sutured to the urethral submucosa with a temporary mattress suture (Fig. 106–10). Tension is adjusted on the Silastic to allow urine flow when the bladder is manually compressed. Urethral pressure profilometry has been used to attain a urethral pressure of 50 to 60 mm Hg. Horizontal mattress sutures are placed through the Silastic strip to maintain proper tension, and the temporary stay sutures are removed.

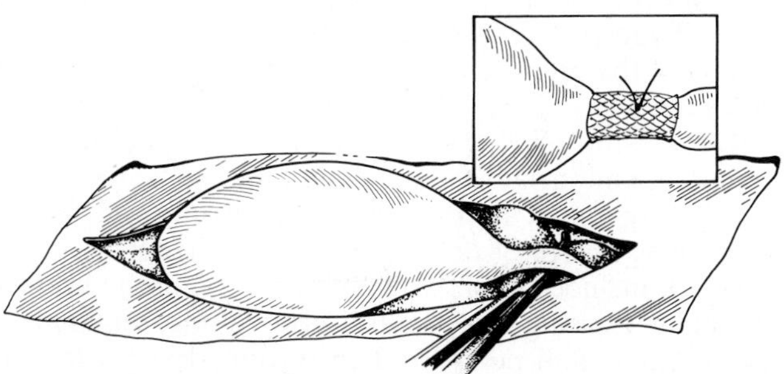

FIGURE 106–10. Placement of a Silastic-Dacron sling around the proximal urethra for urinary incontinence. The Silastic is sutured to the urethra, increasing urinary outflow resistance.

References

1. Anderson SM, Lippincott C: Ureterohysterotomy in the dog. *Vet Surg 19*:55, 1990.
2. Barber D: Postoperative radiography of the urinary system. *Vet Clin North Am Small Anim Pract 14*:31, 1984.
3. Bellah JR: Problems of the urethra—surgical approaches. *Probl Vet Med 1*:17, 1989.
4. Bjorling DE: Traumatic injuries of the urogenital system. *Vet Clin North Am Small Anim Pract 14*:61, 1984.
5. Bjorling DE, Howard PE: Urinary salvage procedures. *Probl Vet Med 1*:93, 1989.
6. Botte RJ: Percutaneous prepubic urinary drainage in normal cats. *Vet Surg 12*:202, 1983.
7. Brearley MJ, Cooper JE: The diagnosis of bladder disease in dogs by cystoscopy. *J Small Anim Pract 28*:75, 1987.
8. Brown NO, et al: Canine urolithiasis: Retrospective analysis of 438 clinical cases. *J Am Vet Med Assoc 170*:414, 1977.
9. Brown SA, Barsanti JA: Disease of the bladder and urethra. *In* Ettinger SJ (ed): *Textbook of Veterinary Internal Medicine.* W.B. Saunders, Philadelphia, 1989, p 2108.
10. Burrows CF, Kolata RJ: Rupture of the canine urinary bladder. *In* Kirk RW (ed): *Current Veterinary Therapy VII.* W.B. Saunders, Philadelphia, 1980, p 1139.
11. Bushby P, Hankes G: Sling urethroplasty for the correction of urethral dilatation and urinary incontinence. *J Am Anim Hosp Assoc 16*:115, 1980.
12. Chew DJ, Dibartola SP: Diagnosis and pathophysiology of renal disease. *In* Ettinger SJ (ed): *Textbook of Veterinary Internal Medicine.* W.B. Saunders, Philadelphia, 1989, p 1893.
13. Christensen GC: The urogenital apparatus. *In* Miller MM (ed): *Anatomy of the Dog.* Philadelphia, W.B. Saunders, 1979, p 554.
14. Christie BA: Anatomy of the urinary tract. *In* Slatter DH (ed): *Textbook of Small Animal Surgery.* W.B. Saunders, Philadelphia, 1985, p 1706.
15. Christie BA: A urethral sling for urinary incontinence in the dog. Proceedings of the 14th Annual Meeting of the American College of Veterinary Surgeons, Knoxville, TN, February 1979.
16. Cooper JE, et al: Cytoscopic examination of male and female dogs. *Vet Rec 115*:571, 1984.
17. Crow SE, Klausner JS: Management of transitional cell carcinomas of the urinary bladder. *In* Kirk RW (ed): *Current Veterinary Therapy VIII.* W.B. Saunders, Philadelphia, 1983, p 1119.
18. Dean PW, Constantinescu GM: Canine ectopic ureter. *Comp Cont Educ 10*:146, 1988.
19. Dean P, et al: Prosthetic sphincter for urinary incontinence: Results in three cases. *J Am Anim Hosp Assoc 25*:447, 1989.
20. Desch JO, Wagner SD: Urinary bladder incisions in dogs—comparison of ventral and dorsal. *Vet Surg 15*:153, 1986.
21. Finco DR, et al: Canine urolithiasis: A review of 133 clinical and 23 necropsy cases. *J Am Vet Med Assoc 157*:1225, 1970.
22. Gahring DR: Surgical management of canine cystic and urethral calculi. *In* Bojrab MJ (ed): *Current Techniques in Small Animal Surgery.* Lea & Febiger, Philadelphia, 1983, p 314.
23. Hobson HP, Bushby P: Surgery of the bladder. *In* Slatter DH (ed): *Textbook of Small Animal Surgery.* W.B. Saunders, Philadelphia, 1985, p 1786.
24. Mason LK, et al: Surgery of ectopic ureters: Pre and postoperative radiographic morphology. *J Am Anim Hosp Assoc 26*:73, 1990.
25. McCarthy TC, McDermaid SL: Prepubic cystoscopy in the dog and cat. *J Am Anim Hosp Assoc 22*:213, 1986.
26. Moreau PM: Neurogenic disorders of micturition in the dog and cat. *Comp Cont Educ Pract Vet 12*:12, 1982.
27. Moreau PM, Lees GE: Incontinence, enuresis, and nocturia. *In* Ettinger SJ (ed): *Textbook of Veterinary Internal Medicine.* W.B. Saunders, Philadelphia, 1989, p 148.
28. Osborne CA, et al: Canine urolithiasis. *In* Ettinger SJ (ed): *Textbook of Veterinary Internal Medicine.* W.B. Saunders, Philadelphia, 1989, p 2083.

29. Osborne CA, et al: Etiopathogenesis and biological behavior of feline vesicourachal diverticula. *Vet Clin North Am Small Anim Pract 17*:697, 1987.
30. Osborne CA, et al: Feline vesicourachal diverticula; biologic behavior, diagnosis and treatment. *In* Kirk RW (ed): *Current Veterinary Therapy X*. W.B. Saunders, Philadelphia, 1989, p 1153.
31. Peacock EE: *Wound Repair*. W.B. Saunders, Philadelphia, 1984, p 438.
32. Pechman RD, et al: Urinary trauma in dogs and cats: A review. *J Am Anim Hosp Assoc 18*:33, 1982.
33. Rosin A, et al: Canine urethral pressure profile. *Am J Vet Res 41*:1113, 1980.
34. Rosin AE, Barsanti JA: Diagnosis of urinary incontinence in dogs: Role of the urethral pressure profile. *J Am Vet Med Assoc 178*:814, 1981.
35. Rosin AH, Ross L: Diagnosis and pharmacological management of disorders of urinary continence in the dog. *Comp Cont Educ 3*:601, 1981.
36. Schwarz PD, Willer RL: Urinary bladder neoplasia in the dog and cat. *Probl Vet Med 1*:128, 1989.
37. Smith CW, et al: Ectopic ureter in the dog—a review of cases. *J Am Anim Hosp Assoc 17*:245, 1981.
38. Stone EA, Mason LK: Surgery of ectopic ureters: Types, methods of correction and postoperative results. *J Am Anim Hosp Assoc 26*:81, 1990.
39. Stone EA, et al: Ureterocolonic anastomosis in ten dogs with transitional cell carcinoma. *Vet Surg 17*:147, 1988.
40. Strafuss AC, Dean MJ: Neoplasms of the canine urinary bladder. *J Am Vet Med Assoc 166*:1161, 1975.
41. Wilson JW, et al: Canine vesicourachal diverticula. *Vet Surg 8*:63, 1979.
42. Wingfield W, Rawlings C: *Small Animal Surgery—An Atlas of Operative Techniques*. W.B. Saunders, Philadelphia, 1979, p 115.
43. Withrow SJ, et al: Intraoperative irradiation of 16 spontaneously occurring canine neoplasms. *Vet Surg 18*:7, 1989.

CHAPTER 107 Surgical Diseases of the Urethra

C. W. Smith

The urethra carries urine from the bladder to the exterior. A male's urethra is relatively long (10 to 35 cm in dogs) and consists of three portions: prostatic, pelvic (membranous), and cavernous (penile). In dogs, the neck of the bladder is very short, whereas in cats, it is extremely elongated.[23] The prostate gland surrounds the proximal portion of a male's urethra at the neck of the bladder.[7] The prostatic portion of the urethra is U shaped and passes through the prostate gland.[7] In dogs, diseases of the prostate gland (hyperplasia, cyst formation, prostatitis, abscess, and carcinoma) may affect this portion of the urethra. The pelvic urethra extends from the prostate gland to the bulb of the penis near the ischial arch.[7] Because of its relationship to the symphysis pubis, this portion of the urethra is vulnerable to injury due to pelvic fractures. The cavernous portion of the urethra begins at the bulb of the corpus spongiosum and extends to the external opening of the penis. The corpus spongiosum and the penile urethra occupy the ventral groove of the os penis.[7] Distension of the urethra in this groove is limited, and urethral obstruction with calculi generally occurs at this level. Fractures of the os penis can cause urethral injury or obstruction.

A female's urethra corresponds to that portion of a male's urethra that lies cranial to the prostatic utricle. In dogs, it is about 0.5 cm in diameter and 7 to 10 cm long. The urethra enters the genital tract approximately 0.5 cm caudal to the vaginovestibular junction. Its dorsal wall is in close apposition to the ventral wall of the vagina. The lumen can expand considerably when under pressure because of its folded mucous membrane.[7] As in males, the close proximity of the urethra to the pubic symphysis makes it vulnerable to injury when pelvic fractures occur. Because of its relationship to the vagina, the urethra may become involved in disease processes in the genital system (vaginitis, vaginal neoplasia).

CONGENITAL OR HEREDITARY LESIONS AFFECTING THE URETHRA

Urethral anomalies are uncommon.[24] Hypospadias, epispadias with exstrophy of the bladder, imperforate urethra, ectopic urethra, urethral aplasia (or agenesis), duplicated urethra, and urethrorectal fistula occur in dogs.[2, 9, 24] I have observed dilatation of the pelvic urethra in a puppy. A few of these conditions, including hypospadias, epispadias with exstrophy of the bladder, and urethrorectal fistula, have been surgically corrected.[2, 8, 9, 24]

Hypospadias

Hypospadias is due to failure of fusion of the urogenital folds and incomplete formation of the penile urethra. Various degrees of this abnormality can occur, with fusion failure occurring anywhere from the penis to the perineal area. In humans, this condition results from inadequate production of androgens by the fetal testes.[21] Differences in the timing and degree of hormonal failure account for the diversity of hypospadias in humans. In dogs, hypospadias is usually associated with failure of fusion of the prepuce and underdevelopment or absence of the penis (Fig. 107–1).

Dogs with hypospadias are seen as puppies with irritated and urine-soaked skin and hair around the urethral opening. Remnants of the incomplete prepuce appear as unsightly defects. Corrective surgery, if performed, includes identifying and preserving the urethral opening, excising the urethral groove and remnants of the prepuce and penis, and castration. Even after surgery, the perineum and ventral abdomen near the urethral opening may become scalded by urine. The prognosis is generally favorable except that patients may be

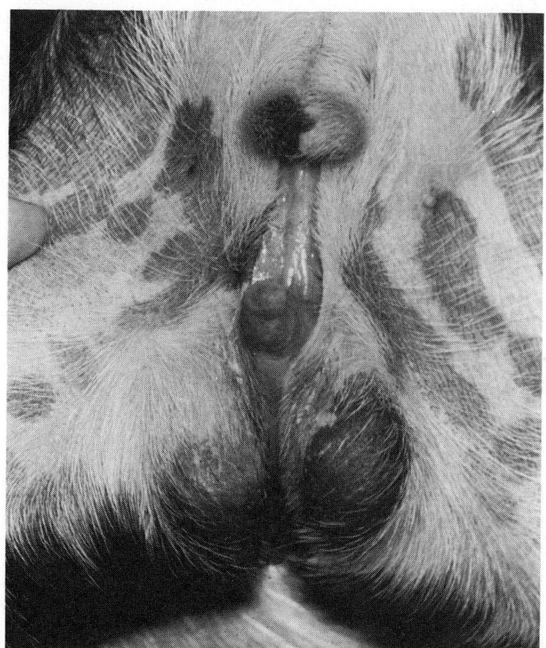

FIGURE 107–1. Canine hypospadias: fusion failure of the urethra, prepuce, and scrotum and underdevelopment of the penis.

more prone to ascending urinary tract infections because of the shortened urethra.

Epispadias

Epispadias is a rarer anomaly that also represents fusion failure. It is manifested as an abnormally located urethral groove along the dorsal surface of the penis. In humans, in whom it is more common, it appears in combination with exstrophy of the bladder, another anomaly. In the latter malformation, the bladder is open midventrally, and the pubic arches fail to unite. The dorsal wall of the bladder thus becomes the ventral body wall, with the ureters discharging urine directly to the exterior.[21] This combination of anomalies has been reported in a dog.[9]

Urethrorectal Fistula

Urethrorectal fistula is a developmental anomaly of the fetal cloaca in which a communication between the urethra and rectum persists.[2, 8, 24] In humans, it is proposed that these fistulas develop as a result of failure of the urorectal septum to completely separate the cloaca into an anterior urethrovesical segment and a posterior rectal segment.[5] They occur twice as frequently in boys as in girls and are associated with an imperforate anus and anomalies of other body systems.[14] In dogs, urethrorectal fistulas have been reported in both sexes. Clinical signs are associated with abnormal micturition, first observed shortly after weaning. Urine passes simultaneously through the urethra and anus. Concurrent cystitis is generally present. Diagnosis is confirmed by physical examination, including rectal examination using a nasal speculum or endoscope, and positive-contrast urethrography, demonstrating leakage of contrast medium from the urethra into the rectum. Surgical correction is performed via ventral pubic symphysiotomy.[2] The pubic symphysis is split with an osteotome and distracted with retractors. The fistula is identified, double ligated, and excised. The symphysis is stabilized using wire. Concurrent medical therapy for cystitis is necessary.

ACQUIRED NONTRAUMATIC LESIONS AFFECTING THE URETHRA

Acquired nontraumatic lesions of the urethra include urethritis and urethral prolapse; obstruction associated with urethral calculi and with stricture formation following inflammation, passage of calculi, and urethral surgery; and neoplasia.

Urethritis

Urethritis as an isolated clinical entity is uncommon. It is generally associated with other inflammatory diseases of the urogenital tract, such as cystitis, prostatitis, or vaginitis. Predisposing factors include trauma, catheterization, urolithiasis, and neoplasia.[30] Therapy for urethritis is directed at controlling infection and eliminating the identifiable factors. Although rare, urethritis can lead to urethral prolapse or stricture formation, necessitating surgical intervention.

Urethral Prolapse

Urethral prolapse has been reported in young male dogs of the brachycephalic breeds.[4, 10] Prolonged sexual excitement and urethral infection may be the cause, although the exact pathophysiology is unknown. Patients are observed to excessively lick the tip of the penis and preputial orifice. Diagnosis is based on observing the protruding mucosa (Fig. 107–2). With a urinary catheter

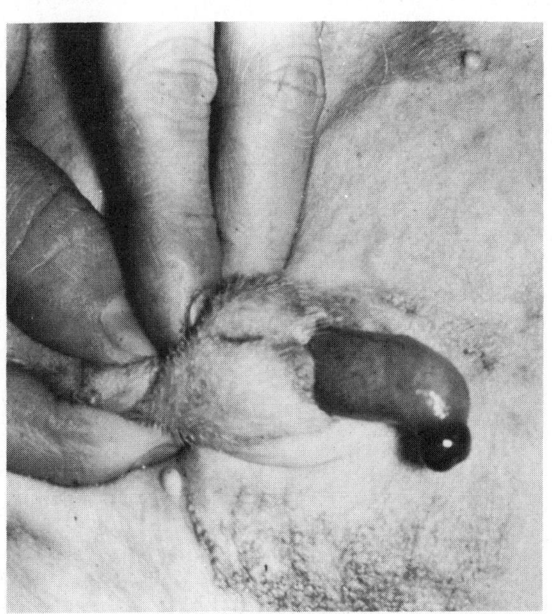

FIGURE 107–2. Prolapse of the penile urethra in a male dog. (Courtesy of Dr. A. G. Schiller.)

in place, the prolapsed urethra is partially incised into the lumen just caudal to the prolapse. The urethra is sutured circumferentially to the tunic of the penis with 4-0 monofilament nylon by alternately incising and suturing. A splinting catheter is usually unnecessary after surgery. Sedation and an Elizabethan collar may be necessary for 3 to 5 days after surgery to prevent self-inflicted trauma. Systemic antibiotics are used to treat urogenital infection when present.

Urethral Obstruction

Obstruction of the urethra is most often due to urethral calculi and stricture formation following inflammation, passage of calculi, and urethral surgery. It may also be the result of a fracture of the os penis, diseases of the prostate, or displacement of the bladder through a perineal hernia.

Urethral Calculi

Urethral calculi are the most common cause of urethral obstruction in male dogs.[4] Less-organized debris causes obstruction in male cats.[25] A detailed discussion of canine and feline urolithiasis may be found in Chapters 108 and 109, respectively. This discussion is limited to determining when surgical intervention is indicated and the surgical procedures used. Urethral obstruction due to calculi may be complete or incomplete and most often occurs just behind the os penis (Fig. 107–3). Clinical signs vary with the degree and duration of obstruction and include dysuria, anuria, hematuria, and distended or turgid abdomen. Signs of uremia may develop if complete obstruction has been present for at least 48 hours.[25] Diagnosis is based on an inability to pass a urethral catheter and radiological demonstration of the presence of stones.

Once the diagnosis has been established, nonsurgical techniques to improve a patient's metabolic status and to alleviate the blockage are attempted before using surgical techniques. Urethral calculi that cannot be moved by either catheterization or urohydropulsion[29] to the exterior or into the bladder require urethral surgery. If the calculi cannot be dislodged, the patient can be anesthetized using general anesthesia or sedation and local anesthesia so that the calculi can be removed via a urethrotomy performed at the obstruction. Cystocentesis and fluid therapy may be necessary to improve a patient's ability to tolerate anesthesia.

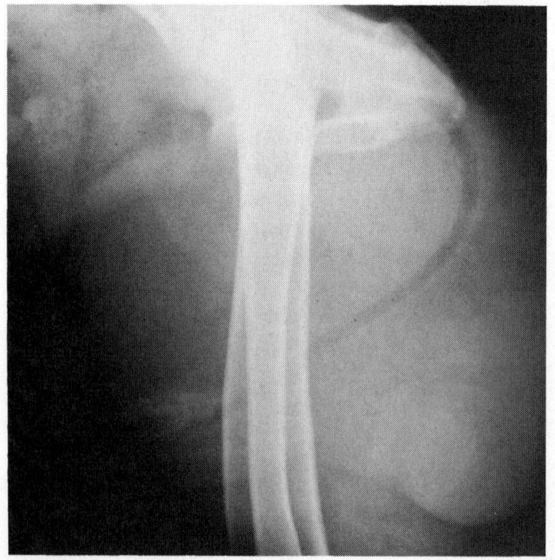

FIGURE 107–3. A lateral radiograph of a male dog with cystic and urethral calculi. Note several calculi in the urethra of the os penis. (Courtesy of Drs. S. Kneller and J. Stowater.)

Urethrotomy/Cystotomy

With a urethral catheter in place to the obstruction, a 3- to 4-cm ventral midline skin incision is made over the obstruction. The subcutaneous tissue is incised down to the retractor penis muscle, which overlies the urethra or the midline. After its fascial attachment is freed, the muscle is retracted laterally to expose the ventral portion of the urethra. A longitudinal incision is made over the calculus (or catheter tip), and the stone is carefully removed. The catheter is advanced, and any remaining calculi are flushed into the bladder with a stream of saline. These calculi and any other cystic calculi are removed via cystotomy. Before cystotomy, radiographs may be necessary to determine whether the urethra is free of calculi and whether any cystic calculi remain.

If the urethra has not been severely traumatized by the calculus or the surgical incision, the urethrotomy can be closed with 4-0 polyglycolic acid or polyglactin 910 sutures using an interrupted pattern. Sutures are anchored in the corpus spongiosum and the urethral mucosa.[2] An indwelling catheter makes it easier to place these sutures carefully, because stricture of the lumen may result if too large a "bite" is taken. If trauma to the urethra is excessive, the urethrotomy incision is not sutured but is allowed to granulate. More postoperative hemorrhage and fibrosis occur when the urethrotomy incision is not sutured.[40, 42] Urine leaks through the wound for several days, and the corpus spongiosum may hemorrhage when the dog urinates or becomes excited.

The major complication associated with urethrotomy is urethral stricture formation. For this reason, a concerted (but gentle) effort is made to move the calculus by catheterization or urohydropulsion before performing urethral surgery. A laparotomy with cystotomy is much less likely to result in complications than is urethrotomy.

Urethrostomy

Creation of a permanent opening into the urethra can be used for (1) calculi that cannot be removed by flushing, (2) animals that cannot be kept free of calculi medically, (3) strictures of the urethra resulting from one or more episodes of prior urethral surgery or trauma, and (4) severe penile trauma when penile amputation is required.

Canine Urethrostomy. In dogs, urethrostomy can be performed in four locations: prescrotal, scrotal, perineal, and prepubic. The location selected is based on the site of obstruction and the surgeon's preference. If a choice exists and if the patient can be castrated, scrotal urethrostomy is recommended. The advantages of a scrotal urethrostomy are that the urethra is wide and more superficial at this location and is surrounded by less cavernous tissue, thus decreasing the possibility of hemorrhage. Obstruction of the proximal urethra may necessitate perineal or prepubic urethrostomy.

A scrotal urethrostomy is performed with the dog in dorsal recumbency (Fig. 107–4). If possible, a catheter is passed to facilitate identification and incision of the urethra. If the dog is intact, castration is performed and the scrotum excised. The retractor penis muscle is isolated and sutured in a lateral position to expose the ventral aspect of the urethra. The urethra is incised for 3 to 4 cm. The periurethral tissue is sutured to the subcutaneous tissue using 4-0 polyglactin 910 or polyglycolic acid in a simple continuous pattern to control hemorrhage and prevent urine leakage. The urethra is sutured to the skin with 3-0 or 4-0 monofilament nylon or polypropylene suture material in a simple interrupted pattern. Skin not sutured to the urethra is closed in the usual way, and the catheter is removed. Complications include hemorrhage from the cavernous tissue for up to 10 days and urethral strictures. Hemorrhage commonly occurs when the animal urinates or becomes excited for 7 to 10 days after surgery. It is usually self-limiting and not large in volume. An Elizabethan collar and sedation are helpful in preventing self-mutilation during the initial healing period. Sedation of the patient at the time of discharge prevents excitement and reduces the risk of hemorrhage.

Feline Urethrostomy. There are many techniques for urethrostomy in male cats,[11, 34] but I prefer perineal urethrostomy using the Wilson and Harrison technique[43, 44] (Fig. 107–5). A patient may be positioned in dorsal or ventral recumbency. A purse-string suture is

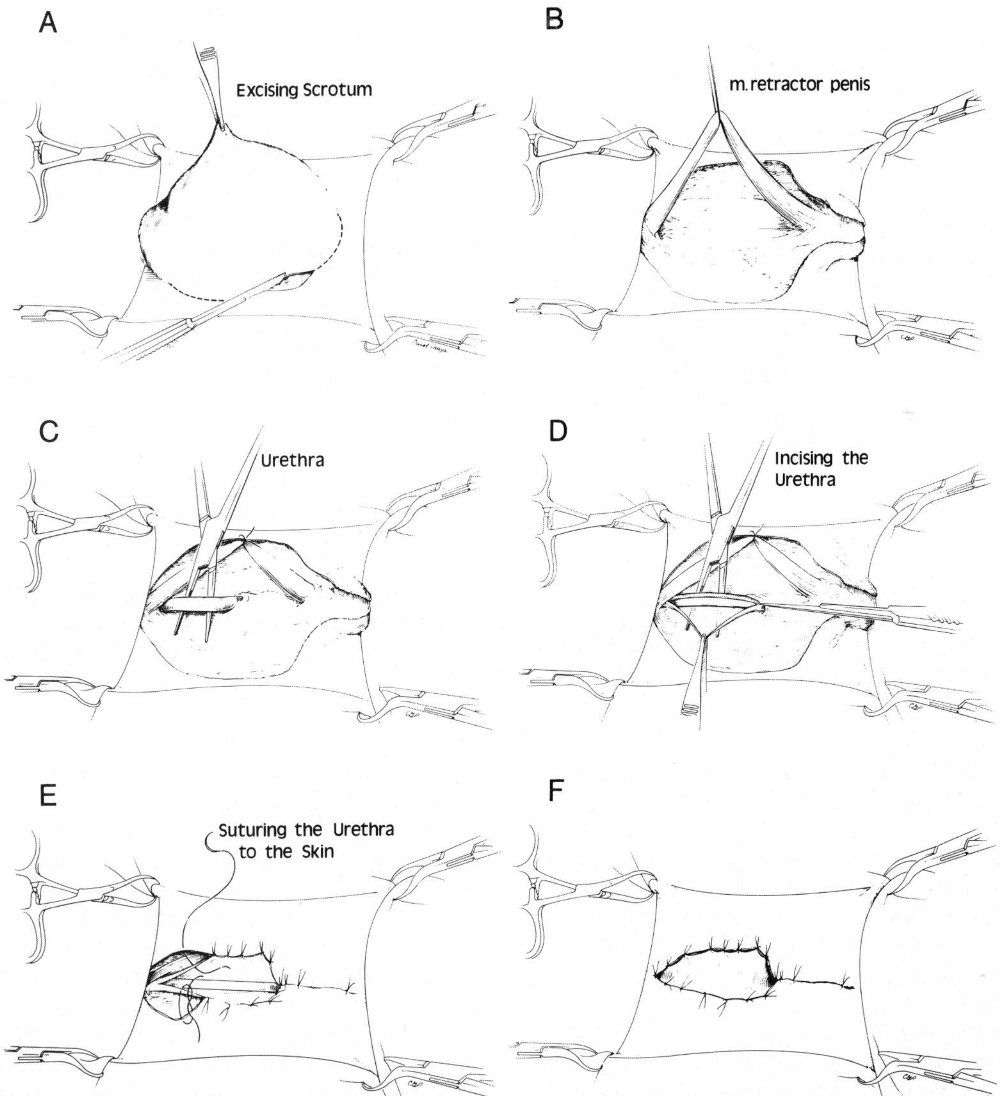

FIGURE 107–4. Scrotal urethrostomy. *A*, An elliptical skin incision is made around the scrotum, which is excised. The dog is castrated. *B*, The retractor penis muscle is isolated and retracted laterally. *C*, The retractor penis muscle is sutured laterally, and the urethra is located. *D*, The ventral aspect of the urethra is incised for 3 to 4 cm. The periurethral tissue is sutured to the subcutaneous tissue. *E*, The urethra is sutured to the skin. *F*, The remaining skin incision is sutured closed.

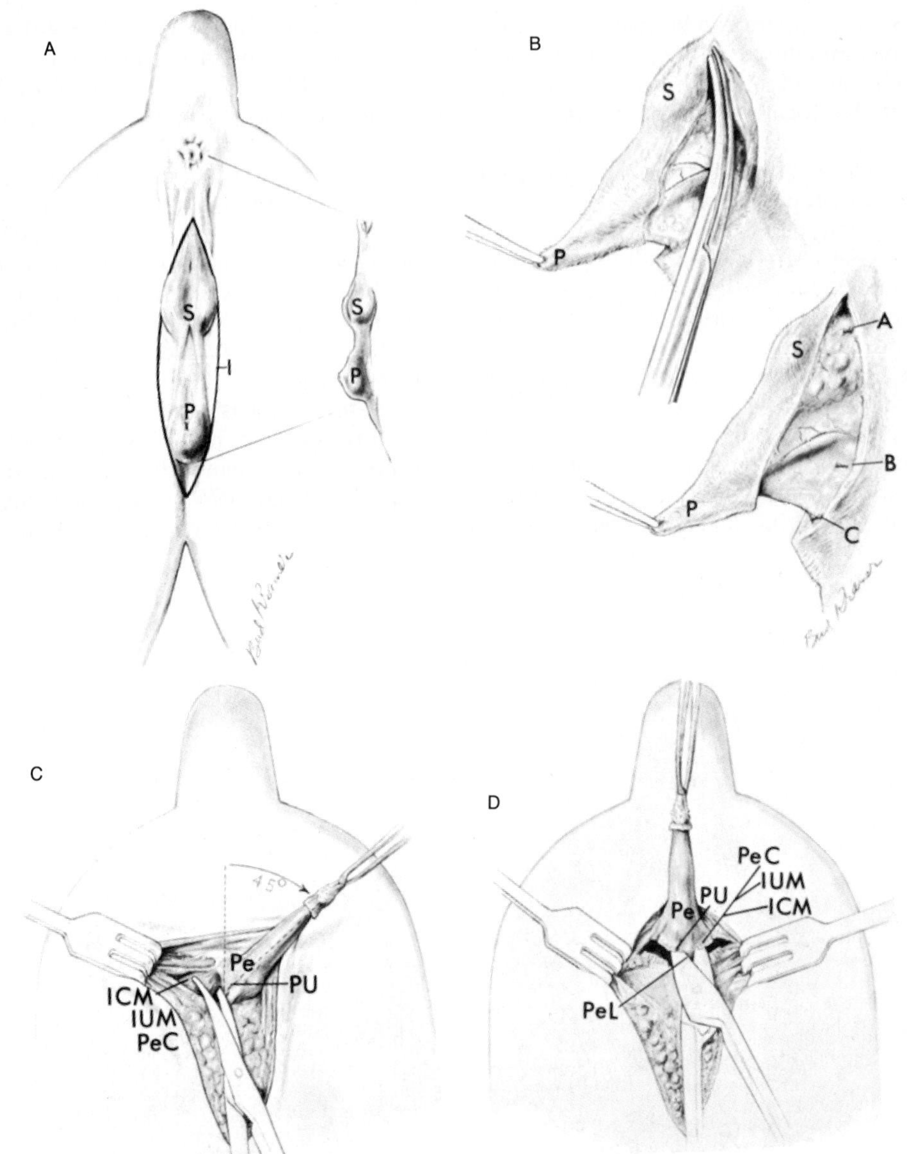

FIGURE 107–5. *A,* Elliptical incision incorporating the scrotum and prepuce. (S, scrotum; P, prepuce; I, skin incision.) *B,* Removal of prepuce and scrotum. (A, caudal scrotal artery; B, cranial scrotal artery; C, dorsal artery and vein of penis, prostatic artery.) *C,* Dissection of the penis from surrounding tissue to its pelvic attachments on the ischium. (ICM, ischiocavernous muscle; IUM, ischiourethral muscle; PeC, crus of penis; Pe, penis; PU, pelvic urethra.) *D,* Incision of the ligament of the penis. (PeL, ligament of penis.)

placed around the anus, an elliptical incision is made around the scrotum and prepuce, and the cat is castrated. The penis is isolated, and the ischiocavernous muscles are exposed by blunt dissection. These muscles are transected at their attachment to the ischium. Incision through the muscle belly causes hemorrhage from the muscle and the underlying crura of the penis. The penis has a fibrous pubic attachment that must also be transected. Careful blunt dissection ventrally and digital elevation of the penis and pelvic urethra from the pelvic floor permit mobilization and posterior displacement of the penis and pelvic urethra. The loose tissue near the penis is carefully excised to expose the retractor penis muscle, bulbocavernous muscle, and bulbourethral glands. The retractor penis muscle is transected near the external anal sphincter muscle, dissected from the urethra, and excised. Care is taken in this dissection to prevent damage to the rectum and pelvic nerves (Fig. 107–6). The penile urethra is incised on its dorsal surface to the bulbourethral glands. In this location, the urethral opening is usually about 4 mm in diameter. The incised pelvic urethra and two-thirds of the penile urethra are sutured to the skin with 4-0 monofilament nylon or polypropylene or 5-0 synthetic absorbable in an interrupted pattern.[16] The remaining urethra and penis distal to the urethrostomy are amputated and discarded. A mattress suture may be placed through the body of the retained penile shaft to control the hemorrhage, and the remaining skin incision is closed. The purse-string suture around the anus is removed. An Elizabethan collar is used to prevent self-mutilation. No indwelling catheter is used postoperatively. Shredded paper may be used

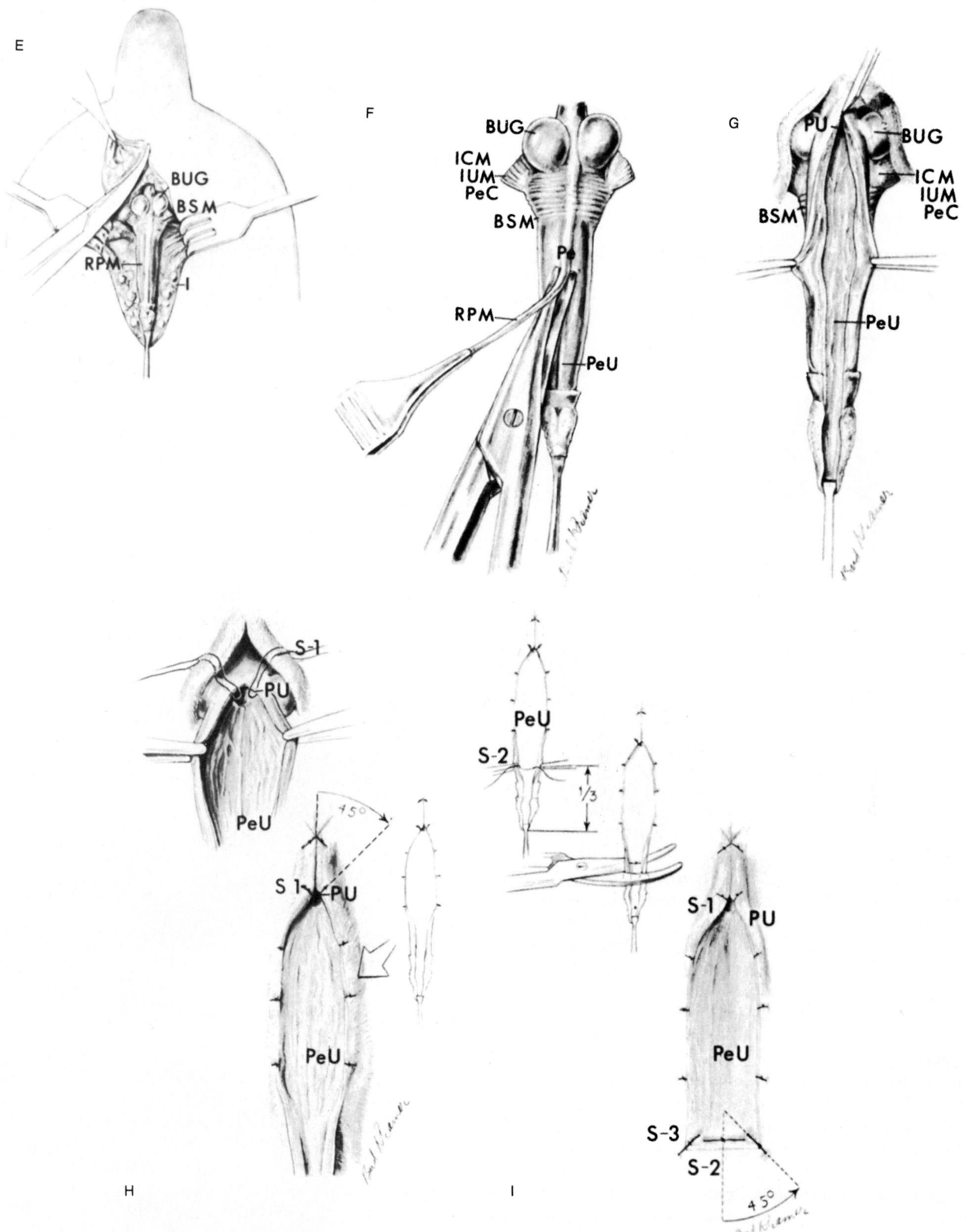

FIGURE 107–5. *Continued E,* Exposure of the retractor penis muscle. (BUG, bulbourethral glands; BSM, bulbocavernous muscle; RPM, retractor muscle of penis.) *F,* Insertion of a probe into penile urethra. (PeU, penile urethra.) *G,* Incision of the penile urethra through the glans penis to the pelvic urethra. *H,* Suture of the pelvic and penile urethral mucosa to the perineal skin. (S-1, initial sutures.) *I,* Placement of through-and-through suture through the body of the penis. (S-1, initial sutures; S-2, through-and-through mattress suture; S-3, mucosa-to-skin sutures.) (From Wilson GP, Kusba JK: Perineal urethrostomy in the cat. *In* Bojrab MJ [ed]: *Current Techniques in Small Animal Surgery.* Philadelphia, Lea & Febiger, 1983; modified from Wilson GP, Harrison JW: Perineal urethrostomy in cats. *J Am Vet Med Assoc 159:*1789, 1971.)

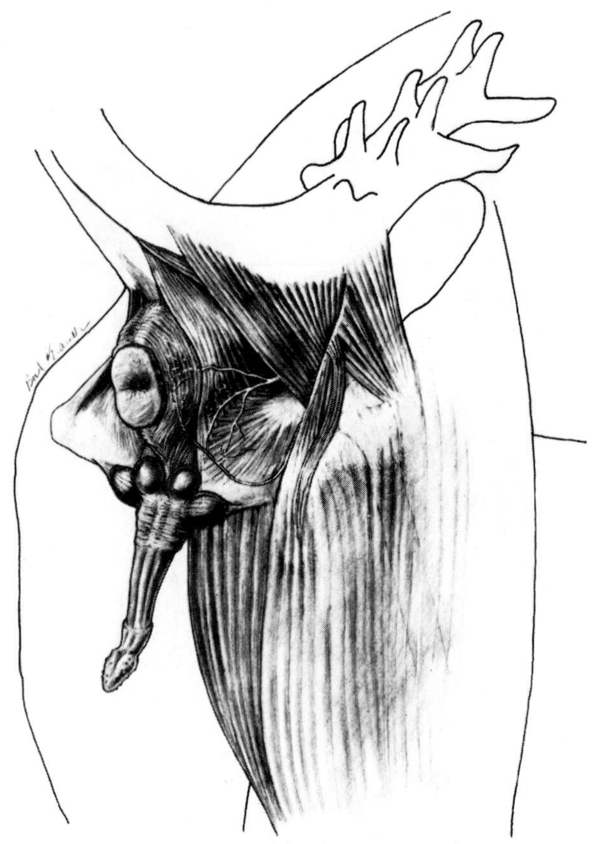

FIGURE 107–6. Pelvic nerves and rectum in relation to the penis and pelvic musculature. (From Wilson GP, Kusba JK: Perineal urethrostomy in the cat. *In* Bojrab MJ [ed]: *Current Techniques in Small Animal Surgery.* 2nd ed. Lea & Febiger, Philadelphia, 1983, pp 325–333.)

instead of litter during healing. Complications include hemorrhage from erectile tissue, wound dehiscence, self-mutilation, cystitis, and urethral stricture (Fig. 107–7).[37]

To treat postoperative strictures, the urethra is freed from surrounding scar tissue and mobilized to permit suturing the healthy urethra to a fresh skin incision. The urethra was usually not adequately mobilized or the pelvic urethra was not incised far enough cranially during the previous operation. When strictures occur more cranially, a prepubic urethrostomy[19] may be necessary. With prepubic urethrostomy, the largest amount of intra-abdominal and pelvic urethra is dissected free, severed distally, and used to provide an adequate length of urethra from the bladder to the ventral abdominal wall. Care should be taken to maintain the urethra in a gentle curve to prevent obstruction. The severed end of the urethra is spatulated and sutured to the ventral abdominal skin.

Urethral Prostheses in Cats. Prosthetic conduits manufactured from steel and Teflon,[17] silicone rubber and Dacron velour,[35] and silicone rubber* alone[33] have been advocated as treatments for urethral stricture and urethral obstruction in cats (Fig. 107–8). The steel and Teflon prosthesis is inserted directly into the bladder to permit flushing and draining, but it promotes cystic calculi in 25 per cent of cases in which maintenance flushing of the prosthesis and bladder has been neglected. The silicone rubber and Dacron prosthesis is sutured to the bladder neck just cranial to the prostate gland, and it replaces the pelvic and penile urethra. Problems with this implant have included perineal fistula, mineral encrustation of the lumen, and rejection as a foreign body. The silicone prosthesis is inserted into the pelvic urethra near the bulbourethral glands. Urine leakage and mechanical irritation have not allowed this prosthesis to remain maintenance free.

A correctly performed perineal urethrostomy remains the surgical method of choice for treating cats with recurrent urethral obstruction.

Neoplasia

Neoplastic processes can involve the urethra, producing partial or complete obstruction. Tumors of the urinary tract are uncommon in cats.[3] In dogs, primary urethral tumors are uncommon but are most likely to occur in females.[38, 39] Clinical signs vary in severity and include mild stranguria to anuria and hematuria. Radiographs, including positive- and double-contrast as well as voiding studies, are important in delineating the location and extent of lesions.[39] Survey radiographs of the abdomen and thorax are made to detect metastatic lesions. Urinary exfoliative cytological study may assist

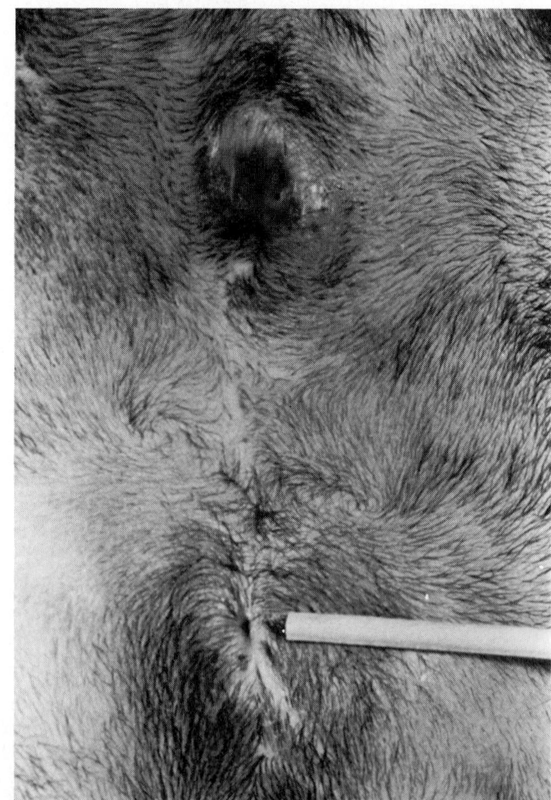

FIGURE 107–7. The perineal area of a cat with a urethral stricture following perineal urethrostomy. Note the pinpoint urethral opening.

*Richards all-silicone urethral shunt tube, Richards Manufacturing Co., Inc., Memphis, TN.

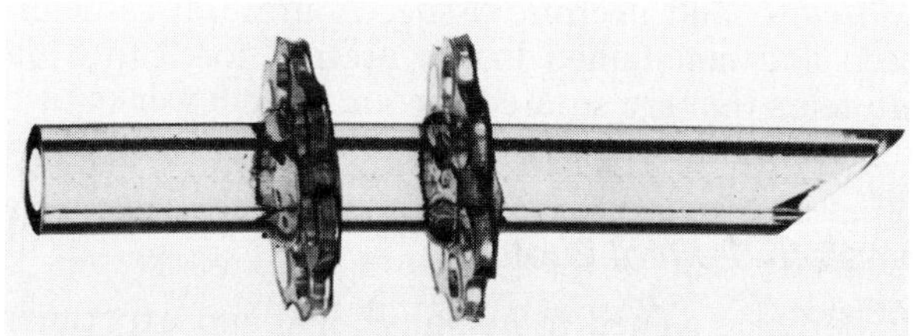

FIGURE 107–8. Richards all-silicone urethral shunt tube.

diagnosis, but more often, excisional or incisional biopsy is necessary. Surgical excision is the treatment of choice when the lesion is discrete but may be impossible when the lesion is diffuse. For diagnostic, prognostic, and chemotherapeutic planning, biopsy is performed on lesions that cannot be resected. For exploratory surgery, the caudal abdominal approach is recommended over the vaginal approach via episiotomy because it permits better observation of the urethra, periurethral tissues, bladder, and regional lymph nodes.[38] For further information about urethral neoplasms, see Chapter 160.

TRAUMATIC LESIONS AFFECTING THE URETHRA

Traumatic lesions of the urethra include contusion, laceration, rupture, and obstruction. Urethral contusions are most often the result of blunt trauma. Urethral lacerations and ruptures are associated with fractures of the pubis and os penis; penetrating wounds caused by knife, gunshot, or bite injuries; and iatrogenic injuries as a result of urethral examination, dilation, catheterization, and surgery on and near the urethra. Acquired urethral obstruction may be due to fractures of the pubis or os penis but can also result from strangulation of the penis by foreign objects (rubber bands), phimosis/paraphimosis, herniation of the bladder into perineal and inguinal areas, and marked prostate enlargement. Unusual causes of urethral obstruction have been described in a dog in which an air gun pellet that had penetrated into the bladder lumen became impacted in the urethra[6] and in a cat in which a plug of hair carried into the bladder by an air gun pellet obstructed the urethra.[1]

The causes of traumatic urethral injuries are many, but the overall incidence is low. In one survey, it was found that the most common urinary tract injury accompanying trauma to the abdomen and pelvis in dogs and cats was ruptured bladder.[27] Less common injuries were ruptured kidney, ruptured urethra, ruptured ureter, and perirenal hematoma. Ruptured urethra was most often associated with pelvic fractures in males, and the injury usually occurred near the urethrovesical junction. The frequency of urinary tract trauma that occurred with blunt pelvic trauma in another survey of 100 cases was 39 percent.[36] Only 5 per cent of these urinary tract injuries involved the urethra, and rupture of the urethra occurred exclusively in male dogs.

Clinical Signs

Clinical signs associated with urethral trauma may be masked by other problems or may be absent. The usual clinical signs include dysuria, anuria, hematuria, pain, fluid in the abdomen, and swelling and discoloration of the skin in the perineal area.[27, 32, 36] Clinical signs vary, depending on the severity of the lesion. Contusion may produce minimal clinical signs, whereas urethral rupture may cause all those listed. Although clinical signs may be helpful when present, their absence does not rule out the presence of urethral trauma. For example, a dog with a urethral tear may void normally. Selcer reported that clinical signs suggestive of urinary tract injury were absent in 59 per cent of pelvic trauma cases with confirmed urinary tract trauma.[36] One-third (13 of 39) of all urinary tract injuries in this series were unsuspected clinically. Sixty-nine per cent (9 of 13) of clinically undetected urinary tract trauma was noted in female dogs. Hematuria was the most frequent clinical sign, but it occurred in only 36 per cent (14 of 39) of dogs with urinary tract trauma. The clinical signs that were consistently associated with urinary tract trauma were dysuria/anuria and external evidence of an abdominal or inguinal hernia.

If the urethra is ruptured, urine leakage produces cellulitis that leads to fistula formation. Peripheral leukocytosis, with cell counts of 50,000 to 100,000/mm^3, may occur when significant local infection is present.[32] Anorectic patients may show signs of dehydration, hypoproteinemia, and hypoglycemia. If the urethra is obstructed, signs of uremia occur.

Diagnosis

Diagnosis is based on a high level of suspicion (abdominal or pelvic trauma), clinical signs, and positive-contrast urethrography. Plain radiographs are rarely diagnostic.[27, 36] Positive-contrast urethrography is performed before catheterization if urethral damage is suspected. Negative-contrast studies with room air are contraindicated because of the potential for development of air emboli.[32] Positive-contrast urethrograms help distinguish incomplete from complete urethral ruptures, which need to be managed differently. An experimental study of dogs with partial or complete division of the penile urethra just cranial to the scrotum revealed extravasation of dye at the site of injury with some dye reaching the bladder in the partial tear group, and extravasation of dye at the site of injury with no dye reaching the bladder in the dogs with complete urethral disruption.[31] A positive-contrast urethrogram usually delineates well the distal boundary of the urethral obstruction or stricture but may not identify its proximal border.

Treatment

Before specific treatment of urethral trauma can be instituted, a patient's general condition is assessed. Shock, anuria, dysuria, uremia, dehydration, and electrolyte imbalances are corrected before the urethra is repaired.

Treatment of urethral trauma takes advantage of the remarkable regenerative ability of the urethral mucosa. The entire length of the urethra will regenerate from a longitudinal strip of mucosa if an intraurethral catheter is maintained for 3 weeks.[41] After complete transection, however, the urethral muscle and mucosa retract. During healing, the intervening space is usually filled by fibroblasts, which produce fibrous connective tissue that contracts during maturation, producing stenosis.[18] Therefore, primary repair to prevent the almost inevitable stenosis or delayed repair to excise it is essential in most cases of complete urethral transection.

Contusions

Specific treatment is based on the type and severity of the injury. Minor urethral contusions and lacerations may heal spontaneously with conservative therapy, including systemic antibiotics and manual assistance in emptying the bladder to prevent urine retention. Healing can sometimes be improved by the placement of a soft, flexible indwelling catheter,* which reduces delay in healing from urine leakage and acts as a urethral splint. The catheter should not be so large that it places undue pressure on the epithelium, because this may interfere with its regeneration.

Lacerations

Lacerations that permit extravasation of urine into the surrounding tissues are explored and sutured with 3-0 or 4-0 polyglactin 910 or polyglycolic acid suture material, and the urine is diverted with an intraurethral catheter for 3 to 5 days. Bite wounds of the extrapelvic urethra are treated similarly, with the addition of a soft Penrose drain to provide drainage for a few days. If gross infection is present, primary closure is delayed. The external wound is allowed to drain for 3 days while the urine is diverted through a urethral catheter. Culture and sensitivity testing and appropriate antibiotic administration are indicated.

Intrapelvic Partial Urethral Rupture

Incomplete rupture of the intrapelvic urethra without impingement by fracture fragments may be treated by diverting urine through the largest urinary catheter that can be comfortably passed and maintained in place for 7 to 21 days (depending on the size of the urethral tear). When passage of the catheter is impossible and a patient cannot tolerate a major surgical procedure, a prepubic cystostomy tube[31] can be placed and maintained until the patient's condition improves. When surgery can be performed, a ventral midline approach for cystotomy and reduction of the fracture fragments may allow visual passage of a urethral catheter across the tear. At this time, suturing the tear may be possible. If fracture fragments are impinging on the urethra, they are reduced and stabilized using wire or other orthopedic techniques. The surgical site is flushed with sterile saline, and in some patients, the pelvic cavity may need further drainage to remove debris resulting from urine leakage, blood clots, and necrotic tissue. A urethral catheter is passed and maintained in the urethra for 3 to 5 days (with tears that are sutured) or for up to 3 weeks (if the tears are left unsutured).

Complete Urethral Rupture

Experience gained in humans[20, 22, 28] and experiments conducted in dogs[17] suggest that, when possible, primary suture repair is the best treatment for complete rupture of the urethra. Through a midline symphysiotomy, the severed ends of the urethra are identified, débrided (1 to 2 mm), and sutured with about six interrupted polyglactin 910, polyglycolic acid, polydioxanone (PDS), or polyglyconate (Maxon), sutures over a urinary catheter, which remains in place for 5 to 7 days. Urethral anastomosis over an indwelling catheter produces less stricture formation and clinical and histopathological derangement than suturing without an indwelling catheter or maintaining an indwelling catheter.[15] With severe trauma to the urethra and periurethral tissue, accumulation of blood, urine, and devitalized tissue may preclude primary suturing. In these cases, delayed urethral repair is indicated. A urinary catheter is passed up the urethra from the penis and directed into the bladder. If necessary, a cystotomy is performed, and a smaller, more rigid catheter is passed from the bladder into the urethra to emerge at the traumatized area. The catheter tip coming from the bladder is tied to the tip of the urethral catheter. The urethral catheter is pulled through the area of urethral damage into the bladder. The catheter is anchored to the prepuce near the urethral orifice. This approximates the severed ends and diverts the urine. Close approximation is extremely important because it may result in healing with an adequate urethral lumen. If a stricture does develop, it is more easily correctable.[28]

The cystotomy incision is closed, the surgical site is irrigated with sterile saline solution, and one or more Penrose drains are placed in the wound. Wire fixation is used to stabilize the symphysiotomy defect, and monofilament nylon, polypropylene, or stainless steel wire is used to close the contaminated laparotomy wound. The intraurethral catheter can be left in place for 3 weeks or until delayed definitive repair is performed. A prepubic cystostomy catheter may also be used to divert urine during healing.[32] The Penrose drains are removed in 3 to 5 days or when drainage subsides. If healing is not satisfactory, definitive repair involving débridement and anastomosis or excision of the stricture and anastomosis can be performed once inflammation subsides.

Urethral Obstruction

Urethral obstruction generally necessitates some temporary measures to decompress the bladder as well as fluid and electrolyte therapy to correct metabolic abnormalities before definitive treatment. Cystocentesis and urinary diversion through catheters, either urethral or prepubic, are helpful lifesaving techniques. If the obstruction is associated with pubic fractures, exploration, reduction, and stabilization of the fracture are required.

*Brunswick Laboratories, St. Louis, MO.

If the urethra is traumatized, it is treated as previously described.

Urethral obstruction from fractures of the os penis (Fig. 107–9) can be treated by reducing the fracture by manipulation and splinting it with a urethral catheter.

Strangulation of the penis by foreign objects such as rubber bands or long hair, if discovered early, may require only removal of the constriction. If the penis becomes gangrenous, penile amputation, castration, and urethrostomy are necessary. Phimosis can lead to paraphimosis with strangulation and necrosis of the penis and urethral obstruction. This also requires penile amputation, castration, and urethrostomy.

Urethral obstruction can occur when the bladder is herniated into the inguinal and perineal regions. The bladder is decompressed by cystocentesis or urethral catheterization and returned to the abdomen. Definitive treatment in these cases is prompt hernia repair. Some degree of urethral obstruction may occur with severe prostatic disease.

Urethral Strictures

Urethral obstruction may be due to stenosis or stricture following urethral trauma or urethral surgery. Extrapelvic urethral strictures are best managed by urethrostomy as discussed earlier. Intrapelvic urethral strictures of 1 cm or less are best treated by resection and anastomosis. Larger defects require heroic measures, such as extrapelvic cystourethral anastomosis[14]; prepubic urethrostomy[19, 45]; or urethral prostheses using silicone rubber, silicone rubber and Dacron,[26] lyophilized human dural tubes,[12] or lyophilized vein homografts.[13] The prostheses serve as a guide for ingrowth of urethral mucosa. Lyophilized vein homograft is the most promising prosthesis. This graft causes very little tissue reaction and consequently little fibrous tissue. The prosthesis became lined with epithelium after 4 to 8 weeks, and eight of nine dogs showed no signs of obstruction during the 6-month follow-up period.[13]

Urethral Trauma Aftercare

Animals treated for urethral trauma often require extensive postoperative nursing care. To maintain urinary catheters without patients' cooperation requires the use of an Elizabethan collar, a body brace, or incorporation of the urethral catheter in an abdominal bandage. Premature removal of the catheter by the patient and subsequent replacement by the clinician can have disastrous consequences. Checking and maintaining the patency of the catheter are essential to ensure proper decompression of the bladder. Frequent urinalysis helps determine the status of the bladder and kidneys. Because of the increased risk of ascending infections with indwelling urinary catheters, closed urinary drainage systems, periodic urine cultures, and appropriate antibiotic therapy are indicated. Wound drains are protected with bandages, their exudate is monitored, and they are removed as soon as drainage subsides. Culturing of the drain detects persistent infection. Proper feeding and hydration encourage healing and speed convalescence.

PREPUBIC URETHROSTOMY

Prepubic urethrostomy results in the creation of a urethrostomy opening on the ventral surface of the abdomen cranial to the pubis and should be considered when an insufficient length of normal urethra is available to perform urethrostomy in one of the more commonly used sites. This technique has been used with considerable success in dogs and cats of both sexes.[3a, 7a, 17a, 17b, 19, 45] In cats and female dogs, the urethrostomy is created on the ventral midline, whereas in male dogs, the opening is placed in a parapreputial position. A technique has also been described in male dogs that results in the creation of a urethrostomy opening within the prepuce.[3a]

A standard surgical incision is made to the caudal abdomen (midline in cats and female dogs and parapreputial in male dogs). As the proximal urethra is identified and isolated, care should be taken to preserve the

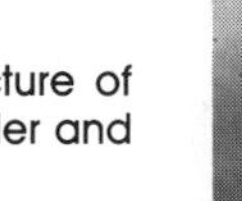

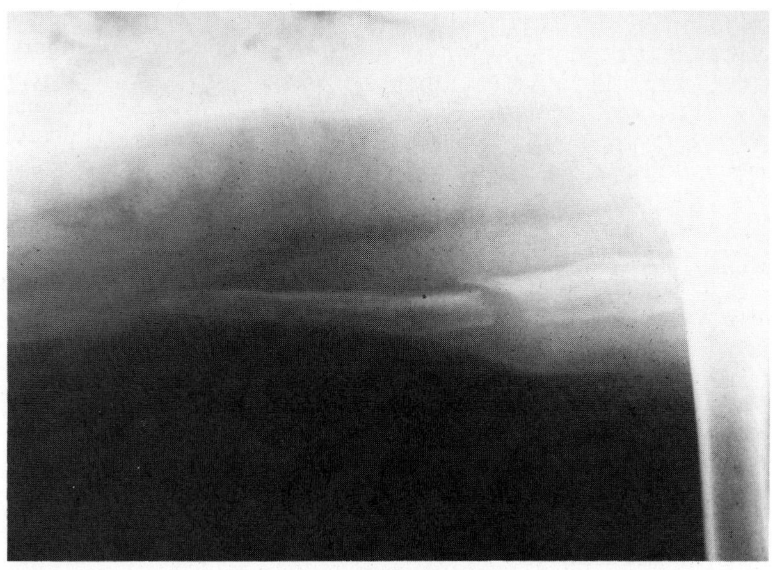

FIGURE 107–9. A lateral radiograph of a fracture of the os penis in a dog. (Courtesy of Drs. S. Kneller and J. Stowater.)

associated innervation and vascular supply. The maximal amount of normal urethra that remains should be retained. In females, the urethra should be severed as near the vagina as possible, and in males, the pelvic urethra should be dissected free of its attachments. The urethra is severed, and the distal end of the proximal portion of the urethra is brought through the abdominal incision.

The location selected for placement of the urethrostomy opening should result in the urethra passing across the abdominal wall in a gentle arc (Fig. 107–10). This prevents kinking of the urethra at the neck of the bladder. The exact location may depend on the length of proximal urethra available and the conformation of the animal. In a male dog with an enlarged prostate gland, a partial prostatectomy may have to be performed to prevent the presence of the bulky prostate gland within the subcutaneous space from interfering with satisfactory positioning of the urethrostomy. An intracapsular partial prostatectomy should be performed, preserving the capsule of the prostate and associated innervation. The adventitia surrounding the urethra is secured to the linea alba or subcutaneous tissues with two interrupted sutures of 3-0 or 4-0 absorbable material. The abdominal wall and subcutaneous tissues are closed in a routine manner, leaving an opening through which the urethra passes without being compressed. One to two centimeters of the urethra should remain exposed (Fig. 107–11). A 5- to 10-mm incision is made on the ventral surface of the urethra, and the wall of the urethra is sutured to the skin with 3-0 or 4-0 monofilament nonabsorbable suture in an interrupted pattern (see Fig. 107–10). The remainder of the skin wound is closed in a standard manner (see Fig. 107–11).

Although the urethra is usually shortened significantly, urinary continence will be maintained if the sphincter mechanism and innervation are preserved. If incontinence occurs, medical treatment, as described elsewhere in this text (see Chapter 103), may be tried. Urine scalding of the skin surrounding the urethrostomy opening has not been a significant problem, even in cats with large, pendulous inguinal fat pads. If this occurs, the skin should be treated with an appropriate ointment or lotion until the animal learns to assume the appropriate posture during micturition. Animals may be predisposed to bacterial cystitis after prepubic urethrostomy, and owners should be warned of this. I have seen urethral obstruction after prepubic urethrostomy owing to stricture of the urethrostomy opening, and urethral obstruction could theoretically occur owing to compression of the urethra as it passes across the abdominal wall or owing to kinking of the urethra as a result of severe shortening of the urethra or selection of an inappropriate site for the urethrostomy opening. There is usually adequate urethral tissue available to revise the surgery, and this should be done.

Prepubic urethrostomy offers a practical treatment alternative when function of the distal urethra is lost. Potential complications limit its application to those cases in which standard techniques for urethrostomy are unsatisfactory.

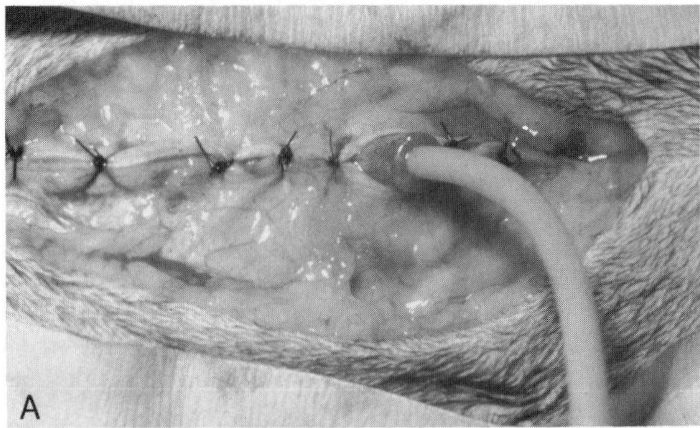

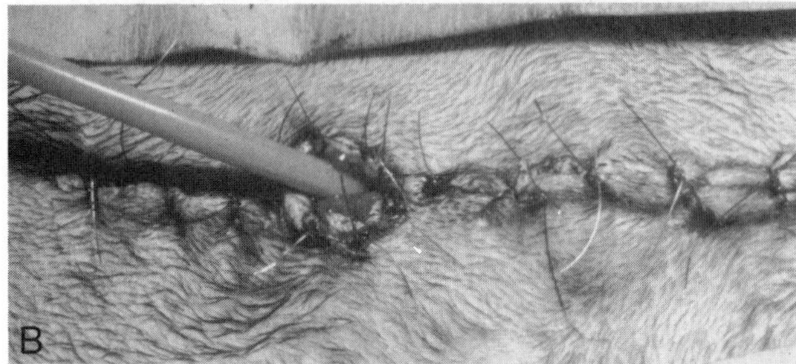

FIGURE 107–11. *A,* After the abdominal wall has been closed, 1 to 2 cm of the urethra remain exposed. *B,* Completed urethrostomy. A catheter is not left in place after surgery. (From Bradley RL: Prepubic urethrostomy. An acceptable urinary diversion technique. *In Problems in Veterinary Medicine: Urogenital Surgical Conditions.* J.B. Lippincott Co., Philadelphia, 1989, p. 120.)

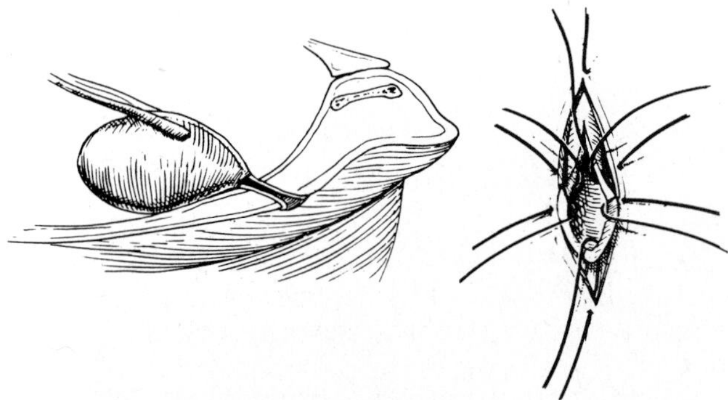

FIGURE 107–10. *A,* The path of the urethra across the abdominal wall should not create an acute angle between the urethra and the bladder. *B,* After an incision is made in the ventral surface of the urethra, the wall of the urethra is sutured to the skin. (From Bjorling DE: Traumatic injuries of the urogenital system. *Vet Clin North Am 14*:61, 1984.)

References

1. Andre PG, Jackson OF: An unusual cause of feline urethral obstruction. *J Small Anim Pract 11*:563, 1970.
2. Archibald J, Owen R ap, R: Urinary system. *In* Archibald J (ed): *Canine Surgery*. 2nd ed. American Veterinary Publications, Santa Barbara, 1974, pp 693–701.
3. Barrett RE, Nobel TA: Transitional cell carcinoma of the urethra in a cat. *Cornell Vet 66*:14, 1976.

3a. Bradley RL: Prepubic urethrostomy. An acceptable urinary diversion technique. *In Problems in Veterinary Medicine: Urogenital Surgical Conditions*. J.B. Lippincott, Philadelphia, 1989, p 120.

4. Brown SG: Surgery of the canine urethra. *Vet Clin North Am 5*:457, 1975.

5. Campbell MF: Anomalies of the genital tract. *In* Campbell MF, Harrison JH (eds): *Urology*. Vol 2. 3rd ed. W. B. Saunders, Philadelphia, 1970, pp 1573–1625.
6. Denny HR: An unusual cause of urethral obstruction in the dog. *J Small Anim Pract 13*:339, 1972.
7. Evans HE, Christensen GC: *Miller's Anatomy of the Dog*. 2nd ed. W. B. Saunders, Philadelphia, 1979, pp 578, 594.
7a. Ford DC: Antepubic urethrostomy in the cat. *J Am Anim Hosp Assoc 4*:145, 1968.
8. Goulden B, et al: Canine urethrorectal fistulae. *J Small Anim Pract 14*:143, 1973.
9. Hobson HP, Ader PL: Exstrophy of the bladder in a dog. *J Am Anim Hosp Assoc 15*:103, 1979.
10. Hobson HP, Heller RA: Surgical correction of prolapse of the male urethra. *Vet Med Small Anim Clin 66*:1177, 1971.
11. Johnston DE: Feline urethrostomy: A critique and new method. *J Small Anim Pract 15*:421, 1976.
12. Kelami A, et al: Replacement of the total resected urethra with alloplastic materials: Experimental studies of dogs. *J Urol 107*:75, 1972.
13. Kjaer TB, et al: Total replacement of part of the canine urethra with lyophilized vein homografts. *Invest Urol 14*:159, 1976.
14. Knecht CD, Slusher R: Extrapelvic anastomosis of the bladder and penile urethra in the dog. *J Am Anim Hosp Assoc 6*:247, 1970.
15. Layton CE, et al: Intrapelvic urethral anastomosis—a comparison of 3 techniques. *Vet Surg 16*:175, 1987.
16. Leighton RL: Surgical procedures. *In* Catcott EJ (ed): *Feline Medicine and Surgery*. 2nd ed. American Veterinary Publications, Santa Barbara, 1975, p 570.
17. Manziano CF, Manziano JR: A bladder prosthesis to relieve urethral blockage in the male cat. *J Am Vet Med Assoc 151*:218, 1967.
17a. McCully R: Antepubic urethrostomy for relief of recurrent urethral obstruction in the male cat. *J Am Vet Med Assoc 126*:173, 1955.
17b. McLaren IG: Prepubic urethrostomy involving transplantation of the prepuce in the cat. *Vet Rec 122*:363, 1988.
18. McRoberts JW, Ragde H: The severed canine posterior urethra: A study of two distinct methods of repair. *J Urol 104*:724, 1970.
19. Mendham JH: A description and evaluation of antepubic urethrostomy in the male cat. *J Small Anim Pract 11*:709, 1970.
20. Meyers RP, Deweerd JH: Incidence of stricture following primary realignment of the disrupted proximal urethra. *J Urol 107*:265, 1972.
21. Moore KL: *The Developing Human*. W. B. Saunders, Philadelphia, 1977, p 231.
22. Morehouse DD, et al: Rupture of the posterior urethra. *J Urol 107*:255, 1972.
23. Nickel R, et al: *The Viscera of the Domestic Mammals*. Verlag Paul Parey, Berlin, 1973, pp 318–328.
24. Osborne CA, et al: Congenital urethrorectal fistula in two dogs. *J Am Vet Med Assoc 166*:999, 1975.
25. Osborne CA, et al: *Canine and Feline Urology*. W.B. Saunders, Philadelphia, 1972, p 319.
26. Palleschi JR, Tanagho EA: Urethral tube graft in dogs. *Invest Urol 15*:408, 1978.
27. Peckman RD: Urinary trauma in dogs and cats: A review. *J Am Anim Hosp Assoc 18*:33, 1982.
28. Pierce JM: Management of dismemberment of the prostatic-membranous urethra and ensuing stricture disease. *J Urol 107*:259, 1972.
29. Piermattei DL, Osborne CA: Nonsurgical removal of calculi from the urethra of male dogs. *J Am Vet Med Assoc 159*:1755, 1971.
30. Polzin DJ, Jeraj K: Urethritis, cystitis, and ureteritis. *Vet Clin North Am 9*:661, 1979.
31. Raney AM: Radiographic findings immediately after urethral rupture: An experimental study and case report. *J Urol 116*:581, 1976.
32. Rawlings CA, Wingfield WE: Urethral reconstruction in dogs and cats. *J Am Anim Hosp Assoc 12*:850, 1976.
33. Rickards DA: The feline urethral shunt. *Feline Pract 6*:48, 1976.
34. Rickards DA, Hinko PJ: Feline urethrostomy: The Cleveland technique. *Feline Pract 4*:41, 1974.
35. Robinette JD: Silicone rubber prostheses for replacement of the urethra in male cats. *J Am Vet Med Assoc 163*:285, 1973.
36. Selcer BA: Urinary tract trauma associated with pelvic trauma. *J Am Anim Hosp Assoc 18*:785, 1982.
37. Smith CW, Schiller AG: Perineal urethrostomy in the cat: A retrospective study of complications. *J Am Anim Hosp Assoc 14*:225, 1978.
38. Tarvin G, et al: Primary urethral tumors in dogs. *J Am Vet Med Assoc 172*:931, 1978.
39. Ticer JW, et al: Positive contrast retrograde urethrography: A useful procedure for evaluating urethral disorders in the dog. *Vet Radiol 21*:2, 1980.
40. Waldron DR, et al: The canine urethra—a comparison of first and second intention healing. *Vet Surg 14*:213, 1985.
41. Weaver RG, Schulte JW: Experimental and clinical studies of urethral regeneration. *Surg Gynecol Obstet 115*:729, 1962.
42. Webber WJ, et al: Comparison of the healing of prescrotal urethrotomy incisions in the dog: Sutured versus nonsutured. *Am J Vet Res 46*:1309, 1985.
43. Wilson GP, Harrison JW: Perineal urethrostomy in cats. *J Am Vet Med Assoc 159*:1789, 1971.
44. Wilson GP, Kusba JK: Perineal urethrostomy in the cat. *In* Bojrab MJ (ed): *Current Techniques in Small Animal Surgery*. 2nd ed. Lea & Febiger, Philadelphia, 1983, pp 325–333.
45. Yoshioka MM, Carb A: Antepubic urethrostomy in the dog. *J Am Anim Hosp Assoc 18*:290, 1982.

CHAPTER 108 Feline Urological Syndrome

S. P. DiBartola and C. A. Tony Buffington

An account of the feline urological syndrome (FUS) was published in 1925.[81] The disorder is common and is characterized by urethral obstruction with sabulous material containing ammoniomagnesium phosphate. The roles of confinement and highly nutritious food have been discussed, as well as the common occurrence in Persian cats. Despite much research on FUS in the past 30 years, there is no consensus about the cause or even the definition of this frustrating disorder that may affect 1 per cent of the feline population. FUS may not be a single disease.[113] It may be considered synonymous with lower urinary tract disease[116–118] or an exclusionary diagnosis reserved for idiopathic lower urinary tract disease in cats.[6] The latter concept does not necessarily imply that FUS is a single disease, but it excludes other lower urinary tract disorders (e.g., bacterial urinary tract infection, urolithiasis, neoplasia, trauma, anatomical defects, and neuromuscular disorders of micturition) that can be ruled out by clinical evaluation. A problem-specific data base for FUS includes urinalysis, bacterial urine culture and sensitivity tests, and plain abdominal radiography.

Contrast radiographic examination of the lower urinary tract is necessary to rule out some lower urinary tract abnormalities (e.g., neoplasia, anatomical defects). The role of anatomical defects such as urachal diverticula has been debated[65, 117, 121, 123, 164] and will not be considered further here.

FUS is defined as idiopathic lower urinary tract disease characterized by dysuria and hematuria with or without urethral obstruction. Urethral obstruction is common in affected male cats and rare in affected females. When present, urethral obstruction in males usually occurs in the penile urethra. This definition excludes urolithiasis, which is characterized by organized concretions in the urinary tract. It implies that a reasonable diagnostic effort has been made to rule out other documented causes of lower urinary tract disease.

The obstructing material typically is unorganized and composed of crystalline and matrix components (Fig. 108–1). The primary crystalloid is struvite (magnesium ammonium phosphate hexahydrate). The origin, composition, and significance of the matrix component are unknown.[119] Using radial immunodiffusion, a unique protein was identified in the urine and urethral plugs of cats with naturally occurring FUS.[132] This protein was not found in the urine of cats with experimentally induced urethral obstruction. The etiological role of this matrix and any constituent mucoproteins in naturally occurring FUS remains unclear.

The majority of cats with signs of lower urinary tract disease have an idiopathic disorder. In a prospective study of 143 cats with hematuria and dysuria, 54 per cent had idiopathic disease.[86, 122] If cats with urethral plugs are included in the idiopathic category, 109 of 143 (76 per cent) had FUS. The question of why the term *canine urological syndrome* has not emerged in clinical veterinary medicine has been posed.[114] The answer seems to lie in the observation that the majority of dogs with signs of lower urinary tract disease do fall into categories that can be identified by a reasonable clinical evaluation. That is, most dogs with signs of lower urinary tract disease have bacterial urinary tract infection, urolithiasis, neoplasia, or some other identifiable disorder.

EPIDEMIOLOGY[161, 162]

The definition of FUS has varied in some studies, making it difficult to compare them. The *incidence* of a disease is the number of new cases per year divided by the average number of individuals in the population at risk throughout the year.[162] Several studies have attempted to determine the incidence of FUS, resulting in estimates of 0.34 per cent (confirmed cases) to 0.52 per cent (suspected cases),[44] 0.60 per cent,[154] 0.64 per cent,[155] and 0.85 per cent.[91] Thus, the incidence of FUS can be concluded to be somewhat less than 1 per cent.

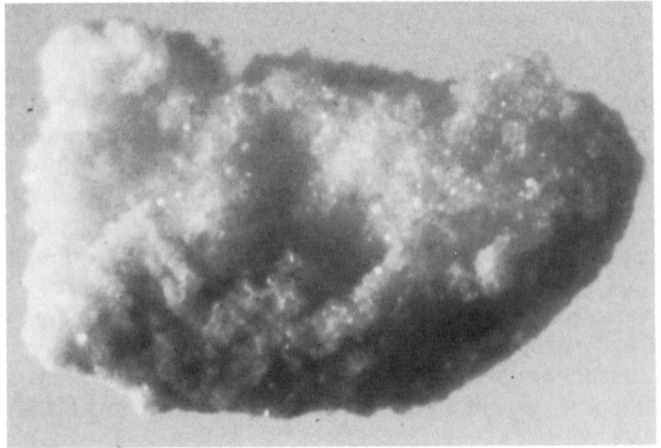

FIGURE 108–1. Urethral plug from a cat with feline urological syndrome.

The ratio of cases of FUS to all cases seen in a clinic or hospital is the *proportional morbidity rate*.[162] The proportional morbidity rate is quite different from incidence because its denominator is biased toward sick animals, those owned by people who are willing and able to bring their pets to veterinarians, and the clinical interests of the veterinarians participating in the study. Estimates of proportional morbidity have ranged from 1 to 6 per cent.[162] A frequently quoted "incidence" of 10 per cent for FUS was actually a proportional morbidity rate.[53, 162] Recurrence rates for FUS are high. In one study, 45 per cent of male cats experienced recurrence within 6 months of an initial episode of obstruction.[10] In another study, the recurrence rate for affected cats without obstruction was 39 per cent within 1 year.[7] Risk factors have been determined by case–control studies that compare the frequency of exposure with certain factors in affected cats and control cats to calculate odds ratios as approximations of relative risk.

Few epidemiological data support a change in the incidence of FUS with time.[162] Likewise, evidence about seasonal trends is conflicting. Some studies have found a higher frequency in winter,[9, 155, 156, 163] and others have found no evidence for seasonal variation.[33] Whether there is geographical variation in the incidence of FUS around the world also is unknown, but the incidence is similar in Great Britain and the United States.[44, 154, 156]

FUS can occur in any breed. Epidemiological studies have demonstrated that Siamese cats have a lower risk and Persian cats a higher risk compared with domestic shorthair cats.[33, 156, 163] It can occur at any age but is unusual in cats less than 1 year old and most frequent between the ages of 2 and 6.[4, 162] The risk for FUS is much greater in males than females when urethral obstruction is considered an essential part of the disorder, compared with FUS without regard to obstruction.[33] When FUS is considered without regard to obstruction, there is no difference in risk between males and females.[71, 156] There is no difference in the diameter of the urethra between castrated and intact male cats[69, 72, 110] nor in the frequency of urethral obstruction when castrated and intact cats were fed a diet that promoted FUS.[35] Adjustment for age is important because both neutering and FUS are age related. When adjusted for age, risk of FUS is greater in castrated males and spayed females than in intact cats.[44, 155, 163] Age at neutering is not important.[126, 155, 160]

Excessive body weight[155, 163] and decreased activity are associated with increased risk for FUS.[44, 126, 155, 158] No increased risk of FUS is noted when multiple-cat households are compared with single-cat households.[44, 126] Horizontally transmitted infectious agents are unlikely to be important in the etiology.

An increased risk of FUS has been reported in cats fed exclusively dry food, and the same or less risk has been observed in those fed canned and other types of foods.[44, 126, 155, 157] An analysis of these data has suggested a dose-response effect on risk with regard to feeding dry food.[161, 162] The risk of FUS increased with the numbers of meals fed per day but was greater with periodic feeding than with *ad libitum* feeding.[44, 155] In one study, cats that only had access to indoor litter pans had almost a four-fold increased risk of FUS compared with cats that urinated outdoors.[155]

FUS-prone cats are 2 to 6 years old, neutered, sedentary, and overweight. They eat dry food, live indoors, and use a litter pan exclusively. Risk factors, however, must be kept in perspective. The incidence of FUS in the cat population is probably less than 1 per cent, whereas many cats kept as companion animals are neutered, sedentary, overweight, kept indoors, and fed exclusively dry food. Furthermore, many commercial cat foods have been reformulated since the original epidemiological studies were conducted.

PATHOGENESIS

The lack of consensus about etiology and results of several epidemiological studies suggests that FUS is a multifactorial disorder.[126, 159, 161] Infectious agents and the relationship of water intake and diet composition to urine volume and struvite crystalluria have received the most attention in studies of pathogenesis.

Infectious Agents

Bacteria

Most cats with lower urinary tract disease do not have bacterial urinary tract infections. This conclusion is based on studies in which quantitative urine cultures were performed on samples collected by cystocentesis at the onset of clinical signs before manipulation of the urethra or initiation of therapy. Bacteria were isolated from urine of 1 of 48 cats;[8] in another study, no bacteria were isolated from the urine.[141] Other studies used qualitative culture techniques or urine samples collected by voiding or catheterization, and bacteria were isolated from 15 to 55 per cent of cats sampled.[33, 113, 131, 165] Furthermore, the nature of the disease being investigated was not always clearly defined in these studies. The role of bacterial urinary tract infection has been reviewed.[92] Results of studies designed to identify fastidious organisms such as *Mycoplasma* and *Ureaplasma* have been negative.[8, 107] Thus, bacterial urinary tract infection is not a primary factor in FUS. Bacterial urinary tract infection is rare in cats, partly because of the high osmolality of feline urine.[95] Bacterial urinary tract infection can be a complicating factor after urethral manipulation, use of indwelling urinary catheters, antibiotic therapy, and perineal urethrostomy.

Viruses

The role of viruses in FUS remains controversial because only one group of investigators has been able to isolate the putative cell-associated herpesvirus and experimentally induce disease in specific pathogen-free cats.[37–39, 129, 133] The strong cellular association of this herpesvirus and the possibility that overt clinical disease may only be manifested in a small number of cats at periodic intervals have been cited as possible reasons for the conflicting results regarding a viral etiology for FUS.[40, 87] Other investigators have been unable to transmit FUS by injecting urine from naturally affected cats into susceptible cats, and viruses have not been recovered from the urine of naturally affected cats in numbers different from normal cats.[8, 56, 73, 107, 146]

The possibility that a virus might be implicated in the etiology of FUS first was suggested when urethral obstruction developed in experimental cats injected with bacteriologically sterile urine from a cat with naturally occurring disease.[127–129] Ultimately, a calicivirus,[128, 133] a syncytium-forming virus,[41] and a cell-associated herpesvirus were isolated.[36] In specific pathogen-free kittens, the cell-associated herpesvirus caused disease by itself, but when combined with the calicivirus, the disease developed more rapidly.[37] Attempts to demonstrate viruses in naturally occurring FUS have been unsuccessful.[8, 35, 56, 73, 107, 146]

Cell-associated herpesvirus was inoculated into the bladder and peritoneal cavities of conventionally reared cats.[86, 87, 122] No signs of lower urinary tract disease developed, and the virus could not be isolated from urine. It was reisolated from bladder explants, and antibody titers were measured in inoculated cats. The cell-associated herpesvirus was antigenically related to bovine herpesvirus 4.[82, 88] Cats with naturally occurring lower urinary tract disease were negative for serum-neutralizing antibodies to the cell-associated herpesvirus.[89] In this same study, antibodies to the cell-associated herpesvirus were detected by indirect immunofluorescence in 31 per cent of cats with naturally occurring lower urinary tract disease and in 23 per cent of control cats.[86]

In one case–control study, no excess risk of FUS was observed in multiple-cat households.[126] This study failed to support a role for horizontally transmitted infectious agents in the etiology of FUS. Evidence to support a primary role for viral agents in the etiology of FUS is insufficient.

Struvite Crystalluria

The urethral plugs in cats with FUS typically contain struvite.[72, 130] In one study, 94 per cent of urethral plugs from cats with lower urinary tract disease were composed of more than 70 per cent struvite.[119] Struvite crystals have been observed in the urine of normal cats and those with FUS.[20, 130] There was no difference in the amount of struvite produced per day by normal or obstructed cats,[130] but struvite production was related to urine pH.[131] The pH range of normal feline urine is 6 to 8, and urine pH of normal cats was no different from cats with FUS.[20, 131] Struvite solubility is reduced in alkaline urine, and struvite crystals were common in urine with pH greater than 6.8.[20, 131] Despite these observations, many cats with FUS have acidic urine at presentation, and the amount of struvite crystalluria does not correlate with the occurrence of FUS. These observations do not preclude a role for struvite crystalluria in FUS, because urinalysis in cats examined for

FUS may not reflect the status of their urine between episodes. Urine pH affects struvite solubility because it determines the amount of phosphate present as HPO_4^{-2}, which releases a proton when it combines with Mg^{++} and NH_4^+ to form struvite.[1] The pKa for the reaction $H_2PO_4^{-1} = H^+ + HPO_4^{-2}$ is approximately 6.8. As urine pH increases above 6.8, the concentration of HPO_4^{-2} and the probability of struvite crystal formation increase.

Periods of high urine pH may allow sufficient time for crystal accretion. Cats maintained on commercial diets may have urine pH values greater than 7 by 4 hours after feeding, but after 12 to 24 hours of fasting, their urine pH typically is less than 7.0.[13, 28, 52, 145, 152] Anorexia develops after urethral obstruction, and affected cats often are presented for treatment more than 24 hours after their last meal. The probability that urine pH is acidic is thus increased. The presence of crystals in acid urine indicates that either the urine is not sufficiently acidified or insufficient time has elapsed for crystals to dissolve. A single determination of acidic urine does not imply that the urine was sufficiently acidic to be undersaturated with struvite before obstruction. The presence of crystals proves it was not.

Diet

The moisture content, mineral composition, nutrient content and digestibility, and caloric density of the diet may be important in the etiology of FUS. These factors influence drinking by cats, as well as urine volume, osmolality, pH, and mineral composition of the urine. Diet ingredients can affect the volume, osmolality, pH, and mineral composition of urine because of their chemical form, extent of gastrointestinal absorption, metabolism, and renal excretion. The method by which cats are fed (i.e., meals or periodic feeding compared with *ad libitum* or continuous feeding) also has been considered for a potential role in the etiology of FUS, based on the possible adverse effect of postprandial alkaline tide on urine pH and struvite solubility.

Moisture Content

Diet moisture content is related to the observation that cats fed dry food drink more water than cats fed canned food but that much of this water contributes to fecal moisture so that urine volume is lower and urine specific gravity higher in cats fed dry food.[2, 54] The urine concentration of all solutes, including potentially calculogenic crystalloids, depends on urine volume. Urine volume is influenced by the water and nutrient content of the diet, by drinking, and by water excretion via feces and the respiratory tract.[3]

Cats fed canned food and meat diets had higher urine volumes and slightly lower urine specific gravity values than cats fed dry food.[153] In this study, the ratio of total water to dry matter intake (TH_2O/DM) was higher in cats fed canned (3.7) than dry diets (2.0 to 2.4). In cats fed canned food, expanded dry food, and nonexpanded dry food, total water intake and urine volume were greatest in the cats fed nonexpanded dry food, whereas urine volume was lowest and fecal water highest in cats fed the expanded dry food.[75] TH_2O/DM was 3.2 on the canned food, 2.8 on the nonexpanded dry food, and 2.3 on the expanded dry food.

Total water intake and urine volume were greatest in cats fed canned and lowest in cats fed dry foods, whereas urine specific gravity was highest in cats fed dry and lowest in those fed canned food.[70] TH_2O/DM was 5.6 on canned, 2.8 on semimoist, and 2.4 on dry food. Cats fed dry food drank more than six times more water than cats fed canned food, but the total daily water intake (drinking water plus water contained in food) was not significantly different between groups.[143] TH_2O/DM was significantly different (3.9 in cats fed canned food versus 2.3 in cats fed dry food). Total water intake was lowest in cats fed dry diets.[78] TH_2O/DM was 1.8 for dry and semimoist food, 2.9 for canned food, and 2.6 for dry food with 4 per cent saline added (41 per cent water). In all of these studies, TH_2O/DM was greater when a canned rather than a dry food was fed to cats. High TH_2O/DM is correlated with low urine specific gravity.[3]

In one study, water content was irrelevant.[136] Total water intake was not significantly different when comparing three dry foods with three canned foods. Urine volume was greater in cats fed canned foods than dry foods, but one canned food with low fat content and digestible energy resulted in urine volume similar to that observed with dry foods. A high-fat, high-calorie diet may prevent FUS. TH_2O/DM for all three canned foods (including the one low in fat) was greater than 4, whereas TH_2O/DM was less than 3 for the dry foods.

The effect of water intake and urine volume on the development of FUS is incompletely understood. Water may be lost through urine, feces, and the respiratory tract, but some studies have measured intake only, and no studies have been controlled for differences in nutrient composition among diets. It is recommended that canned food be fed to cats with FUS to increase TH_2O/DM and decrease urine specific gravity.

Mineral Content

Ash refers to all noncombustible components of a diet and thus includes most of the mineral content without regard to the specific elements present. Ash does not cause FUS. Diets with 8, 22, or 30 per cent bone ash were fed to cats for 10 weeks without adverse effects, except for decreased growth rates.[32] Although some components of ash may be important in the pathogenesis of FUS, the term *ash* itself is of no value.

Dietary minerals that have been examined for their effects on the development of FUS include sodium, magnesium, calcium, and phosphorus. Addition of sodium chloride to the diet increases total water intake in cats.[2, 17, 64, 70] Adding salt to dry foods (3.6 per cent salt on a dry-matter basis) increased TH_2O/DM above 3.[70] Total water intake of cats fed dry food was only 49 per cent of that in cats fed canned food, but increasing the salt content of dry food from 1 to 2.4 per cent resulted in an almost linear increase in water intake.[2] In another study, sodium chloride added to a calculogenic diet doubled water consumption but did not prevent urethral obstruction.[64] The diet may be supplemented with salt to increase water consumption in cats, but it is unclear whether it prevents recurrence of FUS.

The importance of magnesium in the diet has been examined in many studies.* Diets high in magnesium have experimentally produced a disease resembling FUS in cats. Cats developed calculi when fed a diet containing 0.75 to 1.0 per cent magnesium on a dry-matter basis.[25, 102, 134] Calculi developed in cats fed both low and high concentrations of dietary phosphorus, and addition of increased amounts of calcium was protective when either the magnesium or phosphorus content of the diet was increased but not when both were increased.[102]

Taton and colleagues[152] evaluated the effect of magnesium on FUS in the presence or absence of 1.5 per cent ammonium chloride added to dry food containing 0.44 per cent magnesium oxide. The diet containing 1.5 per cent ammonium chloride maintained the urine pH of meal-fed cats at 5.9 ± 0.3, whereas the basal ration resulted in urine pH of 7.0 ± 0.5 (Fig. 108–2). Adding ammonium chloride had no effect on food or water consumption; meal-fed cats eating a commercial ration with 0.16 per cent magnesium but without ammonium chloride had urine pH values 6.6 to 7.6 for 9 hours after feeding. Seven of 12 cats fed a dry food with 0.44 per cent magnesium oxide had two episodes of urethral obstruction, and two developed struvite calculi.[151] Two of 12 cats fed the same diet with 1.5 per cent ammonium chloride each had one episode of obstruction, and one developed struvite calculi. Some cats that developed obstruction or struvite calculi were switched to the diet containing 1.5 per cent ammonium chloride. No further obstructions occurred, and existing struvite calculi dissolved. Previously obstructed cats placed on a commercial dry food containing 0.16 per cent magnesium again developed urethral obstruction. When switched to the diet containing 0.44 per cent magnesium oxide with 1.5 per cent ammonium chloride, no further obstruction occurred. This study demonstrated the effectiveness of 1.5 per cent ammonium chloride in dissolving struvite uroliths in cats fed a calculogenic diet in the presence of dietary magnesium.

*See references 15, 25–27, 50, 72, 80, 99–102, 134, and 151.

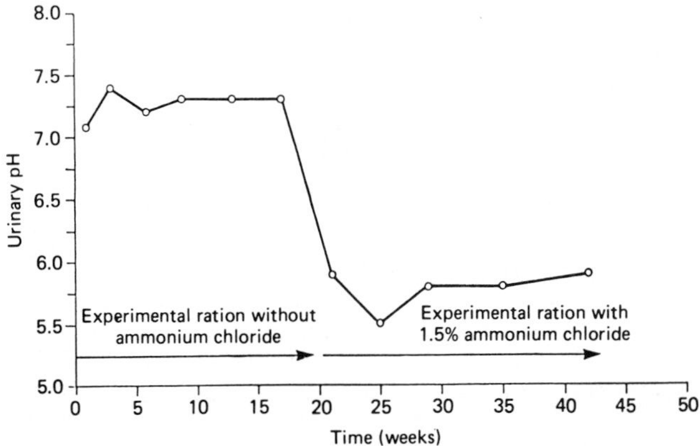

FIGURE 108–2. Effect of ammonium chloride feeding on urine pH in cats. (From Taton GF, et al: Urinary acidification in the prevention and treatment of feline struvite urolithiasis. *J Am Vet Med Assoc 184*: 437, 1984.)

In another study, male cats were fed purified diets with 0.05 per cent magnesium formulated to manipulate systemic acid-base balance.[29] These diets resulted in a mean urine pH of 6.1 in cats when ammonium chloride was added and 7.8 when bicarbonate was added. After 3 months, the urethra of one of the cats fed the bicarbonate-containing diet was obstructed by struvite crystalline material. By the end of 5 months, gross hematuria was evident in all cats fed the bicarbonate-containing diets. These cats were then fed a diet containing 4 per cent ammonium chloride. Hematuria disappeared from all cats, and no further urinary tract problems were observed.

Taken together, these studies suggest that the amount of magnesium found in commercial diets is safe if urine pH is maintained near 6. In contrast, if urine pH is too high, even normal amounts of dietary magnesium may cause increased risk of FUS. When previous studies relating FUS to dietary magnesium were reviewed, magnesium oxide or carbonate had been used as sources of magnesium. This could have affected urine pH as well as magnesium concentration.

To determine if the form of magnesium added had influenced previous experiments, three groups of adult male cats were fed purified diets with 0.05 per cent magnesium in the basal diet or 0.5 per cent in two high-magnesium diets.[15] Cats were fed a basal diet containing 0.05 per cent magnesium as magnesium sulfate or the basal diet with 0.45 per cent magnesium either as the oxide or chloride. In cats fed these diets *ad libitum*, urine pH values were 6.9 ($MgSO_4$), 7.7 (MgO), and 5.7 ($MgCl_2$), whereas meal-fed cats had 3- to 5-hour postprandial urine pH values of 7.5 ($MgSO_4$), 7.6 (MgO), and 6.4 ($MgCl_2$). Results demonstrated that the form of the magnesium salt has a profound effect on urine pH under both meal and *ad libitum* feeding conditions and that results of previous experiments using alkalizing salts of magnesium were confounded by the unrecognized effect of the source of magnesium on urine pH.

The role of magnesium was studied by feeding cats five diets varying in water and magnesium content.[50] Three of these diets were canned, with 0.72, 0.46, and 0.05 per cent magnesium on a dry-matter basis, and two were dry with 0.45 and 0.17 per cent magnesium. In the two high-magnesium canned foods, an attempt was made to correct for the alkalizing effect of added magnesium oxide by neutralizing the food with phosphoric acid. When fed the two high-magnesium canned foods, six of eight cats in each group experienced obstruction despite 12-hour postprandial urine pH values in the range of 5.4 to 7.2. Two dry foods containing 0.45 and 0.17 per cent magnesium without prior neutralization also were fed. Six of eight cats fed the high-magnesium dry diet developed urethral obstruction with 12-hour postprandial urine pH values in the range of 5.5 to 8.3. Cats eating the 0.72 per cent magnesium canned food and those eating the 0.45 per cent magnesium dry food had nearly the same magnesium intake.

None of these models truly represents naturally occurring FUS. The calculi in some studies initially were reported to be nearly devoid of ammonium.[27, 102] The cats formed organized calculi in the bladder and urethra and not the unorganized plugs typical of naturally occurring FUS. Furthermore, calcium and magnesium were added to the diets as the carbonate salts, resulting in higher urine pH, which could have had adverse effects on struvite solubility. In more recent studies, both the obstructing crystalline material and uroliths were composed of struvite.[15, 50, 80, 151] Finally, all commercial cat foods evaluated[26, 43, 100] contain less than 0.3 per cent magnesium, with average values of 0.16 per cent for canned, 0.14 per cent for semimoist, and 0.16 per cent for dry foods.[100] These quantities are much lower than those used in the experimental studies described earlier. The magnesium content of commercial cat foods is fairly consistent.[57]

The effect of dietary mineral salts on urine pH is due to the mineral ions present and to differences in gastrointestinal absorption of cations and anions. Absorption of magnesium and calcium from the gut is less than absorption of the accompanying anion. The absorbed anion also influences acid-base balance. Organic anions, oxides, and hydroxides consume protons during their metabolism to carbon dioxide and water, resulting in generation of bicarbonate and alkalization of the urine. Non-metabolizable anions, such as chloride, absorbed in excess of the accompanying cation are acidifying, because their addition to plasma results in loss of bicarbonate in the feces to maintain electroneutrality. Thus, it is important that minerals added experimentally to the diet have no effect on urine pH. If an acidifying salt of magnesium (e.g., $MgCl_2$) had been the source of dietary magnesium in earlier experiments, it might have been concluded that magnesium protects cats from FUS!

The quantity of magnesium required to saturate urine with struvite at alkaline pH is very small. As pH decreases below 6.4, the amount of magnesium required to saturate the urine with struvite increases exponentially.[14, 16] Conversely, as urine pH increases above 6.9, the amount of struvite that forms in the urine increases markedly.[131] When urine pH is alkaline, the amount of struvite formed in urine is proportional to the dietary magnesium concentration. At urine pH values less than 6.1, struvite does not form regardless of the magnesium concentration of the diet.[14, 16] Thus, the tendency of struvite to form is a function of urine pH. The magnesium content of the diet only becomes important when urine pH is greater than 6.1.

Nutrient Content and Digestibility

Constituents of foodstuffs exert major effects on urine pH. Sulfur-containing amino acids, phospholipids, and phosphoproteins acidify the urine, whereas salts of organic acids alkalinize it.[66] Salts of dietary organic acids, which come primarily from plant material, have an alkalinizing effect.

The effects on urine pH of three ingredients commonly used in commercial cat foods (poultry meal, meat and bone meal, and corn gluten meal) were studied in adult cats.[147] Corn gluten meal substantially reduced urine pH in meal-fed cats. The sulfur amino acid content of corn gluten meal is higher than poultry or meat and bone meal and accounts for the effect of corn gluten meal on urine pH.

The similar magnesium content and lower caloric density of dry foods has led to the suggestion that cats eating dry food of lower caloric density than canned food must consume more food to obtain sufficient calories and in doing so take in more magnesium, thus predisposing them to FUS.[101] Sauer found that urine volume was greatest and urinary magnesium excretion least in cats fed highly digestible diets regardless of whether a dry or canned food was fed.[136, 137] Reduced digestibility also increases fecal volume, resulting in more water in the feces and less in the urine.

Feeding Patterns

Feeding patterns can also affect urine pH. Feeding releases bicarbonate into the extracellular fluid as hydrogen ions are secreted into the lumen of the stomach. This postprandial alkaline tide causes transient alkalinization of the urine and may promote struvite crystal formation. Domestic cats do not eat single large meals when food is continuously available but generally consume 10 to 20 small meals during a 24-hour period.[104] This *ad libitum* feeding pattern attenuates postprandial alkalinization of the urine (Fig. 108–3).[14, 16, 101, 152]

Urine Acidification

A nomogram illustrates the relative importance of determinants of struvite crystallization (Fig. 108–4).[106] Lines A and B show that at pH 7, a tenfold change in magnesium, ammonium, or phosphate concentration changes the negative logarithm of the struvite activity product (pSAP) by one unit. In contrast, a tenfold change (line C) in hydrogen ion concentration changes pSAP by 1.8 log units, corresponding to a 60-fold change in the concentration of any one of its constituent ions. Thus, changing urine hydrogen ion concentration ten-

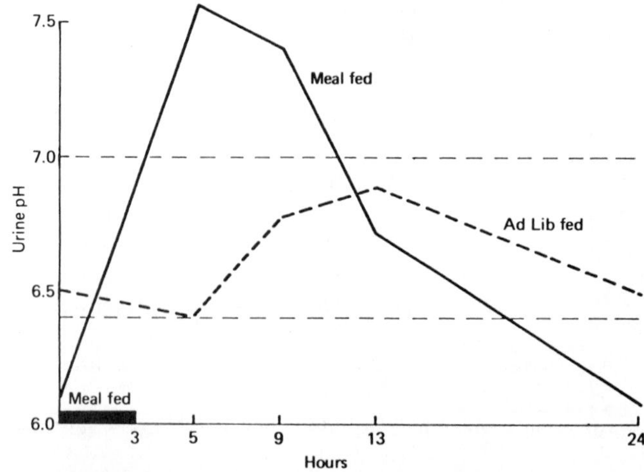

FIGURE 108–3. Variation in urine pH during the day with meals and *ad libitum* feeding conditions. (Modified from Lewis LD, Morris ML: Diet as a causative factor of feline urolithiasis. *Vet Clin North Am* 14:513, 1984.)

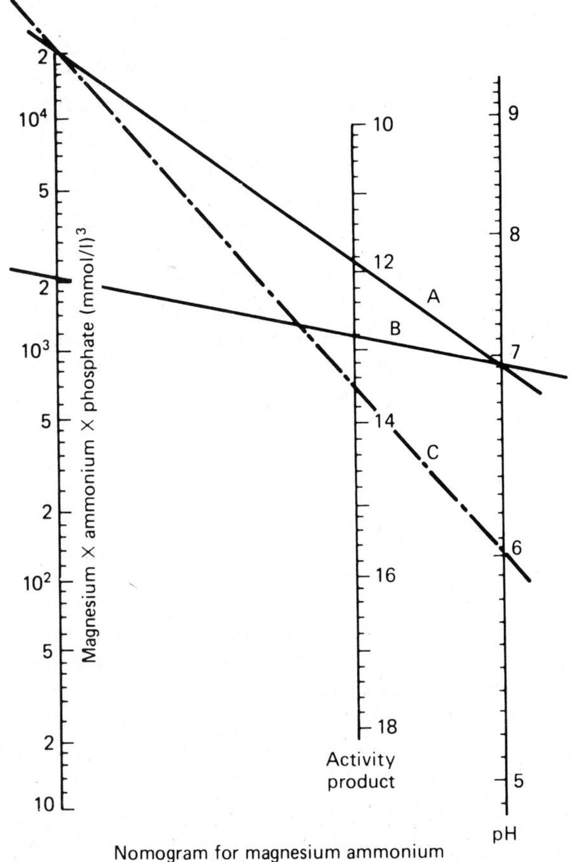

FIGURE 108–4. Nomogram for magnesium ammonium phosphate saturation. (Modified from Marshall W, Robertson WG: Nomograms for the estimation of the saturation of urine with calcium oxalate, calcium phosphate, magnesium ammonium phosphate, uric acid, sodium acid urate, ammonium acid urate and cystine. *Clin Chim Acta 72*:253, 1976.)

fold (1 pH unit) inhibits struvite precipitation six times more effectively than a tenfold change in the concentrations of magnesium, ammonium, or phosphate. A tenfold change in urine magnesium, ammonium, or phosphate concentration is greater than that likely to occur when diets formulated especially to decrease the risk of FUS are substituted for normal diets. The range of urine hydrogen ion concentration that may be produced by dietary manipulation is much greater, at least 1,000-fold (3 pH units).

Acidifying agents have been fed experimentally to determine their effect on urine pH. Chow and colleagues fed cats a calculogenic diet containing 0.75 per cent magnesium as magnesium oxide, and observed that 5 per cent alanine had no effect, 1 per cent *dl*-methionine did not prevent obstruction but prolonged the time until its occurrence, and 15 per cent alanine prevented obstruction.[27] Ammonium chloride (1.67 per cent), 1.67 per cent *dl*-methionine, 6.09 per cent monobasic sodium phosphate, and 4 per cent ascorbic acid were added to dry food of meal-fed cats.[28] Only the ammonium chloride resulted in urine pH of 6 or less 4 hours after feeding and maintained urine pH at 6 during a period of approximately 24 hours. Another previously used acidifier, ethylenediamine dihydrochloride, is ineffective at preventing recurrence of FUS[10] and is a weak urinary acidifier in cats.[48]

Acidification of the urine is not without potential toxicity. When fed experimentally to cats at a dosage of 0.5 to 1.0 g/kg/day (2.8 to 5.5 per cent of diet dry matter), *dl*-methionine caused hemolytic anemia, methemoglobinemia, and Heinz body formation.[105] Methionine (1.5 g/cat/day) has been recommended as a urinary acidifier.[99] For a 3-kg cat eating 60 g of dry matter per day, this constitutes 2.5 per cent of the dry matter. This amount of *dl*-methionine decreases food intake and weight gain in kittens.[42] Therefore, methionine may not be safe to use as the only dietary additive for urinary acidification. Kittens consuming very large amounts of a combination product containing ammonium chloride and *dl*-methionine lost weight, developed neurological abnormalities, and died.[12]

Ammonium chloride also is potentially toxic. Some cats given 1 g/day of ammonium chloride developed anorexia, vomiting, and diarrhea.[103] A diet containing 1.5 per cent ammonium chloride provides a cat approximately 800 mg of ammonium chloride per day. A study of this dosage given as powder or tablet to meal-fed cats showed that 4-hour postprandial urine pH was less than 6.[145] In this study, venous blood pH and bicarbonate concentrations were decreased to values at the lower end of the range reported for normal cats.[112] A combination product supplying 580 mg each of ammonium chloride and *dl*-methionine (equivalent to 0.82 to 1.51 per cent of each compound in the diet) given to meal-fed cats resulted in urine pH of 6, 4 hours postprandially.[144] The effect on venous blood pH and bicarbonate concentrations was more marked than with 800 mg of ammonium chloride alone, but the results were within the normal range.

Ammonium chloride (300 mg/kg or 400 mg/kg) was added to a commercial dry food that normally results in 4-hour postprandial urine pH values of nearly 8.[52] The lower dose did not significantly alter venous blood pH, carbon dioxide pressure, or bicarbonate concentration, and 4-hour postprandial urine pH was not decreased below 6.7 during the 4-week study. The higher dose significantly decreased blood bicarbonate concentration during the course of the study, and 4-hour postprandial urine pH was reduced to approximately 6. Neither dose had significant effects on appetite, body weight, urine specific gravity, or blood ammonia concentrations 30 minutes after feeding.

Additional concerns about chronic acidification are its potentially detrimental effects on renal function and bone development. Dietary potassium content also may be important because chronic metabolic acidosis can cause potassium depletion,[31, 45, 138] which can contribute to renal dysfunction. A syndrome of hypokalemic nephropathy occurs in cats fed an acidifying diet low in potassium.[34] Several cats had metabolic acidosis. Feeding a diet that has marginal amounts of potassium and that also contains excessive acidifying chemicals (e.g., *dl*-methionine) may cause chronic metabolic acidosis and depletion of body potassium stores. Potassium depletion and hypokalemia may lead to renal dysfunction characterized by chronic tubulointerstitial nephritis and increased urinary fractional excretion of potassium, further aggravating potassium depletion.

Acid-base balance is established at a decreased blood bicarbonate concentration during chronic metabolic acidosis by the participation of bone carbonate in the buffering of a chronic acid load. In young, growing,[77] and adult dogs,[18] the addition of ammonium chloride led to demineralization of bone. Chronic acid feeding also affects bone metabolism in both young and adult cats. Diets containing 3 per cent ammonium chloride slowed the growth of young cats, decreased blood pH and bicarbonate concentrations, and lowered urine pH. Urinary calcium excretion increased, and bone demineralization was observed.[13, 14, 16] Similar changes in blood and urine were found in adult cats fed diets containing 1.5 per cent ammonium chloride.[24] Urine pH increases as a function of age in cats fed a constant diet.[13, 14, 16] The onset of increased urine pH at maturity reflects decreased bone mineral accretion. When calcium and dibasic and monobasic hydrogen phosphate precipitate as calcium apatite, hydrogen ions are released, increasing net acid excretion and decreasing urine pH.[21] Skeletal growth in cats is completed by about 16 months of age, near the time when an increased risk of FUS has been described.[161]

If urinary acidifiers are used, the dose must be adjusted carefully for each cat because various diets have different effects on urine pH depending on composition (Fig. 108–5). Acidifying drugs or chemicals should not be added to diets already supplemented with acidifiers or to those that normally result in a urine pH of 6 within 4 hours of feeding. The required dose of acidifier may change if a cat's diet is changed. No specific dosage of acidifier can be considered safe and effective under all conditions. Acidifiers are not used in cats less than 1 year of age, because immature cats normally have acidic urine and addition of acidifiers can lead to failure of normal bone mineralization. Acidifiers are also avoided in older cats with hepatic or renal disease. A cat's urine pH is monitored 4 hours after feeding, and a sufficient amount of acidifier is given to maintain 4-hour postprandial urine pH near 6. When a cat has been treated with an effective dosage for several weeks, a venous blood gas determination or biochemical profile including total carbon dioxide content can be evaluated to be certain that the animal's acid-base status is still normal.

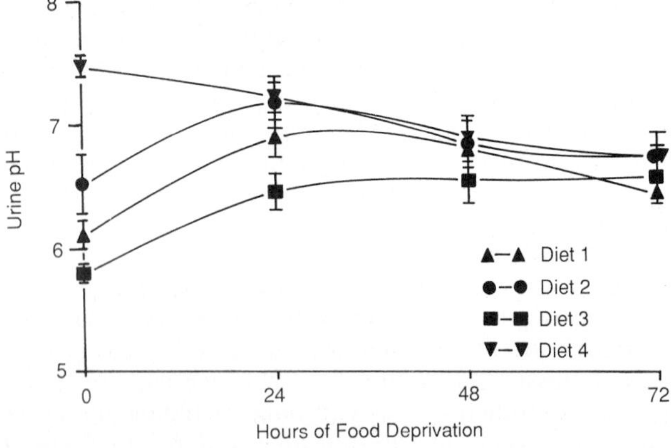

FIGURE 108–5. Effect of food deprivation on urinary pH of adult cats fed four different diets. Diets 1–3 were dry foods with various amounts of ammonium phosphate and calcium chloride, and diet 4 was a canned food. (From Buffington CA: Effects of age and food deprivation on urinary pH in cats. Proceedings of the 3rd Annual Symposium of the European Society of Veterinary Nephrology and Urology. Barcelona, Spain, 1988, pp 60–72.)

Based on the data reviewed in the preceding sections, we recommend that cats with FUS be fed a canned food that is high in digestible energy (greater than 4 Kcal/g dry matter) and contains less than 0.2 per cent magnesium. If a cat is meal-fed, its urine pH is monitored 4 hours after feeding to be sure that it is 6.0 to 6.5. If the urine pH is higher, ammonium chloride is administered with the food.

PATHOPHYSIOLOGY OF OBSTRUCTION

Bilateral ureteral obstruction causes acute renal failure and anuria. Renal blood flow and glomerular filtration rate are markedly decreased after 24 hours of obstruction. In rats, glomerular filtration rate is approximately 20 per cent of normal immediately after relief of obstruction that has been present for 24 hours.[83] If the obstruction is relieved after 24 to 36 hours, glomerular filtration rate returns completely to normal within 1 week.[109] If obstruction lasts longer than 72 to 96 hours, impaired renal function is permanent even after obstruction is relieved.[83]

The postobstructive diuresis that follows relief of obstruction is incompletely understood. Factors that contribute include volume expansion due to fluid administered during the anuric period, accumulation of poorly reabsorbed solutes during the anuric period, and a tubular defect in sodium and water reabsorption.[83] Impaired responsiveness of the distal nephron to antidiuretic hormone may contribute to the defect in urine concentrating ability in obstructive nephropathy. An acidifying defect and increased absolute and fractional excretion of magnesium and phosphorus have also been observed in the urine during the postobstructive phase.

DIAGNOSIS

Anamnesis

The history varies depending on the presence or absence of urethral obstruction. Cats without urethral obstruction are presented for evaluation of *stranguria, pollakiuria*, and *hematuria*. The owner may report that the cat has been in and out of the litter pan frequently, urinating in atypical places such as the bathtub or sink, and excessively grooming its genitalia. Cats with urethral obstruction make frequent unsuccessful attempts to urinate. It is important to determine a cat's posture in the litter pan, because many owners misinterpret the cat's behavior as evidence of constipation. Cats assume a more upright posture during defecation than during urination. The owner is questioned about the caliber of the urine stream, the amount of urine, and the appearance of the urine voided. Owners may observe that the cat strains to urinate but only dribbles urine. Pain is evidenced in some cats by reluctance to move, a hunched-up posture, and a guttural cry. When complete urethral obstruction has been present for more than 48 hours, signs of postrenal uremia such as anorexia, muscle weakness, lethargy, and vomiting occur. Cats die after 72 to 144 hours of complete urethral obstruction.

In an experimental study of urethral obstruction in male cats, clinical signs did not occur until after 24 hours of obstruction. Central nervous system depression, vomiting, weight loss, decreased food intake, decreased water intake, and hypothermia were observed after 48 hours.[49] Dehydration was estimated at 5 to 10 per cent of body weight after 72 hours. The duration of obstruction that resulted in severe clinical signs varied among cats (49 to 92 hours), possibly related to differences in bladder capacity. Severe clinical signs preceded the onset of hyperkalemia.[47]

Physical Findings

Physical examination findings depend on the presence or absence of urethral obstruction. An affected cat without obstruction is not systemically ill and has a small, firm, painful bladder. The bladder is examined for cystic calculi or neoplasia. Cystic calculi can be difficult to palpate because they often are wafer shaped. On the other hand, a small, firm bladder can be mistaken for a cystic calculus.

Physical findings in obstructed cats depend on the duration of obstruction. When a cat has been obstructed for more than 36 to 48 hours, the bladder is firm, distended, and painful, and there is evidence of dehydration (e.g., reduced skin turgor). Confusion can ensue when spontaneous rupture of the bladder has occurred. In this event, the cat is moribund but the bladder cannot be palpated. Fortunately, bladder rupture is rare. If hyperkalemia is present, cardiac arrhythmias may occur. In cats with urethral obstruction and hyperkalemia, heart rates were lower in collapsed cats than in alert ones.[124] Hypothermia is common in cats with prolonged urethral obstruction, and cats should not be placed on cold metal examination tables for prolonged periods. The distal portion of the penis is examined for discoloration and for the presence of a urethral plug that could be dislodged manually.

Laboratory Findings

In cats without urethral obstruction, the complete blood count and serum biochemical determinations usually are normal. The hallmark of FUS on routine urinalysis is hematuria without pyuria.[19] Likewise, bacteriuria usually is not observed. If bacteriuria or abnormal numbers of white blood cells are observed in the sediment, bacterial urinary tract infection is considered and urine culture performed. We routinely culture the urine of cats with lower urinary tract disease. In the absence of pyuria, this is a low-yield diagnostic test, but it ensures that bacterial infection is not overlooked. Urine for culture is collected by cystocentesis, and quantitative techniques are used, because contamination with urethral bacteria results in up to 1,000 colony forming units/ml in normal cats.[98] Results of urine culture usually are negative in cats when samples are taken before urethral manipulation and catheterization.[8, 141] Urine pH often is in the acidic range after anorexia of 24 hours or more.[13, 19, 20, 145] Struvite crystals may be observed in the urine sediment. Their presence is not diagnostic, because they can be observed in the urine of normal cats. Urine specific gravity values often are greater than 1.040. Osbaldiston and Taussig reported values from 1.020 to 1.070 and urine pH values of 5.5 to 8.0 in cats with FUS.[113]

Cats with urethral obstruction may have leukocytosis with a normal distribution of leukocytes or a stress pattern.[19] Increased hematocrit and total plasma protein concentration reflect hemoconcentration. Azotemia, hyperphosphatemia, hypocalcemia, hypermagnesemia, mild hyponatremia, metabolic acidosis with inadequate respiratory compensation, hyperproteinemia, hyperglycemia, and hyperkalemia may occur.[49] Hyperkalemia is the most life threatening, and is due to impaired renal excretion, tissue catabolism, and a transcellular shift of potassium from intracellular to extracellular fluid in response to metabolic acidosis. Hyperglycemia may be due to stress and release of endogenous glucocorticoids. Serum amylase, alkaline phosphatase, and alanine aminotransferase levels are normal.

These abnormalities occur in cats with induced[47, 49] and spontaneous[19] urethral obstruction. After relief of experimental obstruction, hyperkalemia resolved within 24 hours, but azotemia and hyperphosphatemia required 48 to 72 hours to resolve.[49] These findings are clinically useful. If a cat has a normal blood urea nitrogen level, after relief of urethral obstruction, hyperkalemia is not present. After relief of obstruction, cats that survived had polyuria, but nonsurvivors were oliguric. Thus, oliguria after relief of obstruction is an unfavorable prognostic sign. Postobstructive diuresis lasted approximately 3 days in cats with experimentally induced urethral obstruction. Repeated obstruction led to clinical signs of severe illness earlier, possibly because of reabsorption of urine from the damaged bladder mucosa or polyuria causing maximal bladder capacity earlier. In some studies, cats with urethral obstruction had glucosuria, attributed to decreased proximal tubular reabsorption from obstructive nephropathy.[19, 20]

Radiographic Findings[79]

Plain abdominal radiography rules out radiopaque cystic calculi and is part of the data base for cats with lower urinary tract disease. It is difficult to recommend contrast radiographic procedures in all cats with FUS, with the lack of cost–benefit studies.[6] Contrast radiography is reserved for cats with recurrent dysuria.

Pathological Findings

Lesions are limited to the urinary tract and consist primarily of erosion, hemorrhage, edema, and inflammation in the bladder.[108, 111, 113] In one study, cystic lesions could not be correlated with the clinical course.[113]

There is debate about the importance of renal lesions observed in cats with FUS.[90, 113]

TREATMENT*

Treatment of cats with FUS varies depending on the presence and duration of urethral obstruction. Treatment is described for uncomplicated (<24 to 48 hours), complicated (>24 to 48 hours), and uncomplicated unobstructed cases. No therapeutic measures are effective in treating nonobstructed cats with FUS or in preventing recurrence.[7, 125]

Uncomplicated Obstruction (<24 to 48 Hours)

Consideration must first be given to relief of urethral obstruction.[120] Anesthesia is almost always necessary, because cats with urethral obstruction of less than 24 to 48 hours duration usually are not ill. Adequate restraint can be achieved using ketamine (1 to 2 mg/kg IV) or sodium thiamylal (4 to 10 mg/kg IV). Alternatively, a 1:1 mixture of ketamine and diazepam (by volume) can be used at 0.1 ml/kg IV (equivalent to 5 mg/kg ketamine and 0.25 mg/kg diazepam). Acepromazine (0.1 mg/kg), instead of diazepam, can be used with ketamine (1 to 2 mg/kg IV). Tiletamine-zolazepam (Telazol, 1 to 3 mg/kg IV) may also be considered. Cats awaken from sodium thiamylal as a result of redistribution, but ketamine is eliminated primarily by the kidneys. Therefore, recovery may be prolonged if urethral obstruction cannot be relieved, and additional doses of ketamine should not be given. Some clinicians prefer rapidly acting inhalation agents (e.g., halothane, isoflurane) administered via a box.

The distal portion of the penis is examined, and an attempt made to manually dislodge obstructive material. This procedure prevents urethral trauma from catheterization and retrograde flushing. If the obstruction is not located at the tip of the penis, the next step is aseptic passage of a well-lubricated polypropylene urinary catheter (e.g., open-end tomcat catheter) and irrigation of the urethra. Instruments such as a blunt lacrimal or silver abscess cannula may provide more mechanical support but are likely to cause more urethral trauma. The penis is directed dorsally and caudally so that its long axis parallels the vertebral column to eliminate the natural curvature of the urethra.[6] Excessive traction on the penis is avoided because it narrows the urethral lumen.

The urethra is flushed retrograde with 0.9 per cent saline or lactated Ringer solution at room temperature. An acetate buffer (pH 4.5) has been used for irrigation,[74] but it may affect systemic acid-base balance if absorbed from the damaged bladder mucosa of a cat likely to have metabolic acidosis. Likewise, lidocaine is not infused into the bladder, because it can be toxic if absorbed systemically. The catheter can be lubricated with lidocaine gel. Careful attention to aseptic technique and a gentle approach may prevent later complications (e.g., bacterial urinary tract infection, recurrent obstruction due to extraluminal swelling).

The catheter is advanced to the site of obstruction, and retrograde flushing is performed. Simultaneously, an attempt is made to advance the catheter into the bladder. If the attempt is unsuccessful, the distal urethra is occluded and flushing continued to increase intraluminal hydrostatic pressure and force the obstructing material back into the bladder as the catheter is advanced. If hydropulsion is successful, the urethra and bladder are irrigated until the returning fluid is free of blood and crystalline debris. If hydropulsion fails, cystocentesis (using a 1.5-inch, 22- or 23-gauge needle attached via extension tubing to a three-way stopcock and a 20- or 35-ml syringe) is used to decompress the bladder and retrograde flushing is attempted again. Failure necessitates that the clinician rule out extraluminal factors, and contrast radiography may be helpful.[79] If these techniques are unsuccessful, emergency cystotomy with placement of a Foley catheter or perineal urethrostomy is considered.

If obstruction has been relieved by retrograde flushing, an indwelling urinary catheter may be placed,[94] to prevent recurrence, decompress the bladder, and monitor urine output. Indwelling catheterization contributes to continued urethral trauma and ascending bacterial urinary tract infection. An indwelling urinary catheter is not placed if minimal urethral trauma occurs during catheterization, an adequate urine stream is observed, hematuria is minimal, and the bladder returns to normal size after relief of obstruction. Indwelling urinary catheterization is considered if marked urethral trauma occurs during catheterization, an insufficient urine stream is observed, hematuria is severe, or the bladder fails to return to normal size after relief of obstruction. The indwelling urinary catheter is a polyvinyl catheter at least 15 cm long to ensure adequate drainage of the bladder,[96, 97] and it is placed for minimum time, preferably 24 hours or less. The catheter is inserted only until urine flow is observed, usually 9 to 12 cm in male cats.[94]

The duration of indwelling catheterization is minimized, because ascending bacterial urinary tract infection invariably occurs and additional trauma to the urethra and inflammation can contribute to recurrence of obstruction after removing the catheter. The consequences of open indwelling urinary catheterization in cats have been studied.[96, 97, 149] Polyvinyl catheters are more flexible than polypropylene catheters and are significantly less irritating to the urethral mucosa.[96] Indwelling urinary catheterization resulted in bacterial colonization of the bladder within 1 to 3 days, and diuresis increased bacterial counts by removing the antibacterial effect of high urine osmolality. Treatment with ampicillin during indwelling catheterization reduced the frequency of bacterial infection but resulted in highly resistant bacteria in 4 of 12 cats that developed infection despite its use.[97] An Elizabethan collar is required to prevent removal of the catheter. After the catheter is removed, urine is cultured and antibiotic treatment instituted if indicated.

Subcutaneous administration of a balanced electrolyte solution such as lactated Ringer solution at approxi-

*See references 5, 6, 55, 72, 99, 115, and 125.

mately 1.5 to 2 times maintenance (0 to 80 ml/kg/day) promotes diuresis and prevents early recurrence. No benefit was observed with subcutaneous fluid therapy of nonobstructed cats with FUS.[7] The bladder is palpated periodically to detect recurrence of obstruction or bladder hypotony. If the bladder returns to normal size after relief of obstruction, bladder hypotony is unlikely. The bladder is emptied by repeated manual compression if not empty, because some degree of bladder hypotony is likely to be present. Cats resent repeated manual compression of the bladder and can generate marked abdominal muscle tone to resist palpation.

The use of antibiotics after relief of obstruction is controversial. Antibiotics do not prevent ascending bacterial urinary tract infection with an indwelling catheter but result in marked antibiotic resistance of the offending organism.[97] In our opinion, antibiotics should not routinely be used after relief of obstruction. Rather, urine culture is performed after removing an indwelling catheter, and antibiotic therapy is based on urine culture and sensitivity test results. Urinary acidifiers are not used in cats that have been obstructed recently and have metabolic acidosis. Urinary antiseptics containing phenazopyridine[67] or methylene blue[142] are contraindicated because they cause methemoglobinemia and Heinz body hemolytic anemia in cats.

Anti-inflammatory drugs such as glucocorticoids and dimethylsulfoxide (DMSO)[11, 76] are controversial. Glucocorticoids may reduce intramural and periurethral swelling but are catabolic and may aggravate azotemia.[117] DMSO is used in human patients with interstitial cystitis[150] and in cats with FUS,[85] but no controlled studies have been performed. Local instillation of a 25 to 50 per cent solution of DMSO into the bladders of dogs was not associated with detectable side effects.[117] Instillation of 10 per cent DMSO into the bladder has been recommended for cats with chronic lower urinary tract signs refractory to other treatment.[135] Under anesthesia, 10 ml of 10 per cent DMSO is instilled into the bladder, allowed to remain for 10 minutes, and then removed.

Complicated Obstruction (>24 to 48 Hours)[5, 6, 68, 84, 120]

The major therapeutic goals are to correct hyperkalemia, acid-base imbalance, dehydration, and azotemia with appropriate fluid therapy and to relieve obstruction. Initially, blood is drawn for laboratory evaluation. An intravenous catheter is placed, and a crystalloid solution (0.45 per cent sodium chloride with 2.5 per cent dextrose solution) given.[19] A balanced electrolyte solution such as lactated Ringer probably is equally effective despite the fact that it contains 4 mEq/L of potassium.[5, 49] Rehydration is established during the first 4 to 6 hours of hospitalization by rapid intravenous fluid administration. Administration of a balanced electrolyte solution at 50 to 60 ml/kg/hour did not cause pulmonary edema in cats with experimentally induced urethral obstruction.[49] The importance of fluid therapy is emphasized by this study, in which 10 of 13 cats treated only by relief of obstruction died, whereas all 8 cats given parenteral fluids after relief of obstruction survived.[49]

An electrocardiogram is obtained. In cats with urethral obstruction, changes of hyperkalemia included prolonged PR interval, depressed or absent P waves, spiked T waves, prolonged QRS interval, and progressive prolongation of the QT interval.[124] If severe hyperkalemia is suspected, sodium bicarbonate may be administered intravenously. Alkalinization of the extracellular fluid causes a transcellular shift of potassium intracellularly as hydrogen ions leave the cells to titrate the administered bicarbonate. The dose of bicarbonate is calculated as 0.3 × base deficit (milliequivalents) × body weight (kilograms).[19] Half of the calculated dose was administered intravenously, and the remainder infused over 4 to 6 hours. In normal cats, 4 mEq/kg of sodium bicarbonate given intravenously resulted in hypokalemia, hypernatremia, hyperosmolality, and decreased ionized calcium concentrations.[22, 23] We usually use 1 to 2 mEq/kg of sodium bicarbonate, repeated as necessary based on the electrocardiogram and assessment of acid-base balance and serum potassium concentration.

Some clinicians have advocated administration of 0.5 to 1.0 units/kg regular insulin intravenously and 2 g of glucose per unit of insulin to translocate potassium intracellularly,[139] but this therapy is controversial.[46, 140] Relief of obstruction and parenteral administration of a balanced electrolyte solution were sufficient to decrease serum potassium concentration to normal within 24 hours.[47, 49] Therefore, glucose and insulin are not routinely used in the treatment of obstructed cats with hyperkalemia. Another less commonly used technique is to slowly administer 2 to 10 ml 10 per cent calcium gluconate intravenously. This antagonizes the adverse effects of potassium on the myocardium.[84] Routine administration of calcium gluconate is not recommended in the presence of hyperphosphatemia, because soft-tissue mineralization may occur in many organs, including the kidneys.[6] None of these methods has been evaluated experimentally.

Relief of urethral obstruction is performed as described for uncomplicated obstruction. Anesthesia is dangerous in severely depressed or moribund cats and is not used except when necessary to prevent undue urethral trauma. If necessary, the dose of anesthetic must be reduced. Affected cats are hypothermic, and towels or water-circulating heating pads are used to increase body temperature to normal.

An indwelling urinary catheter is placed, and urine output monitored. This approach is recommended because ensuing postobstructive diuresis can be marked, and dehydration occurs if urinary fluid losses are not replaced. As an alternative, frequent body weight determinations can gauge fluid replacement during postobstructive diuresis. This is less accurate but avoids complications of indwelling urinary catheterization.

After normal hydration is restored and hyperkalemia resolved, a balanced electrolyte solution is administered to provide insensible needs (approximately 20 ml/kg/day) plus a volume equal to the daily urine output. Postobstructive diuresis usually lasts 2 to 5 days and is self-limiting. After 24 to 72 hours, blood urea nitrogen and serum creatinine concentrations return to normal, and fluids are gradually decreased to avoid perpetuating diuresis. If the volume administered is inadequate, a cat loses weight, and prerenal azotemia may complicate recovery. If intravenous fluid therapy and urine output monitoring are not possible after the first 24 hours, subcutaneous administration of fluids and serial monitoring of body weight can be used. Urinary acidifiers and nephrotoxic antibiotics (e.g., aminoglycosides) are avoided.

Hypokalemia occurs frequently during postobstructive diuresis and may be treated with supplemental potassium chloride (Table 108–1).[58] If serum potassium concentration is unknown, 20 to 25 mEq potassium chloride is added per liter to prevent hypokalemia.

Unobstructed Cat

There is no evidence that antibiotics are useful in initial treatment of FUS. In one study, FUS was self-limiting in unobstructed cats during a 5-day period, regardless of therapy with chloramphenicol or placebo.[7] Despite this observation, antibiotics are widely used in practice. It is important that clinical studies be properly controlled before concluding that a particular treatment is beneficial, because FUS without obstruction is a self-limiting disorder.[7]

No commercial cat foods cause FUS, nor do any specific foods prevent recurrence of naturally occurring FUS.[6, 7] It is recommended that cats with FUS be fed a canned food that is high in digestible energy (> 4 Kcal/g dry matter) and low in magnesium (< 0.2 percent on a dry-matter basis) on a meal-fed basis. If either the owner or the cat is unwilling to switch to canned food, water can be added directly to the dry food to increase the cat's water intake. Water consumption also may be encouraged by providing fresh water daily and, if necessary, by adding salt to the food. Cats tolerate as much as 4 percent salt in their food.[70, 78]

Cats fed *ad libitum* have less variable urine pH values than cats that are fed meals (Fig. 108–3). One concern about *ad libitum* feeding has been the potential protraction of the alkaline tide.[99–101] In one study, periodic feeding was associated with low urine pH at the same time that urinary mineral concentration, including magnesium, was highest, and this was suggested as a slight advantage for periodic feeding.[51] Urinary acidifiers may not be needed, because some foods promote acidic urine. If a cat is fed meals, urine pH is checked 4 hours after feeding to be sure that it is 6.0 to 6.5. Urine pH of 6.0 to 6.5 within 4 hours of feeding is desirable, and if necessary, ammonium chloride may be administered at the lowest dosage possible to render the urine pH 6.0 to 6.5 within 4 hours of feeding. The required dosage varies depending on the diet but is about 100 to 400 mg/kg/day.[52, 145] Ammonium chloride is given with meals or mixed into the food to antagonize postprandial alkaline tide.

The litter pan is kept clean at all times to encourage frequent urination. Owners are informed of the high recurrence rate of FUS (approximately 40 per cent) and are instructed to observe their cat's urination carefully to detect obstruction early.

TABLE 108–1. POTASSIUM SUPPLEMENTATION DURING POSTOBSTRUCTIVE DIURESIS

Serum K^+ (mEq/L)	mEq KCl to Add to 250 ml Fluid	Maximal Fluid Infusion Rate (ml/kg/hour)
< 2.0	20	6
2.1–2.5	15	8
2.6–3.0	10	12
3.1–3.5	7	16

From Greene RW, Scott RC: Lower urinary tract disease. *In* Ettinger SJ (ed): *Textbook of Veterinary Internal Medicine.* W. B. Saunders, Philadelphia, 1975, p 1572.

COMPLICATIONS OF FELINE UROLOGICAL SYNDROME

Increased Outlet Resistance

Increased outlet resistance is suspected when manual compression of the bladder results in a weak urine stream.[93] It is first necessary to rule out and treat early recurrence of intraluminal obstruction caused by additional crystalline, mucoid, or inflammatory debris. If intraluminal obstruction is not present, extraluminal obstruction caused by edema, inflammation, and hemorrhage is considered. If such changes are likely, an anti-inflammatory dose of glucocorticoids (e.g., 0.5 to 1.0 mg/kg prednisolone) may be beneficial if a cat is not azotemic and does not have bacterial urinary tract infection or an indwelling urinary catheter.

Another extraluminal cause of obstruction is urethral spasm. Treatment of functional outlet resistance can be attempted with alpha-adrenergic blocking drugs such as phenoxybenzamine or acepromazine. The dose of phenoxybenzamine is gradually increased in 2.5-mg increments as necessary from 2.5 mg to 10 mg PO once daily over several days. Alternatively, acepromazine can be given (0.2 mg/kg SC once or twice daily) and, if effective, can be continued at home (1.25 mg PO once daily) for a few days. A large portion of the feline urethra contains striated muscle,[30] and diazepam (2.5 to 5.0 mg PO) may be helpful if this portion of the urethra is responsible for increased outlet resistance. The side effects of phenoxybenzamine include hypotension, reflex tachycardia, and miosis. Acepromazine may cause hypotension and excessive sedation. Diazepam also may cause sedation, but its effects are brief after oral administration.

Propantheline (7.5 mg PO every 72 hours) has been administered for bladder or urethral spasm. It impairs transmission at postganglionic parasympathetic receptors and has little direct effect on smooth muscle.[117] Thus, it has the disadvantage of impairing detrusor contractility despite any beneficial effect it might have to relax urethral smooth muscle. Propantheline was no more effective than a placebo in treatment of unobstructed cats with FUS.[7] There are no other controlled studies of pharmacological manipulation of bladder and urethral tone in cats with FUS. If pharmacological approaches fail, consideration must be given to temporary indwelling catheterization of the bladder.

Detrusor Hypotony

Abnormal detrusor function due to prolonged overdistension of the bladder may be the result of damage to tight junctions between smooth-muscle cells and nerve terminals, thus preventing effective spread of neuronal impulses.[93] Affected cats have large, flaccid bladders that can be expressed manually without excessive force. Detrusor hypotony can be treated with bethanechol (1.25 to 2.5 mg PO TID) for a few days. The side effects of bethanechol include lacrimation, salivation, abdominal cramping, and diarrhea. It is never used with increased outlet resistance unless treatment with phenoxybenzamine has already been instituted. Atropine is the antidote for bethanechol toxicity.

Bacterial Urinary Tract Infection

Bacterial urinary tract infection occurs in 40 to 60 per cent of cats with recurrent urethral obstruction[92] and is a serious complication of indwelling urethral catheterization.[97] It also can complicate perineal urethrostomy because of reduced urethral tone and impaired host defenses.[61] Bacterial urinary tract infection is treated for 2 to 3 weeks with appropriate antibiotics based on urine culture and sensitivity test results.

PERINEAL URETHROSTOMY

Perineal urethrostomy is usually recommended when a male cat experiences repeated episodes of urethral obstruction despite conservative medical treatment directed at prevention. Perineal urethrostomy should not be considered without first performing contrast radiography to rule out another site of obstruction.[79] Perineal urethrostomy prevents recurrence of urethral obstruction in most instances but does not prevent recurrence of clinical signs of lower urinary tract disease. In one study, recurrent dysuria occurred in almost one-third of cats having had perineal urethrostomy.[59]

Bacterial urinary tract infection occurs after perineal urethrostomy.[59, 149] In one study, it was observed in 20 of 75 cats (26 per cent).[149] In another study, bacterial urinary tract infection occurred in 8 of 35 cats (23 per cent) previously treated by perineal urethrostomy.[59] Of the eight cats with documented bacterial urinary tract infection only two had clinical signs of lower urinary tract disease.

Perineal urethrostomy alters urethral pressure profiles in male cats so that protective host defenses may be impaired. The mean maximum urethral closure pressure and mean functional profile length were significantly decreased 1 and 3 weeks after perineal urethrostomy in male cats, and these changes were associated with a loss of periurethral striated muscle activity on electromyography.[62] One year later, urethral closure pressures returned to within the normal range in 11 of 18 cats evaluated, and the loss of striated muscle activity was reversible.[63] Bacterial urinary tract infection was found in 2 of the 11 cats with normal urethral pressure profiles and in 4 of the 7 with abnormal profiles. Alterations in urethral pressure profile after perineal urethrostomy can also be associated with urinary incontinence.[60]

Postoperative strictures may also complicate perineal urethrostomy; most occurred between 2 and 12 weeks after surgery.[148] Postoperative use of indwelling catheters increased the frequency of stricture formation, whereas Elizabethan collars reduced the occurrence.

PREVENTION OF FELINE UROLOGICAL SYNDROME

No studies of specific dietary alterations or drug treatments have been shown to prevent recurrence of naturally occurring FUS in cats. The following conservative recommendations are suggested for unobstructed cats:

1. Change the diet to a canned cat food that is high in digestible energy (>4 Kcal/g dry matter) and less than 0.2 per cent magnesium on a dry-matter basis.
2. Monitor urine pH 4 hours after feeding and add ammonium chloride to the food only as needed to maintain 4-hour postprandial urine pH 6.0 to 6.5.
3. Measure urine specific gravity and consider adding water directly to the food if urine specific gravity is consistently greater than 1.050.
4. Provide fresh water at all times.
5. Clean the litter pan daily.
6. Avoid obesity by limiting caloric intake.

There are no data on cats with naturally occurring disease to support these recommendations.

References

1. Abbona F, Boistelle R: Nucleation of struvite ($MgNH_4PO_4 \cdot 6H_2O$) single crystals and aggregates. *Crystal Res Technol 20*:133, 1985.
2. Anderson RS: Water balance in the dog and cat. *J Small Anim Pract 23*:588, 1982.
3. Anderson RS: Fluid balance and diet. Proceedings of the Kal Kan Symposium for the Treatment of Small Animal Diseases. Kal Kan Foods, Vernon, CA, 1983, pp 19–25.
4. Barker J, Povey RC: The feline urolithiasis syndrome: A review and an inquiry into the alleged role of dry cat foods in its aetiology. *J Small Anim Pract 14*:445, 1973.
5. Barsanti JA, Finco DR: Management of postrenal uremia. *Vet Clin North Am 14*:609, 1984.
6. Barsanti JA, Finco DR: Feline urologic syndrome. *In* Breitschwerdt EB (ed): *Contemporary Issues in Small Animal Practice: Nephrology and Urology*. Churchill Livingstone, New York, 1986, pp 43–74.
7. Barsanti JA, et al: Feline urologic syndrome: Further investigations into therapy. *J Am Anim Hosp Assoc 18*:387, 1982.
8. Barsanti JA, et al: Feline urologic syndrome: Further investigations into etiology. *J Am Anim Hosp Assoc 18*:391, 1982.
9. Bernard MA: Feline urologic syndrome: A study of seasonal influence, frequency of repeat visits and comparison of treatments. *Can Vet J 19*:284, 1978.
10. Bovee KC, et al: Recurrence of feline urethral obstruction. *J Am Vet Med Assoc 174*:93, 1979.
11. Brayton CF: Dimethylsulfoxide (DMSO): A review. *Cornell Vet 76*:61, 1986.
12. Brown JE, Fox LM: Ammonium chloride/methionine toxicity in kittens. *Feline Pract 14*:16, 1984.
13. Buffington CA: Effects of age and food deprivation on urinary pH in cats. Proceedings of the 3rd Annual Symposium of the European Society of Veterinary Nephrology and Urology. Barcelona, Spain, 1988, pp 60–72.
14. Buffington CA: Feline struvite urolithiasis: Effect of diet. Proceedings of the 3rd Annual Symposium of the European Society of Veterinary Nephrology and Urology. Barcelona, Spain, 1988, pp 73–112.

15. Buffington CA, et al: Feline struvite urolithiasis: Magnesium effect depends on urinary pH. *Feline Pract 15*:29, 1985.
16. Buffington CA, et al: The role of diet in feline struvite urolithiasis syndrome. *In* Burger IH, Rivers JPW (eds): *Nutrition of the Dog and Cat.* Waltham Symposium Number 7. Cambridge University Press, Cambridge, MA, 1989, pp 357–380.
17. Burger IH, et al: Nutritional factors affecting water balance in the dog and cat. *In* Anderson RS (ed): *Nutrition of the Dog and Cat.* Pergamon Press, Elmsford, NY, 1980, pp 145–156.
18. Burnell JM: Changes in bone sodium and carbonate in metabolic acidosis and alkalosis in the dog. *J Clin Invest 50*:327, 1971.
19. Burrows CF, Bovee KC: Characterization and treatment of acid-base and renal defects due to urethral obstruction in male cats. *J Am Vet Med Assoc 172*:801, 1978.
20. Carbone MG: Phosphocrystalluria and urethral obstruction in the cat. *J Am Vet Med Assoc 147*:1195, 1965.
21. Chan JCM: The influence of dietary intake on endogenous acid production. *Nutr Metab 16*:1, 1974.
22. Chew DJ, et al: Effect of sodium bicarbonate infusions on ionized calcium and total calcium concentrations in serum of clinically normal cats. *Am J Vet Res 50*:145, 1989.
23. Chew DJ, et al: The effect of sodium bicarbonate infusion on serum osmolality, electrolyte concentrations, and blood gas tensions in cats. *Am J Vet Res 52*:12, 1991.
24. Ching SV, et al: The effect of chronic dietary acidification using ammonium chloride on acid-base and mineral metabolism in the adult cat. *J Nutr 119*:902, 1989.
25. Chow FC: Dietary mineral effects on feline urolithiasis. Proceedings of the Kal Kan Symposium for the Treatment of Dog and Cat Diseases. Kal Kan Foods, Vernon, CA, 1977, pp 36–39.
26. Chow FC, et al: Feline urolithiasis/cat foods: Concentration of calcium, magnesium, phosphate and chloride in various cat foods and their relationship to feline urolithiasis. *Feline Pract 5*:15, 1975.
27. Chow FC, et al: Effect of dietary additives on experimentally-produced feline urolithiasis. *Feline Pract 6*:51, 1976.
28. Chow FHC, et al: Effect of dietary ammonium chloride, dl-methionine, sodium phosphate and ascorbic acid on urinary pH and electrolyte concentrations of male cats. *Feline Pract 8*:29, 1978.
29. Cook NE: The importance of urinary pH in the prevention of feline urologic syndrome. *Pet Food Industry 27*:24, 1985.
30. Cullen WC, et al: Morphometry of the male feline pelvic urethra. *J Urol 129*:186, 1983.
31. DeSousa RC, et al: Renal regulation of acid-base equilibrium during chronic administration of mineral acid. *J Clin Invest 53*:465, 1974.
32. Dickinson CD, Scott PP: Failure to produce urinary calculi in kittens by the addition of mineral salts derived from bone-meal to the diet. *Vet Rec 68*:858, 1956.
33. Dorn CR, et al: Factors affecting risk of urolithiasis-cystitis-urethritis in cats. *Am J Vet Res 34*:433, 1973.
34. Dow SW, et al: Potassium depletion in cats: Renal and dietary influences. *J Am Vet Med Assoc 191*:1569, 1987.
35. Duch DS, et al: The effect of castration and body weight on the occurrence of the feline urological syndrome. *Feline Pract 8*:35, 1978.
36. Fabricant CG, Gillespie JH: Identification and characterization of a second feline herpesvirus. *Infect Immun 9*:460, 1974.
37. Fabricant CG: Herpesvirus induced urolithiasis in specific pathogen-free male cats. *Am J Vet Res 38*:1837, 1977.
38. Fabricant CG: Viruses associated with urinary tract disease. *Vet Clin North Am 9*:631, 1979.
39. Fabricant CG: Herpesvirus induced feline urolithiasis—a review. *Comp Immun Microbiol Infect Dis 1*:121, 1979.
40. Fabricant CG: The feline urologic syndrome induced by infection with a cell-associated herpesvirus. *Vet Clin North Am 14*:493, 1984.
41. Fabricant CG, et al: Feline viruses XI. Isolation of a virus similar to myxovirus from cats in which urolithiasis was experimentally induced. *Cornell Vet 59*:667, 1969.
42. Fau D, et al: Effects of excess methionine in the kitten. *Fed Proc 42*:542, 1983.
43. Feldmann BM, et al: Dietary minerals and the feline urological syndrome. *Feline Pract 7*:39, 1977.
44. Fennell C: Some demographic characteristics of the domestic cat population in Great Britain with particular reference to feeding habits and the incidence of the feline urological syndrome. *J Small Anim Pract 16*:775, 1975.
45. Fettman MJ: Feline kaliopenic polymyopathy/nephropathy syndrome. *Vet Clin North Am 19*:415, 1989.
46. Finco DR: Polemical forum. *J Am Anim Hosp Assoc 12*:675, 1976.
47. Finco DR: Induced feline urethral obstruction: Response of hyperkalemia to relief of obstruction and administration of parenteral electrolyte solution. *J Am Anim Hosp Assoc 12*:198, 1976.
48. Finco DR: Efficacy of ethylenediamine dihydrochloride in dogs and cats. *Am J Vet Res 42*:670, 1981.
49. Finco DR, Cornelius LM: Characterization and treatment of water, electrolyte, and acid-base imbalances of induced urethral obstruction in the cat. *Am J Vet Res 38*:823, 1977.
50. Finco DR, et al: Characterization of magnesium-induced urinary disease in the cat and comparison with feline urologic syndrome. *Am J Vet Res 46*:391, 1985.
51. Finco DR, et al: Food and water intake and urine composition in cats: Influence of continuous versus periodic feeding. *Am J Vet Res 47*:1638, 1986.
52. Finco DR, et al: Ammonium chloride as a urinary acidifier in cats: Efficacy, safety and rationale for its use. *Mod Vet Pract 67*:537, 1986.
53. Foster SJ: The "urolithiasis" syndrome in male cats: A statistical analysis of the problem, with clinical observations. *J Small Anim Pract 8*:207, 1967.
54. Gaskell CJ: Nutrition in diseases of the urinary tract in the dog and cat. *Vet Annu 25*:383, 1985.
55. Gaskell CJ, et al: Clinical management of the feline urological syndrome. *J Small Anim Pract 19*:301, 1978.
56. Gaskell RM, et al: Studies on a possible viral etiology for feline urological syndrome. *Vet Rec 105*:243, 1979.
57. Graser DH, Lewis LD: The consistency of dietary minerals in commercial cat foods and their relationship to feline urolithiasis. *Feline Pract 11*:41, 1981.
58. Greene RW, Scott RC: Lower urinary tract disease. *In* Ettinger SJ (ed): *Textbook of Veterinary Internal Medicine.* W. B. Saunders, Philadelphia, 1975, p 1572.
59. Gregory CR, Vasseur PB: Longterm examination of cats with perineal urethrostomy. *Vet Surg 12*:210, 1983.
60. Gregory CR: Electromyographic and urethral pressure profilometry. *Vet Clin North Am 14*:567, 1984.
61. Gregory CR: The effects of perineal urethrostomy on urethral function in male cats. *Comp Cont Educ Pract Vet 9*:895, 1987.
62. Gregory CR, Vasseur PB: Electromyographic and urethral pressure profilometry: Long-term assessment of urethral function after perineal urethrostomy in cats. *Am J Vet Res 45*:1318, 1984.
63. Gregory CR, et al: Electromyographic and urethral pressure profilometry: Assessment of urethral function before and after perineal urethrostomy in cats. *Am J Vet Res 45*:2062, 1984.
64. Hamar D, et al: Effect of sodium chloride in prevention of experimentally produced phosphate uroliths in male cats. *J Am Anim Hosp Assoc 12*:514, 1976.
65. Hanson JS: Urachal remnant in the cat: Occurrence and relationship to the feline urologic syndrome. *Vet Med Small Anim Clin 72*:1735, 1977.
66. Harrington JT, Lemann J: The metabolic production and disposal of acid and alkali. *Med Clin North Am 54*:1543, 1970.
67. Harvey JW, Kornick HP: Phenazopyridine toxicosis in the cat. *J Am Vet Med Assoc 169*:327, 1976.
68. Hause WR: Management of acute illness in cats. *Mod Vet Pract 65*:359, 1984.
69. Herron MA: The effect of prepubertal castration on the penile urethra of the cat. *J Am Vet Med Assoc 160*:208, 1972.
70. Holme DW: Research into the feline urological syndrome. Proceedings of the Kal Kan Symposium for the Treatment of Dog and Cat Diseases. Kal Kan Foods, Vernon, CA, 1977, pp 40–45.
71. Humphreys J: Incidence of FUS. *Feline Pract 7*:4, 1977.
72. Jackson OF: The treatment and subsequent prevention of struvite urolithiasis in cats. *J Small Anim Pract 12*:555, 1971.
73. Jackson OF: The case against a viral aetiology in feline urolithiasis. *Vet Rec 96*:70, 1975.
74. Jackson OF: The treatment of struvite urethral obstruction in cats using Walpole's acetate buffer solution pH 4.5. *Feline Pract 6*:52, 1976.
75. Jackson OF, Tovey JD: Water balance studies in domestic cats. *Feline Pract 7*:30, 1977.
76. Jacob S: Mode of action and biologic effects of DMSO. *Vet Med Small Anim Clin 77*:365, 1982.
77. Jaffe HC, et al: Ammonium chloride decalcification as modified by calcium intake: The relationship between generalized osteoporosis and osteitis fibrosa. *J Exp Med 56*:823, 1932.
78. Jenkins EE, Coulter DB: Effects of diet on water intake, food intake and feces production in the cat. *Georgia Vet 33*:8, 1987.
79. Johnston GR, Feeney DA: Localization of feline urethral obstruction. *Vet Clin North Am 14*:555, 1984.
80. Kallfelz FA, et al: Urethral obstruction in random source and SPF male cats induced by high levels of dietary magnesium or magnesium and phosphorus. *Feline Pract 10*:25, 1980.
81. Kirk H: Retention of urine and urinary deposits. *In* Kirk H (ed): *The Diseases of the Cat and Its General Management.* Alex Eger, Chicago, 1925, pp 261–267.
82. Kit S, et al: Induction of thymidine kinase activity by viruses with group B genomes: Bovine cytomegalovirus (bovine herpesvirus 4). *Virus Res 4*:197, 1986.
83. Klahr S: Pathophysiology of obstructive uropathy. *Kidney Int 23*:414, 1983.
84. Kolata RJ: Emergency treatment of urethral obstruction in male cats. *Mod Vet Pract 65*:517, 1984.
85. Koller LC: Clinical application of DMSO by veterinarians in Oregon and Washington. *Vet Med Small Anim Clin 71*:591, 1976.
86. Kruger JM: Feline lower urinary tract disease: Etiological role of cell-associated herpesvirus. PhD Thesis, University of Minnesota, 1989.
87. Kruger JM, Osborne CA: The role of viruses in feline lower urinary tract disease. *J Vet Intern Med 4*:71, 1990

88. Kruger JM, et al: Genetic and serologic analysis of feline cell-associated herpesvirus-induced infection of the urinary tract in conventionally reared cats. *Am J Vet Res 50*:2023, 1989.
89. Kruger JM, et al: Viral etiology of feline urologic syndrome: Truth and consequences. Proceedings of the American College of Veterinary Internal Medicine, Washington, D.C., May, 1986, pp 4/3–4/6.
90. Lawler DF, Evans RH: Urinary tract disease in cats: Water balance studies, urolith and crystal analysis, and necropsy findings. *Vet Clin North Am 14*:537, 1984.
91. Lawler DF, et al: Incidence rate of feline lower urinary tract disease in the United States. *Feline Pract 15*:13, 1985.
92. Lees GE: Epidemiology of naturally occurring feline bacterial urinary tract infections. *Vet Clin North Am 14*:471, 1984.
93. Lees GE, Moreau PM: Management of hypotonic and atonic urinary bladders in cats. *Vet Clin North Am 14*:641, 1984.
94. Lees GE, Osborne CA: Use and misuse of indwelling urinary catheters in cats. *Vet Clin North Am 14*:599, 1984.
95. Lees GE, et al: Antibacterial properties of urine: Studies of feline urine specific gravity, osmolality, and pH. *J Am Anim Hosp Assoc 15*:135, 1979.
96. Lees GE, et al: Adverse effects caused by polypropylene and polyvinyl urinary catheters. *Am J Vet Res 41*:1836, 1980.
97. Lees GE, et al: Adverse effects of open indwelling urethral catheterization in clinically normal male cats. *Am J Vet Res 42*:825, 1981.
98. Lees GE, et al: Results of analyses and bacterial cultures of urine samples obtained from clinically normal cats by three methods. *J Am Vet Med Assoc 184*:449, 1984.
99. Lewis LD, Morris ML: Feline urologic syndrome: Causes and clinical management. *Vet Med 79*:323, 1984.
100. Lewis LD, Morris ML: Treatment and prevention of feline struvite urolithiasis. *Vet Clin North Am 14*:649, 1984.
101. Lewis LD, Morris ML: Diet as a causative factor of feline urolithiasis. *Vet Clin North Am 14*:513, 1984.
102. Lewis LD, et al: Effects of various dietary mineral concentrations on the occurrence of feline urolithiasis. *J Am Vet Med Assoc 172*:559, 1978.
103. Lloyd WE, Sullivan DJ: Effects of orally administered ammonium chloride and methionine on feline urinary acidity. *Vet Med 79*:773, 1984.
104. MacDonald ML, et al: Nutrition of the domestic cat, a mammalian carnivore. *Annu Rev Nutr 4*:521, 1984.
105. Maede Y, et al: Methionine toxicosis in cats. *Am J Vet Res 48*:289, 1987.
106. Marshall W, Robertson WG: Nomograms for the estimation of the saturation of urine with calcium oxalate, calcium phosphate, magnesium ammonium phosphate, uric acid, sodium acid urate, ammonium acid urate and cystine. *Clin Chim Acta 72*:253, 1976.
107. Martens JG, et al: The role of infectious agents in naturally occurring feline urologic syndrome. *Vet Clin North Am 14*:503, 1984.
108. McCully RM, Lieberman LL: Histopathology in a case of feline urolithiasis. *Can Vet J 2*:52, 1961.
109. McDougal WS, Wright FS: Defect in proximal and distal sodium transport in postobstructive diuresis. *Kidney Int 2*:304, 1972.
110. Meier FW: Urethral obstruction and stenosis in the male cat. *J Am Vet Med Assoc 137*:67, 1960.
111. Meier FW: Urethroadenocystitis in the male cat. *J Am Vet Med Assoc 151*:1059, 1967.
112. Middleton DJ, et al: Arterial and venous blood gas tensions in clinically healthy cats. *Am J Vet Res 42*:1609, 1981.
113. Osbaldiston GW, Taussig RA: Clinical report on 46 cases of feline urological syndrome. *Vet Med Small Anim Clin 65*:461, 1970.
114. Osborne CA: Forward: Symposium on disorders of the feline lower urinary tract. *Vet Clin North Am 14*:407, 1984.
115. Osborne CA, Lees GE: Feline cystitis, urethritis, urethral obstruction syndrome. *Mod Vet Pract 59*:17, 1978.
116. Osborne CA, et al: Feline urologic syndrome: A heterogeneous phenomenon? *J Am Anim Hosp Assoc 20*:17, 1984.
117. Osborne CA, et al: Medical management of male and female cats with nonobstructive lower urinary tract disease. *Vet Clin North Am 14*:617, 1984.
118. Osborne CA, et al: Redefinition of the feline urologic syndrome: Feline lower urinary tract disease with heterogeneous causes. *Vet Clin North Am 14*:409, 1984.
119. Osborne CA, et al: Epidemiology of naturally occurring feline uroliths and urethral plugs. *Vet Clin North Am 14*:481, 1984.
120. Osborne CA, et al: Immediate relief of feline urethral obstruction. *Vet Clin North Am 14*:585, 1984.
121. Osborne CA, et al: Etiopathogenesis and biological behavior of feline vesicourachal diverticula. *Vet Clin North Am 17*:697, 1987.
122. Osborne CA, et al: Feline lower urinary tract disorders. *In* Ettinger SJ (ed):*Textbook of Veterinary Internal Medicine*. 3rd ed. W. B. Saunders, Philadelphia, 1989, pp 2057–2082.
123. Osborne CA, et al: Medical management of vesicourachal diverticula in 15 cats with lower urinary tract disease. *J Small Am Anim Pract 30*:608, 1989.
124. Parks J: Electrocardiographic abnormalities from serum electrolyte imbalance due to feline urethral obstruction. *J Am Anim Hosp Assoc 11*:102, 1975.
125. Polzin DJ, Osborne CA: Medical prophylaxis of feline lower urinary tract disease. *Vet Clin North Am 14*:661, 1984.
126. Reif JS, et al: Feline urethral obstruction: A case control study. *J Am Vet Med Assoc 170*:1320, 1977.
127. Rich LJ: Feline urethral obstruction, etiological factors and pathogenesis. PhD Thesis, Cornell University, Ithaca, 1969.
128. Rich LJ, Fabricant CG: Urethral obstruction in male cats. *Can J Comp Med 33*:164, 1969.
129. Rich LJ, Fabricant CG: Experimental production of urolithiasis in male cats. *J Am Vet Med Assoc 158*:974, 1971.
130. Rich LJ, Kirk RW: Feline urethral obstruction: Mineral aspects. *Am J Vet Res 29*:2149, 1968.
131. Rich LJ, Kirk RW: The relationship of struvite crystals to urethral obstruction in cats. *J Am Vet Med Assoc 154*:153, 1969.
132. Rich LJ, Norcross NL: Feline urethral obstruction: Immunologic identification of a unique urinary protein. *Am J Vet Res 30*:1001, 1969.
133. Rich LJ, et al: Virus induced urolithiasis in male cats. *Cornell Vet 61*:542, 1971.
134. Rich LJ, et al: Urethral obstruction in male cats: Experimental production by addition of magnesium and phosphate to diet. *Feline Pract 4*:44, 1974.
135. Ross LA: The feline urologic syndrome. Proceedings of the 57th Annual American Animal Hospital Association Meeting, San Francisco, April, 1990, pp 313–315.
136. Sauer LS, et al: Effect of diet composition on water intake and excretion by the cat. *Feline Pract 15*:16, 1985.
137. Sauer LS, et al: Effect of dietary mineral composition on urinary mineral composition and excretion by the cat. *Feline Pract 15*:10, 1985.
138. Scandling JD, Ornt DB: Mechanism of potassium depletion during chronic metabolic acidosis in the rat. *Am J Physiol 252*:F122, 1987.
139. Schaer M: The use of regular insulin in the treatment of hyperkalemia in cats with urethral obstruction. *J Am Anim Hosp Assoc 11*:106, 1975.
140. Schaer M: Polemical forum. *J Am Anim Hosp Assoc 12*:673, 1976.
141. Schecter RD: The significance of bacteria in feline cystitis and urolithiasis. *J Am Vet Med Assoc 156*:1567, 1970.
142. Schecter RD, et al: Heinz body hemolytic anemia associated with use of urinary antiseptics containing methylene blue in the cat. *J Am Vet Med Assoc 162*:37, 1973.
143. Seefeldt SL, Chapman TC: Body water content and turnover in cats fed dry and canned rations. *J Am Vet Med Assoc 40*:183, 1979.
144. Senior DF, et al: Testing the effects of ammonium chloride and *dl*-methionine on the urinary pH of cats. *Vet Med 81*:88, 1986.
145. Senior DF, et al: Effectiveness of ammonium chloride as a urinary acidifier in cats fed a popular brand of canned cat food. *Feline Pract 16*:24, 1986.
146. Shroyer EL, Shalaby MR: Isolation of feline syncytia-forming virus from oropharyngeal swab samples and buffy coat cells. *Am J Vet Res 39*:555, 1978.
147. Skoch ER, et al: Influence of diet on urine pH and feline urological syndrome. Presented at the World Small Animal Veterinary Congress, Barcelona, Spain, 1988.
148. Smith CW, Schiller AG: Perineal urethrostomy in the cat: A retrospective study of complications. *J Am Anim Hosp Assoc 14*:225, 1978.
149. Smith CW, et al: Effects of indwelling catheters in male cats. *J Am Anim Hosp Assoc 17*:427, 1981.
150. Steward BH, et al: The treatment of patients with interstitial cystitis with special reference to intravesical DMSO. *J Urol 107*:377, 1972.
151. Taton GF, et al: Urinary acidification in the prevention and treatment of feline struvite urolithiasis. *J Am Vet Med Assoc 184*:437, 1984.
152. Taton GF, et al: Evaluation of ammonium chloride as a urinary acidifier in the cat. *J Am Vet Med Assoc 184*:433, 1984.
153. Thrall BE, Miller LG: Water turnover in cats fed dry rations. *Feline Pract 6*:10, 1976.
154. Tomey SL, Follis TB: Incidence rates of feline urological syndrome (FUS) in the United States. *Feline Pract 8*:39, 1978.
155. Walker AD, et al: An epidemiological survey of feline urological syndrome. *J Small Anim Pract 18*:283, 1977.
156. Willeberg P: A case-control study of some fundamental determinants in the epidemiology of the feline urological syndrome. *Nord Vet Med 27*:1, 1975.
157. Willeberg P: Diets and the feline urological syndrome: A retrospective case control study. *Nord Vet Med 27*:15, 1975.
158. Willeberg P: Outdoor activity level as a factor in the feline urological syndrome. *Nord Vet Med 27*:523, 1975.
159. Willeberg P: Interaction effects of epidemiologic factors in the feline urological syndrome. *Nord Vet Med 28*:193, 1976.
160. Willeberg P: Animal disease information processing—epidemiologic analyses of the feline urological syndrome. *Acta Vet Scand Suppl 64*:1, 1977.
161. Willeberg P: Epidemiology of feline urological syndrome. *Adv Vet Sci Comp Med 25*:311, 1981.
162. Willeberg P: Epidemiology of naturally occurring feline urologic syndrome. *Vet Clin North Am 14*:455, 1984.
163. Willeberg P, Priester WA: Feline urologic syndrome: Associations with some time, space, and individual patient factors. *Am J Vet Res 37*:975, 1976.
164. Wilson GP, et al: The relationship of urachal defects in the feline urinary bladder to feline urologic syndrome. Proceedings of the Kal Kan Symposium for the Treatment of Dog and Cat Diseases. Kal Kan, Vernon, CA, 1983, pp 125–129.
165. Wooley RE, Blue JL: Quantitative and bacteriological studies of urine specimens from canine and feline urinary tract infections. *J Clin Microbiol 4*:326, 1976.

CHAPTER 109

Medical Treatment of Canine Uroliths

Gregory F. Grauer

Canine urine is frequently supersaturated with organic and inorganic crystalloids. The solubility of crystalloids varies, and during periods of urine supersaturation, sparingly soluble crystalloids may precipitate to form crystals. Although crystalluria may irritate the urinary tract mucosa, the irritation is usually of little consequence unless the crystals are retained in the urinary tract and form uroliths. Uroliths damage the urinary tract mucosa, resulting in inflammation (hematuria, pollakiuria, dysuria/stranguria) and a predisposition to bacterial infection. If uroliths lodge in the ureters or urethra, urine flow may be obstructed.

The incidence of canine urolithiasis is probably between 0.4 per cent and 2.8 per cent in the United States[7, 10] and 1.2 per cent and 2.0 per cent in the United Kingdom.[30, 31] The majority of uroliths in dogs are found in the bladder or urethra, and only 5 to 10 per cent are located in the kidneys or ureters.[7] Uroliths are most frequently observed in dogs between 3 and 7 years old.[5, 7, 10]

Uroliths are named according to mineral content, and in the United States, struvite (magnesium ammonium phosphate) uroliths are the most common type, accounting for approximately 69 per cent of uroliths.[3] Less frequently encountered uroliths include calcium oxalate (10 per cent), urate (7 per cent), silicate (3.5 per cent), cystine (3.2 per cent), and mixed composition (7 per cent).[3] Approximately 95 per cent of urolith weight is crystalline aggregates, and as much as 5 per cent may be an organic matrix made up of protein and mucoprotein complexes.

ETIOLOGY AND PATHOGENESIS

Conditions that contribute to crystallization of crystalloids and urolith formation include a sufficiently high concentration of crystalloids in the urine, adequate time within the urinary tract (urinary retention of crystalloids), a favorable urine pH for crystallization to occur, a nucleation center or nidus on which crystallization may occur, and decreased concentrations of crystallization inhibitors in the urine.[16] High dietary intake of minerals and protein and the ability of dogs to produce highly concentrated urine contribute to urine supersaturation with crystalloid substances. In some cases, decreased tubular reabsorption of crystalloids (e.g., calcium, cystine, and uric acid) or increased production of crystalloids secondary to bacterial infection also contributes to urine supersaturation.

Several theories exist about the pathogenesis of urolith formation. The precipitation-crystallization theory suggests that supersaturation of urine with crystalloids is the primary factor that initiates nidus formation and sustains growth of the urolith. Normal canine urine is supersaturated with several crystalloids. The greater the urine concentration of crystalloids and the less often voiding occurs (e.g., decreased water intake), the greater the chance of urolith formation. Supersaturated urine has a potential energy of precipitation or a driving force favoring crystal formation. The greater the magnitude of supersaturation, the greater the potential for crystallization. Conversely, undersaturated solutions have a potential energy of dissolution, resulting in crystal dissolution at a rate proportional to the degree of undersaturation.

Other theories of urolith formation suggest that substances in urine may promote or inhibit crystal formation. The matrix nucleation theory proposes that an organic matrix substance in urine promotes initial nidus formation. An immunologically unique protein deficient in hydroxyproline may be present in many uroliths and has been termed *matrix substance A*. Additionally, the organic matrix may be composed of albumin, globulin, or Tamm-Horsfall protein. The proteinaceous matrix substance may promote crystallization by providing a surface for crystallization and by binding crystals together, thereby increasing their urinary retention. The crystallization-inhibitor theory suggests absence of a critical inhibitor of crystal formation as the primary factor allowing initial nidus formation. Examples of crystallization inhibitors are citrates, magnesium, glycosaminoglycans, and pyrophosphates. Decreased concentrations of these substances in urine may facilitate spontaneous crystallization and urolith growth. The extent that promoters and inhibitors of crystallization are involved in the pathogenesis of urolith formation is unknown. In all cases, supersaturation of urine with urolith constituents is essential for urolith formation.

Struvite or *magnesium ammonium phosphate* uroliths are the most common uroliths in dogs. Uroliths that are predominantly struvite may also contain a small percentage of calcium phosphate (hydroxyapatite) or calcium carbonate. Urinary tract infection is an important factor predisposing to the formation of struvite uroliths, and *Staphylococcus aureus* and *Proteus* spp. are commonly associated pathogens. These organisms contain urease and are capable of splitting urea to ammonia and carbon dioxide. Hydroxyl and ammonium ions are formed from hydrolysis of ammonia, which reduces hydrogen ion concentrations in urine and results in increased urine pH. Alkaline urine decreases struvite solubility and facilitates crystal formation. The breakdown of urea increases urine concentrations of ammonium and phosphate (owing to increased dissociation of phosphorus) ions, contributing to urine supersaturation. High ammonia concentrations in urine also damage glycosaminoglycans, which protect the urinary mucosa from bacterial pathogen adherence. Additionally, bacterial cystitis increases the amount of organic debris available to serve as a surface for crystallization. Because of the close association with urinary tract infection, struvite uroliths are more frequent in female dogs; 80 to 97 per cent of uroliths in female dogs are struvite.[16] Uroliths in dogs younger than 1 year are also usually struvite.[7, 11]

The pathogenesis of struvite urolith formation in sterile urine is unknown; struvite urolith formation in cats usually occurs without urinary tract infection. Greater urine-concentrating ability and a greater degree of urine supersaturation may be responsible for urolith formation in cats and those dogs without urinary tract infections. Most canine diets are rich in minerals and protein, resulting in urine supersaturation with magnesium, ammonium, and phosphate. In addition, consistently high urine pH in the absence of urinary tract infection (potentially caused by drugs, diet, or renal tubular acidosis) may result in struvite urolith formation.

Struvite uroliths may develop in any breed; those commonly affected include miniature schnauzers, Welsh corgis, dachshunds, poodles, pugs, Pekingese, beagles, and Scottish terriers.[7] The high incidence of struvite uroliths in miniature schnauzers has led to the suggestion of a familial predisposition.[13, 14]

Calcium oxalate uroliths are the most common type in humans; the incidence of calcium oxalate uroliths in dogs is increasing. Calcium oxalate uroliths in dogs are usually the monohydrate (whewellite) rather than the dehydrate (weddellite) form.[17] Factors involved in the pathogenesis of calcium oxalate urolithiasis in dogs are not well understood, but increased concentrations of calcium in the urine may contribute to their formation. Hypercalciuria probably occurs most commonly in dogs postprandially in association with absorptive hypercalcemia.[17] Affected dogs have low to normal parathyroid hormone concentrations and normal urine calcium excretion when fasted. Another potential cause of hypercalciuria is defective tubular reabsorption of calcium. This "renal-leak" hypercalciuria, accompanied by increased parathyroid hormone concentrations, has been observed in one dog with calcium oxalate urolithiasis.[17] Hypercalciuria may also occur secondary to hypercalcemia (e.g., primary hyperparathyroidism, lymphosarcoma, and vitamin D intoxication); however, hypercalcemia-induced hypercalciuria, like renal-leak hypercalciuria, is an infrequent cause of calcium oxalate uroliths.[17] Finally, decreased urine concentrations of citrate, a calcium oxalate crystallization inhibitor, may have a role in some cases of calcium oxalate uroliths in dogs.

Approximately 70 per cent of calcium oxalate uroliths are observed in male dogs, and miniature schnauzers, miniature poodles, Yorkshire terriers, Lhasa apsos, and Shih Tzus are commonly affected.[17] Calcium oxalate uroliths frequently occur in older dogs (mean age is 8 to 9 years), and concurrent urinary tract infection is rare. Calcium oxalate solubility is increased in urine with a pH greater than 6.5, whereas urine pH between 4.5 and 5.5 favors calcium oxalate crystal formation.[17]

Most *urate* uroliths are composed of *ammonium acid urate*; 100 per cent uric acid and sodium urate uroliths are rare in comparison.[29] Uric acid is derived from the metabolic degradation of endogenous purine ribonucleotides and dietary nucleic acids. Dalmatians may have defective hepatic transport of uric acid compared with other dogs, because uric acid conversion to allantoin is decreased even though hepatic uricase concentrations are adequate.[24] Decreased production of allantoin in Dalmatians results in increased urinary excretion of uric acid. Allantoin produced by the oxidation of uric acid by uricase is normally the major metabolite of purine metabolism, and in comparison with uric acid, allantoin is quite soluble in urine. In addition to decreased hepatic metabolism of uric acid, Dalmatians have decreased proximal tubular reabsorption of uric acid, as well as distal tubular secretion of uric acid, both of which augment uric acid and sodium urate concentrations in urine. Urinary uric acid excretion in Dalmatians is approximately ten times that of other dogs;[24] however, increased urinary excretion of uric acid is a predisposing factor rather than a primary cause, because all Dalmatians excrete large quantities of uric acid in their urine but only a small percentage form urate stones. Absence of a crystallization inhibitor may facilitate urolith formation. Glycosaminoglycans in urine may combine with urate salts, resulting in an overall negative charge and reduced crystallization. Ammonia produced by renal tubular cells from glutamine diffuses into the tubular lumen and serves as a buffer for secreted hydrogen ions by the formation of ammonium ions. Ammonium ions are relatively lipid insoluble and are therefore trapped within the tubular lumen. Excretion of both uric acid and ammonium ions is increased secondary to protein ingestion.

Approximately 60 per cent of urate uroliths occur in Dalmatians, and approximately 75 per cent of the uroliths in Dalmatians are urate uroliths.[7] In addition to this breed predisposition, any dog with hepatic insufficiency (e.g., hepatic cirrhosis or a portosystemic shunt) may form ammonium acid urate stones because of increased renal excretion of ammonium urates.[18] Portosystemic shunts are common in miniature schnauzers, Yorkshire terriers, and Pekingese, and ammonium acid urate uroliths are therefore more common in these breeds. Urinary tract infections, especially those with urease-producing bacteria, may facilitate ammonium acid urate crystallization by increasing urine ammonia concentrations. Urinary tract infection may also occur secondary to urolith-induced mucosal irritation. Uric acid crystallization is facilitated in acidic urine, whereas an alkaline pH favors ammonium acid urate crystallization.[29]

Silicate uroliths were first reported in 1976, when crystallographic analysis of uroliths became available. Silicate uroliths frequently but not always assume a jack shape, although not all jackstone uroliths are silicates (ammonium acid urate and struvite uroliths may also be jack shaped).[19] The cause of silicate uroliths is unknown but may be related to dietary intake of silicates, silicic acid, or magnesium silicate. There appears to be a link between formation of silicate uroliths and consumption of large amounts of corn gluten or soybean hulls, which are high in silicates.[6, 22] Many of the reported silicate uroliths have been found in German shepherds and silicate uroliths are much more common in males than females.[19] The mean age of dogs with silicate uroliths is 5.8 years.[19] Alkaline urine increases silicate solubility, and secondary urinary tract infections may occur owing to mucosal irritation caused by the jack-shaped uroliths.

Cystine uroliths occur in dogs with cystinuria, an inherited disorder of renal tubular transport involving cystine and, in some cases, other amino acids (tubular reabsorption of cysteine, the immediate precursor of cystine, and lysine may also be decreased).[18] Plasma cystine concentrations are normal in these dogs, but plasma methionine, a precursor of cystine, may be increased.[4] Plasma cystine is freely filtered through the glomerulus and is normally actively reabsorbed by proximal tubular epithelial cells. If it were not for the relative insolubility of cystine in urine and the potential for urolith formation, cystinuria would be of little consequence. Cystine is most soluble in alkaline solutions, and cystine stones therefore usually form in acidic urine.[25] Not all dogs with cystinuria develop cystine uroliths; cystinuria is therefore a predisposing rather than a primary causative factor. Cystinuria and cystine uroliths are most frequently observed in male dogs, principally dachshunds, but cystinuria has also been reported in basset hounds, English bulldogs, Yorkshire terriers, Irish terriers, and Chihuahuas. For unknown reasons, cystine uroliths do not usually form in immature dogs; the average age at detection is 3 to 5 years.[2] The incidence of cystine urolithiasis in the United Kingdom is ten times that in the United States,[30, 31] probably because of the increased popularity of affected breeds. Urinary tract infections may occur secondarily; however, infection may not be important in the pathogenesis of cystine uroliths.

CLINICAL SIGNS AND DIAGNOSIS

Clinical signs associated with urolithiasis depend on the number, type, and location of the stones within the urinary tract. Most uroliths are located in the urinary bladder, and clinical signs of cystitis (hematuria, pollakiuria, and stranguria/dysuria) are frequently observed. Mucosal irritation is relatively severe with jack-shaped uroliths in comparison with solitary smooth stones; however, mucosal irritation and secondary urinary tract infection are possible with any urolith type or number. In male dogs, smaller uroliths may pass into the urethra, causing partial or complete obstruction with signs of bladder distension and postrenal azotemia (depression, anorexia, and vomiting). Uroliths frequently lodge within a male's urethra at the caudal end of the os penis. Rarely, the urinary bladder or urethra may rupture, resulting in ascites or subcutaneous perineal fluid accumulation and postrenal azotemia. Unilateral renal uroliths may be asymptomatic or associated with hematuria and chronic pyelonephritis. Bilateral renoliths frequently lead to chronic renal failure, especially if associated with pyelonephritis. Urethral uroliths may also be asymptomatic or may be associated with hematuria and abdominal pain. Unilateral obstruction of a ureter often results in unilateral hydronephrosis without evidence of impaired renal function.

Uroliths within the bladder and urethra can often be palpated via the abdomen or rectum; however, a thickened, irritated bladder wall may obscure small uroliths. Palpation of the urinary bladder should be performed before and after voiding, because a full bladder may also obscure uroliths. In male dogs, the urethra should be palpated subcutaneously from the ischial arch to the os penis. Ultrasonography or plain or contrast radiographs of the urinary tract are often necessary to confirm a diagnosis of urolithiasis. Calcium oxalate and struvite uroliths are the most radiodense stones, whereas urate uroliths are relatively radiolucent and may require contrast radiographs for diagnosis. Silicate and cystine uroliths have intermediate radiodensity.

Urinalysis findings in dogs with urolithiasis often suggest urinary tract inflammation (hematuria, pyuria, increased numbers of epithelial cells, and proteinuria). Urine pH varies depending on the stone type and the presence or absence of a concurrent bacterial infection. In general, struvite uroliths are associated with alkaline urine (especially if urease-producing bacteria are present), cystine uroliths with acidic urine, urate and silicate uroliths with neutral to acidic urine pH, and oxalate uroliths with variable urine pH. Crystalluria may be observed, depending on urine concentration, pH, and temperature at which the urine was stored. Although crystalluria may exist without uroliths and uroliths may be present without crystalluria, the identity of the crystals is usually the same as the urolith if the two exist concurrently (Figs. 109–1 through 109–5). Exceptions do occur—for example, silicate or calcium oxalate uroliths may be complicated by a urease-producing bacterial infection, which generates struvite crystals. Bacterial culture and antibiotic sensitivity testing of the urine are performed in all cases of urolithiasis to identify and properly treat any concurrent urinary tract infection. Medical dissolution of uroliths is frequently ineffective if urinary tract infections are not controlled. If a cystotomy is performed, a small piece of bladder mucosa is submitted for bacterial culture, because the urine may be sterile in dogs that were previously treated with antibiotics.

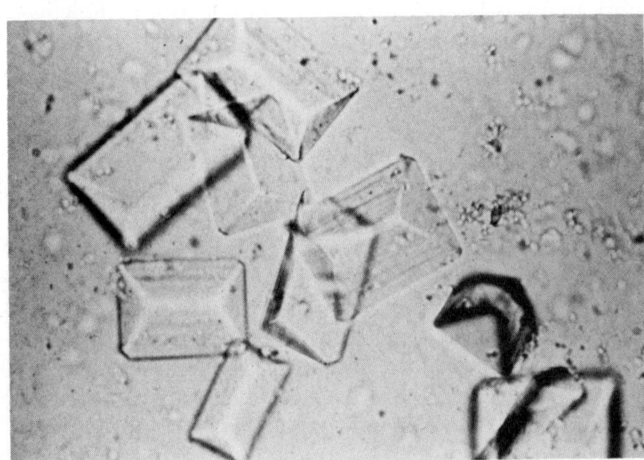

FIGURE 109–1. Struvite crystals in urine sediment. These crystals are normally colorless.

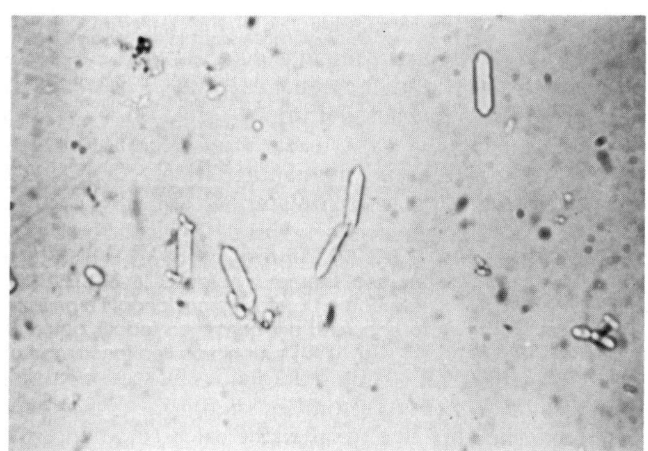

FIGURE 109–2. Monohydrate calcium oxalate crystals in urine sediment. These crystals are normally colorless.

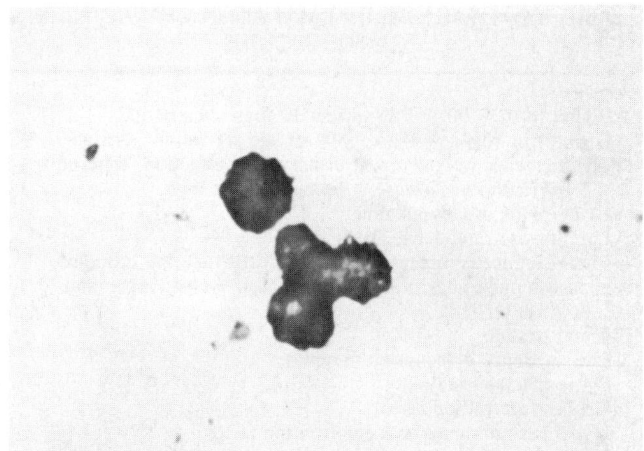

FIGURE 109–4. Ammonium biurate crystals in urine sediment. These crystals are normally dark yellow.

The patient's signalment along with laboratory and radiographic findings are often helpful in determining urolith type (Table 109–1); however, a quantitative urolith analysis is performed if uroliths are passed or removed surgically. Definitive diagnosis of urolith type allows specific measures for dissolution or prevention. Qualitative commercial kit analysis of uroliths is not recommended, because these kits do not detect silicic acid salts, frequently fail to detect calcium-containing uroliths, and give false-positive results for uric acid more than half the time with cystine uroliths.[3]

MEDICAL MANAGEMENT

General principles of treatment include relief of any urethral obstruction and decompression of the bladder, if necessary. This can usually be accomplished by passage of a small-bore catheter, cystocentesis, dislodgment of urethral calculi by hydropulsion,[9, 20, 27] or emergency urethrotomy. Fluid therapy is initiated to restore fluid and electrolyte balance if postrenal azotemia exists. Hyperkalemia is a potentially life-threatening electrolyte disturbance that may occur with postrenal azotemia due to urethral obstruction or of rupture of the urinary bladder or urethra. Bradycardia and electrocardiographic findings of flattened P waves, prolonged PR interval, widened QRS complexes, and tall or spiked T waves suggest hyperkalemia and warrant aggressive treatment. Isotonic saline and sodium bicarbonate or regular insulin followed by glucose are administered intravenously to lower plasma potassium concentrations.[28]

Medical dissolution of struvite, urate, and cystine uroliths is effective (Table 109–2). The choice between surgical removal of uroliths and medical dissolution is not always clear. Disadvantages of surgery include anesthesia, the invasiveness of the procedure (potential surgical complications), the possibility of incomplete removal of uroliths, and persistence of underlying causes. In addition, surgery does not decrease the rate of urolith recurrence. Medical treatment aims to decrease crystalloid concentration in the urine, increase crystalloid solubility in urine, and increase urine volume to produce urine that is undersaturated. The major disadvantage of medical treatment of urolithiasis is the high degree of owner compliance required for several weeks to months. The cost of medical dissolution is comparable to the cost of surgery because multiple

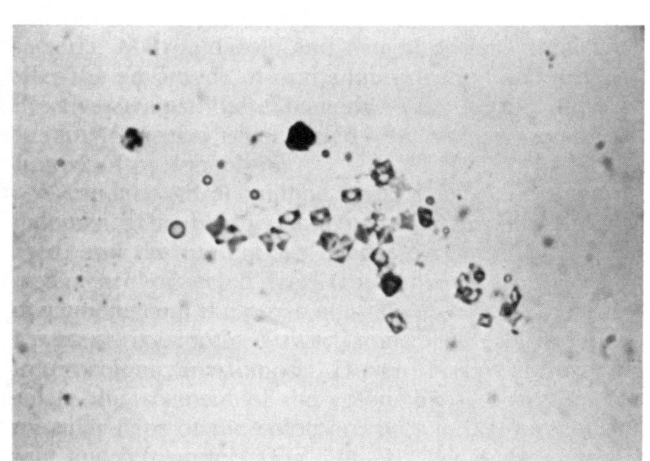

FIGURE 109–3. Dihydrate calcium oxalate crystals in urine sediment. These crystals are normally colorless.

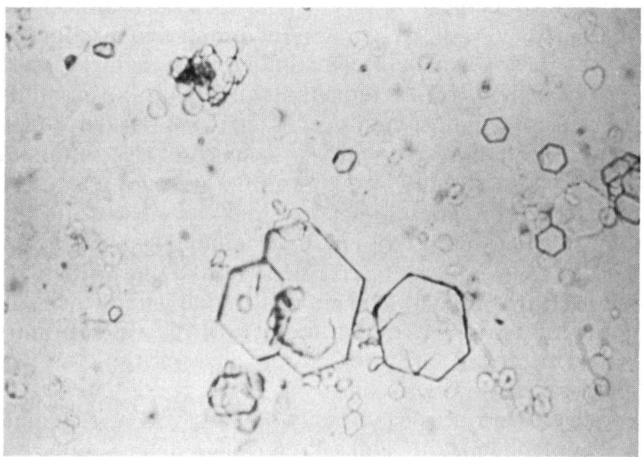

FIGURE 109–5. Cystine crystals in urine sediment. These crystals are normally clear to light yellow.

TABLE 109–1. FACTORS THAT MAY AID IN CHARACTERIZING CANINE UROLITHS

Struvite
- Eighty to 97% of uroliths in female dogs are struvite.
- Uroliths in dogs less than 1 year of age are usually struvite.
- The incidence of concurrent urinary tract infection (especially *Staphylococcus aureus* or *Proteus* spp.) is high.
- Urine pH is usually alkaline.
- Uroliths are radiodense.
- The incidence is increased in miniature schnauzers, poodles, dachshunds, pugs, Pekingese, beagles, Welsh corgis, and Scottish terriers.

Calcium oxalate
- The incidence is increased in males.
- Urine pH is variable.
- Uroliths are radiodense.
- Hypercalcemia may be a contributing factor.
- The incidence is increased in miniature schnauzers, poodles, Yorkshire terriers, Lhasa apsos, and Shih Tzus.

Ammonium acid urate
- The incidence is increased in males.
- Urine pH is usually acid to neutral.
- Urolith radiodensity is variable.
- The incidence is increased in male Dalmatians.
- The incidence is increased in dogs with severe hepatic insufficiency (e.g., portosystemic shunts).

Silicate
- The incidence is increased in males.
- Urine pH is usually acid to neutral.
- Urolith radiodensity is variable.
- The incidence is increased in male German shepherds.
- High dietary intake of silicates probably predisposes (corn gluten and soybean hulls).

Cystine
- The incidence is increased in males.
- Urine pH is usually acidic.
- Urolith radiodensity is variable.
- The incidence is increased in male dachshunds, basset hounds, English bulldogs, Yorkshire terriers, Irish terriers, and Chihuahuas.

urinalyses, bacterial cultures, and radiographs are frequently required for adequate follow-up. Additionally, some uroliths (calcium oxalate and silicate) do not respond to medical dissolution.

General preventive measures that should be used with surgery or medical treatment of uroliths include induction of diuresis and eradication of urinary tract infections. Diuresis lowers urine specific gravity and the urinary concentration of crystalloids. Daily addition of 0.5 to 1.0 g of salt (1 tsp = 3.5 g of sodium chloride) to the diet is usually recommended, although there are exceptions to this recommendation. Hill's Prescription Diet Canine s/d contains large amounts of salt and is not further supplemented.[7] Prevention or dissolution of calcium oxalate and cystine uroliths includes decreased dietary salt, because natriuresis may increase urine calcium and cystine excretion.[12, 17] Maintenance of a urine-specific gravity less than 1.020 is ideal, and dogs are allowed frequent opportunities to void. The urine sediment and pH are monitored frequently, and urinary tract infections are treated quickly on the basis of bacterial culture and sensitivity tests.

Struvite uroliths can usually be dissolved by feeding a calculolytic diet.[1, 23] Hill's Prescription Diet Canine s/d is severely restricted in protein, calcium, phosphorus, and magnesium. It has a high salt content and results in acidic urine.[16] Severe dietary protein restriction reduces hepatic production of urea and decreases urea concentrations in urine and the renal medulla. The result is decreased urea for bacterial urease to act on, as well as decreased medullary hypertonicity and decreased urine-concentrating ability. The average time for struvite urolith dissolution is approximately 12 weeks (the range is 2 weeks to 7 months).[21] Hill's s/d cannot be fed routinely as a maintenance diet and is not used during pregnancy, lactation, growth, or after surgery, because wound healing may be compromised by the ultralow dietary protein.[16] Additionally, because of its high salt content, Hill's s/d is not fed to dogs with congestive heart failure, hypertension, or nephrotic syndrome. Hill's s/d is fed for 30 days after the calculi are no longer palpable or visible radiographically.[16] Hill's s/d diet does not dissolve nonstruvite uroliths and is ineffective if a urinary tract infection persists or anything in addition to the s/d diet is fed. Lack of owner compliance with dietary recommendations (i.e., instructions to feed s/d only) is suggested if serum urea nitrogen concentrations remain greater than 10 mg/100 ml after the diet has been initiated.

In addition to decreasing the concentration of crystalloids in the urine, elimination of any bacterial urinary tract infection is an essential part of the medical treatment of struvite urolithiasis. In some cases, antibiotic treatment alone has resulted in struvite urolith dissolution. If infection is present at the start of treatment, antibiotics are continued throughout the course of medical dissolution, because bacteria may be liberated from a urolith as it dissolves.[24] Antibiotics are selected by urine culture and sensitivity testing, and in severe or

TABLE 109–2. TREATMENT AND PREVENTION OF CANINE UROLITHIASIS

Urolith Type	Treatment Options	Prevention
Struvite	Surgical removal or dissolution: Hill's s/d diet Control infection Urease inhibitor?	Hill's c/d diet Monitor urine pH and urine sediment and treat any infections quickly and appropriately
	Keep urine pH < 6.5, BUN < 10 mg/100 ml, and urine specific gravity < 1.020.	
Calcium oxalate	Surgical removal	Hill's u/d diet Potassium citrate
Urate	Surgical removal or dissolution: Hill's u/d diet Allopurinol, 4–10 mg/kg PO TID Control infection	Hill's u/d diet Allopurinol if necessary
Silicate	Surgical removal	Hill's u/d diet Prevent consumption of dirt
Cystine	Surgical removal or dissolution: Hill's u/d diet D-Penicillamine 15 mg/kg PO BID or *N*-(2-mercaptopropionyl)-glycine (MPG), 15 mg/kg PO BID	Hill's u/d diet Thiol-containing drugs if necessary

BUN, blood urea nitrogen.

persistent urinary tract infections caused by urease-producing bacteria, the urease inhibitor acetohydroxamic acid (AHA) may be added to the treatment regimen.[15] AHA (12.5 mg/kg PO BID) may help dissolve struvite uroliths that are resistant to antibiotics and dietary treatment. Adjunctive treatment with urinary acidifiers (ammonium chloride, 200 mg/kg PO divided TID) is administered in conjunction with Hill's s/d only if the diet fails to maintain the urine pH below 6.5. Medical treatment of sterile struvite uroliths is the same as described earlier, but antibiotics and AHA are unnecessary. Sterile struvite uroliths usually dissolve more rapidly than those accompanying urinary tract infections (the range is 1 to 3 months).[24]

Measures to prevent struvite urolith recurrence include prevention and control of urinary tract infections, maintenance of acidic urine, and decreased dietary intake of calculogenic crystalloids. Hill's Prescription Diet Canine c/d has been recommended as a maintenance diet to prevent struvite urolith recurrence because it is moderately restricted in protein, magnesium, calcium, and phosphorus and results in acidic urine.[16] Because Hill's c/d is mildly restricted in sodium content, 0.5 g of sodium is supplemented daily to increase water consumption and urine production. In dogs with recurrent urinary tract infections, predisposing abnormalities (e.g., urachal remnant or bladder polyp) are ruled out with double-contrast cystography. Silent hyperadrenocorticism may also cause recurrent urinary tract infections. Long-term low-dose prophylactic antibiotic treatment may occasionally be necessary to decrease recurrent urinary tract infections; amoxicillin is used for gram-positive infections, and trimethoprim-sulfonamide or enrofloxacin for gram-negative infections.

Medical treatment for dissolution of oxalate urolithiasis has not been developed. Moderate restriction of protein, calcium, oxalate, and sodium with normal intake of phosphorus, magnesium, and vitamin D is recommended to prevent recurrence of calcium oxalate uroliths. Increased dietary sodium may result in an increase in urinary excretion of calcium and is avoided. Oral potassium citrate may be beneficial for preventing recurrence of calcium oxalate stones. Citrate complexes with calcium, decreasing the urine concentration of calcium, and potassium citrate results in urine alkalinization, which increases the solubility of calcium oxalate. The recommended oral dose of potassium citrate (Urocit-K) for humans is 60 mEq/day divided BID or TID. Thiazide diuretics have been recommended to decrease urinary excretion of calcium; however, studies of dogs have shown inconsistent results, and long-term use of thiazides may increase serum calcium concentrations.[24]

Medical dissolution of urate urolithiasis that is not associated with hepatic insufficiency (e.g., portosystemic shunts) includes a diet low in protein and nucleic acids, alkalization of the urine, xanthine oxidase inhibition, and elimination of urinary tract infections. Hill's Prescription Diet Canine u/d has reduced protein and purine content and results in alkaline urine and has been recommended for urate urolith dissolution and prevention.[16] Similar to Hill's s/d diet, u/d decreases hepatic formation of urea and results in decreased renal medullary hypertonicity and decreased urine-concentrating ability. Because Hill's u/d diet is restricted in salt content, 0.5 to 1.0 g of salt is supplemented daily to increase water consumption and urine production. Additionally, allopurinol, a competitive inhibitor of the enzyme xanthine oxidase that converts hypoxanthine to xanthine and xanthine to uric acid (Fig. 109–6), is administered (10 to 30 mg/kg PO divided BID or TID), and if necessary, sodium bicarbonate or potassium citrate is administered orally to maintain urine pH of 7.[24] Allopurinol is not administered to dogs consuming normal or high-protein diets because it may result in xanthine urolith formation. Similar to the management of struvite uroliths, urinary tract infections are appropriately treated, because urease-producing organisms increase urine ammonium ion concentration and potentiate ammonium urate crystal production. In dogs with urate urolithiasis secondary to severe hepatic insufficiency, the underlying disorder is corrected if possible. If hepatic function can be improved (i.e., surgical correction of a portosystemic shunt) and the urine becomes undersaturated with ammonium and urate ions, urolith dissolution may occur spontaneously. Because low-protein diets and alkalization are not recommended for dogs with hepatic insufficiency, Hill's Prescription Diet Canine k/d is fed to these dogs.

Guidelines for medical dissolution of silicate uroliths are unavailable. Recommendations to decrease recurrence after surgical removal include dietary change,

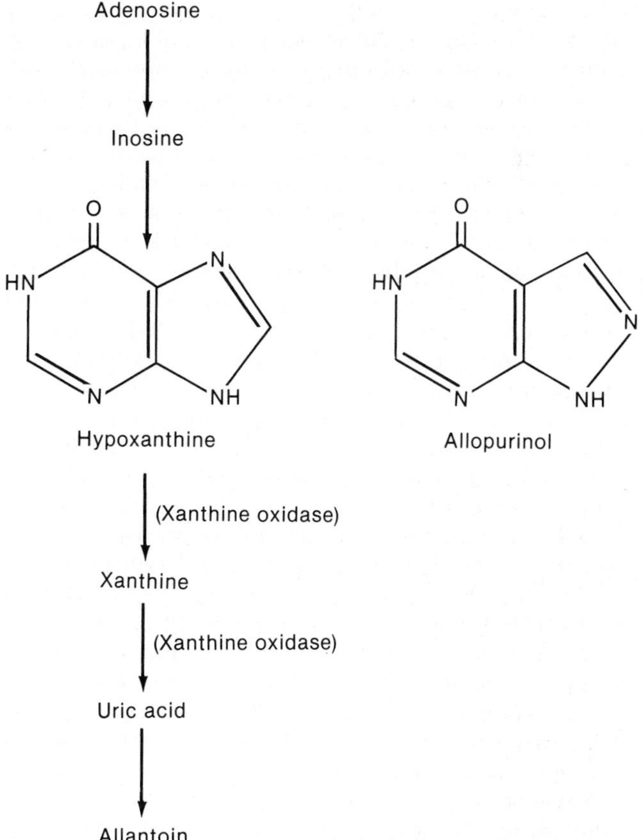

FIGURE 109–6. Metabolism of purine adenosine and a comparison of the structures of hypoxanthine and allopurinol.

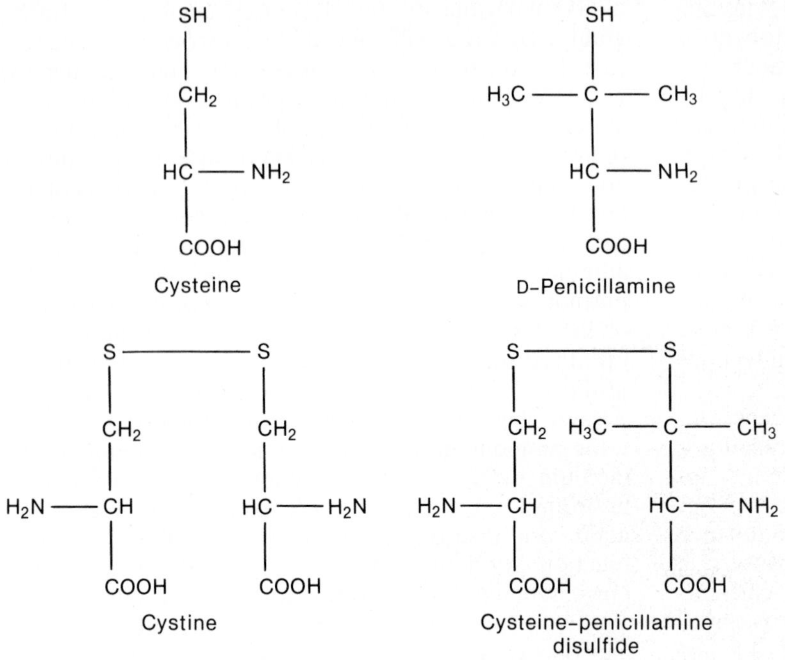

SH | CH2 | HC — NH2 | COOH
Cysteine

SH | H3C — C — CH3 | HC — NH2 | COOH
D-Penicillamine

S — S | CH2 CH2 | H2N — CH HC — H2N | COOH COOH
Cystine

S — S | CH2 H3C — C — CH3 | H2N — CH HC — NH2 | COOH COOH
Cysteine-penicillamine disulfide

FIGURE 109–7. Structures of cystine, cysteine, D-penicillamine, and cysteine-penicillamine disulfide.

augmentation of urine volume, and urine alkalization. Hill's Prescription Diet Canine u/d may be beneficial because it contains low amounts of silicates and results in alkaline urine. Sodium chloride is supplemented at 0.5 to 1.0 g/day. In certain regions, soil may contain high concentrations of silicate, and consumption of dirt is discouraged.

Recommendations for medical dissolution and prevention of cystine uroliths include reduction of dietary protein and methionine, alkalization of urine, and administration of thiol-containing drugs. Hill's Prescription Diet Canine u/d is appropriate because it has a very low protein content, causes urine alkalization, and decreases urine-concentrating ability. Urine pH is maintained at approximately 7.5 with oral potassium citrate. Sodium bicarbonate is avoided, because dietary sodium may enhance cystinuria.[12] D-Penicillamine (15 mg/kg, PO BID, given with food to reduce the potential for nausea and vomiting) forms a disulfide compound with cysteine and reduces the cystine content of the urine (Fig. 109–7). This disulfide compound is 50 times more soluble than cystine in the urine. D-Penicillamine may interfere with surgical wound healing and should not be initiated until 2 weeks after surgery. Other side effects of D-penicillamine may include immune complex glomerulonephritis, fever, lymphadenopathy, and skin hypersensitivity. Another thiol-containing drug, *N*-(2-mercaptopropionyl)-glycine (MPG), increases the solubility of cystine in urine by a disulfide exchange reaction similar to D-penicillamine but with fewer adverse side effects.[26] The recommended dosage of MPG for dogs is 15 mg/kg BID. Thiol-containing drugs are used for cystine urolith prevention if necessary.

Whenever medical dissolution of uroliths is attempted, the patient is re-examined at least monthly. A complete urinalysis is performed, and abdominal palpation performed or radiographs taken to assess urolith size. If urinalysis findings suggest urinary tract infection, a bacterial culture and sensitivity tests are performed and antibiotic treatment initiated or adjusted accordingly. If urolith size is not decreased after 2 months of treatment, owner compliance, control of infection, and urolith type are reassessed and surgical removal considered.

Recurrence rates of urolith formation in dogs of up to 25 per cent have been reported[8] (recurrences are greatest in dogs with urate, calcium oxalate, and cystine uroliths), necessitating appropriate preventive measures and frequent re-evaluations.

References

1. Abdullahi SU, et al: Evaluation of a calculolytic diet in female dogs with induced struvite urolithiasis. *Am J Vet Res 45*:1508, 1984.
2. Bovee KC: Canine cystine urolithiasis. *Vet Clin North Am 16*:211, 1986.
3. Bovee KC, McGuire T: Qualitative and quantitative analysis of uroliths in dogs: Definitive determination of chemical type. *J Am Vet Med Assoc 185*:983, 1984.
4. Bovee KC, et al: Renal clearance of amino acids in canine cystinuria. *Metabolism 23*:51, 1974.
5. Brody RS: Canine urolithiasis: A survey and discussion of 52 clinical cases. *J Am Vet Med Assoc 126*:1, 1955.
6. Brody RS, et al: Silicate renal calculi in Kenyan dogs. *J Small Anim Pract 18*:523, 1977.
7. Brown NO, et al: Canine urolithiasis: Retrospective analysis of 438 cases. *J Am Vet Med Assoc 170*:414, 1977.
8. Brown NO, et al: Recurrence of canine urolithiasis. *J Am Vet Med Assoc 170*:419, 1977.
9. Egger EL, Rigg DL: Treatment of silica urethral obstruction in a dog by retrograde hydropropulsion. *Comp Cont Educ 5*:147, 1983.
10. Finco DR, et al: Canine urolithiasis: A review of 133 clinical cases and 23 necropsy cases. *J Am Vet Med Assoc 157*:1225, 1970.
11. Hardy RM, et al: Urolithiasis in immature dogs. *Vet Med Small Anim Clin 67*:1205, 1972.
12. Jaeger P, et al: Anticystinuria effects of glutamine and of dietary sodium restriction. *N Engl J Med 315*:1120, 1986.
13. Klausner JS, et al: Struvite urolithiasis in a litter of miniature schnauzer dogs. *Am J Vet Res 41*:712, 1980.
14. Klausner JS, et al: Mineral composition of urinary calculi from miniature schnauzer dogs. *J Am Vet Med Assoc 178*:1082, 1981.

15. Krawiec DR, et al: Effect of acetohydroxamic acid on dissolution of canine struvite uroliths. *Am J Vet Res 45*:1266, 1984.
16. Lewis LD, et al: Canine urolithiasis. *In* Lewis LD, et al (eds): *Small Animal Clinical Nutrition III*. Mark Morris Associates, Topeka, KS, 1987, pp 10–11.
17. Lulich JP, et al: Canine calcium oxalate urolithiasis. *In* Kirk RW (ed): *Current Veterinary Therapy X*. W. B. Saunders, Philadelphia, 1989, p 1182.
18. Marretta SM, et al: Urinary calculi associated with portosystemic shunts in six dogs. *J Am Vet Med Assoc 178*:133, 1981.
19. Osborne CA, et al: Canine silica urolithiasis. *J Am Vet Med Assoc 178*:809, 1981.
20. Osborne CA, et al: Nonsurgical removal of uroliths from the urethra of female dogs. *J Am Vet Med Assoc 182*:47, 1983.
21. Osborne CA, et al: Struvite urolithiasis in animals and man: Formation detection and dissolution. *Adv Vet Sci Comp Med 29*:1, 1985.
22. Osborne CA, et al: Etiopathogenesis, clinical manifestations, and management of canine silica urolithiasis. *Vet Clin North Am 16*:185, 1986.
23. Osborne CA, et al: Medical dissolution of canine uroliths: Improving successes, coping with failure. *Proc Am Anim Hosp Assoc Meeting 54*:176, 1987.
24. Osborne CA, et al: Canine urolithiasis. *In* Ettinger SJ (ed): *Textbook of Veterinary Internal Medicine*. W. B. Saunders, Philadelphia, 1989, p 2083.
25. Osborne CA, et al: Medical dissolution and prevention of cystine urolithiasis. *In* Kirk RW (ed): *Current Veterinary Therapy X*. W. B. Saunders, Philadelphia, 1989, p 1189.
26. Pak CYC, et al: Management of cystine nephrolithiasis with alpha-mercaptopropionyl glycine. *J Urol 136*:1003, 1986.
27. Piermattei DL, Osborne CA: Nonsurgical removal of calculi from the urethra of male dogs. *J Am Vet Med Assoc 159*:1755, 1972.
28. Polzin D, et al: Disease of the kidneys and ureters. *In* Ettinger SJ (ed): *Textbook of Veterinary Internal Medicine*. W. B. Saunders, Philadelphia, 1989, p 1962.
29. Senior DF: Medical management of urate uroliths. *In* Kirk RW (ed): *Current Veterinary Therapy X*. W. B. Saunders, Philadelphia, 1989, p 1178.
30. Weaver AD: Canine urolithiasis: Incidence, chemical composition and outcome of 100 cases. *J Small Anim Pract 11*:93, 1970.
31. White EG: Symposium on urolithiasis in the dog. I. Introduction and incidence. *J Small Anim Pract 7*:529, 1966.

SECTION 13

Endocrine System

Thomas D. Scavelli ▪ *Section Editor*

CHAPTER

110 Hypophysectomy

Gert W. Niebauer

Canine hyperadrenocorticism (Cushing's syndrome) was recognized in 1939,[92] marking the beginning of a long Dutch predominance in exploring the pathophysiology and treatment options.[53, 55, 81, 82] Hypophysectomy was investigated in 28 dogs with spontaneous pituitary-dependent hyperadrenocorticism (PDH; Cushing's disease*)[86] and reported as a valuable alternative to adrenalectomy or medical therapy.[53] Few other reports describe hypophysectomy in other centers.[85] This lack of widespread clinical experience is in sharp contrast to the wealth of information on experimental hypophysectomy in dogs and cats, which has a history dating back to the past century.[41] Today, hypophysectomy in dogs is a frequently used experimental procedure worldwide. Surgical knowledge accumulated in experimental studies has not been used on a larger scale in pet animals.

The reasons for scant clinical use of hypophysectomy in veterinary medicine are manifold. Accurate diagnosis of resectable pituitary lesions is challenging and requires hormone radioimmunoassays and computed imaging systems (computed tomography or magnetic resonance imaging). Hypophysectomy is regarded as a difficult neurosurgical procedure with high morbidity and mortality. Traditional alternative treatments for canine PDH are bilateral adrenalectomy, cytotoxic destruction of the adrenal cortex by mitotane o,p′-DDD, and administration of ketoconazole to suppress adrenal steroid synthesis. In the future, hypophysectomy may be established as a routine clinical procedure in dogs, narrowing the gap between veterinary and human neurosurgery. Also, in accordance with the currently expanding understanding of growth hormone–related endocrinopathies in dogs and cats, an extension of the indications for hypophysectomy beyond PDH can be anticipated.[19, 84]

EXPERIMENTAL HYPOPHYSECTOMY

Although experimental hypophysectomies have been performed in many species, cats and dogs were recognized early as the animals best suited for comparative studies. The first published description of hypophysectomy was of dogs in 1886.[41] Two dogs survived 5 and 6 months, respectively. Although no mention was made of whether the hypophysectomies were complete, this relative long survival was an extraordinary achievement, given the standards of surgery at the time. Many attempts to keep hypophysectomized animals alive for long periods failed until 1912.[1] The majority of animals died during or shortly after the procedures, and the few short-time survivors were in such poor condition that the development of endocrinopathies could not be studied, except diabetes insipidus, which develops immediately after hypophysectomy.[4, 5] Advances in pituitary physiology were directly related to the improvement of experimental surgical techniques.

Two main routes of exposure were pursued: intracranial and extracranial. The trans-sphenoidal (transbuccal, transoral, sphenopalatine) approach was the easier and more direct route to reach a dog's or cat's pituitary. Severe hemorrhage from intracranial vascular structures often hampered the efforts. Thermocautery (red-hot iron) and instillation of chromic acid into the sphenoidal bur hole were the early means of destroying the pituitary and providing hemostasis.[90] Surgical and postoperative complications such as brain damage, uncontrollable hemorrhage, infection, palate dehiscence, aspiration pneumonia, and most likely infectious disease such as distemper severely reduced the number of survivors. Although most contemporary physiologists concluded that life, even on a short-term basis, could not be sustained without the pituitary gland,[7, 13, 78, 90] others using similar techniques described dogs[1, 42, 51] and cats[29, 31, 56] surviving hypophysectomy for as long as a few weeks.

Recognizing potential disadvantages of the trans-sphenoidal approach and identifying the surgical technique as the principal reason for poor results, several groups independently embarked on the intracranial approach to the canine hypophysis. Craniotomy with elevation of the temporal lobe to reach the pituitary was followed by higher mortality than the trans-sphenoidal approach.[50, 74] Harvey Cushing, who later pioneered

*Cushing's syndrome is referred to as *Cushing's disease* when caused by a pituitary source, either a tumor or hyperplasia.

hypophysectomy in humans,[38] concluded that the hypophysioprivic status causes death in dogs within a short time.[11, 80] Later, the so-called cachexia hypophysiopriva syndrome was recognized as nothing more than the manifestations of approaching death due to increased intracranial pressure, pneumonia, and other iatrogenic causes.[15]

After 1912, successful hypophysectomies yielded long-term survivors[1, 4, 5]; discovery and definition of the various endocrine functions of the pituitary and hypothalamus rapidly ensued. With few exceptions,[14, 15, 44, 46] these surgical procedures, which included total, partial, and staged hypophysectomies, were performed via the trans-sphenoidal route. Cushing returned the trans-sphenoidal route to favor and developed the classic trans-sphenoidal approach to the human sella turcica.[12, 40] With minor modifications, this approach is the most widely used in humans by neurosurgeons.[49, 63]

The trans-sphenoidal approach to the canine hypophysis is favored and remains unchanged. Morbidity and mortality rates have improved, but the slowly increasing safety record of hypophysectomy is less the result of improved surgical exposure of the pituitary than improved aseptic techniques, antibiotics, and care of experimental animals. The morbidity, though rarely quoted in later experimental studies, was and still is high. The high fatality rates are directly related to intricacies of surgical anatomy: The physical features of dogs vary, distorting the relation of landmarks on the ventral skull to the location of the pituitary and leaving accurate exposure of the hypophyseal fossa to coincidence. The frequent attempts to refine the technique reflect the difficulty in precisely identifying the location of the hypophysis to avoid lacerating vital vascular structures on the base of the skull.[2, 25, 59, 87, 88, 91]

Success of experimental hypophysectomies largely depends on a thorough understanding of the topographical anatomy of the canine skull. Most valuable contributions to the intracranial approach and to trans-sphenoidal hypophysectomy in dogs were published by neurosurgeons.[14, 60] McLean's report[60] on the surgical anatomy of the ventral canine skull and the surgical approaches to the base of the brain is still unsurpassed and likely inspired the first description of experimental hypophysectomy.[58] The Markowitz-Archibald trans-sphenoidal hypophysectomy[57] is the standard method in human-related research.*

Experimental Hypophysectomy in Veterinary Medicine

Veterinary surgeons have just begun to conduct trials to improve clinical hypophysectomy techniques. The stimulus for these efforts lies in the still unsatisfactory safety record of hypophysectomies, in the difficulty in accurately approaching and exposing the pituitary in dogs of various sizes and with diverse skull shapes,[53] and in the uncertainty of achieving and assessing completeness of hypophysectomy.[48, 69] (In experimental surgery, only dogs with mesocephalic skulls are used.)

*See references 8, 21, 23, 24, 43, 45, 64, 70, 83, and 93.

The trans-sphenoidal approach was used in all veterinary studies.[9, 39, 48, 67, 69] In one report, by exploring mandibular symphysiotomy, attempts were made to allow better exposure of the sphenoid bone, especially for use in dolichocephalic dogs.[39] Other studies focused on the question of whether complete hypophysectomy is achievable; microscopically small remnants are likely to remain active when conventional surgical techniques (suction ablation) are used.[48, 69] The common focus of these studies concerns identifying the correct area of trephination in the sphenoid bone without reliable landmarks and with changing skull shapes. This difficulty is the reason for the relatively poor safety record of the procedure and the former recommendation not to attempt hypophysectomies in any but mesocephalic dogs.[20, 53]

The use of radiographic markers as additional landmarks in combination with cranial sinus venography to pinpoint the center of the sella turcica promises to help overcome traditional intricacies of hypophysectomy in dogs.[67]

INDICATIONS FOR HYPOPHYSECTOMY AND DIAGNOSTIC REQUIREMENTS

Large-scale studies have only been performed in dogs. Indications for hypophysectomy, diagnostic approaches, and the technique of trans-sphenoidal hypophysectomy can also be applied to cats. Clinical experience sufficient to recommend hypophysectomy in cats is lacking.

The presence of any primary tumor in the pituitary gland represents a potential indication for hypophysectomy. In general, only pituitary microadenomas (sellar tumors) and functional adenohypophyseal hyperplasia*[61, 75] are amenable to surgical treatment by hypophysectomy.

Most tumors develop in the pars distalis (adenohypophysis); a few arise from the pars intermedia and the infundibulum. Neoplasms originating in the neurohypophysis are rare, as are other intrasellar lesions such as craniopharyngiomas, pituitary cysts, and abscesses.[6, 89]

Neoplasms of the pituitary can be endocrinologically active or silent. Nonfunctional neoplasms (null cell adenomas) cause mass effects only by impinging on adjacent nervous structures such as the optic chiasm, the hypothalamus, or areas beyond. They can cause invagination of the infundibular cavity, dilate the infundibular recess and third ventricle, and increase intracranial pressure directly by expansion or indirectly by obstructing cerebrospinal fluid flow. In dogs, pituitary macroadenomas easily expand dorsally because their growth is uninhibited by the anatomically large hiatus in the sellar diaphragm.[6] Hormonally silent sellar and suprasellar masses can elicit various central nervous signs, with visual deficits developing most frequently. Neurological and ophthalmoscopic examination (papillar

*The term *functional pituitary hyperplasia* is sporadically used in the literature. Clinically and by CT scan, functional pituitary microadenomas and functional pituitary hyperplasia cannot be differentiated. The distinction is of pathophysiological importance only and at present has no impact on therapeutic strategies.

edema) as well as cerebrospinal fluid tap (increased intracranial pressure) can be helpful in localizing mass lesions in the suprasellar area. CT scanning is indispensable in confirming the diagnosis and if surgical resection is attempted. Experience with the excision of large supra- or parasellar tumors is lacking in veterinary medicine, and the majority of such lesions expanding into the hypothalamus or thalamic region probably are nonresectable. Partial ablation of such large masses via the intracranial or trans-sphenoidal route may relieve signs caused by compression and may be beneficial. Radiation therapy (megavoltage photon teletherapy with a cobalt 60 source) causes remission of large pituitary tumors in selected cases.[17] Side effects such as deafness, cranial nerve paralysis, and occasionally cerebral edema occur. Surgery followed by radiation might be the therapeutic avenue of choice in the future, as for large pituitary tumors in human medicine.[33, 34, 66]

In dogs, more than 60 per cent of all neoplastic disorders of the pituitary are endocrinologically active.[6] Adenomas producing excess adrenocorticotropic hormone (ACTH) and eliciting Cushing's disease are the most frequent pituitary disorder in dogs.[62] Approximately two-thirds of all canine adenohypophyseal tumors are microadenomas (<1 cm diameter), the remainder being macroadenomas*[26, 65]; pituitary carcinomas account for less than 3 per cent of all pituitary neoplasms.[6, 65] Thus, nearly 70 per cent of all dogs with PDH have surgically resectable, hyperactive corticotrophs and are definite candidates for hypophysectomy. In dogs with functional macroadenomas (<30 per cent of the dogs with PDH), the benefit/risk evaluation for hypophysectomy has to be considered. In dogs with concomitant signs of Cushing's disease and neurological deficits, the advantage of partial tumor ablation might outweigh the surgical risk. From the diagnostic viewpoint, CT scanning of the sella turcica area is required to differentiate hypophyseal macro- and microadenomas.

Because the pituitary gland does not have a blood-brain barrier, opacification by intravenous contrast is instantaneous.[32] The normal gland as well as macroadenomas usually enhance homogeneously.[27, 28] Microadenomas cannot be seen on CT scans (Figs. 110–1 and 110–2). At present, the likelihood of differentiating pituitary carcinoma from macroadenoma by CT scan cannot be assessed. Preliminary experience suggests no distinction between benign and malignant pituitary tumors on CT scans. Magnetic resonance imaging may allow such differentiation.[73]

Diagnostic steps to evaluate indications for hypophysectomy are summarized (Fig. 110–3). If ACTH stimulation tests or low-dose and high-dose dexamethasone suppression tests or plasma endogenous ACTH measurements or metyrapone suppression tests suggest PDH, pituitary CT scan should be performed. If a macroadenoma is seen, the indication for hypophysectomy is ambiguous. If no pathological changes are visible (microadenomas usually cannot be seen on CT scans), PDH, based on microadenoma or adenohypophyseal hyperplasia, is likely. To confirm the diagnosis, a CT scan or ultrasonography of the adrenal glands is performed. If symmetrical enlargement of both adrenals is present, the diagnosis of PDH caused by resectable pituitary lesions is established and hypophysectomy is indicated. If a CT scan of the sella region cannot be obtained, ultrasonographic assessment of bilateral adrenal enlargement might suffice to justify hypophysectomy; there is a 30 per cent chance of encountering a pituitary macroadenoma (which potentially is nonresectable) and less than 3 per cent probability of a pituitary carcinoma.

In human medicine, hypophysectomy is established as the treatment of choice for adenomatous pituitary lesions producing excess ACTH, growth hormone, thyroid-stimulating hormone, or prolactin.[86] Inoperable tumors or recurring lesions are treated by radiation therapy.[33, 86] For Cushing's disease, in humans, palliative treatment such as adrenalectomy and cytotoxic destruction of the adrenal cortex by o,p′-DDD is regarded as obsolete; total hypophysectomy is avoided in most cases. Exposure of the human adenohypophysis through an usually large, air-filled sphenoidal sinus and microsurgical techniques allow selective ablation of well-demarcated adenomas without damaging pituitary function.

In veterinary medicine, indications for hypophysectomy have only been established for PDH.[53–55, 82] Selective subtotal hypophysectomy or microsurgical ablation of adenomas has not been achieved and will not be possible in the future, based on the anatomy of the canine pituitary (discussed later). Total hypophysectomy in animals remains the only option. Hypophysectomy is superior to the commonly used alternatives: Adrenalectomized animals are rendered addisonian, requiring well-adjusted lifelong mineral and corticosteroid substitution. Medical treatment (o,p′-DDD, ketoconazole) elicits many and often serious side effects, is often ineffective (cyproheptadine, bromocriptine),[76] and frequently has to be discontinued.[3, 26, 52] Hypophysectomy demands only short-term postoperative replacement of vasopressin and lifelong low-dose substitution with corticosteroids and thyroid hormones (discussed later).[23, 24, 34, 37, 47]

Growth hormone supplementation after hypophysectomy is not essential in adult animals. The long-term impact of growth hormone deficit after hypophysectomy remains to be evaluated. I saw mild signs of skin disease (alopecia, scaling) develop in an intact female dog 3 years after hypophysectomy. The signs were reversible by growth hormone supplementation. Lubberink reported skin scaling as frequently occurring 3 to 8 weeks after surgery.[54] On the other hand, somatomedin-C plasma concentrations returned to normal in dogs 1 month after experimental hypophysectomy, despite persistent deficiency of circulating growth hormone, sug-

*The definition of macroadenoma is controversial. Any pituitary neoplasm visible without optical devices during surgery or on necropsy can be regarded as macroadenoma. Some authors define macroadenomas in dogs as lesions >5 mm, others of >1 cm in diameter. The size of the individual animal and the size of its pituitary gland might also affect these distinctions. From a surgical standpoint, we regard any dog with confirmed PDH and a negative contrast-enhanced CT scan as having a microadenoma and any animal with Cushing's disease and a pituitary mass lesion, visible on CT image, as having a macroadenoma (or carcinoma).

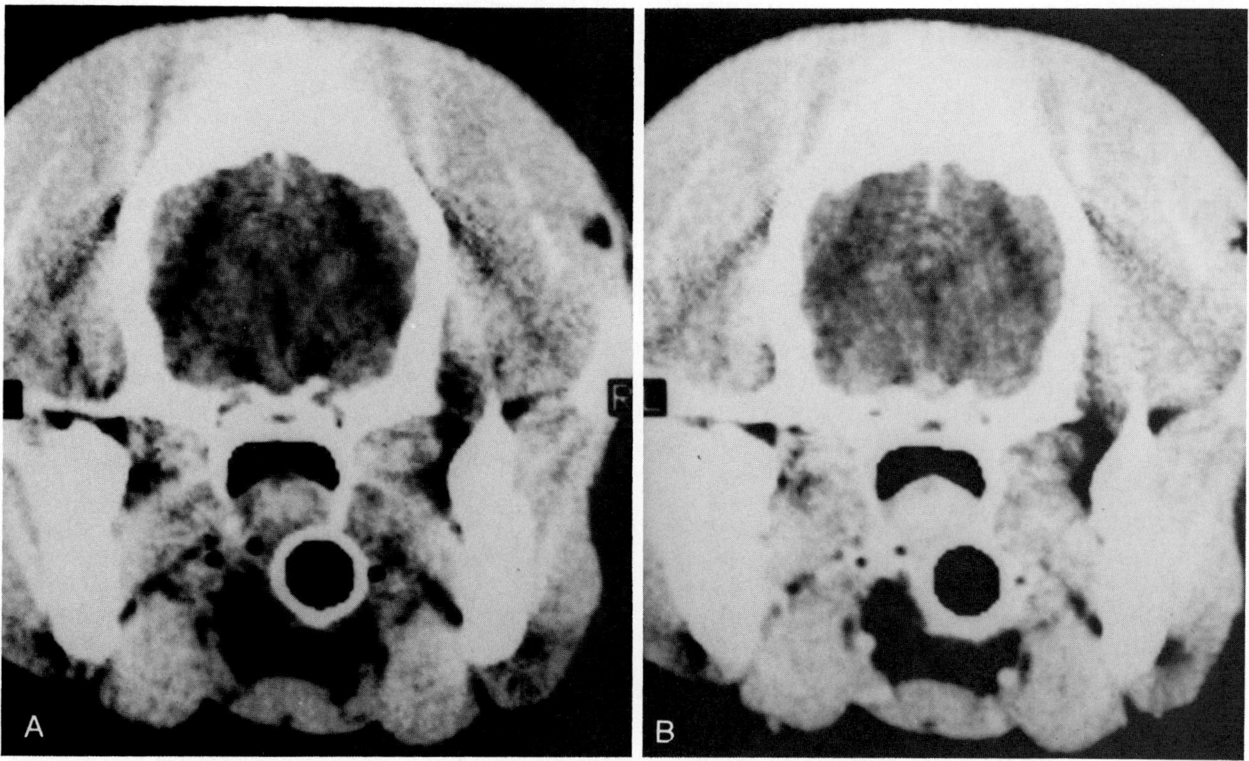

FIGURE 110–1. CT scan of normal canine pituitary gland without (A) and with (B) intravenous contrast enhancement.

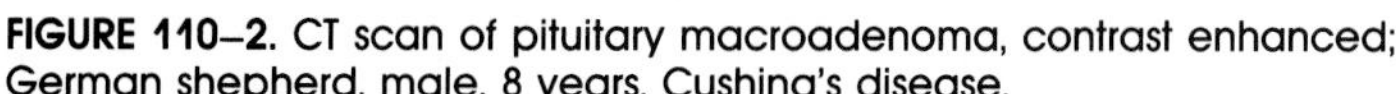

FIGURE 110–2. CT scan of pituitary macroadenoma, contrast enhanced; German shepherd, male, 8 years, Cushing's disease.

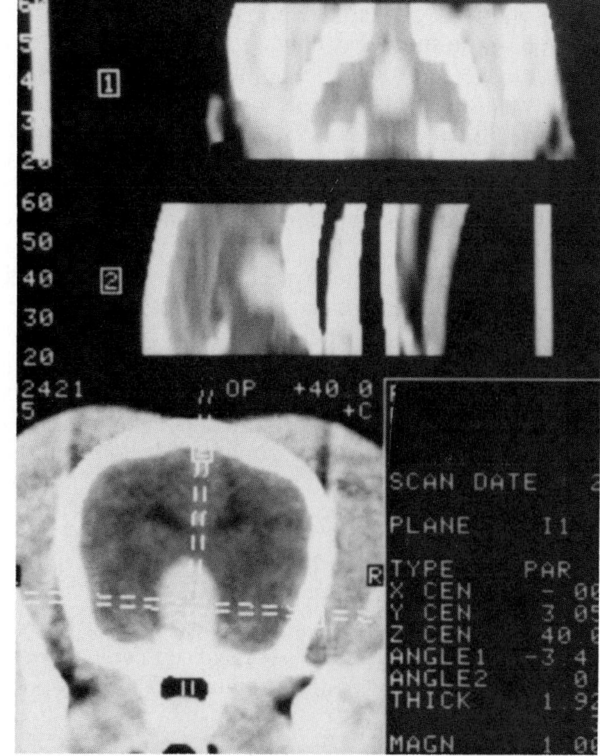

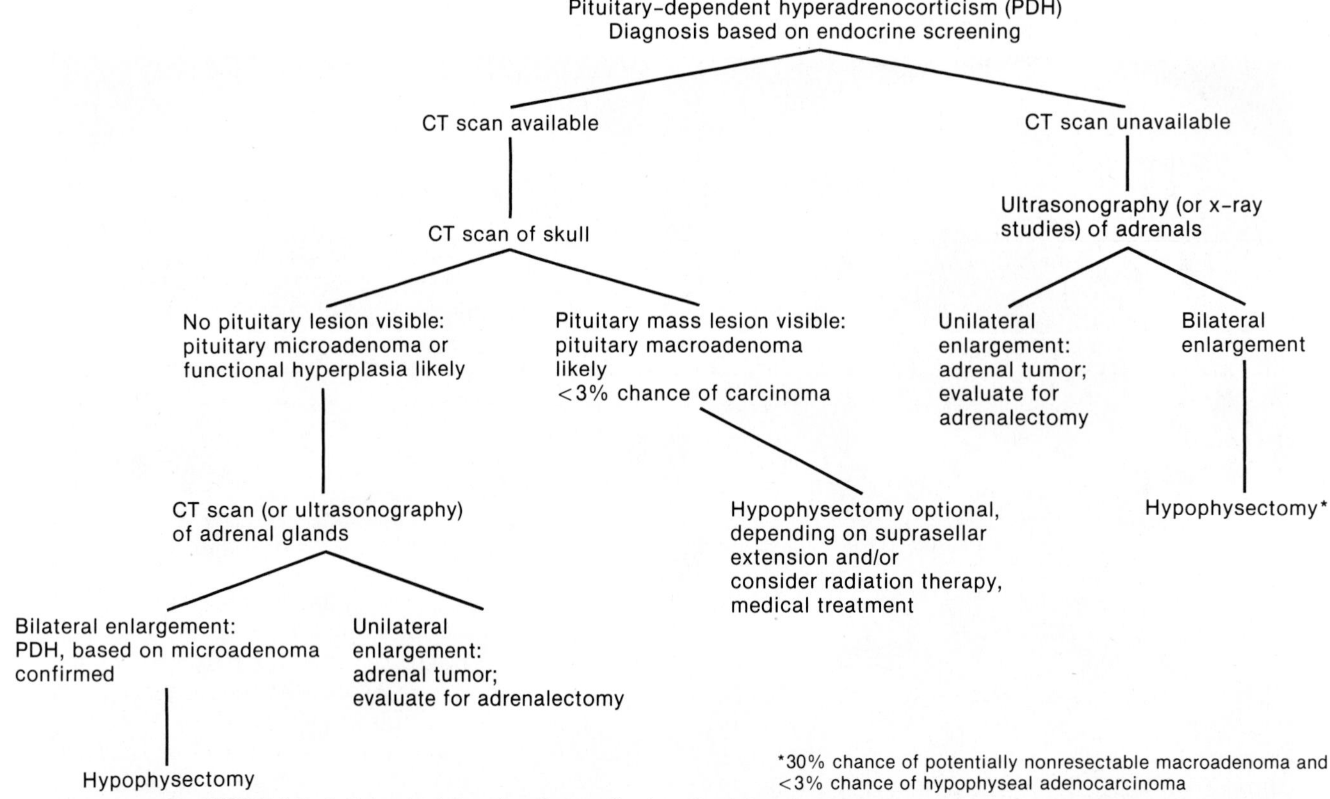

FIGURE 110–3. Flow chart showing diagnostic steps to determine indications for hypophysectomy.

gesting compensatory pituitary-independent regulatory mechanisms.[21]

Diabetes insipidus is transient after hypophysectomy. In dogs, urine-concentrating ability returns to approximately 80 per cent of the preoperative level and remains there within 2 weeks of hypophysectomy.[69] After transection of the supraopticohypophyseal tract, antidiuretic function is restored by hypothalamic centers, making long-term vasopressin substitution unnecessary.[16, 44, 79]

Hypophysectomy renders most animals of both sexes infertile, and the gonads undergo varying degrees of atrophy.[30] In selected valuable breeding animals, this effect is taken into consideration when evaluating treatment options.

An extension of hypophysectomy beyond canine PDH may occur when more data regarding acromegaly and growth hormone–dependent diabetes mellitus become available.[18, 22]

In Cushing's disease, whether the excess ACTH originates from a primary hyperfunction of pituitary corticotrophs or whether the hypophyseal lesion is induced by a dysfunction of higher centers in the central nervous system, causing alterations of corticotropin-releasing factor, is the subject of ongoing research.[10, 36, 77, 86] An answer to this question is unlikely to change the value of hypophysectomy or the indications for it.

Using the technique described next, dogs of any size and with any skull shape (brachycephalic as well as dolichocephalic dogs) are candidates for hypophysectomy.

TRANS-SPHENOIDAL HYPOPHYSECTOMY (NIEBAUER)

Surgical Anatomy

The canine sella turcica is a shallow depression on the dorsal surface of the sphenoid bone. To reach the sella via the trans-sphenoidal route, the soft palate is transected, the mucoperiosteal cover of the sphenoid bone reflected, the sphenoid bone trephined, and the dura mater incised.

The sphenoid bone consists of an outer and an inner layer of dense lamellar bone, with spongy bone containing numerous lacunae in the middle. The thickness of this spongy bone layer varies greatly in dogs of different breeds and ages.

Reliable landmarks to consistently pinpoint the sellar center for sphenoid bone trephination are absent. Dogs lack an air-filled sphenoid sinus, which is a dependable guide to the human pituitary. At surgery, in some older dogs, we have noticed a small equivalent of the sphenoid sinus (likely a remnant of the Rathke pouch), which appears as a somewhat larger, blood-filled lacuna within the spongy bone. If present and identifiable, it can serve as an additional landmark, and the center of the pituitary is found directly dorsal to it.

Three other landmarks on the base of the skull are useful to locate the hypophysis. First, the hamular processes can reliably be palpated in every dog, yet they are helpful for general orientation only. On the skeleton, the sella turcica can be found where a line drawn between the caudal ends of the two hamular processes crosses the midline (Fig 110–4). At surgery, this guideline is only partially helpful. The bony spicules of the hamular processes, which form the caudal ends of the ossa pterygoidea, are covered by muscle (tensor veli palatini) and mucoperiosteum and can only be palpated as relatively flat tubercles. Relying on these points of reference, the center of the hypophysis can be allocated to an area about 5 mm wide—not accurate enough to allow safe trephination.

The second landmark, the intersphenoidal suture, is of questionable value for two reasons. First, it is not identifiable in every dog. The joint between the basisphenoid and the presphenoid closes postpartum and remains clearly visible in young dogs only (intersphenoidal synchondrosis). In middle-aged or older animals, I found this suture often completely ossified and was unable to detect it at surgery. Second, the distance from the center of the sella turcica to the intersphenoidal suture (reported to be 1 cm) is constant only in midsize dogs with mesocephalic skulls.[39] According to body size and skull shape, this distance may vary.

The third landmark to identify the pituitary is the emissary vein. This vein likely occupies the space of the embryonal craniopharyngeal canal and, if clearly identified, can be an excellent landmark. By following the direction of this vein through the sphenoid bone, the center of the pituitary is found. Not unlike the intersphenoidal suture, the emissary vein is an inconsistent finding, especially in older dogs. Also, I have seen dogs in which several veins entered the sphenoid bone through minute nutritional foramina, some of them in the midline or in close proximity to it, mimicking the emissary vein and making identification of the emissary vein impossible.

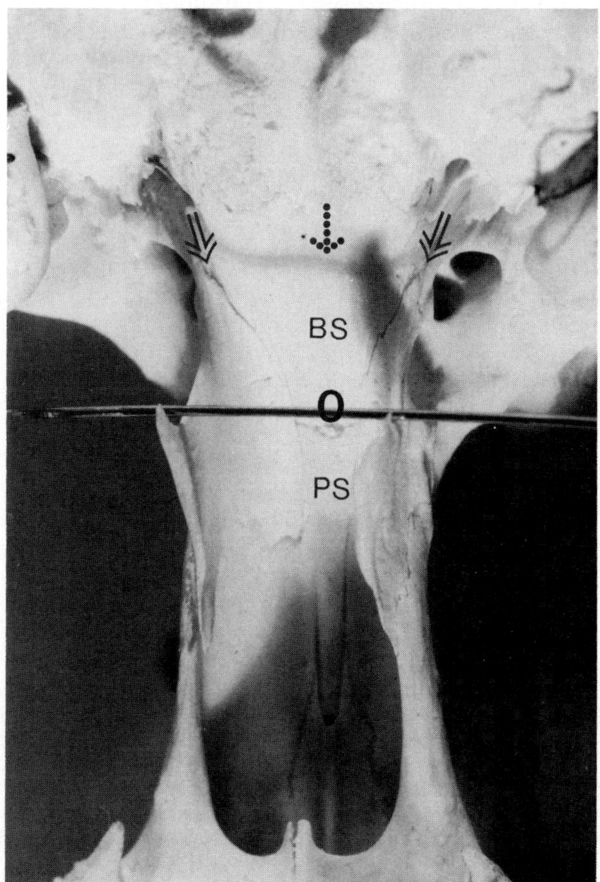

FIGURE 110–4. Landmarks to center trephination over the hypophyseal fossa shown on the base of a mesocephalic skeleton. Line (metal probe) connecting the hamular processes intersects the midline just caudal to the intersphenoidal suture. Ellipse delineates area of (over)-lying hypophyseal fossa. (BS, basisphenoid; PS, presphenoid.) The open arrows point at the caudal apertures of the pterygoid canal (vidian canal). Dotted arrow points rostrally.

Thus, in the surgical technique described later, the use of additional points of reference in the form of radiographic markers combined with a cranial sinus venogram is described. This allows identification of the appropriate location for sphenoid trephination despite the absence of reliable anatomical landmarks. An outline of the vascular anatomy that pertains to venography and hypophysectomy follows.

The cavernous sinus system is located within the extradural space on the interior surface of the sphenoid bone in immediate proximity to the pituitary gland.*[35, 94] These sinuses are the most vulnerable vascular structures during hypophysectomy, and severe, potentially fatal hemorrhage occurs when they are inadvertently lacerated.

Laterally, the pituitary is encircled by the paired, half-moon–shaped cavernous sinuses. During sphenoid bone ostectomy, their medial wall is often visible in the form of a transparent dark-blue membrane. Within the lumina of these sinuses, the internal carotid artery courses caudorostrally. Caudally, the vascular ring around the pituitary gland is closed by the rostral intercavernous sinus, which connects the cavernous sinuses rostral to the dorsum sellae. A small caudal intercavernous sinus extends caudal to the dorsum sellae, forming a small venous circle around the dorsum sellae. On the radiographic image (discussed later), this area should not be mistaken for the hypophyseal fossa. In dogs, the sinus circle around the hypophysis is incomplete rostrally. This narrow area, devoid of larger vascular structures, is located between the pituitary and the optic chiasm. Thus, during surgery, enlargement of an ostectomy site, narrow on the rostrocaudal axis, is permissible in this area only.

The pituitary itself is supplied by a dense network of small surrounding arteries and veins. Most arterial vessels originate from a dorsal hypophyseal artery and follow the infundibular stalk. Some vessels enter or exit the pituitary on its ventral pole and are lacerated as the overlying dura mater is incised. During hypophysectomy, minor hemorrhage from these small bridging pituitary vessels is diffuse and ceases spontaneously (discussed later).

When using conventional surgical techniques (Markowitz-Archibald technique) for pituitary extraction,[57] familiarization with the previously described vascular

---

*For a detailed anatomical description of the canine cranial venous sinus system, see Zimmermann[94]; for the remainder of the intracranial vascular anatomy of dogs, see Habermehl.[35]

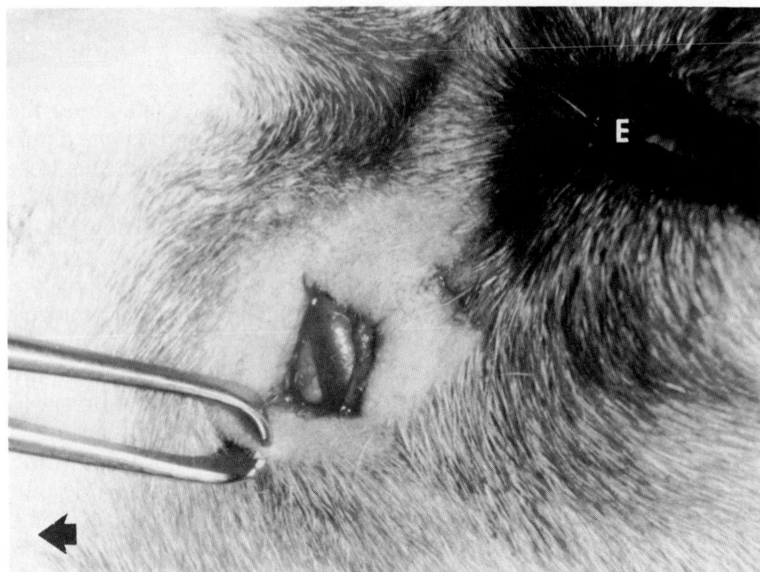

FIGURE 110–5. Cutdown to expose a beagle's left angularis oculi vein for catheterization as preparation for cranial sinus venography. (E, eye, arrow points rostrally.)

anatomy suffices. For using the modified technique described later, the anatomy of some extracranial veins used to perform the sinus venography is important: The angularis oculi vein (Fig. 110–5) is a valveless venous loop, draining via a dorsal (dorsal external ophthalmic vein) and a ventral branch (ventral external ophthalmic vein) and via the orbital fissure into the cavernous sinus system (Fig. 110–6). This extradural venous system is used radiographically to image the venous vascular ring encircling the hypophysis (discussed later).

The pituitary gland lies flat in the hypophyseal fossa, the narrow infundibulum, and the pars tuberalis dorsorostrally, close to the optic chiasm and the caudoventral pole resting on the dorsum sellae. The pars distalis consists of the adenohypophysis and faces entirely the sphenoid sella (Fig. 110–7). The neurohypophysis is enshrouded almost completely by the adenohypophysis. A sheet of dura mater extends from the diaphragma sellae ventrally and covers the entire sellar surface of the pituitary gland. The infundibulum is encircled by dura in a centrally wide-open, ringlike shelf, forming an incomplete diaphragma sellae. The subdural sellar space usually contains cerebrospinal fluid, which leaks as soon as the ventral dura sheet is incised. When suction ablation (the commonly used technique) is used, the pituitary avulses somewhere along the infundibular stalk. The pars tuberalis, containing mainly corticotrophs, extends along the infundibular stalk relatively far dorsally, ending nearly at the hypothalamus. Thus, complete excision of ACTH-producing tissue frequently might not be achievable; however, this anatomical intricacy might be more important in experimental procedures because pituitary microadenomas may not involve the proximal pars tuberalis. By transecting or avulsing the infundibular stalk, the infundibular recess, an extension of the third ventricle, is opened, and additional

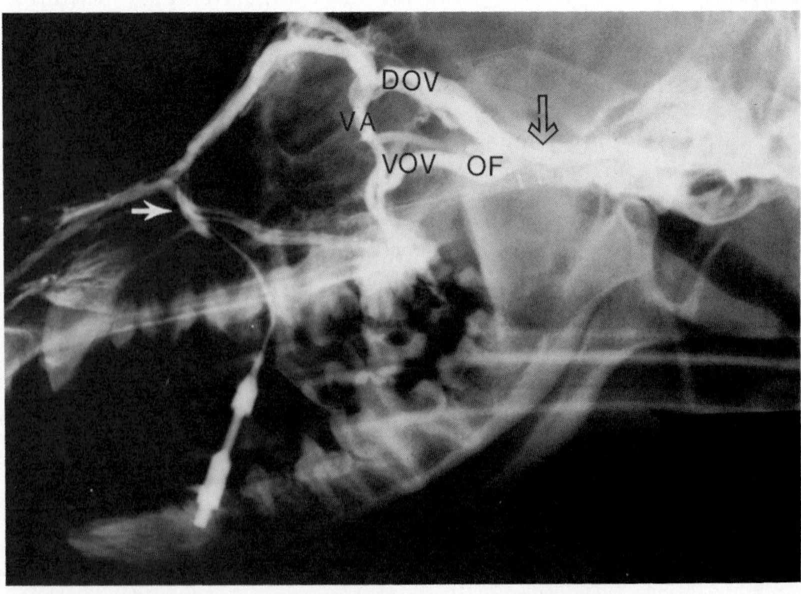

FIGURE 110–6. Lateral view of canine skull after contrast application into the angularis oculi vein unilaterally. White arrow shows injection site, open arrow points to the center of the hypophysis. (OF, orbital fissure; DOV, dorsal external ophthalmic vein and orbital plexus; VOV, ventral external ophthalmic vein; VA, vertical anastomosis between dorsal and ventral [external] ophthalmic veins.)

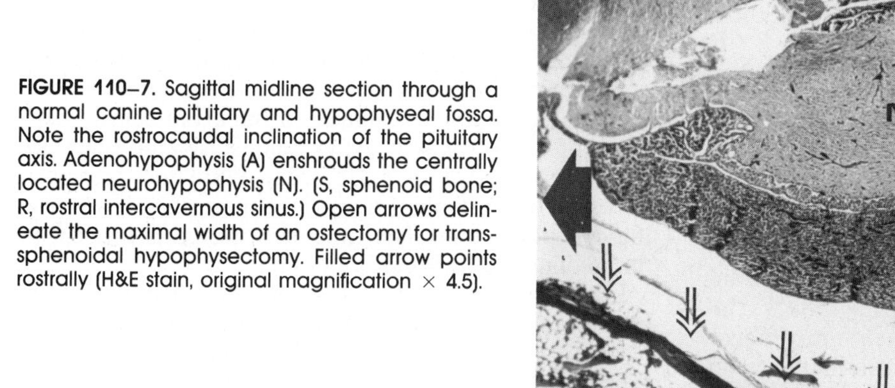

FIGURE 110–7. Sagittal midline section through a normal canine pituitary and hypophyseal fossa. Note the rostrocaudal inclination of the pituitary axis. Adenohypophysis (A) enshrouds the centrally located neurohypophysis (N). (S, sphenoid bone; R, rostral intercavernous sinus.) Open arrows delineate the maximal width of an ostectomy for transsphenoidal hypophysectomy. Filled arrow points rostrally (H&E stain, original magnification × 4.5).

cerebrospinal fluid escapes, though it is often barely noticeable.

The arterial circle of Willis surrounds the hypophysis in a relative wide, subarachnoidal vascular ring on the base of the brain. These vessels are distant enough from the hypophyseal fossa and thus from the surgical field to evade iatrogenic damage under normal circumstances. The proximity of this large vascular ring becomes apparent only after hypophysectomy is completed: A strong pulsation is regularly visible, affecting the torn infundibular stalk and parts of the hypothalamus.

Familiarization with the surgical anatomy of some extracranial structures is important for the success of hypophysectomy as well. Palate dehiscence and iatrogenic keratitis sicca have been observed in some cases (see the later section on complications).[69] These complications are avoidable by using proper surgical techniques based on an understanding of the topographical anatomy.

The soft palate is a strong yet delicate, well-vascularized muscle, covered dorsally by nasal mucosa and ventrally by oral mucosa. Adequate hemostasis and double-layer suture techniques coapting both epithelial layers are essential for proper healing.

Caution must be used during reflection of the mucoperiosteum on the sphenoid bone; a surgeon unfamiliar with the anatomy of the pterygoid canal can damage important nervous and vascular structures. The pterygoid canal (vidian canal) is a furrow in the angle formed by the medial pterygoid plate and the external surface of the sphenoid bone (see Fig. 10–4). This canal, passing caudorostrally on each side of the sphenoid bone, transmits the pterygopalatine artery and nerve. Both structures can be inadvertently damaged at the caudal aperture of the canal, which is located on the skull base just caudal to the hamular processes. Laceration of the vessel can result in substantial hemorrhage. Damage to the pterygopalatine nerve may be permanent and may be succeeded by a secretomotoric deficit to the lacrimal glands of the ipsilateral eye, usually leading to keratitis sicca. The pterygopalatine nerves carry postganglionic (pterygopalatine ganglion) parasympathetic secretomotor fibers that reach the lacrimal nerves via the maxillary and zygomatic nerves.

Instrumentation

In addition to routine instruments, others are recommended. Any surgical drill unit usable for ostectomies, either air driven or electrically powered, can be used. Because self-threading screws (commonly used in restorative dentistry) are recommended as radiographic markers, a dental drill unit* is preferable for both marker placement and sphenoid bone trephination. For the drill, a contra-angle and a straight handpiece are necessary, as well as a set of small (0.425-mm-diameter) gold-coated dental screws.† For the ostectomy, 2- to 4-mm-diameter egg-shaped burs‡ are recommended.

Other instruments include a small hinged Beckman-Weitlaner retractor, a small curette, a dura hook, a fine blunt probe or spatula such as a Stevens tenotomy hook, and conjunctival forceps and scissors.

A vacuum source for suction is mandatory, and Frazier suction tips, preferably of different diameters (between 2 and 4 mm), should be available. Electrocautery is optional. Absorbable suture material (e.g., 3-0 polyglactic acid [Vicryl]) and bone wax§ are needed.

Anesthesia

There are no specific requirements for general anesthesia. Manipulation or drugs significantly increasing

*VC-30 Dental Care Unit, Henry Schein, Inc., Port Washington, NY.

†TMS Link Series, Cat. No. L-511, Whaldent International, New York, NY.

‡Goldies-Dedeco titanium nitride-coated carbide burs, Henry Schein, Inc., Port Washington, NY.

§Bone Wax, Ethicon, Inc., Somerville, NJ.

intracranial pressure are avoided. If resection of a suprasellar mass lesion is attempted, all known precautions to minimize intracranial pressure, such as hyperventilation and administration of mannitol and furosemide, are strongly advised (see Chapter 168).

In any trans-sphenoidal surgery, the endotracheal tube is of smaller diameter than used routinely, given the diameter of the trachea. This narrower tube improves access to the nasopharyngeal area. Tracheostomy for intubation is unnecessary. The endotracheal tube is tied to the lower jaw, leaving the tongue free. During surgery, an assistant can easily move the endotracheal tube to the side and away from the surgical field together with the tongue.

A balanced electrolyte solution is given intravenously during surgery, and a broad-spectrum antibiotic is administered.

Preparation for Surgery

Trans-sphenoidal hypophysectomy is a contaminated surgical procedure. Aseptic technique and avoiding contact of instruments with the teeth or parodontal tissues minimize contamination. Before surgery, the oral cavity is wiped with a surgical sponge soaked in 0.5 per cent chlorhexidine acetate diluted in isopropyl alcohol, followed by spraying with the same disinfectant.

Angularis Oculi Vein Catheterization

The area of the angularis oculi vein (unilaterally) is shaved and routinely prepared for a cutdown procedure, which is preferably performed before positioning the animal for the trans-sphenoidal surgery. Catheterization without surgically exposing the vein is not attempted, because the vein easily rolls away from the needle and is covered by fibers of the levator nasolabial muscle. Once the vein is exposed, gentle handling with forceps facilitates catheterization with an intravenous catheter* pointing caudally (see Fig. 110–5). Because blood flow in either direction is possible in this valveless vein, catheterization pointing rostrodorsally is permissible as well. The catheter is secured with one suture, heparinized, and protected for later use. In general, the right angularis oculi vein is used for angiography because right-sided imaging of the cavernous sinus system with radiographic markers placed to the right of the midline is preferable for right-handed surgeons. If the first attempt at catheterization fails, the opposite vein can be used. Radiographic markers are placed on the same side as the catheter (discussed later).

Surgical Procedure

The recommended procedure consists of three parts: (1) the approach to the sphenoid bone with placement of the radiographic markers, (2) venous sinus angiography, and (3) sphenoid ostectomy with pituitary extraction and closure. For angiography, the animal is transferred to the appropriate location without interrupting anesthesia.

*Abbocath-T20, Abbott Hospitals, Inc., North Chicago, IL.

Part 1: Approach to the Sphenoid Bone, Placement of Radiographic Markers

Dogs are placed in dorsal recumbency with the surgeon seated and facing the head. The mouth is opened maximally with a speculum, and the head is fixed loosely with the palate approximately parallel to the table.

A midline incision is made through the central two-thirds of the soft palate. After hemostasis, the edges are gently retracted with a Beckman-Weitlaner retractor, exposing the nasopharyngeal mucoperiosteum covering the sphenoid bone. The mucoperiosteum is incised on the midline and reflected laterally.

Electrocautery is advantageous for hemostasis. A large area of sphenoid bone has to be exposed to allow placement of radiographic markers well off the midline. Care has to be taken to avoid damage to nerves and vessels entering the pterygoid canal caudolaterally. The sphenoid bone is exposed caudally to a point just beyond the caudal margins of the hamular processes. Minor hemorrhage from various veins perforating the compacta of the sphenoid bone usually occurs. One of these vessels is frequently observed as emanating from the midline and thus might be identified as the emissary vein. In such cases, this vein serves as an excellent landmark leading in direct line to the sellar center (see the earlier section on surgical anatomy). If the intersphenoid suture can be identified, the area of trephination lies just caudal to it. The correct location to start the sphenoid ostectomy can also be approximated by drawing an imaginary line between the hamular processes, which are always easily palpable (see Fig. 110–4). (If the Markowitz-Archibald technique of hypophysectomy is preferred, skip the following section and continue with "sphenoid ostectomy, hypophysectomy and closure.")

When the approximate location of sphenoid trephination has been outlined, radiographic markers are placed into the sphenoid bone close to the area of the anticipated ostectomy site. Using a low-speed dental drill and an appropriate drill bit, three small nonperforating bur holes are drilled to a depth of approximately 2 mm into the exposed sphenoid bone (Fig. 110–8). The holes are placed on a rostrocaudal line 3 to 4 mm off the midline (to the right of the midline for right-handed surgeons, or to the same side as angularis oculi catheter, leaving enough space to allow midline ostectomy later on. All available and identifiable anatomical landmarks are used as a reference to approximate the middle bur hole across the area where the center of the hypophysis can be expected. This is usually accomplished by placing the middle drill hole at the intersection of the paramedian rostrocaudal line and a second imaginary line that connects the hamular processes. The exact location of the middle bur hole is not essential for success. The rostral and caudal bur holes are placed 4 to 5 mm from the middle bur hole. Then, using the same dental drill, three small self-threading screws* (0.425 mm diameter) are placed in the predrilled channels and broken off even with the bone surface. (The screws are intended for permanent placement, and no adverse reactions have been noticed.)

*TMS Link Series, Cat. No. L-511, Whaldent International, New York, NY.

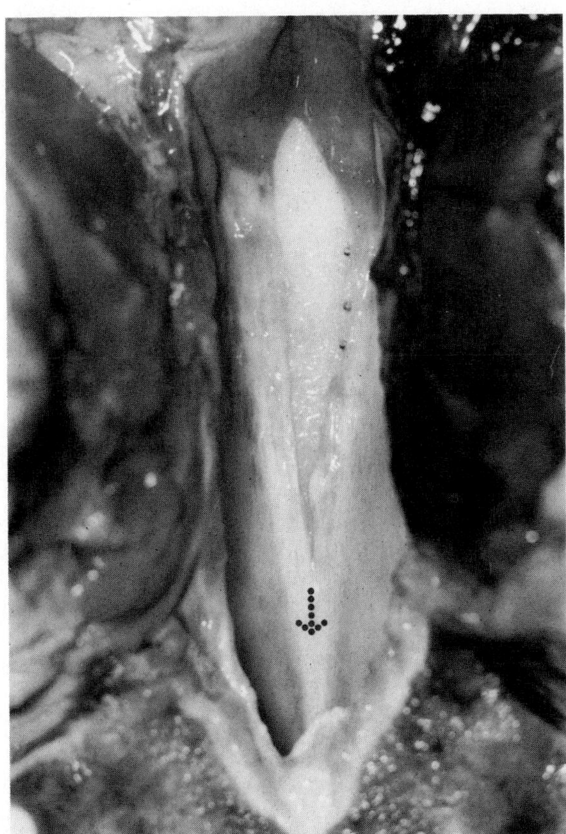

FIGURE 110–8. Placement of radiographic markers (three self-threading dental screws) before ostectomy, shown on a necropsy specimen. The soft palate had been partially resected to facilitate exposure. The nasopharyngeal mucoperiosteum is incised in the midline and reflected over the screws. The sphenoid bone is partially exposed to allow midline ostectomy. Dotted arrow points rostrally.

The instruments are removed, and a chlorhexidine-soaked sponge can be placed over the wound while the dog is repositioned for the radiographic procedure.

Part 2: Venous Sinus Angiography[72]

Animals are placed in sternal recumbency with the head extended and the lower jaw parallel to the plane of the film. Using an extension set attached to the preplaced catheter, 4 to 6 ml (0.2 to 0.3 ml/kg) of contrast medium* is rapidly injected into the angularis oculi vein. During injection, the external jugular veins are compressed with a gauze tourniquet placed around the neck. A single dorsoventral radiograph is taken while the last 1 ml is being injected. The venogram demonstrates unilateral filling of the venous sinus system. The hypophysis is outlined by the cavernous sinus and the rostral intercavernous sinus, which usually enhances across the midline; silhouetting of the opposite cavernous sinus frequently occurs (Figs. 110–9 and 110–10). For accurate identification of the center of the hypophysis, contrast enhancement of the contralateral cavernous sinus is not required.

*Hypaque-76, Winthrop-Breon Laboratories, New York, NY.

Part 3: Sphenoid Ostectomy, Hypophysectomy, Closure

The dog is repositioned for surgery as previously described. A new set of instruments is used. From the radiographs, the ostectomy site is determined by measuring the distance and angles between the center of the hypophysis and the two nearest metal screws. Estimating these distances is sufficient for accurate exposure, because distances in question are only in the millimeter range and at least two screws serve as points of reference.

The ostectomy is begun with the dental drill attached to a straight handpiece and a 2- to 4-mm-diameter egg-shaped bur, depending on the size of the skull (Figs. 110–11 and 110–12). Drilling begins on the midline over the expected center of the hypophysis, and the surgical field is irrigated with saline. The osteotomy is widened slowly and symmetrically. As drilling progresses, orientation can be maintained by continuously viewing the metal screws and assessing their position relative to the drill hole in accordance with the radiographic image. Because of the egg shape of the bur, the ostectomy channel becomes more elliptical as it is deepened. This is helpful in preventing inadvertent damage to the cavernous sinuses. Moderate hemorrhage occurs while drilling the spongy bone. Continuous suction eases the progress, and larger diploic lacunae are sealed with bone

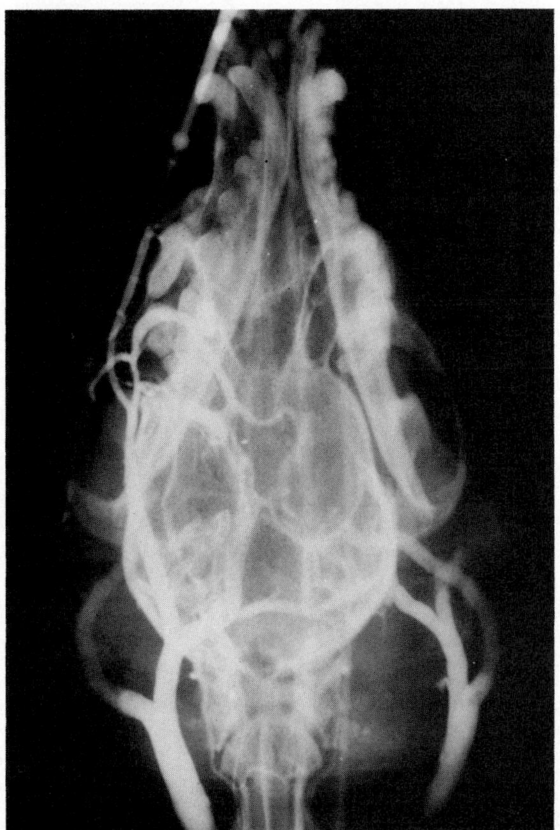

FIGURE 110–9. Dorsoventral view from skull in Figure 110–6 after unilateral injection of contrast medium. The center of the hypophyseal fossa is located on the midline opposite the center screw. (From Niebauer GW, Evans SM: Transsphenoidal hypophysectomy in the dog—a new technique. *Vet Surg 17*:296, 1988.)

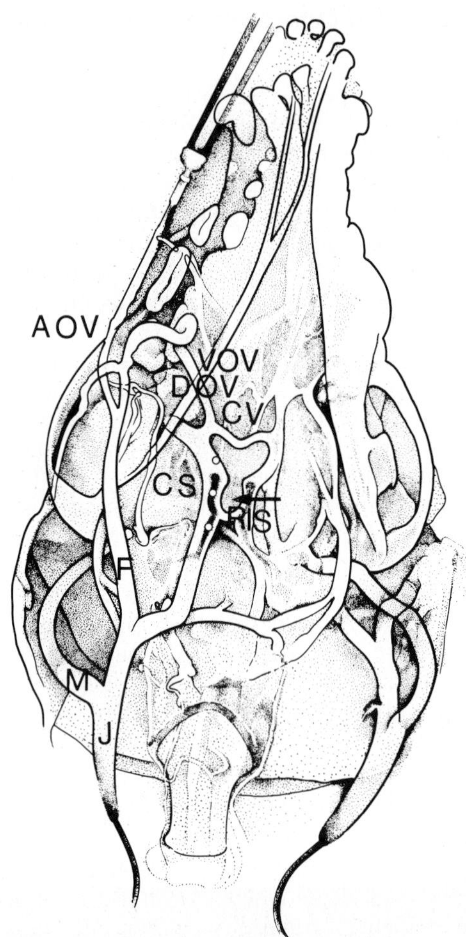

FIGURE 110–10. Schematic drawing of radiograph shown in Figure 110–9. Arrow points to the center of the hypophysis. (AOV, angularis oculi vein; CV, chiasmatic vein [horizontal anastomosis between ventral external ophthalmic veins {VOV}]; CS, cavernous sinus; DOV, dorsal external ophthalmic vein; RIS, rostral intercavernous sinus; F, facial vein; M, maxillary vein; J, external jugular vein.)

wax. When the dorsal cortex is perforated, the yellowish-pink hypophysis can usually be seen through the dura. Pituitary exposure is completed by enlarging the aperture with a small curette. The lateral cavernous sinuses can occasionally be seen as transparent bluish structures on the ostectomy floor. Enlargement of the osseous channel rostrally for 1 to 2 mm is not risky as long as bone chips are broken off with the curette in or near the midline. The hypophysis is covered by dura and does not need to be exposed along its entire length. As soon as the dura is opened in stellate fashion with a dura hook or fine scissors, the pituitary gland usually protrudes into the surgical field and moderate amounts of cerebrospinal fluid leak out. With a fine blunt instrument (i.e., probe or Stevens tenotomy hook), the dural attachments and vascular bridges are loosened or broken. The hypophysis can then be dislodged and partially extracted, stretching the infundibular stalk by applying gentle traction with the suction tip of appropriate diameter (2 to 4 mm). Under ideal circumstances, the stalk can be severed and the entire pituitary harvested for histological studies. A combination of experience and luck is required, and to succeed, careful adjustment of the negative pressure on the suction tip is necessary. The avulsing pituitary frequently disappears in the suction tube. A tissue filter (approximately 150 μm millipore screen) as interphase between the suction tip and the tubing can be used to trap pieces of the aspirated gland for histological study.

Some hemorrhage from vessels supplying the hypophysis occurs. A topical hemostat may be used (e.g., microfibrillar collagen*), although it is not essential. Bleeding ceases spontaneously in most cases by simply occluding the ostectomy hole for 2 to 3 minutes with a surgical sponge soaked in cold saline. Pulsation of the arterial circle of Willis can indirectly be seen as pressure waves are transmitted through the fluid on the floor of the empty sella.

Closure of the ostectomy site is either by direct occlusion with bone wax or by inserting a muscle graft harvested directly from the soft-palate incision. This latter method is preferable, because bone wax is degraded extremely slowly and may cause foreign body reactions or in extreme cases might enhance local osteomyelitis. The small piece of muscle (3 to 4 mm in diameter) is placed into the drill hole and is secured by suturing the mucoperiosteum with one or two loose

*Avitene, nonwoven web form; Alcon, Inc., Humacao, Puerto Rico.

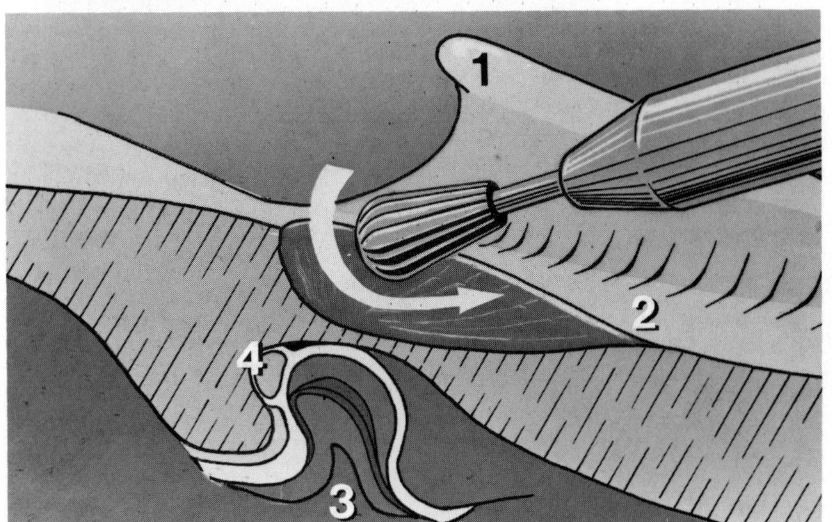

FIGURE 110–11. Sagittal section through part of a mesocephalic canine skull showing the positioning of the drill relative to the hamular process (1). (2, rostral limit of bur grove; 3, hypophysis; 4, rostral intercavernous sinus.)

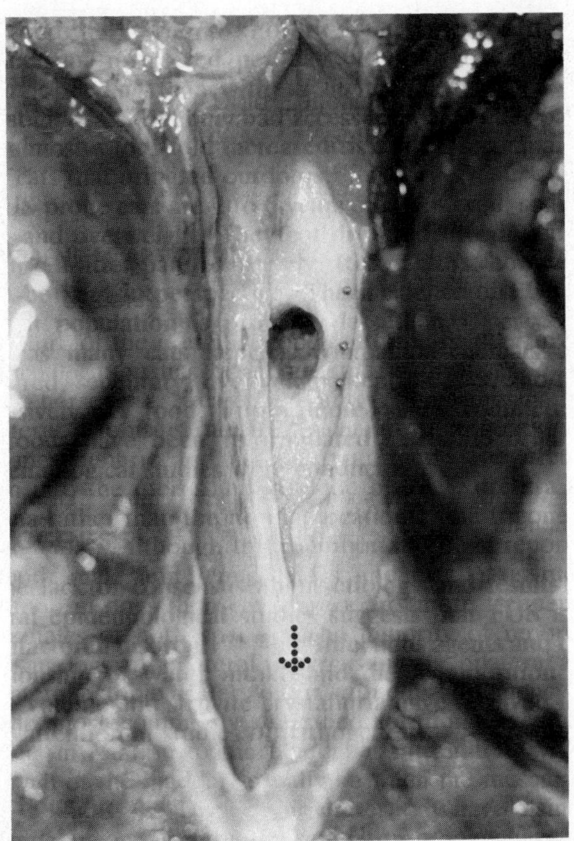

FIGURE 110–12. Skull specimen shown in Figure 110–8 with appropriately sized and centered ostectomy. Dotted arrow points rostrally.

sutures. If the mucoperiosteum tears during exposure of the sphenoid bone, the muscle graft can be held in place with fibrin glue. Instead of muscle, an autologous fat graft can be used.

The soft-palate incision is closed in two layers using absorbable suture material in a simple interrupted pattern. The dorsal layer facing the nasopharynx is sutured first, and the knots are inverted.

Surgical Aftercare

After recovery, food and water are withheld for approximately 24 hours. A balanced electrolyte solution is given intravenously during this period. Monitoring of basic blood parameters, serum electrolytes, and urine specific gravity is recommended for the immediate period of recovery (most animals are middle-aged or older and have suffered Cushing's disease for long periods before surgery).

Immediately after surgery, vasopressin (Pitressin) is given (approximately 0.2 IU/kg IM) every other day and continued for 1 to 2 weeks as necessary. Corticosteroid and thyroid hormone supplementation is initiated shortly after recovery from anesthesia. Each hormone is either injected for the first few postoperative days or given orally. Initial dosage and the dosage for lifelong substitution are the same: prednisolone (or prednisone), 0.2 mg/kg/day; and thyroxine,* 0.02 mg/kg/day.

Antibiotic therapy is continued for at least 1 week after surgery.

Long-Term Endocrine Supplementation

Corticosteroids (prednisone, 0.2 mg/kg) and thyroid hormone* (0.02 mg/kg) are given daily, preferably in the morning. If supplementation is temporarily interrupted (e.g., indigestion, vomiting), no immediate or serious signs of hormone deprivation develop because both the adrenal cortices and thyroid glands continue to secrete low levels of hormones.

Growth hormone substitution is not mandatory, but long-term use might help to prevent the occasionally observed skin scaling and hair loss. At present, the need for such replacement is controversial. Clinical experience is lacking, and growth hormone is difficult to obtain and expensive.

Complications

Severe complications are rare and depend to some degree on the experience of the surgeon. Such complications include severe hemorrhage and iatrogenic damage to the hypothalamus or adjacent central nervous structures. Should either of these complications occur, the damage becomes apparent immediately or during recovery from anesthesia. Survival of such dogs is questionable.

Another major potential complication is dehiscence of the palate incision (usually on the second to fourth day after surgery). Aspiration pneumonia may ensue, and recovery may be hampered severely; the incidence can be minimized by careful suturing and by not placing undue traction on the soft-palate edges when inserting a retractor during surgery. In small dogs, I recommend retention sutures instead of instrument retractors. If palate dehiscence occurs, resuturing is done as soon as possible. Wound retraction and scarring of the soft palate occur readily, making repair without using plastic procedures (split-thickness flap) difficult.

Sphenoid bone osteomyelitis was observed in one dog with experimental hypophysectomy when bone wax was used to occlude the ostectomy site and antibiotics were not administered. Broad-spectrum antibiotic therapy, initiated at or before surgery, is continued for at least 1 week postoperatively. An autologous muscle graft to occlude the sphenoid bur hole is preferred over bone wax.

An uncommon complication (which I observed twice) is keratitis sicca developing as a sequel to iatrogenic damage to fibers of the pterygopalatine nerves (see the earlier section on surgical anatomy). Only undue manipulation beyond the surgical field causes this injury.

Moderate nasal discharge may be observed during the first few postoperative days. The ability to swallow may also be impaired during the immediate postoperative

*Synthetic L-thyroxine (levothyroxine sodium), peroral form, Soloxine, Daniels Pharmaceutical, St. Petersburg, FL; injectable form, Synthroid, Flint Laboratories, Morton Grove, IL.

period as a result of surgical trauma to the nasopharynx and soft palate. It is important to distinguish this transient functional impairment from dysphagia due to palate dehiscence. In general, dogs recover without any complications and function normally the day after hypophysectomy.

Assessment of Completeness of Hypophysectomy

In successfully treated dogs, signs of Cushing's disease begin to diminish shortly after surgery. All signs of the disease are often reversed completely within a few weeks. If signs persist or if recovery is unsatisfactory, endocrine screening tests (described earlier) are repeated. In addition, a growth hormone stimulation test can be performed. Because the anatomical distribution of somatotrophs parallels that of the corticotrophs and is restricted to the adenohypophysis, failure to elicit any response to growth hormone stimulation suggests complete excision of the adenohypophysis.

When macroadenomas have been excised, follow-up CT scans are recommended. This step is especially important when pituitary tissue could not be sampled for histological investigation at surgery. I noted recurrence of PDH in one dog 1 month after surgery; a pituitary carcinoma with widespread brain metastasis was found at necropsy, 3 months after surgery.

ALTERNATIVE SURGICAL APPROACHES: INTRACRANIAL AND PARAPHARYNGEAL ROUTES

Intracranial Transtemporal Approach

The intracranial transtemporal approach to the dog's pituitary has been fully explored experimentally[14, 46, 74] and is indicated for attempted resection of macroadenomas and suprasellar or parasellar pituitary tumors. This approach is not feasible in cats, partly because of their deeper hypophyseal fossa.[14] Although we prefer the trans-sphenoidal approach, we have attempted to reach the pituitary via the transtemporal route and achieved satisfactory exposure.[14, 68, 71]

Dogs are placed in sternal position with the head elevated. In contrast to other intracranial operations, fixation methods have to be used to allow repositioning the head (rotation into the dependent position) during surgery.

The cranial vault is approached routinely via the rostrotentorial route unilaterally, and the temporal muscle is reflected as far ventrally as possible. In some breeds (e.g., brachycephalic dogs), osteotomy of the zygomatic arch is recommended to allow better ventral retraction of the muscle (at closure, the arch can easily be reattached with wire cerclages). Cranial osteotomy involves a large area of the temporal bone, extending as close to the base of the skull as possible (or permissible). The dura is incised, cerebrospinal fluid is allowed to drain, and intracranial pressure is lowered as much as possible by hyperventilation and by medical means. Gravity is used to help expose the base of the brain. Dogs are repositioned by rotating the heads 100° to 140° into an inverted position, with the brain falling away from the base of the skull. The skull remains elevated in relation to the plane of the heart to allow uncongested venous return. Malleable brain spatulas are carefully used to retract the temporal lobe of the brain. If done improperly, this retraction is likely to cause neurological complications. Without retracting the temporal lobe, gravity in combination with lowered intracranial pressure usually allows an adequate view of the infundibular stalk. The oculomotor nerve might bisect the area in question but does not obstruct access to the pituitary with fine instruments. Careful blunt dissection of the vascular and connective tissue attachments of the hypophysis has to follow. Here, in contrast to the trans-sphenoidal approach, where the cavernous sinuses are in dangerous proximity, arteries of the circle of Willis can be inadvertently lacerated. Hemostasis should be meticulous as in any intracranial surgery. Routine closure is accomplished by reattaching the temporal muscle only. Dura closure and replacement of the elevated bone flap are unnecessary.[68]

Parapharyngeal Approach

The parapharyngeal approach was developed experimentally in dogs and reported once.[91] Asepsis is the only advantage of the parapharyngeal route over the trans-sphenoidal approach. However, given the technical improvements of the trans-sphenoidal procedure and the advent of efficient broad-spectrum antibiotics, the parapharyngeal approach offers little advantage. Visibility is limited, and the surgical exposure is inferior to the oropharyngeal approach. Thus, only a short synopsis of the procedure is given.

Initially, the surgical approach is executed like the approach to the tympanic bullae. Then, by blunt midline dissection, a cleavage plane is sought between the mucoperiosteum and the sphenoid bone. The sterility of the procedure (and thereby the value of the procedure) is jeopardized during this phase of dissection, however, because the delicate nasopharyngeal mucosa can be torn easily, exposing the pharynx. The approach is a possible alternative in severe oropharyngeal infections and immunosuppression.

PROGNOSIS

Dogs with pituitary microadenomas or sellar lesions (confirmed by CT scan) are definite candidates for hypophysectomy, and their prognosis is excellent. In successfully treated dogs, recovery is instantaneous and permanent. Endocrine supplementation is easy to accomplish, and metabolic imbalances usually do not occur. Diabetes insipidus is transient and not a prognostic factor.

The size and suprasellar extent of a pituitary neoplasm significantly affect the surgical prognosis. Whether such lesions recur after surgery, to what degree they may recur, or whether they continue to expand is unknown. Fragments of functional tumor that may be dislodged during surgery (incomplete hypophysectomy) may not fully retain their endocrine activity and may continue to grow at a slower rate.

Biopsy, by sampling tissue during surgery, should always be attempted. Pituitary adenocarcinomas, though rare, can easily be mistaken for macroadenomas. Hypophysectomized animals are infertile.

In summary, the size of the sellar lesion, completeness of hypophysectomy, and histological diagnosis are of equal prognostic importance. Accurate assessment of each of these factors is generally the exception rather than the rule. Therefore, in all cases except those with microadenomas and subsequent complete hypophysectomy, the prognosis is guarded.

References

1. Aschner B: Über die Funktion der Hypophyse. *Pflügers Arch Gesamte Physiol 146*:1, 1912.
2. Bennett RJ Jr: A simple method of hypophysectomy in the dog. *Endocrinology 20*:860, 1936.
3. Biewenga WJ, et al: Persistent polyuria in two dogs following adrenocorticolysis for pituitary-dependent hyperadrenocorticism. *Vet Q 11*:193, 1989.
4. Camus J, Roussy G: Polyurie expériéntale par lésions de la base du cerveau. La polyurie dite hypophysaire. *C R Soc Biol 65*:628, 1913.
5. Camus J, Roussy G: Hypophysectomie et polyurie expérimentales. *C R Soc Biol 65*:483, 1913.
6. Capen CC, et al: Neoplasms in the adenohypophysis of dogs. A clinical and pathologic study. *Pathol Vet 4*:301, 1967.
7. Caselli A: Osservazioni sul'ipofisectomia. *Pflügers Arch Gesamte Physiol 73*:385, 1898.
8. Concannon P: Effects of hypophysectomy and of LH administration on luteal phase plasma progesterone levels in the beagle bitch. *J Reprod Fert 58*:407, 1980.
9. Coppa M, et al: Tecnica de hipofisectomia en caninos modificada. *Arch Med Vet 10*:155, 1978.
10. Croughs RM, Koppeschaar HPF: Changing views on the pathogenesis of Cushing's disease in man. *Front Horm Res 17*:78, 1987.
11. Crowe SJ, et al: Experimental hypophysectomy. *Bull Johns Hopkins Hosp 21*:127, 1910.
12. Cushing H: Surgical experiences with pituitary disorders. *JAMA 63*:1515, 1914.
13. Dalla Vedova F: Per la funzione dell'ipofisi; nota preliminaria. *Bol R Acad Med di Roma 29*: 150, 1903.
14. Dandy WE, Reichert FL: Studies on experimental hypophysectomy. I. Effect on maintenance of life. *Bull Johns Hopkins Hosp 37*:1, 1925.
15. Dandy WE, Reichert FL: Studies on experimental hypophysectomy in dogs. III. Somatic, mental and glandular effects. *Bull Johns Hopkins Hosp 62*:122, 1938.
16. Daniel PM, Prichard ML: Studies on the hypothalamus and the pituitary gland. *Acta Endocrinol 80* (Suppl 201):1, 1975.
17. Dow SW, LeCouteur RA: Radiation therapy for canine ACTH-secreting pituitary tumors. *In* Kirk RW (ed): *Current Veterinary Therapy X*. W.B. Saunders, Philadelphia, 1989, pp 1031–1034.
18. Eigenmann JE: Wachstumshormon und insulinähnlicher Wachstumsfaktor beim Hund. *Schweiz Arch Tierheilk 128*:57, 1986.
19. Eigenmann JE: Insulin-like growth factor I in the dog. *Front Horm Res 17*:161, 1987.
20. Eigenmann JE, Lubberink AAME: The pituitary. *In* Slatter D (ed): *Textbook of Small Animal Surgery*. W.B. Saunders, Philadelphia, 1985, pp 1840–1851.
21. Eigenmann JE, et al: The influence of hypophysectomy on NSILA concentrations in the dog: Evidence for partially pituitary-independent regulation. *Acta Endocrinol (Copenh) 86*:498, 1977
22. Eigenmann JE, et al: Elevated growth hormone levels and diabetes mellitus in a cat with acromegalic features. *J Am Anim Hosp Assoc 20*:747, 1984.
23. Eik-Nes K, Brizzle KR: Adrenocortical activity in hypophysectomized dogs. *Am J Physiol 193*:403, 1958.
24. Engeland WC, Gann DS: Splanchnic nerve stimulation modulates steroid secretion in hypophysectomized dogs. *Neuroendocrinology 50*:124, 1989.
25. Essex HE, Astarabadi TM: Transbuccal hypophysectomy in the dog. *Ann Surg 138*:143, 1953.
26. Feldman EC, et al: Therapy for spontaneous canine hyperadrenocorticism. *In* Kirk RW (ed): *Current Veterinary Therapy X*. W.B. Saunders, Philadelphia, 1989, pp 1024–1031.
27. Fike JR, et al: Anatomy of the canine brain using high resolution computed tomography. *Vet Radiol 22*:236, 1981.
28. Fike JR, et al: Computerized tomography of brain tumors of the rostral and middle fossa in the dog. *Am J Vet Res 42*:275, 1981.
29. Friedmann K, Maas N: Über die Exstirpation der hypophysis cerebri. *Berl Klin Wochenschr 37*:1213, 1900.
30. Ganong WF, Hume DM: The effect of graded hypophysectomy on thyroid, gonadal and adrenocortical function in the dog. *Endocrinology 59*:293, 1956.
31. Gemelli A: Sur la fonction de l'hypophyse. *Arch Ital Biol 50*:157, 1908.
32. George AE: Radiologic diagnosis of pituitary tumors. *Semin Reprod Endocrinol 2*:47, 1984.
33. Grigsby PW, et al: Prognostic factors and results of surgery and postoperative irradiation in the management of pituitary adenomas. *Int J Radiat Oncol Biol Phys 16*:1411, 1989.
34. Grigsby PW, et al: Late regrowth of pituitary adenomas after irradiation and/or surgery: Hazard function analysis. *Cancer 63*:1308, 1989.
35. Habermehl KH: Zur Topographie der Gehirngefässe des Hundes. *Zentralb Anat Histol Embryol 2*:327, 1973.
36. Halmi NS, et al: Pituitary intermediate lobe in the dog: Two cell types and high adrenocorticotropin content. *Science 211*:72, 1981.
37. Heap RB, et al: Adrenal secretion rates of C-19 and C-21 steroids before and after hypophysectomy in the pig and the dog. *J Endocrinol 36*:159, 1966.
38. Henderson WR: Pituitary adenomata: Follow-up study of surgical results of 338 cases (Dr. Harvey Cushing's series). *Br J Surg 26*:811, 1939.
39. Henry RW, et al: Transoral hypophysectomy with mandibular symphysiotomy in the dog. *Am J Vet Res 43*:1825, 1982.
40. Hirsch O: Pituitary tumors. A borderland between cranial and transsphenoidal surgery. *N Engl J Med 254*:937, 1956.
41. Horsley V: Functional nervous disorders due to loss of thyroid gland and pituitary body. *Lancet 1*:5, 1886.
42. Houssay BA: Exstirpacion de la hypofisis en el perro. *Endocrinology 2*:497, 1918.
43. Kameda Y, Ikeda A: Immunohistochemical reactions of C-cell complexes in dogs after induced hypercalcemia, antithyroid drug treatment and hypophysectomy. *Cell Tissue Res 208*:417, 1980.
44. Keller AD, et al: Effects of varying degrees of hypophysectomy in the dog. *Arch Pathol 40*:289, 1945.
45. Kemmer FW, et al: Glucoregulatory mechanisms following hypophysectomy in diabetic dogs with residual insulin secretion. *Diabetes 32*:26, 1983.
46. Kendrick MM, Silverberg GD: Transtemporal hypophysectomy in the dog. *Surg Neurol 4*:244, 1975.
47. Lane N, de Bodo RC: Generalized adrenocortical atrophy in hypophysectomized dogs and correlated functional studies. *Am J Physiol 168*:1, 1952.
48. Lantz GC, et al: Transsphenoidal hypophysectomy in the clinically normal dog. *Am J Vet Res 49*:1134, 1988.
49. Laws ER, et al: Transsphenoidal surgery following unsuccessful prior therapy. *J Neurosurg 63*:823, 1985.
50. Livon C: L'hypophyse est-elle un centre réflexe circulatoire? *Mars Med 45*:745, 1908.
51. Lomonaco D, van Rynberk R: Ricerche sulla funzione dell'iposfisi cerebrale. *Riv Mens Neuropat Psichiat 9*:2, 1901.
52. Lorenz MD: Diagnosis and medical management of canine Cushing's syndrome: A study of 57 consecutive cases. *J Am Anim Hosp Assoc 18*:707, 1982.
53. Lubberink AAME: *Diagnosis and Treatment of Canine Cushing's Syndrome*. Drukkereij Elimkwijk, Utrecht, 1977, pp 45–75.
54. Lubberink AAME: Therapy for spontaneous hyperadrenocorticism. *In* Kirk RW (ed): *Current Veterinary Therapy VII*. W.B. Saunders, Philadelphia, 1980, pp 979–983.
55. Lubberink AAME, Rijnberk AD: Hypophysectomy. *In* Kirk RW (ed): *Current Veterinary Therapy V*. W.B. Saunders, Philadelphia, 1974, pp 787–789.
56. Marienesco MG: De la déstruction de la glande pituitaire chez le chat. *Compt Rend Soc Biol 4*:509, 1892.
57. Markowitz J: *Experimental Surgery*. 5th ed. Williams & Wilkins, Baltimore, 1964, pp 581–598.
58. Markowitz J, Archibald J: Transbuccal hypophysectomy in the dog. *Can J Biochem Physiol 34*:422, 1956.
59. Matsuda K, et al: Technique for transpalatal hypophysectomy and electrode implantation into the ventral hypothalamus of the dog. *Endocrinol Jpn 14*:363, 1967.
60. McLean AJ: Transbuccal approach to encephalon in experimental operations upon carnivoral pituitary, pons and ventral medulla. *Ann Surg 88*:985, 1928.
61. McNicol AM: Pituitary morphology in canine pituitary-dependent hyperadrenocorticism. *Front Horm Res 17*:71, 1987.
62. Meijer JC: Canine hyperadrenocorticism. *In* Kirk RW (ed): *Current Veterinary Therapy IX*. W.B. Saunders, Philadelphia, 1986, pp 975–983.
63. Melby JC: Therapy of Cushing disease: A consensus for pituitary microsurgery. *Ann Intern Med 109*:445, 1988.
64. Monos E, et al: The acute effect of hypophysectomy on tissue blood flow and oxygen consumption of the adrenal cortex and medulla in dogs. *Acta Physiol Acad Sci Hung 36*:379, 1969.
65. Nelson RW, et al: Pituitary macroadenomas and macroadenocarcinomas in dogs treated with mitotane for pituitary-dependent hyperadrenocorticism: 13 cases (1981–1986). *J Am Vet Med Assoc 194*:1612, 1989.

66. Nelson PB, et al: Endocrine function in patients with large pituitary tumors treated with operative decompression and radiation therapy. *Neurosurgery 24*:398, 1989.
67. Niebauer GW, Evans SM: Transsphenoidal hypophysectomy in the dog—a new technique. *Vet Surg 17*:296, 1988.
68. Niebauer GW, et al: Evaluation of craniotomy in dogs and cats. *J Am Vet Med Assoc 198*:89, 1991.
69. Niebauer GW, et al: Study of long-term survival after transsphenoidal hypophysectomy in clinically normal dogs. *Am J Vet Res 51*:677, 1990.
70. Okkens AC, et al: Influence of hypophysectomy on the lifespan of the corpus luteum in the cyclic dog. *J Reprod Fertil 77*:187, 1986.
71. Oliver JE Jr: Surgical approaches to the canine brain. *Am J Vet Res 29*:353, 1968.
72. Oliver JE Jr: Cranial sinus venography in the dog. *J Am Vet Radiol Soc 10*:66, 1969.
73. Panciera DL, et al: Magnetic resonance imaging in two dogs with central nervous system disease. *J Small Anim Pract 28*:587, 1987.
74. Paulesco NC: *L'Hypophyse du Cerveau*. Vigot Frères, Paris, 1908.
75. Peterson ME: Pathophysiology of canine pituitary-dependent hyperadrenocorticism. *Front Horm Res 17*:37, 1987.
76. Peterson ME, Drucker WD: Abstract: Advances in the diagnosis and treatment of canine Cushing's syndrome. Proceedings of the 31st Gaines Veterinary Symposium, 1981, pp 17–24. Oct. Baton Rouge, Louisiana.
77. Peterson ME, et al: Immunocytochemical study of the hypophysis in 25 dogs with pituitary-dependent hyperadrenocorticism. *Acta Endocrinol 101*:15, 1982.
78. Pirrone V: Contributo sperimentale allo studio della funzione dell'ipofisi. *Riforma Med 19*:169, 1903.
79. Raisman G: An ultrastructural study of the effects of hypophysectomy on the supraoptic nucleus of the rat. *J Comp Neurol 147*:181, 1973.
80. Redford L, Cushing H: Is the pituitary gland essential to the maintenance of life? *Bull Johns Hopkins Hosp 20*:105, 1909.
81. Rijnberk A, van Wimersma Greidanus TjB: Comparative pathophysiology of regulatory peptides. *Front Horm Res 17*:1, 1987.
82. Rijnberk AD, et al: Spontaneous hyperadrenocorticism in the dog. *J Endocrinol 41*:397, 1968.
83. Roldan AG, et al: The effect of hypophysectomy on ketonemia and liver lipids in pancreatectomized dogs. *Acta Physiol Latinoam 22*:166, 1972.
84. Rutteman GR, et al: Growth hormone and mammary tumors in the dog. *Front Horm Res 17*:173, 1987.
85. Siegel ET, et al: Cushing's syndrome in the dog. *J Am Vet Med Assoc 157*:2081, 1970.
86. Tindall GT, Barrow DL: *Disorders of the Pituitary*. C.V. Mosby, St. Louis, 1986.
87. Tindall GT, et al: Transsphenoidal microsurgery for pituitary tumors associated with hyperprolactinemia. *J Neurosurg 48*:849, 1978.
88. Tiscornia OM, Dreiling DA: Microsurgical ablation of the canine pituitary gland. *Surgery 60*:1077, 1966.
89. Überreiter O: Beitrag zur Diagnostik und Therapie der chirurgischen Krankheiten des Gehirnes und seiner Häute. II. Mitteilung: raumfordernde Prozesse: Tumoren, Pseudotumoren, Parasiten. *Schweiz Arch Tierheilk 99*:51, 1957.
90. Vassale C, Sacchi M: Sulla destruzione della ghiandola pituitaria. *Riv Sper Freniatr 18*:525, 1892.
91. Verdura J, et al: A new technique for aseptic hypophysectomy in the dog. *J Surg Res 3*:174, 1963.
92. Verstraete A, Thoonen J: Twee nieuve gavallen van hypophysaire stoornissen bij den hond. *Vlaams Diergeneesk Tijdschr 8*:304, 1939.
93. Yoshida T, Kondo M: The effect of hypophysectomy and hypophysis-transplantation on the secretion of gut glucagon immunoreactivity and gut glucagon-like immunoreactivity in depancreatized dogs. *Endocrinol Jpn 27*:77, 1980.
94. Zimmermann G: Über die Dura mater encephali und die Sinus der Schädelhöhle des Hundes. *Z Anat Entwicklungsgesch 100*:107, 1936.

CHAPTER 111

Adrenalectomy

Stephen J. Birchard

Adrenalectomy is a challenging surgical procedure performed on animals that are usually at high risk. Hyperadrenocorticism due to a unilateral adrenal tumor and bilateral hyperplasia are the most common indications for surgery. Hyperadrenocorticism causes many metabolic derangements that surgeons and anesthesiologists should recognize (e.g., hyperglycemia, electrolyte abnormalities, hypertension, poor wound healing). Pheochromocytoma, a less common but equally devastating tumor, is another indication for adrenalectomy.[1] The high concentrations of circulating catecholamines associated with pheochromocytoma cause serious cardiovascular problems such as tachycardia and hypertension. Anesthesia and surgery on these animals is also risky. Pheochromocytomas can be aggressive tumors that may invade the lumen of the cranial vena cava, making them difficult to resect.

Surgeons should thoroughly understand the pathophysiology of adrenal diseases that require surgical treatment. Appropriate preoperative and postoperative management is critical to a successful outcome. Recognition of possible complications is important: Hyperadrenocorticism can cause severe muscle wasting and thinning of the skin due to the catabolic effects of excess cortisol. The tissues may have poor tensile strength, retain sutures poorly, heal slowly, and become infected.[8]

ANATOMY

The paired adrenal glands are retroperitoneal, located cranial and medial to the cranial pole of each kidney. A thin capsule surrounds each gland.[3] The right adrenal lies close to the caudal vena cava; its capsule may even be continuous with the tunica externa of the vena cava.[3] When approaching the adrenal glands via a ventral midline laparotomy, medial retraction of the caudal vena cava and caudal retraction of the right kidney are necessary to expose the right adrenal gland. The phrenicoabdominal vein courses over the midventral surface of each adrenal gland; the phrenicoabdominal artery is adjacent to the dorsal aspect of each gland.

The rich vascular supply to the adrenals comes from branches of the aorta and phrenic, renal, accessory renal, lumbar, and phrenicoabdominal arteries.[3] Venous drainage is from the right adrenal vein directly to the vena cava; the left adrenal vein empties into the left renal vein. Adrenal veins may also empty into the phrenicoabdominal veins. Malignant tumors of the adrenal gland occasionally invade these venous structures, complicating removal.

PREOPERATIVE CONSIDERATIONS

Although extensive diagnostic evaluation has probably already been performed to diagnose the adrenal disease, a complete blood count and serum biochemistry profile are repeated the day before surgery. Efforts are made to correct metabolic derangements such as hyperglycemia and fluid and electrolyte imbalances. Hyperalimentation is considered in patients that are malnourished and hypoproteinemic.

Abdominal radiographs may be helpful in localizing an adrenal mass, especially if it is calcified. A study of 23 dogs with adrenal tumors revealed that 57 per cent of them had adrenal calcification.[7] There was little difference in incidence of calcification between adenomas and carcinomas. Hepatomegaly was a consistent radiographic sign of hyperadrenocorticism in these dogs. Thoracic radiographs are obtained to examine the lungs for metastatic disease. Because intravenous invasion by some right-sided adrenal tumors occurs into the caudal vena cava, radiographic contrast studies of the caudal vena cava may be useful. Ultrasonography of the adrenal glands has been useful to delineate the tumor and even predict vascular invasion (Fig. 111–1). Ultrasonography of the liver may also detect evidence of metastasis of the adrenal tumor.

SURGICAL TREATMENT

Monitoring of patients during adrenalectomy is extremely important. Besides routine monitoring of the anesthetic plane, other parameters that should be observed are heart and respiratory rate, electrocardiogram, blood pressure, capillary refill time, and rectal temperature. Intravenous maintenance fluids are given via an indwelling catheter. Periodic blood gas determinations are performed if possible.

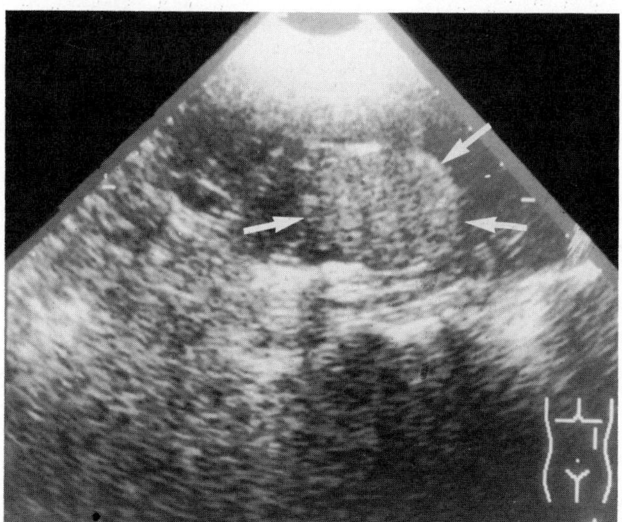

FIGURE 111–1. Ultrasonographic appearance of an adrenal adenoma *(arrows)* in a dog.

Adrenalectomy for hyperadrenocorticism causes a precipitous decline in serum cortisol concentrations. Glucocorticoid replacement is necessary to avoid severe adrenocortical insufficiency. Dexamethasone (0.1 to 0.2 mg/kg) or prednisolone sodium succinate (1.0 to 2.0 mg/kg) is given intravenously immediately after anesthetic induction and repeated immediately postoperatively.[8]

Manipulation of a pheochromocytoma may cause severe tachycardia and hypertension owing to release of catecholamines from the tumor. Close monitoring of an animal's cardiovascular status is important, and treatment with alpha-blocking drugs (phentolamine or propranolol) has been recommended.[11]

Prophylactic antibiotics are considered in severely debilitated animals or those in which a contaminated procedure will be performed in addition to adrenalectomy. The antibiotic (e.g., ampicillin, 20 mg/kg every 8 hours; or cephalothin, 20 mg/kg every 6 hours) is administered intravenously at induction and continued for 24 hours postoperatively.

Surgical Technique

Adrenal glands can be removed by one of two techniques: ventral midline laparotomy or retroperitoneal approach. The ventral midline approach allows exposure of both adrenal glands and other abdominal organs, such as the liver, through one incision. Removal of the dorsally located glands is tedious via the ventral approach. The liver must be significantly retracted, and dehiscence of the ventrally located incision is a potential complication. The retroperitoneal (flank) approach provides adequate exposure of either the right or left gland.[4, 5] However, two incisions are required for removal of both glands, and exposure of other abdominal structures is very limited. Although I prefer the ventral midline approach, both techniques are described.

Ventral Midline Approach

A ventral midline abdominal incision is made from the xyphoid to 4 to 6 cm caudal to the umbilicus. An additional incision is then made in the right or left (depending on the location of the affected adrenal) paracostal skin and musculature to gain additional exposure (Fig. 111–2*A*). Self-retaining retractors are placed to expose the abdominal viscera.

Both adrenal glands are carefully examined (Fig. 111–2*B*). The liver and remaining abdominal viscera are examined and palpated. The vena cava is carefully palpated for tumor extension within its lumen. Large hand-held retractors (malleable or Deaver) are used to retract the liver cranially, kidney caudally, and vena cava medially. Excessive retraction of the caudal vena cava may cause significant reduction in venous return and is done with caution. Large abdominal sponges can be used to cushion these organs and prevent trauma associated with retraction. The phrenicoabdominal vein is ligated and divided, and the adrenal gland is carefully dissected free from surrounding tissues (Fig. 111–2*C*–

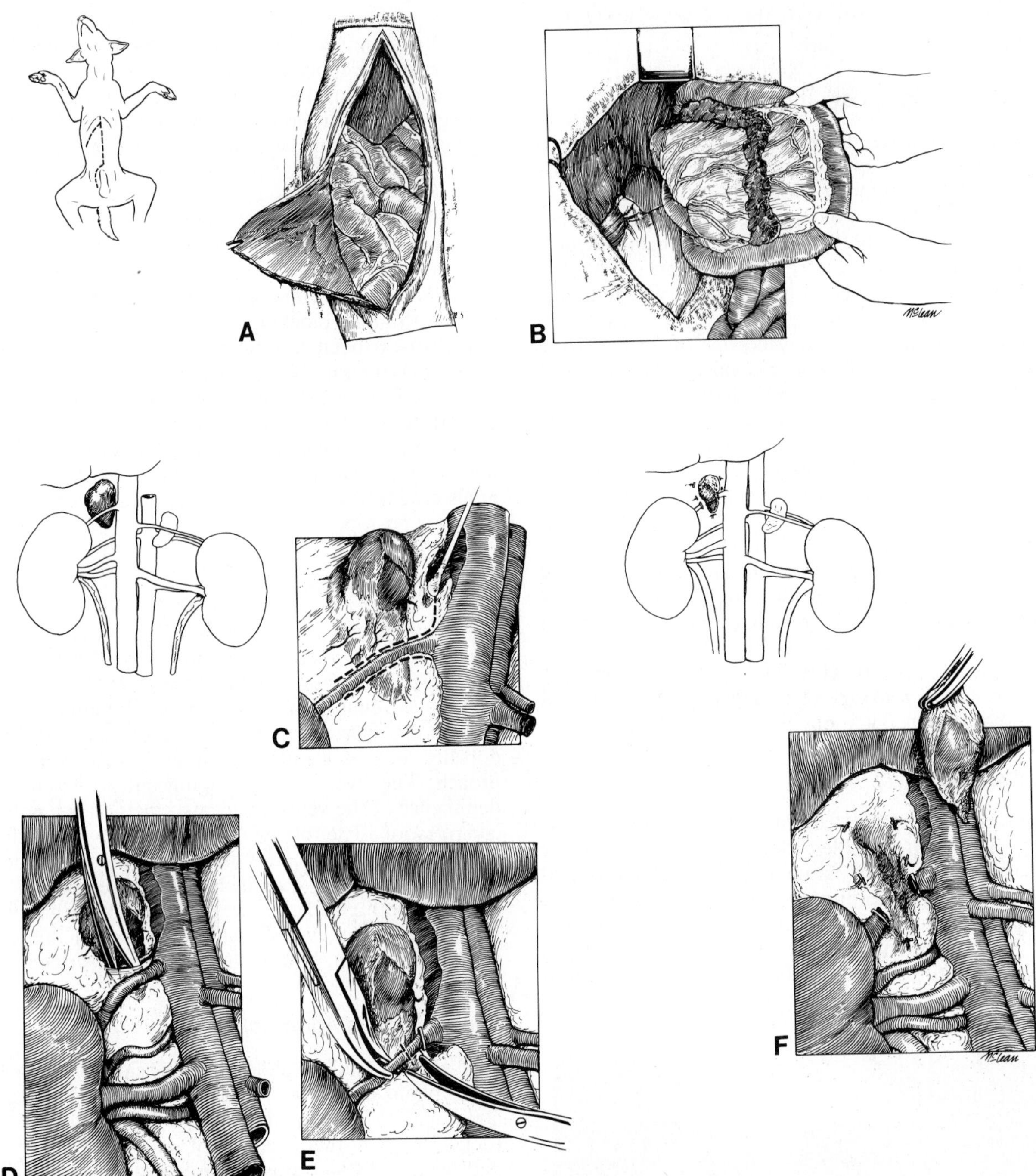

FIGURE 111–2. Surgical technique for adrenalectomy in a dog. *A*, A combined ventral abdominal midline and paracostal approach is made. *B*, Exposure of the adrenal via retraction of the descending duodenum on the right side; descending colon is retracted for exposure of the left adrenal. *C*, The adrenal and phrenicoabdominal vein are dissected. *D* and *E*, Vessels are ligated with hemoclips and divided. *F*, The adrenal is then removed, and the surgical site examined for hemorrhage.

F). Stainless steel hemostatic clips (Ligaclips*) are used for vessel ligation because hand ligatures are difficult in this area. Extensive neovascularization of large adrenal tumors may cause disruption of the normal vascular anatomy of the adrenal and associated kidney (Fig. 111–3). The surgeon should be careful to avoid inadvertently ligating the blood supply to the kidney while removing the adrenal tumor. Care is taken to maintain an intact adrenal capsule during dissection to avoid fragmentation of the tumor and possible seeding of the peritoneal cavity with neoplastic cells (Fig. 111–4). Temporary partial occlusion and incision of the caudal vena cava are necessary to remove tumor thrombus, if present, with subsequent suture closure of the vessel (simple

*Ethicon, Somerville, NJ.

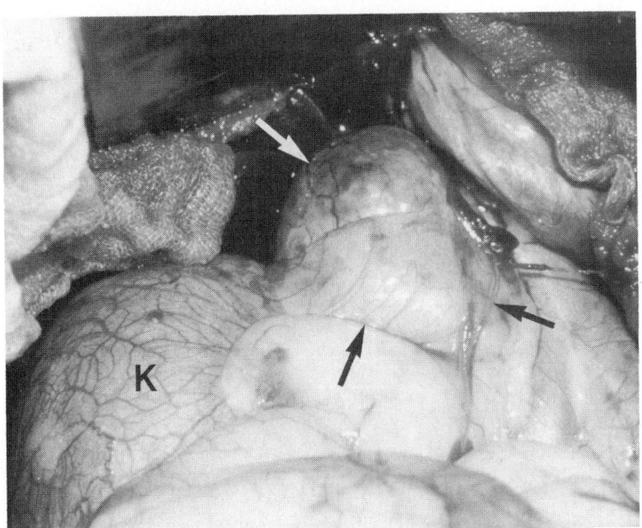

FIGURE 111–3. Intraoperative appearance of an adrenal adenoma *(arrows)* lying craniomedial to the right kidney (K).

continuous 5-0 polypropylene [Prolene*]). This difficult maneuver should be attempted only if a small thrombus is present. Large tumor extensions (Fig. 111–5) are not resectable.

On removal of the gland, the surgical field is carefully examined for hemorrhage. All tissues are submitted for histopathological evaluation. Biopsy of suspicious areas of the liver is also performed. Nonabsorbable sutures are used for wound closure to minimize the chance of dehiscence.

Retroperitoneal Approach

The dog is placed in either right or left lateral recumbency, depending on which gland is to be removed. The caudal thorax and entire lateral abdomen are prepared. A 10-cm dorsal-to-ventral incision is made 1 cm caudal to the last rib.[4] The abdominal muscles are individually incised. The adrenal gland is found within the fatty tissue surrounding it and the kidney. Malleable retractors are used to push the kidney ventrally and expose the adrenal gland. The caudal phrenic vein is ligated and divided. The adrenal gland is dissected free from surrounding tissues, and hemostatic clips are used to ligate the multiple vessels. Babcock forceps can be used with this and the previously described approach to grasp the tissue adjacent to the adrenal and lift it away from the surrounding tissues, making dissection easier.

The abdominal muscles are individually closed with nonabsorbable sutures. The remainder of the closure is routine.

*Ethicon, Somerville, NJ.

Postoperative Care and Complications

Several complications are possible after adrenalectomy. Hemorrhage, fluid and electrolyte imbalances, pancreatitis secondary to iatrogenic trauma, wound infection or pneumonia due to impaired immune system function, and poor wound healing are potential problems. Adrenal insufficiency develops after either bilateral gland removal or unilateral removal for adrenal neoplasia. Glucocorticoids are administered postoperatively (prednisone, 0.5 mg/kg, every 12 hours; or prednisolone, 0.5 mg/kg, every 12 hours). Glucocorticoid therapy is reduced to maintenance levels (prednisone, 0.2 mg/kg every 24 hours; or prednisolone, 0.2 mg/kg every 24 hours) over the next 7 to 10 days.[8] Mineralocorticoid therapy is also necessary after removal of both adrenal glands.[10]

Dogs that have had unilateral adrenal tumors removed should eventually be able to produce endogenous cortisol from the remaining adrenal, allowing discontinuation of glucocorticoid therapy. The decision to stop therapy is based on the results of adrenocorticotropic hormone stimulation tests, and the glucocorticoid is discontinued gradually to prevent a sudden decrease in cortisol concentrations.

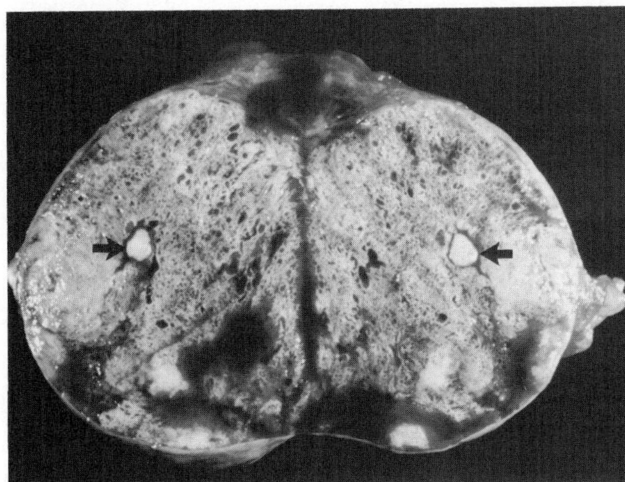

FIGURE 111–4. Adrenal adenoma on cut surface showing an area of calcification *(arrows)*.

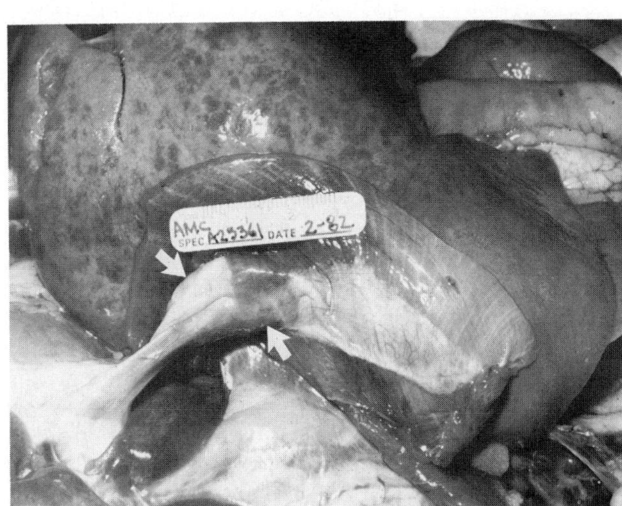

FIGURE 111–5. Postmortem appearance of an adrenal carcinoma in a dog with extension of the neoplasm into the caudal vena cava (arrows). (From Peterson ME, et al: Anesthetic and surgical management of endocrine disorders. *Vet Clin North Am Small Anim Pract* 14:911, 1984.)

Dogs are re-evaluated every 3 to 6 months to check for evidence of recurrence of the adrenal tumor or other associated problems. The prognosis is favorable for benign tumors of the adrenal (adenoma) but poor for malignancies (carcinoma). In one study of 25 dogs with adrenocortical neoplasia, only 3 of 14 dogs with carcinomas were alive 6 months postoperatively.[9] Seven of these dogs were euthanized during surgery because of liver metastasis or vascular invasion of the tumor. Five of 11 dogs with adenoma were alive 6 months postoperatively; 2 of the dogs that died before 6 months died of unrelated causes. The investigators recommended treatment with mitotane (Lysodren) if hyperadrenocorticism persists after adrenalectomy. A subsequent study showed better survival rates after unilateral resection of adenomas (three dogs, life span range: 6.9 to 22 months) and carcinomas (five dogs, life span range: 10.9 to 40 months).[2] The authors of this study concluded that adrenalectomy is the treatment of choice for unilateral lesions. Bilateral adrenalectomy for pituitary-dependent hyperadrenocorticism remains controversial.

Adrenalectomy for adrenal tumors in cats has also been reported,[6] although much less frequently than in dogs. The anatomy of a cat's adrenal glands is similar to that of a dog. The ventral approach is preferred for adrenalectomy in cats.

References

1. Bouayad H, et al: Pheochromocytoma in dogs: 13 cases (1980–1985). *J Am Vet Med Assoc 191*:1610, 1987.
2. Emms SG, et al: Adrenalectomy in the management of canine hyperadrenocorticism. *J Am Anim Hosp Assoc 23*:557, 1987.
3. Hullinger RL: The endocrine system. *In* Evans HE, Christensen GC (eds): *Miller's Anatomy of the Dog*. 2nd ed. W.B. Saunders, Philadelphia, 1979, pp 602–631.
4. Johnston DE: Adrenalectomy via retroperitoneal approach in dogs. *J Am Vet Med Assoc 170*:1092, 1977.
5. Johnston DE: Adrenalectomy in the dog. *In* Bojrab MJ (ed): *Current Techniques in Small Animal Surgery*. 2nd ed. Lea & Febiger, Philadelphia, 1983, pp 386–389.
6. Nelson RW, et al: Hyperadrenocorticism in cats: Seven cases (1978–1987). *J Am Vet Med Assoc 193*:245, 1988.
7. Penninck DG, et al: Radiographic features of canine hyperadrenocorticism caused by autonomously functioning adrenocortical tumors: 23 cases (1978–1986). *J Am Vet Med Assoc 192*:1604, 1988.
8. Peterson ME, et al: Anesthetic and surgical management of endocrine disorders. *Small Anim Pract 14*:911, 1984.
9. Scavelli TD, et al: Results of surgical treatment for hyperadrenocorticism caused by adrenocortical neoplasia in the dog: 25 cases (1980–1984). *J Am Vet Med Assoc 189*:1360, 1986.
10. Schrader LA: Hypoadrenocorticism. *In* Kirk RW (ed): *Current Veterinary Therapy IX*. W.B. Saunders, Philadelphia, 1986, pp 972–977.
11. Trim CM: Anesthesia and the endocrine system. *In* Slatter D (ed): *Textbook of Small Animal Surgery*. Vol II. W.B. Saunders, Philadelphia, 1985, pp 2692–2701.

CHAPTER 112 The Thyroid

Thomas D. Scavelli and Mark E. Peterson

ANATOMY

In dogs and cats, the thyroid gland consists of two distinct lobes adjacent to the first five to eight tracheal rings. In a medium-sized dog, each lobe of the thyroid gland is approximately 5.0 cm long and 1.5 cm wide.[11] In immature dogs and brachycephalic breeds, they are larger. In cats, each thyroid gland lobe is approximately 2.0 cm long and 0.3 cm wide.[5] Two parathyroid glands are associated with each of the two thyroid lobes. The external parathyroid glands are outside the thyroid gland capsule and most often are at the cranial pole of the thyroid gland. The internal parathyroid glands are within the thyroid gland capsule at the caudal and medial aspect of each respective lobe. The external parathyroid is often white or pink and receives most of its vascular supply from branches of the cranial thyroid artery[29] (Fig. 112–1).

The thyroid gland is highly vascular. Most of the blood supply is derived from the cranial thyroid artery, which is a branch of the common carotid artery. In dogs, the caudal thyroid artery unites with the cranial thyroid artery in the loose areolar tissue along the dorsomedial surface of the thyroid gland capsule. The origin of the caudal thyroid artery is the brachiocephalic artery. The caudal thyroid artery is not present in most cats. Venous drainage from each thyroid gland lobe is from the cranial and caudal thyroid veins, which can be located at the corresponding poles within each lobe.

Ectopic thyroid tissue is present in most dogs and cats. This accessory thyroid parenchyma is mainly found in the cervical region but can also be located within the thorax.[6] Carcinoma or adenoma can arise from ectopic thyroid tissue in both dogs and cats. This is especially important in cats when the clinical and laboratory diagnosis of hyperthyroidism has been made but each lobe of the thyroid gland is grossly normal during exploratory surgery. In these cases, the entire cervical region must be inspected and palpated thoroughly. In many cases, the ectopic adenomatous tissue can be located at the thoracic inlet.

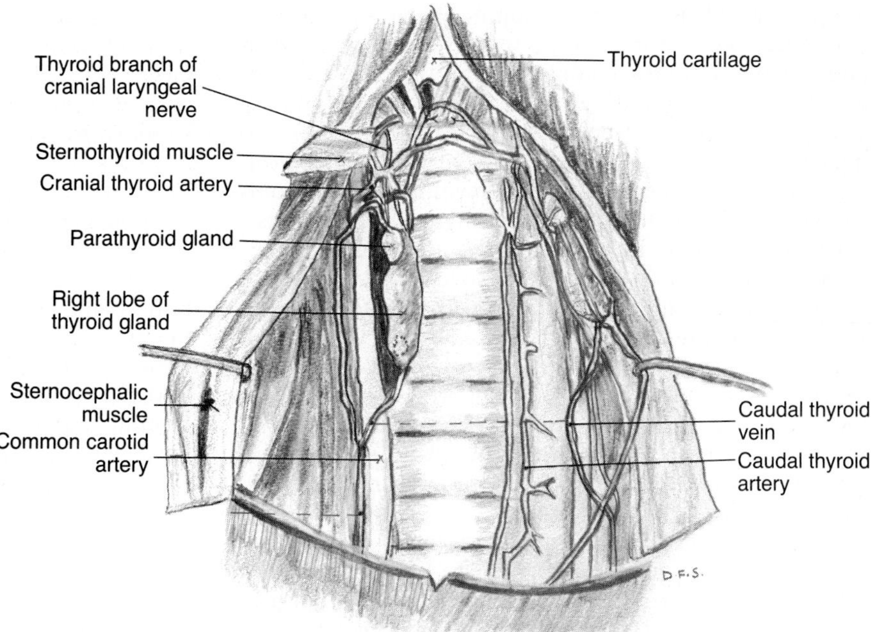

FIGURE 112–1. Ventral view of normal canine cervical anatomy.

THYROID PHYSIOLOGY

Thyroglobulin is a glycoprotein molecule that stores thyroid hormone and its precursors.[44] It is formed within the endoplasmic reticulum of the thyroid follicular cells and is released as colloid into the lumen of the thyroid follicles. The thyroid hormones, triiodothyronine (T_3) and tetraiodothyronine (T_4), are formed when iodine enters the follicular colloid and is united with the tyrosine residues of thyroglobulin.

Once T_3 and T_4 are formed within the follicular lumen, their secretion by the thyroid gland is under the regulatory control of the hypothalamic-pituitary-thyroid feedback mechanism. Thyrotropin (thyroid-stimulating hormone [TSH]) is a glycoprotein produced in the pars distalis of the pituitary gland. TSH stimulates the synthesis of thyroglobulin, T_3, and T_4 in the thyroid follicles. TSH also is the main stimulant for the release of T_3 and T_4 from the follicular colloid into the systemic circulation.[20] The release of TSH from the pituitary gland is under direct control of the neuropeptide thyrotropin-releasing hormone (TRH), which is produced in the hypothalamus. Hypothalamic secretion of TRH occurs in response to low circulating levels of thyroid hormones. Inhibition of TRH secretion occurs with high circulating levels of thyroid hormones or glucocorticoids. Serum T_4 or T_3 concentrations were decreased in approximately 50 per cent of dogs with spontaneous hyperadrenocorticism.[32]

T_3 and T_4 stimulate oxygen use by most metabolically active tissues. T_3 is several times more potent than T_4 in stimulating oxygen use and in binding to cellular proteins.[42] In the euthyroid state, thyroid hormones have an overall anabolic effect on protein metabolism and result in protein synthesis. Conversely, in the hyperthyroid state, these metabolically active hormones have a generalized catabolic effect, with the result being a breakdown of body proteins and fats.

CANINE AND FELINE HYPOTHYROIDISM

Etiology of Hypothyroidism

Abnormally low circulating levels of thyroid hormone are the most common thyroid disorder in dogs. Hypothyroidism results from inadequate production and secretion of thyroid hormone. The specific defect most commonly originates in the thyroid gland; rarely the defect is present in the hypothalamus or pituitary gland. Thyroid dysfunction is termed *primary hypothyroidism,* whereas pituitary and hypothalamic causes are called *secondary* and *tertiary hypothyroidism,* respectively.

Naturally occurring adult primary hypothyroidism is most common in dogs. Sporadic reports describe histological changes in the mature feline thyroid gland that are consistent with primary thyroid dysfunction,[8, 23] but naturally occurring clinical cases have not been identified. Acquired canine primary hypothyroidism is mainly caused by idiopathic follicular atrophy or lymphocytic thyroiditis.[2, 24] Idiopathic thyroid atrophy is a syndrome in which portions of the normal thyroid architecture are replaced by fat cells. The inflammatory reaction within the parenchyma is absent, and the inciting case is unknown. Lymphocytic thyroiditis is an immune-mediated disorder in which the normal thyroid follicles are replaced by lymphocytes and plasma cells.[16] Serological inspection reveals circulating thyroglobulin antibodies, which result in eventual follicular destruction via antigen-antibody complex deposition and cell-mediated activity.[15, 18] The profound inflammatory reaction that occurs with lymphocytic thyroiditis eventually results in thyroid fibrosis.

When hypothyroidism develops in adult cats, the most common cause is iatrogenic removal of the thyroid gland or damage to its blood supply during surgical thyroidectomy.[34] Hypothyroidism is associated with vascular disruption to the remaining thyroid tissue and is usually temporary because the blood supply should be re-established weeks to months after surgery. Hypothyroidism after bilateral thyroidectomy is typically transient because normal thyroid hormone levels are eventually sustained by hypertrophied ectopic thyroid tissue in the neck and thoracic cavity. Iatrogenic hypothyroidism can theoretically also occur after treatment of hyperthyroidism with radioactive iodine or antithyroid medications.

Congenital hypothyroidism is a thoroughly documented syndrome in humans but is infrequent in dogs and cats. The incidence may be higher than the number reported because it may have a role in neonatal mortalities that are never diagnosed. In the limited veterinary reports of hypothyroidism in immature animals, documented causes include iodine organification defects and thyroid dysgenesis.[1, 4, 7, 17, 26] Thyroid gland enlargement (goiter) has occasionally been described in congenital hypothyroidism.[1]

Secondary and tertiary hypothyroidism result from abnormally low production or release of TSH or TRH, respectively. Congenital malformation, tumors, surgical manipulations, and radiation treatment involving the pituitary gland or hypothalamus can result in deficient thyroid hormone production.

Clinical Signs of Hypothyroidism

The major difficulty in diagnosing hypothyroidism is the nonspecific and variable clinical signs in affected animals. Thyroid hormone has a role in the normal cellular function of almost all metabolically active tissues. Thyroid hormone aids in amino acid transport and cellular oxygen consumption within each organ system. Therefore, it is important in the generation of cellular energy throughout the body. The widespread activity of thyroid hormone results in diffuse clinical signs. The brain, testes, uterus, lymph nodes, and spleen are the only individual organs that do not require thyroid hormone for oxygen consumption.[42]

Adult-onset hypothyroidism most frequently afflicts middle-aged medium to large dogs, with no predilection for a particular sex.[2, 28] The golden retriever, Irish setter, Doberman pinscher, dachshund, and cocker spaniel are at increased risk.[28]

Because thyroid hormone's main role is generation of energy throughout the body, many of the clinical signs in hypothyroid animals are manifestations of decreased metabolic rate, which creates lethargy, exercise intolerance, and generalized weight gain. The lower metabolic rate reduces the amount of body heat produced and decreases body temperature. Hypothyroid dogs therefore do not tolerate cold environmental temperatures and are often described as "heat seekers."

Dermatological alterations include alopecia, dry haircoat, thickening of the skin, and hyperpigmentation. This hormonal alopecia is nonpruritic and symmetrical. The alopecia is a result of both a reduction in hair growth and an increase in hair loss via excessive shedding. Mucinous deposits in the dermis can result in focal or diffuse thickening of the skin in some hypothyroid animals.

Peripheral neuropathies have been associated with canine hypothyroidism. Paralysis of the vestibular nerve, facial nerve, and recurrent laryngeal nerve has been clinically linked with hypothyroidism.[2, 19] The exact cause of these peripheral nerve palsies is unknown, but compression by mucinous deposits has been postulated.[2] Theoretically, the neuropathy might be reversible if early diagnosis and treatment were instituted.

Cardiovascular changes associated with hypothyroidism center around alterations in cardiac muscle function.[43] The hypothyroid state can inhibit myocardial function to the point of producing bradycardia and a weak apex beat.[30] Structural cardiac changes with hypothyroidism include thinning of the interventricular septum and the left ventricular free wall.[27] Although these changes in function and structure can occur in animals with severe hypothyroidism, there is no evidence that these cardiac alterations cause heart failure.

One of the more important consequences of hypothyroidism is the potential relationship between low thyroid function and von Willebrand's disease.[41] In humans, endogenous or exogenous elevations in thyroid hormone concentrations cause concurrent increases in the activity of factor VIII and factor VIII-related antigen.[39, 40] Therefore, naturally occurring canine hypothyroidism may result in decreased activity of factor VIII or VIII-related antigen. Impaired function of these clotting factors may predispose to serious bleeding either spontaneously or in association with surgery in dogs with mild or moderate forms of von Willebrand's disease. Clotting function is improved after only a few doses of exogenous thyroid hormone. Dogs that bleed excessively despite thyroid hormone replacement are treated with plasma or whole blood transfusions.

Reproductive dysfunction in hypothyroid bitches is manifested by abnormal estrous cycles, anestrus, abortion, and neonatal mortality.[13] In males, low thyroid levels can result in testicular atrophy, decreased libido, and impaired fertility. Thyroid insufficiency should be considered as having a possible role in canine infertility and thyroid function; both males and females should be evaluated.

Other clinical signs associated with hypothyroidism are diarrhea, constipation, anemia, corneal lipid deposits, disorientation, and grand mal seizures.[2, 10, 22, 31] The ocular and cerebral abnormalities associated with hyperthyroidism are secondary to hyperlipidemia.[3, 31, 21]

Diagnosis of Hypothyroidism

Various laboratory tests are helpful in diagnosing hypothyroidism. The major hematological finding is a normocytic normochromic anemia. This anemia is a result of a lack of bone marrow stimulation caused by the thyroid hormone deficiency and reduced erythropoietin levels.[9] Primary biochemical abnormalities are elevations in serum cholesterol and triglyceride concentrations. Generalized reduction in cell metabolism caused by hypothyroidism results in inhibited clearance and breakdown of primarily cholesterol and, to a lesser extent, triglycerides from the blood.

The most frequently used laboratory tests to diagnose hypothyroidism are serum T_4 concentration and the thyrotropin (TSH) response test. Both tests are based on radioimmunoassay techniques, which quantitate thyroid hormone concentrations via antibody directed against the hormone. T_3 is mainly intracellular; therefore, serum measurement of this hormone is *not* an important indicator of thyroid function. Because T_4 is the major hormone secreted by the thyroid gland, evaluating its concentration in the serum is a valuable indicator of thyroid gland function. Because other nonthyroidal disorders can lower basal serum T_4 values, clinicians should use a dynamic thyroid function test to confirm the diagnosis of primary hypothyroidism. Hyperadrenocorticism, diabetes mellitus, and renal disease falsely lower serum T_4 concentrations.[15, 32] These low values may be due to impaired secretion of thyroid hormone or problems with binding to plasma proteins. The TSH response test is the dynamic test most suitable for general veterinary practice, and its application has been described in detail.[14]

Therapy

Once the diagnosis of hypothyroidism has been confirmed, thyroid hormone supplement must be chosen. Synthetic thyroxine is the most effective drug. In most instances, therapy will be necessary for the remainder of the animal's life. The recommended replacement dose range for T_4 in dogs is 0.02 to 0.04 mg/kg/day.[37] Hormone therapy initially is gradually introduced to the animal, with the total dose being divided into two equal daily doses. After several weeks, most hypothyroid animals can be maintained on once-a-day therapy because the body stores of the hormone are exogenously replaced.

FELINE HYPERTHYROIDISM

Feline hyperthyroidism is one of the more commonly diagnosed endocrine diseases. It is a systemic disorder that results from sustained high circulating levels of T_4 and T_3. The origin of the excessive thyroid hormones is usually adenomatous hyperplasia in one (30 per cent) or both (70 per cent) thyroid glands[12, 35–36] (Fig. 112–2). Carcinoma of the thyroid gland is diagnosed in approximately 1 to 2 per cent of hyperthyroid cats.[45]

Most hyperthyroid cats are middle-aged to old; no breed or sex predilection is noted. The clinical signs in these cats involve many organ systems. Cardiac involvement and an increase in metabolic rate are often the most profound clinical signs. In 205 hyperthyroid cats, clinical findings revealed weight loss (96 per cent), polyphagia (77 per cent), hyperactivity (68 per cent), tachycardia (64 per cent), heart murmur (54 per cent), polyuria (53 per cent), vomiting (49 per cent), diarrhea (31 per cent), voluminous stools (28 per cent), anorexia (28 per cent), panting (28 per cent), muscle tremors (14 per cent), and heart failure (13 per cent).[34, 35] Although most cats with thyrotoxicosis are irritable or hyperexcitable, the reverse occurs in about 10 per cent of cats.

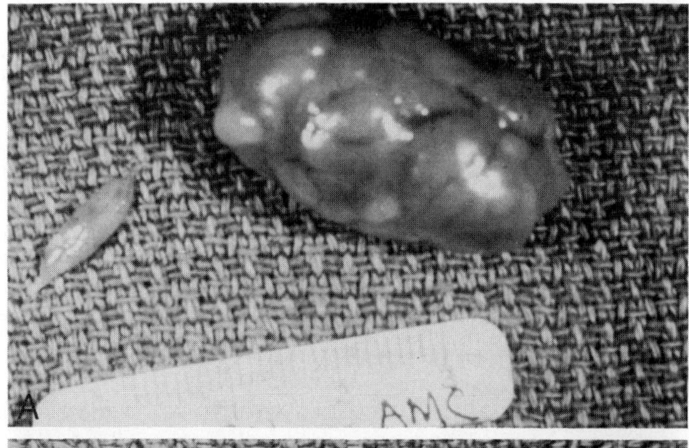

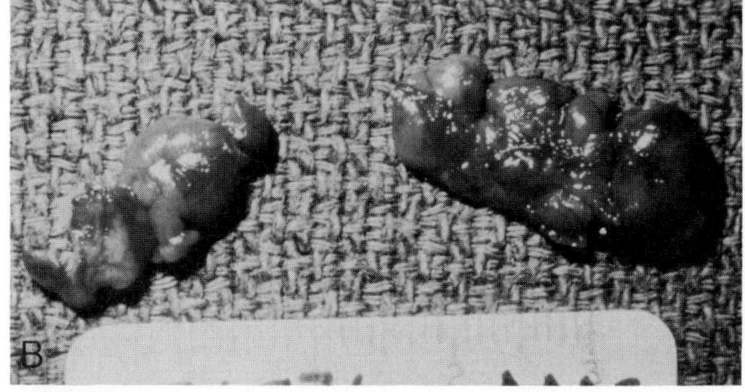

FIGURE 112–2. *A*, Unilateral feline thyroid adenoma. The adenomatous gland is on the right, and the atrophied contralateral gland is on the left. *B*, Bilateral thyroid adenomas.

This form of the disease is called *apathetic hyperthyroidism,* and affected cats display profound depression and weakness as the most obvious features.[35] General body weakness, anorexia, ventral neck flexion, and heart failure are also prominent. This severe depression and heart failure are often due to a secondary cardiomyopathy. In most cases, the cardiomyopathy is hypertrophic; dilated cardiomyopathy occasionally occurs secondary to thyrotoxicosis.

The key to diagnosing this disease on physical examination is gentle, deliberate ventral cervical palpation. Normal thyroid glands are not palpable in cats. In approximately 90 per cent of hyperthyroid cats, the enlarged thyroid glands can be palpated.[35] The head is extended with one hand moving the mandible. As the head is held in extension, the thumb and index finger are placed on the skin at the level of the thoracic inlet and gently advanced cranially toward the larynx. If the thyroid gland is enlarged, it will be felt slipping under the examiner's fingers (Fig. 112–3). This manipulation is performed several times on each side of the cervical midline. In some cases with bilateral thyroid involvement, only one enlarged gland may be palpated, especially if one thyroid is much larger than the contralateral gland and tends to mask its presence. In some cats, one or two affected lobes may descend into the thoracic cavity and escape detection.

Because these are usually elderly sick cats, a complete hemogram and biochemical profile are indicated.[34, 35] A stress hemogram is a common finding, with mature leukocytosis and eosinopenia detected in approximately

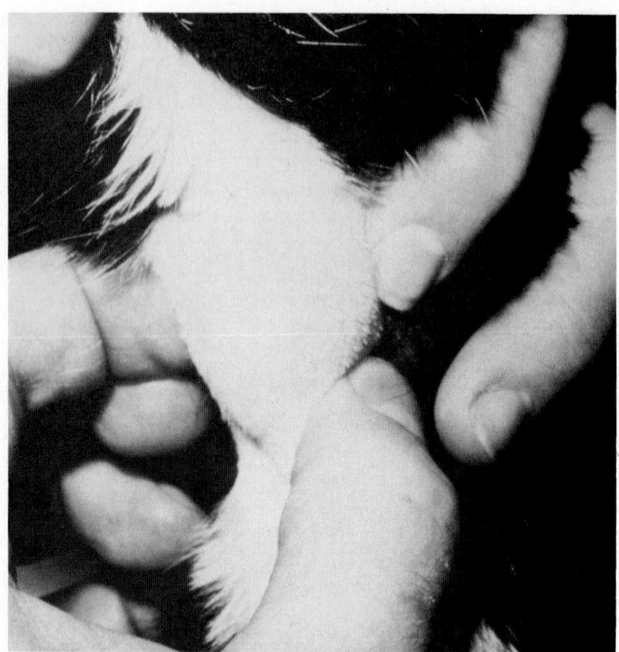

FIGURE 112–3. Palpation technique for thyroid nodules in a cat with the thumb and index finger along the trachea and the head and neck in extension.

45 per cent. Twenty per cent of cats with hyperthyroidism develop moderate erythrocytosis, probably a result of the stimulatory effect of thyroid hormone on bone marrow. Biochemical changes are evident in 50 to 75 per cent of hyperthyroid cats.[12, 35] The abnormal elevations that are most common are alkaline phosphatase (75 per cent), aspartate aminotransferase (65 per cent), lactate dehydrogenase (65 per cent), alanine aminotransferase (55 per cent), total bilirubin (20 per cent), blood urea nitrogen (20 per cent), and inorganic phosphorus (20 per cent).[35] The exact cause of the liver damage is unknown; chronic body wasting, heart failure, and a direct thyrotoxic effect all are possible explanations. As with the changes that occur in the myocardium from excessive circulating thyroid hormone concentrations, those changes that develop in the liver parenchyma are corrected if the hyperthyroid state is successfully treated.

The simplest method to diagnose hyperthyroidism is by determining resting serum concentrations of T_4 or T_3. In most laboratories, the normal range for T_4 is 1 to 4 μg/100 ml, whereas the normal range for T_3 is 10 to 100 μg/100 ml. Some hyperthyroid cats with elevated T_4 values and mild clinical signs have normal T_3 levels. This usually occurs only early in the course of the disease. The presence of concomitant systemic illnesses (i.e., liver or renal disease) can falsely lower circulating thyroid hormone concentrations. In addition, some cats display T_4 levels that vary during the course of a typical day. As a result, if hyperthyroidism is suspected clinically in patients with normal T_4 or T_3 levels, the disease cannot be completely ruled out until concomitant diseases are treated and a TSH response test is performed.

Because high levels of circulating thyroid hormone can lead to hypertrophic changes within the myocardium, a thoracic radiograph is obtained in all suspected cases of feline hyperthyroidism. In 82 hyperthyroid cats with thoracic radiographs, the following changes were detected: cardiomegaly (49 per cent), pulmonary edema (15 per cent), and pleural effusion (15 per cent).[35] Electrocardiographic findings detected with feline hyperthyroidism are mainly sinus tachycardia and increased lead II R-wave amplitude.[33] Changes most commonly seen on echocardiography are left ventricular hypertrophy and left atrial dilation.[3]

Thyroid scanning (imaging) is helpful in treating hyperthyroid cats; this relies on an increased uptake of radioiodine by the overly active thyroid gland. Pertechnetate is rapidly absorbed by the body, and the imaging procedure can be performed rapidly. The goal of thyroid imaging is to determine the extent of the primary disease process and to detect distant metastases. These scans can (1) determine unilateral or bilateral thyroid gland enlargement, (2) detect functional ectopic thyroid tissue, and (3) identify local or distant metastatic lesions from carcinomas of the thyroid gland.

Once the diagnosis of hyperthyroidism has been made, three treatment options are available either to control or remove the adenomatous thyroid gland. These options are antithyroid drugs, radioactive iodine, and surgical thyroidectomy. The preferred treatment depends on the general health of the cat, the surgical experience of the veterinarian, the availability of radioactive products, and the expense of therapy.

Antithyroid drugs inhibit the formation of thyroid hormone and maintain levels of circulating T_3/T_4 at low to normal values; hyperplastic thyroid tissue persists. Methimazole (Tapazole) and propylthiouracil are two antithyroid drugs used to treat hyperthyroid cats. Both are effective in creating a euthyroid state within 2 to 6 weeks, depending on the severity of the hyperthyroidism. Both methimazole and propylthiouracil block thyroid hormone synthesis by preventing the iodination of thyroglobulin and by inhibiting the coupling of iodotyrosyl groups into T_3 and T_4. The advantages of drug therapy are that it is the least expensive treatment option and does not carry the risks associated with anesthesia or surgery. Also, these older cats do not have to be isolated from their home environment and hospitalized for 1 to 2 weeks as when they are treated with a drug such as radioactive iodine. The disadvantages of antithyroid medication are that (1) the abnormal thyroid tissue persists, and this benign disease is never cured, (2) daily medication must be given for the life of the cat, and (3) these drugs can potentially produce mild to serious side effects. Mild side effects like anorexia, vomiting, and lethargy can occur with both methimazole and propylthiouracil. Serious adverse effects are more common with propylthiouracil than methimazole. The most devastating effect of propylthiouracil is a hematological crisis due to immune-mediated hemolytic anemia and thrombocytopenia. Rarely, cats on methimazole can develop severe leukopenia and thrombocytopenia, which reverse when the drug is discontinued. Based on the higher rate of complications and severity of these complications with propylthiouracil, this drug should no longer be the drug of first choice when recommending an antithyroid drug. Methimazole is as effective and safer and therefore is the antithyroid drug of choice.

A therapeutic plan for long-term antithyroid drug therapy (methimazole) is as follows:

1. Begin with an initial dose of 15 mg/day.
2. Monitor T_4 and obtain a complete blood count and platelet count every 2 weeks for the first 2 months.
3. In most cats, the T_4 level is normal within 2 weeks.
4. If little or no decrease in T_4 level occurs after 14 days, increase the dose by 33 to 66 per cent after ensuring that the cat is receiving medication.
5. Once a euthyroid state is reached, decrease the dose to 10 mg/day.
6. Monitor T_4 and obtain a complete blood count, platelet count, and antinuclear antibody at 3-month intervals after the initial 8 weeks of treatment.
7. Serious side effects usually occur during initial treatment but can develop at any time.

Another effective nonsurgical treatment for feline hyperthyroidism is radioactive iodine. ^{131}I is a radioactive isotope that is taken up by the thyroid gland after being given intravenously and is concentrated in the hyperplastic cells. These cells are destroyed by the emission of beta particles. The advantages of this medical alternative are that (1) no surgery or anesthesia is required and (2) normal atrophic thyroid tissue is often spared, and lifetime thyroid hormone maintenance is therefore unnecessary. The disadvantages are that cats must be isolated in a hospital environment for 1 to 2 weeks, possibly leading to anorexia and depression.

In our opinion, radioactive iodine is the best treatment for feline hyperthyroidism when all factors are collectively considered. If nuclear medicine facilities are unavailable, surgical thyroidectomy is then recommended. Long-term antithyroid drug treatment should only be recommended for cats in which hospitalization, anesthesia, and surgery carry a substantial risk.

Before thyroidectomy, a complete blood count, serum chemistry profile, and, when available, a thyroid scan are performed using intravenous technetium-99 as pertechnetate. Most cats are treated preoperatively with methimazole (5 mg PO TID). Methimazole is administered until euthyroidism is achieved, usually 2 to 4 weeks after the onset of drug therapy. Once hyperthyroidism has been reversed, the risks associated with anesthesia are markedly diminished. Propranolol, a beta-adrenergic blocker, is given to cats with significant tachycardia (heart rate >240 beats per minute). Propranolol helps to minimize the hyperexcitability, tachycardia, and arrhythmias associated with hyperthyroidism. Most hyperthyroid cats do not need to be premedicated. Anticholinergic agents (i.e., atropine, glycopyrrolate) may induce tachycardia and are avoided. If a cat is hyperexcitable enough to hinder restraint and anesthetic induction, sedation with acepromazine may be helpful. Acepromazine can be advantageous because it helps prevent the arrhythmias associated with certain anesthetic agents (thiobarbiturates, inhalation gases) and anesthetic hypotension.[37]

Anesthetic induction is most safely administered with agents that do not stimulate catecholamine secretion. Short-acting thiobarbiturates are effective drugs that safely induce anesthesia in hyperthyroid cats and should be followed by intubation and maintenance of general anesthesia with gas anesthetics. Methoxyflurane and halothane are not used because they sensitize cardiac muscle to catecholamine-induced arrhythmias.[37] Isoflurane is the gas anesthetic of choice because it is minimally arrhythmogenic and does not have a significant effect on cardiac output.

Surgical Techniques

Surgical treatment of feline hyperthyroidism is accomplished via extracapsular or intracapsular thyroidectomy. In the extracapsular technique, the entire thyroid gland and capsule are removed without opening the capsule. In the intracapsular technique, the capsule is opened and the thyroid gland is gently teased away from the capsule and removed. In the initial description of the intracapsular technique, the thyroid capsule was left in place and not removed. The modified intracapsular technique involves removal of the thyroid capsule after the gland has been removed.

A ventral midline cervical approach with the neck in slight hyperextension is used. The skin incision extends approximately from the larynx to a point cranial to the manubrium. The sternohyoid and sternothyroid muscles are bluntly separated, and retraction is maintained with a Gelpi self-retaining retractor. The thyroid glands are exposed and removed.

The original feline thyroidectomy technique described in the veterinary literature used a completely extracapsular method. The entire thyroid gland and its capsule were removed without opening the capsule. In this technique, both parathyroids are commonly removed with the entire thyroid gland, and as a result, hypoparathyroidism commonly occurs after surgery. We do not currently recommend this technique for feline thyroidectomy.

Intracapsular dissection entails leaving most or all of the thyroid capsule in place (Fig. 112–4). The thyroid capsule is incised on the ventral surface of the gland in an avascular area, and the incision extended cranially and caudally with scissors so that the entire length of the capsule is opened. The thyroid parenchyma is carefully removed by blunt dissection using small scissors and sterile cotton-tipped applicators. The external parathyroid gland and blood supply are left intact. Small pieces of thyroid capsule are removed if grossly visible fragments of parenchyma are adhered to it, but the majority of the capsule is left in place. Hemostasis is achieved by use of bipolar cautery or ligatures. Because most of the thyroid capsule remains, the main complication is hyperthyroid recurrence.[46] This recurrence is a result of hyperplasia of small nests of adenomatous cells that are adherent to the thyroid capsule but not large enough to be grossly evident.

Modified intracapsular dissection involves removal of most of the thyroid capsule in an attempt to minimize the recurrence rate with the intracapsular technique. After the thyroid parenchyma is removed as described for the intracapsular technique, all thyroid capsule ex-

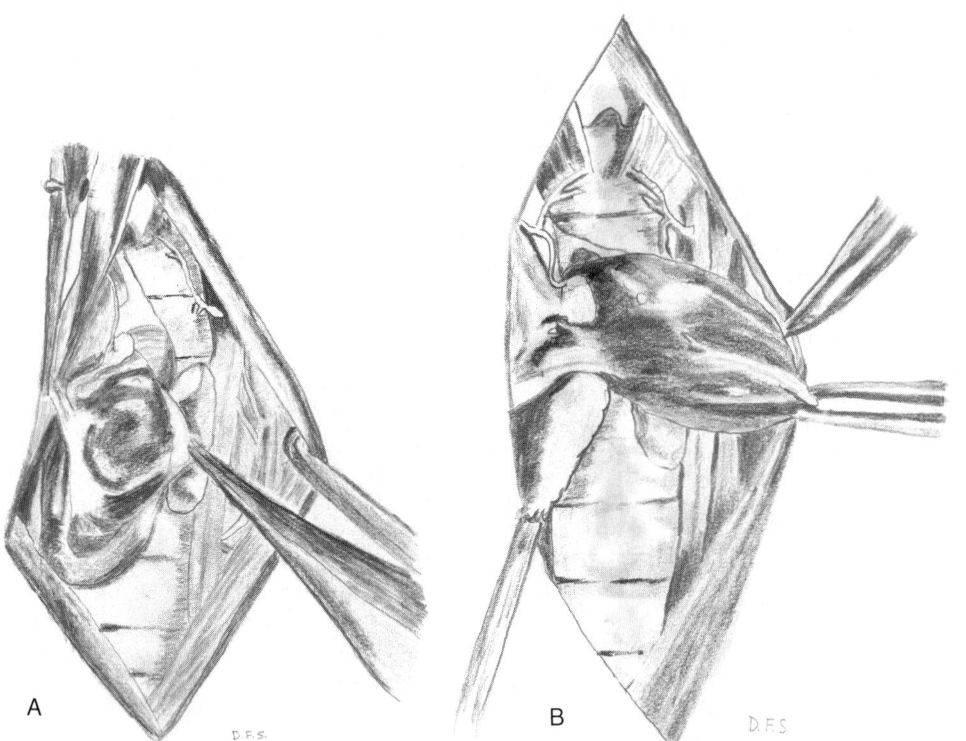

FIGURE 112–4. Intracapsular thyroidectomy technique. *A*, After the capsule is incised along the longitudinal axis of the thyroid gland, the capsule margins are initially peeled off the parenchyma with small tissue forceps. *B*, Sterile cotton applicators are then gently used to tease away the thyroid gland from the capsule. In the modified intracapsular technique, all thyroid capsule, except that immediately adjacent to the external parathyroid gland, is removed.

cept that immediately adjacent to the external parathyroid gland is removed. A small cuff of capsule, along with its blood supply, is left intact adjacent to the external parathyroid gland. Dissection, performed to remove the capsule, is initiated in an area away from the external parathyroid gland. Bipolar cautery and small ligatures are used for hemostasis. Hemorrhage control is critical because a bloody field obstructs pertinent anatomy, including the recurrent laryngeal nerves and parathyroid blood supply.

Modified extracapsular dissection involves removal of the entire thyroid gland and associated capsule without ever opening the capsule (Fig. 112–5). The caudal thyroid vein is ligated or cauterized and transected. Using fine-tipped bipolar cautery forceps, the thyroid capsule adjacent to the external parathyroid gland is cauterized at least 2 mm from the parathyroid gland. Iris scissors are used to cut through the center of the cauterized area. The thyroid gland is further separated by sharp and blunt dissection from the parathyroid gland using iris scissors and sterile cotton-tipped applicators. The dissection caudally frees the thyroid gland from the surrounding tissues, allowing removal of the thyroid gland and its capsule. At that point, the external parathyroid gland remains, with a small section of thyroid capsule and an intact cranial thyroid artery supplying the external parathyroid gland.

Postoperative Complications

There are several potential complications after thyroidectomy, including hypocalcemia, laryngeal paralysis, hyperthyroid recurrence, and hypothyroidism.

Hypocalcemia occurs after inadvertent removal of all four parathyroid glands during bilateral thyroidectomy or as a result of damage to the blood supply of the external parathyroid glands. In the former situation, hypocalcemia may be permanent; in the latter, the hypocalcemia often is reversed when the external parathyroid circulation is re-established over time. In iatrogenic hypoparathyroidism, signs of hypocalcemia usually are noted within 12 to 120 hours postoperatively.[38] Acute hypocalcemia is best treated with intravenous 10 per cent calcium gluconate (0.5 to 1.0 ml/kg, slowly). Once the acute clinical signs (i.e., muscle tremors, seizures) are controlled with this intravenous bolus, 10 ml of 10 per cent calcium gluconate is placed into 250 ml of lactated Ringer solution and dripped at 60 ml/kg/24 hours. Once a cat is stable enough to accept oral medication, both oral calcium and vitamin D are administered. Oral calcium is supplied as calcium lactate (65 mg TID to QID). Vitamin D is supplied as dihydrotachysterol at 0.02 mg/kg/day for 5 days, then 0.01 mg/kg/day for 5 days. A maintenance dose of 0.005 mg/kg/day is given over a 4- to 10-week period. Serum calcium levels are monitored weekly to raise or lower the dose accordingly. Eventually, vitamin D supplementation can usually be discontinued when the parathyroid vascular supply is re-established, in parathyroid vessel injury, or when ectopic parathyroid tissue hypertrophies with time.

Laryngeal paralysis becomes clinically significant when bilateral recurrent laryngeal nerve damage occurs during bilateral thyroidectomy. If at least one of these nerves remains intact and the injury is neuropraxia, laryngeal function should eventually return. If both nerves are transected, laryngeal paralysis is usually permanent.

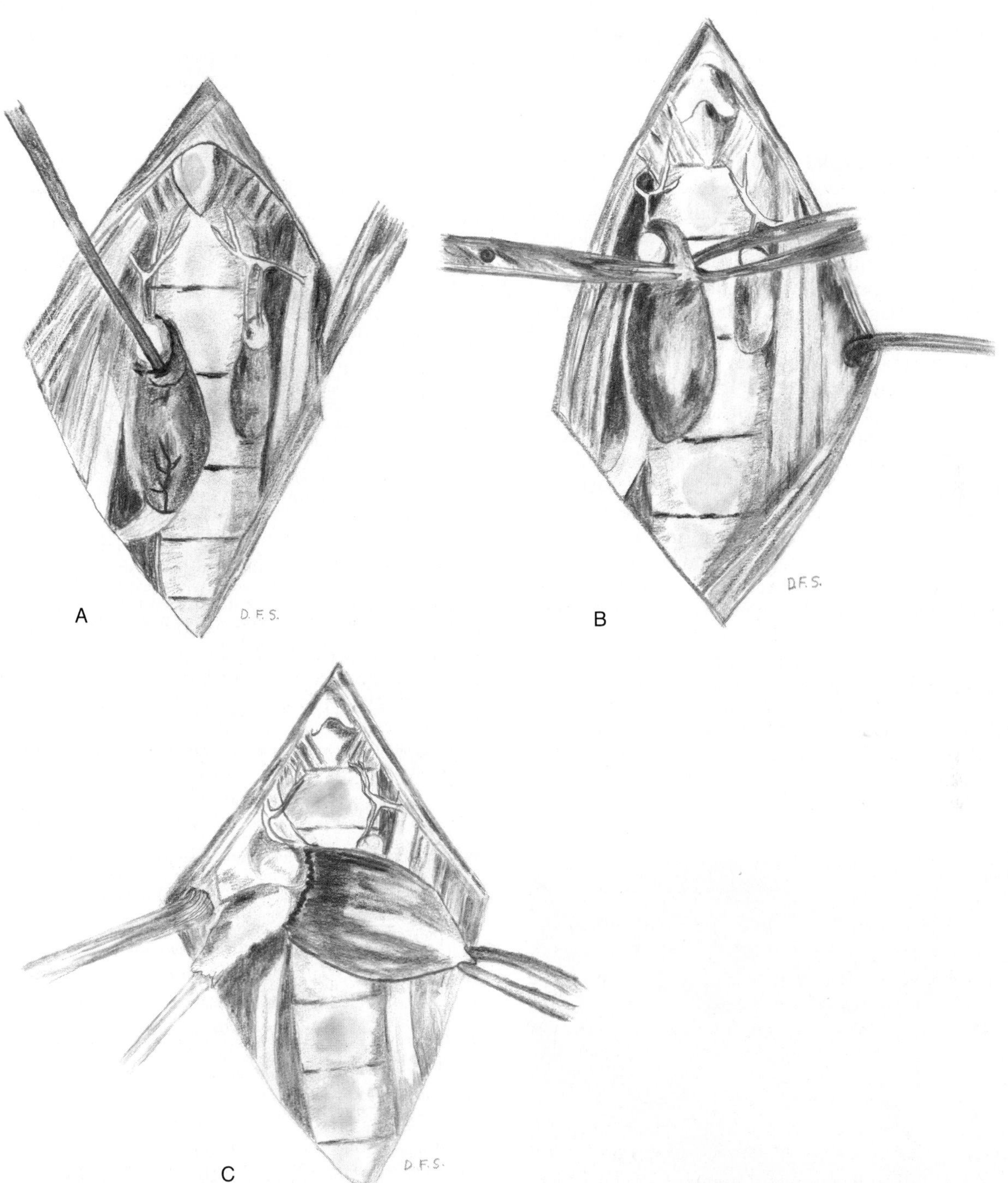

FIGURE 112–5. Modified extracapsular technique. *A,* Bipolar cautery forceps are used to cauterize the thyroid capsule adjacent to the external parathyroid gland. *B,* Iris scissors are used to transect the capsule through the center of the cauterized section. *C,* The thyroid gland is then separated, mainly by blunt dissection, from the parathyroid gland with a sterile cotton-tipped applicator.

Recurrence of hyperthyroidism after bilateral thyroidectomy can be caused by adenomatous changes in ectopic thyroid tissue or more commonly hypertrophy of thyroid remnant cells left behind at the initial site of thyroidectomy. These can be diagnosed by recurrence of elevated serum T_4 levels; the location of the newly hyperplastic thyroid tissue is best defined by a thyroid scan.

CANINE THYROID TUMORS

Most feline thyroid tumors are benign; in dogs, most thyroid tumors are malignant carcinomas. Most of these carcinomas are nonfunctional, with only about 15 per cent producing excessive levels of thyroid hormones.

Because most canine thyroid tumors (approximately 85 per cent) are nonfunctional, they grow slowly and invade the local soft tissues. They are often diagnosed only after growing large enough to be palpated as incidental findings by owners. Most canine thyroid tumors have an abundant blood supply and are locally invasive. These tumors are surgically approached with caution because they are often difficult to resect completely. Their high vascularity results in extensive hemorrhage and local swelling during and immediately after surgery. As a result, anemia and respiratory dysfunction may result after resection of a canine thyroid carcinoma. The surgical margins are often not clean after attempted resection of this invasive type of thyroid carcinoma. As a result, adjuvant therapy using cobalt radiation is recommended by some veterinary institutions to "clean up" the surgical bed.

Clinically, a second, less commonly identified type of thyroid carcinoma is well encapsulated and easier to remove (Fig. 112–6). This group of thyroid tumors does not display the large vascular supply or locally aggressive tissue invasion exhibited by the more commonly identified thyroid neoplasms. Although these tumors are easier to remove, they are still prone to the local recurrences and pulmonary metastasis demonstrated by their more invasive counterpart. The median survival time with surgical resection, in both the encapsulated and invasive group of thyroid carcinomas, is 7 to 8 months.[25]

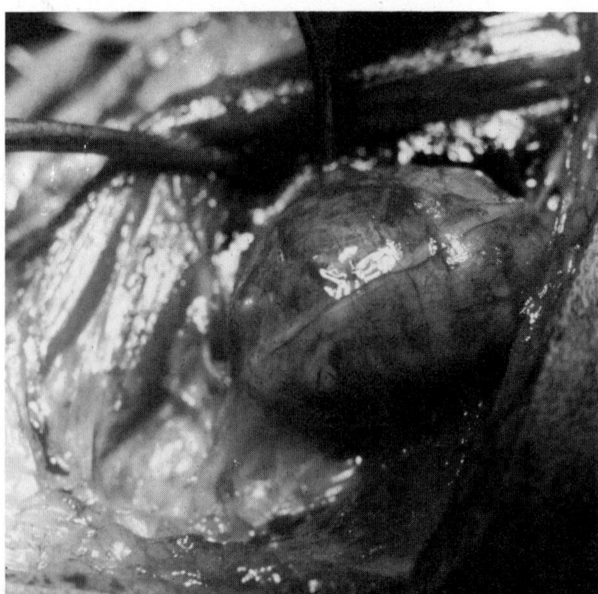

FIGURE 112–6. Ventral cervical region of a dog with a well-encapsulated thyroid carcinoma. This tumor was totally removed with minimal dissection.

References

1. Arnold U: Goitrous hypothyroidism and dwarfism in a kitten. *J Am Anim Hosp Assoc 20*:753, 1984.
2. Belshaw BE: Thyroid diseases. *In* Ettinger SE (ed): *Textbook of Veterinary Internal Medicine*. 2nd ed. W.B. Saunders, Philadelphia, 1983, p 1592.
3. Bond BR, et al: Echocardiographic findings in 103 cats with hyperthyroidism. *J Am Vet Med Assoc 180*:932, 1982.
4. Brouwers J: Goitre et heredite chez le chien. *Ann Med Vet 94*:173, 1950.
5. Carlson AJ: On the cause of congenital goitre (thyroid hyperplasia) in dogs and cats. *Am J Physiol 33*:143, 1914.
6. Carpenter JM: Tumors and tumor-like lesions. *In* Holzworth J (ed): *Diseases of the Cat*. W.B. Saunders, Philadelphia, 1987, p 406.
7. Chastain CB: Congenital hypothyroidism in a dog due to an iodine organification defect. *Am J Vet Res 44*:1257, 1983.
8. Clark ST, Meier H: A clinicopathologic study of thyroid disease in the dog and cat. *Zentral Veterinarmed [A] 5*:17, 1958.
9. Cline MJ, Berlin NI: Erythropoiesis and red cell survival in the hypothyroid dog. *Am J Physiol 204*:415, 1963.
10. Crispin SM, Barnett KC: Arcus lipoides corneae secondary to hypothyroidism in the Alsation. *J Small Anim Pract 19*:127, 1978.
11. Crowe SW, Aronsohn M: The thyroid. *In* Slatter DH (ed): *Textbook of Small Animal Surgery*. W.B. Saunders, Philadelphia, 1985, pp 1865–1874.
12. Feldman EC, Nelson RW: Hyperthyroidism and thyroid tumors. *In* Feldman EC, Nelson RW (eds): *Canine and Feline Endocrinology and Reproduction*. W.B. Saunders, Philadelphia, 1987, p 91.
13. Feldman EC, Nelson RW: Hypothyroidism. *In* Feldman EC, Nelson RW (eds): *Canine and Feline Endocrinology and Reproduction*. W.B. Saunders, Philadelphia, 1987, p 55.
14. Ferguson DC: Thyroid function tests in the dog. *Vet Clin North Am 14*:783, 1984.
15. Gosselin SJ: Biochemical and immunological investigation on hypothyroidism in dogs. *Can J Comp Med 44*:158, 1980.
16. Gosselin SJ, et al: Autoimmune lymphocytic thyroiditis in dogs. *Vet Immunol Immunopathol 3*:185, 1982.
17. Greco DS: Juvenile-onset hypothyroidism in a dog. *J Am Vet Med Assoc 187*:948, 1985.
18. Haines DM: Survey of thyroglobulin autoantibodies in dogs. *Am J Vet Res 45*:1493, 1983.
19. Harvey HJ: Laryngeal paralysis in hypothyroid dogs. *In* Kirk RW (ed): *Current Veterinary Therapy VIII*. W.B. Saunders, Philadelphia, 1983, p 694.
20. Haynes RC, Mural F: Thyroid and antithyroid drugs. *In* Gilman AG, et al (eds): *Goodman and Gilman's The Pharmacologic Basis of Therapeutics*. 6th ed. Macmillan, New York, 1980.
21. Kern TJ, Riis RC: Ocular manifestations of secondary hyperlipidemia associated with hypothyroidism and uveitis in a dog. *J Am Anim Hosp Assoc 16*:907, 1980.
22. Kowalawski K, Kolodej A: Myoelectrical and mechanical activity of stomach and intestine in hypothyroid dogs. *Am J Dig Dis 22*:235, 1977.
23. Lucke VM: A histologic study of thyroid abnormalities in the domestic cat. *J Small Anim Pract 5*:351, 1964.
24. Lucke VM: Thyroid pathology in canine hypothyroidism. *J Comp Pathol 93*:415, 1983.
25. Matthiesen DR, Mullen HS: Problems and complications associated with endocrine surgery in the dog and cat. *Probl Vet Med 2*:627, 1990.
26. Medleau L: Congenital hypothyroidism in a dog. *J Am Anim Hosp Assoc 21*:341, 1985.
27. Miller CW: Echocardiographic assessment of cardiac function in beagles with experimentally produced hypothyroidism. *J Ultrasound Med 3* (suppl):157, 1984.
28. Milne KL, Haynes HM: Epidemiologic features of canine hypothyroidism. *Cornell Vet 71*:3, 1981.
29. Nicholas JS, Swingle WW: An experimental and morphological study of the parathyroid glands of the cat. *Am J Anat 34*:469, 1933.
30. Nijhuis AH: ECG changes in dogs with hypothyroidism. *Tijdschr Diergeneeskd 103*:736, 1978.
31. Patterson JS: Neurologic manifestations of cerebrovascular atherosclerosis associated with primary hypothyroidism in a dog. *J Am Vet Med Assoc 186*:499, 1985.

32. Peterson ME: Effects of spontaneous hyperadrenocorticism on serum thyroid hormone concentrations in the dog. *Am J Vet Res 45*:2034, 1984.
33. Peterson ME: Electrocardiographic findings in 45 cats with hyperthyroidism. *J Am Vet Med Assoc 180*:934, 1982.
34. Peterson ME: Feline hyperthyroidism. *Vet Clin North Am Small Anim Pract 14*:809, 1984.
35. Peterson ME: Feline hyperthyroidism: Pretreatment clinical and laboratory evaluation of 131 cases. *J Am Vet Med Assoc 183*:103, 1983.
36. Peterson ME, Becker DV: Radionuclide thyroid imaging in 135 cats with hyperthyroidism. *Vet Radiol 25*:23, 1984.
37. Peterson ME, Ferguson DC: Thyroid diseases. *In* Ettinger SJ (ed): *Textbook of Veterinary Internal Medicine.* W.B. Saunders, Philadelphia, 1989, pp 1639–1675.
38. Peterson ME, Randolph JF: Endocrine diseases. *In* Sherding RG (ed): *The Cat. Diseases and Clinical Management.* Vol 2. Churchill Livingstone, New York, 1989, pp 1095–1161.
39. Rogers JS: Factor VIII activity and thyroid function. *Ann Intern Med 97*:713, 1982.
40. Rogers RS, Shane SR: Factor VIII activity in normal volunteers receiving oral thyroid hormone. *J Lab Clin Med 102*:444, 1983.
41. Romatowski J: Intercurrent hypothyroidism, autoimmune anemia, and a coagulation deficiency (von Willebrand's disease) in a dog. *J Am Vet Med Assoc 185*:309, 1984.
42. Schaer M: The thyroid gland. *In* Bojrab MJ (ed): *Pathophysiology in Small Animal Surgery.* Lea & Febiger, Philadelphia, 1981, pp 314–319.
43. Skelton CL, Sonnenblick EH: The cardiovascular system. *In* Ingbar SH, Braverman LE (eds): *The Thyroid.* 5th ed. J.B. Lippincott, Philadelphia, 1986, p 1140.
44. Taurog A: Hormone synthesis: Thyroid iodine metabolism. *In* Ingbar SH, Braverman LE (eds): *The Thyroid.* 5th ed. J.B. Lippincott, Philadelphia, 1986, p 53.
45. Turrel JM, et al: Thyroid carcinoma causing hyperthyroidism in cats: 14 cases (1981–1986). *J Am Vet Med Assoc 193*:359, 1988.
46. Welches CD, et al: Occurrence of problems after three techniques of bilateral thyroidectomy in cats. *Vet Surg 18*:392, 1989.

CHAPTER 113

Parathyroid Glands

James A. Flanders

The parathyroid glands regulate the concentration of calcium in the circulation through the actions of parathyroid hormone (PTH). PTH stimulates reabsorption of calcium by the kidneys, mobilization of calcium from bone, and, indirectly, absorption of calcium through the intestine by regulation of vitamin D hydroxylation in the kidneys.

ANATOMY AND VASCULAR SUPPLY

Dogs and cats have four parathyroid glands. Two parathyroid glands are closely associated with each thyroid gland.[47, 85] One parathyroid gland is located within the thyroid parenchyma (internal parathyroid gland), and the other is usually attached to the outer surface of the thyroid capsule (external parathyroid gland). The external parathyroid gland may be present anywhere on the surface of the thyroid gland but is most commonly located at the cranial pole. The elliptical parathyroid glands are approximately 1 mm thick and 5 mm long in both dogs and cats.

The parathyroid glands are surrounded by a thin layer of connective tissue. Most of the parenchyma is composed of a single cell type called the *chief cell.* Chief cells exist in various stages of secretory activity and may also differentiate into a mitochondrion-rich, nonsecretory form called *oxyphil cells.*

The vascular supply of the parathyroid glands is derived from branches of the thyroid arteries and veins. In dogs, the external parathyroid gland is usually supplied by a branch that leaves the thyroid artery before it enters the thyroid gland.[47] Vascular branches that supply the external parathyroid gland in cats may follow a course similar to that in dogs or first pass through the thyroid parenchyma and perforate the thyroid capsule before reaching the parathyroid gland.[47, 72]

EMBRYOLOGY

The external parathyroid glands, along with the thymus, are derived from endodermal tissue of the fetal third pharyngeal pouches. The internal parathyroid glands are derived from the fourth pharyngeal pouches.[86] During fetal development, the parathyroid tissue migrates caudally into the neck. Normally, the parathyroid glands become associated with the thyroid glands in the perilaryngeal region. Fragments of parathyroid tissue may settle in the peritracheal fascia or migrate with the thymus to the thoracic inlet or cranial mediastinum. Ectopic parathyroid tissue is present in 35 to 50 per cent of cats and in 6 to 100 per cent of dogs.[37, 47, 97] Differences in the incidence of ectopic parathyroid tissue are related to the method and extent of dissection by investigators.

PARATHYROID HORMONE

Structure and Synthesis

PTH is synthesized by the chief cells of the parathyroid glands as a 115-amino-acid polypeptide, preproPTH (Fig. 113–1). The first 24 amino acids at the amino terminal are cleaved within the chief cells to yield proPTH. Further intracellular cleavage yields several polypeptides, including intact PTH, an 84-amino-acid polypeptide.[20] Intact PTH has a circulating half-life of less than 5 minutes owing to rapid catabolism by the Kupffer cells of the liver, the renal tubular cells, and osteocytes into several polypeptide fragments (see Fig.

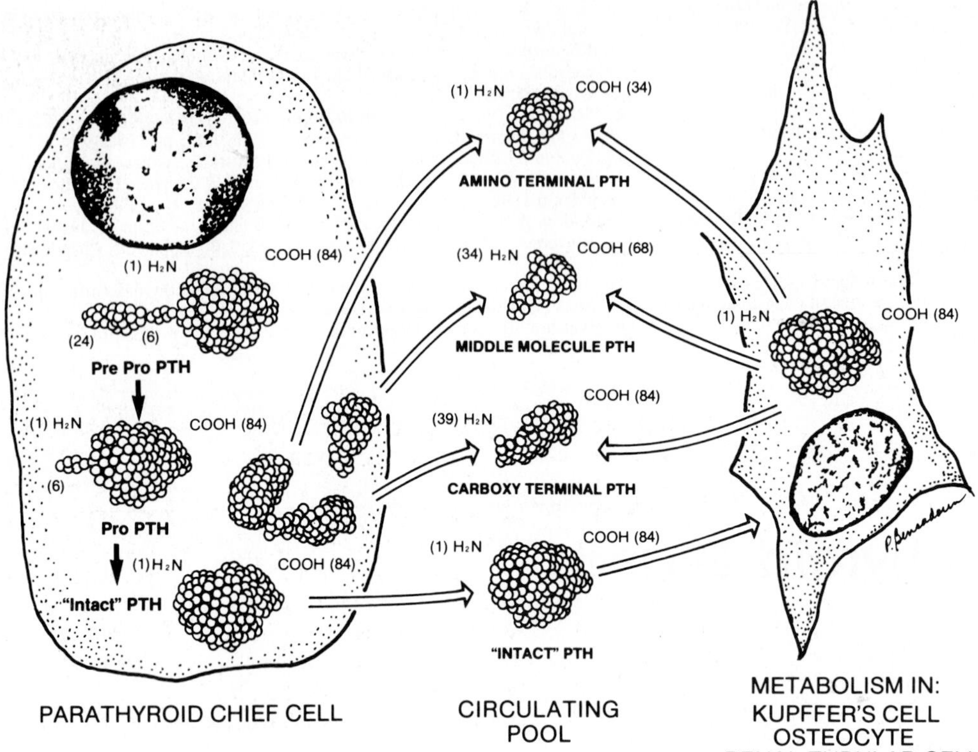

FIGURE 113–1. Metabolism of parathyroid hormone (PTH). "Intact" PTH is synthesized in the parathyroid chief cell and secreted into the circulating pool either in the intact 84-amino-acid form or as small subunits. Circulating intact PTH is cleared from the circulation by enzymatic cleavage in the Kupffer's cells of the liver, osteocytes, and renal tubular cells.

113–1).[54] The most metabolically active portion of PTH consists of the first 24 amino acids at the amino terminal of the molecule (PTH 1-24). Amino-terminal PTH has a short circulating half-life (<5 minutes) owing to glomerular filtration and rapid metabolism by hepatocytes and renal tubular cells. The carboxy-terminal (PTH 39-84) fragment of PTH may have some metabolic activity in bone and the kidneys.[121] Carboxy-terminal and middle molecule (PTH 34-68) fragments are removed from the circulation exclusively by glomerular filtration and have circulating half-lives of approximately 30 minutes in normal dogs.[75] Although all of the PTH fragments are cleared by glomerular filtration, renal failure causes a disproportionate retention of the middle and carboxy-terminal fragments.[35]

Secretion

The parathyroid glands store a small quantity of PTH secretory granules in the chief cells. PTH is rapidly synthesized and released in response to decreases in serum calcium concentration.[20] Serum phosphorus concentration does not have a direct effect on PTH secretion, but high concentrations of phosphorus may depress serum calcium concentration owing to the interaction of calcium with phosphorus in serum.[58] Changes in magnesium concentration also affect PTH secretion similarly to calcium; the response by the parathyroid glands is not as marked.[13]

Physiological Effects

The main function of the parathyroid glands is regulation of the serum calcium concentration. PTH potentiates several systems that conserve calcium within the body (Fig. 113–2). The net effect of PTH secretion is rapid elevation of serum calcium levels. Hypercalcemia is prevented by a negative-feedback loop that inhibits PTH synthesis and secretion.[20] Calcitonin, a hormone secreted from the parafollicular cells of the thyroid gland in response to hypercalcemia, antagonizes some of the

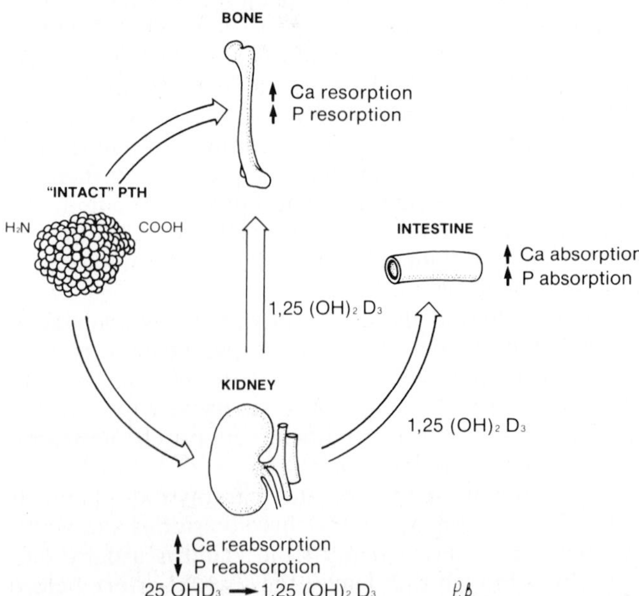

FIGURE 113–2. Parathyroid hormone (PTH) homeostasis. PTH acts directly on the kidneys and bone to increase the serum concentration of calcium. PTH also potentiates the 1-hydroxylation of 25 OHD_3. 1,25 $(OH)_2D_3$ acts on bone and intestine to increase serum calcium concentration.

effects of PTH and helps maintain normal serum calcium levels.

Parathyroid Hormone and Vitamin D Metabolism

Several effects of PTH on calcium homeostasis are mediated by vitamin D. Vitamin D is obtained by either solar irradiation of 7-dehydrocholesterol in the skin or ingestion of food containing vitamin D_2 (plant sources) or D_3 (animal sources).[51] Most vitamin D in the body is vitamin D_3 produced in the skin. A vitamin D-binding globulin transports vitamin D_3 to the liver, where it is hydroxylated to 25-hydroxyvitamin D_3 by microsomal and mitochondrial hydroxylases in hepatocytes.[60] This reaction is substrate dependent and occurs without feedback regulation. A linear relationship exists between the amount of vitamin D_3 introduced into the circulation and the amount of 25-hydroxyvitamin D_3 generated.

PTH controls the next step in vitamin D metabolism, 1-hydroxylation of 25-hydroxyvitamin D_3, which occurs in the mitochondria of the proximal tubules of the kidneys. The end product of renal hydroxylation, 1,25-dihydroxyvitamin D_3 (1,25$(OH)_2D_3$), is the most metabolically active form of vitamin D. It is 100 times more potent than 25-hydroxyvitamin D_3 in promoting bone calcium resorption activity and functions three times faster in promoting calcium absorption through the intestine.[43] The production of 1,25$(OH)_2D_3$ is augmented by PTH and inhibited by increased concentrations of serum calcium, phosphorus, or feedback inhibition from 1,25$(OH)_2D_3$. The 1-hydroxylation of 25-hydroxyvitamin D is reduced by 70 to 80 per cent in the absence of PTH.[61] Calcium deficiency potentiates 1-alpha-hydroxylase activity indirectly by stimulating the secretion of PTH. Phosphorus deficiency directly stimulates 1-alpha-hydroxylase activity.[1]

Feedback inhibition of PTH secretion by the parathyroid glands is provided by 1,25$(OH)_2D_3$. Specific 1,25$(OH)_2D_3$ receptors have been identified on chief cell plasma membranes; binding of these receptors with 1,25$(OH)_2D_3$ results in internalization of the receptor-1,25$(OH)_2D_3$ complex and inhibition of PTH synthesis.[24]

Parathyroid Hormone and Intestinal Calcium Absorption

Effects of PTH on intestinal calcium absorption are mediated through vitamin D. Ingested calcium is absorbed from the gut by two different processes. The first process occurs mainly in the proximal jejunum, is transcellular, and is vitamin D dependent (Fig. 113–3). Calcium is absorbed across the brush border of intestinal mucosal cells along a concentration and electrical gradient. The movement of calcium across the luminal membrane may be potentiated by 1,25$(OH)_2D_3$ by altering membrane composition and structure through changes in phospholipid metabolism.[110] The transcellular movement of calcium is augmented 60-fold by the vitamin D-dependent production of a cytoplasmic calcium-binding protein. Calcium is actively pumped out of the basolateral membrane of the intestinal cell by a vitamin D-responsive calcium-dependent adenosine triphosphatase.[36]

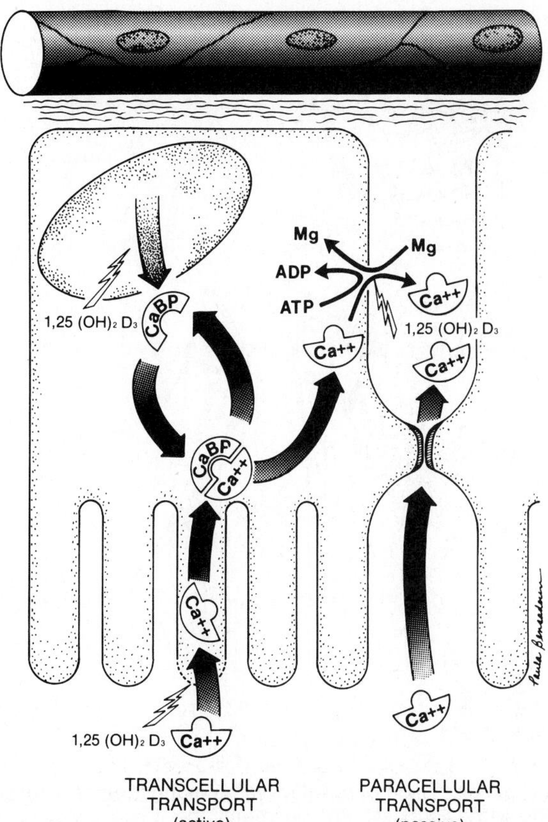

FIGURE 113–3. Intestinal calcium absorption. 1,25 $(OH)_2D_3$ potentiates the absorption of calcium through the intestinal mucosa by altering mucosal cell membrane composition, augmenting production of calcium-binding protein, and increasing the efficiency of calcium-dependent adenosine triphosphatase. Calcium may also pass through the mucosa by passive paracellular transport through tight junctions.

The second process by which calcium is absorbed occurs throughout the small intestine and functions independently of vitamin D.[8] Calcium moves between mucosal cells across gap and tight junctions via a paracellular shunt. Approximately 50 per cent of the ingested calcium absorbed by the intestine passes through the paracellular route.[9] Thus calcium absorption from the intestine does occur in the absence of vitamin D; however, vitamin D potentiates the absorption of calcium, especially at low dietary calcium levels.

Renal Effects of Parathyroid Hormone

PTH has three effects on the the kidneys: It (1) potentiates the renal reabsorption of calcium, (2) increases renal excretion of phosphate, and (3) potentiates the 1-hydroxylation of vitamin D (Fig. 113–4). The effect of PTH on vitamin D metabolism was discussed earlier.

Renal reabsorption of calcium occurs at several sites in the kidneys, with most (50 to 60 per cent) of the

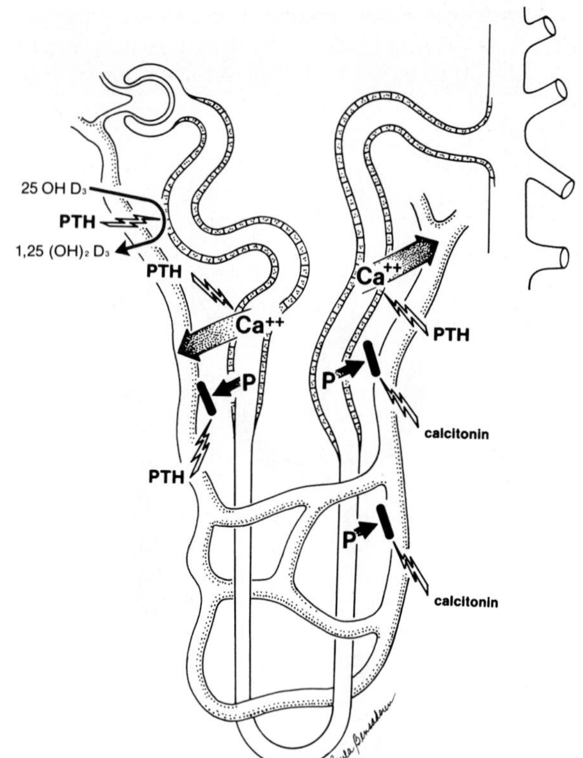

FIGURE 113–4. Action of parathyroid hormone (PTH) and calcitonin on the kidney tubules. PTH augments the 1-hydroxylation of 25 OHD_3 in the proximal tubules. PTH promotes the reabsorption of calcium in both the proximal and distal convoluted tubules. PTH inhibits phosphorus reabsorption in the proximal convoluted tubule and ascending loop of Henle.

reabsorption occurring in the proximal convoluted tubule.[104] The major site of PTH effect on renal reabsorption of calcium is in the distal convoluted tubule.[77, 104] PTH moderates its effects on the kidneys by stimulation of adenyl cyclase with subsequent elevation of cyclic adenosine monophosphate (AMP) levels in the renal tubular cells.[41] The increased cytoplasmic cyclic AMP concentration activates protein kinases, which phosphorylate and thereby either potentiate or inhibit unknown enzyme systems. The phosphorylated enzymes cause increased reabsorption of calcium.

The effect of PTH on renal tubular cells may be influenced by $1,25(OH)_2D_3$. Vitamin D-dependent calcium-binding protein is present in the distal tubular cells, and vitamin D deficiency decreases the amount of intracellular cyclic AMP produced in response to PTH.[34]

Although PTH increases renal reabsorption of calcium, it decreases the reabsorption of phosphorus. This is a homeostatic mechanism that preserves calcium but prevents the calcium-phosphorus solubility product from exceeding saturation limits, thus preventing precipitation of calcium phosphate salts in the soft tissues of the body. PTH inhibits proximal tubular reabsorption of phosphorus through the action of adenylate cyclase activation, similar to the effect of PTH on tubular calcium reabsorption. In regard to phosphorus, cyclic AMP-mediated phosphorylation of intracellular enzymes results in decreased tubular reabsorption.[50]

Parathyroid Hormone and Bone

PTH acts on bone to stimulate the release of calcium and phosphorus from bone mineral stores. Bone minerals are released into the circulation by two mechanisms, osteoclastic bone resorption and osteocyte-mediated release of calcium and phosphorus from an exchangeable pool of bone minerals.[98] PTH effects on bone cells are mediated through the osteoblasts and osteocytes. PTH causes increased metabolic activity in osteoblasts and increased intracellular levels of second messengers such as cyclic AMP, calcium, diacylglycerol, and inositol triphosphate.[46] The increase in osteoblastic intracellular second messengers results in production of many soluble factors that affect surrounding bone cells and bone cell precursors. One factor released from PTH-stimulated osteoblasts causes stimulation of periosteal fibroblasts, which may result in differentiation into osteoblasts.[109] Although production of second messengers in osteoblasts increases after PTH stimulation, many investigators have shown a simultaneous inhibition of collagen and bone matrix component production.[46] PTH-mediated inhibition of bone matrix synthesis is compatible with the calcitropic effects of PTH. New bone matrix requires calcium for mineralization, reducing the availability of calcium for the serum pool.

The effects of $1,25(OH)_2D_3$ on osteoblast proliferation vary with the source of osteoblasts studied; some studies demonstrate an increase in osteoblast number and size, and other studies show no effect on cell number.[46, 74] Osteoblasts are stimulated by $1,25(OH)_2D_3$ to secrete osteocalcin (also called bone *Gla protein*), a noncollagenous protein that has vitamin K-dependent calcium-binding properties via gamma-carboxyglutamic acid similar to the vitamin K-dependent coagulation factors. Osteocalcin and other noncollagenous proteins in bone may coordinate mineralization and control the growth of hydroxyapatite crystals in bone.[67]

Osteoclasts do not have PTH or $1,25(OH)_2D_3$ receptors.[46] Activation of osteoclasts occurs through the action of an osteoclast-stimulating factor released by osteoblasts in response to PTH.[92] Osteoclast-stimulating factor increases the metabolic activity of osteoclasts. Stimulated osteoclasts are more mobile, and bone resorption is markedly increased.

The greatest effect of PTH on acute release of calcium from bone is not the result of an increase in osteoclast activity but an augmentation of calcium release from the exchangeable pool of calcium in bone (Fig. 113–5). The exchangeable pool of calcium is that portion of bone matrix in close proximity to the lacunae and canaliculi of osteocytes.[13] Calcium from the exchangeable pool may be actively transported by osteocytes across a concentration gradient into the blood stream. PTH may augment the movement of calcium out of the exchangeable pool by increasing the osteocyte membrane potential, thus stimulating a calcium "pump."[93] Another theory suggests that the bone fluid in contact with osteocytes contains a soluble form of calcium phosphate crystal such as brushite, which acts as a transition phase between hydroxyapatite and plasma calcium and phosphorus. Brushite is produced by the

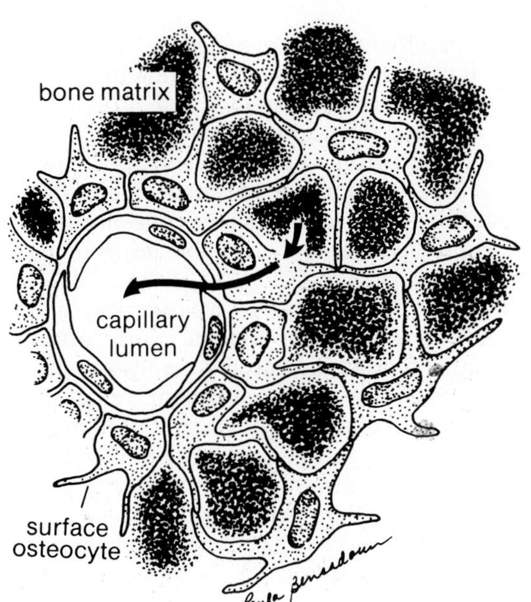

FIGURE 113–5. Parathyroid hormone (PTH) action on the exchangeable pool of calcium in bone. PTH augments the mobilization of exchangeable calcium from bone matrix and into the circulation by action on surface osteocytes.

lining osteocytes and can spontaneously transform into hydroxyapatite or become solubilized, depending on the presence of solubility factors such as acid or noncollagenous proteins produced by the surface osteocytes in response to $1,25(OH)_2D_3$ or PTH.[89]

CALCITONIN

Calcitonin is a 32-amino-acid polypeptide hormone synthesized and secreted by the parafollicular C cells of the thyroid gland.[3] Calcitonin secretion is stimulated by elevations of serum calcium concentration above normal. The presence of calcium in the stomach induces gastrin-mediated calcitonin secretion. Calcitonin reduces serum calcium concentrations to the normal range by antagonizing some of the actions of PTH. The major hypocalcemic effect of calcitonin is inhibition of the bone-resorbing activity of osteoclasts. Under the influence of calcitonin, active osteoclasts withdraw from resorption sites and lose the ruffled cytoplasmic border associated with bone resorption. The action of calcitonin on the kidneys is similar to the effects of PTH (see Fig. 113–4); tubular reabsorption of calcium is augmented, and tubular phosphorus reabsorption is inhibited.[12]

PARATHYROID NEOPLASIA

The most common parathyroid neoplasm in dogs is functional parathyroid adenoma.* Some solitary parathyroid tumors are histologically classified as hyperplasia because of the difficulty in differentiating hyperplastic from adenomatous change.[26] Parathyroid neoplasia is rare in cats.[14] Parathyroid adenomas are usually unilateral and affect only one thyroid-associated parathyroid gland. A functional parathyroid neoplasm involving ectopic parathyroid tissue located in the cranial mediastinum of a dog has been reported.[90] Autonomously functioning chief cells within the neoplastic glands produce and secrete excessive amounts of PTH. The adenomatous tissue remains encapsulated within the thin parathyroid capsule. Two reports have described parathyroid carcinoma in dogs.[4, 90] Neither carcinoma metastasized, but one mediastinal parathyroid carcinoma recurred after excision.

*See references 4, 15, 25, 38, 48, 53, 57, 64, 91, 105, and 115.

Clinical signs associated with functional parathyroid neoplasms (primary hyperparathyroidism) are related to hypercalcemia caused by excessive secretion of PTH. Increased circulating levels of PTH result in increased calcium and phosphorus release from bone, increased calcium reabsorption and increased phosphorus excretion by the kidneys, and increased absorption of calcium and phosphorus through the intestines.

The clinical signs of primary hyperparathyroidism are often subtle and most commonly include polyuria/polydipsia, lethargy, inappetence, and weakness.* Less commonly reported clinical signs include vomiting, stiff gait, pathological fractures, facial deformity, loose teeth, and urolithiasis.[4, 38, 53, 57, 64] One report described seizures attributable to primary hyperparathyroidism.[48]

Polyuria/polydipsia associated with primary hyperparathyroidism may be due to hypercalcemia uncoupling the cyclic AMP response of renal tubular cells to antidiuretic hormone.[15] Renal changes associated with hyperparathyroidism may include interstitial nephritis with normal or decreased glomerular filtration rate and nephrocalcinosis.[104] Elevated serum calcium concentration may decrease glomerular filtration by causing vasoconstriction of the afferent arterioles of the kidney.[54, 66] Vomiting and constipation may be due to decreased excitability of gastrointestinal smooth muscle caused by hypercalcemia.[26] The causes of lethargy, inappetence, and weakness associated with primary hyperparathyroidism are unknown, but metabolic abnormalities associated with hyperparathyroidism such as glucose intolerance, negative nitrogen balance, and increased lysosomal activity may affect muscle strength or gastrointestinal activity.[100]

Hyperparathyroidism produces hypercalciuria, which may predispose to urolithiasis. Chronic administration of exogenous PTH produces calcium phosphate uroliths in dogs.[53] Urolithiasis is a common finding in humans with parathyroid adenomas and has been reported in dogs with parathyroid adenomas.[4, 38, 53, 57, 64] The calculi associated with hyperparathyroidism are most commonly composed of calcium phosphate and may be present in the kidneys, bladder, or urethra.

Although hypercalcemia can cause changes in cardiac electrical activity such as prolongation of the PR interval and shortening of the QT interval, electrocardiographic abnormalities are not commonly reported with canine

*See references 4, 15, 25, 27, 38, 48, 53, 57, 64, 91, 105, and 115.

hyperparathyroidism.[4, 115] One cat with a parathyroid adenoma had cardiac arrhythmias at presentation and died of cardiac arrest.[14]

Increased PTH secretion causes proliferation of osteoblasts and osteoclasts and stimulates bone remodeling sites.[16] The result is augmented bone turnover, with osteoclasia in excess of bone synthesis. Although the number of osteoblasts increases, bone synthesis by the osteoblasts decreases owing to the inhibitory effects of PTH. The radiographic and histological picture of hyperparathyroidism is bone resorption and replacement of resorbed bone by fibrous connective tissue (osteitis fibrosa). Such bony changes occur in humans with primary hyperparathyroidism and in dogs.[4, 38, 57, 64, 105] The skull, maxilla, and mandible are most commonly affected. The mandible and maxilla become soft and pliable as fibrous tissue replaces bone. Some dogs may have deforming proliferations of fibrous tissue in the nose and maxilla. Radiography reveals decalcification of the affected bones; the earliest changes appear as a radiolucency around the teeth as the lamina dura dentis is resorbed. Osteoclastic resorption and demineralization of bone may lead to pathological fractures of long bones or vertebrae. Most dogs with primary hyperparathyroidism do not have clinically obvious skeletal changes, possibly because of early diagnosis before excessive resorption of bone.

Clinical Pathological Changes of Primary Hyperparathyroidism

No consistent abnormalities in the hemogram of dogs with functional parathyroid neoplasms have been reported.[26] Urinalysis may reveal calcium phosphate or calcium oxalate crystals associated with hypercalciuria. Measurement of the fractional excretion of calcium and phosphorus by the kidneys has been reported in two dogs.[15, 26] In both dogs, an increased fractional excretion of phosphorus was noted, but the fractional excretion of calcium was variable. Although PTH acts on the renal tubules to decrease urinary calcium loss, hypercalcemia overwhelms the renal threshold for calcium, and fractional excretion of calcium may be increased.

The most consistent hematological abnormalities associated with primary hyperparathyroidism are hypercalcemia with normo- or hypophosphatemia.[4] In dogs, serum calcium concentrations may be affected by the concentration of serum albumin or protein.[82] Approximately 50 per cent of serum calcium is protein bound, so elevations of serum albumin or protein may elevate total serum calcium measurement. A more accurate measurement of serum calcium can be achieved by measurement of ionized (unbound) calcium. Approximately 45 per cent of serum calcium is ionized, and this fraction is the metabolically active fraction. The remaining 5 per cent is combined with anions such as citrate and phosphate. Measurement of ionized calcium requires specialized equipment. In lieu of ionized calcium measurement, total serum calcium measurement in dogs can be adjusted for variation in protein binding by the following formula derived from a regression analysis of calcium on albumin[82]: Corrected calcium (mg/ml) = measured calcium (mg/100 ml) − albumin (g/100 ml) + 3.5. A formula correcting for total protein binding is not as accurate. The albumin-binding adjustment formula is derived from canine values and is not accurate for cats. The relationship between albumin or protein concentrations and total calcium concentrations in cats is not as predictable, and a reliable adjustment formula cannot be constructed.[31]

Some dogs with primary hyperparathyroidism may have elevations of serum alkaline phosphatase concentration, attributed to increased bone resorption. Chronic hypercalcemia may cause sufficient renal damage to increase serum creatinine and serum urea nitrogen concentrations. In such cases, it may be difficult to distinguish between dogs with primary and secondary hyperparathyroidism without histological examination of the parathyroid glands (see the section on hypercalcemia associated with renal failure).

DIFFERENTIAL DIAGNOSIS OF HYPERCALCEMIA

Several diseases may produce hypercalcemia in dogs (Fig. 113–6). It is obviously important to distinguish among these diseases to provide appropriate treatment.

Hypercalcemia of Malignancy

Nonparathyroid malignancy is the most common cause of hypercalcemia in dogs[80, 112] but is infrequent in cats.[52] Hypercalcemia may be caused by direct destruction of bone by the tumor or tumor metastases. Findings now support the concept that hypercalcemia of malignancy is most often caused by the action of humoral factors produced by nonparathyroid neoplasms.[7, 11, 80] The most commonly reported neoplasms causing hypercalcemia in dogs are lymphosarcoma, adenocarcinoma of the apocrine glands of the anal sacs, and multiple myeloma.[80] Isolated reports have described neoplasms such as squamous cell carcinoma, epidermoid carcinoma of the lung, pancreatic carcinoma, mammary adenocarcinoma, and nasal adenocarcinoma causing hypercalcemia in dogs.[39, 71, 116, 118] In cats, hypercalcemia has been infrequently associated with lymphosarcoma, lymphocytic leukemia, granulocytic leukemia, and erythroleukemia.[18, 23, 120] Hypercalcemia associated with squamous cell carcinoma was noted in two cats.[52]

Approximately one-third of dogs with lymphosarcoma and more than half of dogs with adenocarcinoma of the apocrine glands of the anal sac are hypercalcemic.[14] The factor elaborated by hypercalcemic dogs with lymphosarcoma and adenocarcinoma of the apocrine glands of the anal sac has PTH-like properties, such as increasing renal phosphorus excretion and cyclic AMP production and producing increased bone resorption associated with decreased trabecular bone density and increased osteoclastic osteolysis.[111] The humoral factor does not increase renal calcium reabsorption nor stimulate 1-hydroxylation of 25-hydroxycholecalciferol. It does not cross react with PTH radioimmunoassays.[81] A similar factor has been isolated from many tumors producing hyper-

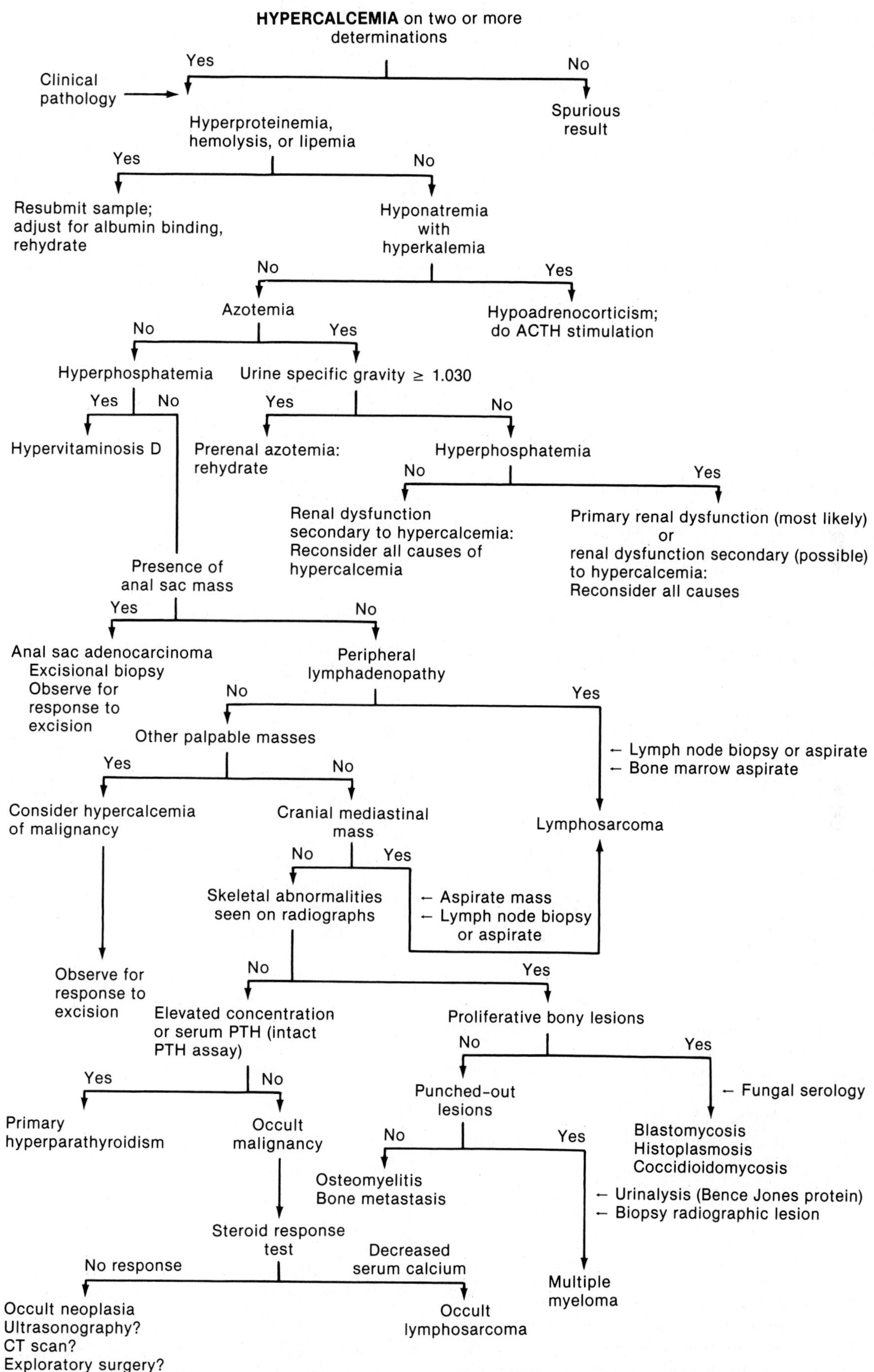

FIGURE 113–6. Algorithm for hypercalcemia. (ACTH, adrenocorticotropic hormone; PTH, parathyroid hormone.)

calcemia in humans and has been called *HHM factor* (humoral hypercalcemia of malignancy factor)[60] or *PTH-like peptide*.[7]

Humoral agents other than the PTH-like peptide may be responsible for hypercalcemia produced by certain neoplasms. Transforming growth factor alpha, interleukin-1, and tumor necrosis factor all are potent stimulators of osteoclast formation and activity and are elaborated by various neoplasms.[84] It is unlikely that osteoclast activation alone produces the hypercalcemia of malignancy; there is a poor correlation between the production of osteoclast-activating factors elaborated by neoplasms and the level of hypercalcemia.[80] No correlation has been found between the number of bone metastases and serum calcium concentration in human patients with cancer.[96] It is likely that the majority of neoplasms producing hypercalcemia produce a PTH-like peptide that may work in concert with other factors to produce hypercalcemia.

Hypercalcemia Associated with Renal Failure

Renal failure is usually associated with increased secretion of PTH and hyperplasia of the parathyroid glands.[19] The cause of renal secondary hyperparathyroidism is a combination of several factors associated with renal failure. Increased serum phosphorus concentration, decreased $1,25(OH)_2D_3$ levels, down-regulation of $1,25(OH)_2D_3$ receptors on the parathyroid glands, skeletal resistance to the calcemic effects of PTH, and elevation of the serum calcium set-point for inhibition of PTH secretion all are associated with uremia.[24] Any of these factors could cause hyperparathyroidism. Despite the presence of increased circulating levels of PTH, hypercalcemia is not common during chronic renal failure. Most dogs and cats with renal failure have normal or low serum calcium concentrations.[10, 27] Hypocalcemia may be attributed to several factors: low levels of $1,25(OH)_2D_3$, which decrease intestinal calcium absorption and decrease the calcemic effect of PTH on bone; a reduction in functional renal tubule cells to reabsorb calcium; and hyperphosphatemia, which decreases calcium owing to the mass action law.[24] The factor that makes some chronic renal failure patients with secondary hyperparathyroidism hypercalcemic whereas most are normocalcemic or hypocalcemic is unknown.[19] No consistent difference in renal or skeletal lesions is noted between patients. A difference may be noted in PTH secretion, PTH effects, or vitamin D response. Thyroparathyroidectomy resulted in eucalcemia in one hypercalcemic dog with renal failure.[27]

Renal secondary hyperparathyroidism most often becomes clinically manifested through changes in the skeleton or soft tissues. Because of the high levels of circulating PTH, bone turnover is increased, resulting in increased osteoclasia and replacement with woven bone or fibrous connective tissue (osteitis fibrosa). Animals with secondary renal hyperparathyroidism may suffer from pathological fractures, loose teeth, and soft mandibles, as do animals with primary hyperparathyroidism.

Hypoadrenocorticism

Approximately 30 to 45 per cent of dogs and 15 per cent of cats with hypoadrenocorticism are hypercalcemic.[94, 95, 114] The cause of the hypercalcemia is unknown; it may be related to elevated serum protein concentration due to dehydration. However, the hypercalcemia is greater than that explained by hyperproteinemia.[95, 114] Hypocalciuria is present in hypoadrenocorticoid patients even though hypercalcemia is present.[94] The hypocalciuria may be due to increased renal reabsorption of calcium. Although calcium is reabsorbed in the proximal tubules of the kidneys along with sodium, the increased reabsorption of calcium remains despite rehydration and an associated decrease in sodium reabsorption. Increased urinary excretion of calcium is reversed with hydrocortisone therapy.[94] Therefore, the absence of corticosteroids may allow increased resorption of calcium. Other investigators found that the hypercalcemia in a human patient with hypoadrenocorticism was due mainly to increased bone resorption. Serum levels of PTH were normal, and $1,25(OH)_2D_3$ concentration was low. Treatment with hydrocortisone resolved the hypercalcemia within 24 hours.[83] Because glucocorticoids may down-regulate osteoclast reactivity to PTH and $1,25(OH)_2D_3$, lack of corticosteroids in hypoadrenocorticism may result in a greater calcemic response from bone.[66, 117]

Hypervitaminosis D

Excessive intake of vitamin D causes hypercalcemia and hyperphosphatemia. Affected animals show clinical signs compatible with hypercalcemia and, in addition, because of the high calcium-phosphate ion product, are susceptible to dystrophic mineralization of soft tissues such as the kidneys, aorta, and bronchi. The most common causes of hypervitaminosis D in dogs and cats are excessive administration of vitamin D-containing dietary supplements, excessive vitamin D therapy for hypocalcemia, ingestion of vitamin D-containing rodenticides,[40, 80] and ingestion of ovine and bovine liver. Vitamin D in supplements is usually in the form of ergocalciferol (vitamin D_2) or cholecalciferol (vitamin D_3). Vitamin D-containing rodenticides have cholecalciferol as the active ingredient.[40] After ingestion, either form of vitamin D is hydroxylated in the liver. Although the 1-hydroxylation of 25-hydroxyvitamin D is modulated by PTH, excessive amounts of 25-hydroxyvitamin D result in increased formation of $1,25(OH)_2D_3$, resulting in hypercalcemia due to increased intestinal absorption of calcium and increased bone turnover. Although 25-hydroxyvitamin D is much less metabolically active than $1,25(OH)_2D_3$, vitamin D toxicity can result in 25-hydroxyvitamin D levels high enough to compete with $1,25(OH)_2D_3$ for vitamin D receptors on target tissue.

Both cholecalciferol and ergocalciferol are lipid soluble and accumulate in liver, muscle, and fat. Because of this accumulation of vitamin D, toxicity can be chronic (weeks) owing to the release of stored vitamin D.[1] Dihydrotachysterol, a synthetic analogue of vitamin D, is commonly used to treat hypocalcemia in small animals.[32] It requires hepatic hydroxylation to become active and is approximately 1/100 as potent as $1,25(OH)_2D_3$.[44] Toxicity involving dihydrotachysterol has short-term effects (3 to 9 days) because dihydrotachysterol is metabolized more rapidly than vitamin D.[1, 44]

Hypercalcemia and Inflammation

Hypercalcemia is an infrequent complication of blastomycosis in dogs.[21, 63] The hypercalcemia is not associated with bone destruction; indeed, few hypercalcemic patients with granulomatous disease have evidence of bone involvement.[21, 62, 65] The hypercalcemia may be due to endogenous production of $1,25(OH)_2D_3$ by macrophages in granulation tissue associated with fungal infection. A similar syndrome occurs in humans with granuloma-producing diseases such as tuberculosis, coccidioidomycosis, and sarcoidosis.[65] The production of $1,25(OH)_2D_3$ by macrophages in patients with sarcoidosis is not under normal negative-feedback regulation.[65]

Why only a minority of patients with granulomatous disease become hypercalcemic is unknown. Several hypotheses such as genetic factors, granuloma mass, or immunological factors have been proposed.[56] Hypercalcemia may occur in patients who have sarcoidosis with elevated levels of 25-hydroxyvitamin D due to high dietary vitamin D intake.[76] Increased substrate would result in high $1,25(OH)_2D_3$ concentrations.

Bacterial infection of bone may be an infrequent cause of hypercalcemia in animals.[79]

EVALUATION OF HYPERCALCEMIC PATIENTS

The differential diagnosis of hypercalcemia in small animals includes primary hyperparathyroidism, secondary renal hyperparathyroidism, hypercalcemia of malignancy, hypervitaminosis D, granulomatous disease, hypoadrenocorticism, and hyperproteinemia (Fig. 113–6).

To establish a diagnosis of hypercalcemia, elevated calcium levels must be present on more than one measurement.

A physical examination is performed initially. Peripheral lymphadenopathy or hepatosplenomegaly may be associated with lymphosarcoma or fungal disease. Careful palpation of the anal sacs may reveal an anal sac adenocarcinoma.

Serum chemistry profile may enable differentiation of other causes of hypercalcemia. Hyperalbuminemia may be the primary cause of mild hypercalcemia in dogs. The adjustment formula for albumin binding of calcium may be used to approximate the actual calcium concentration. If greater precision is needed, ionized calcium concentration can be measured with special ion-specific electrodes.

Hyperkalemia with hyponatremia may suggest hypoadrenocorticism. An adrenocorticotropic hormone stimulation test can confirm the diagnosis of hypoadrenocorticism. Hypercalcemia with hyperphosphatemia and normal renal function is compatible with vitamin D toxicity. Hyperphosphatemia and uremia may signal hypercalcemia associated with renal failure. Renal failure may be the primary cause of hypercalcemia, or renal disease may be secondary to nephrotoxic effects of hypercalcemia caused by some other primary anomaly. Differentiation of primary or secondary renal failure can be difficult. Intense diuresis may decrease hypercalcemia associated with renal failure. Levels of $1,25(OH)_2D_3$ are decreased in primary renal failure (discussed later) and are often normal or elevated with other causes of hypercalcemia.

An elevated serum globulin concentration (monoclonal gammopathy) is present in dogs with multiple myeloma. Urinalysis reveals proteinuria in approximately 35 per cent of dogs with multiple myleoma. Isosthenuria and crystalluria may be present with hypercalcemia due to any cause.

Thoracic and abdominal radiographs are also helpful in determining the cause of hypercalcemia. Cranial mediastinal radiodensity may be compatible with lymphosarcoma affecting the cranial mediastinal lymph nodes; multiple pulmonary radiodensities may represent tumor metastasis or fungal infection. Bone lysis or diffuse osteoporosis is present in 50 per cent of dogs with multiple myleoma.[78] Hepatomegaly and splenomegaly suggest lymphosarcoma. Sublumbar lymphadenopathy may signal lymphosarcoma or metastasis from adenocarcinoma of the apocrine glands of the anal sac.

The chief diagnostic dilemma is in distinguishing between hypercalcemia of malignancy due to occult, nonparathyroid neoplasia and hypercalcemia due to primary hyperparathyroidism. With either condition, affected animals may have nonremarkable findings on physical examination, normal serum chemistry results (other than hypercalcemia), and normal radiographic findings. To help rule out lymphosarcoma, a peripheral lymph node biopsy is performed even if lymphadenopathy is not present. A bone marrow aspirate helps identify intramedullary lymphosarcoma or multiple myleoma.

PTH radioimmunoassay has been validated for dogs,[107] and cats.[30] In one study, a two-site immunoradiometric PTH assay was able to differentiate between normal dogs, dogs with primary hyperparathyroidism, dogs with malignancy, and hypoparathyroid dogs.[106] Dogs with hypercalcemia associated with malignancy had low normal or below normal PTH concentrations. All dogs with histologically confirmed primary hyperparathyroidism had elevated PTH values. Experience using the same PTH assay in human patients has yielded similar results.[87]

Many PTH assays are commercially available; however, when submitting a sample to a laboratory that performs PTH assays, it is essential to select an assay that has been validated for the specific species of animal in question. Antigenic characteristics of PTH may vary between species, or substances in serum may interfere with assay results. It is also important to know which portion of the PTH polypeptide is measured by the assay. Earlier PTH assays measured the carboxy-terminal or the midportion of PTH. These assays are prone to elevate PTH values artificially in the presence of any renal dysfunction, because the carboxy and midportions of PTH are cleared by glomerular filtration. Such PTH assays are acceptable if there is little or no renal dysfunction. A PTH assay that measures the entire PTH polypeptide is less likely to be elevated by decreased glomerular filtration. The PTH assay validated for dogs measures intact PTH.*

Many other diagnostic tests, such as urinary cyclic AMP determination, serum chloride/phosphorus ratio, and fractional excretion of calcium, have been recommended to evaluate hypercalcemic patients.[59] The efficacy of these tests is questionable, and the validation of an intact PTH assay for dogs has made them unnecessary. If primary hyperparathyoidism is suspected on the basis of history, physical examination, and hematological findings, PTH assay is the next step.

SURGICAL TREATMENT OF HYPERPARATHYROIDISM

Surgical excision of neoplastic parathyroid glands is the treatment of choice for primary hyperparathyroidism. No medical treatment causes consistent regression of the neoplastic glands. Although hypercalcemia can be reduced using medical management, hypersecretion of PTH continues, leading to decreased bone mass and osteitis fibrosa.

Preoperative Treatment

Animals with primary hyperparathyroidism usually have mild symptoms and require little preoperative treatment. The hypercalcemia associated with primary hyperparathyroidism is usually not life threatening and is often associated with cardiac arrhythmias.† Because increased serum calcium levels can potentially cause cardiac conduction abnormalities, an electrocardiogram is performed. Animals with primary hyperparathyroidism should be well hydrated. Hypercalcemic damage to renal tubular cells is magnified if glomerular filtration is decreased. Isontonic (0.9 per cent) saline solution is recommended because it contains no calcium and promotes calcium excretion along with the excretion of sodium. If uremia is present, a partial response to diuresis may occur; however, renal response is greater with reduction of serum calcium concentration. The risk of soft-tissue mineralization is minimal in animals with primary hyperparathyroidism, because although the serum calcium concentration is elevated, serum phosphorus concentration is usually low. The risk of soft-tissue calcification is greatest when the product of the serum calcium concentration (in milligrams per 100 ml) multiplied by the phosphorus concentration (in milligrams per 100 ml) is greater than 60.[17]

Patients in a hypercalcemic crisis with severe weakness, vomiting, depression, dehydration, and uremia require emergency management consisting of rapid rehydration with isotonic saline solution. Once the animal is hydrated, furosemide may be administered in high doses (5 mg/kg initially, then 5 mg/kg/hour until the calcium level is lowered) to enhance calciuresis.[17] It is important to maintain hydration during diuretic therapy, or calcium reabsorption in the proximal tubules occurs along with sodium reabsorption. If saline and furosemide diuresis are unsuccessful in lowering calcium concentrations, corticosteroid administration (prednisone, 2 mg/kg) may reduce serum calcium concentration.[26] Early corticosteroid therapy may interfere with diagnosis if the cause of the hypercalcemia is lymphosarcoma. Calcitonin is effective for rapidly reducing serum calcium concentrations. Dosages for dogs and cats have not been established but may be extrapolated from the human dosage of salmon calcitonin (4 to 8 units/kg SC or IM BID to QID).[45] The effects of calcitonin are transient; serum calcium level returns to pretreatment levels within 48 hours after twice-daily treatment in humans. The hypocalcemic effects may be prolonged for as long as 4 days by combining calcitonin treatment with corticosteroid administration.[2] Isolated reports have described the efficacy of calcitonin for treatment of hypercalcemia in dogs and cats, but a study involving a large number of animals has not been published.

Cimetidine, an H_2-receptor blocker, lowers serum calcium and PTH levels in humans with hyperparathyroidism associated with parathyroid neoplasia.[102] Effective dosages were 300 mg PO TID. If the cimetidine was discontinued, hyperparathyroidism recurred. The efficacy of cimetidine treatment for hypercalcemia is controversial; however, several investigators found no response to cimetidine treatment of hyperparathyroidism.[70, 73, 88, 103] The mechanism of action is unknown; cimetidine may inhibit release of PTH or production of PTH precursors. Histamine receptors are present on the surface of parathyroid adenoma cells.[55] Cimetidine treatment of parathyroid adenomas or parathyroid hyperplasia causes consistent enlargement of the affected glands, producing central edema and cytoplasmic enlargement of parathyroid cells.[103] Cimetidine does not lower PTH concentration in patients with secondary hyperparathyroidism or with hypercalcemia of malignancy.[99, 102] It does not decrease PTH concentrations below normal values in humans with primary hyperparathyroidism. Cimetidine given for 8 days before parathyroidectomy reduces postoperative hypocalcemia in human patients.[101] By reducing circulating levels of PTH, cimetidine administration may prevent suppression of the normal parathyroid glands by elevated levels of PTH.

Bisphosphonates, also called *diphosphonates*, are chemical analogues of pyrophosphate that can have profound hypocalcemic effects by inhibiting bone resorption.[33] The chemical structure of bisphosphonates enables a strong binding to hydroxyapatite crystals, preventing both crystal dissolution and formation. Bisphosphonates decrease osteoclast activity after administration for several days.[2]

Bisphosphonates have been used to treat hypercalcemia in humans, and one report described bisphosphonate use for treatment of hypercalcemia in a dog.[42, 69, 105, 108] Bisphosphonates are most effective for treatment of hypercalcemia of malignancy consisting of increased bone turnover.[108] Less efficacy has been observed with

*The validated canine PTH assay is currently available at the endocrinology laboratory, Michigan State University School of Veterinary Medicine.

†See references 4, 15, 25, 38, 48, 53, 57, 64, 91, 105, and 115.

bisphosphonate treatment of hypercalcemia associated with primary hyperparathyoidism[?], because the increased renal reabsorption of calcium is unopposed.[42]

Preoperative Localization of Parathyroid Tumors

It is desirable to identify parathyroid neoplasms preoperatively, not only for planning the surgical approach but also to confirm the diagnosis. Ultrasonography is ineffective in identifying parathyroid tumors in dogs.[4] Computed tomography scanning, magnetic resonance imaging, and dual-isotope thallium-201 chloride-technetium-99m subtraction scanning have been used for identifying parathyroid glands in humans.[22] Carbon-14–labeled amino acids have been used to image the parathyroid glands in rats.[119] Although these techniques may be used in several veterinary centers, cost limits their application for identification of parathyroid tissue in dogs and cats.

Surgical localization of parathyroid tissue may be enhanced with methylene blue.[5, 29, 113] Methylene blue is selectively taken up by the parathyroid glands by an unknown mechanism. Methylene blue is mixed in an appropriate amount of physiological saline solution (250 to 500 ml) to allow administration of 3 mg/kg of methylene blue in a 1-hour period. Maximum-intensity staining occurs in approximately 30 minutes, when the parathyroid glands become slate blue. Adenomatous or hyperplastic glands become more deeply stained than normal or hypoplastic glands.[29] Methylene blue can cause fatal Heinz body anemia in cats. Dogs develop Heinz body anemia from methylene blue at 5 mg/kg but are less likely to suffer from such complications at 3 mg/kg. Heinz body anemia has been reported to occur in dogs given methylene blue at a dose of 3 mg/kg (one fatality), so methylene blue infusion for identification of parathyroid tissue is not without risk.[28, 80]

Parathyroidectomy

Surgical excision of adenomatous or hyperplastic parathyroid glands is the treatment of choice for primary hyperparathyroidism in dogs and cats. The parathyroid glands are exposed through a ventral midline cervical approach using the same technique used to expose the thyroid glands. The external parathyroid glands are usually attached to the capsule near the cranial pole of the thyroid gland. With adenomatous or hyperplastic enlargement, the affected parathyroid gland becomes firm, large (0.5 to 1 cm in length), and nodular (Fig. 113–7). Adenomatous internal parathyroid glands undergo similar changes and are palpable and usually visible through the ventral or dorsal aspect of the thyroid parenchyma. All parathyroid neoplasms reported have involved only one parathyroid gland.* The unaffected glands are of normal size or slightly smaller owing to suppression from elevated PTH concentrations.

Adenomatous external parathyroid glands may be excised by dissection between the parathyroid gland and the thyroid capsule. If there is any question about the completeness of excision or if the internal parathyroid gland is to be excised, partial or unilateral thyroidectomy is indicated. Partial thyroidectomy is performed by transecting the thyroid gland so that the abnormal parathyroid gland is removed along with the surrounding thyroid parenchyma. Hemorrhage from the remaining thyroid parenchyma is controlled by placing several fine mattress sutures along the cut edge. The remaining thyroid parenchyma contains the other ipsilateral parathyroid gland. Although dogs and cats can function normally with only one parathyroid gland, leaving as much parathyroid tissue as possible after parathyroidectomy may help reduce transient postoperative hypoparathyroidism. If a partial thyroidectomy is performed, it is important to preserve the blood supply to the remaining portion of the thyroid gland. The caudal thyroid artery is often absent in cats.

If none of the parathyroid glands are enlarged, there are two possible explanations. The animal may have some other cause of hyperparathyroidism or a neoplasm involving ectopic parathyroid tissue. The surgeon should evaluate both the ventral and the dorsal aspects of the thyroid glands then explore the entire cervical area, particularly along the peritracheal fascia. If no abnormalities are found in the cervical region, then any questionable portions of the evaluation, especially ruling out hypercalcemia due to malignancy, are repeated. If the animal has been carefully evaluated and has elevated concentrations of intact PTH on an assay validated for the species, it is most likely that a neoplasm is involving ectopic parathryoid[?] tissue. If no abnormalities are found in the cervical region, the cranial mediastinum is explored by either splitting the sternum or performing a fourth intercostal space thoracotomy.

If all four parathyroid glands are enlarged, the most likely diagnosis is parathyroid hyperplasia. This condition has been reported as a congenital condition in German shepherd puppies,[105] but without reports of spontaneous hyperplasia in adult dogs or cats. Dogs with renal failure may rarely have secondary parathyroid

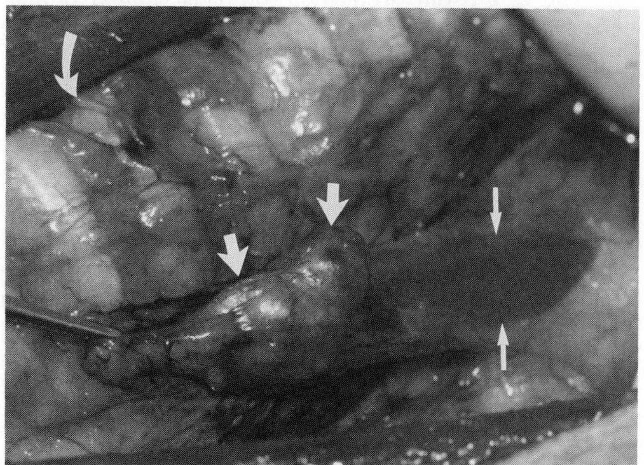

FIGURE 113–7. Parathyroid adenoma *(large arrows)* on the cranial pole of the thyroid gland *(small arrows)* in a dog. The curved arrow points to the trachea.

*See references 4, 15, 25, 38, 47, 48, 53, 64, 91, 105, and 115.

hyperplasia. This condition may be confused with primary hyperparathyroidism only if a patient with parathyroid neoplasia has concurrent renal failure due to either hypercalcemic nephropathy or some other renal disease. If all four parathyroid glands are enlarged, then one to three parathyroid glands may be excised. This reduction in parathyroid mass may reduce the hypercalcemia.

Postoperative Treatment

The most common complication after surgical removal of a parathyroid tumor is postoperative hypocalcemia. In one study, 58 per cent of dogs undergoing excision of a solitary parathyroid tumor developed hypocalcemia.[4] Most of the dogs became hypocalcemic within 1 to 5 days of surgery, and 81 per cent of the dogs becoming hypocalcemic showed signs of tetany.

The major cause of postoperative hypocalcemia is suppression of the remaining parathyroid glands due to negative feedback from chronically elevated PTH concentrations. The suppressed glands require 2 to 3 weeks to begin secreting PTH. Another possible cause of postoperative hypocalcemia is the "hungry bone syndrome," which consists of both hypocalcemia and hypophosphatemia caused by extensive remineralization of a skeleton that was demineralized by hyperparathyroidism.[6] The skeletal demineralization may be present without radiographic changes. Human patients with the hungry bone syndrome have a protracted course of hypocalcemia and require intensive therapy to prevent tetany.[6]

Postoperative hypocalcemia is treated with a combination of vitamin D and calcium supplementation. Severe hypocalcemia is treated with intravenous administration of 15 mg/kg of 10 per cent calcium gluconate (100 mg/ml). The infusion is discontinued if bradycardia is produced. Animals can be maintained on intravenous calcium gluconate by administering 5 mg/kg/hour mixed in maintenance fluids. Calcium gluconate may also be administered subcutaneously if diluted by mixing 1:1 with 0.9 per cent sodium chloride solution.[80]

The vitamin D supplement most commonly used in dogs and cats is dihydrotachysterol. This vitamin D analogue has a more rapid onset of action (3 to 5 days) than vitamin D_3 and does not accumulate in fat. The recommended dose of dihydrotachysterol is 0.02 mg/kg/day given in three divided doses. Starting dihydrotachysterol and oral calcium therapy immediately after surgery may reduce the incidence of postoperative hypocalcemia.[4] The dose is gradually tapered during a 4- to 8-week period, while serum calcium concentration is monitored. Dihydrotachysterol administration can usually be discontinued after 4 weeks. Oral calcium supplementation is given at a dosage of 25 mg/kg/day of elemental calcium. Calcium preparations vary in the concentration of elemental calcium provided per milligram. The oral calcium supplement is decreased during a 4- to 8-week period, depending on the serum calcium concentration. Preoperative treatment with cimetidine reduced the incidence of postoperative hypocalcemia in humans with parathyroid neoplasia.[101] Efficacy in animals is unknown.

Prognosis

The majority of parathyroid tumors are benign and are cured by complete excision. One report described recurrence of a mediastinal parathyroid adenocarcinoma after excision.[90] Most bony lesions caused by chronic hyperparathyroidism resolve after parathyroidectomy. Mild renal disease caused by hypercalcemia often improves after parathyroidectomy.[68]

The cause of parathyroid neoplasia is unknown, and therefore it is unknown if the inciting cause remains after excision of the parathyroid neoplasm. Persistent elevations of PTH were present in 37 per cent of normocalcemic humans after excision of parathyroid adenomas.[49] It is unknown if PTH concentrations remain elevated after excision of parathyroid tumors in dogs or cats. No recurrence of parathyroid neoplasia was noted in dogs monitored for 3 years.[4]

References

1. Adams JS: Vitamin D metabolite-mediated hypercalcemia. *Endocrinol Metab Clin North Am 18*:765, 1989.
2. Attie MF: Treatment of hypercalcemia. *Endocrinol Metab Clin North Am 18*:807, 1989.
3. Aurbach GD, et al: Parathyroid hormone, calcitonin, and the calciferols. *In* Wilson JD, Foster DF (eds): *Williams Textbook of Endocrinology*. 7th ed. W.B. Saunders, Philadelphia, 1985, pp 1137–1217.
4. Berger B, Feldman EC: Primary hyperparathyroidism in dogs: 21 cases (1976–1986). *J Am Vet Med Assoc 191*:350, 1987.
5. Bland KI, et al: Intraoperative localization of parathyroid glands using methylothionine chloride tetremethylthionine chloride in secondary hyperparathyroidism. *Surg Gynec Obstet 160*:42, 1985.
6. Brasier AR, Nussbaum SR: Hungry bone syndrome: Clinical and biochemical predictors of its occurrence after parathyroid surgery. *Am J Vet Med Assoc 84*:654, 1988.
7. Broadus AE, et al: Humoral hypercalcemia of cancer: Identification of a novel parathyroid hormone-like peptide. *N Engl J Med 319*:556, 1988.
8. Bronner F: Intestinal calcium absorption: Mechanisms and applications. *J Nutr 117*:1347, 1987.
9. Bronner F: Calcium absorption. *In* Johnson LR (ed): *Physiology of the Gastrointestinal Tract*. 2nd ed. Raven Press, New York, 1987, pp 1419–1435.
10. Burk RL, Barton CL: Renal failure and hyperparathyroidism in an Alaskan malamute pup. *J Am Vet Med Assoc 172*:69, 1978.
11. Burtis WJ, et al: Humoral hypercalcemia of malignancy. *Ann Intern Med 108*:454, 1988.
12. Capen CC, Martin SL: Calcium-regulating hormones and diseases of the parathyroid glands. *In* Ettinger SJ (ed): *Textbook of Veterinary Internal Medicine*. 2nd ed. W.B. Saunders, Philadelphia, 1983, pp 1550–1591.
13. Capen DD, Weisbrode SE: Hormonal control of mineral metabolism and bone cell activity. *In* Sumner-Smith G (ed): *Bone in Clinical Orthopedics*. W.B. Saunders, Philadelphia, 1982, pp 197–252.
14. Carpenter JL, et al: Tumors and tumor-like lesions. *In* Holzworth J (ed): *Diseases of the Cat: Medicine and Surgery*. Vol 1. W.B. Saunders, Philadelphia, 1987, pp 406–596.
15. Carrillo JM, et al: Primary hyperparathyroidism in a dog. *J Am Vet Med Assoc 174*:67, 1979.
16. Charon SA, et al: Effects of parathyroid hormone on remodeling of iliac trabecular bone packets in patients with primary hyperparathyroidism. *Clin Orthop Rel Res 162*:255, 1982.
17. Chew DJ, Meuten DJ: Disorders of calcium and phosphorus metabolism. *Vet Clin North Am 12*:411, 1982.
18. Chew DJ, et al: Pseudohyperparathyroidism in a cat. *J Am Anim Hosp Vet Med Assoc 11*:46, 1975.
19. Coburn JW, Slatopolsky E: Vitamin D, parathyroid hormone and renal osteodystrophy. *In* Brenner BM, Rector FC (eds): *The Kidney*. 3rd ed. W.B. Saunders, Philadelphia, 1986, pp 1657–1730.
20. Cohn DV, et al: Biosynthesis of proparathyroid hormone and parathyroid hormone. *Am J Med 56*:767, 1974.
21. Dow SW, et al: Hypercalcemia associated with blastomyocosis in dogs. *J Am Vet Med Assoc 188*:706, 1986.
22. Eisenberg H, et al: Parathyroid localization, three-dimensional modeling, and percutaneous ablation techniques. *Endocrinol Metab Clin North Am 18*:659, 1989.

23. Engleman RW, et al: Hypercalcemia in cats with feline-leukemia-virus-associated leukemia-lymphoma. *Cancer 56*:777, 1985.
24. Feinfeld DA, Sherwood LM: Parathyroid hormone and $1,25(OH)_2D_3$ in chronic renal failure. *Kidney Int 33*:1049, 1988.
25. Feldman EC, Krutzik S: Case reports of parathyroid levels in spontaneous canine parathyroid disorders. *J Am Anim Hosp Vet Med Assoc 17*:393, 1981.
26. Feldman EC, Nelson RW (eds): The parathyroid gland–primary hyperparathyroidism. *In* Feldman EC, Nelson RW (eds): *Canine and Feline Endocrinology and Reproduction*. W.B. Saunders, Philadelphia, 1987, pp 328–356.
27. Finco DR, Rowland GN: Hypercalcemia secondary to chronic renal failure in the dog: A report of four cases. *J Am Vet Med Assoc 173*:990, 1978.
28. Fingeroth JM, Smeak DD: Intravenous methylene blue infusion for intraoperative identification of pancreatic islet-cell tumors in dogs. Part II: Clinical trials and results in four dogs. *J Am Anim Hosp Vet Med Assoc 24*:175, 1988.
29. Fingeroth JM, et al: Intravenous methylene blue infusion for intraoperative identification of parathyroid gland and pancreatic islet-cell tumors in dogs. Part I: Experimental determination of dose-related staining efficacy and toxicity. *J Am Anim Hosp Vet Med Assoc 24*:165, 1988.
30. Flanders JA, Reimers TJ: Radioimmunoassay for parathyroid hormone in the cat. *Am J Vet Res 52*:422, 1991.
31. Flanders JA, et al: Adjustment of total serum calcium concentration for binding to albumin and protein in cats: 291 cases (1986–1987). *J Am Vet Med Assoc 194*:1609, 1989.
32. Flanders JA, et al: Feline thyroidectomy: A comparison of postoperative hypocalcemia associated with three different surgical techniques. *Vet Surg 16*:362, 1987.
33. Fleisch H: Bisphosphonates—History and experimental basis. *Bone 8* (Suppl 1):S23, 1987.
34. Forte LR: Regulation of parathyroid hormone receptors. *In* Cooper CW (ed): *Current Research on Calcium-Regulating Hormones*. University of Texas Press, Austin, 1987, pp 41–57.
35. Freitag J, et al: Impaired parathyroid hormone metabolism in patients with chronic renal failure. *N Eng J Med 298*:29, 1978.
36. Ghijsen WE, et al: Regulation of duodenal Ca^{2+} pump by calmodulin and vitamin D-dependent Ca^{2+}-binding protein. *J Physiol 14*:G223, 1986.
37. Godwin MC: The development of the parathyroids in the dog with emphasis upon the origin of accessory glands. *Anat Rec 68*:305, 1937.
38. Goulden BE, MacKenzie CP: Suspected primary hyperparathyroidism in the dog. *N Z Vet J 16*:131, 1968.
39. Grain E: Hypercalcemia associated with squamous cell carcinoma in a dog. *J Am Vet Med Assoc 181*:165, 1982.
40. Gunther R, et al: Toxicity of a vitamin D_3 rodenticide to dogs. *J Am Vet Med Assoc 193*:211, 1988.
41. Habener JF, et al: Parathyroid hormone: Biochemical aspects of biosynthesis, secretion, action, and metabolism. *Physiol Rev 64*:985, 1984.
42. Hamdy NA, et al: Clidronate in the medical management of hyperparathyroidism. *Bone 8* (Suppl 1):S69, 1987.
43. Haussler MR, Brickman AS: Vitamin D: Metabolism, actions, and disease states. *In* Bronner F, Coburn JW (eds): *Disorders of Mineral Metabolism*. Vol II. Academic Press, New York, 1982, pp 360–432.
44. Haussler MR, Cordy PE: Metabolites and analogues of vitamin D: Which for what? *JAMA 247*:841, 1982.
45. Haynes RC, Murad R: Agents affecting calcification: Calcium, parathyroid hormone, calcitonin, vitamin D, and other compounds. *In* Gilman AG, et al (eds): *Goodman and Gilman's The Pharmacological Basis of Therapeutics*. 7th ed. Macmillan, New York, 1985, pp 1517–1543.
46. Huffer WE: Morphology and biochemistry of bone remodeling: Possible control by vitamin D, parathyroid hormone, and other substances. *Lab Invest 59*:418, 1988.
47. Hullinger RL: The endocrine system. *In* Miller ME: *Anatomy of the Dog*. 2nd ed. W.B. Saunders, Philadelphia, 1979.
48. Ihle SL, et al: Seizures as a manifestation of primary hyperparathyroidism in a dog. *J Am Vet Med Assoc 192*:71, 1988.
49. Irvin GL, et al: Parathyroid metabolism after operative treatment of hypercalcemic (primary) hyperparathyroidism. *Surgery 102*:898, 1987.
50. Jacobson H, Knochel JP: Renal handling of phosphorus, clinical hypophosphatemia, and phosphorus deficiency. *In* Brenner BM, Rector FC (eds): *The Kidney*. 3rd ed. W.B. Saunders, Philadelphia, 1986, pp 619–662.
51. Kanis JA: Vitamin D metabolism and its clinical application. *J Bone Joint Surg [Br] 64*:542, 1982.
52. Klausner JS, et al: Hypercalcemia in two cats with squamous cell carcinomas. *J Am Vet Med Assoc 196*:103, 1990.
53. Klausner JS, et al: Calcium urolithiasis in two dogs with parathyroid adenomas. *J Am Vet Med Assoc 191*:1423, 1987.
54. Klee GG, et al: Hypercalcemia. *Endocrinol Metab Clin North Am 17*:573, 1988.
55. Klein I, et al: Human parathyroid adenoma adenylate cyclase: Stimulation by histamine that is blocked by cimetidine. *Metabolism 30*:635, 1981.
56. Kozeny GA, et al: Hypercalcemia associated with silicone-induced granulomas. *N Engl J Med 311*:1103, 1984.
57. Krook L: Spontaneous hyperparathyroidism in the dog: A pathological-anatomical study. *Acta Pathol Microbiol Scand 41* (Suppl 122):27, 1957.
58. Krook L, Lowe JE: Nutritional secondary hyperparathyroidism in the horse. *Pathol Vet 6* (Suppl 1):1, 1964.
59. Kruger JM, et al: Treatment of hypercalcemia. *In* Kirk RW (ed): *Current Veterinary Therapy 9*. W.B. Saunders, Philadelphia, 1986, pp 94–100.
60. Kumar R: The metabolism and mechanism of action of 1,25-dihydroxyvitamin D_3. *Kidney Int 30*:793, 1986.
61. Kurokawa K: Calcium-regulating hormones and the kidney. *Kidney Int 32*:760, 1987.
62. Lee JC, et al: Hypercalcemia in disseminated coccidioidomycosis. *N Engl J Med 297*:431, 1977.
63. Legendre AM: Canine blastomyocosis: A review of 47 clinical cases. *J Am Vet Med Assoc 178*:1163, 1981.
64. Legendre AM, et al: Primary hyperparathyroidism in a dog. *J Am Vet Med Assoc 168*:694, 1976.
65. Lehman J, Gray RW: Calcitriol, calcium, and granulomatous disease. *N Engl J Med 311*:1115, 1984.
66. Levine MM, Kleeman CR: Hypercalcemia: Pathophysiology and treatment. *Hosp Pract 22*:93, 1987.
67. Lian JB, Gundberg CM: Osteocalcin: Biochemical considerations and clinical applications. *Clin Orthop Rel Res 226*:267, 1988.
68. Lins L: Reversible renal failure caused by hypercalcemis. *Acta Med Scand 203*:309, 1978.
69. Ljunbhall S, et al: Comparative effects of calcitonin and clodronate in hypercalcaemia. *Bone 8* (Suppl 1):S79, 1987.
70. Ljunghall S, et al: Cimetidine in primary hyperparathyroidism. *Lancet 2*:480, 1980.
71. MacEwen EG, Siegel SD: Hypercalcemia: A paraneoplastic disease. *Vet Clin North Am 7*:187, 1977.
72. Major RH: Studies on the vascular system of the thyroid gland. *Am J Anat 9*:475, 1909.
73. Mallett RB, et al: Failure of cimetidine to suppress immunoreactive parathyroid hormone and hypercalcaemia in primary hyperparathyroidism. *Postgrad Med J 57*:242, 1981.
74. Malluche HH, et al: Parathyroid hormone and 1,25 vitamin D_3 exert opposite effects on bone. *Adv Exp Med Biol 208*:289, 1985.
75. Martin KJ, et al: The peripheral metabolism of parathyroid hormone. *N Engl J Med 301*:1092, 1979.
76. Mason S, et al: Vitamin D conversion by sarcoid lymph node homogenate. *Ann Intern Med 100*:59, 1984.
77. Massry SG: Renal handling of calcium. *In* Bronner F, Coburn JW (eds): *Disorders of Mineral Metabolism*. Vol II. Academic Press, New York, 1982, pp 189–236.
78. Matus RE, et al: Prognostic factors for multiple myeloma in the dog. *J Am Vet Med Assoc 188*:1288, 1986.
79. Meuten DJ: Hypercalcemia. *Vet Clin North Am 14*:891, 1984.
80. Meuten DJ, Armstrong PJ: Parathyroid disease and calcium metabolism. *In* Ettinger SJ: *Textbook of Veterinary Internal Medicine*. 3rd ed. W.B. Saunders, Philadelphia, 1989, pp 1610–1631.
81. Meuten DJ, et al: Hypercalcemia in dogs with lymphosarcoma: Biochemical, ultrastructural, and histomorphometric investigations. *Lab Invest 49*:553, 1983.
82. Meuten DJ, et al: Relationship of serum total calcium to albumin and total protein in dogs. *J Am Vet Med Assoc 180*:63, 1982.
83. Muls E, et al: Etiology of hypercalcemia in a patient with Addison's disease. *Calcif Tissue Int 34*:523, 1982.
84. Mundy GR: Hypercalcemic factors other than parathyroid hormone-related protein. *Endocrinol Metab Clin North Am 18*:795, 1989.
85. Nicholas JS, Swingle WW: An experimental and morphological study of the parathyroid glands of the cat. *Am J Anat 34*:469, 1925.
86. Noden DM, de Lahunta A: The pharynx and pharyngeal pouches. *In* Noden DM, de Lahunta A: *The Embryology of Domestic Animals*. Williams & Wilkins, Baltimore, 1985, pp 270–278.
87. Nussbaum SR, et al: Highly sensitive two-site immunoradiometric assay of parathyrin, and its clinical utility in evaluating patients with hypercalcemia. *Clin Chem 33*:1364, 1987.
88. Palmer FJ, et al: Cimetidine and hyperparathyroidism. *N Engl J Med 302*:692, 1980.
89. Parfitt AM: Bone and plasma calcium homeostasis. *Bone 8* (Suppl 1):S1, 1987.
90. Patnaik AK, et al: Mediastinal parathyroid adenocarcinoma in a dog. *Vet Pathol 15*:55, 1978.
91. Pearson PT, et al: Primary hyperparathyroidism in a beagle. *J Am Vet Med Assoc 147*:1201, 1965.
92. Perry HM, et al: Conditioned medium from osteoblast-like cells mediate parathyroid hormone induced bone resorption. *Calcif Tissue Int 40*:298, 1987.
93. Peterson DR, et al: Calcium homeostasis: The effect of parathyroid hormone on bone membrane electrical potential difference. *Calcif Tissue Int 37*:307, 1985.
94. Peterson ME, Feinman JM: Hypercalcemia associated with hypoadrenocorticism in sixteen dogs. *J Am Vet Med Assoc 181*:802, 1982.
95. Peterson ME, Randolph JF: Endocrine diseases. *In* Sherding RG (ed): *The Cat: Diseases and Clinical Management*. Churchill-Livingstone, New York, 1989, pp 1095–1161.
96. Ralston S, et al: Hypercalcemia and metastatic bone disease: Is there a causal link? *Lancet 2*:903, 1982.

97. Reed CI, et al: Observations on parathyroidectomized dogs, with particular attention to the regional incidence of tetany, and to the blood mineral changes in this condition. *Am J Physiol 84*:176, 1928.
98. Reeve J, Zanelli JM: Parathyroid hormone and bone. *Clin Sci 71*:231, 1986.
99. Robinson MF, et al: Cimetidine treatment of azotemic secondary hyperparathyroidism. *J Clin Endocrinol Metab 54*:1206, 1982.
100. Shaw JH, et al: Glucose, fat, and protein kinetics in patients with primary and secondary hyperparathyroidism. *Surgery 103*:526, 1988.
101. Sherwood JK, et al: The preoperative use of cimetidine as a means of preventing symptomatic hypocalcemia following a parathyroid operation. *Surg Gynecol Obstet 157*:557, 1983.
102. Sherwood JK, et al: Effect of cimetidine on circulating parathyroid hormone in primary hyperparathyroidism. *Lancet 1*:616, 1980.
103. Sotsiou FC, et al: The effect of cimetidine on parathyroid function and histopathology in primary hyperparathyroidism. *J Pathol 151*:271, 1987.
104. Sutton RA, Dirks JH: Calcium and magnesium: Renal handling and disorders of metabolism. *In* Brenner BM, Rector FC (eds): *The Kidney*. 3rd ed. W.B. Saunders, Philadelphia, 1986, pp 551–618.
105. Thompson LG, et al: Primary hyperparathyroidism in German shepherd dogs: A disorder of probable genetic origin. *Vet Pathol 21*:370, 1984.
106. Torrance AG, Nachreiner R: Intact parathyroid hormone assay and total calcium concentration in the diagnosis of disorders of calcium metabolism in dogs. *J Vet Intern Med 3*:86, 1989.
107. Torrance AG, Nachreiner R: Human-parathormone assay for use in dogs: Validation, sample handling studies, and parathyroid function testing. *Am J Vet Res 50*:1123, 1989.
108. Urwin GH, et al: Treatment of the hypercalcaemia of malignancy with intravenous clodronate. *Bone 8* (Suppl 1):S43, 1987.
109. van der Plas A, Nijweide PJ: Cell-cell interactions in the osteogenic compartment of bone. *Bone 9*:107, 1988.
110. Wasserman RH, et al: Evidence for multiple effects of vitamin D_3 on calcium absorption: Response of rachitic chicks, with or without partial vitamin D_3 repletion, to 1,25-dihydroxyvitamin D_3. *Proc Natl Acad Sci 79*:7939, 1982.
111. Weir EC, et al: Humoral hypercalcemia of malignancy in canine lymphosarcoma. *Endocrinology 122*:602, 1988.
112. Weller RE: Cancer-associated hypercalcemia in companion animals. *Comp Cont Educ 6*:639, 1984.
113. Wheeler MH, Wade JS: Intraoperative identification of parathyroid glands: Appraisal of methylene blue staining. *Am J Surg 143*:713, 1982.
114. Willard MD, et al: Canine hypoadrenocorticism: Report of 37 cases and review of 39 previously reported cases. *J Am Vet Med Assoc 180*:59, 1982.
115. Wilson JW, et al: Primary hyperparathyroidism in a dog. *J Am Vet Med Assoc 164*:942, 1974.
116. Wilson RB, Bronstad DC: Hypercalcemia associated with nasal adenocarcinoma in a dog. *J Am Vet Med Assoc 182*:1246, 1983.
117. Wong GL: Basal activities and hormone responsiveness of osteoclast-like and osteoblast-like bone cells are regulated by glucocorticoids. *J Biol Chem 254*:6337, 1079.
118. Wootton PR, Pearson GR: Hypercalcaemia and malignancy in dogs. *Vet Ann 28*:233, 1988.
119. Wortman JA, et al: Quantitative autoradiography of parathyroid glands in rats with carbon-14-labeled amino acids. *J Nuc Med 28*:1447, 1987.
120. Zenoble RD, Rowland GN: Hypercalcemia and proliferative, myelosclerotic bone reaction associated with feline leukovirus infection in a cat. *J Am Vet Med Assoc 175*:591, 1979.
121. Zull JE, et al: Interaction of parathyroid hormone with its receptors. *In* Cooper CW (ed): *Current research on calcium-regulating hormones*. University of Texas Press, Austin, 1987, pp 31–40.

CHAPTER 114 Surgical Diseases of the Endocrine Pancreas

Roger B. Fingland

Surgical diseases of the endocrine pancreas are uncommon in animals and generally are limited to diseases of the islet cells. A common feature exists between cells of the endocrine system, including pancreatic islet cells, and cells of the autonomic nervous system. These cells arise from neuroectodermal cells of the neural crest and contain membrane-bound secretion vesicles that secrete polypeptide hormones. Cells of the endocrine system and autonomic nervous system are referred to as *APUD* cells because a major cytochemical characteristic of these cells is the capability of *a*mine *p*recursor *u*ptake and *d*ecarboxylation.[5, 29, 37] Tumors arising from APUD cells are called *apudomas*. Apudomas produce clinical signs by secreting excessive quantities of naturally occurring hormones. Because of the relatively simple and interchangeable polypeptide structure of these hormones, apudomas may secrete hormones that are not normally produced in the cell of origin but are secreted by other APUD cells.[5]

Pancreatic beta-cell carcinoma (insulinoma) is the most commonly observed apudoma in veterinary medicine. Other apudomas are exceedingly rare, although non–beta-cell carcinoma (gastrinoma) has been reported in dogs and cats.

PANCREATIC BETA-CELL CARCINOMA

Pancreatic beta-cell carcinomas also are referred to as *insulinomas* and islet cell adenocarcinomas. The term *insulinoma*, although not always correct, is most commonly used and is used here.

Insulinomas are most commonly observed in middle-aged to older dogs. A breed predisposition exists for boxers, German shepherds, standard poodles, Irish setters, and collies.[25, 29, 36] A sex predilection has not been reported. Insulinomas rarely have been reported in cats but are common endocrine tumors in ferrets.[8, 16, 19, 20, 25]

Pathology and Pathophysiology

Insulin-secreting tumors result in hyperinsulinemia and hypoglycemia. Insulin promotes hypoglycemia by decreasing the rate of glucose release from the liver and increasing the uptake of glucose by insulin-sensitive tissues. Neurological signs predominate in hypoglycemic animals because glucose is the primary energy source used by the central nervous system (CNS).[1] Cells of the CNS depend on a constant supply of glucose, and nervous system dysfunction occurs if the blood glucose concentration falls below a critical level. Neuronal glucose use is unaffected by blood insulin concentration, because glucose entrance into neurons of the CNS occurs primarily by diffusion.[8, 25] Other major organ systems, including the heart, kidneys,[5] and liver, also are glucose dependent. Hypoglycemia generally results in clinical signs involving the CNS before signs of other major organ system malfunction become apparent.[8]

Hypoglycemia is a potent stimulus for the release of catecholamines, glucocorticoids, and glucagon, which compensate for hypoglycemia by promoting hepatic glycogenolysis.[13, 28] Thus, clinical signs of hypoglycemia result from both neuroglycopenia (lethargy, weakness, ataxia, bizarre behavior) and stimulation of the sympathoadrenal system (muscle tremors, nervousness, restlessness, hunger).

Clinical signs are related to the rate of development of hypoglycemia rather than the degree of hypoglycemia.[36] Animals with chronic hypoglycemia often tolerate low blood glucose levels (20 to 30 mg/100 ml) and remain asymptomatic, whereas acute moderate hypoglycemia may result in clinical signs.[8, 25] The mechanism allowing animals with chronic low blood glucose levels to remain asymptomatic is not well understood.

Insulinomas are malignant, slow-growing tumors in animals. Early metastasis to the liver, regional lymph nodes, and spleen is common, and the recurrence rate approaches 100 per cent. The pancreatic tumor typically is singular and quite small. Histologically, most insulinomas have an orderly arrangement of cells with few mitotic figures, making microscopic differentiation of malignancy unreliable.[27, 28] The distinction between benign and malignant is based on microscopic evidence of lymphatic and vascular invasion of the primary tumor, the presence of metastases at surgery, and the clinical course of the disease.[2, 27, 28]

Demonstration of hypoglycemia in an animal with episodic weakness does not confirm a diagnosis of insulinoma. Numerous disorders such as hypoadrenocorticism, hepatic lipidosis, hepatic glycogen storage diseases, hepatic cirrhosis, inanition, cachexia, portosystemic shunt, pregnancy toxemia, and hunting dog hypoglycemia may result in hypoglycemia and signs of neuroglycopenia.[25, 28, 29] Hypoglycemia caused by a non–beta-cell, non–insulin-secreting tumor such as lymphosarcoma, hepatoma, hepatocellular carcinoma, and multiple myeloma has been reported and is referred to as *tumor hypoglycemia*.[27, 28]

Diagnosis

A tentative diagnosis of insulinoma is based on demonstration of the Whipple triad: (1) neurological signs associated with hypoglycemia, (2) fasting blood glucose concentration of 40 mg/100 ml or less at the time the animal is symptomatic, and (3) relief of neurological symptoms by feeding or parenteral administration of glucose (Fig. 114–1). The Whipple triad is characteristic of hypoglycemia regardless of etiology and is not specific for insulinoma.[8, 14, 28, 29]

History

Most dogs with insulinomas are symptomatic for several weeks to months before presentation. Astute owners may notice early subtle signs such as nervousness, drowsiness, excitement, hunger, or trembling. Characteristic clinical signs are slowly progressive and episodic and include weakness, depression, disorientation, incoordination, bizarre behavior, seizures or seizure-like activity, and collapse. Clinical signs may be triggered by excitement, stress, exercise, fasting, or eating.[25, 36] Paradoxical postprandial hypoglycemia occurs because insulin release resulting from postprandial hypoglycemia is exaggerated in the presence of an insulin-secreting tumor.[14] Interestingly, clinical signs often are not associated with fasting. Owners typically describe self-limiting generalized seizure activity that lasts between 30 seconds and 5 minutes.[4, 8] Dogs usually are normal between seizures.

Clinical Findings

Physical examination findings generally are nonspecific and subtle. Visual or palpable abnormalities seldom are identified. Dogs with insulinomas frequently are weak and emaciated but occasionally are obese as a result of the anabolic effects of insulin.[8, 14, 17, 25] Weakness, ataxia, seizures, or syncope may be present if the animal is experiencing a hypoglycemic crisis at the time of presentation. Peripheral neuropathy has been reported in dogs with insulinoma.[1, 4, 31] The pathogenesis is speculative. Hyperinsulinism may render peripheral nerves incapable of using fatty acids and amino acids, thus making them dependent on glucose. Alternatively, peripheral neuropathy may represent a paraneoplastic syndrome of pancreatic beta-cell carcinoma.[1]

Radiology

Abdominal and thoracic radiographs seldom contribute because of the small size of the primary tumor and the infrequency of pulmonary metastases. Abdominal ultrasonography should be performed on all animals suspected of having an insulinoma. Ultrasonography often is beneficial in identifying liver metastases and may be helpful in delineating the primary pancreatic mass.

Laboratory Evaluations

Results of a hemogram and urinalysis typically are within the limits of normal in animals with insulinoma. Abnormalities other than a low blood glucose concentration seldom are identified on a serum biochemical profile. Nonfasting blood glucose concentrations frequently are quite low. Twenty-seven of 31 dogs with insulinoma had a nonfasting blood glucose concentration less than 70 mg/100 ml, with an average of 49.8 mg/100 ml.[8] Liver enzyme concentrations may be elevated; however, a correlation has not been found between liver enzyme elevation and the presence of liver metastasis.[25, 29]

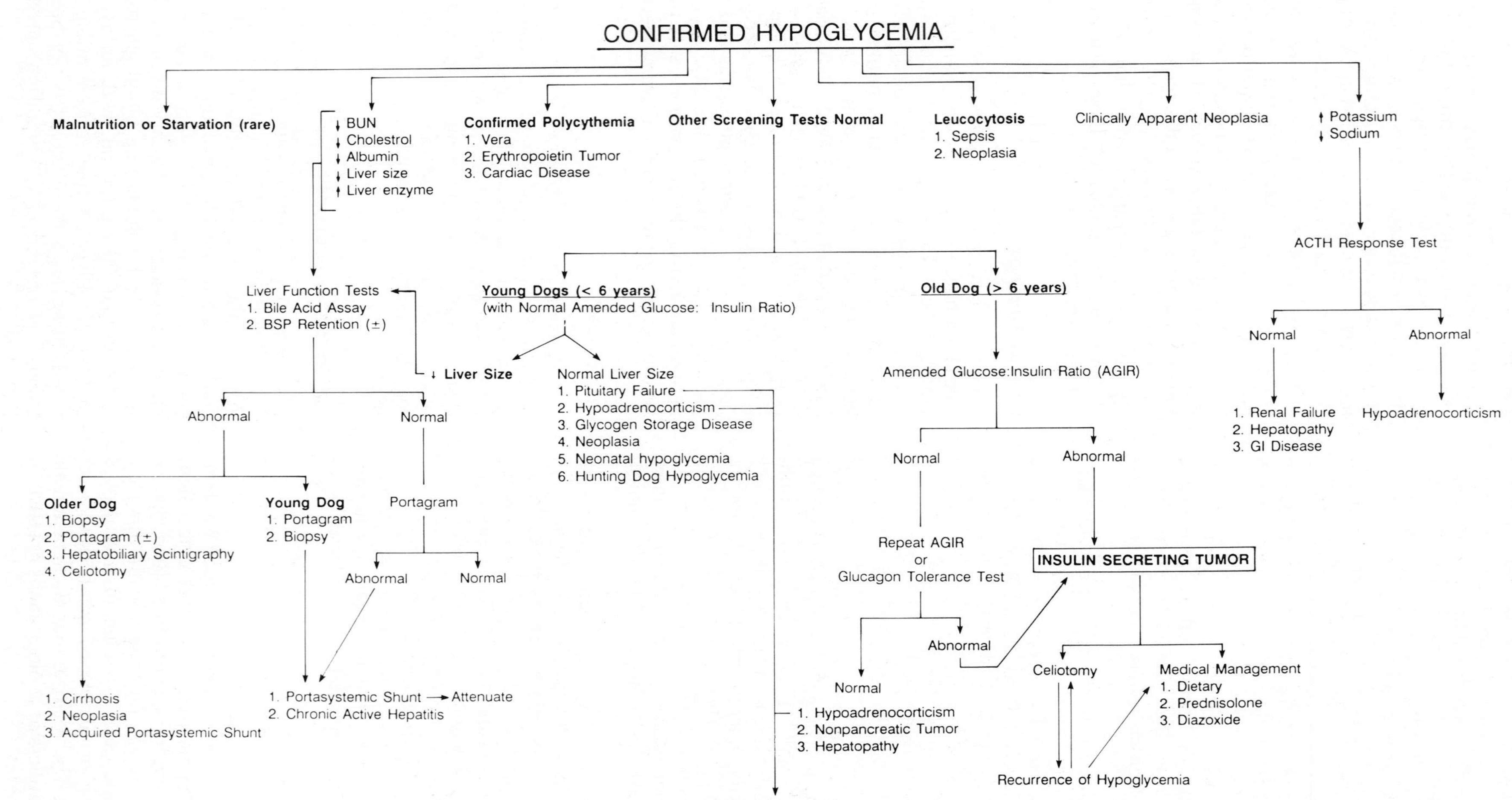

FIGURE 114–1. Diagnostic approach following confirmation of hypoglycemia.

Fasting Blood Glucose

Fasts occasionally are necessary to demonstrate hypoglycemia. Prolonged fasts (i.e., >12 hours) cannot be recommended because profound hypoglycemia may result in life-threatening neuroglycopenia.[8, 17, 29] Fasts of 8 hours or less were successful in demonstrating hypoglycemia in 33 of 35 trials in 31 dogs with insulinoma.[25] Unattended fasts should be avoided. Demonstration of a profoundly low blood glucose concentration after a fast suggests an insulinoma but is not confirmatory.

Plasma Insulin

Plasma insulin concentration is reported in microunits/milliliter of immunoreactive insulin (IRI). Variability exists between laboratories; the IRI level in normal fasted dogs usually is between 5 and 20 uU/ml.[8] To determine IRI levels, an animal is fasted until the blood glucose concentration is less than 60 mg/100 ml, then a blood sample is obtained for glucose and insulin assay.[8]

Animals with insulinoma have persistently elevated IRI levels because hypoglycemia fails to have the normal suppressive effect on insulin secretion if the insulin arises from autonomous neoplastic cells. A high IRI level in association with hypoglycemia (<60 mg/100 ml) strongly suggests insulinoma.[3, 36] Other causes of hypoglycemia generally result in a low or normal IRI level. Animals with insulinomas may have a normal fasting IRI level, owing perhaps to precirculation removal of insulin by the liver.[3, 36] In two studies, 14 of 41 and 4 of 6 dogs with insulinoma had preoperative IRI levels within the normal range.[2, 3] Insulinoma is unlikely in a hypoglycemic animal with a low IRI.

Amended Glucose/Insulin Ratio

Several glucose/insulin ratios have been suggested. The amended glucose/insulin ratio (AGIR) is the most reliable.[17, 25] The AGIR is not used as a sole criterion for diagnosis of insulinoma, because the ability of this test to consistently distinguish between hypoglycemic animals with and without insulinoma has been questioned.[2, 6] The AGIR was abnormal in 41 of 41 dogs with insulinoma, but results are inconsistent.[2, 8, 18, 25]

A blood sample is obtained for glucose and insulin determination when the fasting blood glucose concentration is between 40 and 60 mg/100 ml.[25] The AGIR is determined as follows:

$$\frac{\text{Plasma insulin (uU/ml)} \times 100}{\text{Plasma glucose (mg/100 ml)} - 30}$$

The use of −30 is based on the theory that in normal humans, IRI levels approach zero when the plasma glucose concentration is 30 mg/100 ml or less.[8] A divisor of 1 is used when the plasma glucose concentration is less than 30 mg/100 ml. An AGIR greater than 30 is considered by many to be diagnostic of an insulin-secreting tumor.[8, 25, 27, 29] Equivocal results warrant a repeat test. If the test results remain equivocal, another cause of hypoglycemia should be considered; however, insulinoma cannot be ruled out.[26]

Glucagon Tolerance Test

Provocative tests for insulin secretion are rarely necessary to make a diagnosis of insulinoma in animals.[25, 36] The best-known and most widely used provocative test is the glucagon tolerance test. Administration of glucagon results in an elevation in the blood glucose concentration and stimulates the secretion of insulin by normal and neoplastic beta cells.[25] The glucagon tolerance test may be indicated in hypoglycemic animals that have borderline or inconsistent IRI levels when other diagnostic criteria such as anamnesis, clinical signs, and glucose/insulin ratios are equivocal.[8, 17] A description of the technique and interpretation of the glucagon tolerance test results appears elsewhere.[28]

Preoperative Treatment

Important considerations in the preoperative period are protection from hypoglycemia and clinical signs of neuroglycopenia and maintenance of fluid and electrolyte balance. Frequent assessment of the blood glucose concentration is imperative and easily accomplished with commercially available reagent strips. Euglycemia can usually be maintained by feeding small amounts every 2 to 4 hours. Intermittent intravenous bolus administration of a 50 per cent dextrose solution or continuous infusion of a 10 to 20 per cent dextrose solution may be required to maintain euglycemia. Intracellular shifts of potassium as a result of dextrose infusion may lead to hypokalemia.[14, 36] Serum electrolytes are assessed during dextrose infusion, and potassium supplementation provided as needed. Fluid administration supports pancreatic microvascular circulation and may minimize the development of pancreatitis after surgery. Intravenous fluid administration at twice maintenance rate for 12 hours before, during, and for 24 hours after surgery is recommended.[8, 25, 26]

Acute hypoglycemic crises are treated promptly. A blood sample is obtained for blood glucose determination before therapy. Initial therapy for hypoglycemic seizures is intravenous administration of 2 to 15 ml of 50 per cent dextrose solution.[8, 25] Seizures that do not respond to intravenous dextrose administration are treated with intravenous diazepam or phenobarbital. Animals rarely die during acute hypoglycemic crises, although prolonged, severe hypoglycemia may result in irreversible cerebral lesions.[25]

Food and water are withheld for 12 hours before surgery. Five per cent dextrose solution is administered intravenously during the preoperative fast and surgery. Multiple blood glucose analyses are performed during this time.

Surgical Therapy

Surgical exploration may be necessary to definitively diagnose a pancreatic beta-cell carcinoma. The therapeutic and prognostic value of an exploratory laparotomy justifies surgery when the diagnosis has previously been established.[8, 25] Surgical therapy is considered palliative owing to the almost 100 per cent incidence of recurrence.[28, 36]

A ventral midline abdominal incision is made, and the abdomen is explored. A thorough visual and *gentle* digital inspection of the pancreas is necessary. The liver, duodenum, mesentery, and hepatic, splenic, gastric, duodenum, and cranial mesenteric lymph nodes are evaluated for metastasis. Insulinomas typically are single small (0.5 to 4 cm) yellow to dark-red spherical nodules on the surface of the pancreas.[29] Insulinomas occur in both lobes of the pancreas with equal prevalence.[2, 8, 25, 36] Multiple pancreatic tumors have been reported, so the entire pancreas is evaluated even when a nodule is obvious.[2] The tumor occasionally is within the pancreatic parenchyma and cannot be seen. Palpation of the pancreas is essential but must be gentle to minimize pancreatitis. Rarely, a pancreatic mass cannot be located because the mass is too small or because multiple microscopic tumors are present. If no mass is observed or palpated, half of the pancreas may be resected to remove the portion that contains the tumor.[8]

The goal of surgery is to reduce the tumor mass by removing as much obvious tumor as possible, including metastases to the liver and regional lymph nodes (Fig. 114–2). Reduction in tumor mass frequently results in remission or reduction of clinical signs and improved response to medical therapy. Rarely, pancreaticoduodenectomy and partial gastrectomy followed by gastrojejunostomy and cholecystojejunostomy are necessary. Selective biopsy of tumor tissue followed by appropriate medical therapy may be the preferred treatment in animals with extensive organ involvement. A biopsy of the liver and regional lymph nodes is recommended in all cases. Euthanasia during surgery should not be recommended regardless of the findings because most dogs can be treated medically for several months.[8, 13]

Pancreatic or extrapancreatic nodules occasionally cannot be positively identified as beta-cell carcinoma. Intravenous methylene blue infusion is beneficial in differentiating metastatic nodules from nonmetastatic nodules in dogs.[9, 10, 33] The methylene blue solution is prepared preoperatively by mixing methylene blue in 250 ml of isotonic saline solution to obtain a total dose of 3 mg/kg body weight. Infusion begins approximately 30 minutes before the surgeon expects to begin exploring the abdomen. The entire volume is delivered in 30 minutes. Overhydration of small dogs is avoided by limiting the volume of methylene blue solution infused. Infusing the solution too rapidly may result in excessively rapid excretion and inadequate uptake of the dye by islet cells. Tumor nodules may be differentiated from non–beta-cell tissue by their reddish-violet preferential staining. The mechanism for selective uptake of methylene blue by pancreatic and extrapancreatic islet cells is not known.[9, 10]

Adverse effects of methylene blue infusion include regenerative hemolytic anemia, pseudocyanosis, and staining of floors and animal handling facilities. Regenerative hemolytic anemia may be significant but is transient at the dose recommended.[10] The packed cell volume in four dogs that had methylene blue infusion declined to approximately half the preoperative value.[9] None of the dogs required a blood transfusion, but such therapy may be necessary in some dogs receiving methylene blue infusions. Anesthetists should be advised that pseudocyanosis does occur and necessitates evaluation of other parameters for monitoring patients.[5] Methylene blue is eliminated unchanged by the kidneys. For 48 hours after surgery, animals receiving methylene blue infusions are confined to areas of the hospital that cannot be damaged by the stain. Methylene blue infusion does not increase the risk of postoperative pancreatitis in dogs, although this complication is reported in humans.[9, 10]

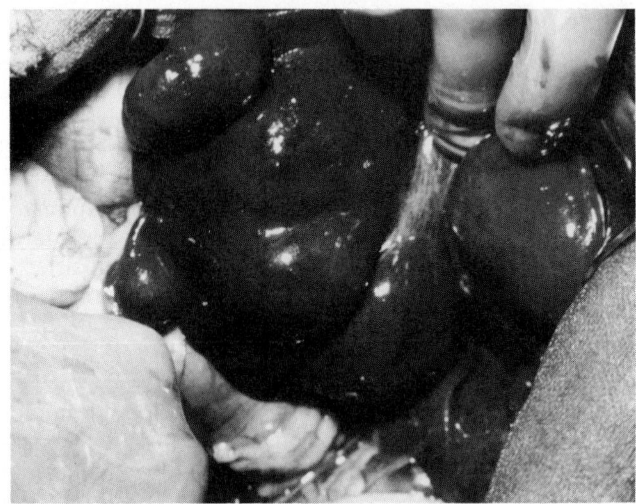

FIGURE 114–2. Operative view showing multiple metastatic nodules in the liver of a dog with insulinoma *(arrows).*

Postoperative Management

Maintenance of normoglycemia and management of iatrogenic pancreatitis are primary considerations in the immediate postoperative period.[36] Frequent blood glucose analyses are essential, and 24-hour monitoring of patients is ideal.

Animals may be hypo-, hyper-, or euglycemic after surgical excision of an insulinoma. Persistent hypoglycemia results from incomplete removal of insulin-secreting neoplastic tissue and is treated as described in the next section on medical treatment. Hyperglycemia may occur after nearly complete removal of insulin-secreting tissue as a result of residual suppression of normal pancreatic beta cells. Transient diabetes mellitus was reported in 5 of 31 dogs that had surgery for insulinoma.[8] Diabetes mellitus that persists after 48 hours may be treated with insulin; however, animals should be loosely regulated to stimulate production of insulin by normal pancreatic beta cells. Postoperative euglycemia is ideal and implies complete or nearly complete removal of neoplastic tissue and normal function of pancreatic beta cells.[28] Postoperative euglycemia does not imply an excellent long-term prognosis.[25]

Postoperative pancreatitis has been reported as a fairly common complication, occurring in 12 of 29 dogs surviving surgery for insulinoma in one report.[21] All dogs that undergo partial pancreatectomy for insulinoma excision are treated for pancreatitis for 24 to 48 hours after surgery. Intravenous fluid therapy and withholding oral food and water are indicated. Water and a bland diet are gradually introduced on the third day after surgery, provided the animal does not have clinical signs of pancreatitis. Therapy continues after 48 hours if clinical signs of pancreatitis persist.

Medical Therapy for Insulinoma

Animals that are euglycemic and symptom free after surgery usually remain so for several months, occasionally for a year or more. Medical therapy is not recommended as long as an animal remains euglycemic. Hypoglycemic signs eventually recur owing to the highly malignant nature of insulinoma in most animals. Animals are either treated medically, or a second exploratory celiotomy is performed when hypoglycemic signs recur.[25–27] Many clinicians prefer to treat animals with recurrent clinical signs medically, because recurrence usually results from widespread metastasis.

Medical therapy of malignant insulinoma consists of dietary, hormonal, and antineoplastic regimens.[36] Each therapeutic method, starting with dietary control, is continued until hypoglycemic signs recur. At that time, another treatment regimen begins without discontinuing the first.[25]

Diet

Hypoglycemic signs can be minimized if a constant source of calories is provided as a substrate for the excess insulin.[25] Feeding three to six small meals per day provides a continuous supply of glucose and avoids the sudden excessive insulin secretion commonly generated by large meals. A carbohydrate-rich diet such as a mixture of canned and dry dog food is recommended.[19] Semimoist dog foods that are high in simple sugars may stimulate insulin secretion by neoplastic beta cells and are avoided.[8, 26] Animals experiencing periods of weakness are fed immediately. Honey, syrup, molasses, and other sugar solutions are avoided if the animal can eat. Sugar solutions reverse acute hypoglycemic crises but predispose an animal to a subsequent episode within 30 to 120 minutes.[8]

Antihormonal Drugs

Glucocorticoids. Glucocorticoid therapy is initiated when dietary management is no longer effective. Glucocorticoids decrease tissue use of glucose by antagonizing the effects of insulin at the cellular level, thereby indirectly increasing the blood glucose concentration. Glucocorticoids directly increase the blood glucose concentration by stimulating hepatic glycogenolysis and promoting hepatic gluconeogenesis.[25, 26] Prednisone is administered orally (0.5 mg/kg/24 hours in divided doses). The dosage may be incrementally increased up to 6 mg/kg/24 hours if clinical signs persist or recur.[25] Signs of hypercortisolism, such as polyuria, polydypsia, polyphagia, or alopecia, are common at the higher dose. The prednisone dose is reduced and diazoxide therapy initiated if dose-related complications occur.

Diazoxide. Diazoxide is a benzothiadiazide diuretic with potent hyperglycemic properties. Diazoxide exerts its hyperglycemic effect by (1) inhibiting the secretion of insulin by blocking emiocytosis of insulin granules, (2) stimulating hepatic gluconeogenesis and glycogenolysis, and (3) decreasing tissue use of glucose by inhibiting cellular uptake of glucose.[25] Diazoxide has no antineoplastic effects and does not impair insulin synthesis.[8]

Diazoxide therapy is indicated when dietary management and glucocorticoids are no longer effective in preventing signs of hypoglycemia. Diazoxide has been used with limited success to control clinical signs in the preoperative period.[18, 21] An initial dosage of 10 mg/kg/day divided into two doses is recommended.[25, 36] The dosage may gradually be increased to a total of 60 mg/kg/day if signs recur or persist. Thiazide diuretics enhance the hyperglycemic effects of diazoxide and may be administered concurrently when diazoxide alone is not effective.

Potential side effects of diazoxide therapy include cataract formation, bradycardia, anemia, thrombocytopenia, diabetes mellitus, sodium and fluid retention, anorexia, vomiting, and diarrhea.[25] Adverse gastrointestinal signs usually can be controlled by administering diazoxide with a meal.

Antineoplastic Drugs

Streptozotocin. Streptozotocin is a naturally occurring nitrosourea isolated from the fermentation cultures of *Streptomyces achromogenes*. Streptozotocin selectively destroys pancreatic beta cells by depressing the pyridine nucleotides nicofinomide-adenine dinucleotide and its reduced form.[8] The drug has potent diabetogenic effects, with the potential to cause overt diabetes mellitus.[26] The dosage of streptozotocin is less than 500 mg/m^2 once every 7 days for two to four treatments. Streptozotocin and fluorouracil in combination are superior to streptozotocin alone in overall rate of response and in rates of complete response in humans with insulinomas.[24] Streptozotocin is extremely nephrotoxic, and its use in animals with recurrent insulinoma cannot be recommended at this time.[22, 23]

Somatostatin. Somatostatin is a tetradecapeptide found in most vertebrate tissues. It inhibits hormone secretion from normal, hyperplastic, and neoplastic endocrine cells. Somatostatin was administered to five dogs with surgically confirmed relapsing insulinoma with moderate to severe clinical signs.[19] Results of this initial study, although mixed, suggest that somatostatin may be useful in treating refractory beta-cell neoplasia in dogs.

Prognosis

The long-term prognosis for dogs with insulinoma is poor. The recurrence rate is nearly 100 per cent. Appropriate and timely surgical intervention and adjunctive medical therapy typically result in survival for 12 to 15 months although 2-year survival has been reported.[8, 17, 18, 21, 25] The prognostic features of 73 dogs with insulinoma were reviewed.[2] Factors of no prognostic value were breed, sex, body weight, clinical signs, duration of clinical signs, preoperative serum glucose concentration, and tumor location within the pancreas. Younger dogs, dogs with distant metastasis, and dogs with higher preoperative serum insulin concentrations had significantly shorter survival times.

GASTRINOMA

In 1955, Zollinger and Ellison described a syndrome in humans of gastric acid hypersecretion, gastrointestinal ulcerations, and a non–beta-cell pancreatic tumor[38] and postulated that an ulcerogenic humoral factor of pancreatic islet origin was responsible. It was later discovered that the pancreatic tumor consisted of cells that secreted large quantities of gastrin. The syndrome, termed the *Zollinger-Ellison syndrome*, was first described in dogs by Jones in 1976.[15]

Pathology and Pathophysiology

Gastrin is a polypeptide hormone that normally is produced by gastrin cells of the antral and duodenal mucosa in response to antral distension and stimulation by amino acids and partially digested proteins.[11, 29] Excessive quantities of gastrin, secreted by the non–beta-cell pancreatic tumor, are responsible for the following characteristic clinicopathological features of Zollinger-Ellison syndrome: (1) hyperplasia and edema of gastric mucosa, (2) hyperchlorhydria, (3) duodenal ulcerations from gastric hyperacidity, (4) villus atrophy and edema of the small intestine, (5) diarrhea with malabsorption due to precipitation of bile salts, interference with chylomicron formation, and damage to intestinal mucosa cells, and (6) steatorrhea due to acid inactivation of pancreatic lipase.[8, 36]

Zollinger-Ellison syndrome is rare in humans and exceedingly rare in animals. The few case reports of gastrinoma in the veterinary literature suggest the condition is more common in middle-aged to older dogs.[12, 29, 32] A sex or breed predilection is not apparent. The biological behavior of gastrinoma is similar in humans and dogs. The disease is insidious in onset, and metastasis to the liver and regional lymph nodes occurs in more than 50 per cent by the time the diagnosis is made.[36]

Gastrinomas may be associated with tumors of other endocrine organs, a condition known as *multiple endocrine neoplasia syndrome* (MEN).[8, 32] MEN type 1, consisting of neoplasia or hyperplasia of pancreatic islets, parathyroids, or pituitary glands, occurs in approximately 25 per cent of humans with Zollinger-Ellison syndrome.[32] C-cell hyperplasia of the thyroid, perhaps due to gastrin stimulation of calcitonin release from C cells, was reported in three of three dogs with gastrinoma.[12] Because gastrin cells are part of the APUD system, gastrinomas may secrete other hormones such as insulin adrenocorticotropic hormone and pancreatic polypeptides as well as gastrin.

Diagnosis

The diagnosis of gastrinoma is based on demonstration of hypergastrinemia and an elevated rate of gastric acid secretion in any animal with typical clinical signs of upper gastrointestinal ulcer disease.[35, 36] A high index of suspicion is necessary to make the diagnosis antemortem.

History

Animals with gastrinoma typically have a 1- to 2-month history of anorexia, weight loss, intermittent diarrhea, depression, vomiting, and hematemesis that is partially responsive or nonresponsive to conservative therapy.[12, 35] A diagnosis of gastric or duodenal ulcers has occasionally been made, and the response to conventional therapy has been poor.

Clinical Findings

Clinical findings are nonspecific and may include weight loss, dehydration, melena, hematemesis, and rarely signs of generalized peritonitis from a perforated ulcer. The animal frequently is severely depressed, emaciated, febrile, and in shock.[19] Signs of epigastric pain, a common symptom in humans, are uncommon in dogs and cannot be elicited on abdominal palpation. Myelofibrosis resulting in generalized bone pain was reported in a Brittany spaniel with gastrinoma.[7]

Radiology

Survey abdominal radiographs often are nondiagnostic. Radiographic signs of localized peritonitis may be present if an ulcer has perforated. Megaesophagus may be apparent on thoracic radiographs if the animal has severe esophagitis. An upper gastrointestinal series may be helpful in establishing a diagnosis based on findings of thickened gastric mucosa, prominent gastric rugal folds, and hypermotility of the small intestine.[35, 36] The stomach may contain a large amount of acidic fluid, which may flocculate the contrast medium.[35]

Laboratory Evaluations

Mild anemia and leukocytosis may be apparent on a hemogram. Hypoproteinemia is a consistent finding in animals with gastrinoma.[8] Hypokalemia, hypochloremia, and metabolic alkalosis occur.[35] Hypocalcemia results from gastrin-stimulated calcitonin secretion. Steatorrhea may be demonstrated by a positive fecal Sudan stain. Fecal occult blood analysis typically is positive. Gastrointestinal bleeding may produce melena and mildly increased blood urea nitrogen levels without a corresponding elevation in serum creatinine concentration from intestinal recycling of urea.[7]

Endoscopy

Endoscopy is performed to evaluate the esophagus, stomach, and duodenum for inflammation and ulceration. Inflammation and erosions of the distal esophagus are often present. Gastroscopy typically reveals prominent, irregular rugal folds despite gastric insufflation, a large quantity of gastric fluid in a fasted animal, and mucosal ulcers or hyperemia, primarily in the antral region.[35, 36] Ulcers may be evident in the proximal duodenum. Gastric biopsy samples are obtained and typically reveal gastric mucosal hypertrophy and chronic gastritis.

Serum Gastrin Level

Demonstration of hyperchlorhydria in conjunction with increased serum gastrin concentration is the most reliable nonsurgical means for establishing a diagnosis of gastrinoma in animals.[8, 35]

A radioimmunoassay test kit for measuring serum gastrin is sufficiently sensitive for use in dogs.[11, 35, 36] Blood samples for serum gastrin analysis are obtained after an overnight fast. Basal serum gastrin levels are 23 to 190 pg/ml in dogs and 28 to 135 pg/ml in cats.[8, 11, 32] Reported basal serum gastrin levels in dogs with gastrinoma range from 360 to 2,780 pg/ml.[8] Greatly elevated serum gastrin levels (i.e., >1,000 pg/ml) are diagnostic of Zollinger-Ellison syndrome.[5]

Provocative tests using oral protein loading, intravenously administered secretion, or intravenously administered calcium gluconate are indicated when basal serum gastrin levels are nondiagnostic.[5, 8] Ingestion of a protein-rich meal results in minimal or no increase in serum gastrin levels in animals with gastrinoma because of the autonomous nature of gastrin secretion by the tumor. Intravenous administration of secretin, 4 U/kg, is the preferred provocative test for gastrin secretion.[8] Secretin results in a slight decrease in serum gastrin levels in normal dogs. In dogs with Zollinger-Ellison syndrome, secretin administration produces a paradoxical increase in serum gastrin levels, with an increase of 200 pg/ml above basal level considered diagnostic.[5] The mechanism for the paradoxical increase in serum gastrin levels is unknown. Intravenous administration of calcium gluconate, 2 mg/kg, results in a minimal increase in serum gastrin in normal dogs but a significant increase in dogs with gastrinoma.[5]

Hypergastrinemia is not pathognomonic for gastrinoma. Conditions that may result in an elevated serum gastrin level include antral G-cell hyperplasia, atrophic gastritis, short bowel syndrome, hyperthyroidism, renal insufficiency, immunoproliferative enteropathy in Basenjis, and gastric dilation/volvulus syndrome.[7, 32] Provocative tests should not result in greatly increased levels in these conditions.

Basal Gastric Acid Secretion

Basal gastric acid secretion levels are determined by placing a pharyngostomy tube in the antral region of the stomach. Dogs do not constantly secrete hydrochloric acid; therefore, basal gastric acid secretion values are almost zero in normal dogs.[12, 35] Fasting basal gastric acid secretion levels are 3 to 15 mEq/hour in dogs with gastrinoma.[32, 34, 35] This test is nonspecific because documentation of gastric hypersecretion of hydrochloric acid suggests hypergastrinemia due to any cause.

Medical Therapy

Medical therapy of gastrinoma involves inhibition of gastrin-stimulated gastric acid secretion with H_2 antagonists such as cimetidine and ranitidine and treatment of ulcer disease. Cimetidine and ranitidine produce temporary subjective clinical improvement in a limited number of dogs.[19, 30, 36] Medical therapy frequently is unsuccessful in the treatment of gastrinoma because of the high incidence of metastasis. The recommended dosage of cimetidine is 5 to 10 mg/kg QID.[19] Ranitidine, a long-acting H_2 antagonist, is administered at a dosage of 10 mg/kg BID. H_2 antagonists bind to histamine receptors on gastric parietal cells and block gastrin-dependent hydrochloride secretion. H_2 antagonists do not decrease the serum gastrin concentration. Cimetidine is beneficial in reducing gastric acid secretion during the period of evaluation and stabilization before surgery in humans with Zollinger-Ellison syndrome.[36] In humans, the effectiveness of H_2 antagonists in patients with Zollinger-Ellison syndrome may decrease with time owing to increased tumor gastrin secretion or tolerance to the drug.[7]

Sucralfate, a sulfated disaccharide that coats ulcerated surfaces in the stomach and duodenum, may be used in animals with gastric or duodenal ulcers. An acid pH is necessary to dissociate sucralfate into its active anions; therefore, the drug is not given during the period 30 minutes before and 2 hours after administration of cimetidine.[7]

The somatostatin analogue SMS201-995 is highly effective in controlling symptoms of gastrinoma in humans.[7] Somatostatin blocks gastric acid production by blocking G-cell gastrin secretion and by directly inhibiting parietal cell hydrogen ion secretion. Use of this drug in one dog yielded promising results.[7]

Surgical Therapy

Surgery is the best therapeutic alternative for animals with gastrinoma. Exploratory celiotomy is the most advantageous method for establishing a diagnosis and allows complete excision or debulking of the tumor mass and evaluation for metastasis. Extensive metastatic disease is often present; however, reducing the tumor mass may enhance the success of medical therapy postoperatively.

A thorough abdominal exploration is performed. The liver, regional lymph nodes, pancreas, duodenum, and mesentery are carefully evaluated for metastatic disease. All grossly visible tumor tissue is resected.[36] The surgical procedure originally recommended by Zollinger and Ellison was total gastrectomy to remove the parietal cells, which are the target cells of gastrin.[38] Tumor excision without gastrectomy is recommended in animals that have a favorable response to medical therapy preoperatively. Total gastrectomy is reserved for animals that are refractory to medical therapy preoperatively. Complications of total gastrectomy include bile reflux, malnutrition, and dysphagia.[7] The technique for partial pancreatectomy and total gastrectomy is described in Chapters 48 and 43.

Postoperative antineoplastic therapy is considered owing to the highly malignant nature of the disease. Streptozotocin is beneficial in approximately 50 per cent of humans with Zollinger-Ellison syndrome.[36]

Prognosis

Valid conclusions regarding long-term survival in dogs with gastrinoma cannot be made because of the limited number of cases reported. The prognosis is poor, and long-term survival seems unlikely.

References

1. Braund KG, et al: Insulinoma and subclinical peripheral neuropathy in two dogs. *J Vet Intern Med 1*:86, 1987.
2. Caywood DD, et al: Pancreatic insulin-secreting neoplasms: Clinical, diagnostic, and prognostic features in 73 dogs. *J Am Anim Hosp Assoc 24*:577, 1988.
3. Caywood DD, et al: Pancreatic islet cell adenocarcinoma: Clinical and diagnostic features in six cases. *J Am Vet Med Assoc 174*:714, 1979.
4. Chrisman CL: Postoperative results and complications of insulinomas in dogs. *J Am Anim Hosp Assoc 16*:677, 1980.
5. Drazner FH: Canine gastrinoma: A condition analogous to the Zollinger-Ellison syndrome in man. *Calif Vet 11*:6, 1981.
6. Edwards DF: It's time to unamend the insulin-glucose ratio. *J Am Vet Med Assoc 188*:951, 1986.
7. English RV, et al: Zollinger-Ellison syndrome and myelofibrosis in a dog. *J Am Vet Med Assoc 192*:1430, 1988.
8. Feldman EC, Nelson RW: Gastrointestinal endocrinology. *In* Feldman EC, Nelson RW (eds): *Canine and Feline Endocrinology and Reproduction*. W.B. Saunders, Philadelphia, 1987.
9. Fingeroth JM, Smeak DD: Intravenous methylene blue infusion for intraoperative identification of pancreatic islet-cell tumors in dogs. Part II: Clinical trials and results in four dogs. *J Am Anim Hosp Assoc 24*:175, 1988.
10. Fingeroth JM, et al: Intravenous methylene blue infusion for intraoperative identification of parathyroid gland and pancreatic islet-cell tumors in dogs. Part I: Experimental determination of dose-related staining efficacy and toxicity. *J Am Anim Hosp Assoc 24*:165, 1988.
11. Gabbert NH, et al: Serum immunoreactive gastrin concentrations in the dog: Basal and postprandial values measured by radioimmunoassay. *Am J Vet Res 45*:2351, 1984.
12. Happe RP, et al: Zollinger-Ellison syndrome in three dogs. *Vet Path 17*:177, 1980.
13. Hill FW, et al: Functional islet cell tumour in the dog. *J Small Anim Pract 15*:119, 1974.
14. Johnson RK: Insulinoma in the dog. *Vet Clin North Am 7*:629, 1977.
15. Jones BR, et al: Peptic ulceration in a dog associated with an islet cell carcinoma of the pancreas and an elevated plasma gastrin level. *J Small Anim Pract 17*:593, 1976.
16. Kaufman J, et al: Pancreatic beta cell tumor in a ferret. *J Am Vet Med Assoc 185*:998, 1984.
17. Kruth SA, et al: Insulin-secreting islet cell tumors: Establishing a diagnosis and the clinical course for 25 dogs. *J Am Vet Med Assoc 181*:54, 1982.
18. Leifer CE, et al: Insulin-secreting tumor: Diagnosis and medical and surgical management in 55 dogs. *J Am Vet Med Assoc 188*:60, 1986.
19. Lothrop CD: Medical treatment of neuroendocrine tumors of the gastroenteropancreatic system with somatostatin. *In* Kirk RW (ed): *Current Veterinary Therapy X*. W.B. Saunders, Philadelphia, 1989.
20. Luttgen PJ, et al: Insulinoma in a ferret. *J Am Vet Med Assoc 189*:920, 1986.
21. Mehlhaff CJ, et al: Insulin-producing islet cell neoplasms: Surgical considerations and general management in 35 dogs. *J Am Anim Hosp Assoc 21*:607, 1985.
22. Meyer DJ: Pancreatic islet cell carcinoma in a dog treated with streptozotocin. *Am J Vet Res 37*:1221, 1976.
23. Meyer DJ: Temporary remission of hypoglycemia in a dog with an insulinoma after treatment with streptozotocin. *Am J Vet Res 38*: 1201, 1977.
24. Moertel CG, et al: Streptozocin alone compared with streptozocin plus fluorouracil in the treatment of advanced islet-cell carcinoma. *N Engl J Med 303*:1189, 1980.
25. Nelson RW: Insulin-secreting islet cell neoplasia. *In* Ettinger SJ (ed): *Textbook of Veterinary Internal Medicine*. W.B. Saunders, Philadelphia, 1989.
26. Nelson RW, Foodman MS: Medical management of canine hyperinsulinism. *J Am Vet Med Assoc 187*:78, 1985.
27. Orsher RW, Eigenmann JE: Pancreas. *Vet Clin North Am 15*:653, 1985.
28. Rogers KS, Luttgen PJ: Hyperinsulinism. *Comp Cont Educ Pract Vet 7*:829, 1985.
29. Rosin E: The pancreas. *In* Gourley IM, Vasseur PB (eds): *General Small Animal Surgery*. J.B. Lippincott, Philadelphia, 1985.
30. Rousseaux CG: Ultrastructure of a canine gastrinoma. *J Comp Path 197*:605, 1987.
31. Shahar R, et al: Peripheral polyneuropathy in a dog with functional islet beta-cell tumor and widespread metastasis. *J Am Vet Med Assoc 187*:175, 1985.
32. Shaw DH: Gastrinoma (Zollinger-Ellison syndrome) in the dog and cat. *Can Vet J 29*:448, 1988.
33. Smeak DD, et al: Intravenous methylene blue as a specific stain for primary and metastatic insulinoma in a dog. *J Am Anim Hosp Assoc 24*:478, 1988.
34. Straus E, et al: Canine Zollinger-Ellison syndrome. *Gastroenterology 72*:380, 1977.
35. Twedt DC, Magne ML: Gastrinoma. *In* Ettinger SJ (ed): *Textbook of Veterinary Internal Medicine*. W.B. Saunders, Philadelphia, 1989.
36. Walshaw R: Surgical diseases of the endocrine pancreas. *In* Slatter DH, (ed): *Textbook of Small Animal Surgery*. W.B. Saunders, Philadelphia, 1985.
37. Willard MD, Schall WD: Apudomas. *In* Kirk RW (ed): *Current Veterinary Therapy VIII*. W.B. Saunders, Philadelphia, 1983.
38. Zollinger RM, Ellison EH: Primary peptic ulcerations of the jejunum associated with islet cell tumors of the pancreas. *Ann Surg 142*:709, 1955.

SECTION 14

Ear

Howard B. Seim III ■ *Section Editor*

CHAPTER

115 The Pinna

Ralph A. Henderson and R. D. Horne

ANATOMY

The auricle (pinna) has a hairless rostrolateral concave surface and a hairy caudomedial convex surface.

The auricular and scutiform cartilage form the external ear canal opening and ear pinna. The large, convoluted auricular cartilage is cone shaped from its origin at the annular cartilage, where it flares to form the pinna distally.

Important surgical landmarks of the auricular cartilage are the helix, anthelix, tragus, antitragus, scapha, and cavum conchae (Fig. 115–1). The helix is the edge of the pinna, and the scapha is the center. A ridge with a prominent tubercle, the anthelix, is on the medial concave aspect of the auricular cartilage at the entrance to the vertical canal. The tragus forms the lateral rim of the vertical canal meatus and is directly opposite the helix. The antitragus is caudal to the tragus and separated from it by the intertragic notch. The funnel-shaped cavum conchae forms the vertical canal and, along with the tragal, antitragal, and anthelicine borders, forms the external auditory meatus (see Fig. 115–1).[3]

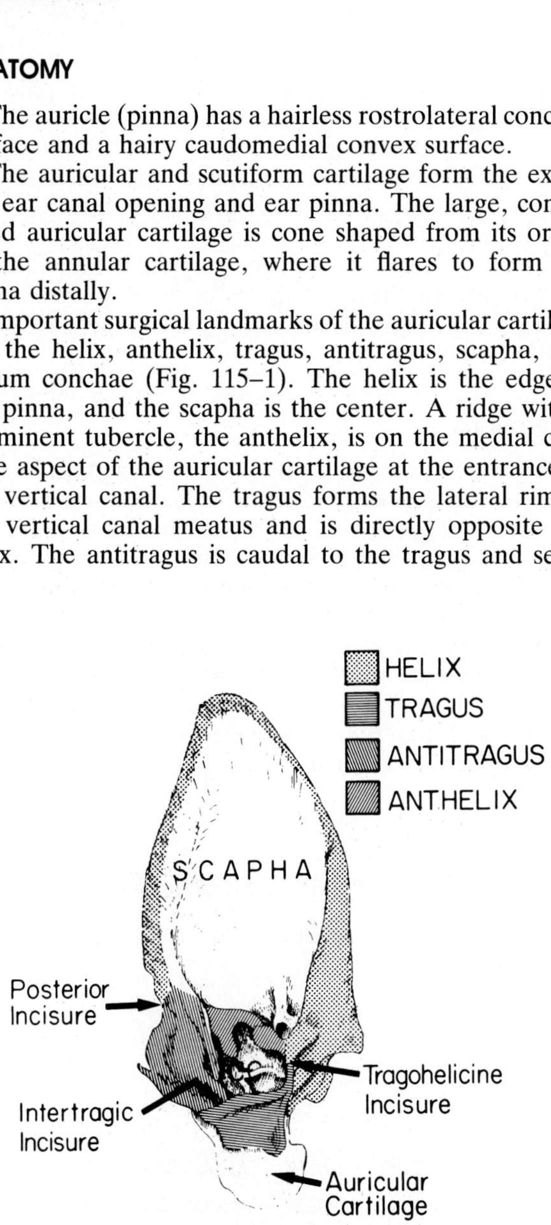

FIGURE 115–1. Anatomy of the concave surface of the auricular cartilage, showing the important anatomical divisions. The intertragic notch and tragohelicine incisure are surgical landmarks.

The boot-shaped scutiform cartilage lies medial to the auricular cartilage and assists in attaching the auricular cartilage to the head. The scutiform is important in correcting ear carriage but not in reconstructive procedures.[9]

The great auricular arteries and veins are branches of the external carotid artery and internal maxillary vein. The lateral, intermediate, and medial vascular rami pass along the convex surface, wrap around the helicine margins, and directly penetrate the scapha to supply the concave epithelium.[3]

The second cervical nerve is the principal caudodorsal sensory innervation on the convex surface, and the auriculotemporal branches of the trigeminal nerve are the principal sensory innervation on the concave surface. The external ear muscles are supplied by the auricular branch (auriculopalpebral trunk) of the facial nerve.[3]

INJURIES

Aural Hematoma

Aural or auricular hematoma is the most common physical injury of the pinna. It is usually self-inflicted by scratching and head shaking. Underlying causes are inflammation, parasites, allergy, and foreign bodies. Hematomas are most apparent on the concave surface of the ear (Fig. 115–2).

The branches of the great auricular artery that penetrate the cartilage are the source of hemorrhage. The hematoma is lined by cartilage on both sides, suggesting fracture or splitting of the cartilage as an etiological factor. Once begun, the bleeding between the cartilages continues until the internal pressure equals the pressure of the feeder arteries. Additional traumatic pressure on the hematoma causes further separation of the tissue and allows hemorrhage to resume. Fibrin is deposited on the walls of the hematoma, leaving a sanguineous seroma. With chronicity, fibrosis and contraction thicken

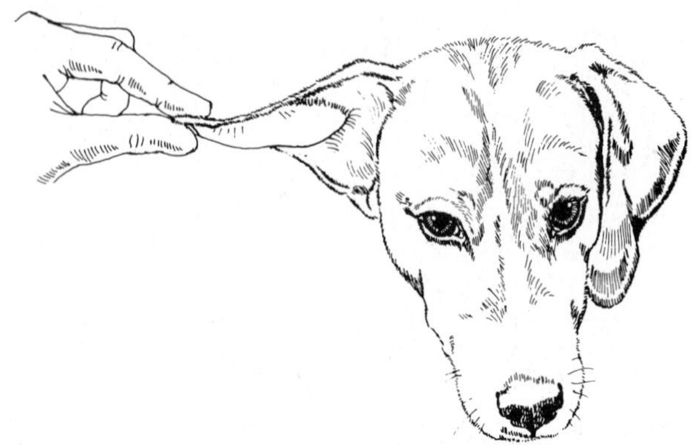

FIGURE 115–2. Auricular hematoma of the concave surface of the ear.

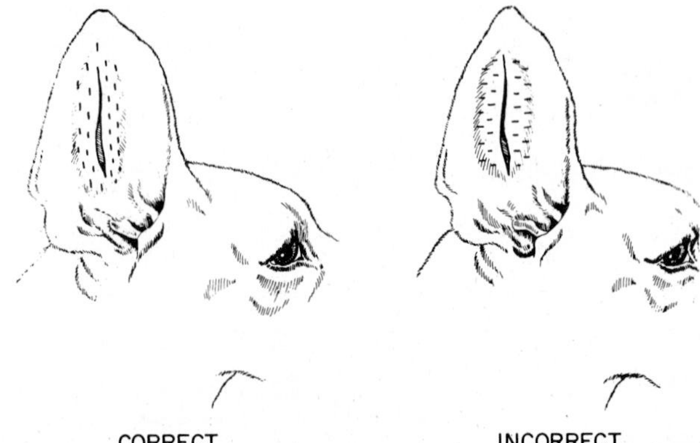

FIGURE 115–3. Sutures to obliterate dead space in an auricular hematoma. Sutures are correctly placed when parallel to and not including the blood vessels. Incorrectly placed sutures can uncorporate vessels and cause avascular necrosis.

and deform the ear. Fibrous reorganization of the ear and secondary "cauliflower" contracture can result.[7, 8]

The therapeutic objectives for an auricular hematoma are to identify the source of irritation, evacuate the hematoma, maintain tissue apposition, reduce fibrin deposition, and prevent recurrence.

Conservative Therapy

Needle aspiration may evacuate the hematoma and restore tissue apposition if used soon after hematoma formation. The contents of the hematoma must be removed aseptically. If the hematoma reforms, repeated aspiration is rarely successful. Cortisone instillation is discouraged because it delays healing and separates the tissues. A pressure bandage is applied after aspiration. Recurrence is common with needle aspiration as the only treatment.

Hematomas in which minimum fibrin is present can be treated by placing a self-retaining disposable teat cannula. The cannula is aseptically placed via a small stab incision in a dependent portion of the hematoma near the ear tip.[10] If continuous drainage is allowed for 2 to 3 weeks, resolution is likely.

Incision

Large, severe, or chronic (thick-walled) hematomas are treated by incision to remove the fibrin and by suturing to reappose the tissue. Hematomas may be opened via straight, cruciate, or S-shaped incisions, depending on the surgeon's preference or the size of the hematoma. Longitudinal contracture is less likely to cause deformity with S-shaped incisions. Because delay may allow the hematoma to enlarge, hematomas are treated immediately after diagnosis.

The incision exposes the hematoma cavity from end to end. The fibrin clot is thoroughly curetted, and the cavity copiously irrigated. Loosely tied mattress sutures are placed through the ear, parallel to the major vessels (Fig. 115–3). The three main great auricular branches are visible on the convex surface and are avoided. To permit drainage, the incision should gape slightly. Sutures are spaced so that no pockets occur to allow reformation. A reinforcing stent such as radiographic film is not usually necessary if correctly placed sutures are not greater than 1 cm in breadth. Sutures tied too tightly cause edema, pain, and surgical failure. Tied sutures should permit insertion of the needle holder tips to the level of the hinge.

A light protective bandage is applied, immobilizing the ear against the dorsum of the head or neck. The bandage is changed after 3 days, and sutures and bandage are removed in 7 to 10 days.

Lacerations

The ears are commonly injured during fights. Regardless of severity, the therapeutic objectives are cleaning, débridement, apposition of tissues, protection, and prevention of secondary infection. The tissues may require sutures for apposition, or second intention healing (contraction and epithelialization) may be adequate.

Three types of lacerations of the ear may be distinguished on the basis of wound depth or structures involved. A laceration may involve one skin surface, the skin and underlying cartilage, or both skin surfaces and the interposed cartilage (Fig. 115–4).

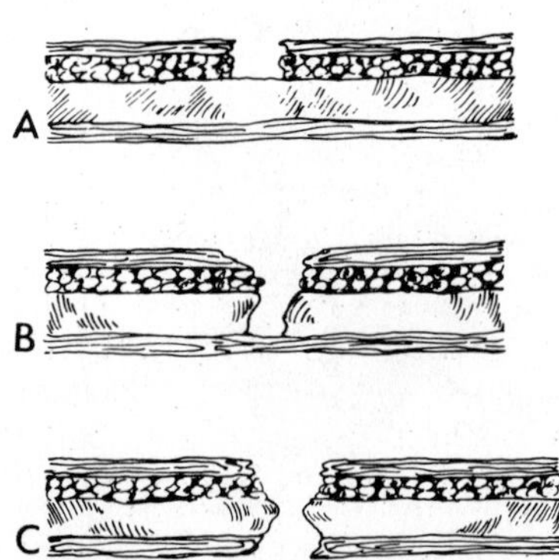

FIGURE 115–4. Lacerations of the ear flaps can include the skin only (*A*, convex surface), skin and cartilage (*B*), or cartilage and both skin surfaces (*C*).

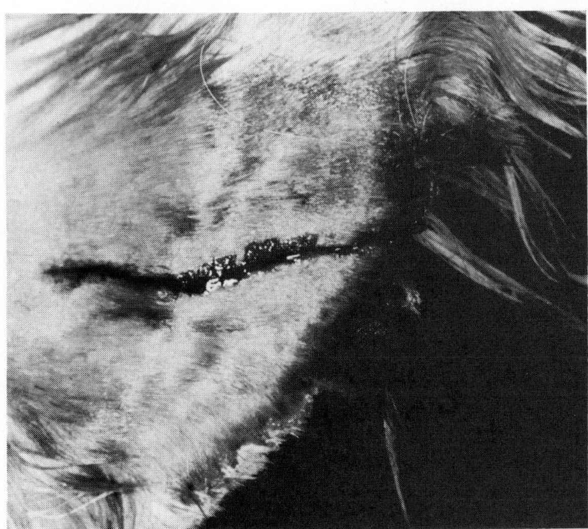

FIGURE 115–5. Lacerations of the concave ear skin superficial to the scapha and helix. The cartilage is intact, and the tissue apposition is excellent because of adherence of skin to the cartilage template.

Skin Wound

Linear lacerations involving only the skin can be sutured (Fig. 115–5) but usually heal adequately by second intention because the rigid cartilaginous template underlying the wound maintains tissue apposition.

Suturing is mandatory when a two- or three-sided flap has been formed (Fig. 115–6). If not sutured, the flap contracts during healing, creating an area that either cannot epithelialize or does so without haired covering. These wounds must be sutured at the margin and through the center of the flap, as with aural hematomas (Fig. 115–7).

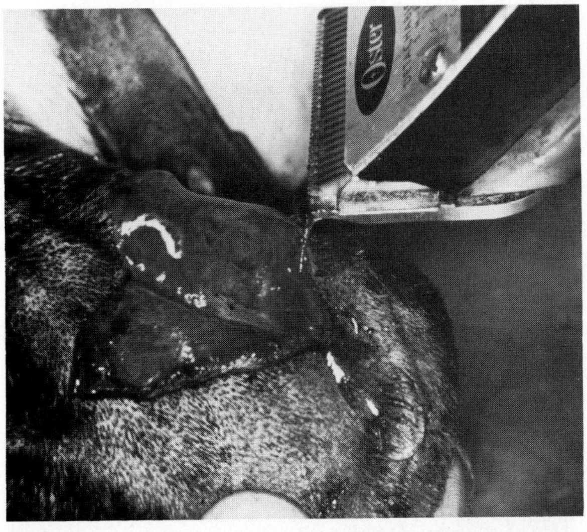

FIGURE 115–6. A traumatically raised pedicle flap on the convex surface of an ear. This wound must be sutured to prevent contracture and a hairless scar (sterile lubricant is present to protect the wound during clipping).

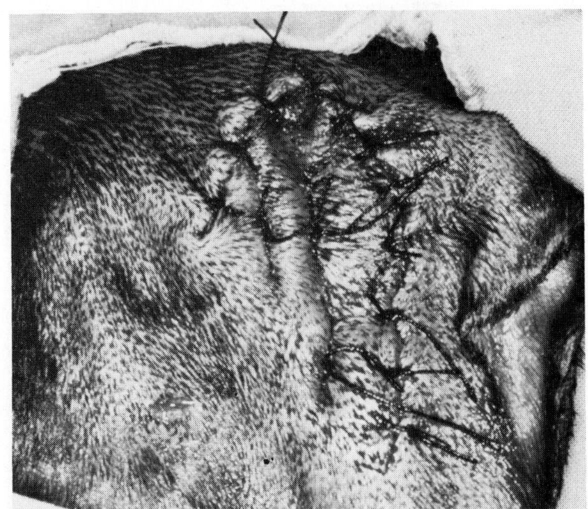

FIGURE 115–7. Sutured pedicle flap shown in Figure 115–6. The dead space has been obliterated with three through-and-through mattress sutures as with aural hematoma obliteration.

Skin and Cartilage Wound

Wounds of the skin and cartilage respond similarly to wounds of skin only, except that in longer wounds, cartilaginous support is lost and healing is delayed until fibrous union occurs. This delay results in malalignment of the cartilage margins and disfigurement of the ear. For best results, the skin is sutured using a vertical mattress pattern with the deeper bite aligning cartilage and the superficial bite aligning skin (Fig. 115–8).

Perforating Wound

Punctures or tears that extend through the pinna but not through the helical border can heal adequately with conservative protection (Fig. 115–9). An improved cosmetic appearance is obtained by suturing, particularly with long tears (Fig. 115–10).

The most serious lacerations are those in which the full thickness of the ear is lacerated through a helical border (Fig. 115–11). When these wounds are left untreated, their margins epithelialize, forming a permanent

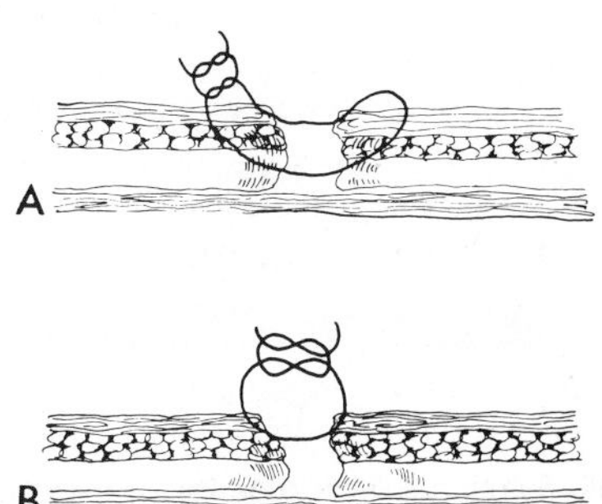

FIGURE 115–8. Suturing partial ear lacerations. *A*, Vertical mattress sutures may be used to align and stabilize the cartilage and skin. *B*, if the cartilage is stable, the wound may be closed with sutures in the skin surface only.

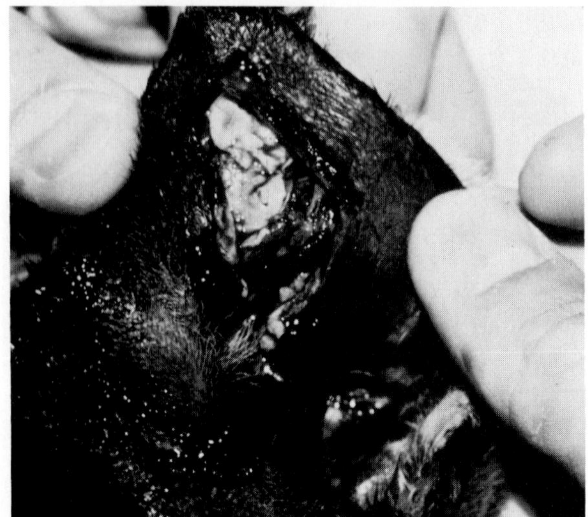

FIGURE 115–9. Contaminated wound through the entire ear but not through the helical border. This wound can be adequately managed with medical débridement and second intention healing. Pendulous-eared dogs may have more tendency toward contractural deformity.

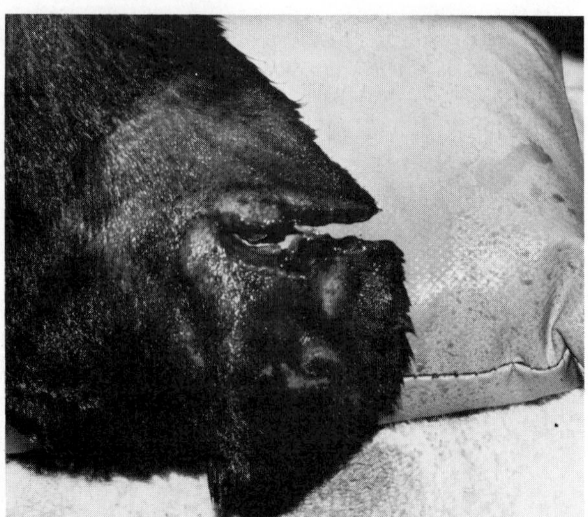

FIGURE 115–11. Auricular full-thickness lacerations through the helical border must be sutured.

defect. Contraction during healing separates the wound edges. Such lacerations should be sutured soon after injury. A line of simple interrupted sutures is placed on each surface, beginning at the helical margin to obtain perfect alignment, or one row of simple interrupted sutures is placed on one side and a vertical mattress suture aligns both skin and cartilage from the other side (see Fig. 115–10).

LOSS OF TISSUE

Inflammatory Lesions

Defects of the pinna can be caused by minor trauma (fissures), ear tip dermatitis, or avulsions. Fissure wounds of the ear begin along the distal helical border and extend for differing lengths toward or into the scapha (Fig. 115–12). They are seen most commonly in pendulous-eared dogs, are caused by continuous abrasion, and are often associated with ear margin seborrhea (e.g., in dachshunds).[6] Because these lesions are chronic, different areas may show different stages of healing.[6] Although dissimilar in cause, the ear tip dermatitis of erect ears caused by biting flies may be similar to ear fissures in effect.

The primary objective is to treat the cause of head shaking. Resolution of chronic skin disease causing ear fissure is less successful. Insect barriers or repellents usually resolve ear tip dermatitis. Though such treatment is rarely necessary, small fissures can be débrided, trimmed, and sutured. Chronic long fissures usually are contracted, making suture apposition of the wound edges impossible; if necessary, they are removed by partial amputation as described later.

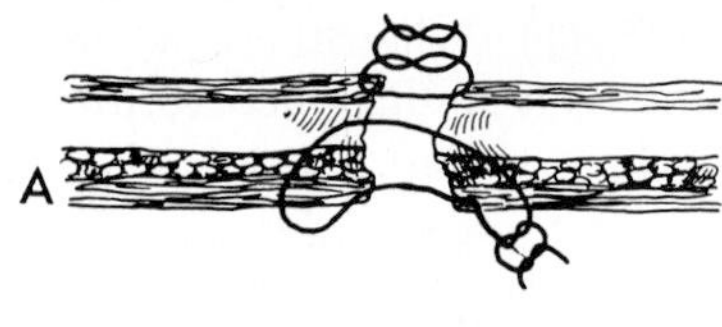

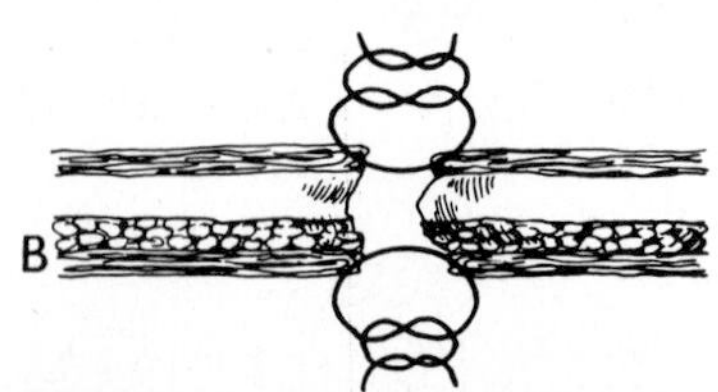

FIGURE 115–10. Suturing full-thickness ear lacerations. A vertical mattress suture may be used to align and stabilize the cartilage and the skin on one side of the ear. *A*, Simple interrupted sutures are placed in the skin on the remaining side of the ear. *B*, The wound may also be closed by simple interrupted sutures placed only through the skin on both ear surfaces.

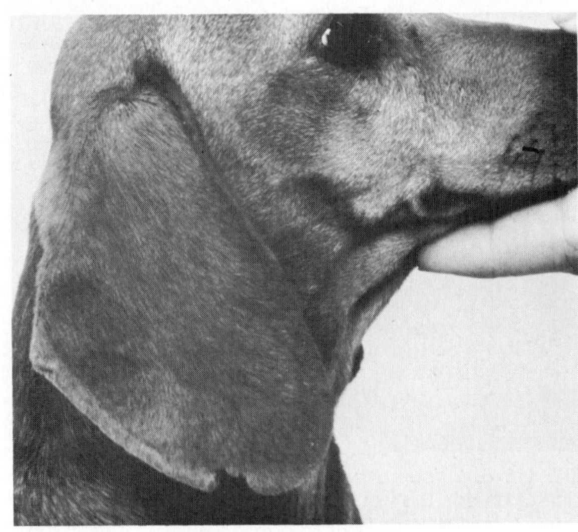

FIGURE 115–12. Ear fissure.

Avulsive Injuries

The margins of untreated avulsion wounds of the pinna heal by contracture and epithelialization. These defects widen as a result of wound contraction. Rarely is the avulsed portion small enough to suture directly without causing obvious cupping or folding of the pinna.

When hemorrhage is controlled, infection is prevented, and wound epithelialization allowed to occur, the result is still an ear with a cosmetic defect. Several methods can be used to correct the defect.

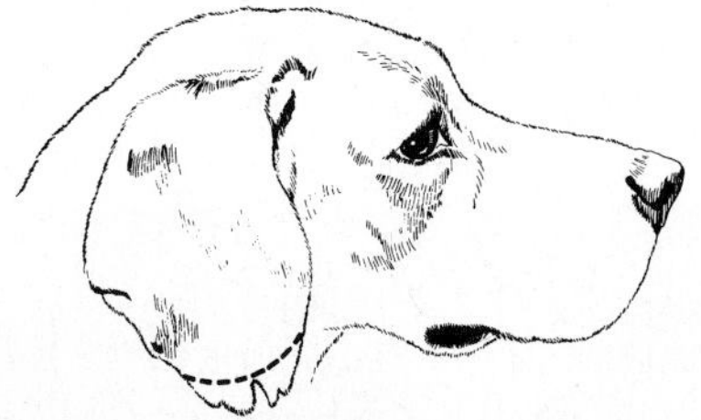

FIGURE 115–13. Partial amputation of auricle. As little tissue as possible is removed during amputation of a portion of the auricle, except when a neoplasm is present.

Partial Amputation

Ears with shallow auricular defects can be cosmetically improved by partial amputation of the auricle. The amputation need not include the apex of the avulsion, and the absolute minimum amount of tissue is excised. The ear is amputated through normal tissue as distally as possible with scissors, curving the wound to approximate normal ear shape (Fig. 115–13). Bleeding vessels are clamped and twisted rather than ligated when possible. The skin edges are apposed by rolling them together with a simple continuous 4-0 suture. The ears must be protected from trauma until completely healed.

Pedicle Flaps

A larger auricular margin defect can be reconstructed by transposing a pedicle flap from the lateral cervicobuccal region. Both the concave and convex epithelial surfaces are replaced.

After aseptic preparation, the margins of defect are débrided and straightened, removing as little tissue as possible. An antibacterial ointment is applied, the ear is bandaged, and the dressing is changed as necessary. At 7 days, the ear epithelium is thicker and more vascular, facilitating acceptance of the pedicle. The skin of the donor cervicobuccal region is loose and vascular, and the direction of hair growth generally resembles that on the convex surface of the ear, except near the ventral midline.

The donor area and the recipient (ear) area are aseptically prepared (Fig. 115–14*A*). The margins of the defect are incised to form two epithelial edges and are sharply but sparingly débrided (Fig. 115–14*B*). The ear is placed on the donor site, and the outline of the auricular defect is inscribed on the donor site. The inscribed area of donor site is incised, extending each incision limb 5 mm farther (Fig. 115–14*C* and *D*). The flap is sutured by beginning at the center of the wound. Postoperatively, a nonadhesive dressing and antibacterial ointment are applied (Fig. 115–14*E*). The ear is bandaged for 2 weeks, and the bandage is changed as necessary.

It is usually possible to complete the transfer of the flap in 2 weeks (Fig. 115–14*F*). Coverage or healing of the medial surface of the pedicle flap may be completed by one of several methods. First, the flap can be severed from the donor site at its base, and a pedicle flap from another site used to cover the concave auricular surface (Fig. 115–15). Second, after the flap is severed, the concave surface can be left to heal by second intention if the area is not too large. Third, the pedicle origin can be incised in the shape of the contralateral defect, folded upon itself, and sutured (Fig. 115–16); however, vascular necrosis may result from crimping vessels supplying the folded flap. Sutures are removed in 10 days, and unhealed surfaces are allowed to heal by second intention (Fig. 115–17).

SOLAR AND COLD INJURIES

Actinic Keratosis of White Feline Ears

The white ears of cats are predisposed to actinic keratosis of the pinnas (solar dermatitis).[6] The skin of the ear tip is exposed to more direct sunlight owing to lack of hair coverage and greater penetration of the erect hair. The initial lesions are a mild sunburn, causing alopecia. When less reduced hair protects the lesion, exposure is increased. During a period of years, the cartilage and overlying skin begin to deform. The skin overlying the helix is frequently ulcerated. The lesion is preneoplastic and may lead to squamous cell carcinoma (Figs. 115–18 and 115–19).

The therapeutic objectives are (1) to decrease the ear's exposure to direct sunlight by keeping the animal indoors during daylight or by applying sunscreen ointment to protect the ear margins and, (2) to amputate progressive ulcerative lesions. Small early lesions may be treated by cryotherapy. Measures to reduce exposure to sunlight are continued after surgery. The protective effect of tattooing the affected area has not been evaluated but may be useful.

Cold Injuries

The auricle is subjected to greater variation in temperature than other parts of the body because of its thinness and dependent position. Cold injury is fairly common in the northern regions of the United States and in Canada. It may occur when the environmental temperature is well above freezing, because of wind chill or exposure to water. In acute cold injury, the auricle feels hard and is unresponsive to painful stimuli. Severe cases undergo avascular necrosis.[8] The frozen portion forms a dry eschar and desquamates. White hair regrows on the margin, but the cosmetic appearance is generally acceptable.

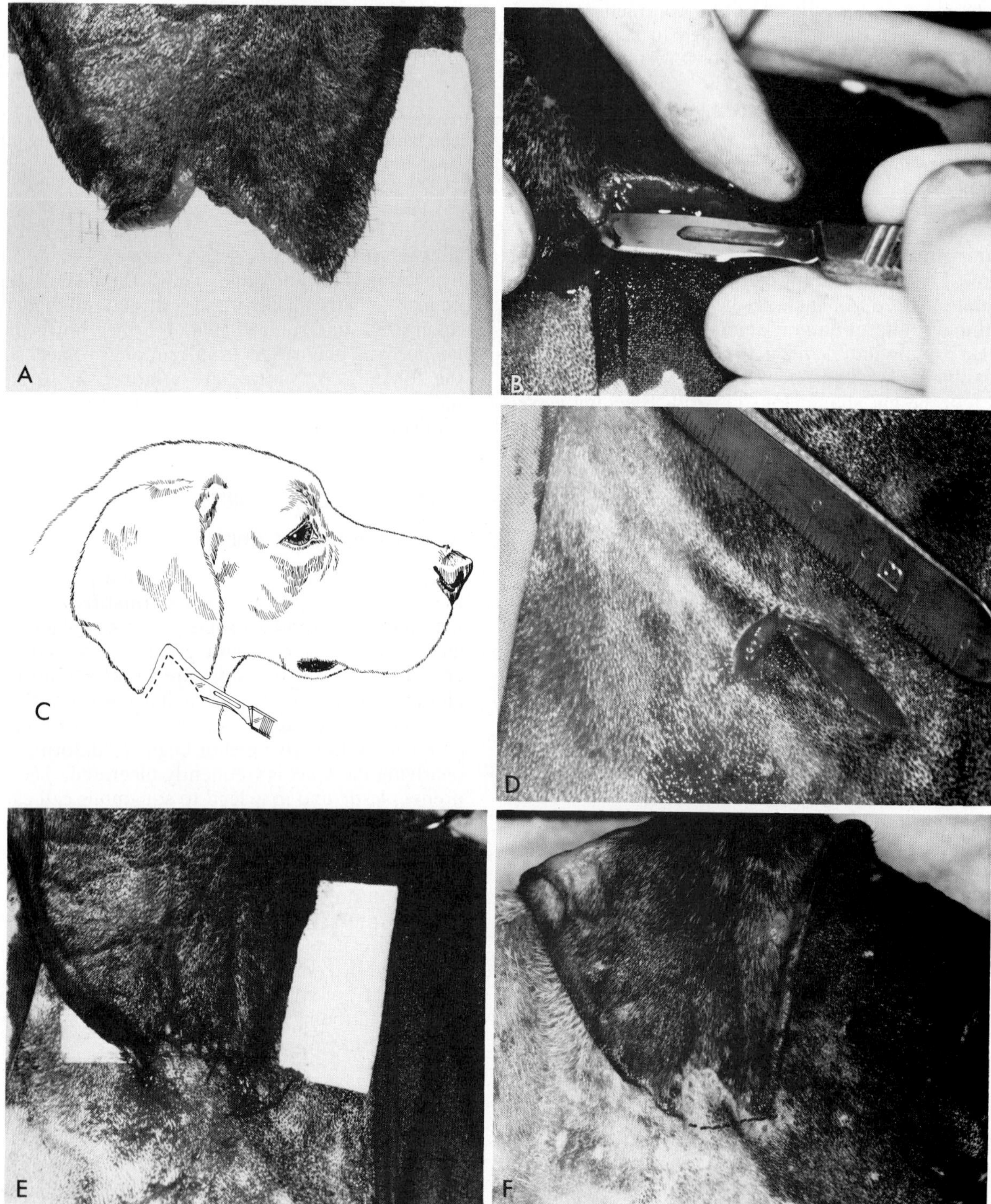

FIGURE 115–14. *A*, Marginal auricular defect to be corrected with a pedicle flap. *B*, Splitting the margin of the defect and débriding the edges. *C*, Ear in position over the cervicobuccal area, with the defect being outlined on the skin. *D*, Pedicle flap formation. The pedicle flap shape is inscribed on the donor site by direct superimposition of the recipient site defect. The incisional lengths are 0.5 cm longer than those of the recipient's margin. *E*, The pedicle is sutured into the defect with simple interrupted sutures. *F*, Two weeks after pedicle transposition. The healed flap is ready for transfer. Proposed line of excision *(dotted line).*

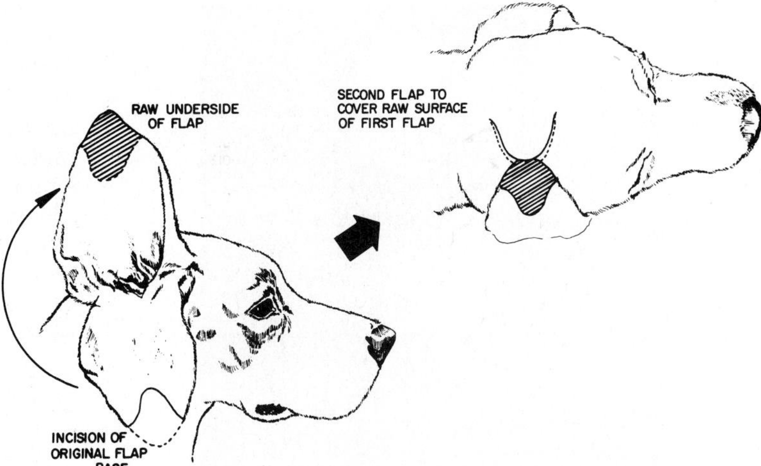

FIGURE 115–15. A technique for completing an auricular defect correction with a second flap.

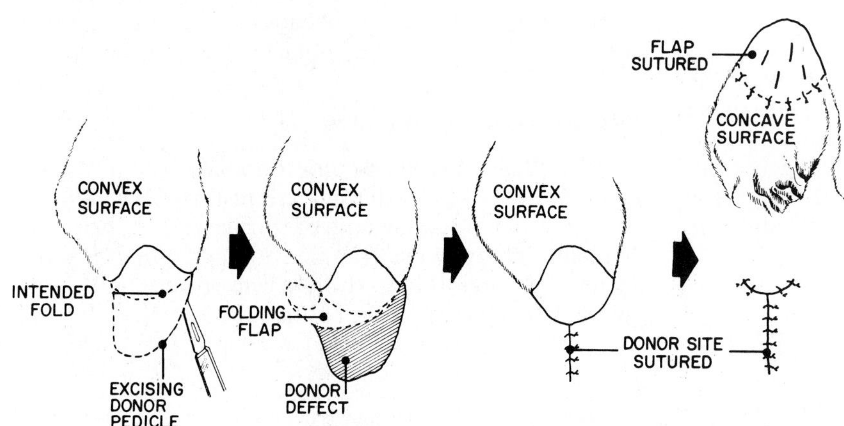

FIGURE 115–16. A second technique for completing an auricular defect correction with a folded pedicle. Vascular kinking and necrosis are more likely with this technique.

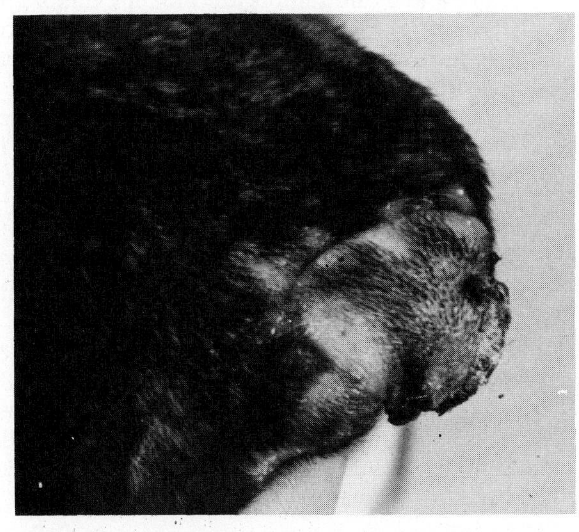

FIGURE 115–17. Completed pedicle flap after 2 weeks (convex surface).

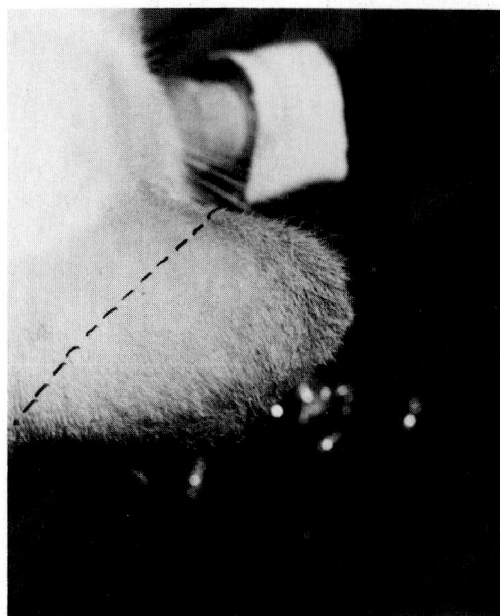

FIGURE 115–18. Feline actinic keratosis. Solar changes (distal to *broken line*), most common on the white ears of cats, are caused by chronic sun exposure.

If gangrene is already apparent, amputation of the line of demarcation is contraindicated because less tissue than expected may slough. The gangrenous area is protected with sterile dressings until sloughing is complete or nonvital tissue is identified. Healed tissues are more susceptible to subsequent cold exposure[8] and may be predisposed to neoplasia.[5]

NEOPLASIA OF THE EXTERNAL EAR

Staging and Diagnosis

Neoplasms arising from the external ear originate from the skin, adnexa, or connective tissue. Neoplasms commonly associated with the external ear include ceruminous gland or sebaceous adenoma or adenocarcinoma, papilloma, squamous cell carcinoma, histiocytoma, mast cell tumor, basal cell carcinoma, and melanosarcoma.

Ceruminous gland tumors are the only tumors unique to the pinna. They arise from apocrine glands of the ear canal and are small, rounded, nodular, or pedunculated lesions with a smooth surface and pinkish color. They remain small but recur readily after incomplete excision. Carcinomas may metastasize to the regional lymph nodes and lungs[5] (see also Chapter 153).

The objectives of treatment are to (1) examine for local or distant spread, (2) identify the histological type, (3) completely excise or destroy the tumor and affected margin, (4) use appropriate adjunctive treatment, and (5) continue periodic observation for recurrence.

Neoplasms that arise in the central portion of the pinna are more common on the convex surface. Small tumors on this surface are easily excised, because the skin is mobile and the skin defect can be closed after undermining. When the skin is undermined for closure, the dissection remains close to the cartilage to avoid vessels. Cartilage may be excised as a deep excision margin because tumors do not easily invade cartilage. Only the skin needs to be sutured. If a tumor has been removed from the concave ear surface and adequate tissue remains for closure, second intention healing under a light bandage usually is cosmetically acceptable. Transposition of a pedicle flap to the medial aspect of the pinna can be used to fill larger defects. Affected portions of the pinna and a margin of normal pinna tissue must be excised to provide local control. Unfortunately, excision is often too timid because of the fear of disfigurement, and the patient suffers metastasis.

DEVELOPMENTAL DEFORMITIES

Developmental deformities of the pinna are uncommon. Excessively small (microtia) or excessively large (macrotia) pinnae may be part of a more widespread deformity. Surgery is rarely indicated.

COSMETIC OTOPLASTY*

Cosmetic otoplasty is performed on the ears of certain breeds to meet breed specifications. There are no medical reasons for these techniques to be performed.

Standards of Ear Trimming

Regardless of the trimming standard, all ears cannot be trimmed alike. Variations are justified depending on the sex of the animal and conformation of the breed. Females generally are trimmed to have a finer ear than males. The ear is cut straight, narrower, and 3 to 6 millimeters shorter; little bell is left. Females of breeds

*Editor's note: This technique is not considered ethical and is illegal in some areas. Local details should be sought.

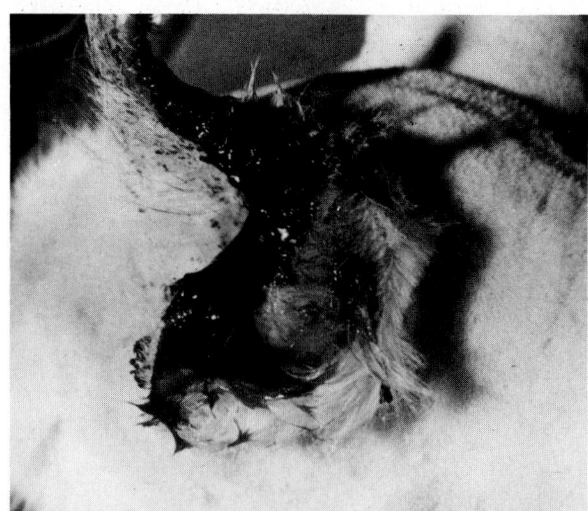

FIGURE 115–19. Squamous cell carcinoma. The contralateral ear of the cat in Figure 115–18 is shown with a squamous cell carcinoma. The lesion is crateriform, appears as a chronic wound, and resulted from chronic solar exposure.

that normally have a broad head, such as the boxer or schnauzer, can carry slightly larger and wider ears than the Doberman or the Great Dane. One should also consider the dog's sire and dam. In females likely to be large and masculine in appearance or thin-boned with fine features and in males likely to be larger and more heavily muscled, the ear trim should be adjusted accordingly.

General Considerations

Trimming the ears of a puppy that is in poor condition is delayed until the puppy's general health improves. Puppies are vaccinated before having their ears trimmed.

Age. A practical age schedule is presented in Table 115–1. Local injection of epinephrine, recommended by some to control bleeding along the incision site, is discouraged owing to its systemic effect. Because 8- to 12-week-old puppies may have insufficient glycogen stores, especially after food restriction, a 5 per cent dextrose in lactated Ringer's intravenous drip is suggested.

Surgical Technique

Instruments such as ear-trimming forms are often not satisfactory because placement is difficult and they usually fail to provide the trim desired. Finely serrated cartilage scissors are essential for the final trimming of the cartilage. With the dog in sternal recumbency and the head raised with a towel placed beneath it, the pinna and top of the head are prepared and draped for aseptic surgery (Figs. 115–20 and 115–21). Tape is placed across the muzzle to hold the head. Small pieces of cotton are placed in the external ear canal.

A triangular skin incision is made just beneath the tragus and antitragus cartilages (see Fig. 115–1) where the ear joins the head; this landmark identifies the point where the ear blends with the head (Fig. 115–22*A*). With one ear extended, a sterile ruler is used to measure

TABLE 115–1. PRACTICAL SCHEDULE FOR EAR TRIMMING IN DOGS

Breed	Age	Ear Length
Schnauzer	10 weeks	⅔ of ear left
Boxer	9–10 weeks	⅔–¾ of ear left
Doberman	8–9 weeks	¾ of ear left
Great Dane	9 weeks or 8–10 kg	¾ of ear left
Boston terrier	4–6 months	Full trim

along the rostral border of the ear, and a small nick is made at the desired length (Fig. 115–22*B*). Both ears are extended fully with the tips together, and a second nick is made in the other ear to ensure identical length (Fig. 115–22*C*).

With one ear pulled forward and held in a stretched position to avoid wrinkling the incision edge (Fig. 115–22*D*), straight Doyen intestinal forceps are placed on the ear, extending approximately two-thirds of the way from the "desired-length" nick to the tragus cartilage. The forceps are placed so that their outside edge is even with the nick at the top of the ear and the natural fold of the ear distally (see Fig. 115–22*D*). After the forceps are placed on both ears, the ears are compared to ensure identical positioning (Fig. 115–22*E*). A straight cut to the junction of the middle and distal one-third of the ear is made with the blade directed toward the edge of the intestinal forceps (Fig. 115–22*F*). The forceps are removed, and bleeding vessels are clamped with mosquito forceps and twisted. A branch of the caudal auricular artery is usually transected one-half of the distance from the ear tip to the tragus cartilage (see Fig. 115–20).

The distal third of the incision is made with finely serrated cartilage scissors. With the part of the ear to remain held in a normal standing position (Fig. 115–22*G*), the incision is continued to blend the distal third of the ear into the dog's head using a smooth, even cut (Fig. 115–22*H*). Rough edges are trimmed, and parts of

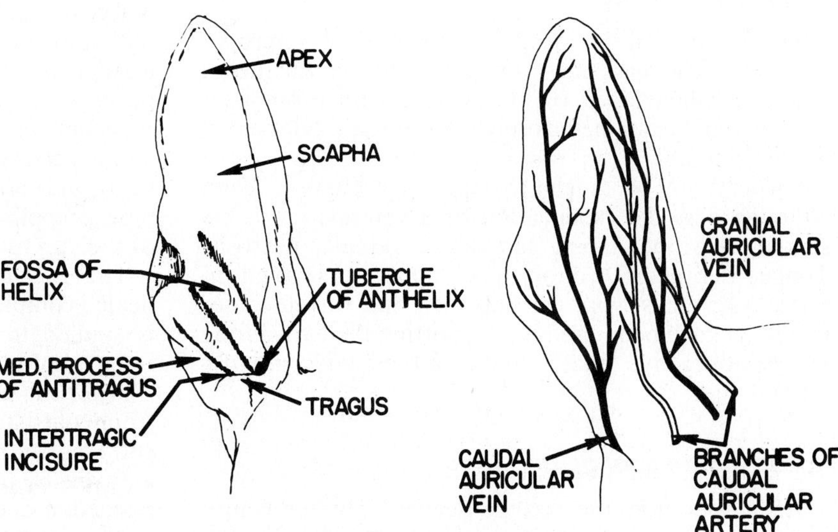

FIGURE 115–20. Anatomy and vasculature of the ear showing the tragus and antitragus cartilages and branches of the caudal auricular vein.

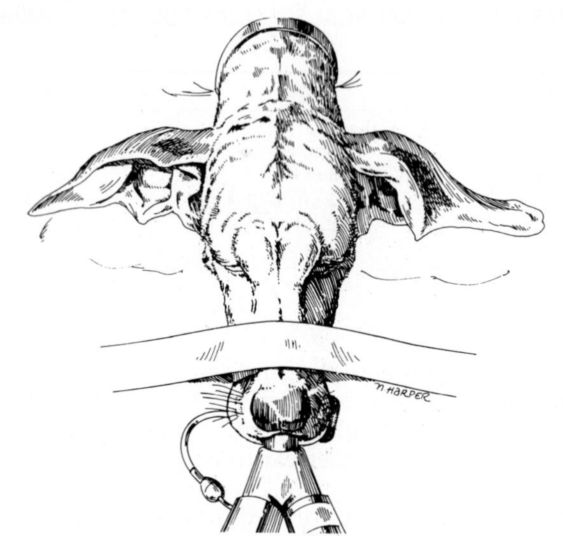

FIGURE 115–21. Proper position of the head to avoid undue pressure on the cervical area. The sandbag should not be placed too far caudally, so it does not put undue pressure on the auricular area.

the tragus and antitragus cartilages are removed to ensure a smooth appearance. The opposite ear is trimmed in the same manner, the ears are compared (Fig. 115–22*I*), and adjustments are made as necessary, usually in only the distal third of the cut.

Interrupted sutures are used to close the skin over the cut portion of the tragus cartilage and the skin defect distal to these cartilages (Fig. 115–23*A* and *B*). The main incision is closed with a simple continuous pattern of monofilament suture, beginning at the ventral aspect of the incision. Placement is from the inside out, so that the loose skin on the outside of the cartilage is rolled over the edge of the cartilage, allowing faster healing and less scar formation. The incision is closed to within 6 to 12 mm of the tip of the ear. The sutures are placed loosely and are left untied at the tips of the ear (Fig. 115–23*C*) to allow for postoperative swelling.

Postoperative Care

Many ears fail to stand out because of improper aftercare. The ears must be pulled above the head, stretched when taped or braced to obtain proper ear carriage, and examined closely for exudates, odors, and malpositioning.

Owners can be taught to tape their puppies' ears, although periodic examination by a veterinarian is essential. Improper taping can cause avascular necrosis. Tongue depressors, cotton-tipped applicators, foam inserts, wire racks, wire ear implants, and various other materials have been used for supporting the ears during the postoperative phase. Successful methods are described next.

Rolled Gauze Sponge and Tape

After operation, the ears are cleaned of blood. Gauze sponges are formed into a cone and placed inside the ear, filling the base of the ear. A strip of gauze is placed along the suture line to prevent tape from touching the incision. With the gauze cone in place and the ear held erect, tape is applied to the ear in a crisscrossing dovetail fashion. A brace formed of adhesive tape in a figure eight around the base of the two ears keeps them parallel to each other (Fig. 115–24). This support is used for about 2 weeks—on for 3 days, off for 1, on for 3 days, and so on. Sutures are removed at 7 to 10 days.

If the ears are not standing at 2 weeks, they are rolled in the direction opposite to that in which they are falling, and the tape is left in place for as long as 5 days at a time.

Cardboard Tube

After the sutures are removed at 7 to 10 days, the ears are held erect by using the cardboard applicator tube of a vaginal tampon with the cotton tampon left in place and the cotton end of the cardboard tube placed in the base of the ear. The ear is pulled or stretched above the head, and the two strips of adhesive tape are used to secure the ear to the tube; one strip is placed around the base of the ear, and the other is placed close to the tip. After 2 weeks, the cardboard tubes are discarded. Air foam with a piece of tape applied inside out is used to fill the bell at the base of the ear. The inside-out tape and a single strip of tape around the base of the ear are used to hold the foam in place. Another strip of tape close to the ear tip holds the ear in a rolled erect position. The foam is used repeatedly as needed until the ears stand permanently; it is changed when the ears become dirty or inflamed and as needed to check progress. The ears are cleaned each time the tapes are changed.

Styrofoam Cups

Immediately after surgery, while the dog is still anesthetized, a stand consisting of three Styrofoam cups, one inside the other, is placed on the dog's head. A notch is cut into the cups at the base of the ears to accommodate the scutiform cartilage. A strip of tape is placed inside out down the side of the cup, over the base, and down the other side. Elastic adhesive bandage is applied to the front and rear edges of the cups to prevent the cups from slipping and rubbing on the head. Ileostomy appliance cement is applied to the medial and lateral surfaces of the ears, which are pulled high on the head and adhered to the cup stand. A final piece of tape is applied vertically on each ear and over the top of the cup to secure the ear in place.

The ears are left in the cup stand until they have healed completely. During this time, antibiotic ointment is applied to the healing edges of the ears for easier removal of scabs.

After the cup stand is removed, the cardboard tubes from coat hangers are used for support. The tubes are cut long enough to extend from the tubercle of the anthelix to just past the end of the ear. The tube is padded at one end with Elasticon and placed in the ear, resting on the shelf formed by the tubercle of the

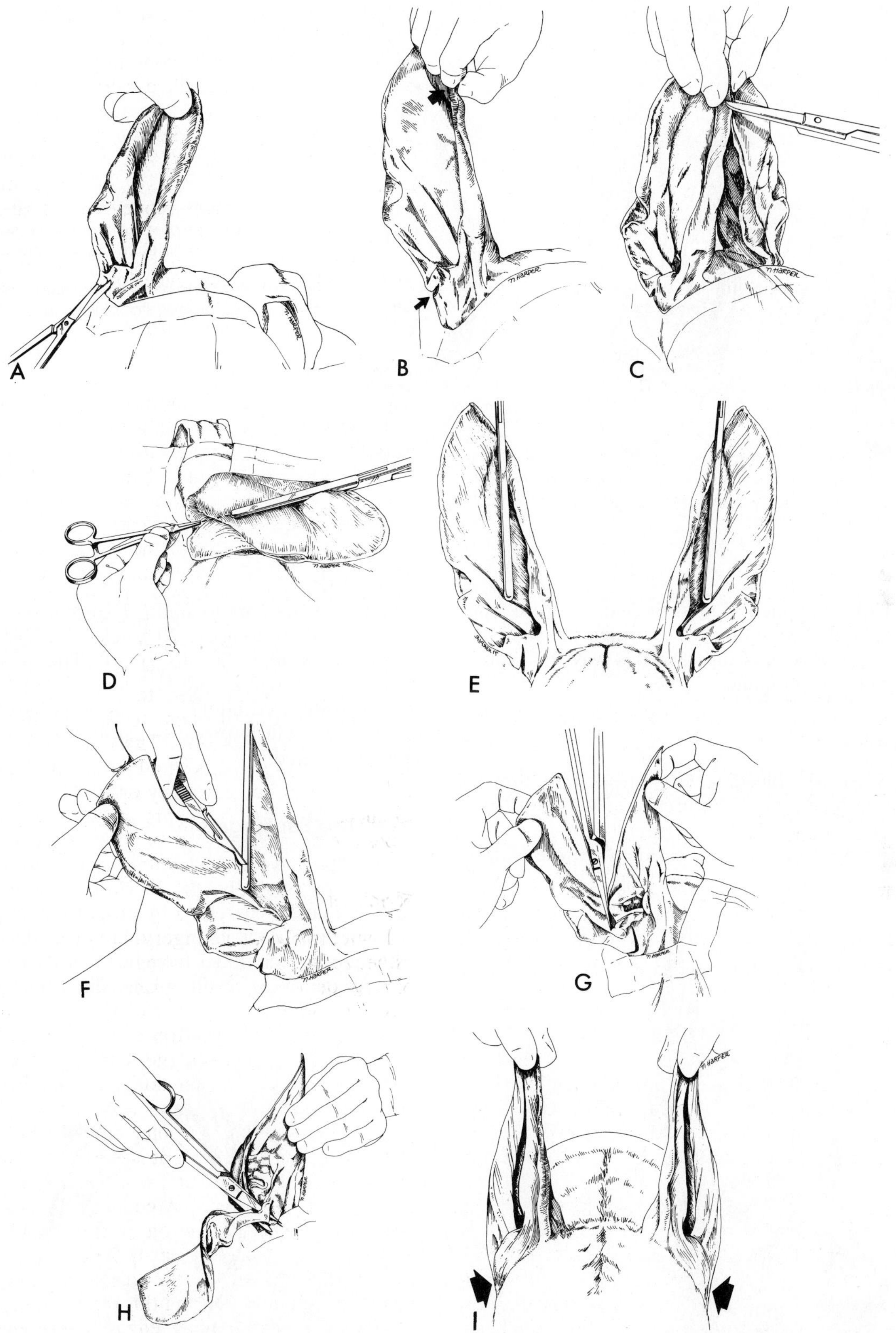

FIGURE 115–22. *A*, Initial skin incision beneath the tragus and antitragus cartilages serves as a future landmark. *B*, Position of the ear for determining the proper length. A small "pinch" mark is made on the rostal border of the ear with the index finger. *C*, Ears extended fully with the tips together. A small incision is made in both ears to ensure identical length. *D*, Position of the ear for placing the intestinal forceps in an identical manner. The broken line follows the natural fold in the ear. *E*, Position of the forceps from a cranial view. The ears should be closely observed to ensure that both forceps are placed in an identical position. *F*, Initial cut outside the forceps, stopping short of the end of the forceps. *G*, Continuation of the incision after removal of the forceps. No attempt is made to put a distinct "bell" in the distal one-third of the ear. *H*, Completion of the incision, blending the ear to the side of the head. Portions of the tragus and antitragus cartilages are removed. The final portion of the incision joins the initial incision (see Fig. 115–27). *I*, Observation of the ears to ensure that both are identical. Additional trimming may be necessary. Notice how the ears blend into the sides of the head *(arrows)*.

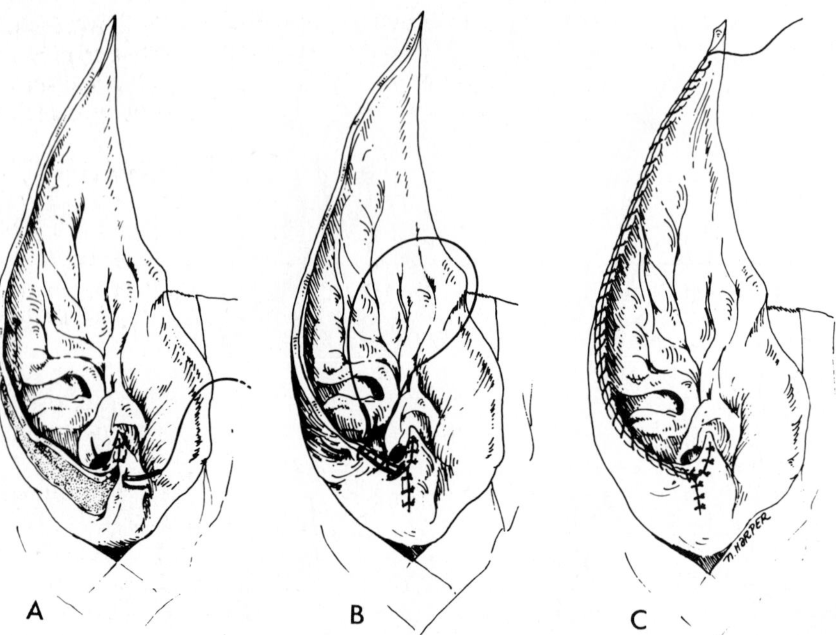

FIGURE 115–23. *A* and *B*, Initial closure with sutures placed through the skin edges only. *C*, Completion of the closure with interrupted sutures placed at the base of the ear and a continuous suture along the edge of the ear, stopping ½ inch from the tip. The suture is left untied.

anthelix. Tape is applied around the ear and tube both at the base and distally and as a bridge between the ears. The ear can remain taped in this way for as long as 2 weeks before retaping.

Complications

During recovery, bleeding is controlled to prevent postoperative hematomas. Sutures should be well tied but not tight.

The most severe problem, at least in the owner's eyes, is failure of the ears to stand. External support may be required for as long as 20 weeks. Despite prolonged efforts, ears may fail to stand. The most common problems are medial and lateral deviation of the tip of the ear (discussed later). Ear supports based inside the ear are particularly prone to cause otitis externa, which must be treated.

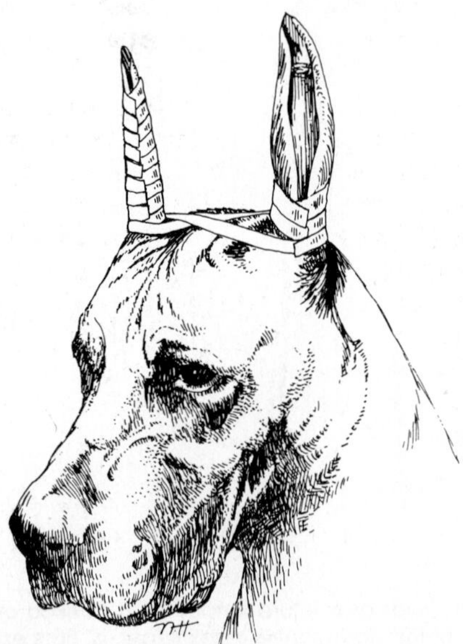

FIGURE 115–24. A 4 × 4 gauze sponge folded tightly in the shape of a cone is placed in the external ear canal. Short strips of 1-inch adhesive tape are placed around the ear. A piece of tape is placed around the top of the head in a figure-eight fashion to hold the ear erect.

Corrective Ear Surgery

Ears that have been trimmed surgically may deviate laterally or medially. If discovered early, faulty ear carriage may be corrected by proper taping procedures, particularly in dogs younger than 6 months.

Numerous techniques have been used to correct faulty ear carriage; most result in only slight improvement.

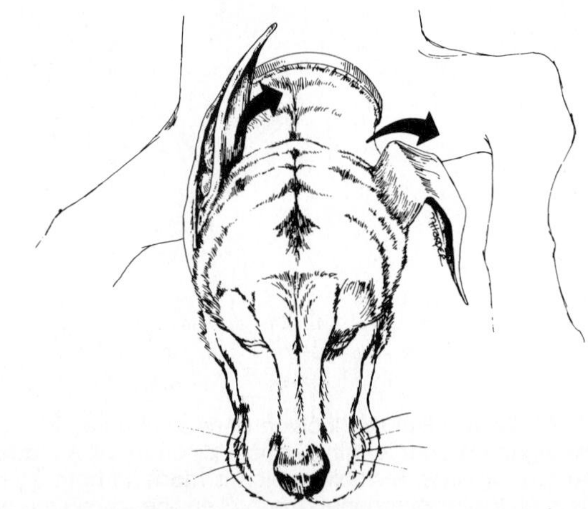

FIGURE 115–25. Position of the head for surgery. Support is provided by placing a sandbag underneath the head. Note the lateral deviation of the left ear and medial deviation of the right ear *(arrows)*.

If the owner and veterinarian are patient and willing to subject the animal to one or more surgical procedures, faulty ear carriage can usually be corrected. The direction of the break in the cartilage, the location of the break, and the position of the scutiform cartilage determine the surgical technique to be used and whether two or more procedures may be necessary.

Conservative Treatment

Conservative treatment must be started as soon as possible. The ear is rolled opposite to the way it is breaking. When the ear is deviated over the top of the head or stands so that it is carried too far medially, it must be rolled away from the dog's head. The ear is grasped and pulled upward as tightly as possible. The index finger is placed in the external ear canal, and the ear is rolled away from the head and around the finger. Starting close to the base of the ear, 1-inch adhesive tape or masking tape in 3- to 5-inch strips is applied to the ear in the same direction as the roll. The tape is carried approximately two-thirds of the way from the base to the tip of the ear. The ear must be stretched tightly, pulling the scutiform cartilage toward the center of the head. Tape is left on the ear for 5 days, and the ear is observed for 1 day to see if improvement has occurred. It is often necessary to replace the tape for another week before faulty ear carriage is corrected. If little improvement is noted after 2 weeks, corrective surgery is necessary.

With a lateral deviation of the ear, the index finger is inserted into the external canal, and the ear is pulled as tightly as possible and rolled toward the center of the head. Again, the tape is applied in the same direction as the roll. The ears look extremely awkward when taped in this position, but the end result is often good.

Surgical Correction

The ears are prepared, and the animal is positioned as for ear trimming (Fig. 115–25).

Medial Deviation. In most instances, only one procedure is necessary. When the ear breaks toward the head, the scutiform cartilage has usually dropped ventrally, and a distinct fold is seen in the cartilage on the medial aspect of the ear (Fig. 115–26*A*).

A longitudinal incision is made through the skin at the junction of the ear and the base of the skull, extending from approximately 6 mm caudal to the rostral edge of the ear to 12 to 16 mm cranial to the border of

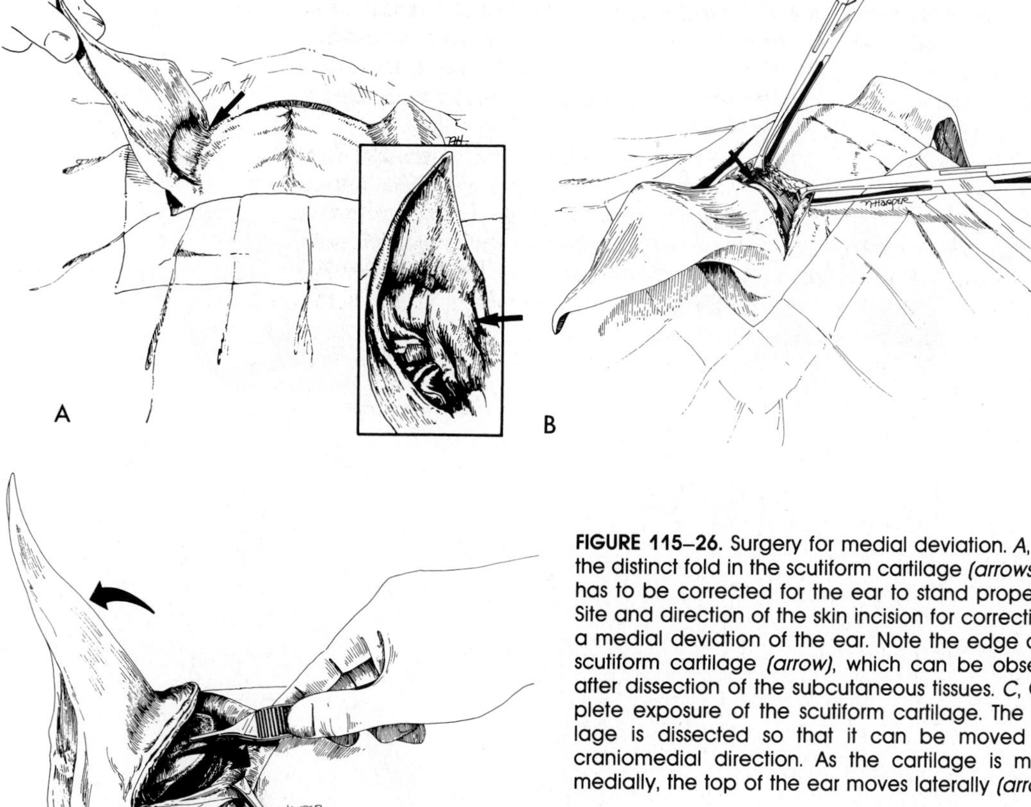

FIGURE 115–26. Surgery for medial deviation. *A*, Note the distinct fold in the scutiform cartilage *(arrows)*. This has to be corrected for the ear to stand properly. *B*, Site and direction of the skin incision for correction of a medial deviation of the ear. Note the edge of the scutiform cartilage *(arrow)*, which can be observed after dissection of the subcutaneous tissues. *C*, Complete exposure of the scutiform cartilage. The cartilage is dissected so that it can be moved in a craniomedial direction. As the cartilage is moved medially, the top of the ear moves laterally *(arrow)*.

the ear (Fig. 115–26*B*). The incision is carried through the subcutaneous tissues, and the scutiform cartilage is exposed by blunt dissection (Fig. 115–26*C*). The cartilage is dissected free of its muscular attachments, pulled medially and slightly rostrally, and sutured to the temporal fascia using 3-0 monofilament nonabsorbable sutures in a horizontal mattress pattern (Fig. 115–27). If this maneuver does not correct the deformity, it is necessary to remove an elliptical piece of skin at the break in the cartilage on the medial aspect of the ear. This procedure is reserved for a later time because it is often unnecessary. The subcutaneous tissues and skin are closed. A gauze sponge rolled into a cone is inserted into the ear. If necessary, a small strip of gauze sponge is placed over the incision site, and the ear is taped from the base to the tip while rolled away from the head.

Lateral Deviation. When the ear sits high on the head and the dog has good control of its base, the only procedure necessary is removal of an elliptical piece of skin on the external surface at the level of the break (Fig. 115–28). The amount of skin to be removed is critical, because it is possible to create a medial deviation if too much is removed.

When the ear breaks at the base of the skull, a more involved surgical procedure is necessary. A longitudinal incision is made at the base of the ear (Fig. 115–28*A*), and the subcutaneous tissues are incised to expose the scutiform cartilage. The cartilage is partially dissected free from its muscular attachments and moved 12 to 16 mm medially and slightly rostrally from its original position, pulling the base of the ear closer to the head. The cartilage is sutured to the temporal muscle fascia with nonabsorbable horizontal mattress sutures. An elliptical piece of skin is removed at the site of the skin incision, the amount of skin removed being determined by the severity of the lateral deviation. In most dogs, removal of 12 to 16 mm of skin, measured at the center of the elliptical incision, is necessary. The skin incision is closed using a vertical mattress suture pattern: A deep bite is taken through the skin on the skull, and the suture material is carried through the subcutaneous tissue, between the skin and scutiform cartilage, partially through the cartilage itself, through the subcutaneous tissue between the skull and the ear, and then through the skin on the ear (Fig. 115–28*B*). The suture is continued by taking shallow bites through the skin edges. Tension is placed on the suture, and the ear is pulled upward. One can determine the amount of tension to be placed on the suture material and the depth of the deep bites of the vertical mattress suture pattern by the position of the ear, which should stand with approximately a 10° lateral deviation (Fig. 115–28*C*). Three such sutures are usually needed to ensure correct ear carriage. Either a vertical mattress or a simple interrupted suture pattern is used to complete the closure of the skin incision. A gauze sponge rolled into a

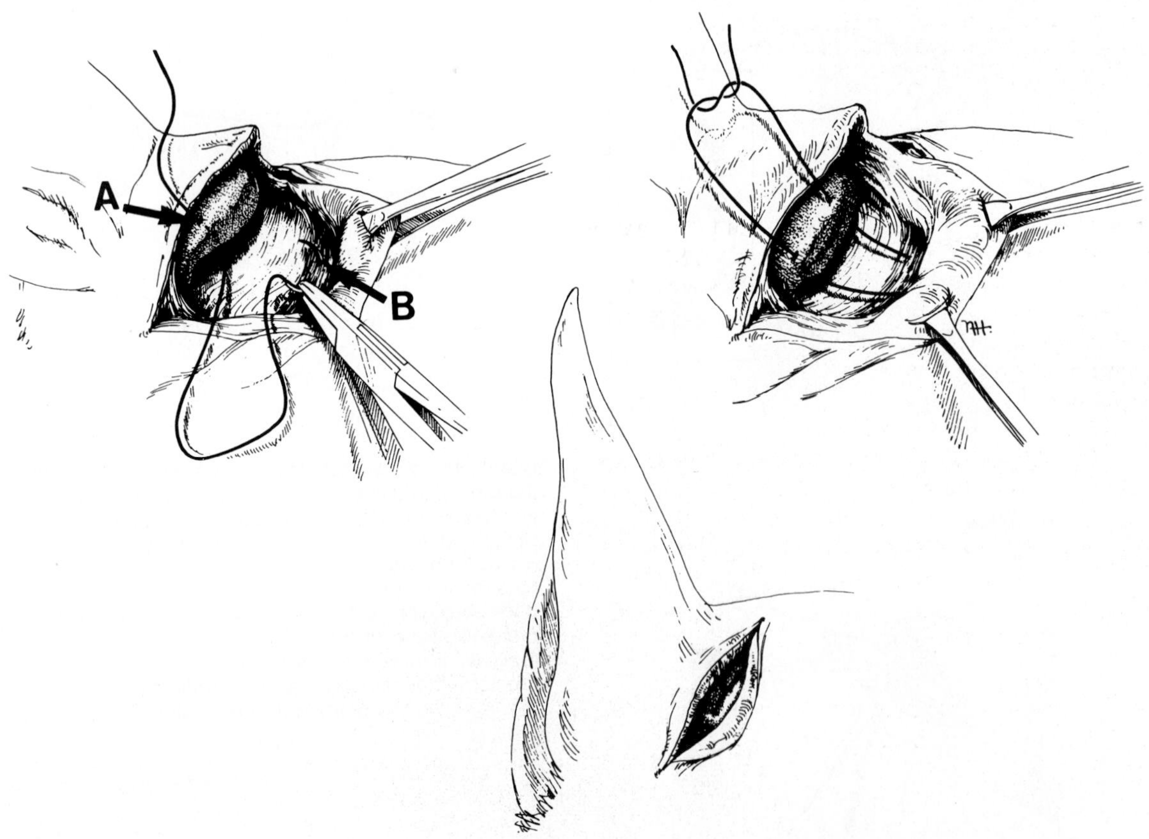

FIGURE 115–27. Proper placement of the mattress suture. The suture is placed through the cartilage and into the temporal fascia using a horizontal mattress suture pattern (A and B). When the suture is tied, the ear assumes the correct position. Closure is routine.

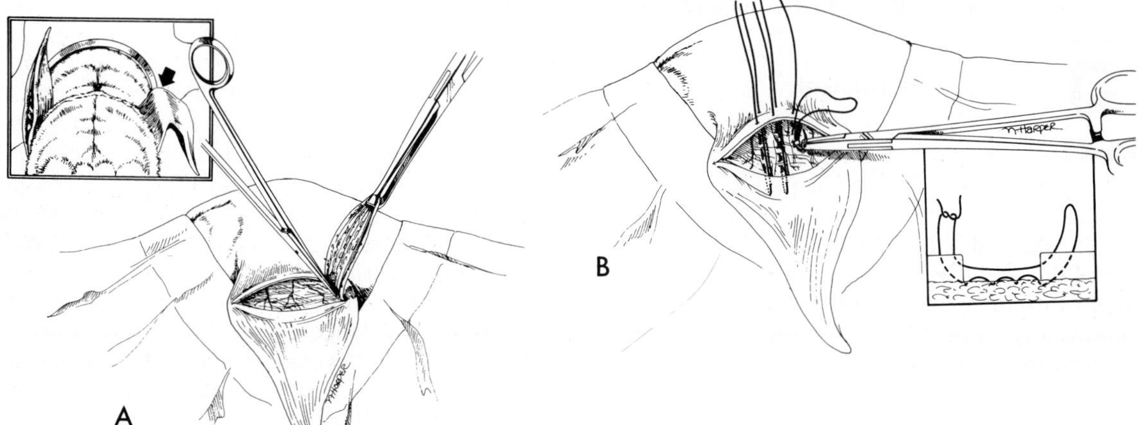

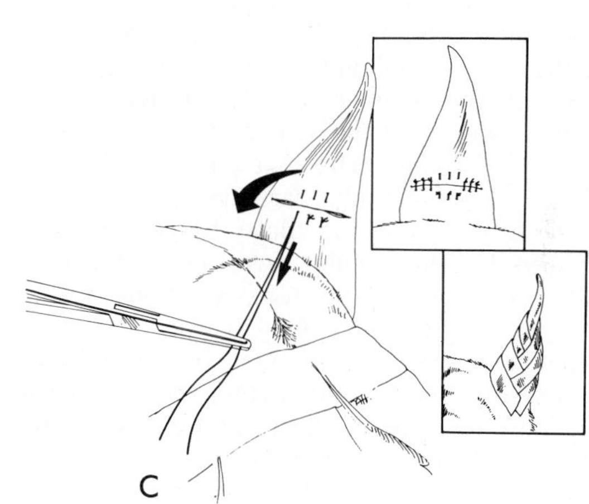

FIGURE 115–28. *A*, Location and direction of the skin incision for correction of a lateral deviation of the ear. Note that the incision is made directly over the "break" in the ear *(inset, arrow)*. The amount of skin to be removed is determined by the severity of the deviation; it is better to remove too little than too much. *B*, Proper placement of three vertical mattress sutures. Note that the deep bite is carried through the subcutaneous tissues *(inset)*. This is perhaps the most important step in the closure and in most instances ensures correction of a lateral deviation. Proper tension on the sutures can be judged by the position of the ear when the sutures are tightened. *C*, Complete closure of the skin defect. Note that the ear stands with approximately a 10° lateral deviation. This is important because scar tissue usually pulls the ear medially. *Lower inset*, The ear is bandaged by placing a gauze sponge rolled in the shape of a cone in the external ear canal. The ear is folded around the sponge from both a cranial and caudal direction. Tape is applied in a "dovetail" fashion. The bandage is left in place for 3 days. In most instances, further bandaging is unnecessary.

cone is placed over the incision site, and the ear is bandaged from the base to the tip (Fig. 115–28*C*).

The ear is left taped for 3 to 5 days and then rebandaged for 5 more days. If the operation has been successful, the ear should be standing in a relatively normal position at 8 to 10 days. If the ear fails to stand properly, it may be necessary to remove another elliptical piece of skin. This "excision" should include the old scar. The skin edges are approximated with either vertical mattress or simple interrupted sutures. The second procedure is delayed for at least 1 month so that results of the initial procedure can be properly evaluated.

References

1. Bostock DE, Owens LN: *Neoplasia in the Cat, Dog and Horse*. Year Book Medical Publishers, Chicago, 1975.
2. Brodey RS, Harvey CE: Atresia of the vertical ear canal in a dog. *J Am Vet Med Assoc 155*:1457, 1969.
3. Cowley F: Treatment of hematoma of the canine ear. *Vet Med/Small Anim Clin 71*:283, 1976.
4. Dorn CR: Epidemiology of canine and feline tumors. *J Am Anim Hosp Assoc 12*:307, 1976.
5. Fraser G, et al: Otitis externa in the dog. *J Small Anim Pract 2*:32, 1961.
6. Getty R, et al: The macroscopic anatomy of the ear of the dog. *Am J Vet Res 17*:364, 1956.
7. Getty RG: The ear. *In* Miller ME, et al (eds): *Anatomy of the Dog*. W.B. Saunders, Philadelphia, 1964.
8. Hardy WD, Jr.: General concepts of canine and feline tumors. *J Am Anim Hosp Assoc 12*:295, 1976.
9. Hayden DW: Squamous carcinoma in a cat with intraocular and orbital metastases. *Vet Pathol 13*:332, 1976.
10. Jabara AG: A mixed tumor and an adenoma both of ceruminous gland origin in a dog. *Aust Vet J 52*:590, 1976.
11. Katsas A, et al: Carcinomas on old frostbites. *Am J Surg 133*:377, 1976.
12. Mueller GH, Kirk RW: Feline solar dermatitis. *In* Muller GH, et al (eds): *Small Animal Dermatology*. 2nd ed. W.B. Saunders, Philadelphia, 1976.
13. Ott RL: Ears. *In* Archibald J (ed): *Canine Surgery*. American Veterinary Publications, Santa Barbara, 1965.
14. Pandy NJ: Experimental production of "cauliflower ear" in rabbits. *Plast Reconstr Surg 53*:534, 1973.
15. Shambaugh GE: *Surgery of the Ear*. 2nd ed. W.B. Saunders, Philadelphia, 1967.
16. Snow JB, Jr.: Surgical disorders of the ears, nose, paranasal sinuses, pharynx, and larynx. *In* Sabiston DC, Jr. (ed): *Davis-Christopher Textbook of Surgery*. 12th ed. W.B. Saunders, Philadelphia, 1981.
17. Vine LL: Corrective ear surgery. *Vet Med/Small Anim Clin 69*:1015, 1974.
18. Wilson JW: Treatment of aural hematoma, using a teat tube. *J Am Vet Med Assoc 182*:1081, 1983.

CHAPTER 116 External Ear Canal

D. J. Krahwinkel

Diseases of the ear canal account for a significant percentage of the problems encountered by small animal practitioners. Proper management of these diseases requires a knowledge of anatomy, physiology, pathophysiology, medical management, and surgical procedures.

ANATOMY AND PHYSIOLOGY

The external ear canal is a funnel-shaped tube of cartilage and bone extending from the external acoustic meatus at the base of the pinna to the tympanic membrane. The function of the canal is to receive and transmit sound waves to the tympanic membrane for the generation of sound. The first part of the canal, formed by the rolled auricular cartilage, joins with the short tube-shaped annular cartilage to complete the canal (Fig. 116–1). The annular cartilage is attached to the auricular cartilage and the temporal bone by ligaments that permit limited mobility of the canal.[7] The vertical portion of the canal (formed by the auricular cartilage) courses ventrally and slightly rostrally before turning medially to form the horizontal canal (formed by a portion of the auricular and the annular cartilage). The horizontal canal terminates in a short osseous external canal that is a projection of the petrous temporal bone.[10] The external meatus of a cat has a more pronounced flare, and the vertical canal tapers ventrally instead of forming a cylindrical tube.[31]

The external ear canal has a cutaneous lining of stratified squamous epithelium with glandular components and hair.[19] Sebaceous glands are located superficially below the epithelial surface, with the tubular apocrine (ceruminous) glands in the deeper layers of the epithelium. Secretions from these glands combined with desquamated epithelium form ear wax. Glands and hairs are numerous in the vertical canal but become sparse in the horizontal portion.

The great auricular artery, a branch from the external carotid, is the arterial blood supply to the ear canal. It arises medial to the dorsal apex of the parotid salivary gland, which overlies the vertical portion of the canal.[10] The vagus nerve supplies sensory innervation to the external canal, and the motor supply is via the facial nerve. The facial nerve leaves the skull through the stylomastoid foramen caudal to the osseous bulla and crosses the ventral surface of the horizontal canal (Fig. 116–1).

OTITIS EXTERNA

Otitis externa has a prevalence of 5 to 20 per cent in dogs and 2 per cent in cats[1] and is the most common ear disease in veterinary practice.[3] In dogs, miniature poodles, cocker spaniels, and fox terriers have the highest incidence, and Himalayan and Persian cats may also be at risk. Dogs 5 to 8 years of age are more prone to otitis; this tendency may reflect an overall increased prevalence of skin disorders. Cats are more affected at 1 to 2 years of age, possibly because of an increased incidence of ear mites. No sex predilection has been described, but otitis peaks in the summer months.[19]

Pendulous and hair-filled ears predispose to otitis.[3,4] Differences in the number and distribution of adnexal structures and overall skin disease may provide better explanations for the breed association.[19]

Etiology

The causes of otitis externa are numerous, and it is most often a multifactorial disease. It is essential to consider each of the etiological agents. The anatomy of the ear and the presence of hair in the canal may predispose to infection. Bacterial pathogens include *Staphylococcus*, *Streptococcus*, *Pseudomonas*, *Proteus*, *Escherichia coli* and *Corynebacterium*.[1,9,10,19] Although otitis may be caused by a single species of bacteria, a combination of organisms are more commonly isolated. Small numbers of gram-positive organisms are cultured from normal ears. Gram-negative bacteria are usually found only in diseased ears.[19] *Staphylococcus* is the most common organism isolated, with *Proteus* the most common gram-negative organism in dogs and *Pasturella* the most common gram-negative organism in cats.

As with bacteria, small numbers of yeasts may be isolated from normal ears.[9,19] If environmental conditions are favorable, these organisms can produce disease. *Malassezia canis* is the most common yeast isolated from otitis cases and may be found alone or in combination with bacteria.[1,19] *Candida* may also be found in diseased ears.

Otodectes cyanotis is a mite that commonly causes otitis in cats and occasionally in dogs.[1,9,19] Other parasites leading to otitis include fleas, spinous ear ticks, *Demodex*, chiggers, and *Cheyletiella*.[19] Irritation due to foreign bodies may produce otitis by creating an environment favorable to opportunistic bacteria and fungi. In certain regions, grass awns (foxtails) are found within the ear canal.

Atopy, food allergy, and contact sensitivities may predispose or cause otitis.[1,9,19] The ear canal is often affected by diseases that cause generalized skin disorders. These diseases may be seasonal or related to diet and topical medications. Metabolic diseases including hypothyroidism and seborrhea may cause severe otitis. The appearance can be that of an oily film or large, soft flakes within the ear canal.[19] Finally, immune-mediated diseases, such as lupus, pemphigus vulgaris, and pem-

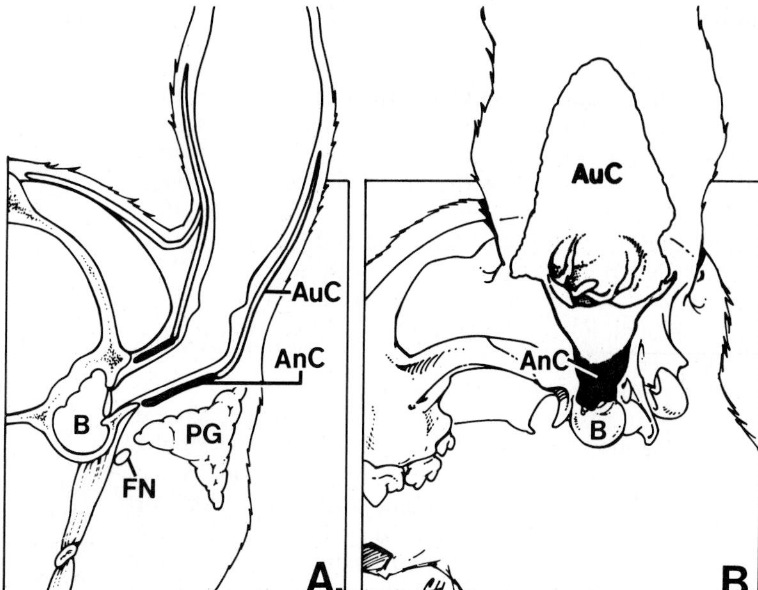

FIGURE 116–1. Transverse *(A)* and lateral *(B)* views of the anatomy of the external ear canal of a dog. (AuC, auricular cartilage; AnC, annular cartilage; PG, parotid salivary gland; FN, facial nerve; B, osseous bulla.)

phigus foliaceous may be manifested as otitis externa.[1,9] As with many cases of otitis, the therapeutic objective is to control these diseases when a cure is not possible.

Pathophysiology

Many cases of otitis are an extension of systemic diseases.[5,24] The inciting causes of otitis externa are varied and in many instances multifactoral. Once the disease begins, its progression is quite similar despite the original etiology.

The inflammatory response with otitis results in damage to the superficial protective stratum corneum of the canal.[9,24] Hyperplasia and hypertrophy of sebaceous and ceruminous glands occur, along with a diffuse cellular infiltration of macrophages, mast cells, lymphocytes, plasma cells, neutrophils, and eosinophils. Moisture, debris, foreign bodies, hair, and glandular secretions are trapped because of the shape of the canal. Retained wax is broken down by the lipolytic action of microorganisms.[9] Erosions and ulcerations occur within the canal, resulting in serum exudates and necrotic debris, which form additional culture media for bacterial proliferation.

Metabolic disorders are associated with increased secretion of free fatty acids.[9] Allergic reactions result in mast cell degranulation and release of lymphokines.[9] Parasites elicit both allergic and mechanical irritation in the canal. Long-standing otitis results in significant hyperplasia of the dermis and epidermis and stenosis of the lumen of the canal.[19] Fibroplasia of the dermis in chronic cases can result in total occlusion of the external auditory meatus. This chronic inflammatory response may give rise to polyps in cats.[19] The tympanic membrane opacifies, scleroses, ulcerates, and eventually ruptures, predisposing to otitis media.

Clinical Signs

Early in this complex disease, clinical signs may be pruritus, manifested by scratching, rubbing the ears, and shaking the head. Mild erythema of the ear canal is noticed. As the disease evolves, the signs become more intense. The animal becomes head shy and exhibits pain when examined. Aural exudate becomes prominent, varying from dry, brown exudate of *Otodectes cyanotis* to a purulent, smelly exudate of bacterial infection. As end-stage disease approaches, the external acoustic meatus becomes completely obstructed with proliferative granulation tissue (Fig. 116–2). Infection and ulceration may erode through the wall of the ear canal and result in a para-aural abscess and fistula.[17,21] In one study, 80 per cent of dogs with end-stage ear disease had one or more dermatological problems, including seborrhea, pyoderma, atopy, or hypothyroidism.[21] Some animals have neurological signs such as facial nerve paralysis, vestibular signs, and head tilt.[22] Severe infection may extend to the temporomandibular joint or surrounding tissues, resulting in pain when opening the mouth.[9] Chronic infection causes calcification of the ear cartilages.[2,6,21,25]

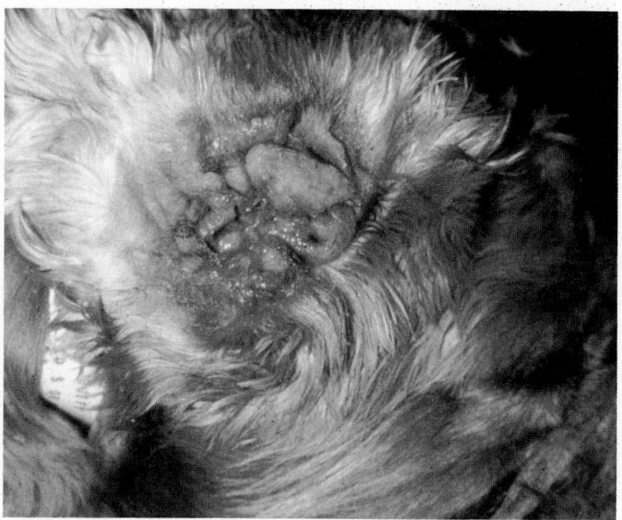

FIGURE 116–2. Cocker spaniel with severe proliferative otitis requiring surgical management.

Diagnosis

The diagnosis of otitis externa is simple. Clinical signs and physical examination reveal the disease. Determining whether the disease is an extension of a systemic disorder or a localized problem may become more difficult. Definitive diagnosis necessitates a thorough examination of the ear, which usually requires sedation or anesthesia, cytological study and culture of the aural exudate, allergy testing, endocrine evaluation, and determination of immune diseases. Although present in high numbers, microorganisms may be opportunistic and disguise the primary systemic cause.

Radiography is of value in some cases to determine the extent of disease. Cartilage calcification may extend to the osseous bulla (Fig. 116–3). Changes in the bulla suggesting severe otitis externa with extension to the middle ear include osseous bulla thickening, lysis, or periosteal reaction and radiodense tympanic cavity (see Chapter 117).[21, 22, 25] Radiographic evaluation may reveal occlusion of the ear canal. Radiographs often fail to demonstrate extension of the disease to the middle ear even when present.[22, 28] Computed tomography or magnetic resonance imaging provides information regarding middle ear involvement.

Examination and Medical Therapy

The first step in proper management of otitis externa is careful examination and evaluation of the ear canal. A ceruminolytic agent applied to the ears a few hours before the examination softens debris and exudate. Deep sedation or light general anesthesia is required for examination and cleaning. Samples are collected for culture and cytological study before adding chemicals to the ear canal. The canal is gently irrigated with warm water or saline to remove exudate and debris. The addition of 0.5 per cent chlorhexidine or 1:100 povidone-iodine to the lavage solution is beneficial for antimicrobial effect but may be toxic to the middle ear if the tympanic membrane is ruptured.[5, 19] Lavage and suction should be under gentle pressure with a soft catheter to avoid rupture of the tympanic membrane. Water propulsion devices are effective in cleaning the canal but can injure the tympanum.[5] Residual debris and foreign bodies are carefully removed with alligator forceps. Suspect neoplasms are examined with the otoscope and sampled with small biopsy forceps.

After the canal is cleaned and dried, specific antimicrobials and anti-inflammatory and drying agents are applied. Definitive treatment depends on the total evaluation of the patient for systemic disease and the results of the ear culture, antimicrobial susceptibility, and cytological study. Some have questioned the value of culture and susceptibility testing for determining proper medication, except for selection of systemic antibiotics.[5] Systemic causes of otitis and many local diseases require both systemic and topical therapy.[19]

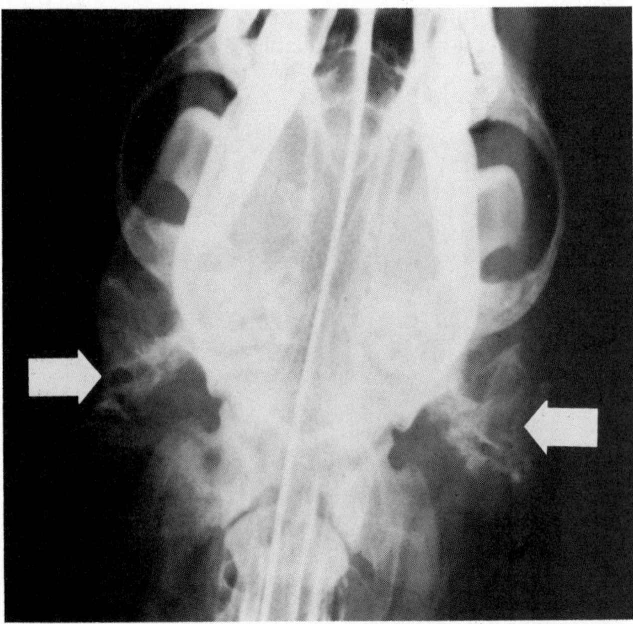

FIGURE 116–3. Radiograph illustrating calcification of the auricular cartilages *(arrows)*.

Surgical Therapy

The importance of surgery in management of otitis externa has long been recognized.[11] Lacroix made famous a procedure for removing a portion of the lateral wall of the canal for drainage of otitis.[14] Zepp improved the procedure by establishing a "drain board" from the lateral wall to maintain horizontal canal patency.[34] Other procedures used in the management of advanced ear canal disease include ablation of the vertical canal and total ear canal ablation with bulla osteotomy.

Lateral Wall Resection (Zepp procedure)

Lateral wall resection is indicated when (1) otitis externa has not responded favorably to proper medical management, (2) otitis externa has recurred despite proper medical management, (3) exposure is needed for biopsy or to remove benign polyps of the canal. (In the first two instances, it is important that irreversible hyperplastic disease has not occurred.)

Lateral wall resection permits drainage of the ear canal and provides ventilation to reduce moisture, humidity, and temperature, all of which favor infection. Surgery improves conditions for treatment but often is not a cure.[3, 8] Proper topical and systemic management must be continued. To depend on lateral wall resection to provide a cure for otitis externa is to invite failure. Numerous reports have documented failure rates of 35 to 47 per cent.[8, 15, 16, 32] The technique is useful when it is performed properly, appropriate medical care is continued, and the procedure is not postponed until irreversible hyperplastic changes have occurred.

Surgical Technique. The ear canal is surgically prepared by thoroughly lavaging with copious amounts of solution as described earlier. If the tympanum is ruptured, chemical solutions are removed from the middle ear with saline lavage. The pinna and skin overlying the ear canal are prepared and positioned with the pinna over the top of the head and the cranial cervical region extended over a "pillow" to elevate the surgical site.

Paired skin incisions are made along the rostral and caudal margin of the vertical canal. They extend ventrally 1.5 times the length of the vertical canal, terminating in a converging manner ventral to the junction of the vertical and horizontal canals. The incisions are joined ventrally and dorsally (Fig. 116–4*A*). The cone-shaped skin flap is dissected and removed. A longitudinal incision is made in the subcutaneous tissue over the vertical canal. The subcutaneous tissue is reflected rostally and caudally to expose the funnel-shaped auricular cartilage. The parotid salivary gland is reflected ventrally to expose the full length of the lateral wall of the vertical canal. Trauma to the parotid gland is avoided. Incisions into the dorsal portion of the parotid gland cause no problems.[15] Paired incisions are made through the rostal and caudal walls of the vertical canal to reflect the lateral half of the vertical canal ventrally (Fig. 116–4*B*). This is best performed by viewing the lumen of the canal and alternately making small rostal and caudal cuts while observing the reflected portion. The incisions are continued ventrally to the ligamentous junction of the auricular and annular cartilages. At this point, the lateral wall bends ventrally with minimal tension. If the cartilages are ossified, they can be removed with rongeurs to permit lateral wall reflection.[3, 6] In my opinion, ears this severely diseased are seldom candidates for lateral wall resection but instead require total ear canal ablation.

The proximal two-thirds of the cartilage flap are excised, and the remaining third is reflected ventrally to form a drain board (or "baffle plate").[15] The drain-board flap is sutured to the ventral skin incision with monofilament nonabsorbable sutures (Fig. 116–4*C*). The epithelial lining may be so friable that the sutures need to be placed through the cartilage. Additional interrupted sutures are used to appose the incised ear canal and skin. Sutures are best placed through the cartilage first and then through the skin. Close attention is given to carefully suturing the rostral and caudal skin margins to the hingepoint. This helps provide an optimum opening of the horizontal ear canal. If any proliferative tissue is found on the medial wall of the vertical canal, on the drain board, or in the opening of the horizontal canal, it is removed with the electroscalpel and permitted to heal by second intention.

Postoperative Care. The primary otitis is treated as determined by previous evaluation. For inflamed and infected ear canals, a topical antibiotic-steroid medication is used. The ears are taped over the head to prevent excessive movements that disrupt the suture line. Prevention of self-mutilation may require bandaging or an Elizabethan collar. Most animals attempt to scratch or rub their ears. Because of the inflamed condition of the tissue, healing is often delayed, and sutures are left in place at least 14 days.

Complications. Failure of lateral wall resection is often related to failure to recognize and treat underlying systemic disease, irreversible changes in the ear canal, failure to drain the horizontal canal properly, strictures of the horizontal canal, presence of concurrent otitis media, failure to perform lateral wall resection correctly, or undue postponement of resection.[8, 12, 15, 16] Exudation of the surgical site may continue for several days postoperatively. Because the surgical site is inflamed and infected, partial dehiscence of the suture line is common.[8] Resuturing is normally unrewarding, and dehiscence is best treated by second intention healing.

Vertical Canal Ablation

Vertical canal ablation is used to salvage a functional horizontal canal when the vertical canal is severely diseased. The procedure combines the advantages of lateral wall resection (drainage, ventilation, and preservation of hearing) with total ear canal ablation (total removal of severely diseased tissue). Vertical canal

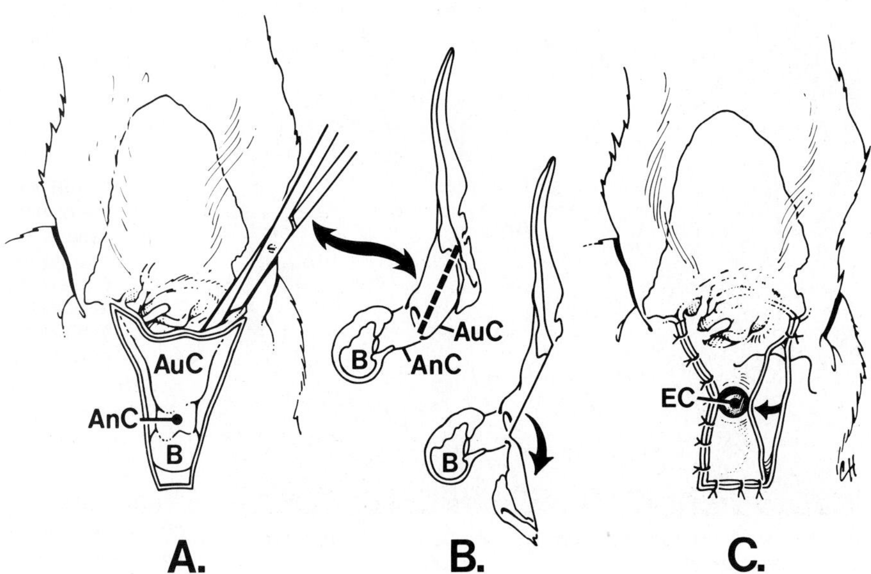

FIGURE 116–4. In performing a lateral wall resection, the skin overlying the canal is removed by making incisions along the rostral and caudal borders of the vertical canal, extending below the level of the horizontal canal. *A*, The dorsal and ventral ends of the incisions are joined and the skin removed. *B*, Heavy scissors are used to incise the rostral and caudal walls of the vertical canal to the level of the annular cartilage, reflecting the lateral half of the vertical canal. *C*, Approximately one-third of the lateral wall is used to create a "drain board," which is sutured to the skin margins. (AuC, auricular cartilage; AnC, annular cartilage; B, osseous bulla; EC, ear canal.)

ablation has certain advantages over lateral wall resection including (1) total removal of vertical canal tissue, (2) less postoperative exudate, (3) less postoperative pain, (4) less incised cartilage, resulting in better healing, and (5) improved cosmetic effect.[26, 29, 30] Indications for vertical canal ablation are irreversible hyperplastic otitis, severe trauma, or neoplasia limited to the vertical canal.[10, 15] Most cases of neoplasia and hyperplastic otitis, however, involve both the vertical and horizontal portions of the ear canal, making this procedure less applicable than total ear canal ablation.

Surgical Technique. Patients are prepared as for lateral wall resection. Paired incisions are made along the rostral and caudal borders of the vertical canal and joined ventrally at the horizontal canal (Fig. 116–5*A*). The dorsal ends of the incisions are joined by transecting the skin and cartilage at the base of the pinna proximal to the opening of the ear canal and dorsal to all diseased tissue. Dissection around the opening of the canal is performed carefully, staying close to the cartilage to avoid damaging the skin or vessels on the medial side of the pinna. The muscular attachments are transected close to the auricular cartilage to free the funnel-shaped vertical canal. The subcutaneous tissue and dorsal portion of the parotid salivary gland are separated and reflected to expose the lateral wall of the vertical canal. Gelpi or Weitlander retractors are useful in spreading the tissue and improving exposure of the surgical field. The dissection is continued in a circular fashion around the entire vertical canal to free it from all muscular and fascial attachments (to the junction of the auricular and annular cartilages). Electrocoagulation is used to control hemorrhage. The canal is transected, and the vertical canal discarded (Fig. 116–5*B*). The opening of the horizontal canal is sutured into the ventral end of the V-shaped incision with simple interrupted monofilament nonabsorbable sutures (Fig. 116–5*C*). The remainder of the wound is closed in a T-shaped manner (Fig. 116–5*D*).

Modification of this procedure includes a baffle plate similar to the drain board of the lateral wall resection formed from the lateral wall of the vertical canal to improve long-term patency of the horizontal canal.[15] Others have reported both dorsal and ventral flaps formed from the lateral and medial walls of the vertical canal.[4, 12] A procedure for a pull-through of the horizontal canal has been described; it avoids a vertical incision and claims a more cosmetic result.[29]

Postoperative Care. Aftercare is similar to that for lateral wall resection, although the wound is less likely to dehisce.[15] Ear carriage may be altered, especially in dogs with erect ears. The surgical site must be protected from self-mutilation by bandage or Elizabethan collar. The horizontal canal must be treated topically or systemically, depending on the cause of the otitis. The hair is regularly clipped from around the opening of the horizontal canal.

Complications. Vertical canal ablation has fewer complications than lateral wall resection.[15] Postoperative stenosis of the horizontal canal may occur but is less likely if the baffle plate is used.[15] Others have reported extremely high success rates with this procedure and its various modifications.[26, 29, 30] If there is doubt that lateral wall resection will result in a cure, then vertical canal ablation or total canal ablation is recommended.

Total Ear Canal Ablation

Total ear canal ablation is a procedure for removal of both vertical and horizontal ear canals. Indications for surgery include (1) chronic end-stage proliferative otitis with obstruction of both vertical and horizontal canals, (2) persistent otitis following lateral wall resection or vertical canal ablation, (3) neoplasia involving the vertical and horizontal canals, (4) collapsed or stenotic horizontal ear canal with or without ossified cartilages, (5) severe trauma to the vertical and horizontal canal, (6) congenital anomalies of the ear canal, (7) para-aural

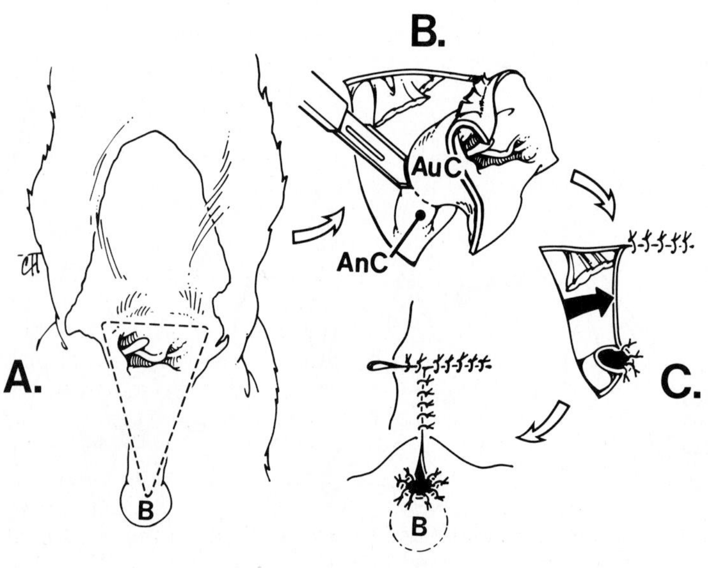

FIGURE 116–5. *A*, A triangular skin incision is made around the opening of the ear and over the vertical canal. *B*, The vertical canal is dissected free from surrounding tissues and transected. *C*, The opening of the horizontal canal is sutured into the ventral end of the skin incision. *D*, The remainder of the skin is sutured in a T-shaped closure. (AuC, auricular cartilage; AnC, annular cartilage; B, osseous bulla.)

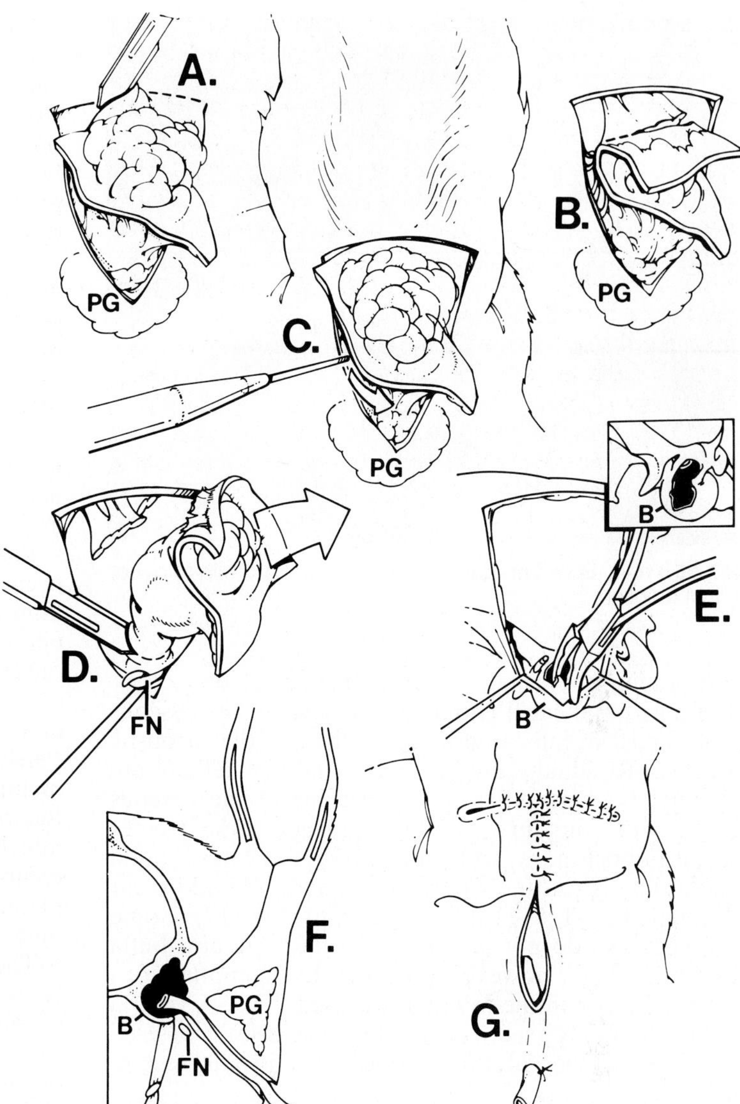

FIGURE 116–6. *A*, A triangular skin incision is made to isolate the ear canal, including all proliferative diseased tissue at the opening of the canal. *B*, The auricular muscles are transected at their attachment to the perichondrium. *C*, The canal is freed by dissecting in a circular fashion, staying close to the cartilage. *D*, The horizontal canal is dissected to the level of the osseous bulla and transected, being careful to avoid damage to the facial nerve. *E*, A lateral bulla osteotomy and curettage is performed. *F*, A Penrose drain is placed into the tympanic cavity and exited ventral to the skin incision. *G*, The skin is sutured in a T-shaped closure, and the drain anchored to the skin. (FN, facial nerve; PG, parotid salivary gland; B, osseous bulla.)

abscessation, and (8) unremitting otitis media.[2, 4, 21, 22, 28, 33] The most common indication is chronic end-stage otitis, encountered in cocker spaniels.[21, 22] Most patients have a history of unresolved otitis externa with repeated medical treatment. Early lateral wall resection or vertical canal ablation may be successful in salvage of the canal. After years of unsuccessful attempts at therapy, end-stage disease develops and the only option is total ear canal ablation. The disease is commonly bilateral, and in many instances, prior surgical procedures have been attempted.[2, 21]

Total ear canal ablation may be contraindicated when otitis media is present because of a lack of drainage pathway of the middle ear.[4, 28] Most animals with end-stage disease have extension of the disease into the middle ear through perforated tympanic membranes but can be successfully managed with total ear canal ablation combined with bulla osteotomy and drainage.[2, 21, 22, 25]

Surgical Procedure. Preparation and positioning are similar to lateral wall resection and vertical canal ablation. Broad-spectrum antibiotics are administered. The initial skin incisions and isolation of the vertical canal are achieved in the same manner as for vertical canal ablation (Fig. 116–6*A*). The dissection is aided by placing self-retaining retractors in the surrounding soft tissue and by grasping the ear canal with a towel clamp for retraction. The auricular muscles are transected at their attachments on the perichondrium (Fig. 116–6*B*). The canal is isolated by dissection in a circular fashion, staying as close to the cartilage as possible (Fig. 116–6*C*). A para-aural abscess or fistula may be encountered, having occurred as a result of infection eroding through the ear canal into the surrounding soft tissue.[17, 25] As the vertical canal is dissected, the auriculopalpebral branch of the facial nerve, the auriculotemporal branch of the trigeminal nerve, and branches of the greater auricular artery and vein may be encountered.[2, 4] As the canal reflects horizontally, the junction of the auricular and annular cartilages may be identified. The facial nerve crosses the caudal and ventral surfaces of the horizontal canal and is gently retracted to avoid damage (Fig. 116–6*D*). The nerve may be trapped in the ossified tissues

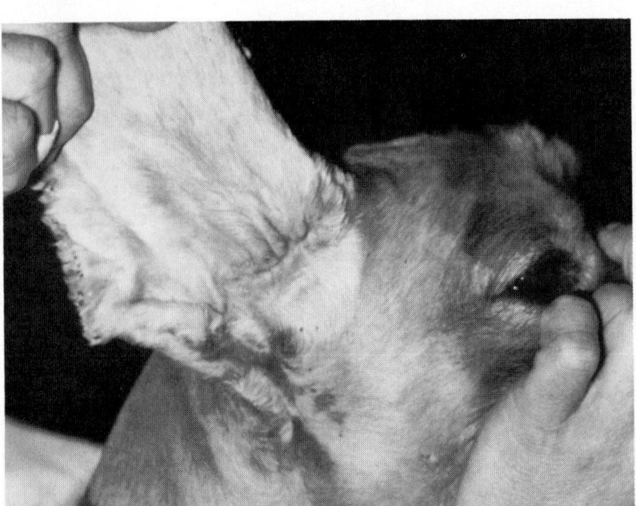

FIGURE 116–7. Excellent cosmetic result is achieved with total ear canal ablation.

surrounding the canal, requiring meticulous dissection. The horizontal canal is freed to the level of the osseous bulla and carefully transected at the external acoustic meatus. Residual canal cartilage and epithelium are completely removed from the opening of the osseous bulla with rongeurs. If not removed, these tissues result in postoperative fistulous tracts. A lateral bulla osteotomy is routinely performed, and the middle ear drained (Fig. 116–*E* and *F*) (see Chapter 117). Some investigators do not recommend routine lateral bulla osteotomy[2, 4, 28]; however, postoperative complications seem fewer when the osteotomy is used.[21, 22, 33] A ventral bulla osteotomy (see Chapter 117) has also been used in place of the lateral approach but is not recommended.[25]

The deep tissues are closed over a drain with absorbable suture, and the skin closed in a T-shaped fashion with a simple interrupted pattern of monofilament nonabsorbable suture (Fig. 116–6*G*). The drain is anchored to the skin with a single skin suture.

Postoperative Care. The ear is placed over the head, and a bandage is used to protect the Penrose drain and surgical site. The bandage is changed daily, and the drain removed when drainage ceases, usually in 3 to 7 days. Additional protection in the form of an Elizabethan collar is used on animals that scratch at their bandage. Antibiotics based on culture and sensitivity results are administered for 7 to 14 days; however, some surgeons believe they are unnecessary.[12] With cellulitis and postsurgical swelling, hot packs are used once or twice daily. Sutures are removed at approximately 10 days. Eye lubricants are used in animals with postoperative facial paralysis. The cosmetic effect of total ear canal ablation is quite good, especially in dogs with pendulous ears (Fig. 116–7).

Complications. Postoperative complications of total ear canal ablation are numerous and frequent.* Most frequently encountered are facial nerve paralysis or neuropraxia, wound drainage or dehiscence, cellulitis and infection, hemorrhage, vestibular disease, hypoglossal nerve dysfunction, deafness, and fistula formation. The overall complication rate is 29 to 82 per cent.[2, 12, 21, 25, 28, 33] Most complications can be prevented by proper surgical technique or are temporary and can be resolved with postoperative care.

Facial and hypoglossal nerve injuries are usually temporary and resolve within 2 weeks, although some are permanent (Fig. 116–8).[3, 21, 22, 25] Vestibular signs, including postural abnormalities, nystagmus, and head tilt, improve with steroids but may take a long time to resolve. They can be prevented by careful surgical technique to avoid damage to the bony labyrinth of the inner ear when curetting the bulla. The hypoglossal nerve and external carotid artery lie ventral to the bulla and are avoided.

Postoperative abscessation or fistulation (which may occur up to 1 year or more after surgery) are due to failure to completely remove all infected cartilage and epithelium of the external ear canal or failure to thoroughly remove all debris and infected tissues from the osseous bulla.[4, 21, 22, 28] Correction requires reoperation and thorough débridement of the remaining tissues. Persistent infection in or around the bulla may be manifested by pain on opening the mouth because of the proximity of the temporomandibular joint to the infected site. Despite the prevalence of postoperative complications, up to 92 per cent of patients are completely relieved of disease, and owner satisfaction is high.[21, 22, 33]

The effect of total ear canal ablation on hearing can be total deafness or no effect at all.[2, 12, 21, 22, 25] These observations have been owners' reports without objective evaluation. Methods to objectively evaluate hearing in dogs have used brain-stem auditory evoked responses.[27] Studies of normal dogs using brain-stem auditory evoked responses demonstrated that hearing qual-

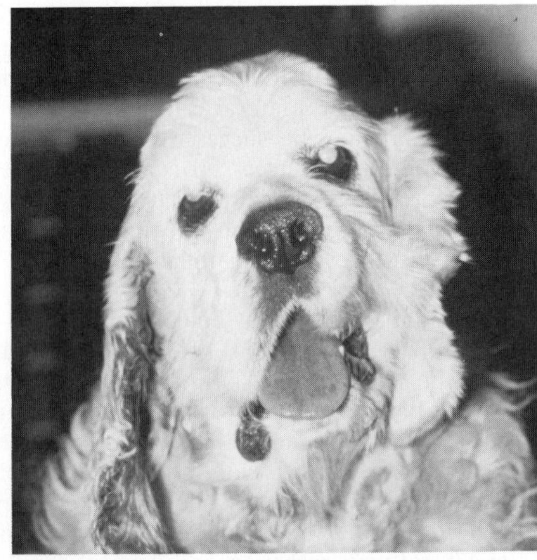

FIGURE 116–8. Facial nerve paralysis following total ear canal ablation evidenced by drooping of the right eyelid and lip.

*See references 3, 4, 21, 22, 25, 28, and 33.

ity was reduced but hearing was not lost.[23] Ten dogs with end-stage ear disease were treated with total ear canal ablation and lateral bulla osteotomy and evaluated by owner observation and brain-stem auditory evoked responses.[13] The results showed that the dogs heard as well or better after surgery than before surgery. Dogs with end-stage ear disease have severely diminished hearing, which is not adversely affected by total ear canal ablation. Hearing is by bone conduction and not by air conduction.

NEOPLASMS OF THE EXTERNAL EAR CANAL

Neoplasms of the ear canal are most common in cats and usually are ceruminous gland carcinoma (Fig. 116–9).[18–20] Squamous cell carcinoma has also been reported.[28] Neoplasms in dogs include malignant melanoma, squamous cell carcinoma, and ceruminous adenocarcinoma.[22, 28] The majority of the tumors are malignant, and 50 per cent are metastatic at the time of diagnosis in the cat.[18, 19] Metastases are most frequent to the local nodes and lungs. The clinical presentation resembles otitis that is usually unilateral. Careful examination and biopsy are required for diagnosis. Lateral wall resection may be required for adequate exposure. Although favorable results have been reported in dogs after surgical treatment by total ear canal ablation,[22] other reports describe surgery alone as usually unsuccessful.[20, 28] Radiation following surgery may improve the prognosis, but adequate confirmatory studies are not available.[18, 20]

Inflammatory polyps of cats are the most common benign lesions.[19] These growths may arise from the epithelial lining of the ear canal or middle ear. The clinical signs mimic otitis externa but may also cause signs of otitis media or pharnygeal obstruction when the polyp extends to the middle ear or pharynx (see Chapter 117). The polyps can often be removed by traction through the external meatus. In other cases, lateral wall resection or bulla osteotomy is required to provide adequate surgical exposure for resection.

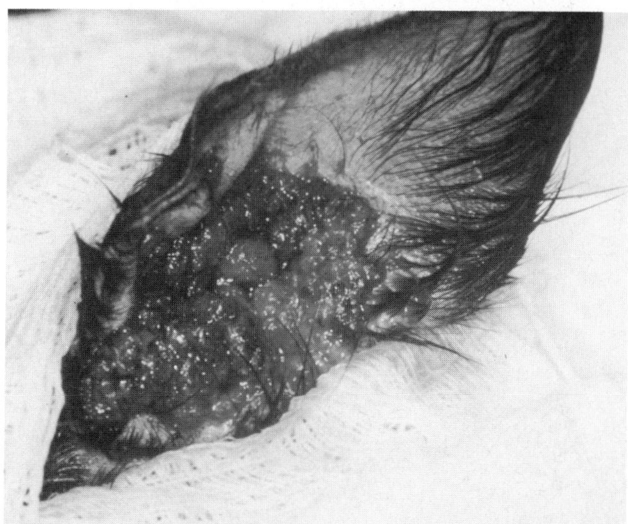

FIGURE 116–9. A ceruminous gland carcinoma growing from the ear canal of a cat.

References

1. August JR: A disease of multifactorial etiology. *Vet Clin North Am 16*:731, 1988.
2. Beckman SL, et al: TECA combining bulla osteotomy and curettage in dogs with chronic otitis externa and media. *J Am Vet Med Assoc 196*:84, 1990.
3. Birchard SJ: The ear. *In* Gourley IM, Vasseur PB (eds): *Small Animal Surgery*. J. B. Lippincott, Philadelphia, 1985.
4. Bojrab MJ, Constantinescu GM: External ear. *In* Bojrab MJ (ed): *Current Techniques in Small Animal Surgery*. 3rd ed. Lea & Febiger, Philadelphia, 1990.
5. Chester DK: Medical management of otitis externa. *Vet Clin North Am 18*:799, 1988.
6. Elkins AD, et al: Surgical management of ossified ear canals in the canine. *Vet Surg 10*:163, 1981.
7. Getty R: The ear. *In* Miller ME (ed): *Anatomy of the Dog*. W.B. Saunders, Philadelphia, 1964.
8. Gregory CR, Vasseur PB: Clinical results of lateral ear resection in dogs. *J Am Vet Med Assoc 182*:1087, 1983.
9. Griffin CE, et al: Diseases of the external ear and pinna. *In* Morgan RV (ed): *Small Animal Practice*. Churchill Livingstone, New York, 1988.
10. Grono LR: The external ear canal. *In* Slatter DH (ed): *Textbook of Small Animal Surgery*. W. B. Saunders, Philadelphia, 1985.
11. Harvey CE: A history of the surgical management of otitis externa in the dog. *Vet Surg* 9:150, 1980.
12. Harvey CE: The ear and nose. *In* Harvey CE, et al (eds): *Small Animal Surgery*. J. B. Lippincott, Philadelphia, 1990.
13. Krahwinkel DJ Jr., et al: Effect of ear ablation in auditory function as determined by brain stem auditory-evoked responses and subjective evaluation. *Vet Surg 18*:70, 1989.
14. Lacroix JV: Surgery for the relief of suppurative otitis. *In* Lacroix JV, Hoskins HP (eds): *Canine Surgery*. North American Veterinarian, Evanston, IL, 1939.
15. Lane JG: Otitis externa. *In* Lane JG (ed): *ENT and Oral Surgery of the Dog and Cat*. John Wright & Sons, Bristol, England, 1982.
16. Lane JG, Little CJL: Surgery of canine external auditory meatus: A review of failure. *J Small Anim Pract 27*:247, 1986.
17. Lane JG, Watkins PE: Para-aural abscess in the dog and cat. *J Small Anim Pract 27*:521, 1986.
18. Legendre AM, Krahwinkel DJ, Jr.: Feline ear tumors. *J Am Anim Hosp Assoc 17*:1035-1037, 1981.
19. Macy DW: The external ear canal. *In* Ettinger SJ (ed): *Textbook of Small Animal Medicine*. W.B. Saunders, Philadelphia, 1989.
20. Madewell BR, Theilen GH: Tumors and tumor-like conditions of epithelial origin. *In* Theilen GH, Madewell BR (eds): *Veterinary Cancer Medicine*. Lea & Febiger, Philadelphia, 1987.
21. Mason KL, et al: Total ear canal ablation combined with lateral bulla osteotomy for end-stage otitis in dogs. *Vet Surg 17*:263, 1988.
22. Matthiesen DT, Scavelli T: Total ear canal ablation and lateral bulla osteotomy in 38 dogs. *J Am Anim Hosp Assoc 26*:257, 1990.
23. Payne JT, et al: Hearing loss in dogs subjected to total ear canal ablation. *Vet Surg 18*:60, 1989.
24. Roth L: Pathologic changes in otitis externa. *Vet Clin North Am 18*:755, 1988.
25. Sharp DJH: Chronic otitis externa and otitis media treated by total ear canal ablation and ventral bulla osteotomy. *Vet Surg 19*:162, 1990.
26. Siemmering GH: Resection of the vertical ear canal for treatment of chronic otitis externa. *J Am Anim Hosp Assoc 16*: 753, 1980.
27. Sims MH: Electrodiagnostic evaluation of auditory function. *Vet Clin North Am 18*:913, 1988.
28. Smeak DD, DeHoff WD: Total ear canal ablation: Clinical results in the dog and cat. *Vet Surg 15*:161, 1986.
29. Tirgari M: Long-term evaluation of the pull-through techniques for vertical canal ablation for the treatment of otitis externa in dogs and cats. *J Small Anim Pract 29*:165, 1988.
30. Tirgari M, Pinniger RS: Pull-through technique for vertical canal ablation for the treatment of otitis externa in dogs and cats. *J Small Anim Pract 27*:123, 1986.
31. Toforoff RJ: Soft tissue surgery. *In* Holzworth J (ed): *Diseases of the Cat*. W. B. Saunders, Philadelphia, 1987.
32. Tufuesson G: Operation for otitis externa in dogs according to Zepp's method. *Am J Vet Res 16*:565, 1955.
33. White RAS, Pomeroy CJ: Total ear canal ablation and lateral bulla osteotomy (TECA/LBO) in the dog: Indications, complications, and long term results in 100 procedures. *Vet Surg 19*:81, 1990.
34. Zepp CP: Surgical technique to establish drainage of the external ear canal and correction of hematoma of the dog and cat. *J Am Vet Med Assoc 115*:91, 1949.

CHAPTER

117 Middle Ear

Howard B. Seim III

Otitis media frequently afflicts dogs. In one survey of 100 patients with otitis externa, 16 percent with acute otitis externa had concurrent otitis media and 50 percent with chronic otitis externa had concurrent otitis media.[9, 29] The most common cause of otitis media is otitis externa[15, 16, 18, 22, 25, 28] thus, middle ear disease should always be suspected in dogs with chronic or recurrent external ear disease. Other less common causes of otitis media include foreign bodies, trauma, neoplasia, or blood-borne pathogens.

ANATOMY AND PHYSIOLOGY

The middle ear consists of the tympanic membrane (eardrum), tympanic cavity (osseous bulla), eustachian tube (auditory canal), and the three auditory ossicles (malleus, incus, stapes) (Fig. 117–1). The tympanic membrane separates the horizontal portion of the external ear canal from the tympanic cavity and consists of a small upper portion, the pars flaccida, and a large lower portion, the pars tensa (Fig. 117–2). The loose pars flaccida extends upward from the lateral process of the malleus to the tympanic notch, forming the upper quadrant of the tympanic membrane. The pars tensa is thin, tough, and glistening. The outline of the manubrium of the malleus usually is clearly visible. Otoscopic examination reveals a portion of the pars flaccida and the caudal quadrant of the pars tensa[18] (Fig. 117–3). It is concave because of the traction on the medial surface by the malleus, one of the three auditory ossicles. The ossicles form a chain from the tympanic membrane to the inner ear and are responsible for amplifying air vibrations that strike the tympanic membrane. These vibrations are transmitted across the middle ear cavity to the inner ear.

Most of the middle ear is composed of the air-filled tympanic cavity (see Figs. 117–1 and 117–2). It is a bony cavity lined with a mucous membrane partially covered by a two-layered columnar ciliated epithelium and partially by a single layer of squamous epithelium.[22] The ventral portion, the part within the osseous tympanic bulla, may be compared in shape to the interior of an eggshell, having an elliptical opening on the side that faces dorsally (see Fig. 117–2). It communicates with the tympanic cavity through this opening.[17] The osseous bulla is thick laterally and rostrally and thin ventrally, caudally, and medially (see Figs. 117–1 and 117–2). In most dogs, it is readily palpable despite its depth.[16]

Several nerves pass through the middle ear, but only two are of clinical significance—the facial and sympathetic nerves. The facial nerve leaves the brain stem in close association with the eighth cranial nerve, travels in the facial canal of the petrous temporal bone, and enters the middle ear cavity.[18] The sympathetic nerve leaves the cranial cervical ganglion, which is located just behind the tympanic bulla, and enters the middle ear cavity.[18]

The eustachian tube, which connects the middle ear to the caudal nasal pharynx, is short in dogs and cats (see Figs. 117–1 and 117–2). It is only 8 mm or less in length and 1 to 2 mm in diameter.[22]

The middle ear defense mechanisms include a mucociliary system and a cellular defense system. The epithelium in the middle ear can actively function in clearing foreign material, as demonstrated experimentally by the rapid clearance of radiopaque material and as observed directly through tympanic membrane perforations.[23] A substance that lowers surface tension has been found in the eustachian tubes of dogs.[5] An infection may decrease production or inhibit the presence of the surface tension-lowering substance, resulting in greater cohesive force between the walls of the eustachian tube, limiting normal clearance.[18]

The cellular defense mechanism present in the middle ear is also important in removing material from the tympanic bulla.[12] Epithelial cells secrete lysosomes to aid in defense. Fibroblasts become active in synthesizing and secreting collagen and ground substance, which participate in protection and repair. Ground substance also constitutes a mechanical barrier against the spread of microorganisms.[18]

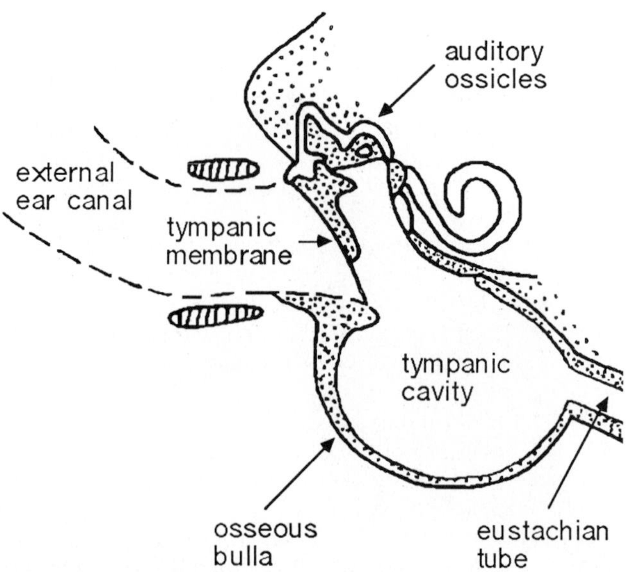

FIGURE 117–1. Middle ear structures. (After Lane, J. G.: *The Complete Manual of Ear Care.* Veterinary Learning Systems Co., Inc. 1986; with permission)

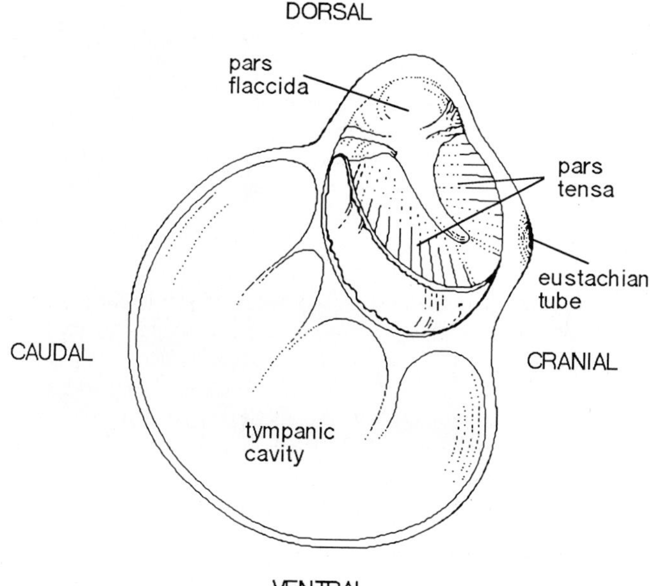

FIGURE 117–2. Relationship of the tympanic membrane to the osseous bulla and tympanic cavity. (After Spreull, J. S. A: Otitis Media in the Dog. In *Current Veterinary Therapy V.* Philadelphia, W.B. Saunders Co., 1976, with permission)

ETIOLOGY AND PATHOGENESIS

Most investigators believe that the most common cause of otitis media is extension of otitis externa, and many cases are overlooked because a careful otoscopic examination is not performed when otitis externa is obvious.[22] The common pathogens cultured from the middle ear include *Staphylococcus* spp., *Streptococcus* spp., *Pseudomonas* spp., *Escherichia coli*, and *Proteus mirabilis*.[18]

Inflammation of the middle ear can be initiated via three routes: across the tympanic membrane, through the eustachian tube, or by hematogenous spread.[22] Extension of otitis externa across the tympanic membrane is the most common route.[15, 16, 18, 22, 25, 28] Debris, hair, foreign bodies, and exudate associated with otitis externa can cause inflammation, necrosis, and rupture of the tympanic membrane, allowing extension of infection into the tympanic cavity.[18] The incidence of infection of the middle ear via the eustachian tube in dogs and cats is low. Cats infrequently develop otitis media through this route as a sequel to upper respiratory tract disease.[11] Infection via hematogenous spread is also uncommon. Trauma, polyps, neoplasms, and foreign bodies in the middle ear can cause inflammation and middle ear disease.

The middle ear has an effective defense mechanism. Any organism capable of eroding or ulcerating the epithelial tissue and tympanic membrane can cause severe pathological changes in the tympanic cavity. Such changes include swelling and occlusion of the eustachian tube, erosion of the mucosal lining of the tympanic cavity, metaplasia of the epithelium of the middle ear to hypersecretory stratified squamous epithelium with variable keratinization, degenerative or proliferative changes of the osseous tympanic bulla, and accumulation of inflammatory debris in the tympanic cavity.[22]

CLINICAL SIGNS

Patients with otitis media generally have signs of otitis externa (see Fig. 117–11). These include discharge from the external ear canal, pawing or rubbing the affected ear, shaking the head, or pain when the head is touched. Some animals may have so much pain that they hold their head tilted because of discomfort rather than because of abnormal vestibular function.[11] Because the facial and sympathetic nerves pass near the middle ear, a facial nerve palsy or Horner's syndrome may occur on the same side as the otitis media. Signs of facial nerve injury include drooping of the ear or lip or inability to move it, drooling of saliva, decreased or absent palpebral reflex, and exposure keratitis. Horner's syndrome is characterized by ptosis, miosis, enophthalmos, and protrusion of the third eyelid.[18] If middle ear infection is chronic or severe enough to cause otitis interna, signs of abnormal vestibular function (head tilt, nystagmus, and ataxia) may occur. Nystagmus frequently disappears after the first week, and ataxia may disappear or be rapidly compensated for, but the head tilt generally remains.[19]

PHYSICAL FINDINGS

A thorough history and physical examination are performed to rule out systemic disorders (i.e., immune-mediated diseases, generalized seborrhea, atopy, and hypothyroidism) that may be contributing to the etiology of the middle ear disease. Patients should also be examined for the presence of facial palsy, Horner's syndrome, exposure keratitis, and vestibular signs. The temporomandibular joints and base of the ear are palpated for swelling or pain. A careful oral and pharyngeal examination is performed to rule out an abscess or mass associated with the eustachian tube. Finally, proper

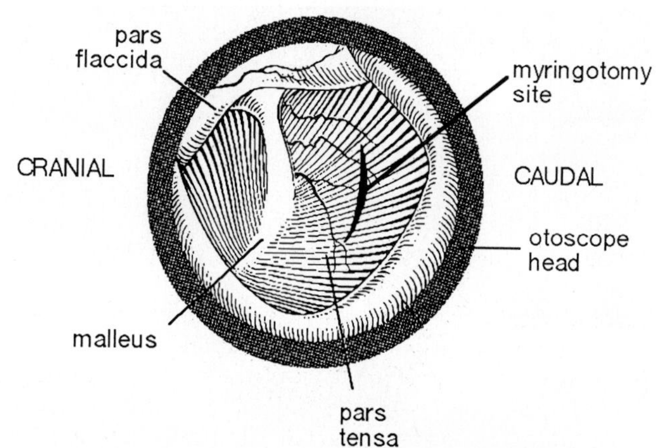

FIGURE 117–3. Otoscopic view of the tympanic membrane of the dog. Note the location of the malleus and myringotomy site. The myringotomy is performed caudal to the malleus. (After Habel, R. E.: In *Applied Veterinary Anatomy.* R. E. Habel Publisher, Ithaca, N. Y., 1981, with permission)

cleaning of the external ear canal facilitates otoscopic examination of the tympanic membrane (see Fig. 117–11). Careful examination of the external ear canal, particularly the tympanic membrane, is helpful in early diagnosis of otitis media (see Fig. 117–3). The normal tympanic membrane is slightly concave, translucent, pearl gray, and glistening. Alteration in its color, tension, or integrity indicates pathological change in the middle ear.

RADIOGRAPHY

Radiographic examination of the osseous bulla may be helpful in establishing a diagnosis of otitis media. Lateral, ventrodorsal, open-mouth, and lateral oblique projections allow adequate observation of the osseous bulla. To obtain the precise positioning required to evaluate the views of the skull, the radiographs must be taken with patients anesthetized and the skull supported.[7]

The normal bulla has an air density within the tympanic cavity. The osseous bulla is normally a thin shell of bone (Fig. 117–4). Radiographic changes in the interior of the bulla compatible with otitis media include the presence of a fluid or bone density. Fluid density may be caused by purulent exudates, granulation tissue, neoplasia, or cellular debris. In patients with chronic otitis media, the tympanic cavity may occasionally be replaced with bone (Fig. 117–5). Radiographic changes in the osseous bulla may be proliferative or lytic (Fig. 117–6). Osseous proliferation or lysis may be seen with neoplasia or osteomyelitis secondary to chronic otitis media.

Although radiographic changes are helpful in establishing a diagnosis of otitis media, these changes may occur late.[8] If the clinical signs and physical findings are compatible with otitis media, with normal radiographs, a presumptive diagnosis of acute otitis media can be made.

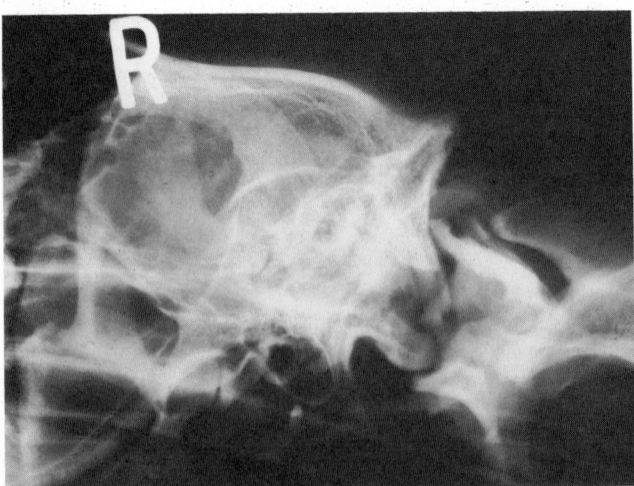

FIGURE 117–4. Right lateral oblique projection of the left bulla of a normal dog. Notice the eggshell appearance of the osseous bulla and the air density of the tympanic cavity.

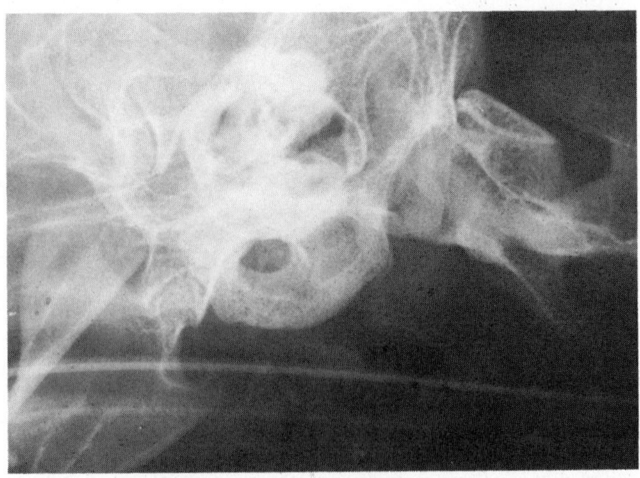

FIGURE 117–5. Lateral oblique projection of the left bulla of a cat with chronic otitis media. The osseous bulla has undergone bony proliferative changes that have resulted in obliteration of the tympanic cavity with bone.

TREATMENT OF OTITIS MEDIA

The goals of treating patients with otitis media are to gain access to the tympanic cavity; remove inflammatory, infected, or foreign debris; perform culture and susceptibility testing; and provide an avenue for adequate ventilation and drainage.[18] These goals can be met by medical or surgical means or both, depending on the chronicity of disease, presence of otitis externa, results of careful otoscopic examination, and radiographic changes present (see Fig. 117–11).

Medical Treatment: Myringotomy

If the tympanic membrane is intact but discolored and bulging, it is incised (myringotomy) to obtain samples

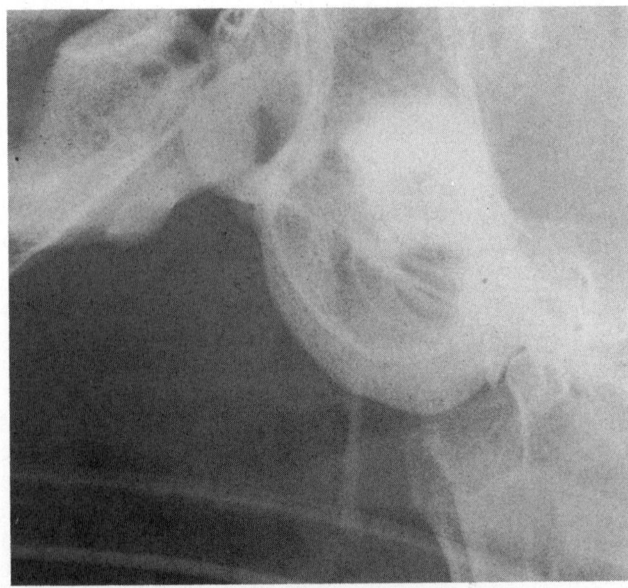

FIGURE 117–6. Lateral oblique projection of the left bulla of a cat with chronic otitis media. Notice the bony proliferation on the ventral aspect of the osseous bulla.

for culture and susceptibility testing and cytological study and to provide drainage from the middle ear cavity. Myringotomy also relieves pain and pressure and provides for lavage and instillation of medication.

Several types of myringotomy have been described.[21] The type most commonly used in veterinary medicine is simple paracentesis.[18] After the external ear canal is thoroughly cleaned (see Chapter 116), a clean otoscope is introduced and the tympanic membrane observed. A blunt probe is directed through the otoscope cone to perforate the tympanic membrane caudal to the malleus (see Fig. 117–3). The probe is removed, and a 20-gauge spinal needle of adequate length is passed through the perforated membrane. A syringe is attached to the spinal needle, and fluid or material from the middle ear cavity is aspirated for cytological study and culture and susceptibility testing. If the fluid is too thick or inspissated to be aspirated, flushing may be required. A metal-tipped suction cannula is inserted through the tympanic membrane next to the spinal needle. A 20-ml syringe is attached to the spinal needle. Sterile physiological saline solution at body temperature is gently flushed into the tympanic cavity and suctioned. Flushing and aspiration are performed until the exudate is completely removed and the saline is clear. Long-term (3 to 6 weeks) systemic antibiotic therapy is instituted based on results of culture and susceptibility testing. Patients that have concurrent otitis externa are treated with local antibiotic preparations.

The disadvantages of myringotomy include poor exposure of the tympanic cavity, poor postoperative drainage, exposure of the middle ear to the external ear canal (particularly in patients with otitis externa), and damage to the delicate middle ear structures. If medical treatment proves ineffective or a neoplasm, inflammatory mass, or foreign body is found, surgical drainage is indicated.

Surgical Treatment

Numerous surgical techniques are used for treatment of otitis media, but only two provide adequate exposure and drainage of the tympanic cavity: lateral bulla osteotomy and ventral bulla osteotomy.

Lateral Bulla Osteotomy

Lateral bulla osteotomy may be performed as a separate procedure or in combination with other procedures involving the external ear canal. When they are performed as a separate procedure,[2, 4] a patient is placed in lateral recumbency with the affected side uppermost. The skin incision is made over the vertical ear canal and extended 1 to 2 cm ventral to the horizontal canal. The subcutaneous tissues are bluntly dissected to reveal the junction between the parotid salivary gland and the ventral aspect of the horizontal ear canal. Further dissection along the most ventral and caudolateral aspect of the horizontal ear canal exposes the facial nerve as it emerges from the stylomastoid foramen. The facial nerve is gently retracted ventrally, exposing the lateral aspect of the bulla. The tissue overlying the bulla is incised with a scalpel blade and elevated with a periosteal elevator.

The bulla may be entered with a Steinmann pin or pneumatic drill. Care is taken to direct the pin or drill in a caudolateral direction to avoid the auditory ossicles and promontory. Once the bulla is entered, rongeurs are used to extend the opening cranially, caudally, and ventrally. Culture and susceptibility testing are performed, and the bulla cavity is gently curetted and irrigated with sterile physiological saline solution. An ingress-egress drain tube system (described later) is placed into the tympanic cavity and secured with 4-0 absorbable suture. The subcutaneous tissue and skin are closed in a routine fashion. The tympanic cavity is lavaged with an appropriate antiseptic or antibiotic based on results of culture and susceptibility testing. The drain is removed in 7 to 10 days.

Many patients with otitis media have concurrent signs of otitis externa and may benefit from combined lateral ear resection and bulla osteotomy. Lateral ear resection is performed as described in Chapter 116, and lateral bulla osteotomy is performed as described earlier.

Patients frequently have otitis media *and* severe obstructive otitis externa or otitis media *and* a previously unsuccessful lateral ear resection. In either case, a total ear canal ablation and lateral bulla osteotomy can be performed.[3, 13, 14, 27] Total ear canal ablation is performed first, allowing exposure of the external acoustic meatus and facial nerve (see Chapter 116). The facial nerve is carefully retracted ventrally, soft tissues surrounding the lateral aspect of the bulla are dissected bluntly, and the periosteum of the osseous bulla is incised and elevated with a periosteal elevator. Rongeurs are used to open the ventral rim of the external acoustic meatus. The osteotomy includes a portion of the lateral and ventral walls of the osseous bulla to provide proper drainage (Fig. 117–7). A bone curette is used to gently remove any remaining epithelium or inflammatory debris from within the bulla. The dorsomedial aspect of the tympanic cavity is avoided to preserve the auditory ossicles and inner ear structures.

After curettage, the tympanic cavity and surrounding soft tissues are copiously lavaged with warm sterile saline. An ingress-egress drainage system is placed to facilitate postoperative lavage and drainage (Fig. 117–8*A*). A 40.6-cm (16-inch) polyethylene or Silastic catheter is fenestrated at its center. The catheter is tunneled from the dorsal aspect of the head into the bulla and exited ventrally. Care is taken to ensure that the fenestration lies within the osteotomy. Fine absorbable suture (4-0) is occasionally needed to fix the fenestrated portion of the tube into the bulla. An alternate method of placing the drain tube system is to enter and exit the tube from a ventral location (Fig. 117–8*B*). I prefer this method because less subcutaneous tunneling is necessary. It is important to suture the fenestrated portion of the drain into the tympanic cavity to prevent premature removal postoperatively. The capacity of the bulla and drain tube is calculated by clamping the exit end of the drain tube and infusing a known quantity of saline

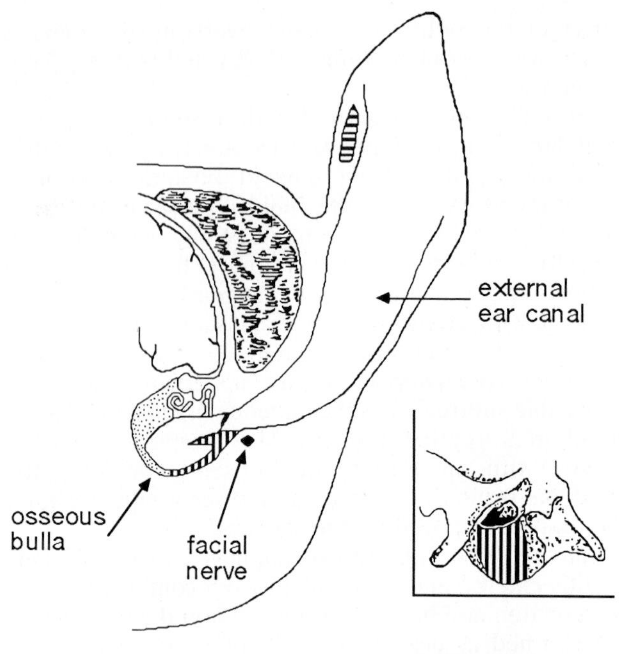

FIGURE 117–7. The middle ear and its relationship to the external ear canal and facial nerve after lateral bulla osteotomy. The insert shows the area of the lateral bulla that is resected to allow adequate exposure and ventral drainage. (After A. Schwarz: Ablation of the External Ear Canal. In *Current Techniques in Small Animal Surgery,* 2nd ed., Lea & Febiger, Philadelphia, 1983, p 104, with permission)

ingress
total ear
canal ablation
osseous
bulla
egress
= drain tube
= osteotomy
A
total ear
canal ablation
osseous
bulla
egress
ingress
= drain tube
= osteotomy
B

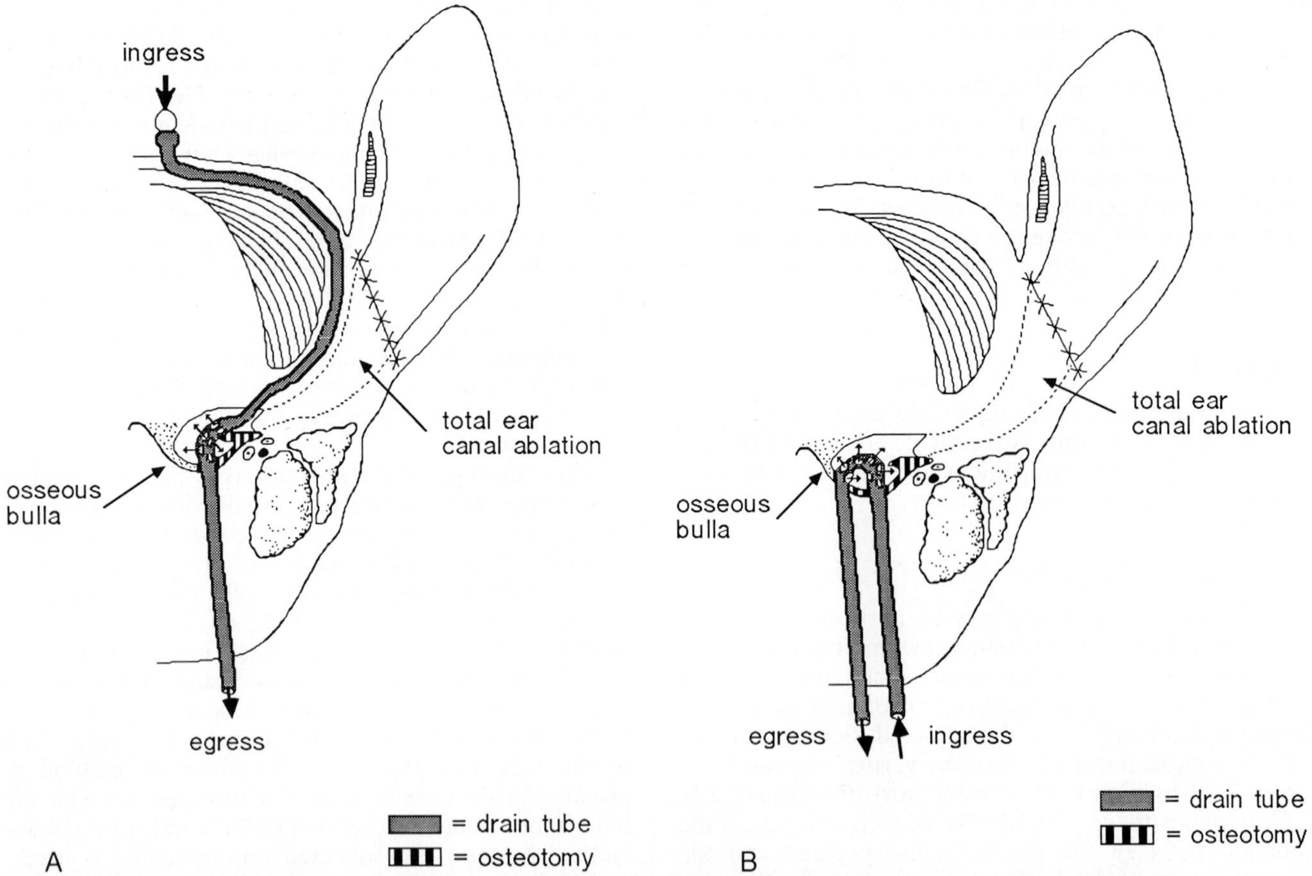

FIGURE 117–8. *A,* Entrance-exit drainage system after total ear canal ablation and lateral bulla osteotomy. The drainage tube is tunneled from the head, through the tympanic cavity, and exited through the cervical region. (After A. Schwarz: Ablation of the External Ear Canal. In *Current Techniques in Small Animal Surgery,* 2nd ed., Lea & Febiger, Philadelphia, 1983, p 104, with permission)

B, Modified entrance-exit drainage system after total ear canal ablation and lateral bulla osteotomy. The drainage tube enters and exits from the cervical region. (After A. Schwarz: Ablation of the External Ear Canal. In *Current Techniques in Small Animal Surgery,* 2nd ed., Lea & Febiger, Philadelphia, 1983, p 104, with permission)

through the entrance of the tube into the tympanic cavity. The tympanic cavity of most dogs and cats has a capacity of 3 to 4 ml. Closure of deep tissues is not performed. Subcutaneous tissue and skin are closed in a routine fashion. The drain tube is secured to the skin.[26]

Antiseptic or antibiotic solutions, based on culture and susceptibility testing, are used to irrigate the bulla. Irrigation is performed as follows: A hemostat is used to occlude the exit end of the drain tube, and the measured solution is injected into the entrance of the drain tube to allow irrigation of the tympanic cavity. Irrigation is repeated two to three times each treatment. The hemostat is removed after each treatment to allow proper drainage. The drain tube is incorporated in a bandage between treatments. The bulla is irrigated three times a day, and the drain remains in place until the defect is filled with granulation tissue, which generally takes 7 to 10 days.[27] Irrigating the tympanic cavity may help remove inflammatory debris, decrease the number of bacteria, and improve the environment for healing.[27]

Results. Few reports discuss the long-term results in patients with acute otitis media treated by lateral bulla osteotomy alone. This is because the majority of patients with otitis media have concurrent otitis externa and generally require multiple procedures.

Patients with end-stage otitis externa and otitis media can be helped by a combination of total ear canal ablation and lateral bulla osteotomy.[3, 4, 13, 14, 27] Total ear canal ablation alone did not provide adequate removal or drainage of infected material or inflammatory debris from the tympanic bulla.[27] Total ear canal ablation in patients with otitis media, performed without bulla osteotomy, may be contraindicated.

A high rate of complications has been reported with total ear canal ablation and lateral bulla osteotomy and is attributed to two main factors: technical difficulty in performing the two procedures and bacterial contamination of the surgical site from contaminated tissues.[14] Complications include facial palsy, wound infection, fistula tract formation, various degrees of hearing loss, and vestibular damage.[3, 13, 14]

The overall long-term success rate of total ear canal ablation and lateral bulla osteotomy is 90 to 95 per cent.[3, 13, 14] If the procedures are performed with adequate knowledge of the regional anatomy and attention to detail, a successful result can be expected.

Ventral Bulla Osteotomy

Ventral bulla osteotomy can also be used to approach the tympanic cavity. It may be performed alone or in combination with other procedures involving the external ear canal. This technique has the advantage of providing improved exposure and more consistent ventral drainage of the tympanic bulla than the lateral bulla osteotomy.[4] With bilateral otitis media, both bullae can be approached without repositioning. The major disadvantages of this technique are the technical difficulty of performing the procedure and repositioning of patients that require concurrent external ear canal surgery (i.e., lateral ear resection or total ear canal ablation).

A patient is placed in dorsal recumbency, and the area surrounding the angle of the jaw is prepared for aseptic surgery. In the majority of dogs and all cats, the bulla can be palpated immediately caudal and slightly medial to the vertical ramus of the mandible. An 8- to 10-cm paramedian skin incision is made just medial to the mandibular salivary gland and centered midway between the angular process of the mandible caudally and the wings of the atlas cranially[4, 15, 20] (Fig. 117–9*A*). The platysma muscle is encountered and incised longitudinally for the length of the skin incision. Blunt dissection is used to separate the digastric muscle from the hyoglossal and styloglossal muscles. Care is taken to

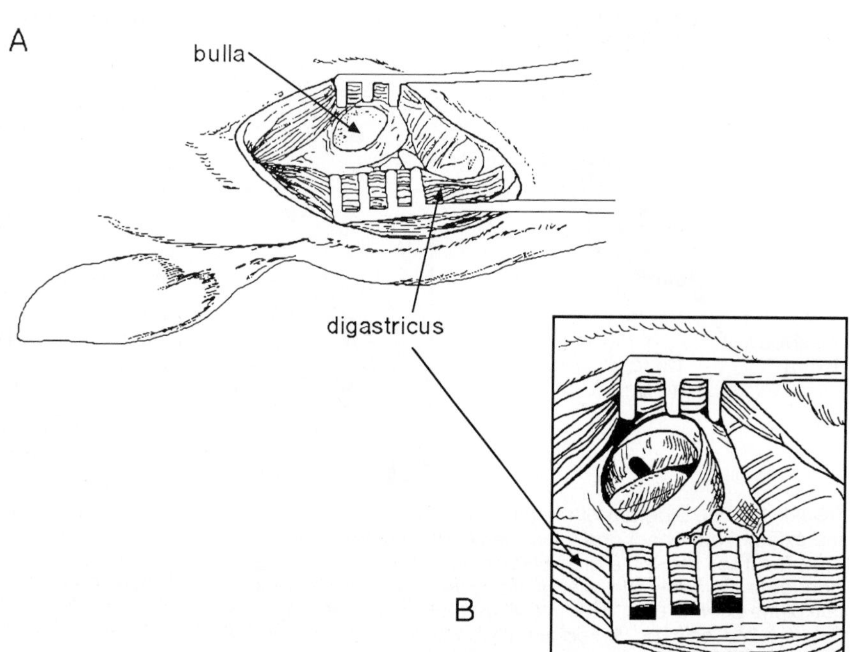

FIGURE 117–9. *A*, Ventral bulla osteotomy. Surgical exposure of the ventral aspect of the osseous bulla. (After Spreull J. S. A.: In *Current Techniques in Small Animal Surgery,* 1st ed. Lea & Febiger, Philadelphia, 1975, with permission)
B, The ventral aspect of the osseous bulla has been removed. The tympanic cavity is explored and irrigated prior to the placement of an ingress-egress drainage system. (After Spreull J. S. A.: In *Current Techniques in Small Animal Surgery,* 1st ed. Lea & Febiger, Philadelphia, 1975, with permission)

identify the hypoglossal nerve, located on the lateral aspect of the hyoglossal muscle. Deep digital palpation in this tissue plane confirms the location of the bulla as a raised rounded structure between the more pointed jugular process of the skull caudally and the angular process of the mandible rostrally.[4] Blunt dissection is continued until the bulla is reached. Careful placement of self-retaining retractors facilitates exposure of the ventral aspect of the bulla, allowing safe entry (Fig. 117–9*B*).

The tympanic cavity may be entered by using a Steinmann pin or pneumatic drill. Care is taken to avoid damaging the dorsal aspect of the tympanic cavity. Once the tympanic cavity has been entered, rongeurs are used to enlarge the opening (Fig. 117–10). The interior of the bulla is examined for foreign bodies, inflammatory debris, or neoplasms. Samples are taken for cytological, microbiological, and histopathological examination. The tympanic cavity is irrigated and suctioned and a bone curette is used to remove the remaining epithelial lining or inflammatory debris.

A similar entrance-exit drainage system is placed as described for lateral bulla osteotomy; however, the tube must enter *and* exit through the ventral cervical skin (see Fig. 117–8*B*). The fenestrated portion of the drain is sutured into the bulla with fine absorbable suture to ensure its position postoperatively. Management of the drain system is as described for lateral bulla osteotomy. The drain is removed in 7 to 10 days.

Results. Results following ventral bulla osteotomy alone are excellent in 90 per cent of reported cases.[4]

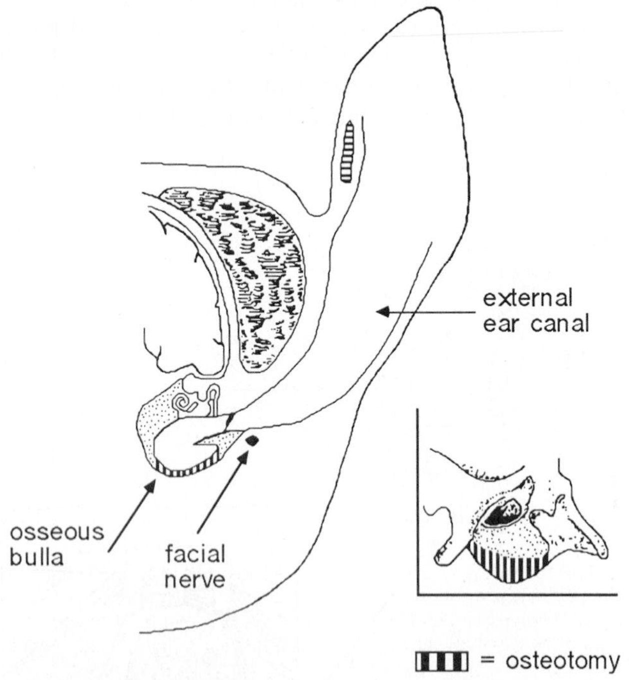

FIGURE 117–10. Diagram of the middle ear and its relationship to the external ear canal and facial nerve after ventral bulla osteotomy. The insert shows the area of the bulla that is resected to allow adequate exposure and ventral drainage. (After A. Schwarz: Ablation of the External Ear Canal. In *Current Techniques in Small Animal Surgery*, 2nd ed., Lea & Febiger, Philadelphia, 1983, p 104, with permission)

This is most likely due to excellent exposure of the tympanic cavity, allowing careful examination of its contents and adequate ventral drainage.

Patients with end-stage otitis externa and otitis media can be helped by a combination of total ear canal ablation and ventral bulla osteotomy.[24] The complications encountered with total ear canal ablation and ventral bulla osteotomy are comparable to those with total ear canal ablation and lateral bulla osteotomy.[24] Valid comparisons of the two techniques are difficult to make; however, the apparent advantages of total ear canal ablation and lateral bulla osteotomy may be that lateral bulla osteotomy affords adequate exposure of the tympanic cavity and patients do not require repositioning after the total ear canal ablation.

NEOPLASMS OF THE MIDDLE EAR

Neoplasia of the middle ear cavity and surrounding structures is uncommon.[10] Clinical signs are generally those of otitis media; however, neoplasms may invade the middle ear, inner ear, and brain, causing severe central nervous system signs. Presumptive diagnosis is made by skull series of radiographs and computed tomography. Definitive diagnosis is made by incisional biopsy. Surgical treatment alone is often unrewarding owing to the anatomical location and invasiveness of the neoplasm. Successful long-term treatment requires adjunctive therapy such as radiation or chemotherapy.

Inflammatory Polyps of the Middle Ear in Cats

Inflammatory polyps are protruding pedunculated growths arising from the mucous membrane secondary to chronic inflammation and local tissue irritation.[6, 10] The lining of the tympanic cavity, auditory canal, and nasopharynx is the site of origin of most inflammatory polyps. The exact cause of the polyps is unknown; however, because of the young age of the majority of patients, a congenital origin has been suspected.

Because of the variable location of the polyps, clinical signs include respiratory stridor, dyspnea, dysphagia, and signs of external or middle ear disease. Diagnosis requires careful oropharyngeal evaluation and otoscopic and radiographic examination of the skull, including the middle ear and nasal cavity.

Treatment of inflammatory polyps is surgical excision. Nasopharyngeal polyps can generally be removed by an oral approach. Polyps involving the external ear canal may require lateral ear resection to expose the origin of the polyp. Polyps originating from the middle ear are approached via ventral bulla osteotomy. The tympanic cavity of a cat contains a septum that separates it into dorsomedial and ventrolateral compartments.[1] This septum is opened to facilitate curettage and drainage of both compartments. Complete excision of inflammatory polyps justifies a favorable long-term prognosis.[6]

SUMMARY

Otitis media occurs frequently in patients with acute or chronic otitis externa. Careful examination of the

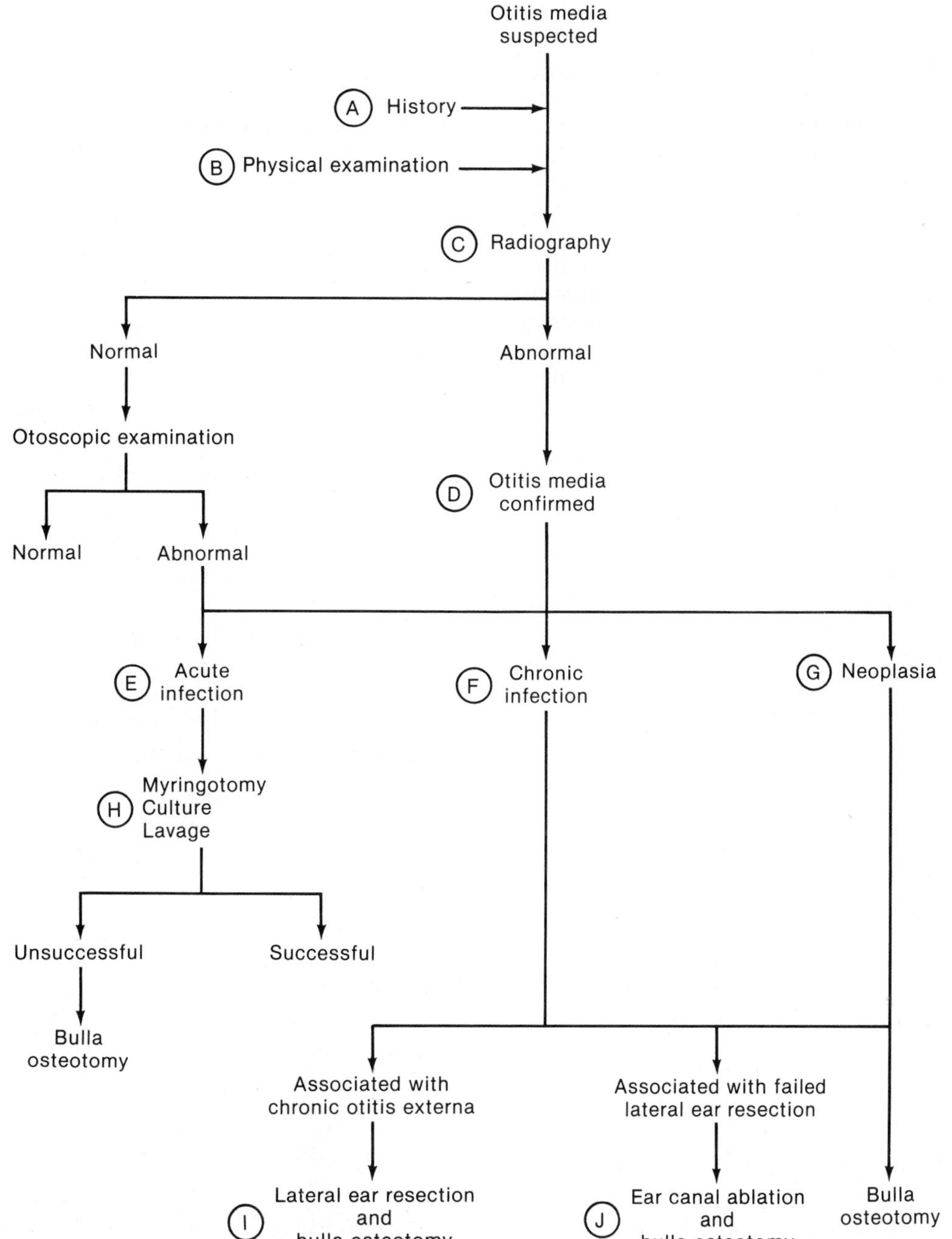

FIGURE 117–11. Otitis media. A, Signs of otitis media include pain, drooping of or inability to move the ear or lip, drooling of saliva, decreased or absent palpebral reflex, keratitis sicca, ptosis, miosis, enophthalmos, protrusion of the nictitating membrane, or signs associated with otitis externa. If the middle ear infection is chronic or severe enough to cause otitis interna, signs of abnormal vestibular function (head tilt, nystagmus, and ataxia) may occur. B, Physical examination may reveal any of the foregoing historical findings as well as pain on palpation of the temporomandibular joint and/or base of the ear. Careful otoscopic examination may reveal abnormalities of the tympanic membrane. C, A skull series of radiographs including lateral, ventrodorsal, open-mouth, and lateral oblique projections should be evaluated. Proliferation or lysis of the osseous bulla or fluid or bone density of the tympanic cavity suggests the presence of otitis media. Although the presence of radiographic changes is helpful in establishing a diagnosis of otitis media, these changes may occur rather late.[8] If the clinical signs and physical findings are compatible with otitis media in the presence of normal radiographic findings, a presumptive diagnosis of acute otitis media should be made. D, Historical findings, physical examination, and radiographic evaluation must be used together to establish a diagnosis of otitis media. E, Patients with acute otitis media may or may not have signs of otitis externa. Careful evaluation of the tympanic membrane may reveal abnormalities in color, tension, or integrity, suggesting pathology of the middle ear. F, Patients with chronic otitis media generally present with signs of otitis externa. Radiographic changes are common. G, Neoplasia of the middle ear is rare. Cats occasionally develop polypoid growths originating from the lining of the tympanic cavity. H, Patients with acute otitis media may be treated by myringotomy, culture and susceptibility testing, irrigation of the tympanic cavity, and local and systemic antimicrobial therapy. If medical therapy proves unsuccessful, bulla osteotomy should be considered. I, Patients with chronic otitis media associated with chronic otitis externa should undergo lateral ear resection and bulla osteotomy. Ventral bulla osteotomy provides excellent exposure of the tympanic cavity, and the approach is more compatible with a lateral ear resection. J, Patients with chronic otitis media associated with an obstructed external ear canal or a failed lateral ear resection should undergo total ear canal ablation and bulla osteotomy. Lateral or ventral bulla osteotomy can be performed with total ear canal ablation. The success rate of either osteotomy procedure is similar; however, total ear canal ablation and lateral bulla osteotomy do not require repositioning the patient.

external ear canal and tympanic membrane and radiographic evaluation of the bulla are necessary to make a definitive diagnosis. Treatment may include medical or surgical techniques dependent on the chronicity of the disease, the presence of otitis externa, the results of otoscopic examination, and the radiographic findings. Surgical exposure of the tympanic cavity is best performed by lateral bulla osteotomy or ventral bulla osteotomy. Depending on the severity of concurrent otitis externa, a combination of external ear canal surgery and bulla osteotomy may be indicated. The prognosis for patients treated early and aggressively is generally favorable.

References

1. Ader PL, Boothe HW: Ventral bulla osteotomy in the cat. *J Am Anim Hosp Assoc 15*:757, 1979.
2. Barrett RE, Rathfon BL: Lateral approach to a bulla osteotomy. *J Am Anim Hosp Assoc 11*:205, 1975.
3. Beckman SL, et al: Total ear canal ablation combining bulla osteotomy and curettage in dogs with chronic otitis externa and media. *J Am Vet Med Assoc 196*:84, 1990.
4. Boothe HW Jr.: Surgical management of otitis media and otitis interna. *Vet Clin North Am Small Amin Pract 18*:90, 1988.
5. Borken EA, Brookler KH: Surface tension lowering substance of the canine eustachian tube. *Ann Otrol Rhinol Laryngol 81*: 268, 1972.
6. Bradley RL, et al: Nasopharyngeal and middle ear polypoid masses in five cats. *Vet Surg 14*:141, 1985.
7. Burk RL, Ackerman N: *Small Animal Radiology: A Diagnostic Atlas and Text*. Churchill Livingstone, New York, 1986.
8. Geary JC: Radiographic aspects of otitis media. *Auburn Vet 21*:71, 1965.
9. Grono LR: Observation on the incidence of otitis externa in the dog. *Aust Vet J 45*:417, 1969.
10. Harvey CE, Goldschmidt MH: Inflammatory polypoid growths in the ear canal of cats. *J Small Anim Pract 19*:669, 1978.
11. Holzworth J: Naturally occurring upper respiratory infection in cats. *J Am Vet Med Assoc 158*:964, 1971.
12. Lim DJ: Functional morphology of the mucosa of the middle ear and eustachian tube. *Ann Otrol Rhinol Laryngol 85* (Suppl):36, 1976.
13. Mason LK, et al: Total ear canal ablation combined with lateral bulla osteotomy for end-stage otitis in dogs; results in thirty cases. *Vet Surg 17*:263, 1988.
14. Matthiesen DT, Scavelli T: Total ear canal ablation and lateral bulla osteotomy in 38 dogs. *J Am Anim Hosp Assoc 26*:257, 1990.
15. McBride RL: Persistent otorrhea in the dog. Proceedings of the 19th Annual Meeting of the AVMA. Toronto, July 1953, pp 247–252.
16. McNutt FW, McCoy JE: Bulla osteotomy in the dog. *J Am Vet Med Assoc 77*:617, 1930.
17. Miller ME, et al: *Anatomy of the Dog*. W.B. Saunders, Philadelphia, 1964.
18. Neer TM, Howard PE: Otitis media. *Comp Cont Educ 4*:410, 1982.
19. Parker AJ, et al: Bulla curettage for chronic otitis media and interna in dogs. *J Am Vet Med Assoc 168*:931, 1976.
20. Rose WR: Bulla osteotomy. *Vet Med Small Anim Clin 72*:1712, 1977.
21. Rose WR: Myringotomy. *Vet Med Small Anim Clin 72*:1646, 1977.
22. Rose WR: Otitis media. *Vet Med Small Anim Clin 71*:1443, 1976.
23. Sade J, et al: Clearance of middle ear effusion by the mucociliary system. *Acta Otolaryngol (Stockh) 79*:277, 1975.
24. Sharp NJH: Chronic otitis externa and otitis media treated by total ear canal ablation and ventral bulla osteotomy in thirteen dogs. *Vet Surg 19*:162, 1990.
25. Shell LG: Otitis media and otitis interna: Etiology, diagnosis, and medical management. *Vet Clin North Am Small Amin Pract 18*:885, 1988.
26. Smeak DD: The Chinese finger trap suture technique for fastening tubes and catheters. *J Am Anim Hosp Assoc 26*:215, 1990.
27. Smeak DD, De Hoff WD: Total ear canal ablation; clinical results in the dog and cat. *Vet Surg 15*:161, 1986.
28. Spreull JSA: Otitis media. *Animal Hospital 2*:89, 1966.
29. Spreull JSA: Treatment of otitis media in the dog. *J Small Anim Pract 5*:107, 1964.

SECTION 15

Musculoskeletal System

Philip B. Vasseur, and Douglas Slatter ■ *Section Editors*

CHAPTER 118

Gait Analysis and Orthopedic Examination

G. Sumner-Smith

THE DIAGNOSIS OF CANINE LAMENESS

Lameness is defined as interference in normal locomotion of an animal, usually involving the propulsion mechanism of one or more limbs. It is often assumed that lameness originates in the skeletal system, but when the cause cannot be found there, attention is directed to other systems, such as the muscular system or neurological system or to referred pain from internal organs. Lameness may be acquired or inherited, the latter resulting from malformation of a system.

Evaluation of lameness requires complete familiarity with normal locomotion.[15] Animals are normally examined in two gaits, walking and trotting. Racing dogs such as greyhounds and Salukis may be examined at their full gait of a gallop to ascertain abnormalities. Some dogs pace, and this gait can be used in place of the trot.

Terms used in the study of locomotion need to be defined. A *stride* is defined as a full cycle from the point when the foot touches the ground (contact point) to when the foot leaves the ground (lift point) and then again touches the ground. The stride is therefore from contact point to contact point (Fig. 118–1). When the foot is on the ground, we speak of the retraction phase (or stance phase), and when the foot is in the air, the protraction phase (or swing phase). When the foot is in the contact phase (retraction), the traction caused by the whole limb on the body ensures that the body moves forward. When the foot is in the swing phase (protraction), the alternate limb is carrying out the propulsion.

It is essential to become familiar with the normal gait, because interference in one or more of these phases suggests lameness in the area affected. Lameness is caused by an animal's attempting to minimize pain, which usually occurs during the contact phase, but protraction can sometimes cause pain and interference with the swing phase.

If an animal is lame while walking, it is advisable to induce it to trot. The trot is as slow as possible to maximize the amount of time that a limb is loaded and hence magnify the signs of lameness.

NORMAL GAITS

Walk (Fig. 118–2)

When an animal walks, four, three, or two legs support it at any one time. Walking is a slow, symmetrical gait in which the legs on one side of the animal perform the same movements as on the other side but half a stride later. Examinations of this gait on a reflecting walkway have shown that the main pad takes the weight first and then the weight is put on the toe pads.

Trot (see Fig. 118–2)

During a trot, the body is supported by two contralateral legs. The forelimbs are free of the ground longer than the hindlimbs, permitting those legs to clear the ground in advance of placement of the hindlimbs.

Pace (see Fig. 118–2)

The pace is a gait in which the limbs of the same side symmetrically support the animal. Some dogs pace nat-

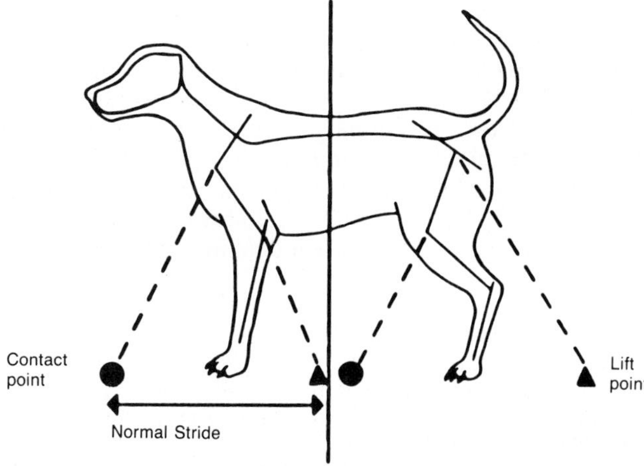

FIGURE 118–1. Contact point and lift point in a normal stride. (From Sumner-Smith G: *Decision Making in Small Animal Orthopaedic Surgery*. B. C. Decker, Philadelphia 1988.)

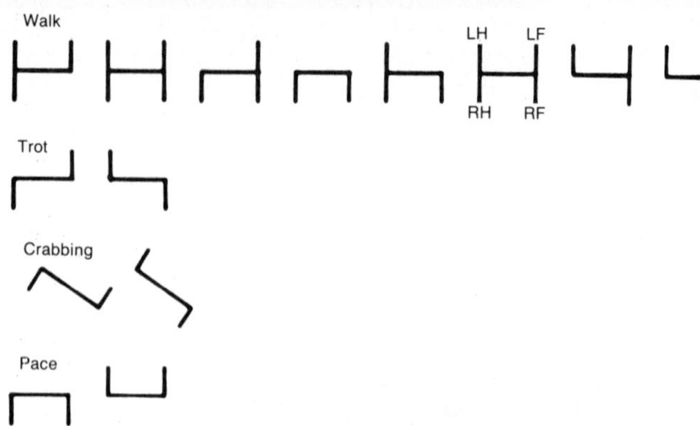

FIGURE 118–2. Gait patterns. (From Sumner-Smith G: *Decision Making in Small Animal Orthopaedic Surgery.* B. C. Decker, Philadelphia, 1988.)

urally, other dogs only trot, and certain individuals both trot and pace.

Joint Angles

When viewing a dog in the middle of a stance phase, it is possible to see the classic joint angles that have been attributed to the limbs; however, considerable variation in these angles is noted in different breeds.

During locomotion, most of the movement of the forelimb takes place between the shoulder blades and the thorax, in the muscle joint known as a *synsarcosis*.[16] At the end of the swing phase, the limb goes into extension and the carpus is also fully extended. When it reaches the end of a retraction or stance phase, the carpus is flexed. Only at the end of both of these phases is any movement seen in the carpus and the elbow (Fig. 118–3).

In the hindlimb, most of the movement takes place at the hip joint[17] (Fig. 118–4). Very little movement occurs in the stifle until the end of the stance phase.

An alteration in joint angles occurs when an animal is lame and the weight is shifted to the other limbs.

QUANTIFICATION OF LAMENESS[18]

It is necessary to have a consistent grading method for lameness to enable clinicians to interpret previously recorded notes and allow colleagues to appreciate whether or not an animal is more lame or less lame than at the previous examination.[1, 2] Although a 1–5 method is used by some clinicians, especially equine veterinarians, I have found the following 1–10 method more useful, particularly when dealing with subtle lameness:

Degrees of Lameness

0: Sound
1: Occasionally shifts weight
2: Mild lameness at a slow trot, none while walking
3: Mild lameness while walking
4: Obvious lameness while walking, but places the foot when standing
5: Degrees of severity
6: Degrees of severity
7: Degrees of severity
8: Degrees of severity
9: Places toe when standing, carries limb when trotting
10: Unable to put the foot on the ground

ORIGIN OF LAMENESS

Lameness may be due to pathology of one or more of the following systems:

Muscles: Rupture or strain of muscle belly or tendon
Bones: Acquired or inherent pathology
Joints: Inflammation and degeneration
Nerves: Nerve entrapment or disruption
Other systems: For example, abdominal pain causing a stilted gait

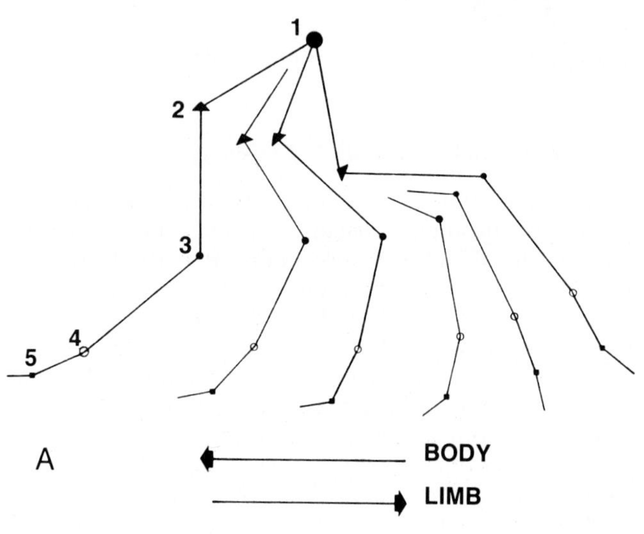

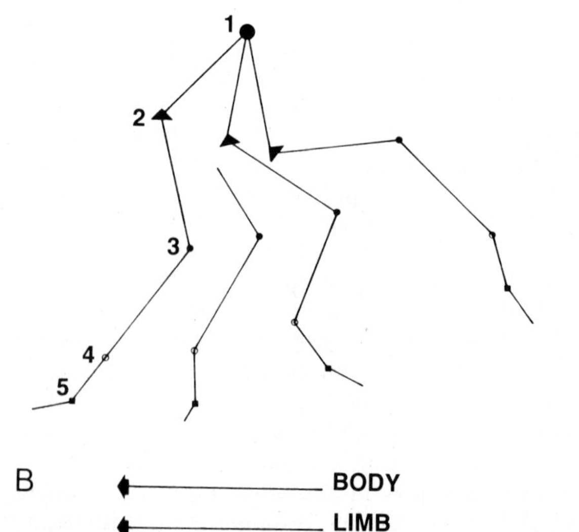

FIGURE 118–3. *A*, Normal goniometric angles of a dog's forelimb during the stance phase (retraction). Pivoting takes place through the synsarcosis of the scapula on the thorax. (1, pivot center of scapula on the thorax; 2, shoulder joint; 3, elbow joint; 4, carpus; 5, metacarpophalangeal joint). *B*, The same forelimb during the swing phase (protraction). (From *Sumner-Smith G: Decision Making in Small Animal Orthopaedic Surgery.* B. C. Decker, Philadelphia, 1988.)

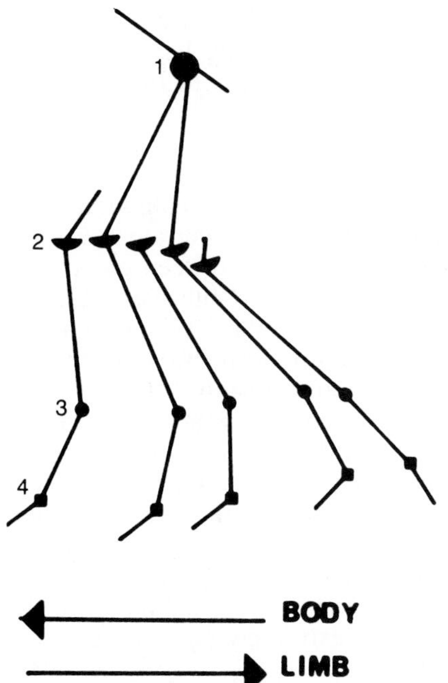

FIGURE 118–4. The normal goniometric angles of the hindlimb during the stance phase. (1, hip; 2, stifle; 3, hock; 4, metatarsal joint.) (From Sumner-Smith G: *Decision Making in Small Animal Orthopaedic Surgery.* B. C. Decker, Philadelphia, 1988.)

Clinicians often have difficulty remembering which limb to watch when the head is dropped. A simple trick is to put an imaginary stone in one's own shoe and then attempt to walk, noting that one spends less time on the painful appendage.

HISTORY

The background history should be available, as well as the immediate history regarding the lameness. It is critical to listen to the owner and to extract from the main remarks and the ancillary comments some idea about what has been observed. One wishes to know the duration of the problem, whether the onset was sudden or gradual, whether an accident preceded the lameness, and whether the lameness only appears at certain times. One should inquire if an incident some time ago might account for the observed outcome.

It is also necessary to know the progress of the lameness; has it evolved to its present state, or is it of an intermittent nature. Does the lameness abate for some time and return unexpectedly? Is the animal more lame at certain times of the day or in certain kinds of weather? Is it particularly lame after exercise or does it "warm out" of the lameness? Is it more affected by having to climb, or does it appear to avoid jumping off even low objects? Is the lameness always in one limb, or does it move around (shifting lameness), producing lameness in different limbs at different times? It is also essential to know if the animal has previously been treated for the condition and if it is currently receiving medication.

One should ascertain the patient's environment to know if the diet may be a cause of the lameness or if the kennel situation could be causing trauma. Information about previous illnesses or accidents is important.

Certain breeds have congenital abnormalities that predispose to lameness. The valgus and plantigrade stance of the forelimbs of a basset hound predisposes to radiocarpal problems. The bowed limbs of a Pekingese predispose to degenerative arthritis of the elbows. Poodles have problems with stifles, and Labradors with hips.

EXAMINATION FOR LAMENESS

When a dog is lame, the swing and stance phases are shortened, abbreviating the time that it can bear weight on the affected limb. Normally, one examines a dog as it moves toward the viewer and then as it goes away, as well as in both lateral directions.*

It is tempting to place the patient on a table and start to palpate. Palpation in the initial stage of investigation is contraindicated. Before seeing an animal move, it is essential to observe it when it is still. One should preferably see it rise, because difficulty in rising may show signs pertaining to the particular area involved. *During the time the history is being taken, the animal is watched because many salient features may emerge when it believes it is not being observed: weight shifting from one limb to another, easing of a joint, and loading one limb more than the other.* If the lameness is not obvious at a slow walk, the animal is induced to trot. Examining a large dog does not usually cause many problems. However, the smaller the dog, the more difficult it is to observe what is happening because the dog's normal locomotion is so rapid. Even at a walk, the legs of a toy breed move so quickly that it is almost impossible to see what is happening. By using the technique of mental slow-motion analysis, one attempts to play back, in one's own mind, what was seen. Next, re-examine the animal to ascertain whether or not the initial impression and the playback were correct. If the impression is confirmed, the examination may be continued; if it is not confirmed, then one should watch the animal move until the site of the lameness has been ascertained. At best, visual examination of dogs with equivocal lameness is diagnostic about 50 per cent of the time.

In cases of hindlimb lameness, the stride length is shortened, and animals carry their head lower to minimize, via a cantilever effect, the amount of weight that is carried on the hindlimb(s).[19] When lame in the hips, a dog shifts weightbearing to the forelimbs and the pelvis is tilted more vertically than normal. If the lameness is unilateral, the pelvis is tilted sideways, and an oscillating motion is seen during locomotion. The oscillation is toward the sound side. When viewed from the rear, particularly if a dog is lame in both hips, the pelvis swivels from side to side. This maneuver minimizes hip motion and instead uses lateral bending of the spine to achieve forward movement. When one hip joint is noticeably worse than the other, the sound limb reaches forward in a quicker manner than the way the unsound

*See references 3–9, 12, and 14.

leg is advanced to the loading position. This movement minimizes weightbearing and pain in the unsound limb. The severity of this sign varies with the degree of lameness.

With lameness in a forelimb, an animal lifts its head when the unsound limb bears weight and drops its head with weightbearing on the sound limb. This may be the actual head movement at that point or may be an impression of dipping the head because the head was lifted when the lame limb was on the ground.

During the examination, observe the length of the swing phase, the duration of the stance phase, the position of the contact point, the position of the lift point, and whether or not the limb is flung forward and carried backward in the normal plane or whether it is abducted or adducted. It is also important to note any alteration in the normal joint angles. A decrease in movement in a joint suggests pain. Note the area of the foot that first contacts the ground. Normally it is the main pad followed by the toe pads: if the opposite occurs, it may denote a lack of desire to fully load the foot. A hatched background, such as a brick wall, often helps assess movement of the head that signals lameness. Additionally, one may be able to see a slight shortening of the contralateral step of an opposite hindlimb when this occurs in the front. The patient hastens to remove the weight from the censored limb, and therefore the swing phase of the sound limb is shortened. It can often cause a misdiagnosis.

Excitement or fear of the visit to the clinic may cause mild lameness to disappear momentarily. It may be necessary to hospitalize the patient to observe it in quieter moments.

Cross Lameness

The term *cross lameness* is acquired from the study of equine lameness; an animal can be lame in the right hindlimb but appear to be lame in the left forelimb. In such situations, the left hind and the right forelimbs, at a trot, propel the animal to a greater degree than the other two limbs, and the cross lameness results as the animal attempts to keep the limbs in phase during the trot—a gait in which the contralateral legs support at the same time. The situation may be compensated by the patient, carrying the sound contralateral limb for one step. The owner reports that when the animal hurries, it occasionally hops on a particular limb; it may be assumed, incorrectly, that that limb is the one causing discomfort.

SPECIFIC TESTS FOR THE EXAMINATION OF LAMENESS

Inspection

Once an animal has been observed in locomotion, it is stood quietly in front of the observer or, if it is small, on the table, and the body inspected. Visual inspection can be very difficult in animals with a long coat but it is invaluable in shorthaired animals. Observe whether or not the musculature is diminished in any part of the body. Note particularly the muscles of the shoulders and the thighs. Their state may be evaluated by standing over the patient and comparing one side with the other.

Palpation

Light palpation and deep palpation are performed. Light palpation is used to ascertain any alteration in the tissues being inspected, and deep palpation determines if pain is present at a particular site. Light palpation is used to search for puffiness of an area, particularly a joint; swelling, whether fluctuating or tense; and an increase in local temperature.

Deep palpation of the bones must be carefully performed because the observer may inadvertently put pressure on either a nerve or muscle, causing discomfort. It is possible to put pressure on most bones without interfering with overlying structures. In a condition such as panosteitis, lesions may be present in more than one bone. The stoicism of some animals and the sensitivity of others can be extremely misleading.

INDIVIDUAL LAMENESSES

This section describes general features of lameness associated with the major joints. Specific disease conditions are addressed in their respective chapters.

Shoulder (Fig. 118–5)

In the shoulder joint, the compression test is particularly helpful.[13] With the joint held in its normal position, the head of the humerus is compressed into the glenoid cavity in three different ways: with slight abduction, with slight adduction, and in a rotational movement during compression. When this is being carried out, the area of the scapular tuberosity and the bicipital bursa is examined at the same time for specific point pain. Pain in the shoulder joint may be intrinsic or extrinsic. Intrinsic pain stems from mechanisms involving the articular surface, and extrinsic pain involves mechanisms in the nearby musculature or structures farther away, which are capable of initiating shoulder pain, such as cervical discs.

When the pain is from intrinsic sources, the movement of the joint is limited. There is an apparent "freezing" of the joint, and that joint's normally minimal contribution to locomotion is taken up by the rest of the limb, particularly the scapula on the thorax. If the lameness is due to an extrinsic condition, movement of the entire shoulder area, not only the joint, is impaired. Muscular conditions causing lameness include infraspinatus contracture, dorsal displacement of the scapula, avulsion of the origin of the biceps brachii, medial displacement of the tendon of origin of the biceps brachii, and partial or complete avulsion of the triceps tendon.[10, 11] In the acute stages, the limb is nonweightbearing, and there is usually displacement of the scapula according to the muscles involved. Loss of musculature and fibrous contraction of the remaining muscle tissue occur with chronicity, impairing joint function. Weightbearing is limited on the injured side, and the animal displays a deformity of

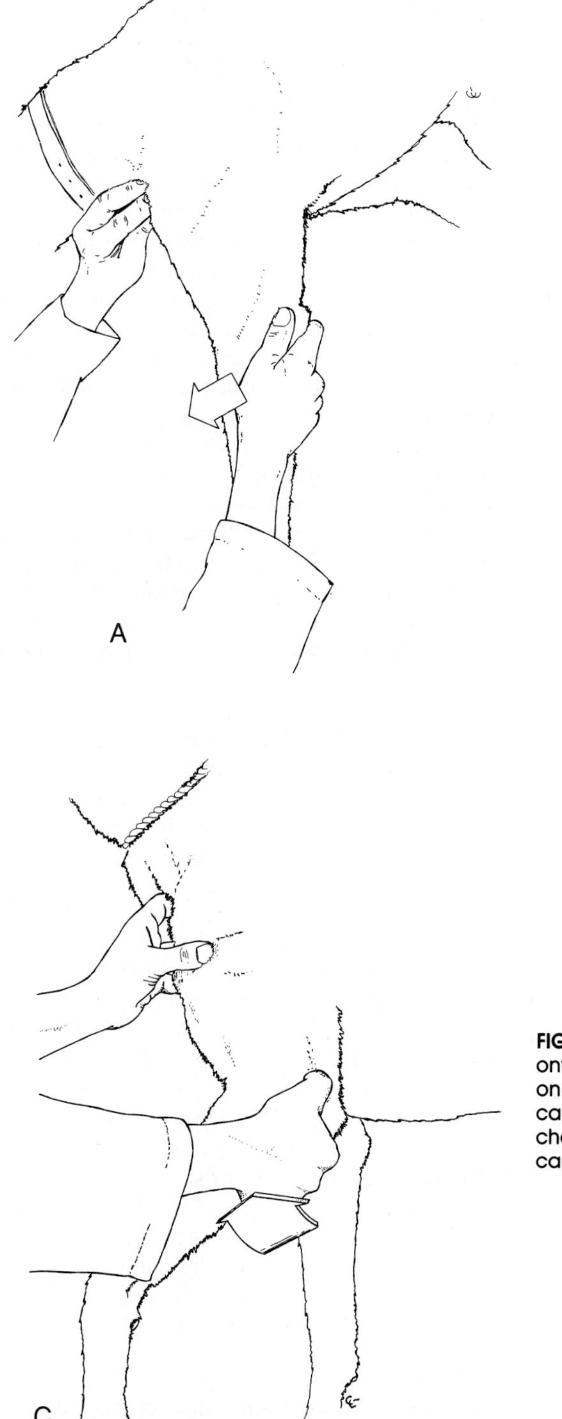

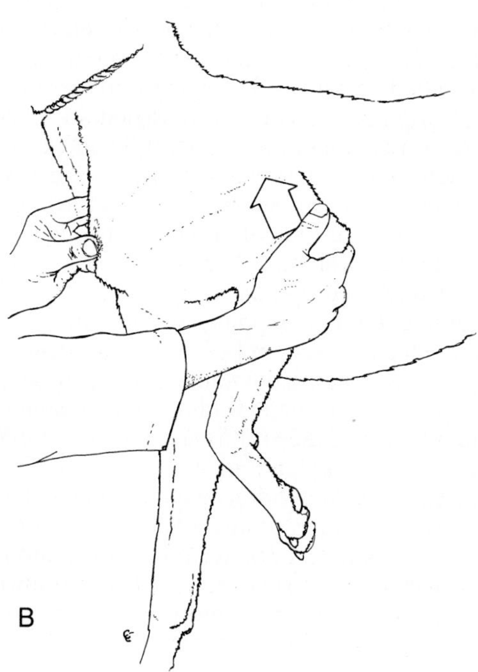

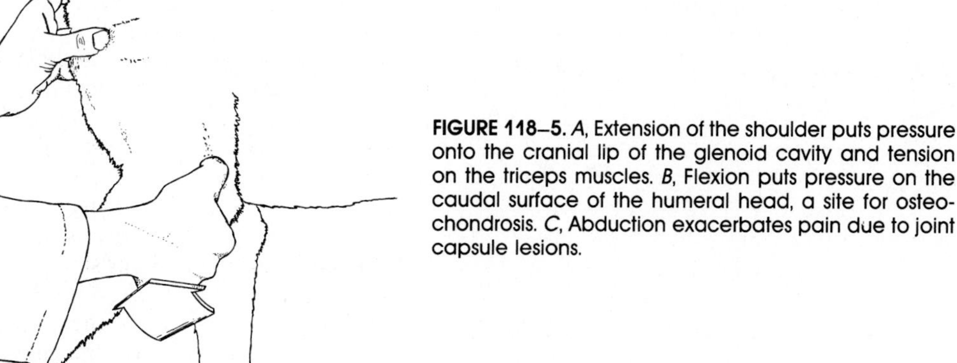

FIGURE 118–5. *A*, Extension of the shoulder puts pressure onto the cranial lip of the glenoid cavity and tension on the triceps muscles. *B*, Flexion puts pressure on the caudal surface of the humeral head, a site for osteochondrosis. *C*, Abduction exacerbates pain due to joint capsule lesions.

the shoulder joint, often with dorsal displacement of the scapula, accompanied by internal rotation. One should ascertain the neurological status of the limb, because acute trauma may have caused brachial plexus damage or damage to peripheral nerves such as the suprascapular nerve.

When the biceps brachii muscle is involved, the lameness may not be greater than a grade 3 or 4 but is variable. Pain may be elicited on flexion and extension of the shoulder joint, and cranial displacement of the humerus may be detectable. Radiographs often demonstrate distal displacement of the supraglenoid tuberosity. Rupture of the transverse humeral ligament permits displacement of the biceps tendon of origin, usually in a medial direction. The animal becomes acutely lame, but this lameness may subside after a few days, becoming exacerbated after prolonged exercise. The displacement may be determined by palpating the area, noting a sensation of the tendon popping in and out of the groove when the leg is flexed and extended, particularly if internal rotation of the scapula and external rotation of the humerus are performed. Radiographic examination is unhelpful because the soft tissues are not visible; one must rely on digital palpation.

Rupture of the triceps tendon may or may not be accompanied by a fracture of the olecranon process. The rupture may be partial, initially seen as a hematoma that gradually resolves. Alternatively, if the rupture was more severe, fibrous tissue formation may cause contracture of the triceps muscle and loss of mass of that muscle. Radiographic examination is only helpful if small fragments have avulsed from the olecranon process.

Humerus

In young dogs, the humerus is a site for panosteitis, and deep pressure on the bone may elicit pain.

Elbow Joints (Fig. 118–6)

Lameness in the elbow is similar to that in the shoulder. Elbow lameness is characterized by reduced joint motion during ambulation. These decreases in the angle of movement are not always total but depend on the severity of the pathology and the stoicism of the animal. Lateral observation of an animal helps distinguish between shoulder and elbow lameness. With elbow lameness, the joint does not fully extend on the end of the stride, and a slight dipping of the head is often seen at the contact point.

Most elbow lameness arises from problems within the joint rather than the surrounding ligaments and tendons (see Chapters 131 and 145C). The joint is examined in flexion and extension to search for any decrease in the range of motion. At the same time, capsular distension or soft-tissue swelling can be palpated. Radiographic examination of the joint may demonstrate luxations, fractures, degeneration, and productive changes. Subtle

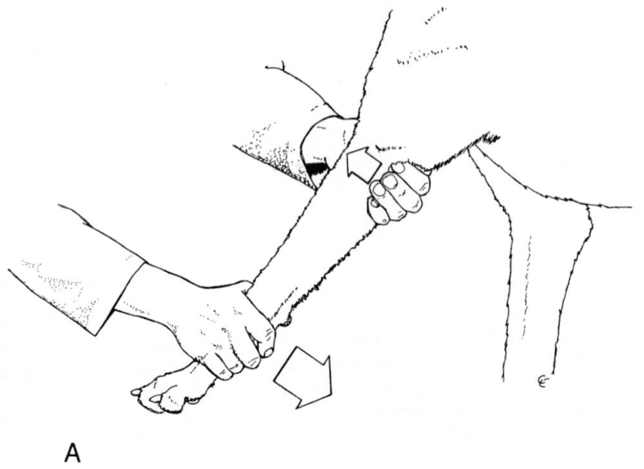

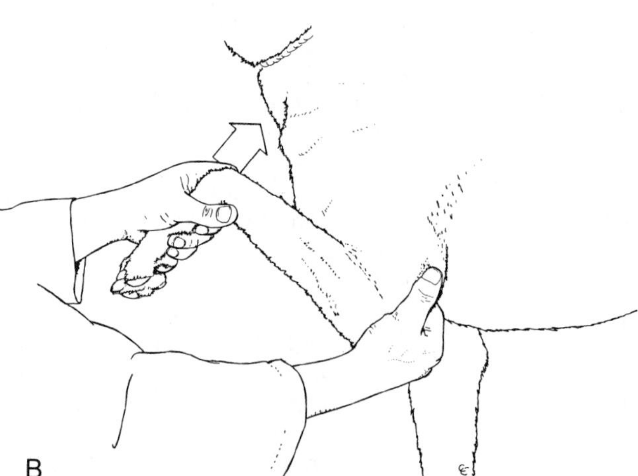

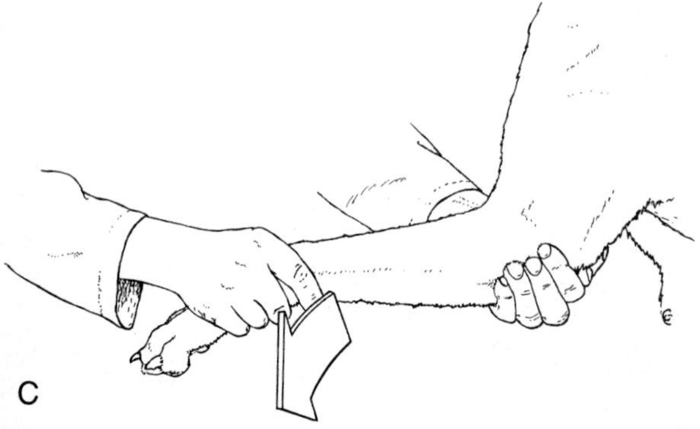

FIGURE 118–6. *A*, Extension creates pain at the site of the anconeal process. *B*, Compression creates pressure on the humeral condyles and the coronoid process and tenses the triceps. *C*, Rotation increases pressure on the coronoid process.

changes require additional projections for accurate evaluation (see Chapters 131 and 145C).

Antebrachium

In young dogs, the antebrachium is a common site of lameness. The growth plates of either the radius or ulna and sometimes both bones are involved. The first sign often is limb deformity, and careful questioning of the owner elicits knowledge of a previous injury. Such injuries can result in partial or complete growth plate closure. These conditions are painful and, if untreated, can produce severe lamenesses due to growth disparity and degenerative joint disease. Examination of the trotting dog often reveals grade 3 to 5 lameness, which can be exacerbated by pressure on the area that is causing the problem.

The radius is a common site for panosteitis, and it is relatively easy to palpate. Confirmation of the diagnosis requires radiography. Panosteitis may cause a shifting lameness, and the signs may disappear from one area and reappear elsewhere.

Fractures of the styloid process of the ulna or radius may be acute and cause severe lameness. With minimal displacement and a fibrous tissue connection, they can be extremely difficult to diagnose. Radiographs may be helpful, but the fracture may not be visible. The area is carefully palpated, and if pain is produced, radiographs are taken at various angles to demonstrate the fracture. The condition can cause extreme pain and can be frustrating to diagnose.

Carpus

When a dog is lame in the carpus, the lameness is rarely visible as the dog moves away from the observer. As the animal moves toward one, it is possible to see the head dipping as the sound limb contacts the ground and the unsound limb is flung forward with an action of the whole leg. Weight is not put on the main footpad, and the animal tends to "toe" as it walks. This is particularly apparent when the animal trots.

Carpal bone injuries are common in racing animals. Subluxation of the joint may be seen in any animal but is particularly common in German shepherds, possibly because of their propensity for leaping before looking and causing hyperextension of the carpus when jumping from heights. Lameness from traumatic radiocarpal luxation is extremely acute, and the area does not bear weight. Unfortunately, these conditions are often incorrectly diagnosed or incorrectly treated, and a clinician may not see a dog until the condition has become chronic. At that time, a plantigrade stance is usually present and diagnosis is not difficult. Stress radiographs are necessary to differentiate radiocarpal, intercarpal, or carpometacarpal subluxation (see Chapter 133).

Metacarpals

Lameness due to problems with metacarpal bones may result from fracture or from subluxation or luxation. Unless the condition is severe, the diagnosis is usually made after radiographic examination, but palpation should suggest the area to be radiographed. In chronic cases, swelling may have subsided but pain may be elicited by local pressure, and during locomotion, the dog gives the impression of "throwing" that area.

Phalanges

Diagnosis of lameness due to a problem in the toes is not usually difficult because of the localized effect that occurs. Acute conditions such as fractures and abscesses cause a dog to carry its leg, whereas chronic cases are reflected by an obvious desire to minimize the load on the foot, and the dog stands with the toe barely touching the ground. Swelling or deformity of the toe is usual, and even if swelling has subsided, local pressure invariably evokes pain. Before proceeding with any type of treatment, radiography is mandatory.

Pelvis

Fractures of the Pelvis

Although pelvic fractures are addressed elsewhere in this text, it is relevant to mention them here for their role in hindlimb lameness. Fracture of the pelvis does not always cause marked deformity and total loss of use of a limb. Mild subluxation of the sacroiliac joint or cracks in the innominate bone may cause transient or persistent lameness due to traction on the lumbosacral nerve roots. The lameness may become chronic. When an injury occurs in any part of the pelvis, a second site of trauma is usually present because the pelvic girdle is in the form of a box. Stiffness, soreness over a site, and conceivably some mild proprioceptive deficit are indications for radiographic examination.

Hip Joint

The bearing surface of the acetabulum is the craniodorsal perimeter and extends forward to a point 45° to the vertical. The bearing surface in the left hip is from 10 o'clock to 1 o'clock and in the right hip from 11 o'clock to 2 o'clock. Pathology of the rest of the acetabulum may cause lameness, but more severe lameness involves the bearing surfaces.

Subluxation (Including Hip Dysplasia)

Hip dysplasia is one of the most common causes of hindlimb lameness. Dogs with hip dysplasia often demonstrate a typical gait pattern (Table 118–1).

TABLE 118–1. HIP DYSPLASIA GAIT PATTERNS

Upright hindlimb
Stiff hindlimb—reaches forward
Low head carriage
Weight carried on hind toe and not the whole foot
Lateral bending of lumbar spine associated with lateral rotation of the pelvis, which is greater on the side that is more painful
Decreased protraction (swing phase)

Marked subluxation is occasionally associated with an audible clicking sound as a dog walks, caused by the femoral head snapping in and out of the acetabulum. The examiner places his or her hands over the greater trochanters and walks along with the dog. Lateral displacement of the greater trochanters during ambulation is readily palpable. Two additional examinations may be carried out to ascertain the amount of subluxation. They may or may not, according to an animal's cooperation, require sedation.

Hip Lift. With the animal resting on its side, grasp the femur in the appropriate hand (left for the left limb) and, keeping the femur parallel with the ground, lift the hip vertically; at the same time, place the fingers of the right hand on the trochanter major. If subluxation is present, the fingers are able to appreciate the trochanter popping up and down. The examiner should practice this maneuver on apparently normal dogs, because after three or four repetitions, it is invariably possible to gain some slight upward movement of the trochanter major. This is because the surface tension exerted by the synovial fluid is broken, and even in a normal dog there is often appreciable but minor upward movement.

Ortolani Sign (Fig. 118–7). With an animal supine, the femurs are pointed vertically, at 90° to the horizontal. The examiner's palms are placed over the flexed stifles, and gentle pressure is exerted toward the ground (or examining table). The thighs are then gently *abducted*, and if the sign is positive, a pronounced movement is felt as the femoral heads click back into the acetabulum. The sign may be positive on one or both sides. This manipulation subluxates the femoral head, and the sudden movement is occasioned by its returning into the depths of the acetabulum. An audible click may or may not be heard. Manipulation of the hip in a nonsedated dog may increase the signs of lameness and assist in confirming the diagnosis.

Stifle Joint

The stifle joint is a common site of lameness in the hindlimb. The signs caused by this lameness are characteristic. In an attempt not to use the joint, greater use is made of the hip joint in the swing phase to permit the animal to cover the necessary distance. The amount of movement in a normal stifle joint is not great except when an animal wishes to lie down. The joint acts as a cushion during locomotion. During the stance phase, from the contact point to the middle of that phase, the amount of loading on the stifle joint increases. When the foot is perpendicular underneath the hip, the load is at its maximum, and if the stifle is the cause of the lameness, the animal fixes the joint and finishes the rest of the stance phase by means of the hip joint. This latter phase is reduced in its excursion.

When the sound leg reaches the lift point, it is carried forward extremely rapidly to minimize the amount of time that the unsound stifle is loaded. "Dipping" of the hip results on the sound side. In severe cases, the carriage of the head is also affected, and it too dips when the opposite forelimb is in the contact phase. In milder cases, discomfort in the stifle joint causes the animal to move the limb continually to ease the load. If the lameness is severe, the animal only puts its toe on the ground.

Lameness in the stifle joint may be accompanied by instability of the joint. The animal usually "toes" the affected leg because it does not wish to load it fully, particularly at the vertical point. If the lameness is confined to the stifle, the limb is swung forward normally. The hock joint usually is fully extended; lameness of the stifle is accompanied by reduced motion in the hock. Bilateral lameness in the stifle joints is often incorrectly assumed to be due to spinal disc disease.

The "drawer sign" is used to test for stability of the cruciate ligament (Fig. 118–8).

Hock Joint

The tarsal joint is a complicated group of joints collectively known as the *hock*. Diagnosis of lameness in the hock is not difficult in severe cases but may be elusive in subtle conditions such as mild osteochondrosis of the talus.

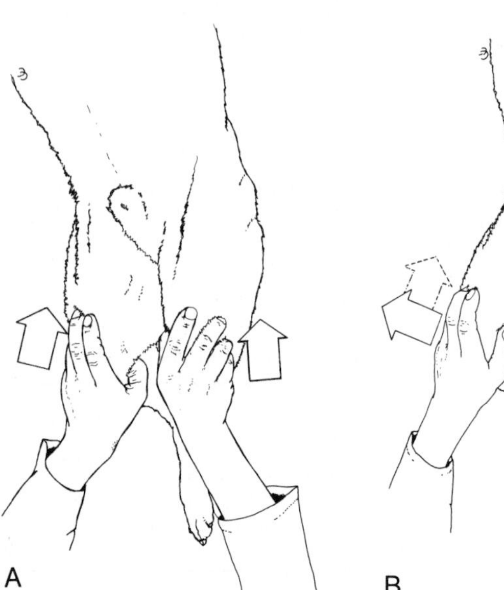

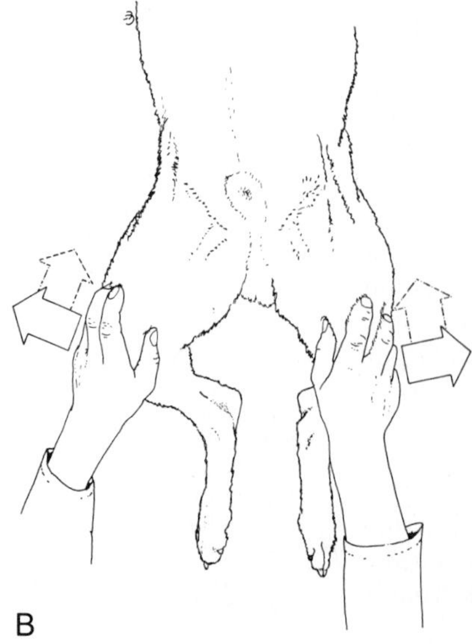

FIGURE 118–7. *A*, The femurs are placed at right angles to the table, and pressure is created by downward displacement. *B*, The limbs are then gently abducted. If joint laxity exists, a sharp click is heard as the femoral heads reseat in the acetabula.

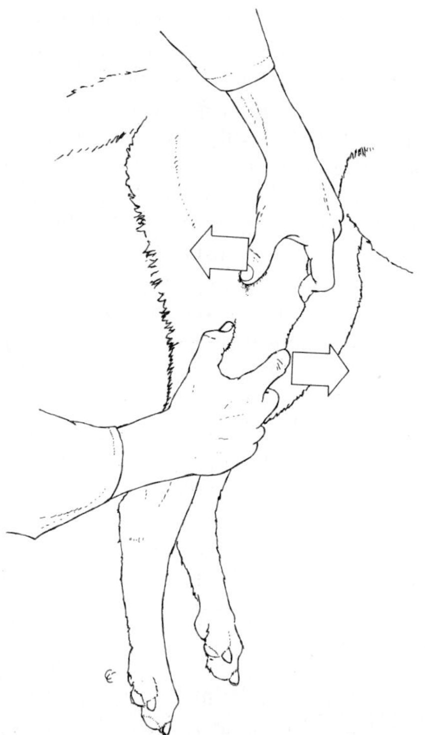

FIGURE 118–8. Cranial drawer test. Excessive displacement of the tibial plateau relative to the femoral condyles is diagnostic of cruciate ligament rupture. Excessive cranial displacement (cranial drawer sign) suggests rupture of the cranial cruciate ligament, whereas excessive caudal displacement (caudal drawer sign) suggests rupture of the caudal cruciate ligament.

Until the end of the stance phase, little movement normally occurs in the hock joint. Should some pathology exist, this movement is further decreased. If the pain is acute, the animal carries the leg completely in a 10:10 lameness. When it does so, the hip and the stifle joint are in a flexed position. With mild hock lameness, the stifle and hip joints move in a normal manner in the swing phase, but there is some resistance to loading when the animal is in the stance phase.

Palpation of the joint is often helpful. With the hock in extension, instability may be ascertained; with it in 90° of flexion, compression may elicit pain.

Lesions of the Spine

Pressure on various areas of the spinal cord may result in lameness due to impaired neurological function in the area supplied. At the same time, either pain or a lack of ability to function may cause lameness. Because the signs may be those of lameness, it is necessary to consider what spinal lesions may cause signs of lameness.

Cervical Spine

Lesions high in the cervical spine, such as in the atlanto-occipital area, may produce anesthesia caudal to the lesion or more commonly may produce exquisite pain. This causes the animal to walk with its head extremely depressed and to take very short steps. Great care should be used in examining such a patient because the lesion may be exacerbated and become irreversible (Fig. 118–9*A*).

Lesions farther down the spine, C3–C7, may produce the classic gait of a "wobbler." This may result from spondylolisthesis or from spinal stenosis; Great Danes and Doberman pinschers are the breeds most commonly affected. With this condition, much may be learned by watching an animal ambulate. Lesions in this area cause an animal to stumble and drag its toes as it walks. These signs may be present in the hindlimbs alone or in all four. In milder cases, the signs may be equivocal, but they may be exacerbated by turning the animal acutely; at that time, staggering becomes more pronounced. If in doubt, a patient is encouraged to trot slowly, and the signs are exacerbated. Lesions low in the cervical spine, such as those in Doberman pinschers, cause patients to walk with a wide-based gait. All four limbs are carried

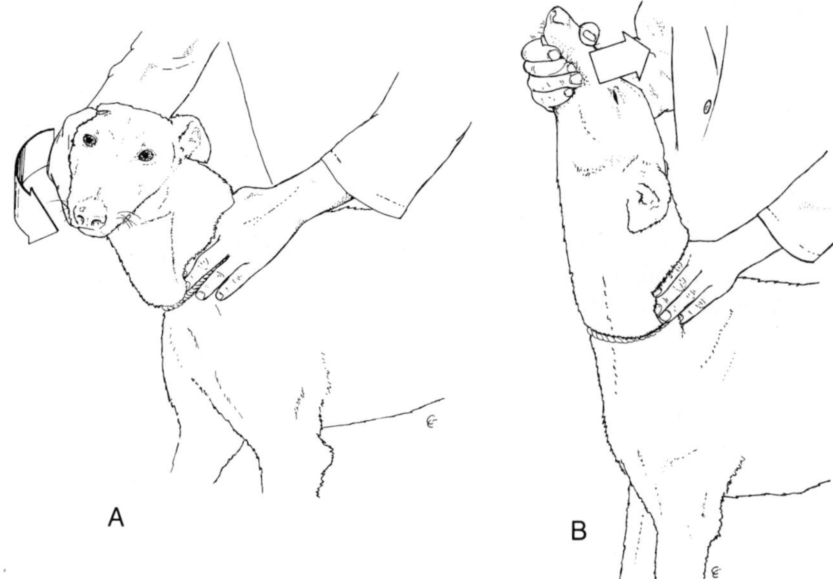

FIGURE 118–9. *A*, By flexing, extending, and rotating the neck, pain due to pathology of the articular facets is exacerbated. *B*, Hyperextension and hyperflexion of the neck are used in elucidating spondylolisthesis with its concurrent neurological sequelae.

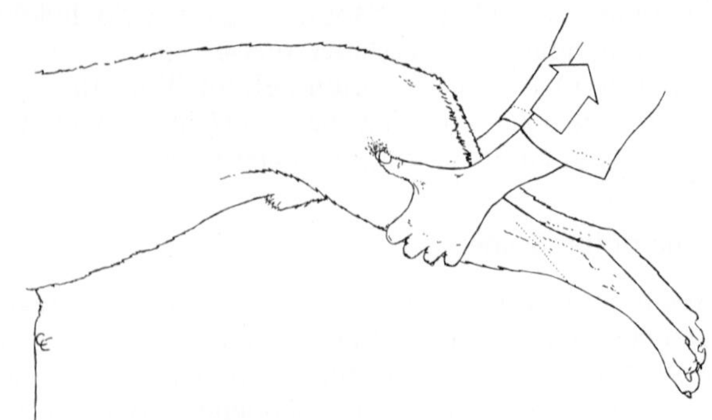

FIGURE 118–10. By elevating the hindquarters and pressing down on the lumbosacral area, pain in that region is increased, indicating that radiographs of the area are desirable.

in slight abduction as the patient attempts to prevent falling sideways. If it is turned in a tight circle, the dog is unable to cross the front limbs, as normally occurs in long-legged dogs when they wish to turn quickly.

In all areas, the signs may be exacerbated by hyperextending the neck. When this is being carried out, it may cause the animal to sit down or to stumble even when in the stationary standing position (Fig. 118–9*B*).

Lesions in the Lumbar Spine

Lesions in the lumbar spine may be due to disc disease, fractures, or neoplasia. Animals with a lesion in the lumbar area have difficulty in rising and show marked shortening of steps. The signs are usually bilateral but occasionally may be unilateral because of the location of the spinal lesion. At the same time, the patient may carry its head low to relieve the weight on its back. Dogs are quite commonly suspected of having lesions of the lumbar spine when the problem is actually the result of bilateral stifle lameness, such as bilateral cranial cruciate ligament rupture.

Lumbosacral Pain

Pain in the lumbosacral area may be due to trauma following an accident, and care should be taken in examining these animals to avoid further subluxation. Pain from these lesions is due to pressure on local nerve trunks. The pressure may or may not cause neurological impairment of the hindlimbs but invariably causes pain.

Chronic lumbosacral pain may be due to nerve entrapment. The pain may be intermittent but is usually progressive. Manipulation of the area, particularly dorsal flexion of the lumbosacral junction, can increase the discomfort and may aid in localizing the pain (Fig. 118–10). A condition termed *cauda equina syndrome* may manifest itself by signs that include difficulty in rising, urinary or fecal incontinence, perineal hyperalgesia or analgesia, paresis of the tail, paresthesia, self-mutilation of the tail and perineal area, and a decrease in the lumbosacral spinal reflexes. These signs vary considerably according to the pathology of the compressive lesion. It is important to distinguish cauda equina syndrome from hip dysplasia; early cases bear some similarity in that the animal is reluctant to rise and to walk upstairs. The two conditions may be differentiated by dorsal flexion of the spine. Unfortunately, radiographs that are positive for hip dysplasia may not rule out involvement of the lumbosacral spine because the diseases may exist concurrently.

References

1. Adrian MJ, et al: Normal gait of the dog: An electrogoniometric study. *Am J Vet Res 27*:90, 1966.
2. Alexander RM: *Animal Mechanics*. Sidwick & Jackson, London, 1968.
3. Arnoczky SP, Tarvin GB: Physical examination of the musculoskeletal system. *Vet Clin North Am Small Anim Pract 11*:575, 1981.
4. Barr ARS, Houlton JEF: Clinical investigation of the lame dog. *J Small Anim Pract 29*:695, 1988.
5. Binnington AG: Lameness work-up. *In* Sumner-Smith G (ed): *Decision Making in Small Animal Orthopaedic Surgery*. B. C. Decker, Philadelphia, 1988, pp 8–9.
6. Campbell J, Stead C: Chronic lameness in dogs. *Practice 5*:124, 1983.
7. Denny HR: *A Guide to Orthopaedic Surgery*. Blackwell Scientific, Oxford, 1980, pp 121–126.
8. Farrow CS: Sprain strain and contusion. *Vet Clin North Am 8*:169, 1978.
9. Foster J: Acute trauma in small animals; 1, Initial assessment and management. *Practice 7*:173, 1985.
10. Gilmore DR: Triceps tendon avulsion in the dog and cat. *J Am Anim Hosp Assoc 20*:239, 1984.
11. Goring RL, et al: Medical displacement of the tendon of origin of the biceps brachii muscle in the racing greyhound. *J Am Anim Hosp Assoc 20*:933, 1984.
12. Leach D, et al: Diagnosis of lameness in dogs: A preliminary study. *Can Vet J 8*:58, 1977.
13. Miller CW: Foreleg lameness in young animals. In Sumner-Smith G (ed): *Decision Making in Small Animal Orthopaedic Surgery*. B. C. Decker, Philadelphia, 1988, pp 12–13.
14. Newton CD, Nunamaker DM: *Textbook of Small Animal Orthopaedics*. J. B. Lippincott, Philadelphia, 1985, pp 125–131.
15. Sumner-Smith G: Normal locomotion. *In* Sumner-Smith G (ed): *Decision Making in Small Animal Orthopaedic Surgery*. B. C. Decker, Philadelphia, 1988, pp 2–3.
16. Sumner-Smith G: Forelimb Action. *In* Sumner-Smith G (ed): *Decision Making in Small Animal Orthopaedic Surgery*. B. C. Decker, Philadelphia, 1988, pp 4–5.
17. Sumner-Smith G: Hindlimb action. *In* Sumner-Smith G (ed): *Decision Making in Small Animal Orthopaedic Surgery*. B. C. Decker, Philadelphia, 1988, pp 6–7.
18. Sumner-Smith G: Lameness. *In* Sumner-Smith G (ed): *Decision Making in Small Animal Orthopaedic Surgery*. B. C. Decker, Philadelphia, 1988, pp 10–11.
19. Sumner-Smith G: Hindlimb lameness. *In* Ford RB (ed): *Clinical Signs and Diagnosis in Small Animal Practice*. Churchill Livingstone, New York, 1988, pp 325–350.

CHAPTER

119 Connective Tissues of the Musculoskeletal System

Adele L. Boskey

Connective tissues serve many functions in the body: They hold it together, organize its compartments, and provide cohesion and internal support. Differing in form and function, the connective tissues, skin, tendons, ligaments, cartilage, bones, teeth, lungs, spleen, capsules and sheaths of muscles, synovium, blood vessels, lungs, and so forth have several common features. All consist of cells, fibers, and nonstructured (amorphous) ground substances; all are derived primarily from mesenchyme; and all show the characteristic presence of banded fibers (collagen) under the light microscope (Fig. 119–1). The thick, ropelike collagen fibrils in tendon, seen at the electron microscopic level (Fig. 119–2*A*), can be contrasted to the random array of thin fibrils of collagen seen around chondrocytes in cartilage (Fig. 119–2*B*). Such variations in the density and arrangement

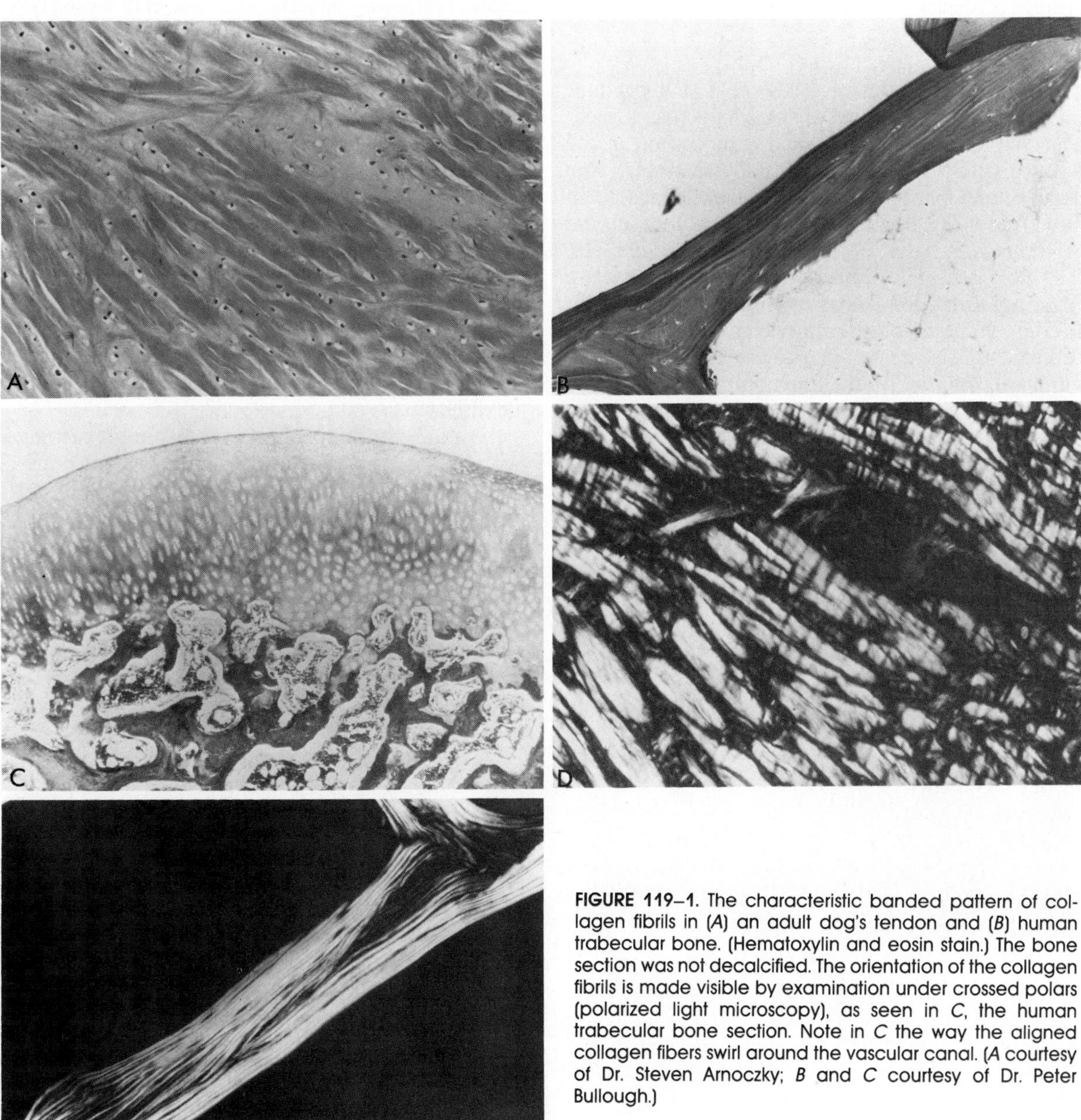

FIGURE 119–1. The characteristic banded pattern of collagen fibrils in (*A*) an adult dog's tendon and (*B*) human trabecular bone. (Hematoxylin and eosin stain.) The bone section was not decalcified. The orientation of the collagen fibrils is made visible by examination under crossed polars (polarized light microscopy), as seen in *C*, the human trabecular bone section. Note in *C* the way the aligned collagen fibers swirl around the vascular canal. (*A* courtesy of Dr. Steven Arnoczky; *B* and *C* courtesy of Dr. Peter Bullough.)

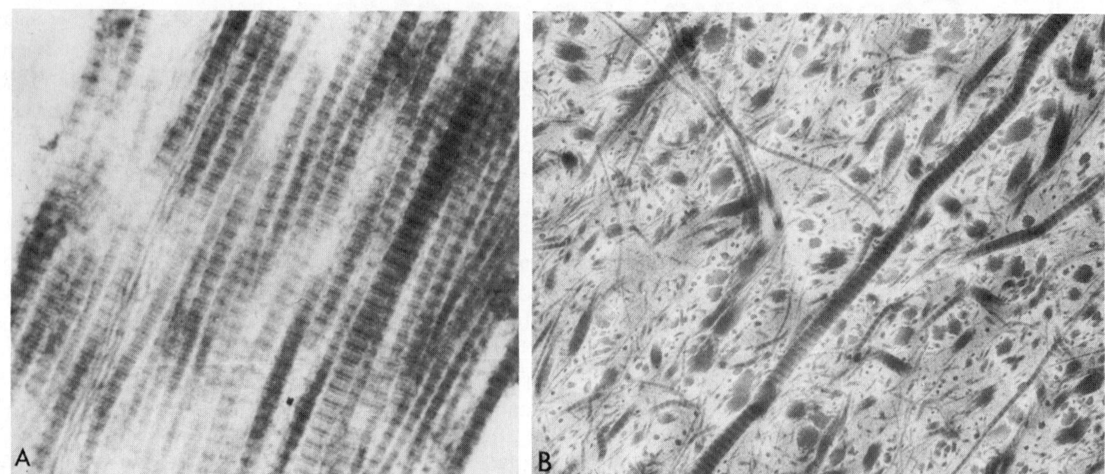

FIGURE 119–2. Transmission electron micrographs show the variations in the arrangement of collagen fibrils in (*A*) tendon and (*B*) cartilage. *A*, Dog tendon. *B*, A chick limb-bud chondrocyte in culture tissue. (*A* courtesy of Dr. Steven Arnoczky; *B* courtesy of Dr. Steven Doty.)

of the collagen fibers relative to the cells that produce them determine the functions of the connective tissues.

In this chapter, the structure and composition of the connective tissues of the musculoskeletal system and their component macromolecules are considered to illustrate (1) how the tissues perform their function and (2) the molecular bases of connective tissue diseases. Muscles, not generally considered to be connective tissues, contain intracellular as opposed to extracellular fibrous components. Because muscle cells do secrete an extracellular matrix containing connective tissue elements and are essential for the functioning of the skeletal system, they are also considered in this chapter.

Tissues that provide tensile strength (i.e., the ability to withstand stress) contain long, parallel bundles of fibers. The ability of ligaments and tendons to stretch depends on the presence of both collagen and another protein—rubbery, expansible elastin. Two- and three-dimensional networks of fibers exist in the tissues that serve protective functions. The periosteum, which covers the surface of bone; the perichondrium, which coats the cartilage surface; and the membrane fibrosa of the joint capsule all are both elastic and resistant to tensile forces. These tissues contain considerably more nonfibrous ground substance than the other connective tissues. Even more complicated patterns of fibers are found in tissues such as the arterial walls and healing incised wounds, which are exposed to pulsing fluids and lesser stresses and thus require greater flexibility. In these tissues, relatively short fibers appear in a circular arrangement in close contact with elastin fibers and smooth muscle. In cartilage, the collagen fibrils are spaced farther apart, with a more random orientation to provide mechanical strength and resilience while giving the tissue flexibility.

Hyaline cartilage[26] is a semitransparent cartilage found at the bone/joint surface, on the ventral ends of ribs, and in the respiratory system (Fig. 119–3*A*). It is extremely flexible owing to the presence of high-molecular-weight macromolecules known as *proteoglycans*. Hyaline cartilage contains a high proportion of water (more than 70 per cent of the tissues' wet weight). The other principal molecular components of hyaline cartilage are collagen (15 to 20 per cent of wet weight) and proteo-

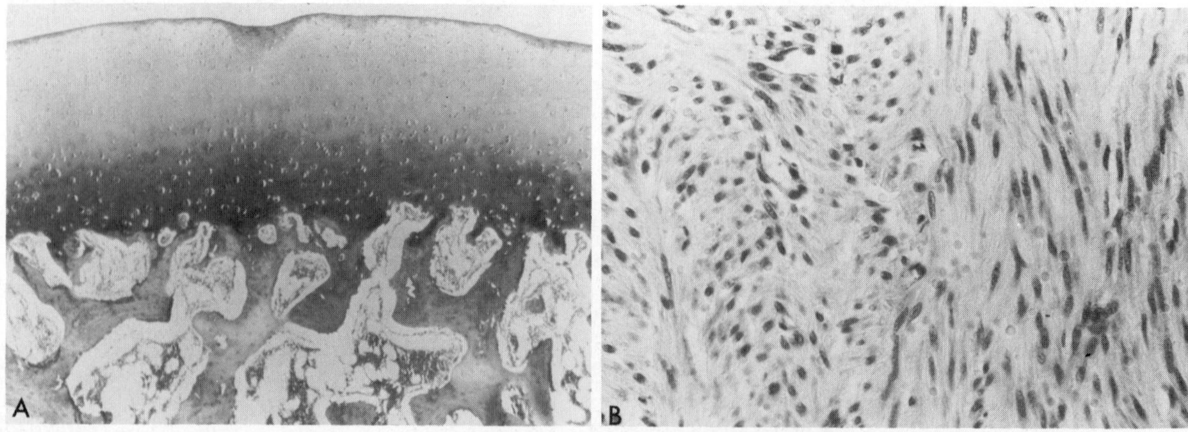

FIGURE 119–3. Light micrographs showing (*A*) hyaline cartilage and (*B*) fibrocartilage in an adult dog. *A*, The articular cartilage was stained with toluidine blue to reveal the territorial distribution of proteoglycans. *B*, The medial meniscus was stained with hematoxylin and eosin. (Courtesy of Dr. Steven Arnoczky.)

glycans (2 to 10 per cent of wet weight). Elastic cartilage, such as that found in the external ear, has even greater elasticity and opacity than hyaline cartilage. Fibrocartilage (Fig. 119–3*B*), found in the intervertebral discs and in close association with joints, contains denser collagen fibers and proteoglycans similar but not identical to those in hyaline cartilage. The functional differences between these cartilages are due to the different interactions between proteoglycans, collagen, and other matrix components within these tissues and to the different types of collagens in these tissues.

The "synovial system," consisting of articular cartilage, synovial membrane, and synovial fluid, contains various tissue types crucial to the functioning of the joints.[10, 17] The synovial cells (fibroblasts and chondrocytes) within the synovial membrane secrete and synthesize hyaluronic acid, a heteropolymer of *N*-acetylglucosamine and glucuronic acid. The presence of large (3 mg/ml)[17] quantities of the highly charged hyaluronic acid in the synovial fluid allows it to provide lubrication and nutrition to the joints. The synovial membrane also regulates the entry and egress of fluids and macromolecules into the cartilage. Loss of integrity of components of the synovial system, caused by inflammation, sepsis, or other causes of proteolysis, is a major component of the etiology of arthritis.[3, 18]

Bones and teeth are mineralized connective tissues[5, 14] that differ from the other connective tissues because they contain calcium phosphate mineral crystals (hydroxyapatite), which are deposited in an oriented fashion on the collagen fibers. The calcium phosphate mineral crystals make the tissue strong and rigid, providing the capacity for locomotion and protection. These crystals also provide a storage site for mineral deposition and are key in controlling mineral ion homeostasis.

COMPOSITION OF THE CONNECTIVE TISSUES

All connective tissues are composed of cells, extracellular fibers, and ground substance (the nonstructured components of the matrix). The principal cells producing connective tissue matrices are fibroblasts. These long, spindle-shaped cells stretch across bundles of collagen fibers. Fibroblasts are closely related to the chondrocytes, which produce cartilaginous matrices; the osteoblasts, which produce bone matrix; and the odontoblasts, which produce dentin matrices. Numerous other cells (macrophages, synovial cells, adipose cells, mast cells, monocytes, lymphocytes, plasma cells, and muscle cells) also produce connective tissue elements.

Collagen

The major fibrous component synthesized by connective tissue cells is collagen.[31, 36] Because of its unique fibrous structure, collagen provides tensile strength and integrity. Collagen is the most abundant mammalian protein, accounting for 20 to 50 per cent of the dry weight of an adult's long bones, 67 to 71 per cent of the dry weight of skin, and 87 to 92 per cent of the dry weight of tendons. Collagen is also a blood vessel constituent; thus it is found in low levels in all tissues.

At least 13 different types of collagens have been identified.[31] These collagens vary in size, structure, and the ability to form aggregates. However, all contain (to variable extents) three tightly coiled polypeptide chains known as *alpha chains*. The alpha chains are twisted about one another in a triple-helix configuration. Most of the connective tissue collagens form supermolecular aggregates (fibrils and fibers). The stability of individual fibrils (sets of collagen molecules aligned in a quarter-staggered array) and fibers (groups of collagen fibrils) is increased by the presence of intramolecular and intrafibrillar cross-links.

The individual alpha chains of the collagen molecules, for the most part, consist of the repeating tripeptide $(Gly\text{-}X\text{-}Y)_n$. Glycine, accounting for one-third of all the constituent amino acids, is the only amino acid small enough to fit in the center of the collagen triple helix. Proline, alanine, hydroxyproline, and hydroxylysine occur frequently in the X and Y positions. Hydroxylysine is frequently glycosylated with galactose or with glucose and galactose.

The most abundant class of connective tissue collagen is type I. It is found in skin, bones, tendons, and ligaments. Type I collagen consists of two identical alpha chains and one alpha chain of different amino acid composition. Type II collagen is the principal collagen of cartilage, the nucleus pulposus, and vitreous humor. Details on the structure and composition of these and other collagens and their association in collagen heteropolymers has been reviewed elsewhere.[31]

Collagen biosynthesis[36] (Table 119–1) begins with processing of the collagen gene. The collagen genes[32] are very complex; thus transcription of collagen DNA into mRNA is a multistep process involving the cleavage and splicing of numerous fragments. Translation of the mRNA produces individual polypeptide chains (pre-pro-alpha-chains), which are much larger than the individual alpha chains in the collagen molecule and structurally different from them. At least nine enzymatically catalyzed post-translational modifications and several reactions that probably occur spontaneously are needed to hydroxylate, glycosylate, and process the triple-helix molecule into insoluble extracellular fibrils.

A defect in any of these steps, whether it is inherited or caused by specific inhibition of a single step, could cause serious widespread changes in the properties of the collagen fibrils and the connective tissues that contain them. Study of the defects present in animals with the so-called collagen diseases has provided much of the current knowledge of the functions of the components of the collagen molecule.[25, 38, 42]

Errors in formation of messenger ribonucleic acids from collagen genes, defects in the type I collagen gene itself, and abnormalities in gene frequency all have been associated with various forms of osteogenesis imperfecta, a heterogeneous group of connective tissue diseases characterized by bone fragility.[36] Introduction of simian virus (SV40) genes into the mouse genome (transgenic mice) has provided verification of the osteogenic defects associated with expression of an abnormal collagen gene.[25, 42] Disruption of the host collagen genome provided several models of osteogenesis imperfecta.

TABLE 119–1. COLLAGEN BIOSYNTHESIS

	Enzymes and Cofactors	Product and Function	Associated Diseases	Notes
Intracellular events				
Transcription and translation of collagen mRNAs	All enzymes needed for eukaryotic transcription and translation	Soluble, extended collagen pre-pro-alpha chains	Osteogenesis imperfecta, Ehlers-Danlos IV	Simultaneous for alpha 1 and alpha 2 of type I collagen
Post-translational modification Hydroxylation of proline	4-Prolyl hydroxylase: oxygen, iron, ascorbic acid, α-ketoglutarate; 3-prolyl hydroxylase: same cofactors	Gly-Pro-4-OHPro. Forms hydrogen bonds, which stabilize triple helix Gly-3-OHPro-Pro	Scurvy (vitamin C deficiency)	Essential for the formation of stable collagen Amount of OHPro varies with tissue
Hydroxylation of lysine	5-Lysyl hydroxylase; same cofactors	Gly-X-5-OH-Lys glycosylated	Hydroxylsine deficiency disease; osteogenesis imperfecta	
Glycosylations	Collagen UDP galactosyl transferase Mn^{+2} collagen UDP glucosyltransferase, Mn^{+2}	Gly-X-5-OH-Lys | Gal | Glc	Diabetes mellitus	
	Mannose transferase	Mannose in nonhelical region	Osteogenesis imperfecta	C-terminal propeptide
Self-assembly	Disulfide reductase	Soluble triple helix–procollagen		Reductase activity parallels prolyl hydroxylase
Extracellular events				
Cleavage of propeptides	N-procollagen peptidase; C-procollagen peptidase	Insoluble collagen molecule	Ehlers-Danlos VII Dermatosporaxis	Sites differ in different collagen types
Packing of collagen		Fibrils	Ehlers-Danlos I; dominant Ehlers-Danlos (cats, mink, dogs)	Formation of active aldehydes
Cross-link formation				Number of cross-links increases with age
Aldehyde formation	Lysyloxidase oxygen, Cu^{+2}	Allysine/hydroxylysine	Lathyrism (β-aminopropionitrile); penicillamine; X-linked cutis laxa; aneurysm (mice); Menke's kinky hair; alkaptonuria	
Aldol condensation Aldimine formation Rearrangement	Spontaneous	Intra- and interchain Schiff bases and aldol condensation products		

mRNA, messenger ribonucleic acid; UDP, uridine diphosphate.

Such transgenic animals in which viral DNA or specific DNA clones not normally expressed in the animal are injected into embryonic stem cells promise to provide models[38] of many connective tissue diseases.

While the individual alpha chains are being synthesized, within the cell, before triple-helix formation, specific proline and lysines are hydroxylated in a series of reactions requiring molecular oxygen, iron, α-ketoglutaric acid, and vitamin C (ascorbic acid). This may explain the connective tissue abnormalities encountered in animals with scurvy (vitamin C deficiency). After hydroxylation and glycosylation of the alpha chains, the final step in the intracellular processing of collagen is self-assembly into a triple-helix molecule.

Secretion of the collagen molecule from the cell, which occurs only after triple-helix formation, is followed by the enzymatic cleavage of the N- and C-terminal nonhelical domains of the molecule. In the absence of the procollagen peptidase(s) (e.g., in dermatosporaxis), the collagen fibrils formed are so soluble that skin and joints are extremely flexible and hyperextensible. As the collagen fibrils assemble in the extracellular space, they are stabilized by inter- and intramolecular cross-links. Aldehydes, formed by the copper-dependent oxidative deamination of lysine and hydroxylysine residues, spontaneously react with other aldehydes (aldol condensation) or free-NH_2 groups (aldimine formation), gradually forming three-dimensional cross-links. Blockage of aldehyde formation (either inherited or induced by the chelation of copper ions) can produce bone deformities (lathyrism), joint dislocations, and aortic aneurysms as a direct result of the inability of the collagen to cross-link.

Elastin

The other fibrous component of the connective tissue matrix is elastin.[39] This rubber-like component of elastic ligaments, blood vessels, skin, and lungs accounts for only a small amount of the matrix in nonextensible tissues (based on wet weight, 2.6 per cent elastin versus 32 per cent collagen in tendon) and a major proportion of the matrix of deformable tissues (32 per cent elastin versus 7 per cent collagen in certain ligaments such as the ligamentum nuchae). Skeletal ligaments contain less elastin (5 to 10 per cent wet weight) and more collagen than the specialized liagments). In contrast to the highly oriented, regularly arranged collagen fibrils, elastin generally occurs in a compacted nonstructured (amorphous) form that is rubbery and soft and can be extended to double its length. In fact, elastin isolated from tendon can be extended 100 times before it breaks, whereas tendon collagen breaks after expanding to 5 times its length. Thus, initial expansion of the tissue is energetically easier because small forces can easily extend the soft elastic fibers, and the coiled collagen does not resist expansion. As the tissue extends and the collagen straightens, the load is transferred to the collagen and the tissue stiffens.

Like collagen, elastin contains a high percentage of glycine (27 per cent). Elastin is more hydrophobic than collagen and hence is more insoluble. The repeating unit in elastin is a pentapeptide, distinct from the Gly-X-Y tripeptide of collagen. Elastin contains no hydroxylysine and little hydroxyproline. Elastin is similar to collagen in that it is synthesized in a high-molecular-weight soluble form. After conversion to tropoelastin, lysyl oxidase, the same copper-dependent enzyme required for collagen aldehyde formation, causes the majority of the lysines of elastin to be oxidatively deaminated. Spontaneous reaction of specific active lysyl aldehydes results in the formation of two cross-linked amino acids peculiar to the elastin structure (desmosine and isodesmosine). Cross-links stabilize the compact (or random) structure of elastin, making this compact structure the energetically more favorable one to which the molecule always returns after expansion.

Proteoglycans

The high-molecular-weight proteoglycans[19, 31, 34] (Fig. 119–4), with their component acidic glycosaminoglycans, provide resilience and flexibility to the connective tissue matrix (Fig. 119–5). Although proteoglycan structure differs among the connective tissues[19] all proteoglycans consist of a protein core to which glycosaminoglycans are covalently attached. The individual glycosaminoglycans are large anionic molecules consisting of repeating disaccharides—one acidic sugar (glucuronic or iduronic acid) and one basic monosaccharide (2-amino 2-deoxyglucose or galactose), which is made anionic by *N*-acetylation or *N*- or *O*-sulfation. In many but not all tissues, the proteoglycans form aggregates of gigantic molecular weight by associating with hyaluronic acid. These aggregates, owing to their high charge density and branched configuration, are responsible for the viscoelastic, semipermeable nature of cartilage, synovium, and the intervertebral discs. Modification of proteoglycan structure has marked effects on tissue properties. For example, abnormalities in cartilage ultrastructure are associated with proteoglycan modification in osteoarthritis,[18] in enzyme-treated cartilages,[12] and in animals with genetic abnormalities in proteoglycan synthesis.[27, 33, 43]

Matrix Proteins

Improved methods for isolating and characterizing proteins from the connective tissue matrix have led to the identification of numerous noncollagenous matrix proteins in the connective tissues. These proteins, which include glycoproteins, phosphoproteins, gamma-carboxylated proteins, and proteolipids, are less abundant than collagen but are believed to have important roles in their component tissues.

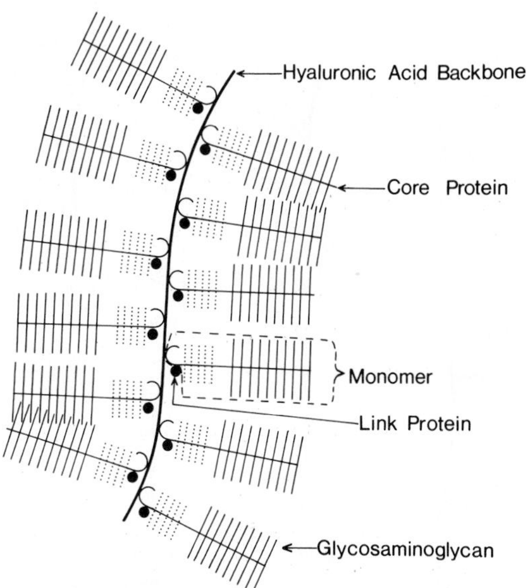

FIGURE 119–4. Diagram of a typical proteoglycan aggregate. The hooked end of the core protein contains a hyaluronate binding region, which facilitates interaction of proteoglycan monomers with the hyaluronic acid backbone. The link proteins stabilize this interaction. Individual repeating disaccharides—the glycosaminoglycans, keratin sulfate, and (in cartilage, predominantly) chondroitin sulfate—are covalently linked to serine groups on the core protein.

Glycoproteins, as distinct from proteoglycans, are protein compounds that contain no large repeating sugar units and therefore tend to have a high protein/sugar ratio. Among the less abundant but important connective and related tissue glycoproteins are fibronectin,[24] laminin (basement membranes),[29] osteopontin (bone sialoprotein),[13] and chondronectin (cartilage).[22] Each of these proteins functions *in vitro* to regulate cell adhesion, motility, or alignment.

Osteonectin,[13] a phosphorylated glycoprotein synthesized by bone as well as other nonconnective tissue cells, is a calcium-binding protein that avidly binds to both collagen and bone mineral. Osteocalcin[20] (bone gla protein), which contains γ-carboxyglutamic acid residues formed in a vitamin K-dependent reaction, is the most abundant noncollagenous protein in rodent and bovine bones. A role for this protein in osteoclast recruitment has been suggested.[16]

Phosphoproteins are extremely important in calcifying connective tissues. In bone and dentin, for example, bone phosphoprotein and phosphophoryn, phosphoryl ated proteins closely associated with collagen fibrils,[15] have been implicated in the initiation of mineralization.[6, 15]

Also synthesized by connective cells,[21] and accumulated in calcified matrices are peptide growth factors,[41] which regulate the proliferation and differentiation of

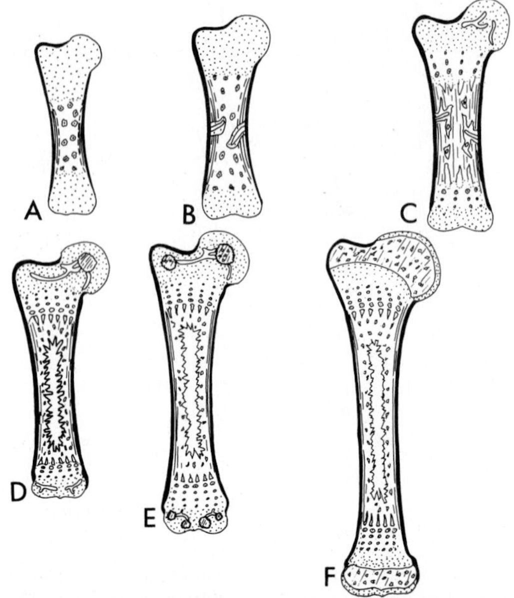

FIGURE 119–5. The embryonic (A–C) and neonatal (D–E) development of long bones. *A*, Initially the long bone is predominantly cartilaginous. Calcifying hypertrophic chondrocytes in the center of the bones are surrounded by a thin collar of cancellous periosteal membranous bone (primary ossification center). *B*, As development proceeds, there is vascular invasion of the calcified cartilage. Hyaline cartilage persists at the proximal and distal ends of the bone. *C*, Vascular invasion is followed by the deposition of endochondral bone on the calcified matrix, and epiphyseal capillaries begin to invade the hyaline cartilage. *D*, At birth, a secondary ossification center within the hyaline cartilage and a central marrow cavity appear, surrounded by newly formed compact bone. *E*, With further development, the cartilaginous matrix narrows and more compact bone is laid down. *F*, A well-defined growth plate then appears in the proximal and distal epiphysis. Growth in width occurs by periosteal bone formation, whereas longitudinal growth occurs by endochondral ossification.

these cells. Some of these growth factors have also been implicated in cartilage and bone disease.[3]

ANATOMY AND PHYSIOLOGY OF SPECIALIZED CONNECTIVE TISSUES

Bone

Bone forms an essential part of the locomotor system, acting as lever arms during motion and resisting the force of gravity. Bones also protect and support adjacent tissues and organs. In addition to these mechanical functions, bones serve an important chemical function, providing a reservoir for mineral ion homeostasis.[14]

Bone consists of several functionally distinct regions. At the articulating surfaces is articular cartilage. Surrounding the entire bone is a membranous structure, the periosteum. Lining the area enclosing the cartilage (capsule) of the joints and also lining tendon sheaths, providing nutrition and lubrication to the articular cartilage while serving as a protective barrier, are the synovial membranes. Below the articular cartilage, in the epiphysis, lies the secondary center of ossification, and below that, in growing animals, the physis, or growth plate. Woven lamellar cancellous bone lies below the physis in a metaphysis, and the compact cortical bone surrounds a marrow cavity in the diaphyseal region.

Three principal cell types are found in all bones: osteoblasts, osteoclasts, and osteocytes. The osteoblasts—round, plump cells with abundant endoplasmic reticulum—are the bone cells responsible for synthesizing the matrix. They are found on the surface of bone-forming regions, known as haversian systems, which surround blood vessels within the matrix of woven bone. Once encased in mineral, these osteocytes do not die but rather communicate via long processes with other mineral-encased cells and with unencased cells. Osteoclasts,[30] the large (20 to 100 nm in diameter) multinucleated cells with ruffled borders that lie on the surface of the mineralized matrix, are directly responsible for removing the mineral and matrix (bone resorption).[2] In healthy bone, the activities of the osteoclasts and osteoblasts are coupled (via protein factors released from the bone); thus resorption stimulates new bone formation. The ability of bone to adapt its architecture and external form by resorption and reformation in response to stresses (Wolff's law) is one of the unique properties of this tissue.[14]

The component of the extracellular bone matrix that distinguishes it from other connective tissue matrices and enables it to perform its unique functions is the mineral. The mineral found in bone is an analogue of the naturally occurring mineral hydroxyapatite, $Ca_{10}(PO_4)_6(OH)_2$.[5, 14] Bone mineral crystals, in contrast to the large (centimeters to meters) geological apatite crystals, are extremely small (200 to 400 Å in largest dimension). The microscopic crystals found in bone mineral, as a consequence of their small size, tend to be more soluble than geological apatites and to contain more impurities than pure hydroxyapatite crystals. Bone mineral is in equilibrium with body fluids, and demineralization of bone (resorption) occurs when the intake of minerals (calcium, magnesium, phosphorus) necessary for bone formation is inadequate (as in vitamin D-deficiency rickets) or when loss of mineral ions is excessive (as in hyperparathyroidism). Regulation of the serum concentration of minerals (homeostasis), via control of bone formation and resorption, is principally controlled by three substances: parathyroid hormone, calcitonin, and vitamin D.[11, 28, 37]

Bone Formation

Bone forms and grows, for the most part, by the transformation of cartilage into an ossified structure. In an embryo, mesenchymal cells condense to form a cartilage model, which later transforms into bone (see Fig. 119–5). The cells in this cartilage model differentiate into chondroblasts, which secrete a cartilaginous matrix. Cell division by chondrocytes, developed as the chondroblasts were trapped within the matrix they themselves secreted, and apposition of new chondrocytes from the periosteum allow growth of this primitive bone form. Formation of a calcified osseous collar (periosteum) is followed by vascular invasion, resulting in the formation of a secondary ossification center, which becomes the diaphysis and metaphysis of bone. The epiphyseal plate,[23] or growth plate (Fig. 119–6), extends from the resting or reserve cell zone to the zone of calcified cartilage. In the resting cell zone, cells are widely spaced and show less frequent mitosis. Each of these cells divides to form another stem cell and a proliferating cell. Proliferating cells divide rapidly, lining up in long columns. The columns of cells are separated by wide partitions of cartilage matrix, the synthetic product of these cells. As the columns of cells approach the metaphyseal area, the cells enlarge, forming hypertrophic cells. In the lower half of the hypertrophic cell zone, cartilage calcification begins. All these cells are viable, and each cell type produces matrix proteins; however, the characteristics of these proteins differ from zone to zone (discussed later). The cell progression from resting to hypertrophic is fairly rapid, taking only 10 days in a growing rat.[23] After cartilage calcification, the invasion of blood vessels is associated with the removal of calcified cartilage and the deposition of woven bone (primary spongiosa). This woven bone is subsequently remodeled to yield cortical bone with a well-developed marrow cavity. Longitudinal growth proceeds via endochondral ossification, the conversion of the rapidly growing cartilage in the physis (area between primary and secondary ossification centers) into calcified cartilage and bone. The cartilage of the original model persists at the articular surface and as discs of cartilage (physis) separating the two calcifying regions.

The process of endochondral ossification, which also occurs in fracture healing, can be understood most easily in terms of the changes in the epiphyseal growth plate. The mitochondria[7] of the chondrocytes in the proliferating zone contain numerous electron-dense calcium-phosphate granules, whereas the cells in the more distal zone of provisional calcification contain few such granules. The disappearance of calcium phosphate from the mitochondria at the time that mineral crystals first appear in the extracellular matrix suggests a causal relationship between intra- and extracellular deposits. It is in the lower half of the hypertrophic zone that calcification commences.[35] Much of the first mineral to appear outside the chondrocytes is associated with membrane-bound bodies called *extracellular matrix vesicles*.[1, 4, 44] These vesicles, rich in the enzyme alkaline phosphatase, may provide a preferential site for mineral deposition within the growth plate, as well as in other mineralizing tissues. Whether the vesicles are the site of the first mineral deposits or whether they are only situated close to those sites is still debated.[35]

Along with changes in morphology and cell metabolism[7] are alterations in the composition of the growth plate matrix, which may be associated with initial calcification.[35] Type X collagen,[40] produced only by hypertrophic cells, and the C propeptide of type II collagen, chondrocalcin, accumulate at sites of initial calcification along with proteoglycan.[35] Changes in proteoglycan structure, content, and focal distribution also occur.[8, 35]

Initial cartilage calcification[44] appears to involve the formation of alkaline phosphatase–rich extracellular matrix vesicles, modification of the proteoglycan-rich matrix, an increase in the extracellular calcium and phosphorus ion product, and the interaction of matrix proteins with the newly forming mineral. Some of these matrix proteins serve to orient the mineral and regulate the size of the crystals. Although different cell types and matrix proteins are found in the other mineralizing tissues, the events involved in initial mineralization are similar.

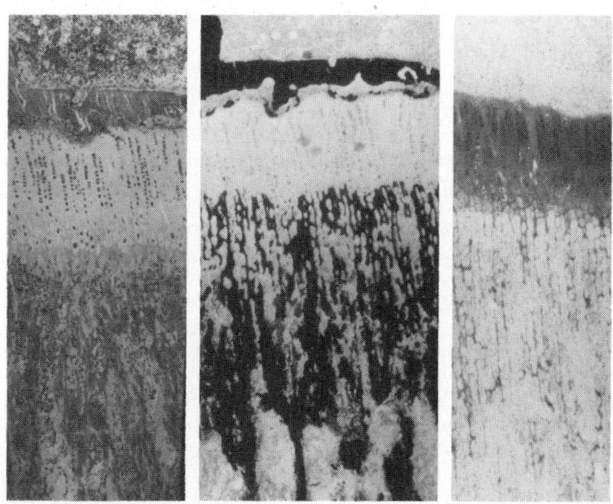

FIGURE 119–6. Growth plate of a 21-day-old rat, nondecalcified section, stained with hematoxylin and eosin (*left*), von Kossa stain (*center*), and safranin O (*right*). The cells of the growth plate extend from the bony spicules in the proximal area to the newly forming mineral spicules in the distal metaphyseal region. The widely spaced small cells at the top of the growth plate are the resting, or reserve, cells. These cells then line up in columns (columnar or proliferating cells) and begin to swell (hypertrophic cells). Calcification, shown in the von Kossa–stained section, occurs around the lowest hypertrophic cells. It is in this region that safranin O staining for proteoglycans is diminished. Staining for proteoglycans persists well into the calcified regions.

Muscle[9]

Fibrous proteins are found intracellularly as well as in the extracellular matrix. Motion of single cells and whole tissues, as well as motion of organelles within the cells, depends on these intracellular proteins, called the *cytoskeletal proteins* because of their location (cytoplasmic) and structure (insoluble and fibrous). The cytoskeletal proteins are those fibrous elements that hold the cell intact, maintain its shape, and provide it with contractible, locomotive, and adhesive properties. First characterized in muscle cells but known to exist in some form in all eukaryotic cells, the cytoskeleton consists, in order of decreasing size, of thick filaments (40 to 45 nm in diameter), microtubules (24 to 25 nm in diameter), intermediate filaments (10 to 20 nm in diameter), and thin filaments (5 to 8 nm in diameter).

The microtubules, consisting of fibrous tubulin polymers and associated regulatory proteins, traverse the cytoplasm of all cells as continuous structures and are involved in mitosis. The intermediate filaments, which differ in structure and composition in different tissues, are responsible for maintaining cell structure and anchoring the nucleus during mitosis. Microfilaments, consisting predominantly of actin, are essential for cell motility and, via interactions with matrix proteins (such as fibronectin), for cell-matrix interactions. The thick filaments contain myosin, a protein first isolated from muscle.

In the muscle cell, bundles of thick filaments, held in place by intermediate filaments,[29] interact with thin filaments (actin), contracting and producing mechanical work. The contractile proteins of the muscle cells produce work in the form of motion, sustenance of weight, balance, propulsion of blood, regulation of temperature, secretion, and excretion.

Three types of muscle are found in vertebrates: skeletal, cardiac, and smooth. Skeletal muscle, also called *striated* because of its light microscopic appearance, is attached to the bones by tendons and controls the voluntary movement of these bones. Cardiac muscle is similar in appearance to striated muscle, but the heart muscle is not under voluntary control. Smooth muscle, which for the most part is not under voluntary control, lacks striations of the other muscle types. Examples of smooth muscles are the muscles of the intestinal wall, bile ducts, and blood vessels.

Cells (sarcomeres) of striated muscles are the best characterized. Microscopic examination of these cells demonstrates characteristic features. Each cell (2 to 3 cm in length) is surrounded by a membrane, the sarcolemma or plasmalemma. Discrete connections exist between this membrane and the fibrous elements of the cells. Tendons are attached to the outer surface of this membrane. The integrity of the plasmalemma is essential for maintaining the electrical potential that controls the contractile process.

Within the boundaries of the cell membrane are the sarcoplasm (muscle cell cytoplasm), numerous cell nuclei, and mitochondria. The mitochondria, by the process of oxidative phosphorylation, produce the energy source of the cell, adenosine triphosphate (ATP). ATP is hydrolyzed during contraction to give adenosine diphosphate (ADP), inorganic phosphate, and energy. In the resting muscle, ADP can be reconverted to ATP by reaction with creatine phosphate.

The Contractile Process

The contractile process depends on interaction of four proteins: myosin, actin, troponin, and tropomyosin, with ionic calcium. Myosin is unique among the connective tissue fibrous proteins in that it is the only fibrous protein with enzymatic activity. Each myosin molecule consists of two long alpha-helical rods coiled about each other, each ending in a globular region. The ATPase activity of myosin resides in a globular head at the end of the molecules. Various proteins that regulate enzymic activity are associated with the globular regions.

Within the thick filaments, the myosin molecules are arranged tail to tail in a 1.5-μm-long cigar-shaped structure decorated with projections (globular heads) along its entire length. These thick filaments interdigitate with the actin-containing thin filaments to form the muscle fibers. It is this combination of fibers that gives striated muscle its characteristic appearance. The swiveling or oarlike movements of the myosin cross-bridges toward the actin filaments result in shortening of the fibers (contraction).

Actin is a globular protein found in numerous cells. It polymerizes to form a fibrous structure that resembles twisted two-stranded beads. Filamentous actin has the unique ability to activate the release of ADP from its binding site on the globular myosin heads. Thus, interaction of myosin head groups with actin thin filaments results in activation of the multistep reaction in which ATP binds to myosin, forms an activated complex, and is rapidly hydrolyzed but not released. The release of ADP is substantially slower and requires interaction with actin.

The trigger for the start of this set of reactions is calcium. After transmission of an electrical signal, calcium ions flow into the cell, where they interact with troponin, a globular protein that has specific binding sites for this ion and for another protein, tropomyosin. Tropomyosin sits in the groove formed by the twisting chains of actin. Binding of calcium ions to troponin causes a series of conformational changes that allow tropomyosin to slide into the groove, permitting the myosin heads to interact with two actin subunits. After release of ADP, the myosin heads return to their original positions. After binding of a new ATP molecule, the muscle cell is ready for another calcium ion-triggered contraction.

References

1. Anderson HC: Vesicles associated with calcification in the matrix of epiphyseal cartilage. *J Cell Biol 41*:58, 1969.
2. Baron R: Molecular mechanisms of bone resorption by the osteoclast. *Anat Res 224*:317, 1989.
3. Bird TA, Saklatvala J: Identification of a common class of high affinity receptors for both types of porcine interleukin-1 on connective tissue cells. *Nature 324*:263, 1986.
4. Boskey AL: Models of matrix vesicle calcification. *Inorg Perspect Biol Med 2*:51, 1979.
5. Boskey AL: Current concepts of the physiology and biochemistry of calcification. *Clin Orthop 167*:225, 1981.
6. Boskey AL: Noncollagenous matrix proteins and their role in mineralization. *Bone Mineral 6*:111, 1989.
7. Brighton CT, Hunt RM: The role of mitochondria in growth plate calcification as demonstrated in a rachitic model. *J Bone Joint Surg 60*:630, 1978.
8. Buckwalter JA, et al: Changes in proteoglycan aggregates during cartilage mineralization. *Calcif Tissue Int 411*:228, 1987.
9. Burke JM, Ross R: Synthesis of connective macromolecules by smooth muscle. *Int Rev Connect Tissue Res 8*:119, 1979.
10. Castor CW: The physiology of the synovial cell and its contribution to disease processes. *In* Holt PJL (ed): *Current Topics in Connective Tissue Disease*. Churchill Livingstone, New York, 1975, p 1.
11. Christakos S, et al: Vitamin D-dependent calcium binding proteins: Chemistry distribution, functional considerations, and molecular biology. *Endocrinol Rev 10*:3, 1989.
12. Engfeldt B, et al: Effect of papain on bone. I. Histologic, autoradiographic, and microradiographic study on young dogs. *Arch Pathol 68*:600, 1959.
13. Fisher LW, et al: Purification and partial characterization of small proteoglycans I and II, bone sialoproteins I and II, and osteonectin from the mineral compartment of developing human bone. *J Biol Chem 262*:9702, 1987.
14. Glimcher MJ: On the form and function of bone: From molecules to organs. *In* Veis A (ed): *The Chemistry and Biology of Mineralized Connective Tissues*. Elsevier/North Holland, New York, 1982, p 617.
15. Glimcher MJ: Mechanism of calcification: Role of collagen fibrils and collagen-phosphoprotein complexes *in vitro* and *in vivo*. *Anat Rec 224*:139, 1989.
16. Glowacki J, Lian JB: Impaired recruitment and differentiation of osteoclast progenitors in osteocalcin depleted bone implants. *Cell Differ 21*:247, 1987.
17. Greiling H, et al: Interaction of synovial cells and synovial fluid with cartilage. *In* Keuttner K, et al (eds): *Articular Cartilage Biochemistry*. Raven Press, New York, 1986, p 195.
18. Hamerman D: The biology of osteoarthritis. *N Engl J Med 320*:1322, 1989.
19. Hassell JR, et al: Proteoglycan core protein families. *Ann Rev Biochem 55*:539, 1986.

20. Hauschka PV, et al: Osteocalcin and matrix Gla protein—vitamin K-dependent proteins in bone. *Physiol Rev 69*:990, 1989.
21. Hauschka PV, et al: Growth factors in bone matrix: Isolation of multiple types by affinity chromatography on heparin-sepharose. *Biol Chem 261*:12665, 1986.
22. Hewitt AT, et al: Isolation and partial characterization of chondronectin, an attachment factor for chondrocytes. *J Biol Chem 257*:2330, 1982.
23. Hunziker EB, et al: Quantitation of chondrocyte performance in growth-plate cartilage during longitudinal bone growth. *J Bone Joint Surg 69*:162, 1987.
24. Hynes RO: Fibronectin and its relation to cellular structure and behavior *In* Hay ED (ed): *Cell Biology of the Extracellular Matrix*. Plenum, New York, 1981, p 295.
25. Jaenisch R: Transgenic animals. *Science 240*:1468, 1988.
26. Karpati G: Muscle: Structure, organization, and healing. *In* Cruess RL, (ed): *The Musculoskeletal System. Embryology, Biochemistry, and Physiology*. Churchill Livingstone, New York, 1982.
27. Kimato K, et al: Absence of proteoglycan core protein in cartilage from the cmd/cmd (cartilage matrix deficiency) mouse. *J Biol Chem 256*:6961, 1981.
28. Koshy KT: Vitamins D: An update. *J Pharm Sci 71*:137, 1982.
29. Lazarides E: Intermediate filaments, a chemically heterogeneous, developmentally regulated class of proteins. *Ann Rev Biochem 51*:219, 1982.
30. Marks SC Jr: The origin of osteoclasts: Evidence, clinical implications and investigative challenges of an extra-skeletal source. *J Oral Pathol 12*:226, 1983.
31. Mayne R: Cartilage collagens: What is their function, and are they involved in articular disease. *Arthritis Rheum 32*:241, 1989.
32. Ohkubo H, et al: Isolation and characterization of overlapping genomic clones covering the chicken alpha 2 (type I) collagen gene. *PNAS US 77*:7059, 1980.
33. Orkin RW, et al: Defects in the cartilaginous growth plates of brachymorphic mice. *J Cell Biol 73*:287, 1977.
34. Poole AR: Proteoglycans in health and disease: Structures and functions. *Biochem J 236*:1, 1986.
35. Poole AR, et al: Cartilage macromolecules and the calcification of cartilage matrix. *Anat Rec 224*:167, 1989.
36. Prockop DJ, et al: The biosynthesis of collagen and its disorders. *N Engl J Med 301*:13, 1979.
37. Raisz LG, Kream BE: Regulation of bone formation. *N Engl J Med 309*:29, 1983.
38. Ruther U, et al: Deregulated *c-fos* expression interferes with normal bone development in transgenic mice. *Nature 325*:412, 1987.
39. Sanberg LB, et al: Elastin structure biosynthesis, and relation to disease states. *N Engl J Med 304*:577, 1981.
40. Schmidt TM, Conrad HE: A unique low molecular weight collagen secreted by cultured chick embryo chondrocytes. *J Biol Chem 257*:12444, 1982.
41. Sporn MB, Roberts AB: Peptide growth factors are multifunctional. *Nature 332*:217, 1988.
42. Stacey A, et al: Perinatal lethal osteogenesis imperfecta in transgenic mice bearing an engineered mutant pro-alpha 1(I) collagen gene. *Nature 10*:332, 1988.
43. Wilkstrom B, et al: Morphological studies of the epiphyseal growth zone in the brachymorphic (bm/bm) mouse. *Virchows Arch* [B] *47*:167, 1984.
44. Wuthier RE: A review on the primary mechanism of endochondral calcification with special emphasis on the role of cells, mitochondria and matrix vesicles. *Clin Orthop Rel Res 169*:219, 1982.

CHAPTER 120 Fracture Biology and Biomechanics

Don Hulse and Bill Hyman

Long bones are subjected to physiological and nonphysiological forces. Nonphysiological forces occur in unusual situations such as automobile accidents, gunshot injuries, or falls. They can be transmitted to bone directly and may easily exceed the ultimate strength of bone, giving rise to a fracture. Physiological forces are generated by weightbearing, muscle contraction, and associated physical activity. They are transmitted to the bone through the joint surfaces and muscle contraction. Physiological forces are uniaxial (tension or compression) and can give rise to torsional and bending moments. Physiological forces do not commonly exceed the ultimate strength of bone and are not responsible for bone fractures except in unusual cases.

The physiological force of weightbearing occurs as the feet make contact with the ground. Simultaneously, the ground responds with an equal but opposite reaction referred to as the *ground reaction force*. The magnitude of the ground reaction force varies proportionately with body acceleration and the distribution of body weight carried by the foot at impact (force = mass × acceleration). In addition to magnitude, the time during which the foot is in contact with the ground is important in determining the effect of the force. Therefore, impulse (rapid) loading can have a different effect from the same force applied slowly. In dogs, during slow walking, the ground reaction force has been measured to equal 30 per cent of the body weight with each forelimb and 20 per cent of the body weight with each rear limb. However, due to acceleration and impulse loading, the ground reaction force may increase to five times or more body weight at a fast trot or a run or when landing from a jump. The ground reaction force causes axial compression, bending moments, and torsional moments in the bone. These moments must be balanced by muscle contraction to control motion and maintain equilibrium.

A bending moment occurs when a force causes an object to bend about an axis, and a torsional moment occurs when a force causes an object to rotate about an axis (Fig. 120–1). A bending or torsional moment is the product of a force times the moment arm (lever arm) over which it acts. The moment arm is equal to the perpendicular distance from the line of action of the force to the point where the moment acts (e.g., when the front foot strikes the ground, a primarily vertical ground reaction force is produced). The perpendicular distance from the line of action of the ground reaction force to the carpal joint is the moment arm. The product of the ground reaction force and the moment arm is the bending moment that causes the foot to bend cranially about the carpal joint. The moment of the ground reaction force acting at the carpal joint is balanced by muscle contraction to maintain equilibrium. Because of relatively short moment arms (lever arms), muscles must

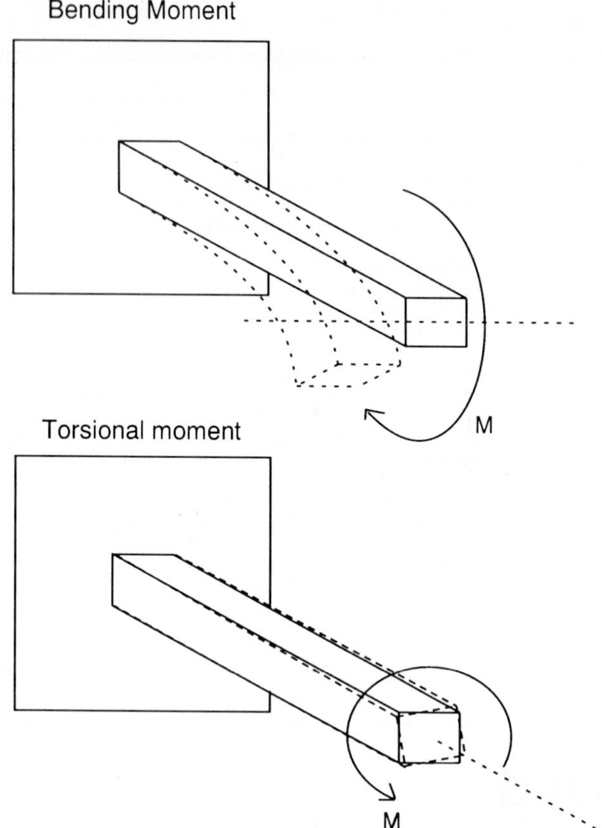

FIGURE 120–1. A bending moment where the beam is being bent downward about the horizontal axis. The lower illustration represents a torsional moment where the beam is being twisted about a longitudinal axis.

exert considerable force to maintain equilibrium. For example, if the ground reaction force in a retriever is 30 kg and the perpendicular distance from the vertical line of action of the ground reaction force to the radiocarpal joint (moment arm) equals 10 cm, the bending moment causing cranial bending of the joint is 300 kg-cm. If the moment arm of the lateral ulnar muscle (distance from the accessory carpal bone to the radiocarpal joint) is 2 cm, the muscle would need to contract with a force of 150 kg to balance the moment of the ground reaction force (Fig. 120–2). Although the sum of all the moments is zero at equilibrium (in this case, the ground reaction force balanced by the contraction of the lateral ulnar muscle), there remains a net force generated by muscle contraction and the ground reaction, which is transmitted to the long bones via the joint surface. Although this model is oversimplified, one can begin to appreciate how very large loads are created and transmitted to the bones through the joints.

The sum of the physiological forces is transmitted to the bones via the joint surfaces and causes axial compression, axial tension, bending moments, and torsional moments on the column of bone (for simplicity, bending moments and torsional moments are referred to as *bending* or *torsion* through the remainder of the text). The percentage of the joint load transmitted as axial compression or bending is determined by the point and direction of force application at the articular surface relative to the column of bone, the normal curvature of the bone, and limb position. If the force is applied eccentric (off center) to the bony column, both compression and bending occur; a force applied concentric (in line) with the bony column produces compression. Bones loaded more eccentrically (femur, humerus) are subject to greater bending; bones loaded more concentrically carry a greater compressive force (Fig. 120–3). A second factor that determines the amount of bending versus axial compressive force is the normal curvature of the bone. Although the radius and tibia are loaded through a joint surface that is more in line with the longitudinal axis of the bony column and are subject to compressive loading, the normal curvature of these bones results in significant bending loads. In fact, *in vivo* strain analysis has shown that 85 to 89 per cent of the predominant physiological internal stress in most bones is derived from bending. The only long bone found to be loaded primarily in compression is the equine metacarpus.

Torsion arises from the twisting of the body when the foot is firmly planted on the ground. Muscle forces also contribute significantly to torsion because their points of attachment are peripheral to the axis of rotation of the bone. The axis of rotation of the bone generally corresponds to the center of the marrow cavity. As such, muscle contraction occurs with a moment arm (lever arm), which is the distance from the center of the marrow cavity to the point of muscle attachment onto the cortical surface. The force of muscle contraction results in a torsional moment (force × moment arm), which causes rotation of the bony column. This is most significant when the line of muscle force is perpendicular to the longitudinal axis of the bone, as with the iliopsoas

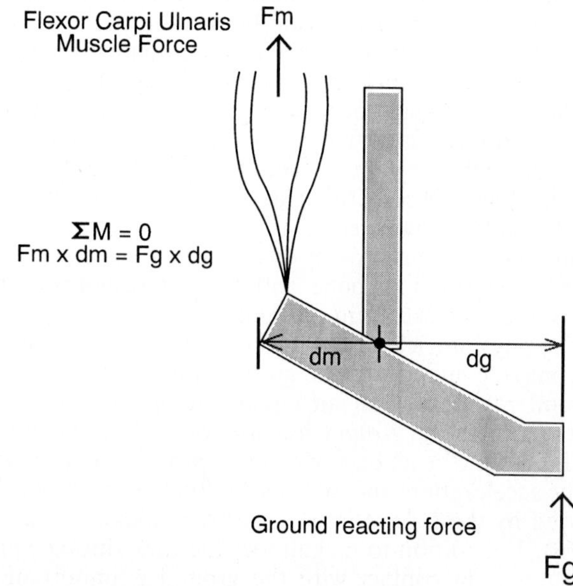

FIGURE 120–2. Balance of moments generated about the carpal joint. The ground reaction force (Fg) acts about the moment arm (dg), causing a cranial bending moment (Fg × dg). To maintain normal posture, this moment must be balanced by a moment generated from contraction of the flexor carpi ulnaris (Fm × dm).

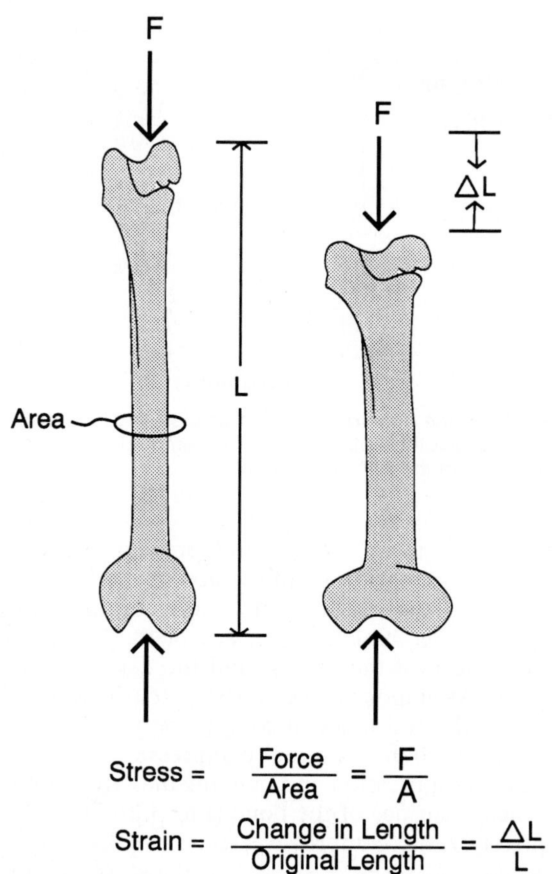

FIGURE 120–3. Internal stresses and internal strains within the bony column. Internal stress is a function of the applied force divided by the cross-sectional area, whereas internal strain is derived by dividing the change in length by the original length.

muscle and external rotators of the hip joints. The clinical importance in this example is significant external rotation associated with proximal femoral fractures.

Axial forces and moments applied to any structure deform from the original shape, and local forces are produced within the structure. If the local force intensities and deformations are determined for a specified area of the bone, the force intensities are referred to as *internal stresses* and the deformations as *internal strains*. Internal stresses have the dimensions of force/cross-sectional area, and internal strains are equal to the change in length/original length (Fig. 120–4). Internal stresses and strains are considered to be normal if they are directed perpendicular to a cross-sectional surface of bone. They are referred to as *shear stress and strain* if they are directed obliquely or parallel to a cross-sectional surface of bone. At any point in the bone, the nature of the stresses depends on what cross-sectional surface is being examined.

The four primary physiological forces are (1) axial compression, (2) axial tension, (3) bending, and (4) torsion. Each of these alone or in combination results in a complex pattern of internal stresses and strains within the bone. The normal stresses and strains are associated with tension and compression at a cross-sectional surface, whereas shear stress and strain are directed obliquely or parallel to cross-sectional surfaces of the bone. When a fracture occurs, these internal stresses and strains are present at the fracture line. Internal shear stress and tensile stress damage fragile tissues crossing the fracture gap. Internal stresses and strains can be neutralized with stabilizing devices.

When the joint force is evenly distributed over the articular surface and in line (concentric) with the column of bone, axial compression of the bone occurs. The resulting internal stresses and strains are (1) compression stress parallel to the column of bone, which causes shortening; (2) tensile strain perpendicular to the column of bone, which would cause expansion; and (3) shear stress oblique to the column of bone, which causes shortening and lateral displacement (Fig. 120–5). Clinically, the perpendicular tensile strain arising from axial compression is not important because expansion of the bone is unlikely. However, the compressive and shear stresses are significant and cause collapse of a comminuted or oblique fracture if not resisted.

Axial tension is the direct result of muscle contraction at a point of insertion. The resulting internal tensile stress must be resisted by orthopedic implants to prevent significant separation of the fracture surfaces. Axial tension is the only physiological force of significance in certain fracture types, such as fractures of the greater trochanter, olecranon, and tibial crest. These injuries are treated by the tension band principle, which applies pins and wire or bone plates and screws to resist internal tensile stress.

When a significant component of the joint force is transmitted eccentrically to the column of bone, bending occurs. It may result from the joint surface being eccen-

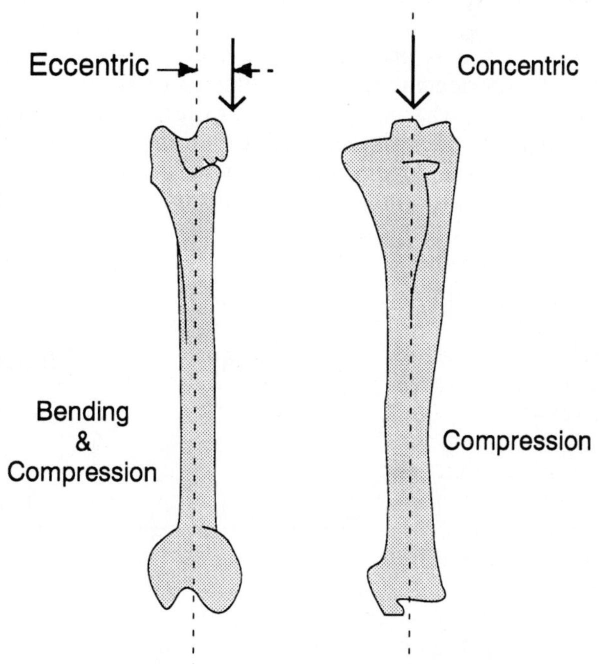

FIGURE 120–4. Eccentric or concentric loading of bony columns. If the joint load application is not in line with the column of bone (femur), then a bending moment is produced. If the joint load is in line with the center of the bony column, an axial load is produced.

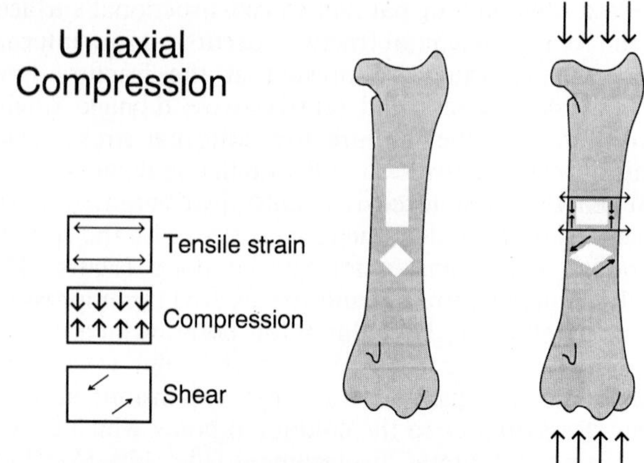

FIGURE 120–5. The internal stresses associated with an axial compressive load. Note the change in relationship of the rectangular and diamond-shaped boxes. Shear stress occurs at an oblique angle to the long axis of bone with uniaxial compression.

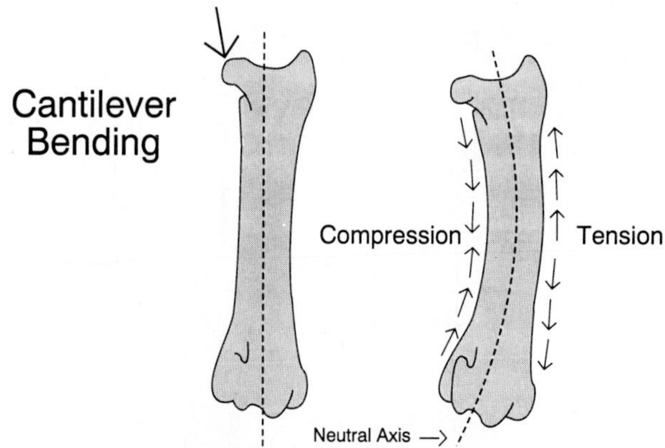

FIGURE 120–6. The generation of compression and tension surfaces of bone associated with bending. Maximal compression and tension occur at the surface of the bone.

tric to the column of bone (e.g., proximal femur) or from the normal curvature of the bone (e.g., radius). When a structure such as bone undergoes bending, internal tensile stress is produced on the convex surface and internal compressive stress is produced on the concave surface. The magnitude of these compression and tension stresses increases as the distance from the neutral axis increases. In proceeding from the concave surface toward the convex surface, the neutral axis is the point within the structure where compressive stress ends and tensile stress begins (Fig. 120–6). It is the point where there is zero axial stress and roughly corresponds to the center of the marrow cavity. The maximum tensile stress is present at the periosteal surface on the convex surface of the bone, and maximal compressive stress is present on the concave surface. The surface experiencing tension is referred to as the *tension band surface*, whereas the surface experiencing primary compressive stress is referred to as the *compression surface*. Tensile stress can pull apart fracture surfaces. It is important to know the tension band surface of each long bone to resist tension and prevent fracture gap widening. The tension band surface of the femur is the craniolateral surface. It is the craniolateral surface of the tibia, the craniolateral surface of the humerus, the cranial surface of the radius, and the caudal surface of the ulna. As important as resisting tensile stress from bending is the resistance of compression on the concave surface of the bone. Internal compression stresses arise from axial compression and bending and are additive on the concave surface of the bone (Fig. 120–7). Failure to adequately resist compressive stress results in collapse of the cortical surface, such as collapse of the medial cortical surface (medial buttress) associated with a comminuted femoral fracture.

Torsion causes internal shear stress perpendicular to the long axis of bone. The result is rotational deformation and lateral displacement of the fracture surface. Torsion also causes internal tensile and compressive stress oblique to the longitudinal axis of the bone (Fig. 120–8). Clinically, internal shear stress arising from rotational instability can cause delayed union or nonunion of a transverse fracture. Internal tensile stress must be resisted to prevent separation of an oblique or spiral fracture.

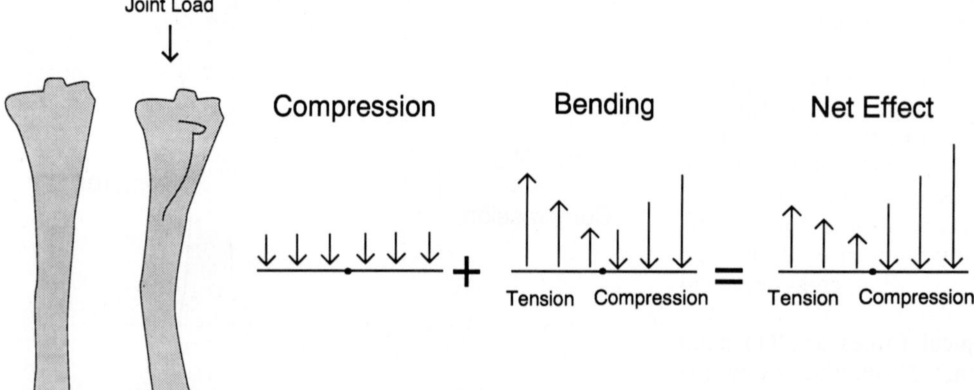

FIGURE 120–7. Most bones are subject to both axial compression and bending. The additive effect of this type of loading is depicted in the diagram. A net decrease in tension on the tension surface and a net increase in compression on the compression surface equal the applied uniaxial compressive force.

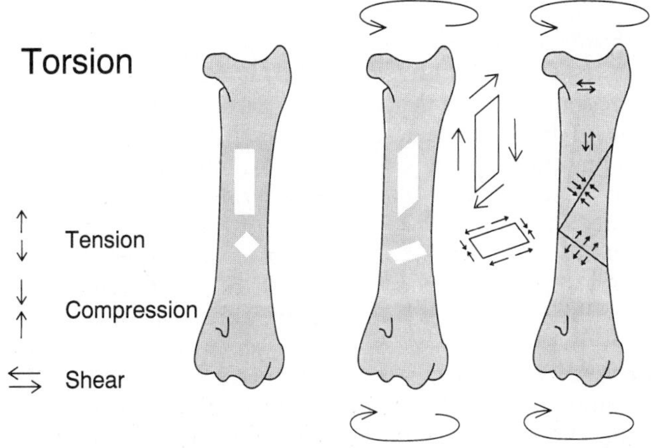

FIGURE 120–8. The internal stresses associated with torsion. Note the change in relationship between the sides of the rectangular and diamond-shaped boxes. Shear stress occurs perpendicular to the long axis of the bone, and tensile stress occurs in a spiral oblique pattern around the surface of the bone.

Although it is convenient to categorize these physiological forces and subsequent internal stresses, clinically the bones experience combined axial compression, axial tension, bending, and torsional loading. An appreciation of the normal and shear stresses and strains generated by physiological forces, coupled with the knowledge of an implant's ability to resist these stresses, is important for optimal fracture management.

Bones function in locomotion as kinematic links with lubricated joints, which allow coordinated movement through muscle contraction. Bone also supports and protects soft tissues and maintains mineral homeostasis. It is a true composite material, formed from collagen and hydroxyapatite; the strength and stiffness of bone are greater than either collagen or hydroxyapatite alone. Collagen prevents the stiff apatite from undergoing brittle fracture, and apatite prevents flexible collagen from excess deformation. Except for minor variations, all bone is formed of identical material. Macroscopically, two distinct structures are recognized: cortical and cancellous bone. The major differences between cortical and cancellous bone are the relative porosity and structural dimensions of each. Cortical bone has from 5 to 30 per cent porosity, and cancellous bone has from 30 to 90 per cent porosity. Mechanically, the two most important properties of bone are its strength and stiffness; these properties are described in both structural and material terms (e.g., the difference in the tensile strength and stiffness of a tibia from a poodle and a Great Dane). As bones are subjected to increasing loads, they deform until failure occurs. The larger bone from a Great Dane deforms less at a given load and ultimately fails at a larger load than a smaller bone from a poodle. A force/deformation curve can be developed to represent the structural properties of the two bones (Fig. 120–9). Structural properties depend not only on the material composition but also on the dimensions of each bone. Important geometric dimensions are cross-sectional area, distribution of bone about the neutral axis (shape), and length of the bone. If we normalize bones by considering force per unit area (stress), each bone has similar characteristics. When the dimensions of each bone are normalized by accounting for cross-sectional area and length, a stress/strain curve can be produced to represent the material properties of each bone (see Fig. 120–9). As a structure, strength is defined as the ultimate load a bone can withstand before breaking; as a material, strength is defined as the ultimate stress at which the material breaks. To determine the structural and material stiffness of each bone, further examination of the force/deformation and stress/strain curves is necessary. Initially, each bone reacts to a given force in a linear manner—deformation is directly related to the amount of force. This section of the curve is also called the *elastic region*, because when the force is removed, the bone returns to its original shape. The point at which the force causes permanent change in shape is referred to as the *yield point*. At this point, deformation remains when the force is removed. In living bone, permanent deformation generally means

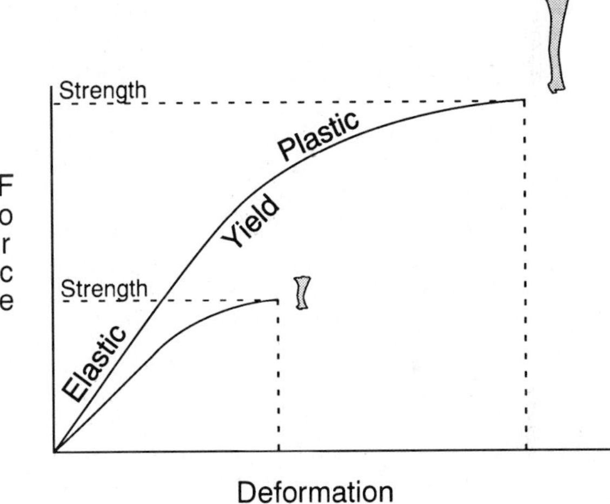

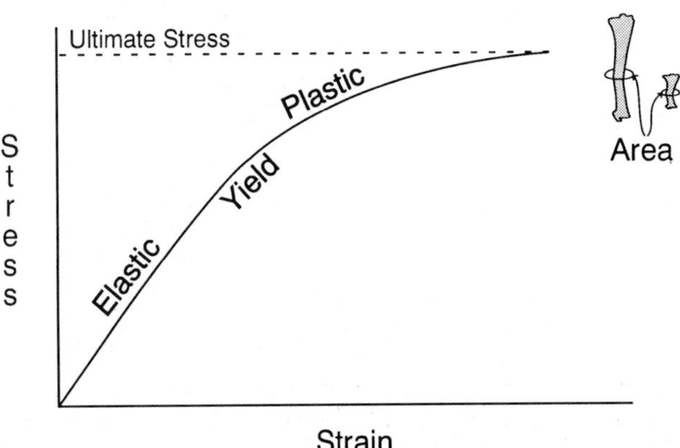

FIGURE 120–9. A force-deformation curve representing structural properties and a stress-strain curve representing material properties of bone. The elastic region, yield point, and plastic region of each curve are shown. The stiffness is represented by the slope of the force-deformation curve in the elastic region. The modulus is the slope of the stress-strain curve in the elastic region.

microstructural damage. The section of the curve from the yield point to where the bone breaks is called the *plastic region*, and the *point of failure* is the ultimate load or ultimate stress. The structural stiffness is the slope of the force/deformation curve within the elastic region. Similarly, the material stiffness (modulus) is the slope of the stress/strain curve in the elastic region. The greater the slope (steepness) of the curve, the greater the structural or material stiffness of the bone.

The area enclosed beneath the force/deformation or stress/strain curve represents the energy absorbed by the bone before failure. Strength and stiffness of bone are related to the magnitude of force and the rate at which the force is applied. If bone is loaded at a very high rate, as with the impact of an automobile or a gunshot injury, both stiffness and strength to failure increase. When this occurs, the amount of energy absorbed before the bone fractures is significantly increased (Fig. 120–10). When energy is released at fracture, bone fragmentation and significant trauma of the surrounding soft tissues occur. Materials such as bone, whose energy absorption depends on the applied loading rate, are *viscoelastic*. The clinical significance of this property of bone is that considerable energy release and tissue trauma can be expected with high-velocity injuries. Bone is also an *anisotropic material*—strength and stiffness are related to the direction of loading. The strength and stiffness of bone are greatest if the bone is loaded parallel to the osteon orientation. Long bones are better able to resist loads applied parallel to the longitudinal axis (osteon orientation) of the diaphysis than loads applied perpendicular to the bone axis.

The various loading modes to which bones are subjected (compression, bending, and torsion) lead to specific fracture patterns. Because bone is weakest when subjected to shear stress or tensile stress, failure occurs within the zones of high shear and tensile stress. Bones subject to compressive loads generally fail obliquely to the longitudinal axis corresponding to the plane of maximum internal shear stress (see Fig. 120–5). Bending loads initiate a transverse fracture corresponding to the high internal tensile stress on the convex surface of the bone (see Fig. 120–6). A small fragment may occur on the compression surface of the bone, initiated at the zone of high internal shear stress. If compression and bending occur at the same time, the internal shear stress (due to net compression) is accentuated on the concave surface, resulting in a larger "butterfly" fragment or comminution of the concave surface (see Fig. 120–7). Torsional loads create internal shear stress parallel to the column of bone and can initiate a fracture at the point of maximal shear stress (see Fig. 120–8). The fracture is propagated in a spiral fashion around the circumference of the bone, corresponding to the zone of maximal internal tensile stress. Clinically, fractures may be simple low-energy fractures in which the failure force can be deduced, or more commonly, the fracture pattern is more complex because of combinations of loads.

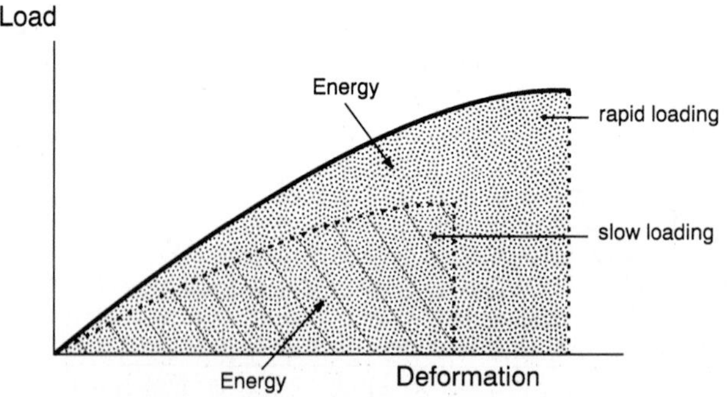

FIGURE 120–10. With rapid loading, the ultimate strength and stiffness of bone increase. The energy absorbed before fracture and release into the soft tissue is represented by the area under the curve. As can be seen, a high-velocity impact releases considerably more energy to the soft tissue than a low-velocity injury.

Because locomotion is vital for survival, nature has provided repair mechanisms that unite fractures and enable an animal to return to full function. After a fracture, the morphological features of repair tissue depend on a number of factors; two of these are the vascular and mechanical environment at the fracture site. When healing of a fracture occurs, the principal components of the normal afferent vascular system (nutrient artery, metaphyseal and periosteal arteries) are enhanced. In addition, the area receives a temporary new blood supply that is entirely distinct from normal. This is termed the *extraosseous blood supply of healing bone* and is derived from the surrounding soft tissues. Although the normal afferent vascular system returns to its dominant position as stability allows, the extraosseous blood supply is important in the initial stages of healing. Gentle reflection of soft tissues during open reduction of a fracture is vital for preservation of early nutrient supply to the pluripotential cells near the fracture site.

Biomechanically, the interfragmentary strain theory proposes that pluripotential cells are responsive to local deformation within the fracture gap. Different tissue cells are able to withstand specified levels of deformation (stretching) beyond which they are unable to survive. Granulation tissue can withstand 100 per cent deformation before failure. Cartilage and fibrous tissue tolerate 10 per cent deformation, and bone tolerates 2 per cent deformation before failure. The fracture ends and the tissue within the fracture gap are subject to high deformation when stabilization is not adequate. The only tissue that can survive this environment is granulation tissue. However, as healing progresses, two mechanisms take place to reduce strain within the gap. First, osteoclastic resorption of the fragment ends increases the gap width. Because normal strain is equal to the change in length/original length, increasing the gap length reduces the amount of local strain within the fracture gap. Second, the granulation tissue gradually becomes more fibrous, improving stability and reducing movement between the bone fragments. Stability reduces the degree of interfragmentary deformation, allowing tissues with lower tolerance to deformation and greater inherent stiffness to survive within the fracture gap. Interfragmentary deformation is eventually reduced to the point where bone survives and unites the fragment ends. Surgical implants alter the local environment by providing stability to reduce interfragmentary deformation. However, the implant may be incapable of providing complete restoration of load-carrying capacity, necessitating postoperative restriction of activity. The use of an implant must be balanced with the fact that vascular injury occurs with surgery. Strict attention to the principles of atraumatic surgery must be followed for optimal results.

Bony union can occur by two different repair mechanisms: (1) direct healing (osteonal reconstruction) and (2) indirect healing (intermediate callus formation). The effectiveness of the implant in providing stability, coupled with the biological environment at the fracture surface, determines whether bony union occurs directly or indirectly.

Direct healing occurs through osteonal remodeling of the cortex and may be classified as primary osteonal or secondary osteonal reconstruction:

- Direct healing: primary osteonal reconstruction
  - Contact healing
  - Gap healing
- Secondary osteonal reconstruction
- Indirect healing: Intermediate callus formation

Primary osteonal reconstruction occurs with anatomical alignment of the fracture ends and absolute stability. The morphological appearance between the fractured ends is characterized by areas of contact and areas where small gaps of different widths are present. Primary osteonal reconstruction is further subdivided into contact healing and gap healing. Contact healing occurs in the zones of cortical bone contact and is characterized by osteonal remodeling across the fracture plane (Fig. 120–11). In preparation for osteonal remodeling, cutting cones are formed at the ends of the osteons nearest the fracture. Osteoclasts line the spearhead of the cutting cone for bone resorption, and osteoblasts line the rear of the cutting cones in preparation for bone formation. Bone resorption and bone formation occur simultaneously as the cutting cones advance and cross the fracture plane from one fragment to the other at a rate of 50 to 80 μm/day. Gap healing occurs in the small fragment gaps between contact zones. Although the bone is not in direct apposition, absolute stability is provided by the contact zones on either side of the gap. Interfragmentary deformation must be less than 2 per cent, and the gap width must not exceed approximately 1 mm for gap healing to occur. The gap is initially filled by blood vessels and loose connective tissue. After approximately 2 weeks, the vascular supply is established and osteoblasts deposit lamellar bone in the gap between the fragment ends. The new lamellar bone fills the gap but is oriented perpendicular to the fragment ends. The initial connection between the new bone and existing bone of the fragment ends is poor, making this area mechanically inferior. In 3 to 4 weeks, cutting cones are formed by new osteons within the gap and by osteons present within the pre-exsiting bone near the fragment ends. Cutting cones originating from both the gap and

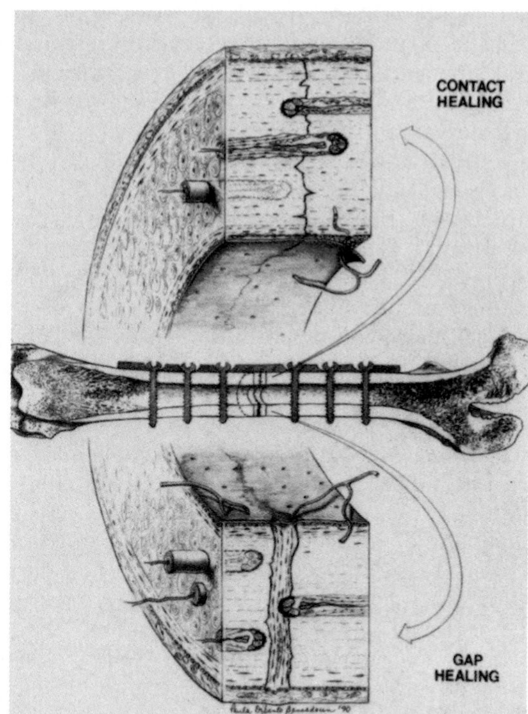

FIGURE 120–11. Types of primary bone healing under conditions of rigid stability. (1) Contact healing: Following fracture reduction and stabilization, no gap was present between fracture fragments in the cortical bone under the plate. Bony union and haversian remodeling occur simultaneously. (2) (Small) gap healing: Following fracture reduction and stabilization, a small gap (<800 μm was present between the fracture fragments in the cortex opposite the plate. Layers of bone have been laid down on the two fracture surfaces, filling the gap with transversely oriented lamellar bone. Gap bone is removed and replaced by longitudinally oriented osteons through haversian remodeling. (Editor's note: For purposes of describing bone healing, this figure is correct; however, the artist's rendition of plate application on the medial side of the femur is technically incorrect—correct plate application is on the lateral side of the femur.) (From Kaderly, R: Primary bone healing. *Semin Vet Med Surg* 6:22, 1991.)

the fragment ends cross the fracture plane to unite the new lamellar bone within the gap to the fragment ends (see Fig. 120–11). With time, the new lamellar bone in the gap becomes longitudinally oriented and re-establishes the anatomical and mechanical integrity of the cortex.

Osteonal remodeling can also occur with callus and is termed *secondary osteonal reconstruction*. This type of healing takes place with pin and wire stabilization of long oblique fractures as well as with bone plates and external fixator stabilization. With this method, the implant does not provide the stability necessary to reduce the deformation within the fracture gap to a level necessary for direct deposition of bone. Areas within the fracture plane are subject to instability and initially high levels of interfragmentary strain. Within these zones, bone resorption of the fragment ends occurs, lengthening the fracture gap and reducing interfragmentary strain. Simultaneously, external callus is formed and stabilizes the fragment ends. The implant does provide the stability necessary for rapid bridging of the fracture line by external callus. Once the external callus unites, the deformation within the fracture gap is reduced to the extent that bone tissue can survive between the fragment ends. If the fracture gap is small, osteonal reconstruction of the cortex proceeds as for gap healing, described earlier. If the fracture gap is too wide, if the vascular supply is impaired, or if interfragmentary deformation does not allow for survival of osseous tissue, indirect bone healing occurs.

Indirect bone healing occurs when osseous tissue is formed through transformation of fibrous tissue or cartilage (Fig. 120–12). This occurs when interfragmentary deformation, impairment of blood supply, or the width of the fracture gap does not allow direct formation of lamellar bone. Tissues that can survive within the fracture environment are initially deposited and subsequently prepare the fracture gap for survival of bone cells. The stages of indirect bone healing have been divided into inflammation, soft callus, hard callus, and remodeling.

Inflammation begins immediately after fracture and persists until initiation of fibrous tissue or cartilage formation. At fracture, the blood vessels are disrupted, with hemorrhage and hematoma formation. The function of the hematoma is controversial. Some believe the hematoma simply acts as a spacer and must be removed for healing to occur, whereas others believe the hematoma provides a scaffold and source of cells for the formation of granulation tissue. The appearance of granulation tissue marks the beginning of the soft callus. Granulation tissue matures into fibrous tissue or fibrocartilage, depending on local environmental conditions. Fibrous tissue forms at the periphery of the external callus, where blood supply is abundant. Toward the center of the callus, between the fragment ends, where blood supply is limited, fibrocartilage forms. The amount of callus formed directly depends on the degree of motion—the greater the instability, the greater the diameter of the internal and external callus. The farther the external callus is deposited from the center of the bone (neutral axis), the greater the ability of the damaged bone to resist bending and rotation. Both soft callus tissues have sufficient mechanical properties to bridge the fracture but not to decrease the local deformation to a level conducive to osteoblast survival.

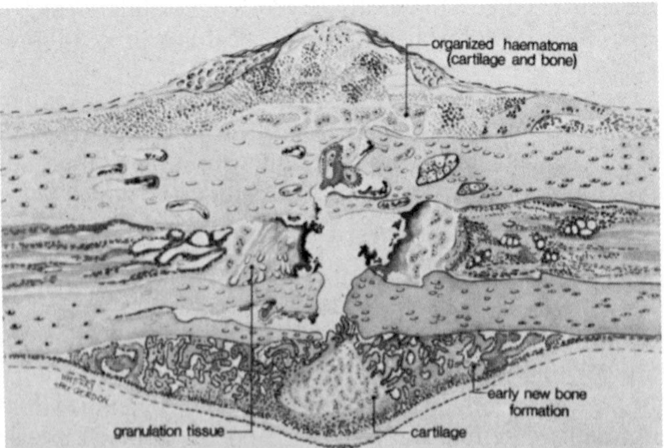

FIGURE 120–12. Early repair. There is organization of the hematoma, early primary new bone formation in subperiosteal regions, and cartilage formation in other areas. (From Newton, N: *Textbook of Small Animal Orthopaedics.* J. B. Lippincott, Philadelphia, 1984, p 36.)

To further increase stiffness of the fracture environment, mineralization begins and signifies the beginning of the hard callus. In fibrocartilage, mineralization of the matrix progresses from the fragment ends to the center of the fracture gap. In fibrous tissue, mineralization occurs between the collagen fibrils to become fiber bone. Mineralized fibrous tissue and fibrocartilage have the structural strength and stiffness to limit the gap deformation to acceptable levels to allow bone formation to begin. Fibrocartilage undergoes endochondral ossification where osteoid is deposited on the scaffold of mineralized cartilage and mineralized fiber bone. The mineralized fibrous tissue and fibrocartilage are gradually replaced to form cancellous bone. The structural stiffness and strength of the cancellous callus are sufficient for a return to function once complete bridging has occurred. The healed bone at this time has a greater diameter than normal and may be misshaped. However, the cancellous structure is not permanent. Over the ensuing months or years, through the stage of remodeling, the cancellous bone is changed to longitudinally oriented lamellar bone and the bone contour is restored.

The method of bone healing is determined by the stability given by the implant and by biological factors. Different implants are able to prevent compression, bending, and rotation to different degrees. For example, intramedullary pins resist bending only. Rotation and compression are not adequately prevented in most cases. When properly applied to a simple fracture, bone plates and screws act with the bone to form a composite that exhibits strength and stiffness resembling normal bone. As the fracture becomes more fragmented, the plate and bone cannot act as a functional composite, markedly reducing the strength and stiffness of the osteosynthesis. External fixators can be assembled to provide strength and stiffness similar to bone plates and screws. In addition, a surgeon has the flexibility to destabilize the osteosynthesis as healing progresses. All implants, when used properly, can result in direct healing (primary or secondary osteonal reconstruction of the cortex).

The biomechanical properties and methods of application for each implant are discussed in subsequent chapters. Some of the biological factors that are important include the age and size of the patient, type and location of the fracture, whether the fracture is stabilized through closed or open reduction, the presence of multiple fractures, high-velocity versus low-velocity injury, and whether the injury is an open or closed fracture. Clinical factors include a patient's and a client's compliance, postoperative limb function desired, available equipment, and experience of the surgeon. The method of fixation is chosen by evaluating the radiograph to determine the areas of tensile and shear deformation, knowledge of the stabilization properties and principles of application for each implant, and consideration of the biological and clinical factors described.

GLOSSARY OF RELEVANT TERMS

Axial force: A force applied in one direction and distributed evenly over the surface of the loaded structure. Units of measure: kilograms, newtons.

Moment arm (lever arm): The perpendicular distance from the line of action of a force to the point where the moment is to be calculated. Unit of measure: meter.

Bending moment of force: A force that tends to bend a bone about an axis perpendicular to its long axis. The product of the force and a moment arm. Unit of measure: newton-meter.

Torsion moment of force (torque): A force that tends to twist a bone about its longitudinal axis. The product of a force and the moment arm. Unit of measure: newton-meter.

Ground reaction force: Force exerted in response to the foot contacting the ground. It is equal to but in the opposite direction of the force generated by foot contact. Units of measure: kilograms, newtons.

Internal stress: Local force intensity experienced by a finite area of the bone surface. The average stress is equal to the total force/cross-sectional area. Unit of measure: newtons/mm^2.

Internal strain: Local deformation of a finite area of bone. Equal to the change in length/original length (normal strain); or a change in angle relative to the original angle (shear strain). Expressed as percentage.

Neutral axis: When the bone undergoes bending, the neutral axis is the point of zero stress within the bone that corresponds to the point of transition from compression stress to tensile stress.

References

1. Carter DR, Spengler DM: Biomechanics of fractures. *In* Sumner-Smith G (ed): *Bone in Clinical Orthopedics*. W.B. Saunders, Philadelphia, 1982, pp 305–334.
2. Nordin M, Frankel V: *Biomechanics of the Musculoskeletal System*. 2nd ed. Lea & Febiger, Philadelphia, 1989, pp 3–27.
3. Perren S: Primary bone healing. *In* Bojrab MJ (ed): *Pathophysiology in Small Animal Surgery*. Lea & Febiger, Philadelphia, 1981, pp 519–527.
4. Perren S, Rahn BA: Biomechanics of fracture healing. 1: Historical review and mechanical aspects of internal fixation. *Orthop Surv* 2:108, 1978.
5. Radin EL: *Practical Biomechanics for the Orthopedic Surgeon*. John Wiley & Sons, New York, 1979, pp 43–89.
6. Rahn BA. Bone healing. Histologic and physiologic concepts. *In* Sumner-Smith G (ed): *Bone in Clinical Orthopedics*. W.B. Saunders, Philadelphia, 1982, pp 335–386.

CHAPTER 121

Emergency Management of Fractures

Lawrence W. Anson

INITIAL MANAGEMENT

Traumatic musculoskeletal injury is a common problem in companion animal practice. A rapid but careful initial physical examination should be conducted to assess the patient (Fig. 121–1). Primary attention is given to life-threatening injuries. Priorities are establishing a patent airway, securing hemostasis, and providing circulatory support. Thereafter, constant reassessment of a patient's response to treatment is required. After a patient is stabilized, re-examination, including assessment of the thoracic and abdominal cavities, is completed. Fluid or free air within the thorax, detected by radiography, may require further diagnostics and therapeutic intervention. The central and peripheral nervous systems are closely evaluated for injuries that may influence the prognosis. After soft-tissue problems have been identified and decisions made about necessary treatment, musculoskeletal injury can be addressed.

Orthopedic injuries have been divided into three groups in an effort to establish priorities for treatment.[1] In the first group are those injuries requiring immediate intervention. These include fractures with the potential for injury to the central nervous system, such as depressed skull fractures and spinal fractures/luxations. Their management is discussed in the section on the nervous system. Also included in group I are open fractures. Medical and surgical management of open fractures is discussed in subsequent paragraphs.

The injuries in group II include luxations, intra-articular fractures, and physeal fractures. Treatment of these injuries may be safely delayed for 1 to 2 days. Definitive treatment of group III injuries, which include closed long-bone shaft fractures, nonarticular pelvic fractures, scapular fractures, and metacarpal/tarsal fractures, may also be delayed.

These groupings should only be considered as guidelines. Individual circumstances may dictate different case management. Complete re-examination of patients is performed frequently to identify occult injuries and to alter medical care in response to changes in an animal's condition.

CLOSED FRACTURES

Initial assessment of a fracture includes an appraisal of whether it is closed or open (Fig. 121–2). Closed

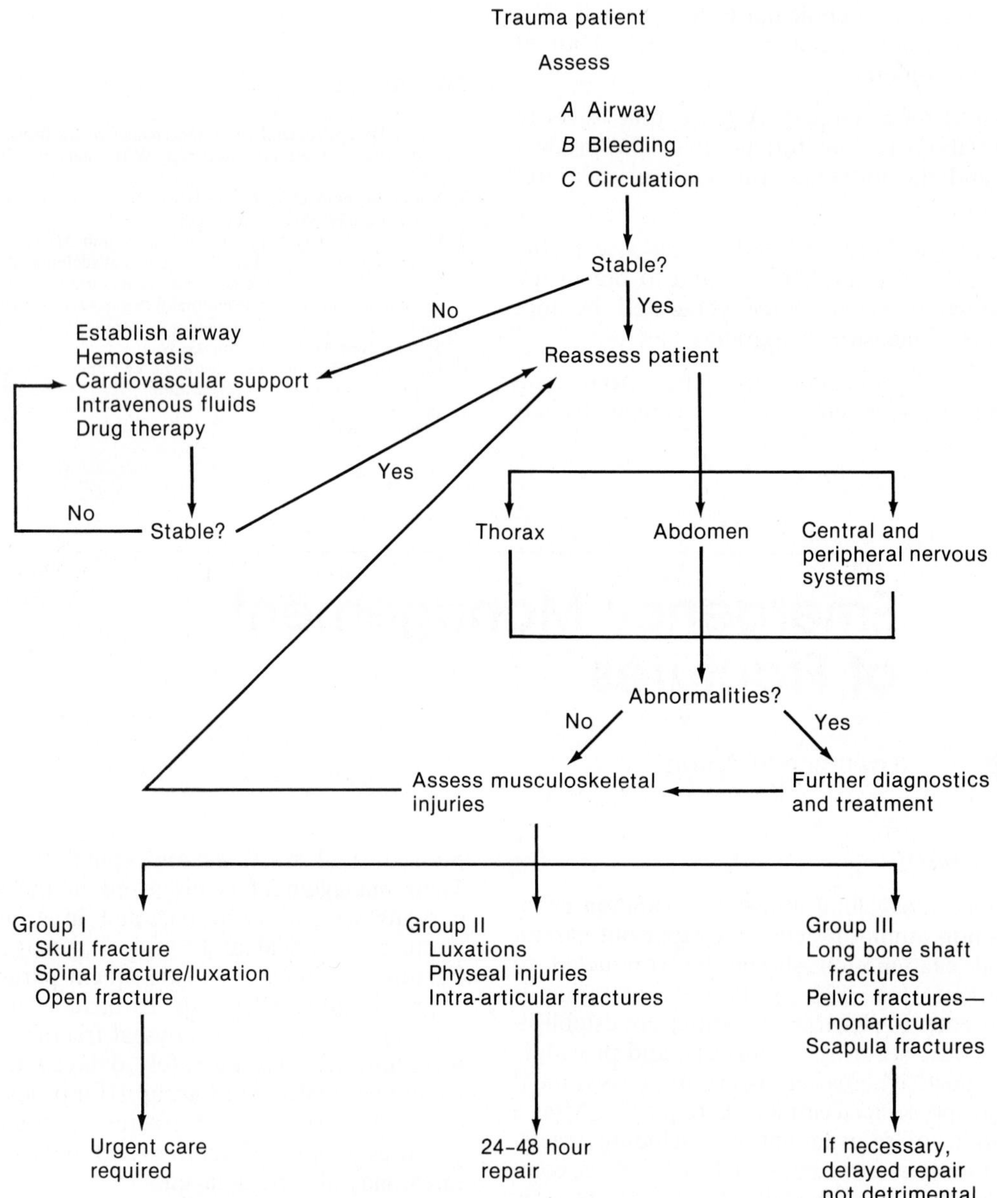

FIGURE 121–1. Algorithm for assessing traumatic musculoskeletal injuries.

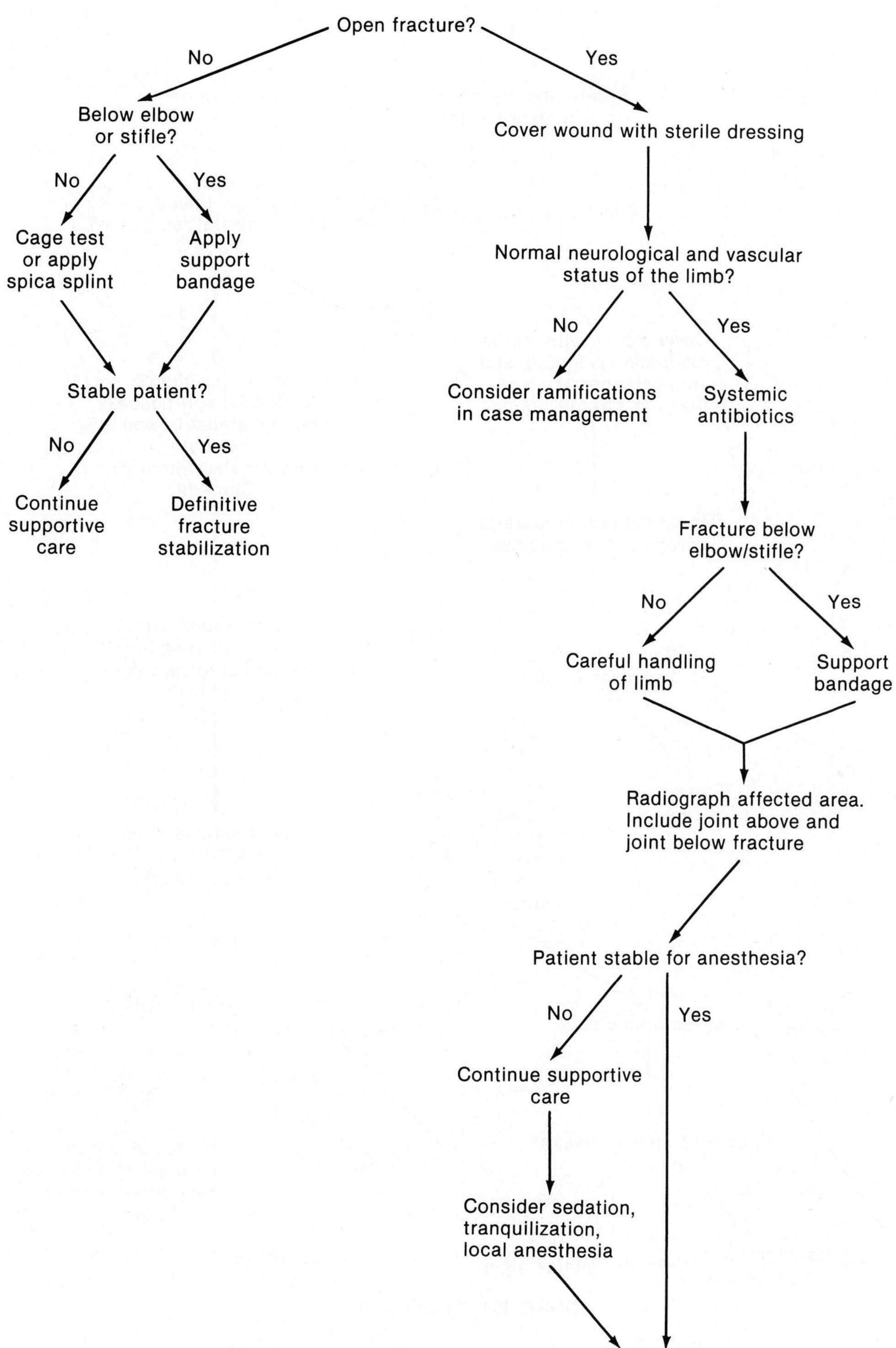

FIGURE 121–2. Algorithm for assessing and treating fractures.

Illustration continued on following page

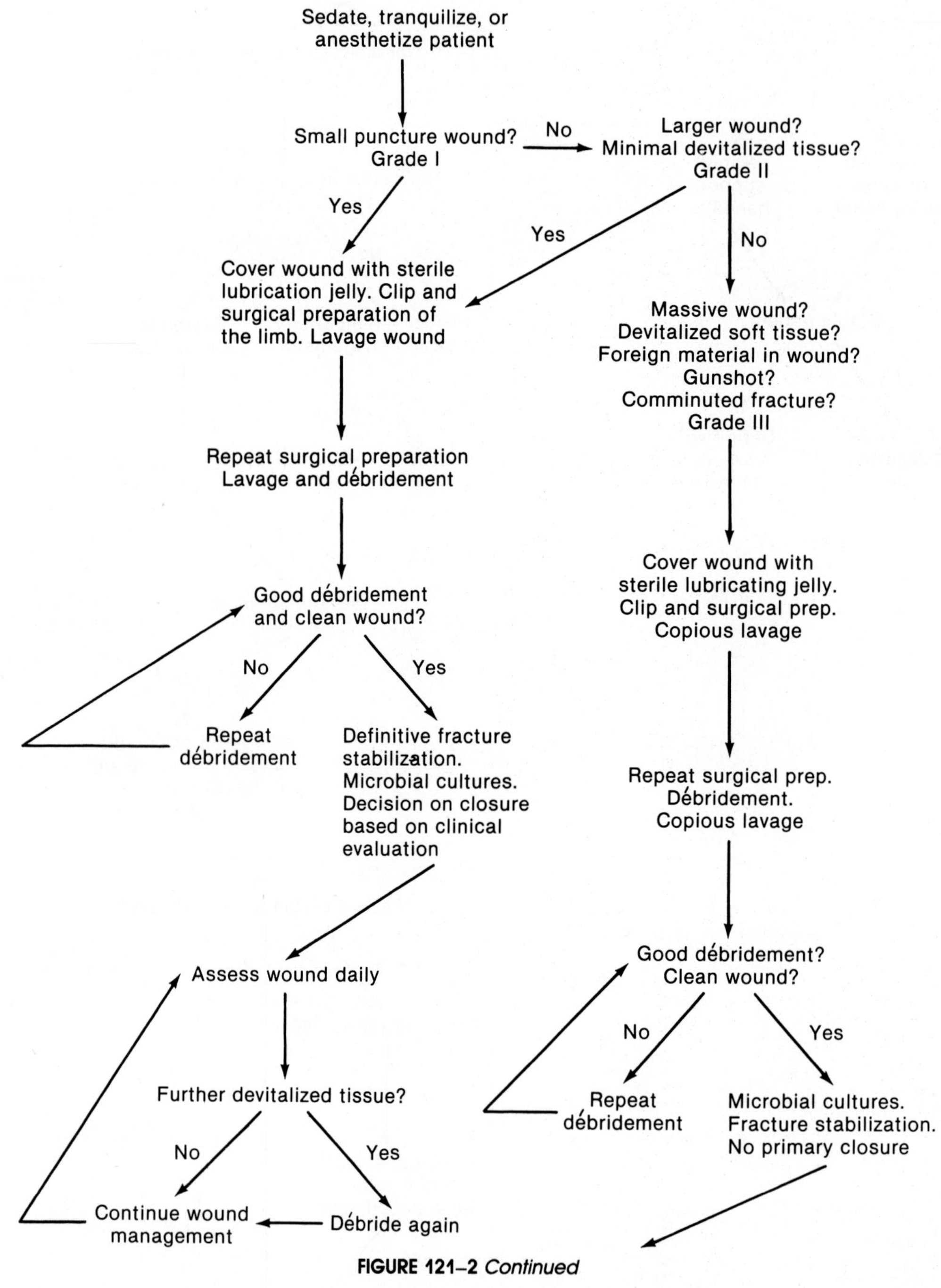

FIGURE 121–2 *Continued*

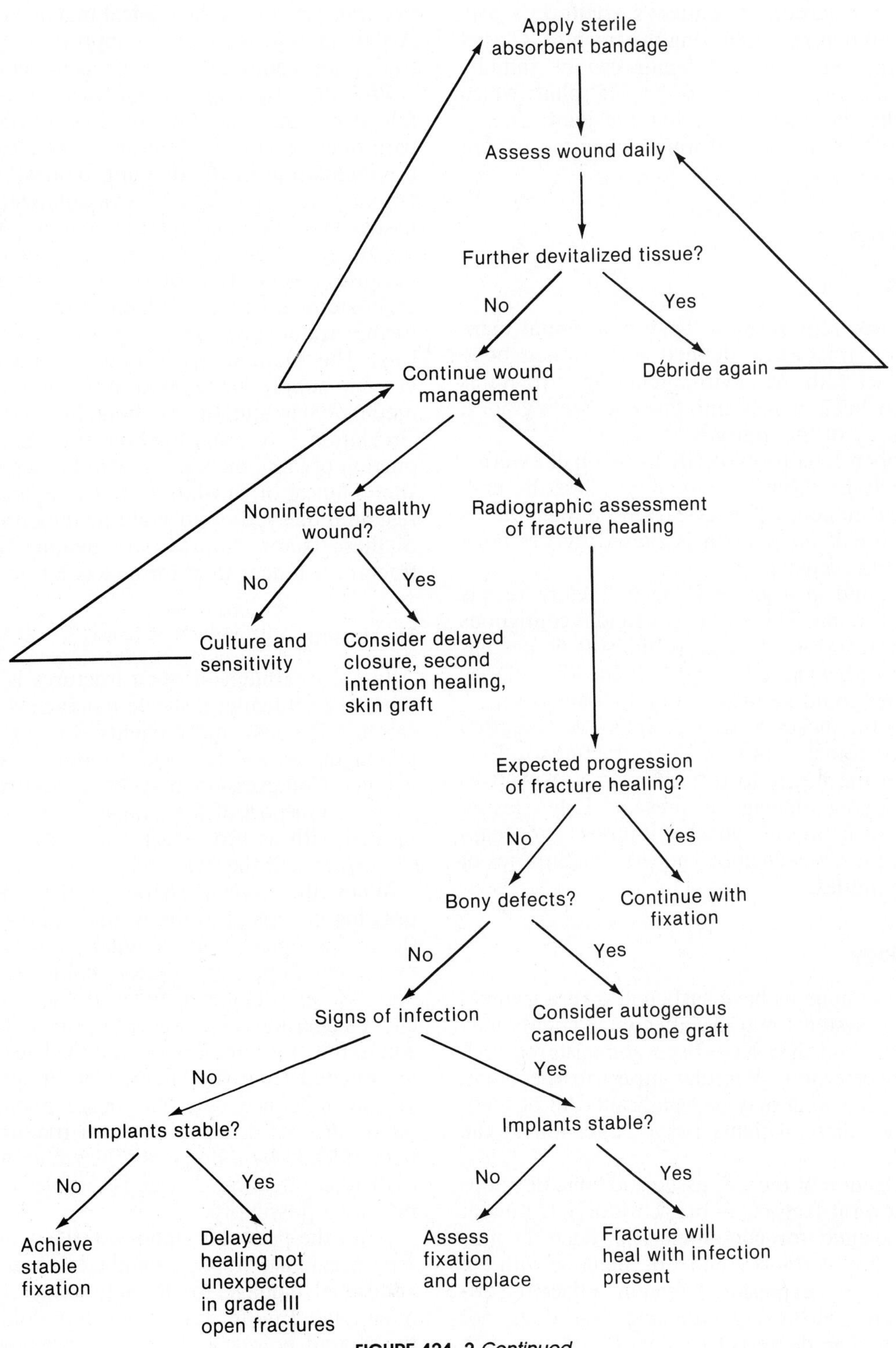

FIGURE 121–2 *Continued*

fractures below the elbow or stifle may benefit from temporary external support. A padded support bandage lessens the chance of additional soft-tissue trauma and may prevent a closed fracture from becoming open. Edema formation may be decreased and thus make the surgical approach easier. A patient's comfort is also increased by temporarily stabilizing the fracture. Closed fractures of the humerus and femur can be initially treated with cage rest or by use of a spica splint, which immobilizes the shoulder or coxofemoral joint. Definitive fracture repair can be performed when the patient is stable.

OPEN FRACTURES

Classification

Open fractures require more aggressive initial management. Open fracture is defined as a broken bone that is in contact with the environment. Open fractures have arbitrarily been divided into three separate grades, based on severity of the injury.[8]

A grade I open fracture typically has a small external wound that may be difficult to identify unless the limb is carefully examined. If necessary, the haircoat is clipped. The break in the skin is caused by the bone penetrating to the outside.

The skin wound in a grade II open fracture results from external trauma. This variable wound is contiguous with the fracture. More damage to the soft tissues has occurred than with a grade I fracture. Some low-velocity gunshot injuries could be included in this category.

Grade III is the most severe open fracture. The often high degree of comminution of these fractures reflects the severity of the injury to the soft tissues. Extensive skin and soft-tissue damage is present. Examples of grade III open fractures are gunshot injuries from weapons with high muzzle velocities and shearing injuries of the distal extremities.

Pathophysiology

Many of these animals have sustained severe trauma. Multiple organ systems may be affected. Patients may be hypovolemic and may have been administered high doses of corticosteroids. Vascular injury to the bone, muscle, fascia, and skin may be significant. All of these factors increase these patients risk of infection at the fracture site.

Whether infection of the soft tissue and bone develops depends on several factors. A break in the integument provides an avenue for contamination. Bacteria may reach the fracture by direct contact of the bone with the environment or by extension from an adjacent soft-tissue infection.[6] However, contamination does not equal infection. The degree of trauma, correlating with the fracture grade, is important in the development of an infection. The viability of the skin, soft tissue, and bone is decreased. Vascular occlusion isolates the injured tissues from the body's defense mechanisms and circulating antibiotics. Establishment of bone infection is aided by coexisting damage to the periosteal tissue, periosteum, bone, and bone marrow.[6] An animal's resistance to bacterial infection may be decreased because of effects on host defense mechanisms. In this situation, less virulent bacteria may be more likely to cause infection. A final factor that determines whether infection will develop is the clinical management of the case. A patient who is treated inappropriately is more likely to develop complications such as infection.

Prolonged healing of open fractures is to be expected for several reasons. Greater energy dissipation occurs with open fractures, resulting in greater impairment of the circulation in surrounding tissues.[3] Impaired circulation causes a delay in revascularization of the soft tissues and bone and retards healing. A second reason for delayed union is loss of the fracture hematoma, because organization of the hematoma is one of the early steps in healing.[3] Open reduction of the fracture further traumatizes the soft tissues and increases blood loss. The method of fixation can further disrupt the vascular supply to the bone. Intramedullary pins impede medullary circulation, and bone plates disturb periosteal circulation.[11] Internal fixation also results in the introduction of large metallic foreign bodies into the fracture site. Clinical or subclinical infections may occur, with a resultant delayed or aberrant healing process.[13] Because of these factors, the average healing time of an open fracture is longer than for a closed fracture.

Treatment

Initial treatment of open fractures is often begun by the owner. Ideally, a sterile bandage is placed over the wound. Because most clients do not have access to bandaging materials, a clean cloth is used to cover the wound. Compression may be used to control hemorrhage. Transport of the animal to the hospital is accomplished with as little risk of injury as possible to both the owner and the pet.

When the animal arrives at the hospital, a sterile dressing is applied to the wound. Careful assessment of the neurological and vascular status of the limb is extremely important. Questionable vascularity of the limb or abnormal neurological function may affect a client's decision on treatment options. The environment where the injury took place and the source of the trauma are elicited from the client. Certain situations can obviously influence decisions made about case management, such as an open humeral fracture as a result of being kicked by a horse and hence an attendant risk of clostridial infection or a gunshot injury, when litigation may be a possibility.

After the patient is stabilized, the wound is inspected. Any previously applied bandage is removed. To avoid additional damage to the soft tissues, the limb is not manipulated more than necessary. Poking and probing the wound before a clinician is prepared to débride it increase the risk of nosocomial infections and are avoided.

Because open fractures are contaminated, administration of an antibiotic is appropriate case management. Knowledge of bacteria commonly isolated from patients with osteomyelitis is used as a guide in selecting an appropriate antibiotic. Gram-positive isolates commonly found are the coagulase-positive *Staphylococcus* spp. and *Streptococcus* spp.[4, 12, 14] Gram-negative organisms are *Escherichia coli, Proteus* spp., *Pasteurella* spp., and *Pseudomonas* spp.[4, 12, 14] Mixed infections also may be found.[4, 12, 14] Severe soft-tissue injury with associated devitalized muscle mass, damage to vascular supply, and hence decreased oxygen content in the tissues may create a local environment where anaerobic bacteria flourish.[5] Intravenous administration of a broad-spectrum antibiotic that achieves therapeutic levels in both bone and soft tissue, such as a cephalosporin, should be considered.[10]

Depending on the disposition and condition of the patient, a support bandage may be applied for temporary fracture stabilization. If the fracture is proximal to the elbow or stifle, a support bandage is contraindicated unless the shoulder or hip joint is also immobilized. With proximal fractures, an inappropriately applied bandage may act as a pendulum, resulting in exacerbation of the injury. Tranquilization and gentle handling of the limb may be a better option than a bandage.

Radiographic evaluation of the fracture includes a minimum of two views, lateral to medial and cranial to caudal, and includes the joints above and below the fracture. The radiographs are carefully assessed for signs such as fissures, which may affect fracture management.

Radiographs and initial débridement of the wound may not require chemical restraint of the animal. However, definitive débridement of the wound and fracture stabilization will require some type of anesthetic management. Depending on a patient's condition, options may include local anesthesia or regional anesthesia such as an epidural. Neuroleptanalgesia could also be considered. If a patient is in stable condition, general anesthesia may be indicated.

Adequate débridement of the wound is critical in the treatment of open fractures. In an effort to convert a contaminated wound to a clean one, adherence to aseptic technique cannot be overemphasized. Cap, mask, and gloves should be worn and sterile instruments used. To prevent hair from entering the wound while the limb is being clipped, sterile lubrication jelly is used to cover the wound. After surgical preparation of the limb, copious lavage of the wound is performed. Gross contamination is washed away or removed with débridement of the tissues.

Lavage can be accomplished with a 35-ml syringe and an 18-gauge needle.[9] A satisfactory solution for lavage is sterile isotonic saline either with or without 0.05 per cent chlorhexidine.[15]

Initial débridement involves the use of sharp dissection to remove obviously devitalized soft tissue. Undermining the wound edges is avoided. After this stage is complete, the surgeon should repeat the surgical preparation, reglove, and perform the final débridement, again using copious lavage. Surgical exposure should be adequate for thorough débridement, but extensive soft-tissue dissection is avoided. Because of the potential for litigation with gunshot fractures, bullets are saved.

Culture and sensitivity testing are performed. A prospective study in humans concluded that infection was correlated with the organisms in the wound at the end of débridement, not at the beginning.[7] In light of these findings, culture and sensitivity test results should be obtained when the débridement is finished.

Débridement of bone is usually performed during stabilization of the fracture. All bone that remains in the fracture is carefully cleaned. The potential for sequestrum formation is of primary clinical concern. Guidelines for débriding bone are as follows: Small pieces that have no soft-tissue attachment may be removed. If a piece of bone with no soft-tissue attachment is integral to the reconstruction of the fracture, an attempt is made to salvage it. Bone fragments with soft-tissue attachments are left in the fracture site whether or not they are incorporated into the fracture repair.

Fracture Fixation

Definitive stabilization of the fracture is carried out as soon as possible. Benefits to be gained are an increase in a patient's comfort and easier management of open wounds. Stabilization improves blood supply to the tissues, facilitates healing, and promotes resistance to infection.

Coaptation devices are rarely used except as temporary support or on stable fractures with easily managed soft-tissue wounds. Casts and splints make wound care difficult. Frequent changes result in excessive movement of the fracture. Skin with tenuous blood supply is not placed under a restrictive cast or splint.

Intramedullary pins may be used in grade I and II open fractures if adequate stabilization is achieved. The potential exists to contaminate the medullary cavity. The risk with adequately débrided wounds is probably low.

Rigid fixation is provided by bone plates and screws. Their use is indicated in grades I and II. The extensive soft-tissue dissection required for their placement makes plates less attractive as an option for grade III fractures.

In many grade III open fractures, external fixators are ideal. The pins may be placed away from the fracture site and the traumatized soft tissue, preserving blood supply and aiding wound care. In some cases, circumstances may dictate limb amputation as the most expedient treatment.

After fracture stabilization, a decision must be made about wound closure. Influencing factors are the time since injury, the environment in which the injury occurred, the fracture grade, the degree of soft-tissue injury, and the adequacy of the débridement. If the advisability of wound closure is in doubt, management as an open wound is appropriate. Well-débrided, clean grade I and II fractures are candidates for primary closure. Requirements include adequate vascularity, no tension or dead space, and no devitalized tissue. If dead space is excessive, then closed suction drains can be used with a primary closure.

Grade III open fractures are rarely closed primarily. Delayed closure or second intention healing is the method of choice. After final débridement and culture, the wound is covered with a sterile dressing. Saline-soaked gauze sponges may be used to keep the tissues moist and aid in débridement. Bandage changes are made as required for appropriate wound management. Repeated débridement, if required, is an advantage of managing a case in this manner. If large cortical bone defects are present, the use of a delayed cancellous bone auto graft, after the wound is covered with granulation tissue, helps speed union of the fracture.[2] With delayed closure or second intention healing, frequent re-evaluation of the patient is required to respond to changes in the wound.

More detailed information about the management of specific fractures, bone grafting, osteomyelitis, and wound management may be found in other chapters of this text.

References

1. Aron DN: Emergency management of the musculoskeletal trauma patient. *Comp Cont Educ Pract Vet 4*:220, 1982.
2. Bardet JF, et al: Open drainage and delayed autogenous cancellous bone grafting for treatment of chronic osteomyelitis in dogs and cats. *J Am Vet Med Assoc 183*:312, 1983.
3. Brown PW: The open fracture. Cause, effect and management. *Clin Orthop 96*:254, 1973.
4. Caywood DD, et al: Osteomyelitis in the dog: A review of 67 cases. *J Am Vet Med Assoc 172*:943, 1978.
5. Evarts CM, Mayer PJ: Complications. *In* Rockwood CA Jr, Green DP (eds) *Fractures in Adults.* 2nd ed. J.B. Lippincott, Philadelphia, 1984, pp 219–279.
6. Kahn DS, Pritzker KPH: The pathophysiology of bone infection. *Clin Orthop 96*:12, 1973.
7. Merritt K: Factors increasing the risk of infection in patients with open fractures. *J Trauma 28*:823, 1988.
8. Muller ME, et al: Compound fractures in the adult. *In* Muller ME, et al (eds): *Manual of Internal Fixation. Technique Recommended by the AO-Group.* Springer-Verlag, New York, 1970, pp 211–219.
9. Ndikuwera J, Winstanley EW: High pressure pulsatile lavage and high pressure syringe lavage in the treatment of contaminated wounds in dogs. *J Small Anim Pract 26*:3, 1985.
10. Patzakis MJ, et al: Use of antibiotics in open tibial fractures. *Clin Orthop 178*:31, 1983.
11. Rhinelander FW: Blood supply of healing long-bones. *In* Newton CD, Nunamaker DM (eds): *Textbook of Small Animal Orthopaedics.* J.B. Lippincott, Philadelphia, 1985, pp 39–58.
12. Smith CW, et al: Osteomyelitis in the dog: A retrospective study. *J Am Anim Hosp Assoc 14*:589, 1978.
13. Smith MM, et al: Bacterial growth associated with metallic implants in dogs. *J Am Vet Med Assoc 195*:765, 1989.
14. Stead AC: Osteomyelitis in the dog and cat. *J Small Anim Pract 25*:1, 1984.
15. Swaim SF, Lee AH: Topical wound medications: A review. *J Am Vet Med Assoc 190*:1588, 1987.

CHAPTER 122

Methods of Internal Fracture Fixation

General Principles

David J. DeYoung and Curtis W. Probst

Fracture repair in small animals is divided into three categories: closed reduction with external support, internal fixation alone, and internal fixation with secondary external support. The last category is further divided into internal fixation with minimal reliance on external support and internal fixation with heavy reliance on external support (Fig. 122–1). In this section, internal fixation as the sole means of fracture repair is discussed. However, the level of stability achieved with internal fixation may be inadequate, and secondary external support is often necessary. A surgeon should strive to maintain fracture alignment and stability with internal implants and rely on external support only when necessary. When fracture stability depends too heavily on external support, the incidence of complications increases dramatically. This situation most often arises from the improper choice of primary fixation.

Too often, the immediate goal of fracture repair is to maintain anatomical reduction and fixation until the body's healing mechanisms restore the structural continuity of the bone. If one only considers bone union in fracture repair, long-term or permanent disabilities may develop because of soft-tissue complications (Fig. 122–2). Adhesions restrict or prevent the normal gliding motion in adjacent muscles and tendons. Joints of the affected limb may also stiffen because of capsular fibrosis and contracture, and disuse atrophy of articular cartilage may ensue.[18] These disabling soft-tissue complications, collectively referred to as *fracture disease*, must be avoided during fracture repair and healing. Because the objective in fracture repair is early return of the injured limb to full function, soft tissue as well as bone must be considered. Early return to function is achieved by anatomical reconstruction of the bone with stable internal fixation and strict adherence to the basic principles of surgery, especially atraumatic soft-tissue handling and preservation of blood supply to the bone. Satisfaction of these criteria precludes the use of restrictive coaptation devices and promotes early use of the muscles and joints of the affected limb. Stable internal fixation of fractures is achieved by two basic methods: insertion of intramedullary pins and application of bone plates.

CHOICE OF FIXATION

The method of fracture repair is based on the type and location of the fracture, the size and age of the animal, the number of bones or limbs involved, and

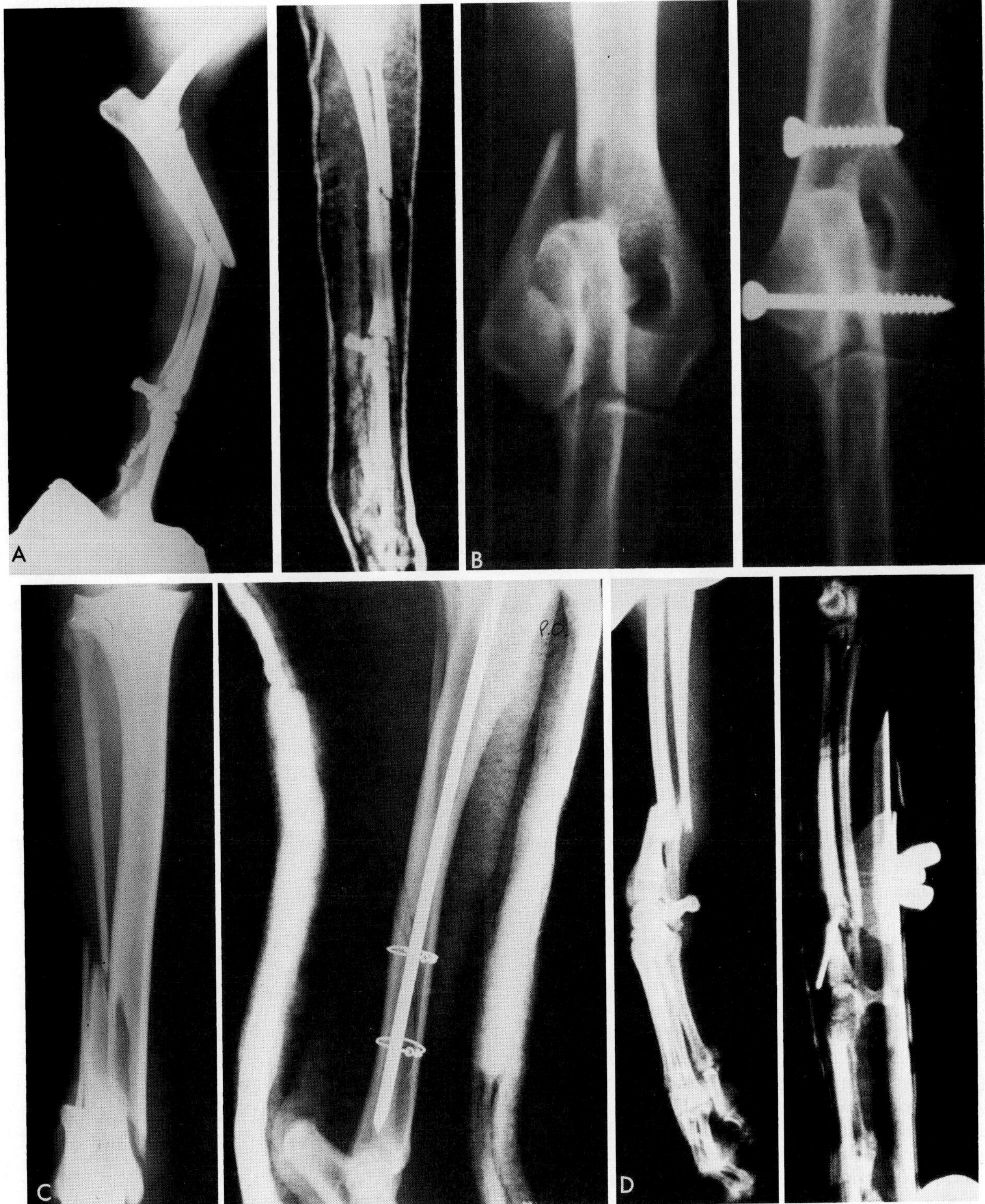

FIGURE 122–1. Three categories of fracture repair. *A*, Closed reduction with external support. *B*, Internal fixation alone. Internal fixation with secondary external support: *C*, minimal reliance on external support and *D*, heavy reliance on external support.

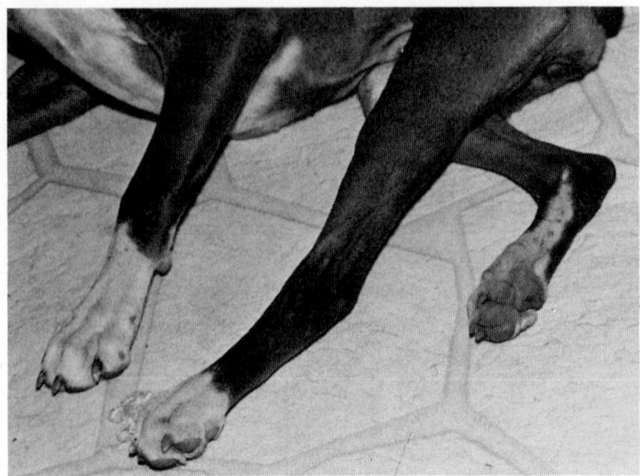

FIGURE 122–2. Fracture disease. Adhesions, capsular fibrosis, and contracture secondary to fracture repair, resulting in hyperextension and permanent disability of the limb.

concurrent soft-tissue disease. Other factors to consider include the animal's behavior and environment, the owner's cooperation during the convalescent period, and the animal's expected level of performance after bone union. Cost, surgical expertise, and the availability of equipment and technical assistance must be considered. The initial plan of fracture management is based on sound medical judgment. Deviation from this plan because of economics or lack of expertise, equipment, or technical assistance may compromise the outcome. It is better to provide the optimum in fixation or to offer referral to a specialist than to compromise the principles of fracture repair. What begins as an apparently simple case may become a long, unpleasant ordeal.

Size, age, and temperament of the animal are obvious factors in selecting the correct implant. Fractures in small or medium-sized animals may be adequately stabilized with intramedullary pins. If one considers other factors, this type of fixation may not be adequate. A small animal that is 12 years of age and housed outdoors without restriction of activity may require the more stable fixation provided by a bone plate. A properly applied bone plate withstands such an animal's additional activity and provides stability during the longer healing time required in geriatric animals. In addition, a plate may be indicated when a disease process such as a fracture, dislocation, or even arthritis is present in another limb. The resulting early return to full function of the fractured limb enables the animal to walk sooner and allows the application of an Ehmer sling or similar device to another limb.

The type and location of a fracture may dictate using one implant over another. For instance, it is technically easier to apply a bone plate to a pelvic fracture than to attempt fixation with alternative methods. Not only is the resulting stability much greater, but the return to function is almost immediate. Conversely, some fractures do not readily lend themselves to bone plate application. Metaphyseal and epiphyseal fractures may not leave enough bone length to allow adequate plate fixation. Also, plate fixation of a fracture in an epiphysis with remaining growth potential arrests growth.

A fracture associated with extensive soft-tissue damage may require stabilization with an external skeletal fixator.*[20] Surgical dissection of such a fracture may cause further devitalization of tissues, delayed healing, or wound infection. Application of an external skeletal fixator stabilizes the bone until the soft tissues heal, at which time additional fixation may be undertaken.

FRACTURE FORCES

In addition to the preceding criteria, it is necessary to consider the forces acting on the fracture site when selecting an implant (see Chapter 120). When force is applied to a limb during weightbearing, the load is transmitted along the bone, resulting in stresses that tend to malalign or disrupt the fracture site. These stresses are also present without weightbearing because of muscle tension.

For most purposes in clinical orthopedics, it is sufficient to consider four basic forces. These are rotational, bending, and shearing forces and fragment apposition (Fig. 122–3). The last is not a true fracture force, but it is necessary to consider fragment apposition during implant selection. A fixation device, whether it involves external or internal stabilization, must neutralize inherent forces acting on that particular fracture to prevent motion at the fracture site. It is not necessary for these forces to cause gross displacement of the fracture segments to adversely affect healing. Slight undetectable movement can impede the growth of small capillary buds across the fracture site. This vascular ingrowth is enhanced by stable fixation.[11, 14, 16, 23] Lack of revascularization accounts for nonunion in fractures with anatomical reduction and seemingly adequate fixation. If fracture forces are neutralized, soft-tissue structures are preserved, vascular integrity is maintained, and infection is prevented, optimal conditions have been established for fracture healing.

Before surgical reconstruction of a fractured bone, the radiographic appearance of the fracture fragments

*Kirschner Medical Corporation, Timonium, MD.

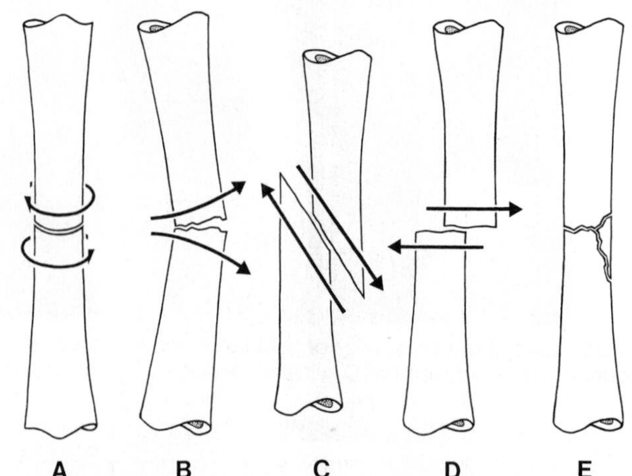

FIGURE 122–3. Basic fracture forces. *A*, Rotation. *B*, Bending. *C*, Angular shear. *D*, Horizontal shear. *E*, Fragment apposition.

is analyzed. By observing the nature of the fracture fragments, the forces acting at the fracture site are predicted and an implant that will neutralize them is selected.

Rotational force is present in all fractures. Rotation is most often a problem in transverse or slightly oblique long-bone fractures that do not interdigitate. Anatomically reduced fracture fragments that interdigitate have some ability to resist rotation, especially when compressed by implants or muscle contraction. Rotation at the fracture site may cause delayed union or nonunion and can result in rotational deformities of the limb distal to the fracture site (Fig. 122–4).

Bending results from eccentric axial loading, the presence of a cortical defect on the compression side, or both. The common tendency is to use inadequate fixation where *bending forces* predominate. If the implants are unable to withstand the bending forces, implant failure (i.e., plate bending, pin breakage) and loss of reduction may occur. The angulation resulting from the implant failure further potentiates the bending force because of increased eccentric loading. A common error in fracture fixation is application of an external coaptation device as secondary support for a femoral or humeral fracture. These devices seldom provide additional support for the implants and may be detrimental because the top of a cast or the bar of a Schroeder-Thomas splint can act as a fulcrum to enhance bending forces (Fig. 122–5).

Shearing force is most commonly associated with an oblique fracture. Shearing force causes the two bone ends to slide relative to each other in a direction parallel to their plane of contact. Shear force exists even in a simple transverse fracture. The fracture ends tend to slide by each other in a horizontal plane. This horizontal shearing force is most frequently a problem when a single intramedullary pin is used for fixation. Shearing forces can have devastating effects on a fracture; every effort is made to neutralize the impact of shear on the fracture site.

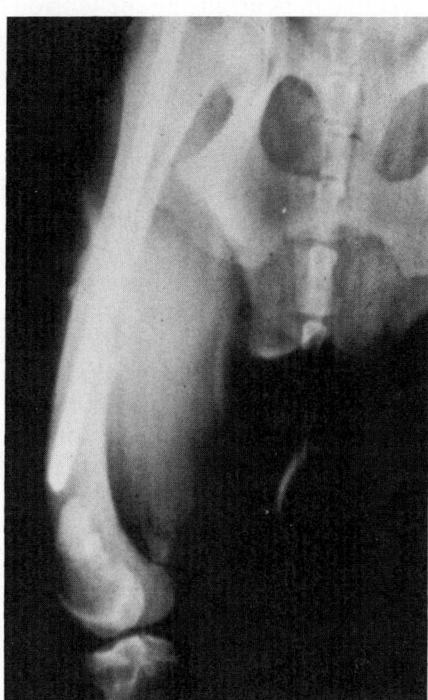

FIGURE 122–4. Rotational deformity. As a result of rotation at the fracture site, the distal fracture segment is rotated 90° in relation to the proximal fracture segment.

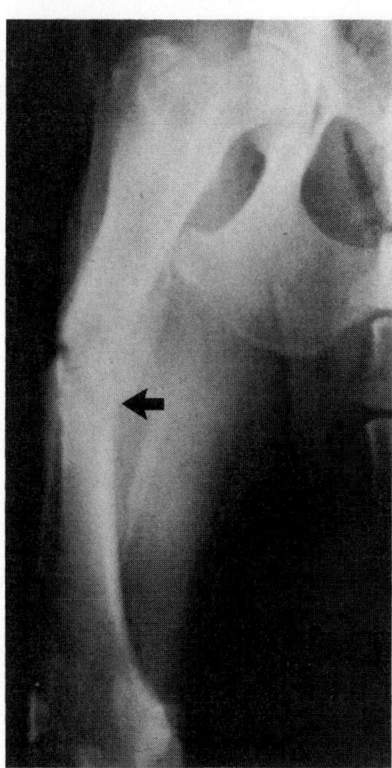

FIGURE 122–5. Enhancement of bending force resulting from use of a Schroeder-Thomas splint. In this fracture, the bar of the splint was acting as a fulcrum at the fracture site.

Fragment apposition is not a true fracture force. It is important to maintain fragment apposition in comminuted fractures, because anatomical cortical contact helps the implants withstand rotational, shearing, and bending forces at the fracture site. After fracture repair, tremendous forces act on the reduced fracture fragments. Fixation of fracture fragments is as secure as possible, because the fragments contribute to fracture stability. Failure to maintain fragment apposition may cause failure of fixation. Such fixation is most critical when a less stable type of primary fixation is used (Fig. 122–6).

It is difficult to classify each implant's ability to neutralize fracture forces because of the various fracture types. However, some generalizations can be made (Table 122–1). A particular implant may be effective in neutralizing a force, but such effectiveness does not ensure a successful repair with that implant alone (e.g., cerclage wire or lag screws).

The ability of a single intramedullary pin to counteract horizontal or angular shearing force depends on the size of the pin in relation to the medullary cavity. If the pin is smaller than the medullary cavity, shearing may occur, resulting in horizontal movement or over-riding of fracture segments. If the pin diameter equals that of the medullary cavity, shearing forces are effectively counteracted. Because most bones are not perfect cylinders, the pin rarely fills the medullary cavity of both fracture

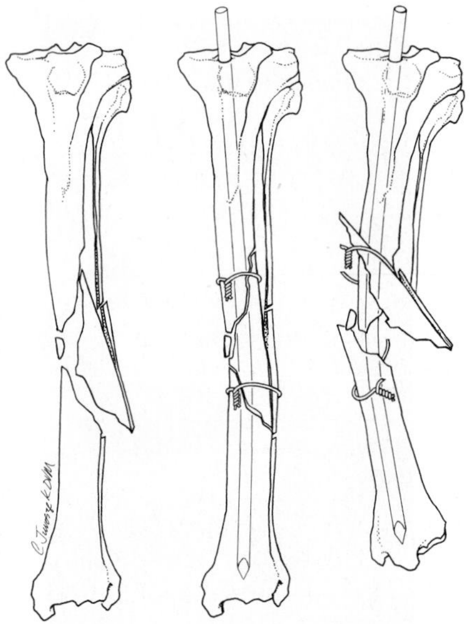

FIGURE 122–6. Fragment apposition. Failure of the primary fixation device as a result of loss of fragment apposition.

segments. Either supplemental fixation or an alternative means of repair is required to neutralize the shearing forces.

The ability of an intramedullary pin to resist bending force is directly proportional to its diameter as well as to the ratio of the pin diameter to the medullary diameter. As the medullary diameter becomes excessively large, it is difficult to counteract the bending force solely with an intramedullary pin. It may be necessary to add supplemental fixation such as an external fixation device to resist the bending forces. An alternative means of fixation such as a bone plate may be a better choice in this instance.

Rotation is not effectively counteracted by a single intramedullary pin, regardless of its size.[21] The cortical purchase at the end of the bone is insufficient to prevent rotation of the bone segments around the pin. Rotational forces may be counteracted by interlocking of fragments and by compression caused by internal and external loading forces.[17] With the exception of a two-piece fracture, intramedullary pins do not maintain fragment apposition.

TABLE 122–1. ABILITY OF VARIOUS IMPLANTS TO NEUTRALIZE FRACTURE FORCES

Implant	Rotational Force	Bending Force	Shearing Force	Fragment Apposition
Single intramedullary pin	−	+	−	−
Multiple intramedullary pins	+	+	−	−
Bone plate	+	+	+	+
External fixator	+	+	+	−
Cerclage wire	(+)	(+)	(+)	+
Lag screw	(+)	(+)	(+)	+

+, neutralization achieved; −, neutralization not achieved; (+), neutralization achieved but devices must be protected by another implant to minimize failure.

When using intramedullary pins, special care must be taken to counteract rotation, shear, and bending forces. If these criteria cannot be met, supplemental fixation must be used or an alternative implant chosen. The use of multiple intramedullary pins aids in counteracting rotational forces.[8, 21] Multiple pins provide additional fixation in the cancellous bone of the distal end of the bone and emerge from separate points in the proximal end of the bone.[7] In addition, the net effect of multiple pins is increased diameter of the implant in relation to the medullary canal. This arrangement resists bending and horizontal shearing forces. The use of multiple intramedullary pins is called *stack pinning*.[7]

Properly applied, bone plates provide the most stable form of fracture fixation. They neutralize rotational, shearing, and bending forces and maintain apposition of multiple fragments. Plates also increase the stability of fracture repair through axial loading or compression of the bone fragments. As with other devices, success depends on selection and proper application of an implant of appropriate size.

Lag screws and cerclage wire are effective in achieving fragment apposition, but their ability to maintain reduction under clinical loading conditions is poor. Their primary function is to maintain fragment apposition to facilitate application of the primary implant. These forms of fixation are most often applied to stabilize oblique fractures or to maintain reduction of fragments. In these instances, shearing forces predominate and frequently result in failure of lag screw or cerclage wire fixation. Once fracture reduction has been achieved with lag screws or cerclage wires, the forces acting at the fracture site are neutralized with a bone plate or external fixator. Failure to realize the inherent weakness of these devices or improper application of them is a common cause of fracture failure.

Wire is effective in neutralizing the tension or distracting force that occurs at an apophysis such as the tibial tubercle, olecranon process, or trochanter major. A tension band device consisting of two parallel pins and a figure-eight wire is used to repair fractures or osteotomies of these apophyses.

Various modifications of external skeletal fixators can be used for primary fracture fixation or as secondary fixation (see Chapter 123). In either case, these devices are effective in neutralizing fracture forces.[2, 3, 9, 21] Applied to the tension side of a bone, a unilateral external fixator aids in counteracting bending forces and is an effective antirotational device. In addition, when applied to an oblique or comminuted fracture as secondary fixation, the splint protects lag screws or cerclage wires from shearing forces, although not as effectively as a bone plate.[21]

SURGICAL CONSIDERATIONS

During open reduction, strict aseptic conditions must be maintained. A patient's hair is carefully removed from a wide area surrounding the surgical site, and the skin prepared with an effective surgical germicide. It is advantageous in long-bone fracture repair to prepare and drape a patient so the entire limb is accessible during surgery to facilitate manipulation of the limb and inspection of limb alignment during reduction. Impervious stockinette covering the limb can be sutured or clipped to the wound edges to minimize wound contamination from the surrounding skin. A nonwoven or felted paper moisture barrier drape is used to prevent wound contamination resulting from bacterial penetration.[22]

Atraumatic tissue handling is essential to minimize complications and promote early return to function. Meticulous attention to hemostasis is important to reduce the amount of blood left in the wound. Blood clots provide an excellent culture medium to support bacterial growth and may delay wound healing by preventing tissue apposition. Frequent wound lavage with warm saline or Ringer's solution helps promote a healthy wound environment by preventing tissue desiccation.[12] Wound lavage also mechanically removes bacteria, blood, and other debris from the surgical site. Every effort must be made to preserve the blood supply to fracture fragments, because bone healing and resistance to infection depend on adequate vascular supply.[12]

THEORY AND TECHNIQUE OF INTRAMEDULLARY PINNING

Equipment

Round Steinmann pins are available in various sizes. The most commonly used pins are 9 and 12 inches in length and 1/16 to 1/4 inch in diameter. Smaller pins, called Kirschner wires, are available in diameters of 0.028, 0.035, 0.045, and 0.062 inch. These smaller pins are useful in auxiliary fixation devices such as tension bands and as intramedullary pins in small bones. Both types of pins are available with several different points on either one or both ends. The double-pointed pins are the most versatile and economical to use because they can be inserted retrograde or can be cut in half and both ends used. Intramedullary pins are available with chisel, trocar, and threaded trocar points (Fig. 122–7). Nonthreaded trocar points are the most commonly used for intramedullary pinning because of their ability to penetrate cortical bone. Threaded trocar-point intramedullary pins are more difficult to insert and offer no advantage over nonthreaded points.[10] Threaded pins are weaker at the thread shaft junction and are prone to break at this point. Chisel-pointed pins have a broad, flat point that resists cortical penetration. This can be advantageous when pins are driven from the metaphyseal portion of soft bone into the diaphysis. The chisel point is less apt to engage the opposite cortex and leave the medullary canal prematurely.

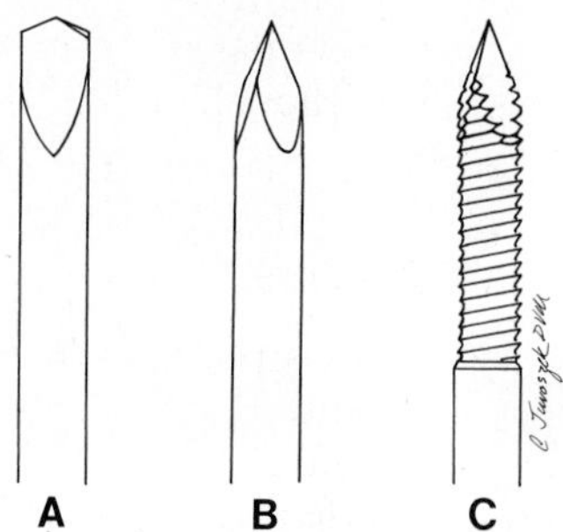

FIGURE 122–7. Steinmann intramedullary pin points. *A*, Chisel. *B*, Trocar. *C*, Threaded trocar.

A pin chuck is required to insert the pins into the bone, and a pin cutter is necessary to cut them to the proper length. Because intramedullary pinning does not always result in adequate fracture stability, auxiliary fixation devices such as cerclage wire and external fixator components should be available. As with any type of fracture repair, alignment and fixation of the fragments are facilitated by bone forceps.

Principles of Intramedullary Pinning

One or more pins are inserted into the medullary canal to maintain fracture alignment and stability until union occurs. The pins can be placed by the closed or open technique. The closed method avoids surgical exposure and is applicable to stable fractures of palpable long bones. An open approach may expedite fracture repair and cause less soft-tissue damage. The open method offers the advantages of direct exposure and manipulation of the bone fragments and allows application of auxiliary fixation such as cerclage wire. It also provides the opportunity to test and visually assess the degree of stability achieved.

Angular stability, or resistance to bending, is achieved by stable anchorage of the pin in the cortical or cancellous bone of the proximal and distal ends of the bone.[17] Theoretically, bending and horizontal shearing are prevented when the pin diameter equals the medullary diameter at the fracture site. Because of the natural curvature of most long bones and variations in cross-sectional diameter, the pin rarely fills the medullary canal.[17] Therefore, bending and horizontal shearing forces may cause motion at the fracture site. Filling the medullary canal at the fracture site may be undesirable, because the pin interferes with medullary blood supply. It also complicates application of a secondary fixation device, such as an external fixator. A good compromise is to select a pin diameter that occupies approximately 60 to 70 per cent of the medullary cavity. Rotational stability depends on muscular compression and inherent stability resulting from interdigitation of the fracture fragments. Anatomical reduction of fracture fragments helps resist rotation. These concepts re-emphasize the importance of stable fixation of comminuted fragments with cerclage wire of sufficient strength to withstand the forces acting on the fracture. Cerclage wire should seldom be smaller than 20 gauge even for the smallest animals.

It is important to recognize when the limitations of a single pin have been exceeded. It may become necessary to use a multiple-pin technique or to add secondary fixation, such as an external fixator. It is inadvisable to combine external coaptation splints with internal skeletal fixation because of the fulcrum effect and restriction of limb use. Intramedullary pinning techniques are restricted to small and medium-sized animals. The large and giant breeds have such a large medullary cavity that standard round pins are unable to maintain adequate alignment and stability. The size and weight of these large animals generate forces that cannot be counteracted by Steinmann pins; therefore, plate and screw fixation is generally required.

Technique of Application

Only the open method of fracture repair is described because it is more commonly used. The extent to which an approach is developed depends on the severity of the fracture. A simple transverse fracture requires only enough exposure to allow placement of reduction forceps on each fracture fragment. A long oblique or comminuted fracture requires more extensive exposure. Greater exposure facilitates fragment alignment and application of cerclage wires. Despite the additional time required for the approach and closure, a liberal exposure can result in decreased surgical time and better reduction and stability. Inadequate surgical exposure necessitates excessive retraction of the soft tissues, causing unnecessary trauma.

After exposure, the pin may be inserted into the bone via either a normograde or retrograde technique. With the normograde technique, the pin is started into the bone from an external landmark and advanced to the fracture site. With the retrograde method, the pin is started from the fracture site and advanced up the marrow cavity through the cortex and out of the skin. The pin chuck is removed and placed on the proximal end of the pin, and the pin retracted until the distal point is level with the fracture site. Regardless of the method used, the proximal bone fragment is firmly held with bone forceps to prevent rotation as the pin is advanced. The pin is inserted into the medullary canal with steady pressure and back-and-forth quarter turns of the pin chuck. The pin chuck is placed in the palm of the hand while rotating the pin, to put the pin in line with the center of axial rotation of the wrist and prevent wobbling as the pin is rotated.

Once the pin has been placed in the proximal fragment, the bone is anatomically reduced with the aid of bone forceps and held in reduction while an assistant seats the pin into the distal fracture segment. It is helpful for the person seating the pin to place the free hand around the distal portion of the bone to provide counterpressure. If the fracture is oblique, the fragments are reduced and alignment is maintained with cerclage wires or a reduction clamp before seating the pin. If the pin is seated without anatomical reduction, adjustments in alignment may be difficult, because the pin may have different axial alignment in each of the two fracture segments. If the fracture is comminuted, the fragments are anatomically reduced, and reduction maintained with cerclage wire or reduction clamps while the pin is seated in the distal fragment. A comminuted fracture is reconstructed first to a two-piece fracture, then the two remaining pieces are reduced.

After reduction, the pin is inserted into the distal segment until resistance is felt on the pin chuck. The chuck is removed, and a pin of equal length is placed beside the intramedullary pin to measure the distance of penetration into the distal fragment. Extreme caution must be used to avoid penetrating the adjacent joint with the pin. Postoperative radiographic examination is necessary to document reduction and implant position.

Once the pin is seated in the distal fracture segment, the reconstructed bone is stressed to evaluate stability. Adjacent joints are also flexed and extended to determine if the pin is interfering with normal joint motion. Inspect the entire limb for rotational and angular alignment. Gross examination of the limb is facilitated if the entire leg has been aseptically prepared and pulled through the drape before surgery. If any malalignment or instability is present, the fragments are correctly aligned and additional fixation applied. Two common techniques are to add additional intramedullary pins or a two- or four-pin unilateral external fixator (Fig. 122–8). The additional intramedullary pin may be added by the normograde method, or if its use was anticipated, it may be passed retrograde before fracture reduction.

Application of a two-pin unilateral external fixator is a simple and effective means of providing additional fixation. This device can be applied after closure. Application before closure allows visual evaluation of its effectiveness. The fixator clamps are available in three sizes, the small and medium sizes being used in small animals. The pins are inserted through the skin and soft tissues and into the bone with the aid of a pin chuck. The pins are advanced through both cortices until the entire point protrudes through the far cortex. If the external fixator pin strikes the intramedullary pin, the fixator pin often can be driven past the intramedullary pin by slight cranial or caudal angling. The pins are placed at the proximal and distal extremities of the bone to be most effective and to avoid placement in the

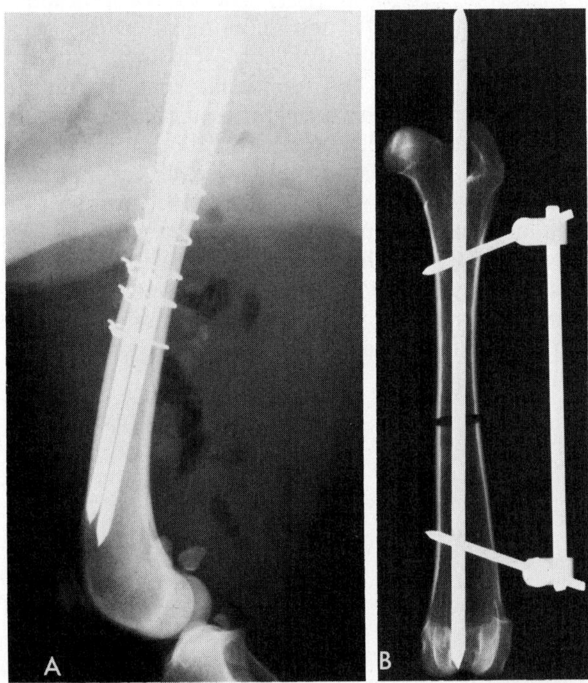

FIGURE 122–8. When instability occurs after single intramedullary pin insertion, additional stability may be achieved with multiple intramedullary pins (*A*) or the addition of a two-pin unilateral external fixator (*B*).

incision.[2] The pins are inserted at an angle of 70° to the long axis of the bone,[2] to prevent the external fixator from being pulled out. It is important to insert the pins in the same axial plane when viewed from the end of the bone.[2] After placement, the pins are connected by a single connecting bar and held securely with two fixator clamps. Before tightening the clamps, final adjustments are made in the fracture alignment and manual compression is applied to the bone. At this time, fracture stability is evaluated. If instability or a cortical defect is noted, more rigid fixation can be achieved by the addition of one or more external fixator pins in each fracture fragment.[21] Regardless of the number of pins, they can usually be connected by a single connecting bar. This can be accomplished by placing the additional clamps on the bar and inserting the additional pins through the clamps and on into the bone. This ensures all four pins are in the same plane (Fig. 122–9). The unilateral external skeletal fixators are useful for providing secondary support to intramedullary pins, especially in upper extremities.

Surgical Anatomy and Landmarks for Pin Placement

Femur

The femoral shaft is exposed from a lateral approach centered over the fracture site.[15] One obvious characteristic of the femur is the firm attachment of the adductor muscle to the caudal cortex. The fibers of this muscle blend with the periosteum and provide an important source of extraosseous blood supply to the healing fracture. Care is taken to avoid stripping this important vascular supply away from the bone. Adductor muscle attachment to any major fragments is left intact to promote rapid incorporation of these fragments. The correct use of a wire passer minimizes the amount of muscle separation required to place cerclage wire around the bone.

Pin insertion in the femur is from the proximal end. The pin is inserted through the skin and underlying soft tissues, sliding along the medial surface of the trochanter major into the trochanteric fossa. At this point, the pin is inserted into the medullary cavity and down to the fracture site (Fig. 122–10). The pin chuck is held in axial alignment with the bone. During retrograde pin insertion, the hip is held in slight extension and the leg is adducted to minimize soft-tissue penetration and avoid the sciatic nerve as the pin emerges from the bone proximally.[13] Normograde pin insertion requires more skill but has the advantages of trapping less soft tissue while avoiding the sciatic nerve and facilitates cutting the pin shorter.[13] A shorter pin minimizes seroma formation and decreases discomfort.

Because of the cranial bowing of the canine femur, the intramedullary pin engages the cranial cortex near the patella. If an attempt is made to seat the pin the remaining distance, the pin may inadvertently enter the stifle joint (Fig. 122–11 *A*). To avoid this, the distal fracture segment is angled slightly cranial to direct the pin caudally in the distal segment. The caudal angulation allows the pin to be seated into the cancellous bone of the femoral condyles (Fig. 122–11*B*). If it is not clear in which direction the pin is traveling, a lateral radiograph is made before final pin seating. A second intramedullary pin alongside the seated pin may give erroneous information, resulting in penetration of the stifle joint. Once the pin has been seated in the distal fragment, it is cut off proximally as short as possible while still allowing retrieval. If the pin is left too long, tissues are traumatized as it moves back and forth during ambulation. The trauma can result in seroma formation over the pin and lead to disuse of the limb during convalescence.

If the animal suddenly stops using the limb and shows

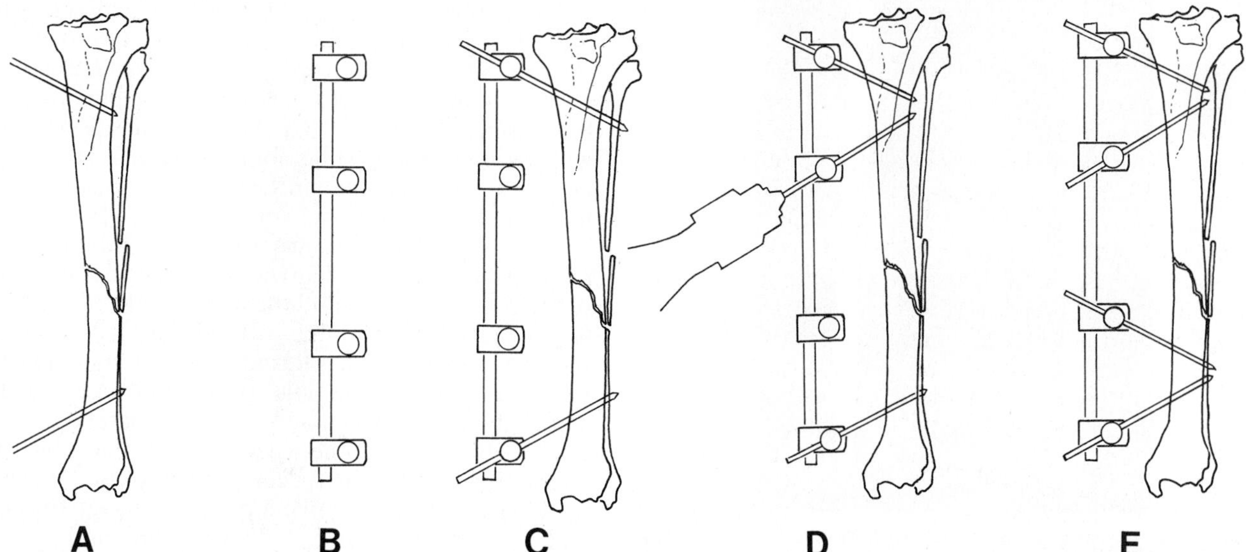

FIGURE 122–9. Four-pin unilateral external fixator. *A*, The proximal and distal pins are inserted first. The connecting bar and single clamps are assembled (*B*) and connected to the pins (*C*). *D*, The third and fourth pins are inserted into the bone, through the clamp holes in the same plane as the first two. *E*, Final adjustments are made in fracture alignment, and the clamps are tightened.

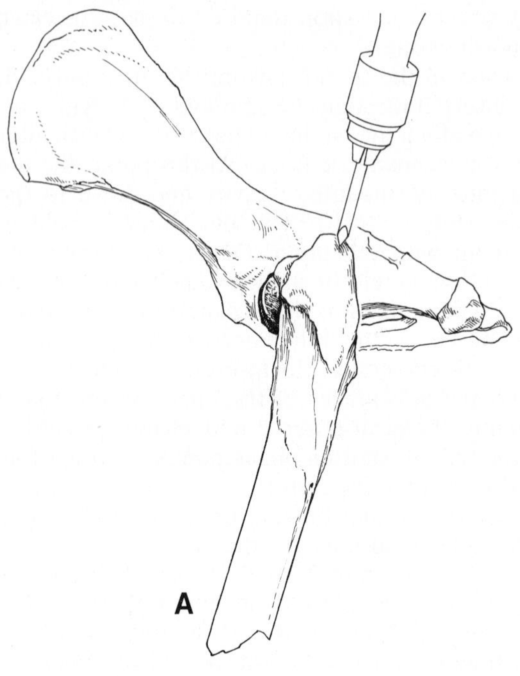

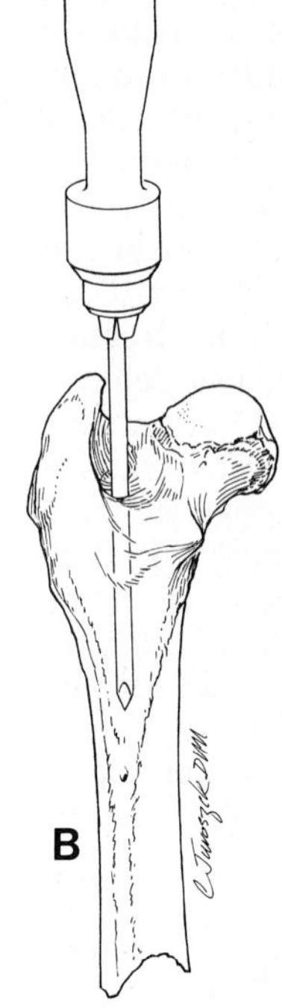

FIGURE 122–10. Normograde pin placement in the femur. *A*, The pin is inserted through the skin and soft tissues to the trochanter major. The pin is then "walked" medially until it slides into the trochanteric fossa. *B*, The pin is inserted into the medullary cavity and aimed down the femoral shaft.

signs of unusual pain or a proprioceptive deficit, entrapment of the sciatic nerve is suspected. During flexion of the hip joint, it is possible for the pin to engage the sciatic nerve. Extreme flexion of the hip is common in cats because of their grooming habits and in dogs as they scratch their ears. This complication may necessitate careful surgical exploration of the area to remove the pin, if possible, or replacement of the nerve to its normal position and shortening of the pin. If exploration of the pin is undertaken for nerve impingement, the leg is prepared for surgery in a normal walking position. A hanging leg preparation may result in additional nerve damage. Entrapment or damage to the sciatic nerve has led to amputation of the limb because of nerve paralysis and self-mutilation.

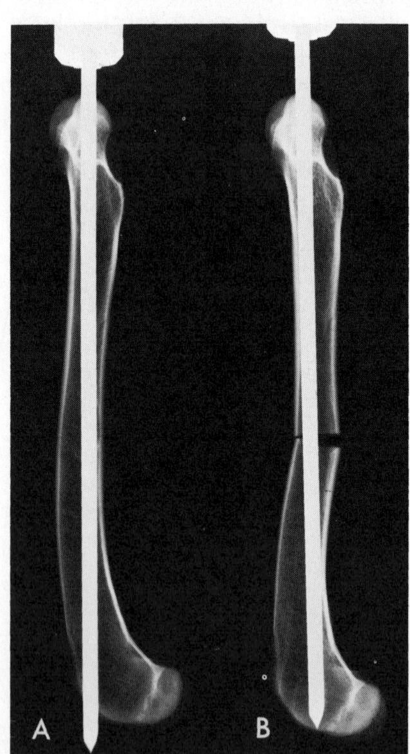

FIGURE 122–11. Pin placement in the distal end of the femoral shaft. *A*, A pin seated in the intact or anatomically reduced femur engages the cranial cortex. *B*, A pin seated in the distal end of the femur following cranial angulation of the distal fracture segment. The pin is directed caudally into the cancellous bone.

Tibia

The entire shaft of the tibia can be exposed from a medial approach.[15] The incision is centered over the fracture site and extended proximally and distally according to the extent of the fracture. The pin must never be passed retrograde from the fracture site because it will emerge in the stifle joint, resulting in extensive destruction of articular cartilage, cruciate ligaments, and menisci, as well as permanent disability (Fig. 122–12). The proper point of pin insertion is on the medial side of the tibial tubercle, halfway between the attachment of the patellar tendon and the cranial edge of the medial femoral condyle (Fig. 122–13). The pin is started with the stifle joint in the flexed position and advanced toward the shaft of the tibia. If the pin is inserted at too acute an angle, it may emerge from the lateral or caudal cortex. Because of the curvature of the tibia, it is necessary for the pin to curve as it passes down the medullary canal. Too large a pin may engage the cortex and leave the bone rather than bending and following the medullary cavity. If a large pin is required, it is helpful to insert a smaller pin first, then remove it and pass the larger pin through the established guide hole.

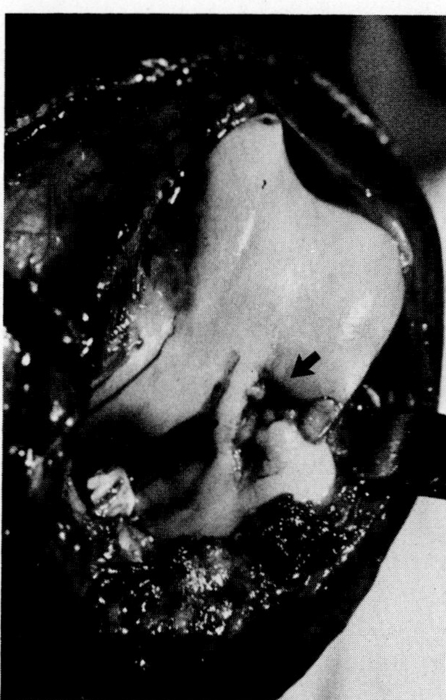

FIGURE 122–12. Damage to the articular cartilage of the femur (*arrow*), resulting from a pin placed retrograde from the fracture site in a tibia. Similar damage can result from not cutting the intramedullary pin short enough.

The base of the medial malleolus is the landmark for distal pin placement. Because the tip of the malleolus protrudes beyond the articular surface of the tibia, it is necessary to measure this distance from the craniocaudal radiograph and use that point as a reference for seating the pin (Figs. 122–14 and 122–15). Once the pin is properly seated, the proximal end is cut off short enough so that its end does not damage the articular cartilage of the femoral condyles during extension of the joint (see Figs. 122–12 and 122–15). One successful method is to seat the pin to the desired point, then retract it 5 to 7 mm and cut it off close to the tibia. At this time, the distal aspect of the limb is held firmly to provide counterpressure while the pin is driven the remaining 5 to 7 mm with a mallet and center punch device (Fig. 122–16). The pin should not be countersunk below the surface of the tibia, or retrieval is difficult.

Unilateral external fixators for secondary fixation are applied to the medial aspect of the bone.[2] The device is well tolerated in this position; it should be wrapped to prevent unnecessary trauma to the opposite limb.

Humerus

The humerus is a difficult bone to approach because of the location and direction of the musculature and the close proximity of major nerves to the surgical site. Careful consideration must be given to selecting the appropriate surgical approach for a fracture of the humerus. The proximal aspect of the shaft is approached through a lateral skin incision.[15] The distal portion of the shaft can be approached either medially or laterally.[15] If it is necessary to extensively reconstruct the condylar region of the humerus, an osteotomy of the olecranon process is performed to expose the intercondylar region of the joint and the caudal surface of the distal aspect of the humerus.[15] The caudal and lateral approaches can be combined to provide access to the

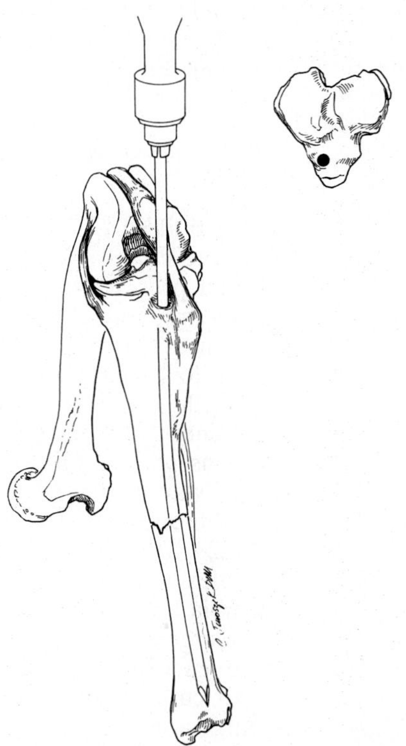

FIGURE 122–13. Normograde pin placement in the tibia. The point of pin insertion in the tibia is on the medial side of the tibial tubercle, halfway between the attachment of the patellar tendon and the cranial edge of the medial femoral condyle.

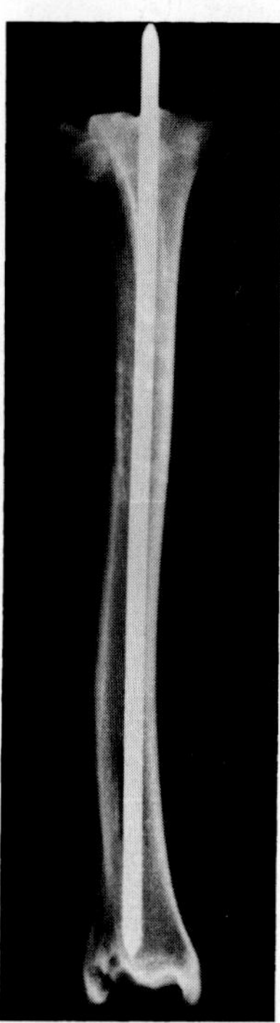

FIGURE 122–14. When the tip of the medial malleolus is used as a guide in final pin placement in the tibia, the distance from the tip of the malleolus to the joint surface must be considered.

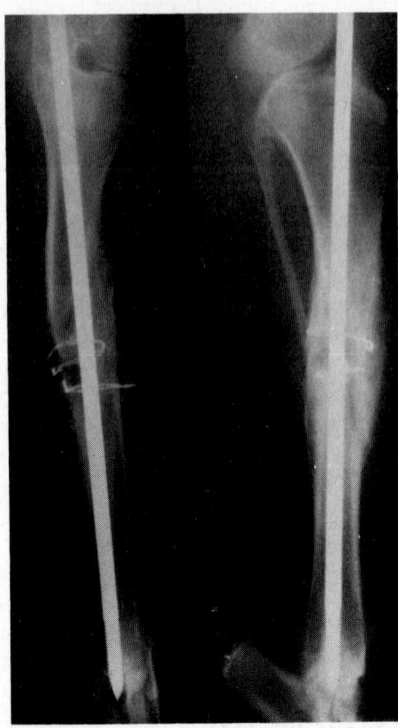

FIGURE 122–15. Intramedullary pin cut too long, resulting in contact of the pin with the femoral condyle (see Fig. 122–12). Notice also that the distal tip of the pin was incorrectly placed; it extends through the joint to the tip of the medial malleolus.

entire humerus for fractures involving multiple sites of the humeral shaft and condyles.

Pins can be inserted into the humerus by either the normograde or the retrograde method. The landmark for normograde insertion is the cranial crest of the proximal aspect of the greater tubercle (Fig. 122–17). If the retrograde method is chosen, care must be taken to avoid entering the shoulder joint. The pin is started at the medial cortex of the proximal fracture segment and aimed laterally as it passes up the medullary cavity. This angle directs the pin toward the greater tubercle and also positions it near the medial cortex at the fracture site. The medial location is advantageous, because the pin must be directed down into the medial aspect of the distal humeral condyle to avoid the elbow joint and gain the best anchorage. The pin is directed medially because the medial portion of the condyle is larger and in direct axial alignment with the shaft (Fig. 122–18*A*). The size of the medullary cavity in the medial portion of the condyle is the limiting factor in selecting pin size. When seating the pin, one must ascertain that the pin is entering the medial condyle, or it will enter the joint instead. It is sometimes helpful to bend the end of the pin slightly medially before inserting it in the distal fragment (see Fig. 122–18*A*). With the tip of the pin bent, the pin is inserted with shorter rotations of the chuck to ensure that the point stays directed medially. The distal fragment may also be angled slightly laterally as the pin is advanced. The pin can be advanced until it just penetrates the distal cortex of the medial condyle. Radiographic confirmation of pin placement requires a craniocaudal view to determine whether it is in the joint or the medial aspect of the condyle.

A unilateral external fixator can be applied to the lateral aspect of the humerus for secondary fixation. If the fracture is in the distal shaft, a three-pin external fixator may be necessary. The distal fixator pin can be placed across the condyles. When only one fixator pin is used in the distal fragment, the stability of this three-pin configuration can be augmented by increasing the size of the distal fixator pin to the diameter of the connecting bar. A double connecting clamp is used to

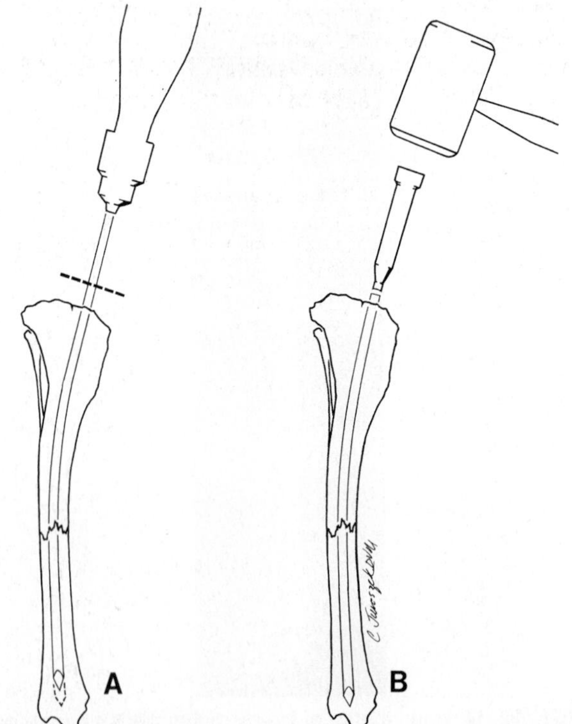

FIGURE 122–16. *A*, The pin is seated to the desired level, retracted, and cut. *B*, The pin is then driven to its previous position.

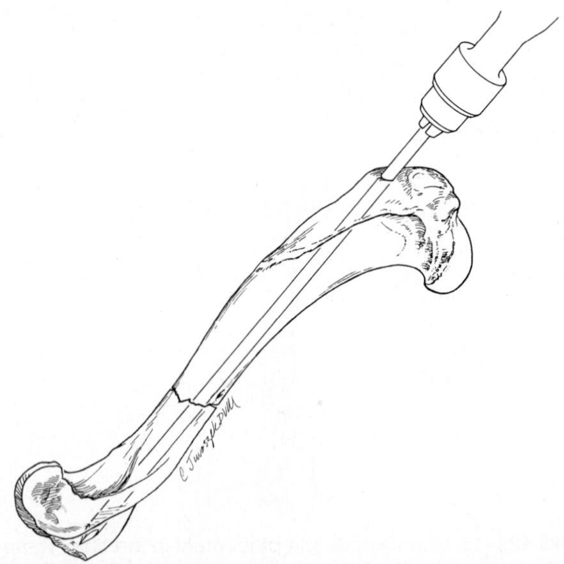

FIGURE 122–17. The landmark for normograde insertion of an intramedullary pin in the humerus is the cranial crest of the proximal aspect of the greater tubercle.

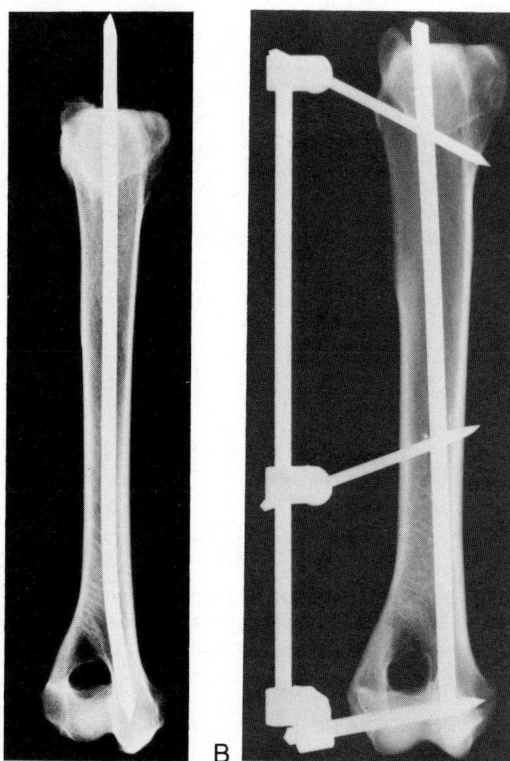

FIGURE 122–18. *A*, The distal pin point is seated into the medial aspect of the humeral condyle. In this example, the end of the pin was curved slightly medially to facilitate placement in the medial condyle. *B*, A three-pin unilateral external fixator using an oversized partially threaded pin and a double connecting clamp distally.

attach the fixator pin to the connecting bar. The transcondylar fixator pin must be placed perpendicular to the bone and is prone to inadvertent removal. Force required for pullout can be increased by predrilling an undersized pilot hole, then threading a partially threaded fixator pin across the condyles (Fig. 122–18*B*). In fractures of the distal portion of the humerus, it is often desirable to insert a cross pin from the lateral epicondyle proximally into the medial cortex of the shaft for additional fixation.

Radius and Ulna

Because of the anatomical configuration of the radius, it is impossible to pass an intramedullary pin retrograde from the fracture site without the pin entering the adjacent joints. A pin can be inserted into the radius with a normograde technique. This specialized pinning method is discussed later along with Rush pinning. Simple fractures of the radius and ulna in small and medium-sized dogs are frequently managed with external casts. Fractures of the distal portion of the radius and ulna in toy breeds are prone to nonunion. Unilateral external fixators are recommended in all but very young animals. If plate fixation is used in these toy breeds, a plate is chosen that is not too stiff. The veterinary cuttable plate* is useful for distal radius fractures in toy breeds. If the plate does not allow loading of the bone, nonunion may result. Oblique and comminuted fractures of the radius in large dogs are best stabilized with bone plates or unilateral or bilateral external fixators rather than with intramedullary pins. It is occasionally necessary to pin the ulna to provide additional support for implants in the radius (Fig. 122–19) or for primary fixation of a fracture involving the articular surface of the trochlear notch. The proximal aspect of the ulna is exposed through a caudal approach, and the distal portion through a caudolateral approach.[15] The pin can be inserted by either a retrograde or a normograde technique. In a normograde technique, the pin is started in the top of the olecranon process, centered over the medullary cavity. As the pin is advanced, the lateral curvature of the proximal aspect of the ulnar shaft must be palpated and the pin aligned accordingly. If this curvature is not accounted for, the pin may exit from the bone medially, just distal to the elbow joint. Before pin insertion, it is necessary to examine a radiograph to determine whether a medullary cavity exists at the fracture site and to choose a pin that fits. Frequently, only small pins are used in the ulna, even in large dogs.

*Synthes USA, Paoli, PA.

Advantages and Disadvantages of Intramedullary Pinning

Pins are less costly to purchase, are less time-consuming to use, require less exposure, and are easier to implant and remove than bone plates. These advantages must be considered along with the disadvantages of less

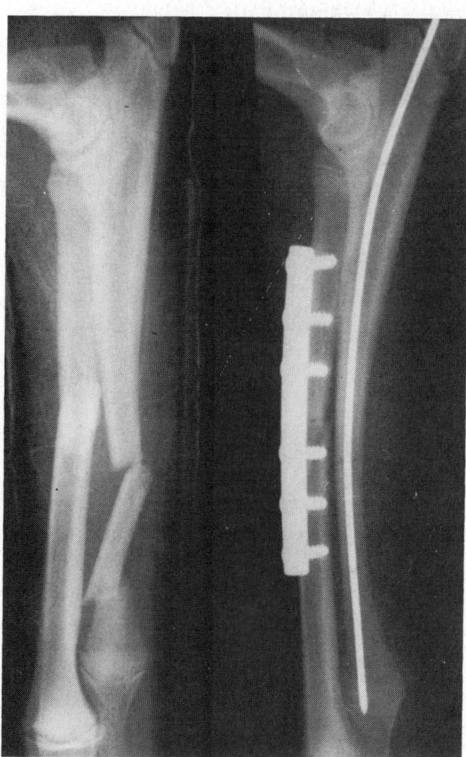

FIGURE 122–19. An intramedullary pin inserted in the ulna to maintain reduction of a segmental ulnar fracture and to provide additional support for the plated radial fracture.

stable fixation, slower return to function, secondary bone union, and more involved aftercare. These are generalizations that do not apply to all individuals or situations. With experience, bone plate application may be as fast as pin fixation, even with a simple fracture. After bone plate fixation, return to function is almost immediate, few follow-up examinations are required, and the chance of a successful outcome is greater.

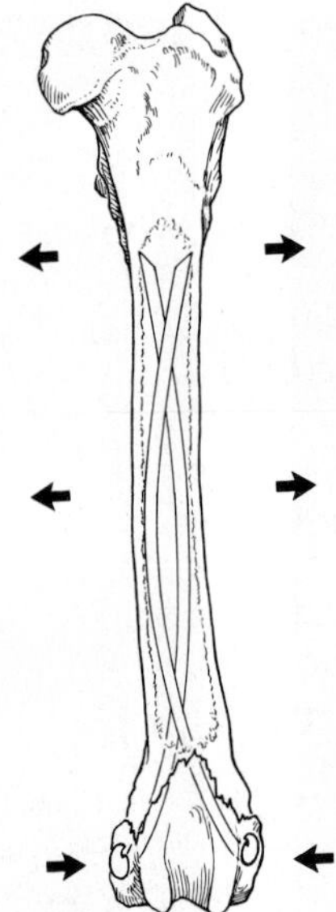

FIGURE 122–20. When properly inserted, Rush pins provide three-point fixation under spring-loaded tension. Arrows show the direction of the tension at the three points of fixation.

Postoperative Management

After surgery, fracture alignment and implant placement are evaluated by two radiographic views. Examination of postoperative radiographs not only allows assessment of the surgery but also provides documentation of implant positioning and fracture alignment for comparison with follow-up radiographs during the healing phase.

In many cases, a compression bandage may be beneficial to reduce or prevent swelling immediately after surgery. It is usually removed before discharge. Most animals with uncomplicated fractures can be discharged 1 to 2 days after surgery. At discharge, it is beneficial to provide the client with written instructions outlining the convalescent period. These notes should include instructions for medications, diet, bandage care, exercise restrictions, and dates for follow-up examinations. The client is told to restrict the animal's activity to leash exercise only until further instructed. It is advisable to prevent small dogs from jumping from furniture. The client may need to purchase a cage or to confine the animal to an appropriate room when it is alone or at night. Regardless of size, it is best to avoid stairs unless the animal is restrained with a leash.

After intramedullary pinning and external fixator application, the animal is rechecked in 10 to 14 days for suture removal. At this time, the limb is evaluated for return of function, and joints adjacent to the fractured bone are assessed for range of motion. The point where the pin emerges from the bone is examined for swelling or evidence of pin migration. If physical examination fails to reveal any problems, radiographic evaluation is unnecessary. The external fixator is examined for broken or bent pins and for skin irritation resulting from improper positioning of the connecting clamps.

Implants are removed at 3 to 4 weeks after surgery in a puppy and at 6 to 16 weeks in an adult. Implant removal is based on function, palpation of the fracture site, and radiographic confirmation of bone union. External fixators are removed 2 to 4 weeks after surgery, depending on the age of animal and the type of fracture. Removal can be done without anesthesia or tranquilization if the connecting bar is removed and each pin is pulled out in the same plane in which it was inserted. Removal of the intramedullary pin usually requires anesthesia. This also allows careful palpation of the fracture site before and after pin removal.

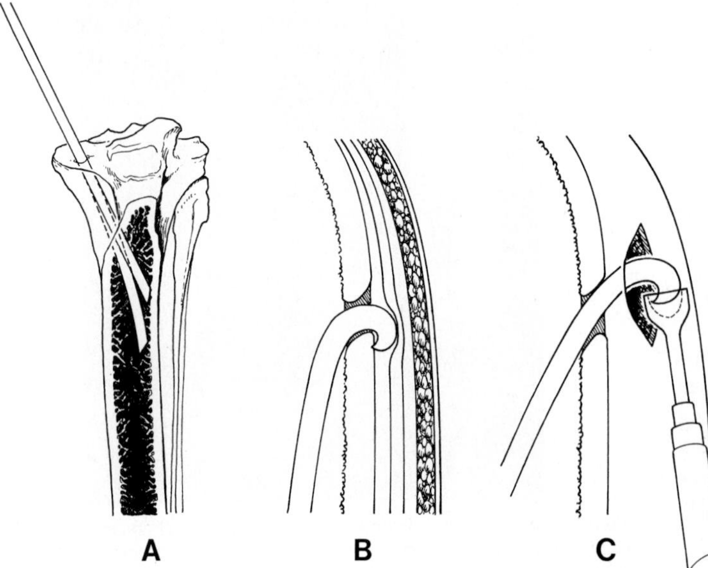

FIGURE 122–21. *A*, The point of the Rush pin is beveled to allow it to slide along the inner cortex with less chance of penetration. *B*, The opposite end of the pin is hooked to engage the cortex (*B*) and facilitate removal (*C*).

THEORY AND TECHNIQUE OF RUSH PINNING

Equipment

Rush pins are designed to be driven into bone to provide three-point fixation under spring-loaded tension (Fig. 122–20).[17, 25] The point of a Rush pin has a single bevel, which allows it to be deflected off the far cortex and to slide along the inner cortical surface (Fig. 122–21*A*). The opposite end of the pin is hooked to grasp the outer cortex, preventing migration into the bone and facilitating removal (Fig. 122–21*B* and *C*). The pins are available in four different diameters: 3/32 inch, 1/8 inch, 3/16 inch, and 1/4 inch. Each pin diameter is supplied in several different lengths. Equipment required for insertion includes an awl to start a guide hole, a driver-extractor, and a mallet (Fig. 122–22). Smaller pins can be made from Steinmann pins or Kirschner wires with chisel points. The Steinmann pin is bent until a tight loop is formed at the required length, and one arm of the pin is cut off close to the loop so a hook is formed (Fig. 122–23).[6]

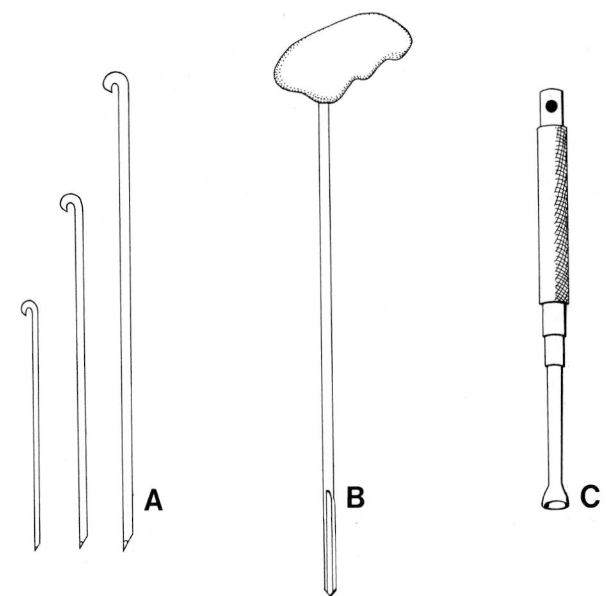

FIGURE 122–22. *A*, Three sizes of Rush pins. *B*, The large awl used to start a guide hole. *C*, The driver-extractor tool.

Principles and Technique of Application

Rush pinning technique is restricted to fractures in the metaphyseal regions of bones. The pins are inserted into the metaphysis at an acute angle, passing obliquely through the cancellous bone and into the medullary cavity, to the fracture site. Because the flat point of a Rush pin does not cut well through cortical bone, a guide hole is made with an awl reamer or a Steinmann pin of the same diameter. The angle of insertion of the pin is critical to avoid penetrating the opposite cortex and to provide adequate spring-loaded tension. Rush pins are inserted at a 30° angle to the axial plane of the bone for optimum results (Fig. 122–24*A*). The angle should not be greater than 40°, because penetration of the opposite cortex may occur. If the angle is less than 20° spring-loaded tension is inadequate.

In most cases, two pins are used, one started on each side of the smaller fragment. After both pins are started, the fracture is held in reduction while the pins are alternately driven into the large fracture segment (Fig. 122–24*B*). Pins are driven across the fracture site, glance off the opposite cortex, and cross back toward the near cortex. It is helpful to bend the pins into a slight curve before insertion; called "prestressing," this helps prevent penetration of the opposite cortex. The end result is three-point fixation of the bone under spring-loaded tension without complete filling of the medullary cavity. To ensure spring-loaded tension, the shape of the bone must be considered when prebending the pin. The shape of the bone in relationship to the pin determines whether the pin acts merely as an intramedullary pin or as a dynamic Rush pin with three-point fixation (Fig. 122–25). This technique, when properly applied, is effective in resisting major fracture forces. Rush pins do not sufficiently counteract these forces if applied to a diaphyseal fracture.

Indications for Use

Fractures most commonly repaired with this technique are transverse fractures of the proximal humeral, prox-

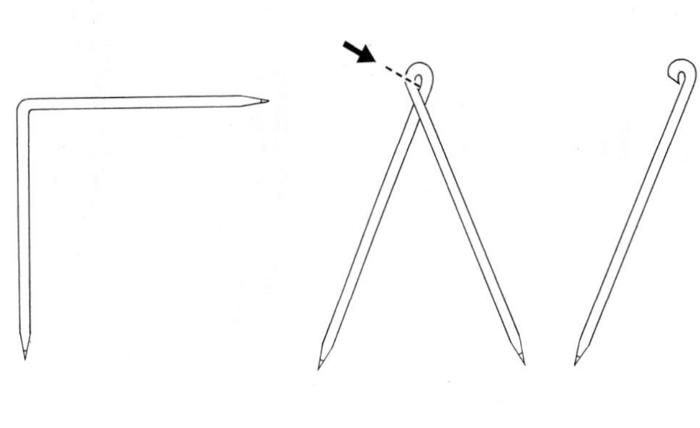

FIGURE 122–23. A Rush pin can be made from a chisel-pointed Steinmann pin by forming a tight loop at the desired length. One arm of the pin is then cut off close to the loop so a hook is formed.

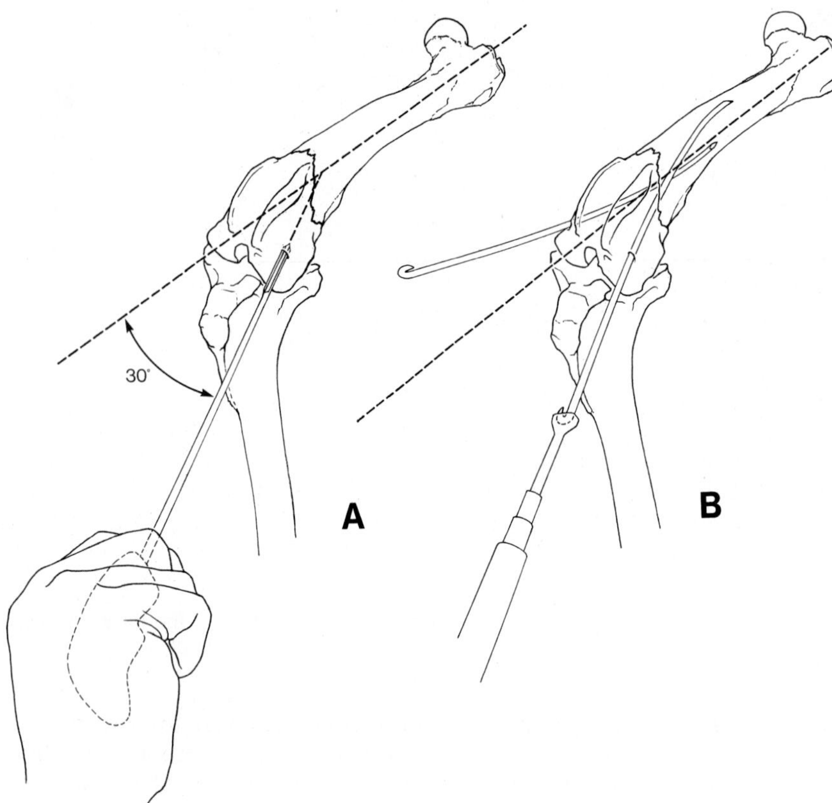

FIGURE 122–24. *A*, The appropriate size awl is used to start the guide hole at a 30° angle to the long axis of the bone. *B*, Once both pins have been started, they are alternately driven into the opposite fracture segment with the aid of the driver-extractor tool and a mallet.

imal tibial, and distal femoral metaphyses. Modifications of the Rush technique are frequently used to repair fractures in the metaphysis and diaphysis of metacarpal and metatarsal bones, as well as the radius. In these instances, the only similarity to the Rush technique often is the method of pin insertion. Because these bones have articular cartilage surfaces on both ends and no convenient prominences for pin insertion, the Rush method of pinning is the only acceptable means of gaining access to the medullary canal. Use in these cases may require external coaptation to partially neutralize the forces acting at the fracture site.

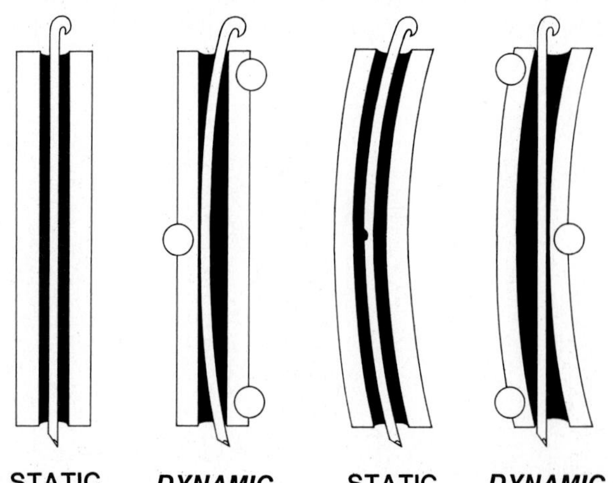

FIGURE 122–25. The shape of the bone in relation to the pin determines whether the pin merely acts as a static intramedullary pin or as a dynamic Rush pin.

When Rush pins are used to repair epiphyseal fractures in growing animals, premature closure of the growth plate may occur. Experimental use of Rush pins across the distal femoral epiphysis in normal puppies with no fracture resulted in premature closure and significant shortening of the limb if the pins were not removed. If the pins were removed 4 weeks after implantation, growth retardation did not occur.[19] Pins can be removed at 1 month, because these fractures heal rapidly.

Postoperative Management

Management after Rush pinning is the same as for intramedullary pinning. Because of the close proximity of metaphyseal fractures to the joint, it is advantageous to encourage early use of the limb to minimize joint stiffness. Pressure bandages are not used for longer than 1 or 2 days, especially with epiphyseal fractures in young growing animals. The tremendous healing response in these animals often results in fibrous adhesions of the adjacent soft tissues, leading to a stiff joint, which can be a serious and debilitating complication. If the stifle joint of a growing animal becomes locked in hyperextension, the animal is unable to advance the limb and bear weight; therefore, self-rehabilitation does not occur (see Fig. 122–2).

THEORY AND TECHNIQUE OF BONE PLATING

The primary objective in fracture treatment is to return the injured limb to full function. Fracture disease is avoided through early active limb use, made possible by stable internal fixation without coaptation. A complete understanding of fracture forces is necessary to counteract these forces properly with bone plates and screws. A properly applied bone plate counteracts bending, rotational, and shearing forces and apposes fragments.

Specialized training and equipment are required to apply bone plates properly. A complete set of instruments, a full range of implants, and knowledge of their use are necessary before fracture repair is attempted. A less than thorough understanding of bone plating principles and techniques or a lack of equipment usually results in an unfavorable outcome of fracture repair. A plate may be used on any fracture when there is enough bone length on each side of the fracture site to adequately attach the plate. The ASIF* system is used to illustrate the principles, but the same principles can be applied to any plating system.

Interfragmentary Compression

Compression was initially thought to stimulate bone healing, because compressed fractures healed without visible callus.[11, 23] Compression, however, has no osteogenic properties. Compression of fractures increases fracture stability through frictional impact loading and narrowing the gap between fragments, providing optimum conditions for direct bone union.[1, 24] One of the features of bone healing under compression is that the removal of necrotic bone and the laying down of new bone can take place simultaneously and within a few cells distance of each other.[24] There is no net resorption of bone in this type of bone healing.[24]

Fracture compression can be achieved through interfragmentary compression with lag screws or axial compression with a plate. Interfragmentary compression can be accomplished with either cortical or cancellous bone screws, although a screw has a lag effect only when it gains purchase in the far cortex and not in the cortex adjacent to the screw head. Because the cortical screw is fully threaded, the hole near the screw head must be overdrilled so the threads will not engage the near cortex. The overdrilled hole is called the *glide hole*, and the hole in the far cortex is called the *thread hole*. If a cortical screw is used as a lag screw and a glide hole is not created in the near cortex, the screw threads maintain the fracture gap and compression does not occur (Fig. 122–26). The cortical screw can be easily removed from cortical bone after fracture healing because it is fully threaded.[1]

Cancellous screws have relatively thin core diameters and wide threads. They are available as either partially threaded screws, having a nonthreaded portion near the head and threads near the tip, or as fully threaded screws. The partially threaded screws are supplied with two different thread lengths (Fig. 122–27). The cancellous screw is used in soft cancellous bone of the metaphysis and epiphysis. The bone in these areas has a thin cortical shell unlike the thicker cortex of diaphyseal bone. If cancellous screws are used in diaphyseal bone, they usually cannot be removed because cortical bone grows right up to the threadless shaft of the screw. If removal is attempted, the threads cannot cut a path through the threadless cortex, and the excessive torque generated may break the screw. To achieve interfragmentary compression with a cancellous screw, it is important that only the smooth shank be within the near fragment and that the entire threaded portion be within the far fragment (Fig. 122–28). If threads are present on both sides of the fracture, the threads maintain the fracture gap and compression cannot occur.[1, 18] Unlike cortical screws, cancellous screws in cancellous bone do not require tapping for the entire length of the hole. Only the first few millimeters of the hole are tapped to facilitate starting the screw. As the screw is advanced into the cancellous bone, the trabeculae are tightly compressed, resulting in greater holding power.[1]

*Association for the Study of Internal Fixation, Synthes Ltd. (USA), Wayne, PA.

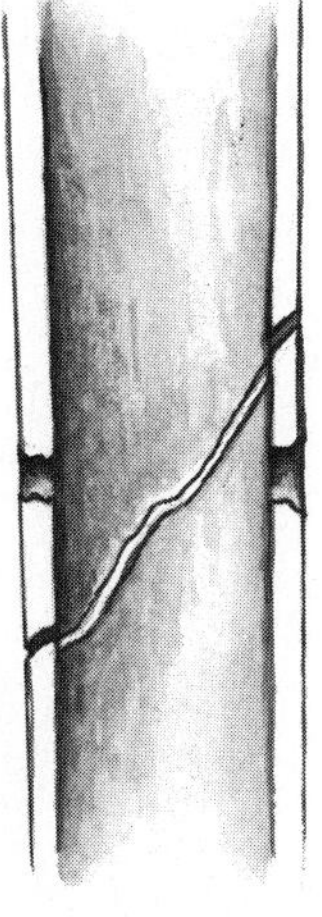

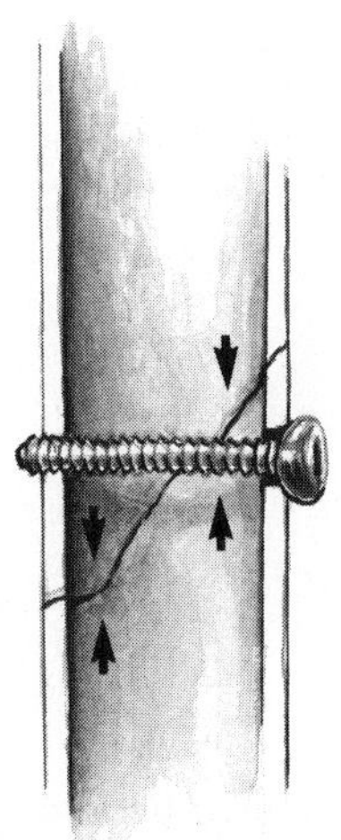

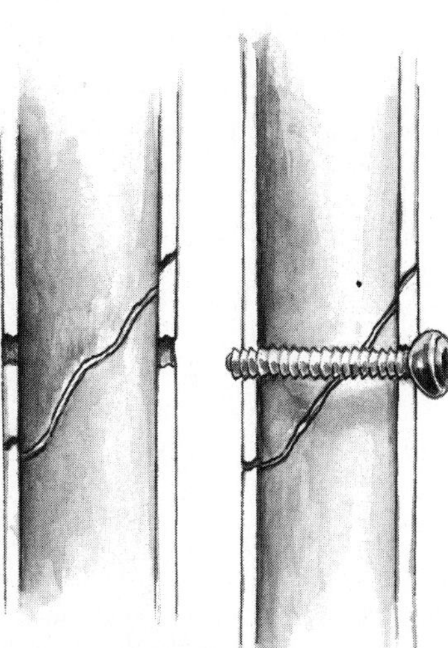

CORRECT
A

INCORRECT
B

FIGURE 122–26. *A*, Compression of two fragments with a screw can occur only when the hole in the cortex adjacent to the screw head is at least as large as the outer diameter of the thread. This hole is called the *glide hole*. The thread glides through this hole and engages only the opposite cortex in the thread hole. When the screw head contacts the cortex, interfragmentary compression is achieved. *B*, The screw cannot compress if both cortices are drilled and tapped, because the screw threads maintain the fracture gap. Either the bone or screw will break before there is the slightest approximation of the fragments.

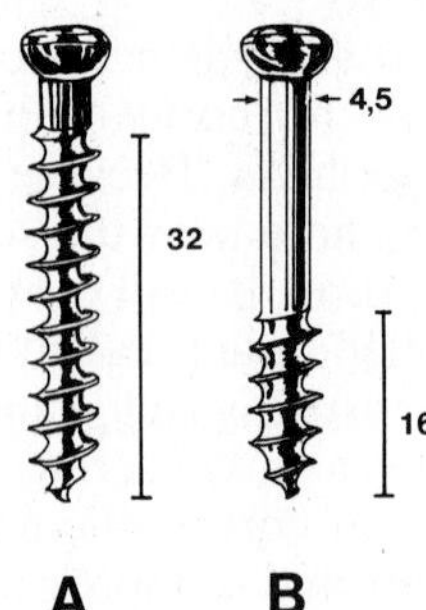

FIGURE 122–27. Two 6.5-mm ASIF cancellous screws with a 4.5-mm shaft. *A*, 32-mm thread. *B*, 16-mm thread.

To achieve evenly distributed interfragmentary compression, the screw is centered in the middle of both fragments (Fig. 122–29). If the screws are placed eccentrically, they produce shear instead of pure compression, resulting in loss of reduction (Fig. 122–30). To achieve interfragmentary compression of a butterfly fragment, the screw is inserted to bisect the angle subtended between a line perpendicular to the long axis of the bone and one perpendicular to the fracture plane (Fig. 122–31).[1, 2] Because lag screws are ineffective in neutralizing fracture forces, they are rarely used as the sole means of fixation in diaphyseal fractures. The primary function of a lag screw is to provide fragment apposition through interfragmentary compression. The resulting fracture alignment and stability must be protected against the forces acting on the fracture with a bone plate. Such a plate is called a *neutralization plate*.

Screws are available with either self-tapping threads or non–self-tapping threads. It was thought that self-tapping screws provided poor holding power because their insertion caused bone necrosis, resulting in the screw's being embedded in fibrous tissue rather than bone. This is incorrect. The advantage of the non–self-tapping screw does not lie in its greater holding power but in the ease and precision with which it can be inserted into bone.[18]

Principles of Bone Plate Application

Bone plates are available in various sizes and shapes for different fractures. Selection is based on many factors, including the size of animal, bone involved, degree of comminution, presence of fissures, and location of the fracture within the bone. Plates should be large enough to neutralize the forces acting at the fracture site but not too stiff for the bone. If the plate is too stiff, complications may occur. The fracture may not heal, or union may be delayed. A new fracture may occur at the junction of the plate and the more elastic bone. The bone may atrophy because the plate prevents the normal physiological stress necessary for maintaining normal bone composition. General guidelines have been

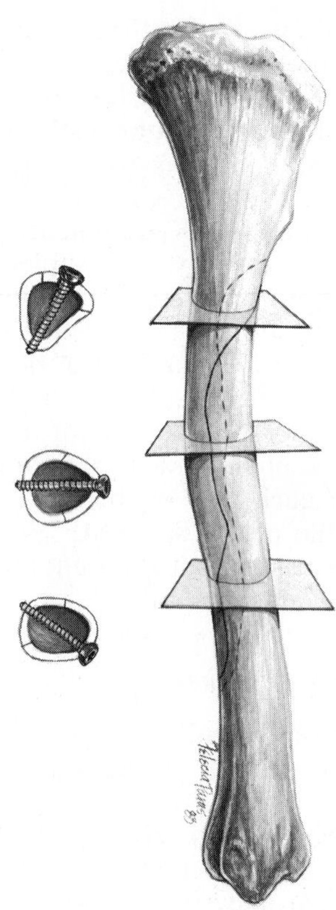

FIGURE 122–29. The orientation of lag screws used to compress an oblique fracture is shown. *Cross sections*, ideally, the screws are placed through the middle of both fragments to achieve maximal compression.

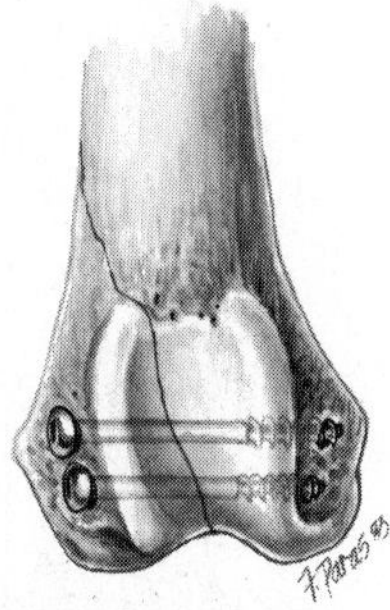

FIGURE 122–28. Interfragmentary compression has been achieved with two cancellous screws. Note that the threads are present in the far fragment only. Compression will not occur if the threads are present on both sides of the fracture line. Washers may be necessary in young animals to prevent the screw head from sinking into soft cancellous bone.

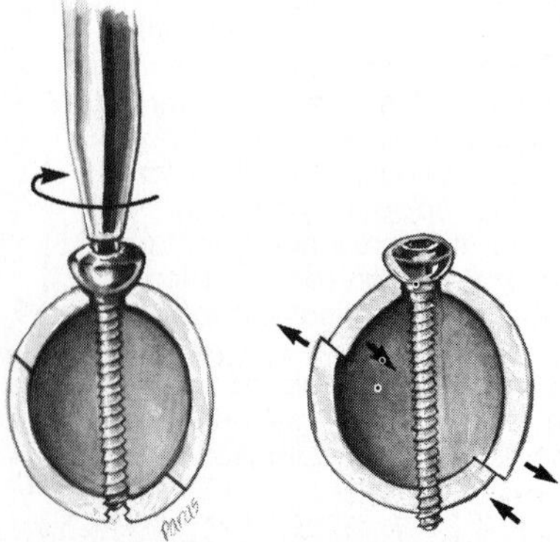

FIGURE 122–30. The effect of an eccentrically placed screw is shown. As the screw is tightened, it produces shear instead of pure compression, resulting in loss of reduction.

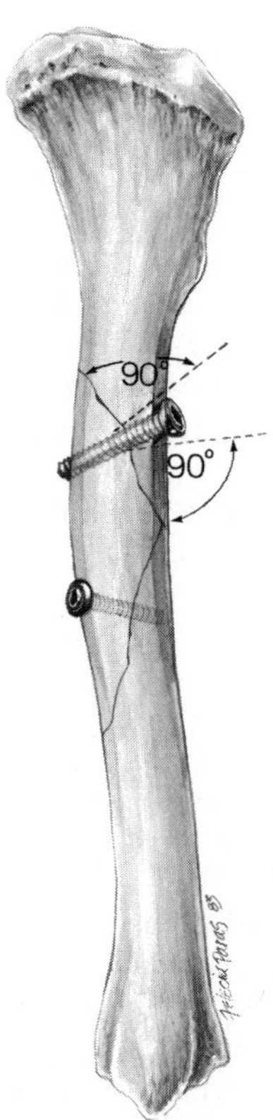

FIGURE 122–31. Lag fixation of a single butterfly fragment is shown. The screws have been inserted in such a way that they bisect the angle subtended by the perpendiculars dropped to the fracture plane and to the long axis of the bone.

suggested for selecting the proper size bone plate on the basis of an animal's weight.[2]

There are three types of plates: straight, special, and angled. Straight plates are used for the diaphysis, special plates for the epiphysis and metaphysis, and angled plates for the proximal and distal regions of the femur.[1] Straight plates are the most commonly used plates in veterinary surgery because they can be contoured easily and used in most areas. In the AO system, plates are available in 2.0-mm, 2.7-mm, 3.5-mm, and 4.5-mm sizes, denoting the screw size used with each plate. The 3.5-mm and 4.5-mm plates are available in narrow and broad widths. Most straight plates are available with oval holes only. Tubular plates are a specialized type of straight plate available in 2.7-mm, 3.5-mm, and 4.5-mm sizes, with oval holes.

The dynamic compression plate is an improvement over the original round-hole plate. The special geometry of its oval screw holes has increased the potential uses of the plate. The dynamic compression plate does not require a tension device for axial compression and can be used to compress fractures without additional surgical exposure. Compression is achieved through eccentric placement of the screws in the oval holes of the plate. Because of the sloping design of the screw holes, the plate moves as the screw head is seated. Movement of the plate results in axial compression. Drilling of the eccentric holes is done with the aid of a special drill guide, called a *load guide*. When compression is not desired, a neutral load guide is used. It is also possible to angle screws in any direction through the oval holes.[1] These two features of the dynamic compression plate make it a more versatile and popular implant than the original round-hole plate.

Semitubular plates can be used as self-compressing plates, but they are only 1 mm thick and easily deformable. Because they are so easily deformable, they should be used as tension band plates when the only deforming forces are those of tension. The advantage of tubular plates is their ability to provide rotational stability by close adaptation to bone and by digging their edges into the bone. Their disadvantage is that the screw heads protrude deeply through the screw holes and may shatter the underlying cortex. The stability of tubular plates is considerably greater than that of other straight plates of equal thickness. The eccentric placement of screws in the oval holes accounts for the self-compressing properties of the plate.[1] The major indication for tubular plates is for fractures of the radius and ulna. However, regular straight plates function equally well.

A plate's ability to provide rigid fixation is directly proportional to its distance from the fulcrum of the bending moment.[1] At least six cortices should be firmly engaged by screws on either side of the fracture.[1, 18] Deviation from this rule may be necessary, depending on the location of the fracture, because the bone might not be long enough beyond the fracture to engage six cortices. More screws may be placed on each side of the fracture if the animal is normally active and the ability of the owner to confine the animal postoperatively is uncertain.

Screws in a fracture or fissure line may result in distraction of fragments, worsening of the fissure, or stripping of the screw threads, necessitating screw removal. Placing a short screw through only one cortex or leaving a screw hole empty may be necessary to avoid this problem (Figs. 122–32 and 122–38).

Plates are contoured to the original shape and curvature of the particular bone. They must be bent and twisted to fit the bone properly, requiring a bending press or bending irons. A radiograph of the normal opposite limb is useful as a template for contouring the plate. Malleable templates that can be easily bent and twisted with the fingers are available to facilitate contouring the plate (Fig. 122–33).[1, 2] An improperly contoured plate causes loss of fracture alignment when it is applied to the bone.

A plate can serve various functions, depending on the manner in which it is used. It may act as a tension band plate if it is placed on the tension side of a weightbearing bone such as the lateral femur. It may act as a neutralization plate if it is used to protect a comminuted area that has been reconstructed with lag screws. It may also function as a buttress plate if it is used to bridge a diaphyseal defect.[1, 2] With a tension band, tensile forces are counteracted and converted into compressive forces. Every eccentrically loaded bone is subjected to bending stresses, resulting in a distribution of stresses with tension on the convex and compression on the concave side of the bone (Fig. 122–34). To restore the load-bearing capacity of an eccentrically loaded bone, tensile forces must be absorbed by the tension band (plate), and the

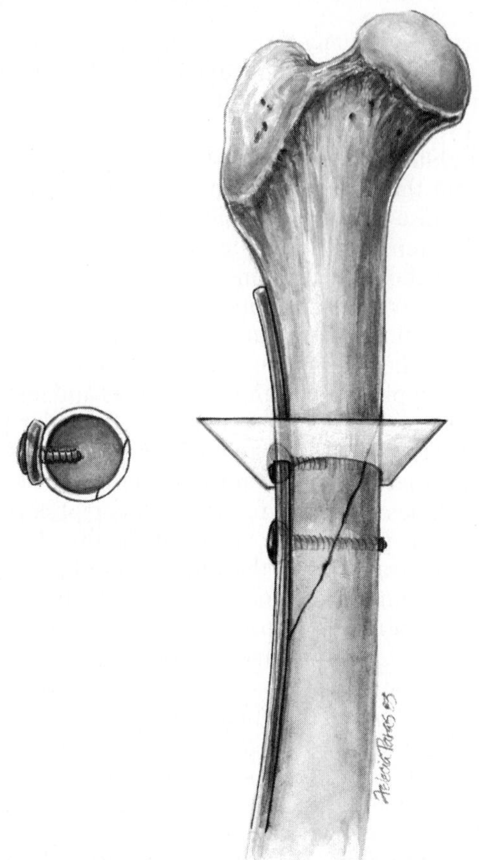

FIGURE 122–32. A short screw through the plate is used to prevent the screw from entering the fracture line.

bone itself must be able to withstand axial compression. Plates used as tension bands are intended to convert tensile forces of eccentrically loaded bones, such as the femur, into compressive forces (Fig. 122–35*A*). If a plate is placed on a side of the bone where compressive forces predominate, it cannot act as a tension band to stabilize the fracture. The plate may be unable to withstand or counteract the bending forces on the compression side of the bone, fatigue under cyclic loading, and break (Fig. 122–35*B*). If a plate is applied to the lateral side of the femur and a portion of the medial cortex is absent, the requirements of the tension band plate have not been met because the bone cannot absorb compression.[1]

In vivo strain analysis indicates that the tension band side of the femur or tibia is craniolateral and that of the humerus is craniomedial; plates are not always applied to these areas.[1, 19] The tension band side of weightbearing bones may change, depending on the phase of stride. The tension band side of a fractured bone (e.g., humerus) may vary, depending on the location of the fracture within the bone. These factors, as well as the difficulty of the surgical approach, are considered when deciding where the plate is to be applied to the bone. Plates are usually applied to the medial aspect of the tibia, because the lateral approach is more difficult. The femur is usually plated on the lateral side rather than on the craniolateral aspect so that the plate will not interfere with gliding of the quadriceps muscle. The humerus may be plated caudally, medially, cranially, or laterally, depending on the fracture location and the surgeon's preference. The radius is usually plated cranially, and the proximal aspect of the ulna may be plated caudally, laterally, or medially. When the true tension side of a bone is not plated, stability relies heavily on the inherent strength of the plate to overcome the forces caused by axial loading.

Tension band plates are usually used to repair transverse or short oblique two-piece fractures and nonunited fractures. Theoretically, a plate applied to a bone on its tension side acts as a tension band when tension is applied during weightbearing. The tension in the plate results in axial compression of the bone. To maintain axial compression during periods of rest as well as activity, the plate must be prebent so that after it is applied, it is under tension.[1] If a straight plate is applied to a straight bone, a gap occurs in the opposite cortex as tension is applied to the plate. To overcome this, the plate must be prebent or contoured to a slight convexity at the fracture site. When a contoured plate is applied, the opposite cortices come in contact and a slight gap occurs in the cortices under the plate. As axial compression is generated by applying tension to the plate, the cortices under the plate come in contact and compressive forces are evenly distributed across the entire fracture surface (Fig. 122–36). A similar effect is obtained when a plate is applied to a concave bone such as the femur (Fig. 122–37).[1, 24]

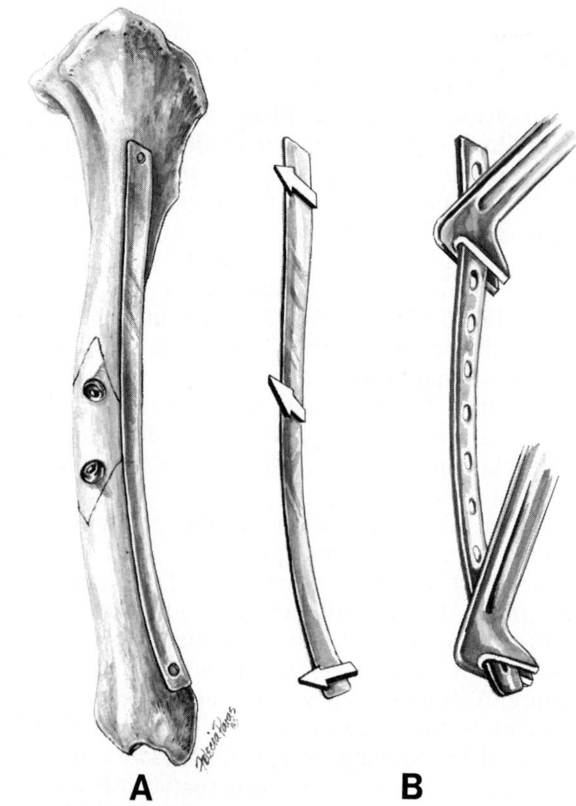

FIGURE 122–33. *A*, After reduction and lag screw fixation of the fracture, a malleable template is contoured to the shape of the bone. *B*, The contoured malleable plate serves as a template for contouring the bone plate.

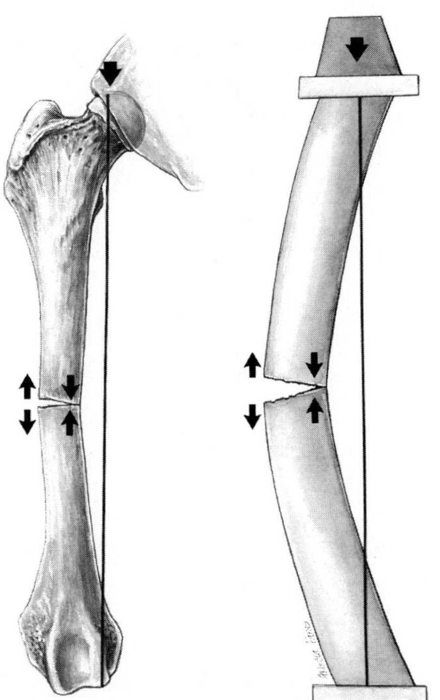

FIGURE 122–34. Long bones are subjected to eccentric loading. The femur, for example, can be compared to a bent column. As the load is applied, tension on the convex side and compression on the concave side of the column result.

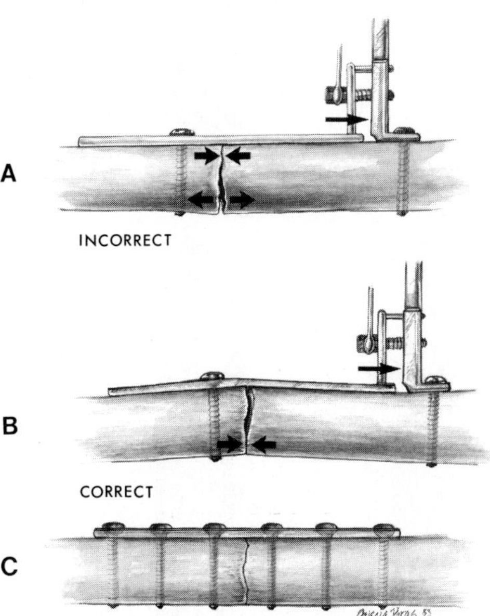

FIGURE 122–36. *A*, The result of applying a straight plate to a straight bone. As tension is applied to the plate, a gap forms in the cortices opposite the plate. *B*, As the prebent plate is applied to the bone, the opposite cortices come in contact, and a slight gap develops in the cortices under the plate. *C*, As the remaining screws are inserted and tension is applied to the plate, the cortices under the plate come in contact, and the compressive force is evenly distributed across the entire fracture surface.

Neutralization plates are used to stabilize comminuted fractures in which the butterfly fragments have been reconstructed with lag screws. Screw fixation alone provides poor resistance to shearing forces from axial loading or weightbearing, necessitating protection of the comminuted area with a plate. This is by far the most common function of plates. Because such a plate neutralizes bending, rotational, and shearing forces that are acting on the fracture, it is called a *neutralization plate*. First, the comminuted fracture is reduced and fixed with lag screws, and then a carefully contoured plate is applied to the two main fragments (Fig. 122–38). When a plate is applied as a neutralization plate, it must be

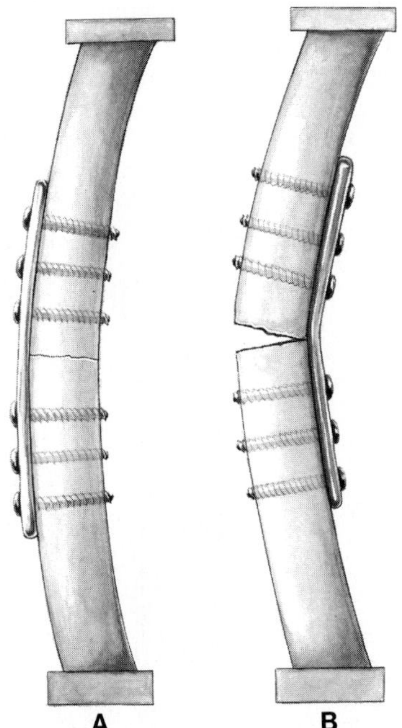

FIGURE 122–35. *A*, The result of a plate applied to the convex side of the column. The plate converts the tensile forces into compressive forces. *B*, The result of a plate applied to the concave side of the column. The plate cannot convert the tensile forces but is subject to bending forces and would soon fatigue and break.

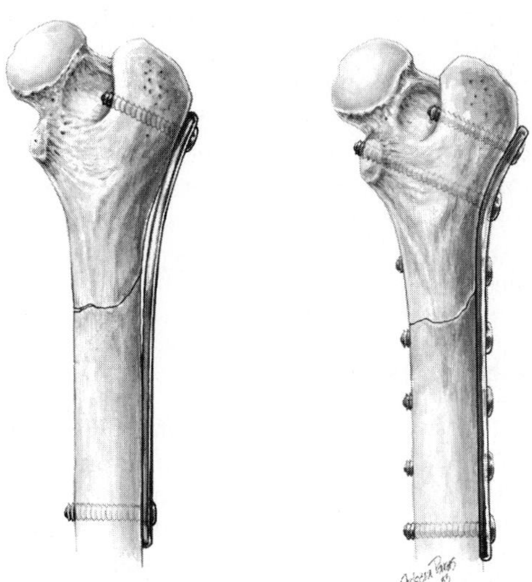

FIGURE 122–37. The effect of applying a straight plate to a concave bone. Although the plate has been contoured, it is straighter than the underlying cortex, and a 1- to 2-mm gap remains between the plate and the bone at the fracture. Application of the plate results in compression of the opposite cortex.

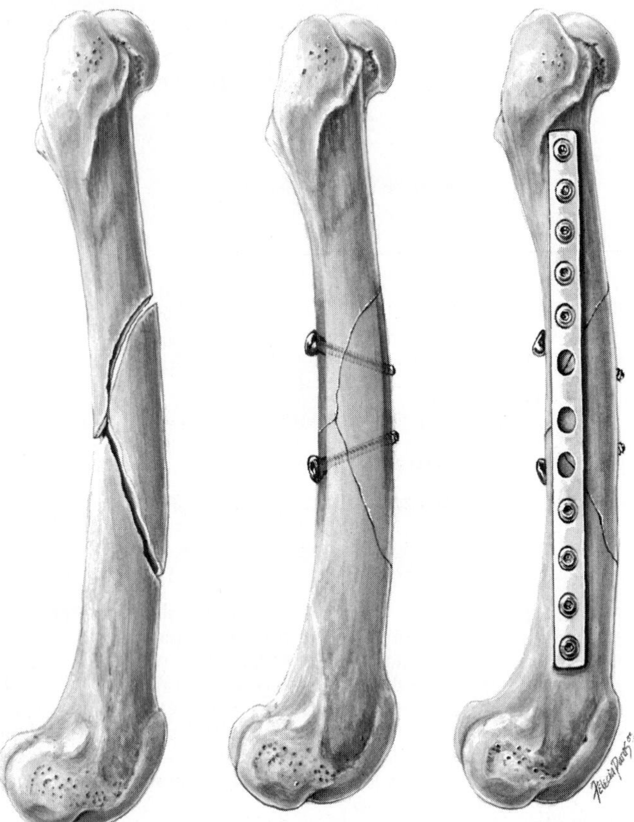

FIGURE 122–38. The use of a neutralization plate to protect the lag screw fixation of a comminuted area. The fracture is first reduced and stabilized with lag screws, and the plate is then applied to the two main fragments. Note that three screw holes have been left empty to keep screws from entering fracture lines.

prebent to prevent gaps from forming in the cortices opposite the plate. Lag screws can be inserted through the plate when necessary.[1, 18] Even in short oblique fractures, one oblique lag screw is inserted through the plate to increase stability (Fig. 122–39).[1]

In animals, a buttress plate is primarily used to bridge a diaphyseal defect filled with cancellous bone graft while the graft is being incorporated (Fig. 122–40).[1] The plate must be carefully adapted to the shape of the bone because it is functionally designed to distract and support, not to compress. Its function is to prevent the fracture from collapsing until the diaphyseal defect can be filled with new bone. A buttress plate is never applied under tension.[1]

Postoperative Treatment

Achieving stable internal fixation is only one aspect of fracture management. The postoperative and convalescent care is important to allow healing of the fracture before failure of the implant and to promote early function of the injured limb. After stable fracture fixation with a bone plate, the affected limb can be placed in a light support wrap, which helps prevent postoperative swelling and reduce any swelling present before the fracture repair. Prevention of postoperative swelling is beneficial in promoting early use of the limb. The

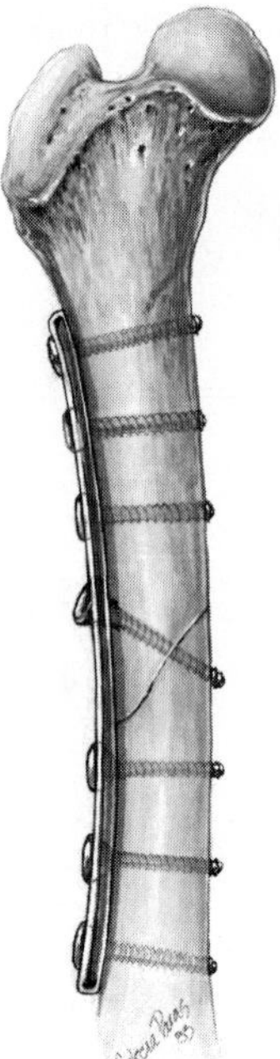

FIGURE 122–39. A lag screw inserted obliquely across a short oblique fracture. This procedure increases stability by creating interfragmentary compression.

animal is encouraged to use the limb as soon as possible to maintain muscle tone and gliding function of muscles and tendons and to prevent fibrous adhesions from forming, thus preventing fracture disease. The early postoperative period must be closely supervised to prevent excessive activity that may result in implant failure.

Clients are advised how to care for convalescing pets properly. An animal's activity must be restricted until the fracture has healed. The owner must be made aware that the animal should begin using the affected limb normally long before the fracture has completely healed.

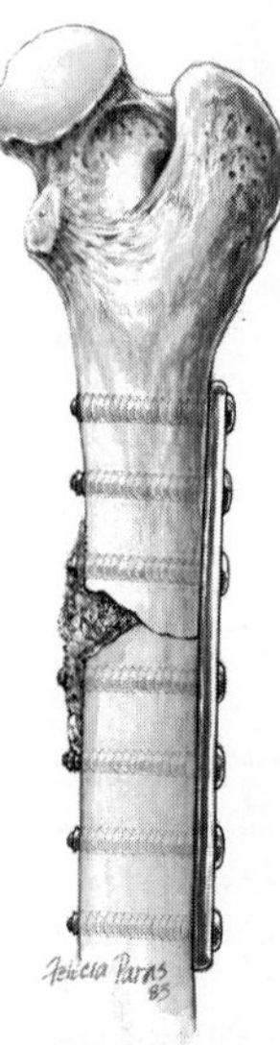

FIGURE 122–40. The use of a buttress plate to bridge a diaphyseal defect filled with cancellous bone graft. The function of the buttress plate is to support the bone fragments until the graft can be incorporated into the fracture.

Unsupervised activity during this period may result in implant failure. The animal is periodically returned to the hospital for follow-up radiographs to assess fracture healing.

Stress Protection and Implant Removal

Plate removal is advised after bone union, not only because of possible corrosion but also because bone under a plate never becomes physiologically or biomechanically normal. Cortical osteopenia occurs in the bone directly underneath the plate. The explanation for the osteopenia appears related to interference with periosteal blood flow under the plate.[23] Also, the rigid plate prevents the bone from responding to normal physiological stimuli because of the difference in the modulus of elasticity between the bone and the implant.[23] If a plate is too stiff, thinning of the underlying cortices may result. Because this response, known as *stress protection*, is partially the result of improper implant selection, it is important not to "overplate" a fracture.

Implants are not removed before the architecture of the bone has become radiographically normal. The prestress of the implant slowly dissipates as bone healing and remodeling take place, and some loosening of the implant may occur. This is an advantage because it results in physiological loading of the bone and with it a return to normal architecture. Complete bone remodeling generally takes 12 to 18 months.[1]

There are some exceptions to the rule of implant removal.[1, 2] Plates are usually not removed from healed pelvic fractures, because stress protection of this bone seldom occurs. Plates are seldom removed from humeral fractures if there is no evidence of stress protection. The approach is difficult, and the likelihood of damaging major nerves is increased because they are more difficult to identify in the scar tissue that forms after fracture repair. Single screws in the metaphysis or epiphysis need not be removed.[1, 2] Plates are often not removed from old animals.

A diaphysis loses 50 per cent of its torsional resistance from the insertion or removal of just a single screw. Experiments have shown that this reduction in strength lasts 1 to 2 months.[4, 5] Long bones must be protected from excessive stress after implant removal. An animal's activity must be restricted for 8 to 12 weeks after plate removal to prevent refracture of the bone.

References

1. Brinker WO, et al (eds): *Manual of Internal Fixation in Small Animals*. Springer-Verlag, New York, 1984.
2. Brinker WO, et al (eds): *Small Animal Orthopedics and Fracture Treatment*. 2nd ed. W.B. Saunders, Philadelphia, 1990.
3. Brinker WO, et al: Stiffness studies on various configurations and types of external fixators. *J Am Anim Hosp Assoc 21*:280, 1985.
4. Brooks DB, et al: The biomechanics of torsional fractures: The stress concentration effect of a drill hole. *J Bone Joint Surg 52*:507, 1970.
5. Burstein AH, et al: Bone strength: The effect of screw holes. *J Bone Joint Surg 54*:1143, 1972.
6. Campbell JR: The technique of fixation of fractures of the distal femur using Rush pins. *J Small Anim Pract 17*:323, 1976.
7. Chaffee VW: Multiple (stacked) intramedullary pin fixation of humeral and femoral fractures. *J Am Anim Hosp Assoc 13*:599, 1977.
8. Dallman MJ, et al: Rotational strength of double-pinning techniques in repair of transverse fractures in femurs of dogs. *Am J Vet Res 51*:123, 1990.
9. Egger EL: Static strength evaluation of six external skeletal fixation configurations. *Vet Surg 12*:130, 1983.
10. Howard PE, Brusewitz GH: An *in vitro* comparison of the holding strength of partially threaded vs. nonthreaded intramedullary pins. *Vet Surg 12*:119, 1983.
11. Kaderly RE: Primary bone healing. *Semin Vet Med Surg 6*:21, 1991.
12. Nunamaker DM: Management of infected fractures. *Vet Clin North Am 5*:259, 1975.
13. Palmer RH, et al: Relationship of femoral intramedullary pins to the sciatic nerve and gluteal muscles after retrograde and normograde insertion. *Vet Surg 17*:65, 1988.
14. Perren SM: Primary bone healing. *In* Bojrab MJ (ed): *Pathophysiology in Small Animal Surgery*. Lea & Febiger, Philadelphia, 1981.
15. Piermattei DL, Greeley RG: *An Atlas of Surgical Approaches to the Bones of the Dog and Cat*. 2nd ed. W.B. Saunders, Philadelphia, 1979.
16. Rhinelander FW: Blood supply of healing long bones. *In* Newton CD, Nunamaker DM (eds): *Textbook of Small Animal Orthopedics*. J.B. Lippincott, Philadelphia, 1985.
17. Rudy RL: Principles of intramedullary pinning. *Vet Clin North Am 5*:209, 1975.
18. Schatzker J: Concepts of fracture stabilization. *In* Sumner-Smith AG (ed): *Bone in Clinical Orthopaedics*. W.B. Saunders, Philadelphia, 1982.
19. Stone EA, et al: Effect of Rush pins on the distal femoral growth plate of young dogs. *Am J Vet Res 42*:261, 1981.
20. Toombs JP: Principles of external skelatal fixation using the Kirschner-Ehmer splint. *Semin Vet Med Surg 6*:68, 1991.
21. Vasseur PB, et al: Evaluation of fixation devices for prevention of rotation in transverse fractures of the canine femoral shaft: An *in vitro* study. *Am J Vet Res 45*:1504, 1984.
22. Whyte W: The role of clothing and drapes in the operating room. *J Hosp Infect 11*:2, 1988.
23. Wilson JW: Vascular supply to normal bone and healing fractures. *Semin Vet Med Surg 6*:26, 1991.
24. Winstanley EW: Aspects of compression treatment of fractures. *Vet Res 95*:430, 1974.
25. Wolf EF: Rush pins in veterinary orthopedics—a review. *J Am Anim Hosp Assoc 11*:756, 1975.

Cerclage Wiring and Tension Band Fixation

Anthony D. Pardo

The use of wire in veterinary orthopedic surgery continues to remain popular owing to its versatility, ease of use, and economical nature. Virtually every small animal general practice equipped to perform basic internal fixation of fresh fractures should have the minimal equipment and implants needed to apply the basic forms of wire fixation—namely full-cerclage, hemicerclage, and tension band fixation. Although wire fixation does provide for stable adjunct fixation in a number of fracture situations, proper adherence to the principles for its use is paramount to minimize the chances for fixation failure and fracture nonunion.

An early report of the use of cerclage wire in small animal fracture repair warned of the possibility of nonunion associated with these implants.[12] Fixation failures were suggested as a result of vascular compromise in the underlying cortical bone and subsequent wire loosening. More recent clinical reports contradict this finding and suggest that cerclage wires have a secure place in the repair of long-bone fractures.[7, 29, 31] Basic research support for the use of wire for internal fixation was provided by investigations of the vascular response of canine bone to fracture and fracture healing with stainless steel wires and other implants.[16, 17] These studies and others,[9, 13, 18, 25, 28, 30] confirmed that cortical vascularity is maintained under wire cerclage and that uncomplicated bone healing can be expected after proper application of these devices.

Considerable attention has also been given to various aspects of wire application such as the amount of tension developed in wire by various instruments and surgeons,[3, 19, 27] comparisons of looped and twisted knot-securing systems,[3, 19, 27] the effects on wire tension of bending and cutting the twisted knot,[19] comparisons of alternative materials used for cerclage,[8, 21, 26] and effects of cerclage devices on biomechanical properties of cortical bone.[6] Cerclage devices have excellent merit and should have an important role in the internal fixation of fractures in small animals. The majority of failures that occur can be readily ascribed to violations of the principles of proper wire use.

MATERIALS

As with most orthopedic implants, surgical wire is made of 316L stainless steel, which is an alloy of iron, chromium, nickel, molybdenum, and other metals, having favorable handling characteristics and excellent corrosion resistance.[11] Orthopedic wire can be purchased in a number of diameters, as preformed looped wire, and on wire spools. Wire sizes are commonly given in gauges with conversion measurements in millimeters (Table 122–2). Wire sizes from 0.64 to 1.25 mm (22 to 16 gauge) are most commonly used in small animal orthopedics. Sizes smaller or larger than this are either too weak to counteract fracture forces or are difficult to work with, respectively. More specific size recommendations are discussed later.

Besides stainless steel wire, numerous other materials have been investigated and used for cerclage of long-bone fractures in both humans and dogs. Nylon band cerclage (nylon cable ties) has been used with success for cerclage of long-bone fractures in elderly people with osteoporosis to avoid collapse of the underlying weakened cortex or as an adjunct to plate and screw fixation.[15, 23] Biomechanical testing of these nylon bands *in vitro* has identified a number of concerns about their likely stability *in vivo*. In the dry state, only bands of at least 7.6-mm width were capable of equaling the tensile strength of a 1.2-mm-diameter steel wire. Prior soaking in saline for 24 hours or steam autoclaving resulted in a significant loss of tensile strength as a result of increased pliability of the band or brittleness of the locking mechanism, respectively.[8, 21] After a 24-hour saline soak, only the 7.6-mm-wide bands could withstand peak loads equal to those generated in 0.8-mm (20 gauge) twisted-knot stainless steel wire.[8] Ethylene oxide sterilization did not adversely affect the biomechanical properties of the nylon bands. Thus, the performance of these nylon bands *in vivo*, in the presence of body fluids and significant weightbearing loads, must be questioned. Nevertheless, these systems have been used with success in humans for temporary intraoperative fixation of fractures as well as adjunctive fixation for comminuted fractures in osteoporotic bone.[20, 23]

Other materials that are infrequently used in human surgery, such as titanium cable and braided polyester tape,[21] have little application in animals as a replacement for stainless steel wire cerclage.

TABLE 122–2. CONVERSION OF SURGICAL WIRE SIZES

Suture Material Size	Gauge	Size in Inches	Size in Millimeters
6–0	40	0.0031	0.079
6–0	38	0.0040	0.102
5–0	35	0.0056	0.142
4–0	34	0.0063	0.160
4–0	32	0.0080	0.203
3–0	30	0.0100	0.254
2–0	28	0.0126	0.320
0	26	0.0159	0.404
1	25	0.0174	0.455
2	24	0.0201	0.511
3	23	0.0226	0.574
4	22	0.0254	0.643
5	20	0.0320	0.813
7	18	0.0403	1.016
—	16	0.0492	1.25

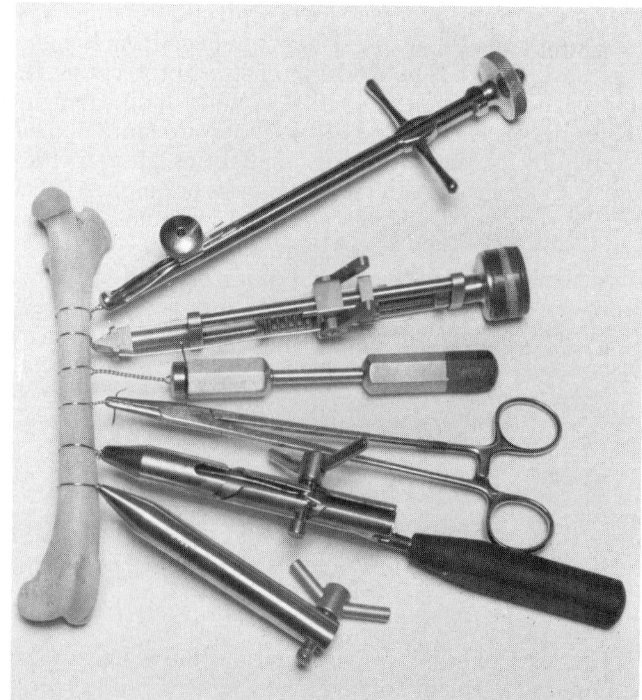

FIGURE 122–41. Several of the commonly used wire tighteners and twisters. From top to bottom: Shifrin wire tightener, Rhinelander wire tightener-twister, Richards standard wire twister, wire-twisting forceps, ASIF loop wire tightener, and Richards loop wire tightener. The Shifrin and Rhinelander wire twisters separate the acts of tightening the wire and twisting the knot. The two loop wire tighteners require the use of wires with a preformed eye on one end.

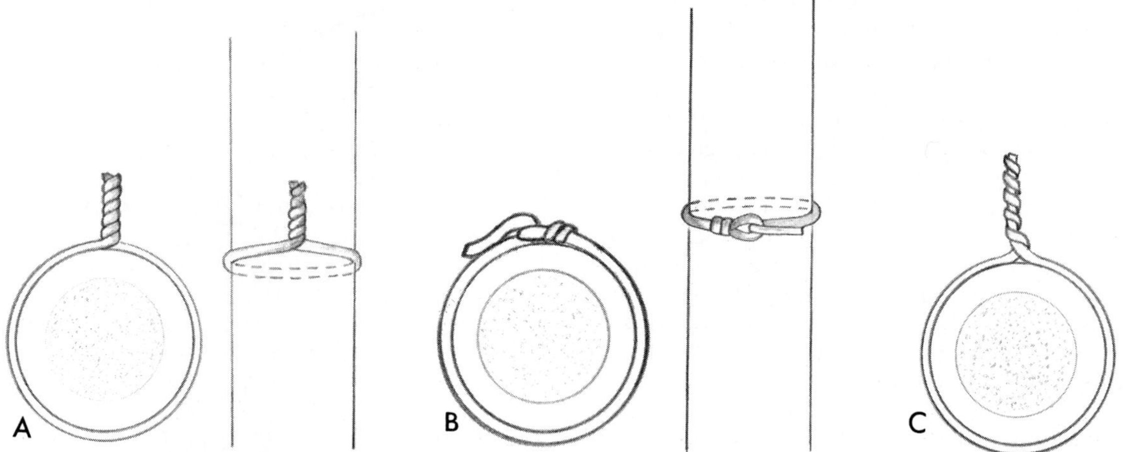

FIGURE 122–42. Twist (*A*) and loop (*B*) wire knots. In twist knots, the wires twist on each other. An incorrect twist knot (*C*) slips more easily because one wire twists around the other.

INSTRUMENTS FOR WIRE APPLICATION

Application of wires to bones can be performed easily with a few simple instruments. Because orthopedic wire is rarely used as a sole method of fixation and is frequently used in conjunction with intramedullary pins and Kirschner wires, a Jacob handchuck and key, an air drill or electric drill, and an assortment of pins are necessary. Various instruments are available to tighten and secure the wire around the bone (Fig. 122–41). Some instruments secure the wire with a loop-type knot, whereas others create a twisted knot (Fig. 122–42). Because stability is one of the factors critical to the successful use of cerclage wire in fracture fixation, the surgeon must apply the wire tightly and secure it with a knot that will maintain that level of compression through the postoperative period.

Two basic types of knots are used to secure the wire in tension—a looped knot and a twisted knot (see Fig. 122–42). The looped knot cerclage is applied by passing the free end of the wire around the bone and through the preformed eye of the wire strand. The instrument then tightens and secures the wire in a two-step process. During the first step, the instrument pulls the wire tight. Then, while maintaining tension on the wire, the surgeon bends the wire 180° back on itself to complete the securing process (Fig. 122–43). With this technique, the processes of creating tension in the wire and securing the knot are performed independently. In contrast, with the exception of the Rhinelander and Shifrin wire tigh-

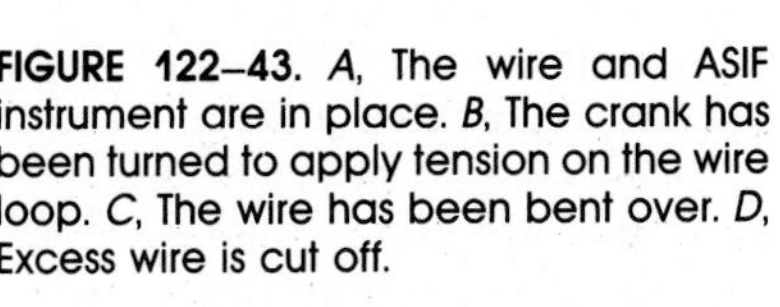
FIGURE 122–43. *A*, The wire and ASIF instrument are in place. *B*, The crank has been turned to apply tension on the wire loop. *C*, The wire has been bent over. *D*, Excess wire is cut off.

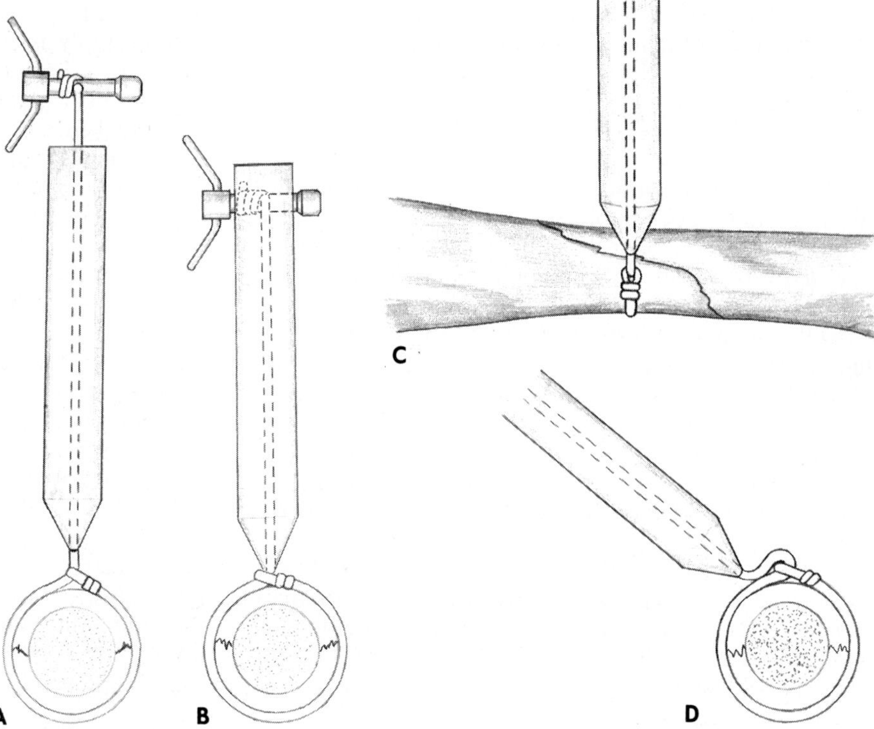

teners (see Fig. 122–41), the instruments that create a twist-type knot do so by creating tension and twisting the wire at the same time. This movement leads to a decrease in the amount of static tension developed in the twisted wire compared with the looped wire. Several studies have shown that a twisted-knot cerclage develops only 40 to 60 per cent of the static tension in a looped-knot wire of comparable size.[3, 19] On the other hand, when subjected to dynamic testing, twisted knots were superior at resisting slippage and developed a significantly greater tensile load than looped wires.[19, 25] Looped knots failed by unbending, whereas twisted knots failed by untwisting. During dynamic testing of twisted wires, maximal tensile loads were reached after significant displacement of the simulated fracture had occurred (several millimeters) and at a point where fixation failure of a clinical fracture would most likely result.[27]

Another consideration that may have a role in the choice of wire type is the effect that cutting and bending a twisted knot has on static tension in the wire. Studies have shown that cutting the twisted knot to a length of three twists can result in up to a 21 per cent loss of tension on the wire.[19] Furthermore, if the knot is then bent over to minimize trauma to the overlying soft tissues, a further loss of 30 to 70 per cent of the tensile strength may be experienced.[19] This loss of tension does not occur in the looped wire because it is already bent flush with the bone and is not affected by cutting. If a twisted knot is used, tension loss may be minimized by bending the wire down to the bone while the last twist is applied or by leaving the twist unbent after cutting.

It is difficult to choose one securing technique over the other without compromising one factor or the other (i.e., static tension versus knot strength). In clinical practice, either a looped knot or twisted knot may be successfully used to secure full-cerclage, hemicerclage, or tension band wires. Many surgeons prefer the looped-knot cerclage system because of its ease of application and greater interfragmentary compression.

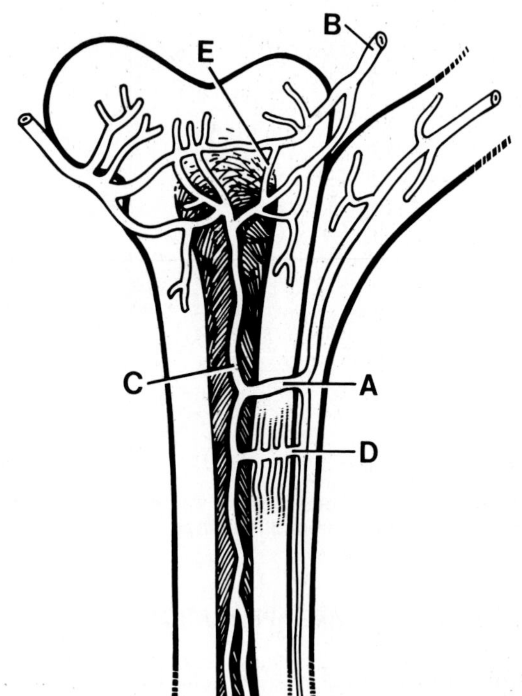

FIGURE 122–44. Schematic representation of the normal afferent vascular supply to a mature long bone. (A, nutrient artery of the diaphysis; B, metaphyseal arteries; C, medullary artery; D, periosteal arteriole; E, anastomosis between the metaphyseal and diaphyseal medullary vessels.) The diaphyseal nutrient artery (A) and metaphyseal arteries (B) anastomose (E) to form the major medullary artery (C), which supplies the cortex. Centrifugal blood flow from the medullary blood vessels supplies the entire cortex except in areas of dense fibrous attachments, where periosteal blood vessels (D) may supply the outer third of the cortex.

INFLUENCE OF WIRE IMPLANTS ON BONE HEALING

To achieve bone union after fracture, adequate stabilization and blood supply are essential. In the absence of either of these, bone healing may be compromised, and delayed union or nonunion results. Thus, it is important to consider the effects of wire implants on cortical bone and callus vascularity during fracture healing.

The blood supply to normal long bones consists of three major subdivisions: the afferent, efferent, and intermediate vascular systems.[5, 16–18, 28] The afferent or arterial blood supply of long bones is derived from three major sources: the nutrient artery of the diaphysis, the metaphyseal vessels, and the periosteal arterioles (Fig. 122–44). In normal bone, most of cortical blood flow is derived from medullary vessels, which result from anastomosis of the principal nutrient artery and metaphyseal vessels. Arterial blood from these medullary vessels flows centrifugally from the medulla through the cortex to supply most of the diaphyseal cortex. Vascular contribution to the intact cortex by periosteal vessels is minimal except in areas of dense muscular and fibrous attachments. Even in these areas, periosteal arterial blood supply is probably limited to the outer third of the cortex. The efferent or venous system also drains in a centrifugal manner from the medullary cavity to the periosteal surface through large emissary veins and vena communicans paralleling the nutrient artery. The intermediate vascular system of bone is unique in that the capillary-sized vessels are confined within cortical bone, travel a limited distance longitudinally in the cortex (1 to 2 mm), and do not directly supply nutrients to the cellular elements of the cortex. Microscopic canaliculi connect capillary-sized vessels in haversian and Volkmann canals to the lacunar osteocytes and deliver nutrients to those cells.

After fracture, loss of the medullary blood vessels results in a transient shift in blood supply to the cortex from a medullary- to extraosseus-derived, centripetal blood flow to the healing callus.[16–18, 28] With adequate stabilization, rapid restoration of the medullary vessels occurs within the first few weeks, and a centrifugal blood flow pattern to the cortex is re-established. At this point, the dominant blood supply to the endosteal, intercortical uniting, and periosteal callus is once again derived from the medullary arteries (Fig. 122–45). Tight application

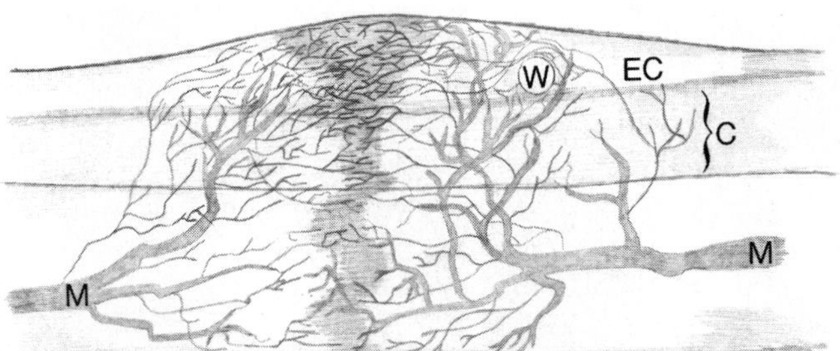

FIGURE 122–45. Medullary vessels (M) penetrate the cortex (C) and supply blood to the external callus (EC). The vasculature will be unimpeded by the presence of a wire (W) tight on the cortex.

of small-diameter wire implants to the periosteal surface of the cortex does not impair or alter this pattern of blood supply to the healing fracture. Several reasons can be given for this observation[10, 18, 28]:

1. Extraosseus vessels and medullary-derived vessels supplying the cortex and external callus are directed perpendicular to the bone and readily grow around the wires.
2. Periosteal venous and arterial systems do not typically travel longitudinally on the bone surface, where they might become strangled by wire.
3. The intracortical capillaries are protected from compression by the surrounding bone.
4. Intracortical, longitudinal blood flow is limited to 1 or 2 mm, minimizing collateral avascularity from the overlying wire.

Wide bands applied tightly to the cortex (e.g., Parham-Martin bands) are reputed to interfere with the extraosseus arterial blood supply to the cortex and venous drainage from the periosteal surface and thus result in detrimental cortical avascularity.[16] Microangiographic studies now suggest that in intact bone, placement of encircling nylon or metal bands does not result in avascularity of the underlying cortex.[9, 13] Unfortunately, these studies did not address the effects of these wide bands on cortical revascularization after fractures accompanied by a transient loss of both the medullary and extraosseus blood supply. Most investigators discourage the use of these bands in fracture repair.[10, 18]

Concurrent use of other implants does affect revascularization of fractured cortical bone. Intramedullary devices that do not completely fill the medullary cavity allow re-establishment of the medullary blood supply and thus do not interfere with fracture healing. Medullary reaming or complete filling of the medullary canal by implants adversely affects the re-establishment of a medullary blood supply to the fracture site and delays the healing process.

GENERAL INDICATIONS

Fractured bones and metal implants are subjected to a number of forces that may result in displacement of the fracture segments. Figure 122–46 illustrates the major forces acting across a fracture. To effectively neutralize the respective forces of tension, shear, rotation, and bending, the surgeon must choose the correct wire configuration and the proper implant to complement that wire. In general, wire is best able to maintain fragment apposition in long oblique fracture planes, thus reducing shear and rotational forces. Additional stabilization in the form of intramedullary pins, bone plates, or external skeletal fixation is necessary to decrease the bending forces acting on the wire implant. In combination with Kirschner wires, figure-eight wire is effective in counteracting tensile forces and converting them to compressive forces.

FULL-CERCLAGE WIRES

Indications

Full cerclage implies the use of wire loops that completely encircle the diaphysis of the bone. They are best suited for uniform, cylindrical long bones such as the femur, tibia, and humerus, where they are commonly used in combination with intramedullary pins. Full-cerclage wires are often used around long oblique and spiral fractures of the diaphysis, where they serve to counteract shear, rotational, and angular forces and provide compression across the fracture line. Generally, these fractures should be sufficiently oblique to allow the use of multiple wires to minimize the chances of cerclage wire failure (Fig. 122–47). Full-cerclage wire may be used in repair of comminuted fractures of the diaphysis in selected cases when anatomical fragment reconstruction is possible. Wire is always used in combination with additional implant devices in these cases.

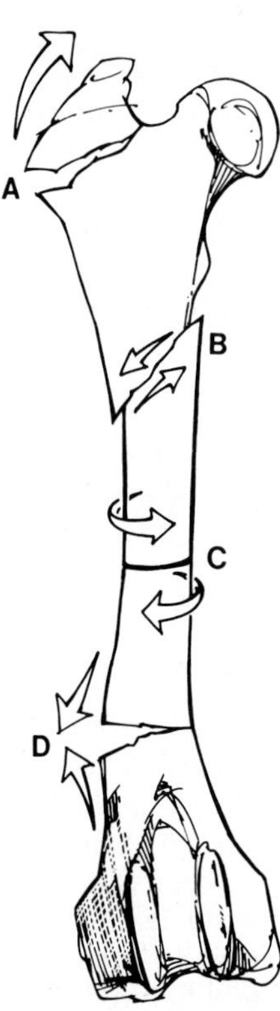

FIGURE 122–46. The typical forces that act along fracture lines. (A, tension or distraction; B, shear; C, rotation; D, bending.)

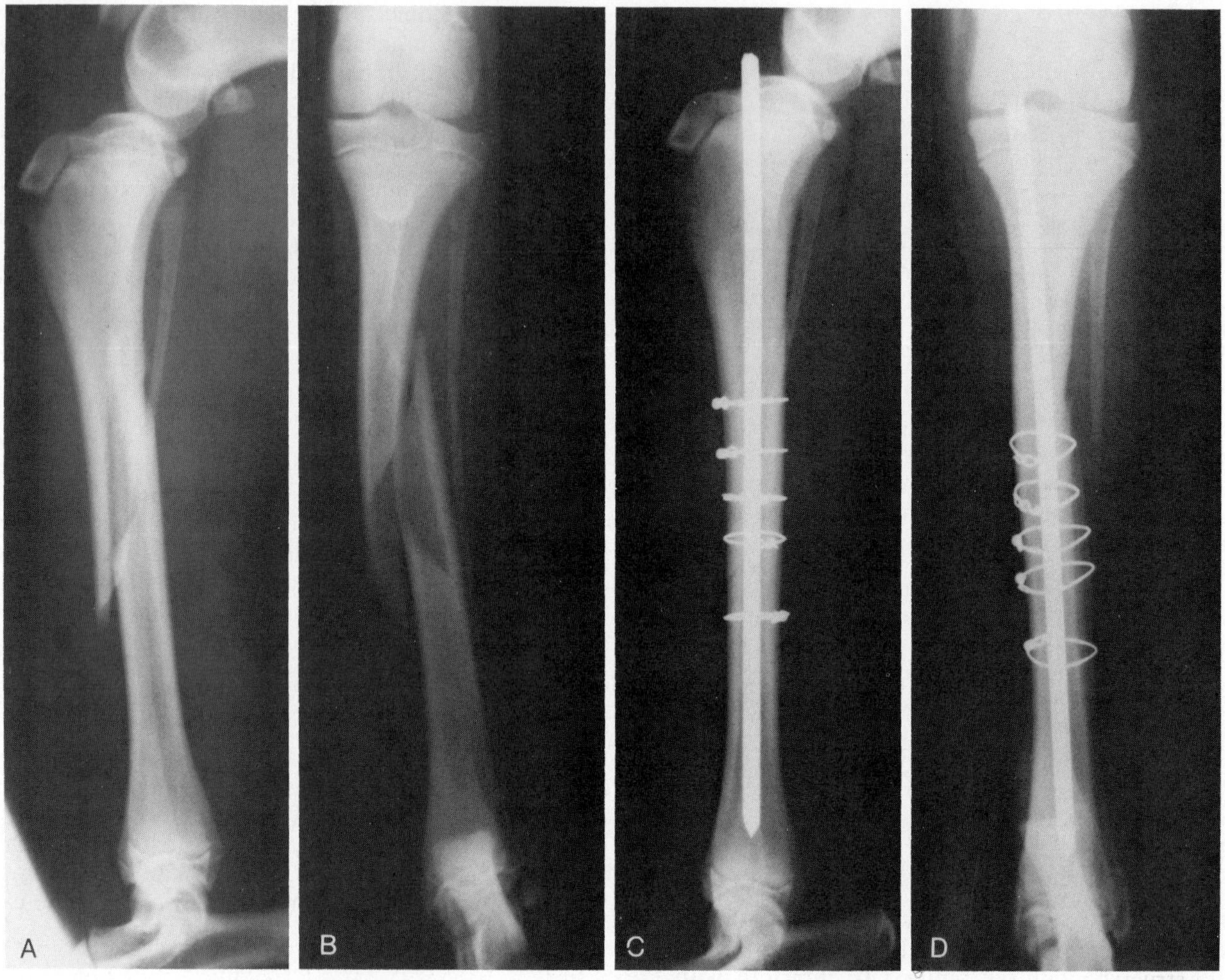

FIGURE 122–47. *A* and *B*, Lateral and craniocaudal views of a closed spiral tibial fracture in a 5-month-old dog. *C* and *D*, Postoperative films showing repair using a normograded single intramedullary pin and five full cerclage wires. The fracture is anatomically reduced. Four wires encircle the main fracture, and one stabilizes a fissure fracture in the distal segment. The wires are 1 cm apart, perpendicular to the bone shaft and tight against the cortex.

Full-cerclage wire may be used around longitudinal undisplaced fissure fractures in the main fracture segments before attempting reduction or application of intramedullary devices to prevent further distraction or propagation of these fissures into complete fractures (Fig. 122–48). Additionally, full-cerclage wire may occasionally be used around a bone-plated diaphysis to protect tenuous screw purchase in soft or immature bone, as well as over open plate holes in areas of comminution.

Principles of Application

Adherence to the basic principles of cerclage wire application is paramount if fixation failure is to be avoided. Wires must be applied tightly and directly against the periosteum. In areas of muscular or fascial attachments, a wire passer (Fig. 122–49) may be used to place the wire directly against the bone with minimal soft-tissue dissection while avoiding entrapment of tissues beneath the wire. Compression of soft tissues under the wire leads to ischemic necrosis and atrophy, which then result in loosening of the wire. Wires should be placed directly over periosteum, if present. Excessive periosteal stripping is unnecessary and undesirable, especially in immature bone, where excessive periosteal callus formation may result.

Wire should be of sufficient size to withstand the forces generated in the fracture during the healing period. Orthopedic wire in sizes 0.64 and 0.8 mm (22

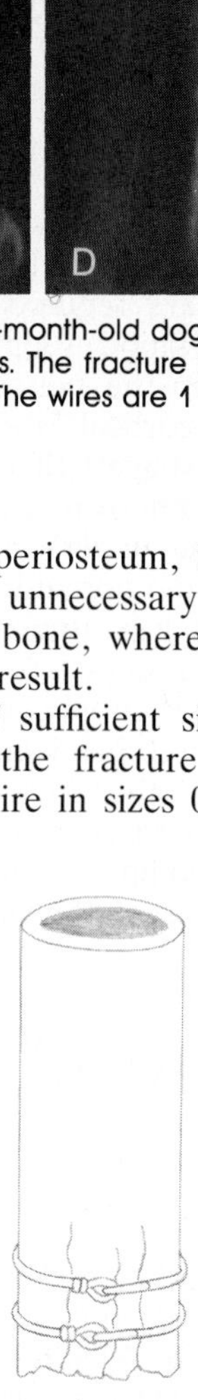

FIGURE 122–48. Full-cerclage wires are used to hold fissures in a barrel-stay fashion.

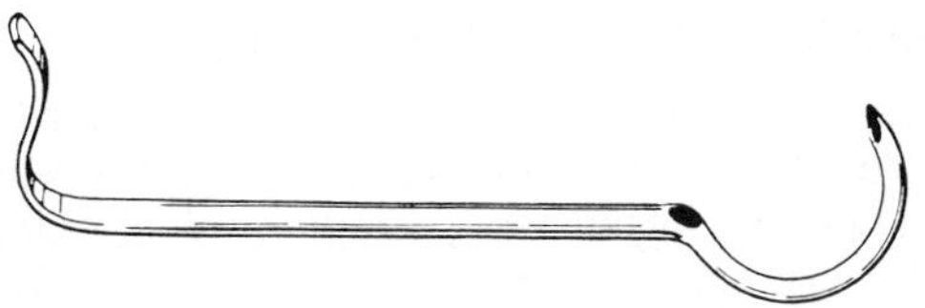

FIGURE 122–49. Wire passer. This instrument makes it possible to insert the cerclage wire around the bone with minimum soft-tissue detachment. (From Brinker WO, et al: *Handbook of Small Animal Orthopedics and Fracture Treatment.* 2nd ed. W.B. Saunders, Philadelphia, 1990.)

and 20 gauge) is generally used for fractures in cats and small dogs. Fractures in medium-sized and larger dogs are usually repaired using 0.8-mm (20-gauge) and 1.0- to 1.25-mm (18- to 16-gauge) diameter wire, respectively. Wire sizes smaller than these are subject to premature failure and are not used routinely.

Tight application of the wire helps ensure adequate compression of the fracture site and stability of the repair. The two basic methods of wire tightening and fixation, looped knot and twisted knot, were discussed previously (see Figs. 122–42 and 122–43). Looped-knot wire-tightening instruments generate a greater final tension in the wire than twisted knot devices, but twisted knots provide greater resistance to knot slippage.[3, 19, 27] If twisted knots are used, the excess wire must be cut off, resulting in up to a 21 per cent loss of tension.[19] The resulting twisted knot may be left perpendicular to the bone surface if overlying soft-tissue protection is adequate. Alternatively, the knot may be bent down flush with the bone surface to protect nearby neurovascular structures and skin. Up to 70 per cent of the tension in the wire may be lost during the bending maneuver, and the wire knot may be weakened.[19] If the wire is to be bent over, it is best to do this when forming the last one-half twist in the knot. Excess wire beyond three twists is removed with wire cutters.

Wire cerclage is placed perpendicular to the long axis of the bone. If placed obliquely to the bone shaft, the previously tight wire may shift to a position perpendicular to the bone's long axis, resulting in a loose wire (Fig. 122–50). The conical shape of diaphyseal bone near the metaphyses may result in slippage of a full-cerclage wire to the narrower area of the bone, with loosening. This loss of fixation may be avoided by preplacing a K wire across the shaft or grooving the cortex with a file or scalpel blade in the desired location of the cerclage wire. As the wire is tightened, it either nestles in the precut groove or slides up against the transverse K wire, preventing further slippage down the flared bone (Fig. 122–51).

A common error in pin and wire repair of fractures is failure to use a sufficient number of cerclage wires for fixation. In general, a minimum of two cerclage wires is used for repair of oblique or spiral fractures. If a single wire is used, it may serve as a fulcrum for motion of the fracture segments, with subsequent loss of fixation or delayed union. Full-cerclage fixation is only considered for oblique fractures whose length is at least two times the diameter of the bone shaft. Cerclage wires are placed approximately 1 cm apart throughout the length of the fracture, starting a minimum of 5 mm from the proximal and distal fracture ends (Fig. 122–52). Cerclage wires must not lie within a fracture line nor cross a cortical defect created by the loss of a bone fragment. In general, all cerclage wires are placed after reduction of the fracture but before placement of any intramedullary devices. Wires should be checked for tightness after fracture fixation is complete by firmly pushing against them with an instrument. Any movement of the wire along the shaft denotes looseness and warrants replacement with a new wire.

Removal of full-cerclage wires after fracture healing is usually not necessary in dogs and cats unless complications result from their presence. In immature animals, periosteal callus formation frequently results in these wires becoming surrounded by bone, making their removal almost impossible. Fortunately, there does not appear to be any significant stress protection of the underlying bone by these implants, nor is appositional growth retarded by their presence. The resulting thickening of the cortex under the implant does result in a

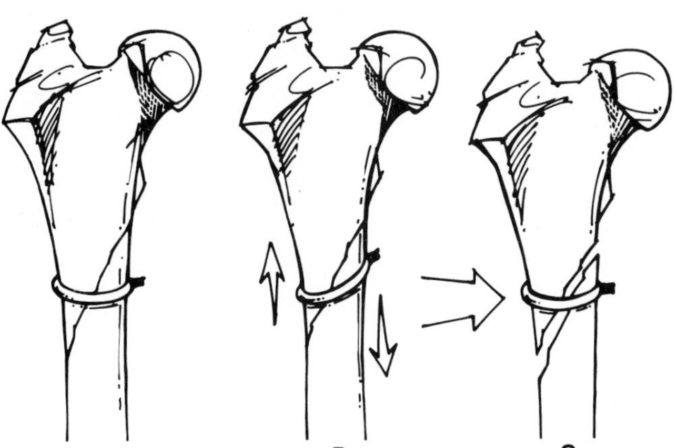

FIGURE 122–50. *A*, Wire that is placed perpendicular to the bone shaft will remain tight. *B*, Wire placed obliquely across the shaft will tend to slip to a perpendicular position with motion and result in a loss of fracture apposition (*C*).

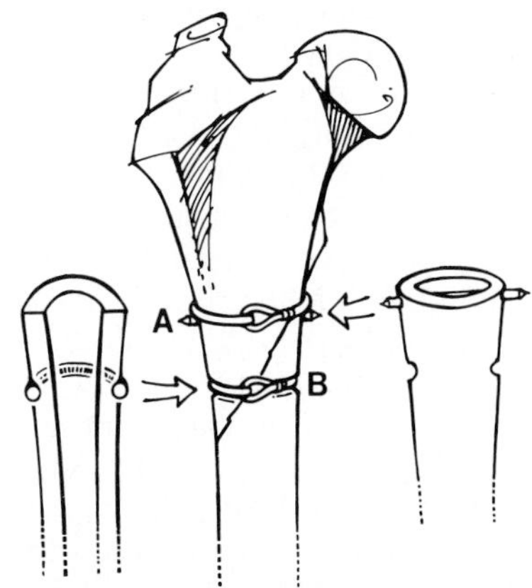

FIGURE 122–51. Full-cerclage wires can be prevented from slipping down the conical regions of the diaphysis by tightening the wire against a transverse K wire placed through the shaft (A) or by notching the cortex slightly (B) in the desired location for the wire.

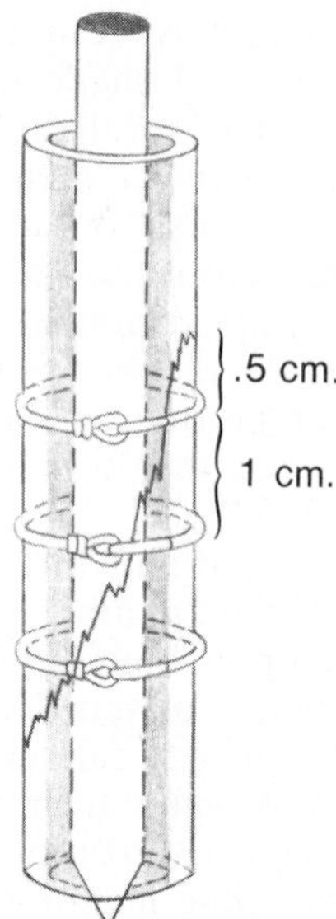

FIGURE 122–52. This long oblique fracture is repaired with three full-cerclage wires.

temporary increase in stiffness and loss of torsional strength in immature canine diaphyseal bone, returning to normal by 12 weeks after surgery.[6] Wire removal after uncomplicated fracture healing is not performed in small animal patients.

INTERFRAGMENTARY WIRES

Cerclage wire placed through holes in the cortex, partially around the bone shaft, and across a fracture line is referred to as an *interfragmentary wire*. These wires may be placed in a number of configurations including figure-eight, horizontal mattress, or simple interrupted patterns across transverse fractures of the diaphysis to neutralize rotational forces that are not controlled by intramedullary devices. Interfragmentary wiring, or hemicerclage, is also commonly used as a method of reduction and fixation of fractures of the scapula, mandible, maxilla, and occasionally the pelvis. The wire provides reduction and compression across the fracture site. Interfragmentary wires are commonly used in combination with other implants such as bone plates, screws, or intramedullary pins.

The ability of various interfragmentary wire configurations to provide rotational stability to a transverse diaphyseal fracture has been investigated.[2] The results of that study showed that a cruciate mattress pattern provided better control of rotation in the fracture model than either horizontal mattress or simple interrupted patterns. Increasing the overall distance of the interfragmentary wire from the fracture resulted in a loss of rotational stability in the cruciate and horizontal mattress patterns. Tightening each arm of the mattress patterns separately with a twisted knot resulted in better compression of the fracture than if the wire was twisted in only one location. Hemicerclage wires (simple interrupted pattern) provided minimal control of rotational forces in the transverse fracture model and are not recommended.

Figure-Eight Antirotation Wires

Figure-eight wires help neutralize rotational forces and provide interfragmentary compression when correctly applied to transverse diaphyseal fractures (Fig. 122–53). To maximize control of rotation, transverse portions of the wire must be as close to the fracture as possible without risking fragmentation of the edge. Transverse holes are drilled perpendicular to the long axis of the bone, approximately 1 cm away from the fracture ends, using a drill bit or small K wire. Ideally, the holes are placed so that the finished wire lies on the tension surface of the bone with the wires crossing the fracture at a 90° angle to each other. Separate strands of wire are placed through each of the drilled holes and crossed at the fracture site. The fracture is reduced, and an intramedullary pin is driven down the shaft and seated in the distal metaphysis. The wire is tightened and secured using a separate twisted or looped knot for each arm of the cruciate pattern.

Care is taken to avoid overtightening the wire to prevent distraction of the fracture fragments on the opposite side of the bone. Use of two separate wire strands and two knots is recommended over weaving a single strand of wire in a figure-eight with a single securing knot. This ensures a more uniformly tightened wire and less chance of metal fatigue due to excessive manipulation.

Hemicerclage Wire

The use of simple interrupted hemicerclage wires in long-bone fractures is best reserved for reduction and stabilization of small fragments and short oblique fractures in combination with intramedullary pins. Because they consist of only one wire strand, hemicerclage wires are effective in neutralizing shearing or rotational forces in only one direction. Hemicerclage wires are frequently used in the repair of mandibular fractures and other fractures of the flat bones.[4, 24]

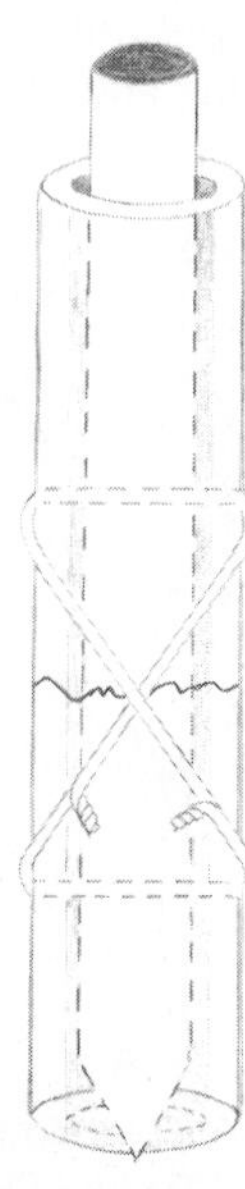

FIGURE 122–53. A figure-eight antirotation wire applied to a transverse irregular fracture.

Hemicerclage wire is placed through holes drilled through the cortex on each side of the fracture. For best control of rotation and shear forces, the fracture should be oblique and should interdigitate well, and the wire should cross perpendicular to the fracture line. In a transverse diaphyseal fracture, a figure-eight wire results in better fixation. Before the wire is tightened, the fracture is reduced and the intramedullary pin is advanced into the distal fragment. The wire is then tightened and secured (Fig. 122–54).

If tightening the hemicerclage wire results in distraction of the opposite cortex of the bone, a second hemicerclage wire may be placed and tightened on that side. For many transverse long-bone fractures in large dogs, bone plating results in a more stable repair and reliable return to function than combined use of intramedullary pins and interfragmentary wires.

TENSION BAND WIRES

Indications

The engineering principle of the tension band may be used in the repair of certain fractures and osteotomies to convert tensile and distractive forces into compressive forces across the fracture line. The principles of the tension band wire can be applied to any fracture or osteotomy in which the pull of muscles, tendons, or ligaments results in distraction of a bone fragment away from the parent bone. When the tension band wire is applied to the tension surface of the fracture, it exerts a tensile force equal in magnitude and 180° opposite to the distracting force created by the muscle, tendon, or ligament. The force vector generated by these two opposing forces results in compression across the fracture (Fig. 122–55). If properly applied, a tension band wire repair allows for early postoperative mobilization, with excellent compression and stability of the fracture.[1, 22]

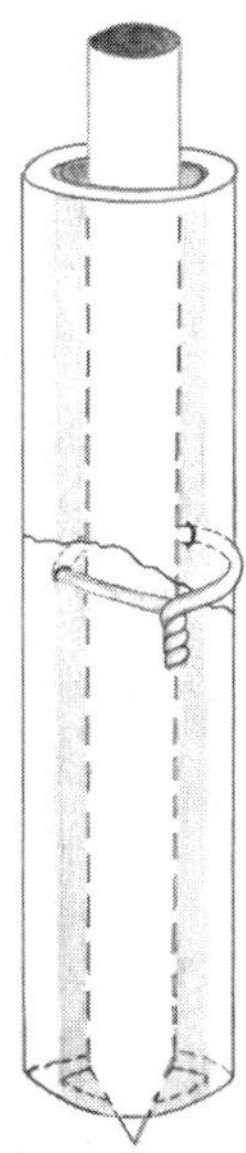

FIGURE 122–54. A hemicerclage wire can be applied to a transverse irregular or short oblique fracture.

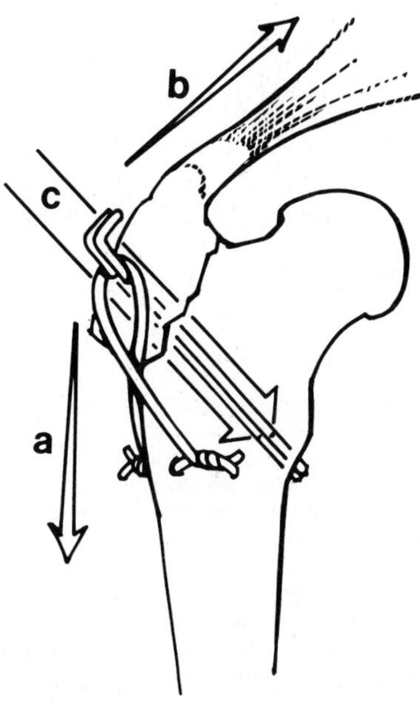

FIGURE 122–55. Schematic representation of the tension band principle applied to a fracture of the greater trochanter of the femur. The tensile force (a) in the wire is directed opposite to the distracting force (b) resulting from the pull of the gluteal muscles. The resultant force vector (c) is directed perpendicular to the fracture along the K wires, causing compression of the fracture.

Tension band repair is indicated for the following fractures and osteotomies: greater trochanter of the femur, tibial tuberosity, medial and lateral malleoli of the tibia/fibula, tuber calcis, tuber ischii, supraglenoid tubercle, scapular acromion, greater tubercle of the humerus, olecranon, patella, and various avulsions or osteotomies of collateral ligaments.

Principles of Application

A similar approach is used to apply this technique to fractures and osteotomies. The fracture is reduced, and two Kirschner wires (0.035 to 0.062 inch) are driven from the tip of the bone fragment across the fracture and into the parent bone. Two K wires are usually necessary to provide rotational stability of the fracture, although in extremely small fragments, a single small K wire may suffice. The K wires are directed perpendicular to the fracture, parallel to each other, and must engage the opposite cortex for maximum stability (Fig. 122–56). A small hole is drilled transversely through the cortex on the diaphyseal side, approximately the same distance from the fracture line as the height of the reduced fragment. Wire (0.64 to 1.0 mm in diameter) is passed through the drill hole and around the proximal ends of the K wires in a figure-eight pattern. The wire must lie in contact with bone and against the pins over the bone fragment without interposed soft tissues to prevent subsequent loosening. Twist knots are created on each side of the figure-eight, and the knots are tightened simultaneously to distribute tension evenly throughout the wire.[1] Two loop knots may be applied, but this is a cumbersome process requiring simultaneous use of two loop tighteners. A single loop knot may be

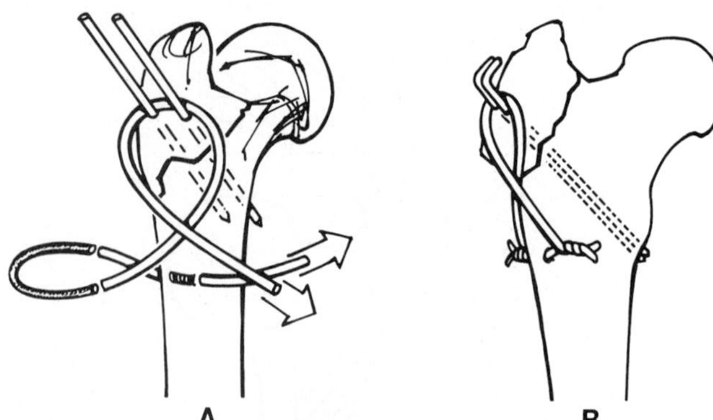

FIGURE 122–56. Application of a tension band wire. *A*, The fracture is reduced and secured with two small K wires placed through the fragment, perpendicular to the fracture line, and through the metaphysis, engaging the opposite cortex. A figure-eight wire is placed through a hole in the cortex and around the pins, leaving a loop on one side and the two free ends on the other. *B*, The finished tension band wire repair. The loop and the free ends in the wire have been tightened independently with twist knots, and the K wires bent over and trimmed.

used satisfactorily, although tension on the wire is less evenly distributed than with two knots. The knots are bent down against the bone, and excess wire is removed. The proximal ends of the K wires are bent over and cut short to minimize soft-tissue irritation. Reduction and fixation of the fracture with a lag screw and K wire has been described as an alternative to the use of two K wires for repair of olecranon osteotomies in dogs.[14]

In the repair of transverse patellar fractures, one or two small K wires and a tension band cerclage wire are placed along the cranial (tension) surface of the bone. Alternatively, a single cerclage wire may be placed through holes drilled transversely through the cranial surface of the proximal and distal aspects of the patella, and the free ends twisted tight. During weightbearing, flexion of the stifle results in compression of the fracture and reduction of the articular surface of the patella.

Removal of tension band implants is indicated in mature animals only if the metal causes soft-tissue irritation or if implant loosening occurs. In performing surgical approaches in immature animals, tenotomies are often preferable to osteotomies to avoid damage to open physes. If a tension band repair must be performed across an open physis, removal of the figure-eight wire is recommended after 4 weeks to decrease the risk of premature physeal closure.

COMPLICATIONS

Most complications encountered with the use of cerclage wire generally result from one or more violations of the described principles of proper wire use.[29] Inappropriate choice of fracture for cerclage application, too few cerclage wires, undersized wires, loosely applied wires, and inadequate ancillary fixation may contribute to fixation failure and nonunion. Failure should not be blamed on the inadequacies of the wire implants but instead on the poor judgment of the surgeon. Used properly in appropriate cases, wire implants are valuable.

References

1. Birchard SJ, Bright RM: The tension band wire for fracture repair in the dog. *Comp Cont Educ 3*:37, 1981.
2. Blass CE, et al: Mechanical properties of three orthopedic wire configurations. *Am J Vet Res 46*:1725, 1985.
3. Blass CE, et al: Static and dynamic cerclage wire analysis. *Vet Surg 15*:181, 1986.
4. Brinker WO, et al: *Handbook of Small Animal Orthopedics and Fracture Treatment*. 2nd ed. W.B. Saunders, Philadelphia, 1990.
5. Brookes M: *The Blood Supply of Bone*. Butterworths, London, 1971.
6. Ellison GW, et al: The effects of cerclage wiring on the immature canine diaphysis. A biomechanical analysis. *Vet Surg 11*:44, 1982.
7. Hinko PJ, Rhinelander FW: Effective use of cerclage in the treatment of long-bone fractures in dogs. *J Am Vet Med Assoc 166*:520, 1975.
8. Kirby BM, Wilson JW: Knot strength of nylon-band cerclage. *Acta Orthop Scand 60*:696, 1989.
9. Kirby BM, Wilson JW: Effect of circumferential bands on cortical vascularity and viability. *J Orthop Res 9*:174, 1991.
10. Liska WD: Wires in long bone fracture repair. *In* Slatter D (ed): *Textbook of Small Animal Surgery*. W.B. Saunders, Philadelphia, 1985, pp 2003–2014.
11. Muller ME, et al: *Manual of Internal Fixation*. 3rd ed. Springer-Verlag, New York, 1991.
12. Newton CD, Hohn RB: Fracture non-union resulting from cerclage appliances. *J Am Vet Med Assoc 164*:503, 1974.
13. Nyrop KA, et al: Vascular response of the equine radius to cerclage devices. *Vet Surg 19*:249, 1990.
14. Palmer RH, et al: A combined tension band and lag screw technique for fixation of olecranon osteotomies. *Vet Surg 17*:328, 1988.
15. Partridge AJ, Evans PE: The treatment of fractures of the shaft of the femur using nylon cerclage. *J Bone Joint Surg [Br] 64*:210, 1982.
16. Rhinelander FW: The normal microcirculation of diaphyseal cortex and its response to fracture. *J Bone Joint Surg 50A*:784, 1968.
17. Rhinelander FW: Circulation in bone. *In* Bourne GH (ed): *The Biochemistry and Physiology of Bone*. Academic Press, New York, 1972, pp 2–77.
18. Rhinelander FW, Wilson JW: Blood supply to developing, mature, and healing bone. *In* Sumner-Smith G (ed): *Bone in Clinical Orthopedics*. W. B. Saunders, Philadelphia, 1982, pp 81–158.
19. Rooks RL, et al: *In vitro* cerclage wiring analysis. *Vet Surg 11*:39, 1982.
20. Schmidt TL, Davis WM: Intraoperative use of nylon bands in fracture fixation. *Clin Orthop 154*:341, 1981.
21. Shaw JA, Daubert HB: Compression capability of cerclage fixation systems. A biomechanical study. *Orthopedics 11*:1169, 1988.
22. Simeone L: Dynamic cerclage in traumatology. *Ital J Orthop Traumatol 13*:73, 1987.
23. Tountas AA, et al: The partridge nylon cerclage: Its use as a supplementary fixation of difficult femoral fractures in the elderly. *J Orthop Trauma 4*:299, 1990.
24. Umphlet RC, Johnson AL: Mandibular fractures in the dog. A retrospective study of 157 cases. *Vet Surg 19*:272, 1990.
25. Wilson JW: Effect of cerclage wires on periosteal bone in growing dogs. *Vet Surg 16*:299, 1987.
26. Wilson JW: Knot strength of cerclage bands and wires. *Acta Orthop Scand 59*:545, 1988.
27. Wilson JW, et al: Resistance of cerclage to knot failure. *J Am Vet Med Assoc 187*:389, 1985.
28. Wilson JW: Vascular supply to normal bone and healing fractures. *Semin Vet Med Surg (Small Anim) 6*:26, 1991.
29. Withrow SJ: Use and misuse of full cerclage wires in fracture repair. *Vet Clin North Am 8*:201, 1978.
30. Withrow SJ: Vascular and bone response to full cerclage wires. *In* Bojrab MJ (ed): *Pathophysiology in Small Animal Surgery*. Lea & Febiger, Philadelphia, 1981, pp 869–871.
31. Withrow SJ, Holmberg DL: Use of full cerclage wires in the fixation of 18 consecutive long-bone fractures in small animals. *J Am Anim Hosp Assoc 13*:735, 1977.

CHAPTER

123

External Skeletal Fixation

General Principles

Erick L. Egger

External skeletal fixation is a means of stabilizing fractures or joints using percutaneous fixation pins that penetrate the bone cortices internally and are connected together externally to form an external frame. The device consists of pins and connecting elements to complete the frame (Fig. 123–1). It provides stable fixation of bone fragments with minimal additional damage to soft tissues and osseous vascularity while avoiding the need for implants in the fracture site or immobilization of adjacent joints. It is particularly useful in those open or highly comminuted fractures with poor circulation that require prolonged fixation. The low cost and reusability of many of the components are advantages for most practices and clients. Ease of application and a wide spectrum of indications make the fixator useful for veterinarians in general practice.

HISTORY AND DEVELOPMENT

Parkhill[36] first described the use of external skeletal fixation in humans in 1897. Lambotte[29] used a design similar to current devices in 1907. In the 1930s, Anderson, Hoffmann, and Stader (a veterinarian) developed the designs that are still the basis of many devices in use today.[21] Ehmer[18] modified a human design specifically for veterinary use in the late 1940s. During World War II, many external skeletal fixation splints were incorrectly applied to human casualties under battle conditions. A high incidence of pin tract infection and nonunion resulted.[40] Consequently, external skeletal fixation was discouraged as a form of fracture management until a rebirth of interest in the 1970s. Much effort is currently being devoted to improving both equipment and techniques of application.[1, 3, 20]

FIXATOR NOMENCLATURE AND CHARACTERISTICS

Nomenclature of the external fixation device is based on components used and their geometric arrangement.[21, 25]

Simple Fixators

The simplest fixators consist of relatively rigid fixation pins attached to longitudinal connecting bars or frames. Fixation pins that pass through one side of the limb and both bone cortices are called *half pins*. They can be connected together to form a type I (half-pin) splint. Type I configurations can be used on the humerus or femur to avoid interfering with the body wall. They can also be positioned to avoid soft-tissue injuries on the lower limbs. With proper application techniques, all fixation pins can be attached to a single connecting bar (Fig. 123–1). This type I single connecting bar configuration provides adequate stability for treating most relatively stable simple fractures in small animals.[7, 12] For large animals or less stable fractures, a second connecting bar can be added to the same fixation pins (Fig. 123–2), creating a double connecting bar configuration that nearly doubles the splint's resistance to compressive forces.[13] Two single connecting bar splints can be applied parallel to and at 60° to 90° of axial rotation to each other. The ends of the connecting bars are joined to form a triangular cross section. The resulting biplanar type I configuration (Fig. 123–3) is more resistant to craniocaudal bending forces than even full-pin uniplanar splints.[14] It can be applied to very proximal or distal fractures because its biplanar design allows an adequate number of fixation pins to obtain good stability. Double connecting clamps can be used with an additional connecting bar to bridge between two pin splints placed in each fragment. This double-clamp type I configuration (Fig. 123–4) is highly adjustable after placement. The double clamp itself is quite weak, resulting in minimal resistance to compressive forces.[7, 12] Consequently, its usefulness is limited to very rapidly healing fractures such as corrective osteotomies.

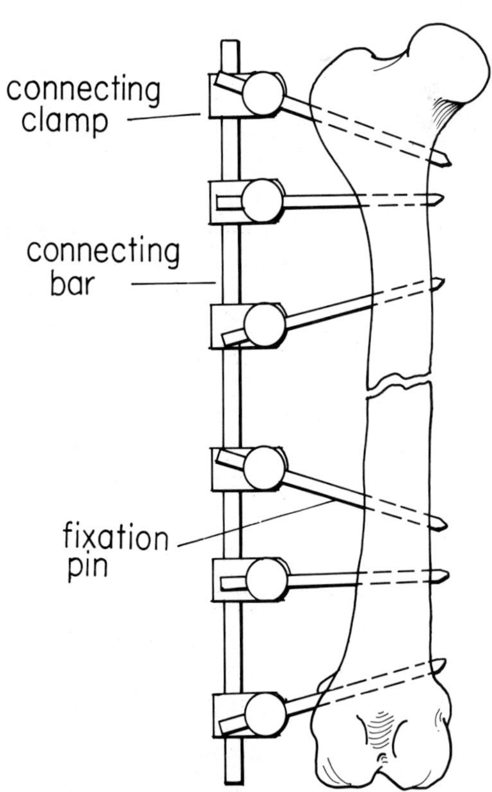

FIGURE 123–1. Components of an external fixation apparatus identified on a single connecting bar type I (half-pin or unilateral) configuration.

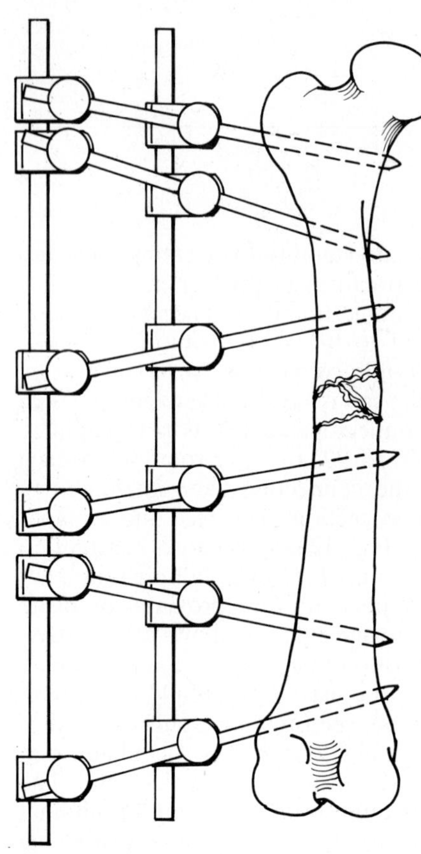

FIGURE 123–2. Double connecting bar type I configuration.

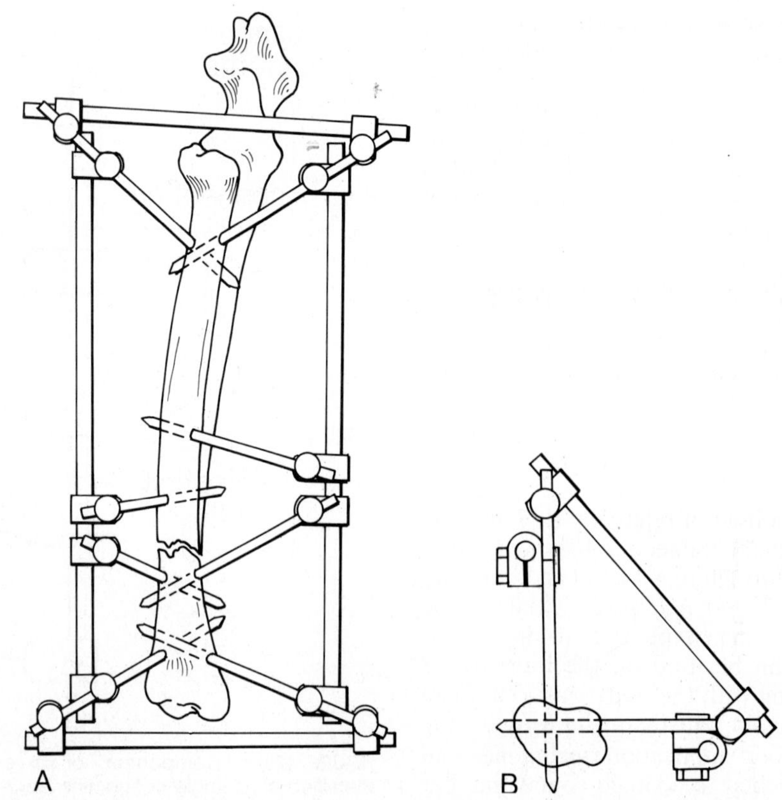

FIGURE 123–3. Biplanar type I configuration *A*, Frontal view. *B*, Cross-sectional view.

Fixation pins that pass through both sides of the limb and the bone are called *full pins*. The pins can be connected together to form a type II (full-pin) splint (Fig. 123–5). Type II configurations are very resistant to compressive forces.[7, 12] They can be used on relatively unstable fractures. To avoid interference with the body wall, they are limited to use below the elbow or the stifle.

Because it can be difficult to get all of the fixation pins to line up on both sides of the limb without a pin guide, many surgeons modify the type II splint by using only one full pin in each fragment with additional half pins for adequate stability (Fig. 123–6).

A type I and a type II splint can be combined to form a type III (trilateral) frame (Fig. 123–7). Type III configurations are the most rigid of currently used configurations and are roughly ten times more resistant to axial compression than type I splints.[12] Consequently, they are used for highly unstable or infected fractures, nonunions, and arthrodesis when prolonged rigid fixation is needed.

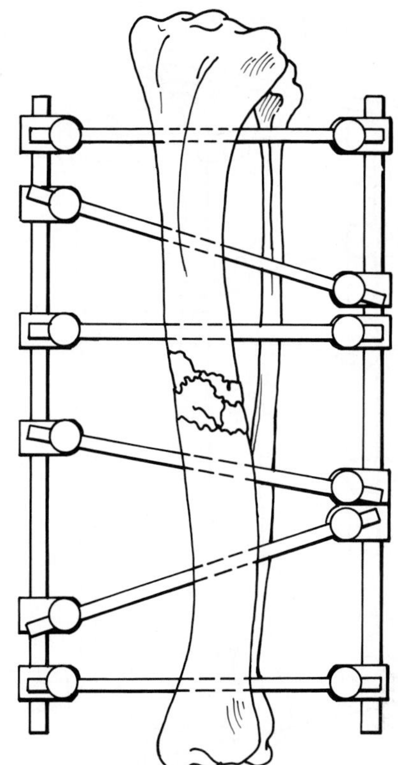

FIGURE 123–5. Type II (full-pin or bilateral) configuration.

Circular Fixation (see Chapter 123B)

Circular (ring) fixators use small-diameter flexible Kirschner wires instead of rigid fixation pins. These wires are driven through the bone fragments at perpendicular angles and attached under tension to rigid rings. The rings are then connected together with three adjustable longitudinal rods (Fig. 123–8). Circular fixators

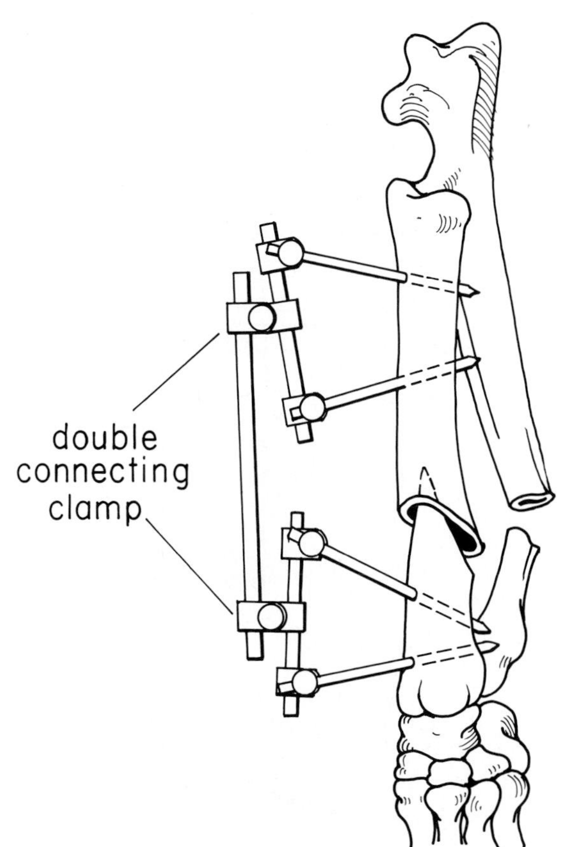

FIGURE 123–4. Double-clamp type I configuration.

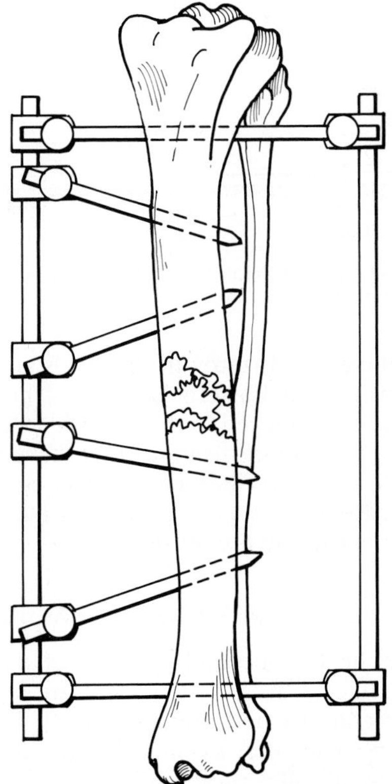

FIGURE 123–6. Modified type II configuration, in which only two fixation pins are applied as full pins, making application easier.

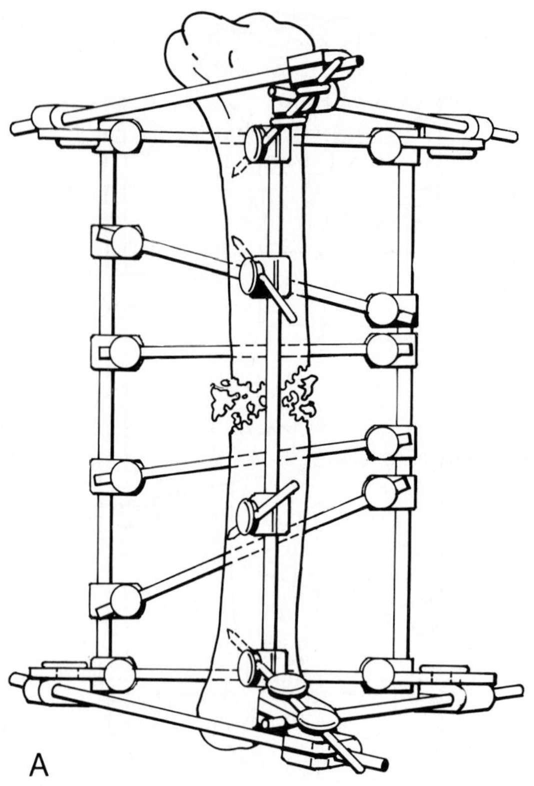

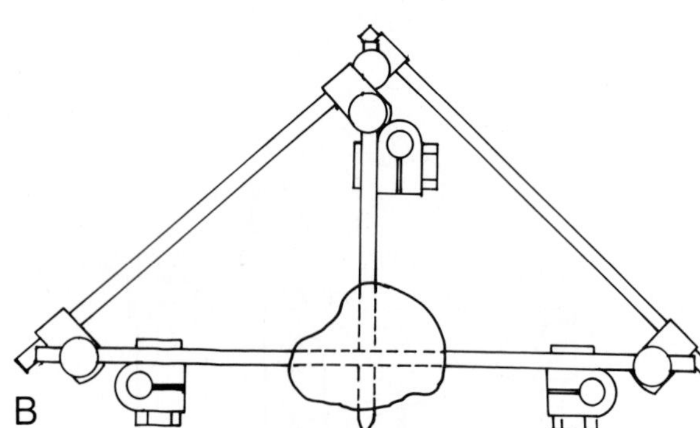

FIGURE 123–7. Type III (trilateral configuration. *A*, Frontal view. *B*, Cross-sectional view.

were developed by Ilizarov in the 1940s and have been used extensively in Eastern Europe.[21] They have only recently been introduced to the English-speaking world. In addition to fracture fixation, they have great application potential for limb lengthening and deformity correction. Reports of veterinary application are beginning to appear in the literature.[30]

FRACTURE HEALING WITH EXTERNAL FIXATION

Fracture healing depends on the character of the fracture itself and the rigidity of fracture fixation. Generally, a fracture treated with a relatively flexible fixator that allows some interfragmentary motion heals with more periosteal callus proliferation.[46] One millimeter of induced axial micromotion improved the healing of ovine tibial osteotomies.[19] Conversely, a well-reduced fracture stabilized with very rigid fixation often heals with direct crossing of the fracture by osteons and little periosteal callus formation. Many studies have shown this pattern of healing results in faster return of strength.[31, 38, 45, 46] No single best method of fracture healing exists for all fractures. The ease with which the rigidity of external skeletal fixation can be adjusted allows a clinician to manipulate the mechanical environment that directs this healing process.

The current trend in human orthopedics is toward some degree of interfragmentary motion or loading.[24] One such strategy (called *dynamization*) involves modification of an initially rigid frame to allow axial compressive loading of the fracture with physiological weightbearing once early healing has occurred.[11] This enhances hypertrophy and remodeling of the fracture while providing protection from excessive stress that might cause refracture. This concept is most useful in those unstable fractures that initially require rigid fixation to maintain reduction. Around 6 weeks after surgery is the optimal time for dynamization of fractures in dogs,[16, 17] removing the connecting bars and pins from one side of a type II or type III splint or removing alternate fixation pins of a type I splint.

The rate of fracture healing is variable. A simple fracture in a young dog commonly heals in 6 weeks, whereas a complex comminuted fracture in a mature dog may require as long as 6 months or more. Loss of sharpness in detail of the fracture edges is the earliest sign of fracture healing. Clinical healing is determined by the loss of discernible fracture lines and the development of bony continuity in at least three of four cortices on two radiographic views.

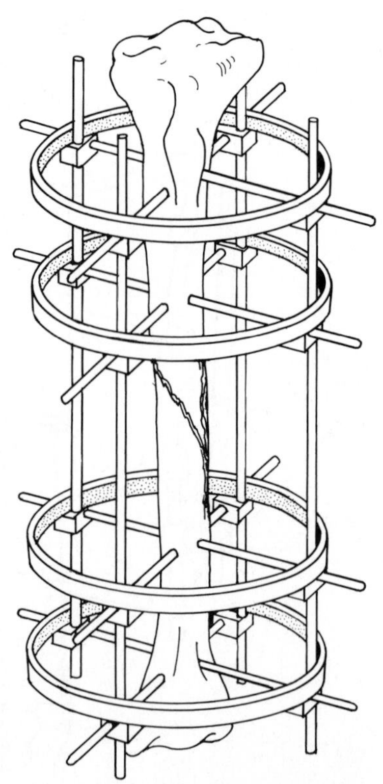

FIGURE 123–8. Circular or ring fixator as developed by Ilizarov.

EXTERNAL FIXATION DEVICES AND EQUIPMENT

The most common external skeletal fixation device used in veterinary orthopedics is manufactured by Kirschner Medical Company.* Three sizes are useful for small animal application (Fig. 123–9). The small apparatus is appropriate for use on cats, dogs up to approximately 8 to 10 kg, some exotic pets, and raptors. The medium apparatus is the most commonly used and is appropriate for most dogs. The large apparatus has been redesigned based on the human tibial frame. It is useful on large dogs and other larger animals. The basis of the apparatus is the connecting clamp that holds the fixation pin to the connecting bar. The clamps are expensive but are manufactured of stainless steel and are reusable. Connecting bars must be the correct diameter (1/8 inch, small; 3/16 inch, medium; 5/16 inch, large) for the clamp. The clamps allow for variation in fixation pin size. The small device uses 3/32 inch or smaller, medium uses 1/8 inch or smaller, and large uses 5/32 inch or smaller diameter fixation pins. Threaded fixation pins are available in those sizes; however, nonthreaded pins are more economically created by using double-pointed Steinmann pins cut in two. We prefer to use a low-speed power drill for pin insertion. A variable-speed 3/8-inch electric drill with a cord works well but requires gas sterilization. Extended chucks and drill shrouds that can be autoclaved are available for rechargeable drills and can be obtained at moderate cost.† A nut wrench (both open ended and spin tite are useful) and pin cutter are needed for application of a Kirschner apparatus. Human external fixator systems can be applied to large veterinary patients,[35] but their expense precludes widespread veterinary use.

Another form of external fixation that was originally described for use in treating human mandibular fractures[33] and is being increasingly used for veterinary patients[23, 41] replaces the connecting bar and clamps with a column of methyl methacrylate. This is commonly known as an *acrylic-pin splint* (Fig. 123–10). The strength and stiffness of these splints directly depend on the diameter of the acrylic column. For all described configurations, an acrylic column diameter of 3/4 inch provides at least as much support as the standard medium (3/16-inch-diameter steel connecting bar) Kirschner apparatus.[44] Methacrylate is available as dental molding acrylic (1 pound makes at least ten splints).

*Kirschner Medical Co., Timonium, MD.
†Animal Clinic Products, Montgomery, AL.

PRINCIPLES OF APPLICATION

External skeletal fixation is easy to use, but close adherence to several principles improves results and reduces postoperative problems.

One of the most important advantages of external skeletal fixation is that it can be applied with little additional damage to vascularity and the healing process. Closed reduction of the fracture minimizes such damage. Closed reduction may not provide adequate fracture reduction or alignment, particularly with complex fractures or fractures located proximal to the elbow or stifle joint. Delayed union, nonunion, or malunion can result.[28] I prefer a limited open approach for better fracture alignment and reduction. A limited open approach also allows placement of autogenous cancellous bone graft into fracture defects. This graft is usually collected from the fractured limb, using the craniolateral humeral greater tubercle for forelimb fractures and the medial aspect of the proximal tibia for hindlimb fractures.

External fixation is only as effective as the pin contact with bone.[10] Because premature loosening of fixation pins is the most common cause of postoperative problems and even fixation failure,[2, 20] attention to pin design and application is essential. Both clinically and experimentally, threaded pins offer a firm grip on bone[2, 3] and increase stiffness of the fixator.[5] Threaded pins used in veterinary medicine are manufactured by cutting threads

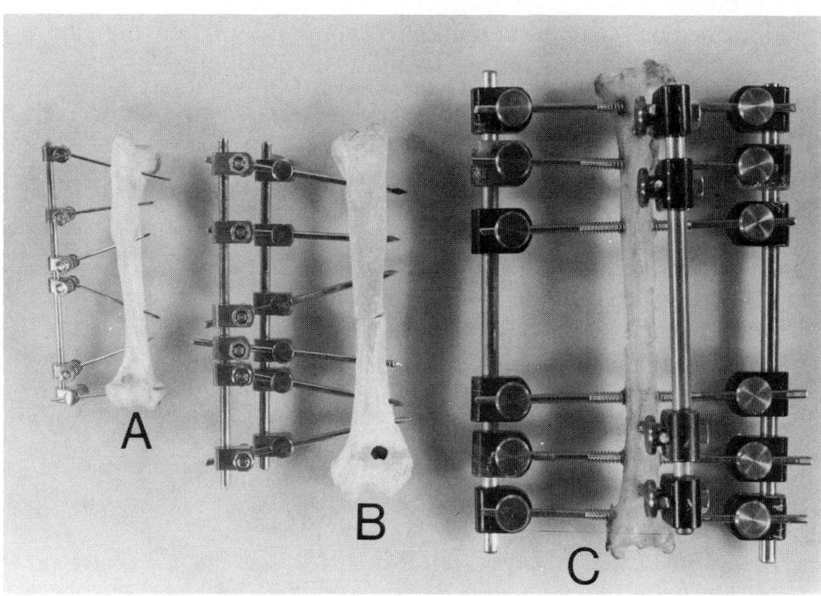

FIGURE 123–9. Small (*A*), medium (*B*), and large (*C*) Kirschner apparatus.

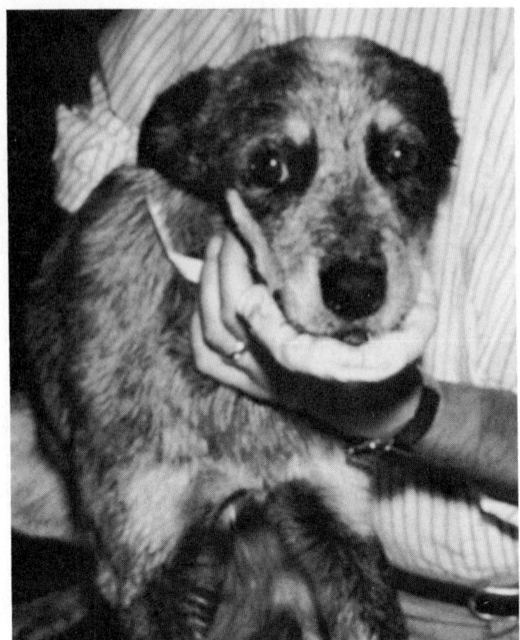

FIGURE 123–10. Acrylic-pin fixator applied to mandibular fracture.

into the shaft, resulting in a decreased core diameter. Consequently, these pins have a tendency to break or bend at the junction of the threaded and nonthreaded shaft.[3] A new half-pin design (sold by Kirschner* as the Ellis pin) (Fig. 123–11), which is threaded only far enough to engage the far cortex, offers five to seven times the resistance to pullout of nonthreaded pins while maintaining all of their resistance to bending[3] and is about twice the cost of nonthreaded pins. Alternatively, pins with enhanced threads "raised" over a constant shaft diameter (Turner half pins and Bonnell full pins†) have excellent pullout resistance and bending strength (Fig. 123–12). They are expensive (at least five times the cost of nonthreaded pins owing to the complicated manufacturing process) and often require predrilling a pilot hole.[2] Consequently, I often use one of these raised-thread pins in each fragment, with the balance nonthreaded or Ellis pins to reduce costs.

The diameter of the fixation pins is based on the diameter of the bone. If the pin diameter is too small, the pins are too flexible and allow excessive motion with potential loss of fracture reduction. If the pin diameter is too large, the bone is weakened and pin hole fracture may result.[8] A pin diameter about 20 percent of the bone diameter is usually suitable.

The method of pin insertion is important. In the past, hand-chuck placement has been advocated to avoid thermal necrosis of bone due to frictional heat.[2, 6, 32] Wobbling with a hand chuck can result in oversized pin holes and pin loosening. Furthermore, hand placement in cortical bone is hard work, commonly resulting in less than the optimal number of pins being used. Direct power insertion is preferable. Direct slow-speed (150 rpm or less) power drill placement does not result in significant temperature elevation or premature pin loosening in canine diaphyseal bone.[15] Excess pressure and high speed are avoided. Predrilling the pin hole with a slightly smaller twist bit (about 90 percent pin diameter) is a commonly accepted technique in human orthopedics and might be considered in very dense bone such as the olecranon.[2]

Before pins are placed, the fracture is approximately reduced so excessive skin tension does not develop against the pins when final reduction is achieved. When pins are inserted, they are placed through small separate skin incisions. This method decreases the tendency for soft tissues to wrap up around the rotating pin and reduces the incidence of skin necrosis. The pins are not placed through the approach incisions because that makes closure difficult. When possible, the fixation pins should not penetrate large muscle masses and areas of extensive soft-tissue motion because this is a common cause of poor postoperative limb use and serum drainage from the pin tract. The pins are placed through the widest diameter of the bone to provide the most strength and to avoid cracking the bone. Even when applying a half-pin splint, the pins are driven so the tip completely penetrates the far cortex. The triangular shape of the pin tip makes incompletely penetrating pins loosen.

If nonthreaded pins are used, they are placed at a divergent angle to each other to maintain a mechanical grip on bone. An angle of 30° to 40° between the outermost pins placed in each fragment offers the best compromise between pin strength and bone grip.[9]

The number of pins placed in each fragment affects the stiffness of the fixator. Mechanical studies on a type II fixator found that increasing from two to three pins per fragment resulted in a 66 percent increase in axial stiffness, and increasing to four pins per fragment resulted in an additional 33 percent increase.[5] Using more than four pins per fragment had relatively little effect on stiffness.

Increasing the number of pins avoids overloading the bone surrounding each pin.[9] Overloading causes microfractures, and the subsequent bone resorption results in premature pin loosening. A minimum of three and

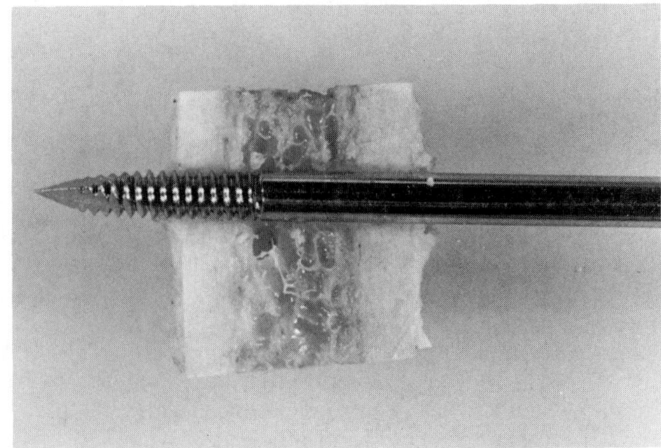

FIGURE 123–11. Ellis pin with its short threaded portion places the stress riser junction within the protected medullary canal.

*Kirschner Medical Co, Timonium, MD.
†Zimmer, Warsaw, IN.

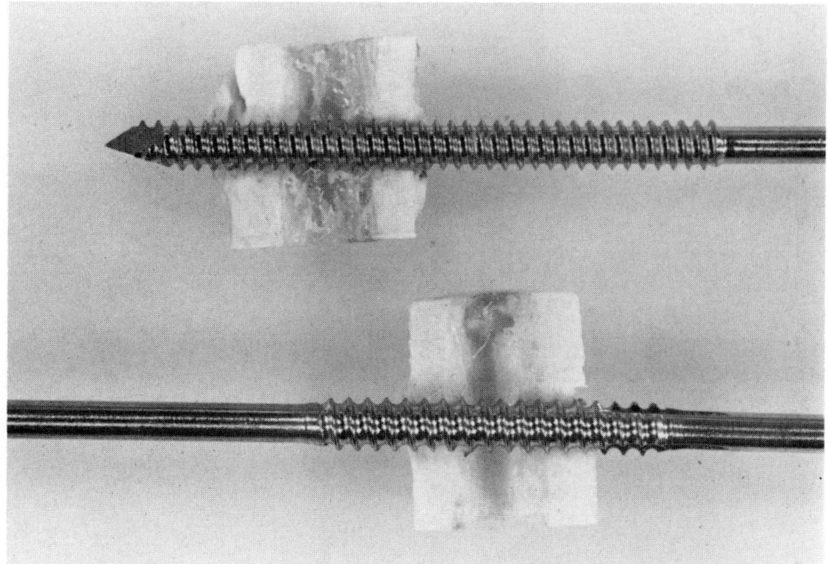

FIGURE 123–12. Raised thread pin designs (Turner half pin and Bonnell full pin) offer enhanced bone holding and maximum bending strength.

preferably four pins on each side of a fracture is preferable. These pins are best spread over the length of the fractured bone to distribute the disruptive forces and maintain maximum fixator strength.[39]

In oblique and comminuted fractures, interfragmentary fixation such as lag screws and cerclage wires can be used to improve reduction. The manipulation required to apply these devices may damage vascularity and retard healing. In addition, rigid interfragmentary devices are not used with a flexible frame configuration, because they concentrate stress,[22] causing further fragmentation of the fracture. I prefer divergent Kirschner wires (Fig. 123–13). These wires can be applied with minimal additional soft-tissue damage, and they provide adequate stabilization without the stress-concentrating effect.

As the frame is constructed, the positioning of the connecting bar must be considered. Some distance must be left between the skin and the bar to allow for swelling and callus formation without encroachment of skin on the clamps. Increasing this distance significantly reduces the stiffness and strength of the frame. A good compromise is about 2 to 3 cm for a medium-sized dog.[1] This distance is scaled to the size of the patient and the location of the device.

GENERAL PROCEDURE FOR FIXATOR APPLICATION

1. Fracture is approximately reduced by either closed manipulation or through a limited open approach minimizing soft-tissue damage.
2. The most proximal and distal fixation pins are driven through small skin incisions into the two fragments at appropriate angles (Fig. 123–14 *A*).
3. Connecting clamps and a connecting bar are slid onto the end pins, with the anticipated number of "open" clamps in the middle (Fig. 123–14*B*).
4. The fracture is reduced. With an open approach, bone clamps facilitate manipulation and reduction. In selected comminuted or oblique fractures, interfragmentary fixation may be used to hold fragments in place.
5. The connecting bar is positioned far enough from the body to allow for swelling and callus formation

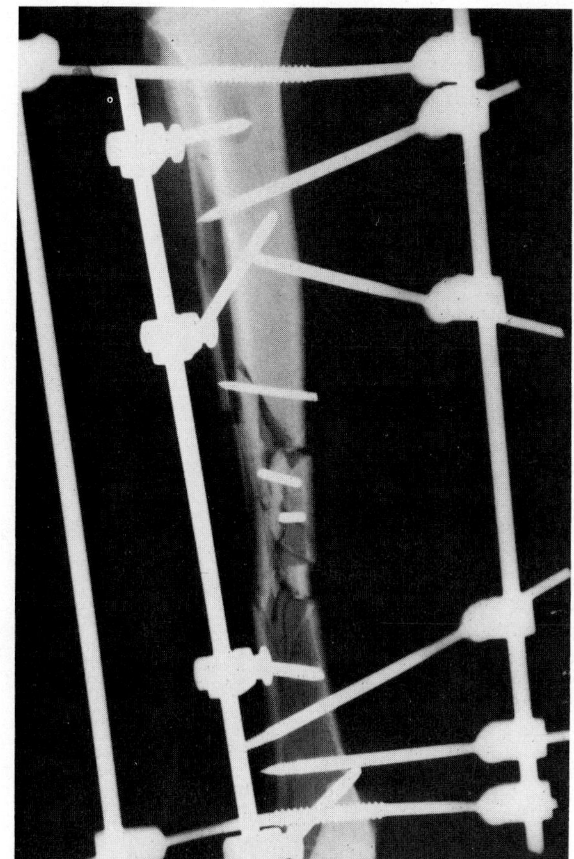

FIGURE 123–13. Divergent Kirschner wires used to maintain interfragmentary reduction.

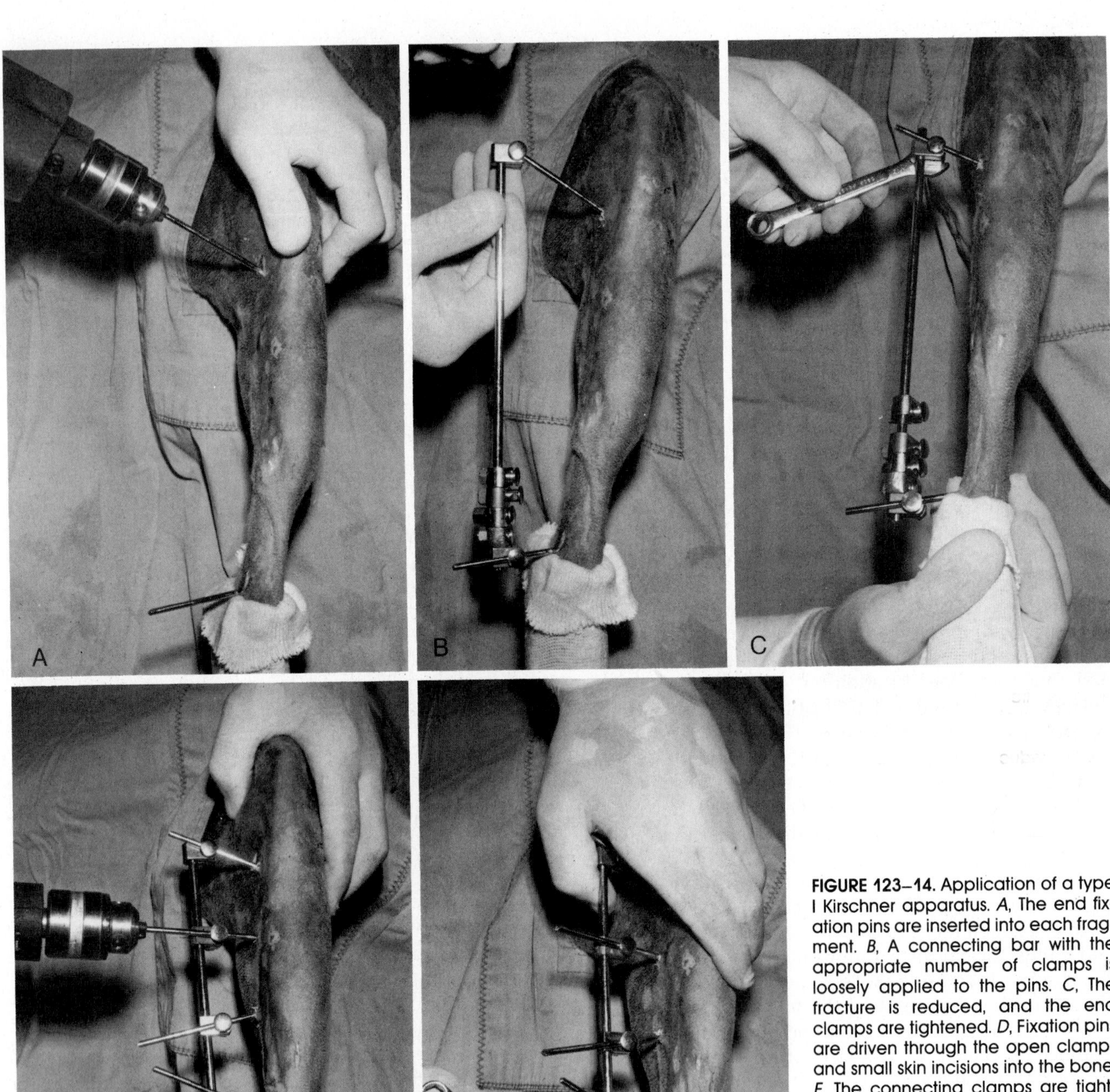

FIGURE 123–14. Application of a type I Kirschner apparatus. *A*, The end fixation pins are inserted into each fragment. *B*, A connecting bar with the appropriate number of clamps is loosely applied to the pins. *C*, The fracture is reduced, and the end clamps are tightened. *D*, Fixation pins are driven through the open clamps and small skin incisions into the bone. *E*, The connecting clamps are tightened as each pin is driven.

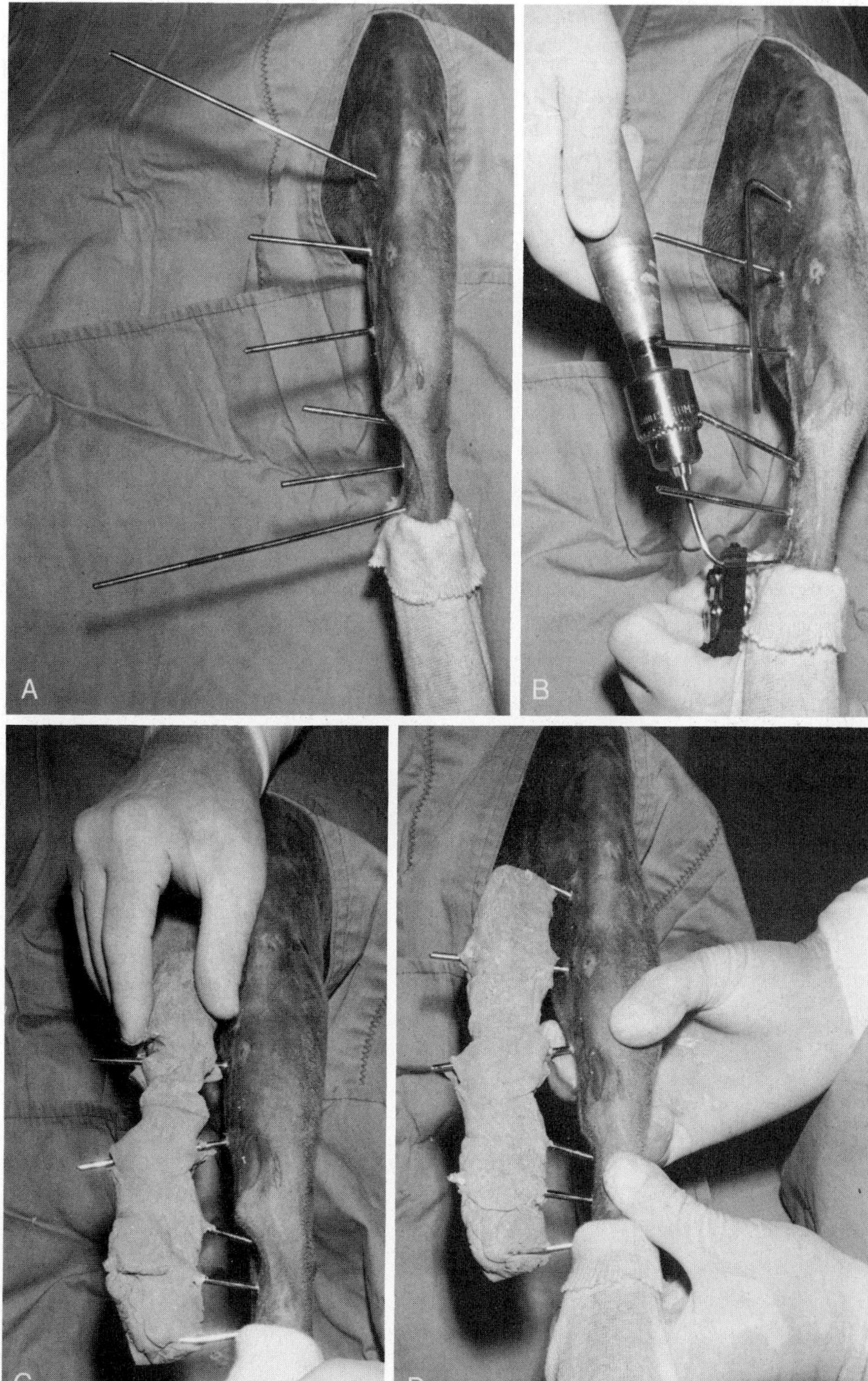

FIGURE 123–15. Application of an acrylic-pin splint with closed reduction. *A*, Fixation pins are inserted at divergent angles. *B*, Several of the pins are bent to lie parallel to the bone. *C*, Acrylic is molded to form a connecting column incorporating all pins. *D*, Fracture is reduced and held until acrylic sets.

without encroachment of the skin on the clamps, and the end clamps are tightened (Fig. 123–14*C*).

6. If a more rigid configuration is required, a second connecting bar can be "stacked" on top of the first to create a double connecting bar type I half-pin splint. Distal to the elbow or stifle, the second bar can be added to the opposite end of full pins to form a type II configuration.

7. The remaining fixation pins are driven through the open clamps at appropriate angles (Fig. 123–14*D*).

8. The clamps are tightened as each pin is placed (Fig. 123–14*E*).

9. If desired, a second half-pin splint is applied at roughly 90° axial rotation to the first to create a biplanar configuration.

10. With an open approach, the fracture site is thoroughly lavaged and an autogenous cancellous bone graft is inserted in any remaining fracture defects. The approach incision is closed or, if indicated, packed open to heal by second intention or until delayed closure is desired.

11. Excessive fixation pin length is removed with a pin cutter.

12. Postoperative radiographs are always taken to assess fracture reduction and fixation.

TECHNIQUE FOR ACRYLIC-PIN SPLINT APPLICATION

To create an acrylic-pin splint, the appropriate number of fixation pins are inserted in the fragments as previously described (Fig. 123–15*A*). They are not required to be in planar alignment. One or more of the pins are bent to lie parallel with the bone an appropriate distance (usually 3 to 4 cm) from the skin (Fig. 123–15*B*). For application after closed reduction, the nonsterile methyl methacrylate (dental molding* or hoof repair†) acrylic is mixed until it becomes doughy (3 to 4 minutes). The acrylic is molded to form a connecting column incorporating all pins (Fig. 123–15*C*). The fracture is then reduced and held until the acrylic sets (8 to 10 minutes) (Fig. 123–15*D*). With open reduction, the fracture is temporarily stabilized with connecting clamps and bars placed farther away from the skin on a few of the pins (Fig. 123–16*A*). The approach incision can be closed and the fracture radiographed to ensure adequate reduction. The acrylic is mixed and molded to the pins as before (Fig. 123–16*B*). Once the methacrylate has set, the connecting clamps, bar, and excessive fixation pin length can be removed (Fig. 123–16*C*). Alternatively, sterile methyl methacrylate (bone cement)‡ can be used with an open approach, negating the need for the temporary connecting clamps and bars. Sterile bone cement is used for implanting total joint replacements. Two or three packs may be needed for some fractures. Alternatively, commercial kits for creating acrylic-pin external fixation have been developed comparable to the small and medium Kirschner apparatus.§

*Orthodonic Resin, L. D. Caulk Co., Milford, DE.
†Technovit, Jorgensen Labs, Loveland, CO.
‡Simplex P, Howmedica, Rutherford, NJ.
§APEF System, Ganthier Medical Inc., Rochester, MN.

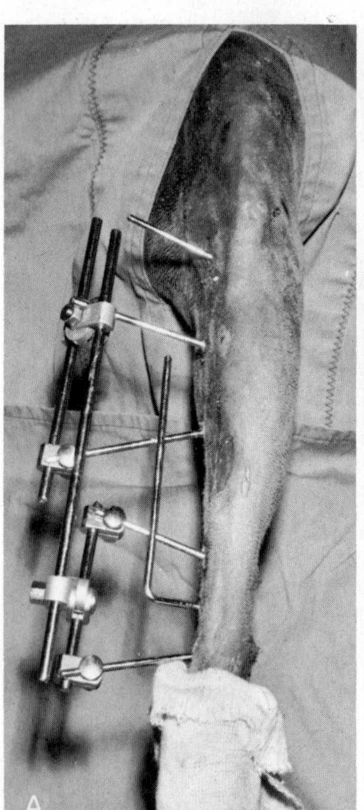

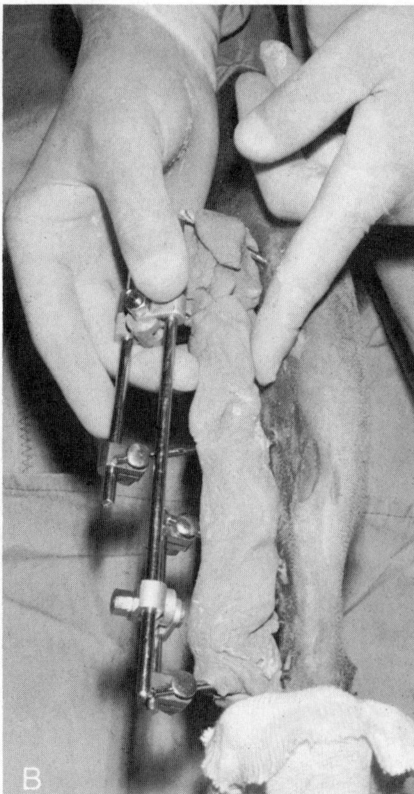

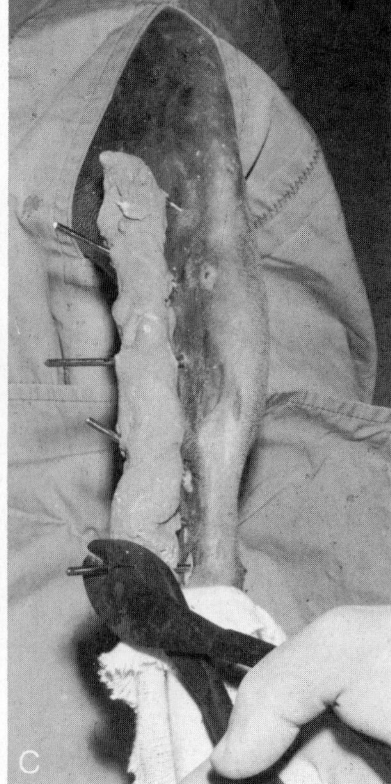

FIGURE 123–16. Application of an acrylic-pin splint with an open approach. *A*, Reduction is temporarily stabilized using connecting clamps with connecting clamps and bars placed farther away from the body. *B*, Acrylic is molded to form the connecting column. *C*, Once acrylic has set, the clamps, bars, and excess pins are removed.

ORIENTATION OF EXTERNAL FIXATORS ON SPECIFIC LONG BONES

Humerus. Application of external skeletal fixation to the humerus usually requires a minimal open approach for adequate reduction. Type I splints are usually oriented laterally, with the proximal pins placed cranial to the deltoid muscle while the distal pins can be placed through the condyle, avoiding the supracondylar foramen and the radial nerve. Biplanar type I splints are oriented cranially and laterally.

Radius. The radius can be stabilized with external skeletal fixation after either open or closed reduction. Uniplanar type I splints are usually oriented laterally for proximal fractures, cranially for small bones, or medially for distal fractures, although any of these orientations are acceptable to avoid penetrating and interfering with soft-tissue injuries. Biplanar type I splints are oriented cranially and laterally for proximal fractures or cranially and medially for distal fractures. Type II splints are usually applied from medial to lateral.

Femur. Femoral fractures require an open approach to obtain adequate reduction. Only type I uniplanar splints applied from the lateral aspect are used to avoid muscle entrapment and stifle joint stiffening. A second connecting bar can be applied to the half pins if needed for fixator strength.

Tibia. Tibial fractures can be reduced using open or closed methods. Uniplanar type I splints are best applied from the medial aspect to minimize soft-tissue penetration but can be applied either cranially or laterally if necessary to avoid soft-tissue wounds. Type II splints are placed from medial to lateral. Biplanar type I or type III splints use cranially and medially or laterally oriented pins. Proximal pins are placed in the wider and stronger caudal aspect of the tibia.

INDICATIONS FOR CLINICAL USE OF EXTERNAL FIXATION

Adjuncts to Other Internal Fixation

External skeletal fixation may be used for ancillary support of other forms of internal fixation. It can be effective in controlling axial rotation and, to some degree, axial collapse of the fracture site when used with intramedullary pins. A two-pin type I splint has traditionally been used for this purpose,[6] although my experience suggests that using three pins significantly decreases the incidence of premature pin loosening and loss of fixation. This supplementary fixation can usually be removed in 3 to 5 weeks, when the callus becomes sufficiently organized to control rotation.

Simple Fractures

Although simple fractures can be treated with many techniques, external fixation may be a wise choice in certain instances. A patient with multiple fractures becomes ambulatory much faster than with coaptation. The ease of implant removal and ability to avoid stress protection allow faster return to athletic function than does plating.

Comminuted Fractures

Severely comminuted fractures may be treated with external fixation when more exacting reconstruction is impossible (Fig. 123–17). External fixation requires minimal bone for fixation and can span large defects. Care is taken to avoid damage to osseous vascularity, because healing relies on early callus formation. Consequently, a closed reduction or limited open reduction with massive cancellous bone autograft is necessary. Overall joint alignment but not necessarily perfect fracture reduction is sought. A relatively rigid configuration is initially applied to neutralize disruptive forces. Dynamization after early fracture healing has occurred (6 to 10 weeks) is considered to enhance callus hypertrophy and remodeling.

Open, Gunshot, and Infected Fractures

External fixation has the advantage of not invading the fracture site and spreading contamination or infection. The fixation pins can usually be applied away from the affected area, lessening the chance of premature bone lysis and early implant failure, which could result in nonunion. External fixation is particularly useful for stabilizing severe open-wound fractures because it supports the fracture and soft-tissue vascularity while preserving access to the traumatized area for continued treatment. Gunshot-induced fractures often combine the problems of severe comminution and bone loss with significant contamination and severe soft-tissue vascular damage (Fig. 123–18). Moderate débridement followed by rigid external fixation, cancellous bone autografting, and packing the wound open is indicated. Repeated débridement may be required every 2 to 4 days as the healing process delineates viable from necrotic tissue. Treatment of fractures with established infections requires removal of unstable hardware, sequestra (necrotic, infected bone fragments), and infected proliferative scar tissue. Rigid external fixation to allow revascularization is applied, avoiding the infected wound as much as possible. The wound is thoroughly lavaged and packed open to allow repeated lavage and débridement. Cancellous grafting may be delayed for 10 to 14 days to allow granulation tissue to cover the fracture ends and provide vascularity for the graft.

Mandibular Fractures

External fixation has the advantage of being able to avoid the placement of implants in open wounds and infected alveolar sockets. Mandibular fractures are often comminuted and open into the mouth.[43] The use of external fixation allows preservation of remaining vascular supply to the multiple small fragments. An acrylic-pin splint works well, particularly for bilateral mandibular fractures (see Chapter 142).

Nonunions

Nonunions can be described as hypertrophic or atrophic. In hypertrophic nonunions, the bone is capable

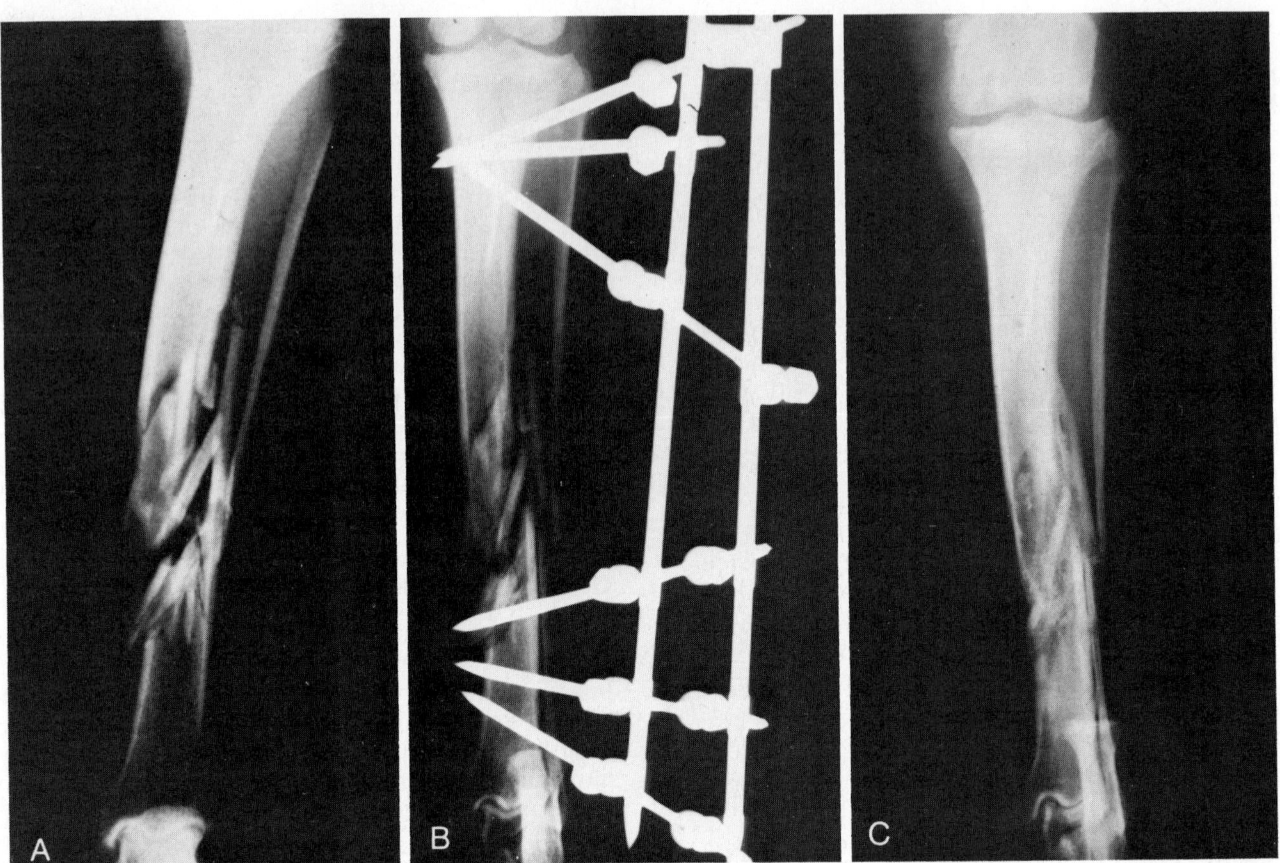

FIGURE 123–17. Severely comminuted tibial fracture in a large dog. *A*, Preoperative radiograph. *B*, Postoperative appearance with double connecting bar type I fixator. *C*, Final radiographic appearance 20 weeks after fracture and 6 weeks after fixator removal.

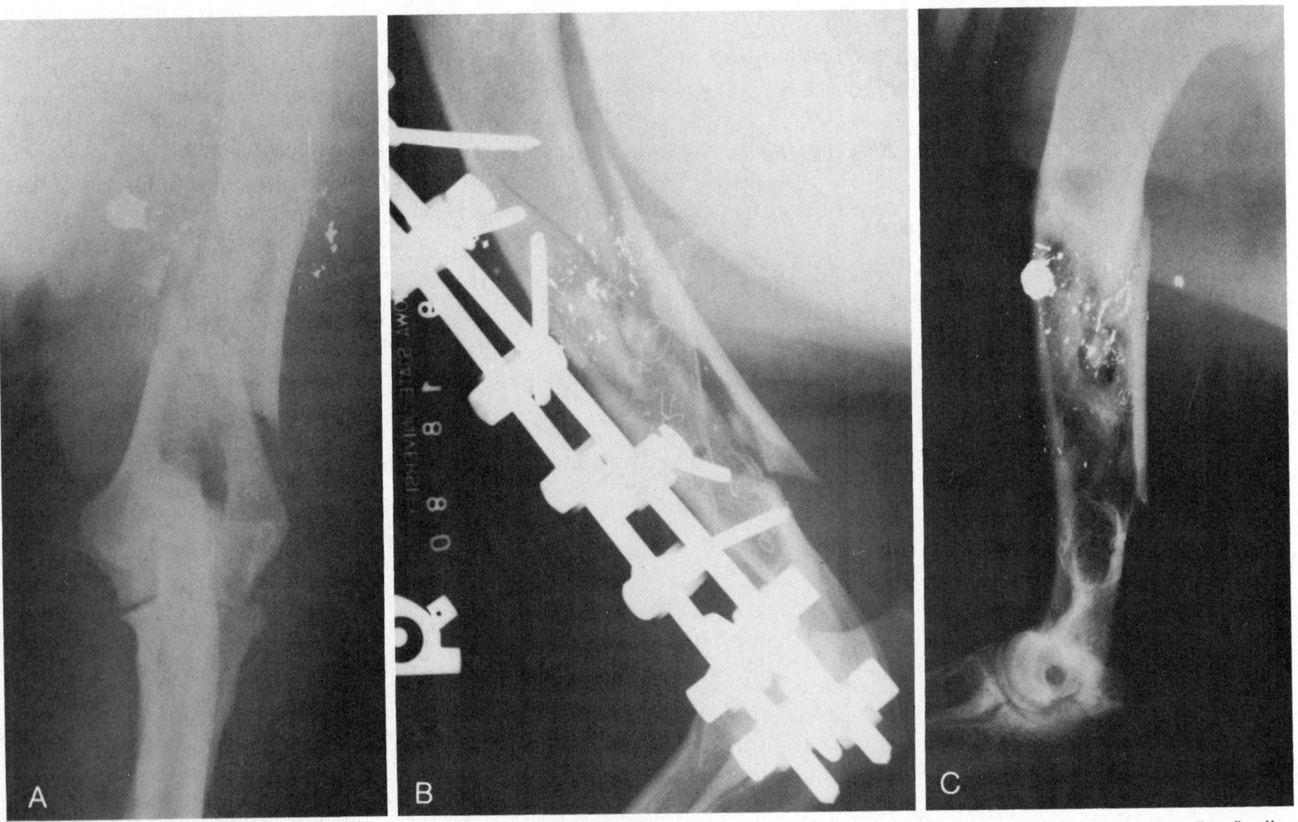

FIGURE 123–18. Distal humeral gunshot fracture in an Irish setter. *A*, Preoperative appearance. *B*, Postoperative radiograph after fixation. *C*, Final appearance 24 weeks after fracture and 8 weeks after fixator removal.

of biological reaction (healing) when the proper environment exists. Stabilization is all that is usually necessary and can be provided with reduction and application of rigid fixation (Fig. 123–19). Atrophic nonunions have lost the capacity of biological reaction. This type is most commonly encountered in fractures of hypovascular areas, such as distal radius and ulna, in miniature breeds that have poor leg use when treated with external coaptation or when a previous operation has resulted in loss of fragment vascularity and fracture stability. Treatment requires open reduction, removal of unstable hardware, decortication of avascular bone, opening of the medullary canal, and packing with cancellous bone graft to stimulate vascular proliferation and callus production. External fixation can be used to provide necessary stabilization while allowing the bone-stimulating stress of weightbearing.

Transarticular Stabilization

External fixation is being increasingly used for transarticular stabilization. It is ideal for cases of ligamentous rupture associated with adjacent soft-tissue injury. The ligament may be repaired or replaced with a prosthesis and protected by the external fixator while treatment of the open wound continues (Fig. 123–20). The connecting bars can be bent to the desired joint angle to facilitate fixator application and minimize frame bulk.[4, 34, 42] The fixation is usually maintained for 3 to 6 weeks, depending on severity of injury. Range of motion exercises are recommended to restore joint motion after fixator removal.

Transarticular external fixation may be used to help protect articular or periarticular fractures from weightbearing forces. Note that intra-articular fractures require anatomical reduction and fixation with an interfragmentary compression device such as a lag screw to avoid degenerative joint changes. Because of their metaphyseal location, such fractures heal quickly, so the transarticular portion of the fixator can usually be removed after 4 to 8 weeks. Physical therapy is needed to attain maximum joint function. External fixation may also be used for arthrodesis of certain joints. It is especially useful in cases with severe soft-tissue damage or infection, when the use of internal fixation would be less desirable. The principles of arthrodesis are followed: removal of articular cartilage, cancellous bone grafting, and prolonged fixation requiring multiple pins and a rigid configuration.

Growth Deformities

External fixation is a very effective means of treating growth deformities, particularly of the radius and ulna. To correct an angular deformity in a mature dog, oblique osteotomies of the deformed bones are performed at the level of greatest deviation.[6] The tip of the distal segment is impacted into the medullary cavity of the proximal segment to provide additional stability. The external fixator is applied (a full-pin configuration) and adjusted until adequate correction is obtained. A distraction splint can be used in the dynamic treatment of a progressive growth deformity. The circular fixators

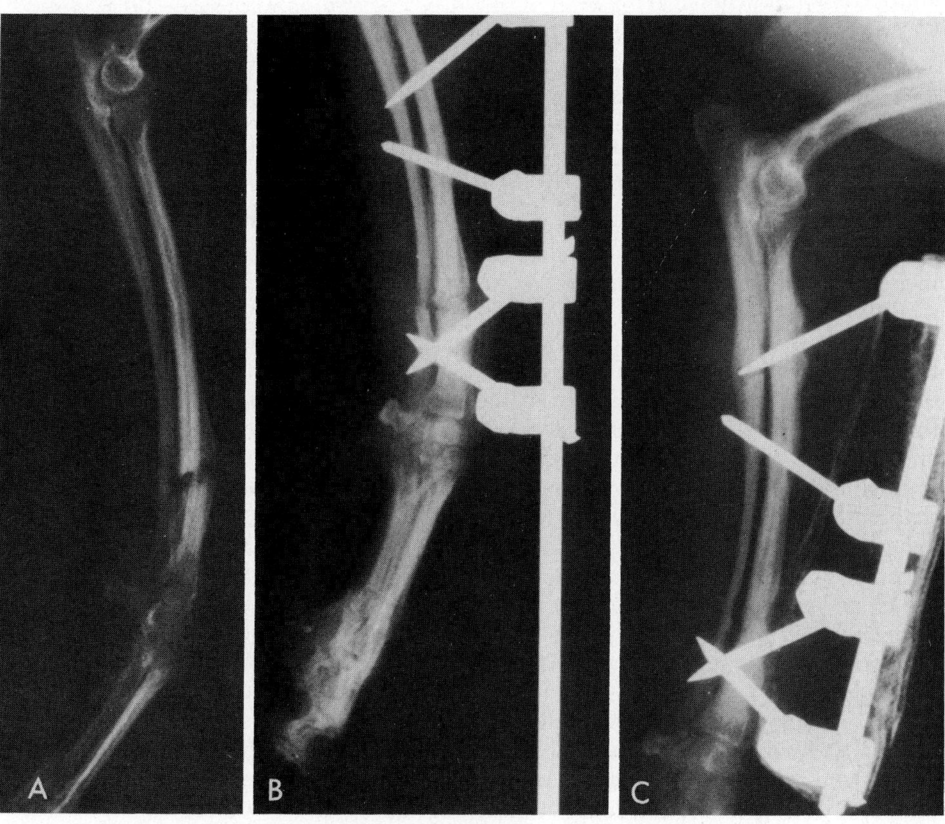

FIGURE 123–19. Distal radial and ulnar fracture in a Yorkshire terrier that had been treated with a cast for 4 weeks. *A*, Preoperative radiograph showing the periosteal proliferation denoting hypertrophic nonunion. *B*, Postoperative appearance after application of a type I fixator. *C*, Radiograph demonstrating solid healing eight weeks after surgery. (From Whittick WG: Canine Orthopedics. 2nd ed. Lea & Febiger, Philadelphia, 1990. Reprinted with permission.)

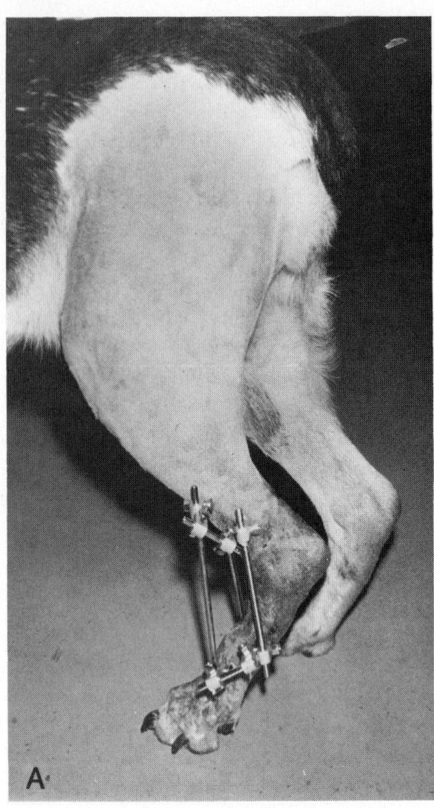

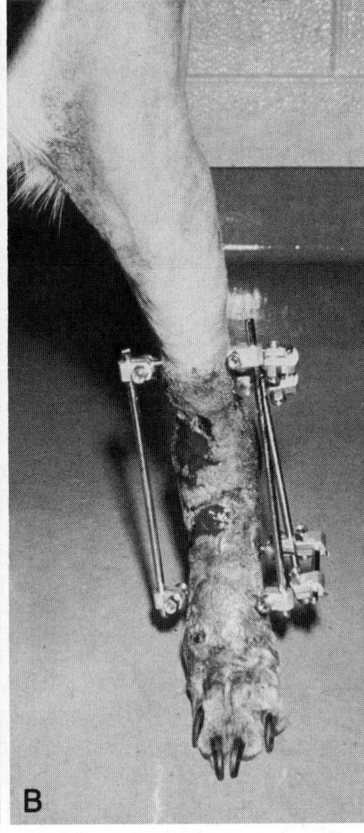

FIGURE 123–20. *A* and *B*, Transarticular fixator supporting soft-tissue repair of tibial tarsal avulsion injury. (From Whittick WG: Canine Orthopedics. 2nd ed. Lea & Febiger, Philadelphia, 1990. Reprinted with permission.)

(Ilizarov) have potential here.[26] The prematurely fused bone is surgically osteotomized, and external fixation is applied. After a lag phase of 4 to 7 days, the fixator is elongated daily. Research suggests a distraction rate of 1 mm/day divided into 0.5-mm increments every 12 hours results in primary bone regeneration[27] (see Chapter 123B).

POSTOPERATIVE MANAGEMENT OF EXTERNAL FIXATION

Hospital Care

After surgery, long-bone fractures are placed in a compressive (Robert Jones) bandage to protect the incision and minimize swelling. Any open wounds or incisions are covered with a sterile nonadherent dressing, and roll cotton or cast padding is packed around the pins and under connecting bars. Additional cotton or padding is rolled on the leg from the toes to above the injury. The padding is compressed with elastic gauze and fixed with tape. In most cases, this bandage is removed after 2 to 5 days. With open fractures or with severe soft-tissue injury, the wound is often débrided, lavaged, and rebandaged every 2 to 3 days until it is covered with granulation tissue. Because of the stability the fixator provides, such frequent bandage changes can be performed without traumatizing early vascular proliferation and callus formation. When the compressive bandage is no longer necessary, it is replaced with a gauze and tape cover that envelopes the connecting clamps and bars of the fixator. This cover protects the animal and the owner from the sharp ends of the fixation pins and decreases the incidence of catching the apparatus on fixed objects (Fig. 123–21). The cover is applied so it does not contact the skin but allows air circulation around the skin–pin interface. The use of antibiotics with external fixation is still controversial.[37] Broad-spectrum antibiotics are indicated for contaminated open or infected fractures until culture and sensitivity testing can direct more specific therapy. Furthermore, because of the soft-tissue trauma attending even most closed fractures, a broad-spectrum antibiotic for 4 to 7 days after surgery is recommended until the body defenses are mobilized.

Home Care and Follow-up

Most animals treated with external fixation can be released to the owner within 2 to 4 days after surgery. The animal is released with instructions to limit exercise to leash walking and to take particular care to avoid fences or other similar open structures that might catch the apparatus. The apparatus is protected with a tape cover until the device is removed. The owners are instructed to inspect the apparatus daily and are advised to expect a small amount of dry crust to develop at the skin–pin interface. Although a great diversity of opinion exists about proper pin care,[1, 37] I advise minimal or no cleaning of pin sites. Voluminous serous or serosanguineous discharge may signal a serious problem and is dealt with as discussed later (see the section on potential complications). Patients return for a recheck after 10 to 14 days for suture removal and to evaluate loose clamps. Further rechecks are performed at 3- to 4-week intervals, depending on the anticipated rate of healing, or sooner if problems develop.

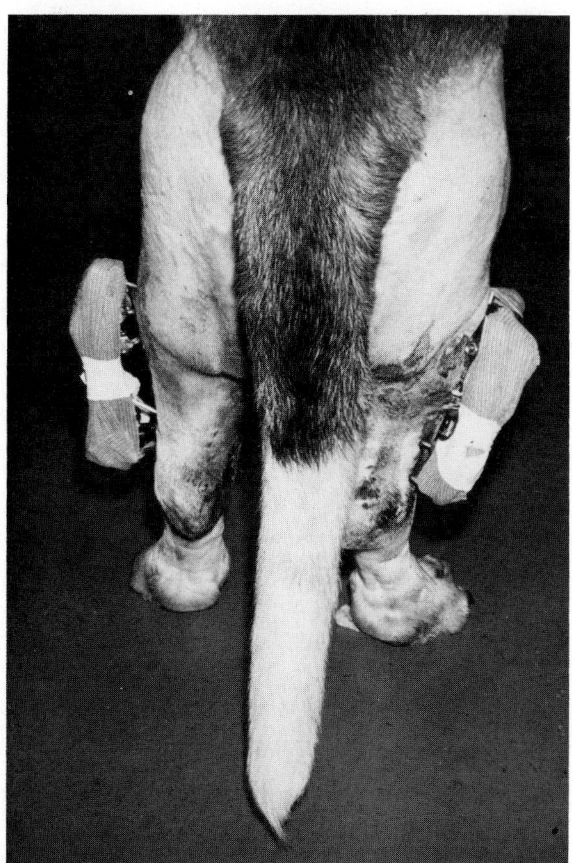

FIGURE 123–21. After removal of the compressive wrap, gauze and tape are used to protect the splint.

Removal of External Fixation

When fracture healing is deemed clinically complete, the fixator can usually be removed with minimal or no sedation. The connecting clamps and bars are removed, and the fixation pins are pulled using a hand chuck or pin puller in a twisting motion. If threaded pins were used, they must be "unscrewed" (a Jacob hand chuck works well for this). Full pins are removed by cutting off and cleaning one end and pulling through the other. After pin removal, a small amount of serosanguineous fluid often drains from the pin site, which can be cleaned with hydrogen peroxide. The pin holes should not be sutured closed. Restriction of activity for 6 to 8 weeks is indicated while the fracture remodels and bone hypertrophies.

ECONOMIC MANAGEMENT OF EXTERNAL FIXATION

Most of the expense of a complex fixator is the cost of the connecting clamps, which can be reused many times. I control cost by charging a client the expense of replacing the entire apparatus when the patient is discharged. The client is then refunded 75 per cent of the clamp costs if clamps are returned in usable condition. Twenty-five per cent of the cost is retained as a user fee. This plan seems to work well because it encourages clients to return for follow-ups and keeps the loss of equipment to a minimum. Also, the refund often offsets charges for follow-up visits and radiographs.

POTENTIAL COMPLICATIONS AND THEIR MANAGEMENT

The most common complication of fracture repair with external skeletal fixation is drainage around the fixation pins.[20] This is often caused by excessive skin and soft-tissue movement or tension against the pins. Careful placement of the pins through nondisplaced soft tissue and avoiding large muscle masses minimize this problem. In some locations, such as the distal femur, soft-tissue movement against the pins is unavoidable, and some drainage is to be expected. Activity restriction and periodically cleaning the pin site with 2 per cent hydrogen peroxide are recommended.

Loosening of the fixation pin at the pin–bone interface commonly results in drainage and infection of the pin tract (Fig. 123–22). Once a pin becomes loose, the only effective treatment is removal. The drainage usually resolves rapidly. Aside from the nuisance of drainage, loosening of pins may decrease leg use. If too many pins loosen too quickly, stability may be lost and nonunion develops. In those cases, additional fixation pins must be inserted to maintain adequate stability. Although this usually requires general anesthesia, it can be done by closed insertion of a new pin at a new site. The use of 3 or 4 threaded pins per fragment prevents most pin loosening and subsequent drainage or infection.

An uncommon problem is iatrogenic fracture through the fixation pin holes. This usually occurs when oversized fixation pins are used, when fixation pins are placed too close together, or when fixation pins are placed in fissure fractures. Unrestricted postoperative activity can also result in fractures through pin holes, particularly if the holes are enlarged by loose pins. Such problems are managed by repositioning pins in intact bone.

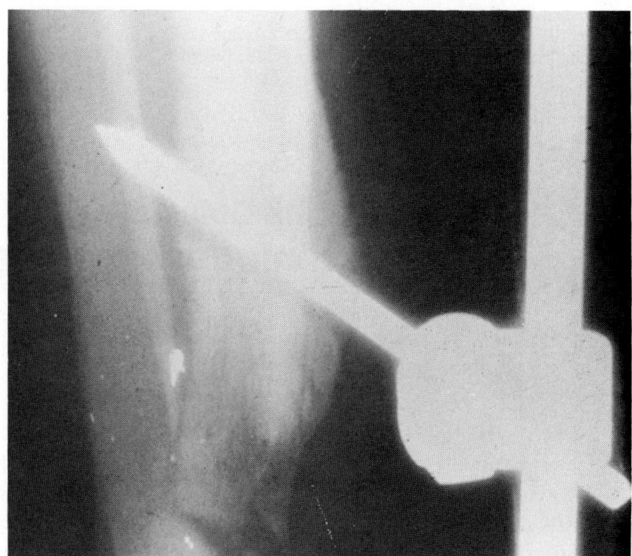

FIGURE 123–22. Radiographic appearance of bone lysis. There is periosteal proliferation around the pin, which denotes loosening.

References

1. Aron DN, Toombs JP: Updated principles of external skeletal fixation. *Comp Cont Educ 6*:845, 1984.
2. Aron DN, et al: Primary treatment of severe fractures by external skeletal fixation: threaded pins compared with smooth pins. *J Am Anim Hosp Assoc 22*:659, 1986.
3. Bennett RA, et al: Comparison of the strength and holding power of 4 pin designs for use with half-pin (type I) external skeletal fixation. *Vet Surg 16*:207, 1987.
4. Bjorling DE, Toombs JP: Transarticular application of the Kirschner-Ehmer splint. *Vet Surg 11*:34, 1982.
5. Briggs BT, Chao EYS: The mechanical performance of the standard Hoffman-Vidal external fixation apparatus. *J Bone Joint Surg, 64A*:566, 1982.
6. Brinker WO, Flo GL: Principles and application of external skeletal fixation. *Vet Clin North Am 2*:197, 1975.
7. Brinker WO, et al: Stiffness studies on various configurations and types of external fixators. *J Am Anim Hosp Assoc 21*:801, 1985.
8. Chao EYS: Biomechanics of external fixation. *In* Brooker AF, et al (eds): *Principles of External Fixation*. Williams & Wilkins, Baltimore, 1983, pp 165–199.
9. Chao EYS, Pope MH: The mechanical basis of external fixation. *In* Seligson D, Pope MH (eds): *Concepts in External Fixation*. Grune & Stratton, New York, 1981, pp 13–39.
10. Coombs R: Introduction. *In* Coombs R, et al (eds): *External Fixation and Functional Bracing*. Orthotext, London, 1989, p xix.
11. De Bastiani G, et al: The treatment of fractures with a dynamic axial fixator. *J Bone Joint Surg [Br] 66*:538, 1984.
12. Egger EL: Static strength evaluation of six external skeletal fixation configurations. *Vet Surg 12*:130, 1986.
13. Egger EL, et al: Use of the type I double connecting bar configuration of external skeletal fixation on long bone fractures in dogs: A review of 10 cases. *J Am Anim Hosp Assoc 22*:57, 1986.
14. Egger EL, et al: Type I biplanar configuration of external skeletal fixation: Application technique in nine dogs and one cat. *J Am Vet Med Assoc 187*:262, 1985.
15. Egger EL, et al: Effect of fixation pin insertion on the bone-pin interface. *Vet Surg 15*:246, 1986.
16. Egger EL, et al: Canine osteotomy healing when stabilized with decreasingly rigid fixation compared to constantly rigid fixation. *Trans Orthop Res Soc 11*:473, 1986.
17. Egger EL, et al: Effects of destabilizing rigid external fixation on healing of unstable canine osteotomies. *Trans Orthop Res Soc 13*:302, 1988.
18. Ehmer EA: Bone pinning in fractures of small animals. *J Am Vet Med Assoc 110*:14, 1944.
19. Goodship AE, Kenwright J: The influence of induced micromovement upon the healing of experimental tibial fractures. *J Bone Joint Surg [Br] 67B*: 650, 1985.
20. Green ST: *Complications of External Skeletal Fixation: Causes, Prevention, and Treatment*. Charles C Thomas, Springfield, IL, 1981, p 20.
21. Green ST: History of external fixation. *In* Coombs R, et al (eds): *External Fixation and Functional Bracing*. Orthotext, London, 1989, pp 59–65.
22. Green ST: Combined internal and external fixation. *In* Coombs R, et al (eds): *External Fixation and Functional Bracing*. Orthotext, London, 1989, pp 233–238.
23. Greenwood KM, Creagh GB: Biphase external skeletal splint fixation of mandibular fractures in dogs. *Vet Surg 9*:128, 1980.
24. Halloran WX: Motion. *In* Coombs R, et al (eds): *External Fixation and Functional Bracing*. Orthotext, London, 1989, pp 9–12.
25. Hierholzer G, et al: External fixation—classification and indications. *Arch Orthop Trauma Surg 92*:175, 1978.
26. Ilizarov G: Angular deformities with shortening. *In* Coombs R, et al (eds): *External Fixation and Functional Bracing*. Orthotext, London, 1989, pp 359–375.
27. Ilizarov G: The tension-stress effect on the genesis and growth of tissues: The influence of the rate and frequency of distraction. *Clin Orthop Rel Res 239*:263, 1989.
28. Johnson AL, et al: Radial and tibial fracture repair with external skeletal fixation. Effects of fracture type, reduction, and complications on healing. *Vet Surg 18*:367, 1989.
29. Lambotte A: *L'intervention operatoire dans les fracteurs*. Lamartins, Brussels, 1907.
30. Latte Y: Treatment of radius curvus by Ilizarov apparatus. *Trans Vet Orthop Soc 16*, 1989.
31. Lewallen DG, et al: Comparison of the effects of compression plates and external fixators on early bone healing. *J Bone Joint Surg [Am] 66A*:1084, 1984.
32. Matthews LS, et al: The thermal effects of skeletal fixation-pin insertion in bone. *J Bone Joint Surg [Am] 66A*:1077, 1984.
33. Morris JH: Biphase connector, external skeletal splint for reduction and fixation of mandibular fractures. *J Oral Surg 2*:1382, 1949.
34. Morshead D, Leeds EB: Kirschner-Ehmer apparatus immobilization following Achilles tendon repair in six dogs. *Vet Surg 13*:11, 1984.
35. Olds R, Green SA: Hoffmann's external fixation for arthrodesis and infected nonunions in the dog. *J Am Anim Hosp Assoc 19*:705, 1983.
36. Parkhill C: A new apparatus for the fixation of bones after resection and in fractures with a tendency to displacement. *Trans Am Surg Assoc 15*:251, 1897.
37. Prinz H, et al: Pin-track infection. *In* Coombs R, et al (eds): *External Fixation and Functional Bracing*. Orthotext, London, 1989, pp 149–152.
38. Schenk RK, Willenegger H: Zum Histologischen Bild der sogenannten Primarheilung der Knochenkompakta nach experimentellen Osteotomien am Hund. *Experientia 19*:593, 1963.
39. Shearer J, Egan J: Computerized analysis of pin geometry. *In* Coombs R, et al (eds): *External Fixation and Functional Bracing*. Orthotext, London, 1989, pp 129–137.
40. Siris I: External pin transfixation of fractures; an analysis of eighty cases. *Ann Surg 120*:911, 1944.
41. Staumbaugh JE, Nunmaker DM: External skeletal fixation of comminuted maxillary fractures in dogs. *Vet Surg 2*:72, 1982.
42. Toombs JP, et al: Angled connecting bars for transarticular application of Kirschner-Ehmer external fixation splints. *J Am Anim Hosp Assoc 25*:213, 1989.
43. Umphlet R, Johnson A: Mandibular fractures in the dog: A retrospective study of 157 cases. *Vet Surg 19*:272, 1990.
44. Willer RL, et al: A comparison of stainless steel versus acrylic for the connecting bar of external skeletal fixators. *J Am Anim Hosp Assoc 27*:541, 1991.
45. Williams EA, et al: The early healing of tibial osteotomies stabilized by one-plane or two-plane external fixation. *J Bone Joint Surg [Am] 69A*:355, 1987.
46. Wu JJ, et al: Comparison of osteotomy healing under external fixation devices with different stiffness characteristics. *J Bone Joint Surg [Am] 66A*:1258, 1984.

The Ilizarov External Ring Fixator: Principles, Techniques, and Uses

A. D. Elkins and M. Morandi

In 1951, Ilizarov started using simple metal components and bicycle wires connected to a circular external frame with nuts, bolts, and rods. The wires were 1.5 to 1.8 mm in diameter and were manually tensioned using primitive clamps attached to the rings. The device was a modification of several other external fixators that were popular at that time in Russia and Europe. The device was initially used for fracture management; by adding hinges to the threaded connector rods, Ilizarov was able to correct angular and rotational deformities as well. Anecdotally, it was reported that one of Ilizarov's patients accidentally turned the connecting rod of the fixator apart in "distraction" rather than in "compression." When viewing subsequent radiographs, Ili-

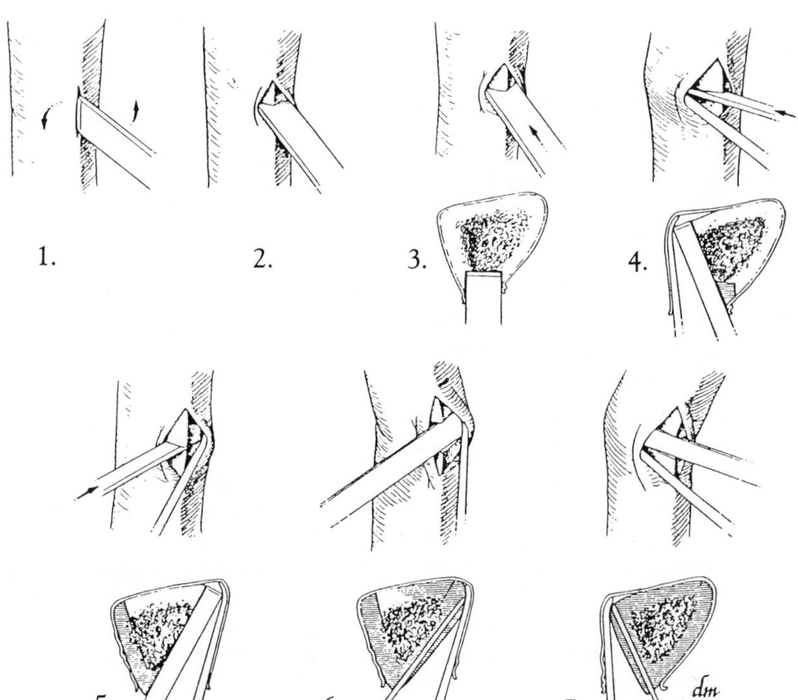

FIGURE 123–23. During corticotomy, the osteotome does not penetrate the marrow space but cuts only the cortex, leaving the medullary supply intact. (Courtesy of Medicalplastic s.r.l., Milan, Italy, and Smith and Hephew Richards, Memphis, TN.)

zarov observed that new bone had formed in the osteotomy gap that had formed by distraction of the fixation device. Ilizarov recognized the potential of this finding and began using the fixator for simultaneous correction of leg length discrepancies and angular and rotational deformities.

Ilizarov developed this new concept of distraction osteogenesis and described the formation of new bone under the law of tension-stress.[3] This law states that gradual traction on living tissue creates stresses that stimulate and maintain regeneration and active growth of certain tissues. Bone subjected to gradual traction becomes metabolically activated. Natural osteogenesis occurs at a rate of 50 to 100 μm/day within growing bones but at the rate of only 12 μm/day in mature bones.[1, 5–7] Adequate blood supply to the bone is the most important factor in determining the degree of this regeneration process.

Ilizarov's original technique for distraction osteogenesis involved a corticotomy and stable fixation. Corticotomy, as opposed to osteotomy, is removal of the cortex only, leaving the intramedullary blood supply intact (Fig. 123–23).[4] The periosteum is elevated and preserved during the corticotomy. Using this technique, one can direct bone growth and modify its shape in all directions, like a plastic tube. Corticotomy is performed in the metaphysis, which is more vascular than diaphyseal bone. The corticotomy is placed at a distance from the nutrient artery and does little damage to the adjacent soft tissue because it is performed through a small skin incision. The undifferentiated mesenchymal cells of the bone marrow, not damaged by the corticotomy, become osteoblasts and subsequently form osseous tissue without an intermediate cartilaginous phase. For this to occur, a constant displacement force, averaging 1 mm/day, is applied, orienting the osseous cells in the direction of the tensile stress. After corticotomy, a period of 3 to 7 days is allowed for local bridging of the gap by fibrous tissue. Gradual traction is then applied to stimulate ossification during the elongation period.[2]

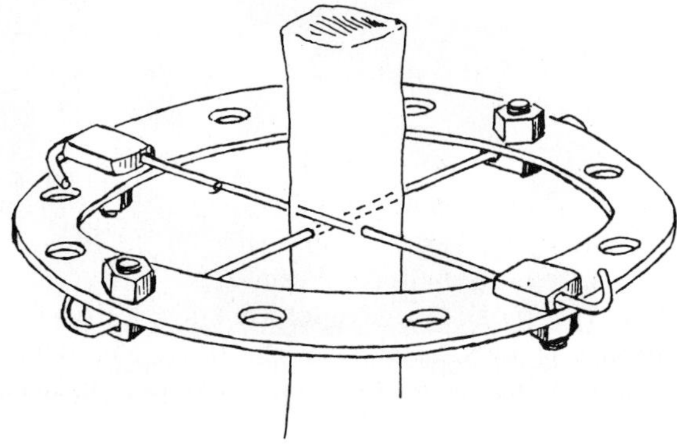

FIGURE 123–24. Two small K wires (1.5 to 1.8 mm) are placed both proximal and distal to the corticotomy site. These wires are parallel to the joint and approximately 90° to each other. Note that one wire is above the ring and the other wire below the ring. (Courtesy of Medicalplastic s.r.l., Milan, Italy, and Smith and Hephew Richards, Memphis, TN.)

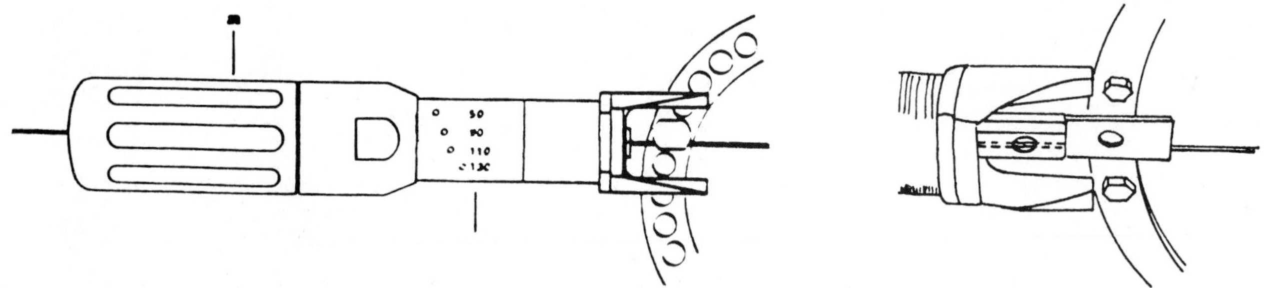

FIGURE 123–25. The wires are tensioned to 90 kg of tension with a dynamometric wire tensioner. (Courtesy of Medicalplastic s.r.l., Milan, Italy, and Smith and Hephew Richards, Memphis, TN.)

Although Ilizarov's original research suggested that corticotomy must be performed, Zembo and colleagues repeated Ilizarov's experiments and reported no difference in vascularity or regenerated bone formation in animals undergoing osteotomy or corticotomy, as long as the periosteum was left intact.[11]

The technique of application for the Ilizarov fixator is simple, but more elaborate designs require careful and detailed preoperative planning. In general, two small Kirschner wires (1.5 to 1.8 mm) are placed both proximally and distally to the corticotomy site (Fig. 123–24). The wires are smaller foreign bodies than conventional external fixation pins, can be placed in virtually any location, and are less likely to cause fissure fractures in the bone fragments. The risk of thermal necrosis is minimized by the small diameter and the type of point (bayonet shape). The wires are placed parallel to the respective joints and approximately 90° to each other (see Fig. 123–24). The wires can be easily repositioned in the bone, if the proper direction or angulation is not obtained initially. The wires are fastened to the rings and tensioned to 90 kg of tension with a dynamometric wire tensioner* (Fig. 123–25). Inadequately tensioned transfixation wires can cause pain and lack of weight-bearing and may arrest osteogenesis by allowing a bridge to form prematurely. The rings are placed around the limb, one parallel to the other to form a cylinder, with the axis of the tubular bone in the center. The position of the rings can be modified in all directions by adjusting the threaded rods or the hinges. Compression, distraction, angulation, translation, and rotation can be corrected with the apparatus. The Ilizarov technique has been used in human orthopedics for such conditions as tibial nonunions, infected pseudoarthrosis, limb lengthening, angular limb deformities, complex fractures, and bone transport in areas of bone loss.[8–10]

The tension in the pins provides the basis for the stability of the fixator.[3] The stability of the fixation eliminates torsional and sliding movements while maintaining some axial microelasticity. The number of pins placed through the bone, the tension applied to the pins, the number of rings, the distance between the

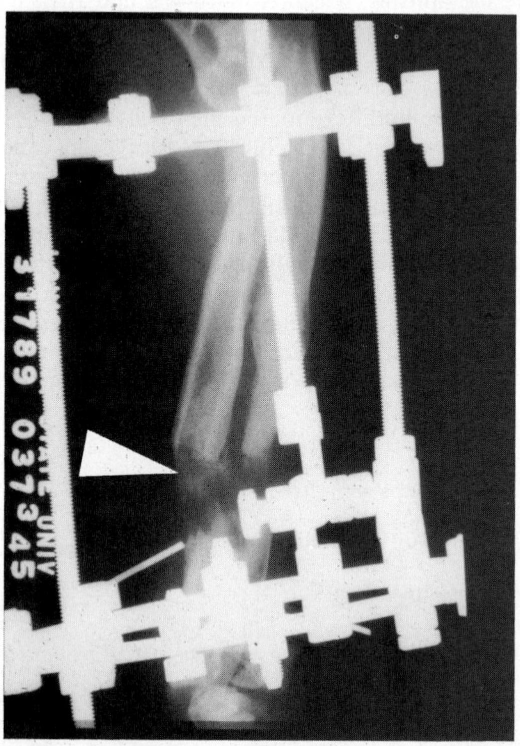

*Wire Tensioner, Medicalplastic, Milan, Italy.

FIGURE 123–26. Radiograph of radial lengthening 3 weeks postoperatively. The arrow notes the regenerated bone in the distraction gap.

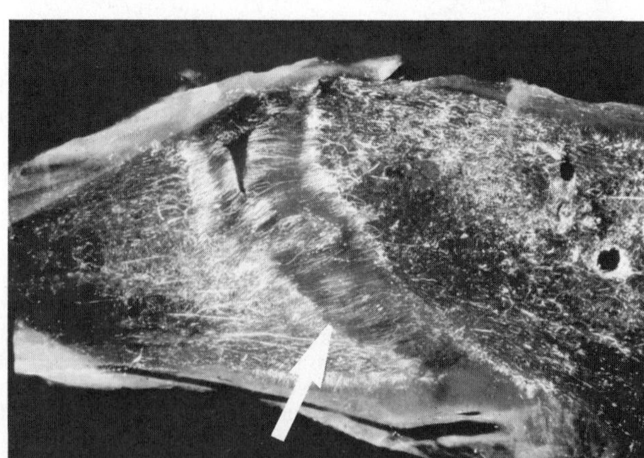

FIGURE 123–27. Barium-infused microangiogram of regenerated bone after 35 days of distraction. The arrow notes the parallel alignment of the vessels and new bone trabeculae in the direction of the tension-stress force.

rings and the surface of the skin, and the distance between each ring all influence stability. Biomechanical testing of the Ilizarov fixator revealed that torsional and shearing rigidity are equal to that of other external fixators, whereas axial rigidity is less than 80 per cent of the other fixators.[4] In the lower extremity, the force of weightbearing during walking is transmitted through the pins directly to the bone. There are no eccentric forces, or "bypass" effects but instead an axial, "elastic" stability allowing for micromovements.[4]

A lag period between corticotomy and distraction is important to allow osteogenic and chondrogenic cells time to organize and proliferate. The rate of distraction is likewise critical. At too slow a rate, the osteotomy or corticotomy heals prematurely during the distraction period. At too rapid a rate, the vascular supply to the bone is disrupted and nonunion results. Ilizarov described the ideal rate of distraction to be 1 mm/day divided into 2 to 4 distraction periods.[3]

Radiographically, the new bone can be recognized in the gap formed by bone distraction by 3 weeks postoperatively (Fig. 123–26). The level of osteogenic activity within the distraction zone depends on the degree of stability of the fixator and the amount of damage to the bone marrow, periosteum, and nutrient vessels occurring at the time of corticotomy.[3] The regenerated bone that develops within the distraction zone under optimal conditions resembles an epiphyseal growth plate with its orientation of trabeculae parallel to the direction of elongation (Fig. 123–27). Parallel columns of osteoid that turn into lamellar bone extending in both directions from the 2- to 4-mm-wide central "growth zone" are seen on histological study. However, unlike the epiphyseal plate, regenerated bone created under optimal conditions by the tension-stress effect develops without the formation of an intermediate cartilaginous step but develops directly from the fibrous tissue. If instability exists at the corticotomy site, the regenerated bone goes through the intermediate cartilaginous step much like endochondral ossification. Therefore, osteogenesis under the influence of the tension-stress effect shares some of the features of both endochondral and intramembranous ossification.[3] Electron microscopy of the regenerated bone in the distraction gap shows that an inflammatory reaction follows the corticotomy, as occurs in

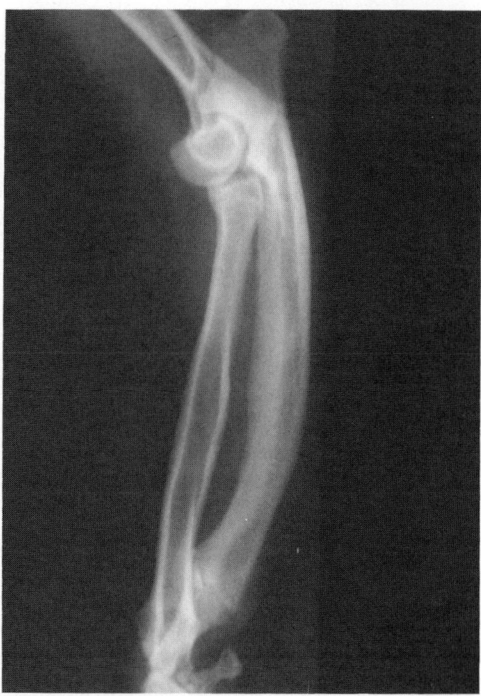

FIGURE 123–29. Lateral radiograph of the dog in Figure 123–28 showing caudal bowing with thickening of the ulna and subluxation of the radial-humeral joint. This was due to growth retardation of the distal radial physis.

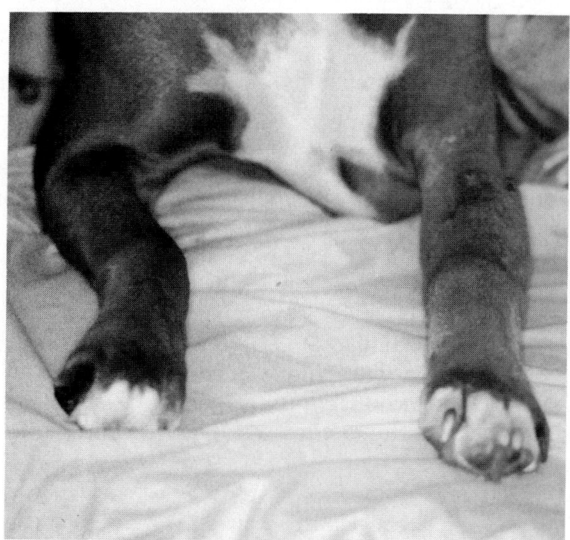

FIGURE 123–28. Frontal view of 6-month-old boxer with a fracture of the right forelimb at 3 months of age.

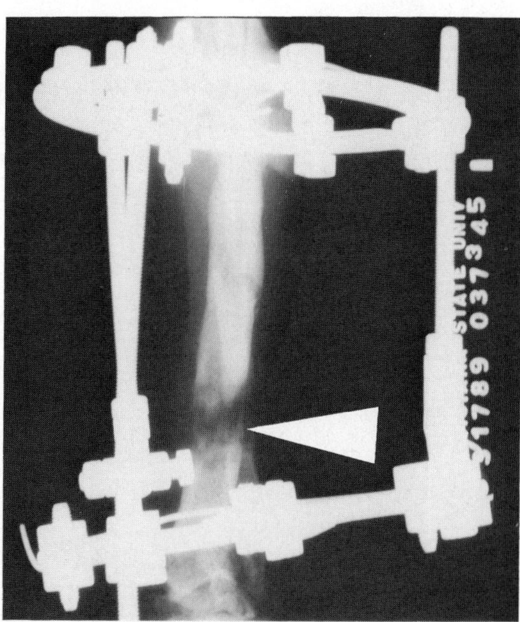

FIGURE 123–30. Craniocaudal radiograph of the dog in Figure 123–28 after 45 days of distraction at the rate of 0.5 mm twice daily. The arrow notes the regenerated bone in the distraction gap.

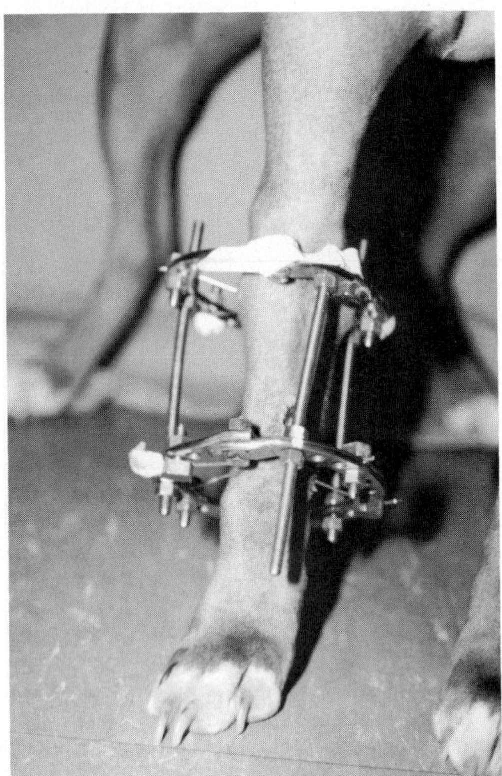

FIGURE 123–31. Frontal view of the dog in Figure 123–28 taken 60 days postoperatively, before fixator removal. Note correction of the angular deformity.

fracture healing. Once distraction begins, fibroblast-like cells appear in the distraction gap, with their long axes parallel to the vector of elongation.[3] After the distraction period, the Ilizarov fixator is maintained in a neutral phase for 4 to 6 weeks to allow maturation of the regenerated bone. The direction of distraction may be reversed during this neutral phase to actually achieve compression at the osteotomy or corticotomy site.

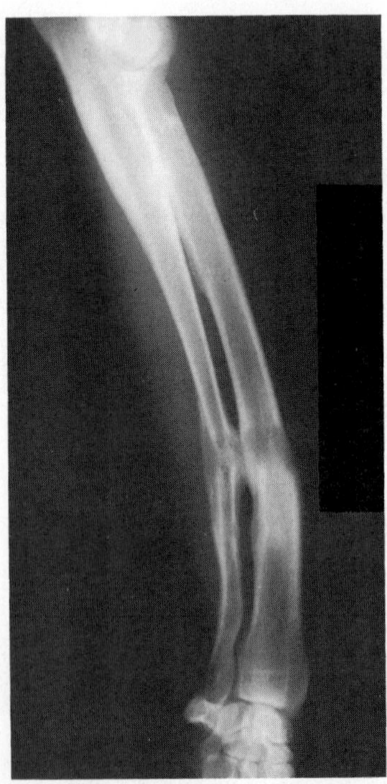

FIGURE 123–32. Lateral radiograph of the dog in Figure 123–28, 6 months postoperatively. Note the maturing regenerated bone and correction of the radial-humeral subluxation.

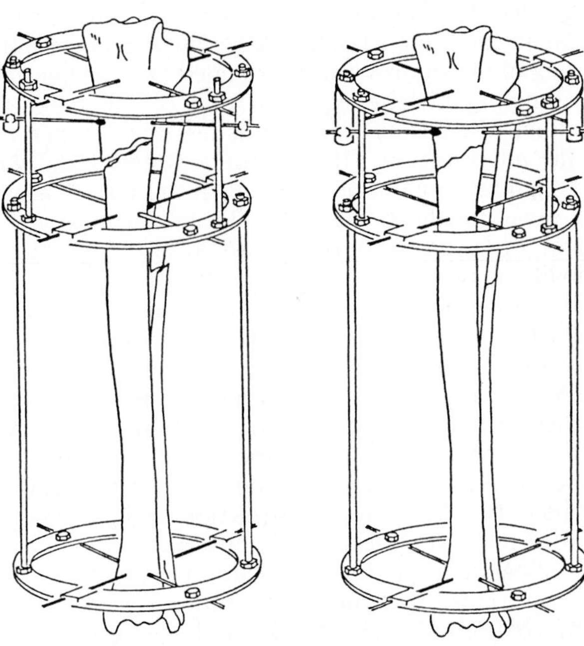

FIGURE 123–33. The Ilizarov fixator applied to a proximal tibial fracture. By the use of three rings and proper placement of the wires, the fragments are reduced and stabilized while healing. (Courtesy of Medicalplastic s.r.l., Milan, Italy, and Smith and Hephew Richards, Memphis, TN.)

SUMMARY

The Ilizarov ring fixator, when properly applied, stabilizes bone fragments in all planes while allowing enough axial micromotion to stimulate osteogenesis.[3] The use of thin tensioned wires to secure the bone fragments to the rings minimizes damage to the soft tissue, periosteum, and marrow blood supply while allowing weightbearing. These small wires may be placed close to the joint surface without fear of creating fractures. The Ilizarov technique enables veterinary surgeons to correct angular limb deformities while simultaneously increasing limb length. We found it difficult to perform a true corticotomy in dogs. There appears to be no difference in the rate or quality of bone formation in the distraction gap with either corticotomy or osteotomy. One of the major uses of the Ilizarov external fixator in veterinary orthopedics will be to correct limb shortening, especially in the forelimbs of large dogs with physeal damage and angular deformity (Figs. 123–28 through 123–32). The device is currently also being used for fracture repair near joints and for limb salvage procedures to replace bone loss due to tumors, fractures, or bone cysts (Fig. 123–33).

References

1. Aronson J, et al: Mechanical induction of osteogenesis. *Ann Clin Lab Sci* *18*:195, 1988.
2. Aronson J, et al: The histology of distraction osteogenesis using different external fixators. *Clin Orthop* *241*:106, 1989.

3. Ilizarov GA: The tension-stress effect on the genesis and growth of tissues. *Clin Orthop 238*:249, 1989.
4. Ilizarov GA, et al: Experimental studies of bone lengthening. *Exp Khir Anesth 14*:3, 1969.
5. Jowsey J, et al: Quantitative microradiographic studies of normal and osteoporotic bone. *J Bone Joint Surg [Am] 47A*:785, 1965.
6. Lee WR: Appositional bone formation in canine bone: A quantitative microscopic study using tetracycline markers. *J Anat 98*:665, 1964.
7. Lee WR, et al: Calcium accretion and bone formation in dogs. *J Bone Joint Surg [Br] 47B*:157, 1965.
8. Morandi M, et al: The Ilizarov transosseous osteosynthesis method: A treatment for infected pseudarthrosis and bone defects. Proceedings of the International Conference on the Ilizarov Techniques for Management of Difficult Skeletal Problems, 1987, pp 28–29.
9. Tajana GF, Morandi M: Distraction osteogenesis in man with circular external fixation. Proceedings of the 13th International Conference on Hoffman External Fixation, Mayo Clinic Foundation, Rochester, MN. May 1989, p 71.
10. Tajana GF, et al: Comparative analysis of distraction osteogenesis in dog and man using circular external fixation. Proceedings of the 13th International Conference on Hoffman External Fixation, Mayo Clinic Foundation, 1989, p 21.
11. Zembo MM, et al: Radiographic analysis of regenerate bone formation following tibial distraction osteosynthesis by the method of Ilizarov with a circular external fixator in a canine model. Proceedings of the 13th International Conference on Hoffman External Fixation, Mayo Clinic Foundation, 1989, p 10.

CHAPTER 124

External Coaptation

Charles E. DeCamp

External splinting preceded surgical reduction and internal fixation of fractured bone by thousands of years. Hippocrates, in 350 B.C., established many of the basic principles of closed treatment for fractured bone. He recommended that "two strong men" pull in opposite directions to reduce the fractured bone before bandages were applied and made rigid with waxes and resins.[10] Despite advances in surgical care of fractures, coaptation has a continuing role. External coaptation may serve as temporary support or first aid, as secondary support after surgical intervention, or as the primary support and stabilization for selected fractures. Although scientific knowledge of wound and fracture biology progresses, we must not neglect the "art" of constructing a proper splint. Rigid materials such as splint rod, fiber glass, and plaster provide strength required in external coaptation but also may endanger the splinted limb if used improperly. In choosing between the various types of bandages, slings, splints, and casts, it is important first to consider the conflicting basic principles of bandaging versus external coaptation. The challenge to a practitioner who has a diverse knowledge of orthopedic disease and a wide variety of orthopedic bandages is to balance a patient's need for bandaging with the strict requirements for bone splinting.

PRINCIPLES OF AN ORTHOPEDIC BANDAGE

A well-padded bandage is almost always comfortable to the animal wearing it and provides sufficient support for stabilization of many orthopedic conditions during healing. If a fracture is present, too much padding within a splint or cast may allow movement of bone fragments at a fracture site and be detrimental to healing. Too little padding in a splint or cast may also cause complications. If a rigid cast with minimal padding is applied to a heavily traumatized limb and soft-tissue inflammation is not properly anticipated, poor vascular supply may develop and lead to pressure ulceration of the skin and underlying structures. Complete necrosis of the extremity under the bandage may result in the loss of the limb (see Fig. 124–3*C*). It is of utmost importance, when selecting external coaptation, to consider the state of the soft tissue and decide which coaptation appliance will best stabilize the limb.

An orthopedic bandage serves many useful functions that can augment and support the healing processes of soft tissue and bone. The four primary functions of a bandage are protection, absorption of draining material, compression of soft tissue, and stabilization.[9] Protection of the soft tissue is necessary to prevent external contamination with bacteria if an open wound is present. Animal patients are notorious for licking their wounds, and a protective bandage prevents bacterial contamination and also may prevent serious self-mutilation due to licking and biting. Absorptive qualities of a bandage limit accumulation of exudates and decrease wound infection.[9] Compression of soft tissue by the bandage further helps to limit the development of exudates within "dead space" and reduces fluid accumulations (hematoma, seroma, edema) that may affect healing. Heavy cotton padding compressed with elastic gauze is used in many bandages for absorptive and compressive qualities, but it also limits mobility of an affected limb.

PRINCIPLES OF EXTERNAL COAPTATION

Internal fixation of a fracture may best be described as "bone splinting." External coaptation is thought of as "limb splinting."[5] An external splint depends on compressive or tensile properties of soft tissue in the affected limb to augment stability at a fracture site, whereas internal fixation depends less on soft tissue to provide stability.[7, 8] A Schroeder-Thomas splint uses traction to maintain fracture reduction. The tension on the muscle mass at the fracture site also helps provide fragment stability for optimal bone healing. If a Schroeder-Thomas splint is inappropriately applied without traction to a fractured limb, a less stable result is achieved.

Fracture Forces

Four mechanical forces may develop at a fracture site: bending, rotation, compression or shear, and distraction.[1, 2] The forces acting on a particular fracture are considered before choosing coaptation as a suitable method of treatment. Different methods of external coaptation vary in their ability to counteract fracture forces and stabilize an injury. Bending and rotational forces are adequately neutralized in most fractures by a cast, as long as the joints above and below the injury are immobilized.[1, 2] Compressive or shear forces are difficult to neutralize with a cast.[1, 2] If an oblique or comminuted fracture is present, a cast may be inadequate to neutralize a shear force, and loss of fracture reduction may develop when the animal bears weight on the limb. A Shroeder-Thomas splint may effectively reduce shear force at the fracture but may be less effective than a cast at reducing other fracture forces. Distraction forces at a fracture site, such as those in olecranon fractures or fractures of the greater trochanter of the femur, are caused by muscle tension and are poorly neutralized by external coaptation. As an adjunct to internal fixation, a sling to prevent weightbearing may be more effective than splinting in reducing muscle tension and distraction.

GUIDELINES FOR COAPTATION

Fractures and soft-tissue injuries that require external coaptation are variable, and no single set of rules can be adequate to describe all uses of coaptation.

Basic Guidelines

Fracture Reduction

Minimally displaced stable fractures are best suited to healing by external coaptation. Reduction of fracture fragments does not improve after a cast or splint has been applied and so must be achieved before application. Most animals will not allow extensive manipulation of a fracture site without struggling and thus upsetting improvements already achieved. General anesthesia is usually required if significant manipulations are needed for fracture reduction, but even with anesthesia, closed fracture reduction rarely results in perfect fragment apposition. Fracture forces or soft-tissue interposition may prevent exact reduction without surgical intervention. Further loss of reduction may develop after anesthesia recovery when the animal is awake and bearing weight. Radiography must be used to ensure that fracture reduction remains adequate for healing. If sufficient fracture reduction cannot be maintained by closed methods, surgical intervention for reduction and fixation must be considered. Adequate reduction for fracture healing varies with the type of fracture and the patient. A juvenile patient, with greater healing potential than an adult, may tolerate greater fragment displacement without developing delayed or nonunion healing. A "50 per cent rule" has been applied to fracture reduction and external coaptation. Cortical positioning of fracture ends should have 50 per cent contact to expect fracture healing. Such rules are often self-defeating, and a practitioner who routinely accepts 50 per cent reduction as adequate in fracture repair will be disappointed with the healing that results. Successful bone healing is far more likely to occur if perfect reduction is the goal for every fracture.

Fracture Alignment

Although perfect reduction may be impossible with closed reduction in some fractures, care must be taken to ensure proper limb alignment. Fracture fragments are positioned so that the approximate anatomical relationship of the joint above and below the injury is maintained. Failure to align bone fragments with respect to the joints of the limb may result in rotational or angular malunion severe enough to cause functional gait abnormality and lameness from secondary degenerative joint disease. "Nonfunctional" malunion fractures require surgical correction with osteotomy and internal fixation to restore a pain-free gait. It is important to avoid this consequence by careful attention to limb alignment at the initial placement of coaptation.

Standing Position

An animal is usually restrained or anesthetized in lateral recumbency for placement of external coaptation. Splints, bandages, and casts are applied so that the limb is maintained in a neutral standing position. Stiffness of joints commonly develops secondary to trauma, surgery, and immobilization of a limb. If a joint has been positioned in a standing position for coaptation, the animal will bear weight on the limb while the splint is in place and after splint removal. If joint stiffness is present after splint removal, walking on the limb often helps to relieve the signs. If a limb is stiff in an abnormal position, the animal may be unable to bear weight even after the splint is removed. Adhesions between muscle, tendons, and bone may limit a joint's range of motion. It is important to mobilize a joint as soon as possible during fracture healing to help prevent loss of function.

Joint Above and Below

A basic principle in external coaptation is that the joints above and below a fracture must be immobilized. Consequently conventional splints and casts are adequate for fractures below the elbow or stifle but not above. A conventional full-leg cast does not extend proximally beyond midhumerus or midfemur. Immobilization of the shoulder or hip joint is not effective unless a spica splint or cast is constructed. Use of a conventional cast or splint as treatment for a femoral or humeral fracture is contraindicated. A modified spica splint may be constructed to immobilize the shoulder or hip joint in addition to the more distal joints. Such splints provide temporary immobilization of femoral and humeral fractures and may be useful before internal fixation.

CHOOSING APPROPRIATE EXTERNAL COAPTATION

Choice of an external coaptation device that best suits a patient's needs is determined by numerous patient and environmental factors (Fig. 124–1). If severe soft-tissue inflammation is expected, a temporary well-padded splint is more beneficial to the soft tissue than a rigid, thinly padded cast. A rigid cast may be placed several days or weeks later when the threat of severe inflammation has subsided. Some conditions, such as infected wounds associated with a fracture, require access for local wound treatment. If the wound is small, a window may be cut into the bandage or cast for treatment. If the wound is large, temporary splinting with a reinforced padded bandage or a bivalved cast provides better access to the wound. The amount of weightbearing and joint mobility desired also affects the choice of coaptation. If weightbearing on the affected limb is not desired and

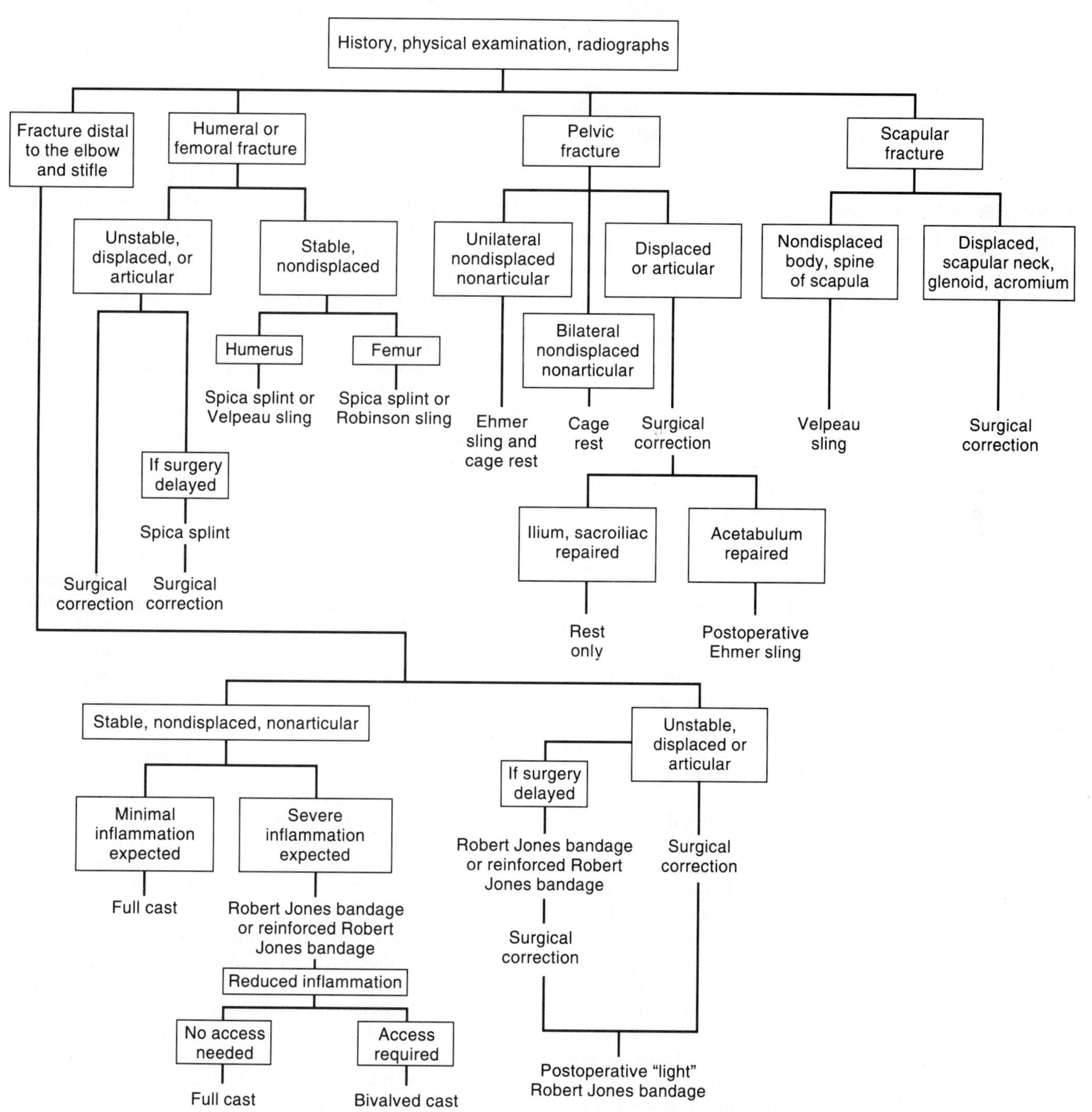

FIGURE 124–1. Algorithm for choosing coaptation (or not) for suspected fractures.

the limb does not need to be splinted or bandaged, a sling may be selected to prevent leg use. Casts and splints generally allow weightbearing on the limb but rigidly immobilize the involved joints. Rigid immobilization of the joints is not desired after surgical fracture repairs or after many soft-tissue joint surgeries. A soft, well-padded bandage may be more appropriate than a cast or splint when moderate weightbearing and joint mobility are desired. When external coaptation provides the primary stabilization of a fracture, rigid immobility of the limb is required and a full cast provides better stability than well-padded splints or slings. The choice of coaptation device may also be affected by the probability of client and animal compliance. Some animals will not tolerate coaptation without self-mutilation or are so vicious that they make routine cast or splint management a dangerous experience. Some owners are so disinterested in their pet's welfare that routine cast monitoring and care are impossible. Whether the compliance problem is animal or human in origin, rigid internal fixation may be more appropriate.

BANDAGES, SPLINTS, SLINGS, AND CASTS

Robert Jones Bandage

The Robert Jones bandage and its modifications are the most widely used coaptation bandages in veterinary orthopedics. The bulk and mild compression of a Robert-Jones bandage provide support and reduce swelling. Tissue heals with less tension at sutured margins, and the animal's comfort is usually dramatically improved. Well padded with bulk cotton and compressed with successive layers of elastic gauze and tape, a Robert Jones bandage provides excellent temporary support for an injured extremity before or after surgical intervention. A Robert Jones bandage extends from the toes to midhumerus or femur and so may be used to provide temporary support of fractures or dislocations at or below the elbow and stifle joints. Adequate immobilization of a fracture is achieved to prevent worsening of fracture displacement and further injury to the soft tissues by sharp bone fragments. Immobilization by a Robert Jones bandage is inadequate as primary stabilization for a fracture. Thick cotton padding loosens after application and contributes to instability at the fracture site. Loosening of the bandage also increases mobility of the joints and may actually be desirable after some joint surgeries.

The limb is prepared for application of a Robert Jones bandage by completing necessary wound care and covering open wounds with a nonadherent dressing. Tape stirrups are essential to prevent the bandage from slipping beyond the toes. The stirrups are constructed from adhesive tape of width appropriate to the size of the animal (1/2 inch, small dog or cat; 1 inch, large dog). Strips of tape are applied to either the cranial and caudal or medial and lateral surfaces of the extremity, to extend from the carpus or tarsus to 3 to 6 inches beyond the toes (Fig. 124–2*A*). No circumferential bands of tape are applied, because they may obstruct vascular supply.[4] Cotton padding is prepared by unrolling the 12-inch roll from its paper backing, rerolling the 12-inch roll without the paper, and tearing the 12-inch cotton roll into two 6-inch-wide rolls. The narrower width provides better conformation of the bandage to the limb. Beginning at the toes, the cotton padding is wrapped around the limb and continued proximally to the level of the midshaft femur or humerus (Fig. 124–2*B*). The cotton padding is overlapped by approximately 50 per cent on itself and is rolled proximally and distally until sufficient bulk is established. The toenails of the two middle toes remain barely visible at this point, allowing later access for evaluation. Elastic gauze is applied to the cotton padding, beginning again with the toes. With strong, even pressure to compress the cotton, at least two or three layers of gauze are applied to the bandage to achieve the smooth, even tension required (Fig. 124–2*C*).

At the proximal and distal ends of the bandage, the gauze is tucked into the bandage to give the bulk cotton a neat appearance and prevent it from fraying and falling out of the bandage. If the bandage is sufficiently compressed, it sounds like a ripe watermelon when tapped with a finger.[3, 4] The tape stirrups that extend from the bandage are inverted and stuck to the outer surface of the elastic gauze. Elastic tape is used to cover the entire bandage (Fig. 124–2*D*). Caution must be exercised, especially in smaller dogs and cats, to avoid applying the elastic tape with excessive tension. It is possible to overcompress a Robert Jones bandage and obstruct vascular supply.

The Robert Jones bandage is a safe bandage, and few complications occur with its use. Clients must be advised to observe the toes for swelling or abrasion (Fig. 124–3 *A*). The bandage is kept dry by covering it with plastic sheeting if the animal is to be walked during wet conditions. A wet bandage rapidly causes acute moist dermatitis that is difficult to treat without bandage removal. With proper care, a Robert Jones bandage is easily maintained by a pet owner for several weeks. Some loosening of the bandage always develops within several hours or days. Loosening may be acceptable after some soft-tissue operations but is unacceptable if the bandage is providing temporary support of a fracture. For optimal compression and stabilization, a Robert Jones bandage is changed every few days or reinforced with rigid splint material.

Light or Modified Robert Jones Bandage

A light or modified Robert Jones bandage is applied in similar fashion to the Robert Jones bandage, except that much less cotton padding is used (Fig. 124–4*A*). Cast padding may be substituted for roll cotton. Less immobilization of the limb is achieved because the reduced padding is more flexible. This bandage is indicated whenever a lightly compressing support wrap is needed to reduce soft-tissue edema, but not in circumstances requiring rigid stability. It is commonly used after cruciate ligament stabilization or exploratory joint operations at or below the stifle or elbow. A light Robert Jones bandage is contraindicated for temporary support of a fracture but may be used after internal fixation to reduce swelling of the soft tissue without rigidly immobilizing the joints of a limb.

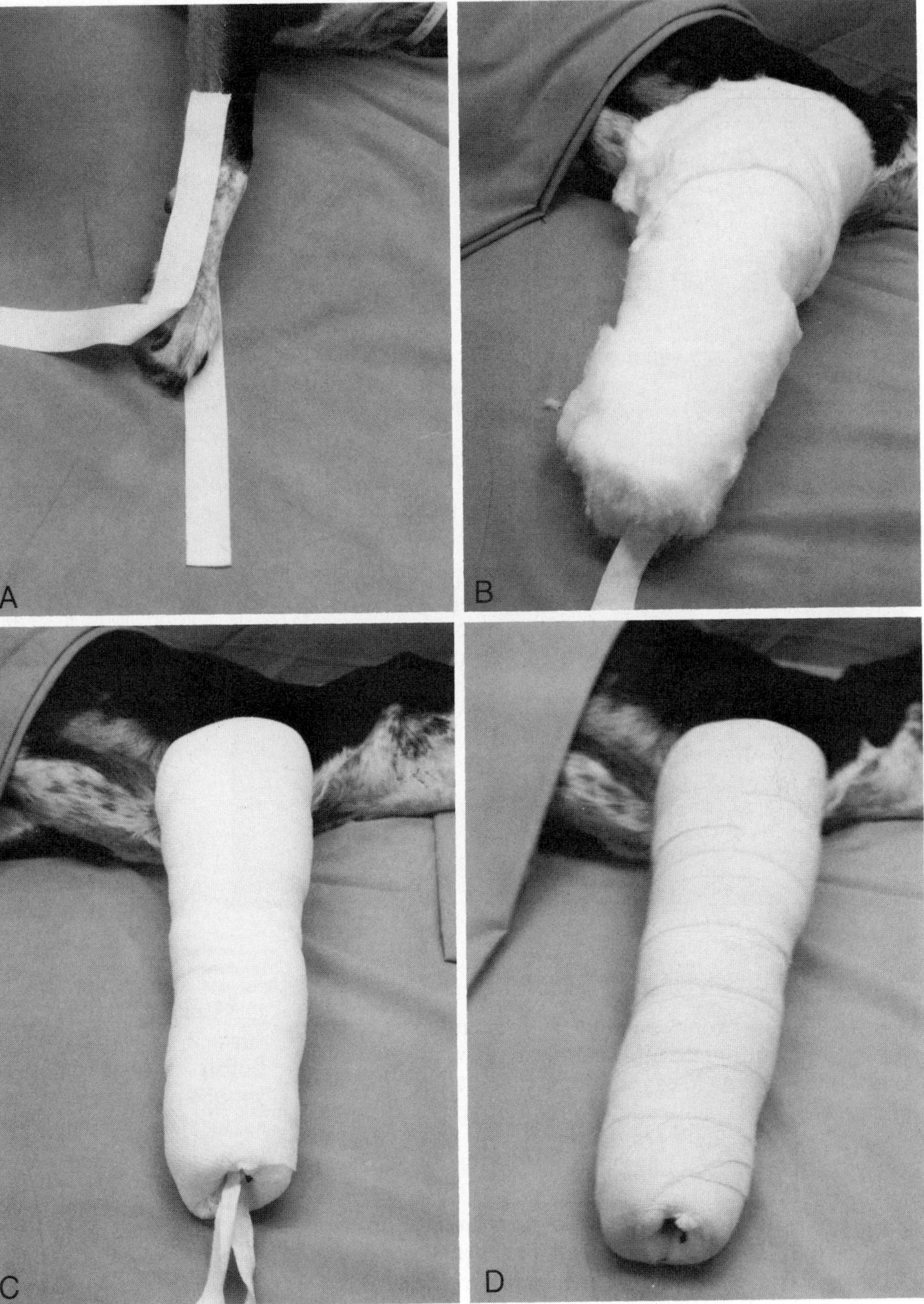

FIGURE 124–2. The Robert Jones bandage. *A*, Tape stirrups are applied to the medial and lateral surface of the leg. *B*, Roll cotton is wrapped loosely to provide bulk to the bandage. *C*, The cotton roll is compressed with elastic gauze to provide stiffness and compression. *D*, Stirrups have been inverted, and the bandage is covered with elastic tape.

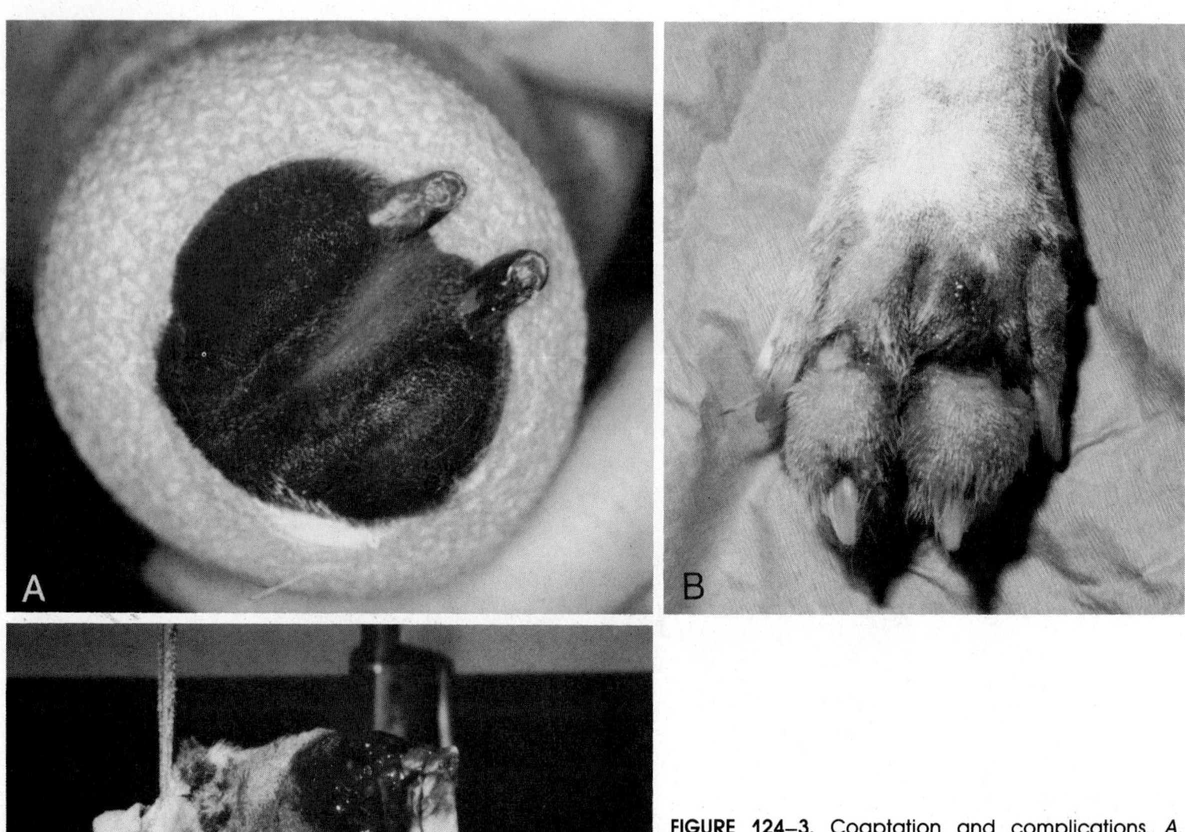

FIGURE 124–3. Coaptation and complications. *A*, These toes have become swollen from protruding too far from a bandage. Note that the toenails have spread apart. *B*, Lacerated toes after weightbearing in a short, poorly padded cast. *C*, Complete necrosis of the foot after encasing the limb in a cast without anticipation of inflammation from the soft-tissue wound.

Reinforced Robert Jones Bandage

A light Robert Jones bandage is frequently reinforced with rigid material to enhance immobilization of the joints. The advantage of reinforcing a light Robert Jones is that the large bulk and weight of a conventional Robert Jones bandage are avoided. The improved stability and the reduced bulk of a reinforced Robert Jones bandage make it an excellent choice for temporary stabilization of a fracture before surgery or as adjunctive external coaptation for a tenuous internal repair. A reinforced Robert Jones bandage does not provide sufficient stabilization for primary fixation of a fracture.

Reinforcement material is generally applied to the bandage on top of the cotton padding and elastic gauze and covered with elastic tape (Fig. 124–4*F*). A light Robert Jones bandage is easily reinforced with aluminum splint rod bent to conform to the lateral or medial surface of the bandage (Fig. 124–4*E*). This is commonly described as a *lateral* splint. Other materials may also be used as reinforcement. Three to five layers of a fiberglass casting tape may be applied to the caudal or lateral surface of the bandage and covered with elastic tape before drying (Fig. 124–4*D*). Preformed metal or plastic spoon splints or metasplints may be applied to the caudal surface of the bandage and covered with elastic tape (Fig. 124–4*B* and *C*). In the forelimb, a spoon splint does not immobilize the elbow joint and is not used as definitive fixation for injuries above the carpus. In the hindlimb, a spoon splint does not extend above the tarsus without modification and does not immobilize the tibiotarsal joint. Unless the injury is confined to the metatarsus or distal tarsal joints, other splinting methods are used.

Spica Splint

A spica splint envelopes the affected limb and torso of an animal to immobilize the shoulder or hip joint in

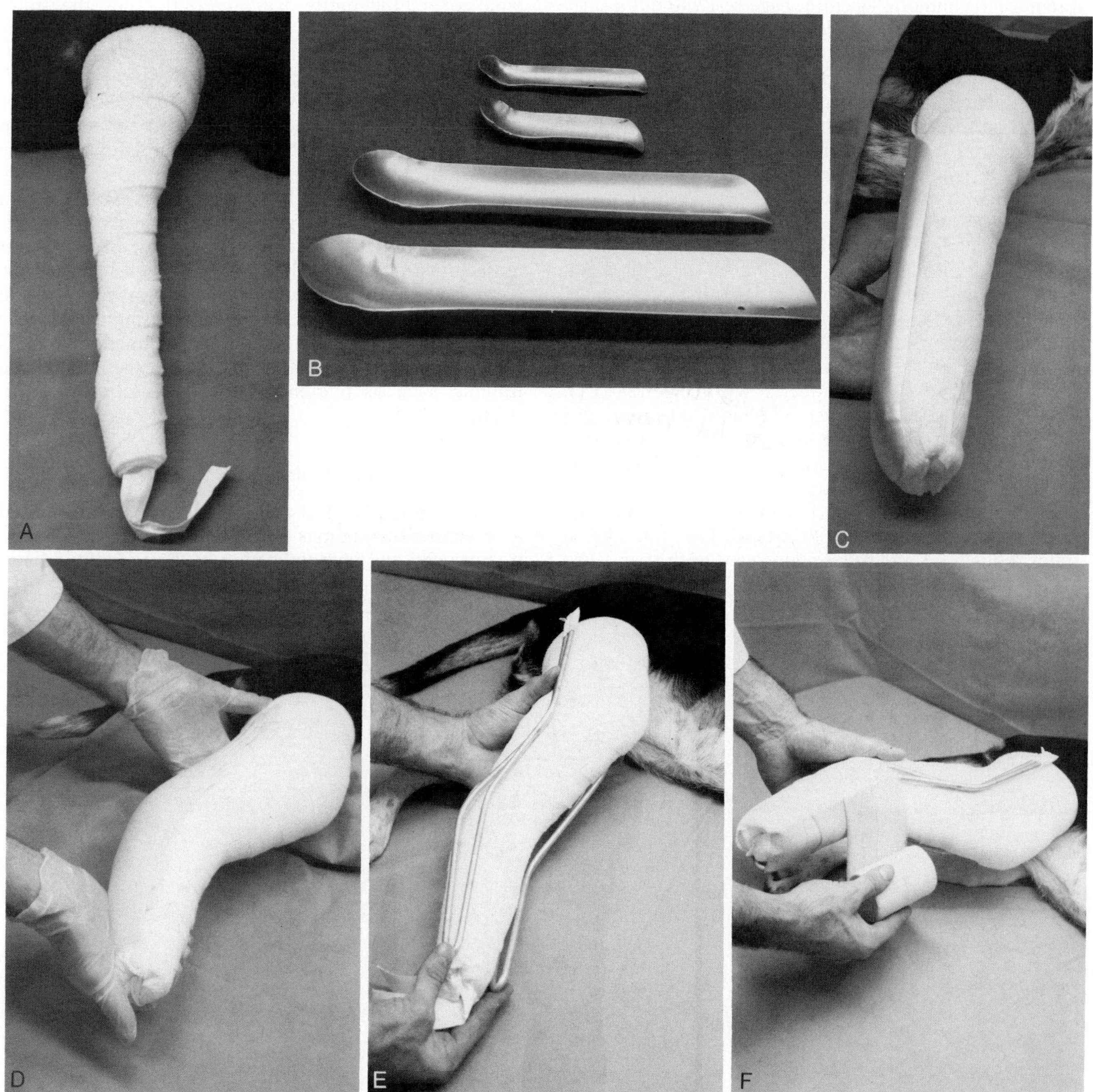

FIGURE 124–4. Modifications of the Robert Jones bandage. *A*, Less roll cotton or cast padding is used to construct a "light" Robert Jones bandage. *B*, Spoon splints are available in many sizes and forms. *C*, Spoon splint reinforcement of a light bandage. *D*, Cast material may be applied to any surface of the bandage. *E*, Splint rod reinforcement. *F*, Reinforcing material is fixed to the bandage with elastic tape.

addition to the more distal joints of the extremity. Because the shoulder or hip joint is immobilized in a spica, this splint may be used as temporary preoperative support of humeral and femoral fractures. Most femoral and humeral fractures are usually too displaced to use the spica splint as primary fixation. For animals suffering a femoral or humeral fracture, cage rest without a spica splint is acceptable if surgical repair is not delayed. If surgical repair must be delayed because of additional injuries or because the animal must be transported to a referral center, a spica splint is applied to reduce subsequent soft-tissue trauma from the fracture. A greenstick fracture of the humerus or femur occasionally is seen in a young puppy or kitten. It may then be appropriate to use a spica splint as primary fixation.

Construction of a spica splint is begun similarly to a light Robert Jones, except that no tape stirrups are necessary. Cotton padding is wrapped onto the limb, beginning with the toes and progressing proximally. When the axilla or inguinal area is reached, cotton padding is wrapped around the animal's torso several times, caudal to the contralateral limb and alternating cranial and caudal to the affected limb (Fig. 124–5*A*). Elastic gauze is wrapped onto the limb, beginning distally and progressing in the same manner as the cotton padding. The gauze compresses and conforms the cotton padding but does not provide sufficient strength to immobilize the joints. The bandage is reinforced with splint rod or fiber-glass casting tape (Fig. 124–5*B*). If splint rod is used, the rod is conformed to the bandaged leg from the toes to the dorsal midline and back down to the toes on the same side. If casting tape is chosen, the tape is folded on itself to provide a lateral splint of four to six layers from the toes to the dorsal midline of the animal. Both conformed splint rod and casting tape may be used as reinforcement for the bandage. Elastic tape covers the entire bandage and holds the splint material in place (Fig. 124–5*C*). If a spica splint is properly constructed, the limb and torso are immobilized and moved as a single unit.

Spica splints generally cause few complications because they are well padded and used for short-term temporary splintage. They do not slip down the leg because if properly constructed, the splint is firmly attached to the torso. Occasional abrasions develop in the axilla or inguinal region. Dogs and cats have difficulty walking at first with a spica splint in place, but most adjust and can walk reasonably well within a few days. Care must be taken, especially in applying the forelimb spica splint, to avoid compressing an animal's thorax and compromising respiratory function. This is especially true if an animal has pre-existing thoracic trauma, such as pneumothorax or pulmonary contusions.

Schroeder-Thomas Splint

Aluminum splint rod and bandage material are used in a Schroeder-Thomas splint to provide traction at a fracture site and immobilization of the joints in a limb.

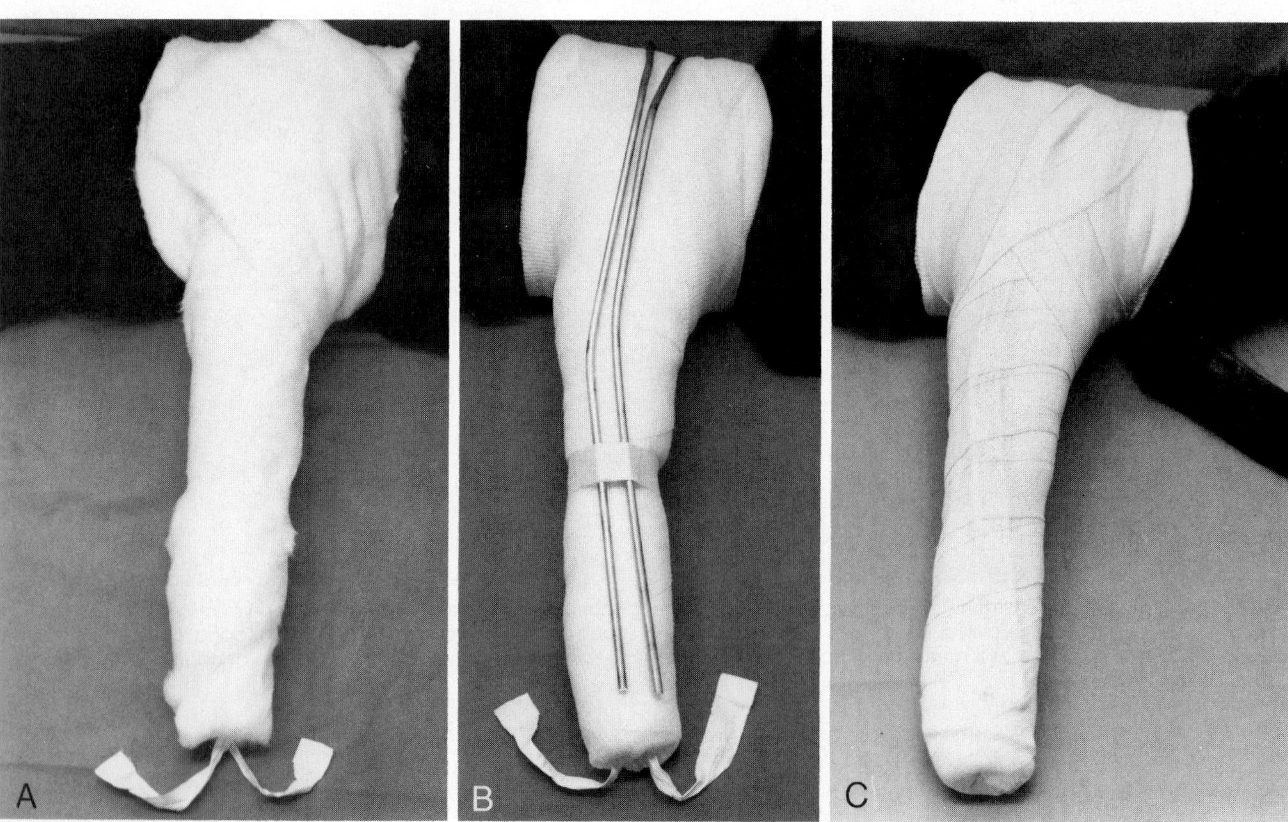

FIGURE 124–5. Spica splint. *A*, Roll cotton incorporates the thorax and the limb. *B*, Elastic gauze compresses and conforms the bandage. Splint rod or cast material extends from the toes to midline to reinforce the splint. *C*, Completed spica splint.

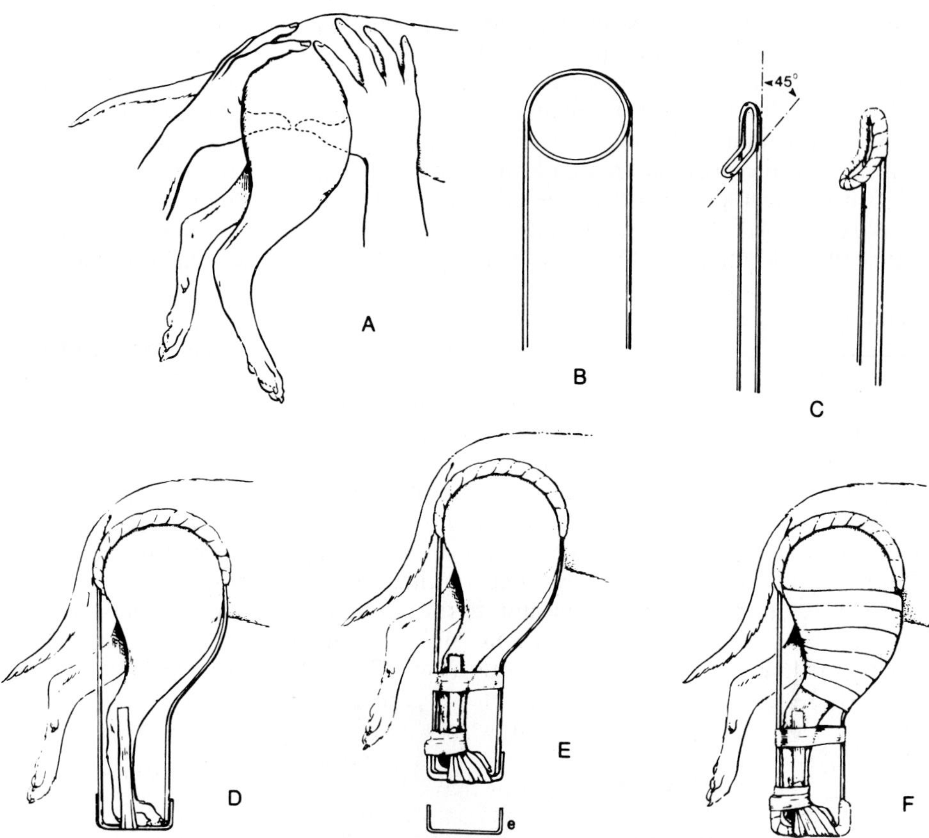

FIGURE 124–6. Schroeder-Thomas splint. After the diameter of the thigh is approximated (*A*), the aluminum rod is bent, forming one and one-half circles (*B*). *C*, The lower half of the ring is bent at a 45° angle to accommodate the thickness of the thigh; cotton or cast padding is added, followed by gauze and tape. *D* and *E*, With the splint pushed firmly into the inguinal region, the cranial rod is bent to the approximate angulation of the limb with the toes in a standing position. The foot is anchored with adhesive tape. *E*, If the dog weighs more than 25 pounds, a walking bar is applied. *F*, A layer of cotton is placed around the upper leg, then anchored to the cranial bar with a layer of gauze and tape. (From Flo GL: Fractures: Classification, diagnosis and treatment. *In* Brinker WO, et al. [eds]: *Handbook of Small Animal Orthopedics and Fracture Treatment.* W. B. Saunders, Philadelphia, 1983.)

This splint has been widely used in the past for small animals, but its indications have become progressively fewer.[3] The Schroeder-Thomas splint may be used as primary fixation for selected minimally displaced midshaft fractures of the radius, ulna, and tibia. Because the Schroeder-Thomas splint does not adequately immobilize the shoulder or hip joint, it is not used to stabilize fractures of the humerus or femur. Bending forces from the encircling rod and rotational forces on the fracture site make this splint inadequate for most fractures of the femur and humerus. A Schroeder-Thomas splint may be used to provide limb immobilization after joint surgery, but because it provides no compression of the soft tissue, a light or reinforced Robert Jones bandage is commonly chosen in its place.

The following is a description for construction of a Schroeder-Thomas splint for a hindlimb (Fig. 124–6).[3] A forelimb construction is similar, with some modification of the splint rod because of the different angulation of the leg. General anesthesia is advised if traction is to be applied at a fracture site. The animal is placed in lateral recumbency with the affected leg approximating a standing position. The diameter of the uppermost thigh is approximated by encircling the thigh with both hands. Aluminum splint rod (1/8 inch, 3/16 inch, or 3/8 inch) is bent to form a circle of the same diameter as the thigh. The bending is continued until one and one-half circles have been formed and both ends of the splint rod are parallel and facing the same direction. The lower half of the circle is bent at a 45° angle toward the midline of the animal to relieve pressure from the medial thigh. The entire ring is well padded with cotton roll or cast padding and covered with gauze and tape. The leg is passed through the ring, and the splint is firmly pushed into the inguinal area. Note that the ventral aspect of the ring passes the femur at the midshaft level. If this splint is used for a femoral fracture, this portion of the ring acts as a fulcrum and applies a bending force to the fracture when the animal is in lateral recumbency or abducting the limb. With the ring firmly pushed into the inguinal area, the limb is maintained in a standing position (do not extend the stifle), and the cranial bar is bent to the contour of the leg without touching it. The bar is bent at the toes so that the foot is kept in a standing position. The caudal bar is left straight until it is bent to accommodate the foot and overlap with the cranial bar. The overlapping cranial and caudal bars are wrapped with adhesive tape to fix their relative position and provide a platform for the foot. The foot is anchored to the platform of splint rod along the caudal aspect of the splint with multiple vertical and slightly angled strips of adhesive tape. The following steps are important if traction is to be applied to the region of the tibial shaft. Horizontal strips of adhesive tape are used to anchor the proximal and distal metatarsus to the caudal straight splint rod. In medium-sized animals, this region is first padded lightly with cast padding and elastic gauze before applying the horizontal strips. Cast padding or cotton roll encircles the limb from midtibia to above the stifle joint. The upper leg is then fixed to the cranial bar with elastic gauze and adhesive tape. By pulling the stifle joint cranially and proximally, limited traction is applied to the tibial region. A walking bar is applied to the base of the splint. The entire splint may be covered with adhesive or elastic tape if desired.

Routine splint care is essential after applying a Schroeder-Thomas splint. The limb is carefully inspected for abrasions in the inguinal area and for pressure necrosis of skin of the toes and at the metatarsus. If the tape loosens from the foot or metatarsus, traction is lost and repair or replacement of the splint is indicated.

Velpeau Sling

A Velpeau sling maintains the carpus, elbow, and shoulder joints in a flexed position and prevents weightbearing on the forelimb (Fig. 124–7*A*). A Velpeau sling immobilizes the shoulder joint and is used as primary or adjunctive stabilization for shoulder luxations, bicipital bursitis, minimally displaced fractures of the scapula and proximal humerus, and conditions of the distal forelimb if nonweightbearing is desired.

Application of the sling is easiest if the animal is awake and gently supported in a standing position on three legs by an assistant. General anesthesia may be used in a fractious patient, with the animal positioned in lateral recumbency with the affected side up. Cast padding encircles the carpus and paw, with the joint in moderate flexion. This padding prevents overflexion of the paw. The carpus, elbow, and shoulder are flexed and held in position while the cast padding is wrapped around the torso to completely cover the flexed forelimb. The padding is typically wrapped caudal to the contralateral limb; it is necessary to alternate the wrap cranial and caudal to the contralateral limb in dogs that are likely to step out of their sling. This is especially true of young energetic dogs with relatively nonpainful conditions, such as bicipital bursitis. Gauze and elastic tape are used successively to cover the padding. A small (3-cm) window is cut into the lateral surface of the bandage for daily assessment of the toes and foot.

A Velpeau sling is a comfortable bandage and if properly applied causes few complications. Abrasions may develop where the bandage touches the opposite

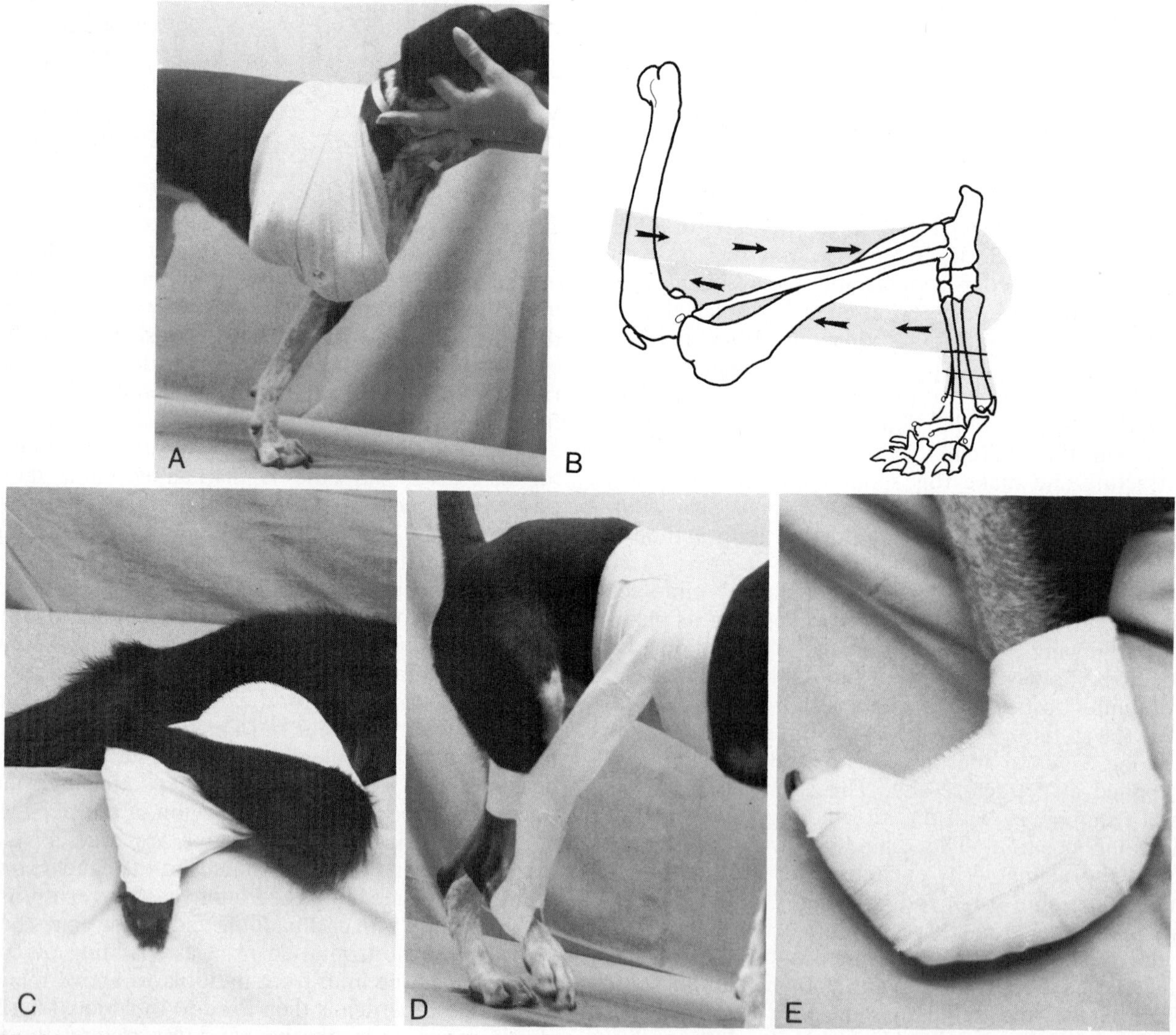

FIGURE 124–7. Slings to prevent weightbearing. *A*, Velpeau sling. *B*, Direction for fabrication of an Ehmer sling. *C*, Completed Ehmer sling. *D*, Pelvic limb (Robinson) sling. *E*, Carpal flexion bandage.

axilla and may be avoided by careful observation and removal of excessive bandage material. Care is taken in application of the sling not to compress the animal's thorax or to compress the flexed carpus and paw with gauze and elastic tape. Undue compression of the bandage material or pre-existing vascular obstruction of the paw may result in necrosis of the skin and underlying structures.

Ehmer Sling

An Ehmer sling is used to prevent weightbearing on a pelvic limb and to maintain a limited degree of internal rotation of the hip and abduction of the limb. It is commonly used as primary coaptation after closed reduction for craniodorsal coxofemoral luxation. Internal rotation of the hip rotates the femoral head beneath the dorsal rim of the acetabulum to help prevent reluxation of that joint. Unfortunately, internal rotation of the hip joint is not rigidly fixed with this sling, and reluxation of the joint can and does occur. An Ehmer sling is also commonly used as adjunct stabilization for coxofemoral luxations after surgical correction and to prevent weightbearing after internal repair of acetabular and femoral fractures.

A small amount of cast padding is first wrapped around the metatarsus to prevent skin necrosis in this area. Gauze is next wrapped around the metatarsus and continued to extend over the metatarsus and around the medial side of the stifle joint while holding the stifle and tarsus flexed (Fig. 124–7*B*). Gauze is continued over the cranial and lateral aspects of the stifle joint, keeping the sling as high as possible on the upper thigh. The gauze is continued medially to the tarsus and back over the dorsum of the metatarsus. Several layers of gauze are added, following the same path. Elastic tape is used to cover the gauze and also to overlap onto the skin by approximately 1 inch. A properly constructed Ehmer sling has no circumferential bands around any aspect of the limb, except for the initial padding of the metatarsus (Fig. 124–7*C*).

An Ehmer sling may be maintained for 2 weeks after its application. The sling must be carefully observed for complications. Abrasions or pressure necrosis of the skin may develop over the cranial thigh or the medial tarsus. The toes and foot must be carefully observed for swelling or other signs of vascular interference. Although serious complications are rare, they may be devastating. If serious complications arise, the sling is changed or removed completely. The most common problem with an Ehmer sling is that it slips from the stifle and becomes nonfunctional. If recurrent slippage develops, a belly band may be constructed of gauze and tape. The sling is fixed to the belly band to improve abduction and to help stabilize the stifle with internal rotation. This is especially useful in cats, which have very mobile skin over the stifle and are difficult to maintain in an Ehmer sling.

Pelvic Limb Sling

A pelvic limb sling (Robinson sling) prevents weightbearing on the hindlimb but allows relatively free movement of the joints (Fig. 124–7*D*).[6] It is only rarely used as primary stabilization of an injury but serves as an excellent adjunct to surgical repair. The sling may be used to prevent stress on healing fractures of the femur and tibia and is also used after coxofemoral and stifle joint operations.

Elastic gauze and adhesive or elastic tape are applied to the abdomen and caudal thorax to create a 4-inch-wide circumferential band that anchors the sling to the torso. A long strip of 3-inch adhesive tape, sized to the animal, is doubled over on itself to create a strip of tape with no adhesive showing. The midpoint of the tape strip is passed around the metatarsus, with the two loose ends parallel and pointing cranially. The strip is secured to the metatarsus by wrapping additional tape around the strips cranial to the foot, encircling the foot. Additional padding (cast padding and gauze) may be applied to the metatarsal region before this step, if desired. The loose ends of the tape strip are brought dorsally and cranially, one on each side of the affected limb. Both strips are fixed to the circular abdominal band on the same (affected) side. They are secured dorsally on the anchoring band with sufficient tension to raise the foot from the ground by 2 to 4 inches. Several wraps of adhesive tape are sufficient to secure the strips to the anchoring band. Additional adhesive tape is used to connect the two main strips of tape behind the tibia to prevent slippage of the sling. The pelvic limb sling may easily be maintained for several weeks without causing complications.

Carpal Flexion Bandage

A carpal flexion bandage prevents weightbearing on the forelimb and firmly flexes the carpus to relieve tension from the flexor tendons.[2] It is most commonly used to shield stress from tendon repairs after traumatic laceration and to prevent weightbearing for other orthopedic repairs of the forelimb.

To construct a carpal flexion bandage, the carpus is flexed and then wrapped with cast padding and gauze. Flexion is maintained by wrapping 1-inch elastic tape in a circular pattern from the paw to the distal radius. The entire bandage is covered with wider adhesive or elastic tape (Fig. 124–7*E*).

A carpal flexion bandage provides excellent protection of flexor tendon repairs in the forelimb. Caution is required when using this bandage in the presence of generalized carpal soft-tissue injury. If the carpus is maintained in an extreme flexed position for too long, adhesions that are strong enough to prevent extension of the carpus may form. To avoid permanent contracture of the carpus, limited extension is returned within 3 to 4 weeks after surgery by lengthening the circular bands to allow partial or complete extension.

Hobbles

Hobbles are circumferential tape strips constructed to allow weightbearing on the hindlimbs and walking but prevent abduction of the limbs at different levels. Tarsal hobbles are placed just above the tarsus and provide mild support and assistance in walking to animals recovering from pelvic trauma. Tarsal hobbles prevent abduction of the limb at the tarsus but do not prevent abduction of the stifles and distal femur. With traumatic caudoventral coxofemoral luxation, abduction of the stifles must be avoided to prevent reluxation. Stifle hobbles should be constructed after closed reduction or internal repair of this injury.

Tarsal hobbles are constructed by doubling adhesive tape to form a strip of sufficient length without any adhesive surface showing. The strip is loosely wrapped around both hindlimbs above the tarsus, with enough space between the legs to allow walking but prevent abduction. The strip encircles both limbs and is secured to itself with adhesive tape. The hobbles are secured from slipping by wrapping additional tape between the legs, effectively entrapping each individual limb (Fig. 124–8*A*).

Stifle hobbles are made similarly but, without modification, tend to slip distally. To prevent slipping, an additional strip of tape is doubled over to cover its adhesive surface and is fixed to the lateral and cranial surface of the stifle hobble. The tape strip is directed dorsally over the back of the dog, cranial to the pelvis, and brought down to the opposite limb to be fixed to the lateral and cranial aspect on the other side of the hobble. This additional strip of tape prevents the stifle hobbles from slipping distally and therefore prevents stifle abduction (Fig. 124–8*B*).

Full Leg Cast

A cast is a limb splint constructed with light padding and casting tape applied circumferentially to rigidly enclose an extremity (Fig. 124–9). The stability achieved is adequate fixation for healing of many fractures and joint conditions. A full leg cast encloses the limb from the toes to the midshaft humerus in the forelimb or midshaft femur in the hindlimb. It is impossible to extend the cast any more proximally because of soft-tissue impingement in the axilla or inguinal regions. The shoulder and hip joints are not immobilized in the conventional full leg cast, effectively limiting the use of casts for fractures below the level of the elbow or stifle joint. Casts are most effective in treating minimally displaced stable fractures of the radius, ulna, tibia, and fibula in young, fast-healing animals. They may be used for adjunctive fixation of internal fixation. Displaced fractures may be treated with a cast if the fracture is properly reduced and aligned before applying the cast. Many badly displaced fractures may be impossible to maintain in reduction without surgical intervention. For instance, a cast applied to a midshaft oblique tibia fracture may be inadequate to overcome shearing forces at the fracture site during weightbearing. If reduction cannot be maintained by the cast, surgical intervention is indicated rather than risking a delayed union. A cast is never used to rigidly enclose a fracture site when extensive soft-tissue damage has occurred and severe

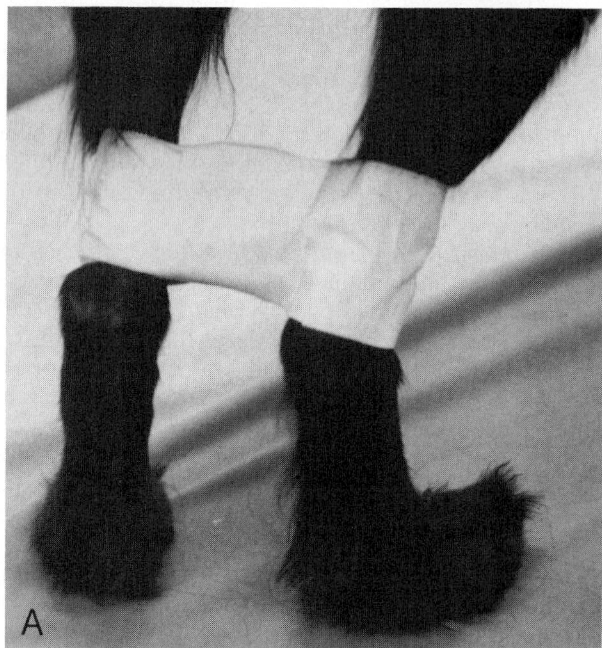

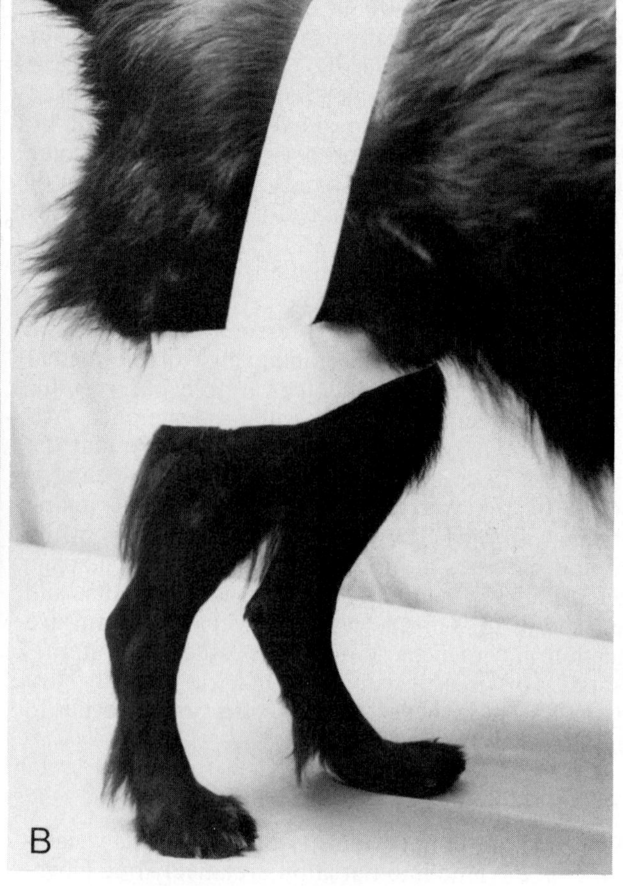

FIGURE 124–8. Hobbles. *A*, Tarsal hobbles. *B*, Stifle hobbles. Note that additional pelvic tape strip prevents distal slippage.

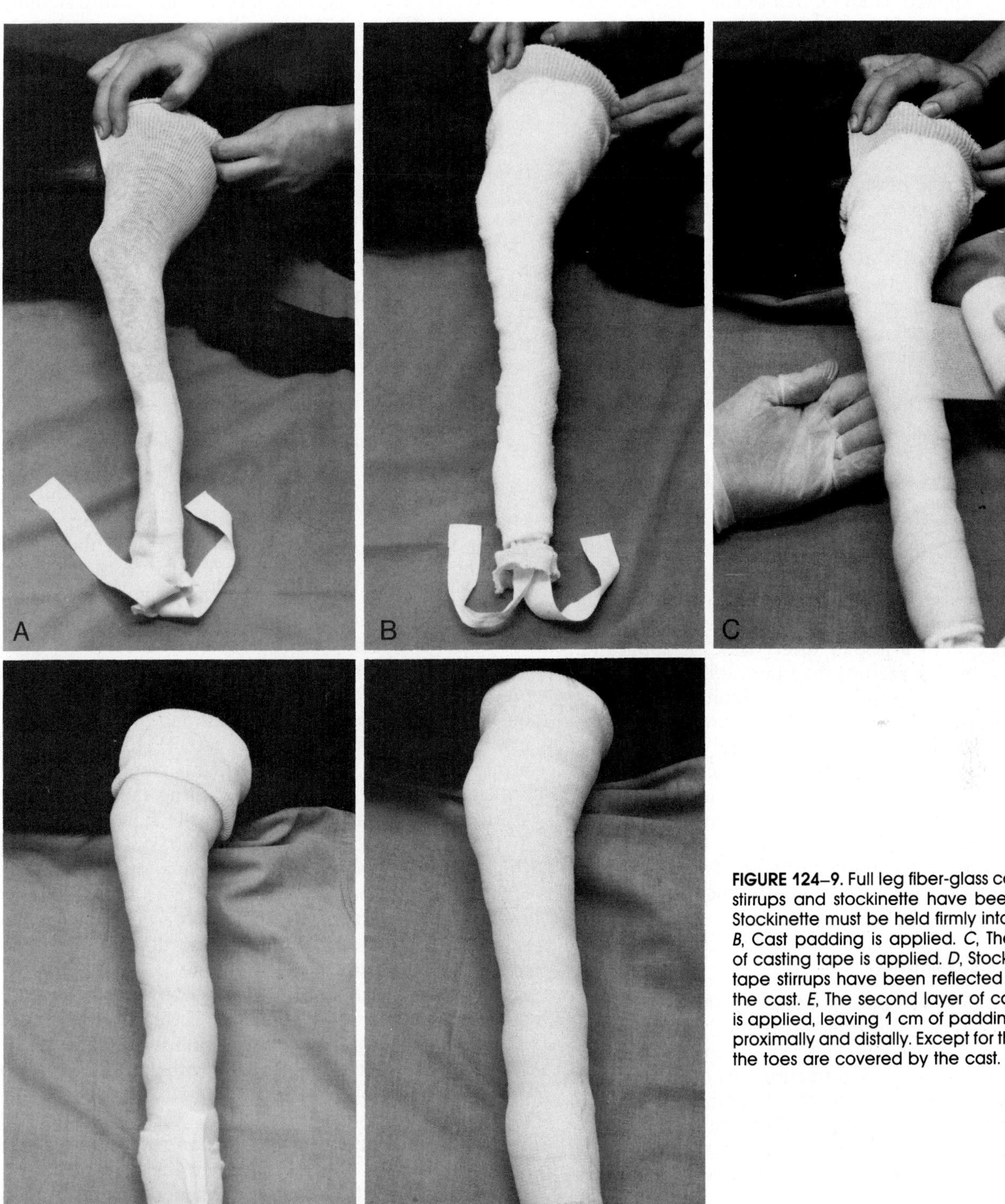

FIGURE 124–9. Full leg fiber-glass cast. *A*, Tape stirrups and stockinette have been applied. Stockinette must be held firmly into the axilla. *B*, Cast padding is applied. *C*, The first layer of casting tape is applied. *D*, Stockinette and tape stirrups have been reflected back onto the cast. *E*, The second layer of casting tape is applied, leaving 1 cm of padding exposed proximally and distally. Except for the toenails, the toes are covered by the cast.

inflammation is expected. Swelling can be sufficient to cause vascular obstruction and necrosis of the limb (see Fig. 124–3*C*). A more heavily padded bandage or splint is then used temporarily until swelling is reduced and a cast may be applied safely. Open wounds are not covered by casts unless frequent changes are anticipated or unless a "window" is cut into the cast for local treatment of the wound. Large cast windows affect stability of the coaptation.[2]

Cast Materials

Casts made from plaster-impregnated casting tape are strong and inexpensive. Several disadvantages of plaster casting tape have made the newer resin-impregnated casting tapes more desirable for veterinary use. Dogs are especially prone to soil or wet a cast. Plaster loses strength when wet and does not dry well if soaked. Moist dermatitis and tissue maceration may develop if the cast is not properly dried or changed. Plaster casts are heavy and may impede movement in small dogs or cats. Because plaster is relatively radiopaque, assessment of bone healing with radiographs may require cast removal.

Newer synthetic casting tapes are fiber-glass or polyester fabrics impregnated with water-activated polyurethane resin. They are lightweight, extremely strong, impact resistant, and radiolucent and do not lose significant strength when wet. Most manufacturers do not suggest allowing fiber-glass casts to get wet. If an accident occurs, fiber-glass casts may be carefully and thoroughly dried with a hot-air drier. Ease of application and conformability are less than desirable with some of the older fiber-glass products, but handling characteristics of the material have now been improved. Extensible fiber-glass fabric has greatly improved the ability of synthetic casting tape to conform to the anatomy of a dog's leg. Silicone has been added to the polyurethane resin to reduce the tacky feel of uncured resin. The single most persistent criticism of synthetic casting tape is the expense. Polyurethane-impregnated fiber-glass casting tapes cost far more (6 to 10 times) than plaster casting tape.

Method of Application

For most dogs and cats, general anesthesia is advised for closed fracture reduction and application of the cast. The animal is placed in lateral recumbency with the affected leg up. Slow, even traction and digital pressure directed by radiographs of the fracture are used to reduce and align the fracture. With the limb carefully supported, tape stirrups are applied to the medial and lateral surfaces of the foot. A one-layer cast stockinette is applied from the toes to as high on the limb as possible (see Fig. 124–9*A*). The stockinette exceeds the cast both proximally and distally by 1 to 2 inches to enable the material to be folded over later in the procedure. Doughnuts may be constructed by cutting holes in small pads made of cast padding. They are applied to the accessory carpal bone and the olecranon of the front limb or to the calcaneus of the hindlimb to help prevent pressure ulceration on these structures.

Beginning with the toes, cast padding is wrapped around the leg and proximally by overlapping the previous layer by one-third to one-half. The doughnuts are fixed in place beneath the cast padding. Padding does not exceed two layers thick, if optimum fracture stability is desired. Gloves are worn to protect the operator's hands from resin of the synthetic casting tape. Casting tape is selected for the animal, based on its size—2 inch for cats and small dogs and 3 inch for medium-sized to large dogs. The casting tape is immersed in cold water and squeezed several times to facilitate water penetration into the roll. Excess water is squeezed from the roll, and the tape is immediately applied to the limb (Fig. 124–9*B*). It is important to work quickly because most fiber-glass casting tapes set in 5 to 7 minutes. Beginning at the toes, the casting tape is wrapped around several times to begin the cast. The cast encloses the toes, but the end is left open for evaluation of the two middle toes. If any portion of a toe extends distally beyond the cast, tissue maceration may develop during weightbearing (see Fig. 124–3*B*). As an added precaution to avoid damage to the toes, cast padding extends about 1 cm beyond the casting tape.

Casting tape is rapidly applied with moderate pressure up the leg, with about 50 per cent overlap of the preceding wrap. Care is taken to avoid wrinkles in the casting tape as it is worked over major angulations of the limb. As the casting tape is applied to the thigh or the upper forelimb, additional tension is used to compress the larger muscle mass. At the proximal limit of the cast, the casting tape is terminated about 1 cm from the end of the cast padding. After one layer of casting tape has been applied, the ends of the stockinette are quickly reflected back over the cast and the tape stirrups inverted and adhered to the cast (Fig. 124–9*C*). If bivalving the cast is anticipated, this step is postponed until after the second wrap of casting tape. A second layer of casting tape is applied in the same way as the first, covering the tape stirrups and stockinette ends (Fig. 124–9*D*). Note that two layers of casting tape applied with 50 per cent overlap create four layers on cross section of the cast, sufficient for weightbearing in small to medium-sized dogs. Larger dogs require four to six layers to allow weightbearing.

Specific instructions are given to owners to ensure proper cast care after application. The cast must be kept clean and dry to prevent acute dermatitis underneath it. The end of the cast is covered with heavy plastic to prevent wetting when the animal is walked outside. The proximal and distal edges of the cast are examined frequently to check for skin abrasion. If pressure ulceration of the skin develops under the cast, the only external manifestations may be lameness and a fetid odor from developing exudates. The toes are monitored daily for swelling that might signal vascular obstruction. If cast complications develop, the cast is changed or removed. If properly maintained, a cast may be left intact for about 1 month in an adult animal. In a rapidly growing animal, full leg casts are changed every 2 weeks. Radiographs are taken monthly to assess fracture healing, or sooner if the cast must be changed.

Cast Removal

An oscillating cast saw is required for removal of fiber-glass casts. Because of the considerable noise and vibrations generated by this instrument, a mild tranquilizer is administered. The cast is cut on two sides for removal, either medial and lateral or cranial and caudal. The cast saw is used to cut the cast with an up-and-down cutting action rather than a side-to-side sawing motion to minimize skin lacerations.

Modifications of Casts

Half Cast. A half cast is shorter than a full leg cast and does not extend above the elbow or stifle. Also called a *walking cast*, a half cast is indicated in minimally displaced fractures of the metacarpus and metatarsus and to immobilize various carpal and tarsal conditions. Some have advocated use of a half cast for tibial and radial fractures, where the cast relies on muscle compression rather than immobilization of the joints to stabilize a fracture site.[7, 8] Extreme care should be used in selecting appropriate radial and tibial fractures to treat with a half cast. This cast is used only for relatively stable nondisplaced fractures, in which rotational forces at the fracture site are already effectively neutralized (intact fibula or ulna).

Walking Bar. A walking bar may be applied to any cast by contouring aluminum splint rod to the end of the cast and taping it in place (Fig. 124–10*A*). A walking bar prevents direct weightbearing on the toes and may be useful in treating metacarpal or metatarsal injuries or to help prevent cast-induced abrasions of the toes if the cast is too short.

Bivalved Cast. Changing a cast frequently to examine the limb is usually contraindicated. Excessive movement at the fracture may cause loss of fracture reduction and delay healing. Newer fiber-glass casting tape is radiolucent and allows radiographs to be taken to check fracture reduction and healing without removing the cast. Some conditions of soft tissue require more frequent access to the limb for wound care and assessment. Pre-existing soft-tissue trauma or complications from a previously applied cast, such as severe skin ulceration, may require frequent rebandaging and therefore cast changes. Small windows may be cut into the cast for limited access to a wound or to relieve pressure on an area (e.g., the point of the calcaneus). If a major wound is present, bivalving the cast allows frequent cast changes without the added expense of new casting tape at each change. If bivalving a cast is anticipated, the stockinette and tape stirrups are not incorporated into the casting tape but taped to the outer surface of the cast.

To bivalve a cast, an oscillating cast cutter is used to cut through the casting tape along the medial and lateral sides of the cast (Fig. 124–10*B*). When it is time to change the cast, the two halves of the cast are removed intact. After local wound care is completed, new cast

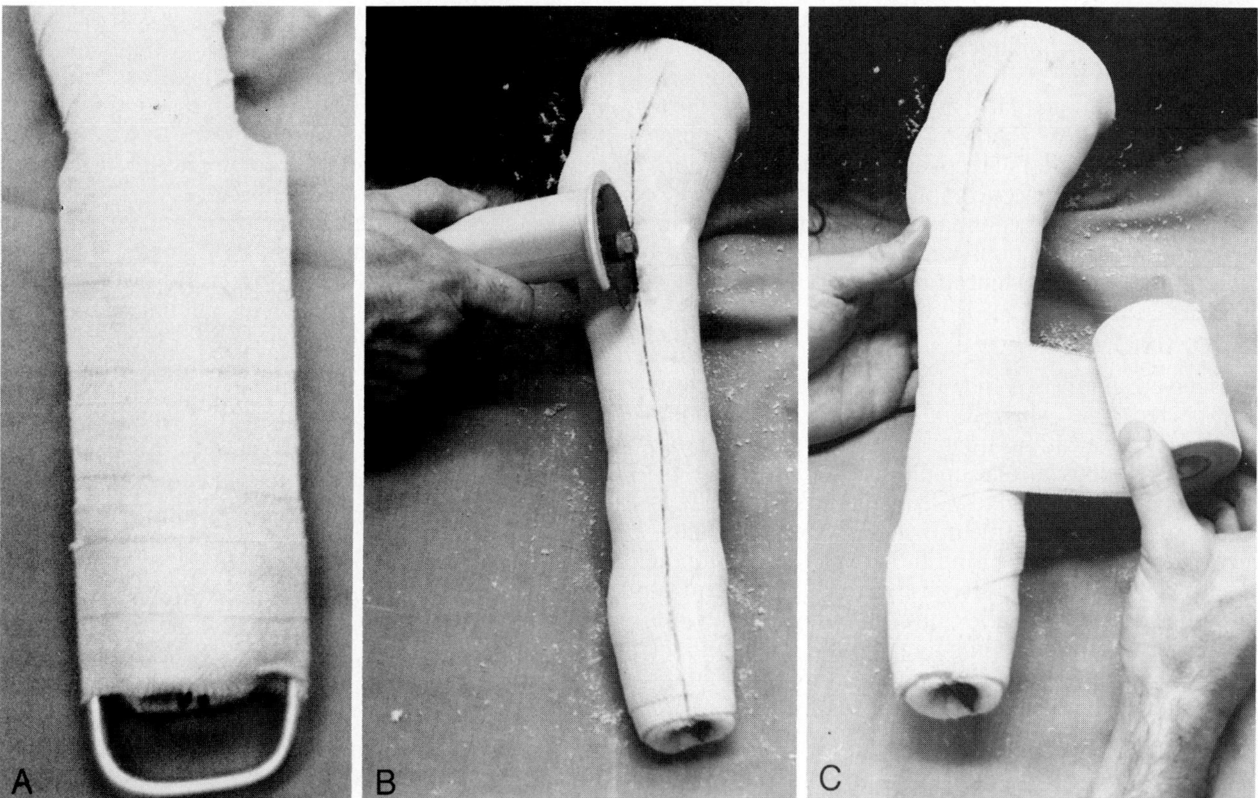

FIGURE 124–10. Modifications of the cast. *A*, A walking bar has been applied to prevent any weightbearing on the toes. *B*, An oscillating saw is used to "bivalve" the cast if frequent changes are required for wound care. *C*, The bivalved cast is taped closed after wound care is completed and new padding has been applied.

padding is applied to the limb, and the original halves of the cast are reused. Slight modification of the original cast may be made with the cast cutter to help fit the cast to the new padding. Cutting off the sharp corners of each half of the cast often helps with the fitting. A bivalved cast is covered with elastic tape until the next cast change (Fig. 124–10*C*).

References

1. Arnoczky SP, Stoll SG: External coaptation. Proceedings of the 46th Annual Meeting of the American Animal Hospital Association, New Orleans, April 1979.
2. Arnoczky SP, et al: External coaptation and bandaging. *In* Slatter DH (ed): *Textbook of Small Animal Surgery*. W. B. Saunders, Philadelphia, 1985.
3. Brinker WO, et al: *Handbook of Small Animal Orthopedics and Fracture Treatment*. W. B. Saunders, Philadelphia, 1983.
4. Nunamaker DM: Methods of closed fixation. *In* Newton CD, Nunamaker DM (eds): *Textbook of Small Animal Orthopaedics*. J. B. Lippincott, Philadelphia, 1985.
5. Prieur WD, Sumner-Smith G: Bone splinting. *In* Brinker WO, et al (eds): *Manual of Internal Fixation in Small Animals*. Springer-Verlag, New York, 1984.
6. Robinson GW, McCoy L: A pelvic sling for dogs. *In* Bojrab MJ (ed): *Current Techniques in Small Animal Surgery*. Lea & Febiger, Philadelphia, 1975.
7. Sarmiento A: A functional below-the-knee cast for tibial fractures. *J Bone Joint Surg 49A*:855, 1967.
8. Smith GK: Biomechanics pertinent to fracture etiology, reduction, and fixation. *In* Newton CD, Nunamaker DM (eds): *Textbook of Small Animal Orthopaedics*. J. B. Lippincott, Philadelphia, 1985.
9. Swaim SF: *Surgery of Traumatized Skin: Management and Reconstruction in the Dog and Cat*. W. B. Saunders, Philadelphia, 1980.
10. Wu KK: *Techniques In Surgical Casting and Splinting*. Lea & Febiger, Philadelphia, 1987.

CHAPTER 125 Delayed Union, Nonunion, and Malunion

Robert E. Kaderly

The goal of fracture treatment is complete functional recovery of the injured limb as quickly as possible. A delayed union prolongs a patient's discomfort and disability, but eventual satisfactory union of the fracture is usually possible. A nonunion limits limb use because of the loss of normal skeletal support at the pseudoarthrosis. A malunion that has caused significant shortening, angulation, or rotation of the limb likewise prevents complete functional recovery. Most delayed union, nonunion, and malunion complications are directly related to conservative treatment or nontreatment of fractures, orthopedic infections, technical errors in fracture fixation, and errors in clinical judgment.

DELAYED UNION

A delayed union is a fracture that has not healed in the expected time when compared with other similar fractures (type, location) treated similarly in comparable patients. Metaphyseal and epiphyseal fractures are expected to heal more rapidly than diaphyseal fractures because of the greater fracture surface area, the abundance of cancellous bone, and the greater circulation at the ends of long bones.[16] Because periosteal and endosteal tissues are more proliferative in young animals,[19] a properly treated fracture in a 6-month-old animal might unite in 6 weeks whereas the same fracture in a mature animal might require 12 weeks or more. A delayed union infers that the fracture healing process is continuing but at a less than optimal rate.

Pathophysiology and Pathology

Prolongation of the fracture healing process has been associated with local physical factors and systemic factors (see Chapter 120 for a review of fracture healing). Physical factors at the fracture site include instability, vascular impairment, large fracture gaps, interposed soft tissues, infection, and inappropriate use of skeletal implants. Rigid stabilization of bone fragments is one prerequisite for primary bone healing. Instability causes mechanical damage to delicate vessels and prevents resorption cavities from crossing the fracture site and developing into "spot welds" of mature osteons.[28] In secondary bone healing, the processes of vascularization of the soft callus, callus ossification, and anastomosis of damaged intramedullary vessels are impaired by motion at the fracture site. Although fracture healing can overcome a considerable amount of bending, compression, and some tension at the fracture site, shear and torsion disrupt the uniting fibroblastic network.[34] The degree of instability at the fracture site influences the method of callus ossification and is inversely proportional to the rate of callus ossification. Little instability at the fracture site allows bone to form directly in the callus by osteogenic cells; with greater instability, fibroblasts first form fibrous tissue that undergoes necrosis, mineralizes, and is replaced by bone; with even greater instability, chondrocytes first form cartilage, and the slow process of endochondral ossification is begun.

Vascular impairment at the fracture site may also be a result of injury to adjacent soft tissues at the time of fracture formation or during open reduction and internal fixation. The soft tissues surrounding a fracture provide the periosteal callus with the extraosseous blood supply of healing bone.[25] Fractures occurring in bones poorly covered by muscle (radius, tibia) normally heal more slowly because the available source of vessels for recruitment into the healing process is limited. Avascular bone fragments delay healing and must be revascularized to undergo resorption or incorporation into the fracture callus. Generalized impairment of limb circulation may be present because of remote vascular damage, concurrent systemic disease, old age, or limb immobilization. Limb immobilization results in various degrees of disuse muscle atrophy and osteoporosis.

Large gaps at a fracture site due to poor reduction, severe comminution, or bone loss increase the time required for bridging callus to unite and stabilize the main fracture fragments. Muscle, fascia, or other soft tissues may be interposed in large gaps between fracture fragments (particularly during attempts at closed reduction) or become incorporated into large gaps during healing. Interposed soft tissue prevents rigid stability, maintains the fracture gap, and acts as a barrier to bridging callus formation.

Infection at the fracture site delays the healing process by promoting tissue ischemia and necrosis. During the inflammatory response, bacteria and inflammatory cells die, proteolytic enzymes are released, local pH decreases, ossified tissue is demineralized and resorbed, purulent debris accumulates, and greater ischemia and tissue necrosis ensue. Necrotic bone is resorbed or sequestered, and the fracture gap enlarges. Open fractures and open repair of closed fractures are the most common causes of osteomyelitis in small animal orthopedics.[9, 33] In one retrospective study of humans, the incidence of delayed union was twice as high in open fractures as in closed, and the incidence of nonunion was four times higher in open fractures than in closed.[41]

Noninfectious nonsuppurative osteomyelitis may occur around metal implants as a result of metal corrosion, use of dissimilar metals, or an allergic reaction to the foreign material (metallosis). Bony lysis and implant loosening may prolong fracture healing.

Inappropriate use or technical errors involving skeletal implants often contribute to delayed fracture healing. Full-cerclage or hemicerclage orthopedic wire applied too loosely allows micromotion of the fragments and results in bone resorption. A cerclage wire placed in a fracture line or migrating into it also allows micromotion and interferes with bridging callus formation.[22] Very large rigid implants (particularly bone plates) assume the forces of weightbearing normally borne by the fractured limb, sometimes resulting in "stress shielding" osteoporosis and prolonged bone remodeling.[8]

Several systemic factors have also been implicated in delayed fracture healing. Cortical alloimplants from nonmatched donors cause immune reactions, which delay fracture healing and graft incorporation.[5] Nutritional disturbances, avitaminosis, diseases involving calcium and phosphorus metabolism, pre-existing osteomalacia or osteoporosis, and cancer cachexia can interfere with osteoid mineralization.[26] A fundamental disturbance in the production or differentiation of mesenchymal stem cells into sufficient quantities of osteoblasts or chondroblasts is also suspected in some cases.[15]

Histological Characteristics

Delayed union is characterized by abundant periosteal and endosteal callus and vigorous intracortical remodeling. The original fracture hematoma is replaced with fibrous connective tissue and fibrocartilage (Fig. 125–1). Intramembranous bone formation and endochondral bone formation occur simultaneously in different areas. Osteoblasts are present and are actively depositing osteoid on the surface of collagen fiber bundles (intramembranous bone formation). Avascular zones of fibrocartilage are found more centrally in areas of compression. Fibrocartilage mineralization and eventual endochondral bone formation occur if bone healing continues.

Clinical Signs and Diagnosis

The diagnosis of a delayed union is a matter of degree. A delayed union may be described as a fracture that is relatively stable, will likely end in clinical union, but is healing at a less than optimal rate. A delayed union

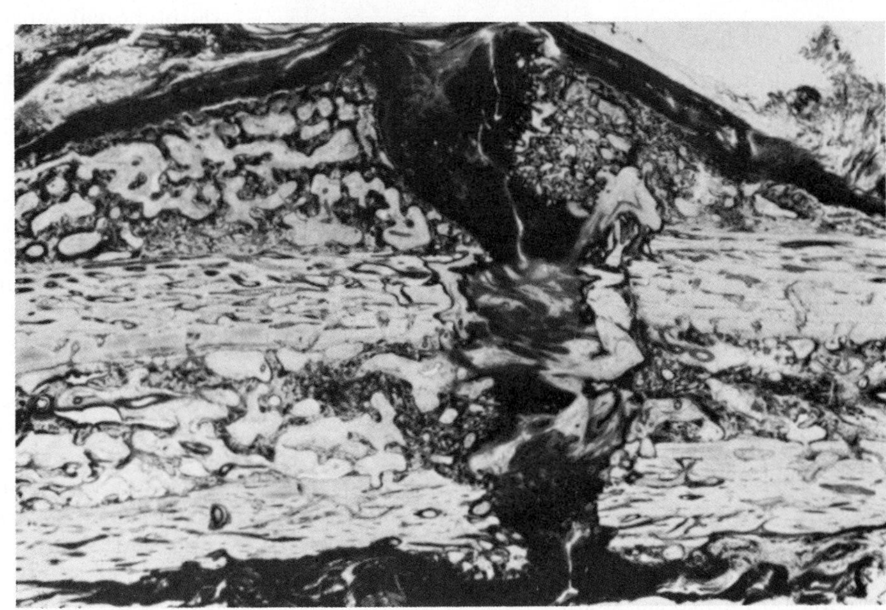

FIGURE 125–1. Histological characteristics of an experimentally induced *delayed nonunion.* Nonbridging woven bony callus is present; vigorous intracortical remodeling is occurring at the ends of the fracture fragments. Interfragmentary tissue consists of areas of fibrous tissue and fibrocartilage. (×7) (From Schenk RK, Müller J, Willenegsen H: Nonunion: The histologic picture. *In* Sumner-Smith G [ed]: *Bone in Clinical Orthopaedics.* W. B. Saunders, Philadelphia, 1982, p. 445.)

may also be described as a fracture that is grossly unstable and will likely end in nonunion (i.e., the healing process ceases). After the expected period of time for the completion of normal fracture healing has elapsed, the clinical signs of persistence of pain, warmth and instability at the fracture site, the animal's reluctance to use the limb, and the presence of disuse muscle atrophy may suggest that fracture healing is progressing but union is delayed.

Several procedures may be performed to determine more objectively the stage of fracture healing and to differentiate delayed union from nonunion. A comparison of sequential radiographs taken at 4- to 6-week intervals should show progression of healing. Radiographic characteristics of ongoing fracture healing include limited bone resorption at the fracture site, periosteal new bone formation somewhat proximal and distal to the fracture site, periosteal and endosteal bridging callus, and bridging callus mineralization. The medullary cavity remains open at the fracture site throughout the healing process (Fig. 125–2).

Bone scintigraphy (radionuclide imaging) also may be used to evaluate suspected delayed unions and nonunions. Injected radiopharmaceutical concentrates at sites of hypervascularity, osteogenesis, and active bone remodeling.[20] In normal fracture healing, increased radiopharmaceutical uptake reaches a peak 1 to 3 months after injury and declines to normal by about 12 months.[17] In humans, a persistent photopenic area ("cold spot") occurring at the fracture site within 4 weeks of injury suggests delayed union, nonunion, or sequestrum formation.[30]

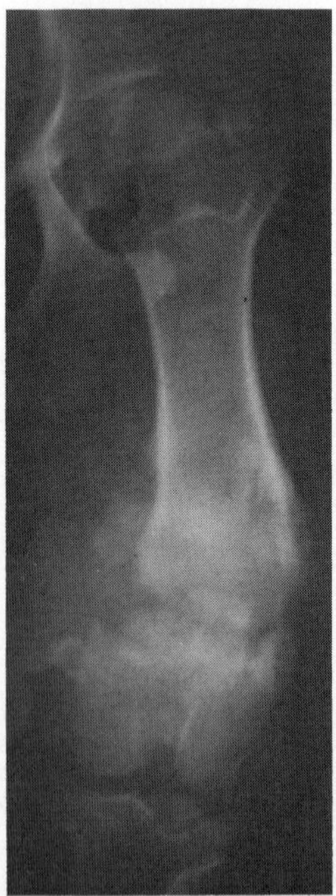
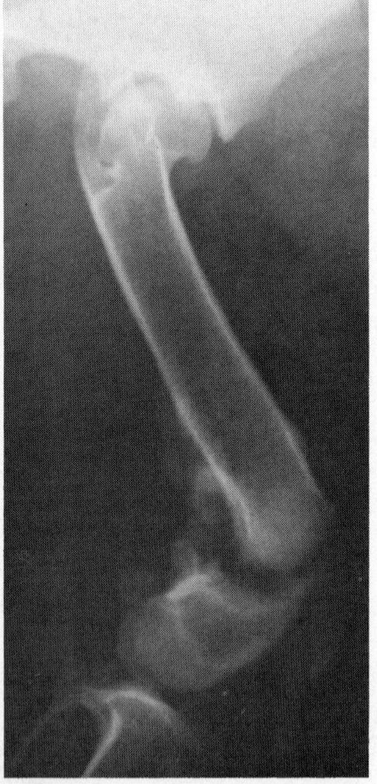

FIGURE 125–2. Six-week-old delayed union of a supracondylar fracture of the left femur in a young basset hound that had been treated initially by external coaptation. Even in the presence of considerable instability, proliferative ossified callus caudally suggests an osteogenic response sufficient to bridge the fracture gap and eventually form a malunion.

Osteomedullography involves the instillation of contrast medium into the medullary cavity of the distal fracture fragment. A series of radiographs are made at 1-second intervals for 5 seconds. In normal fracture healing, continuity of contrast medium across the fracture is radiographically apparent within 3 weeks of fracture treatment. Delayed union with the potential for eventual union is also characterized by a positive osteomedullograph.[23]

Clinical Treatment

After physical examination and radiography, reasons for a delay in the fracture healing process are often obvious. Part of the treatment plan includes correcting the cause of the delayed union.

Noninfected Delayed Unions (Fig. 125–3)

Surgical intervention is indicated for delayed unions in which the main fracture fragments are significantly malaligned and cannot be adequately realigned by closed reduction. If malalignment has continued for several weeks and over-riding or angulation is severe, open reduction may be difficult. If malalignment is a result of implant failure or loosening, the original implants are removed. Gentle use of a fracture distractor and incision of the tissues within the fracture site permit distraction and alignment of the fragments. Fibrous or cartilaginous tissue within the fracture gap need not be excised if adequate reduction and rigid stabilization with compression can be achieved.[27] Dynamic compression bone plating, bone plating using a compression jig, and a rigid external fixator configuration in a compression mode are options.

Surgical intervention is also indicated in adequately aligned delayed unions in which skeletal implants have loosened, significant instability is present at the fracture site, and conservative treatment may end in nonunion. Surgical treatment need not always involve exposure of the fracture site. The addition of an external fixator to a rotationally unstable fracture in which an intramedullary pin was used often allows union. If rotational instability of a femoral, tibial, or humeral fracture is due to a single small loose-fitting intramedullary pin, closed insertion of additional small intramedullary pins (stacked pinning) may be successful.[36] Compression is applied to the fracture before tightening the external fixator clamps or seating the stacked intramedullary pins to increase friction between fragments and reduce interfragmentary strain. A loose bone plate is firmly reattached or replaced with a new compression plate attached to the bone by screws placed through new screw holes. A loose bone plate can occasionally be firmly reattached by substituting cancellous screws for some of the original cortical screws.

Delayed unions involving aligned main fracture fragments may be treated conservatively if skeletal implants have remained firmly attached to the bone fragments, instability at the fracture site is minimal, no obvious signs of osteomyelitis are present, and a united fracture in 8 to 12 additional weeks is highly probable. Activity

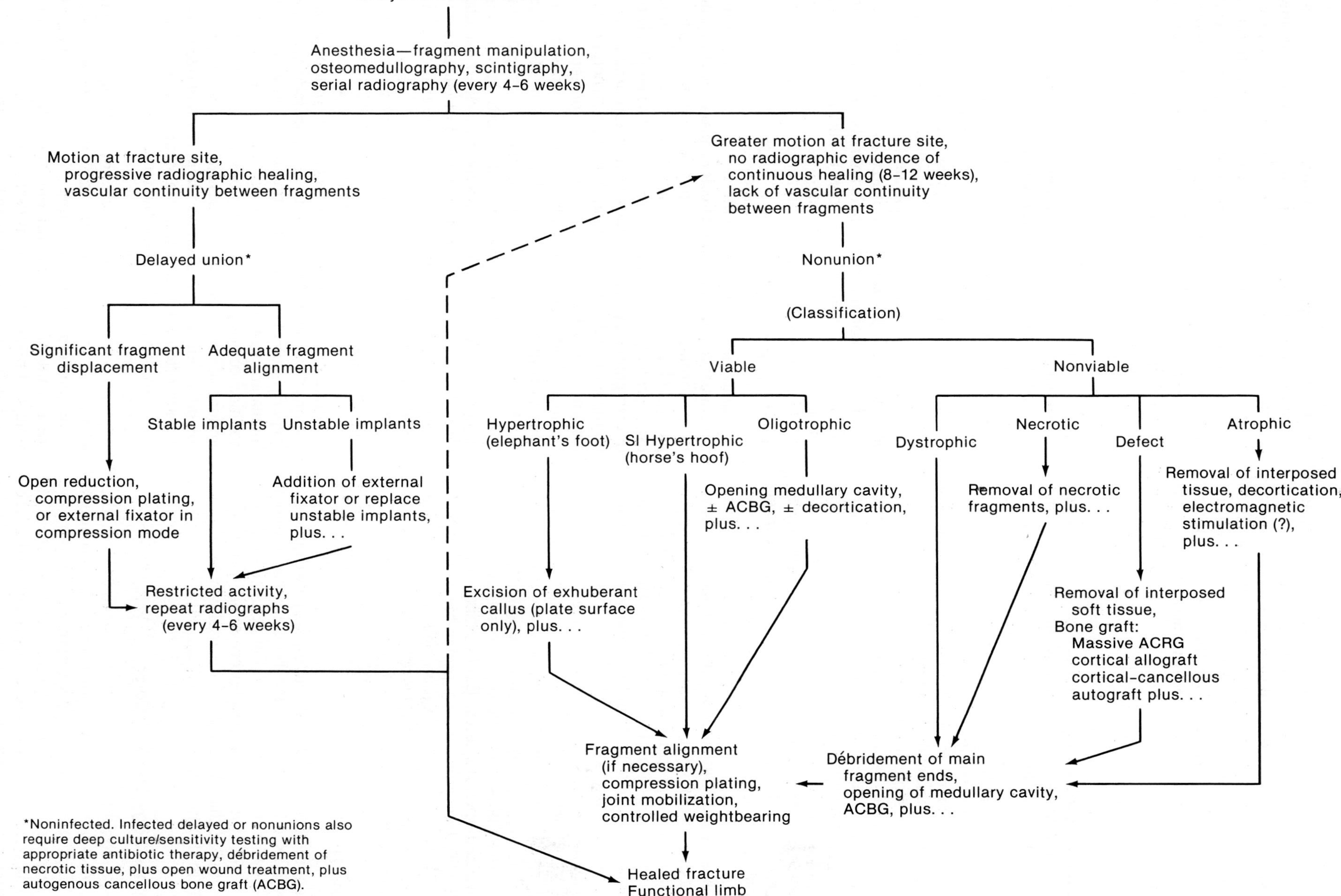

FIGURE 125–3. Pathogenesis and treatment principles of delayed union and nonunion.

must be restricted to cage rest and short leash walks until clinical union. The use of nonweightbearing slings that allow frequent passive physical therapy may enhance the chances of fracture union. Other delayed unions may be stimulated by placing the limb in a well-fitted splint or cast and inducing stress at the fracture site through controlled weightbearing activity.

Infected Delayed Unions (see Chapter 126)

Fracture healing has been shown to progress to union in the presence of infection if fracture fragments are rigidly immobilized.[45] Osteomyelitis directly delays the healing process by altering the microenvironment at the fracture site and indirectly by contributing to fracture fragment instability from implant loosening due to bone necrosis at the bone–implant interface.

Surgical treatment is indicated in infected delayed unions that radiographically demonstrate unstable implants and large sequestra. Deep culture and sensitivity testing, débridement of necrotic soft tissues, sequestrectomy, and rigid skeletal fixation with interfragmentary compression are indicated. The fracture site may then be treated as an open wound and grafted with autogenous cancellous bone after resolution of the osteomyelitis.[3] Alternatively, initial treatment may include cancellous bone grafting and primary wound closure.

Delayed unions that radiographically demonstrate mild osteomyelitis but no evidence of bone sequestra, draining fistula, or implant loosening may be treated conservatively. Appropriate conservative treatment consists of performing deep bacterial culture (using a Jamshidi bone biopsy needle[24]) and sensitivity tests, administering 6 to 8 weeks of antibiotic therapy based on sensitivity tests results, severely restricting exercise until clinical union has occurred, and radiographic re-evaluation every 2 to 4 weeks. The importance of stable rigid implants for an extended healing period suggests the use of bone plates and screws as initial treatment in most infected open fractures. External fixators that use threaded fixation pins may be preferable in grade III open fractures. Threaded fixation pins are superior to smooth pins in remaining firmly fixed at the bone–pin interface for extended periods.[2, 4]

NONUNION

A nonunion is an ununited fracture usually characterized by a pseudoarthrosis at the fracture site. Without surgical intervention, eventual union is highly doubtful because the fracture healing process has ceased. A delayed union that is healing at a very slow rate may be difficult to distinguish from nonunion.

Pathophysiology and Pathology

Several conditions contribute to nonunion, but the exact causes are unknown.[10] Bone reacts early to injury by developing a primary callus response. The primary callus response wanes after approximately 2 weeks if contact between the collars of callus is not made. The formation of an external bridging callus is also a finite response that apparently is important in stimulating the induction of osteogenic repair tissue.[21] Persistent interfragmentary instability is responsible for an increased mass of fracture callus, but motion inhibits initiation of interfragmentary fibrocartilage mineralization.[29] Until matrix mineralization occurs, interfragmentary fibrocartilage remains an avascular tissue—a barrier to the penetration of vascular resorptive channels necessary for resumption of endochondral ossification. As in delayed union instability, impaired circulation, large gaps, interposed soft tissue, and infection are major factors in decreasing interfragmentary bridging. In a large series of nonunions in human patients, nonunion occurred more commonly when fractures were open or infected, segmental (with impaired blood supply to the segmental fragment), severely comminuted, insecurely fixed, immobilized for an insufficient period of time, treated by ill-advised open reduction, or distracted by traction or by a plate and screws.[7] The description of nonunion as being "a failure of the surgeon rather than a failure of osteogenesis" is true in most cases.[39] The common locations of nonunion in small animals are radius-ulna (60 per cent), tibia (25 per cent), and femur (15 per cent).[37]

Histological Characteristics

Nonunions, compared with delayed unions, often have an increased amount of callus at the fracture site. Bone formation may be in progress in the walls of periosteal and endosteal callus on each fragment; however, *bridging* ossification is not present. The persistent interfragmentary tissue consists of a uniform zone of nonmineralized fibrocartilage. Vascular structures and evidence of active bone turnover are present at the fragment ends, but vascular resorptive canals do not penetrate the nonmineralized fibrocartilage (Fig. 125–4). Fissures may be present in the interfragmentary fibrocartilage, later showing coalescence into a joint space.[29] In older nonunions, a synovium-lined pseudarthrosis may be present, and at the end of each fracture fragment, the medullary cavity may be sealed over with ossified endosteal callus.

Classification

Nonunions may or may not be capable of a biological response and have been classified accordingly as viable (hypervascular) or nonviable (avascular).[40] Viable nonunions are subclassified as hypertrophic, slightly hypertrophic, or oligotrophic, depending on the relative amount of callus present. *Hypertrophic nonunions* ("elephant's foot") have abundant hypervascularized callus and are often related to fractures that have been destabilized by premature removal or loosening of the skeletal fixation device. *Mildly hypertrophic nonunions* ("horse's hoof") have an inadequate amount of callus, and mild sclerosis of the fragment ends; they typically occur with moderate rotational instability. *Oligotrophic nonunions* are devoid of visible callus but are still capable of a biological response. Fibrous tissue containing blood vessels may be present between the fragments, but the ends

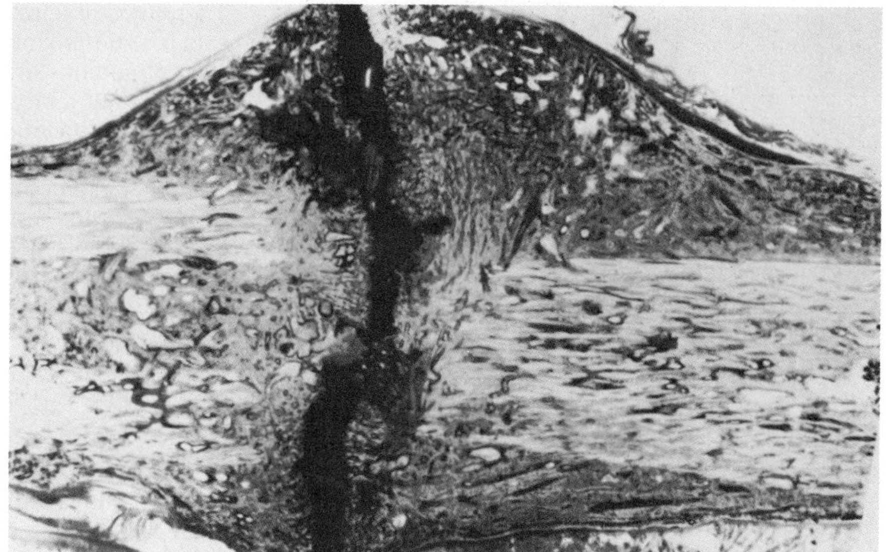

FIGURE 125–4. Histological characteristics of an experimentally induced *nonunion.* Nonbridging compact bony periosteal, endosteal, and intracortical callus is present across the fracture fragment ends. A uniform zone of fibrocartilage occupies the fracture gap. (×7) (From Schenk RK, Müller J, Willenegsen H: Nonunion: The histologic picture. *In* Sumner-Smith G [ed]: *Bone in Clinical Orthopaedics.* W. B. Saunders, Philadelphia, 1982, p. 445.)

of the fragments eventually round off, undergo resorption, and decalcify. These nonunions occur with major displacement or distraction of the fracture fragments.

Nonviable nonunions are subclassified as dystrophic, necrotic, defect, or atrophic. *Dystrophic nonunions* are characterized by an intermediate fragment that has healed to only one main fragment. The poorly vascularized intermediate fragment is incapable of stimulating a sufficient osteogenic response to bridge the gap with the second major fragment. *Necrotic nonunions* are associated with comminuted fractures in which major fragments are avascular or poorly vascularized and eventually die. The necrotic fragments do not become incorporated in the fracture callus. *Defect nonunions* result from the loss of a significant section of bone at the fracture site. At the time of injury, large fragments may be lost through open wounds. Defects may also result from resorption of necrotic fragments or removal or excision of fragments during surgery. *Atrophic nonunions* are sequelae to the other three types of nonviable nonunions. Significant bone resorption at the fragment ends, loss of all vascularity and osteogenic activity, and osteoporosis characterize these nonunions.

Clinical Signs and Diagnosis

The clinical signs of nonunion differ from delayed union. Motion at the fracture site is usually greater, and movement of the main fracture fragments is often painless or only mildly uncomfortable. Partial weightbearing on the affected limb is not unusual; however, limb deformity and muscle atrophy are present.

Radiographic characteristics of nonunion may include a variable amount of nonbridging periosteal and endosteal callus, interfragmentary radiolucency, sclerosis and smoothing of the ends of the fracture fragments, mineralized tissue sealing over the medullary cavity, and (particularly in older nonunions) a pseudarthrosis (Fig. 125–5). Necrotic bone fragments are more radiodense than viable fragments and may show sequestration and involucrum formation. Instability at the nonunion may be documented by stress radiography.

Bone scintigraphy and osteomedullography (see the earlier section on diagnosis of delayed union) may be helpful.

Clinical Treatment

Noninfected Nonunions

The mere presence of a nonunion does not dictate clinical treatment. A reasonable chance of achieving relief of discomfort, improved limb function, and correction of limb deformity should accompany any chosen treatment. Nontreatment may be the preferred choice in an older sedentary animal with a minimally displaced chronic nonunion that has formed a relatively stable, functional, and painless pseudarthrosis.

The principles of nonunion treatment differ from the general principles of fracture treatment only in their emphasis. Restoring fragment stability by rigid internal or external skeletal fixation, reducing the fracture gap by fragment alignment and compression of interfragmentary tissues, and stimulating vascularity and osteogenesis by the use of débridement, bone grafting, and decortication all are important in encouraging fracture healing in all nonunions (see Fig. 125–3). With hypertrophic viable nonunions, removal of interfragmentary tissue (nonmineralized fibrocartilage) is not necessary.[27] Only enough periosteal callus is removed to create a flat cortical surface for secure plate fixation. With slightly hypertrophic and oligotrophic viable nonunions, the ends of each main fragment may be sealed over with a confluence of ossified endosteal callus. Surgical incision into the interfragmentary tissue and opening the medullary cavity of each fragment before reduction, compression, and rigid stabilization allow intramedullary vessels to anastomose across the fracture. Although oligotrophic nonunions are capable of a biological response, in addition to the previously mentioned procedures, débridement of the fragment ends and packing

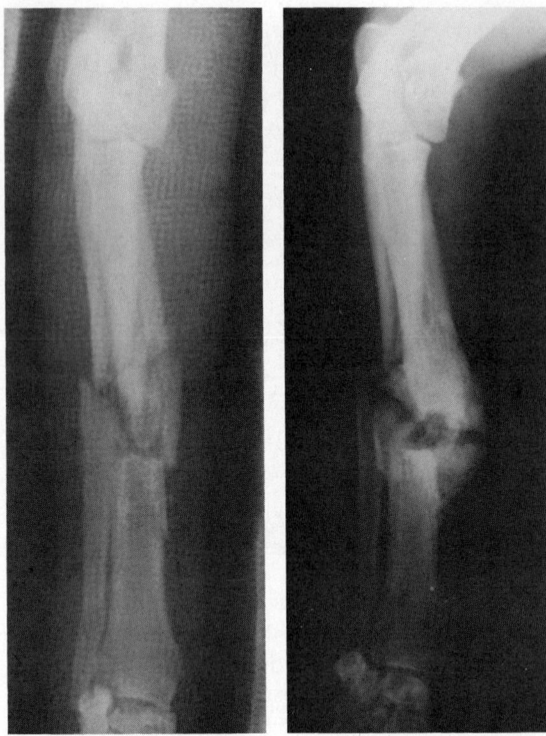

FIGURE 125–5. Original fracture and 12-week re-evaluation of a comminuted diaphyseal fracture of the right radius and ulna in a Labrador retriever. Initial fracture treatment had involved the application of a poorly conforming fiber-glass cylinder cast, which resulted in the formation of a nonunion. A pseudoarthrosis was present at the fracture site at the time of surgical intervention.

the fracture gap with generous amounts of autogenous cancellous bone improve the chance of union.

The treatment of nonviable nonunions is challenging because of the presence of necrotic bone, severely compromised blood supply, significant bone loss, and poor osteogenic potential at the fracture site. All nonviable nonunions benefit from débridement of the ends of the fracture fragments, opening the medullary cavity if necessary, and packing the fracture site with autogenous cancellous bone. Necrotic nonunions require removal of all avascular bone fragments. Defect nonunions or large defects created by the removal of necrotic fragments often require large volumes of autogenous cancellous bone or autogenous corticocancellous bone (ilial wing, rib chips) to fill the defect, as well as the use of strong buttress plates.[38] Collagen sponge is useful as a cylindrical retainer for holding cancellous bone chips in large cortical defects.[18] Resection of the fragment ends, use of a well-fitting segmental cortical alloimplant, and compression at both ends of the graft may be considered if the defect nonunion is not infected.[32] Atrophic nonunions may benefit from decortication or electromagnetic stimulation.[10] Electromagnetic therapy has been used sparingly in small animal orthopedics because of its impracticality. The devices are expensive and relatively cumbersome, and treatment of up to 12 hours per day for 3 to 6 months may be required for a beneficial effect.[10, 11, 35]

The treatment of nonunion of the metaphysis or epiphysis requires additional considerations. Because of their close proximity to a joint, metaphyseal or epiphyseal nonunions are often associated with joint stiffness; malaligned joint surfaces; hypertrophied synovium, cartilage, or bone; intra-articular adhesions; and loss of cancellous bone. Arthrotomy, alignment of the joint surface, and débridement of hypertrophied or restrictive intra-articular tissues is often necessary to re-establish an acceptable range of joint motion. The importance of prompt postoperative physical therapy emphasizes the need for strong skeletal stabilization. T-shaped or L-shaped plates, double-hook (intertrochanteric osteotomy) plates, or reconstruction plates may be used to immobilize the smaller juxta-articular fragment.

Infected Nonunions

Nonunions are frequently the result of previously infected fractures. Motion and infection are synergistic in establishing a self-perpetuating cycle of tissue destruction, fibrosis, and instability at the fracture site. Restoring rigid stability to the fracture fragments by replacing loose skeletal fixation devices is the first consideration in interrupting this destructive cycle. As with infected delayed unions, deep cultures are taken before antimicrobial therapy, and all necrotic bone and soft tissue at the fracture site are débrided. Depending on the severity of the infection, the fracture gap may be packed with autogenous cancellous bone and closed immediately, or the site may be treated as an open wound followed by cancellous bone grafting after granulation tissue has covered the exposed bone.[3] After union, skeletal implants are removed to resolve residual osteomyelitis.

MALUNION

A malunion is a fracture that has healed in an abnormal position, usually causing various degrees of functional impairment of the limb. Limb shortening, angulation, or rotation may cause improper balance or abnormal gait; uneven distribution of weight across the joint may cause degenerative arthritis, and movement of an adjacent joint may be restricted.

Pathophysiology and Pathology

Malunions often result from spontaneous healing of untreated fractures or fractures that have been treated improperly. With untreated fractures, the fragments become displaced because of the contraction of damaged muscles that span the fracture, the weight of the distal limb, or the animal's attempt to use the injured limb. Malunions resulting from improperly treated fractures are caused by either inaccurate reduction or ineffective immobilization during healing. Adequate alignment may be lost during application of a cast or splint. Valgus malalignment commonly occurs during cast application of radius and ulna or tibial fractures if the suspended injured limb is uppermost; a varus correction must be made while the cast is still moldable. A loose cast due to improper application or subsequent to the resolution of underlying soft-tissue swelling may also be responsible for loss of reduction.

Classification (Fig. 125–6)

Malunions may be classified according to the type of displacement that the main fracture fragments have undergone. *Over-riding malunions* involve long fragments that have been pulled past each other but remain axially and rotationally aligned. *Angular malunions* demonstrate significant deviation from axial alignment, and *rotational malunions* exhibit torsional deformity. Most malunions seen clinically are a combination of over-riding, angular, and rotational displacement. Poorly reduced intra-articular fractures or premature loss of intra-articular stabilization results in *intra-articular malunions*.

Clinical Treatment

The cause of the malunion, the severity of the disability, and the remodeling potential of the affected bone all are factors to be considered in determining the best course of clinical treatment (Fig. 125–6). Immature animals possess exceptional bone remodeling potential, which eventually may result in restoration of nearly normal form and function (Fig. 125–7). Surgical treatment of malunion is indicated if, by performing the surgical procedure, significant functional improvement can be expected. Correction of a deformity resulting from malunion for cosmetic reasons alone is rarely justified. The degree of deformity does not always correspond to the degree of disability. Because of the normal angulation in major joints of the forelimb and hindlimb of small animals, increasing joint extension can often compensate for over-riding malunions that have caused mild to moderate limb shortening. Dogs can compensate for up to 20 per cent femoral shortening by decreasing the standing angle of the contralateral stifle.[14] Craniocaudal angular malunions in which adjacent joint surfaces remain parallel may not require surgical correction. Slight deformity near a joint or mild

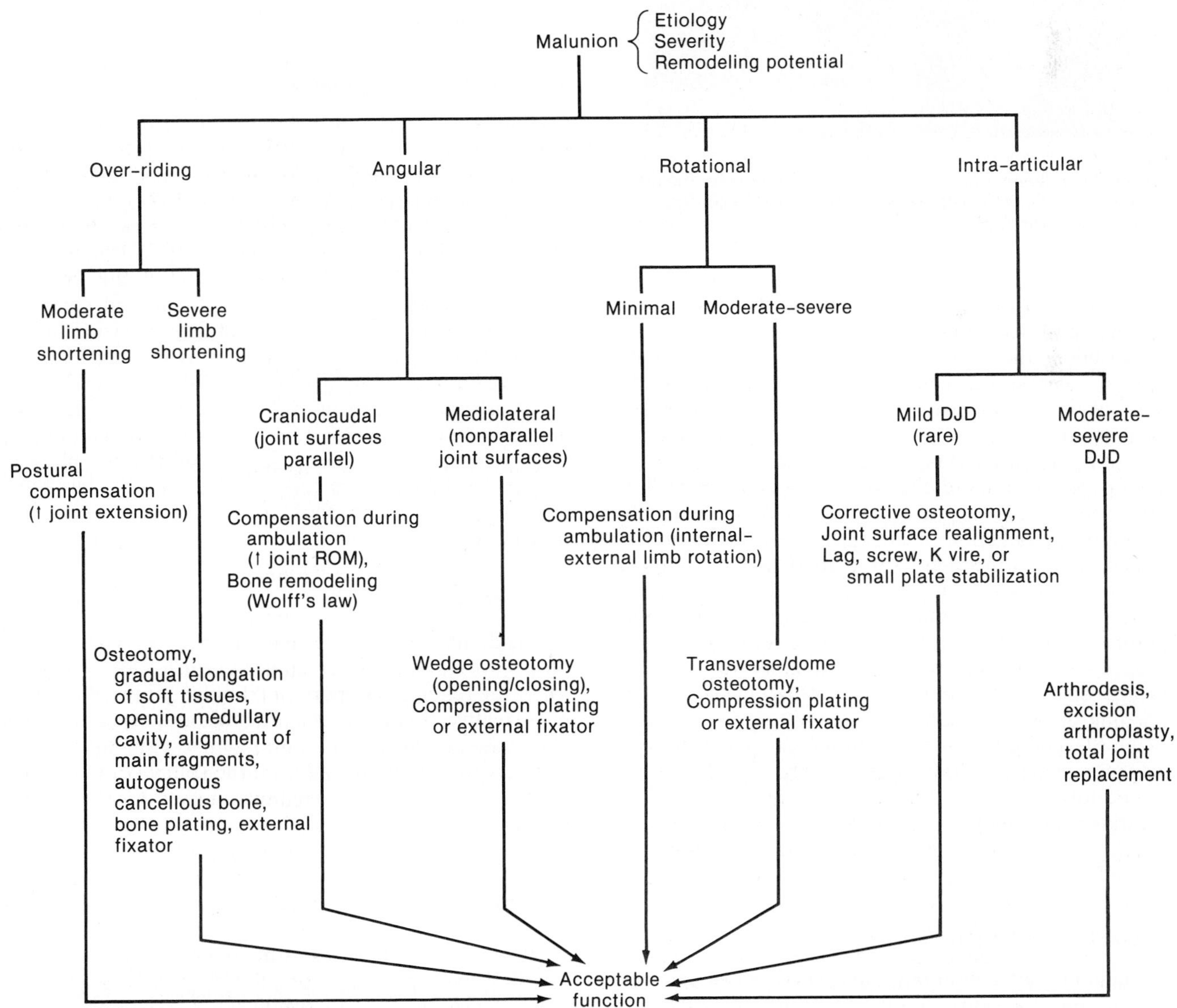

FIGURE 125–6. Types of malunions and principles of treatment. (DJD, degenerative joint disease; ROM, range of motion.)

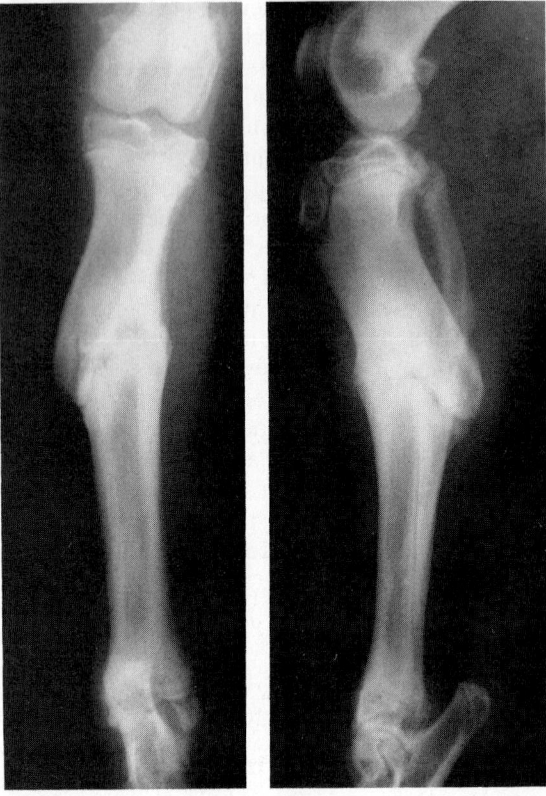

FIGURE 125–7. Spontaneous healing of a transverse right tibial fracture in a 6-month-old mixed-breed dog in angular malunion. Remodeling has improved the angulation of the major segments; however, the stifle and talocrural joint surfaces are not parallel.

rotational deformity may be severely debilitating and require surgical treatment.

Malunions that cause significant disability require osteotomy, gentle distraction of the soft tissues, débridement of the fracture ends and opening of the medullary cavities, alignment of the main fragments, and application of rigid fixation. Gaps created at the osteotomy site during realignment are filled with autogenous cancellous bone. After osteotomy of severely over-riding or angular malunions, elongation of contracted soft tissues may be difficult without the aid of a fracture distractor. Forceful use of the distractor can severely damage soft tissue and bone, resulting in compartment syndrome, vascular impairment, muscle fibrosis, "fracture disease" neurapraxia, and fracture. Angular malunions with varus or valgus deformity (mediolateral displacement) require opening or closing wedge osteotomy to prevent subsequent degenerative arthrosis from unequal forces on articular cartilage. Transverse or dome osteotomy may be performed for correction of moderate to severe rotational malunions.[25] The following examples of malunions are commonly encountered in small animal orthopedics.

Malunions of the Hindlimb

Malunions of conservatively treated pelvic fractures that narrow the pelvic canal and cause tenesmus, constipation, or obstipation require corrective osteotomy, partial hemipelvectomy, or spreading of the pelvic symphysis with a cortical bone graft. Acetabular malunions due to poor reduction or conservative treatment eventually result in degenerative arthrosis.[6] Excision arthroplasty or total hip replacement is usually necessary in severely debilitated animals. Malunions of the proximal femur resulting in coxa valga, coxa vara, or abnormal femoral anteversion may be corrected by varus or valgus intertrochanteric osteotomy (with derotation if necessary) to prevent coxofemoral subluxation, hip dysplasia, or patellar luxation. Severe shortening of the femoral shaft increases the normal standing angle of the stifle and causes hyperextension of the hock. Restoring length by osteotomy and alignment of the fragments must be performed gradually to avoid sciatic or femoral neurapraxia, quadriceps fibrosis or tie-down, and vascular compromise. Varus or valgus malunion of the tibia requires opening or closing wedge osteotomy or oblique osteotomy to prevent subluxation and degenerative arthrosis of the stifle or talocrural joint. Derotational osteotomy is indicated for rotational malunions of the tibia to prevent patellar luxation or cranial cruciate ligament rupture.

Malunions of the Forelimb

Angular malunion of the scapula may require corrective osteotomy, excision arthroplasty of the scapular glenoid, or glenohumeral arthrodesis, depending on the severity of the degenerative changes present.[12, 13] As with femoral malunions, lengthening procedures for aligning humeral malunions must be performed gradually to avoid damage to the nerves of the brachial plexus. Intra-articular malunions of humeral condylar fractures usually cause severe disability. Excision of the radial head or elbow arthrodesis may be necessary to improve limb function. Malunions of the radius and ulna or synostosis between the radius and ulna in a growing animal may cause elbow joint or carpal subluxation, as with growth deformities involving premature physeal closure.[1] If ligamentous support of the carpus has been lost, pancarpal arthrodesis plus corrective osteotomy may be necessary.

Other Malunions

Mandibular malunions may require corrective osteotomy to restore proper dental occlusion or condylectomy for relief of temporomandibular joint pain. After conservative treatment of vertebral body fractures, late neurological impairment or radicular pain may result from encroachment of callus on the spinal cord or spinal nerves. Decompressive laminectomy or foraminotomy is indicated.

References

1. Alexander JW, et al: Malformation of canine forelimb due to synostosis between the radius and ulna. *J Am Vet Med Assoc 173*:1328, 1978.
2. Aron DN, et al: Primary treatment of severe fractures by external skeletal fixation: Threaded pins compared with smooth pins. *J Am Anim Hosp Assoc 22*: 659, 1986.

3. Bardet JF, et al: Open drainage and delayed autogenous cancellous bone grafting for treatment of chronic osteomyelitis in dogs and cats. *J Am Vet Med Assoc 183*:312, 1983.
4. Bennett RA, et al: Comparison of the strength and holding power of 4 pin designs for use with half pin (type I) external skeletal fixation. *Vet Surg 16*: 207, 1987.
5. Bos G, et al: The effect of histocompatibility matching on canine frozen bone allografts. *J Bone Joint Surg [Am] 65-A*: 89, 1983.
6. Boudrieau RJ, Kleine LJ: Nonsurgically managed caudal acetabular fractures in dogs: 15 cases (1979–1984). *J Am Vet Med Assoc 193*:701, 1988.
7. Boyd HB, et al: Observations on non-union of the shafts of the long bones, with a statistical analysis of 842 patients. *J Bone Joint Surg [Am] 43-A*:159, 1961.
8. Bradley GW, et al: Effects of flexural rigidity of plates on bone healing. *J Bone Joint Surg [Am] 61-A*:866, 1979.
9. Caywood DD, et al: Osteomyelitis in the dog: A review of 67 cases. *J Am Vet Med Assoc 172*:943, 1978.
10. Crenshaw AH: Delayed union and nonunion of fractures. *In* Edmonson AS, Crenshaw AH (eds): *Campbell's Operative Orthopaedics*. 6th ed. Vol 1. C. V. Mosby, St. Louis, 1980, pp 761–820.
11. Day L: Electrical stimulation in the treatment of ununited fractures. *Clin Orthop 161*:54, 1981.
12. Fowler JD, et al: Scapulohumeral arthrodesis: Results in seven dogs. *J Am Anim Hosp Assoc 24*:667, 1988.
13. Franczuszki D, Parkes LJ: Glenoid excision as a treatment in chronic shoulder disabilities: Surgical technique and clinical results. *J Am Anim Hosp Assoc 24*:637, 1988.
14. Franczuszki D, et al: Postoperative effects of experimental femoral shortening in the mature dog. *J Am Anim Hosp Assoc 23*:429, 1987.
15. Frost HM: *Bone Remodelling and Its Relationship to Metabolic Bone Disease*. Charles C Thomas, Springfield, IL, 1973.
16. Gross PM, et al: Measurement of blood flow to bone and marrow in experimental animals by means of the microsphere technique. *J Bone Joint Surg [Am] 63-A*1028, 1981.
17. Henry WB, et al: Feline model for the study of frozen osteoarticular hemijoint transplantation: Qualitative and quantitative assessment of bone healing. *Am J Vet Res 46*:1714, 1985.
18. Johnson AL, et al: Evaluation of collagen as a retainer for autogenous cancellous bone used in repair of full thickness cortical bone defects. *Vet Surg 16*:146, 1987.
19. Kita K, et al: Changes in bone marrow blood flow with aging. *J Orthop Res 5*: 569, 1987.
20. Lamb CR: Bone scintigraphy in small animals. *J Am Vet Med Assoc 191*:1616, 1987.
21. McKibbin B: The biology of fracture healing in long bones. *J Bone Joint Surg [Br] 60-B*:150, 1978.
22. Newton CD, Hohn RB: Fracture nonunion from cerclage appliances. *J Am Vet Med Assoc 164*:503, 1974.
23. Paranen J, Ponto L: Osteomedulloangiography: A method of estimating the consolidation prognosis of tibial shaft fractures. *Clin Orthop 161*:8, 1981.
24. Powers BE, et al: Jamshidi needle biopsy for diagnosis of bone lesions in small animals. *J Am Vet Med Assoc 193*:205, 1988.
25. Rhinelander FW: The normal microcirculation of diaphyseal cortex and its response to fracture. *J Bone Joint Surg [Am]50-A*:784, 1968.
26. Robbins SL, Cotran RS: The musculoskeletal system—bones. *In Pathologic Basis of Disease*. 2nd ed. W. B. Saunders, Philadelphia, 1979, pp 1477–1513.
27. Rosen H: Compression treatment of long bone pseudoarthrosis. *Clin Orthop 138*:154, 1979.
28. Schenk RK: Histology of fracture repair and nonunion. *AO Bulletin*. Buchdruck-Offset Paul Haupt AG, Bern, Switzerland, 1978.
29. Schenk RK, et al: Nonunion: The histologic picture. *In* Sumner-Smith G (ed). *Bone in Clinical Orthopaedics*. W. B. Saunders, Philadelphia, 1982, pp 415–427
30. Selcer BA: Imaging: Bone. *Vet Radiol 24*:243, 1983.
31. Sikes RI, et al: Dome osteotomy for correction of long bone malunions: Case reports and discussion of surgical technique. *J Am Anim Hosp Assoc 22*:221, 1986.
32. Sinibaldi KR: Evaluation of full cortical allografts in 25 dogs. *J Am Vet Med Assoc 194*:1570, 1989.
33. Smith CW, et al: Osteomyelitis in the dog: A retrospective study. *J Am Anim Hosp Assoc 14*:589, 1978.
34. Sumner-Smith G, Bishop H: Nonunion: Pathogenesis and treatment. *In* Sumner-Smith G (ed) *Bone in Clinical Orthopaedics*. W. B. Saunders, Philadelphia 1982, pp 399–415.
35. Taylor RA: Electrically-induced osteogenesis: A review. *J Am Anim Hosp Assoc 20*:435, 1984.
36. Vasseur PB, et al: Evaluation of fixation devices for prevention of rotation in transverse fractures of the canine femoral shaft: An *in vitro* study. *Am J Vet Res 45*:1504, 1984.
37. Vaughan LC: A clinical study of nonunion fractures in the dog. *J Small Anim Pract 5*:173, 1964.
38. Walter MC, et al: Treatment of severely comminuted diaphyseal fractures in the dog, using standard bone plates and autogenous cancellous bone graft to span fracture gaps: 11 cases (1979–1983). *J Am Vet Med Assoc 189*:457, 1986.
39. Watson-Jones R: Fractures and joint injuries. *Clin Orthop 105*:4, 1974.
40. Weber BG, Cech O: *Pseudoarthrosis: Pathology, Biomechanics, Therapy, Results*. Hans Huber Medical Publisher, Berne, Switzerland, 1976.
41. Wilber MC, Evans EB: Fractures of the femoral shaft treated surgically. *J Bone Joint Surg [Am] 60-A*:489. 1978.

CHAPTER 126 Orthopedic Infections

Mark M. Smith

Wound infections in orthopedic surgery usually result from contamination of open fractures or from open fracture repair, resulting in osteomyelitis and soft-tissue infection. Osteomyelitis is inflammation of bone and its marrow contents.[36] The majority of infections are caused by bacteria; fungi are occasionally involved, and parasites and viruses rarely.[11] Chronic osteomyelitis may result from sequestra or contamination of implants. Young dogs may develop osteomyelitis from hematogenously delivered bacteria. Septic arthritis can occur as a postoperative complication, by wounds or hematogenous contamination.[11, 14]

ANTIBIOTIC THERAPY IN ORTHOPEDIC INFECTIONS

Clinicians must anticipate which bacteria are likely to be present in a particular wound and must be aware of the spectrum, pharmacokinetics, side effects, and cost of available antibiotics. Pharmacokinetic data for antibiotic uptake in bone and joint fluid are derived from single-dose studies in normal animals. Pathological factors can alter the minimum inhibitory concentration (MIC) of antibiotics. These factors include tissue fluid pH, number and type of white blood cells, local glucose and protein levels, fluid viscosity, and oxygen tension.[9]

Basic Principles

Knowledge of the antibiotic spectrum and of the normal microbial flora of skin, soil, and the hospital environment provides the basis for empirical selection of antibiotics.[9]

Penetration of bone and joint cavities by the antibiotic is critical for eradication of infection. Most antibiotics achieve acceptable MIC levels in synovial fluid and bone. Aminoglycosides are less effective in hypoxic or acidotic conditions and in the presence of polymorphonuclear leukocytes and may be ineffective for some bone or joint infections.[27]

Duration of antimicrobial therapy is consistent with the severity of the disease process. Bone infections are generally slow to resolve, and antibiotic therapy is commonly necessary for weeks or months.[27]

Prophylactic Use of Antibiotics

Prophylactic therapy is considered in all clean orthopedic procedures involving implantation of foreign materials and in arthroscopy. The timing of administration and choice of antibiotic are important. Maximum tissue concentration of the antibiotic is necessary during the vulnerable period between skin incision and closure. Antibiotics administered 3 hours or more before contamination may select for resistant organisms. Single-dose intravenous prophylaxis 20 minutes before the incision is the present practice in human orthopedics.[34] Antibiotic administration later than 3 to 5 hours after contamination is ineffective.

Coagulase-positive and coagulase-negative *Staphylococcus* spp. are the most common pathogens associated with orthopedic procedures. Cefazolin, a first-generation cephalosporin, is a bactericidal drug that is effective against staphylococcal organisms. It has a relatively long half-life (1.8 hours) and achieves excellent penetration into bone (25 per cent of blood levels when given intravenously).[9, 52] Penicillins are not as desirable in orthopedic surgery because of poor penetration into bone and an inadequate spectrum against coagulase-negative *Staphylococcus epidermidis*.

Tourniquet application may necessitate administration of greater doses of antibiotics to achieve adequate tissue concentrations. In humans, the cefazolin dose is doubled and administered 20 minutes before the procedure.[10]

Synovial fluid antibiotic kinetics parallel serum antibiotic kinetics for most antibiotics.[5, 27] After peak serum antibiotic concentration is reached, a concentration gradient is established with the synovium. The antibiotic's ability to enter synovial fluid depends on molecular size and inflammation-dependent changes in synovial permeability. Synovial fluid protein concentration and polymorphonuclear leukocyte number positively correlate with the severity of inflammation, demonstrating that antibiotics can readily enter synovial fluid in the presence of inflammation. As the inflammatory process resolves, synovial fluid antibiotic levels may decrease correspondingly. Adequate concentrations of antibiotic are attained in synovial fluid after systemic administration, eliminating the need for direct intra-articular injection. Locally injected antibiotics may cause chemical synovitis, further compounding the pathological process.[20, 37]

ACUTE HEMATOGENOUS OSTEOMYELITIS

Clinical Findings

In dogs, acute hematogenous osteomyelitis most often affects neonates or young individuals. The source of infection may be the umbilicus[36]; however, older, immature dogs may develop the disease after umbilical closure. The history often includes focal infection or more generalized disease. Clinical signs include fever, malaise, and nonweightbearing lameness. Morbidity ranges from lameness to severe debilitation. Physical examination findings include soft-tissue swelling over the involved bone; it may fluctuate if purulent exudate has extended through the periosteum. Multiple sites of infection are not unusual, so a thorough physical examination is mandatory.

Pathophysiology

Hematogenous bacterial infections in immature dogs generally localize in metaphyseal areas, possibly because of turbulent blood flow in the transitional area between metaphyseal capillaries and venous sinusoids. Bacterial emboli cause inflammation and microthrombi formation, producing an ischemic environment that is conducive to bacterial proliferation.[40] Septic arthritis associated with acute hematogenous osteomyelitis occurs when a portion of the metaphysis is intra-articular.[28]

In neonates, acute hematogenous osteomyelitis may involve the epiphysis and joint cavity, possibly because of vascular connections between the epiphysis and metaphysis. After the physes close, extensive anastomoses form between epiphyseal and metaphyseal vessels. Therefore, in adult animals, hematogenous osteomyelitis localizes in periarticular subchondral bone; involvement of diaphyseal bone is rare.[7]

Bacterial infection causes inflammation, resulting in hyperemia, increased vascular permeability, diapedesis of phagocytic cells, and extravasation of serum protein, antibodies, complement, and fibrin. Increased intramedullary pressure causes vascular thrombosis and necrosis of trabecular bone, as well as metaphyseal abscess formation.

The host immune response may "wall off" the infection and form a chronic abscess.[39] Purulent material is surrounded by connective tissue that separates normal bone from the granulation tissue lining the abscess. Progressive abscessation denotes an unsuccessful immune response. Purulent exudate accumulates, pressure increases, and exudate enters cortical bone along the path of least resistance, through haversian and Volkmann canals. Increased cortical porosity secondary to inflammation and increased osteoclastic activity aids in dissemination of the exudate (Fig. 126–1). Exudate reaching the outer cortex elevates the periosteum, further compromising cortical blood supply, and may lead to sequestrum formation.[29] Sequestra are avascular seg-

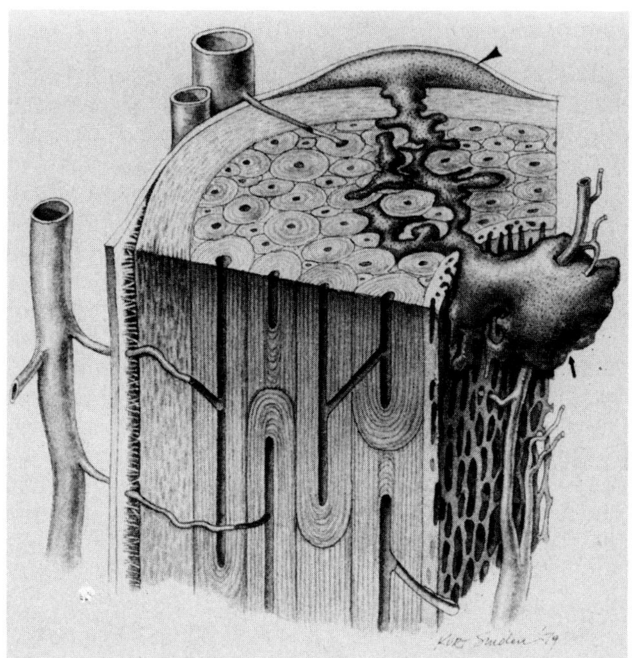

FIGURE 126–1. The manner in which an infectious process in the medullary canal (*arrow*) permeates the cortex and collects beneath the periosteal membrane (*arrowhead*). (From Resnick D, Niwayama G: Osteomyelitis, septic arthritis, and soft tissue infection: The mechanisms and situations. *In* Resnick D, Niwayama G [eds]: *Diagnosis of Bone and Joint Disorders.* W. B. Saunders, Philadelphia, 1988.)

ments of bone surrounded by purulent exudate and eventually isolated by fibrous tissue and new bone originating from the cambium layer of the periosteum. The new, highly vascular bone surrounds the sequestrum and is called the *involucrum*. Although the involucrum isolates the infection, it also prevents the immune system and antibiotics from reaching sequestered bone, acting as a bacterial nidus for reinfection and chronic osteomyelitis.

Subchondral osteomyelitis in mature animals remains intramedullary because of tight adherence of periosteum to a thick cortex.[29] Subperiosteal abscessation can occur in Volkmann canals and rupture through the periosteum, causing contiguous soft-tissue infection and draining tracts to the skin surface. The periosteal blood supply is minimally affected, making sequestra formation rare. Therefore, the hallmarks of late-onset acute hematogenous osteomyelitis are bone destruction, osteoporosity, and periosteal new bone formation. These changes are evident radiographically and must be differentiated from the bony changes associated with neoplasia.[51]

Diagnosis

A tentative diagnosis of acute hematogenous osteomyelitis is based on a history of prior infection and physical findings. The white blood cell count is usually elevated. Radiographs demonstrate only soft-tissue swelling for the first 2 to 3 weeks; thereafter, areas of lysis and new bone production involving the metaphysis become apparent.[23] Technetium scintigraphy demonstrates increased uptake of the isotope at sites of infection and is useful in the early stages.[12] Fine-needle aspiration of fluctuant areas may yield positive cultures if samples are obtained before antibiotic administration. Gram-positive organisms such as *Staphylococcus* or *Streptococcus* spp. are most likely. In human patients, more than 50 per cent of blood cultures are positive for gram-positive organisms, primarily *Staphylococcus*.[51] Similar data are not available for animals with acute hematogenous osteomyelitis; however, blood cultures are indicated when an animal is systemically ill.

Treatment

A broad-spectrum bactericidal antimicrobial, such as a cephalosporin, is administered intravenously for 3 to 5 days, until culture and sensitivity test results are available. If the bacteria cannot be identified, continued administration of the antibiotic is based on the animal's clinical response. A favorable initial response permits an oral antibiotic, which should be continued for 4 weeks.[50] Limb immobilization is not recommended because of deleterious effects on joint cartilage. Fluid therapy, nutritional supplementation, and analgesics may be needed.

Palpable abscesses are drained and débrided, and culture specimens obtained before copious lavage. If débridement is adequate, closure over a drain can be considered. If the adequacy of débridement is in doubt, the wound is left open.

Extension of infection into a joint is a surgical emergency (treatment of septic arthritis is discussed later).

OSTEOMYELITIS FROM EXOGENOUS SOURCES

Acute Osteomyelitis

Clinical Findings

Acute osteomyelitis is usually a complication of open fracture repair, and clinical signs are generally apparent after 5 to 7 days. Animals are febrile and often have leukocytosis. Surgical wounds are edematous, red, and warm. The animal may not bear weight on the limb, and the surgical site is painful.

Pathophysiology

Development of infection at the fracture site depends on the integrity of the soft tissues, the virulence of the contaminating organism, and the ability of the host to mount an effective immune response. Adequate blood supply is essential to deliver nutrition, oxygen, cellular components of the immune response, and antibiotics. The trauma associated with the initial injury and surgical repair causes significant disruption of blood supply, making these animals less capable of eliminating contaminating organisms. Internal fixation devices further disrupt blood supply and provide a large metallic foreign body for bacterial adherence and proliferation.[22] Hematoma, devitalized soft tissues, and avascular bone are an excellent medium for bacterial proliferation. Bacterial by-products, enzymes of leukocyte origin, and lowered tissue pH further damage tissue and degrade bone matrix. Extension of the infection into the cortex through haversian and Volkmann canals further occludes vascular supply and destroys cellular components in their lacunae.

Diagnosis

A history of recent fracture repair and evidence of wound infection (swelling, heat, drainage) suggest acute osteomyelitis. Radiographs demonstrate proliferative new bone and occasionally gas in soft tissues. Sequestra may be suspected, but they generally do not become visible radiographically for several weeks or months. Fine-needle aspirates from the fracture site or exudate from draining tracts are submitted for culture and sensitivity testing.

Treatment

Aggressive early intervention is necessary to prevent the development of chronic osteomyelitis. The fracture must be stable; if implants are not providing stabilization, they must be removed. External fixation devices are often indicated to provide stabilization and minimize soft-tissue damage. Broad-spectrum bactericidal antibiotics (e.g., cefazolin) are administered intravenously. Antibiotic protocols are modified depending on culture results and clinical response. The duration of antibiotic administration varies among individual patients. It has been demonstrated in human patients with acute osteomyelitis that antibiotic administration for a minimum of 30 days is associated with low recurrence.[16]

In most cases, the surgical wound is opened for débridement, lavage, and drainage. If débridement is thorough and the tissues appear healthy, the wound is closed over a drain. Low-vacuum closed suction systems minimize ascending contamination and provide effective drainage. Drainage systems are cared for aseptically and removed when fluid accumulation has subsided, usually in 3 to 5 days. Open wound management with delayed closure may be necessary in severely infected wounds.

Chronic Osteomyelitis

Chronic osteomyelitis usually results from inadequate treatment of acute osteomyelitis; it may also develop from cryptic infections associated with metallic prostheses.[8, 11, 22, 31]

Clinical Findings

Moderate to severe atrophy is present in the affected limb, and a draining tract is usually present. The drainage generally subsides with administration of antibiotics but invariably returns when the medication is discontinued. Pain at the fracture site and the amount of weightbearing are variable and depend on whether or not the fracture has united. Episodes of systemic illness can occur and probably represent septicemia.

Diagnosis

The history and physical findings are sufficient to make a tentative diagnosis. Radiographic signs include new bone production with areas of lysis, extensive remodeling, and often the presence of a sequestrum (Fig. 126–2).[46] Cultures from draining tracts are usually polymicrobic and do not necessarily include the causative organisms. Bacteria able to cause osteomyelitis often produce a mucopolysaccharide substance that enables adherence to various surfaces.[8, 19, 22, 31] This property enhances virulence by isolating bacteria from the immune system and decreasing exfoliative properties, thus limiting isolation of these bacteria. Specimens obtained directly from sequestra and devitalized tissue provide more accurate culture results. Antibiotics are not given for at least 24 hours before sample collection. Samples are submitted for aerobic and anaerobic culture and sensitivity testing.[24, 25]

Treatment

Chronic osteomyelitis is a surgical disease, with antimicrobial chemotherapy an integral part of the treatment regimen.[36] Aggressive débridement of necrotic tissue includes sclerotic bone that may be occluding the

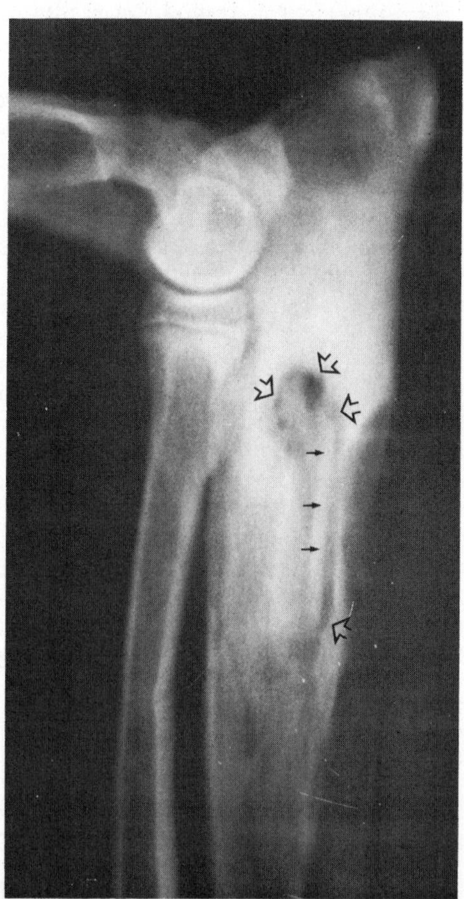

FIGURE 126–2. Lateral radiograph of a canine ulna showing evidence of osteomyelitis consisting of a sequestrum (*closed arrows*) and involucrum (*open arrows*).

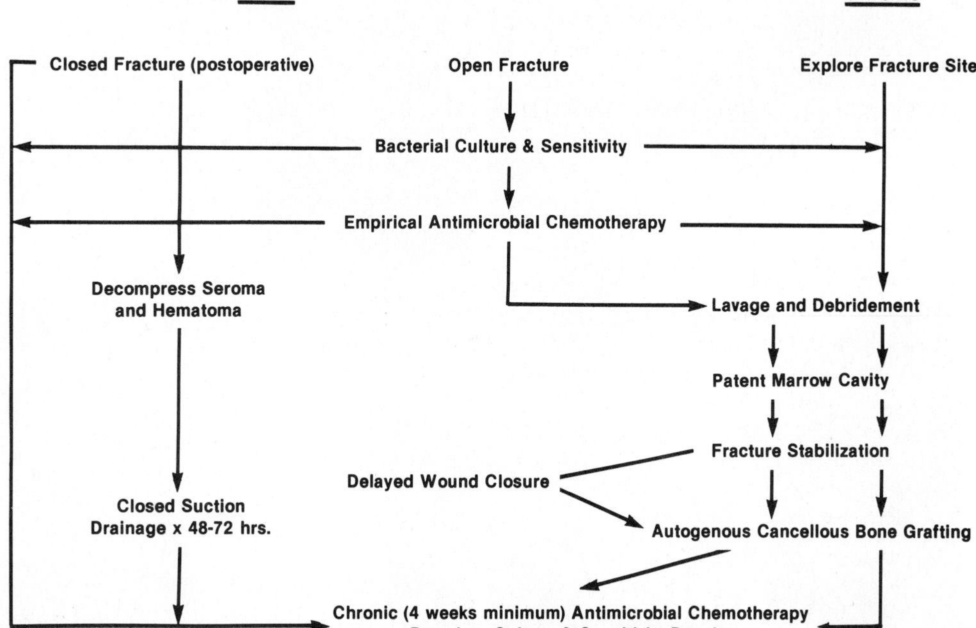

FIGURE 126–3. The decision-making process in treatment of acute and chronic osteomyelitis in dogs and cats.

medullary cavity.[35] Stabilization of the fracture is essential, if it has not already united. With significant soft-tissue infection, external fixators are preferred because they can be applied with minimal disruption of blood supply.[15, 41] If the soft tissues are healthy and the surgical procedure has consisted primarily of sequestrectomy and débridement of the fistulous tract, plate fixation may be considered. Intramedullary pins are contraindicated because they do not provide adequate stability and may permit extension of the infection throughout the medullary cavity. All implants are ultimately removed, if possible, because they harbor organisms and potentially contribute to fracture-associated sarcoma.[44, 45]

After débridement and stabilization, the wound is copiously lavaged with warm saline or a solution containing 0.25 per cent chlorhexidine. Cancellous bone autografts are extremely effective in promoting union and filling bony defects. They are always used for nonunions unless excessive exudation is expected, in which case grafting can be carried out later.[39] If antiseptics or antibiotics have been included in the lavage solution, the wound is thoroughly lavaged with warm saline alone before implantation of the cancellous graft.[21] If débridement has been complete and dead space can be eliminated, the wound is closed primarily. If exudation is expected to continue or débridement has been incomplete, the wound can be left partially open or a closed suction drainage system can be placed.

Postoperatively, nursing care and physical therapy are of great importance. Drains are managed aseptically and removed when drainage has subsided. The affected limb is manipulated through range of motion exercises at least three times daily. Warm compresses can be applied to promote vascularity, facilitate drainage, and keep the wound clean. If recumbent, the animal must be moved frequently to prevent pressure sores. Nutritional status and fluid balance are carefully monitored. Whirlpool baths and brief exercise periods make the animal more comfortable and encourage use of the limb. Only in severe chronic cases, with irreversible muscle damage and joint stiffness, is amputation necessary. Complications include refractory osteomyelitis, nonunion, and restricted joint motion. Repeated cancellous autografting generally results in union, provided that the fracture is stable. Refractory infections usually resolve with removal of implants and appropriate antimicrobial therapy. Aggressive physical therapy, especially swimming exercise, improves joint motion and muscle strength (Fig. 126–3).

FUNGAL OSTEOMYELITIS

Coccidioidomycosis (*Coccidioides immitis*) occurs in the southwestern United States, and inhalation of arthrospores can cause respiratory tract infection, which then disseminates to other organ systems within 2 to 5 months.[3, 36] Bone infection occurs in approximately 50 per cent of infected patients and is characterized by increased bone density, proliferative new bone arising from the periosteum, bone lysis, and joint involvement (Fig. 126–4). Serological and intradermal sensitivity tests may provide positive results, circumventing bone biopsy and fungal culture. Bone biopsy may be necessary to rule out neoplasia and provides an excellent sample for culture (the organism grows on Sabouraud media). Treatment consists of long-term administration of antifungal drugs such as amphotericin B or ketoconazole.* The prognosis is guarded.

Other fungal agents that can cause osteomyelitis include *Blastomyces dermatitidis, Histoplasma capsulatum, Cryptococcus neoformans*, and *Aspergillus fumigatus*.

---

*Editor's note: Various new antifungal agents are in the clinical testing stage and may improve results.

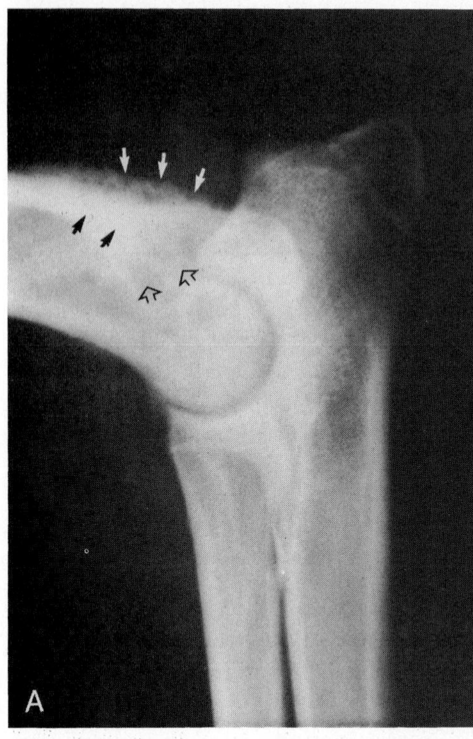
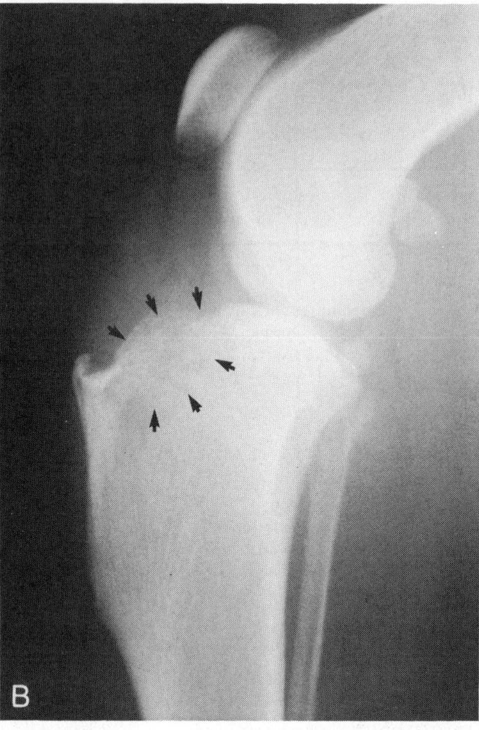

FIGURE 126–4. Coccidioidomycosis in a dog. *A*, The elbow radiograph shows increased bone density (*closed arrows*), bone lysis (*open arrows*), and new bone arising from the periosteum (*white arrows*) in the distal humeral metaphyseal area. *B*, The stifle shows bone lysis of the proximal tibia (*closed arrows*).

Some of these agents are more prevalent in different areas. Differential diagnosis requires culture and intradermal or serological testing. Nocardiosis (*Nocardia* spp.) is a respiratory tract infection that can spread hematogenously to bone.[36, 43] The organism is also present in soil and can cause infection in open fractures. The clinical course and radiographic signs suggest chronic suppurative osteomyelitis. The diagnosis is based on Gram stain and culture. Treatment is long-term antimicrobial therapy based on culture and sensitivity testing.

SEPTIC ARTHRITIS

Septic arthritis is a potentially devastating bacterial infection secondary to joint contamination from hematogenous or exogenous routes.[4] The latter are most common and include injuries, surgical procedures, and intra-articular injections. Potential sources of hematogenously derived bacteria are the respiratory or digestive tracts, umbilicus, and endocardium.[11, 30]

Clinical Findings

Septic arthritis is usually monoarticular. The joint is swollen, painful, and warm, and rectal temperature is often elevated. The limb either does not bear weight or is markedly lame.

Pathophysiology

Contamination of the synovium results in hyperemia and edema, with infiltration by polymorphonuclear leukocytes. Inflammation of the synovium, capillary rupture, and focal areas of necrosis promote extravasation of fibrin, clotting factors, polymorphonuclear leukocytes, and proteinaceous serous fluid into the joint.[4] The polymorphonuclear leukocytes are responsible for the purulent appearance of the fluid, and their presence marks the beginning of irreversible cartilage destruction. Synovial cells and polymorphonuclear leukocytes phagocytize bacteria and release lysosomal enzymes and enzymatic by-products that break down cartilage matrix and expose collagen fibrils to further enzymatic destruction. Synovial fluid dynamics and cartilage nutrition are impaired by the inflammatory process. These factors, combined with mechanical trauma due to joint movement, result in severe fragmentation of collagen fibrils. Fibrin deposition on denuded cartilage surfaces exacerbates the process by chemotactically attracting polymorphonuclear leukocytes, which release additional enzymes. Granulation tissue from the synovium may contribute to joint destruction by penetrating and undermining the joint surface. Loss of the joint surface allows inflammatory cells and bacteria to invade subchondral bone, causing suppurative osteomyelitis. The latter is particularly serious because subchondral bone destruction is followed by healing, with granulation tissue and eventual fibrous ankylosis. Calcification of this tissue causes bony ankylosis and complete loss of joint function. Therapeutic intervention before cartilage destruction is imperative.[2, 33]

Diagnosis

A tentative diagnosis is based on clinical findings. Definitive diagnosis is based on evaluation of joint fluid obtained via arthrocentesis. Abnormal findings include increased numbers of polymorphonuclear leukocytes (40,000/mm^3 to 100,000/mm^3 or greater), bacteria, and increased turbidity or purulent appearance. Direct culture of synovial fluid is commonly negative, so synovial fluid samples are immediately placed into blood culture medium to facilitate growth and culture.[33]

Early radiographic signs are related to effusion and soft-tissue swelling. With progression of sepsis, radiographic signs include bone lysis, joint surface irregularity, and subluxation. Nuclear scintigraphy provides earlier diagnostic information than conventional radiographs.[12, 23, 26] Referral to veterinary centers with nuclear medicine capability should be considered for patients with equivocal clinical signs.

Treatment

Therapy is directed at minimizing cartilage destruction. Antimicrobial chemotherapy begins immediately after arthrocentesis for cytological study and culture. Intravenous administration of a broad-spectrum bactericidal drug such as a cephalosporin is indicated pending culture and sensitivity test results. The fluoroquinolones are potent broad-spectrum antimicrobials that are effective for chronic osteomyelitis and septic arthritis in humans.[13, 17, 18, 47] They may provide an alternative to the cephalosporins for dogs with septic arthritis. Antibiotics are continued for a minimum of 4 weeks.

Joint lavage is essential to remove cellular and enzymatic constituents. In young animals, decompression is particularly important to reduce pressure and preserve epiphyseal vascularity. Needle aspiration and lavage do not adequately remove deleterious materials from the joint and may cause iatrogenic cartilage damage. Arthrotomy, surgical débridement, and copious lavage are indicated for (1) postoperative joint infections, (2) septic joints untreated for 72 hours or more, (3) joints that have not responded to 72 hours of conservative treatment, and (4) penetrating wounds involving a joint.[5] The joint is lavaged with large volumes of isotonic solution to remove fibrin clots, purulent exudate, and foreign material. The use of antibiotic and antiseptic solutions for lavage is controversial. Antiseptic solutions may cause chemical synovitis.[1, 32] Each case must be considered individually, and for infections caused by extremely resistant organisms, the potential advantages of antibiotics or antiseptics in the lavage solution may outweigh the hazards.

Fibrin and necrotic synovium must be removed because they act as a nidus for bacterial growth and may lead to a refractory condition. Bilateral arthrotomy aids in exposure of joint surfaces and access for lavage and drainage. An entrance-exit joint-flushing system allows for further lavage during the postoperative period and is considered for animals with severe infections and extensive tissue devitalization. Such systems are difficult to maintain in animals, and open wound management is an effective alternative.[32]

Parenteral antibiotics, daily aseptic bandage changes, and hospitalization are recommended during the first postoperative week. Daily wound inspection allows assessment of the infection, lavage of blood clots and exudate, and passive range of motion exercises to facilitate drainage (Fig. 126–5).

INFECTION ASSOCIATED WITH PROSTHETIC IMPLANTS

Total hip replacement is frequently performed in dogs, and infection is a catastrophic complication that generally requires removal of the prosthesis and polymethyl methacrylate bone cement.

Clinical Findings

Animals may be systemically ill or have only intermittent pain and lameness. The severity of the clinical signs depends on the number and virulence of the pathogen, the host environment, and route of infection.[42] In humans, *Staphylococcus intermedius* often causes systemic illness, whereas *S. epidermidis* has a more indolent course.

Pathophysiology

In humans, individuals having had previous surgery at the site of the implant have a higher incidence of infection than in first-time operations. Other factors that increase the risk of infections are obesity, aging, malnutrition, diabetes mellitus, corticosteroid administration, and rheumatoid arthritis. Wound hematoma and seroma, disruption of fascial planes, ischemia, and wounds in diabetic or steroid-treated patients provide environments for rapid proliferation of pathogens. Hematogenous infection provides fewer organisms at the bone–cement interface.

Infection usually occurs in osseous tissue adjacent to the foreign body (Fig. 126–6).[42] Because most total joint replacements in veterinary medicine are cemented, infection occurs at the bone–cement interface. Contamination can occur from endogenous or exogenous sources. In humans, 20 to 40 per cent of infections around prostheses are thought to arise from endogenous contamination.[42] Endogenous contamination has not been documented in dogs but theoretically could result from bacteremia associated with dental procedures or urinary tract infections and other such sources. Exogenous contamination occurs during surgical procedures and probably causes the majority of infections after total hip procedures in dogs. Studies of humans demonstrate that most infections around prosthetic implants are caused by a single pathogen, and *Staphylococcus* organisms are cultured in approximately 50 per cent.

Metallic prosthetic devices and cement are foreign substances that render a wound more susceptible to infection. Foreign bodies decrease the quantity of bacteria necessary to establish infection and provide a site for bacterial adherence that is functionally sequestered from the immune system and antibiotics.[22, 44] Cement in unpolymerized form inhibits phagocytic and complement function *in vitro*.[38] *In vivo* polymerized cement decreased the number of bacteria required to cause osteomyelitis.

The interaction between host and bacteria may enhance virulence. Fibronectin, a connective tissue and plasma glycoprotein, aids adherence of *Staphylococcus* to cement *in vivo* and may be a factor in development

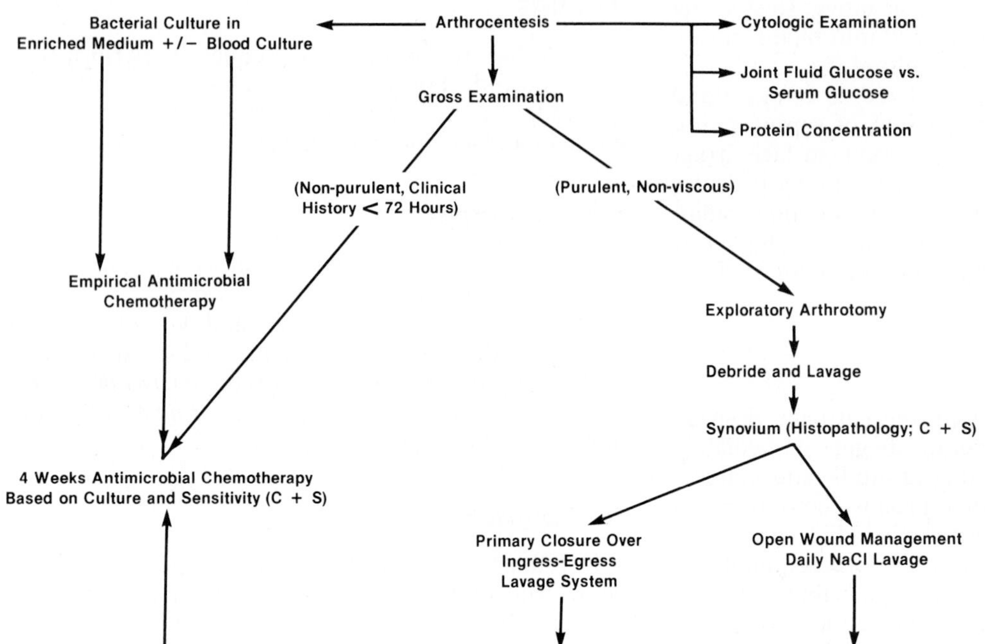

FIGURE 126–5. Treatment of septic arthritis in dogs and cats.

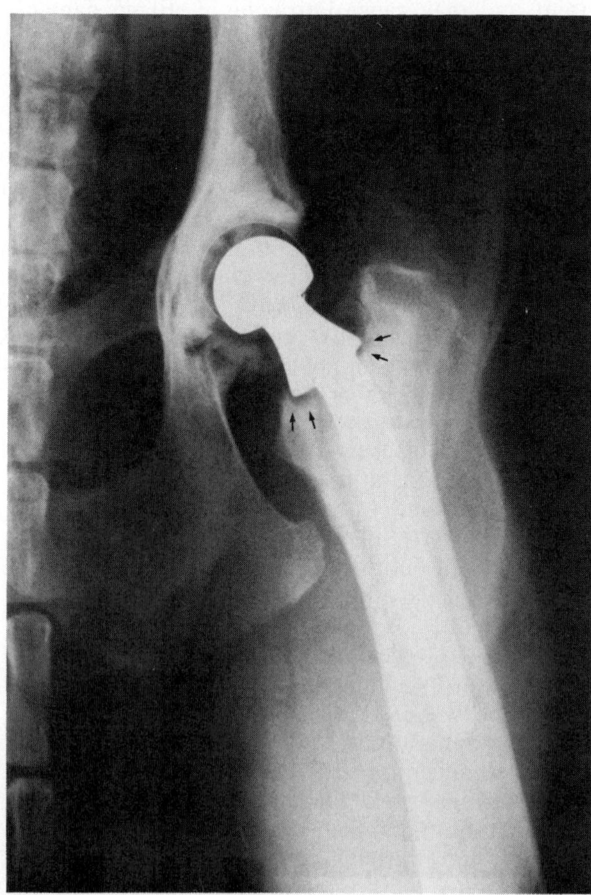

FIGURE 126–6. Osteomyelitis associated with total hip replacement in a dog. A ventrodorsal radiograph of the left prosthetic coxofemoral joint shows bone lysis of the proximal femur adjacent to the femoral component (*closed arrows*).

of sepsis.[48, 49] Certain bacteria produce a mucopolysaccharide biofilm on prosthetic devices. Biofilm formation may alter the local environment in favor of bacteria by concentrating nutrients and protecting microbes from surfactants, opsonic antibodies, phagocytes, and antimicrobial agents.[22] Bacterial biofilms allow the persistence of infection despite appropriate antimicrobial chemotherapy. These infections may become cryptic, with clinical signs occurring years after implantation. Débridement at the bone–cement interface is necessary to prevent recurrence of infection after removal of the prosthesis.

Diagnosis

Persistence of lameness after total joint replacement in the absence of technical errors should alert the clinician to the possibility of infection. Serial radiographs are helpful in showing bone lysis and loosening of the prosthesis at the bone–cement interface. Joint aspiration under aseptic conditions is required to isolate the infecting bacteria. The pathogens may be fastidious or anaerobic, requiring special transport and culturing techniques. Tests include a direct smear (Gram stain); aerobic, anaerobic, mycobacterial, and fungal culture; and sensitivity testing. Joint fluid is analyzed as discussed earlier for septic arthritis.

Therapy

Early infections are treated aggressively by immediate incision, débridement, and primary closure over closed suction drainage, which is maintained for 2 to 3 days. Broad-spectrum bactericidal antibiotics are given intravenously until culture and sensitivity test results are available. Salvage of prosthetic arthroplasty is most feasible if the bone–cement interface is intact and the causative agent is highly sensitive to antimicrobial agents.[6, 42]

Protracted infections require extensive débridement and removal of all foreign material including cement. Closure over closed suction drainage or open wound management may be required. Delayed reimplantation of a prosthesis is performed in humans after a minimum of 6 weeks of intravenous antimicrobial chemotherapy. In dogs, this is impractical.

References

1. Bertone AL, et al: Effect of four antimicrobial lavage solutions on the tarsocrural joint of horses. *Vet Surg 15*:305, 1986.
2. Blinkhorn RJ, et al: Punch actinomycosis causing osteomyelitis of the hand. *Arch Intern Med 148*:2668, 1988.
3. Brodey RS, et al: Disseminated coccidioidomycosis in a dog. *J Am Vet Med Assoc 157*:926, 1970.
4. Brown GS, Newton CD: Infectious arthritis and wounds of joints. *In* Newton CD, Nunamaker DM (eds): *Textbook of Small Animal Orthopaedics*. J. B. Lippincott, Philadelphia, 1985.
5. Brown MP, et al: Kanamycin sulfate in the horse: Serum, synovial fluid, peritoneal fluid, and urine concentrations after single-dose intramuscular administration. *Am J Vet Res 42*:1823, 1981.
6. Callaghan JJ, et al: Reimplantation for salvage of the infected hip: Rationale for the use of gentamicin-impregnated cement and beads. *In The Hip: Proceedings of 14th Open Scientific Meeting of the Hip Society*. C. V. Mosby, St. Louis, 1986.
7. Caywood DD, et al: Osteomyelitis in the dog: A review of 67 cases. *J Am Vet Med Assoc 172*: 943, 1978.
8. Costerton JW, Marrie TJ: Mode of growth of bacterial pathogens in chronic polymicrobial human osteomyelitis. *J Clin Microbiol 22*:924, 1985.
9. Cunha BA: Antibiotics in orthopedic infections. *In* Schlossberg D (ed): *Orthopedic Infection*. Springer-Verlag, New York, 1988.
10. Cunha BA, et al: Penetration of cephazolin and cefradine into bone in patients undergoing total knee arthroplasty. *Infection 2*:80, 1984.
11. Daly WR: Orthopedic infections. *In* Slatter DH (ed): *Textbook of Small Animal Surgery*. W. B. Saunders, Philadelphia, 1985.
12. Demopulous GA, et al: Role of radionuclide imaging in the diagnosis of acute osteomyelitis. *J Pediatr Orthop 8*:558, 1988.
13. DesPlaces N, Acar JF: New quinolones in the treatment of joint and bone infections. *Rev Infect Dis 10*:5179, 1988.
14. Dubey L, et al: Osteomyelitis secondary to trauma or infected contiguous soft tissue. *Pediatr Infect Dis J 7*: 26, 1988.
15. Egger EL, Greenwood KM: External skeletal fixation. *In* Slatter DH (ed): *Textbook of Small Animal Surgery*. W. B. Saunders, Philadelphia, 1985.
16. Fitzgerald RH, et al: Bacterial colonization of wounds and sepsis in total hip arthroplasty. *J Bone Joint Surg [Am] 55A*:1242, 1973.
17. Fong IW: The role of fluoroquinolones in the management of skin, soft tissue, and bone infections. *Clin Invest Med 12*:44, 1989.
18. Fong IW, et al: Bone penetration of enoxacin in patients with and without osteomyelitis. *Antimicrob Agents Chemother 32*:834, 1988.
19. Geissler WB, Purvis JM: Hematogenous osteomyelitis and septic arthritis in children: A ten year review. *J Miss State Med Assoc 30*:71, 1989.
20. Goldenberg DL, et al: Treatment of septic arthritis: Comparison of needle aspiration and surgery as initial modes of joint drainage. *Arthritis Rheum 18*:83, 1975.
21. Gray JC, Elves MW: Osteogenesis in bone grafts after short-term storage and topical antibiotic treatment. *J Bone Joint Surg [Br] 63B*:441, 1981.
22. Gristina G, Costerton JW: Bacterial adherence and the glycocalyx and their role in musculoskeletal infection. *Orthop Clin North Am 15*:517, 1984.
23. Gupta NC, Prezio JA: Radionuclide imaging in osteomyelitis. *Semin Nucl Med 18*:287, 1988.
24. Hall BB, et al: Anaerobic osteomyelitis. *J Bone Joint Surg [Am] 65A*:30, 1983.
25. Hall BB, et al: Anaerobic septic arthritis and osteomyelitis. *Orthop Clin North Am 15*:505, 1984.
26. Hoffer PB, Newmann RD: Gallium and infection. *In* Gottschalk A, et al (eds): *Diagnostic Nuclear Medicine*. Williams & Wilkins, Baltimore, 1988.
27. Hughes SPF, Fitzgerald RH Jr: *Musculoskeletal Infections*. Year Book Medical Publishers, Chicago, 1987.
28. Juhn A, et al: Subacute osteomyelitis presenting as bone tumors. *Orthopedics 12*:245, 1989.
29. Kahn DS, Pritzker KPH: The pathophysiology of bone infection. *Clin Orthop Rel Res 96*:12, 1973.
30. Koch DB: Management of infectious arthritis in the horse. *Comp Cont Educ 1*:545, 1979.
31. Mayberry-Carson K, et al: Bacterial adherence and glycocalyx formation in osteomyelitis experimentally induced with *Staphylococcus aureus*. *Infect Immun 43*:825, 1984.
32. McIlwraith CW: Treatment of infectious arthritis. *Vet Clin North Am 5*:363, 1983.
33. Montgomery RD, et al: Comparison of aerobic culturette, synovial membrane biopsy, and blood culture medium in detection of canine bacterial arthritis. *Vet Surg 18*:300, 1989.
34. Neu HC: Cephalosporin antibiotics as applied in surgery of bones and joints. *Clin Orthop 190*:50, 1984 .
35. Nunamaker DM: Management of infected fractures–osteomyelitis. *Vet Clin North Am 5*:259, 1975.
36. Nunamaker DM: Osteomyelitis. *In* Newton CD, Nunamaker DM (eds): *Textbook of Small Animal Orthopaedics*. J. B. Lippincott, Philadelphia, 1985.
37. Orsini JA: Strategies for treatment of bone and joint infections in large animals. *J Am Vet Med Assoc 185*:1190, 1984.
38. Petty W, et al: The influence of skeletal implants on incidence of infection: Experiments in a canine model. *J Bone Joint Surg [Am] 67A*:1236, 1985.
39. Resnick CS, Resnick D: Pyogenic osteomyelitis and septic arthritis. *In* Traveras J, Ferucci J (eds): *Radiology, Diagnosis, Imaging, Intervention*. J. B. Lippincott, Philadelphia, 1986.
40. Resnick D, Niwayam G: *Diagnosis of Bone and Joint Disorders*. W. B. Saunders, Philadelphia, 1981.
41. Roe SC, et al: Placement of multiple full pins for external fixation: Technique and results in four dogs. *Vet Surg 14*:247, 1985.
42. Salvati EA, Brause BD: Infection of orthopedic prosthesis. *In* Schlossberg D (ed): *Orthopedic Infection*. Springer-Verlag, New York, 1988.
43. Small G: Systemic mycoses. *J Am Vet Med Assoc 155*:2002, 1969.
44. Smith MM, et al: Bacterial growth associated with metallic implants in dogs. *J Am Vet Med Assoc 195*:765, 1989.
45. Stevenson S, et al: Fracture-associated sarcoma in the dog. *J Am Vet Med Assoc 180*:1189, 1982.

46. Tumeh SS, et al: Chronic osteomyelitis: The relative roles of scintigrams, plain radiographs, and transmission computed tomography. *Clin Nucl Med 13*:710, 1988.
47. Ulf Westblom T, et al: Successful oral treatment of methicillin-resistant *Staphylococcus aureus* osteomyelitis using ciprofloxacin. *Am J Med 85*:884, 1988.
48. Vandaux PE, et al: Absorption of fibronectin onto polymethylmethacrylate and promotion of *Staphylococcus aureus* adherence. *Infect Immun 45*: 168, 1984.
49. Vandaux P, et al: Foreign-body infection: Role of fibronectin as a ligand for the adherence of *Staphylococcus aureus* adherence. *J Infect Dis 150*:546, 1984.
50. Waldvogel FA: Acute osteomyelitis. *In* Schlossberg D (ed): *Orthopedic Infection*. Springer-Verlag, New York, 1988.
51. Waldvogel FA, et al: Osteomyelitis: A review of clinical features, therapeutic considerations and unusual aspects. *N Engl J Med 282*:198, 1970.
52. Williams DN, et al: Bone and serum concentrations of five cephalosporin drugs: Relevance to prophylaxis and treatment in orthopedic surgery. *Clin Orthop 179*:253, 1983.

CHAPTER 127 Bone Grafting

Sharon Stevenson

A properly applied bone graft is often the critical factor differentiating a successful fracture repair from a nonunion or the possibility of a limb salvage procedure from the need for an amputation. Considerable data have accumulated since bone grafts were introduced in 1915[1] and the principles of bone grafting have been well established. Early grafts provided mechanical stability, but since the development of metal implants, bone grafts have been valued more as a scaffold for the ingrowth of new host bone[7] and a source of osteogenic cells and inductive factors.[80] Many types of grafts are available, each with its own advantages and disadvantages. The most commonly used bone graft in veterinary surgery is the fresh cancellous autograft, which has the advantages of histocompatibility, live cells, and excellent osteogenic and inductive potential. If the graft must provide mechanical stability or fill large defects, cortical bone is preferable. Cortical bone is often collected and preserved for convenience and to reduce the immunogenicity of foreign donor cells implanted into the host. The various methods of preservation have different effects on the properties of a bone graft and its rate of incorporation by the host.

This chapter discusses the various histological types of grafts and their normal incorporation. The methods of preservation of bone grafts and their effects on incorporation and antigenicity are presented. The specific indications for bone grafts in veterinary surgery are detailed, and the preferred techniques for harvesting and handling bone grafts are addressed.

BONE GRAFT TERMINOLOGY

The term *graft* implies the transfer of living tissue, whereas *implant* refers to nonviable material placed in the body. Implants also can be nonbiological materials, such as metal or ceramic, in addition to dead bone (e.g., frozen or freeze-dried cortical bone). The next aspect of description refers to the origin of a graft. A graft moved from one site to another within the same individual is an *autograft*, described by the adjectives *autologous, autogenous*, or *autochthonous*. An *allograft* (adjective: *allogeneic*) is tissue transferred between two genetically different individuals of the same species. A *xenograft* is tissue of one species implanted into a member of a different species (adjective: *xenogeneic*).

Bone grafts can constitute wholly cancellous bone, wholly cortical bone, corticocancellous bone, or bone and articular cartilage (osteochondral). Fresh cancellous bone or bone marrow added to a preserved alloimplant constitutes a *composite* graft.

Bone grafts can be fresh or preserved. Fresh grafts may be vascularized grafts, transferred with their blood vessels, which are then anastomosed to vessels at the recipient site. The more common fresh bone graft is the free graft. It is not vascularized and depends on the ingrowth of host vessels for cellular nutrition.

Bone grafts may be preserved by freezing, freeze-drying, irradiation, autoclaving, or chemical preservation. Cell death results from all these techniques, and the graft functions mainly as a space filler and scaffold for ingrowth of new host bone. Maintenance of sterility is of primary concern with any preservation method.

FUNCTIONS OF BONE GRAFTS

Osteogenesis

Osteogenesis refers to bone formation with no indication of cellular origin. When new bone is formed on or about a graft, it may be either of graft origin (i.e., from cells that survived the transfer and are capable of forming bone) or from cells of host origin. Surface cells on cortical and cancellous grafts that are properly handled can survive and produce new bone.[24] This early bone formed by viable graft cells is often critical in callus formation during the first to 4 to 8 weeks after surgery. Cancellous bone, with its very large surface area covered by quiescent lining cells or active osteoblasts, has potential for more graft-origin new bone formation than does cortical bone. Host mesenchymal cells may be recruited to form bone and cartilage by the process of osteoinduction. Differentiation of mesenchymal cells may be modulated by bone morphogenic protein,[49] osteogenin, osteoblast inductive factor, transforming growth factor-beta (TGF-β), or a host of other bioactive factors. Research findings imply that cytokines have important roles in bone and bone graft physiology (e.g., interleukin-1 [IL-1] stimulates bone resorption).[22] Osteoclasts are the effector cells in this process, but the effect is mediated by osteoblasts after IL-1 binds to them.[76] IL-1 has been identified as one of the factors termed *osteoclast activating factor*.[14] IL-1 also stimulates osteoblast activity[23, 63] and prostaglandin E (PGE) production by bone cells and fibroblasts. TGF-β is present in high concentrations in the bone matrix[78] and is released during resorption.[9] TGF-β stimulates osteoblasts *in vitro*,[9] angiogenesis,[61] and the formation of granulation tissue.[64] Both TGF-β and platelet-derived growth factor stimulate bone resorption, mediated by PGE_2.[75] Platelet-derived growth factor is produced by bone cells[57] in addition to platelets and macrophages.[78] Tumor necrosis factor-alpha stimulates bone resorption and inhibits bone formation *in vitro* by yet unknown mechanisms.[6] Finally, PGE_2 is produced by polymorphonuclear leukocytes, platelets, osteoblasts, osteoclasts, endothelial cells, fibroblasts, and other cells.[26] Its synthesis is stimulated by cytokines produced by cells of the inflammatory response. PGE_2 participates in the inflammatory response as a negative feedback control for the production of lymphokines. Exposure to PGE_2 increases the number, size, and ruffled borders of osteoclasts.[33, 56] Osteoblasts are targets for PGE activity; PGE stimulates bone formation *in vivo*,[51] but the response is dose dependent *in vitro*.[65]

Mechanical Support

When placed in large defects resulting from trauma or *en bloc* resection of neoplastic bone and stabilized with internal fixation, bone grafts and implants act as weightbearing space fillers or struts and as scaffolds for the ingrowth of new host bone.[7] The three-dimensional process of ingrowth of sprouting capillaries, perivascular tissue, and osteoprogenitor cells from the recipient bed into the structure of an implant or graft is termed *osteoconduction*. Osteoconduction may result from osteoinduction (e.g., in a fresh cortical autograft) or may occur without active participation of the implant, as with porous ceramic or mineral apatite implants.

FACTORS AFFECTING INCORPORATION OF BONE GRAFTS AND IMPLANTS

The factors that affect the incorporation of bone grafts and implants can be divided into two categories: those resulting from surgical technique and those related to graft and implant immunogenicity and method of preservation.

Surgical Technique

The first and foremost requirement for successful incorporation of any graft is *stability*. Small cancellous autografts may be osteogenic enough for cells to divide, produce new bone, and eventually stabilize themselves by callus formation, but cortical grafts of any type fail when inadequately fixed.[31, 67, 70] Small vascular buds are unable to penetrate the cortex and begin resorption of haversian systems because of the trauma of persistent movement. Without this invasion of vessels, no new bone can be formed, and sequestration results. This finding has been proved experimentally in dogs,[70] and veterinary clinical reports confirm the absolute need for rigid internal fixation with large cortical grafts.[31, 60, 70]

Postoperative infection is also catastrophic and usually requires graft removal or even amputation for resolution.[31, 50] It is inadvisable to insert a large alloimplant in a contaminated or previously operated site. Cancellous autograft may be used to great advantage in the treatment of osteomyelitis,[12, 74] provided certain guidelines are followed (see the later section on indications for bone grafts/implants).

Graft/Implant Immunogenicity and Methods of Preservation

Differences in incorporation are noted in fresh allografts compared with fresh autografts and also in alloimplants preserved by various methods, even under optimal conditions of sterility and stability. Because osteocytes, chondrocytes, and marrow cells display histocompatibility antigens and humoral and cellular immune responses to donor histocompatibility antigens occur experimentally and clinically, the immune response is thought to modulate graft/implant revascularization and remodeling. Matching for histocompatibility antigens favorably affects incorporation of fresh and frozen canine allografts.[71–73]

INCORPORATION OF BONE GRAFTS/IMPLANTS

Incorporation is a partnership between the recipient site and the bone graft, each providing unique and indispensable contributions.[17] The graft provides a small but critically important population of cells (if it is fresh), bioactive bone-inducing factors present in the matrix such as bone morphogenetic protein (osteoinduction),[80] and a suitable structural shape to support new host bone formation (osteoconduction). The host provides the inflammatory response and ensuing fibrovascular stroma, which eventually revascularize the graft. Anything that interferes with the ingrowth of vessels or the availability of osteoprogenitor cells adversely influences the bone graft.[17]

Incorporation of bone grafts has recognized phases, just as in fracture healing.[52, 83] Radiology, histology, bone scintigraphy, and biomechanical testing are used to measure and evaluate incorporation of bone grafts.[46] Care is necessary when evaluating scintiscans, because even a thin layer of osteoblasts and new bone on the surface of an otherwise dead cortical graft gives positive findings on scintiscan.[5] A positive scan, when performed in the first week after implantation of a vascularized graft, suggests microvascular patency and the probability that the osteocytes and osteoblasts are alive. Radiology is helpful in evaluating the incorporation of cancellous autografts clinically; it is less helpful with large alloimplants of cortical bone because the denseness of the cortical implant makes subtle changes difficult to see. Because the radiographic appearance and biomechanical strength of the graft reflect the cellular events taking place, histological incorporation is described and related to results of other methods of evaluation. New methods of bone imaging that may be useful in evaluating bone grafts include scanning acoustic microscopy,[86] magnetic resonance imaging, and dual-photon absorbiometry.[4]

Cancellous Autografts

Phase I Inflammation. Inflammatory changes occur within minutes to hours of the surgical procedure, and many of the cells die, particularly osteocytes in trabecular lacunae. Multiple vascular buds infiltrate the transplant bed, and lymphocytes, plasma cells, and mononuclear cells appear throughout the area. By the second week, the inflammatory process subsides, fibrous granulation tissue becomes increasingly dominant in the area, and osteoclastic activity increases.[7] Phase I lasts up to 1 week in cancellous autografts.

Phase II and III: Revascularization and Osteoinduction. Revascularization of cancellous grafts commences as early as 2 days after implantation under favorable circumstances.[62] Host vessels, osteoblasts, and osteoblast precursors can easily infiltrate the porous graft from the periphery toward the center. Because osteoclast precursors are blood borne, the ingrowth of host vessels marks the beginning of graft resorption.

During this phase of graft incorporation, the host immune system becomes sensitized to donor antigens. Autografts do not elicit an immune response, but allografts or alloimplants may be sufficiently immunogenic to stimulate a humoral and cellular response that slows or even blocks subsequent incorporation. Revascularization of cancellous autografts is usually complete by 2 weeks.

Phase IV: Osteoconduction. As vascular invasion of the cancellous graft proceeds, primitive mesenchymal cells differentiate into osteogenic cells. Osteoblasts line the edges of dead trabeculae and deposit a seam of osteoid that eventually surrounds a central core of dead bone. The radiodensity of the transplanted area initially increases. Subsequently, the graft is remodeled (i.e., the new host bone and entrapped cores of necrotic bone are gradually resorbed by osteoclasts). At this point, the overall radiodensity of the cancellous transplant decreases. Concurrently, hematopoietic marrow elements accumulate within the transplanted bone. Because necrosis of bone does not alter its mechanical strength,[15] the cancellous graft is first strengthened by the addition of new bone. As remodeling proceeds, the mechanical strength of the transplanted area returns to normal.[7] The period of osteoconduction and remodeling may last up to several months in a cancellous autograft; it may persist for years in large alloimplants (Fig. 127–1).

Phase V: Mechanical. The final phase of bone graft incorporation rarely occurs in cancellous autografts because they usually are completely resorbed and replaced by viable new bone.[7] During this phase, nonviable, nonresorbed grafted material remains and functions in a mechanical, weightbearing, or stress-transmitting fashion. The percentage of the graft or implant that remains in original form is variable but may approach 90 per cent in humans.[79] Grafts are remodeled in response to the same mechanical stimuli (i.e., Wolff's law) as normal skeletal bone.[45] A graft placed subcutaneously or as an onlay graft is often completely resorbed with little or no new bone apposition[5] because the graft is not mechanically stressed. Conversely, when a graft is placed as a weightbearing strut in a long-bone segmental defect, it

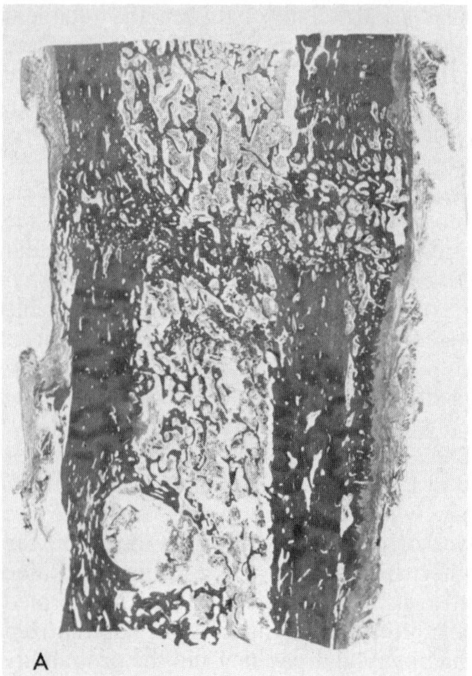

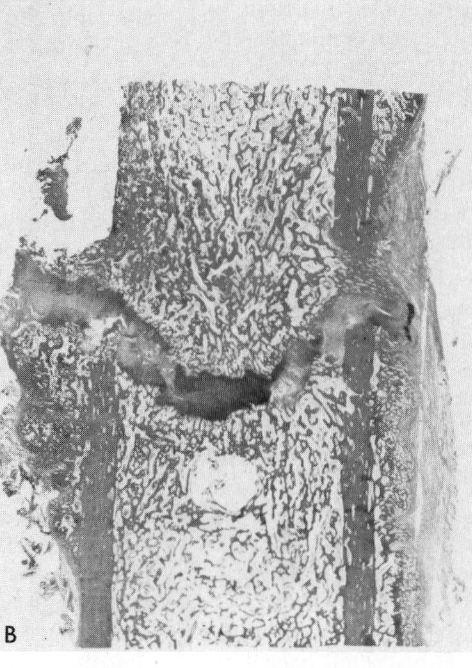

FIGURE 127–1. The effect of cancellous bone grafts on gap healing in femoral diaphyses. The femurs were osteotomized with an oscillating bone saw, a 3-mm wafer of bone was removed, and the bones were stabilized with 4.5-mm broad dynamic compression plates. *A*, A femur in which the 3-mm gap was packed with cancellous autograft. At 6 weeks after operation, the gap is bridged by bone tissue and remodeling is evident. *B*, When the gap is left empty, the space fills with fibrous connective tissue, cartilage, or fibrocartilage (the dark tissue). These tissues may eventually mineralize and be replaced with osseous tissue, but the bone is unstable much longer than when a cancellous bone graft is inserted.

is remodeled like the normal segment that it replaced, both spatially and temporally.

Cortical Autografts

Inflammatory changes noted after implantation of a cortical autograft do not vary significantly from those after placement of cancellous autologous bone. Revascularization of cortical autografts is much slower. Complete revascularization usually requires at least twice the time required for cancellous transplants.[7] This delay in complete revascularization may be attributed to the structure of cortical bone, because vascular penetration of the transplant is the result of peripheral osteoclastic resorption and vascular infiltration of Volkmann and haversian canals.[15]

A second major difference between the incorporation of cortical and cancellous autografts is that repair of cortical grafts is first initiated by osteoclasts[15] rather than by osteoblasts. Resorption of cortical bone at 2 weeks after transplantation was significantly greater than resorption of normal bone, increased until the sixth week, and gradually declined to nearly normal levels by the end of 1 year.[15, 59] Radiographically, an increase in lucency is noted, and the graft is significantly weaker than normal bone. This mechanical weakness first becomes measurable at 6 weeks after transplantation and persists at least 6 months in canine segmental fibular autografts. New bone formation proceeds slowly, and the strength of the transplant returns to normal by 1 year,[15] even though 40 per cent of the necrotic graft bone remains. The radiographic appearance may not correlate well with actual mechanical strength, which complicates the clinical decision of metal implant removal. Additionally, although resorption proceeds independently of the general metabolic state, apposition of new bone is influenced by the anabolic state of the animal, by drugs such as methotrexate and doxorubicin (Adriamycin), and by radiation therapy.[15, 19] Grafts in animals treated with these drugs or radiation demonstrate significantly less new bone formation while resorption continues normally, compared with untreated controls. These parallel processes result in grafts that are significantly weaker than control untreated grafts.[59]

The fifth or mechanical phase of bone graft incorporation is predominantly a feature of cortical grafts and implants. Although resorption is more active in cortical grafts than in the rest of the skeleton for up to 1 year, the osteoconductive remodeling process does not continue until all the grafted bone is removed and replaced by new host bone, as in cancellous grafts. Necrotic haversian canals are enlarged by osteoclasts; resorption consistently involves only osteonal systems and does not remove interstitial lamellae. These unreplaced necrotic lamellae account for the graft matrix that remains at 8 weeks postoperatively. Because dead bone matrix is as strong as live bone matrix, this mixture of graft interstitial lamellae and new host osteons is as strong as control segments of bone.[15] The mechanical weakness noted during early phases of graft incorporation is directly related to the porosity that occurs during remodeling. It is not known whether necrotic interstitial lamellae are ever completely removed.

Vascularized Grafts

Vascularized grafts are not commonly used in veterinary clinical practice because of the technical difficulty of microvascular anastomoses and the expensive equipment required for microsurgery. Experimental work has clarified techniques and incorporation of vascularized bone autografts in dogs.[5, 21, 67] When the vessels are successfully anastomosed and the graft suffers only transient surgical ischemia, more than 90 per cent of osteocytes survive the transplantation procedure. Graft-host union occurs quickly,[21] and resorption followed by osteoconduction and remodeling, as consistently observed in free cortical grafts, is not noted. Correct microvascular techniques as well as rigid internal fixation are important for successful incorporation of vascularized grafts.[21] Successful transplantation of vascularized rib grafts into segmental femoral defects and of vascularized entire knee joints[21] has been achieved in dogs. Because the vascular tree of the graft is anastomosed directly to the recipient, vascularized allografts and implants are probably more immunogenic than are nonvascularized allografts. Sensitization of the recipient is predominantly a response to donor cell surface histocompatibility antigens.[73]

Osteochondral Grafts

Two major types of osteochondral grafts are used: very thin "shell" grafts (articular cartilage plus 2 to 8 mm of subchondral bone) and massive grafts that may include the entire metaphysis, epiphysis, and articular cartilage of a long bone.[50] Shell grafts are generally used for joint resurfacing in the treatment of trauma or arthritis. Shell *autografts* are incorporated quickly and completely when fixation is adequate. The subchondral bone retains its supportive function throughout replacement, so no distortion of the articular surface occurs.[50] Shell allografts are subject to late pannus formation, and humoral antibodies to donor antigens have been identified. Massive osteochondral grafts are almost always frozen alloimplants and are used in limb salvage procedures following *en bloc* tumor excision[47, 50] or massive trauma.[28] Although experimental massive autografts function quite well, both experimental and clinical massive alloimplants show late complications, including subchondral bone collapse, cartilage erosion and fibrillation, luxations, and fractures of the grafts.[71, 72] It was originally thought that cartilage was not antigenic,[25] but chondrocytes do display histocompatibility antigens, and components of cartilage matrix can stimulate a humoral and cellular immune response in dogs receiving osteochondral allografts.[84, 85] Because the appearance of antibodies and cells that are specific for cartilage matrix components corresponds temporally to destructive pannus formation by the synovium, it is now thought that the immune response is important in long-term cartilage allograft survival and function.[85, 85]

Fresh Cancellous and Cortical Allografts

A lymphoplasmacytic infiltrate quickly surrounds fresh allografts. Although the initial ingrowth of new host vessels may occur quite rapidly, these vessels are quickly surrounded by inflammatory cells, become occluded, and undergo hyaline degeneration.[7, 27] Subsequently, progressive necrosis of graft cells occurs. The remodeling of both cortical and cancellous allogeneic bone is delayed,[7] although a second phase of osteogenesis may be initiated by the host approximately 4 weeks after transplantation.[7, 27] This second phase of osteogenesis in allografts is not as successful as osteogenesis in autografts and results in little remodeling and osteoconduction.[7] Cortical allografts remain significantly weaker than cortical autografts at least 6 months after transplantation.[7] After 1 year, sufficient osteoconduction has occurred for allografts and autografts to be biomechanically and structurally similar, although more unremodeled, necrotic bone is noted in allografts.[7, 27] Variations in this pattern have been noted, ranging from absolute rejection with fibrous tissue encapsulation to incorporation only slightly slower than that of autografts. These variations in host-allograft interaction are probably due to differences in graft immunogenicity and host responsiveness. The incorporation of vascularized allografts resembles vascularized autografts while cyclosporine is being administered, but recipients respond to donor antigens and incorporation is stopped within 3 weeks after cessation of cyclosporine administration.[73]

Primarily because of graft immunogenicity and the ensuing slowness or lack of incorporation, fresh allografts are only marginally satisfactory,[7] and preserved alloimplants are preferred by most surgeons. Any method of preservation results in death of cells; however, some preserved alloimplants are still immunogenic, probably owing to intact antigens present on the surface of necrotic cells. Ideally, a method of preservation preserves the implant's ability to stimulate osteogenesis while eliminating its antigenicity. Many of the methods that adequately reduce the immunogenicity also destroy the ability of the implant to induce new bone formation; revascularization and accompanying resorption are often markedly impaired. Sterility is of primary concern with any method of preservation because of catastrophic effects of infection on implant incorporation.

Boiled, Autoclaved, Deproteinized, and Merthiolated Alloimplants

Although these methods remove most of the immunogenicity of alloimplants, they also remove the capacity for osteoinduction.[7] Treated bone is resistant to revascularization and remodeling by the host. Because of these experimental observations, as well as extremely poor clinical results, these methods of preservation are rarely used.[7] After an operating room mishap, autologous bone is occasionally autoclaved and reinserted in a fracture site. Although probably not antigenic, the autoimplant is very slowly revascularized and remodeled and requires absolute stability for a much longer period than the usual fresh fracture. Successful clinical use of autoclaved segments of neoplastic and traumatized bone has been reported.[7, 11]

Decalcified Bone

Bone decalcified by hydrochloric acid retains its osteoinductive capacity, probably because of the persistence of bone morphogenic protein.[54, 79] This bone has little strength and cannot be used as a weightbearing strut. Reports on its revascularization and remodeling are conflicting.[7] Although probably preferable to boiling, autoclaving, deproteinizing, and merthiolation, decalcification as a means of implant preservation has largely been replaced by freezing and freeze-drying.

Frozen Alloimplants

Frozen alloimplants are less immunogenic than fresh allografts[71] and retain the ability to induce osteogenesis.[7] Although revascularization and remodeling are delayed compared with fresh autografts, resorption and osteoconduction occur more rapidly and completely in frozen implants than in fresh allografts.[27] When stable, even massive frozen alloimplants are incorporated well and have been clinically satisfactory in cats and humans.[30, 50] Less favorable results have been noted in dogs, probably because of inadequate fixation.[31]

Freeze-Dried Alloimplants

The freeze-drying process does not hinder implant incorporation, because freeze-dried autologous bone is repaired like fresh autologous bone.[8] The use of freeze-dried alloimplants, although more successful than fresh allografts, results in significantly increased nonunions compared with autografts.[8] Freeze-drying alters the mechanical properties of the bone, resulting in microfractures and brittleness. Implants must be carefully handled and protected with internal fixation devices.[7] Long-term complications of freeze-dried alloimplants are similar to those of frozen alloimplants and include fatigue fractures, nonunion or delayed graft-host union, and occasionally complete implant resorption.[7]

Ethylene Oxide Sterilized Alloimplants

Ethylene oxide sterilized allografts incorporate satisfactorily.[37, 39] It is not known how ethylene oxide sterilization affects the antigenicity or the bone inductive properties of the graft. No cells survive the sterilization process.

Synthetic Graft Materials

Both polymers and ceramics are used to repair bony deficiencies.[32] Polymers such as polylactic acid and polyglycolic acid prepared as sheets or spheres have been used to support ceramics or cancellous bone grafts and to fill defects. Polymers have no mechanical strength, and neither ceramics nor polymers are osteoinductive.

Ceramics are brittle and are not used in weightbearing high-stress areas without sufficient support.[43] As a carrier for bone inductive agent or bone cell chemotactic factor or as a bone expander in combination with a bone graft, both polymers and ceramics may be useful.

Large defects of cortical bone also heal after implantation of autogenous cancellous bone retained by a collagen sponge[40] and after implantation of powdered demineralized bone matrix.[20] Both of these materials have no mechanical strength but are highly osteoinductive.

Summary

Fresh autologous cancellous bone is incorporated the most rapidly of any graft; it contributes to osteogenesis both by survival of graft cells and by induction of new bone formation at the graft site. Fresh autogenous cortical bone is incorporated more slowly because of its dense structure; osteoclasts must carve openings through necrotic haversian systems to allow revascularization. Fresh allogeneic bone is subject to attack by the immune system of the recipient; thus, its course of incorporation is less predictable but is certainly slower and less complete than that of autografts. Preserved alloimplants are useful when they retain some osteoinductive capacity while being minimally immunogenic. The preserved alloimplants are not very biologically acceptable and are poorly incorporated. Ceramics and coral skeletons may be adequate osteoconductors but are currently experimental.

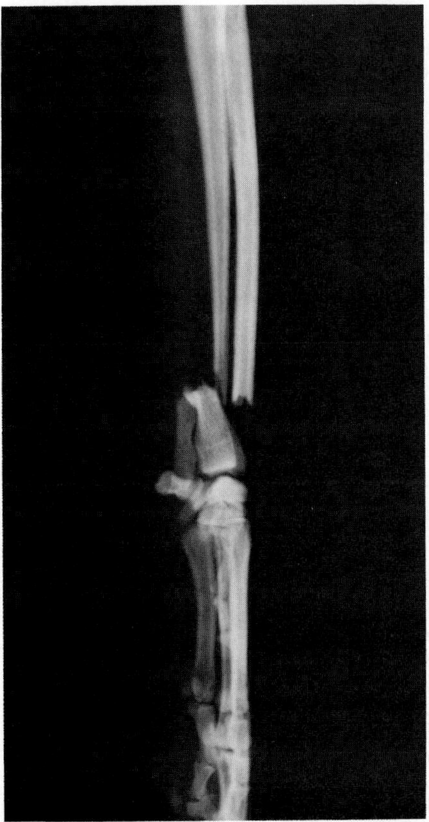

FIGURE 127–2. This distal radial fracture in a 3-kg dog was treated by external coaption, resulting in nonunion. An autogenous cancellous graft and internal fixation would probably have provided sufficient stability and osteogenic stimulus to successfully unite this slowly healing fracture.

INDICATIONS FOR BONE GRAFTS AND IMPLANTS

If rapid formation of large amounts of new bone is required (e.g., for an arthrodesis or for defects in a reconstructed comminuted fracture), cancellous autografts are clearly superior to allografts of any kind. When the graft functions primarily as a weightbearing strut and can be stabilized with internal fixation for a relatively long period, allogeneic material is an acceptable alternative to autologous bone.

In general, the two principal indications for bone grafts are to enhance healing and to replace bone lost through trauma or surgical resection.[34] These indications are not mutally exclusive: In a severely comminuted fracture, both characteristics may be desirable.

Enhancement of Healing in Comminuted or Retarded Fractures

All comminuted fractures benefit from a graft of autologous cancellous bone because they frequently have avascular fragments that are resorbed. Additionally, it is not always possible to achieve stable internal fixation. Thus, early and vigorous production of new bone originating from and stimulated by fresh autologous cancellous bone is helpful.[34] The mechanical stability provided by this early callus may prevent fatigue and eventual failure of a metal implant. Even simple fractures of bones known to be slow to heal (e.g., the distal radius in small dogs) benefit from the osteogenesis provided by a cancellous autograft (Fig. 127–2). Cancellous grafts are useful to augment healing of screw holes after plate removal.[48]

Arthrodesis

When an arthrodesis is performed, for whatever reason, it is of utmost importance to achieve a stable bony union of the joint surfaces as quickly as possible. The usefulness of autogenous cancellous and corticocancellous bone has been confirmed by numerous clinical reports[55] and by an experimental study.[42] When carpi were stabilized with rigid internal fixation, significantly more new bone formation and bone remodeling were seen in grafted than nongrafted joint spaces.[42] The autografts were well incorporated by 8 weeks after surgery. This early production of new bone with an accompanying increase in mechanical stability may permit early removal of external coaptation devices.

Nonunions

Although the majority of nonunions following fractures of long bones in dogs are proliferative and are adequately treated by rigid internal fixation with compression if possible,[68] avascular and infected nonunions profit greatly from internal fixation augmented by an autologous cancellous bone graft. Avascular nonunions often occur in the distal radius or ulna of small dogs and in other bones with poor blood supply. Sclerotic bone ends are curetted to bleeding bone, if possible, and an abundance of fresh autologous cancellous bone is packed into the nonunion site to enhance osteogenesis. This principle has been confirmed experimentally: Fresh autologous grafts stimulated renewed osteogenesis in delayed union.[66]

Cancellous autografts may also be used to advantage in the treatment of infected nonunions.[53] The nonunion site is débrided, sequestra are removed, and open irrigation drainage with an appropriate antibiotic solution is performed if possible.[53] When healthy granulation tissue forms and minimal purulent exudate is present, internal fixation and bone grafting may be carried out. Rigid fixation is an absolute requirement. Only fresh autogenous cancellous bone is useful in treating infected nonunions or other bone infections, because all other grafts and implants sequester.

Contaminated and Infected Fractures: Osteomyelitis

Cancellous autografts are important in treatment of open, contaminated fresh fractures.[58] They have great potential for revascularization and may be applied in any area at the initial débridement and stabilization, provided the surrounding soft tissues are viable and adequately vascularized. The graft is not covered with skin or muscle and may be protected with a sterile petroleum jelly gauze dressing, followed by a bandage. If the graft fails, it is resorbed or expelled through the wound, and sequestration is not usually a problem. If the soft-tissue bed is poorly vascularized or inadequate, delayed grafting is preferable to immediate grafting. The wound is débrided, protected, and left to granulate for approximately 14 days. When the bed of the wound is filled with healthy granulation tissue, the granulation tissue may be trimmed back around the bone and the graft inserted. Sterile petroleum jelly gauze and a dressing are applied. Although the graft may initially appear to be dead, vascularization occurs in several weeks. If sufficient contraction and epithelialization of the skin do not occur, skin may be grafted over the revascularized bone graft.[58]

Cancellous autografts may also be extremely useful in treating chronic osteomyelitis.[12, 74] Chronic bone infections often result in large areas of avascular bone and dense scar tissue, which can be impenetrable barriers to antibiotics administered parenterally. When all sequestra, avascular bone, and scar tissue are removed, the large cavity that results is slow to fill with new bone and is easily reinfected. A one-stage procedure is recommended: adequate débridement and lavage of the infected tissue followed by implantation of large amounts of cancellous autologous bone.[74] Appropriate antibiotics are given during and after surgery. In all procedures involving implantation of fresh cancellous autologous bone into an infected or contaminated bed, care is taken to avoid contamination of the donor site. Donor sites are draped separately and new gloves and separate clean sets of surgical instruments are used. Alternatively, the bone graft may be collected before approaching the infected site and stored in blood-soaked sponges (see the later section on harvesting and handling of grafts and implants).

Bone Loss

Relatively large segments of bone may be lost through trauma or surgical excision of tumors, cysts, or shattered fracture fragments. When the defect is not segmental and when the bone retains sufficient mechanical strength for weightbearing, the defect may be packed with autogenous cancellous bone (e.g., curettage and grafting of a Brodie abscess).[44] Large segmental defects require internal or external fixation and a cortical graft. Autologous rib grafts, together with plate fixation, have been used to repair comminuted fractures in dogs.[82] This technique requires two consecutive surgical procedures with the accompanying morbidity, and many surgeons prefer to use alloimplants to replace shattered diaphyseal bone.[29–31, 36, 60, 81] The bones most commonly repaired with an allograft are the femur, humerus, and tibia.[30, 60] Allograft replacement of extremely comminuted diaphyseal segments is successful in cats[29, 30, 81] but less so in dogs.[30] The surgical procedure, although not more difficult than a standard osteosynthesis, requires extreme attention to detail.[31] Adequate stability *must* be achieved, the wound must be free of infection, and maximal host–implant contact at the interface is desirable.[31, 70] Several clinical and experimental[3, 13] reports have emphasized the importance of packing the implant–host interface with profuse amounts of cancellous autologous bone. This cancellous autograft stimulates host revascularization and osteogenesis and enhances incorporation of the alloimplant.

A highly comminuted fracture occasionally involves the joint surface, creating a difficult clinical problem. Although somewhat experimental, preserved or fresh osteochondral alloimplants/grafts may be used to replace the destroyed fragment and retain joint function.[28] Careful attention should be paid to graft-host joint surface congruity and asepsis. Although articles in the veterinary[28] and human[50] literature report good short-term clinical results with this technique, long-term results are unknown. Experimental work suggests that an immune response to cartilage matrix antigens may occur, with accompanying pannus formation and cartilage destruction.[84, 85]

Osteochondral or cortical alloimplants are also used to fill defects following *en bloc* tumor excision (see Chapter 147).[47, 50] Alloimplants have also been used to correct malunions. For example, when the pelvic canal is narrowed by malunion of pelvic fractures, a symphysiotomy may be performed, the cut edges gently separated, and the space filled with an alloimplant.[16] The same principle could be applied to long-bone malunion fractures, which require bone stock to fill surgically created defects.

HARVESTING AND HANDLING OF GRAFTS AND IMPLANTS

Certain principles of graft handling must be followed to ensure optimum osteogenesis and incorporation at the recipient site and minimum morbidity at the donor site.

The first set of rules is designed to promote maximal survival of cells on the surface of the graft. A key consideration is the selection of a donor site with a large population of surface cells. The most commonly selected sites in dogs are the proximal tibia and humerus for fresh cancellous bone and the iliac crest or rib for fresh corticocancellous bone. Once an appropriate site has been selected, the surgeon must harvest the graft with minimum trauma.[2]

Oscillating bone saws are avoided when harvesting cancellous or corticocancellous grafts. Their use is associated with a marked temperature rise in adjacent bone, cell death, and retarded osteogenesis.[2, 35] In one experiment in rats, radial diaphyseal segmental osteotomies produced with oscillating saws became nonunions, whereas the same segmental fractures produced with bone-cutting forceps healed well.[35] If the use of power tools is unavoidable, they are cooled with saline lavage during use, the edges kept well sharpened, and excessive speeds avoided (1,500 rpm maximum).[2]

Large drill bits or pins can be used to open the cortex to collect cancellous bone. If a larger opening is needed, the hole is lengthened along the longitudinal axis of the bone, keeping the corners rounded. This technique mechanically weakens the donor bone the least.[10] A square hole cut with an oscillating saw is undesirable because it not only has edges of dead bone due to thermal necrosis but also weakens the bone significantly.[10]

Once the donor bone has been removed, numerous precautions must be taken to prevent the death of surface cells. Exposing the graft to air for 30 minutes kills a significant number of cells. Immersion in saline inhibits osteogenesis, and exposing the grafts to antibiotic powders is absolutely contraindicated.[24] Irrigation of the recipient bed before graft placement with dilute solutions of bacitracin (25 to 50 units/ml) and polymyxin B sulfate (25 to 50 μg/ml) is permissible.[25] The use of antibiotic solutions after graft implantation is controversial and is probably best avoided. The optimum technique is to harvest the graft immediately before use and to transfer the graft directly into the recipient bed. If this is not possible because of risk of contamination of the donor site with bacteria or tumor cells, it is best to wrap the graft in a moistened blood-soaked sponge. The graft can be placed in a metal bowl, covered with additional saline-soaked sponges, and held for 3 to 4 hours if necessary. If the graft is held for a short time in a blood-soaked sponge on the instrument table, it is wise to attach large forceps to the sponge so that it is not inadvertently discarded.

Attention must also be paid to the recipient bed. Asepsis, hemostasis, and atraumatic technique are crucial. Additionally, several key steps are taken to promote effective diffusion of nutrients. First, prevent the interposition of dead space, hematoma, or necrotic tissue between the graft and the bed. Second, place cancellous portions of the graft next to cancellous portions of the bed. Third, do not pack the graft so tightly that diffusion is impossible. Fourth, the importance of stable fixation of the grafted area has already been mentioned but cannot be overemphasized.

The recipient bed may also be affected by previous treatment. For example, after radiation therapy, vascularization is usually poor and excessive amounts of fibrous connective tissue may be present. Cancellous autografts have been used successfully in previously irradiated tissue, but cortical grafts or implants are not recommended. Chemotherapy, corticosteroid therapy, malnutrition, and debility affect incorporation.

Bone Graft Collection

Autografts

The medial aspect of the proximal tibia and the craniolateral aspect of the proximal humerus are easy to approach surgically and yield large amounts of cancellous bone.[12, 34, 41] Corticocancellous bone may be collected from the iliac crest or a rib.[69] Iliac crest bone is especially helpful when fusing joints, because the flat pieces may be wedged into the joint spaces to help stabilize the joint. Autogenous rib grafts require a moderately complicated collection procedure and are useful in segmental defects and in the repair of comminuted fractures. The ninth or tenth ribs are the easiest to harvest because there is little overlying muscle. The cranial ribs are straighter but more difficult to approach.

Allografts/Alloimplants

Potential donors are carefully screened for pre-existing bacterial, viral, metabolic, or neoplastic disease. Osteochondral tissues may be removed up to 24 hours after death and remain biologically useful if the cadaver has been properly refrigerated.[10] Aseptic technique is critical in implant collection unless some method of sterilization (irradiation, ethylene oxide) is used. Touch swabs or tissue blocks of the harvested bone (outer surface and medullary cavity) and donor site are cultured for aerobic and anaerobic organisms. Bones are double wrapped before freezing. Pathogens, as well as tissue, are preserved by freezing and freeze-drying. An infection rate of 7 per cent or less has been reported in human alloimplant recipients, about twice the incidence of infection in patients receiving fresh cancellous autografts.[77] If an individual bone culture is positive, that graft is discarded. If 25 per cent of cultures from a given donor are positive, all tissue harvested from that donor is discarded.[19] Although antibiotic solutions during harvest or storage are not recommended, the implant may be thawed or reconstituted in a dilute antibiotic solution (e.g., penicillin, polymyxin, bacitracin), and a brief regimen of broad-spectrum systemic antibiotic administration is prudent.

The chosen method of storage dictates handling and packaging of grafts. If fresh implantation is desired, allografts may be held in a humidified atmosphere at 37°C in tissue culture medium supplemented with 20 per cent autologous serum for 24 to 48 hours. If stored, each packaged graft is radiographed and marked with the name of the bone (indicating right or left), donor identification, date of harvest, and any additional pertinent information. The recommended temperature for storage of frozen grafts is −70°C, although −20°C has been used satisfactorily. Autolysis may occur at warmer temperatures (−10°C), because bone does not freeze at these temperatures. However, successful use of alloimplants stored in conventional freezers (−10°C) has been reported.[30] The period of safe storage by freezing is unknown; the current recommendation is no longer than 2 years. Frozen implants are thawed quickly in warm physiological solutions just before use. Chondrocyte viability is important in maintaining the integrity of transplanted hyaline cartilage and is protected when implants are frozen. The articular surface is immersed in 10 per cent sterile glycerol or dimethyl sulfoxide for 30 minutes; the graft implant is refrigerated for 18 hours, then frozen. This technique results in 40 per cent chondrocyte viability when the implants are quickly thawed.[18]

The use of 84 per cent ethylene oxide at room temperature and pressure, polyethylene wrapping material, and storage at −20°C for no longer than 6 months is recommended for these implants.[38]

References

1. Albee FH: *Bone Graft Surgery*. W.B. Saunders, Philadelphia, 1915.
2. Albrektsson T: The healing of autologous bone grafts after varying degrees of surgical trauma. *J Bone Joint [Br] 62B*:403, 1980.
3. Bacher JD, Schmidt RE: Effects of autogenous bone on healing of homogenous cortical bone grafts. *J Small Anim Pract 21*:235, 1988.
4. Becker EJ, Griffiths HJL: Diagnostic imaging in orthopaedic disorders. *In* McCollister Evarts C (ed): Surgery of the Musculoskeletal System. 2nd ed. 1989, pp 199–225.
5. Berggren A, et al: Bone scintigraphy in evaluating the viability of composite bone grafts revascularized by microvascular anastomoses, conventional autogenous bone grafts, and free non-revascularized periosteal grafts. *J Bone Joint Surg 64A*:799, 1982.
6. Bertolini DR, et al: Stimulation of bone resorption and inhibition of bone formation *in vitro* by human tumour necrosis factor. *Nature 319*:516, 1986.
7. Burchardt H, Enneking WF: Transplantation of bone. *Surg Clin North Am 58*:403, 1978.
8. Burchardt H, et al: Freeze-dried allogeneic segmental cortical bone grafts in dogs. *J Bone Joint Surg 60A*:1082, 1978.
9. Centrella M, et al: Transforming growth factor B is a bifunctional regulator of replication and collagen synthesis in osteoblast-enriched cell cultures from fetal rat bone. *J Biol Chem 262*:2869, 1987.
10. Clark CR, et al: The effect of biopsy-hole shape and size on bone strength. *J Bone Joint Surg 59A*:213, 1977.
11. Coupland BR: Experimental bone grafting in the canine: The use of autoclaved autogenous normal tibial bone. *Can Vet J 10*:170, 1969.
12. deOliveira JC: Bone grafts and chronic osteomyelitis. *J Bone Joint Surg [Br] 53B*:672, 1971.
13. Desch JP, et al: Combination of a cortical allograft with a cancellous autograft in the canine tibia. *Vet Surg 11*:84, 1982.
14. Dewhurst FE, et al: Purification and partial sequence of human osteoblast activating factor: Identity with interleukin 1B. *J Immunol 135*:2562, 1985.
15. Enneking WF, et al: Physical and biological aspects of repair in dog cortical bone transplants. *J Bone Joint Surg 57A*:232, 1975.
16. Evans I: Use of an allogeneic bone graft to enlarge the pelvic outlet in a cat. *Vet Med Small Anim Clin 75*:218, 1980.
17. Friedlaender GE: Current concepts review: Bone grafts. *J Bone Joint Surg 69A*: 786, 1986.
18. Friedlaender GE: Current concept review. Bone banking. *J Bone Joint Surg 64A*: 307, 1983.
19. Friedlaender GE, Mankin HJ: Bone banking: Current methods and suggested guidelines. *In* Murray DG (ed): AAOS: Instructional Course Lectures. Vol 30. C.V. Mosby, St Louis, 1982, pp 36–55.
20. Gepstein R, et al: Bridging large defects in bone by demineralized bone matrix in the form of a powder. *J Bone Joint Surg 69A*:984, 1987.
21. Goldberg VM, et al: Transplantation of the canine knee joint on a vascular pedicle. *J Bone Joint Surg 62A*:414, 1980.
22. Gowen M, Mundy GR: Actions of recombinant interleukin 1, interleukin 2, and interferon- on bone resorption *in vitro*. *J Immunol 136*:2478, 1986.
23. Gowen M, et al: Stimulation of the proliferation of human bone cells *in vitro* by human monocyte products with IL-1 activity. *J Clin Invest 75*:1223, 1985.
24. Gray JC, Elves MW: Early osteogenesis in compact bone isografts: A quantitative study of the contributions of the different graft cells. *Calcif Tissue Int 29*:225, 1979.
25. Gray JC, Elves MW: Osteogenesis in bone grafts after short-term storage and topical antibiotic treatment. *J Bone Joint Surg [Br] 63B*:441, 1981.
26. Harvey W, Bennett A: Prostaglandins in bone resorption. CRC Press, Boca Raton, FL, 1988.
27. Heiple KG, et al: A comparative study of the healing process following different types of bone transplantation. *J Bone Joint Surg 45A*:1593, 1963.
28. Helphrey ML, Stevenson S: Osteoarticular allogeneic bone grafting in dogs. *Vet Surg 9*:83, 1980.
29. Hendricksen P: Entire segment bone transplant in a cat. *J Am Vet Med Assoc 174*:826, 1979.
30. Henry WB, Wadsworth PL: Diaphyseal allografts in the repair of long bone fractures. *J Am Anim Hosp Assoc 17*:525, 1981.
31. Henry WB, Wadsworth PL: Retrospective analysis of failures in the repair of severely comminuted long bone fractures using large diaphyseal allografts. *J Am Anim Hosp Assoc 17*:535, 1981.
32. Hollinger JO, Battistone GC: Biodegradable bone repair materials. *Clin Orthop Rel Res 207*:290, 1986.
33. Holtrop ME, et al: Abstract: The response of osteoclasts to prostaglandin and osteoclast activating factor as measured by ultrastructural morphometry. *In* Horton JE, et al (eds): *Proceedings of the Mechanisms of Localized Bone Loss. Calcif Tissue* IRL, Washington, D.C., 1977, pp 13–20, 1978.
34. Hulse DA: Pathophysiology of autologous cancellous bone grafts. Comp *Cont Educ 2*:136, 1988.
35. Jacobs RL, Ray RD: The effect of heating on bone healing. *Arch Surg 104*:687, 1972.
36. Johnson AL: Principles and practical application of cortical bone grafting techniques. *Comp Cont Educ 10*:906, 1980.
37. Johnson AL, Stein LE: Morphologic comparison of healing patterns in ethylene oxide sterilized cortical allografts and untreated cortical autografts in the dog. *Am J Vet Res 49*:101, 1988.
38. Johnson AL, et al: Effect of ethylene oxide sterilization and storage conditions on canine cortical bone harvested for banking. *Vet Surg 16*:418, 1987.
39. Johnson AL, et al: Ethylene oxide sterilization of cortical bone for bone banking. *Vet Surg 15*:49, 1986.
40. Johnson AL, et al: Evaluation of collagen as a retainer for autogenous cancellous bone used in repair of full thickness cortical bone defects. *Vet Surg 16*:146, 1987.
41. Johnson KA: Cancellous bone graft collection from the tibia in dogs. *Vet Surg 15*:334, 1986.
42. Johnson KA, Bellenger CR: The effects of autologous bone grafting on bone healing after carpal arthrodesis in the dog. *Vet Rec 107*:126, 1980.
43. Kitsugi T, et al: Bonding behavior of a glass-ceramic containing apatite and wollastonite in segmental replacement of the rabbit tibia under load-bearing conditions. *J Bone Joint Surg [Am] 71A*:264, 1989.
44. Knecht CD, et al: Treatment of Brodie's abscess by means of bone autograft. *J Am Vet Med Assoc 158*:492, 1971.
45. Kushner A: Evaluation of Wolff's law of bone formation. *J Bone Joint Surg 22*:589, 1940.
46. Lamb CR: Bone scintigraphy in small animals. *J Am Vet Med Assoc 196*:1616, 1987.
47. LaRue SM, et al: Limb sparing treatment for canine osteosarcoma. *J Am Vet Med Assoc 195*:1734, 1989.
48. Lesser AS: Cancellous bone grafting at plate removal to counteract stress protection. *J Am Vet Med Assoc 189*:696, 1986.
49. Lindholm TS, Urist MR: A quantitative analysis of new bone formation by induction in composite grafts of bone marrow and bone matrix. *Clin Orthop Rel Res 150*:288, 1980.
50. Mankin HJ, et al: Massive resection and allograft transplantation in the treatment of malignant bone tumors. *N Engl J Med 294*:1247, 1976.
51. Marks SC Jr, Miller SC: Local infusion of prostaglandin E stimulates mandibular bone formation *in vivo*. *J Oral Pathol 17*:500, 1980.
52. McKibbin B: The biology of fracture healing in long bones. *J Bone Joint Surg [Br] 60B*:150, 1978.
53. Meyer S, et al: The treatment of infected non-union of fracture of long bones. *J Bone Joint Surg 57A*:836, 1975.
54. Mitzutani J, Urist MR: The nature of bone morphogenetic protein (BMP) fractions derived from bovine bone matrix gelatin. *Clin Orthop Rel Res 171*:213, 1982.
55. Moore RW, Withrow SJ: Arthrodesis. *Comp Cont Educ 3*:319, 1981.
56. Nefussi JR, Baron R: PGE_2 stimulates both resorption and formation in bone *in vitro*:Differential responses of the periosteum and the endosteum in fetal rat long bone cultures. *Anat Rec 211*:9, 1985.

57. Nemeth GG, et al: Growth factors and their role in wound and fracture healing. *In* Barbul A, et al (eds): *Growth Factors and Other Aspects of Wound Healing: Biological and Clinical Implications*. Alan R. Liss, New York, 1988, pp 1–17.
58. Nunamaker DM: Treatment of open fractures in small animals. Comp *Cont Educ 1*:66, 1979.
59. Pelker RR, et al: Effects of Adriamycin and methotrexate on fracture healing biomechanics. *Trans Orthop Res Soc 8*:186, 1983.
60. Phillips L, et al: Cortical bone allografts. *Comp Cont Educ 10*:1167, 1988.
61. Rappolee DA, et al: Wound macrophages express TGF-a and other growth factors *in vivo*:Analysis by mRNA phenotyping. *Science 241*:708, 1988.
62. Ray RD: Vascularization of bone grafts and implants. *Clin Orthop Rel Res 87*:43, 1972.
63. Rifas L, et al: Macrophage-derived growth factors for osteoblast-like cells and chondrocytes. *Proc Natl Acad Sci USA 81*:4558, 1984.
64. Roberts AB, et al: Transforming growth factor type B: Rapid induction of fibrosis and angiogenesis *in vivo* and stimulation of collagen formation *in vitro*. *Proc Natl Acad Sci USA 83*:4167, 1986.
65. Rodan GA, Martin TJ: Role of osteoblasts in hormonal control of bone resorption—a hypothesis. *Calcif Tissue Int 33*:349, 1981.
66. Rokkanen P, et al: Subcortical cancellous bone grafting (Phemister-Charnley) in the treatment of delayed union. *Injury 2*:185, 1971.
67. Sauer HD, Schoettle H: The stability of osteosyntheses bridging defects. *Arch Orthop Trauma Surg 95*:27, 1979.
68. Schenk RK, et al: Experimentell-histologisher Beitrag zur Entstehung und Behandlung von Pseudarthrosen. *Hefte Unfallheilkd 94*:15, 1967.
69. Schlenker JD, et al: A new flap in the dog containing a vascularized rib graft—the latissmus dorsi myocutaneous flap. *J Surg Res 29*:172, 1980.
70. Sinibaldi KR: Evaluation of full cortical allografts in 25 dogs. *J Am Vet Med Assoc 194*:1570, 1989.
71. Stevenson S: The immune response to osteochondral allografts in dogs. *J Bone Joint Surg 69A*:573, 1987.
72. Stevenson S, et al: The fate of articular cartilage following transplantation of fresh and cryopreserved, tissue antigen matched and mismatched osteochondral allografts in dogs. *J Bone Joint Surg 71A*:1297, 1989.
73. Stevenson S, et al: Interactions among immunosuppression, immune response and histomorphometry in canine fibular vascularized and nonvascularized segmental allografts. *Trans Orthop Res Soc 14*:272, 1989.
74. Sudmann E: Treatment of osteomyelitis by free grafts of cancellous autologous bone tissue. *Acta Orthop Scand 50*:145, 1979.
75. Tashjian AH, et al: PDGF stimulates bone resorption via a PG-mediated mechanism. *Endocrinology 111*:118, 1982.
76. Thompson BM, et al: Osteoblasts mediate IL-1 stimulation of bone resorption by rat osteoblasts. *J Exp Med 164*:104, 1986.
77. Tomford WW, et al: A study of the clinical incidence of infection in the use of banked allograft bone. *J Bone Joint Surg 63A*:244, 1981.
78. Triffitt JT: Initiation and enhancement of bone formation: A review. *Acta Orthop Scand 58*:673, 1987.
79. Urist MR: Bone transplantation. *In* Urist MR (ed): *Fundamental and Clinical Bone Physiology*. J. B. Lippincott, Philadelphia, 1980, pp 331–368.
80. Urist MR, et al: The bone induction principle. *Clin Orthop 53*:243, 1967.
81. Wadsworth PL, Henry WB: Entire segmental cortical bone transplant. *J Am Anim Hosp Assoc 12*:741, 1976.
82. Walker RG: Rib grafts in the repair of comminuted fractures in the dog. *Vet Rec 79*:350, 1966.
83. White AA, et al: The four biomechanical stages of fracture repair. *J Bone Joint Surg 59A*:188, 1977.
84. Yablon IG, et al: Matrix antigens in allografts. I. The humoral response. *Clin Orthop Rel Res 168*:243, 1982.
85. Yablon IG, et al: Matrix antigens in allografts. II. The cell-mediated response. *Clin Orthop Rel Res 172*:277, 1983.
86. Zimmerman MD, et al: The evaluation of bone remodeling about orthopaedic implants with ultrasound. *J Orthop Res 7*:607, 1989.

CHAPTER 128

Scapula

Robert B. Parker

Although the scapula is infrequently fractured, its anatomical location is very important. The scapula is a relatively flat, thin bone that acts as a support for the entire thoracic limb. The flatness of the body and spine precludes the use of standard intramedullary pins for fixation.[4] Important osseous landmarks include the body, with associated supraspinatus and infraspinatus fossae; the spine, with its prominent distal acromion process; and the articular glenoid cavity, with the supraglenoid tuberosity and scapular neck (Fig. 128–1).

Because of the scapula's location, trauma sufficient to produce a scapular fracture can easily produce concomitant injury. It is important to assess each patient for cervical and rib fractures, shoulder luxations, thoracic trauma (pneumothorax and pulmonary injury), brachial plexus trauma, and suprascapular nerve trauma.

Proper radiographic positioning is essential to fully evaluate the extent of scapular injury. General anesthesia or heavy sedation is required for a patient's comfort and cooperation. Caudocranial and mediolateral views are the minimum requirement for a complete study. When a patient is positioned for the craniocaudal view, the sagittal plane of the thorax is rotated approximately 30° away from the affected limb to help prevent confusing overlap of bony densities (Fig. 128–2). The mediolateral view is obtained with the patient in lateral recumbency with the affected leg adjacent to the film. The scapula is extended approximately 45°, placing it over the caudal cervical area and preventing superimposition of the sternum and ribs.

Fractures of the scapula are classified according to their location: (1) fractures of the body and spine, including the acromion process; (2) fractures of the neck; and (3) fractures involving the glenoid cavity, including fractures of the supraglenoid tuberosity. A fracture treatment algorithm summarizes treatment options (Fig. 128–3).

FRACTURES OF THE SCAPULAR BODY

Because of protection afforded by the thorax and lateral supporting musculature, fractures of the scapular body are often displaced minimally. A midbody transverse fracture often occurs with minimal medial displacement of the distal segment. Pain with minimal crepitus can be elicited over the scapula, and an incongruity of the scapular spine may be palpated. These fractures are best treated by restricting activity for 3 to 4 weeks and

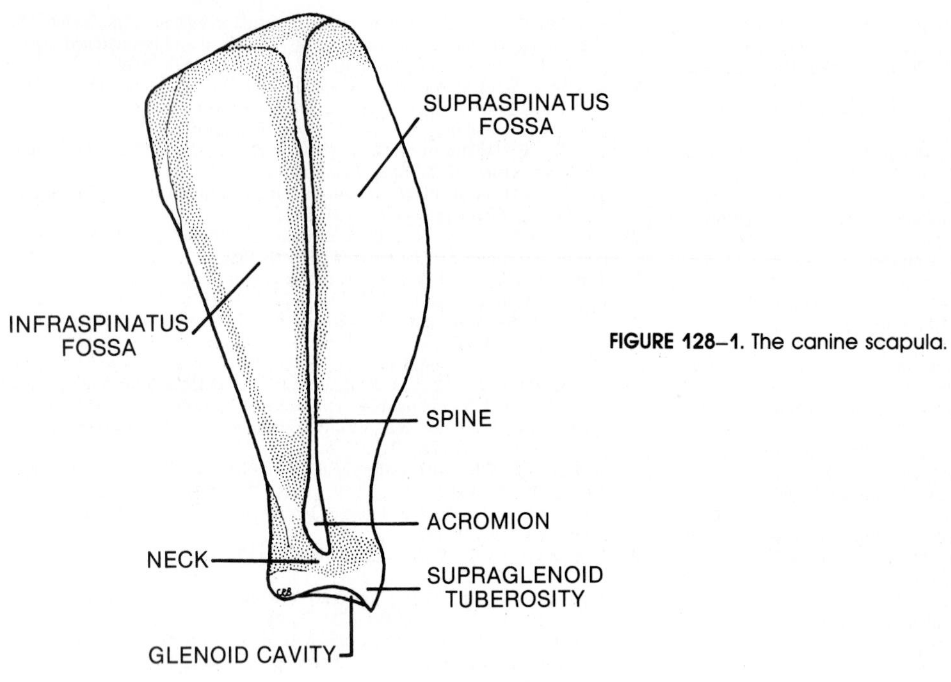

FIGURE 128–1. The canine scapula.

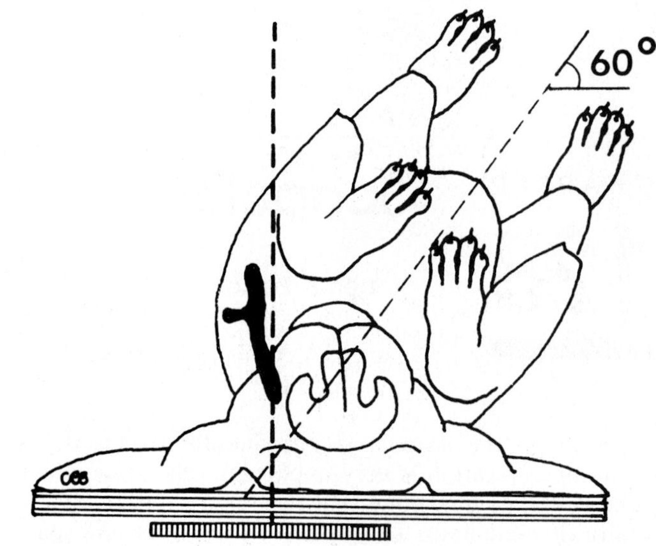

FIGURE 128–2. Rotation of the sagittal plane 30° to obtain a proper caudocranial radiograph.

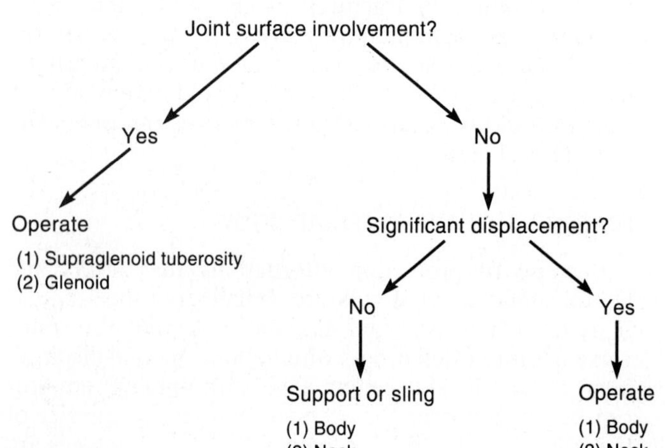

FIGURE 128–3. Scapular fracture management algorithm.

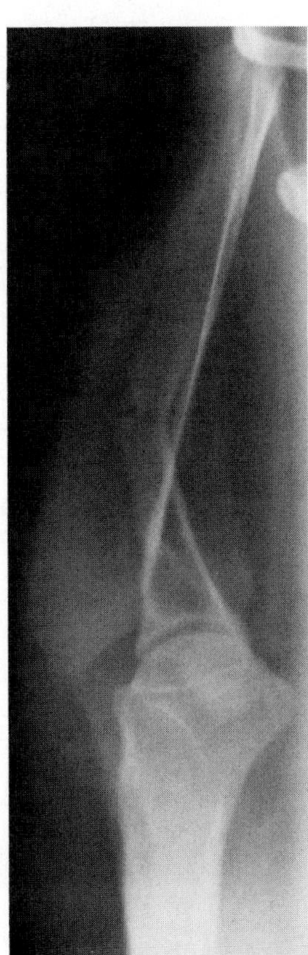

FIGURE 128–4. Caudocranial radiograph of a minimally displaced scapular body fracture treated with a Velpeau sling.

applying scapular support bandages or Velpeau slings (Fig. 128–4). The prognosis for full function is excellent.

Comminuted fractures of the scapular body with minor displacement can be treated by either closed or open methods. Because the blood supply to the scapula is extensive, healing of scapular fractures is generally excellent. Open reduction and internal fixation are indicated for scapular body fractures exhibiting severe instability or displacement or when the displacement is cosmetically unacceptable (Fig. 128–5). The distal fragment frequently over-rides medially and proximally, with the fracture site of the proximal fragment impinging on the shoulder joint area (Fig. 128–6). Healing in this position could result in limited shoulder function.

The scapular body is approached through a lateral incision over the scapular spine. Incision of the deep fascia over the spine allows cranial retraction of the trapezius and omotransversarius muscles and caudal retraction of the spinous portion of the deltoid muscle. The supraspinatus and infraspinatus muscles are elevated from the spine and body and retracted.

After reduction, stabilization can be achieved with wire, small bone plates, or small fixation pins. Depending on the size of the animal, 18- to 22-gauge wire can be used as twisted wire sutures or in a mattress pattern through preplaced holes in each fragment. A figure-eight tension band placed through holes in the spine may enhance fixation.[7] Depending on stability, the fixation may be supplemented with a scapular support bandage or a Velpeau sling.

Bone plates and screws can also be used to stabilize scapular body fractures. Because the scapular body is thin, the plate is wedged into the angle formed by the body and spine (Fig. 128–7). An inverted semitubular plate may conform well to this area.[5] The resulting oblique direction of the screws allows slightly more bone purchase in the thicker bone at the base of the spine. Plates can also be placed directly on the spine to provide stability to scapular body fractures (Fig. 128–8). Plastic (polyvinylidine fluoride) plates have been used for stabilization of comminuted scapular body fractures.[2] Although they provide less rigid fixation than stainless steel plates, their ease in modification and conformability to bone have been cited as desirable features.

Regardless of the technique used, the surgeon should be careful to prevent iatrogenic trauma to the brachial plexus and thorax from pins and drill bits.

FRACTURES OF THE ACROMION

Although infrequently encountered as a primary fracture, nonunion of the acromion process may occur secondary to inadequate repair of an acromion osteotomy after a lateral approach to the shoulder. Affected animals generally have a weightbearing lameness with pain on palpation of the acromial process. The acromion serves as the origin of the acromial head of the deltoid muscle; therefore, constant muscle pull distracts the fragment, and internal fixation is recommended.

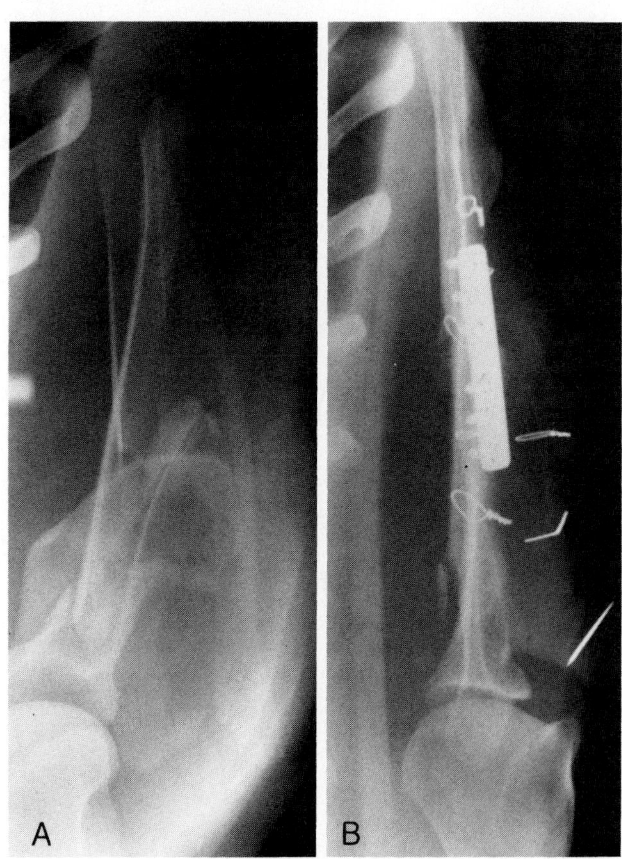

FIGURE 128–5. Preoperative (*A*) and postoperative (*B*) views of a displaced comminuted fracture with marked instability treated with a combination of a bone plate, wire sutures, and fixation pins.

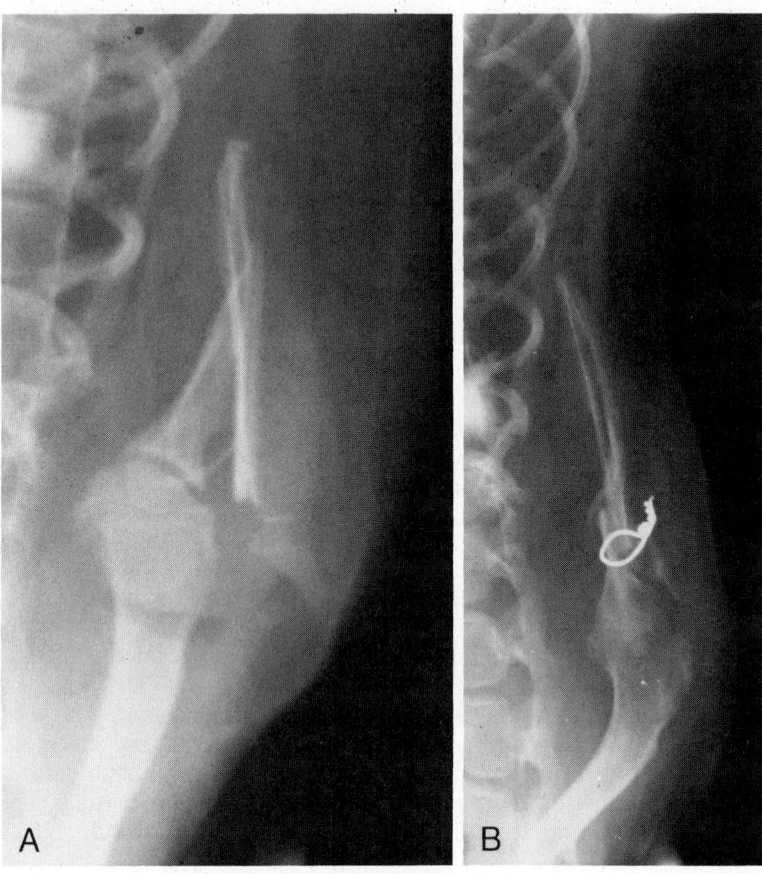

FIGURE 128–6. Preoperative (*A*) and postoperative (*B*) views of a scapular body fracture with proximal medial displacement treated with a single wire suture and a Velpeau support.

The acromion is approached through a lateral incision centered over the acromial process. Incision of the deep fascia of the spine allows caudal retraction of the spinous head of the deltoid muscle. The distal fracture fragment is ventrally displaced and is found attached to the origin of the acromial head of the deltoid muscle. After reduction, fixation can be achieved with twisted stainless steel wire sutures or a small pin and tension band (Fig. 128–

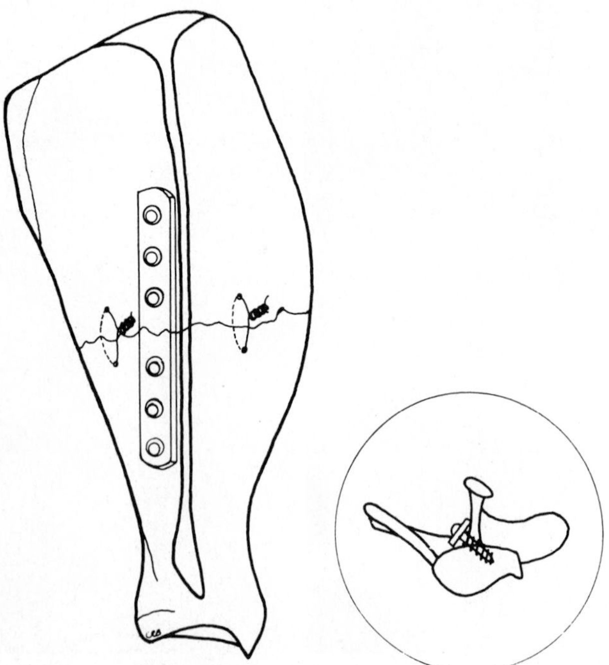

FIGURE 128–7. Wire and plate fixation of a scapular body fracture. *Inset*, Oblique pin position.

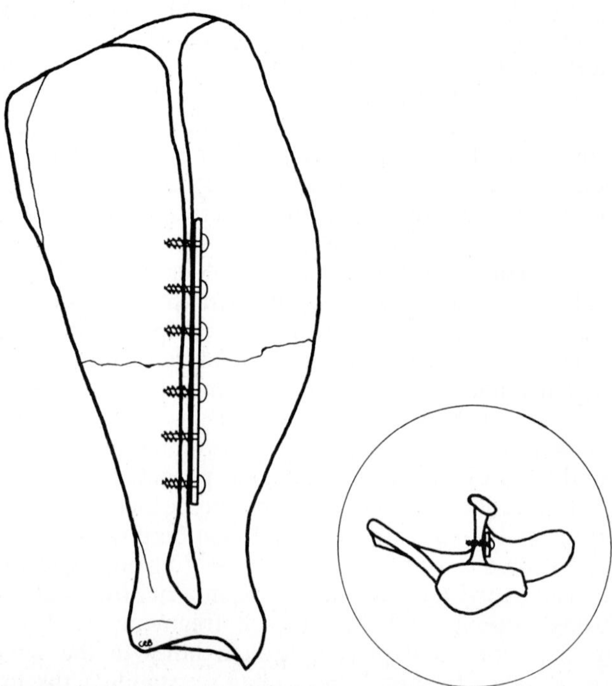

FIGURE 128–8. Plate application on the scapular spine for stabilization of a scapular body fracture.

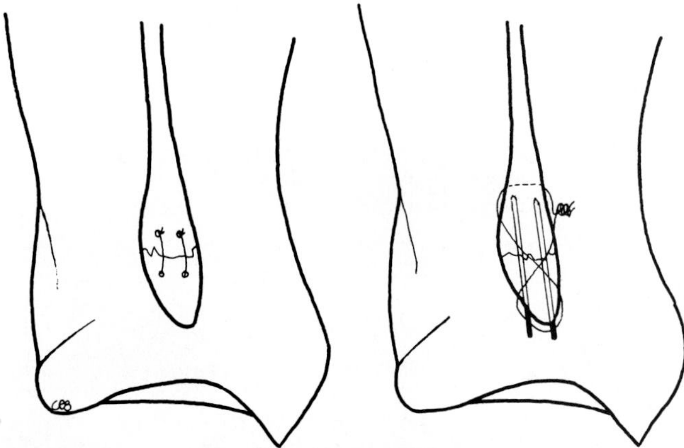

FIGURE 128–9. Fractured acromion repaired with either wire sutures or a pin and tension band.

9). The distal fragment may be too small to accommodate two drill holes for the wire sutures; therefore, a small pin and tension band may be more appropriate.

If fixation is secure, postoperative bandages or slings are not necessary, and the prognosis for full recovery is excellent.

FRACTURES OF THE SCAPULAR NECK, GLENOID, AND SUPRAGLENOID TUBEROSITY

Fractures in this area frequently are severely displaced and may involve the articular surface of the glenoid. Patients are presented with a nonweightbearing lameness, and pain and crepitus are palpable on manipulation of the shoulder joint. Because these fractures usually are severely displaced and are in close proximity to the shoulder joint, open reduction and internal fixation are indicated to prevent exuberant callus formation and possibly limited shoulder function. Articular involvement is also an indication for anatomical reduction and rigid fixation.

Surgical exposure of the scapular neck and glenoid requires knowledge of the regional anatomy and a willingness to expose as much as necessary to reduce these often difficult fractures. A lateral approach to the shoulder is performed by osteotomy of the acromion process.[6] A curved incision is made over the shoulder joint, starting proximally at the midportion of the spine and continuing distally over the lateral midshaft of the humerus. After incision of the deep fascia over the spine, the omotransversarius and trapezius muscles and the spinous head of the deltoid muscles are retracted. The acromion is osteotomized to allow distal retraction of the acromial head of the deltoid muscle. Sufficient bone should remain attached to the muscle to allow subsequent fixation to the spine. The supraspinatus and infraspinatus muscles are retracted to expose the neck area, or more commonly, either one or both of these muscles are freed from their humeral insertions to allow maximum retraction. Lateral and caudal exposure is gained by infraspinatus or teres minor tenotomy. To allow proximal retraction of the supraspinatus muscle, the greater tubercle of the humerus is osteotomized. Care is taken to identify and protect the suprascapular nerve. After reduction and fixation are complete, closure is begun in layers. The greater tubercle is repaired with a pin and tension band. The infraspinatus and teres minor tenotomies are repaired with either a horizontal mattress or locking loop suture pattern of nonabsorbable suture material. The acromial osteotomy is fixed with a pin and tension band, and the remainder of the closure is routine.

Stabilization of scapular neck fractures can be difficult. After reduction, initial stability can be maintained with a small Steinmann pin or K wire inserted in the supraglenoid tuberosity and driven obliquely across the fracture (Fig. 128–10). The scapula thins proximally, and care is taken to prevent pin penetration of the medial cortex. A second cross pin can be introduced from the posterior aspect across the fracture site. Excellent stability in this area can also be achieved with small bone plates (Fig. 128–11).

Fractures involving the articular surface can be particularly challenging, and the principles of anatomical reduction with rigid internal compression fixation must be followed. With a T fracture of the scapular neck and the glenoid, the articular fragments are initially reduced and secured with a lag screw. The resulting two-piece fracture is managed as described for scapular neck fractures (Fig. 128–12). Avulsion fractures of the supraglenoid tuberosity are displaced by the pull of the biceps brachii muscle (Fig. 128–13). After exposure and anatomical reduction, these fractures are stabilized with a lag screw or a pin and tension band (Fig. 128–14).[1]

If stable fixation has been achieved, early limited weightbearing or passive range-of-motion exercises are

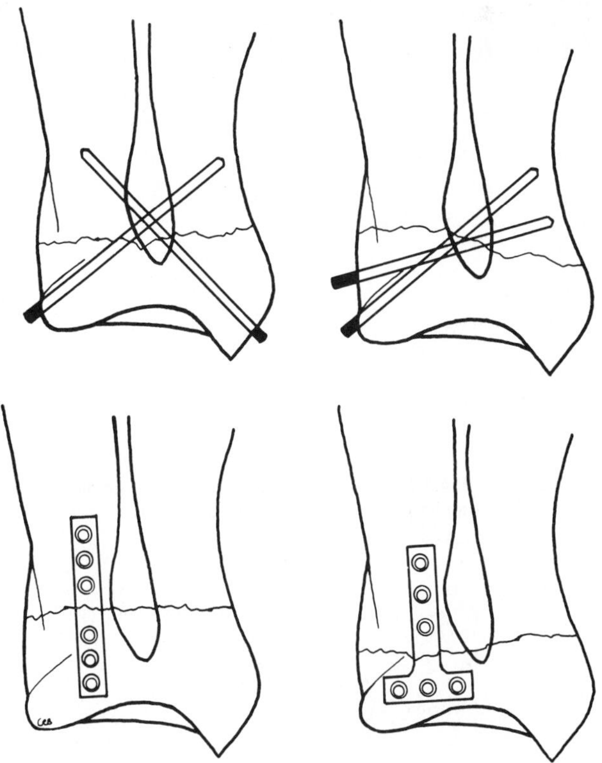

FIGURE 128–10. Various methods for stabilization of scapular neck fractures.

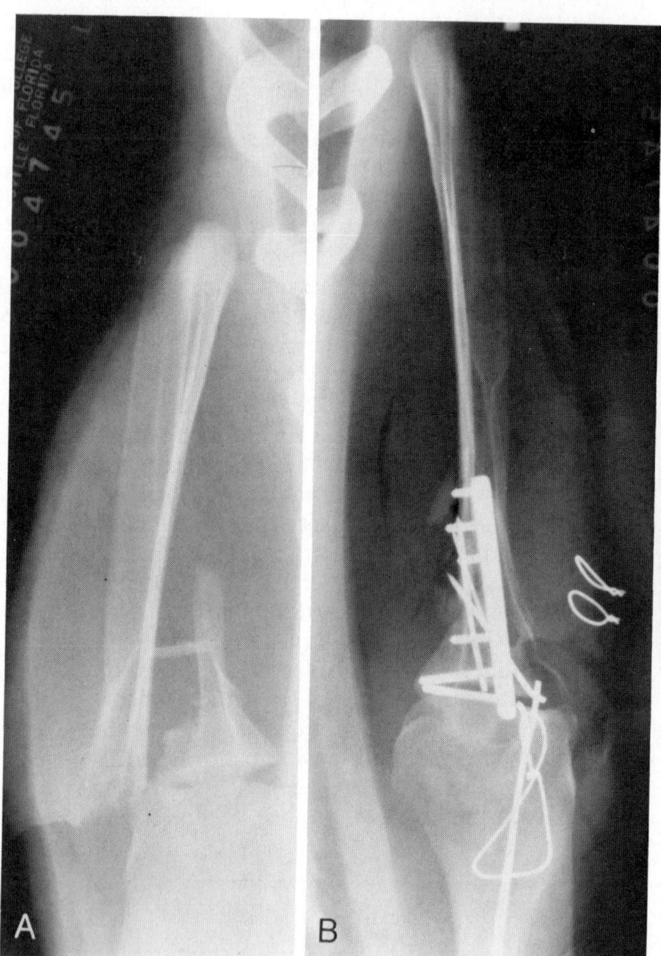

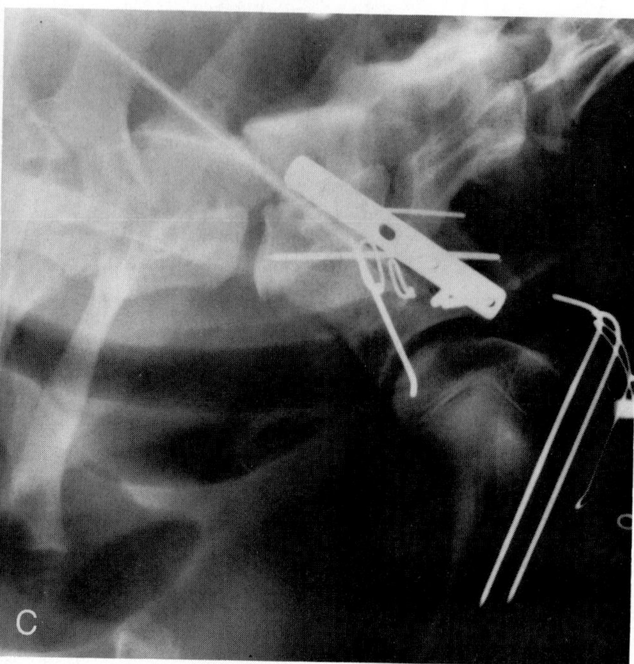

FIGURE 128–11. Preoperative (*A*) and postoperative (*B* and *C*) radiographs of a displaced scapular neck fracture stabilized with a bone plate and K wires. Note the greater tubercle and acromial osteotomies used in the surgical approach.

FIGURE 128–12. A T fracture of the scapular neck repaired with an interfragmentary lag screw and two crossed pins.

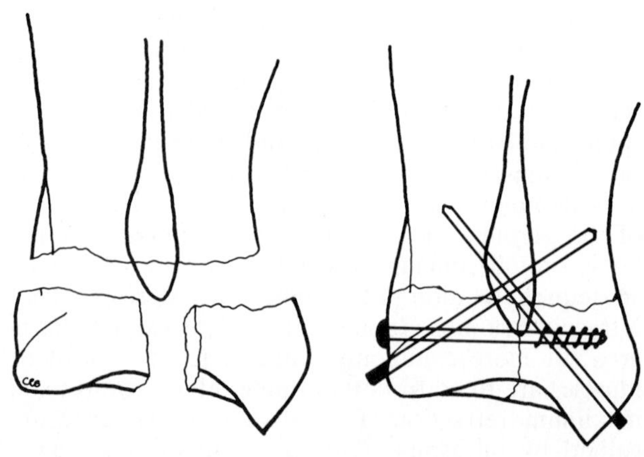

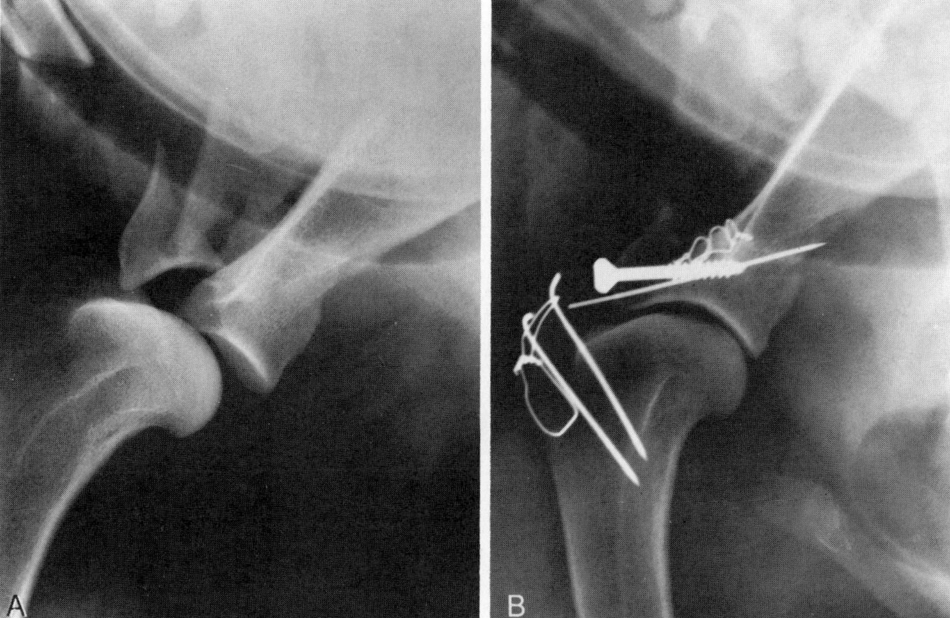

FIGURE 128–13. Preoperative (*A*) and postoperative (*B*) radiographs of a fractured supraglenoid tuberosity treated with an interfragmentary lag screw and an antirotational pin. Note the greater tubercle and acromion osteotomies.

encouraged. If necessary, a scapular support bandage may be applied for 10 to 14 days.

SCAPULAR DISLOCATION

The ventral serratus muscle is a large muscle mass that covers the caudal half of the lateral thoracic wall and inserts on the proximal medial aspect of the scapula. It is the major muscular support for the scapula and thoracic limb. Rupture of this muscle can occur secondary to trauma. The resulting clinical signs are dramatic, with marked upward displacement of the scapula (Fig. 128–15). If the distal limb is adducted, the proximal part of the scapula displaces laterally. Affected animals generally are not in pain but do have a characteristic gait abnormality.

Surgical repair is usually necessary for a functional and cosmetic result. Closed reduction and a tight Velpeau sling have been reported as a successful treatment for acute dislocations in cats.[4] Primary wire support is also an effective method of repair.

A wire suture from the caudal margin of the scapula around the fifth, sixth, or seventh rib can be used as primary repair or as a supplement to soft-tissue repair. After the scapula is replaced in its normal position, a skin incision is made caudal to the scapular spine. The caudal margin of the scapula is palpated, and a small portion of the teres major muscle is elevated. The fifth, sixth, or seventh rib is palpated, and a small portion is subperiosteally isolated. A loop of 20-gauge stainless steel wire is passed around the rib, taking care not to enter the thorax. The free ends are passed through holes drilled through the caudal scapula and are twisted on the lateral surface.[3] The torn soft tissues are reapposed, and closure is routine.

A Velpeau sling, a shoulder spica coaptation splint, or a scapular bandage is used for 3 weeks postoperatively.

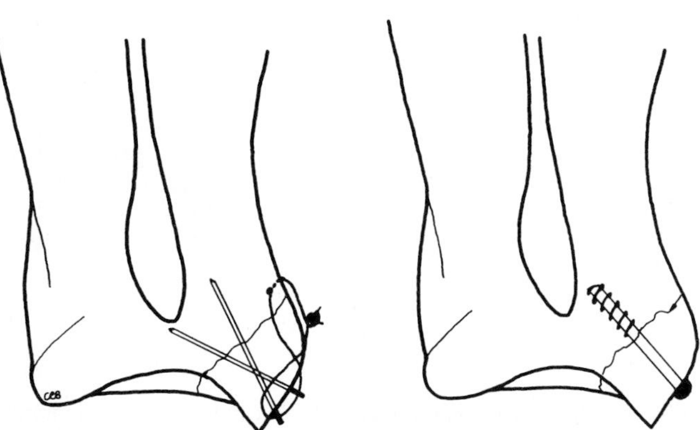

FIGURE 128–14. A supraglenoid tuberosity fracture repaired with a pin and tension band or an interfragmentary lag screw.

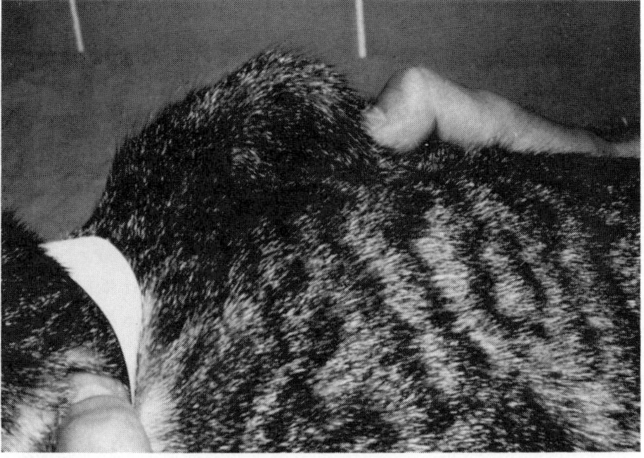

FIGURE 128–15. Clinical appearance of a cat with a scapular dislocation. (Courtesy of Dr. R. L. Leighton.)

References

1. Brinker WO, et al: *Handbook of Small Animal Orthopedics and Fracture Treatment*. W.B. Saunders, Philadelphia, 1983, pp 134–137.
2. Caywood D, et al: The use of a plastic plate for repair of a comminuted scapular body fracture in a dog. *J Am Anim Hosp Assoc 13*:176, 1977.
3. Leighton RL: Luxation of the scapula. *In* Bojrab MJ (ed): *Current Techniques in Small Animal Surgery*. Lea and Febiger, Philadelphia, 1975, pp 497–499.
4. Newton CD: Fractures of the scapula. *In* Newton CD, Nunamaker DM (eds): *Textbook of Small Animal Orthopaedics*. J. B. Lippincott, Philadelphia, 1985, pp 333–342.
5. Piermattei DL: Fractures of the scapula. *In* Brinker WO, et al (eds): *Manual of Internal Fixation in Small Animals*. Springer-Verlag, New York, 1984, pp 125–134.
6. Piermattei DL, Greeley RG: *An Atlas of Surgical Approaches to the Bones of the Dog and Cat*. 2nd ed. W. B. Saunders, Philadelphia, 1979, pp 63–71.
7. Straw RC: Repair of scapular fractures. *In* Bojrab MJ (ed): *Current Techniques in Small Animal Surgery*. 3rd ed. Lea & Febiger, Philadelphia, 1990, pp 736–740.

CHAPTER 129 Luxation of the Scapulohumeral Joint

Philip B. Vasseur

Scapulohumeral luxation is unusual in dogs and very rare in cats.* This chapter refers exclusively to dogs. The majority of luxations are either medial or lateral; cranial and caudal types have been reported but occur much less often.† The cause is often traumatic disruption of the supporting elements of the joint; however, congenital medial luxation in small dogs has been associated with capsular laxity and insufficiency of the glenoid cavity.[5, 11, 12]

SURGICAL ANATOMY

The scapulohumeral joint is supported by its joint capsule and associated glenohumeral ligaments and by the short, powerful tendons that insert about the proximal humerus ("cuff tendons").[18] The latter tendons are the insertions of the supraspinatus muscle cranially, the subscapularis medially, and the infraspinatus and teres minor laterally and caudolaterally, respectively. This muscle-tendon complex has been termed the *rotator cuff* in humans.

The joint capsule attaches to the scapula immediately proximal to the glenoid rim and forms a loose sleeve that is especially voluminous caudally. Distally it attaches to the humerus several millimeters below the articular surface of the humeral head. A portion of the capsule encloses the origin of the biceps brachii tendon and extends distally into the intertubercular groove. The capsule also forms sleeves around the cuff tendons, and these outpocketings of the synovium can be seen if distended with contrast material during arthrographic examinations.

The glenohumeral ligaments are collateral supporting structures on the deep surface of the medial and lateral joint capsule (Fig. 129–1). Both ligaments invaginate into the joint cavity and are enveloped by synovial membrane. The medial ligament consists of cranial and caudal components; the lateral ligament is a solitary band wider at its origin and becoming narrower at its insertion on the humerus.

*See references 1, 2, 5, 11, 12, 17, and 19.

†See references 3–6, 10–12, 17, and 19.

LATERAL SCAPULOHUMERAL LUXATION

Lateral luxation of the scapulohumeral joint is a traumatic injury occurring most often in large dogs.[4, 5, 11, 17, 19] The mechanism of injury is not known, but adduction of the limb may be necessary to luxate the humeral head laterally. It has been shown experimentally and observed in clinical patients that lateral luxation is attended by rupture of both the lateral joint capsule with its glenohumeral ligament and the tendon of the infraspinatus.[17, 18]

Clinical Findings and Diagnosis

Clinical signs and physical examination are sufficient for a tentative diagnosis. The affected limb is carried in flexion, and the foot may be internally rotated. Pain and crepitation are noted on manipulation of the shoulder, and the greater tubercle of the humerus can be palpated

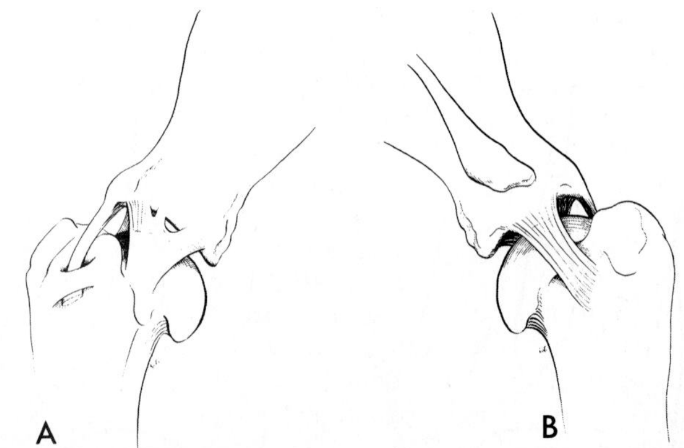

FIGURE 129–1. *A*, Medial glenohumeral ligament. *B*, Lateral glenohumeral ligament. (Redrawn with permission from Evans HE [ed]: *Miller's Anatomy of the Dog*. 3rd ed. WB Saunders, Philadelphia, 1993.)

lateral to its normal position. A complete neurological examination is essential to detect possible injury to the brachial plexus. Radiographs of the shoulder are necessary to confirm the diagnosis and to detect fractures or excessive wearing of the glenoid rim. If the luxation is intermittent, stress radiographs, with the limb held in adduction, may be required to demonstrate the instability.

Treatment

If the injury has occurred within the previous 5 to 7 days, closed reduction and splintage are often successful. After induction of general anesthesia, the limb is held in extension, and the head of the humerus is pressed medially while counterpressure is applied to the neck of the scapula. Closed reduction is generally not difficult; however, the joint should remain reduced during gentle flexion and extension maneuvers. If the joint tends to reluxate easily, the prognosis for successful closed reduction is guarded. If the reduction is stable, the limb is immobilized using a spica splint for 10 to 14 days (see Chapter 124).

More chronic injuries (> 1 week) or very unstable joints require surgical reduction and stabilization. Fracture of the glenoid cavity or biceps tendon avulsion may occur concurrently with traumatic lateral luxation; such injuries also require open reduction and fixation.

Numerous surgical techniques have been used to stabilize lateral luxations. One of the first techniques was a modification of a procedure that had been used in humans, in which a Teflon band is passed through drill holes in the proximal humerus and scapular spine.[1] A similar technique using a strip of skin was described by Vaughn.[19]

I prefer to use the biceps brachii tendon to provide lateral collateral support to the joint. The procedure was first described by Hohn and colleagues and is a modification of a procedure used in humans.[11] The skin incision is placed over the craniolateral joint surface. It extends distally, just medial to the midline of the humerus, and ends at the midshaft.[11, 15] After incision and retraction of the subcutaneous tissue with the skin, the brachiocephalicus muscle is identified and retracted medially following a fascial incision along its lateral margin. The superficial pectoral muscle is freed from the humerus from its proximal border distally to the distal communicating vein, which crosses the muscle. The deep pectoral is similarly incised to free its entire insertion. The proximal portion of the deep pectoral muscle underlies the supraspinatus muscle, which must be isolated and retracted to permit full exposure of the deep pectoral insertion. After elevation and retraction of the pectoral muscles, the fascial attachments between the deep pectoral and supraspinatus muscles are divided sufficiently to allow retraction of the supraspinatus. The transverse humeral ligament is incised, and the biceps tendon freed from surrounding fascia and the joint capsule.

An osteotomy of the greater tubercle is required to reflect the supraspinatus tendon and allow transfer of the biceps tendon to the lateral side of the proximal humerus (Fig. 129–2). The tendon is placed into a preformed groove in the lateral humeral cortex and anchored with staples or a screw and spiked washer. The greater tubercle is reattached with a tension band apparatus or a screw, and the joint capsule closed with absorbable suture material. The superficial and deep pectoral muscles are sutured to the fascia of the deltoid muscle. The remaining fascial layers, subcutaneous tissues, and skin are closed separately. Strict confinement is required for 2 to 3 weeks postoperatively, during which time passive range of motion exercise is beneficial. Short leash walks are started 2 weeks after surgery, and activity is gradually increased depending on individual progress.

Prognosis and Complications

Six of seven dogs with lateral luxations corrected by means of the biceps tendon translocation procedure regained normal use of the limb.[17] In their original report of the technique, Hohn and colleagues described four dogs, all of which regained complete function.[11]

Dogs with secondary degenerative joint changes may have persistent lameness, requiring analgesic medication or, in severe cases, arthrodesis (see Chapter 140).[7, 9]

MEDIAL SCAPULOHUMERAL LUXATION

Medial luxation can occur in any size dog, but is more common in small breeds.[6, 11] In large dogs, traumatic disruption of the subscapularis muscle and medial joint capsule is the cause of the instability.[17, 18] In small dogs and toy breeds, congenital or developmental laxity results in medial instability, and the condition is often bilateral. In some dogs, a malformed and hypoplastic glenoid cavity is present, and reduction is not possible.

Clinical Findings and Diagnosis

Acutely traumatized dogs carry the affected limb in flexion with the foot rotated outward. Pain is associated with extension of the shoulder, and the greater tubercle may be palpated medial to its normal position. Dogs with chronic luxations may not appear to be in pain. A thorough neurological examination is essential.

Small dogs with nontraumatic medial luxation may have intermittent or constant lameness. The joint may often be easily reduced and reluxated with manipulation and is not painful. Dogs with severe malformation of the glenoid usually do not bear weight and hold the affected limb in flexion.

Radiographic examination of dogs with traumatic luxations is important to verify the diagnosis and check for concurrent fractures, especially of the glenoid cavity. Radiographs of the shoulder in small dogs with chronic luxations may show considerable secondary degenerative changes, including erosion of the medial glenoid rim (Fig. 129–3). In some small dogs, however, the luxation is intermittent and secondary changes are very minor. In these dogs, stress radiographs may be necessary to demonstrate the instability. Severe dysplasia of the glenoid cavity may be present, in which case reduc-

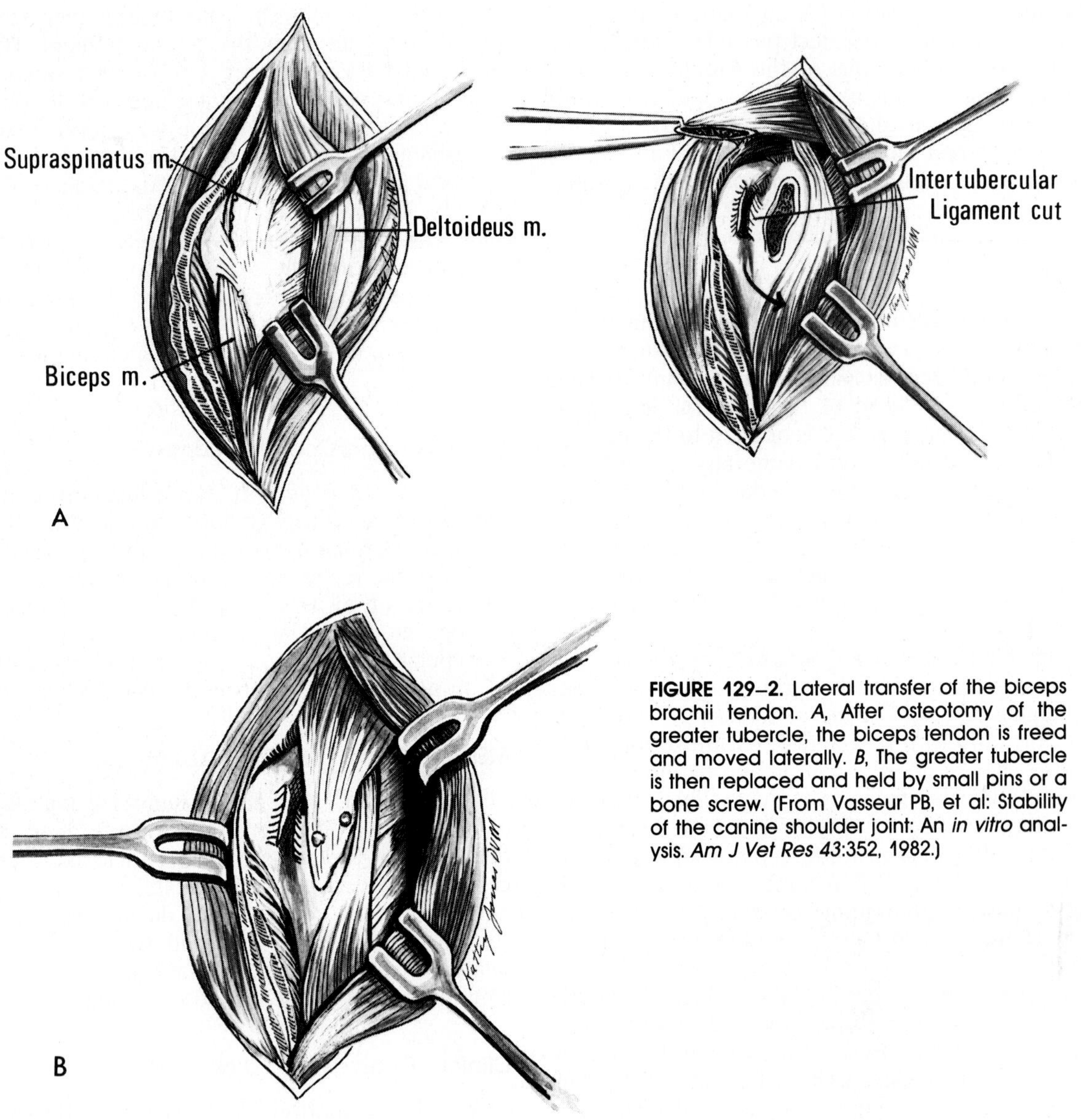

FIGURE 129–2. Lateral transfer of the biceps brachii tendon. *A*, After osteotomy of the greater tubercle, the biceps tendon is freed and moved laterally. *B*, The greater tubercle is then replaced and held by small pins or a bone screw. (From Vasseur PB, et al: Stability of the canine shoulder joint: An *in vitro* analysis. *Am J Vet Res 43*:352, 1982.)

tion is not possible (Fig. 129–4). Such findings obviously influence the prognosis and the type of surgical correction required.

Treatment

Conservative care of acute traumatic medial luxations consists of closed reduction and placement of the limb in a Velpeau-type sling for 2 weeks. This type of sling distracts the humeral head laterally (see Chapter 124). Unstable reductions and fractures involving the articular surfaces require surgical intervention.

Chronic luxations in small dogs may cause only intermittent lameness with minimal secondary degenerative changes. Decisions regarding surgical stabilization in these types of cases must be made on the basis of age, general health, and the severity of the disability. Nonweightbearing lameness associated with severe dysplasia of the glenoid cavity in small dogs requires arthrodesis or resection arthroplasty to restore limb use.[16]

In 1968, Ball modified Vaughn's procedure for lateral luxations to stabilize a medial luxation in a dog using a nylon prosthesis.[3] Hohn and colleagues described medial transfer of the biceps tendon to provide medial collateral support to the joint.[11]

In the Hohn procedure, the initial approach, with retraction of the pectoral muscles, is identical to that used for lateral luxations. The leg is then rotated outward, and the subscapularis muscle is elevated and detached from the lesser tubercle.[14] The tendon of the coracobrachialis muscle lies craniomedially and is retracted with the subscapularis. Tissues over the intertubercular groove and the transverse humeral ligament are transected, and the dorsal joint capsule surrounding the biceps brachii tendon is incised to allow mobilization of the tendon. A crescent-shaped osteotomy is made in the lesser tubercle, with the bottom of the crescent following the contour of the humeral head. The flap of bone is elevated, with the hinged portion being craniodorsal. A small amount of cancellous bone is curetted from beneath the flap, the luxation is reduced, and the tendon is fitted into the groove beneath the bone flap

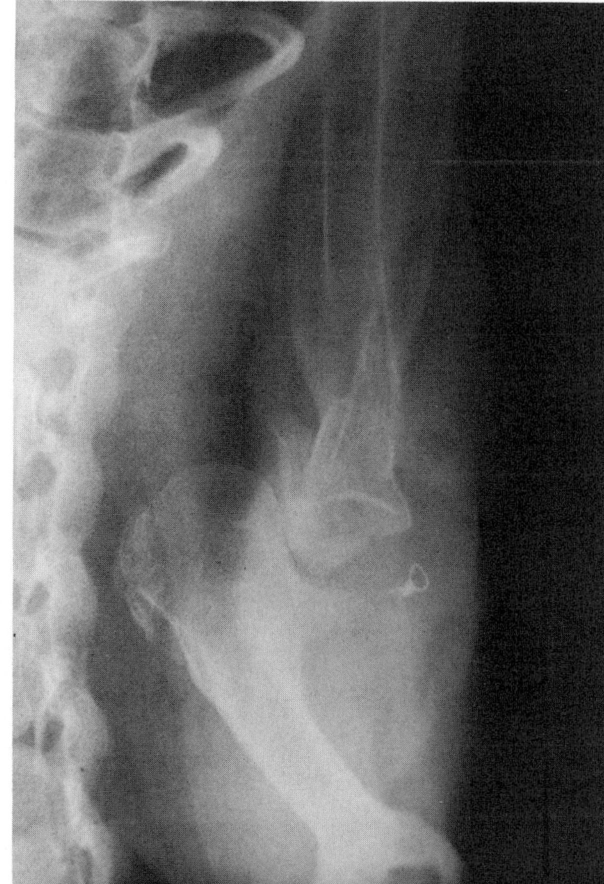

FIGURE 129–3. Craniocaudal radiographic projection of a chronic shoulder luxation in a 9-year-old Chihuahua. A pseudoarthrosis has formed between the lateral aspect of the humerus and the medial aspect of the glenoid cavity, with extensive secondary joint disease.

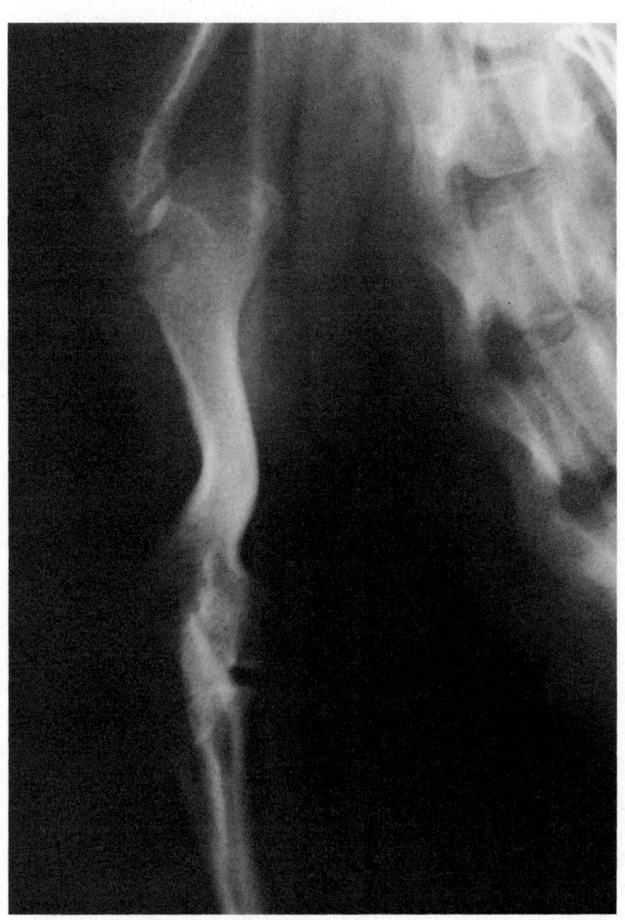

FIGURE 129–4. Craniocaudal radiographic projection of the left shoulder joint of a 7-month-old Chihuahua. Note the medial luxation of the humeral head and the dysplastic appearance of the gleniod cavity. (From Vasseur PB: Arthrodesis for congenital medial luxation of the shoulder. *J Am Vet Med Assoc, 197*:50, 1990.)

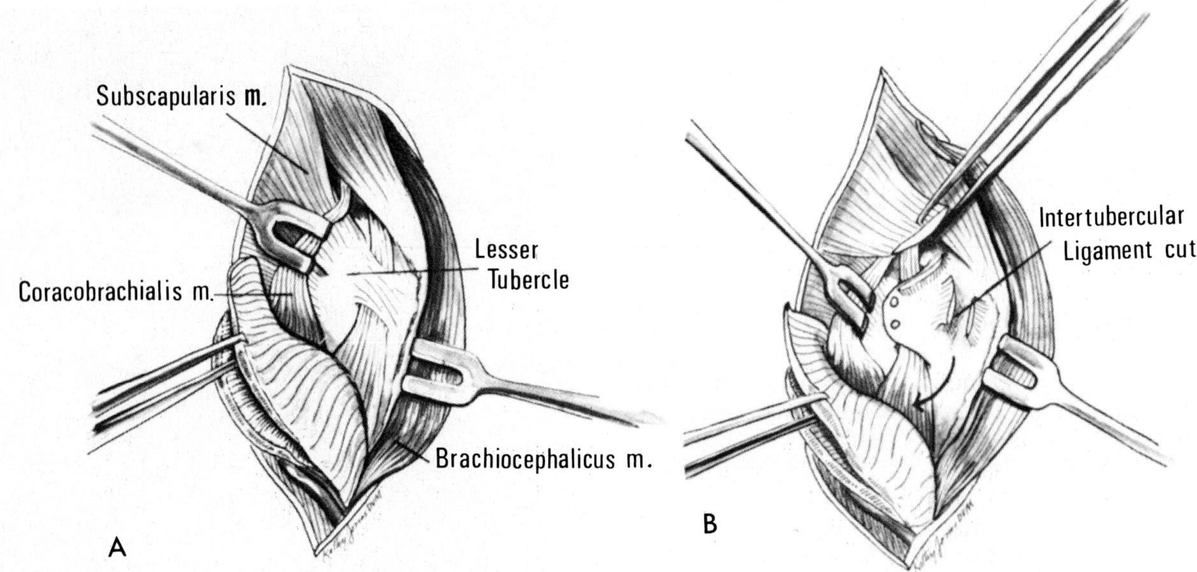

FIGURE 129–5. Medial transfer of the biceps brachii tendon. *A,* Retraction of the pectoral muscles permits observation of the biceps tendon and the lesser tubercle. *B,* A flap is made in the lesser tubercle, and the biceps tendon is transferred into a trough underneath the flap, which is then secured with two small pins. (From Vasseur PB, et al: Stability of the canine shoulder joint: An *in vitro* analysis. *Am J Vet Res 43*:352, 1982.)

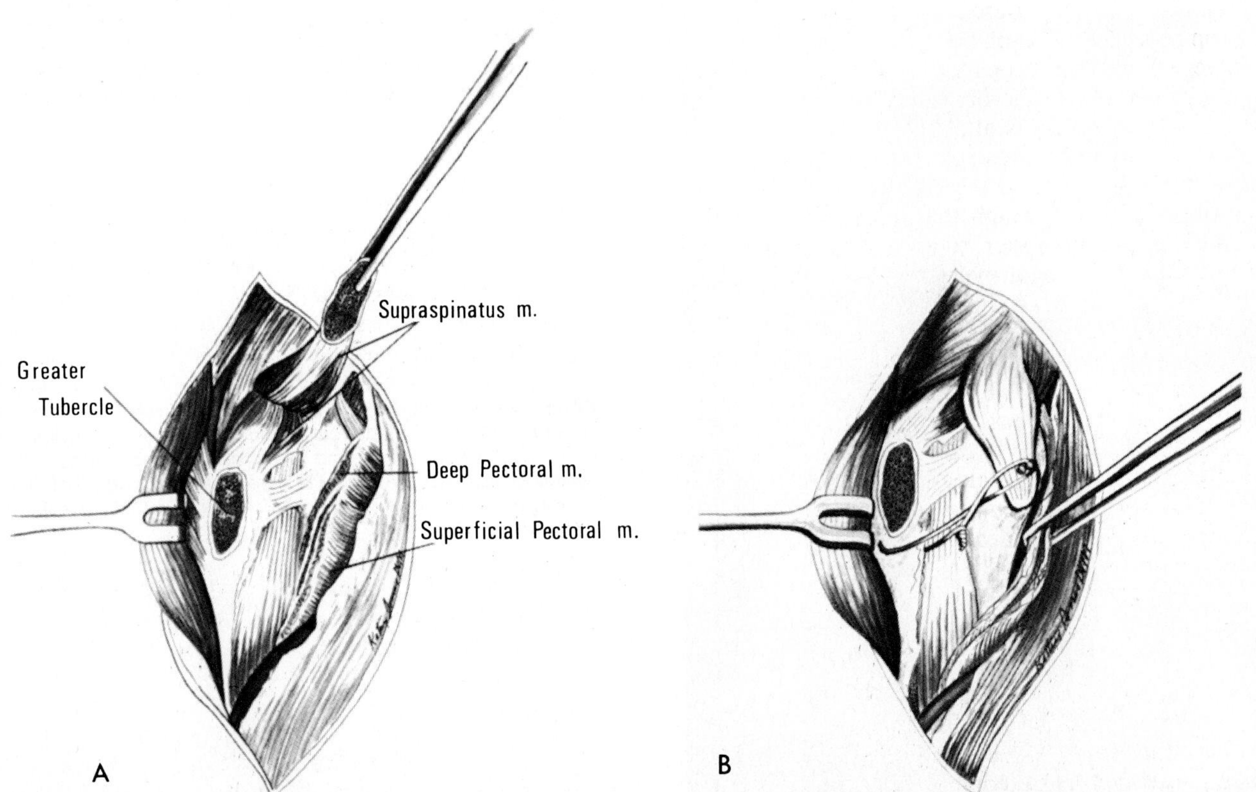

FIGURE 129–6. *A,* Osteotomy of the proximal greater tubercle allows mobilization of a portion of the supraspinatus muscle. *B,* The bone fragment is moved to the area of the lesser tubercle and stabilized using a tension band apparatus. (From Vasseur PB, et al: Stability of the canine shoulder joint: An *in vitro* analysis. *Am J Vet Res 43*:352, 1982.)

(Fig. 129–5). The flap is secured with two Kirschner wires.

The medial joint capsule is reefed with heavy chromic gut, and the subscapularis muscle is advanced and sutured near the insertion of the deep pectoral using mattress sutures. Both pectoral muscles are attached to the deltoid and deep brachial fascia. The brachiocephalicus muscle is sutured to the brachial fascia, and the subcutaneous and skin layers are closed separately. The leg is placed in a Velpeau-type sling for 7 to 10 days.

Transfer of a portion of the supraspinatus insertion and reefing of the medial joint capsule have been advocated for luxations when the biceps tendon has been damaged or when tendon transfer has been unsuccessful.[4]

The approach to the joint is identical to that for a biceps brachii tendon translocation.[14] The medial joint structures are imbricated, and if the transverse humeral ligament or tendon of the biceps brachii has been damaged, it is repaired to maintain function of the muscle and prevent lameness.

With the leg in an extended position, an osteotome is positioned on the crest of the greater tubercle. It is directed so that the medial line of the incision is parallel to the humeral border of the transverse humeral ligament, and the lateral line is positioned just cranial to the infraspinatus tendon. The cut splits the tendon of the supraspinatus so that approximately half remains attached to the base of the greater tubercle (Fig. 129–6).

The tendon of the supraspinatus is carefully split dorsally only to the extent that the free end can reach the area of the lesser tubercle. If the tendon is split too far, proper tension cannot be maintained. An area on the lesser tubercle is prepared by removing the outer cortex with an osteotome or drill. The severed portion of the greater tubercle is attached to the prepared site with two Kirschner wires. A hole is drilled in the humeral crest just distal to the osteotomy site. A tension band wire is placed through the hole, then around the pins, and tightened. After routine closure, the leg is immobilized in a Velpeau-type sling for 7 to 10 days.

Arthrodesis may be indicated for severe congenital glenoid dysplasia, severe secondary degenerative joint disease, and in joints in which prior attempts at stabilization have failed. In small dogs, a single screw placed through the scapular neck and into the proximal humerus provides adequate fixation (Fig. 129–7).[16] Larger dogs require plate fixation along the scapular spine and proximal humerus (see Chapter 140).[7, 9]

Alternatives to arthrodesis include resection of the glenoid[8, 13] and amputation.

Prognosis

In evaluating medial translocation of the biceps tendon, one study reported satisfactory results in 11 of 12 dogs,[17] another in 10 of 11 dogs.[11] In the latter report, the one unsatisfactory outcome was attributed to a worn and shallow glenoid.

Scapulohumeral arthrodesis provides good to excellent use of the limb in the majority of animals

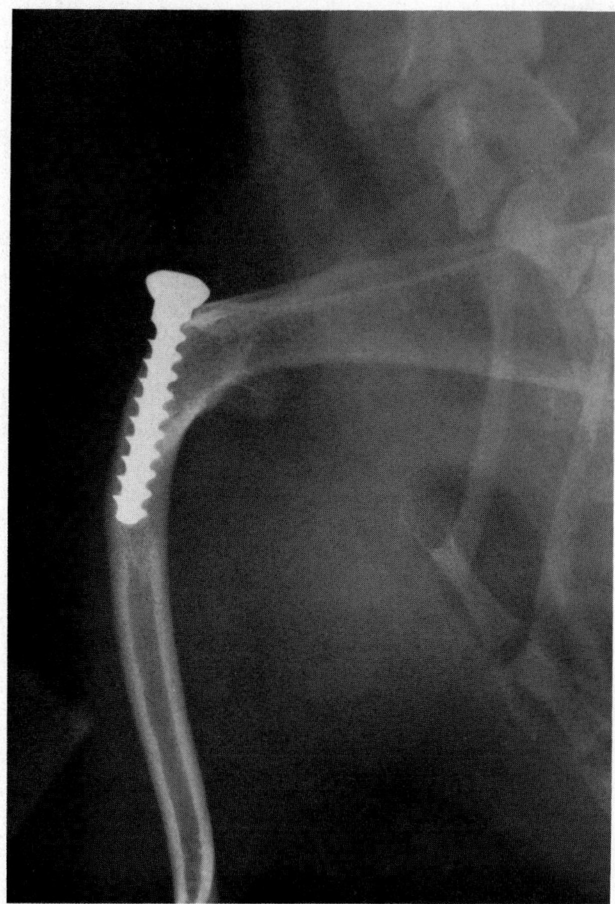

FIGURE 129–7. Lateral radiographic projection of the left shoulder taken 8 months after arthrodesis for congenital medial luxation with gleniod dysplasia (same case as in Fig. 129–4). The dog had almost normal use of the leg. (From Vasseur PB: Arthrodesis for congenital medial luxation of the shoulder. *J Am Vet Med Assoc* *197*:50, 1990.)

studied.[8, 13] My experience has been that arthrodesis in small dogs provides consistently good results, whereas in larger dogs the results are variable and difficult to predict. Excision of the glenoid cavity provided excellent results in two of ten dogs and good results in the remaining eight dogs.[8] Some reduction in range of motion, muscle atrophy, and slight climb shortening were noted in all limbs postoperatively.

CRANIAL SCAPULOHUMERAL LUXATION

Cranial luxation of the shoulder is rare and is associated with trauma.[6] Physical and radiographic examinations confirm the diagnosis. Animals with cranial luxation described in the literature required surgical intervention for correction of the instability.

Surgical Technique

The approach to the shoulder for open reduction of a cranial luxation is identical to that for a lateral luxation.[15] After osteotomy of the greater tubercle, a groove is made *in the osteotomy site* deep enough to accommodate the tendon of the biceps brachii. The tendon is mobilized by incising the transverse humeral ligament and the dorsal joint capsule and is placed in the groove beneath the greater tubercle. The joint capsule is closed, and the greater tubercle is fixed in place with a tension band apparatus or lag screw. The remaining closure is routine. The limb is supported using a spica splint for 10 days.

CAUDAL SCAPULOHUMERAL LUXATION

Caudolateral or caudodistal luxation is rare. Imbrication or reefing of the joint capsule works well in affected animals. An approach is made to the caudolateral region of the shoulder joint, and the joint capsule is imbricated with Lembert sutures of heavy chromic gut. The limb is supported in a nonweightbearing sling for 10 days.

References

1. Alexander JE: Open reduction and fixation of shoulder luxation. *Small Anim Clin 2*:379, 1962.
2. Alexander JW: Orthopedic conditions of the forelimb. *Am Anim Hosp Assoc Proc 48*:311, 1981.
3. Ball DC: A case of medial luxation of the canine shoulder joint and its surgical correction. *Vet Rec 83*:195, 1968.
4. Craig E, et al: Treatment of shoulder joint luxations. *In* Bojrab MJ (ed): *Current Techniques in Small Animal Surgery*. 3rd ed. Lea & Febiger, Philadelphia, 1990, pp 740–748.
5. DeAngelis MP: Luxations of the shoulder joint. *In* Bojrab MJ (ed): *Current Techniques in Small Animal Surgery*. Lea & Febiger, Philadelphia, 1975, pp 499–504.
6. DeAngelis MP, Schwartz A: Surgical correction of cranial dislocation of the scapulohumeral joint in a dog. *J Am Vet Med Assoc 156*:435, 1970.
7. Fowler D, et al: Scapulohumeral arthrodesis: Results in seven dogs. *J Am Anim Hosp Assoc 24*:667, 1988.
8. Franczuszki D, Parks LJ: Glenoid excision as a treatment in chronic shoulder disabilities: Surgical technique and clinical results. *J Am Anim Hosp Assoc 24*:637, 1988.
9. Herron MR: Abstract: Scapulo-humeral arthrodesis: An evaluation of two techniques in 33 cases. *Vet Surg 18*:78, 1989.
10. Hinko PJ: Recurrent shoulder luxation. *Canine Pract 4*: 46, 1977.
11. Hohn RB, et al: Surgical stabilization of recurrent shoulder luxation. *Vet Clin North Am 1*:537, 1971.
12. Lippincott CL: Reefing of the shoulder joint. A technique to surgically restore the integrity of a luxated scapulohumeral articulation in the dog. *Vet Med Small Anim Clin 66*:695, 1971.
13. Piermattei DL, Blass CE: Resection of the glenoid rim and humeral head. *In* Bojrab MJ (ed): *Current Techniques in Small Animal Surgery*. 3rd ed. Lea & Febiger, Philadelphia, 1990, pp 748–749.
14. Piermattei DL, Greeley RG: *An Atlas of Surgical Approaches to the Bones of the Dog and Cat*. 2nd ed. W. B. Saunders, Philadelphia, 1979, pp 72–75.
15. Piermattei DL, Greeley RG: *An Atlas of Surgical Approaches to the Bones of the Dog and Cat*. 2nd ed. W. B. Saunders, Philadelphia, 1979, pp 76–77.
16. Vasseur PB: Arthrodesis for congenital medial luxation of the shoulder. *J Am Vet Med Assoc 197*:50, 1990.
17. Vasseur PB: Clinical results of surgical correction of shoulder luxation in dogs. *J Am Vet Med Assoc 182*:503, 1983.
18. Vasseur PB, et al: Stability of the canine shoulder joint: An *in vitro* analysis. *Am J Vet Res 43*:352, 1982.
19. Vaughn LC: Dislocation of the shoulder joint in the dog and cat. *J Small Anim Pract 8*:45, 1967.

CHAPTER 130

Fractures of the Humerus

Marvin L. Olmstead

The humerus is the largest bone of the thoracic limb.[2] The proximal end of the humerus consists of the greater tubercle and humeral head. The articular surface of the humeral head is twice as large as the glenoid cavity of the scapula. Just in front of the humeral head lies a large craniolateral projection, the greater tubercle. The shaft of the bone extending distally is relatively flat and has a convex curve along its cranial surface. The caudal surface has a corresponding concave curvature. The medial side of the shaft is relatively straight except for a flare toward the proximal and distal ends of the bone. The most prominent feature of the lateral surface is the musculospiral groove and the ridge of the anconeal line. The intertubercular groove is found between the greater tubercle and the lesser tubercle in the proximal humerus. The shaft flows distally into the humeral condyle, which includes the articular area and the adjacent fossae. The radial fossa is found cranially just above the articular surface of the condyle, and the olecranon fossa is present caudally. The supratrochlear foramen allows communication between the two fossae in all but small humeri, where it is not present. The humeral condyle is divided into medial and lateral portions. Laterally, the capitellum of the humerus provides an articular surface for the radial head to contact and the trochlea articulates with the trochlear notch of the ulna, thus forming the elbow joint. The lateral epicondyle, or extensor epicondyle, of the humerus is an easily identified lateral prominence of the distal humerus. Just cranial and slightly distal to the epicondyle is a depression, the extensor fossa, which is an important landmark when placing a screw for intercondylar fractures. The medial epicondyle, or flexor epicondyle, is larger than the lateral epicondyle. The flexor and extensor designations that are placed on these epicondyles denote the action of the muscles that originate at the respective epicondyles. Although the shaft of the humerus is surrounded by a number of large muscles, the greater tubercle proximally and the epicondyles distally are easily palpable because they have relatively little muscle coverage. The brachial muscle, which lies within the musculospiral groove, is important because the radial nerve passes on its distal lateral

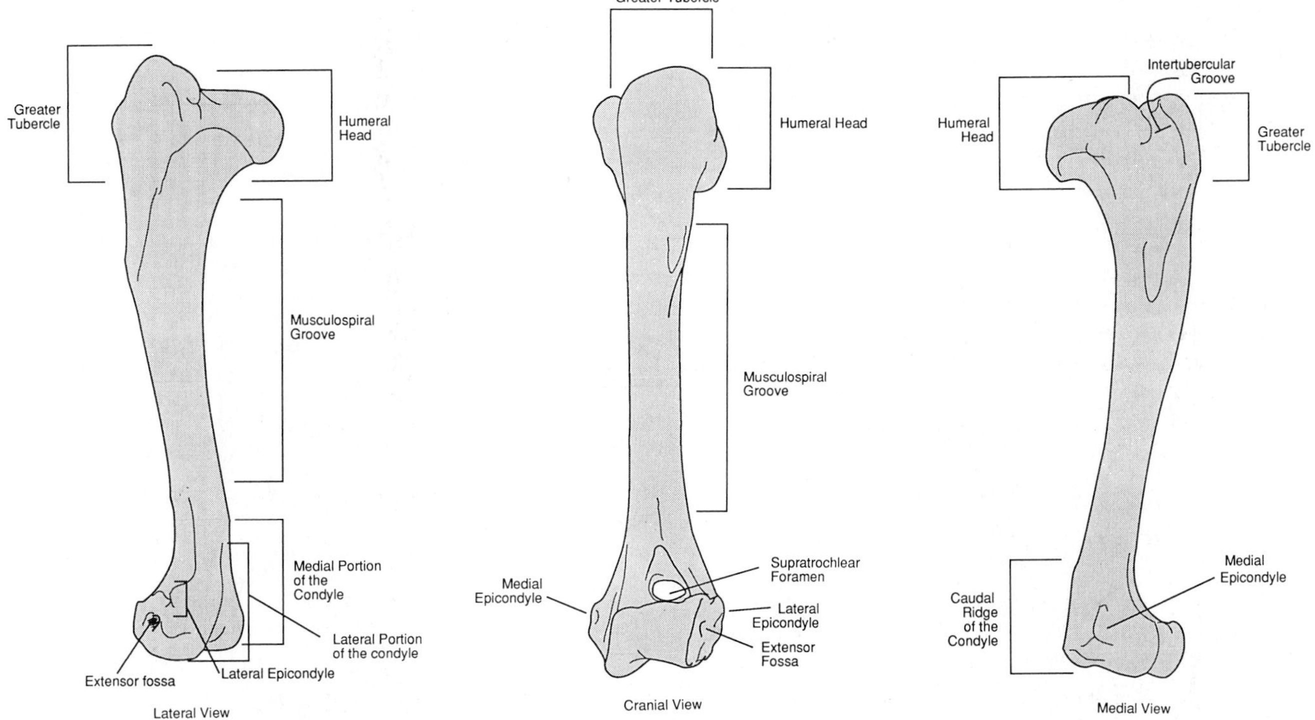

FIGURE 130–1. Structures or areas of surgical significance.

surface. Because many fractures occur in this portion of the shaft of the bone, the radial nerve is always in danger when a humeral fracture occurs. Although the incidence of radial nerve injuries is low, the radial nerve is always checked when a humeral fracture is present. Other nerves of the brachial plexus may also be injured when a humeral fracture occurs, and thus a complete forelimb neurological evaluation is indicated with this type of injury. On the medial side of the limb, the median, ulnar, and musculocutaneous nerves, along with the brachial artery, parallel the shaft of the humerus throughout its length. The location of the humerus in relation to the thoracic cavity makes it imperative that the chest be evaluated with auscultation and radiographs when humeral fractures occur. Depending on the method of fixation chosen and the location of the fracture, the previously mentioned structures are important when stabilizing humeral fractures (Figs. 130–1 and 130–2).

FIXATION TECHNIQUES

The circumstances under which a humeral fracture can be managed using an extended lateral splint (spica) or a Velpeau bandage occur very infrequently. They include minimally displaced nonarticular fractures in very young animals. External splintage of humeral fractures for more than 2 or 3 weeks may cause severe restriction of elbow motion and must be avoided. The difficulty in adequately splinting the humerus, the propensity for loss of elbow motion, and the unstable nature of most humeral fractures dictate the need for internal fixation in most of these fractures.

Internal fixation of humeral fractures is accomplished using plates, screws, orthopedic wire, intramedullary pins, external fixators, or a combination. Because these are the mainstays of fracture fixation, some general points regarding their application to the humerus must be considered.

Intramedullary Pinning

Intramedullary pin fixation of the humerus may be performed either open or closed. Closed fracture fixation is limited to those cases that are neither complex nor greatly displaced. An animal with this fracture often is young, so rapid healing and good remodeling can be expected. To perform a closed reduction, the intramedullary pin is introduced through a small skin incision at a point just distal to the proximal edge of the greater tubercle. This pin is driven distally toward the medial portion of the humeral condyle or just above the supratrochlear foramen. No matter what the fixation technique, general anesthesia, strict asepsis, and a thorough knowledge of implant application and anatomical landmarks are essential. The conditions under which closed pinning can be successful are infrequent.

Open reduction is the most frequent manner in which humeral fractures are handled. Specific approaches are discussed at appropriate points later in this chapter. Intramedullary pins may be introduced either retrograde or normograde with a hand chuck or power pin driver. Generally, only one pin that is about two-thirds the diameter of the medullary canal at its narrowest point is used. When a pin is driven normograde, a small incision is made just distal to the proximal edge of the

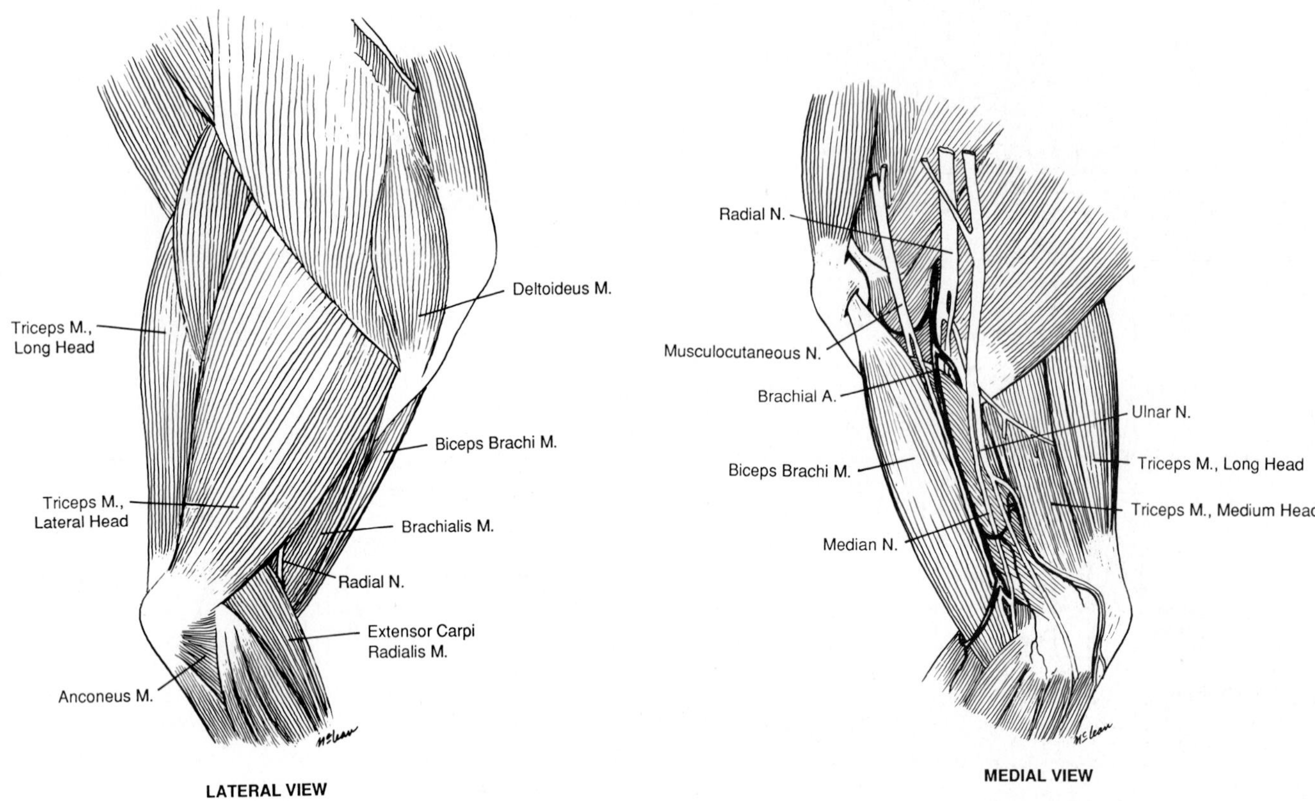

FIGURE 130–2. Important muscles and surgically significant nerves and arteries around the humerus.

greater tubercle. The pin is inserted at that site, aiming it slightly medially. The pin is driven distally until it seats in the medial portion of the humeral condyle or just above the supratrochlear foramen, depending on the location of the fracture (Fig. 130–3). When a pin is driven retrograde in the proximal fragment, it is aimed so that it will exit just distal to the proximal edge of the greater tubercle. The pin is driven proximally until an adequate amount is exposed to allow application of the hand chuck or driver. The pin is then withdrawn proximally until its distal tip is just visible at the fracture line. The fracture is reduced, and the pin is driven toward either the medial portion of the humeral condyle or the supratrochlear foramen. The pin should never penetrate through the bone above the supratrochlear foramen or it may become an irritant when the elbow is extended.

If the pin is driven retrograde in the distal segment, care is taken to ensure that it is aligned parallel with the caudal edge of the medial portion of the humeral condyle (Fig. 130–4). This edge is very straight and provides a reliable anatomical landmark for placement of a pin in this direction. The pin is driven out the most distal edge of the medial portion of the epicondyle and withdrawn until its proximal tip is at the level of the fracture line. The fracture is reduced, and the intramedullary pin driven proximally until it exits just distal to the proximal edge of the greater tubercle. The distal point of the intramedullary pin should be cut off so that the pin is square at this end. With the hand chuck or

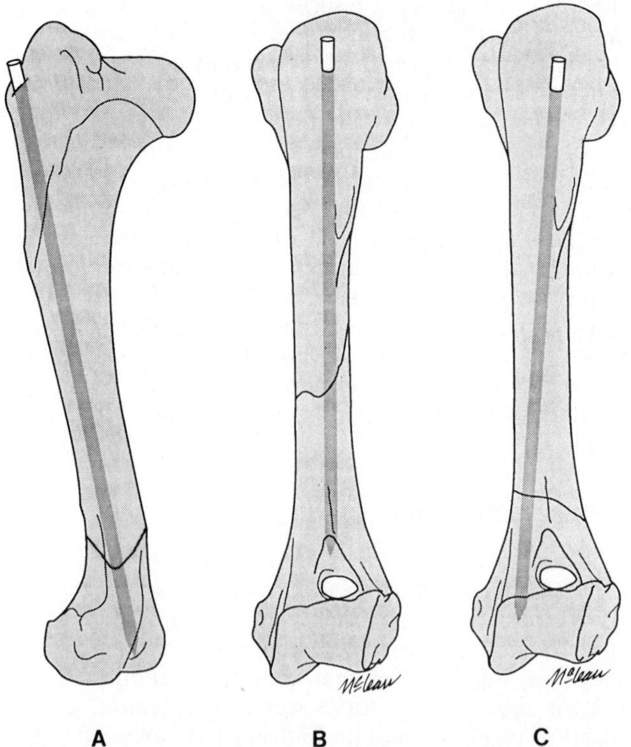

FIGURE 130–3. An intramedullary pin used in repair of a shaft fracture (*A*) enters the bone at a point just distal to the proximal edge of the greater tubercle and is seated (*B*) just proximal to the supratrochlear foramen or (*C*) in the medial portion of the humeral condyle depending on the fracture's location.

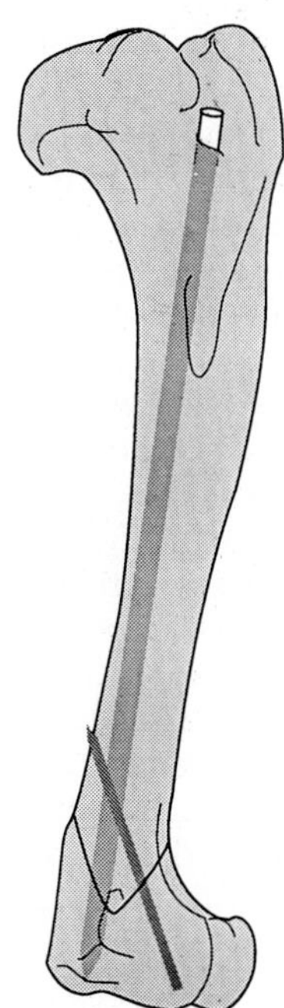

FIGURE 130–4. When supracondylar fractures are stabilized with intramedullary pins, the pin that traverses the length of the bone is parallel with the caudal edge of the medial portion of the humeral condyle.

driver on the portion of the pin extending from the proximal segment of bone, the pin is withdrawn until it is flush with the distal edge of the medial portion of the humeral condyle. In all cases, the intramedullary pin is cut off proximally, close to the point where it leaves the bone near the greater tubercle. Just enough pin is left out to allow removal later.

It is sometimes advantageous to place a second pin in the medullary canal. If two pins are to be used, the size of the first pin is reduced to not greater than half the diameter of the medullary canal. Stacked pins may be of the same or different sizes. When stacking two or more pins in the humerus, the pins may be placed either normograde or retrograde. It is often necessary to pull the proximal end of the pin not being driven into the distal bone segment out of the way of the hand chuck or driver. Once one of the pins is seated in the distal segment, the rest of the pins can be seated.

Intramedullary pin fixation often needs some form of auxiliary support such as cerclage wire or external fixators to stabilize the fracture. The decision to add auxiliary support to intramedullary pin fixation depends on fracture stability after the pins have been applied and the forces that will act on the fracture site during the postoperative period.

Plate Fixation

Bone plates, when applied to the humerus, as with any other bone, may have one of four functions: (1) neutralization, (2) buttress, (3) static compression, and (4) dynamic compression.[1, 5] The function of a plate is not determined by its shape but by how it is used to stabilize a fracture and to some extent by the fracture's configuration or position in the bone. A plate has neutralization function when the fracture has been anatomically reconstructed with lag screws either through or outside the plate, and the plate is used to protect that reconstruction (Fig. 130–5). A buttress plate either prevents fracture segments in a joint from shifting in position or it bridges a significant cortical defect in a shaft fracture (Fig. 130–6). For a plate to have static compressive function, compression must have been applied to the fracture line at surgery (Fig. 130–7). This can be achieved by using either a compression jig, which attaches to the end of the plate, by loading one or more screws in the plate through a specially designed plate hole, or by bending the plate in such a manner that when the screws are tightened, compression is achieved at the fracture line (prestressing the plate). Dynamic compression is achieved when a plate is applied on the tension side of the bone and the force created by muscle pull or weightbearing causes cyclic compression along the fracture line (Fig. 130–8).

Bone plates can be placed on any surface of the humerus; therefore, position of the plate depends on the location of the fracture and the surgeon's preference (Fig. 130–9). Cranial placement of the plate works well for very proximal fractures and can be used for fractures of the shaft that allow at least two and preferably three screws placed above and below the fracture line. Cranial application is limited distally on the shaft because the biceps muscle makes it difficult to achieve exposure that allows placement of the screws in the distal third of the humeral shaft. The lateral surface of the humerus is used for fractures from the proximal third distally. The difficulty in placing a plate laterally arises in contouring the plate properly. The plate must not only be bent to

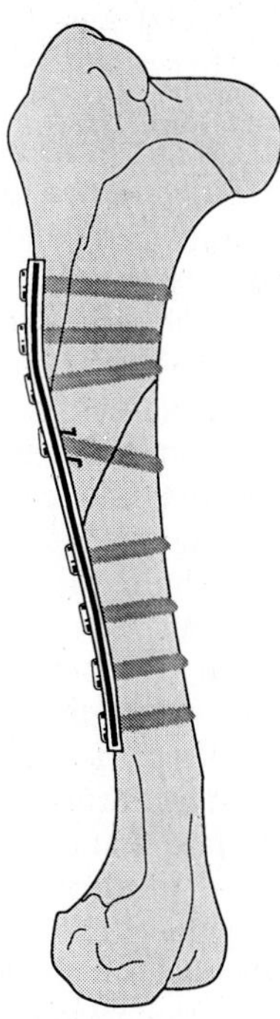

FIGURE 130–5. A plate has neutralization function when the fracture is anatomically reconstructed with lag screws and the plate protects those screws from the forces that act at the fracture site. In the illustration, the fourth most distal plate screw is a lag screw. Lag screws may be placed either through or outside the plate.

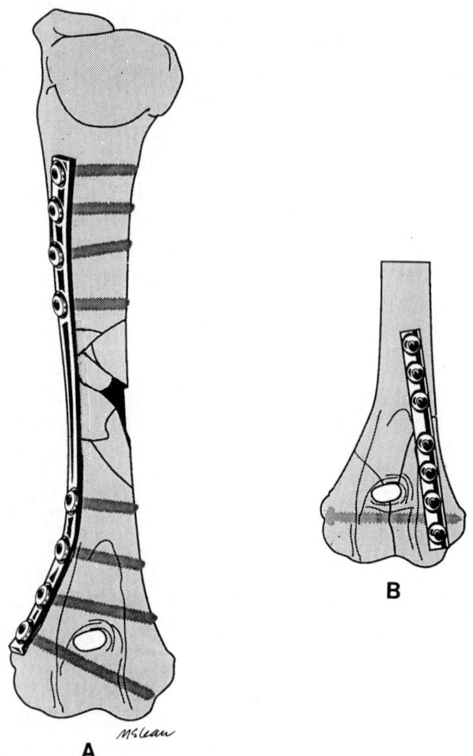

FIGURE 130–6. Plates have buttress function (*A*) if they bridge an area of bone deficit or (*B*) prevent a joint surface from collapsing.

accommodate for the flare of the lateral portion of the humeral condyle but must be twisted to match the sloping surface of the musculospiral groove. Also, when placing a plate laterally, the brachial muscle with the radial nerve must be freed and moved cranially and caudally as screws are placed. It is imperative that the radial nerve be protected with gentle tissue handling. Caudal placement of plates is generally reserved for distal intra-articular and supracondylar fractures. Although the plate can be placed caudally throughout the length of the humerus, exposure is limited proximally. Contouring the plate for placement on the caudal aspect of the bone is not difficult, because this area of the bone is relatively straight. The plate is placed along the caudal edge of the medial portion of the humeral condyle and extended proximally along the caudal humeral shaft. This position allows long screws to be placed in the medial portion of the humeral condyle, giving firm fixation for fractures in this area. However, when doing this, care must be taken to see that the plate does not interfere with the anconeal process as it progresses through a range of motion. The narrow width of the caudal edge of the medial portion of the humeral condyle limits the size of plate that can be used in this area. Bone plates also require little contouring when they are placed on the medial side of the humerus. Although a plate can be placed throughout the length of the medial side of the humerus, the location of vital neurovascular structures demands a thorough knowledge of the anatomy of this area to avoid compromising important structures. To place the plate proximally also requires incising the insertion of the pectoral muscles to gain adequate exposure. If the plate is placed on the medial surface as distally as possible, care is taken in positioning the screws so that they do not penetrate the articular surface of the humerus. It may be necessary to angle screws obliquely toward the cranial humerus to avoid having threads exposed in articular cartilage.

A number of points must be considered when placing screws within the plate. To maintain axial alignment of the plate, at least two screws are placed on either side of the fracture line. If the fracture is midshaft and adequate bone is available, at least three screws are used on either side of the fracture line to give greater assurance that the forces acting at the fracture line are negated. Cortical screws are adequate in most instances; in large dogs, near the proximal end of the bone, cancellous screws may be placed in the humeral head as long as they do not penetrate the articular surface. Generally, screws are placed perpendicular to the plate's surface. Depending on the fracture and location of the plate, it may be necessary to angle the screws. This can only be done if the screw hole design allows it.

External Fixators

External fixators are placed on the lateral side of the bone to keep them from interfering with limb function

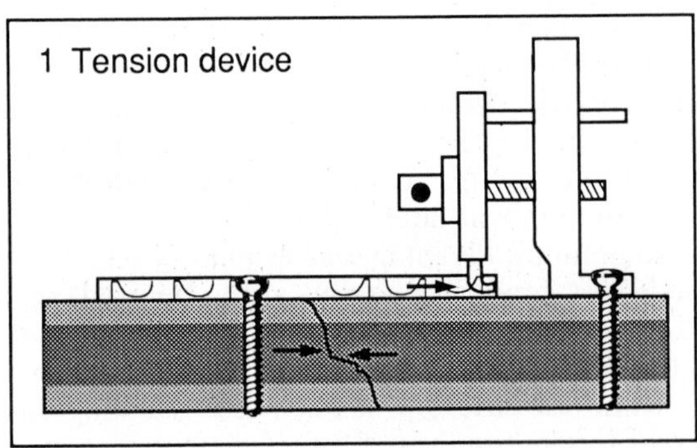

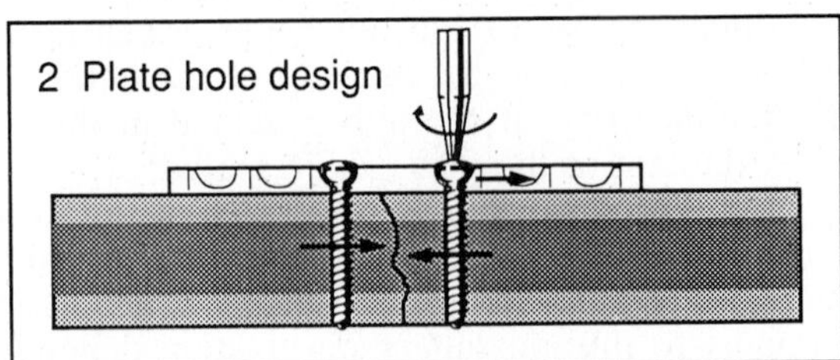

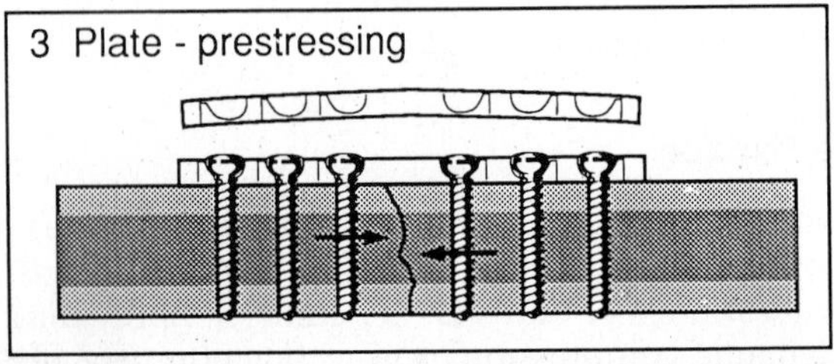

FIGURE 130–7. Three ways a plate can be used to maintain static compression at a fracture site: 1, with the use of a compression device or jig; 2, by using the specially designed plate holes; or 3, by prestressing the plate.

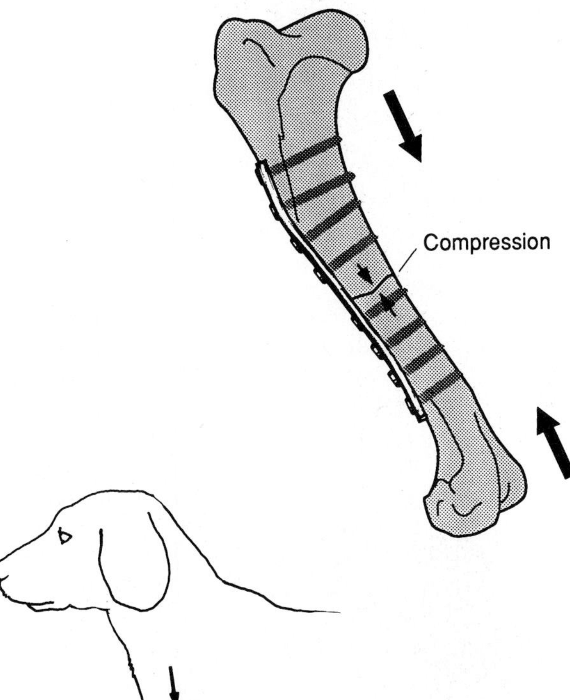

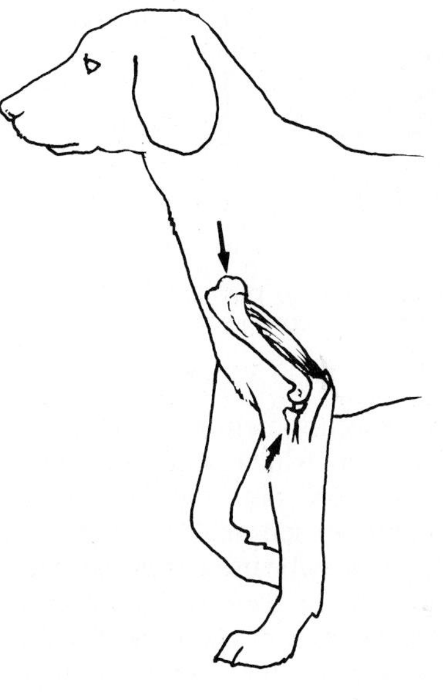

FIGURE 130–8. Dynamic compression is achieved when a plate is applied to the tension side of the bone and muscle pull or weightbearing causes cyclic compression along the fracture line.

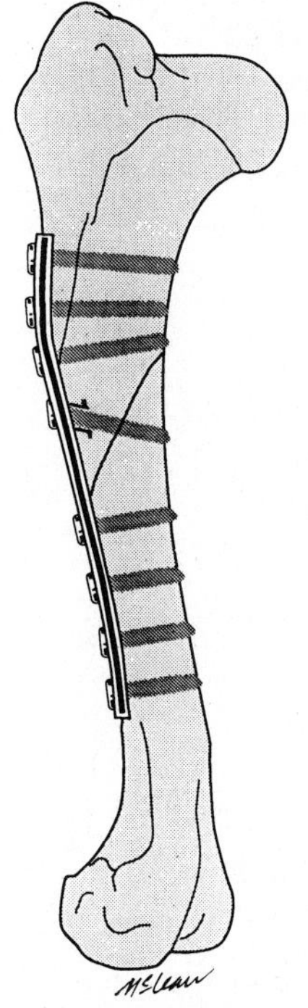

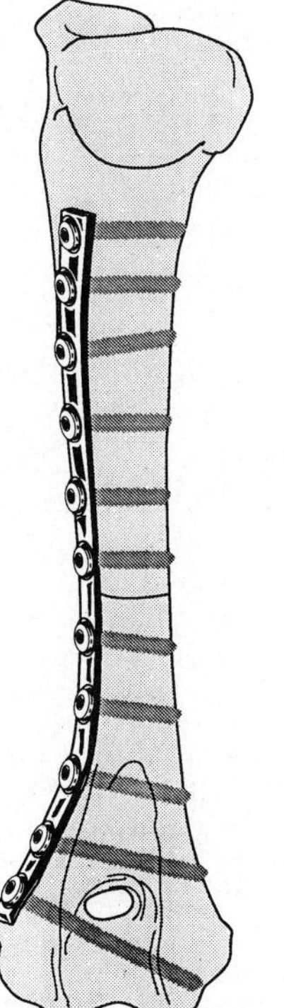

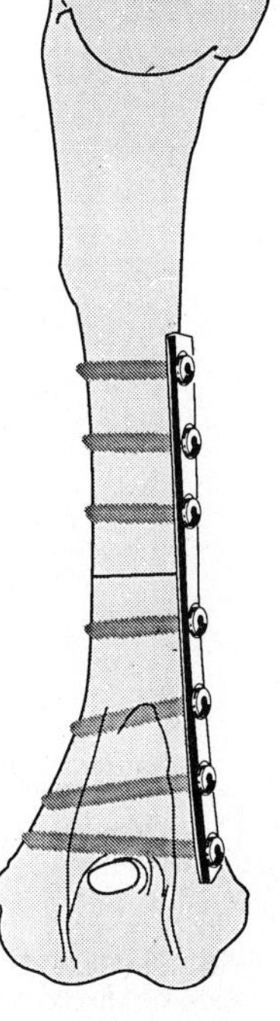

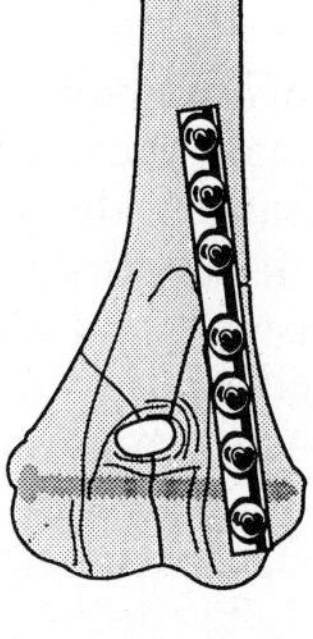

FIGURE 130–9. Bone plates are placed on all four surfaces of the humerus.

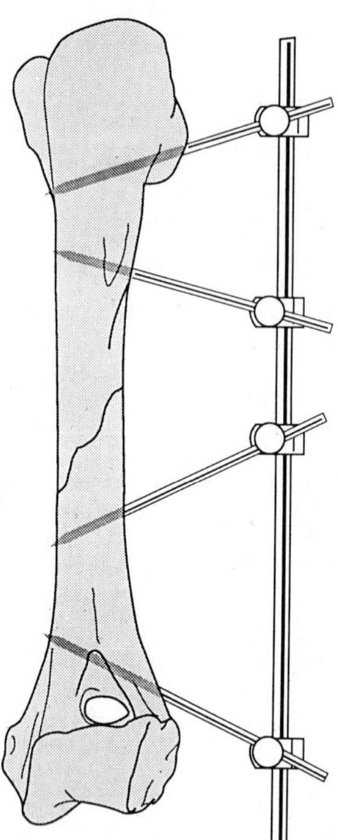

FIGURE 130–10. An external fixator is positioned from lateral to medial on the humerus in a type I configuration.

and because anatomy prevents them from being placed medially. The type I fixator, which penetrates one skin level and two cortices of bone with the fixation pin, is the primary type of fixation used on the humerus (Fig. 130–10). External fixators may be used as primary means of fracture fixation but more frequently are used as auxiliary fixation in combination with intramedullary pins. When using the external fixator as primary fixation, at least two and preferably three fixation pins are placed in each main segment of bone. The pin is angled between 30° and 45° to the long axis of the bone. This angle can be difficult to achieve with the distal pins because of conformation of the bone. If the fracture allows it, the pin is angled above the supratrochlear foramen. If the fracture is too distal to allow placement of the pin above the supratrochlear foramen, it may be necessary to place the most distal pin parallel with the joint surface in the capitum and the trochlea (Fig. 130–11). In large dogs with highly comminuted fractures, Turner hip pins have been used in place of the standard ⅛-inch fixation pin.[3] The large threads of the Turner hip pin make the implant more stable. For the strongest configuration, all of the fixation pins are connected to one bar. If necessary, the configuration can be further strengthened by adding a second connecting bar. When combined with an intramedullary pin, the external fixator negates rotation by providing a fixed connection between the proximal and distal fragments (Fig. 130–12). It is also useful in helping prevent collapse of the fragments.

Auxiliary Fixation

Orthopedic wire, small intramedullary pins, and bone screws are most frequently used as auxiliary support in combination with the previously described methods of fixation. These implants reduce and stabilize fragments anatomically but are generally not strong enough by themselves to be relied on for primary fixation of fractures. The exception to this is a fracture of the lateral humeral condyle, discussed later.

When orthopedic wire is used as a full-cerclage wire, it should be large enough to be applied tightly (Fig. 130–13). Full-cerclage wires are placed perpendicular to the long axis of the bone. At least two wires are used to stabilize a complete fracture line. To use full-cerclage wires, the fracture line is at least two and a half times the diameter of the bone. The fracture is generally reduced with bone clamps, and the wire is placed. Care is taken in placing the wire to ensure that soft-tissue attachments to bone are minimally disrupted. While the wire is being tightened, even tension is provided if the wire is being twisted. The loop of wire that passes around the bone is not allowed to rotate out of its perpendicular orientation to the long axis. Tension is maintained on the wire until it contacts the bone's surface. Once the bone surface is engaged, tension can be released and the surgeon's hand rolls in the same direction as the twist, thus laying the twisted ends of the wire flush with the bone. The twists can be cut off, leaving three or four twists at the end. Maintaining the full-cerclage wires perpendicular to the long axis of the bone keeps them at the smallest diameter possible and helps prevent loosening. These wires are at least 1 cm away from the fracture line and at least 1 cm apart. A hemicerclage wire is a wire that is passed through two holes that are drilled on either side of the fracture line.

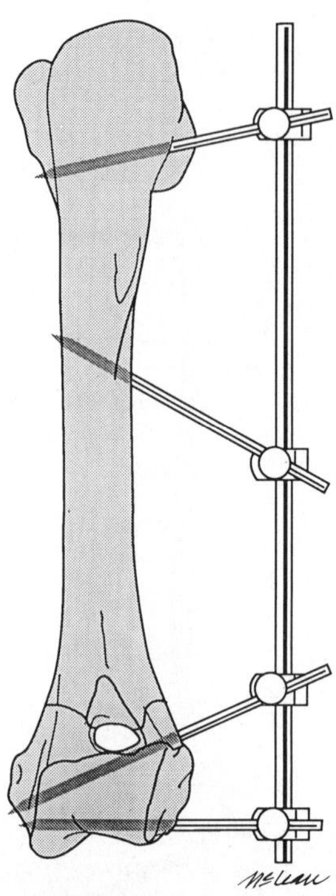

FIGURE 130–11. For stabilization of very distal fractures with an external fixator, it is necessary to place the most distal fixation pin parallel to the joint surface.

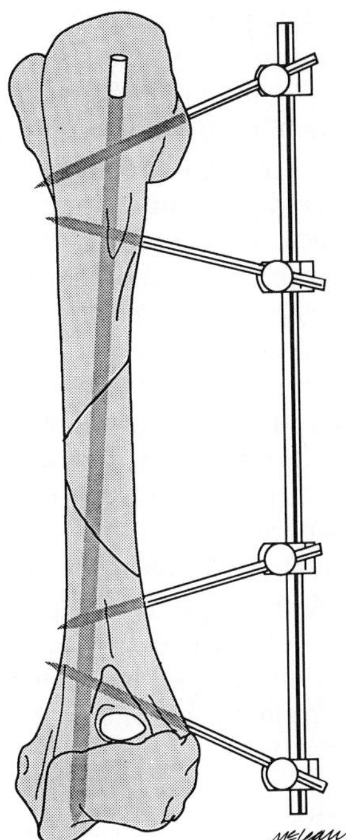

FIGURE 130–12. Combining the external fixator with an intramedullary pin is necessary in some cases to overcome rotation forces and prevent collapse of the fracture.

The ends are twisted together, forming a simple interrupted suture in the bone. Hemicerclage wires are best applied perpendicular to the fracture line to minimize shear forces and provide maximum stability.

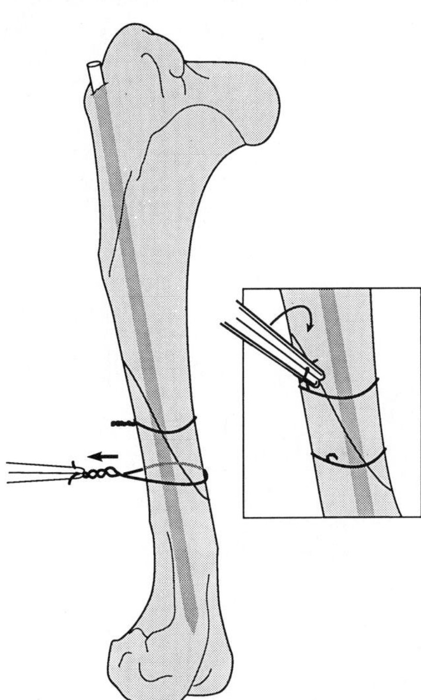

FIGURE 130–13. When applying a cerclage wire, even tension is maintained on the wire while it is twisted to the bone surface. The wire is also positioned perpendicular to the bone's long axis. Care is taken to ensure that the wire does not rotate out of its perpendicular orientation while being twisted. After the wire has tightly engaged the bone, tension on the wire is released and the surgeon's wrist follows the same direction as the twist, laying the twisted wire against the bone.

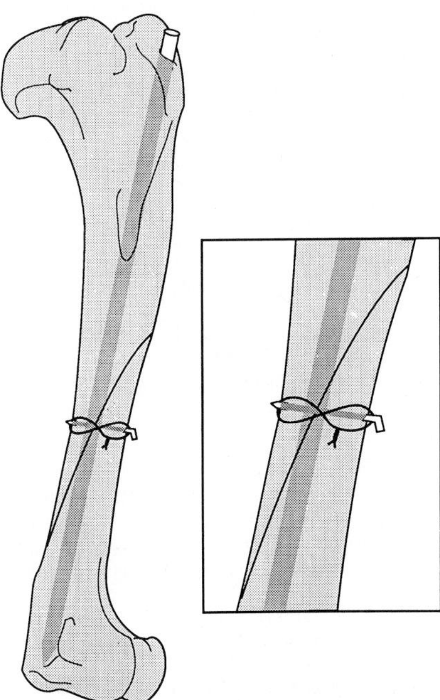

FIGURE 130–14. The figure-eight skewer pin is applied by driving a Kirschner wire through both bone segments so that the tip of the pin just penetrates the far segment. A wire is anchored in a figure-eight pattern around the pin. The pin is bent over and cut off.

In the figure-eight skewer pin technique, a Kirschner wire is driven through both segments of bone and a wire is placed in a figure-eight pattern on the outside of the bone, using the exposed tips of the Kirschner wire as anchor points (Fig. 130–14). The pin is driven through the bone until just enough of the pin is exposed through the farthest fragment to allow wire to be looped around it. Once the figure-eight wire is tightened, the long end of the pin that is in the chuck is bent over and cut off. The bend in the pin helps prevent migration. This type of fixation can be placed either perpendicular to the long axis of the bone or perpendicular to the fracture line. In a long oblique fracture, one or two skewer pins are very effective at eliminating shear motion and rotational instability. The figure-eight wire captures the bone segments, and the Kirschner wire provides more rigid fixation than malleable orthopedic wire.

Bone screws are generally used as auxiliary fixation when bone plates are applied. Because a bone screw fills so much of the medullary cavity, it is difficult to incorporate intramedullary pinning and bone screws together in shaft stabilization. Bone screws may function as lag and position screws when used as auxiliary fixation (Fig. 130–15). For details of lag screws, see Chapter 122.

A position screw does not allow a segment to collapse inward. Because of the straight orientation of some fracture lines, placement of a lag screw would cause the fracture segment to collapse. If there is a question about whether a screw with lag function would cause the fragment to collapse, the security of the screw can be tested before placement by first putting pointed reduction forceps in the same position as the proposed lag screw. If the fragment collapses when the forceps are tightened, a position screw is used. If compression is

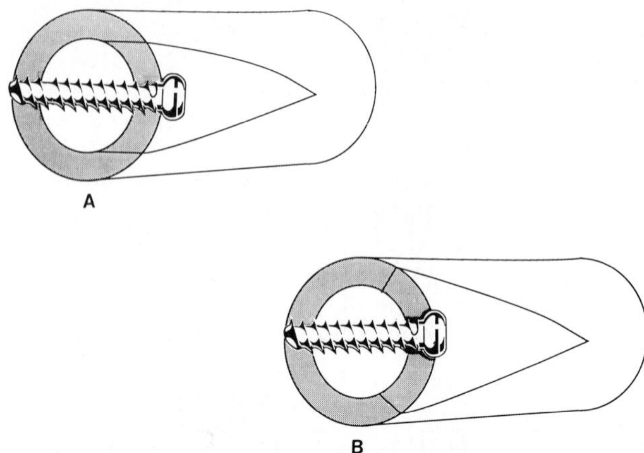

FIGURE 130–15. (*A*) Bone screws with threads purchasing bone in both fragments maintain fragment relationships and have position function. (*B*) Bone screws that only purchase bone in the far cortex provide interfragmentary compression and have lag function.

achieved with the pointed reduction forceps, a lag screw is used. The position screw purchases bone on both sides of the fracture line and is used to maintain position of a fragment.

PROXIMAL HUMERAL FRACTURES

Fractures of the greater tubercle are relatively uncommon. They are simply approached by reflecting the brachiocephalic muscle and sometimes the superficial and deep pectoral muscles from their insertion. A fracture of the greater tubercle is sometimes created by performing an osteotomy as part of an approach to the scapulohumeral joint.

The age of the animal is a determining factor in choosing a method of fixation. In adult animals, intramedullary pins, lag screws, or tension bands may be used to stabilize fracture segments (Fig. 130–16). In growing animals, only intramedullary pins can be used because tension bands and lag screws cause premature closure of the physis of the greater tubercle. When using intramedullary pins, two or three are inserted at divergent angles, starting from the proximal portion of the greater tubercle, and driven distally into the medullary cavity. Tension band wire is created by first fixing the greater tubercle to the main body with two intramedullary pins. A hole is drilled in the cranial surface of the distal segment perpendicular to the long axis of the bone. This hole is just large enough to allow the tension band wire to pass through it. The wire is passed around the two pins at the point where they enter the greater tubercle, and the two free ends are twisted tightly together. The intramedullary pins are bent toward the muscle and cut off. Lag screws that are placed in the greater tubercle are positioned perpendicular to the fracture line. At least two lag screws are used to prevent rotation of the fragment. Mechanically, the most appropriate method of fixation of the greater tubercle is with the tension band technique.

Because of the size of the humeral head, fractures are rare. Intramedullary pins, lag screws, or a combination can be used to stabilize the humeral head. After reduction, divergent intramedullary pins are inserted from cranial to caudal, stabilizing the two segments. It is important that the pins do not penetrate the humeral head. Lag screws are used in adult animals. The lag screws are positioned perpendicular to the fracture line. If only one lag screw is inserted, an antirotational pin is used with the lag screw. Either cortical or cancellous screws can be used as lag screws. Lag screws should never penetrate the articular surface.

Fractures just below the greater tubercle and humeral head can be repaired using intramedullary pins or bone plates. Intramedullary pinning is reserved for relatively simple fractures. After reduction of the fracture segments, one or two pins are introduced at the greater tubercle and driven distally into the intramedullary canal. Bone plates are applied along the cranial surface of the humerus. At least two screws are positioned above the fracture line, making it necessary to use a T plate for fracture repair (Fig. 130–17). If possible, a lag

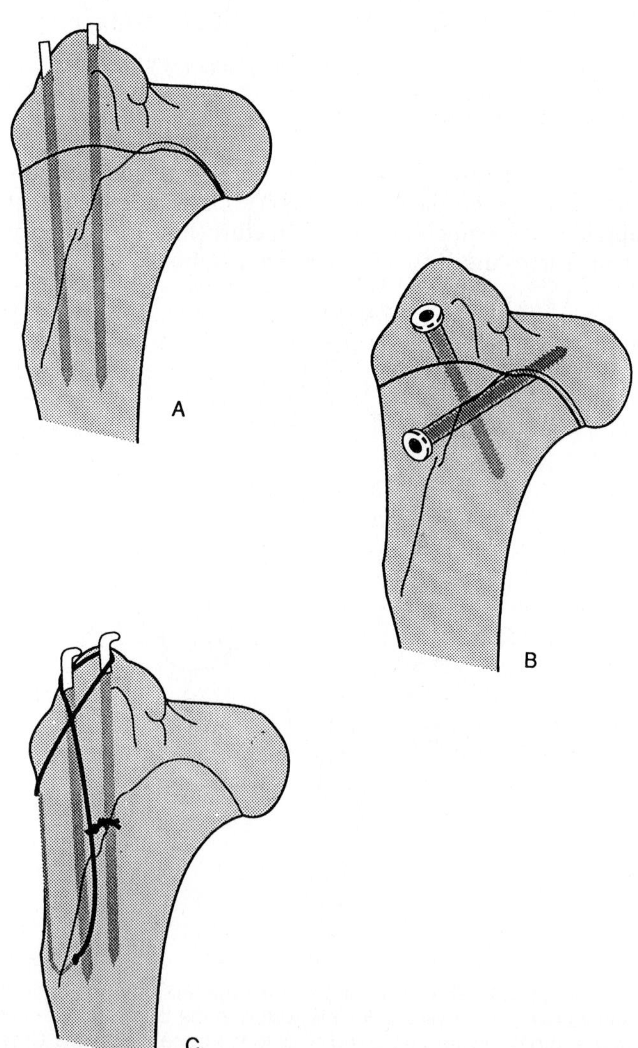

FIGURE 130–16. Proximal humerus fractures in adult animals are stabilized with (*A*) intramedullary pins, (*B*) lag screws, or (*C*) a tension band. In immature animals with open growth plates, only intramedullary pins are used.

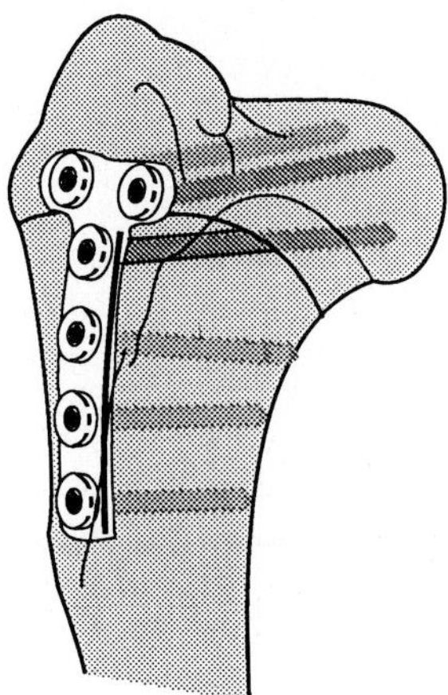

FIGURE 130–17. Proximal humerus fractures are sometimes repaired with a T plate. In some instances, a lag screw is placed in the head of the humerus.

screw is placed through a plate hole distal to the fracture line or outside the plate from the distal fragment into the humeral head to stabilize the fracture.

SHAFT FRACTURES

Fractures of the shaft of the humerus are common owing to the tapering configuration of the bone, making this part relatively weaker than the proximal end. The shaft of the humerus is approached laterally by reflecting the triceps caudally and the brachiocephalicus and the superficial pectoral muscles cranially and medially. The brachial muscle and its accompanying radial nerve are isolated and identified because it is usually necessary to work on either side of these structures. From medially, the triceps is reflected caudally and the biceps cranially. The median and ulnar nerves are identified and protected during the medial approach.

Intramedullary pins, external fixators, and bone plates are the primary methods of fixation for humeral shaft fractures. Lag screws and orthopedic wires are auxiliary methods of fixation.

Intramedullary pins may be inserted either normograde or retrograde. The distal position of the pin is determined by the position of the fracture in the shaft. The closer the distal end of the fracture line is to the supracondylar portion of the humerus, the greater the indication for placing the pin in the medial portion of the humeral condyle. Placing the pin in this portion of the humerus can be difficult because the medullary canal is relatively small; the pin extends down the canal parallel to the caudal medial edge of the humeral condyle. The small size of the medullary cavity in the medial humeral condyle limits the size of intramedullary pins that can be used. This limitation does not compromise fracture repair. With fractures that do not end close to the supracondylar area, it is possible to have the distal placement of the pin end at a point just above the supratrochlear foramen. Less accurate proximal alignment of the pin is required, and a larger pin can be used than when the pin must traverse the full length of the humerus. It is possible to stack two or more pins in the humerus, especially if the pins are seated above the supratrochlear fossa. This arrangement allows some rotational stability, but auxiliary methods of fixation are usually necessary.

It is generally not possible to use intramedullary pins alone to repair humeral shaft fractures. Two-piece fractures that interdigitate and need no additional support are the exception. Because of the spiral configuration of the humeral shaft, two-piece fractures are often spiral or oblique. Shear and rotational forces thus must be neutralized. Along with an intramedullary pin, two full-cerclage wires applied to spiral or oblique fractures that are two and a half times bone diameter may be adequate. However, the marked variation in size of the humeral shaft may make it difficult for even properly placed cerclage wires to maintain their position without sliding down the bone. Although notching the cortex with a bone file is sometimes used to minimize wire slippage, the notch acts as a stress riser and may weaken the bone. Wire security is always tested before closure, and wires that have loosened are replaced. A figure-eight skewer wire is a good alternative to full-cerclage wires for spiral or oblique fractures. It cannot slide and keeps fragments locked together.

Lag screws are difficult to combine with an intramedullary pin because both implants often must occupy the same space to be properly applied. If there is no interference between implants, this method is acceptable.

With more complex fractures, the fragments are reduced and stabilized, when possible, with a combination of cerclage wires and intramedullary pins. An external fixator can be used in addition; a single pin above and below the fracture line is all that is needed to provide necessary stability. Depending on the type of fracture and the age of the animal, the external fixator is kept in place for 2 to 6 weeks. Intramedullary pins stay in place until radiographic evidence shows that the fracture is completely healed.

When a fracture is so severely comminuted that it cannot be reconstructed (e.g., a bullet wound), one treatment option is to stabilize the bone with *only* an external fixator. This allows limited exposure or occasionally no exposure to the fracture while maintaining general length and alignment of the bone. These fractures must undergo indirect bone healing. The external fixator frame must be secure enough to maintain its position throughout the healing process. It is impossible to apply a type II frame to the humerus, and a type I frame that has two to three pins each in the proximal and distal segments must be used. In large dogs, it is advisable to apply double external bars to the fixator to increase rigidity. Strong threaded pins can be used to ensure secure bone purchase throughout the healing period (see Chapter 123). As healing progresses, based on clinical and radiographic evaluation, the fixator can be destabilized by removing the second external bar. Destabilization can be achieved by removing one pin from either the proximal or distal bone segment or one from both. At least two pins remain in each segment until the fracture is healed.

Bone plates are an effective method of shaft fracture stabilization. By providing rigid internal fixation, they allow early ambulation. Most surgeons prefer to apply plates either cranially or laterally, but medial plate application is gaining acceptance. Caudal application is not favored, except for distal fractures, because of the difficulty in adequate exposure and the fact that this is a compression surface in the humerus. Plate application requires anatomical contouring of the plate. The cranial and medial sides are the easiest to contour to, and the lateral, because of its curves and slopes, is the hardest. Whenever possible, the fracture segments are reconstructed with lag screws and stabilized with a plate and screws. In some cases, it is not possible to use lag screws because of severe comminution or fragment configuration. Then the plate may be applied to just the proximal and distal segments to maintain bone length and joint alignment. Small pins or orthopedic wire may be used to align the fragments if care is taken to preserve blood supply to the bone.

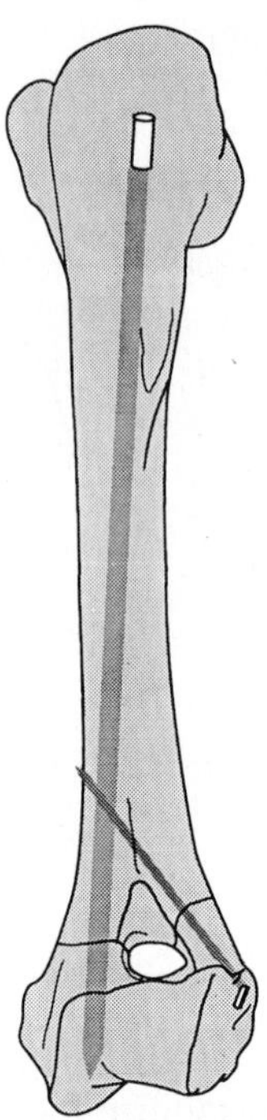

FIGURE 130–18. Two-piece supracondylar fractures can be stabilized with two intramedullary pins. One pin traverses the length of the bone from just below the greater tubercle to the medial portion of the condyle. The other pin is placed lateral to medial starting distal and caudal to the lateral epicondyle.

SUPRACONDYLAR FRACTURES

A patient's age often dictates the method of treatment used on supracondylar fractures of the humerus. Bone plates, intramedullary pins, or external fixators can be used on adult animals, whereas animals with growth potential should be treated only with intramedullary pins. Bone plates or external fixators that span the physis cause premature closure, whereas a smooth intramedullary pin that is positioned parallel with physeal cell columns does not inhibit growth.

Two intramedullary pins can be used to stabilize two-piece fractures (Fig. 130–18). The first intramedullary pin is driven from the fracture surface in the medial portion of the humeral condyle out the most distal end of the condyle. This pin is aligned parallel to the caudal edge of the condyle. The pin is withdrawn distally until it is below the fracture's surface. The fracture is reduced, and the pin is driven into the proximal segment until it exits at or near the greater tubercle. Enough of the pin is exposed to allow a chuck to be placed on the pin at the proximal end. The alignment of the distal segment is checked, because the lateral portion of the condyle can often be rotated out of alignment. If this has happened, the malalignment is corrected before setting the second pin. Starting at a point just caudal to the lateral epicondyle, a small pin is driven from lateral to medial across the fracture line. This pin usually penetrates the medial cortex in the metaphysis. If the pin is small enough and its angle of insertion steep enough, the pin may divert when it contacts medial endosteal bone and follow the medullary canal. In such cases, it is not necessary to make the pin exit the bone proximally. Once the second pin is seated, the distal end of the first pin is cut off, and the pin is withdrawn from the proximal end until the squared-off distal end of the pin is flush with the most distal end of the bone. The proximal end of the first pin is cut short enough to allow the skin to slip over the pin but left long enough to allow pin removal after the fracture is healed.

Two-piece fractures or comminuted fractures in adult dogs can be plated (Fig. 130–19). Whenever possible, lag screws are used to reconstruct comminuted fractures before the plate is applied. Cerclage wires may be needed to rebuild some fractures. Care is taken to locate and protect the radial nerve as wire is passed around the bone. The plate is placed on the medial portion of the humeral condyle, either along its caudal edge or on its medial aspect just behind the epicondyle. When placing the plate caudally, the screws are driven from caudal to cranial. Because this plate is on the edge of the bone and close to the olecranon, size selection is critical. A relatively small plate provides adequate stability in most cases. Long screws can be used in the distal segment because the full cranial-to-caudal length of the condyle can be used. A plate placed on the medial face of the condyle may be larger than one placed on the caudal edge, but distal screw placement is more difficult because the risk of compromising joint movement is greater with a misplaced intra-articular screw. It may be necessary to angle the distal screws forward to keep them in the condyle.

External fixators are rarely used to stabilize this fracture because of their relative inability to resist rotational forces. External fixators are usually used with intramedullary pins. These fractures often are comminuted so that stability, joint alignment, or bone lengths are at risk of compromise. One or two pins above and below the fracture lines in a type I frame along with an intramedullary pin that traverses the length of the bone are often all that is needed to provide adequate stabilization. When possible, properly applied cerclage wires are used to reduce bone fragments. It is often possible to remove the external fixator in 4 to 6 weeks when it is used with a pin.

FRACTURES OF THE CONDYLE

Fractures of the lateral portion of the humeral condyle are frequent in immature animals and occasional in adults. Adult cocker spaniels have a higher than expected incidence of these fractures.[6] In immature dogs, this fracture is the most commonly encountered Salter IV fracture. Because the fracture is intra-articular, it is critical that anatomical reduction of the fracture be achieved.

The cranial lateral approach provides adequate exposure. The lateral head of the triceps is reflected caudally, and the lateral epicondyle identified. The extensor carpi radialis and the extensor digitorum communis muscles are incised at their origin along the ridge of the lateral epicondyle. The joint capsule is incised across its dorsal condylar insertion and along the epicondyle. Retraction of the joint capsule exposes the cranial aspect of the articular portion of the condyle.

An interfragmentary lag screw and an antirotation implant are used to stabilize fractures of the lateral portion of the humeral condyle (Fig. 130–20). The lag screw provides interfragmentary compression and maintains alignment at the joint surface. Either cortical or cancellous bone screws are used for the lag screw. The glide hole for the lag screw is started in the center of the extensor fossa that is just cranial and ventral to the lateral epicondyle and drilled parallel to the surface of the condyle. It exits in the center of the condyle. The orientation of the glide hole is critical because it dictates the alignment and thus the exit point of the thread hole. This hole can be drilled from the outside inward before the fracture is reduced, but the fragment must be firmly secured during the drilling process to ensure correct alignment. Drilling this hole from the inside out requires extra manipulation of the fragment and added tissue disruption to adequately expose the surface of the condyle. The glide hole can also be drilled after the fragments are reduced, but care must be taken to ensure that the glide hole crosses the fracture line but does not penetrate too far into the far fragment where the thread hole is to be drilled. Once the glide hole is established, the fracture segments are reduced and the thread hole drilled. An ideally placed thread hole exits the bone at or near the medial epicondyle. Approximately one and one-half threads of the screw protrude from the bone at the epicondyle. The proper length lag screw is inserted and tightened. As the tightening is done, the head of the screw should not sink into the bone. If the bone is so soft that the head does sink into the bone, a washer is used with the screw. As the final tightening of the screw is done, the proximal portion of the fragment is checked for anatomical reduction.

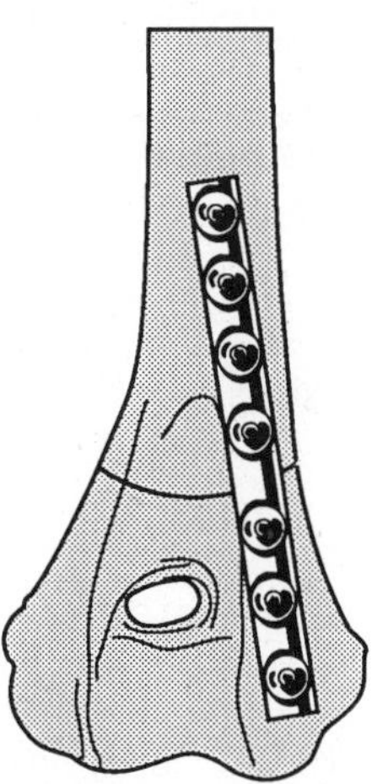

FIGURE 130–19. A bone plate placed on the caudal aspect of the medial portion of the humeral condyle stabilizes some supracondylar fractures.

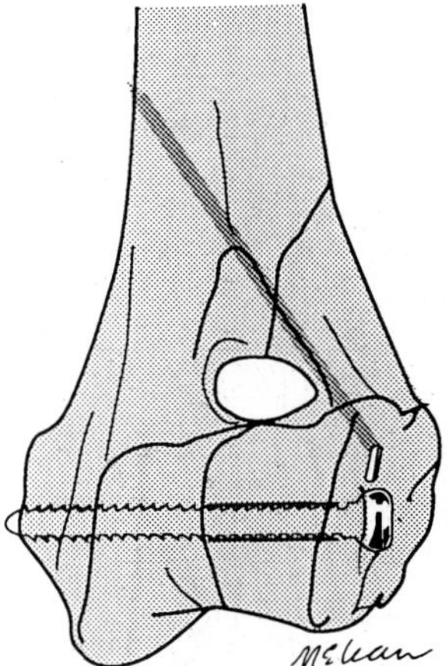

FIGURE 130–20. A fracture of the lateral portion of the humeral condyle is best repaired with a transcondylar lag screw and an intramedullary pin for rotational stability.

Stabilization of the proximal portion of the fracture segment eliminates rotation of the segment and provides added stability to the fracture repair. The antirotation implant may be either an additional lag screw if the proximal portion of the fragment is long enough or a small intramedullary pin. Lag screws are placed perpendicular to the fracture line. The small intramedullary pin is inserted caudal to and slightly proximal to the lateral epicondyle. It is directed parallel with the shaft of bone connecting the lateral condyle and the main shaft of bone. The pin just exits the bone in the medial metaphysis and is bent over and cut off, leaving a short ending hook.

Fractures involving only the medial condyle are uncommon. As with fractures of the lateral portion, they are repaired with lag screws and an antirotation implant. A medial approach is used, and the glide hole is drilled from the medial epicondyle to the center of the condyle. When the screw is implanted, the tip exits in the depression cranial and ventral to the lateral epicondyle. Antirotation implants are inserted medial to lateral.

When both the medial and lateral portions of the condyle are involved, the fracture is referred to as a *T* or *Y* fracture, based on its configuration. These fractures usually occur in adult animals. They commonly are approached through a transolecranon osteotomy. The osteotomy is from just proximal to the anconeal process,

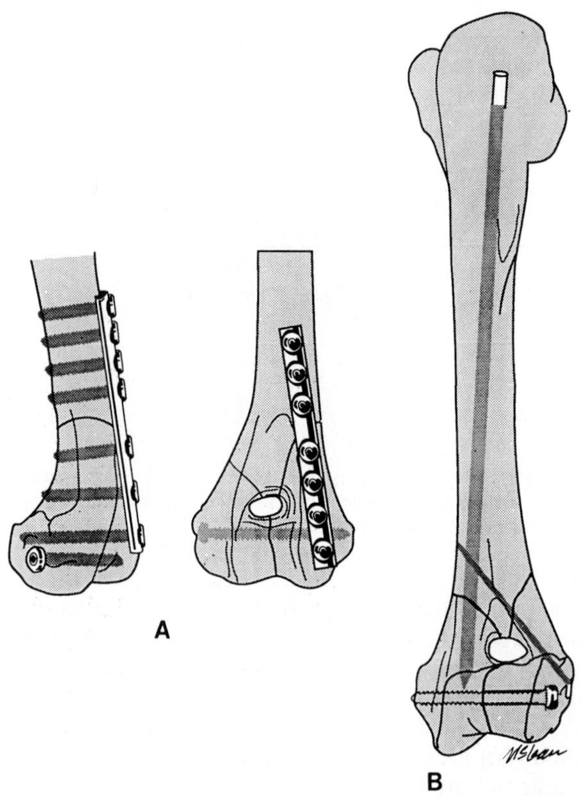

FIGURE 130–21. Intracondylar T or Y fractures are repaired with an intracondylar lag screw and either (*A*) a plate or (*B*) intramedullary pins.

angling distally on the caudal ulna to a point halfway between the level of the radial head and the tip of the anconeal process. All of the insertion of the triceps is included on the proximal fragment. A tension band is used to reduce the osteotomy. In young animals, a tenotomy is performed at the triceps insertion to avoid trauma to the proximal ulnar physis. Medial and lateral approaches may be combined through one slightly extended skin incision for reduction and stabilization. Although combining approaches may give a more limited exposure to the joint surface, it is my experience that animals return to function faster and more fully than with the trochanteric osteotomy. With either approach, the ulnar nerve on the medial side of the limb is identified and protected. On the lateral side, the radial nerve needs protection if the fracture extends proximally.

The first step in reducing these fractures is to use a lag screw to make the condylar segments one anatomically reconstructed piece. The fracture can then be treated like a supracondylar fracture using either intramedullary pins with or without external fixators or bone plates (Fig. 130–21). In rare instances, in large dogs or giant breeds with severely comminuted fractures, it may be necessary to apply a plate to both the caudal portion of the medial part of the condyle and the lateral surface of the lateral portion of the lateral condyle. The majority of intercondylar fractures can be adequately repaired with a single plate and axillary fixation. Plating provides the most rigid fixation, allowing early passive physical therapy and controlled weightbearing. This is important when dealing with elbow fractures because of that joint's tendency to stiffen when traumatized.

CONCLUSION

Fractures of the humerus generally require open reduction and internal fixation if the animal is to return to normal function with a healed bone. Knowledge of the anatomy of the humerus and its adjacent structures is essential for a successful approach to a given fracture. Once exposed, the fracture must be appropriately reduced and stabilized to allow the bone to heal. During the healing process, the animal's activity must be controlled so that excessive stress is not applied to the bone. Most fractures heal without complication, and patients return to acceptable function.

References

1. Brinker WO, et al (eds): *Manual of Internal Fixation in Small Animals*. Springer-Verlag, New York, 1983.
2. Evans HE, Christensen GC (eds): *Miller's Anatomy of the Dog*. 2nd ed. Philadelphia, W.B. Saunders, 1979.
3. Hulse DA: Personal communication, 1989.
4. Jackson DA: Management of humeral fractures. *In* Bojrab MJ (ed): *Current Techniques in Small Animal Surgery*. 3rd ed. Philadelphia, Lea & Febiger, 1990, pp 756–770.
5. Olmstead ML, Newton CD: Principles of fracture treatment. *In* Harvey CE, et al (eds): *Small Animal Surgery*. J.B. Lippincott, Philadelphia, 1990, pp 561–587.
6. Vannini R, et al: Humeral condylar fractures caused by minor trauma in 20 adult dogs. *J Am Anim Hosp Assoc 24*:355, 1988.

CHAPTER 131

Elbow Luxation

J. Komtebedde and Philip B. Vasseur

Elbow luxation can be congenital or can be acquired as a result of trauma. Because the elbow is inherently a very stable joint, acquired luxations are relatively uncommon. Congenital luxations are unusual in dogs and are unreported in cats. Because of the rarity of these disorders in cats, this chapter refers exclusively to dogs. Elbow luxation as a result of premature radial or ulnar physeal closure is discussed elsewhere in this text (see Chapter 132).

SURGICAL ANATOMY

The elbow is a ginglymoid or hinge joint that is a composite of three articulations: humeroradial, humeroulnar, and proximal radioulnar.[5] The humeral condyle can be divided into several parts. The capitulum articulates with the head of the radius, and the trochlea articulates with the trochlear notch of the ulna. The lateral and medial epicondyles are the origins of the extensor and flexor muscles of the antebrachium, respectively, and also serve as the proximal attachment sites of the lateral and medial collateral ligaments. The olecranon fossa articulates with the anconeal process of the ulna during extension beyond 90° (Fig. 131–1).

The humeroradial joint transmits most of the weight supported by the elbow articulation. The humeroulnar joint restricts the movement of the elbow primarily to a sagittal plane. The proximal radioulnar joint allows for a limited degree of rotation. Medial and lateral translation and varus/valgus movements are limited by the collateral ligaments and the protrusion of the anconeal process into the olecranon fossa.

The joint capsule is common to all three articulations. The collateral ligaments each have two components (cranial and caudal crura), which attach to the proximal radius and ulna, respectively. The annular and the oblique ligament are the other ligaments of the elbow joint (Fig. 131–2).

The ulnar and median nerves traverse the medial aspect of the elbow joint under the antebrachial fascia. After crossing the medial epicondyle, the ulnar nerve passes between the ulnar head of the flexor carpi radialis and flexor digitorum superficialis muscles. At the flexor surface of the elbow, cranial to the epicondyle, the median nerve dips laterally under the pronator teres muscle together with the median artery. The radial nerve bifurcates into deep and superficial branches proximal to the elbow joint. The deep branch lies under the extensor carpi radialis muscle, and the superficial branch divides into two components that extend distally on the medial and lateral borders of the cephalic vein.

TRAUMATIC ELBOW LUXATION

The elbow joint is inherently stable owing to the configuration of the humeroulnar joint and the presence of periarticular ligamentous structures. Therefore, fractures of the distal humerus and proximal radius and ulna are more common than elbow luxations.[2, 3] Depending on the mechanism of injury, fracture-dislocations such as the Monteggia fracture may occur. When luxations do occur, the radius and ulna invariably luxate laterally, because of the restraining effect of the prominent medial epicondylar ridge of the humerus.

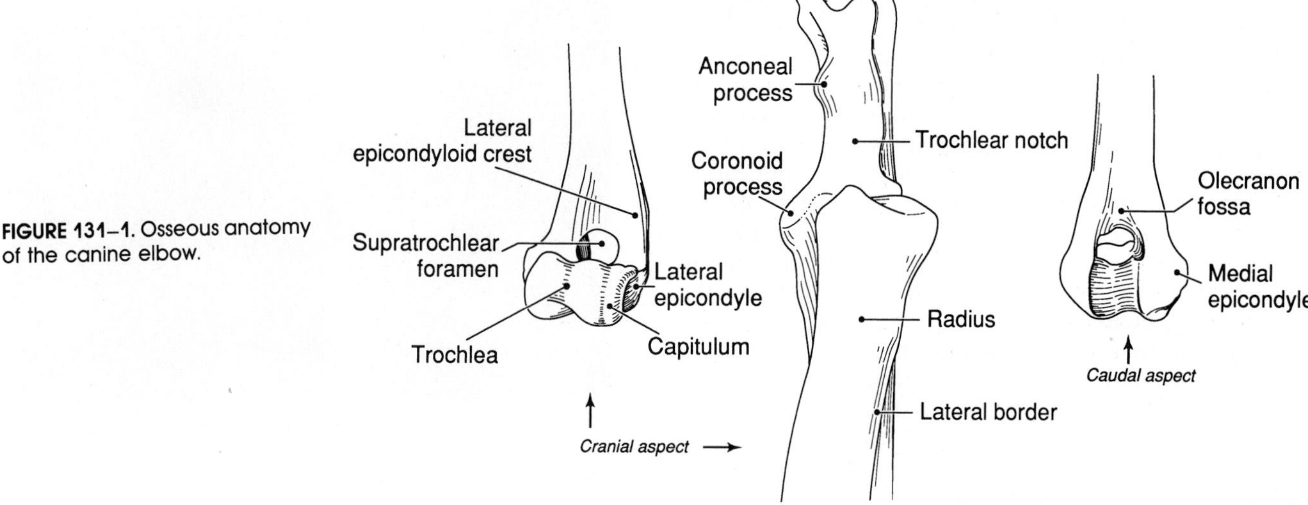

FIGURE 131–1. Osseous anatomy of the canine elbow.

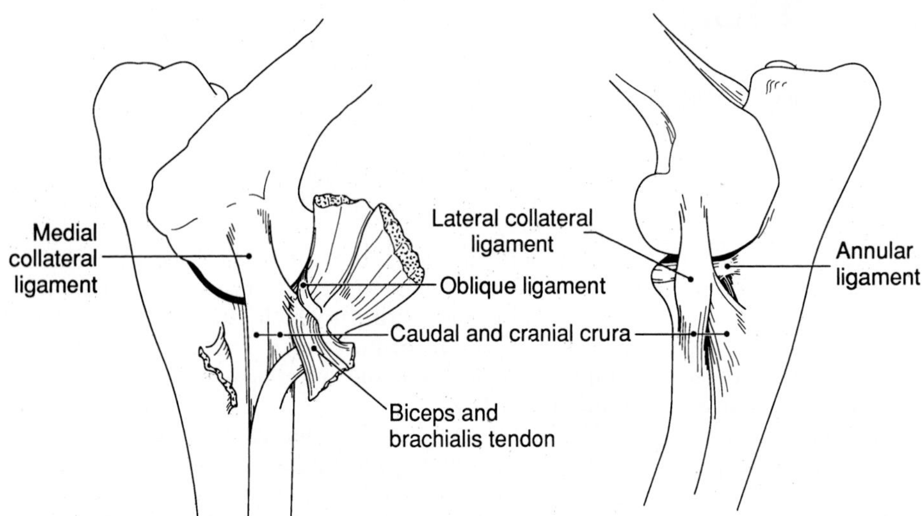

FIGURE 131–2. Arthrology of the canine elbow.

Complete luxation is associated with rupture or avulsion of the attachments of one or both collateral ligaments and the joint capsule. In more severe injuries, the origins of the flexor or extensor muscles may be ruptured or avulsed from the humeral condyle as well.

Diagnosis

In most cases of traumatic elbow luxation, the client describes a history of recent injury, with the dog having been hit by a car or involved in a dog fight. If other organ systems have not been seriously affected, the primary complaints are that the animal is not using the affected leg and that the leg is swollen and painful in the region of the elbow.

Examination of the affected leg usually reveals (1) a nonweightbearing lameness with the elbow in slight flexion, (2) abduction and external rotation of the antebrachium, (3) "widening" of the elbow with an indistinct lateral epicondyle but a distinct radial head laterally, (4) lateral position of the olecranon in relation to the humeral condyle, and (5) marked pain.[3] Neurological function is usually normal, based on the presence of skin sensation and voluntary withdrawal. With chronic luxations, the pain is less severe, and crepitus may suggest secondary osteoarthrosis.

Radiographs are required to document the presence or absence of fractures and in chronic luxations to determine the degree of osteoarthrosis. The craniocaudal projection demonstrates lateral displacement of the radius and ulna, and in complete luxations, the radius and ulna may be displaced proximally by the force of the triceps muscle. The anconeal process is located either in the olecranon fossa or lateral to the lateral epicondyle. Avulsion fractures of the attachment of the collateral ligaments are suspected when a separate bony density is present on the craniocaudal projection (Fig. 131–3). Chronic luxations show various degrees of secondary osteoarthrosis. Thoracic radiographs and additional tests such as a complete blood count, serum chemistry profile, and urinalysis are advisable before anesthesia and surgical intervention.

Management (Fig. 131–4)

In acute cases, every effort is made to achieve a closed reduction as soon as the animal can be safely anesthetized, because the results are generally quite satisfactory.[2] Closed reduction is often difficult to achieve,

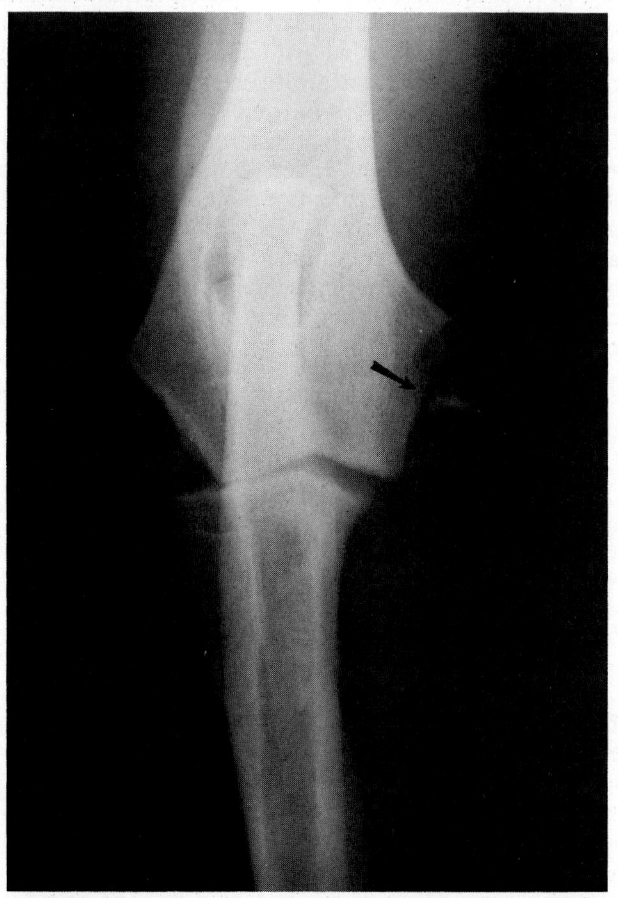

FIGURE 131–3. Craniocaudal radiograph of an acute lateral elbow luxation, made after closed reduction. Note the separate bony density denoting an avulsion fracture of the medial collateral ligament (*arrow*).

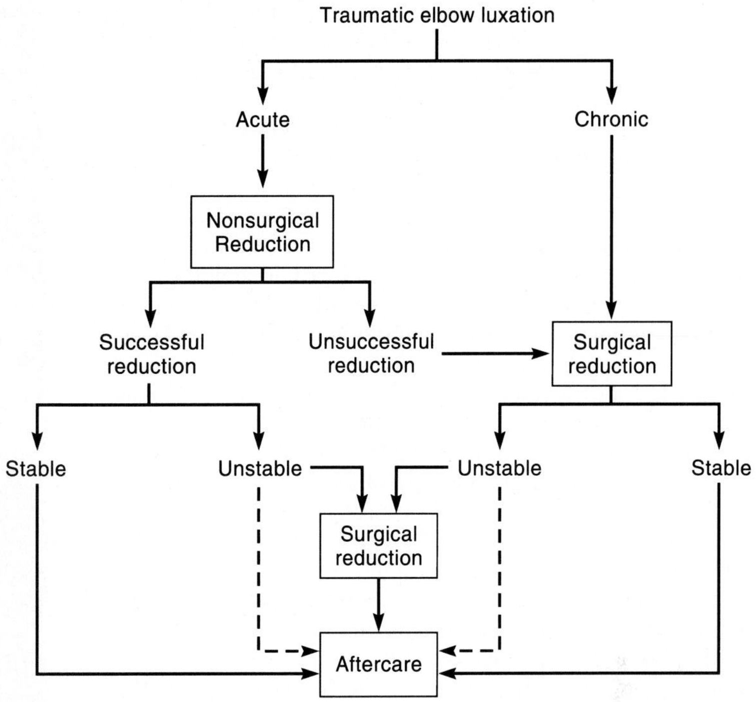

Traumatic elbow luxation → Acute; Chronic
Acute → Nonsurgical Reduction → Successful reduction; Unsuccessful reduction
Unsuccessful reduction → Surgical reduction
Chronic → Surgical reduction
Successful reduction → Stable; Unstable
Surgical reduction → Unstable; Stable
Unstable → Surgical reduction → Aftercare
Unstable - - → Aftercare
Stable → Aftercare

FIGURE 131–4. Algorithm depicting the alternatives and decision-making process in cases of traumatic elbow luxation. Broken lines indicate alternative treatments that depend on physical findings and other factors, as described in the text.

however, because of the powerful muscle forces involved and the complex configuration of the elbow articulation. General anesthesia with sufficient muscle relaxation is essential, and suspending the limb from a drip stand for 5 minutes before attempted reduction is helpful. Neuromuscular blockade may also facilitate reduction. The technique for closed reduction depends on the location of the anconeal process. The objective is to "hook" the anconeal process into the olecranon fossa and use it as a fulcrum to facilitate reduction. If the anconeal process is still in the olecranon fossa, the limb is extended slightly to fix the anconeal process in position. The antebrachium is abducted and rotated internally; pressure is exerted on the lateral aspect of the radial head to achieve reduction. If the anconeal process is positioned lateral to the epicondyle, it can usually be reduced into the olecranon fossa by markedly flexing the elbow, combined with internal rotation and abduction of the antebrachium. Placement of a towel clamp or Lewin bone clamp through the skin and into the olecranon can provide caudal distraction of the ulna and thereby facilitate positioning of the anconeal process into the olecranon fossa, if necessary. Once the anconeal process is reduced, the luxation can be further reduced as described.

If nonsurgical reduction is successful, the integrity of the collateral ligaments is evaluated to determine if further treatment is necessary. The elbow and carpus are flexed to 90°, and the antebrachium rotated. With an intact lateral collateral ligament, internal rotation is limited to 60°; with an intact medial ligament, external rotation should not exceed 40°.[3] Manipulation of the extended elbow into varus and valgus is another test that is a simple and reliable means for assessing collateral stability. Postreduction radiographs are indicated to evaluate congruency of the joint surfaces and the presence or absence of subluxation. Radiographic evidence of subluxation should be interpreted carefully, because it has been shown in humans that subluxation can be purely secondary to muscle relaxation during anesthesia.[7] Collateral ligament injury is common with elbow luxations, and a judgment must be made after closed reduction about whether or not surgical reconstruction of the collateral ligaments is warranted. With marked varus or valgus instability, reconstruction is indicated. If, on the other hand, the postreduction instability is considered mild and the radiographs demonstrate only minimal subluxation, conservative treatment is indicated, especially if the animal is a companion and not an athletic or working dog.

Open Reduction and Stabilization. Open reduction is necessary when closed reduction is not possible or when luxation has recurred after a closed reduction. Chronic luxations are often impossible to reduce closed because of the associated fibrosis and muscle contracture. Surgical stabilization, including reconstruction of the collateral ligaments, is indicated if marked instability follows open reduction, particularly in cases in which closed reduction has failed and in chronic luxations that have a propensity for reluxation. If surgical exploration reveals that the joint surfaces are badly damaged, arthrodesis can be considered.

For reduction, a caudolateral approach is used.[12] The skin incision is placed just caudal to the epicondyle, extending from the distal third of the humerus to the proximal third of the radius and ulna. If the anconeal muscle has not been lacerated by the injury, a myotomy may be used to open the joint. Less hemorrhage is encountered if the muscle can be elevated from the olecranon using subperiosteal dissection. The articular cartilage is inspected, and the antebrachium manipulated so that the anconeal process is levered over the lateral epicondylar ridge and engages the olecranon fossa. Sufficient muscle relaxation and the placement of a clamp on the olecranon facilitate reduction. If overriding and muscle contraction are severe, a blunt instrument can be used as a lever to gently force the radius/ulna medially. This can be damaging to the joint surface, however, and should be avoided if possible. A femoral distraction device can be used to achieve reduction in difficult cases.* The external fixation screws are placed into the distal humerus and proximal ulna, and the device opened enough to permit reduction of the humeroradial joint. After reduction, the joint is thoroughly lavaged and elbow stability assessed. If marked instability and a tendency for reluxation are noted, the collateral ligament is reconstructed.

Several types of collateral ligament repair can be used, depending on location and type of injury: primary repair with augmentation or ligament replacement with nonabsorbable suture material.[2, 3] The lateral collateral ligament can be exposed through the caudolateral approach described earlier. The proximal portions of the common and lateral digital extensor muscles are identified, and the remnants of the ligament can be found under them. Primary repair of the body or end of the ligament is accomplished by reapposing the injured ends with nonabsorbable suture material, using a locking loop pattern. Care is taken to avoid the deep branch of the radial nerve. The distal end of the ligament can be reattached to the annular ligament and surrounding fibrous tissue. The proximal end can be reattached to the epicondyle by passing a suture through a predrilled transverse tunnel in the epicondyle or around a screw and washer in the epicondyle. Avulsion fractures of the proximal or distal attachments can be repaired with a small lag screw or by a modified tension band device (Fig. 131–5). To replace a collateral ligament, screws with washers are placed in the sites of attachment of the ligament to the humeral epicondyle and radial neck. Heavy nonabsorbable suture material is looped over each screw using a figure-eight pattern. Surgical stabilization of the medial collateral ligament is performed similarly but through a medial incision.

The flexor or extensor muscle groups are occasionally avulsed from their attachments to the humeral epicondyles. Generally, they can be sutured to periosteum and fibrous tissue. Severe soft-tissue injury is associated with significant instability and a guarded prognosis. When soft-tissue repair does not provide adequate stabilization and reluxation is likely, an external fixator may be placed across the joint to maintain reduction during the phase of soft-tissue healing. It is removed after 7 days to permit range of motion exercises. Some loss of motion is to be expected.

After surgical reduction and stabilization, joint stability is evaluated and postoperative radiographs are taken to evaluate anatomical alignment and placement of metallic implants. A soft padded bandage from midhumerus downward is applied for 24 to 48 hours to minimize postoperative swelling.

*ASIF Femoral Distractor, Synthes Ltd., Paoli, PA.

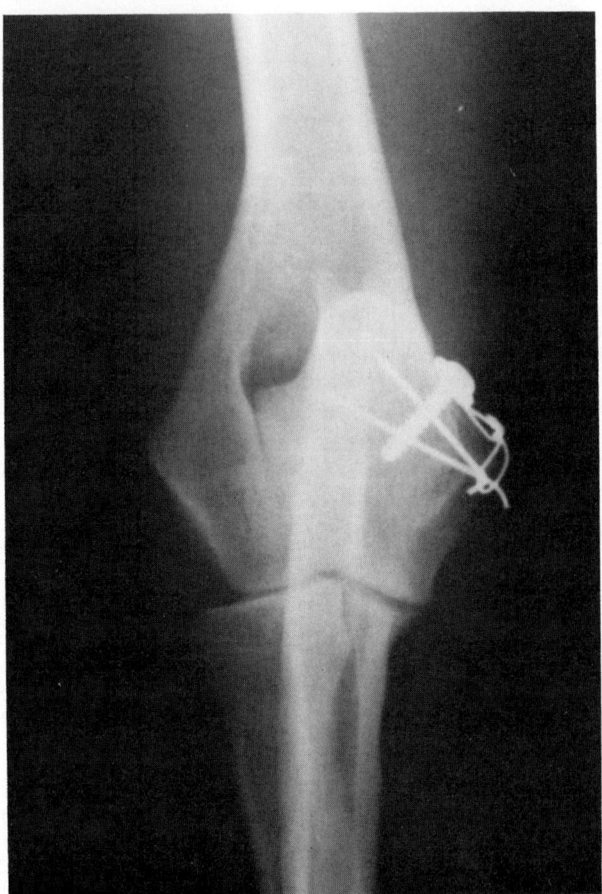

FIGURE 131–5. Postoperative radiograph demonstrating internal fixation of an avulsion fracture of the proximal attachment of the medial collateral ligament.

Aftercare

Aftercare varies depending on the severity of injury, type of repair, and owner compliance.[2, 3] In humans, prolonged immobilization exceeding 21 days is strongly associated with unsatisfactory results (flexion contracture, continued pain).[9] Also, clinical evidence in humans shows that early mobilization is safe and does not increase the risk of reluxation.[9] The benefits of early motion for injured cartilage have been well established. Gentle passive motion should be started as soon as possible.

In dogs with residual instability or muscle injury, a well-padded spica splint is applied to the forelimb and maintained for 7 to 10 days postoperatively. After it is removed, the client is instructed to initiate passive range of motion exercise and keep the dog strictly confined. In dogs with stable reductions, an alternative program that provides immediate motion is preferred. Two days after surgery, a nonweightbearing carpal flexion bandage is applied to prevent weightbearing. Gentle passive motion exercise is started as soon as possible. After 10 days, the nonweightbearing bandage is removed and the animal allowed to use the leg while its activity is still restricted for another 3 weeks. Passive motion is continued during this period or even longer.

Postoperative complications include reluxation, infection, decreased range of motion, and secondary osteoarthrosis. The prognosis after traumatic elbow luxation depends on the severity of cartilage and soft-tissue damage, duration before repair, degree of stabilization achieved, and owner compliance.[2, 3] The prognosis is good to excellent for luxations of less than 1 week when a stable closed reduction has been achieved and physical rehabilitation is started early. If the reduction requires surgery, especially external fixation, the prognosis is less favorable because secondary osteoarthrosis may develop and cause intermittent lameness. Chronic or recurrent luxations have a guarded prognosis because of the usual severity of degenerative joint disease.[2]

CONGENITAL ELBOW LUXATION

Information about congenital elbow luxation is limited because of its infrequent occurrence. The classic form of the disease is characterized by lateral rotation of the ulna and internal rotation of the antebrachium; the radiohumeral joint is relatively unaffected. This form of congenital elbow luxation occurs most commonly in small breeds of dogs: Yorkshire terrier, Boston terrier, miniature poodle, Pekingese, miniature pinscher, Pomeranian, pug, and Chihuahua. It has also been reported in the cocker spaniel, English bulldog, Shetland sheepdog, collie, and crossbreeds.[1, 4, 8, 10] The cause of the disorder is unknown. It has been hypothesized to be the result of an embryonic failure in the formation of intra-articular ligaments with hypoplasia of the medial collateral ligament,[1] although this etiology has been questioned.[10]

A second type of elbow luxation has been reported in puppies, characterized by caudolateral displacement of the radial head, with the ulna in a relatively normal position.[4] The condition occurs mostly in large dogs. The condition may be caused by trauma or asynchronous growth of the radius and ulna, but affliction shortly after birth or within the first weeks of life suggests a congenital lesion.[4] The heritability of either form of congenital elbow luxation is undefined.

Congenital luxation of the elbow also can occur in association with generalized joint laxity (arthrodysplasia). Multiple skeletal deformities, especially ectrodactyly, can be present in affected individuals.[1, 6, 11]

Lateral Rotation of the Ulna

Diagnosis

Afflicted puppies are usually between 4 and 22 weeks old when taken to a veterinarian. A front leg deformity sometimes was observed at birth or soon after birth; other times a lameness of several weeks duration is the presenting complaint.

Affected puppies have a characteristic posture and gait.[4, 10, 13] The elbow is held flexed, with the antebrachium markedly pronated. With bilateral involvement, the front legs may almost cross and the dog bears weight on the caudomedial aspect of the elbows and antebrachium. Palpation reveals prominent lateral displacement of the olecranon and triceps tendon, with moderate to severe muscle atrophy. Pain and crepitation are generally absent. Ulceration of the skin is sometimes present, secondary to the abnormal weightbearing.

Significant radiographic findings include lateral displacement and cranial rotation of the proximal ulna, relatively normal position of the radial head, and narrowing of the radial neck (Fig. 131–6). In more severe cases, malarticulation of the humeroradial joint with dysplasia of the proximal radial epiphysis may be present. Osteoarthrosis is not commonly observed on radiographic examinations.[8]

Management

When discussing management options for congenital elbow luxation with a client, the possible hereditary etiology and the palliative nature of available treatments need to be clearly addressed. If a dog is able to ambulate reasonably well without pain, conservative management may be the best option. Surgical treatment provides good long-term clinical results if the procedure is performed when the dog is younger than 4 months. The surgical approach is determined primarily by the age of the dog at the time of diagnosis.

Closed Reduction and Percutaneous Fixation. This approach is usually successful in dogs that are less than 4 months old, because degenerative changes have not developed and the joint can be manipulated into reasonable reduction. After induction of anesthesia and aseptic preparation of the leg, reduction is accomplished by applying pressure to the lateral surface of the olecranon, forcing it caudally and medially into the olecranon fossa.[10, 13] Counterpressure on the medial surface of the humerus is necessary, and considerable force may be required to achieve adequate positioning of the olecranon. The surgeon should be patient and not try to achieve complete reduction immediately. Care must be taken not to fracture the olecranon, because affected dogs are quite small and the bone relatively weak.

After reduction is achieved, it is maintained using either a transarticular pin or a modified external fixator. With transarticular pinning, one or two K wires or small Steinmann pins are driven from the caudal aspect of the olecranon into the humeral condyle and distal metaphysis. The pins are cut flush with the skin (Fig. 131–7).[13] The modified external fixator consists of two small pins that are placed transversely through the distal humeral condyle and the olecranon. Elastic bands are placed over a padded caudal splint from the lateral aspect of the olecranon pin to the medial aspect of the humeral pin to achieve medial rotation of the ulna.[10] Aftercare with the external fixator is more involved than with the transarticular pin method.

Open Reduction and Stabilization. Chronic changes in older dogs are more difficult to reduce and have a less favorable prognosis. A caudolateral approach is generally satisfactory; however, if more exposure is needed, an olecranon osteotomy is indicated. To reduce a chronic luxation, useful techniques include lateral

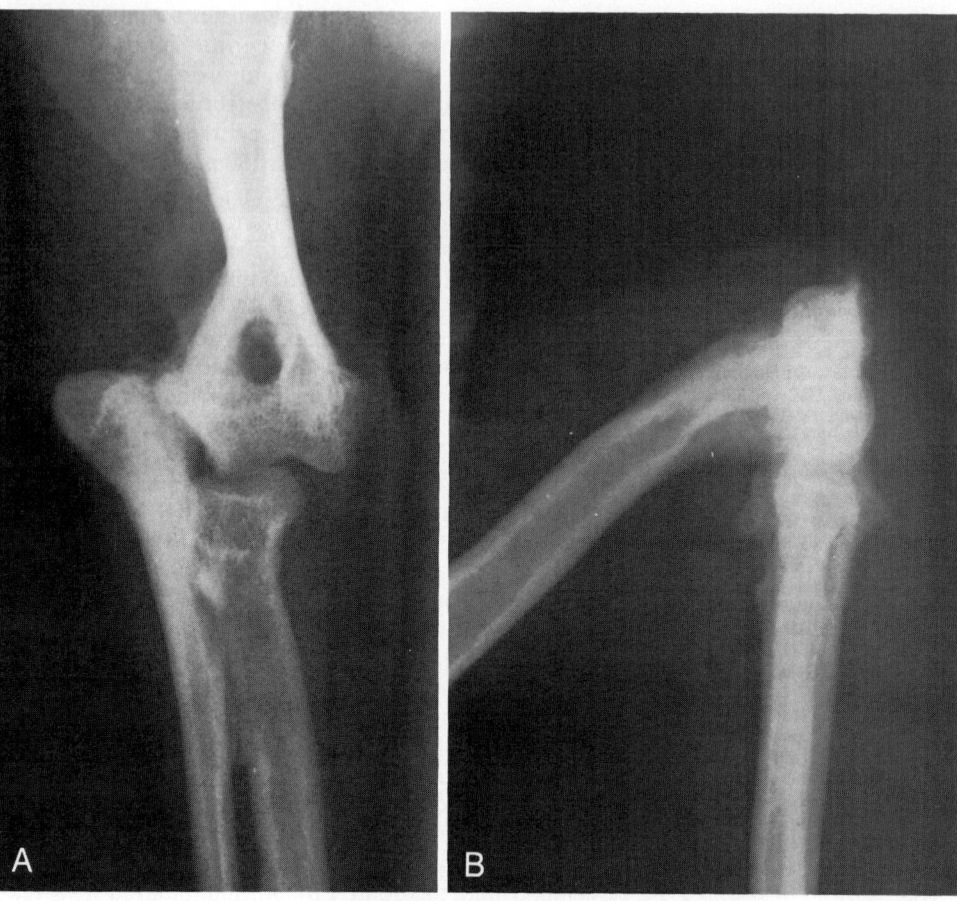

FIGURE 131–6. Craniocaudal (*A*) and lateral (*B*) radiographs of a chronic congenital elbow luxation. Note the lateral rotation of the proximal ulna.

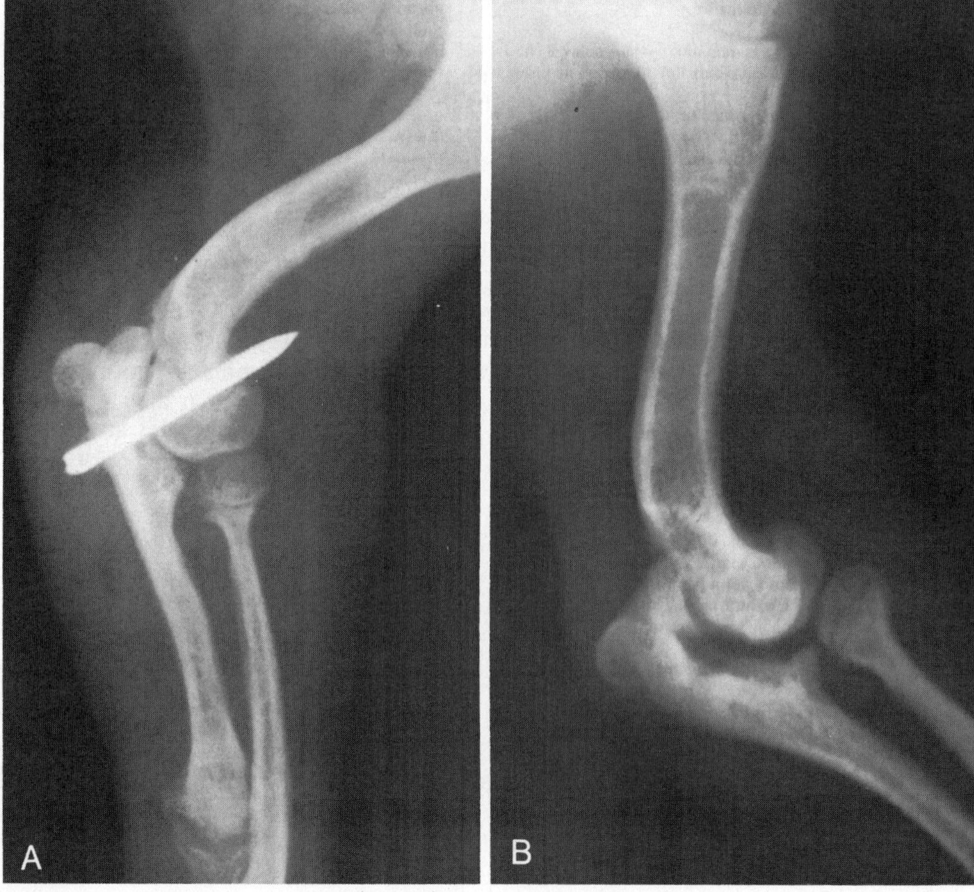

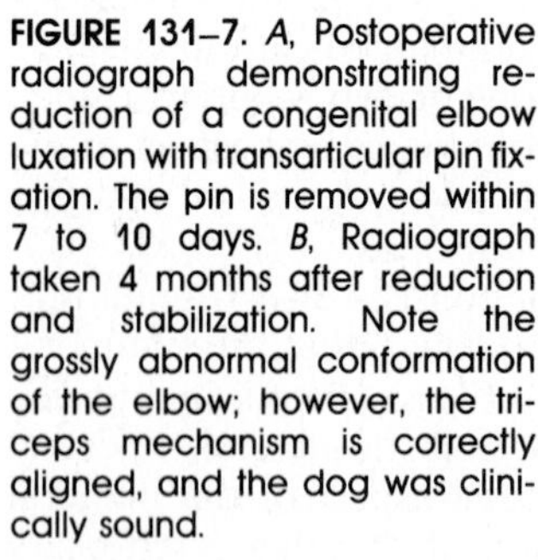

FIGURE 131–7. *A*, Postoperative radiograph demonstrating reduction of a congenital elbow luxation with transarticular pin fixation. The pin is removed within 7 to 10 days. *B*, Radiograph taken 4 months after reduction and stabilization. Note the grossly abnormal conformation of the elbow; however, the triceps mechanism is correctly aligned, and the dog was clinically sound.

releasing incisions, capsulotomy, desmotomy (lateral collateral ligament), and anconeus myotomy.[4, 10]

After reduction, stabilization can be achieved by (1) transarticular pinning, (2) external fixators, (3) olecranon transposition, (4) reconstruction of the trochlea and trochlear notch, (5) collateral ligament reconstruction, and (6) medial imbrication.[4, 10] If the trochlea and trochlear notch are fairly congruent, lateral release, medial imbrication, and medial olecranon transposition are usually sufficient to maintain reduction. The presence of severe degenerative joint disease is an indication for arthrodesis or amputation. Postoperative radiographs are taken to judge joint alignment and implant positioning.

Aftercare

A well-padded spica splint is applied for 7 to 10 days. Exercise is restricted for 4 to 6 weeks. If a modified external fixator is used, frequent evaluations of the pins and bandage are necessary. Transarticular pins and external fixators are removed after 7 days, and activity is strictly limited for an additional 4 to 6 weeks. Physical therapy is started as soon as possible.

Complications include reluxation, infection, secondary osteoarthrosis, and physeal arrest. A normal joint does not develop after reduction and stabilization, but satisfactory function of the affected leg(s) usually can be achieved with early successful reduction. If repair is done late and osseous changes are severe, the prognosis is guarded.

Caudolateral Luxation of the Radial Head

Diagnosis

Affected puppies show mild or no suppination of the antebrachium, and the olecranon is in a normal position. A valgus deformity may be present at the carpus. The radial head is palpable on the lateral aspect of the elbow. Pain and crepitation are not present in young dogs, and the lameness is not nearly as severe as in dogs affected with lateral rotation of the ulna. Radiographs are necessary to document the abnormal position of the radial head and to evaluate the physes. The distal ulnar physis may appear abnormal, implying that retarded growth at this physis may have a role in this disease.

Management

If the condition is not severe, a conservative approach may be satisfactory. The dog is examined at 2- to 3-week intervals for evaluation of limb conformation and lameness, and radiographs are made to verify elbow joint congruity and continued growth, especially at the distal ulnar physis.

In cases of complete luxation of the humeroradial joint, surgical reduction and stabilization are required. In young dogs, a lateral approach to the radial head is

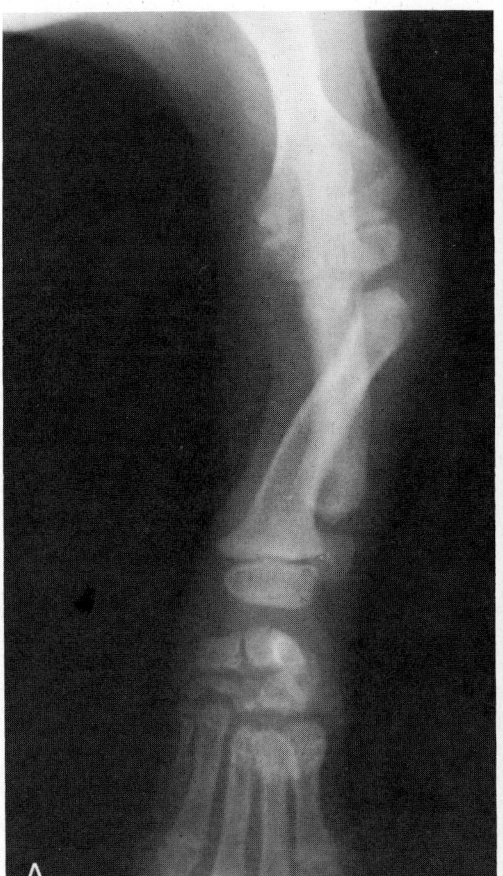

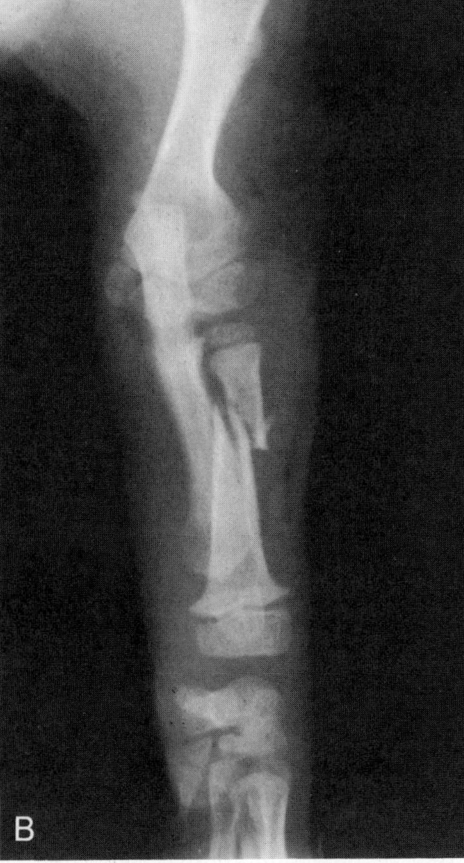

FIGURE 131–8. *A*, Radiograph of an 8-week-old Jack Russell terrier with caudolateral luxation of the radial head. *B*, Postoperative radiograph demonstrating oblique osteotomy of the proximal radius and reduction of the humeroradial joint.

followed by oblique osteotomy of the radius, distal to the proximal physis. The osteotomy is necessary to permit manipulation of the proximal radius. The humeroradial joint is reduced, and nonabsorbable suture material is used to imbricate the lateral collateral ligament and joint capsule (Fig. 131–8). A light padded bandage is applied for 5 to 7 days to minimize limb use and protect the surgical site. If the distal ulnar physis is abnormal, consideration should be given to concurrent osteotomy of the ulna, with periosteal resection and implantation of a fat graft to retard healing. In the latter circumstance, more prolonged and substantial coaptation (spica bandage) is necessary postoperatively for 2 to 3 weeks. Older dogs with secondary changes do not carry as favorable a prognosis, and more aggressive surgical correction is necessary. Osteotomy of the radius and fixation of the proximal radius to the ulna are generally satisfactory in restoring joint alignment.[4] Postoperatively, a carpal flexion bandage is used for 2 to 3 weeks to minimize limb use and permit simultaneous passive motion of the joint.

References

1. Bingel SA, Riser WH: Congenital elbow luxation in the dog. *J Small Anim Pract 18*:445, 1977.
2. Bone DL: Chronic luxations. *Vet Clin North Am 17*:923, 1987.
3. Campbell JR: Luxation and ligamentous injuries of the elbow of the dog. *Vet Clin North Am 1*:429, 1971.
4. Campbell JR: Congenital luxation of the elbow of the dog. *Vet Annu 19*:229, 1979.
5. Evans HE, Christensen GC (eds): *Miller's Anatomy of the Dog*. 2nd ed. W.B. Saunders, Philadelphia, 1979.
6. Fox MW: Polyarthrodysplasia (congenital joint luxation) in the dog. *J Am Vet Med Assoc 145*:1204, 1964.
7. Josefsson BO, et al: Surgical versus non-surgical treatment of ligamentous injuries following dislocation of the elbow joint. *J Bone Joint Surg [Am] 69A*:605, 1987.
8. Kene ROC, et al: The radiological features of congenital elbow luxation/subluxation in the dog. *J Small Anim Pract 2*:621, 1982.
9. Melhoff TL, et al: Simple dislocation of the elbow in the adult. *J Bone Joint Surg [Am] 70A*:244, 1988.
10. Milton JL, Montgomery RD: Congenital elbow dislocation. *Vet Clin North Am 17*:873, 1987.
11. Montgomery M, Tomlinson J: Two cases of ectrodactyly and congenital elbow luxation in the dog. *J Am Anim Hosp Assoc 21*:781, 1985.
12. Piermattei DL, Greeley RC: An atlas of surgical approaches to the bones of the dog and cat. W.B. Saunders, Philadelphia, 1979.
13. Withrow SJ: Management of a congenital elbow luxation by temporary trans-articular pinning. *Vet Med Small Anim Clin 72*:1579, 1977.

CHAPTER 132

Fractures of the Radius and Ulna

Erick L. Egger

Fractures of the radius and ulna represent a significant proportion (17 to 18 per cent) of all fractures in cats and dogs.[35] The high incidence of delayed union and nonunion,[9, 28] carpal hyperextension and stiffness,[33] and growth deformities[22] reflects the potential complexity of treating these fractures.

FRACTURES OF THE OLECRANON

The olecranon is the proximal extremity of the ulna, which serves as the attachment and lever arm for the triceps, the powerful extensor muscles of the elbow. Consequently, complete fractures of the olecranon result in severe proximal displacement of the fragment away from the ulna (Fig. 132–1). Because external coaptation is unable to control the distractive pull of the triceps, open reduction and internal fixation are indicated. Olecranon fractures may be nonarticular or may extend into the elbow joint through the trochlear (semilunar) notch. These fractures are surgically exposed via a caudal approach, which subperiosteally elevates the flexor carpi ulnaris and extensor carpi ulnaris muscles to expose the olecranon and ulnar shaft.[36] For articular fractures, the anconeus muscle and joint capsule can also be incised to expose the interior of the joint.[36] Extending the elbow decreases the pull of the triceps muscle, facilitating fracture reduction. Perfect reduction of any articular components is necessary to avoid secondary arthritis. The fracture can be fixed by several methods.

The tension band wire technique uses monofilament

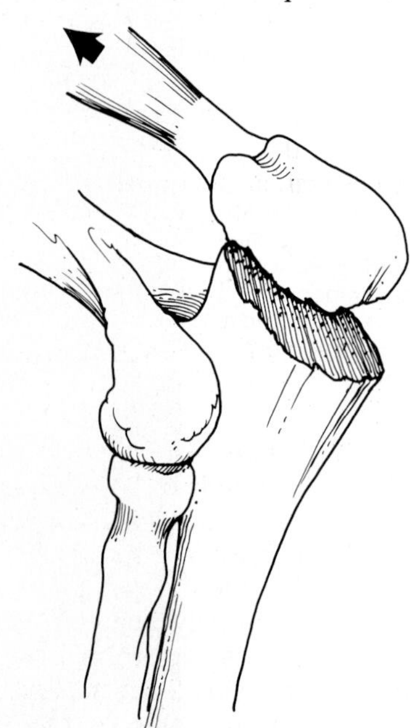

FIGURE 132–1. Fracture of the olecranon with proximal displacement of the fragment due to distractive pull of the triceps muscle.

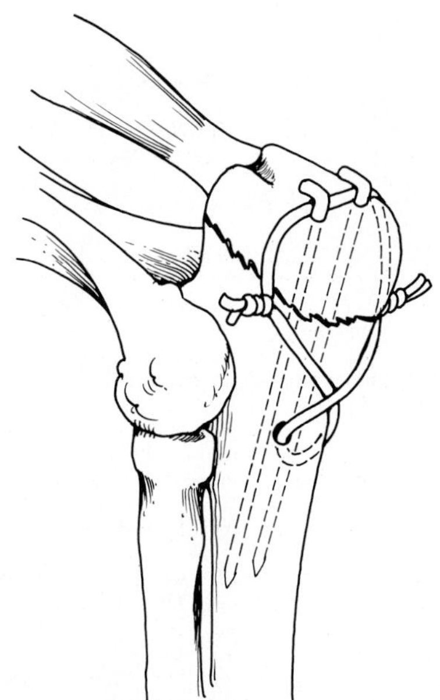

FIGURE 132–2. Pin and tension band repair of olecranon fracture demonstrating how the pull of the triceps muscle is converted into dynamic compression of the fracture.

orthopedic wire to convert the pull of the triceps muscle into dynamic compression of the fracture (Fig. 132–2). Two Kirschner wires or small (up to 3/32 inch in diameter) Steinmann pins are used to reduce the fracture and control rotation. The pins are parallel and oriented medially and laterally. They are started on the proximal tip of the olecranon and driven across the fracture to penetrate the cranial cortex of the ulnar shaft distal to the trochlear notch. A transverse hole is made from medial to lateral in the caudal ulna, approximately the same distance distal to the fracture as the length of the olecranon fragment. Monofilament stainless steel wire is used for the tension band. Twenty-gauge wire is used in cats and small dogs, and 18-gauge wire is used on any larger animal. A single tightening twist is made in the center of a 25-cm length of the wire. One end is passed through the hole in the ulna. The center of the wire crosses behind the caudal ulna, and the opposite end is threaded under the triceps tendon and around the cranial aspect of the pins. The free ends of the wire are then twisted together to form a figure-eight pattern. The two twists are alternately tightened until the wire is snug and the caudal aspect of the fracture is reduced. The wire should not be overtightened or the cranial aspect of the fracture gap will open. The extra wire is cut off, leaving three to four twists. The ends are bent over to lie flat on the bone. The ends of the pins are bent over to form hooks, cut off, and rotated cranially over the wire. They should be countersunk into the triceps tendon to avoid damage to the overlying soft tissues. The pins and wire are not routinely removed.

A screw can be used in lag fashion to stabilize an olecranon fracture. However, the mechanical pull of the muscles will be at a right angle to the screw shaft, predisposing to cycling stresses and failure of the screw (particularly if perfect reduction and compression of the fracture are not achieved). Consequently, a tension band wire should be applied to protect the screw from bending forces. In addition, a small Kirschner wire should be placed parallel to the screw to prevent rotation (Fig. 132–3). A clinical review of this screw and wire technique for repair of ulnar osteotomies found a significantly lower associated morbidity than with the classic pin and wire technique.[34]

Comminuted olecranon fractures can be stabilized by applying a plate along the caudal ulnar shaft. In this location, the plate acts as both a tension band to resist the pull of the triceps and a buttress to resist fracture collapse (Fig. 132–4).[4] Lateral placement of the plate has also been described.[7] Although this lateral orientation may be less effective as a tension band, it provides more buttress support for extremely unstable fractures. Also, lateral application is technically easier in smaller animals. The proximal fragment must be large enough to accept at least two screws. Alternatively, in large dogs, the double-hook plate* may be used on short fragments.[2] Care must be taken to avoid placing screws through the articular surface of the trochlear notch.

Postoperative management depends on stability of the repair. A Robert Jones compressive bandage may be used for a few days to limit swelling. A traumatized elbow joint stiffens quickly if immobilized. Joint motion must be encouraged with either controlled walking or passive range of motion exercises. If a good tension band effect was achieved, additional support is not needed. If bony defects persist after surgery or if fixation is tenuous, a carpal flexion bandage is considered.[27] This bandage allows active motion of the elbow while preventing weightbearing and can be left on for several weeks to allow early fracture healing (Fig. 132–5).

PROXIMAL ULNAR FRACTURE WITH LUXATION OF THE RADIAL HEAD

Proximal ulnar fracture with luxation of the radial head is known as the Monteggia lesion in the human

*Robert Mathup Co., Bettlach, Switzerland.

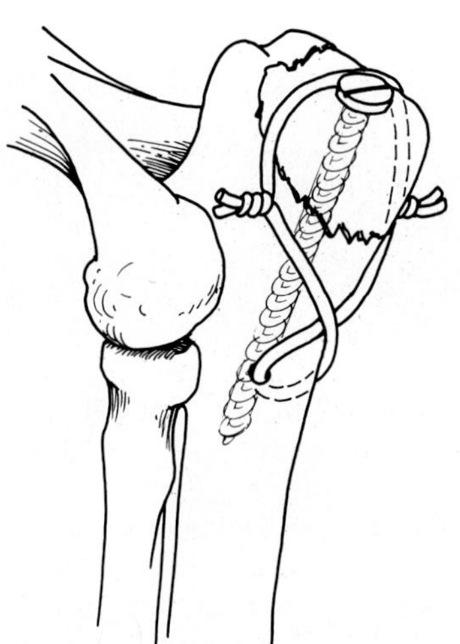

FIGURE 132–3. Olecranon fracture repaired with lag screw and tension band wire fixation.

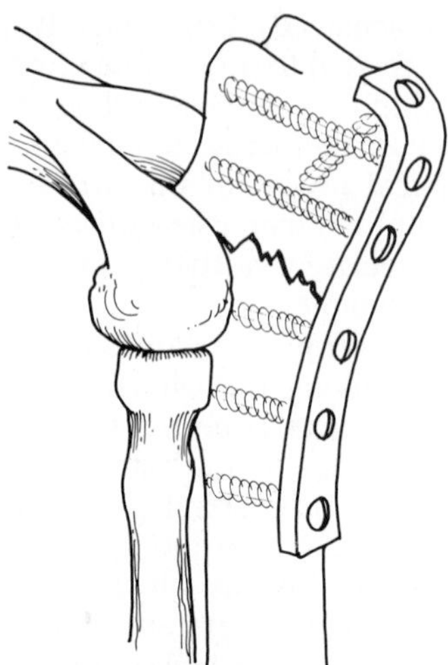

FIGURE 132–4. Olecranon fracture repaired with a caudally oriented bone plate that acts as both a buttress and tension band.

literature.[44] The ulnar fracture can occur anywhere from the trochlear notch to the midshaft of the ulna. The radial head usually displaces cranially and proximally. In small animals, the syndrome is thought to be caused by a severe blow to the caudal aspect of the ulna when the antebrachium is extended and bearing weight.[42] A high incidence of concurrent radial head chip fractures (39 per cent) has been reported.[42]

Treatment depends on the fracture configuration and the clinician's preference. Nonoperative closed reduction and external coaptation are not recommended because of the decreased elbow joint range of motion and delayed ulnar healing that commonly result.[42] The syndrome can be divided into those cases in which the ulnar fracture is proximal and the annular ligament has ruptured and those cases in which the ulnar fracture is relatively distal and the ligament remains intact. In either situation, rapid swelling, muscle spasm, and fibrous proliferation necessitate early treatment. A caudal approach to the ulna is often adequate if the radial head reduces with manipulation.[36] A craniolateral approach[45] is used if the radial head cannot be relocated because

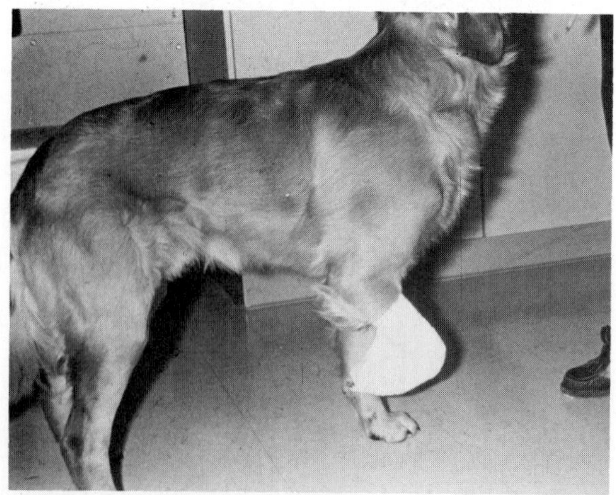

FIGURE 132–5. Carpal flexion bandage, which prevents weight-bearing but allows shoulder and elbow joint motion.

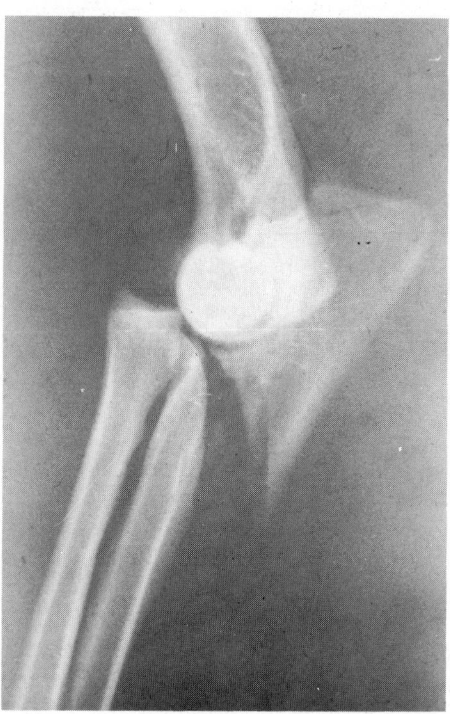

FIGURE 132–6. Monteggia fracture in which the proximal annular ligament remained intact, maintaining the normal relationship of the ulnar shaft and the radial head.

of either debris and fibrous tissue in the joint or muscle contraction and over-riding. This approach allows débridement of the joint and levering of the radial head back into place. With comminuted ulnar fractures, the radial head should be reduced first to assist in the reduction and alignment of the ulnar fragments.

If the annular ligament remains intact, as is often the case when the ulnar fracture occurs at the base or into the trochlear notch, the relationship of the radial head and the ulnar shaft remains normal (Fig. 132–6). Reduction of the ulnar fracture occurs only with reduction of the radial head luxation. Stable fixation of the ulna fracture with pins and tension band wire or bone screws and plate stabilizes the radial head reduction.

If the annular ligament is ruptured, the radial head separates from the proximal ulnar shaft. This occurs when the ulnar fracture is distal to the annular ligament (Fig. 132–7). Treatment requires not only reduction and stabilization of the fracture but also approximation and fixation of the normal radial and ulnar relationship. The ligament ends can occasionally be identified and sutured primarily. A high incidence (32 per cent) of radial head reluxation has been reported with primary ligament repair.[42] Consequently, supplemental support is recommended. Orthopedic wire can be applied in interfragmentary fashion around the radius and through a hole in the ulna (Fig. 132–8). Bone screws or threaded pins can be used to transfix the radius to the ulna either in interfragmentary lag fashion or by extending the fixation screws used in plating the ulnar fracture into the radius (Fig. 132–9). A postoperative compressive bandage (Robert Jones) is used for several days to control swelling, but early range of motion exercises are necessary to avoid elbow stiffness.

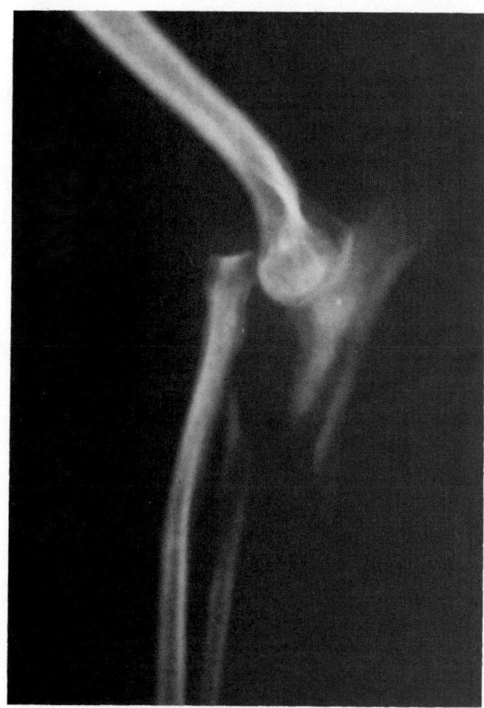

FIGURE 132–7. Monteggia fracture in which the ulnar fracture is distal to the proximal annular ligament and the ligament has ruptured. Note the separation of the radial head and the ulnar shaft.

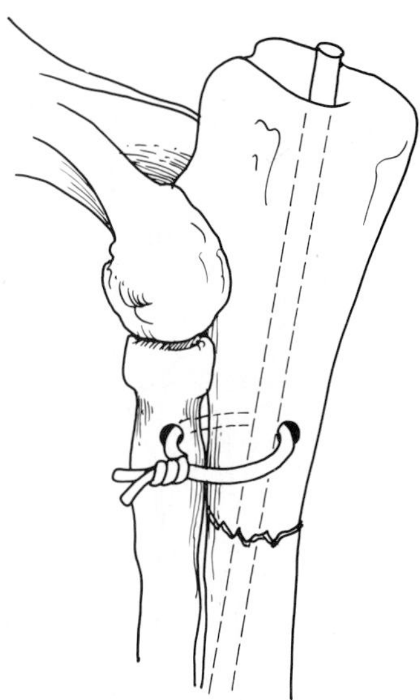

FIGURE 132–8. Interfragmentary wire stabilization of the radius and ulna and intramedullary pin fixation of the ulnar fracture for treatment of a Monteggia fracture.

FRACTURES OF THE RADIAL HEAD

Fractures of the radial head are uncommon because the anatomy of the elbow joint predisposes to fractures of the lateral humeral condyle, sparing the radius.[15] When fractures of the head occur, they usually involve the articular surface. Meticulous reduction and stable internal fixation are necessary to prevent secondary arthritis and joint stiffness. The fracture is approached through a lateral skin incision. The deep exposure depends on the location and extent of the fracture. Craniolateral exposure is obtained by incising the origin and distal medial retraction of the common digital extensor muscle.[45] Lateral exposure is obtained by osteotomizing the lateral humeral epicondyle and by distal reflection of the collateral ligament and extensor tendons.[35] Caudolateral exposure is obtained by incising the origin and by caudal distal retraction of the lateral ulnar and anconeus muscles.[36] Once the fracture is exposed and reduced, stabilization can take one of two forms.

The ideal method of radial head fixation is an intrafragmentary lag screw. Splitting of the fragment can be reduced by countersinking the screw head. A Steinmann pin or Kirschner wire may be needed to control rotation of the fragment around the screw (Fig. 132–10). If screws are unavailable or are too large for fixation without splitting the fragment, stabilization can be achieved with multiple Kirschner wires placed at divergent angles. Optimum reduction and compression of the fracture are accomplished with bone-holding clamps,

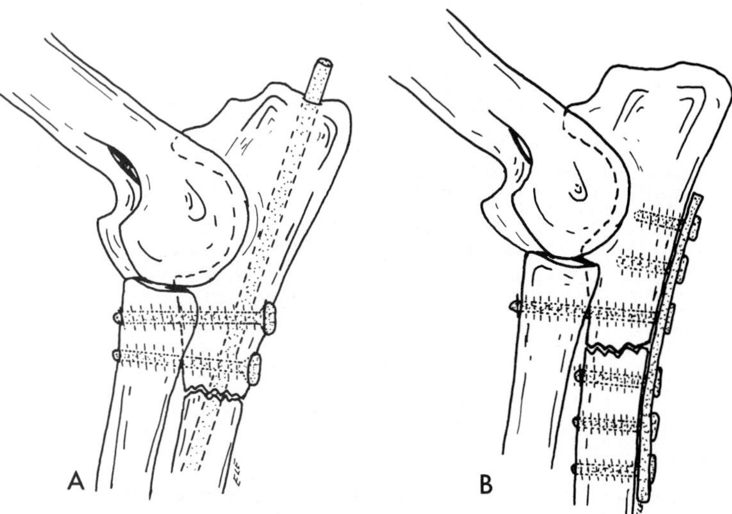

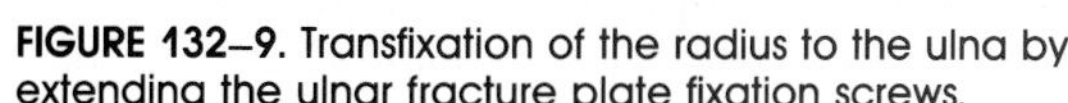

FIGURE 132–9. Transfixation of the radius to the ulna by extending the ulnar fracture plate fixation screws.

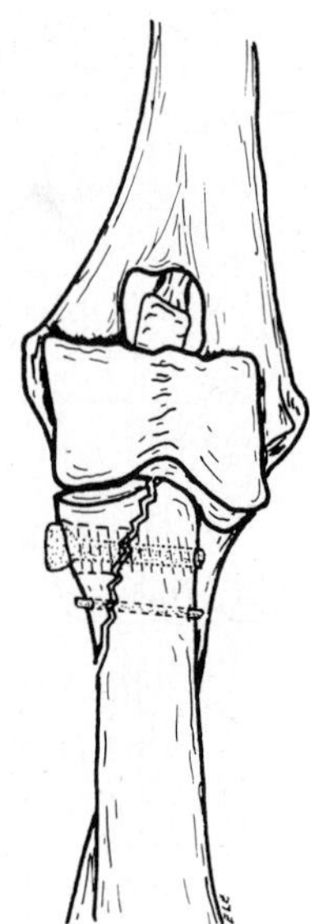

FIGURE 132–10. Lag screw and antirotational interfragmentary pin fixation of a radial head fracture.

because driving the K wires does not improve reduction or provide compression. At least two and preferably three or more K wires are placed at maximally divergent angles to prevent the fragment from rotating or sliding along the wire (Fig. 132–11). The K wires are usually driven from the smaller fragment into the larger until they penetrate the far cortex to prevent loosening and migration, which would result in loss of fracture fixation. Closure is achieved by suturing the incised tendon origins or reattaching the humeral epicondyle with a lag screw or pins and tension band wire. As with trochlear fractures, a delay in weightbearing, depending on the stabilization obtained, may be desired.

If the fracture is chronic, with severe articular damage, or is not reconstructible owing to severe comminution, a salvage procedure may be necessary. Resection

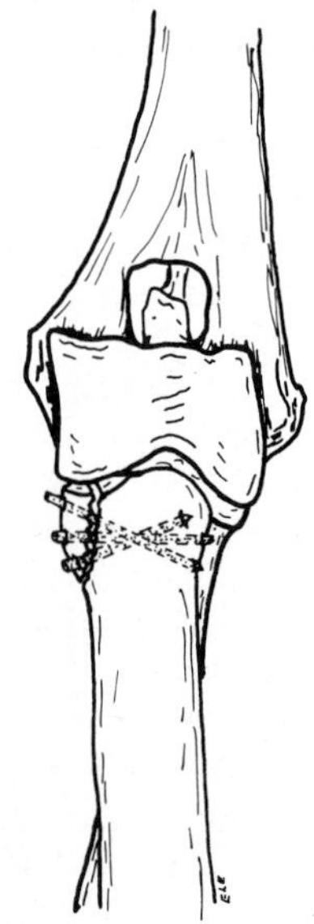

FIGURE 132–11. Divergent Kirschner wire fixation of a radial head fracture.

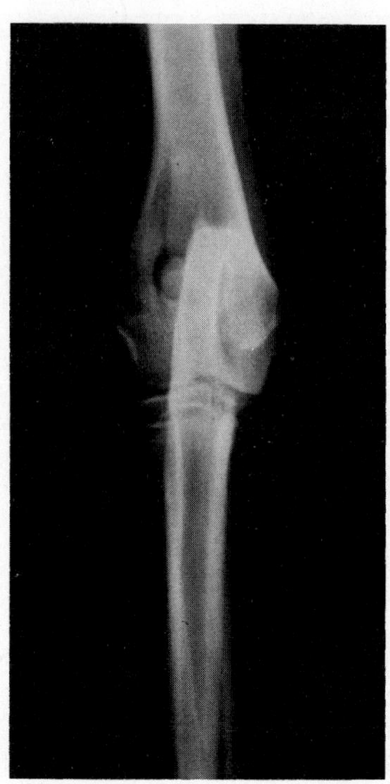

FIGURE 132–12. Fracture separation of the proximal radial physis.

of the radial head has been described as treatment for lateral luxation of the radial head secondary to growth deformities in small dogs.[24] This technique has also been cited as a potential method of treating radial head fractures.[37] Care should be taken to protect the radial nerve, and placing a free autogenous fat graft into the resection site seems to improve clinical results.[12] In larger, more athletic dogs, an elbow arthrodesis should be considered.

FRACTURE/SEPARATION OF THE PROXIMAL RADIAL PHYSIS

A fracture through the proximal radial physeal plate is rare in young dogs (Fig. 132–12). It may be associated with lateral elbow luxation.[4] Closed reduction followed by immobilization in extension with a splint for 7 to 10 days may be possible, particularly with elbow luxation that can be reduced. Open reduction through a craniolateral approach is performed if closed reduction is unsuccessful.[45] The radial head can be fixed in place with one or two Kirschner wires started at the articular edge and driven distally through the growth plate into the metaphysis (Fig. 132–13). If the animal is actively growing, the Kirschner wires are placed as perpendicular to the physis as possible to avoid impeding growth. The K wires are usually removed after healing occurs, in 2 to 3 weeks. The owner is warned of possible premature physeal closure, and the animal is periodically monitored for signs of growth deformity.

FRACTURES OF EITHER THE RADIAL OR ULNAR SHAFTS

Fractures of the radial or ulnar shafts with continuity of the other bone occur relatively often, particularly in

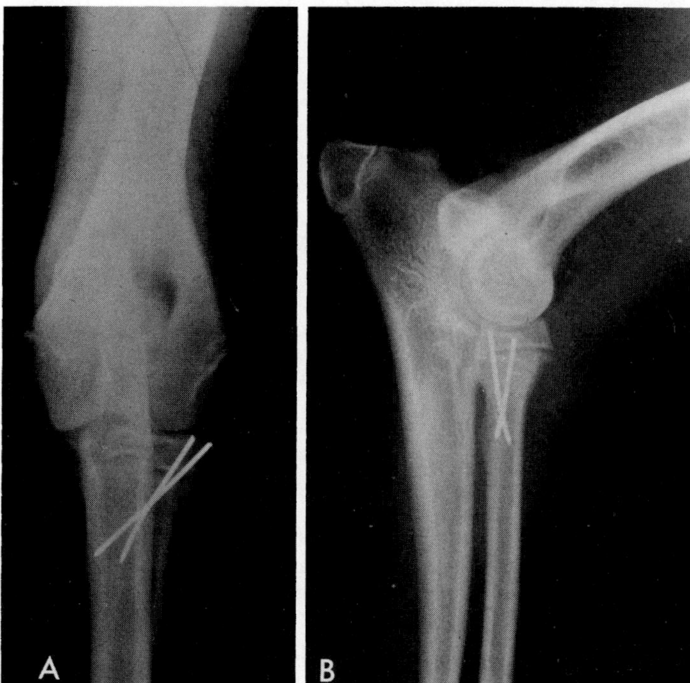

FIGURE 132–13. *A* and *B*, Fixation of a fracture separation of the proximal radial physis with two Kirschner wires.

young animals, with nonvehicular trauma such as horse kicks, bite wounds, and low-velocity gunshot injuries.[35] Because severe displacement of the fragments rarely occur, two views with high-quality radiographs are often needed for diagnosis (Fig. 132–14). Treatment with external coaptation in the form of a cast or splint is satisfactory in nearly all cases.

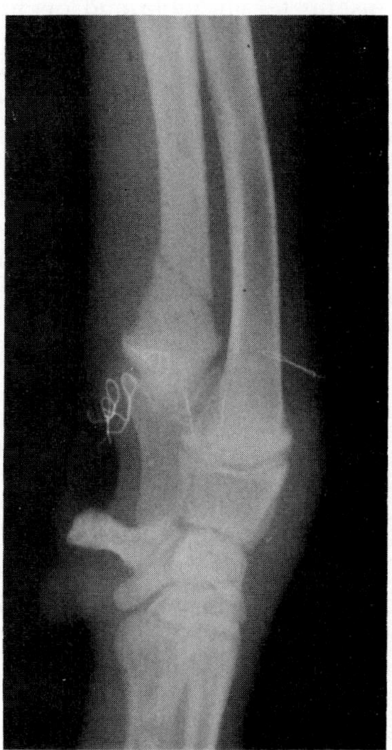

FIGURE 132–14. A minimally displaced ulnar fracture and intact radius.

SHAFT FRACTURES OF BOTH THE RADIUS AND ULNA

Fractures of both the radius and ulna are common.[36] Selection of a fixation technique depends on a patient's age and size, axial stability of the fracture, concurrent musculoskeletal injuries, and the condition of associated soft tissues. An algorithm is presented to aid in this selection (Fig. 132–15).

Transverse or short oblique fractures are resistant to axial compressive forces once reduced (stable). These fractures can often be treated with closed manipulation and external coaptation. Reduction is facilitated by early treatment (within 24 to 48 hours) and complete muscle relaxation with adequate anesthesia. Reduction can be facilitated using the "toggling" technique. The fracture angle is accentuated, and the fracture ends apposed. Straightening the fracture angle then toggles the ends together to complete reduction. Adequate reduction is usually considered to be at least 50 per cent fracture end alignment as the *worst* finding on two standard orthotopic radiographic views (Fig. 132–16). Although some cranial or caudal angulation is acceptable, valgus or varus (lateral or medial) angulation is carefully avoided because it can result in secondary arthritis from abnormal weightbearing. The reduced fracture can be stabilized with external coaptation in the form of a cylinder cast or Thomas splint. Specifically for antebrachial fractures, casts need to extend from the toes proximally to midway between the elbow and the point of the shoulder. Slight flexion of the carpal region may preclude the carpal hyperextension commonly seen after cast treatment in young animals.[33] The cast can often be cut down to distal of the elbow after early fracture consolidation in 4 to 6 weeks, allowing elbow motion

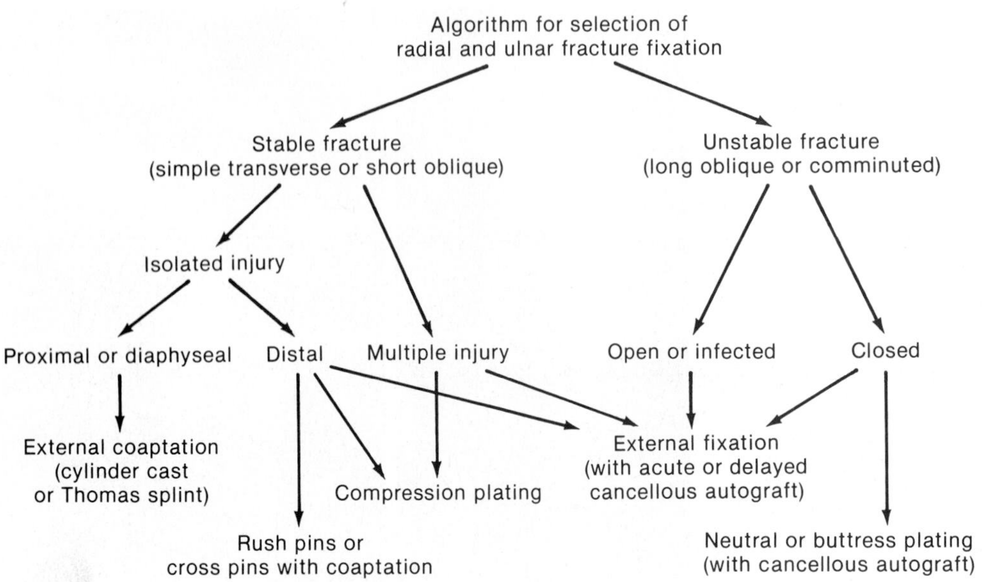

FIGURE 132–15. Algorithm for selection of radial and ulnar fracture fixation techniques.

and improving leg use. The cast is kept dry and monitored daily by the owner for swelling, chewing, and abrasions. Initially, weekly rechecks are suggested. The Thomas splint can be an effective means of coapting certain antebrachial fractures if properly applied. Thomas splints commonly hold the limb with the joints in excessive extension. Also, the splint makes ambulation difficult, and secondary decubital sores and abrasions are common. Primary treatment of antebrachial fractures with posterior or lateral splintage, either handmade or preformed (Mason Metasplint), is usually insufficiently stable and is discouraged. External coaptation of antebrachial fractures in toy and miniature canine breeds has been associated with a high rate (75 per cent) of nonunions and malunions.[28] Nonoperative manipulation of such small bones into reduction is difficult to achieve and maintain. Consequently, coaptation is not recommended in these animals.

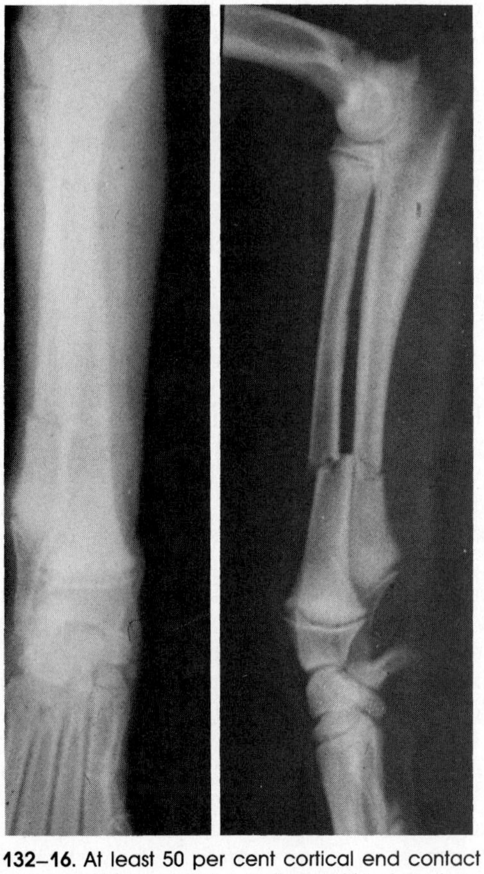

FIGURE 132–16. At least 50 per cent cortical end contact in both craniocaudal and lateromedial radiographic views is necessary for adequate closed reduction of antebrachial fractures.

External skeletal fixation can be used as an effective means of treating most antebrachial fractures and is particularly useful for unstable and open fractures. A fixator can be applied after either a closed reduction or with an open approach. Although a shorter fracture healing time has been reported with closed reduction,[23] an open approach improves fracture reduction and decreases the incidence of malunion. If open reduction is required, it is limited to just a few centimeters in length through a dorsal approach. The skin is incised just medial to the cephalic vein, and the extensor muscles retracted laterally.[36] The principles of external skeletal fixation are described in Chapter 123. The specific configuration to be used depends on the inherent stability and location of the fracture.[13] Relatively stable simple fractures can be treated with type I half-pin splintage applied to the cranial or medial aspect of the radius. Unstable comminuted or open fractures with large defects are best treated with a biplanar frame or type II full-pin splintage. A biplanar configuration allows pin fixation in two planes (Fig. 132–17), so it can be used on very short fragments where other forms of fixation do not have adequate bony purchase.[14] Type III (trilateral) splintage offers maximum resistance to fracture collapse and thus is particularly useful for highly comminuted or infected fractures that require prolonged fixation.[16] As in other methods of fixation, if open reduction of a comminuted fracture leaves defects, a

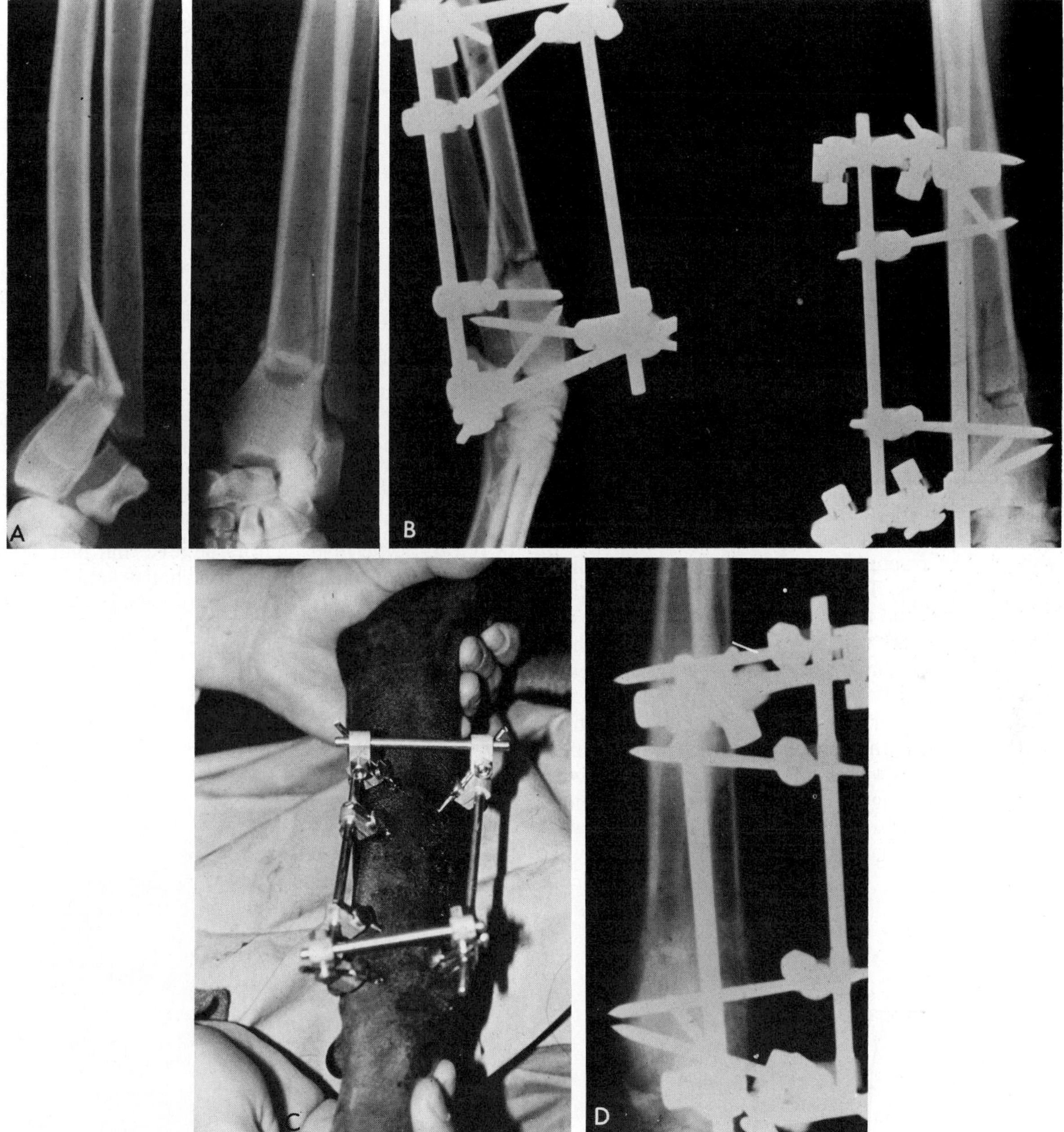

FIGURE 132–17. *A*, A distal radius and ulna fracture. *B*, Fixation with a biplanar, type I external fixator. *C*, Appearance of the fixator. *D*, Healed fracture 11 weeks after surgery.

cancellous autograft from the humeral greater tubercle is used to stimulate early callus formation.

Intramedullary pinning of radial fractures has for many years been an accepted method of treating antebrachial fractures. However, complications are common (80 per cent) for several reasons.[28] The small, oval medullary canal limits pin size and consequently the resistance of the repair to bending forces. Intramedullary pins are not inherently resistant to axial compression, so their use on unstable fractures frequently results in fracture collapse. Pin placement damages the endosteal blood supply of a bone notorious for avascular nonunions, particularly in small breeds.[9] Finally, insertion of a pin is difficult without damaging or limiting joint function. Intramedullary pinning of the radius is not recommended, because other more mechanically and biologically suitable means of fixation are commonly available.

Distal antebrachial fractures can be treated with Rush pin or cross-pin fixation of the radius. Rush pins avoid major damage to either the endosteal blood supply or the carpal joint (Fig. 132–18), but their application requires specialized equipment and can be difficult, particularly in smaller dogs. One report described treating simple oblique, distal metaphyseal fractures using cross pins and a cerclage wire with external casting.[18] Although the use of a single cerclage wire is generally discouraged,[17] in this situation, the coaptation controls bending forces while the internal fixation provides fracture stability. The fracture is reduced and temporarily held with bone forceps. The cerclage wire is applied and tightened to compress the fracture. The first pin is inserted through both cortices perpendicular to the fracture line. A second is inserted at a divergent angle to the first (Fig. 132–19).

Shaft fractures of the radius can be treated with bone screws and plates using the principles described in Chapter 122. Plating offers very stable fixation and allows immediate weightbearing, which is particularly useful in managing polytrauma with multiple limb injuries. Plating is also useful in managing distal radial and ulnar fractures in very small dogs because these fractures commonly heal slowly and can develop into atrophic nonunions if treated with coaptation or other methods that do not encourage normal weightbearing.[9, 28] Likewise, plating can be used to treat nonunions once they develop. Some investigators believe that plating is indicated for treatment of antebrachial fractures in immature dogs when external coaptation may result in hyperextension.[33] Plates are generally applied to the cranial surface of the radius through a cranial approach to the antebrachium.[36] The fracture is compressed to achieve maximum stability, either by applying tension on the

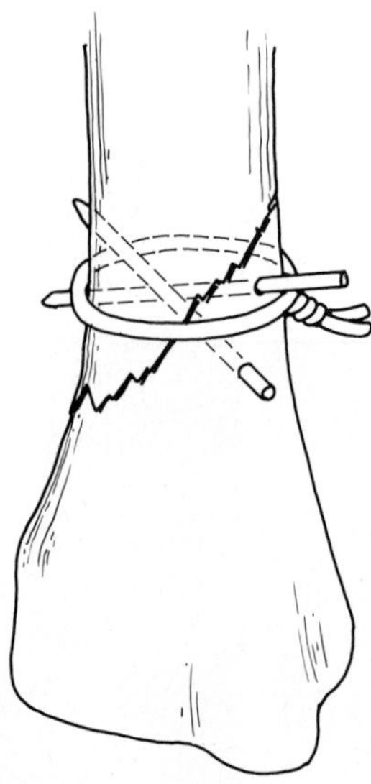

FIGURE 132–19. Fixation of a distal oblique antebrachial fracture with two cross pins and a cerclage wire.

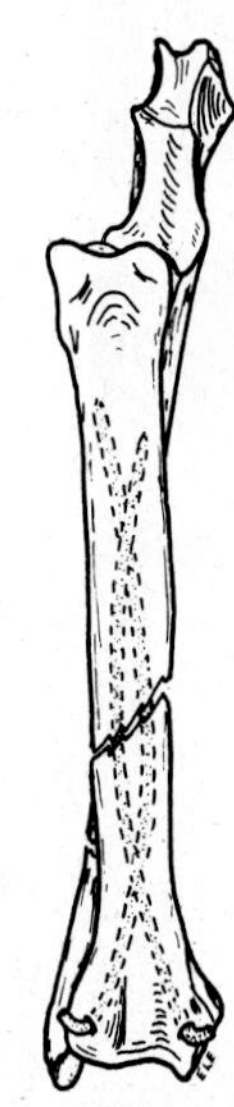

FIGURE 132–18. Fixation of a fractured distal radius and ulna using the flexible Rush pin technique.

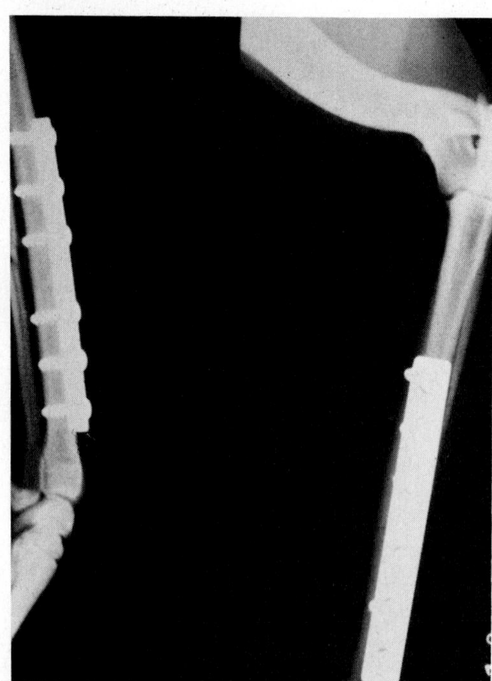

FIGURE 132–20. Compression plate fixation of a radial fracture, which allows early return of weightbearing.

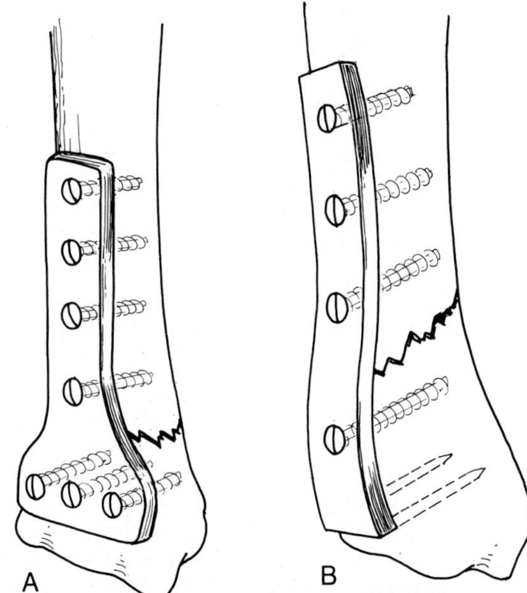

FIGURE 132–21. *A*, T-plate fixation of a very distal radial fracture allows adequate fixation of the short fragment by transverse screw orientation. *B*, Double-hook plate fixation of a similar distal fracture for larger dogs.

plate or by the use of interfragmentary screws (Fig. 132–20). For extremely distal fractures, a T plate that allows placement of two screws in the transverse plane is useful in cats and small dogs (Fig. 132–21), and a double-hook plate can be used in large dogs.[2] Cortical defects are packed with a cancellous autograft from the greater tubercle of the humerus. When treating a nonunion, avascular sclerotic bone is resected, the fracture ends of the medullary cavity are opened to allow vascular ingrowth, and a copious cancellous graft is added to induce callus formation. Removal of the plate is considered after the fracture has healed to avoid stress protection and cold sensitivity, approximately 5 to 14 months after fixation in mature dogs.[3] Refracture after plate removal varies, but less rigid plate designs reduce occurrence.[6, 11]

Interfragmentary or cerclage wires may help stabilize radial fractures. They do not control bending and should not be used as the primary means of fixation.[17] Passing the wires between the radius and ulna can be difficult, and the wires should not encompass both the radius and ulna because some motion persists and the wires loosen.

Simple antebrachial fractures are usually treated by primary fixation of the radius. Ulnar shaft fractures can also be stabilized to provide alignment and ancillary support of highly comminuted radial fractures. An intramedullary pin can be driven normograde down from the olecranon, and interfragmentary wire can be used to control rotation (Fig. 132–22).

FRACTURE SEPARATION OF THE DISTAL RADIAL PHYSIS

Fracture separations of the distal radial physis (Fig. 132–23), much like proximal physeal separations, can often be treated by closed reduction and external coaptation. If open reduction is needed, stabilization with small pins or Kirschner wires placed perpendicular to the physis is usually adequate (Fig. 132–24). A caudal splint may be applied for 10 to 14 days to control rotation and limit use of the limb. The pins are removed

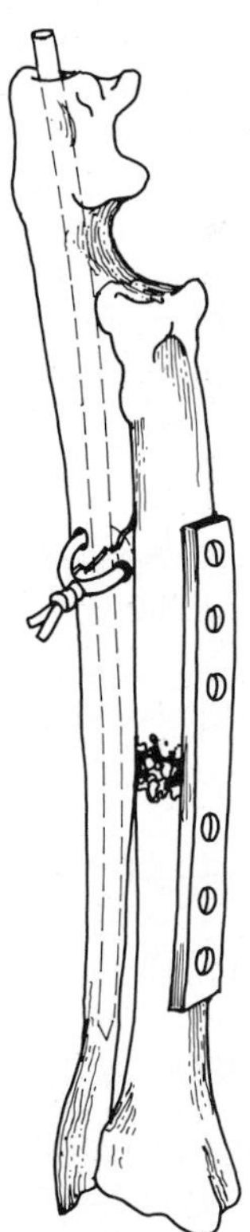

FIGURE 132–22. Fixation of a simple ulnar fracture with an intramedullary pin and interfragmentary wire to provide alignment and supplementary support of a highly comminuted, unstable radial fracture.

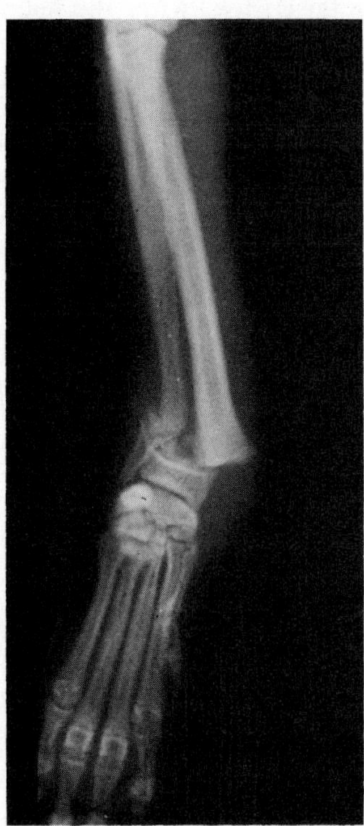

FIGURE 132–23. Fracture separation of the distal radial physis.

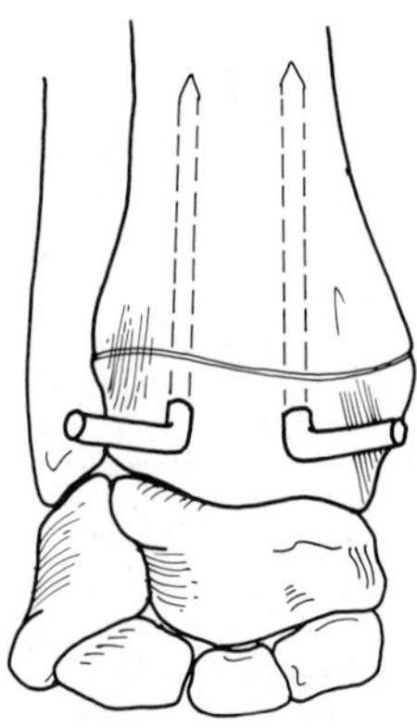

FIGURE 132–24. Fixation of a distal radial physis separation with two small pins oriented perpendicular to the growth plate.

in 3 to 4 weeks. As with proximal physeal injuries, the owner is advised of the possibility of premature physeal closure and secondary growth deformity.

FRACTURES OF THE DISTAL RADIUS AND ULNA

Major fractures into the radial articular surface can be treated with an interfragmentary lag screw or multiple divergent Kirschner wires as described for radial head fractures (Fig. 132–25). Avulsion fractures of either the radial or ulnar styloid processes result from pull on the corresponding collateral ligament (Fig. 132–26). Consequently, these fractures must be accurately reduced and stabilized to regain normal antebrachial carpal joint stability. The pin and tension band wire technique for treating olecranon avulsions works well in these cases. When treating radial avulsions, the pins are most stable when driven from the fragment across the medullary cavity into the far cortex. After the figure-eight wire is placed, the pins are cut, bent over, and buried in the collateral ligament (Fig. 132–27). A single pin is used to stabilize the fracture and to hook the tension band wire when treating ulnar avulsions (Fig. 132–28). Postoperative bandaging may be used to protect the repair, and exercise is restricted until the fracture heals. Pin and wire removal is indicated if they become loose or irritate the soft tissues after the fracture heals.

GROWTH ABNORMALITIES OF THE ANTEBRACHIUM

Deformities of the foreleg can occur for various reasons. The two-bone system of the antebrachium is predisposed to deformity caused by continued growth of one bone after premature growth cessation of the other. The bones normally elongate through the process of endochondral ossification, which occurs in the growth plate or physis.[39] The first layer of the physis adjacent to the epiphysis is called the *resting zone*. Cells in the resting zone are randomly arranged and are responsible for the production and storage of matrix and nutrients used by the other zones of the physis. The *proliferative zone* is adjacent to the resting zone and shares the same biochemical composition. The cells in the proliferative zone continuously replicate and produce new cartilage. As the new cartilage is produced, the older cartilage is "pushed" toward the metaphysis. The chondrocytes in the cartilage progressively mature, palisade, and hypertrophy in the *hypertrophic zone* as they progress away from the proliferative zone. Finally, the cartilage calcifies as the chondrocytes degenerate in the zone of *provisional calcification*. Chondroclasts and osteoblasts carried on invading metaphyseal capillary beds then replace the cartilage with bone. Closure of a physis occurs when the germinal cell layer stops producing new cartilage and the existing cartilage proceeds to hypertrophy, ossify, and be remodeled into bone. Premature closure of the distal ulnar physis is a recessive inheritable trait in Skye terriers,[30] and growth deformities have been seen with retardation of endochondral ossification in giant-breed dogs, possibly associated with osteochondrosis or nutritional deficiencies.[24] The most common cause of premature growth cessation is trauma to one of the physeal plates.[5] These injuries to the physis have been classified into five groups by Salter and Harris, based on the fracture's anatomical configuration.[41] A transverse fracture through the weak region of the hypertrophied and degenerating cartilage, which is being

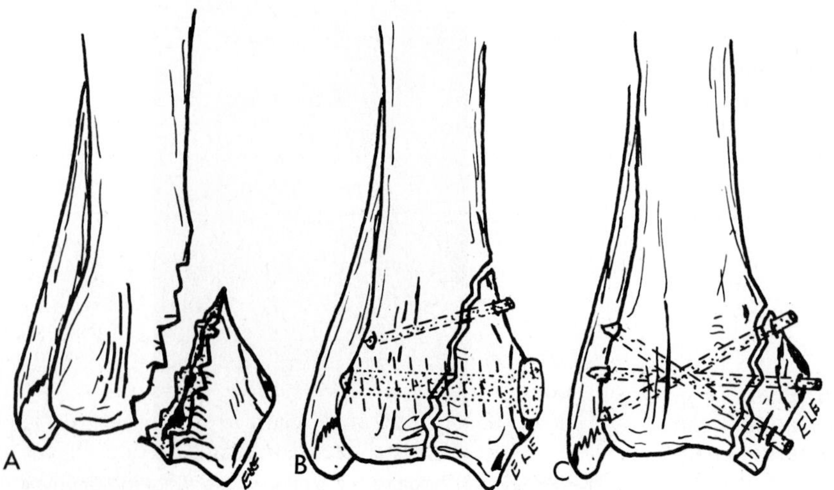

FIGURE 132–25. *A*, A distal radial articular fracture. *B*, Fixation with a lag screw and antirotational cross pin. *C*, Fixation with multiple divergent Kirschner wires.

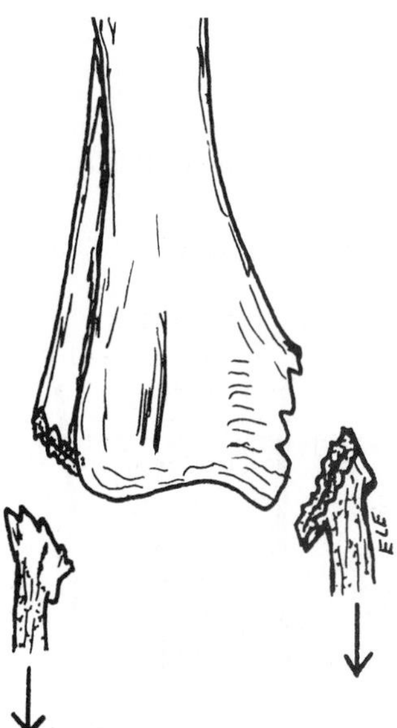

FIGURE 132–26. Avulsion fractures of the radial and ulnar styloid processes caused by traction from the corresponding collateral ligaments.

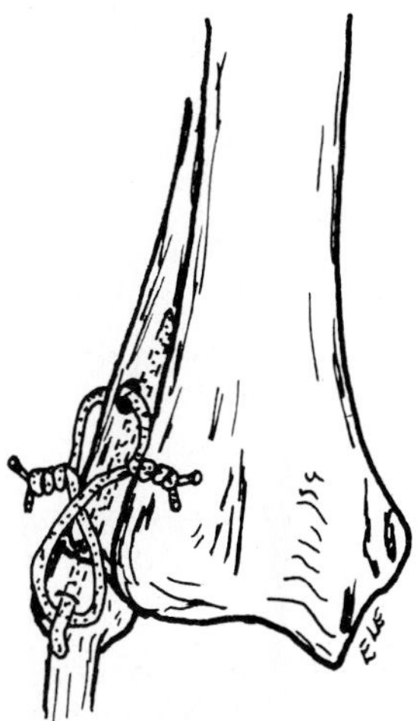

FIGURE 132–28. Fixation of an ulnar styloid avulsion fracture with a single pin and a tension band wire.

invaded by capillaries and chondroclasts, is called a Salter I fracture (slipped epiphysis) (Fig. 132–29*A*). A similar fracture that extends into the metaphyseal bone is called a Salter II (Fig. 132–29*B*). A fracture that is partially through the hypertrophied cartilage and extends through the germinal cell layer into the epiphysis is called a Salter III (Fig. 132–29*C*). A Salter IV fracture begins in the metaphysis and extends through the physis and epiphysis and into the joint (Fig. 132–29*D*). A Salter V fracture is a crushing injury to the chondroblastic cell layer (Fig. 132–29*E*). A Salter V fracture is not apparent on radiographic examination and often occurs with other injuries or Salter fractures. Consequently, Salter V fractures frequently are not diagnosed at the time of injury.

Fractures that damage the germinal cell layer have a higher incidence of premature growth cessation (closures).[41] Consequently, a Salter V crushing injury has a high incidence of premature closure. The prognosis for normal growth is also affected by the severity of fracture displacement.[31] This suggests that displacement causes damage to the vascular supply of the germinal cell layer. If sufficient vascular impedance occurs, cartilage production ceases and premature physeal closure ensues.

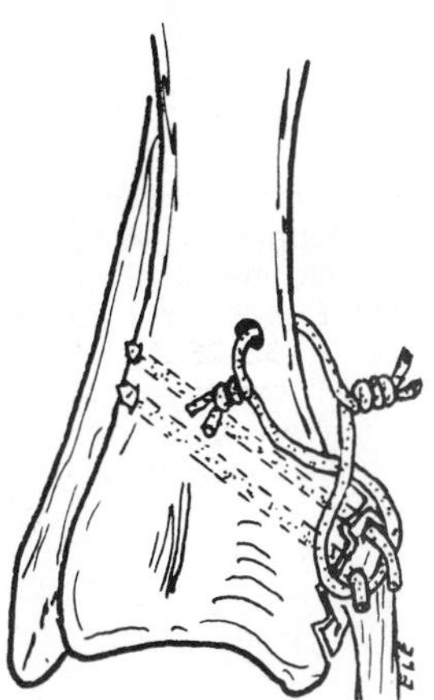

FIGURE 132–27. Fixation of a radial styloid avulsion fracture with two pins and a tension band wire.

Growth deformities of the canine antebrachium can result from injury to any one of three physes: distal ulnar, distal radial, or proximal radial. Each of these injuries has a specific set of resultant deformities, which are discussed independently. Not all of the changes associated with each physeal closure are seen in every clinical case. Angular deformities are seen more in the longer-limbed dogs, whereas shorter-limbed dogs develop more severe joint malarticulations. The age of the animal at the time of premature closure also affects the relative degree of deformity and joint malarticulation, perhaps because of the variation in stiffness of bone with age and the duration of altered growth until maturity. Growth deformities usually have a history of progressive limb angulation or lameness 3 to 4 weeks after forelimb trauma. Owners occasionally are unaware of the causative trauma. Growth deformities in cats are quite uncommon; congenital agenesis of the radius has been reported.[1]

Premature Closure of the Distal Ulnar Physis

The incidence of premature closure or fusion resulting in growth deformities is greatest in the distal ulnar growth plate of dogs.[32] This may be due to the conical configuration of the distal ulnar physis. A transverse force applied to a horizontal physis (e.g., distal radius) results in a Salter I fracture through the hypertrophied cartilage. A transverse force applied to the distal ulna compresses one side of the cone, causing damage to the germinal layer of chondroblasts in the proliferative zone (Salter V fracture), cessation of cartilage production, and premature closure.

Growth deformities that result from premature distal ulnar physeal closure are particularly severe because this physis contributes 75 to 85 per cent of ulnar longi-

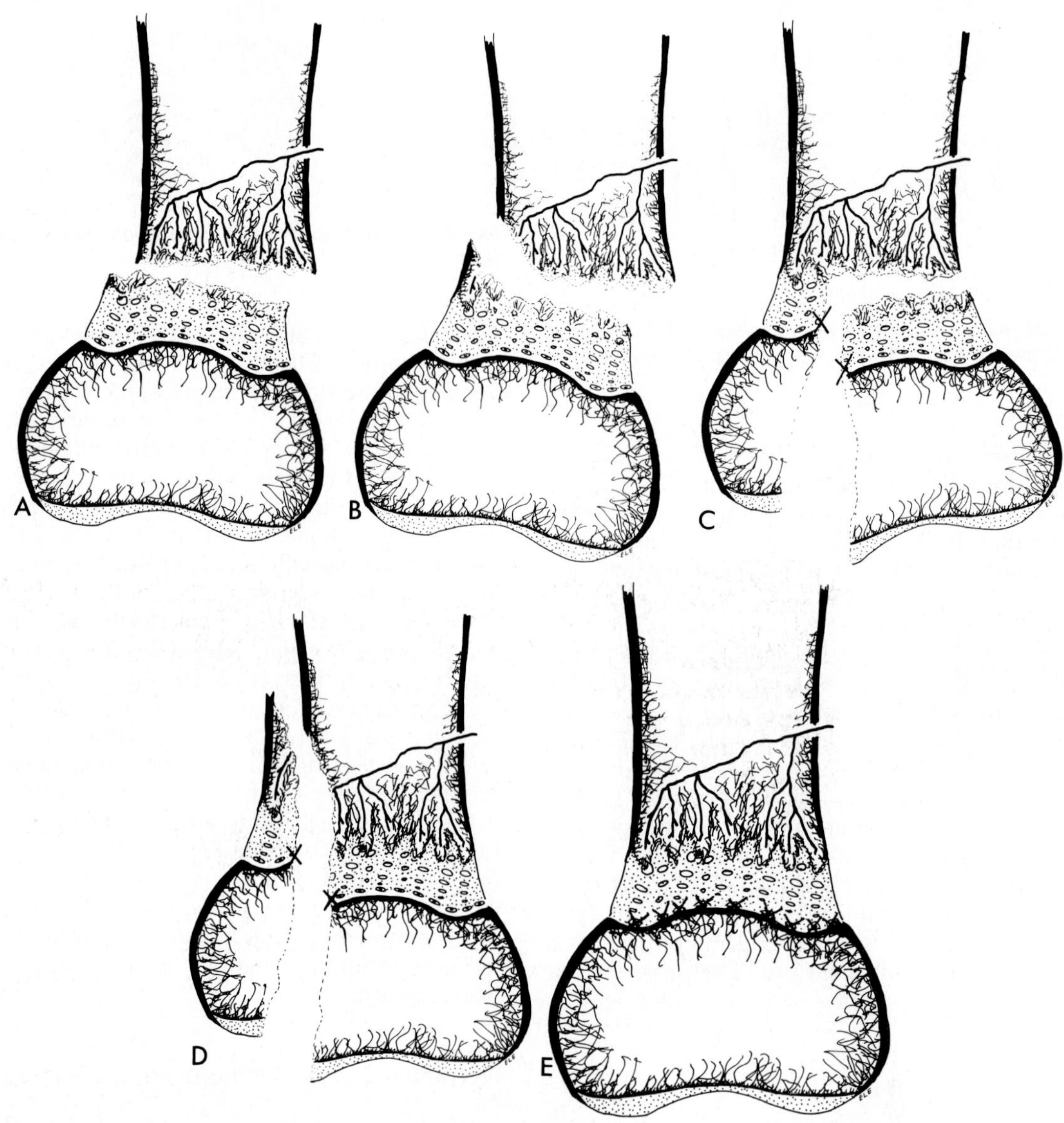

FIGURE 132–29. *A*, A Salter I fracture cleaves transversely through the region of cartilage hypertrophy and degeneration. *B*, A Salter II fracture cleaves transversely through the hypertrophied cartilage and extends into the metaphysis. *C*, A Salter III fracture cleaves transversely through the hypertrophied cartilage and extends through the proliferative zone into the epiphysis. *D*, A Salter IV fracture cleaves longitudinally from the metaphysis through the physis and epiphysis into the joint. *E*, A Salter V fracture crushes germinal chondroblastic cell layer.

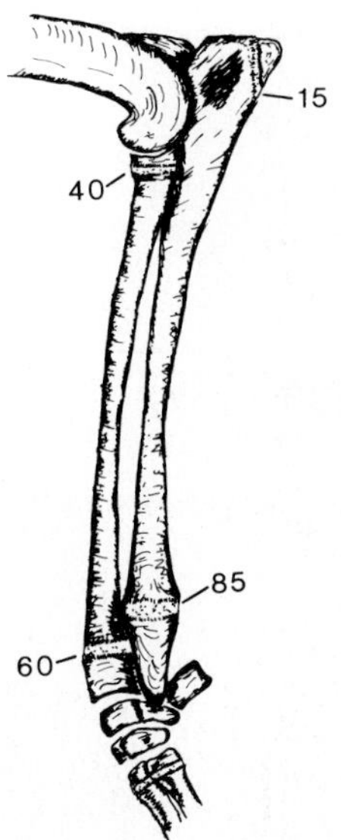

FIGURE 132–30. The relative contributions of the physes to the longitudinal growth of the radius and ulna.

tudinal growth (Fig. 132–30).[5] The characteristic deformities reflect the two-bone anatomy of the forelimb. The ulna extends from a medial position at the elbow, obliquely across the long axis of the forelimb to a lateral position at the carpus, slightly caudal to the radius. Once the physis has fused, ulnar growth ceases and the ulna behaves like a retarding strap twisted around the radius. As the radius continues to grow, it bows away from the ulna. Three deformities of the radius result: lateral deviation (valgus), cranial bowing (curvus), and external rotation (supination) (Fig. 132–31). This discrepancy in growth results in caudolateral subluxation of the radial carpal joint, which causes stretching of the medial soft-tissue supporting structures. The radial head may also push the humeral condyles out of the trochlear notch of the ulna. Abnormal articulations resulting in irreversible degenerative osteoarthritis in the antebrachial carpal joint and the elbow are common sequelae. The net effect of the retarding strap effect of the ulna and the radial deformities is a relative shortening of limb length compared with the contralateral normally growing limb (Fig. 132–32). The appropriate treatment for antebrachial deformities due to premature ulnar closure depends on the patient's age and remaining growth potential.

Treatment of Distal Ulnar Physeal Closure in Immature Dogs

Animals that have a significant amount of radial growth potential remaining (usually less than 5 to 6 months of age) are treated with a technique that relieves the restraining effect of the ulna and allows the radius continued growth. Ulnar release permits lengthening of the limb and can result in partial correction of existing deformity.[43] This self-correction has been attributed to accelerated physeal growth on the concave side of the bone once the retarding strap is removed.[25] The simplest of these techniques is a segmental ulnar ostectomy, which can easily be performed through a caudal approach to the ulna.[36] Approximately 2 cm of the distal ulnar metaphysis is removed using an oscillating bone saw or Gigli wire. To prevent bony bridging of the gap and reformation of the restraining band, all of the associated periosteum must also be removed.[10] In addition, some investigators suggest implanting a free autogenous fat graft into the ostectomy site.[8] The interposed fat retards bone union by acting as a barrier to vascular invasion and secondary osteoblastic proliferation (Fig. 132–33).[46] An ample quantity of fat is carefully harvested from a separate incision over the gluteal region. The graft should be one piece and carefully handled to avoid trauma, which might result in necrosis. This fat is placed

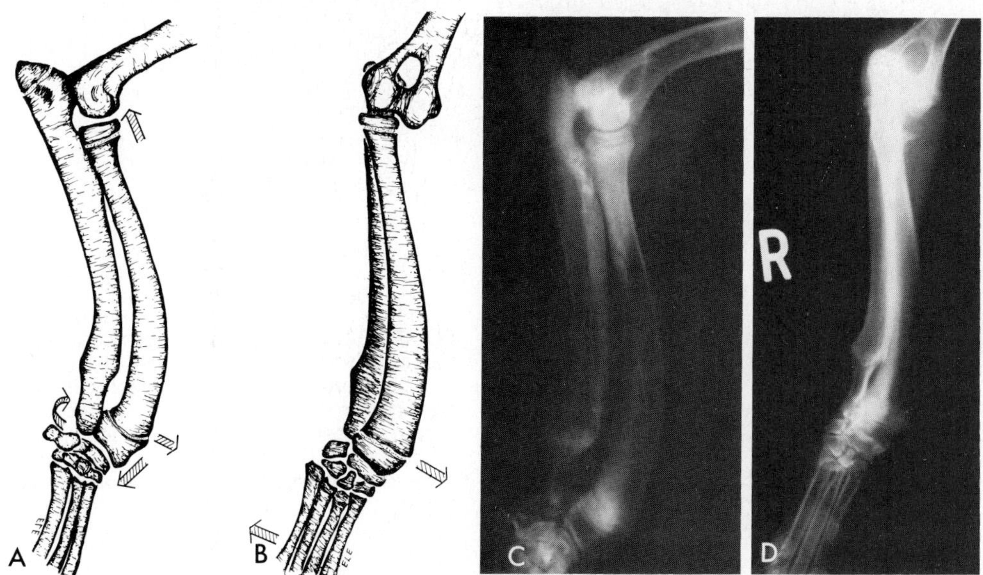

FIGURE 132–31. *A* to *D*, Valgus, cranial bowing (curvus), and external rotation (supination) deformities that occur after premature closure of the distal ulnar physis and continued radial growth.

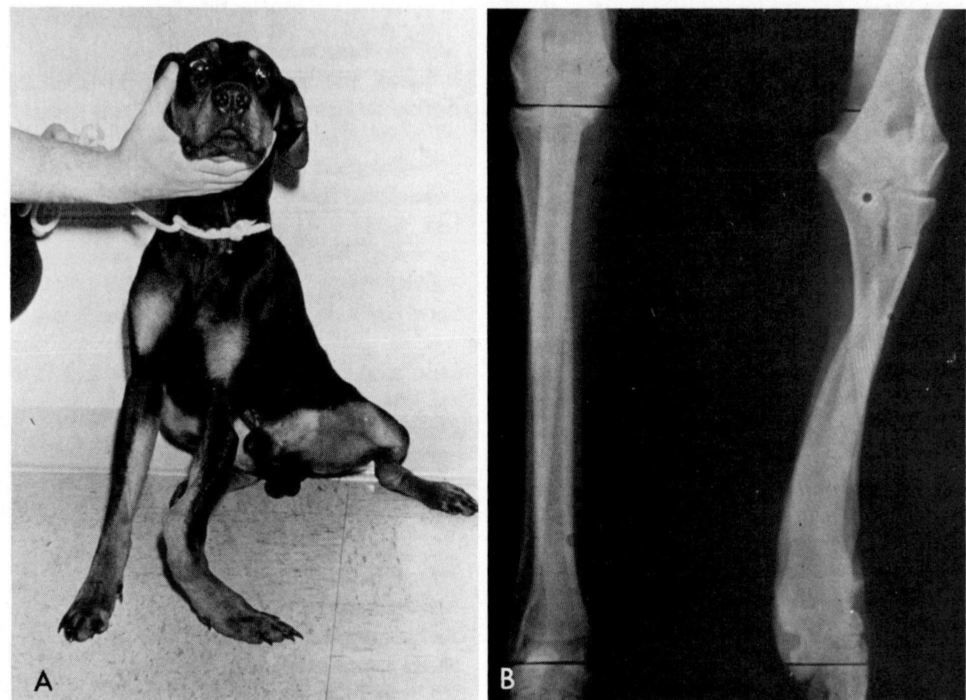

FIGURE 132–32. *A* and *B*, The absolute and functional relative shortening of leg length caused by premature closure of the distal ulnar physis.

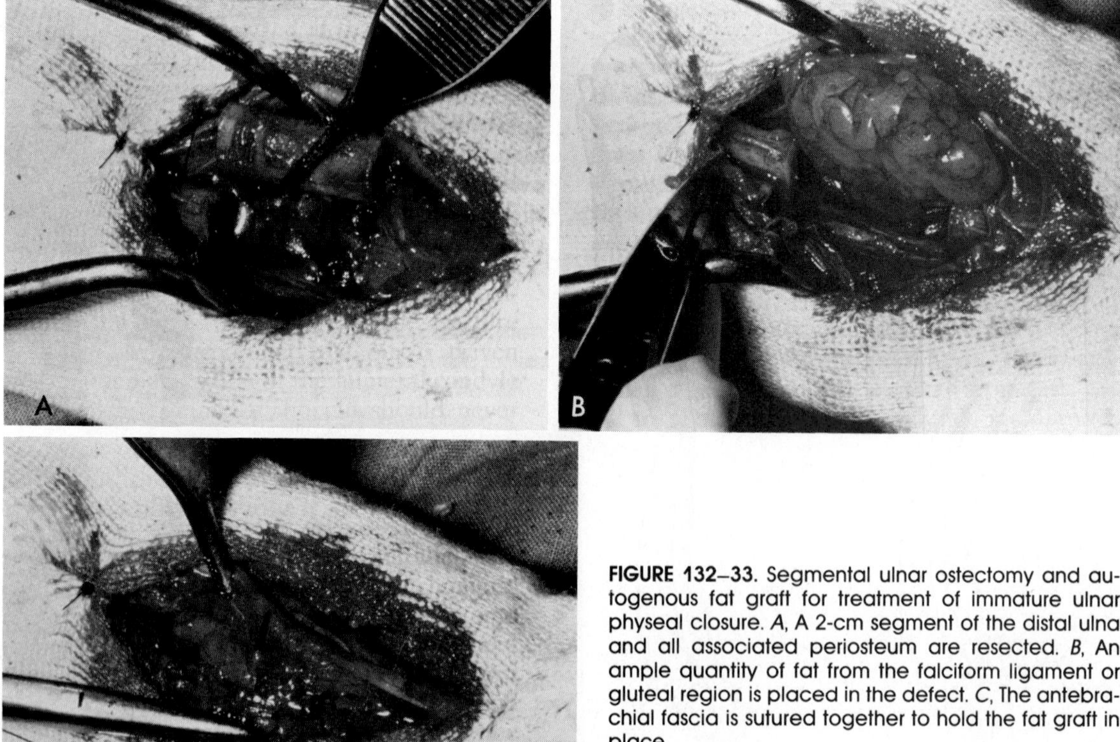

FIGURE 132–33. Segmental ulnar ostectomy and autogenous fat graft for treatment of immature ulnar physeal closure. *A*, A 2-cm segment of the distal ulna and all associated periosteum are resected. *B*, An ample quantity of fat from the falciform ligament or gluteal region is placed in the defect. *C*, The antebrachial fascia is sutured together to hold the fat graft in place.

in the ulnar defect, and the deep antebrachial fascia is sutured together to hold the graft in place.

The prognosis for adequate long-term function and completeness of spontaneous straightening obtained with segmental ulnar ostectomy depended on both the severity of the deformity and the remaining growth potential of the radius.[43] Young puppies (median age of 5 months) with a valgus deformity of more than 25° and dogs near growth completion (median age of 6.5 months) with valgus deformities of more than 13 ° did not adequately respond to just a segmental ulnar ostectomy and required further definitive surgical treatment.

In summary, *early* diagnosis and dynamic treatment of premature ulnar closure offers the best prognosis for normal leg length, straightness, and function.

Definitive Correction of Ulnar Physeal Closure in Mature Dogs

If bone growth has ceased, definitive treatment is indicated. This treatment consists of two components if needed. The first is correction of the angular and rotational deformities. Several techniques for corrective osteotomy are available.[40] Whichever technique is used for angular deformity treatment, the correction is performed at the point of greatest curvature to provide the desired articular alignment with the best overall limb straightening (Fig. 132–34). Angular correction at another point in the limb yields an S-shaped antebrachium.

Oblique osteotomies stabilized with external skeletal fixation result in some restoration of leg length, can be applied to short and irregular fragments, and allow significant adjustment of alignment during surgery.[40] The limb is prepared and draped so the elbow, carpus, and paw can be palpated and manipulated during surgery. A traditional double connecting clamp type I (unilateral) configuration can be used; I prefer the modified type II configuration for its greater stability[13] and application technique, which assists osteotomy alignment (Fig. 132–35). The most proximal and distal fixation pins are driven in full-pin fashion from lateral to medial, parallel to the elbow and antebrachial carpal joints, respectively. The lateral surface of the ulnar shaft is approached through a small longitudinal incision.[36] The bone is cut with an oscillating saw or osteotome, and the incision is closed. The cranial surface of the radius is approached through a separate longitudinal incision.[36] An oblique osteotomy is performed with a saw at the level of greatest deformity and parallel to the radial carpal joint line. The appropriate connecting clamps and bars necessary for a type II full-pin splint configuration are loosely attached to the fixation pins. The distal point of the proximal radial fragment is impacted into the medullary cavity of the distal fragment. The cranial bowing, valgus, and particularly the external rotation are manually corrected and checked by flexing the elbow and antebrachial carpal joints. The connecting clamps on the proximal and distal fixation pins are tightened. The intermediate pins are then driven either as half pins or full pins through the remaining open connecting clamps. The clamps are tightened, and incisions closed. External skeletal fixation can also be used to stabilize very short fragments by using a biplanar configuration.[14]

Cuneiform wedge ostectomies provide a wide, flat surface for fragment contact, significantly contributing to fixation stability and bone healing.[40] Although a wedge ostectomy does not increase the anatomical limb length, correction of the valgus deformity increases the functional length of the limb. The cuneiform ostectomy is a wedge with an angle in both the craniocaudal plane and the mediolateral plane. The angle of these wedges can be determined by drawing perpendicular lines to the long axis of the proximal and distal fragments (Fig. 132–36). Exsanguination of the limb with a sterile elastic wrap and a tourniquet applied above the elbow reduces hemorrhage and improves surgical visibility results in significantly increased postoperative swelling. The measured angles are translated into a single three-dimensional wedge, which is created by performing two ostectomies that intersect at the caudolateral cortex of the radius. The ulna is cut to remove its restraining effect. The resected radial wedge is closed to reduce the angular deformities, and the external rotation corrected by internally rotating the distal fragment and paw. If the fragments are adequate in length, the osteotomy is stabilized with a standard bone plate and screws.[20]

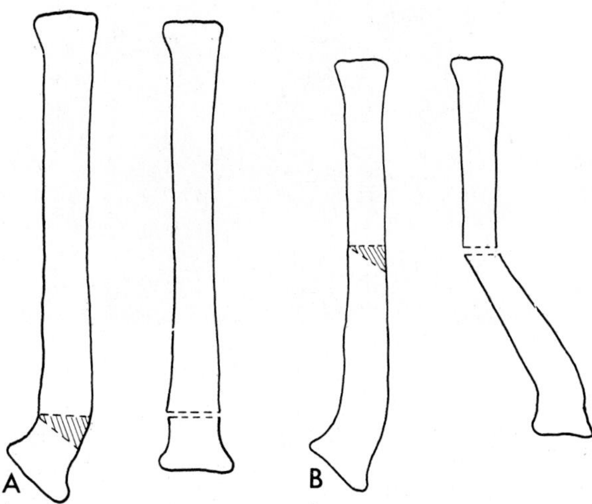

FIGURE 132–34. *A*, Location of a corrective osteotomy at the level of greatest curvature to achieve maximum correction. *B*, The S-shaped antebrachium that results from performing the osteotomy at another level.

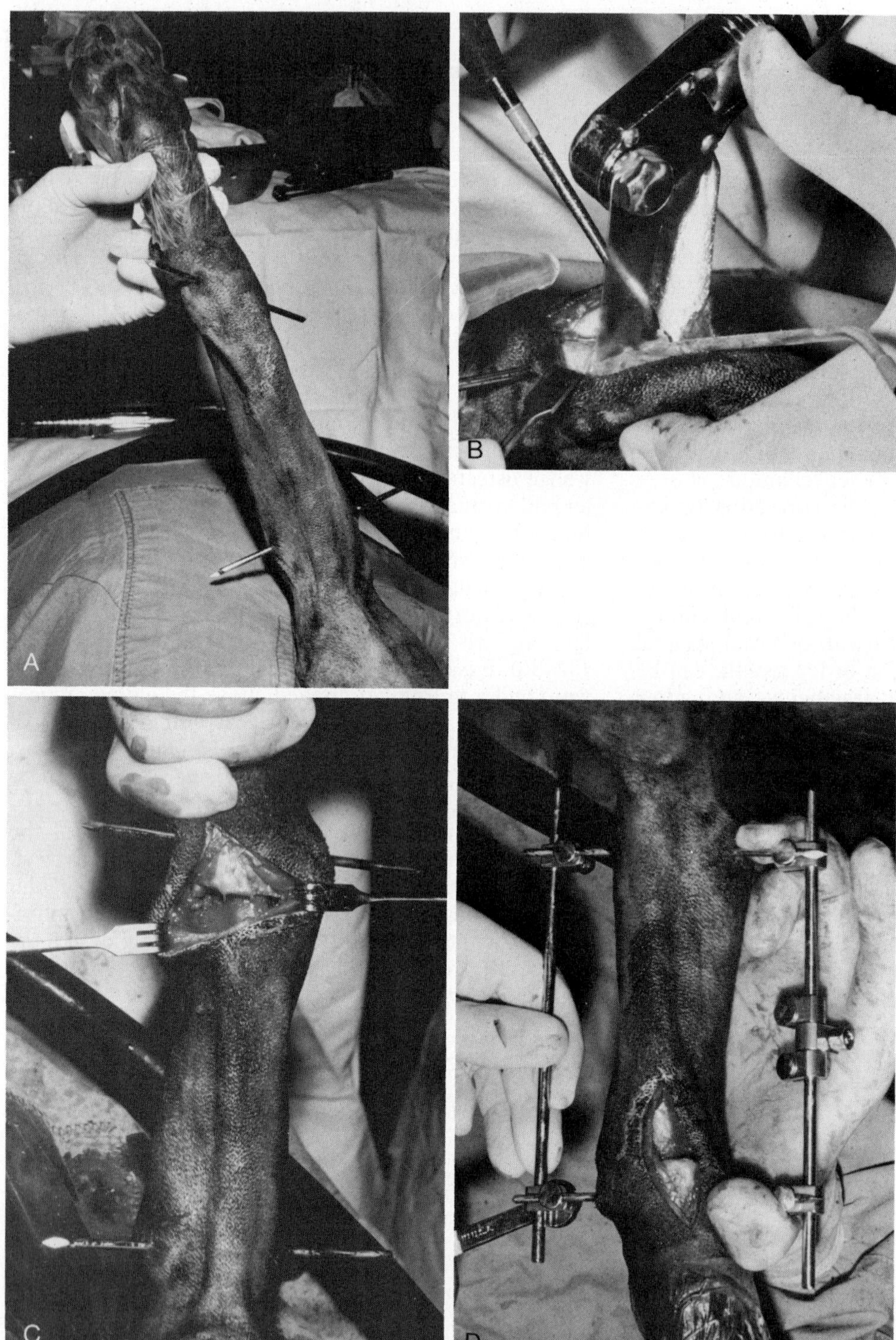

FIGURE 132–35. Oblique osteotomy for definitive correction of a premature ulnar physeal closure. *A*, The most proximal and distal fixation pins are inserted parallel to the rotational axis of the elbow and antebrachial-carpal joints, respectively. *B*, Transverse ulnar and oblique radial osteotomies are performed at the level of greatest deformity. *C*, The distal spike of the proximal fragment is impacted into the medullary canal of the distal fragment, and correction of the deformity is obtained by manipulating the two fixation pins into parallel alignment. *D*, Connecting bars, clamps, and additional fixation pins are applied to create a type II external fixator.

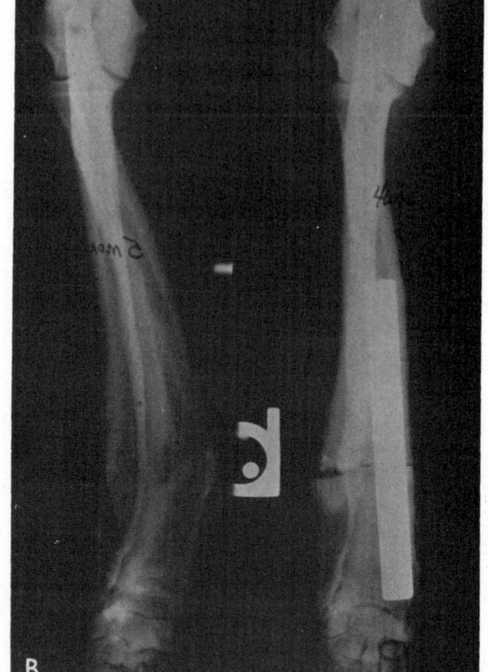

FIGURE 132–36. *A*, Determining the appropriate angle for correcting deformities by wedge ostectomy. *B*, The ostectomy can be stabilized with a bone plate and screws if the fragments are adequate in length. (*B* courtesy of Dr. S.G. Stoll.)

Alternatively, a T plate or double-hook plate can be used.

The second component of treating a mature deformity is treatment of the humeroulnar subluxation by repositioning the elbow articular components. Because the affected limb is already shortened, lengthening of the ulna is more appropriate than shortening the radius. One report describes using a dynamic proximal ulnar osteotomy for this purpose (Fig. 132–37).[19] A caudal approach is made to the shaft of the ulna and the trochlear notch.[35] In severe cases, the elbow joint is examined for fibrosis and osseous proliferation, which is resected or remodeled. A 30° oblique ulnar osteotomy is performed with an oscillating bone saw or Gigli wire, starting just distal to the coronoid and extending proximally toward the caudal ulnar cortex. The osteotomy usually widens spontaneously from the muscular and ligamentous pull, but a periosteal elevator may be needed to break down the interosseous ligament. A small intramedullary pin is inserted normograde from

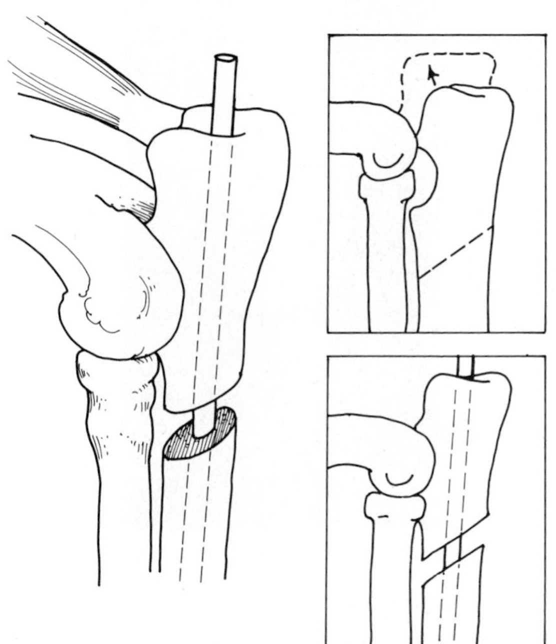

FIGURE 132–37. Dynamic proximal ulnar osteotomy performed for realignment of the elbow joint articulation.

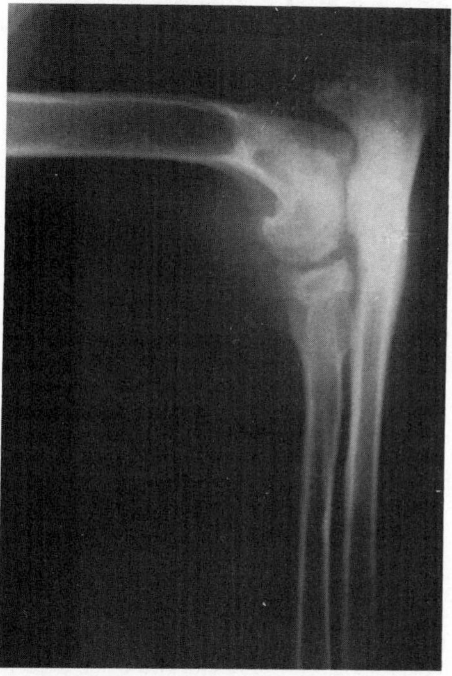

FIGURE 132–38. Elbow malarticulation from distal displacement the radial head caused by premature closure of the proximal radial physis.

the olecranon across the osteotomy. This ensures axial alignment while allowing continued osteotomy distraction and elbow realignment. Early postoperative elbow joint motion is encouraged to maximize elbow mobility and articular remodeling.

Premature Radial Physeal Closure

Either the proximal or the distal radial physis can prematurely cease growing and cause antebrachial abnormalities.[5] Premature closure of the proximal radial physis with continued ulnar growth results in malarticulation of the elbow joint, characterized by widening of the radial to humeral space and the humeral to anconeal joint space (Fig. 132–38). Severe malformation of the articular components with secondary arthritis rapidly develops. Decreased longitudinal growth causes shortening of the limb relative to the normal limb in some cases. The abnormalities that result from premature closure of the distal radial physis can be quite variable (Fig. 132–39). If ulnar growth continues, the elbow malarticulation just described for proximal clo-

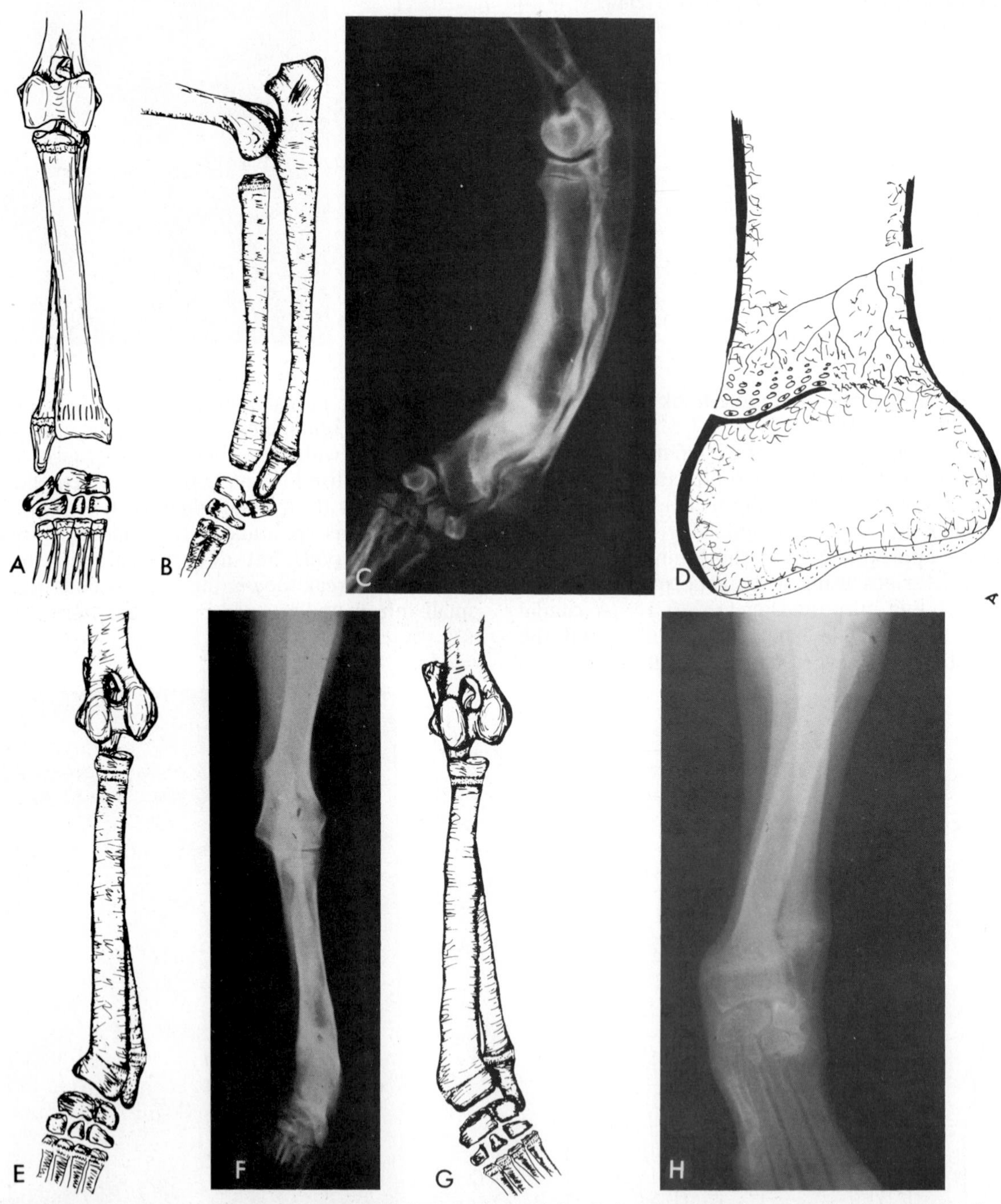

FIGURE 132–39. Abnormalities resulting from premature closure of the distal radial physis. *A*, Radial carpal joint malarticulation. *B* and *C*, Caudal radial and ulnar bowing. *D*, Angular deformity from asymmetrical premature closure of a physis and continued growth of the balance. *E* and *F*, Varus angular deformity from premature closure of the medial side of the distal radial physis. *G* and *H*, Valgus deformity from premature closure of the lateral side of the distal radial physis.

sures is common. If a complete symmetrical premature closure of the physis occurs, the limb may remain straight and develop a widened radial carpal joint space, or a caudal bow may develop in both the radius and ulna. More commonly, the physeal closure is asymmetrical, with bony bridging on one side of the physis and continued growth of the opposite. Premature closure of the medial side of the physis causes a varus angular deformity and occasionally inward rotation of the manus. Premature closure of the lateral side of the physis causes valgus angular deformity and external rotation, characteristic of premature distal ulnar physeal closure with which it is often concurrent.

Treatment of Radial Physeal Closure in Immature Dogs

Dynamic treatment of radial growth deformities before closure of the distal ulnar and remaining radial growth plate has three objectives: maintaining alignment of the elbow articular components, developing maximum antebrachial length, and correcting or preventing angular deformities. With complete symmetrical or advanced asymmetrical physeal closures, these objectives are met by progressive spreading of a radial osteotomy. A Kirschner[38] or Charnley[26] apparatus has been used for this purpose. However, the ring fixator designs (Fig. 132–40) are better suited for this application because of their ability to be adjusted simultaneously in all planes and rotation.[29] After the appropriate fixation pins are placed, the radius is osteotomized through a cranial approach,[36] at the point of greatest curvature. The fixation device is completed, and the osteotomy is spread to the limits of the surrounding soft tissues. Complete reduction of elbow malarticulation and angular deformity is not immediately necessary. These corrections are continued as the apparatus is distracted. Research with dogs using a ring fixator found a distraction rate of 1 mm a day to be optimal for elongation and regeneration of new bone.[21] A greater frequency of distraction gave the best results, and four times a day was suggested.[21] Excessive spreading tension should not be put on the fixation at any one time, because the bones are soft and the fixation pins can cut through the bone. The leg should be frequently examined radiographically to evaluate elbow reduction and ulnar physeal status. The fixation device may have to be replaced if extended spreading is required for more than 6 to 8 weeks. External support is maintained for several weeks after the external skeletal fixation device is removed, while the radius strengthens.

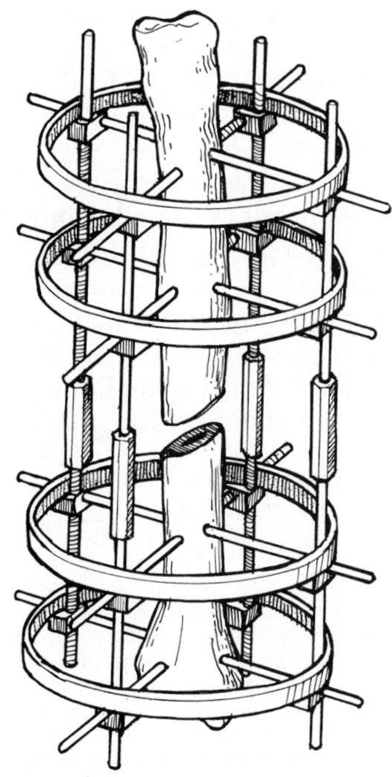

FIGURE 132–40. Ring fixator used for simultaneous limb lengthening and deformity correction.

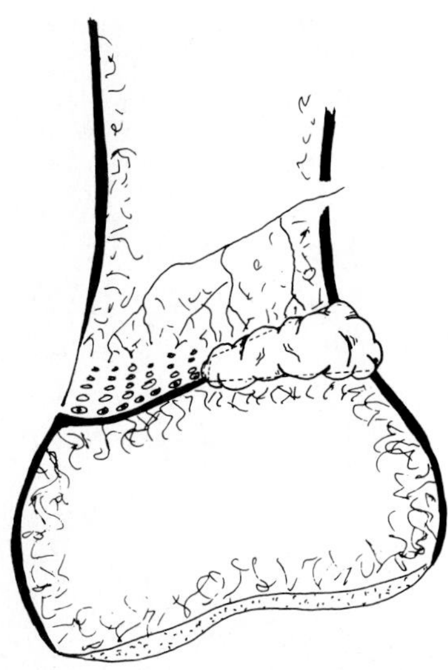

FIGURE 132–41. Treatment of an asymmetrical premature closure by bony bridge resection and implantation of an autogenous fat graft.

Segmental ostectomy of the radius has been described as a simpler means of obtaining radial length if the ulna is still growing.[22] As described for ulnar ostectomy, a 2-cm length of the radius and periosteum is removed. The continued pull of the ulna results in radial elongation and elbow joint realignment. Although no problems with fracture of the ulna were noted,[22] postoperative support and careful restriction of activity are advised until the ulna hypertrophies enough for full weightbearing. At maturity, the ostectomy site may require cancellous autografting and fixation to obtain radial union.*

Early asymmetrical closure of the distal radial physis can be treated by resection of the osseous bridge and imposition of an autogenous fat graft.[46] The margins of the osseous bridge are determined by palpation with a 25-gauge needle. The bone bridge is resected with a curette, and the defect packed with a fat graft obtained from the flank (Fig. 132–41). The graft is held in place

*Section editor's note: My experience with partial radial ostectomy in young puppies has been disappointing. Ulnar growth is insufficient to maintain length, and radioulnar synostosis is a consistent complication.

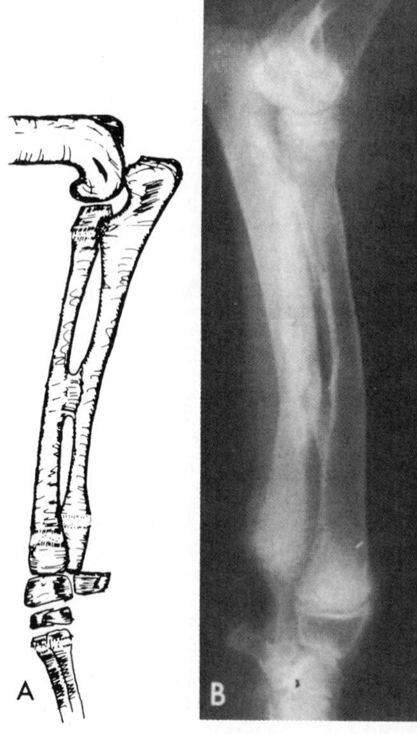

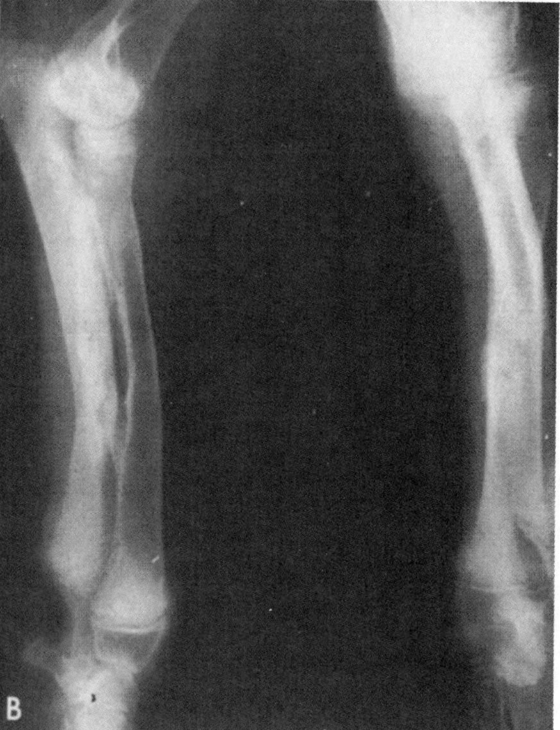

FIGURE 132–42. Elbow malarticulation and arthritis secondary to synostosis of the radius and ulna.

by suturing the adjacent soft tissues over the area. Significant remaining angular deformities may need to be treated with a corrective osteotomy.

Definitive Treatment of Radial Physeal Closure in Mature Dogs

Definitive treatment of premature radial physeal closures realigns elbow articular components and straightens angular deformities. The elbow can be realigned by spreading an osteotomy of the radius. Exploration of the elbow joint may be needed to resect excessive fibrous tissue and remodel osseous malformation and proliferation. After distraction of the osteotomy and realignment of the elbow articular components, the osteotomy is stabilized with an external fixator as described for immature radial physeal closures. Correction of angular deformities can usually be accomplished simultaneously by locating the lengthening osteotomy at the point of greatest curvature and progressively straightening the limb as it is lengthened.

Synostosis of the Radius and Ulna in Growing Dogs

Synostosis of the radius and ulna is not a disease of the physeal growth plates but a restriction in the relative proximal movement of the ulnar shaft that normally occurs during growth.[5] This movement reflects the virtually total contribution to ulnar length by the distal ulnar physis, while the contribution to radial length is nearly equal between the proximal and distal radial growth plates. When this movement is restricted, a relative overgrowth of the proximal radius occurs, with proximal displacement of the humeral condyles and trochlear notch deformation (Fig. 132–42). Significant shortening, angular deformity, or antebrachial carpal joint alterations usually do not occur. The strong pull of the distal ulnar growth through the radioulnar ligament apparently stimulates additional growth from the distal radial physis.[5] Synostosis of the radius and ulna is usually associated with a bridging callus following inadequate reduction of a fracture of the radius and ulna. Internal fixation devices such as fixation pins or bone screws that transfix both bones when treating fractures can also cause this.

Treatment of synostosis is removal of the restricting element and realignment of the elbow joint. Transfixing pins or screws are removed. Bridging callus can be resected, and the defect filled with an autogenous fat graft to prevent reformation. A dynamic proximal ulnar osteotomy is performed to treat the elbow malarticulation.[19] The osteotomy defect is implanted with an autogenous fat graft if the animal is still growing.

References

1. Alexander JW: Agenesis of the radius. *In* Slatter DH (ed): *Textbook of Small Animal Surgery*. W.B. Saunders, Philadelphia, 1985, pp 2316–2317.
2. Bellah JR: Use of a double hook plate for treatment of a distal radial fracture in a dog. *Vet Surg 16*:278, 1987.
3. Brinker WO, et al: Removal of bone plates in small animals. *J Am Anim Hosp Assoc 11*:577, 1975.
4. Brinker WO, et al: *Handbook of Small Animal Orthopedics and Fracture Treatment*. 2nd ed. W. B. Saunders, Philadelphia, 1990, pp. 197–208.
5. Carrig CB, Wortman JA: Acquired dysplasias of the canine radius and ulna. *Comp Cont Educ 3*:557, 1981.

6. Chapman MW, et al: Compression-plate fixation of acute fractures of the diaphyses of the radius and ulna. *J Bone Joint Surg [Am] 71A*:159, 1989.
7. Clark DM: Treatment of open comminuted intraarticular fractures of the proximal ulna in dogs. *J Am Anim Hosp Assoc 23*:331, 1987.
8. Craig E: Autogenous fat grafts to prevent recurrence following surgical correction of growth deformities of the radius and ulna in the dog. *Vet Surg 10*:69, 1981.
9. DeAngelis MP, et al: Repair of fractures of the radius and ulna in small dogs. *J Am Anim Hosp Assoc 9*:436, 1973.
10. DeCamp CE, et al: Periosteum and the healing of partial ulnar ostectomy in radius curvus of dogs. *Vet Surg 15*:185, 1986.
11. Deluca PA, et al: Refracture of bones of the forearm after the removal of compression plates. *J Bone Joint Surg [Am] 70A*:1372, 1988.
12. Dieterich HF: Personal communication, 1983.
13. Egger EL: Static strength evaluation of six external skeletal fixation configurations. *Vet Surg 12*:130, 1983.
14. Egger EL, et al: Type I biplanar configuration of external skeletal fixation: Application technique in nine dogs and one cat. *J Am Vet Med Assoc 187*:262, 1985.
15. Evans HE, Christensen GC: *Miller's Anatomy of the Dog*. 2nd ed. W. B. Saunders, Philadelphia, 1979, pp 182–185.
16. Foland ML, Egger EL: Application of type III of external skeletal fixation. A review of 23 clinical fractures in 20 dogs and 2 cats. *J Am Anim Hosp Assoc 27*:193, 1991.
17. Gambardella PC: Full cerclage wires for fixation of long bone fractures. *Comp Cont Educ 2*:665, 1980.
18. Gambardella PC, Griffiths RC: A technique for repair of oblique fractures of the distal radius in dogs. *J Am Anim Hosp Assoc 20*:429, 1984.
19. Gilson SD, et al: Treatment of humeroulnar subluxation with a dynamic proximal ulnar osteotomy; a review of 13 cases. *Vet Surg 18*: 114, 1989.
20. Hurov L: Surgical correction of acquired forelimb growth deformities in an immature doberman pinscher by multiple osteotomies and radial plating: A case report. *J Am Anim Hosp Assoc 19*:659, 1983.
21. Ilizarov GA: The tension-stress effect on the genesis and growth of tissues: Part II. The influence of the rate and frequency of distraction. *Clin Orthop Rel Res 239*:263, 1989.
22. Johnson AL: Correction of radial and ulnar growth deformities resulting from premature physeal closure. *In* Bojrab MJ (ed): *Current Techniques in Small Animal Surgery*. 3rd ed. Lea & Febiger, Philadelphia, 1990, pp. 793–801.
23. Johnson AL, et al: Radial and tibial fracture repair with external skeletal fixation; effects of fracture type, reduction, and complications on healing. *Vet Surg 18*:367, 1989.
24. Johnson KA: Retardation of endochondral ossification at the distal ulnar growth plate in dogs. *Aust Vet J 57*:474, 1981.
25. Karaharju EO, et al: Remodeling by asymmetrical epiphyseal growth. *J Bone Joint Surg [Br] 58B*:122, 1976.
26. Knecht CD, Bloomberg MS: Distraction with an external fixation clamp (Charnley apparatus) to maintain length in premature physeal closure. *J Am Anim Hosp Assoc 16*:873, 1980.
27. Kraus KH: Carpal flexion bandage. *In* Bojrab MJ (ed): *Current Techniques in Small Animal Surgery*. 3rd ed. Lea & Febiger, Philadelphia, 1990, p 911.
28. Lappin MR, et al: Fractures of the radius and ulna in the dog. *J Am Anim Hosp Assoc 19*:643, 1983.
29. Latte Y: Treatment of radius curvus by Ilizarov apparatus. *Trans Vet Orthop Soc 16*:1989.
30. Lau RE: Inherited premature closure of the distal ulnar physis. *J Am Anim Hosp Assoc 14*:690, 1978.
31. Lombardo SJ, Harvey JP: Fractures of the distal femoral epiphyses, factors influencing prognosis: A review of thirty-four cases. *J Bone Joint Surg [Am] 59A*:742, 1977.
32. Marretta SA, Schrader SC: Physeal injuries in the dog: A review of 135 cases. *J Am Vet Med Assoc 182*:708, 1983.
33. McLain DL, Brown SG: Fixation of radius and ulna fractures in the immature dog and cat; a review of popular techniques and a report of eight cases using plate fixation. *Vet Surg 11*:140, 1982.
34. Palmer RH, et al: A combined tension band and lag screw technique for fixation of olecranon osteotomies. *Vet Surg 17*:328, 1988.
35. Phillips IR: A survey of bone fractures in the dog and cat. *J Small Anim Pract 20*:661, 1979.
36. Piermattei DL, Greeley RG: *An Atlas of Surgical Approaches to the Bones of the Dog and Cat*. 2nd ed. W. B. Saunders, Philadelphia, 1979, pp 106–113.
37. Putnam RW, Archibald J: Excision of canine radial head. *Mod Vet Pract 49*:32, 1968.
38. Robertson JJ: Application of a modified Kirschner device in the distraction mode as a prevention of antebrachial deformities in early physeal closure. *J Am Anim Hosp Assoc 19*:345, 1983.
39. Robertson WW: Newest knowledge of the growth plate. *Clin Orthop Rel Res 253*:270, 1990.
40. Rudy RL: Corrective osteotomy for angular deformities. *Vet Clin North Am 1*:549, 1971.
41. Salter RB, Harris WR: Injuries involving the epiphyseal plate. *J Bone Joint Surg [Am] 45A*:587, 1963.
42. Schwarz PD, Schrader SC: Ulnar fracture and dislocation of the proximal radial epiphysis (Monteggia lesion) in the dog and cat: A review of 28 cases. *J Am Vet Med Assoc 185*:190, 1984.
43. Shields Henney LH, Gambardella PC: Premature closure of the ulnar physis in the dog: A retrospective clinical study. *J Am Anim Hosp Assoc 25*:573, 1989.
44. Sisk TD: Fractures. *In* Edmonson AS, Crenshaw AH (eds): *Campbell's Operative Orthopedics*. 6th ed. C.V. Mosby, St. Louis, 1980, pp 690–693.
45. Turner TM, Hohn RB: Craniolateral approach to the canine elbow for repair of condylar fractures or joint exploration. *J Am Vet Med Assoc 176*:1264, 1980.
46. Vandewater A, Olmstead ML:Premature closure of the distal radial physis in the dog: A review of eleven cases. *Vet Surg 12*:7, 1983.
47. Vandewaer A, et al: Partial ulnar ostectomy with free autogenous fat grafting for treatment of radius curvus in the dog. *Vet Surg 11*:92, 1982.

CHAPTER 133

Carpus and Digits

Curtis W. Probst and Darryl L. Millis

The carpus and digits are complex structures. The tendency is to treat fractures and ligament injuries of the carpus and digits conservatively with external coaptation and hope for a favorable outcome. This may be successful in small, inactive dogs but rarely restores full function in large dogs. Displaced articular fractures lead to degenerative joint disease. Soft tissues may break down, leaving the joint unstable and resulting in degenerative joint disease. Surgical treatment of many injuries of the carpus and digits may provide a more favorable outcome.

ANATOMY

Carpal Bones

The carpus consists of seven carpal bones arranged in two rows, plus a small medial sesamoid bone in the tendon of the abductor pollicis longus muscle. The radial, ulnar, and accessory carpal bones compose the proximal row, and the first, second, third, and fourth carpal bones make up the distal row (Fig. 133–1).

The radial carpal bone is located on the medial aspect of the proximal row and articulates with the radius and

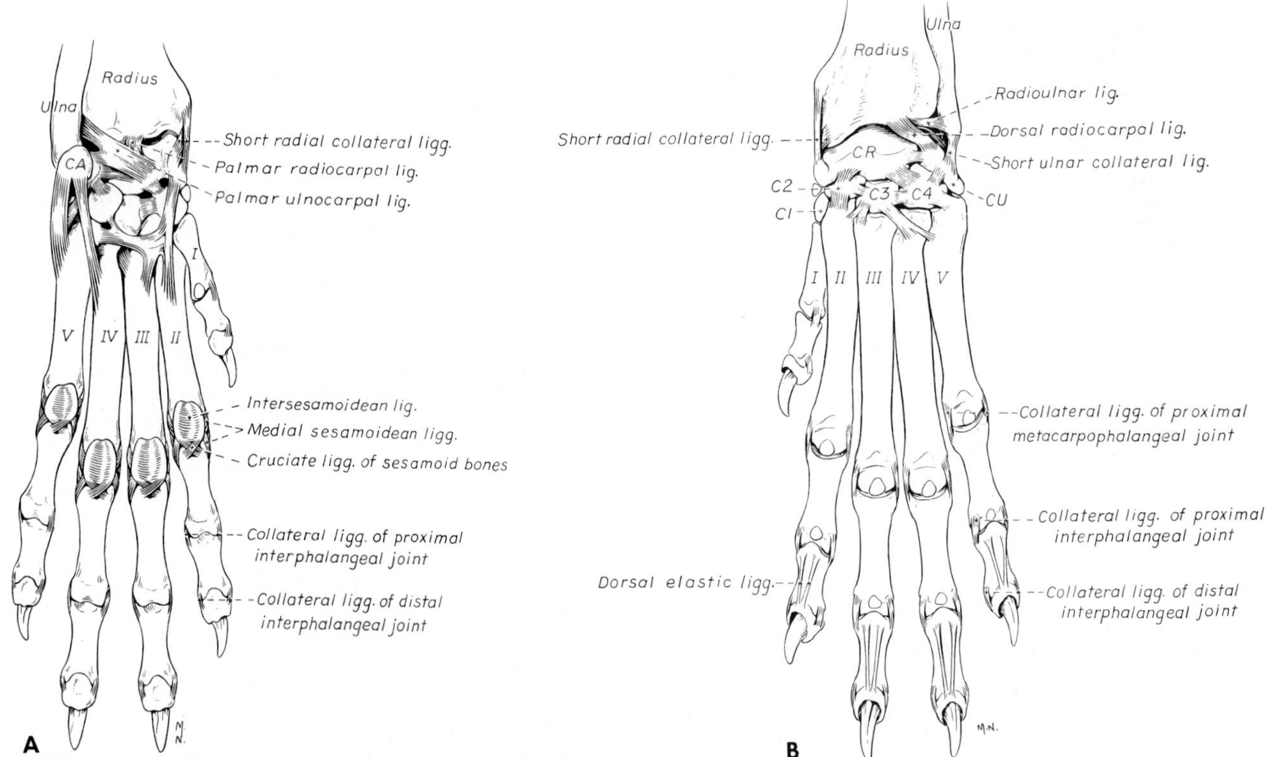

FIGURE 133–1. *A*, Deep ligaments of left forepaw, palmar aspect. (CA, accessory carpal; I to V, metacarpals.) *B*, Bones and Ligaments of left forepaw, dorsal aspect. (CR, radial carpal; CU, ulnar carpal; C1 to C4, first, second, third, fourth carpals; I to V, metacarpals.) (From Evans HE, et al: *Miller's Anatomy of the Dog.* 2nd ed. W.B. Saunders, Philadelphia, 1979, pp 250, 251.)

all the numbered carpal bones.[11] The radial carpal bone is formed by the fusion of the radial, intermediate, and central carpal bones. These are apparent by 4 weeks of age and are fused by 3 to 4 months in dogs.[7]

The ulnar carpal bone lies laterally in the proximal row. It articulates with the radius and ulna proximally, the fourth carpal and fifth metacarpal bones distally, and the accessory carpal bone on the palmar surface. The accessory carpal bone has two centers of ossification, which fuse by 3 to 6 months.[7]

The numbered carpal bones articulate distally with the corresponding metacarpal bones except for the fourth carpal, which articulates with both the fourth and fifth metacarpal bones.

Carpal Joints

The antebrachiocarpal joint, located between the distal radius and ulna and the proximal row of carpal bones, permits the greatest amount of flexion and extension in the carpus. The middle carpal joint, between the two rows of carpal bones, allows some flexion and extension. The carpometacarpal joint, between the distal row of carpal bones and the metacarpal bones, allows little motion. The intercarpal joints are between the individual carpal bones of each row. Movement in the intercarpal joints is limited.

Carpal Ligaments

The ligaments of the carpus are short, and no continuous collateral ligament spans all three joints (see Fig. 133–1). The short radial collateral ligament, with straight and oblique portions, originates from the styloid process and inserts on the medial and palmaromedial surfaces of the radial carpal bone. The short ulnar collateral ligament extends from the ulnar styloid process to the ulnar carpal bone. The flexor carpi ulnaris inserts on the proximal edge of the accessory carpal bone. Two ligaments originate from the distal border of the accessory carpal bone and insert on metacarpals IV and V. The joint capsule provides support on the dorsal and palmar aspects of the carpus. Superficial and deep sleeves of collagenous tissue, with flexor tendons between, fuse medially and laterally to form short collateral ligaments.[11]

The flexor retinaculum (transverse palmar carpal ligament) attaches laterally to the accessory carpal bone and medially to the styloid process of the radius and the radial and first carpal bones (Fig. 133–2). This structure has superficial and deep parts and forms the palmar aspect of the carpal canal, which contains tendons, vessels, and nerves. The thick palmar carpal fibrocartilage crosses the palmar surface of the carpal bones and attaches to all except the accessory carpal bone. It is especially thick distally and has strong attachments to the distal row of carpal bones and proximal metacarpals III, IV, and V. It forms the deep surface of the carpal canal and serves as the origin for most muscles of the digits.[11]

Metacarpal Bones

The metacarpal bones are numbered I to V from medial to lateral (see Fig. 133–1). Each consists of a proximal base, a middle body, and a distal head.

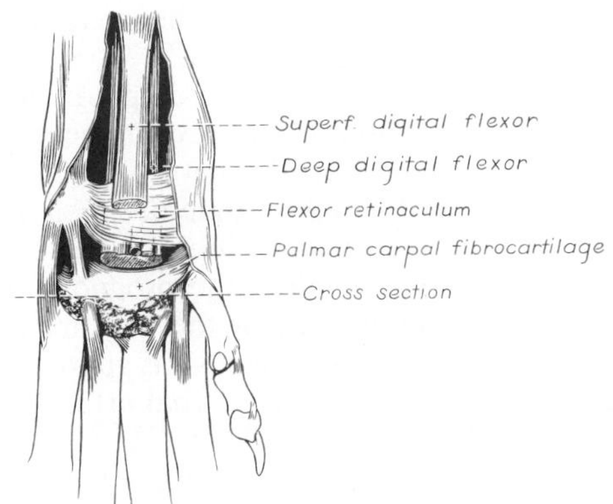

FIGURE 133–2. Superficial ligaments of left carpus, palmar aspect. (From Evans HE, et al. *Miller's Anatomy of the Dog.* 2nd ed. W.B. Saunders, Philadelphia, 1979, p 249.)

Metacarpal I articulates proximally with the first carpal bone and distally with its proximal phalanx and a single palmar sesamoid bone. Metacarpal I has only a proximal physis, whereas metacarpals II to V also have distal physes.[7] Metacarpals II through V are weight-bearing. Each articulates proximally with one or more numbered carpal bones as well as the adjacent metacarpal bones. Distally, the heads articulate with a proximal phalanx and two palmar sesamoid bones. These sesamoids are numbered 1 to 8 from medial to lateral.[3] Metacarpals II to V each have a single dorsal sesamoid, which articulates with the dorsal head. The bodies of the metacarpal bones have relatively thick cortices, which thin toward the bases and heads.

Metacarpal Muscles, Tendons, and Ligaments

The flexor carpi radialis muscle inserts on the proximal palmar surfaces of metacarpals II and III, whereas the extensor carpi radialis inserts on the dorsal surfaces.

The abductor pollicis longus inserts on the proximal medial aspect of metacarpal I. The interosseous muscles originate from the palmar surfaces of the bases of the metacarpal bones.

Support to the metacarpophalangeal joints is provided by the joint capsule, lateral collateral ligaments, intersesamoidean ligaments, tendons of insertion of the interosseous muscles, and lateral, medial, distal, and cruciate sesamoidean ligaments[11] (see Fig. 133–1).

Phalangeal Bones, Joints, and Ligaments

Each main digit consists of proximal, middle, and distal phalanges. The rudimentary first digit has only proximal and distal phalanges. The proximal interphalangeal and distal interphalangeal joints are formed by the proximal and middle and by the middle and distal phalanges, respectively.

Two elastic dorsal ligaments extend from the proximal dorsal aspect of the middle phalanx to the dorsal ungual crest of the distal phalanx. These ligaments keep the claws passively retracted and normally allow the claws to touch the ground only when tension is overcome by the flexor digitorum profundus muscles.[11]

FRACTURES

Radial Carpal Bone

History and Clinical Signs

Fractures of the radial carpal bone are rare. They occur most often in working dogs (e.g., sled dogs and field trial dogs) during heavy exertional activity. These fractures are usually the result of jumps or falls but may result from direct trauma.[3, 4, 6, 9, 16]

Fractures of the radial carpal bone are usually chips or slabs involving the articular surfaces. Clinical signs depend on the severity of the fracture and degree of displacement. The lameness is severe initially but may subside in a few weeks. A dog may be sound when rested but lame after exercise.[3, 4, 6, 9, 16]

Diagnosis

Physical Examination. Soft-tissue swelling of the carpus may be slight if the fracture is not displaced or more extensive if the fragments are severely displaced. In chronic fractures, soft-tissue thickening around the joint may be more noticeable because of synovitis and arthritis. If the fracture fragments are large and displaced, crepitus and pain may be elicited by palpating the carpus.[3, 4, 6, 9, 16]

Radiographs. The diagnosis requires a high index of suspicion, especially if the fracture is not displaced. High-quality radiographs are essential. Dorsopalmar, mediolateral, and oblique views are often required. Fractures of the radial carpal bone include chip fractures, dorsal slab fractures (Fig. 133–3*A*), body fractures (Fig. 133–4*A*), or avulsion fractures of the medial palmar prominence.

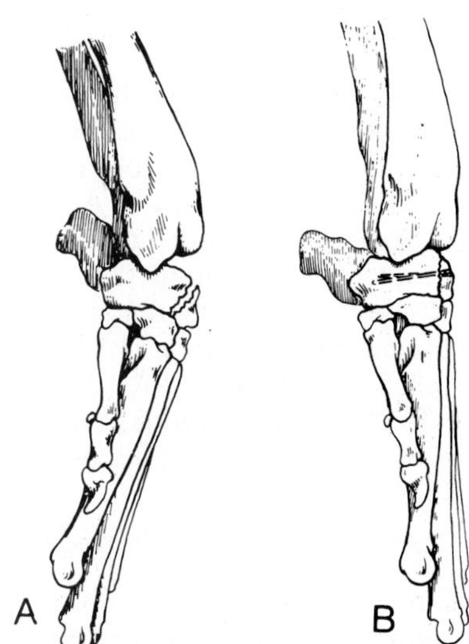

FIGURE 133–3. *A*, Dorsal slab fracture of the radial carpal bone. *B*, Radial carpal bone fracture fragments also may be secured by two or more K wires countersunk beneath the surface of the articular cartilage or bone. (From Brinker WO, et al: *Handbook of Small Animal Orthopedics and Fracture Treatment.* W.B. Saunders, Philadelphia, 1990, p 212.)

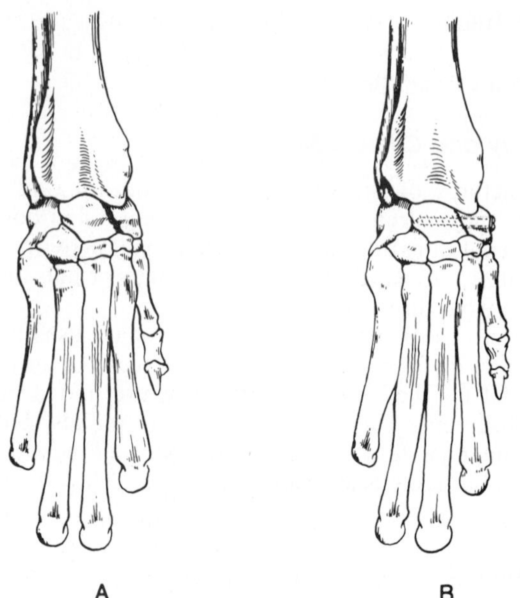

FIGURE 133–4. *A*, Oblique fracture through the body of the radial carpal bone. *B*, Lag screw fixation with a screw inserted from the medial surface of the radial carpal bone. The screw is placed through the insertions of the radial collateral ligaments. In this position, the screw head does not interfere with joint motion. (From Brinker WO, et al: *Handbook of Small Animal Orthopedics and Fracture Treatment*. W.B. Saunders, Philadelphia, 1990, p 213.)

Treatment

Undisplaced or incomplete fractures may heal if the leg is coapted for 6 to 8 weeks. Either a cast or Mason metasplint may be used to immobilize the carpus.[3, 4, 6, 9, 16]

If the fragments are displaced, surgery is indicated. Use of a tourniquet during surgery enhances visibility and increases the likelihood of accurate fracture reduction. The approach used depends on the fracture, but most fractures may be exposed with a dorsal or dorsomedial approach.

If the fragment is large, it may be reattached with a lag screw (Fig. 133–4*B*) or K wires (Fig. 133–3*B*). The screw is placed so that the head does not interfere with the articular surface. K wires may be countersunk below the cartilage or bone. As with any articular fracture, anatomical reduction is required. Small chip fractures are excised if they cannot be reattached. The defect usually fills in with fibrocartilage.[3, 4, 6, 9, 16]

Carpal arthrodesis is indicated for comminuted radial carpal bone fractures and chronic radial carpal bone fractures with degenerative joint disease.[3, 4, 6, 9, 16]

Aftercare, Complications, and Prognosis

If the fracture has been treated with internal fixation, the joint is supported with a molded palmar splint for 6 to 8 weeks. A dog's exercise is restricted until radiographic evidence illustrates fracture healing. If the carpus has been fused, the joint is supported with a splint and the dog's activity is restricted until the arthrodesis is complete. If the fracture fragments have been excised, the joint is supported in a padded bandage for 2 weeks. The dog's activity may gradually be increased during the 4 weeks after bandage removal.[3, 4, 6, 9, 16]

The main complication of radial carpal bone fracture is degenerative joint disease, the development and prognosis for which depend on the nature of the fracture, quality of repair, and length of time between injury and treatment. If the fracture lends itself to accurate reduction and rigid internal fixation, the prognosis is favorable. If the bone is eburnated or the fracture is chronic and arthritis is present, the prognosis is guarded or poor. These cases are best treated by carpal arthrodesis.

Accessory Carpal Bone

History and Clinical Signs

Fractures of the accessory carpal bone are uncommon except in racing greyhounds. Most accessory carpal bone fractures in greyhounds occur in the right leg. Racing in a counterclockwise direction is a contributing factor in these fractures. As a dog rounds the turns, all of the body weight is placed on the right front leg, and a fracture occurs. These fractures are classified as avulsion fractures. Other accessory carpal bone fractures usually result from a jump or fall.[3, 4, 6, 9, 12, 16]

In racing dogs, clinical signs are usually not apparent until the day after the injury. The dog shows a slight lameness, and swelling around the accessory carpal bone may be observed. The lameness and swelling usually subside with rest but return when the dog exercises again.[3, 4, 6, 9, 12, 16]

Diagnosis

Physical Examination. Slight hyperextension of the carpus may occur with distal ligamentous avulsion fractures. There may be decreased range of motion and pain on flexion of the joint. Conversely, normal range of motion exists with proximal tendinous avulsion fractures, along with increased soft-tissue swelling and pain on extension.[6]

Radiographs. An extended mediolateral radiograph distracts the fragments and enhances visibility of the fracture.[6]

Accessory carpal bone fractures in racing greyhounds have been classified into five types.[12] A type I fracture is an avulsion fracture of the distal margin of the articular surface of the accessory carpal bone at the origin of ligaments connecting the accessory carpal bone to the ulnar carpal bone (Fig. 133–5). A type II fracture is defined as an avulsion fracture of the proximal margin of the articular surface of the accessory carpal bone at the insertion of the ligaments from the distal ulna and radius (see Fig. 133–5). Type II fractures occur only in combination with type I fractures. A type III fracture is an avulsion fracture at the distal palmar end of the accessory carpal bone at the origin of the two palmar ligaments that insert on metacarpals IV and V (see Fig. 133–5). A type IV fracture is an avulsion fracture at the tendinous insertion of the flexor carpi ulnaris at the proximal palmar surface of the accessory carpal bone (see Fig. 133–5). A type V fracture is a comminuted fracture of the accessory carpal bone (see Fig. 133–5).[12]

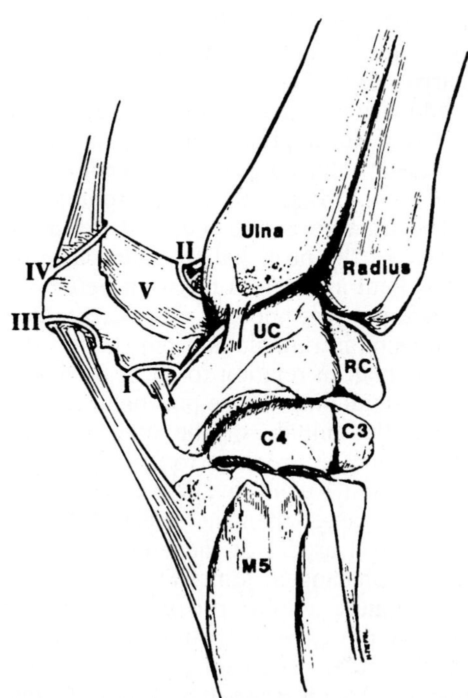

FIGURE 133–5. Classification of accessory carpal bone fractures. Lateral aspect of canine carpus (UC, ulnar carpal bone; RC, radial carpal bone; C3, third carpal bone; C4, fourth carpal bone; M5, fifth metacarpal bone), illustrating type I, II, III, and IV fractures of the accessory carpal bone. Type V are comminuted fractures. (From Johnson KA: Accessory carpal bone fractures in the racing greyhound. Classification and pathology. *Vet Surg 16*:61, 1987.)

Treatment

Splints or casts rarely result in complete healing of avulsion fractures (i.e., types I to IV). Internal fixation of comminuted fractures (i.e., type V) is rarely feasible; these fractures are most often treated by casting the carpus in 20° of flexion.[3]

The surgical treatment of accessory carpal bone avulsion fractures depends on the size of the fragment. If the fragment is too small to be reattached, it is excised. When the fragment is excised, successful healing depends on the ligaments becoming reattached to the bone by scar tissue. If such healing has insufficient strength, the accessory carpal bone becomes unstable and degenerative joint disease results.[3] An animal may not return to racing with this treatment.[3]

If the fragments are large enough, they may be reattached with small lag screws, divergent K wires, or a pin and tension band wire (Fig. 133–6).

Aftercare, Complications, and Prognosis

The carpus is supported with a splint or cast after internal fixation of the fracture. The carpus is flexed approximately 20° while applying the splint or cast. External coaptation is maintained for 4 to 6 weeks. The dog's exercise is restricted for an additional 4 to 6 weeks. Activity is gradually increased during the next 4 weeks.

For a comminuted fracture treated with a cast, the cast is maintained until there is radiographic evidence of healing. The carpus is supported with a splint for 2 to 4 weeks after excising small fracture fragments. Activity is restricted for an additional 4 weeks after removing the splint or cast.

The prognosis for accessory carpal bone fractures depends on the type of fracture, method of treatment, and anticipated use of the dog. At one institution, less than 50 per cent of the greyhounds treated by excision of the fracture fragment won a race afterward.[3] Repair of these fractures is a more rational approach to treatment, but there are insufficient data to support a definitive prognosis.[3]

Ulnar and Numbered Carpal Bones

Fractures of the ulnar and numbered carpal bones are rare. Such fractures are usually small chips on the dorsal surface of the bones. Affected dogs may exhibit a mild intermittent lameness with mild joint effusion. These fractures are difficult to diagnose because the small fragments are difficult to see radiographically. Multiple oblique radiographic views are often necessary to demonstrate them. Treatment consists of removing the fragment and curetting the damaged articular surface to stimulate fibrocartilage formation.[3] The carpus is supported with a padded bandage for 2 weeks after surgery. Exercise is restricted for an additional 2 to 4 weeks.

Metacarpal Bone Fractures

History and Clinical Signs

Metacarpal bone fractures occur most commonly in young dogs or cats that have been stepped on or have had the foot trapped under a rigid object.[14] Fractures may involve one or more metacarpal bones. Animals usually do not bear weight and are lame.

Diagnosis

Physical Examination. Animals with metacarpal fractures have soft-tissue swelling, pain, and crepitus over

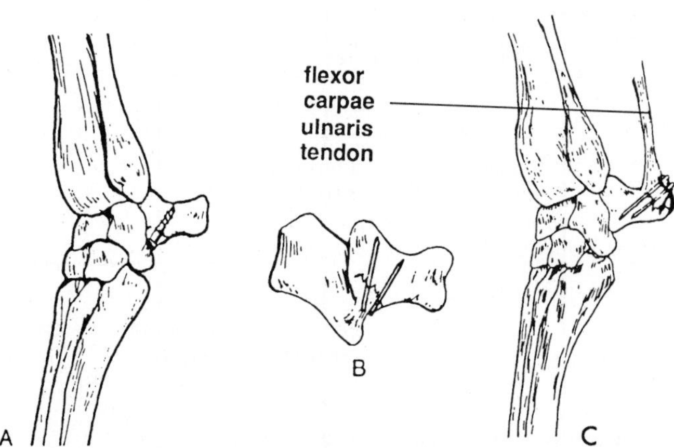

FIGURE 133–6. *A* and *B*, Avulsion fracture of the base of the accessory carpal bone repaired with a compression screw *(A)* or Kirschner wires *(B)*. *C*, Fracture of the free end of the accessory carpal bone repaired with Kirschner wires and a tension band. (From Earley TD: Carpal and tarsal injuries. *In* Bojrab MJ [ed]: *Current Techniques in Small Animal Surgery*. 3rd ed. Lea & Febiger, Philadelphia, 1990, p 873.)

the fracture site. The skin is examined closely for penetrating wounds suggesting an open fracture. Varus or valgus deformities may be present if metacarpals II or V are fractured.[3]

Radiographs. Lateral and dorsopalmar radiographs are examined carefully for degree of displacement, type of fracture (especially the degree of comminution and whether it is an open or closed fracture), and articular involvement.[13] Rarely, oblique lateral radiographs may be helpful in further delineating fractures.

Treatment

Treatment may be achieved with a cast or splint if only one or two metacarpal bones are fractured with mild displacement and if one of the main weightbearing bones (III or IV) is intact (Fig. 133–7).[3, 10, 14, 18] The remaining intact bones act as internal splints to aid alignment. Coaptation allows palpation of the toes for swelling and extends beyond the toes to minimize weightbearing and palmar displacement of the fractures. An aluminum rod as a walking bar helps distribute weightbearing forces if a cast is used. Preformed metal splints are easy to apply and accomplish similar objectives.

Internal fixation is performed if more than two metacarpals are fractured, both metacarpals III and IV are fractured, severe displacement or comminution exists, articular surfaces are involved, or the base of metacarpal II or V is fractured.[3, 10, 14, 18] Pins and wires in a tension band or lag screws may be used to repair basilar fractures of metacarpals II and V.[3]

Intramedullary pins may be used to repair metacarpal shaft fractures. Normograde pin insertion involves flexing the metacarpophalangeal joint while inserting the pin in the distal fragment, away from the articular surface. The fracture is reduced, and the pin is driven into the base of the proximal fragment. The distal end of the pin is bent away from the joint and cut short.

Retrograde pin placement is also acceptable.[3, 18] One problem in using intramedullary pins is that the medullary canal is small in relation to cortical width, thereby necessitating small pins. These pins bend easily and may exit through the middle of the metacarpophalangeal joint rather than just proximal to it if retrograded.

One technique to avoid this problem involves drilling a hole one size larger than the selected intramedullary pin on the dorsal aspect of the bone just proximal to the metacarpophalangeal joint (Fig. 133–8).[2] The hole is drilled obliquely, aiming proximally. The tip of the intramedullary pin is bent slightly and retrograded distally from the fracture site until the bent tip passes out of the hole. The pin is grasped and partially pulled out, the fracture is reduced, and the pin is driven into the base of the proximal fragment. The distal pin end is bent proximally and cut short. This technique avoids entering the metacarpophalangeal joint and causing degenerative joint disease.

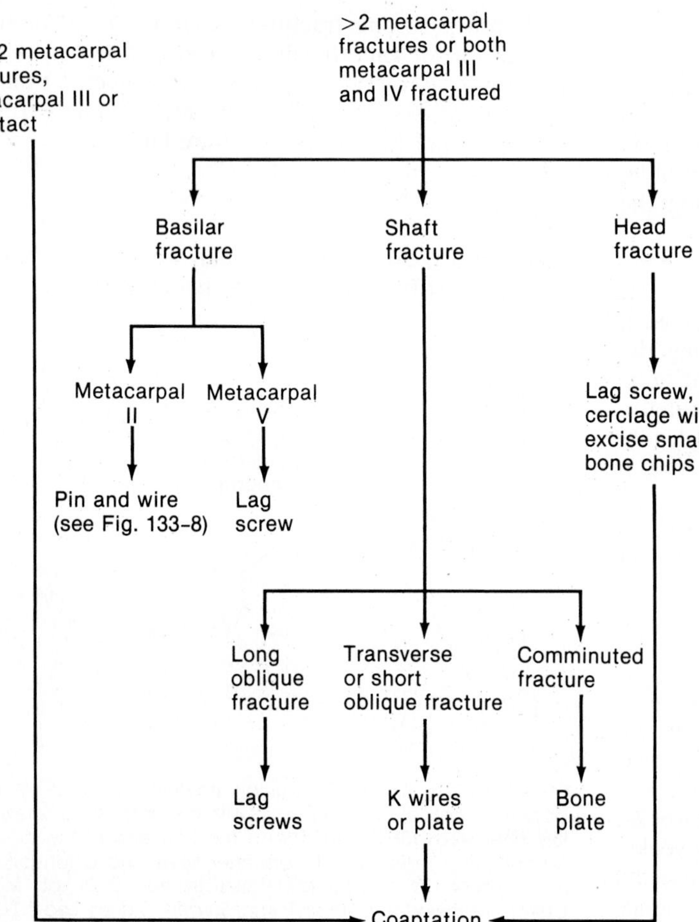

FIGURE 133–7. Treatment of metacarpal (MtC) bone fractures.

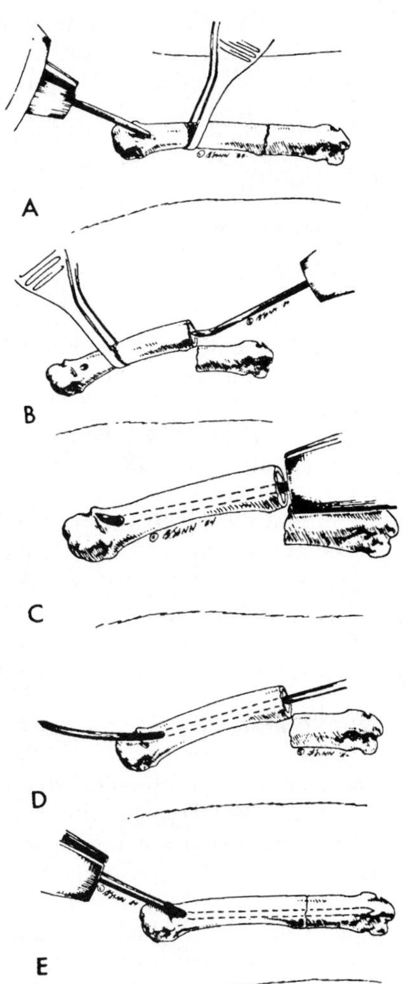

FIGURE 133–8. An alternative technique for intramedullary pin fixation of metacarpal fractures. *A*, Drill a hole in the dorsal aspect of the distal end of the metatarsal bone. *B*, Retrograding the pin from the fracture site with the tip oriented dorsally. *C* and *D*, Passing a bent pin tip through the dorsal drill hole. *E*, Driving the pin into the proximal segment after fracture reduction. (From Benedetti TL, et al: A technique for intramedullary pinning of metatarsals and metacarpals in dogs and cats. *J Am Anim Hosp Assoc 22*:150, 1986.)

Small bone plates, screws, and cerclage wire have been used and are particularly applicable for repair of comminuted fractures.[3]

Fractures of the head are rare and result in metacarpophalangeal instability. A lag screw or hemicerclage wire passed through small holes in the bone may be used to repair these fractures. Small chips are excised. If chronic lameness due to degenerative joint disease occurs, amputation of the digit provides pain relief.[3]

Aftercare, Complications, and Prognosis

All metacarpal fractures are coapted in a molded palmar splint or cast until healed, usually about 6 weeks. The animal's activity is restricted for another 4 weeks, and fixation devices, especially pins, are usually removed after healing is complete.

Complications of metacarpal fracture repair include osteomyelitis, malunion, nonunion, degenerative joint disease, and chronic lameness.[13]

The prognosis for metacarpal fractures is generally favorable if adequate reduction, alignment, and fixation are achieved. One study reported a less favorable prognosis if articular surfaces are involved, the fracture segments are greatly displaced, or the fractures are highly comminuted.[13]

Sesamoid Bones

History and Clinical Signs

Sesamoid fractures are uncommon but may be noted in large working dogs or show dogs. Sesamoid fractures are caused by excessive tension on the digital flexor tendons, such as during jumping. Sudden lameness occurs but rapidly subsides.[3] The dog may show lameness only after strenuous exercise. Because the lameness subsides with rest, animals are often not evaluated until the injury is chronic.

Diagnosis

Physical Examination. Affected animals usually are not lame unless they have exercised just before they are presented. Slight swelling of the affected metacarpophalangeal joint may be noted. Firm pressure on the palmar surface of the affected joint often elicits a pain response from the dog.

Radiographs. High-detail radiographs are required to diagnose these fractures. Oblique views may also be helpful. The second and seventh sesamoids are most commonly fractured.[3] Fractures of the sesamoids associated with the third or fourth digits also occur.

Some dogs have bipartite sesamoids, so one should carefully examine the radiographs and compare them with radiographs of the opposite side before making the diagnosis. Bipartite sesamoids have smooth margins compared with fractured sesamoids. Dogs with bipartite sesamoids do not feel pain on palpation of the metacarpophalangeal joints.

Treatment

Acute fractures may be treated by splinting the distal leg. Some fractures heal sufficiently, but many require surgery later.[3] Because owners may not seek veterinary care initially, many fractures are already chronic when the diagnosis is made. All lame dogs with chronic fractures are treated surgically.[3]

Surgical treatment consists of removal of the fracture fragments.[3,4] If the fracture is in the middle of the bone, both pieces are removed. If the fracture is near one end of the sesamoid, the smaller piece is removed (providing it is less than one-third of the total bone) and the larger piece is left.

Aftercare and Prognosis

A snug padded bandage is applied to the distal limb and is maintained for 7 to 10 days. The prognosis for surgically treated fractures is favorable.[3]

Phalanges

History and Clinical Signs

Phalangeal fractures are common. They are caused by trauma, usually unseen by owners. Lameness is pronounced, and a dog may carry the affected leg.

Diagnosis

Physical Examination. The affected digit is swollen. Firm palpation of the digit elicits a pain response from the dog. Crepitus is rarely palpated, and radiographs are required to confirm the diagnosis.

Radiographs. The dorsopalmar view of the foot is the most helpful, but oblique views may be obtained. The first and second phalanges are most commonly fractured (Fig. 133–9). The third phalanx is rarely fractured.

Treatment

Most fractures are treated with a splint or short cast. One may consider internal fixation (i.e., lag screws or small plates) for intra-articular fractures or for fractures in performance animals. The surgical exposure is simple because the bone is immediately beneath the skin.[3] The internal repair is protected with external coaptation.

Aftercare, Complications, and Prognosis

External coaptation is maintained for 4 to 6 weeks if it is the only treatment. If internal fixation has been used, the external coaptation is removed in 3 to 4 weeks. Exercise is restricted to leash walks until fracture healing is complete.

Degenerative joint disease may occur after an intra-articular fracture, even if internal fixation is used. Amputation of the affected digit may be necessary if the animal is symptomatic.

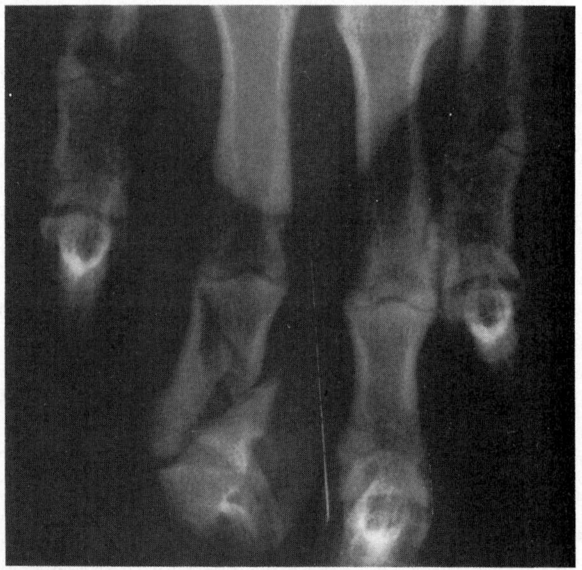

FIGURE 133–9. A comminuted fracture of the second phalanx of the third digit.

The prognosis for nonarticular fractures is favorable. The prognosis for articular fractures is more guarded, especially in performance animals. The prognosis after amputation of one digit is favorable.

LIGAMENTOUS INJURIES

Radial/Ulnar Collateral Ligaments

History and Clinical Signs

The radial collateral ligaments are more commonly injured than the ulnar collateral ligaments. The radial collateral ligaments are under constant tension because as a dog stands, the foot is in a slight valgus position. Injuries of the ulnar collateral ligaments are reportedly less serious because they are not subject to as much tension.[3]

Most injuries to carpal ligaments result from jumps or falls, but some are due to vehicular trauma. Animals usually carry the affected leg. Variable carpal swelling is present.[3]

Diagnosis

Physical Examination. The area of instability can be localized by palpation. The integrity of the collateral ligaments may be assessed by manipulating the carpus to place valgus and varus stresses on the carpus. This is done with the carpus in extension and flexion. Palpation of the contralateral carpus for comparison may be helpful.[3, 8, 10]

Radiographs. Nonscreen or high-detail screen radiographs are necessary to confirm the diagnosis. Several views are often necessary. These may include craniocaudal, lateral, oblique, and stressed positions. Widening of the joint space on the affected side may be seen on the stress views. Radiographs of the opposite carpus may be obtained for comparison if necessary.[3, 8, 10]

Treatment

Primary repair of the radial collateral ligament may be possible in acute injuries. It is important to repair both the straight and oblique parts.[3, 8] Suture repair of the ligaments followed by appropriate splinting may be adequate,[8] but reinforcing such a repair with synthetic material is advisable.[3]

A medial incision is made directly over the radial styloid process. Bone tunnels are drilled into the medial aspect of the distal radius and the radial carpal bone (Fig. 133–10). Nonabsorbable suture material is passed through the holes and tied to mimic the straight and oblique parts of the collateral ligament (see Fig. 133–10).[3] Success has been reported using autogenous tissue such as the flexor carpi radialis tendon to replace the collateral ligaments.[8]

Aftercare, Complications, and Prognosis

The carpus is immobilized with a palmar splint for 4 to 6 weeks. A padded bandage may be used for an additional 2 to 4 weeks. The dog's activity is restricted

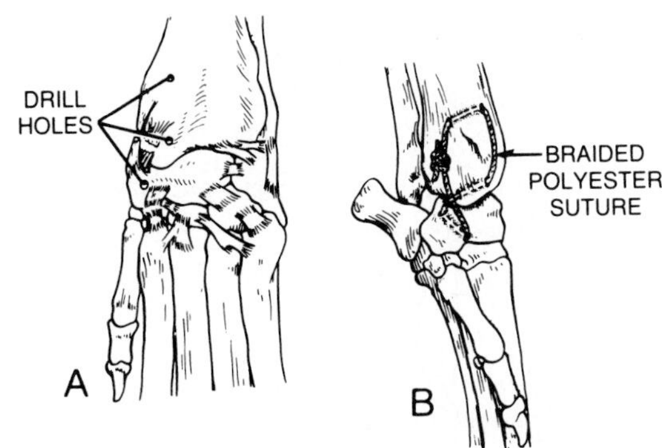

FIGURE 133–10. Synthetic braided suture is threaded through bone tunnels placed in the radial carpal bone and radius to simulate both the long and short ligaments. (From Brinker WO, et al: *Handbook of Small Animal Orthopedics and Fracture Treatment.* W.B. Saunders, Philadelphia, 1990, p 521.)

for an additional 2 to 4 weeks. The prognosis depends on the intended use of the dog, the length of time between injury and treatment, and the amount of degenerative joint disease.

Palmar Ligaments and Palmar Fibrocartilage

History and Clinical Signs

Rupture of the palmar carpal ligaments and palmar fibrocartilage is commonly referred to as a *hyperextension injury* and is one of the more common carpal injuries. It typically results from a jump or fall, although the client may not witness the injury. It is often thought that carpal hyperextension is the result of tendon injury, but tendons have only a minor role in supporting the palmar aspect of the carpus.[3]

Affected animals may not bear weight, especially for the first few days after injury. If weight is placed on the affected leg, the carpus is hyperextended, and in severe cases, the accessory carpal pad may touch the ground.

Diagnosis

Physical Examination. The affected carpus may be swollen. Manually extending the carpus (i.e., stressing the palmar ligaments) reveals the area of instability. Forcing a dog to stand on the leg produces the typical stance of carpal hyperextension.

Radiographs. A stressed lateral view is the most helpful in determining the level of injury. One should try to determine what joint is involved to select the appropriate treatment (Fig. 133–11). The distribution of joint involvement has been reported as antebrachiocarpal, 10 and 31 per cent; middle carpal, 50 and 22 per cent; and carpometacarpal, 40 and 47 per cent.[3, 15]

Treatment

Splinting the carpus is usually not rewarding because randomly oriented scar tissue does not have sufficient strength to support the stress placed on the carpus. If attempted, it is reserved for acute cases of mild hyperextension at the antebrachiocarpal joint in small dogs. If such treatment fails, arthrodesis may be performed later.[3]

Surgical treatment is usually more successful. Although some success in primary repair of these injuries has been reported,[8] carpal arthrodesis is the most common treatment of carpal hyperextension. Although panarthrodesis of the carpus can be used to treat all carpal hyperextension injuries, partial arthrodesis may be better for injuries involving the middle carpal and carpometacarpal joints and to maintain function of the antebrachiocarpal joint. Appropriate treatment depends on the joint involved.

If hyperextension injury is at the antebrachiocarpal joint, panarthrodesis of the carpus is recommended. Although technically possible to fuse the antebrachiocarpal joint only, it is not recommended because the increased stress placed on the distal carpal joints predisposes them to injury.[3]

Panarthrodesis or partial arthrodesis of the carpus is usually performed with a tourniquet in place. The skin incision for panarthrodesis is centered on the dorsal midline and extends from the distal third of the radius to the distal metacarpal bones. The common digital extensor tendon is retracted laterally, and the extensor carpi radialis tendon is retracted medially. The insertion of the extensor carpi radialis tendon on the third metacarpal bone is severed. The adductor pollicis longus

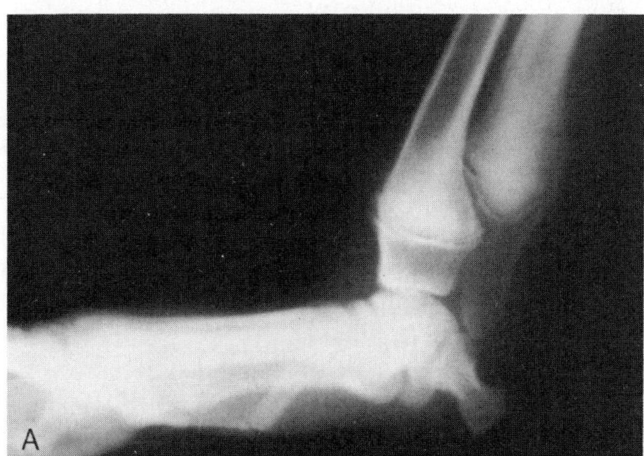

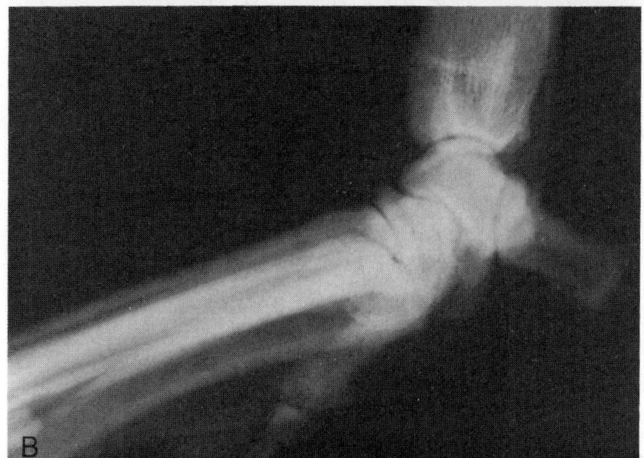

FIGURE 133–11. *A,* A stress radiograph showing a hyperextension injury involving the radiocarpal joint. *B,* A stress radiograph showing a hyperextension injury involving the middle carpal joint.

tendon is transected to expose the dorsal surface of the radius. The joint capsule covering the dorsal surface of the carpus is removed. The carpus is flexed, and the articular cartilage is removed from all three joint levels with a curette or high-speed bur. A cancellous bone graft is harvested from the proximal humerus and placed into the joint spaces. A bone plate (usually seven holes) is bent to provide 10° to 15° of carpal extension. The plate is applied to the dorsal surface of the radius and the dorsal surface of the third metacarpal bone so that three screws are placed into each bone. An additional screw is placed into the radial carpal bone if possible (Fig. 133–12). It is important to make sure the foot is aligned properly while applying the plate. The branch of the extensor carpi radialis tendon that is severed from its insertion on metacarpal III is sutured to the branch inserting on metacarpal II. A technique for plating the palmar surface of the carpus has been described.[5]

The approach for partial arthrodesis is the same as for panarthrodesis, except that the incision need not begin so far proximally and the joint capsule of the antebrachiocarpal joint is not removed. After the articular cartilage is removed from the middle carpal and carpometacarpal joints, the cancellous bone graft is placed into these joints. A T plate can be applied to the radial carpal bone and to the third metacarpal bone (Fig. 133–13), or K wires may be inserted from metacarpals III and IV into the radial carpal bone (Fig. 133–14).

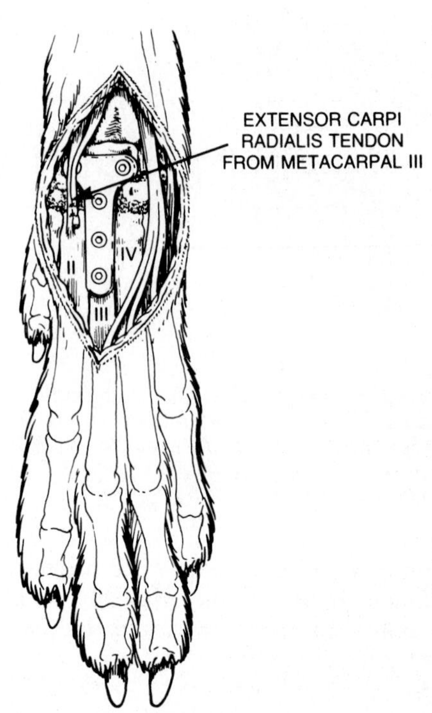

FIGURE 133–13. Partial arthrodesis of the carpus using T-plate fixation. The plate is attached to the distal end of the radial carpal bone, the screws angling proximally. The tendon of the extensor carpi radialis inserting on metacarpal III has been transposed to metacarpal II and is sutured there. (From Brinker WO, et al: *Handbook of Small Animal Orthopedics and Fracture Treatment.* W.B. Saunders, Philadelphia, 1990, p 531.)

Aftercare, Complications, and Prognosis

A molded palmar splint is applied to the leg after surgery. The splint is maintained until the arthrodesis has completely healed. We usually do not remove the bone plate or K wires after healing is complete.

Complications after carpal arthrodesis are few. Swelling of the foot may occur and is closely monitored. Keeping tourniquet time to a minimum and applying the splint immediately after wound closure help minimize foot swelling. Slight varus or valgus angulation of the carpus may be noticed when the drapes are removed, but this rarely causes a functional problem.

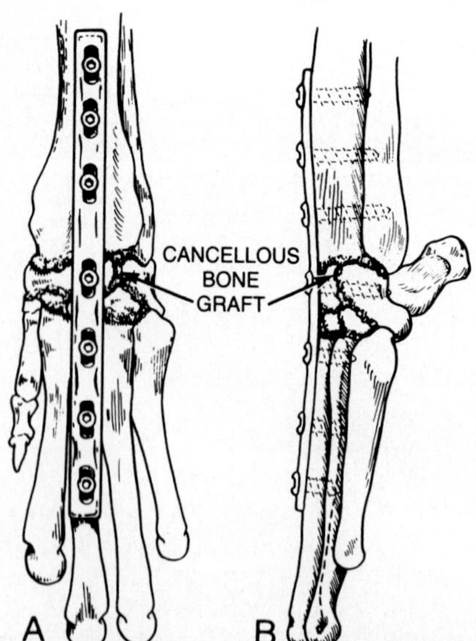

FIGURE 133–12. A pancarpal arthrodesis using a seven-hole bone plate. One screw is placed into the radial carpal bone if possible. (From Brinker WO, et al: *Handbook of Small Animal Orthopedics and Fracture Treatment.* W.B. Saunders, Philadelphia, 1990, p 535.)

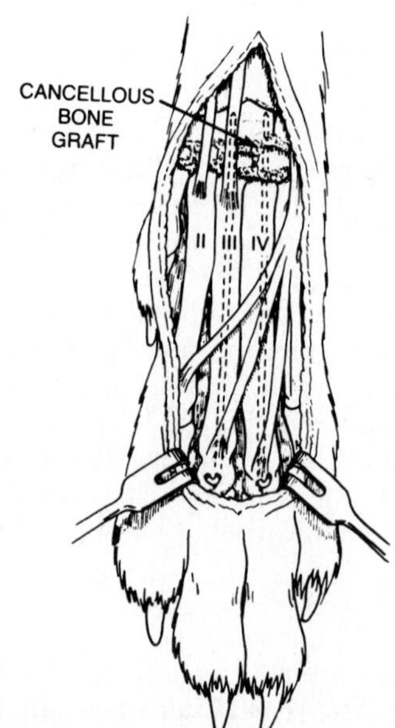

FIGURE 133–14. Partial arthrodesis of the carpus with pin fixation. (From Brinker WO, et al: *Handbook of Small Animal Orthopedics and Fracture Treatment.* W.B. Saunders, Philadelphia, 1990, p 529.)

The prognosis after partial or complete carpal arthrodesis is favorable. Dogs compensate well for the loss of carpal motion.

FLEXOR TENDON LACERATIONS

History and Clinical Signs

Severance of the digital flexor tendons is generally the result of laceration by sharp objects. Hemorrhage may be profuse, and the skin and other surrounding soft tissues are commonly traumatized.[14] The superficial and deep digital flexor tendons insert on the proximal ends of the second and third phalanges, respectively.[11] These tendons, particularly the deep digital flexor tendon, maintain the toes in the proper position with respect to the digital footpads and the walking surface of the foot.

Diagnosis

In acute tendon laceration, the cut ends of the tendons may be visible. Laceration of the superficial digital flexor tendon may have little functional or physical consequence. However, complete severance of both the superficial and deep digital flexor tendons results in palmigrade positioning of one or more digits, especially during weightbearing. Chronic injury may result in ulceration of the pads and interdigital areas. Injuries to the deep digital flexor tendon or both tendons resulting in flattening of the digits or chronic damage to the foot require surgical treatment.

Treatment

Acute lacerations of the flexor tendons with minimal contamination may be definitively repaired if surgery is performed within 4 to 6 hours. Older injuries or those that are severely contaminated or infected are treated by surgical débridement and proper open wound management until the tissues are healthy. It may be helpful to tag the ends of the severed tendons with colored suture material to facilitate later identification.

Anastomosis of the severed tendon is performed using standard tendon repair techniques, including the use of appropriate tendon suture patterns.[14] A tourniquet is helpful in maintaining hemostasis. The location of the laceration may require transection of the flexor retinaculum to achieve proper exposure. After anastomosis of the severed tendons, this ligament is sutured.

Chronic lacerations are more difficult to repair because of the damage to surrounding soft tissues and the amount of fibrous scar tissue present. The severed tendon ends may be difficult to locate, and anastomosis is complicated by contraction of the tendon ends. Repair of tendons is performed as described earlier, but tendon lengthening techniques or grafts may be necessary to reappose tendon ends.

Aftercare, Complications, and Prognosis

The limb is immobilized in a cast or padded splint in a flexed position for 3 to 4 weeks after surgery. Laceration of both flexor tendons may require immobilization for 6 to 8 weeks. The splint or cast is changed at least every 2 weeks and kept clean and dry. The toes are checked daily for swelling. After splint removal, exercise is restricted to leash walks only for 6 to 8 weeks, followed by a gradual return to normal activity.

Complications include breakdown of the repair as a result of excessive tension on the anastomosis, infection, and adhesions of the tendons to surrounding soft tissues. The prognosis for acute injuries with minimal tension on the anastomosis is generally favorable but for massive injuries with excessive tension or chronic injuries is guarded to poor.

SHEARING INJURIES

History and Clinical Signs

Shearing injuries occur most commonly as a result of vehicular trauma. The medial or lateral aspect of the carpus is trapped under a car tire while braking. The pavement acts as an abrasive and grinds away soft tissues, bone, tendons, and ligaments. Complete loss of all supporting structures and exposure of joint surfaces may occur.

Diagnosis

Physical Examination. The limb is carefully evaluated for evidence of neurological or circulatory damage. If the distal limb is cold or deep pain is absent, the prognosis for salvaging the foot is guarded.

Radiographs. Although damage may be adequately assessed during physical examination, radiographs determine the amount of bone loss and whether other fractures exist. Varus or valgus stress radiographs may be necessary to determine the extent of collateral ligament damage.

Treatment

The tendency is to attempt primary closure of the wound. This is avoided because the wounds are grossly contaminated or infected. Rather, meticulous débridement is done immediately, and all devitalized tissue and foreign material are removed. Copious irrigation with sterile saline is important. Débridement is performed under as sterile conditions as possible to prevent nosocomial infections. After débridement and lavage, the wound is cultured and appropriate systemic antibiotic therapy begun. The wound is covered with a sterile dressing, and a Robert Jones bandage applied.

Initially, daily bandage changes are performed under sterile conditions. Further débridement is performed as necessary. Discomfort is usually minimal because the cutaneous nerve supply is often destroyed. As the amount of wound discharge diminishes, the interval between bandage changes may be increased. In general, a healthy bed of granulation tissue begins forming in 5 to 7 days. After the wound is completely covered with healthy granulation tissue and infection is controlled, definitive stabilization of the joint may be performed.

Occasionally, no surgical stabilization of the joint is necessary because the granulation tissue and fibrous tissue formed during wound healing provide sufficient support of the joint. If this treatment is elected, a splint may be applied to provide additional support of the joint. The splint provides support without interfering with bandage changes. The cost and time required for this treatment must be compared with that of surgical treatment.

Surgical stabilization may be provided by using bone screws, washers, suture material, and remaining tendons and ligaments to fashion prosthetic collateral ligaments (Fig. 133–15).[10] If severe injury prevents the use of prosthetic collateral ligaments or if comminuted articular fractures are present, arthrodesis of the joint is indicated as the primary treatment.

Aftercare, Complications, and Prognosis

A soft wrap is applied to the limb for 2 to 6 weeks to provide some support. Exercise is restricted for 4 to 6 weeks and gradually increased thereafter. Osteomyelitis, implant failure, and breakdown of repair are possible complications. Properly treated, many of these injuries heal well. Amputation is only considered if the injury is extremely severe or if neurological or circulatory function is absent in the distal extremity.

CARPAL LAXITY SYNDROME IN YOUNG DOGS

History and Clinical Signs

A carpal laxity syndrome that is not associated with trauma has been described in young dogs.[1, 17] It generally occurs in 8- to 16-week-old puppies and is characterized by a palmigrade stance, increased range of motion of the carpus, and a valgus position of the carpus when bearing weight. Doberman pinschers, German shepherds, and Great Danes are predisposed to this condition. Although the cause is unknown, one or several pups in a litter may be affected. In one study, no consistent trends were detected in relation to diet, but the majority of affected animals were raised on smooth concrete surfaces or in small enclosures.[1]

The changes in joint mobility may result from changes in the ability of the digital flexor muscles to support the carpus. The relative lack of exercise of affected pups may result in decreased muscle tone and joint hyperextension.[17]

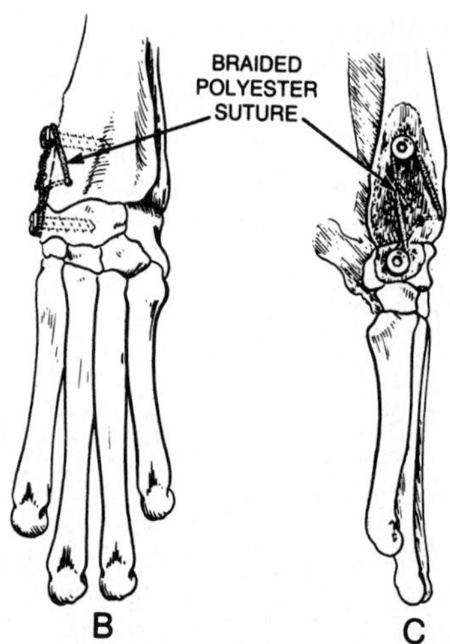

FIGURE 133–15. Prosthetic collateral ligament following a shearing injury of the carpus. (From Brinker WO, et al: *Handbook of Small Animal Orthopedics and Fracture Treatment.* W.B. Saunders, Philadelphia, 1990, p 523.)

Treatment and Prognosis

The treatment for this condition is to provide mild to moderate free exercise on grass or other supporting surfaces. Severe cases may benefit from a light support wrap to protect the palmar surface of the carpus; however, prolonged use of rigid splints may retard muscle development. Patients generally respond in 2 to 6 weeks, with no apparent long-term deficits.

DIGIT AMPUTATION

Indications

Digit removal is commonly performed in dogs and cats for severely comminuted fractures, intra-articular fractures, chronic sprains, irreparable luxations, severe shearing injuries, neoplasia, chronic infections, and degenerative joint disease. The reason for amputation determines the level of amputation. More radical resection is indicated for infectious and neoplastic processes. Amputation at the metacarpophalangeal joint or higher is preferred in these cases, whereas amputation at the proximal or distal interphalangeal joint may be adequate for traumatic or degenerative conditions. The surgical principles are similar regardless of the level of amputation.

Surgical Technique

Thorough surgical preparation of the area is difficult because of the toenails and pads. Washing the foot and placing it in a wrap consisting of gauze sponges soaked in dilute chlorhexidine solution the night before surgery may reduce bacterial numbers. A tourniquet placed just before incising the skin aids in hemostasis. The digital pad is preserved when amputation is performed at the distal interphalangeal joint but is removed for more proximal amputations.

For a distal phalangeal amputation, a transverse skin incision is made, completely encircling the base of the nail but preserving the digital pad. The joint is disarticulated by incising the extensor and flexor tendons and the collateral ligaments. The distal second phalanx is removed to allow more soft tissues to be interposed between the bone end and skin. The pad is sutured to the skin using a simple interrupted pattern.[3]

More proximal amputations are performed by making an inverted Y-shaped incision over the area with the stem of the Y on the dorsal aspect of the digit. The two arms of the Y join on the palmar aspect of the digit proximal to the digital pad. The stem of the Y may be made on the side of the foot if amputating the second or fifth digits. The digital arteries and veins are ligated.

The extensor and flexor tendons and the collateral ligaments are sharply incised, and the digit removed. The distal end of the remaining bone is removed. The palmar sesamoid bones are removed when amputation is performed at the metacarpophalangeal joint. The subcutaneous tissues and skin are sutured using a simple interrupted pattern.[3]

Aftercare

A padded bandage is placed on the foot for 7 to 10 days. Exercise is restricted for 3 weeks postoperatively. Prognosis is generally favorable if only one digit is removed. Lameness may result if more than two digits are removed or if both the third and fourth digits are removed.

References

1. Alexander JW, Earley TD: A carpal laxity syndrome in young dogs. *J Vet Orthop 3*:22, 1984.
2. Benedetti TL, et al: A technique for intramedullary pinning of metatarsals and metacarpals in cats and dogs. *J Am Anim Hosp Assoc 22*:149, 1986.
3. Brinker WO, et al: *Handbook of Small Animal Orthopedics and Fracture Treatment*. W. B. Saunders, Philadelphia, 1983, pp 167–183, 386–400.
4. Brinker WO, et al: *Manual of Internal Fixation in Small Animals*. Springer-Verlag, New York, 1984, pp 190.
5. Chambers JN, Bjorling DE: Palmar surface plating for arthrodesis of the canine carpus. *J Am Anim Hosp Assoc 18*:875, 1982.
6. Dee JF: Radial carpal bone fracture and luxation. *In* Sumner-Smith G (ed): *Decision Making in Small Animal Orthopedic Surgery*. B. C. Decker, Philadelphia, 1988, p 64.
7. de Lahunta A, Habel RE: *Applied Veterinary Anatomy*. W. B. Saunders, Philadelphia, 1986, pp 96–117, 137–139.
8. Earley TD: Canine carpal ligament injuries. *Vet Clin North Am 8*:183, 1978.
9. Earley TD: Carpal and tarsal injuries. *In* Bojrab MJ (ed): *Current Techniques in Small Animal Surgery*. 3rd ed. W. B. Saunders, Philadelphia, 1990, pp 871–873.
10. Early TD, Dee JF: Trauma to the carpus, tarsus, and phalanges of dogs and cats. *Vet Clin North Am 10*:717, 1980.
11. Evans HE, Christensen GC: *Miller's Anatomy of the Dog*. 2nd ed. W. B. Saunders, Philadelphia, 1979, pp 90–197, 248–254.
12. Johnson KA: Accessory carpal bone fractures in the racing greyhound: Classification and pathology. *Vet Surg 16*:60, 1987.
13. Manley PA: Distal extremity fractures in small animals. *J Vet Orthop 2*:38, 1983.
14. Newton CD, Nunamaker DM: *Textbook of Small Animal Orthopaedics*. J. B. Lippincott, Philadelphia, 1985, pp 387–391.
15. Parker RB, et al: Pancarpal arthrodesis in the dog: a review of forty-five cases. *Vet Surg* 1981;10:35–43.
16. Piermattei DL, Wind A: Orthopedic problems of the lower limbs. *Proc Am Anim Hosp Assoc 44*: 341–350, 1977.
17. Shires PK, et al: Carpal hyperextension in two-month-old pups. *J Am Vet Med Assoc 186*:49, 1985.
18. Wind A: Fractures of the metacarpal (metatarsal) bones. *Proc Am Anim Hosp Assoc 43*:346, 1976.

CHAPTER 134

Pelvic Fractures

C. W. Betts

Fractures of the pelvis result from trauma but differ considerably in the degree of osseous and soft-tissue damage. Rarely, a pathological fracture may occur secondary to a pelvic bone tumor. Most fractures result from vehicular injuries, and many dogs sustain significant damage to other tissues. Other causes of pelvic fracture include dog fights, gunshot wounds, and blunt trauma. Approximately 25 per cent of all fractures involve the pelvis.[5] The majority of pelvic fractures are multiple because of the boxlike configuration of the pelvis and the short, strong musculotendinous support of the osseous structures. In 299 dogs with pelvic fractures, iliac fractures constituted 18.2 per cent; pubic fractures, 28.2 per cent; acetabular fractures, 14.6 per cent; ischial fractures, 23.1 per cent; and sacroiliac dislocations, 15.9 per cent.[48] Because of the tendency toward multiple fractures and the degree of trauma necessary to fracture the pelvis or cause a fracture-dislocation, adjacent soft tissue and surrounding organ systems must be carefully evaluated.

In pelvic fractures in humans, unrelenting extraperitoneal hemorrhage is the primary cause of death and is second only to skull fracture as the most common fatal bone injury.[15]

Injury to the genitourinary organs is suspected in a patient with pelvic fracture if the patient is unable to void or has hematuria or a bloody urethral discharge. Injury to the bladder may occur by perforation or sudden compression, which may cause rupture by a rapid increase in intravesicular pressure.[45] Rupture of the urethra is more common in male dogs.[48] Spontaneous pressure-elicited micturition occurs more readily in females because of the short, wide pelvic urethra, in contrast to the longer, narrow penile urethra of males. Ureteral avulsion and urinary bladder rupture occur with equal frequency in males and females.[36]

Open fractures of the pelvis in humans are associated with a high mortality rate.[41] A laceration near a pelvic fracture suggests an open fracture even if the laceration does not always provide direct access to the fracture site. Perineal and perianal lacerations also imply an open fracture and probable fecal contamination of the fracture hematoma.[24] Infection in the retroperitoneal hematoma resulting in subsequent septicemia is the most common cause of late death after pelvic fracture in humans.[15]

In addition to direct injury or perforation, the compressive force transmitted to the pelvic viscera may injure the bladder, perineal urethra, rectum, lumbosacral nerve roots, and hypogastric vessels. The rectal wall is less susceptible to rupture or tearing by compression forces than the perineal skin, but when it occurs, the tear frequently is just inside the anus, where the rectum is fixed and less distensible.[2] The rectum may also be injured by compression against the sacral promontory and by perforation of intruding bone edges. Sensory and motor function in the extremities may be lost either by lumbosacral nerve root avulsions or by sciatic nerve injury due to acetabular fractures.[39] Sciatic nerve injury was recorded in 2 of 45 dogs with pelvic fracture.[28] With severe pelvic trauma, a check for adjacent soft-tissue damage and multiple organ injury is indicated. Traumatic rupture of the diaphragm, spleen, or liver and severe contusion of the kidneys are encountered with pelvic injuries. In 604 patients with pelvic fractures, an average of 3.1 concomitant injuries were sustained by the 71 patients that died, compared with 1.0 for survivors.[34]

Although the history is usually straightforward, it is important to inquire whether the dog had urinated shortly before being hit. Perforation or laceration is still a concern, but rupture from intravesicular pressure change is unlikely. If the dog did not urinate before the accident or the owner is unsure of the circumstances, one should ask whether the dog has urinated since injury. The ability to urinate does not preclude bladder or urethral damage, but voiding a normal amount of clear urine is incompatible with serious injury to the urinary tract.

Dogs often support their weight and even walk despite a major pelvic fracture, especially if it is bilateral. With unilateral fractures, the hindlimb on the affected side may be carried. The owner is asked whether the dog has been able to support weight on all four limbs or just three or has refused to stand. By the time the dog is brought to the veterinarian, it may be reluctant to support weight because of musculoskeletal pain, so an accurate history is important.

PHYSICAL EXAMINATION

Patients that have sustained trauma of sufficient magnitude to fracture the pelvis are exposed to a high risk of associated injuries.[9, 44] A thorough physical examination is required. In 26 human patients in whom pelvic fracture was the primary cause of death, 93 per cent were in shock or had clinical evidence of hypovolemia at admission; 18 patients (69 per cent) exsanguinated from their pelvic fractures (within an average of 9 hours) after hospital admission.[34]

Extensive palpation and manipulation of the pelvis are unnecessary, because diagnostic radiographs are taken. Pelvic asymmetry can be determined by comparative palpation of the iliac crests, greater trochanters, and ischial tuberosities. The relative positions of these three bony prominences to one another in the os coxae may provide diagnostic information. These prominences normally form a shallow angle, with the long arm of the angle between the iliac crest and the greater trochanter and the short arm between the greater trochanter and the ischial tuberosity. A greater trochanter that is difficult to palpate and seems medially displaced, with crepitus, decreased rotation, and pain elicited by manipulation suggests an impacted acetabular fracture. Dorsal and cranial displacement of the greater trochanter is associated with a coexisting craniodorsal hip luxation, whereas dorsal displacement alone is more compatible with a femoral neck fracture, capital physeal separation, or a combination of femoral head or neck fracture and avulsion of the greater trochanter. Cranial displacement of the iliac crest occurs with sacroiliac separations and sacral fractures. Instability of the sacroiliac joints can often be detected by applying medial and caudal pressure. A fracture of the iliac shaft with cranial displacement of the caudal segment shortens the distance between the iliac crest and the greater trochanter. An isolated ischial fracture may shorten the distance between the ischial tuberosity and the greater trochanter and may facilitate hyperextension of the stifle by effectively lengthening the hamstrings, but withdrawal may be impaired. The upper limb is carefully elevated, and the groin area is inspected for lacerations and bruising. Severe bruising and inability to palpate the ventral abdominal wall occur with rupture of the prepubic tendon or avulsion fracture of the pubis. These patients are checked carefully for inguinal and femoral ring hernias.

Finally, a rectal examination is gently performed. If this procedure is unusually painful for the animal, a sacral or coccygeal fracture is suspected. Blood on the examining finger is presumptive evidence of rectal injury. During rectal palpation of a male dog, the prostate is sought; if it is not palpable, a tear in the pelvic urethra may be assumed.[24] If perineal lacerations are present, they should be closely inspected but not deeply probed to avoid recurrence of bleeding.

Evidence of genitourinary damage is confirmed by radiography. A retrograde urethrogram is obtained before catheterization of the bladder. If the urethra is lacerated or separated, catheterization may introduce infection into the pelvic hematoma, add to the trauma of the injured urethra, and fail to reveal an incomplete urethral injury. If the urethra is intact, a cystogram is performed, including a postevacuation film. Intravenous pyelography is used to evaluate the upper urinary tract.[45] If the urinary system is intact but blood is found in the urine, urinalysis is indicated.

Once the general examination is over, the animal is carefully raised to a standing position. Most of the weight on the rear limbs is borne by the examiner. Conscious proprioception is evaluated, but musculoskeletal pain may render the test useless. The most important criterion is the presence of pain in the distal extremity, acknowledged by cerebral recognition. Femoral and sciatic responses are checked. The absence of sensation in the lateral digits implies sciatic injury due to nerve root avulsion, sacroiliac luxation, acetabular fracture, or a proximal third femoral fracture. Anesthesia of the medial digit and inability to lock the stifle in extension are evidence of femoral nerve injury and possibly a lower lumbar fracture.

A complete data base is obtained for any dog that has sustained major pelvic fractures. Death due to hemorrhage is seldom documented in dogs with pelvic fractures at referral institutions. It is doubtful that such dogs are referred, and dogs that die of trauma seldom undergo necropsy. Pelvic fracture patients that require abdominal exploration for associated injuries usually have evidence of extensive sublumbar extravasation and retroperitoneal hemorrhage with occasional free blood in the abdominal cavity. A complete blood count and serum chemistry measurements are performed.

Radiographic examination is performed after a thorough history has been obtained, a physical examination performed, and laboratory samples taken. Most dogs experience minimal discomfort when radiographed in lateral recumbency. It may be necessary to permit the dog to lie on its back with the hips and stifles flexed and the limbs abducted in a frogleg position to obtain a ventrodorsal view. If necessary, a lateral decubital view with a horizontal beam can be used to assess the upper hemipelvis. Thoracic and abdominal radiographs are taken at this time if necessary. If a dog is in severe pain and difficult to position, wait until it has been stabilized and can be sedated or anesthetized to obtain diagnostic pelvic radiographs.

ASSESSMENT

Pelvic fractures are repaired to decrease the morbidity associated with multiple injuries and lengthy hospitalization. The choice of surgical intervention or conservative therapy is based on experience and radiographic interpretation.

One must keep postural influence on muscle pull and bony displacement in mind when assessing radiographs taken soon after trauma, particularly if a dog is anesthetized. Encroachment on the pelvic canal by a segmental fracture of the ilium and ischium is much more pronounced when the limbs are abducted for the ventrodorsal view. When evaluating the lateral view of an acetabular fracture, a wider fracture gap and more ventral displacement of the ischial tuberosity are seen on films taken with the involved hip flexed than with the hip in a neutral or extended position.

TREATMENT PLAN

Conservative Therapy

Conservative treatment is used for animals with little or no displacement of the fracture segments, an intact acetabulum, and essentially intact continuity of the pelvic ring.[6] The pelvic girdle provides an effective muscular sling for minimally displaced fractures. The abundant soft-tissue covering ensures adequate blood supply. Conservatively treated pelvic fractures almost always heal. Unfortunately, many pelvic fractures are treated conservatively because of the tired old axiom that "the fractures will heal and your dog will be a functional pet." If one critically assesses these dogs months and years after injury, many are not functioning as well as expected. The fractures have healed, but dogs with segmental fractures now have obstipation (Fig. 134–1) and, less frequently, dysuria. If pelvic encroachment becomes established, breeding females may experience dystocia or need Cesarean section. Dogs with cranially displaced iliac shaft fractures or sacroiliac luxations may have a noticeable gait abnormality that is unacceptable for a performance animal. Dogs with significantly displaced acetabular fractures, especially with an impacted femoral head, frequently develop severe secondary degenerative joint disease. When such dogs are subjected to femoral head and neck excision for the impaction fracture, the results are usually disastrous, with virtual fusion resulting. Patients *correctly selected* for conservative management of pelvic fractures generally do well.

A successful conservative regimen consists of confinement, comfortable quarters, restricted and supervised exercise, and attention to hydration, alimentation, urination, and defecation. A padded area with easy access to water and food is provided. Because of musculoskeletal pain due to the fracture, dogs lie continuously on the unaffected side and may develop decubital ulcers. Hydrotherapy helps relieve aches and pains from bruised muscles and healing areas.

A simple rehabilitation program is initiated to keep the owner involved in the pet's care and aware of its progress. Warm compresses, flexion and extension exercises, and early assisted ambulation decrease the convalescent period.

Some simple supportive measures can be taken to reduce motion at the fracture site and the chance of additional trauma. The easiest to provide is firm footing to prevent slipping and abduction injuries. A simple tape hobble around the hocks restricts mobility and prevents severe abduction/adduction independent of the opposite limb. A bandage roll can be taped between the stifles and the hocks hobbled in slight adduction to maintain lateral leverage on fractures displaced medially. Animals bound in this fashion need close supervision and nursing care. Because daily digital levering of medially displaced segments is ineffectual, painful for the animal, and potentially dangerous (iatrogenic rectal laceration), it is not recommended.

An animal with a minimally displaced unilateral caudal acetabular fracture with an intact contralateral hemipelvis is a candidate for a nonweightbearing sling. A figure-eight (Ehmer) sling is not necessary, because a neutral position of the hip is preferred. Also, the Ehmer sling must be put on very carefully, because pressure sores are common over the cranial aspect of the thigh and the caudal metatarsus owing to tension necessary to internally rotate the hip. The sling is maintained for 10 to 14 days, the toes are checked carefully for swelling during this time, and the dog is gradually returned to normal activity during the following 2 to 3 weeks.

Renal function is monitored and assisted if necessary. Water intake may be limited because of reluctance to move around, and urination may be difficult because of inability to posture and reluctance to break house training. For the same reasons, constipation may develop, necessitating enemas, laxatives, or suppositories.

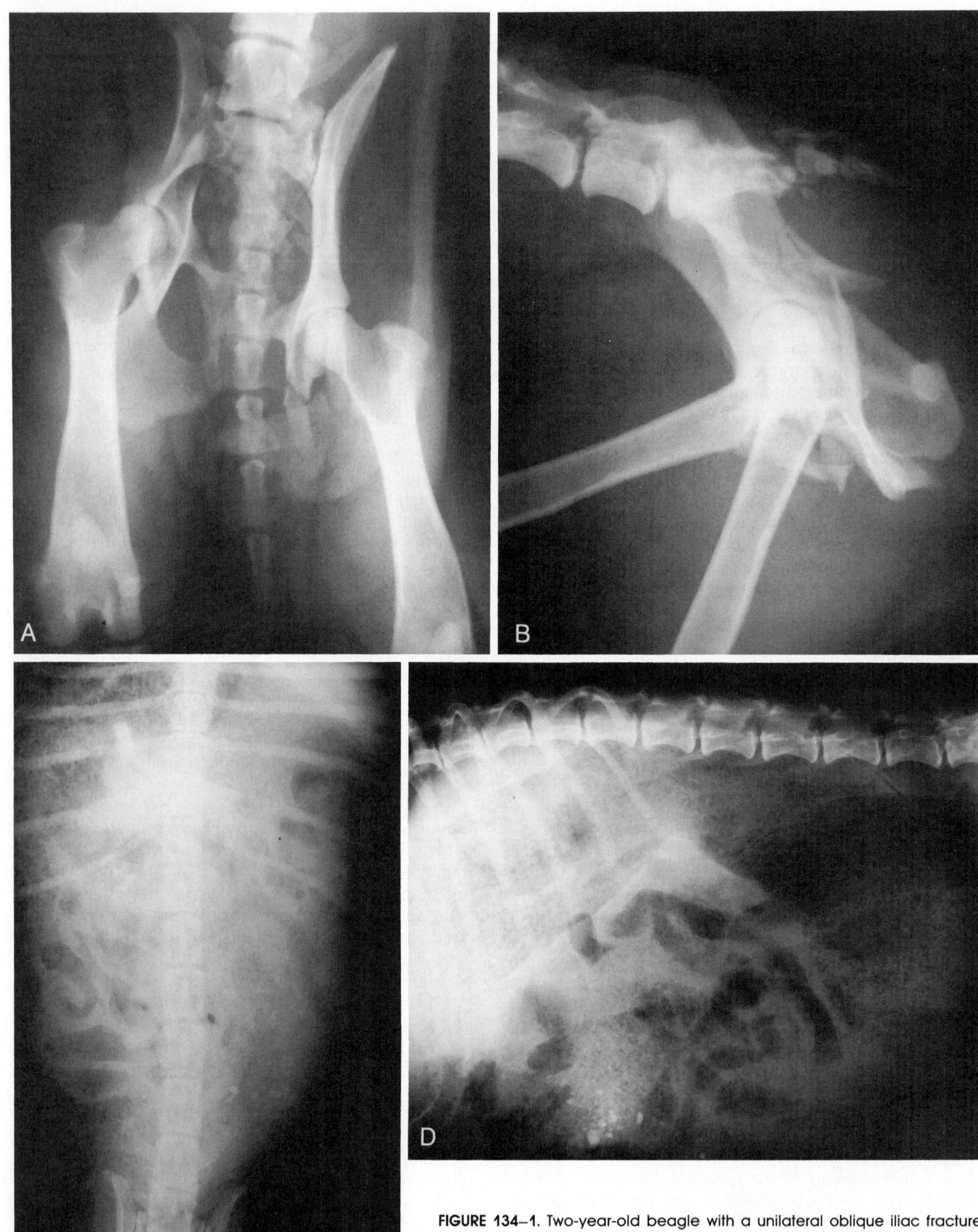

FIGURE 134–1. Two-year-old beagle with a unilateral oblique iliac fracture with medial displacement and a sacrococcygeal fracture/separation. Because of economic constraints, the dog was treated conservatively. Ventrodorsal *(A)* and lateral *(B)* views. Two years later, the dog had chronic obstipation and an acquired megacolon. *C*, The healed fracture with medial encroachment on the pelvic canal and the distended colon are seen on the ventrodorsal view. *D*, The megacolon is obvious on the lateral view.

Surgical Therapy

The criteria for prompt surgical intervention are (1) marked decrease in the size of the pelvic canal, (2) fracture of the acetabulum (displacement of articular surfaces), (3) instability of the hip (fracture of the ilium, ischium, and pubis on the same side; segmental or Malgaigne fracture), and (4) unilateral or bilateral instability, particularly if accompanied by coxofemoral dislocation or other limb fractures) (see Figs. 134–2 and 134–4).[7]

Early surgical treatment of pelvic fractures in dogs was performed with intramedullary pins, wire sutures, and the Kirschner fixation splint.[11, 22] The combination of external fixators, primarily the Hoffman apparatus, and the Swiss system of internal fixation has markedly improved the results of pelvic surgery in humans.[25, 41, 42]

Fortunately, the pelvic anatomy of dogs is more suitable for application of plates and screws. External fixators, excluding the Kirschner device, are too expensive for veterinary surgery. Pin and wire fixation does work, but the highest percentage of success occurs with bone plates and screws.[7, 14]

Early surgical treatment of pelvic fractures is encouraged. Concomitant pelvic stabilization may reduce damage to the lumbosacral plexus, diminish hemorrhage, and prevent further genitourinary trauma.[41] Because of the extent of pre-existing soft-tissue injury in animals with multiple fractures, surgical and anesthetic risks are increased. It is incumbent on the surgeon to select for initial repair the area that provides the most benefit to the patient if further surgery must be delayed. Surgical repair is attempted as soon as feasible for the condition of the animal, preferably within 4 days of injury.[7] Each additional day considerably increases the effort and iatrogenic trauma necessary for repair. After 8 or 9 days, reduction of major iliac shaft fractures in large dogs is almost impossible.

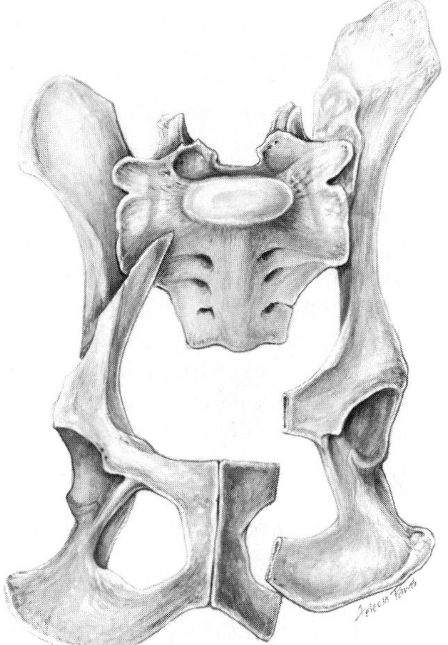

FIGURE 134–2. Iliac and ischial fractures have resulted in instability of the hip joint. The opposite hemipelvis is unstable because of the cranial sacroiliac displacement.

Iliac Fractures

Iliac fracture is one of the more commonly encountered pelvic fractures. The basic tenets of internal fixation apply—namely, anatomical reduction, stable fixation, and early return to function. The majority are oblique iliac shaft fractures with retention of the sacroiliac joint by the cranial segment. The cranial and ventral aspect of the cranial segment occasionally is also fractured, with ventral displacement from the pull of the sartorius and tensor fascia muscles. The caudal segment includes the acetabulum. With an accompanying fracture of the pubis and ischium, the fracture is classified as a segmental fracture. Because these fractures often result from vehicular accidents, the shearing force generated in a cranial direction may result in extreme cranial displacement of the caudal segment. Such fractures are difficult to reduce after 4 to 5 days, especially if the injuries are bilateral. The caudal segment is more commonly displaced medially, increasing the likelihood of sciatic or sacral nerve injury. If the fracture is not repaired, the resulting callus further reduces the size of the pelvic canal. Because the free segment includes the coxofemoral joint, motion occurs at the fracture site with weightbearing, which prolongs pain, delays healing, and stimulates callus formation.

If surgery is ill advised because of associated multiorgan injury or is not an economically feasible alternative, conservative treatment can be used. Confinement is essential. With concomitant adductor muscle and pubic symphysis injuries, a simple tape hobble prevents further abduction injury. Segmental fractures with medial displacement may be gently manipulated and partially reduced per rectum with the animal under general or epidural anesthesia.[37] The reduction can be maintained by placing a roll of cotton or foam rubber proximally between the thighs and taping the stifles together to provide leverage against the roll, creating a fulcrum effect. This support is maintained for 8 to 10 days to ensure early collagen deposition and initial fibrous tissue strength. If possible, sling support is provided twice a day for extended periods. Because of established behavior habits, many dogs are reluctant to void indoors. This reluctance is further complicated by an inability to stand. Activity is restricted and supervised for 3 more weeks after the roll is removed. In dogs with segmental fractures, tape hobbles are used for 1 or 2 weeks after the roll is removed.

With long oblique fractures of the iliac shaft, satisfactory results can be obtained by pinning from dorsal to ventral at right angles to the fracture site. For more transverse iliac shaft fractures, a leverage pinning technique can be used by starting the pins on the medial aspect of the iliac crest, placing them antegrade to the level of the acetabulum without invading the joint. The sacroiliac joint provides a stable fulcrum against which to lever the caudal segment laterally to prevent medial displacement. Placing intramedullary pins is facilitated by using a power drill. Bowing the pin with slight leverage against the drill allows the point of the pin to follow the curvature of the bone. Two to three pins should be used to provide additional stability against bending forces with transverse iliac shaft fractures (Fig.

134–3) and to counteract the shearing forces that predominate with oblique fractures.

The prevailing preference among veterinary orthopedic surgeons is bone plate and screw fixation for iliac fractures.[7, 8, 14, 33, 40] Long oblique fractures in large dogs can occasionally be rigidly fixed with two to three lag screws, but plate application is usually necessary (Fig. 134–4). One lag screw is insufficient unless combined with plate fixation. The latter provides maximum stability (Fig. 134–5). Three cancellous lag screws placed from ventral to dorsal in a cranial direction across oblique iliac fractures in cadaveric hemipelves provided stiffer and stronger fixation than lateral plate fixation.[43]

The lateral approach to the ilium is recommended over the dorsal approach (Fig. 134–6). It provides access through muscle separation and subperiosteal elevation rather than transection of muscle.[7, 8, 19, 29] If necessary, the middle gluteal muscle can be entirely elevated from all but the dorsum of the ilium. The deep gluteal muscle is elevated as necessary from the caudal segment. Once adequate exposure is achieved, reduction requires a combination of levering, traction, and rotation.[7] Kern or Lewin bone-holding forceps or a large towel clamp applied to the crest of the ilium provides a handle for cranial traction. Lewin or Vulsellum bone-holding forceps or a towel clamp can be applied to the greater trochanter, taking care to avoid the sciatic nerve (Fig. 134–7), to aid in caudal retraction of the acetabular component of segmental fractures. An intramedullary pin can also be placed normograde into the femur, and the Jacobs chuck used for a handle on the caudal segment. When the ischial component is continuous with the acetabulum, caudal retraction is gained by securing a grasp on the ischial tuberosity with Lewin or Kern forceps. A Steinmann pin placed in ventral to dorsal direction can also be used as a point of purchase for caudal traction on the ischium. Self-retaining retractors (Gelpi, Weitlaner, pediatric Beckman) are useful in freeing the surgeon's and assistant's hands while maintaining adequate exposure. In long oblique fractures, bone forceps can be applied dorsally to ventrally at a right angle to the fracture line. By placing cranial force on the cranial segment and caudal force on the caudal segment, the caudal segment can be "walked" caudally into reduction. Once reduction is achieved, the self-retaining forceps (Kern, Speed-lock, Verbrugge) clamped from dorsal to ventral across the segments maintain reduction during plate application. An awareness of the proximity of the sciatic nerve to the medial aspect of the body of the ilium during placement of bone clamps is essential (see Fig. 134–7).

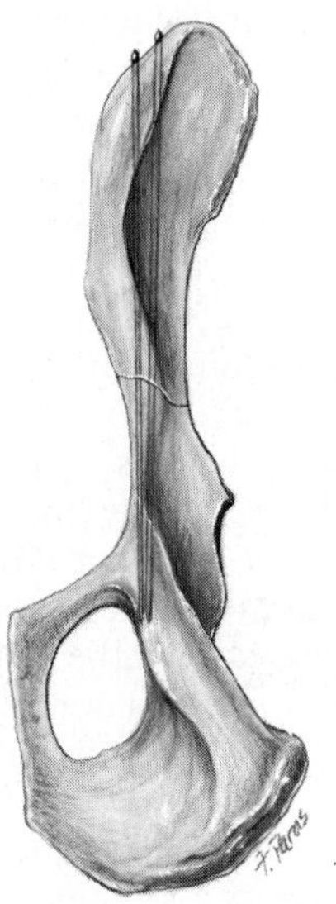

FIGURE 134–3. Leverage pinning has been used to repair a relatively transverse iliac shaft fracture.

The dynamic compression plating system or lag screws are recommended for maximum stability. The plate is contoured in excess of the normal concavity of the ilium to ensure as wide a pelvic canal as possible. Anatomical reduction is desirable, but stable fixation and restoration of the normal pelvic canal diameter are higher priorities. The plate is fixed to the caudal segment first to take advantage of the stable cranial segment for levering the caudal segment laterally (Fig. 134–8). If the plate is secured to the cranial segment first, the caudal segment has to be held up to the overcontoured plate; this maneuver is difficult because the caudal segment is the mobile segment. Dynamic compression plates (2.7 and 3.5 mm) are routinely used, depending on the size of the animal. The 2-mm plate can be used on cats and small dogs (Fig. 134–9).

Closure is routine, and postoperative care is minimal. A nonweightbearing sling is unnecessary. Standard wound management is followed. Exercise is limited and supervised for 3 to 4 weeks after surgery, then normal exercise is gradually resumed. Radiographs are taken 4 to 6 weeks after surgery to evaluate fracture healing.

Acetabular Fractures

Open reduction is indicated for acetabular fractures of the cranial and middle thirds of the articular surface. Most weightbearing occurs on the cranial two-thirds of the acetabulum. Cranial and medially displaced caudal third fractures are repaired because the caudal buttress of the acetabulum is usually in contact with the femoral head.

Minimally displaced fractures, especially of the caudal third of the dome, are treated by confining the dog for 3 or 4 weeks. Preferably, a nonweightbearing sling is used with confinement to minimize motion at the fracture site. The sling maintains the hip joint in a neutral position, and no attempt is made to internally rotate or flex the hip as with the Ehmer sling. The sling is maintained for 10 to 14 days to ensure early healing of soft tissue and initial callus. The sling is removed, physical therapy is initiated, and supervised activity is started. Owners are advised that some degree of secondary degenerative joint disease will develop. In 15 dogs with nonsurgically treated caudal third acetabular fractures, evaluated from 6 to 67 months after injury, 13 dogs had radiographic evidence of moderate to severe osteoarthrosis. Twelve dogs had decreased range of motion or pain in the affected hip, and seven dogs were lame.[3] Surgical repair of these fractures is difficult, and

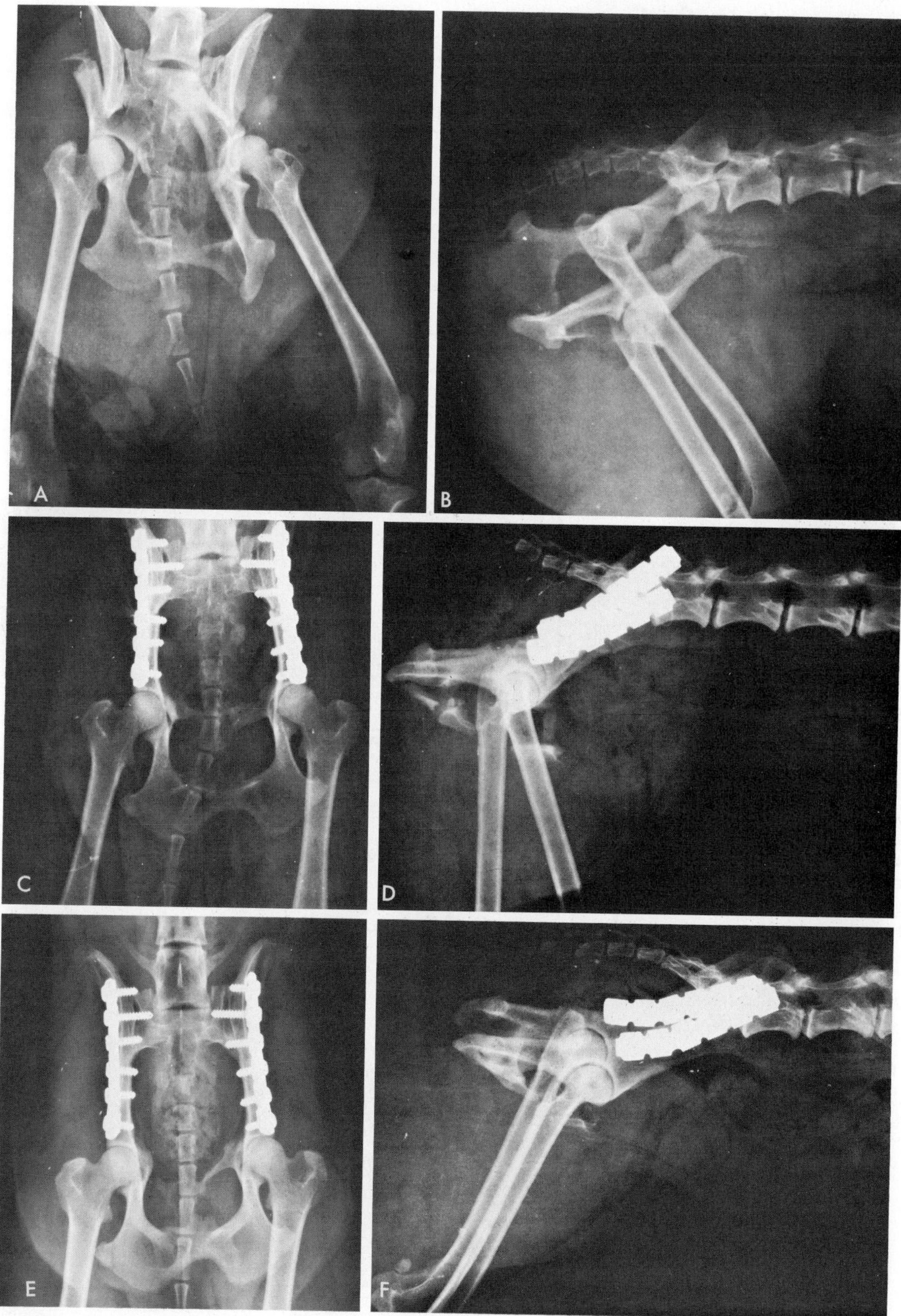

FIGURE 134–4. Seven-year-old poodle with iliac shaft fractures. This case demonstrates the versatility of ASIF reconstruction plates. *A* and *B*, Preoperative ventrodorsal and lateral views. *C* and *D*, Postoperative ventrodorsal and lateral views. *E* and *F*, Ventrodorsal and lateral views taken 10 months after operation. (Courtesy of Dr. Ulrike Matis.)

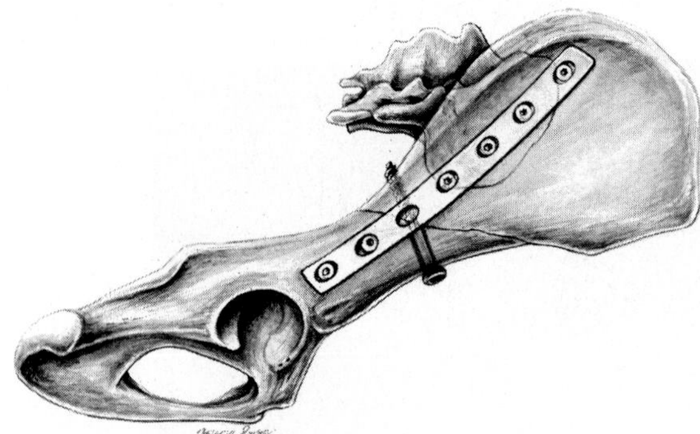

FIGURE 134–5. An oblique iliac shaft fracture has been maximally stabilized with an interfragmentary lag screw and a dynamic compression plate.

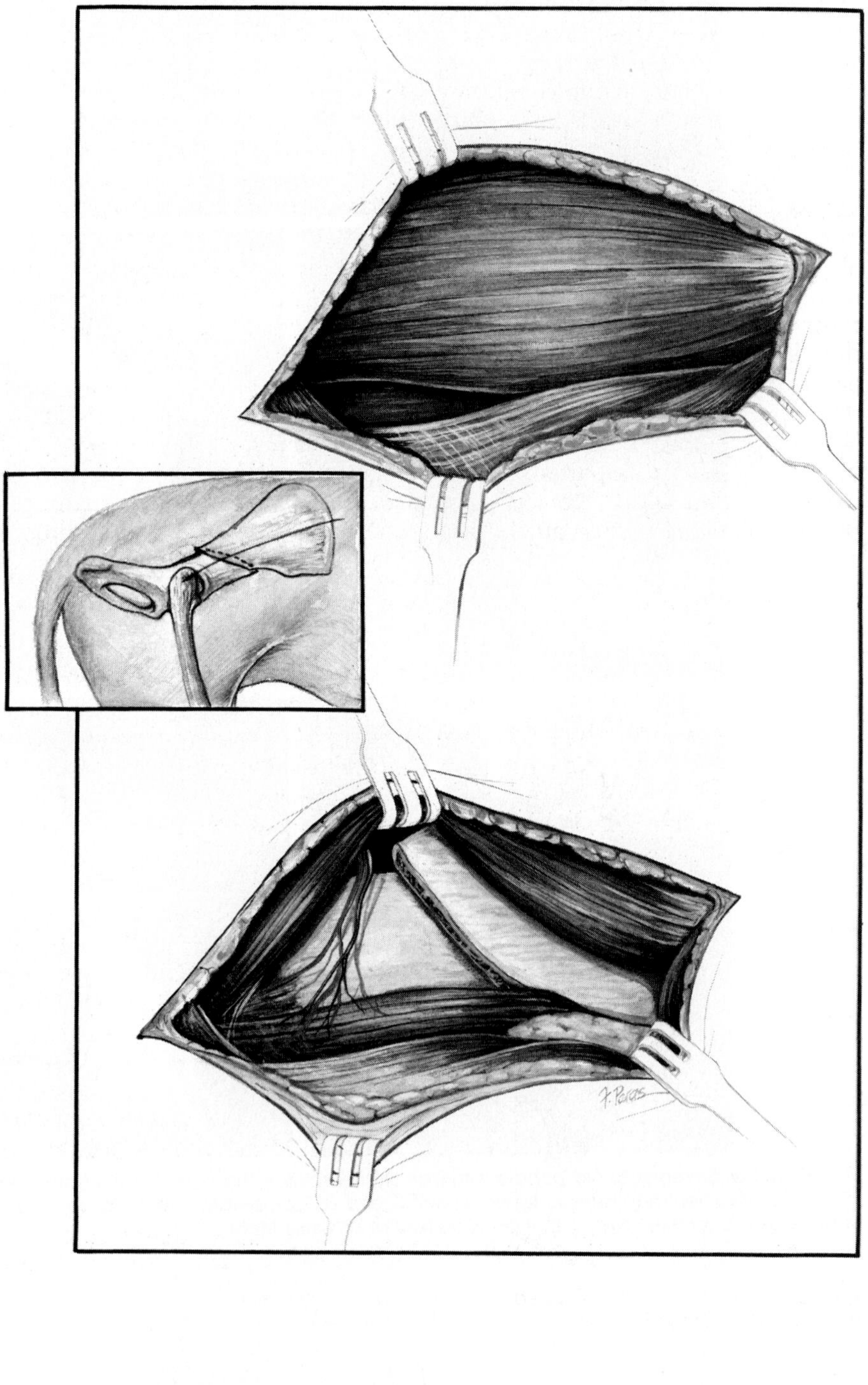

FIGURE 134–6. The lateral approach using a gluteal roll-up method is advocated for iliac shaft fractures.

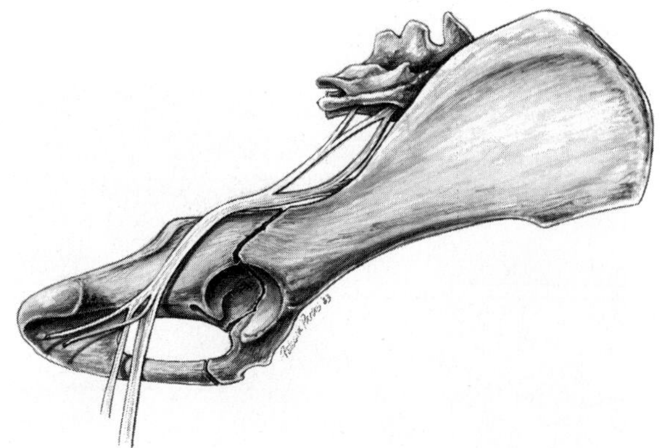

FIGURE 134–7. The sciatic nerve courses just caudal to the acetabulum.

most surgeons treat them conservatively. In 26 racing greyhounds with stress fractures of the acetabulum, the two dogs with surgically repaired fractures successfully returned to competitive racing. Only one dog treated conservatively returned to competitive racing.[46]

Open reduction and fixation of acetabular fractures pose a challenge. The prognosis depends on the type of fracture, the amount of damage to the weightbearing surface, the degree of persistent displacement or incongruity of the articular surface, and the presence or absence of other pelvic fractures.[42] Whenever dislocation or instability of fracture segments is present, surgical repair is advised to decrease the severity and extent of the osteoarthritis that inevitably develops. Crepitus is usually felt when the hip is manipulated.[7] Regardless of the plan, the priority sequence is the patient first, the limb second, and the fracture third. With concomitant limb injury, more important fractures may pre-empt definitive repair of the acetabular fracture. An attempt is always made to first repair the fracture that affords a patient the most benefit.

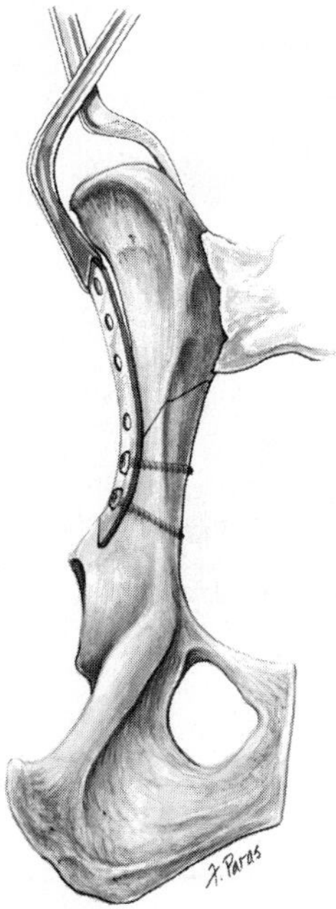

FIGURE 134–8. The plate is secured first to the caudal segment, then to the cranial segment.

Acetabular fractures have been classified into four groups according to the course of the fracture line[20, 21]—cranial, central, caudal, and comminuted (Fig. 134–10). Central transacetabular fractures occur most commonly, with comminuted transacetabular fractures second in frequency.[17] In addition to standard views, an oblique lateral view with the upper unaffected limb abducted and pulled caudally prevents superimposition of structures and aids in defining comminuted acetabular fractures. When available, tomograms or computed tomography scans are helpful in determining articular surface involvement of comminuted fractures and aid in determining the feasibility of surgical repair.

The principles and goals of articular surgery are anatomical reduction of the articular surfaces, rigid reduction, and early return to full function. These principles must be adhered to for successful results with repair of acetabular fractures. To achieve them, adequate exposure of the fracture site and the ability to maneuver the fragments while protecting soft-tissue structures are imperative. Most surgeons prefer the dorsal approach by trochanteric osteotomy (Fig. 134–11).[6, 20, 21, 29, 47] A muscle separation technique that provides exposure of the dorsal acetabular rim through caudal retraction of the superficial gluteal muscle, cranial retraction of the middle gluteal muscle, and elevation of the deep gluteal muscle has been described.[44] The advantages of this technique are less tissue trauma and decreased operative time. Additional exposure for caudal acetabular fractures can be obtained by incising the conjoined insertion of the internal obturator and gemelli muscles. Insertions of the external obturator and quadratus femoris muscles are left intact. The gemelli muscles are elevated subperiosteally with the internal obturator muscle. Opening the bursa under the internal obturator muscle provides maximal use of the external rotators as a soft-tissue retractor for the sciatic nerve. Elevation of the internal rotators exposes the cranial half of the ischium. Reduction of the cranially displaced ischial component of an acetabular fracture is facilitated by a Z-plasty release of the sacrotuberous ligament.[38] The approach selected should provide adequate exposure for that particular fracture while minimizing soft-tissue trauma, especially to the sciatic nerve.

Reduction can be difficult because of limited access to the fracture fragments for application of bone clamps. Cranial traction can be obtained by grasping the iliac

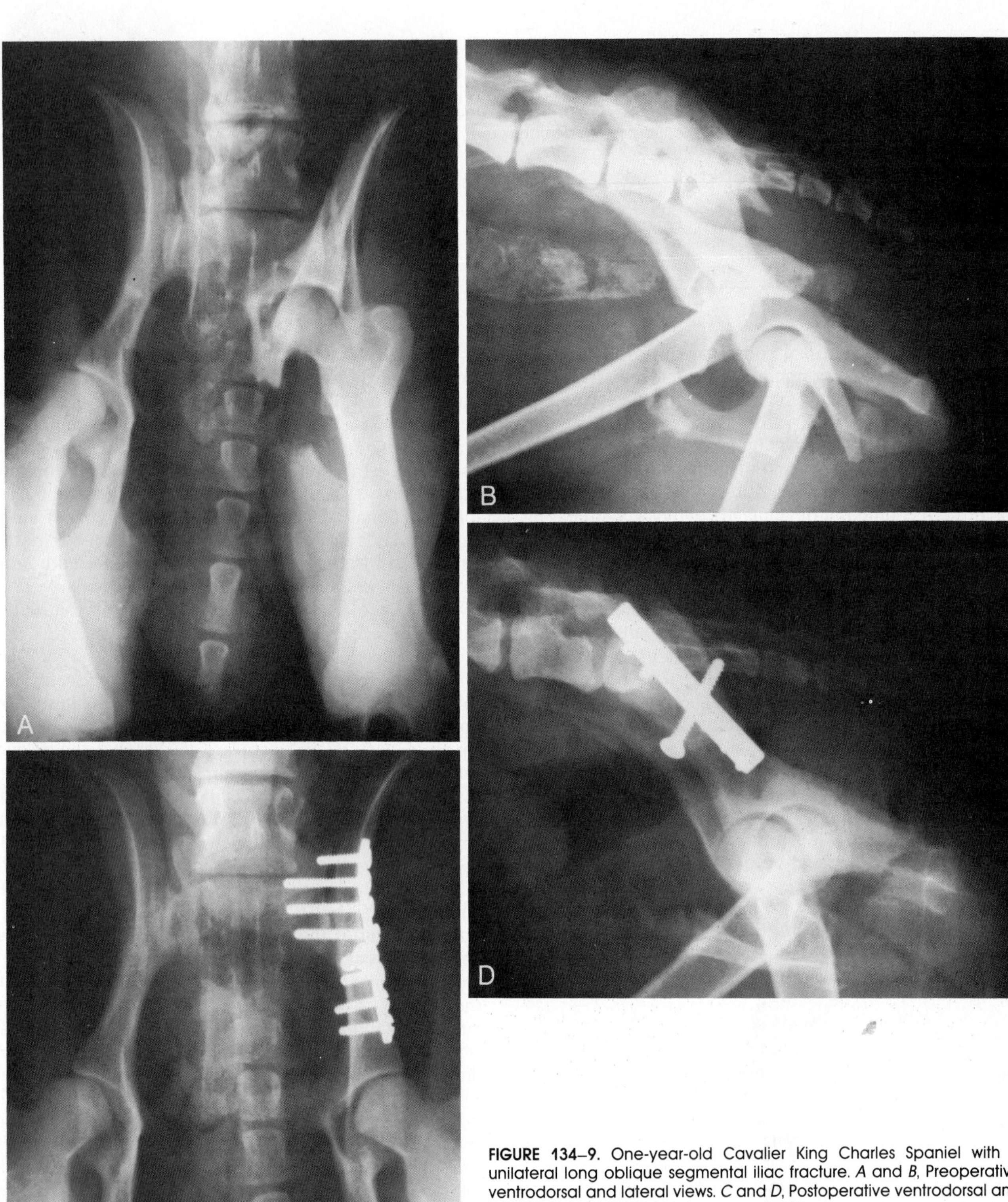

FIGURE 134–9. One-year-old Cavalier King Charles Spaniel with a unilateral long oblique segmental iliac fracture. *A* and *B*, Preoperative ventrodorsal and lateral views. *C* and *D*, Postoperative ventrodorsal and lateral views of plate plus lag screw fixation.

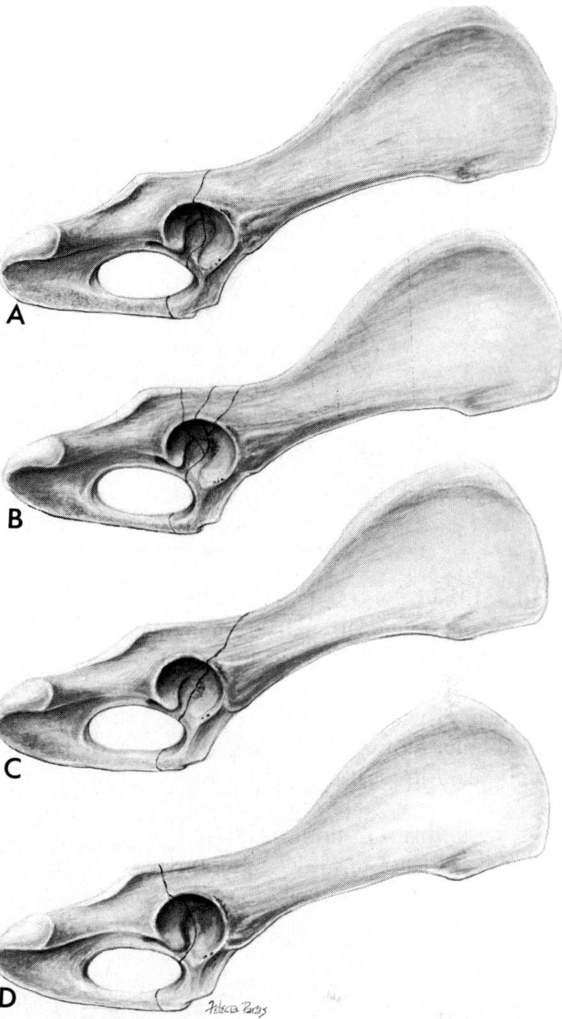

FIGURE 134–10. Acetabular fractures. *A*, Central. *B*, Comminuted. *C*, Cranial. *D*, Caudal.

crest with Lewin or towel forceps. Caudal retraction of the caudal segment can be accomplished by grasping the ischial tuberosity with Lewin or towel forceps or by placing a Steinmann pin through the ischial tuberosity from ventral to dorsal, and by using a Jacobs chuck as a handle. With additional dissection, Kern or speed-lock bone forceps can be applied to the caudal ischium, improving medial and lateral leverage and rotation. If the cranial ischium is exposed, bone forceps can be placed just cranial and caudal to the acetabulum, but extreme care must be used not to stretch or compress the sciatic nerve excessively. When the femoral head is impacted through the medial acetabulum, lateral traction on the proximal femur is necessary. The greater trochanter can be grasped with Lewin or vulsellum bone forceps, or a Steinmann pin can be placed normograde into the proximal femur with a Jacobs chuck used as a handle for lateral leverage. Reduction forceps can also be placed on the distal portion of the dome cranially by spanning the greater trochanter. Once reduction is achieved, temporary reduction can be maintained by placing Kirschner wires across the fracture. A lag screw is used as a component of the final fixation whenever the fracture is sufficiently oblique.

Plate and screw fixation consistently yields the best results. Pins are difficult to place in acetabular fractures and may not provide stable fixation. Also, pins may loosen before fracture healing has occurred.[6] Interlocking stable fragments can be stabilized with bone screws and orthopedic wire used as a tension band.[6, 18] Multiple pin fixation or screw and wire fixation as a tension band can be incorporated with methyl methacrylate bone cement instead of plating.[32] The ASIF mini and small fragment sets have marked the turning point in repair of acetabular fractures in animals.[16] The finger plates are readily adaptable to the contours of a dog's acetabulum and include either straight, L-shaped, or T-shaped configurations. Although seldom used, the smaller miniplates provide secure fixation for fractures in animals too small for the finger plates. With ASIF reconstruction plates, contouring of acetabular plates has been markedly simplified (Fig. 134–12). Also, precontoured horseshoe-shaped acetabular plates (2.0 and 2.7 mm) are available and adaptable to many fractures and sizes of patients.[1, 4] For large and giant-breed dogs, the 2.7-mm and 3.5-mm dynamic compression plates may be more appropriate. Because the plate is applied to the tension side of the acetabulum, a small plate is strong enough for weightbearing forces unless a defect is present that would subject the plate to cyclic bending stress with weightbearing. Thus, it is advisable to inspect the articular side of the fracture as well as the dome to avoid a

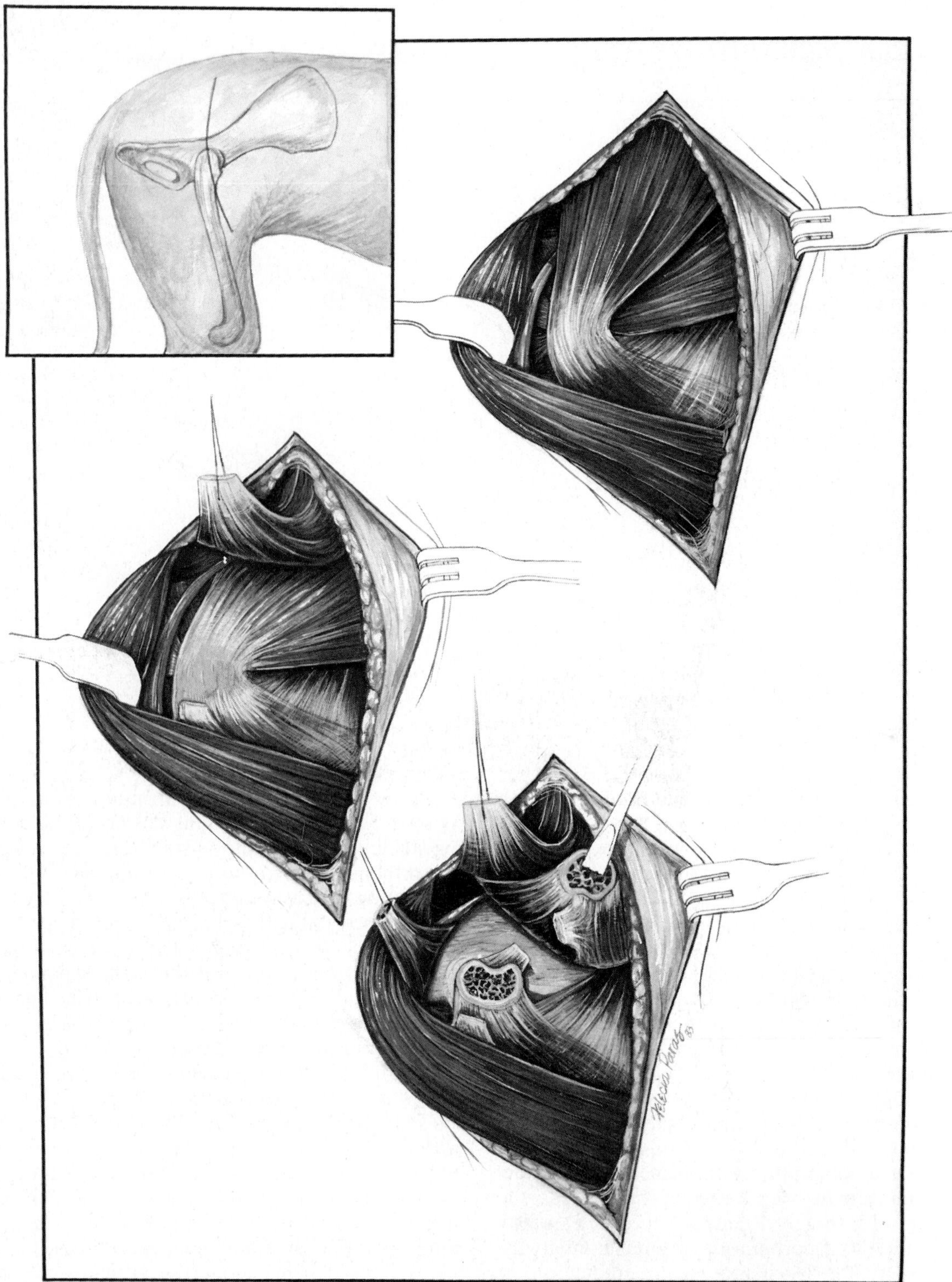

FIGURE 134–11. The trochanteric osteotomy approach is advocated for acetabular fractures.

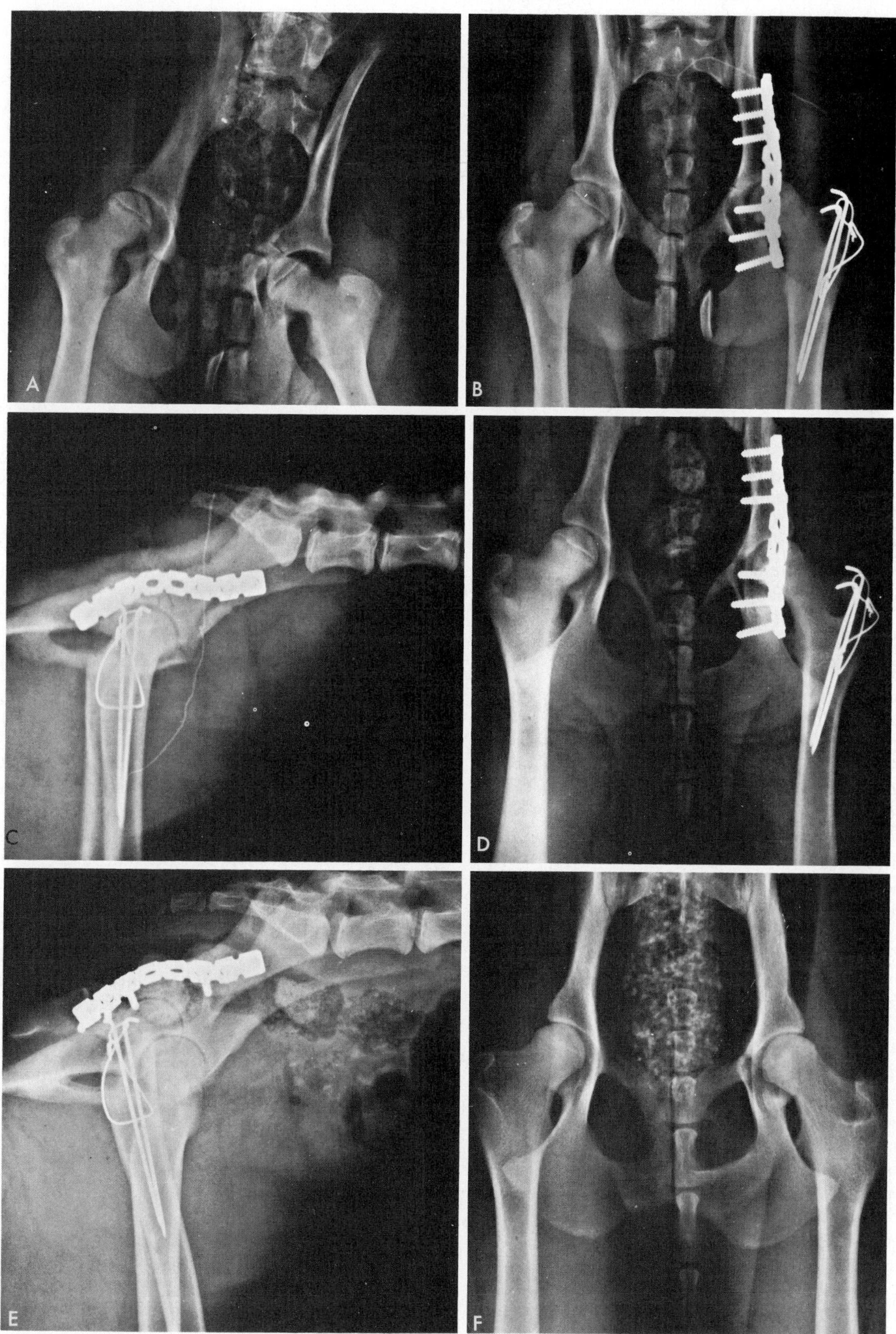

FIGURE 134–12. Acetabular fracture in a 6-month-old German shepherd-type mixed-breed dog that was repaired using an ASIF reconstruction plate. *A*, Preoperative ventrodorsal view. *B* and *C*, Postoperative ventrodorsal and lateral views. *D* and *E*, Ventrodorsal and lateral views taken 10 weeks after operation. *F*, Ventrodorsal view taken 2 years after operation. (Courtesy of Dr. Ulrike Matis.)

fracture gap at the articular surface due to undercontouring of the plate. Fibrin, clots, and bone fragments or debris are removed from the joint. Because weightbearing occurs primarily on the cranial two-thirds of the dome, congruency between the femoral head and the cranial articular surface is imperative. The tendency is for the caudal segment to be slightly dorsally displaced at the cartilaginous labrum owing to an inability to rotate the caudal segment laterally and ventrally. This position is preferable to ventral displacement of the caudal segment, thus interfering with weightbearing on the cranial segment.

Because of traumatic or iatrogenic joint capsule disruption, secure closure of the joint capsule may be difficult. Mattress patterns with nonabsorbable monofilament suture are recommended. Secure joint capsule closure decreases or eliminates the subluxation seen on the radiographs taken immediately after surgery. The remaining wound closure proceeds sequentially to ensure re-establishment of tissue planes and a stable hip joint. A nonweightbearing sling is advised for 10 to 14 days after operation, unless additional injuries make this impractical. Close confinement and supervised exercise are important. After the sling is removed, relative confinement and leash walks only are continued for an additional 2 weeks. During the first 24 to 48 hours after operation, neuropraxia may be evident as a consequence of excessive sciatic nerve retraction. Urination is monitored, because walking and posturing are difficult with the affected limb in a sling. Occasionally, catheterization or bladder expression is necessary. The sling is kept clean and dry to avoid unnecessary changes. A slight amount of swelling is usual and can be relieved by massaging the foot and getting the dog up frequently. Follow-up radiographs are taken to assess fracture healing 4 to 6 weeks after operation. Range of motion, crepitus, and elicitable pain are evaluated.

Segmental iliac fractures with an acetabular fracture can be repaired with a single reconstruction plate. Precontouring the plate to a representative pelvis decreases operative time.[27] Postoperative care is similar to care for isolated acetabular fractures.

Ischial Fractures

Isolated ischial fractures are uncommon and seldom need surgical repair. When ischial fractures accompany other pelvic fractures, stabilization and reduction of the major fragments usually result in acceptable reduction and stabilization of the ischial fracture.[6] When the ischial fragment is large and isolated from the rest of the pelvis, the resulting instability justifies correction. Conservative therapy consists of confinement and a nonweightbearing sling in a neutral position. Flexion of the hip or stifle causes caudal and distal displacement of the ischial fragment because of the pull on the origin of the hamstring muscles. The loss of caudal stability may cause hyperextension of the stifle and delayed healing of the fracture if the dog is allowed to bear weight and walk.

The caudal approach to the hip and cranial ischium is used.[6, 29, 38] Fixation is achieved by an intramedullary pin, wire sutures, or small bone plates. Fractures of the ischial tuberosity can be repaired with bone screws (Fig. 134–13). Fractures caudal to the external rotators can be reduced through a modified perineal approach. This approach works well for decompression of the sciatic nerve compressed by craniomedially displaced ischial fractures.

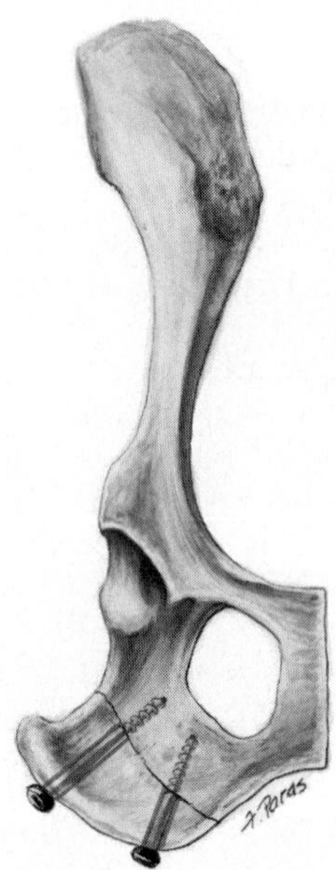

FIGURE 134–13. A substantial fracture of the ischium has been repaired with lag screws.

Sacroiliac Joint Fracture-Luxation

Unilateral separation of the sacroiliac joint is much more common than bilateral luxation.[6, 30, 35] Because of the geometry of the pelvis, unilateral displacement cannot occur without associated fractures or a pelvic symphyseal separation. Surgery is indicated for fractures with marked instability, pain, or bilateral instability.[6, 18]

A dorsal approach to the iliac crest is used, with ventral reflection of the middle gluteal muscle and medial retraction of the sacrospinalis to expose the sacroiliac joint. The cranial gluteal artery, vein, and nerve are avoided where they pass from medial to lateral over the caudodorsal iliac spine to enter the middle gluteal muscle. The articular surface of the ilium is just ventral to the caudal half of the dorsal iliac crest. A diagonal from the dorsal to the ventral iliac spine also bisects the body of the sacrum. Reduction is accomplished by caudal displacement of the ilium, which can be facilitated by having the anesthetist hold the forelimbs or by tying the forelimbs. Bone-holding forceps can be applied to the cranial iliac crest, but lateral leverage on the greater trochanter or ischial tuberosity is needed to overcome the associated medial displacement of the caudal portion of the hemipelvis. When the ilium is reduced, visual access to the sacroiliac joint is limited. A mosquito hemostat can be used to palpate the reduction indirectly. Preplacement of a vertical Kirschner wire in the sacral wing and the dorsal iliac crest at the midpoints of the respective articulations provides a reference point for reduction. Temporary reduction can be maintained with a Kirschner wire. For small dogs and cats, the Kirschner wire is usually left in place after fixation is secured with a single lag screw, but the K wire contributes minimally to elimination of rotational forces.[31] In larger dogs, placement of two lag screws is possible. The angle of drilling is about 20° from dorsal to ventral to gain purchase in the body of the sacrum and to direct the screw below the vertebral foramen. Two screws correctly placed provide stronger fixation than one screw placed correctly. In both instances, use of the largest screw possible maximizes the strength of repair.[12, 31]

Before drilling, a safe depth for drilling is estimated, by checking the ventrodorsal radiograph to prevent entry into the spinal canal during placement of lag screws. If the opposite hemipelvis or sacroiliac joint is intact, a transiliac bolt can be placed to decrease shearing forces and pullout of lag screws (Fig. 134–14).[3] A transiliac bolt is indicated for markedly overweight dogs, in impacted fractures of the sacrum, and in some bilateral fractures. An alternative to the transiliac bolt for unilateral hemipelvis displacement is wiring of the pelvic symphysis after the sacroiliac luxation is reduced and stabilized. A common mistake with fixation of sacroiliac luxations is securing the ilium into the body of L7. If the fixation is stable and no neurological damage occurs, reoperation is not worthwhile. The anatomical landmarks for ideal bone screw placement have been established.[13] Placing a single large lag screw at least 50 per cent into the body of the sacrum provides superior results to placing two lag screws more superficially (Fig. 134–15).[12] A single lag screw that penetrates only the wing of the sacrum seldom holds. I prefer to predrill the sacrum then overdrill the ilium and use a fully threaded screw. This facilitates drilling into the sacral body. The ventral approach is also advocated, especially for simultaneous repair of a coexisting iliac body fracture.[26] Stabilization of bilateral sacroiliac luxations with a single large trans-sacral bone screw is effective[23] and obviates placement of bone screws bilaterally.

After operation, a dog is in much less pain and can be rehabilitated more quickly. Exercise is limited for 4 to 6 weeks to decrease mechanical force on the screws and to permit a strong soft-tissue repair, because bone-to-bone union does not occur. Dogs are observed for sciatic nerve dysfunction after operation, because the sciatic nerve passes just ventral to the lateral aspect of the body of the sacrum. Sacral nerve injuries may be evidenced by abnormal urination or defecation. Sacral fractures are less frequent. Exposure and reduction are more difficult. It is critical to place the lag screws in the sacral body to achieve sufficient fixation (Fig. 134–16).

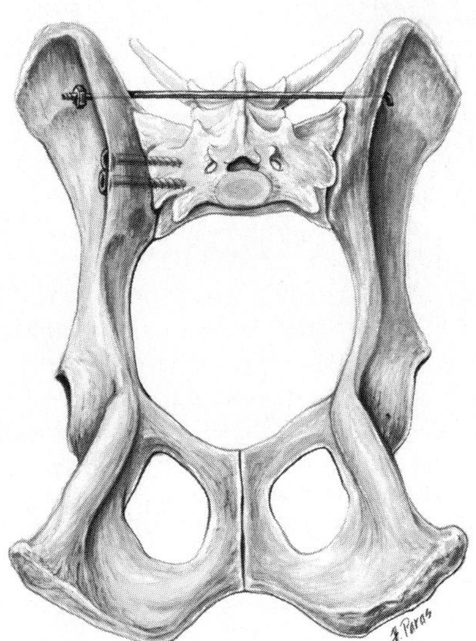

FIGURE 134–14. A transiliac bolt has been placed to augment the lag screw fixation of the sacroiliac luxation.

Pubic Fractures and Pelvic Symphyseal Separation

Pubic fractures commonly accompany other pelvic fractures. Stabilization of the major segments usually provides adequate reduction and stability for the pubic fractures. Damage to the genitourinary system may result from pubic bone fracture or separation-displacement of the pelvic symphysis. Marked cranial displacement of the pubic brim suggests an avulsion fracture associated with the prepubic tendon. In these cases, the inguinal and groin area usually is severely bruised. Caudal ventral hernias are common with this particular injury.

Surgical repair, if necessary, is effected by wiring the fragments together. Exposure is gained through an open approach to the ventral surface of the pelvic symphysis. This can be combined with a caudal celiotomy for repair of prepubic tendon injuries or other caudal abdomen injuries. The obturator nerve is avoided in fractures involving the obturator foramen. Malleable retractors can be placed under bone fragments during drilling, to protect underlying soft-tissue structures. Maximum stability can be achieved with finger plating if fragment size is sufficient.

COMPLICATIONS OF PELVIC FRACTURES

Major complications may arise during conservative or surgical treatment of pelvic fractures. They stem from associated soft-tissue or multiorgan trauma. The importance of a thorough history and physical examination cannot be overemphasized. Serial monitoring of vital functions for several days is equally important. Traumatic myocarditis may not appear for 48 to 72 hours after trauma. Because of the strong muscular support of the pelvis, surgical intervention is needed within 2 to 4 days of injury. Reduction, especially in large dogs, becomes increasingly difficult with each passing day. Unfortunately, pulse deficits, a ruptured bladder, and occasionally a diaphragmatic hernia may not be diagnosed initially. Peripheral nerve injury is always a concern with craniomedial displacement of iliac bone fragments and cranial displacement of the ilium with sacroiliac fracture-dislocation. In one series, 11 per cent of dogs and cats with these injuries had peripheral nerve injury. Eighty-one per cent had good or excellent limb function 16 weeks after the peripheral nerve injury was sustained.[22]

Surgical complications include hemorrhage and nerve trauma. One must take care when using power drills and bone taps to avoid penetrating or lacerating adjacent structures, including the sciatic nerve, cranial and caudal gluteal arteries, urethra, and rectum.

Postoperative complications result from inadequate reduction, implant failure, sciatic nerve damage, and

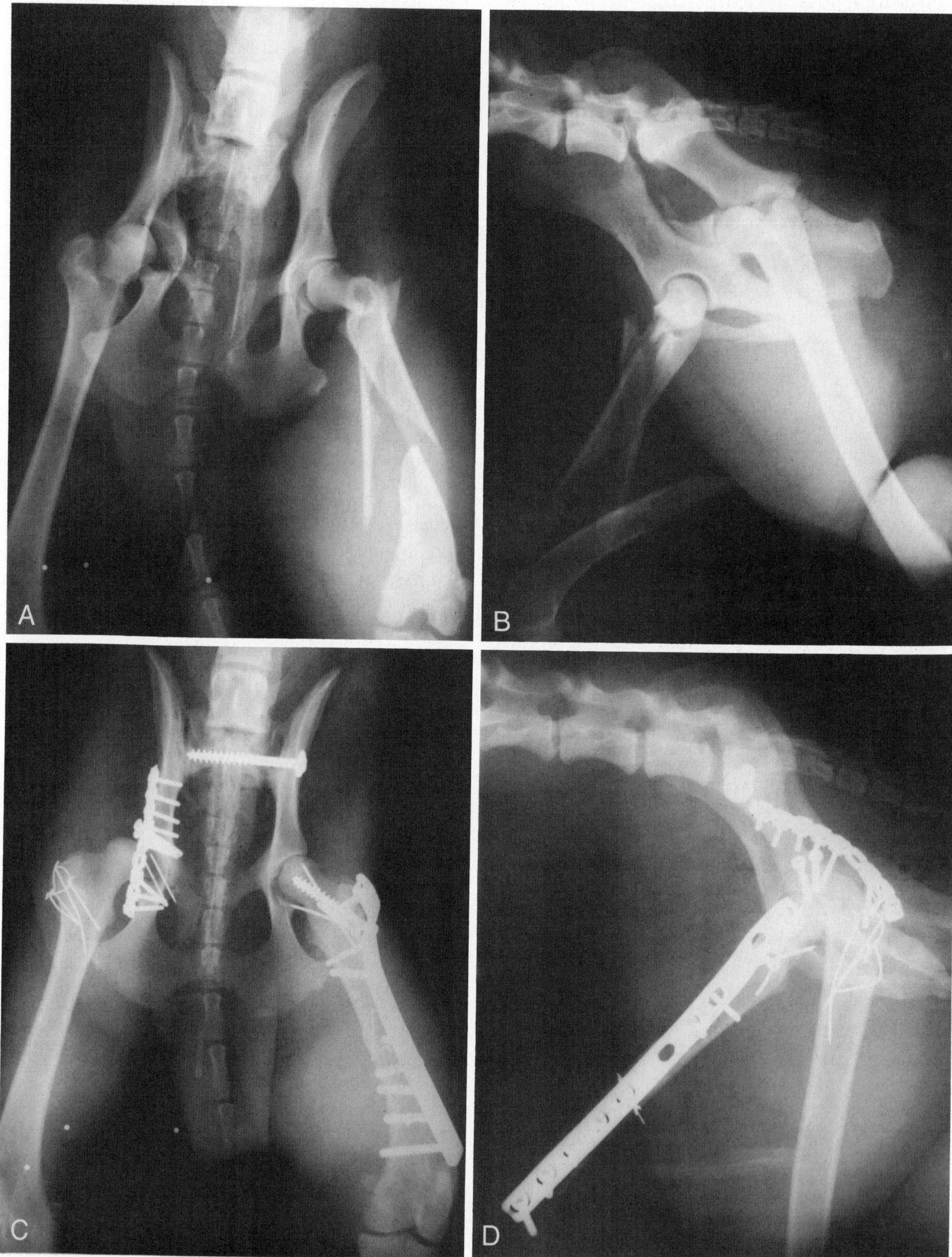

FIGURE 134–15. One-year-old golden retriever with a comminuted acetabular fracture of one hemipelvis, a sacroiliac luxation of the contralateral hemipelvis, and a comminuted femoral shaft fracture with a basilar femoral neck fracture. *A* and *B*, Preoperative ventrodorsal and lateral views. *C* and *D*, Postoperative ventrodorsal and lateral views. Note the placement of the 6.5-mm cancellous lag screw in the sacrum. (Courtesy of Drs. Thomas George and Michael Flynn.)

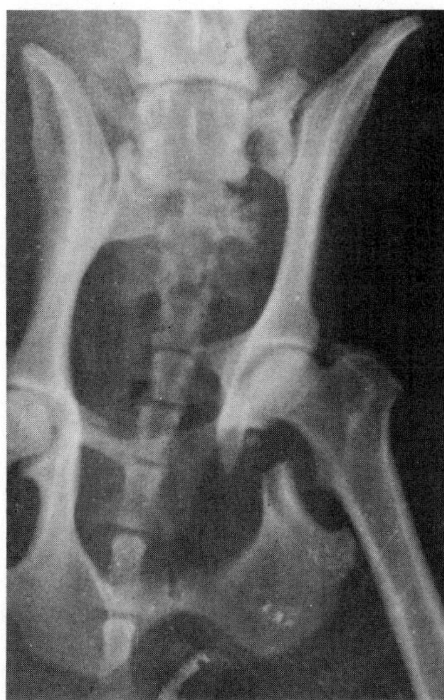

FIGURE 134–16. Sacral fracture. Animals with these injuries must be carefully evaluated for neurological damage.

rarely osteomyelitis. Surgical intervention to relieve acquired sciatic nerve entrapment secondary to callus formation caudal to the acetabulum is seldom successful. In one study, only one dog of six returned to normal function after neurolysis.[10] Nonunion seldom occurs, but malunion due to conservative treatment or inadequate surgical reduction can result in obstipation, dysuria, and dystocia (see Fig. 134–1). Reduction in pelvic diameter can be corrected by pubic symphisiotomy and insertion of an allograft to widen the pelvic canal.

ADVANTAGES OF PELVIC FRACTURE REPAIR

Dogs with repaired pelvic fractures convalesce and rehabilitate more rapidly and completely than those treated conservatively. Musculoskeletal function is better in surgically treated dogs. Clients are generally pleased with the results, and hospitalization and nursing care are less than required for conservative treatment. An important factor is the reduced morbidity from concomitant injuries and associated complications such as pressure sores, pulmonary problems in recumbent animals, and urine or fecal soilage. Postoperatively, an animal that has minor musculoskeletal discomfort is much easier to treat and more responsive to therapy than one that has major fractures and is recumbent.

References

1. Anson LW, et al: Clinical evaluation of canine acetabular fractures stabilized with an acetabular plate. *Vet Surg 17*:220, 1988.
2. Berman AT, Tom L: Traumatic separation of the pubic symphysis with associated fatal rectal tear: A case report and analysis of mechanism of injury. *J Trauma 14*:1010, 1974.
3. Boudrieau RJ, Kleine LJ: Nonsurgically managed caudal acetabular fractures in dogs: 15 cases (1979–1984). *J Am Vet Med Assoc 193*:701, 1988.
4. Braden TD, Prieur WD: New plate for acetabular fractures: Techniques of application and long-term follow-up evaluation. *J Am Vet Med Assoc 188*:1183, 1986.
5. Brinker WO: Fractures of the pelvis. *In* Archibald J (ed): *Canine Surgery*. 2nd ed. American Veterinary Publications, Santa Barbara, 1974.
6. Brinker WO: The pelvis. *In* Bojrab MJ (ed): *Current Techniques in Small Animal Surgery*. Lea & Febiger, Philadelphia, 1975.
7. Brinker WO, et al: Fractures of the pelvis. *In Handbook of Small Animal Orthopedics and Fracture Treatment*. 2nd ed. WB Saunders, Philadelphia, 1990.
8. Brown SG, Biggart JF: Plate fixation of ilial fractures in the dog. *J Am Vet Med Assoc 167*:472, 1975.
9. Bryan WJ, Tullos HS: Pediatric pelvic fractures: A review of 52 patients. *J Trauma 19*:799, 1979.
10. Chambers JN, Hardie EM: Localization and management of sciatic nerve injury due to ischial or acetabular fracture. *J Am Anim Hosp Assoc 22*:539, 1986.
11. Clark JH: Repairing pelvic fractures. *Mod Vet Pract* 31, 1967.
12. DeCamp CE, Braden TD: Sacroiliac fracture-separation in the dog. A study of 92 cases. *Vet Surg 14*:127, 1985.
13. DeCamp CE, Braden TD: The surgical anatomy of the canine sacrum for lag screw fixation of the sacroiliac joint. *Vet Surg 14*:131, 1985.
14. Denny HR: Pelvic fractures in the dog: A review of 123 cases. *J Small Anim Pract 19*:151, 1978.
15. Flint LM Jr, et al: Definitive control of bleeding from severe pelvic fractures. *Ann Surg 189*:709, 1979.
16. Heim U, Pfeiffer KM: *Small Fragment Set Manual Technique: Recommended by the ASIF Group*. Springer-Verlag, New York, 1974.
17. Herron MR: Sacroiliac luxations: Methods of closed repair. *Feline Pract* 46, 1976.
18. Herron MR: Screw-wire fixation of acetabular fractures. *Canine Pract* 48, 1977.
19. Hohn BH, James JM: Lateral approach to the canine ilium. *J Am Anim Hosp Assoc 2*:111, 1966.
20. Hulse DA: Acetabular fractures. *In* Bojrab MJ (ed): *Current Techniques in Small Animal Surgery*. 2nd ed. Lea & Febiger, Philadelphia, 1983.
21. Hulse DA, Root CB: Management of acetabular fractures: Long term evaluation. *Comp Cont Educ 2*:189, 1980.
22. Jacobson A, Schrader SC: Peripheral nerve injury associated with fracture or fracture-dislocation of the pelvis in dogs and cats: 34 cases (1978–1982). *J Am Vet Med Assoc 190*:569, 1987.
23. Kaderly RE: Stabilization of bilateral sacroiliac fractures-luxations in small animals with a single trans-sacral screw. *Vet Surg 20*:91, 1991.
24. Maull KI, et al: The deep perineal laceration—an injury frequently associated with open pelvic fractures: A need for aggressive surgical management. *J Trauma 17*:685, 1977.
25. Mears DC, Fu F: External fixation in pelvic fractures. *Orthop Clin North Am 11*:465, 1980.
26. Montavon PM, et al: Ventrolateral approach for repair of sacroiliac fracture-dislocation in the dog and cat. *J Am Vet Med Assoc 186*:1198, 1985.
27. Ost PC, Kaderly RE: Use of reconstruction plates for the repair of segmental ilial fractures involving acetabular comminution in four dogs. *Vet Surg 15*:259, 1986.
28. Phillips IR: A survey of bone fractures in the dog and cat. *J Small Anim Pract 20*:661, 1979.
29. Piermattei DL, Greely RC: *An Atlas of Approaches to the Bones of the Dog and Cat*. 2nd ed. W. B. Saunders, Philadelphia, 1979.
30. Pond MJ: Sacroiliac luxation. *In* Bojrab MJ (ed): *Current Techniques in Small Animal Surgery*. Lea & Fegiber, Philadelphia, 1975.
31. Radasch RM, et al: Static strength evaluation of sacroiliac fracture-separation repairs. *Vet Surg 19*:155, 1990.
32. Renegar WR, Griffith RC: The use of methyl methacrylate bone cement in the repair of acetabular fractures. *J Am Anim Hosp Assoc 13*:582, 1977.
33. Robins GM, et al: The plating of pelvic fractures in the dog. *Vet Res 93*:550, 1973.
34. Rothenberger DA, et al: Major vascular injuries secondary to pelvic fractures: an unsolved clinical problem. *Am J Surg 136*:660, 1978.
35. Ryan WW: Sacroiliac luxation. *In* Bojrab MJ (ed): *Current Techniques in Small Animal Surgery*. 2nd ed. Lea & Febiger, Philadelphia, 1983.
36. Selcer BA: Urinary tract trauma associated with pelvic trauma. *J Am Anim Hosp Assoc 18*:785, 1982.
37. Singleton WB: Limb fractures in the dog and cat. V. Fractures of the hind limb. *J Small Anim Pract 7*:163, 1966.
38. Slocum B, Hohn RB: A surgical approach to the caudal aspect of the acetabulum and the body of the ischium in the dog. *J Am Vet Med Assoc 167*:65, 1975.
39. Stone HH, et al: Massive crushing pelvic injuries. *Am Surg 34*:869, 1968.
40. Tarvin GB: Management of pelvic fractures. *In* Bojrab MJ (ed): *Current Techniques in Small Animal Surgery*. 2nd ed. Lea & Febiger, Philadelphia, 1983.
41. Tile M: Pelvic fractures: Operative versus nonoperative treatment. *Orthop Clin North Am 11*:423, 1980.
42. Tile M: Fractures of the acetabulum. *Orthop Clin North Am 11*:481, 1980.

43. VanGundy TE, et al: Mechanical evaluation of two canine iliac fracture fixation systems. *Vet Surg 17*:321, 1988.
44. Wadsworth PL, Henry WB: Dorsal surgical approach to acetabular fractures in the dog. *J Am Vet Med Assoc 165*:908, 1974.
45. Weems WL: Management of genitourinary injury in patients with pelvic fractures. *Ann Surg 189*:717, 1979.
46. Wendelberg K, et al: Stress fractures of the acetabulum in 26 greyhounds. *Vet Surg 17*:128, 1988.
47. Wheaton LG, et al: Surgical treatment of acetabular fractures in the dog. *J Am Vet Med Assoc 162*:385, 1973.
48. Wingfield WE: Lower urinary tract injuries associated with pelvic trauma. *Canine Pract* 26, 1974.

CHAPTER 135

The Hip Joint

Paul A. Manley

ANATOMY

The hip is a ball-and-socket joint in which a hemispherical femoral head fits into an ellipsoid acetabular socket within the pelvic bone. The anatomical configuration of this joint permits a wide range of motion while providing maximum stability. The anatomical components function collectively in development and maintenance of hip congruency.[30, 34]

The proximal femur includes the head, the neck, and three trochanters. The neck is the continuation of the femoral diaphysis, and its length is controlled by endochondral growth of the capital growth plate. Premature arrest of this growth plate leads to a short femoral neck and subluxation of the hip joint.[8] The femoral neck joins the shaft of the femur at an angle of 146.2° (SD 4.8°) (Fig. 135–1).[35–37] This angle has been called the *cervicofemoral angle* or the *angle of inclination* and may be defined as the angle formed at the intersection between the femoral neck axis and the femoral shaft axis on a ventrodorsal radiograph.[28] This measurement depends on the technique of measurement, positioning, and the angle of femoral torsion.[35] As the angle of femoral torsion increases, the apparent angle of inclination increases. An increased apparent angle of inclination may be due to increased femoral torsion, an actual increase in inclination, or a combination of both.[23] When the angle of inclination is corrected for femoral torsion, the range has been reported as 137° to 155°, with a mean of 144.7°.[61] The angle between the plane of the femoral condyles and the axis of the femoral neck is the torsion or declination angle.[34] In dogs, the axis of the femoral neck normally projects cranial to the transcondylar plane (Fig. 135–2). The angle of torsion is positive and is called *anteversion*. Similarly, if the axis projects caudally, the angle of torsion is negative and called *retroversion*. The normal angle ranges from +12° to +40°, with a mean of +27° when measured by direct radiographic technique.[65] This method is subject to error owing to positional variation. The radiographic cross-sectional view of the medullary cavity can be seen with a number of different femoral positionings, each resulting in a different angle of femoral torsion. This may be due in part to the cranial-caudal bowing of the femoral diaphysis.[23] A more accurate method, using *in vitro* testing, reveals a femoral torsion of 5.4° +/− 4.82°.[23] However, this method has not been duplicated *in vivo*. A method of indirect measurement using trigonometry and biplanar radiography has demonstrated a normal femoral torsion angle of 18° to 47°, with a mean of 31°.[61] The angle of inclination is not a factor in the development of hip dysplasia in dogs, although some dogs with

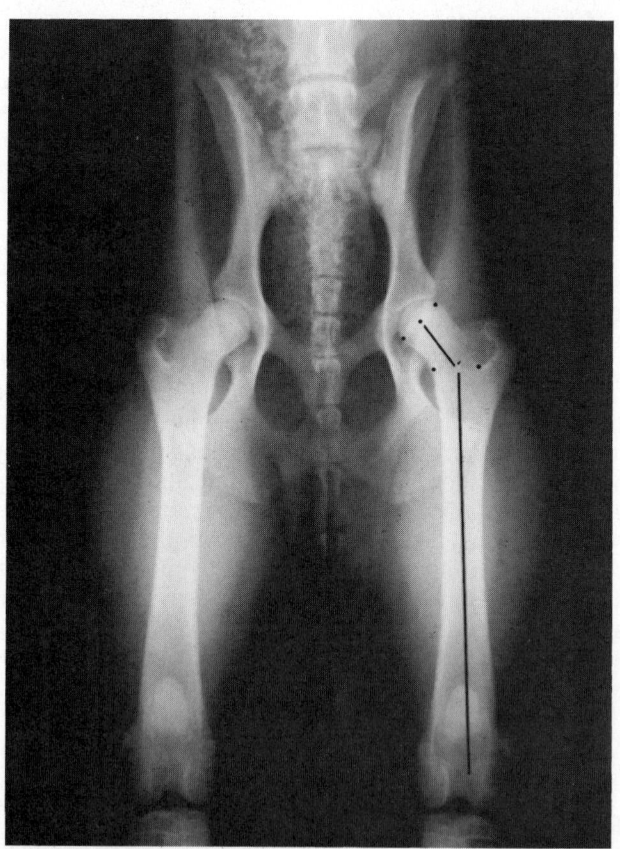

FIGURE 135–1. Ventrodorsal radiographic view of a dog's pelvis with normal hip conformation, demonstrating the technique for measuring the cervicofemoral angle or angle of inclination (From Hauptman J, et al: Angles of inclination and anteversion in hip dysplasia in the dog. *Am J Vet Res 46*:2033, 1985.)

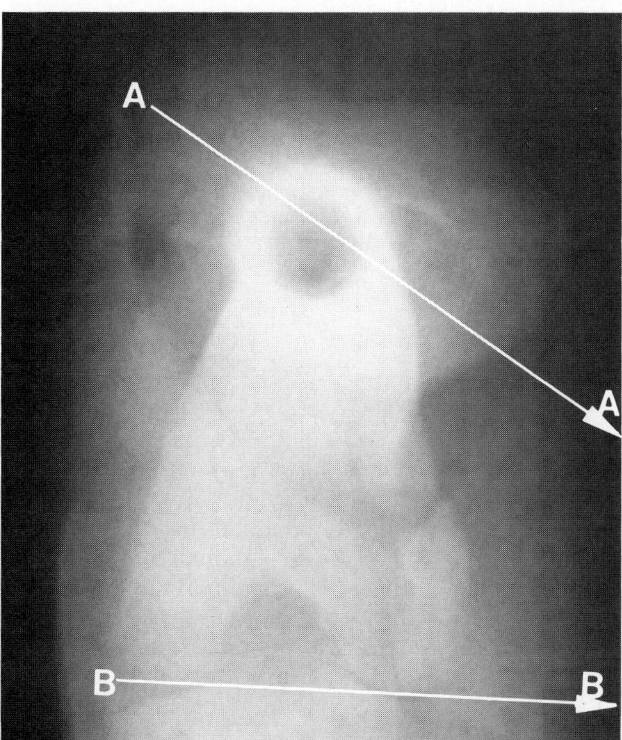

FIGURE 135–2. Radiographic view of a dog's femur, demonstrating a direct method of measuring the angle of femoral torsion. Line A is drawn through the axis of the femoral neck, bisecting the femoral head. Line B is drawn parallel to the caudal surface of the distal femoral condyles. The angle formed by the intersection of these two lines represents the angle of femoral torsion or anteversion. (From Nunamaker DM, et al: Femoral neck anteversion in the dog: Its radiographic measurement. *J Am Vet Radiol Soc 14*:45, 1973.)

hip dysplasia have an increased angle of inclination.[23, 56] Based on calculations using a mathematical model of canine gait, an increased angle of inclination or subluxation of the femoral head has been associated with an increase in hip joint forces.[2] The significance of these forces in the generation of pathological changes in the hip joint has not been described. The importance of angle of femoral torsion in the development of canine hip dysplasia is controversial. Some reports suggest that femoral torsion increases in dysplastic dogs as it does in humans affected with congenital hip dysplasia. It is not clear whether these increases are primary or secondary to hip dysplasia.[23]

The femoral head is hemispherical and forms a cap for the femoral neck. Articular cartilage covers most of the femoral head and is derived from the epiphysis. On the caudal aspect of the femoral head, the articular cartilage extends along the femoral neck toward the trochanteric fossa (Fig. 135–3). The fovea capitis is a depressed area on the caudomedial aspect of the femoral head that is devoid of articular cartilage. The fovea is the point of attachment for the ligament of the head of the femur (round ligament).[30] The ligament is not round but is flat and extends from the fovea to the acetabular fossa of the acetabulum, where it blends with the periosteum and the transverse acetabular ligament. The ligament of the head of the femur is important in the acute stability of the hip joint; as an elastic structure, it is subject to stretching and hypertrophy, which is evident with chronic subluxation of the hip.[55, 59, 85] As the ligament hypertrophies, it may contribute to hip joint instability by increasing the intra-articular volume.[55] The margins of articular cartilage are joined by synovial membrane, which is reflected from the joint capsule onto the femoral neck.

The greater trochanter is the largest of the three femoral trochanters and serves as the point of insertion of the deep gluteal, middle gluteal, and piriformis muscles.[30] The greater trochanter is connected to the femoral neck dorsally by a ridge of bone called the *transverse line* (Fig. 135–4). The trochanteric fossa is a depression located caudal to this ridge and medial to the greater trochanter (see Fig. 135–3). The fossa serves as the point of insertion for the gemelli, internal obturator, and external obturator muscles. The lesser trochanter is a triangular projection of bone located at the base of the caudomedial aspect of the femoral neck. The intertrochanteric crest on the caudal aspect of the greater trochanter curves caudomedial to terminate at the lesser trochanter (see Fig. 135–3). The third trochanter is located 1 to 2 cm distal to the apex of the greater trochanter on its lateral aspect. It is the point of insertion for the superficial gluteal muscle.[30]

The acetabulum is formed from contributions of the ilium, pubis, ischium, and acetabular bones.[30] These four bones fuse in the 12th postnatal week to form a socket that continues to develop in response to the presence of the femoral head.[85] The fit of the femoral head within the acetabulum can be estimated from a ventrodorsal radiograph of the pelvis by measuring the Norberg angle.[63] This angle is defined by a line con-

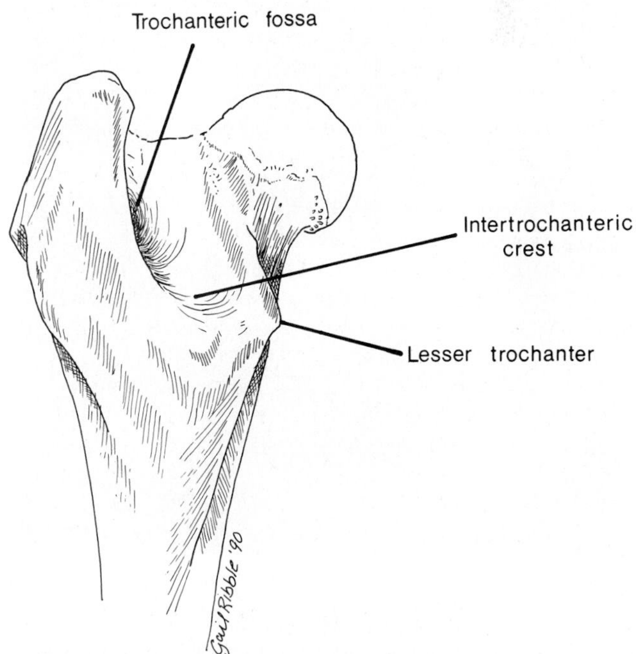

FIGURE 135–3. The caudal aspect of the femoral head, femoral neck, and proximal femoral diaphysis. The articular cartilage on the caudal aspect of the femoral head extends toward the trochanteric fossa. The intertrochanteric crest curves toward the lesser trochanter.

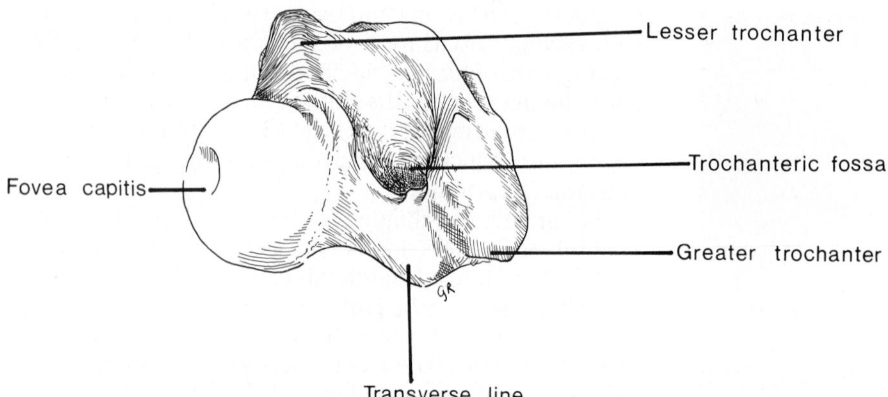

FIGURE 135–4. The dorsocaudal aspect of the femoral head, neck, and proximal femoral diaphysis. The fovea capitis, the transverse line, the greater trochanter, the trochanteric fossa, and the lesser trochanter are shown.

necting the centers of the femoral heads and a second line from the centers of the femoral heads to the cranial acetabular rims. An angle less than 105° indicates displacement of the femoral head relative to the acetabulum and implies hip dysplasia (Fig. 135–5). The Orthopedic Foundation for Animals subjectively evaluates this angle as part of their grading procedure for hip dysplasia. The mouth of the acetabulum is normally directed caudally and laterally. The lunate surface is the horseshoe-shaped portion of the acetabulum normally covered by articular cartilage. A prominent buttress of bone exists to reinforce the dorsal and cranial aspect of the lunate surface (Fig. 135–6). Combined with a thickened subchondral bone in the craniodorsal region of the acetabulum, this buttress accommodates the normally high craniodorsal stresses.[35] The acetabular fossa is a thin, depressed nonarticular area at the center of the horseshoe that serves as a point of attachment for the ligament of the head of the femur. The transverse acetabular ligament is a fibrocartilaginous ligament that is located at the ventral aspect of the acetabular fossa. This ligament extends across the open end of the acetabular fossa to embrace the ventral aspect of the femoral head. The acetabular labrum is the continuation of this ligament as a fibrocartilage annulus attached to the periphery of the acetabulum. These fibrocartilage structures effectively increase the depth of the acetabulum and the stability of the hip joint. In hip dysplasia, subluxation of the femoral head may cause premature wear and tear of the dorsal acetabular labrum and the articular cartilage of the dorsal lunate surface.[82]

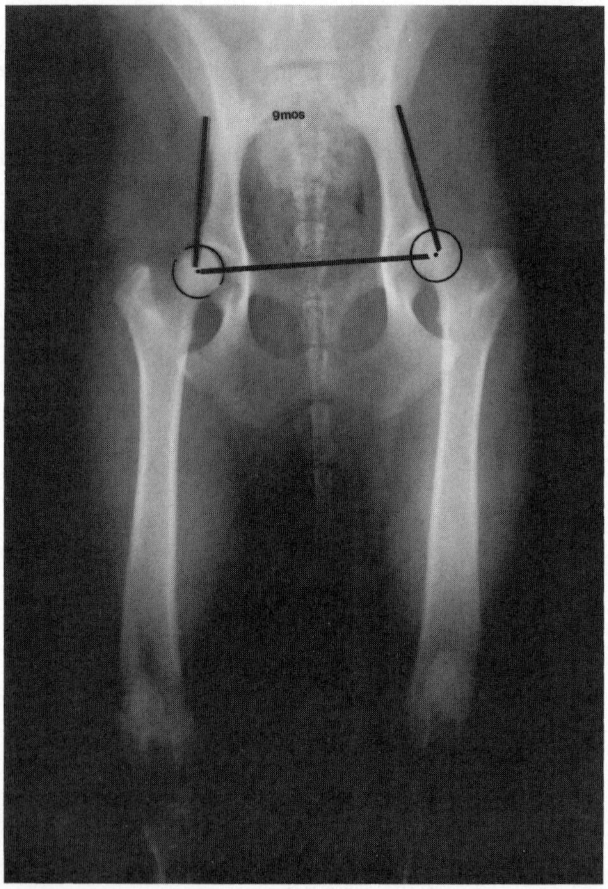

FIGURE 135–5. Ventrodorsal radiograph of the pelvis of a 9-month-old dog, demonstrating subluxation of the femoral heads. The Norberg angle is formed by a line connecting the centers of the femoral heads and a line from each femoral head center to its respective cranial acetabular rim. An angle of less than 105° is considered abnormal. (From Norberg I: The Norberg method of assessing hip dysplasia. *In* Douglas S, Williamson H [ed]: *Veterinary Radiological Interpretation.* Lea & Febiger, Philadelphia, 1970, pp 109–111.)

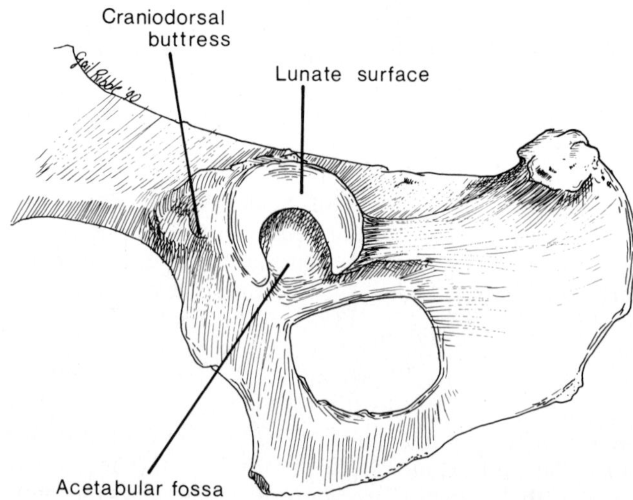

FIGURE 135–6. The lateral aspect of the canine acetabulum. The lunate surface, the craniodorsal buttress, and the acetabular fossa are represented.

The joint capsule is a thick, tight cuff covering the femoral head and enclosing the hip joint. Cranially, the entire femoral neck is covered by capsule. Dorsally, the capsule extends along the transverse line. Caudally, the trochanteric crest and a portion of the femoral neck remain extracapsular. In one study of 25 hip joints from mature Labrador retrievers with normal hip conformation, the volume of joint fluid was 0.26 ml (range: 0.05 to 0.80).[55] In dysplastic dogs, the volume of joint fluid increased to 18 ml (mean: 2.52 ml).[55] The joint capsule of the hip is important in maintaining the femoral head within the socket.[59] In congenital hip dysplasia in humans, the capsule is elongated.[43] It is not clear whether the elongation is primary or secondary to the subluxation.[43, 47]

The blood supply to the joint capsule, the femoral neck, and the femoral epiphysis of immature dogs arises from the lateral and medial circumflex femoral arteries, with a minor supply from the caudal gluteal artery. These three vessels form an extracapsular arterial ring that supplies the entire circumference of the hip joint. The lateral circumflex artery gives rise to the dorsal and cranial portion of the ring, the medial circumflex femoral artery gives rise to the ventral and caudal portion, and the caudal gluteal gives rise to a small portion near the trochanteric fossa. The arteries of the extracapsular ring pierce the joint capsule and give rise to a series of ascending cervical arteries (retinacular arteries), which ascend the femoral neck within the synovial reflection of the joint capsule.[49, 83] These ascending arteries cross over the periphery of the capital growth plate and enter the femoral head as the epiphyseal arteries. The dorsal and ventral epiphyseal arteries form an intraosseous arcade to supply the femoral head (and the proliferative zone of the capital growth plate in immature dogs). Although an arterial supply is evident within the ligament of the head of the femur, it supplies little of the femoral epiphysis (Fig. 135–7).[49, 83] The medial circumflex femoral artery gives rise to the nutrient artery, which enters the femur on its caudal aspect between its proximal and middle thirds. The nutrient artery becomes the metaphyseal artery to the proximal femur and the femoral neck. In immature animals (before closure of the capital growth plate), the metaphyseal artery does not cross the capital growth plate. Once the growth plate closes, the metaphyseal artery anastomoses with the epiphyseal artery to supply the capital epiphysis. An increase in joint fluid, subluxation of the femoral head, trauma to the femoral neck, or fracture of the capital growth plate may result in irreversible damage to the blood supply in this region, with concomitant developmental changes in the hip joint.[44, 49, 57, 85]

The acetabular side of the hip joint receives its blood supply from the iliolumbar, lateral circumflex femoral, cranial gluteal, caudal gluteal, and medial circumflex femoral arteries. The iliolumbar gives rise to the nutrient artery of the ilium, which is responsible for most of the intraosseous vascular supply to the acetabulum.[49]

The hip joint is surrounded by several large muscle groups that are important in support, stability, and locomotion.

The flexors of the hip include the iliospoas, the tensor fascia lata, the articularis coxae, the rectus femoris, and the sartorius muscles.[30] The iliopsoas is the principal flexor in humans and is vital in dogs.[34] The articularis coxae is a small muscle and has an insignificant role in flexion and internal rotation of the hip. The sartorius and the rectus femoris muscles indirectly flex the hip through their action at the stifle joint.[30, 34]

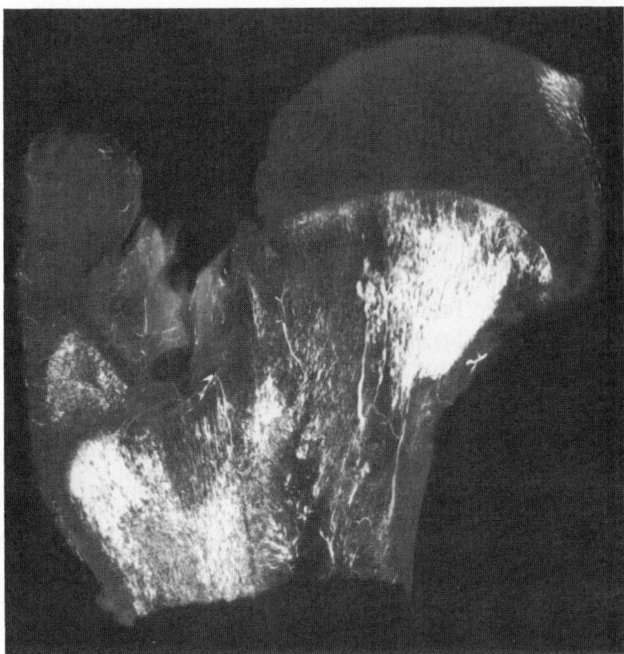

FIGURE 135–7. A microangiogram of the femoral head and neck of a 2-month-old dog. The ascending cervical arteries have been severed, resulting in devascularization of the femoral head; the arterial supply of the ligament of the head of the femur is evident but does not contribute to the vascularity of the head of the femur.

The extensors of the hip provide the largest muscle mass in the hip and include the gluteals, piriformis, quadratus femoris, biceps femoris, semitendinosus, semimembranosus, gracilis, and adductor muscles.

The external rotators include the internal obturator, external obturator, gemelli, quadratus femoris, and iliopsoas. Transection of the external rotators results in some internal rotation of the hip and stifle and abnormal carriage of the hindlimb. The internal rotators and abductors of the femur include the gluteal muscles and tensor fascia lata. The adductors of the femur include the adductor longus, adductor magnus et brevis, pectineus, and gracilis.

SURGICAL APPROACHES TO THE HIP

The approach to the hip joint is dictated by the degree of exposure required for a specific surgical procedure. A craniolateral approach allows access to the cranial aspect of the femoral neck and head and the cranial third of the acetabulum. This approach might prove suitable for a femoral head and neck excision but may be unsuitable for an acetabular fracture of the caudal third of the joint.

Craniolateral Approach

The craniolateral approach or modified craniolateral approach is the most commonly used approach to the hip joint of dogs and cats. It allows exposure of the caudal aspect of the ilial body, cranial third of the acetabulum, and cranial and dorsal aspects of the femoral head and neck. Simple modification of this approach can dramatically increase exposure of the hemipelvis.

The skin incision is made just cranial to the greater trochanter and the cranial aspect of the proximal femur. The incision extends proximally toward the dorsal midline and distally to the mid-diaphysis of the femur.[35, 76] The incision may be a straight line bordering the cranial aspect of the femur or may have a gentle dorsocranial curve centered over the greater trochanter (Fig. 135–8). The subcutaneous tissue is sharply or bluntly dissected until the superficial fascia of the biceps femoris muscle is identified. The fascia is incised along the cranial border of the biceps to the distal limit of the skin incision, and the biceps is retracted caudally to reveal the tensor fascia lata, fascia lata, and superficial gluteal muscle (Fig. 135–9). The fascia lata is incised distally over the vastus lateralis and proximally between the tensor fascia lata and the superficial gluteal muscles. Retraction of the tensor fascia lata cranially and the superficial gluteal caudally exposes the hip joint, which is bordered dorsally by the middle and deep gluteal muscles, cranially by the rectus femoris muscles, and laterally by the vastus lateralis muscle (Fig. 135–10). Retraction of these muscles permits exposure of the cranial joint capsule. This can be verified by placing an index finger over the capsule and extending and flexing the hip. One should be able to palpate the cranial and dorsal aspect of the acetabular rim and the femoral head. Exposure to the dorsal aspect of the joint capsule is enhanced by performing a tenotomy of the insertion of the cranial portion of the deep gluteal at the greater trochanter (Fig. 135–11).[76] Both the middle and the deep gluteals may be retracted caudally after tenotomies of their insertions to maximize the exposure of the dorsal aspect of the hip joint.[76] The capsule is incised from the dorsal acetabular rim in a distal direction, parallel to the femoral neck. The articularis coxae is a small muscle that extends over the cranial joint capsule. It is usually cut when the joint capsule is entered and does not require repair. Further exposure of the joint is possible by incising the capsule parallel to the acetabular rim in a T shape. Retraction of the cut edges of the joint capsule allows exposure of the femoral head and neck and cranial acetabulum. Elevation of the origins of the vastus lateralis, intermedius, and medialis exposes the distal insertion of the joint capsule on the cranial femoral neck (see Fig. 135–11).[17] This modification may be helpful when performing femoral head and neck excisions, allowing access for complete excision of the femoral neck.

Before closure, the joint is lavaged with sterile saline or lactated Ringer's solution. The joint capsule is closed with absorbable or nonabsorbable sutures using an interrupted pattern. Preplacing the sutures is often helpful in closing the capsule. Partial tenotomies may be closed with either absorbable or nonabsorbable interrupted mattress sutures. The vastus muscles are sutured to their remnants or to the cranial insertion of the joint capsule on the femoral neck. The fascial layers are closed with continuous absorbable suture. Subcutaneous and intradermal tissues are closed with continuous absorbable suture.

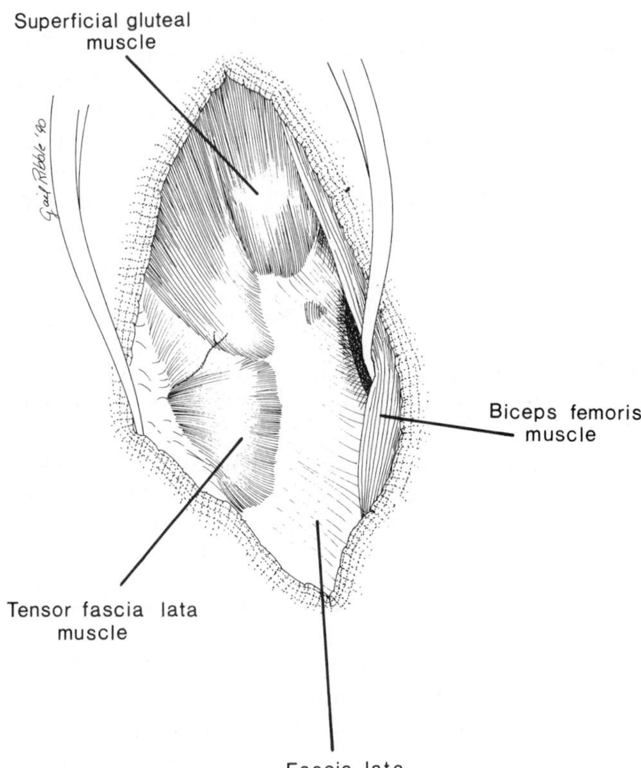

FIGURE 135–9. A craniolateral approach to the proximal femur and the hip joint. The superficial fascia of the biceps femoris is incised, and the biceps muscle is retracted by Gelpi forceps. The tensor fascia lata muscle, the fascia lata, and the superficial gluteal muscle are deep to the biceps.

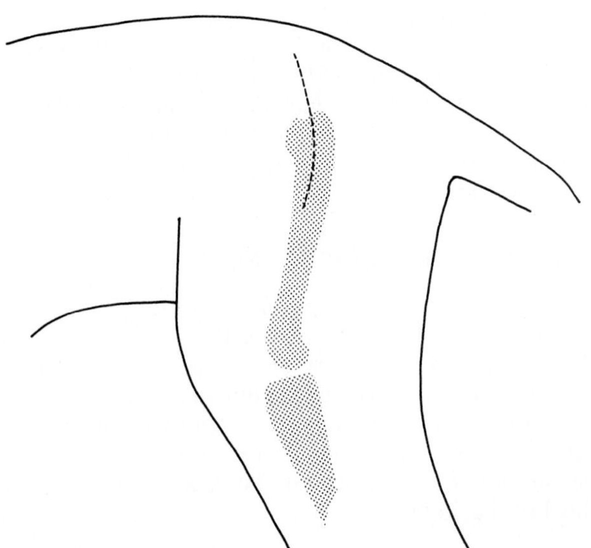

FIGURE 135–8. The position of a skin incision over the proximal femur. In this case, the skin incision curves gently over the greater trochanter.

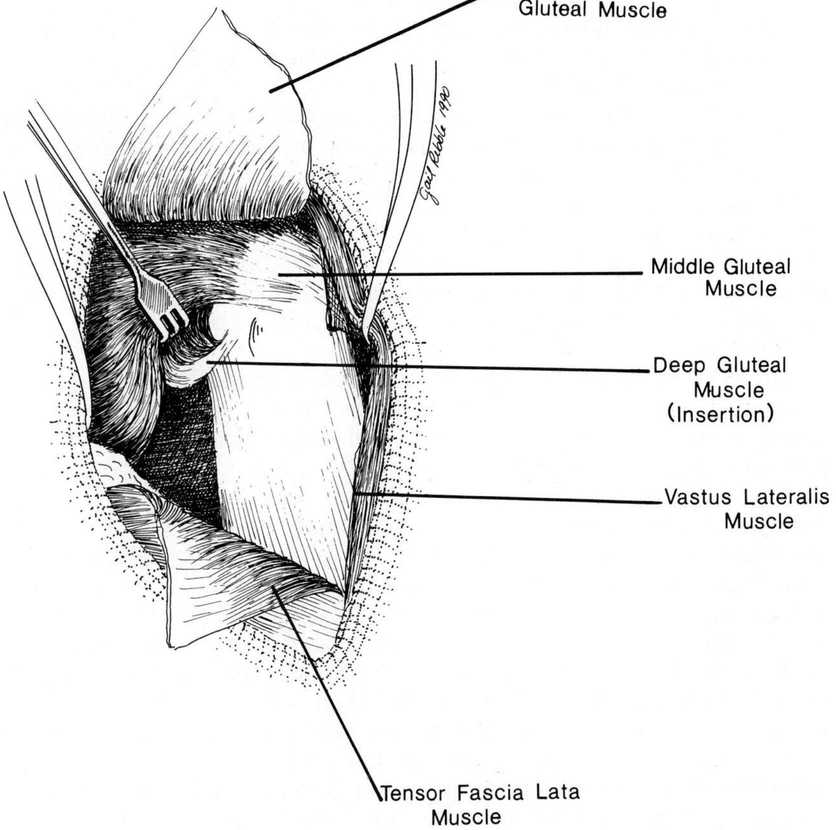

Superficial Gluteal Muscle

Middle Gluteal Muscle

Deep Gluteal Muscle (Insertion)

Vastus Lateralis Muscle

Tensor Fascia Lata Muscle

FIGURE 135–10. Deeper dissection of the proximal femur and the hip joint. The tensor fascia lata and superficial gluteal muscles are incised and retracted. The middle gluteal muscle is retracted with a Senn retractor, exposing the tendon of insertion of the deep gluteal muscle. The vastus lateralis muscle covers the lateral aspect of the femur.

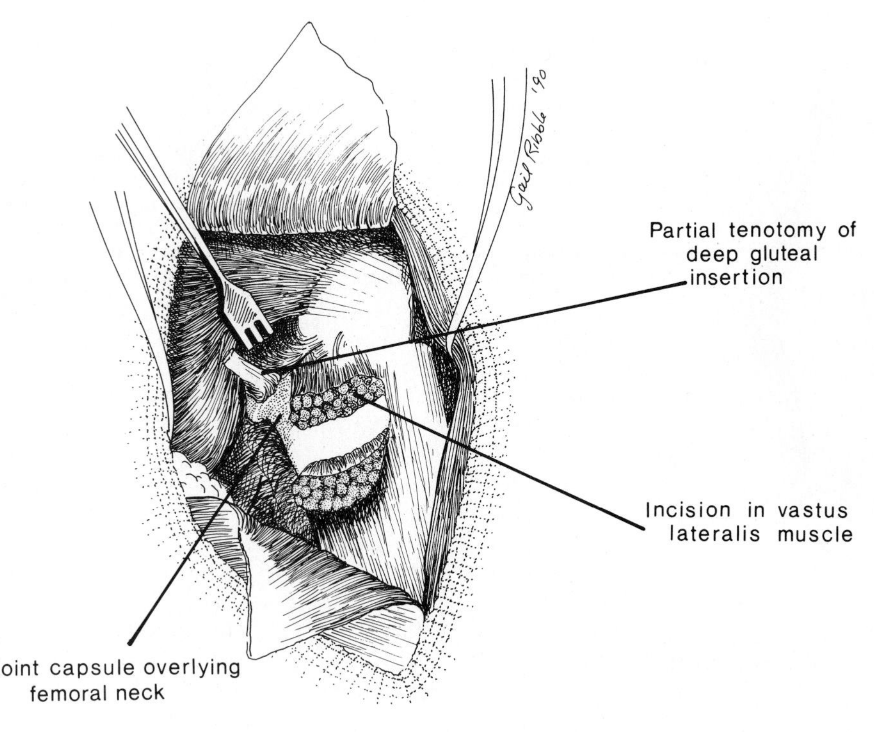

FIGURE 135–11. Partial tenotomy of the insertion of the deep gluteal muscle on the greater trochanter. The vastus lateralis muscle is incised close to its attachment along the femoral neck. This aids in the exposure of the coxofemoral joint through the craniolateral approach.

Modifications of the Craniolateral Approach

Dorsal exposure of the hip joint can be enhanced by performing tenotomies of the insertions of the middle and deep gluteals or by osteotomy of the greater trochanter.[16, 76] Either procedure allows access to the entire acetabulum and the cranial and dorsal aspects of the femoral head and neck. The initial exposure is as for the craniolateral approach. The superficial gluteal may be retracted caudally or tenotomized at its insertion on the third trochanter. In the latter, the superficial gluteal can be retracted dorsally and caudally to expose the entire greater trochanter, revealing the insertions of the middle and deep gluteal muscles.

Tenotomy of the Middle and Deep Gluteal Muscles. If the gluteal muscles are tenotomized, their insertions on the greater trochanter are isolated and incised with tendinous tissue retained on both sides of the incision.[76] The tendon of insertion of the deep gluteal is located on the cranial greater trochanter, and division of its tendon is easily seen. The tendon of insertion of the middle gluteal is located dorsally on the greater trochanter, and the tendon is covered by an extension of muscle fibers over the trochanter. The tendon is not easily seen, but transection close to the trochanter ensures tendinous tissue on both sides (Fig. 135–12). The deep gluteal usually adheres to the joint capsule, necessitating dissection to expose the joint fully. The capsule is opened with a simple vertical or T incision.

Closure of the capsule is as for the craniolateral approach. The tendons of the deep and middle gluteal are closed with nonabsorbable suture in an interrupted mattress pattern. Two or more sutures are placed in each tendon. The superficial gluteal is closed with either absorbable or nonabsorbable suture in an interrupted pattern. All other aspects of the closure are similar to the craniolateral approach.

Osteotomy of the Greater Trochanter. Osteotomy of the greater trochanter can be performed once the middle and deep gluteal have been isolated. The osteotomy is commonly performed with a Gigli wire, an osteotome, or an oscillating saw (Fig. 135–13). If a Gigli wire is used (my personal preference), curved Kelly forceps are passed under the gluteal muscles from cranial to caudal, and the wire is grasped and pulled down to the junction between the trochanteric line and the greater trochanter. Further exposure of the caudal part of the acetabulum can be facilitated by including the gemelli and obturators in the osteotomy. If this is desirable, the Gigli wire must be passed under these muscles.[74] Alternatively, these muscles may be transected after osteotomy of the trochanter.[35] A caudal approach has been described, in which the external rotators are transected without tenotomy of the gluteal muscles. This is a common approach in humans and is useful for total hip arthroplasty. In dogs, this approach offers limited exposure of the caudal aspect of the acetabulum and, without tenotomy of the gluteals or osteotomy of the greater trochanter, has limited application.[35] After osteotomy, the deep gluteal is elevated from the joint capsule and the capsule is opened.

The greater trochanter is reattached using two Kirschner wires and a tension band, a lag screw, or figure-eight wire.[35, 74, 76] The external rotators are reattached

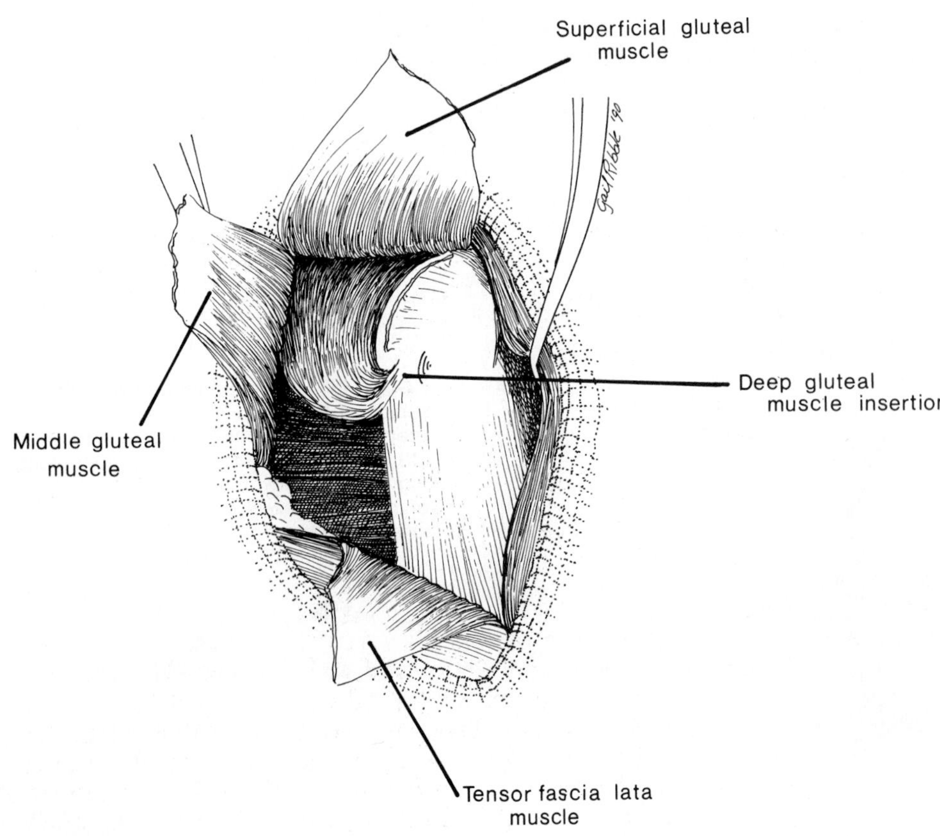

FIGURE 135–12. Transection of the tendon of insertion of the middle gluteal muscle. The deep gluteal tendon of insertion is seen and is transected as in Figure 135–11, revealing the greater trochanter and the craniolateral and dorsal aspects of the joint capsule.

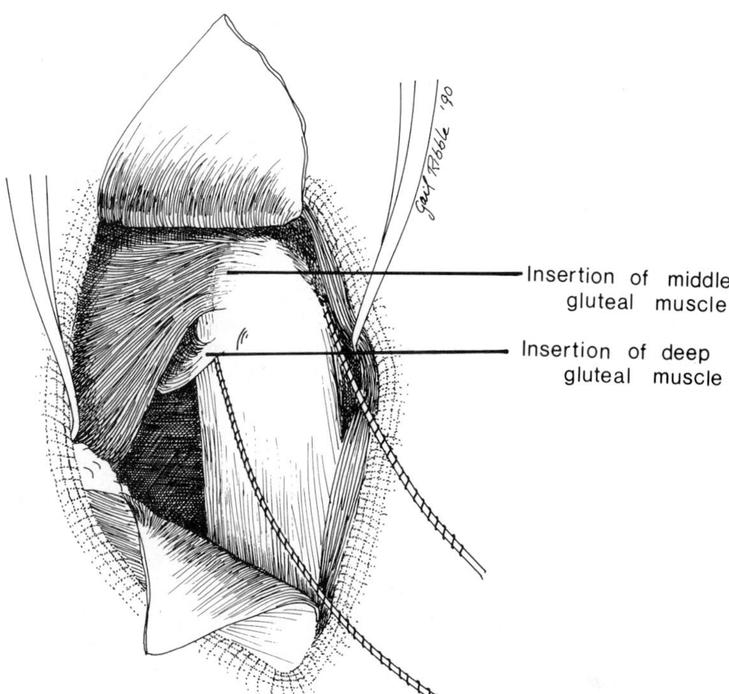

FIGURE 135–13. Passage of a Gigli wire under the tendons of the middle and deep gluteal muscles.

using a mattress or Bunnell suture into the trochanteric fossa or alternatively passing a suture through drill holes extending from the trochanteric fossa to the craniolateral aspect of the proximal femur.[35] The remainder of the closure is similar to the gluteal tenotomy approach.

Dorsal Approach

The dorsal approach, or more correctly the dorsal intergluteal approach, provides limited exposure of the dorsal acetabular rim. It is useful for acetabular fractures in the middle to caudal third of the acetabulum but provides inadequate exposure of the cranial acetabulum.

A curved skin incision is made from the dorsal iliac spine, over the greater trochanter, to the proximal third of the diaphysis of the femur. Skin and subcutaneous fat are undermined, and the cranial border of the biceps femoris muscle and the fascia overlying the superficial gluteal muscle are identified. The gluteal fascia is incised to allow caudal retraction of the superficial gluteal and biceps muscles. The sciatic nerve is identified and gently retracted with a Penrose drain. The belly of the middle gluteal is retracted cranially, and a periosteal elevator is used to elevate the deep gluteal from the ischiatic spine toward the acetabulum.[23] The joint capsule can be incised either horizontally or vertically.

The joint capsule is closed with interrupted sutures. It may not be possible to suture the deep gluteal to its origin. If not, it is placed in position and allowed to heal by granulation.[76] The gluteal fascia is closed with absorbable sutures in a continuous pattern. Closure of subcutaneous tissue and skin is routine.

Ventral Approach[35, 76]

The ventral approach offers limited access to the ventral aspect of the femoral neck and head and the ventral aspect of the acetabular fossa. It offers little advantage over the craniolateral approaches, although it has been recommended for femoral head and neck excision in cats and small dogs and for exploration of caudoventral hip luxations.

MANAGEMENT OF HIP DYSPLASIA

Canine hip dysplasia is a complex disease characterized by primary hip joint laxity in immature animals, resulting in malarticulation and secondary development of degenerative joint disease (see Chapter 145). The available treatments for hip dysplasia vary widely and depend on the age of the animal, desired function, pathological condition of the joint, and financial resources of the owner (Fig. 135–14). For convenience, it is common to divide the treatment categories into conservative and surgical. The surgical category may be further subdivided into palliative, preventive, and salvage procedures.

Conservative Therapy

A recommendation of conservative therapy in the management of hip dysplasia may be made in immature animals after the diagnosis of hip joint laxity has been verified by physical examination and subluxation of the femoral head has been confirmed by radiographic examination. Similarly, it may be recommended in mature animals with evidence of compromised hip joint function associated with advanced degenerative changes. It is seldom the first recommendation to an owner; however, financial considerations may dictate its practicality. In immature dogs, discomfort may be associated with an unstable joint or with a stable joint with early degenerative changes.[102] In mature dogs, discomfort is usually associated with advanced degenerative changes (Fig.

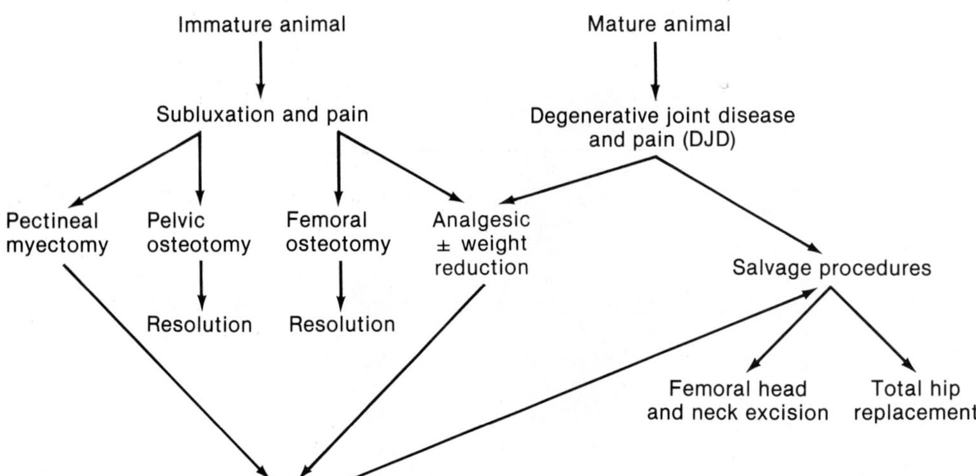

FIGURE 135–14. An algorithm demonstrating the possible treatments for a dog with hip dysplasia.

135–15). The primary goals of therapy are to alleviate discomfort and maintain function. Many dogs may live a reasonably comfortable life despite advanced degenerative joint disease.[4] If an animal is overweight, recommendations include weight loss to decrease the load across the hip joints.[35] A balanced diet is fed to the animal, and vitamin and mineral supplements are discouraged.[7] The judicious use of analgesics may help ameliorate pain. Although analgesics may alleviate pain, they do not alter the degenerative changes that occur in the coxofemoral joint.[102] Nonsteroidal anti-inflammatory drugs (NSAIDs) are the most widely recommended analgesics in the treatment of dysplasia. Acetylsalicylic acid is given (10 to 20 mg/kg PO TID) as necessary. Other orally administered NSAIDs, including phenylbutazone and meclofenamic acid, have been recommended.[102] All NSAIDs have a potential side effect of gastrointestinal irritation and generally are administered with a small quantity of food.* Studies have shown that several NSAIDs suppress proteoglycan synthesis in the articular cartilage matrix and may accelerate matrix degradation.[14] Polysulfated glycosaminoglycan (Adequan) has gained favor in therapy of degenerative joint disease. It is composed of alternating chains of hexosamine and hexuronic acid and incorporates itself into the matrix of articular cartilage after intra-articular or systemic injection.[29] Adequan has a net chondroprotective effect, in part due to its ability to inhibit the catabolic enzymes and neutral proteases that have been associated with degenerative joint disease.[42] Adequan has not received approval by the Food and Drug Administration for use in companion animals.

Nonconcussive exercise such as swimming may help maintain muscle mass and joint function without overstressing the hip joints. Highly traumatic exercises including running and jumping may exacerbate discomfort and are not usually recommended. Passive physiotherapy, including gentle massaging of muscles and flexion and extension exercises, may offer some benefits.[102] Forced abduction and extension of the hindlimbs have been recommended in dogs from 6 to 16 weeks of age as a treatment for joint instability. A single report claims

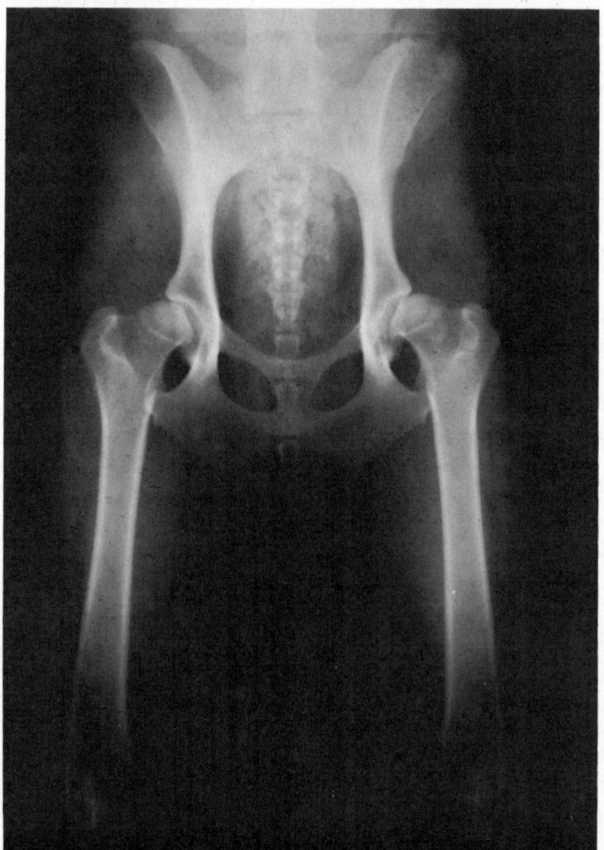

FIGURE 135–15. A ventrodorsal radiographic view of the pelvis of the dog in Figure 135–5 at 3 years of age, showing extensive degenerative changes involving the coxofemoral joints. This dog was presented for exercise intolerance and lameness.

Section Editors' note: NSAIDs other than aspirin and phenylbutazone may be highly toxic in dogs and are not recommended.

excellent results with repetitive abduction and extension of the femur in the treatment of coxofemoral laxity.[18] Unfortunately, clinical reports have not been substantiated by long-term follow-up.[102]

Surgical Therapy

Palliative

Transection of the pectineal muscle or tendon has been recommended for the treatment of hip dysplasia in dogs and cats.[13, 38, 75] Generally, this procedure has found merit in immature animals with pain due to subluxation and little or no evidence of degenerative joint changes. The procedure does not improve joint stability, and the effect is temporary. An unstable joint eventually progresses to an osteoarthritic joint, and pain usually recurs. Performance of myotomy versus myectomy or tenectomy seems to have little bearing on the ability of this operation to reduce discomfort. The clinical benefits of this procedure are difficult to predict but generally are related to the degree of degenerative changes in the hip joint at surgery.[102] In animals with an unstable joint and mild degenerative changes, the results are favorable. As the degenerative changes become more severe, the results of this procedure are inconsistent.

The purpose of a pectineal myectomy is to release one of the adductor muscles and allow increased abduction of the femur.[3] Theoretically, spasm of the pectineal muscle could create an upward force on the femoral head, driving it against the dorsal acetabular rim.[3, 79, 102] Although pectineal muscle fiber hypotrophy has been verified in dogs with hip dysplasia, a cause-and-effect relationship has not been established.[46] This procedure is not recommended as a substitute for a corrective osteotomy; however, it may provide temporary relief from pain.

The procedure is usually performed bilaterally with an animal in dorsal recumbency and the femurs flexed and abducted. The pectineal muscle can be easily palpated as a taut band on the medial aspect of the thigh. When performing a myectomy, a skin incision is made directly over the muscle, extending from the pubic bone to the middle third of the femoral diaphysis. The femoral artery and vein are located cranial to the pectineal muscle. The subcutaneous tissue is bluntly dissected to expose the belly of the muscle. It may be necessary to retract the sartorius cranially to see the distal extent of the muscle. The proximal caudal femoral artery and vein cross the medial aspect of the pectineal muscle just proximal to its myotendinous junction. A small branch of the artery and vein enter the distal portion of the muscle and must be ligated. The entire muscle can be transected and removed by cutting through the tendinous portion distally and by stripping the muscle proximally. The muscle can be sharply dissected or elevated from its proximal origin on the prepubic tendon and ileopectineal eminence of the pubic bone. Alternatively, dissection of the tendinous portion is performed distal to the proximal caudal femoral artery and vein, and the tendon is completely transected. Subcutaneous tissue and skin are closed with a simple continuous or interrupted pattern. A seroma occasionally forms near the pectineal muscle 3 to 5 days after surgery, usually as a result of inadequate hemostasis. Management of the seroma is conservative. Redevelopment of a tight band on the medial aspect of the thigh indicates incomplete transection of the tendinous portion of the pectineal muscle.[102]

Preventive Procedures

Reconstructive osteotomies of the femur or pelvis have been advocated to increase the stability of the hip joint in immature animals by bringing the femur and acetabulum into closer apposition. Secondarily, these procedures prevent the development or slow the progression of degenerative changes in the hip joint by providing a more congruent articulation. A femoral osteotomy can be performed to place the proximal femur in a varus position (angle of inclination < 145°) and to correct excess anteversion. A pelvic osteotomy allows rotation of the acetabulum over the femoral head to increase dorsal coverage.

Intertrochanteric Osteotomy. *Femoral osteotomy* is usually performed in the intertrochanteric region to correct the angle of inclination or the angle of femoral torsion.[35, 64, 80, 101] A decrease in the angle of inclination to a varus position decreases the hip joint force and abductor force,[2] allowing better centering of the femoral head within the acetabulum and decreasing the abnormal loading of the dorsal acetabular rim that is evident with subluxation.[78, 80] The procedure is recommended in young growing dogs that have radiographic evidence of subluxation and have either an increased angle of inclination or an increased angle of femoral torsion or both. It is not recommended as the treatment of choice in animals that have subluxation and severe acetabular dysplasia.[35, 101] Femoral osteotomy is most effective if performed before the development of degenerative changes in the hip joint.[101] The procedure is recommended at the level of the lesser trochanter so that the femoral malformation can be corrected proximally, without changing the shape of the femoral diaphysis.[101] Midshaft femoral osteotomies to correct excess femoral torsion are not successful.[64]

The angle of inclination and angle of femoral torsion can be calculated from the ventrodorsal and lateral radiographs (see Fig. 135–1).[61] A valgus deformity of the femoral neck (inclination angle > 145°) can be corrected by removing a wedge from the proximal femoral metaphysis to create a cervicofemoral angle of 135°,[80, 101] placing the femoral neck and head in a slight varus position.[2, 78, 79] Excess anteversion or retroversion can be corrected by derotation of the proximal segment to the desired angle. A shortened femoral neck can be corrected by moving the distal femoral segment laterally in relation to the femoral head and neck.[80] Calculating desired angles of inclination and femoral torsion before surgery allows preplanning and prebending of implants, thus expediting the surgical procedure.

The surgical technique of intertrochanteric osteotomy has been adequately described and illustrated.[35, 79, 80, 101]

A skin incision is made over the lateral aspect of the femur, extending from the level of the greater trochanter to the middle third of the femur. Subcutaneous tissue is undermined, and the fascia lata and biceps femoris muscle are identified. An incision is made along the cranial border of the biceps in the fascia lata. The biceps is retracted caudally, and the fascia lata is retracted cranially to expose the lateral femur. The superficial gluteal is identified and transected close to its insertion on the third trochanter. The vastus lateralis is identified and elevated from the craniolateral proximal femur. A transverse femoral osteotomy is performed just proximal to the lesser trochanter. A second osteotomy is performed proximal to the transverse osteotomy to remove a wedge of bone and to correct the angle of inclination. Derotation of the proximal segment at this time corrects abnormal femoral torsion (internal rotation of the proximal segment corrects excess anteversion). A double-hook plate, a blade plate, or a dynamic compression plate is used to secure the osteotomy (Fig. 135–16).[64, 101] The double-hook plate has been specifically designed for intertrochanteric osteotomies in dogs.[79] The instrumentation that accompanies this plate facilitates accurate wedge osteotomy and stable fixation of the proximal femur.[80, 101] Closure of the soft tissues is routine. Postoperatively, the animal is confined to leash walking for 4 to 6 weeks. Swimming may be helpful in the convalescent period as a form of active physiotherapy.[101] If the procedure is to be performed bilaterally, the second operation is planned approximately 1 month after the first. Complications associated with this procedure include infection, implant failure, and progression of degenerative joint disease. The latter appears related to the degree of degenerative changes at surgery.[101]

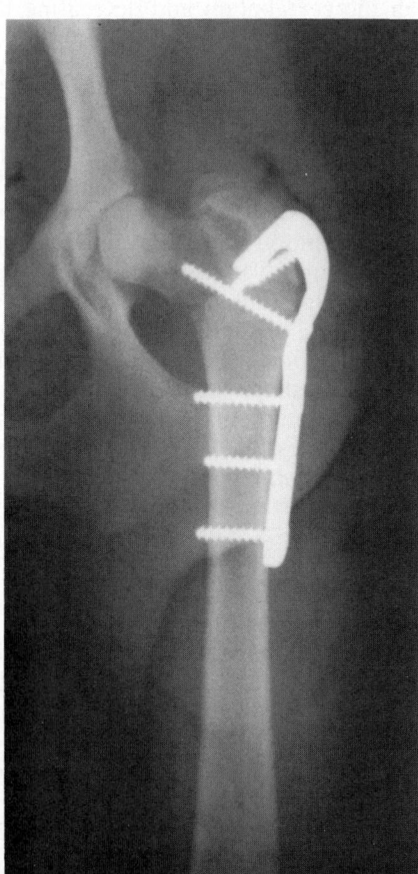

FIGURE 135–16. Ventrodorsal radiographic view of the femur, demonstrating an intertrochanteric osteotomy that has been stabilized with a hook plate.

Pelvic Osteotomy. An *osteotomy* is performed on the *ilium, ischium,* and *pubis* so that the acetabular segment of the pelvis can be rotated over the top of the femoral head to increase its dorsal coverage. The optimum rotation has not been determined; however, it is readily accepted that excessive rotation compromises extension and abduction of the hindlimb by impinging the femoral neck on the acetabular rim.[87, 90] Rotation of the acetabulum by 60° places the dorsal aspect of the femoral head into the nonarticular portion of the acetabulum (acetabular fossa) and is not desirable.[93] The amount of rotation necessary to cover the femoral head adequately has been calculated from radiographs,[87] estimated by measuring the angles of reduction and subluxation on physical examination,[89] and determined by direct observation at surgery.[86, 90] Acetabular rotation of 20° to 30° is adequate for most cases, except for those with extreme subluxation.[89] Pelvic osteotomy alone is not recommended if there is an increase in the angle of inclination or femoral torsion. A femoral osteotomy is first necessary to correct these abnormalities. As in a femoral osteotomy, a pelvic osteotomy appears to be most effective in young growing animals with subluxation and minimal evidence of degenerative changes in the hip joint.[86, 89] The procedure has been recommended in mature animals with minimal degenerative changes and has been used in animals with severe osteoarthritis. The results have been less encouraging in these latter two situations.[89]

Two basic techniques and several variations are used for performing pelvic osteotomy in dogs.* The first technique uses an ischial osteotomy with or without a pubic osteotomy and a "stair-step" ilial osteotomy.[39, 41, 86, 87] The angle of the horizontal cut in the stair-step osteotomy is thought by some to be critical in determining the rotation of the acetabular segment.[41, 86, 87] However, the final position of the acetabular segment is controlled more by the surgeon than by the angle of the horizontal cut.[77] Regardless of the variation in technique, lateralization and rotation of the acetabular segment by the stair-step method appears to increase the angle of anteversion of the acetabulum.[77] The acetabular segment is maintained in position with a screw or a cerclage wire. The advantage of this method is that it can be performed through one incision site. The disadvantage is that the degree of acetabular rotation may be limited and the fixation of the ilial osteotomy is not rigid. Transplantation of the greater trochanter has been recommended as an adjunct to this method, presumably to decrease the forces acting on the hip joint.[70, 87] The value of lateral and distal transfer of the greater trochanter in altering the load on the hip joint has been inadequately studied.

In the second method of pelvic osteotomy, a separate

*See references 39, 41, 77, 86, 87, 89, 90, and 93.

incision is used to create a pubic osteotomy or a subtotal pubic ostectomy, an ischial osteotomy, and a straight ilial osteotomy.[35, 89, 90] This procedure allows greater control over the rotation of the acetabular segment and more rigid stabilization of the ilial osteotomy. Removing a portion of the pubic bone decreases reduction of the pelvic canal diameter compared with a simple pubic osteotomy. Finally, the development of a stepped plate permits lateralization of the acetabular segment that is impossible with a standard straight plate.[89]

This procedure is a modification of a previously described technique.[89] The animal is positioned in lateral recumbency with the affected limb free draped. The limb is abducted, and an incision is made on the medial aspect of the thigh over the insertion of the pectineal muscle. The muscle is elevated from the ileopectineal eminence, and the pubic bone is identified. An oscillating saw is used to transect the pubic bone laterally at the iliopectineal eminence and medially at the pubic tubercle. The pubic bone is removed and placed in a blood-soaked sponge for later use. The site is closed routinely. The second incision is a vertical incision, performed in the perineal area midway between the ischial tuberosity and the anus. After blunt dissection of the subcutaneous tissue, the muscles are elevated from the dorsal and ventral surfaces of the ischium until the caudal obturator foramen is palpated. A reciprocating bone saw is used to cut the ischium from the lateral limit of the obturator foramen to a point midway between the ischial tuberosity and the medial angle of the ischial tuberosity. The ischial incision is packed with a saline-soaked sponge until later in the procedure. The third incision is a ventrolateral approach to the ilium.[76] A skin incision is made from the ventral aspect of the iliac crest to the third trochanter of the femur. The muscles are separated and retracted until the body of the ilium is identified. The deep gluteal muscle is elevated from the ilium by subperiosteal dissection. Care is taken to preserve the cranial gluteal artery, vein, and nerve. Cranial exposure of the body of the ilium and the caudal wing is enhanced by elevating the middle gluteal from the ventral aspect of the iliac spine. The iliac muscle is elevated from the medial aspect of the body of the ilium just caudal to the sacroiliac junction. An osteotomy is performed in the body of the ilium, caudal to the sacroiliac joint and either perpendicular to the long axis of the hemipelvis or perpendicular to a pin that runs from the ischial tuberosity to the ventral third of the iliac crest. A malleable retractor is placed between the iliac muscle and the medial surface of the ilium to protect the sciatic nerve during osteotomy of the ilium. The acetabular segment of the hemipelvis can be rotated by grasping the caudal fragment of the ilium and the lateral fragment of ischium with bone forceps to achieve dorsal coverage of the femoral head. This can be verified by palpation of the coxofemoral joint while the acetabular segment is held in the desired position. Once adequate coverage has been achieved, a 2.7- or 3.5-DC Plate or Reconstruction Plate* is twisted to the desired angle and applied to the ilium (Fig. 135–

*Synthes, Paoli, PA.

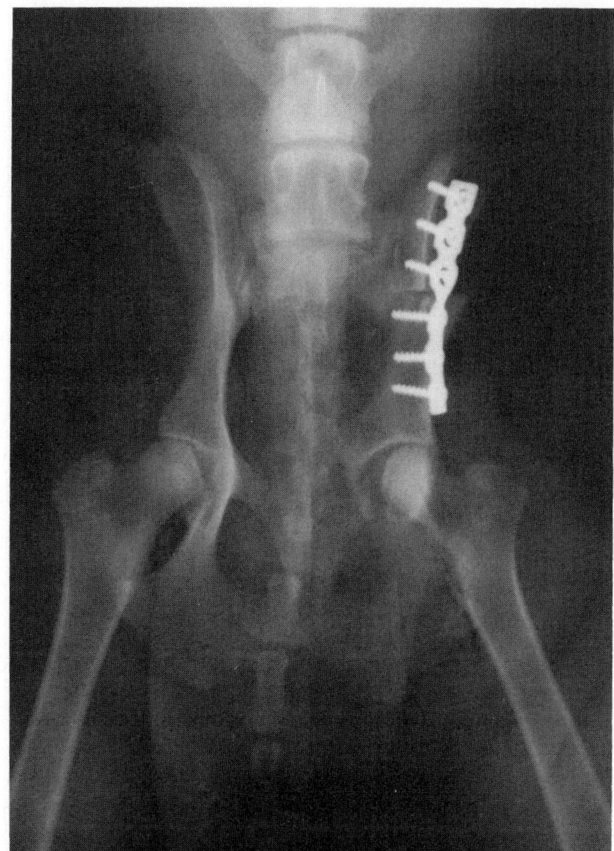

FIGURE 135–17. Ventrodorsal radiographic view of a dog's pelvis immediately after a triple pelvic osteotomy. The ilial osteotomy has been stabilized with a 3.5-mm reconstruction plate. The plate has been twisted at its midpoint.

17). Alternatively, a Canine Pelvic Osteotomy Plate* with a preformed angle of 20°, 30°, or 45° can be used (Fig. 135–18). Small pieces of pubic bone are placed between the ilial fragments as an autogenous corticocancellous graft. Holes may be drilled on either side of the ischial osteotomy site to accommodate wire fixation of the ischium. The ischial and ilial incisions are closed routinely.[35, 89] Postoperative care is similar to that for femoral osteotomy. Passive physiotherapy is encouraged postoperatively, but active physiotherapy is limited to leash walking for 4 to 6 weeks and swimming as soon as the incision allows. Complications with this procedure include implant failure, infection, continual progression of degenerative changes, and limitation of extension and abduction of the hip.

Other surgical procedures that have been described for dysplastic animals include acetabuloplasty, femoral neck lengthening, and biocompatible osteoconductive polymer shelf arthroplasty. *Acetabuloplasty* is a procedure in which multiple osteotomies are performed around the acetabulum so that the acetabulum can be directed laterally and ventrally to increase dorsal coverage of the femoral head.[15] This operation is technically demanding and has little benefit over pelvic osteotomy.

*Slocum Enterprises, Eugene, OR.

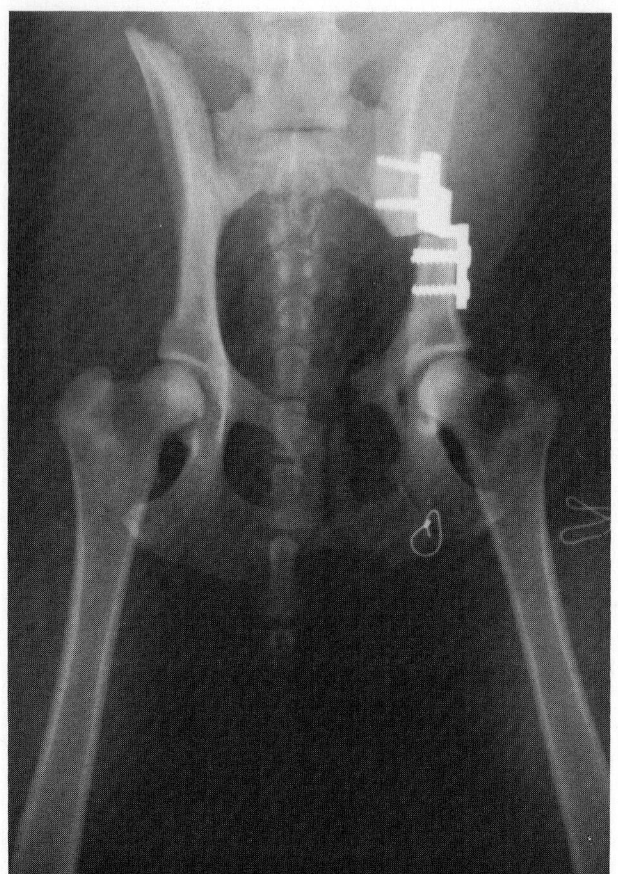

FIGURE 135–18. Ventrodorsal radiographic view of a dog's pelvis after a triple pelvic osteotomy (TPO). A canine pelvic osteotomy plate has been used on the ilial osteotomy.

Femoral neck lengthening has been proposed for dysplastic dogs that have shortened femoral necks or abnormal angles of femoral torsion. An osteotomy is performed in the proximal femur, extending from the transverse line to the proximal or middle third of the femoral diaphysis. The osteotomy is separated, and preformed wedges are placed to keep the osteotomy spread apart. This procedure allows medial and varus positioning of the femoral head and neck.[88] It is relatively new, and data regarding its effectiveness are insufficient. Dogs that sustain capital physeal fractures before 7 months of age often develop coxofemoral subluxation secondary to premature closure of the capital physis.[57] In this select group, the procedure may have indications; however, unless a large number of dysplastic dogs have shortening of the femoral neck, this procedure seems to offer little benefit over the intertrochanteric osteotomy. *Biocompatible osteoconductive polymer shelf arthroplasty* has been proposed as a method of extending the acetabular rim of the pelvis to accommodate a subluxated femoral head. A biocompatible osteoconductive polymer is attached to the dorsal brim of the acetabulum with a single bone screw. Theoretically, this acts as a scaffold for bone ingrowth and lateral extension of the dorsal brim. However, the shelf is nonarticular, and continued wear of the femoral head is anticipated. At best, this procedure might offer temporary relief from the discomfort associated with subluxation, but it is not a substitute for pelvic osteotomy.

Salvage

Femoral Head and Neck Excision. Femoral head and neck excision or excision arthroplasty is a salvage procedure in the coxofemoral joint for hip dysplasia; degenerative joint disease; Legg-Calvé-Perthes disease; irreparable fractures of the femoral head, neck, or acetabulum; recurrent luxations; and failed total hip replacements.[99] If the procedure is correctly performed, a painful articulation can be converted to a pain-free false joint.[35] Although long-term follow-ups on clinical cases have been evaluated subjectively through client questionnaires and physical examinations, the degree of pain associated with the procedure is unclear.[9, 25, 26, 31] Most reports describe evidence of some long-term functional impairment, which may vary from a mild lameness after excessive exercise to intermittent nonweightbearing.[9, 25, 26, 31] Muscle atrophy, limb shortening, and reduction of hip extension are commonly observed, even after extended follow-up periods.[25, 58] The average time to leg use after the surgery is approximately 5 weeks.[9, 62] Return to normal function may take considerably longer. When femoral head and neck excision was performed on dogs with normal hip conformation, objective gait analysis revealed that the dogs had not returned to normal function 16 weeks after the procedure.[58]

Femoral head and neck excision is a viable salvage procedure, with limitations. One should not expect an affected joint to function normally afterward. Providing the physical demands placed on the animal are not extreme, adequate functional results for the majority of patients can be expected.[9, 35, 62] Cats and small dogs may function better than larger dogs,[31, 35, 99] although the size of the animal may not be an important factor in the success of this procedure.[9, 62] A smooth ostectomy site is critical in creating a pain-free fibrous articulation.[9, 31, 35, 62, 99] Radiographic evaluations do not necessarily correlate with clinical results. Bone-to-bone articulation is avoided because it has been associated with lameness.[26] Interpositional materials have been recommended to decrease bone-to-bone contact and to improve the recovery rate. These materials include joint capsule, fat, fascia, and deep gluteal and biceps femoris muscle slings. Although subjective evaluations of muscle slings have been encouraging,[9, 10, 24, 53, 54] objective assessment of function has not demonstrated conclusive benefits from their use.[58]

A craniolateral approach to the hip joint is used most often for femoral head and neck excision.[31, 35, 58, 99] Other approaches have been described, including modifications of the craniolateral approach with a gluteal tenotomy or a trochanteric osteotomy and a ventral approach.[16, 21, 76] Once the joint capsule has been exposed through the craniolateral approach, it is incised parallel to the long axis of the femoral neck and reflected from its insertion on the femur. Most of the cranial aspect of the femoral neck can be exposed by reflecting the joint capsule cranially and dorsally and the vastus muscles ventrally and distally. If the ligament of the head of the femur is intact, it is transected with a scalpel, periosteal elevator, or heavy curved scissors.[35] The femur is externally rotated, luxating the femoral head from the acetabulum. Incision of the medial and ventral attachments of the joint capsule to the femoral neck may be necessary to luxate the femoral head completely. The femur is rotated so that the patella is perpendicular to the table. An Army-Navy retractor is positioned between the femoral neck and the acetabulum to provide stabilization during the osteotomy. The line of osteotomy extends from the medial greater trochanter (transverse line) to a point just proximal to the lesser trochanter. The osteotomy is performed in a cranial to caudal direction, angled from medial to lateral to remove the entire femoral neck (Fig. 135–19).[99] An oscillating saw or sharp osteotome is recommended for the osteotomy. Regardless of the instrument used, the osteotomy site should be smooth and rough spots removed with rongeurs or a bone rasp.[35, 99] The incision site is flushed with sterile saline or lactated Ringer solution. If sufficient joint capsule remains, it is closed over the acetabulum with interrupted or continuous absorbable sutures. If a muscle flap is used, it is secured to the proximal femur as described.[10, 24, 53, 54] Evidence is not available to support the use of a muscle flap. The vastus group are resutured to their origin or may be sutured to the joint capsule or the insertion of the deep gluteal muscle if the origin has been elevated. The deep gluteal muscle is closed with an interrupted mattress suture. Closure is routine.

Postoperatively, passive physiotherapy consisting of gentle flexion and extension is begun as soon as the animal allows it. Analgesics may be necessary in the immediate postoperative period to control pain. Swimming and slow leash walking are encouraged within the first week. Animals that have had chronic lameness before surgery have a slower recovery, presumably because of muscle atrophy and joint fibrosis.[31] Active and passive physiotherapy is essential in functional rehabilitation. Shortening of the limb, patella luxation, muscle atrophy, limitation of hip extension, recurrent lameness, and exercise intolerance are associated complications.[25, 99]

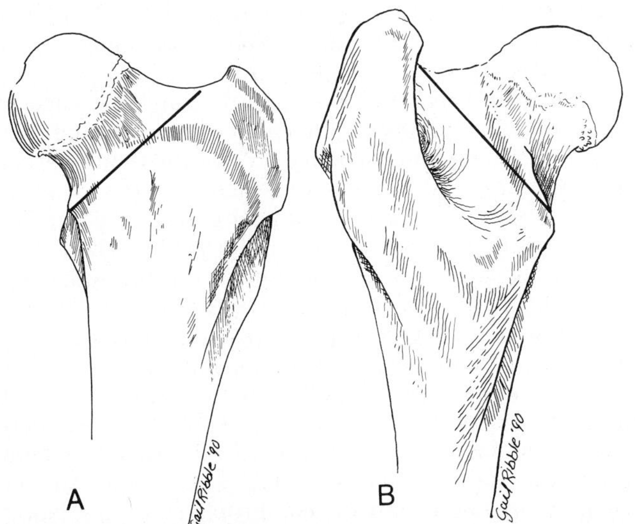

FIGURE 135–19. The cranial *(A)* and caudal *(B)* aspects of the proximal femur, showing the relative position of the osteotomy line for a femoral head and neck excision.

Total Hip Replacement. Total hip replacement has been an accepted practice in humans for more than 30 years, since its initial experimental use in dogs.[32] The procedure has become a viable alternative to femoral head and neck excision for the treatment of degenerative joint disease, hip dysplasia, chronic hip luxation, and irreparable fractures of the coxofemoral joint in medium-sized to large dogs. A high incidence of dislocation, infection, and implant loosening initially raised questions about its clinical applicability in dogs.[5, 52] Improvements in implant design, implant materials, and surgical technique have resulted in decreased complications and cautious acceptance of the procedure in dogs.* Total hip replacement is generally recommended for large athletic dogs or performance animals, in which femoral head and neck excision may be less successful.[25, 31, 62, 99] Total hip replacement is used with less success for revision of failed femoral head and neck excision.

The technique for performing cemented total hip replacement is a modification of previously described techniques.[69, 73] A craniolateral approach is performed on the affected hip joint. Elevation of the origins of the vastus muscles and partial tenotomy of the deep gluteal muscle (see Fig. 135–11) enhances exposure of the cranial aspect of the femoral neck. In a revision of a failed femoral head and neck excision or total hip replacement, a modification of the craniolateral approach is preferred, either by performing a gluteal tenotomy or trochanteric osteotomy (see Figs. 135–12 and 135–13). An incision is made in the joint capsule so that it may be reflected from the neck of the femur. The femoral head is luxated and rotated approximately 90° so that an osteotomy can be performed. In total hip replacement, a trial femoral prosthesis is placed so that the stem is adjacent and parallel to the diaphysis of the femur. The collar of the trial prosthesis is positioned at the base of the femoral neck just proximal to the lesser trochanter. An electroscalpel is used to mark the position of the collar on the femoral neck, and the trial prosthesis is removed. An osteotomy is performed along this line from cranial to caudal and medial to lateral as for femoral head and neck excision (see Fig. 135–19). The medial to lateral angulation of the osteotomy allows correction of the angle of femoral torsion and helps ensure that the femoral prosthesis is not placed with excess anteversion. The femur is externally rotated, and different femoral reamers are used to prepare the femoral canal for the endoprosthesis. The reamers are placed as far laterally as practical, possibly requiring removal of a portion of the transverse line. This ensures central reaming of the medullary canal and aids in neutral positioning of the femoral prosthesis. The largest trial prosthesis that easily fits into the femoral medullary canal is fitted. The trial prosthesis is not excessively anteverted (cranial-caudal plane) and is in a neutral position in the lateral-medial plane (neither varus nor valgus). Minor adjustments can be made by correcting

*See references 40, 50, 52, 67–69, 71, and 73.

the femoral neck ostectomy. The trial prosthesis is removed, and the femur is rotated back to a neutral position. A medium Hohmann retractor is placed with its tip under the ventral edge of the acetabulum, and the femur is retracted caudally. A Gelpi retractor is placed in the acetabulum so that the tips retract the cranial and caudal edges of the joint capsule. An acetabular reamer (Protek*) is used to remove all articular cartilage from the lunate surface of the acetabulum. All soft tissue and remnants of ligament are removed with a rongeur. The acetabular cup is inserted into the prepared bed and fitted. Most of the acetabular component should be covered by the acetabular rim. Removal of the pegs on the undersurface of the prosthetic cup generally facilitates coverage. Although more aggressive reaming allows the acetabular component to sit deeper, preservation of subchondral bone in the acetabular bed is important for a stable bone–cement interface.[20] Multiple holes are placed in the subchondral bone with a 000 bone curette. The acetabulum and femoral canal are lavaged with a pulsating suction lavage unit (Pulsovac-Zimmer†) to remove loose bone debris.[20]

The acetabulum is packed with a dry sponge while the bone cement is mixed. One gram of unsuspended cephalexin (Keflex) is ground to a fine powder and mixed with 20 g of polymethyl methacrylate. The two powders are mixed in the same bowl, and 20 ml of methyl methacrylate monomer is added. The cement is mixed for 2 minutes, and approximately 4 ml of cement is placed into a medullary plug syringe (Johnson & Johnson‡) and injected into the medullary canal of the femur. The femur is suctioned just before this injection. The plug is injected 2 to 3 cm distal to the tip of the trial prosthesis. The level of the injection is predetermined by placing the trial prosthesis next to the medullary plug syringe. The Hohmann retractor is replaced under the ventral edge of the acetabulum, and the femur is retracted. Once the cement has attained a doughy state and will not stick to a surgical glove, it is hand packed into the acetabular bed. Before hand packing, the acetabulum is flushed and suctioned. The acetabular implant is placed in the acetabular bed using the positioner to ensure a neutral or mildly retroverted position. Correct positioning of the acetabular implants is paramount in the long-term success of this procedure (Fig. 135–20).[50, 67, 71] Excess cement is removed without dislodging the acetabular component. After the cement has hardened, the positioner and retractors are removed and the femur is rotated to expose the medullary canal. The femoral canal is suctioned and lavaged while a second batch of cement is mixed. One gram of Keflex is finely ground and mixed with 40 g of cement. The monomer is added and mixed as before. After 3 minutes, the cement is poured into a cement gun (Johnson & Johnson‡) and injected into the medullary canal, starting distally and gradually removing the gun proximally from the ostectomy site. Using a polyethylene rod, the cement is tamped into the medullary canal. The femoral prosthesis is placed in a neutral position in the femoral canal (Fig. 135–21). Excess cement is removed, and the prosthesis is held firmly until the cement hardens. The surgery site is flushed with copious amounts of sterile saline. The components are reduced, and the joint is fully extended and flexed to check for luxation of the components. If the components have been placed properly, the head does not easily luxate from the cup. The joint capsule is closed with an interrupted nonabsorbable suture. All other tissues are closed as for femoral head and neck excision.

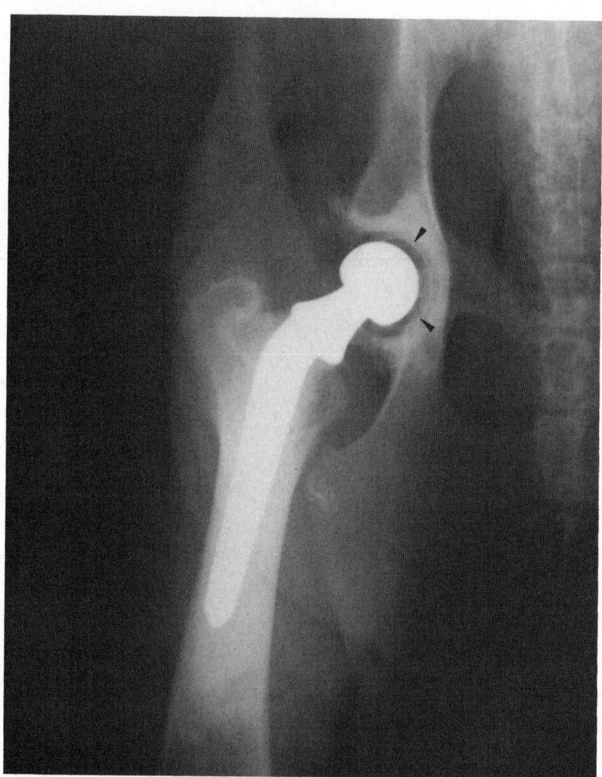

FIGURE 135–20. Ventrodorsal radiographic view of a dog's coxofemoral joint after total hip replacement. The position of the acetabular component is determined by the position of the radiopaque wire. In this case, the acetabular cup has been placed in a neutral position relative to the longitudinal axis of the acetabulum.

Postoperatively, the dog is kept in a large cage or small run for 48 hours. The animal is towel supported when walking on any slippery surface for the first week after surgery, and activity is restricted to leash walking only for 4 to 6 weeks. The animal is rechecked at 7 to 10 days and at 3 months using radiography. Thereafter, the animal is checked at 6 months, at 1 year, and yearly to document progressive radiographic changes.[50, 60] The most common complications in order of importance are loosening of implants, dislocations, and infections (Fig. 135–22). In a study of 174 total hip replacements in dogs, 3.5 per cent became loose, 2.9 per cent dislocated, and 1.2 per cent became infected.[67] The risk of infection is reduced by meticulous operative technique and increased operative experience. Prophylactic antibiotics are used parenterally to cover the period of surgery and are mixed with the bone cement. Dislocations can be

*Synthes, Paoli, PA.
†Pulsovac-Zimmer, Warsaw, IN.
‡Johnson & Johnson Orthopedics, New Brunswick, NJ.

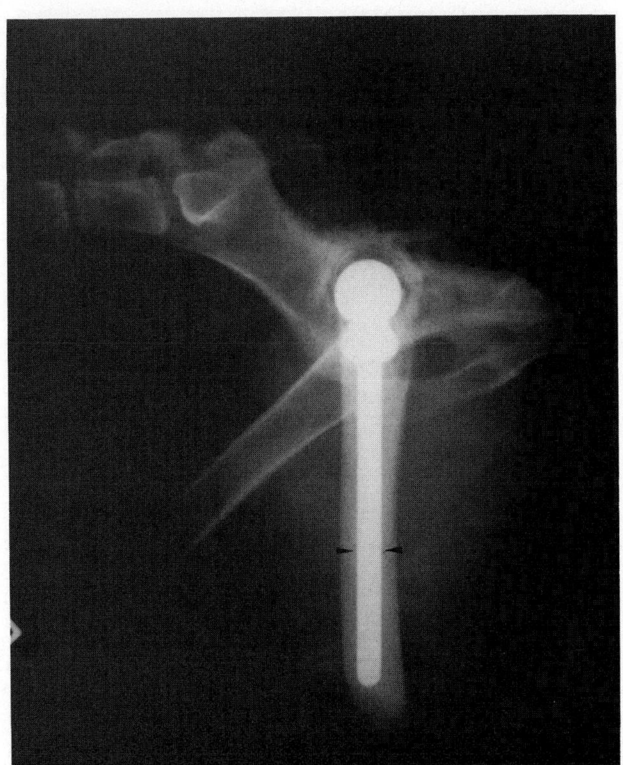

FIGURE 135–21. Lateral radiographic view of a dog's coxofemoral joint after total hip replacement. The femoral prosthesis is located in the middle of the medullary canal in a neutral position.

reduced by ensuring proper positioning of the acetabular and femoral prostheses.[50, 67] Methods to reduce the incidence of component loosening include pressurization of the cement, centrifugation of the cement, precoating the implant with polymethyl methacrylate, conservative reaming of the acetabulum, and pulsatile suction and lavage.[84] Some of these methods have been incorporated in the present technique.

Implants for total hip replacement have been secured to the host bone with acrylic cement. Despite newer cementing techniques, failures have been observed at the cement–bone or cement–implant interface in humans and dogs.[60, 67, 71, 72, 81] In humans, femoral or acetabular loosening may approach 30 per cent of patients observed for more than 10 years.[84] Infection, thermal necrosis of bone during cement polymerization, operative trauma, implant micromotion, poor cementing technique, increased activity of the patient, and load mismatching between the cement, bone, and implant are implicated as reasons for implant loosening.[19, 60] A fixation system that gradually transmits load from the implant to the surrounding bony structure might offer considerable advantages over the altered biomechanical environment that occurs with cemented fixation.[66] Uncemented total hip replacement relies on tissue ingrowth into the implant to provide a stable fixation.[11] Histological and biomechanical evaluation of uncemented total hip replacement supports the concept that bony ingrowth of the prosthesis allows a more physiological transfer of load from implant to bone.[11, 96–98] Despite the theoretical evidence to support the superiority of uncemented total hip replacement, long-term clinical trials are not available to verify this hypothesis. Although much of the experimental work for uncemented replacement has been performed in dogs, there is little clinical evidence to support loosening as a major complication in canine total hip replacement.[67, 68, 71] This may be partly because of the differences between quadripedal and bipedal gait, a dog's shorter life span relative to a human's, or the inability of clinicians to detect low-grade hip pain and subtle lameness in a dog. Further clinical and experimental work is necessary before definitive conclusions can be made about the applicability of uncemented total hip replacement.

HIP DISLOCATION

The hip is the most commonly luxated joint in small animals. The most common cause of acquired hip luxation is trauma, with motor vehicle accidents accounting for approximately 60 per cent.[6, 27] The majority of hip luxations are craniodorsal, presumably because of the type of injury and contraction of the gluteal muscles, which are strong extensors and abductors of the hip joint. The hip occasionally luxates caudoventrally, with displacement of the femoral head into the obturator foramen, or rarely caudodorsally. Caudoventral luxations are more commonly associated with falls.[94] The hip may also luxate medially, in association with an

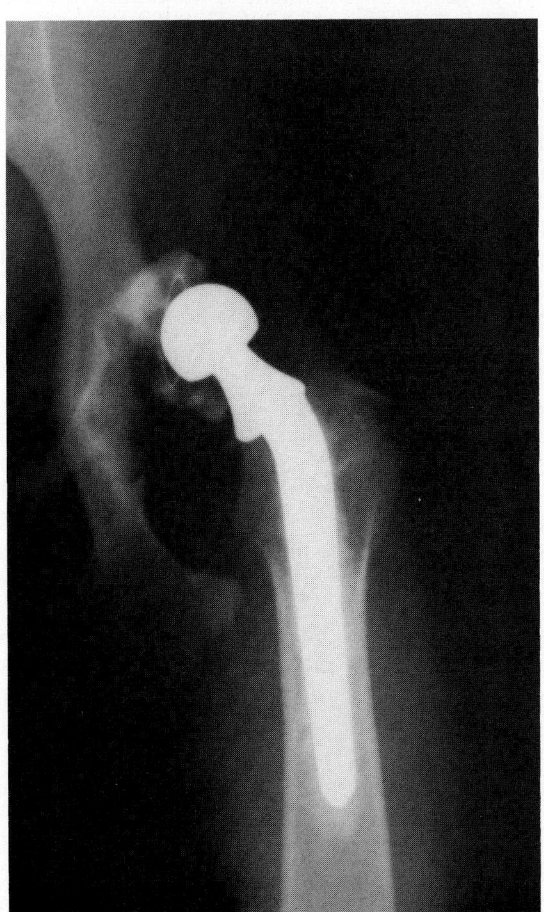

FIGURE 135–22. Ventrodorsal radiographic view of a dog's coxofemoral joint, showing luxation of the acetabular component 8 months after total hip replacement. The radiopaque material surrounding the wire is bone cement.

acetabular fracture.[35] The extent of soft-tissue damage that occurs with luxation depends on traumatic forces, direction of luxation, and duration of the luxation before definitive treatment. Invariably, the ligament of the head of the femur and the joint capsule are torn, permitting luxation. Damage to the supporting musculature of the coxofemoral joint is variable. The deep gluteal muscle is closely applied to the dorsal joint capsule and is often damaged in dorsal luxations. Avulsion of the ligament from the femoral head may include a fragment of bone. Erosion of the articular cartilage of the femoral head is commonly associated with chronic luxation and rubbing of the femoral head against the ilium.[95]

Hip luxation is suspected when an animal has a nonweightbearing lameness of the hindlimb and a history of trauma. The limb is usually held adducted, with some external rotation if the luxation is craniodorsal.[35, 95] If the luxation is caudoventral, the limb is usually held abducted, with internal rotation.[94] Physical examination may reveal pain and crepitus on flexion and extension of the hip joint. In a craniodorsal luxation, dorsal displacement of the greater trochanter may be palpated in reference to the ischial tuberosity and the cranial dorsal iliac spine. Comparison with the unaffected side often reveals a disparity in position of the greater trochanters. Placing the thumb between the greater trochanter and ischial tuberosity and externally rotating the femur causes impingement of the thumb in a normal hip.[35, 95] Caudal extension of the hindlimbs may suggest a relative shortening of the affected limb if the luxation is craniodorsal. If the luxation is caudoventral, the affected limb may seem longer than the contralateral hindlimb, and because of medial displacement, the greater trochanter is difficult to palpate.[94] Radiographic examination is necessary to confirm the diagnosis. Ventrodorsal and lateral projections are made to evaluate luxation; the presence or absence of avulsion fractures of the femoral head; concomitant femoral neck, femoral head, or acetabular fractures; and degenerative joint disease (Fig. 135–23).[95]

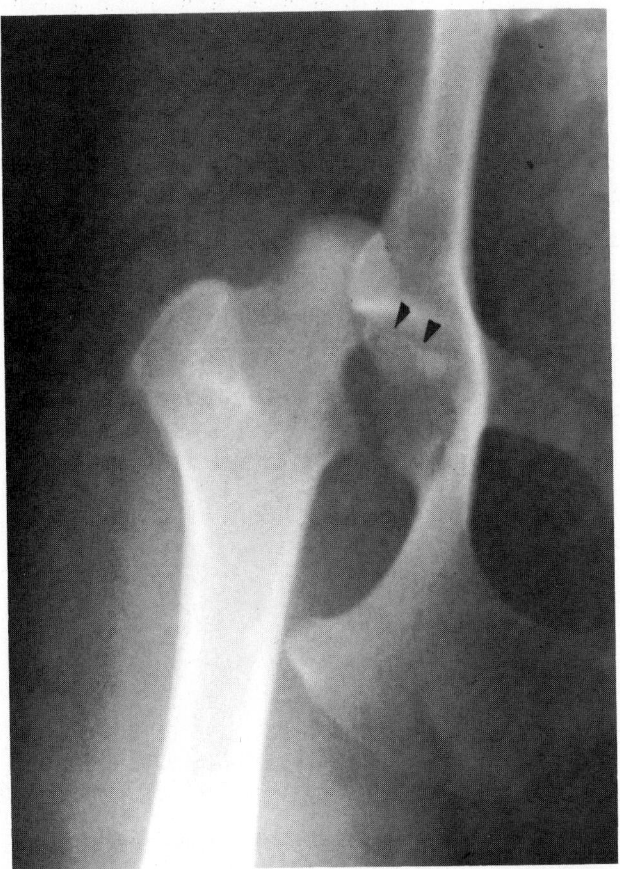

FIGURE 135–23. Ventrodorsal radiographic view of a dog's coxofemoral joint, showing dislocation of the femoral head. The arrows point to a fragment of the femoral head within the acetabulum. This was a fragment from the fovea capitis.

Many methods have been described to treat hip luxation (Fig. 135–24). *Closed reduction* is the treatment of choice for most cases of acquired hip luxation.[94] Indications for open reduction include avulsion fractures of the femoral head; fractures of the femoral neck, greater trochanter, or acetabulum; and unsuccessful closed reductions. Advanced hip dysplasia or degenerative joint disease may preclude successful closed reduction. A survey of 127 cases of hip luxation revealed success in 65 per cent of dogs and 69 per cent of cats treated by closed reduction. Other studies describe success rates of 35 to 53 per cent for closed reductions.[6, 12] The majority of successful closed reductions are performed within 10 days of luxation.[27] If the luxation is not treated, a false joint forms, resulting in various degrees of dysfunction.[12]

The animal is anesthetized and placed in lateral recumbency with the affected limb uppermost. For a craniodorsal luxation, the affected limb is externally rotated and pulled distally so that the femoral head can be internally rotated into the acetabulum.[35] The hip is fully extended and flexed to ensure that it is firmly seated; external rotation of the hip is avoided because it causes reluxation. Reluxation that occurs during flexion and extension usually suggests the presence of soft tissue in the acetabulum. This may consist of remnants of the ligament of the head of the femur, joint capsule, or hematoma. A second attempt at closed reduction is performed. If this is unsuccessful, open reduction is indicated. If the closed reduction is successful, the limb is placed in an Ehmer sling or a flexion bandage and postreduction radiographs are obtained. The bandage remains in place for 7 to 10 days, at which time it is removed and the hip is moved through a full range of motion to ensure continued reduction. Strict leash walking is recommended for 4 to 6 weeks after bandage removal. In caudoventral luxation, reduction is achieved by applying traction and abduction to the distal femur while forcing the proximal femur in a lateral direction. Caudoventral luxations are not reduced by forcing them into a craniodorsal luxation, because this causes unnecessary trauma to soft tissues. An Ehmer sling is not necessary after closed reduction of a caudoventral luxation.[94]

De Vita pinning has been recommended to augment closed reduction, if the original luxation is craniodorsal. A properly placed De Vita pin acts as a dorsal and lateral extension of the acetabular rim. An advantage of this technique is that it allows early mobilization of

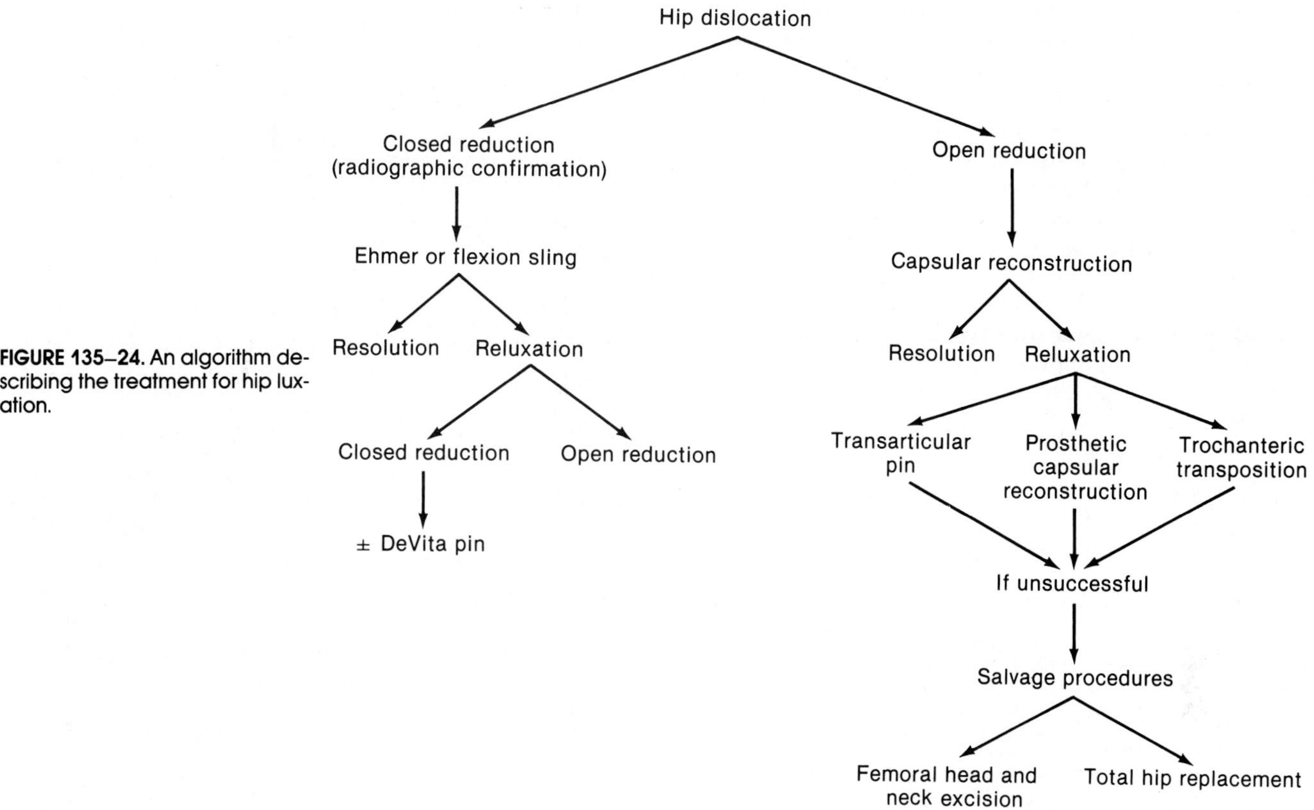

FIGURE 135–24. An algorithm describing the treatment for hip luxation.

the limb. An intramedullary pin is placed ventral to the ischial tuberosity, dorsal to the femoral neck, and into the ventral aspect of the wing of the ilium.[27, 35] The pin is left in place for 4 to 6 weeks.[51] Despite proper placement of the pin, reluxation and early pin migration are major complications associated with this procedure.[27] Threaded pins are less susceptible to migration.[27, 51]

Open reduction is usually performed through a craniolateral approach to the hip joint. A modification of the craniolateral approach with a gluteal tenotomy or trochanteric osteotomy can be performed for greater exposure. A craniolateral or ventral approach is used for caudoventral luxations. Regardless of the approach, the joint capsule is identified and preserved. An incision may be necessary in the joint capsule to débride the acetabulum of hematoma, fibrous tissue, or remnants of the ligament of the head of the femur. The femur is externally rotated, and remnants of its ligament are incised. The femur is retracted distally and internally rotated so that the femoral head is repositioned in the acetabulum. Flexion and extension of the hip joint verify seating of the femoral head. The capsule is closed with preplaced nonabsorbable sutures using a simple interrupted or mattress pattern. If portions of the capsule cannot be reconstructed, the origin of the vastus lateralis and insertion of the deep gluteal can be used to support the existing tissue. Closure of all other structures is routine. If the deep gluteal muscle is torn, attempts are made to repair it. After skin closure, the hip is supported in an Ehmer sling or flexion bandage for 7 to 10 days. Capsulorrhaphy is often the only method necessary to treat hip luxations.[12]

A *prosthetic capsule reconstruction* has been advocated when the capsule and gluteal musculature have been severely compromised by the luxation.[48] A craniolateral approach with a trochanteric osteotomy is performed. Two screws and washers are placed in the dorsal acetabular rim, one cranial and one caudal to the femoral head. A third screw and washer are placed in the trochanteric fossa. Heavy nonabsorbable sutures are placed in a figure-eight pattern from the acetabular screws to the femoral screw, with the limb held in slight abduction. Closure is routine, and an Ehmer sling or flexion bandage is maintained for 7 to 10 days after surgery.[99] Twenty-one cases treated with this technique had no reluxation, and 65 per cent of patients had good to excellent use of the limb on follow-up examination; the majority were recurrent or chronic luxations.[48]

Relocation of the greater trochanter has been recommended as a method of increasing the tension in the gluteal musculature to abduct and internally rotate the hip.[22, 70] A craniolateral approach with an osteotomy of the greater trochanter is performed. The limb is held in abduction, and the greater trochanter is relocated distal and caudolateral to its original position and held in place with pins and a tension band wire or screws.[1] After closure of the incision, the limb is maintained in an Ehmer sling or flexion bandage for 7 to 10 days. This technique is useful only if the gluteal muscles are intact.

Transarticular pinning has been recommended when the joint capsule is severely damaged and recurrent luxation occurs with flexion and extension of the hip. A pin is drilled from the area of the third trochanter through the fovea of the femoral head and through the acetabular fossa. The pin can be palpated by an assistant as its tip protrudes into the pelvic canal.[8, 45] Closure of the soft tissues is routine, and the limb is maintained in a flexion bandage for 10 to 14 days. At that time, the pin is removed and passive physiotherapy is instituted by flexion and extension of the hip. One report discourages the use of this procedure in animals that have concurrent intra-articular fractures or hip dysplasia. In this study, satisfactory hindlimb function was preserved in 80 per cent of patients.[45]

In recurrent luxation, after open and closed methods of treatment or when irreparable femoral head or acetabular fractures are present, a salvage procedure (femoral head and neck excision or total hip replacement) is recommended.

References

1. Alexander JW: Coxofemoral luxation in the dogs. *Compendium 4*:575, 1982.
2. Arnoczky SP, Torzilli PA: Biomechanical analysis of forces acting about the canine hip. *Am J Vet Res 42*:1581, 1981.
3. Bardens JW, Hardwick H: New observations on the diagnosis and cause of hip dysplasia. *Vet Med Small Anim Clin 63*:238, 1968.
4. Barr ARS, et al: Clinical hip dysplasia in growing dogs: The long term results of conservative management. *J Small Anim Pract 28*:243, 1987.
5. Bartel DL, et al: Biomechanical considerations in the design of a canine total hip prosthesis. *J Am Anim Hosp Assoc 11*:553, 1975.
6. Basher AWP, et al: Coxofemoral luxation in the dog and cat. *Vet Surg 15*:356, 1986.
7. Bennett D: Hip dysplasia and ascorbate therapy: Fact or fancy? *Semin Vet Med Surg 2*:152, 1987.
8. Bennett D, Duff SR: Transarticular pinning as a treatment for hip luxation in the dog and cat. *J Small Anim Pract 21*:373, 1980.
9. Berzon JL, et al: A retrospective study of the efficacy of femoral head and neck excisions in 94 dogs and cats. *Vet Surg 9*:88, 1980.
10. Bjorling DE, Chambers JN: The biceps femoris flap and femoral head and neck excision in dogs. *Compendium 8*:359, 1986.
11. Bobyn JD, et al: The effect of proximally and fully porous-coated canine hip stem design on bone remodeling. *J Orthop Res 5*:393, 1987.
12. Bone DL, et al: Traumatic coxofemoral luxation in dogs. Results of repair. *Vet Surg 13*:263, 1984.
13. Bowen JM, et al: Progression of hip dysplasia in German shepherd dogs after unilateral pectineal myotomy. *J Am Vet Med Assoc 161*:899, 1972.
14. Brandt KD, Slowman-Kovacs S: Nonsteroidal antiinflammatory drugs in treatment of osteoarthritis. *Clin Orthop 213*:84, 1986.
15. Brinker WO: Corrective osteotomy procedures for treatment of canine hip dysplasia. *Vet Clin North Am 1*:467, 1971.
16. Brown RE: A surgical approach to the coxofemoral joint. *North Am Vet 34*:420, 1953.
17. Brown SG, Rosen H: Craniolateral approach to the canine hip: A modified Watson-Jones approach. *J Am Vet Med Assoc 159*:1117, 1971.
18. Candlin FT: The diagnosis and treatment of hip dysplasia: One point of view. *J Am Anim Hosp Assoc 8*:323, 1972.
19. Chandler HP, et al: Total hip replacement in patients younger than thirty years old. *J Bone Joint Surg (AM) 63A*:1426, 1987.
20. Cornell CN, Ranawat CS: The impact of modern cementing techniques on acetabular fixation in cemented total hip replacement. *J Arthroplasty 1*:197, 1986.
21. DeAngelis M, Hohn RB: The ventral approach to excision arthroplasty of the femoral head. *J Am Vet Med Assoc 152*:135, 1968.
22. De Angelis M, Prata R: Surgical repair of coxofemoral luxation in the dog. *J Am Anim Hosp Assoc 9*:13, 1973.
23. Dueland DJ: A study of femoral torsion with respect to canine hip dysplasia. Master's Thesis, Cornell University, 1981, pp 1–95.
24. Dueland RT: Deep gluteal muscle transfer in excision arthroplasty in dogs. *Mod Vet Pract 65*:860, 1984.
25. Duff R, Campbell JR: Long term results of excision arthroplasty of the canine hip. *Vet Rec 101*:181, 1977.
26. Duff R, Campbell JR: Radiographic appearance and clinical progress after excision arthroplasty of the canine hip. *J Small Anim Pract 19*:439, 1978.
27. Duff SRI, Bennett D: Hip luxation in small animals: An evaluation of some methods of treatment. *Vet Rec 111*:140, 1982.
28. Dunlap K, et al: A new method of determination of torsion of the femur. *J Bone Joint Surg (AM) 35A*:289, 1953.
29. Enislidis AC: The distribution in tissue of tritium-labelled glycosaminoglycane polysulfate on intra-articular injection. *Med Welt 3*:733, 1972.
30. Evans HE, Christensen GC (eds): *Miller's Anatomy of the Dog*. W.B. Saunders, Philadelphia, 1979.
31. Gendreau C, Cawley AJ: Excision of the femoral head and neck: The long-term results of 35 operations. *J Am Anim Hosp Assoc 13*:605, 1977.
32. Gorman HA: A new prosthetic hip joint. *Milit Med 121*:91, 1957.
33. Gorman HA: Hip joint prostheses. *Vet Scope 7*:3, 1962.
34. Harty M: Anatomy of the hip joint. *In* Tronzo RG (ed): *Surgery of the Hip Joint*. Lea & Febiger, Philadelphia, 1973, pp 45–78.
35. Hauptman J: The hip joint. *In* Slatter DH (ed): *Textbook of Small Animal Surgery*. W.B. Saunders, Philadelphia, 1985, pp 2153–2179.
36. Hauptman J, et al: Angles of inclination and anteversion in hip dysplasia in the dog. *Am J Vet Res 46*:2033, 1985.
37. Hauptman J, et al: The angle of the canine femoral head and neck. *Vet Surg 8*:74, 1979.
38. Henry JD: A modified technique for pectineal tendonectomy in the dog. *J Am Vet Med Assoc 163*:465, 1973.
39. Henry WB, Wadsworth PL: Pelvic osteotomy in the treatment of subluxation associated with hip dysplasia. *J Am Anim Hosp Assoc 11*:636, 1975.
40. Hoefle WD: A surgical procedure for prosthetic total hip replacement in the dog. *J Am Anim Hosp Assoc 10*:269, 1974.
41. Hohn RB, Janes JM: Pelvic osteotomy in the treatment of canine hip dysplasia. *Clin Orthop 62*:70, 1969.
42. Howell DS, et al: Effect of glycosaminoglycan polysulfate ester on proteoglycan-degrading enzyme activity in an animal model of osteoarthritis. *In* Otterness I, et al (ed): *Advances in Inflammation Research* Raven Press, New York, 1986, pp 197–206.
43. Howarth B: Development of present knowledge of congenital displacement of the hip. *Clin Orthop 125*:68, 1977.
44. Hulse DH, et al: Revascularization of femoral capital fractures following surgical fixation. *J Vet Orthop 2*:50, 1980.
45. Hunt CA, Henry WB: Transarticular pinning for repair of hip dislocation in the dog: A retrospective study of 40 cases. *J Am Vet Med Assoc 187*:828, 1985.
46. Ihemelandu EC, et al: Canine hip dysplasia: Differences in pectineal muscles of healthy and dysplastic German shepherd dogs when two months old. *Am J Vet Res 4*:411, 1983.
47. Ippolito E, et al: Histologic, histochemical and ultrastructural studies of the hip joint capsule and ligamentum teres in congenital dislocation of the hip. *Clin Orthop 146*:246, 1980.
48. Johnson ME, Braden TD: A retrospective study of prosthetic capsule technique for the treatment of problem cases of dislocated hips. *Vet Surg 16*:346, 1987.
49. Kaderly RE, et al: Intracapsular and intraosseous vascular supply to the mature dog's coxofemoral joint. *Am J Vet Res 44*:1805, 1983.
50. Konde LJ, et al: Radiographic evaluation of total hip replacement in the dog. *Vet Radiol 23*:98, 1982.
51. Leeds EB, Renegar WR: The use of the De Vita pin in the multitraumatized canine patient with a concurrent coxofemoral luxation. *J Vet Orthop 1*:35, 1979.
52. Lewis RH, Jones JP: A clinical study of canine total hip arthroplasty. *Vet Surg 9*:20, 1980.
53. Lippincott CL: Excision arthroplasty of the femoral head and neck utilizing a biceps femoris muscle sling. Part two: The caudal pass. *J Am Anim Hosp Assoc 20*:377, 1984.
54. Lippincott CL: Improvement of excision arthroplasty of the femoral head and neck utilizing a biceps femoris muscle sling. *J Am Anim Hosp Assoc 17*:668, 1987.
55. Lust G, et al: Intra-articular volume and hip joint instability in dogs with hip dysplasia. *J Bone Joint Surg (AM) 62A*:576, 1980.
56. Lust G, et al: Canine hip dysplasia: Concepts and diagnosis. *J Am Vet Med Assoc 187*:638, 1985.
57. Manley PA: Femoral neck shortening associated with premature closure of the capital growth plate, unpublished data, 1992.
58. Mann FA, et al: A comparison of standard femoral head and neck excision and femoral head and neck excision using a biceps femoris muscle flap in the dog. *Vet Surg 16*:223, 1987.
59. Michaels G, Matles AL: The role of the ligament teres in congenital dislocation of the hip. *Clin Orthop 71*:199, 1970.
60. Mjoberg B, et al: Mechanical loosening of total hip prostheses. *J Bone Joint Surg (Br) 68B*:770, 1986.
61. Montavon PM, et al: Inclination and anteversion angles of the femoral head and neck in the dog. *Vet Surg 14*:277, 1985.
62. Montgomery RD, et al: A retrospective comparison of three techniques for femoral head and neck excision in dogs. *Vet Surg 16*:423, 1987.
63. Norberg I: The Norberg method of assessing hip dysplasia. *In* Douglas S, Williamson H (eds): *Veterinary Radiological Interpretation*. Lea & Febiger, Philadelphia, 1970, pp 109–111.
64. Nunamaker DM: Surgical correction of large femoral anteversion angles in the dog. *J Am Vet Med Assoc 165*:1061, 1974.
65. Nunamaker DM, et al: Femoral neck anteversion in the dog: Its radiographic measurement. *J Am Vet Radiol Soc 14*:45, 1973.
66. Oh I, Harris WH: Proximal strain distribution in the loaded femur. *J Bone Joint Surg [Am] 60A*:75, 1978.
67. Olmstead ML: Total hip replacement in the dog. *Semin Vet Med Surg 2*:131, 1987.
68. Olmstead ML, et al: A five year study of 221 total hip replacements in the dog. *J Am Vet Med Assoc 183*:191, 1983.

69. Olmstead ML, et al: Technique for canine total hip replacement. *Vet Surg 10*:44, 1981.
70. Papavasiliou VA: Lateral and distal transfer of the greater trochanter. *Clin Orthop 207*:198, 1986.
71. Parker RB, et al: Canine total hip arthroplasty: A radiographic correlation of clinical results in 20 cases. *J Am Anim Hosp Assoc 20*:105, 1984.
72. Paterson M, et al: Loosening of the femoral component after total hip replacement. *J Bone Joint Surg [Br] 68B*:392, 1986.
73. Paul HA, Bargar WL: A modified technique for canine total hip replacement. *J Am Anim Hosp Assoc 23*:13, 1987.
74. Paul HA, et al: Approach to the canine coxofemoral joint, body of the ilium and ischium by osteotomy of the greater trochanter. *J Am Anim Hosp Assoc 23*:71, 1987.
75. Peiffer RL, Blevins WE: Hip dysplasia and pectineus resection in the cat. *Feline Pract 4*:40, 1974.
76. Piermattei DL, Greeley RG: *An Atlas of Surgical Approaches to the Bones of the Dog and Cat.* W.B. Saunders, Philadelphia, 1979.
77. Pijanowski GJ, et al: *In vitro* analysis of two canine pelvic osteotomy techniques. *Vet Surg 10*:139, 1981.
78. Prieur WD: Coxarthrosis in the dog: Part 1: Normal and abnormal biomechanics of the hip joint. *Vet Surg 9*:145, 1980.
79. Prieur WD: Double hook plate for intertrochanteric osteotomy in the dog. *Synthes Bull 1*:1, 1984.
80. Prieur WD: Intertrochanteric osteotomy. *In* Bojrab MJ (ed): *Current Techniques in Small Animal Surgery*. Lea & Febiger, Philadelphia, 1990, pp 667–670.
81. Radin EL, et al: Changes in the bone-cement interface after total hip replacement. *J Bone Joint Surg [Am] 64A*:1118, 1982.
82. Riser WH: The dog as a model for the study of hip dysplasia. *Vet Pathol 12*:234, 1975.
83. Rivera LA, et al: Arterial supply to the canine hip joint. *J Vet Orthop 1*:20, 1979.
84. Rothman RH, Hozack WJ: *Complications of Total Hip Arthroplasty*. W.B. Saunders, Philadelphia, 1988, pp 1–177.
85. Schoenecker PL, et al: A dynamic canine model of experimental hip dysplasia. *J Bone Joint Surg [Am] 66A*:1281, 1984.
86. Schrader SC: Triple pelvic osteotomy of the pelvis and trochanteric osteotomy as a treatment for hip dysplasia in the immature dog: The surgical technique and results of 77 consecutive operations. *J Am Vet Med Assoc 189*:659, 1986.
87. Schrader SC: Triple pelvic osteotomy of the pelvis as a treatment for canine hip dysplasia. *J Am Vet Med Assoc 178*:39, 1987.
88. Slocum B: Femoral neck lengthening. *In The Cutting Edge in Veterinary Orthopedics*. Slocum Enterprises, Eugene, 1988, pp 1–4.
89. Slocum B, Devine T: Pelvic osteotomy in the dog as treatment for hip dysplasia. *Semin Vet Med Surg 2*:107, 1987.
90. Slocum B, Devine T: Pelvic osteotomy technique for axial rotation of the acetabular segment in dogs. *J Am Anim Hosp Assoc 22*:331, 1986.
91. Slocum B, Hohn RB: A surgical approach to the caudal aspect of the acetabulum and the body of the ischium in the dog. *J Am Vet Med Assoc 167*:65, 1975.
92. Stauffer RN: Ten-year follow-up study of total hip replacement. *J Bone Joint Surg [Am] 64A*:983, 1982.
93. Tarvin GB, Pijanowski GJ: Letter to the editor: Triple osteotomy of the pelvis. *J Am Vet Med Assoc 179*:4, 1982.
94. Thacher C, Schrader SC: Caudal ventral hip luxation in the dog: A review of 14 cases. *J Am Anim Hosp Assoc 21*:1, 1985.
95. Tomlinson JL: Reduction of coxofemoral luxations. *In* Bojrab MJ (ed): *Current Techniques in Small Animal Surgery*. Lea & Febiger, Philadelphia, 1990, pp 670–676.
96. Turner TM, et al: A comparative study of porous coating in a weight-bearing total hip arthroplasty model. *J Bone Joint Surg [Am] 68A*:1396, 1986.
97. Vanderby R, et al: A micromotion comparison of cemented and porous ingrowth total hip replacements in a canine model. *Trans Orthop Res Soc 35*:577, 1989.
98. Vanderby R: Strain adaptation in the canine after total hip replacement, unpublished data.
99. Vasseur PB: Femoral head and neck ostectomy. *In* Bojrab MJ (ed): *Current Techniques in Small Animal Surgery*. Lea & Febiger, Philadelphia, 1990, pp 674–682.
100. Wadsworth PL, Henry WB: Dorsal surgical approach to acetabular fractures in the dog. *J Am Vet Med Assoc 165*:908, 1974.
101. Walker TL, Prieur WD: Intertrochanteric femoral osteotomy. *Semin Vet Med Surg 2*:117, 1987.
102. Wallace LJ: Canine hip dysplasia: Past and present. *Semin Vet Med Surg 2*:92, 1987.

CHAPTER 136

Fractures of the Femur

J.L. Milton

Because of the proximity of the femur to the trunk, the heavy surrounding musculature, and the complexity of many fractures, adequate alignment and stabilization are difficult if not impossible to achieve by external fixation. The high incidence of internal fixation as the preferred treatment is reflected in studies that report the femur as the most common site of nonunion and osteomyelitis.[6, 7, 24, 38] This high rate of complications demonstrates inadequacies in commonly used methods of repair and frequency of errors in surgical judgment, especially in respect to surgical treatment of complicated femoral fractures.

EMERGENCY TREATMENT

Because of the heavy surrounding muscle mass and the difficulty in immobilizing the proximal segment and the hip, temporary support or stabilization with a padded bandage (Robert Jones), coaptation splint, or a Schroeder-Thomas splint is not indicated in most cases. Restriction of activity by cage confinement is the most prudent method for protecting the fracture and surrounding soft tissue from further injury.

PROXIMAL FEMUR

Anatomical Features

The proximal end (metaphysis-epiphysis) is composed of the femoral head and neck, the tractional epiphyses (greater, lesser, third trochanters), and the subtrochanteric area (Fig. 136–1). The femoral head and most of the neck are enclosed or covered by the joint capsule. The femoral neck projects obliquely from the shaft in a dorsomedial and slightly cranial direction. The angles of inclination (approximately 130° to 145°) and anteversion (approximately 30°) vary with the method of determination and the age and breed of dog.[3, 22, 33] The cortex of the neck is thickened ventrally (calcar) to resist weightbearing forces. The trochanters serve as muscle

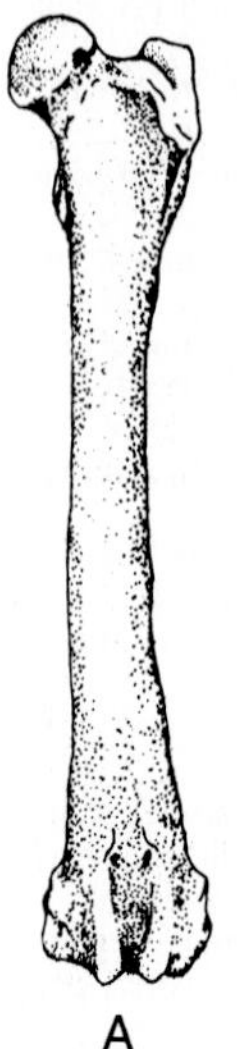

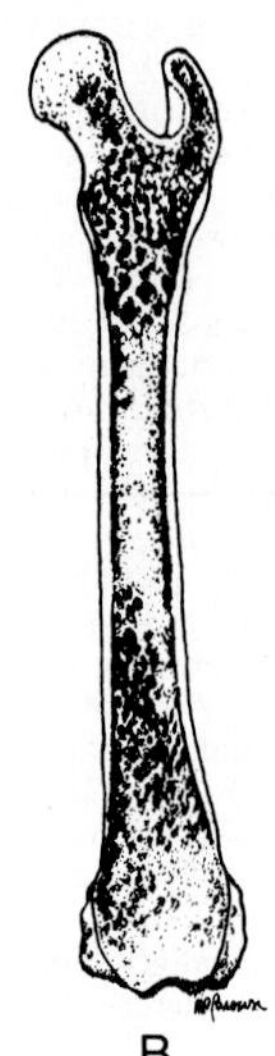

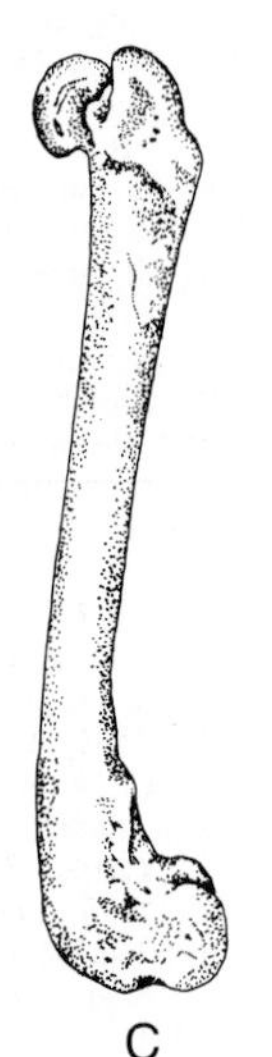

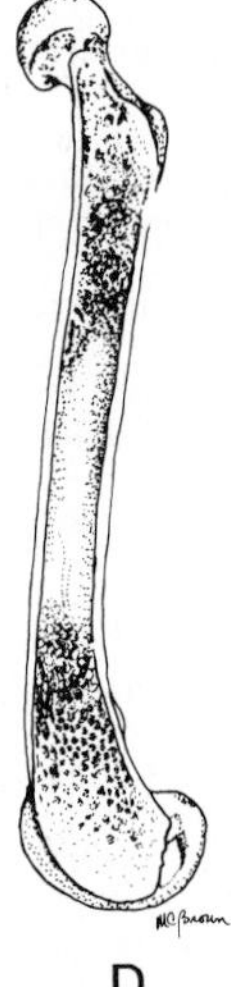

FIGURE 136–1. Conformation and structure of typical, well-proportioned dog's femur. *A*, Cranial view. *B*, Frontal section. *C*, Lateral view. *D*, Sagittal section.

attachment sites and are subject to tractional forces: greater trochanter—middle, deep gluteals, piriform; lesser trochanter—iliopsoas; third trochanter—superficial gluteal. The caudal hip muscles (external rotators) insert in the trochanteric fossa.

Blood Supply

The proximal femur, with its numerous muscle attachments and predominately cancellous bone composition, has a rich blood supply. However, the blood supply to the femoral head, because of the vascular pattern, is limited and subject to disruption with traumatic injury (Fig. 136–2).

The blood supply to the canine femoral head (capital epiphysis) is derived primarily from the lateral and medial circumflex femoral arteries, with limited contribution from the caudal gluteal artery.[4, 25, 34] Branches of these vessels ascend the femoral neck in the joint capsule (ascending cervical or retinacular arteries), cross the physis, and immediately enter the epiphysis (epiphyseal branches). The femoral neck is supplied by branches of these ascending cervical arteries (extraosseous supply) and by ascending branches of the nutrient artery (intraosseous supply). Because of the physeal barrier and the absence of epiphyseal penetration by arteries in the ligament of the head, the capital epiphysis in immature animals totally depends on the ascending cervical arteries for a blood supply.

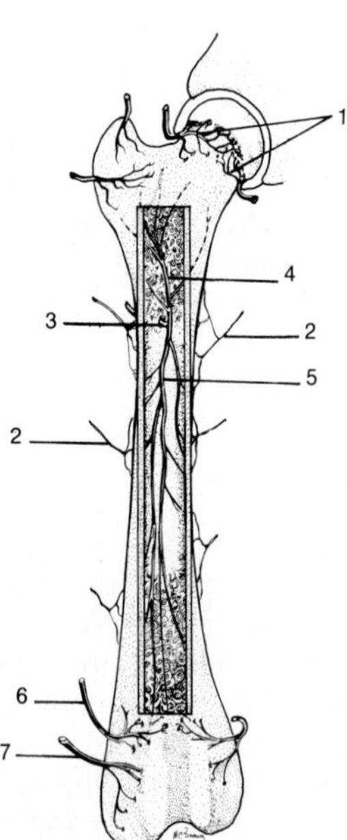

FIGURE 136–2. Blood supply to femur, cranial view (1, ascending cervical arteries; 2, periosteal arteries; 3, nutrient artery; 4, ascending branch nutrient artery; 5, descending branch nutrient artery; 6, distal metaphyseal artery; 7, distal epiphyseal artery.)

Growth

The physes of the femoral head and greater trochanter contribute approximately 30 to 40 per cent of the longitudinal growth of the femur. The exact time of physeal closure varies, with most studies reporting beginning closure at approximately 6 months and complete closure between 9 and 12 months.[9, 33, 40] From a clinical viewpoint, the time of closure is not nearly as important as the percentage of remaining growth at any given age. At 5 months, 80 per cent of the proximal femoral physeal growth is completed, and by 7 months, 95 per cent of skeletal growth is completed.[33]

The femoral head physis is primarily responsible for growth of the femoral neck, and the trochanteric physis for growth of the subtrochanteric metaphyseal region with some contribution to the femoral neck. Experimental fusion or retardation of growth from the femoral head or greater trochanter physis produced proximal deformity but little alteration in total length of the femur.[15, 42] Deformities and complications caused by premature closure of the proximal physes are described in the discussion of fractures of the capital physis and the greater trochanter (Fig. 136–3).

Fracture Classification

In the following discussion, proximal femoral fractures are divided into capital epiphyseal (femoral head), cap-

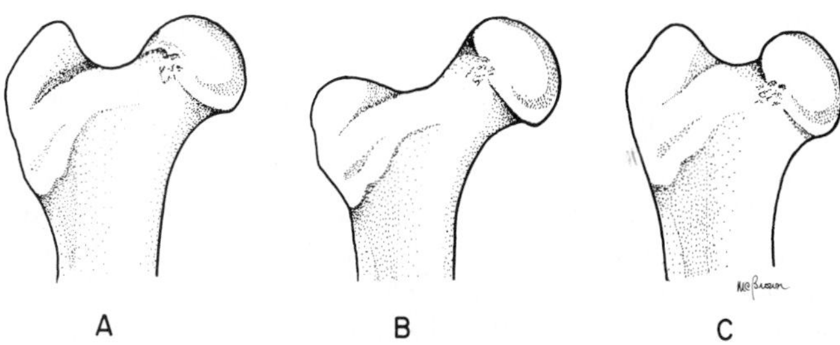

FIGURE 136–3. Development of proximal femur. *A*, Normal. *B*, Premature closure of trochanteric physis. *C*, Premature closure of capital physis.

ital physeal, femoral neck, trochanteric, subtrochanteric, and multiple (Fig. 136–4). Intertrochanteric fractures occur between the greater trochanter and lesser trochanter. They are rare in small animals, are treated in a similar manner to femoral neck or subtrochanteric fractures, and are not described as a specific entity.

Surgical Approaches

The femoral head and neck are adequately exposed through the craniolateral approach to the hip. Exposure can be increased by tenotomy of the deep gluteal muscle and reflection of the origin of the vastus lateralis. With capital physeal and femoral neck fractures, incision through the joint capsule to expose the head facilitates reduction, orientation of the fracture segments, and evaluation of pin placement. Dorsal approach to the hip by osteotomy of the greater trochanter provides the greatest exposure but is rarely needed.[31] Fractures of the greater trochanter and subtrochanteric region are exposed by a lateral approach to the proximal femur.[31]

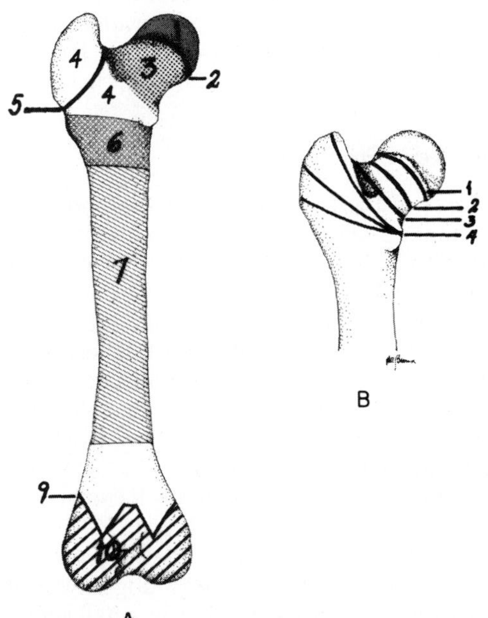

FIGURE 136–4. *A*, Anatomical classification of femoral fracture. (1, capital epiphyseal [femoral head]; 2, capital physeal; 3, femoral neck; 4, intertrochanteric; 5, greater trochanter; 6, subtrochanteric; 7, diaphyseal [shaft]; 8, distal metaphyseal; 9, distal physeal; 10, distal epiphyseal.) *B*, Anatomical classification of femoral neck fractures including intertrochanteric fractures. (1, subcapital; 2, transcervical; 3, basilar; 4, intertrochanteric.)

Capital Epiphyseal Fractures (Avulsion Fractures of Femoral Head)

Avulsion fractures of the femoral head occur most often with coxofemoral luxations in immature animals (Fig. 136–5). In most cases, the small, predominately cartilaginous segment is simply excised with the attached ligament of the head of the femur before reduction of the femoral head. Rarely the avulsed segment is large, with substantial subchondral bone. In these cases, excision of the fragment leaves a major defect in the ventral third to half of the femoral head and predisposes the joint to arthritic changes. Alternative treatment considerations include internal fixation, excision arthroplasty, and hip prosthesis. Internal fixation is preferred, but the procedure is technically demanding. Techniques of internal fixation include compression screw fixation, multiple small pin fixation, and a combination of the two (see Fig. 136–5). Excellent or good results in four of five cases treated by compression screw and Kirschner wire or Smilley nail fixation were reported.[41] With rigid internal fixation, accurate anatomical alignment, and proper postoperative care, the prognosis is favorable. Excision arthroplasty or total hip reconstruction is recommended in fractures that have failed or developed severe degenerative joint disease.

Capital Physeal Fractures

The physis is the weak point of the immature skeleton, and trauma frequently results in fractures at this site rather than dislocation. Capital physeal fractures are the most common fracture of the proximal femur and are observed in animals between 4 and 11 months of age, with the highest incidence between 6 and 8 months.[11, 13, 30] Most are Salter-Harris type I.

Avascular necrosis of the femoral head is uncommon when the fracture is treated properly by internal fixation.[11, 13, 23, 30] Excision arthroplasty is most justified with chronic injuries and in complex fractures with comminution of the head or neck or both. Internal fixation is not delayed, because remodeling of the neck produces an incongruent, unstable reduction (Fig. 136–6).[13, 26]

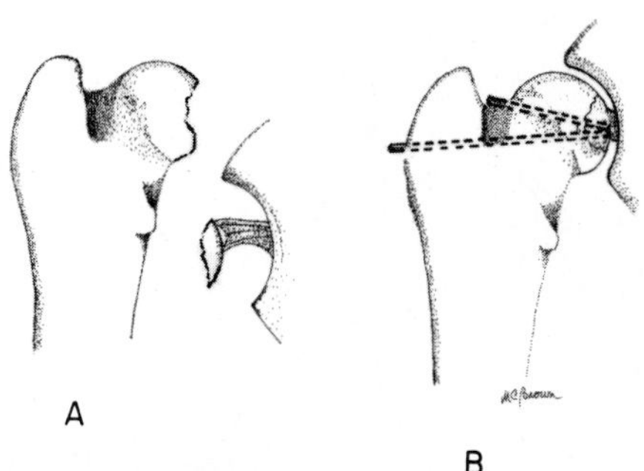

FIGURE 136–5. *A*, Coxofemoral luxation with avulsion fracture of the capital epiphysis (femoral head). *B*, Fixation with two Kirschner wires. *C*, Interfragmentary compression fixation with a bone screw.

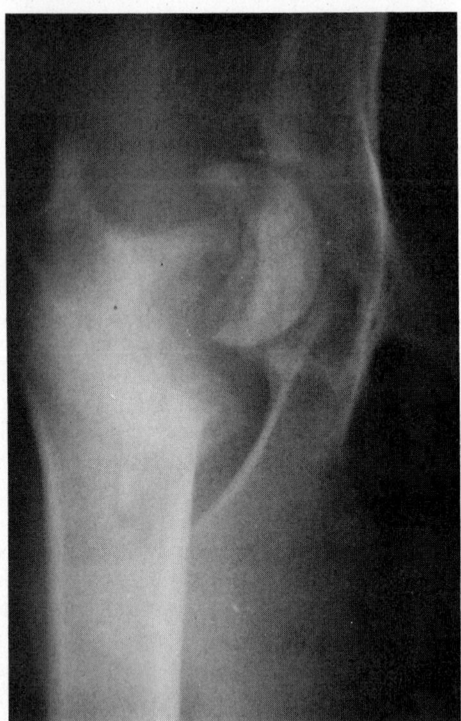

FIGURE 136–6. Chronic untreated capital physeal fracture shows gross resorption of femoral neck, limited remodeling of femoral head, and degenerative changes in the acetabulum.

Multiple small pins or Kirschner wires are most frequently used to stabilize the small epiphyseal segment (femoral head) and offer a simple, comparatively atraumatic technique (Fig. 136–7).[2, 13] Compression screw fixation has been advocated to increase stabilization and promote revascularization.[23, 30] Compression of the physis in an actively growing animal younger than 5 months may promote physeal closure and deformity of the proximal femur.

At least two Kirschner wires (0.45 to 0.62 inch) are inserted through the neck and into the head. Retrograde and normograde techniques of pin placement have been described. With the normograde technique, pins are inserted from the lateral aspect of the proximal femur

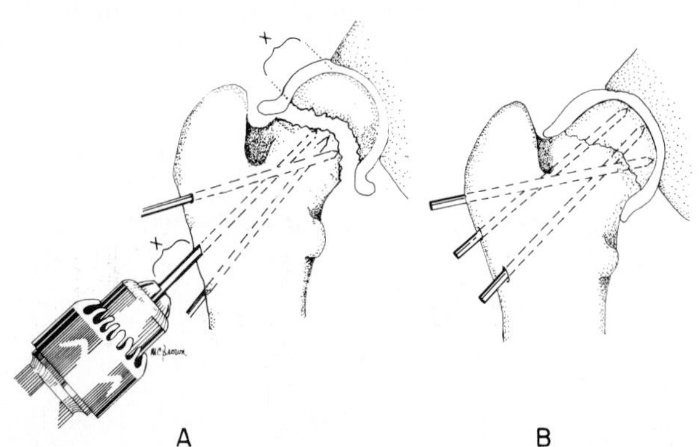

FIGURE 136–7. Capital physeal fracture treated with multiple Kirschner wires. *A*, Kirschner wires inserted in normograde manner. *B*, Fracture is reduced, and pins are seated into the subchondral bone.

into the neck to the level of the fracture (Fig. 136–7*A*). Pin placement is examined at the fracture site, the fracture is reduced, and the pins are driven into subchondral bone of the femoral head (Fig. 136–7*B*). Examination of pin placement at the fracture site is optional, and reduction of the femoral head may precede insertion of the pins. The pins are directed into different segments of the femoral head. With retrograde technique, the pins are drilled from the fracture through the femoral neck to emerge along the lateral aspect of the proximal femur. The pins are retracted to the level of the fracture; the fracture is reduced, and the pins are seated into the head. The articular surface is checked for pin penetration by subluxation of the head and visual inspection or by movement of the joint.

The technique of compression screw fixation is similar to that described for femoral neck fractures (Fig. 136–8). With capital physeal fractures, the glide hole is drilled through the greater trochanter and femoral neck (near segment) before reduction of the fracture.

The prognosis for bone healing and a return to satisfactory function is favorable but guarded for normal development of the femoral head and neck. Bone healing is observed in 3 to 6 weeks. Factors that influence the prognosis include remaining growth potential (age of the animal), type of fracture, degree of fracture displacement (soft-tissue damage), and technique and accuracy of treatment. Premature closure of the physis is usually observed within 3 weeks and may cause a shortened femoral neck, coxa vara, and elongation of the greater trochanter (see Fig. 136–3*C*). These changes are most prominent in animals with significant growth potential (younger than 5 months) and may lead to malformation and degeneration of the hip. Resorption of the outer margins of the femoral neck (apple-core appearance) is common on radiographic examination between 3 to 6 weeks after surgery but has not caused clinical problems.[13, 23]

Femoral Neck Fractures

Fractures of the femoral neck occur predominately in mature animals. Femoral neck fractures are subdivided according to specific location into subcapital, transcervical, and basilar (see Fig. 136–4*B*) and according to their relationship to the joint capsule into intracapsular (medial) and extracapsular (lateral). These subdivisions are of little clinical value because all neck fractures are treated by similar surgical techniques. Most fractures are basilar and frequently accompany trochanteric and subtrochanteric fractures.

Techniques using lag screws or Kirschner wires are used for internal fixation (see Figs. 136–7 and 136–8). Compression screw fixation offers the most rigid stabilization and is preferred in large dogs. Multiple small pins provide satisfactory fixation in small and medium-sized animals. Femoral head and neck excision is always an option and is most indicated in irreparable comminuted fractures.

Specific steps in the compression screw technique vary according to a surgeon's preference and type of screw used, but the end result of thread purchase in only the

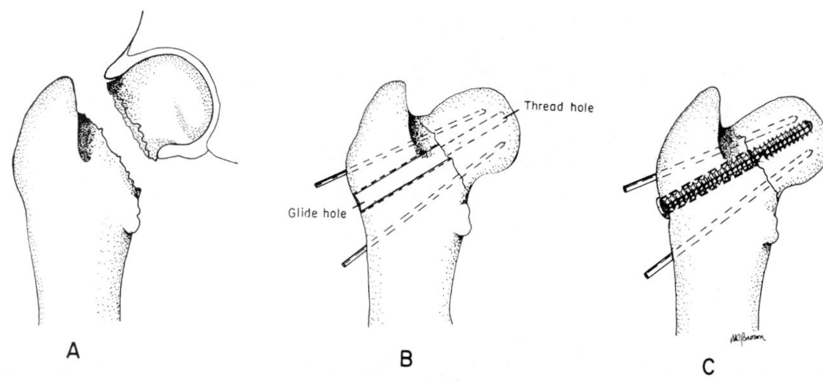

FIGURE 136–8. *A*, Basilar fracture of the femoral neck. *B*, Initial fixation with one or two Kirschner wires; glide hole and thread hole created for interfragmentary compression with *(C)* a fully threaded bone screw.

far segment (head) and a glide hole in the near segment is common to all techniques (see Fig. 136–8). Reduction of the fracture before drilling the screw hole aids in positioning and aiming the drill into the femoral neck and head. Once reduced, the fracture is stabilized with one or two Kirschner wires placed eccentrically through the neck and head (see Fig. 136–8*A*). To ensure proper direction of the drill, a small pilot hole can be drilled and enlarged after evaluation of placement, a C-shaped drill guide can be used, or a guide pin can be placed adjacent to the femoral neck and head. The thread hole is drilled from the region of the third trochanter through the central core of the neck and into the head. The drilling depth can be estimated by measurements taken from a parallel course along the exposed cranial aspect of the head, neck, and greater trochanter. For a full-threaded screw, a glide hole is created in the outer (near) segment by enlarging the channel to the diameter of the screw. The length of the hole (glide plus thread) is measured with a depth gauge, and 2 to 4 mm is subtracted from the measurement to allow for compression at the fracture and sinking of the screw head. The thread hole in the far segment (head) is tapped for a non–self-tapping screw; the entrance is beveled with a countersink, and the screw is inserted. An alternative technique involves drilling of the glide hole first (normograde or retrograde), followed by reduction of the fracture, stabilization with Kirschner wires, and drilling the thread hole (see Fig. 136–8*B*).

The technique for fixation with multiple Kirschner wires or small pins is similar to that described previously for capital physeal fractures (see Fig. 136–7). The fracture is usually reduced before normograde insertion of the pins. With a stable anatomical reduction, the prognosis for a return to normal function is favorable.

Greater Trochanter Fractures

Fractures of the greater trochanter are uncommon and occur most frequently at the physis in conjunction with capital physeal fractures. This fracture in mature animals may occur with fractures of the femoral neck or dislocations of the hip (Figs. 136–9 and 136–10). The greater trochanter is subjected to tractional forces from the gluteal muscles and compression forces from the vastus lateralis muscle. Although fixation with a compression screw or multiple small pins and tension band wire is recommended, interfragmentary compression is not always required to provide adequate stabilization of this broad-based angular fracture of trabecular bone.

Fractures in immature animals are treated satisfactorily with multiple Kirschner wires directed diagonally into the medial cortex of the proximal metaphysis and diaphysis (see Fig. 136–9*B*). Tension band wire is optional but should be used to increase stabilization when needed without fear of producing substantial functional disturbances due to premature closure of the physis.[15, 21] In mature animals, interfragmentary compression with multiple pins and tension band wire or a compression screw is recommended (see Fig. 136–9*C*).

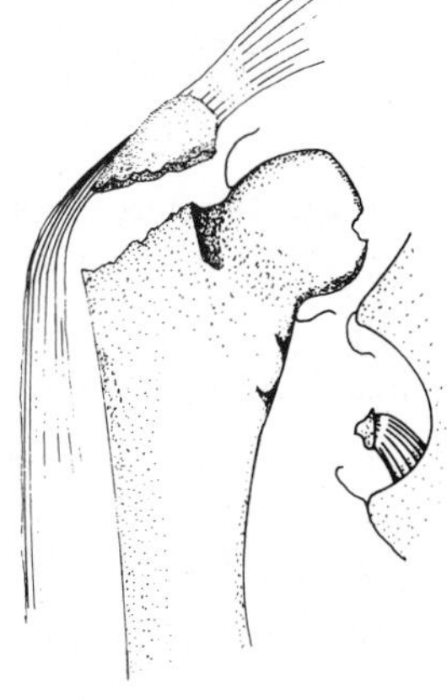

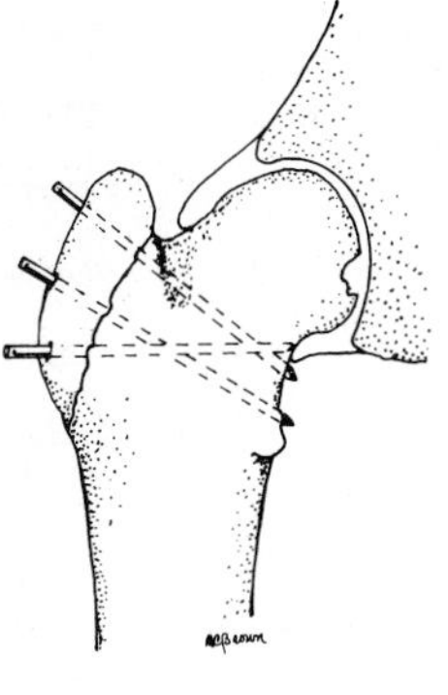

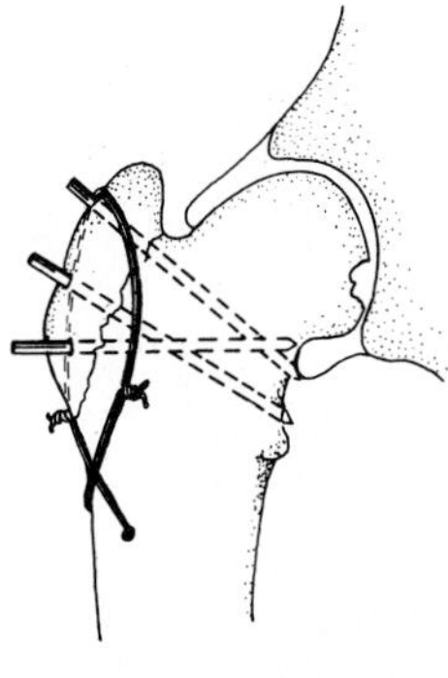

FIGURE 136–9. *A*, Fracture of the greater trochanter with coxofemoral luxation and small avulsion fracture of the femoral head. *B*, Excision of the bone fragment and ligament, reduction of the hip, and fixation of the greater trochanter with three Kirschner wires. *C*, Additional fixation with tension band wiring.

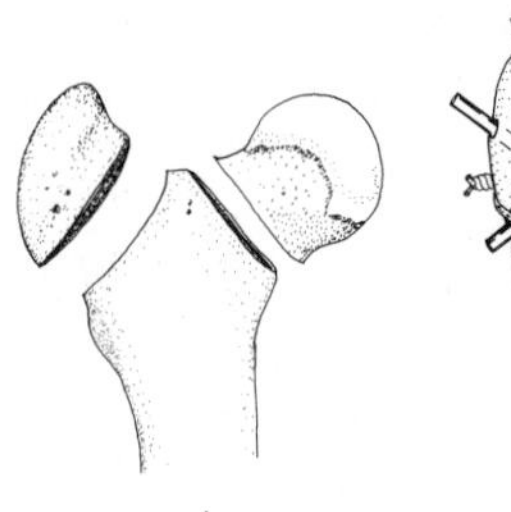

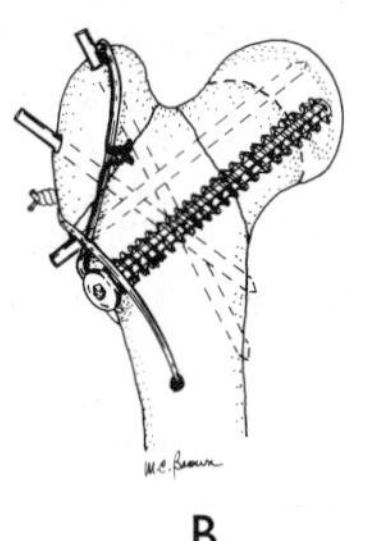

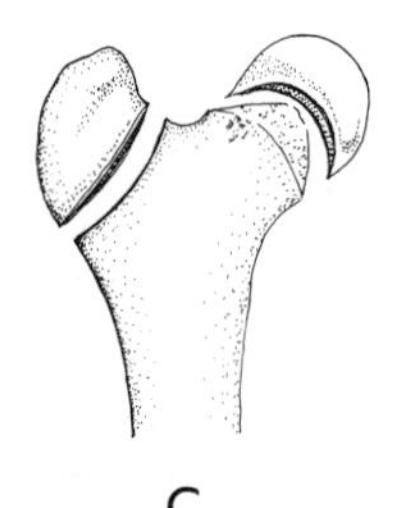

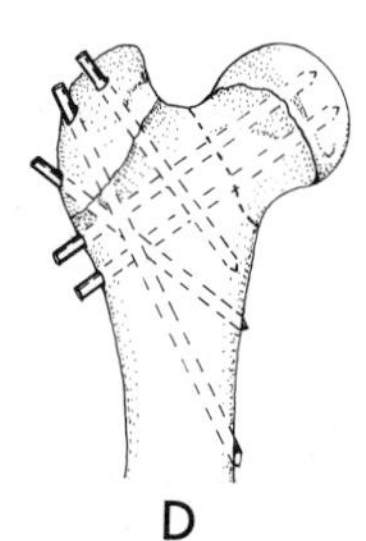

FIGURE 136–10. *A*, Fracture of the greater trochanter and femoral neck. *B*, Repair with multiple pins, tension band wiring, and a compression screw. *C*, Fracture of the greater trochanter and capital physis. *D*, Repair with multiple pins.

The prognosis for a return to normal function is favorable, but guarded for normal development of the greater trochanter in immature animals. Deformities reported from premature closure of the trochanteric physis include shortened trochanter, coxa valga, and elongated or narrowed femoral neck (see Fig. 136–3*B*).[15, 21, 42] These changes generally do not affect limb function.

Subtrochanteric Fractures

Subtrochanteric fractures are uncommon and are most often observed with multiple fractures of the proximal femur (Fig. 136–11). Repair of such fractures can be difficult because of the frequency of comminution, involvement of the femoral neck, comparatively short proximal segment, large medullary canal, and tapered contour of the subtrochanteric region.

Bone plating techniques (compression, neutralization, buttress) provide rigid stabilization of the fracture and are especially indicated in large dogs and comminuted fractures (Fig. 136–11*C*). The plate is contoured over the greater trochanter to provide adequate screw purchase in the short proximal segment. Screw purchase can be increased by placing the plate so that one screw is inserted into the femoral neck and by bending the proximal end of the plate over the greater trochanter so the most proximal screws are directed distally and medially into the base of the femoral neck. Comminuted segments are stabilized before application of the plate with transcortical pins and cerclage wire, hemicerclage wire, or compression screws.

Intramedullary fixation has more application in simple transverse, oblique, and spiral fractures, especially in small and medium-sized animals. In this metaphyseal fracture, with a short proximal segment and large medullary canal, a single intramedullary pin provides little resistance to rotation, compression, and shear forces. Multiple (stack) pins or pins used according to Rush pin principles provide more stable fixation. Various wiring techniques (figure-eight, cerclage, hemicerclage) and transcortical pins are used to improve stabilization or provide fixation of comminuted segments (Fig. 136–11*B*). In this flared proximal metaphyseal region, intramedullary pins do not completely fill the medullary canal, and transcortical pins are used to increase fixation and points of anchorage for cerclage wires. A type I external pin splint may be used for additional fixation, especially in comminuted fractures.

With simple fractures, a stable anatomical reduction, and proper aftercare, the prognosis for a return to normal function is favorable. Comminuted fractures offer the greatest challenge and have a more guarded prognosis.

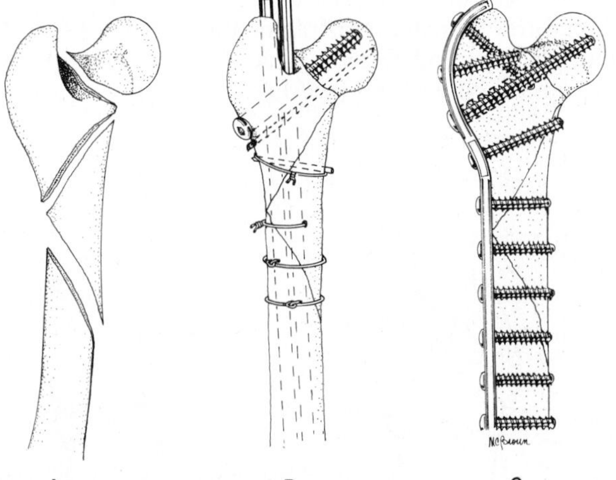

FIGURE 136–11. *A*, Comminuted fracture of the proximal femur involving the subtrochanteric area and femoral neck. *B*, Repaired with compression screw fixation of neck fracture, axial alignment with multiple pins; fragment stabilization with cerclage wires and transcortical pin. *C*, Repaired by bone plating (neutralization). Note plate positioning to accommodate screw fixation in femoral neck.

Multiple Fractures

Multiple fractures of the proximal femur, involving various combinations of femoral head and neck, greater trochanter, and subtrochanteric-intertrochanteric fractures, are treated by combining the various techniques described for each of the individual fractures (see Figs. 136–10 and 136–11).

Postoperative Care

Exercise is restricted to controlled (leash) activity for 3 to 4 weeks. A figure-eight bandage or nonweightbearing sling is considered when rigid fixation has not been achieved.

FEMORAL DIAPHYSIS

Anatomical Features

The tubular diaphysis is composed almost entirely of cortical bone with little trabecular support. In dogs, the diaphysis has a slight cranial bow, but in cats, it is comparatively straight (see Fig. 136–1). The central two thirds is fairly uniform in diameter, with its narrowest point (isthmus) located proximally. The shaft is free of muscle attachments except along the caudal border (facies aspera), where the adductor muscle attaches.

Proximally and distally, the shaft flares to form the metaphysis; cortical bone thins, and trabecular bone progressively increases in density. Weightbearing forces transmitted between the medially positioned femoral head and the caudally positioned condyles create compression forces caudomedially and tension forces craniolaterally.

Blood Supply

The blood supply is similar to that of other long bones, with the major contribution from the nutrient artery (branch of the medial circumflex femoral) (see Fig. 136–2). In mature animals, the periosteal blood supply is minimal and is most evident along the facies aspera. Vascular injury due to trauma and surgical manipulation is a major factor in the development of nonunion or osteomyelitis or both.[32]

Growth

The diaphysis grows in length by endochondral ossification from the proximal and distal physes. The distal physis contributes most (60 to 70 per cent) of the longitudinal growth. Large intramedullary pins that penetrate the distal physis of immature animals with substantial remaining growth (dogs younger than 4 to 5 months) may cause growth disturbances by creating an osseous bridge across the physis.[27] However, a study of femoral shortening by mid-diaphyseal ostectomy revealed that normal mature dogs can withstand up to a 20 per cent loss of total femoral length without significant alteration of limb function.[17]

Circumferential growth occurs by intramembranous osteogenesis from the periosteum. Cerclage wires do not interfere with appositional growth but can cause alterations in the normal mechanical properties of growing diaphyseal bone that could predispose to fracture during the first 8 weeks after application.[14] This predisposition to fracture has not been a clinical problem.

Fracture Classification

Three general groups of fractures occur: transverse, oblique/spiral, and comminuted. Open fractures are rare because of the heavy surrounding musculature. The type of fracture is important in considering the forces that must be neutralized by internal fixation (see Chapter 120).

Surgical Approach

The femoral diaphysis is exposed by a lateral approach.[31] The extent of exposure varies with the type of fracture and the method of treatment (e.g., simple transverse versus comminuted, and retrograde pinning versus bone plating). The approach can be combined with various approaches to the hip and the stifle to expose the entire length of the femur.

Treatment of Diaphyseal Fractures

Diaphyseal fractures of the femur are noted for substantial displacement and over-riding of the fracture segments. The distal segment is usually displaced and pulled caudomedially into the adductor and hamstring muscle groups by the gastrocnemius muscle, and the proximal segment is pulled cranially and rotated externally by the iliopsoas and external hip rotators. Comminuted fragments from the cranial portion of the diaphysis have little if any muscle attachment, and fragments from the caudal portion retain firm attachment to the adductor muscle.

Alignment and stabilization necessary for rapid bone healing and return to function are difficult if not impossible to achieve using external splintage. Conservative treatment (Schroeder-Thomas splint, coaptation splints, cage rest) usually results in side-to-side healing, deformity, and substantial shortening of the limb. Although not the ideal method of treatment, conservative treatment may produce acceptable functional results when recommended internal fixation techniques are not accepted by the owner. Caution must be observed with immobilization of the limb in immature animals because irreversible muscle and stifle joint changes may develop (hyperextended stifle, quadriceps contracture).

Transverse Fractures

Intramedullary pinning is a practical and economical method of treating transverse diaphyseal fractures of the femur, but the detrimental force of rotation is not neutralized with single-pin fixation. Type I external fixators (see Chapter 123) are the most effective technique for controlling rotation (Fig. 136–12*A–D*). An alternative technique is to use multiple intramedullary pins.[8] Küntscher nails are useful in humans, but the relatively thin cortex in dogs precludes reaming and negates the potential advantage of increased endosteal contact.

Compression plating is most indicated in large mature dogs but is considered in any mature animal in which a rapid return to normal function is desirable (Fig. 136–12*E*). With transverse fractures, the fracture gap is decreased or eliminated; bone-to-bone contact is established at the fracture, and the plate and screws are under minimal stress. Return to function and bone healing are rapid. With proper operative technique and patient care, complications are rare.

Oblique/Spiral Fracture

With oblique and spiral fractures, satisfactory alignment and stabilization can be achieved by combining various internal fixation techniques (Fig. 136–13).

Intramedullary pinning combined with transcortical pins and full-cerclage or hemicerclage wire is the simplest method of treatment and provides adequate sta-

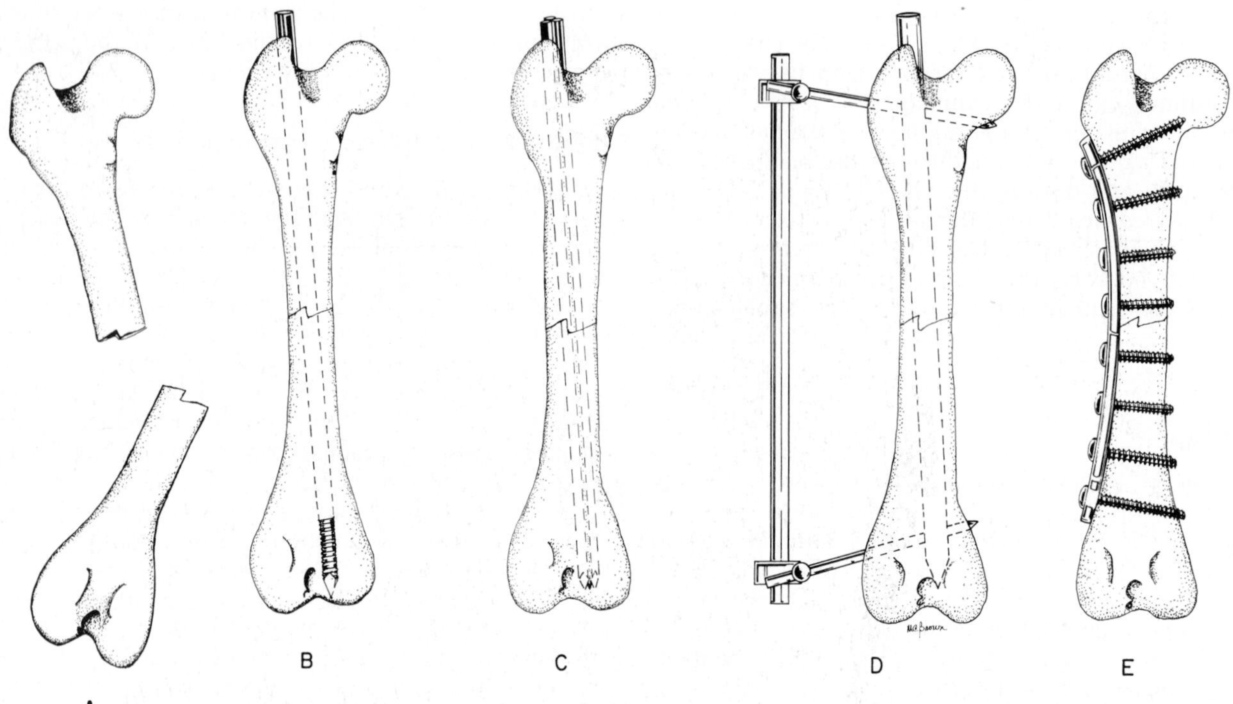

FIGURE 136–12. *A*, Transverse midshaft fracture. *B*, Repaired with single intramedullary pins. *C*, Multiple (stack) pinning. *D*, Single intramedullary pin with additional fixation from a two-pin, type I external pin splint and figure-eight wire. *E*, Bone plate (compression).

bilization in many cases (Fig. 136–13*B*). Axial stabilization (bending) is provided by the intramedullary pin and compression; shear and rotation forces are neutralized by full-cerclage and hemicerclage wires. Transcortical pins (0.45 to 0.062 inch) increase stabilization and serve as points of anchorage for full-cerclage or figure-eight wires. Complete filling of the medullary canal with the intramedullary pin is not critical when fixation can be supplemented with an adequate number of wires and transcortical pins (short oblique versus long spiral fracture).

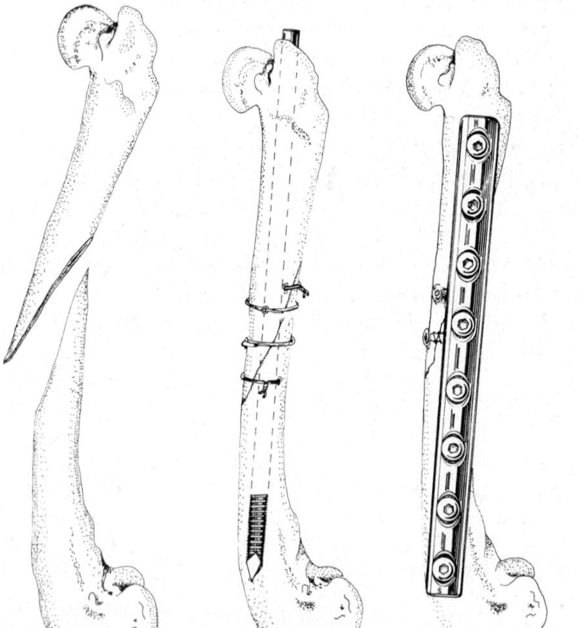

FIGURE 136–13. *A*, Oblique/spiral diaphyseal fracture. *B*, Repaired with single intramedullary pin and full-cerclage and hemicerclage wires. *C*, Bone plate and compression screws (neutralization).

Interfragmentary compression screws, used in conjunction with a bone plate (neutralization plating), provide rigid fixation and accurate alignment with minimal fracture gap (Fig. 136–13*C*). Compression screw placement, inside or outside the plate, is dictated by the plane of fracture.

Independent use of compression screws, cerclage wires, and transcortical pins has been advocated in the treatment of long spiral fractures. The use of these techniques in animals is not recommended because the strength of fixation is inadequate to allow early activity.

Comminuted Fractures

Comminuted fractures of the femoral diaphysis often have small fragments that are difficult to align accurately and stabilize completely (Fig. 136–14). These complex fractures require sophisticated repair techniques capable of resisting compression, shear, rotation, and bending. Rebuilding the fracture so that all fragments are accurately aligned and gaps are eliminated is often impossible. Malalignment and substantial osseous defects decrease stabilization and shift stresses from the bone to the appliance, predisposing to failure. Inadequate fixation, extensive soft-tissue damage, and a loss of periosteal and medullary blood supply predispose this type of fracture to nonunion or osteomyelitis or both.

Intramedullary fixation supplemented with full-cer-

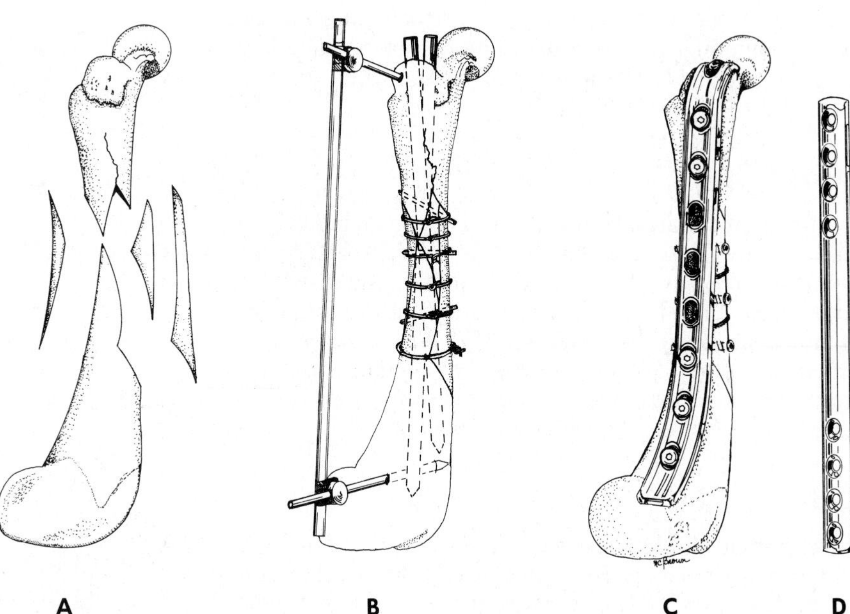

FIGURE 136–14. *A*, Comminuted diaphyseal fracture. *B*, Repaired with multiple (stack) intramedullary pins, cerclage wires, transcortical pins, and two-pin type I external pin splint. *C*, Repaired with a bone plate (buttress), compression screws, and full-cerclage wires. *D*, Bone lengthening plate, without screw slots in central portion, provides greater strength.

clage wires, as well as transcortical pins, may be used to treat comminuted femoral diaphyseal fractures. Compression forces are not completely neutralized and may cause collapse. Stabilization can be improved by using multiple pins. Additional support can be provided with a type I external pin splint (Fig. 136–14*B*). Best results with pin and wire fixation are expected when the fragments are large enough to permit anatomical reconstruction.

Bone plating provides the most rigid fixation and is most indicated in mature dogs of large and giant breeds (Fig. 136–14*C*). Screws, wires, and pins used for fragment reduction are placed in a way that does not interfere with plate positioning. Fixation of the plate with at least three screws (cortices) in each main segment is desirable and often requires a plate that extends most of the bone length. The plate is positioned so that fracture gaps and fissure lines do not interfere with screw purchase. Vacant screw slots create weak points in the plate and contribute to plate fatigue and failure. When reconstruction of the fracture is incomplete and large defects remain, a bone lengthening plate with a solid central portion can be used to provide increased implant strength (Fig. 136–14*D*).[18]

In highly comminuted fractures that cannot be reconstructed, a segmental diaphyseal allograft can be used with compression bone plating. One study reported a 96 per cent successful result in dogs (see Chapter 127).[37]

Cancellous bone grafts promote healing of comminuted diaphyseal fractures and are considered mandatory when substantial gaps are present. Multiple grafting procedures may be required to obtain union across large defects.

A number of variables affect the prognosis, including signalment, severity of comminution, surgical technique (time, sterility, trauma, alignment, fixation), and patient care. A guarded prognosis is rendered in most cases. Best results are achieved in young animals and when bone fragments are large.

Postoperative Care

Postoperative care is very important and is most critical with comminuted fractures. Restriction to house and leash activity is recommended for at least 4 to 6 weeks. Uncontrolled activity is not allowed until radiographic examination demonstrates adequate bone healing.

External support with a Schroeder-Thomas splint or other splinting methods is rarely beneficial in providing additional stabilization of the fracture. Splints increase postoperative management responsibilities and, without proper care, increase complications.

DISTAL FEMORAL FRACTURES

Anatomical Features

The distal femur is composed of the metaphysis, epiphysis, and in immature animals the physis (see Figs. 136–1 and 136–4). The diaphysis flares to form the metaphysis, cortical bone thins cranially, and trabecular bone progressively increases in density. The physis has an irregular W shape from both a craniocaudal and mediolateral perspective and creates four osseous protuberances from the metaphysis and four corresponding depressions in the epiphysis (see Fig. 136–16*A*). With physeal fractures, the caudal protuberances are commonly fractured and included with the epiphyseal segment (Salter-Harris type II).[1, 19] The epiphysis is composed of a trochlea and two condyles and is covered, for the most part, by joint capsule or articular cartilage. The comma-shaped condyles extend caudal to the long axis of the femur. In chondrodysplastic breeds, the distal portion of the epiphysis is flatter and the condyles project more caudally. The collateral ligaments attach to the epicondyles, and the cruciate ligaments attach in the intercondylar fossa. The tendons of the long digital extensor and popliteal muscles pass within the joint capsule to attach to the cranial and lateral aspect of the lateral condyle, respectively. The gastrocnemius muscle, with its medial and lateral sesamoid bones (fabellae), originates from the caudal aspect of the distal metaphysis.

Blood Supply

Sufficient collateral circulation to the distal metaphysis and epiphysis is provided by the nutrient artery and branches of the popliteal, caudal femoral, and geniculate arteries so that vascular insufficiency following trauma is not a problem (see Fig. 136–2). With most physeal fractures (type II), the metaphyseal segment displaces cranially and is stripped of its superficial vessels but the epiphyseal vessels generally remain intact.

Growth

Although all studies agree that most of the longitudinal growth occurs from the distal physis, the exact percentage reported varies from 60 to 75 per cent. Likewise, the time for physeal closure is variable, with reported ages ranging from 6 to 14 months.[9, 33, 40] More important than the time of physeal closure is the remaining growth potential at the time of physeal injury. Riser studied femoral growth in greyhounds and found the most rapid growth period was between 3 and 5 months and 80 per cent of the growth occurred by 5 months, with 95 per cent by 7 months.[33]

Fracture Classification

Fractures of the distal femur are classified as metaphyseal, physeal, and epiphyseal (see Fig. 136–4). Physeal fractures are further divided according to the classification of Salter and Harris.[35]

A rigid classification is difficult to establish because of the anatomical and structural differences between mature and immature animals. The term *supracondylar* has referred to both metaphyseal and physeal fractures. In this discussion, supracondylar fractures are considered low metaphyseal fractures (physeal region) in mature animals. Although classified as metaphyseal fractures, they are repaired with the same methods as Salter-Harris type I or II physeal fractures. Intercondylar or condylar fractures of mature animals involve the epiphysis but have similar location and methods of repair as Salter-Harris type III or IV physeal fractures.

Surgical Approach

The lateral approach to the stifle provides satisfactory exposure for repair of most distal femoral fractures and can be extended proximally to expose the diaphysis.[31] Isolated fracture of the medial condyle can be exposed by a medial approach to the stifle. Reflection of the medial collateral ligament by osteotomy of the medial epicondyle increases exposure and facilitates repair.[12]

Metaphyseal Fractures

Metaphyseal fractures occur most frequently in mature animals but are not a common fracture. Transverse and mildly comminuted fractures are most common at this junctional area between the (cortical) diaphysis and (cancellous) epiphysis (Fig. 136–15). The short distal segment and the large medullary canal present problems in stabilization for both intramedullary pinning and bone plating.

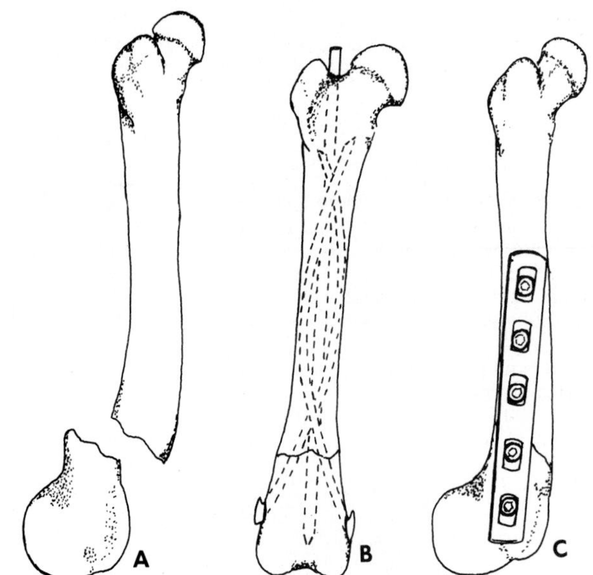

FIGURE 136–15. *A*, Transverse fracture of distal metaphysis. *B*, Repaired with Rush pins and single intramedullary pin. *C*, Repaired with a bone plate (compression).

A single pin, multiple pins, and Rush pins are used for intramedullary fixation (Fig. 136–15*B*). Adequate stabilization and pin seating are difficult, particularly with single-pin fixation and with transverse and comminuted fractures. Over-reduction of the short distal segment facilitates pin seating in the condyles, but the resultant malalignment of the fracture may decrease stabilization. Multiple pins or pins used according to the Rush pin principles provide greater stabilization and are preferred over a single pin. A type I external pin splint may be used to provide additional fixation.

Bone plating provides the most rigid fixation and is the preferred method of repair for large dogs and for transverse and comminuted fractures (Fig. 136–15*C*). Plate fixation to the short distal segment with three screws may be impossible, and cancellous bone screws are generally used because of the thin cortex and abundant trabecular bone.

The metaphysis has a rich blood supply and source of osteogenic cells. With adequate stabilization of the fracture, bone healing occurs very rapidly. Improper seating of a single intramedullary pin with inadequate stabilization is a common cause of complications.

Physeal Fractures

Physeal fractures occur in immature animals between 3 and 11 months of age, with the greatest incidence between 5 and 8 months. Most physeal fractures in dogs are Salter-Harris type II (Fig. 136–16). Cats have a high occurrence of Salter-Harris type I. Types III and IV are rare in both species. Type V, compression fractures,

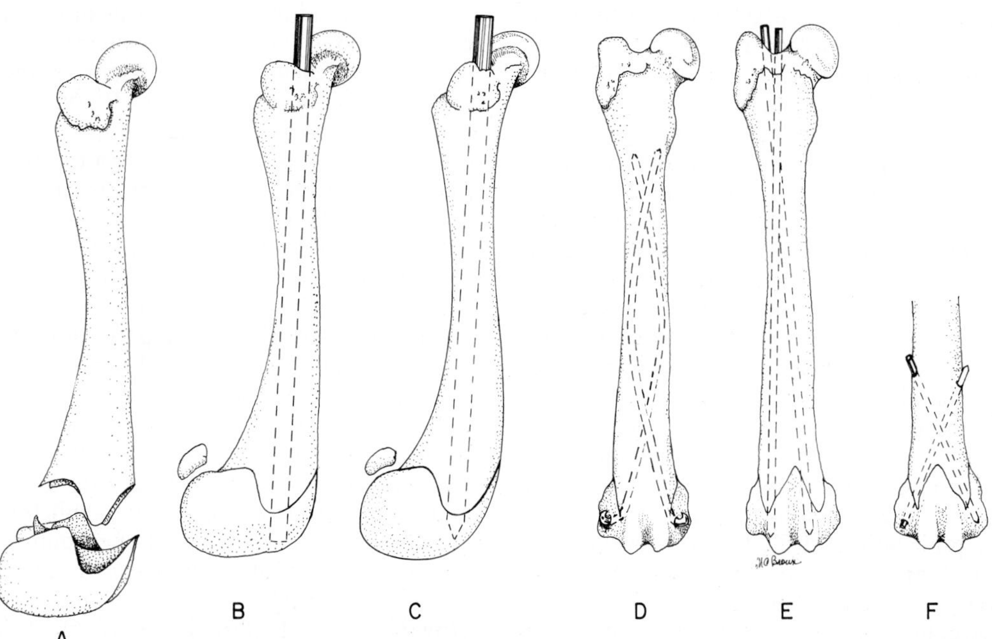

FIGURE 136–16. *A,* Distal Salter-Harris type I, II physeal fracture. Repaired with normograde intramedullary pinning *(B),* retrograde intramedullary pin *(C)*; Rush pinning *(D)*; double pinning *(E)*; and cross pinning *(F).*

may occur in conjunction with any of the other physeal fractures and contribute to growth retardation. The degree of retardation is related to the age of the animal, the method of repair, and the amount of trauma to the physis (type of fracture) and surrounding soft tissue.*

Salter-Harris Types I and II and Supracondylar Fractures

The method of treatment should provide sufficient stabilization to allow early use of the leg and should have minimal effect on physeal growth. Anatomical reduction of the fracture is preferred. Over-reduction has been suggested to increase pin seating in the short epiphyseal segment but is not recommended. The protuberances from the metaphyseal segment interdigitate with the corresponding fossae in the epiphyseal segment and contribute to stabilization. Reduction may be difficult to achieve, especially in chronic fractures. Aggressive manipulation of the epiphyseal segment with bone forceps and traumatic levering techniques may cause significant physeal and articular cartilage damage and should be avoided if possible.

Internal fixation is usually required. Popular methods include single intramedullary pin, double intramedullary pins, Rush pins, and cross pins (see Fig. 136–16). Other reported fixation techniques include type I external pin splints, bone plates, bone screws, staples, and orthopedic wire. External immobilization with a flexion (Ehmer) sling and Schroeder-Thomas splint has been used successfully, but irreversible joint and muscle changes (quadriceps contracture, hyperextended stifle) are major concerns.†

*See references 1, 5, 10, 19, 20, 27, 36, and 39.

†See references 1, 10, 16, 20, 28, 29, and 36.

Interference with growth is a consideration in immature animals with substantial remaining potential, but its importance overall has probably been overemphasized. Premature closure of the physis commonly occurs as a result of initial trauma regardless of the method of treatment; most physeal fractures occur in animals over 5 months of age that have achieved 80 per cent of their skeletal growth; dogs can lose at least 20 per cent of their total femoral length without substantial functional impairment.[10, 17, 20, 33] In dogs younger than 4 to 5 months, interference with growth is a factor in selecting the method of repair.

A single smooth pin, placed centrally through the physis, interferes minimally with bone growth.[27] Stabilization of the fracture is aided by accurate reduction and interlocking of the metaphyseal and epiphyseal segments. Single intramedullary pins are most indicated in small to medium-sized animals and in animals 3 to 4 months of age with substantial remaining growth. Pin insertion may be normograde or retrograde (Fig. 136–16*B* and *C*). With the normograde technique, reduction of the fracture before insertion of the pin facilitates proper pin position and direction. To ensure maximum anchorage in the epiphysis, the pin is inserted into the trochlea just above the intercondylar notch and directed along the caudal aspect of the metaphysis and diaphysis. After the pin has exited the trochanteric fossa proximally, the distal end is cut adjacent to the articular cartilage and is retracted into subchondral bone. Removal of the trocar point provides uniform pin fixation throughout the entire length of the epiphyseal segment and yields maximum seating. Damage to the articular cartilage at the pin entrance site has not caused significant problems. Retrograde pin placement avoids any damage to the articular cartilage, allows observation of pin placement in the metaphyseal segment, but does not provide maximum seating in the short epiphyseal segment. Adequate seating in the epiphysis is promoted by directing the pin along the caudal aspect of the metaphysis and medullary canal. The pin is removed in 3 to 6 weeks, after radiographic evidence of healing.

Double pins, Rush pins, and cross pins provide more than one point of fixation, increasing stabilization (Fig. 136–16*D* through *F*). These techniques are especially indicated for fractures in large dogs. With the double-pinning technique, the pins are inserted retrograde into the medial and lateral aspect of the metaphyseal segment so that seating occurs in the medial and lateral condyles. Pin protrusion from the trochanteric fossa facilitates removal after healing. Rush pins and cross pins are inserted in a normograde manner after reduction of the fracture. With both techniques, the opposing pins intersect above the fracture. Rush pins are started in the epiphyseal segment just cranial to the lateral and medial epicondyles. A pilot hole is drilled at approximately a 30° angle to the long axis of the bone, and the pin is contoured to accommodate reflection off the opposite cortex and movement up the medullary canal. Steinmann pins can be used in a similar manner to Rush pins. Cross pins are started at a similar site to Rush pins or can be inserted from the metaphyseal segment into the condyles. Small nonthreaded Kirschner wires (0.062 inch) are used and should penetrate the metaphyseal segment well above the fracture. Additional stabilization can be provided by using more than two pins. The distal ends of the pins are retracted or set flush with the condyles to avoid soft-tissue irritation. Rush pins and cross pins are not removed routinely.

The age of the animal and the rich blood supply and osteogenic tissue contribute to rapid bone healing. Premature closure of the physis is common and may be promoted by surgical repair. Uniform shortening of the femur rarely causes substantial impairment of function. Complications (quadriceps contracture, hyperextended stifle) due to voluntary or forced immobilization of the stifle are of most concern.

Salter-Harris Types III and IV and Intercondylar Fractures

Salter-Harris types III and IV and intercondylar fractures of mature animals are treated in the same manner. These fractures are rare in both age-groups but are more common in mature animals. The collateral and cruciate ligaments remain attached to the fractured condyle and maintain some degree of alignment. Poor-quality radiographs may fail to demonstrate intercondylar fractures.

Simple intercondylar fractures most often involve the medial condyle. Multiple Kirschner wires, compression screws, and various combinations of the two are used for fixation (Fig. 136–17*A* and *B*). Multiple pins provide sufficient fixation in immature animals and small dogs and cats. Compression screw fixation provides the most rigid fixation and is necessary for fractures in medium and large dogs.

Fractures of both condyles (T-Y) are treated by intercondylar fixation with compression screws or Kirschner wires and fixation of the repaired epiphyseal segment to the metaphysis with Rush pins, double pins, or cross pins (Fig. 136–17*C* and *D*). Fragmentation of the articular cartilage frequently occurs with these fractures. Small cartilage fragments are discarded. Large fragments with a subchondral component are reduced and fixed with 0.035- to 0.045-inch Kirschner wires. The cut ends of the wires are seated into subchondral bone.

The prognosis for rapid bone healing and return of function is favorable. Few cases are reported. With simple intercondylar fractures in animals with substantial growth potential, partial closure of the physis and deformity of the distal femur are a concern. Premature closure of the physis is expected with T-Y fractures in immature animals. Malalignment and unstable fixation of these articular fractures contribute to development of degenerative joint disease.

Epiphyseal Fractures

Intercondylar or condylar fractures have been described with Salter-Harris types III and IV fractures. Transcondylar fractures of the epiphysis are rare and occur most frequently in mature chondrodysplastic dogs. These fractures traverse the epiphysis (condyles) close to the intercondylar notch and involve the trochlear groove. An intercondylar component (T fracture) and fragmentation of the trochlear ridges are often present but may not be visible with radiography. Close proximity to the intercondylar notch prevents intercondylar stabilization with a compression screw. Fixation is achieved with multiple Kirschner wires placed through the articular surface of the condyle and into the metaphysis. The pins are set below the articular cartilage. Articular cartilage fragments with substantial subchondral bone are fixed in a similar manner.

Isolated fractures of the epiphysis occur with ligament and tendon injuries. Ruptures of the cruciate and collateral ligaments and popliteus and long digital extensor tendons frequently produce avulsion fractures in young animals.

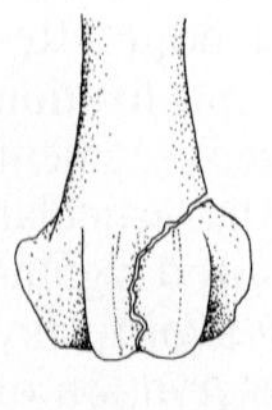

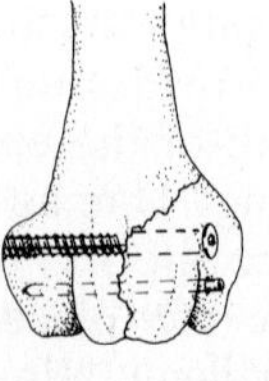

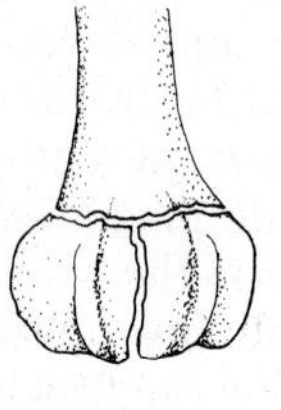

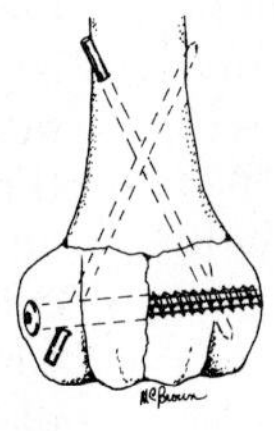

FIGURE 136–17. *A*, Simple intercondylar or Salter-Harris type III, IV fracture. *B*, Repaired with Kirschner wires and compression screw. *C*, Combined fracture (T) of both condyles. *D*, Repaired with a compression screw and cross pins.

Postoperative Care

House or cage confinement and leash activity are recommended for 3 to 4 weeks. Passive movement of the stifle and controlled weightbearing are encouraged. External support and immobilization of the limb are not recommended because of complications (quadriceps contracture, hyperextended stifle) associated with immobilization of the stifle in immature animals.

References

1. Alcantara PJ, Stead AC: Fractures of the distal femur in the dog and cat. *J Small Anim Pract 16*:649, 1975.
2. Anderson WD, et al: Method for treatment of fractures of the femoral neck in the dog: An experimental study. *J Am Vet Med Assoc 122*:158, 1953.
3. Bardet JF, et al: Measurement of a femoral torsion in dogs using a biplanar method. *Vet Surg 12*:1, 1983.
4. Bassett FH, et al: Normal vascular anatomy of the head of the femur in puppies with emphasis on the inferior retinacular vessels. *J Bone Joint Surg [Am] 51A*:1139, 1969.
5. Berg RJ, et al: Evaluation of prognostic factors for growth following distal femoral physeal injuries in 17 dogs. *Vet Surg 13*:172, 1984.
6. Caywood DD, et al: Osteomyelitis in the dog: A review of 67 cases. *J Am Vet Med Assoc 8*:943, 1978.
7. Cechner PE, et al: Fractures repair failure in the dog: A review in 20 dogs. *J Am Anim Hosp Assoc 13*:613, 1977.
8. Chaffee VW: Multiple (stacked) intramedullary pin fixation of humeral and femoral fractures. *J Am Anim Hosp Assoc 13*:599, 1977.
9. Chapman WL: Appearance of ossification centers and epiphyseal closure as determined by radiographic technique. *J Am Vet Med Assoc 147*:138, 1965.
10. Culvenor JA, et al: Closure after injury of the distal femoral growth plate in dogs. *J Small Anim Pract 19*:549, 1978.
11. Daly WR: Femoral head and neck fractures in the dog and cat: A review of 115 cases. *Vet Surg 7*:29, 1978.
12. Daly WR, Tarvin GB: Medial epicondyle osteotomy as an approach to repair of medial femoral condyle fractures in the dog. *Vet Surg 10*:113, 1981.
13. DeCamp CE, et al: Internal fixation of femoral capital physeal injuries in dogs: 40 cases (1979–1987). *J Am Vet Med Assoc 194*:1750, 1989.
14. Ellison GW, et al: The effect of cerclage wiring on the immature canine diaphysis: A biochemical analysis. *Vet Surg 11*:44, 1982.
15. Ewald FC, Hirohashi K: Effect of distal transfer of the greater trochanter in growing animals. *J Bone Joint Surg [Am] 51A*:1139, 1973.
16. Franczuski D, et al: The use of paired pins in the fixation of distal femur fracture in the dog and cat. *J Am Anim Hosp Assoc 22*:173, 1986.
17. Franczuski D, et al: Postoperative effects of experimental shortening in the immature dog. *J Am Anim Hosp Assoc 23*:429, 1987.
18. Frey AJ, Olds R: A new technique for repair of comminuted diaphyseal fractures. *Vet Surg 10*:51, 1981.
19. Grauer GR, et al: Incidence and mechanism of distal femoral physeal fractures in the dog and cat. *J Am Anim Hosp Assoc 17*:579, 1981.
20. Hardie EM, Chambers JN: Factors influencing the outcome of distal femoral fracture fixation: A retrospective study. *J Am Anim Hosp Assoc 20*:927, 1984.
21. Hauptman J, Butler HC: Effect of osteotomy of the greater trochanter with tension band fixation on femoral conformation in beagle dogs. *Vet Surg 8*:13, 1979.
22. Hauptman J, et al: The angle of inclination of the canine femoral head and neck. *Vet Surg 8*:74, 1979.
23. Hulse DH, et al: Revascularization of femoral capital physeal fractures following surgical fixation. *J Vet Orthop 2*:50, 1981.
24. Hunt JM, et al: The complications of diaphyseal fractures following surgical fixation. *J Small Anim Pract 21*:103, 1980.
25. Kaderly RE, et al: Extraosseous vascular supply to the mature dog's coxofemoral joint. *Am J Vet Res 43*:1208, 1982.
26. Lee R: Proximal femoral epiphyseal separation in the dog. *J Small Anim Pract 11*:669, 1976.
27. Makela EA, et al: The effect of a penetrating biodegradable implant on the growth plate. *Clin Orthop Rel Res 241*:300, 1989.
28. Milton JL, et al: Cross-pinning: A simple technique for treatment of certain metaphyseal and physeal fracture of long bones. *J Am Anim Hosp Assoc 16*:891, 1980.
29. Neimeyer KH, Hoffer RE: Rush pin repair of distal fracture of long bones in the dog. *J Am Vet Med Assoc 159*:1433, 1971.
30. Nunamaker DM: Repair of femoral head and neck fractures by interfragmentary compression. *J Am Vet Med Assoc 163*:569, 1973.
31. Piermattei DL, Greeley RG: *An Atlas of Surgical Approaches to the Bones of the Dog and Cat*. 2nd ed. W. B. Saunders, Philadelphia, 1979.
32. Rhinelander FW, Wilson JW: The blood supply of developing mature and healing bone. *In* Sumner Smith G (ed): *Bone and Clinical Orthopedics*. W. B. Saunders, Philadelphia, 1982, pp 82–158.
33. Riser WH: Growth and development of the normal canine pelvis, hip joints and femurs from birth to maturity: A radiographic study. *J Vet Radiol Soc 2*:24, 1973.
34. Rivera LA, et al: Arterial supply to the canine hip joint. *J Vet Orthop 1*:20, 1979.
35. Salter RB, Harris WR: Injuries involving the epiphyseal plate. *J Bone Joint Surg [Am] 45A*:587, 1963.
36. Shires PK, Hulse DA: Internal fixation of physeal fractures using the distal femur as an example. *Comp Cont Educ Pract Vet 11*:854, 1980.
37. Sinibaldi KR: Evaluation of full cortical allografts in 25 dogs. *J Am Vet Med Assoc 194*:1570, 1989.
38. Smith CW, et al: Osteomyelitis in the dog: A retrospective study. *J Am Anim Hosp Assoc 14*:589, 1979.
39. Stone EA, et al: Effect of Rush pins on the distal femoral growth plate of young dogs. *Am J Vet Res 42*:261, 1981.
40. Sumner-Smith G: Observations on epiphyseal fusion of the canine appendicular skeleton. *J Small Anim Pract 7*:303, 1966.
41. Vernon FF, Olmstead ML: Femoral head fractures resulting in epiphyseal fragmentation: Results of repair in five dogs. *Vet Surg 12*:123, 1983.
42. Weissman SL, et al: Growth of the upper end of the femur: Experimental investigation in the rabbit. *Acta Orthop Scand 45*:225, 1974.

CHAPTER 137 Stifle Joint

Philip B. Vasseur

ANATOMY AND BIOMECHANICS

Stifle joint disorders are a frequent cause of hindlimb lameness. The accuracy of diagnosis and the effectiveness of therapy depend on detailed knowledge of the anatomy and function of joint components.

The stifle is a complex hinge joint with two functionally distinct articulations. Weightbearing occurs primarily through the articulation between the femoral and tibial condyles. The femoropatellar articulation greatly increases the mechanical efficiency of the quadriceps muscle group and facilitates extensor function.

The stifle joint capsule has three distinct cavities that intercommunicate (Fig. 137–1).[64] The largest joint cavity is between the patella and femur; the other two are between the femoral and tibial condyles. A sac protrudes from the patellar joint cavity proximally underneath the quadriceps tendon. Other subpouches connect the fem-

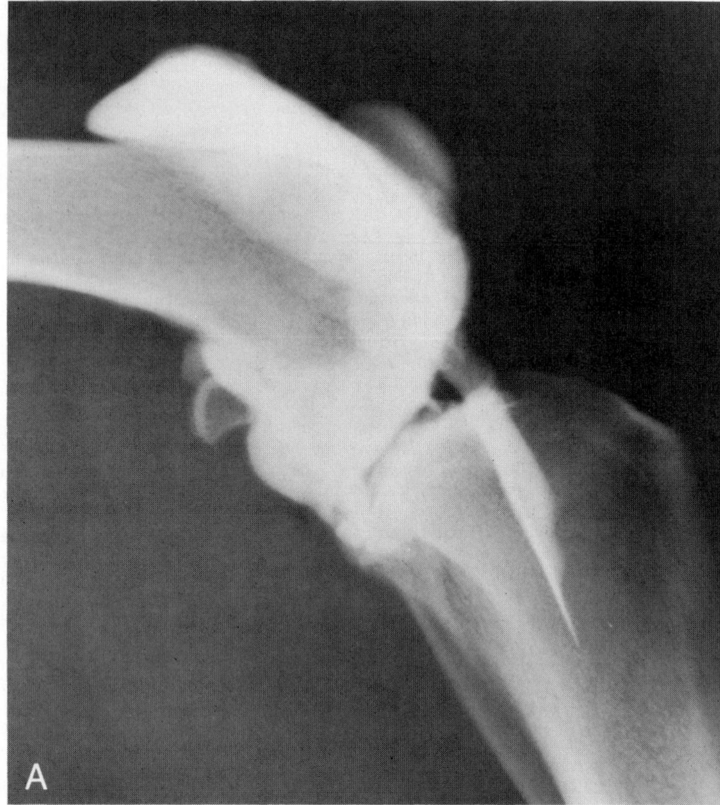

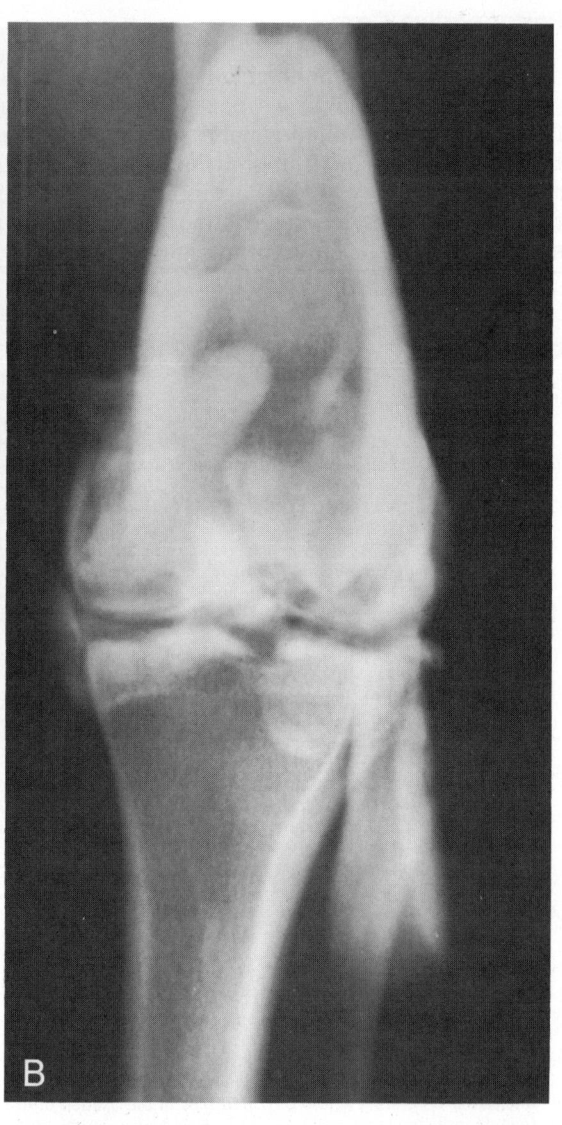

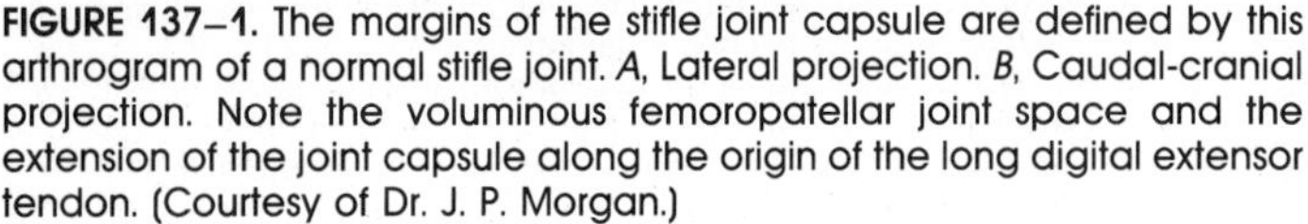

FIGURE 137–1. The margins of the stifle joint capsule are defined by this arthrogram of a normal stifle joint. *A*, Lateral projection. *B*, Caudal-cranial projection. Note the voluminous femoropatellar joint space and the extension of the joint capsule along the origin of the long digital extensor tendon. (Courtesy of Dr. J. P. Morgan.)

orotibial joint cavity with the fabellae, the long digital extensor tendon, and to a limited extent the popliteal tendon. The joint capsule is structurally reinforced by a fibrous retinaculum and by the tendons and ligaments that span the joint. Distal to the patella, the synovial and fibrous layers of the joint capsule are separated by the infrapatellar fat body.[64] Displacement of the infrapatellar fat body is visible on radiographs and suggests thickening of the joint capsule or joint effusion.

The lateral and medial menisci are semilunar fibrocartilage structures interposed between the articular surfaces of the femur and tibia. In cross section, the menisci are wedge shaped, with the thicker border located peripherally and with attachments to the joint capsule. The menisci are each anchored to the tibial plateau by cranial and caudal meniscotibial ligaments, and the lateral meniscus has an attachment to the femur, called the *femoral ligament of the lateral meniscus* or *meniscofemoral ligament* (Fig. 137–2).[64] The small transverse or intermeniscal ligament unites the cranial meniscotibial ligaments. The intermeniscal ligament is an important landmark because it overlies the tibial attachment of the cranial cruciate ligament and may be used to anchor grafts used for cranial cruciate ligament reconstruction.[97]

The meniscal ligaments have been referred to as *horns*, and that section of the meniscus extending between the horns is called the meniscal *body*.[142] Structurally, the horns and body differ. The horns are oval in cross section, the body triangular. Hyalinized areas are much more frequent in the body than in the horns. The collagen of the horns is organized into discrete bundles separated by loose connective tissue septa, whereas collagen of the body is arranged in a herringbone pattern. No septa are present in the body. The meniscal horns are richly supplied with blood vessels and nerves, including large myelinated fibers that apparently terminate in the horns, whereas the body is almost completely devoid of blood vessels and nerves.[142] Only the peripheral 10 to 15 per cent of the meniscal body is supplied by a vascular synovial plexus arising from the joint capsule (Fig. 137–3).[95] The central zone of the meniscal body is nourished by diffusion of synovial fluid. The functions of the menisci include (1) energy absorption and stress transfer across the joint, (2) stabilization of the joint by deepening the articular surfaces of the tibial

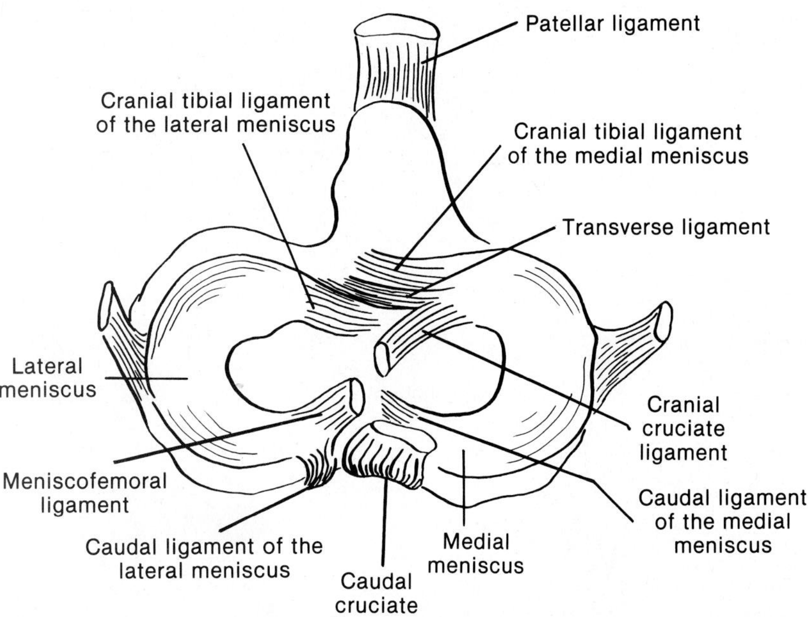

FIGURE 137–2. The meniscotibial ligaments. The caudal portion of the lateral meniscus is also attached to the femur and is more mobile than the caudal portion of the medial meniscus. The transverse or intermeniscal ligament joins the cranial poles of the two menisci and overlies the insertion of the cranial cruciate ligament.

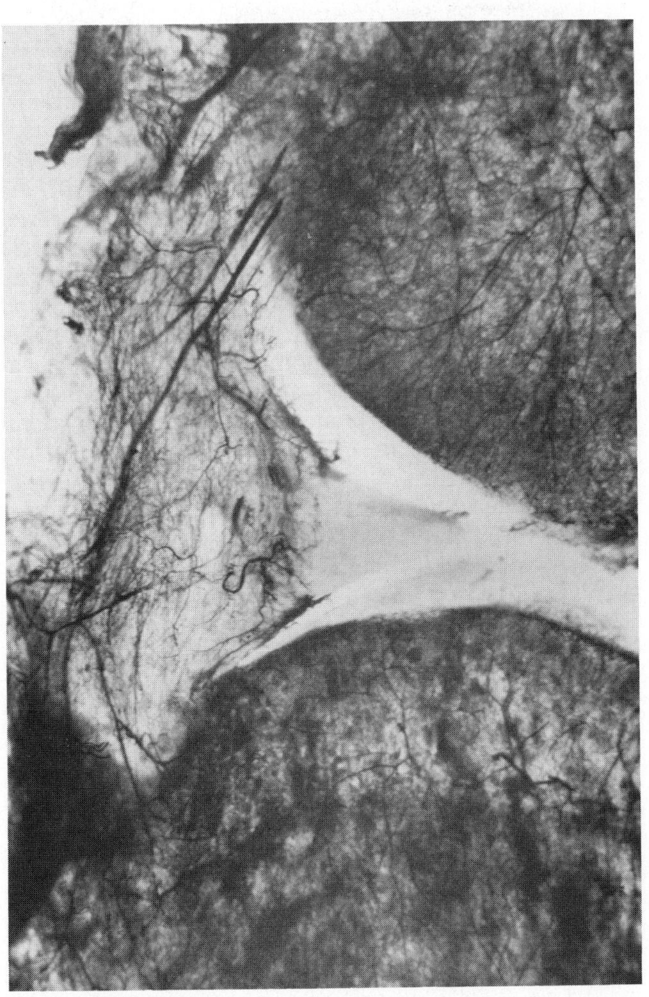

FIGURE 137–3. Transverse section of a medial meniscus after arterial perfusion with India ink and tissue clearing. Note that the synovial attachments provide blood supply to the peripheral third of the meniscus; the inner two-thirds is devoid of blood supply. (Courtesy of Dr. Steve Arnoczky.)

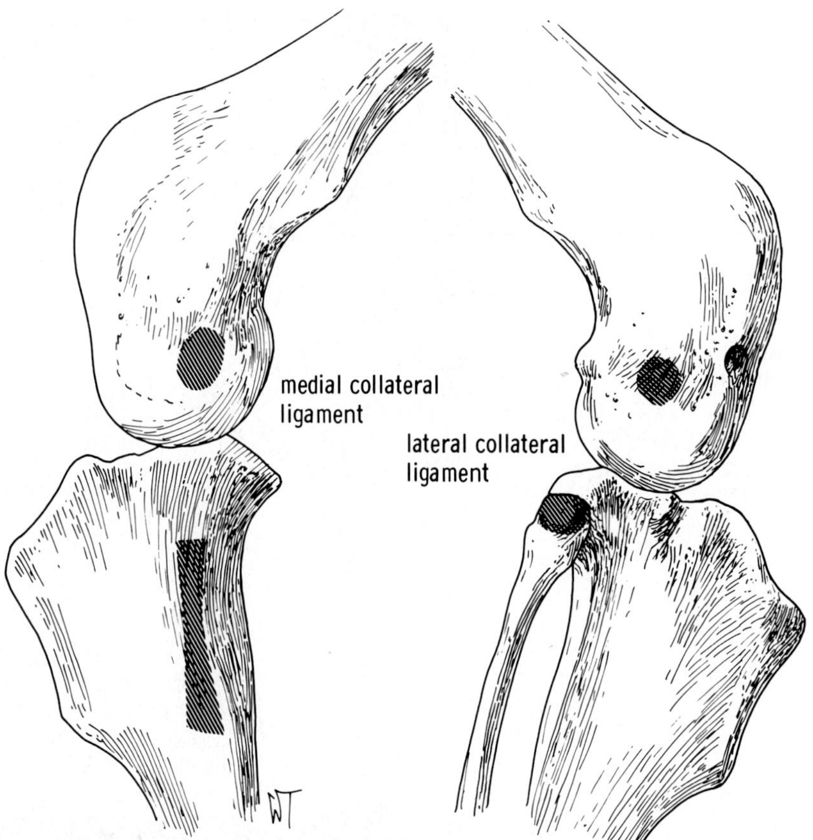

FIGURE 137–4. Schematic illustration of the origin and insertion sites of the collateral ligaments. Note the extensive tibial attachment of the medial collateral ligament. (From Vasseur PB, Arnoczky SP: Collateral ligaments of the canine stifle joint: Anatomic and functional analysis. *Am J Vet Res 42*:1133, 1981.)

plateau, (3) lubrication of the joint, and (4) prevention of synovial impingement between the articular surfaces of the femur and tibia.* The menisci in the normal standing position transmit approximately 65 per cent of the weightbearing load.[115] Innervation of the meniscal horns suggests that the menisci have a sensory function that may aid in joint proprioception and protect the joint from excessive loading, possibly through reflex arcs involving the regional musculature.[142]

The primary ligamentous support of the stifle joint is provided by the femorotibial ligaments, which are the medial and lateral collateral ligaments and the cranial and caudal cruciate ligaments. The collateral ligaments unite with and provide some support to the joint capsule; however, they are entirely extra-articular. The cruciate ligaments invaginate the joint capsule from the caudal aspect of the joint and are covered by a layer of synovial membrane; thus, they are intra-articular but extrasynovial.

The medial collateral ligament arises from an oval area of the medial femoral epicondyle (Fig. 137–4). This ligament blends with and forms a strong attachment to the joint capsule and medial meniscus.[209] As the ligament extends distally across the medial tibial condyle, it passes superficial to the tibial insertion of the semimembranosus muscle and inserts over a large rectangular area of the proximal medial tibia. A fluid-filled bursa is generally present between the medial collateral ligament and the tibia, suggesting translational movement between the ligament and bone surfaces (Fig. 137–5). The cranial border of the medial collateral ligament remains taut throughout a normal range of motion; however, the caudal portion becomes lax in flexion (Fig. 137–6).

The origin of the lateral collateral ligament is an oval area just proximal to the origin of the popliteal muscle on the lateral femoral epicondyle (Fig. 137–4). The ligament passes superficial to the popliteal tendon and extends caudodistally to insert on the fibular head. Only loose connective tissue joins the lateral collateral ligament to the joint capsule, and there are no distinct attachments to the lateral meniscus.[209] The entire lateral collateral ligament is lax in flexion, becoming taut during extension (Fig. 137–7).

The collateral ligaments are primarily responsible for limiting varus (lateral collateral ligament) and valgus (medial collateral ligament) motion of the tibia.[209] Their effect is most pronounced in extension; as the stifle joint flexes, the cruciate ligaments become stressed by varus or valgus loads and are increasingly important in limiting varus and valgus motion.[131]

The cranial and caudal cruciate ligaments are named for their respective tibial insertion sites. The primary blood supply to the cruciate ligaments arises from the synovial tissues that ensheathe the ligaments rather than from sources arising at osseous attachment sites.[17] The infrapatellar fat body and soft tissues caudal to the joint are important sources of vessels (Fig. 137–8). The central core of the midsection of each ligament is less vascularized.[17, 212]

The caudal cruciate ligament arises within the intercondyloid fossa from the lateral aspect of the medial

*See references 11, 20, 44, 57, 95, 142, and 150.

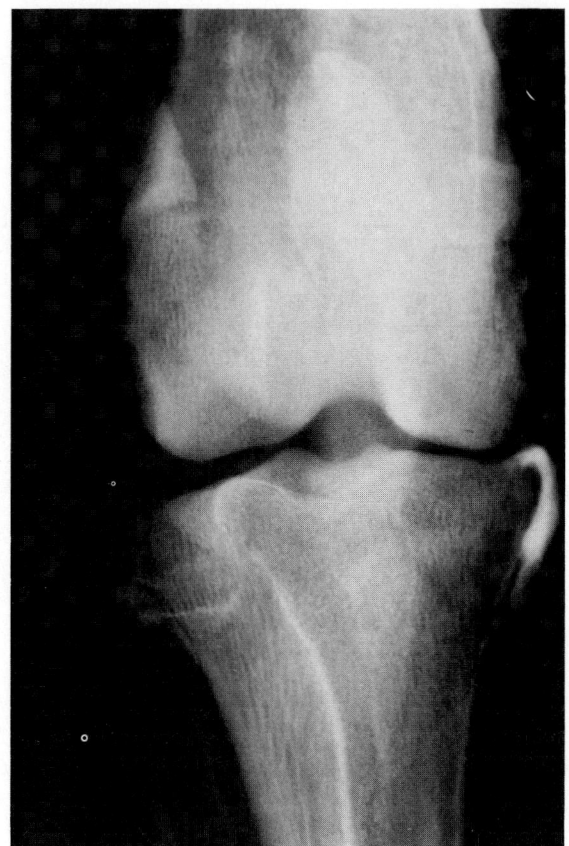

FIGURE 137–5. Radiograph of the stifle joint in which the bursa underneath the medial collateral ligament has been injected with radiopaque contrast material. (From Vasseur PB, Arnoczky SP: Collateral ligaments of the canine stifle joint: Anatomic and functional analysis. *Am J Vet Res 42*:1133, 1981.)

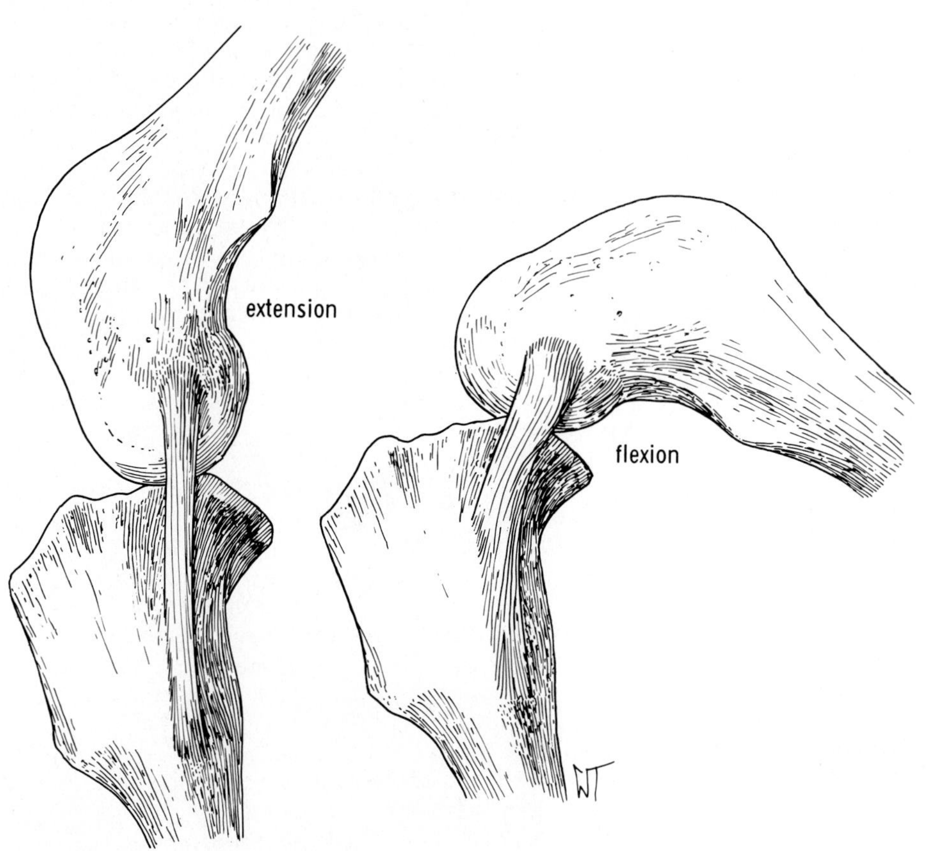

FIGURE 137–6. The medial collateral ligament in flexion and extension. The caudal portion becomes lax in flexion, whereas the cranial portion remains taut. (From Vasseur PB, Arnoczky SP: Collateral ligaments of the canine stifle joint: Anatomic and functional analysis. *Am J Vet Res 42*:1133, 1981.)

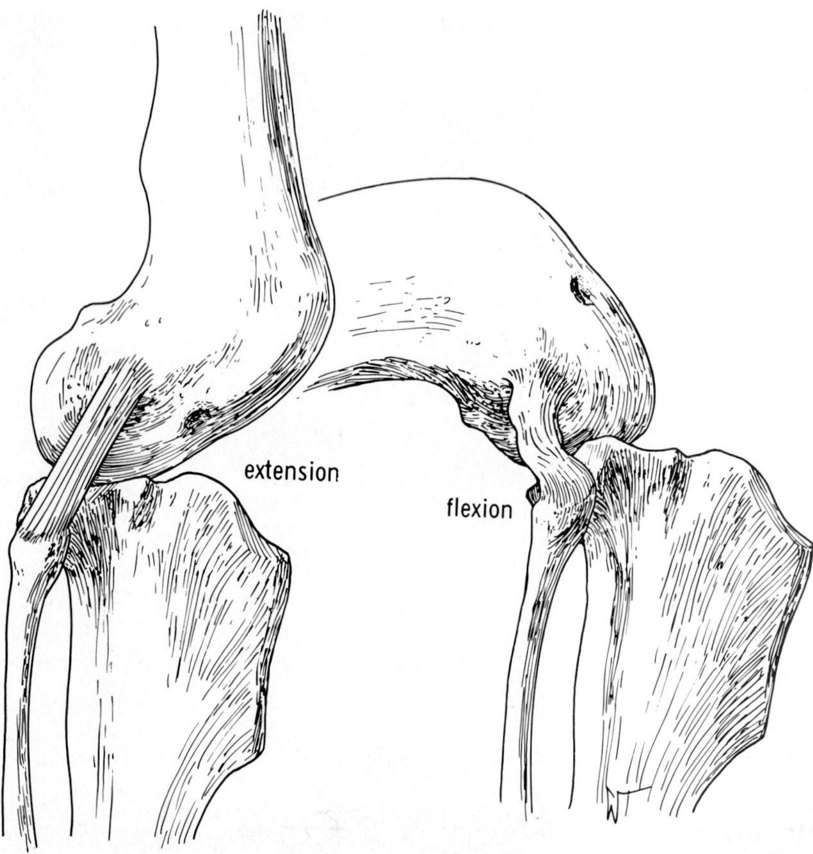

FIGURE 137–7. The lateral collateral ligament in flexion and extension. The entire ligament becomes lax in flexion. (From Vasseur PB, Arnoczky SP: Collateral ligaments of the canine stifle joint: Anatomic and functional analysis. *Am J Vet Res 42*:1133, 1981.)

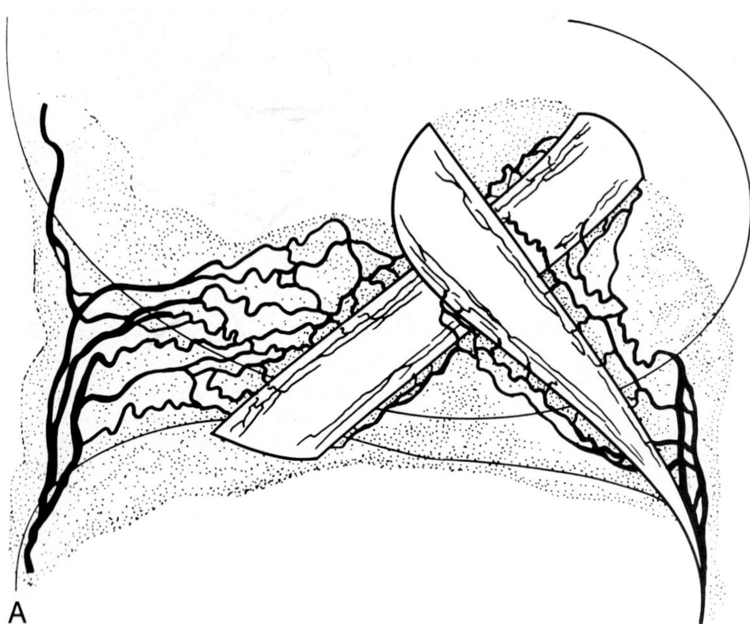

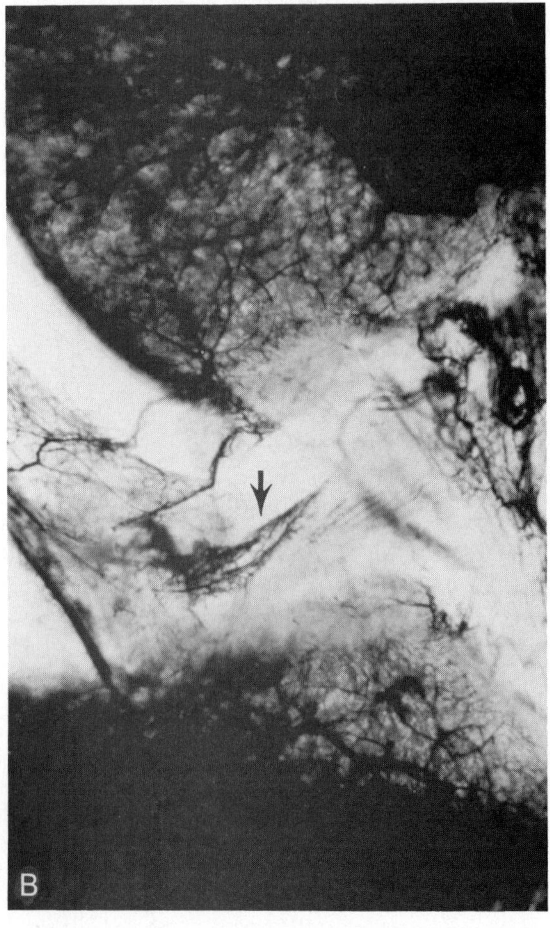

FIGURE 137–8. Blood supply to the cruciate ligaments. *A*, Schematic illustration showing the primary source of blood supply coming from the surrounding soft tissues. The vessels ramify over the surface of the ligaments and penetrate to form an endoligamentous blood supply. *B*, Sagittal section of a stifle joint following perfusion with India ink and tissue clearing. Vessels from the infrapatellar fat body are shown over the surface of the cranial cruciate ligament *(arrow)*. (Courtesy of Dr. Steve Arnoczky.)

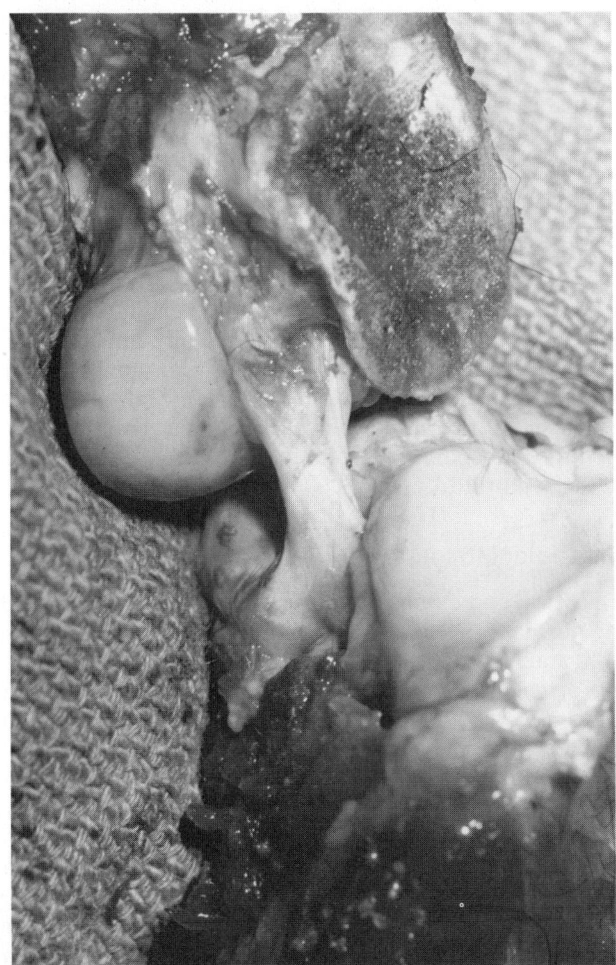

FIGURE 137–9. The caudal cruciate ligament and its attachments to the lateral surface of the medial femoral condyle and the caudal border of the tibial plateau. The lateral femoral condyle has been removed.

femoral condyle and extends caudodistally to the lateral edge of the popliteal notch of the tibia (Fig. 137–9). It is separated into two functional components.[9] The relatively larger cranial portion is taut in flexion and lax in extension, and the caudal portion is taut in extension and lax in flexion. The caudal cruciate ligament prevents caudal translation of the tibia relative to the femur (caudal drawer motion) and helps limit internal rotation of the tibia by twisting together with the cranial cruciate ligament.[9] The caudal cruciate ligament is a secondary restraint to hyperextension and helps to limit varus/valgus motion in the flexed joint.[11, 131]

The cranial cruciate ligament arises within the intercondyloid fossa from the caudomedial part of the lateral condyle of the femur and extends diagonally across the intercondyloid fossa to the cranial intercondyloid area of the tibia (Fig. 137–10). The cranial cruciate ligament also has been divided into two functional components, a craniomedial band and a larger caudolateral portion.[9, 87] Differences in the mechanical properties of each subunit have been reported, with the craniomedial band providing the most resistance to cranial drawer motion at 30° and 60° of flexion.[36, 81] The craniomedial band is taut throughout the range of motion, and the caudolateral portion is taut in extension but lax in flexion. These general concepts are of importance in the diagnosis of partial tears of the cranial cruciate ligament, but they oversimplify the complex structure and functional relationships of the ligament. The cranial cruciate ligament is composed of numerous 20-μm-wide bundles of collagen fibers separated by columns of cells in fibrous capsules.[41] These bundles are grouped into fascicles of various sizes enclosed by thin membranous sheets that form single or multiple layers between fascicles.[41, 227] Blood vessels and nerves are found within these interfascicular membranes, presumably to provide protection from shearing stresses that may accompany normal function.[41, 110] Fascicles are visible grossly and generally extend from origin to insertion without crossing or interweaving (Fig. 137–11).[41] The entire ligament spirals laterally about 90° between attachment sites. The twist in the ligament results in the gross appearance of two fairly distinct "bands," especially in flexion (Fig. 137–12). If the ligament is untwisted, it is more uniform in appearance. During joint motion, sequential tightening of certain fascicles and relaxation of others occurs, constantly maintaining joint stability throughout a range

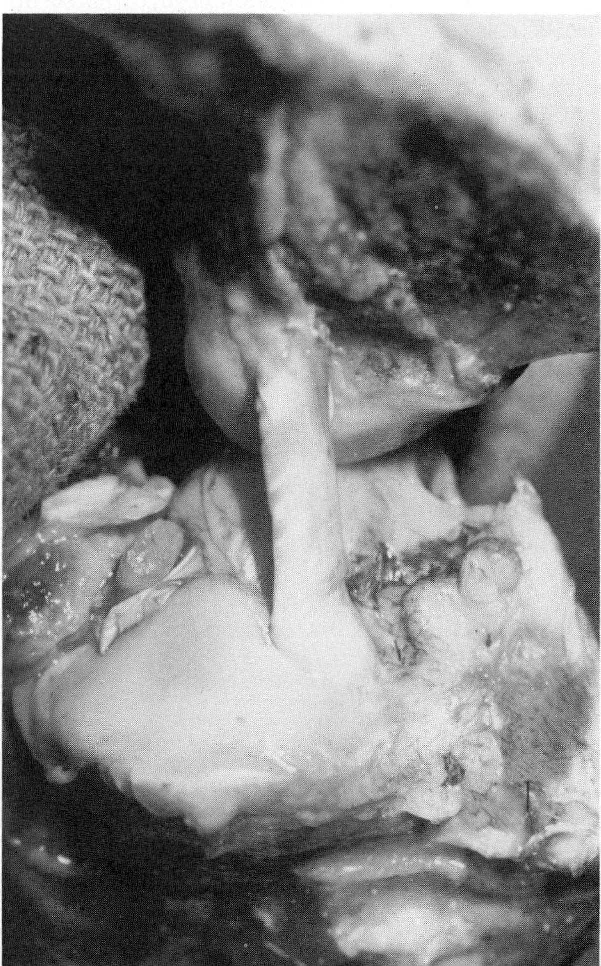

FIGURE 137–10. The cranial cruciate ligament and its attachments to the medial surface of the lateral femoral condyle and the cranial portion of the tibial plateau. Note the broad tibial insertion site, which lies underneath the intermeniscal ligament. The medial femoral condyle has been removed.

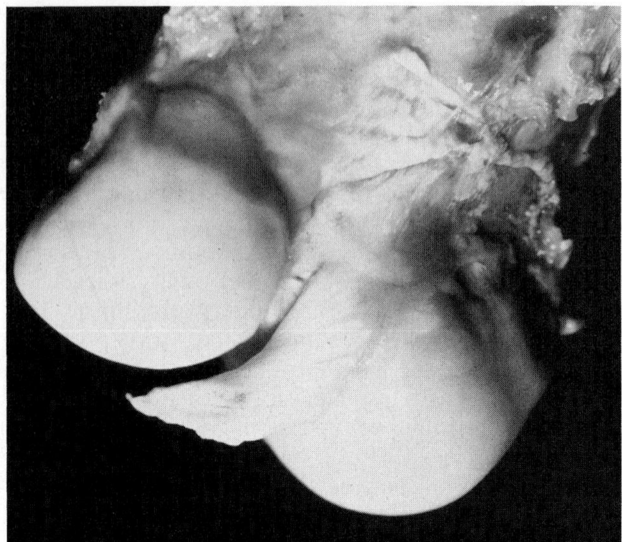

FIGURE 137–11. The femoral attachment site of the cranial cruciate ligament, showing the numerous fascicles that make up the ligament.

of motion.[217] At osseous attachment sites, a transitional zone of fibrocartilage and mineralized cartilage minimizes stress concentration by allowing a gradual change in stiffness.[8] The transitional area is divided into four zones.[43]

Mechanoreceptors and various afferent nerve fibers are present within the cranial cruciate ligament,[104, 185, 186, 196, 230] and forces that cause strain within the ligament result in simultaneous contraction of the caudal thigh muscles and relaxation of the quadriceps muscle group.[196] This is interpreted as a protective feedback mechanism, because quadriceps contraction increases strain within the ligament and hamstring contraction reduces strain.[7, 125, 169] Similar responses were also obtained in humans with cranial cruciate ligament–deficient knee joints, suggesting that an alternative reflex arc unrelated to cranial cruciate ligament receptors helps maintain joint integrity.[196]

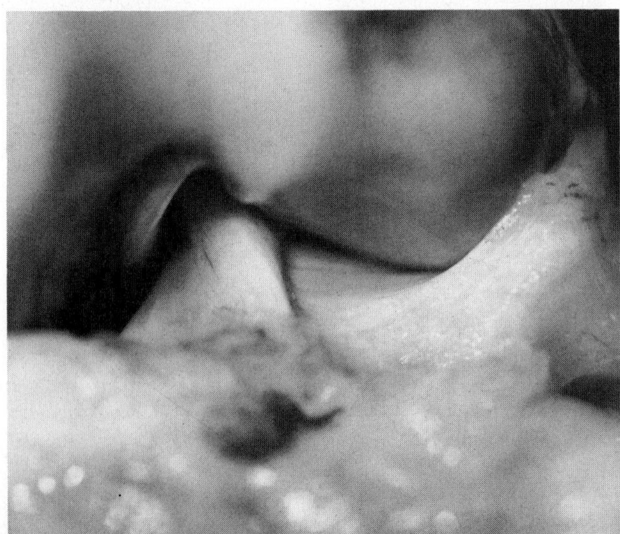

FIGURE 137–12. The cranial cruciate ligament, showing the outward spiral of the ligament, creating the appearance of two distinct bands.

The cranial cruciate ligament is the primary restraint against cranial drawer motion and hyperextension.[9, 87] It also limits internal rotation of the tibia by twisting against the caudal cruciate ligament. The cranial cruciate ligament prevents excessive varus or valgus motion of the tibia in the flexed stifle joint.[131]

The medial and lateral femoropatellar ligaments are narrow bands of loose fibers that partially blend with the overlying femoral fascia.[64] They extend from the patella to the respective fabella medially and laterally. The lateral ligament is usually visible; however, the medial ligament often blends with femoral periosteum and is not discernible. These ligaments combine with the more substantial femoral fascia to support the patella in the femoral trochlea.

Stifle Joint Motion

Flexion and extension occur in the sagittal plane, with the normal range of motion being about 140°.[124] Because of ligamentous constraints and the complex geometry of the articulations involving the femoral and tibial condyles and the menisci, in particular the irregular contours of the femoral condyles, simple uniplanar rotation about a stationary axis does not occur.* With flexion, the lateral collateral ligament relaxes and allows the lateral femoral condyle to displace caudally, resulting in internal rotation of the tibia. Conversely, during extension, the lateral collateral ligament tightens and causes the lateral femoral condyle to move cranially, resulting in external rotation of the tibia. This sequence of rotational movement that occurs during flexion and extension has been termed the *screw home* mechanism in humans.[11] A small amount of craniocaudal motion also occurs in the sagittal plane as a result of the cam shape of the femoral condyles. The femoral condyles roll caudally with flexion and cranially with extension, relative to the tibial plateau.[95]

Slight varus (medial) and valgus (lateral) movement of the tibia occurs in the transverse plane. The collateral ligaments are responsible for limiting this motion in the extended joint; with flexion, the cruciate ligaments also contribute to the control of varus and valgus motion.[131, 209]

Excessive joint motion is prevented not only by the ligamentous constraints of the stifle joint but also by a complex system of reflex arcs that involves the major muscle groups around the stifle.[196]

CRANIAL CRUCIATE LIGAMENT RUPTURE

Rupture of the cranial cruciate ligament is frequently associated with hindlimb lameness in dogs. Much has been learned about this ligament since the first report in 1926, yet the cause of rupture is often unknown and the optimum mode of treatment remains controversial.

Cranial cruciate ligament rupture may be purely traumatic, occurring in a young large dog and associated

*See references 11, 62, 128, 143, 144, 191, and 225.

with an acute history and distinct traumatic event. A small percentage of these dogs avulse a bony insertion of the ligament rather than tear the ligament within its substance; the tibial attachment site fails more often than the femoral.[95] The majority of dogs with cranial cruciate ligament rupture have a more chronic course without a history of distinct trauma. The primary complaint may be acute lameness, but further questioning often reveals that the lameness has been episodic and related to bouts of vigorous exercise. Physical and radiographic examination generally confirms chronic degenerative changes in the affected stifle joint.

Epidemiology and Pathogenesis

Rupture of the cranial cruciate ligament occurs in large breeds of dogs more often than in small breeds, with the rottweiler, bull mastiff, and chow chow particularly at risk.[218] Acute traumatic ligament rupture most often occurs in dogs less than 4 years of age[26]; dogs with the syndrome of chronic lameness and degenerative joint disease usually are between 5 and 7 years of age.[192] There is a trend for small dogs (<15 kg) to rupture the ligament later in life (>7 years of age) than large dogs.[208, 218] Numerous clinical studies have reported a higher incidence of rupture in females than males.[24, 54, 75, 195] This trend has been confirmed by an epidemiological study that found the incidence of cranial cruciate ligament rupture in spayed females to be 3.26 per cent versus 1.74 per cent in intact females and 1.52 per cent in intact males.[218] Ovariectomy in rats decreases the elastin content and fiber diameter in the hip joint capsule, and sex hormones may affect collagen metabolism.[188] The effect of chronic hypoestrogenemia on the metabolism and mechanical properties of the cranial cruciate ligament in dogs is unknown.

The strength of a dog's cranial cruciate ligament deteriorates with aging, correlating with loss of fiber bundle organization and metaplastic changes of cellular elements (Fig. 137–13).[11, 212] These changes are more pronounced and occur at an earlier age in large dogs, perhaps helping to explain the occurrence of rupture earlier in life than in small breeds.[212] Ligament deterioration is more marked in the central core of the ligament, and this is related to a paucity of blood supply.[2, 11, 201, 212, 229] Relative lack of vessels in the central core has not been correlated with oxygen tensions or metabolic abnormalities within that region.

These degenerative changes are naturally occurring aging processes that develop in all dogs; thus, other factors must be involved in causing ligament rupture. The rupture can be purely traumatic in young dogs with apparently normal ligaments. Poor physical conditioning may contribute to ligament rupture in these cases,[26, 95] in that strong and properly conditioned muscles about the knee are important in protecting intra-articular structures from excessive stresses.[169, 196] Many large dogs do not receive regular conditioning exercise but instead are allowed intermittent episodes of exuberant physical activity.

Abnormal conformation of the limb is implicated as a cause of degenerative joint disease (postural arthrosis) and excessive stresses within the ligament, thereby causing chronic deterioration and eventual rupture.[11, 179] Abnormal tibial conformation is associated with cranial cruciate ligament rupture in dogs,[167] and rupture of various ligaments in broiler fowl are associated with abnormal conformation.[59] Internal rotation of the tibia or hyperextension of the stifle theoretically causes excessive loading of the cranial cruciate ligament. Conformation or undefined factors may be heritable. I have observed cranial cruciate ligament rupture, often bilateral, in a high percentage of the offspring of certain rottweiler bitches; the ruptures have occurred before 2 years of age in affected individuals.

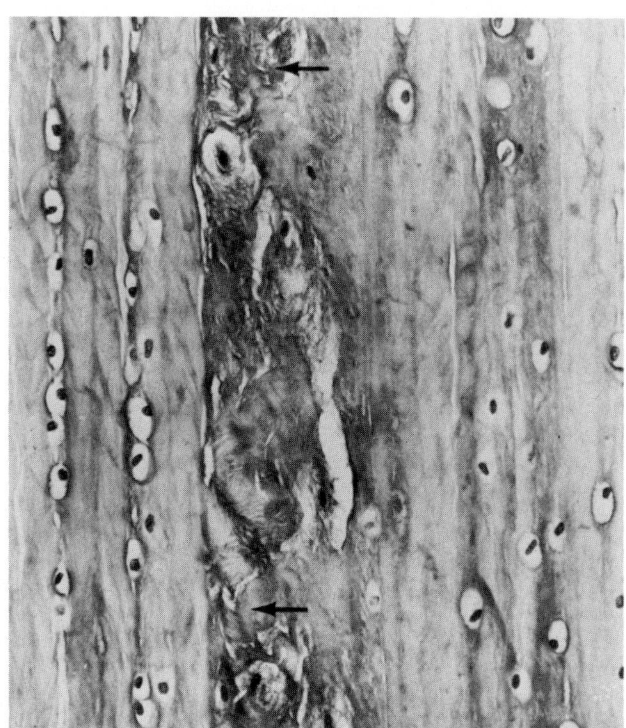

FIGURE 137–13. Sagittal section through the cranial cruciate ligament in a 7-year-old dog, showing small acellular areas, early chondroid metaplasia of surviving fibroblasts, and failure to maintain collagen fibrils within primary collagen bundles *(arrows)*. (H&E stain, × 225.) (From Vasseur PB, et al: Correlative biomechanical and histologic study of the cranial cruciate ligament in dogs. *Am J Vet Res 46*:1842, 1985.)

Dogs with cranial cruciate ligament rupture frequently are overweight. Obesity causes further loading of what may be a compromised ligament and is likely to be a contributing factor in many dogs.

Anticollagen antibodies and immune complexes have been detected in the synovial fluid and sera of dogs with cranial cruciate ligament rupture, and immune mechanisms may have a role.[137, 138] Collagenase is elevated in dogs with naturally occurring rupture and in normal rabbits after severance.[4, 136] Collagenase degrades ligaments and tendons and may be produced by cartilage cells in response to chemical mediators released by macrophages.[172, 206] At diagnosis, the majority of dogs with rupture have a noninflammatory arthropathy, with total white blood cell counts in the synovial fluid less than 5000/mm^3 in 92 per cent of the dogs.[80]

Partial tears of the cranial cruciate ligament are diagnosed with increasing frequency.[30, 182, 202, 203] Partial tears in dogs consistently progress to complete rupture of the ligament, usually within 1 year of the onset of lameness.[26] Partial tears are also associated with greater joint inflammation, as measured by total white blood cell counts in the synovial fluid.[80] Bennett and colleagues proposed the term *cruciate disease* to describe the clinical syndrome of lameness, joint effusion, osteoarthrosis, and progressive deterioration of the cranial cruciate ligament.[26] Joint instability may not be palpable early in the course but usually becomes apparent as the ligament undergoes progressive failure.[26] Partial tears are thus not a distinct entity but an early sign of a disease that eventually results in complete ligament disruption. This concept is important for several reasons. When a partial tear is explored surgically, a decision has to be made about the intact portion of the ligament. I have often found that the remaining ligament tissue is not structurally sound but appears stretched and easily ruptures when manipulated. It is clearly indicated to remove the entire ligament and proceed with reconstruction. In some, the remaining ligament is grossly normal, and a veterinary surgeon has reported successful augmentation of the remaining tissue as a treatment for partial tears.[202] Augmentation is not indicated if the intact portion of the ligament is pathological. Sectioning of either the craniomedial or caudolateral portions of the ligament did not result in clinically detectable instability, and if abnormal cranial drawer motion is present clinically, either the entire ligament is torn or the intact portion has undergone significant disruption.[87]

Clinical Signs and Diagnosis

The diagnosis of cranial cruciate ligament rupture is based on a history of lameness and physical examination findings. Dogs with acute traumatic ligament rupture are severely lame and occasionally do not bear weight on the affected limb. The lameness gradually subsides, and by 3 to 5 weeks after injury the dog has a mild to moderate limp. Muscle atrophy is not dramatic but develops with time. The joint is generally not sensitive to routine manipulation; elicitation of the cranial drawer sign often causes pain. The key to diagnosis of traumatic ruptures is to verify a truly acute onset of lameness, usually with a definite history of injury, and if the joint is examined within a few weeks of injury, the presence of minimal or no degenerative joint disease in the affected stifle.

Dogs with chronic cruciate disease have a more insidious history of lameness, often intermittent and exacerbated by physical activity. The affected joint is thickened, especially medially, and has radiographic evidence of degenerative joint disease. The frequency of bilateral disease is as high as 31 per cent.[26] Cranial instability may be difficult to elicit because of periarticular fibrosis, especially if the ligament is partially torn. Some degree of abnormal movement usually can be detected, especially if the dog is sedated or anesthetized. Joint effusion is invariably present.

It is useful to observe the dog carefully during history taking and before physical examination. Difficulty rising, subtle weight shifts during standing, and limb positions during rest can indicate which limb is involved and suggest the severity of the problem. The stress of physical examination often causes the animal to become tense and fearful, and subtle abnormalities become undetectable.

Physical Examination

After observing the dog at rest, have the client walk and trot the dog to observe conformation and gait. A bowlegged conformation, internal rotation of the tibia, or straight stifles increase suspicion of cruciate disease. After the limb primarily involved is determined, the orthopedic examination is carried out, examining the affected limb last (see Chapter 118). The best tools for diagnosis of cranial cruciate ligament rupture are your hands. I prefer to perform the initial examination with the dog standing on the floor, because dogs are generally less stressed than by being held down on a table and the standing position facilitates comparison with the opposite side. The examination begins with the least stressful manipulations and gradually proceeds to those that may elicit pain (e.g., cranial drawer test).

The general contour of the limb is palpated, with attention given to muscle mass and sites of pain, always comparing with the opposite side. The shape and size of the medial aspect of the stifle joint are particularly important. Dogs with chronic cranial cruciate ligament rupture have thickening of the medial joint capsule that is readily detected by palpation. Joint effusion is evaluated by careful palpation of the joint space on either side of the patellar tendon and compared with the opposite side (a substantial number of dogs are bilaterally affected). In a normal joint, the edges of the patellar tendon are sharp and distinct; when joint effusion is present, the capsule bulges on either side of the tendon and the margins of the tendon are obscured. The stifle joint is gently moved through a range of motion, with attention given to crepitation, pain, and clunks or clicks that suggest meniscal damage. The lack of a clicking sound on physical examination does not imply that the meniscus is normal, because there is little correlation between physical findings and meniscal pathology detected during exploratory arthrotomy. During examination, isolate manipulations to the stifle joint. Concurrently stressing the hip or hock joints can give misleading results if lesions are present in either joint.

Cranial drawer motion may be detected by the cranial drawer test or the tibial compression test. The cranial drawer test can be performed with a dog standing or in lateral recumbency, as preferred by the examiner; a tranquilizer or occasionally general anesthesia is required in nervous dogs or dogs in pain. It is critical that the examiner's fingers be placed on distinct bony landmarks to perform this test (Fig. 137–14). The cranial drawer test is performed with the stifle in extension and in about 30° of flexion to aid detection of partial tears.

With complete tears of the cranial cruciate ligament, abnormal cranial drawer motion is noted in both the extended position and in flexion. Often the craniomedial

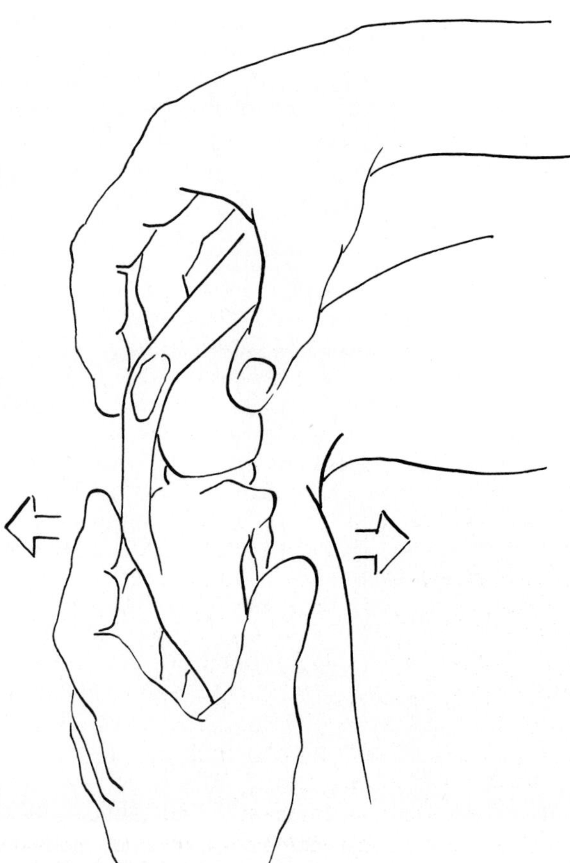

FIGURE 137–14. The cranial drawer examination. Note placement of the fingers directly on bony prominences (patella and lateral fabella with one hand, tibial crest and fibular head with the other). The joint should be tested in full extension and in 30° of flexion.

band of the ligament is torn, leaving the caudolateral portion intact.[182, 202, 203] The caudolateral portion is taut in extension, therefore preventing cranial tibial displacement. Abnormal cranial drawer motion is evident in flexion because the caudolateral portion is relaxed. Isolated rupture of the caudolateral portion occurs and can confuse diagnosis because the intact craniomedial portion prevents detection of drawer motion, regardless of joint position. The latter cases are typical of partial tears in that degenerative joint changes, although present, are often mild, and the medial meniscus usually is normal. The lameness in these dogs can be chronic, with histories of moderate to severe lameness for more than 1 year, and associated muscle atrophy.

A short cranial drawer motion (1 to 3 mm) with an abrupt stop is often detected in young dogs and is normal. Comparison with the opposite side determines if the motion is abnormal. The cranial drawer test often causes pain, even in normal dogs, and this should not be misinterpreted as a sign of pathological lesions within the joint.

The tibial compression test can also be carried out with a dog standing or in lateral recumbency with the affected limb uppermost. The stifle joint is held in *slight* flexion, and the hock is flexed and extended with one hand while the other palpates the tibial tuberosity for cranial subluxation (Fig. 137–15). The cranial drawer test is more reliable; examiners with small hands find the tibial compression test easier to perform in large dogs.

Radiographic Examination

In dogs with partial tears of the cranial cruciate ligament, cranial drawer motion may be difficult to detect, and high-quality radiographs are important in demonstrating joint effusion and often early signs of degenerative joint disease (Fig. 137–16). Both stifle joints are radiographed for comparison. Degenerative joint disease in the contralateral stifle may be of prognostic value, suggesting an increased likelihood of cranial cruciate ligament rupture compared with dogs with normal contralateral joints.[58] Radiographs may also demonstrate the bone fragment in younger dogs with avulsion injuries and may show cranial subluxation of the tibial plateau relative to the femoral condyles.

Evaluation of the Intercondyloid Fossa

In humans and in dogs with chronic instability associated with cranial cruciate ligament rupture, the inter-

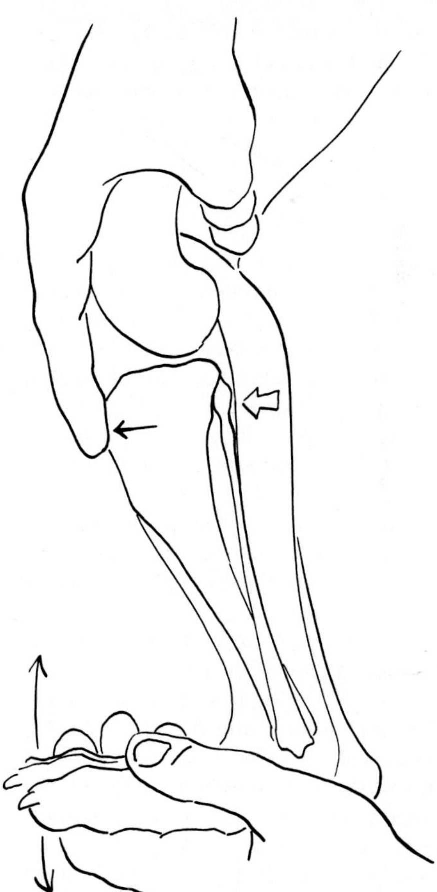

FIGURE 137–15. Tibial compression test. With the stifle joint in *slight* flexion, the hock is dorsiflexed, placing the gastrocnemius muscle under tension. If the cranial cruciate ligament is torn, the femur displaces caudally with simultaneous cranial subluxation of the tibia. The popping back and forth of the tibial tuberosity in association with hock motion is palpated with the index finger.

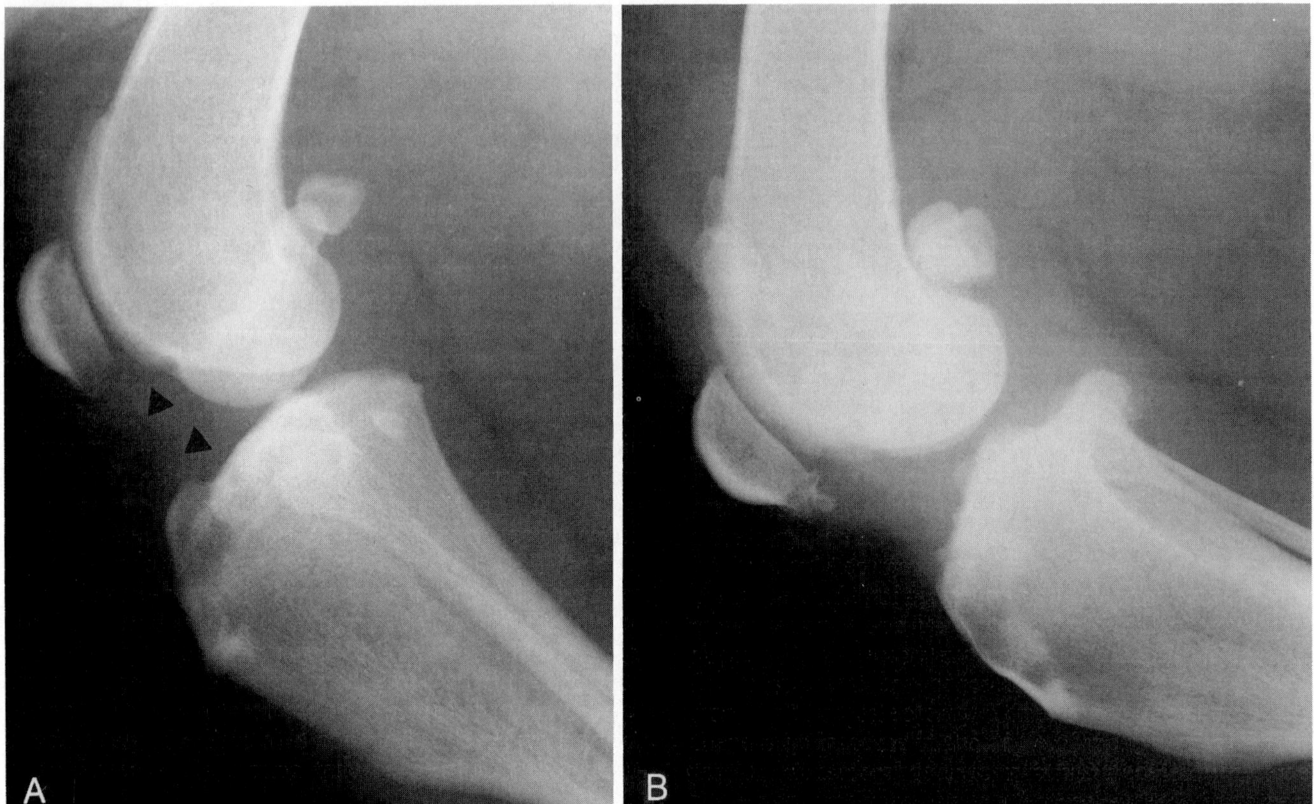

FIGURE 137–16. Radiographic examination of a stifle joint with partial tearing of the cranial cruciate ligament. *A*, Lateral view made when the dog was 18 months old. Note the presence of joint effusion causing cranial displacement of the infrapatellar fat body *(arrows)*. A small osteophyte has formed on the distal pole of the patella; otherwise, the joint is normal. *B*, Lateral view made when the dog was 2½ years old. Note the marked progression of degenerative joint disease (marginal osteophytes, effusion, sclerosis). At this time, the dog had a complete rupture of the cranial cruciate ligament.

condyloid fossa ("intercondylar notch") consistently undergoes narrowing associated with development of osteophytes within the fossa.[69, 210] In humans, the anterior and occasionally posterior aspect of the notch are widened to prevent impingement of grafts used for cranial cruciate ligament reconstruction.[88, 117, 141, 175] Magnetic resonance imaging illustrates the ligament in humans and may be useful to document notch impingement of intra-articular grafts (Fig. 137–17).[93] Congenital narrowing or malformation of the intercondyloid fossa has been incriminated as a possible cause of rupture involving the cranial cruciate ligament itself or grafts used for reconstruction.*

The notch is not seen well on standard cranial-caudal or caudal-cranial projections of the stifle.[211] It is readily observed by placing a dog in sternal recumbency, flexing the hip and stifle joints, and directing the radiographic beam perpendicular to the femoral condyles (Fig. 137–18). The importance of notch stenosis relative to intra-articular reconstruction of the cranial cruciate ligament in dogs is unknown. Radiographic assessment of the intercondylar notch in dogs with ligament rupture reveals consistent and often marked stenosis (Fig. 137–19).

*See references 6, 69, 77, 92, 109, 140, and 197.

Clinical Pathology

Joint fluid analysis is generally unrewarding because the majority of dogs with cranial cruciate ligament rupture have synovial fluid white blood cell counts less than 5,000/mm^3, consistent with chronic degenerative joint disease.[26, 80] The cells are generally mononuclear; large numbers of polymorphonuclear cells suggest immune-mediated joint disease (see Chapter 144). Dogs with partial tears may have elevated total white blood cell counts (mononuclear) in synovial fluid[80]; therefore, arthrocentesis and joint fluid analysis may be valuable in diagnosis of minimal instability but with other signs associated with partial tearing of the cranial cruciate ligament (lameness, joint effusion, pain).

Serum chemistry and hematology findings are normal in dogs with cranial cruciate ligament rupture.

Meniscal Injury

Injury to the medial meniscus is frequently associated with cranial cruciate ligament rupture. Dogs with partial tears have a low frequency of meniscal damage (5 of 25 dogs).[182] With chronicity, the frequency of meniscal damage increases and is as great as 80 per cent in dogs with complete tears.[75]

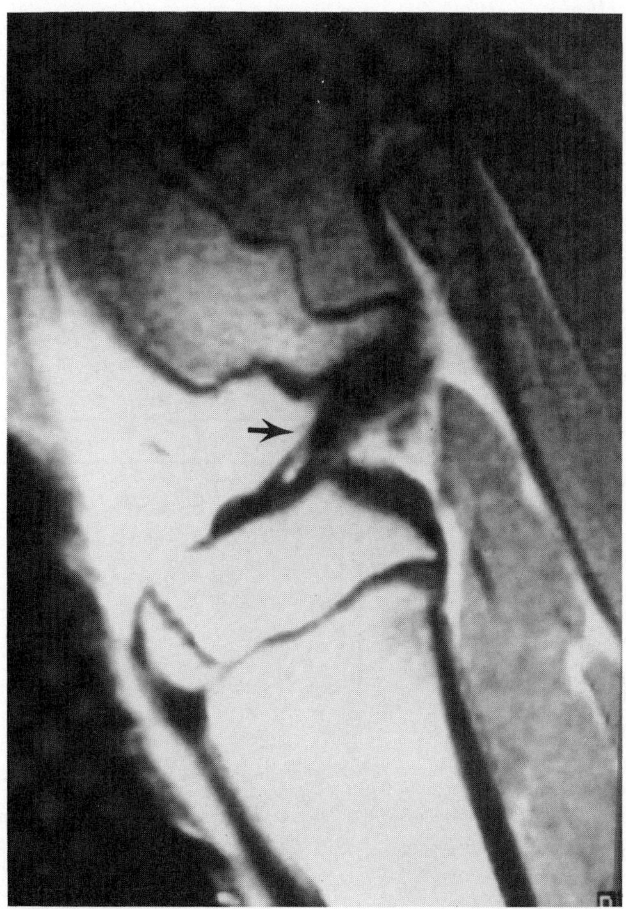

FIGURE 137–17. Magnetic resonance imaging of the anterior cruciate ligament *(arrow)* in a human knee. (Courtesy of Dr. Steve Howell.)

Mechanism of Meniscal Damage

Loss of the cranial cruciate ligament results in cranial subluxation of the tibia, which occurs repetitively with joint motion. The medial meniscus is firmly bound to the tibial plateau by meniscal ligaments, whereas the lateral meniscus is relatively mobile. When the tibia subluxates cranially, the caudal portion of the medial meniscus becomes wedged between the medial femoral condyle and the tibial plateau, causing excessive compressive and shear forces within the meniscus.[95] The most common injury resulting from this malarticulation is a longitudinal tear in the substance of the caudal body.[72, 95, 165] The inner margin of the torn meniscus often displaces cranially and centrally, remaining attached at either end, forming the so-called bucket-handle tear. The displaced portion can snap back and forth underneath the medial femoral condyle and is the cause of the clunking or clicking sound occasionally heard during manipulation of the joint or when the animal is walking.[95] In some instances, the entire caudal portion of the meniscal body may detach from its capsular attachments and flip back and forth under the femoral condyle.[72] Although the caudal portion of the meniscus can luxate cranially without having lost its capsular attachments,[199] marked displacement of the caudal body in a patient with rupture of the cranial cruciate ligament is pathological, and the unstable portion of the meniscus is excised.

Meniscal lesions may be difficult to detect grossly, accentuated by the difficulty of surgically exposing the medial meniscus. One study reported horizontal cleavage lesions on the underside of 20 per cent of 180 menisci excised from human patients and emphasized the importance of careful examination of the entire meniscus.[84] Ultrasonography and magnetic resonance imaging techniques have been used successfully in human patients to evaluate meniscal pathology[101, 116, 184, 187] and may be useful in animals.

Malformation of the menisci can occur (discoid meniscus); such malformations are of no clinical significance.[10]

The Effect of Meniscectomy

Removal of the medial meniscus causes an inflammatory state within the joint cavity and increased degenerative changes in adjacent bone and cartilage.[25, 44, 57, 111, 120, 151] Deterioration of joint cartilage is characterized histologically by fibrillation, swelling, fissures, cell proliferation, clustering, cell nesting, and even necrosis. Biochemical changes include proteoglycan loss, proteoglycan disaggregation, and an increase in proteoglycan synthesis. As a result of increased hydration, the main structural fibers of articular cartilage, composed of type II collagen, are exposed to increased biomechanical forces. The minor collagens (e.g., type IX collagen) may stabilize proteoglycan-type II interaction, thus preserving some degree of mechanical integrity.[120] Because the deleterious effects of medial meniscectomy are pro-

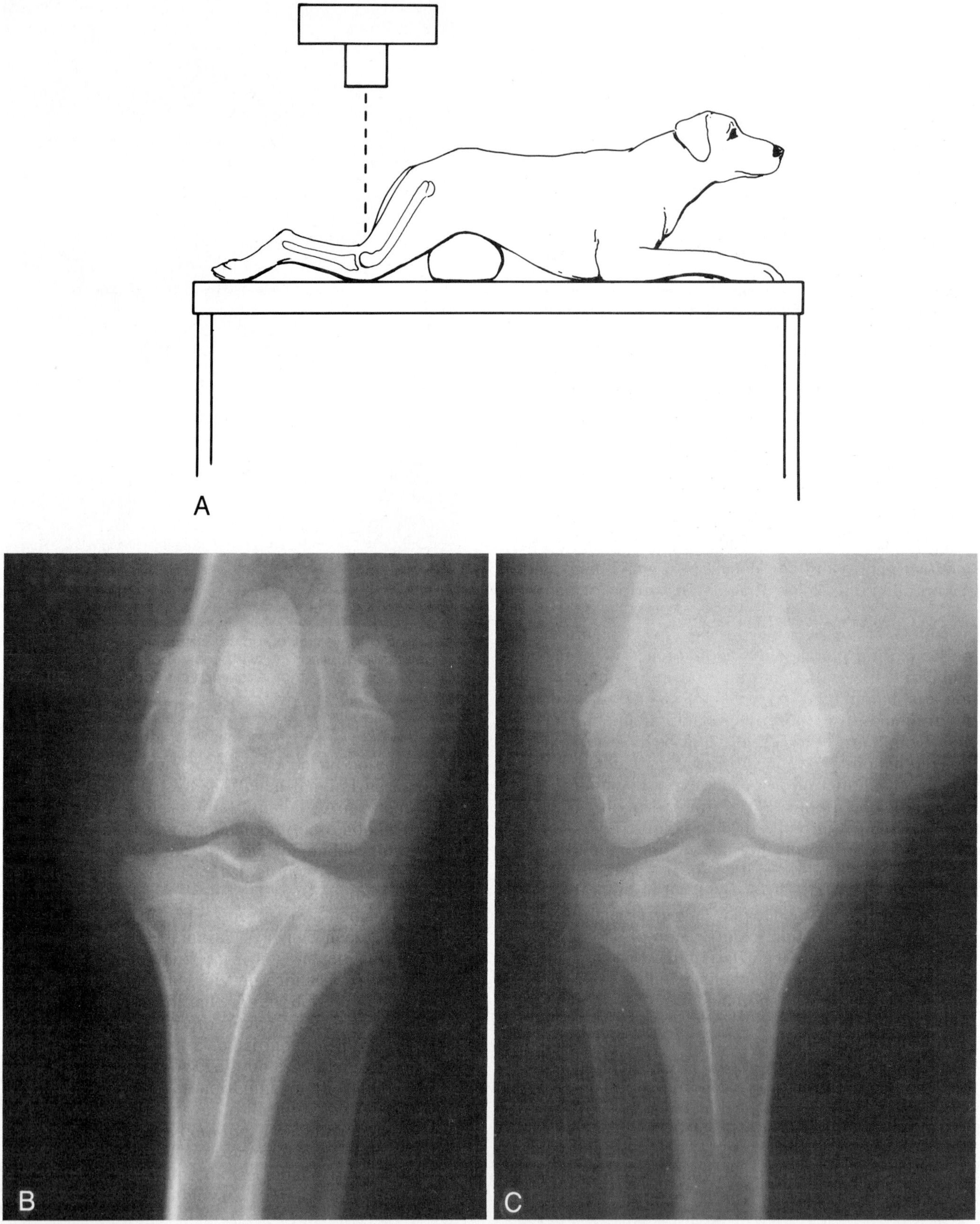

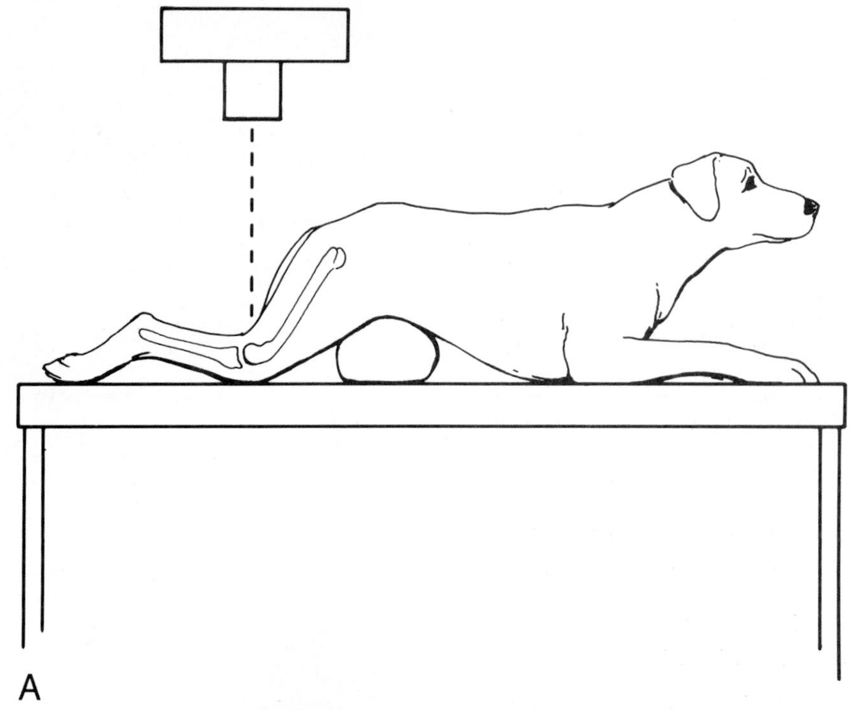

B

C

FIGURE 137–18. *A*, Schematic illustration of proper positioning for obtaining radiographs of the intercondylar notch. The dog is positioned in sternal recumbency with a sandbag used to elevate the abdomen. The hip is slightly extended, and the x-ray beam directed perpendicular to the femoral condyles. *B*, Standard caudal-cranial view of the stifle joint. The intercondylar notch is not seen well. *C*, Notch view of the stifle joint, made as described in *A*.

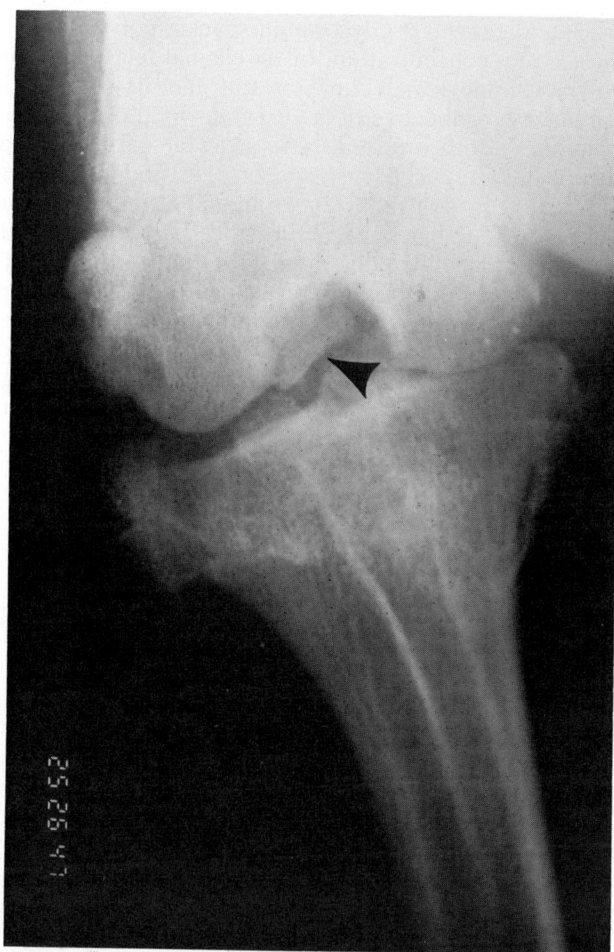

FIGURE 137–19. Notch view of the stifle joint in a dog with chronic instability secondary to rupture of the cranial cruciate ligament. Narrowing is associated with osteophyte production from the lateral margin of the intercondylar notch *(arrow)*.

portional to the amount of meniscus removed, as little of the meniscus as possible is removed.[44, 111, 120] Systemic administration of glycosaminoglycan polysulfate provided some protection to the articular cartilage of the meniscectomized compartment in beagles.[83]

Meniscal regeneration occurs after complete meniscectomy in humans and dogs.[55, 76, 151] The regenerated structure offers some protection to the joint surface that is covered.[11] Regeneration is not uniform and does not prevent degenerative sequelae.

Primary repair of meniscal lesions is not feasible because of the chronic nature of the injuries in dogs and the fact that the meniscus is avascular throughout much of the body. Acute peripheral tears healed well when repaired, whereas radial tears that were sutured together healed with fibrovascular scar filling the gap created when the repair site spread apart. This change in meniscal geometry was reflected in significant alterations in mechanical function, because radial repairs resembled complete meniscectomies with regard to changes in articular contact area and hoop strain behavior.[135]

A method for facilitating repair of avascular areas of the meniscus is by providing vascular access channels.[14, 95] The perimeters of the menisci are perfused with blood vessels derived from the synovial membrane. By making a full-thickness radial cut in the meniscal body, a "path" is created to allow fibrovascular tissue to reach areas of meniscal damage and allow reformation of fibrocartilaginous tissue. The clinical application of this technique has not been established, and the study of the healing of radial lesions[135] raises concern about the possible deleterious consequences of creating radial defects in the meniscal body.

Defects within the avascular portion of the meniscal body that were filled with exogenous fibrin clot healed through proliferation of fibrous connective tissue that eventually modulated into fibrocartilaginous tissue.[20] The fibrin clot acts as a chemotactic and mitogenic stimulus for reparative cells and provides a scaffolding for repair.

The use of meniscal allografts and collagen-based prostheses for meniscal replacement has produced encouraging results.[19, 200, 226]

Guidelines for Meniscectomy

Clinical management of meniscal injuries is controversial. Major meniscal injuries, such as large bucket-handle tears, cause lameness, and the damaged segment should be excised. Routine removal of the entire medial meniscus has been advocated, based on the rationale that progressive meniscal deterioration occurs in all dogs with cranial cruciate ligament rupture, and degenerative changes in the meniscus may not be evident.[74] Conversely, investigators have reported good to excellent results when the menisci were left in place in most or all of the dogs operated on.[54, 56] Preservation of the meniscus is clearly beneficial given the degenerative sequelae associated with its removal. Meniscectomy adversely affected the prognosis after surgery for rupture of the cranial cruciate ligament.[66] Leaving in place menisci that are grossly normal is not without risk; the most common cause of lameness in dogs that have had prior surgery for cranial cruciate ligament rupture is a damaged meniscus.[195] The frequency of lameness developing in dogs that had a grossly normal medial meniscus left intact has not been documented; in my experience, it is uncommon (<10 per cent).

Based on these considerations, the following guidelines for meniscectomy can be given:

1. The meniscus is protective of joint cartilage and is preserved if it is grossly normal.
2. Damaged portions of the meniscus are excised because they can cause lameness. Vascular access channels may improve healing of lesions in the avascular zone but also may alter the mechanical function of the remaining meniscus.

Treatment

Decisions about the nature of therapy in dogs with rupture of the cranial cruciate ligament are influenced by the animal's age, body size and weight, intended use (e.g., active hunting dog versus sedentary house pet), concurrent orthopedic or medical problems, economic considerations, and anticipated owner compliance.

Conservative (i.e., nonsurgical) therapy is recommended for cats. Eighteen of 18 cats examined after a mean follow-up period of 20.5 months became clinically normal without surgical intervention.[181] The mean duration before regaining normal limb function was 4.8 weeks, with a range of 1 to 16 weeks. A clinical report described three cats with concurrent cranial cruciate ligament rupture and cardiomyopathy; two died in the immediate postoperative period, and the third died 2 weeks after surgery.[103]

Small dogs (i.e., < 15 kg) often do well without surgical intervention. Twenty-four of 28 dogs (86 per cent) that weighed 15 kg or less were clinically normal or improved after a mean follow-up period of 36.6 months.[208] Pond and Campbell reported a 90 per cent success rate in nonsurgical treatment of dogs weighing less than 20 kg.[164] Strande monitored the clinical behavior of normal dogs after severance of the cranial cruciate ligament.[201] Of three dogs that weighed less than 15 kg, two were walking normally within 6 months, and the other was graded as 1 to 2 on a lameness scale of 0 to 4 (0 = no lameness). The same investigator studied the performance of clinical patients that were not operated on, and 8 of 11 small dogs (73 per cent) were free of lameness after an average period of 5.5 months. Based on the latter studies, it is prudent to wait for at least 6 to 8 weeks before recommending surgery for small dogs. These dogs are older at diagnosis and are often obese, with concurrent medical problems. Small dogs that are lame for 6 weeks after diagnosis and show no improvement often have meniscal tears and are operated on for meniscectomy and joint stabilization.

Conservative therapy is basically restriction of activity to short leash walks, weight reduction, and the use of analgesics as needed. A more organized program of physical therapy including range of motion exercises and swimming has been useful in the few cases in which it has been practical; unfortunately, such active involvement in the rehabilitation of the pet is impossible for many clients.

Large dogs (> 15 to 20 kg) clearly benefit from surgical therapy. In 46 of 57 (81 per cent) large dogs (> 15 kg) with cranial cruciate rupture treated conservatively, lameness persisted or worsened during a follow-up period of 10.2 months.[208] Three of three large dogs that had their ligament severed as a control population remained lame after 6 months.[201] In the latter study, only 6 of 20 large dogs that had clinical cranial cruciate ligament rupture and were treated conservatively became sound.

Medical Treatment

Intra-articular sodium hyaluronate injection significantly reduced articular cartilage damage in dogs after section of the cranial cruciate ligament.[183] The beneficial effects could have been due to a direct effect on the cartilage; it is possible that hyaluronic acid might act on the synovial membrane and limit the inflammatory response. Glycosaminoglycan polysulfuric acid ester improved cartilage viability and reduced collagenase levels in dogs with experimental severance of the cranial cruciate ligament.[3] Glycosaminoglycan polysulfate reduced the concentration of lysosomal elastase from polymorphonuclear leukocytes and may be of value in minimizing connective tissue breakdown in osteoarthritic joints.[22] Both oral and intra-articular corticosteroids significantly reduced cartilage erosion and osteophyte production in dogs with experimental severance of the cranial cruciate ligament.[155] Electron micrographic study of the cartilage demonstrated that the corticosteroids had not caused cell inhibition or death, and no deleterious effects were noted in normal controls. These findings suggest that there is considerable potential for reduction of pathological joint lesions in dogs through pharmacological manipulation of the intra-articular environment. Further research and clinical trials are necessary before application of these therapies in clinical patients.

Surgical Methods of Joint Stabilization

Numerous surgical procedures have been designed to restore stability and minimize secondary degenerative joint disease.* Although limb function can be improved in the majority of dogs by using various techniques, none of the procedures has proved clearly superior to any other; a study of the factors affecting the prognosis after surgery for cranial cruciate ligament rupture found that the type of surgical procedure had little influence on the eventual outcome.[66] The common denominator to all of these procedures may be enhancement of periarticular fibrosis, with stabilization coming at the expense of range of motion.[121] The latter mechanism explains the reported success of techniques such as pin firing.[113, 118] The true test of a reconstructive procedure is whether or not it prevents the development of secondary degenerative joint disease. Unfortunately, published studies indicate that degenerative joint disease progresses despite a satisfactory clinical result.[26, 75, 210]

Three basic surgical methods are used for restoring stability in a joint with cranial cruciate ligament rupture: (1) The ligament can be repaired primarily, including suture techniques for midsubstance tears or tension band fixation of bony avulsion injuries. (2) The ligament can be replaced or reconstructed using various materials, and these techniques are classified as intra-articular or intra-capsular methods. (3) The joint can be stabilized by transposition of periarticular structures or placement of suture materials outside of the joint. The latter methods are classified as extra-articular or extra-capsular.

Primary Repair. Primary repair of midsubstance cranial cruciate ligament tears is not feasible in dogs. The ability of the ligament to heal directly with scar tissue is limited; the ligament stumps invariably atrophy, accompanied by collagen degradation. In rabbits, cranial cruciate ligament degeneration after ligament severance was related to an increased concentration of collagenase in the synovial fluid.[4] Hyaluronan improved healing of lacerations of the ligament in rabbits[219] and may be of

*See references 15, 50, 52, 53, 56, 65, 71, 75, 89, 90, 113, 118, 126, 127, 158, 173, 190, 195, and 201.

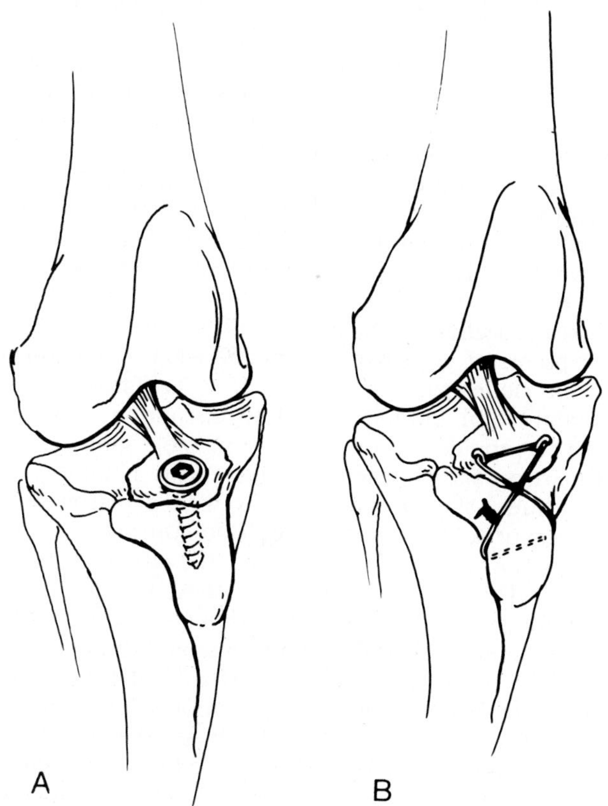

FIGURE 137–20. Schematic illustration of repair methods for avulsion fractures of the tibial attachment of the cranial cruciate ligament. *A*, Screw fixation. *B*, Tension band fixation.

value in acute lacerations that can be securely sutured. Even if primary repair were technically and biologically feasible, veterinarians rarely see dogs immediately after rupture, and rupture is pathological in many instances. Repair of a healthy ligament would be difficult enough; repair of a ligament that has undergone chronic degeneration is inadvisable. In humans with acute tears, the ligament can be sutured and is usually augmented with additional tissues or synthetic materials. The results after such repair are controversial.[5]

Avulsion Injuries. Dogs with acute avulsion injuries of a cranial cruciate ligament attachment site can be treated effectively by tension band repair or screw fixation of the avulsed segment, provided that the piece of bone is large enough to support the implant (Fig. 137–20).[61, 95, 168] Suture fixation of these injuries can be attempted if the bone fragment is small or friable, but I found the latter method unsuccessful in two large dogs. Tenuous repairs are supported by extracapsular stabilization and coaptation of the limb for 2 to 3 weeks.

Intra-articular Reconstruction: General Principles

Graft Selection. The ligament may be reconstructed using biological tissues (autograft, allograft, xenograft), synthetic material, or a combination of biological tissue and synthetic material (composite grafts). Composites often include autogenous patellar tendon supported by Dacron or polyglycolic acid. After implantation of biological grafts, considerable graft strength is lost.[47] It is desirable to begin with a graft that is at least as strong or stronger than the tissue to be replaced.

Reconstructions that use a muscle-tendon unit, such as the semimembranosus, to replace the ligament or duplicate its function are termed *dynamic* repairs because of the potential for active muscle contraction in response to joint loads. Critical studies have failed to document any advantage to this type of repair.[1, 176]

The most frequently used materials for reconstruction are autografts consisting of patellar tendon, fascia lata, or combinations of the two. Tension testing of canine patellar tendon–based grafts demonstrated abrupt failure of central and medial third grafts but sequential failure of the laterally based graft.[107] None of the autograft systems approached the stiffness, maximum load, and energy absorbed to maximum load of the normal ligament. The central and lateral autografts were stiffer, had greater maximum loads, and absorbed more energy to maximum load than the medial autograft. The maximum load sustained by central and lateral autografts was approximately 29 per cent of that sustained by the contralateral cranial cruciate ligament. The medial autograft sustained only 10 per cent of the cranial cruciate ligament value.

Autogenous tissues are used because of the convenience of harvesting the graft directly from the patient and lack of immune response. The major disadvantage of autografts is inferior stiffness and strength in comparison with the cranial cruciate ligament. Clinically, donor site morbidity is negligible; experimental removal of the central third of the canine patellar tendon caused a 10 per cent loss of length and marked reduction in strength and stiffness of the remaining tendon for 6 months after excision.[34]

Allograft tissues are advantageous in that larger quantities can be harvested from donor animals so that the graft can be made stronger, and they obviate the need to sacrifice host tissues.[189, 213] The immune response to allogeneic tendon and ligament tissue is minimized by deep freezing, and most allografts are harvested in a sterile manner and stored at −70°C before implantation.[130, 189, 205] The immune response to allogeneic bone is reduced but not eliminated by deep freezing and may have a role in the response to bone-ligament-bone allografts.[112, 119] Ethylene oxide sterilization of allografts used for ligament reconstruction is not recommended; one report described human patients with persistent joint effusion and inflammation associated with toxic byproducts of ethylene oxide, apparently released from the allograft.[102]

Numerous reports describe satisfactory results using frozen allogeneic tissue, without a significant immune response to the graft.[18, 100, 139, 189, 215] Deep-frozen allografts did elicit an immune response, which was measurable only in the synovial fluid of the operated joint.[213] The inconvenience of collection and storage of allografts has limited their use in veterinary surgery, especially because a clear advantage over autogenous grafts has not been demonstrated. Bovine xenografts have been used in dogs and in humans, with generally unsuccessful results.[132, 207]

Synthetic materials offer the convenience of "off-the-shelf" availability, lack of morbidity associated with graft harvest, and the ability to custom design a prosthesis with appropriate mechanical properties.[231] Some synthetic materials are intended to be permanent, such as Gore-Tex* and some Dacron prostheses, or to function as scaffolds, allowing fibrous tissue ingrowth and eventual replacement by host tissue. Carbon fiber is an example of the latter type; extensive investigations in dogs and other species suggest that carbon fiber is unsatisfactory for ligament reconstruction.[23, 53, 157, 198]

Dacron prostheses have been studied extensively in dogs, with mixed results.[31, 65, 82, 89, 178] Dacron composite grafts and the use of synovial membrane to shield the ligament and facilitate fibrous ingrowth have provided encouraging results experimentally.[27, 204] Fibroblast seeding of a Dacron graft accelerated and improved fibrous ingrowth.[31] Unfortunately, synthetic grafts are often expensive and are unproven in clinical veterinary practice.

Graft Placement. The normal cranial cruciate ligament is a complex structure composed of numerous fascicles, each with independent sites of origin and insertion. Individual fascicles or groups of fascicles are tensed or relaxed, depending on joint position. Grafts used for reconstruction are cords or sheets of tissue with more discrete points of anchorage. If the distance between those points changes during joint motion, the graft simultaneously lengthens or shortens. Excessive lengthening could overstress the graft or cause fixation failure, whereas shortening causes the graft to become lax and compromises joint stability. Considerable effort has been expended to determine so-called isometric points of attachment that maintain the same relative distance as the joint moves.† The location of the femoral attachment site is more critical than the tibial site.[29, 38, 91, 180] The recommended tibial attachment site is within the craniomedial area of the tibial attachment site of the ligament, whereas the most frequent recommendation for the femoral attachment site is proximal and caudal within the origin of the cranial cruciate ligament. The latter studies have primarily used human cadavers, with grafts placed through tunnels in the femur and tibia. Problems with drill tunnels include fraying of the graft at the margin of the tunnel and difficulty in consistently locating the tunnel in an isometric location.‡ The optimum locations for drill tunnels in dogs are undetermined.

The alternative to a femoral drill hole is to place the graft over the top of the lateral femoral condyle.[16] Although contradictory reports have been published on the isometry of the over-the-top location for intra-articular grafts,[91, 129, 132, 145, 156] both the original technique and modifications have been used successfully.[15, 51, 52, 190] Reports describe reduced graft excursion in human knees when a trough is placed in the femoral condyle to lower the graft position slightly.[129, 156]

Graft Tension. The relationship between tension applied to the graft and joint stability depends on the length and stiffness of the graft. This relationship is complicated by the fact that graft tension decreases within minutes by stress relaxation.[47] A study using human cadaveric knees demonstrated that the mean graft load necessary to restore normal stability was as follows: patellar tendon, 16 newtons; semitendinous, 38 newtons; and iliotibial band, 61 newtons.[33] Yoshiya and colleagues, in a dog model, reported decreased vascularization of the graft when higher graft loads were applied at the time of tensioning (39 newtons versus 1 newton).[228] The optimum prefixation graft tension has not been studied clinically.

Graft Fixation. In the immediate postoperative period, the points of graft fixation are the weakest component of the bone-graft-bone system.[47, 79] To facilitate early rehabilitation and minimize graft disruption, it is advisable to provide the most secure possible graft fixation. Robertson and colleagues compared the holding power of sutures, staples, and a screw with a plastic spiked washer or a screw with a metallic soft-tissue plate.[174] The screw fixation systems had the greatest holding power. The screw and spiked washer system has been used for fixation of a patellar tendon fascia lata autograft to the femur in dogs.[97, 190] Lameness and draining tracts over the screw have been reported.[177] If a screw and spiked washer fixation is used, removal 2 to 3 months postoperatively is recommended.[94] Another secure system of fixation is a looped graft placed around a screw.[79]

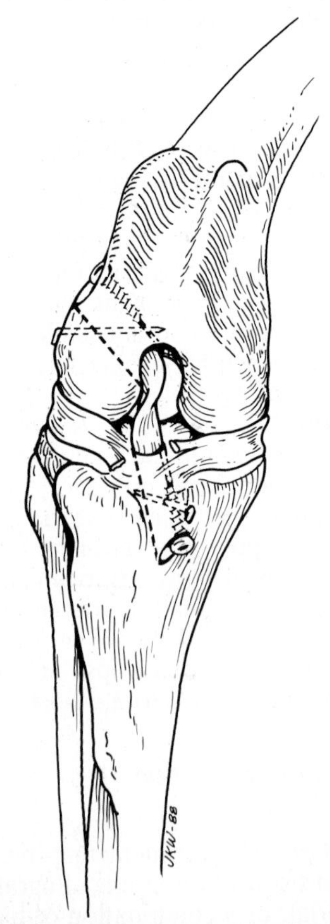

FIGURE 137–21. Schematic illustration of interference screw fixation for bone-ligament-bone grafts. (From Vasseur PB, et al: Anterior cruciate ligament allograft transplantation in dogs. *Clin Orthop* *269*:295, 1991.)

*W. L. Gore and Associates, Flagstaff, AZ.
†See references 29, 38, 40, 91, 129, 145, 156, and 180.
‡See references 29, 38, 40, 91, 132, 145, and 180.

Bone plugs placed within tunnels can be fixed securely using interference screw fixation (Fig. 137–21).[170] If graft tissue is left attached to its anatomical origin (e.g., patellar tendon anchored to the tibial tuberosity), the attachment site is secure, with the additional advantage of gradual stress transfer from graft to bone. The disadvantage of pedicled grafts is that the point of attachment is not isometric.

"Notchplasty." Osteophytes consistently form on the inner margin of the lateral femoral condyle, forming a "ledge" (Fig. 137–22). Removal of this new bone and reshaping of the cranial margins of the intercondylar notch is referred to as a *cranial notchplasty*.[78, 117, 175] A 6-mm bone gouge is used to remove the bulk of new bone, followed by a small bone rasp to smooth and contour the condylar margin (Fig. 137–23). Care is taken not to damage the origin of the caudal cruciate ligament in the proximal notch. Generally, the osteophytes are soft and easily removed; however, the bone may be more dense in chronic cases. Cranial notchplasties are effective in facilitating passage of intra-articular grafts through the intercondylar notch and in preventing graft impingement during extension.

Intra-articular Reconstruction: Operative Methods

Regardless of the operative technique, it is critical that the joint be explored for evaluation of the cartilage surfaces, inspection of menisci, and notchplasty in intra-articular repairs.

Preparation of Patients. With an animal in lateral recumbency and the affected limb uppermost, the hair is clipped from the hock proximally to the dorsal midline, including the entire circumference of the limb. The skin is prepared aseptically, and the limb draped to allow full manipulation during the operation. Water-impervious stockinette is recommended. Cefazolin (20 mg/kg) or oxacillin (30 mg/kg) is given intravenously after the induction of general anesthesia and continued every 6 hours intravenously for 24 hours.

Paatsama developed the classic intra-articular operation for use in dogs, using autogenous fascia lata routed through drill holes in the femur and tibia.[149] The procedure is a modification of one for use in humans.[35] The procedure has subsequently been modified by Paatsama[152] and by Rudy[179] (Fig. 137–24).

Disadvantages of the Paatsama procedure include the tensile strength weakness of the graft; inconsistent location of bony tunnels, causing nonisometric graft placement; and possible abrasion at the graft–tunnel interface. A comparison of the Paatsama procedure and an extra-articular procedure revealed breakage of the fascia lata graft in 10 of 26 stifles.[127] Only four of the ten dogs were lame, and periarticular fibrosis may have been the primary stabilizing factor in both groups of dogs (intra- and extra-articular groups).

Dickinson and Nunamaker Procedure. Dickinson and Nunamaker described successful results using a simplified modification of the Paatsama procedure.[56] After isolation of the graft and joint exploration (see Fig. 137–24), the graft is left pedicled to the craniolateral tibia and placed directly into the joint and through a drill tunnel in the lateral femoral condyle. The graft is made long enough so that it can be brought around the lateral femoral condyle and sutured back to itself and the lateral fibrous joint capsule (Fig. 137–25). Using this technique, the investigators reported good (28) or excellent (58) clinical results in 86 of 89 (97 per cent) of dogs.

Over-the-Top Procedures. Placing intra-articular grafts over the proximal and caudal aspect of the lateral femoral condyle in the over-the-top position results in consistent graft placement and is technically easier than

Text continued on page 1840

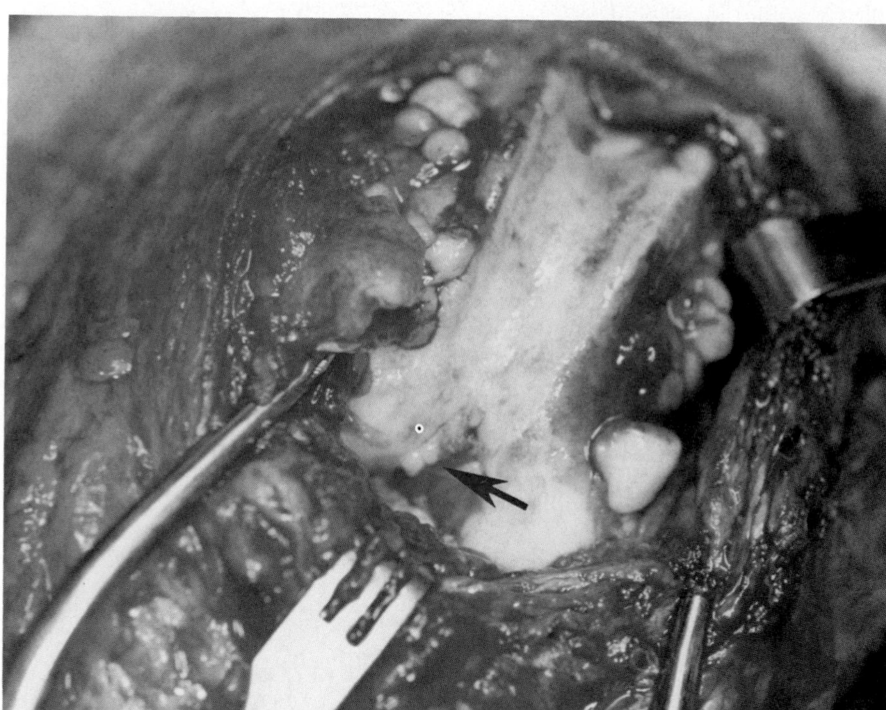

FIGURE 137–22. Osteophyte formation on the lateral margin of the intercondylar notch *(arrow)* of a dog with chronic instability associated with cranial cruciate ligament rupture.

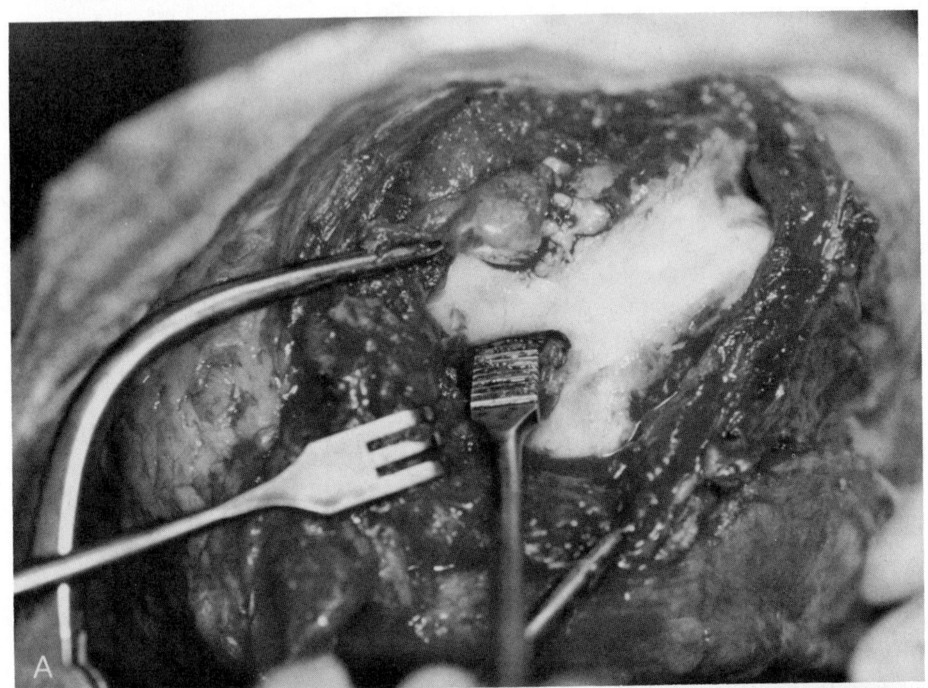

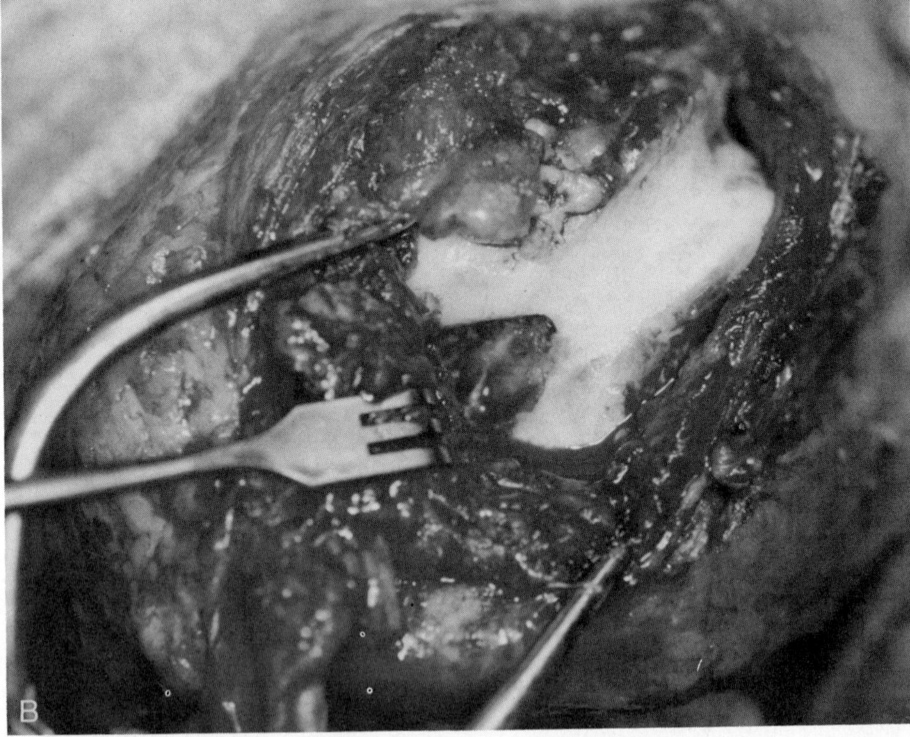

FIGURE 137–23. Notchplasty procedure. *A*, The new bone is removed using a 6-mm bone gouge with care taken not to damage the caudal cruciate ligament, and a small bone rasp is used to smooth the condylar margin. *B*, Appearance after notchplasty. Compare with Figure 137–22 (same patient) and Figure 137–24*E*.

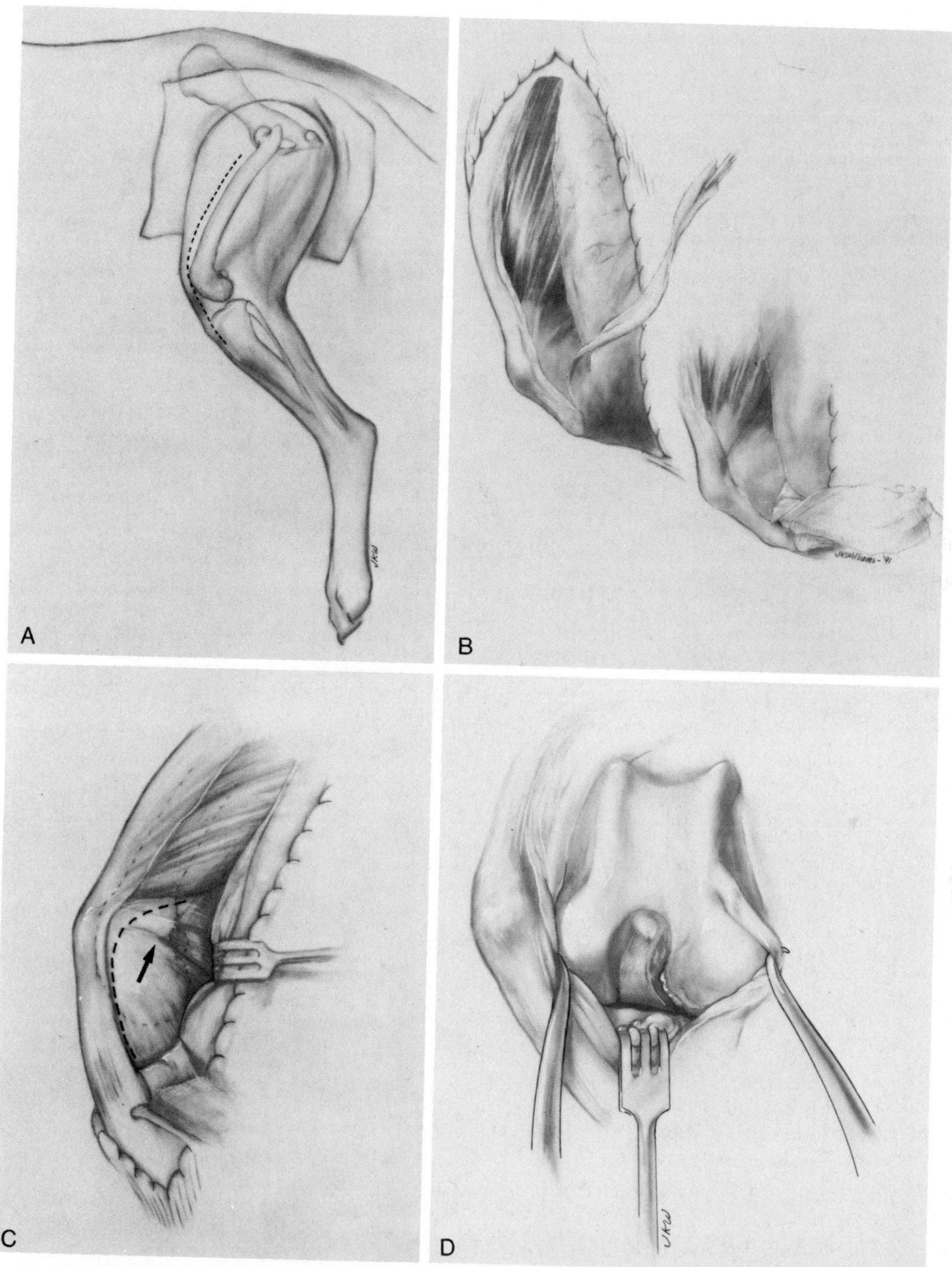

FIGURE 137–24. *A*, Skin incision used to initiate the modified Paatsama procedure for reconstruction of the cranial cruciate ligament. The incision is placed cranial to the biceps femoris muscle and extends from the base of the greater trochanter to a point just distal to the tibial tuberosity on the craniolateral aspect of the joint. *B*, The subcutaneous tissue is cleared from the fascia and sutured or clipped to the stockinette. A fascial graft 1.5 to 2.5 cm in width is constructed by making parallel incisions in the fascia lata, leaving the graft pedicled to the lateral margin of the tibial plateau. The graft is wrapped in saline-moistened gauze to prevent dehydration. *C*, The biceps fascia is reflected caudally, exposing the lateral aspect of the joint capsule and margin of the vastus lateralis muscle. A curved arthrotomy is made, taking care not to cut the vastus lateralis (broken line). A small muscle slip extending from the gastrocnemius to the vastus lateralis *(arrow)* is consistent and must be cut. *D*, After medial luxation of the patella, intra-articular exposure is greatly facilitated by placement of small Gelpi retractors between the patellar tendon and the tendon of the long digital extensor, and by retraction of the infrapatellar fat body using a Miller-Senn retractor. Marginal osteophytes along the femoral trochlea are removed using a rongeur if they are large and irregular and interfere with femoropatellar joint motion. A fine rasp is useful to smooth the underlying bone surface after osteophyte removal.

Illustration continued on following page

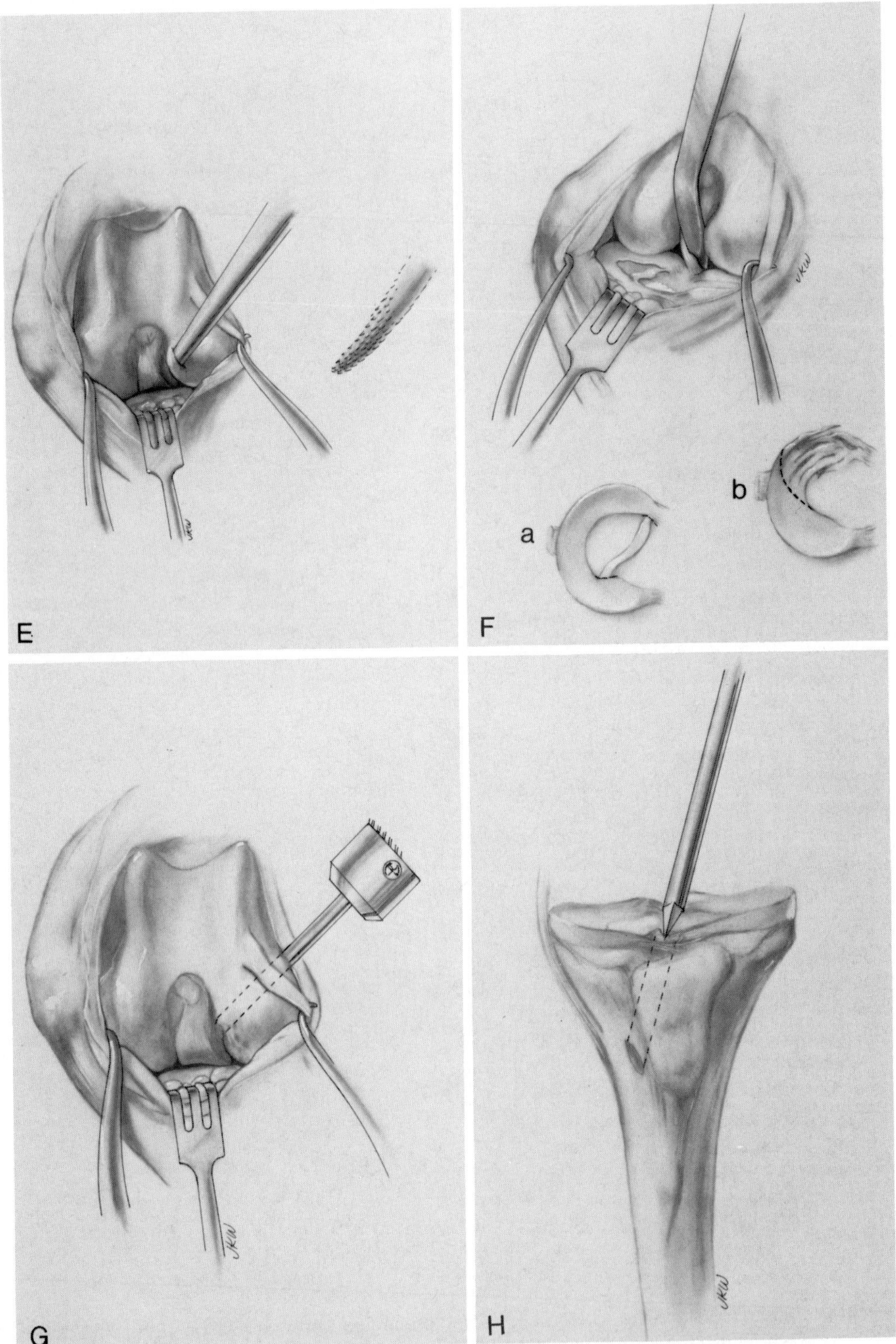

FIGURE 137–24 ***Continued*** *E*, Proliferative new bone is removed from the lateral margin of the intercondylar notch using a small bone gouge, and the condylar margin smoothed using a bone rasp *(inset)*. *F*, Exposure of the medial meniscus is accomplished by placing a baby Hohmann retractor over the caudal margin of the tibial plateau and using it as a lever to elevate the femoral condyles. A moistened sponge placed over the cartilage surface of the femur is useful to prevent damage caused by the retractor. A curved mosquito forceps can be used for the same purpose if a Hohmann retractor is not available. Bucket-handle tears of the medial meniscus are excised by cutting the cranial and caudal attachments of the damaged segment *(a)*. Diffuse damage to the caudal pole of the medial meniscus is treated by excision of either the caudal body of the meniscus or by complete meniscectomy *(b)*. *G*, A tunnel is made in the lateral femoral condyle using a Steinmann pin, directed from the lateral cruciate ligament origin to the area of cranial cruciate ligament attachment to the condyle. A common error is to make this tunnel exit too cranially; a drill guide is useful to ensure proper tunnel orientation. *H*, A Steinmann pin is used to make a tunnel from the tibial attachment site of the cranial cruciate ligament, exiting on the medial surface of the proximal tibia.

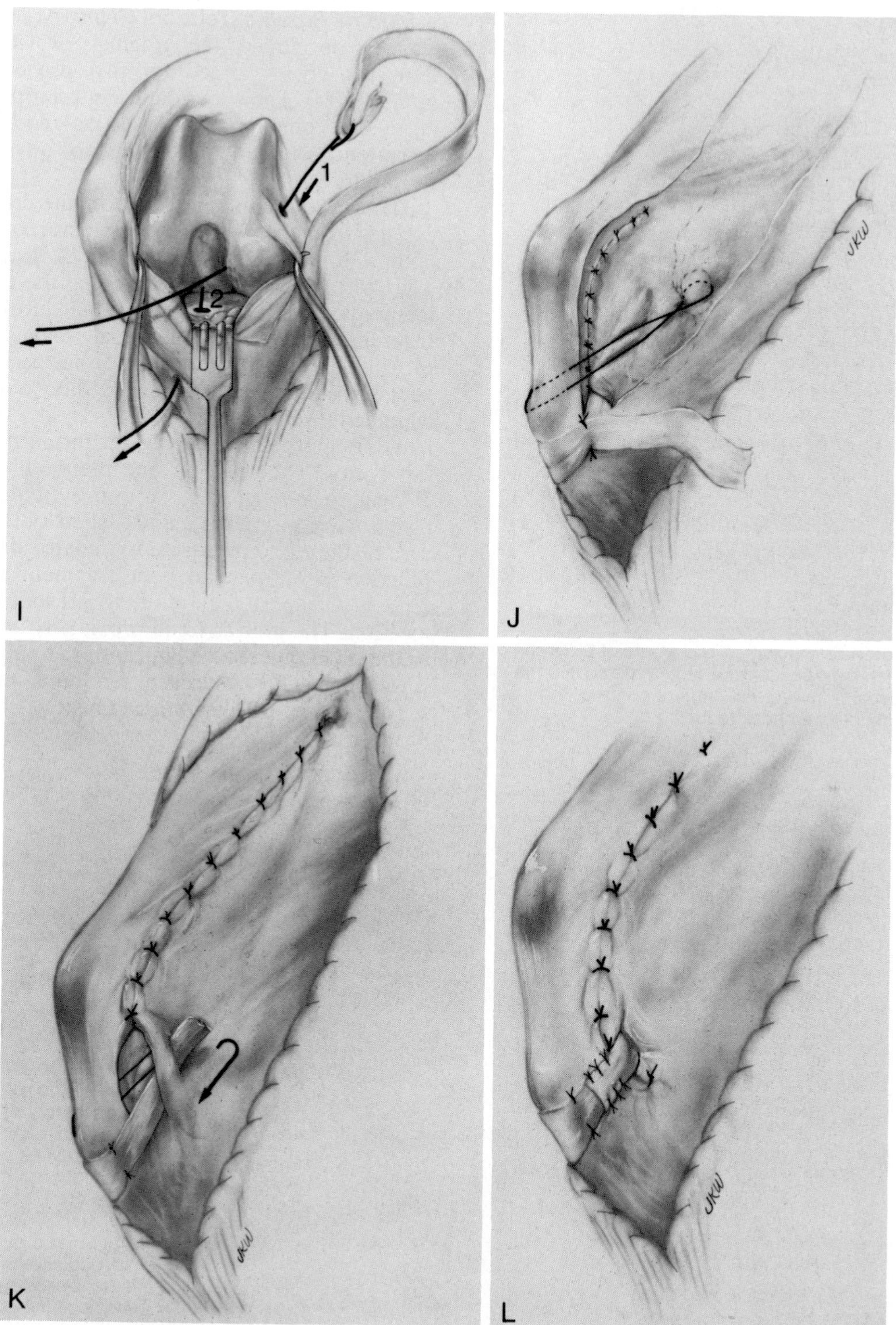

FIGURE 137–24 *Continued* *I*, The graft is passed first through the femoral tunnel (1) and then the tibial tunnel (2) to exit the proximal medial tibia. A looped wire is useful to facilitate graft passage. *J*, The graft is pulled over the cranial surface of the tibial tuberosity and held with sutures. An imbrication suture (DeAngelis technique) is placed from the lateral fabella to the distal patellar tendon, using monofilament nonabsorbable material. *K*, The fascia is imbricated using interrupted Lembert sutures, and the graft is passed through a small incision in the distal fascia to exert tension on the biceps femoris *(arrow)*. *L*, The graft is sutured to itself, and the remaining fascial defect closed with interrupted sutures.

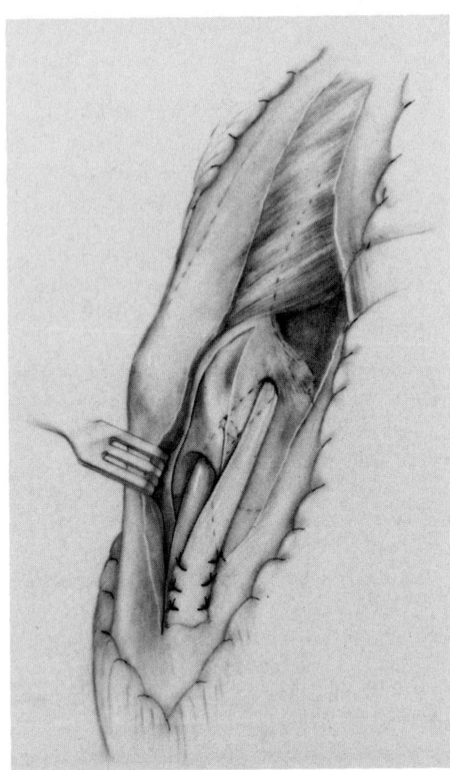

FIGURE 137–25. Fascia lata autograft procedure of Dickinson and Nunamaker in which a laterally based graft is routed into the joint and through a tunnel in the lateral femoral condyle. The graft is made long enough to suture back to itself.

creating bone tunnels. An *in vitro* study found that over-the-top placement provided a more biomechanically sound repair than extra-articular stabilization.[16]

Medial Patellar Tendon Graft. Arnoczky and colleagues developed the original over-the-top procedure for dogs,[15] based on two procedures used in humans.[108, 123] The superior strength properties of patellar tendon compared with fascia lata, combined with the consistency of graft placement, are advantages of this procedure.

The skin incision is placed over the cranial thigh and extends from the midshaft of the femur, over the patellar tendon, to the craniolateral aspect of the proximal tibia. The graft is constructed by incising the patellar tendon longitudinally, isolating the medial third of the tendon from the tibial tubercle proximally over the patella and proximolaterally to incorporate the fascia lata. A parallel incision is made in the medial joint capsule and extended proximally (Fig. 137–26*A*). The total graft length is approximately twice the distance from the tibial tuberosity to the patella, and the width approximately 1½ cm in a large dog. A wedge of patellar bone is osteotomized from the medial aspect of the patella, with care taken not to penetrate to the articular surface. The junction of the patellar bone fragment and quadriceps tendon is harvested carefully to prevent rupture at this location. The graft is freed proximally and left pedicled to the tibial tubercle. As much of the fat pad as possible is left attached to the distal tendon to maximize blood supply and revascularization potential. The joint is ex-

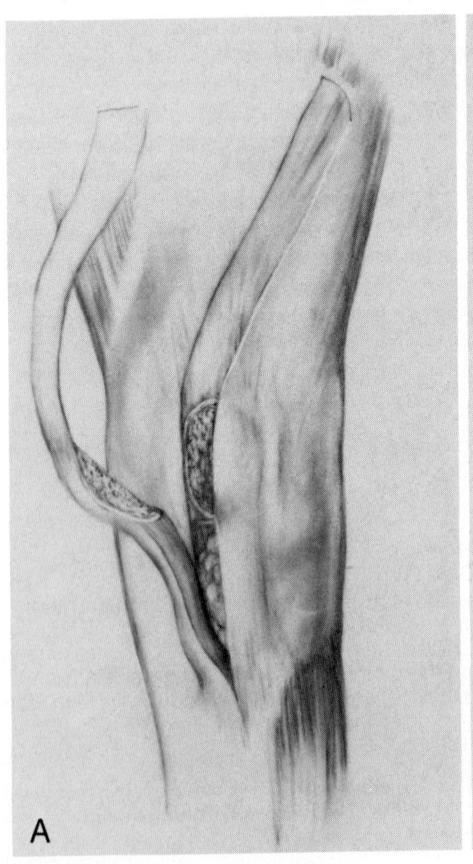

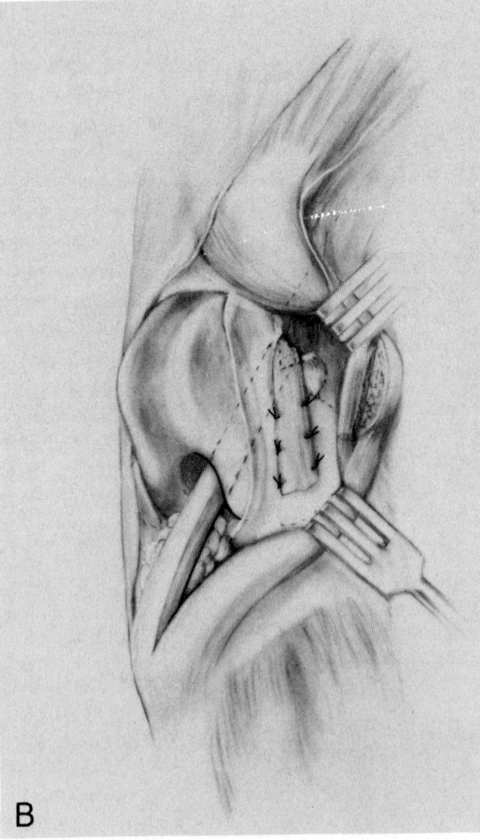

FIGURE 137–26. *A*, The original over-the-top procedure of Arnoczky uses a graft composed of the medial third of the patellar tendon, a portion of the patella, and fascia lata proximal to the patella. *B*, The graft is routed through the joint, medial to the remaining patellar tendon, over the lateral femoral condyle, and sutured to the dense periosteum on the lateral surface of the condyle.

plored through the medial arthrotomy incision, which is lengthened as needed to permit lateral luxation of the patella and exposure of the lateral femoral condyle. An incision is made in the lateral femorofabellar fascia, and a curved hemostat is passed into the intercondylar notch, lateral to the caudal cruciate ligament. The tip of the graft is grasped in the forceps and pulled through the joint. The graft is pulled taut and sutured to the periosteum and lateral collateral ligament (Fig. 137–26*B*). The arthrotomy is closed with interrupted sutures, and the remaining tissues apposed in layers.

Four-in-One Over-the-Top Procedure. This technique is a modification of Arnoczky's original procedure and uses fascia lata rather than patellar tendon, and the intra-articular graft is supported by an extra-articular lateral stabilizing suture (Fig. 137–27).[30] This procedure eliminates technical difficulties associated with osteotomy of the patella, as required in the Arnoczky technique, but sacrifices the superior strength of patellar tendon grafts.

The technique combines the stabilizing effects of four procedures: The caudal sartorius and biceps muscles are advanced to create caudal traction on the tibia; a lateral imbrication suture prevents drawer motion and protects the intra-articular graft; closure of the fascial defect imbricates the lateral retinaculum; and the fascial strip replaces the cranial cruciate ligament.

Hulse Procedure.[97] An autogenous graft composed of the lateral third of the patellar tendon and a portion of the lateral retinaculum is routed lateral to the patellar tendon under the intermeniscal ligament, and over the top of the lateral femoral condyle. The strength properties of the graft and its performance in dogs have been studied experimentally.[37, 107] Clinical studies have reported good to excellent results in more than 90 per cent of the dogs.[52, 190] I modify the original procedure by creating a trough in the femorofabellar fascia, by making the graft long enough to extend back to the patellar tendon, creating an extracapsular support, and by placement of a lateral imbrication suture* to support the graft in the early postoperative period (Fig. 137–28).

The Hulse procedure is advantageous in that it uses a relatively strong graft (29 per cent of the breaking strength of the cranial cruciate ligament),[107] and the graft is anchored under the intermeniscal ligament at the anatomical insertion site of the cranial cruciate ligament. The modifications described here provide extra-articular reinforcement to the graft by placement of an imbrication suture and a fascial strip anchored to the lateral joint capsule. Placing the graft within a trough between the fabella and femur lowers the femoral fixation site, which should improve the isometricity of graft placement.[129, 156]

Extra-Articular Reconstruction: Operative Methods

Extra-articular procedures are generally easier to perform and therefore quicker than intra-articular procedures. Fibular head transposition is a notable exception because it is a technically demanding operation. Ultimate joint stabilization after most extra-articular repairs is due to accentuation of periarticular fibrosis.[30] Although extra-articular procedures have been considered particularly advantageous for use in smaller dogs, fibular head transposition and the Flo imbrication have been successfully used in large dogs as well.[30, 32, 71, 134, 195] Concerns about the healing of autogenous tissues within the intra-articular environment of stifle joints with chronic degenerative joint disease has led to increased interest in extra-articular methods of joint stabilization.[30] However, documentation that the intra-articular environment is detrimental to the healing of autogenous graft tissue has not been published.

As with intra-articular procedures, it is important to open the joint to inspect the menisci and articular cartilage and to remove large osteophytes before the stabilization procedure. Débridement of ligament stumps and notchplasty are not required with extra-articular techniques.

Tightening of the lateral retinaculum (imbrication) was first reported by Childers, who placed Lembert sutures in the lateral fascia over the stifle joint.[39] McCurnin and colleagues[127] and Pearson and associates[154] modified the technique by repositioning and increasing the number of Lembert sutures and adding medial imbrication for additional support. DeAngelis and Lau further improved the technique by providing firm anchorage to the sutures, proximally to the dense connective tissue around the lateral fabella and distally to the patellar tendon.[50] With their technique, only one or two sutures are necessary to provide stabilization (Fig. 137–24*J*).

Further modification of the lateral imbrication approach was described by Gambardella and colleagues,[75] who included three sutures anchored to the distal patellar tendon, one from the lateral fabella and two from the lateral collateral ligament (Fig. 137–29).

One of the most frequently used extra-articular procedures[71] includes both lateral and medial imbrication sutures. The procedure has been modified and is called the *three-in-one* technique (Fig. 137–30).[30]

When braided, nonabsorbable sutures are used for this procedure, formation of draining tracts over the sutures occurred in 21 per cent of the cases.[60] Soaking the sutures in a chlorhexidine solution before implantation may help reduce the frequency of draining tracts.[30]

Fibular Head Transposition. This technique uses the lateral collateral ligament to resist cranial translation and internal rotation of the tibia (Fig. 137–31). The use of autogenous tissue with a stable attachment at either end is a clear advantage over imbrication methods that use suture materials. Additionally, being a vascularized connective tissue, the lateral collateral ligament may hypertrophy in response to the presumably increased stresses imposed by its altered position. An *in vitro* study using cadaver joints demonstrated that fibular head transposition provided greater stiffness, less laxity, and less decay per test than patellar tendon or fascia lata over-the-top repairs or lateral suture imbrication.[153] Good to excellent clinical results have been reported in

Text continued on page 1846

*Maxon, Davis and Geck, Wayne, NJ.

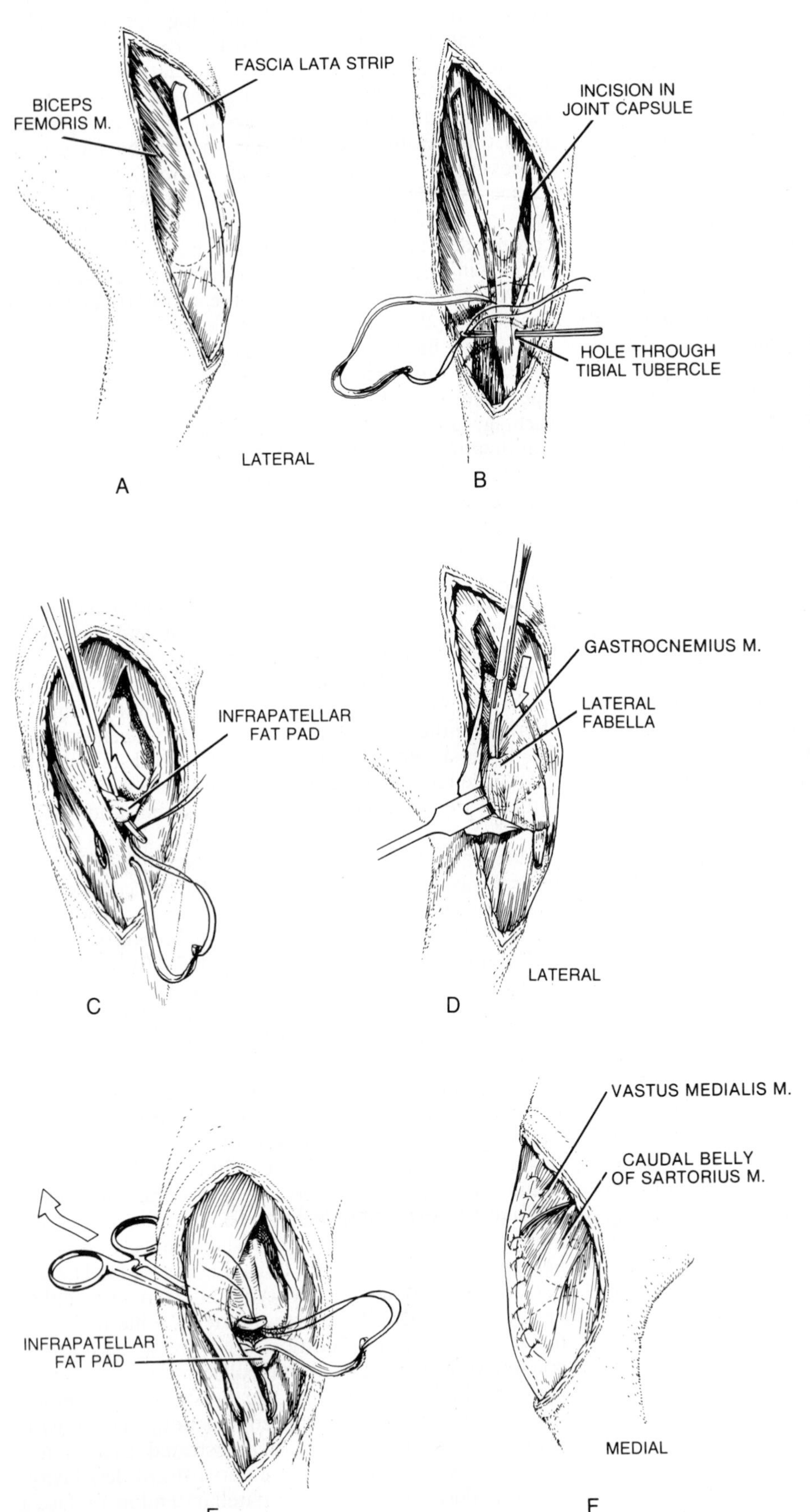

FIGURE 137–27. Four-in-one over-the-top procedure. *A*, A lateral skin incision is followed by a medial arthrotomy to inspect the joint and menisci. A laterally based strip of fascia lata, 1.5 to 2.0 cm wide and two to three times the length from the midpatella to the tibial tuberosity, is created for use as an intra-articular graft. *B*, A 4.0 to 5.0-mm (5/32 to 3/16 inch) hole is drilled through the tibial tuberosity, and an eyed needle or twisted wire is used to pull the graft through the hole from lateral to medial, using a piece of suture material as a leader. *C*, The graft is then routed under the fat pad and into the joint using curved forceps. *D*, The fascia lata is retracted caudally to expose the lateral fabella, and mosquito forceps are passed medial to the fabella, through the caudal joint capsule, and into the intercondylar notch, lateral to the caudal cruciate ligament. *E*, The suture material is grasped in the forceps, and the graft drawn through the joint and over the top of the lateral femoral condyle. *F*, The caudal belly of the sartorius is included in the closure of the medial arthrotomy to increase tension in the muscle and aid joint stabilization. The insertion of the caudal belly of the sartorius muscle is partially detached from the tibia, then sutured with the joint capsule and medial fascia to the patellar tendon as far proximally as the patella. From that point proximally, the sartorius is not included in the closure.

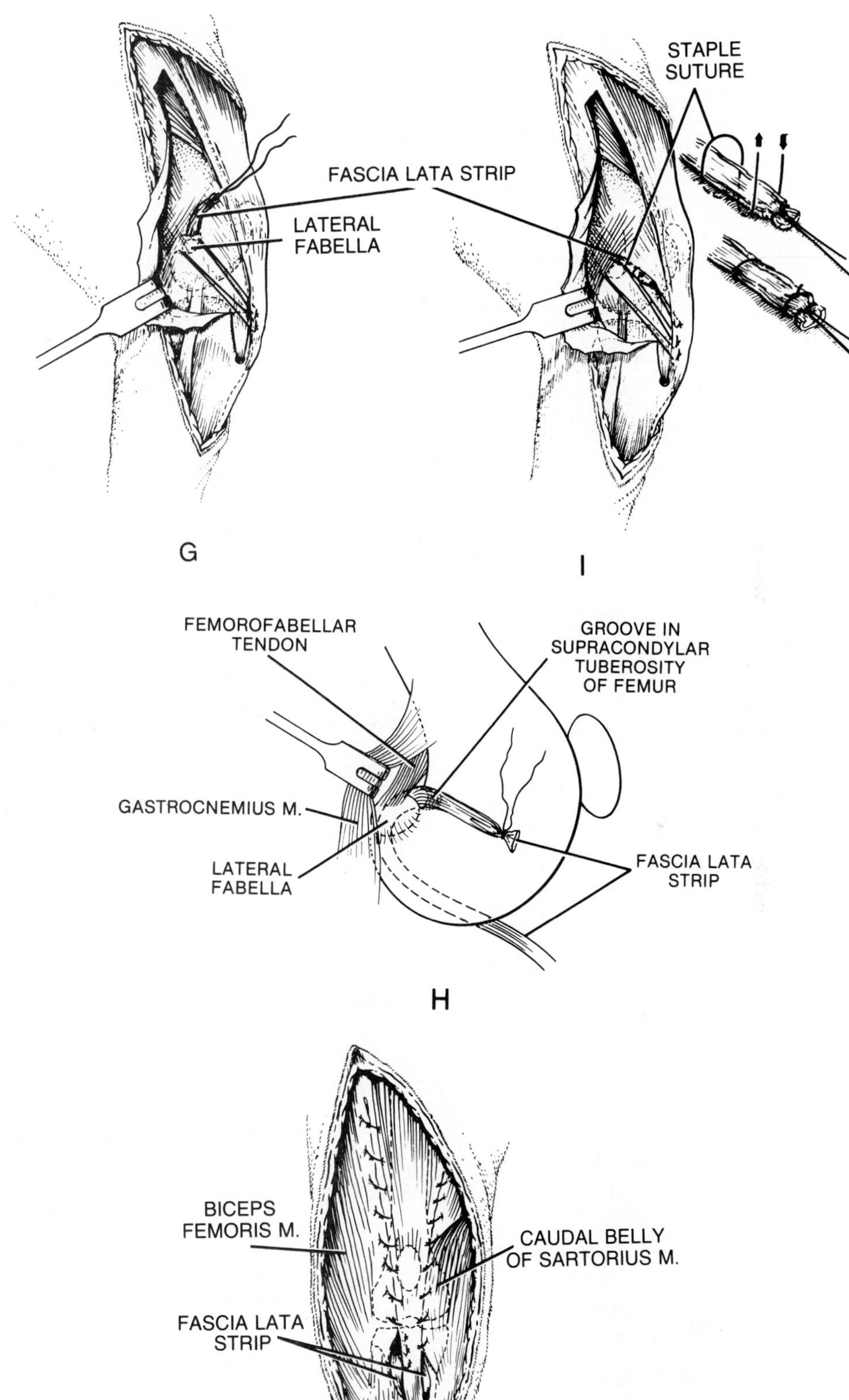

FIGURE 137–27 ***Continued*** *G*, Two sutures of number 2-4 nonabsorbable material are placed from the lateral fabella to the distal patellar tendon and tied tightly to eliminate cranial instability and protect the graft. *H*, The femorofabellar fascia just proximal to the lateral fabella is elevated, and a groove formed in the underlying cortex using a rasp, rongeur, or bone file. *I*, The fascial strip is pulled underneath the femorofabellar fascia and anchored with a staple suture *(inset)*. *J*, The lateral fascial defect is closed, thereby imbricating the lateral retinaculum. (From Brinker WO, et al: *Handbook of Small Animal Orthopedics and Fracture Treatment.* 2nd ed. W.B. Saunders, Philadelphia, 1990, pp 406–407.)

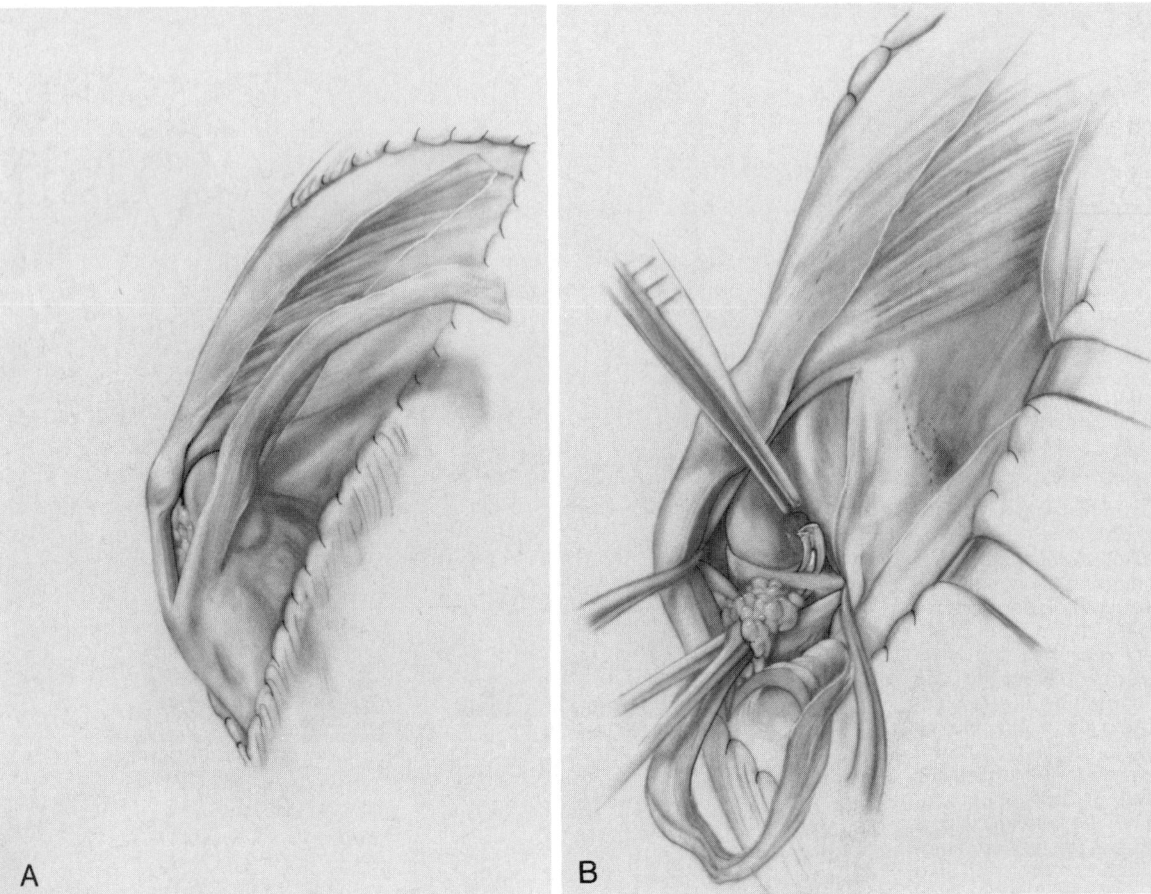

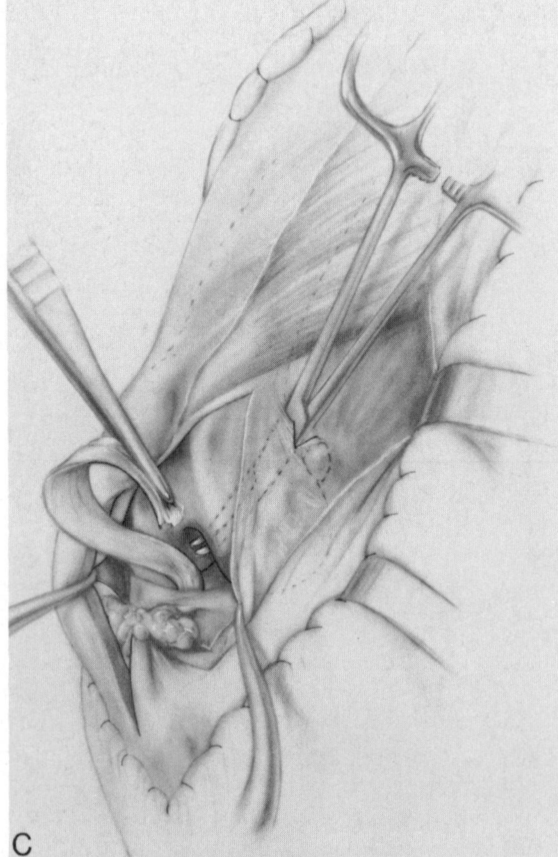

FIGURE 137–28. Modified Hulse under-and-over procedure. *A*, The skin incision is the same as for the Paatsama procedure (see Fig. 137–24*A*). The graft is created by freeing the lateral third of the patellar tendon and a portion of the fibrous retinaculum of the joint capsule and extending the incisions proximally into the fascia lata cranial to the biceps femoris muscle. The graft is freed proximally, dissected from underlying attachments, and wrapped in moistened gauze. *B*, A lateral arthrotomy is used to explore the joint cavity and evaluate the intercondylar notch and menisci. Curved mosquito forceps are passed underneath the fat pad and intermeniscal ligament, and the jaws opened and closed to create a passageway for the graft. The proximal tip of the graft is grasped in the forceps and passed into the joint cavity. The graft is pulled through using thumb forceps, taking care not to twist the graft. *C*, An incision is made in the lateral femorofabellar fascia, and a hemostat passed through the caudal joint capsule and into the intercondylar notch, lateral to the caudal cruciate ligament.

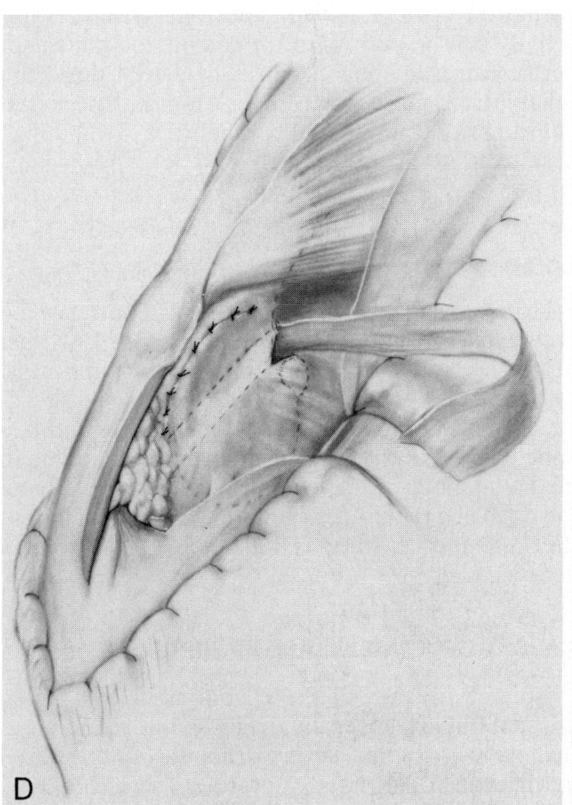

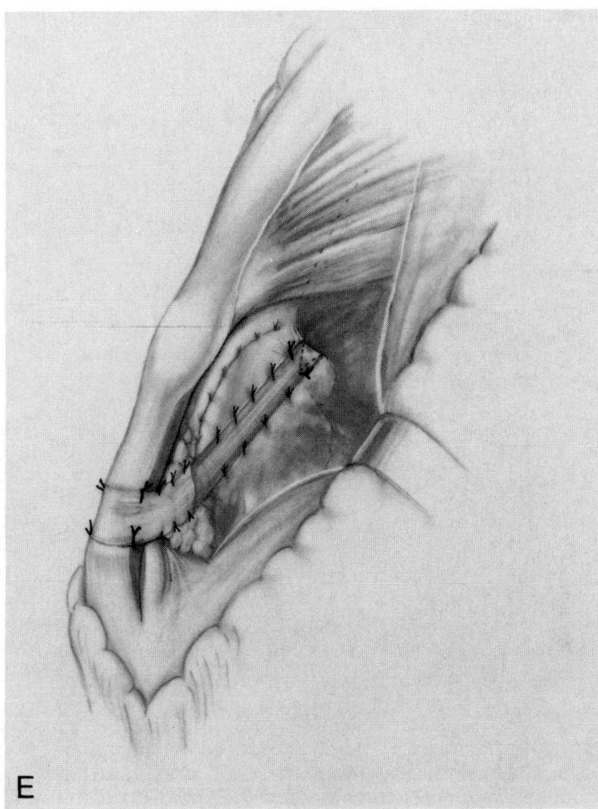

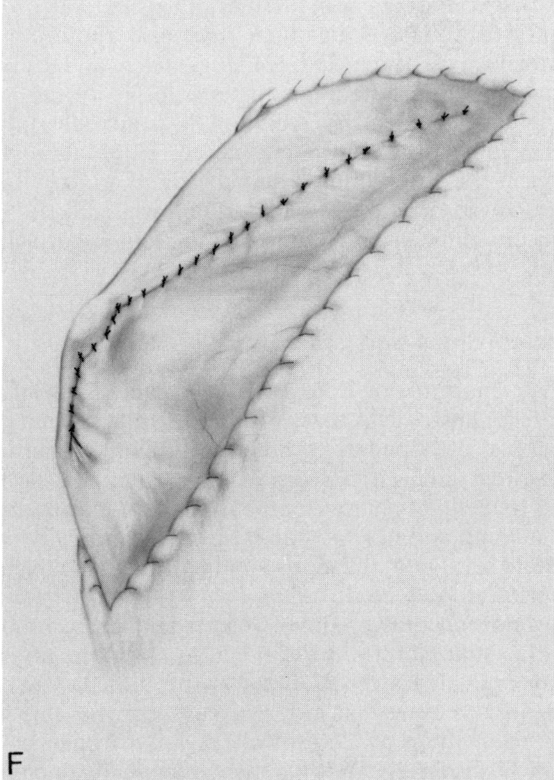

FIGURE 137–28 ***Continued*** *D*, The graft is grasped within the forceps and pulled over the lateral femoral condyle; it is not anchored at this time. The synovial joint capsule is closed with absorbable suture material, and an imbricating suture of size 1 or 2 Maxon is placed from the lateral fabella to the distal portion of the patellar tendon (see Fig. 137–24*J*). This suture eliminates cranial instability and provides temporary protection of the graft. Tightening the suture at this stage stabilizes the joint and eliminates the need to pull excessively on the graft to abolish drawer motion. *E*, The graft is placed within the femorofabellar space, pulled snug, and anchored with two or three sutures of size 0 Maxon. The end of the graft is passed underneath and around the distal insertion of the patellar tendon and sutured back to itself. Interrupted sutures of absorbable material are used to anchor the graft to the lateral aspect of the joint capsule. *F*, The fascial defect is closed using size 2-0 to 0 Maxon, providing additional lateral imbrication, and the remaining closure is routine.

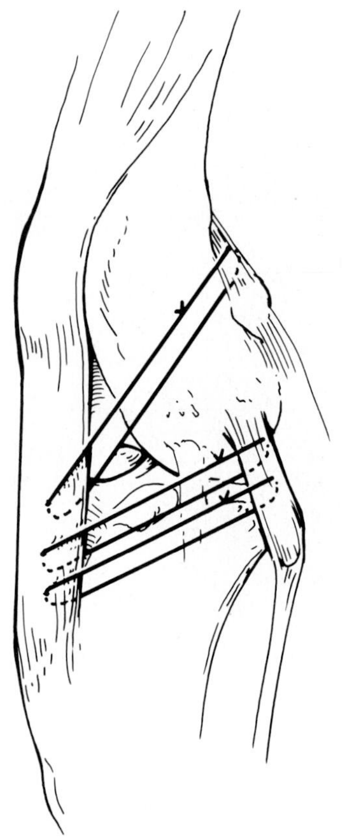

FIGURE 137–29. Extracapsular lateral imbrication technique of Gambardella. Nonabsorbable sutures are used, one from the proximal femorofabellar fascia and two from the lateral collateral ligament all of which are anchored to the distal patellar tendon.

more than 90 per cent of dogs whose stifle joints were stabilized with this technique.[134, 195]

Reported complications with fibular head transposition include fibular head fracture (12.5 per cent) and seroma formation (7.5 per cent).[134] Like other extra-articular procedures, fibular head transposition inhibits internal tibial rotation by tightening lateral supporting structures and creating a hinge-type joint.[153] Internal rotation of the tibia is an inherent component of stifle joint motion and is caused by the geometric configuration of the femoral and tibial joint surfaces. With repeated joint motion and physiological loading, some degree of cranial-caudal joint laxity recurs and is probably related to development of internal tibial rotation and stretching of the lateral imbrication.

Postoperative Management

I routinely apply a modified Robert Jones bandage to minimize swelling and protect the wound for 48 hours postoperatively. Although more prolonged external coaptation is desirable to reduce stress on the graft and graft fixation sites, the deleterious effects of joint immobilization (muscle atrophy, cartilage degeneration, intra-articular scarring) outweigh potential advantages.[147, 163] Fibular head transposition is advantageous in that the graft itself (lateral collateral ligament) and its fixation are considerably more stable than suture techniques and many of the intra-articular graft fixations. Regardless of the method of stabilization, dogs are restricted to short leash walks for at least 6 weeks after surgery. Gradually increasing levels of activity are permitted until 12 weeks postoperatively, when full activity can be permitted for companion animals. High-performance animals, such as field trial dogs, must be rehabilitated more slowly, over a 6-month period, before entering full training and competition. Swimming is the best exercise to strengthen muscles and regain joint motion.

Complications

Experienced veterinary surgeons report few postoperative complications. Infections occur in 1 to 2 per cent of the cases, and an injury or overexertion occasionally causes breakdown of the repair within the first 1 to 2 weeks. If a dog does well postoperatively and becomes lame again months or years later, damage involving the medial meniscus is almost always the cause. Removal of the damaged meniscus is generally successful in resolving the lameness; further stabilization of the joint is not necessary.

CAUDAL CRUCIATE LIGAMENT RUPTURE

Isolated injuries of the caudal cruciate ligament are unusual but are generally diagnosed in young large dogs that have sustained severe trauma.[105] The most likely mechanism for isolated rupture is a direct blow to the cranial tibia, causing a caudal drawer motion and overloading of the ligament. If the joint is extended during injury, a collateral ligament may also rupture.[63] In a retrospective study, 2 of 14 dogs with caudal cruciate ligament rupture had concurrent rupture of the medial collateral ligament.[105] Additional orthopedic injuries, not involving the stifle joint, were present in 7 of the 14 dogs in the latter study. Bony avulsions were evident in 5 of 12 dogs in which radiographs were taken.[105] The majority of avulsions occur from the femoral attachment site.[30, 49, 63, 105, 114]

Clinical Signs and Diagnosis

The majority of dogs with caudal cruciate ligament rupture have a history of major trauma and often multiple orthopedic problems. Hindlimb lameness is consistent and varies from a mild weightbearing lameness to complete nonweightbearing. Pain may be evident on manipulation of the stifle joint. It is critically important to evaluate the entire animal so that concurrent injuries are detected.

Abnormal drawer motion is evident on examination of the stifle joint; however, differentiation of caudal from cranial drawer motion can be difficult. Accurate diagnosis requires an index of suspicion for this injury and recognition of a "neutral" position from which the tibia is displaced. With intact cruciate ligaments, the tibial tuberosity forms a distinct prominence on the cranial surface of the stifle joint. Loss of the cranial cruciate ligament can cause cranial subluxation and protrusion of the tibial tuberosity, whereas rupture of

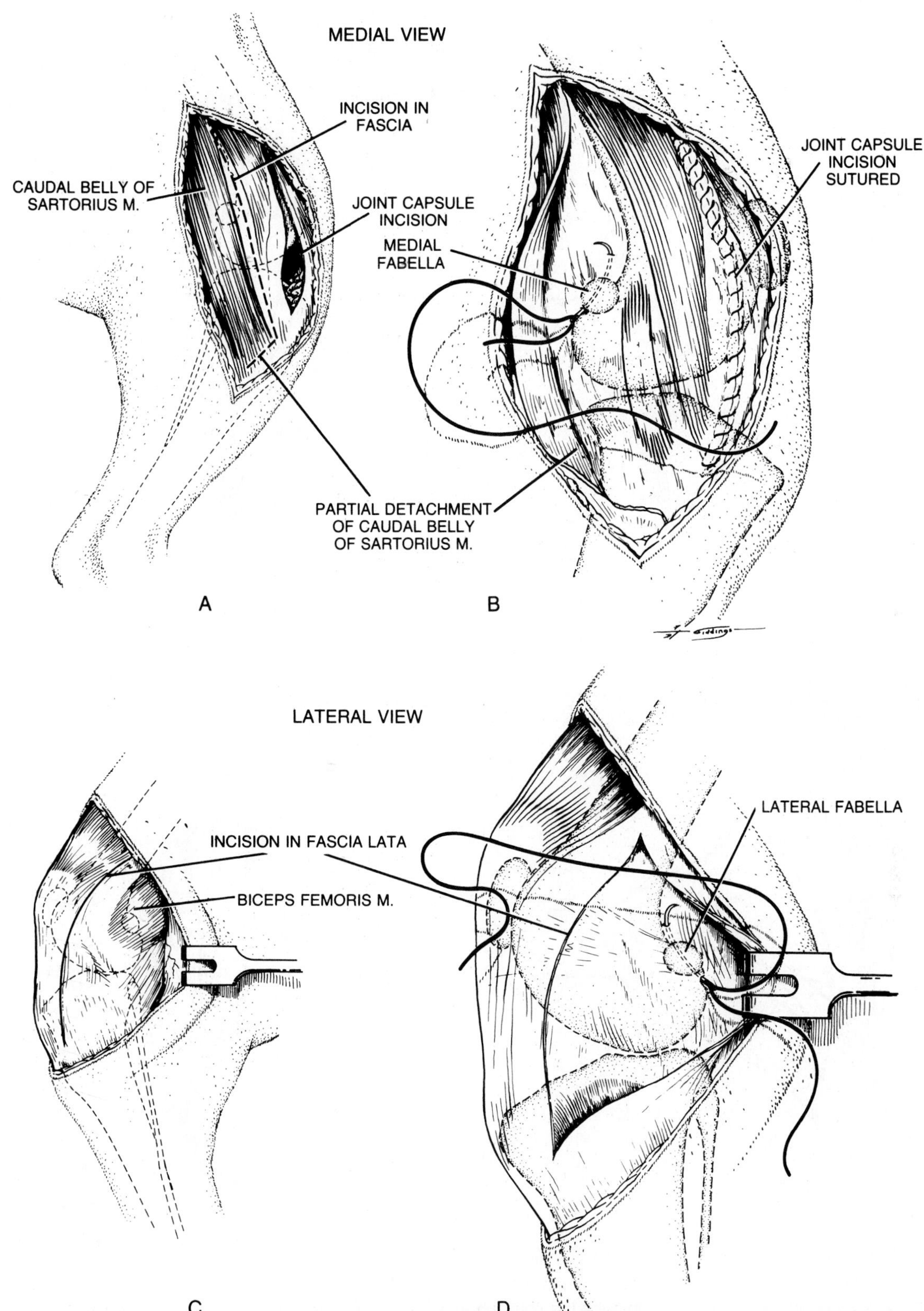

FIGURE 137–30. Three-in-one procedure of Flo. *A*, After a craniomedial skin incision and medial arthrotomy for joint inspection, the fascia is incised along the cranial border of the caudal belly of the sartorius, partially freeing it from its tibial attachment. *B*, The joint capsule incision is closed, and braided polyester suture (size 0-1 for small dogs, 1-4 for larger dogs) is passed behind the medial fabella. *C*, The skin is retracted laterally, and an incision is made in the fascia over the lateral aspect of the joint. *D*, The biceps femoris is retracted caudally to expose the lateral joint capsule and the lateral fabella. A double length of heavy polyester suture (as in *B*) is passed around the lateral fabella. The suture is cut near the needle to leave two independent strands.

Illustration continued on following page

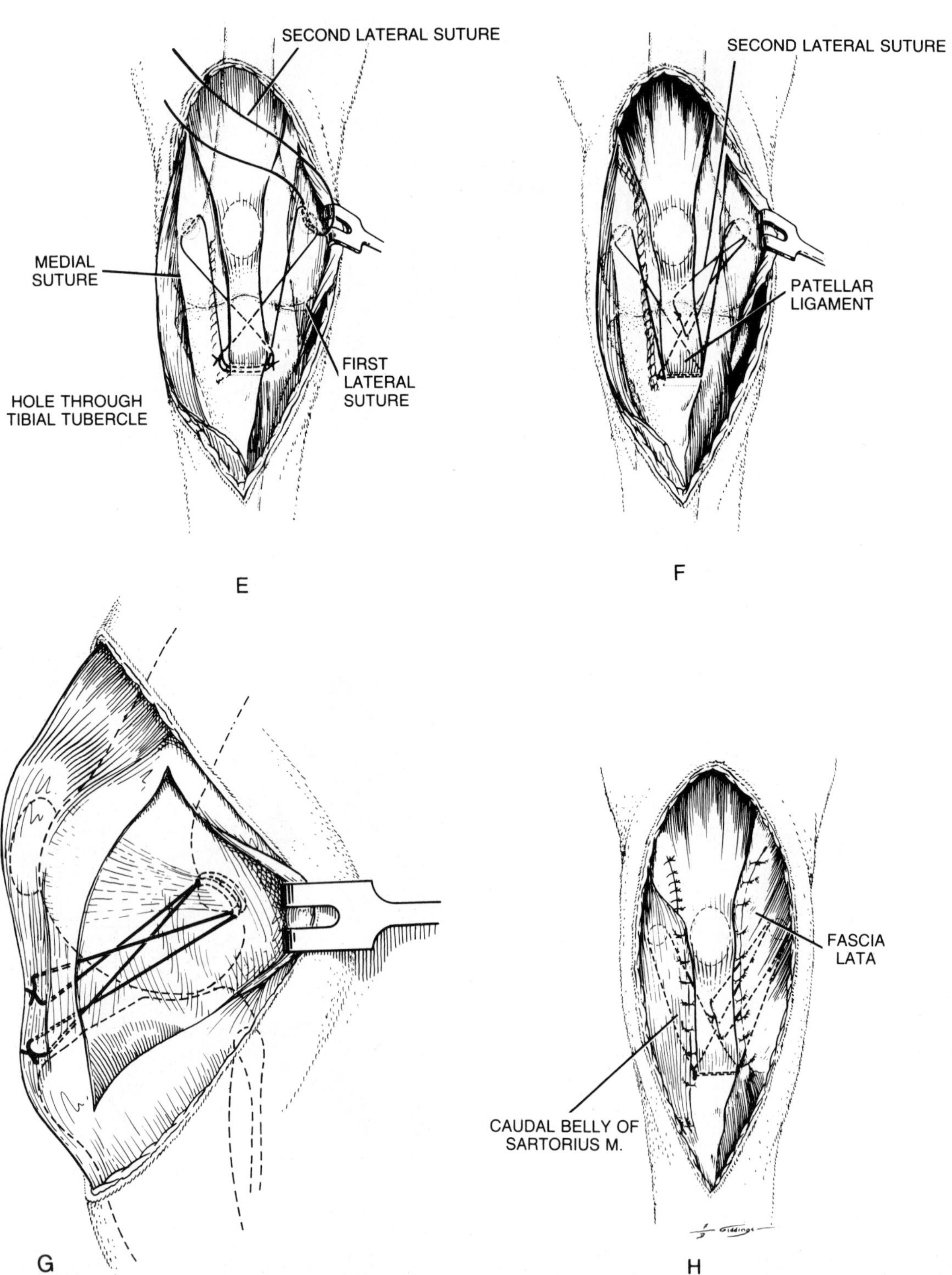

FIGURE 137–30 ***Continued*** *E*, A hole is drilled through the tibial tubercle close to the attachment of the patellar tendon, and the medial suture and one of the lateral sutures are passed through the hole. *F*, With the joint in slight flexion, the sutures are tightened sufficiently to eliminate joint laxity; the lateral suture is tied before the medial one is tightened. The second lateral suture is placed through the midportion of the patellar tendon to further imbricate the joint. *G*, Lateral view. Rather than place the sutures through a hole in the tibial tuberosity, they all can be attached to the distal patellar tendon, as shown. *H*, The detached portion of the caudal sartorius is sutured with the medial fascia to the patellar tendon proximally to the level of the patella. From that point proximally, the sartorius is not included in the medial fascial closure. The fascia lata is overlapped laterally to place the biceps muscle under increased tension. (From Brinker WO, et al: *Handbook of Small Animal Orthopedics and Fracture Treatment*. 2nd ed. W.B. Saunders, Philadelphia, 1990, pp 401–402.)

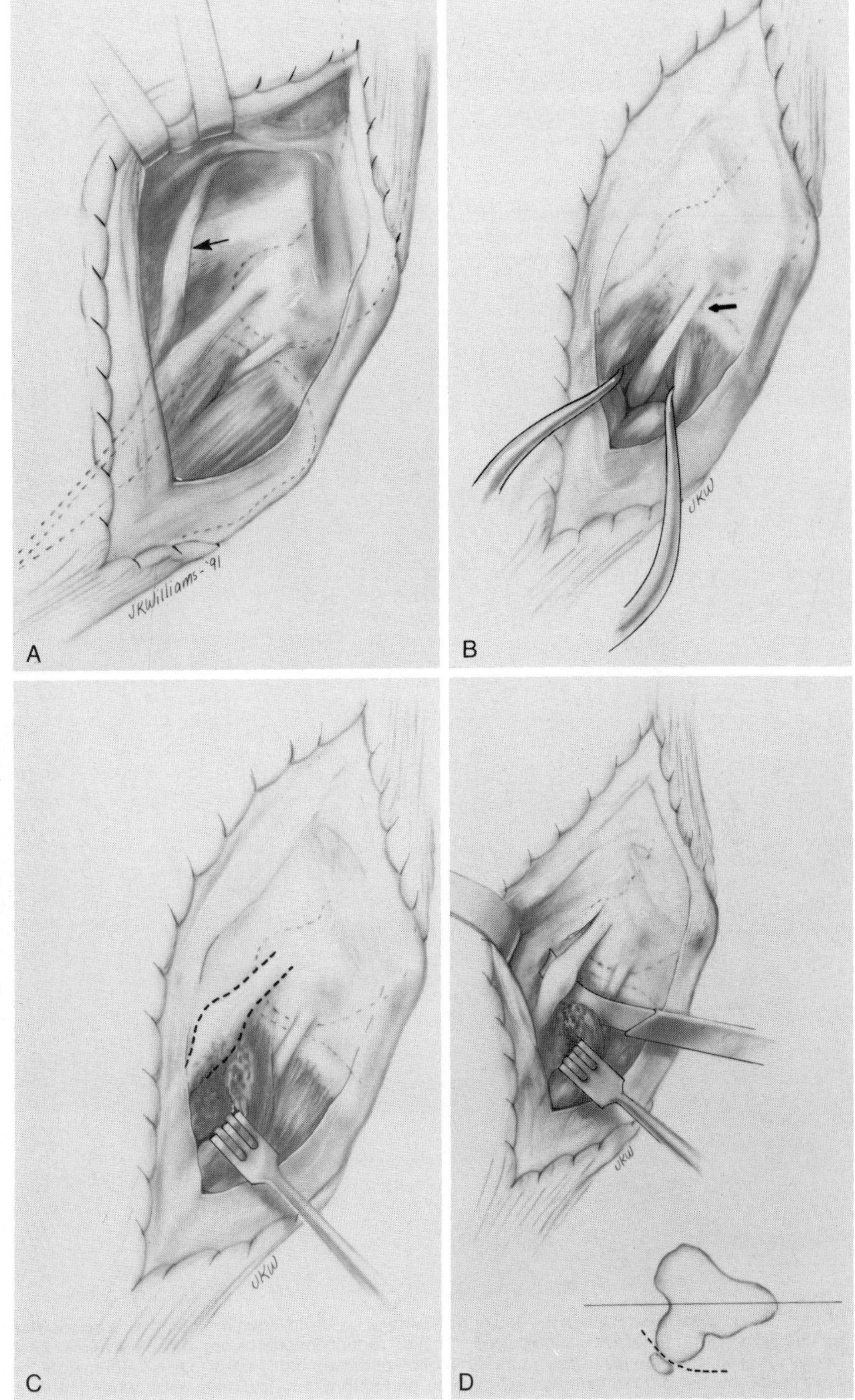

FIGURE 137–31. Fibular head transposition. *A*, A lateral skin incision and lateral arthrotomy are used to inspect the joint and resect damaged menisci, if necessary. The fascia lata and biceps femoris muscle are retracted caudally exposing the fibular head, lateral collateral ligament, and underlying muscles. This fascial incision should be extended distally 3 to 4 cm from the tibial plateau to provide adequate exposure of the muscles arising from the proximal tibia. The fibular nerve must be identified and protected. The nerve obliquely crosses the lateral head of the gastrocnemius muscle and then passes between the flexor hallucis longus caudally and the peroneus longus muscle cranially, to enter the muscles of the cranial part of the crus *(arrow)*. *B*, The peroneus longus muscle is separated from the tibialis cranialis muscle, which is further elevated from the proximal tibia until the tendon of the long digital extensor is exposed *(arrow)*. Small Gelpi retractors are invaluable to aid in retraction during this stage of the operation. *C*, The peroneus longus is retracted cranially, and the lateral collateral ligament is isolated by making longitudinal incisions cranial and caudal to the ligament (broken lines). The peroneus longus has a partial attachment to the fibular head, which often must be elevated. *D*, The fibular head is mobilized by severing the ligaments that attach the fibular head to the tibia. These attachments can be diffuse, and considerable fibrous tissue may be present in dogs with chronic instability. The fibular head is not directly lateral to the tibia but is at the caudolateral margin of the tibial plateau *(inset)*, so the dissection must proceed at an angle between the fibular head and the tibia. Failure to appreciate this orientation frequently results in fractures of the fibular head. A curved meniscus knife is shown dissecting the attachments between the tibia and fibular head.

Illustration continued on following page

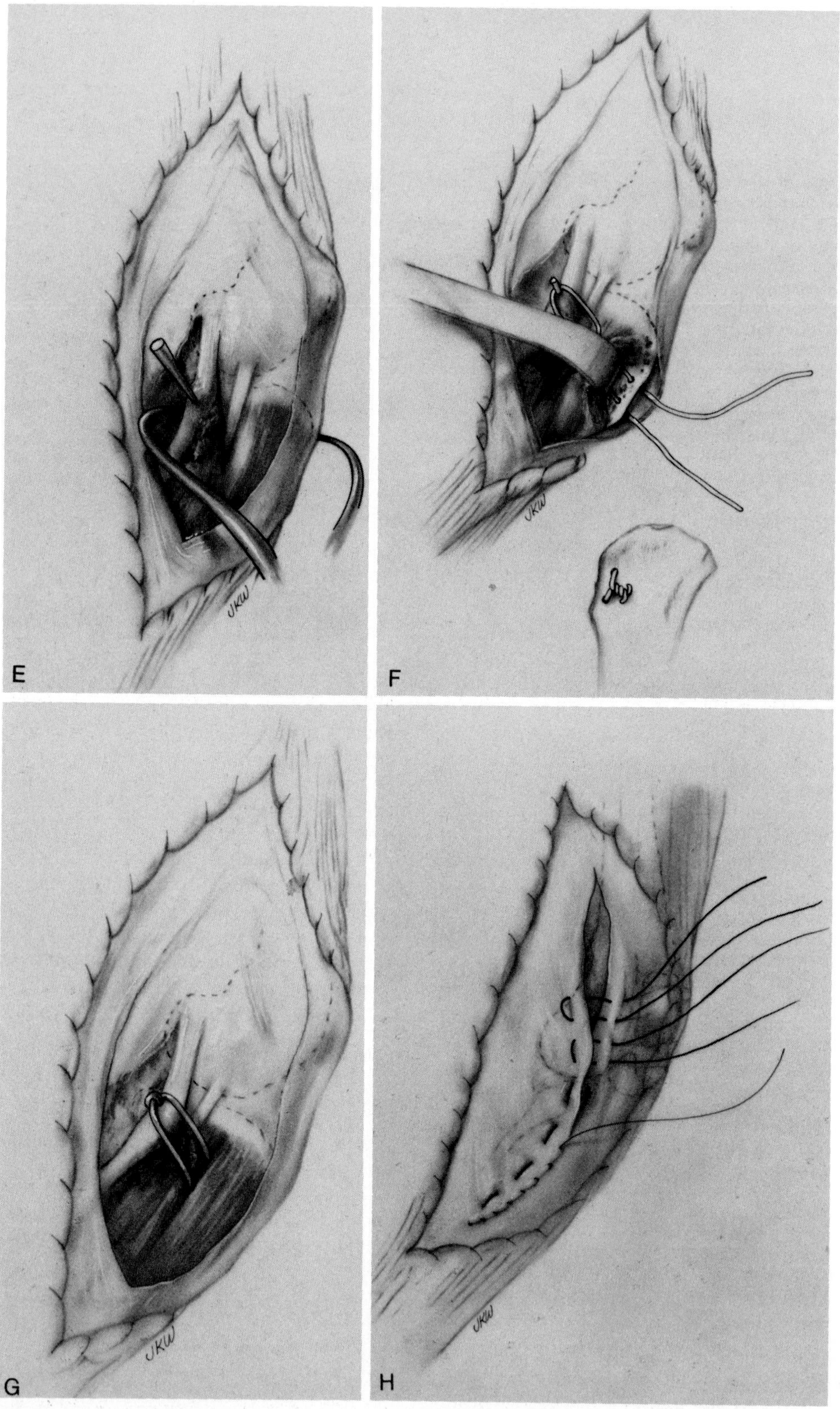

FIGURE 137–31 ***Continued*** *E*, When the fibular head/lateral collateral ligament complex is adequately mobilized, a Kirschner wire is driven into the fibular head to facilitate manipulation. Pointed reduction forceps are extremely helpful at this point to hold the fibular head in a cranial location while the joint is tested for elimination of drawer motion. The joint is held in slight flexion, *with the tibia rotated externally*, while the fibular head is manipulated into position and held with reduction forceps. When the joint is stable, the Kirschner wire is driven into the tibia to fix the fibular head in position. *F*, Two holes 2 mm in diameter are drilled into the tibial tuberosity, and an 18- or 20-gauge wire passed through the holes, underneath or through the tibialis cranialis muscle and around the pin, with the free ends exiting the medial surface of the tibial tuberosity. The wire is twisted tight enough to abolish any remaining drawer motion, then cut and bent over *(inset)*. *G*, The Kirschner wire is then bent over and driven flush with the fibular head using a pin set. *H*, The biceps fascia is advanced and sutured to the cranial fascia using a vest-over-pants pattern to imbricate and further stabilize the joint. The free edge of biceps fascia is sutured to underlying fascia using a continuous pattern, and the remaining closure is routine.

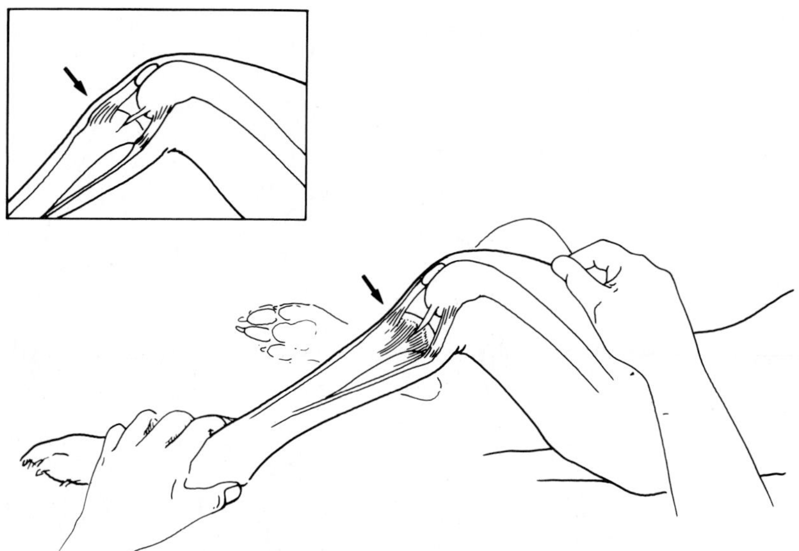

FIGURE 137–32. Tibial sag caused by rupture of the caudal cruciate ligament. Caudal displacement of the tibial tuberosity results in a flat or even concave appearance of the cranial surface of the stifle joint, compared with the normally prominent appearance of the tibial tuberosity.

the caudal cruciate ligament results in caudal tibial displacement and reduced prominence of the tibial tuberosity, or "tibial sag" (Fig. 137–32). It is important to observe the position of the tibial tuberosity in animals with abnormal cranial-caudal displacement. With caudal cruciate ligament rupture, the tibia is often subluxated caudally because of the pull of the hamstring muscles. When the joint is first examined, it may appear that cranial drawer motion is present because the tibia displaces cranially, when in fact it is simply being reduced into a normal position. It is also helpful to note the position of the fingers while testing drawer motion. If the thumb placed behind the fibular head begins in a position caudal to the thumb over the lateral fabella, it is likely that the tibia is caudally displaced because of caudal cruciate ligament rupture, and cranial tibial motion is actually reduction into a normal position. In these circumstances, a sharp and distinct endpoint to the drawer motion suggests an intact cranial cruciate ligament and supports the diagnosis of caudal cruciate ligament rupture.

Radiographs of the stifle joint are necessary to detect fractures or avulsion fragments and to evaluate degenerative joint disease in chronic cases.

Treatment

The paucity of cases of isolated caudal cruciate ligament rupture makes recommendations about treatment unreliable. All reports of clinical caudal cruciate ligament rupture describe attempts at surgical stabilization of the joint.[49, 105, 114] The results of surgical correction are good and bear little correlation to the type of repair technique or the degree of stabilization achieved.[105] Two studies using normal dogs showed that severance of the caudal cruciate ligament caused temporary lameness, and degenerative joint changes were minimal after 6 months.[85, 165] In a retrospective study of clinical patients, 4 of 14 dogs with caudal cruciate ligament rupture had been lame for 3 months or longer; 2 of the 4 dogs were operated on and were available for follow-up examination 6 months and 7 years postoperatively, respectively, and both regained a clinically normal gait.[105]

Given that caudal cruciate ligament severance causes minimal pathology within the stifle joint and that dogs studied experimentally all recovered a normal gait, it seems prudent to recommend a trial period of at least 1 month before surgical stabilization of joints with tears of this ligament, especially in cats, smaller dogs, geriatric individuals, or those with significant medical problems. For active large dogs, especially working and hunting dogs, joint exploration is recommended to inspect the menisci, cranial cruciate ligament, and articular surfaces. Acute avulsion injuries (from the femur) are operated on immediately because secure fixation of the avulsed segment is generally feasible, thus restoring normal function. Extra-articular stabilization procedures are recommended for tears of the caudal cruciate ligament. The prognosis with surgical stabilization is favorable.

Surgical Techniques

Avulsion Injuries. Avulsion fractures most commonly occur from the femoral attachment site. Exposure is readily accomplished through a lateral arthrotomy, and fixation using a lag screw, divergent Kirschner wires, or wire suture is recommended (Fig. 137–33). Avulsion from the tibial attachment site is stabilized using the same techniques; exposure is more difficult and requires an approach to the caudomedial compartment of the joint.[160]

Tears of the Caudal Cruciate Ligament. A procedure for extra-articular stabilization is illustrated in Figure 137–34.[30, 49] Stabilization on the medial side of the joint includes imbrication of the caudomedial joint capsule and placement of a large imbricating suture from the proximal patellar tendon through a hole in the caudomedial corner of the tibia. On the lateral side, the caudal joint capsule is imbricated with mattress sutures, and another large imbricating suture is placed from the proximal patellar tendon through a hole in the fibular head. Additional support is supplied by a fascia lata

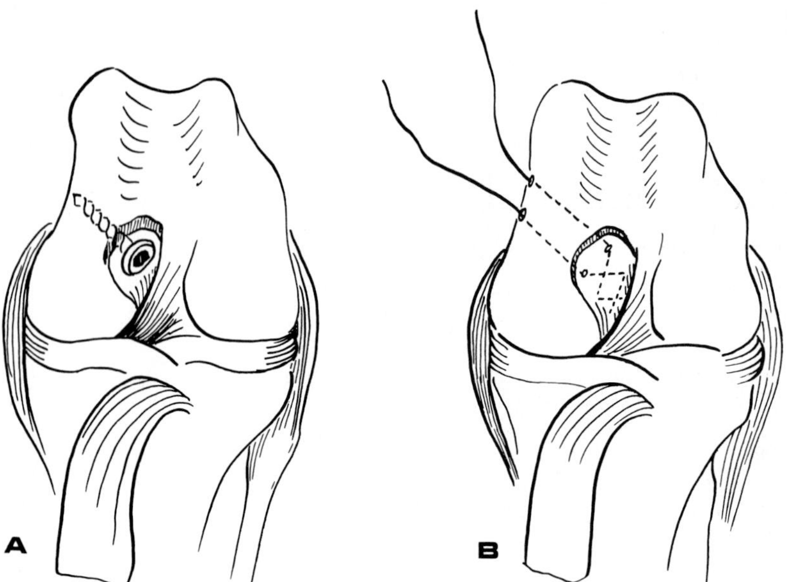

FIGURE 137–33. Fixation techniques for avulsion fractures of the femoral attachment of the caudal cruciate ligament. *A*, Lag screw fixation. *B*, Nonabsorbable suture fixation.

transfer, which is pedicled at the proximal aspect of the patella and anchored to the fibular head. The imbricating sutures and fascia lata are placed to resist caudal drawer motion.

Aftercare. A padded bandage is applied for 48 hours postoperatively to minimize swelling and protect the wound. Exercise is restricted to short leash walks for 3 weeks; passive range of motion exercise is helpful during this period. After 3 weeks, longer walks and limited free activity are permissible. Full athletic activity is not permitted until 3 months after surgery.

COLLATERAL LIGAMENT INJURIES

Isolated collateral ligament injuries are unusual. More often, collateral ligament injury is a component of a "deranged" or luxated stifle joint in which multiple ligaments and often menisci are damaged. I have diagnosed isolated rupture of the medial collateral ligament in sight hounds used for coursing competitions.

Injuries that damage ligament fibers are termed *sprains*. First-degree sprains are mild and cause minimal instability. Second-degree sprains involve stretching and

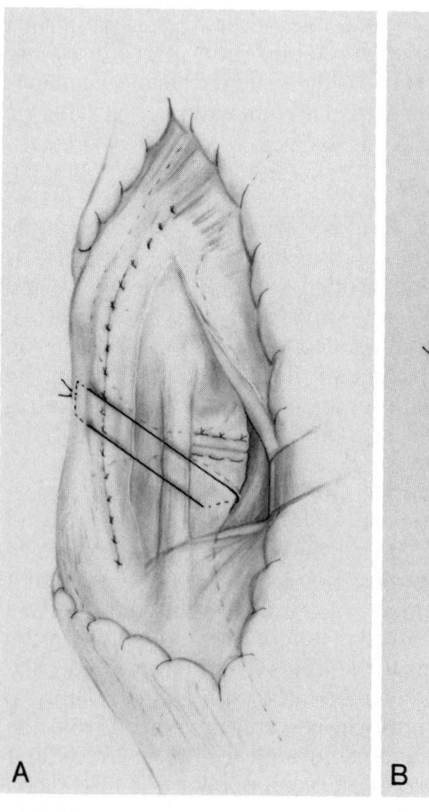

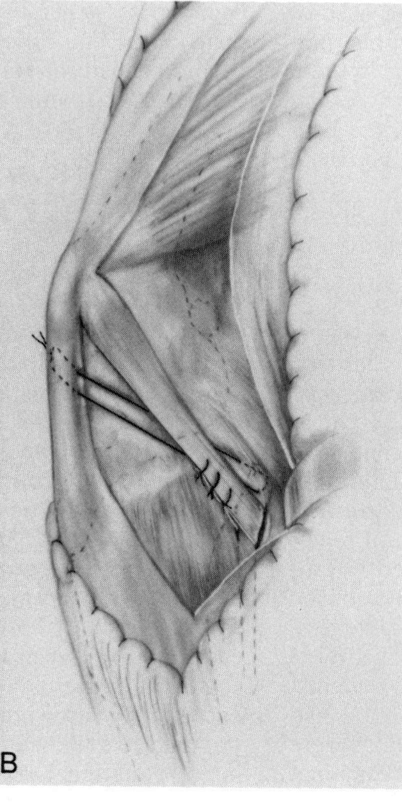

FIGURE 137–34. Extra-articular stabilization method for intrasubstance tears of the caudal cruciate ligament. *A*, A craniomedial skin incision is followed by a medial arthrotomy to permit inspection of the cruciate ligaments and menisci. The caudal belly of the sartorius is partially detached and retracted caudally, permitting imbrication of the caudomedial joint capsule and exposure of the caudal tibial plateau. A heavy nonabsorbable suture (1 or 2 polypropylene) is placed from the patellar tendon, just distal to the patella, through a hole in the caudomedial corner of the tibial plateau, and tightened to eliminate caudal drawer motion. *B*, The skin is retracted laterally, the biceps fascia is incised, and the biceps femoris muscle retracted caudally, exposing the lateral joint capsule, lateral collateral ligament, and fibular head. The capsule is imbricated caudal to the ligament using 2-0 absorbable suture material and a heavy nonabsorbable suture (1 or 2 polypropylene) is placed from the patellar tendon, just distal to the patella, through a hole in the fibular head, and tightened to further stabilize the joint. The latter imbrication suture can be augmented with a flap of fascia lata pedicled at the proximal patella.

tearing of ligament fibers and some degree of instability, although the ligament is grossly intact. Third-degree sprains are complete ruptures of the ligament.[46, 67] Grading the degree of instability helps establish the severity of ligament injury and organize treatment.

Clinical Signs and Diagnosis

Patients usually have a history of acute trauma and lameness, which may be severe, depending on the degree of injury. The animal may have only a mild limp, depending on the time after injury. The stifle joint is usually tender, and various degrees of swelling are present over the involved ligament.

Medial Collateral Ligament

The valgus stress test is used to evaluate the medial collateral ligament. With the stifle joint extended, one hand is used to stabilize the femur and palpate the medial joint line while the other hand is used to abduct the tibia, thereby applying a valgus stress (Fig. 137–35). The medial joint space opening, as well as the stiffness of the motion limit (soft or hard endpoint), is estimated and compared with the contralateral joint. When the medial collateral ligament is completely torn, increased external tibial rotation is possible with the stifle flexed.[30]

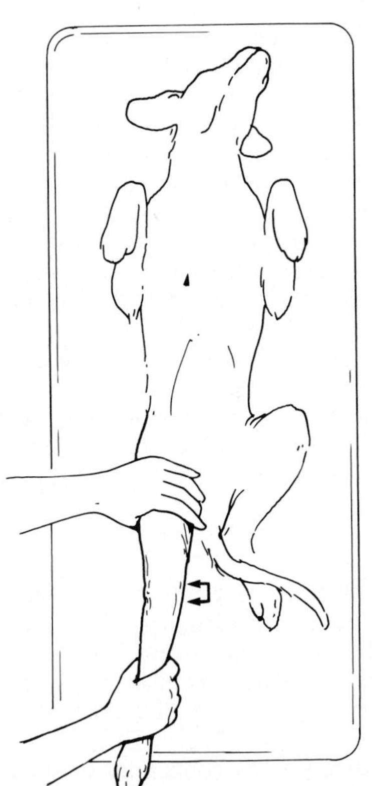

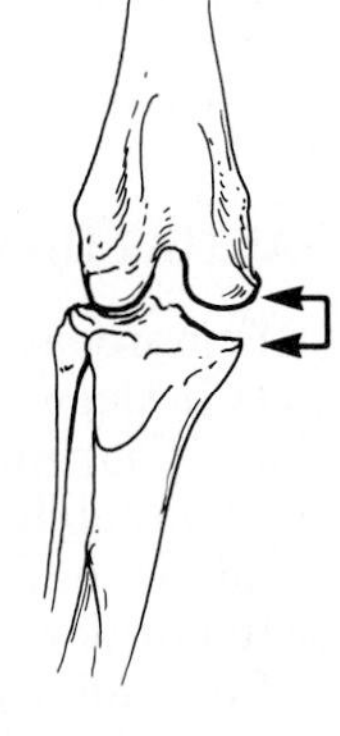

FIGURE 137–35. Valgus stress test for evaluation of the medial collateral ligament. With the joint held in extension, the tibia is abducted, thereby stressing the ligament and opening the medial joint space. Isolated rupture of the ligament causes only slight increases in valgus angulation. Marked valgus instability indicates a combined injury involving the medial collateral ligament and one or both cruciate ligaments.

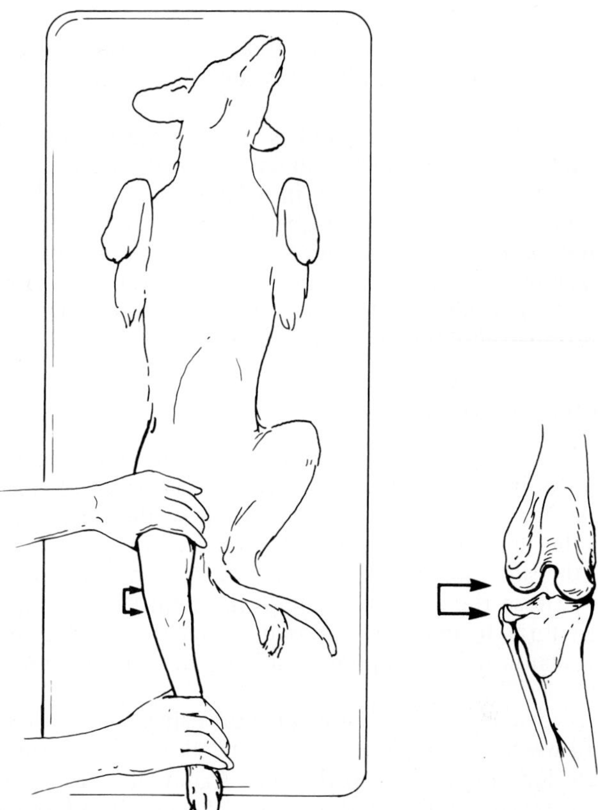

FIGURE 137–36. Varus stress test for evaluation of the lateral collateral ligament. With the joint held in extension, the tibia is adducted, thereby stressing the ligament and opening the lateral joint space. Isolated rupture of the ligament causes only slight increases in varus angulation. Marked varus instability suggests a combined injury involving the lateral collateral ligament and one or both cruciate ligaments.

Lateral Collateral Ligament

The varus stress test is used to evaluate the integrity of the lateral collateral ligament. With the stifle joint held in extension, one hand stabilizes the femur and simultaneously palpates the lateral joint line. The other hand is used to adduct the tibia, thereby applying a varus stress to the joint (Fig. 137–36). The lateral joint space opening, as well as stiffness of the motion limit, is estimated and compared with the contralateral joint.

Radiographs are useful to detect avulsion injuries and determine the presence of degenerative joint disease. Stress radiographs can be taken to document the instability.

Treatment

Because no clinical studies have investigated isolated collateral ligament injuries in dogs, recommendations for treatment are based on clinical experience and research literature. The concept of primary repair of torn collateral ligaments has been supported by experimental studies,[42, 146] and immediate surgical repair of second- and third-degree injuries in active large dogs has been recommended.[30] In humans, conservative treatment of isolated medial collateral ligament tears has been successful,[86, 99] and numerous animal studies involving complete severance of this ligament have demonstrated that conservative treatment of isolated ligament injury produced better results than surgical repair and immobilization.[73, 222–224]

Based on the latter studies, it is recommended that isolated tears of either collateral ligament be managed conservatively. One week in a lateral splint is advised to limit excessive movement, followed by 6 weeks of limited activity (leash walks only). If lameness and instability persist, ligament reconstruction is advised. Acute avulsion injuries with substantial bone fragments are repaired immediately.

Operative Techniques

A medial or lateral parapatellar incision is made, depending on the ligament involved. The medial collateral ligament is exposed by incision of the deep fascia of the thigh along the cranial border of the caudal belly of the sartorius muscle. The muscle is retracted caudally to expose the medial collateral ligament.[160] The lateral collateral ligament is exposed by incision and caudal retraction of the aponeurosis of the biceps femoris muscle.[159]

Avulsion fragments are repaired using a small screw and washer, a small screw and spiked washer, or divergent Kirschner wires. If the bony fragment is disrupted, a screw and spiked metal plate may be considered to stabilize the ligament attachment site (Fig. 137–37). Intrasubstance tears can be sutured using a locking loop pattern; however, these repairs are invariably tenuous, especially in chronic cases, and the suture repair is protected with a screw and figure-eight support (Fig. 137–38).

The joint is protected in a lateral splint for 1 week after surgery, followed by 6 weeks of restricted activity (leash walks only). The prognosis after repair of isolated collateral ligament tears is favorable.

STIFLE LUXATION

Stifle luxation, or derangement of the stifle, refers to severe injuries in which numerous ligaments, the joint capsule, and often the menisci have been damaged. The most common combination of injuries is both cruciate ligaments and the medial collateral ligament.[21] Because stifle luxation is the result of a severe trauma, it is imperative that animals be completely examined for additional injuries. Thoracic radiographs are important to rule out contusions, pneumothorax, rib fractures, and diaphragmatic hernia.

Diagnosis is based on thorough palpation of the joint under general anesthesia. Because multiple ligaments are involved, the results of palpation can be confusing. It is helpful to hold the joint in extension and gently apply varus and valgus stresses to test the collateral ligaments. Drawer motion is tested with the joint held in slight flexion and neutral rotation. Confirmation of which structures are damaged requires joint exploration. Radiographs are helpful to identify avulsion fractures, and stress views can be used to document instability.

Cats and small dogs have been successfully treated using transarticular pinning to provide temporary stabilization.[216] The most frequent complication was pin migration. Splintage of the limb in a Schroeder-Thomas splint for 3 to 4 weeks also has been successful in cats.[221] Extra-articular suture techniques and joint immobilization via external fixation were successful in 12 dogs and 1 cat.[21] Meticulous reconstruction of damaged ligaments followed by external splintage also has been successful in restoring limb function, even in large dogs.[30, 96]

Operative Technique

Joint exposure must provide for access to both the medial and lateral compartments. The skin incision is started laterally over the distal femur, curves across the patellar tendon, and extends distally over the proximal medial tibia.[161] A lateral arthrotomy is used to inspect the joint surfaces, cruciate ligaments, and meniscal attachments. If the injury is recent, the menisci usually are not damaged, but their ligamentous attachments to the tibia and joint capsule may be ruptured.[30] Meniscal attachments are sutured with 3–0 monofilament absorbable suture material. In large dogs, I reconstruct the cranial cruciate ligament with an autogenous patellar tendon/fascia lata graft.[97, 190] The collateral ligaments, if ruptured, are repaired as described previously. If the caudal cruciate ligament is ruptured, extra-articular stabilization is provided using heavy monofilament suture material, as described previously. The joint capsule is carefully imbricated to provide additional stabilization, and the remaining wound closed routinely.

The limb is protected in a lateral splint for 2 weeks, followed by exercise restriction (leash walks only) for an additional 4 weeks. Passive range of motion exercise and whirlpool therapy are helpful in the early postoperative period. The prognosis is favorable, considering the severity of these injuries. The joints lose some range of motion but become quite stable as the result of extensive periarticular fibrosis within 8 to 12 weeks after surgery. The owners can expect good limb function; however, some degree of degenerative joint disease develops, and occasional stiffness and mild lameness are common.

Chronic severe derangement of the stifle joint with advanced osteoarthrosis is best managed by arthrodesis (see Chapter 140) or amputation (see Chapter 141).

PATELLAR LUXATION

Femoropatellar instability is a common cause of lameness in dogs. The condition varies from complete, irreducible luxation of the patella and severe lameness to mild instability without associated clinical signs. The luxation may be intermittent, lateral or medial, traumatic or developmental.

The most common diagnosis is congenital or developmental medial patellar luxation in small dogs. Medial patellar luxation in large dogs is now a relatively frequent diagnosis.[30] A grading scheme for medial patellar luxation is described (Table 137–1). Cats also develop patellar luxation, usually medial, but much less commonly than dogs.[70, 106, 122] The luxation in cats is generally

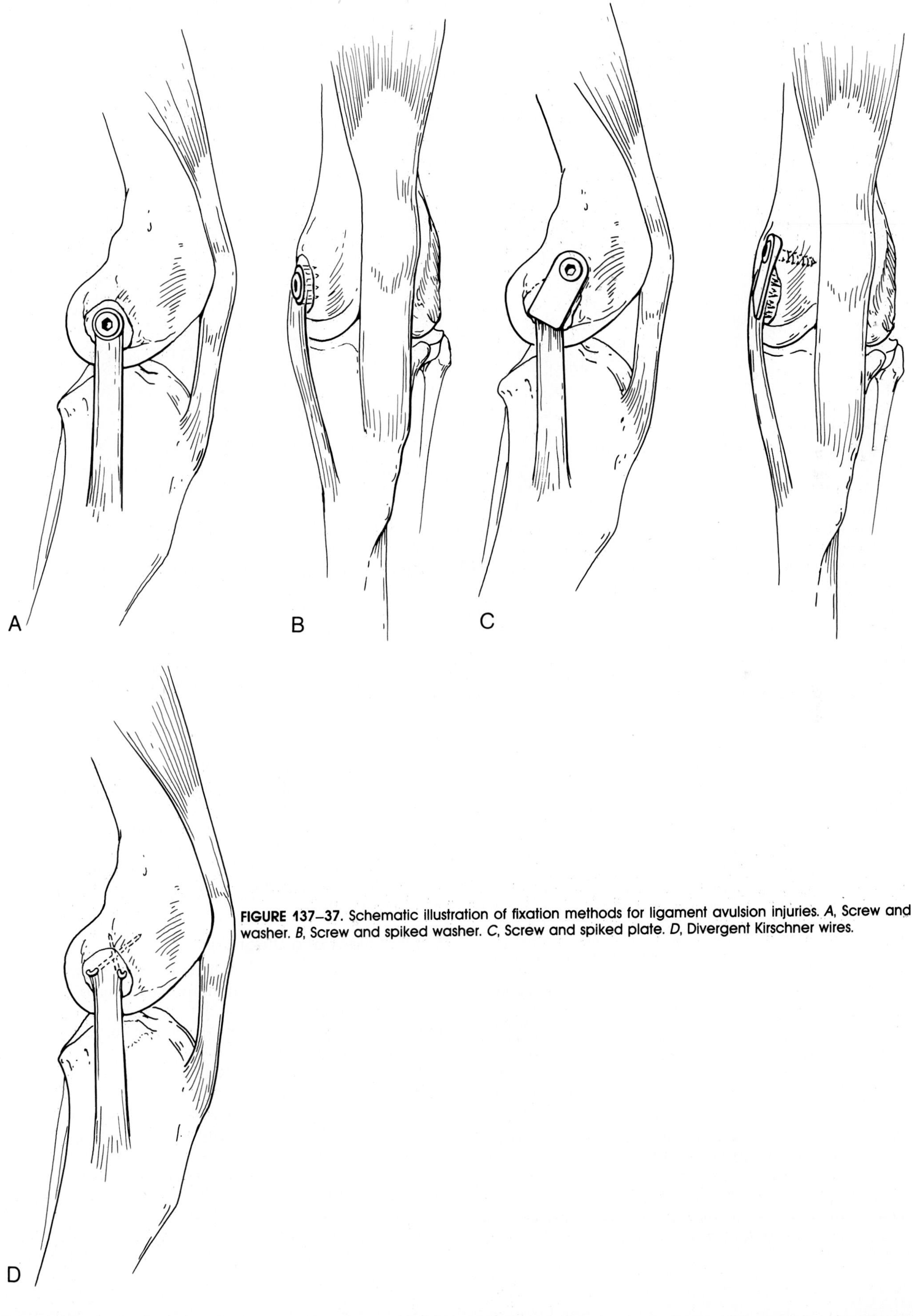

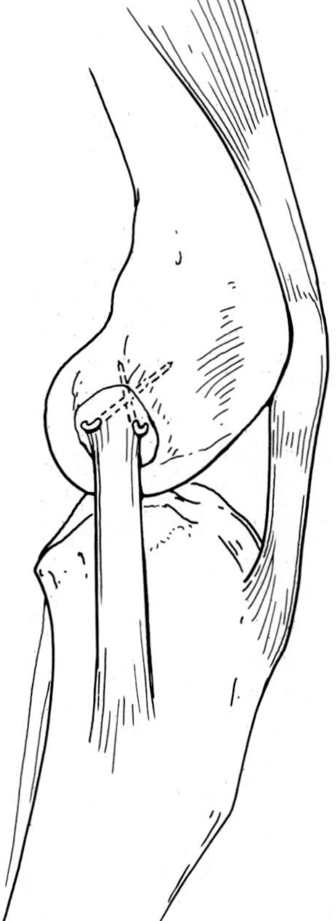

FIGURE 137–37. Schematic illustration of fixation methods for ligament avulsion injuries. *A*, Screw and washer. *B*, Screw and spiked washer. *C*, Screw and spiked plate. *D*, Divergent Kirschner wires.

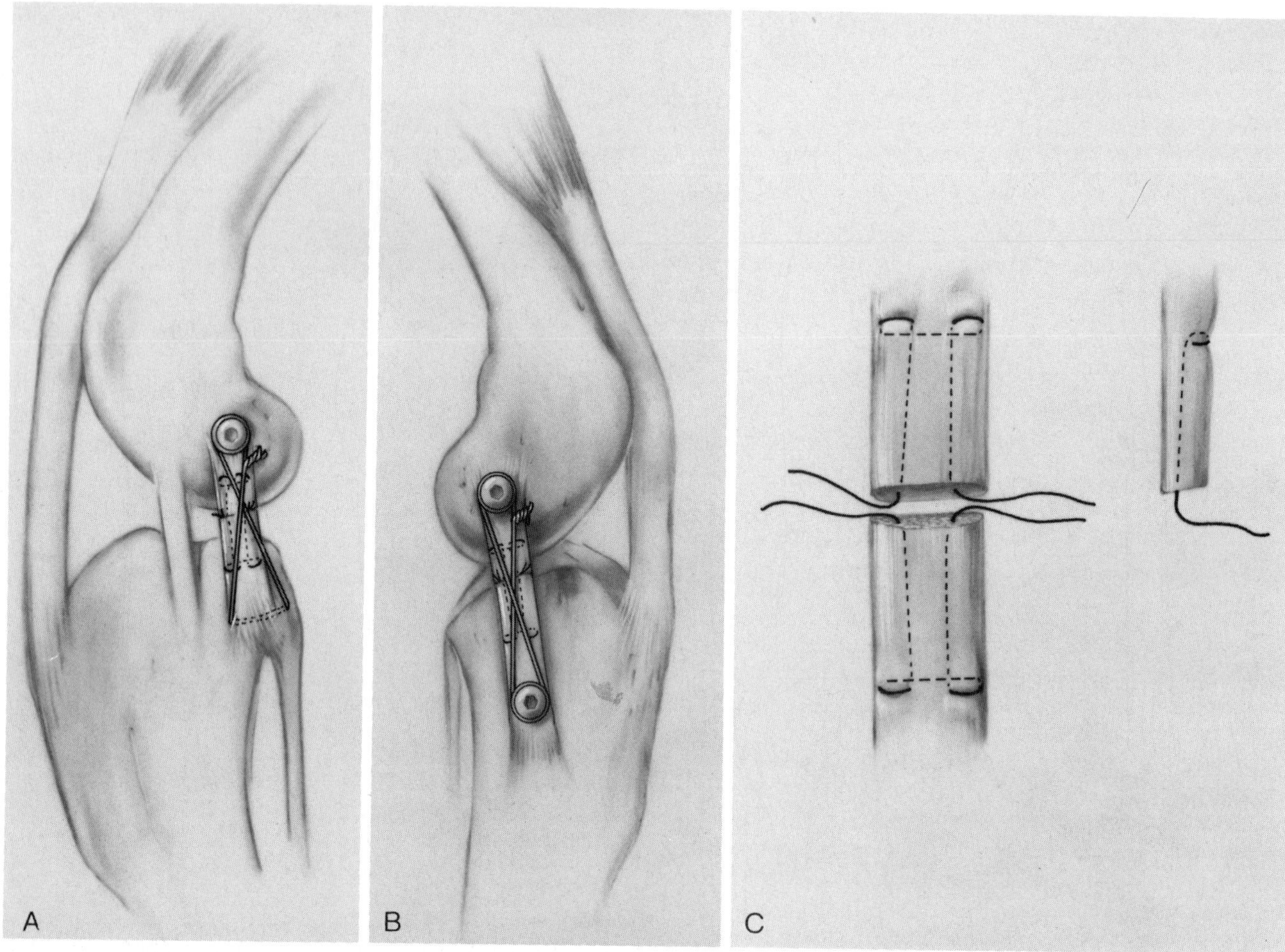

FIGURE 137–38. Locking loop suture repair of intrasubstance tears of the collateral ligaments, protected by figure-eight wire suture. *A*, Lateral collateral ligament. *B*, Medial collateral ligament. *C*, Locking loop pattern for tendon and ligament repair. Note that the transverse bite must be superficial to the longitudinal suture strands for the repair to be effective.

TABLE 137–1. GRADING SYSTEM FOR MEDIAL PATELLAR LUXATION

Grade 1:	The patella can be luxated medially when the stifle joint is held in full extension. There is no crepitation or bony deformity. Clinical signs are not present or occur very infrequently.
Grade 2:	Spontaneous luxation occurs with clinical signs of a nonpainful, "skipping" type of lameness. Mild deformities develop, consisting of internal rotation of the tibia and abduction of the hock. This condition may progress to a Grade 3 luxation with associated cartilage erosion on the patellar and trochlear surfaces.
Grade 3:	The patella is permanently luxated but can be manually reduced. More severe bony deformities are present, including marked internal tibial rotation and an S-shaped curve of the distal femur and proximal tibia. A shallow trochlear groove may be palpable. The client often complains of an abnormal, "crouched" gait rather than intermittent lameness, because the dog often uses the leg in a semiflexed, internally rotated position. The condition is often bilateral.
Grade 4:	This is a severe condition with permanent, nonreducible luxation of the patella. The tibia is rotated from 60° to 90° relative to the sagittal plane. If not corrected early in life, severe bony and ligamentous deformities develop and are often not reparable.

From Singleton WB: The surgical correction of stifle deformities in the dog. *J Small Anim Pract 10*:59, 1969.

intermittent and associated with a mechanical, nonpainful lameness. Surgical correction is recommended if lameness is frequent.

Lateral luxation in small dogs is rare and is usually congenital. Lateral patellar luxation in large dogs or giant breeds is often a distinct syndrome associated with severe limb deformities and carries a much more guarded prognosis.

Clinical Signs and Diagnosis

Acute traumatic patellar luxation may be medial or lateral and is associated with nonweightbearing lameness and pain on manipulation of the joint. These signs gradually subside and may be mild in an animal with chronic luxation.

The clinical signs associated with congenital or developmental medial patellar luxation vary with the degree or grade of luxation (see Table 137–1). Grade 1 luxations are an incidental finding during routine physical examination but may cause lameness after vigorous exercise. Grade 2 luxations cause intermittent lameness associated with luxation of the patella. The lameness resolves spontaneously with patellar reduction. The owner often comments that the dog suddenly skips and carries the leg without apparent pain, flexes and extends

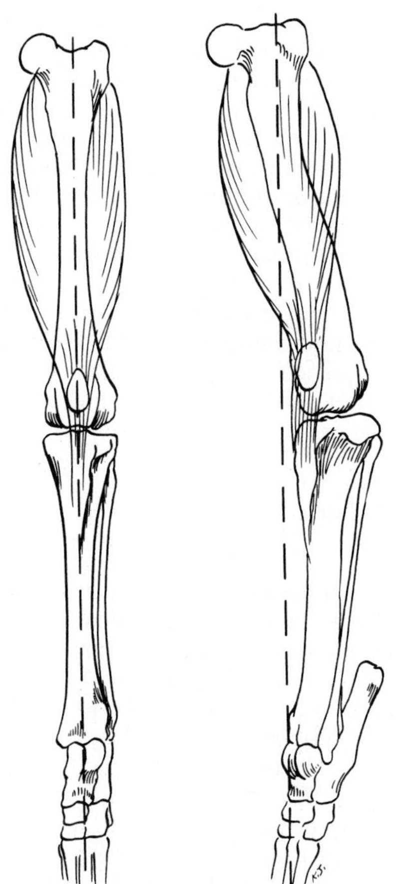

FIGURE 137–39. The bony changes associated with medial patella luxation. Note the varus deformation of the proximal femur and marked internal rotation of the tibia. A normal limb is shown on the left.

the joint several times, and bears weight again. Grade 3 medial patellar luxation is associated with more severe bony deformities, including lateral bowing and internal rotation of the tibia (Fig. 137–39). Coxa vara is associated with this condition,[166] but we did not observe this deformity in 34 dogs.[220] Lameness may be mild with grade 3 luxation or not present at all. It is common to discover grade 3 luxation during a routine physical examination of an older dog that has never been lame. Some dogs develop a marked lameness with grade 3 medial patellar luxation. This may be associated with progressive cartilage erosion from the surfaces of the patella and medial ridge of the femoral trochlea. Acute lameness in a dog with chronic luxation is usually caused by rupture of the cranial cruciate ligament. Grade 4 medial patellar luxation is a severe condition characterized by marked internal rotation and lateral bowing of the tibia. Affected animals develop a crablike posture and gait that can be debilitating. Some dogs can barely walk and must be carried by their owners.

Lateral patellar luxation occurs rarely in small dogs and may cause an acute, painful lameness. More often, it is a component of a severe limb deformity in large dogs and giant breeds, characterized by coxa valga, excessive anteversion of the femoral neck, hypoplasia of the vastus medialis, medial bowing of the femur and tibia (genu valgum), and external rotation of the foot (Fig. 137–40).[148] These animals have a crouched posture, awkward gait, and generally unthrifty appearance.

Physical Examination

Careful physical examination is necessary to characterize the patellofemoral instability and rule out cranial cruciate ligament rupture. The animal is observed at a walk and trot to evaluate overall conformation and gait. First examine the stifle joint with the animal standing, to facilitate comparison with the contralateral joint and to judge the influence of quadriceps muscle contraction. One hand is placed over the patella, and the other hand used to pick up the tibia and place the joint through a range of motion. Patellar tracking is evaluated, and the presence of crepitation or pain is noted. Spontaneous luxation is easily detected as a snapping or popping sensation. With the joint in extension, the patella is isolated between the thumb and index fingers and pushed medially and laterally. In a normal joint, the patella may subluxate slightly but does not luxate.

Radiography

Radiographs can document the luxation and are useful to determine the extent of bony deformity and degen-

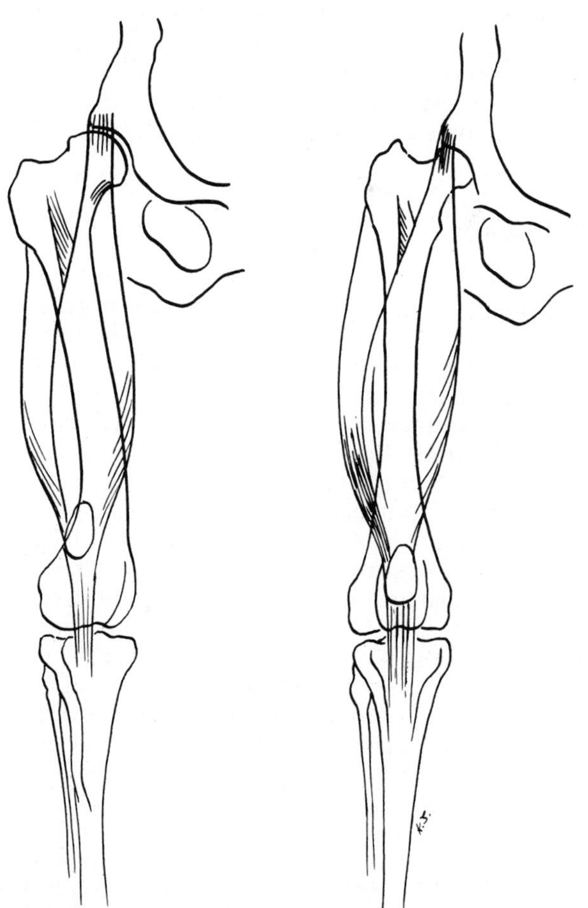

FIGURE 137–40. The bony deformities associated with lateral patellar luxation. Note the valgus deformity of the proximal femur and external rotation of the stifle. These dogs often have a knock-kneed appearance when affected bilaterally. A normal limb is shown on the right.

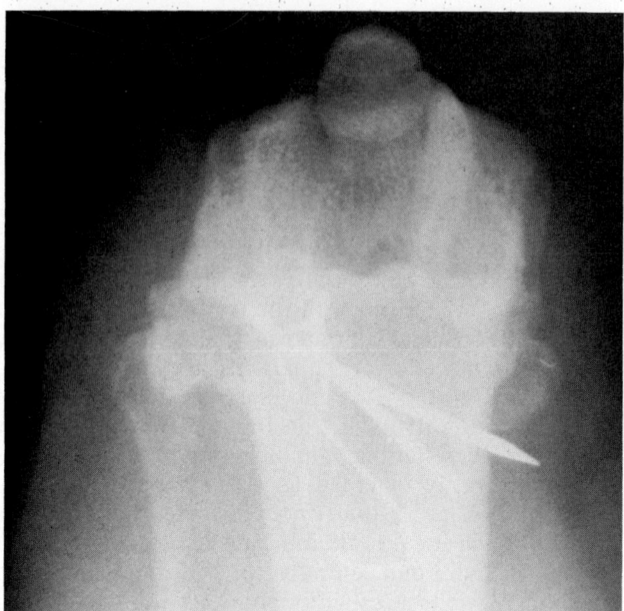

FIGURE 137–41. Skyline radiographic projection of the femoropatellar joint after surgical correction of medial patellar luxation in a 30-kg dog. This projection provides an improved view of patellar position within the trochlea, compared with conventional lateral and cranial-caudal views.

erative joint changes. Dogs with intermittent luxation may be reduced during positioning, and the radiographs appear normal. Skyline views of the distal femur are useful both pre- and postoperatively to evaluate the depth and contour of the femoral trochlea (Fig. 137–41).

Treatment

Because patellar luxations vary greatly in the degree of pathology present and the potential for degenerative sequelae, it is imperative to individualize the treatment for each patient. Several situations are clear-cut. Grade 1 medial patellar luxation without clinical signs is managed conservatively; if lameness develops, the dog is reevaluated. Grade 4 medial patellar luxation is corrected surgically early in life to prevent severe bony deformity and disability. Traumatic luxations are repaired by suturing the respective fascial defect (medial or lateral).

The gray zones involve small dogs with grade 2 or grade 3 medial patellar luxation and only occasional lameness. These dogs generally have mild degenerative joint disease, and it does not markedly progress; routine surgical correction is not recommended. Medial patellar luxation is associated with internal tibial rotation and may cause excessive stress within the cranial cruciate ligament and predispose to rupture. The incidence of such rupture in dogs with medial patellar luxation has not been studied specifically. In 34 dogs (52 stifles) with medial patellar luxation monitored for a mean of 3.6 years, unilateral cranial cruciate ligament rupture occurred in 2 dogs.[220] I do not believe it is justified to operate on dogs with medial patellar luxation based solely on the desire to prevent cranial cruciate ligament rupture. The primary criterion for operating on these dogs is the frequency of lameness and disability. If lameness is frequent and a major concern for the owner, the luxation is corrected. If the lameness is mild and infrequent, surgery is discussed and offered as an option if the problem worsens. The combination of medial patellar luxation and cranial cruciate ligament rupture causes significant disability and is surgically corrected if the dog is otherwise sound.

Lateral patellar luxation, when associated with severe limb deformities, is a complex disorder with a guarded prognosis. It is imperative to educate owners about the nature of the limb deformities and not embark on an expensive sequence of operations unless an owner is fully committed and knowledgeable about potential complications.

Surgical Methods

Surgical correction of patellar luxation requires realignment of the extensor mechanism and stabilization of the patella in the femoral trochlea. Extensor realignment is accomplished through transfer of the tibial tuberosity or rotation of the tibia, and the patellofemoral joint is stabilized by deepening the femoral trochlea via various "trochleoplasty" or "sulcoplasty" procedures. Because patellar luxation causes tightening of the capsular tissues on the side of the luxation and stretching of the tissues opposite the luxation, appropriate releasing incisions and imbrication techniques are usually necessary to achieve neutral tracking of the patella in the femoral trochlea.

Trochleoplasties. The simplest method for deepening the femoral trochlea is to remove the articular surface and 1 to 2 mm of subchondral bone using a rongeur or high-speed bur (*abrasion trochleoplasty*, Fig. 137–42). The surface is smoothed with a bone rasp. An experimental study showed that such defects fill with well-vascularized, highly cellular, loose connective tissue that reorganized with time into dense fibrous connective tissue that resembled fibrocartilage.[133] Scanning electron micrographic examination revealed that the surface was irregular. Clinical reports suggest that the latter technique is highly successful as a component of surgical correction of medial patellar luxation in small dogs.[12, 13, 48, 171, 214, 220]

Resurfacing the subchondral bone defect using autogenous periosteal grafts has been described.[98] The grafts produced fibrocartilage within 4 weeks, compared with 40 weeks in ungrafted controls. The grafted stifles had less patellar cartilage damage than controls.

Another technique that deepens the trochlear surface while maintaining the hyaline cartilage is called *recession trochleoplasty*.[28, 194] A small saw is used to cut a V-shaped wedge in the femoral trochlea. Additional subchondral bone is removed either by making additional cuts with the saw or by rongeur treatment of the underlying bone. The articular wedge is then replaced into the defect in a recessed position (Fig. 137–43). Pressure from the patella and the friction generated between the graft and subchondral bone preclude the need for internal fixation. The procedure is easier in large dogs but can be performed in dogs as small as

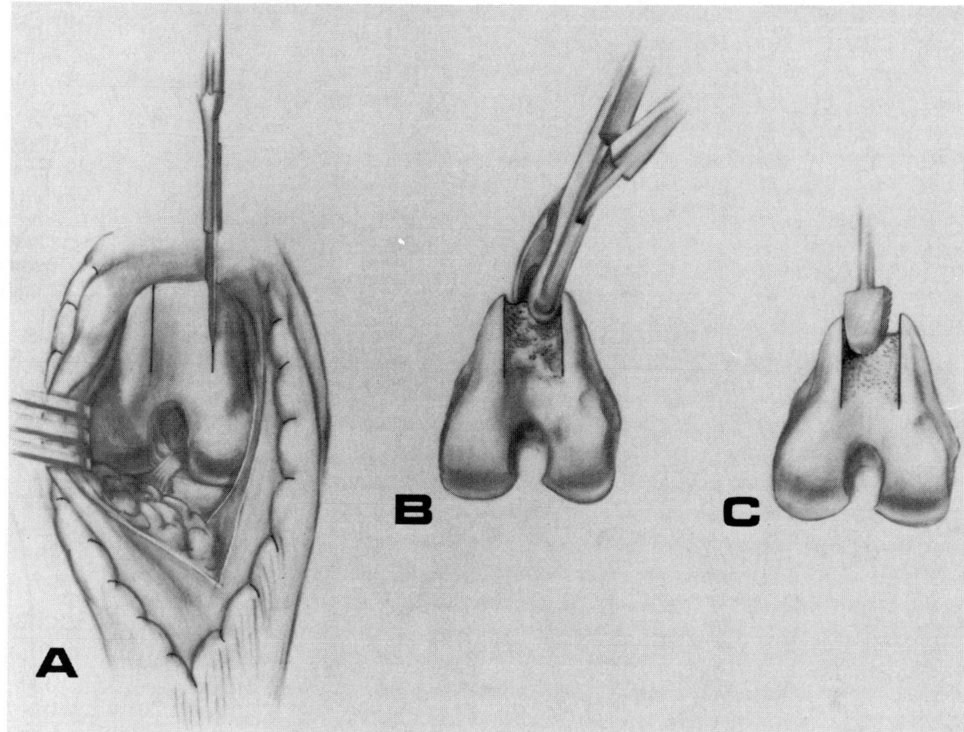

FIGURE 137–42. Abrasion trochleoplasty. *A,* A number 15 scalpel blade is used to define the area of cartilage removal. *B,* A rongeur or high-speed bur is used to remove the cartilage and 2 to 3 mm of subchondral bone. *C,* The surface is smoothed with a bone rasp. Approximately half of the patellar height should remain above the trochlear margin.

3 to 5 kg. I prefer this technique over the abrasion trochleoplasty because dogs use the limb sooner.

A simpler technique can be used to recess the articular surface in dogs less than 6 months old. In young dogs, the cartilage can be separated from the underlying subchondral bone. Scalpel incisions are made proximally and along the trochlear ridges, and the cartilage surface is elevated using a periosteal elevator (Fig. 137–44). After 2 to 3 mm of subchondral bone is removed with a bone curette or rasp, the cartilage flap is replaced. The articular surface is recessed so that approximately half of the patella protrudes above the level of the trochlear ridge.

Tibial Tuberosity Transposition. Movement of the tibial tuberosity changes the alignment of the extensor mechanism relative to the femoral trochlea; it can be used to correct medial or lateral patellar luxations. Most commonly, the tuberosity is moved to a lateral position to correct medial patellar luxation (Fig. 137–45).

The tuberosity can be moved medially to correct lateral patellar luxation; the operation is similar to that described earlier except for the lack of muscle coverage on the medial aspect of the proximal tibia. Release of the lateral capsular tissues is routinely performed to free the patella and facilitate realignment of the extensor mechanism.

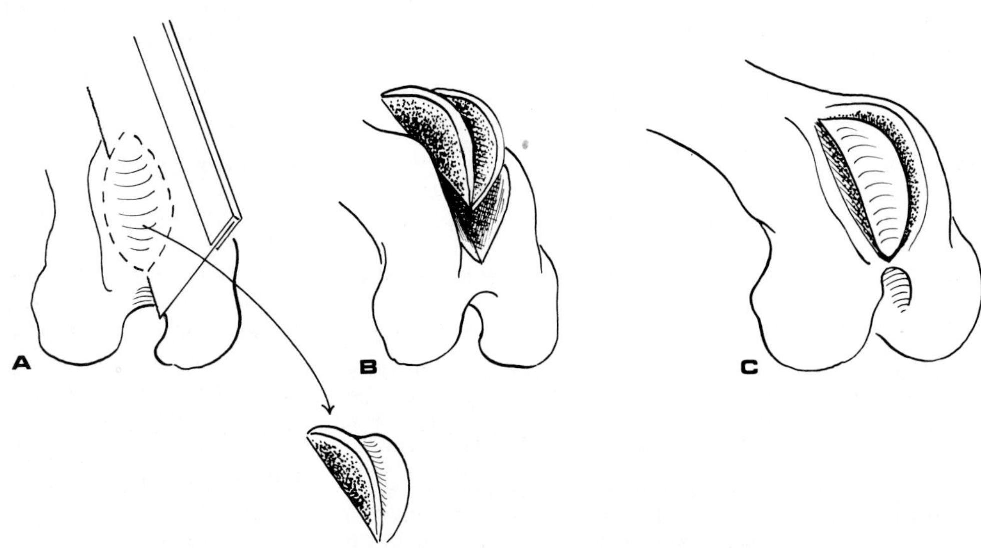

FIGURE 137–43. Schematic illustration of trochlear wedge resection technique for improving patellofemoral stability. *A,* Cuts are made with a small saw, starting at the trochlear ridges. *B,* Underlying bone is removed by making additional saw cuts or by using a rongeur or high-speed bur. *C,* The wedge is replaced in a recessed position, thereby permitting deeper seating of the patella within the trochlea.

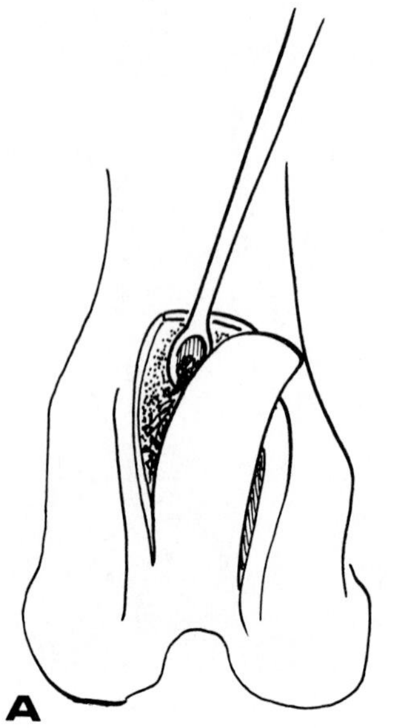

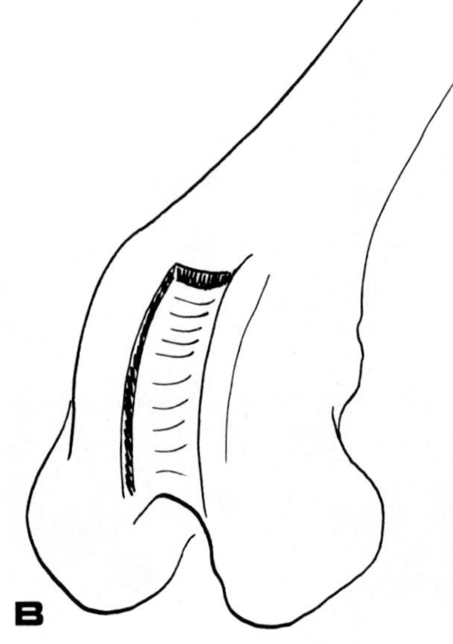

FIGURE 137–44. Trochlear chondroplasty. This technique is possible only in dogs younger than 6 months. *A*, A cartilage flap is outlined using a number 15 scalpel blade, and a sharp periosteal elevator is used to undermine the cartilage and form a hinged flap. A rongeur or curette is used to remove 2 to 3 mm of subchondral bone. *B*, The flap is replaced, and the stability of patellofemoral reduction is evaluated. More bone can be removed if necessary. Fixation of the flap is not necessary.

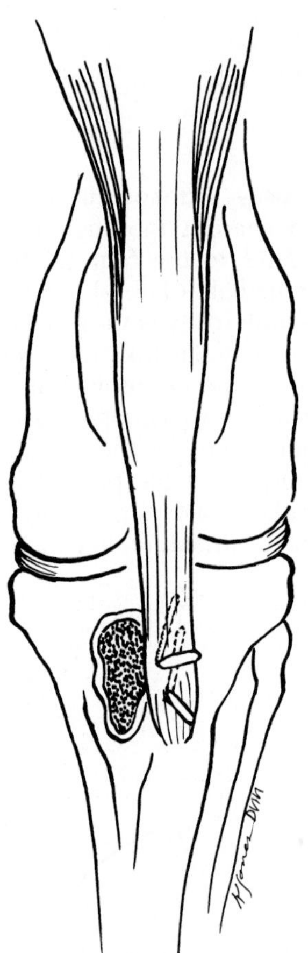

FIGURE 137–45. Lateral transplantation of the tibial tuberosity for medial patella luxation. The cranial tibial muscle is elevated from the lateral surface of the proximal tibia, and an osteotome is positioned to remove the insertion site of the patellar tendon. The tuberosity is cut with the osteotome, taking care to leave the distal soft-tissue attachments. The lateral edge of the cut surface can be removed with rongeurs or a bone rasp to facilitate stable seating of the tuberosity in a lateral position. The tuberosity is fixed in position using one or two small Kirschner wires. The position of the tuberosity (degree of lateral rotation) is determined for each individual case. It is important to release the medial fascia as needed to minimize tension and facilitate neutral tracking of the patella. Distal displacement of the tuberosity can cause malarticulation and should be avoided.

Antirotational Techniques. Rotational deformity of the tibia is often a component of the patellar luxation complex. Correction of the rotation is desirable in a young animal that has remodeling potential. In older animals, however, the entire limb has developed abnormally, with permanent bony and ligamentous abnormalities. Simply rotating the tibia medially or laterally does not correct these problems.

Tibial rotation can be corrected by placement of heavy nonabsorbable suture material from a fabella (lateral fabella for medial patellar luxation, medial fabella for lateral patellar luxation) to the tibial tuberosity or distal patellar tendon (Fig. 137–46). Fibular head transposition causes external rotation of the tibia and is useful in dogs with medial patellar luxation. These techniques are especially advantageous in dogs with combined medial patellar luxation and cranial cruciate ligament rupture, because they reduce cranial-caudal laxity and correct rotation. The suture techniques are not permanent corrections, and I use them only as ancillary support to more definitive corrections. Because of its secure fixation, fibular head transposition (combined with recession trochleoplasty) can be used in active large dogs that have a bowlegged, bulldog type conformation with combined cranial cruciate ligament rupture and medial patellar luxation.

Aftercare and Prognosis

In most cases, a well-padded wrap is maintained for 7 to 10 days and removed along with the skin sutures. The animal is restricted to short leash walks for 3 to 5 weeks, and the owner is encouraged to provide passive range of motion exercises. Recurrence of the luxation is generally due to inadequate correction, such as failure to move the tibial tuberosity.

The prognosis is favorable for small dogs with grade 2 or 3 medial patellar luxation. Large dogs with medial patellar luxation also do well if the luxation is corrected before severe cartilage erosion has occurred. Grade 4 luxations can be successfully corrected in dogs less than 4 to 6 months of age; after that time, the bony and ligamentous deformities become severe and the prog-

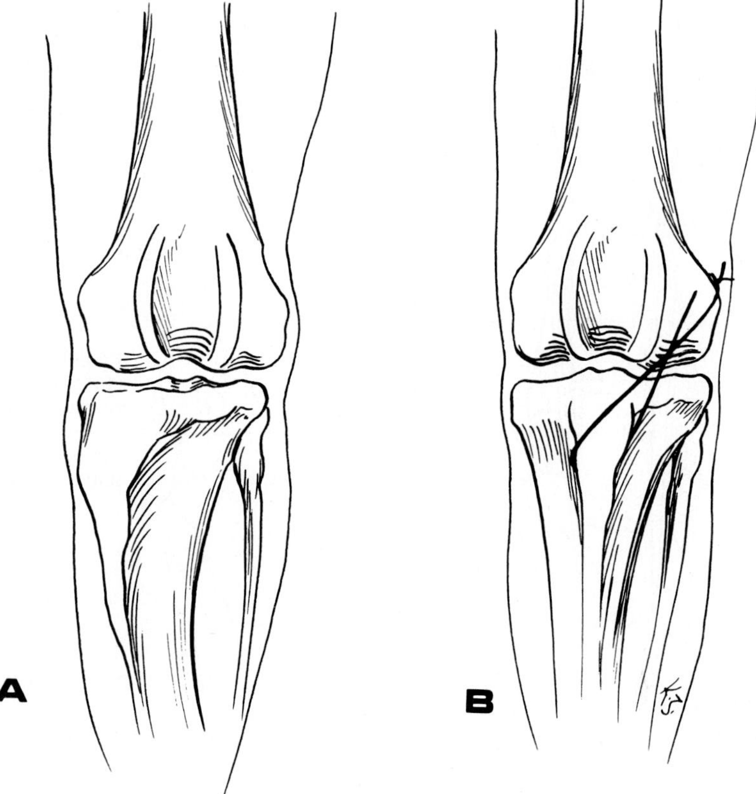

FIGURE 137–46. Antirotational suture for correction of medial patellar luxation. Nonabsorbable material is placed around the lateral fabella and through a hole in the tibial crest. *A*, Before suture replacement. *B*, After tightening suture.

nosis is guarded. Uncomplicated lateral patellar luxation carries a favorable prognosis; if it occurs as a component of a severe limb deformity as described previously, the prognosis is guarded.

PATELLAR FRACTURES AND PATELLAR TENDON INJURIES

Patellar fractures are uncommon and are usually the result of a direct blow. Patellar tendon tears are also unusual, and the cause is often unknown. A direct wound can cause tendon laceration, or the tendon may rupture when quadriceps contraction occurs simultaneously with forced knee flexion. The lameness is often severe, and physical examination reveals marked pain over the site of injury. Patellar tendon rupture is suggested by dorsal displacement of the patella. It is imperative in all such cases to carefully examine the stifle joint for concurrent injuries to the ligaments and menisci.

Patellar fractures require tension band fixation to overcome the distracting forces of the quadriceps muscles. Conservative treatment results in nonunion of the bone and secondary fracture disease in the limb, with a correspondingly worse prognosis. Patellectomy is strictly a salvage procedure for highly comminuted fractures and should be avoided if at all possible because of the critical importance of the patella in providing extensor power to the stifle.

Repair of Patellar Fractures

A combination of tension band fixation and cerclage wiring provided superior stabilization for simple patellar fractures and is recommended (Fig. 137–47).[45] The sta-

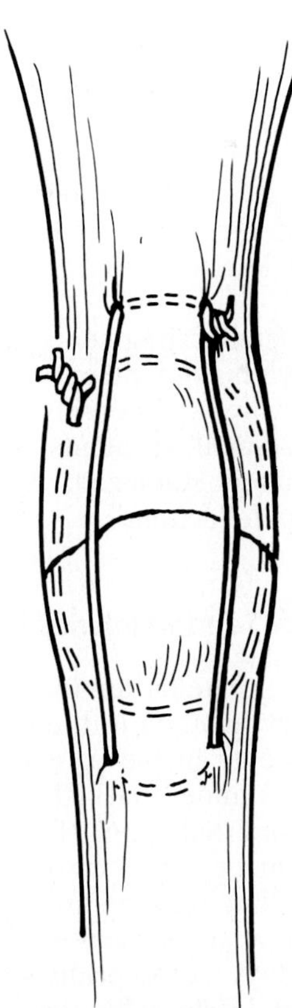

FIGURE 137–47. Tension band and cerclage wire fixation of patellar fractures. The patella is reduced and held with a circumferential cerclage wire passed in a purse-string fashion close to the bone. To complete the fixation, a second wire is passed through the quadriceps tendon, looping cranially across the patella to act as a tension band. Eighteen-gauge wire is used for large dogs, 20 gauge for smaller dogs and for cats.

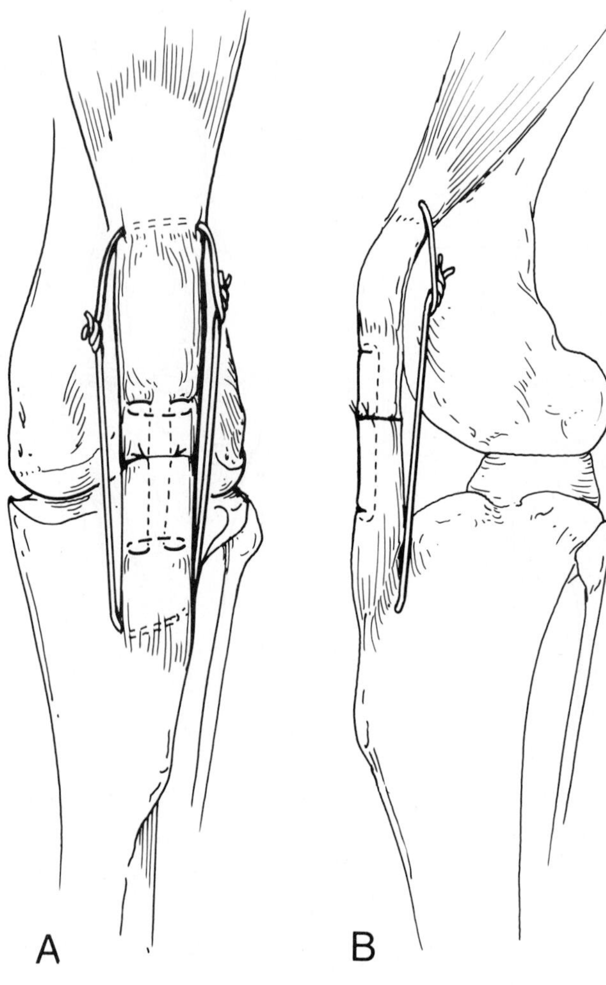

FIGURE 137–48. Repair of patellar tendon ruptures. Monofilament wire (18 gauge for large dogs, 20 gauge for small dogs and for cats) is placed proximal to the patella and through a hole in the tibial tuberosity and tightened sufficiently to appose the tendon ends without tension. A locking loop pattern with 2-0 or 0 nonabsorbable suture is used to complete the repair. *A*, Cranial view. *B*, Lateral view.

ble fixation offered by this method is important because it allows early controlled mobilization of the knee, preventing the deleterious effects of prolonged immobilization.

Comminuted patellar fragments are stabilized using small Kirschner wires, and the entire patella is encircled with a cerclage wire and tension band apparatus as described earlier. Small fragments are discarded if they cannot be adequately stabilized. A marginal repair is accepted before patellectomy.

Repair of Patellar Tendon Injuries

Primary repair of patellar tendon injuries is necessary to restore extensor function to the stifle and to prevent degenerative sequelae in the patellofemoral joint. Because the tendon is under marked tension, the repair is protected by an internal splint (Fig. 137–48).[68] Severe tendon defects can be augmented by suturing autogenous tensor fascia lata into the area of the defect.[68]

A well-padded wrap is maintained until suture removal 7 to 10 days postoperatively, and exercise is restricted to short leash walks for 4 to 6 weeks. The wire eventually breaks, often causing lameness, and then requires removal. The prognosis for isolated patellar tendon injuries is favorable.

AVULSION INJURIES

Avulsion injuries involving the long digital extensor, gastrocnemius and related fabellae, and popliteal tendon of origin are unusual and generally require surgical management (see Chapter 146).

References

1. Adelaar RS, et al: Dynamic musculotendinous transfer to replace the anterior cruciate ligament in the dog. *J Bone Joint Surg [Br] 65B*:650, 1983.
2. Alm A, et al: The anterior cruciate ligament. A clinical and experimental study on tensile strength, morphology and replacement by patellar ligament. *Acta Chir Scand 445*(Suppl):5, 1974.
3. Altman RD, et al: The effect of glycosaminoglycan polysulfuric acid ester on articular cartilage in experimental arthritis. *J Rheumatol 14*:127, 1987.
4. Amiel D, et al: Injury of the anterior cruciate ligament: The role of collagenase in ligament degeneration. *J Orthop Res 7*:486, 1989.
5. Amiel D, et al: Cruciate ligaments: response to injury. *In* Daniel DM, et al (eds): *Knee Ligaments: Structure, Function, Injury, and Repair*. Raven Press, New York, 1990, pp 365–377.
6. Anderson AF, et al: Analysis of the intercondylar notch by computed tomography. *Am J Sports Med 15*:547, 1987.
7. Arms SW, et al: The biomechanics of anterior cruciate ligament rehabilitation and reconstruction. *Am J Sports Med 12*:8, 1984.
8. Arnoczky SP: Anatomy of the anterior cruciate ligament. *Clin Orthop 172*:19, 1983.
9. Arnoczky SP, Marshall JL: The cruciate ligaments of the canine stifle: An anatomical and functional analysis. *Am J Vet Res 38*:1809, 1977.
10. Arnoczky SP, Marshall JL: Discoid meniscus in the dog: A case report. *J Am Anim Hosp Assoc 13*:569, 1977.

11. Arnoczky SP, Marshall JL: Pathomechanics of cruciate and meniscal injuries. *In* Bojrab MJ (ed): *Pathophysiology in Small Animal Surgery*. Lea & Febiger, Philadelphia, 1981, pp 590–603.
12. Arnoczky SP, Tarvin GB: Surgery of the stifle—the patella (Part II). *Comp Cont Educ 2*:200, 1980.
13. Arnoczky SP, Tarvin GB: Surgical repair of patellar luxations and fractures. *In* Bojrab MJ (ed): *Current Techniques in Small Animal Surgery*. Lea & Febiger, Philadelphia, 1990, pp 714–721.
14. Arnoczky SP, Warren RF: The microvasculature of the meniscus and its response to injury. An experimental study in the dog. *Am J Sports Med 11*:131, 1983.
15. Arnoczky SP, et al: The over-the-top procedure: A technique for anterior cruciate ligament substitution in the dog. *J Am Anim Hosp Assoc 15*:283, 1979.
16. Arnoczky SP, et al: Biomechanical evaluation of anterior cruciate ligament repair in the dog: An analysis of the instant center of motion. *J Am Anim Hosp Assoc 13*:553, 1977.
17. Arnoczky SP, et al: Microvasculature of the cruciate ligament and its response to injury. *J Bone Joint Surg [Am] 61A*:1221, 1979.
18. Arnoczky SP, et al: Replacement of the anterior cruciate ligament using a patellar tendon allograft. *J Bone Joint Surg [Am] 68A*:376, 1986.
19. Arnoczky SP, et al: Meniscal replacement using a cryopreserved allograft. An experimental study in the dog. *Clin Orthop 252*:121, 1990.
20. Arnoczky SP, et al: Meniscal repair using exogenous fibrin clot. *J Bone Joint Surg [Am] 70A*:1209, 1988.
21. Aron DN: Traumatic dislocation of the stifle joint: Treatment of 12 dogs and one cat. *J Am Anim Hosp Assoc 24*:333, 1988.
22. Baici A, et al: Inhibition of human elastase from polymorphonuclear leucocytes by a glycosaminoglycan polysulfate (arteparon). *Biochem Pharmacol 29*:1723, 1980.
23. Barclay SM, Barclay WP: Filamentous carbon fiber prosthesis for cranial cruciate ligament replacement in the dog. *Cornell Vet 74*:3, 1984.
24. Barnes AJ: Rupture of the anterior cruciate ligament of the dog: A survey from practices in the Kent region BSAVA. *J Small Anim Pract 18*:55, 1977.
25. Bendele AM: Progressive chronic osteoarthritis in femorotibial joints of partial medial meniscectomized guinea pigs. *Vet Pathol 24*:444, 1987.
26. Bennett D, et al: A reappraisal of anterior cruciate ligament disease in the dog. *J Small Anim Pract 29*:275, 1988.
27. Berry JL, et al: Evaluation of Dacron-covered and plain bovine xenografts as replacements for the anterior cruciate ligament. *Clin Orthop 236*:270, 1988.
28. Boone EG, et al: Trochlear recession wedge technique for patellar luxation: An experimental study. *J Am Anim Hosp Assoc 19*:735, 1983.
29. Bradley J, et al: Orientation of the cruciate ligament in the sagittal plane. A method of predicting its length-change with flexion. *J Bone Joint Surg [Br] 70B*:94, 1988.
30. Brinker WO, et al: Diagnosis and treatment of orthopedic conditions of the hindlimb. *In* Brinker WO, et al (eds): *Handbook of Small Animal Orthopedics and Fracture Treatment*. W. B. Saunders, Philadelphia, 1990, pp 341–470.
31. Brody GA, et al: *In vitro* fibroblast seeding of prosthetic anterior cruciate ligaments. A preliminary study. *Am J Sports Med 16*:203, 1988.
32. Budsberg SC, et al: Force plate analysis before and after stabilization of canine stifles for cruciate injury. *Am J Vet Res 49*:1522, 1988.
33. Burks RT, Leland R: Determination of graft tension before fixation in anterior cruciate ligament reconstruction. *Arthroscopy 4*:260, 1988.
34. Burks RT, et al: Biomechanical and histological observations of the dog patellar tendon after removal of its central one-third. *Am J Sports Med 18*:146, 1990.
35. Burnett QM II, Fowler PJ: Reconstruction of the anterior cruciate ligament: Historical overview. *Orthop Clin North Am 16*:143, 1985.
36. Butler DL, et al: Location-dependent variations in the material properties of anterior cruciate ligament subunits. *Proc Orthop Res Soc 37*:234, 1991.
37. Butler DL, et al: Biomechanics of cranial cruciate ligament reconstruction in the dog II. Mechanical properties. *Vet Surg 12*:113, 1983.
38. Bylski-Austrow DI, et al: Anterior cruciate ligament replacements: A mechanical study of femoral attachment location, flexion angle at tensioning, and initial tension. *J Orthop Res 8*:522, 1990.
39. Childers HE: New methods for cruciate ligament repair. II: Repair by suture technique. *Mod Vet Pract 47*:59, 1966.
40. Clancy WG, et al: Anterior cruciate ligament reconstruction using one-third of the patellar ligament, augmented by extra-articular tendon transfers. *J Bone Joint Surg [Am] 64A*:352, 1982.
41. Clark JM, Sidles JA: The interrelation of fiber bundles in the anterior cruciate ligament. *J Orthop Res 8*:180, 1990.
42. Clayton ML, Weir GJ: Experimental investigations of ligamentous healing. *Am J Surg 98*:373, 1959.
43. Cooper RR, Misol S: Tendon and ligament insertion: A light and electron microscopic study. *J Bone Joint Surg [Am] 52A*:1, 1970.
44. Cox JS, et al: The degenerative effects of partial and total resection of the medial meniscus in dogs' knees. *Clin Orthop 109*:178, 1975.
45. Curtis MJ: Internal fixation for fractures of the patella. A comparison of two methods. *J Bone Joint Surg [Br] 72B*:280, 1990.
46. Daniel DM: Diagnosis of a ligament injury. *In* Daniel DM, et al (eds): *Knee Ligaments: Structure, Function, Injury and Repair*. Raven Press, New York, 1990, pp 3–10.
47. Daniel DM: Principles of knee ligament surgery. *In* Daniel DM, et al (eds): *Knee Ligaments: Structure, Function, Injury and Repair*. Raven Press, New York, 1990, pp 11–29.
48. DeAngelis M, Hohn RB: Evaluation of surgical correction of canine patellar luxation in 142 cases. *J Am Vet Med Assoc 156*:587, 1970.
49. DeAngelis MP, Betts CW: Posterior cruciate ligament rupture. *J Am Anim Hosp Assoc 9*:447, 1973.
50. DeAngelis MP, Lau RE: A lateral retinacular imbrication technique for the surgical correction of anterior cruciate ligament rupture in the dog. *J Am Vet Med Assoc 157*:79, 1970.
51. Denny HR, Barr ARS: An evaluation of two "over the top" techniques for anterior cruciate ligament replacement in the dog. *J Small Anim Pract 25*:759, 1984.
52. Denny HR, Barr ARS: A further evaluation of the "over-the-top" technique for anterior cruciate ligament replacement in the dog. *J Small Anim Pract 28*:681, 1987.
53. Denny HR, Goodship AE: Replacement of the anterior cruciate ligament with carbon fibre in the dog. *J Small Anim Pract 21*:279, 1980.
54. Denny HR, Minter HM: The long term results of surgery of canine stifle disorders. *J Small Anim Pract 14*:695, 1973.
55. DeYoung DJ, et al: Experimental medial meniscectomy in dogs undergoing cranial cruciate ligament repair. *J Am Anim Hosp Assoc 16*:639, 1980.
56. Dickinson CR, Nunamaker DM: Repair of ruptured anterior cruciate ligament in the dog: Experience of 101 cases, using a modified fascia strip technique. *J Am Vet Med Assoc 170*:827, 1977.
57. DiStefano VJ: Function, post-traumatic sequelae and current concepts of management of knee meniscus injuries: A review article. *Clin Orthop 151*:143, 1980.
58. Doverspike M, Vasseur PB: Contralateral cranial cruciate ligament rupture: incidence in 114 dogs. *J Am Anim Hosp Assoc*, in press.
59. Duff SRI: Further studies on knee ligament failure in broiler breeding fowls. *J Comp Pathol 96*:485, 1986.
60. Dulisch ML: Suture reaction following extra-articular stifle stabilization in the dog. I. A retrospective study of 161 stifles. *J Am Anim Hosp Assoc 17*:569, 1981.
61. Dunbar AD: Screw fixation for cranial cruciate ligament avulsion in a dog. *Mod Vet Pract 66*:119, 1985.
62. Dye SF, Cannon WD Jr: Anatomy and biomechanics of the anterior cruciate ligament. *Clin Sports Med 7*:715, 1988.
63. Egger EL: Caudal cruciate ligament repair. *In* Bojrab MJ (ed): *Current Techniques in Small Animal Surgery*. Lea & Febiger, Philadelphia, 1990, pp 701–708.
64. Evans HE, Christensen GC: *Miller's Anatomy of the Dog*. W. B. Saunders, Philadelphia, 1979, pp 257–264.
65. Fallon RK, Tomlinson JL: Abstract: Permanent prosthetic cranial cruciate ligament. *Vet Surg 14*:54, 1985.
66. Fallon RK, Tomlinson JL: Abstract: Prognostic indicators in 80 consecutive cases of cranial cruciate ligament rupture: a prospective study. *Vet Surg 15*:118, 1986.
67. Farrow CS: Sprain, strain, and contusion. *Vet Clin North Am 8*:169, 1978.
68. Farrow CS, Newton CD: Ligamentous injury (sprain). *In* Newton CD, Nunamaker DM (eds): *Textbook of Small Animal Orthopaedics*. J. B. Lippincott, Philadelphia, 1985, pp 843–851.
69. Feagin JA Jr, et al: The anterior cruciate ligament: Radiographic and clinical signs of successful and unsuccessful repairs. *Clin Orthop 164*:54, 1982.
70. Flecknell PA, Grudffydd-Jones TJ: Congenital luxation of the patellae in the cat. *Feline Pract 9*:18, 1979.
71. Flo GL: Modification of the lateral retinacular imbrication technique for stabilizing cruciate ligament injuries. *J Am Anim Hosp Assoc 11*:570, 1975.
72. Flo GL, DeYoung D: Meniscal injuries and medial meniscectomy in the canine stifle. *J Am Anim Hosp Assoc 14*:683, 1978.
73. Frank C, et al: Medial collateral ligament healing—a multidisciplinary assessment in rabbits. *Am J Sports Med 11*:379, 1983.
74. Gambardella PC: Personal communication, 1990.
75. Gambardella PC, et al: Lateral suture technique for management of anterior cruciate ligament rupture in dogs: A retrospective study. *J Am Anim Hosp Assoc 17*:33, 1981.
76. Gibson A: Regeneration of the internal semilunar cartilages after operation. *Br J Surg 19*:302, 1931.
77. Girgis FG, et al: The cruciate ligaments of the knee joint. Anatomical, functional and experimental analysis. *Clin Orthop 106*:216, 1975.
78. Good L, et al: Intercondylar notch measurements with special reference to anterior cruciate ligament surgery. *Clin Orthop 263*:185, 1991.
79. Good L, et al: Load tolerance, security, and failure modes of fixation devices for synthetic knee ligaments. *Clin Orthop 253*:190, 1990.
80. Griffin DW, Vasseur PB: Synovial fluid analysis in dogs with cranial cruciate ligament rupture. *J Am Anim Hosp Assoc 28*:277, 1992.
81. Guan Y, et al: Contribution of anterior cruciate ligament subunits during anterior drawer in the human knee. *Proc Orthop Res Soc 37*:589, 1991.
82. Gupta BN, Brinker WO: Anterior cruciate ligament prosthesis in the dog. *J Am Vet Med Assoc 154*:1057, 1969.
83. Hannan N, et al: Systemic administration of glycosaminoglycan polysul-

phate (Arteparon) provides partial protection of articular cartilage from damage produced by meniscectomy in the canine. *J Orthop Res 5*:47, 1987.
84. Hansen FW: Underside lesions of the meniscus. *Acta Orthop Scand 49*:610, 1978.
85. Harari J, et al: Evaluation of experimental transection and partial excision of the caudal cruciate ligament in dogs. *Vet Surg 16*:151, 1987.
86. Hastings DE: The non-operative management of collateral ligament injuries of the knee joint. *Clin Orthop 147*:22, 1980.
87. Heffron LE, Campbell JR: Morphology, histology and functional anatomy of the canine cranial cruciate ligament. *Vet Rec 102*:280, 1978.
88. Higgins RW, Steadman JR: Anterior cruciate ligament repairs in world class skiers. *Am J Sports Med 15*:439, 1987.
89. Hinko PJ: The use of a prosthetic ligament in repair of the torn anterior cruciate ligament in the dog. *J Am Anim Hosp Assoc 17*:563, 1981.
90. Hohn RB, Miller JM: Surgical correction of rupture of the anterior cruciate ligament in the dog. *J Am Vet Med Assoc 150*:1133, 1967.
91. Hoogland T, Hillen B: Intra-articular reconstruction of the anterior cruciate ligament. An experimental study of length changes in different ligament reconstructions. *Clin Orthop 185*:197, 1984.
92. Houseworth SW, et al: The intercondylar notch in acute tears of the anterior cruciate ligament: A computer graphics study. *Am J Sports Med 15*:221, 1987.
93. Howell SM: Personal communication, 1991.
94. Hulse DA: Personal communication, 1991.
95. Hulse DA, Shires PK: The stifle joint. *In* Slatter DH (ed): *Textbook of Small Animal Surgery*. W. B. Saunders, Philadelphia, 1985, pp 2193–2235.
96. Hulse DA, Shires PK: Multiple ligament injury of the stifle joint in the dog. *J Am Anim Hosp Assoc 22*:105, 1986.
97. Hulse DA, et al: A technique for reconstruction of the anterior cruciate ligament in the dog: Preliminary report. *Vet Surg 9*:135, 1980.
98. Hulse DA, et al: Resurfacing canine femoral trochleoplasties with free autogenous periosteal grafts. *Vet Surg 15*:284, 1986.
99. Indelicato PA: Non-operative treatment of complete tears of the medial collateral ligament of the knee. *J Bone Joint Surg [Am] 65A*:323, 1983.
100. Jackson DW, et al: Cruciate reconstruction using freeze dried anterior cruciate ligament allograft and a ligament augmentation device (LAD). *Am J Sports Med 15*:528, 1987.
101. Jackson DW, et al: Magnetic resonance imaging of the knee. *Am J Sports Med 16*:29, 1988.
102. Jackson DW, et al: Intraarticular reaction associated with the use of freeze-dried, ethylene oxide-sterilized bone-patella tendon-bone allografts in the reconstruction of the anterior cruciate ligament. *Am J Sports Med 18*:1, 1990.
103. Janssens LAA, et al: Anterior cruciate ligament rupture associated with cardiomyopathy in three cats. *Vet Comp Orthop Traumatol 4*:35, 1991.
104. Johansson H, et al: Activity in receptor afferents from the anterior cruciate ligament evokes reflex effects on fusimotor neurones. *Neurosci Res 8*:54, 1990.
105. Johnson AL, Olmstead ML: Caudal cruciate ligament rupture: A retrospective analysis of 14 dogs. *Vet Surg 16*:202, 1987.
106. Johnson ME: Feline patellar luxation: A retrospective case study. *J Am Anim Hosp Assoc 22*:835, 1986.
107. Johnson SG, et al: System behavior of commonly used cranial cruciate ligament reconstruction autografts. *Vet Surg 18*:459, 1989.
108. Jones KG: Reconstruction of the anterior cruciate ligament. A technique using the central one-third of the patellar ligament. *J Bone Joint Surg [Am] 45A*:925, 1963.
109. Keiffer DA, et al: Anterior cruciate ligament arthroplasty. *Am J Sports Med 12*:301, 1984.
110. Kennedy JC, et al: Tension studies of human knee ligaments. *J Bone Joint Surg [Am] 58A*:350, 1976.
111. King D: Regeneration of the semilunar cartilage. *Surg Gynecol Obstet 62*:167, 1936.
112. Kliman M, et al: Orthotopic bone transplantation in mice. III. Methods of reducing the immune response and their effect on healing. *Transplantation 31*:34, 1981.
113. Knecht CD: Evolution of surgical techniques for cruciate ligament rupture in animals. *J Am Anim Hosp Assoc 12*:717, 1976.
114. Knecht CD, et al: Repair of avulsion of the caudal cruciate ligament in a dog using a bone screw. *J Am Anim Hosp Assoc 12*:784, 1976.
115. Krause WR, et al: Mechanical changes in the knee after meniscectomy. *J Bone Joint Surg [Am] 58A*:599, 1976.
116. Laine HR, et al: Ultrasound in the evaluation of the knee and patellar regions. *J Ultrasound Med 6*:33, 1987.
117. Lambert KL: Vascularized patellar tendon graft with rigid internal fixation for anterior cruciate ligament insufficiency. *Clin Orthop 172*:85, 1983.
118. Lambert RD: Electrosurgical treatment for cranial cruciate ligament rupture. *Mod Vet Pract 60*:557, 1979.
119. Langer F, et al: The immunogenicity of fresh and frozen allogeneic bone. *J Bone Joint Surg [Am] 57A*:216, 1975.
120. Lanzer WL, Komenda G: Changes in articular cartilage after meniscectomy. *Clin Orthop 252*:41, 1990.
121. Leighton RL: Repair of ruptured cruciate ligament with whole thickness skin. *Small Anim Clin 1*:246, 1961.
122. Leighton RL: Repair of bilateral medial patellar luxation in a cat. *Feline Pract 8*:23, 1978.
123. Macintosh DL: Acute tears of the anterior cruciate ligament: Over-the-top repair. Proceedings of the Academy of Orthopaedic Surgeons, Dallas, 1974.
124. Mann FA, et al: Manual goniometric measurement of the canine pelvic limb. *J Am Anim Hosp Assoc 24*:189, 1988.
125. Markolf KL, et al: Direct measurement of resultant forces in the anterior cruciate ligament. *J Bone Joint Surg [Am] 72A*:557, 1990.
126. McCurnin DM, Sceli DE: Surgical treatment of ruptured cranial cruciate ligament in the dog. *Vet Med/Small Anim Clin* 1183, 1975.
127. McCurnin DM, et al: Clinical and pathologic evaluation of ruptured cranial cruciate ligament repair in the dog. *Am J Vet Res 32*:1517, 1971.
128. McLeod WD: The biomechanics and function of the secondary restraints to the anterior cruciate ligament. *Orthop Clin North Am 16*:165, 1985.
129. Melhorn JM, Henning CE: The relationship of the femoral attachment site to the isometric tracking of the anterior cruciate ligament graft. *Am J Sports Med 15*:539, 1987.
130. Minami A, et al: Effect of the immunological antigenicity of the allogeneic tendons on tendon grafting. *Hand 14*:111, 1982.
131. Monahan JJ, et al: *In vivo* strain patterns in the four major canine knee ligaments. *J Orthop Res 2*:408, 1984.
132. Montgomery RD, et al: Comparison of over-the-top and tunnel techniques for anterior cruciate ligament replacement. *Clin Orthop 231*:144, 1988.
133. Moore JA, Banks WJ: Repair of full-thickness defects in the femoral trochlea of dogs after trochlear arthroplasty. *Am J Vet Res 50*:1406, 1989.
134. Mullen HS, Matthiesen DT: Complications of transposition of the fibular head for stabilization of the cranial cruciate-deficient stifle in dogs: 80 cases (1982–1986). *J Am Vet Med Assoc 195*:1267, 1989.
135. Newman AP, et al: Mechanics of meniscal repair in a canine model (Abstract). *Am J Sports Med 15*:404, 1987.
136. Niebauer GW, Lubec G: Kie kollagenaseaktivitat beim kreuzbandrib des hundes und ihre hemmung in vitro. *Zentralbl Veterinarmed [A] 27*:628, 1980.
137. Niebauer GW, Menzel EJ: Immunological changes in canine cruciate ligament rupture. *Res Vet Sci 32*:235, 1982.
138. Niebauer GW, et al: Antibodies to canine collagen types I and II in dogs with spontaneous cruciate ligament rupture and osteoarthritis. *Arthritis Rheum 30*:319, 1987.
139. Nikolaou PK, et al: Anterior cruciate ligament allograft transplantation. Long-term function, histology, revascularization, and operative technique. *Am J Sports Med 14*:348, 1986.
140. Norwood LA, Cross MJ: The intercondylar shelf and the anterior cruciate ligament. *Am J Sports Med 5*:171, 1977.
141. O'Brien W, et al: Femoral intercondylar notch impingement on anterior cruciate ligament substitutes (AOSSM abstract). *Am J Sports Med 15*:627, 1987.
142. O'Connor BL: The histological structure of dog knee menisci with comments on its possible significance. *Am J Anat 147*:407, 1976.
143. O'Connor JJ, et al: Geometry of the knee. *In* Daniel DM, et al (eds): *Knee Ligaments: Structure, Function, Injury, and Repair*. Raven Press, New York, 1990, pp 163–199.
144. O'Connor JJ, et al: Mechanics of the knee. *In* Daniel DM, et al (eds): *Knee Ligaments: Structure, Function, Injury, and Repair*. Raven Press, New York, 1990, pp 201–237.
145. Odensten M, Gillquist J: Functional anatomy of the anterior cruciate ligament and a rationale for reconstruction. *J Bone Joint Surg [Am] 67A*:257, 1985.
146. O'Donoghue DH, et al: Repair of knee ligaments in dogs. I. The lateral collateral ligament. *J Bone Joint Surg [Am] 43A*:1167, 1961.
147. Ogata K, et al: The intra-articular effect of various postoperative managements following knee ligament repair: An experimental study in dogs. *Clin Orthop 150*:271, 1980.
148. Olmstead ML: Lateral luxation of the patella. *In* Bojrab MJ (ed): *Pathophysiology in Surgery*. Lea & Febiger, Philadelphia, 1981, pp 638–640.
149. Paatsama S: Ligamentous injuries of the canine stifle joint. A clinical and experimental study. Master's Thesis, Helsinki, Finland, 1952.
150. Paatsama S: The structure and histopathology of the canine meniscus. *Am J Vet Res 15*:495, 1954.
151. Paatsama S: Regeneration of the canine meniscus. *Nord Vet Med 7*:953, 1955.
152. Paatsama S: Ein Weiterer Beitragzu Den Kniegelenksoperatonen Beim Hund. Proceedings of the 17th World Veterinary Congress, 1963.
153. Patterson RH, et al: Biomechanical stability of four cranial cruciate ligament repair techniques in the dog. *Vet Surg 20*:85, 1991.
154. Pearson PT, et al: Lembert suture technique to surgically correct ruptured cruciate ligaments. *J Am Anim Hosp Assoc 7*:1, 1971.
155. Pelletier JP, Pelletier JM: Protective effects of corticosteroids on cartilage lesions and osteophyte formation in the Pond-Nuki model of osteoarthritis. *Arthritis Rheum 32*:181, 1989.
156. Penner DA, et al: An *in vitro* study of anterior cruciate ligament graft placement and isometry. *Am J Sports Med 16*:238, 1988.
157. Person MW: Prosthetic replacement of the cranial cruciate ligament under arthroscopic guidance. A pilot project. *Vet Surg 16*:37, 1987.
158. Pichler ME, et al: The fascia lata as a replacement for the cranial cruciate ligament: Two new surgical techniques. *J Am Anim Hosp Assoc 18*:779–784, 1982.

159. Piermattei DL, Greeley RG: *An Atlas of Surgical Approaches to the Bones of the Dog and Cat*. W. B. Saunders, Philadelphia, 1979, pp 172–173.
160. Piermattei DL, Greeley RG: *An Atlas of Surgical Approaches to the Bones of the Dog and Cat*. W. B. Saunders, Philadelphia, 1979, pp 174–175.
161. Piermattei DL, Greeley RG: *An Atlas of Surgical Approaches to the Bones of the Dog and Cat*. W. B. Saunders, Philadelphia, 1979, pp 168–169.
162. Piermattei DL, Greeley RG: *An Atlas of Surgical Approaches to the Bones of the Dog and Cat*. W. B. Saunders, Philadelphia, 1979, pp 166–167.
163. Piper TL, Whiteside LA: Early mobilization after knee ligament repair in dogs: an experimental study. *Clin Orthop 150*:277–282, 1980.
164. Pond MJ, Campbell JR: The canine stifle joint. I. Rupture of the anterior cruciate ligament. An assessment of conservative and surgical treatment. *J Small Anim Pract 13*:1–10, 1972.
165. Pournaras J, et al: The significance of the posterior cruciate ligament in the stability of the knee. An experimental study in dogs. *J Bone Joint Surg 65B*:204–209, 1983.
166. Putnam RW: Patellar luxation in the dog. 1968, Thesis.
167. Read RA: Deformity of the proximal tibia in dogs. *Vet Rec 111*:295–298, 1982.
168. Reinke JD: Cruciate ligament avulsion injury in the dog. *J Am Anim Hosp Assoc 18*:257–264, 1982.
169. Renstrom P, et al: Strain within the anterior cruciate ligament during hamstring and quadriceps activity. *Am J Sports Med 14*:83–87, 1986.
170. Reznick AM, et al: Optimizing interference fixation for cruciate ligament reconstruction. *Proc Orthop Res Soc 15*:519, 1990.
171. Richards CD: Surgical correction of medial patellar luxation: Tibial crest transplantation and trochlear arthroplasty. *Vet Med Small Anim Clin 70*:322, 1975.
172. Ridge SC, et al: Induction of the synthesis of latent collagenase and latent neutral protease in chondrocytes by a factor synthesized by activated macrophages. *Arthritis Rheum 23*:448, 1980.
173. Roberts HM, et al: Caudal capsulorrhaphy for the correction of cranial cruciate ligament rupture in the dog. *Rhod Vet J 8*:46, 1977.
174. Robertson DB, et al: Soft tissue fixation to bone. *Am J Sports Med 14*:398, 1986.
175. Rosenberg TD, et al: Arthroscopic cruciate repair and reconstruction: An overview and descriptions of technique. *In* Feagin JA Jr (ed): *The Crucial Ligaments*. Churchill Livingstone, New York, 1988, pp 409–423.
176. Roth JH, et al: Intra-articular reconstruction of the anterior cruciate ligament with and without extra-articular supplementation by transfer of the biceps femoris tendon. *J Bone Joint Surg [Am] 69A*:275, 1987.
177. Roush JK, et al: Chronic osteomyelitis associated with orthopedic implants and cranial cruciate repair in three dogs. *J Am Vet Med Assoc 196*:1123, 1990.
178. Rubin RM, et al: Prevention of knee instability. Experimental model for prosthetic anterior cruciate ligament. *Clin Orthop 113*:212, 1975.
179. Rudy RL: Joints of the hindlimb (cruciate ligament injuries). *In* Archibald J (ed): *Canine Surgery*. American Veterinary Publications, Santa Barbara, 1974, pp 1142–1152.
180. Sapega AA, et al: Testing for isometry during reconstruction of the anterior cruciate ligament. *J Bone Joint Surg [Am] 72A*:259, 1990.
181. Scavelli TD, Schrader SC: Nonsurgical management of rupture of the cranial cruciate ligament in 18 cats. *J Am Anim Hosp Assoc 23*:337, 1987.
182. Scavelli TD, et al: Partial rupture of the cranial cruciate ligament of the stifle in dogs: 25 cases (1982–1988). *J Am Vet Med Assoc 196*:1135, 1990.
183. Schiavinato A, et al: Intraarticular sodium hyaluronate injections in the Pond-Nuki experimental model of osteoarthritis in dogs II. Morphological findings. *Clin Orthop 241*:286, 1989.
184. Schils JP, et al: Diagnostic imaging of ligamentous injuries of the knee. *In* Daniel DM, et al (eds): *Knee Ligaments: Structure, Function, Injury, and Repair*. Raven Press, New York, 1990, pp 461–480.
185. Schultz R, et al: Mechanoreceptors in human cruciate ligament. *J Bone Joint Surg [Am] 66A*:1072, 1984.
186. Schutte MJ, et al: Neural anatomy of the human anterior cruciate ligament. *J Bone Joint Surg [Am] 69A*:243, 1987.
187. Selby B, et al: Sonography in the detection of meniscal injuries of the knee: evaluation in cadavers. *AJR 149*:549, 1987.
188. Shikata J, et al: Experimental studies of the elastic fiber of the capsular ligament: Influence of ageing and sex hormones on the hip joint capsule of rats. *Connect Tissue Res 7*:21, 1979.
189. Shino K, et al: Replacement of the anterior cruciate ligament by an allogeneic tendon graft. *J Bone Joint Surg [Br] 66B*:672, 1984.
190. Shires PK, et al: The under-and-over fascial replacement technique for anterior cruciate ligament rupture in dogs: A retrospective study. *J Am Anim Hosp Assoc 20*:69, 1984.
191. Shoemaker SC, Daniel DM: The limits of knee motion. *In* Daniel DM, et al (eds): *Knee Ligaments: Structure, Function, Injury, and Repair*. Raven Press, New York, 1990, pp 153–161.
192. Singleton WB: Observations based upon the surgical repair of 106 cases of anterior cruciate ligament rupture. *J Small Anim Pract 10*:269, 1969.
193. Singleton WB: The surgical correction of stifle deformities in the dog. *J Small Anim Pract 10*:59, 1969.
194. Slocum B, et al: Wedge recession for treatment of recurrent luxation of the patella. *Clin Orthop 164*:48, 1982.
195. Smith GK, Torg JS: Fibular head transposition for repair of cruciate-deficient stifle in the dog. *J Am Vet Med Assoc 187*:375, 1985.
196. Solomonow M, et al: The synergistic action of the anterior cruciate ligament and thigh muscles in maintaining joint stability. *Am J Sports Med 15*:207, 1987.
197. Souryal TO, et al: Bilaterality in anterior cruciate ligament injuries: Associated intercondylar notch stenosis. *Am J Sports Med 16*:449, 1988.
198. Steyn DG: An experimental study on the use of a carbon fibre prosthesis for the repair of the cranial cruciate ligament in the dog. *J S Afri Vet Assoc 55*:23, 1984.
199. Stone EA, et al: Folding of the caudal horn of the medial meniscus secondary to severence of the cranial cruciate ligament. *Vet Surg 9*:121, 1980.
200. Stone KR, et al: Future directions. Collagen-based prostheses for meniscal regeneration. *Clin Orthop 252*:129, 1990.
201. Strande A: *Repair of the Ruptured Cranial Cruciate Ligament in the Dog*. Williams & Wilkins, Baltimore, 1967.
202. Strom H: Partial rupture of the cranial cruciate ligament in dogs. *J Small Anim Pract 31*:137, 1990.
203. Tarvin GB, Arnoczky SP: Incomplete rupture of the cranial cruciate ligament in a dog. *Vet Surg 10*:94, 1981.
204. Townley CO, et al: The free synovial graft as a shield ior collagen ingrowth in cruciate ligament repair. *Clin Orthop 197*:266, 1985.
205. Turner WD, et al: An *in vitro* study of the structural properties of deep-frozen versus freeze-dried, ethylene oxide-sterilized canine anterior cruciate ligament bone-ligament-bone preparations. *Clin Orthop 230*:251, 1988.
206. van der Kraan PM, et al: Development of osteoarthritic lesions in mice by "metabolic" and "mechanical" alterations in the knee joints. *Am J Pathol 135*:1001, 1989.
207. Van Steensel CJ, et al: Failure of anterior cruciate ligament-reconstruction using tendon xenograft. *J Bone Joint Surg [Am] 69A*:860, 1987.
208. Vasseur PB: Clinical results following nonoperative management for rupture of the cranial cruciate ligament in dogs. *Vet Surg 13*:243, 1984.
209. Vasseur PB, Arnoczky SP: Collateral ligaments of the canine stifle joint: Anatomic and functional analysis. *Am J Vet Res 42*:1133, 1981.
210. Vasseur PB, Berry CR: Progression of stifle osteoarthrosis following reconstruction of the cranial cruciate ligament in 21 dogs. *J Am Anim Hosp Assoc*, *28*:129, 1992.
211. Vasseur PB, Koblik P: Radiographic and surgical evaluation of the intercondyloid fossa in dogs with rupture of the cranial cruciate ligament. *J Am Vet Med Assoc*, submitted for publication.
212. Vasseur PB, et al: Correlative biomechanical and histological study of the cranial cruciate ligament in dogs. *Am J Vet Res 9*:1842, 1985.
213. Vasseur PB, et al: Replacement of the anterior cruciate ligament with a bone-ligament-bone anterior cruciate ligament allograft in dogs. *Clin Orthop 219*:268, 1987.
214. Vierheller RC: Surgical correction of patellar ectopia in the dog. *J Am Vet Med Assoc 134*:429, 1959.
215. Webster DA, Werner FW: Freeze-dried flexor tendons in anterior cruciate ligament reconstruction. *Clin Orthop 181*:238, 1983.
216. Welches CD, Scavelli TD: Transarticular pinning to repair luxation of the stifle joint in dogs and cats: A retrospective study of 10 cases. *J Am Anim Hosp Assoc 26*:207, 1990.
217. Welsh RP: Knee joint structure and function. *Clin Orthop 147*:7, 1980.
218. Whitehair J, Vasseur PB: Epidemiology of cranial cruciate ligament rupture in dogs. *J Am Vet Med Assoc*, in press.
219. Wiig ME, et al: The early effect of high molecular weight hyaluronan (hyaluronic acid) on anterior cruciate ligament healing: An experimental study in rabbits. *J Orthop Res 8*:425, 1990.
220. Willauer CC, Vasseur PB: Clinical results of surgical correction of medial luxation of the patella in dogs. *Vet Surg 16*:31, 1987.
221. Wind AP: Personal communication, 1991.
222. Woo S L-Y, et al: New experimental procedures to evaluate the biomechanical properties of healing canine medial collateral ligaments. *J Orthop Res 5*:425, 1987.
223. Woo S L-Y, et al: The response of ligaments to injury: Healing of the collateral ligaments. *In* Daniel DM, et al (eds): *Knee Ligaments: Structure, Function, Injury, and Repair*. Raven Press, New York, 1990, pp 351–364.
224. Woo S L-Y, et al: Treatment of the medial collateral ligament injury. 2. Structure and function of canine knees in response to differing treatment regimens. *Am J Sports Med 15*:22, 1987.
225. Woo S L-Y, et al: Fundamental studies in knee ligament mechanics. *In* Daniel DM, et al (eds): *Knee Ligaments: Structure, Function, Injury, and Repair*. Raven Press, New York, 1990, pp 115–134.
226. Wood DJ, et al: Replacement of the rabbit medial meniscus with a polyester-carbon fibre bioprosthesis. *Biomaterials 11*:13, 1990.
227. Yahia LH, Drouin G: Microscopical investigation of canine anterior cruciate ligament and patellar tendon: Collagen fascicle morphology and architecture. *J Orthop Res 7*:243, 1989.
228. Yoshiya S, et al: Graft tension in anterior cruciate ligament reconstruction. An *in vivo* study in dogs. *Am J Sports Med 15*:464, 1987.
229. Zahm H: Die ligamenta decessata in gesunden und arthrotischen kniegelenk des hundes. *KleintierPraxis 10*:38, 1965.
230. Zimney M, et al: Mechanoreceptors in the human anterior cruciate ligament. *Anat Rec 214*:204, 1986.
231. Zoltan DJ, et al: Synthetic and allograft anterior cruciate ligament reconstruction. *Clin Sports Med 7*:773, 1988.

CHAPTER

138 Fractures of the Tibia and Fibula

Ann L. Johnson and E.G. Boone

Fractures of the tibia result from trauma. Most fractures of the tibia include the fibula, although the fibula is frequently ignored in treatment unless the stability of the stifle or hock is jeopardized. Fractures of the tibia account for 20 per cent of fractures.[9, 10, 14] Motor vehicle accidents are responsible for a large percentage.[10] Other causes of fractured tibias include gunshots, fights, falls, and unknown trauma. Skeletal tumors may predispose the bone to fractures.

Two hundred thirty-five dogs and cats with tibial fractures were studied over 5 years.[2, 3] Three fractures were of the proximal tibia, 195 were of the tibial diaphysis, and 43 were of the distal tibia. Several animals sustained bilateral tibial fractures. Animals younger than 1 year accounted for 100 per cent of the proximal tibial fractures, 55 per cent of the diaphyseal fractures, and 41 per cent of the distal tibial fractures. The right and left tibias were equally affected. Proximal fractures included avulsions of the tibial tubercle and separation of the proximal physis. Diaphyseal fractures included transverse (14 per cent), spiral and oblique (44 per cent), comminuted (34 per cent), and segmental fractures (3 per cent). Distal tibial fractures included metaphyseal (9 per cent), physeal (30 per cent), epiphyseal (2 per cent), and malleolar, including the fibula (58 per cent). Twelve per cent of tibial diaphyseal fractures and 37 per cent of distal tibial fractures were open. Open fractures and comminuted fractures occurred more frequently in animals older than 1 year.

ANATOMY

The tibia articulates proximally with the femur, distally with the tarsus, and on its lateral side both proximally and distally with the fibula.[11] The proximal end is relatively flat and triangular, with the articular surface in its caudal half. The cranial process is the tibial tuberosity, which provides insertion for the patellar ligament. The tibial tuberosity continues distally as the cranial border of the tibia, before tapering into the diaphysis. The proximal tibial metaphysis is relatively flat medially but concave laterally and caudally. The mid-diaphysis is cylindrical. The shaft is slightly S shaped when viewed cranially and laterally. The distal end of the tibia is flared slightly in a medial to lateral direction. The distal epiphysis forms the medial malleolus, which is the proximal attachment of the medial collateral ligament of the hock joint.

The fibula is a long, flat compressed bone on the lateral side of the tibia.[11] Its proximal end is enlarged to form the fibular head, which articulates with the lateral tibial condyle. It serves as the distal attachment of the lateral collateral ligament of the stifle. The fibular diaphysis is thin but widens distally at the epiphysis, which articulates with the tibial tarsal bone. The distal end is the lateral malleolus and provides proximal attachment for the lateral collateral ligament of the hock.

The tibia has two growth plates proximally and one distally. The first proximal one contributes 40 per cent of the length of the tibia and closes between 6 and 11 months of age. The second proximal growth plate forms the tibial tuberosity and closes at the same time. The distal physis contributes 60 per cent of the tibial length and closes at 5 to 8 months of age. The proximal fibula closes at 6 to 10 months of age, and the distal fibula fuses at 5 to 8 months of age.[6]

In adults, the main afferent artery is the caudal tibial artery, which enters the medullary canal through the nutrient foramen in the caudolateral edge at the junction of the proximal and middle thirds. Within the medullary canal, it divides into proximal and distal branches that anastomose with metaphyseal branches at each end. Terminal branches of the metaphyseal arteries enter the proximal and distal extremities of the medullary cavity to anastomose with terminal branches of the ascending and descending arteries. These anastomoses are important because they permit the metaphyseal arteries to sustain medullary arterial supply when the principal nutrient artery has been ruptured by fracture or surgery. These medullary anastomotic arteries supply the inner two-thirds of the tibial cortical circulation. Periosteal arterioles, especially at fascial or ligamentous attachments, supply the outer third of the cortical circulation.[13]

The principal efferent venous drainage is via the large emissary veins through the nutrient foramen, with secondary drainage through cortical venous channels into periosteal vessels and periosteal capillaries that are in continuity with cortical lamella.[13]

SURGICAL TREATMENT

Diagnosis of tibial fractures is by physical and radiographic examination. Affected animals usually do not bear weight on the injured limb and have palpable swelling and crepitation at the fracture site. Two radiographic views of the tibia, including the stifle and the hock, confirm the diagnosis and identify the fracture type. Because of the frequency of multiple organ injury sustained during trauma of sufficient force to cause fractures, the animal is evaluated carefully.[1, 9, 10, 14] Preoperative treatment includes careful cleaning of open wounds and application of a Robert Jones bandage to protect the fracture and surrounding soft tissues and prevent or reduce limb swelling before surgery.

The method of reduction and fixation is determined preoperatively. Applicable reduction and fixation techniques include closed reduction with external coaptation or an external fixation splint and open reduction with fixation using pins and orthopedic wire, an external fixation splint, or plate and screws. Selection of method depends on the type and location of the fracture, signalment of the animal, additional skeletal injuries, and the surgeon's familiarity with the various types of fixation equipment and fixation techniques.

If antibiotics are indicated because of an open fracture or anticipation of a lengthy, complicated procedure, a broad-spectrum antibiotic is administered intravenously at anesthetic induction and continued parenterally for at least 48 hours after surgery until the results of culture and sensitivity testing are known.

The primary surgical approach to the tibia is a cranial medial incision parallel to the tibial crest and extending the length of the tibia. Minimal muscle covers the medial aspect of the tibia, and dissection is continued through the fascia, avoiding the medial saphenous vein and nerve crossing the middle to distal thirds of the tibial diaphysis (Fig. 138–1). The medial and lateral malleoli are exposed using medial and lateral skin incisions directly over the malleoli.

A soft padded bandage is applied postoperatively to protect the surgical wound and prevent excessive swelling of the limb. The bandage is changed as needed for about 5 days. Warm compresses or hydrotherapy may reduce limb swelling. Daily physical therapy of the hock and stifle increases range of motion and decreases postoperative edema. The animal is confined, and exercise is limited for 4 to 6 weeks. Postoperative and follow-up radiographs are evaluated for alignment of the fracture, positioning of implants, and healing activity. Bridging callus or loss of visible fracture lines on the radiograph is an indication to allow increased activity. Fixation removal is recommended when the fracture is healed and no longer needs support. Time to fixation removal varies with the age of the dog, type of fracture, and fixation.

FRACTURE FIXATION TECHNIQUES IN IMMATURE ANIMALS

Immature animals sustain physeal fractures, greenstick fractures, transverse fractures, spiral or oblique fractures, segmental fractures, and comminuted fractures. They sustain more greenstick and segmental fractures and fewer comminuted and open fractures than adults.[2] Fixation devices in immature animals include casts and splints, intramedullary pins, Kirschner wires, orthopedic wire, external fixation, and for selected fractures plates and screws. Immature animals heal faster and have fewer problems with osteomyelitis and nonunions. Disruption of growth is a possibility, and limb shortening and angular deformities are potential complications.

Avulsion of the Tibial Tuberosity

Avulsion of the tibial tuberosity through the proximal physis results in proximal displacement of the tuberosity and is reduced and stabilized to restore function of the quadriceps muscle and extension of the stifle. Open reduction is necessary. Fixation after open reduction consists of a ligament-to-bone suture technique, two Kirschner wires, wire sutures, or a tension band wire (Fig. 138–2).

Physeal Fractures of the Proximal and Distal Tibia

The proximal tibial physeal fracture is usually a Salter type I or II fracture, although rarely a Salter III or IV may occur.[4] With a Salter I or II fracture, the epiphysis may be displaced caudolaterally to the tibial diaphysis and collateral ligaments may be injured. Reduction of the fracture is essential for both normal appearance and function.

Open reduction and internal fixation are usually required for treatment of the physeal fracture. In addition, the proximal fibular fracture may need to be stabilized with a small Kirschner wire (Fig. 138–3) to stabilize the tibial plateau and stifle. Kirschner wires or an intramedullary pin is recommended for fixation of the physeal fracture. Lag screw fixation may be used in nearly mature dogs, in which interference with growth is minimal (see Fig. 138–3).

The distal tibial physeal fracture is also usually a Salter type I or II fracture. Closed reduction may be achieved if treatment is begun early enough and the

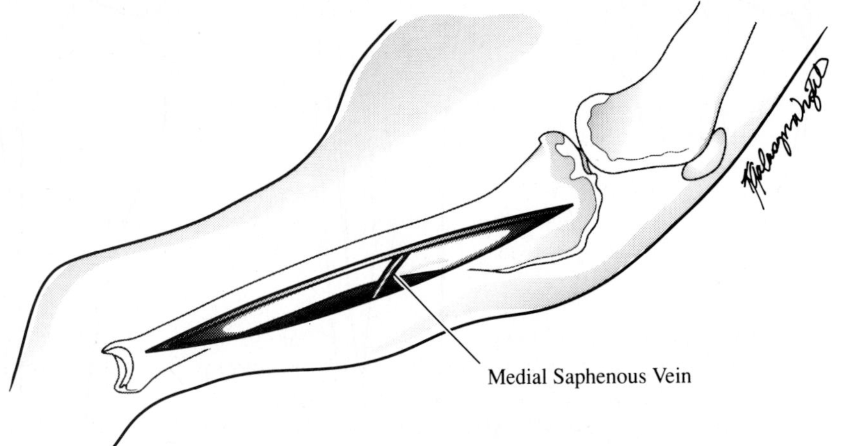

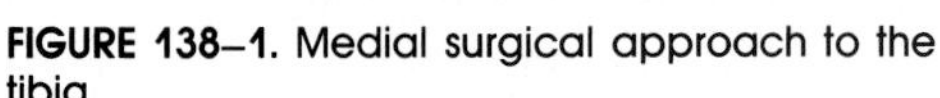
FIGURE 138–1. Medial surgical approach to the tibia.

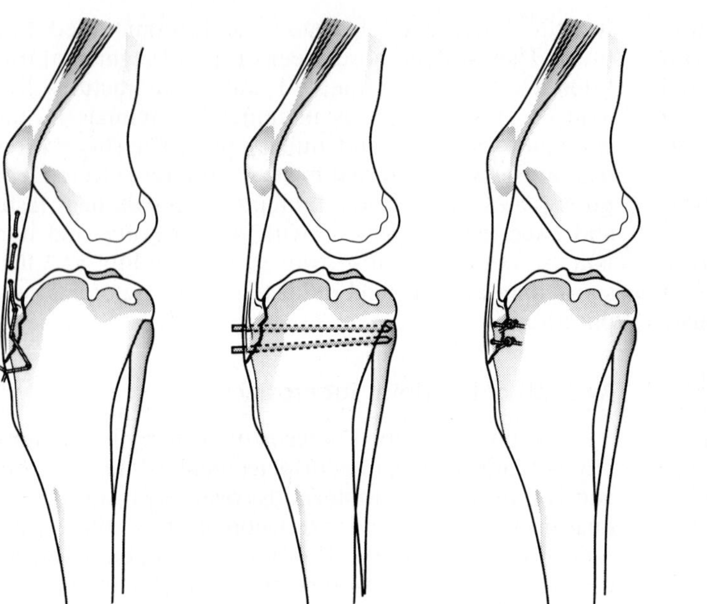

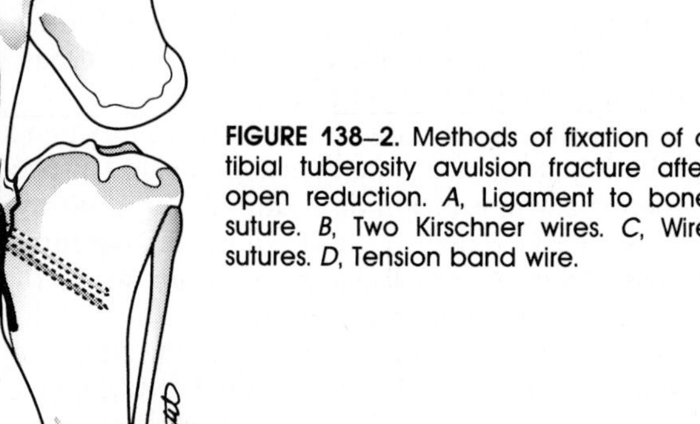

FIGURE 138–2. Methods of fixation of a tibial tuberosity avulsion fracture after open reduction. *A*, Ligament to bone suture. *B*, Two Kirschner wires. *C*, Wire sutures. *D*, Tension band wire.

fracture is stabilized with a cast. If open reduction is necessary, fixation is by Kirschner wires (Fig. 138–4).

Fracture of the Diaphysis of the Tibia

Greenstick or incomplete fractures of the tibia require minimal reduction with care to avoid angular deformities after reduction. The fracture is stabilized with a cast or splint for 3 to 4 weeks.

Transverse or short oblique fractures may be reduced with open or closed manipulation. If closed reduction is successful, a cast or external fixation splint is applied (Fig. 138–5). If open reduction is required, an intramedullary pin and half-pin fixation splint, an external fixation splint, or a plate may be used to stabilize the fracture (Fig. 138–5). It is difficult to control rotational forces at the transverse fracture site with a single intramedullary pin, with or without orthopedic wire.

Spiral or Long Oblique Fractures of the Tibial Diaphysis

It is difficult to achieve a stable closed reduction of spiral or long oblique fractures because of the tendency for the fracture to over-ride; consequently, open reduction and internal fixation are usually necessary to achieve optimum reduction. Intramedullary pinning with rotational stability achieved with multiple cerclage wires or Kirschner wires with figure-eight orthopedic wire is effective for these fractures (Fig. 138–6). Correct placement of the intramedullary pin is important to avoid interfering with the stifle joint. The pin is started from

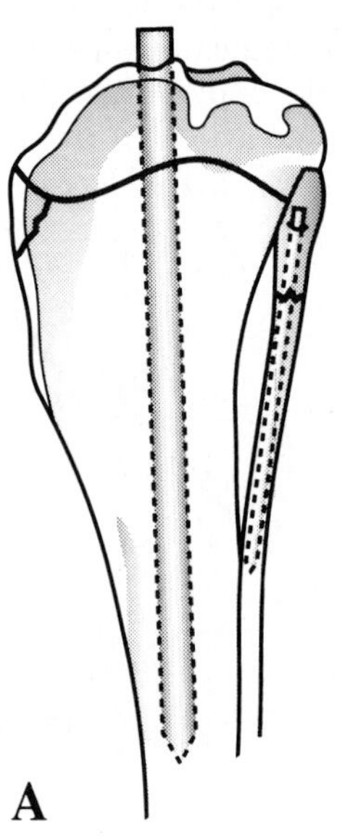

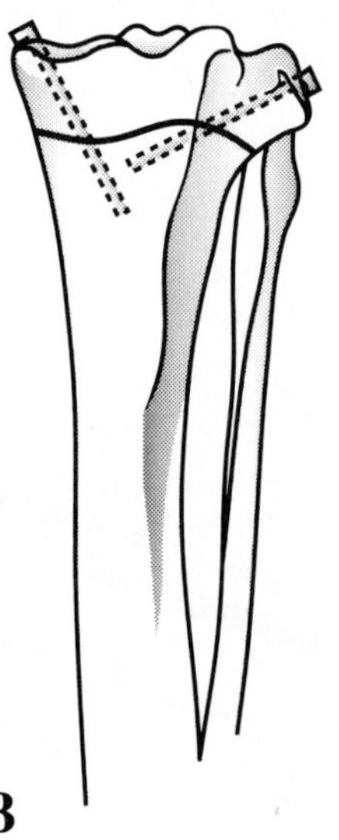

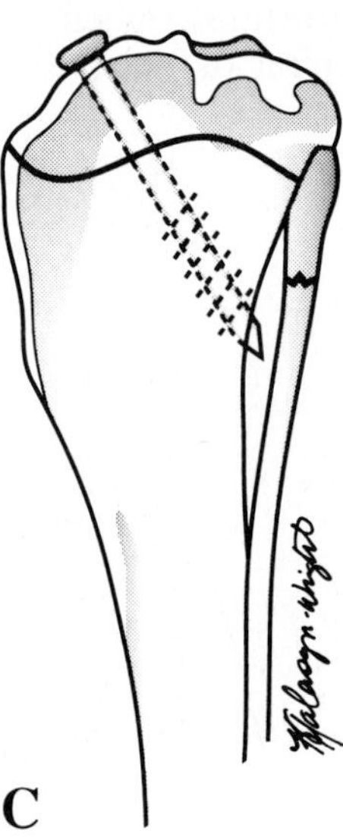

FIGURE 138–3. Methods of fixation of a proximal tibial physeal fracture. *A*, Intramedullary pin. *B*, Two Kirschner wires. *C*, Lag screw fixation.

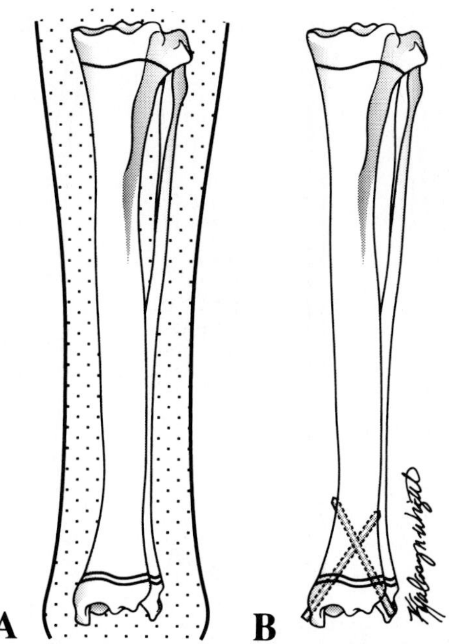

FIGURE 138–4. Methods of fixation of a distal tibial physeal fracture. *A*, Cast. *B*, Two Kirschner wires.

the medial aspect of the proximal end of the tibia, where it is inserted through the skin and penetrates the bone at a point midway between the tibial tuberosity and the medial tibial condyle on the medial ridge of the tibial plateau (Fig. 138–7). A small enough pin is chosen to allow the pin to traverse the curve of the medullary canal without disrupting the reduction of the fracture (see Fig. 138–7). A smaller-diameter pin also allows placement of Kirschner wires through the diaphysis of the tibia at the fracture line.

Comminuted and Segmental Fractures of the Diaphysis of the Tibia

The method of fixation of comminuted or segmental fractures depends on the direction of the fracture lines. Oblique or spiral fracture lines are treated by reduction and interfragmentary compression with cerclage wire or lag screws. Transverse fracture lines are treated with an external fixation splint or a plate. Axial stability is achieved using intramedullary pins, an external fixation splint, or a plate (Fig. 138–8). The objective of reducing and stabilizing a comminuted fracture is to reduce and stabilize the fragments until a two-piece fracture remains and can be reduced and treated as a simple fracture. Severely comminuted fractures (e.g., gunshot injuries) may have small pieces that cannot be reduced or stabilized. In these fractures, aligning the stifle and hock joints, distracting the tibia to normal length, and bridging the fracture with an external fixation splint or a plate functioning as a buttress plate are the best way to stabilize the fracture (Fig. 138–9). Precontouring the plate to match a cranial-caudal radiograph of the normal tibia helps maintain normal contour and length of the fractured tibia. Closed reduction or open reduction of tibial diaphyseal fractures for fixation with a bilateral external fixation splint can be achieved by first placing the proximal and distal transfixation pins parallel to their respective joints and in the transverse plane. A fracture distractor* is applied to the transfixation pins on one side of the limb, usually the concave side of the fracture. The fracture is distracted until length is normal or the fracture is reduced. Reduction is held by stabilizing the fixation pins with a connecting bar placed on the opposite side of the limb. The fracture distractor is

*Synthes, Paoli, PA, USA.

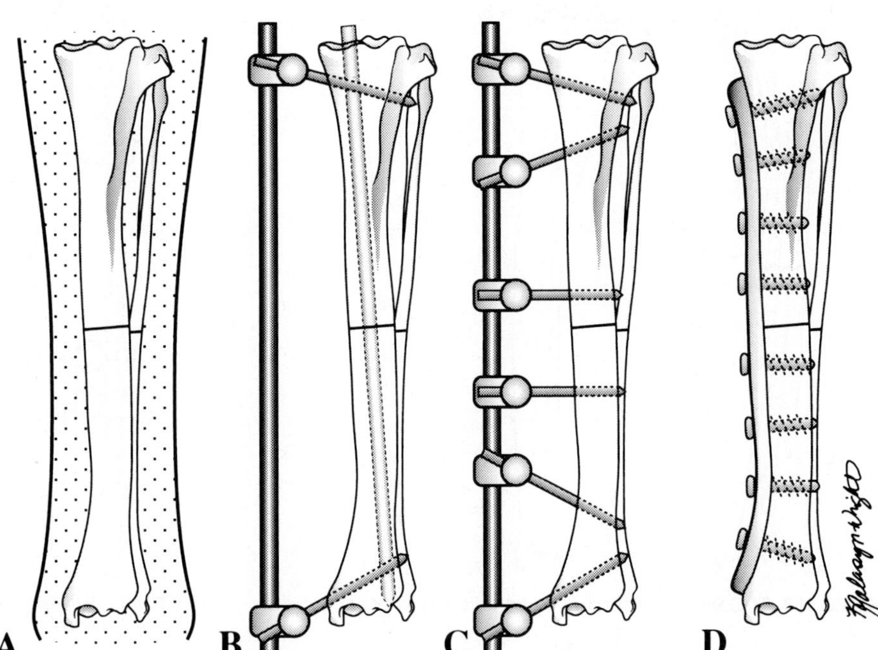

FIGURE 138–5. Methods of fixation of a transverse diaphyseal fracture. *A*, Cast. *B*, Intramedullary pin and two-pin unilateral external fixation splint. *C*, External fixation splint. *D*, Plate and screws.

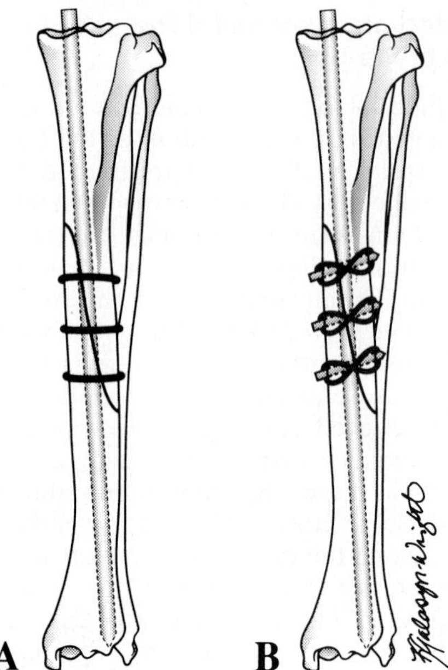

FIGURE 138–6. Methods of fixation of a spiral diaphyseal fracture. *A*, Intramedullary pin and cerclage wires. *B*, Intramedullary pin, Kirschner wires, and figure-eight orthopedic wire.

removed, and the bilateral splint is constructed (Fig. 138–10). If the fracture is opened for reduction, a cancellous bone graft is placed in the fracture gap and at fracture lines immediately before closure of the surgical wound.

Tibia

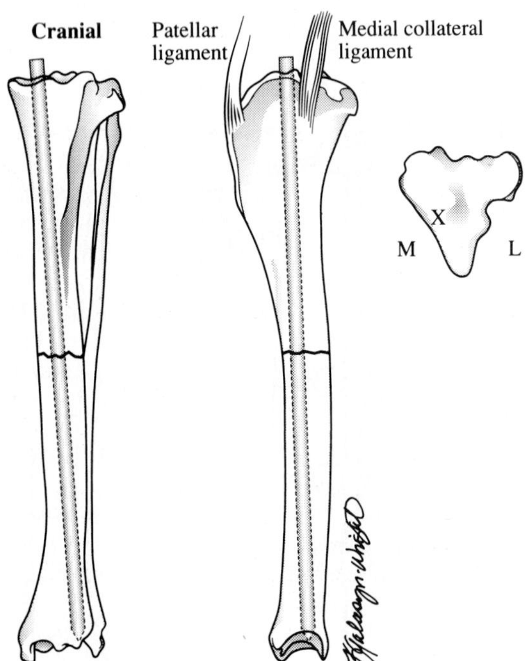

FIGURE 138–7. Correct placement of an intramedullary pin in the tibia.

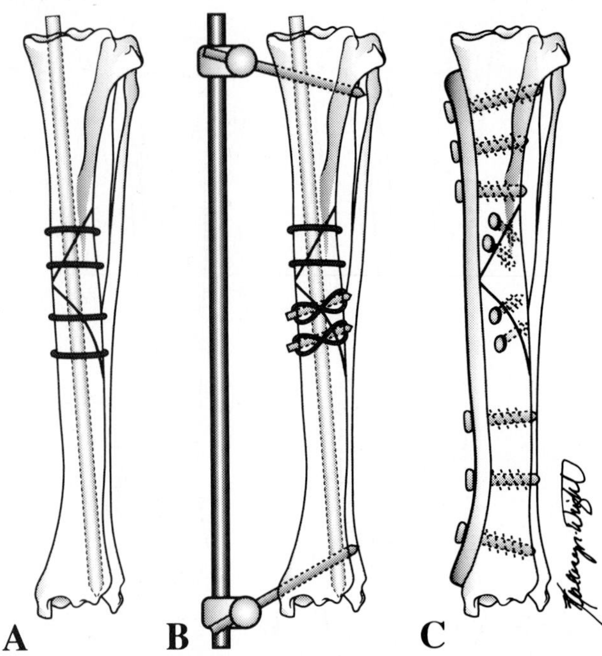

FIGURE 138–8. Methods of fixation of a comminuted tibial fracture. *A*, Intramedullary pin and cerclage wire. *B*, Intramedullary pin, cerclage wire, Kirschner wires with figure-eight orthopedic wire and a two-pin unilateral external fixation splint. *C*, Lag screw and neutralization plate.

FRACTURE FIXATION TECHNIQUES IN MATURE ANIMALS

Mature animals usually sustain fractures of the diaphysis, including transverse, spiral or oblique, and comminuted fractures. Mature animals sustain more com-

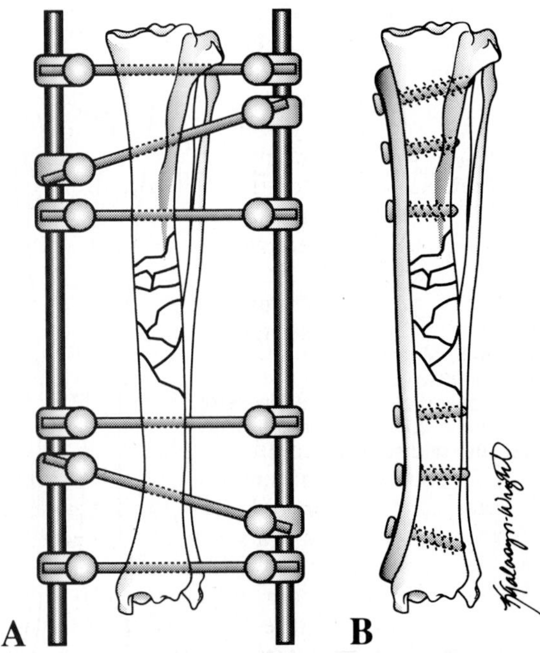

FIGURE 138–9. Methods of fixation of a severely comminuted tibial fracture. *A*, Bilateral six-pin external fixation splint. *B*, Buttress plate.

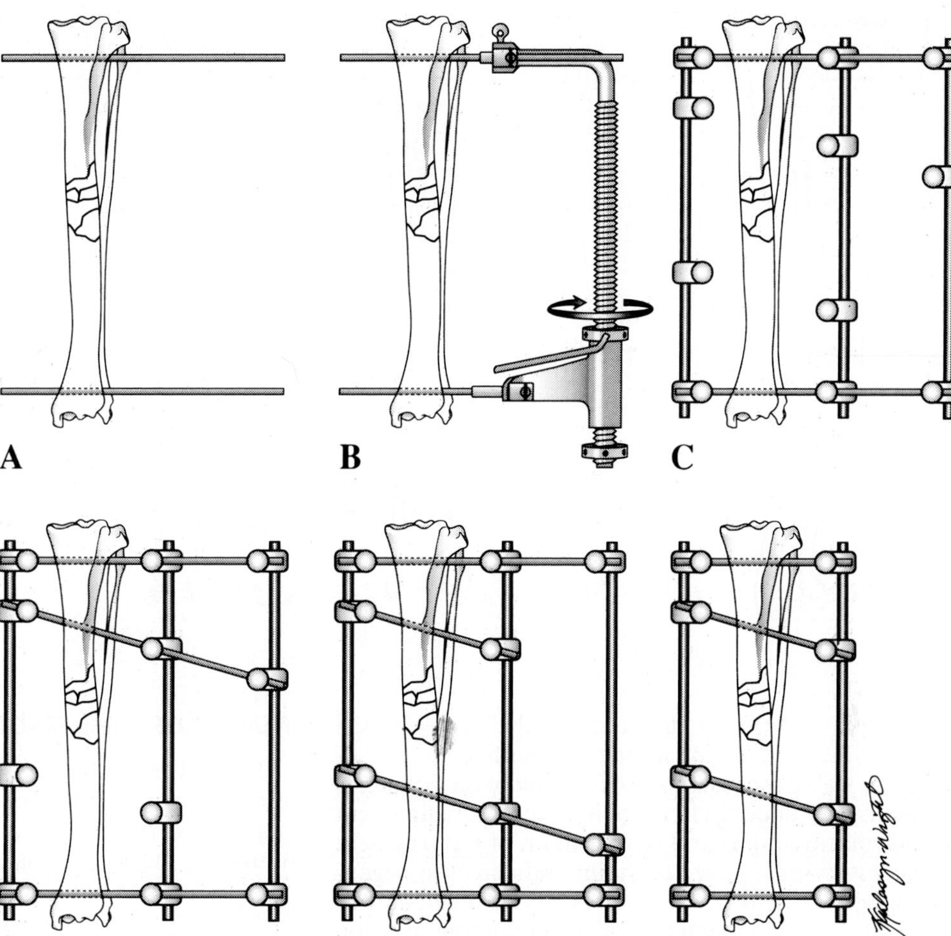

FIGURE 138–10. Use of the fracture distractor and bilateral external fixation splint for reducing and stabilizing a tibial fracture.

minuted and open fractures than do immature animals.[2] Mature animals are subjected to more shearing injuries and malleolar fractures.[3] Fixation devices used for mature animals include intramedullary pins, Kirschner wires, orthopedic wire, external fixation splints, and plates and screws. Casts may be used if closed reduction is stable. The applicability and stability of the bilateral external fixation splint to the tibia make this fixation technique attractive for treatment of open fractures in mature animals. Older animals heal more slowly and have a greater risk of osteomyelitis and nonunions. The increase in healing time and complication rate reflects not only the age of the animal but also the severity of the fracture and the use of rigid fixation.[2]

Fractures of the Proximal Tibia

Fractures of the proximal tibial metaphysis and epiphysis are infrequent in mature animals. Fractures are usually transverse or short oblique through the metaphysis. Casting is applicable if a stable closed reduction is possible. If open reduction is necessary, fixation is achieved by using an intramedullary pin supplemented by Kirschner wire and figure-eight orthopedic wire fixation. Crossed Kirschner wires or cancellous lag screws may also be used, although additional external support may be required (Fig. 138–11). Fractures of the proximal fibula require stabilization if stifle stability is impaired by disruption of the lateral collateral ligament. The fibular head may be secured to the tibia with a bone screw and Teflon washer (see Fig. 138–11).

Fractures of the Diaphysis of the Tibia

Diaphyseal fractures in mature animals are treated like those in immature animals (see Figs. 138–5 through 138–10). The increased frequency of open fractures affects selection of fixation devices. Open fractures are contaminated and must be rigidly stabilized to prevent infection. Loose implants and avascular bone fragments contribute to osteomyelitis and nonunion. External fixation splints are excellent for treating open fractures because the pins do not disrupt the fracture site. The splint can rigidly stabilize the main fracture fragments and allow open access to soft-tissue injuries. Rigid external fixators permit joint motion and limited use of the limb; these are major advantages over cast fixation. In addition, the entire fixation device is easily removed when the fracture is healed. Rigid internal fixation can also be used in infected fractures as long as stability of the fracture site is achieved and implants are removed after healing.

Fractures of the Distal Tibia

Fractures of the distal tibia in mature animals usually involve the malleoli, either as fractures of the malleoli

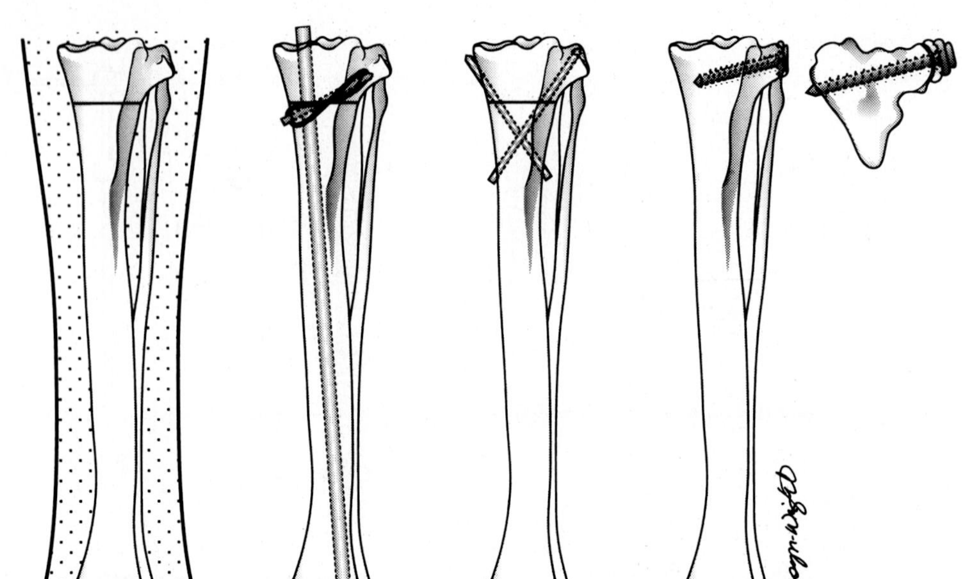

FIGURE 138–11. Methods of fixation of a proximal tibial fracture (*A–C*) and a proximal fibular fracture (*D*). *A*, Cast. *B*, Intramedullary pin, Kirschner wire, and figure-eight orthopedic wire. *C*, Two Kirschner wires. *D*, Screw with Teflon washer.

or as shearing injuries that remove the malleoli (see Chapter 139 for shearing injuries of the hock). Loss of malleolar stability causes loss of function of the collateral ligaments and talocrural instability. Accurate alignment of malleolar fractures and rigid fixation of the fragment are necessary to stabilize the joint and decrease degenerative joint disease.[3, 4] Fractures of the malleoli are usually treated with open reduction and internal fixation using either a tension band device or lag screw (Fig. 138–12). External coaptation or transarticular external fixation is used as necessary to support internal fixation of the fracture.

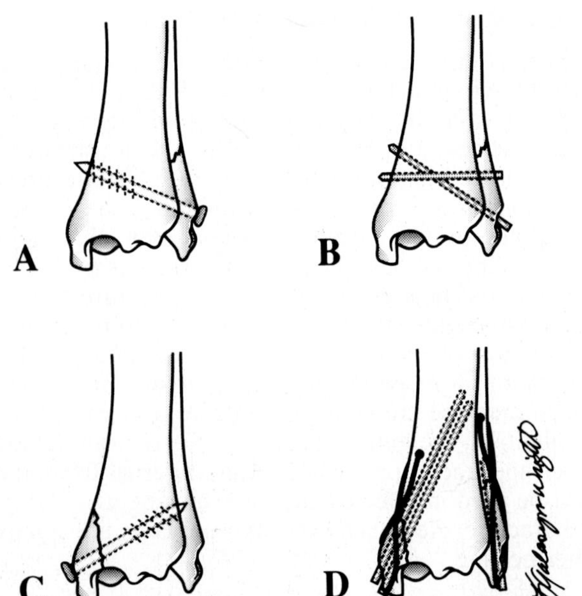

FIGURE 138–12. Methods of fixation of malleolar fractures. *A*, Lag screw. *B*, Kirschner wires. *C*, Lag screw. *D*, Tension band wire.

HEALING OF TIBIAL FRACTURES

Physeal fractures heal quickly, with either continued production of cartilage or cessation of growth and bridging of the physis with bone (Fig. 138–13). In either situation, the fracture is stable within 3 to 4 weeks and implants can be removed. If the physis is still functional, the implants are removed to eliminate further interference with growth.[4]

Tibial diaphyseal fractures in immature animals varied in time to healing from 3.95 ± 0.98 weeks for cast fractures, to 7.12 ± 2.04 weeks for pinned and wired fractures, to 10.5 ± 3.65 weeks for plated fractures. Healing times for the tibial diaphysis in mature animals were similar for fractures treated with a cast at 3.65 ± 1.38 weeks but were significantly increased to 13.29 ± 8.54 weeks for pinned fractures and 19.38 ± 10.25 weeks for plated fractures.[2] In tibial and radial fractures treated with external fixation, the mean time to fixation removal was 10 weeks and to unsupported weightbearing was 11 weeks.[8] Type and location of fracture, method of reduction, and accuracy of reduction were evaluated to determine their effects on healing time. Although none had a significant effect, the trend was toward longer healing times with open fractures and shorter healing times with closed reduction.[8]

Rate and type of healing depend on the location of the fracture, type of fixation used, and stability achieved at the fracture site. Primary union occurs when there is absolute stability and contact between fracture segments. This is achieved with implants that cause compression of the fracture site such as lag screws, cerclage wire, tension band wire, and a dynamic compression plate (Fig. 138–14).[12] Primary union has also been documented when rigid external fixation is applied to a fracture that is anatomically reduced.[8] As fixation becomes less rigid, bone union occurs through callus production and remodeling (Figs. 138–15 through 138–

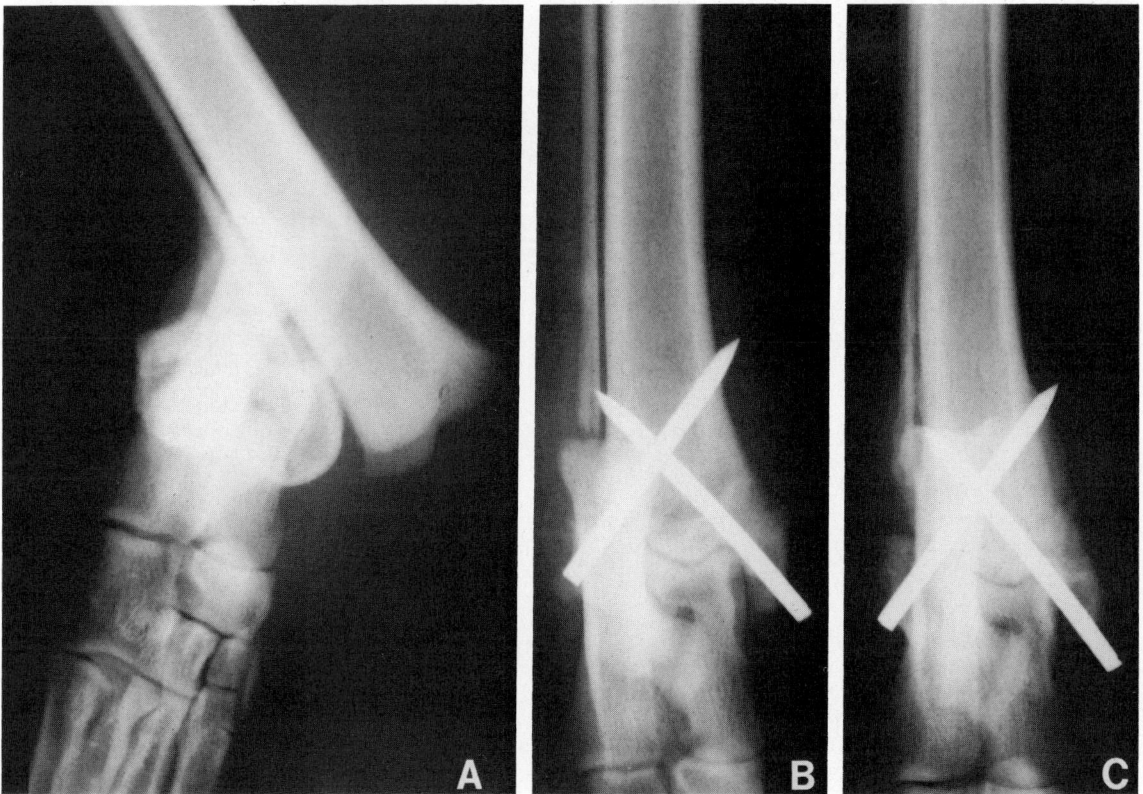

FIGURE 138–13. *A*, A distal tibial physeal fracture. *B*, Postoperative fixation with Kirschner wires. *C*, Five weeks after surgery.

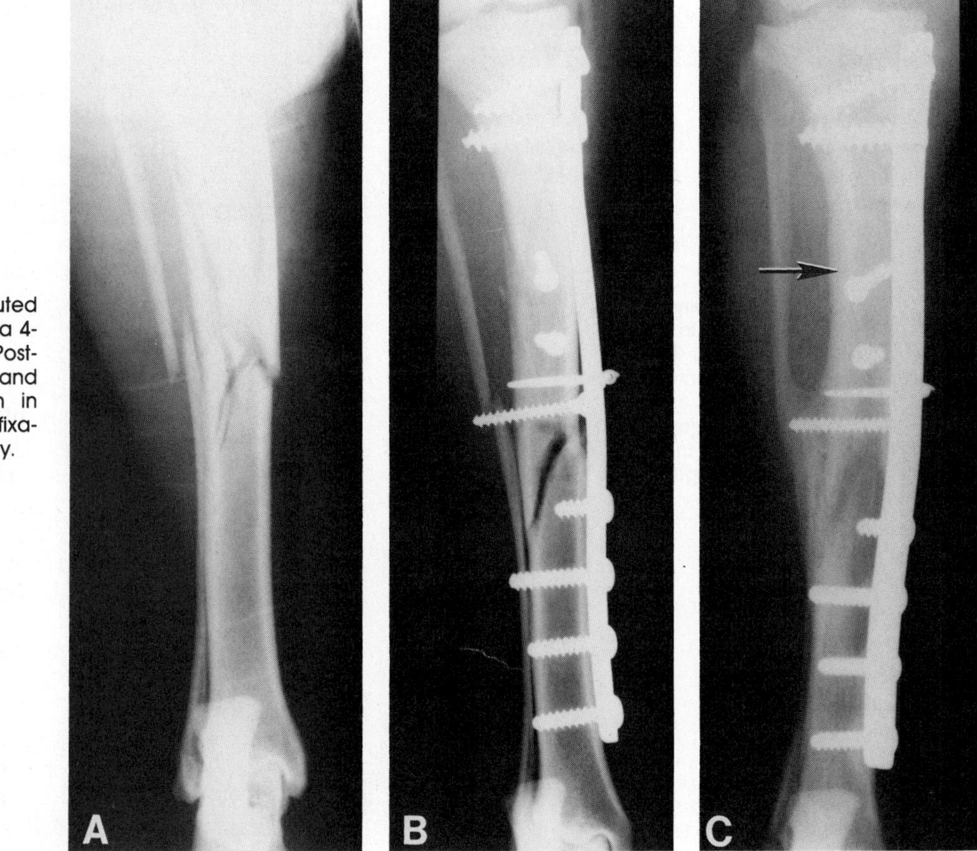

FIGURE 138–14. *A*, A comminuted fracture of the tibial diaphysis in a 4-year-old Labrador retriever. *B*, Postoperative fixation with plate and screws. *C*, Primary bone union in areas of compression and rigid fixation *(arrow)* 20 weeks after surgery.

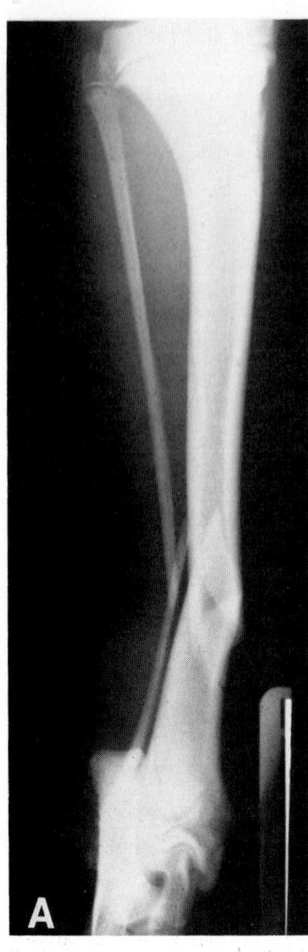

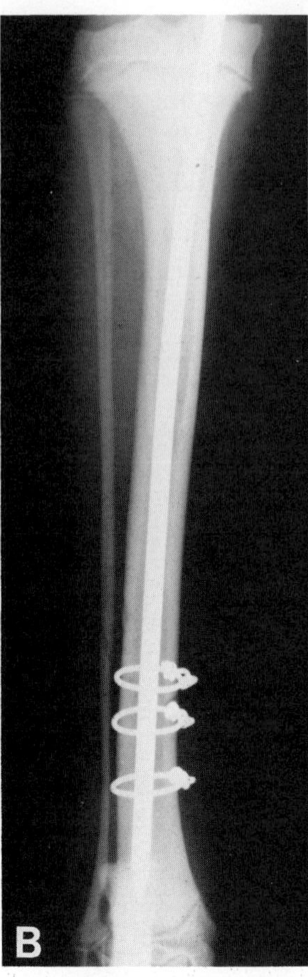

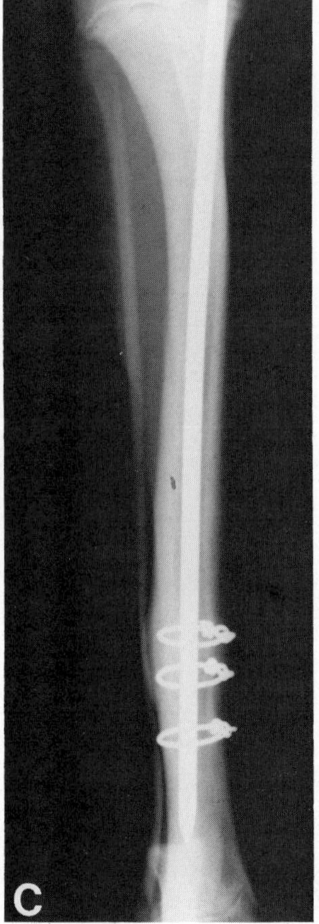

FIGURE 138–15. *A*, Simple fracture of the tibial diaphysis in a 6-month-old Afghan hound. *B*, Postoperative fixation with an intramedullary pin and cerclage wires. *C*, Minimal periosteal callus, reflecting the stability of the fixation, 7 weeks after surgery.

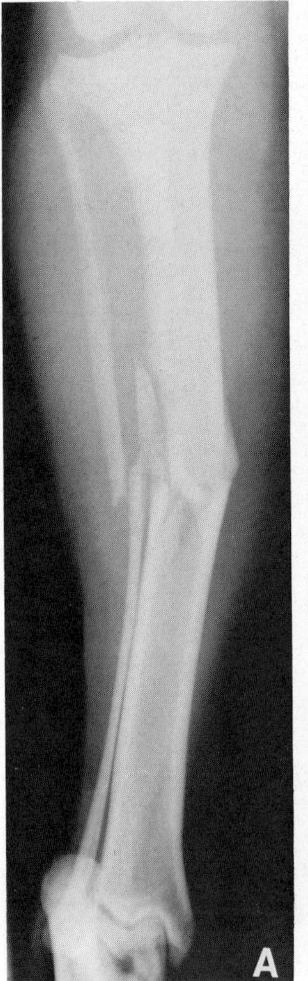

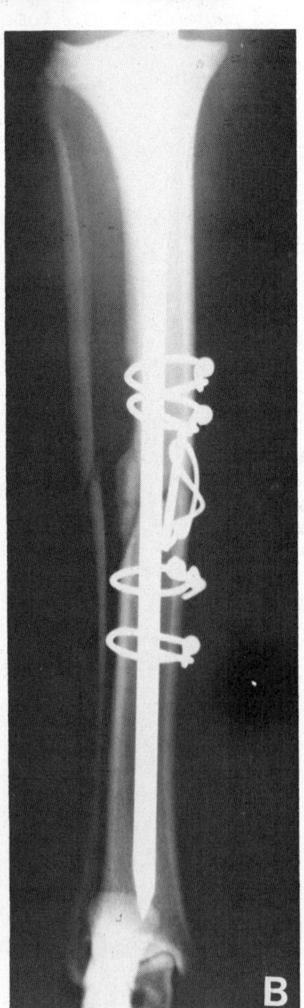

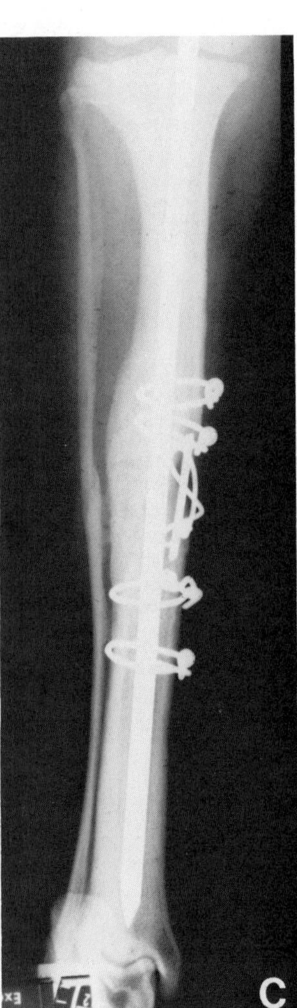

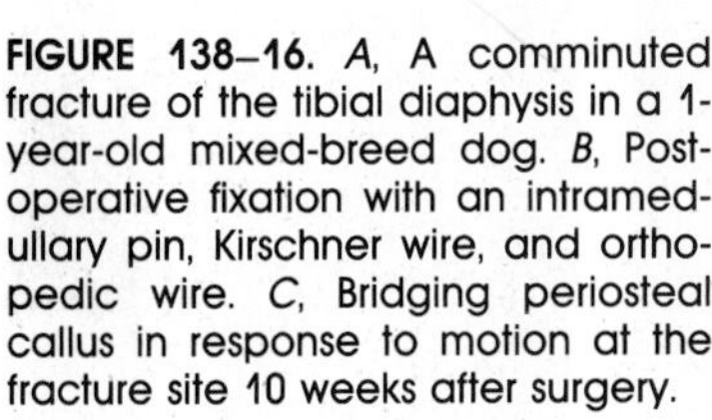

FIGURE 138–16. *A*, A comminuted fracture of the tibial diaphysis in a 1-year-old mixed-breed dog. *B*, Postoperative fixation with an intramedullary pin, Kirschner wire, and orthopedic wire. *C*, Bridging periosteal callus in response to motion at the fracture site 10 weeks after surgery.

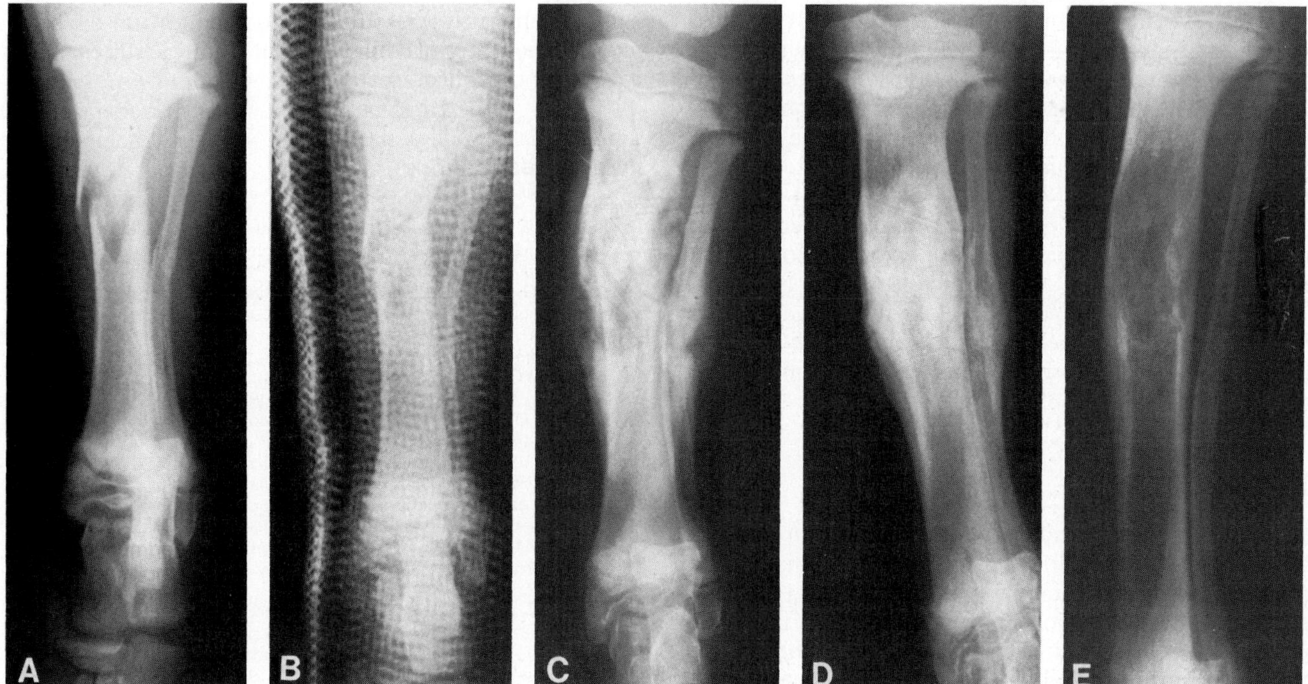

FIGURE 138–17. *A*, A fracture of the tibial diaphysis in a 2-month-old Old English sheepdog. *B*, Postoperative fixation with a cast. *C*, 11 days after fixation. *D*, 25 days after fixation. *E*, Remodeling of periosteal callus 47 days after fixation.

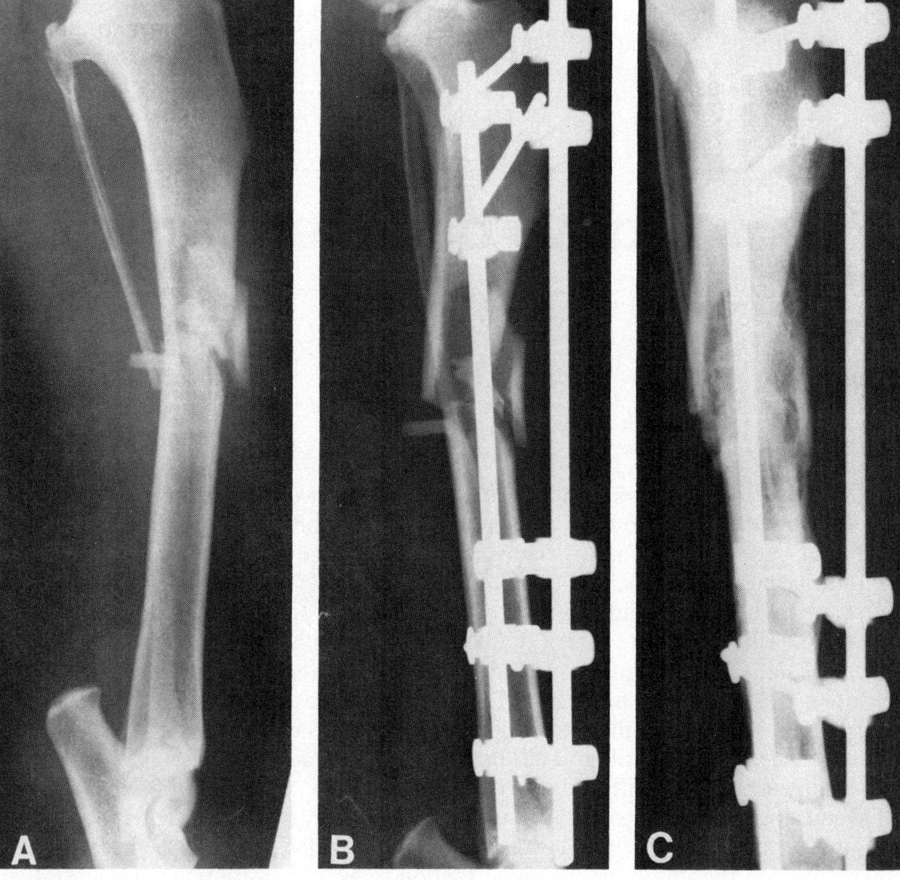

FIGURE 138–18. *A*, A comminuted fracture of the tibial diaphysis in a 4-year-old Irish setter. *B*, Postoperative fixation with a bilateral external fixation splint. *C*, Bridging periosteal and endosteal callus 9 weeks after surgery.

17).[12] Bridging periosteal callus allows implant removal earlier than with primary bone union. This effect is partially responsible for the shorter healing times reported for fractures stabilized with pins and wires compared with compressive fixation. Fractures stabilized with external fixators and not anatomically reconstructed heal by callus formation. In some animals, the callus is more endosteal in origin and minimal periosteal callus is observed (Fig. 138–18).[8]

In the tibia, most implants are removed after healing of the fracture. Pins may interfere with function of the stifle. Plates have little soft-tissue covering and may cause irritation of the soft tissues or may conduct cold or heat to the bone. Cerclage wire and screws are only removed if associated with loosening of the implant or infection.

COMPLICATIONS

Complications associated with tibial fracture repair are similar to those reported for long-bone diaphyseal fracture repair and include infection, implant failure, delayed union, nonunion and malunion, and impaired function of the limb.[5,7] Causes of these problems are instability, improper reduction, wound contamination, or interference with adjacent joints by implants.[7]

Nonunion occurs in approximately 4 per cent of tibial fractures.[2,8] The cause usually is instability, in some cases complicated by osteomyelitis. Extremely rigid fixation coupled with a large fracture gap may result in nonunion if adequate cancellous bone grafting is not used.[8] Malunions result in angular or rotational deformities and are usually associated with severely comminuted fractures in which the cortex cannot be anatomically reconstructed. Attention to position of the limb and relationship of the adjacent joint surfaces helps avoid this complication.

References

1. Bertoy RW, et al: Organ system injury and postoperative complications in dogs and cats with two long bone fractures: A matched case design. *Vet Comp Orthop Trauma 2*:140, 1989.
2. Boone EG, et al: Fractures of the tibial diaphysis in dogs and cats. *J Am Vet Med Assoc 188*:41, 1986.
3. Boone EG, et al: Distal tibial fractures in dogs and cats. *J Am Vet Med Assoc 188*:316, 1986.
4. Brinker WO, et al: *Handbook of Small Animal Orthopedics and Fracture Treatment*. W. B. Saunders, Philadelphia, 1983, pp 110–122.
5. Caywood DD, et al: Osteomyelitis in the dog: A review of 67 cases. *J Am Vet Med Assoc 172*:943, 1978.
6. DeKleer VS: Development of bone. *In* Sumner Smith G (ed): *Bone in Clinical Orthopedics*. W. B. Saunders, Philadelphia, 1982, pp 1–81.
7. Hunt JM, et al: The complications of diaphyseal fractures in dogs: A review of 100 cases. *J Small Anim Pract 21*:103, 1980.
8. Johnson AL, et al: Radial and tibial fracture repair with external skeletal fixation: Effects of fracture type, reduction, and complications on healing. *Vet Surg 18*:367, 1989.
9. Kolata RJ, Johnston DE: Motor vehicle accidents in urban dogs: A study of 600 cases. *J Am Vet Med Assoc 167*:938, 1975.
10. Kolata RJ, et al: Patterns of trauma in urban dogs and cats: A study of 1000 cases. *J Am Vet Med Assoc 164*:499, 1974.
11. Miller ME, et al: *Anatomy of the Dog*. 2nd ed. W. B. Saunders, Philadelphia, 1979, pp 210–215.
12. Rahn BA: Bone healing: Histologic and physiologic concepts. *In* Sumner Smith G (ed): *Bone in Clinical Orthopedics*. W. B. Saunders, Philadelphia, 1982, pp 335–386.
13. Rhinelander FW: Tibial blood supply in relation to fracture healing. *Clin Orthop Rel Res 105*:34, 1974.
14. Spackman CJA, et al: Thoracic wall and pulmonary trauma in dogs sustaining fractures as a result of motor vehicle accidents. *J Am Vet Med Assoc 185*:975, 1984.

CHAPTER 139 Tarsus and Metatarsus

R. A. Taylor and Jon F. Dee

ANATOMY

The tarsus consists of seven bones arranged in two transverse rows. Only the talus articulates with the tibia and fibula. The tarsus is more than three times longer than the carpus.[7] The trochlea of the talus (Fig. 139–1) is formed by a medial and lateral trochlear ridge. The groove and ridges deviate laterally about 25° from the sagittal plane. This configuration allows the hindlimb to be thrust lateral to the forelimb when a dog gallops. The trochlea of the talus fits into reciprocal grooves that form the cochlea of the tibia. The distal articular head of the talus articulates with the central tarsal bone.

The calcaneus is the largest tarsal bone. The proximal half of the bone is the tuber calcanei and provides attachment for the common calcaneal tendon. The calcaneus articulates with the talus via three articular facets. The medial articular facet is on the dorsomedial side of the calcaneus for articulation with the medial surface of the talus. The dorsal articular surface fits a comparable surface on the talus. The distal articular facet is the smallest articular facet and is confluent with a small facet for the central tarsal bone. The calcaneus articulates distally with the fourth tarsal bone.

The central tarsal bone articulates with all tarsal bones and lies in the medial part of the tarsus between the proximal and distal rows. The central tarsal bone acts as a buttress for the other tarsal bones.[5]

The first, second, and third tarsal bones articulate with the central tarsal bone proximally and their respective metatarsal bones distally. The third tarsal bone is much larger and also articulates with the fourth tarsal bone on its lateral surface.

The fourth tarsal bone is as large as both the central

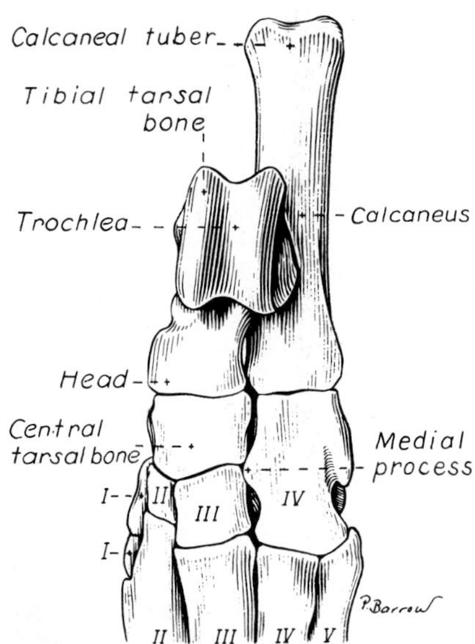

FIGURE 139–1. Bony anatomy of the canine tarsus. (From Evans HE [ed]: *Miller's Anatomy of the Dog.* 3rd ed., W. B. Saunders, Philadelphia, 1993, p 219.)

tarsal bone and the third tarsal bone combined. It articulates proximally with the calcaneus and distally with the fourth and fifth metatarsal bones. It articulates with the central tarsal bone and the third tarsal bone on its medial surface. The tuberosity of the fourth tarsal bone is a palpable landmark located on the midplantar aspect of the bone.

Two plantar sesamoid bones may be associated with the tarsometatarsal articulation. The lateral plantar tarsometatarsal sesamoid bone is present in 50 per cent of greyhounds. A smaller medial sesamoid, called the *intra-articular tarsometatarsal sesamoid*, is present in 27 per cent of greyhounds[13] (Fig. 139–2). These bones are rare in other breeds.

The first metatarsal bone is small and may be fused with the first tarsal bone.[7] The remaining metatarsal bones (II through V) are similar in size and shape. These bones articulate distally with their respective digits. At each metatarsophalangeal joint, on the plantar aspect of the joint, is a pair of small sesamoid bones known as the *medial* and *lateral proximal sesamoids*. Smaller dorsal sesamoids are also found at each metatarsophalangeal articulation. The first digit, when present, is known as the *dewclaw*.

Tarsal Joints

The tarsocrural joint is the articulation between the tibia and talus (Fig. 139–3). The talocalcaneal joint is the articulation between the talus and calcaneus. The talocalcaneocentral joint is the joint formed between the talus, calcaneus, and central tarsal bones. The articulation between the calcaneus and fourth tarsal bone forms the calcaneoquartal joint. The centrodistal joint is formed between the central tarsal bone and the first, second, and third tarsal bones. The tarsometatarsal joints are formed between the second, third, and fourth tarsal bones and the second, third, fourth, and fifth metatarsal bones.

The tarsal joints are composite articulations. Collectively, the tarsus functions as a ginglymus, or hinge joint, which provides more than 90 per cent of the total joint mobility. This action occurs principally in the talocrural joint. Some side movement is possible from the collective tarsal joints; however, the vertical joints between individual tarsal bones are rigid.

Ligamentous Support of the Tarsus and Metatarsus

The tarsus is supported by medial and lateral collateral ligaments. They originate from the medial and lateral malleoli and are composed of a short and a long part. The short portion of the medial collateral ligament attaches distally to the talus and then extends distally with the long portion to attach to the first tarsal and metatarsal bones.

The short portion of the lateral collateral ligament attaches to the talus and calcaneus. These bands are at right angles to the long part of the lateral collateral ligament and are located under the long part.[7] The long part of this ligament is attached to the fifth metatarsal bone.

The plantar ligaments are better developed than those on the dorsal side, allowing them to withstand the tensile stresses placed on the joint. These plantar ligaments are

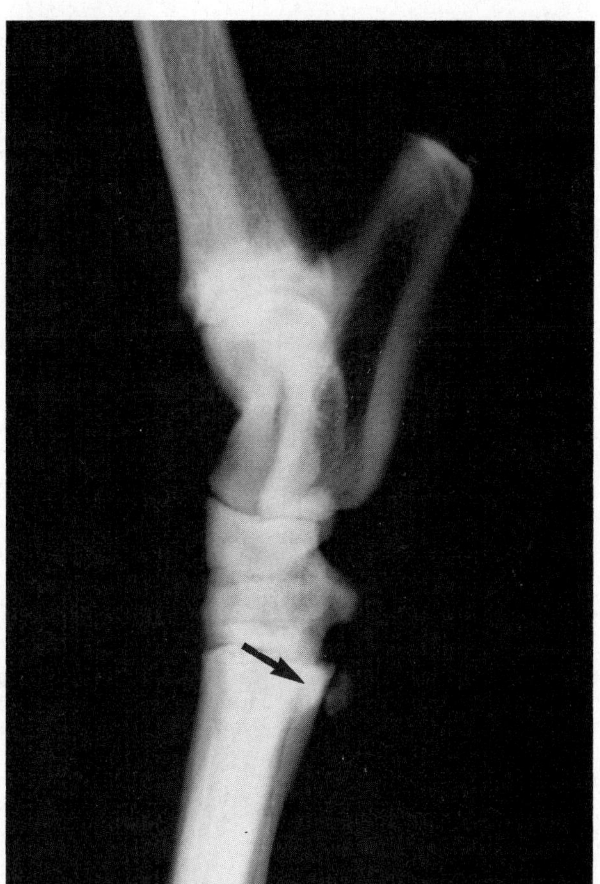

FIGURE 139–2. Lateral radiograph of the left tarsus and metatarsus of a greyhound. Arrows point to the larger lateral plantar tarsometatarsal sesamoid bone and the smaller intra-articular tarsometatarsal sesamoid bone.

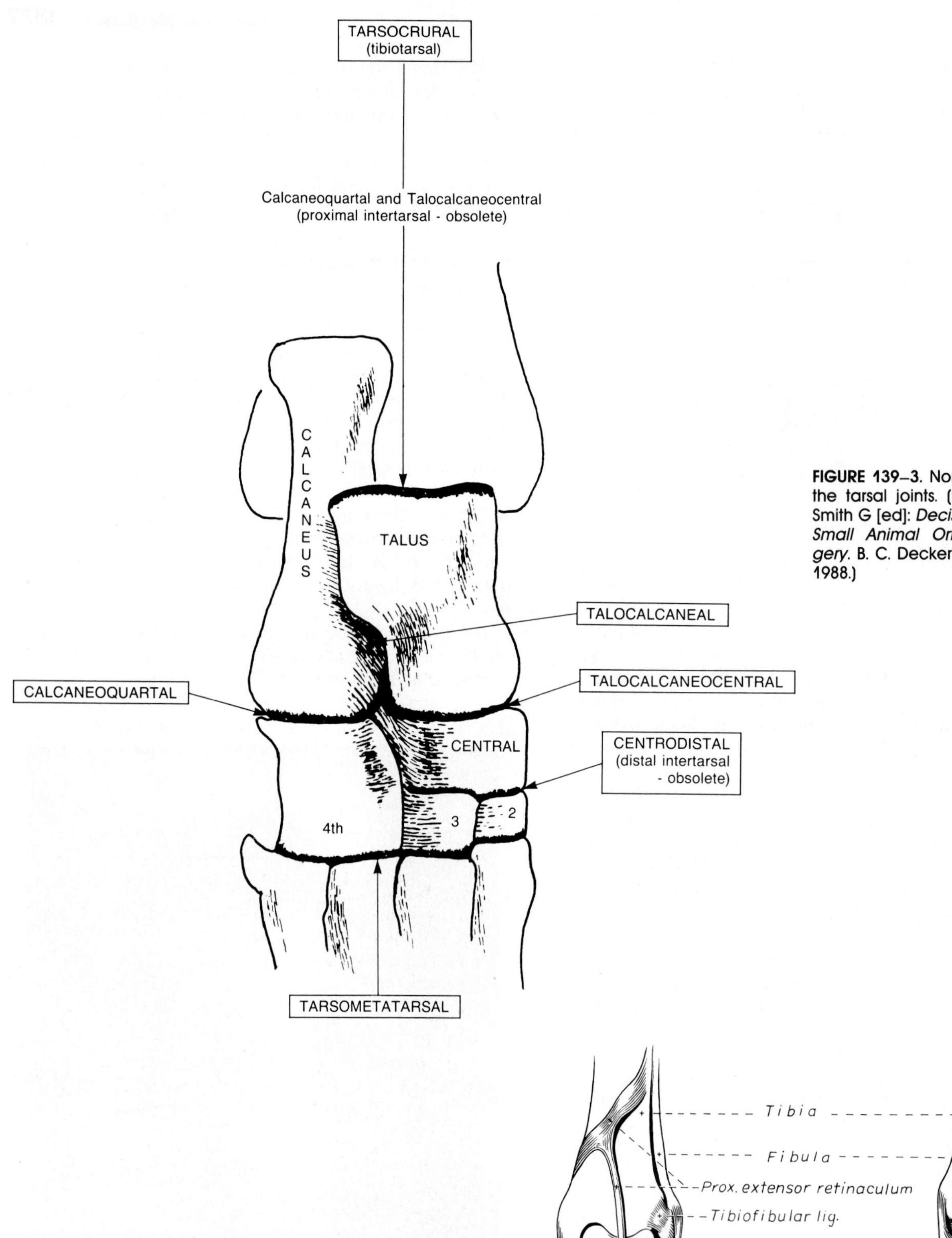

FIGURE 139–3. Nomenclature of the tarsal joints. (From Sumner-Smith G [ed]: *Decision Making in Small Animal Orthopedic Surgery.* B. C. Decker, Philadelphia, 1988.)

FIGURE 139–4. Ligaments of the tarsus. (From Evans HE [ed]: *Miller's Anatomy of the Dog.* 3rd ed. W. B. Saunders, Philadelphia, 1993, p 265.)

distinct. One ligament extends from the base of the calcaneus to the fourth tarsal bone and then to the bases of the fourth and fifth metatarsal bones (middle plantar ligament) (Fig. 139–4). A second ligament leaves the plantar surface of the sustentaculum tali and attaches to the central tarsal bone on its way to the tarsometatarsal joint capsule (medial plantar ligament). A third plantar ligament leaves the caudolateral surface of the calcaneus and unites with the long lateral collateral ligament before attaching to the base of the fifth metatarsal bone (lateral plantar ligament).

The ligament between the talus and calcaneus is named the *talocalcaneal ligament*.[11]

Dorsally, numerous short ligaments unite the talus with the third and fourth tarsal bones, and the talus, central tarsal bone, second tarsal bone, and third tarsal bone.

Three lateral and four medial joint sacs are noted. Communication exists between the talocrural joint, the talocalcaneal joint, the calcaneoquartal joint, and the talocalcaneocentral joint. The centroquartal, centrodistal, and tarsometatarsal joints intercommunicate.[7]

Blood Supply and Innervation

The cranial tibial artery becomes the dorsal pedal artery at the talocrural joint.[7] This artery is found within the proximal transverse ligament and closely parallels the distal course of the long digital extensor tendon. It supplies the dorsal and lateral aspect of the tarsus. The plantar branch of the saphenous artery supplies the medial and plantar aspects of the tarsus. Venous drainage occurs via the medial and lateral saphenous veins.

The tibial nerve passes medial to the calcaneal tuber to become the medial and lateral plantar nerves. The saphenous nerve supplies the dorsal and plantar innervation to the medial aspect of the tarsus. The superficial peroneal nerve supplies the dorsal aspect of the tarsus.

EVALUATION OF THE TARSUS AND METATARSUS

Physical examination of the tarsus and metatarsus is performed systematically. The region is scrutinized for swelling or abnormal joint angles. Each tarsal and metatarsal bone is carefully palpated, and range of motion is noted. The joints are stressed in mediolateral, dorsoplantar, and rotary planes. In some injuries, sedation or general anesthesia is necessary for complete evaluation.

The findings on physical examination dictate the radiographic views necessary to confirm the presence of bony or ligamentous injury. Standard lateral and dorsoplantar views often are inadequate and are complemented with stress views and oblique views when necessary (Figs. 139–5 and 139–6). Using stress radiography, a controlled force is applied on a joint to demonstrate an abnormal spatial relationship between two or more of its components. Stress radiography is especially helpful to demonstrate ligamentous injury in the hock[8, 12] and can help identify osteochondritic lesions of the talus dome.

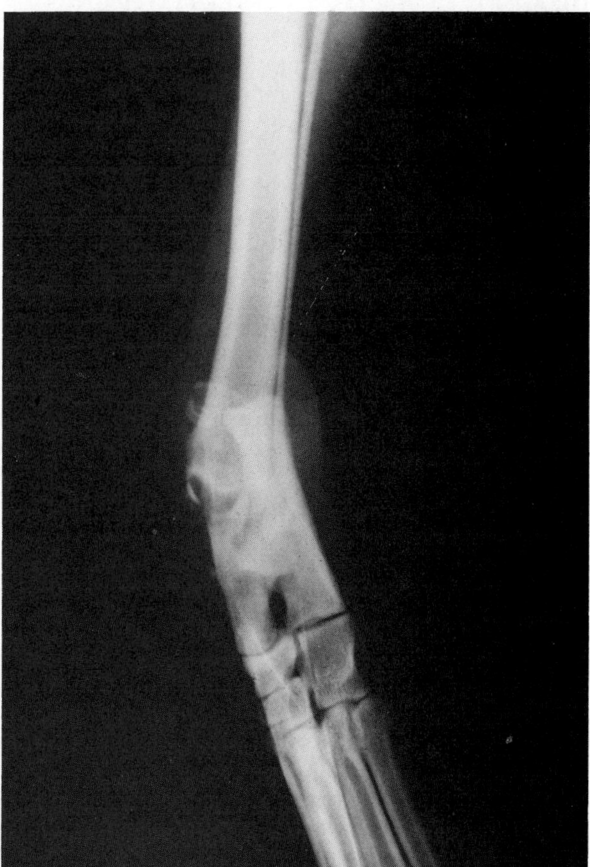

FIGURE 139–5. A stressed dorsoplantar view demonstrating medial collateral ligament rupture.

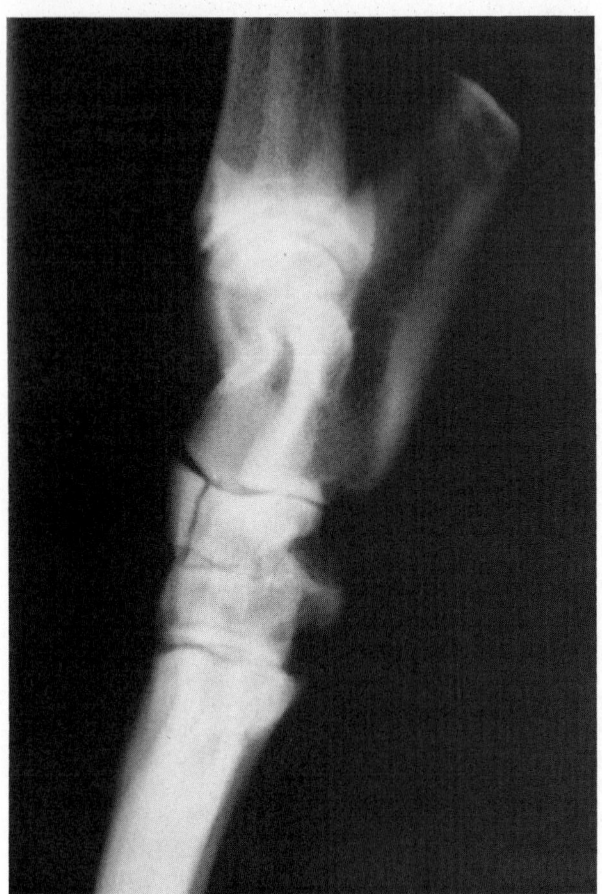

FIGURE 139–6. A lateral view of the central tarsal bone illustrating a subtle type I fracture.

LUXATIONS OF THE TARSUS AND METATARSUS

The most common luxations involve the tarsocrural joint. These are debilitating injuries that respond poorly when handled conservatively. Reconstructive surgery and in some cases arthrodesis are required to provide tarsocrural stability.

Because both collateral ligaments originate from their respective malleoli, fracture of either malleolus results in a tarsocrural subluxation or luxation (Fig. 139–7). Medial malleolar fractures occur more commonly; the short components of the collateral ligaments may occasionally avulse independently of the long components. Small fragments must be excised, and the remaining soft tissues sutured. Larger fragments are reattached with pins and figure-eight tension band fixation. Lateral malleolar fractures are repaired in a similar way, and when possible a small pin is passed antegrade into the fibula.

Tarsocrural luxations are frequently the result of traumatic rupture of either the medial or lateral collateral ligaments. It is helpful to examine each ligament to assess the integrity of the short and long components of the collateral ligaments. The tarsus is flexed to examine the lateral collateral ligament. In this position, the long portion of the ligament is relaxed and the short segment is taut. The foot is twisted inward to assess the integrity of the short portion of the lateral collateral ligament. With the tarsus extended, the long portion is taut and the short portion is relaxed.[6] A varus stress is applied to assess the integrity of the long portion of the lateral collateral ligament. When the tarsus is flexed, the short portion of the medial collateral ligament is taut. Applying a valgus stress demonstrates integrity of this ligament. The long portion of the medial collateral ligament is taut when the tarsus is extended, and a valgus stress is used to examine this portion.

Transected ligaments can be treated by primary suture repair using nonabsorbable suture. Either a Bunnell-Mayer or locking loop suture pattern can be used.

In many cases, primary repair of the torn and frayed ligament is either impossible or fails to provide adequate support. Prosthetic material attached to bone screws placed in the tibia and the talus or calcaneus is indicated when ligament reconstruction is impossible (Fig. 139–8).

Aron[1] has demonstrated the advantage of a double prosthetic replacement in tarsocrural luxations. Placing two bone screws distally to anchor the prosthetic ligament more closely mimics the support of the short and long portion of the collateral ligament.

For shearing injuries of the medial collateral ligament, the proximal screw may be placed in the area of the former medial malleolus, and for a lateral collateral ligament shear injury, a screw is placed in the area of the former lateral malleolus. It is important to angle the screws proximally 15° to avoid entering the joint space or injuring the cochlea of the tibia. A cranial-to-caudal bone tunnel may be used in the appropriate malleolus as an alternative to a bone screw for a fixation point for the suture material in animals with intact malleoli. For

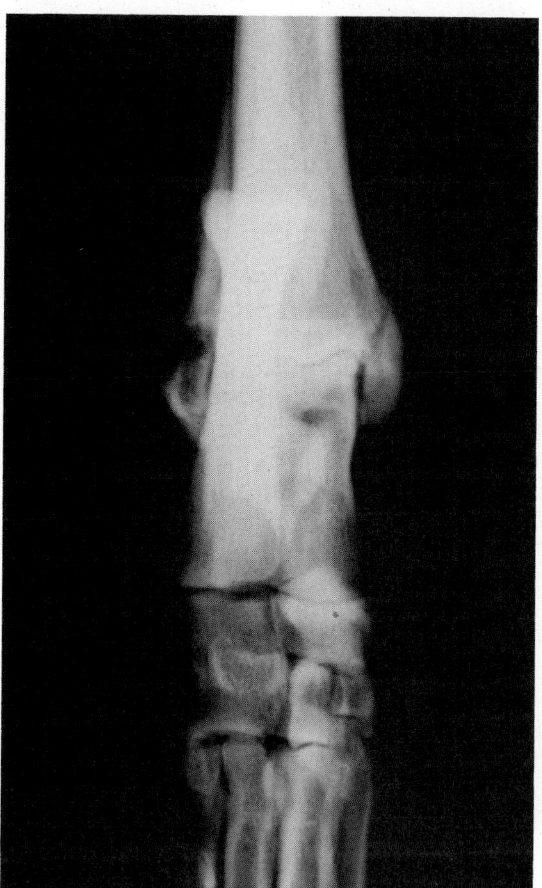

FIGURE 139–7. Dorsoplantar radiographic view of a medial malleolar fracture.

the medial short ligament insertion site, the screw is placed in the proximoplantar quadrant of the medial trochlear face of the talus.

For lateral luxations, the insertion site for the short ligament prosthesis is proximal and plantar to the articular aspect of the tuber calcanei. The long ligament insertion site is the tubercle located at the dorsal extent of the base of the calcaneus.[1] Figure 139–9 illustrates a double prosthetic repair of a medial collateral ligament rupture.

SHEAR INJURIES OF THE TARSUS

Shear injuries of the tarsus invariably contain dirt, rocks, asphalt, hair, and often feces. Shear injuries require aggressive débridement, joint and soft-tissue lavage, and bacterial culture before attempted primary closure. Most shear wounds are left open to drain and allowed to heal by second intention and contraction. Wet to dry bandages are changed daily, and the injured part must be immobilized. An external fixator can be used to immobilize the joints. When possible, bacterial cultures are obtained at initial débridement; a broad-spectrum antimicrobial regimen is indicated. As the wounds heal and drainage decreases, definitive repair of the ligamentous instability can be undertaken.

PROXIMAL PLANTAR INTERTARSAL LUXATION

Proximal plantar intertarsal luxations are a result of damage to the plantar ligaments (Fig. 139–10). Disruption of the calcaneoquartal and talocalcaneocentral joints occurs. These injuries respond poorly to conservative management because the damaged ligaments are on the tension band side of the tarsus. Motion results in continuous destructive forces. This injury, although reported in many breeds, most commonly occurs in greyhounds.

Injuries of the plantar ligaments may avulse bone chips from the plantar process of the central tarsal bone or from the base of the calcaneus. Repair of this injury consists of primary arthrodesis of the calcaneoquartal joint by pin and figure-eight tension band wire. With severe instabilities, arthrodesis of the talocalcaneocentral joint may also be accomplished. The tarsus is coapted in a position of function for 6 to 8 weeks. In greyhounds, this injury is debilitating, and despite successful arthrodesis, few dogs return to racing.

DORSAL PROXIMAL INTERTARSAL SUBLUXATION

This is a subtle hyperextension injury, and patients are able to bear weight (Fig. 139–11). Little soft-tissue swelling occurs. Diagnosis is confirmed with stress radiographs demonstrating dorsal opening of the joint space. Most have a medial or lateral component. In performance animals, this subluxation is best treated by primary arthrodesis of the talocalcaneocentral or the calcaneo-

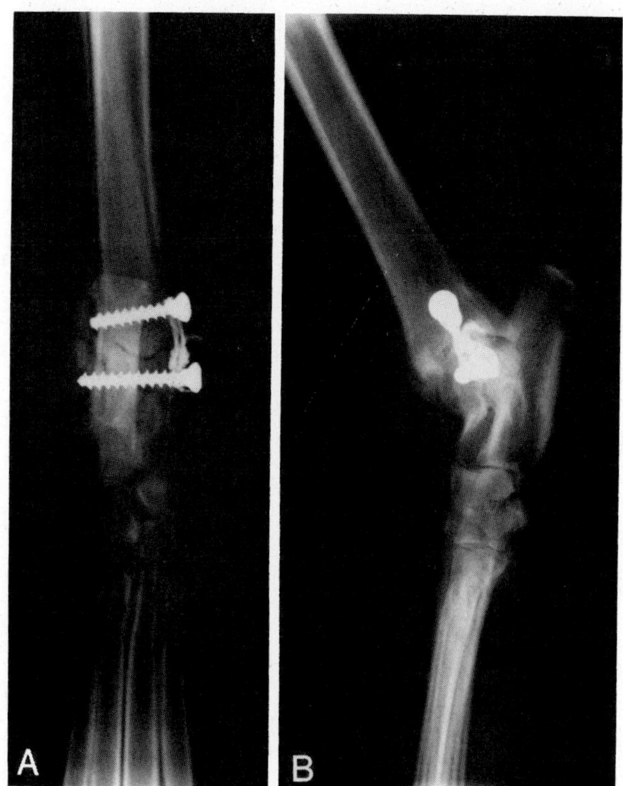

FIGURE 139–8. Radiographs of a medial collateral rupture repaired with two screws and braided suture material, taken 10 years postoperatively.

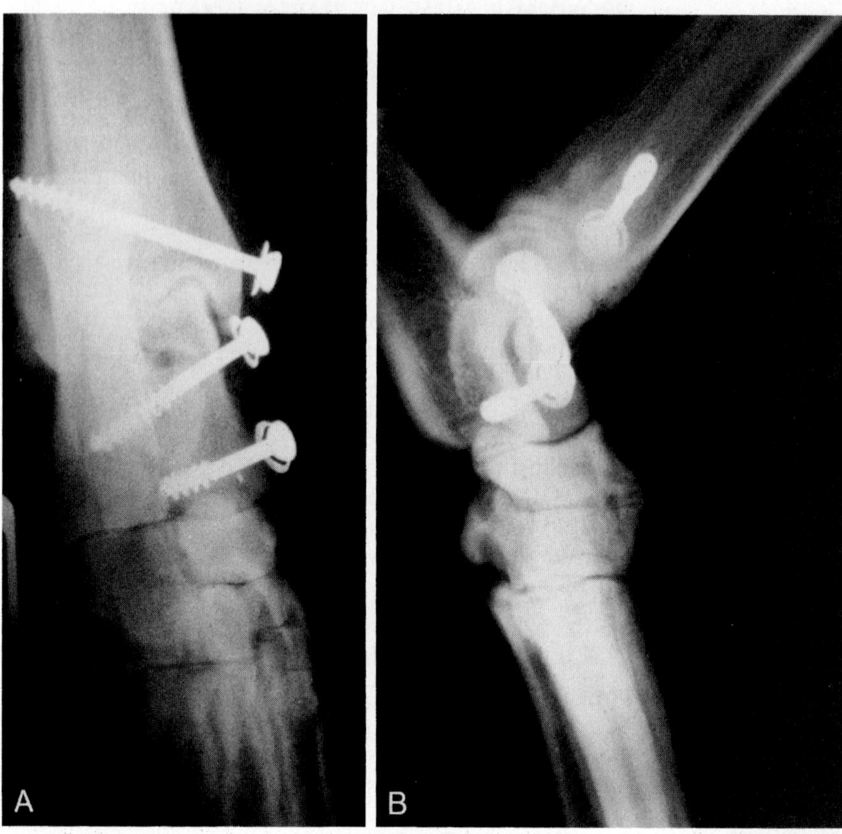

FIGURE 139–9. Radiographs illustrating double prosthetic repair of a medial collateral ligament rupture. Repair included screws, spiked washers, and braided polypropylene suture.

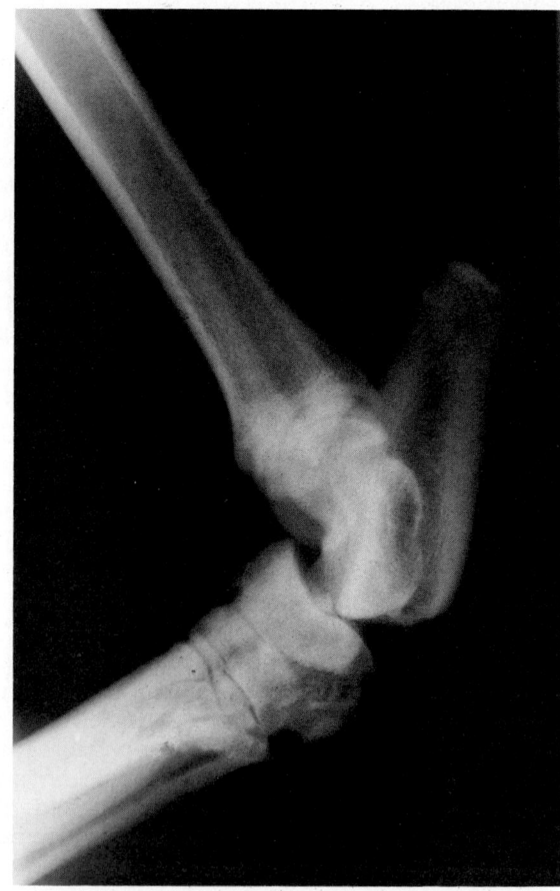

FIGURE 139–10. Proximal plantar subluxation.

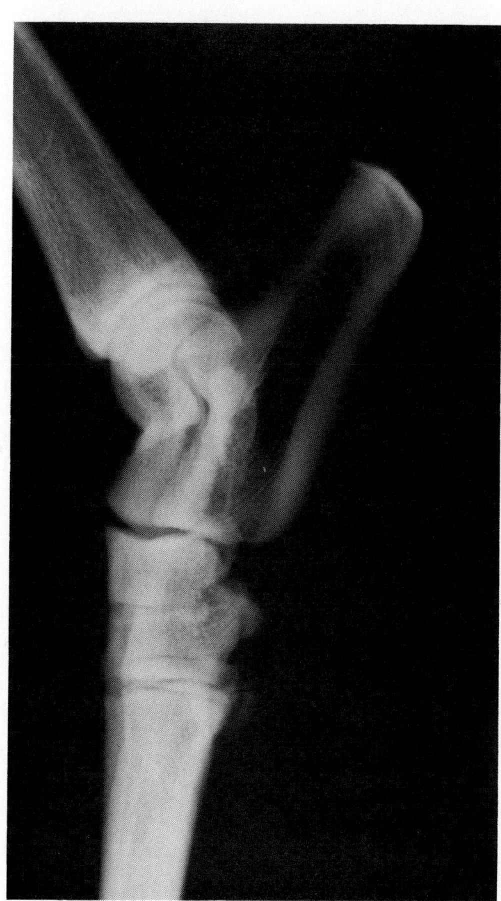

FIGURE 139–11. Dorsal proximal intertarsal luxation.

quartal joints. Bone screws are lagged from the head of the talus through a small portion of the central tarsal bone and into the fourth tarsal bone or from the base of the calcaneus into the fourth tarsal bone, respectively.

In nonperformance animals, some dorsal proximal intertarsal luxations can be treated successfully by coaptation for 6 to 8 weeks.

TARSOMETATARSAL JOINT SUBLUXATION

Tarsometatarsal joint subluxations can be either dorsal or plantar. Physical examination and stress radiography are required for diagnosis. Plantar subluxations are more common despite thicker and stronger ligaments. Primary arthrodesis is recommended in most cases. The use of crossed pins for a dorsal instability and a pin and figure-eight tension band wire or a lateral bone plate is ideal for plantar tarsometatarsal arthrodesis. This can also be accomplished with antegrade pins and a tension band wire after removal of articular cartilage. A high-speed bone bur can be used to cut a trough in the distal dorsal cortex of each metatarsal bone. Appropriate pins are driven antegrade into the distal row of tarsal bones. The affected limb is coapted for 6 to 8 weeks, using radiography to assess healing of the arthrodesis site.

TARSOCRURAL ARTHRODESIS

Tarsocrural arthrodesis is indicated for failed reconstructions, irreparable soft-tissue injuries, severely comminuted articular fractures, and crippling degenerative joint disease. The joint is approached medially either by incising the medial collateral ligaments or by osteotomy of the medial malleolus. Before insertion of an autogenous cancellous bone graft, all articular cartilage of the tibial cochlea and talus condyles is removed. The angle of arthrodesis is 135° for dogs and 120° for cats. Arthrodesis is accomplished by lagging a screw from the dorsolateral aspect of the distal tibia through the body of the talus. A second screw is lagged through the dorsomedial aspect of the distal tibia through the body of the talus to seat in the lateral plantar aspect of the base of the calcaneus. Arthrodesis can also be accomplished with multiple Kirschner wires in small dogs and cats. A lag screw can be placed from the plantar aspect of the talus into the distal tibia. Bone plates and external fixators can also be used for arthrodesis.[10] Bending the external bars of an external fixator to approximate normal joint angles more closely has been reported.[3a] This technique provides better stability and greater ease of application. The arthrodesis is splinted for 6 to 8 weeks and monitored radiographically until arthrodesis is successful.*

FRACTURES OF THE CALCANEUS

Calcaneal fractures are common in racing greyhounds and rare in other breeds. In greyhounds, calcaneal fractures are associated with either central tarsal fractures or disruption of the plantar ligaments, resulting in proximal plantar intertarsal luxation. Ost and colleagues[11] reported 51 calcaneal fractures and found that fractured calcaneal fragments were associated with the insertion of tendons and ligaments. They hypothesized that a central tarsal fracture caused the head of the talus to be displaced distally into the fracture gap of the central tarsal bone, with talocalcaneal subluxation. Tension from the common calcaneal tendon and loss of dorsomedial support by the talus and central tarsal bone place abnormal stress on the calcaneus and plantar ligaments. Relief of the accumulated forces on the lateral and plantar aspect of the tarsus can occur by fracture of either the fourth tarsal bone or the calcaneus. Tensile forces created by the pull of the common calcaneal tendon are transmitted through the calcaneus via the plantar ligaments. Excessive tensile forces exceeding the strength of the calcaneus cause avulsion of the middle plantar ligament, and plantar proximal intertarsal subluxation occurs.

The type of calcaneal fracture dictates the treatment method. Steinmann pins, tension band wiring, and lag screws are most commonly used. Neutralization plates and cerclage wires have also been used to repair calcaneal fractures.

*Section Editors' Note: Pantarsal arthrodesis using a dorsally placed compression plate has been consistently successful and has eliminated the complications associated with lag screw arthrodesis of the tarsocrural joint.

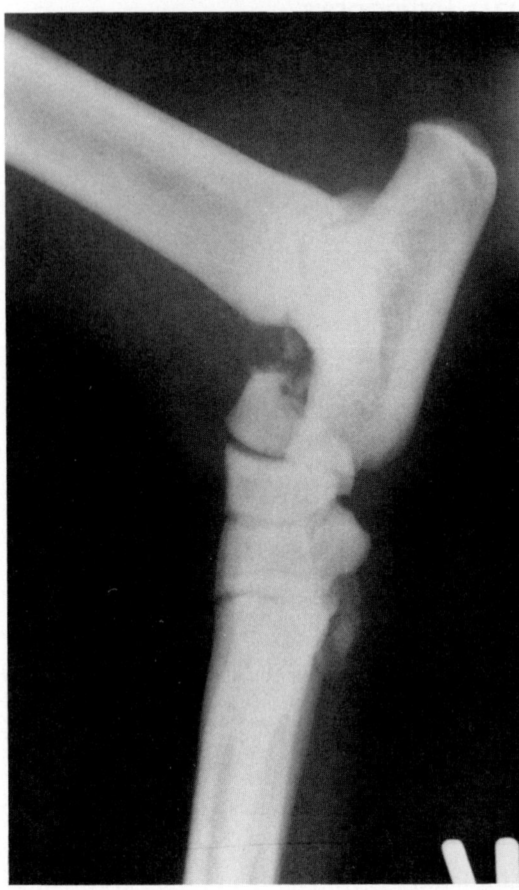

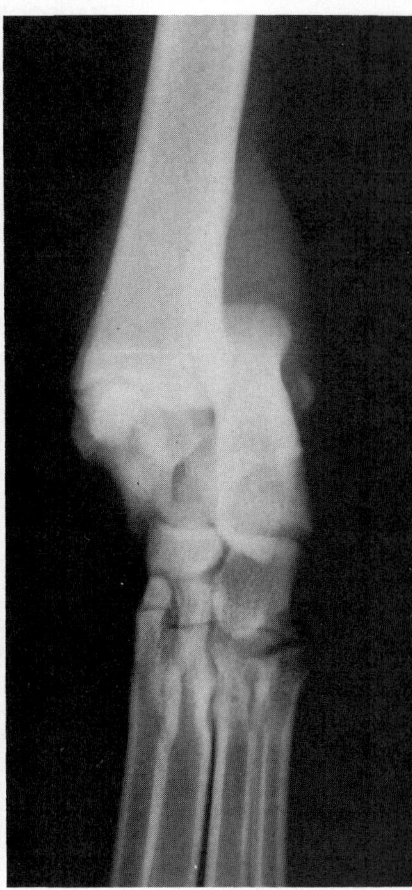

FIGURE 139–12. Radiographs illustrating a talar neck fracture.

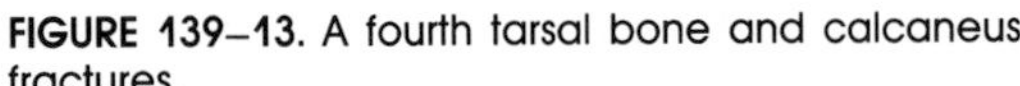

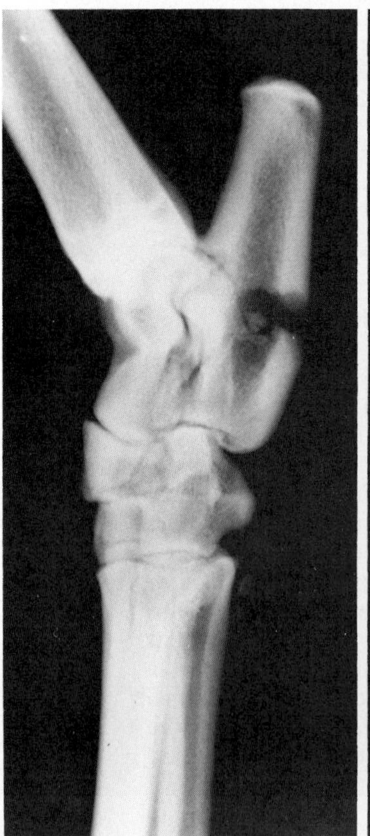

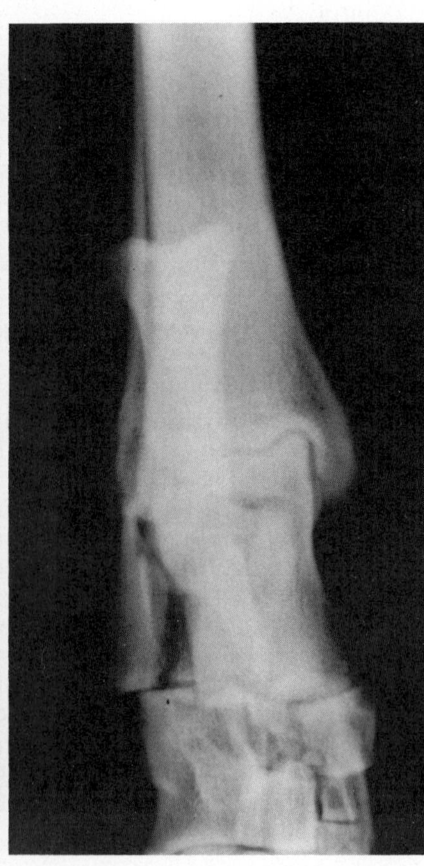

FIGURE 139–13. A fourth tarsal bone and calcaneus fractures.

TALUS FRACTURES

Isolated talus fractures are rare. Talar head fractures may be encountered with central tarsal fractures. This type of fracture is repaired by lag screw fixation (Fig. 139–12).

Talar fractures in pets often result from trauma. Intra-articular body fractures are surgically repaired and usually can be approached by osteotomy of the appropriate malleolus. Osteochondral fragments of the talus dome, unassociated with osteochondrosis, can be reattached with Kirschner wires that are subsequently countersunk. The use of absorbable polyglycolic pins to reattach these fractures has been limited in dogs. The prognosis for head and neck fractures associated with central tarsal fractures is fair to good. The prognosis for intra-articular fractures of the body is guarded owing to the potential for degenerative joint disease.

CENTRAL TARSAL FRACTURES

Central tarsal fractures are most commonly reported in racing greyhounds but do occur in other breeds.[9] In dogs racing counterclockwise, compressive forces are concentrated in the right tarsus. Central tarsal fractures frequently show radiographic evidence of compression, subluxation, and comminution but are rarely open. Once the buttress action of the central tarsal bone is lost, the talocalcaneocentral joint collapses. With many severe central tarsal fractures, simultaneous fracture of the fourth tarsal bone and the calcaneus may occur. Second tarsal bone fractures may also be combined with severe central tarsal fractures (Fig. 139–13).

Central tarsal fractures have been graded according to the fracture type and amount of displacement (Fig. 139–14). Diagnosis of type I and type II fractures is by "point pain" over the central tarsal bone as well as by radiography. Undisplaced fractures may be attended by little apparent lameness. It is easy to overlook type I fractures, and a high index of suspicion is helpful for detection. Repair of type I and type II fractures requires one 2.0- or 2.7-mm cortical screw placed in lag fashion. These fractures are coapted for 4 weeks, and the prognosis is excellent.

Type III fractures are rare and require the use of one 4.0-mm partially threaded cancellous bone screw for fixation. The fracture is held immobilized and lagged into the body of the fourth tarsal bone.

Type IV fractures usually have many small posterior comminutions in addition to the two major fragments. Surgical repair consists of a 4.0-mm partially threaded cancellous bone screw lagged into the body of the fourth tarsal bone. A second 2.0- or 2.7-mm cortical screw placed in lag fashion is used to secure the anterior fragment. It is advisable to use two bone-holding forceps to reduce both fractures simultaneously before screw placement is attempted. The prognosis for type IV fractures is favorable.

Type V fractures are usually externally coapted or internally stabilized to salvage the animal for breeding purposes.

A titanium central tarsal implant has been used to replace a type V central tarsal fracture.[14] The implant was tolerated well, and the animal was able to return to racing. Further investigational work is needed for this type of prosthesis. Figure 139–15 presents a decision algorithm for handling central tarsal fractures.

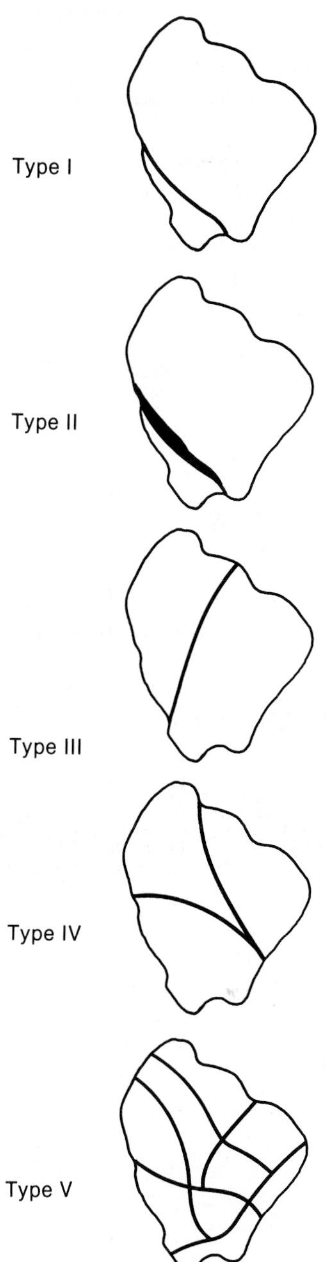

FIGURE 139–14. Dorsal views of the central tarsal bone, with heavy lines indicating fracture lines.

SECOND, THIRD, AND FOURTH TARSAL FRACTURES

Fractures or luxations of the second tarsal bone are rare and most commonly accompany severe central tarsal fractures. Isolated fractures or subluxations are treated with lag screw fixation to the third tarsal bone. Small screws (2 mm) are recommended.

Third tarsal fractures may be isolated. When they are acute, slight swelling and point pain may be present; when chronic, they exhibit periosteal new bone formation. Anterior slab fractures are secured with a 2.0- or

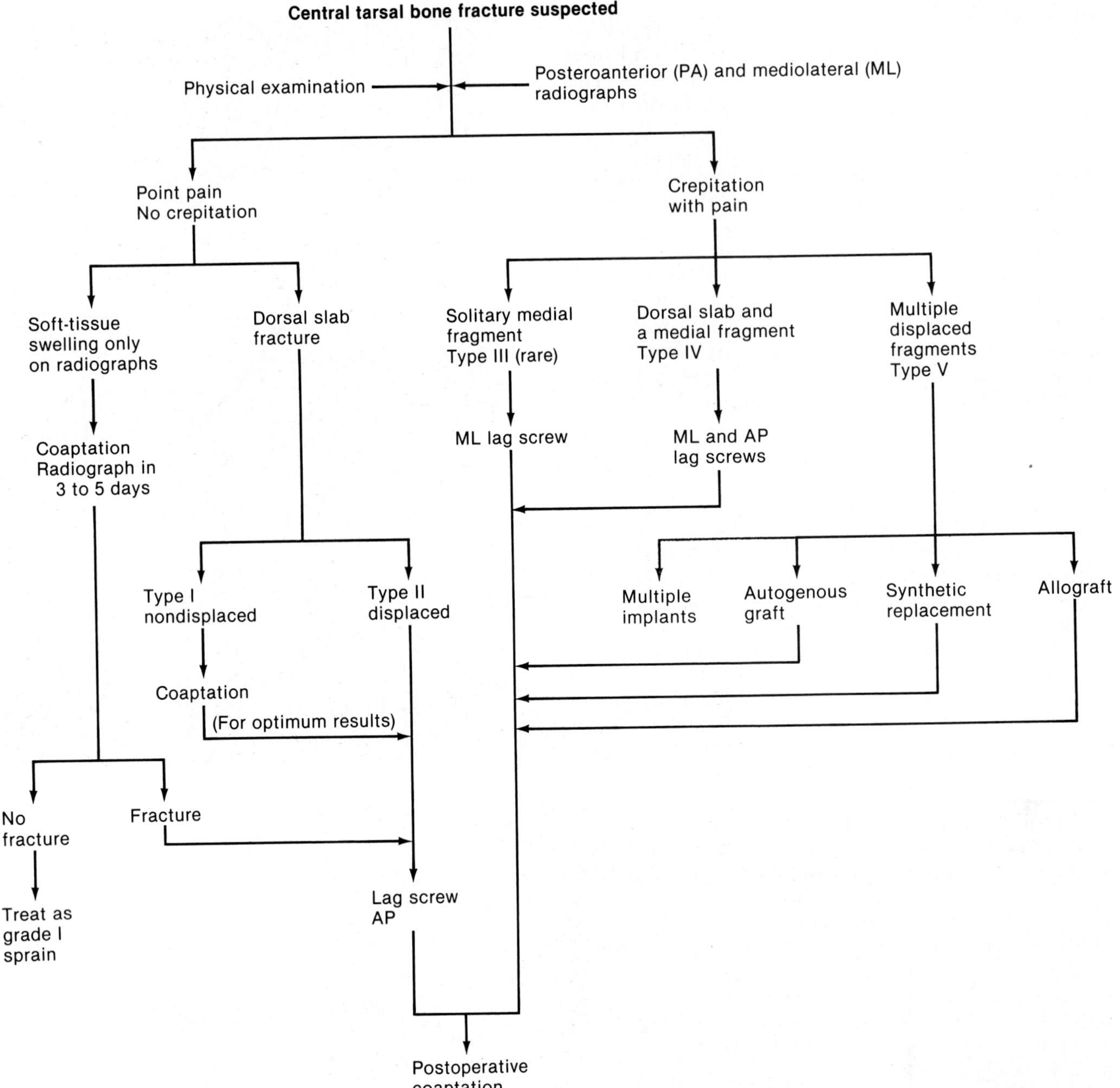

FIGURE 139–15. Algorithm for central tarsal fractures. (From Sumner-Smith G [ed]: *Decision Making in Small Animal Orthopedic Surgery.* B. C. Decker, Philadelphia, 1988.)

2.7-mm cortical bone screw placed in lag fashion (Fig. 139–16).

Most fourth tarsal fractures occur in conjunction with central tarsal fractures. Approximately 40 per cent of greyhounds[3] with central tarsal fractures have a compression fracture of the fourth tarsal bone. Repair of fourth tarsal fractures is indirectly achieved by repairing the central tarsal bone fracture.

METATARSAL FRACTURES

Metatarsal fractures usually cause an acute nonweight-bearing lameness with various amounts of swelling, crepitus, and pain. Radiographs can confirm the diagnosis; oblique views occasionally help outline stress fractures of one metatarsal bone. Undisplaced fractures may be treated with coaptation for 4 to 6 weeks. When severe displacement occurs or when multiple bones are fractured, internal fixation is indicated. Lag screws, cerclage wires, and retrograded Kirschner wires can be used effectively.[2] Veterinary Cuttable Plates[4]* have revolutionized the repair of multiple metatarsal bone fractures in racing greyhounds (Fig. 139–17).

FRACTURES OF THE SESAMOID BONES

Fracture of the plantar sesamoids occurs primarily in greyhounds. When presented acutely, mild soft-tissue swelling and point pain are noted over the plantar aspect of the affected metatarsophalangeal joint. Chronic fractures are evidenced by soft-tissue proliferation and decreased range of motion of the affected joint. Detailed

*Synthes, Paoli, PA.

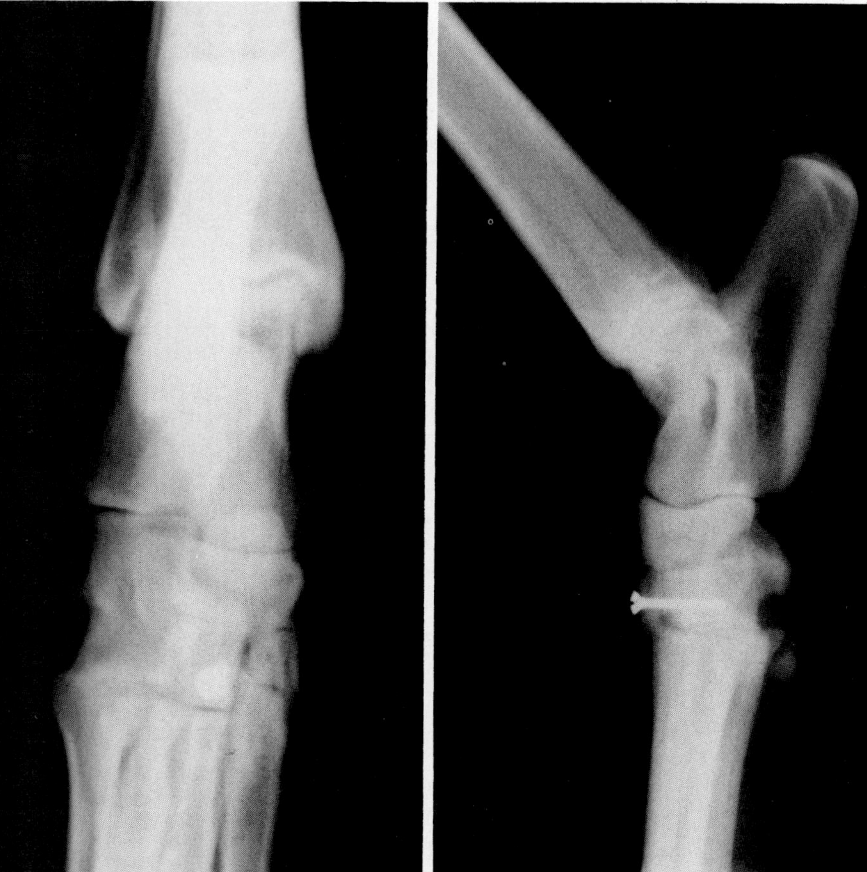

FIGURE 139–16. Radiographs of a third tarsal fracture repaired with a 2-mm lag screw.

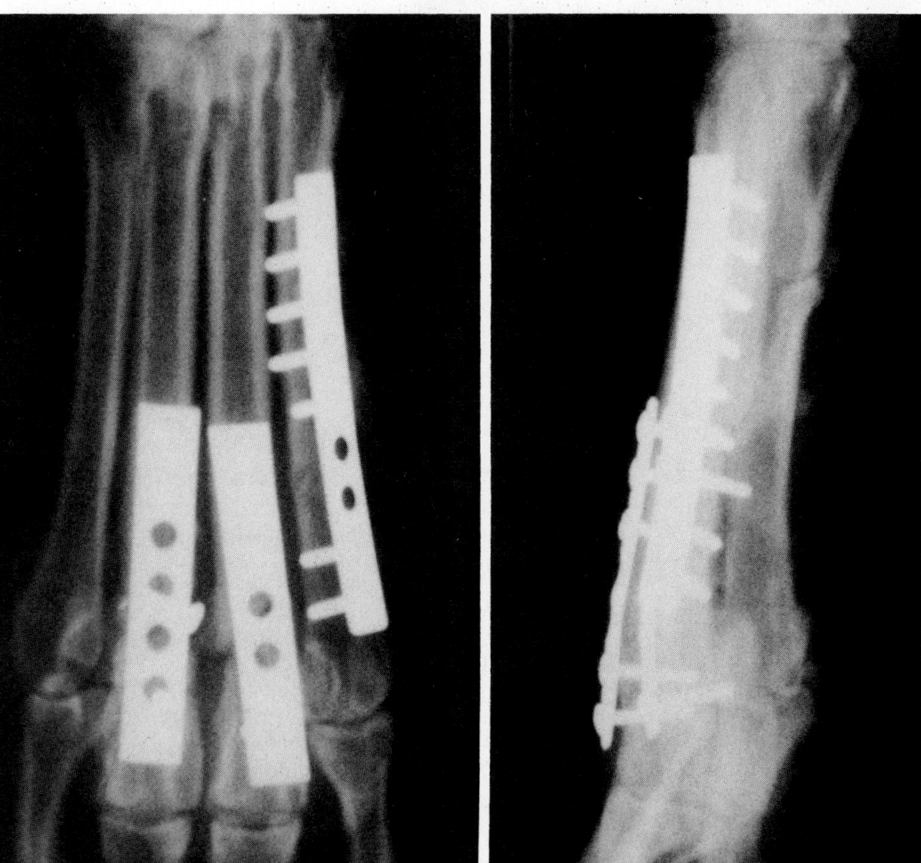

FIGURE 139–17. Veterinary Cuttable Plates used to repair multiple metatarsal fractures.

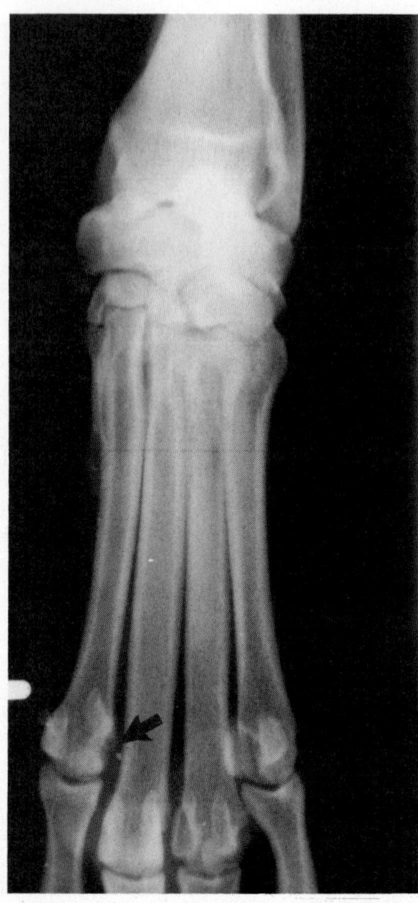

FIGURE 139–18. Sesamoid fracture at the articulation of the second metacarpophalangeal joint *(arrow)*.

radiographs are necessary to identify these fractures (Fig. 139–18). Removal of the comminuted bone fragments is indicated because the fragments are too small for repair. The prognosis for return to racing is favorable.

References

1. Aron DN: Prosthetic ligament replacement for severe tarsocrural joint instability. *J Am Anim Hosp Assoc 23*:41, 1987.
2. Bellenger CR, et al: Fixation of metacarpal and metatarsal fracture in greyhounds. *Aust Vet J 59*:205, 1981.
3. Boudrieau RJ, et al: Central tarsal bone fractures in the racing greyhound. *J Am Vet Med Assoc 184*:12, 1984.

3a. Brinker WO, Piermattei DL, Flo GL: *Handbook of Small Animal Orthopedics and Fracture Treatment.* 2nd ed. W. B. Saunders, Philadelphia, 1990, p 452.

4. Bruse S, et al: Internal fixation with a veterinary cuttable plate in small animals. *Vet Comp Orthop Traumatol 1*:40, 1989.
5. Dee JF: Fractures in the racing greyhound. *In* Bojrab MJ (ed): *Pathophysiology in Small Animal Surgery*. Philadelphia, Lea & Febiger, 1981.
6. Ellison GW: Conditions of the tarsus and metatarsus. *In* Slatter DM (ed): *Textbook of Small Animal Surgery*. W. B. Saunders, Philadelphia, 1985.
7. Evans HE, Christensen GC (eds): *Miller's Anatomy of the Dog*. 2nd ed. W. B. Saunders, Philadelphia, 1979.
8. Farrow CS: Stress radiography: Applications in small animal practice. *J Am Vet Med Assoc 181*:777, 1982.
9. Gitz R: What is your diagnosis? (central tarsal fracture in a dog). *J Am Vet Med Assoc 193*:2, 1988.
10. Olds R, Green S: Hoffman's external fixation for arthrodesis and infected non-unions in the dog. *J Am Anim Hosp Assoc 19*:705, 1983.
11. Ost PC, et al: Fractures of the calcaneus in the racing greyhound. *Vet Surg 16*:53, 1987.
12. Owens JM, et al: Roentgenology of joint trauma. *Vet Clin North Am 8*:419, 1978.
13. Wood AKW, McCarthy PH: Radiographic and anatomic observations of plantar sesamoid bones at the tarsometatarsal articulation of greyhounds. *Am J Vet Res 45*:2158, 1984.
14. Yocham GD, et al: Central tarsal implant in a racing greyhound. *J Am Vet Med Assoc 193*:7, 1988.

CHAPTER 140

Arthrodesis

Arnold S. Lesser

Arthrodesis is the removal of motion from a joint by fusion of the opposing surfaces into a solid bony unit. It is usually performed as a salvage procedure to restore use to a painful or unstable joint that is unresponsive to more conservative treatment. Arthrodesis is indicated when continued motion of the joint is counterproductive mechanically or physiologically and a less drastic, more anatomical repair is not possible.

There are alternatives to arthrodesis. Total joint replacement with a prosthesis is commonly used in human medicine but is still relatively new to veterinary clinical practice. Ablation such as a femoral head and neck excision arthroplasty can be used for the coxofemoral and scapulohumeral joint but rarely in other joints. A third alternative is allogenic osteochondral joint replacement, in which both the bone and cartilaginous structures are transplanted to replace a diseased joint. This procedure is still in the experimental stages but, if perfected, holds some exciting prospects for joint surgery.

GENERAL INDICATIONS

Fusion of a joint is usually performed to relieve a painful condition due to instability or inflammatory disease. Instability induces pain because of the abnormal motion and stresses placed on the soft tissues and nerves surrounding the joint. Pain is relieved by rigid support provided by arthrodesis. Inflammation of a joint is termed *arthritis*. As a clinical entity, arthritis is not a simple disease but one with various manifestations, subtypes, and causes. It is also the most common indication for arthrodesis. Arthritic pain is caused by abnormal wear on both hard and soft tissues, combined with the release of inflammatory products, proteolytic enzymes, prostaglandins, and other agents. Much of this pain is centered in the joint capsule and adjacent soft tissues. By obliterating the joint, arthrodesis arrests this process.

The most common indications for arthrodesis in veterinary medicine can be divided into three categories: traumatic, developmental, and congenital. Traumatic injuries to joints consist of both fractures and ligamentous disruptions with or without dislocation. They include fractures involving a joint surface in which a primary repair leads to chronic instability, degenerative joint disease, and pain. Examples include (1) shearing injuries and fracture-dislocations of the hock or carpus with major bone and ligament loss and (2) severely comminuted condylar fractures of the distal humerus and femur, especially in miniature breeds. In either case, it may be impossible to recreate a functional joint with a primary fracture repair. Postfracture osteomyelitis and malunions also fit into this category.

The major developmental diseases can be included under the heading *arthritis* and are further subdivided into idiopathic or secondary degenerative joint disease, septic arthritis, and immune-mediated arthritis (rheumatoid or polyarthritis).

Congenital elbow luxations and stifle deformities that are not amenable to primary reconstruction are examples of indications for arthrodesis.

A fourth category is the use of arthrodesis to improve the mechanics of a limb rather than to relieve pain and instability—for example, arthrodesis of the carpus for radial nerve paralysis or the talocrural joint in conjunction with a muscle transfer for ischial paralysis.

GENERAL PROCEDURE

The actual surgical procedure, regardless of the joint, involves certain principles. Stability is of prime importance, even more so in arthrodesis than fracture fixation because the mechanical structures of a limb are designed to provide and maintain motion at this location. Therefore, the body is working against maintaining immobility at the fixation point. Factors to be overcome are the longer lever arm provided by the long bones adjacent to the joint and the anatomical arrangement of the muscles and tendons spanning the joint. The type of fixation and the surgical technique are critical, and the use of compression, which provides more rigid fixation, is desirable. Plates, screws, cross pins, tension band wire, and external pin splints used alone or in combination, plus external coaptation, are the common devices used to accomplish rigid fixation.

The articular cartilage is removed down to bleeding subchondral bone to enhance bone contact and facilitate early union. Rasps, curettes, osteotomes, or an air drill or oscillating saw can be used for this purpose. If an angular or rotational deformity exists, it can be corrected at this time by removing a suitable amount of bone. It is also possible to contour the opposing surfaces to provide maximum bone-to-bone contact and enhance stability.

For added insurance, autogenous cancellous bone grafts are used to shorten healing time and to fill in small defects in the opposing surfaces. When additional bone is required, cortical onlay or inlay grafts from the rib or ilium can also be used. Cancellous autografts provide osteoinducement, some viable osteoblasts, and a scaffold for ingrowth of new blood vessels via creeping substitution.

Normal angles for different joints have been reported, but the simplest method of determining the correct angle is to measure the opposite normal limb during weight-bearing. This angle may have to be adjusted if there will be shortening caused by the procedure. The more obtuse the angle (the straighter the limb), the longer the limb; conversely, the more acute the angle (more bend), the shorter the limb will be. Therefore, the surgeon can adjust the final length of the limb by varying the angle of the fused joint. If it is necessary to remove bone to fuse a joint like the stifle, the final angle should be more obtuse to make up for any shortening. The angle can be measured during surgery with a sterile goniometer, preplaced pins, or a prebent template.

GENERAL COMPLICATIONS

When a point of motion is obliterated via arthrodesis, increased stress is transferred to adjacent bones and joints. This is especially true in the carpus and vertebrae. Fusion of the antebrachiocarpal joint without fusion of the adjacent intercarpal joints results in degenerative joint disease of the latter. When performing arthrodesis on a midlimb joint, these stresses are transferred to the long bones themselves, increasing the risk of fracture, especially in large active dogs. The ends of plates and screw holes act as stress risers, further increasing the risk of fracture. Therefore, plates are removed after fusion is complete and the limbs protected, or exercise is restricted until the screw holes have filled in.

Other possible causes of failure are infection, insufficient fixation, or insufficient removal of cartilage. Any technical error such as poor plate placement or too small or too short a plate can cause implant failure.

SHOULDER

Indications

Shoulder problems requiring arthrodesis are not common. However, any condition causing severe arthritis and intractable pain can be considered an indication for arthrodesis. Included are intra-articular fractures, osteochondritis dissecans, and chronic luxations in miniature breeds.

Procedure

Once the shoulder joint is exposed, the articular cartilage on both sides of the joint is removed. Cancellous bone graft can be placed between the opposing surfaces, and the joint can be temporarily stabilized at

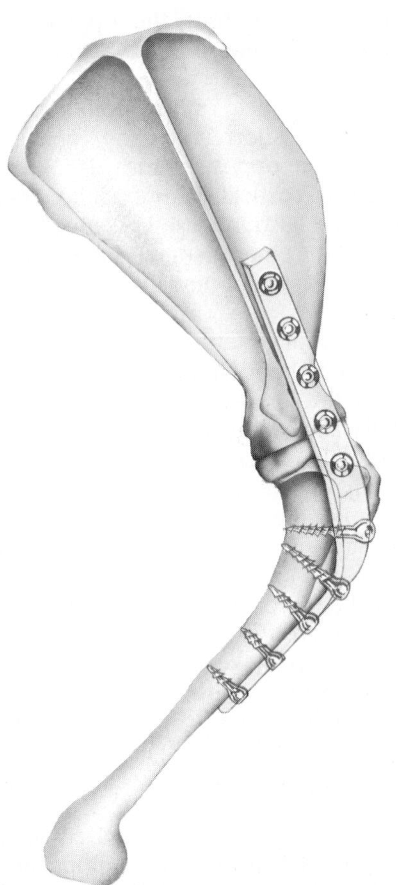

FIGURE 140–1. A longer plate angled to engage the base of the spine should be used because of the thin bone of the scapula.

the proper angle with a Kirschner wire. The most stable fixation is provided by a bone plate, which is strongly recommended in large and medium-sized dogs. The plate is placed along the cranial aspect of the spine of the scapula and angled just slightly caudally to take advantage of the thickened bone where the spine arises from the body of the scapula. Because the bone is relatively thin, a longer plate with more screws than usual is used. Distally, the plate can be bent and slightly twisted to lie along the craniolateral aspect of the humerus (Fig. 140–1).

An alternative technique for cats and smaller dogs is the use of Kirschner wires across the joint. One or two K wires can be placed from the scapular neck into the proximal humerus, and then one or two more can be run from the humerus into the scapular neck. The cranial aspect of the shoulder joint is the tension band side because of the normal angle between the axis of the humerus and scapula. Therefore, a figure-eight wire placed over the pins cranially adds compression during weightbearing. Even so, it is recommended to add a fiberglass spica extending over the shoulder until bony union is achieved. The spica is added insurance even when a plate is used.

Complications

Where it crosses under the deltoid tuberosity, the suprascapular nerve must be isolated and protected to avoid injury to it. Another problem is loosening of the plate where it attaches to the scapula because of the poor bone stock.

ELBOW

The most common indication for arthrodesis of the elbow is degenerative joint disease, which in this joint usually is secondary to trauma (fractures and luxations) or developmental diseases such as ununited anconeal process, fragmented coronoid process, osteochondritis dissecans, or premature closure of the distal radius or ulnar growth plates.

Condylar fractures, especially comminuted Y or T fractures, can be difficult to treat and can lead to degenerative joint disease if the postoperative alignment or final healing is not perfect. This is particularly true in miniature breeds, which have very little bone stock to hold the implants (Fig. 140–2).

The elbow is also prone to loss of motion after any fracture through or adjacent to the joint. When a joint loses motion, normal nutrition of the cartilage is adversely affected and degeneration can ensue, requiring arthrodesis (Fig. 140–3).

Congenital and traumatic fracture luxations (Fig. 140–4) that cannot be stabilized while preserving motion are indications for arthrodesis.

Procedure

Because of its configuration, the elbow is a difficult joint to fuse. In medium-sized and large dogs, affixing

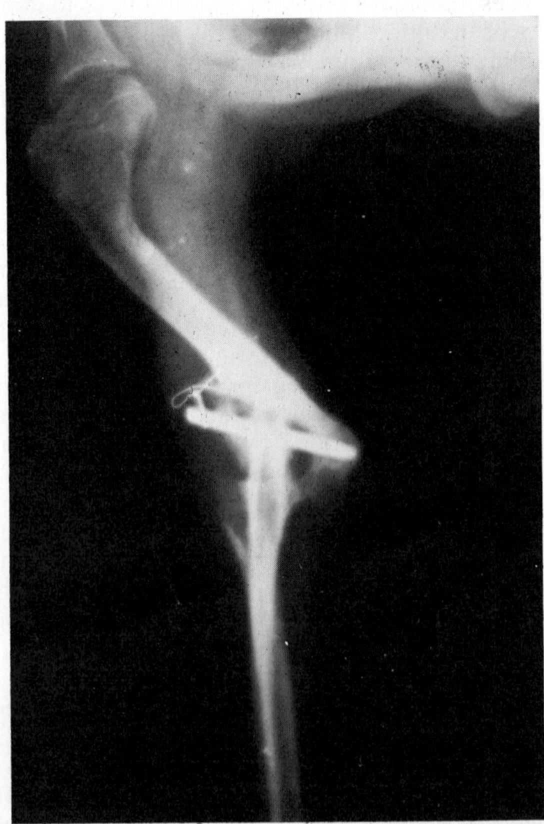

FIGURE 140–2. A comminuted lateral condylar fracture that collapsed after surgical repair in a 2-kg Yorkshire terrier. The resulting malunion with valgus deformity and subluxation is a candidate for arthrodesis.

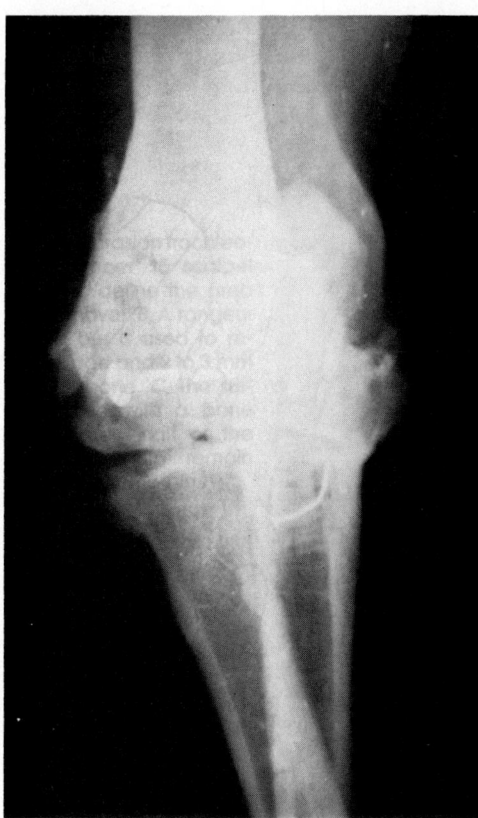

FIGURE 140–3. An old distal humeral fracture that has ankylosed. If the animal is in pain, an arthrodesis is indicated.

a plate along the caudal aspect of the humerus and ulna is the best method (Fig. 140–5). Fortunately, the caudal aspect of the elbow is the tension band side. However, the olecranon must be osteotomized to allow the plate

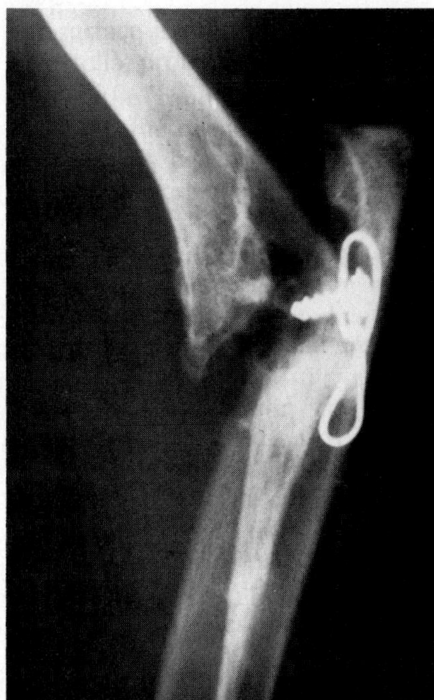

FIGURE 140–4. An old elbow fracture-luxation in which a primary repair to re-establish the elbow joint failed. There is now so much bone atrophy that only a fusion will produce a stable foreleg.

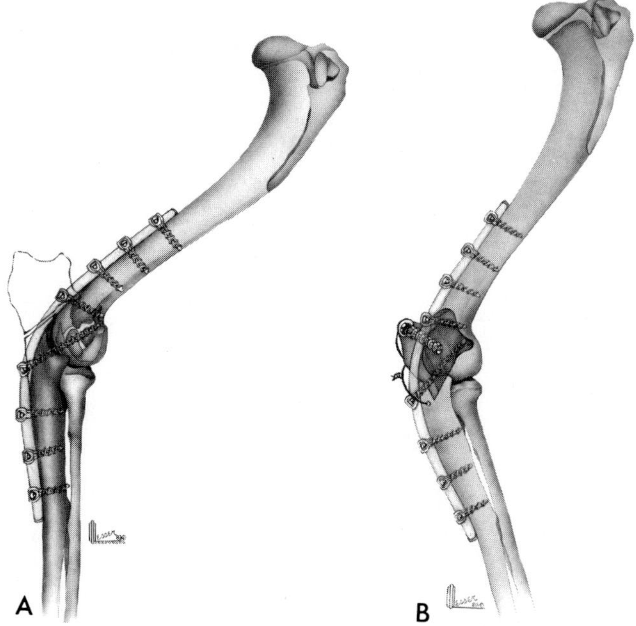

FIGURE 140–5. *A*, The plate is placed on the caudal aspect (tension side) of the elbow with a minimum of three screws in the humerus and three screws in the ulna. Screws crossing the arthrodesis should be placed under compression. *B*, The olecranon can be sacrificed as graft and the triceps sutured down, or it can be attached to the humerus on either side of the plate with a screw and tension band wire.

to achieve close contact with both the humerus and the ulna. The angle at which the olecranon is osteotomized can be determined by continuing a line parallel to the caudal aspect of the humerus across the olecranon, with the joint held at the proposed angle (Fig. 140–6). This position improves contact for the plate as it crosses the joint. The olecranon can be reattached to the ulna or humerus with a screw and tension band wire. An alternative method is to use the olecranon as graft material and suture the triceps tendon to tissue in the same area. Besides the olecranon osteotomy, it may be necessary to incise the lateral collateral ligament and elevate the origins of the extensor muscles from the lateral humeral condyle to provide exposure for removal of the cartilage from the distal humerus, radial head, and coronoid process. These structures should be contoured to provide areas of close contact. The ulnar nerve runs on the medial aspect of the elbow in this area and is identified and protected.

The angle of the arthrodesis can be measured in surgery with the use of preplaced K wires and a goniometer. The pins are placed at premeasured angles to the humerus and ulna, so they become parallel when these bones form the proper angle (Fig. 140–7). Another method is to radiograph one leg at the desired angle and prebend an old plate or plate template to the proper angle by comparing it with the x-ray film. When the plate is placed on the bones, the joint will be at the measured angle. If the actual plate to be used is prebent, the holes may not line up optimally. The bones can then be maintained in this position with a pin through the ulna into the humerus. The angle of the fusion can be predetermined by measuring the opposite leg. The av-

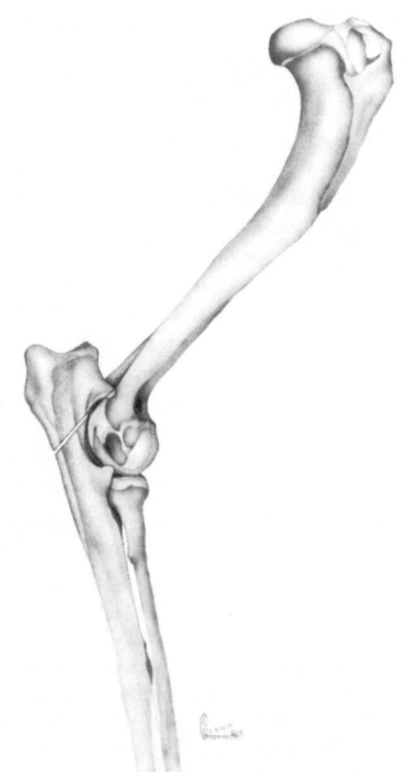

FIGURE 140–6. The olecranon is osteotomized at an angle parallel to the caudal aspect of the humerus to facilitate plate placement.

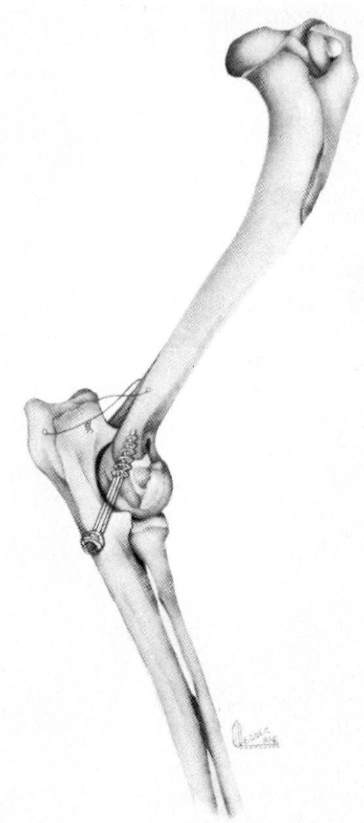

FIGURE 140–8. In small or toy breeds, a compression screw can be used to fuse the elbow with the assistance of a figure-eight wire. When possible, a plate should be used owing to the superior stability produced.

erage angle of the elbow is approximately 130° to 150°. This angle may be increased to increase leg length or vice versa.

The triceps muscles can be elevated to allow caudal placement of the plate. A minimum of three screws (six cortices) are used in the humerus and ulna, respectively, and one or more lag screws can be placed across the fusion site for additional interfragmentary compression. A self-compressing plate with nine or ten holes is adequate for a 30- to 35-kg dog.

In cats or small dogs, other methods of fixation combining pins, screws, and wire can be used. A screw can be placed under compression from the olecranon across the joint and up the humeral shaft (Fig. 140–8).

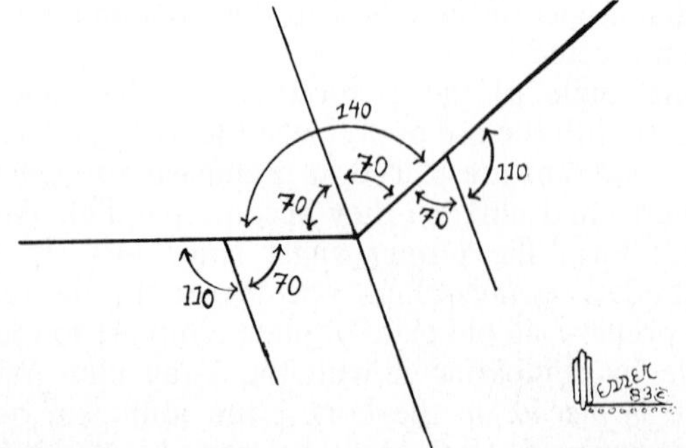

FIGURE 140–7. The surgeon can calculate the angle of arthrodesis at operation by placing pins at set angles in the humerus and ulna. If the angle of arthrodesis is 140°, placing the pins at 70° (one-half of 140°) to these bones, with the angle facing the elbow, will make the pins parallel when the elbow is at 140°.

In addition, a figure-eight wire should be placed from the olecranon to the humerus to oppose flexion of the elbow with weightbearing. A triceps tenotomy is used for exposure. Cross pins can be substituted for the screw, but then there are no compressive forces across the joint, and any motion at the fusion site encourages migration of the pins. With these techniques, a full cast is necessary for added protection, and it is left on until there is evidence of bone union. There is no reason why a small plate cannot be used in these cases, because it provides superior fixation. If the plate fixation is proper, only a padded bandage is necessary for a few weeks, but a cast gives added insurance.

External pin splints such as a Kirschner-Ehmer apparatus can be used either as a secondary support for one of the methods described or as the primary fixation device. If it is used alone, a full splint is applied using multiple external bars with the pins protruding through both sides of the limb. The protruding transosseous pins are connected, and one or two bars are used to oppose flexion of the joint by connecting the proximal and distal pins. This method is not as adaptable in the elbow as in the tarsocrural joint because of the thicker muscles and the interference of the chest wall with the medial pins and bar.

Whenever sufficient stability is questionable, an external cast or splint is added because there is no concern for loss of joint motion as there is for loss of fixation. The length of time casts and splints should remain in place depends on the quality of the internal fixation and the size and activity of the patient. When in doubt, the safest policy is to leave the external support on until there is radiographic evidence of healing. Six weeks is the average time.

Complications

Insufficient stability and infection are common causes of failure, especially if a plate is not used. If a plate is used on a large, active dog, fracture of the radius and ulna or humerus may occur at the end of the plate, where a stress riser occurs because of the difference in the elasticity between the plate and bone. It is recommended that the plate be removed once fusion is complete.

CARPUS

Indications

The most frequent indications for arthrodesis of the carpus are hyperextension injuries and fracture luxations, especially old injuries (Fig. 140–9). Many of these luxations are no longer reducible or, if so, are very unstable because of accompanying ligament damage. Casting alone is often insufficient—especially in large dogs with hyperextension injuries that may have been incurred from falls or leaping from heights or moving vehicles. Other surgical reconstructive procedures have been reported, but arthrodesis is consistently effective. The antebrachiocarpal joint may be spared or included in the arthrodesis, depending on the extent of the trauma (see Chapter 133). If the luxation or fracture is at the middle carpal or carpometacarpal joints only and the ligamentous structures of the accessory carpal bone are intact, it is possible to fuse these joints only, sparing the antebrachiocarpal joint. However, if the antebrachiocarpal joint is fused, the other joints of the carpus must be included, or secondary degenerative joint disease will develop in the latter, causing pain. Even when the antebrachiocarpal joint is not included in the arthrodesis, some loss of motion often occurs.

As in any joint, severe degenerative joint disease or other arthritic condition unresponsive to medication is an indication for fusion. Rheumatoid arthritis is especially prevalent in the carpal joint, and in advanced cases these joints become very unstable as a result of ligament damage (Fig. 140–10). Affected dogs have clinical signs similar to hyperextension injuries but without any history of trauma. This condition more frequently affects small dogs.

Another indication for carpal fusion is peripheral nerve damage. If the patient can support weight on the leg but lands on the dorsal surface of the paw, arthrodesis can improve this condition. However, most of these animals suffer from brachial plexus injuries, and too many muscles are affected for arthrodesis to be helpful. In simple radial paralysis, other treatments are available, but fusion can be considered.

Another situation in which carpal fusion may be necessary is nonunion of fractures of the radius and ulna in miniature breeds. Severe bone atrophy precludes simple handling of these cases. Fusion of the carpus provides adequate bone distal to the fracture to anchor plates or external pin splints in conjunction with cancellous autografts. The other general indications mentioned earlier also apply to the carpal joint.

Procedure

In a pancarpal arthrodesis, all three joints—antebrachiocarpal (radiocarpal), middle carpal, and carpometacarpal—are included. The common forms of fixation are external pin splints, cross pins, and plates. The cartilage of all involved joints, including the middle carpal, must be removed. It is necessary to incise the carpal fascia, each individual capsule, and some of the short intercarpal ligaments to accomplish this. It is then also possible

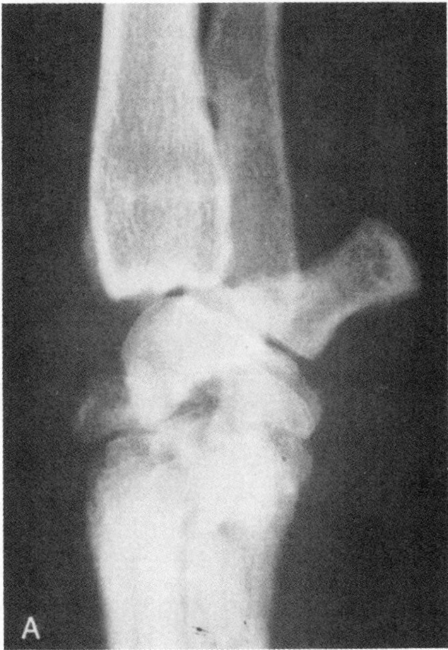

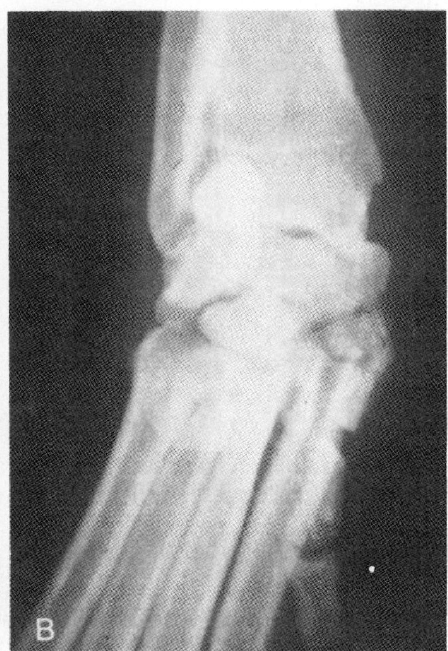

FIGURE 140–9. *A* and *B*, Multiple fractures of the carpal bones. If the ligamentous structures of the accessory carpal bone are also ruptured, pancarpal arthrodesis is indicated. These animals are presented with hyperextension of the carpus.

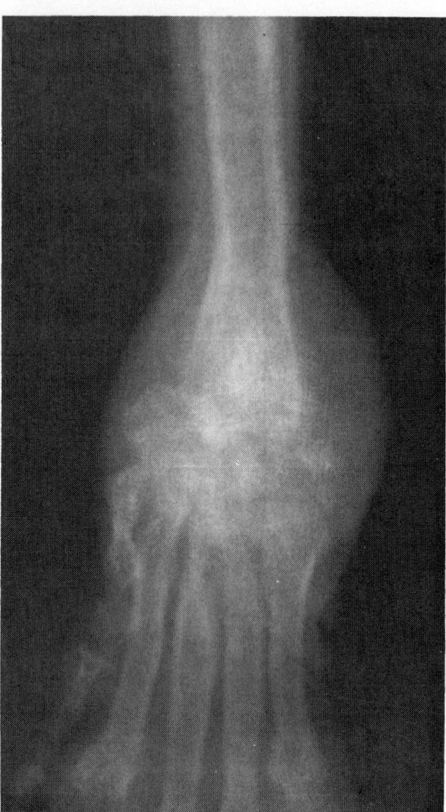

FIGURE 140–10. Rheumatoid arthritis in a miniature breed dog. There is often multiple joint involvement, and the disease is progressive, so a successful arthrodesis may only be palliative.

to pack all of these joints with cancellous bone graft. If cross pins are used, they enter from the proximal third of the second or fifth metacarpal bone, cross the three joints, and exit from the ulna or radius, respectively. The pins emerge proximal to the flare of the distal radius medially and exit from the ulna at the same level laterally (Fig. 140–11). Starting the pins proximally ensures a proper bite in these bones. The bone of the carpus is very hard, and power equipment is helpful in placing these pins. However, the dense bone may cause excessive heat production during pin insertion under power, leading to heat necrosis and early loosening of the pins. The use of a plate is superior. Most reports recommend placing the plate on the cranial (dorsal) aspect of the radius and carpus. This position allows the simplest approach but places the plate on the compression side rather than the tension side.

An approach for placing the plate on the palmar aspect has been reported (Fig. 140–12). This procedure has the advantage of placing the plate on the tension side of the bones but does require a more difficult and time-consuming approach. The minimum surgical exposure time reported was 30 minutes.

When the dorsal approach is used (Fig. 140–13), the only deeper structures encountered are the cephalic and accessory cephalic veins and the extensor tendons. The extensor carpi radialis can be transected, exposing the intercarpal and carpometacarpal joints for curettage. The tendon of the abductor pollicis longus can be transected or retracted. The following screws are placed: three in the radius (six cortices), one in the radial carpal bone to pull this section up to the plate, and three more in the third or fourth metacarpal bone. The plate is bent to provide 5° to 15° of extension. Leaving the plate straight causes excess stress of the metacarpophalangeal joint and should be avoided.

A dynamic compression plate has the advantage of providing compression between screw holes and therefore between the multiple joint surfaces. Plates also provide rigid support and are well tolerated for the prolonged healing periods required for fusions. Cross pins and external pin splints require more postsurgical care. Therefore, as in the elbow, plates are the first choice in carpal arthrodesis. External pin splints are effective when extensive soft-tissue damage is present.

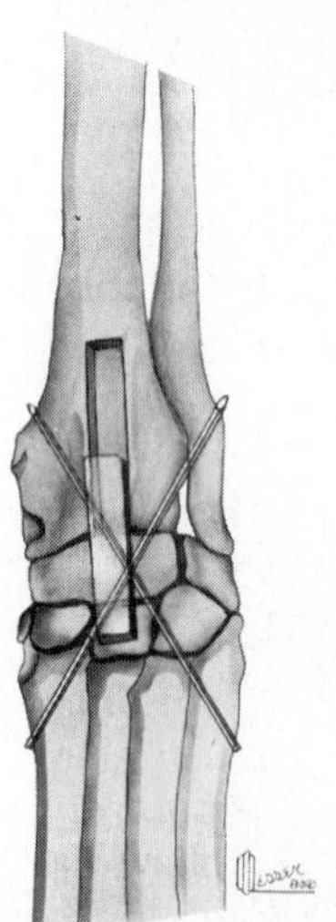

FIGURE 140–11. The use of crossed pins combined with an inlay graft formed from a slot in the distal radius and advanced into a bed cut into the carpal bones.

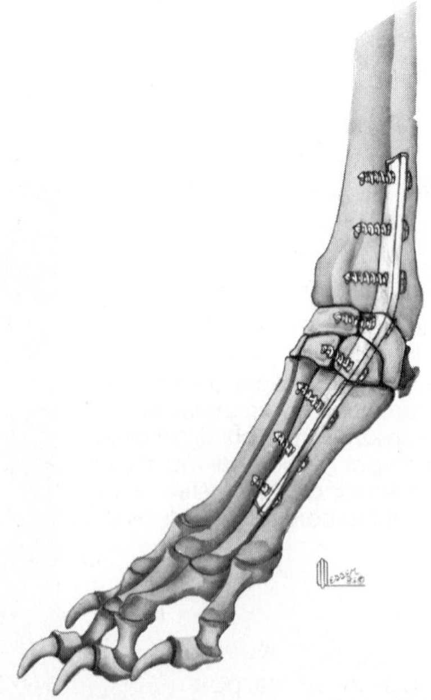

FIGURE 140–12. A plate placed on the caudal surface of the radius and palmar surface of the metacarpals places the plate on the tension side of the joint but requires a more difficult approach.

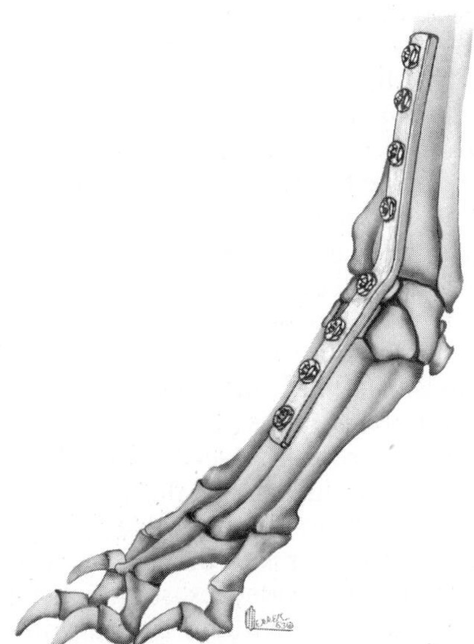

FIGURE 140–13. The preferred method of pancarpal arthrodesis is a plate with at least three to four screws in the radius, one in the radiocarpal bone, and three more in the third or fourth metacarpal bone. The carpus is placed in 5° to 15° of extension.

If the antebrachiocarpal joint and its ligaments are not injured and the accessory carpal bone and its attached ligaments are intact, a partial arthrodesis can be performed. Injuries of the middle carpal or carpometacarpal joints and disruption of the palmar carpal fibrocartilage are common indications for this procedure (Fig. 140–14). A simplified procedure using cancellous bone graft and a cast alone with no internal fixation has been reported. A T plate extending from metacarpal II or III to the radial and ulnar carpal bones can be used, with the cross of the T being proximal. Two other procedures are acceptable: (1) cross pins emerging from the carpal bones rather than the radius or (2) two or three pins driven up the second, third, and fourth metacarpal bones via the metacarpophalangeal joint and across the metacarpocarpal joint into the carpal bones (Fig. 140–15).

Cancellous bone is good insurance with any arthrodesis, but onlay or inlay grafts are especially suitable at the carpus. A rectangular section of ilium, rib, or distal radius can be placed in a slot formed across the antebrachiocarpal or intercarpal joints. Cortical grafts are especially suited to fusion of the carpus in atrophic nonunion of the radius and ulna in toy breeds. Sections of rib or ilium can be used to span the atrophied bone and carpal joint. The fixation is provided by two or three K wires above and below the fracture, protruding from both sides of the leg and connected with bars of methylmethacrylate. The carpus is fused in these cases because not enough bone stock remains on either side of the fracture in the radius and ulna.

Complications

Fusion of the antebrachiocarpal joint without fusion of the intercarpal or carpometacarpal joints leads to degenerative joint disease of the latter owing to increased stress imposed on these structures. Failure of arthrodesis is commonly due to infection, incomplete cartilage removal, or technical error in size or placement of the implants. Plates in this area are often removed to prevent osteolysis of the carpal bones due to stress protection. Also, cranially placed plates have very little soft-tissue cover and may cause discomfort from temperature changes or proximity to the overlying skin.

STIFLE

Indications

Degenerative disease of the stifle is usually secondary to ligament injuries, the two most common of which are old, chronic anterior cruciate ruptures and severe traumatic derangements (Fig. 140–16). In the latter, numerous structures are torn and primary reconstructive procedures may be unsuccessful, or excessive cartilage damage may require arthrodesis. With chronic cruciate tears, the degree of secondary degenerative joint disease determines whether primary repair or arthrodesis is attempted. Open fractures involving the stifle and accompanied by cartilage damage or bone and cartilage loss are another indication (Fig. 140–17). Another indication is "fracture disease" (Fig. 140–18). Although this disease can affect any joint, it most commonly occurs in the stifle and usually in young dogs treated for femoral fractures. The quadriceps is tied down to the callus, restricting motion of the stifle and leading to atrophy of the muscles and bones and fibroplasia of the capsule. All motion is eventually lost, and if the joint becomes painful, arthrodesis in a functional position is recommended.

Procedure

In the stifle, it is necessary to remove the cruciates and both menisci along with the articular cartilage.

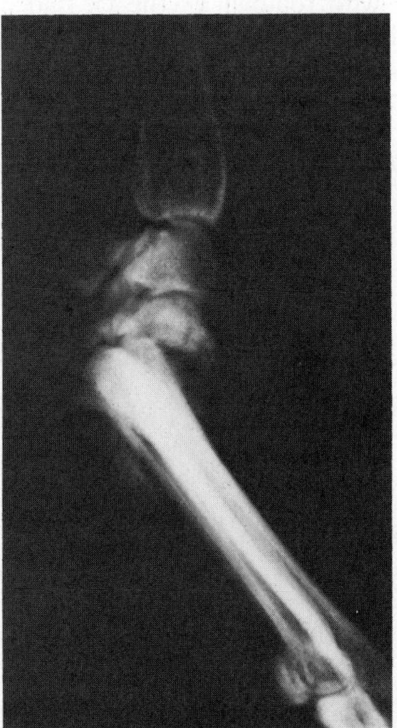

FIGURE 140–14. In this example, the antebrachiocarpal joint and the ligaments of the accessory carpal bone are uninjured. Fusion of the carpometacarpal joints alone is sufficient.

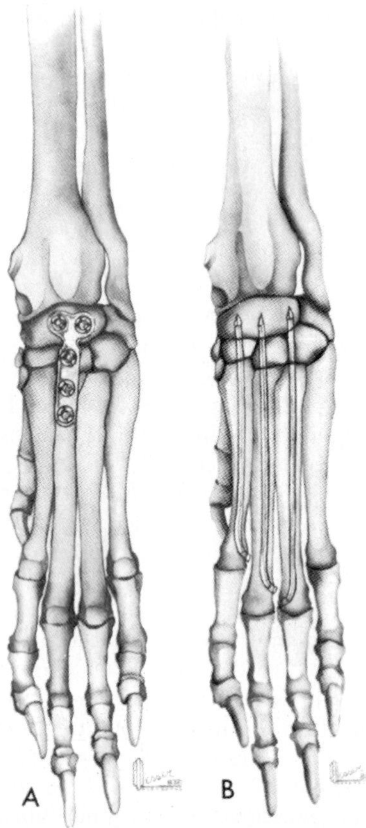

FIGURE 140–15. Partial carpal injuries can be treated by fusing the involved joints excluding the antebrachiocarpal joint. *A*, The use of a T plate. *B*, Intramedullary pins placed through slots in the distal metacarpals and driven up into the radial and ulnar carpal bones. Three or four pins can be used, depending on the size of the patient.

Excision of the straight patellar ligament from the tibial crest along with removal of the fat pad provides easy access to those structures. Besides removing the cartilage, contouring the ends of the tibia and femur is recommended to provide close bone contact. The angles at which the ends are cut are important because they determine the final angle of fusion. Both angles are determined with a sterile goniometer or wires before the cuts are made. An oscillating saw works better than curettes or a bur for this purpose. After the cuts are complete, a Steinmann pin is placed from the medial aspect of the tibia across the joint proximally and out the lateral femoral condyle. This pin holds the joint at the proper angle. If cross pins or cross screws are to be the method of fixation (small dogs or cats), then either a second pin is inserted from the medial femoral condyle to the lateral tibial cortex or a hole is drilled in the same manner, and a screw is placed from the tibia to the femur (distal to proximal). The flare of the tibial plateau laterally does not provide reliable purchase for the threads. Either cancellous screws or overdrilling the first hole provides compression across the fusion. The first pin is then replaced by another compression screw (Figs. 140–19 and 140–20). If the pins are not replaced with screws, it may be necessary to add figure-eight wire (18 or 20 gauge) over the ends of the pins medially and laterally to create added stability and compression. Casts, splints, or external pin splints are used in addition to these methods for extra support until healing is evident.

The use of a plate on the cranial aspect of the femur and tibia is the best method for larger dogs and smaller patients as well (Fig. 140–21). The patella is removed or displaced to one side or the other. The quadriceps muscle is elevated subperiosteally to allow placement of the plate on the cranial cortex of the femur, and the plate is contoured over the cranial aspect of the tibia. The tibial crest and tibial tuberosity are removed to provide a flat bed for better plate contact. At least three to four screws are placed in the diaphysis of the femur and tibia, respectively. Any screws between these should compress the opposing surfaces. A pin is used for temporary fixation to hold the joint at the proper angle

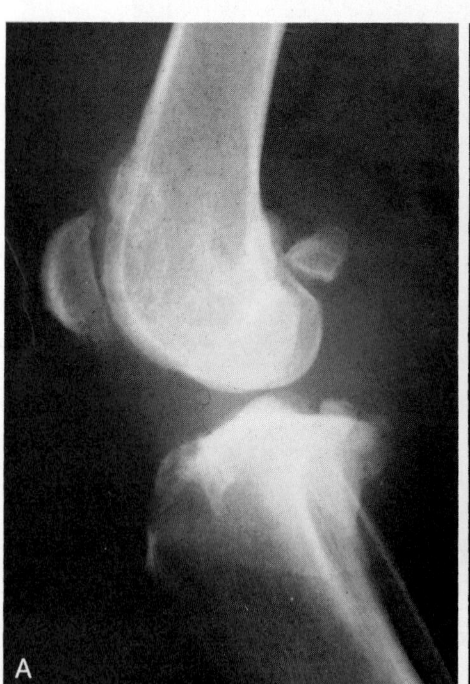

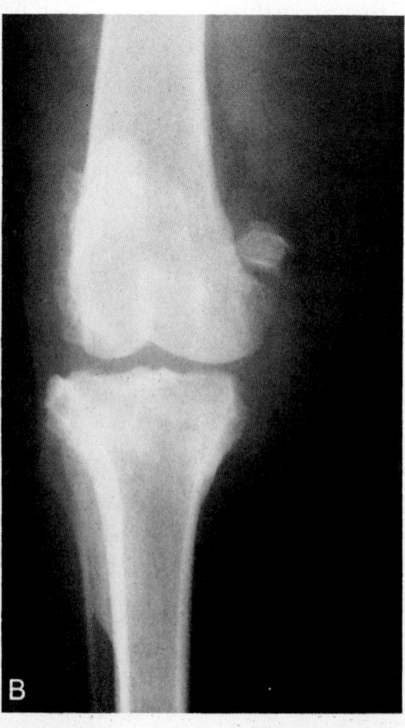

FIGURE 140–16. *A* and *B*, Degenerative joint disease of the stifle is often secondary to unrepaired ligamentous injuries, especially long-standing cranial cruciate tears. If there is significant pain and disuse unresponsive to medication, an arthrodesis is indicated.

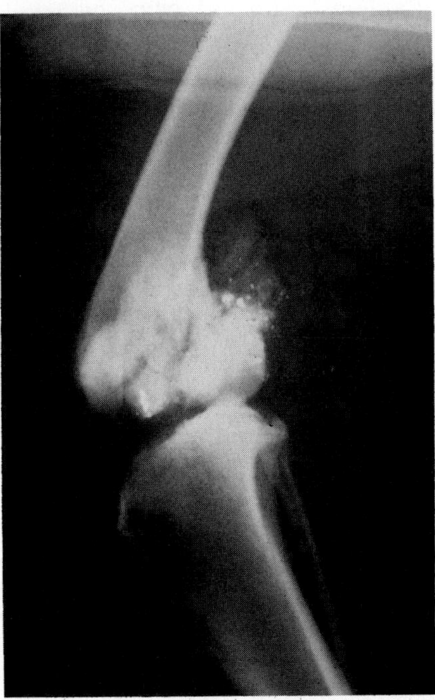

FIGURE 140–17. A gunshot wound causing severe comminution of the distal femur not amenable to a primary repair is a candidate for arthrodesis.

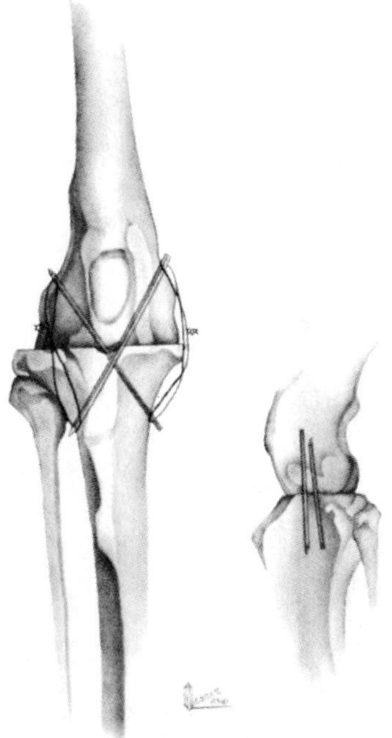

FIGURE 140–19. If crossed pins are used to fuse the stifle, then an 18- or 20-gauge wire should be added around the pins to produce compression across the arthrodesis for added stability.

while the plate is attached. The joint is prepared in the manner discussed previously, and the subchondral bone from the excised tibial and humeral condyles and cancellous autograft can be placed between the bone ends before compressing them.

The angle is calculated from the opposite leg, the average angle being 125° to 150°. Because a significant amount of bone is removed, it is usually necessary to fuse the leg in a straighter angle to regain length.

External pin splints are adaptable to this joint, either alone or in combination with internal pins or screws. If used alone, more than two pins are used above and below the joint along with multiple bars as described

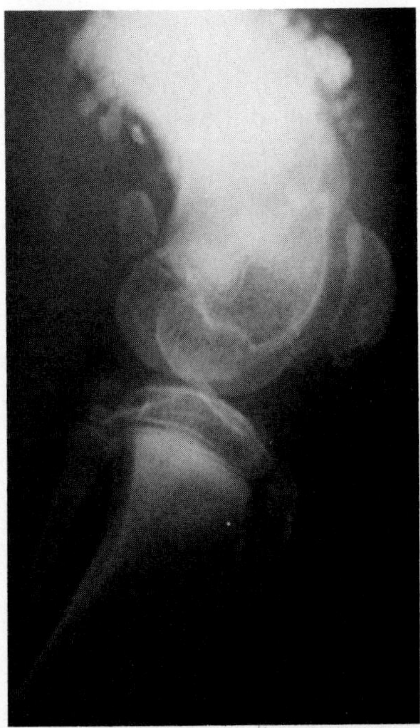

FIGURE 140–18. An untreated femoral fracture in a young dog, leading to immobility of the stifle, atrophy of bone, and fibroplasia of the joint capsule. This limb was fixed in full extension, and the dog could not place the leg properly. Arthrodesis at a normal angle plus fracture fixation would return this limb to function. Attempts at returning motion to these joints are often unrewarding.

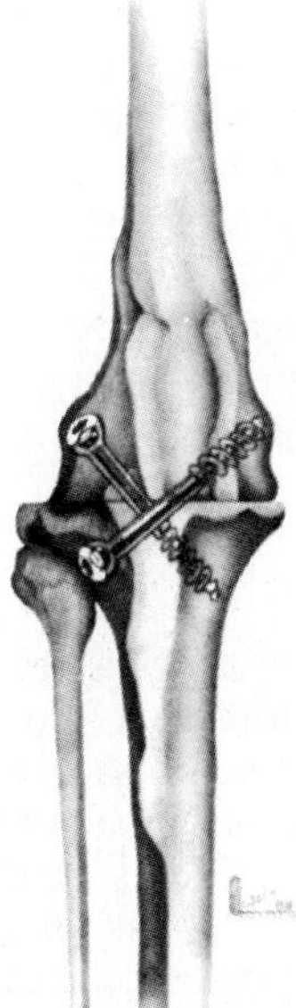

FIGURE 140–20. The stifle can be fused with two compression screws. It is important to start the screw that runs from the lateral aspect of the tibia to the medial condyle of the femur from distal to proximal. If the screw is run the opposite way, there is insufficient bone on the lateral aspect of the proximal tibia for the threads to engage.

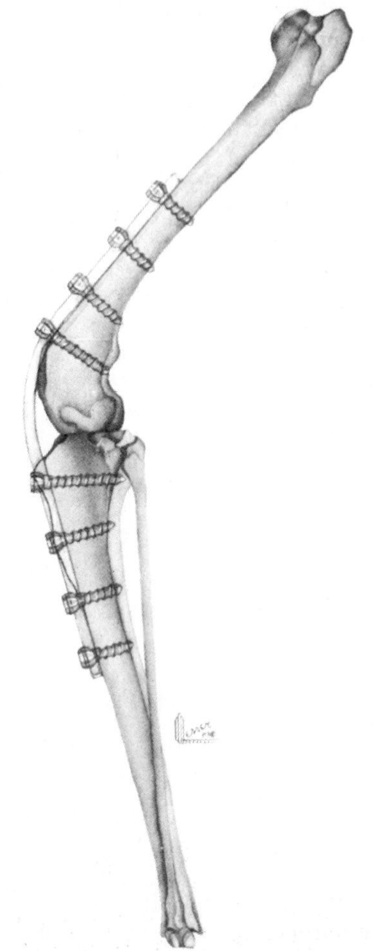

FIGURE 140–21. The favored method of arthrodesis of the stifle is a plate on the cranial aspect of the joint. The tibial crest and possibly part of the trochlea can be removed to improve the seating of the plate. The excised section of the tibial crest is shown overlapping the plate.

previously. In humans, the joint is fused at 180°, and these splints are the most commonly used method of fixation. In dogs and cats, the standing angle of the stifle ranges from 125° to 150°. Therefore, compression can be applied across the joint, but extra bars must be placed to buttress against flexion. The problem with external pin splints in such instances is the inability to place a bar on the medial aspect of the femur for added strength.

Complications

Fusion of the stifle creates a very long lever arm and therefore excessive forces at the arthrodesis site. To overcome this, the plate must cover almost half of the femur and tibia. Too short a plate and poor bone contact are the most common causes of technical failure. The long lever arm creates a risk of fracture at the plate ends. Therefore, the plate should eventually be removed and the limb protected for 3 to 4 weeks longer.

HOCK

Indications

The tarsal joints are subject to traumatic injury as well as degenerative disease (Fig. 140–22). One of the most common traumatic injuries encountered in this joint is the shearing fracture that may occur when the leg has been dragged along the road by a car, causing significant loss of soft tissue and bone. The collateral ligaments and most of the malleolus are lost in these injuries, leaving the joint open and devoid of soft-tissue coverage and stability. The medial aspect is more frequently affected than the lateral. These wounds usually heal without active signs of infection, and sufficient fibroplasia often occurs to stabilize the joint without further surgery. However, if instability remains and simple replacement of the appropriate collateral ligament is insufficient, pantarsal arthrodesis is indicated. Severe fracture luxations of the tarsocrural, middle tarsal, or tarsometatarsal joints also occur and can be treated with fusions of the involved joints alone (Fig. 140–23). Rupture of the plantar ligament also requires fusion of one or more of these latter joints.

Rupture of the calcaneal ligament not amenable to suture because of either severe trauma to the ligament or fragmentation of the calcaneus (Fig. 140–24) can be treated by fusion of the talocrural joint.

Rheumatoid arthritis or polyarthritis also commonly affects the hock, and as with the carpus, arthrodesis can be used as a palliative treatment. Osteoarthritis or septic arthritis, if severe enough, can require arthrodesis. Degenerative joint disease from an osteochondritis dissecans lesion of the talus is one such situation.

A unique indication for fusion of the talocrural joint is its use in conjunction with muscle transfer for the treatment of ischial nerve paralysis. In this case, the fusion positions the foot properly and removes a point of motion along the path of the transferred tendon.

Procedure

The simplest method of removing motion from the talocrural joint is driving a Steinmann pin up through the sustentaculum tali of the fibular tarsal bone, through

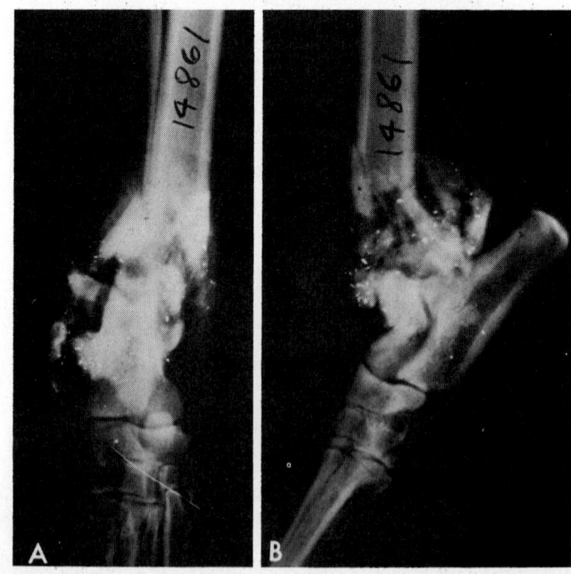

FIGURE 140–22. *A* and *B*, A severe intra-articular fracture of the hock, where a primary repair is not feasible. Gunshot wounds are often responsible for this type of injury, which requires arthrodesis.

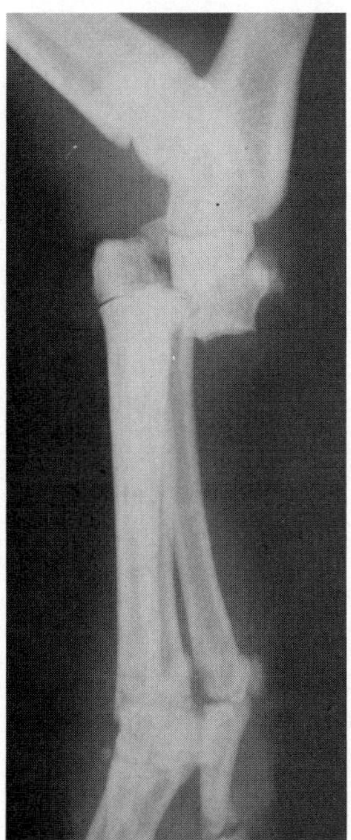

FIGURE 140–23. In this injury in which the talocrural joint is spared, it is only necessary to fuse the joints involved.

the tibial tarsal bone, and up the medullary cavity of the tibia. If the cartilage is not removed and the pin is removed within weeks, not months, this provides a temporary support. If the pin is left *in situ* for months or years, fibroplasia of the capsule and surrounding tissues creates an ankylosed or fibrosed joint. If the cartilage is removed, true arthrodesis can occur; however, the pin does not create compression across the fusion site, and more efficient alternatives are available.

In small and medium-sized dogs and cats, a compression screw from the sustentaculum tali into the medullary cavity of the tibia provides stable fixation as long as the threads of the screw can obtain sufficient bone contact (Fig. 140–25). Once the medulla is wider in diameter than the shaft of the screw, this technique does not suffice, and the screw must be anchored in the cortex of the tibia. The screw can be placed in either direction, proximally from the medial malleolus of the tibia through the tibial tarsal bone and exiting from the fibular tarsal bone or vice versa (Fig. 140–26). In either case, it is recommended that orthopedic wire (18 or 20 gauge) be passed from the calcaneus to the caudal cortex of the tibia to support the talocrural joint against flexion. This helps prevent the screw from moving and should be used whenever a screw is used alone. In addition, to facilitate screw placement, a small guide wire is passed first to hold the joint in the proper alignment for drilling and tapping for the screw. This pin can be removed or left in place or replaced with a larger pin for additional stability.

Another technique is the use of a plate along the cranial aspect of the tibia and tarsal bones. (*Section Editors' Note:* Pantarsal arthrodesis using a dorsally positioned compression plate [similar to pancarpal arthrodesis] is the most effective technique for severe tibiotarsal derangements.) As in the carpus, this is not the tension side, so a cast or splint is added even when the plate is used and always when a screw and wire are used until the joint is solidly fused.

External pin splints can be used either as the primary or secondary method of fixation. In the hock, it is best to place the pins through with bars both medially and laterally. A minimum of two pins are placed in the tibia, another pin in the tibial tarsal bone, and two more

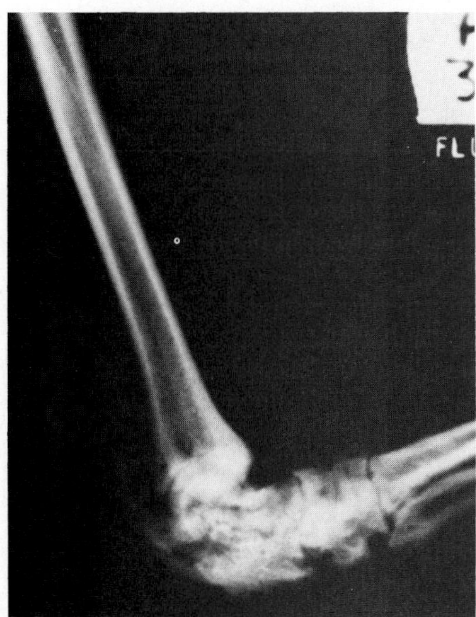

FIGURE 140–24. The collapse of the calcaneus due to osteomyelitis allowed avulsion of the calcaneal tendon. Because the lever arm of the fibular tarsal bone is gone, reattachment of the calcaneal tendon may not be effective. Arthrodesis of the talocrural joint would accomplish the same goal of relieving the plantigrade stance of the animal.

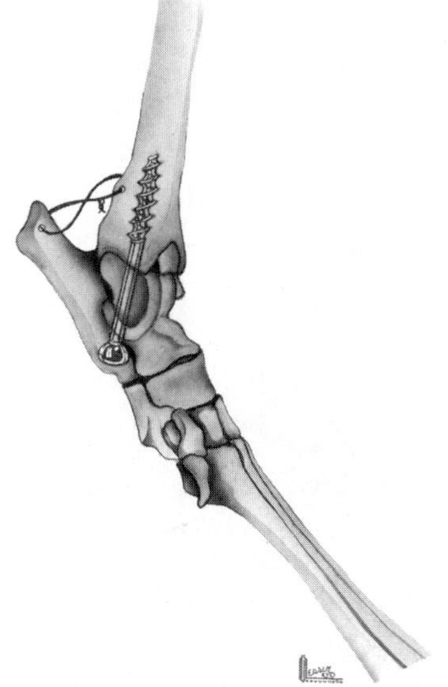

FIGURE 140–25. A screw can be placed from the fibular tarsal bone through the tibial tarsal bone up into the medullary canal of the tibia. Once the medullary canal becomes wider than the screw, this placement is no longer viable. A figure-eight wire is placed for support and to prevent flexion of the hock during weightbearing.

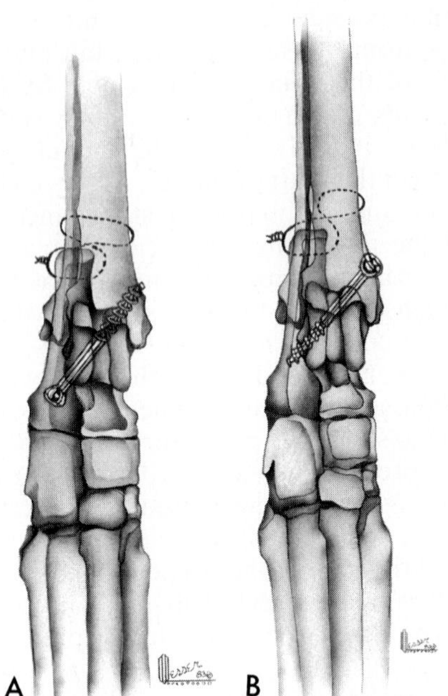

FIGURE 140–26. The screw can also be placed from the fibular tarsal bone to emerge from the medial maleolus *(A)* or the opposite, from proximal to distal *(B)*. A wire is placed as shown in Figure 140–25.

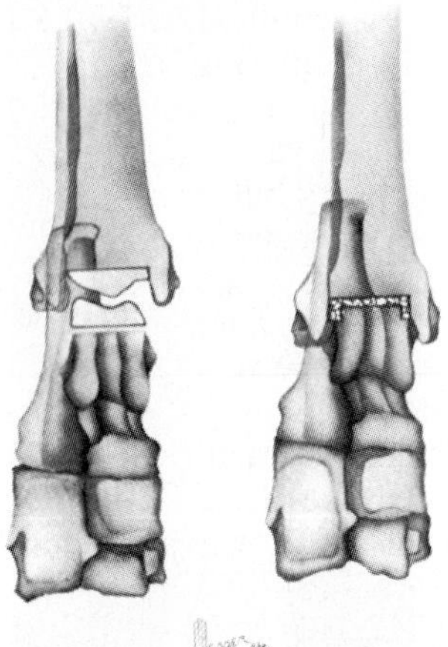

FIGURE 140–28. When the articular cartilage is being removed, it is advantageous to shape the opposing surfaces to produce the most stable configuration possible. In the talocrural joint, two congruent rectangular surfaces can be shaped and then filled with cancellous bone to create optimum bone-to-bone contact.

either in the middle tarsal bone and the metatarsals or both in the metatarsals. The bars support the joint against flexion during weightbearing (Fig. 140–27).

Crossed Steinmann pins can be used in larger dogs. They are placed from the tibial tarsal and fibular tarsal bones across the joint to emerge from the lateral and medial cortex of the distal tibia, respectively. Care must be taken not to distract the joint surfaces while driving the two pins. On the contrary, it is beneficial to have an assistant place compressive forces across the joint as the pins are driven.

When removing the cartilage from the talocrural joint, it is especially important to produce two congruent surfaces. Use of a curette, bur, or miniature oscillating saw allows the surgeon to create a flat plateau on the trochlea of the tibial tarsal bone and a rectangular depression of the distal tibia. The latter is accomplished by removing the intermediate ridge of the distal tibial articular surface along with the cartilage from the lateral

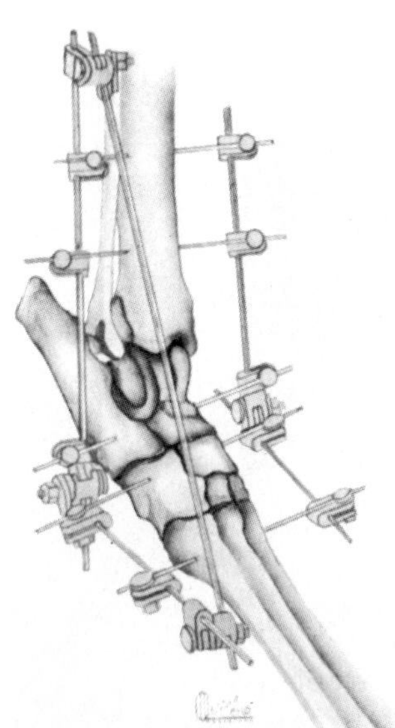

FIGURE 140–27. An external splint such as a Kirschner-Ehmer apparatus is well adapted for use in fusing the hock. Compression should be placed across the talocrural joint, and another bar (or bars) should be added to support against flexion.

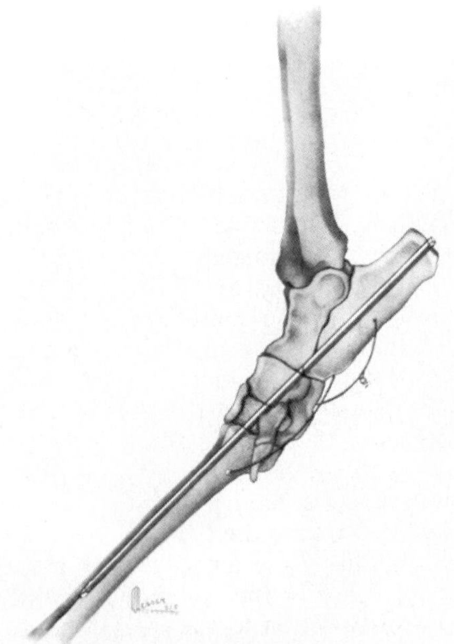

FIGURE 140–29. Luxation of the tarsometatarsal joint can be treated with an intramedullary pin and tension band wire. The wire can extend from a hole drilled in the fibular tarsal bone as illustrated or alternatively from around the promixal end of the pin before it crosses to enter the proximal metatarsals.

aspect of the medial malleolus. These locking surfaces create additional stability (Fig. 140–28). Cancellous graft is used to fill in gaps and speeds healing of the fusion.

The standing angle varies from 130° to 150° for the hock of an average dog but does differ between individuals of different conformation. Therefore, measuring the opposite leg is still the most reliable method of determining the proper angle. The angle for cats has been reported to be 115° to 125°.

When an injury involves just the intertarsal or tarsometatarsal joints (e.g., fractures or luxations), only the affected joints need be fused. In one method, a Steinmann pin is inserted down the fibular tarsal bone, through the fourth tarsal bone, into the third or fourth metatarsal bone. This is reinforced with a figure-eight wire (18 to 20 gauge) extending from either (1) the proximal end of the pin or (2) a hole in the calcaneus or tuber calcus to a hole through the proximal metatarsal bones (Fig. 140–29). This wire acts as a tension band. An alternative technique is to place a plate on the lateral surface of the fibular tarsal bone across to the fifth metatarsal bone. At least four screws are placed in the metatarsal bone. A padded bandage rather than a cast or splint is often all that is necessary in these latter two procedures. Cancellous graft is also recommended for fusions of the tarsometatarsal joint.

Complications

In talocrural fusions, fracture of the screw or pin due to fatigue stress is of concern, and protection with a splint or cast along with the wire previously mentioned is recommended. Once the fusion is solid, the risk decreases, but the screw can be removed if desired. Insufficient removal of the cartilage and insufficient stability are the most common causes of failure. For this reason, it is recommended that a cast be kept on until union is achieved.

References

1. Chambers JN, Bjorling DE: Palmar surface plating for arthrodesis of the canine carpus. *J Am Anim Hosp Assoc 18*:1875, 1982.
2. Gambardella PC, Griffiths RC: Treatment of hyperextension injuries of the canine carpus. *Comp Cont Educ 4*:127, 1982.
3. Johnson KA: Carpal arthrodesis in dogs. *Aust Vet J 56*:515, 1980.
4. Johnson KA, Bellenger CB: The effects of autologous bone grafting on bone healing after carpal arthrodesis in the dog. *Vet Rec 107*:126, 1980.
5. Miller MC, et al: *Anatomy of the Dog*. W.B. Saunders, Philadelphia, 1964, pp 231–261.
6. Newton CD, Nunamaker DM: *Textbook of Small Animal Orthopaedics*. J.B. Lippincott, Philadelphia, 1985, p 565.
7. Olds RB: Arthrodesis. *In* Bojrab MJ (ed): *Current Techniques in Small Animal Surgery*. Lea & Febiger, Philadelphia, 1975, pp 542–548.
8. Slocum B: Partial carpal fusion in the dog. *J Am Vet Med Assoc 180*:1204, 1980.
9. Stoll SG, et al: A technique for tibiotarsal arthrodesis utilizing cancellous bone screws in small animals. *J Am Anim Hosp Assoc 11*:185, 1975.

CHAPTER 141 Amputations

Joseph P. Weigel

Indications for amputation include severe trauma, ischemic necrosis, intractable orthopedic infection, severe disability due to unmanageable arthritis, paralysis, congenital deformity, and neoplasia. However, veterinary surgeons should also consider the adaptability and suitability of the individual animal to amputation and the owner's view of the animal's disabled condition. Preoperative assessment of metastasis by chest radiography in neoplasia is a factor in determining an animal's suitability for surgery. Placing a sling on the affected leg and observing the animal's ability to function on three legs help determine the animal's adaptability. The veterinarian should advise amputation when medically and humanely feasible but should also demonstrate concern for and attention to the owner's wishes. Decisions to amputate based on financial factors or a decision to euthanize instead of amputate must be respected by the veterinarian and handled with great sensitivity and concern. Although the final decision is the owner's right, it is our responsibility and challenge to guide clients to a proper decision. Owners' reported responses to limb amputation have been favorable.[3, 6]

GENERAL CONSIDERATIONS IN AMPUTATION SURGERY

Level of Amputation

In forelimb amputation, scapular removal is faster and easier than shoulder disarticulation. If the scapula is left in shorthaired dogs, muscle atrophy allows bony prominences of the scapula to be seen, creating a cosmetically unacceptable appearance to some owners. Removal of the scapula may render the chest wall more susceptible to blunt trauma.

In the rear limb, amputation at midthigh leaves a stump that can protect the male genitalia and is also easier to perform than disarticulation at the hip. In any case, it is advisable to perform the amputation through normal tissue well above the diseased area and proximal enough in the limb to avoid leaving a dangling, useless stump.

Amputation Through the Joint Versus Amputation Through the Bone

It is generally advisable to amputate through the bone, thereby allowing the bone end to atrophy. If the limb is severed through the elbow or stifle joint, the articular epiphysis remains without atrophy while soft tissue atrophies, leaving inadequate coverage of the bone and rendering it susceptible to trauma. When the limb is removed at the shoulder or hip joint, sufficient soft tissue remains to protect the bone.

Division of Muscles

Muscles may be severed at origins or insertions or divided through the belly. Electroincision is helpful in controlling hemorrhage.

Division of Vessels

Major arteries are double ligated with nonabsorbable inert suture material. The artery and vein are not ligated together to avoid the formation of an arteriovenous fistula. Veins may be singularly ligated with nonabsorbable suture. Attention is given to the level of arterial division to guard against necrosis of parts of the stump.

The artery is generally ligated first to allow blood to drain from the limb through intact veins. This technique helps preserve vascular volume, electrolytes, and protein. With diseased limbs that pose a possibility of disseminating the disease by surgical manipulation, it is advisable to ligate the vein first and the artery immediately afterward.

Division of Nerves

Neuromas after amputation are not generally a problem. As a consequence, there are no special concerns about severance of nerves. Nerve trunks are severed by sharp dissection while held in mild tension.

Closure of the Stump

Correct closures start with a properly planned amputation. Extensive dissection of the subcutaneous space results in dead space that is difficult to close. The bone end must be adequately covered with viable muscle. When muscle is sutured, the fascial covering and not the muscle itself is used to hold the suture. Seromas, common sequelae to amputation surgery, can be prevented by gentle technique, effective hemostasis, secure closure of fascial planes, elimination of dead space, and avoidance of extensive subcutaneous dissection.

PHYSIOLOGICAL CONSIDERATIONS

Preoperative evaluation of a patient's physiological status is important when a major amputation is planned. Complete hematological evaluation with a biochemistry and electrolyte panel is advisable. When a limb is removed, a large amount of tissue with fluid, electrolytes, and red blood cells is lost. This loss becomes more important when a patient is in poor preoperative condition or the diseased limb has increased blood flow and inflammation. Intravenous fluid administration during the operation is necessary to maintain hydration and blood pressure. Postoperative monitoring is essential to the recognition and treatment of shock.

TECHNIQUES*

Foreleg Amputation by Shoulder Disarticulation[4]

The lateral skin incision is curved, starting in the region of the major tubercle of the humerus and extending caudodistally, half of the length of the brachium and then being redirected caudoproximally to end in the caudal point of the axillary space. A straight medial incision connects the cranial and caudal points of the lateral incision. The skin distal to the incision is dissected free of its subcutaneous attachments down to the elbow joint on both the lateral and medial sides. The cephalic vein is ligated and divided as it passes cranially under the cleidobrachialis muscle. The axillobrachial vein is divided and ligated as it branches from the cephalic. The cleidobrachialis muscle is lifted from its insertion on the distal end of the humeral crest. The acromial portion of the deltoid muscle is lifted from its insertion on the deltoid tuberosity and reflected proximally. The brachial fascia is incised distally along the border of the lateral head of the triceps muscle distally to the olecranon. The triceps tendon is fully isolated and transected just above the olecranon (Fig. 141–1).

Attention is next directed to the medial side of the leg. The superficial pectoral muscles are severed from their insertion on the crest of the major tubercle. The deep pectoral muscle, now visible, can be separated from its insertion on the minor and major tubercles of the humerus and the medial fascia of the brachium. The cutaneous trunci muscle, which passes lateral to the vasculature and nerves, is severed and reflected to expose the main neurovascular structures. The brachial artery is isolated, double ligated, and divided between its deep brachial branch and bicipital branch. The brachial vein is separately ligated and incised at the same level. The median and ulnar nerves, caudal to the brachial artery, are sharply transected. The radial nerve is severed as it passes lateral to the brachial artery and into the accessory and medial heads of the triceps muscle. The musculocutaneous nerve is transected as it passes cranial to the nerves and vessels just described. The cranial circumflex humeral artery is divided as it branches from the proximal portion of the brachial artery. The severed vessels and nerves are retracted so that the combined insertion of the latissimus dorsi, teres major, and cutaneous trunci muscles can be lifted from the teres tuberosity of the humerus. The fascia along

*All anatomical references from Evans HE, Christensen GC: *Miller's Anatomy of the Dog*. 2nd ed. W.B. Saunders, Philadelphia, 1979.

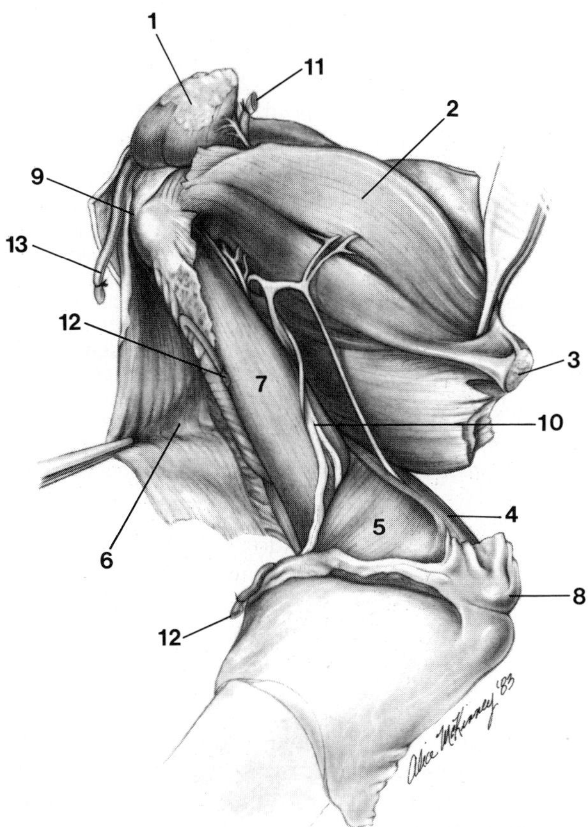

FIGURE 141–1. Lateral dissection of the left thoracic limb. (1, deltoid muscle [acromial portion]; 2, triceps muscle [lateral head]; 3, triceps tendon; 4, anconeus muscle; 5, extensor carpi radialis muscle; 6, cleidobrachialis muscle; 7, brachial muscle; 8, olecranon process of the ulna; 9, major tubercle of the humerus; 10, radial nerve; 11, axillobrachial vein; 12, cephalic vein; 13, omobrachial vein.)

the cranial border of the tensor fasciae antebrachii muscle is incised distally and retracted caudally. The division between the medial and accessory heads and the lateral and long heads of the triceps muscle is exposed. The triceps muscle is bluntly separated so that the medial and accessory heads are left with the amputated limb. The medial and accessory heads are severed distally from the common tricipital tendon.

The branches of the collateral ulnar artery, supplying the distal portion of the triceps, are severed as they enter the long head of the triceps. Branches of the radial nerve to the lateral and long heads are transected. The deep brachial artery is still intact and supplies the lateral and long heads of the triceps muscle. The axillobrachial vein is divided and ligated again as it terminates in the axillary vein (Fig. 141–2).

The final step is division of the muscles close to the joint. This dissection is started by severing the insertion of the supraspinatus muscle from the major tubercle of the humerus. The joint capsule is incised along with the muscle. The insertions of the infraspinatus and teres minor muscles are severed from the humerus. After the aponeurosis of the lateral head of the triceps muscle is lifted from the humeral crest, the incision in the lateral joint capsule is continued caudally and around the joint to the medial side, where the subscapular muscle is severed from its insertion on the minor tubercle of the humerus. The incision is continued cranially, severing the tendon of origin of the coracobrachial muscle. Amputation is complete when the tendon of origin of the biceps brachii muscle is transected (Fig. 141–3).

The stump is closed by suturing the triceps tendon cranially to the fascia of the superficial pectorals. The fascia of the supraspinatus and deltoid muscles is sutured

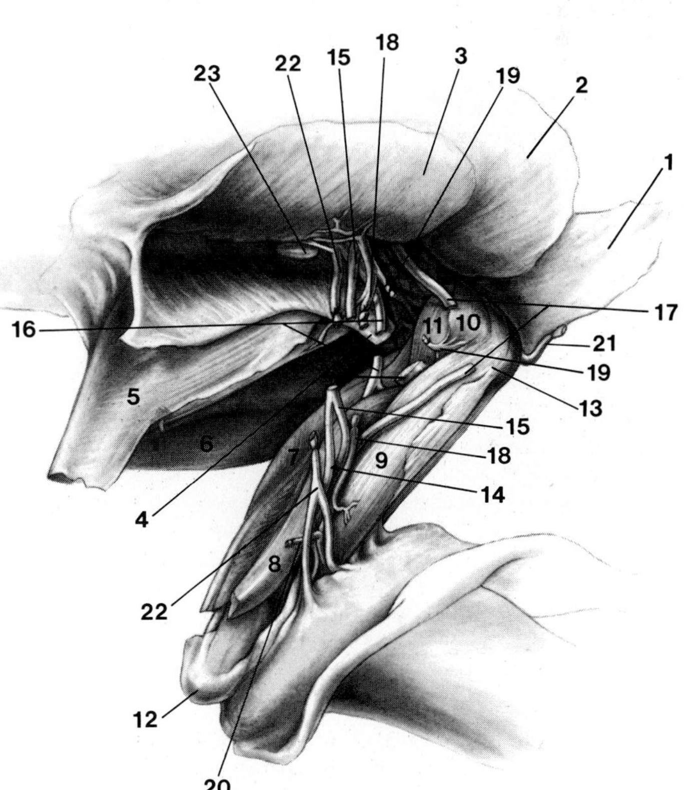

FIGURE 141–2. Medial dissection of the left thoracic limb. (1, cleidobrachialis muscle; 2, superficial pectoral muscle; 3, deep pectoral muscle; 4, combined insertion of the latissimus dorsi muscle, teres major muscle, and cutaneous trunci muscle; 5, triceps muscle [long head]; 6, triceps muscle [lateral head]; 7, triceps muscle [accessory head]; 8, triceps muscle [medial head]; 9, biceps brachii muscle; 10, subscapularis muscle; 11, coracobrachialis muscle; 12, olecranon process of the ulna; 13, major tubercle of the humerus; 14, ulnar nerve; 15, median nerve; 16, radial nerve; 17, musculocutaneous nerve; 18, brachial artery; 19, cranial circumflex humeral artery; 20, collateral ulnar artery; 21, cephalic vein; 22, brachial vein; 23, axillary lymph node.)

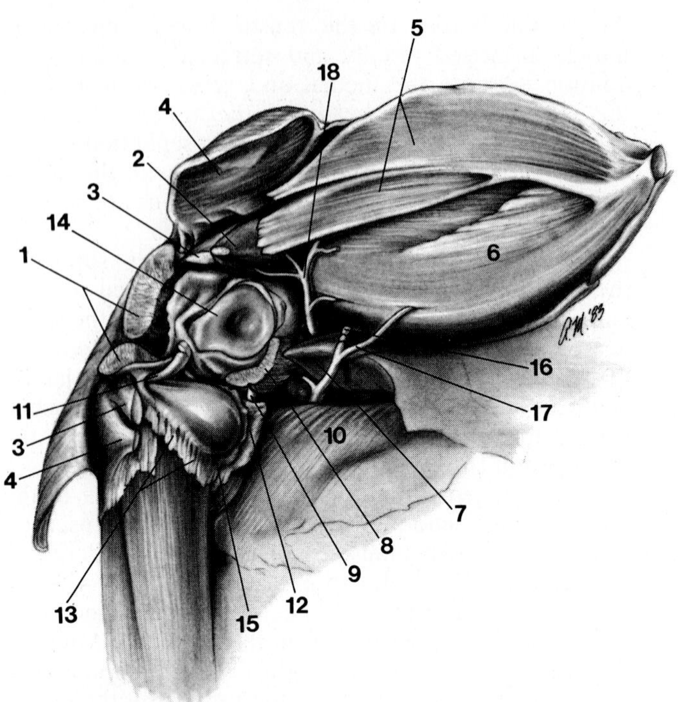

FIGURE 141–3. Dissection around the left shoulder joint, caudolateral view. (1, supraspinatus muscle; 2, teres minor muscle; 3, infraspinatus muscle; 4, deltoideus muscle [acromial portion]; 5, triceps muscle [lateral head]; 6, triceps muscle [long head]; 7, combined insertion of the latissimus dorsi muscle, teres minor muscle, and cutaneous trunci muscle; 8, subscapularis muscle; 9, tendon of the coracobrachialis muscle; 10, deep pectoral muscle; 11, partially severed tendon of origin of the biceps brachii muscle; 12, tendon of insertion of the subscapularis muscle; 13, joint capsule; 14, glenoid cavity of the scapula; 15, head of the humerus; 16, brachial artery [reflected proximally]; 17, deep brachial artery; 18, caudal circumflex humeral artery.)

to the fascia of the cleidobrachialis muscle. The subcutaneous tissue and skin are closed in a routine fashion.

Foreleg Amputation with Removal of the Scapula[2]

The skin incision is started several centimeters above the dorsal border of the scapula and is extended distally along the spine of the scapula to the shoulder joint. At this point, a circumferential incision around the shoulder joint starts and ends. Laterally, the cephalic vein is ligated and divided as it passes deep to the cleidobrachialis muscle. A deep incision along the cranial edge of the spine of the scapula severs the origin of the omotransversarius muscle and the cervical part of the

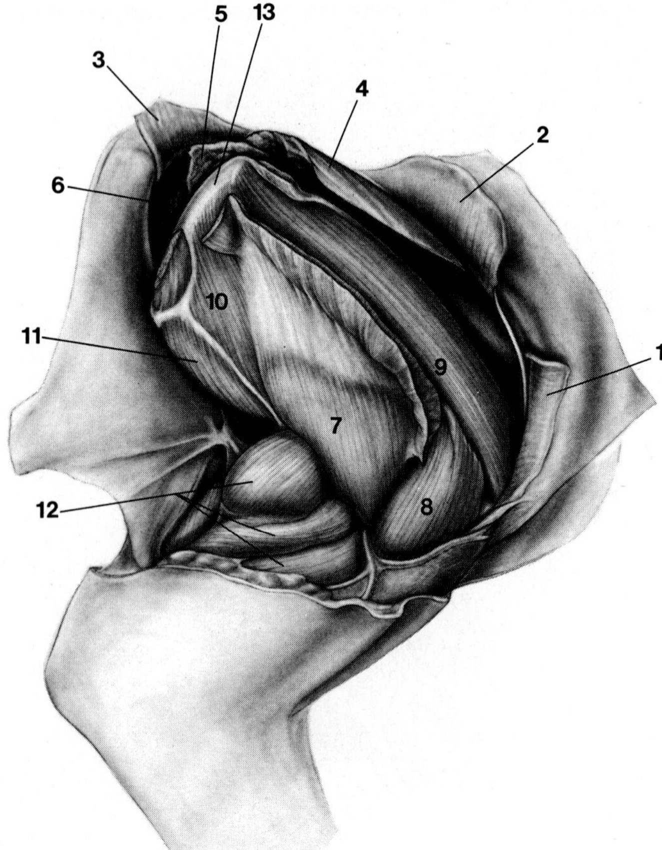

FIGURE 141–4. Lateral dissection of the right thoracic limb. (1. omotransversarius muscle; 2, trapezius muscle [cervical part]; 3, trapezius muscle [thoracic part]; 4, rhomboideus muscle [cervical portion]; 5, rhomboideus muscle [thoracic portion]; 6, latissimus dorsi muscle; 7, deltoid muscle [spinous portion]; 8, deltoid muscle [acromial portion]; 9, supraspinatus muscle; 10, infraspinatus muscle; 11, teres major muscle; 12, triceps muscle; 13, dorsal border of the scapula.)

trapezius muscle. This incision is continued dorsally around the spine of the scapula and far enough distally to sever the thoracic part of the trapezius muscle. The insertion of the rhomboideus muscle can be separated from the dorsomedial border of the scapula (Fig. 141–4). The origin of the ventral serratus muscle (1.5 to 2.0 cm thick) is lifted from the facies serrata of the scapula, allowing the scapula to be partially abducted from the body. In the caudal aspect of the axillary space, the intermuscular fascia is bluntly dissected, exposing the combined insertion of the latissimus dorsi, teres major, and cutaneous trunci muscles on the teres tubercle of the humerus. The insertion of these muscles is severed proximal to the level where the teres major joins the common insertion. The thoracodorsal artery and vein are separately ligated and divided. The thoracodorsal nerve is also cut. The axillary lymph node or nodes are exposed along the dorsal border of the deep pectoral.

With the scapula held in abduction and its cranial border rotated medially, the axillary artery can be isolated, double ligated, and divided between the origin of the external and lateral thoracic arteries. The lateral thoracic artery is ligated and divided from the axillary artery. The brachial and axillary veins are individually ligated and divided. In a caudal-to-cranial direction, the median, ulnar, radial, axillary, subscapular, and suprascapular nerves are transected. The musculocutaneous nerve lies deep to these nerves and is transected before it enters the biceps brachii muscle. Branches of the superficial cervical artery, including the suprascapular artery, can be ligated and divided at this time. With the nerves and vessels divided, the scapula can be further abducted, exposing the ventral musculature (Fig. 141–5). The deep pectoral muscle is separated from its insertion on the major and minor tubercles of the humerus and the medial brachial fascia. The superficial pectorals are separated from the crest of the humerus. When the cleidobrachialis muscle is severed, the amputation is complete (Fig. 141–6).

The fascia of the deep pectoral muscle is sutured to the scalenus muscle and the ventral border of the latissimus dorsi muscle. The fascia of the cleidobrachialis muscle is sutured to the fascia of the superficial pectorals. The fascia of the trapezius and omotransversarius muscles is sutured to the dorsal border of the latissimus dorsi muscle. The skin and subcutaneous tissues are closed.

Foreleg Amputation Through the Humerus[1]

Amputation through the humerus is simple and fast but is restricted to cases in which the abnormality is distal to the elbow. The lateral skin incision is begun on the cranial aspect of the brachium, curved distally to just above the elbow, then directed caudoproximally to the caudal aspect of the brachium. A straight medial

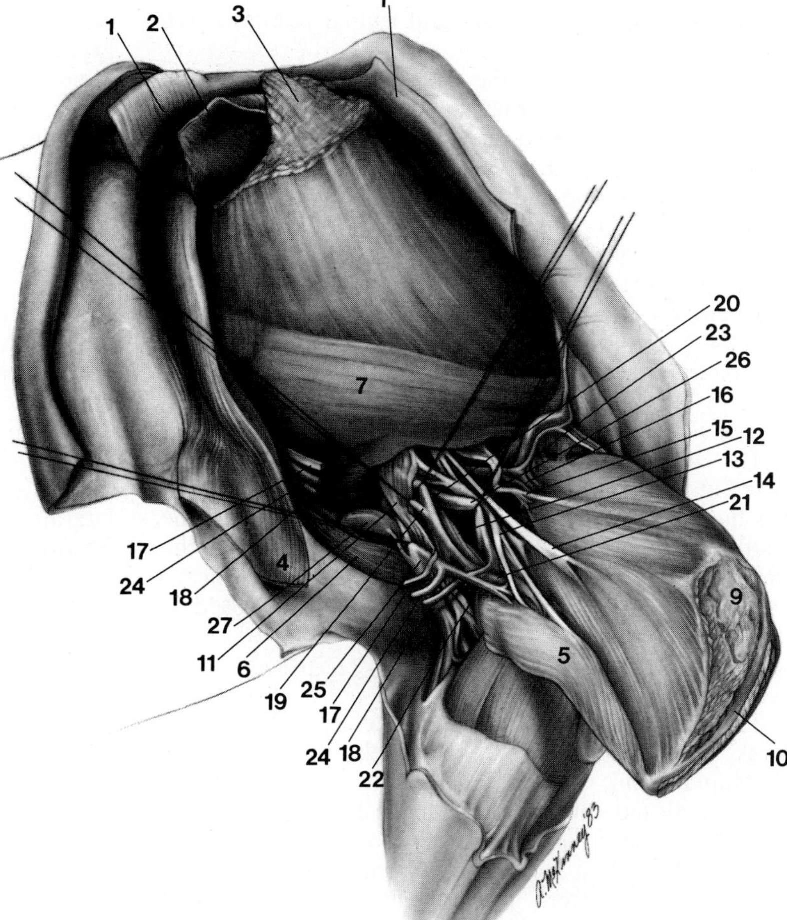

FIGURE 141–5. Dissection of the right thoracic limb with the scapula abducted. (1, trapezius muscle; 2, rhomboideus muscle; 3, ventral serratus muscle; 4, severed insertion of the latissimus dorsi and cutaneous trunci muscle; 5, teres major muscle; 6, deep pectoral muscle; 7, scalenus muscle; 8, rectus thoracis muscle; 9, facies serrata of the scapula; 10, dorsal border of the scapula; 11, ulnar and median nerve trunk; 12, radial nerve; 13, axillary nerve; 14, subscapular nerve; 15, suprascapular nerve; 16, musculocutaneous nerve; 17, thoracodorsal nerve; 18, thoracodorsal artery; 19, lateral thoracic artery; 20, axillary artery; 21, subscapular artery; 22, brachial artery; 23, superficial cervical artery; 24, thoracodorsal vein; 25, brachial vein; 26, axillary vein; 27, axillary lymph node.)

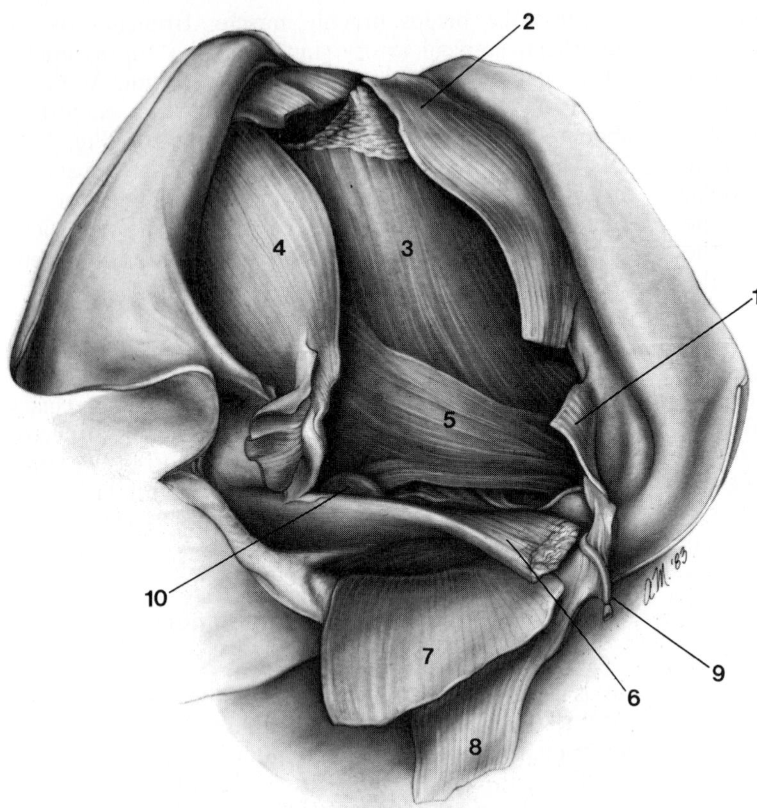

FIGURE 141–6. Final dissection of the right thoracic limb. (1, omotransversarius muscle; 2, trapezius muscle; 3, ventral serratus muscle; 4, latissimus dorsi muscle; 5, scalenus muscle; 6, deep pectoral muscle; 7, transverse superficial pectoral muscle; 8, descending superficial pectoral muscle; 9, cephalic vein; 10, axillary lymph node.)

incision connects the cranial and caudal points of the lateral incision.

On the medial side, the brachial artery, identified caudal to the biceps brachii muscle, is double ligated and divided proximal to the collateral ulnar artery. The brachial vein is separately ligated and divided at the same level. The median, ulnar, and musculocutaneous nerves are sharply divided.

The triceps tendon with the tensor fascia antebrachii muscle is isolated from the brachial fascia on the medial side and from the anconeus muscle on the lateral side and then transected from the olecranon. The brachial and biceps brachii muscles are severed from their insertions just distal to the elbow. The cephalic vein is ligated and divided, and the radial nerve is severed.

The distal and middle third of the humeral shaft is exposed by lifting the brachiocephalicus muscle from the humeral crest. The bone is cut in the middle of the shaft. The humeral stump is covered by suturing the distal end of the triceps to the brachial and biceps brachii muscles. The subcutaneous tissues are closed.

Rear Leg Amputation Through the Femur[5]

The lateral skin incision is semicircular, starting in the flank, extending distally to the patella, and ending at the tuber ischii. The medial skin incision, connecting the cranial and caudal points of the lateral incision, is also semicircular but extends only to midfemur. In the cranial lateral skin incision, a branch of the superficial circumflex iliac artery may be encountered. The skin distal to the incision on both sides of the thigh is reflected down to the stifle joint. The caudal belly of the sartorius muscle is transected midway through the belly. The gracilis muscle is transected at the same level. The femoral artery and vein are dissected free from the fascia. The saphenous nerve, which is closely associated with the femoral artery, is isolated and divided between the proximal caudal femoral artery and the saphenous artery. The femoral vein is ligated at the same level. The vascular stumps are retracted, and the musculotendinous portion of the pectineal muscle is transected down to the bone. Before the quadriceps muscle group is transected, the descending genicular arterty is ligated and separated from the femoral artery. The cranial belly of the sartorius muscle and the quadriceps muscle group are transected just proximal to the patella (Fig. 141–7).

Lateral dissection is started by incising the aponeurosis of the biceps femoris muscle, the fascia lata, and the belly of the biceps femoris muscle parallel to the lateral skin incision. A branch of the distal caudal femoral artery or a muscular branch directly from the femoral artery to the biceps femoris muscle may be encountered. The articularis genus muscle is not included with the quadriceps dissection. The biceps femoris muscle is retracted dorsally, and the ischial nerve is isolated and severed at the major trochanter (Fig. 141–8).

The remaining muscles are transected at midfemur, starting with the abductor cruris caudalis, then the semitendinosus, the two bellies of the semimembranosus, and finally the adductor muscle. After the proximal part of the adductor muscle is partially lifted from the bone, the femur is cut at the junction of its middle and proximal thirds (Fig. 141–9).

The distal end of the quadriceps muscle group is

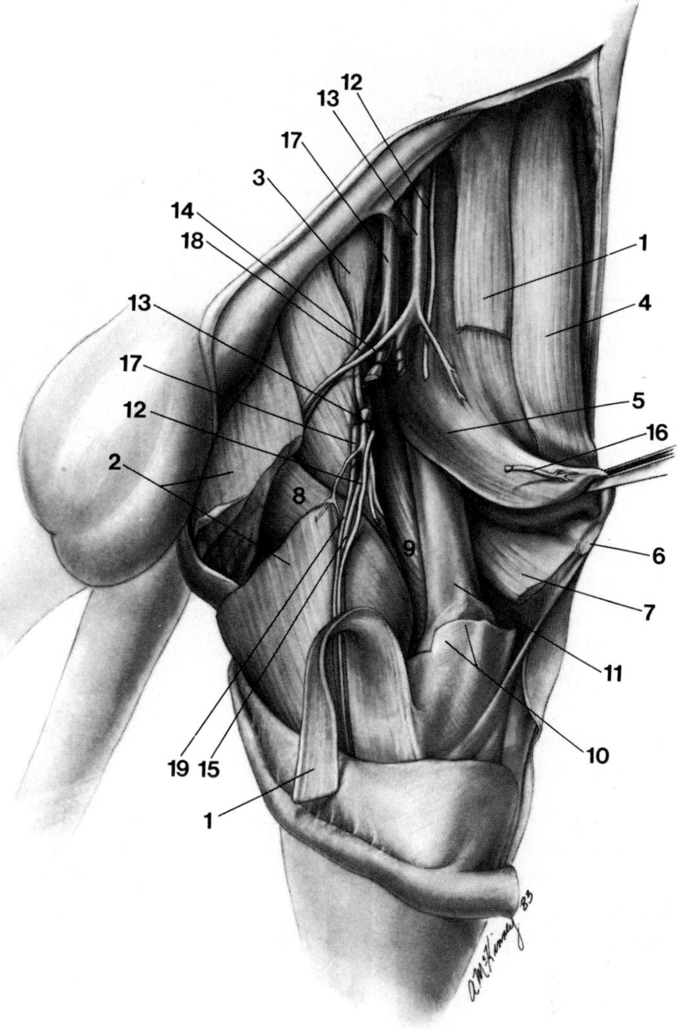

FIGURE 141–7. Medial dissection of the left pelvic limb. (1, sartorius muscle [caudal belly]; 2, gracilis muscle; 3, pectineal muscle; 4, sartorius muscle [cranial belly]; 5, vastus medialis muscle; 6, quadriceps tendon; 7, vastus lateralis muscle; 8, semimembranosus muscle; 9, adductor muscle; 10, joint capsule [stifle]; 11, femur; 12, saphenous nerve; 13, femoral artery; 14, proximal caudal femoral artery; 15, saphenous artery; 16, descending genicular artery; 17, femoral vein; 18, proximal caudal femoral vein; 19, saphenous vein.)

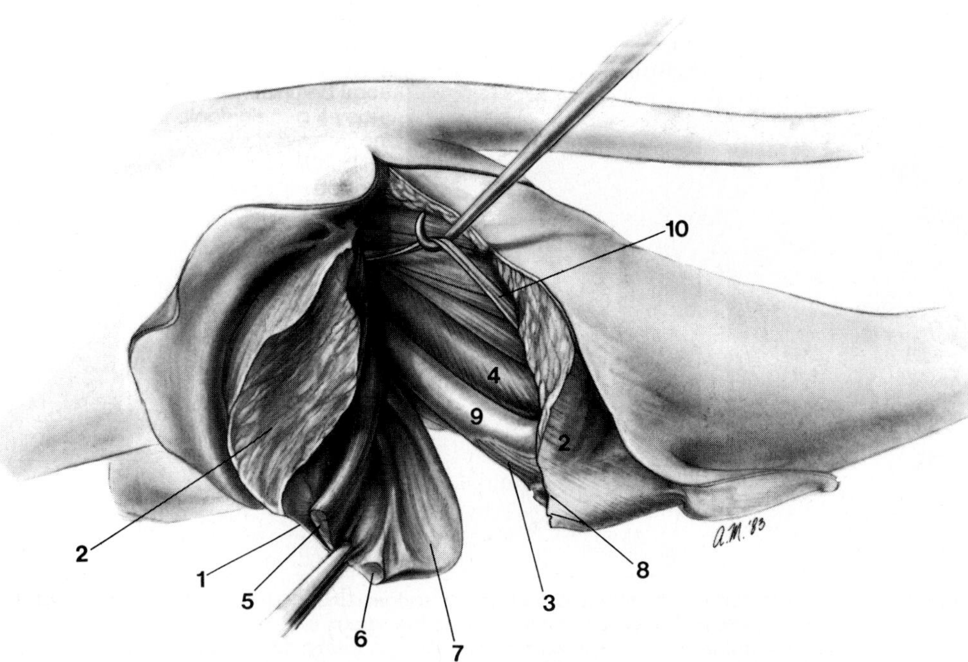

FIGURE 141–8. Lateral dissection of the left pelvic limb. (1, fascia lata and aponeurosis of the biceps femoris muscle; 2, biceps femoris muscle; 3, articularis genus muscle; 4, adductor muscle; 5, vastus lateralis muscle; 6, quadriceps tendon; 7, vastus medialis muscle; 8, joint capsule [stifle]; 9, femur; 10, ischial nerve.)

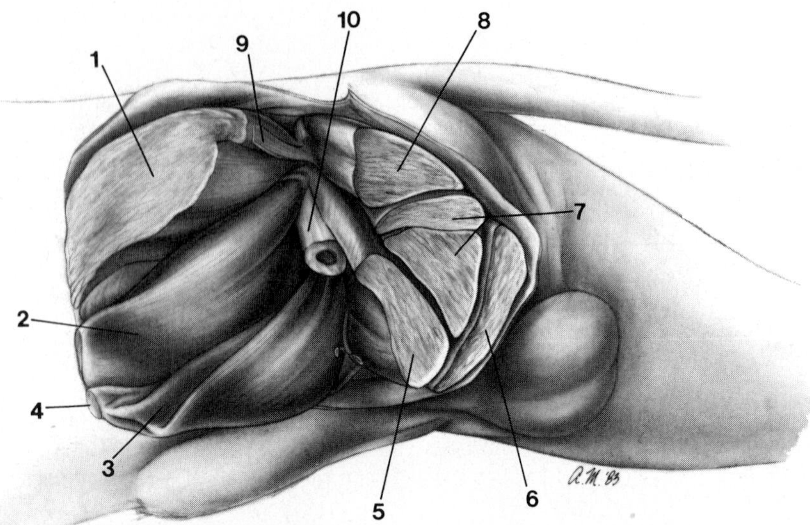

FIGURE 141–9. Final dissection of the rear leg left pelvic limb. (1, biceps femoris muscle; 2, vastus lateralis muscle; 3, vastus medialis muscle; 4, quadriceps tendon; 5, adductor muscle; 6, gracilis muscle; 7, semimembranosus muscle; 8, semitendinosus muscle; 9, abductor cruris caudalis muscle; 10, femur.)

brought caudally and sutured to the adductor muscle. The biceps femoris muscle is sutured to the gracilis muscle medially. The caudal sartorius muscle is sutured to the fascia lata. The skin and subcutaneous tissues are closed.

Amputation of the Pelvic Limb by Disarticulation of the Hip[5]

The lateral skin incision is semicircular, starting in the flank, extending to midfemur, and ending at the tuber ischii. By passing just distal to the inguinal fold, the medial skin incision parallels the fold connecting the cranial and caudal points of the lateral skin incision. The skin distal to the incision is reflected to facilitate anatomical identification. The dissection is begun on the medial side by exposing the femoral artery and vein as they leave the vascular lacunae. The femoral artery is double ligated and divided proximal to the origin of the lateral circumflex femoral artery and vein. The femoral vein is divided and ligated at the same level. The superficial circumflex iliac artery is also ligated. Both the cranial and caudal bellies of the sartorius muscle are transected approximately 2 cm from their origin on the iliac crest and ventral spines of the ilium. The pectineal, gracilis, and adductor muscles are cut at the same level. The medial circumflex femoral artery and vein are ligated and divided as they pass lateral to the pectineal

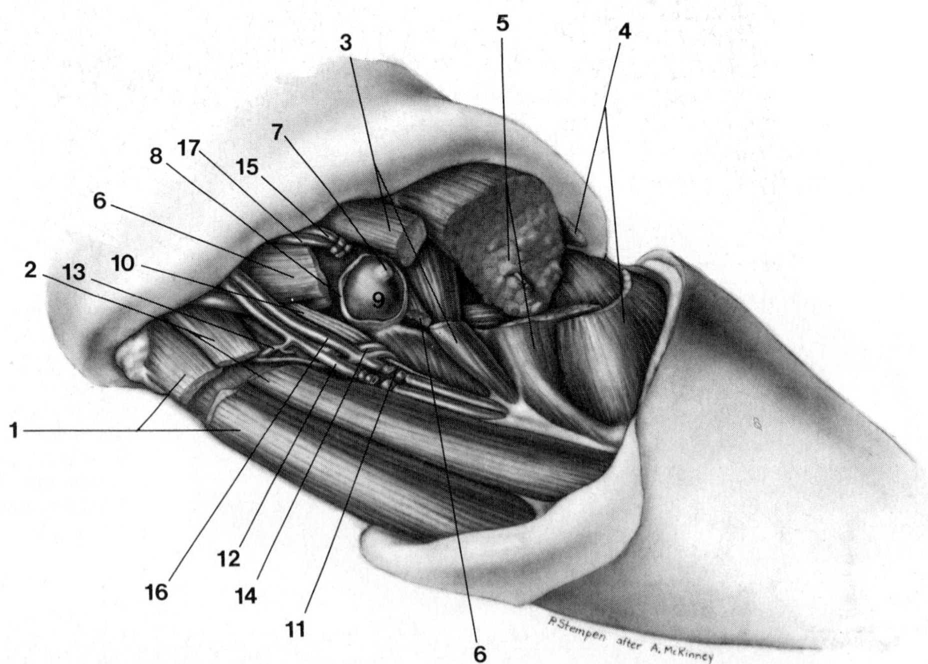

FIGURE 141–10. Medial dissection of the right pelvic limb. (1, sartorius muscle [cranial belly]; 2, sartorius muscle [caudal belly]; 3, pectineal muscle; 4, gracilis muscle; 5, adductor muscle; 6, iliopsoas muscle; 7, ligament of the head of the femur; 8, joint capsule [hip]; 9, head of the femur; 10, femoral nerve; 11, saphenous nerve; 12, femoral artery; 13, superficial circumflex iliac artery; 14, lateral circumflex femoral artery; 15, medial circumflex femoral artery; 16, femoral vein; 17, medial circumflex femoral vein.)

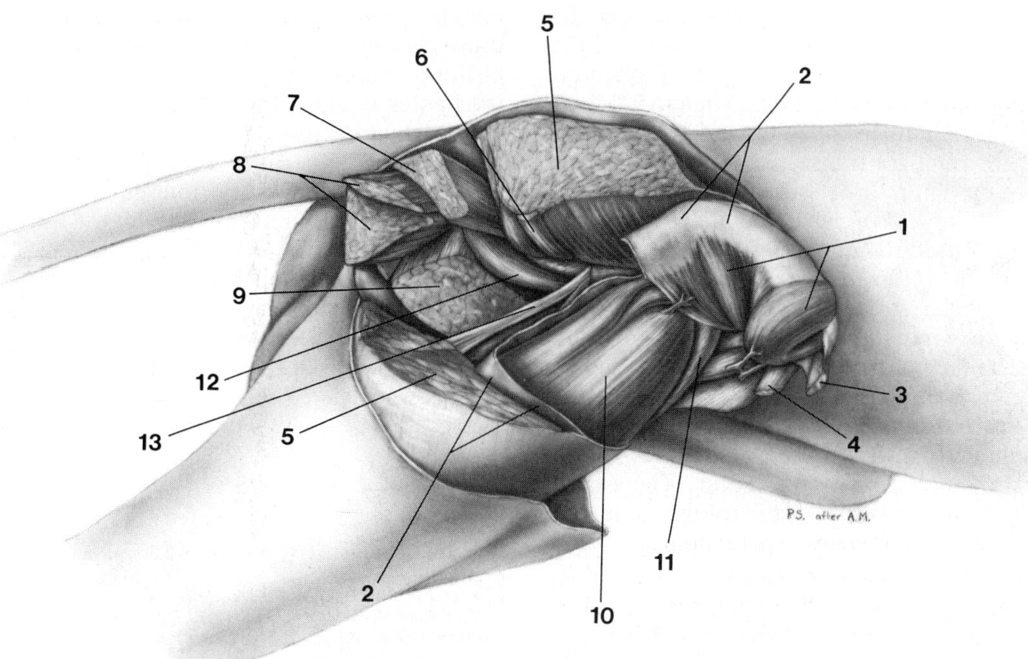

FIGURE 141–11. Lateral dissection of the right pelvic limb. (1, tensor fasciae latae muscle; 2, fascia lata; 3, sartorius muscle [cranial belly]; 4, sartorius muscle [caudal belly]; 5, biceps femoris muscle; 6, abductor cruris caudalis muscle; 7, semitendinosus muscle; 8, semimembranosus muscle; 9, adductor muscle; 10, vastus lateralis muscle; 11, rectus femoris muscle; 12, quadratus femoris muscle; 13, ischial nerve.)

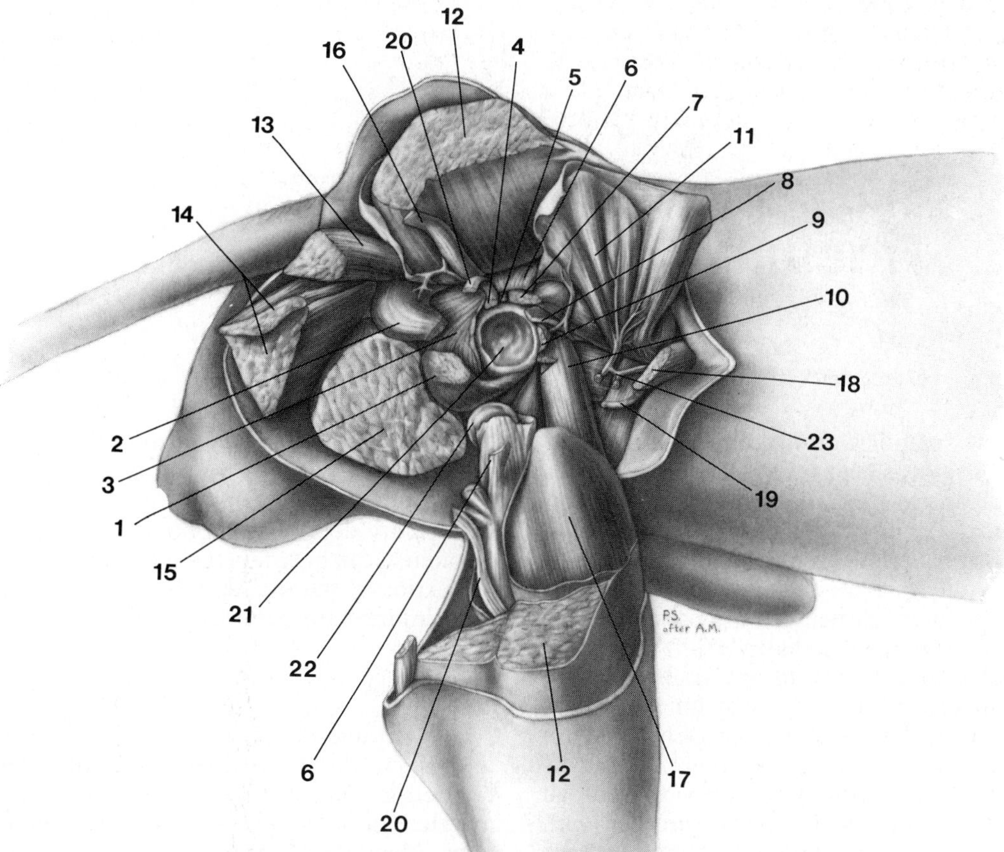

FIGURE 141–12. Final dissection of the right pelvic limb. (1, adductor longus muscle; 2, quadratus femoris muscle; 3, external obturator muscle; 4, internal obturator muscle; 5, gemelli muscle; 6, superficial gluteal muscle; 7, middle gluteal muscle; 8, deep gluteal muscle; 9, articularis coxae muscle; 10, partially severed origin of the rectus femoris muscle; 11, tensor fasciae latae muscle; 12, biceps femoris muscle; 13, semitendinosus muscle; 14, semimembranosus muscle; 15, adductor muscle; 16, abductor cruris caudalis muscle; 17, vastus lateralis muscle; 18, sartorius muscle [cranial belly]; 19, sartorius muscle [caudal belly]; 20, ischial nerve; 21, acetabulum; 22, head of the femur; 23, superficial circumflex iliac artery.)

muscle. The iliopsoas muscle is exposed and can be lifted from its insertion on the trochanter minor of the femur and retracted cranially, exposing the saphenous and femoral nerves, which are severed. The medial joint capsule is incised cranially to caudally, and the ligament of the head of the femur is transected (Fig. 141–10).

Dissection of the lateral side is begun by transecting the tensor fasciae latae muscle at the junction of the proximal and middle thirds of the femur. This incision is carried through the biceps femoris and abductor cruris caudalis muscles. The surgeon returns to the cranial aspect of the leg to incise the fascia lata and lift it from the shaft of the femur to expose the greater trochanter. The biceps femoris muscle and tensor fasciae latae muscles are retracted dorsally, exposing the semitendinosus and semimembranosus muscles, which are transected in the proximal third of the femur. The ischial nerve is exposed and severed distal to the branches supplying the semimembranosus, semitendinosus, and biceps femoris muscles (Fig. 141–11).

The hip is placed in flexion and abduction, exposing the quadratus femoris muscle, which is lifted from its insertion just proximal to the trochanter tertius of the femur. With the leg in the same position, the external rotators are severed as they enter the trochanteric fossa. The rotators include the internal obturator, external obturator, and gemelli muscles. The hip is abducted and flexed with some internal rotation, and the gluteal muscles transected. The superficial gluteal muscle is transected first, followed by the middle gluteal and piriform muscles. The last muscle to be cut from the trochanter is the deep gluteal. The dorsal joint capsule and articularis coxae muscle are transected, completely freeing the femur from the joint cavity of the acetabulum. The rectus femoris muscle is removed from its origin on the iliopubic eminence of the ilium, completing the amputation (Fig. 141–12).

Closure is accomplished by suturing the fascia of the biceps femoris muscle to the gracilis muscle and, if necessary, to the semimembranosus or semitendinosus muscles. The tensor fasciae latae can be sutured to the iliopsoas muscle. The subcutaneous tissue and skin are closed.

References

1. Bone DL, Aberman HM: Forelimb amputation in the dog. *J Am Anim Hosp Assoc 24*:525, 1988.
2. Borzio F: Amputation of the foreleg of the dog. *In* Bojrab MJ (ed): *Current Techniques in Small Animal Surgery*. Lea & Febiger, Philadelphia, 1975.
3. Carberry CA, Harvey HJ: Owner satisfaction with limb amputation in dogs and cats. *J Am Anim Hosp Assoc 23*:227, 1987.
4. Leighton RL: Amputation of the foreleg of the dog. *In* Bojrab MJ (ed): *Current Techniques in Small Animal Surgery*. Lea & Febiger, Philadelphia, 1975.
5. Slocum B: Amputation of the canine pelvic limb. *In* Bojrab MJ (ed): *Current Techniques in Small Animal Surgery*. Lea & Febiger, Philadelphia, 1975.
6. Withrow SJ, Hirsch VM: Owner response to amputation of a pet's leg. *Vet Med Small Anim Clin 74*:332, 1979.

CHAPTER 142 Skull and Mandibular Fractures

Erick L. Egger

An animal with a mandibular or skull fracture usually has been subjected to significant trauma. Although a client may express great concern over a bloody mouth, a dropped jaw, or facial swelling, the clinician must perform a thorough physical examination of other systems to evaluate life-threatening injuries. Particularly with maxillary fractures, partial airway obstruction can occur and may necessitate immediate oxygen therapy or emergency tracheostomy. As with any traumatic incident, the patient is carefully evaluated for shock and pulmonary injuries and treated appropriately.[5] Also, a significant but cryptic injury such as spinal column or acetabular fracture may significantly alter the overall prognosis and an owner's willingness to proceed with therapy. A gauze or leather muzzle may temporarily be used to reduce open bilateral mandibular or maxillary fractures and minimize exposure of bone. Many dogs with such injuries must breathe through their mouth because of nasal hematoma and swelling. Muzzling may produce excitement and hyperthermia and exacerbate airway obstruction—such devices must be used with care. Because the majority of mandibular and many skull fractures are open, these animals are routinely placed on systemic broad-spectrum antibiotics, and wounds are débrided and fractures stabilized as soon as the animal can be safely anesthetized. Thorough physical evaluation of the mouth and radiographic evaluation of bony injuries are better performed at that time.

ANESTHESIA

General anesthesia is required in nearly all patients to evaluate the injury adequately. Injectable drugs can be used for induction, oral evaluation, application of a muzzle, and even wiring of simple symphyseal separations. Maintenance of anesthesia with inhalant agents is preferable in most animals requiring significant surgery. This allows adequate evaluation and treatment. More importantly, by using an inflatable cuffed endotracheal tube, aspiration of blood or lavage fluid is avoided. The endotracheal tube can hinder manipulation in the oral cavity and prevents closing the mouth to check reduction by alignment of the canine teeth. Consequently, the tube is commonly rerouted to exit through a pharyngostomy.

Pharyngostomy Intubation (Fig. 142–1)

Anesthesia is induced, and oral intubation is performed as usual. The hair is clipped, and the skin caudolateral to the angle of either mandible is aseptically prepared. By oral palpation, the piriform fossa of the lateral pharynx caudal to the mandible is tented up. An incision approximately one and one-half times the diameter of the tube is made through the skin into the pharynx either just cranial or just caudal to the hyoid bone. Forceps are passed through the incision from the outside to grasp the cuff inflation tube and pull it to the outside. The endotracheal tube adapter is detached from the tube, and the cranial end of the tube is pulled through the incision using forceps passed from the exterior. The tube is reattached to the adapter and the anesthetic circuit. After surgery and recovery from anesthesia, the cuff is deflated and the tube is pulled out through the pharyngostomy incision. The skin incision is usually left unsutured to heal by second intention.

GENERAL SURGICAL CONSIDERATIONS

Intraoral approaches have the fewest complications,[15] probably because of the great vascularity and healing potential of the mucous membrane compared with skin. The oral cavity is prepared as aseptically as possible using a nonirritating dilute antiseptic solution. A detergent-based scrub should not be used. Fracture reduction and fixation can often be accomplished through the oral wound. Extension of the wound by incising and elevating the mucosa to expedite exposure is a compromise, with damage to the healing potential, and is limited as much as possible.

Any foreign material is removed, and nonviable tissues débrided. Bone with significant soft-tissue attachment may contribute to callus formation and is retained even if it cannot be rigidly fixed. Likewise, teeth, even if partially involved in the fracture, are left in place because they provide stability and aid alignment.[21]

Although mandibular fractures heal well,[21] if significant bone loss has occurred or defects remain after fracture reduction, autogenous cancellous bone grafts are used to fill the gaps and induce bone formation. Cancellous autograft tissue is easily collected from the greater tubercle of the humerus. For difficult fractures, the graft is collected as the first stage of surgery, before contamination of instruments and the surgical field. Once fixation is complete, the fracture site is copiously lavaged with an isotonic solution and the bone graft gently packed into the defect. If the fracture is grossly infected or avascular, the grafting procedure may be delayed for 10 to 14 days to allow granulation tissue to

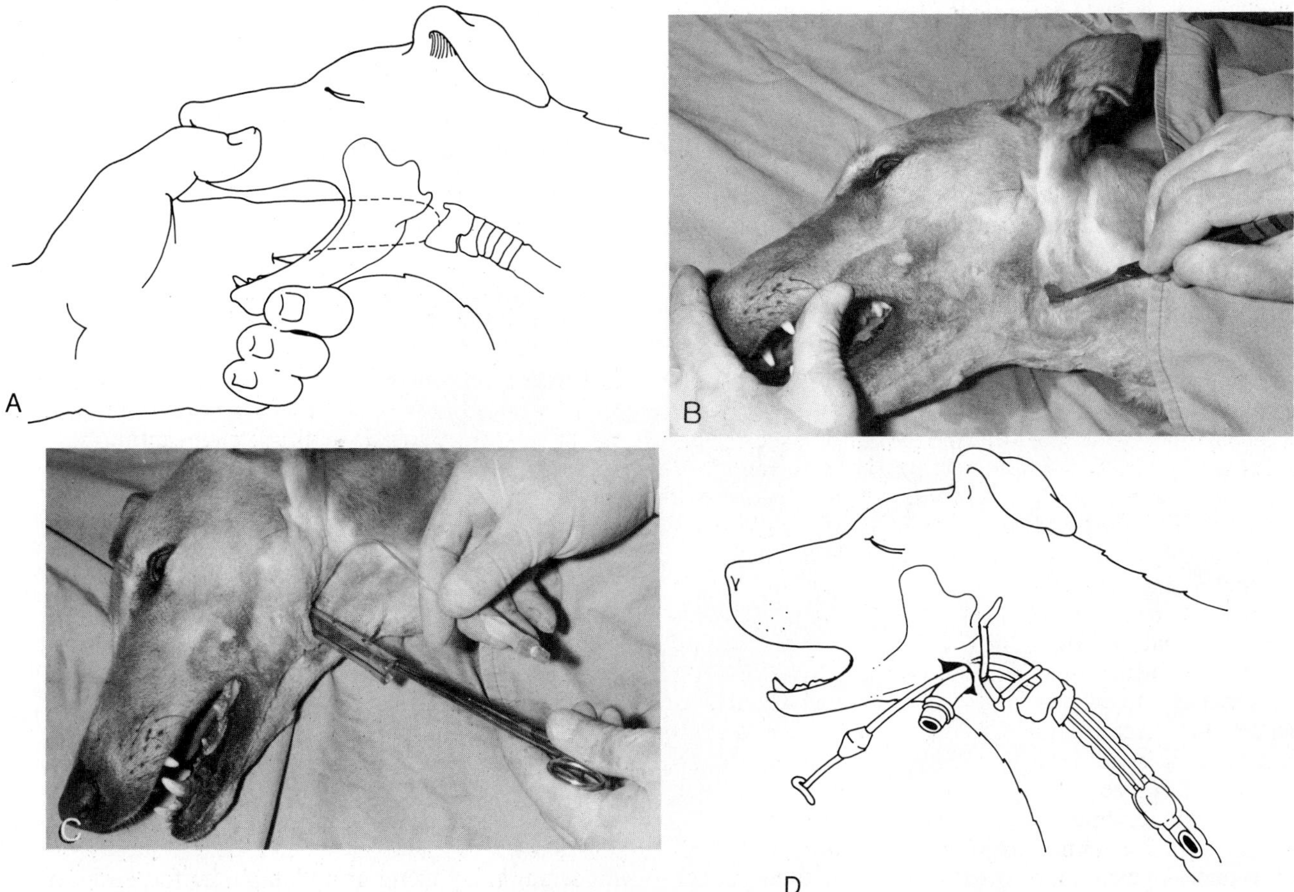

FIGURE 142–1. Technique for pharyngostomy intubation. *A*, A finger is used to identify and elevate the piriform fossa of the pharynx. *B*, An incision is made through the skin into the pharynx. *C*, Forceps are used to pull first the cuff inflation tube, then the adapter end of the tube itself, through the incision. *D*, Final location of the tube.

biologically débride and revascularize the region. Granulation tissue provides a better recipient bed and increases the graft's osteogenic effectiveness. Wounds and incisions are sutured only if thoroughly débrided and if closure can be accomplished without tension. A monofilament nonabsorbable or slowly absorbable synthetic suture material is recommended. A ventral or lateral skin incision may be necessary to expose the fracture adequately. If the approach communicates with an open oral lesion, delayed skin closure or closure over a drain is considered to decrease infection.

POSTOPERATIVE TREATMENT

The care necessary after mandibular and oral cavity skull fractures depends on the type of fixation applied. If rigid stabilization is achieved, relatively few restrictions are made other than feeding soft foods until the fractures heal. If less than optimal fixation is obtained, the repair may be supplemented with a muzzle and pharyngostomy tube used to supply nutrition for 3 to 4 weeks while early fracture healing occurs. This approach is useful if large defects in soft-tissue coverage of bone remain after surgery and may be combined with daily lavage of the oral cavity with saline. An Elizabethan collar may be necessary to prevent the patient from disturbing the fixation (particularly a muzzle or external fixator) but can usually be removed after inflammation subsides. Because the majority of these fractures are open, antibiotic therapy is appropriate and reduces the incidence of infection.[21] Initial broad-spectrum coverage followed by specific drug selection based on culture and sensitivity testing obtained at surgery is ideal.

MANDIBULAR FRACTURES

Two related reports[21, 22] found that canine mandibular fractures were relatively uncommon, accounting for about 3 per cent of the total number of canine fractures. Although approximately 15 per cent of fractures in cats involve the mandible, the majority were symphyseal separations. Most mandibular fractures were traumatically induced (89 to 100 per cent) and open (65 to 70 per cent). However, a significant number of mandibular fractures in dogs (11 per cent) occurred during dental extractions. Malocclusion was the most common significant complication of mandibular fractures in dogs (35 per cent), followed by infection (27 per cent) and delayed union (7 per cent). The need for attention to reduction and proper wound treatment to obtain optimal results is thus emphasized.

Mandibular Symphyseal Fracture/Separation

The majority of these injuries are actually separations of the mandibular syndesmosis and heal by fibrous rather than bony callus.[21, 22] Fixation does not need to be extremely rigid or prolonged; 3 to 4 weeks is usually sufficient. A single stainless steel wire (18 to 22 gauge) encircling the rostral mandibular rami just behind the canine teeth works well. Each end of the wire can be passed under the gingiva with a hypodermic needle to exit the skin on the ventral midline (Fig. 142–2*A*). The ends are twisted together as the fracture is manipulated and held in reduction (Fig. 142–2*B*). The excess wire is cut off, leaving two to three twists. The wire can be removed by cutting the intraoral segment between the canine teeth and pulling the twists ventrally. This wire fixation can be augmented with interfragmentary cross pins or a screw in large dogs or if the injury involves fracture of the incisor area.[6]

Mandibular Body Fractures

The body of the mandible extends from the symphysis caudally to the vertical ramus and includes the alveoli

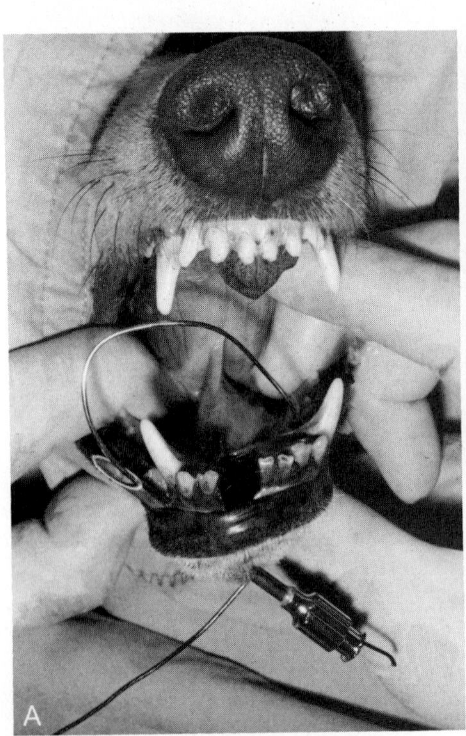

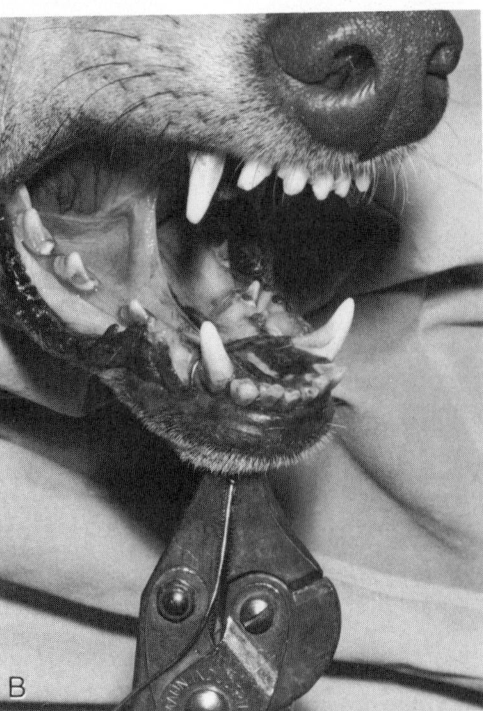

FIGURE 142–2. Placement of an encircling wire for treatment of symphyseal separation. *A*, Hypodermic needle is used to pass the stainless steel wire under the gingiva just behind the canine teeth to exit the skin on the ventral midline. *B*, The wire ends are twisted together as the separation is held in reduction.

for all teeth. Consequently, mandibular body fractures often involve alveoli, exposing tooth roots.[21,22] Although bone cannot heal directly to tooth roots,[12] leaving teeth in place assists reduction and fixation of the fracture. If a tooth becomes nonviable, it can easily be removed later.

Treatment

Selection of treatment for mandibular fractures depends on many factors, including soft-tissue injuries, fracture configuration, economics, and clinician preference. The relationship of these fractures to the choice of treatment is depicted (Fig. 142–3).

External Coaptation (Muzzles)

A tape muzzle can be used to treat relatively stable midbody unilateral fractures. A muzzle maintains fracture reduction by holding the upper and lower canine teeth interlocked.[6] It provides limited mechanical support but relies on the opposite intact mandibular ramus and maxilla to act as splints. A muzzle works well if the soft tissues are relatively healthy and fracture healing potential is good, as in young animals. It can also be used as ancillary support to limit excessive loading if surgical fixation is marginal. A muzzle does not work well on rostral fractures, in cats, or in brachycephalic dogs. Muzzles are usually applied under general anesthesia without oral intubation so that dental alignment can be used for fracture reduction. If nutrition is maintained orally, a gap large enough for the tongue to be extended (0.5 to 1.5 cm) is left between upper and lower incisors to allow the patient to lap liquefied gruels and water. The mouth can be held entirely shut if a pharyngostomy tube is used. Nonelastic tape ½ to 2 inches wide is used. Details of application are illustrated (Fig. 142–4). The muzzle can be maintained for several months if needed but requires conscientious skin cleaning to avoid contact dermatitis.

Interarcade Wiring

Interarcade wiring consists of bilateral loops of wire passed between the mandible and maxilla.[8] It can maintain dental occlusion for many patients such as cats and brachycephalic dogs when muzzles cannot. Depending on the location of the injury, the wires are passed through transverse holes in the alveolar ridge just caudal to the canine teeth or between the roots of the last

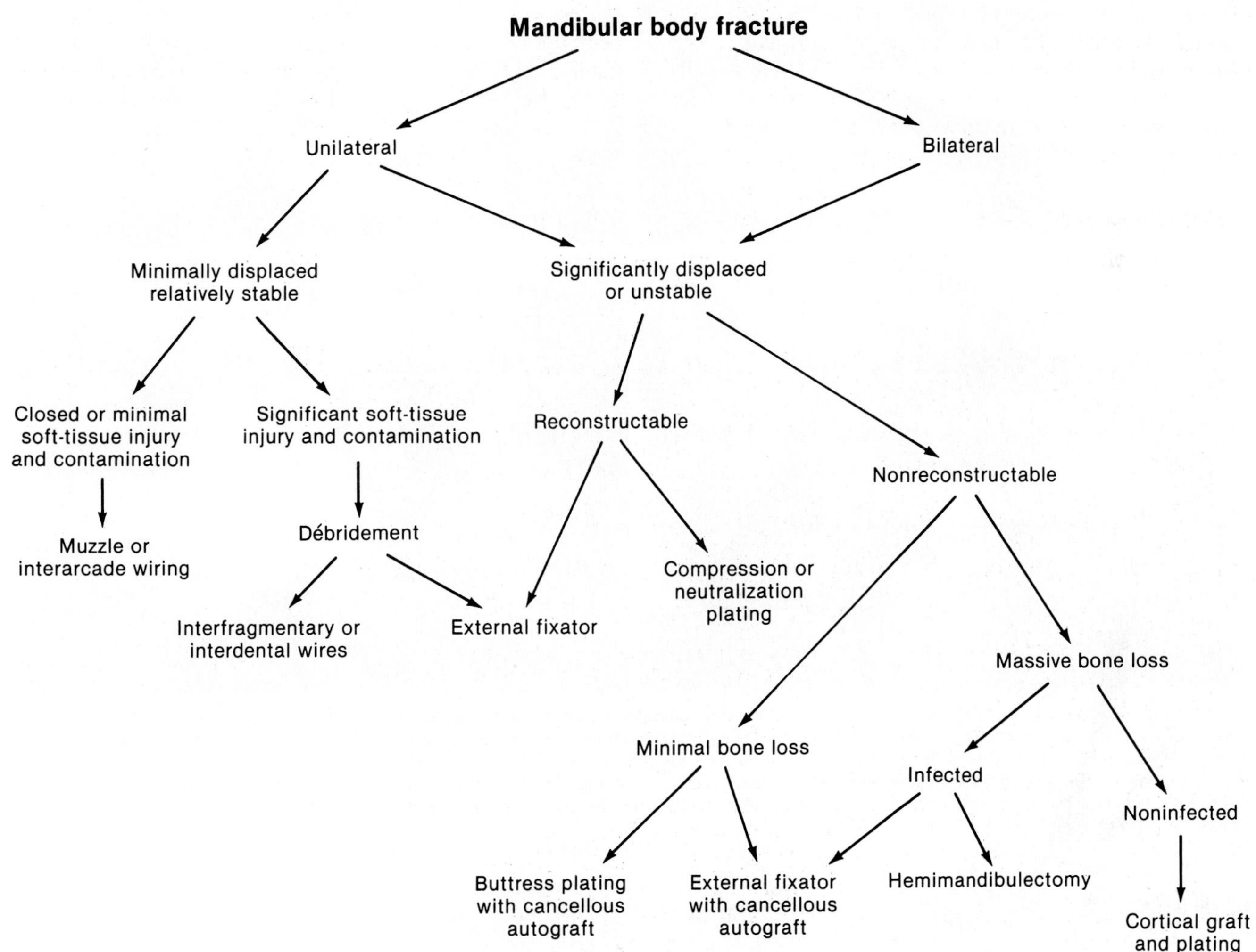

FIGURE 142–3. Mandibular body fracture treatment.

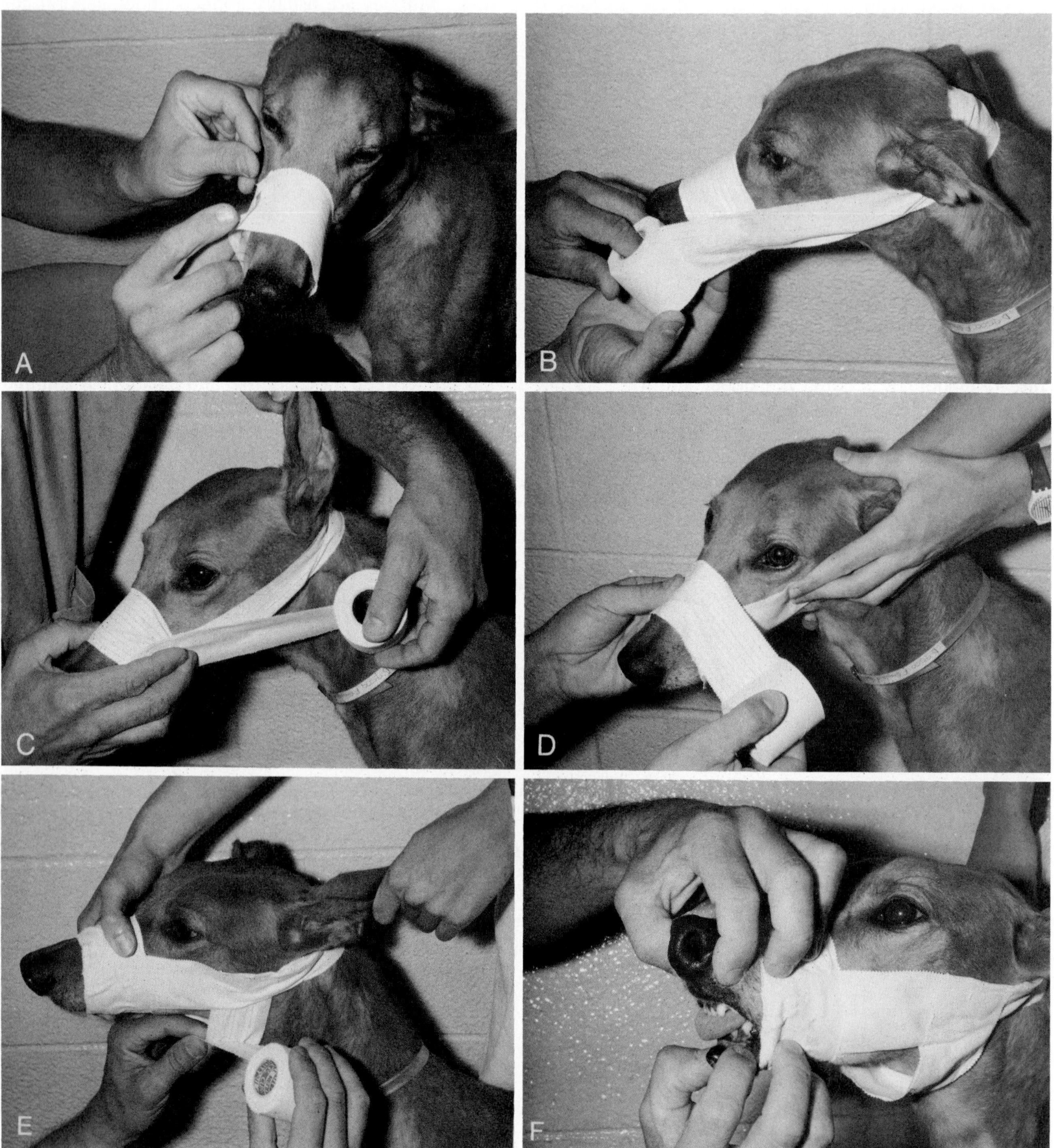

FIGURE 142–4. Application of a tape muzzle. *A*, First a loop of tape, adhesive surface out, is applied around the muzzle. *B*, A second piece of tape is then attached, adhesive side out, to the first loop starting on one side, passing caudal to the ears, and back to the other side of the loop. *C*, A third piece of tape is applied directly over the second with the adhesive side in. *D*, The fourth tape is then placed directly over the first, around the muzzle with the adhesive side in. *E*, Finally, a chin strap is applied as before to prevent the muzzle from being pulled over the ears. *F*, The canine teeth must interdigitate for stabilization, but a space can be left between the incisor teeth to allow lapping of liquids.

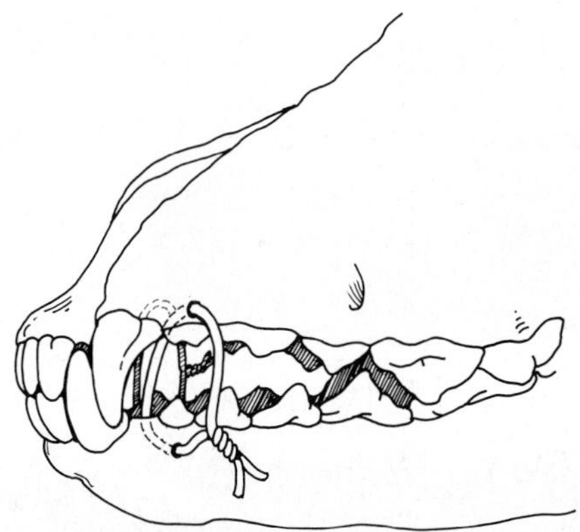

FIGURE 142–5. Intra-arcade wiring can be used when muzzles cannot be applied. Bilateral wire loops are passed through holes in the mandible and maxilla and tightened enough to maintain occlusion yet allow prehension of liquids and soft foods.

maxillary premolar and first mandibular molar teeth (Fig. 142–5). A 0.045- to 0.062-inch Kirschner wire and hand chuck are used to create the holes, and 22- to 18-gauge monofilament stainless steel wire used for the loops. The wires are twisted, tightening the loops to provide stable occlusal alignment. As with muzzles, if enough space is left between the incisor teeth, nutrition may be maintained by allowing the patient to lap a liquid gruel. Alternatively, a pharyngostomy tube may be used.

Intraoral Splints

Intraoral splints for treatment of mandibular fractures have been reported.[10] The splint is generally constructed of partially cured dental acrylic, which is molded to the shape of the sublingual space once the fracture has been reduced. When completely cured, the acrylic is attached with multiple wire loops that encircle the mandible or adjacent teeth. My experience with this technique has been disappointing because the splint tends to accumulate food and exudation in open fracture sites,[15] complicating postoperative care and contributing to poor healing.

Interdental Wiring

Selected simple transverse mandibular body fractures can be managed with simple interdental wiring techniques.[6] Teeth must be intact and solid. Two teeth rostral and two caudal to the fracture are encircled to provide firm anchorage. Eighteen- to 22-gauge monofilament stainless steel wire is passed through holes in the gingiva at the neck of the tooth. The holes can be created using a hypodermic needle or small Kirschner wire. The wire is applied in a simple loop or a figure-eight pattern. The wire is tightened by twisting just enough to keep the alveolar border of the fracture closed when a ventrally directed force is applied to the incisor region (Fig. 142–6*A*), resulting in *dynamic* compression and increased stability of the fracture with loading. The temptation to overtighten the wire must be avoided because this causes opening of the ventral mandibular border (Fig. 142–6*B*).

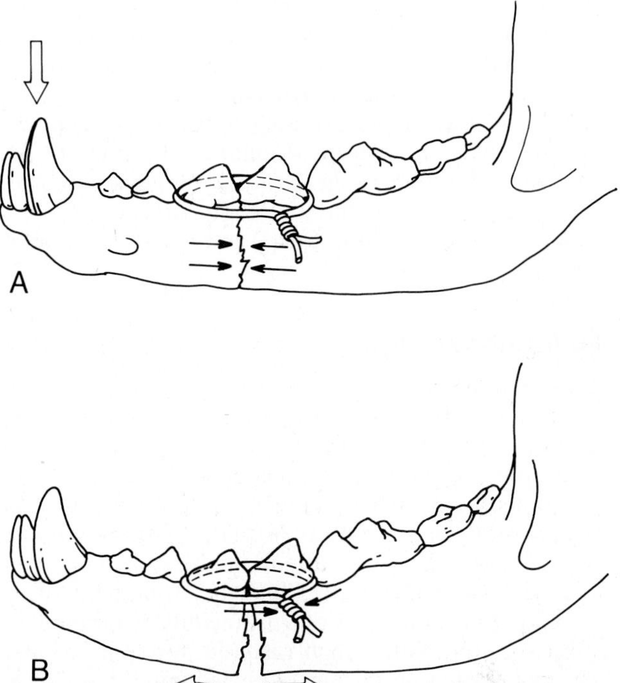

FIGURE 142–6. Fixation of a simple transverse mandibular body fracture with interdental wiring. *A*, The wire loop is passed around two teeth cranial and two teeth caudal to the fracture. The wire is tightened just enough to maintain reduction with ventrally directed load applied to the incisor region. *B*, Overtightening the wire causes distraction of the ventral mandibular border.

Interfragmentary Wire

Interfragmentary wire can be used to stabilize simple transverse or short oblique mandibular fractures, particularly if the opposite mandible is intact to act as a splint.[6, 15] If significant comminution exists or bone loss has occurred, adequate reduction is difficult and malocclusion commonly results.[21] There is also danger of damaging osseous vascularity from direct manipulation without gaining adequate stability, leading to delayed union or nonunion. Monofilament stainless steel wire of adequate strength (18 or 20 gauge) should be used. A simple interrupted loop results in the most effective tightening and fracture fixation (Fig. 142–7). Placing at least two wires across each fracture line greatly increases

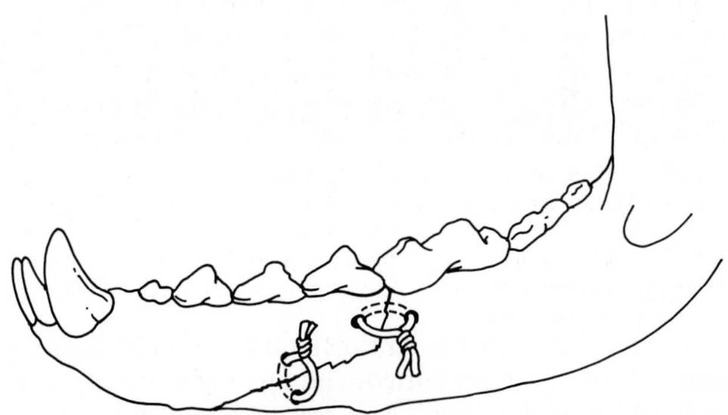

FIGURE 142–7. Use of two interfragmentary wire loops to stabilize a simple midmandibular body fracture. Note both wires are oriented perpendicular to the fracture line, and one is placed as close to the alveolar border as possible.

stability. One of the wires is placed as close as possible to the alveolar border, which is the tension band side of the mandible.[3] Wire is passed through holes created with 0.045- to 0.062-inch Kirschner wires in a hand chuck or a power drill, avoiding tooth roots. The wire loops are oriented as perpendicular to the fracture line as possible to minimize shear forces. Gingiva may need to be elevated to allow the wire to lie adjacent to bone. The wire is twisted, bent down, and cut short to minimize mucosal irritation.

Intramedullary Pins

Intramedullary pins have commonly been used to stabilize mandibular fractures.[3] The technique is difficult, and the results are often disappointing.[4] The curved, narrow shape of the medullary canal and tooth roots limits the diameter of pin that can be inserted and consequently the stability of fixation. Experimentally, intramedullary pinning resulted in delayed healing compared with plate fixation.[18] Clinically, treatment of canine mandibular fractures by intramedullary pinning has been associated with a high rate (58 per cent) of malocclusion or nonunion due to malalignment.[21] Consequently, *intramedullary pinning as the primary fixation of mandibular fractures is not recommended.*

Screw and Plate Fixation

Properly applied plate fixation provides excellent stabilization of complex and even bilateral mandibular body fractures.[15] Plates function differently depending on the biomechanics of the fracture and the technique of application. With simple fractures, tension can be applied to the plate, compressing the fracture and increasing stability. More communited fractures may first be reconstructed with interfragmentary fixation such as lag screws and wires. The reconstruction is then protected from disruptive forces with a plate applied in the neutral mode. Finally, a plate may function as a buttress device to keep a nonreconstructable fracture or one with significant bone loss from collapsing. Adhering to the principles of plating can be difficult owing to the complex shape of the bone and the presence of tooth roots, which limit screw placement. The use of human reconstruction plates* allows three-dimensional contouring and better fitting of the plate to the bone with improved fracture reduction (Fig. 142–8). This plate design also has more holes per unit length and can be cut to the desired length to obtain the minimum four cortices per fracture fragment. Although the tension side of the mandible is along the alveolar border, plates are often applied through lateral or ventral approaches to avoid tooth roots and the mandibular nerve.[17]

External Fixators

An external fixator is an excellent method of treating complex, highly comminuted, and open mandibular fractures with bone loss because it can provide rigid stability

*Synthes, Monument, CO.

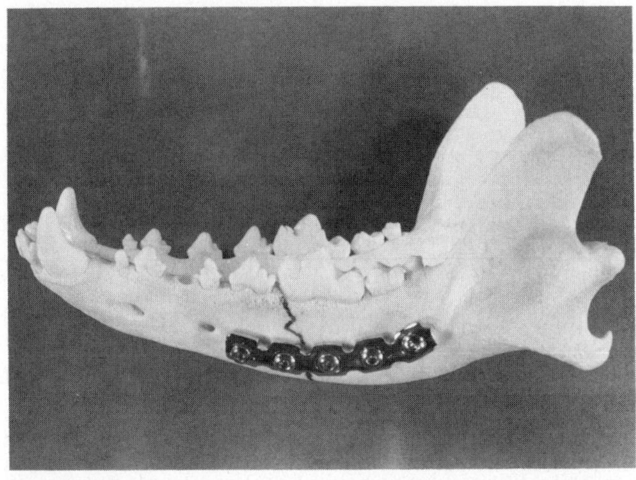

FIGURE 142–8. Use of a mandibular reconstruction plate for fracture fixation allows contouring in all planes. The result is optimal fit of the plate to the complex shape of the mandible and reduction of the fracture.

without requiring implants in open fracture wounds. The Kirschner* apparatus works well in many situations.[2] I use more acrylic pin splints in which an acrylic column replaces the connecting bar and clamps, because they are easily contoured to treat bilateral and multiple fractures. Their fixation pins can be moved and angled in any direction to avoid tooth roots and foramina. A commercial device designed for human application† can be used for some canine patients.[7] It is expensive and limited to use on larger dogs. Similar inexpensive splints can be made by hand molding dental (Orthodontic Resin‡) or hoof repair (Technovit§) acrylic to form the connecting column. Bench testing has shown that such splints can be constructed to obtain the stability desired.[23] As a guideline, an acrylic column 1.5 to 2.5 cm in diameter is adequate for medium to large dogs. Principles of application follow those for any external fixator (Fig. 142–9). A minimum of two and preferably three pins should be used per fracture fragment. Threaded pins prolong pin–bone interface integrity. The pins can be wedged between tooth roots but are not driven through them. The free ends of the pins are generally bent or notched to improve acrylic purchase. Although ancillary interfragmentary fixation can be used, rapid fracture healing by limiting fragment exposure and maintaining osseous soft-tissue attachments is important. A cancellous autograft is applied if osseous defects persist. Postoperatively, patients can be fed a normal soft diet (canned or moistened dry food). The skin and apparatus are cleaned to prevent food accumulation and skin excoriation. Once the fracture has healed, the apparatus is removed by cutting each pin between the acrylic and skin to remove the bar and withdrawing the pins individually. Alternatively, the bar can be cut between pins with an oscillating cast cutter

*Kirschner Medical Co., Tinmonium, MD.
†Walter Lorenz Surgical Instruments, Inc., Jacksonville, FL.
‡L. D. Caulk Co., Milford, DE.
§Dr. Jorgensen Laboratories, Loveland, CO.

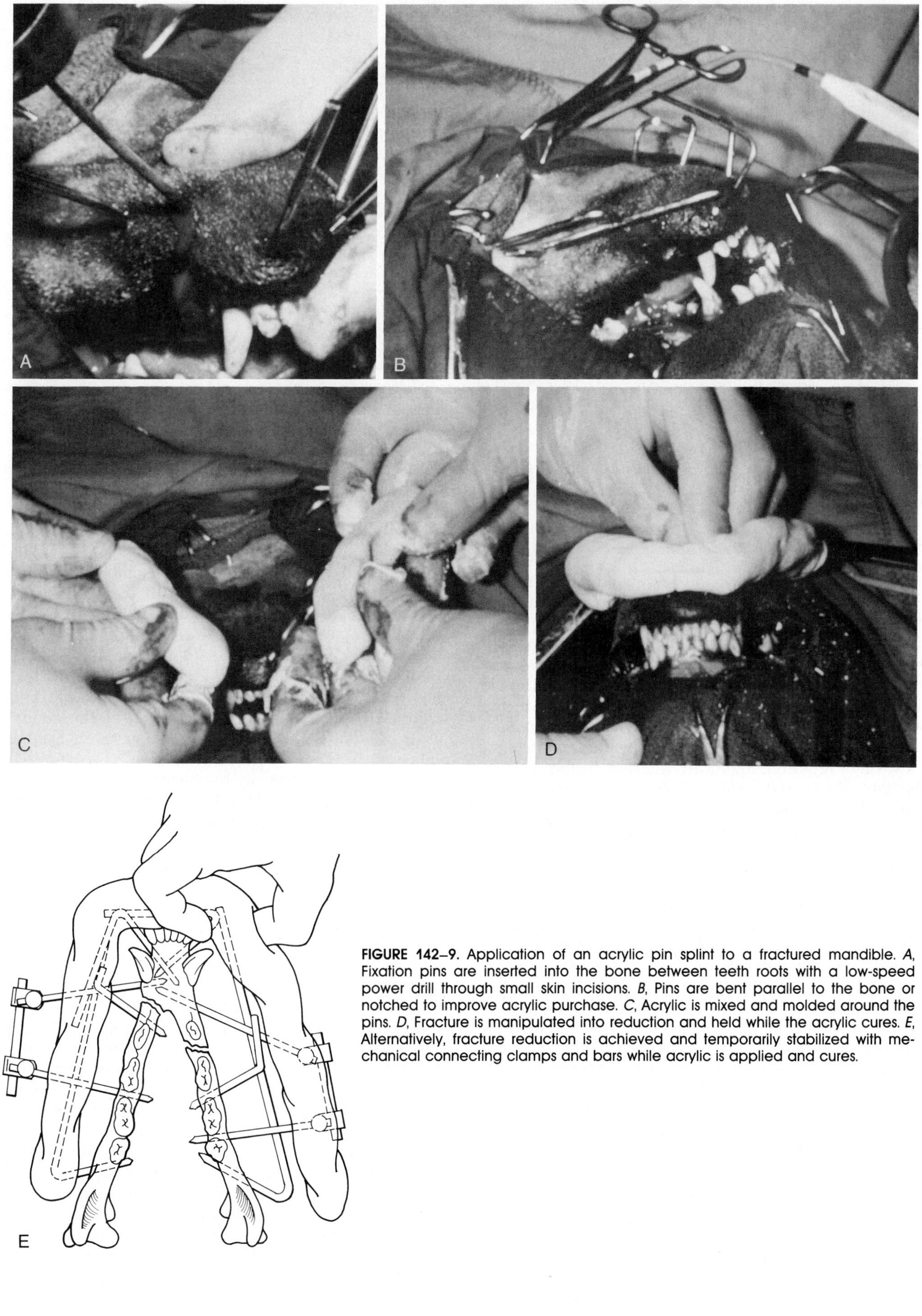

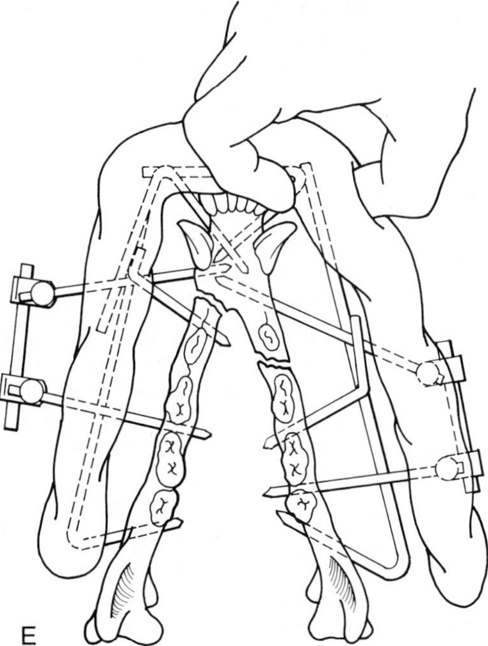

FIGURE 142–9. Application of an acrylic pin splint to a fractured mandible. *A*, Fixation pins are inserted into the bone between teeth roots with a low-speed power drill through small skin incisions. *B*, Pins are bent parallel to the bone or notched to improve acrylic purchase. *C*, Acrylic is mixed and molded around the pins. *D*, Fracture is manipulated into reduction and held while the acrylic cures. *E*, Alternatively, fracture reduction is achieved and temporarily stabilized with mechanical connecting clamps and bars while acrylic is applied and cures.

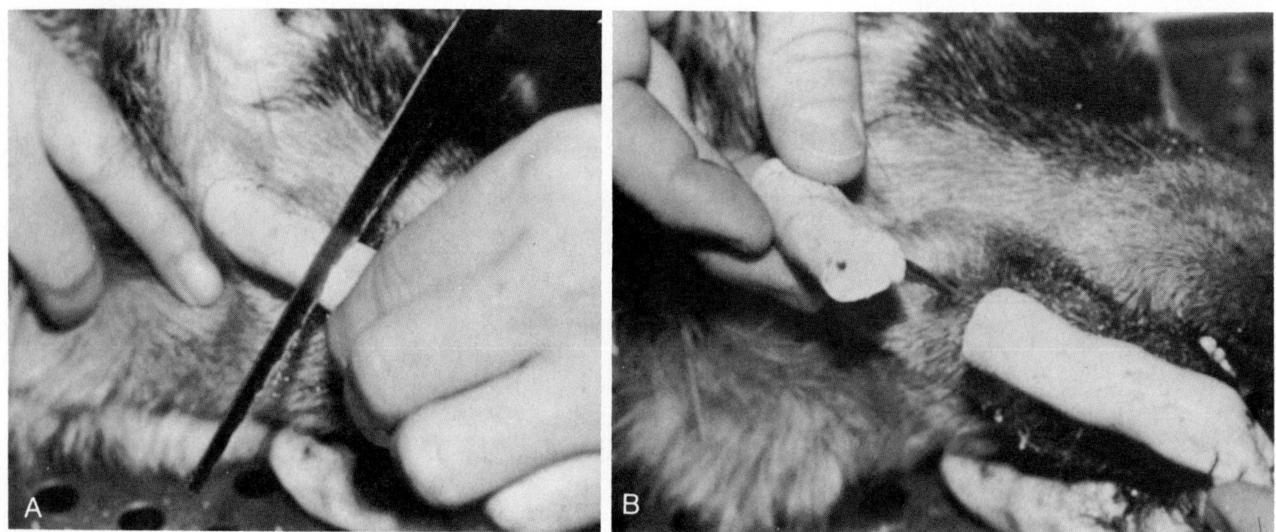

FIGURE 142–10. Removal of an acrylic pin splint after fracture healing. *A*, Cutting through the acrylic bar between pins with a hacksaw blade. *B*, Twisting out segment of bar with one pin.

or hacksaw and each pin with bar segment removed individually (Fig. 142–10).

Partial Mandibulectomy

Partial mandibulectomy and hemimandibulectomy for the treatment of neoplastic conditions have resulted in good return to function.[24] Consequently, this technique can be used as a salvage procedure for nonunion associated with intractable infection and bone loss.[15, 24] Enough bone is resected to remove all abnormal tissue and to allow tension-free closure of soft tissue over the resection stumps. Attempts at stabilizing the remaining bone with internal fixation have resulted in implant loosening, requiring removal. Internal fixation is not recommended, and medial drift of the mandible is minimal.[24]

Caudal Mandibular Fractures

Fractures of the vertical ramus and condylar regions are difficult to expose because of the surrounding musculature.[17] Cortical bone of the mandible in these areas is thin, limiting purchase of bone screws or external fixation pins. Consequently, most of these fractures are treated conservatively with tape muzzles or interarcade wiring to maintain proper dental occlusion.[6, 21] If internal fixation is required, interfragmentary wires or small angled plates applied in oral or lateral approaches can be used.[11, 14]

Intra-articular fractures of the temporomandibular joint can be exposed through a lateral approach.[17] These fractures are difficult to stabilize, so conservative treatment is commonly used.

If significant arthritic changes develop and limit mastication, condylectomy can be performed later.[9] An osteotome, bone-cutting forceps, or an oscillating saw can be used to remove the condyle. Adequate bone is resected to prevent contact between the temporal bone and mandible. A pseudoarthrosis develops and generally allows good return to function. Analgesics and chewy foods may be used to encourage motion of the joint.

TEMPOROMANDIBULAR JOINT LUXATIONS

Temporomandibular joint luxations may occur as isolated injuries or in association with mandibular fractures.[6, 15, 20] The mandibular condyle can displace either rostrally or caudally relative to the mandibular fossa of the temporal bone. If the luxation is unilateral and the condyle displaces rostrally, the mandibular canine teeth shift rostrally and away from the side of the luxation relative to the maxillary canine teeth. If the condyle luxates caudally, the mandibular canines shift caudally and toward the side of the luxation. The injury is examined radiographically to confirm luxation direction and rule out fracture. Although standard ventral dorsal and lateral views adequately demonstrate the joint in dogs, 20° of rotation is required in cats to observe the joint on the lateral projection.[20] Most temporomandibular luxations can be reduced with closed manipulation (Fig. 142–11). In the standard technique, a wooden dowel (pencil for cats) is placed transversely in the back of the mouth between the last molars to act as a fulcrum.[6] The rostral mandible and maxilla are squeezed together to distract the condyle ventrally. The mandible is pulled rostrally or pushed caudally to move the condyle into place. Multiple manipulations may be required to obtain reduction. Some joints are stable after closed reduction, but many reluxate if not supported. Consequently, I palpate the joint and provide additional support if instability is apparent. A muzzle is adequate in many dogs, but interarcade wiring works better, particularly in cats. The periarticular tissues fibrose well, and the joint becomes stable. Consequently, support is needed for only 7 to 14 days. Open reduction and stabilization by suture imbrication of the joint capsule can be accomplished in many patients when closed reduction is unsuccessful. Delay in treatment can result in significant condylar cartilage damage, requiring condylar resection.[9]

SKULL FRACTURES INVOLVING THE ORAL CAVITY

Palatine Fractures

Palatine fractures may have minimal clinical signs, epistaxis, or oral bleeding.[1, 13] Nondisplaced fractures usually require no treatment or simple suturing of the mucosal tear. Displaced longitudinal fractures of the palate can be treated with interdental wire loops placed between corresponding right and left canine and last molar teeth (Fig. 142–12). In cats, large simple interrupted sutures of absorbable material can also be used to stabilize these injuries.

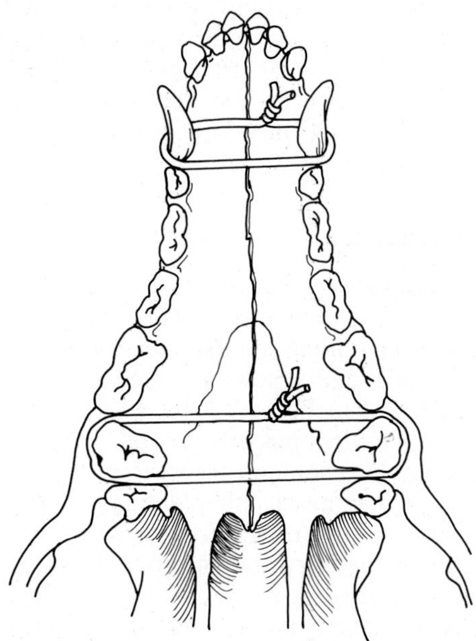

FIGURE 142–12. Interdental wiring between the maxillary canine and molar teeth to treat longitudinal fractures of the hard palate.

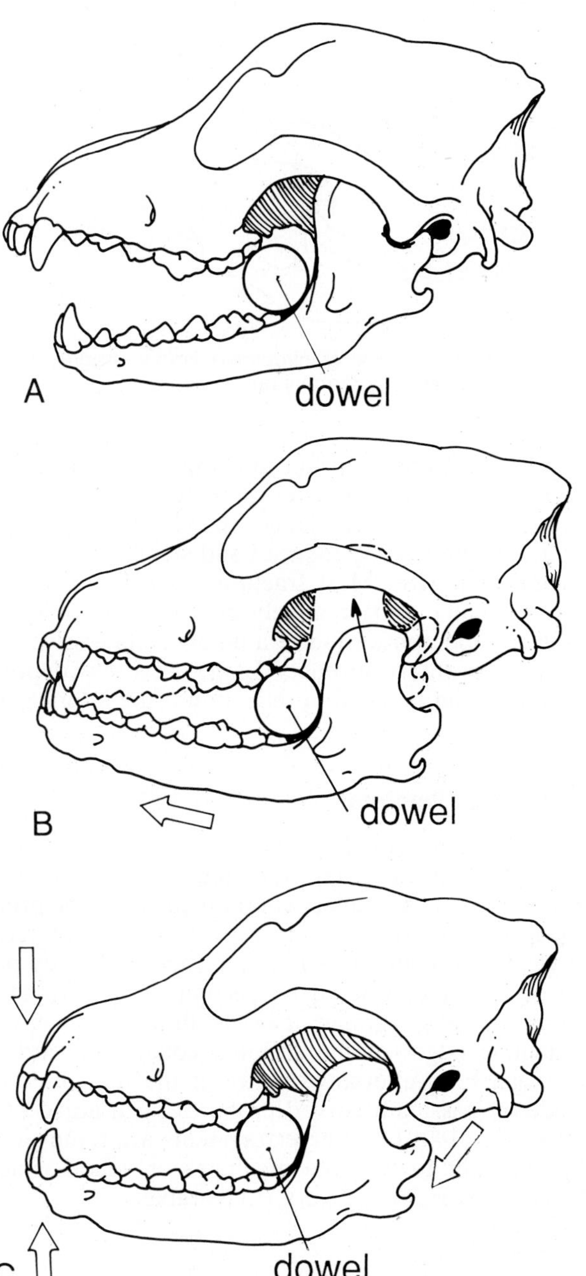

FIGURE 142–11. Technique for closed reduction of a caudal temporomandibular luxation. *A*, A wooden dowel is placed transversely between the last upper and lower molars. *B*, The rostral mandible and maxilla are squeezed together to distract the condyle ventrally. *C*, The mandible is then pulled forward (or pushed caudally for cranial luxations) to move the condyle back into the mandibular fossa of the temporal bone. Multiple manipulations may be required to obtain reduction.

Fractures of the Maxilla and Premaxilla

Fractures of the premaxilla and maxilla extending into the oral cavity are treated like mandibular fractures. Obtaining adequate dental occlusion is the therapeutic goal. These bones have even thinner cortices than the mandible, but they do heal quickly with minimal support. Consequently, tape muzzles or interarcade wires are used if stabilization is required.

Avulsion Fractures

Avulsion fractures of alveolar bone and teeth that still have mucosal or gingival attachments are reduced and

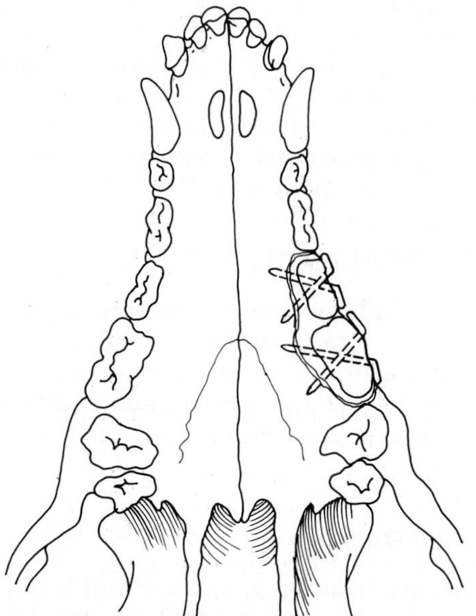

FIGURE 142–13. Use of divergent Kirschner wires to stabilize avulsion fractures of the alveolar bone and associated teeth.

stabilized. One technique involves driving small divergent Kirschner wires through the fragment into the hard palate (Fig. 142–13).[6] If the fragment is missing or nonviable and an opening into the nasal cavity results, a mucosal flap is advanced to prevent an oronasal fistula.[1]

Transverse Fractures

Transverse maxillary and palatine fractures may have minimal clinical signs or gross instability of the rostral skull. If the dorsal nasal and maxillary bones are intact, they act like a hinge, allowing excellent reduction of fractures. These can be stabilized with interdental or interfragmentary wires placed perpendicular to the fracture line. Complete bilateral transverse fractures of the maxilla and of the nasal and palatine bones result in gross instability of the rostral fragment.[1, 19] A combination of interfragmentary and interdental wires may be used if the fractures are fairly simple. If fracture comminution is significant, perfect reconstruction with wire is probably impossible, and fracture collapse may result in distortion and malocclusion. An acrylic pin splint can be applied in many such cases using interarcade alignment of the canine teeth to establish proper dental occlusion.[19] The application technique is similar to that described for mandibular fractures. Because of the thin bone involved, pin size is limited to small-diameter (0.045-inch) Kirschner wires appropriate for cats and small dogs, whereas 3/32-inch pins may be large enough for even big dogs. A greater number of pins (four to six per fragment) are used.

Zygomatic Arch Fractures

Nondisplaced fractures of the zygomatic arch may have severe swelling of the periorbital soft tissues; however, surgical intervention is not necessary.[6] Medially displaced fractures of the arch may interfere with mastication or displace the globe.[1, 6] Elevation, alignment, and stabilization with interfragmentary wires suffice for simple fractures. If more severe comminution precludes reconstruction of the fracture or the fracture has healed in malalignment, resection of the arch is indicated.[13] Exposure is accomplished through a skin and platysma muscle incision directly over the bone.[17] The palpebral nerve and transverse facial vessels are adjacent and must be avoided.[13]

EXTRAORAL SKULL FRACTURES

Extraoral skull fractures may be extracranial or intracranial. In either case, concussion and secondary cerebral edema may cause central nervous system depression. Emergency medical care including corticosteroids, mannitol, and ventilation with oxygen may be necessary.[5]

Extracranial Fractures

Extracranial fractures may have soft-tissue swelling and bony crepitus or subcutaneous emphysema if a

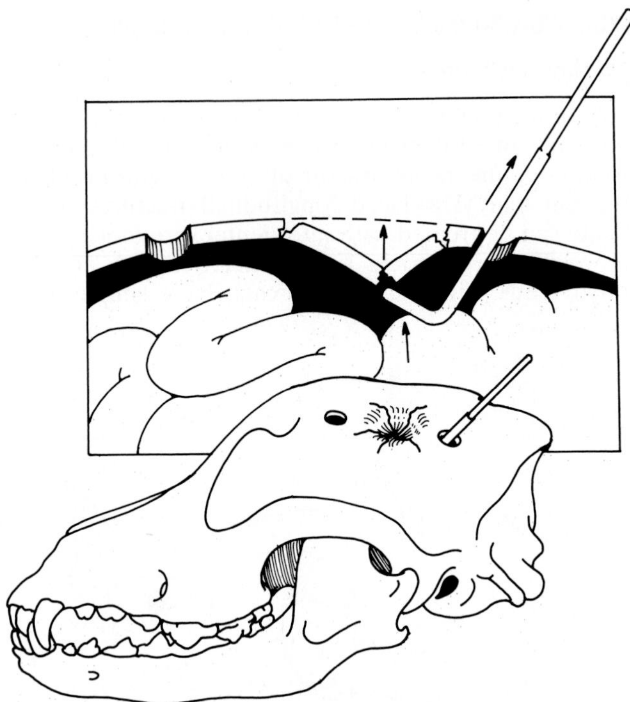

FIGURE 142–14. Elevation of intracranial fracture fragments with a curved probe through adjacent bur holes.

fracture fragment has penetrated the frontal sinus. These fractures rarely require surgical intervention unless they invade the orbit and endanger the globe. In such cases, the fragments can be reduced and stabilized with interfragmentary wire. Most fractures into the dorsal sinus can be treated conservatively by aspiration of the emphysema and application of a mildly compressive dressing to prevent recurrence. Large, severely depressed fragments can be fixed in reduction using interfragmentary wires.

Intracranial Fractures

The large temporal muscles and thick cortices of the skull make intracranial fractures rare. Treatment of concussion and secondary cerebral edema is the primary concern. Nondisplaced linear fractures do not require surgical treatment. A depression fracture directly pressing on the brain should be decompressed. Direct elevation of the fragment may be difficult because the remaining edges of the cranium collapse inward with leverage.[13] An alternative is to lift the fragments from inside by passing a curved probe through adjacent bur holes (Fig. 142–14).[16] Free fragments are removed taking care not to tear the meninges or venous sinuses. The prognosis for recovery is favorable.

References

1. Bone DL: Maxillary fractures. *In* Bojrab MJ (ed): *Current Techniques in Small Animal Surgery*. 3rd ed. Lea & Febiger, Philadelphia, 1990, pp. 883–890.
2. Brinker WO, Flo G: Principles and application of external skeletal fixation. *Vet Clin North Am* 5:197, 1975.

3. Brinker WO, et al: Fractures and dislocations of the upper and lower jaw. *In* Brinker WO, et al (eds): *Handbook of Small Animal Orthopedics and Fracture Treatment*. W. B. Saunders, Philadelphia, 1983, pp 184–194.
4. Cechner PE: Malocclusion in the dog caused by intramedullary pin fixation of mandibular fractures: two case reports. *J Am Anim Hosp Assoc 16*:79, 1980.
5. Chrisman CL: Management of head injury patients. *J Am Anim Hosp Assoc 40*:328, 1973.
6. Dulisch ML: Skull and mandibular fractures. *In* Slatter DH (ed): *Textbook of Small Animal Surgery*. W. B. Saunders, Philadelphia, 1985, pp 2286–2295.
7. Greenwood KW, Creach GB: Biphasic external skeletal splint fixation of mandibular fractures in dogs. *Vet Surg 9*:128, 1980.
8. Lantz G: Interarcade wiring as a method of fixation for selected mandibular injuries. *J Am Anim Hosp Assoc 17*:599, 1981.
9. Lantz G, Cantwell HD: Unilateral mandibular condylectomy: Experimental and clinical results. *J Am Anim Hosp Assoc 18*:883, 1982.
10. Latimer KE, et al: Emergency stabilization of jaw fractures in a dog using acrylic splints. *Vet Med Small Anim Clin 72*:1029, 1981.
11. Leighton RL, Wolf AM: Treatment of a subcondylar fracture of the mandible in a cat by open reduction and wire fixation. *Feline Pract 9*:30, 1979.
12. Neal D, et al: Morbidity associated with teeth in the line of mandibular fractures. *J Oral Surg 36*:859, 1978.
13. Newton CD: Fractures of the skull. *In* Newton CD, Nunamaker CM (eds): *Small Animal Orthopedics*. J. B. Lippincott, Philadelphia, 1985, pp 287–295.
14. Nibley W: Treatment of caudal mandibular fractures: A preliminary report. *J Am Anim Hosp Assoc 17*:555, 1981.
15. Nunamaker DM: Fractures and dislocations of the mandible. *In* Newton CD, Nunamaker CM (eds): *Small Animal Orthopedics*. J. B. Lippincott, Philadelphia, 1985, pp 297–305.
16. Oliver JE: Craniotomy, craniectomy, and skull fractures. *In* Bojrab MJ (ed): *Current Techniques in Small Animal Surgery*. Lea & Febiger, Philadelphia, 1975, pp 359–363.
17. Piermattei DL, Greeley RG: *An Atlas of Surgical Approaches to the Bones of the Dog and Cat*. 2nd ed. W. B. Saunders, Philadelphia, 1979, pp 28–32.
18. Roush JK, Wilson JW: Healing of mandibular body osteotomies after plate and intramedullary pin fixation. *Vet Surg 18*:190, 1989.
19. Stambaugh JE, Nunamaker DM: External skeletal fixation of comminuted maxillary fractures in dogs. *Vet Surg 11*:72, 1982.
20. Ticer JW, Spencer CP: Injury of the feline temporomandibular joint: Radiographic signs. *J Am Vet Radiol Soc 19*:146, 1978.
21. Umphlet RC, Johnson AL: Mandibular fractures in the dog: A retrospective study of 157 cases. *Vet Surg 19*:272, 1990.
22. Umphlet RC, Johnson AL: Mandibular fractures in the cat: a retrospective study. *Vet Surg 17*:333, 1988.
23. Willer RL, et al: A comparison of stainless steel versus acrylic for the connecting bar of external skeletal fixators. *J Am Anim Hosp Assoc 27*:541, 1991.
24. Withrow SJ, Holmberg DL: Mandibulectomy in the treatment of oral cancer. *J Am Anim Hosp Assoc 19*:273, 1983.

CHAPTER 143 Degenerative Joint Disease

Alan J. Lipowitz

Degenerative joint disease (DJD, osteoarthritis) is a disease of the cartilage of joints. Primary clinical signs are joint pain, altered gait, limited range of motion of the affected joint, and various amounts of effusion and local inflammation. The disease affects many species of animals and has been observed in fossil dinosaur skeletons 200 million years old.[56] It is the most common chronic joint disease of humans.[13]

PATHOGENESIS

DJD in man is a heterogeneous group of disorders with many etiological factors that result in a common final pathway leading to changes in cartilage integrity.[13, 37] DJD has primary and secondary etiologies. This classification has also been used for DJD of animals. The term *idiopathic DJD* is now preferred rather than *primary DJD* because it is likely that specific forms of the disease are due to specific causes that have not been identified.[37] In secondary DJD, alterations of articular tissues are the consequence of known factors and conditions affecting joints. Secondary DJD in humans is divided into several categories—traumatic, metabolic, endocrine, congenital/developmental, calcium deposition disease, neuropathic, and other conditions of bone and joints. Although idiopathic and secondary DJD are classified separately, the ultimate changes in joint tissue integrity are the same. The difference is that in some cases the causes are known and in others they are not.

A current theory on the etiopathogenesis of DJD describes two major causes leading to the final common pathway.[26] One cause is the application of abnormal stresses placed on normal joint tissues, and the other assumes that normal loading forces are being transmitted through the joint but that the joint tissues are abnormal (Fig. 143–1).

PATHOLOGY

Cartilage loss, especially in areas of increased load, subchondral bony sclerosis, marginal osteophytosis, and variable synovial membrane inflammation are among the major morphological changes in a joint affected with DJD (Figs. 143–2 and 143–3). Significant biochemical changes in the cartilage include an increase in water content, an increase in space between collagen fibers with a concomitant reduction in their size, alterations in the synthetic functions of chondrocytes, and a reduction in concentration of matrix proteoglycan (PG).[5] The increase in cartilage hydration may be due to an alteration in the weave of the collagen network. Change in the collagen network, with a dilution of PG, produces a deterioration of the cartilage matrix and changes in the mechanical properties of the cartilage. Deformation under loading is increased, and there is less elastic return and consequently more contact pressure on subchondral bone. Surface fissures and fibrillation are the result[22] (Fig. 143–4).

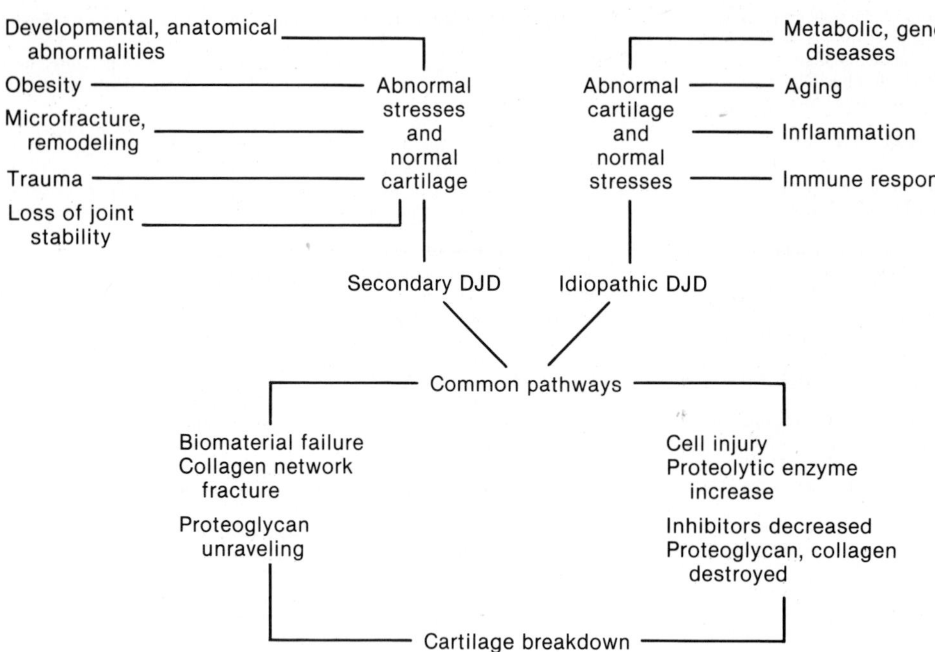

FIGURE 143–1. Etiopathogenesis of degenerative joint disease (DJD). Common final pathways leading to cartilage breakdown. (Adapted from Howell DS: Pathogenesis of osteoarthritis. *Am J Med 80*[Suppl 4B]:24, 1986.)

The reduction in matrix concentration of PG occurs even though the concentration of collagen remains unchanged. The progressive decrease in PG content is directly correlated with the severity of the disease. This loss occurs with increased PG synthesis, suggesting an accelerated rate of PG breakdown.[49] Degradative enzymes intrinsic to cartilage are responsible for the PG catabolism.[51] Although total glycosaminoglycan content of affected cartilage is diminished, not all components are equally affected. When compared with normal cartilage, there is a relative decrease in keratin sulfate and an increase in chondroitin 4-sulfate such as is found in normal young or immature cartilage. Collagenases have also been found in articular cartilage affected by DJD, and their levels have also been correlated with disease severity.[14]

Synovial membrane changes associated with DJD vary from mild to moderate inflammation. These changes include synovial cell hypertrophy and hyperplasia, plasma cell and lymphocytic infiltration, and increased vascularization of the subsynoviocytic tissues. Subsynovial fibrosis is also a common feature.[33]

Deposition of immunoglobulins and complement in the cartilage and synovial membrane of experimentally induced DJD suggests the role that immune-mediated reactions may have in the development and perpetuation of joint inflammation.[40] Studies of the antigenic capacity of cartilage PG and articular collagen have shown that immune-mediated reactions contribute to the pathophysiological changes of DJD. In rabbits, cellular immunity to PG and types I, II, and III collagen was evident.[8] The immune response to collagen was nonspecific, whereas the immunity to PG correlated with the severity of the DJD lesions. Autoimmunity to native type II collagen has also been found in people with several different types of noninflammatory osteoarticular syndromes.[19] Other clinical studies in humans have provided evidence of immune complex deposition in the

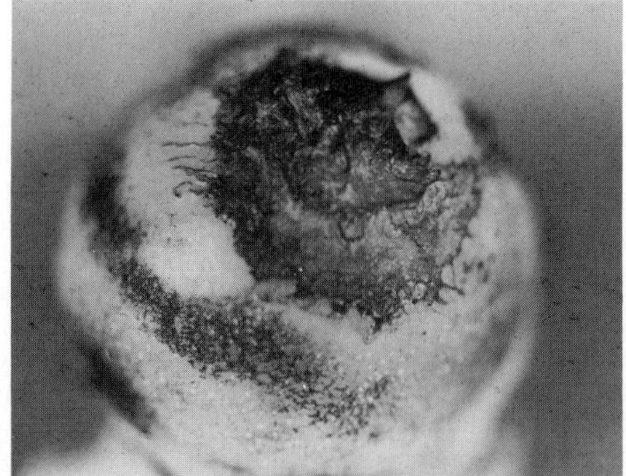

FIGURE 143–2. Femoral head of a dog with degenerative joint disease. The cartilage surface has been painted with India ink to illustrate areas of fissuring, pitting, and cartilage erosion.

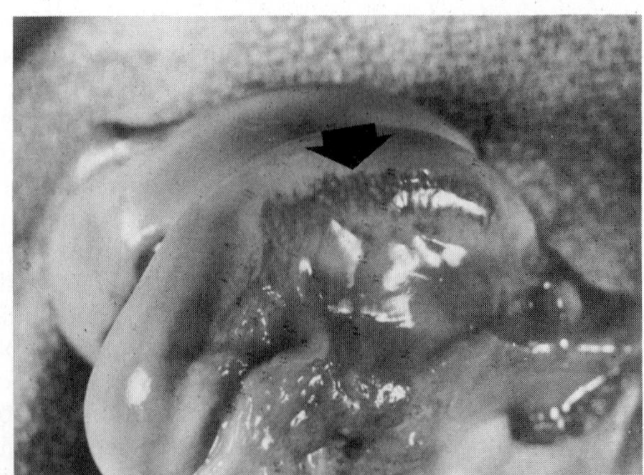

FIGURE 143–3. The medial femoral condyle of a dog 3 weeks after transection of the anterior cruciate ligament. Note the area of hyperemia at the attachment of the synovial membrane *(arrow)*.

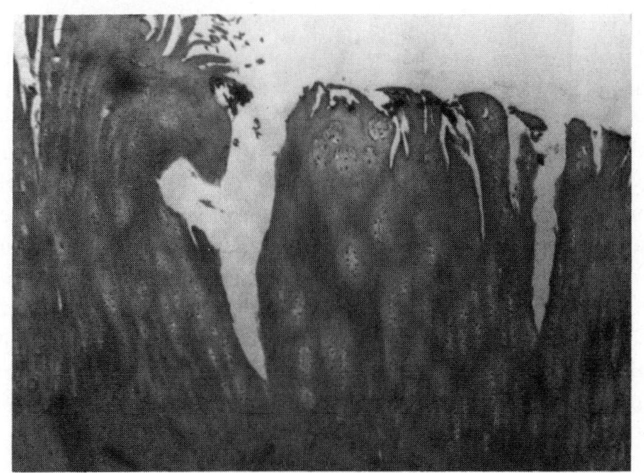

FIGURE 143–4. Fibrillated articular cartilage illustrating clefts within the matrix. (H&E, ×40).

tissues of joints affected by DJD.[25, 28] Although the exact role of specific immune responses in the pathogenesis of DJD is not fully explained, there is little doubt that autoimmunity and the phagocytosis of immune complexes leading to the release of substances deleterious to the affected joint have important roles in the pathogenesis of DJD.[9, 27]

Antibodies to homologous type I and type II collagen have been found in the serum and synovial fluid of dogs that have DJD secondary to rupture of the cranial cruciate ligament,[43] and a cartilage matrix glycoprotein has been identified in the serum and synovial fluid of some dogs with experimentally induced DJD.[15] In addition, C1q-binding immune complexes have been found in the serum and synovial fluid of dogs with DJD secondary to cranial cruciate ligament rupture.[42] In contrast, a correlation could not be found between serum concentrations of keratan sulfate and cartilage changes in dogs with DJD secondary to experimental transection of the cranial cruciate ligament.[7] This information further defines the immunological processes associated with DJD and may soon lead to specific laboratory tests that can detect DJD in its earliest stages.

CLINICAL PRESENTATION

Animals affected with DJD are usually presented because of lameness or change in gait. Many conditions of dogs produce changes in limb use, and they must be differentiated from those producing DJD.[58] A detailed, carefully taken history and thorough physical examination including a neurological assessment are a part of every examination for lameness. Careful questioning of the owner should accompany the actual physical examination. It must be determined when the lameness was first noticed and under what circumstances. It is important to determine whether the animal has a local or systemic condition that may manifest as lameness or joint disease. Did a traumatic incident or unusual experience precede the lameness? The pattern of joint involvement, if any, must be determined. In what order, if any, did the joint involvement occur? Is the involvement self-limited, migratory, or progressive? *Migratory* indicates that the condition subsides in one joint only to begin in another. *Progressive* means that the first joint remains affected and additional joints become involved.

Previous treatments, their effects, and how long they were given must be determined. Side effects or adverse reactions to therapy are also noted.

Signalment is combined with the information gleaned from the physical and neurological examinations to establish a list of tentative differential diagnoses. In some cases, more than one condition may be contributing to lameness and gait abnormality. For example, many older German shepherds with degenerative myelopathy frequently have coxofemoral DJD secondary to hip dyplasia.

PHYSICAL EXAMINATION

All body systems are evaluated in an animal being examined for lameness (see Chapter 118). Neurological evaluation must be included. Gait and limb function are assessed by observing the animal as it walks, trots, or runs. The gait assessment examination is conducted on a nonslippery floor surface. Useful information on limb function may be obtained by observing the animal as it goes up and down stairs. Examination of the affected limb includes palpation of the musculature and joints and a comparison with the opposite normal limb.[58] It is advisable to examine and palpate the normal limb first so that a reference may be established. Placing the animal in lateral recumbency with the limbs to be palpated uppermost allows limbs and joints to be examined and manipulated more easily than if the animal were standing. Muscles are examined for swelling, atrophy, and tears at their origins or attachments and in the substance of the muscle belly. Lymph nodes, such as the popliteal and axillary, are identified.

The bones of each limb are palpated for enlargements, pain, and loss of continuity. The major joints of the forelimb (shoulder, elbow, carpus) and the hindlimb (hip, stifle, tarsus) are carefully palpated and manipulated. Each joint is manipulated through its full range of motion, which can be measured with a goniometer. The vibratory sensations of crepitus, if present, must be noted. Crepitation often suggests osteophyte formation or articular cartilage damage. The ligamentous and tendinous structures of each joint are assessed for integrity and laxity. Joint effusion is usually not a prominent feature of DJD, although slight increases in synovial fluid volume are often present. Palpable joint enlargement is more common in chronic cases of DJD and varies with the degree of periarticular soft-tissue fibrosis, joint capsule thickening, and osteophyte formation. The intercarpal, intertarsal, and phalangeal joints are also evaluated for range of motion, stability, enlargement, and effusion.

RADIOGRAPHIC EXAMINATION

Once the affected joints have been identified, radiographs are taken to determine the relative degree of degenerative change. It is important to obtain high-

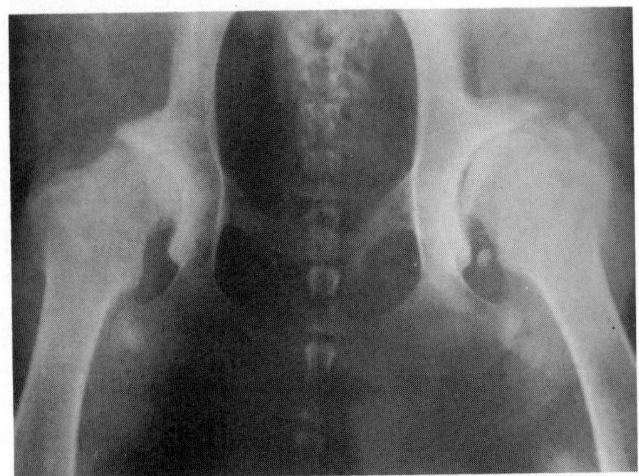

FIGURE 143–5. Ventrodorsal radiographic view of the pelvis and coxofemoral joints of a dog with severe degenerative joint disease. Note the subchondral bony sclerosis, joint space narrowing, and periarticular osteophyte formation.

quality radiographs of the joints in at least two standard views. The patient's position is important when the radiographs are made, and sedation or anesthesia may be necessary to obtain compliance. Special radiographic views or joint positions, such as oblique views of the tarsus or flexed lateral positions of the elbow, may be helpful in identifying the extent of degenerative change.

The characteristic radiographic features of DJD include subchondral bony sclerosis, subchondral cyst formation, joint space narrowing, and intra-articular or periarticular osteophyte formation[39] (Figs. 143–5 and 143–6).

Subchondral bony sclerosis is more common in chronic DJD. Radiographically, it appears as a homogeneous radiodense area beneath the articular cartilage of the affected joint. This dense area may occur in response to increased stress on the subchondral bone, which was normally shared by the articular cartilage.

Subchondral cysts are not commonly found in DJD in dogs and cats, although they often occur in large animals.[39] The so-called subchondral cysts of DJD are not true cysts because they lack a definitive capsule. They are fluid- or mucus-filled spaces in the subchondral bone resulting from microfractures of the subchondral trabeculae in response to increased mechanical stress. With time, the trabecular spaces created by the fractures coalesce and a cyst-like space is created. Radiographically, these lesions appear as rounded lucent areas surrounded by a thin layer of sclerotic subchondral bone.

Narrowing of joint space width is a fairly consistent radiographic feature of DJD, especially in chronic cases.[39] This is due to a loss of articular cartilage, allowing the more radiodense subchondral bone to come in closer contact and giving the appearance of a narrower joint space. However, the radiographic appearance of the joint space is affected by a patient's position, assumption of a weightbearing or nonweightbearing position when the radiograph was made, joint effusion, and the integrity of the ligamentous structures of the affected joint. For example, dogs with hip dysplasia and DJD of the coxofemoral joints have joint effusion, which affects the radiographic relationship between the femoral head and the acetabulum.[35, 36] In such cases, joint space width appears radiographically quite different before and after arthrocentesis.

Osteophytes are often present in joints affected by DJD. They form in the periarticular region of the joint at the attachments of the synovial membrane and appear radiographically as bony spurs or outgrowths arising from the margins of the articular surface.[38] Their presence implies abnormal activity within or adjacent to the affected joint. Osteophytes in association with DJD are most often seen radiographically in the hip, stifle, shoulder, and elbow joints.

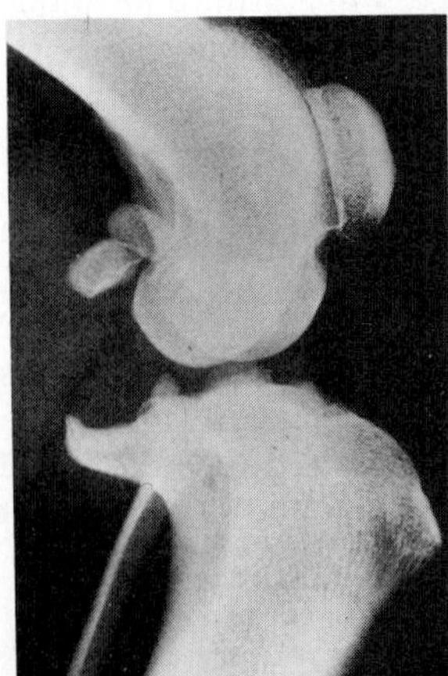

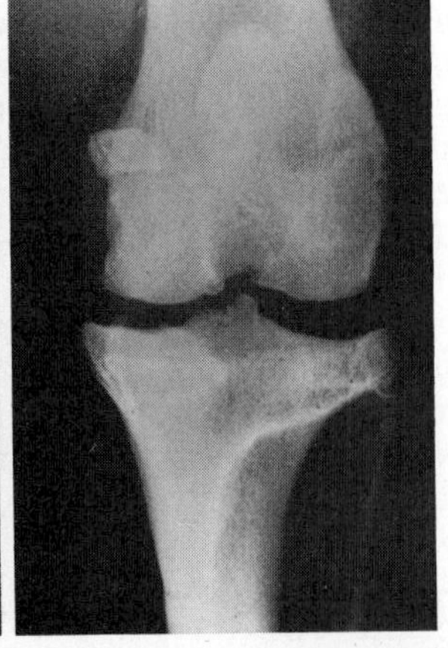

FIGURE 143–6. Lateral and craniocaudal radiographic views of the stifle joint of a dog 6 months after cranial cruciate ligament transection. Note the osteophytes at the joint margins and in the intercondylar notch.

CLINICAL LABORATORY FINDINGS

Results of a complete blood count, urinalysis, and serum chemistry studies are usually within normal limits in cases of DJD unless other conditions exist. Results of rheumatoid factor tests and lupus erythematosus clot tests are negative, as is the search for antinuclear antibodies. A decrease in synovial fluid viscosity due to a reduction in hyaluronic acid concentration, an increase in synovial fluid volume, and increased numbers of mononuclear phagocytic cells in the synovial fluid often confirm the presence of a low-grade intra-articular inflammatory process.[52, 54] Total white blood cells in the synovial fluid rarely exceed 5,000/mm^3.

TREATMENT

The goals in treating DJD are to alleviate discomfort, prevent or at least retard the development of further degenerative changes, and restore affected joints to as nearly normal and pain-free function as possible. Rest and physical therapy are used to decrease the inflammation in the affected joints and to strengthen the supporting structures of the joint.

Surgical treatment with medical and physical therapy may be beneficial, especially in patients with secondary DJD. How these treatment modalities are applied depends on the severity of the DJD, the joints involved, and an owner's expectations about the function of the patient. Each patient with DJD is different, and each should be treated with an individualized regimen.

Surgical therapy in dogs is directed at correcting the inciting cause of DJD. It includes stifle joint stabilization after rupture of the cranial cruciate ligament, pelvic osteotomy or intertrochanteric osteotomy in cases of DJD secondary to hip dysplasia, or procedures to correct patellar luxations. In severe cases of DJD, arthrodesis may be considered. In humans, newer surgical approaches in the treatment of DJD aimed at altering the course of the underlying disease have included removal of abnormal tissue[17] or grafting normal tissue to the affected joint.[10, 70]

Rest and Physical Therapy

Rest and physical therapy decrease inflammation in an affected joint and strengthen the supporting structures of the joint. Controlled exercise is used to maintain muscle tone and prevent fibrosis of periarticular tissues. Stressful activity is kept to a minimum, and an animal's tolerance of activity judged carefully. Walking the patient on a leash several times a day is advisable initially. As a patient responds and if no untoward effects develop, such as reluctance to walk, stiffness or soreness after the activity, or changes in gait patterns, longer walks are begun. More strenuous activities can be introduced as a patient gains strength. Medical therapy includes various drugs that act to reduce inflammation and provide analgesia.

Drug Therapy

No drug or combination of drugs now available can consistently prevent or reverse the pathological changes in DJD. Nonsteroidal anti-inflammatory drugs (NSAIDs) are administered primarily for the symptomatic relief of clinical signs by their analgesic and anti-inflammatory activities. Examples of these drugs include aspirin, ibuprofen, indomethacin, and meclofenamate. These drugs and other NSAIDs exert their actions by inhibiting the synthesis or release of prostaglandins. In general, these drugs seem to be effective while blood levels are maintained; withdrawal is usually followed by a recurrence of joint discomfort. Although effective in moderating the inflammation of DJD, NSAIDs are symptomatic treatments only.

Nonsteroidal Anti-Inflammatory Drugs

Aspirin (acetylsalicylic acid) is the basic drug for the treatment of DJD. When used with care, it can be effective and relatively free of side effects. Aspirin affects various metabolic processes and enzyme systems. In contrast to the opiates, aspirin acts peripherally rather than centrally as an analgesic. Mild to moderate peripheral pain is relieved by the ability of aspirin to block the effect of inflammatory mediators such as bradykinin.[12] The action of aspirin as an anti-inflammatory agent is due to its ability to inhibit prostaglandin synthesis.[61]

Sufficient doses must be used to obtain adequate results. An oral aspirin dosage of 25 mg/kg every 8 hours produces and maintains therapeutic serum salicylate concentrations in normal dogs.[34] Once the desired effects have been obtained, the amount of drug and its frequency of administration may be reduced. Doses reaching 50 mg/kg may produce emesis.[69] Vomiting can occur at lower doses as well and may be prevented by administering the drug with food. Plain aspirin given at therapeutic doses can cause petechiae and linear hemorrhages of the gastric mucosa. Products containing aspirin and magnesium-aluminum hydroxide do not produce gastric lesions when given at therapeutic doses.[34] Cimetidine given at an oral dose of 7.5 mg/kg does not prevent gastric mucosal hemorrhage in dogs given plain aspirin orally at 35 mg/kg every 8 hours.[4]

At therapeutic doses, aspirin is virtually free of serious side effects. Gross overdoses may produce hyperthermia, severe acid-base and electrolyte disturbances, renal hemorrhage, convulsions, and coma.[12] Treatment for these acute and severe problems includes gastric lavage to remove unabsorbed drug, urine alkalization with sodium bicarbonate to enhance renal excretion of salicylate, and peritoneal dialysis to remove salicylates from the plasma.[12]

In dogs, the most common side effects are vomiting and melena. Other toxic manifestations include skin eruptions, edema, gastrointestinal bleeding and ulceration, hypoprothrombinemia, and deafness. Seizures caused by aspirin overdosing have been reported in dogs.[60] Withholding medication alleviates these problems.[12]

Phenylbutazone has been used successfully in some animals for symptomatic treatment of DJD. Its mechanism of action is similar to aspirin. It is given orally in dosages ranging from 0.5 mg to 1.0 mg/kg every 8 hours. Bone marrow depression is the most serious of its side effects. Animals on long-term treatment are periodically evaluated with hemograms. Gastric and duodenal ulcers, malaise, pruritus, rashes, and renal dysfunction are the side effects in humans.

Ibuprofen given orally in a total dose of 15 mg/kg divided into three daily doses and indomethacin in an oral dose of 1.0 to 1.25 mg/kg divided into two or three daily doses have been suggested for the treatment of DJD in dogs.[48] Both drugs may cause gastrointestinal problems.*

Although there are many NSAIDs, there are no studies of efficacy in dogs. In humans, few data show that any of the newer compounds are superior to aspirin in effectiveness when the object of therapy is an immediate anti-inflammatory effect.[67]

Side Effects of NSAIDs. Attention has been directed at the potential effects that aspirin and other NSAIDs may have on renal function as a result of their prostaglandin inhibitory activities. Prostaglandins E_2, $F_{2\alpha}$, I_2, and thromboxane A_2 are the major biologically active prostaglandins that affect the kidneys. With respect to renal function, these compounds are produced by specialized structures in the kidneys and are active only

---

**Editor's note*: Toxic effects of ibuprofen in dogs may be severe or fatal. Its use is not recommended.

locally. The target structures of these prostaglandins include intrarenal arterioles, efferent arterioles, the glomeruli, and the distal tubules. The direct consequences of their effects include an increase or decrease (depending on the active compound) in renal vascular perfusion, an increase in filtration rate, an increase in sodium excretion, an increase in renin release, and interference with antidiuretic hormone action.[20]

Some reports have described the deleterious effects of NSAIDs on renal function in humans. However, in most of these cases, underlying renal disease was present before the NSAIDs were taken.[20, 59] NSAIDs exert few if any deleterious effects on renal function in conscious, healthy animals.[59] In contrast, it has been shown that inhibition of prostaglandin synthesis decreased renal blood flow in dogs made hypotensive by hemorrhage,[23] caval obstruction,[44] or intravenous administration of endotoxin.[24] Indomethacin and ibuprofen significantly decreased glomerular filtration rate and effective renal plasma flow in dogs with experimental peritonitis.[16] In addition, inhibition of furosemide-induced natriuresis by acetylsalicylic acid has been demonstrated in pentobarbital-anesthetized dogs but not in conscious dogs.[3] However, permanent renal injury of clinical significance was not noted in these studies. Still, use of NSAIDs should be closely monitored in animals with existing renal, liver, or heart disease and in patients with volume contraction such as produced by diuretics, sepsis, or anesthesia.[59]

Gastric ulceration and hemorrhage are well-recognized side effects of NSAIDs. Mucosal permeability to acid, active ion transport, blood flow, mucus secretion, epithelial restitution, and prostaglandin synthesis are important factors in preventing gastric mucosal damage from its own secreted acid.[18] NSAIDs cause mucosal damage by adversely affecting these defenses; the net effect of NSAIDs is to make the gastric mucosa more susceptible to the damaging effects of acid in the lumen. NSAID-produced gastrointestinal lesions have been described in dogs, the severity varying with the dosage and duration of administration.* Various agents, including enteric coating, buffering, antacids, and H_2 receptor antagonists, have been used to overcome the gastric irritating effects of these drugs.[4, 55] None has been completely successful. A prostaglandin E_1 analogue has been successful in preventing gastric lesions in dogs when given simultaneously with orally administered aspirin.[29, 30] This drug now holds the most hope for preventing NSAID-produced gastrointestinal lesions.

Normal aging processes alter one's ability to handle drugs. The absorption, distribution, biotransformation, tissue and receptor responses, and excretion of a drug vary depending on the age of the subject. In people, it is generally recognized that the elderly, especially those older than 75 years, are more susceptible to the side effects of drugs.[57] Drug absorption in the elderly is altered by changes in gastrointestinal blood flow, delayed gastric emptying, and decreased gastric acid production.[2] The elderly also have decreases in total body water and reduced serum albumin and thus have fewer drug binding sites and the potential for displacement of more free drug. Decreases also occur in hepatic blood flow, hepatic mass, and glomeruli, with decreased tubular function and renal plasma flow.[31] Similar detailed information about the effects of aging on organ function in older dogs is not available. It is prudent to assume that older dogs are more susceptible to the side effects of NSAIDs as are older people.

Several NSAIDs reduce PG synthesis in organ cultures of normal canine articular cartilage, and the inhibition of PG synthesis produced by salicylate is greater in osteoarthritic cartilage *in vitro* and *in vivo* than in normal cartilage.[45, 47] The effects of salicylates in reducing PG synthesis equally affect normal chondrocytes and those from osteoarthritic cartilage when the cells are isolated from their extracellular matrices.[62] Also, PG synthesis was reduced in the cartilage of immobilized joints in dogs given oral aspirin compared with the cartilage from nonimmobilized joints in the same dogs. The same oral doses of aspirin had no effect on PG synthesis in the cartilage of normal dogs.[46] The clinical ramifications of these findings are undetermined.

Corticosteroids and Other Drugs

Corticosteroids are potent anti-inflammatory agents that may be beneficial in some animals with DJD. They should be reserved for those cases unresponsive to NSAIDs. Steroids for the treatment of DJD are given in low doses and for short periods. Prednisolone may be given parenterally at a dose of 1 to 2 mg/kg, followed by an oral maintenance dosage of 0.5 to 1.0 mg/kg once daily. The lowest possible maintenance dosage is established, such as alternate-day or every-third-day administration of 0.5 to 1.0 mg/kg.

Intra-articular injection of steroids has been used in humans and animals for the treatment of DJD. Pain relief and return of joint function depend on the steroid used, dose, frequency of administration, affected joint, and degree of joint disease.[6] Repeated injections of corticosteroid into the joints of rabbits depressed the synthesis of collagen and PG and caused degeneration of the articular cartilage.[41] In contrast, orally administered prednisolone and intra-articular triamcinolone protected against cartilage lesions, osteophyte formation, and synovial membrane inflammatory changes when given to dogs at the time their cranial cruciate ligaments were transected to create stifle DJD.[50] Also, intra-articular triamcinolone significantly reduced the degenerative changes produced by joint injection of iodoacetate in the knees of guinea pigs.[68] The intra-articular injections of steroids in these studies did not produce cartilage lesions in normal joints. These studies suggest that when properly used, systemic and intra-articular steroids may be of benefit in certain cases of DJD.

As noted, conventional medical therapy of DJD consists primarily of administering drugs that have analgesic and anti-inflammatory properties. While bringing relief of signs, they do little to promote "chondroprotection"—that is, cartilage repair or inhibition of further cartilage breakdown. Studies of an extract of bovine

*See references 11, 27, 32, 53, 55, and 63–66.

lung and tracheal tissue in experimentally created DJD in dogs have been encouraging.[1] Perhaps the future of DJD therapy lies not in developing drugs that provide symptomatic relief but in producing those that stimulate cartilage regeneration and repair.

References

1. Altman RD, et al: Prophylactic treatment of canine osteoarthritis with glycosaminoglycan polysulfuric acid ester. *Arthritis Rheum 32*:759, 1989.
2. Bender AD: Effect of age on intestinal absorption. *J Am Geriatr Soc 16*:1331, 1968.
3. Berg KJ, Lowe D: Inhibition of furosemide-induced natriuresis by acetylsalicylic acid in dogs. *Scand J Clin Lab Invest 37*:125, 1977.
4. Boulay JP, et al: Effect of cimetidine on aspirin-induced gastric hemorrhage in dogs. *Am J Vet Res 47*:1744, 1986.
5. Brandt KD: Osteoarthritis. *Clin Geriatr Med 4*:279, 1988.
6. Brandt KD: Treatment of osteoarthritis. *In* McCarty DJ (ed): *Arthritis and Allied Conditions*. 11th ed. Lea & Febiger, Philadelphia, 1989.
7. Brandt KD, Thonar E J-M: Lack of association between serum keratan sulfate concentrations and cartilage changes of osteoarthritis after transection of the anterior cruciate ligament in the dog. *Arthritis Rheum 32*:647, 1989.
8. Champion BR, Poole AR: Immunity to homologous type III collagen after partial meniscectomy and sham surgery in rabbits. *Arthritis Rheum 25*:274, 1982.
9. Cooke TDV: Significance of immune complex deposits in osteoarthritic cartilage. *J Rheumatol 14*(Suppl 14):77, 1987.
10. Czitrom AA, et al: Bone and cartilage allotransplantation. *Clin Orthop 208*:141, 1986.
11. Daehler M: Transmural pyloric perforation associated with naproxen administration in a dog. *J Am Vet Med Assoc 189*:694, 1986.
12. Davis LE: Clinical pharmacology of salicylates. *J Am Vet Med Assoc 176*:65, 1980.
13. Davis MA: Epidemiology of osteoarthritis. *Clin Geriatr Med 4*:241, 1988.
14. Ehrlich MG: Degradative enzyme systems in osteoarthritic cartilage. *J Orthop Res 3*:170, 1985.
15. Fife RS, et al: Changes in cartilage matrix glycoprotein in serum and synovial fluid of dogs with experimental osteoarthritis. *Clin Res 45*:920, 1986.
16. Fink MP, et al: Effects of nonsteroidal antiinflammatory drugs on renal function in septic dogs. *J Surg Res 36*:516, 1984.
17. Friedman MJ, et al: Preliminary results with abrasion arthroplasty in the osteoarthritic knee. *Clin Orthop 182*:200, 1984.
18. Fromm D: How do nonsteroidal antiinflammatory drugs affect gastric mucosal defenses? *Clin Invest Med 10*:251, 1987.
19. Garbrecht FC, et al: Autoimmunity to articular collagen in patients with osteoarticular syndromes. *J Rheumatol 13*:517, 1986.
20. Garella S, Matarese RA: Renal effects of prostaglandins and clinical adverse effects of nonsteroidal antiinflammatory agents. *Medicine 63*:165, 1984.
21. Goldberg VM, Kresina TF: Immunology of articular cartilage. *J Rheumatol 14*(Suppl 14):73, 1987.
22. Hamerman D: The biology of osteoarthritis. *N Engl J Med 320*:1322, 1989.
23. Henrich WL, et al: The role of renal nerves and prostaglandins in control of renal henodynamics and plasma renin activity during hypotensive hemorrhage in the dog. *J Clin Invest 61*:744, 1978.
24. Henrich WL, et al: Dissociation of systemic and renal effects in endotoxemia; prostaglandin inhibition uncovers important role of renal nerves. *J Clin Invest 69*:691, 1982.
25. Herman JH, et al: Lymphokines: Potential role in the immunopathogenesis of osteoarthritis. *Semin Arthritis Rheum 11*(Suppl 1):115, 1980.
26. Howell DS: Pathogenesis of osteoarthritis. *Am J Med 80*(Suppl 4B):24, 1986.
27. Hurley JW, Crandal LA: The effects of salicylates upon the stomach of dogs. *Gastroenterology 46*:36, 1964.
28. Jasin HE: Autoantibody specificities of immune complexes sequestered in articular cartilage of patients with rheumatoid arthritis and osteoarthritis. *Arthritis Rheum 28*:241, 1985.
29. Katz LB, et al: Rioprostil prevents gastric bleeding induced by nonsteroidal antiinflammatory drugs in dogs and arthritic rats. *J Rheumatol 13*:887, 1986.
30. Katz LB, et al: Selective gastric lesion properties of rioprostil, a prostaglandin E_1 analog in rats and dogs. *J Pharmacol Exp Ther 242*:927, 1987.
31. Lasagna L: Drug effects as modified by aging. *J Chronic Dis 3*:567, 1956.
32. Lev R, et al: Effects of salicylates on the canine stomach: A morphological and histochemical study. *Gastroenterology 62*:970, 1972.
33. Lipowitz AJ, et al: Synovial membrane changes after experimental transection of the cranial cruciate ligament in dogs. *Am J Vet Res 46*:1166, 1985.
34. Lipowitz AJ, et al: Serum salicylate concentrations and endoscopic evaluation of the gastric mucosa in dogs after oral administration of aspirin-containing compounds. *Am J Vet Res 47*:1586, 1986.
35. Lust G, et al: A relationship between degree of laxity and synovial fluid volume in coxofemoral joints of dogs predisposed for hip dysplasia. *Am J Vet Res 41*:55, 1980.
36. Lust G, et al: Intra-articular volume and hip joint instability in dogs with hip dysplasia. *J Bone Joint Surg [Am] 62A*:576, 1980.
37. Mankin HJ, et al: Workshop on the etiopathogenesis of osteoarthritis. Proceedings and recommendations. *J Rheumatol 13*:1127, 1986.
38. Marshall JL: Periarticular osteophytes: Initiation and formation in the knee of the dog. *Clin Orthop 62*:37, 1967.
39. Morgan JP: *Radiology in Veterinary Orthopedics*. Lea & Febiger, Philadelphia, 1972, pp 185–186.
40. Moskowitz RW, Kresina TF: Immunofluorescent analysis of experimental osteoarthritic cartilage and synovium: Evidence for selective deposition of immunoglobulin and complement in cartilaginous tissue. *J Rheumatol 13*:391, 1986.
41. Moskowitz RW, et al: Experimentally induced corticosteroid arthropathy. *Arthritis Rheum 13*:236, 1970.
42. Niebauer GW, Menzel EJ: Immunological changes in canine cruciate ligament rupture. *Res Vet Sci 32*:235, 1982.
43. Niebauer GW, et al: Antibodies to canine collagen type I and II in dogs with spontaneous cruciate ligament rupture and osteoarthritis. *Arthritis Rheum 30*:319, 1987.
44. Oliver JA, et al: Participation of the prostaglandins in the control of renal blood flow during acute reduction of cardiac output in the dog. *J Clin Invest 67*:229, 1981.
45. Palmoski MJ, Brandt KD: Effect of salicylate on proteoglycan metabolism in normal canine articular cartilage *in vitro*. *Arthritis Rheum 22*:746, 1979.
46. Palmoski MJ, Brandt KD: Aspirin aggravates the degeneration of canine joint cartilage caused by immobilization. *Arthritis Rheum 25*:1333, 1982.
47. Palmoski MJ, et al: Marked suppression by salicylate of the augmented proteoglycan synthesis of osteoarthritic cartilage. *Arthritis Rheum 23*:83, 1980.
48. Pederson NC, Pool R: Canine joint disease. *Vet Clin North Am 8*:465, 1978.
49. Pelletier JP, Martel-Pelletier J: Cartilage degradation by neutral proteoglycanases in experimental osteoarthritis. *Arthritis Rheum 28*:1393, 1985.
50. Pelletier JP, Martel-Pelletier J: Protective effects of corticosteroids on cartilage lesions and osteophyte formation in the Pond-Nuki model of osteoarthritis. *Arthritis Rheum 32*:181, 1989.
51. Pelletier JP, et al: Canine osteoarthritis: Effects of endogenous neutral metalloproteoglycanases on articular cartilage proteoglycans. *J Orthop Res 6*:379, 1988.
52. Perman V: Synovial fluid. *In* Kaneko J (ed): *Clinical Biochemistry of Domestic Animals*. 3rd ed. Academic Press, New York, 1980.
53. Phillips BM: Aspirin-induced gastrointestinal microbleeding in dogs. *Toxicol Appl Pharmacol 24*:182, 1973.
54. Pond MJ: Normal joint tissues and their reaction to injury. *Vet Clin North Am 1*:523, 1971.
55. Rainsford KD: Current concepts of the mechanisms of side effects of nonsteroidal antiinflammatory drugs as a basis for establishing research priorities. An experimentalist's view. *J Rheumatol 15* (Suppl 17):63, 1988.
56. Rodman GP (ed): Primer on the rheumatic diseases. *JAMA 224*(Suppl):78, 1973.
57. Roth SH: Pharmacologic approaches to musculoskeletal disorders. *Clin Geriatr Med 4*:441, 1988.
58. Roy WEF: Examination of the canine locomotor system. *Vet Clin North Am 1*:53, 1971.
59. Rubin SI: Nonsteroidal antiinflammatory drugs, prostaglandins, and the kidney. *J Am Vet Med Assoc 188*:1065, 1986.
60. Schubert TA: Salicylate-induced seizures in a dog. *J Am Vet Med Assoc 185*:1000, 1984.
61. Short CR, Beadle RE: Pharmacology of antiarthritic drugs. *Vet Clin North Am Small Anim Pract 8*:401, 1978.
62. Slowman-Kovacs SD, et al: Effects of salicylates on chondrocytes from osteoarthritic and contralateral knees of dogs with unilateral anterior cruciate ligament transection. *Arthritis Rheum 32*:486, 1989.
63. Spyridakis LK, et al: Ibuprofen toxicosis in a dog. *J Am Vet Med Assoc 188*:918, 1986.
64. Stanton ME, Bright RM: Gastroduodenal ulceration in dogs: Retrospective study of 43 cases and literature review. *J Vet Intern Med 3*:238, 1989.
65. Taylor LA: Aspirin-induced gastrointestinal lesions in the dog. *J Am Vet Med Assoc 152*:617, 1968.
66. Thomas MB: Piroxicam-associated gastric ulceration in a dog. *Comp Cont Educ 10*:1004, 1987.
67. Wilkens RF: The use of nonsteroidal antiinflammatory agents. *JAMA 240*:1632, 1978.
68. Williams JM, Brandt KD: Triamcinolone hexacetonide protects against fibrillation and osteophyte formation following chemically induced articular cartilage damage. *Arthritis Rheum 28*:1267, 1985.
69. Yeary RA, Brandt RJ: Aspirin dosages for the dog. *J Am Vet Med Assoc 167*:63, 1975.
70. Zarnett R, Salter RB: Abstract: The cellular origin and evolution of hyaline-like cartilage produced by free periosteal grafts under the influence of continuous passive motion. *Trans Orthop Res Soc 11*:270, 1986.

CHAPTER 144

Immune-Mediated Joint Diseases

Patrick E. Hopper

Arthritis, an inflammatory disease of the joints, is characterized by cellular infiltrates and inflammatory changes in the synovial membrane and synovial fluid. The causes of inflammatory arthropathies are diverse and are categorized into two basic groups: infectious (septic) and noninfectious (nonseptic). Noninfectious inflammatory arthropathies include the immune-mediated arthritides, which are subdivided into nonerosive (nondeforming) and erosive (deforming) arthritis (Table 144–1).

Immune-mediated arthritides have been identified in dogs and cats, although the incidence is relatively low in cats.[7, 26] The cause of immune-mediated arthritides is unknown. Independent of their diverse origins, a type III (immune complex) hypersensitivity reaction is involved in the pathogenesis of the synovitis. Clinical manifestations are due to persistent inflammatory reactions that are the result of the deposition and phagocytosis of immune complexes and release of damaging lysosomal enzymes within the synovial membrane.

The immune-mediated arthritides are a heterogeneous group of diseases; however, considerable overlap exists with respect to clinical, laboratory, radiological, and pathological features. Therefore, a distinct description of these diseases is difficult, and clinically it is necessary to evaluate several factors collectively before making a definitive diagnosis.

CANINE NONEROSIVE ARTHRITIS

Idiopathic polyarthritis is the most common form of immune-mediated joint disease.[8, 49] The cause and source of the immune complexes are unknown. The disease can occur at any age in either sex, although most occurs in young adults between 1 and 3.5 years of age. Any breed, as well as mongrels, can be affected, particularly large breeds (German shepherd, Doberman pinscher) and various sporting breeds (Labrador and golden retrievers, Irish setter).

TABLE 144–1. SUBCLASSIFICATION OF IMMUNE-MEDIATED NONINFECTIOUS INFLAMMATORY ARTHROPATHIES

Erosive arthritis
Rheumatoid arthritis
Nonerosive arthritides
Idiopathic polyarthritis
Systemic lupus erythematosus
Polyarthritis/polymyositis syndrome
Plasmacytic-lymphocytic synovitis
Arthritis associated with chronic infectious diseases
Enteropathic arthritis
Hepatopathic arthritis
Arthritis associated with malignant neoplasia
Drug-induced arthritis

Systemic lupus erythematosus (SLE) is characterized as a multisystemic disease with various clinical manifestations, with immunological abnormalities that include autoimmunity (type II reaction) and immune complex (possibly nuclear antigen and antinuclear antibody [ANA]) hypersensitivity.[40] The cause of SLE is unknown, although genetics, immunoregulatory defects, and viral infection have been implicated in dogs.[29–31, 41, 51] SLE in dogs has no age predilection (8 months to 14 years), but females and certain breeds (German shepherds, collies, Shetland sheepdogs, beagles, and poodles) may be predisposed.[18, 21, 55]

Plasmacytic-lymphocytic synovitis and polyarthritis/polymyositis syndromes have been identified in dogs.[11, 49] The synovitis in plasmacytic-lymphocytic arthritis primarily affects the stifle joints in various breeds. The polyarthritis/polymyositis syndrome occurs most often in young adults of spaniel breeds. The cause of both of these conditions is unknown. They are classified as immune-mediated disorders based on histological characteristics and immunofluorescence studies of the synovium, absence of identifiable microorganisms, and response to immunosuppressive therapy. Increased concentrations of immune complexes within the synovial fluid and serum may accompany plasmacytic-lymphocytic synovitis.[46]

There appears to be no age, breed, or sex predilection for the remaining nonerosive arthritides. In sterile arthritis associated with chronic infections remote from the joints, the infectious process may provide the antigenic stimulus for immune complex formation.[1, 8, 48]

The gastrointestinal tract can be associated with an inflammatory joint disease, also referred to as *enteropathic arthritis*. In humans, this type of polyarthritis is recognized as a complication of ulcerative colitis and regional enteritis.[15, 39] A similar relationship has been recognized in dogs with fulminating enterocolitis and ulcerative colitis.[7, 8, 49] The pathogenesis of enteropathic arthritis is unknown, but it is postulated that the inflamed bowel may result in an increased permeability to either potential antigens or unknown toxins that may have some effect on the synovium. A common etiology may also be shared by the inflamed bowel and joints. Hepatopathic arthropathy, a type of enteropathic arthritis, has been associated with chronic active hepatitis and cirrhosis in humans and dogs.[38, 49] The antigenic material passing from the bowel into the portal circulation is probably not phagocytized by the tissue macrophages in the liver, thus allowing access to the general circulation.

Neoplastic processes in other parts of the body have been associated with polyarthritis.[7, 8, 49] The pathogenesis of this type of arthritis is probably multifactorial, and again, an immune complex disease arising from tumor antigens and antibodies may participate.

Drug-induced arthritis has been recognized infrequently.[19, 23, 49, 60] Canine allergic drug reactions most often are associated with cutaneous manifestations. Although any breed of dog can become sensitized to a drug, Doberman pinschers and Weimaraners are at greater risk for developing sulfadiazine-induced allergies.[19, 23, 60] In humans, certain drugs (procainamide, hydralazine, sulfonamides, propranolol, quinidine) induce polyarthritis and an SLE-like syndrome.[24] Drugs may act directly as complete antigens by attaching to plasma proteins and causing the development of circulating drug-antibody complexes. Alternatively, they may act as haptens by binding with host proteins of cell walls to produce new antigens.[61]

Clinical Presentation

Independent of the type of immune-mediated joint disease, the clinical features are similar and include fever (persistent or episodic), inappetence/anorexia, and malaise accompanied by lameness of varying severity. The primary complaint occasionally is chronic lameness without any systemic signs. Joint disease and clinical manifestations tend to be cyclical: the onset is acute, and improvement can be spontaneous. The arthritic manifestations range from overt lameness to subtle signs of generalized weakness. A single (monoarticular, pauciarticular) or shifting (pauciarticular, polyarticular) leg lameness may be observed. Dogs with polyarticular involvement show generalized stiffness (arched back, stilted gait) after rest or exercise and may exhibit difficulty rising and lying down, predominantly involving the hindquarters. Generalized pain and behavioral changes, such as aggression and increased irritability, are often observed when affected dogs are handled. Some severely affected dogs, particularly small or toy breeds, refuse to stand, walk, or exercise. In these instances, appreciation of the joint disease is difficult and often overlooked.

The presence of a nonerosive immune-mediated polyarthropathy cannot always be determined by physical examination. If all limbs are not carefully palpated in a dog presented for lameness in a single limb, a polyarticular disease may not be appreciated. In addition to pyrexia (103° to 106°F [39.4° to 40.8°C]), tachypnea and peripheral lymphadenopathy are common. Regardless of the type of immune-mediated arthritis, distal extremities and stifle joints are most commonly affected. Synovial distension, pain, soft-tissue swelling, or heat in one or more of the joints is a physical finding more frequently associated with acute febrile states. In more chronic forms, swelling and heat are often absent and only subtle signs of discomfort or joint capsule thickening are detectable. Spinal hyperesthesia, involving the neck and back, is a consistent clinical feature. In some cases, muscle pain and joint pain may be difficult to differentiate. In severely affected dogs, the disease can be debilitating, resulting in generalized muscle atrophy and weight loss. Disproportionate atrophy of the temporal and masseter muscles is often observed.

Specific immune-mediated arthritides cannot be distinguished based on clinical presentation alone. Joint disease tends to be the sole manifestation in idiopathic polyarthritis. The clinical manifestations in dogs with SLE are diverse and depend on organ involvement, but polyarthritis is the most common finding (60 to 90 per cent) and frequently the primary presenting complaint.[18, 21, 41, 48, 55] Skin and mucocutaneous lesions are prevalent in SLE (43 per cent) but not necessarily a concurrent finding with polyarthritis.[55] Various cutaneous manifestations are also common features of drug-induced arthritis. Less common physical abnormalities found in dogs with SLE include respiratory (pleuritis), gastrointestinal (vomiting, diarrhea), muscular (myositis), neurological (meningitis, myelopathy), cardiac (myocarditis), or vascular (edema) disorders. In plasmacytic-lymphocytic synovitis, the stifle joint is primarily affected, leading to degeneration of the cruciate ligaments and instability. The signs of arthritis associated with other disease processes may be a minor or major manifestation of the overall disease syndrome. Monoarticular and pauciarticular involvement of the carpi and tarsi are the most frequent musculoskeletal findings, and bilateral symmetry may not be apparent. Additional clinical signs may be present and depend on the body system and disease process involved. A thorough physical examination and history, including previous therapy and travel, often help in recognizing infectious and other secondary immune-mediated arthritides.

Clinical Pathology

Anemia is infrequent in most nonerosive arthritides, the exception being canine SLE (20 to 35 per cent). Nonregenerative anemia is the predominant type of anemia in canine SLE, instead of an autoimmune hemolytic anemia.[21, 48, 55] A positive Coombs' test in dogs with SLE is associated with hemolytic and nonhemolytic anemias.[48, 55] In nonerosive arthritides, elevated concentrations of fibrinogen (acute phase protein) and increases in the erythrocyte sedimentation rate are consistent. Mild to marked leukocytosis and absolute neutrophilia are common in acute febrile attacks, although the leukogram can be normal. In such cases, hyperfibrinogenemia may precede leukocyte changes. Leukopenia and thrombocytopenia are rare findings in most dogs with polyarthritis. Most often, leukopenia (28 per cent) and thrombocytopenia (12 per cent) are present in dogs with SLE.[55] Autoantibodies directed against leukocytes are detected by the antiglobulin consumption test, and platelets are detected by the platelet factor-3 test.[10, 62]

Serum chemistry profiles are either normal or show variable decreases in albumin and absolute or relative increases in serum globulin. In patients with these abnormalities, serum electrophoresis is valuable to confirm hypoalbuminemia and demonstrate elevations in alpha$_2$- and gamma-globulins. Mild nonspecific increases in liver enzymes (serum alkaline phosphatase, alanine transaminase, and aspartate transaminase) can also be noted, whereas marked elevations may be present in hepatopathic arthritis. Creatine phosphokinase or aldolase concentrations may be elevated if polymyositis is present. Blood chemistry abnormalities reflecting multisystemic involvement suggest SLE or infectious processes, such as bacterial endocarditis.

Findings on urinalysis are unremarkable. Detection of proteinuria is compatible with SLE and present in approximately 50 per cent of the cases.[18, 21, 48, 55] Proteinuria is also present in most cases of polyarthritis associated with bacterial endocarditis and frequently is accompanied by hematuria and renal casts.[12]

Synovial fluid analysis is essential to establish and differentiate between inflammatory and noninflammatory arthropathies. Arthrocentesis of multiple joints, both clinically affected and asymptomatic, is recommended because multiple joints are often pathologically but not clinically affected, and analysis from a single joint occasionally is inconclusive. Therefore, analysis of synovial fluid is the single most helpful test to establish the presence, severity, and distribution of joint involvement in inflammatory joint diseases. Collection of fluid and approaches for arthrocentesis are described elsewhere.[22, 59]

The volume of synovial fluid is often increased in patients with joint capsule distension. Pathological joints sometimes are difficult to aspirate or yield small (normal) quantities of synovial fluid. Normal synovial fluid is colorless to slightly yellow, transparent, and very viscous. Affected joints show variable discoloration and increased turbidity as a consequence of increased cellularity. Viscosity is assessed by observing the fluid as it is expelled slowly from a needle. Normal fluid forms a long (>2.5 cm) "string" between the needle and a glass slide before the drop separates. In addition, the drop on the slide should remain spherical rather than disperse over the slide. A thin, runny consistency or the inability to form a long string suggests a deficiency in polymerized hyaluronic acid or dilution from excess serum. Nonerosive arthritides generally have low viscosity. These samples may also clot on exposure to air (fibrinogen clot test) if not mixed with an anticoagulant (EDTA) for cytologic examination. This is because fibrinogen and other clotting factors are absent in normal but present in inflammatory synovial fluid. Hyaluronic acid is degraded by EDTA, therefore heparin is preferred for the mucin clot test. The mucin clot test indirectly determines the extent of polymerization of hyaluronic acid. A poor, friable, or nonexistent mucin clot is usually observed.

Nucleated cell counts in nonerosive immune-mediated arthropathies are moderately or markedly increased, ranging from 3,000/μl to 100,000/μl or more (reference range, <3,000/μl).[8, 10, 11, 48] Neutrophils (nontoxic) are the predominant cell type, ranging from approximately 30 per cent to 100 per cent (average 80 per cent) of nucleated cells (reference, <12 per cent and frequently ≤5 per cent).[8, 10, 11, 48] An increased number of neutrophils suggests inflammation of the synovial membrane and has no differentiating diagnostic value for specific inflammatory arthritides. Generally, more severely inflamed joints contain a greater concentration of nucleated cells and a correspondingly greater percentage of neutrophils. Lymphocytes and large mononuclear cells with phagocytic potential account for the remainder of nucleated cells. Lupus erythematosus cells are found on rare occasions and are diagnostic of SLE.[37] These cells should not be confused with leukophagocytic macrophages or neutrophils containing phagocytosed particulate material (probably nucleic acid).

Immune-mediated nonerosive arthritides, excluding SLE, are negative for both rheumatoid factor (RF) and fluorescent ANA (FANA) or have positive titers at insignificant levels. Lupus erythematosus cell preparations and FANA are available to test for the presence of antinuclear antibodies. The lupus erythematosus cell phenomenon is a nonspecific and insensitive test found only in a low percentage of SLE affected dogs. Thus, lupus erythematosus cell preparations are not routinely performed. Indirect FANA is the most specific and sensitive serological test for SLE. Dogs with SLE occasionally have low or negative (seronegative lupus) FANA titers. FANA is not specific for SLE, and low titers can be found in a number of chronic infectious, inflammatory, and neoplastic disorders. In dogs, bacterial endocarditis accompanied by polyarthritis has been documented, resulting in the production of circulating autoantibodies, including FANA and RF.[13] A positive FANA test result therefore should be interpreted with caution and correlated with clinicopathological, pathological, and immunopathological findings. Geographic location or other clinical signs, in addition to polyarthritis, may require serological testing for chronic infectious diseases and include occult dirofilariasis, coccidioidomycosis, Lyme disease, ehrlichiosis, and Rocky Mountain spotted fever.*

Microbiological (bacterial and *Mycoplasma* spp.) examinations of synovial fluid and synovial membranes are negative, the exception being chronic infections associated with polyarthritis. In chronic infections associated with polyarthritis, both infectious and noninfectious arthritis may coexist. Infected joints occasionally have positive synovial membrane but negative synovial fluid cultures.[12] In experimentally induced infectious arthritis, culture of synovial fluid incubated 24 hours in blood culture medium was more reliable than synovial membrane biopsy.[42] Therefore, synovial biopsy is not justified for culture due to the risk of anesthesia and associated trauma unless a synovial specimen is also indicated for histopathological and immunofluorescence examinations. Negative cultures should not be interpreted as evidence that an infectious disease is not present elsewhere in the body. If joint cultures are negative and an underlying infectious process is still suspected (i.e., bacteremia or bacterial endocarditis), isolation of the organism from blood is considered diagnostic. Blood cultures are positive (50 to 88 per cent) and less commonly urine cultures (35 to 45 per cent) are positive in dogs with bacteremia, bacterial endocarditis, or discospondylitis.[12, 16] Other infectious agents, such as *Borrelia burgdorferi* (Lyme disease) and rickettsial organisms, are difficult to culture, and determination of antibody titers is at present the most useful diagnostic test.[20, 36]

---

*See references 3, 5, 17, 25, 28, 33, 36, 48, and 57.

Radiographic Findings

Radiographic findings in immune-mediated nonerosive arthritides are usually normal or limited to nonspecific signs of soft-tissue swelling and joint distension. Even in chronic cases, radiographic signs are minimal: increased periarticular soft-tissue density due to fibrosis, periosteal bone proliferation at ligament or joint capsule attachments, and secondary degenerative joint disease. Consequently, radiographic joint surveys often do not contribute to differentiation between the inflammatory joint diseases, including the early stages of rheumatoid and septic arthritis. However, radiographic joint surveys should not be excluded from the initial examination, because the inflammatory process can be superimposed on a joint already affected with osteoarthritis.

Pathology and Immunopathology Features

Synovial membrane biopsies (surgical arthrotomy and needle biopsy[22]) help confirm chronic active inflammation and identify immunoglobulins, complement, and fibrinogen deposits within the synovium. Affected synovium is thickened, congested, and edematous on gross examination. The pathological changes are similar for the immune-mediated arthritides; however, the histopathological features of synovitis can be variable. Pannus formation, destruction of cartilage and bone (marginal erosion), and villus hypertrophy are not common features. The synovitis is characterized by an inflammatory infiltrate in the supporting layer composed of lymphocytes, plasma cells, macrophages, and neutrophils in various proportions. The predominant cells identified can be either mononuclear cells or neutrophils, involving the more superficial areas of the supporting layer or a mixture of both. The exception is plasmacytic-lymphocytic synovitis, which is characterized by an intense plasmacytic-lymphocytic infiltrate and can be associated with minimal subchondral erosions and villus hypertrophy.[49] Fibrin deposits are present in most immune-mediated cases of arthritis, and vasculitis is sometimes seen.

Immunofluorescence examination usually identifies IgG- or IgM-producing plasma cells within the synovium. Macrophages, synovial lining cells, and sometimes blood vessel walls contain immunoglobulin and complement deposits.[8, 10, 11] With renal, skin, or muscle involvement, appropriate biopsy samples should be obtained for histopathological and immunofluorescence examinations.

Diagnosis

Diagnosis of immune-mediated nonerosive arthritis is based on the history, clinical signs, radiological and pathological features, and clinicopathological findings. Fever and joint pain are usually unresponsive to acetylsalicylic acid (aspirin) or antibiotics, although apparent clinical improvement may be observed owing to the cyclical nature of the disease. A diagnosis of idiopathic polyarthritis can be made when serological abnormalities are absent or detected at insignificant levels, bacterial cultures are negative, and evidence of an underlying disease process is absent. The criteria for diagnosis of the polyarthritis/polymyositis syndrome are similar to those of idiopathic polyarthritis, with the addition of polymyositis. Definitive diagnosis of polyarthritis/polymyositis syndrome is confirmed by histopathologic evidence of myositis (necrosis, phagocytosis and mononuclear cell infiltrate), because clinical signs may be difficult to distinguish from joint pain and muscle enzymes may not be reliable indicators of muscle damage.

The diagnosis of SLE in dogs can be exceedingly difficult because of the marked variability in clinical manifestations and laboratory findings. SLE is a multisystemic disease, and simultaneous or sequential involvement of more than one body system should be evident.[58] The presence of two or more main clinical features stated earlier constitutes multisystemic involvement. Pyrexia, lethargy, and inappetence are minor nonspecific features that are not regarded as multisystemic involvement. Central to the diagnosis of canine SLE is the demonstration of a significantly high ANA titer in the blood. Antibodies directed against blood cells and immune complex deposits in tissue biopsy specimens consistent with the clinical involvement should be demonstrable. If all criteria are satisfied, *definite* canine SLE is diagnosed. When one major sign is present with a positive ANA result, the diagnosis of *probable* canine SLE is justified because involvement of more than one body system may take time. There is disagreement about the justification of probable SLE without the presence of ANA.[10, 18, 55, 61] Approximately 10 per cent of humans with SLE are ANA negative; however, other autoantibodies, besides ANA, directed against soluble tissue antigens can be demonstrated.[35, 50]

A diagnosis of polyarthritis associated with a chronic infective disease process elsewhere in the body depends on finding a sterile arthritis and identifying an infectious agent remote from the joints. Urinary and respiratory tract infections and bacterial endocarditis are most frequently identified.[8, 48] Severe periodontitis, occult dirofilariasis, discospondylitis, and chronic actinomycosis have also been described. Arthritis is often the only presenting clinical sign because many of these infections are not clinically obvious. Chronic and subacute bacterial endocarditis present the most difficulty in differentiating infectious from noninfectious immune-mediated arthritis. Bacterial endocarditis is considered in all dogs with unexplained fevers, lameness, cardiac murmur, and multisystemic involvement compatible with circulating immune complexes or embolic phenomena. Affected dogs can be any age (range, 1 to 10 years), breed, or sex, although male dogs of large breeds and sporting breeds have an increased risk.[12, 16, 49] The pattern of joint involvement is pauciarticular and asymmetrical. Specific joints involved are most often large proximal joints and intervertebral disc spaces. Diagnosis is made on clinical features and positive bacterial cultures from blood, urine, and synovial fluid or membrane specimens. The diagnosis can be particularly difficult when bacterial examinations are negative or when serum autoantibodies are identified. The diagnosis of bacterial endocarditis with septic emboli can be supported by finding bony destruction radiographically, microscopic synovial abscesses, and negative immunofluorescence of involved muscle or kidney specimens.

The overlying enteric, hepatic, or neoplastic disease process associated with arthritis is usually apparent and generally precedes or coincides with the onset of lameness. Enteropathic arthritis is diagnosed by detecting an inflammatory bowel disease, such as chronic ulcerative colitis or fulminating enterocolitis, concurrently with sterile arthritis. Hepatopathic arthritis is substantiated when chronic active hepatitis or cirrhosis is identified histologically and no other cause of polyarthritis is found. The presence of any malignancy remote from the joints should be suspected as causing sterile arthritis until proved otherwise. Occult or latent neoplastic processes are difficult to diagnose. Polyarthritis is the major clinical manifestation in such cases and may not be confirmed until postmortem examination.

Plasmacytic-lymphocytic synovitis in dogs is usually not diagnosed before surgical intervention for cranial cruciate ligament rupture. Gonitis and synovial effusion usually precede ligament rupture by weeks or months. Synovial fluid analysis before surgery can be misleading as to the underlying cause of gonitis. The total nucleated cell count is not dramatically increased, and mononuclear cells are the predominant cell type. These findings are also consistent with degenerative joint disease or acute trauma. At surgery, abnormal synovium and synovial fluid are observed, but marginal erosions of subchondral bone and pannus formation, usually identified with rheumatoid arthritis (RA), are absent or minimal. Histologically, the synovitis is characterized by marked diffuse plasmacytic and lymphocytic infiltrations. These findings are similar to those observed in RA but differ significantly in intensity from those in spontaneous cranial cruciate ligament rupture and degenerative joint disease of dogs. If these changes are not appreciated at the time of surgery and the synovitis is not controlled by drug therapy, the success of surgical stabilization is doubtful. Arthrocentesis should be performed on multiple joints to rule out other immune-mediated polyarthritides.

Drug-induced arthritis is suspected if the use of any drug is accompanied by a sterile arthritis with or without various dermatological lesions. The most common drugs incriminated are antibiotics, especially sulfonamides and penicillins. In Doberman pinschers with sulfadiazine-induced allergies, clinical signs were delayed 10 to 21 days after initial treatment.[19, 60] However, re-exposure to the sulfa component in this breed reproduced the allergic reactions within 1 to 16 hours. Thus, prior drug history as well as current therapy may be significant. Further support of a drug-induced arthritis is the disappearance of clinical signs 2 to 7 days after drug withdrawal.

It should be clear that no single clinical finding or test result is pathognomonic for any specific type of inflammatory joint disease. A specific diagnosis is most often substantiated by elimination of other causes of polyarthritis. The many similarities shared by inflammatory joint diseases, particularly the immune-mediated forms, should emphasize the importance of a systematic approach and careful interpretation of all test results (Fig. 144–1).

Treatment

The treatment of immune-mediated nonerosive arthritis depends on the primary disease identified. The arthritis generally resolves spontaneously if treatment of the infectious, gastrointestinal, hepatic, or neoplastic disease is successful. Persistent arthritis may necessitate administration of glucocorticoids. In some geographic areas canine ehrlichiosis and borreliosis infections are associated with a nonerosive polyarthritis indistinguishable from immune-mediated nonerosive polyarthritides.[5, 17, 28, 33, 36, 57] For this reason, doxycycline (10 mg/kg once daily) is recommended while awaiting (5 to 7 days) serological test results for suspected infectious disorders. If clinical signs persist or partially improve and synovial fluid abnormalities persist, an infectious cause is unlikely and an immune-mediated polyarthritis is more certain. In addition to rest and confinement, idiopathic polyarthritis, SLE, plasmacytic-lymphocytic synovitis, and polyarthritis/polymyositis syndrome are treated with glucocorticoids or combination immunosuppressive drugs.

Prednisone or prednisolone is administered orally at a dosage of 2 to 4 mg/kg (100 mg/m^2 body surface area) in divided doses for 2 weeks. After 2 weeks, the dog is re-evaluated. Clinical signs and physical examination, although helpful, should not be the basis for adjusting glucocorticoid dosage or adding immunosuppressive drugs to the treatment protocol. As in the diagnosis of inflammatory joint disease, arthrocentesis and cytological examination of synovial fluid are essential in evaluating the response to treatment. Those joints containing the most dramatic synovial fluid abnormalities can be monitored and used as reference points on subsequent rechecks. When synovial fluid is normal but minor joint problems persist, a comparison of serial radiographs may aid in determining the extent of joint dysfunction due to degenerative joint disease and ligamentous changes.

Treatment is modified depending on whether or not the disease is in remission. Remission is the resolution of clinical abnormalities and the absence of inflammatory changes in the synovial fluid. Remission is observed within 2 to 4 weeks if prednisolone alone is to be successful. If remission has occurred, prednisolone is reduced by 50 per cent at 2-week intervals until maintenance dosage (1 mg/kg every other morning) is attainable. Synovial fluid volume diminishes during remission, making the collection of synovial fluid more difficult. Prednisolone can usually be safely reduced if a dog is clinically stable but synovial fluid cannot be obtained. In such cases, the measurement of fibrinogen, if previously elevated, may be of value in determining a patient's clinical status. Any degree of inflammation in synovial fluid is considered as active disease; therefore, medication is not reduced or discontinued. If remission has been maintained, alternate-day therapy (1 mg/kg) is continued for an additional 1 to 2 months and rechecks extended to once a month. If complete remission has

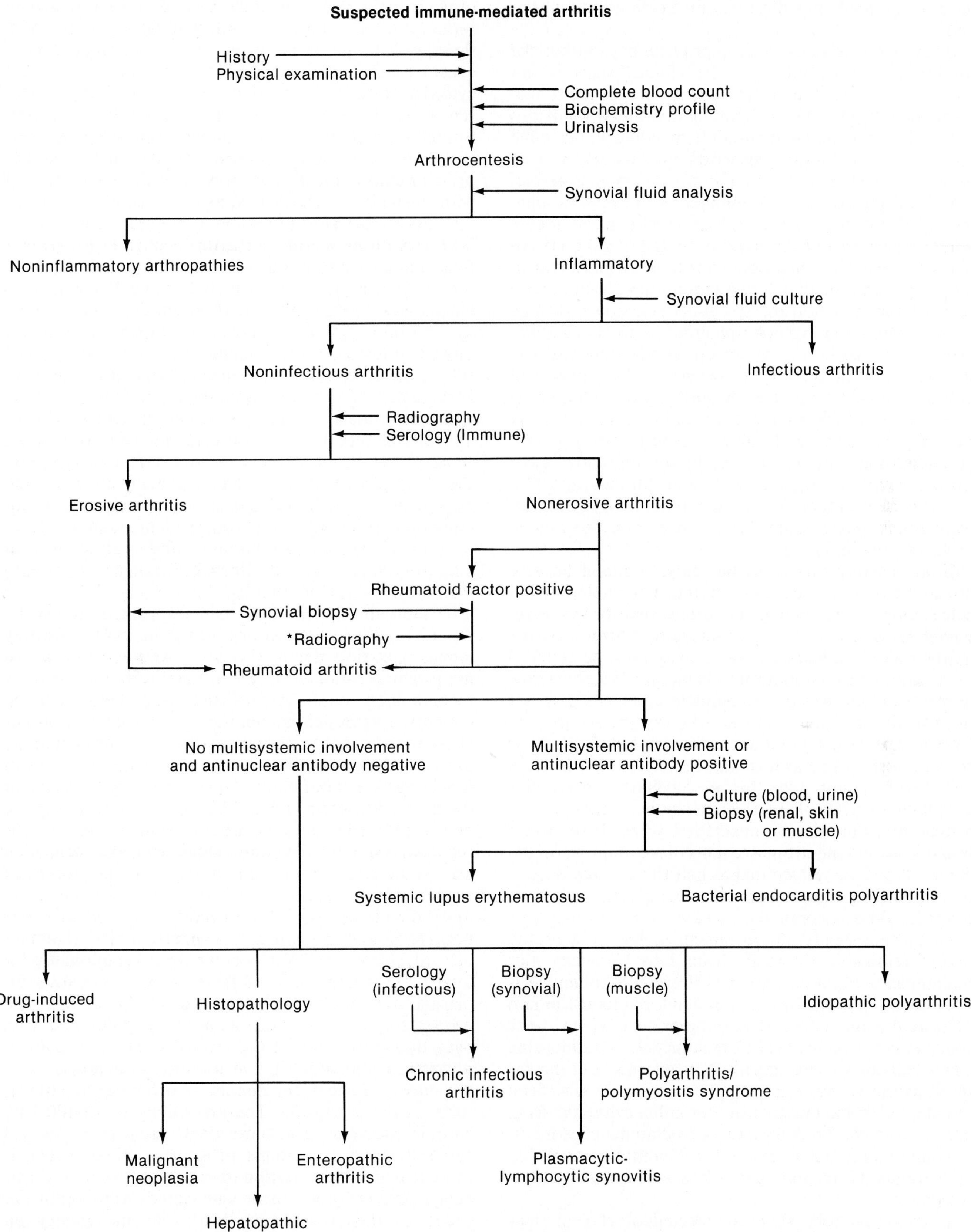

FIGURE 144–1. Algorithm for suspected immune-mediated arthritis. Ideally, synovial membrane biopsy samples are taken and subjected to histological and immunofluorescence examinations to differentiate between immune-mediated arthritides and RA. However, RA is rare, and the pathological changes for the various types of immune-mediated nonerosive arthritides are similar. Synovial fluid analysis is as informative. The exceptions are suspected bacterial endocarditis, polyarthritis, and plasmacytic-lymphocytic synovitis.

*Serial radiographic evaluations of affected joints may be necessary in some cases of rheumatoid arthritis (RA) because evidence of bony destruction may not be apparent for weeks to months.

been maintained after this time, medication is discontinued.

If, after the second week, improvement in either the joint fluid abnormalities or the clinical signs is not substantial, combination therapy (glucocorticoid and cytotoxic drug) is started. Combination therapy can also be used as the initial treatment, avoiding undesirable effects from high-dose glucocorticoid therapy. It may also be used when more rapid improvement is desirable. I prefer a glucocorticoid combined with cyclophosphamide. The dosage of cyclophosphamide is 50 mg/m^2 body surface area given orally once daily on 4 consecutive days or on alternate days for a week. This constitutes one cycle of therapy. Azathioprine (Imuran) can be used for induction therapy, but remission may take longer than when cyclophosphamide is used. Azathioprine is less toxic and preferred for the few cases in which long-term therapy is necessary. The dosage of azathioprine is 50 mg/m^2 body surface area given orally once daily. Chlorambucil (Leukeran, 2 mg/m^2 body surface area daily) and 6-mercaptopurine (Purinethol, 50 mg/m^2 body surface area daily) are alternative cytotoxic drugs that have met with some success.[49] A glucocorticoid is administered simultaneously with cytotoxic drugs at the same dosage or at half the dosage outlined previously.

Bone marrow toxicity is the most common adverse effect of the cytotoxic drugs. Therefore, complete blood cell counts are recommended every week or two until complete remission is achieved. Cytotoxic drugs, particularly cyclophosphamide, occasionally must be reduced or discontinued temporarily owing to bone marrow suppression, even though complete remission has not been achieved. The cytotoxic drug dose is reduced by 25 per cent if the white blood cell count falls to 6,000/μl or the platelet count is less than 125,000/μl. If the white blood cell count falls below 5,000/μl (neutrophils <2,500/μl) or the platelet count below 100,000/μl, cytotoxic drugs are discontinued for 1 week. If the white blood cell and neutrophil counts have improved, the cytotoxic drug is reinstituted at half the original dose.

Combined immunosuppressive therapy at the highest tolerable dose is continued as long as active disease is present and steady improvement is seen. The time before remission can range from 2 to 16 weeks. For maintenance therapy, the dose of cyclophosphamide is not changed and therapy is extended for at least 1 month after remission. However, azathioprine is given every other day at the dose used for induction. Azathioprine can usually be alternated with a glucocorticoid (1 mg/kg) on consecutive days. If complete remission has been maintained at the end of 1 or 2 months, cytotoxic drugs are withdrawn. Prednisolone, at maintenance dose, is continued for 2 to 3 more months. If complete remission is maintained after this time, the glucocorticoid is withdrawn.

If abnormal joint fluid is detected or clinical signs reappear during maintenance therapy, remission may be re-established by using combined immunosuppressive drug therapy. It has been my experience that abnormal joint fluid usually precedes clinical signs and consists predominantly of mononuclear cells. Thus, active disease or relapse is not ruled out by finding fewer numbers of neutrophils than detected on initial presentation. The same cytotoxic drug can be selected again for induction therapy. Therapy is adjusted, as previously described, except that maintenance therapy of prednisolone and cytotoxic drugs is extended for 3 to 4 months after remission. Periodic urine cultures (monthly) are performed during long-term immunosuppressive therapy. If therapy is necessary for more than 5 months, azathioprine or chlorambucil is used. Neither drug is associated with sterile hemorrhagic cystitis and is rarely associated with bone marrow suppression at maintenance dose.

Dogs with idiopathic polyarthritis have been successfully treated with prednisolone and auranofin. The recommended dosage is 0.05 to 0.2 mg/kg PO BID to a maximum of 9 mg/day. Renal (proteinuria), hematological (thrombocytopenia, hemolytic anemia), dermatological (pruritus, rash, stomatitis), and gastrointestinal side effects may develop during chrysotherapy with auranofin.[34, 56] Therefore, a complete blood count, platelet count, urinalysis, and serum creatinine determination are recommended to monitor drug-induced side effects. Watery diarrhea was the only side effect observed in the dogs described. The diarrhea resolved when the dosage of auranofin was lowered or withdrawn. Combination therapy with auranofin (Ridaura), an oral form of gold therapy (chrysotherapy), and a glucocorticoid may provide a safe and effective alternative to combination cytotoxic drug therapy.[56]

The prognosis for idiopathic polyarthritis is usually favorable. Glucocorticoid therapy alone can successfully induce remission in many cases.[8, 49] Patients not responding to glucocorticoid therapy usually respond favorably to combined immunosuppressive drug therapy. In all patients, recurrence is common (30 per cent to 50 per cent) for a variable period of time after drug therapy has been discontinued. Treatment for indefinite periods is necessary in about half of these patients with recurrent disease. The prognosis for SLE is guarded, depending on the extent of the systemic involvement, and poor if renal involvement develops. Dogs with SLE can often achieve long-term remission on alternate-day therapy of a glucocorticoid, and some may achieve long-term remission without drugs. Prolonged therapy for an ANA-positive dog in remission is unsubstantiated. Humans with SLE may be ANA positive and asymptomatic for long periods without drug therapy. The prognosis for plasmacytic-lymphocytic synovitis is favorable with proper surgical repair to stabilize the joint and with drug therapy to control the synovitis. The prognosis of polyarthritis/polymyositis syndrome is guarded. The presence of concurrent muscle involvement apparently worsens the prognosis. The arthritides associated with chronic infectious, gastrointestinal, and hepatic diseases generally have a favorable prognosis, although relapse can occur if the underlying disease is not resolved. The prognosis for those cases associated with neoplastic processes depends on the particular malignancy involved, but the prognosis is usually poor.

CANINE EROSIVE ARTHRITIS

Canine RA is a chronic progressive inflammatory joint disease characterized by erosive, destructive changes within the joints. The cause is unknown, although the disease is regarded as an immune-mediated polyarthropathy. Both cellular and immune (types II, III, and IV hypersensitivity) interactions are involved in the pathogenesis of the joint inflammation and destruction.[61, 66, 67] The synovitis is probably caused by immune complex (type III) reactions involving an unidentified antigen complex with specific antibodies, RF, and complement.[67] Immune complexes isolated from RA effusions are composed almost entirely of RFs (anti-IgG) of the IgG and IgM classes.[63] The IgG-RFs seem to be particularly important because they can activate complement and stimulate monocytes to release prostaglandins and mononuclear cell factors. In turn, mononuclear cell factors stimulate collagenase and prostaglandin production by synovial cells.[43, 63] Therefore, these unique antibodies (IgG-RFs) can contribute to inflammation and destruction in RA. In dogs, RA is a rare form of joint disease affecting predominantly medium and small breeds, with no apparent sex predilection.[2, 9, 44, 47] The onset of clinical signs in dogs ranges from 8 months to 13 years, although most dogs are between 4 and 7 years.[2, 9, 44, 47]

Polyarthritis of greyhounds has been described as a specific entity for which the cause and pathogenesis are unknown.[27] It has been subclassified as an immune-mediated erosive polyarthropathy.[49] However, this polyarthritis most closely resembles idiopathic nonerosive polyarthritis (negative serological and microbiological examinations) with evidence of severe cartilage degeneration. The cartilage changes described were often seen in the absence of pannus formation; however, pannus at the margins of the joints was often present but not as extensive as in RA.[27] Subchondral bone was only minimally affected, and erosion at the margins of the articular surfaces was noted to a limited extent.[27] In addition, idiopathic nonerosive polyarthritis has been described in a greyhound.[6] *Mycoplasma spumans* was isolated from the joint fluid of a young greyhound with polyarthritis.[4] The type of inflammatory arthropathy observed in greyhounds remains to be determined, as well as any predisposition in this breed. The remainder of this section pertains to RA in dogs.

Clinical Presentation

Canine RA is characterized by a shifting leg lameness and generalized stiffness, particularly after rest. The onset of lameness is usually gradual. The clinical manifestations can be episodic or intermittent and increase in frequency and duration with each relapse. Simultaneous involvement of multiple joints is present in most cases, generally in a bilaterally symmetrical fashion. Some dogs have difficulty in walking and exhibit an inability to sit or lie down without extreme discomfort or effort. In addition to lameness, signs of systemic illness are observed and include fever, lethargy, and inappetence/anorexia. In chronic stages, signs of systemic illness are often absent. Persistent, progressive joint problems are the main complaint.

In the early stages of RA, fever and lymphadenopathy accompany signs of joint disease. The signs of joint disease include pain, effusion, and soft-tissue swelling within and around joints. Crepitation and reduction of joint motion are observed. Spinal pain is rarely detected. The most commonly affected joints differ slightly from the nonerosive arthritides and include the carpus, stifle, elbow, hip, and tarsus.[2, 9, 14, 44, 47] However, the most severely affected joints are the carpal, tarsal, and interphalangeal joints. Joint instability with angular deformity and degenerative changes develops with chronicity. Generalized muscle atrophy may be evident. Subcutaneous nodules (rheumatoid nodules), a distinguishing feature of RA in humans, are rarely noted in dogs.[9]

Clinical Pathology

Hematological changes are usually not specific and include low-grade anemia (normocytic, normochromic), elevated erythrocyte sedimentation rate, and fibrinogenemia. In general, the leukogram is normal and a few cases show leukocytosis or leukopenia.[9, 44, 47]

Although serum chemistry profiles are usually unremarkable, the albumin/globulin ratio is significantly lower in most dogs. Serum alkaline phosphatase and sometimes alanine transaminase and aspartate transaminase levels are elevated. Proteinuria may be detected; otherwise, the results of the urinalysis are negative.

Synovial fluid samples are generally discolored (yellow) and turbid. Excessive amounts of synovial fluid may be present. Fibrin clot test results can be positive, and viscosity is usually decreased. The mucin clot is typically poor and friable. Total nucleated cell counts are increased (average, 30,000/μl; range, 6,000 to 85,000/μl), with a predominance of neutrophilic leukocytes (average, 75 per cent; range, 20 to 95 per cent).[9] Degenerative neutrophils and free nuclear material are regularly noted. Cytoplasmic inclusions (phagocytized immune complexes) in macrophages and neutrophils (ragocytes) are commonly seen in humans with RA but rarely in dogs. Microbiological examinations (bacterial, *Mycoplasma* spp.) of synovial fluid and synovial membrane are negative.

The incidence of positive RF tests in canine RA ranges from 25 to 70 per cent, depending on the sensitivity of the specific test system.[9, 47, 61, 65] The titers of RF in dogs with RA are also comparatively lower than in humans. The methods for detecting RF reflect the presence of IgM antibody (IgM-RF), the most common RF in humans with RA. In canine RA, the predominant RF is IgG (IgG-RF).[65] This may explain, in part, the high prevalence of seronegative RA in dogs. The presence of RF is not specific for canine RA. Any chronic disease, infectious (bacterial endocarditis) or noninfectious, associated with persistent antigen exposure and immune complex production, can potentially result in low positive titers.[61] Moreover, significant titers of RF have been detected in 5 per cent of the normal dog population.[44] Most dogs with RA are negative for FANA. An insignificant FANA titer can be found in some dogs as well as humans without excluding the diagnosis of RA.[9, 47, 52]

Radiographic Findings

The earliest radiographic findings include joint capsule distension and periarticular swelling. The most significant and characteristic radiographic feature of RA is the presence of bony erosions or loss of trabecular bone density in the epiphyses or individual bones (carpus, patella, sesamoids) of the joints.[9, 14, 44, 47] The destructive lesions are progressive and occur in the subchondral or juxta-articular bone. These features are seen radiographically as poorly demarcated or discrete ("punched-out") radiolucent foci of various sizes. The carpal, stifle, metacarpo/metatarsophalangeal, and tarsal joints are frequently affected.[9, 14, 44, 47] In some early cases, it may be weeks or months before radiographic evidence of bone destruction appears. Changes in joint spaces (widening or narrowing) may be apparent. In advanced stages, subluxation, luxation, and ankylosis are seen radiographically. The joint instability, as a result of cartilage, ligament, and capsular damage, may also lead to secondary degenerative joint disease.

Histopathology and Immunopathology

Gross examination of affected joints shows a discolored and proliferated synovium and loss of articular cartilage.[9, 54] Histologically, the synovitis is characterized by hyperplasia of superficial synovial cells, fibrin deposits, villus hypertrophy, and a marked inflammatory infiltrate dispersed throughout the supporting layer of the synovium. The infiltrate consists predominantly of lymphocytes and plasma cells with macrophages. Neutrophilic cell infiltrates are usually sparse, but they may be a more prominent feature in some cases of canine RA.[54] Excessive granulation tissue arising from the synovium may extend over and attach to the articular surface (pannus formation) or infiltrate under cartilage and subchondral bone. Pannus and infiltration of cartilage and subchondral bone lead to erosion of the articular cartilage at the margins of affected joints. Immunofluorescence examination shows fibrin deposits and deposits of immunoglobulins and complement within macrophages.[9]

Diagnosis

No single test can diagnose canine RA, including the presence of RFs in the blood. The diagnostic criteria for RA in humans should be applied to canine RA (Table 144–2) until in-depth studies of dogs are available.[9, 47, 53] In dogs, only the *classic* (seven criteria) and *definite* (five criteria) forms of RA are diagnosed. Criteria 1 through 5 are nonspecific and compatible with many nonerosive immune-mediated arthritides. It is recommended that at least two of criteria 7, 8, and 10 should be satisfied as well. These criteria are the most differentiating in RA. Furthermore, the diagnosis of canine RA is substantiated by exclusion of other causes of inflammatory polyarthritis.

TABLE 144–2. CRITERIA FOR THE DIAGNOSIS OF CANINE RHEUMATOID ARTHRITIS

1. Stiffness after rest
2. Pain or tenderness in at least one joint
3. Swelling in at least one joint
4. Swelling of at least one other joint within 3 months
5. Symmetrical joint swelling
6. Subcutaneous nodules over bony prominences or extensor surfaces or in juxta-articular regions
7. Destructive radiographic changes typical of rheumatoid arthritis
8. Positive agglutination test for serum rheumatoid factor
9. Poor mucin precipitate from synovial fluid
10. Characteristic histopathological changes in the synovial membrane
11. Characteristic histopathological changes in nodules

Classic rheumatoid arthritis is diagnosed when seven of the criteria are satisfied. *Definite* rheumatoid arthritis is diagnosed when five of the criteria are satisfied. Arthritis manifestations, criteria 1 through 5, must be present for at least 6 weeks.

*Data from the American Rheumatoid Association for the diagnosis of rheumatoid arthritis in human beings.[53]

Treatment

In human beings, RA is without specific therapy, and treatment with various drugs remains empirical.[32] Aspirin and other nonsteroidal anti-inflammatory drugs, considered the first line of therapy in human RA, are ineffective or palliative at high dosages (25 to 35 mg/kg every 8 hours) in dogs.[9, 44, 45, 47] This is probably because most dogs with RA have advanced disease at the time of diagnosis, and their clinical course is rapidly progressive. The use of systemic corticosteroids as a single agent may provide dramatic initial improvement, but this response usually cannot be sustained even at higher doses. If articular erosions have already occurred, most humans with RA require combined-drug treatment with gold or antimalarial (hydroxychloroquine) drug therapy.[32] Controlled trials have established the effectiveness of methotrexate and sulfasalazine in humans.[49a] The efficacy of these drugs for the treatment of RA in dogs has not been established, with the exception of gold. Gold salt therapy, alone or in combination with prednisolone, has been effective in some cases of canine RA.[9, 45] The recommended dose of gold sodium thiomalate (Myochrysine) and aurothioglucose (Solganol) is 1 mg/kg/week IM.[34] Although anaphylactic reactions in treated dogs have not been observed, a test dose (0.25 mg/kg) of gold salt is recommended before a therapeutic dose. As with oral gold therapy, dogs receiving parenteral gold should be monitored for signs of kidney dysfunction and hematological abnormalities at least every 2 weeks. If clinical improvement is observed, gold can be tapered by decreasing the frequency of administration and maintaining the same dose of 1 mg/kg. One major disadvantage of chrysotherapy is the delay (6 to 12 weeks) in apparent clinical improvement.[34, 45] Humans with refractory RA are candidates for immunosuppressive drug therapy, particularly cyclophosphamide or azathioprine. If severe joint damage is not already present, combination drug therapy with cyclophosphamide and prednisolone may be effective in controlling RA in some dogs.[47]

Unfortunately, the prognosis for canine RA is poor. The most common cause of death is euthanasia.[61] Clinical remission in most dogs is incomplete, and lameness, particularly stiffness, persists. In a few cases, the joint disease does not progress and remains static. Despite therapy, most dogs develop progressive joint disease leading to various degrees of instability and ankylosis and eventually to deformity and incapacitation.

References

1. Aho K, et al: HL-A 27 in reactive arthritis following infection. *Ann Rheum Dis 34* (Suppl 1):29, 1975.
2. Alexander JW, et al: Rheumatoid arthritis in the dog: Clinical diagnosis and management. *J Am Anim Hosp Assoc 12*:727, 1976.
3. Armstrong PJ, Dibartola SP: Canine coccidioidomycosis: A literature review and report of eight cases. *J Am Anim Hosp Assoc 19*:937, 1983.
4. Barton MD, et al: Isolation of *Mycoplasma spumans* from polyarthritis in a greyhound. *Aust Vet J 62*:206, 1985.
5. Bellah JR, et al: *Ehrlichia canis*-related polyarthritis in a dog. *J Am Vet Med Assoc 189*:922, 1986.
6. Bennett D: Joint disease. *In* Chandler EA, et al (eds): *Canine Medicine and Therapeutics*. 2nd ed. Blackwell Scientific Publications, Oxford, 1984, pp 167–205.
7. Bennett D: Naturally occurring models of inflammatory polyarthropathies in the domestic dog and cat. *Br J Clin Pract 40*:3, 1986.
8. Bennett D: Immune-based non-erosive inflammatory joint disease of the dog. 3. Canine idiopathic polyarthritis. *J Small Anim Pract 28*:909, 1987.
9. Bennett D: Immune-based erosive inflammatory joint disease of the dog: Canine rheumatoid arthritis. *J Small Anim Pract 28*:779, 1987.
10. Bennett D: Immune-based non-erosive inflammatory joint disease of the dog. 1. Canine systemic lupus erythematosus. *J Small Anim Pract 28*:871, 1987.
11. Bennett D, Kelly DF: Immune-based non-erosive inflammatory joint disease of the dog. 2. Polyarthritis/polymyositis syndrome. *J Small Anim Pract 28*:891, 1987.
12. Bennett D, Taylor DJ: Bacterial endocarditis and inflammatory joint disease in the dog. *J Small Anim Pract 29*:347, 1987.
13. Bennett D, et al: Bacterial endocarditis with polyarthritis in two dogs associated with circulating autoantibodies. *J Small Anim Pract 19*:185, 1978.
14. Biery DN, Newton CD: Radiographic appearance of rheumatoid arthritis in the dog. *J Am Anim Hosp Assoc 11*:607, 1975.
15. Bowen GE, Kirsner JB: The arthritis of ulcerative colitis and regional enteritis. *Med Clin North Am 49*:17, 1965.
16. Calvert CA, Greene CE: Bacteremia in dogs: Diagnosis, treatment and prognosis. *Comp Cont Educ Pract Vet 8*:179, 1986.
17. Cowell RL, et al: Ehrlichiosis and polyarthritis in three dogs. *J Am Vet Med Assoc 192*:1093, 1988.
18. Drazner FH: Systemic lupus erythematosus in the dog. *Comp Cont Educ Pract Vet 2*:243, 1980.
19. Giger U, et al: Sulfadiazine-induced allergy in six doberman pinschers. *J Am Vet Med Assoc 186*:479, 1985.
20. Greene RT, et al: Clinical and serologic evaluations of induced *Borrelia burgdorferi* infection in dogs. *Am J Vet Res 49*:752, 1988.
21. Grindem CB, Johnson KH: Systemic lupus erythematosus: Literature review and report of 42 new canine cases. *J Am Anim Hosp Assoc 19*:489, 1983.
22. Hardy RM, Wallace LJ: Arthrocentesis and synovial membrane biopsy. *Vet Clin North Am Small Anim Pract 4*:449, 1974.
23. Harvey RG: Sterile polyarthritis in Weimaraners following administration of sulfadiazine-trimethoprim for pyoderma. *Vet Rec 120*:537, 1987.
24. Hess EV (ed): Drug-induced lupus. Proceedings of the Kroc Foundation Conference. *Arthritis Rheum 24*:979, 1981.
25. Hibler SC, et al: Rickettsial infections in dogs. Part I. Rocky Mountain spotted fever and Coxiella infection. *Comp Cont Educ Pract Vet 10*:856, 1985.
26. Hopper PE, Vasseur PB: Feline immune-mediated inflammatory joint disease: A study of 23 cases. Submitted *Am J Vet Intern Med*, 1992
27. Huxtable CR, Davis PE: The pathology of polyarthritis in young greyhounds. *J Comp Pathol 86*:11, 1976.
28. Kornblatt AN, et al: Arthritis caused by *Borrelia burgdorferi* in dogs. *J Am Vet Med Assoc 186*:960, 1985.
29. Lewis RM: Evidence for a virus in canine systemic lupus erythematosus. *In* Glynn LE, Schlamberger HD (eds): *Experimental Models of Chronic Inflammatory Diseases*. Springer-Verlag, New York, 1977, p 71.
30. Lewis RM, Schwartz RS: Canine systemic lupus erythematosus. Genetic analysis of an established breeding colony. *J Exp Med 134*:417, 1971.
31. Lewis RM, et al: Canine systemic lupus erythematosus. Transmission of serologic abnormalities by cell-free filtrates. *J Clin Invest 52*:1893, 1973.
32. Lightfoot RW: Treatment of rheumatoid arthritis. *In* McCarty DJ (ed): *Arthritis and Allied Conditions*. 11th ed. Lea & Febiger, Philadelphia, 1989, pp 772–782.
33. Lissman BA, et al: Spirochete-associated arthritis (Lyme disease) in a dog. *J Am Vet Med Assoc 185*:219, 1984.
34. Long RE: Potential of chrysotherapy in veterinary medicine. *J Am Vet Med Assoc 188*:539, 1986.
35. Maddison PJ, et al: Serologic findings in patients with "ANA-negative" systemic lupus erythematosus. *Medicine 60*:87, 1981.
36. Magnarelli LA, et al: Clinical and serologic studies of canine borreliosis. *J Am Vet Med Assoc 191*:1089, 1987.
37. Miller JB, et al: Synovial fluid analysis in canine arthritis *J Am Anim Hosp Assoc 10*:393, 1974.
38. Mills PR, Sturrock RD: Clinical associations between arthritis and liver disease. *Ann Rheum Dis 41*:295, 1982.
39. Moll JM: Inflammatory bowel disease. *Clin Rheum Dis 11*:87, 1985.
40. Monier JC, et al: Antibody to soluble nuclear antigens in dogs (German shepherds) with a lupus-like syndrome. *Dev Comp Immunol 2*:161, 1978.
41. Monier JC, et al: Clinical and laboratory features of canine lupus syndromes. *Arthritis Rheum 23*:294, 1980.
42. Montgomery RD, et al: Comparison of aerobic culturette, synovial membrane biopsy, and blood culture medium in detection of canine bacterial arthritis. *Vet Surg 18*:300, 1989.
43. Nardella FA, et al: Self-associating IgG rheumatoid factors stimulate monocytes to release prostaglandins and mononuclear cell factor that stimulates collagenase and prostaglandin production by synovial cells. *Rheumatol Int 3*:183, 1983.
44. Newton CD, et al: Rheumatoid arthritis in dogs. *J Am Vet Med Assoc 168*:113, 1976.
45. Newton CD, et al: Gold salt therapy for rheumatoid arthritis in dogs. *J Am Vet Med Assoc 174*:1308, 1979.
46. Niebauer GW, Menzel EJ: Immunological changes in canine cruciate ligament rupture. *Res Vet Sci 32*:235, 1982.
47. Pedersen NC, et al: Noninfectious canine arthritis: Rheumatoid arthritis. *J Am Vet Med Assoc 169*:295, 1976.
48. Pedersen NC, et al: Noninfectious canine arthritis: The inflammatory, nonerosive arthritides. *J Am Vet Med Assoc 169*:304, 1976.
49. Pedersen NC, et al: Joint diseases of dogs and cats. *In* Ettinger SJ (ed): *Textbook of Veterinary Internal Medicine Diseases*. 3rd ed. W.B. Saunders, Philadelphia, 1989, pp 2329–2377.

49a. Pinals RS, et al: Sulfasalazine in rheumatoid arthritis. A double-blind placebo-controlled trial. *Arthritis Rheum 29*:84, 1981.

50. Provost TT, Reichlin M: Antinuclear antibody-negative systemic lupus erythematosus. *J Am Acad Dermatol 4*:84, 1981.
51. Quimby FW, et al: Characterization of a retrovirus that cross reacts serologically with canine and human systemic lupus erythematosus. *Clin Immunol Immunopathol 9*:194, 1978.
52. Rochmis PG, et al: Native DNA binding in rheumatoid arthritis. *Ann Rheum Dis 33*:357, 1974.
53. Ropes MW, et al: 1958 Revision of diagnostic criteria for rheumatoid arthritis. *Ann Rheum Dis 33*:357, 1974.
54. Schumacher HR, et al: Synovial pathologic changes in spontaneous canine rheumatoid-like arthritis. *Arthritis Rheum 23*:412, 1980.
55. Scott VW, et al: Canine lupus erythematosus. 1. Systemic lupus erythematosus. *J Am Anim Hosp Assoc 19*:481, 1983.
56. Serra DA, White SD: Oral chrysiotherapy with auranofin in dogs. *J Am Vet Med Assoc 194*:1327, 1989.
57. Stockham SL, et al: Canine granulocytic ehrlichiosis in dogs from central Missouri: A possible cause of polyarthritis. *Vet Med Rev 6*:3, 1985.
58. Tan EM, et al: Revised criteria for the classification of systemic lupus erythematosus. *Arthritis Rheum 25*:1271, 1982.

58a. Tugwell P, et al: Methotrexate in rheumatoid arthritis. *Ann Intern Med 110*:581, 1989.

58b. Weinblatt ME, et al: Efficacy of low-dose methotrexate in rheumatoid arthritis. *N Engl J Med 312*:818, 1985.

59. Werner LL: Arthrocentesis and joint fluid analysis: Diagnostic applications in joint diseases of small animals. *Comp Cont Educ Pract Vet 1*:855, 1979.
60. Werner LL, Bright JM: Drug-induced immune hypersensitivity disorders in two dogs treated with trimethoprim-sulfadiazine: Case reports and drug challenge studies. *J Am Anim Hosp Assoc 19*:783, 1983.
61. Werner LL, Halliwell REW: Diseases associated with autoimmunity. *In* Chandler EA, et al (eds): *Canine Medicine and Therapeutics*. 2nd ed. Oxford, Blackwell Scientific Publications, 1984, p 270.
62. Wilkins RJ, et al: Immunological mediated thrombocytopenia in the dog. *J Small Anim Pract 29*:347, 1980.
63. Winchester RJ: Characterization of IgG complexes in patients with rheumatoid arthritis. *Ann NY Acad Sci 256*:73, 1975.
64. Wolfe JH, Halliwell REW: Total hemolytic complement values in normal and diseased dog populations. *Vet Immunol Immunopathol 1*:287, 1980.
65. Wood DD, et al: A latex test for canine rheumatoid factor. *Vet Immunol Immunopathol 1*:103, 1980.
66. Zvaifler NJ: Etiology and pathogenesis of rheumatoid arthritis. *In* McCarty DJ (ed): *Arthritis and Allied Conditions*. 11th ed. Lea & Febiger, Philadelphia, 1989, pp 659–673.
67. Zvaifler NJ: Rheumatoid synovitis. An extravascular immune complex disease. *Arthritis Rheum 17*:297, 1974.

CHAPTER

145

Other Orthopedic Diseases

Hip Dysplasia in Dogs

George Lust

Malformation of the hip in dogs, or canine hip dysplasia, is a developmental not a congenital disorder of the coxofemoral joints. The disease is a serious medical problem because hip osteoarthritis, restricted joint mobility, pain, and lameness are associated with it. A similar disease occurs in humans, gorillas, bears, horses, cattle, and cats. However, hip dysplasia is most prevalent among dogs. It is particularly common in large breeds such as Saint Bernards, Alaskan malamutes, bulldogs, boxers, collies, Doberman pinschers, rottweilers, German shepherds, golden retrievers, huskies, Labrador retrievers, Old English sheepdogs, pointers, and standard poodles, but the smaller breeds are not spared. Perhaps the smaller dogs, as well as cats, have less stress on their joints and thus have no obvious symptoms. Dogs and bitches are affected with similar frequency, although one study[12] identified more females with the disease.

The etiopathogenesis of hip dysplasia in dogs is not well understood and has been frustrating to study. Research during the past 20 years has not elucidated the essential nature of the disease. A genetic basis has been identified, but the pattern of inheritance is multifactorial not simple mendelian genetics. Because diagnosis based on pelvic radiography can accurately identify the presence or absence of the abnormality only in adults, control of canine hip dysplasia has been limited. Because of ignorance about the pathogenesis and the lack of a specific early marker, a precise breeding program for control of canine hip dysplasia is not available.

Several other reviews can be consulted for other perspectives.[23, 28, 37, 40] The focus of this chapter is on the pathogenesis of hip dysplasia; a discussion of therapy for hip dysplasia or osteoarthritis is not included here (see Chapters 135 and 143).

CLINICAL SIGNS AND DIAGNOSIS

Clinical Signs

Decreased activity and various degrees of joint pain are early manifestations. These signs are often first observed between the ages of 4 months and 1 year. Young dogs can have a swaying and unsteady gait. They may draw their hindlimbs forward, perhaps to redistribute some weight to their forelegs. Affected dogs often run with both hindlegs moving together, the so-called gait of bunny hopping.

As the disease progresses, a dog may have difficulty in rising from a sitting or lying position, and stairs are difficult to climb. Affected dogs may exhibit pain when an affected hip joint is manipulated. In most cases, pain limits movement of the joint. The disease is progressive and can be crippling, but some dogs have little apparent discomfort despite abnormalities in their joints. Running and intense activity aggravate the condition and can reveal signs of the disease.

Radiography

Observation and physical examination can arouse suspicion of hip dysplasia; however, the diagnosis of hip dysplasia is established by radiographic examination with the dog under general anesthesia or deep sedation to ensure proper positioning. A ventrodorsal pelvic radiograph is made with the dog's hindlimbs extended to their maximum position, with the femurs parallel to each other and to the spine.[28, 39] The patellae are superimposed over the sagittal plane of the femoral condyles of the stifle by rotating the stifles inward. The pelvis must be positioned symmetrically so that the obturator foramina appear of equal size. Radiographs taken with a dog in that standard position can reveal abnormalities that cannot be detected in other positions. Disease-free hip joints have well-formed femoral heads that fit congruently into the acetabula (Fig. 145–1*A*). In large dogs, the center of each femoral head should be located medial to the cranial edge of the acetabulum, and more than 50 per cent of the projected area of the femoral head should be shadowed by the dorsal rim of the acetabulum.[23, 28, 39]

Coxofemoral joints of pups that later become dysplastic appear structurally disease free at birth. It is not yet possible to conclude definitively that an abnormality does or does not exist in hip joints at birth, but none has been reported.[23, 28, 37] The initial radiographic diagnosis can sometimes be made as early as 10 to 12 weeks but frequently is made between 5 and 9 months of age (Fig. 145–2). Studies have provided data that the initial radiographic diagnosis of hip dysplasia is made most frequently at about 6 months of age in susceptible dogs.[16, 29] At this age, many dogs that appeared disease free on x-ray examination had intra-articular pathological changes.[29] By 1 year of age, 70 to 80 per cent of susceptible dogs have radiographic signs of dysplasia.

The joint is considered dysplastic when the femoral head conforms poorly to the acetabulum (Fig. 145–1*B*). Increased joint space is commonly observed, and structural abnormalities can be detected in the acetabula and femoral heads. Subluxation, or partial displacement, of the femoral heads from the acetabula is the hallmark of canine hip dysplasia. In early and radiographically mild forms of dysplasia, hip joints have some subluxation of femoral heads.[23] When the center of a femoral head is directly caudal to the cranial edge of the acetabulum, the severity of hip dysplasia is rated moderate; if dislocated further, the hip dysplasia is rated severe.[23, 25, 26]

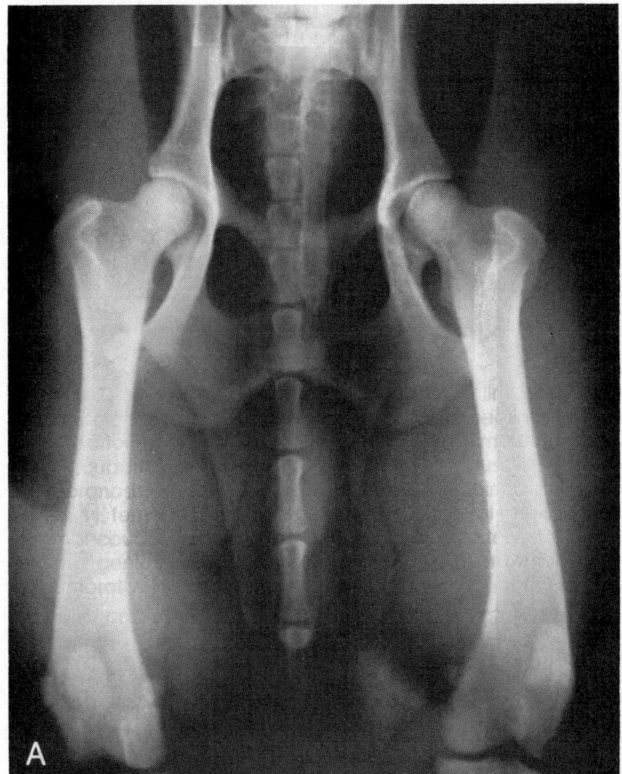

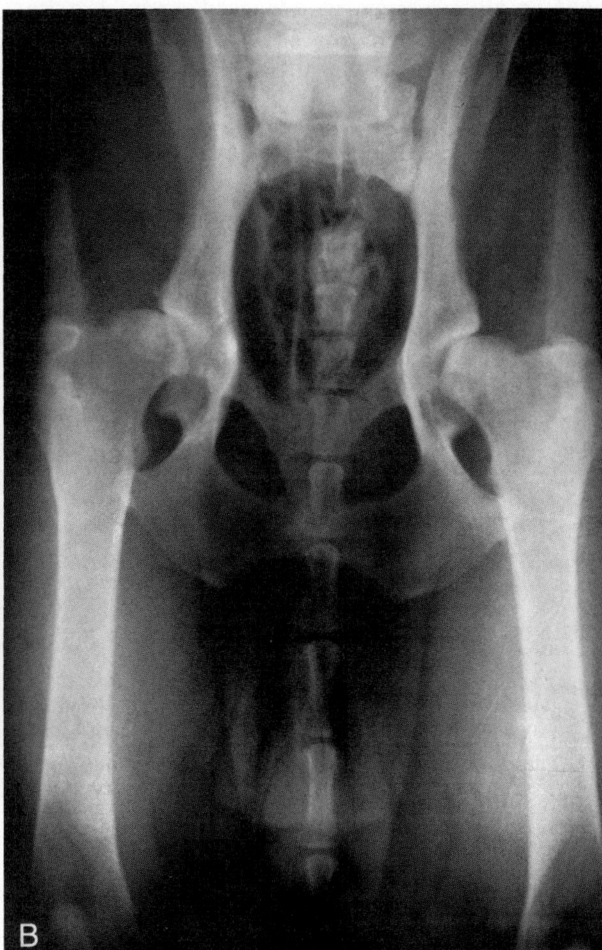

FIGURE 145–1. Pelvic radiographs taken in the legs-extended standard position. *A*, Three-year old male Labrador retriever with disease-free (also called *normal*) coxofemoral joints. Positioning was not ideal in that the patella of the left stifle was not properly rotated medially. Note that the centers of the femoral heads are medial to the cranial edge of the acetabula. *B*, Five-year old male Labrador retriever with advanced hip dysplasia. Note that the centers of the femoral heads are subluxated (partially displaced laterally); femoral heads and acetabula have bone proliferation (osteophytes) and remodeling.

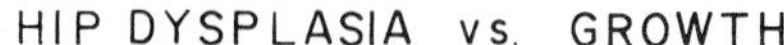

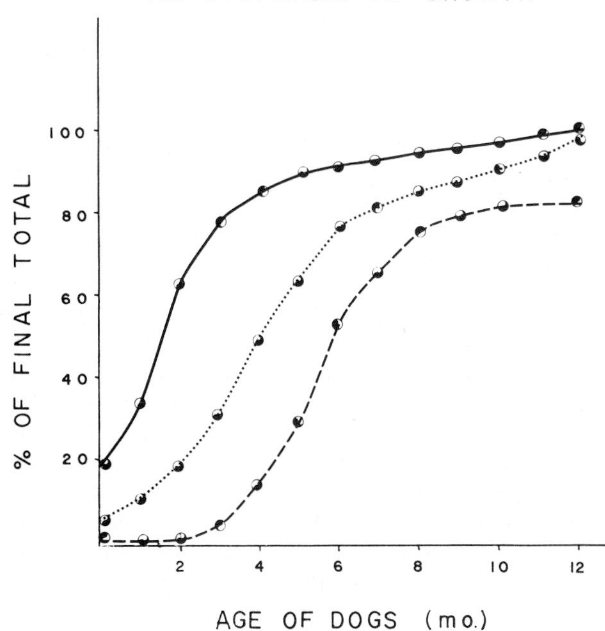

FIGURE 145–2. The relationship between weight gain, length of femurs, and the occurrence of hip dysplasia. A group of 55 Labrador retrievers from 11 litters of pups in which bitches and sires had hip dysplasia were examined. The data are presented as the percentage of each parameter versus age of the growing pups. The top (solid) line represents the average length of the femurs; the middle (dotted) line represents the average weight of the pups; and the lower curve *(broken line)* represents the percentage of dogs with hip dysplasia on standard pelvic radiographic examination.

Osteophytes are observed in advanced cases. Radiographic changes characteristic of hip dysplasia sometimes cannot be detected until a dog is 2 years old. The changes often are subtle and can be detected only by an experienced radiologist. In studies of German shepherds and Labrador retrievers, about 40 per cent of dogs disposed to hip dysplasia had radiographic evidence of dysplasia at 6 months of age, 70 to 80 per cent at 1 year of age, and about 90 per cent at 2 years.[16, 29] It is not known at what age the disease begins and whether asymptomatic changes occur in all dogs at about the same age, to be observed on a radiograph later. For practical purposes, canine hip dysplasia can be defined as radiographic evidence (dog in the standard hip extended position) of subluxation of the femoral heads at any age or the presence of subluxation and secondary bone changes in the region of the hip joint of a 2-year-old dog.

The conventional hip-extended position for radiographic examination is unnatural and exerts constraints on the joint capsule, the round ligament, and muscles, perhaps "tightening" some abnormal joints. It is because of this concern that another position was used[2, 35]; anesthetized dogs were placed with their hindlimbs nearly perpendicular to the tabletop, and a distraction force applied to the femurs. A different concern is that incipient disease may not be evident when the radiographic examination is performed on a young dog. Some consideration also should be given to the concept that canine hip dysplasia may be the most prominent manifestation of a disease affecting several joints and that examination of the hips alone does not disclose disease in other joints. About 15 per cent of adult dogs without visible lesions on radiographic examination had mild degenerative joint disease at necropsy.[29] It is unknown whether pelvic radiographs taken of dogs older than 2 years or even 3 years would be more useful in establishing a dog's disease-free status.

Joint Laxity

A characteristic feature of hip dysplasia is joint instability. An objective of research is to ascertain the role of joint laxity in the development of dysplastic hips. Laxity is the opposite of tightness. In the context of canine hip dysplasia, it refers to the degree of motility of the femoral head within the acetabulum and the joint capsule. According to conventional wisdom, laxity favors the development of hip dysplasia. The cause of increased laxity in the pathogenesis is unknown, but data suggested that the laxity is associated with mild synovitis and increases in the volume of the round ligament and synovial fluid.[23] Some anesthetized dogs have increased coxofemoral joint laxity on palpation but appear normal on radiographic examination.[23–26, 29, 35] An anatomical basis for this inconsistency has not been identified, but possible explanations include how precisely the animal is positioned, the force used during palpation, and depth of anesthesia.

Palpation for joint laxity in young dogs is not reliable to predict hip dysplasia.[24] Attempts to quantify the extent of hip joint laxity by measuring the distance of external displacement of the greater trochanter at palpation did not increase the usefulness of palpation.[23] Manipulation of a joint, or palpation, is a subjective procedure. An extension of the palpation method is the use of a distractive force, in conjunction with an object between the thighs to displace femoral heads during pelvic radiographic examination.[2, 13, 35] This approach is attractive and has been the subject of investigation.[2, 35] To estimate the extent of laxity, Smith and colleagues[35] measured the distance in millimeters between the center of the femoral head and the acetabulum. This was done by superimposing circle gauges on the cortical margins of the acetabulum and the femoral head to determine the respective geometric centers. Bellkoff and associates[2] measured the percentage of the femoral head medial to the cranial acetabular rim. Both of these quantitative measurements and the Norberg angle[25, 26] are useful in a number of situations when it is necessary to assess the extent of subluxation of femoral heads on pelvic radiographs. Preliminary data of Smith and colleagues[35] and of my own studies suggested that the hip joints of some pups appeared normal on the standard radiographs but had abnormal femoral head displacements by the new method and may later become dysplastic. The dogs must be observed for several years to determine whether those with greater joint laxity are, indeed, more susceptible to hip dysplasia than their counterparts with relatively tight joints. Although this concept appears reasonable to detect various degrees of joint laxity, the relationship between subluxation of a femoral head on a pelvic radiograph obtained in the conventional legs-extended position and the "forced" laxity with hind legs either extended or almost perpendicular to the table remains undefined, especially in young growing dogs. The exact relationship between increased laxity observed by the force methods and the other signs of disease, or the lack thereof, observed with the legs-extended position is unclear and needs to be explained. For this reason, the forced laxity procedures[2, 35] should be regarded as experimental and unproven. To establish their usefulness in hip dysplasia diagnosis, they require standardization and follow-up studies for correlation with the conventional pelvic radiographic method. If indeed the canine and human disease have a similar pathogenesis and if capsular and ligamentous laxity have a critical role in the progression of canine hip dysplasia, a method for measuring hip joint laxity in young dogs would be useful. In human pediatric orthopedic medicine, palpation for laxity and the Ortolani "click" have long been used to diagnose hip dysplasia in newborn infants.[38]

Blood-Based Diagnostic Test

An early blood marker for hip dysplasia clearly is a desirable goal. The attainment of such a test probably is not within the immediate reach of veterinary medical science because no clear-cut biochemical or metabolic difference between disease-free and dysplastic dogs has been identified. Some biochemical differences in the cartilage and synovial fluid of affected joints have been reported.[3, 4, 6] Despite extensive research,[20] a diagnostic blood test for the disease is not available.

The ability to predict development of hip dysplasia in

an individual dog would be useful in devising methods for early disease modification, for genetic screening and counseling, and eventually for prevention of the disease. Some progress has been made in describing genetic factors disposing human beings to rheumatoid arthritis[27] and to osteoarthritis.[18, 31] Restriction fragment length polymorphism (RFLP) linkage analysis has been used to identify the genes involved in the etiopathogenesis of these joint diseases. Because hip dysplasia in dogs has a strong genetic basis, it is plausible to reason that RFLP linkage analysis of the DNA from dogs susceptible to dysplasia can be used in that endeavor and thus facilitate identification of DNA fragments (DNA obtained from white blood cells) corresponding to the hip dysplasia phenotype.

NATURE OF DISEASE

Genetics

Hip dysplasia in dogs has a hereditary basis.[12, 14, 19, 21, 40] The pattern of inheritance suggests that more than one gene is involved, but the number is unknown. It is considered to be a polygenic or quantitative trait with the expression being determined by an interaction of genetic and environmental factors.[21] The practical implication is that breeding dogs for desirable traits such as good temperament or large size may result in the unwitting selection of animals susceptible to hip dysplasia. Many offspring of dogs with hip dysplasia also become dysplastic.[23] Likewise, sound dogs are more likely to be born to parents with disease-free hips.[12, 14, 19, 40] Thus, the incidence of hip dysplasia can be reduced by selecting for breeding only dogs that have disease-free hips as assessed by standard radiographic examination. Selective breeding has led to some decrease in occurrence, but the disease has not been eliminated.[5, 23, 40] A major problem is that we do not know the cause of hip dysplasia. Also, a dog with normal hip joints may have one or more characteristics that result in hip dysplasia only when they occur in concert with certain other characteristics in another dog, and it is well known that parents with phenotypically normal hips may have dysplastic progeny.[21, 22, 40] Many dogs used for breeding are not examined by pelvic radiography, and whether they are disease free or dysplastic is not known.

Many investigators involved with the genetics of this disease accept that hip dysplasia is a quantitative trait with a heritability of between 0.25 and 0.40.[12, 14, 19, 21, 40] The breeding records from German shepherds, Labrador retrievers, rottweilers, boxers, and golden retrievers have been examined, and it was concluded that dysplastic offspring can occur in any type of mating.[40] The more disease free the parents, the more normal, on average, were their progeny.[21, 22, 40] On a population basis, breeding normal males to normal females resulted in 64 to 81 per cent normal dogs and 19 to 36 per cent dysplastic offspring. For dysplastic-dysplastic matings, 7 to 37 per cent of offspring were normal and 63 to 93 per cent were dysplastic.[40] From these considerations, it cannot be concluded that such matings produce only disease-free offspring, even when both parents are free of hip dysplasia. Despite this uncertainty, it is advisable to breed only disease-free dogs to reduce the incidence and severity of hip dysplasia in the canine population.

Progression of Abnormalities in Hip Joints

The basic nature of hip dysplasia, as well as the identity of the tissues that are affected first and how the initial defect results in the development of the disease, is not clear. Coxofemoral joints of pups that later become dysplastic are structurally and functionally disease free at birth. No obvious anatomical abnormalities are found in the bones of the hip joints of growing dogs that are destined to develop hip dysplasia. For example, the occurrence of the disease is unrelated to the degree of inclination of the femoral head with reference to the shaft of the femur or the degree of rotation of the femoral head about the shaft of the femur—the "anteversion angle" (torsion angle).[1, 10, 11, 23] Formation of a disease-free hip joint does require close congruity between the femoral head and the acetabulum. When dysplasia develops, this fails to occur. Hip dysplasia in dogs is a developmental discontinuity of the femoral head and the acetabulum. This relationship between the articulating surfaces allows excessive movement of the femoral head. The effect is to damage, mildly inflame, and eventually weaken the hip joint. Early in the development of disease, the amount of synovial fluid is increased, and the round ligament that binds the femoral head to the acetabulum becomes hypertrophied. The normally smooth articular cartilage that covers the ends of bones to facilitate low-friction motion between surfaces deteriorates. Proliferative synovitis is present in the synovial lining cells, and the joint capsule becomes thickened.[23, 28, 29, 37] At this stage of the disease, often before radiographic evidence of joint disease is present, there is a direct relationship between the combined intra-articular volume (i.e., of the round ligament plus synovial fluid) and the extent of hip joint laxity.[25, 26] In more advanced stages of disease, synovitis and cartilage loss are increased, capsule thickening continues, bone changes occur and osteophytes form on the acetabulum and femoral head, and muscles in the region of the hip atrophy.[23, 28, 37]

It is likely that the pain associated with canine hip dysplasia in its early stages results from stretching or tearing of fibers in the joint capsule and the round ligament. The pain associated with advanced disease is that of osteoarthritis. Pain-sensing (nociceptive) fibers are present in the joint capsule, round ligament, fat pads, subsynovium, and periosteum. Articular cartilage is aneural.

Multiple Joint Involvement

Hip dysplasia, as the name implies, is usually considered to be an abnormality restricted to the tissues of the hip joints. Although pain and disability are often greatest in the hip joint, either unilaterally or bilaterally, several other joints also may be diseased in an affected dog. The vertebral joints, mandibular joints, stifle, shoulder, and elbow joints are frequently affected.[29] In one study of young dogs that were genetically disposed

TABLE 145–1. DEGENERATIVE JOINT DISEASE (OSTEOARTHRITIS) IN THREE JOINTS OF YOUNG AND ADULT DOGS

Group and Age	Hip Joints	Stifle Joints	Shoulder Joint	Multiple Joints Bilaterally –	Multiple Joints Bilaterally +
		Percentage of Dogs Affected			
A: 0.5 years ± 0.1 (n = 92)	71	22	38	40	67
B: 3.1 years ± 1.8 (n = 24)	88	38	29	54	83
C: 4.1 years ± 1.4 (n = 16)	63	25	50	38	56
D: 10.7 years ± 3.2 (n = 100)	52	36	37	32	70

Dogs in groups A, B, and C were Labrador retrievers; dogs in group D were represented by many different breeds. Disease in dogs of groups A, B, and D was substantiated at necropsy. Disease in group C dogs was diagnosed radiographically. Data are expressed as percentage of dogs with disease in that joint. Joints were classified as either disease free or osteoarthritic. Evidence of disease was as described by Olsewski and colleagues.[29] Multiple joints represented two or more joints per dog, either excluding (−) or including (+) dogs with the same joint affected bilaterally. The number of dogs examined in each group is listed in parenthesis.

to hip dysplasia, about 30 per cent also had pathological changes in the shoulder and stifle joints (Table 145–1). The changes including mild synovitis, increased synovial fluid volume, and degeneration of the articular cartilage appeared in some shoulder or stifle joints before intra-articular changes were observed in coxofemoral joints.[29] The occurrence of advanced osteoarthritic changes such as thickened capsules, osteophytes, and loss of cartilage in shoulder and in stifle joints of older dogs suggested that disease is progressive in these joints (see Table 145–1). The increased volume of synovial fluid and the mild synovitis in the shoulder joints of some of the young dogs would be expected to result in increased shoulder joint laxity similar to the increased laxity observed in hip joints. These observations taken together suggest that disease may develop intra-articularly in several joints including the hip and that hip dysplasia represents the most conspicuous sign of the disease. A possible explanation for the high frequency of hip involvement may be that coxofemoral joints with mild synovitis and increased volume of synovial fluid progress from inapparent increased laxity to subluxation of femoral heads on a radiograph because the hip joints have little horizontal support in weightbearing.[23, 29, 30]

Other considerations of possible relevance to hip dysplasia are consistent with multiple joint involvement. The hormones estrogen, growth hormone, insulin, and relaxin individually have been causally implicated as mediators of hip dysplasia.[32] Further studies will help to substantiate if one or more hormones has a role in hip dysplasia development. At this time, there is no compelling evidence to suggest that estrogens have such a role.[8, 36] However, in one study,[36] relaxin concentrations were increased in the blood and in the milk of postparturient dysplastic bitches compared with normal bitches. It is plausible to reason that if a hormone were involved in the pathogenesis of this disease, it would exert a systemic effect, and several joints would consequently be affected.

Growth Patterns

Several reports in the literature suggested that the development of hip dysplasia can be influenced by food consumption. Nutritional supplements have no proven benefit. Investigators have proposed that the time of appearance and the rate of progression of hip dysplasia can be affected by the rate of weight gain of a dog.[9, 22, 24, 33] Weight gain as a result of increased food consumption accelerated; conversely, slowing weight gain by reducing food during the first several months of life delayed the appearance or diminished the severity of dysplasia. These conclusions on the relationship between food consumption and hip dysplasia development were based on preliminary studies using a relatively small number of animals per trial, and the statistical significance of the data was not assessed.

A study using 48 growing pups provided data that strongly supported the concept that retarded weight gain of pups as a result of restricted food consumption significantly decreased the extent of subluxation of femoral heads in those dogs eating the restricted amount of diet.[17] Twenty-four of the dogs were fed 25 per cent less food from 8 weeks of age to 2 years. The results were statistically significant ($P<0.05$) and implied that restricted food consumption lessened the severity of hip dysplasia and even prevented its occurrence.[17]

It has been proposed[21, 22] that susceptible dogs made "normal" by dietary restriction would in effect have "masked" the disease and can yield dysplastic progeny. It was reasoned that radiographically normal dogs possibly carrying the undesired genes for hip dysplasia can be identified by using high food consumption.[22] The strategy is to force the expression of dysplasia in pups being considered for breeding by stimulating food consumption and possibly other practices. The concept is that such a procedure can reveal the potential for disease in apparently disease-free parents.

Role of the Acetabulum

A "shallow" acetabulum on radiographic examination has been reported to be associated with hip dysplasia.[23, 28, 30, 37] Neither a temporal sequence for the shallow acetabulum in dysplasia development nor a cause for it in the first place has been established. However, in a preliminary study in my laboratory, this subject was examined using Labrador retrievers. The triradiate cartilage of acetabula fused earlier, at 5 months of age on average, in Labrador retriever pups with a rapid weight gain due to ingesting superoptimal quantities of food. The closure of acetabular growth plates was delayed to

7 months of age in pups gaining weight at a slowed rate. The growth plates of femoral heads in these pups fused at about 10 months of age. We postulated[23] that early fusion of the triradiate bones of the acetabula results in disparities of bone development leading to hip dysplasia. Consistent with this concept were the data of a report by Delgado-Baeza and colleagues[7] suggesting that surgically induced fusion of the triradiate acetabular growth plates in newborn rats caused subluxation of femoral heads and hip dysplasia. Further studies will help to clarify the relationship between acetabular development and canine hip dysplasia.

Muscle Involvement

Based on observations that hip dysplasia is associated with a reduction in the bulk of pelvic muscles, Riser[33] proposed that hip dysplasia develops as a sequel to alterations in the function of pelvic muscles. Other investigators alternatively postulated that pelvic muscle abnormalities, such as a loss of muscle mass, represented secondary changes during dysplasia, occurring as a sequel to a yet unidentified intrinsic abnormality in the hip joints. The role of muscle mass in development of dysplasia has not been defined well and requires more research for a better understanding. Another related observation was that canine hip dysplasia involves dysfunction of neurones and myofibers.[15] Abnormal myofiber composition in pectineal muscles of 8-week-old pups was identified before other changes in the hip joints were found. The investigators suggested that examination of the myofibers of pectineal muscles in 2-month-old pups be used to predict development of hip dysplasia. This interesting and promising prospect has not yet been exploited further. However that may be resolved, susceptible dogs have developed hip dysplasia despite pectineal myectomy.[15] Pelvic muscle abnormalities have been further implicated in that unilateral hip dysplasia was induced in young pups by cast immobilization of a leg with the stifle in total extension, resulting in hypertrophy of the pectineal muscle.[34]

COMPARISON WITH HIP DYSPLASIA IN HUMANS

Malformation of hip joints has been identified in many other species of mammals, both domesticated and wild. However, only the disease in humans has been the subject of extensive research, and a vast literature exists. A comprehensive review of the natural history of hip dysplasia in humans was published by Weinstein.[38] The onset of hip dysplasia in the human population, in part, follows a different course than the disease in dogs, but the progression of intra-articular changes and the clinical manifestations of the two diseases have many similarities. Despite the fact that hip dysplasia in humans has been the focus of numerous investigations, its cause also is unknown.

Four differences between the human and the canine diseases can be considered: the frequency, the age of onset and diagnosis, the sex distribution, and the obvious difference that humans are bipedal and dogs are quadrapedal. Although exact numbers vary slightly from study to study, it is generally accepted that between two and ten babies per 1,000 live births have hip dysplasia,[38] whereas in dogs the incidence of disease can be greater than 50 per cent in many breeds.[40] A notable exception in the frequency of the disease in humans was reported for the Navajo Indians and the Lapps, who before abandoning the use of baby cradle boards, which forced the babies' legs into an extended position, had a frequency many times higher (25 to 52 per 1,000 live births) than in the overall human population. The second difference is that in children, the diagnosis in most cases can be made by using manipulation and palpation of the hip joints shortly after birth; in dogs, most cases of hip dysplasia develop between 4 and 12 months of age, and diagnosis by palpation has been unreliable. Third, in children, females account for about 80 per cent of the cases of congenital dysplasia of the hip, whereas in dogs both sexes are affected equally often. Finally, a curious paradox in regard to the method of ambulation may be relevant to an understanding of hip dysplasia. Children, who walk bipedally, spend much of their early life with their legs flexed and abducted, whereas pups, who walk quadrapedally, slide about with their legs extended for about 3 weeks after birth.

Evidence suggests that genetic factors have a role in the human condition, in that affected parents have children with hip dysplasia and siblings frequently have the disease. For normal hip joint development to occur, a delicate, genetically determined balance between growth of the triradiate articular bone and a well-seated femoral head is required.[38] The intrauterine environment apparently influences the development of the hip joint in several ways. It has been reported that first-born children have an increased frequency of hip dysplasia and are more frequently delivered in breech positions (legs first). In congenital hip dysplasia, the incidence of breech presentation has been reported to be about 20 per cent. It is striking that babies born in the breech position have a much higher incidence of hip dysplasia and that twice as many females as males are born in this position.[38] The frequency of breech births is not known for the canine population, but dogs and bitches are affected with dysplasia with about equal frequency.

References

1. Bardet JF, et al: Measurement of femoral torsion in dogs using a biplanar method. *Vet Surg 12*:1, 1983.
2. Bellkoff SM, et al: Development of a device to measure canine coxofemoral joint laxity. *Vet Comp Orthop Traumatol 1*:31, 1989.
3. Burton-Wurster N, Lust G: Synthesis of fibronectin in normal and osteoarthritic articular cartilage. *Biochim Biophys Acta 800*:52, 1984.
4. Burton-Wurster N, Lust G: Deposition of fibronectin in articular cartilage of canine osteoarthritic joints. *Am J Vet Res 46*:2542, 1985.
5. Corley EA, Hogan PM: Trends in hip dysplasia control: Analysis of radiographs submitted to the OFA; 1974–1984. *J Am Vet Med Assoc 187*:805, 1985.
6. Cullis-Hill D, Ghosh P: The role of hyaluronic acid in joint stability—a hypothesis for hip dysplasia and allied disorders. *Med Hypotheses 12*:171, 1987.
7. Delgado-Baeza E, et al: Experimental acetabular dysplasia associated with a lesion of the triradiate cartilage. *Clin Orthop Rel Res 234*:75, 1988.
8. Edqvist LE, et al: Blood plasma levels of progesterone and oestradiol in the dog during the oestrus cycle and pregnancy. *Acta Endocrinol 78*:554, 1975.
9. Gustafsson PO, et al: Skeletal development of greyhounds and German shepherds dogs and their offspring. *Acta Radiol 334*(Suppl):81, 1975.

10. Hauptman J, et al: The angle of inclination of the canine femoral head and neck. *Am Coll Vet Surg 8*:75, 1979.
11. Hauptman J, et al: Angles of inclination and anteversion in hip dysplasia in the dog. *Am J Vet Res 46*:2033, 1985.
12. Hedhammar A, et al: Canine hip dysplasia: Study of heritability in 401 litters of German shepherd dogs. *J Am Vet Med Assoc 174*:1012, 1979.
13. Henry JD, Park RD: Wedge technique for demonstration of coxofemoral joint laxity in the canine. Proceedings of the Canine Hip Dysplasia Symposium Workshop Orth Found Anim, 1972, pp 117–126.
14. Hutt FB: Genetic selection to reduce the incidence of hip dysplasia in dogs. *J Am Vet Med Assoc 175*:1041, 1967.
15. Ihemelandu EC, et al: Canine hip dysplasia; differences in pectineal muscles of healthy and dysplastic German shepherd dogs when two months old. *Am J Vet Res 44*:411, 1983.
16. Jessen CR, Spurrell FA: Radiographic detection of canine hip dysplasia in known age groups. Proceedings of the Canine Hip Dysplasia Symposium Workshop Orth Found Anim 1972, pp 93–100.
17. Kealy RD, et al: Effects of reduced food on subluxation of femoral heads in growing dogs. *J Am Vet Med Assoc*, in press.
18. Knowlton RG, et al: Genetic linkage of the type II procollagen gene (COL2A1) to primary osteoarthritis associated with a mild chondrodysplasia. *N Engl J Med*, in press.
19. Leighton EA, et al: A genetic study of canine hip dysplasia. *Am J Vet Res 38*:241, 1977.
20. Leipold HR, et al: Canine serum keratan sulfate and hyaluronate concentrations—relationship to age and osteoarthritis. *Arthritis Rheum 32*:312, 1989.
21. Lust G, Farrell PW: Hip dysplasia in dogs; the interplay of genotype and environment. *Cornell Vet 67*:447, 1977.
22. Lust G, et al: An improved procedure for genetic selection against hip dysplasia in dogs. *Cornell Vet 68*(Suppl):42, 1978.
23. Lust G, et al: Canine hip dysplasia; concepts and diagnosis. *J Am Vet Med Assoc 187*:638, 1985.
24. Lust G, et al: Development of hip dysplasia in dogs. *Am J Vet Res 34*:87, 1973.
25. Lust G, et al: A relationship between degree of laxity and synovial fluid volume in coxofemoral joints of dogs predisposed for hip dysplasia. *Am J Vet Res 41*:55, 1980.
26. Lust G, et al: Intra-articular volume and hip joint instability in dogs with hip dysplasia. *J Bone Joint Surg [Am] 62A*:576, 1980.
27. McDaniel DO, et al: Analysis of RFLP in rheumatic disease. *Rheum Dis Clin North Am 13*:353, 1987.
28. Morgan JP, Stephens M: *Radiographic Diagnois and Control of Canine Hip Dysplasia*. Iowa State University Press, Ames, IO, 1985.
29. Olsewski JM, et al: Degenerative joint disease: Multiple joint involvement in young and mature dogs. *Am J Vet Res 44*:1300, 1983.
30. Olsson SE: Canine hip dysplasia. *In* Kirk R (ed): *Current Veterinary Therapy*. 5th ed. W. B. Saunders, Philadelphia, 1980, pp 802–806.
31. Palotie A, et al: Predisposition to familial osteoarthrosis linked to type II collagen gene. *Lancet 1202*:924, 1989.
32. Paatsama SP, et al: Somatotropin, thyrotropin and corticotropin hormone induced changes in the cartilage and bones of young dogs. *J Small Anim Pract 12*:603, 1971.
33. Riser WH: The dog as a model for the study of hip dysplasia. *Vet Pathol 12*:229, 1975.
34. Schoenecker PL, et al: A dynamic canine model of experimental hip dysplasia. *J Bone Joint Surg [Am] 66A*:1281, 1984.
35. Smith GK, et al: New concepts of coxofemoral joint stability and development of clinical stress-radiographic method for quantitating hip joint laxity in the dog. *J Am Vet Med Assoc 196*:59, 1990.
36. Steinetz BG, et al: Plasma relaxin levels in pregnant and lactating dogs. *Biol Reprod 37*:719, 1987.
37. Wallace LJ: Canine hip dysplasia: Past and present. *Semin Vet Med Surg 2*:92, 1987.
38. Weinstein SL: Natural history of congenital hip dislocation and hip dysplasia. *Clin Orthop Rel Res 225*:62, 1987.
39. Whittington K, et al: Report of the panel on canine hip dysplasia. *J Am Vet Med Assoc 139*:791, 1961.
40. Willis MB: Hip dysplasia. *In Genetics of the Dog*. Howell Book House, New York, 1989, pp 144–179.

Osteochondrosis

Curtis W. Probst and Spencer A. Johnston

Osteochondrosis is a well-described yet incompletely understood systemic disease of endochondral ossification affecting humans, dogs, swine, horses, cattle, chickens, and turkeys. The term *osteochondrosis* describes a disease that affects the normal endochondral ossification of the growth plates, be they epiphyseal, metaphyseal, or apophyseal.[61] Osteochondritis dissecans (OCD), the clinical manifestation of osteochondrosis with which veterinarians are most familiar, denotes a dissecting lesion between bone and articular cartilage. *Osteochondritis* is a misnomer because it implies inflammation of bone and cartilage, a rare condition.[16, 42, 48] The term has become so well entrenched that although a misnomer, it allows description of the clinical disease entity.

Loose bodies in joints, particularly the human knee, were identified as early as 1726.[39] Throughout the 19th and early 20th centuries, theories of the origin of these loose bodies included trauma, spontaneous necrosis, and cartilage proliferation of the periarticular synovial tissue.[39] Konig's description of OCD (1887) centered around a possible cause (i.e., necrosis) as an alternative to trauma or in conjunction with it.[2]

Since osteochondrosis was reported in the canine humeral head,[7] clinical reports have dominated the literature, and relatively few population and histopathological studies have been performed.

PATHOPHYSIOLOGY

Normal Anatomy

Mature epiphyseal articular (i.e., hyaline) cartilage differs markedly from the cartilage of the physeal growth plate. The articular cartilage can be divided into three regions (Fig. 145–3).[13, 28, 36, 42] The most superficial region lies immediately under the articular surface and consists of the lamina splendens and gliding zone. The lamina splendens is a region of filamentous proteins to which bind proteinaceous material important in providing lubrication for the joint surfaces.[36] The cells of the gliding zone are parallel to the surface because of the orientation of collagen fibers in this region.[13, 36] The middle region consists of cells arranged perpendicular to the surface and includes the transitional and radial zones. The transitional zone is an important region of cell activity and interstitial growth that allows the articular cartilage to cover the epiphysis.[13, 36] The radial zone is characterized by cells lined up in irregular columns. This alignment of cells is due to the orientation of collagen fibers (i.e., perpendicular to the surface and subchondral bone) in this region.[13, 36] The deep region consists of calcified cartilage and subchondral bone that supports the articular cartilage. The deep zone is the region where vascular invasion of calcified tissue occurs and

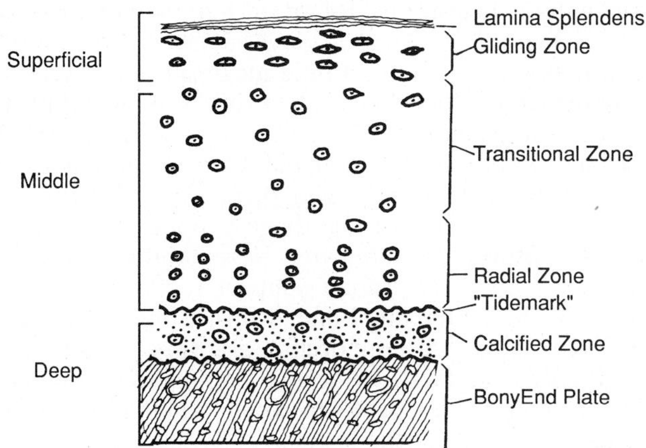

FIGURE 145–3. Regions and zones of mature articular cartilage. Note the tidemark that separates calcified from noncalcified tissues. It is at this level that cleavage occurs in osteochondritis dissecans. (Modified from Mankin HJ: The articular cartilages. *In* Newton CC, Nunamaker DM [eds]: *Textbook of Small Animal Orthopedics.* J.B. Lippincott, Philadelphia, 1985.)

endochondral ossification follows.[28] The deep region is separated from the middle region by a thin line known as the *tidemark* (see Fig. 145–3). Histologically, the tidemark separates noncalcified tissue from calcified tissue.[12, 36]

The tidemark is not present in young animals and develops near maturity. More than one tidemark may be present in older animals.[36] The tidemark is visible owing to altered uptake of stain.[36] It is unknown why the tidemark has its unique staining characteristics because there is no difference in the constitution of this region and the surrounding tissue.[36] The tidemark may consist of a change in direction of collagen fibers as they pass from the middle to the deep region and become embedded in calcified tissue.[36] Such an organization of tissue may allow for protection against shear stress forces.[36] The tidemark is significant because at this level the separation of calcified and noncalcified tissue occurs in osteochondritis.[12]

Normal Growth

The normal process of longitudinal bone growth of dogs is endochondral ossification.[13] This entire process begins with the embryonic limb bud that differentiates into a cartilaginous model for the future bone. As capillaries enter and supply the perichondrium surrounding the cartilage model, osteoblasts form and begin to lay down bone. This process continues until a primary ossification center is formed. The bone model now contains a central elongating portion that consists of bone (i.e., the primary ossification center) with cartilaginous ends. These cartilaginous zones are the anlage for the developing epiphysis.

The chondrocytes of the epiphyseal anlage mature into osteoblasts and form secondary centers of ossification. The epiphysis develops a bony centrum surrounded by cartilage. The cartilage facing the synovial lumen becomes articular cartilage, and the cartilage facing the metaphysis becomes the physeal growth plate. Both the epiphyseal and physeal growth plates provide cartilaginous sources for growth. The physeal growth plate, which consists of the zones of resting, proliferating, maturing, and calcifying cartilage, remains until skeletal maturity, when osteocyte replacement overtakes chondrocyte renewal and growth ceases. The epiphysis remains covered by articular cartilage throughout normal life.

The articular cartilage must grow as the epiphysis grows. It is believed that the growing articular cartilage may actually be divided into two layers, the articular and epiphyseal layers (Fig. 145–4).[28] The articular layer is the more superficial component and consists of the future region extending from the lamina splendens to the radial zone. This layer is responsible for expansion of the articular surface as growth occurs. The deeper epiphyseal portion, which includes the future calcified zone, actually functions as a proliferative portion and cartilaginous model for endochondral ossification similar to the maturing and calcifying portions of the metaphyseal growth plate.[28] Vascular buds invade the columnar arrangement of cells in this second layer, and calcification ensues, resulting in the production of epiphyseal bone.

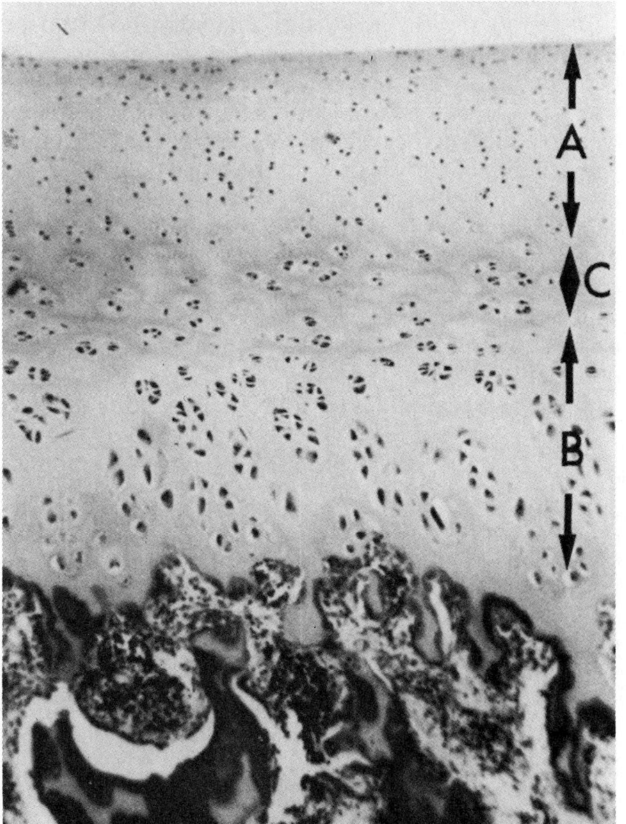

FIGURE 145–4. Immature articular cartilage of a synovial joint. (A, articular layer, which is the future superficial and middle regions; B, epiphyseal layer, which is the future deep region; C, a region of increased acidophilia that may be similar to the zone of resting cartilage of the physis.) (From Kincaid SA, Van Sickle DC: Bone morphology and osteogenesis: Potential for disease. *Vet Clin North Am 13*:3, 1983.)

Pathology

Osteochondrosis is marked by a disturbance in the normal differentiation of cartilage during endochondral ossification, resulting in thickening of the articular epiphyseal complex.[47] The primary lesion in OCD is a dissecting intracartilaginous separation between the calcified and noncalcified tissues.[12, 37] There are four gradations of the lesion,[14] from the mildest, grade I, in which the articular surface is grossly normal yet a small defect is noted in the subchondral bone, to grade IV, with vertical fracture of the articular cartilage and separation of the cartilage flap from the underlying bone (Fig. 145–5). This separated articular fragment is referred to as a *joint mouse*. Grade IV is the most common form of osteochondrosis. Osteochondrosis in animals is not painful until a fissure reaches the articular surface of the cartilage; diagnosis of grades I to III OCD is rarely made in dogs because of lack of clinical signs.[44]

The possibility of cartilage separation from subchondral bone without communication with the articular surface is consistent with radiographically identifiable lesions not associated with clinical signs. Radiographically, osteochondrosis is identified as a radiolucent zone along the articular margin of the bone. The radiolucent zone is due to bone growth around a local site of retardation of ossification and cartilage.[2] Radiographic evidence of osteochondrosis is often bilateral in animals with unilateral signs.

In 29 dogs with OCD, the separation occurred between calcified and noncalcified tissue along the tidemark and rarely involved the subchondral bone.[12] There was no association with bony necrosis. The fragments were of thickened cartilage. Some fragments contained viable bone, but it was thought that bone only developed in those separated fragments that had a blood supply originating from vascularized fibrous attachments to the underlying marrow of the defect bed. The cartilage fragments were larger than the corresponding bed from which they were derived, because fragments are nourished by synovial fluid and may continue to grow once detached.

An increased amount of lipid is found in the cartilage flap with OCD lesions.[30] Based on staining properties of retained nonmineralized cartilage, delayed cartilage calcification may be due to a lipid metabolism defect.

Articular cartilage normally exhibits poor ability to replace and repair itself. When cartilage suffers a partial-thickness injury, no bleeding and relatively little necrosis results, owing to low oxygen demand of this tissue.[36] Because blood supply to cartilage is poor, little inflammation ensues. Chondrocytes have limited ability to produce matrix and cannot support repair.[13, 36] Repair occurs if the underlying bone, with its blood supply, is involved. When bleeding occurs, a fibrin clot forms and eventually is replaced by fibrous granulation tissue and fibrocartilage. The degree to which healing occurs depends on the size of the lesion.

In experimental studies in ponies, 3-mm defects were filled with fibrocartilage by 9 months, and 9-mm defects were incompletely filled.[11] The larger the defect, the more likely the animal is to have persistent lameness, and the larger the lesion, the more likely the opposite joint surface is to develop a "kissing" lesion. The development of kissing lesions opposite an articular cartilage defect is due to lack of normal physiological compression of the cartilage opposite the defect,[54] which is necessary to maintain healthy articular cartilage.[54]

The tissue reaction to cartilage separation varies in severity proportional to the gross pathological grading. Beneath the cleft, an active repair process is noted, with granulation tissue production, fibrogenesis, and osteoblast and osteoclast activity. Necrosis is not observed in the naturally occurring disease in dogs.[12] The reparative process of osteochondrosis is related to the size of the osteochondral defect and the time from the development of the defect.

During the repair process, subchondral bone formation occurs at the base of the granulation tissue bed but stops at the tidemark.[36] The reparative fibrous granulation tissue undergoes chondrification and even develops some hyaline cartilage.[13, 36] Continuous passive motion during healing may encourage hyalinization of the reparative fibrocartilage.[58] Fibrocartilage begins degeneration within 1 year and leads to secondary osteoarthritis due to release of breakdown products.[23]

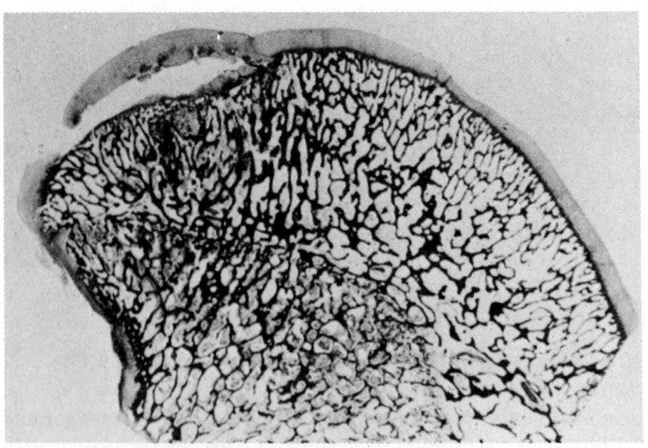

FIGURE 145–5. Sagittal section of the proximal humeral head, demonstrating intracartilaginous cleavage with flap formation (From Milton JL: Osteochondritis dissecans in the dog. *Vet Clin North Am 13*:117, 1983.)

Pathogenesis

The pathogenesis of osteochondrosis is a disturbance of articular/epiphyseal cartilage growth and endochondral osteogenesis. It is due to slow ossification of cartilage in the deep zone.[47] In addition to increased articular cartilage thickness, chondrocytes of cartilage in this region had an irregular arrangement and were abnormal along the line of cleavage.[47] The normal process of endochondral ossification of the deep cartilage ceases. Articular cartilage thickening leads to poor diffusion of nutrients from the synovial fluid to the deep zones of the articular cartilage.[41] This leads to abnormal metabolism and function of the deep chondrocytes and, with some trauma, separation of the calcified and abnormal noncalcified tissues.

Once the articular cartilage dissects free from the underlying calcified tissue, the lesion of OCD has formed.

Vertical fracture of articular cartilage is a later manifestation in pathogenesis of OCD.[12, 14] If trauma sufficient to cause vertical fracture of the articular cartilage does not occur, the cartilage flap may reattach to the underlying subchondral bone because blood is present in the separation space as a result of bleeding from subchondral bone. This blood allows deposition of fibrin and permits undifferentiated mesenchymal cells to invade the area, leading to reattachment of the cartilage to the underlying bone.[28, 34]

If vertical fracture of cartilage does occur, motion between the flap and subchondral bone is present. Synovitis results from irritation, with pain ensuing. Healing does not take place because of this motion and the presence of synovial fluid between the cartilage flap and bone. Healing occurs only if the fragment is stabilized or removed.

The amount of trauma necessary to cause flap formation depends on the amount of cartilage thickening. Trauma does not have to be severe to cause separation of cartilage and bone.[29]

Etiology

The etiology of osteochondrosis in animals is most likely multifactorial. The disease process involves traumatic, environmental, and constitutional aspects. Numerous theories regarding the nature of the disease have been put forth. The one major difference between osteochondrosis in dogs and humans is that ischemia, which occurs in humans, is not noted in animals.[12, 61]

The canine shoulder joint (i.e., proximal humerus) has been the most frequently studied site for naturally occurring OCD. The articular cartilage of the caudal humeral head is normally thicker than the surrounding articular cartilage because of the normal incongruity of the scapulohumeral joint.[29] Increased articular cartilage thickness allows greater distribution of force over a larger area of the subchondral bone.[29] The thickness of the cartilage is derived from the two layers of the articular epiphyseal cartilage, particularly the epiphyseal layer, which undergoes slow ossification. The caudal medial aspect of the humeral head develops more slowly than the remaining area, and this discrepancy allows for greater exposure to microtrauma and may have a role in the separation between cartilage and bone.[9] The incongruity of the joint may lead to persistent mild trauma of thickened cartilage and eventually separation of cartilage and bone.[14, 41]

The process of ossification of the epiphysis may be under hormonal influences. Histological increases in cartilage thickness occur in animals given excessive somatotropin or thyrotropin.[46] Excessive administration of these hormones resulted in a condition similar to OCD. Testosterone also stimulates epiphyseal growth and acts synergistically with growth hormone.[37] Estrogen has the opposite effect, encouraging calcification of cartilage.[37] These observations may account for greater predilection for males to develop osteochondrosis than females.

Overnutrition is directly related to the frequency of osteochondrosis in pigs.[45] Rapid growth secondary to overnutrition results in increased cartilage thickness.[24, 45] Free feeding in young Great Danes leads to multiple skeletal abnormalities and cartilage disturbances, including osteochondrosis.[24] These anomalies were due to excessive dietary calcium, which resulted in hypercalcitoninism, inhibiting cartilage maturation.[24] In swine and poultry, osteochondrosis can be reduced by restricted feeding.[45] Dogs presumably would similarly benefit from normal diet and a slower rate of growth. A familial tendency for development of OCD exists, but definitive studies showing inheritability have not been completed.[12, 31, 40]

These findings are insufficient to explain why some animals develop clinical lesions of osteochondrosis. Trauma may have a major role in the etiology of the disease, and several models have been developed to test the hypothesis.[46] Trauma, either direct or indirect, is an acknowledged cause of OCD in humans.[39] Osteochondrosis and OCD are often caused by normal stress on abnormally developing bone.[18]

Species, Breed, and Age Distribution

Osteochondrosis is most frequently encountered in immature dogs whose mature weight is greater than 25 kg.[34, 43, 44, 57, 65] The breeds most commonly affected are the Labrador and golden retriever, rottweiler, Great Dane, Saint Bernard, German shepherd, and Bernese mountain dog, although all large dogs and giant breeds may develop the disease. Factors such as genetics and breed popularity influence the breed incidence.*

Clinical signs become apparent between 4 and 12 months of age, although the pathological process starts much earlier.[36]

OSTEOCHONDRITIS DISSECANS OF THE SHOULDER

Signalment

Lesions of the shoulder joint usually involve the caudal central aspect of the humeral head articular cartilage, although lesions of the glenoid occur. Although this disease most frequently occurs in large dogs,† it also affects small and medium-sized breeds.[17, 22, 26, 31]

The age at which animals are presented for treatment varies. Ages ranging from 3 months to 5 years have been reported,‡ although 75 per cent of cases in one study were presented between 5 and 10 months of age.[55]

Males are more commonly affected than females (2 to 5:1).[14, 51, 63] The incidence of bilateral disease is reported to range between 20 and 85 per cent.[12, 51, 55, 63] Right and left legs are involved with equal frequency.[63]

Clinical Signs

The most common clinical sign is a mild to moderate unilateral front leg lameness. It is unusual for dogs to show bilateral front leg lameness, even when both shoulders are affected.[19, 25, 51, 55] The lameness improves

*See references 34, 36, 42, 43, 57, 65, and 69.
†See references 5, 22, 25, 27, 51, 55, 63, and 68.
‡See references 5, 19, 22, 25, 27, 32, 51, 55, 63, and 68.

after rest and is worse after exercise. Dogs typically stand with the affected leg somewhat externally rotated and the elbow adducted. Joint capsule effusion is seldom palpated because of the overlying musculature. Some atrophy of the supraspinatus and infraspinatus muscles may be present, but it is seldom marked unless the lameness has been severe and protracted.

Extreme flexion and extension of the shoulder joint usually elicit a pain response. Flexion and extension of the shoulder may produce an audible click. Because breeds of dogs presented for shoulder OCD are the same breeds that are typically presented for elbow disorders, one should not overly flex and extend the elbow while examining the shoulder to minimize the chance of confusing elbow pain with shoulder pain.

Diagnosis

The history and physical examination lead to a presumptive diagnosis of OCD, but shoulder radiographs are necessary to confirm the diagnosis (Fig. 145–6). Mediolateral projections of both shoulders are obtained. Most can be diagnosed with this lateral view because the lesion is usually located in the central portion of the caudal aspect of the humeral head. The lesion occasionally is located more lateral or medial to the center of the humeral head. In these cases, obtain two additional lateral views, one while internally rotating the leg and the other while externally rotating the leg. The cranial-caudal radiographic view of the shoulder is difficult to obtain in an awake dog and offers little additional information.

The typical OCD lesion of the caudal humeral head appears radiographically as a flattened radiolucent defect in the subchondral bone immediately beneath the articular cartilage (Fig. 145–7). A mineralized cartilage flap or joint mice may be seen (Fig. 145–8). Joint mice may migrate into the tendon sheath of the biceps brachii (see Fig. 145–8). Contrast arthrography can be helpful in confirming the presence of joint mice within the biceps tendon sheath (Fig. 145–9) and in diagnosing articular cartilage defects.[32, 46]

Treatment

Conservative

Conservative therapy consisting of strict rest with or without analgesics has been recommended for some patients.[4, 22, 25, 32, 37, 68] Analgesics are used sparingly because they do not help the lesion heal and may cause a dog to become more active by minimizing pain. Because most dogs with bilateral disease do not require surgery on both legs, conservative therapy may have a place in the management of shoulder OCD.

We use conservative therapy (i.e., 4 to 6 weeks of strict rest) if the owner is reluctant to have surgery performed on the dog. The owner is asked to return the dog for surgery if there is no improvement during that time or if the lameness worsens. Conservative therapy can also be used if the dog is less than 7 months old, has mild lameness of short duration, and has a small radiographic lesion. I do not recommend conservative therapy if the dog is older than 7 months, if the lameness is severe or protracted, or if a radiographically demon-

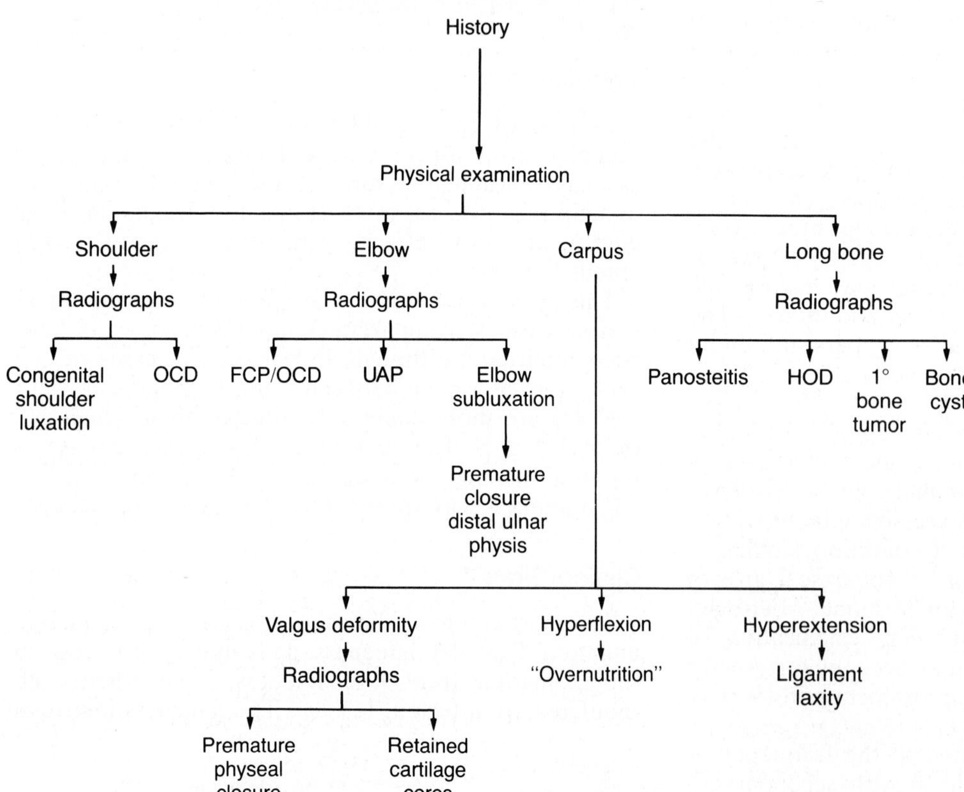

FIGURE 145–6. Front leg lameness in young dogs. (OCD, osteochondritis dissecans; FCP, fragmented coronoid process; UAP, ununited anconeal process; HOD, hypertrophic osteodystrophy.)

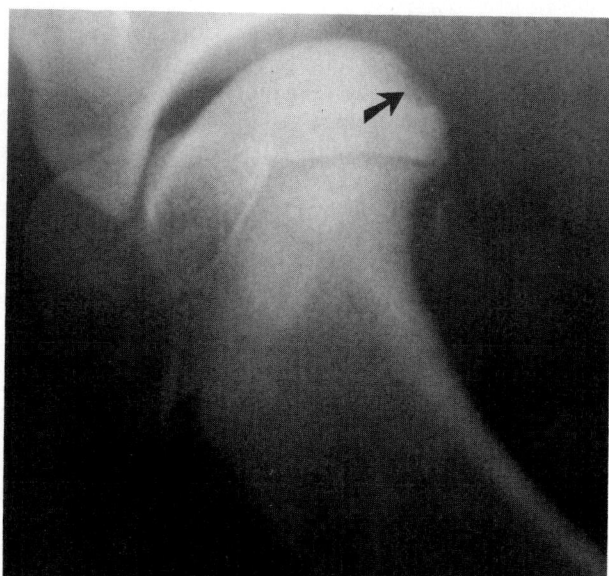

FIGURE 145–7. The arrow points to the characteristic radiolucent defect seen with osteochondritis dissecans of the caudal humeral head.

strable joint mouse or mineralized cartilage flap is present.

One author recommends analgesics and forced strenuous activity.[43] The objective is to dislodge the cartilage flap and thus facilitate healing. The cartilage flap may fall into the caudal cul-de-sac of the joint capsule and become resorbed. We do not recommend this treatment because many dogs we have treated surgically had part or all of the flap dislodged and were still lame. There is no assurance that the loose flap will be resorbed rather than nourished by synovial fluid and begin to grow.[55] Free cartilage fragments in the joint may contribute to degenerative joint disease.[22, 37]

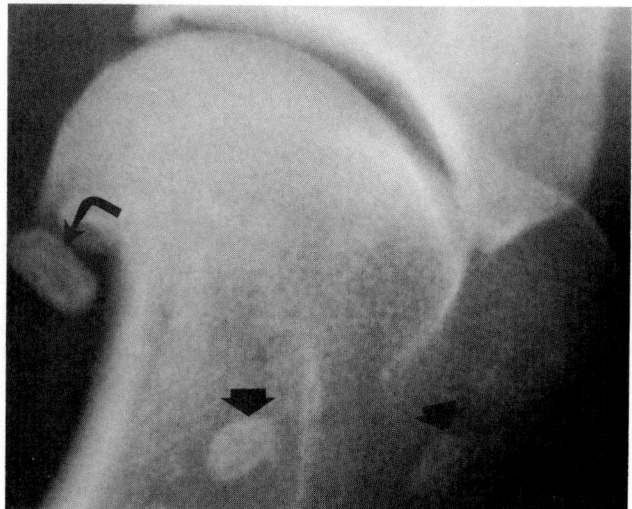

FIGURE 145–8. The curved arrow points to a joint mouse in the caudal cul-de-sac of the shoulder joint. Joint mice are formed from osteochondritis dissecans flaps that have become dislodged from the humeral head. Because the tendon sheath of the origin of the biceps brachii tendon communicates with the shoulder joint, it is possible for joint mice *(straight arrows)* to migrate into the tendon sheath.

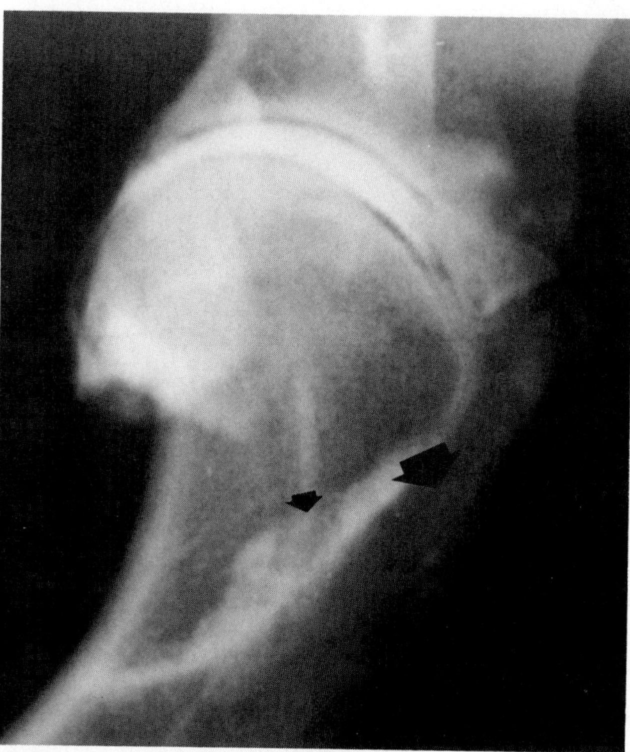

FIGURE 145–9. A contrast arthrogram has been performed on the same shoulder as in Figure 145–8. The small arrow points to a filling defect in the biceps tendon sheath caused by one of the joint mice. The large arrow points to the other joint mouse in the biceps tendon sheath.

Surgical

Surgical treatment produces the most rapid return to function and minimizes degenerative joint disease.* The objectives of surgery are to remove all loose cartilage fragments, including joint mice, and to stimulate the articular surface defect to heal by fibrocartilage formation.

Although many approaches to the scapulohumeral joint have been described,† only three are detailed here. Regardless of approach, the animal is positioned in lateral recumbency with the affected leg uppermost. The leg is suspended and prepared for aseptic surgery. It is then draped using a hanging limb draping procedure.[49]

Surgical Anatomy. The origins and insertions of the following muscles are important: omotransverse, acromial and spinous heads of the deltoid, teres minor, infraspinatus, and lateral and long heads of the triceps. The location of the caudal circumflex humeral vessels, the axillobrachial vein, the bifurcation of the cephalic vein, and the muscular branches of the axillary nerve are important.

Craniolateral Approach. A curved skin incision is begun at the distal third of the scapular spine and is continued distally along the scapular spine and the cranial border of the acromial head of the deltoid muscle, extending to the proximal third of the humerus (Fig. 145–10). The subcutaneous fat and fascia are

*See references 5, 19, 22, 25, 27, 32, 37, and 63.

†See references 5, 8, 10, 19, 21, 25, 27, 32, 49, 51, 53, 55, 60, and 66.

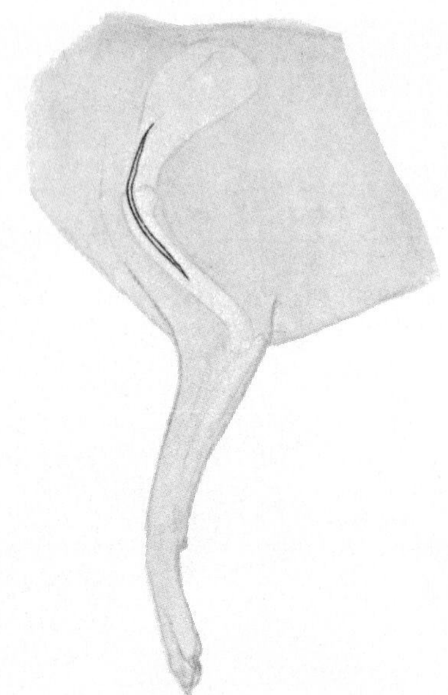

FIGURE 145–10. A curved skin incision is begun at the distal third of the scapular spine and is continued distally along the scapular spine and the cranial border of the acromial head of the deltoid muscle. The incision is stopped at the proximal one-third of the humerus. (From Piermattei DL, Greeley RG: *An Atlas of Surgical Approaches to the Bones of the Dog and Cat.* 2nd ed. W.B. Saunders, Philadelphia, 1979, p 67.)

incised along the same line as the skin. Excessive undermining of the skin is avoided. The deep fascia along the cranial border of the acromial head of the deltoid muscle is incised (Fig. 145–11). The acromial head of the deltoid muscle is retracted caudally, exposing the tendon of insertion of the infraspinatus muscle. The tendon of insertion of the teres minor muscle is more difficult to identify and is located distal and caudal to the infraspinatus tendon. A tenotomy of the infraspinatus tendon is performed about 5 mm from its humeral insertion (Fig. 145–12). A stay suture may be placed into the proximal portion of the tendon before performing the tenotomy. The infraspinatus muscle and the acromial head of the deltoid muscle are retracted caudally, exposing the joint capsule. Partial tenotomy of the origin of the acromial deltoid may aid exposure. The joint capsule is incised parallel to the rim of the glenoid and midway between the glenoid rim and the humeral head (Fig. 145–13). Once the humeral head has been exposed, the shoulder must be extended and the humerus internally rotated to reveal the lesion (Fig. 145–14).

The joint capsule is closed with interrupted absorbable sutures. The infraspinatus tendon is reattached using nonabsorbable suture in a Bunnell-Mayer or locking loop pattern. The deep fascia and subcutaneous fat layers are apposed with interrupted absorbable sutures. The skin edges are apposed with absorbable sutures in a subcuticular pattern. Interrupted nonabsorbable sutures are used for skin closure. During closure, care is taken to eliminate dead space by tacking down each layer.

This approach provides good exposure of the humeral head but limited exposure of the caudal joint compartment[49] and may limit removal of joint mice from the caudal cul-de-sac of the joint.

Caudolateral Approach. A curved skin incision is begun at the distal third of the scapular spine and is continued distally along the caudal border of the scapular spine between the acromial and spinous heads of the deltoid muscle (Fig. 145–15). The bifurcation of the cephalic vein marks the distal limit of the incision. The subcutaneous fat and fascia are incised along the same line as the skin. Skin edges are retracted, exposing the deep fascia (Fig. 145–16). The fascial division between the spinous and acromial heads of the deltoid muscle is identified (see Fig. 145–16). (It is important not to confuse the caudal edge of the tendon of origin of the acromial head as this division.) The spinous head of the deltoid muscle is separated from the scapular spine and

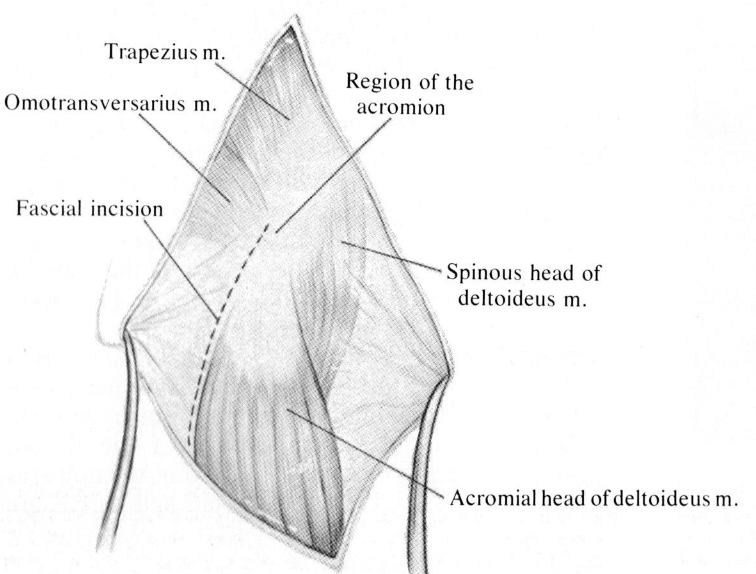

FIGURE 145–11. The deep fascia along the cranial border of the acromial head of the deltoid muscle is incised. (From Piermattei DL, Greeley RG: *An Atlas of Surgical Approaches to the Bones of the Dog and Cat.* 2nd ed. W.B. Saunders, Philadelphia, 1979, p 67.)

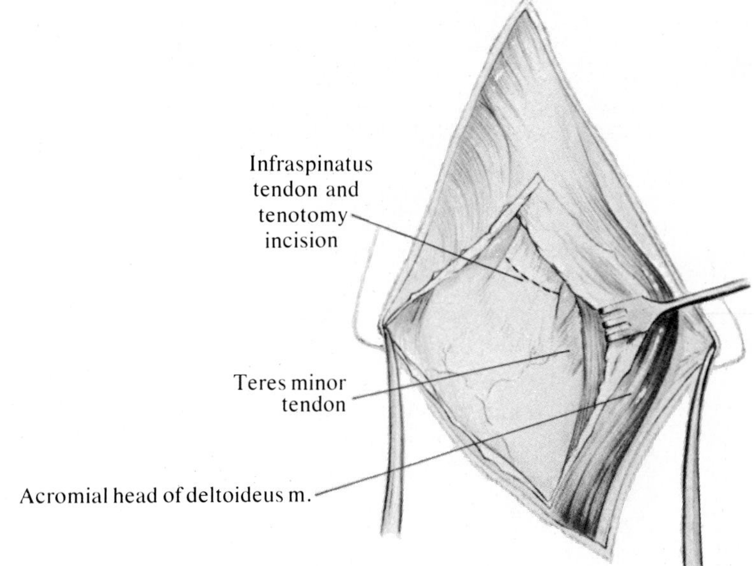

FIGURE 145–12. The acromial head of the deltoid muscle is retracted caudally, exposing the tendon of insertion of the infraspinatus muscle. A tenotomy of the infraspinatus tendon is performed about 5 mm from its humeral insertion. (From Piermattei DL, Greeley RG: *An Atlas of Surgical Approaches to the Bones of the Dog and Cat.* 2nd ed. W.B. Saunders, Philadelphia, 1979, p 67.)

the acromial head by incising sharply along this fascial separation (Fig. 145–17). Small vessels between the spinous and acromial heads of the deltoid muscle are encountered and ligated. The spinous head is retracted caudally, and the acromial head is retracted cranially (Fig. 145–18). The infraspinatus and teres minor muscles, the caudal circumflex humeral vessels, and the muscular branches are identified (Fig. 145–18). The humeral head can be felt just cranial and distal to the teres minor muscle. The teres minor and infraspinatus muscles are bluntly undermined and retracted craniodorsally. It is not necessary to incise the muscular branches of the axillary nerve, because they can be retracted. The joint capsule is incised parallel to the glenoid rim and midway between it and the humeral head. Stay sutures are placed through the joint capsule to aid retraction (Fig. 145–19). Distal retraction of the joint capsule helps protect the muscular branches of the axillary nerve and caudal circumflex humeral vessels during exploration of the joint (see Fig. 145–19). To expose the lesion, the shoulder is extended and the humerus internally rotated (Fig. 145–20).

The joint capsule is closed with interrupted absorbable sutures. The teres minor, infraspinatus, and deltoid fascia are apposed with interrupted absorbable sutures. The subcutaneous fat and skin are apposed as described

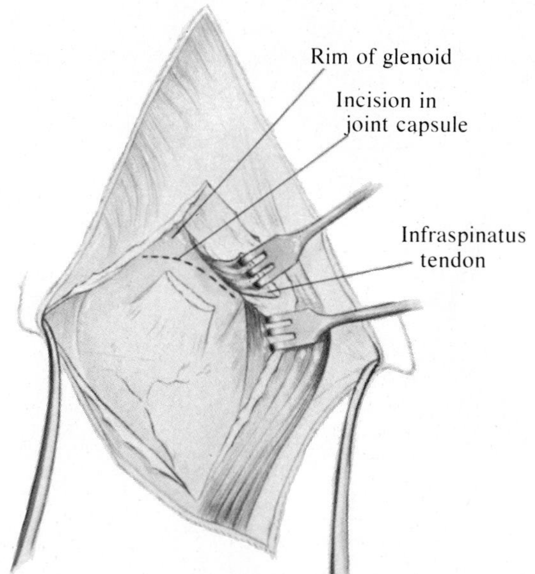

FIGURE 145–13. The joint capsule is incised parallel to the rim of the glenoid and midway between the glenoid rim and the humeral head. (From Piermattei DL, Greeley RG: *An Atlas of Surgical Approaches to the Bones of the Dog and Cat.* 2nd ed. W.B. Saunders, Philadelphia, 1979, p 67.)

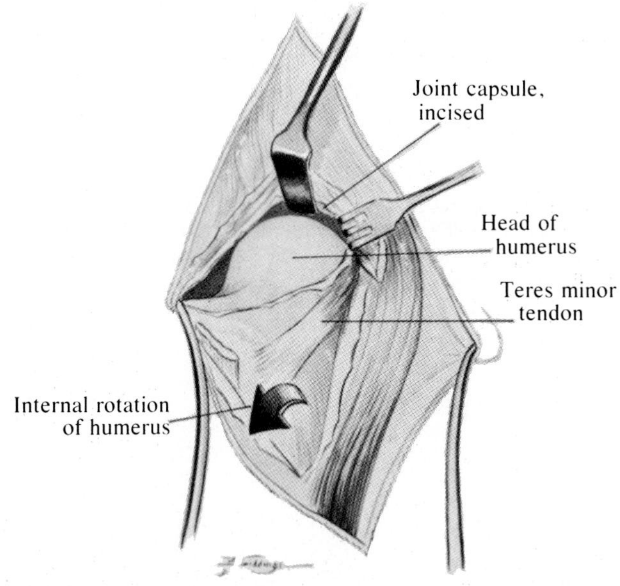

FIGURE 145–14. Once the humeral head has been exposed, the shoulder must be extended and the humerus internally rotated to expose the osteochondritis dissecans lesion. (From Piermattei DL, Greeley RG: *An Atlas of Surgical Approaches to the Bones of the Dog and Cat.* 2nd ed. W.B. Saunders, Philadelphia, 1979, p 67.)

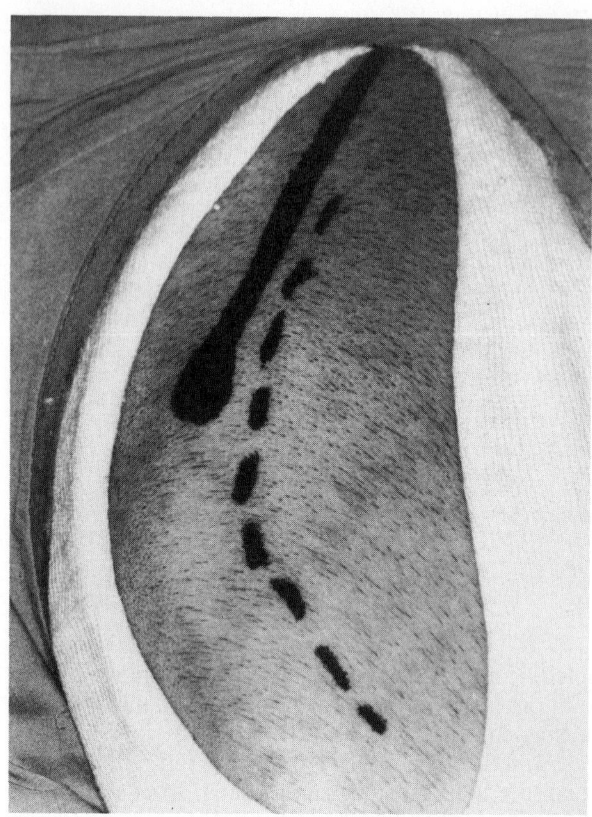

FIGURE 145–15. A curved skin incision *(broken line)* is begun at the distal third of the scapular spine and is continued distally along the caudal border of the scapular spine and between the acromial and spinous heads of the deltoid muscle.

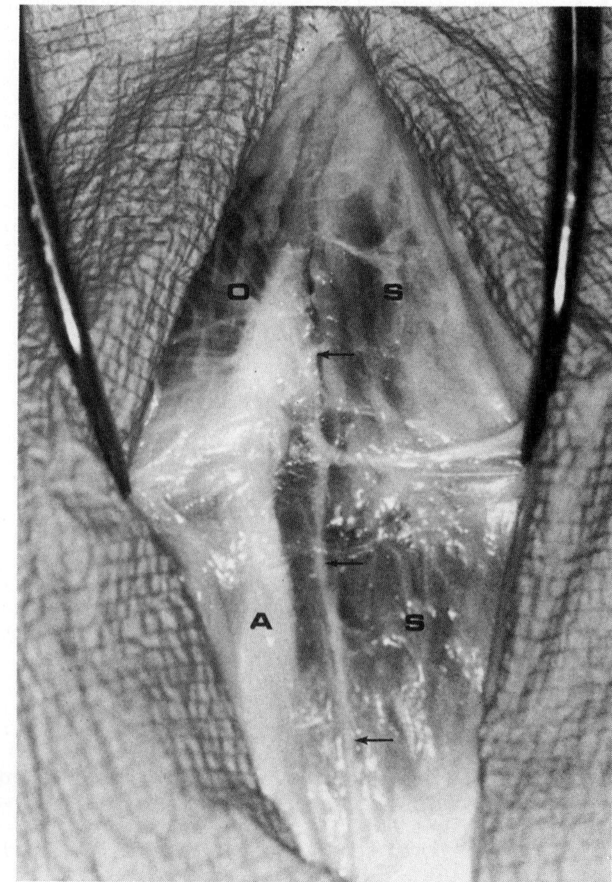

FIGURE 145–16. The skin edges are retracted exposing the omotransversarius muscle (O) and the acromial (A) and spinous (S) heads of the deltoid muscle. The arrows show the fascial division between the two heads of the deltoid muscle.

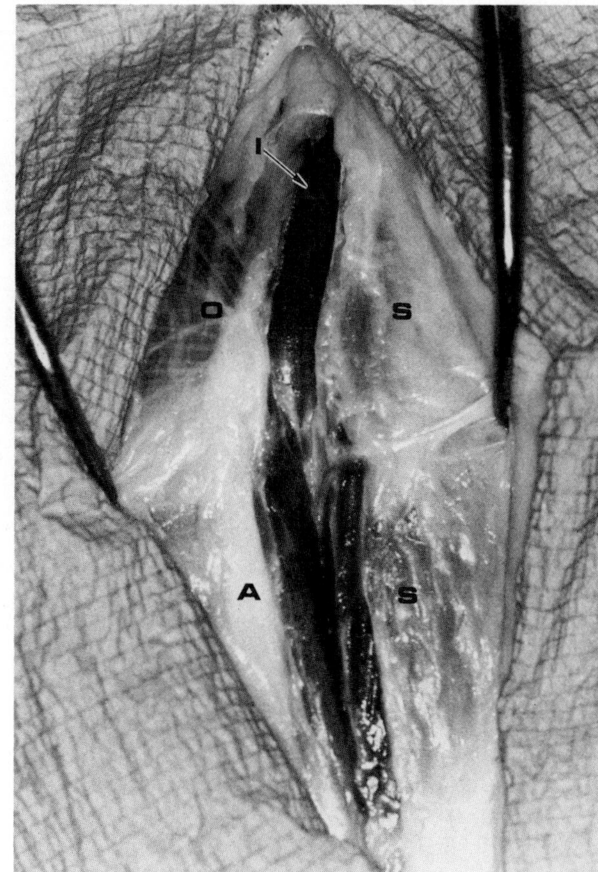

FIGURE 145–17. The spinous head (S) of the deltoid muscle is separated from the scapular spine and the acromial head (A) by incising sharply along the fascial separation. The infraspinatus muscle (I) can be seen beneath the spinous head of the deltoid muscle. (O, omotransversarius muscle.)

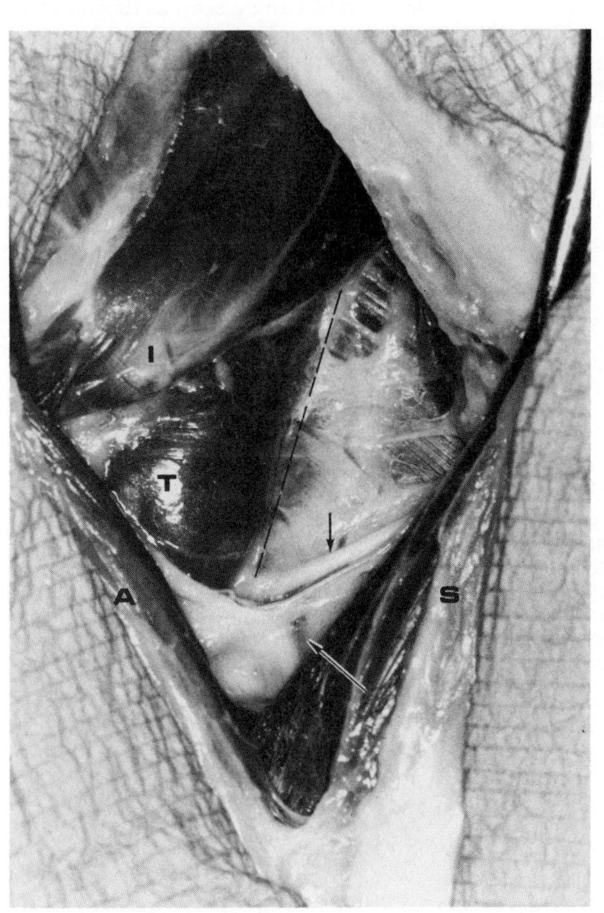

FIGURE 145–18. The spinous head (S) of the deltoid muscle is retracted caudally and the acromial head (A) is retracted cranially, exposing the infraspinatus muscle (I) and the teres minor muscle (T). The teres minor and infraspinatus muscles are bluntly undermined *(broken line)*. The small black arrow points to the muscular branch of the axillary nerve. The long arrow points to the caudal circumflex humeral vessel.

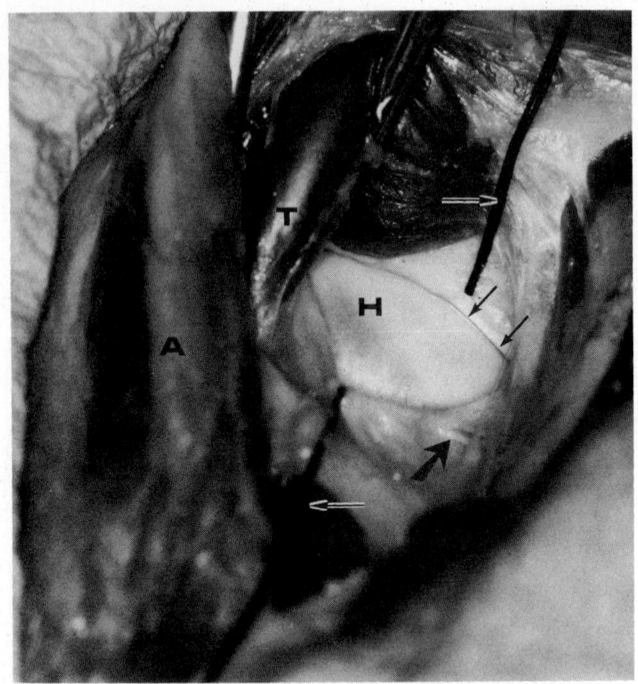

FIGURE 145–19. The teres minor muscle (T) has been retracted craniodorsally, and the joint capsule was incised parallel to the glenoid rim *(small black arrows)*. Stay sutures *(black-and-white arrows)* have been used to retract the joint capsule. The muscular branch of the axillary nerve and the caudal circumflex humeral vessel *(large black arrow)* have been protected by ventral retraction of the joint capsule. (H, humeral head; A, acromial head of the deltoid muscle.) (From Probst CW, Flo GL: Comparison of two caudolateral approaches to the scapulohumeral joint for treatment of osteochondritis dissecans in dogs. *J Am Vet Med Assoc 191*:1102, 1987.)

for the craniolateral approach. Dead space is eliminated by tacking down successive layers.

This approach allows for exposure of approximately 50 per cent of the articular surface of the humeral head and permits inspection of the caudal and medial aspects of the joint.[51]

Caudal Approach. A skin incision is begun at the midpoint of the caudal scapular border and continued parallel to the scapular spine along the caudal edge of the spinous head of the deltoid muscle, ending at the caudal border of the proximal humerus (Fig. 145–21). The subcutaneous fat and fascia are incised along the same line as the skin. The skin is retracted to expose the spinous head of the deltoid muscle and the lateral and long heads of the triceps muscle. The caudal circumflex humeral vessels, the axillobrachial vein, and branches of the axillary nerve can be seen as they emerge from beneath the spinous head of the deltoid muscle (Fig. 145–22). The spinous head of the deltoid is bluntly undermined distal to the axillary nerve and caudal circumflex humeral vessels. The latter is protected during the dissection. The spinous head is retracted cra-

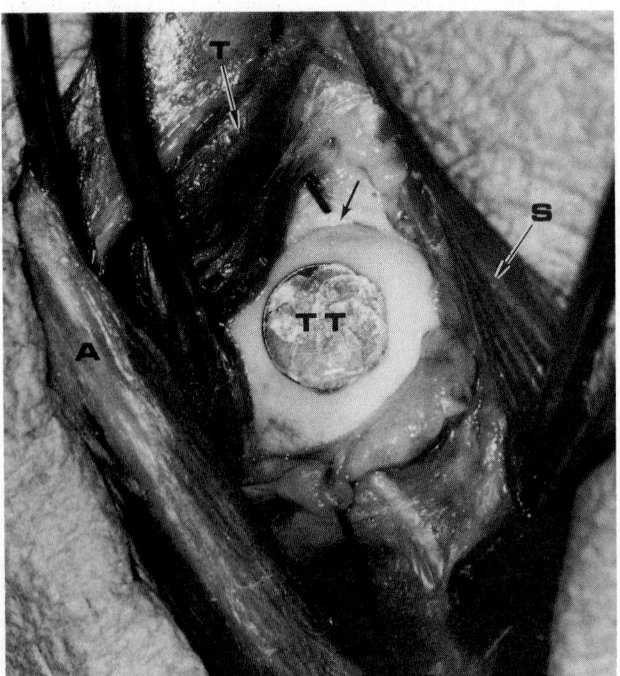

FIGURE 145–20. The humerus has been rotated internally and adducted, and the scapulohumeral joint has been extended. (TT, location of a typical osteochondritis dissecans lesion.) The black arrow indicates the glenoid rim, which may limit complete exposure of a cartilage flap. (A, acromial head of the deltoid muscle; T, teres minor muscle; S, spinous head of the deltoid muscle.) (From Probst CW, Flo GL: Comparison of two caudolateral approaches to the scapulohumeral joint for treatment of osteochondritis dissecans in dogs. *J Am Vet Med Assoc 191*:1102, 1987.)

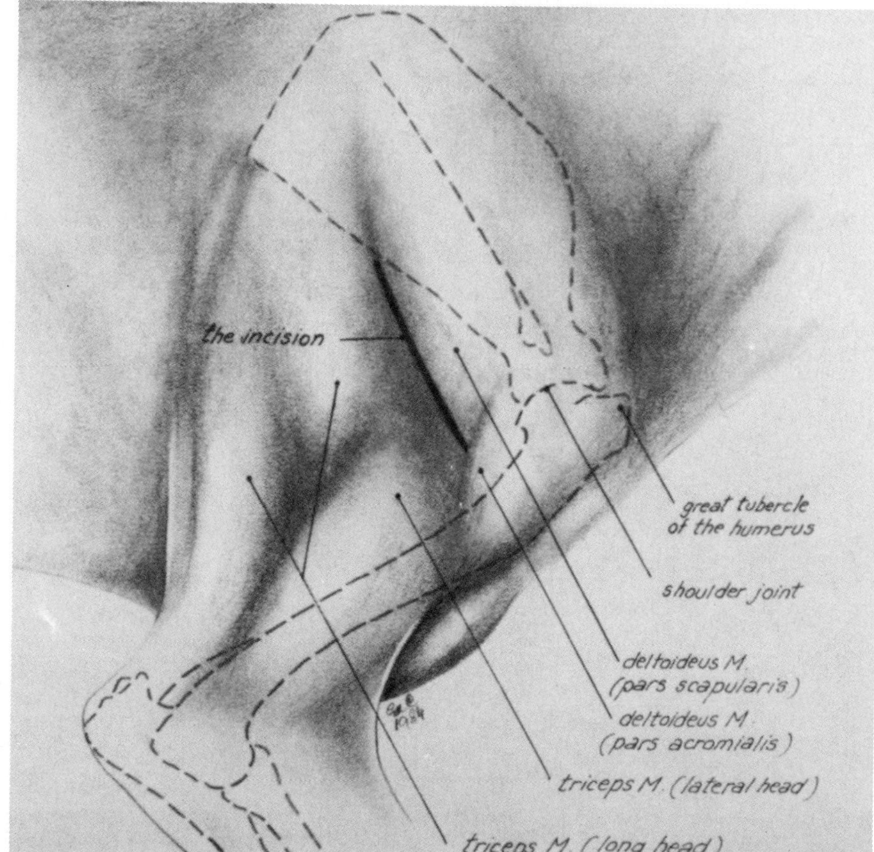

FIGURE 145–21. Lateral view of the right shoulder region of a dog, showing pertinent landmarks and the position of the skin incision for the caudal approach to the scapulohumeral joint. (From Tomlinson J, et al: Caudal approach to the shoulder joint in the dog. *Vet Surg 15*:295, 1986.)

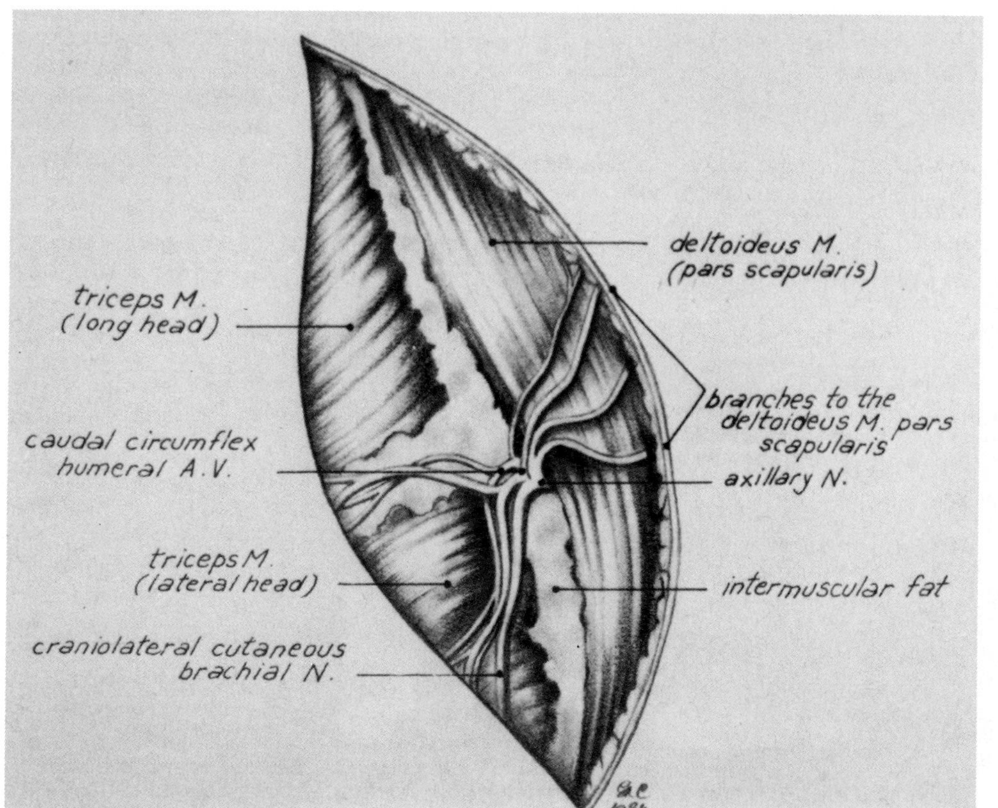

FIGURE 145–22. Lateral view of the shoulder region, demonstrating the separation between the deltoid and triceps muscles. The caudal circumflex humeral artery and vein and axillary nerve emerge at the level of the separation of the long and lateral heads of the triceps brachii muscle. Care must be taken to preserve these structures. (From Tomlinson J, et al: Caudal approach to the shoulder joint in the dog. *Vet Surg 15*:296, 1986.)

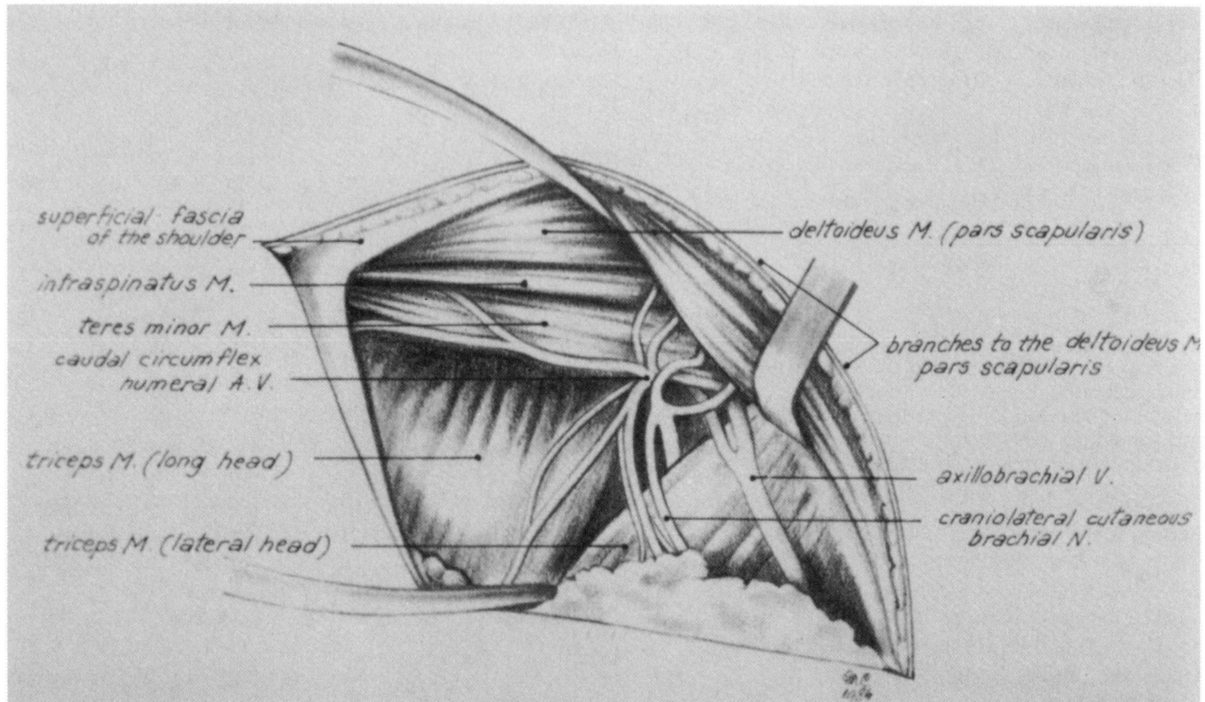

FIGURE 145–23. Caudal-to-cranial view of the shoulder after further separation of the deltoid and triceps brachii muscles. The teres minor and infraspinatus muscles are visible. (From Tomlinson J, et al: Caudal approach to the shoulder joint in the dog. *Vet Surg 15*:297, 1986.)

nially, exposing the teres minor and infraspinatus muscles (Fig. 145–23). The teres minor muscle is bluntly undermined while retracting the axillary nerve and caudal circumflex humeral vessels caudally and dorsally. Craniodorsal retraction of the teres minor muscle exposes the joint capsule (Fig. 145–24). The joint capsule is incised parallel to the glenoid rim and midway between it and the humeral head. The shoulder joint is extended, and the humerus is internally rotated to expose the lesion (Fig. 145–25).

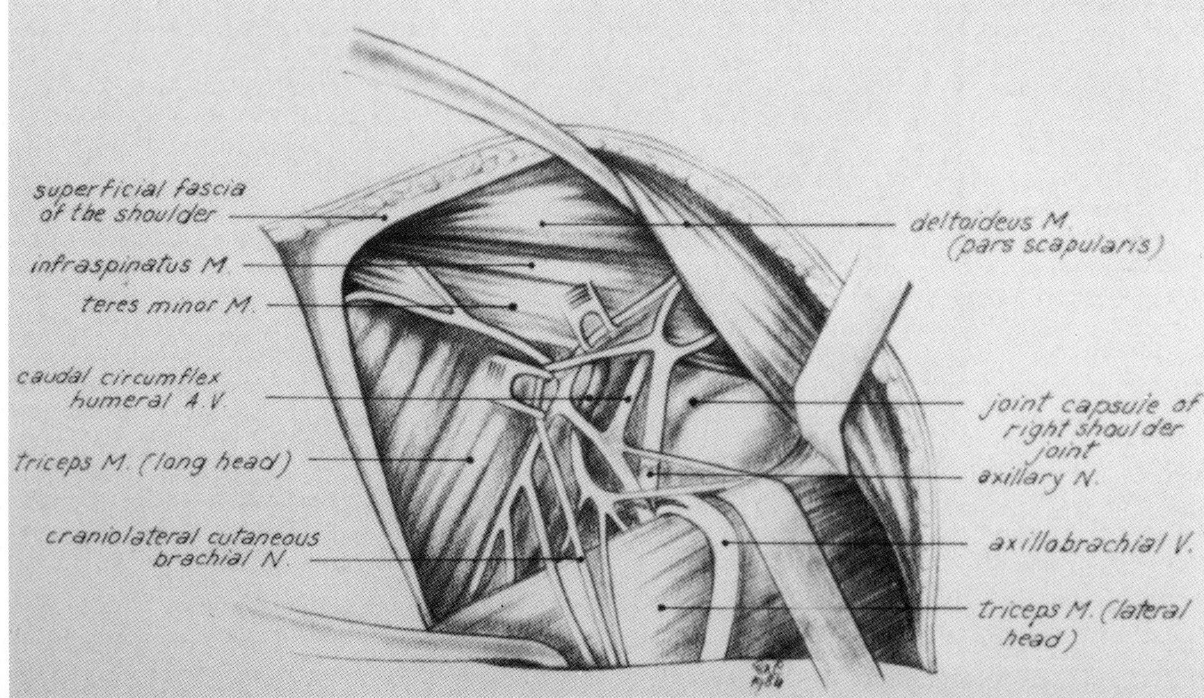

FIGURE 145–24. Caudal-to-cranial view of the surgical area. The joint capsule has been exposed after dissection under and retraction of the teres minor muscle. The caudal circumflex artery and vein and axillary nerve are carefully retracted dorsally and caudally to increase exposure of the joint capsule. (From Tomlinson J, et al: Caudal approach to the shoulder joint in the dog. *Vet Surg 5*:297, 1986.)

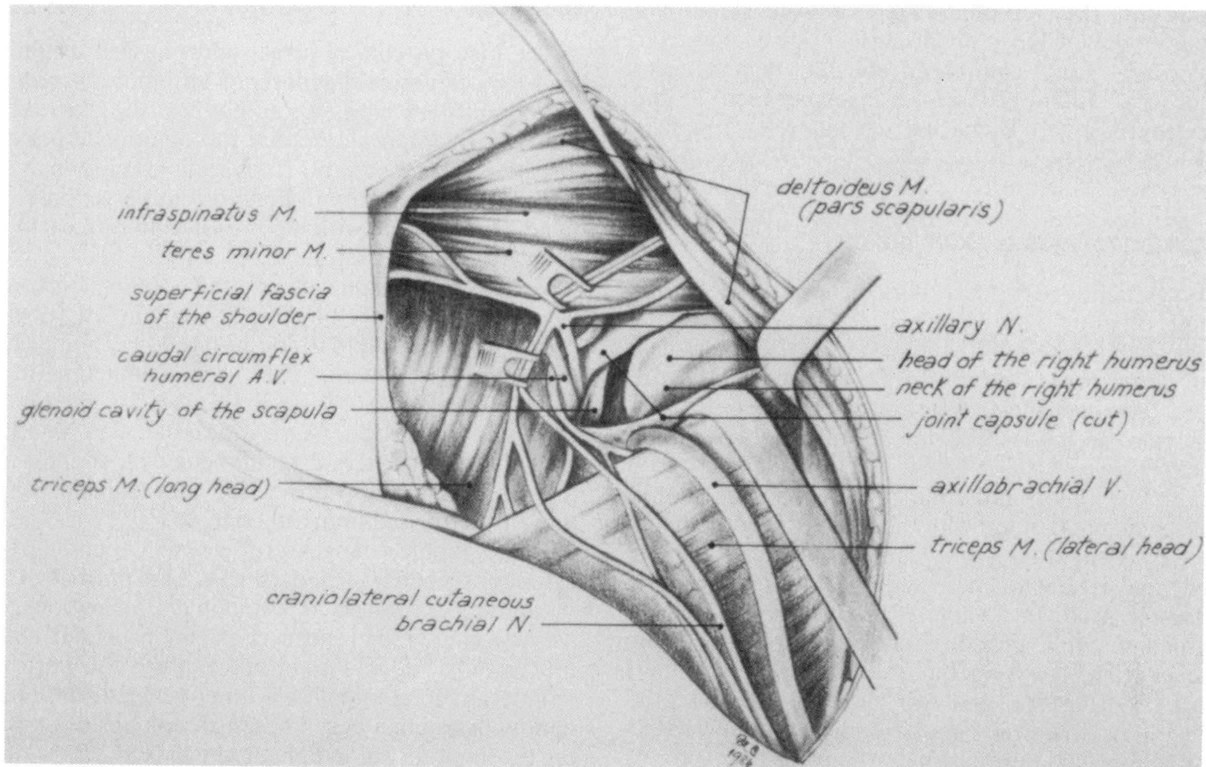

FIGURE 145–25. Caudal view of the humeral head after incision of the joint capsule. Rotation with adduction and extension of the humerus exposes the osteochondritis dissecans lesion. (From Tomlinson J, et al: Caudal approach to the shoulder joint in the dog. *Vet Surg 15*:298, 1986.)

The joint capsule is closed with interrupted absorbable sutures. The teres minor and deltoid muscles are allowed to return to normal positions. The deltoid fascia is sutured to the triceps fascia with interrupted absorbable sutures. The subcutaneous fat and skin are apposed, and dead space is eliminated.

This approach provides good exposure of the caudal aspect of the humeral head and joint capsule. Access to the medial compartment of the shoulder joint is also attained.[66]

Removal of the Cartilage Flap. Regardless of the approach, the cartilage flap is removed. All or a portion of the flap usually is still attached at the craniomedial extent of the lesion. The flap can be detached with a periosteal elevator, scalpel, or curette. It is important to remove all of the loose articular cartilage around the periphery of the lesion with a small bone curette. The margins of the remaining articular defect are left perpendicular to the joint surface because beveling the margins results in a larger defect that takes longer to heal and is more likely to cause a concurrent lesion in the glenoid cavity.[31]

We do not recommend routine, vigorous curettage of the subchondral bone beneath the cartilage flap. In some patients, the reparative fibrocartilage has already begun to form. To curette such a lesion delays the healing process. Forage (i.e., drilling multiple holes into subchondral bone) offers an alternative to curettage. If the subchondral bone is pale and sclerotic, curettage is necessary but removal of subchondral bone is minimized. Forage also may be useful. The joint is lavaged with sterile saline before closure.

Aftercare, Complications, and Prognosis. Most patients can be discharged the day after surgery. Bandaging is not necessary. Owners are instructed to restrict the dog's exercise to leash walks for the next 4 weeks. The skin sutures are removed in 7 to 10 days.

The most common complication after surgical exposure of the shoulder joint is seroma formation.[10] The incidence of seroma formation has been reported to be 0, 6, and 18 per cent.[27, 51, 66] The exact cause of seroma formation is unknown, but several factors contribute, including failure to restrict the dog's activity, inadequate hemostasis, excessive undermining of the skin, and failure to eliminate dead space. Inadequate closure of the joint capsule is not a factor in seroma formation.[59]

The prognosis after surgical treatment is good to excellent.[5, 22, 51, 66] Most dogs return to normal within 4 weeks of surgery. Older dogs with chronic lameness and degenerative joint disease have a more guarded prognosis.

OSTEOCHONDRITIS DISSECANS OF THE ELBOW

Signalment

The signalment is the same as in dogs with OCD of the shoulder and occurs most frequently in large dogs.[6, 16, 21, 44, 50, 52] The disease is most prevalent in Bernese mountain dogs and in golden and Labrador retrievers.[44]

The age at which dogs are presented for examination varies. Ages ranging from 4 months to 12 years are reported, and most dogs are less than 1 year old.[6, 16, 44, 52] Some dogs are asymptomatic (or lameness is not noticed) until they are older; therefore, one should not rule out elbow OCD simply because a dog is mature.

Males are more commonly affected than females (2:1).[6, 16, 44, 52] Bilateral disease ranges between 20 and 50 per cent.[6, 16, 44, 52] Right and left elbows are equally involved.[6, 16, 52]

Clinical Signs/Physical Examination

An owner may report that the dog appears stiff in the morning or after periods of rest. Lameness is usually present but may be mild or intermittent. The lameness is worse after vigorous exercise. Owners may not notice bilateral lameness and seek veterinary advice only if the dog sustains an injury. It is important not to be misled by the history.

Muscle atrophy is not consistent on physical examination. A dog may stand with the affected elbow slightly adducted. A slight lateral swelling of the elbow may be present and is due to increased synovial fluid volume and joint capsule thickening. Crepitus may be felt on joint manipulation. Flexion and extension of the elbow may elicit pain. It is sometimes difficult to determine if the pain is from the elbow or shoulder. Because the signalment and clinical signs of dogs with elbow OCD and shoulder OCD are similar, it may be necessary to radiograph both the elbow and shoulder.

Diagnosis

The history, clinical signs, and physical examination lead to a tentative diagnosis of an elbow disorder, but radiographs are necessary to confirm the diagnosis (see Fig. 145–6). *Both* elbows are radiographed because the disease is often bilateral. Early radiographic changes are subtle, so high-quality radiographs are essential.[6, 21, 44] A tabletop technique with high-resolution rare earth intensifying screens is preferable.[44]

Several radiographic views are necessary for complete evaluation of the elbow.[21, 44] A mediolateral view is obtained by placing the dog in lateral recumbency with the elbow downward. The joint is maximally flexed during film exposure so that most of the anconeal process can be seen. A craniocaudal view is obtained with the dog in sternal recumbency. A slightly medial oblique craniocaudal projection may enhance observation of the medial humeral condyle.[21, 44]

Radiographic changes are varied, depending on the extent of secondary osteoarthritis. One of the first visible radiographic changes is osteophyte formation on the nonarticular cranial surface of the proximal anconeal process.[6, 44, 50] One should not confuse the normal craniolateral and craniomedial tuberosities of the proximal ulna with osteophytes. These osteophytes are best seen on the lateral radiograph of the flexed elbow. Osteophytes are also frequently seen on the proximal radial

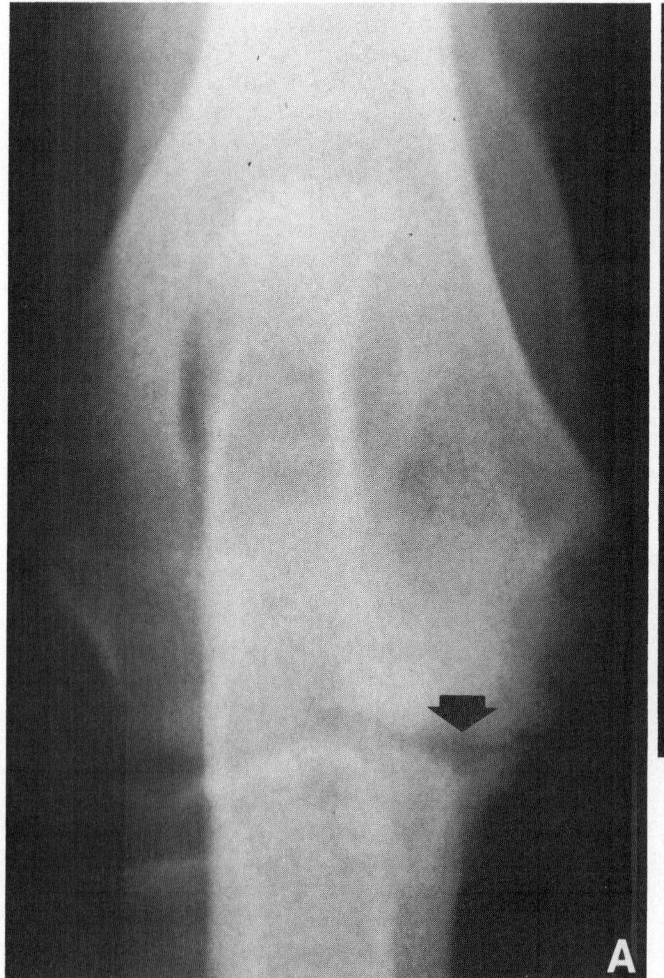

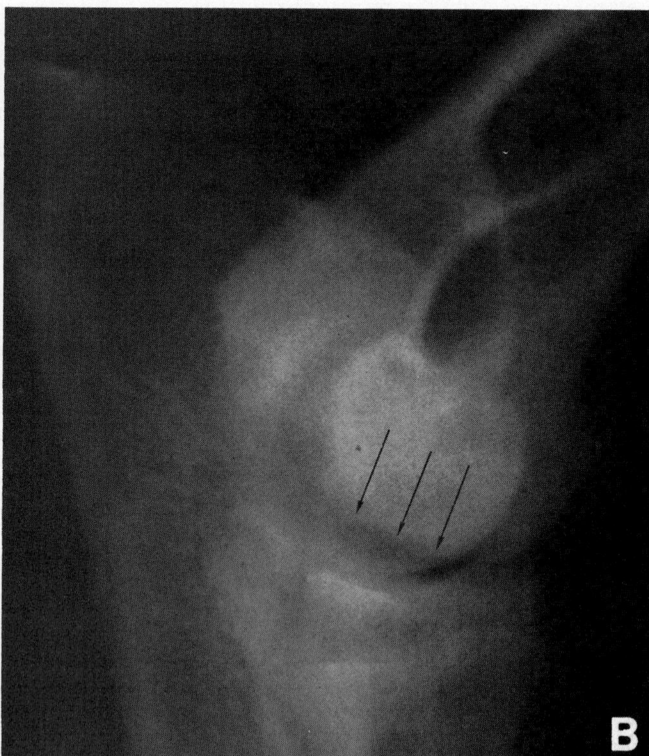

FIGURE 145–26. Craniocaudal *(A)* and lateral *(B)* radiographic views of a dog's elbow. The arrows point to a radiolucent area in the medial condyle of the humerus that is an osteochondritis dissecans lesion.

head, medial humeral condyle, and medial coronoid process. These radiographic changes are nonspecific and represent secondary degenerative joint disease. Many dogs with elbow degenerative joint disease suffer from a general incongruity of the joint termed *elbow dysplasia* (see the last section of this chapter).

Specific radiographic changes are not seen in every patient. A radiolucent defect may be noted in the medial humeral condyle (Fig. 145–26). This lucency is best observed in a craniocaudal, slightly medial oblique projection with the elbow in about 30° of flexion.[44] If the defect is large, it may also be visible on a lateral projection as a flattening of the articular surface of the medial condyle (see Fig. 145–26). In most cases, the radiographic changes of OCD of the elbow are not diagnostic; definitive diagnosis often requires exploratory arthrotomy.

Treatment

Treatment consists of a medial arthrotomy and removal of the cartilage flap. A simple medial approach without tenotomy or osteotomy provides excellent exposure of the elbow joint.[16, 52]

Surgical Anatomy

Locations of the pronator teres and flexor carpi radialis muscles and branches of the brachial artery and median nerve near the joint are important.

Surgical Approach

The dog is positioned in dorsal recumbency and tilted slightly toward the affected side. A sandbag is positioned lateral to the leg so that the lateral aspect of the elbow rests on the sandbag after the leg is draped (Fig. 145–27). A curved 6- to 8-cm skin incision is begun just proximal to the medial humeral epicondyle (Fig. 145–28). The antebrachial fascia is incised along the same line as the skin incision, exposing the pronator teres and flexor carpi radialis muscles (Fig. 145–29). Fascia between these muscles is incised, and the muscles are separated and retracted. The branch of the median nerve that passes obliquely beneath the pronator teres and flexor carpi radialis muscles is identified (Fig. 145–30). A horizontal incision is made through the joint capsule and medial collateral ligament (Fig. 145–31). The median nerve passes close to the craniomedial aspect of the joint and is avoided. A stay suture is placed in the distal joint capsule to aid in retraction. The antebrachium is abducted against the sandbag to open the medial aspect of the joint, thus exposing the trochlea humeri (see Fig. 145–31).

The cartilage flap is removed from the medial aspect of the humeral condyle as described for the shoulder joint (see Fig. 145–31). The joint is lavaged with sterile saline before closure. The medial collateral ligament is reapposed with nonabsorbable suture using a locking loop tendon suture or horizontal mattress pattern. The median nerve is avoided during closure. Joint capsule, antebrachial fascia, and subcutaneous tissue are apposed with synthetic absorbable suture using a simple interrupted pattern.

Aftercare, Complications, and Prognosis

The wound is covered with a sterile dressing, and a padded bandage is applied to the leg. The bandage remains in place until the sutures are removed in 10 to 14 days. Dogs can usually be discharged from the hospital the day after surgery. Clients are instructed to restrict the dog's activity to leash walks for 4 weeks.

The only complication is seroma formation. If the

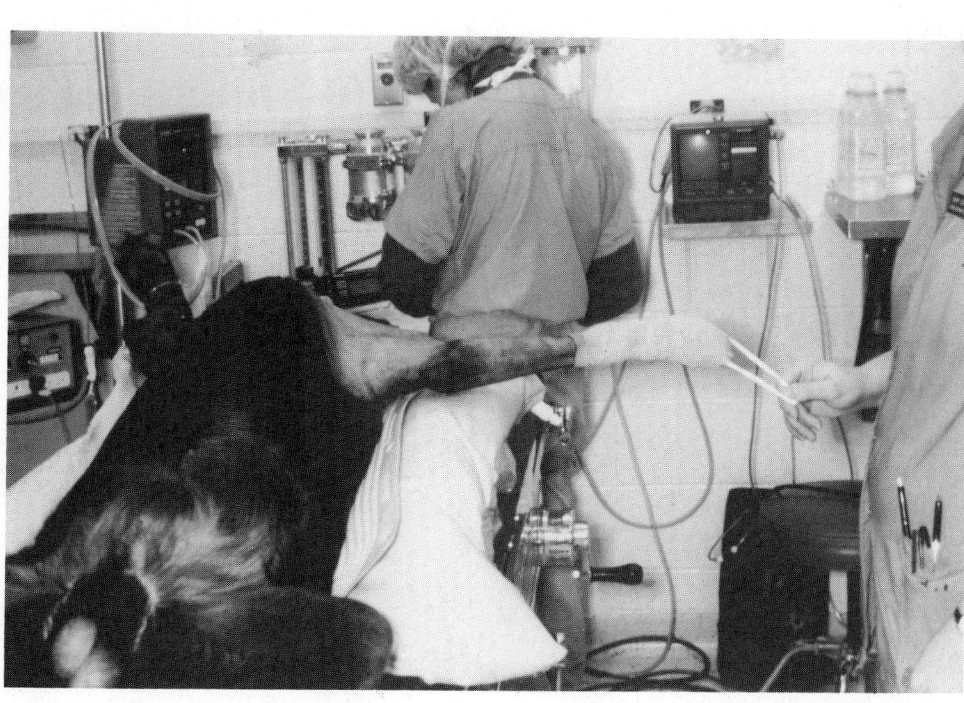

FIGURE 145–27. The dog is in dorsal recumbency and tilted slightly toward the affected side. A sandbag can be positioned laterally to the leg so that the lateral aspect of the elbow rests on the sandbag after the leg is draped. (This photo was taken before draping to demonstrate the positioning.)

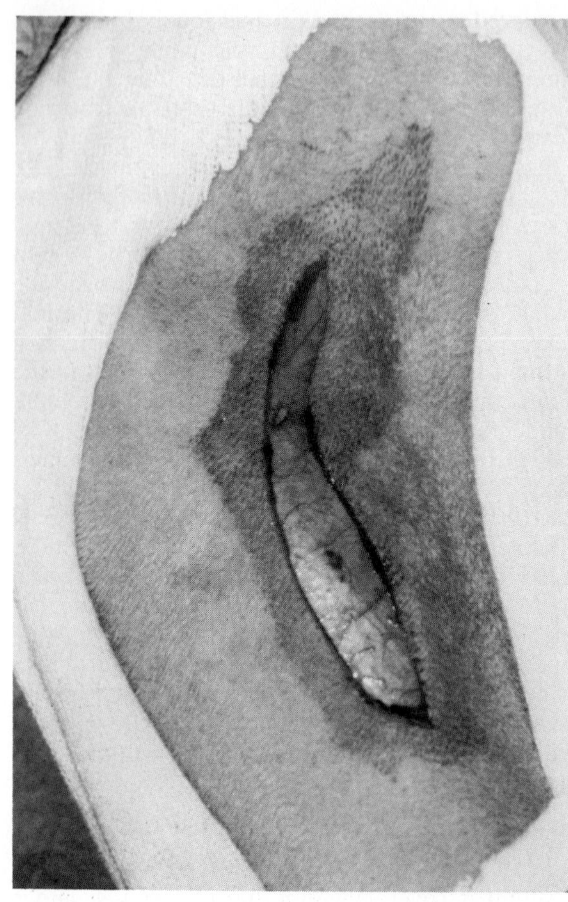

FIGURE 145–28. A 6- to 8-cm curved skin incision has been made on the medial aspect of the elbow, beginning at the medial epicondyle.

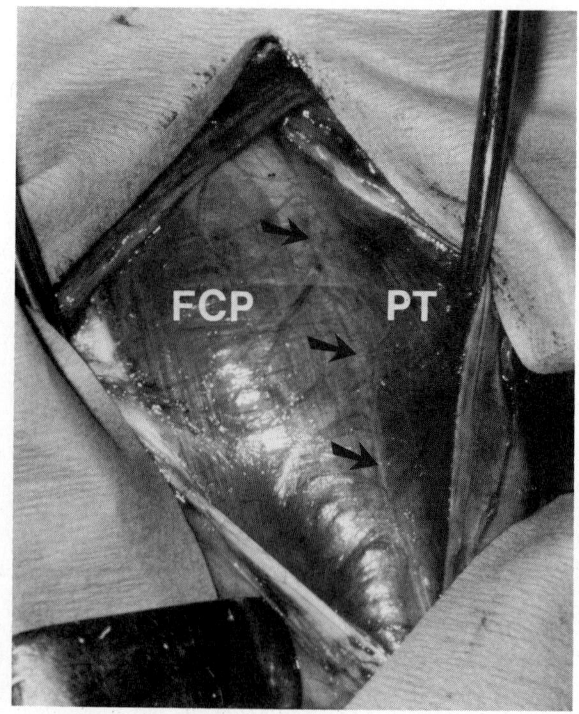

FIGURE 145–29. The antebrachial fascia is incised along the same line as the skin, thus exposing the pronator teres (PT) and flexor carpi radialis (FCR) muscles. The arrows point to the division between these muscles. (From Probst CW: Fragmented medial coronoid process and osteochondritis dissecans of the elbow. *Comp Anim Pract* 2:30, 1988.)

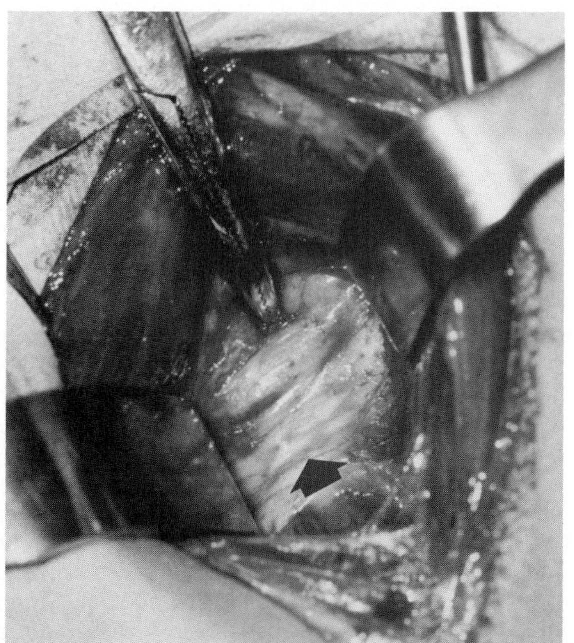

FIGURE 145–30. The fascia between the pronator teres and flexor carpi radialis muscles has been incised, and these muscles retracted. The hemostat points to the joint space. The arrow points to the median nerve as it courses distally to the elbow joint. (From Probst CW: Fragmented medial coronoid process and osteochondritis dissecans of the elbow. *Comp Anim Pract 2*:30, 1988.)

bandage remains in place and the dog's activity is restricted, seroma formation is uncommon.

The prognosis after surgery depends on the size of the lesion and the severity of the secondary osteoarthritis present at treatment. Generally, young dogs with small lesions and minimal secondary osteoarthritis have a favorable prognosis. Dogs with more severe lesions, more severe osteoarthritis, and concurrent fragmented medial coronoid have a more guarded prognosis. Most dogs improve clinically after surgery, but the osteoarthritis may progress.

OSTEOCHONDRITIS DISSECANS OF THE STIFLE

Signalment

Although OCD occurs much less commonly in the stifle than in the shoulder or elbow, it also afflicts young large dogs.[8, 15, 33, 38] Males are more commonly affected than females.[15, 38]

Clinical Signs

The main clinical sign is lameness. The onset of lameness is insidious, and the lameness worsens with exercise. The owners are frequently only aware of a unilateral lameness even though both stifles are affected. Dogs with bilateral disease may assume a couched stance.[38]

Mild muscle atrophy may be present, particularly in the more chronic cases. A slight joint effusion is often present. Pain and occasional crepitus or an audible click may be elicited on manipulation.[8, 15, 38]

Diagnosis

A diagnosis of OCD of the stifle cannot be confirmed by physical examination. Joint effusion, muscle atrophy, pain, and crepitus could be associated with various causes of osteoarthritis of the stifle. Mediolateral and caudocranial radiographic views of the stifle are necessary to confirm the diagnosis (Fig. 145–32).

A flattened area on the weightbearing surface of the femoral condyle and joint mice may be seen on the mediolateral view (Fig. 145–33). It is difficult but not impossible to determine from the mediolateral view which femoral condyle is involved. The fossa of the long digital extensor tendon can be used to determine which is the lateral condyle. The caudocranial view can help reveal which condyle is involved if the lesion can be seen (see Fig. 145–33). The lesion may not always be visible in this view and should not be confused with the superimposed extensor fossa.[38]

Bilateral lesions occur in 72 per cent of cases.[38] The medial femoral condyle alone was involved in 4 per cent.[38] The lesion was located in the medial femoral condyle in 80 per cent in one human study.[35] Most of the lesions in dogs occur in the lateral femoral condyle.[15, 33, 38]

Treatment

The treatment of stifle OCD is similar to treatment in other joints. If the lesion is located in the lateral

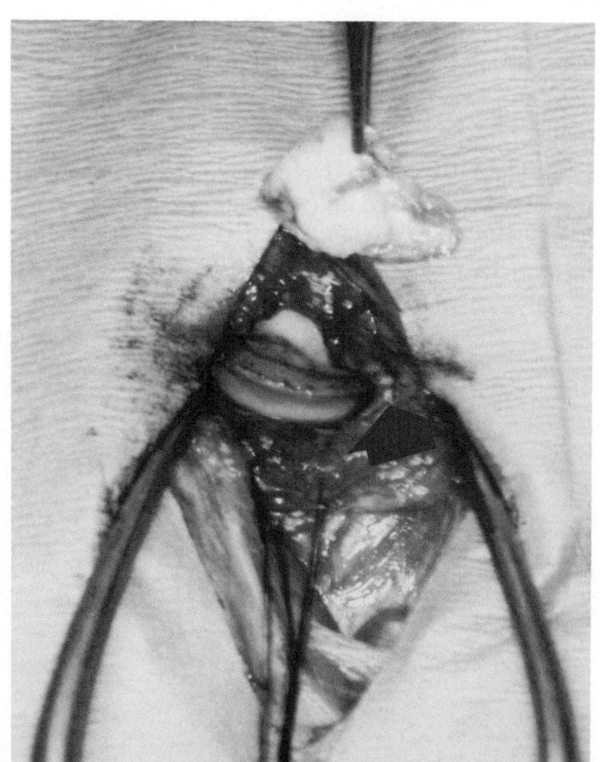

FIGURE 145–31. A horizontal incision has been made through the joint capsule and medial collateral ligament *(arrow)*. A stay suture has been used to retract the joint capsule distally. The antebrachium has been abducted to open the medial aspect of the joint, exposing the trochlea humeri. A large cartilage flap has been removed from the weightbearing surface of the medial humeral condyle.

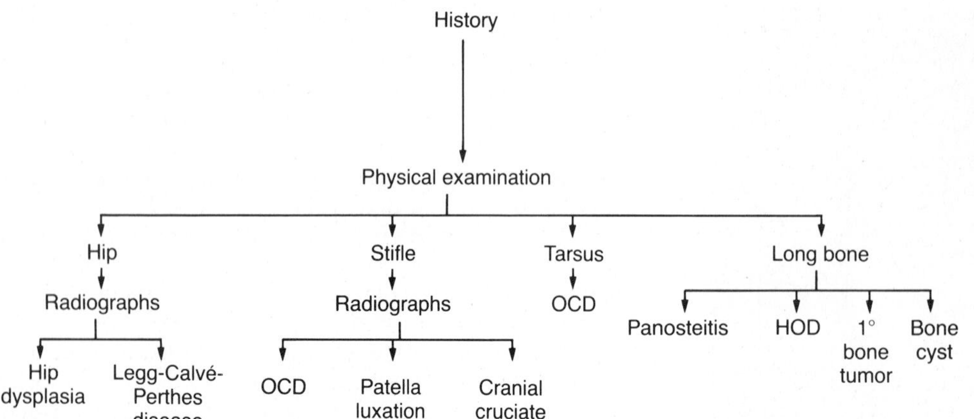

FIGURE 145–32. Algorithm for rear leg lameness in young dogs. (OCD, osteochondritis dissecans; HOD, hypertrophic osteodystrophy.)

femoral condyle, a lateral arthrotomy is performed. A medial arthrotomy is performed for medial condylar lesions. The surgical anatomy and approaches to the stifle are described elsewhere.[49]

All joint mice and loose cartilage flaps are removed (Fig. 145–34). As with all OCD defects, the articular margins are left perpendicular to the articular surfaces. If reparative fibrocartilage has not formed, lightly curette the defect or drill holes into the subchondral bone with a K wire (Fig. 145–35). The joint is flushed with sterile saline before closure. Joint capsule, biceps or sartorius fascia, and subcutaneous tissue are apposed with synthetic absorbable sutures using a simple interrupted pattern.

Aftercare, Complications, and Prognosis

The wound is covered with a sterile dressing, and a modified Robert Jones bandage is applied. The dog usually can be discharged from the hospital the day after surgery. The bandage and skin sutures can be removed in 10 to 14 days. Activity is restricted to leash walks for 4 weeks.

The prognosis depends on the extent of the degenerative joint disease and size of the lesion.[38] As with OCD of the elbow, the degenerative joint disease of the stifle progresses. Dogs with small lesions and late onset of clinical signs have the best prognosis.[38] Dogs with large lesions, advanced degenerative joint disease, and early onset of clinical signs have a worse prognosis.[38]

OSTEOCHONDRITIS DISSECANS OF THE TARSUS

Signalment

OCD of the tarsus also occurs in large dogs and is most commonly reported in rottweilers and Labrador retrievers.[1, 40, 56, 57, 64, 66] Although most dogs are less than 1 year old when initially presented,[1, 40, 56, 57, 64, 66] one study reports an age range of 5 to 48 months.[64] Females seem to be more commonly affected (2:1), although large studies are unavailable.[1, 40, 56, 57, 64, 66]

Clinical Signs

Hindlimb lameness is the most common clinical sign. Hyperextension of the tarsocrural joint is common. Joint

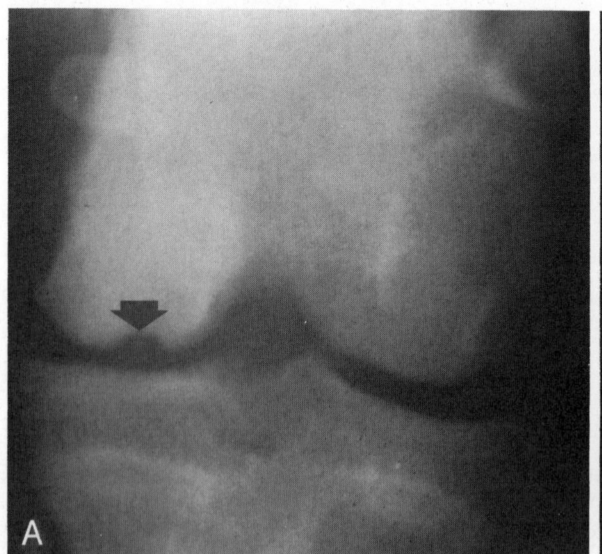

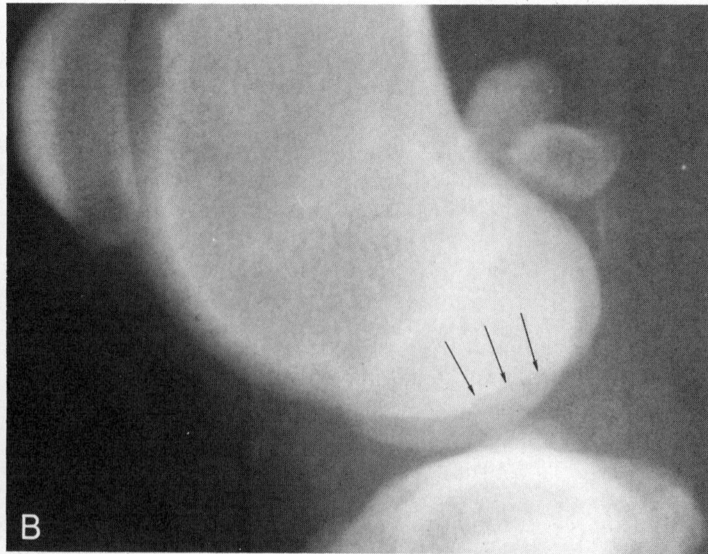

FIGURE 145–33. Caudocranial *(A)* and lateral *(B)* radiographic views of a dog's stifle. The arrows point to a flattened area on the weigtbearing surface of the medial femoral condyle.

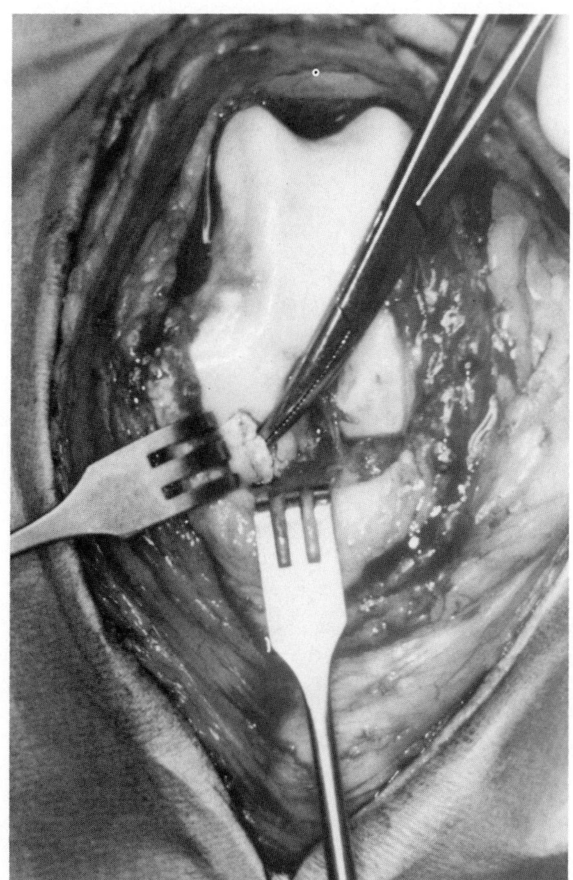

FIGURE 145–34. A medial arthrotomy of the stifle has been performed, and the patella has been luxated laterally. The hemostat is pointing to a loose cartilage flap in the weightbearing surface of the medial femoral condyle.

effusion and tarsal thickening are often present, especially on the medial side of the joint. Decreased range of motion may be noted, especially in flexion. Pain may be elicited on joint manipulation. Crepitus is occasionally present.*

Diagnosis

Confirmation of OCD of the talus depends on high-quality radiographs. The craniocaudal projection is most helpful in diagnosing OCD of the medial trochlear ridge of the talus (Fig. 145–36).[56, 67] The mediolateral or oblique views are most helpful in diagnosing OCD of the lateral trochlear ridge, because the calcaneus is superimposed over the lateral trochlear ridge, in the craniocaudal view (see Fig. 145–36).[56, 67] Flexed mediolateral and craniocaudal views may also aid in the diagnosis.[40] Both hocks are radiographed because the disease often occurs bilaterally.[8, 64]

Radiographic abnormalities include a radiolucent or flattened area involving either trochlear ridge (occasionally both) and a widened joint space.[40, 64] A widened joint space is more common with lesions involving the medial trochlear ridge. Soft-tissue swelling is invariably present, and degenerative joint disease develops in chronic cases.

*See references 1, 8, 40, 56, 57, 64, and 66.

Treatment

The most common treatment used for OCD of the tarsus has been removal of the cartilage flap or joint mice with or without curettage of the subchondral bone.[40, 56, 57, 64] An alternative to curettage of the subchondral bone is drilling holes into the subchondral bone.[1] This technique allows neovascularization without disturbing cartilage elements that may be present.[1]

The talus may be exposed by osteotomy of the medial malleolus[62] or lateral malleolus. These techniques offer the advantages of excellent exposure and preservation of the collateral ligaments of the tarsus. The medial malleolar osteotomy is technically demanding, and the articular cartilage of the distal tibia is disrupted, contributing to osteoarthritis.

Medial and lateral approaches to the talus that do not require osteotomy or desmotomy have been evaluated.[3, 20] These approaches offer exposure of most of the talus, but a malleolar osteotomy may still be required to expose large lesions of the medial trochlear ridge.*

Aftercare, Complications, and Prognosis

The wound is covered with a sterile dressing before applying a support bandage. If an osteotomy has been performed, a rigid splint is used to support the internal repair for 4 to 6 weeks. Activity is restricted for 4 to 6

*Editor's note: For medial lesions, an approach caudal to the malleolus has proved satisfactory. Lateral lesions require osteotomy of the lateral malleolus for adequate exposure.

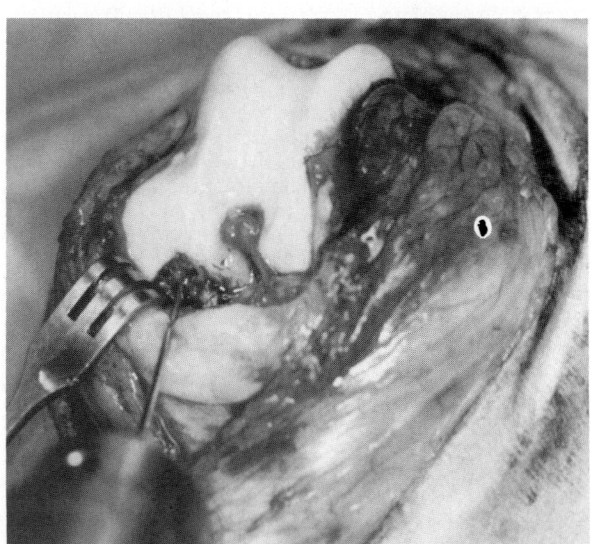

FIGURE 145–35. The same view as in Figure 145–34, but after removal of the cartilage flap. Holes are drilled into the subchondral bone using a hand chuck and K wire. The holes allow the subchondral bone to bleed but do not enlarge the defect.

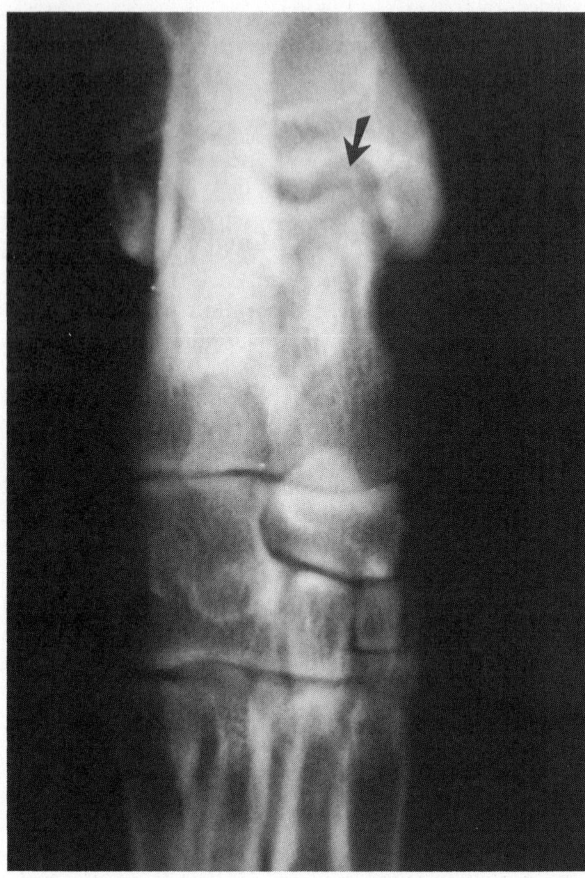

FIGURE 145–36. Craniocaudal radiographic view of dog's tarsus. The arrow points to an osteochondritis dissecans lesion involving the medial trochlear ridge of the talus. The lateral trochlear ridge of the talus is difficult to see because of superimpositon of the calcaneus.

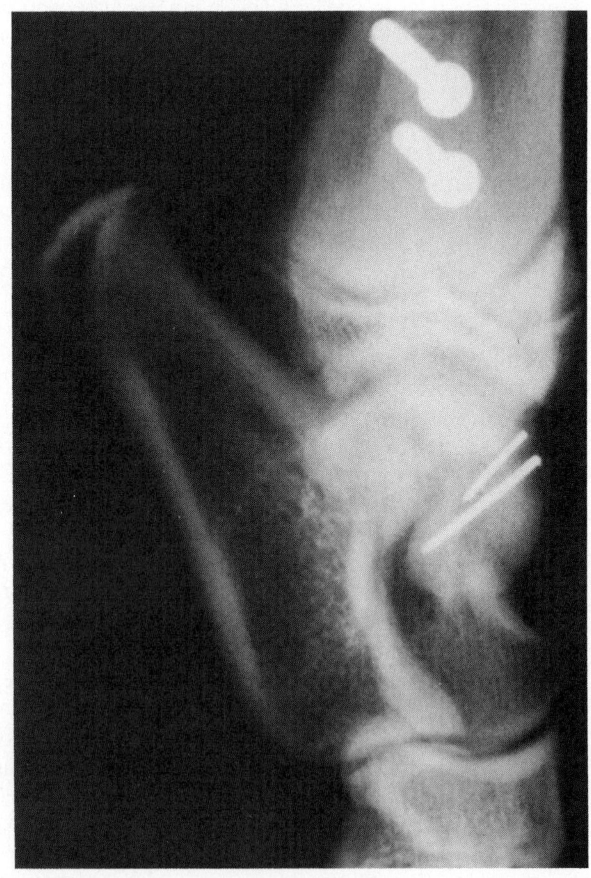

FIGURE 145–37. Lateral radiographic view of a dog's tarsus. A large osteochondral fragment of the lateral trochlear ridge of the talus has been reattached with two divergent K wires. The wires were countersunk below the level of the articular cartilage. An osteotomy of the fibula was used to expose the talus, and it has been repaired with two lag screws.

weeks after surgery (8 to 10 weeks if an osteotomy has been performed).

No common complications are associated with this procedure. A potential complication of an osteotomy procedure is failure of the osteotomy to heal owing to unstable fixation.

The goal of surgical treatment is to limit or halt the progression of osteoarthritis and lameness associated with OCD of the tarsus. Surgical removal of the lesion did not modify progression of osteoarthritic changes.[64] Removal of the cartilage flap may accentuate joint instability and contribute to osteoarthritis.[40] A more rational approach is to reattach the cartilage fragments,[67] which might be feasible in patients with large cartilage flaps or with osteochondral fragments (Fig. 145–37).

The long-term prognosis for OCD of the talus is guarded. Most reports suggest that osteoarthritis tends to progress.[56, 57, 64] The prognosis is generally favorable if the lesions are small and treated early.

References

1. Aron DN, et al: Free chondral fragment involving the lateral trochlear ridge of the talus in a dog. *J Am Vet Med Assoc 186*:1095, 1985.
2. Barrie HJ: Osteochondritis dissecans 1887–1987: A centennial look at Konig's memorable phrase. *J Bone Joint Surg [Br] 69B*:693, 1987.
3. Beale BS, Goring RL: Exposure of the medial and lateral trochlear ridges of the talus in the dog. Part I: Dorsomedial and plantaromedial surgical approaches to the medial trochlear ridge. *J Am Anim Hosp Assoc 26*:13, 1990.
4. Berzon JL: Osteochondritis dissecans in the dog: Diagnosis and therapy. *J Am Vet Med Assoc 175*:796, 1979.
5. Birkeland R: Osteochondritis dissecans in the humeral head of the dog: Comparison of results achieved with conservative and surgical treatment. *Nord Veterinaremed 19*:294, 1967.
6. Boudrieau RJ, et al: Osteochondritis dissecans of the elbow in the dog. *J Am Anim Hosp Assoc 19*:627, 1983.
7. Brass W: Über die Osteochondrosis des Hundes. *Tierarztl Umsch 11*:200, 1956.
8. Brinker WO, et al: *Handbook of Small Animal Orthopedics and Fracture Treatment*. W. B. Saunders, Philadelphia, 1983, pp 326, 337, 366.
9. Carrig CB, Morgan JP: Microcirculation of the humeral head in the immature dog. *J Am Vet Radiol Soc 15*:28, 1974.
10. Cechner PE, Knecht CD: Approach to the canine shoulder without myotomy, osteotomy, or tenotomy. *J Am Anim Hosp Assoc 15*:753, 1979.
11. Convery FR, et al: The repair of large osteochondral defects: An experimental study in horses. *Clin Orthop 82*:253, 1972.
12. Cordy DR, Wind AP: Transverse fracture of the proximal humeral articular cartilage in dogs (so called osteochondritis dissecans). *Pathol Vet 6*:424, 1969.
13. Cormack DH: *Ham's Histology*. 9th ed. J. B. Lippincott, Philadelphia, 1987.
14. Craig PH, Riser WH: Osteochondritis dissecans in the proximal humerus of the dog. *J Am Vet Radiol Soc 6*:40, 1965.
15. Denny HR, Gibbs C: Osteochondritis dissecans of the canine stifle joint. *J Small Anim Pract 21*:317, 1980.
16. Denny HR, Gibbs C: The surgical treatment of osteochondritis dissecans and ununited coronoid process in the canine elbow joint. *J Small Anim Pract 21*:323, 1980.
17. Dingwall JL, et al: Osteochondritis dissecans in a miniature poodle. *Mod Vet Pract 53*:47, 1972.
18. Duthie RB, Houghton GR: Constitutional aspects of the osteochondroses. *Clin Orthop 158*:19, 1981.
19. Faulkner RT: Osteochondritis dissecans of the shoulder joint: Its surgical treatment. *Vet Med Small Anim Clin Nov*:1709, 1980.
20. Goring RL, Beale BS: Exposure of the medial and lateral trochlear ridges of the talus in the dog. Part II: Dorsolateral and plantarolateral surgical approaches to the lateral trochlear ridge. *J Am Anim Hosp Assoc 26*:19, 1990.
21. Goring RL, Bloomgerg MS: Selected developmental abnormalities of the canine elbow: Radiographic evaluation and surgical management. *Comp Cont Educ Pract Vet 5*:178, 1983.
22. Griffiths RC: Osteochondritis dissecans of the canine shoulder. *J Am Vet Med Assoc 153*:1733, 1968.
23. Hamerman D: The biology of osteoarthritis. *N Engl J Med 320*:1322, 1989.
24. Hedhammer A, et al: Overnutrition and skeletal disease: An experimental study in growing great Dane dogs. *Cornell Vet 64*(Suppl 5):1, 1974.
25. Hohn RB: Osteochondritis dissecans of the humeral head. *J Am Vet Med Assoc 163*:69, 1973.
26. Johnson KA, Dennis KA: Osteochondritis dissecans in a beagle. *Aust Vet J 54*:364, 1978.
27. Jones DGC, Vaughan LC: The surgical treatment of osteochondritis dissecans of the humeral head in dogs. *J Small Anim Pract 11*:803, 1970.
28. Kincaid SA, Van Sickle DC: Bone morphology and postnatal osteogenesis: Potential for disease. *Vet Clin North Am 13*:3, 1983.
29. Kincaid SA, Van Sickle DC: Regional histochemical and thickness variations of adult articular cartilage. *Am J Vet Res 42*:428, 1981.
30. Kincaid SA, et al: Lipids of normal and osteochondritic cartilage of the immature canine humeral head. *Am J Vet Res 46*:1060, 1985.
31. Knecht CD: Osteochondrosis of the shoulder and stifle in 3 of 5 border collie littermates. *J Am Vet Med Assoc 170*:58, 1977.
32. Lau RE, Shumway JD: Osteochondrosis of the humeral head. *Canine Pract 6*:26, 1979.
33. Leighton RL: Surgical treatment of osteochondritis dissecans of the canine stifle. *Vet Med Small Anim Clin 76*:1733, 1981.
34. Lenehan TM, Van Sickle DC: Canine Osteochondrosis. *In* Newton CD, Nunamaker DM (eds): *Textbook of Small Animal Orthopedics*. J. B. Lippincott, Philadelphia, 1985, pp 981–997.
35. Linden B: Osteochondritis dissecans of the femoral condyles: A long term follow up study. *J Bone Joint Surg [Am] 59A*:769, 1977.
36. Mankin HJ: The articular cartilages. *In* Newton CD, Nunamaker DM (eds): *Textbook of Small Animal Orthopedics*. J. B. Lippincott, Philadelphia, 1985, pp 90–103.
37. Milton JL: Osteochondritis dissecans in the dog. *Vet Clin North Am 13*:117, 1983.
38. Montgomery DR, et al: Osteochondritis dissecans of the canine stifle. *Comp Cont Educ Pract Vet 11*:1199, 1989.
39. Nagura S: The so-called osteochondritis dissecans of Konig. *Clin Orthop 18*:100, 1960.
40. Olson NC, et al: Osteochondritis dissecans of the tarsocrural joint in three canine siblings. *J Am Vet Med Assoc 176*:635, 1980.
41. Olsson SE: General and aetiologic factors in canine osteochondrosis. *Vet Q 9*:268, 1987.
42. Olsson SE: Morphology and physiology of the growth cartilage under normal and pathologic conditions. *In* Sumner-Smith G (ed): *Bone in Clinical Orthopedics*. W. B. Saunders, Philadelphia, 1982, p 159.
43. Olsson SE: Osteochondrosis in the dog. *In* Kirk RW (ed): *Current Veterinary Therapy VI*. W. B. Saunders, Philadelphia, 1977, pp 880–886.
44. Olsson SE: The early diagnosis of fragmented coronoid process and osteochondritis dissecans of the canine elbow joint. *J Am An Hosp Assoc 19*:616, 1983.
45. Olsson SE, Reiland S: The nature of osteochondrosis in animals. Summary and conclusions with comparative aspects on osteochondrosis dissecans in man. *Acta Radiol 358*:299, 1978.
46. Paatsama S, et al: Etiological factors in osteochondritis dissecans. *Acta Orthop Scand 46*:906, 1975.
47. Paatsama S, et al: A study of osteochondritis dissecans of the canine humeral head using histological, OTC bone labelling, microradiographic and microangiographic methods. *J Small Anim Pract 12*:603, 1971.
48. Pappas AM: Osteochondrosis dissecans. *Clin Orthop 158*:59, 1981.
49. Piermattei DL, Greedley RG: *Atlas of Surgical Approaches to the Bones of the Dog and Cat*. 2nd ed. W. B. Saunders, Philadelphia, 1979, pp 3–11, 62–71, 164–162.
50. Probst CW: Fragmented medial coronoid process and osteochondritis dissecans of the elbow. *Comp Anim Pract 2*:27, 1988.
51. Probst CW, Flo GL: Comparison of two caudolateral approaches to the scapulohumeral joint for treatment of osteochondritis dissecans in dogs. *J Am Vet Med Assoc 191*:1101, 1987.
52. Probst CW, et al: A simple medial approach to the canine elbow for treatment of fragmented coronoid process and osteochondritis dissecans. *J Am Anim Hosp Assoc 25*:331, 1989.
53. Rehmel RA: Approach to the shoulder. *In* Wingfield WE, Rawlings CA (eds): *Small Animal Surgery*. W. B. Saunders, Philadelphia, 1979, pp 176–181.
54. Richardson DW, Clark CC: Biochemical changes in articular cartilage opposing full- and partial-thickness cartilage lesions in horses. *Am J Vet Res 51*:118, 1990.
55. Robins GM: Osteochondritis dissecans in the dog. *Aust Vet J 54*:272, 1978.
56. Robins GM, et al: Osteochondritis dissecans of the lateral ridge of the trochlea of the tibial tarsal bone in the dog. *J Small Anim Pract 24*:675, 1983.
57. Rosenblum GP, et al: Osteochondritis dissecans of the tibio-tarsal joint in the dog. *J Small Anim Pract 19*:759, 1978.
58. Salter RB, et al: The biological effect of continuous passive motion on the healing of full thickness defects in articular cartilage. *J Bone Joint Surg [Am] 62A*:1232, 1980.
59. Schiller AG, et al: Surgical treatment of osteochondrosis dissecans without suturing the joint capsule. *Vet Med Small Anim Clin 70*:50, 1978.
60. Schulman AJ, et al: Longitudinal myotomy of the acromial head of the

deltoid: A modified approach for the surgical treatment of osteochondritis dissecans in the dog. *J Am Anim Hosp Assoc 22*:475, 1986.
61. Siffert RS: Classification of the osteochondroses. *Clin Orthop 158*:10, 1981.
62. Sinbaldi KR: Medial approach to the tarsus. *J Am Anim Hosp Assoc 15*:77, 1979.
63. Smith CW, Stowater JL: Osteochondritis dissecans of the canine shoulder joint: A review of 35 cases. *J Am Anim Hosp Assoc 11*:658, 1975.
64. Smith MM, et al: Clinical evaluation of dogs after surgical and nonsurgical management of osteochondritis dissecans of the talus. *J Am Vet Med Assoc 187*:31, 1985.
65. Story EC: Prognostic value of arthrography in canine shoulder osteochondrosis (osteochondritis) dissecans. *Vet Clin North Am 8*:301, 1978.
66. Tomlinson J, et al: Caudal approach to the shoulder joint in the dog. *Vet Surg 15*:294, 1986.
67. Van Ee RT, et al: Osteochondritis dissecans of the lateral ridge of the talus in a dog. *J Am Vet Med Assoc 193*:1284, 1988.
68. Vaughan LC, Jones DGC: Osteochondritis dissecans of the head of the humerus in dogs. *J Small Anim Pract 9*:283, 1968.
69. Wissler J, Sumner-Smith G: Osteochondrosis in the elbow joint in the dog. *J Am Anim Hosp Assoc 13*:349, 1977.

Elbow Dysplasia

A. P. Wind

The term *elbow dysplasia* was introduced to describe generalized osteoarthrosis of the elbow joint in which the anconeal process was ununited in some but not all affected joints. Later, fragmentation of the medial coronoid process of the ulna and osteochondritis dissecans of the humeral condyle were associated with this arthrosis. These three diseases have been described as individual entities. Their occurrence, clinical signs, and various surgical treatments have been well documented.* The importance of a genetic predisposition has been appreciated.†

The breeds primarily afflicted are of intermediate size and heavy set, with a high incidence in the Bernese mountain dog, rottweiler, German shepherd, golden retriever, and Labrador retriever. Other breeds affected are the Newfoundland, Saint Bernard, mastiff, springer spaniel, Australian shepherd, chow chow, Sharpei, Shetland sheepdog, and some terrier breeds.

PROPOSED ETIOLOGIES

Because the occurrence of the three diseases overlaps, a common etiology has been sought. Olsson proposed that all three diseases are manifestations of osteochondrosis.[20, 21] Other studies have discounted the primary role of osteochondrosis and implicated joint incongruity caused by underdevelopment of the ulnar trochlear notch.[30–32] Implications for a common etiology for elbow dysplasia include:

1. The presence of similar incongruity in different forms of elbow dysplasia
2. Overlap in breeds and dogs within these breeds with different forms of elbow dysplasia
3. The relatively frequent combination of fragmentation of the medial coronoid process with osteochondritis dissecans of the humeral condyle, and ununited anconeal process with a fragmented or otherwise damaged medial coronoid process
4. Different forms of elbow dysplasia in the elbows of the same animal

The theory of articular incongruity as a primary cause of fragmentation of the medial coronoid process, ununited anconeal process, or osteochondritis dissecans of the elbow is best understood by a comparison of the anatomical and radiographic appearance of normal and affected joints.

*See references 1, 3, 4, 7–10, 12, 14, 15–22, and 24–29.
†See references 2, 5, 6, 11, 13, 21, and 31.

GROSS ANATOMY

Normal Elbow Joint

The normal radioulnar joint surface is characterized by a smooth transition from the ulnar trochlear notch onto the horizontal articular surface of the radius and from the medial downward slope of the radius onto the medial coronoid process (Fig. 145–38). The main radial articulation is horizontal, whereas the ulnar articulation slopes downward. This implies that the radius is the main weightbearing bone and that the ulna serves more as a lever arm for the extensor muscles of the elbow joint. Compared with the coursing breeds, heavier-set breeds have a relatively larger proximal ulna and a slightly larger, wider, less steeply sloping medial coronoid process. This anatomy may suggest an increase in the weightbearing function of the ulna in these breeds.

The articular cartilage of the ulnar trochlear notch extends medially and laterally to the attachment of the joint capsule, with only a slight thinning of this cartilage along the lateral aspect of the notch. The uninterrupted continuity of this cartilage implies that the entire ulnar trochlear notch is in close contact with the articular cartilage of the olecranon fossa and the humeral trochlea.

The main weightbearing surface of the humerus in the elbow joint is the humeral trochlea, which articulates with both the radius and the ulna. Only the cranially sloping lateral part of the radial head articulates with the head of the humerus.

Dysplastic Elbow Joint

In an elbow joint with fragmentation of the medial coronoid process or osteochondritis dissecans, the medial coronoid process and the distal edge of the ulnar trochlear notch frequently lie slightly above the level of the adjoining radius, creating a step between the radius and the ulna and causing incongruity within the joint. The height of the step may vary from barely noticeable

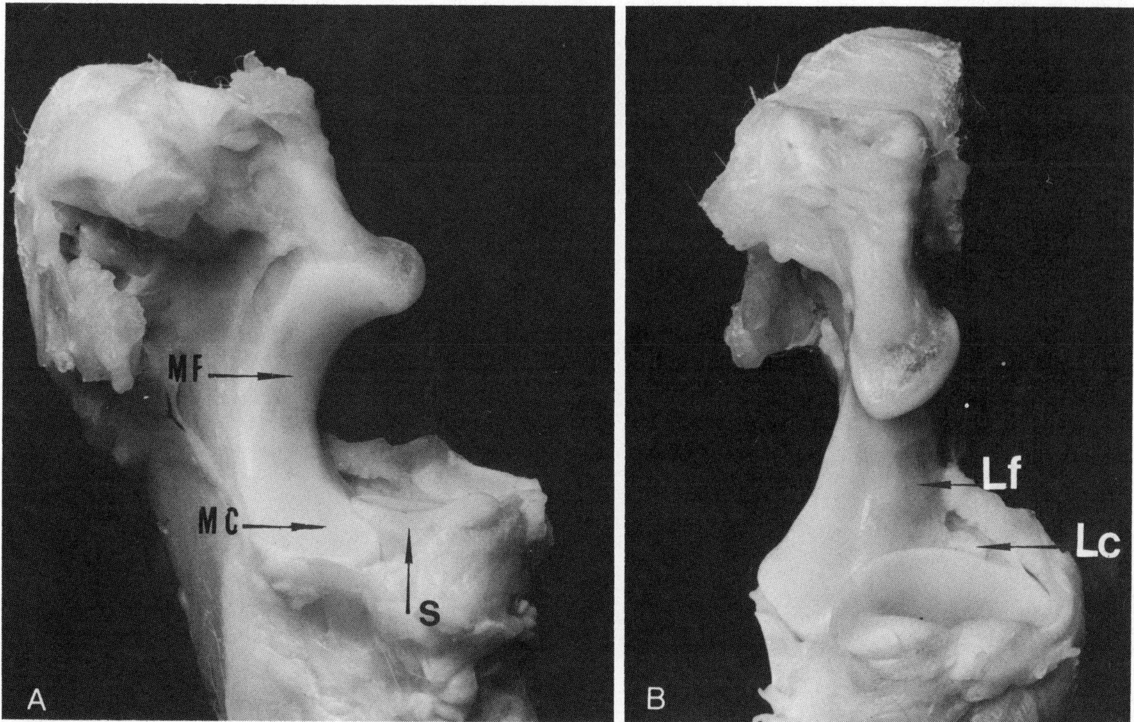

FIGURE 145–38. *A*, Gross morphology of normal left elbow joint, medial view. (MF, medial flange of ulnar trochlear notch; MC, medial coronoid process; S, downward slope of radial articulation.) Note smooth transition from the ulnar trochlear notch onto the radius. *B*, Gross morphology of normal left elbow joint, cranial view. (Lf, lateral flange of ulnar trochlear notch; Lc, lateral coronoid process.) Note smooth transition from the downward slope of radial articulation onto the medial coronoid process. Some thinning of trochlear notch articular cartilage is visible just above lateral-flange arrow. (Reprinted with permission from Wind AP: Elbow incongruity and developmental elbow diseases in the dog: Part I. *J Am Anim Hosp Assoc 22:*712, 1986.)

to a distance of 3 to 4 mm. This may mean that either the radius is too short or the ulnar trochlear notch has a smaller than normal diameter. Whatever the reason, it seems likely that weightbearing forces on the ulna are increased, causing excessive loading of the medial coronoid process (especially its lateral edge) and the distal edge of the trochlear notch, leading to fragmentation (Fig. 145–39). The fragment is often the size of a rice grain or larger and may be attached cranially to the annular ligament. Incomplete fragmentation in the form of chondral or subchondral fissures can also occur. In severely affected joints, the entire process may be fractured. A superficial to deeply grooved "kissing" lesion may be present on the humeral articular surface opposite the coronoid fragment.

Joint surface incongruity may not always be grossly

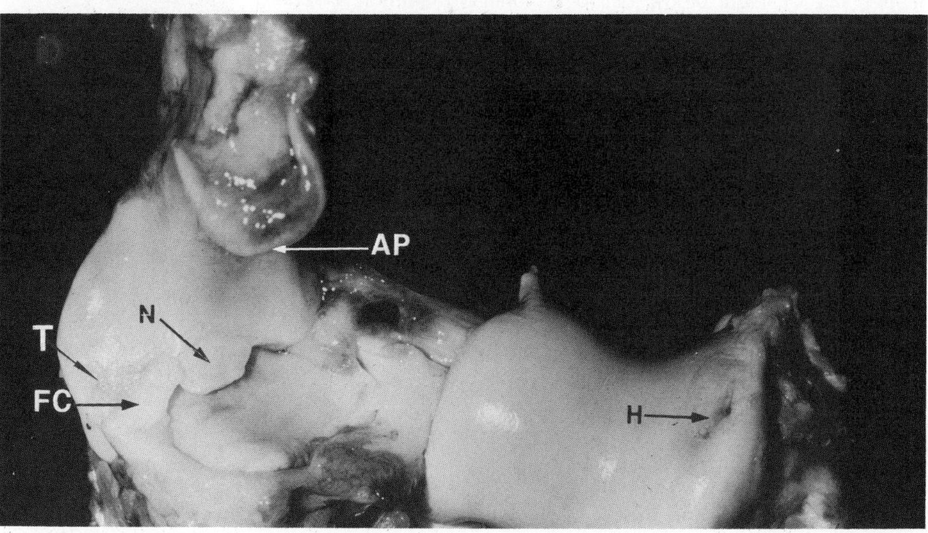

FIGURE 145–39. Left elbow joint of 11-month-old Bernese mountain dog. (AP, anconeal process; N, fragmented distal edge of ulnar trochlear notch; FC, fragmented lateral edge of medial coronoid process; T, soft and unossified tip of medial coronoid process; H, osteochondritic lesion of humeral articular cartilage opposite central and medial aspects of medial cornoid process.) Note the step between the distal edge of the ulnar trochlear notch and the radius. (Reprinted with permission from Wind AP: Elbow incongruity and developmental elbow diseases in the dog: Part I. *J Am Anim Hosp Assoc 22:*712, 1986.

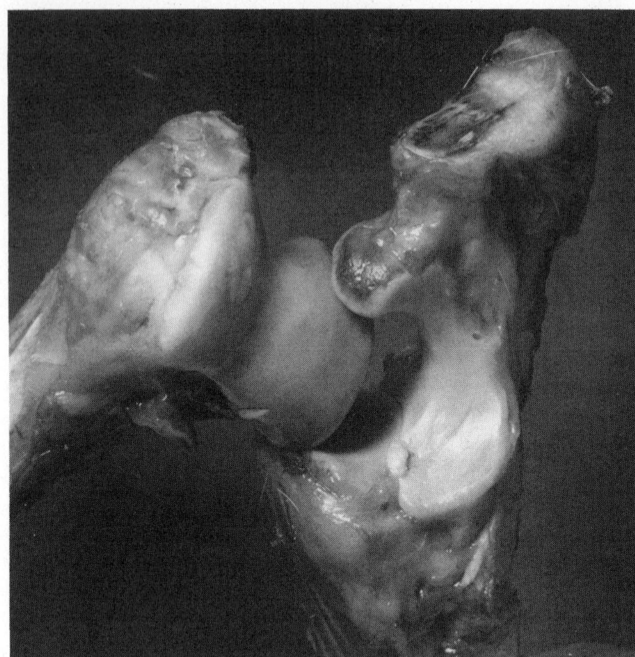

FIGURE 145–40. Right elbow joint of 6-month-old Labrador retriever. OCD lesion visible on the medial aspect of the humeral trochlea opposite the center of the medial coronoid process. The medial coronoid process is broad and flat, with little downward medial slope. Its lateral edge is fractured. The center of the distal edge of the ulnar trochlear notch lies above the level of the radius.

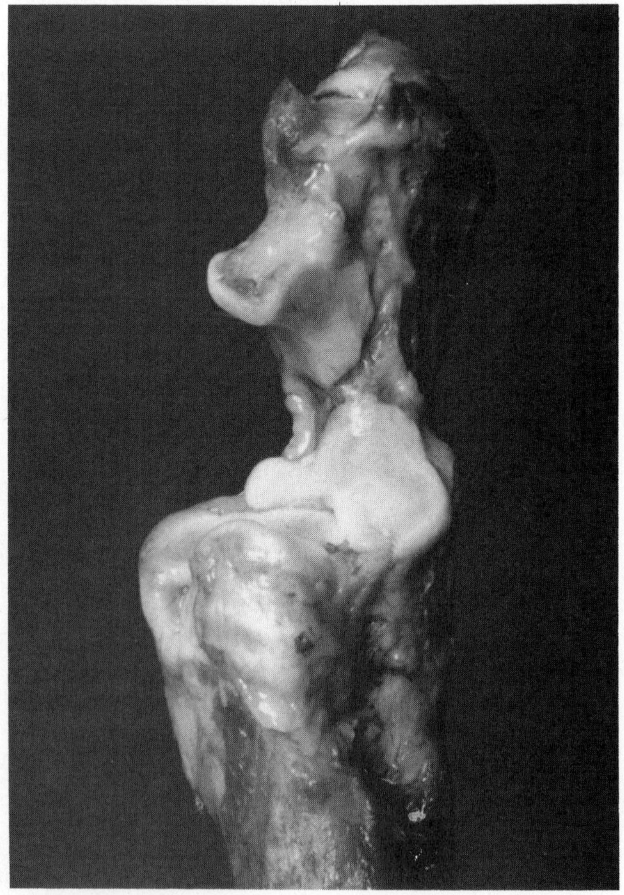

FIGURE 145–41. Right elbow joint of 6-month-old German shepherd. Note complete loss of the central articular cartilage of the ulnar trochlear notch, a step between the entire distal edge of the trochlear notch and radius, and fragmentation of the lateral edge of the medial coronoid process. Also note that the entire medial coronoid process lies above level of the radius and that its articular surface is broad and flat with little downward medial slope.

evident at examination. This may be due to compensatory adjustments during growth, tending to minimize unequal growth rates between the articular and metaphyseal physes of the humerus, radius, and ulna (compatible with the retarded growth of the radius in response to premature closure of the distal ulnar physis). In joints with an ununited anconeal process, this incongruity may not be noticeable either; instead, there may be a distal displacement of the medial coronoid process. Evidence of damage to the medial coronoid process is frequent, however, suggesting that incongruity was present originally but that the nonunion allowed a distal shift of the ulnar trochlear notch.

In joints with osteochondritis dissecans (Figs. 145–39 and 145–40), this lesion is usually more medial than the kissing lesion and lies opposite the central and medial aspects of the medial coronoid process. Loosened pieces of cartilage may migrate cranially into the radial fossa.

In many affected elbows, especially after the age of 6 months, the articular cartilage of the center and lateral flange of the ulnar trochlear notch is interrupted or entirely absent (Fig. 145–41). A loss of contact stresses between the central and lateral aspects of the ulnar trochlear notch and the humeral trochlea is implied.

Secondary osteoarthrosis becomes evident after the age of 6 to 7 months. Osteophytes and articular lipping develop in the following order: dorsal edge of the anconeal process, lateral epicondylar ridge, rim of the medial flange of the ulnar trochlear notch and medial coronoid process, cranial medial edge of the head of the radius, and medial aspect of the humeral condyle. In severe cases, generalized osteophytosis is present.

The early appearance of osteophytes on the anconeal process and the lateral epicondylar ridge (i.e., lateral edge of olecranon fossa), as well as the frequent finding of loss of central or lateral articular cartilage of the ulnar trochlear notch, suggests that the anconeal process skews medially within the olecranon fossa during flexion, resulting in traction on the lateral joint capsule and causing loss of contact between the lateral aspect of the ulnar trochlear notch and the humeral trochlea. This medial skewing may be evident clinically as "paddling" (i.e., supination of the forelegs on flexion), which is frequently observed in affected dogs.

RADIOGRAPHIC APPEARANCE

Normal Elbow Joint (Fig. 145–42)

A normal elbow joint is characterized by congruity (i.e., small, even joint spaces between humerus, radius, and ulna). On the lateral view, the center of the ulnar trochlear notch and the radius lie on a continuous arc. The medial coronoid process is well ossified by the age of 6 months, and its radiographic outline clearly defined.

Dysplastic Elbow Joint

The radiographic appearance of dysplastic elbows is characterized by incongruity and sequential osteoarthrosis (Figs. 145–43 through 145–46). On a lateral radiograph taken at the age of 6 months, the following may be noticed:

1. Increased humeroulnar joint space in the central area of the ulnar trochlear notch
2. Increased humeroradial joint space
3. A break in the normal continuous arc between the ulnar trochlear notch and the radial articulation, with the distal edge of the ulnar trochlear notch lying a step above the level of the radius
4. Cranial displacement of the humerus on the radius
5. Incomplete or irregular outline of the medial coronoid process
6. Mild increase in bone density at the distal end of the ulnar trochlear notch
7. Early osteophytosis at the dorsal aspect of the anconeal process

On the craniocaudal view, an increased humeroradial and decreased humeroulnar joint space or a joint space that is irregular in width may be seen.

In young dogs, increased stress on the medial coronoid process delays ossification and may result in a poorly outlined process. This does not mean that the process has fragmented. Direct radiographic observation of the fragment is usually not possible because it normally lies between the main part of the coronoid process and the radius and is obscured by overlying shadows. When the fragment involves the entire tip of the process, it may be visible on the lateral view. (The sesamoid in the annular ligament and lying craniolateral to the radius should not be confused with a coronoid fragment.) If the kissing lesion opposite the medial coronoid fragment is deep, it may be visible as a small bony defect on the medial aspect of the humeral trochlea.

Osteochondritis dissecans can usually be seen on an accurately taken craniocaudal radiograph as a flat triangular radiolucent area on the medial articular edge of the humeral trochlea (see Fig. 145–44). On a lateral view, it may create a flattening of the medial caudoventral edge of the humeral trochlea (see Fig. 145–44*A*).

One of the first signs of stress within the elbow joint is increased bone density at the distal end of the trochlear notch. This increase in bone density may be due to subchondral sclerosis, osteophytosis of the medial flange of the ulnar trochlear notch, or both. Subsequent signs include osteophytes on the dorsal aspect of the anconeal process and on the lateral epicondylar ridge and lipping of the medial aspect of the medial coronoid process and the cranial aspect of the radial head. Depending on the degree of incongruity (and age), mild to severe generalized osteoarthrosis may be present. As mentioned earlier, incongruity may not always be obvious. This is also true radiographically, and these forms of elbow dysplasia are usually associated with lesser degrees of osteoarthrosis (Fig. 145–47*A* and *B*).

CAUSES OF INCONGRUITY

The incongruity observed between the distal edge of the ulnar trochlear notch, including the medial coronoid process, and the radius suggests either asynchronous growth of the radius and ulna or insufficient development of the ulnar trochlear notch.

Measurements of radial and ulnar length have demonstrated a statistically significant relative increase in

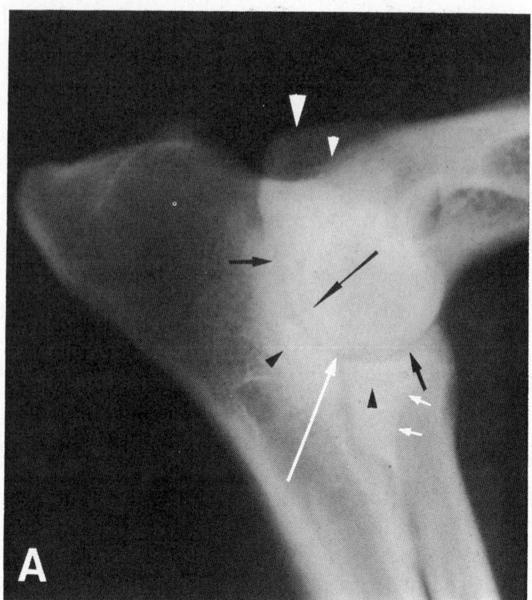

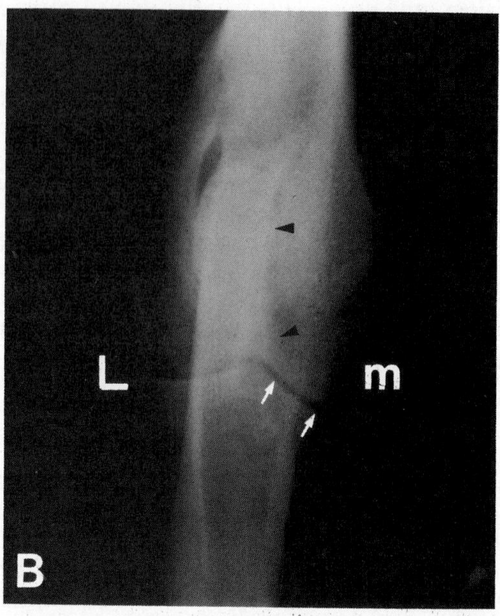

FIGURE 145–42. *A*, Radiograph of a normal elbow joint, lateral view. Three partial concentric joint spaces are visible: Joint space between the center of the ulnar trochlear notch and the center of the humeral trochlea *(long black arrow)*; joint space between the lateral flange of the ulnar trochlear notch and the lateral aspect of the humeral trochlea *(small black arrows)*; and joint space between the medial flange of the ulnar trochlear notch with the medial coronoid process and medial aspect of the humeral trochlea *(black arrow heads)*. The joint spaces are small, even, and congruent. The small white arrowhead points to the lateral epicondylar ridge. The large white arrowhead points to the medial epicondylar ridge. Small white arrows point to the cranial outline of the medial coronoid process. The long white arrow points to the distal edge of the ulnar trochlear notch or lateral coronoid process. The center of the ulnar trochlear notch and the radial articular surface appear to lie on a continuous arc. *B*, Radiograph of normal elbow joint, craniocaudal view. (L, lateral aspect; M, medial aspect.) White arrows point to the medial coronoid process. Black arrowheads point to the medial edge of the medial ulnar trochlear flange. Note the small, even joint spaces.

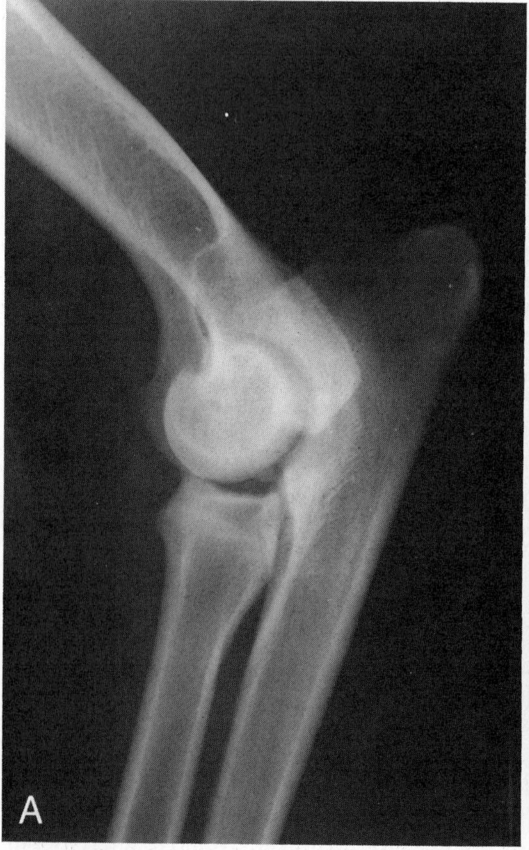

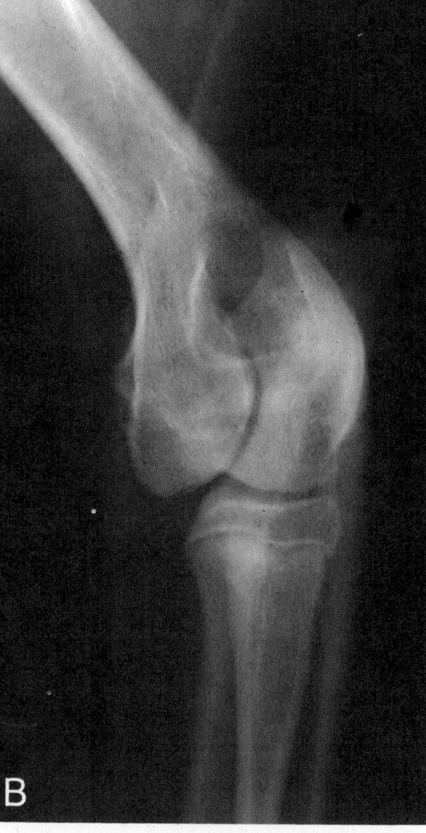

FIGURE 145–43. *A*, Lateral radiograph of elbow joint depicted in Figure 145–39. Severe joint incongruity is present, with a large step between the distal edge of the ulnar trochlear notch and the radius and cranial displacement of the humerus on the radius. The medial coronoid process fragment and a trochlear notch edge fragment are visible in the widened humeroradial joint space. The outline of the medial coronoid process is blunted (unossified tip). New bone production at dorsal joint capsule attachment of anconeal process is causing elongation of the process. Moderate increased bone density is seen at the distal end of the ulnar trochlear notch. *B*, Oblique craniocaudal radiograph of elbow joint depicted in Figure 145–39. Osteochrondritis dissecans lesion visible on the articular surface of the medial aspect of the humeral trochlea.

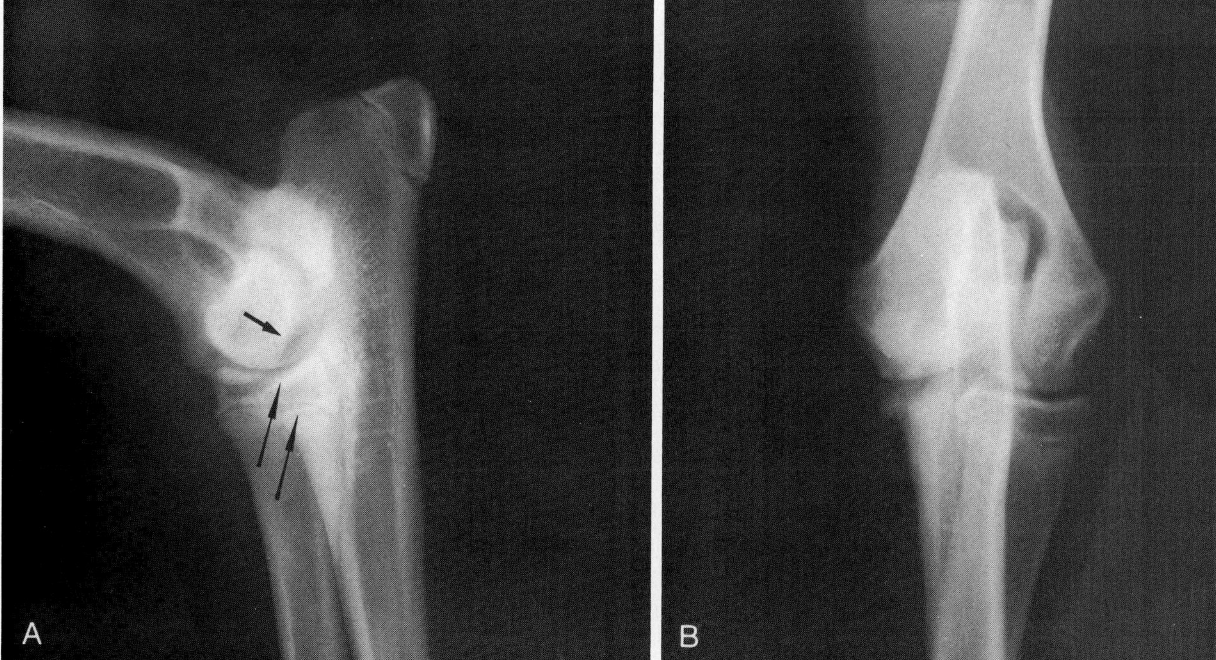

FIGURE 145–44. *A*, Lateral radiograph of elbow of 6-month-old Labrador retriever depicted in Figure 145–40. The proximal radial physis is still clearly visible. Long black arrows point to the articular surface and physis of the cranially downward sloping lateral aspect of the radial head. Note flattening of the medial aspect of the humeral trochlea *(short black arrow)*. Also visible are increased bone density at the distal end of ulnar trochlear notch and osteophytosis of the anconeal process and lateral epicondylar ridge. The medial coronoid process is poorly outlined (most likely because of incomplete ossification). The medial coronoid fragment is not visible. *B*, Craniocaudal view of elbow depicted in Figure 145–40. Note the irregular radiolucent area (osteochondritis dissecans lesion) of the medial aspect of the humeral trochlea and lipping of the medial coronoid process. The medial coronoid fragment itself is not visible (lies in middle of joint). Joint spaces are wide and irregular.

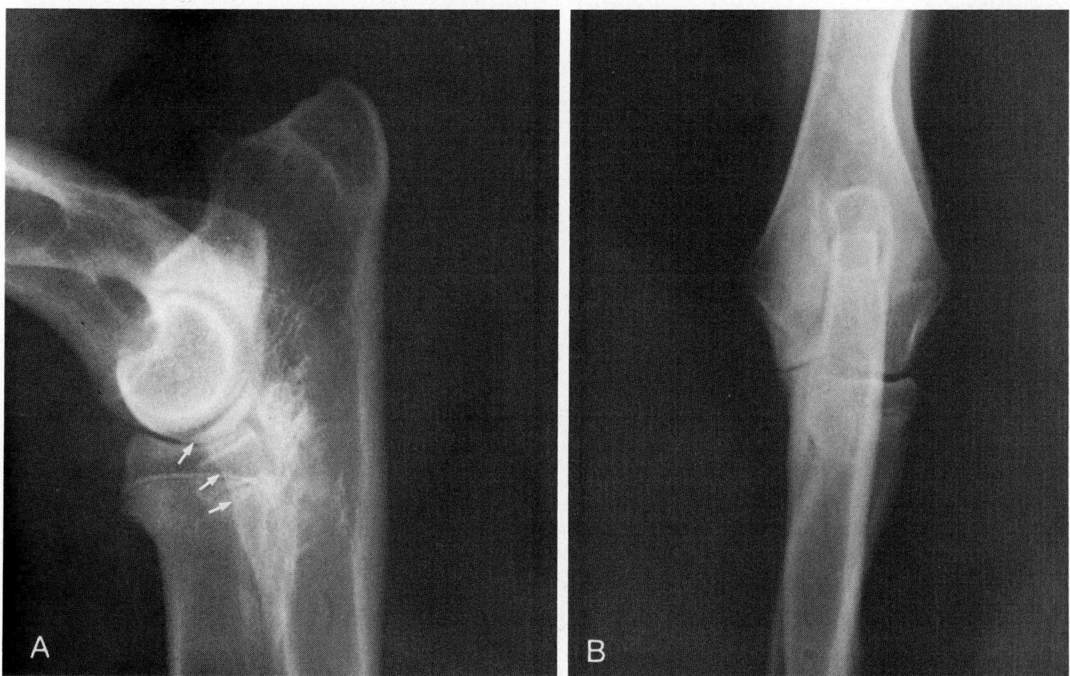

FIGURE 145–45. Lateral and craniocaudal radiographs of elbow of 6-month-old German shepherd depicted in Figure 145–41. Note the proximal position of the medial coronoid process *(white arrows)*, unequal width of joint spaces, and increased bone density at the distal end of the ulnar trochlear notch.

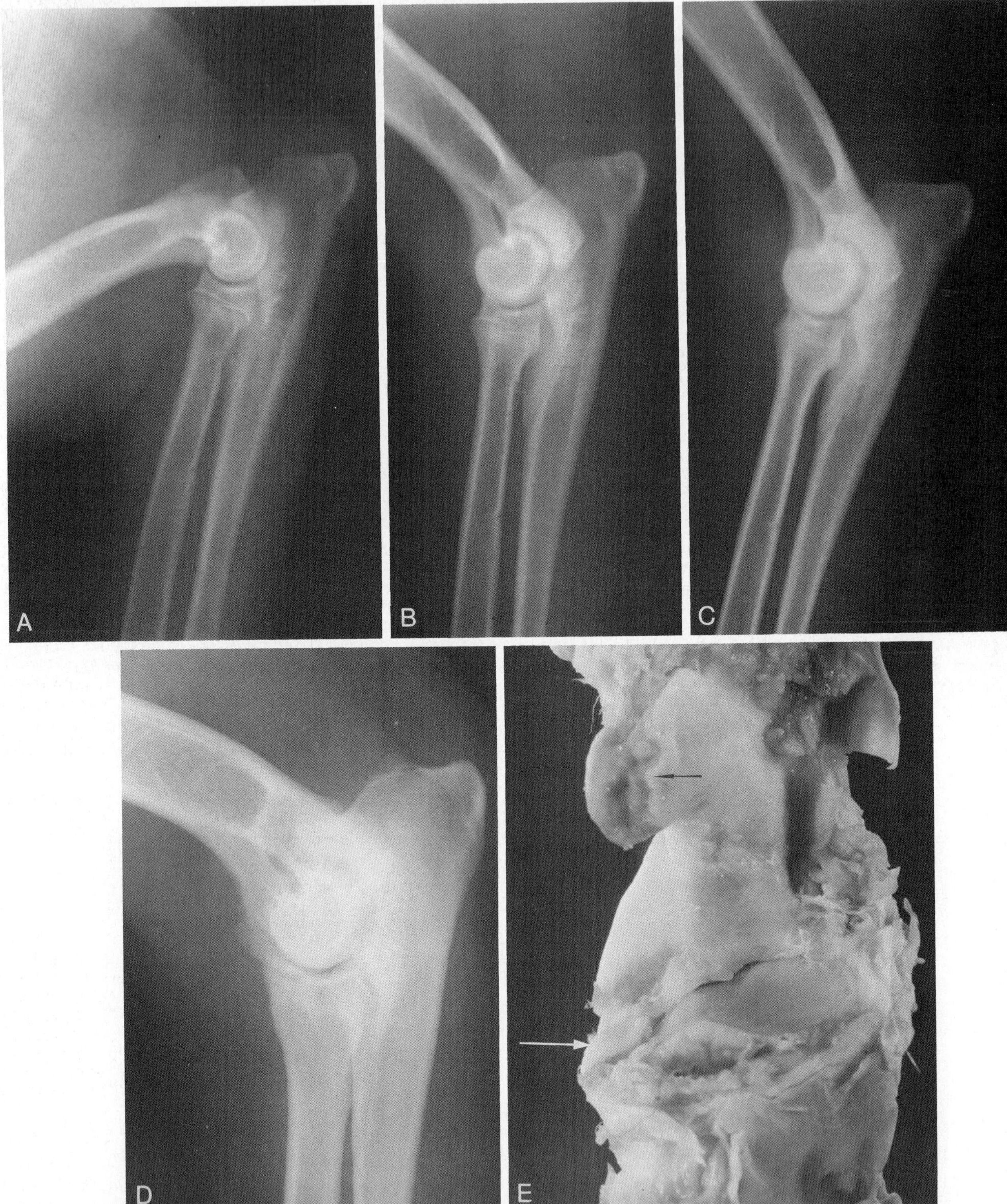

FIGURE 145–46. Lateral radiographs of left elbow joint of a Bernese mountain dog. *A*, At 6 months of age. Note the increased and irregular width of the humeroradial joint space and the step between the distal edge of the ulnar trochlear notch and radius. The medial coronoid process is well outlined, but there is evidence of joint stress in the form of diffuse increase in bone density around the ulnar trochlear notch. *B*, At age 7 months. Note irregular joint spaces, cranial displacement of the humerus on the radius, decreased distinctness of the medial coronoid process with a suggestion that the tip is fractured, increased bone density around the ulnar trochlear notch, and beginning ostophytosis of the anconeal process and lateral epicondylar ridge. *C*, At age 8 months. As described in *B* but more obvious. There is also lipping of the cranial edge of the radius. *D*, At age 18 months. Further progression of osteoarthrosis. *E*, Gross pathology of right elbow joint at 18 months of age. Black arrow points to a ridge of osteophytes along the lateral dorsal aspect of the anconeal process. White arrow points to fractured medial coronoid process.

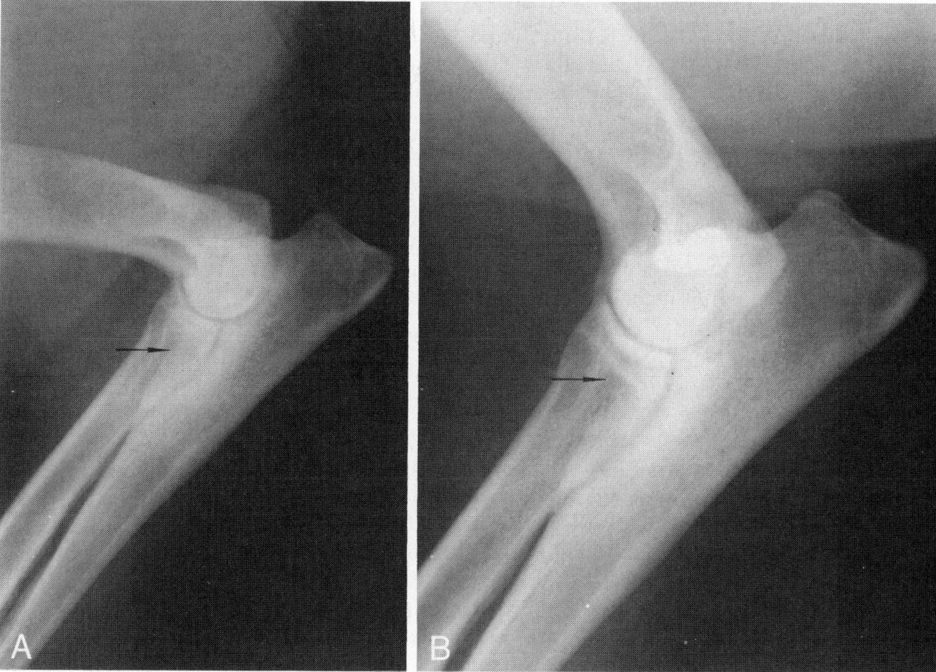

FIGURE 145–47. Radiographs of left elbow of 3-year-old Labrador retriever. The dog had been intermittently lame in left front leg for more than a year. There was slight muscle atrophy. On surgical exploration of the elbow joint, an incomplete fracture of the cranial and lateral edge of the medial coronoid process was found. A slight tap with an osteotome at the cranial end of the fracture line caused complete fracture. The fragment was removed, and lameness disappeared. *A*, Preoperative lateral view: Joint spaces appear small, even, and congruous. Primarily noticeable is the increase in bone density at the distal end of the ulnar trochlear notch and beyond and the radiolucent area in the base of the medial coronoid process *(black arrow)*. The fragment is barely visible above radiolucent area. *B*, Postoperative view. The fragment has been removed via an osteotomy of the medial epicondyle.

length of the proximal ulna in breeds with elbow dysplasia.[31] Length ratios (proximal ulna to radius) in sight hounds ranged from 0.17 to 0.19 and in affected breeds from 0.19 to 0.23.

The "step" between the distal edge of the ulnar trochlear notch and the articular surface of the radius is at most 5 mm. This degree of incongruity, although compatible with lagging radial growth, is insufficient to explain the relative increase in length of the proximal ulna. It is possible that lagging radial growth may constitute a portion of the relative increase in size of the proximal ulna; comparison of relative proximal ulnar measurements of affected animals with those of nonaffected animals within the same breed did not show a consistent increase in the affected animals. Another contradictory finding is the radiographic appearance. Instead of an increase in the joint space between the anconeal process and humerus, as noted with traumatic premature closure of either of the radial physes, this joint space usually appears narrower.

An alternative explanation is underdevelopment of the ulnar trochlear notch, resulting in a notch with too small a curvature to encompass the humeral trochlea. The increase in the relative size of the proximal ulna in affected (heavier) breeds most likely represents an adaptation to accommodate an ulnar trochlear notch of sufficient size to encompass a larger humeral trochlea. Because the ulnar trochlear notch surrounds the humeral trochlea to a considerable extent, the rate of bone production by the articular epiphyseal growth plate of the ulnar trochlear notch needs to be a great deal more rapid than the growth rate of the humeral trochlea. Failure to keep pace with the growth of the humeral trochlea may be the underlying cause of the observed incongruity.

EFFECTS OF AN UNDERDEVELOPED ULNAR TROCHLEAR NOTCH

The presumed underdevelopment of the ulnar trochlear notch and its resulting incongruity become evident between the ages of 4 and 6 months, when the skeleton is incompletely ossified and a separate center of ossification for the anconeal process may still be present. Depending on the degree of underdevelopment and the breed involved, the effect may be

1. Osteoarthrosis only
2. Fracture, fragmentation, or fissure of the medial coronoid process (and maybe the distal end of the ulnar trochlear notch) due to increased weightbearing forces on too high a process
3. Ununited anconeal process in dogs in which a separate center of ossification is still present after the onset of incongruity. This nonunion is most likely due to micromovement of the cartilage bridge between the separate center of ossification and the olecranon (movement caused by too tight a fit between the anconeal process and humerus)
4. Osteochondritis dissecans of the medial aspect of the humeral trochlea due to interference with endochondral ossification caused by excessive pressure generated by too high a medial coronoid process
5. Combinations of the above

CLINICAL FINDINGS

Affected dogs are frequently lame or have an abnormal gait, the latter especially when both elbows are involved. This gait may be characterized by excessive supination of the front paws. This is not pathognomonic, however, because many apparently normal dogs of affected breeds supinate also. The animal may hold the elbows out or tucked in and often stands with its feet rotated out. Manipulation of the elbow may be resented. The presence of crepitation can be misleading because crepitation may be detected in some normal elbows. Effusion may be palpable beneath anconeal and extensor muscles and may be more pronounced after activity. In chronic cases, thickening of the joint capsule, increased prominence of the medial humeral epicondyle, and muscle atrophy are present. In severe cases, the dog sits or lies down much of the time and plays for shorter periods than other dogs its age. Some dogs can barely walk around the block.

DIAGNOSIS

In young dogs (5 to 7 months), the diagnosis is primarily based on clinical signs and radiographic evaluation. Radiographs are made of both elbows to allow comparison, especially of subtle findings, and to check for the presence of bilateral elbow dysplasia, which is common. Correct radiographic technique is critical for making the diagnosis. Radiographs are taken with tabletop technique. A setting of 15 mAs and 50 kVp with a Dupont Extremity System and Dupont 4L film is useful. I prefer the following views:

1. A "long" lateral of the elbow joint, which includes the elbow, the radius and ulna, and the carpal joint. The radiograph is taken with the animal in lateral recumbency with the object leg down and the elbow extended to an inside angle of 100° to 120°. The paw is held in relaxed supination. The elbow joint is in an exactly lateral position. The x-ray beam is centered on midradius. This projection allows examination of radial and ulnar physes and verifies the degree of forearm rotation. Moderate supination of the paw places the medial coronoid process parallel to the cassette for optimum observation.
2. Craniocaudal view. The animal is positioned on its sternum with the object leg in maximum extension and mild supination. The olecranon is in the exact center. The x-ray beam is angled 10° to 20°, depending on degree of elbow extension. This view allows evaluation of joint spaces and examination of the humeral trochlea for osteochondritis dissecans.
3. A flexed lateral of the elbow joint (inside angle $< 90°$) may be advisable to differentiate an ununited anconeal process from a humeral condylar physis or to increase the visibility of the anconeal process and the lateral epicondylar ridge to check for osteophytes.

In *mature* dogs, the diagnosis of elbow dysplasia (with fragmented coronoid or osteochondritis dissecans) is easier than in young dogs because of the presence of osteoarthrosis, especially osteophytosis of the anconeal process. A flexed lateral radiograph is most useful, especially if the examination is requested for the purpose of registration.

TREATMENT (see the section on ununited anconeal process)

Therapy may be surgical or conservative, depending primarily on the degree of osteoarthrosis. Moderation of exercise and strict weight control are important for all dogs with elbow dysplasia. Intermittent use of analgesics may be required, depending on the severity of the condition. Aspirin is recommended (10 to 20 mg/kg BID). Phenylbutazone is prescribed if aspirin is not effective; its initial use is supervised because of the possibility of bone marrow suppression. Because severe ulceration of the gastrointestinal tract can occur in dogs given nonsteroidal anti-inflammatory drugs, careful monitoring is indicated.

Joint incongruity causes cartilage damage and osteoarthrosis. The severity and rate of progression of this arthrosis depend on the degree of incongruity. When the incongruity is minor, secondary lesions (osteochondritis dissecans, fragmentation of the medial coronoid process, or ununited anconeal process) do not occur and osteoarthrosis is of no significance. With greater incongruity, osteochondritis dissecans, fragmentation of the medial coronoid process, and ununited anconeal process are common, and both the incongruity and the lesions contribute to the severity of the osteoarthrosis.

The onset of pain is usually between 4 and 6 months of age and is in part due to joint fluid entering subchondral bone either via osteochondritis dissecans, chondral fissures or fragmentation of the medial coronoid process, or chondral and physeal fissures within a separate center of ossification of the anconeal process. *In situ* movement of the bony or cartilaginous fragments prevents healing of the exposed subchondral or subphyseal bone, and the pain persists but diminishes with time. The fragments are a constant irritant, causing more severe lameness and more rapid progression of osteoarthrosis. Surgical removal of the fragments is recommended before development of severe arthrosis. *Clients should be made aware of the progressive nature of the disease and that improvement but not normality is to be expected.* The possible coexistence of other developmental diseases (e.g., hip dysplasia) should be determined to advise the owner more accurately. Owners of performance dogs are warned that their expectations should be limited.

SURGICAL CANDIDATES

All immature dogs with fragmentation of the medial coronoid process, osteochondritis dissecans, or an ununited anconeal process are surgical candidates, dogs with slight to moderate incongruity and minimal osteoarthrosis having the most favorable prognosis. Even those with marked incongruity and large lesions benefit from surgery because of the decrease in pain. The degree of osteoarthrosis may be severe enough by the age of 2 years to decrease exercise tolerance considerably and warrant intermittent analgesics. Nevertheless, most affected dogs manage to cope with the problem by limiting their exercise and by weight control.

Dogs that have a combined ununited anconeal process and fragmentation of the medial coronoid process have the worst prognosis. Even with surgery, crippling lameness is usually present by the age of 4 to 5 years; the lameness is often unresponsive to exercise limitation, weight control, or drug therapy.

Mature dogs with mild to moderate osteoarthrosis may also be considered for surgery. Dogs with severe osteoarthrosis (i.e., with stable but painful elbow joints) are not operated on because interference with this stability may aggravate rather than diminish the problem. Analgesic medication or arthrodesis is considered for these patients.

SURGICAL PROCEDURES (see a later section in this chapter for surgical removal of ununited anconeal process)

Removal of Fragmentation of the Medial Coronoid Process or Osteochondritis Dissecans of the Humeral Condyle or Both

Adequate exposure with minimal morbidity is achieved by a medial approach to the medial compartment of the elbow joint. Exposure for the arthrotomy can be gained by separation of the flexor muscles and capsulotomy or via an osteotomy of the medial humeral epicondyle.[15, 19, 23] The choice of technique is a matter of personal preference, although better exposure is gained with an osteotomy. Rigid fixation of the epicondyle provides immediate stability and minimizes the need for coaptation postoperatively, compared with capsulotomy and severance of the collateral ligament.

Approach Via the Medial Collateral Ligament

A curving incision is started proximal to the medial epicondyle and extended to the center of the antebrachium. The subcutis and superficial and deep antebrachial fascia are incised along the same line. Retraction of the deep fascia exposes the pronator teres and the flexor carpi radialis muscles. One to 2 cm distal to the epicondyle and at the cranial edge of the pronator teres, the median nerve, artery, and vein are isolated and retracted with a Penrose drain. The fascia is incised between the pronator teres and flexor carpi radialis, which are separated and held with a Gelpi retractor. Be careful to preserve a branch of the median nerve passing between these muscles. The joint capsule and collateral ligament are incised, parallel to the joint space. The radius and ulna are abducted and pronated to open the medial joint and allow inspection of the medial coronoid process and medial aspect of the humeral trochlea. Adequate exposure requires excellent lighting, hemostasis, and retraction. Loose or partially fissured coronoid fragments are removed, as well as an osteochondritis dissecans flap if present. The resulting defects are gently curetted. The joint is lavaged with saline before closure. The medial collateral ligament is carefully reapposed with nonabsorbable suture material while the antebrachium is held in adduction. Antebrachial fasciae, subcutis, and skin are closed in a routine manner. Postoperatively, the incision is covered with a sterile dressing, and a modified Robert Jones bandage is maintained until the sutures are removed 10 to 14 days later. Exercise is restricted for 3 to 4 weeks, with a gradual return to normal activity.

Approach Via Osteotomy of the Medial Humeral Condyle

A curving incision is started cranial and proximal to the medial humeral epicondyle and extended caudal to the epicondyle to the center of the antebrachium. The subcutis, distal end of the medial omobrachial fascia, and antebrachial fasciae are incised along the same line. Care is taken when incising the omobrachial fascia to avoid damaging the ulnar nerve, which is isolated and retracted with a Penrose drain. Areolar tissue and fat are dissected from the epicondyle to delineate the osteotomy site clearly. The fascia and joint capsule between the flexor carpi radialis muscle and the digital flexors are incised to the deep flexor's origin on the epicondyle. The osteotomized epicondyle includes the origins of the pronator teres and flexor carpi radialis muscles. For this, an osteotome of 10 to 12 mm width is usually necessary. The first cut is made parallel and cranial to the tendon of the deep digital flexor, perpendicularly into the bone from medial to lateral. The second cut is at a cranial right angle to the first cut, starting at its proximal end and directed perpendicularly into the bone. The depth of the cuts is approximately 5 to 6 mm. The third cut is made directly cranial to the origin of the pronator teres muscle and perpendicular to the cranial end of the second cut. This cut is made obliquely into the bone and directed caudally.[23] The osteotomized epicondyle with pronator teres, flexor carpi radialis, and medial collateral ligament is retracted distally after cutting capsular attachments. The joint is inspected, and any coronoid fragments or osteochondritis dissecans flap removed and the defects curetted. Before closure, the joint is lavaged with saline.

The osteotomized epicondyle is reattached at its original site with a lag screw or tension band device. To prevent fracture of the osteotomized fragment when a lag screw is used, a small drill bit is used to predrill the fragment before drilling the glide hole with a larger drill bit. A metal washer is recommended to distribute force more evenly. If the piece fragments, a locking loop or Bunnell-Mayer tendon suture can be placed just below the fragments to reattach the tendons and collateral ligament to the humerus via a bone tunnel drilled through the humerus proximal to the osteotomy site. The fascial incisions, subcutis, and skin are closed in separate layers.

Postoperatively, the incision is covered with a sterile dressing and the leg is placed in a light padded bandage for 48 hours. Exercise restriction is advised for 3 weeks, followed by gradual return to normal activity.

Combined Medial Approach to Fragmentation of the Medial Coronoid Process or Osteochondritis Dissecans and Ununited Anconeal Process

In some animals, fragmentation of the medial coronoid process or osteochondritis dissecans occurs together with an ununited anconeal process. In these, the ununited anconeal process can be removed via the caudomedial compartment combined with an exploration of the craniomedial compartment.

The incision is the same as described earlier for osteotomy of the medial humeral epicondyle. The craniomedial compartment is exposed as described previously, via muscle separation or epicondylar osteotomy. After closure of the craniomedial compartment, the caudomedial compartment is approached by retracting the ulnar nerve cranially and incising the brachial fascia along the cranial border of the medial head of the triceps. The triceps is undermined and retracted caudally, and the caudal border of the medial epicondylar crest is palpated. Attachments of the anconeal muscle and joint capsule are incised parallel to the crest, leaving a 2- to 4-mm margin for closure. Because the medial epicondylar crest extends farther caudally than the lateral one, a slightly larger incision than the one used in the lateral approach is necessary. After the anconeal process is removed and the joint is lavaged, the joint capsule and anconeal muscle are sutured and the remainder of the incision is closed routinely. Postoperative care is the same as described previously.

Bilateral Involvement of the Elbow Joints

When surgery is indicated for both joints, they can be operated on at the same time because use of the legs after surgery is not impaired to the extent that a dog is unable to walk.

PROGNOSIS

In moderately affected dogs, with or without surgery, weight control and the animal's natural inclination to limit its exercise allow the animal to cope with this problem. Working dogs are frequently limited in their performance. In severely affected dogs, it is often a crippling disease.

HEREDITY OF ELBOW DYSPLASIA

Studies of German shepherds[5] and rottweilers[11] have demonstrated that elbow dysplasia is an inherited disease. The study of 207 rottweilers showed that about 40 per cent of the offspring were affected when 2 affected dogs were mated, whereas the percentage of affected offspring was 12.5 and 0, respectively, when one or none of the parents were affected.

A study of 616 rottweilers[13] showed that the rottweiler as a breed had a genetic predisposition, that certain stud dogs had a higher percentage of affected offspring, and that the likelihood of elbow dysplasia was 1.8 times higher in the offspring of matings in which one or both parents were affected than in the offspring of nonaffected parents. This study also showed that males in this breed were 1.5 times more likely to be affected than females.

In a study comparing the occurrence of elbow dysplasia in 77 Bernese mountain dogs and in 30 dogs of other Swiss mountain breeds (Entlebucher, Appenzeller, and Grossen Schweizer), 27.9 per cent of the Bernese mountain dogs were affected, compared with 10 per cent of the other breeds.[2]

In a radiographic study of elbows of 825 middle-sized and large dogs, the incidence of elbow dysplasia was determined. Elbow dysplasia was strongly breed specific statistically and was found primarily in intermediate and heavy-set breeds compared with sight hounds and setter breeds.[31, 32]

IMPLICATIONS AND RECOMMENDATIONS

Elbow dysplasia is a polygenetic heritable disease, as is hip dysplasia. Radiographic examination of breeding stock for hip dysplasia has been carried out by the Orthopedic Foundation for Animals since the 1950s. Excluding radiographically affected animals from breeding has considerably diminished the incidence of this disease. Mating of normal phenotypes may still produce dysplastic pups, because the parents carry genes for dysplasia (genotypically affected). Better control of this type of genetic disease requires knowledge of the disease incidence in offspring. This implies (1) registration of normal as well as affected individuals and (2) access to this information for analysis.

The Orthopedic Foundation for Animals is a closed registry regarding affected dogs and gives out information only on "normals" to parties other than the breeder (owner). The registry data are incomplete because radiographs of affected animals are frequently not submitted, since a breeder or owner may not want to spend the money then be unable to use the report to sell offspring.

A fully open registry for hip dysplasia and lately for elbow dysplasia has been developed in Sweden, sponsored by the Swedish Kennel Club. It is the only registry that can definitely show evidence of a marked decrease in the frequency of a disease as a result of development and use of an open data base. It has been successful because the program evaluates the radiographic status of a given dog, records the radiographic status of progeny, and makes information available to prospective breeders and buyers. Both phenotypic and genotypic information are combined in the disease control program. A similar open registry has been started in Norway to combat elbow dysplasia.

In this country, efforts are under way to start an open registry for hip and elbow dysplasia. Successful development of such a registry requires a great deal of education and cooperation on the part of breeders, dog owners, and veterinarians. Breeders, especially of breeds at risk, are advised to have their breeding stock examined not only for hip dysplasia but also for elbow dysplasia. Affected animals are sterilized, and when new breeding stock is to be introduced, a great effort is made to ascertain the elbow status of not only the dog but also its dam, sire, siblings, and half siblings.

References

1. Berzon JL, Quick CB: Fragmented coronoid process: Anatomical, clinical, and radiographic considerations with case analyses. *J Am Anim Hosp Assoc 16*:241, 1980.
2. Bienz HA: Klinische und Radiologische Untersuchungen uber den Fragmentierten processus coronoideus medialis im ellbogengelenk des berner sennenhundes und der anderen sennenhunde rassen. Dissertation, University of Zurich, Zurich, Switzerland, 1985.
3. Carlson WD, Severin GA: Elbow dysplasia in the dog. *J Am Vet Med Assoc 138*:295, 1961.
4. Cawley AJ, Archibald J: Ununited anconeal processes of the dog. *J Am Vet Med Assoc 134*:454, 1959.
5. Corley EA: Elbow dysplasia in the German shepherd dog. Dissertation, Colorado State University, Fort Collins, CO, 1966.
6. Corley EA, et al: Genetic aspects of canine elbow dysplasia. *J Am Vet Med Assoc 153*:543, 1969.
7. Grondalen J: Arthrosis with special reference to the elbow joint of young rapidly growing dogs. I. A review of the literature. *Nord Veterinaermed 31*:62, 1979.

8. Grondalen J: Arthrosis with special reference to the elbow joint of young rapidly growing dogs. II. Occurrence, clinical and radiographical findings. *Nord Veterinaermed 31*:69, 1979.
9. Grondalen J: Arthrosis in the elbow joint of young rapidly growing dogs. III. Ununited medial coronoid process of the ulna and osteochondritis dissecans of the humeral condyle. *Nord Veterinaermed 31*:520, 1979.
10. Grondalen J: Arthrosis in the elbow joint of young rapidly growing dogs. VI. Interrelation between clinical, radiographical and pathoanatomical findings. *Nord Veterinaermed 34*:65, 1982.
11. Grondalen J: Arthrosis in the elbow joint of young rapidly growing dogs. VII. Occurrence in the rottweiler breed. *Nord Veterinaermed 34*:76, 1982.
12. Grondalen J, Grondalen T: Arthrosis in the elbow joint of young rapidly growing dogs. V. A pathoanatomical investigation. *Nord Veterinaermed 33*:1, 1981.
13. Grondalen J, Lingaas F: Arthrosis of the elbow joint among rottweiler dogs. Results from investigations into hereditary disposition. *Tydschr Diergeneesk* (Suppl)*113*:498, 1988.
14. Grondalen J, Rorvik AM: Arthrosis in the elbow joint of young rapidly growing dogs. IV. A follow up investigation of operated dogs. *Nord Veterinaermed 32*:212, 1980.
15. Henry SB, et al: Medial approach to elbow joint with osteotomy of medial epicondyle. *Vet Surg 9*:46, 1979.
16. Herron MR: Ununited anconeal process: A new approach to surgical repair. *Mod Vet Pract 51*:30, 1970.
17. Ljunggren G, et al: The elbow dysplasias in the dog. *J Am Vet Med Assoc 148*:887, 1966.
18. Mason TA, et al: Osteochondrosis of the elbow joint in young dogs. *J Small Anim Pract 21*:641, 1980.
19. McCurnin DM, et al: A medial approach to the canine elbow joint. *J Am Anim Hosp Assoc 12*:475, 1976.
20. Olsson SE: En ny typ av armbagsledsdysplasi hos hund? *Svensk Veterinartidning 26*:152, 1974.
21. Olsson SE: Lameness in the dog: A review of lesions causing osteoarthrosis of the shoulder, elbow, hip, stifle and hock joints. *Am Anim Hosp Assoc Proc 1*:363, 1975.
22. Olsson SE: The early diagnosis of fragmented coronoid process and osteochondritis dissecans of the canine elbow joint. *J Am Anim Hosp Assoc 19*:616, 1983.
23. Piermattei DL, Greeley RG: *An Atlas of Surgical Approaches to the Bones of the Dog and Cat.* 2nd ed. W. B. Saunders, Philadelphia, 1979, pp 102–105.
24. Sinibaldi K, Arnoczky SP: Surgical removal of the ununited anconeal process in the dog. *J Am Anim Hosp Assoc 11*:192, 1975.
25. Stevens DR, Sande RD: An elbow dysplasia syndrome in the dog. *J Am Vet Med Assoc 165*:1065, 1974.
26. Stiern RA: Ectopic sesamoid bones at the elbow (patella cubiti) of the dog. *J Am Vet Med Assoc 128*:498, 1956.
27. Tirgary M: Clinical, radiographical and pathological aspects of ununited medial coronoid process of the elbow joint in dogs. *J Small Anim Pract 21*:595, 1980.
28. Van Sickle DC: The relationship of ossification to canine elbow dysplasia. *J Am Anim Hosp Assoc 2*:24, 1966.
29. Vaughan LC: Congenital detachment of the processus anconaeus in the dog. *Vet Rec 74*:309, 1962.
30. Wind AP: Incidence and radiographic appearance of fragmented coronoid process (in the Bernese mountain dog). *California Veterinarian 36*:19, 1982.
31. Wind AP: Elbow incongruity and developmental elbow diseases in the dog: Part I. *J Am Anim Hosp Assoc 22*:711, 1986.
32. Wind AP, Packard ME: Elbow incongruity and developmental elbow diseases in the dog: Part II. *J Am Anim Hosp Assoc 22*:724, 1986.

Ununited Anconeal Process

Christopher Thacher

DEFINITION

Ununited anconeal process (UAP) in dogs is encountered most frequently in juvenile large dogs, in which the anconeal process fails to undergo bony fusion to the ulnar diaphysis. The anconeal process may remain attached by fibrous tissue or it may become physically separated, producing instability and secondary degenerative joint disease.

HISTORICAL ASPECTS AND NOMENCLATURE

Ununited anconeal process was first reported by Stiern (1956), who described ectopic sesamoid bones, or "patella cubiti," in the elbow joints of three related German shepherds that had been presented for forelimb lameness.[22] In 1959, Cawley and Archibald used the term *ununited anconeal process* to describe 11 cases in German shepherds.[2] Eleven dogs with what was termed *elbow dysplasia*, which included UAP, were reported in 1961 by Carlson and Severin.[1] Six cases described as "congenital detachment of the processus anconeus" were reported in 1962.[24] Subsequent reports have described radiographic, anatomical, and etiological aspects of UAP.[3, 4, 8, 14, 23]

Although the term *ununited anconeal process* was coined in 1959 by Cawley and Archibald, who correctly identified the anatomical defect and location of the bone fragment, it was a number of years before the term was accepted. The initially proposed terms *ectopic sesamoid* and *patella cubiti* were dismissed as being anatomically inappropriate.[2] Patella cubiti is a rare condition, first reported in humans, in which the proximal epiphysis of the ulna is detached from the parent bone and incorporated into the tendon of the triceps muscle. The condition is rare in dogs.[14] The term *elbow dysplasia* further confused the issue.[1] Carlson and Severin considered UAP to be a frequent but not necessarily constant feature of a syndrome characterized by forelimb lameness and osteoarthritis of the elbow. The specific role of the anconeal process in the pathogenesis of the condition was unclear. In 1966, the same investigators, in association with Ljunggren, presented a classification scheme for elbow dysplasia.[14] UAP, along with patella cubiti and ununited medial epicondyle of the humerus, were considered as categories of elbow dysplasia. In an alternate classification for elbow dysplasia proposed in 1974 by Stevens and Sande, elbow dysplasia was divided into three different subgroups: (1) separation at an epiphyseal plate (including UAP, ununited medial humeral epicondyle, and patella cubiti), (2) congenital luxations of the elbow, and (3) premature closure of the epiphyseal plates.[21] Herron (1971) and Sinibaldi and Arnoczky (1975) suggested that the term *elbow dysplasia* was nonspecific and not to be used in conjunction with UAP.[12, 19] Current research, however, suggests that UAP may be a component of a more generalized elbow disorder for which the term *elbow dysplasia* would be appropriate (see the previous section of this chapter).

ANATOMY

The anconeal process forms the proximal aspect of the trochlear notch, and during extension, the process fits into the olecranon fossa of the humerus. The anconeal process thus aids in stabilizing the foreleg in an extended, weightbearing posture.[7, 11] The anconeal process has no muscular or ligamentous attachments, and it is enclosed entirely within the joint capsule of the elbow.[5, 24]

Cawley and Archibald (1959) hypothesized that the anconeal process was a fourth center of ossification in some breeds.[2] This was confirmed by Van Sickle, who compared the ossification of the ulna of the German shepherd and greyhound.[23] Radiographic and histological analyses demonstrated that the anconeal process is initially composed of cartilage, but at 11 to 12 weeks of age, several small centers of ossification appear and gradually coalesce into a single center separated from the ulna by a plate of cartilage. In greyhounds, bony fusion was complete by 14 to 15 weeks, but in German shepherds, it required 16 to 20 weeks.

ETIOLOGY AND PATHOGENESIS

In initial reports describing UAP, the affected animals all were German shepherds, and many were closely related.[1, 2, 22, 24] Heredity was assumed to be a major etiological factor. A breeding program involving German shepherds, some with normal elbows and some with elbow dysplasia (including individuals with and without UAP) found that a dominant, non–sex-linked gene or genes was a factor in the etiology and that environmental influences were of little significance.[3, 4] Other studies have implicated hormonal factors, metabolic defects, nutritional deficiencies, and acute or chronic trauma as etiological factors.[2, 6, 9, 21]

UAP, along with fragmented coronoid process and osteochondritis dissecans, may be a manifestation of osteochondrosis.[16] Osteochondrosis is a systemic disease that inhibits calcification of cartilage matrix during endochondral ossification, leading to thickened cartilage with necrosis and fissure formation in the deeper layers. Osteochondrosis could weaken the attachment of the anconeal process to the ulna and, with the stress of weightbearing, could lead to failure of the process to unite with the ulna. Underdevelopment of the trochlear notch may cause excessive stress on the developing anconeal process and cause nonunion (see the previous section of this chapter).

The UAP may be attached to the ulna by fibrous tissue or it may be completely separated from the parent bone,[11] producing lateral instability. Instability and the presence of a free fragment of bone within the joint lead to irritation, abnormal wear, and secondary degenerative joint disease.* Early changes include joint effusion, disruption of the cartilage in the semilunar notch, joint capsule thickening, and periarticular osteophyte production. Loss of cartilage and eburnation of subchondral bone, remodeling of the process, and joint capsule thickening with reduced range of motion are noted in chronic cases.

*See references 1–3, 6–8, 11, 14–16, 19, 21, 22, and 24

The German shepherd was the first breed in which UAP was described.[1, 2, 22, 24] By 1968, however, UAP had been identified in Saint Bernards, Irish wolfhounds, basset hounds, Newfoundlands, bloodhounds, Labrador retrievers, Great Danes, French bulldogs, pointers, Great Pyrenees, weimeraners, and dachshunds.[4, 13, 14] Classic UAP is a disease of large to giant breeds of dogs, and a separate center of ossification for the anconeal process has been documented in a number of these breeds. In chondrodystrophic breeds, premature closure of the distal ulnar physis causes caudal subluxation of the proximal ulna and shearing stress on the anconeal process.[11] Anconeal separation in these breeds should be considered as a type of fracture rather than classic UAP.

CLINICAL SIGNS AND DIAGNOSIS (Fig. 145–48)

Because the anconeal process may not fuse to the diaphysis of the ulna until 4 to 5 months of age, the diagnosis of UAP is premature if made before a dog is 4½ to 5 months old.[23] The usual age of presentation is 6 to 12 months, but affected dogs may not exhibit clinical signs until they are much older.[15, 19, 22] Major trauma could cause a shearing fracture of the anconeal process in an otherwise normal canine elbow, but older dogs with UAP invariably have moderate to severe degenerative joint disease, suggesting a chronic disease process. Lameness in mature dogs with UAP may be a sign of progressive degenerative joint disease, or a fibrous union may have become destabilized by a minor traumatic event.[15] UAP is bilateral in 20 to 35 per cent of affected dogs.[1, 2, 8, 19, 24] In most cases with bilateral involvement, however, one side is clinically worse than the other. Males are affected more frequently than females (2:1),[1, 8, 19, 24] possibly because of the more rapid growth and greater size of male dogs.

Intermittent lameness exacerbated by exercise is the most frequent presenting complaint. The lameness usually becomes evident between 6 and 12 months of age. When the disease is present in both elbows, the lameness may be shifting or may even be difficult to detect when both elbows are equally affected. The lameness is more insidious and progressive in older dogs because of the progressive nature of the osteoarthritic changes. Careful questioning of the owner, however, may reveal a history of mild lameness when the dog was younger.

Gait examination reveals a weightbearing lameness, often with abduction of the elbow and external rotation of the foot. Effusion is present early in the course of the disease, and joint capsule thickening becomes predominant with time. Extension and flexion of the elbow elicit pain and crepitation. Atrophy of the muscles of the affected forelimb may be noticeable. It may be possible to palpate the loose process by pressing on either side of the triceps tendon.[24]

Definitive diagnosis is made by radiographic examination. A radiolucent line separating the anconeal process from the diaphysis of the ulna in a dog older than 5 months is diagnostic of UAP. The anconeal process is obscured by the medial epicondyle of the humerus in the standard lateral view of the elbow, so a flexed lateral view is important to observe the process adequately

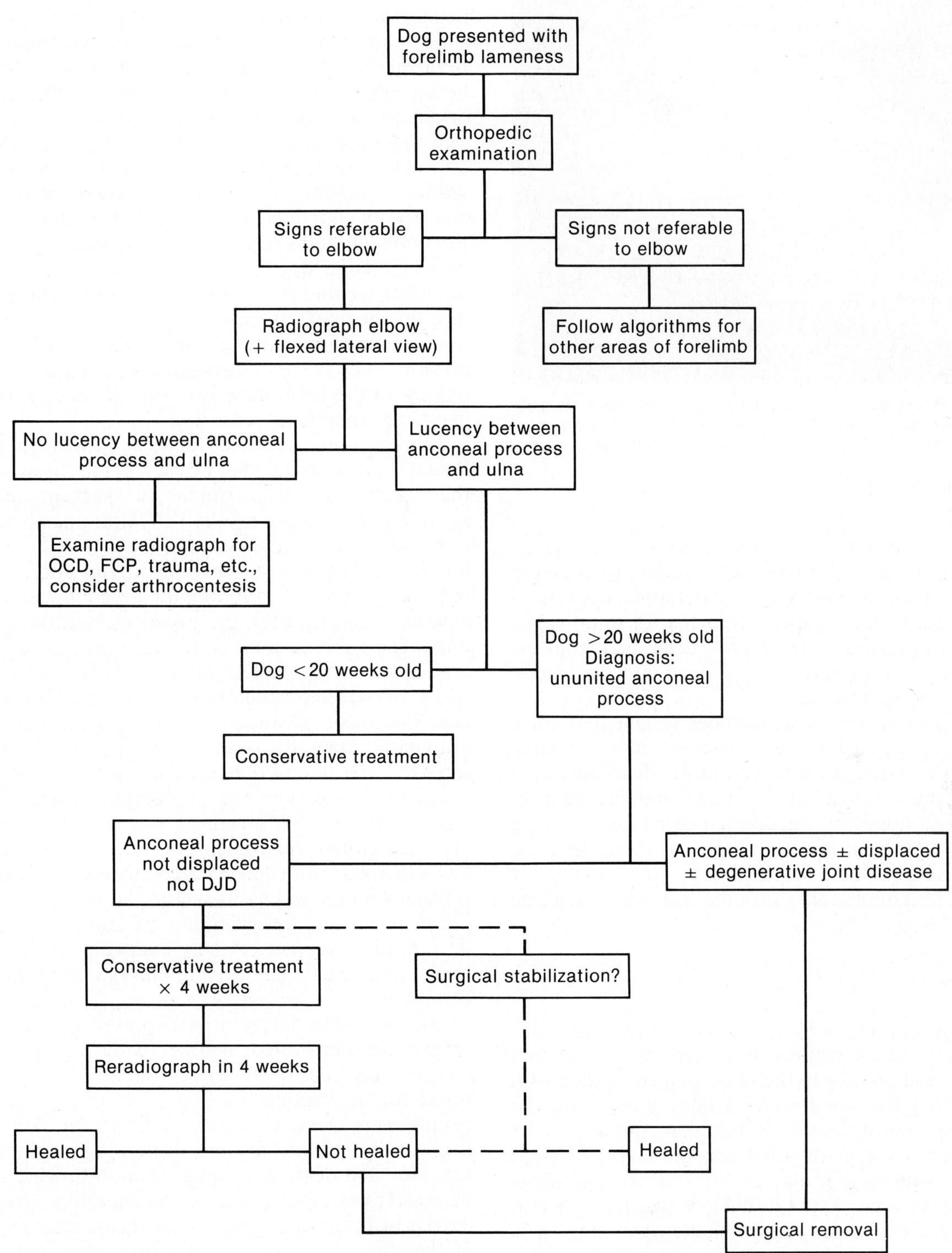

FIGURE 145–48. Diagnostic process and therapeutic alternatives for dogs with ununitied anconeal process. (OCD, osteochondritis dissecans; FCP, fragmented coronoid process; DJD, degenerative joint disease.)

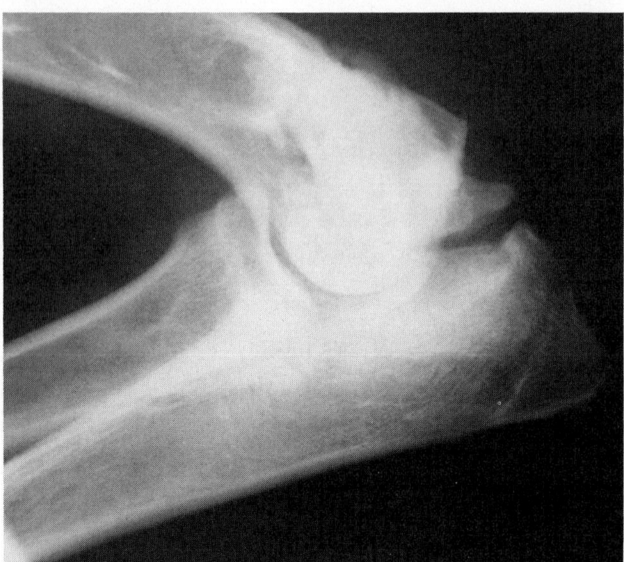

FIGURE 145–49. Flexed lateral projection of the left elbow of a 10-month-old German shepherd presented for left forelimb lameness of 6 weeks duration. The ununited anconeal process is clearly visible.

(Fig. 145–49). Periarticular osteophytes and remodeling changes are observed on the craniocaudal projection in chronic cases. Both elbows are radiographed because of the frequency of bilateral involvement. In some cases, the anconeal process is significantly separated from the ulna, to the point of appearing wedged into the olecranon fossa of the humerus.[18]

The differential diagnosis includes fragmented coronoid process, osteochondritis dissecans of the medial portion of the condyle, osteochondritis dissecans, panosteitis, trauma (including fractures and ligamentous injuries), and osteoarthritis due to other causes. Young large dogs may have more than one of these diseases, and even though one of them may be immediately obvious, the radiographs and the patient should be evaluated for the others.

TREATMENT

Treatment options include conservative management, removal of the anconeal process, or surgical stabilization of the anconeal process to the ulna. In a young dog with a process that has not formed a bony union with the ulna in the appropriate time but that appears to be stable via a fibrous union, strict rest and immobilization of the limb with a splint or cast for 4 weeks may allow bony union to occur.[11] If the UAP is discovered as an incidental finding in an asymptomatic older dog, it is appropriate not to intervene surgically unless clinical signs develop.

Chondrodystrophic breeds, especially the bassett hound, may exhibit elbow pain and very slight displacement of the anconeal process as a result of early closure of the distal ulnar physis. In such cases, surgical sectioning of the radioulnar ligament may relieve the stress on the anconeal process and allow fusion to occur. If the process is displaced and unstable, excision is recommended.

Lag screw fixation of the anconeal process has been described.[10, 11] The rationale for fixation is to maintain the original anatomy of the elbow joint as closely as possible, thus reducing the instability and secondary degenerative joint disease. The surgical approach is similar to that described later for anconeal process removal, but the incision may need to be slightly larger because greater exposure is required. The technique originally described driving the screw from the process into the ulnar diaphysis. Union should occur within 6 to 10 weeks, although delayed healing and persistent nonunion are common.[11] In younger dogs, the screw head has been sheared off as a result of continued growth. Recommendations have been made either to delay fixation until the dog is 9 to 10 months old or to use a modified technique of driving the screw from the ulna into the anconeal process.[12, 18] If the anconeal process is not anatomically reduced, interference with elbow extension may occur. Remodeling changes and osteophytes on the ulna, humerus, and the anconeal process itself can complicate reduction.

Surgical removal of the process through a modified lateral approach to the elbow is the most common therapy because it is simple to perform and yields generally satisfactory results.[17–20] After anesthetic induction and surgical preparation of the affected limb, a skin incision is begun just proximal to the lateral humeral epicondyle, curved to follow the epicondylar crest, and extended distally over the proximal portion of the radius. The subcutaneous fascia is incised to expose the cranial border of the lateral head of the triceps muscle, which is retracted caudally, exposing the anconeal muscle. The anconeal muscle and underlying joint capsule are incised along the origin of the muscle on the caudal aspect of the lateral epicondylar crest, and the incision is enlarged to expose the caudolateral compartment of the elbow and the anconeal process. The process is grasped with towel forceps or Ochsner forceps while any soft-tissue attachments are transected. Hemorrhage is usually minor and easily controlled with pressure. The joint capsule and overlying muscle and fascia are closed in a routine manner. A soft padded bandage may be applied for several days to minimize swelling and seroma formation.

The prognosis after surgical removal is favorable if surgery is performed before extensive degenerative changes have occurred. In a series of 19 elbows monitored for an average of 19.5 months postoperatively, results were good to excellent in 15 elbows, with an average 3.5 weeks to return to full weightbearing.[19] Crepitus and decreased range of motion were detected in most joints, but stasis of degenerative changes occurred in 15 elbows. The osteoarthritic changes present at the time of surgery are not reversible and continue to progress slowly. Some investigators believe that the benefit produced by surgical removal is temporary and that lameness returns.[13]

References

1. Carlson WD, Severin GA: Elbow dysplasia in the dog. A preliminary report. *J Am Vet Med Assoc 138*:295, 1961.
2. Cawley AJ, Archibald J: Ununited anconeal processes of the dog. *J Am Vet Med Assoc 134*:454, 1959.

3. Corley EA, Carlson WD: Radiographic, genetic, and pathologic aspects of elbow dysplasia. *J Am Vet Med Assoc 147*:1651, 1965.
4. Corley EA, et al: Genetic aspects of canine elbow dysplasia. *J Am Vet Med Assoc 153*:543, 1968.
5. Evans HE, Christensen GC: *Miller's Anatomy of the Dog*. 2nd ed. W.B. Saunders, Philadelphia, 1979.
6. Fox SM, et al: Developmental anomalies of the canine elbow. *J Am Anim Hosp Assoc 19*:605, 1983.
7. Goring RL, Bloomberg MS: Selected developmental abnormalities of the canine elbow: Radiographic evaluation and surgical management. *Comp Cont Educ Pract Vet 5*:178, 1983.
8. Hanlon GF: Additional radiographic observations on elbow dysplasia in the dog. *J Am Vet Med Assoc 155*:2045, 1969.
9. Hayes HM, et al: Epidemiologic observations of canine elbow disease (emphasis on dysplasia). *J Am Anim Hosp Assoc 15*:449, 1979.
10. Herron MR: Ununited anconeal process: A new approach to surgical repair. *Mod Vet Pract 51*:30, 1970.
11. Herron MR: Ununited anconeal process in the dog. *Vet Clin North Am 1*:417, 1971.
12. Herron MR: Ununited anconeal process. *In* Bojrab MJ (ed): *Current Techniques in Small Animal Surgery*. Lea & Febiger, Philadelphia, 1975, pp 526–529.
13. Lenehan TM, Van Sickle DC: Ununited anconeal process. *In* Newton CD, Nunamaker DM (eds): *Textbook of Small Animal Orthopedics*. J.B. Lippincott, Philadelphia, 1985, pp 999–1006.
14. Ljunggren G, et al: The elbow dysplasias in the dog. *J Am Vet Med Assoc 148*:887, 1966.
15. Mitten RW, Hoefle WD: Ununited anconeal process: Unusual presentation in two dogs. *J Am Anim Hosp Assoc 14*:595, 1978.
16. Olsson S: Congenital and hereditary diseases. *In* Bojrab MJ (ed): *Pathophysiology in Small Animal Surgery*. W.B. Saunders, Philadelphia, 1981, pp 610–611.
17. Piermattei DL, Greeley RG: *An Atlas of Surgical Approaches to the Bones of the Dog and Cat*. 2nd ed. W.B. Saunders, Philadelphia, 1979.
18. Sinibaldi KR: Ununited anconeal process. *In* Bojrab MJ (ed): *Current Techniques in Small Animal Surgery*. Lea & Febiger, Philadelphia, 1983, pp 719–722.
19. Sinibaldi KR, Arnoczky SP: Surgical removal of the ununited anconeal process in the dog. *J Am Anim Hosp Assoc 11*:192, 1975.
20. Snavely DA, Hohn RB: A modified lateral surgical approach to the elbow of the dog. *J Am Vet Med Assoc 169*:826, 1976.
21. Stevens DR, Sande RD: An elbow dysplasia syndrome in the dog. *J Am Vet Med Assoc 165*:1065, 1974.
22. Stiern RA: Ectopic sesamoid bones at the elbow (patella cubiti) of the dog. *J Am Vet Med Assoc 128*:498, 1956.
23. Van Sickle DC: The relationship of ossification to canine elbow dysplasia. *J Am Anim Hosp Assoc 2*:24, 1966.
24. Vaughan LC: Congenital detachment of the processus anconeus in the dog. *Vet Rec 74*:309, 1962.

Perthes' Disease

Mark M. Smith

Necrosis of the proximal femoral epiphysis occurs in children and in immature small dogs. More descriptive terms for the disease include *aseptic necrosis of the femoral head, coxa plana*, and *coxa magna*. Because the articular cartilage becomes thickened, it has also been described as a form of osteochondrosis.[13] The radiographic and histological appearance of the disease is similar in humans and dogs; however, the predilection for males in humans has not been observed in dogs. Perthes' disease in dogs is usually unilateral, and a higher than expected incidence is noted in the Manchester terrier, miniature pinscher, poodle, Lakeland terrier, West Highland white terrier, and Cairn terrier.[4, 10, 11]

CLINICAL SIGNS AND DIAGNOSIS

Dogs with Perthes' disease become lame, usually between 4 months and 11 months of age. The onset may appear acute; however, muscle atrophy is invariably present in the affected leg, suggesting a more chronic history. The lameness is progressive for 1 to 2 months, then may become static. The leg usually bears weight, but periods of carrying the leg, especially when running, are not unusual. When bilateral, the lameness may be shifting or persistently worse on one side or the other. Manipulation of the hip evokes pain and guarding, although crepitation is usually absent. Muscle atrophy is most apparent in the hamstring and gastrocnemius muscles. The primary differential diagnosis in young dogs is medial patella luxation, which may occur as an incidental finding. The presence of thigh muscle atrophy and pain in the hip will distinguish Perthes' disease from medial patella luxation.

Mild forms of the disease may occur, and clinical signs may not be severe enough to provoke veterinary attention. Dogs with chronic Perthes' disease have mild muscle atrophy and radiographic signs of chronic degenerative joint disease. In older dogs with chronic Perthes' disease, rupture of the cranial cruciate ligament is the primary differential diagnosis, especially if the onset is acute.

A tentative diagnosis of Perthes' disease is based on the history and physical findings and confirmed by radiographic examination. Early radiographic signs include irregular densities within the metaphysis and discrete radiolucent areas within the epiphysis. These findings generally precede lameness, thus clinical patients invariably have more advanced changes, including deformity of the epiphysis, thickening of the femoral neck, and increased width of the joint space (Fig. 145–50). More chronic and severe cases demonstrate collapse and fragmentation of the femoral head with periarticular new bone formation. The diagnosis of Perthes' disease is confirmed by radiographic findings that include deformity of the epiphysis, thickening of the femoral neck, and increased width of the joint space.

PATHOPHYSIOLOGY

The cause of Perthes' disease is unknown. Histological findings suggest that the disease is the result of infarction of epiphyseal and metaphyseal bone, including the physis.[17] Histopathological changes are divided into three stages.[1, 2, 12] Initially, the femoral head remains spherical without collapse or repair changes during the stage of necrosis. Articular cartilage and chondrocytes have a normal histological appearance with no clefting

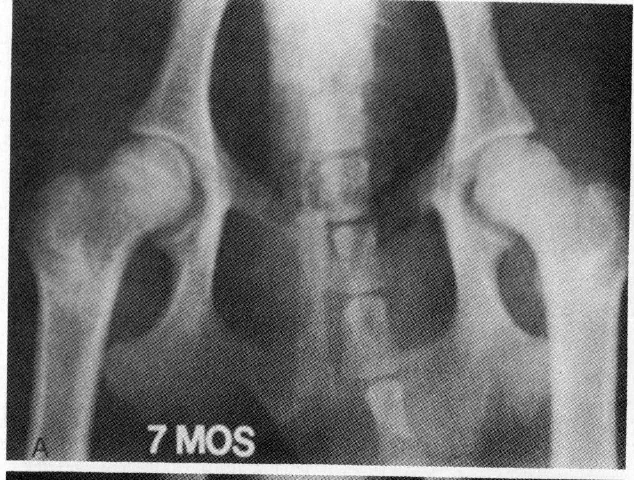

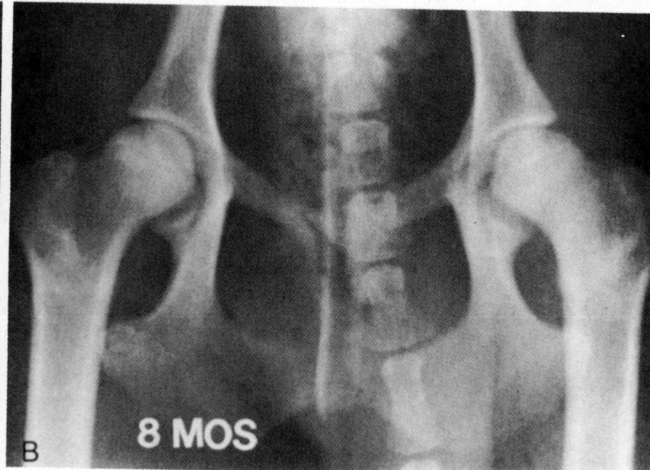

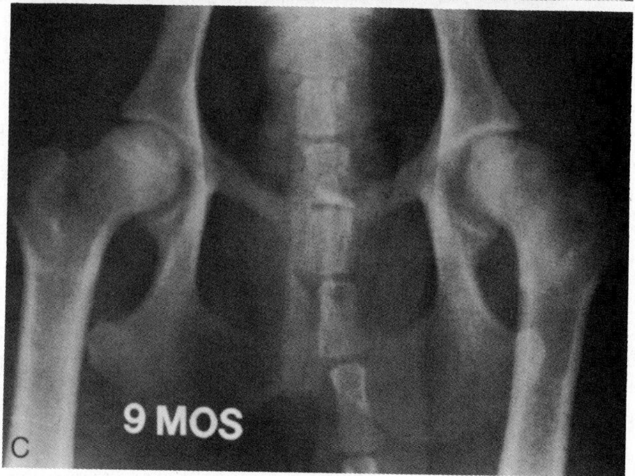

FIGURE 145–50. Radiographic changes of Perthes disease in a Manchester terrier. *A*, At 7 months of age, increased density is apparent in the left proximal femoral metaphysis the dog was clinically normal at this time. *B*, At 8 months, slight collapse of the left epiphysis is apparent, and the dog became lame on the left hindlimb 2 weeks after this radiograph was made. *C*, At 9 months of age, the left epiphysis has collapsed and marked thickening of the femoral neck is seen. (From Vasseur PB, et al: Mode of inheritance of Perthes' disease in Manchester terriers. *Clin Orthop 244*:281, 1989).

or fibrillation. Necrosis is evidenced by decreased numbers of lacunar osteocytes and marrow elements. Granulation tissue surrounds the bony trabeculae. Growth plate chondrocytes and cellular components of enchondral ossification are normal. Trabecular thickening is present in the metaphyseal area (Fig. 145–51). Collapse of the epiphysis and repair of epiphyseal bone indicate early repair. The articular cartilage is thickened, furrowed, and clefted as a result of subchondral bone collapse. Pannus is evident at the periphery of the articular cartilage. The central epiphyseal area has necrotic trabeculae and debris. Peripheral epiphyseal areas undergo revascularization and repair. The growth plate is disrupted by invasion of fibrovascular repair tissue. Osteonecrotic metaphyseal bone interrupts enchondral ossification. In the advanced repair stage, the articular cartilage remains thickened, with multiple clefts and infolding in addition to fraying of superficial cartilage layers and cloning of chondrocytes. The epiphysis is deformed, growth plate architecture is lost, and subchondral spaces contain necrotic debris surrounded by fibrovascular tissue and osteoclasts (Fig. 145–52).

Metaphyseal lesions are related to vascular disruption of a common blood supply to the epiphysis and metaphysis.[14, 17] Epiphyseal bone is slower to revascularize because of a more tenuous primary blood supply. Weightbearing stress results in collapse and fragmentation of the epiphysis, further delaying healing.[3] Metaphyseal healing is relatively advanced owing to extensive collateral and adjacent circulation. Therefore, in the later stages of the disease, chronologically similar lesions in the metaphysis and epiphysis are less apparent radiographically in the metaphysis because healing is more advanced.

Vascular alteration may be related to trauma or predisposing anatomical factors. Toy poodles have a subsynovial blood supply to the femoral epiphysis, compared with an intraosseous system in larger mongrel dogs. The subsynovial location of vessels in toy poodles may increase their susceptibility to ischemia with increased intra-articular pressure.[8, 15] Likewise, in children, transient synovitis was investigated as a cause of increased intra-articular pressure that could inhibit venous flow from the epiphysis. Several studies have failed to demonstrate a causal relationship between Perthes' disease and transient synovitis.[5, 7, 9] Endocrine imbalance has been considered as a cause of Perthes' disease in dogs,[11] but the asymmetrical nature of the disease makes it unlikely.[13]

Perthes' disease in Manchester terriers has a multifactorial inheritance pattern with a high degree of heritability, as in humans.[6, 17]

TREATMENT

Conservative therapy consisting of strict cage rest or a nonweightbearing sling is an option for dogs with minimal clinical and radiographic changes (Fig. 145–53).

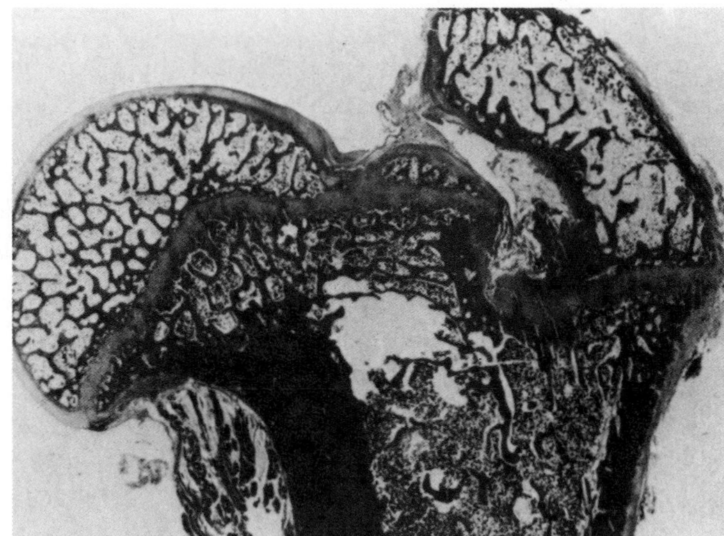

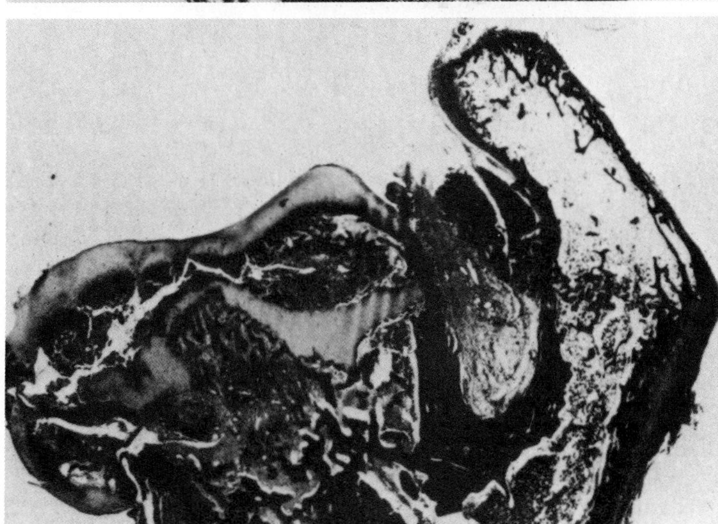

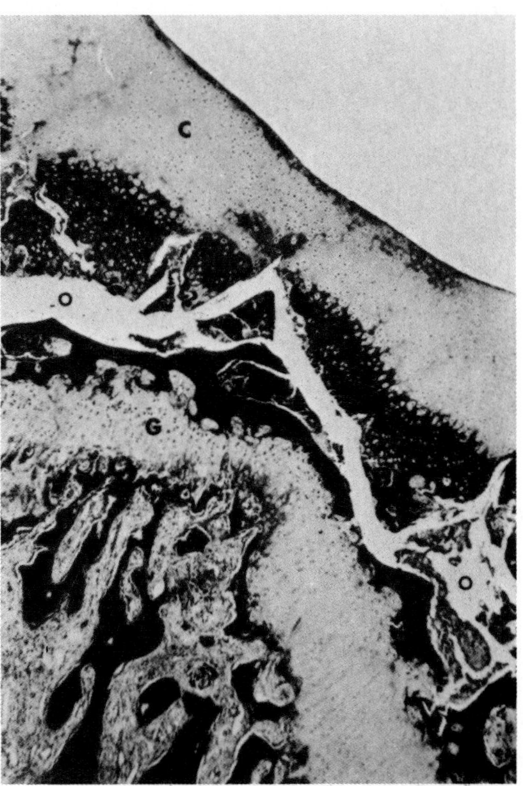

FIGURE 145–51. *Top left,* Normal femoral head (trichrome stain, ×6). *Bottom left,* This left femoral head shows changes of collapse of the epiphysis, widening of the metaphysis, and irregular width of the growth plate (trichrome stain, ×6). *Top right,* The articular cartilage (C) is of variable thickness and has lost its normal sphericity. Only a few necrotic remnants of the bony epiphysis remain in the subchondral space (O). The growth plate (G) appears viable although irregular in thickness (trichrome stain, ×40). (From Mickelson MR, et al: Legg-Calve-Perthes disease in dogs: A comparison to human Legg-Calve-Perthes disease. *Clin Orthop 157*:287, 1981.)

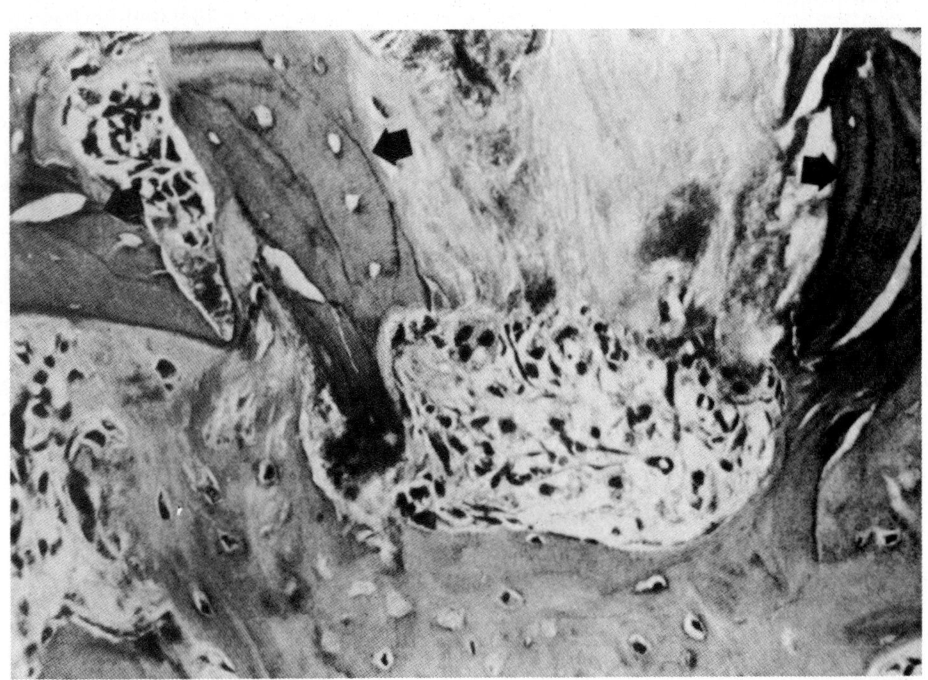

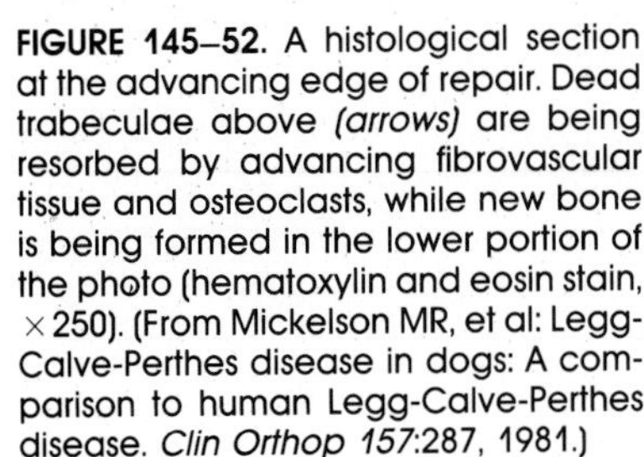

FIGURE 145–52. A histological section at the advancing edge of repair. Dead trabeculae above *(arrows)* are being resorbed by advancing fibrovascular tissue and osteoclasts, while new bone is being formed in the lower portion of the photo (hematoxylin and eosin stain, ×250). (From Mickelson MR, et al: Legg-Calve-Perthes disease in dogs: A comparison to human Legg-Calve-Perthes disease. *Clin Orthop 157*:287, 1981.)

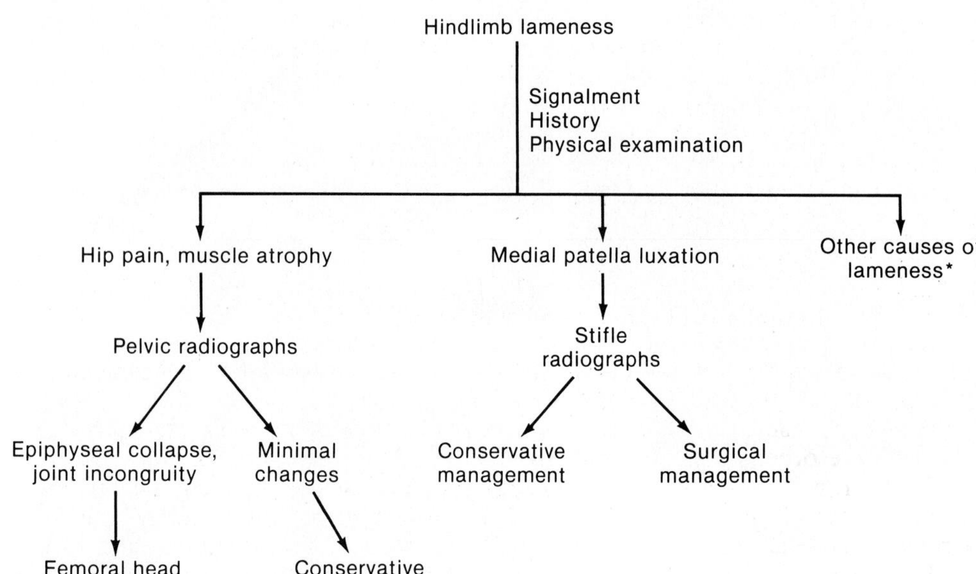

FIGURE 145–53. Treatment of Perthes' disease in dogs. Most dogs require femoral head ostectomy for satisfactory resolution of the clinical signs. The operation should not be delayed, because recovery is prolonged in dogs with chronic degenerative changes and severe muscle atrophy.

*See Chapter 119 for a detailed work-up of lameness.

Unfortunately, most dogs with clinical signs associated with Perthes' disease are relatively severely affected, and surgical treatment is required.

Femoral head and neck ostectomy is recommended for dogs with lameness and radiographic signs of femoral head collapse and joint incongruity. The surgery is a salvage procedure; with dedicated owner compliance and physical therapy, the prognosis for pain-free ambulation is favorable.

The surgical technique is described in Chapter 135. The key to success postoperatively is vigorous physical activity to encourage use of the limb.[16] Dogs that have been chronically lame before surgery have a more prolonged recovery; 6 to 12 months sometimes must elapse before the muscle mass returns and lameness resolves. Conservative therapy is not pursued for more than 1 month unless progress is made.

References

1. Bohr HH: On the development and course of Legg-Calve-Perthes disease (LCPD). *Clin Orthop 150*:30, 1980.
2. Catteral A, et al: A review of the morphology of Perthes' disease. *J Bone Joint Surg [Br] 64B*:269, 1982.
3. DeNatale JS, et al: Mechanical behavior of the femoral head in Legg-Perthes disease. *Biomater Med Devel Artif Organs 9*:19, 1981.
4. Gamberdella PC: Legg-Calve-Perthes in dogs. *In* Bojrab MJ (ed): *Pathophysiology in Small Animal Surgery*. Lea & Febiger, Philadelphia, 1981, pp 625–630.
5. Gershuni DH, et al: The questionable significance of hip tamponade in producing osteonecrosis in Legg-Calve-Perthes syndrome. *J Pediatr Orthop 3*:280, 1983.
6. Hall DJ: Genetic aspects of Perthes' disease. *Clin Orthop 209*:100, 1986.
7. Kallio P, et al: Transient synovitis and Perthes disease. *J Bone Joint Surg [Br] 68B*:808, 1986.
8. Kemp HBS: Perthes' disease in rabbits and puppies. *Clin Orthop 209*:139, 1986.
9. Landin LA, et al: Transient synovitis of the hip. *J Bone Joint Surg [Br] 69B*:238, 1987.
10. Lee R, Fry PD: Some observations on the occurrence of Legg-Calve-Perthes (coxa plana) in the dog, and an evaluation of excision arthroplasty as a method of treatment. *J Small Anim Pract 10*:309, 1969.
11. Ljunggren GL. Legg-Perthes in the dog. *Acta Orthop Scand Suppl 95*:1, 1967.
12. Mickelson MR, et al: Legg-Calve-Perthes in dogs: A comparison to human Legg-Calve-Perthes disease. *Clin Orthop 157*:287, 1981.
13. Nunamaker DM: Legg-Calve-Perthes disease. *In* Newton CD, Nunamaker DM (eds): *Textbook of Small Animal Orthopaedics*. J.B. Lippincott, Philadelphia, 1985, pp 949–952.
14. Rivera LA, et al: Arterial supply to the canine hip joint. *J Vet Orthop 1*:20, 1979.
15. Singleton WB, Jones EL: The experimental induction of subclinical Perthes' disease in the puppy following arthrotomy and intracapsular tamponade. *J Comp Pathol 89*:57, 1979.
16. Vasseur PB: Femoral head and neck ostectomy. *In* Bojrab MJ (ed): *Current Techniques in Small Animal Surgery*. 3rd ed. Lea & Febiger, Philadelphia, 1990, pp 674–683.
17. Vasseur PB, et al: Mode of inheritance of Perthes' disease in Manchester terriers. *Clin Orthop 244*:281, 1989.

Miscellaneous Orthopedic Diseases

P. A. Manley and J. Amundson Romich

PANOSTEITIS

Panosteitis is a spontaneously occurring self-limiting disease of unknown cause affecting young large or giant breeds of dogs.[3, 61, 89, 90] The disease involves the diaphyseal and metaphyseal areas of long bones and is characterized by medullary enostosis and occasionally subperiosteal new bone formation.[61] It is most common in German shepherds[16, 96, 97] but has also been reported in the bassett hound, Scottish terrier, Great Dane, Saint Bernard, Doberman pinscher, German shorthaired pointer, Irish setter, Airedale, golden retriever,

Labrador retriever, Samoyed, and miniature schnauzer.[16, 44, 56, 77, 93]

Panosteitis is not a primary bone disease but a disease of the fatty bone marrow, with secondary effects involving bone.[61, 97] The disease is initially characterized by degeneration of medullary adipocytes near the nutrient foramen.[61, 97] In response to this cellular degeneration, stromal cells that line the medullary vascular sinusoids proliferate. These cells lay down osteoid and within the medullary cavity form a nidus that becomes calcified and expands to reach the endosteal surfaces.[97] The nidus continues to grow proximally and distally within the medullary cavity. Increased congestion within the vascular sinusoids may accompany new bone production, and a secondary endosteal and periosteal response is stimulated.[97] New bone is eventually resorbed, and hematopoietic and fatty bone marrow are reestablished.[61, 97] Thirty days after the onset of the disease process, hematopoietic marrow replaces lamellar bone, and radiographically, the medullary cavity begins to clear. By 60 to 90 days, the hematopoietic marrow has differentiated into fatty bone marrow and the bone and bone marrow have returned to their normal radiographic appearance.[97]

An etiological agent for canine panosteitis has not been identified, although various causes have been suggested. These include bacterial and viral osteomyelitis, hereditary predisposition, transient vascular abnormalities, allergic reactions, metabolic abnormalities, parasite migration, autoimmune reactions following viral infections, hyperestrinism, and stress.[16, 61, 96, 97] Canine panosteitis may occur concurrently with other skeletal diseases. It is important to differentiate the history and clinical signs of panosteitis from other diseases affecting young growing animals (Fig. 145–54).

Clinical signs usually occur in large dogs between 5 and 12 months of age but have been documented as early as 2 months of age and as late as 5 years.[16] Males are more commonly affected; if encountered in females, panosteitis is usually associated with the first estrus.[44, 97] Affected animals have acute lameness ranging from slight to severe without a history of trauma. The lameness may be persistent or intermittent and involve one or more limbs.[16, 96] The disease usually begins in the front limbs, the ulna being the most commonly affected long bone. Other bones likely to be involved in panosteitis include, in descending order of prevalence, the radius, humerus, femur, and tibia.[97] The disease com-

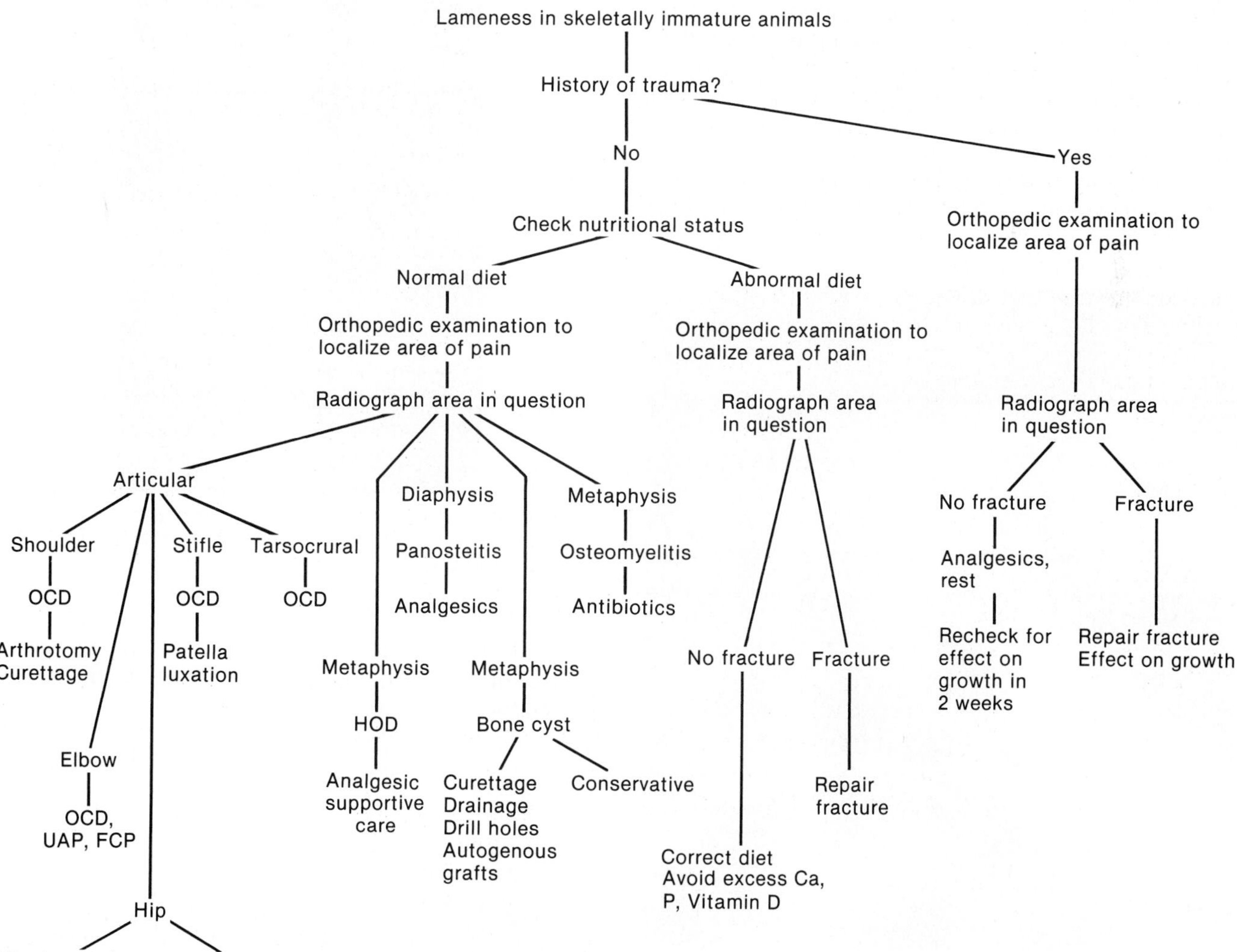

FIGURE 145–54. Diagnosis and treatment of lameness in immature dogs. (OCD, osteochondritis dissecans; UAP, ununited anconeal process; FCP, fragmented coronoid process; LCP, Legg-Calvé-Perthes disease; HOD, hypertrophic osteodystrophy.)

monly resolves in one location only to shift to another. This cycle typically occurs at 2- to 3-week intervals, with short lapses between episodes.[16] The intervals between successive episodes increase as the animal matures.[61] Recurrence of the disease in a previously affected bone is uncommon.[16] Physical examination reveals discomfort associated with deep palpation of the affected area.[3, 16, 61] The animal may also have a history of intermittent fever, lethargy, and anorexia and may show evidence of muscle atrophy. These signs are usually secondary to pain. Clinical signs usually resolve by the time the animal reaches 18 to 20 months of age.

Diagnosis of panosteitis is confirmed by radiography. Although the earliest radiographic abnormality is increased radiolucency in the region of the nutrient foramen, this is rare. Histologically, the radiolucency represents the initial cellular degeneration within the fatty marrow and the subsequent vascular proliferation. At this stage, the bone may be extremely sensitive to deep palpation owing to vascular congestion within the medullary sinusoids.[97] The earliest recognizable radiographic abnormality is an increase in intramedullary density.[3, 61] In the early stages, this increased density is unifocal and has indistinct margins (Fig. 145–55). Histologically, this represents the initial calcification of the newly formed bone.[97] As the disease progresses, multiple foci of increased radiodensities coalesce within the medullary cavity. The endosteal surface may become indistinct as the radiodensity spreads toward each metaphysis (Fig. 145–56). The periosteal response is most often mild. In later stages of the disease, areas of increased radiodensity within the medullary canal regress, although the sclerosis may remain apparent for several months.[3]

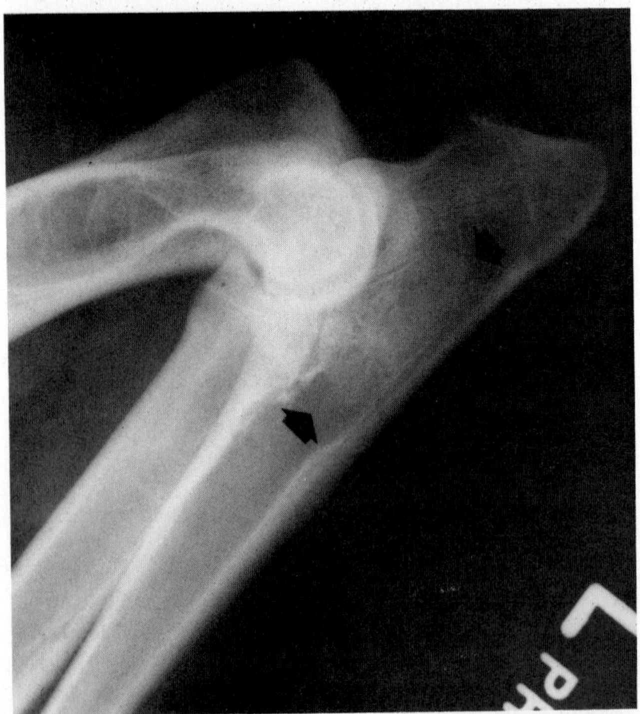

FIGURE 145–55. Panosteitis in the proximal ulna of an immature German shepherd. Note the increase in medullary density representing calcification of the fatty marrow *(arrow)*.

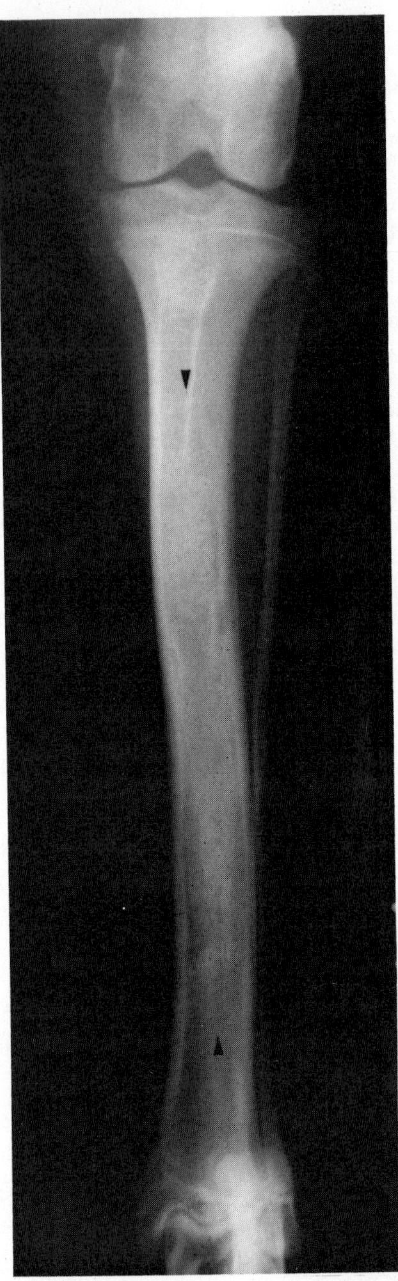

FIGURE 145–56. Panosteitis in the tibial diaphysis of an immature Labrador retriever. The margins are indistinct, and the limits of the lesion are depicted by the two arrows.

There is no correlation between radiographic signs, degree of lameness, and amount of pain elicted on palpation.[3, 61]

Treatment consists of supportive care and analgesics to alleviate discomfort. We recommend buffered aspirin (10 to 20 mg/kg PO TID). If gastrointestinal upset occurs or aspirin is ineffective, other nonsteroidal anti-inflammatory drugs may be considered; however, dogs are very sensitive to many of these drugs, and caution must be implemented in their use (see Chapter 143). We do not recommend steroids for prolonged periods in young growing animals.

The prognosis for return to full function is excellent; however, it is important to counsel owners about the cyclical nature of the disease so that they do not become frustrated with its prolonged course. Complications are seldom noted.

HYPERTROPHIC OSTEODYSTROPHY

Hypertrophic osteodystrophy is a developmental disease of immature large and giant breeds of dogs in which the metaphyseal area of long bones becomes swollen and painful. The distal radius and ulna are the bones most commonly affected, although all long bones are susceptible.[2] The disease occurs in the Great Dane, Irish wolfhound, Saint Bernard, borzoi, boxer, Dalmatian, Irish setter, weimaraner, German shorthaired pointer, Doberman pinscher, German shepherd, Labrador retriever, collie, greyhound, bassett hound, and some terrier breeds.[40, 46, 59, 80]

Although the pathogenesis is obscure, this disease exerts its major effect in the region of the growth plate and adjacent metaphysis of long bones. A disturbance of the metaphyseal blood supply leads to a failure or delay in ossification of the hypertrophic zone of the metaphyseal growth plate. The hypertrophic zone may become elongated and extend into the metaphyseal trabeculae. Inflammation, hemorrhage, necrosis, fracture, and extensive remodeling are prominent in the trabeculae adjacent to the metaphyseal growth plate. Fracture of the trabeculae may cause a secondary lifting of the periosteum with subsequent production of new bone that may encircle the metaphyseal area.[59] Periosteal reaction is an inconsistent finding with hypertrophic osteodystrophy and may represent a different grade of the disease.[58]

The cause of hypertrophic osteodystrophy is unknown. Vitamin C deficiency has remained a popular theory because of reports of low vitamin C levels in urine and serum of some affected animals.[19, 34, 59, 94] Because dogs are able to synthesize vitamin C in their liver and intestines, a deficiency may actually reflect an inability to properly use the vitamin C present.[3, 47] Clinically, vitamin C supplementation in affected animals has not met with universal success.[11, 47] Massive dietary supplementation has been associated with development of this disease; however, this is not a consistent finding.[46, 78] An infectious etiology has also been proposed.[40, 106] Aspects of the clinical and pathological signs associated with hypertrophic osteodystrophy bear similarities to an infectious process.[59] At this time, an organism has not been isolated. Reports linking hypertrophic osteodystrophy to an upper respiratory infection have not been based on isolation of a specific pathogen.[58] A single report in the literature related hypertrophic osteodystrophy to a hereditary predisposition.[40]

Most affected animals are presented between 2 and 8 months of age. Clinically, the presentation may vary from a slight limp to a nonweightbearing lameness. Depending on this presentation, the metaphyseal regions of the long bones may be swollen, warm, and painful when touched (Fig. 145–57). Severely affected animals may be systemically ill and have a history of depression and anorexia with clinical findings of pyrexia and weight loss. The disease is usually bilaterally symmetrical and episodic. Reports of a response to a particular therapy may actually be a reflection of the episodic nature of hypertrophic osteodystrophy.[58]

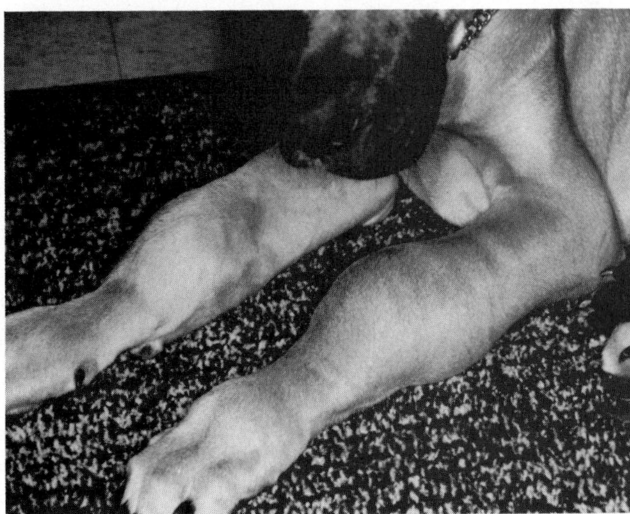

FIGURE 145–57. Hypertrophic osteodystrophy in a 5-month-old Great Dane. Note the extensive swelling at the distal antebrachium.

The diagnosis is confirmed by radiographic examination. In the early stages of the disease, an irregular radiolucent line may be apparent in the metaphyses adjacent to the growth plate (Fig. 145–58). This represents necrosis and resorption of metaphyseal trabeculae.[59] The metaphyseal growth plate may be normal throughout the course of the disease or may show irregular widening associated with delayed ossification of the hypertrophic zone. Subperiosteal new bone formation may be localized to the area adjacent to the metaphyseal growth plate or may be so extensive that it involves all of the metaphysis and some of the diaphysis (Fig. 145–59).

Treatment of hypertrophic osteodystrophy is largely supportive. Buffered aspirin is recommended for relief of discomfort. In severely debilitated animals, parenteral fluid and electrolyte therapy may be necessary. Attentive nursing care is paramount in successful management of these patients. If an affected animal is being fed an improper diet, this is corrected. Oversupplementation of the diet with vitamins and minerals is avoided, and based on current literature, vitamin C therapy is not advised. Antibiotics may be indicated for treatment of secondary infections.

The prognosis is good to excellent for animals with only mild lesions but is guarded for severely affected animals. If an animal reaches maturity (many are euthanized owing to morbidity), spontaneous remissions are possible.

In mild cases, disturbance of normal metaphyseal growth is not a problem. Premature growth arrests are likely in the most severely affected animals. Dynamic or definitive correction of angular deformities or shortened long bones may be needed. Complications may be indirectly associated with hypertrophic osteodystrophy. In severely moribund animals, secondary bacterial infections (pneumonia, cystitis) and decubital ulcers may

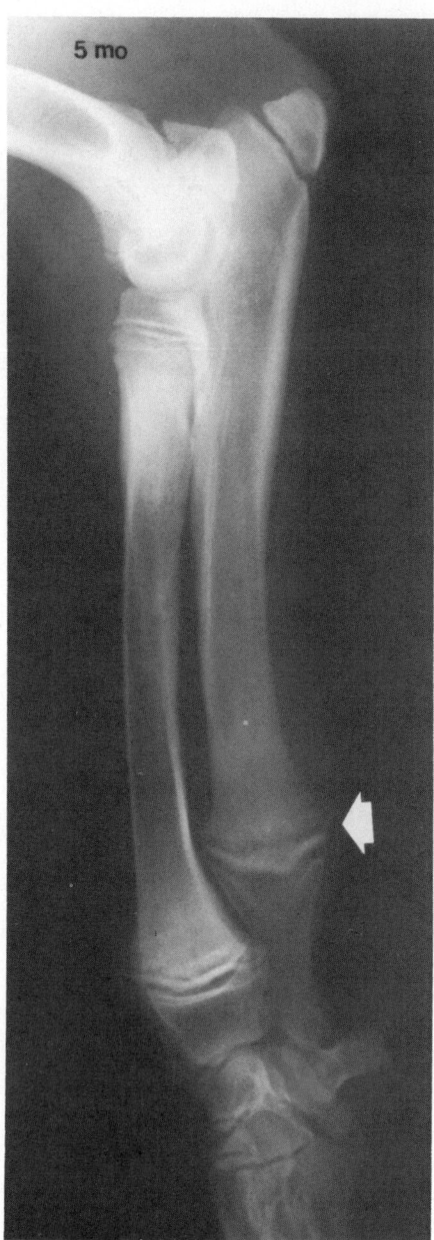

FIGURE 145–58. Hypertrophic osteodystrophy. The arrow points to an irregular radiolucent line located just proximal to the growth plate of the distal ulna.

develop if the animal is recumbent for a prolonged period.

HYPERTROPHIC OSTEOPATHY

Hypertrophic osteopathy is a secondary pathological disease process characterized by bilateral symmetrical swellings primarily affecting the distal portions of all four limbs. Initially, soft-tissue swelling predominates; however, as the disease progresses, a diffuse periosteal reaction may involve the majority of bones in the limbs.[60] The disease most commonly occurs in humans and dogs, but it has been noted in cats, horses, cows, mink, and nonhuman primates.[24, 62, 63, 66, 84, 104] The disease was first described in the veterinary literature in the 1920s in a dog with tuberculosis.[102, 107]

Pulmonary osteoarthropathy, hypertrophic pulmonary osteoarthropathy, and *hypertrophic pulmonary osteopathy* are names given to this condition because of its association with some form of pulmonary disease. Metastatic pulmonary lesions are most commonly linked with this condition; however, primary pulmonary neoplasia, chronic bronchopneumonia, pulmonary abscesses, and pulmonary tuberculosis have been reported.[57, 85, 95, 103, 107] Other intrathoracic diseases such as dirofilariasis, spirocercosis, blastomycosis, foreign bodies, rib tumors, and endocarditis may predipose to development of hypertrophic osteopathy.[23, 29, 91, 98] Dogs suffering from bladder tumors (especially rhabdomyosarcoma) and adenocarcinoma of the liver have also been reported to develop the condition; therefore, the pulmonary portion of the name has been eliminated.[43, 102]

The pathogenesis of hypertrophic osteopathy is not understood. Because the majority of cases are associated with underlying pulmonary disease, the pathogenesis is believed to be related to these pulmonary disturbances. The precise cause is unknown, however. The most popular theory suggests that increased peripheral blood flow results from the pulmonary disease. The increase in blood flow results in congestion of many connective tissue structures, including periosteal tissue. The peri-

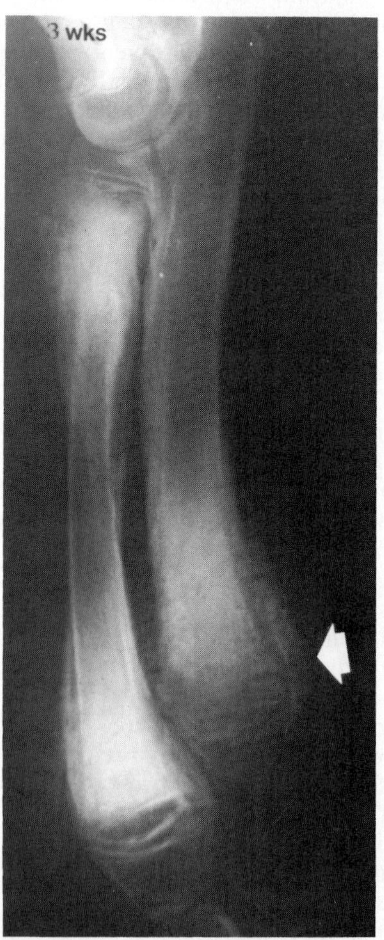

FIGURE 145–59. Hypertrophic osteodystrophy. Note the periosteal response extending from the distal radius and ulna and from the proximal radius. The periosteal response is located adjacent to the metaphyseal growth plate. This film was taken 3 weeks after Figure 145–58.

osteum responds by laying down new bone on the cortical surfaces.[38] The mechanism responsible for this increased peripheral blood flow is believed to be neural in origin. Afferent nerves involved with the primary lesion join the vagus or intercostal nerves. Irritation of the afferent pathways may stimulate a nervous reflex that is mediated by the vagus, the intercostal nerves, or some other afferent pathway, resulting in increased peripheral blood flow.[3, 60] Support for this theory is demonstrated by rapid regression in the clinical signs of hypertrophic osteopathy after surgical removal of the primary thoracic lesion or section of the vagus nerve.[60, 100]

The majority of affected animals are presented for sudden or gradual onset of swelling and lameness involving all four limbs. This condition occurs most often in middle-aged animals because of the associated increased risk of neoplasia. Physical examination reveals firm swellings of the distal portion of all four limbs that are warm and sometimes painful when palpated. Systemic signs may be associated with the primary lesion.

Radiographic examination of the appendicular skeleton reveals bilateral symmetrical periosteal reactions affecting all bones of the limbs. Early in the condition, the metacarpal and metatarsal bones may be primarily affected. As the disease progresses, however, the more proximal long bones and many of the joints become involved. The periosteal reaction may be smooth and regular or rough and aggressive (Fig. 145–60). Soft-tissue swelling is seen in the areas of periosteal proliferation. Radiography should include plain films of the thoracic cavity to check for pulmonary involvement and contrast abdominal studies and ultrasonography to rule out abdominal disease.

Treatment involves removal or elimination of the primary lesions. Surgical removal of tumors and granulomas or medical therapy for dirofilariasis and Spirocera infection should result in resolution of hypertrophic osteopathy. Clinical signs should resolve within 1 to 2 weeks of treatment. Resolution of the bony lesions may take months.[49, 53]

The prognosis depends on the underlying disease process and the ability to eliminate the primary lesion surgically or medically. Complications are usually associated with the primary disease.

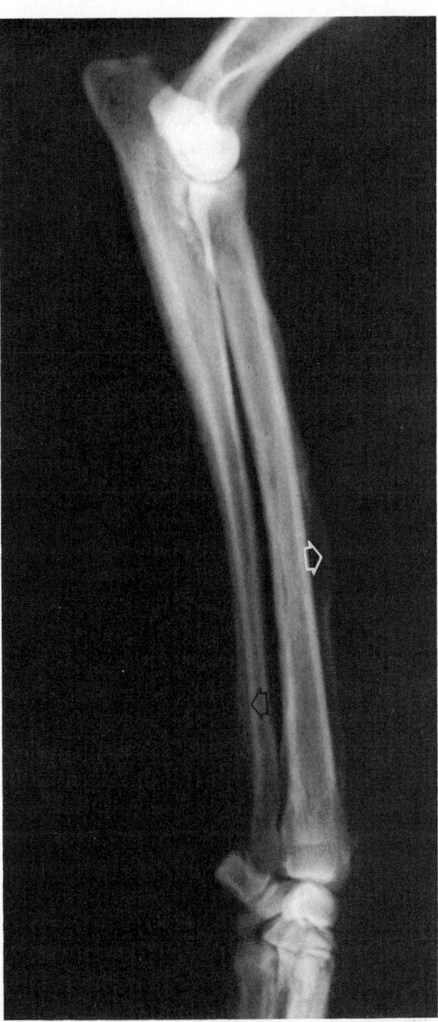

FIGURE 145–60. Hypertrophic osteopathy. Note both rough and smooth periosteal reactions involving the diaphysis of the radius and ulna.

HYPERPARATHYROIDISM (see also Chapter 113)

Parathyroid hormone (PTH) is synthesized by the chief cells of the parathyroid gland in response to decreased serum calcium concentration. This hormone exerts its major effect on target cells in the bone, kidneys, and intestines. In bone, PTH mobilizes calcium from skeletal reserves by stimulating osteoclastic and osteocytic bone resorption.[27, 42] In the kidneys, PTH inhibits renal tubular phosphate resorption, resulting in increased urinary phosphate excretion.[18] PTH has only a minor role in calcium retention in the distal convoluted tubules.[27] In addition, PTH stimulates the hydroxylation of 25-hydroxycholecalciferol to 1,25-dihydroxycholecalciferol in the renal mitochondria. This is the active form of vitamin D, which is responsible for stimulating intestinal calcium absorption. These combined functions allow PTH to maintain normal calcium/phosphorus homeostasis.[41]

Primary hyperparathyroidism and secondary hyperparathyroidism result in increased PTH production and release, with increased resorption of cortical bone. Primary hyperparathyroidism is an unusual condition occurring most often with hyperplasia or neoplasia of the parathyroid glands. Secondary hyperparathyroidism is a more common disease in dogs and may be associated with renal disease or a nutritional deficiency.[3]

Renal secondary hyperparathyroidism may be encountered in older animals with chronic renal failure or in younger animals with congenital renal insufficiency. Renal secondary hyperparathyroidism results from the kidneys' inability to excrete phosphorus and to convert 25-hydroxycholecalciferol to its active metabolite. Hyperphosphatemia indirectly lowers blood calcium, whereas a decrease in the active form of vitamin D decreases intestinal absorption of calcium; both result in hypocalcemia.[27]

The predominant clinical signs reflect the severity of the renal disease: vomiting, dehydration, polydipsia, and depression. Skeletal involvement may be most apparent in the bones of the skull and jaw. Resorption of alveolar bone and loss of lamina dura dentes may occur early in the disease, with loosening of the teeth and mastication problems.[27] Other bones in the skull may become soft and pliable and may be susceptible to pathological fractures. Long bones are less affected; however, pathological fractures may occur with relatively minor trauma.[27]

Diagnosis is made on clinical signs, serum chemistry studies, urinalysis, and radiography. Blood test results may show elevated blood urea nitrogen and creatinine levels. Serum calcium levels may be within the normal range owing to bone resorption. Radiography of the abdomen may reveal small kidneys. Radiography of the skeletal system may delineate diffuse demineralization of the rami of the mandible/maxilla, with loss of lamina dura dentes and localized radiolucent areas, diffuse demineralization of other bones involved, and pathological fractures (Fig. 145–61).

Treatment is directed toward slowing the progression of kidney disease and restoring kidney function, and includes supportive therapy, dietary protein restriction (high quality, low quantity), phosphate binding gels, and various treatments for anemia and acidosis. Supplementation with calcium (gluconate or lactate) and vitamin D may decrease the severity of the skeletal lesions.[27] The prognosis is guarded, depending on the stage of kidney disease.[20] Complications may be associated with renal failure or with secondary effects on the skeletal system. Delayed fracture union is anticipated.

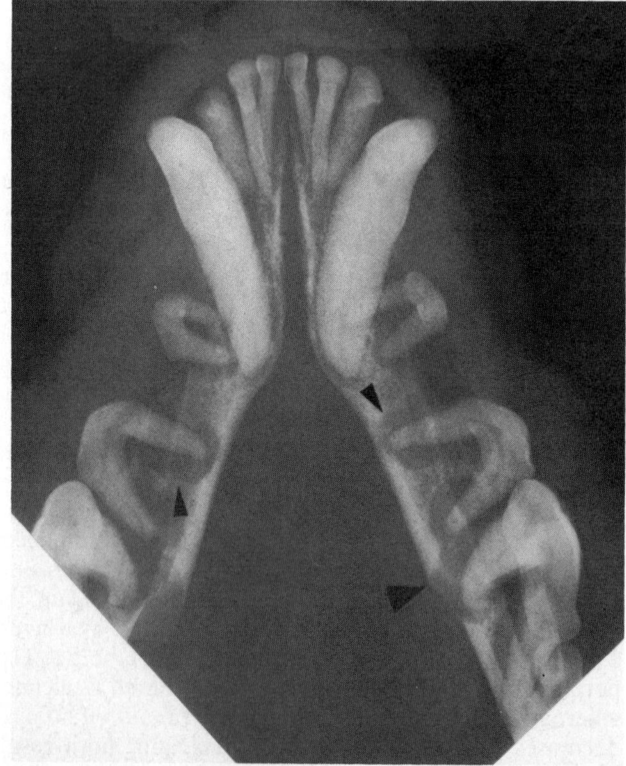

FIGURE 145–61. Renal secondary hyperparathyroidism. Note the radiolucent areas around the teeth, typical of alveolar resorption *(small arrows)*. The large arrow points to a pathological fracture on the left side of the mandible.

Nutritional secondary hyperparathyroidism is a metabolic disorder in which PTH is increased as a result of a nutritionally induced hypocalcemia, hyperphosphatemia with normal or low calcium levels, or inadequate amounts of vitamin D. The disease develops in young puppies and kittens fed a predominantly meat diet, which is high in phosphorus and low in calcium and has an imbalanced calcium/phosphorus ratio.[27, 54] Young animals may develop the disease in only a few weeks, whereas adult animals may consume a deficient diet for several months before they develop hyperparathyroidism.

Young animals are often presented with a reluctance to move, lameness, or an incoordinated gait.[27] Palpation of the bones may elicit discomfort, and pathological fractures may be obvious because of abnormal curvatures in the limbs. In adult animals, clinical signs are usually related to resorption of the bones of the skull and mandible, as in renal secondary hyperparathyroidism.

Diagnosis involves radiographs and a thorough dietary history. Radiographically, the cortices of the long bones are thin owing to increased resorption, and the medullary cavity may appear abnormally wide. Loss of lamina dura dentes and evidence of multiple pathological fractures may be seen. Laboratory test results for renal function are within normal limits. Serum calcium and phosphorus levels may be normal or abnormal.[27]

Treatment involves correcting the dietary mineral imbalance and confining the animal to reduce the chances of further pathological fractures. Dietary calcium/phosphorus ratio during the healing phase is maintained at 2:1. Improvement of the skeletal condition during dietary supplementation may be monitored radiographically.[55] It may take 8 to 10 weeks for fractures to heal and for the cortical thickness to return to normal. After treatment is complete, the diet is formulated to maintain the calcium/phosphorus ratio at 1.2:1.0.[27] The prognosis is favorable if the condition is treated before the development of significant skeletal deformities. Complications are generally associated with delayed fracture union or with malunions.

VITAMIN D DEFICIENCY (RICKETS AND OSTEOMALACIA)

Rickets and osteomalacia are diseases that result from an inadequate supply of cholecalciferol or vitamin D. Rickets occurs in growing animals before growth plate closure, whereas osteomalacia occurs in adult animals after growth plate closure.[3] These diseases occur rarely in dogs and cats because of the natural availability of vitamin D. Cholecalciferol is present in small amounts in most pet foods and can be synthesized by the action of sunlight on 7-dehydrocholesterol in the epidermis of the skin.[52] The liver and kidneys hydroxylate vitamin D to its active metabolite, 1,25-dihydroxycholecalciferol, which is responsible for calcium and phosphorus absorption from the intestine.[6, 17, 27, 41] Young animals need 1,25-dihydroxycholecalciferol for normal maturation of the metaphyseal growth plates. Mineralization of the matrix in the hypertrophic zone of the metaphyseal growth plates does not occur without adequate vitamin D. Rickets is a disease of immature animals; it results in failure of transformation of the cartilage component of the growth plate to primary spongiosa.[3, 27] In adult animals, vitamin D is necessary to permit the osteoclasts and osteocytes to respond to PTH to allow bone resorption.[27, 32] Calcium homeostasis cannot be maintained and newly formed osteoid cannot be mineralized in osteomalacia.[3, 27]

In rickets and osteomalacia, affected animals may be presented for a wide variety of skeletally induced abnormalities, which may include lameness, difficulty getting up, a stiff gait, bowing of limbs, pathological fractures, or sudden paralysis. Historical evidence may suggest an inadequate diet or a housing situation that does not allow the animal to be exposed to sunlight. Alternatively, a diet high in mineral oil may prevent absorption of calcium and phosphorus.[3] Radiographic signs may be similar to hyperparathyroidism and commonly include radiolucent cortical bone due to poor mineralization and a loss of lamina dura dentes. Pathological fractures may also be seen.

Treatment consists of repair of fractures and correction of dietary habits. Feeding a nutritionally balanced commercially prepared growth ration is recommended. Vitamin D supplementation may initially be necessary to correct overt deficiencies but should not exceed 500 IU/kg of diet or 10 to 20 IU/kg of body weight daily.[68] Lactose, which promotes intestinal absorption of calcium independent of vitamin D, improves endochondral growth and bone development and mineralization in rats.[64] Although no data have been collected for dogs, this treatment may prove beneficial.

The prognosis for vitamin D deficiency is favorable if the pathological fractures have not resulted in irreparable damage. Complications are usually related to pathological fractures.

CRANIOMANDIBULAR OSTEOPATHY

Craniomandibular osteopathy is a non-neoplastic proliferative bone disease affecting primarily the flat bones of the skull (especially the mandible, tympanic bullae, and occipital bone). One or more of these bones may be affected, and the lesions are usually bilateral and symmetrical. The disease predominately afflicts Scottish terriers and West Highland white terriers; however, it has been documented in the Boston terrier, English bulldog, cairn terrier, Laborador retriever, Great Dane, Doberman pinscher, and boxer.* The animals are usually affected between 3 and 6 months of age.

In craniomandibular osteopathy, mandibular lamellar bone is resorbed and juvenile bone (woven bone or primary spongiosa) is produced.[74, 80] The woven bone is coarse, with fibers running in unregimented directions. The medullary cavity of the mandible eventually becomes filled with this primitive bone. Normal bone may sometimes be deposited, but woven bone tends to dominate the histological picture.[51] At skeletal maturity, the woven bone may be replaced by more mature bone, but the bone rarely reverts to its normal condition.[4, 74, 82]

*See references 9, 26, 45, 79, 87, 99, and 101

The cause of craniomandibular osteopathy is unknown. It has been compared with osteitis deformans (Paget's disease), a bone disease of humans.[5, 51] Osteitis deformans is characteristically polyostotic but may rarely occur in a monostotic form and may involve the bones of the skull. Histologically, Paget's disease bears some similarities to craniomandibular osteopathy; however, clinically it occurs in patients over 40 years of age.[1] The occurrence of craniomandibular osteopathy in select breeds of dogs and littermates may suggest a genetic basis, although a mode of inheritance has not been established.[4] No sex predilection is noted.

Animals are usually presented because of pain associated with opening the mouth. Other symptoms include lethargy, anorexia, pyrexia, excess salivation, lymphadenopathy, temporal muscle atrophy, weight loss, and dehydration.[3, 81] Physical examination may reveal a firm swelling of the mandible that is bilaterally symmetrical. Attempts to open the mouth may be unsuccessful in an unsedated animal. Even under general anesthesia, the mouth may only open a few centimeters.

Diagnosis is confirmed by radiographic examination of the skull. Radiographs demonstrate bilaterally symmetrical periosteal lesions involving the mandible and temporal bones.[81] The periosteal reaction may be so extensive that function of the temporomandibular joints becomes severely compromised (Fig. 145–62). At skeletal maturity (usually 11 to 13 months of age), the proliferative lesions become static and the edges of affected bones become smooth. Occasionally, there is evidence of a periosteal reaction in the metaphyseal regions of long bones reminiscent of the lesions in hypertrophic osteodystrophy.[81]

Craniomandibular osteopathy is a self-limiting dis-

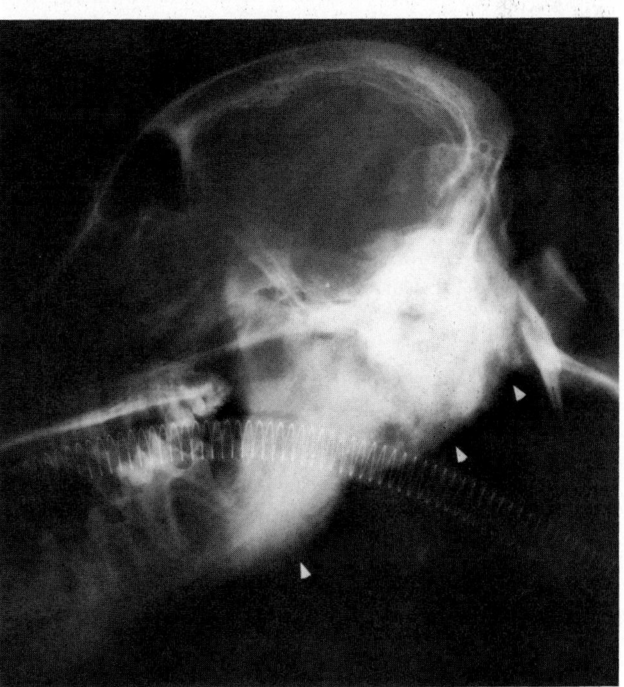

FIGURE 145–62. Craniomandibular osteopathy in a West Highland white terrier. The arrows point to the extensive periosteal reaction along the ventral aspect of the mandible and around the tympanic bulla.

ease. Treatment is directed at relieving discomfort and supporting the animal until the disease regresses. Analgesics may be given to relieve pain. Steroids have also been advocated by some.[81, 87] Some animals may require a pharyngostomy tube to maintain proper nutrition. Surgical attempts to reduce bone mass have not resulted in improvement.[74]

The prognosis for this disease depends on the degree of bony involvement. Severe involvement may compromise an animal's ability to sustain itself nutritionally. Complications usually involve an animal's inability to open its mouth. Resection of the condyloid process of the mandible or a partial hemimandibulectomy can be considered in severely affected dogs.

OSTEOCHONDRODYSPLASIA

Osteochondrodysplasia is an abnormality of cartilage or bone growth and development.[50] This is a general classification for constitutional disorders of the human skeleton that has been applied to domestic animals.[21, 48, 50] Breeders' selection of certain traits as desirable has resulted in the development of many achondroplastic and hypochondroplastic breeds.

Achondroplasia, which literally means "failure of cartilage growth," is characterized by a proportionate short-limbed dysplasia that is evident at birth. This is an autosomal dominant trait. Histologically, endochondral ossification of all long bones is retarded, resulting in shortened and deformed limbs. The axial skeleton has numerous defects; a shortened maxilla (relative mandibular prognathism), stenotic nares, a small foramen magnum, and often hemivertebrae.[50] The bulldog, Boston terrier, pug, Pekingese, Japanese spaniel, and Shih Tzu are achondroplastic.

Hypochondroplasia is similar to achondroplasia; however, the changes in the appendicular and axial skeleton are less severe. The skull may appear normal, but premature chondroid metaplasia of the nucleus pulposus of the intervertebral discs is noted. The limbs are shortened and deformed and in some cases may be susceptible to disproportionate growth (Fig. 145–63). The dachshund, basset hound, beagle, Welsh corgi, Dandie Dinmont terrier, Scottish terrier, and Skye terrier are hypochondroplastic.[50]

Other types of nonselected heritable bony defects may periodically become apparent in certain breeds. The mode of inheritance is generally autosomal recessive or polygenic.[21, 50] Dwarfism has been reported in the Scottish terrier, Alaskan malamute, Samoyed, Labrador retriever, English pointer, Norwegian elkhound, Great Pyrenees, and Scottish deerhound. The skeletal defects usually involve the appendicular skeleton and specifically the metaphyseal growth plates of long bones. Disorganization of the proliferative zone, abnormalities within the hypertrophic zone, and subsequent defects of primary and secondary spongiosa are often observed on histological section.[21, 22, 103]

Affected animals are presented because the owner or breeder has noticed skeletal deformities at some time after birth. The deformities most often appear in the appendicular skeleton but as previously noted may also occur in the axial skeleton. Affected young animals may have difficulty walking because of obvious skeletal deformities. Littermates may also be affected.[21]

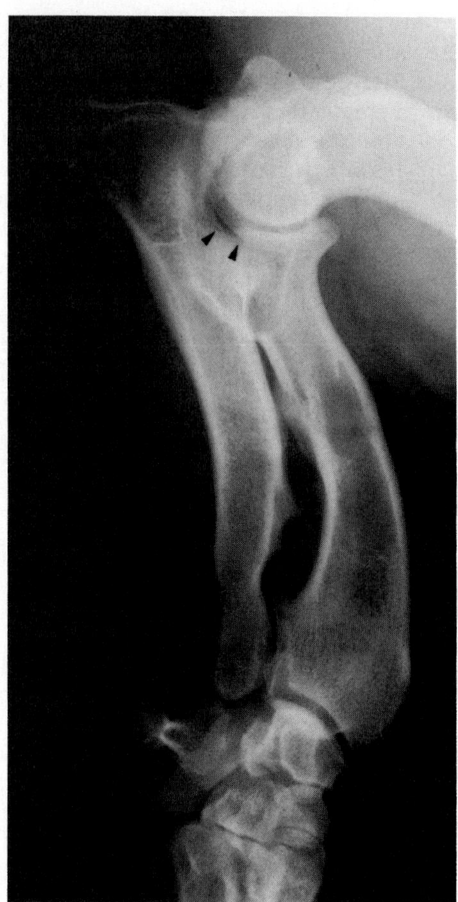

FIGURE 145–63. Disproportionate growth between the radius and ulna in a mature bassett hound. The arrows point to a widening of the ulnohumeral articulation.

Diagnosis is based on clinical findings, radiography, and occasionally growth plate biopsy.[22] Radiographs typically demonstrate abnormalities in the metaphyseal growth plate, including a wide physeal line, retained endochondral core, and irregularities in normal ossification. The long bones appear shorter than normal and are often bowed. The radius and ulna may be more severely affected owing to the asynchronous growth of paired bones.[21, 50]

In most instances that involve severe skeletal deformities, treatment is unrewarding. Complications usually result from these deformities and become apparent as an animal matures.

RADIAL AGENESIS

Hemimelia is a rare disease of animals in which one of the paired bones is congenitally absent. The radius is the most commonly affected bone, followed by the tibia.[50] Radial agenesis (aplasia) has been reported in cats, dogs, rats, chickens, and goats.[7, 10, 12, 105] The condition is most often unilateral but may be bilateral.

Long-bone anomalies have been described in offspring of rats fed zinc- or manganese-deficient diets. Similarly, manganese- or copper-deficient diets fed to chickens

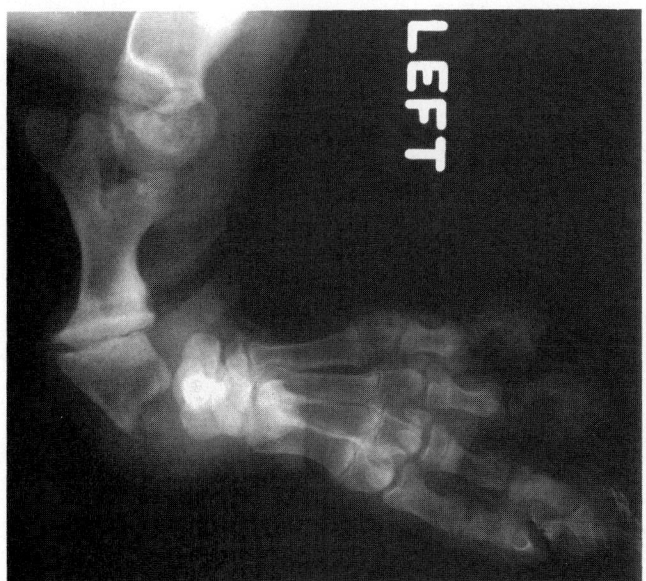

FIGURE 145–64. Radial agenesis. Note complete absence of the radius with subluxation of the ulnocarpal joint.

have produced long-bone agenesis.[10] Radial agenesis affecting several offspring in a litter of cats, lends credibility to a hereditable cause.[92] Other suggested causes of hemimelia include intrauterine compression, inflammation, maternal nutritional deficiencies, irradiation, vaccines, and drugs.[76]

An animal affected with radial agenesis is usually presented shortly after birth for deformity of the front limb resulting in compromised gait. Physical examination reveals a rotational deformity of the forelimb, with limitation of flexion and extension at the elbow and the carpus.

Radiographic examination reveals complete or partial agenesis of the radius with a compensatory increase in the diameter of the ulna.[50] Subluxation or luxation of the humeroulnar and ulnocarpal joint may be evident (Fig. 145–64).

Amputation of the affected limb is the treatment of choice for unilateral lesions. If the limb is not amputated, ulceration of the carpus may develop when the animal drags the limb.[72] Euthanasia may be necessary if the animal is bilaterally affected.

BONE CYSTS

Simple bone cysts are benign fluid-filled structures that occur uncommonly in dogs. They may appear in only one bone (monostotic) or in many bones (polyostotic) in the same animal.[39, 86] They most often affect the metaphysis and the diaphysis of long bones. They contain a clear, sterile, serosanguineous fluid and have a connective tissue lining.[31, 86] Monostotic bone cysts have been reported in the distal ulna, distal radius, distal femur, and distal humerus of dogs.[13, 39, 67] Cysts have been reported in medium-sized to large dogs.[39, 71, 83, 86]

The cause of simple bone cysts is unknown. The most plausible theory appears to involve venous obstruction in the metaphyseal area with secondary osteolysis of bone due to the expansile nature of the cyst. A report of polyostotic bone cysts in Doberman pinschers suggests a hereditary predisposition.[28, 86]

Solitary bone cysts generally occur in animals younger than 1 year. Animals either have no clinical signs referable to the cystic lesion or are presented with a history of lameness. Pain, swelling, and joint stiffness may be evident in the area of the bone cyst.[39] If a pathological fracture is present, the animal may show acute exacerbation of the lameness.

Radiographic examination reveals a radiolucent defect with cortical thinning and mild osseous expansion in the metaphyseal or diaphyseal region of the long bone. The cyst usually has a homogeneous radiolucent appearance (unicameral) but may have thin bony partitions that appear to divide it into compartments (multicameral).[31, 86] Because of the cortical thinning, pathological fractures are commonly associated with bone cysts (Fig. 145–65).[75, 86]

Drainage, curettage, and autogenous grafting have been recommended as treatments for bone cysts.[86] Excellent clinical results have also been reported with a technique using multiple drill holes.[31] Cyst fluid is collected for cytological and bacteriological evaluation to rule out an infectious agent. Pathologic fracture through the cyst may necessitate immobilization.[86] The prognosis is favorable if the cyst or pathological fracture does not interfere with normal growth.

Aneurysmal bone cysts are expansile osteolytic lesions composed of large vascular sinusoids separated into compartments by thin-walled connective tissue stroma. These cysts are non-neoplastic but may be locally aggressive.[14] They have been reported in cats, dogs, horses, and humans.[14, 39] The pathogenesis and cause are unknown, but trauma and disruption of the normal hemodynamics of the vascular bone marrow are plausible theories.[75]

Radiographs reveal an expansile radiolucent lesion that is often trabeculated giving a soap-bubble appearance.[14] There may be extensive destruction of bone with little bone production. The differential diagnosis includes primary or metastatic bone neoplasia and solitary bone cysts. Surgical excision is the treatment of choice. Radiation therapy has also been recommended.[14] In the metaphyseal and epiphyseal areas of long bones, complete resection may be difficult without compromising limb function. Limb amputation or resection with autograft or allograft replacement may be indicated.

MULTIPLE CARTILAGINOUS EXOSTOSES

Multiple cartilaginous exostoses are a proliferative disease of bone and cartilage in which partially ossified protrusions arise from the cortical surfaces of bones. Only bones formed by endochondral ossification are involved. The disease has been reported in dogs, horses, and cats.* In dogs, the vertebrae, ribs, and long bones are most frequently affected.

In humans, multiple cartilaginous exostoses are hereditary and associated with malignant transformation

*See references 8, 15, 25, 30, 35–37, 65, 70, 73, and 88.

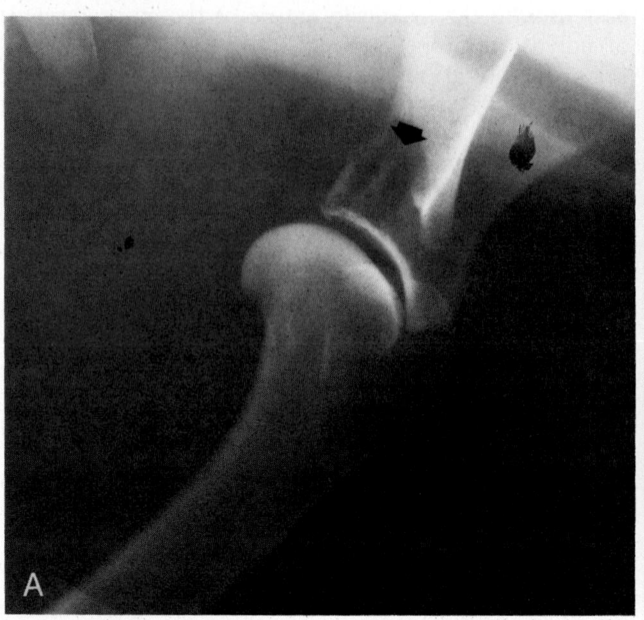

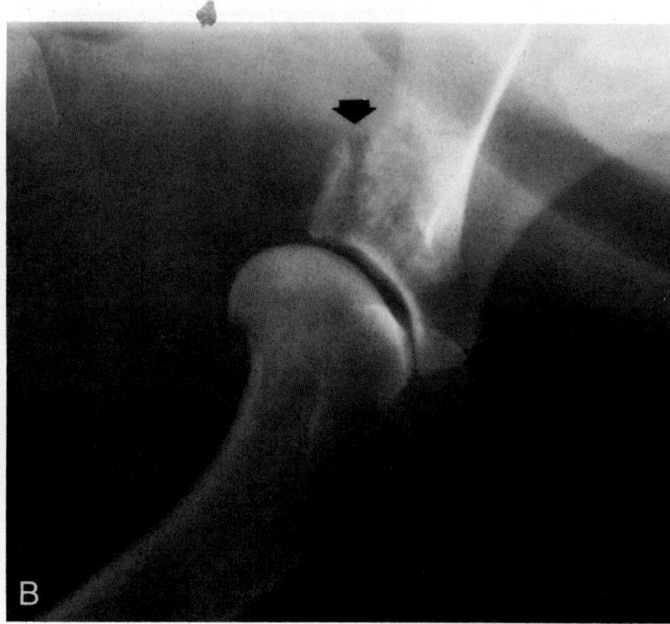

FIGURE 145–65. *A*, Monostotic bone cyst in the distal scapula of a 5-year-old female golden retriever. The cyst appears divided by a bony trabecula *(arrow)*. *B*, The same bone 1 month later. A pathologic fracture is seen along the caudal aspect of the scapula. The margins of the bone cyst are indistinct owing to bone remodeling around the fracture site.

in approximately 5 per cent of patients.[75] In dogs, a familial tendency has been reported[30, 37] and the disease has been linked to chondrosarcoma and osteosarcoma.[8, 33, 69] The cause of multiple cartilaginous exostoses is believed to be displacement of chondrocytes from the metaphyseal growth plate and their subsequent differentiation into cartilage and bone. This usually occurs in a juxtacortical position near the metaphyseal growth plate of long bones but has been observed in the diaphyseal area.[3, 69] The growth of the exostoses usually stops when the metaphyseal growth plate closes.

The disease commonly occurs in dogs younger than 18 months, with no breed or sex predilection. The disorder may not be clinically apparent except for the presence of one or more bony nodules over the long bones, ribs, or vertebrae. Alternatively, the animal may have intermittent or progressive lameness if the bony lesions interfere with the functions of tendons, ligaments, or neurovascular structures.[3] Biopsy of the affected area reveals hyaline cartilage in various stages of differentiation, trabecular bone, and cortical bone.[36]

Radiographically, bony masses appear to arise from the cortical surfaces of bones of the appendicular and axial skeleton (except the skull).[3] The masses may appear large with smoothly contoured edges or may be multilobulated.[36, 69]

Treatment varies with the extent of the lesions. If the lesions are not actively growing, the treatment may be palliative. Surgical excision may be indicated if the lesion interferes with function. The prognosis depends on the extent of skeletal involvement. Solitary lesions in a young, skeletally mature dog at a surgically accessible site have a favorable prognosis. Chronic lesions may transform to bone neoplasia. Because of the unpredictable nature of the disease, periodic radiographic evaluation is advised to assess any change in size or shape of the lesion.

References

1. Aegerter E, Kirkpatrick JA: *Orthopedic Diseases*. W.B. Saunders, Philadelphia, 1975.
2. Alexander JW: Hypertrophic osteodystrophy. *Canine Pract 5*:48, 1978.
3. Alexander JW: Orthopedic diseases. *In* Slatter DH (ed): *Textbook of Small Animal Surgery*. W.B. Saunders, Philadelphia, 1985.
4. Alexander JW: Selected skeletal dysplasias: Craniomandibular osteopathy, multiple cartilaginous exostoses, and hypertrophic osteodystrophy. *Vet Clin North Am Small Animal Pract 13*:55, 1983.
5. Alexander JW, Kallfelz FA: A case of craniomandibular osteopathy in a Labrador retriever. *Vet Med Small Anim Clin 70*:560, 1975.
6. Allen LH: The role of nutrition in the onset and treatment of metabolic bone disease. *Nutrition Update 1*:263, 1983.
7. Alonso RA, et al: An autosomal recessive form of hemimelia in dogs. *Vet Rec 110*:128, 1982.
8. Banks WC, Bridges CH: Multiple cartilaginous exostoses in a dog. *J Am Vet Med Assoc 129*:131, 1956.
9. Battershell D: Craniomandibular osteopathy. *J Am Vet Med Assoc 155*:1735, 1969.
10. Baum KH, Hull BL: Radial agenesis and ulnar hypoplasia in two caprine kids. *J Am Vet Med Assoc 186*:170, 1985.
11. Bennett D: Nutrition and bone disease in the dog and cat. *Vet Rec 98*:313, 1976.
12. Betts CW: Agenesis of the radius. *In* Bojrab MJ (ed): *Pathophysiology in Small Animal Surgery*. Lea & Febiger, Philadelphia, 1981.
13. Biery DN, et al: Bone cysts in the dog. *J Am Vet Radiol Soc 17*:202, 1976.
14. Biller DS, et al: Aneurysmal bone cyst in a rib of a cat. *J Am Vet Med Assoc 190*:1193, 1987.
15. Blevins WE, Cantwell HD: Osteochondromatosis: A cause of pelvic asymmetry in dogs. *J Vet Ortho 2*:31, 1980.
16. Bohning R, et al: Clinical and radiologic survey of canine panosteitis. *J Am Vet Med Assoc 156*:870, 1970.
17. Boris A, Hurley J: Relative activities of some metabolites and analogs of cholecalciferol in stimulation of tibia ash weight in chicks otherwise deprived of vitamin D. *J Nutr 107*:194, 1977.
18. Borle AB: Calcium and phosphate metabolism. *Ann Rev Physiol 36*:361, 1974.
19. Bosch F, et al: A case of Barlow's disease in the dog—first description in Chile. *Vet Med Rev 2*:371, 1971.
20. Breitschwerdt E: Acute renal failure. *In* Morgan R (ed): *Handbook of Small Animal Practice*. Churchill Livingstone, New York, 1988.
21. Breur GJ, et al: Clinical, radiographic, pathologic, and genetic features of osteochondrodysplasia in Scottish deerhounds. *J Am Vet Med Assoc 195*:606, 1989.
22. Breur GJ, et al: Percutaneous biopsy of the proximal humeral growth plate in the dogs. *Am J Vet Res 49*:1529, 1988.
23. Brockus CW, Hathocock JT: Hypertrophic osteopathy associated with pulmonary blastomycosis in a dog. *Vet Radiol 29*:184, 1988.

24. Brodey RS: Hypertrophic osteoarthropathy in the dog: A clinicopathologic survey of 60 cases. *J Am Vet Med Assoc 159*:1242, 1971.
25. Brown RJ, et al: Multiple osteochondroma in a Siamese cat. *J Am Vet Med Assoc 160*:433, 1972.
26. Burk RL, Broadhurst JJ: Craniomandibular osteopathy in a Great Dane. *J Am Vet Med Assoc 169*:635, 1976.
27. Capen CC: Calcium-regulating hormones and metabolic bone disease. *In* Newton CD, Nunamaker DM (ed): *Textbook of Small Animal Orthopaedics*. J.B. Lippincott, Philadelphia, 1985.
28. Carrig CB, Seawright AA: A familial canine polyostotic fibrous dysplasia with subperiosteal cortical defects. *J Small Anim Pract 10*:397, 1969.
29. Caywood DD, et al: Hypertrophic osteopathy associated with a bronchial foreign body and lobar pneumonia in a dog. *J Am Vet Med Assoc 186*:698, 1985.
30. Chester DK: Multiple cartilaginous exostoses in two generations of dogs. *J Am Vet Med Assoc 159*:895, 1971.
31. Chigira M, et al: The aetiology and treatment of simple bone cysts. *J Bone Joint Surg [Br] 65B*:633, 1983.
32. DeLuca HF, Schnoes H: Vitamin D: Recent advances. *Ann Rev Biochem 52*:411, 1982.
33. Doige CE, et al: Chondrosarcoma arising in multiple cartilaginous exostoses in a dog. *J Am Anim Hosp Assoc 14*:605, 1978.
34. Dueland RT: Hypertrophic osteodystrophy. *In* Kirk RW (ed): *Current Veterinary Therapy V*. W.B. Saunders, Philadelphia, 1974.
35. Finnie JW, Sinclair IR: Multiple cartilaginous exostoses in the dog. *J Small Anim Pract 22*:597, 1981.
36. Gambardella PC, et al: Multiple cartilaginous exostoses in the dog. *J Am Vet Med Assoc 166*:761, 1975.
37. Gee BR, Doige CE: Multiple cartilaginous exostoses in a litter of dogs. *J Am Vet Med Assoc 156*:53, 1970.
38. Gerbode F, et al: Experimental hypertrophic osteoarthropathy. *Surgery 60*:1030, 1966.
39. Goldschmidt MH, Biery DN: Bone cysts in the dog. *In* Newton CD, Nunamaker DM (eds): *Textbook of Small Animal Orthopaedics*. J.B. Lippincott, Philadelphia, 1985.
40. Grondalen J: Metaphyseal osteopathy (hypertrophic osteodystrophy) in growing dogs: A clinical study. *J Small Anim Pract 17*:721, 1976.
41. Guyton AC: *Textbook of Medical Physiology*. W.B. Saunders, Philadelphia, 1981.
42. Habener JF: Regulation of parathyroid hormone secretion and biosynthesis. *Ann Rev Physiol 43*:211, 1981.
43. Halliwell WH, Ackerman N: Botryoid rhabdomyosarcoma of the urinary bladder and hypertrophic osteoarthropathy in a young dog. *J Am Vet Med Assoc 165*:911, 1974.
44. Hardy WD, Stockman WS: Clinicopathologic conference. *J Am Vet Med Assoc 154*:1600, 1969.
45. Hathcock JT: Craniomandibular osteopathy in an English bulldog. *J Am Vet Med Assoc 81*:389, 1982.
46. Hedhammar A, et al: Overnutrition and skeletal disease: An experimental study in growing Great Dane dogs. *Cornell Vet 64*(Suppl 5):1, 1974.
47. Holmes JR: Suspected skeletal scurvy in the dog. *Vet Rec 74*:801, 1962.
48. International nomenclature of constitution diseases of bone. *Ann Radiol 26*:457, 1983.
49. Jaffe HL: Pulmonary hypertrophic osteoarthropathy. *In* Jaffe HL (ed): *Metabolic, Degenerative, and Inflammatory Diseases of Bones and Joints*. Lea & Febiger, Philadelphia, 1972.
50. Jezyk PF: Constitutional disorders of the skeleton in dogs and cats. *In* Newton CD, Nunamaker DM (eds): *Textbook of Small Animal Orthopaedics*. J.B. Lippincott, Philadelphia, 1985.
51. Jubb KVF, Kennedy PC: *Pathology of Domestic Animals*. Academic Press, New York, 1970, pp 59–62.
52. Kallfelz F: Skeletal and neuromuscular diseases. *In* Lewis L (ed): *Small Animal Clinical Nutrition III*. Mark Morris, Topeka, 1982.
53. Kelly MJ: Long-term survival of a case of hypertrophic osteopathy with regression of bony changes. *J Am Animal Hosp Assoc 20*:439, 1984.
54. Krook L: Metabolic bone diseases in dogs and cats. Proceedings of the 38th Annual Meeting of the American Animal Hospital Association, 1971, pp 350–355.
55. Krook L: Reversibility of nutritional osteoporosis: Physiochemical data on bone from an experiemntal study in dogs. *J Nutr 101*:233, 1971.
56. LaCroix JA: Diagnosis of orthopedic problems peculiar to the growing dog. *Vet Med 65*:229, 1970.
57. Leighton RL, Olson S: Hypertrophic osteoarthropathy in a dog with a pulmonary abscess. *J Am Vet Med Assoc 150*:1516, 1967.
58. Lenehan TM: Hypertrophic osteodystrophy. Presented at the 17th Annual Veterinary Forum, Chicago, 1989.
59. Lenehan TM, Fetter AW: Hypertrophic osteodystrophy. *In* Newton CD, Nunamaker DM (eds): *Textbook of Small Animal Orthopaedics*. J.B. Lippincott, Philadelphia, 1985.
60. Lenehan TM, Fetter AW: Hypertrophic osteopathy. *In* Newton CD, Nunamaker DM (eds): *Textbook of Small Animal Orthopaedics* J.B. Lippincott, Philadelphia, 1985.
61. Lenehan TM, et al: Canine panosteitis. *In* Newton CD, Nunamaker DM (eds): *Textbook of Small Animal Orthopaedics*. J.B. Lippincott, Philadelphia, 1985.
61a. Meier H, et al: Hypertrophic osteodystrophy associated with disturbance of vitamin C synthesis in dogs. *J Am Vet Med Assoc 130*:483, 1957.
62. Merritt AM, et al: Hypertrophic pulmonary osteopathy in a steer. *J Am Vet Med Assoc 159*:443, 1971.
63. Meuten DJ, Rendano VT: Hypertrophic pulmonary osteoarthropathy in a mare with a dysgerminoma. *J Equine Med Surg 2*:445, 1978.
64. Miller SC, et al: Dietary lactose improves endochondral growth and bone development and mineralization in rats fed a vitamin D-deficient diet. *J Nutr 118*:72, 1988.
65. Morgan JP, et al: Hereditary multiple exostoses in the horse. *J Am Vet Med Assoc 140*:1320, 1962.
66. Nafe LA, et al: Hypertrophic osteopathy in a cat associated with renal papillary adenoma. *J Am Animal Hosp Assoc 17*:659, 1981.
67. Ninth annual seminar, American College of Veterinary Pathologists, Chicago, 1968.
68. *Nutrient Requirements of Dogs*. Publication 0–309–03496–5, National Academy of Sciences. National Academic Press, Washington, DC, 1985.
69. Owen LN, Bostock DE: Multiple cartilaginous exostoses with development of a metastasizing osteosarcoma in a Shetland sheepdog. *J Small Anim Pract 12*:507, 1971.
70. Owen LN, Nielsen SW: Multiple cartilaginous exostoses (diaphyseal aclasis) in a Yorkshire terrier. *J Small Anim Pract 9*:519, 1968.
71. Owen LN, Walker RG: Osteitis fibrosa cystica of the radius of an Irish wolfhound. *Vet Rec 75*:40, 1963.
72. Pederson NC: Surgical correction of a congenital defect of the radius and ulna of a dog. *J Am Vet Med Assoc 153*:1328, 1968.
73. Pool RR, Carrig CB: Multiple cartilaginous exostoses in the cat. *Vet Pathol 9*:350, 1972.
74. Pool RR, Leighton RL: Craniomandibular osteopathy in a dog. *J Am Vet Med Assoc 154*:657, 1969.
75. Resnich D, et al: Tumors and tumor like lesions of bone: Imaging and pathology of specific lesions. *In* Resnich D, Niwayama G (eds): *Diagnosis of Bone and Joint Disorders*. W.B. Saunders, Philadelphia, 1988.
76. Richardson DC: Radial agenesis. *J Vet Orthop 1*:39, 1979.
77. Riedesel DH: Eosinophilic panosteitis of young dogs. *Iowa State Univ Vet 1*:29, 1969.
78. Riser WH: Radiographic differential diagnosis of skeletal diseases of young dogs. *J Am Vet Radiol Soc 5*:15, 1964.
79. Riser WH: What is your diagnosis? Craniomandibular osteopathy in a Labrador puppy. *J Am Vet Med Assoc 148*:1543, 1966.
80. Riser WH, Newton CD: Craniomandibular osteopathy. *In* Newton CD, Nunamaker DM (eds): *Textbook of Small Animal Orthopaedics*. J.B. Lippincott, Philadelphia, 1985.
81. Riser WH, Shirer JF: Normal and abnormal growth of the distal foreleg in large and giant dogs. *J Am Vet Radiol Soc 6*:50, 1965.
82. Riser WH, et al: Canine craniomandibular osteopathy. *J Am Vet Radiol Soc 8*:23, 1967.
83. Rothman M, Schnelle GB: Brodie's abscess in a Great Dane. *North Am Vet 30*:591, 1949.
84. Ryder-Davies P, Hime JM: Hypertrophic pulmonary osteoarthropathy in a gibbon. *J Small Anim Pract 13*:655, 1972.
85. Schlotthauer CF, Millar JAS: Hypertrophic pulmonary osteoarthropathy in association with pulmonary neoplasia in dogs. *J Am Vet Med Assoc 119*:442, 1951.
86. Schrader AC, Burk RL: Bone cysts in two dogs and a review of similar cystic bone lesions in the dog. *J Am Vet Med Assoc 182*:490, 1983.
87. Schulz S: A case of craniomandibular osteopathy in a boxer. *J Small Anim Pract 19*:749, 1978.
88. Shupe JL, et al: Multiple exostoses in horses. *Mod Vet Pract 51*:34, 1970.
89. Stead AC, et al: Panosteitis in dogs. *J Small Anim Pract 24*:623, 1983.
90. Stogdale L: Panosteitis. *Vet Pract* 7, 1981.
91. Susanek SJ: Hypertrophic osteopathy. *Comp Cont Educ 4*:689, 1982.
92. Swalley J, Swalley M: Agenesis of the radius in a kitten. *Feline Pract 8*:25, 1978.
93. Tandy J, Haywood S. A case of panosteitis. *Vet Rec 100*:287, 1977.
94. Teare JA, et al: Ascorbic acid deficiency and hypertrophic osteodystrophy in the dog: a rebuttal. *Cornell Vet 69*:384, 1979.
95. Thrasher JP: Hypertrophic pulmonary osteoarthropathy in dogs. *J Am Vet Med Assoc 139*:441, 1961.
96. Turnier JC, Silverman S: A case study of canine panosteitis: Comparison of radiographic and radioisotopic studies. *Am J Vet Res 39*:1550, 1978.
97. Van Sickle DC, Hohn RB: Selected orthopedic problems in the growing dog. Monograph, American Animal Hospital Association, 1975, p 20.
98. Vulgamott JC, Clark RG: Arterial hypertension and hypertrophic pulmonary osteopathy associated with aortic valvular endocarditis in a dog. *J Am Vet Med Assoc 177*:243, 1980.
99. Watkins JD, Bradley R: Craniomandibular osteopathy in a Labrador puppy. *Vet Rec 79*:262, 1966.
100. Watson ADJ, Porges WL: Regression of hypertrophic osteopathy in a dog following unilateral intrathoracic vagotomy. *Vet Rec 93*:240, 1973.
101. Watson ADJ, et al: Craniomandibular osteopathy in Doberman pinschers. *J Small Anim Pract 16*:11, 1975.
102. White EG: Osteoarthropathy in dogs. *J Am Vet Med Assoc 101*:202, 1942.
103. Whitebread TJ, et al: An inherited enchondrodystrophy in the English pointer dog. *J Small Anim Pract 24*:399, 1983.

104. Wilton GS, Graesser FE: Hypertrophic pulmonary osteoarthropathy in a mink. *Can Vet J 8*:77, 1967.
105. Winterbotham EJ, et al: Radial agenesis in a cat. *J Small Anim Pract 26*:393, 1985.
106. Woodard JC: Canine hypertrophic osteodystrophy. A study of the spontaneous disease in littermates. *Vet Pathol 19*:337, 1982.
107. Woolridge GH, Holmes JWH: Pulmonary tuberculosis in the dog with complications involving bones of the limbs. *Vet Rec 49*:508, 1937.

CHAPTER

146 Muscles and Tendons

Mark Bloomberg

Injuries to muscles and tendons of small animals are a diagnostic challenge. Such injuries are often masked by more severe injuries such as fractures or dislocations. Unless the musculotendinous injury is severe enough to be disabling or is presented in the acute stages, the animal may show few clinical signs. Most musculotendinous injuries do not require surgical intervention; instead, careful postdiagnostic treatment, including physical therapy, and gradual return to training or normal activity are necessary.

Injuries to muscles and tendons are categorized into the (1) muscle belly, (2) musculotendinous junction, (3) tendon, and (4) tendon at its origin or insertion. The basic principles of healing, types of injuries, and surgical repair are discussed and applied to specific muscle and tendon injuries.

SKELETAL MUSCLE

Injuries to skeletal muscles are not as dramatic as tendon injuries.[18] Bruised (contused) or partially ruptured muscles are common. A thorough history and physical examination including detailed palpation of the animal's musculature are necessary to pinpoint the damaged muscles. Severe muscle or musculotendinous ruptures or tears are unusual yet are more easily diagnosed in their acute stages because of dramatic clinical signs.

If lameness caused by isolated muscle injuries persists for longer than 24 hours, additional injuries should be suspected.[18] Although the animal may be sound at a walk, the effects of muscle injury may be more readily discernible at a faster gait. This fact is important to remember when examining racing or working animals.

Anatomy

In mammals, skeletal muscles account for approximately one-third to one-half of total body weight.[20] A skeletal or striated muscle fiber is made up of long cylindrical fibers formed into bundles. The significance of any injury to muscle relates to changes in the individual fibers. Connective tissue sheaths support each individual fiber (endomysium), fiber bundle (perimysium), and the entire muscle (epimysium).[26] The fibrous connective tissue septa contain blood vessels and nerve fibers. They bind and integrate the action of the individual fibers and simultaneously allow freedom of motion between individual muscle components and muscles.[43] A muscle fiber is composed of individual myofibrils, the basic unit of muscle. The myofibrils are interconnected by the sarcoplasm and retinaculum, which provide the connecting link for transmission of impulses from the sarcolemmal sheath to the myofibril.

Skeletal muscles are attached by connective tissue to bone or cartilage. These connective tissue attachments may be a cordlike tendon or a flat aponeurosis. Some muscles attach directly to periosteum via fleshy appendages. The proximal fixed portion of muscle is its origin, and the immovable distal point of attachment is its insertion. The expanded fleshy part of a muscle is its belly; the origin is the head; and minor insertions are called *slips*.[20]

A muscle contraction is initiated by a nerve impulse traveling through a motor nerve fiber (axon) to the muscle fiber. Each axon serves several muscle fibers. Neuromuscular units are known as *motor units*. The more motor units per muscle fiber, the greater the precision of movement of the muscle. The more muscle fibers, the stronger the muscle.[20]

Healing of Skeletal Muscle

Myofibrils can regenerate if not strangulated by extensive fibrous tissue.[47] Healing between muscle ends by fibrous protein synthesis is not as desirable as regeneration of myofibrils. If the sarcolemmal nuclei are destroyed, regeneration does not take place. If they survive, their reaction to injury is rapid and effective. If the endomysial support of the fibers is not destroyed, new fibers replace degenerated ones, and long stretches of muscle may be reconstructed. If the endomysial tube has been destroyed, the growing bud becomes a multinucleated club, which may be successful in sprouting branches, depending on the amount of obstruction by fibrous tissue or hemorrhage. Undifferentiated cells adjacent to muscle fibers may form myoblasts and contribute to muscle regeneration.[47]

Muscle Injuries

Minor injuries to muscles can be divided into contusions, strains, and lacerations. Contusions frequently accompany traumatic injury. Unless the contusion is massive, treatment is usually unnecessary. Owing to hematoma formation, a massive contusion results in excessive inflammation and edema that can result in marked muscle dysfunction requiring treatment. Treatments for muscle contusions depend on whether the injury is acute (within 24 hours) or chronic. Initial first aid consists of immobilization and cold compresses. After 24 hours, therapy consists of warm water compresses or baths, regional compressive wraps, protective bandaging, and immobilization.[21] Systemic administration of antibiotics is reserved for massive contusions that have caused muscle necrosis. Nonsteroidal anti-inflammatory drugs are preferred over systemic corticosteroids.

A strained muscle is the result of overstretching or overuse of any part of the muscle-tendon unit, causing structural alterations, pain, and lameness.[21] The treatment of muscle strains is similar to that of muscle contusions, consisting primarily of enforced rest. Topical or systemic administration of nonsteroidal anti-inflammatory agents along with hydrotherapy hastens return of function.

The treatment of muscle lacerations depends on whether the injury is acute or chronic or if there is potential for loss of function because of fibrous healing. Before conservative therapy or surgical repair of a lacerated muscle, the basic principles of the treatment of open wounds should be followed. Wounds are irrigated with copious amounts of isotonic fluid and adequately débrided. Sutures are placed in the muscle sheaths rather than the muscle fibers themselves. Synthetic monofilament nonabsorbable sutures placed in an interrupted horizontal mattress pattern are preferred to reduce adhesion formation (Fig. 146–1*A*). Synthetic absorbable suture materials such as polydioxanone (PDS*) or polyglyconate (Maxon†) may be used because they are monofilament and retain tensile strength for an adequate period. If the muscle sheath has been severely damaged or if it is necessary to reappose a deeply lacerated muscle belly, muscle fibers can be apposed with interrupted horizontal mattress sutures placed deep into the muscle bellies and reinforced with rubber or Silastic tubing or buttons to prevent sutures from pulling out (Fig. 146–1*B*).[9, 14, 43]

Surgical transection of a muscle belly may be necessary for surgical exposure (e.g., transection of the teres minor for approach to the shoulder joint or the brachial muscle for exposure of the distal humerus). In flat muscle bellies, the incision parallels the muscle fibers, as in a grid incision, to avoid postoperative complications affecting use of the limb.[9] Muscles with round bellies may have to be cut transversely. If the muscle is transected, subsequent repair follows the guidelines described later under treatment of muscle rupture.

*Ethicon, Inc., Somerville, N J.
†Davis-Geck, Inc., Manati, PR.

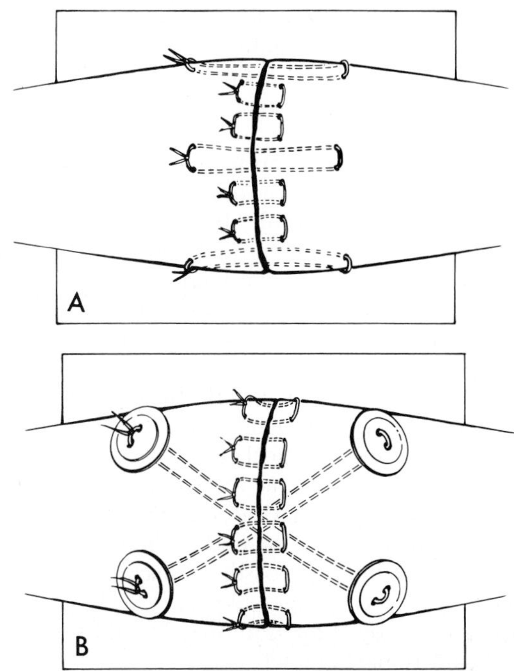

FIGURE 146–1. Suture techniques for anastomosis of muscle. *A*, Interrupted horizontal mattress sutures placed deep and superficially in an attempt to penetrate any available fascial sheaths within the muscle. *B*, Interrupted horizontal mattress sutures have been bolstered by the addition of button tension sutures. (Modified from Milton JL, Henderson RA: Surgery of muscles and tendons. *In* Bojrab MJ [ed]: *Current Techniques in Small Animal Surgery.* 2nd ed. Lea & Febiger, Philadelphia, 1983.)

Muscle Rupture

Rupture of muscle may be partial or complete. The cause of muscle rupture is a powerful active contraction of a flexor motor unit at the same time that forced passive extension occurs.[47] Muscle is a highly differentiated tissue that is more resistant to trauma than tendon. Complete ruptures are unusual in small animals, except for the diaphragm and abdominal muscles.[9] Muscle ruptures are reported more frequently in racing greyhounds as a result of strenuous athletic activity. Such injuries include ruptures of the gracilis, triceps, and gastrocnemius muscles.[16, 26, 58] Rupture of the ventral serratus occurs in cats and dogs.[28, 43] Joint dislocations and fractures can cause rupture of adjacent musculature.[43]

It is often difficult to differentiate between partial and complete muscle rupture. Muscular injuries may show signs of local tenderness, subcutaneous ecchymosis, swelling, and lameness. Chronic injuries may show lameness and muscle atrophy. A higher percentage of muscle ruptures occur at the musculotendinous junction than through the fleshy belly.[9]

Incomplete ruptures usually do not require operative repair. An acutely injured muscle may initially be treated with immobilization and cold packs. Immobilization with a modified Robert Jones dressing for 2 to 3 weeks, followed by 2 or 3 weeks of restricted activity, may be all that is necessary. Immobilization prevents excessive movement and further separation of the torn muscle to allow optimal muscle cell regeneration and to minimize scar tissue formation. Although excessive movement is undesirable during the healing process, restricted activity is encouraged to minimize formation of adhesions.

If complete or partial rupture of a muscle is difficult to determine, the damaged muscle can be explored through a small skin incision. It is better to make an early diagnosis of a muscle rupture and repair it than to attempt resection of scar tissue later.

Complete rupture of a muscle, either midsubstance (belly) or musculotendinous, resulting in loss of function or a crippling injury is an indication for reparative surgery. Clinical signs vary with the severity of the muscle damage and the significance of the particular muscle injured. Initial clinical signs are acute onset of lameness or altered gait and localized signs of inflammation. A palpable gap may be noted between the ends of the muscle belly, accompanied by hematoma formation. The loss of integrity of the muscle belly is often termed *dropped muscle* (Fig. 146–2).[18, 43] Diagnosis of a ruptured muscle by palpation may be difficult if the muscle sheath remains intact.

Delay in surgical repair of a ruptured muscle permits extensive fibrous tissue synthesis in and around the muscle ends.[47] New connective tissue forms rapidly between the severed ends of the muscle belly, causing a fibrous scar. If the muscle heals in a shortened position, the range of motion is decreased. With physical therapy and active and passive movement, scar tissue can remodel and elongate but not without serious loss of strength.[43]

Surgical Repair of Ruptured Muscle

Care is taken in handling muscle. If additional exposure is needed, the skin incision is lengthened. If muscles need to be separated further, their origins or insertions can be carefully freed by sharp dissection, osteotomy, or subperiosteal elevation. It is preferable to elevate the periosteum with the muscle attached, allowing the periosteum to return to its original position when the muscle is replaced.

Severed muscles are reattached as soon as possible after the diagnosis is made, by anatomical alignment of the muscle ends with an end-to-end anastomosis. Muscles are subject to longitudinal forces, which, combined with the inherently weak suture-holding power of muscle, contribute to sutures pulling out when tension is applied. The severed muscle ends are carefully inspected

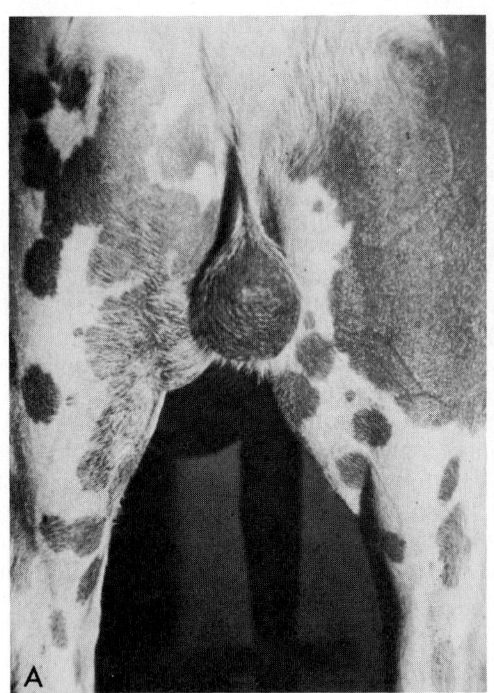

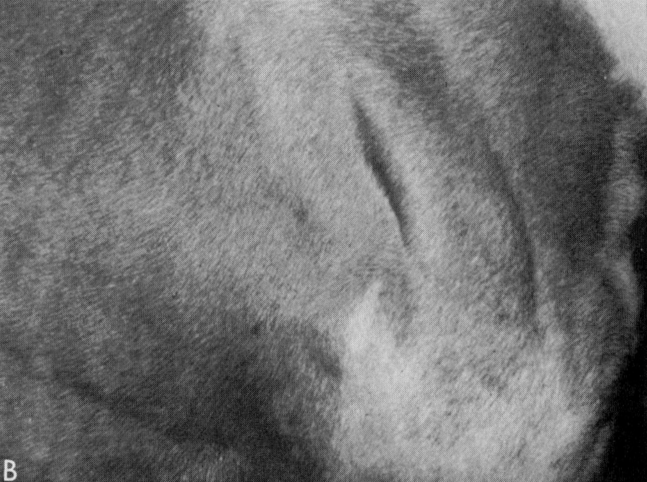

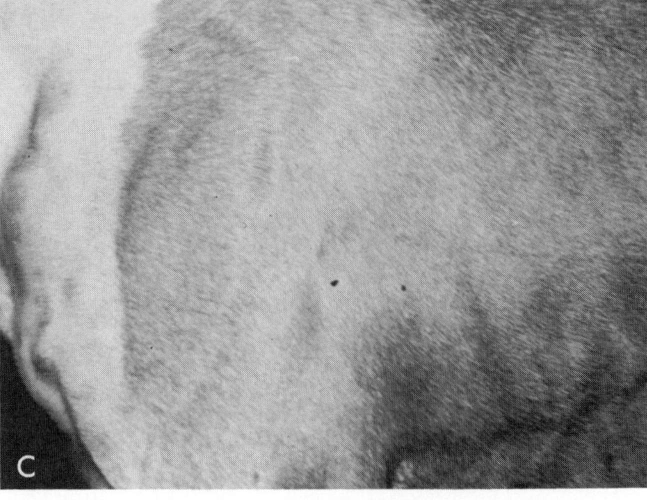

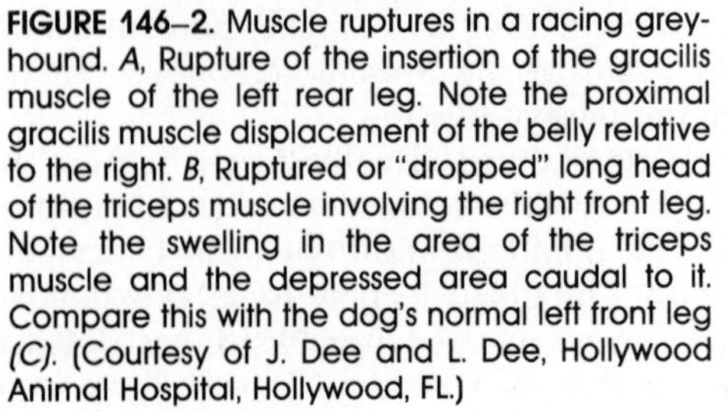

FIGURE 146–2. Muscle ruptures in a racing greyhound. *A*, Rupture of the insertion of the gracilis muscle of the left rear leg. Note the proximal gracilis muscle displacement of the belly relative to the right. *B*, Ruptured or "dropped" long head of the triceps muscle involving the right front leg. Note the swelling in the area of the triceps muscle and the depressed area caudal to it. Compare this with the dog's normal left front leg (*C*). (Courtesy of J. Dee and L. Dee, Hollywood Animal Hospital, Hollywood, FL.)

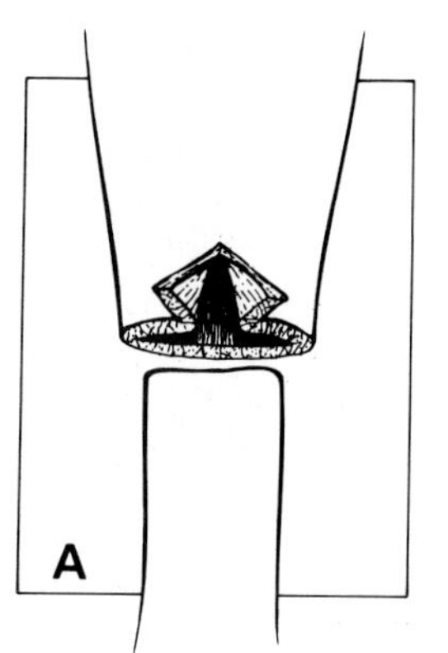

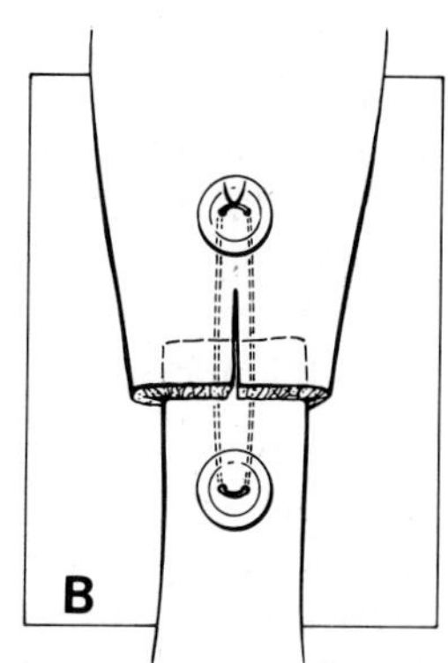

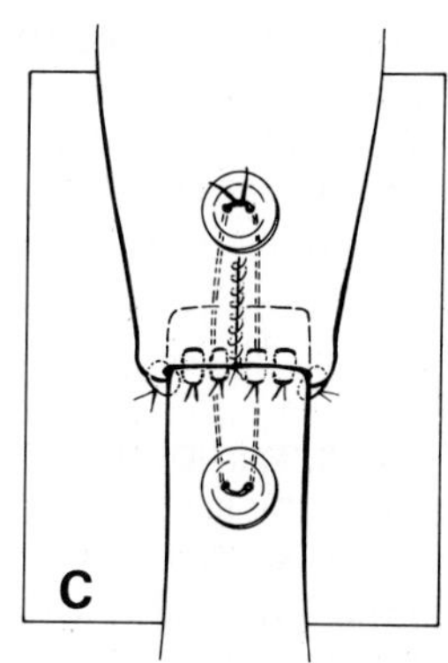

FIGURE 146–3. Anastomosis of muscle at musculotendinous junction. *A*, The muscle has been slit for 2 to 3 cm, creating a bed for implantation of the end of the tendon. *B*, The tendon end has been implanted in the bed and secured with button tension sutures. *C*, After implantation, the fascial sheath of the muscle has been sutured to the paratenon of the tendon with simple interrupted horizontal mattress sutures of nonabsorbable material. (Modified from Braden TD: Tendon and muscles. *In* Bojrab MJ [ed]: *Current Techniques in Small Animal Surgery.* 2nd ed. Lea & Febiger, Philadelphia, 1983.)

for deep fascial layers, which may provide holding power for sutures. Muscles may be uni-, bi- or multipennate, which means that one or more tendons pass alongside the muscle or invade it.[20] These tendons also provide solid tissue for sutures.

The ends of the ruptured muscle may be approximated with large horizontal mattress sutures of a nonabsorbable nonreactive material such as nylon, polypropylene, or polyester fiber. These sutures are tightened until the muscle edges are together. To help prevent sutures from pulling out, the suture material can be tied over stents, buttons, fascia, or rubber or Silastic tubing to distribute tension. These can be used alone or in conjunction with intramuscular sutures (see Fig. 146–1).[9, 14, 43] Once the edges of the muscle are apposed, the muscle sheath at the anastomotic site is sutured circumferentially with horizontal mattress sutures of a nonabsorbable material smaller than the intramuscular sutures. With small muscles or flat, sheetlike muscles, two buttons or stents used as tension absorbers are sufficient.

Postoperatively, it is important that the affected muscle be immobilized for 2 to 3 weeks, followed by gradual return to activity and physical therapy over 4 to 6 weeks. The prognosis for complete return of function for working or racing dogs is guarded.[18] With or without surgical intervention, postoperative sequelae such as atrophy, fibrosis, and various degrees of dysfunction may result. Surgical resection of scar tissue (cording) followed by muscle-to-muscle anastomosis may restore function if combined with physical therapy.[34] Muscle can be freed from surrounding adhesions to restore function. Scarred muscle that severely restricts joint motion can be excised if that particular muscle is not essential to normal function of the limb.[42]

Musculotendinous rupture is more common than rupture of the muscle belly. Grossly, less hemorrhage and hematoma formation occur than with injuries involving the muscle belly. Clinically there is less pain and swelling.[18] The severity of the rupture and the function of the involved muscle determine the clinical signs and treatment. Diagnosis of musculotendinous rupture may be difficult because separation of the segments is usually not palpable as the rupture occurs over a broad area and portions of the tendon and muscle sheath may remain intact. A diagnosis of musculotendinous rupture is supported by conformational changes and lameness caused by loss of muscle function.[43]

If the rupture is complete, immediate surgical repair is indicated. When the muscle and tendon are of similar size, the ends can be approximated as described for muscle tears. If a disparity exists in size of the tendon and muscle, the tendon can be implanted into the end of the muscle for 2 to 3 cm (Fig. 146–3),[9] by slitting the muscle for 2 to 3 cm halfway through its depth.[8, 13] Postoperative care is as for repair of muscles.

SPECIFIC MUSCLE INJURIES

Rupture of the Ventral Serratus Muscle

Trauma to the forelimb may result in rupture of all or part of the ventral serratus muscle and cause upward displacement of the scapula (see Chapter 128).[28, 43]

Rupture of the Gracilis Muscle

Rupture of the gracilis muscle ("dropped muscle") is commonly seen in racing greyhounds.[14, 18, 22, 27] It also occurs in foxhounds and German shepherds.[34]

The gracilis muscle is a sheetlike muscle on the medial surface of the thigh. It arises from the pelvic symphysis and inserts along the entire length of the tibial crest. At its insertion, it sends a part of its crural fascia as a reinforcing band to the calcaneal tendon. The caudal part of the gracilis muscle is the portion that attaches to the tuber calcis.[20] The caudal part of the gracilis is an important extensor of the tarsus.[22] The function of the gracilis muscle is adduction of the thigh and extension of the hip. Rupture of the muscle is characterized by a hematoma on the medial surface of the thigh (see Fig. 146–2*A*). Injuries to the gracilis muscle result in various degrees of lameness depending on the severity of the injury. If this condition is diagnosed immediately after injury, surgical intervention is indicated. A small incision is made over the medial thigh and reattachment of the muscle ends, or for a musculotendinous tear, attachment of the tendon of origin or insertion is performed with interrupted horizontal mattress sutures of monofilament nonabsorbable suture material.

If this condition remains undiagnosed or untreated, a fibrous scar or cording develops on the caudomedial midthigh. Muscle fibrosis may result in a contracture of the rear leg and a distinct rear leg lameness because of inability to extend the stifle. Surgical release of the contracture is the treatment of choice. Partial resection of the fibrous tissue bands may cause recurrence of the contracture. It is best to remove the entire muscle and fibrotic tissue, followed by physical therapy to ensure complete range of motion of the stifle joint.[34]

Rupture of the Long Head of the Triceps

Rupture of the long head of the triceps occurs mostly in racing greyhounds (see Fig. 146–2*B* and *C*), although it has occurred in connection with intratendon steroid injections.[17] As with any muscle tear or rupture, a cold compress, ice pack, or cold spray is applied to the area soon after injury.[18] Prompt surgical intervention is indicated to reattach the fleshy ends of the belly of the long head of the triceps. The area is immobilized by bandages for 2 weeks, followed by gradual return to activity. Dogs with this injury heal with rest and moderate exercise (to prevent adhesions) without surgical repair. They may return to racing but drop one or two grades at the track.[18]

Rupture of the Achilles Mechanism

The Achilles mechanism is composed of five muscles that have three tendinous components forming the common calcaneal or Achilles tendon (Fig. 146–4*A*).[52] The gastrocnemius muscle arises by distinct medial and lateral heads from the supracondylar tuberosities of the femur. A sesamoid bone or fabella is located within each muscle head at the point of origin. The medial and lateral heads fuse distally to form a large tendon that inserts on the tuber calcanei. The tendon of the gastrocnemius is the major component of the common calcaneal tendon. The other two tendinous components are formed by the tendon of the superficial digital flexor muscle and a common tendon of the biceps femoris, gracilis, and semitendinosus muscles. The primary function of the Achilles mechanism is to extend the tibiotarsal joint while flexing the stifle and digits.[20]

Muscular or musculotendinous rupture of the Achilles mechanism primarily afflicts mature dogs of working and racing breeds.* A typical history includes trauma when the animal jumps and lands on its rear legs. One report described rupture caused by parasitic disease of the gastrocnemius muscles.[46] The condition may be bilateral and is manifested as tarsal hyperflexion and stifle hyperextension due to inability to extend the tarsus, the degree of which depends on the severity and completeness of the disruption. A diagnosis of Achilles mechanism injury is based on postural changes and flaccidity of the calcaneal tendon (Fig. 146–5). Complete musculotendinous separation can mimic a separation of the tendon itself. Careful palpation of the gastrocnemius muscle and calcaneal tendon reveals inflammatory changes near the musculotendinous junction. Standing or stress radiographs assist in diagnosis of musculotendinous injury, because all three musculotendinous units must be disrupted before excessive tarsal hyperflexion is present.[52, 53]

*See references 7, 10, 43, 44, 53–55, 57, 59, 60, 62.

The origin of the lateral or medial head of the gastrocnemius muscle may avulse or tear as a result of hyperextension of the stifle.[16, 53] The result may be nonweightbearing lameness accompanied by palpable pain and swelling caudal to the distal femur. Extension of the stifle causes discomfort. Radiographic evaluation of the stifle reveals distal displacement of the fabella (Fig. 146–6). If the position of one or both fabellae is in question, compare their location with those of the opposite stifle. The superficial digital flexor muscle is also avulsed if the lateral fabella is displaced.

This is a surgically treatable condition requiring reattachment of the head of the gastrocnemius muscle, especially if clinical signs are severe. The surgical approach to the head of the gastrocnemius muscle is made through a parapatellar skin incision, depending on whether the avulsion is of the lateral or medial head. The incision may extend from the distal third of the femur to the tibial tuberosity. After the subcutaneous tissues are undermined; further dissection depends on whether a lateral or medial approach was chosen. Laterally, the biceps femoris muscle is separated from the vastus lateralis muscle and retracted caudally. Medially, the insertion of the caudal head of the sartorius muscle is incised and retracted caudally. In either instance, the underlying capsular tissue is incised to expose the respective supracondylar area of the femur. The torn heads of the gastrocnemius muscle and superficial digital flexor muscle can be found with careful dissection. A fabella is palpable in the head of the gastrocnemius muscle. If possible, the torn muscle is reattached with

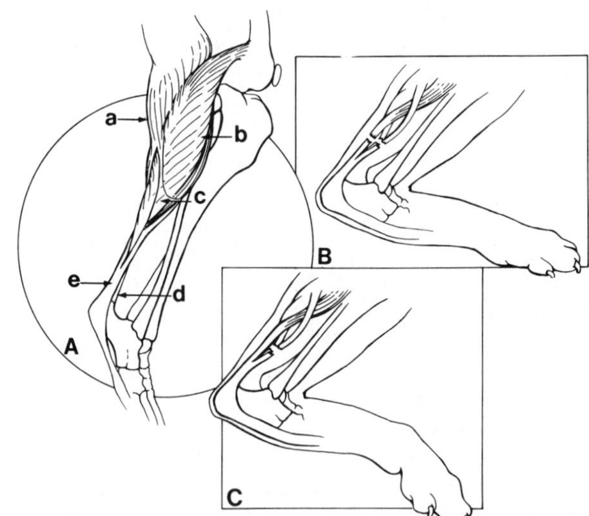

FIGURE 146–4. Rupture of the gastrocnemius tendon and common tendon of the biceps femoris, gracilis, and semitendinosus muscles. *A*, Lateral view of Achilles mechanism: a, semitendinosus muscle; b, gastrocnemius muscle; c, superficial digital flexor muscle; d, tendon of the gastrocnemius muscle; e, common tendon of the biceps femoris muscle, gracilis muscle, and semitendinosus muscle. *B*, Note hyperflexion of the hock with complete rupture of the common calcaneal tendon. *C*, On weightbearing, the hock not only drops but the digits flex, demonstrating that the superficial digital flexor tendon is intact. (Modified from Reinke JD, Kus SP: Achilles mechanism injury in the dog. *Comp Cont Educ* 8:639, 1982.)

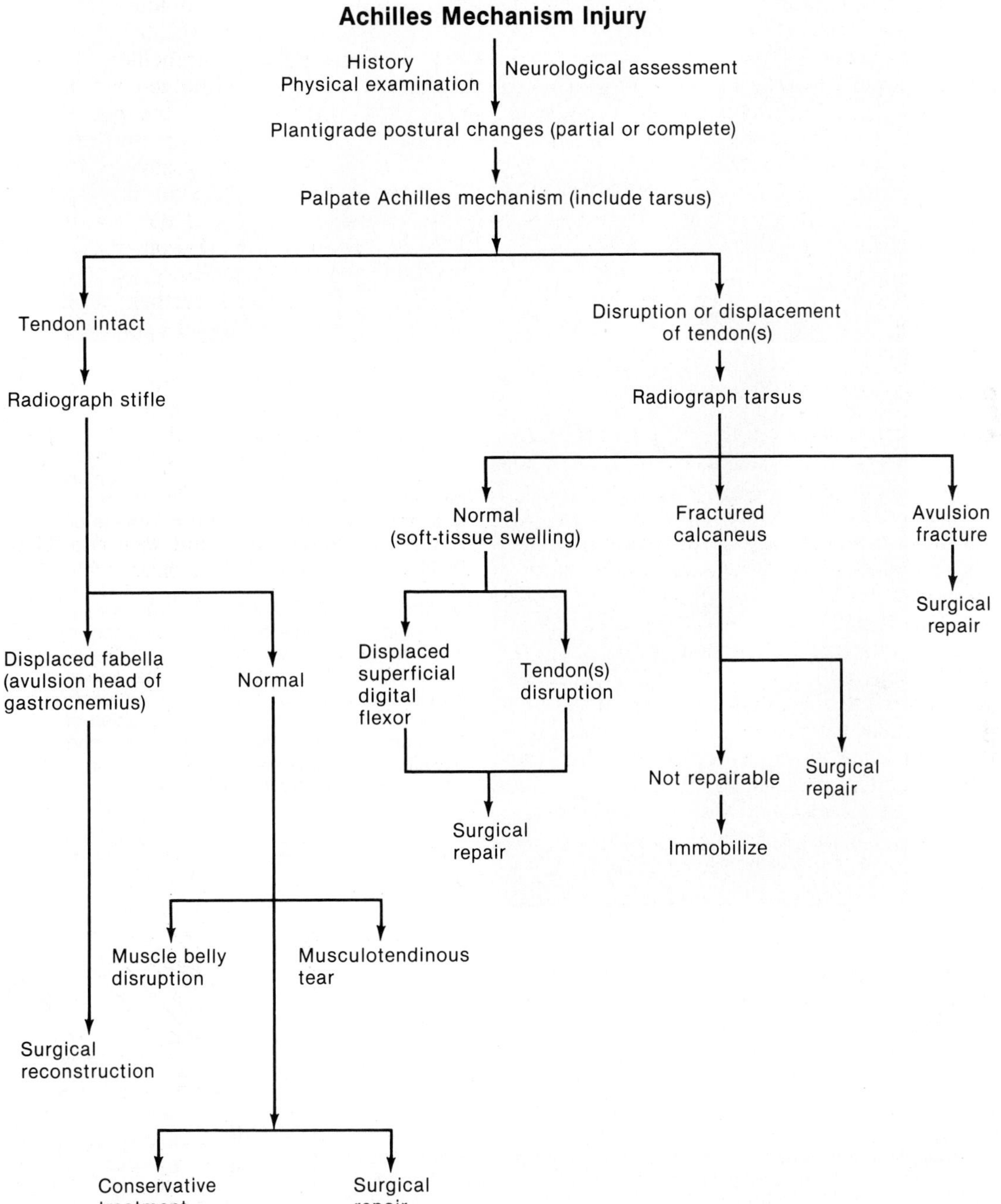

FIGURE 146–5. This algorithm should be used for differential diagnosis and treatment of injuries of the Achilles mechanism in dogs.

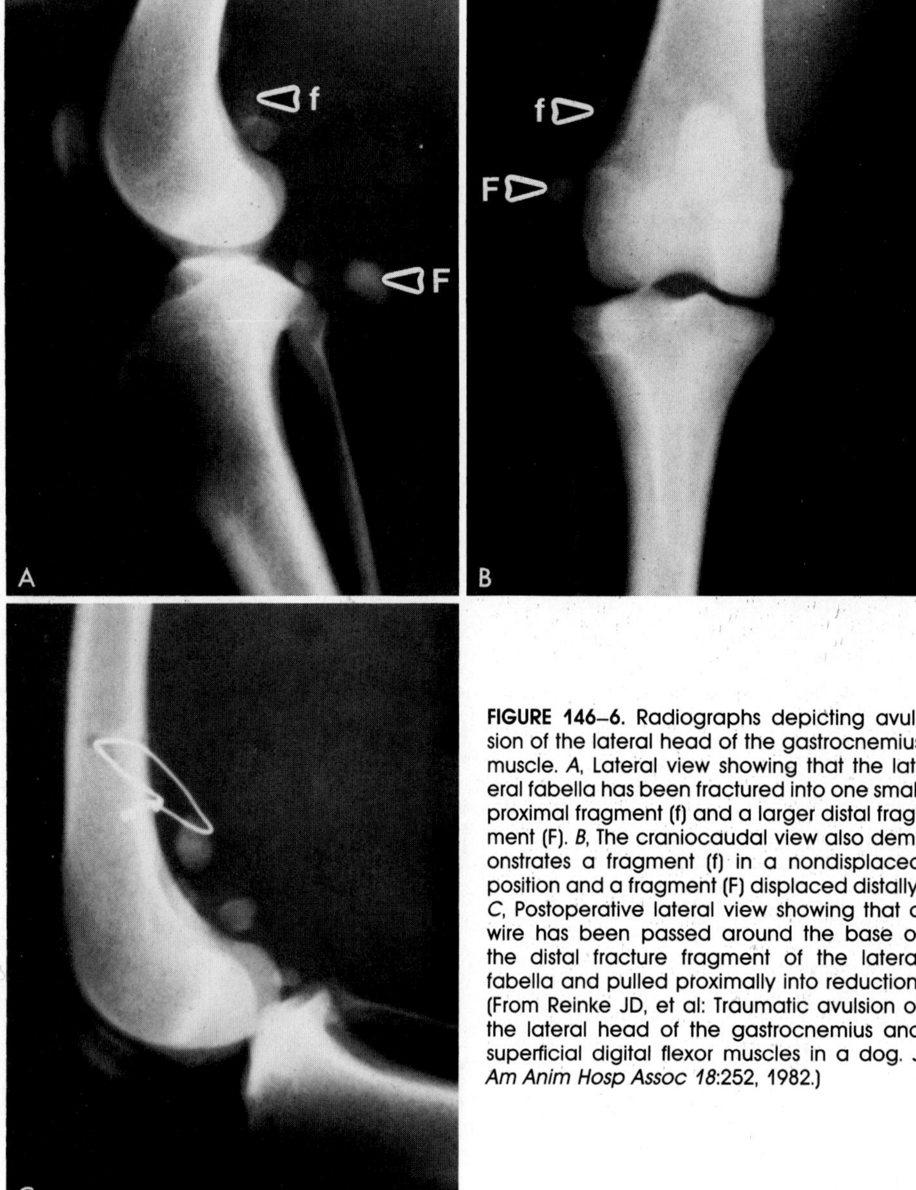

FIGURE 146–6. Radiographs depicting avulsion of the lateral head of the gastrocnemius muscle. *A*, Lateral view showing that the lateral fabella has been fractured into one small proximal fragment (f) and a larger distal fragment (F). *B*, The craniocaudal view also demonstrates a fragment (f) in a nondisplaced position and a fragment (F) displaced distally. *C*, Postoperative lateral view showing that a wire has been passed around the base of the distal fracture fragment of the lateral fabella and pulled proximally into reduction. (From Reinke JD, et al: Traumatic avulsion of the lateral head of the gastrocnemius and superficial digital flexor muscles in a dog. *J Am Anim Hosp Assoc 18*:252, 1982.)

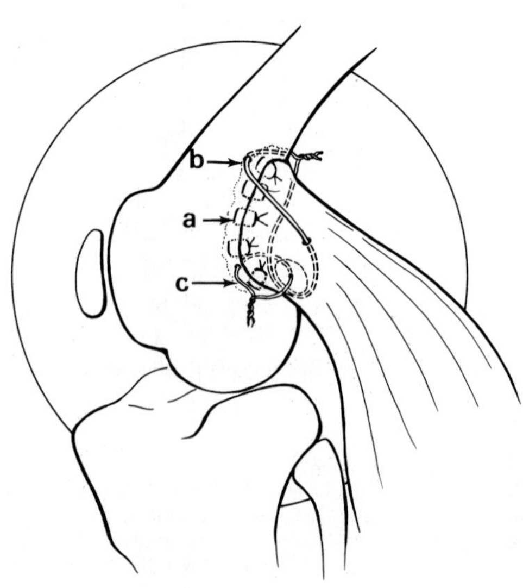

FIGURE 146–7. Depiction of various methods of repair of an avulsion of the head of the gastrocnemius muscle. The muscle may be reattached by primary suture of the tendinous tissue of origin (a), figure-eight wire suture around the fabella and through a drill hole in the distal femur (b, see also Fig. 146–6*C*), wire suture through the caudodistal femur and the fabella (c), or any combination of these methods.

nylon or polypropylene suture in a mattress, figure-eight, or alternative pattern (Fig. 146–7). This involves drilling a hole in the distal femur 2 to 3 cm proximal to the origin of the head of the gastrocnemius muscle. An 18- to 20-gauge stainless steel wire is passed through this hole and either through or around the avulsed fabella and tied on itself. Placement of the stifle in slight flexion aids in reducing the avulsed muscle. For 2 to 3 weeks postoperatively, the leg is placed in a full leg cast or Schroeder-Thomas splint, with the stifle in slight flexion. After external coaptation is removed, exercise is restricted for an additional 2 to 3 weeks.

Acute cases of musculotendinous rupture of the Achilles mechanism are treated surgically by apposition of the muscle-tendon junction. It is important to prevent stress on the anastomotic site by rigid immobilization of the tarsus and the stifle. The musculotendinous junction is approached through a skin incision directly over the caudal aspect of the middle third of the tibia. The proximal muscle and tendon are anastomosed, as described earlier (Fig. 146–8). Rigid internal fixation can be accomplished by a number of methods, including the insertion of a bone screw[7–9] or intramedullary pin[12] from the tuber calcanei into the distal tibia, or with external pin splintage spanning the tibiotarsal joint.[24] A self-tapping lag screw is used to prevent soft tissues caudal to the distal tibia from getting caught in the bone tap and to allow adjustment of the extension of the tarsus. Any of these internal fixation devices should be supplemented with casts, splints, or coaptation bandages. The external support is removed in 4 to 6 weeks and the internal fixation between 6 and 8 weeks postoperatively. Such an injury can be successfully treated without surgery if the stifle is placed in partial flexion and the tarsus in partial extension. This is best accomplished with a Schroeder-Thomas splint, external pin splintage, or full leg cast.[43, 44]

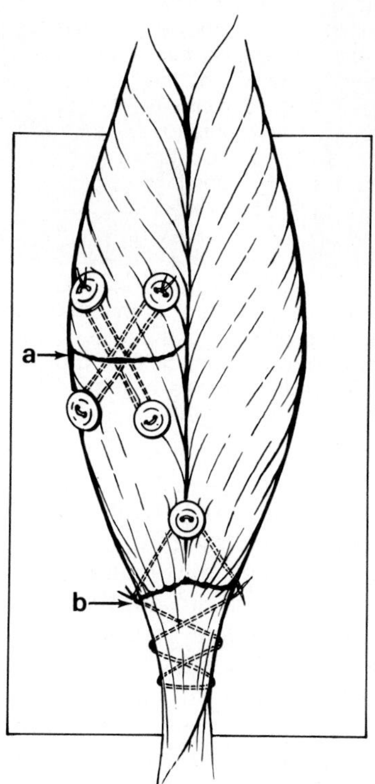

FIGURE 146–8. Surgical repair of a rupture of the belly of the gastrocnemius muscle using tension button technique (a). Musculotendinous rupture of the distal end of the gastrocnemius muscle repaired with button tension technique and Bunnell-Mayer suture pattern (b). (Modified from Reinke JD, Kus SP: Achilles mechanism injury in the dog. *Comp Cont Educ 8*:639, 1982.)

If an injury to the musculotendinous junction of the Achilles mechanism is not recognized or treated during the acute phase, the animal may be presented with a chronic injury or one that has failed to heal with conservative treatment. Chronic injuries can be treated by shortening the calcaneal tendon to re-establish function of the gastrocnemius and superficial digital flexor muscles. The tendon can be shortened by doubling over, plication, or resection of a portion of it.[9, 13, 38] Resection of the fibrous scar at the musculotendinous junction is extremely traumatic and unnecessary and causes a weaker repair. The tarsus is stabilized as described previously. Postoperative care is identical to that of musculotendinous anastomosis.

Rupture of the belly or fleshy portion of the gastrocnemius muscle is unusual.[44, 46] Although in one report the muscle healed spontaneously, it had been immobilized for 4 weeks in a Schroeder-Thomas splint.[44]

The superficial digital flexor can rupture at its musculotendinous junction.[10, 53] The clinical signs and treatment are identical to avulsion of the head of the gastrocnemius muscle.[43]

Other specific muscles that may rupture in working or racing animals include the tensor fasciae latae, rhomboideus thoracis, origin of the infraspinatus, origin of the pectorals, insertion of the biceps brachii, sartorius, origin of pectineus, and origin of the external abdominal oblique and longissimus muscles.[18, 43]

Muscle Contractures and Fibrosis

Muscle contractures are due to damage to muscle fibers, nerves, and blood vessels. Tissue damage causes irreversible fibrosis, adhesions, and contracture and often lameness ranging from minor changes in gait to complete loss of limb function.[43] The causes of muscle damage may be (1) circulatory insufficiency due to arterial or venous obstruction (i.e., Volkmann contracture and subfascial hematoma), (2) a response to parasitic or protozoan infections or autoimmune diseases, such as dirofilariasis, toxoplasmosis, and eosinophilic myositis, and (3) the result of injuries, fractures, and mismanagement of orthopedic problems.[34] Muscle contractures resulting in clinical lameness include those of the quadriceps, infraspinatus, semitendinosus, and gracilis muscles.

Infraspinatus Muscle Contracture

Contracture of the infraspinatus muscle has been described primarily in hunting dogs.[30, 48, 59] The animal shows pain in the shoulder during or soon after exercise.[48] The history may include trauma with acute onset of lameness that gradually subsides.[43] Although the lameness may decrease, it is accompanied by a characteristic gait that demonstrates persistent outward rotation, adduction of the elbow, and abduction of the distal limb with a carpal "flip." This gait abnormality develops 2 to 4 weeks after the initial injury, as a result of contracture of the infraspinatus muscle. Limited range of motion of the shoulder and abduction of the humerus are also noted. Disuse atrophy of the shoulder may develop when surgical treatment is delayed. It is usually unilateral but may occur bilaterally.

The exact cause is unknown, but it appears to be a primary muscle disorder rather than neurological in origin. Histologically, affected tissues show degeneration and atrophy of skeletal muscle with fibrous tissue replacement.[48] This observation agrees with the theory that an injury causes incomplete rupture of the infraspinatus muscle, leading to fibrosis and contracture.

Surgical treatment consists of a caudolateral approach to the affected shoulder joint.[49] The affected infraspinatus muscle appears fibrotic, with atrophy of the belly of the muscle. Blunt and sharp dissection is used to free the musculotendinous area of the scarred, fibrotic muscle from where it crosses the scapulohumeral joint. Once the fibrous tissue is freed from the joint capsule, it is incised either in the tendon or musculotendinous portion of the infraspinatus. A distinct popping noise may be heard when the fibrous tissue is severed, and the forelimb immediately is more easily adducted. All evidence of fibrous contracture is incised, and the range of motion of the shoulder joint is improved. Postoperatively, the animal is allowed restricted exercise for 1 to 2 weeks. The affected front leg is not immobilized after surgery. The prognosis for full recovery is excellent.

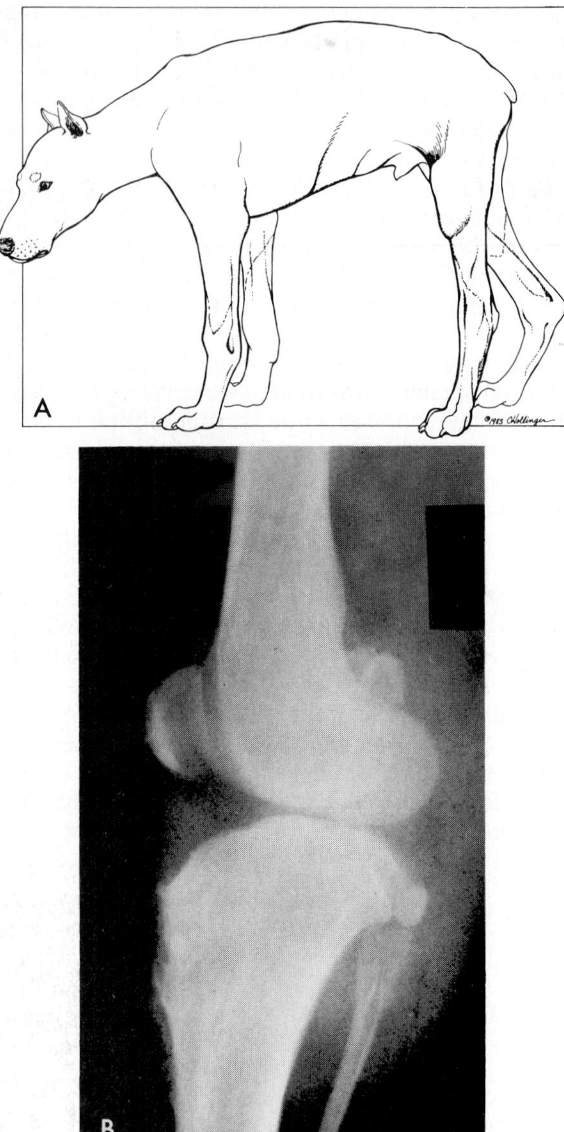

FIGURE 146–9. *A*, Quadriceps muscle contracture illustrated by the hyperextension (genu recurvatum) of this dog's right rear leg. *B*, Lateral radiographic projection of the stifle of a dog with quadriceps contracture after open reduction of a proximal diaphyseal femoral fracture. Note the degree of hyperextension and bony proliferation in and around the stifle.

Quadriceps Muscle Contracture

Contracture of the quadriceps muscle has been recognized in humans and animals for many years.[14, 34, 43, 47, 59, 61] It can occur with distal femoral fractures in young dogs. It is most often associated with inadequate fracture repair, osteomyelitis, or overzealous handling of tissues surrounding the femur in conjunction with prolonged immobilization in extension.[59] Congenital quadriceps contracture has been described in puppies.[14, 43, 54] Not all muscles of the quadriceps group may be affected.[34] Joint stiffness develops initially as a result of adhesions between the quadriceps muscle and the distal femur. With time, the affected leg is held in marked extension to such an extent that the knee may be bent backward in genu recurvatum (Fig. 146–9), with the hock extended. The affected leg essentially becomes a "walking stick" for the animal, with little use in locomotion. The cranial thigh becomes atrophied, taut, and cordlike and essentially tied to the femur. As the condition becomes chronic, the pathological changes become more complex; degenerative changes and fibrosis occur periarticularly and intra-articularly.

Numerous surgical procedures are advocated for treatment of quadriceps contracture.[14, 34, 43, 59] Restoration of motion in the stifle joint is achieved by (1) breaking down adhesions between the quadriceps muscle group and distal femur, (2) loosening adhesions in and around the femorotibial joint, (3) lengthening the quadriceps mechanism, and (4) releasing adjacent extensors of the stifle (e.g., sartorius and tensor fasciae latae).[42] Whatever surgical procedure is chosen, the prognosis remains very guarded for complete return of function of the stifle. Because of the tendency for adhesions to re-form postoperatively, it is critical that the owner recognize the need for postoperative physical therapy.

Surgical procedures described for release of the contracture include partial quadriceps myotomy,[34] Z-myoplasty,[43] and freeing of adhesions and implantation of ophthalmic Gelfilm between the quadriceps and distal femur.[63] The treatment varies with severity of the contracture and often incorporates a combination of surgical techniques.

A lateral approach to the stifle and femur is made through a generous skin incision.[49] The quadriceps adhesions are freed from the femur. This may require removal of excessive bony callus from the distal femur. The incision is extended into the stifle joint capsule to free patellar adhesions and improve joint flexibility. It may be necessary to perform a medial arthrotomy and carry the incision proximally along the caudal border of the vastus medialis. Once the quadriceps muscle group has been mobilized, the patella is luxated medially to allow forcible flexion of the stifle. Manipulation of the stifle is continued with the patella reduced. Care is taken when forcibly flexing the stifle in immature animals not to avulse the tibial tuberosity or proximal tibial epiphysis. If adequate range of motion (20° to 40° flexion) cannot be restored, various lengthening procedures such as a Z-plasty or a sliding myoplasty are necessary.

A Z-myoplasty is performed by isolating the cordlike bands of the quadriceps group and releasing all adhesions to the femur. A Z incision is made in the fibrotic muscle to include any medial or lateral bands. The stifle is flexed as much as possible. The muscle flaps created by Z-plasty incision are transposed and sutured together with a monofilament nonabsorbable suture.

An alternative and equally successful procedure is a sliding myoplasty.[43] The surgical approach and exposure are the same as for a Z-myoplasty. The cranial belly of the sartorius is incised near its insertion on the patella. The rectus femoris is isolated and transected near the patella, avoiding the neighboring femoral nerve and cranial femoral artery. The vastus group is isolated as a unit and elevated from their origin on the proximal femur. The stifle is moved through a range of motion, allowing the vastus to slide beside the rectus femoris. As in the previous procedure, the stifle is flexed until it reaches a functional angle. The vastus group is sutured to the rectus femoris and cranial belly of the sartorius with simple interrupted or horizontal mattress sutures of a monofilament nonabsorbable suture material.

Postoperatively, regardless of the surgical procedure used; the stifle is kept in flexion with either a figure-eight bandage, Robinson sling, or external pin splintage for 4 to 5 days. The external support is removed on day 5 or 6, and passive flexion and extension performed. The first postoperative manipulation of the stifle is best accomplished while the animal is under general anesthesia or heavy sedation. The external support is not reapplied, but the stifle is subjected to passive extension and flexion exercises three to five times per day thereafter. Exercise is encouraged, and when the dog can bear weight on the limb with it held in slight flexion, passive physical therapy is discontinued.

The surgical procedure is a success if it returns the animal to 50 to 75 per cent use of the affected limb. If the outcome is unsatisfactory, alternatives include arthrodesis of the stifle or amputation of the affected limb.

Fibrotic Myopathy

Fibrotic myopathy of various muscles occurs in horses, cats, dogs, and humans.[37, 45] It involves the supraspinatus, gracilis, quadriceps, and semitendinosus muscles of dogs and the semitendinosus muscle of cats.[37] The pathogenesis of this condition is unclear at this time. Fibrotic myopathy may be the result of primary neuropathy or myopathy, frequent intramuscular injections, exercise-induced or acute trauma, or congenital causes. Histologically, the muscle fibers are replaced with dense collagenous connective tissue, resulting in a taught fibrous band. Needle electromyography may reveal no electrical activity that supports the clinical presence of a nonpainful, mechanical lameness.[45]

Fibrotic myopathy of the semitendinosus muscle is the condition most frequently reported.[45] The semitendinosus muscle extends the hip, stifle, and tarsal joints and flexes the stifle when the limb does not bear weight. Affected dogs have lameness characterized by external rotation of the hock and internal rotation of the stifle as the rear limb is carried forward.[37] The foot undergoes a characteristic flipping motion at the end of each forward stride.

Surgical release of fibrotic muscle is the recommended treatment for fibrotic myopathy; it has met with limited success. The surgery usually consists of tenotomy, myotenotomy, Z-plasty, or complete excision of the fibrotic tissue. Surgical release restores normal range of motion of the affected limb. Immediately postoperatively, the lameness is usually absent. Within a few months of surgery, the fibrous band usually gradually returns along with an accompanying degree of lameness.[39, 45] The prognosis for treatment of fibrotic myopathy must remain guarded. If the lameness is not disabling, surgery is not advised.

Myositis Ossificans

Myositis ossificans occurs in similar locations in humans and animals. It is classified as generalized, progressive, or localized and has been reported as having a predilection for the muscles around the hip joints.[39] The exact pathogenesis is unknown, but the localized form may be the result of a local initiating factor resulting in proliferation of mesenchyme to bone. Proposed causes of myositis ossificans include an infectious process, ossification of hematoma, and trauma (tearing of the periosteum with release of osteoblasts and metaplasia of soft tissues).[50] The lesions may involve tissues other than muscle and may be inflammatory.[39] An animal may exhibit chronic lameness with subsequent muscle atrophy, possible neurological deficits, and pain after exercise. Calcification usually occurs 2 to 4 weeks after trauma. Radiographically, the lesion may be a well-defined calcified mass with a central transparency (Fig. 146–10). Histologically, the lesions consist of zonal proliferation of cellular fibrous tissue, osteoid tissue, and immature bone.

Tumors of Muscle (see Chapter 161)

MUSCLE BIOPSY

It may be necessary to evaluate muscle tissue histopathologically to differentiate neurological, neoplastic, parasitic, or degenerative disease processes. The sample of muscle tissue is isolated between two stay sutures,

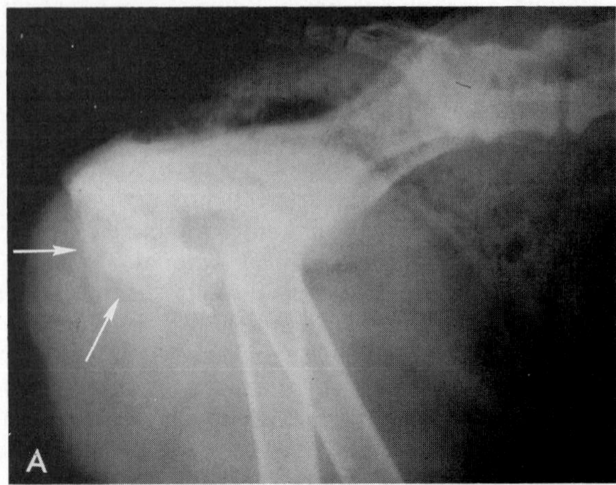

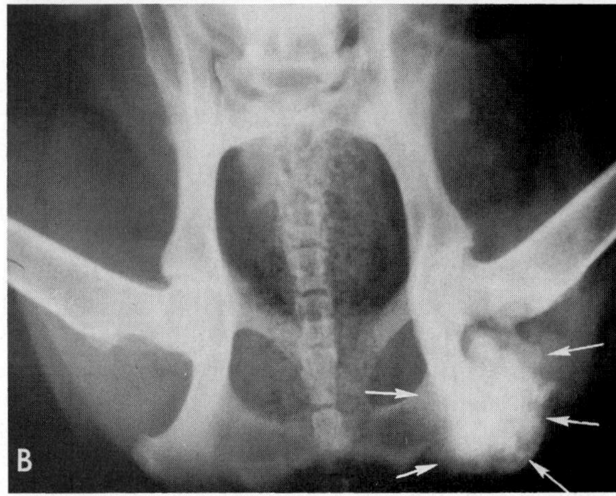

FIGURE 146–10. Lateral *(A)* and ventral *(B)* dorsal views of the pelvis of an adult Doberman pinscher, depicting a well-defined calcified mass typical of myositis ossificians involving the ischial tuberosity *(arrows)*. Surgical excision of the calcified tissue resulted in recovery with no recurrence. (Courtesy of Dr. Robert Parker, University of Florida, Gainesville, FL.)

excised, and stretched by wedging the sutures in clefts made in a wooden tongue depressor. This method prevents contracture and damage to the myofibrils. The sample is wrapped in a moist saline sponge and fixed immediately in solutions such as glutaraldehyde or paraformaldehyde or frozen in liquid nitrogen.[38]

HEREDITARY MYOPATHY OF LABRADOR RETRIEVERS

An inherited condition of Labrador retrievers is characterized by generalized muscle atrophy, abnormal flexion posture of neck, and a stiff hopping gait.[32, 42] It is transmitted by a single autosomal recessive gene. As early as 3 to 4 months of age clinically affected animals may show signs that are aggravated by cold, exercise, and stress.[11]

The diagnosis of hereditary myopathy is based on signalment, clinical signs, mild or moderate elevation of serum creatinine phosphokinase levels, electrophysiology, and muscle biopsy. Electromyography of skeletal muscle reveals abnormal spontaneous potentials characterized by fibrillation potentials, positive sharp waves, and high-frequency bizarre wave activity. A muscle biopsy sample shows disseminated fiber atrophy and multifocal presence of giant fibers, necrosis, many fibers with internal nuclei, fiber splitting, and type 2 fiber depletion.[11]

The differential diagnosis includes polymyositis, myotonic myopathy, hyperadrenocorticism, toxoplasmosis, myasthenia gravis, and glycogen storage diseases. The clinical signs stabilize at 6 to 12 months of age. There is no effective treatment, but dogs have a normal life span.[10]

TENDONS

Anatomy

Tendons are dense, irregular collagenous tissues composed of fibroblasts, parallel collagen fibers embedded in a ground substance, and extracellular fluid.[19] The fibroblasts or tenocytes are the only cells in tendons. The collagen fibers are arranged in fascicles, or bundles, which are surrounded by a woven mesh of loose areolar connective tissue called *endotenon*. The endotenon permits some longitudinal movement of the collagen bundles and carries all blood vessels, lymphatic vessels, and nerves. The entire tendon is covered by a fine connective tissue sheath called the *epitenon*, which is continuous on its undersurface with the endotenon. The epitenon is continuous on its outside surface with the *paratenon*. The paratenon covers and separates tendons from each other and facilitates free gliding of the tendon. In areas of local pressure on the tendon, the paratenon forms a tendon synovial sheath.

The vascular supply to tendons enters at three major locations. The proximal third of the tendon is supplied by vessels entering at the musculotendinous junction. The middle third of the tendon is supplied by extrinsic vessels passing longitudinally in the paratenon or synovial sheath. The distal third of the tendon is supplied by vessels entering at the osseous tendon insertion. The vessels within the tendon running between the fascicles or tendon bundles (intrinsic vessels) supply the collagen bundles and anastomose freely with each other and the extrinsic vessels.[15]

The vascularity of tendons depends on their location. Paratenon-covered tendons are more vascular than synovium-sheathed tendons. The degree of vascularity is important in healing.[19]

Tendon Healing

An important factor is whether a tendon heals without formation of adhesions to adjacent tissues, resulting in decreased gliding function. Tendon injuries are often accompanied by injury to surrounding soft tissues or bone. Consequently, healing does not take place in an isolated environment. The adhesions that develop are part of the healing process, resulting in the healing of the tendon and its surrounding tissues according to the principles of "one wound—one scar."[47] The healing process of tendons can be divided into paratenon-covered tendons and sheathed tendons. This division is necessary because of the greater role the paratenon and its extrinsic blood supply have in healing than does the intrinsic blood supply of the sheathed tendons. The cells of the mature tendon are spindle-shaped tenocytes, which have little capacity for reproduction or production of collagen.[9]

Healing in a paratenon-covered tendon depends less on intrinsic blood supply, because undifferentiated fibroblasts and capillary buds from the paratenon invade the damaged area between the tendon ends. The fibroblasts synthesize collagen. As the ground substance increases outside the fibroblast, the collagen polymerizes into fibrils. During the first week of injury, the healing tissue becomes visible as thin wavy fibers deposited randomly in and around the tendon wound. During the second week, the vascular reaction reaches its peak, as do fibroblastic proliferation and collagen production. During the third and fourth weeks, collagen fibers near the tendon ends become more longitudinally oriented. Collagen fibers in the center of the healing wound remain unorganized and perpendicular to lines of stress.[47]

The final stage of tendon healing involves secondary remodeling. A reduction in mass occurs as the collagen remodels and the tensile strength increases owing to the high degree of organization along the lines of stress. The collagenization continues until about 20 weeks, when little histological difference is noted between scar tissue and tendon. As movement and function return, the adhesions are weakened and remodeled.[19, 41, 47]

The importance of adhesions in tendon surgery relates to restoration of gliding function. Prevention of adhesions is paramount in human hand surgery but much less so in small animals. A more practical approach to minimizing tendon adhesion formation is the use of proper surgical technique, passive mobilization, and proper postoperative care.[23]

The return of sufficient tensile strength may be more important than gliding function in veterinary surgery.[19] Postoperative care must be based on proper suture techniques, postoperative immobilization, and gradual return to activity. During the first 4 to 5 days after surgical repair, the tendon ends soften, resulting in loss of holding power. During the next 2 weeks, the strength of repair gradually increases during the initial fibroplasia and collagen stages, at which time the strength is primarily due to the suture material. The suture pattern may be more important than the suture material.[58] Immobilization of the tendon repair site during the first 3 weeks postoperatively is critical to prevent increases in separation of the tendon ends with resulting invasion of excessive scar tissue and decreased tensile strength. It appears that the ideal postoperative immobilization period is 2 to 3 weeks, followed by 3 weeks of restricted activity, then gradual return to normal activity.[9]

General Principles of Tendon Surgery

Basic principles of asepsis and atraumatic handling of tissues are followed. The goal is to minimize adhesion formation (tenodesis) and restore as much gliding function as possible. An essential part of tendon surgery is careful and meticulous planning of the surgical procedure. Skin incisions are not made directly over the tendon but parallel to the proposed surgical site or curved over the tendon so the healing skin wound does not adhere to the tendon repair (tenorrhaphy) site. Maintenance of hemostasis is complete and may be accomplished by pressure from moist sponges, electrocautery used in moderation, or a tourniquet. Tourniquets work well on distal extremities of animals.

To minimize adhesions, all tissues are handled as gently as possible. The tissues are kept moist with sterile saline. The tendon segments are handled by gloved fingers, by straight needles placed through the tendon, or by skin hooks. If the ends of the tendon must be grasped by forceps for traction or suture placement, the traumatized end of the tendon is excised after sutures have been secured.[9, 13, 14] The results are best when the tendon ends are perfectly apposed.

Although the suture material and pattern for tendon surgery may vary based on a surgeon's preference, the shape of the tendon, and the particular technique used, basic principles must always be followed.* The suture material is inert, strong, easy to pass through tissues, and nonabsorbable.

Such suture materials include stainless steel wire, braided polyester fiber, monofilament nylon, and polypropylene. Although stainless steel wire has maximum knot security, it can be difficult to work with and breaks with fatigue. Polyester fiber is a multifilament suture requiring many knots for security, thus decreasing its desirability. Monofilament nylon and polypropylene are the most desirable sutures for repair of tendons. The size of the material depends on the size of the tendon; thus the largest size that comfortably passes through the tendon is used.[9] The most commonly used suture patterns are the horizontal mattress, Bunnell, and Bunnell-Mayer (Fig. 146–11).[9, 13] The locking loop (Kessler-Mason-Allen) and the modified Kessler are superior because they are less constrictive to the intrinsic blood supply and provide greater tensile strength than Bunnell sutures (Fig. 146–12).[1, 57]

The three-loop pulley suture for tendon repair provides greater tensile strength and resistance to gap formation than the locking loop patterns in *in vitro* studies (Fig. 146–13).[4]

Krackow and colleagues[31] and Lin and associates,[38] respectively, have described two promising new variations on the locking loop-type suture pattern. Further studies are needed to evaluate the effect of these suture patterns.

Surgical Repair of Severed Tendons

The majority of tendon injuries in small animals are related to lacerations rather than rupture. Unless the injury is chronic and tendon segments have severely contracted or the injury has devitalized large segments of tendon, primary end-to-end tenorrhaphy is the best method for restoration. The repair is performed with minimal delay in those wounds that have little trauma

*See references 1, 9, 13, 14, 41, 52, 56, and 58.

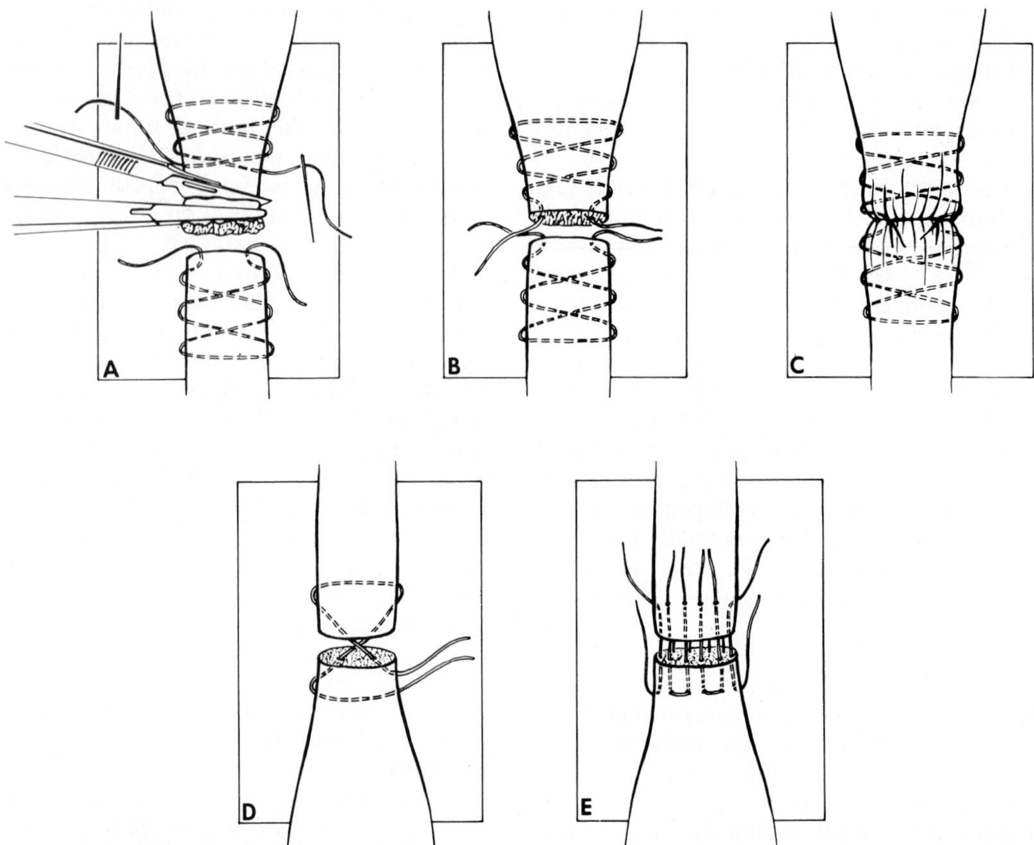

FIGURE 146–11. Suture technique for end-to-end anastomosis. *A, B,* and *C,* Bunnell-Mayer technique. *D,* Bunnell technique. *E,* Interrupted horizontal mattress suture technique.

and contamination. If the 4- to 6-hour period for primary closure has passed or if contamination is severe, an alternative approach is taken. This period for primary closure can be extended with thorough débridement and copious lavage if trauma and contamination are minimal and adequate soft tissue and blood supply surround the surgical site.

If primary anastomosis of the tendon ends is undertaken, the wound is thoroughly cleaned and débrided and tendon stumps exposed. When tendons are cut, the proximal segment retracts as muscles contract. If the proximal stump cannot be located in the wound, further enlargement of the wound can be avoided by making a small incision proximal to the site of injury. The proximal tendon stump can be located through this wound; then, by placing a suture through the end of the tendon, it can be carried subcutaneously along the tendon bed to emerge at the surgical site for reattachment.[14] Traction can be maintained on the tendon segments by placing straight needles transversely through the tendon proximal and distal to the proposed suture pattern.

If too much time has elapsed since the injury, if the tissue is infected or grossly contaminated, or if the surrounding soft tissues are too severely traumatized to provide adequate blood supply, repair is delayed. The wound is thoroughly débrided, and a small piece of colored suture material placed in the ends of the tendon stumps. The leg is immobilized to reduce separation of the tendon segments. These sutures act as markers so that after healing of the wound and resolution of the infection, secondary tendon repair may be attempted.[14, 47] Successful repair of tendon lacerations in an infected wound has been reported but is not encouraged because of wound breakdown and excessive adhesion formation.[6]

The technique and suture pattern provide anatomical apposition of the tendon segments and adequate strength for healing. No one suture pattern is satisfactory in all instances. In small animals, the end-to-end pattern is used because it maintains the original length and diameter of the tendon and is simple to perform. Techniques such as the overlapping side-to-side or fish mouth provide a stronger anastomosis but require longer tendon lengths (Fig. 146–14). Round or semiround tendons 2 cm or more in length are anastomosed by the locking loop (modified Kessler) or three-loop pulley suture patterns.

Regardless of the suture pattern used, the next step is to close the paratenon with a simple interrupted, simple continuous, or horizontal mattress suture of a fine monofilament nonabsorbable suture material.

If the tendon stumps are too short for these techniques, the Bunnell technique may be used, with a simple continuous suture in the paratenon placed 45° to the tendon. Other suture patterns are better suited for short, flat, or aponeurotic tendons. An interrupted hor-

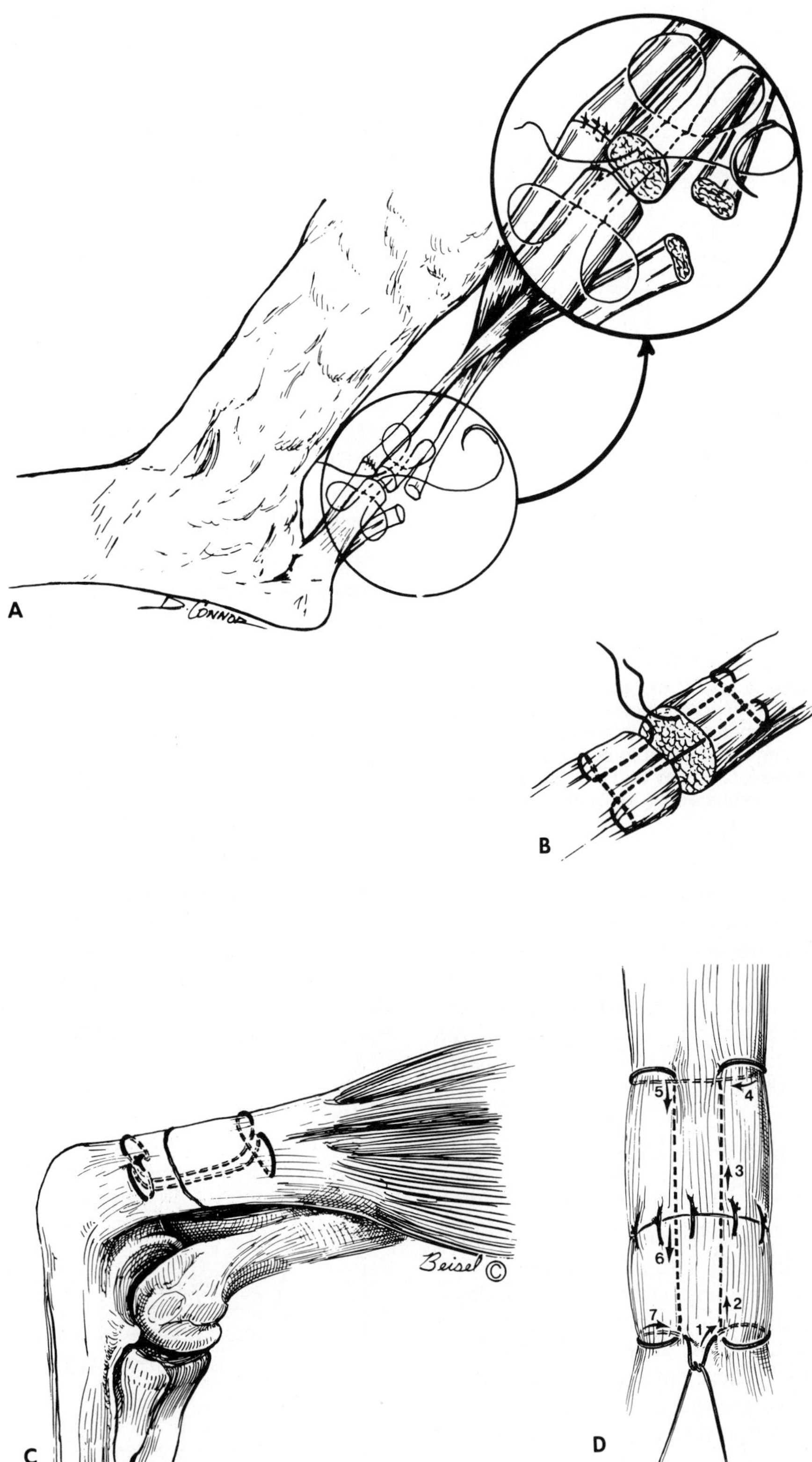

FIGURE 146–12. *A* and *B*, Locking loop (Kessler-Mason-Allen) suture technique. *C* and *D*, Modified Kessler suture. These two suture patterns can be used for end-to-end tendon anastomosis. It is important that the transverse segment of either suture pattern pass just superficial to the two longitudinal segments of the suture *(D)*. *(A* and *B* from Tomlinson J, Moore R: Locking loop tendon suture use in repair of five calcanean tendons. *Vet Surg 3*:105, 1982. *C* and *D* from Aron DN: A "new" tendon stitch. *J Am Anim Hosp Assoc 17*:587, 1981.)

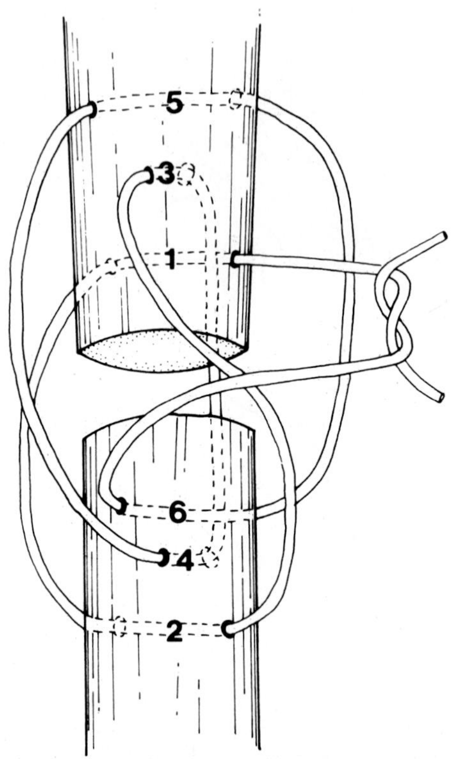

FIGURE 146–13. Three-loop pulley suture pattern. The initial loop is made when needle passes 1 and 2 are placed in a near-far pattern. The three continuous horizontal mattress sutures or loops are positioned in separate planes approximately 120° apart. Each loop is tightened before tying the knot. (From Berg RJ, Egger EL. *In vitro* comparison of the three-loop pulley and locking loop suture patterns for repair of canine weightbearing tendons and collateral ligaments. *Vet Surg 15*:107, 1986.)

izontal mattress suture may be used as well as the buttonhole overlapping suture. The disadvantages of this latter suture are that it requires excessive tendon length, a small portion of tendon is exposed, sutures are not buried, and the area of repair is bulky. Because the tendon ends overlap, this technique is contraindicated when a tendon passes through a synovial sheath.

Tendon Lengthening and Shortening

Tendon Lengthening

Lengthening may be indicated for contracture of a tendon or muscle tendon unit with chronic lameness or a conformation defect. In young, actively growing dogs, contracture or laxity of a muscle-tendon unit may be due to parasitism, malnutrition, dietary imbalances, or improper environment.[43] These animals may have buckling or dropping of the carpus or tarsus. Initial treatment is to correct the cause. Surgical intervention is necessary only in severe cases.

Before determining whether a tendon-lengthening procedure is necessary, the status of the muscle-tendon unit is assessed. If the muscle is unnecessary, a simple tenotomy or tenectomy can be performed as for infraspinatus muscle contracture.[43] When function must be preserved, the tendon should be lengthened. The most common technique for lengthening a tendon is the Z-tenotomy (Fig. 146–15*A* and *B*). This involves a half-section splitting of the tendon. An elongated Z incision is made in the tendon, first by splitting it longitudinally and then by incising the ends of the incision in opposite directions. The split ends of the tendon are separated the desired distance but left overlapping so that the anastomosis is a side-to-side rather than end-to-end repair. This provides stronger, more rapid healing. The tendon ends are apposed with an interrupted horizontal mattress suture pattern, followed by closure of the paratenon in a simple continuous pattern. Other methods of tendon lengthening include oblique splitting and gliding, accordion, and Lange techniques (Fig. 146–15*C* through *E*).[9, 14, 55]

Specific clinical indications for tendon lengthening include quadriceps, Achilles (common calcaneal), superficial and deep flexor, and flexor carpi ulnaris tendon contractures.[14]

Tendon Shortening

The most common indication for tendon shortening is improper healing of tendons after injury, especially if they have healed while the joint is hyperextended or hyperflexed. Excessive strain during growth may cause breakdown of supporting structures, with stretching of the tendon. An Achilles mechanism injury may cause improper healing of the gastrocnemius muscle-tendon junction or tendon, excessive tendon length, and hyperflexion of the tarsus. A similar situation can arise with improper healing of the superficial and deep flexor tendons of the forelimb.[14]

A tendon can be shortened by a number of methods, but the technique chosen should not involve a tenotomy because of the morbidity of anastomotic breakdown (Fig. 146–16). Hoffa's method of tendon shortening is easy and reliable but less applicable in tendons that are thickened and scarred (Fig. 146–16*A*).[9] If the sutures loosen prematurely, the tendon may lengthen again. A

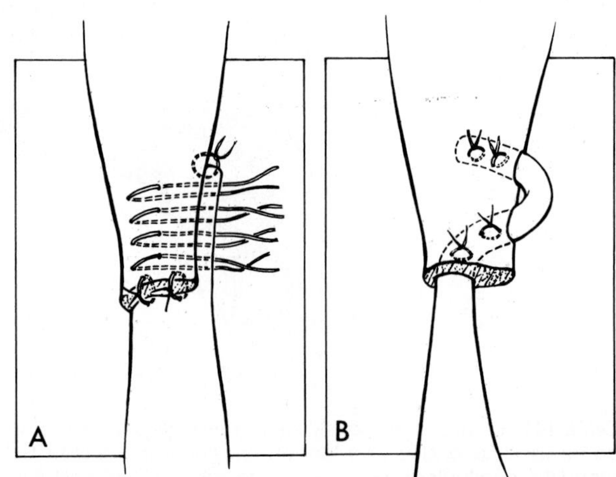

FIGURE 146–14. Overlapping techniques for tendon anastomosis may be used when tendon ends are long enough. *A*, Side-to-side. *B*, Fish mouth.

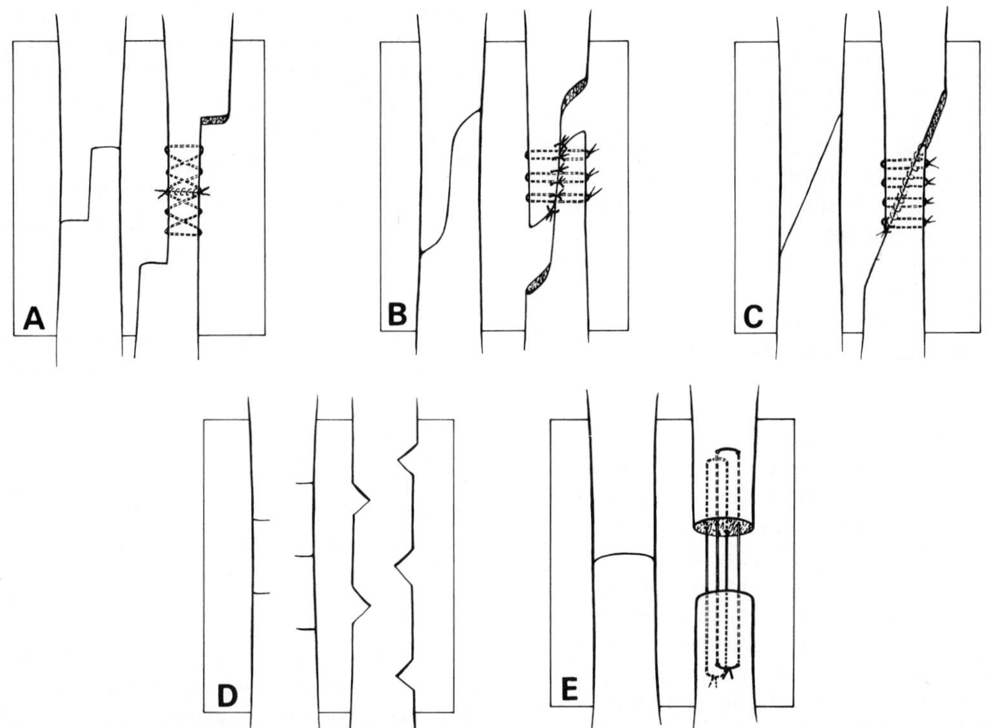

FIGURE 146–15. Various tendon lengthening techniques: *A*, Z-tenotomy. *B*, Modification of the Z-tenotomy. *C*, Oblique section and gliding. *D*, Accordion partial tenotomy. *E*, Lange method. (Modified from Butler HC: Tendon, muscle and fascia. *In* Archibald J (ed): *Canine Surgery*. 2nd ed. American Veterinary Publications, Santa Barbara, CA, 1974.)

tendon can also be shortened by doubling over the tendon on itself and using horizontal mattress sutures to secure the overlap (Fig. 146–16*B*). Other techniques for shortening tendons include a Z-tenectomy, in which an area of the Z incision is excised (Fig. 146–16*C*) or a simple tenectomy of a transverse section of the tendon followed by an end-to-end anastomosis (Fig. 146–16*D*).

Postoperative care includes internal or external immobilization of the limb until gradual return to activity can be initiated.

Tendon Grafting

Tendon grafts are rarely indicated or performed in small animal surgery.[43] A tendon graft is indicated when the tendon has been so severely damaged that tenorrhaphy is impossible or when generalized tenodesis is present and tenolysis is not possible.[9] Regardless of the type of graft, survival of a tendon graft depends on adequate nutrition.[19] Although both autografts and allografts have been described in humans, use in animals is limited by availability.

An excellent source of donor tissue to replace a portion of tendon in small animals is the tensor fascia lata.[9, 10] After an adequate length of tensor fasciae latae is harvested, it is rolled into a tube and anastomosed to the tendon ends using a Bunnell-Mayer or Bunnell suture pattern. Postoperative care of tendon grafts is similar to other tenorrhaphy procedures, except that the period of immobilization is extended by 3 weeks.[10]

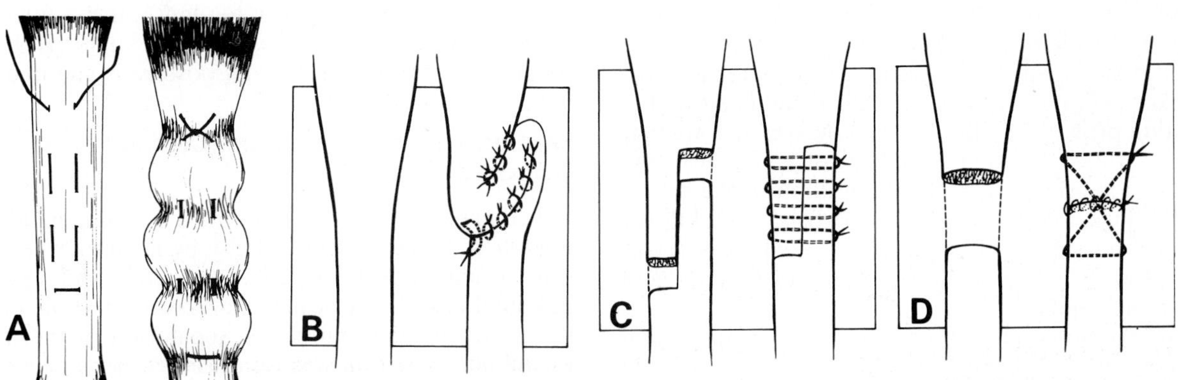

FIGURE 146–16. Tendons may be shortened using the following techniques: *A*, Hoffa method. *B*, Doubling over. *C*, Z-tenectomy. *D*, Segmental tenectomy. (Modified from Butler HC: Tendon, muscle and fascia. *In* Archibald J (ed): *Canine Surgery*. 2nd ed. American Veterinary Publications, Santa Barbara, CA, 1974.)

Tenolysis

Surgical release of tendon adhesions (tenodesis) is called *tenolysis*. Tendon adhesions are of little concern in small animals unless they involve a gliding tendon such as the digital flexors or have resulted in severe contracture. The critical factor is the extent of the tenodesis rather than the tissues attached.[9] To restore a soft-tissue layer between the movable and immovable scar, fascia, fat, or subcutaneous tissue can be used. If such tissues are not available, paratenon can be used. Although tenolysis after superficial burns, severe contusions, closed fractures, and soft-tissue injury has a high success rate, the same does not hold true for tenolysis after tendon repair.[9]

After trauma to soft tissues or bones, adhesions of tendons to these structures during the healing process may occur, especially if the paratenon remains unanastomosed or there is no soft tissue to incorporate between immovable and movable scar.[9] A paratenon transplant is indicated. The best source of paratenon in small animals is the calcaneal tendon. The paratenon is carefully harvested from around the calcaneal tendon and kept from contracting and adhering to itself by stay sutures placed at the corners of the transplant. The paratenon transplant is sutured to any existing paratenon and not the tendon. If paratenon is not available for suturing, loose fascia around the muscle and tendon junction is used. A fine monofilament nonabsorbable suture is used for attaching the transplant.

SPECIFIC TENDON INJURIES

Severed Digital Flexor Tendons

Severance of the digital extensor and flexor tendons of small animals commonly accompanies laceration of the skin. Trauma to the digital extensor tendons is of less concern because of the many anastomoses after they branch from the main tendon. If function after trauma to the digital extensors or flexors is normal, surgical intervention is not warranted. If loss of function is noted at a later date, a secondary repair can be performed.[9, 61]

More commonly, the lacerations occur on the plantar surface of the carpus and tarsus, resulting in severance of all or part of the superficial and deep digital flexor tendons.[5, 9, 43, 59] The superficial and deep digital flexor tendons insert on the proximal end of the second and third phalanges, respectively. The function of these tendons is to maintain the toes in proper position in relation to the digital and metacarpal or metatarsal pads. The flexor action of these tendons is maintained by the lubrication provided by the synovial sheaths and annular ligaments, which function as pulleys to change direction of the tendon. Because of the duplication of the digital flexor tendons, severance of the superficial digital flexor alone may have little effect on posture, whereas severance of the deep digital flexor results in flattening of one or more digits.[59]

The most common locations of severance of the digital flexor tendons are above and below the metatarsal and metacarpal pads.[43] An injured animal is often presented with profuse hemorrhage and accompanying soft-tissue damage. By having the dog stand on the affected leg or by pushing its foot hard against the palm of the hand, changes in posture of the digits can be detected.[59] The metacarpal or metatarsal pads may be excoriated if a chronic postural defect has been caused by previous digital flexor tendon injury.

The site of the laceration as well as the direction and size of the wound may be helpful in determining which structures have been damaged. If the cut is across the back of the metatarsus or metacarpus, both digital flexors may be severed. If the wound is small, only a portion of the digital flexors may be damaged. If the wound is extremely deep, the muscles beneath the tendons may also be severed.

Postural defects, such as flattening of one or more digits or elevation of the toes, are an indication for surgical exploration. Because the deep digital flexor tendon is of primary importance in posture of the toe, injuries to the superficial and deep digital flexor tendons in the metacarpal and metatarsal area and deep digital flexor near the digit require surgical treatment.

Surgical exposure of the digital flexors in the metacarpal and metatarsal areas is not difficult. A tourniquet enhances the exposure and results in less tissue trauma. Tendon ends are anastomosed as described earlier for tendon repair. Adequate soft tissues are available to cover the surgical repair.

Lacerations of the deep digital flexor tendon near the phalanges may damage annular ligaments and synovial sheaths. The tendon ends are much more difficult to expose because they may retract into the synovial sheaths beneath the annular ligament and superficial digital flexor tendon. The thick footpads and short ends of the severed tendons may require the annular ligament to be excised to expose the proximal segment if flexion and milking of the proximal tissue do not expose the tendon end.[38] After tenorrhaphy, damaged annular ligaments or synovial sheaths are sutured. The smaller the dog or cat, the more difficult are identification and reattachment of the tendon ends. Postoperative management is similar to that of other tendon injuries in that the metacarpus or metatarsus is immobilized in slight flexion for at least 3 weeks.

Chronic injuries are more difficult to treat in that the soft tissues on the plantar surface of the foot may be heavily scarred. The tendon ends can be reattached as described earlier, but large defects often remain. These defects in the digital flexor tendons can be filled with tendon grafts, fascial grafts, or suture material, but the prognosis for return to normal posture is guarded.[43]

Severed Achilles Mechanism (Common Calcaneal Tendon)

The major cause of rupture of the common calcaneal tendon is direct trauma, usually by a sharp object. The skin wound may be small, horizontal, and anywhere proximal to the tuber calcanei.[55] Damage to the belly of the gastrocnemius muscle or separation at the musculotendinous junction was discussed earlier.*

*See references 6, 8, 10, 14, 43, 44, 53, 55, 57, 59, 60, and 62.

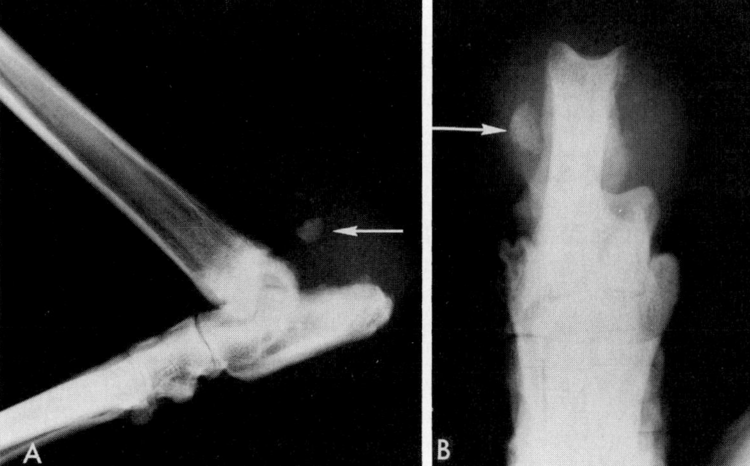

FIGURE 146–17. Lateral *(A)* and skyline *(B)* views of the tarsus of a dog with chronic avulsion of the calcaneal tendon. Note the avulsed bone fragments *(arrows)* and hyperflexed tibiotarsal joint *(A)*.

Clinical signs of injury include tarsal hyperflexion and stifle hyperextension. If the superficial digital flexor is severed, the paw becomes more plantigrade than normal. Diagnosis is aided by having the animal bear weight on the leg. These postural changes along with flaccidity of the tendon on flexion of the hock confirm the diagnosis (see Fig. 146–5). If the superficial digital flexor tendon remains intact, the animal assumes a dropped-hock posture with flexion of the digits. Thorough palpation of the Achilles tendon mechanism is indicated to locate the injury. If no skin wound is present, avulsion of the tendon from the proximal calcaneus, with or without a piece of bone, is suspected. Radiographs of the stifle and tarsus are always taken, along with stress films if indicated (Fig. 146–17).[52]

Surgical repair of the severed calcaneal tendon should occur as soon after injury as possible. Restoration of gliding function is not of extreme importance. Surgical correction can be undertaken in open contaminated wounds if proper débridement is practiced.[6] The calcaneal tendon is approached through a lateral skin incision that may incorporate the previous skin wound. After thorough débridement of the wound, a primary tenorrhaphy is performed on each of the three tendon components. A locking loop (Kessler) or three-loop pulley suture pattern may be used (see Figs. 146–12 and 146–13), and the wound closed as described previously.

It is common to find the calcaneal tendon avulsed from the tuber calcanei (Fig. 146–18). The tendon is reattached by first placing the suture in the proximal portion of the tendon. At least two sutures are inserted so that all three major tendons of the common calcaneal tendon are included (see Fig. 146–12). Two holes are drilled in the tuber calcanei. The two ends of the suture are passed through the drill holes, the tendon approximated to its insertion, and the suture tied. The soft tissues surrounding the calcaneus are sutured to the tendon of insertion with simple interrupted sutures to prevent the tendon from sliding to one side of the tuber calcanei (see Fig. 146–18).

Avulsion of a piece of the calcaneus (epiphysis in immature animals) may occur along with the tendon. In this instance, the piece of bone along with its tendon of insertion is reattached with a bone screw or pin and tension band wire.

As in chronic injuries, primary end-to-end tenorrhaphy may not be possible because of tendon retraction or tendon damage. Defects in the common calcaneal tendon have been repaired with tensor fasciae latae,[10] transposition of the deep digital flexor,[40] and carbon fiber implants.[60]

Postoperatively, the hock is immobilized in a semiextended position for 3 to 4 weeks using a full cast or external fixator, followed by 3 weeks of limited activity in a modified Robert Jones dressing. In large or obese dogs, additional internal immobilization of the tibiotarsal joint can be accomplished by an 18-gauge stainless steel wire placed in a figure-eight between the tuber calcanei and the distal caudal tibia or a bone screw between the tuber calcanei and the distal tibia, with the tibiotarsal joint at a functional angle (135°). Any internal immobilization device is removed approximately 6 weeks after surgery.[6, 9]

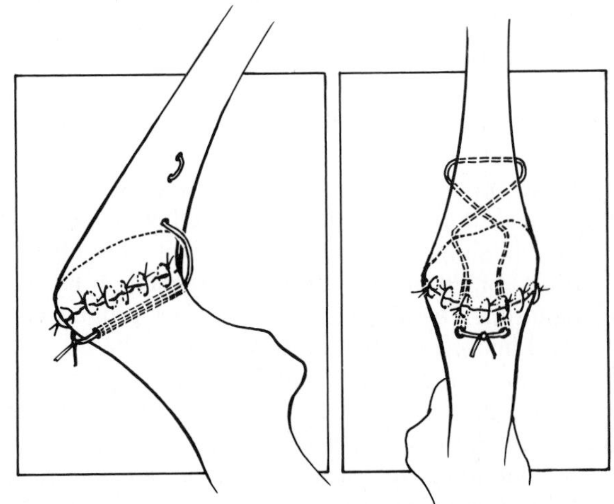

FIGURE 146–18. Repair of an avulsion of the calcaneal tendon from the tuber calcanei. A Bunnell suture has been woven through the tendon and then continued through two drill holes in the calcaneus and tied to itself. Sutures should be placed in the paratendinous tissue to enhance collateral stability of the tendon.

One technique for repair of Achilles tendon ruptures in humans and dogs does not use immobilization of the tibiotarsal joint for acute and chronic injuries.[37] The tendon ends are primarily anastomosed with a nonabsorbable suture, followed by insertion of a tension suture of Dacron vascular graft or 4-mm polyester suture passed through a drill hole in the tuber calcanei and looped through the musculotendinous junction. Dogs walk plantigrade immediately after surgery but regain normal use of the limb within 3 weeks.

The prognosis for functional recovery is favorable in all except large dogs. Unsatisfactory hyperflexion of the hock may result because of failure to immobilize the tibiotarsal joint properly or too early a return to normal activity.[59]

Displacement of the superficial digital flexor tendon has been described as a separate clinical entity[2, 5, 53] (see Chapter 139).

TENDON TRANSPOSITION OR RELOCATION

Transposition or relocation of a tendon is carried out to alter the function of a muscle—for example, anastomosis of a flexor tendon to an extensor tendon with nerve paralysis. Such relocations are also indicated to stabilize a joint (e.g., relocation of the greater trochanter in the surgical treatment of luxation of the coxofemoral joint or transposition of the sartorius muscle for stabilization of the stifle).

One of the more rewarding surgical procedures is transposition of the tendon of a flexor muscle to treat paralysis of the extensors of the carpus (radial nerve) and tarsus (peroneal nerve). The indications and methods for such surgical techniques have been described in detail.[3, 35]

INJURIES OF TENDONS AT ORIGIN OR INSERTION

It is common for injuries to occur at the tendon-bone or cartilage junction, where the tendon of origin or insertion blends with the periosteum and collagen fibers of the bone or cartilage. Collagen fibers of the tendon that blend with the bony substances are called *Sharpey's fibers*.[26] The extrinsic vascular supply of the tendon is continuous with the periosteum at the tendon-bone junction.[43]

Because most tendons insert or originate near the metaphyseal region of long bones, a rich vascular supply promotes healing. These injuries consist of avulsion of the origin or insertion, often accompanied by bone fragmentation (avulsion fracture). The prognosis for successful healing of such injuries is good, based on the rich vascular supply of the metaphyseal region of the bone and the fact that this type of injury is more common in immature animals.[42] Many of the injuries occur at traction epiphyses, resulting in delayed healing and malunions because of constant motion and muscle contraction.

Three basic types of tendon-bone injuries occur: (1) separation of tendon from bone, (2) avulsion fractures, and (3) avulsion of a small piece of bone with the tendon.[42] Once a diagnosis has been made, there should be no delay in surgical correction.

If little tissue remains adjacent to the bone, a drill hole is placed at the site of tendon insertion or origin and a horizontal mattress, Bunnell, or modified Kessler suture used to reattach the avulsed segment. If a small fragment of bone has been avulsed with the tendon, it can either be discarded or left with the tendon. If the bone segment is large enough, the suture can pass through it or it can be secured with Kirschner wires or a small bone screw.

Traction epiphyses are common sites of avulsion fractures, especially in young large dogs. The sites include the greater trochanter, tibial tuberosity, greater tubercle of the humerus, tuber calcanei, and supraglenoid tubercle. The medial malleolus of the tibia, distal fibular epiphysis, distal ulnar epiphysis, and proximal ulnar epiphysis (olecranon) may also be affected with similar disorders. Although the cause may be traumatic, the injuries are usually not severe and may be overlooked initially until presented as chronic. Avulsions of tendons and fractures involving the pressure epiphyses usually involve a superficial layer of bone and cartilage[43] (e.g., avulsion of the long digital extensor and popliteal tendon).

These injuries frequently are near the metaphysis and are closely associated with joints. Besides having detectable lameness, injured animals may resist manipulation and palpation of the joint nearest the site of injury. Radiographs may confirm the tendon separation and are especially helpful in detecting abnormal location of a sesamoid bone or epiphysis. Displacement of the avulsed bony segment may be subtle; radiographs of the opposite limb are taken for comparison.

SPECIFIC TENDON AVULSION INJURIES

Avulsion of the Tendon of Origin of the Long Digital Extensor

The long digital extensor muscle is located on the proximal cranial tibia. It is partially covered by the cranial tibial muscle medially and long peroneal muscle laterally. The tendon of origin arises from the extensor fossa of the lateral condyle of the femur and passes distally through the muscular groove on the craniolateral aspect of the tibia to blend with its muscle belly. The tendon inserts on the extensor process of the third phalanges of digits two through five. The long digital extensor muscle extends the digits and flexes the tarsus.[20]

This injury occurs primarily in immature large dogs.[2, 12, 33, 43, 56, 59] Injured animals have a weightbearing lameness and pain on manipulation of the affected stifle. Some lateral soft-tissue swelling may be noticed. Clinically, this condition should not be confused with a ruptured or avulsed cranial cruciate ligament or osteochondrosis of the femoral condyles. Radiographs of the affected stifle reveal an avulsed segment of bone and cartilage near the extensor fossa of the lateral femoral condyle. The lateral radiographic view best demonstrates the lesion (Fig. 146–19). In a very immature animal, the avulsed segment may consist primarily of

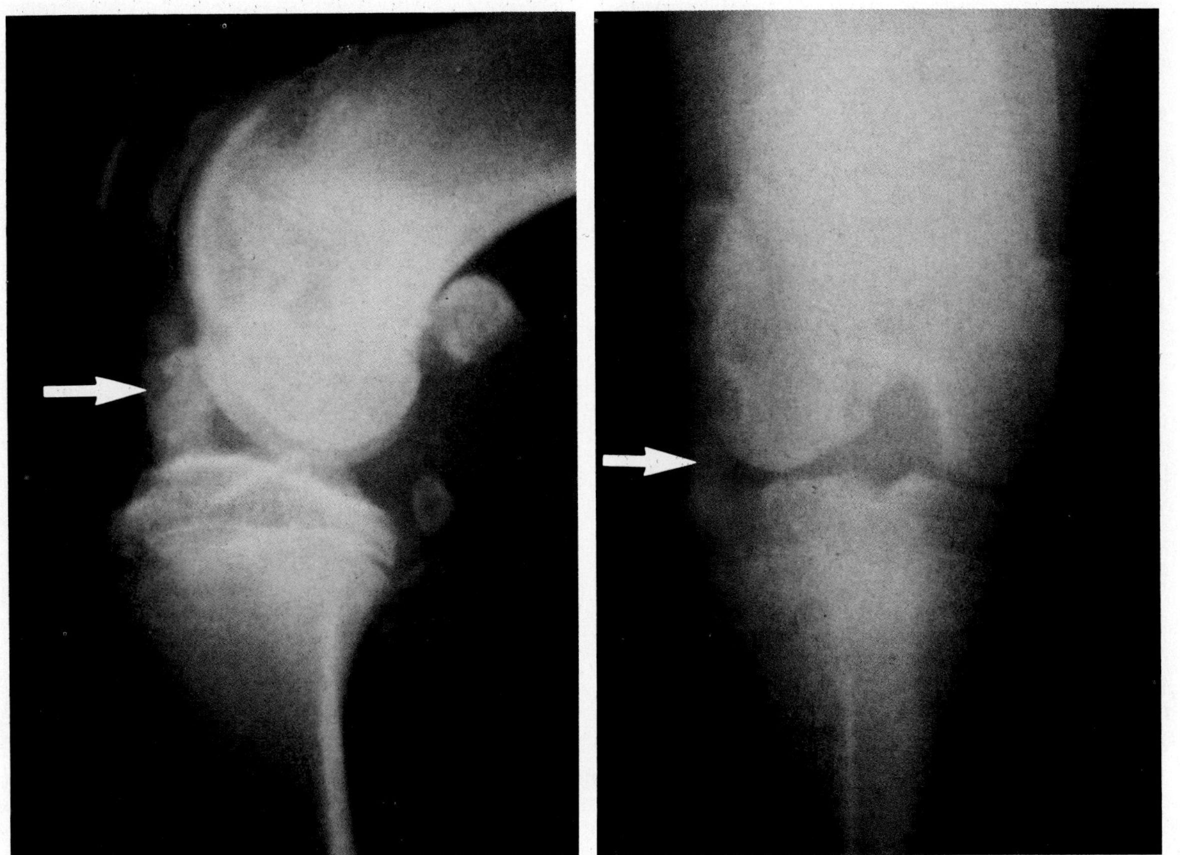

FIGURE 146–19. Lateral *(A)* and craniocaudal *(B)* views of the stifle of a 7-month-old Great Dane. Note a calcified density in the anterolateral aspect of the stifle joint *(arrow)*. (From Lammerding JJ, et al: Avulsion fracture of the origin of the extensor digitorum longus muscle in three dogs. *J Am Anim Hosp Assoc 12*:764, 1976.)

cartilage and may not be visible radiographically. In either case, the diagnosis is confirmed by exploratory arthrotomy.

The treatment of choice is reattachment of the avulsed bone to its origin on the lateral femoral condyle. The surgical approach is a lateral approach to the stifle.[49] The avulsed segment of bone and tendon is reattached with bone screws. Use of a spiked washer with the bone screw assists in securing the soft tissues surrounding the bone fragment.

The avulsed portion of bone may be too small for screw fixation. In addition, chronic injuries may not allow positioning of the avulsed bony segment in the extensor fossa. The bone fragment may be left in place or excised, and a fresh bed prepared on the lateral femoral condyle. The avulsed segment can be wired or stapled in place. If no bone remains attached to the avulsed tendon, it can be sutured to the joint capsule near its point of penetration.

Postoperatively, fixation is protected for 2 weeks by placing the affected limb in a Schroeder-Thomas splint, full-length cast, or modified Robert Jones dressing. The animal is gradually returned to normal activity over a 3- to 4-week period after the external support is removed. The prognosis for return of function of the affected limb is excellent.

Avulsion of the Origin of the Popliteal Muscle[43, 51]

The popliteal muscle is covered by the gastrocnemius muscle and superficial digital flexor muscle as it lies on the lateral surface of the joint capsule of the stifle and proximal tibia. It arises by a long tendon from the lateral femoral condyle just medial to the lateral collateral ligament of the stifle. Its tendon contains a sesamoid bone. The tendon continues caudally and lateral to the lateral meniscal cartilage to its muscle belly on the caudal proximal tibia. The popliteal muscle flexes the stifle and inwardly rotates the leg.[20]

The clinical signs are similar to other stifle injuries, such as avulsion of the long digital extensor tendon. The diagnosis is confirmed by radiographs of the affected stifle, which reveal distal displacement of the popliteal sesamoid bone that may also be accompanied by a bone fragment positioned caudal to the point of attachment of the popliteal tendon (Fig. 146–20).[43]

Treatment requires surgical reattachment of the avulsed tendon through a lateral approach. Reflection of the biceps femoris muscle caudally reveals the lateral collateral ligament, joint capsule, popliteal tendon, and lateral head of the gastrocnemius muscle. Reattachment of the avulsed tendon and its accompanying bone frag-

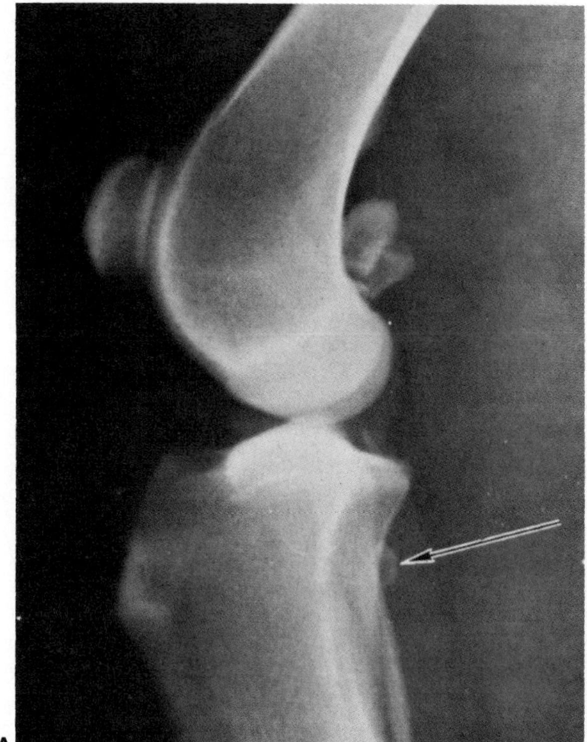

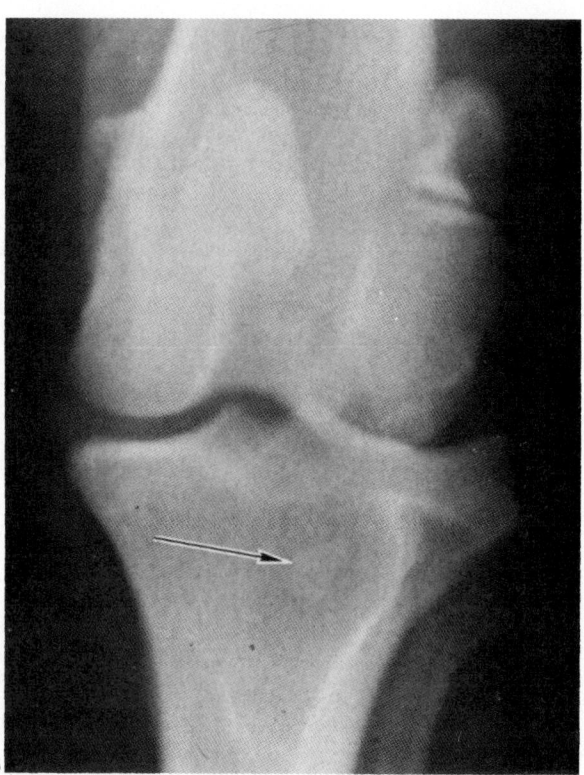

FIGURE 146–20. Lateral *(A)* and craniocaudal *(B)* radiographs of the stifle, showing distal displacement of the sesamoid bone of the popliteal tendon *(arrow)*. (From Pond MJ, Losonsky JM: Avulsion of the popliteus muscle in the dog: A case report. *J Am Anim Hosp Assoc 12:*60, 1976.)

ment is accomplished with a small cortical bone screw with or without a spiked washer (Fig. 146–21). Postoperative care is like that for an avulsed long digital extensor tendon.

Avulsion of the Lateral or Medial Head of the Gastrocnemius Muscle

This injury occurs in the fox terrier,[16] German shepherd,[59] and Labrador retriever.[43] The lateral and medial heads of the gastrocnemius muscle originate from the lateral and medial supracondylar tuberosities, respectively, of the femur. Each head of the gastrocnemius muscle has a sesamoid (fabella) located in its tendon of origin.[20] The lateral and medial fabellae articulate with the femoral condyles and are bound to them by ligamentous tissue.

Clinical diagnosis is based on hyperflexion of the hock with weightbearing. Radiographs of the affected stifle reveal distal displacement of the fabella. Surgical repair of the avulsion is the treatment of choice and was described earlier under rupture of the common calcaneal tendon.

Avulsion of the Origin of the Biceps Tendon

The biceps brachii muscle is a long muscle on the cranial surface of the humerus. Its tendon of origin arises on the supraglenoid tuberosity, and the muscle completely spans the humerus to insert on the proximal ends of the radius and ulna. The transverse humeral ligament holds the tendon of origin in the intertubercular groove by spanning the greater and lesser tubercles. The function of the biceps brachii is to flex the elbow and extend the shoulder.[20]

Avulsion of the origin of the biceps tendon occurs primarily in large dogs 4 to 8 months old.[43] The clinical signs include weightbearing lameness and pain or discomfort on flexion and extension of the shoulder. Treatment of choice is surgical reduction of the tendon and accompanying avulsed piece of bone (Fig. 146–22). The scapulohumeral joint is exposed through a craniomedial approach.[49] Lateral retraction of the supraspinatus muscle reveals the avulsed tubercle of the scapula. Care is taken to avoid damage to the suprascapular nerve. The tendon of origin and the tubercle are aligned after placing the scapulohumeral joint in extension. The tubercle is attached to the glenoid of the scapula with a pin and tension band wire or small bone screw.

Postoperative care consists of bandaging with the shoulder extended and the elbow flexed. The external support is removed at the end of 2 weeks, and the animal's activity is restricted to leash exercise for 3 to 4 weeks. The prognosis for return to normal function is excellent only if the avulsed bone has been securely fastened. In my experience, any fixation other than with a bone screw or pin and tension band wire will fail.

Bicipital Tenosynovitis

Inflammation of the tendon of origin and bursa of the biceps brachii is called *bicipital tenosynovitis*. Inflam-

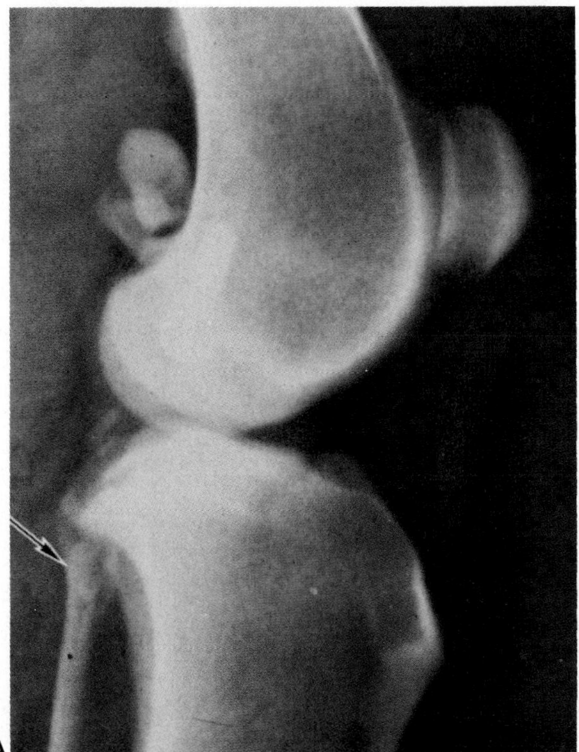

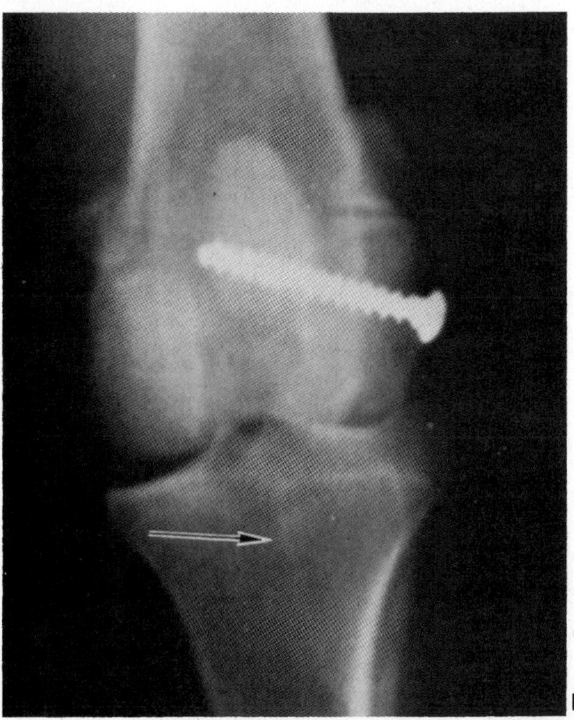

FIGURE 146–21. Lateral *(A)* and craniocaudal *(B)* radiographs of the stifle shown in Figure 146–20, taken immediately postoperatively. A bone screw has been placed in the lateral condyle of the femur. The arrow points to the sesamoid bone, which is located more proximally than noted preoperatively. (From Pond MJ, Losonsky JM: Avulsion of the popliteus muscle in the dog: A case report. *J Am Anim Hosp Assoc 12*:60, 1976.)

mation of the tendon may be caused by excessive stress, acute or chronic, or may be associated with the synovitis resulting from osteochondritis of the humeral head. The shoulder joint communicates with the bicipital bursa, and "joint mice" can become lodged adjacent to the tendon in the intertubercular groove.

Clinical signs include forelimb lameness that may be acute or chronic. Acute pain may be caused by local pressure applied directly to the bicipital tendon and bursa.

Acute bicipital tenosynovitis manifests by hyperemia of the bursa wall and subsequent effusion. As the condition becomes chronic, synovial hyperplasia of the bursa, chondromalacia of the intertubercular groove, osteophytosis of the margins of the intertubercular groove, and metastatic calcification of the bicipital tendon develop.[29]

Initial treatment of bicipital tenosynovitis includes limited activity and nonsteroidal anti-inflammatory medications. Injection of intrasynovial long-acting corticosteroids yields temporary relief in severe cases. The use of corticosteroid injections remains controversial. If corticosteroids are injected into the synovial sheath or shoulder joint, the patient must be rested for a prolonged period. Injections are given no more frequently than every 2 weeks, and treatment should not exceed two injections.[29]

In refractory cases, the treatment of choice is surgical obliteration of the bursa and transposition of the biceps tendon. This procedure is performed through a craniomedial approach to the shoulder. The biceps tendon is transected at its origin. The bicipital bursa is excised. The tendon is passed through a drill hole in the greater tubercle of the humerus and sutured on itself.[29]

Unusual Tendon Avulsions

Numerous rare injuries involving avulsion of tendons of origin or insertion have been described, such as (1) avulsion of the medial epicondyle of the humerus,[59] (2) rupture or avulsion of the triceps tendon from the olecranon,[17] (3) avulsion of the insertion of the biceps brachii muscle and brachial tendons from the proximal ulna,[43] and (4) avulsion of the insertion of the extensor carpi radialis tendon from the proximal metaphysis of metacarpals II and III.[43]

TENDON DISPLACEMENT

Displacement of a tendon from its normal position can impair limb function and result in clinical lameness. The cause of such displacement is usually traumatic, but the injury frequently remains unnoticed in the acute stages.

Displacement of the Tendon of Origin of the Long Digital Extensor

Two cases of caudal displacement of the long digital extensor have been described.[2, 59] Both were in young

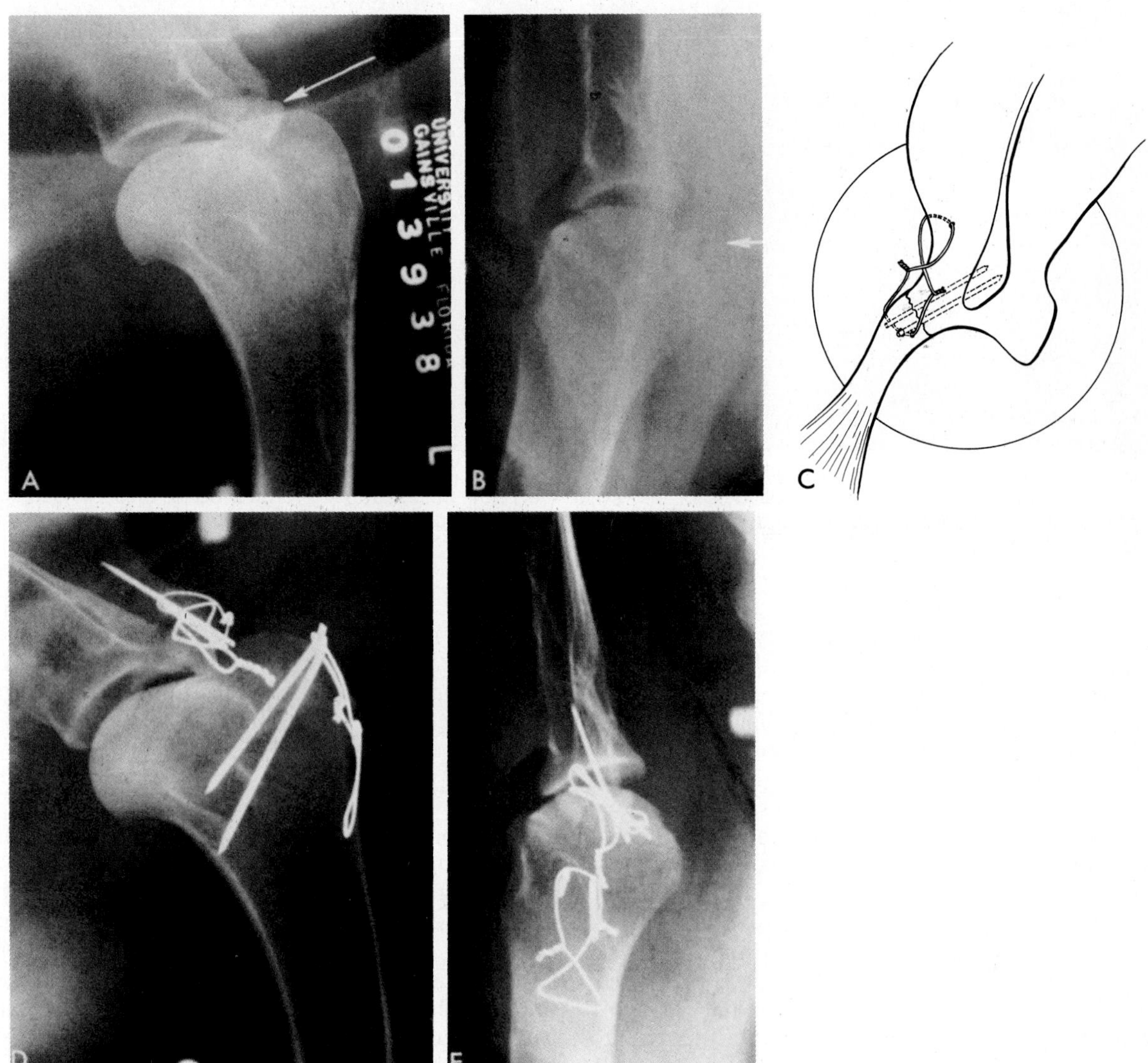

FIGURE 146–22. *A* and *B*, Lateral and craniocaudal radiographs of the scapulohumeral joint of a mature Doberman pinscher. The arrow points to the accompanying avulsion of the supraglenoid tubercle with the origin of the biceps brachii muscle. *C*, Repair technique for avulsion of the origin of the biceps brachii muscle with pin and tension band wire. *D* and *E*, Postoperative lateral and craniocaudal radiographs depict repair of the avulsion with a pin and tension band wire technique. Note that surgical exposure was enhanced after osteotomy of the greater tubercle of the humerus. The osteotomy was also repaired with a pin and tension band wire.

animals exhibiting severe chronic lameness.[59] On flexion and extension of the stifle, the tendon of origin snaps out of the muscular groove on the craniolateral proximal tibia.[43, 59] Surgical treatment involved creating a stainless steel wire or staple roof over the muscular groove in the tibia to prevent displacement of the tendon.[2]

Displacement of the Superficial Digital Flexor Tendon

Medial displacement of the tendon of the superficial digital flexor of the rear limb is described in Chapter 139.

Displacement of the Tendon of Origin of the Biceps Brachii

Medial displacement of the tendon of origin of the biceps brachii muscle has been reported in a border collie,[2] miniature poodle,[43] and greyhound.[25]

The lameness is usually weightbearing and chronic. Manipulation of the shoulder joint elicits pain and discomfort. Careful palpation over the craniomedial aspect of the joint shows medial slipping of the biceps tendon during flexion. On extension of the shoulder, the tendon often returns to its normal location. Extension of the elbow with the shoulder partially flexed may also produce slipping of the tendon.[2]

The biceps tendon is approached through a craniomedial skin incision over the shoulder.[49] With the shoulder in extension, the biceps tendon is replaced into the groove. If the groove is shallow, it can be enlarged or deepened with a bone curette or rongeurs. Any remnants of the synovial sheath are sutured over the tendon with a nonabsorbable monofilament suture material. Additional fixation in the form of mattress sutures, wire staples, or a bone plate can be placed over the groove between the greater and lesser tubercles, forming a roof over the tendon.[2, 25, 40]

Postoperative care consists of strict confinement with no exercise for 2 weeks. No external support for the limb is necessary. This period is followed by 3 to 4 weeks of leash exercise only. The animal is gradually returned to normal activity. The greyhound mentioned earlier returned to successful competitive racing 4 months after surgical treatment.[25]

References

1. Aron DN: A "new" tendon stitch. *J Am Anim Hosp Assoc 17*:587, 1981.
2. Bennett D, Campbell JR: Unusual soft tissue orthopaedic problems in the dog. *J Small Anim Pract 20*:27, 1979.
3. Bennett D, Vaughn LC: The use of muscle relocation techniques in the treatment of peripheral nerve injuries in dogs and cats. *J Small Anim Pract 17*:99, 1976.
4. Berg RJ, Egger EL: *In vitro* comparison of the three loop pulley and locking loop suture patterns for repair of canine weightbearing tendons and collateral ligaments. *Vet Surg 15*:107, 1986.
5. Bernard MA: Superficial digital flexor tendon injury in the dog. *Can Vet J 18*:105, 1977.
6. Bloomberg MS, et al: Repair of severed Achilles tendon in a dog: A case report. *J Am Anim Hosp Assoc 12*:841, 1977.
7. Bone DL, Gavin MD: Myositis ossificans in the dog: A case report and review. *J Am Anim Hosp Assoc 21*:135, 1985.
8. Braden TD: Musculotendinous rupture of the Achilles apparatus and repair using internal fixation only. *Vet Med Small Anim Clin 69*:729, 1974.
9. Braden TD: Tendons and muscles. *In* Bojrab MJ (ed): *Current Techniques in Small Animal Surgery*. Lea & Febiger, Philadelphia, 1975.
10. Braden TD: Fascia lata transplants for repair of chronic Achilles tendon defects. *J Am Anim Hosp Assoc 12*:800, 1976.
11. Braund KG: Hereditary myopathy in Labrador retrievers. *Calif Vet 39*:18, 1985.
12. Brinker WD, et al: *Handbook of Small Animal Orthopedics and Fracture Treatment*. W.B. Saunders, Philadelphia, 1983.
13. Bunnell S: Primary repair of severed tendons: The use of stainless steel wire. *Am J Surg 47*:502, 1940.
14. Butler HC: Tendon, muscle, and fascia. *In* Archibald J (ed): *Canine Surgery*. 2nd ed. American Veterinary Publications, Santa Barbara, 1974.
15. Caplan HS, et al: Intrinsic vascularization of tendons. *In* American Academy of Orthopaedic Surgeons: *Symposium on Tendon Surgery in the Hand*. C. V. Mosby, St Louis, 1975.
16. Chaffee VW, Knecht DC: Avulsion of the medial head of the gastrocnemius in the dog. *Vet Med Small Anim Clin 70*:929, 1955.
17. Davies JV, Clayton-Jones DG: Triceps tendon rupture in the dog following corticosteroid injection. *J Small Anim Pract 23*:779, 1982.
18. Dee JF, et al: Injuries of high performance dogs. *In* Whittick WG (ed): *Canine Orthopedics*. 2nd ed. Lea & Febiger, Philadelphia, 1974.
19. Early TD: Tendon disorders. *In* Bojrab MJ (ed): *Pathophysiology of Small Animal Surgery*. Lea & Febiger, Philadelphia, 1981.
20. Evans HE, Christensen GC: *Miller's Anatomy of the Dog*. 2nd ed. W.B. Saunders, Philadelphia, 1979.
21. Farrow CS: Sprain, strain and contusion. *Vet Clin North Am 8*:169, 1979.
22. Frandson RD, Davis RW: "Dropped muscle" in the racing greyhound. *J Am Vet Med Assoc 126*:468, 1955.
23. Gelberman RH, et al: Flexor tendon repair. *J Orthop Res 4*:119, 1986.
24. Gleeson LN: Treatment of traumatic lesions of tendo-Achilles by joint fixation with a Stader splint. *Vet Med 41*:442, 1946.
25. Goring RL, et al: Medial displacement of the tendon of origin of the biceps brachii muscle in the racing greyhound. *J Am Anim Hosp Assoc 20*:933, 1984.
26. Ham AW: *Histology*. 8th ed. J.B. Lippincott, Philadelphia, 1980.
27. Hickman J: Greyhound injuries. *J Small Anim Pract 16*:455, 1975.
28. Hoerlein BF, et al: Upward luxation of the canine scapula: A case report. *J Am Vet Med Assoc 136*:258, 1960.
29. Hohn RB, Harrison JW: II. The pectoral limb. Bicipital tenosynovitis. Proceedings of the 42nd Annual Meeting of the American Animal Hospital Association, Cincinnati, OH, April, 1975, p 428.
30. Hufford T, et al: Contracture of the infraspinatus muscle and surgical correction in two dogs. *J Am Anim Hosp Assoc 11*:613, 1975.
31. Krackow KA, et al: A new stitch for ligament-tendon fixation. *J Bone Joint Surg [Am] 68A*:764, 1986.
32. Kramer JW, et al: A muscle disorder of Labrador retrievers characterized by deficiency of type II muscle fibers. *J Am Vet Med Assoc 169*:817, 1976.
33. Lammerding JJ, et al: Avulsion fracture of the origin of the extensor digitorum longus muscle in 3 dogs. *J Am Anim Hosp Assoc 12*:764, 1976.
34. Leighton RL: Muscle contractures in the limbs of dogs and cats. *Vet Surg 10*:132, 1981.
35. Lesser AS, Soliman SS: Experimental evaluation of tendon transfer for the treatment of sciatic nerve paralysis in the dog. *Vet Surg 9*:72, 1980.
36. Levy M, et al: A method of repair of Achilles tendon rupture without cast immobilization. *Clin Orthop 187*:199, 1984.
37. Lewis DD: Fibrotic myopathy of the semitendinosus muscle in a cat. *J Am Vet Med Assoc 193*:240, 1988.
38. Lin GT, et al: Biomechanical studies of running suture for flexor tendon repairs in dogs. *J Hand Surg 13A*:553, 1988.
39. Liu SK, Dorfman HD: A condition resembling human localized myositis ossificans in two dogs. *J Small Anim Pract 17*:371, 1976.
40. Malnati GA: Deep digital flexor tendon transposition for rupture of the calcanean tendon in a dog. *J Am Anim Hosp Assoc 17*:451, 1981.
41. Mason ML, Allen HS: The rate of healing of tendon. An experimental study of tensile strength. *Ann Surg 113*:424, 1941.
42. McKerrell RE, Braund KG: Hereditary myopathy in Labrador retrievers: Clinical variations. *J Small Anim Pract 28*:479, 1987.
43. Milton JL, Henderson PA: Surgery of muscles and tendons. *In* Bojrab MJ (ed): *Current Techniques in Small Animal Surgery*. 2nd ed. Lea & Febiger, Philadelphia, 1983.
44. Mitchell M: Spontaneous repair of a ruptured gastrocnemius muscle in a dog. *J Am Anim Hosp Assoc 16*:513, 1980.
45. Moore RW, et al: Fibrotic myopathy of the semimembranosus muscle in four dogs. *Vet Surg 10*:169, 1981.
46. Parker RB, Cardinet GH: Myotendinous rupture of the Achilles mechanism associated with parasitic myositis. *J Am Anim Hosp Assoc 20*:115, 1984.
47. Peacock EE, Van Winkle WV: *Surgery and Biology of Wound Repair*. 2nd ed. W.B. Saunders, Philadelphia, 1976.
48. Pettit GD, et al: Studies on the pathophysiology of infraspinatus muscle contracture in the dog. *Vet Surg 7*:8, 1978.
49. Piermattei DL, Greeley RG: *An Atlas of Surgical Approaches to the Bones of the Dog and Cat*. 2nd ed. W.B. Saunders, Philadelphia, 1979.
50. Pollock S, et al: Clinical significance of trauma, myositis ossificans, and

malignant mesenchymoma in the dog: Report of an unusual case. *J Am Anim Hosp Assoc 14*:237, 1978.
51. Pond MJ, Lasonsky JE: Avulsion of the popliteus muscle in the dog: A case report. *J Am Anim Hosp Assoc 12*:60, 1976.
52. Reinke JD, Kus SP: Achilles mechanism injury in the dog. *Comp Cont Educ 4*:639, 1982.
53. Reinke JD, et al: Traumatic avulsion of the lateral head of the gastrocnemius and superficial digital flexor muscles in a dog. *J Am Anim Hosp Assoc 18*:252, 1982.
54. Rudy RL: Stifle joint. *In* Archibald J (ed): *Canine Surgery*. 2nd ed. American Veterinary Publications, Santa Barbara, 1974.
55. Smith KW: Achilles tendon surgery for correction of hyperextension of the hock joint. *J Am Anim Hosp Assoc 12*:848, 1976.
56. Srugi S, Adamson JE: A comparative study of tendon suture material in dogs. *Plast Reconstr Surg 50*:31, 1972.
57. Tomlinson J, Moore R: Locking loop tendon suture use in repair of five calcanean tendons. *Vet Surg 11*:105, 1982.
58. Urbaniak JR, et al: Tendon suturing methods: Analysis of tensile strength. *In* American Academy of Orthopedic Surgeons: *Symposium on Tendon Surgery of the Hand.* C. V. Mosby, St Louis, 1975.
59. Vaughn LC: Muscle and tendon injuries in dogs. *J Small Anim Pract 20*:711, 1979.
60. Vaughn LC, Edwards GB: The use of carbon fibers (Grafil) for tendon repair in animals. *Vet Rec 102*:287, 1978.
61. Vaughn LC, Faull WB: Correction of a luxated superficial digital flexor tendon in a greyhound. *Vet Rec 67*:335, 1955.
62. Vierheller RC: Surgical repair of severed tendons and ligaments in the dog. *Mod Vet Pract 53*:35, 1972.
63. Wright JR: Correction of quadriceps contractures. *Calif Vet 34*:7, 1980.

CHAPTER 147 Limb-Sparing Surgery for Dogs with Bone Neoplasia

Rodney C. Straw and Stephen J. Withrow

Osteosarcoma is the most common primary bone tumor in humans and dogs.[15, 20, 21] Amputation is the traditional surgical treatment in both species but is considered only palliative because occult metastatic disease is not treated by surgery. The 1-year survival is 10 per cent for dogs, and the 5-year survival is 20 per cent for people with osteosarcoma when surgery is the only treatment.[5, 15, 35, 38]

Limb-sparing surgery aims to provide a functional pain-free limb for the patient after removal of the local disease without adversely affecting survival. Humans undergoing limb-sparing procedures are often treated with chemotherapy while they wait for custom-made endoprostheses to be designed and manufactured.[2] This chemotherapy is called *neoadjuvant chemotherapy* by some; other names include *induction chemotherapy, preoperative chemotherapy*, and *protochemotherapy*.[13, 14] Neoadjuvant chemotherapy may "down stage" the tumor and make surgery easier. Limb-sparing surgery involves local tumor removal with marginal or wide margins.[9, 19] The bone or joint removed is usually replaced with a metal endoprosthesis, an allograft, or a combination of the two. Function in most patients has been good,[25] and chemotherapy has improved survival. Laboratory studies and clinical trials suggest delivery of chemotherapy before removal of primary tumors has survival benefits for patients.[3, 12, 18, 30, 32, 43] Reported 5-year survival for humans is now 50 per cent or better at many centers.[33, 34]

Previous attempts with various agents to treat micrometastatic disease in dogs with osteosarcoma have been unsuccessful.[8, 16, 24, 27] Reports suggest that cisplatin (Platinol) either alone or in combination with doxorubicin (Adriamycin) improves survival in dogs with osteosarcoma.[26, 32, 38] Neoadjuvant or adjuvant cisplatin chemotherapy with surgery is currently recommended for dogs with osteosarcoma. Most dogs tolerate limb amputation well, and owners are generally pleased with function and appearance.[6, 44] In certain instances, limb sparing is preferred, such as for extremely large dogs, dogs with concurrent orthopedic or neurological disorders, or dogs with owners who refuse amputation. For these dogs, limb-sparing surgery may be a viable alternative to amputation. In the few early reports of limb-sparing surgery in tumor-bearing dogs, follow-up information was limited.[39, 42] Two more detailed reports and a review describe limb sparing in larger numbers of dogs.[22, 37, 40] This chapter describes our experience with limb-sparing surgery for bone tumors in 80 dogs (Table 147–1).

CASE SELECTION

Dogs with osteosarcoma or other primary neoplasms of the appendicular skeleton may be candidates for limb-sparing procedures. Suitable dogs have their primary tumors clinically confined to one appendicular site with no more than 50 per cent of the length of the bone

TABLE 147–1. DOGS WITH PRIMARY BONE TUMORS TREATED WITH LIMB SPARING BETWEEN JANUARY 1985 AND DECEMBER 1989*

Site of Tumor Excised	Number of Dogs
Distal radius	52
Proximal humerus	13
Ulna	5
Distal femur	5
Distal tibia	3
Proximal tibia	1
Distal humerus	1
Total	80

*Colorado State University.

affected as determined radiographically. Selected dogs with multiple myeloma or skeletal lymphoma may have their affected limbs spared using combined chemotherapy and radiation therapy. Surgery for these dogs may be necessary to repair pathological fractures, but large *en bloc* resections and allograft replacement are rarely indicated.

Histological diagnosis is made from biopsy material, preferably obtained by a closed technique using a Jamshidi bone marrow biopsy needle.* The biopsy site is selected carefully. Two radiographic projections of the limb are evaluated before biopsy. Biopsy is performed while the dog is anesthetized, and strict aseptic technique is used. The skin incision is made with consideration of possible subsequent treatment, so the biopsy tract and potential seeding of tumor cells can be removed at surgery. Closed needle biopsy accurately retrieves diagnostic material in 80 to 90 per cent of affected animals if two samples are taken and one includes the center (usually lytic) zone of the tumor. Specific details of biopsy technique are described elsewhere.[28] Ideally, the biopsy is performed by the same person who performs the limb-sparing procedure to allow optimal positioning and minimal biopsy tract contamination. A veterinary pathologist who is well experienced in bone neoplasia and needle core biopsy greatly enhances the accuracy of results.

In addition to biopsy of the primary site, tumor staging includes radiography of the affected limb, regional lymph node palpation with fine-needle aspiration cytological evaluation performed if lymphadenopathy is detected, and thoracic radiography using dorsoventral and both lateral projections. Bone survey radiography is also useful.[23] This includes lateral radiographs of all bones (ventrodorsal of pelvis is preferred) using the standard technique appropriate for the region radiographed. The incidence of second bone lesions detected by bone survey radiography in dogs with osteosarcoma at presentation is 6.4 per cent, which is a higher yield than the incidence of pulmonary metastasis detected by thoracic radiography in the same dogs (4 per cent).[36]

All dogs with osteosarcoma that we treated with limb-sparing procedures have had stage II-B disease.[10, 11] All have had high histological grade primary tumors (B) that have extended through the bone cortices and into adjacent soft tissue (II). Suitable candiates for limb-sparing surgery must otherwise be in good health and have good cardiac, renal, and bone marrow function to tolerate surgery and adjuvant chemotherapy.

Location of the primary tumor is an important consideration in case selection because dogs with primary tumors in the hindlimbs generally do not function as well after limb-sparing surgery as dogs with tumors in the front limbs.[22] Primary tumors around the elbow are rare; we have treated only one case with elbow fusion with good functional results. Proximal femoral lesions have been treated with a proximal femoral allograft and concomitant total hip replacement.[41] Knee fusions have had poor functional results, but custom metallic total knees can be fashioned for dogs to fit into an allograft. Distal tibial tumors can be resected with fusion of the tarsal joint, but infection rates are prohibitively high. Considering the generally excellent function of dogs with rear leg amputation and the high complication rate with limb-sparing surgery in the rear leg, we rarely use salvage procedures for tumors of the femur or tibia. The most suitable dogs for limb sparing are those with tumors in the distal radius. These dogs generally function well, and the period of postoperative rehabilitation is generally shorter than for dogs undergoing limb-sparing surgery for proximal humeral tumors.

ADJUVANT TREATMENT

One of the potential advantages of administering preoperative chemotherapy is reduction in the size and extent of the primary tumor, permitting less extensive, cosmetically acceptable, and function-sparing surgery. Dogs with long-bone osteosarcoma have extension of tumor outside the medullary canal into adjacent soft tissue and periarticular structures. Wide surgical margins are impossible to achieve if limb function is to be preserved, especially in tight compartments such as the distal radius. If effective preoperative treatment is delivered to the tumor, marginal margins (i.e., excision at the level of the tumor pseudocapsule) may allow removal of all residual viable local tumor.

High-dose radiation (36 to 52 Gy) delivered to the affected limb before limb-sparing surgery in dogs, without systemic chemotherapy, resulted in an unacceptably high local complication rate and did not control metastatic disease.[40] Some form of systemic therapy is important for control of micrometastatic cancer in these dogs.

Cisplatin delivered intra-arterially to the tumor-bearing leg with or without external beam irradiation is a viable preoperative treatment. Angiography is performed to identify tumor blood supply. Cisplatin is delivered at 70 mg/m^2 body surface area in an artery proximal to the vessel supplying the tumor via a catheter inserted in the femoral artery (for front leg primaries). This is repeated in 3 weeks. Angiograms performed before limb-sparing surgery, 3 weeks after the second chemotherapy, usually demonstrate decreased tumor vascularity. The change to a hypovascular tumor generally correlates with a high percentage of tumor necrosis when the excised tumor is evaluated histomorphometrically.

Evaluation of the response of the primary tumor by determining percentage of necrosis is a valuable determinant of the effectiveness of preoperative treatment in people.[1, 2, 7, 17, 31, 42] If the percentage of tumor necrosis is low, the response is considered inadequate and the postoperative chemotherapeutic regimen is modified.[31] Percentage of tumor necrosis has been evaluated in resected specimens from dogs with osteosarcoma undergoing various preoperative treatments.[29] Mean percentage of tumor necrosis was as follows: untreated tumors (n = 94) 27 per cent, radiation therapy alone (n = 23) 82 per cent, two doses of intra-arterial cisplatin

*American Pharamaseal Co., Valencia, CA.

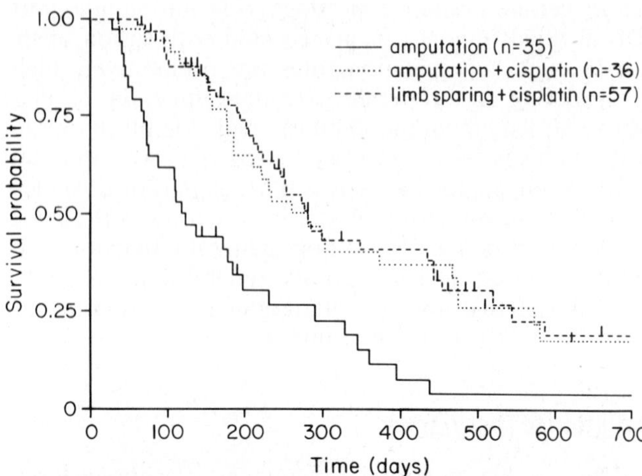

FIGURE 147–1. Kaplan-Meier survival curves for dogs with appendicular osteosarcoma treated with limb-sparing surgery or amputation and receiving cisplatin chemotherapy compared with dogs treated with amputation without chemotherapy. (From Straw RC, et al: Management of canine appendicular osteosarcoma. *Vet Clin North Am 20*:1157, 1990.)

at 70 mg/m^2 dose (n = 14) 45 per cent, two doses of intravenous cisplatin at 70 mg/m^2/dose (n = 6) 24 per cent, two doses of intra-arterial cisplatin at 70 mg/m^2/dose and radiation therapy (n = 45) 82 per cent, and 10 doses of intravenous cisplatin at 10 mg/m^2/dose and radiation therapy (n = 8) 78 per cent. No significant difference was noted between percentage of tumor necrosis in untreated osteosarcoma compared with intravenous cisplatin alone, but a significant increase in percentage of tumor necrosis was present in all other groups. Percentage of tumor necrosis was strongly correlated with local tumor control, because 91 per cent of dogs with greater than 90 per cent tumor necrosis had local control, whereas 78 per cent of dogs with 80 to 89 per cent tumor necrosis had local tumor control and only 30 per cent of dogs with less than 79 per cent tumor necrosis had local control. Because those dogs with radiation as part of their preoperative treatments had higher mean percentage of tumor necrosis, radiation in combination with chemotherapy may have a role in the management of osteosarcoma.

Fifty-seven dogs with osteosarcoma have been treated preoperatively with cisplatin (with or without radiation) before limb-sparing surgery. Comparing survival of these dogs with survival when cisplatin was used with amputation (n = 36), no significant difference is noted. Dogs receiving cisplatin and either limb-sparing procedures or amputation had longer survival times than dogs treated with amputation alone (n = 35) (Fig. 147–1). Limb-sparing operations do not adversely affect survival in selected dogs with appendicular osteosarcoma. Overall, limb function has been satisfactory, with approximately 80 per cent of dogs experiencing good to excellent limb function. Timing of drug administration, route of administration, total cumulative dose effect of new adjuvants and combination chemotherapy and other multimodal treatments are yet to be fully evaluated in dogs with osteosarcoma.

SURGICAL TECHNIQUE

A second-generation cephalosporin antibiotic is administered intravenously immediately preoperatively, during surgery, and for 24 hours afterward. Strict attention is paid to the principles of aseptic technique. A wide area is clipped of hair and thoroughly prepared for surgery. A cloth stockinette is applied, and adhesive waterproof draping material is put over the stockinette. The skin is sewn to the drapes after the primary incision is made.

For a distal radius site, the dog is placed in lateral recumbency, with the affected limb elevated. A skin incision is made on the dorsolateral aspect of the leg from a point just distal to the elbow to just proximal to the metacarpophalangeal joint. Soft tissue is dissected to the level of the tumor pseudocapsule. The individual extensor tendons are not isolated or retracted from the tumor. Care is taken not to enter the tumor. The extensor carpi radialis muscle is transected proximal to the tumor, and the distal part of this muscle and its tendon are removed with the tumor. The common digital extensor tendon usually is closely involved with the tumor pseudocapsule and is also removed with the mass. The bone is cut with an oscillating bone saw 3 to 5 cm proximal to the proximal radiographic margin of the tumor. The distal margin is usually at the radiocarpal joint, although various amounts of carpal bones can be removed. The joint capsule is incised, keeping close to the proximal row of carpal bones. For tumors that have extension to the ulna, the ulna is also cut with a bone saw and the distal third removed with the tumor. Computed tomography is helpful in determining the limits of

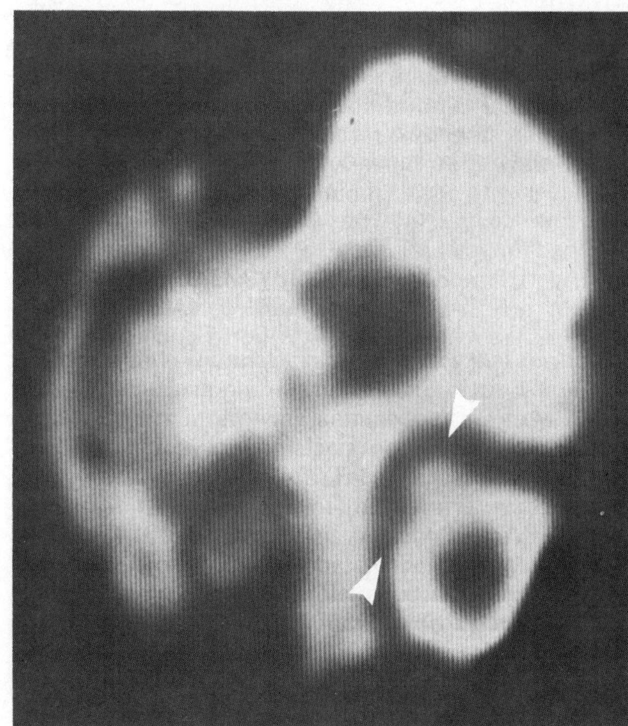

FIGURE 147–2. Computed tomogram of an osteosarcoma of the distal radius. Extension to the ulna is shown by arrows.

tumor extension (Fig. 147–2). Care is taken to preserve as much vasculature as possible, especially on the palmar surface. Large vessels associated with the tumor are ligated and divided. Surgical hemostatic staples* are helpful for deep vessel occlusion. The specimen is radiographed for partial evaluation of margins then submitted for histological evaluation, including assessment of completeness of surgical margins and percentage of tumor necrosis.

A fresh-frozen cortical allograft[41] is thawed in 1 L of an antibiotic/saline solution,† the articular cartilage is removed, the graft is cut to fit, and the medullary cavity reamed to remove fat and cellular debris. The articular cartilage of the proximal carpal bones is removed, and the allograft is stabilized using ASIF principles (Fig. 147–3). A dynamic compression plate (4.5 mm narrow or broad) with a minimum of three screws proximal and four screws distal to the graft is used. Some dogs with narrow metacarpal bones require 3.5-mm screw placement with washers to prevent the screw heads from falling through the plate. Alternatively, a 3.5-mm broad dynamic compression plate can be used with 3.5-mm

*Surgiclip, United States Surgical Corp., New York, NY.

†Neomycin, 1 g; polymixin B, 500,000 U; potassium penicillin, 5,000,000 U.

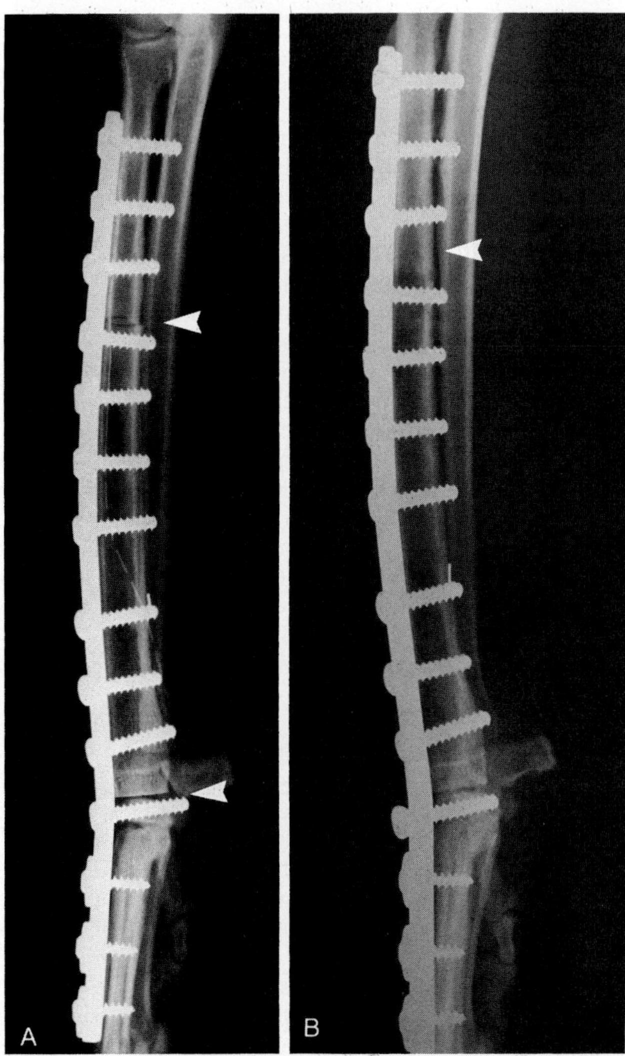

FIGURE 147–4. *A*, Postoperative radiograph of a limb-sparing procedure to remove an osteosarcoma of the distal radius in a 9-year-old female mixed-breed dog. Arrows depict the proximal and distal limits of the allograft. The dog also received two intra-arterial doses of cisplatin. *B*, Radiographic appearance of the same limb 3 months after surgery. Note healing of the proximal graft–host interface *(arrow)*. This dog was still alive and free of disease 9 months after surgery, with excellent limb function.

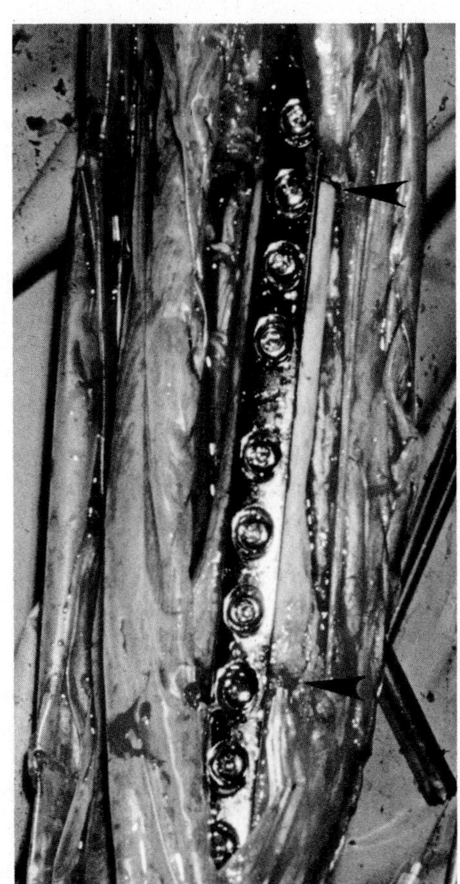

FIGURE 147–3. Intraoperative photograph of a distal forelimb after tumor removal. Allograft *(arrows)* is stabilized using a 4.5-mm dynamic compression plate.

screws. The plate extends distally to a level just proximal to the metacarpophalangeal joint (Fig. 147–4).

With new surgical garments, gloves, and instruments, autogenous cancellous bone graft is procured from the proximal humeral metaphysis or iliac crest and is packed around the host–bone interfaces. A closed suction drain is inserted, and the wound is closed. The leg is supported in a padded bandage. The drain is removed the day after surgery in most cases. To prevent self-mutilation (licking) after surgery, Elizabethan collars are used as necessary. No external splint or cast is used, and most dogs function well soon after surgery. Postoperative swelling can be considerable but usually resolves by 2 weeks. Although exercise is limited for the first 3 to 4 weeks to allow soft tissues to heal, no extensive exercise restriction need apply after this time. It is important that limb use be encouraged even early after surgery to prevent flexure contracture of the digits. Continuation of postoperative antibiotics is controversial, and we have no proof that it is a help or a hindrance in preventing infection.

The principles of resection are the same for other sites; however, because of abundant soft tissue in the area, wider margins are often attained with proximal humerus resections. A lateral approach is made to the proximal humerus via an incision that extends from the proximal spine of the scapula to the distal humerus. Care is taken to identify and protect the radial nerve. It is usually possible to preserve the cephalic vein. The scapulohumeral joint is disarticulated after first incising the transverse band of the intertubercular groove, which allows the biceps brachii to be retracted. Depending on the extent of the tumor, a variable amount of normal musculature is removed with the specimen. Usually included are the spinous head of the deltoid muscle and portions of the infraspinatus, teres minor, and brachial muscles. The ostectomy is performed in the humeral diaphysis about 3 to 5 cm distal to radiographically evident tumor.

Articular cartilage is removed from the glenoid, and the supraspinatus muscle is subperiosteally elevated from the spine of the scapula. A frozen humeral cortical allograft is prepared by thawing and removing the medullary contents and articular cartilage. A 4.5-mm dynamic compression plate that extends from the proximal spine of the scapula to the distal humerus is bent to fuse the shoulder at approximately 90° of flexion. The plate lies on the cranial aspect of the humerus. At least three cortical screws must have purchase in the distal host humerus (Fig. 147–5). It is preferable to make the allograft about 1 to 2 cm shorter than the excised specimen to avoid restriction of elbow flexion. The allograft is held in compression. The biceps brachii is relocated in the intertubercular groove of the allograft. It is usually difficult to attach the pectoral muscle system to the allograft or implant, but failure to relocate the insertion of these muscles is not a problem. A closed suction drainage system is placed in the wound before closure.

Dogs usually show variable signs of radial nerve palsy for the first week after surgery but generally start placing the limb within that week. Passive range of motion of the elbow and physiotherapy begin as early as possible to prevent ankylosis. By about 3 weeks after surgery, the function of the operated limb is usually good, and dogs learn to lengthen the stride by advancement of the scapula rather than shoulder joint extension. Toe dragging has been a problem in some dogs and is related to an overlong allograft, an inappropriate arthrodesis angle, or both. A leather boot can be applied to protect the toes.

RESULTS

Limb-sparing surgery for dogs with primary bone tumors is still in its infancy. At this early stage, in carefully selected cases, limb function can be maintained without adversely affecting survival.[22] Overall function has been satisfactory, with approximately 80 per cent of dogs experiencing good to excellent limb function.[22] Dogs receiving the same dose of cisplatin with either amputation or limb-sparing operations have the same probability of survival.[37] With two intra-arterial doses of cisplatin with or without radiation therapy before limb-sparing procedures, the median survival for dogs is 52 weeks. This is significantly longer than 19.8 weeks when amputation is the only treatment.[35]

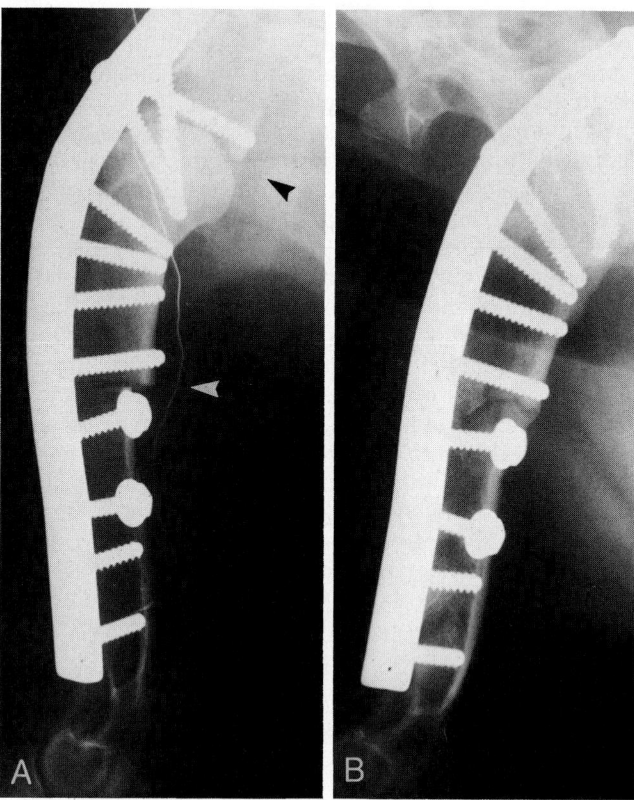

FIGURE 147–5. *A*, Postoperative radiograph of a limb-sparing procedure to remove an osteosarcoma of the proximal humerus in a 7-year-old male golden retriever. Arrows depict the proximal and distal limits of the allograft. *B*, Radiographic appearance of the same limb 9 months after surgery. Note healing of both the proximal and distal graft–host interfaces. This dog was still alive and free of disease 15 months after surgery, with good limb function.

COMPLICATIONS

The local recurrence rate after limb sparing is approximately 20 per cent, but 70 per cent of these dogs can be salvaged with further surgery (amputation or local resection). Local recurrence of osteosarcoma is rarely the cause of death or euthanasia. The infection rate is approximately 30 per cent, but the limb is preserved in 70 per cent of these dogs when treated with long-term antibiotics. For distal radius sites, if the ulna is still present, prognosis for recovery from infection is good. For humeral sites and distal radial sites where the ulna has been removed at the time of limb sparing, however, the prognosis for saving the leg is poor. Surgical intervention is necessary in some cases and includes removal of the radial allograft so the dog bears weight on the plate and ulna, removal of the allograft and replacement with an antibiotic-impregnated cement spacer, placement of antibiotic-impregnated cement beads, or allograft removal and replacement with cancellous autograft (modified Papineau technique).[4] Infection of proximal humeral allografts generally results in amputation because allograft removal is not an option.

Another complication of limb-sparing surgery has been screw loosening in the allograft and host bone. For the radial location, this is radiographically evident from 3 to 9 months postoperatively. The cause is presumed to be related to "normal" revascularization and resorption (creeping substitution) of the allograft. During the healing phase, screws may loosen in the allograft and result in further loosening in the host bone owing to lack of rigid stability. No further surgery is generally performed, and "tightening up" loose screws is not helpful. Replacement of loose screws with larger ones or removal of noncrucial screws can be attempted. Plate removal often results in fracture through the allograft because complete incorporation is not achieved.

Shoulder fusions for proximal humeral lesions place tremendous stress on the distal humeral host bone. Spiral fractures of this bone may develop. Some limbs can be resalvaged with a second plate or cerclage wires, but some require amputation.

CONCLUSIONS

Although limb-sparing surgery is still evolving in veterinary medicine, it is now established as a viable option to amputation in selected dogs with primary bone tumors. Important prerequisites include a dedicated owner and clinician. Limb-sparing surgery is part of an involved multimodal approach and demands close liaison between surgeon, chemotherapist, radiologist, radiation therapist, and pathologist. Major complications include recurrence of local disease due to inadequate excision or preoperative treatment, infection, implant/allograft failure, and failure of adjuvant treatment to control systemic disease.

Research continues to decrease the risk of major complications and improve survival of dogs with primary appendicular bone tumors while maintaining good limb function. Neoadjuvant intra-arterial cisplatin delivered to the primary tumor on two occasions 21 days apart beginning 42 days before operation is appropriate for most dogs. It is extremely rare for the primary tumor not to respond and even less likely for it to progress with the use of intra-arterial cisplatin. Postoperative chemotherapy is also indicated, and depending on the percentage of tumor necrosis in the resected specimen, intravenous cisplatin is recommended every 21 days for four postoperative treatments.

References

1. Ayala AG, et al: The pathologist's role in the diagnosis and treatment of osteosarcoma in children. *Hum Pathol 15*:258, 1984.
2. Bacci G, et al: Neoadjuvant chemotherapy for osteosarcoma of the extremity. *Clin Orthop Rel Res 24*:268, 1987.
3. Bell RS, et al: Timing of chemotherapy and surgery in a canine osteosarcoma model. *Cancer Res 48*:5533, 1988.
4. Bissonette KW: Modified Papineau technique for infected limb salvage cases. Proceedings of the Veterinary Cancer Society, Raleigh, NC, Oct, 1989, p 72.
5. Brodey RS, Abt DA: Results of treatment in 65 dogs with osteosarcoma. *J Am Vet Med Assoc 168*:1032, 1976.
6. Carberry CA, Harvey JH: Owner satisfaction with limb amputation in dogs and cats. *J Am Anim Hosp Assoc 23*:227, 1987.
7. Chuang VP, et al: The therapy of osteosarcoma by intra-arterial cis-platinum and limb preservation. *Cardiovasc Intervent Radiol 4*:229, 1981.
8. Colter SM, Parker LM: High dose methotrexate and leucovorin rescue in dogs with osteogenic sarcoma. *Am J Vet Res 39*:1943, 1978.
9. Ennecking WF: A system of staging musculoskeletal neoplasms. *Clin Orthop Rel Res 204*:9, 1986.
10. Ennecking WF: Staging of musculoskeletal neoplasms. *In* Uhthoff HK (ed): *Current Concepts of Diagnosis and Treatment of Bone and Soft Tissue Tumors*. Springer-Verlag, New York, 1984, pp 1–21.
11. Ennecking WF, et al: A system for surgical staging of musculoskeletal sarcoma. *Clin Orthop 153*:106, 1980.
12. Fisher B, et al: Effect of local or systemic treatment prior to primary tumor removal on the production and response to serum growth-stimulating factor in mice. *Cancer Res 49*:2002, 1989.
13. Frei E III: Clinical cancer research: An embattled species. *Cancer 50*:1979, 1982.
14. Frei E III: What is in a name—neoadjuvant. *J Natl Cancer Inst 80*:1088, 1988.
15. Goorin AM, et al: Osteosarcoma: Fifteen years later. *N Engl J Med 313*:1637, 1985.
16. Hamilton HB, et al: Effect of RA233 on metastasis in dogs with osteosarcomas. *Am J Vet Res 48*:1380, 1987.
17. Jaffe N, et al: Osteosarcoma: Intra-arterial treatment of the primary tumor with cis-diamine-dichloroplatinum-II (CDP): Angiographic, pathologic and pharmacologic studies. *Cancer 51*:402, 1983.
18. Kalifa C, et al: Osteosarcoma—an attempt to reproduce T-10 protocol in a single institution. *Proc Am Soc Clin Oncol 4*:236, 1985.
19. Lane JM, Glasser DB: Staging, margins and functional end results of bone tumor surgery. *In* Coombs R, Friedlaender G (eds): *Bone Tumor Management*. Butterworth, Boston 1987, pp 307–312.
20. Lane JM, et al: Osteogenic sarcoma. *Clin Orthop Rel Res 204*:93, 1986.
21. LaRue SM, Withrow SJ: Tumors of the skeletal system. *In* Withrow SJ, MacEwan EG (eds): *Clinical Veterinary Oncology*. J.B. Lippincott, Philadelphia, 1989, pp 234–252.
22. LaRue SM, et al: Limb-sparing treatment for osteosarcoma in dogs. *J Am Vet Med Assoc 195*:1734, 1989.
23. LaRue SM, et al: Radiographic bone surveys in the evaluation of primary bone tumors in dogs. *J Am Vet Med Assoc 5*:514, 1986.
24. Madewell BR, et al: Amputation and doxorubicin for treatment of canine and feline osteogenic sarcoma. *Eur J Cancer 4*:287, 1978.
25. Mankin HJ, et al: Osteoarticular and intercalary allograft transplantation in the management of malignant tumors of bone. *Cancer 50*:613, 1982.
26. Mauldin GN, et al: Canine osteosarcoma treated by amputation versus amputation and adjuvant chemotherapy using doxorubicin and cisplatin. *J Vet Intern Med 2*:177, 1988.
27. Meyer JA, et al: Canine osteogenic sarcoma treated with amputation and MER: An adverse effect of splenectomy on survival. *Cancer 49*:1613, 1982.
28. Powers BE, et al: Jamshidi needle biopsy for diagnosis of bone lesions in small animals. *J Am Vet Med Assoc 193*:205, 1988.
29. Powers BE, et al: Per cent tumor necrosis as a predictor of treatment response in canine osteosarcoma: A comparison between untreated tumors and tumors after radiation therapy, chemotherapy or the combination. *Cancer 67*:126, 1991.
30. Rosen G: Neo-adjuvant chemotherapy for osteogenic sarcoma. A model for treatment of malignant neoplasms. Recent Results. *Cancer Res 103*:148, 1986.
31. Rosen G, et al: Preoperative chemotherapy for osteogenic sarcoma: Selection of postoperative adjunct chemotherapy based on the response of the primary tumor to preoperative chemotherapy. *Cancer 49*:1221, 1982.
32. Shapiro W, et al: Use of cisplatin for the treatment of appendicular osteosarcoma in dogs. *J Am Vet Med Assoc 4*:507, 1988.
33. Sisson MA: Current concepts review: Limb salvage for osteosarcoma. *J Bone Joint Surg [Am] 70A*:307, 1988.
34. Sisson MA, et al: Limb salvage treatment versus amputation for osteosarcoma of the distal end of the femur. *J Bone Joint Surg [Am] 68A*:1331, 1986.
35. Spodnick GJ, et al: Prognosis for dogs with appendicular osteosarcoma treated by amputation alone: 162 cases (1978–1988). *J Am Vet Med Assoc 200*:995, 1992.
36. Straw RC, et al: Letter: Radiographic bone surveys. *J Am Vet Med Assoc 195*:1458, 1989.
37. Straw RC, et al: Management of canine appendicular osteosarcoma. *Vet Clin North Am 20*:1141, 1990.
38. Straw RC, et al: Amputation and cisplatin for treatment of canine osteosarcoma. *J Vet Intern Med 5*:205, 1991.

39. Theilen GH, et al: Treatment of canine osteosarcoma for limb preservation using osteotomy—adjuvant radiotherapy and chemotherapy (a case report). *Vet Med Small Anim Clin 72*:179, 1977.
40. Thrall DE, et al: Radiotherapy prior to cortical allograft limb sparing in dogs with osteosarcoma: A dose response assay. *Int J Radiat Oncol Biol Phys 18*:1351, 1990.
41. Vasseur P: Limb preservation in dogs with primary bone tumors. *Vet Clin North Am 17*:889, 1987.
42. Winkler K, et al: Neoadjuvant chemotherapy of osteosarcoma: Results of a randomized cooperative trial (COSS-82) with salvage chemotherapy based on histological tumor response. *J Clin Oncol 6*:329, 1988.
43. Winkler K, et al: Neoadjuvant chemotherapy for osteogenic sarcoma: Results of a cooperative German/Austrian study. *J Clin Oncol 2*:617, 1984.
44. Withrow SJ, Hirsch VM: Owner's response to amputation of a pet's leg. *Vet Med Small Anim Clin March 74*:332, 1979.

SECTION 16

Oncology

Dennis D. Caywood ■ *Section Editor*

CHAPTER

148

Biology of Neoplastic Disease

Wallace B. Morrison, Mary Ann Vonderhaar, and Ralph C. Richardson

A vast number of biochemical, genetic, immunological, and anatomical changes occur in cells and tissue as they change from normal to neoplastic. Many characteristics of a normal cell, including growth patterns, are determined both genetically and by the surrounding present and past microenvironment. Neoplastic cells are transformed so they are less affected by their immediate microenvironment and neighboring cells. They grow autonomously without regard for normal intracellular and intercellular regulatory mechanisms. Tumor cells may also gain new properties such as altered cell surface antigens and receptors and enzyme activity and produce peptide and polypeptide hormones.

ETIOLOGY OF NEOPLASIA IN DOGS AND CATS

Various extrinsic and intrinsic causes of neoplasia have been identified.[23, 24] Extrinsic causes include ultraviolet and ionizing radiation, tumor viruses, and chemical carcinogens. Intrinsic causes include diet, hormone effects, genetic predisposition, and age. Individual causes in naturally occurring tumors are often difficult to assess because of overlapping intrinsic and extrinsic influences. In many cases, the cause is unknown. The process of malignant transformation secondary to extrinsic, intrinsic, or unknown causes is discussed later in this chapter.

Irradiation

In experimental circumstances, dogs exposed to ionizing radiation develop many different types of neoplasia. For example, dogs exposed to ^{226}Ra, ^{228}Ra, ^{90}Sr, or ^{239}Pu by intravenous injection develop bone and soft-tissue sarcomas.[24] Inhalation of ^{144}Ce, ^{90}Sr, or ^{239}Pu results in sarcomas and carcinomas of the lung.[24] Injection of ^{226}Ra or ^{144}Ce results in myeloproliferative disorders and leukemia.[24] These experimental findings bear little relevance to induction of spontaneous tumors in dogs, because the doses and the routes of exposure do not realistically reflect normal circumstances.

Although natural exposure to high concentrations of radionuclides is unlikely, exposure to ultraviolet radiation is a common, well-recognized cause of cutaneous squamous cell carcinoma in white cats, white-faced cattle, and possibly collies and Shetland sheepdogs. White cats and white-haired areas (especially ear tips and nose) of multicolored cats are susceptible to chronic inflammatory dermatitis that is exacerbated by exposure to direct sunlight. These inflammatory lesions may evolve to squamous cell carcinoma. Poorly pigmented skin posterior to the planum nasale in dogs may be susceptible to a similar progression of a focal chronic inflammatory dermatitis to squamous cell carcinoma. The prevalence of solar-induced skin tumors is higher in cats than in dogs.[37]

Oncogenic Viruses

The most clinically important oncogenic virus is feline leukemia virus (FeLV). FeLV contains an enzyme known as *reverse transcriptase* (RNA-dependent DNA polymerase) that can copy viral RNA into double-stranded DNA, which can then be integrated into an infected cell's genome. This non-native DNA contains one or more transforming genes whose protein products induce normal cellular oncogenes to mediate malignant transformation. FeLV is the cause of lymphoma, leukemia, and myeloproliferative disease in cats.[23, 24]

Another, less important oncogenic virus is feline sarcoma virus. This virus causes (in the presence of FeLV as a helper virus) multicentric fibrosarcoma in young cats. Feline sarcoma virus is not associated with solitary fibrosarcomas of older cats.

Oncogenic DNA viruses also cause tumors. DNA viruses are either enveloped double-stranded herpesviruses or naked double-stranded papovaviruses or adenoviruses. DNA viruses contain transforming genes whose expression leads to tumor development.[23] In dogs, a DNA papovavirus causes multiple wartlike lesions on oral mucous membranes and the tongue (oral papillomatosis). A papovavirus is also suspected of causing cutaneous papillomas in dogs.

Diet, Hormones, and Prostaglandins

The influence of diet on the development of many neoplasms is well accepted.[48, 49] Epidemiological studies with corroborating rodent studies have linked diet to the pathogenesis of human neoplasms.[2, 6, 47, 48] One of the most suspicious components of diet in mammary tumor development is fat. Body size (obesity) is a closely associated risk factor for tumor development.[48]

The precise relationship between dietary fats and mammary tumorigenesis is unclear. Diets high in fats may influence gut flora to increase deconjugation and reabsorption of steroid hormones that may initiate or promote neoplasia. The small amount of estrogens normally synthesized by gut flora may be enhanced by diets high in fat. Excess dietary fat and obesity are associated with lower levels of the globulins that normally bind sex hormones, resulting in higher concentrations of unbound (active) sex hormone available at target organs for initiation or promotion of malignancy.[48]

Excess dietary fat and obesity may increase the synthesis of prolactin. Studies in animal models suggest that prolactin contributes to mammary tumor development. It has not been established that prolactin secretion has a role in human mammary tumor development. Circumstantial evidence suggests a role for prolactin in canine mammary neoplasia, based on the finding of higher pituitary prolactin concentrations in bitches with mammary neoplasia than in normal intact bitches.[41] As in women, no definitive role for prolactin in mammary tumor development has been established in dogs.

Prostaglandin synthesis may be an important factor in promoting the effects of dietary fat on the risk of mammary tumors.[6] Diets high in linoleic acid are particularly suspect. Prostaglandins are derived from linoleic acid and are synthesized in large amounts by some human mammary neoplasms. The etiological role for prostaglandins is unclear. Prostaglandins probably do participate in some tumor initiation and promotion by regulating cell proliferation, differentiation, and components of the immune system.

Most human and laboratory research dietary studies have focused on the risk for developing mammary neoplasia, not on survival time. No comparable canine studies have assessed the effects of dietary fats on mammary tumor risk. Data from epidemiological studies suggest a longer median survival time after mastectomy for dogs fed low-fat diets (less than 39 per cent, total calories from fat sources). When the diets of dogs with malignant mammary tumors were characterized by the percentage of total calories derived from fat and protein, the median survival time for dogs fed low-fat (< 39 per cent of total calories), high-protein (> 27 per cent of total calories) diets was 3 years. The median survival time for dogs fed low-fat diets with medium amounts of protein (23 to 27 per cent of total calories) was 1.2 years. The median survival time for dogs fed a low-fat, low-protein (< 23 per cent of total calories) diet was 0.5 years.[40]

Chemical Carcinogens

The role of chemical carcinogens in the development of human and animal neoplasms has been extensively studied. Workers in different occupations (painters, farmers, rubber manufacturing workers, hairdressers, truck drivers, and others), exposed to various chemicals, have higher rates of bladder cancer than the general population.[12]

Dogs have been used as experimental models for bladder carcinogenesis and in evaluating the risks of exposure to aromatic amines. The total dose of carcinogen necessary to produce bladder tumors in dogs with aromatic amines is considerably less if given in small amounts for extended periods.[12] This dose and exposure frequency is significant because pet dogs exposed to topical insecticides, particularly flea and tick dips, have been found to have an increased risk of transitional cell carcinoma of the bladder. The risks of developing bladder tumors were highest among dogs receiving more than two applications per year. In the same study, the risk of topical insecticide-associated bladder tumors in pet dogs was enhanced by obesity.[12]

Various active ingredients are found in flea and tick dips, including organophosphates, carbamates, pyrethrins, and pyrethroid compounds. Many pyrethrin and pyrethroid insecticides contain complex chemical synergists that enhance insecticidal activity. Label substances identified as inert ingredients (which may represent up to 96 per cent of many products) are actually petroleum distillates, aromatic petroleum solvents, polyethers, and xylene, which are potential carcinogens.[12]

THE CELL CYCLE AND ITS RELATIONSHIP TO THE TREATMENT OF NEOPLASIA

Normal and rapidly dividing cell populations, such as those in bone marrow and intestinal mucosa, are frequently dose limiting because many cytotoxic drugs and ionizing radiation have their greatest effect on proliferating cells. Normal cells and neoplastic cells cycle through the same phases of cellular activity that precede and follow mitosis.[42]

The cell replication cycle is divided into discrete phases. At the beginning of the completion of mitosis, cells enter a phase of RNA and intracellular protein synthesis (G_1), which precedes the synthesis of DNA. After this, cells enter a phase of DNA synthesis (S). As cells cease to synthesize DNA, they enter another phase of RNA and intracellular protein synthesis (G_2), which occurs immediately before mitosis (M). The G_1 and G_2 phases occur in the gaps (G = gap) between the events of mitosis and DNA synthesis. The duration of S, G_2, and M is fairly constant. In mammalian cells, M phase is consistently brief (30 to 90 minutes), S phase is usually long (8 to 30 hours), and G_2 is brief (approximately 60 minutes). The duration of the G_1 phase varies greatly. The term G_0 has been introduced for cells that are not in cycle but are able to be recruited into the cycle in the G_1 phase. Cells in G_0 are sometimes referred to as *resting* or *nondividing*.[34, 43]

Tumor tissue is extremely heterogeneous with respect to the proportion of cells in any portion of the cycle. The percentage of cells from different human tumors in S phase can vary from 4 to 24 per cent.[42] In a flow cytometric analysis of 82 cases of canine malignant lymphoma, the proportion of cells in S phase varied from 2.27 to 24.30 per cent.[16] The distribution of cells cycling within a tumor may have important implications for therapy, because active cell division is necessary for sensitivity to cytotoxic drugs and ionizing radiation. Many drugs used for chemotherapy are more active in specific phases. Dogs with malignant lymphoma having an increase in cells in S phase or S plus G_2M phases of the cell cycle have shorter first remissions after chemotherapy with doxorubicin hydrochloride than dogs with fewer cells in the same phases of the cell cycle.[16]

Rapidly growing tumors tend to be most sensitive to cytotoxic drug therapy. Some drugs such as the antimetabolite group (e.g., methotrexate) and the vinca alkaloids (e.g., vincristine sulfate) have lethal effects against rapidly dividing cells only. Anthracyclines (e.g., doxorubicin) and most alkylating agents (e.g., cyclophosphamide) have some activity against slowly proliferating cells but are much more active against rapidly dividing cells.[42]

Most antineoplastic drugs and ionizing radiation have cytotoxic effects at different phases of the cycle. Antimetabolite and anthracycline drugs have maximum cytotoxic effects in S phase. Vinca alkaloids also have action in S phase but are most active in M phase. Alkylating drugs and ionizing radiation have two periods of maximum activity, one near transition between G_1 and S phases and one for G_2 phase or M phase.[43]

Regulation and Growth of Normal Cells

Proto-oncogenes are normal genes that control the production of the growth regulatory substances that regulate many of the processes associated with normal cell division, proliferation, and differentiation.[35] The majority of growth regulatory substances are peptide growth factors that stimulate cell proliferation by binding to specific cell surface receptors.[4, 35, 38]

A cascade of biochemical events, initiated by a growth factor, signals the nucleus for proliferation to begin. When a growth factor binds to a surface receptor, the receptor becomes transiently activated and in turn causes activation of other proteins in the growth stimulatory pathway through the production of various second messengers. Ultimately, these signals are transmitted to the cell nucleus, where expression of specific proto-oncogenes and genes is induced, resulting in cell division.[4, 38]

Growth factors are secreted by cells and interact with specific membrane-bound glycoprotein receptors that function as transducers of signals generated by them. Most growth factors are multifunctional and act on a broad range of target cells. Under differing circumstances, the same growth factor may stimulate or inhibit cell proliferation. As a result, a cell's response to a growth factor varies under influences from the extracellular environment. Some normal growth factors for cells such as insulin, insulin-like growth factor, platelet-derived growth factor, epidermal growth factor, transforming growth factors alpha and beta, and the T-lymphocyte growth factor (interleukin-2) are also involved in carcinogenesis.[4, 7, 38]

Growth factors may act as self-stimulants (autocrine), stimulants of nearby cells (paracrine), or stimulants of distant cells (endocrine). Autocrine secretion of growth factors by neoplastic cells is important in uncontrolled growth of tumor cells.[38] If a cell can produce its own growth factors or receptors for them, or if a cell can alter the postreceptor signaling pathway for a growth factor, it may have a growth advantage over other cells that are subject to external regulation.

Signal Transduction

Signal transduction is the process of cellular expression of a proto-oncogene following the interaction of a growth factor with a cell membrane receptor. The best characterized mechanisms of signal transduction involve beta-adrenergic receptors and the signal transducers adenylate cyclase and transducin. Beta-adrenergic receptors are coupled to membrane-bound transducing proteins known as *G proteins* because they bind guanine nucleotides (guanosine triphosphate and guanosine diphosphate). When stimulated by a receptor protein, the G proteins are activated and other intracellular messenger systems are either activated or deactivated. With the beta-adrenergic receptor, the activated G protein stimulates adenylate cyclase, resulting in increased intracellular concentrations of the prototypical second-messenger cyclic adenosine monophosphate (AMP). Second-messenger molecules like cyclic AMP directly or indirectly cause specific intracellular events.[7]

Other common mechanisms of signal transduction involve cellular kinases and phosphatases that add or remove phosphate groups from intracellular enzymes that change cellular growth. Phosphorylation of intracellular enzymes by kinases can dramatically alter enzymatic activity and cellular growth. Kinases may be activated directly by stimulated receptors or indirectly by second messengers such as cyclic AMP generated by G protein–dependent pathways.[7, 8, 26, 35]

The activation of a kinase known as *maturation promoting factor* is the immediate trigger for cell division. During the cellular events preceding mitosis, a protein activator of maturation promoting factor known as *cyclin* gradually increases in its intracellular concentration until maturation promoting factor becomes active and cell division begins. At this point, the cyclin is abruptly degraded, mitosis is completed, and the whole cycle repeats.[26]

NEOPLASTIC TRANSFORMATION AND GROWTH OF CELLS

Oncogenes are derived from normal proto-oncogenes and are either altered or overexpressed versions of their normal cellular proto-oncogene counterparts. Because proto-oncogenes are normal constituents of a cell's genetic complement, they become pathological only when their structure or control is disturbed by oncological events. The term *proto-oncogenes* is confusing and misleading because it incorrectly implies that they reside in the genome for the sole purpose of expressing the malignant phenotype, when they are essential to normal activity such as cell division.[4, 35]

Oncogenes are genes that are capable of inducing or maintaining cell transformation to a malignant phenotype. Oncogenes can be activated from proto-oncogenes by such processes as insertional mutagenesis (the insertion of foreign DNA sequences into a defined genetic locus from, for example, a retrovirus), chromosomal rearrangements (often involving the *c-myc* locus), and by point mutations (*ras* oncogenes are activated by mutations in specific DNA codons).[3, 4, 7, 35]

Oncogenes encode for the synthesis of oncoproteins, which are similar to the normal products of the proto-oncogenes except they have lost important regulatory constraints on their activity and do not need external activation.[7] When oncoproteins replace normal proteins in signal transduction, oncogenesis may occur. It is not clear when oncogenes act in the cell cycle, but they may prevent cells from returning to normal after division.[26] The *ras* family of oncogenes, which is one of the most frequently identified oncogenes in human and animal tumors, functions through unregulated G-protein activation.[35, 45, 51]

Oncogenes act in a dominant manner if expression of one transforming allele contributes to the neoplastic phenotype. Loss of antioncogenes from a cell's karyotype can promote cell growth, with results similar to activation of a growth-promoting oncogene. Antioncogenes, also known as *tumor-suppressing* genes, regulate cell growth.[4, 8, 44]

The existence of antioncogenes was first suggested by hybridization experiments. The fusion of a normal cell with a malignant cell frequently resulted in a benign hybrid. This observation supports the idea that transformation of a normal cell to a malignant cell often involved the loss of antioncogenes that were restored to the neoplastic cell after fusion with a normal partner. This suggests that malignancy is a recessive trait that follows loss of antioncogenes. For example, retinoblastoma is a heritable tumor in humans that results from a homozygous deletion (Rb gene) that allows uncontrolled growth of the mutated cells.[4, 8, 45]

Many descriptions of tumor development involve a time-dependent multistep (initiation and progression) process.[8] The first step of initiation may be associated with various stimuli, such as viral, environment, or dietary influences that activate a dominant oncogene or inactivate a pair of recessive antioncogenes.

The events involved in progression of neoplasia are less clear. The genetic alterations that initiate the malignant phenotype are not necessarily involved in progression. This is why activated oncogenes are not always detected in advanced neoplasia.[8]

Amplification of proto-oncogenes (an increased number of copies of the proto-oncogene in the cancer cell genome) has been implicated in progression of the neoplastic phenotype. Amplification of proto-oncogenes is an occasional feature of a diverse group of tumors and a recurrent abnormality of specific proto-oncogenes in particular tumors.[3, 4, 35, 51] The *c-myc, L-myc,* and *N-myc* oncogenes are important components of amplified DNA in several human tumors.[4] The exact causes of gene amplification are obscure, but amplification has only been detected in cells that have taken at least some of the steps toward neoplastic growth.[4]

Metastasis

Neoplasms are composed of subpopulations of cells that differ in growth rate, karyotype, surface receptors, susceptibility to cytotoxic drugs, and other biological characteristics. They can also have subpopulations that form early in the development of the primary tumor and that have the ability for metastasis.[21] For a cell to metastasize successfully, it must leave the primary tumor (or a metastatic site), invade local host tissue, enter into and survive in circulation, arrive at a distant vascular bed, enter into the parenchyma and interstitium of a tissue, and multiply to form a metastatic colony.[9, 21] As a result of these demanding requirements, not all cells can successfully metastasize.

The transition from an *in situ* to a locally invasive neoplasia is accompanied by angiogenesis.[9–11, 40] Angiogenesis is the development of new blood vessels that may serve the nutritional needs of a growing tumor or may support and assist invasion into adjacent normal tissue.[10, 14, 21] An enzyme known as *collagenase type IV* and other enzymes such as heparinase and cathepsins make it easier for cells to penetrate the often defective basement membrane of newly formed blood vessels within the primary tumor. Distant metastases can develop when cancer cells enter the general circulation as single cells or in clumps. Single cells or clusters of cells in circulation can attach to intact endothelium or to exposed areas of subendothelial basement membrane.[21] Clumps of tumor cells, often aggregated with fibrin, host leukocytes, or host platelets, can embolize precapillary venules. Tumor cells that attach to venule or capillary endothelium induce rapid retraction of endothelial cells, exposing basement membrane to which the cells can then adhere via surface matrix receptors. The retracted endothelial cells are free to migrate over the tumor cells and isolate them from the circulation. Tumor cells degrade the basement membrane over a period of 8 to 24 hours by secreting various proteases and collagenases (including collagenase type IV). Tumor cell pseudopodia penetrate the basement membrane and the cell becomes "extravasated" into the surrounding tissue.[20, 21, 35]

Endothelial retraction also occurs after arterial localization. Intra-arterial tumor colonies may grow large enough to fill the vessel and damage endothelium, thereby exposing basement membrane for additional cell attachment. Tumor cells extravasated to an extravascular location can proliferate into colonies, but angiogenesis must occur before they can grow to larger than 0.5 mm.[10]

Because neoplasms generally lack a well-developed lymphatic system, their cells communicate with lymphatic channels only at the tumor periphery and not within the tumor mass.[14, 21] Neoplastic cells that do enter lymphatic channels are carried to lymph nodes and quickly (within 10 to 60 minutes) leave by efferent lymphatics. Cells that enter the lymphatic network frequently enter the systemic venous drainage via numerous lymphatic-hematogenous communications. Regional lymph nodes thus do not function as true mechanical barriers to neoplastic cell dissemination.[21]

Although patterns of metastasis vary widely, the most frequent localization of metastasis is likely to be in the first capillary bed encountered by the circulating cells. Metastases from some types of tumors demonstrate an organ trophism because not all patterns of metastasis can be predicted from anatomical patterns alone.[21]

Many oncogenes have been associated with the genetic and biochemical events that lead to tumor growth, invasion, and metastasis. *In vitro* studies have demonstrated the *ras* family of oncogenes capable of inducing the metastatic phenotype.[4, 21] Activation of *N-ras* allele in a dog with radiation-induced acute nonlymphocytic leukemia has been described.[25] Increased expression of the *H-ras* oncogene is correlated with lymph node metastasis in human breast carcinoma.[51]

Amplification of the *HER-2/neu* oncogene is correlated with metastatic human breast carcinoma.[5, 18, 39] In one study of 189 primary human breast neoplasia specimens, *HER-2/neu* was amplified in 30 per cent of the tumors and amplification was a significant predictor for overall survival, time to relapse, estrogen receptor status, size of primary tumor, and number of axillary lymph nodes positive for metastasis.[39] Overexpression (increased amounts of gene product) of *HER-2/neu* and *c-myc* is common in canine mammary carcinoma and melanoma cell lines and suggests these genes may be involved in alteration of growth regulation and neoplasia.[1]

Metastasis from Cancer of Unknown Primary Origin

Tumors of unknown primary origin are metastases from a primary tumor that cannot be detected. A useful clinical definition of tumor of unknown primary origin is a biopsy-proven malignancy without a demonstrable source of a primary neoplasm as determined by medical history, physical examination, complete blood count, serum biochemical analysis, urinalysis, thoracic and abdominal radiographs, and where indicated prostatic massage, bronchoalveolar lavage, cerebrospinal fluid analysis, ophthalmic examination, and endoscopic investigations. Computed tomographic and magnetic resonance scans also fail to identify the primary neoplasm in patients with tumors of unknown primary origin.

Although derived from different tissues of origin, these tumors have important common biological characteristics. They display a marked degree of malignancy and metastasis early in primary development when the tumor is still small. The primary tumor may subsequently involute or retain its initial small size because of a slow growth rate while the metastatic sites proliferate aggressively.[28]

These tumors are malignant from the outset (type II progression) rather than evolving from benign to malignant (type I progression). Although many canine tumors such as oral melanoma and osteosarcoma are type II progressors in that no definitive premalignant lesions have even been identified, tumors of unknown primary origin differ from these tumors because they have no demonstrable primary site and do not retain any pattern of metastatic spread that would be dictated by the organ from which they arose. Once such a tumor is identified, there is no way to predict when or where additional metastases will appear.[29]

Carcinoma is the most frequent of such tumors in dogs. Affected dogs are usually 7 years or older, large (> 18 kg), physically impaired at the time of diagnosis, and affected with various nonspecific clinical signs such as weakness, cough, pain, and anorexia. Survival is poor.[29]

NEOPLASTIC CELL ADAPTATIONS TO SURVIVE CHEMOTHERAPY

Successful chemotherapy for malignant neoplasia is frequently made impossible by the development of drug resistance. Resistance of neoplastic cells to chemotherapy may be acquired after exposure to cytotoxic drugs or may be a property of the cells from the onset of malignant transformation (*de novo* resistance). Neoplastic cell populations that exhibit acquired drug resistance are at first responsive to chemotherapy, but the initial clinical remission is followed by an untreatable relapse. Tumors that exhibit *de novo* resistance are, by definition, refractory to treatment with cytotoxic drugs and carry a poor prognosis.[30]

Cellular resistance to individual drugs usually depends on circumvention of a specific intracellular process that is targeted by the drug. In single-drug resistance, the mechanism is usually not effective for different classes of cytotoxic drugs. Mechanisms of single-drug resistance include decreased uptake by drug-specific transport mechanisms, decreased activation of pro-drugs, changes in target enzymes, alterations in cellular metabolism and repair mechanisms, and increased inactivation. Gene mutation and amplification account for some of these mechanisms.[31]

Multidrug Resistance

Multidrug resistance occurs when acquired resistance to a single drug simultaneously confers resistance to classes of drugs that are structurally and functionally different. Multidrug resistance is a difficult clinical problem. Although structurally and functionally dissimilar, drugs associated with multidrug resistance all are hydrophobic compounds derived predominantly from plants and fungi.[17, 31] A major mechanism of multidrug resistance in some neoplastic cells involves the increased expression of a specific gene *(Mdr-1)* that codes for the expression of a 170-kilodalton plasma membrane glycoprotein known as *P glycoprotein* (Pgp).[17, 19, 31, 36]

Structural analysis of Pgp reveals that it forms an adenosine triphosphate (ATP)-binding transmembrane pore through which it actively effluxes drugs.[17] Drug uptake and release studies of cells with multidrug resistance have shown that they can acquire, by overexpression of *Mdr-1*, the ability to pump drugs out of the cell without changing the rate of drug entry into the cell. Doxorubicin, vinblastine, dactinomycin, and colchicine enter cells by passive diffusion but are actively effluxed when resistance develops.[36]

It is assumed that resistant tumor cells expressing the multidrug-resistant phenotype possess an enhanced form of a normal cellular protective mechanism. The same transport mechanism provides protection to normal cells by the efflux of environmental toxins.[17, 31] Just how a single Pgp molecule can recognize and bind various types of substrates and how multidrug-resistant cells express different patterns of cross-resistance is unclear. Pgp is highly conserved among distantly related species and is a member of a superfamily of transport proteins.[17] A similar molecule mediates multidrug resistance in the malaria-causing parasite *Plasmodium falciparum*.[17, 31]

The clinical consequences of the overexpression of Pgp with respect to determining a patient's sensitivity to chemotherapy is not completely understood. In some studies, the amount of Pgp is higher in tumor biopsy samples obtained after relapse from chemotherapy than before treatment.[17] The full significance of Pgp expression with respect to clinical response is undetermined.

Some drugs such as verapamil can reverse multidrug resistance *in vitro*. Verapamil is a calcium channel antagonist that binds to Pgp to inhibit drug efflux. Unfortunately, the concentrations of verapamil needed to reverse multidrug resistance *in vivo* result in excessive clinical toxicity.[13, 17, 31]

The recognition of Pgp has advanced the understanding of neoplastic cells exhibiting multidrug resistance. Although Pgp is not the only mechanism of multidrug resistance, it is generally accepted as important in chemotherapy failure.[17, 31]

PARANEOPLASTIC SYNDROMES

Paraneoplastic syndromes are diverse systemic disorders associated with neoplasia but due to noninvasive actions of a tumor. Paraneoplastic syndromes are unrelated to size, location, metastasis, or physiological activities of the tissue of origin and may precede or accompany the inciting tumor (Table 148–1).[29] The incidence of paraneoplastic syndromes among animal patients with neoplasia is unknown, but approximately 75 per cent of human patients experience paraneoplastic syndromes at some time during the disease.[33] The recognition of a paraneoplastic syndrome is important because (1) the observed abnormality may represent a hallmark of a specific tumor and facilitate early diagnosis and treatment; (2) it may help quantify and monitor the response to therapy; and (3) it may aid in the evaluation of tumor recurrence or disease progression.[33]

Paraneoplastic syndromes frequently result from the inappropriate production of peptide and polypeptide hormones by tumor cells that are released into the circulation and cause unphysiological effects at distant target organs. This phenomenon is sometimes referred to as *ectopic hormone production*. These effects are often mediated by cells that constitute the APUD (amine precursor uptake and decarboxylation) cell system. The APUD cell system is a diffuse system of neuroendocrine cells that shares a common capacity for peptide and polypeptide secretion. Tumors containing functional APUD cells (apudomas) may produce single or multiple hormones so that a wide variety of clinical syndromes are possible.

Neoplasia-Associated Hypercalcemia

Neoplasia-associated hypercalcemia is characterized by persistent elevations of serum calcium (> 12 mg/100ml). Clinical signs are related to the role of calcium in normal physiology (maintaining stability and excitability of neuronal membranes and in the contractility of smooth, skeletal, and cardiac muscle). Hypercalcemia can result in mental depression, mental weakness, anorexia, vomiting, and various arrhythmias. Calcium nephropathy and renal failure may follow hypercalcemia if the calcium and phosphorus product (total serum calcium multiplied by serum phosphorus) exceeds 70. Polyuria with a compensatory polydipsia may be an early sign of hypercalcemia because calcium ions decrease the sensitivity of the distal convoluted tubules and collecting ducts to antidiuretic hormone.[30]

Measured serum calcium concentrations may need to be adjusted after considerations of blood pH and total protein. Because approximately half of the total serum calcium is nonionized and bound to albumin, hypoalbuminemia lowers the normal upper limit of serum calcium by relatively increasing the unbound form. Acidosis disturbs this equilibrium between nonionized and ionized calcium (bound and unbound) in favor of the ionized form. Total serum calcium based on serum albumin concentration and total protein concentration may be corrected according to the following formulas[27, 28]:

$$\text{Corrected serum Ca} = \text{measured Ca} - \text{albumin} + 3.5$$

$$\text{Corrected serum Ca} = \text{Ca} - (0.4 \times \text{total protein}) + 3.5$$

Neoplasia-associated hypercalcemia has been described with various benign and malignant conditions in veterinary patients. The most common tumors associated with hypercalcemia are malignant lymphoma, apocrine gland adenocarcinoma of the anal sac, multiple myeloma, and parathyroid adenoma. The general mechanism involved in the pathogenesis of neoplasia-associated hypercalcemia as a paraneoplastic syndrome (not due to direct lysis of bone or bone marrow) is inappropriate production of circulating humoral factors by neoplastic cells, causing osteoclastic bone reabsorption. Factors that different investigators have identified as causing hypercalcemia include parathormone-like, vitamine D–like, osteoclast activating factors, and prostaglandins (E type).[27, 29, 30]

The mechanism of hypercalcemia in dogs with malignant lymphoma is unclear. In some cases it is hormonally mediated, whereas in others it may result from production of a locally acting bone-reabsorbing factor. Proposed bone-reabsorbing factors include prostaglandins and a family of proteins known collectively as *osteoclast activating factors*.[27] The humoral factor responsible for hypercalcemia in dogs with malignant lymphoma has been tentatively identified as a 50,000-dalton protein that interacts with parathyroid hormone receptors and has potent adenyl cyclase stimulating activity.[47]

Hypercalcemia associated with apocrine cell adenocarcinoma of the anal sac is purely humoral because resection of the tumor results in normocalcemia and local or metastatic recurrence results in recurrent hypercalcemia.[27] The humoral factor causing hypercalcemia in dogs with apocrine cell adenocarcinoma is a potent stimulator of adenyl cyclase activity and is a large

TABLE 148–1. SOME PARANEOPLASTIC SYNDROMES OF DOGS AND CATS

Paraneoplastic Syndrome	Major Inciting Tumor Type	Species Affected
Hypercalcemia	Malignant lymphoma	Dog, cat
	Apocrine cell carcinoma of anal sac	Dog
	Parathyroid tumor	Dog
	Multiple myeloma	Dog
	Mammary adenocarcinoma	Dog
	Others	
Altered coagulability		
Platelet dysfunction	Multiple myeloma	Dog
Hyperheparinemia	Mast cell	Dog, cat
Disseminated intravascular coagulation	Hemangiosarcoma	Dog
	Thyroid carcinoma	Dog
	Others	
Hypoglycemia	Pancreatic islet cell tumor	Dog, cat
	Leiomyoma	Dog
	Others	
Eosinophilia	Fibrosarcoma	Dog
	Others	
Anemia	Sertoli cell tumor	Dog
	Various leukemias	Dog, cat
	Hemangiosarcoma	Dog
	Others	
Gastroduodenitis	Pancreatic nonislet cell tumor (Zollinger-Ellison)	Dog, cat
	Mast cell	Dog, cat
	Others	
Hyperviscoscity	Multiple myeloma	Dog
	Malignant lymphoma	Dog
	Mammary adenocarcinoma	Dog
	Others	
Polycythemia	Renal carcinoma	Dog
	Renal lymphoma	Dog
	Fibrosarcoma	Dog
	Others	
Immune complex disease	Lymphocytic leukemia	Dog
	Others	
Hypertrophic osteopathy	Primary lung tumors	Dog
	Metastatic lung tumors	Dog
	Esophageal carcinoma	Dog
	Rhabdomyosarcoma of bladder	Dog
	Others	
Neutrophilic leukocytosis	Fibrosarcoma	Dog
	Liposarcoma	Dog
	Others	
Bone marrow failure	Sertoli cell tumor	Dog
	Ovarian carcinoma	Dog
Myasthenia gravis	Thymoma	Dog, cat
Fever	Various tumors	Dog, cat
Hyperadrenal corticism	Pancreatic islet cell	Dog
Anorexia/cachexia	Various tumors	Dog, cat
Diencephalic syndrome	Astrocytoma	Dog
Nephrotoxicity	Multiple myeloma	Dog
	Others	

70,000-dalton protein.[47] Hypercalcemia associated with multiple myeloma results from osteolysis caused by the elaboration and local action of bone-reabsorbing factors.[26]

Hypercalcemia associated with parathyroid adenoma results from an overproduction of an appropriate hormone (parathyroid hormone) for the tumor type rather than secretion of a hormone that is inappropriate for the tumor tissue type.

Hypoglycemia

Hypoglycemia caused by neoplasia is most commonly associated with insulinoma but does occur with other types of tumors. Any large mesenchymal tumor may cause hypoglycemia by mechanisms that include the production of insulin-like substances, excessive glucose consumption by the tumor, concurrent hepatic disease, and malnutrition.[29]

Hypoglycemia with insulinoma has detectable elevations of serum insulin. The amended glucose-to-insulin (AGIR) ratio is helpful in demonstrating the presence of an insulin-secreting tumor:

$$\text{AGIR} = \frac{\text{Serum insulin (uU/ml)} \times 100}{\text{Serum glucose (mg/100 ml)} - 30}$$

If the serum glucose level is 30 or less, a value of 1 is used in the denominator. Insulin-secreting tumors are characterized by an AGIR of more than 30. The AGIR may be elevated in dogs with sepsis or nonpancreatic tumors.[46]

Hypertrophic Osteopathy

Hypertrophic osteopathy occurs secondary to malignant and nonmalignant diseases in the thorax or abdomen. Most cases are due to metastatic or primary neoplastic pulmonary disease. In dogs, hypertrophic osteopathy is more commonly associated with primary lung tumors than with metastatic tumors when the incidence of metastatic tumors relative to primary lung tumors is considered. Rhabdomyosarcoma of the bladder without metastases and carcinoma of the liver with foci of pulmonary atelectasis also result in hypertrophic osteopathy.[15, 30, 42]

Clinical signs usually include a history of gradual or occasionally sudden onset of lameness and reluctance to move. All four limbs are usually affected simultaneously. Duration of signs before diagnosis ranges from 1 day to 7 months. Hypertrophic osteopathy is characterized by a rapid increase in peripheral blood flow to the distal extremities, stimulating connective tissue and periosteal proliferation. These proliferative changes are responsible for the clinical signs.[15, 42]

The cause is unknown, but several mechanisms have been proposed. Hypertrophic osteopathy develops, at least in part, as a result of neural afferent component. Afferent impulses, traveling in the vagus and intercostal nerves from the lesion to the central nervous system, may be responsible for initiating development. There is at least one case report of resolution of hypertrophic osteopathy after vagotomy. Another possible explanation involves localized neural hypoxia from shunting of blood caused by the tumor, resulting in a reflex osteopathy. A hormonal cause has also been proposed.[15, 42]

Treatment has included lobectomy, tumor removal, vagal resection, intercostal nerve resection, and chemotherapy.[15] Treatment failure is usually related to recurrence of the tumor or metastases.

Hyperviscosity Syndrome

Hyperviscosity syndrome is usually associated with monoclonal gammopathies in patients with multiple myeloma. As the amount of an abnormal protein in the serum increases, the serum viscosity increases. Clinical signs are related to altered central nervous system function, such as ataxia, dementia, depression, and coma. Retinopathies with engorgement of retinal vessels, retinal hemorrhages, and congestive heart failure have also been reported in dogs. In one survey, hyperviscosity syndrome accompanied 20 per cent of monoclonal gammopathies. Abnormal serum proteins may be macroglobulins or myeloma-type proteins. Specific immunoglobulins involved may be IgM, IgG, or IgA. Although IgA is a small molecule, it can polymerize into larger proteins. Bleeding episodes may result from the antagonistic effects of the abnormal proteins on platelet aggregation and release of platelet factor 3.[29, 30, 33]

Treatment is directed at control of the inciting tumor. Emergency phlebotomy may be performed with concurrent replacement of blood with an equal volume of isotonic fluids.

Fever

Fever is a paraneoplastic syndrome that accompanies many types of neoplasia. When fever is a paraneoplastic syndrome, it is usually low grade and unresponsive to antibiotics. Fever associated with malignancy is due to production of interleukin-1 (endogenous pyrogen) by macrophages or tumor cells, acting on the hypothalamus to increase local synthesis of prostaglandins. The normal set-point of the hypothalamus is raised, and physiological responses such as peripheral vasoconstriction diminish heat loss and result in fever. Drugs that inhibit prostaglandin synthesis may mask the presence of malignancy by inhibiting fever.[29, 33]

Altered Coagulability

Hypocoagulable and hypercoagulable states can accompany neoplasia. Alterations in normal hemostasis usually accompany tumors that cause platelet dysfunction, disseminated intravascular coagulation, or heparin excess.

Platelet dysfunction is occasionally noted in patients with neoplasia and is most frequently observed with gammopathies from multiple myeloma. Abnormal varities or amounts of serum proteins may adhere to platelets and interfere with their normal function, causing hemorrhage.[29]

Mast cell tumors, especially multiple or invasive tumors, are associated with hyperheparinemia. Excessive heparin production may cause prolonged bleeding time and complicate hemostasis after biopsy or surgery.[30]

Disseminated intravascular coagulation may occur as a consequence of almost any serious systemic disease and results in hemorrhage from the combined effects of platelet consumption (thrombocytopenia), clotting factor consumption, and increased amounts of fibrin degradation products (anticoagulant effect). With neoplasia, it is often associated with tumors that are rich in tissue thromboplastin, such as the liver, thyroid and prostate tumors. Hemangiosarcoma is frequently associated with disseminated intravascular coagulation in dogs. In a patient with extensive neoplasia and disseminated intravascular coagulation, the prognosis is usually poor.

Hemorrhagic Gastroduodenitis

Histamine from mast cell tumors in dogs and cats stimulates specific receptors (H_2) on gastric parietal cells, resulting in stimulation of hydrochloric acid production. Excess gastric and duodenal acidity can cause inappetence and vomiting secondary to mucosal ulceration.

Pancreatic nonbeta-cell tumors in dogs and cats that inappropriately secrete gastrin (Zollinger-Ellison syndrome in humans) may cause gastric and duodenal ulceration. Both tumor types can lead to life-threatening gastric and duodenal bleeding and serosal perforation.

Symptomatic treatment with an H_2-receptor antagonist like cimetidine or ranitidine, combined with a surface protectant such as sucralfate, may palliate symptoms, but prompt treatment of the inciting tumor is usually necessary to relieve clinical signs. If an H_2-receptor antagonist is administered with sucralfate, the sucralfate should be given first because it needs an acid environment to become active.[29]

Misoprostol is a synthetic prostaglandin E_1 that has antisecretory and cytoprotective properties that may be of use in treating gastric and duodenal ulceration. Misoprostol is used in humans to alleviate gastric and duodenal ulceration induced by nonsteroidal anti-inflammatory drugs.[50] Our preliminary experience with misoprostol in treatment of mast cell tumor–associated gastric ulceration is encouraging. A dosage of 6 mg/kg every 12 hours is recommended.

Cachexia

Metabolic alterations in lipid, protein, and carbohydrate metabolism alone or in combination with other factors (impaired digestion and absorption, concurrent anorexia, and external nutrient loss in effusion, exudate, urine, and stool) may result in a net energy loss to the host although adequate calories are consumed. Profound weight loss in patients with neoplasia under these circumstances is known as *cancer cachexia*.[33, 44]

Neoplastic cell metabolism may be characterized by incomplete aerobic metabolism that, for normal cells, yields energy via the Krebs cycle. Metabolism via alternate anaerobic pathways (Cori cycle) consumes far more energy than is produced. Under normal aerobic conditions, 1 mole of glucose is metabolized to 36 moles of ATP (energy) via the Krebs cycle. When neoplastic cells metabolize glucose anaerobically, only 2 moles ATP and a surplus of lactate are produced. Inefficient anaerobic metabolism requires large amounts of glucose that deprive normal cells of glucose they need. The surplus lactate is converted back to glucose in the liver by a pathway that consumes 12 moles of ATP to convert 1 mole of lactate to 1 mole of glucose. Serum lactate concentrations in dogs with malignant lymphoma are significantly higher than in normal dogs. The same study found serum insulin concentrations greater than those of normal dogs in response to an intravenous glucose tolerance test.[44]

Protein catabolism may be a prominent part of cancer cachexia. Amino acids derived from host proteins are used for tumor protein synthesis and, in addition to lactate, gluconeogenesis.[33] Depletion of body fat can be dramatic. Increases in host lipolysis and oxidation of lipids for energy lead to a severe loss of body fat.[33, 44]

Diencephalic Syndrome

The diencephalic syndrome is an uncommon paraneoplastic syndrome of dogs and human infants. It is characterized by a diencephalic tumor (often as astrocytoma or other glial cell tumor) that is accompanied by dysfunction of the hypothalamus, hypophysis, and autonomic nervous system. In addition, high serum concentration of growth hormone results in severe lipolysis and weight loss despite the intake of adequate calories. Paradoxically, acromegaly is not a clinical feature of this syndrome even though serum growth hormone concentration may be markedly elevated.[32]

References

1. Ahern TE, et al: C-myc and HER-2/neu proto-oncogene over-expression and restriction fragment length polymorphisms in canine tumors and tumor-derived cell lines. Proceedings of the 9th Annual Conference, Veterinary Cancer Society, Raleigh, N.C., Oct. 1989, pp 81–82.
2. Albanes D: Total calories, body weight and tumor incidence in mice. *Cancer Res 47*:1987, 1987.
3. Bishop JM: The molecular genetics of cancer. *Science 235*:305, 1987.
4. Burck KB, et al: Oncogenes: An introduction to the concept of cancer genes. Springer-Verlag, New York, 1988.
5. Cline MJ, et al: Proto-oncogene abnormalities in human breast cancer: Correlations with anatomic features and clinical course of disease. *J Clin Oncol 5*:999, 1987.
6. Cohen LA, et al: Dietary fat and mammary cancer. II. Modulation of serum and tumor lipid composition and tumor prostaglandins by different dietary fats: Association with tumor incidence patterns. *J Natl Cancer Inst 77*:43, 1986.
7. Druker BJ, et al: Oncogenes, growth factors, and signal transduction. *N Engl J Med 321*:1383, 1989.
8. Dulbecco R: Cancer progression: The ultimate challenge. *Int J Cancer 4(Suppl)*:6, 1989.
9. Fidler IJ, Hart IR: Biologic diversity in metastatic neoplasms. Origins and implications. *Science 217*:998, 1982.
10. Folkman J: Tumor angiogenesis. *Adv Cancer Res 43*:175, 1985.
11. Furcht LT: Critical factors controlling angiogenesis: Cell products, cell matrix, and growth factors. *Lab Invest 55*:505, 1986.
12. Glickman LT, et al: Epidemiologic study of insecticide exposures, obesity, and risk of bladder cancer in household dogs. *J Toxicol Environ Health 28*:407, 1989.
13. Gottesman M, Pastan I: Clinical trials of agents that reverse multidrug resistance. *J Clin Oncol 7*:409, 1989.
14. Gullino PM, Grantham F: The vascular space of growing tumors. *Cancer Res 24*:1727, 1964.
15. Hahn KA, Richardson RC: Cisplatin chemotherapy: An effective method of controlling metastatic malignant mesenchynoma and hypertrophic osteopathy in a dog. *J Am Vet Med Assoc 195*:351, 1989.
16. Hamilton TA: Prognostic value of flow cytometric DNA analysis of canine lymphoma. Proceedings of the 10th Annual Conference, Veterinary Cancer Society, Auburn, Ala., Nov. 1990, p 63.
17. Juranka PF, et al: P-glycoprotein: Multidrug-resistance and a superfamily of membrane-associated transport proteins. *FASEB J 3*:2583, 1989.
18. Kolata G: Oncogenes give breast cancer prognosis. *Science 235*:160, 1987.
19. Kramer RA, et al: Role of glutathione redox cycle in acquired and *de novo* multidrug resistance. *Science 241*:694, 1988.
20. Lapis K, et al: Endothelization of embolised tumor cells during metastasis formation. *Clin Exp Metastasis 6*:73, 1988.
21. Liotta LA, Stetler-Stevenson WG: Principles of molecular cell biology of cancer: Cancer metastasis. *In* DeVita VT, et al (eds): *Cancer: Principles and Practice of Oncology*. 3rd ed. J.B. Lippincott, Philadelphia, 1989, pp 98–115.
22. Liotta CA: Tumor invasion and metastasis: Role of the extracellular matrix. *Cancer Res 46*:1, 1986.
23. MacEwen EG: Cancer overview: Epidemiology, etiology, and prevention. *In* Withow SJ, MacEwen EG (eds): *Clinical Veterinary Oncology*. J.B. Lippincott, Philadelphia, 1989, pp 3–15.
24. Madewell BR, Theilen GH: Etiology of cancer in animals. *In* Theilen GH, Madewell BR (eds): *Veterinary Cancer Medicine*. 2nd ed. Lea & Febiger, Philadelphia, 1987, pp 13–25.
25. Madewell BR, et al: Ras proteins detected and discriminated in canine neoplasms by selective use of antisera. Proceedings of the 9th Annual Conference, Veterinary Cancer Society, Raleigh, N.C., Oct. 1989, pp 85–86.
26. Marx JL: The cell cycle coming under control. *Science 245*:252, 1989.
27. Matus RE, Weir ED: Hypercalcemia of maliganancy. *In* Kirk RW, Bonagura JD (eds): *Current Veterinary Therapy X*. W.B. Saunders, Philadelphia, 1989, pp 928–933.
28. Morrison WB: Paraneoplastic syndromes. Proceedings of the 57th Annual Meeting of the American Animal Hospital Association, San Francisco, Cal., Mar. 1990, pp 466–468.
29. Morrison WB: Paraneoplastic syndromes of the dog. *J Am Vet Med Assoc 175*:559, 1979.
30. Morrison WB, Hahn K: Cancers of unknown primary origin. Proceedings of the 8th Annual Veterinary Medical Forum, American College of Veterinary Internal Medicine, Auburn, Ala., Nov. 1990, pp 411–413.

31. Moscow JA, Cowan KH: Multidrug resistance. *J Natl Cancer Inst 80*:14, 1989.
32. Nelson RW, et al: Diencephalic syndrome secondary to intracranial astrocytoma in a dog. *J Am Vet Med Assoc 179*:1004, 1981.
33. Ogilvie GK: Paraneoplastic syndromes. *In* Withrow SJ, MacEwan EG (eds): *Clinical Veterinary Oncology*. J.B. Lippincott, Philadelphia, 1989, pp 29–38.
34. Pardee AB: Principles of cancer biology: Biochemistry and cell biology. *In* DeVita VT, et al (eds): *Cancer: Principles and Practice of Oncology*. 2nd ed. J.B. Lippincott, Philadelphia, 1985, pp 3–22.
35. Park M, VandeWoude GF: Principles of molecular cell biology of cancer: Oncogenes. *In* DeVita VT, et al (eds): *Cancer: Principles and Practice of Oncology*. 3rd ed. J.B. Lippincott, Philadelphia, 1989, pp 45–66.
36. Pastan I, Gottesman M: Multidrug resistance in human cancer. *N Engl J Med 316*:1388, 1987.
37. Richardson RC, Elliot GS: The biology of neoplastic disease. *In* Slatter DH (ed): *Textbook of Small Animal Surgery*. W.B. Saunders, Philadelphia, 1985, pp 2360–2369.
38. Roberts AB, Sporn MB: Principles of molecular cell biology of cancer: Growth factor related to nutrition. *In* DeVita VT, et al (eds): *Cancer: Principles and Practice of Oncology*. 3rd ed. J.B. Lippincott, Philadelphia, 1989, pp 67–80.
39. Salmon DJ, et al: Human breast cancer: Correlation of relapse and survival with amplification of the HER-2/neu oncogene. *Science 235*:177, 1987.
40. Schirrmacher V: Cancer metastasis: Experimental approaches, theoretical concepts, and impacts for treatment strategies. *Adv Cancer Res 43*:1, 1985.
41. Shofer FS, et al: Histopathologic and dietary prognostic factor for canine mammary carcinoma. *Breast Cancer Res Treat 13*:49, 1989.
42. Susaneck SJ, Macy DW: Hypertrophic osteopathy. *Comp Cont Educ 4*:689, 1982.
43. Tannock IF: Principles of cell proliferation: Cell kinetics. *In* DeVita VT, et al (eds): *Cancer: Principles and Practice of Oncology*. 3rd ed. J.B. Lippincott, Philadelphia, 1989, pp 3–13.
44. Vail DM, et al: Alterations in carbohydrate metabolism in canine lymphoma. *J Vet Intern Med 4*:8, 1990.
45. Weinberg RA: Oncogenes, anti-oncogenes, and the molecular basis of multistep carcinogenesis. *Cancer Res 49*:3713, 1989.
46. Weir EC: Malignancy associated hypercalcemia. Proceedings of the 4th Annual Veterinary Medical Forum, Vol II, Washington, D.C., 1986, pp 13–68.
47. Wheeler SL: Tumors of the endocrine system. *In* Withrow SJ, MacEwan EG (eds): *Clinical Veterinary Oncology*. J.B. Lippincott, Philadelphia, 1989, pp 253–282.
48. Willett WC, MacMahon B: Diet and cancer: An overview (second of two parts). *N Engl J Med 310*:697, 1984.
49. Willett WC, et al: Dietary fat and the risk of breast cancer. *N Engl J Med 316*:22, 1987.
50. Wilson DE: Antisecretory and mucosal protective actions of misoprostol: Potential role in the treatment of peptic ulcer disease. *Am J Med 83*:2, 1987.
51. Yokota J, et al: Alterations of *myc, myb*, and *ras*^{Ha} proto-oncogenes in cancers are frequent and show clinical correlation. *Science 231*:261, 1986.

CHAPTER 149

Diagnosis of Neoplasia

Wallace B. Morrison, Terrance A. Hamilton, Kevin A. Hahn, Ralph C. Richardson, and Wolfgang Janas

SAMPLE COLLECTION

A diagnosis of neoplasia cannot be made on clinical or radiographic findings alone. A portion of the suspected neoplasm must be removed and examined microscopically. A biopsy is required to confirm a diagnosis of malignancy. Biopsies also provide information for planning therapy.

If a biopsy is to provide useful information, proper technique must be used to obtain an adequate sample. Biopsies may be as simple as collection and analysis of accumulated fluid or as complex as removing tissue for evaluation during involved surgical procedures. In general, it is prudent to evaluate any tissue cytologically before initiating a more invasive procedure. After cytological examination, tissue is submitted for histopathological evaluation for definitive diagnosis. Incisional or excisional biopsy may be used, but the latter is preferable.

Risk to the patient in biopsy procedures should be avoided. Uncontrollable hemorrhage is the most serious complication.[26] Clotting tests and correction of hemostatic abnormalities are conducted before biopsy. A clotting abnormality is an absolute contraindication for biopsy of most organs and tissues except bone marrow. A second contraindication is improper or damaged biopsy instruments, which may preclude procurement of an adequate sample.[26] Repeated attempts to obtain a sample compound the risk of complications. The person performing the biopsy should be familiar with the procedure.[26] Study and practice are essential before attempting biopsy techniques on patients to enhance procurement of adequate specimens and minimize the risk of postbiopsy complications. Although risk may be present, it must be kept in perspective. The value of the information obtained through biopsy often outweighs the potential negative aspects of the procedure.

Fine-Needle Aspiration and Cytological Study

Cytological examination of cells from effusion or masses is useful diagnostic procedure. Samples for cytological evaluation can be easily collected from many epithelial structures, body cavities, and internal organs. Guidance by ultrasonography, fluoroscopy, and endoscopy has greatly improved fine-needle aspiration sampling of deep structures.

Cytological interpretation of fine-needle aspirates may not yield a definitive diagnosis but may discriminate between a benign and malignant process. Cytological interpretations often require histopathological confirmation. In one study comparing cytological versus histopathological interpretations in 147 canine skin tumors, 74 per cent could be correctly identified by cytological examination.[8]

Potential risks following fine-needle aspiration biopsy include fistula formation, bleeding, spreading of infection, and tumor seeding, but the technique is rarely associated with morbidity. Any negative consequences of fistula formation or tumor seeding can be minimized if the aspiration is planned so that the needle track can be removed during subsequent surgical excision. As with other biopsy procedures, a contraindication for fine-needle aspiration biopsy is severe coagulopathy. Of all the biopsy techniques available, fine-needle aspiration poses the least risk to patients with bleeding potential if a small-diameter needle is selected and the tissues are disturbed as little as possible.

The technique of cell collection is simple. Cells are removed from a lesion with a 22- or 25-gauge needle using negative pressure created with a syringe. The needle length depends on the location and accessibility of the lesion. The most direct path to the lesion is chosen. It is not necessary to prepare the area extensively if a dermal, subcutaneous, or submucosal mass is to be aspirated, because this technique is no more invasive than an injection. Alcohol swabbing of the skin and parting of hair facilitate collection from superficial masses without complications. If intrathoracic or intra-abdominal masses are aspirated, a small area of skin is clipped and prepared as for surgery. If the lesion is palpable, it is localized and stabilized with one hand while the other hand guides the needle, with syringe attached, through the skin into the lesion. Negative pressure is created by drawing back on the syringe plunger. Using a jabbing motion, the needle is passed through several secants of the lesion. The movement of the needle is rapid to prevent diluting the sample with peripheral blood. The tip of the needle should not leave the lesion during the negative pressure phase. If it does, cells may be aspirated from surrounding tissues or the needle may pass completely through the lesion and pull air through the needle into the syringe. Negative pressure is released before removing the needle from the lesion. The sample may appear in the barrel of the syringe but is usually present in the lumen of the needle. After the needle is detached, the syringe is filled with air, the needle reattached, and the air used to force the needle contents onto several glass slides.

Once the sample is collected, processing may be accomplished in a number of ways. The most common method of evaluating cytological specimens is by light microscopy. Fluids of low viscosity are prepared for microscopic examination by using a conventional blood smear technique. Viscous fluids are prepared by a "squash" technique, in which a drop of the sample is placed on a glass slide.[31] A second glass slide is placed on top of the sample. The sample spreads between the two slides. Downward pressure on the top slide is usually not necessary. More viscous fluids require gentle pressure, but excessive pressure is avoided to prevent alteration of microscopic structure of the sample by causing disruption or destruction of the cells. The cohesive effect of the fluids causes the slides to cling together. The slides are drawn apart by sliding the top slide away from the bottom slide, leaving a smear of cells and fluid in a monolayer. After air drying, slides prepared in such a manner are ready for staining.

Cytological criteria for malignancy include a predominance of large monomorphic cells of various sizes and recognition that the cells are ectopic to the tissue of origin. Nuclear features characteristic of malignancy include a high but variable nuclear/cytoplasmic ratio and variability in nuclear size, shape, and number. Nuclei of malignant cells often contain prominent and multiple nucleoli, abnormal mitotic figures, and irregular or coarse chromatin patterns. Cytoplasmic characteristics are not of great value in determining malignancy but can be useful for assessing the degree of differentiation and for identifying cytoplasmic granular and secretory products that suggest a specific cell type or tissue of origin. To diagnose malignancy, a minimum of three or four criteria must be prominently displayed within a high proportion of cells examined. Highly anaplastic tumors may contain many abnormalities simultaneously. Criteria for malignancy are summarized in Table 149–1.[6, 20]

Some malignant tumors, such as canine thyroid carcinoma, are difficult to diagnose by fine-needle aspiration biopsy because they are highly vascular and cytologically resemble peripheral blood. It may also be difficult to diagnose a neoplasm cytologically when concurrent inflammation is present because hyperplastic changes in cells associated with inflammation can mimic malignancy. In inflamed tumors, cytological malignancy must be interpreted cautiously, and histopathological confirmation of the lesion is recommended.[6, 20]

The cytological interpretation often cannot be highly specific, but classification of cells as epithelial, mesenchymal, or round-cell origin is usually possible. Epithelial cells exfoliate in clusters, and the shape of individual cells may reflect a specific epithelial type (squamous, cuboidal, columnar). Foamy, vacuolated, or markedly distended cytoplasm or acinus-like formation suggests a glandular origin. Nuclei of epithelial cells are round. Mesenchymal cells are more likely to exfoliate individually rather than in clusters, although in highly cellular specimens clumps may be observed. Individual mesenchymal cells are spindle-shaped. Identification of extracellular matrix material such as mucin or osteoid associated with mesenchymal cells may provide clues for diagnosing specific malignant tumors such as myxosarcoma or osteosarcoma. Identification of intracellular pigment granules allows an easy and specific diagnosis of melanocytic tumors.[6, 20] Round-cell tumors (lymphoma, mast cell, histiocytoma, transmissible venereal tumor, extramedullary plasmacytoma, and Merkel cell tumor) exfoliate as single cells and lack the elongated

TABLE 149–1. CYTOLOGICAL CRITERIA OF MALIGNANCY

Criteria
General criteria
Highly cellular specimen of a single cell type
Pleomorphism but many large cells
Ectopic cell population
Nuclear criteria
High nuclear/cytoplasmic ratio
Variation in nuclear size, shape, and number
Prominent nucleoli
Variation in nucleoli size, shape, and number
Abnormal mitotic figures
Irregular and/or coarse chromatin

shape of mesenchymal cells. Aspirates of round-cell tumors are usually cellular and often have specific features that allow identification.[6, 20]

Most cytological specimens are stained with Romanowsky stains such as Wright and Diff-Quik* stains. Romanowsky stains provide adequate differential staining for the majority of specimens. Users of Diff-Quik stain must remember that cytoplasmic granules within mast cells occasionally fail to stain and that staining time may need to be extended to two to three times longer than for peripheral blood smears. Papanicolaou and Sano trichrome stains provide excellent nuclear detail but require immediate fixation in either 95 per cent ethanol, a commercial cytological fixative, or unscented hair spray.[6, 20]

Unfortunately, the more immature (undifferentiated) a cell is, the more difficult it is to identify its cell line or tissue of origin. This is especially true of acute leukemias. The use of cytochemical stains greatly enhances the accuracy of diagnoses of acute leukemias because cytochemical staining patterns of leukemic cells are similar to their normal counterparts and often allow identification of what would otherwise be unidentifiable blast cells. Cytochemical staining patterns of leukemic cells for dogs and cats are summarized in Table 149–2.[5, 11, 17, 41]

Transtracheal Aspiration and Tracheal Washing

Transtracheal aspiration is used to obtain cytology and microbiology samples from the bifurcation of the trachea or one of the mainstem bronchi.[31] Aspiration is performed through the cricothyroid ligament, which is palpated as a small notch within the larynx. The site is clipped and prepared as for surgery. Local anesthesia is administered to prevent excessive struggling during the procedure. A long indwelling intravenous catheter capable of sliding through a needle is used. It must be long enough to reach the tracheal bifurcation. The needle is introduced through the cricothyroid ligament and angled down into the trachea. The catheter is gently threaded into the trachea, and the needle withdrawn. Sterile saline (3 to 10 ml) is injected from a 12- to 30-ml syringe into the trachea, and negative pressure is applied. Air, mucus, and some fluid are drawn into the syringe. The syringe may be disconnected, the excess air expelled, and the aspiration repeated several times. The patient usually coughs during the process, so the procedure must be done quickly to prevent the catheter tip from being coughed up into the pharynx.

*Diff-Quik, American Scientific Products, McGaw Park, IL.

Bone Marrow Biopsy

Any unexplained abnormality in peripheral blood and the possibility of neoplastic infiltration of bone marrow are potential indications for a bone marrow biopsy.[28] Although biopsies performed on thrombocytopenic animals may result in slight postbiopsy hemorrhage, thrombocytopenia is not an absolute contraindication to bone marrow biopsy, and hemorrhage usually can be controlled by digital pressure.

A number of bone marrow needle types are available (15 to 18 gauge, 1 to 1½ inches), and all provide satisfactory results. The Illinois sternal needle* (Fig. 149–1) has a guard screwed over the needle, preventing accidental overpenetration during insertion. Its ample hub size and guard provide a handle for the operator to use to penetrate dense cortical bone. It is available in a 15-gauge 1-inch adult size for large animals and an 18-gauge 1-inch pediatric size for smaller animals.

The most common sites for bone marrow sampling in small animals include (1) the wing of the ilium, dorsally or laterally, (2) the greater tubercle of the proximal humerus, and (3) the trochanteric fossa of the proximal femur. Because the character of samples obtained from active bone marrow sites is similar regardless of location,

*V. Mueller Co., Chicago, IL.

TABLE 149–2. CYTOCHEMICAL REACTIONS IN CELLS FROM LEUKEMIC ANIMALS

Leukemia	Chloracetate Esterase	Nonspecific Esterase	Periodic Acid-Schiff	Peroxidase	Sudan Black	Leukocyte Alkaline Phosphatase
Erythroleukemia	+/−	+/−	+/−	+/−	+	+/−
Acute lymphoblastic leukemia	−	+/−	−	−	−	−
Acute megakaryocytic leukemia	−	−	+	−	−	−
Acute monocytic leukemia	−	+	+	+/−	+/−	−
Acute myelogenous leukemia	+	−	+	+/−	+/−	+
Acute myelomonocytic leukemia	+/−	+	+/−	+	+	+

+, positive; −, negative; +/−, weakly or occasionally positive.

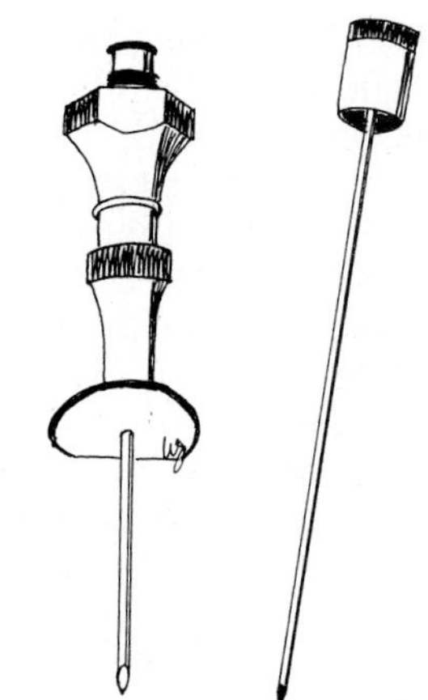

FIGURE 149–1. Illinois sternal needle with stylet.

selection of a specific site is often determined by personal preference.

The biopsy site is clipped and prepared for surgery. Local anesthesia of the periosteum accompanied by manual restraint of the patient is usually adequate. Local anesthetic is injected using a 22-gauge needle of the same length as the biopsy needle. This serves as a probe to determine whether the biopsy needle can reach the chosen site and also provides the operator with a mental image of the anatomical relationships involved. A small amount of local anesthetic agent (0.25 to 0.5 ml) is injected into the periosteum in a circle approximately 1 cm in diameter. A small incision with a number 11 scalpel blade aids passage of the biopsy needle through the skin. The needle, with stylet in place, is pushed through a tiny incision in the skin and overlying muscle onto the bone. With gentle pressure, the needle is rotated to create a small notch on the surface of the bone. Moderate pressure is applied, and the needle is firmly seated into the bone by clockwise and counterclockwise rotations. Once solidly seated, the bevel of the needle is usually in the marrow cavity. The stylet is removed, and a 10- to 12-ml syringe is attached. Vigorous negative pressure is applied. Aspiration usually causes transient pain by stimulating sensory nerve endings in the endosteum. This response generally denotes that the tip of the needle is in the marrow cavity. As soon as red marrow appears in the hub of the syringe, negative pressure is released. It is essential to discontinue aspiration as soon as the marrow appears in the syringe to minimize dilution of the sample with peripheral blood.

After aspiration, the syringe is removed, leaving the needle in place until adequate smears are prepared. Small drops of the marrow are expelled onto glass slides and smeared using the squash technique described earlier. These smears must be made as soon as possible after the marrow is aspirated. The sample clots within 10 to 30 seconds because the speed of clotting is increased by the release of thromboplastin from damaged cells. If too large a drop is expelled onto the slide, it is difficult to make a well-prepared monolayer smear. If this occurs, standing the slide on end and allowing the sample to run down the slide permits pulling another slide across only one portion, making a thin smear. Bone marrow material that remains after slide preparation may be allowed to clot and the clot placed into a container of suitable fixative for histopathological examination. If an adequate sample is to be procured, the pain response on aspiration should be observed, the smear should be a monolayer with a feathered edge, and fat globules and bone spicules should be found in the smear. If these criteria are met, the needle may be removed. Before submitting them for evaluation, representative slides can be stained and examined microscopically. If marrow particles (bone spicules and fat) and megakaryocytes can be identified, the sample is generally adequate for evaluation. If not, another biopsy may be indicated.

A bone marrow core biopsy can be taken from any of the sites used for bone marrow aspiration. These cores are usually taken with a Jamshidi biopsy needle* (Fig. 149–2). The Jamshidi needle has a uniform tubular configuration except for a tapered distal tip. The tip is beveled and has a sharp cutting edge. The tip of the Jamshidi needle allows the core sample to expand in the shaft, preventing compression of the sample and facilitating removal of the core from the bone. The proximal end has an adapter for a syringe, permitting its use as an aspiration needle as well.

To obtain a biopsy sample with a Jamshidi needle, the needle is seated, with stylet in place, into the cortical bone. The stylet is removed, and the needle slowly advanced 1 to 2 cm with a rotating motion. Depth of penetration can be gauged by positioning the thumb at a point 1 to 2 cm from the skin on the shaft of the needle or by inserting the stylet and observing its displacement. After the needle has been advanced to an appropriate depth, it is rotated 360° in one direction several times to twist the core loose at its base. The needle and bone core are removed from the bone. The core is gently pushed out of the needle with a wire probe inserted in the distal cutting end and out the

*Kormed, Inc., Minneapolis, MN.

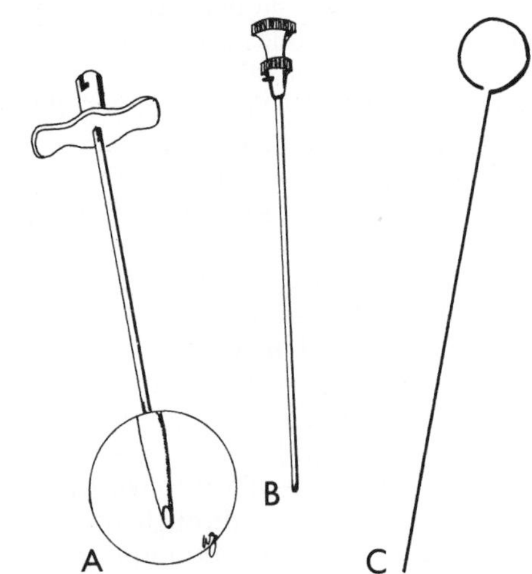

FIGURE 149–2. *A*, Jamshidi biopsy needle illustrating conical shape of the tip. *B*, Stylet. *C*, Wire probe to push sample out of the needle.

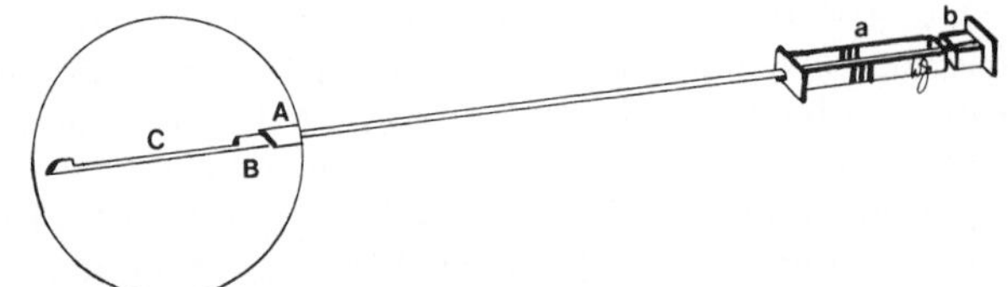

FIGURE 149–3. Disposable Tru-Cut biopsy needle. (A, Outer cannula with plastic handle [a]; B, obturator-specimen rod with plastic handle section [b]; C, specimen notch.)

proximal hub end. The core is not pushed from the hub end because of the narrow conical tip. The sample is placed between two glass slides and gently rolled back and forth to prepare slides for cytological examination. The core can be placed into a container of suitable fixative.

Lymph Node Biopsy

Local or generalized lymph node enlargement is an indication for lymph node biopsy.[29] Before biopsy, lymph nodes are carefully palpated. The specific areas of involvement and the consistency of the nodes are evaluated. Soft and fluctuant nodes may suggest significant suppuration or necrosis. Abnormally firm or fixed nodes may contain neoplastic or inflammatory elements. Lymph nodes involved in an acute inflammatory process may be quite painful, whereas nodes affected with chronic inflammatory or neoplastic disorders usually are not painful. Several methods of biopsy are available.

Fine-needle aspiration is the quickest and easiest procedure for biopsy of lymph nodes. It can be performed on nodes of any size provided they can be adequately localized and stabilized by palpation. Deeper lymph nodes can be reached with the aid of ultrasonography or radiography.

Lymph nodes can be removed by surgical excision, which provides the largest and perhaps the best possible specimen for examination. The need for general anesthesia and the time required to excise a lymph node make this surgery uncommon. In lieu of excision, a lymph node specimen can be obtained with a needle biopsy technique. Needle biopsy instruments can be used on the same lymph nodes accessible to aspiration. The disadvantages of a needle biopsy are the small amount of tissue procured, lack of direct observation for needle placement, and the chance of missing a focal lesion. The instrument most commonly used for this method is the Tru-Cut disposable biopsy needle* (Fig. 149–3).

The Tru-Cut needle biopsy technique must be well understood to obtain the best results.[26, 39] Local anesthesia is generally sufficient, but sedation or general anesthesia may be necessary for restraint and control of pain if deep tissues are sampled. The skin over the biopsy site is clipped and prepared for surgery. A small incision facilitates passage of the needle through the skin. The Tru-Cut needle is introduced through the skin to the lymph node capsule with the obturator specimen rod fully retracted within the outer cannula. If the lymph node is large enough and in a relatively safe area, a thrusting technique may be used. After the capsule is penetrated, the outer cannula is kept stationary and the obturator specimen rod is thrust into the lymph node by pushing forward on its handle section. If the node is smaller than the specimen notch or in a hazardous location, the thrusting technique is not used. Instead, the capsule is penetrated and the needle advanced through the lymph node to its distal edge. While the obturator specimen rod is kept stationary, the outer cannula is slowly drawn back to the proximal edge, taking care not to pull it out of the capsule. In either case, without moving the obturator specimen rod, the outer cannula is advanced forward over the specimen notch with a quick thrust to cut and trap the biopsy specimen in the specimen notch. The needle is withdrawn from the body with the specimen (Fig. 149–4). The tissue sample can be gently teased out of the specimen notch with a sterile hypodermic needle and fixed in formalin.

If desired, direct impressions can be made for cytological examination. The tissue can be placed on a glass slide, and another slide can be gently touched to the tissue. A hypodermic needle or fine-toothed forceps may also be used to lift and move the tissue around. In

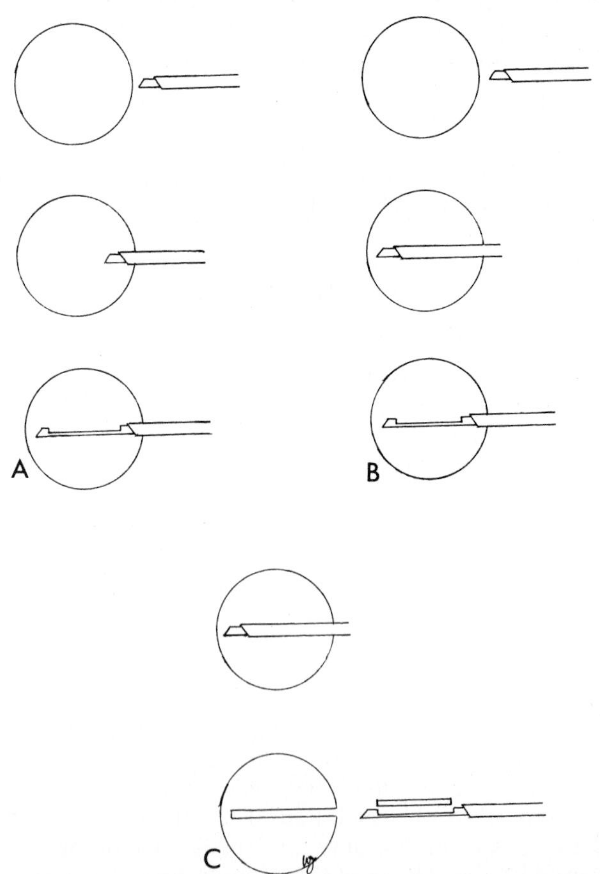

FIGURE 149–4. Tru-Cut penetration methods. *A*, In larger lesions, penetrate capsule and then thrust obturator-specimen rod forward. *B*, In smaller lesions, penetrate through capsule to far edge of lesion and pull back outer cannula to near edge. *C*, Cut specimen and remove.

*Travenol Laboratories, Inc., Deerfield, IL.

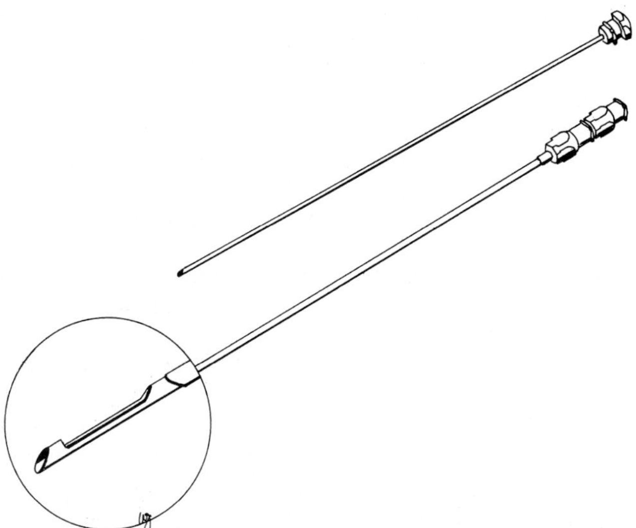

FIGURE 149–5. Lee biopsy needle. Note the combination cutting (notch) and suction (lumen) features.

any case, great care must be taken in handling the tissue. It is generally wise to obtain multiple samples if cytological and histopathological specimens are to be prepared. Hemorrhage is usually the only postbiopsy complication and can be minimized by applying digital pressure and possibly a pressure dressing to the area.

Percutaneous Lung Biopsy

The Lee needle* and the Tru-Cut needle are effective for obtaining small portions of lung tissue. The Lee needle is similar to the Tru-Cut needle but is smaller and has suction capabilities through the inner cutting needle (Fig. 149–5). Assisted by radiographic and sometimes fluoroscopic imaging, cells or tissue may be obtained from affected areas of the lung. Tru-Cut needles (see the previous section on lymph node biopsy) are used for large solid masses in the thorax. The Lee biopsy needle, which combines aspirating action with cutting action, may be used to sample aerated lung tissue.

The technique for obtaining aerated tissues is straightforward. After the Lee needle is placed, negative pressure is applied, and the inner needle is withdrawn while the outer cannula is held steady, thus severing the tissue and drawing it into the suction device (e.g., 50-ml syringe or vacuum pump). The outer cannula may be withdrawn and the process repeated, allowing numerous specimens to be collected across the sampled area. Complications of lung biopsy include pneumothorax and hemoptysis. The procedure is not completed if gross blood is aspirated. If hemoptysis develops, the patient is restrained with the sampled side down. Patients are closely observed for dyspnea secondary to pneumothorax or hemothorax for 12 to 24 hours after all lung biopsies.

Bone Biopsy

A large core of bone may be removed using a Michele trephine† (Fig. 149–6), or a small core may be obtained with a Jamshidi biopsy needle (see the earlier section on bone marrow biopsy). Power-driven trephines are available but are not recommended for obtaining biopsy samples because the heat associated with the high speed burns the specimen. Hand-driven trephines give some idea of bone density and strength. Large core techniques require general anesthesia and normal clotting parameters.

The lesion to be sampled is first located radiographically, and the area of interest is determined. The site is clipped and prepared for surgery. An incision of the skin and underlying musculature is generally needed to accommodate a large trephine. The trephine, with stylet in place, is inserted through the skin incision and advanced through the muscle to the bone. The stylet is removed, and the trephine is advanced into the bone to an appropriate depth, using a rotating motion. The depth can be gauged by using the calibrations on the shafts of large trephines or by inserting the stylet and observing its displacement. Once the appropriate depth is obtained, the trephine is rotated 360° in one direction several times and rocked back and forth to break the core loose at its base. The trephine and core samples are removed from the bone, and the sample gently expelled by the stylet. Because there is no mechanism to hold the sample in the end of the large trephines, it may occasionally be difficult to remove the core from the bone. Holding a thumb over the proximal end of the trephine and creating a vacuum or applying lateral torque during withdrawal may be helpful.

The sample is placed between two glass slides and gently rolled back and forth to prepare it for cytological examination. The core can then be placed into a container of suitable fixative for histopathological examination. Postbiopsy hemorrhage often results from large core biopsies.

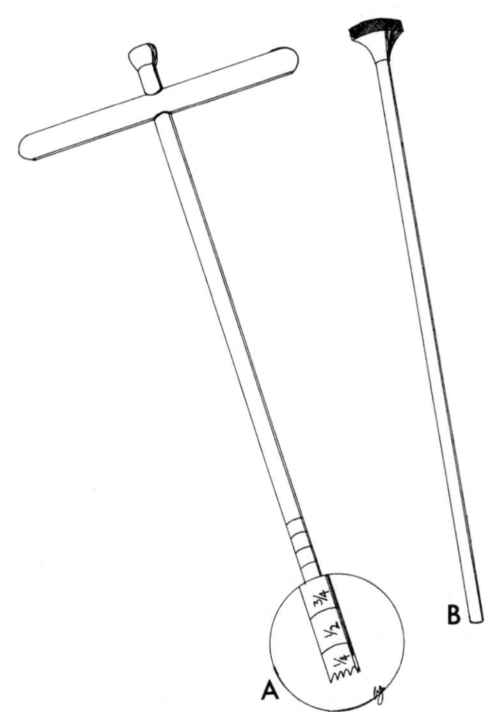

FIGURE 149–6. *A*, Michele trephine illustrating cutting saw-toothed tip. *B*, Stylet.

*Unique Industries, Memphis, TN.
†V. Mueller Co., Chicago, IL.

Incisional and Excisional Biopsies

Cytological evaluation of tumor samples can be helpful in reaching a tentative diagnosis and planning additional diagnostic procedures, but histopathological examination is usually necessary to establish a definitive diagnosis. An incisional or excisional biopsy is required.

Incisional biopsies may be used in any tumor but are most frequently of value in large soft-tissue neoplasms. A wedge of tissue is taken from an area that will be removed during a later excision or that lies within the treatment field if nonsurgical therapy such as radiation is to be applied. Care is taken so that the biopsy does not create new tissue planes. The wedge is large enough to ensure a representative sample of tumor. Infected and necrotic areas are avoided. If possible, a junction of tumor and normal tissue is sampled.

Excisional biopsy is nearly always the procedure of choice if a surgical biopsy is indicated. The surgical margins of an excised tumor should extend at least 1 cm around and deep to the mass. If the tumor is a suspected mast cell tumor or hemangiopericytoma, a 3-cm margin is recommended to excise all infiltrating cells.

HISTOPATHOLOGY

For prognostic purposes, it is important to know whether a tumor is benign or malignant. The histopathological cellular criteria for malignancy are similar to the criteria used in cytological evaluation; however, histopathology allows for examination of the neoplasm's architecture and growth pattern (invasiveness).

Malignant tumors often exhibit marked pleomorphism. Numerous and abnormal mitotic figures are often scattered throughout the tissue section. Cell cohesiveness and cell-to-cell contact are decreased, and there is an increased tendency for cells to migrate away from their site of origin. Malignant cells often invade the surrounding tissues, lymphatics, and blood vessels. It is this process of invasion that leads to metastasis, which is the hallmark of malignancy.

In addition to providing a diagnosis, histopathological examination can frequently be used to provide important prognostic information. The histopathological grade of a tumor may predict clinical behavior. Low-grade malignancies frequently are slowly progressive and may be treated by local therapy such as surgery. High-grade malignancies are frequently invasive, rapidly growing, and metastatic in their behavior. Histopathological grading is generally determined by criteria of tumor differentiation, mitotic index, necrosis, and blood vessel invasion.[3]

Histopathological grading of canine mast cell tumors has prognostic significance and is based on the degree of differentiation of the individual cells. The more differentiated a mast cell is, the better the prognosis. In a study of dogs with mast cell tumors, 6 per cent with undifferentiated tumors were alive at 15 months, 44 per cent with moderately differentiated (intermediate grade) mast cells were alive at 15 months, and 83 per cent with well-differentiated tumors were alive 15 months after their diagnosis.[27] Criteria for histopathological grading have been defined for several other tumor types, including canine lymphoma and canine mammary carcinoma.[32, 35]

Mitotic index is of prognostic significance in canine soft-tissue sarcomas. In one study of sarcomas in dogs, tumors with a mitotic index of nine or more mitotic figures at a magnification of 400× had a median survival time of 49 weeks and recurrence rate of 62 per cent, whereas tumors with a mitotic index of less than nine mitotic figures at the same magnification had a median survival time of 118 weeks and a recurrence rate of only 25 per cent.[2]

Microscopic examination of cut margins of tissue is a common way to determine if a tumor has been completely excised. The presence of neoplastic cells at a surgical margin can influence the decision about the need for further surgery or adjunctive therapy such as radiation or chemotherapy. If no neoplastic cells are visible at the margins of the biopsy specimen, clinicians usually assume that the excision is complete. Incomplete excision is assumed if neoplastic cells extend to the biopsy margin. The report of "clean" surgical margins may provide a misleading interpretation of the completeness of surgical excision. It is important to remember that pathologists examine only a small section of tissue relative to the volume excised. To conclude that all margins are free of neoplastic infiltration based on the evaluation of a 5- to 6-μm slice of a portion of the tumor may lead to an erroneous conclusion (Fig. 149–7*A–C*). It is easy to understand how false interpretations can occur with excision of tumors that spread irregularly along fascial planes or that have small clusters of neoplastic cells invading surrounding tissues. Examination of different tissue planes of a biopsy specimen can lead to different conclusions about the completeness of the surgical excision. A false report of a clean surgical margin would likely delay appropriate additional therapy and have a negative influence on the outcome of any therapy.

Inaccurate histopathology reports can also result from inflamed tumors. Inflammation can obscure the true tumor morphology, causing the pathologist to render an inaccurate diagnosis. A knowledge of the biological behavior of a tumor coupled with high-quality specimen submission is the most useful approach to determine the need for additional therapy.

IMMUNOHISTOCHEMISTRY

Anaplastic or undifferentiated tumors represent a diagnostic challenge. Identification of the tissue of origin of an undifferentiated tumor is important in determining prognosis and planning treatment. Immunohistochemistry, using either monoclonal or polyclonal antibodies, can be helpful when the tissue of origin of a tumor cannot be determined with standard stains.[25] Various characteristic cytoplasmic markers in normal tissues, when identified in undifferentiated neoplastic tissue, help to determine origin. The presence or absence of intermediate filaments is one of the more important classes of tumor markers.[34] Intermediate filaments are filamentous proteins that are ultrastructurally recogniz-

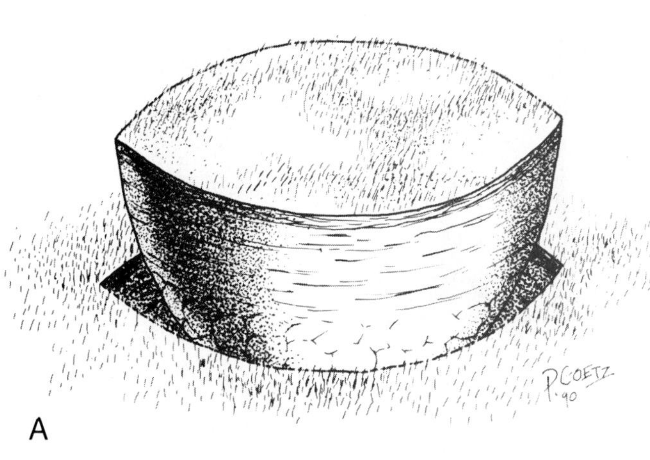

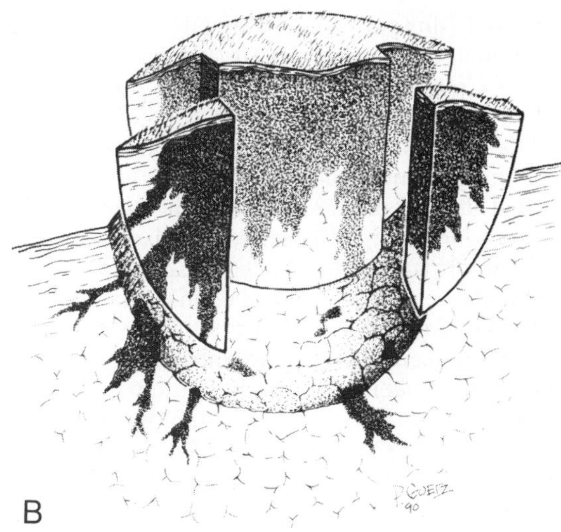

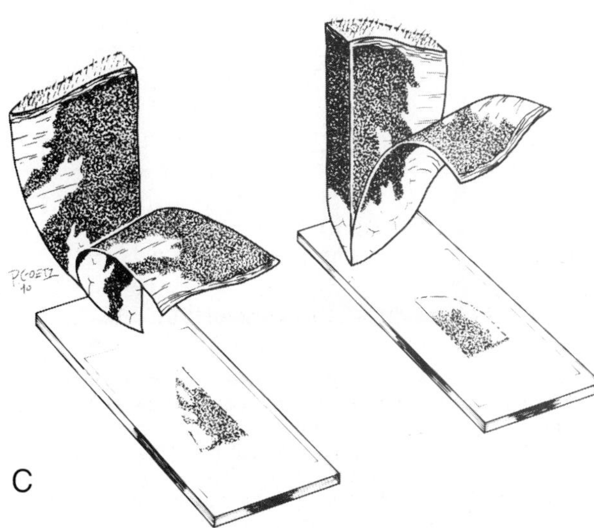

FIGURE 149–7. *A*, A representation of a portion of skin containing an invasive neoplasm after surgical excision. *B*, The same neoplasm *(shaded area)* after formalin fixation and initial trimming. *C*, Only a 5- to 6-μm slice of a portion of a tumor is mounted and examined. If tissue from the right side of the specimen is examined, excision will appear complete. Examination of the left side of the specimen will reveal tumor cells extending to the biopsy margin. The choice of what portion of a tumor is considered "representative" is subjective and may lead to erroneous conclusions about the completeness of an excision.

able as straight or slightly curved filaments 8 to 10 nm in diameter. They are intermediate in size between two other cytoskeletal structures: the microfilaments that are approximately 6 nm in diameter and composed of actin, and the microtubules that are about 25 nm in diameter.[25]

A large family of intermediate filaments, known as *cytokeratin filaments*, are typical of epithelial cells and carcinomas. Nineteen subclasses of cytokeratin filaments, ranging from 40 to 68 kilodaltons, have been identified with monoclonal antibodies.[25, 34] Epithelial tissue and tumors of epithelial origin (carcinomas) stain positive for various cytokeratin filaments with the appropriate monoclonal antibody and standard immunohistochemical techniques such as the avidin-biotin-peroxidase complex method.

Distinct intermediate filaments are found in other tissues and are useful in identifying undifferentiated tumors. Glial fibrillary acidic protein is present in glial cells and gliomas. Neural filaments are diagnostic of neural cells and some types of neuroendocrine tumors. Vimentin is an intermediate filament that is typical of mesenchymal cells and their derived tumors such as melanomas and other nonepithelial neoplasms. Desmin is an intermediate filament that is characteristically present in muscle cells and in most tumors derived from muscle cells.[25, 34] Kappa and lambda light chains are excellent markers for detecting canine B-cell lymphomas and plasmacytomas.[34] Neuron-specific enolase and S-100 protein are often present within amelanotic melanomas. The combined use of vimentin, S-100 protein, and neuron-specific enolase is useful in distinguishing amelanotic melanoma from other undifferentiated round-cell tumors in dogs.[34]

FLOW CYTOMETRY

Flow cytometry measures various cellular, physical, and biochemical properties such as size and cytoplasmic granularity. Cells can be labeled with monoclonal antibodies or fluorescing dyes so that various cell surface antigens may be detected. Flow cytometric analysis of tumor cell DNA may be performed on either fresh living cells in suspension or formalin-fixed and paraffin-embeded archival specimens.[36]

The quantification of DNA is a well-characterized and widely used flow cytometric technique. Cells are stained so that the degree of fluorescence is directly proportional to the DNA content. A normal resting lymphocyte has a normal (diploid) amount of DNA. If the lymphocyte is stimulated to proliferate, it contains twice the amount of DNA (tetraploid) immediately before mitosis.

Ploidy is defined as cell DNA content and is expressed as DNA index (the ratio of DNA content of the G_0/G_1 cells in the abnormal population to the G_0/G_1 cells in a normal diploid population).[22] Tumor cell DNA content is of prognostic significance for survival of many humans with tumors such as breast cancer, colon cancer, multiple myeloma, acute lymphoblastic leukemia, and others.[22, 30] A limited number of flow cytometric studies of DNA content of cells from spontaneously occurring canine tumors have been performed. Rutteman and colleagues analyzed 57 canine mammary tumors for DNA ploidy but were unable to determine any prognostic significance for survival. An association was observed between degree of malignancy and aneuploidy (abnormal DNA content).[33]

Human lymphoma patients with a high percentage of malignant cells in S phase and G_2/M phase have a poorer prognosis than those with less-proliferative tumors.[22] In a study of 82 paraffin-embedded samples of canine lymphoma analyzed by flow cytometry, samples containing cells predominately in G_2/M phase correlated with a median survival of 11 weeks compared with a median survival of 31 weeks for dogs with less-proliferative tumors (Fig. 149–8*A* and *B*). Multiploid samples (samples with more than one abnormal stem cell line) were also associated with a poor prognosis (median survival of 9 weeks).

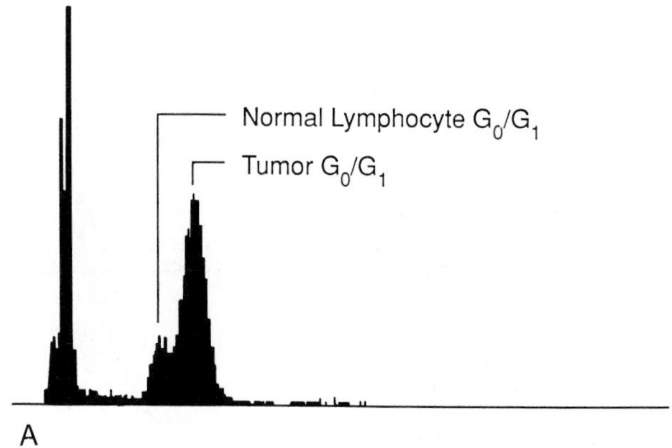

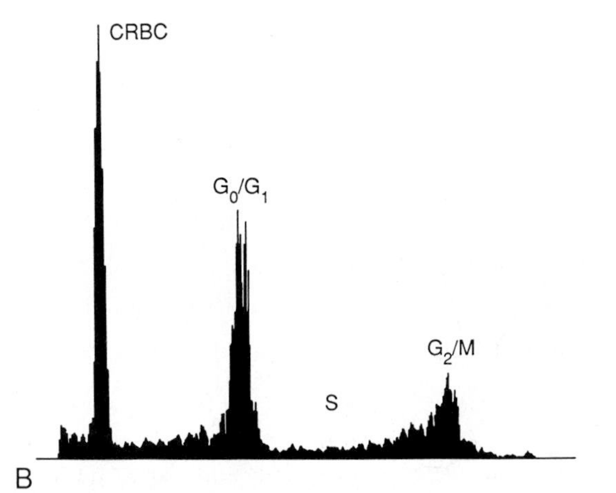

FIGURE 149–8. *A*, A histogram derived from the flow cytometric analysis of a fine-needle aspirate of a canine lymph node diagnosed as lymphoma. The aneuploid tumor peak is evident on the far right, and the normal diploid peak (from the normal lymphocyte population of the lymph node and from peripheral blood contamination) is seen on the left. *B*, A histogram derived from the flow cytometric analysis of a formalin-fixed and paraffin-embedded canine lymphoma specimen showing the relative distribution of cells in different phases of the cell cycle. The peak at the far left of each histogram represents the DNA of chicken red blood cells (CRBC) that are used as a standard.

MOLECULAR CYTOGENETICS

Cytogenetic and molecular biological analysis of tumor cells has become an integral part of diagnosis and clinical staging in humans with neoplasia.[18] These techniques are also being used more commonly in veterinary oncology for the same purposes.[9, 10] Chromosome changes present before therapy disappear when patients enter remission. Cells with an abnormal karyotype (similar to the initial karyotype) return with relapse.[9]

The most common abnormality found in veterinary and human tumors is gene rearrangement. One gene is removed from continuity with another gene, resulting in overexpression of the "moved" gene.[18] The gene involved in the rearrangement is not abnormal. However, regulation of expression is abnormal and results in excessive synthesis of the gene product (a protein) at an inappropriate time.[37] Lymphoma develops when the *c-myc* proto-oncogene is repositioned (translocated) near the immunoglobulin gene in the human, mouse, cat, dog, and chicken.[7, 24] The immunoglobulin gene promotes transcription of the *c-myc* proto-oncogene, which serves as a strong promoter for additional DNA transcription. This process stimulates cell growth and division and can be seen by differential staining of chromosomes (banding). The RNA and DNA isolated from a tumor biopsy specimen can be analyzed to determine the presence or absence of physical rearrangements, amplifications, additions, deletions of genes, and variations in gene size and expression.

Gene amplification and overexpression of *c-myc* have been reported in more than one-third of human solid tumor types, including lung, stomach, breast, colon, and neuroblastoma, and in primary tumors from persons with acute promyelocytic leukemia, chronic myelocytic leukemia, and Burkitt's lymphoma.[40] Amplification of *c-myc* correlates with aggressiveness of primary or disseminated carcinomas and sarcomas.[40] Investigations suggest a strong correlation between structural alteration or overexpression of *c-myc* and prognosis in humans.[1] The *c-myc* proto-oncogene has been identified and is amplified and overexpressed in 100 per cent of canine mammary neoplasms and 78 per cent of canine melanomas grown *in vitro*.[1, 21] In cats, the *c-myc* proto-oncogene is associated with feline leukemia virus.[23] Feline *c-myc* is homologous with avian and murine *c-myc*, which are directly involved in promoting lymphoma.

Advanced high-grade malignancies commonly have increased numbers of chromosomes (aneuploidy). Abnormal chromosome numbers (therefore abnormal

DNA content) can provide diagnostic and prognostic information. In one canine study, aneuploidy and supernumerary metacentric chromosomes were found in 8 of 10 and 5 of 10 leukemic dogs, respectively.[9] In a study of nine cats with leukemia (four lymphocytic, two myelogenous, one monocytic, one myelomonocytic, one eosinophilic), chromosome abnormalities such as double minute chromosomes, tetrasomy, or trisomy were common.[10]

Future applications of cytogenetics and molecular biology in veterinary oncology may include preferential screening of breeds predisposed to malignancy, such as boxers, to determine factors responsible for tumorigenesis.

SAMPLE COLLECTION

Bronchoalveolar Lavage

Bronchoalveolar lavage is a technique in which the alveoli and smaller airways of a portion of lung are bathed with saline, allowing exfoliated cells to be collected through a bronchoscope. The saline and suspended cellular and acellular material can be analyzed cytologically and, when appropriate, biochemically, immunologically, and microbiologically. The technique is a valuable adjunct to thoracic radiography and tracheal washings in the diagnosis of various infectious, inflammatory, and neoplastic conditions affecting the lungs.[14]

The technique in dogs and cats is performed under general anesthesia. With the patient in sternal recumbency, a bronchoscope is directed to the area of lung to be sampled and is wedged into an airway. A quantity of sterile saline (5 to 25 ml, depending on the size of the patient) is passed through the biopsy port of the bronchoscope with a syringe and immediately aspirated. Lavage fluid often appears foamy because of the presence of surfactant. Cytological examination of lavage fluid can be performed after centrifugation.

Bronchoalveolar lavage is not the same as tracheal washings. The two techniques provide different data because the cells recovered by each technique are from different regions of the respiratory tract. Cells recovered in tracheal wash fluid represent those in large airways. Cells recovered by bronchoalveolar lavage are from deep in the lung parenchyma.

Bronchoalveolar lavage frequently yields a cytological diagnosis of deep parenchymal disease when more invasive techniques such as lung biopsy by fine-needle aspiration or open thoracotomy are inappropriate. The sensitivity and specificity of bronchoalveolar lavage fluid analysis can be useful in clinical management of patients with tumors and in performing clinical trials when accurate staging is essential for evaluating new protocols.[15] In a study of 21 dogs with lymphoma, 12 of 21 dogs had evidence of pulmonary involvement with lymphoma based on bronchoalveolar lavage fluid cytology. Nine of the 12 positive dogs and all of the negative dogs had radiographic evidence of either normal pulmonary parenchyma or only mildly increased interstitial densities. In none of the 21 dogs examined was tracheal wash fluid cytological evaluation helpful in determining pulmonary involvement with lymphoma.

IMAGING

Creating diagnostic images with x-rays, ultrasound, computed tomography, magnetic resonance, and scintigraphy has become increasingly sophisticated and important in detecting, diagnosing, and monitoring treatment responses in patients with tumors. Image resolution, contrast, and distortion determine the value of the different imaging techniques in clinical assessment, staging, and re-evaluation. Diagnostic imaging assists in evaluation by helping to assess the margins of a neoplasm with respect to size, metastasis, and degree of invasiveness. The sensitivity and specificity of each imaging technique vary, and as a result, the ability to clearly distinguish tissue margins differs.

Survey radiographs provide excellent spatial resolution compared with other modalities of imaging; however, contrast discrimination between normal and neoplastic soft tissue is poor. Invasiveness and tissue architecture cannot be assessed, and soft-tissue structures in contact with one another cannot be distinguished as separate entities if they have the same physical density (Fig. 149–9*A* and *B*). Definitive characterization of parenchymal disease requires histopathological review.

Medical gray scale ultrasonography can be used to create images of a tumor and provide more information about soft-tissue architecture and size than is available from survey radiographs alone. Ultrasonography does not define spatial resolution as well as radiography because images are displayed as anatomical reconstructions of a tissue slice made by the ultrasound beam.[4, 12, 16] Sharp definitions of the far margins of a mass are limited by the heterogeneity of echoic and anechoic signals from many composite structures (Fig. 149–9*C*).[12] Ultrasonography cannot image through bone or air, so it is not possible to image the brain, spinal cord, lung, or an air-filled gastrointestinal tract directly.[16] Diffuse and focal parenchymal disease can be determined but not definitively characterized. Definitive characterization of parenchymal disease requires biopsy. Abdominal fluid does not interfere with the creation of an ultrasonographic image as it does with standard radiographs. Cystic structures can usually be identified with ultrasonography, and machines with Doppler capabilities can determine and assess blood flow. Image quality and tissue orientation rely heavily on the skill of the ultrasonographer.

Computed tomography allows excellent contrast discrimination among different tissue types. Two-dimensional images can be constructed in the dorsal, sagittal, and transverse planes for determining accurate tumor measurements. The physical density of a tumor may be compared with normal tissues to provide information on size or degree of invasiveness. As with ultrasonography, spatial resolution is poor with computed tomography because only one slice of tissue at a time is available for examination, but the unique cross-sectional imaging ability of computed tomography makes it possible to detect soft tissues independent of overlying bony structures (Fig. 149–9*D*).[12]

Magnetic resonance imaging, for the same reasons as for ultrasonography and computed tomography, is characterized by poor spatial resolution, but it has contrast

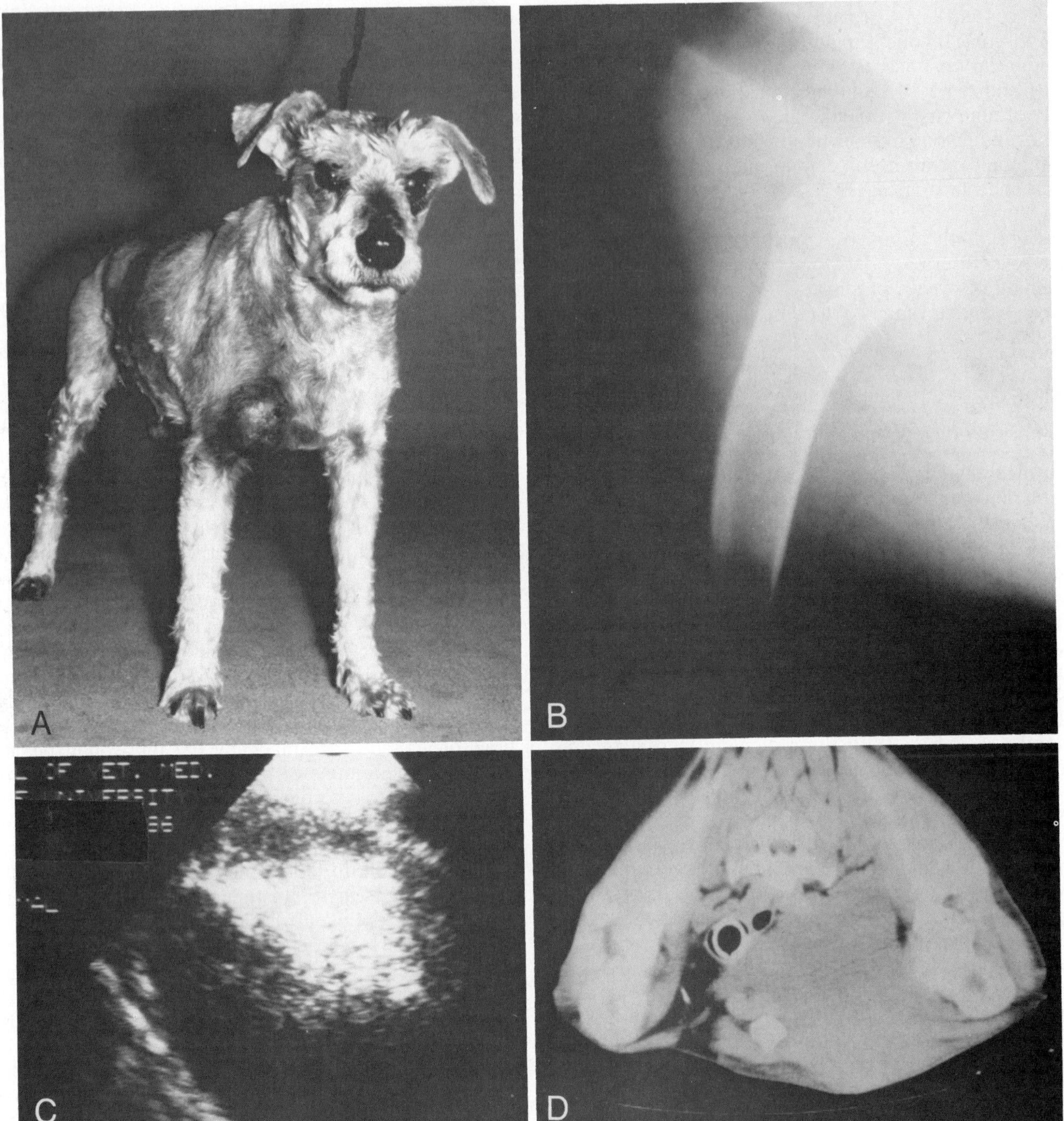

FIGURE 149–9. *A*, A photograph of dog with a hemangiopericytoma in the area of the right shoulder. *B*, This radiograph of the shoulder area of the same dog fails to delineate normal from neoplastic soft tissue. *C*, An ultrasonographic image of the hemangiopericytoma. The bright area in the center of the image is the tumor. There is no clear distinction of the margins of the tumor. *D*, A computed tomographic image of the shoulder area. The margins of the tumor are easily seen, revealing its invasive nature.

capabilities superior to computed tomography. The major advantage of magnetic resonance imaging over computed tomography is in diagnostic evaluation of the central nervous system.[12, 19]

Scintigraphic images are made by using a gamma camera to detect the amount of a radiopharmaceutical agent that distributes to the tissue under study. Facilities for scintigraphy are available at numerous veterinary schools and at several private veterinary medical facilities. The use of scintigraphy in evaluating dogs and cats with thyroid disease is well documented.[38] Nuclear medicine has many other diagnostic uses, including biliary scans, bone scans, assessment of ventricular performance, liver and spleen scans, lung perfusion scans, and others.

Bone scintigraphy is more sensitive than survey radiography for detecting primary and secondary bone tumors. Subtle abnormalities in bone attributed to early metastasis may not be easily recognized with survey radiography but may be identified with scintigraphy and

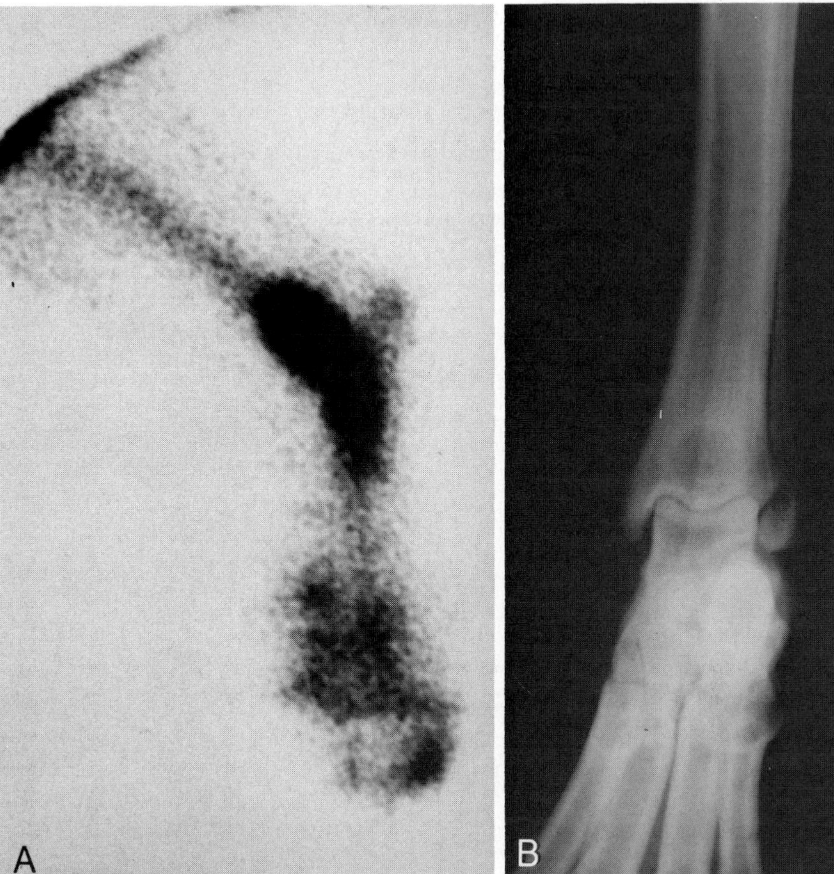

FIGURE 149–10. *A*, A bone scintigraph of the distal left tibia of a dog with metastatic osteosarcoma. An area of increased isotope uptake is seen in the distal tibia. The primary tumor was located in the proximal right humerus. Clinical signs were limited to lameness of the right forelimb. *B*, A radiograph of the left hock showing a circular area of lysis in the distal tibia. This lesion was subsequently confirmed histologically as osteosarcoma.

confirmed with specific radiographs and bone biopsy.[13] Skeletal metastasis can be detected earlier with scintigraphy than with radiography because scintigraphic images depend more on the bone remodeling that develops before the structural changes detected with radiography.[13] In a study of 25 dogs with appendicular or axial osteosarcoma, 14 had scintigraphically enhanced sites beyond the primary tumor site, with 7 of the 14 sites subsequently being histopathologically confirmed as osteosarcoma (Fig. 149–10*A* and *B*).[13]

Inflammation, trauma, and neoplasia can account for scintigraphic enhancement of bone; therefore, scintigraphy does not differentiate benign from malignant bone disease. Scintigraphically suspicious sites should be radiographed and biopsy performed to establish a definitive diagnosis.[13]

References

1. Ahern TE, et al: C-myc and Her-2/NEU proto-oncogene overexpression and restriction fragment length polymorphism in canine tumors and tumor-derived cell lines. Proceedings of the 9th Annual Conference, Veterinary Cancer Society, Raleigh, NC, Oct, 1989.
2. Bostock DE, Dye MT: Prognosis after surgical excision of canine fibrous connective tissue sarcomas. *Vet Pathol 17*:581, 1980.
3. Coindre JM, et al: Histopathologic grading in spindle cell soft tissue sarcomas. *Cancer 61*:2305, 1988.
4. Feeney DA, et al: Two-dimensional, gray-scale ultrasonography for assessment of hepatic and splenic neoplasms in the dog and cat. *J Am Vet Med Assoc 184*:68, 1984.
5. Focklawn NR, Kociba GJ: Cytochemical characterization of feline leukemic cells. *Vet Pathol 23*:155, 1986.
6. French TJ: General diagnostic cytology: Inflammation, hyperplasia, neoplasia. Proceedings of the 8th Annual Veterinary Medical Forum, American College of Veterinary Internal Medicine, Washington, DC, May, 1990.
7. Freytag SO: Enforced expression of the c-myc oncogene inhibits cell differentiation by precluding entry into a distinct predifferentiation state in G_0/G_1. *Molec Cell Biol 8*:1614, 1988.
8. Griffiths GL, et al: Fine needle aspiration cytology and histologic correlation in canine tumors. *Vet Clin Pathol 13*:7, 1984.
9. Grindem CB, Buoen LC: Cytogenetic analysis of leukaemic cells in the dog. A report of 10 cases and a review of the literature. *J Comp Pathol 96*:626, 1986.
10. Grindem CB, Buoen LC: Cytogenetic analysis in nine leukaemic cats. *J Comp Pathol 101*:21, 1989.
11. Grindem CB, et al: Cytochemical reactions in cells from leukemic dogs. *Vet Pathol 23*:103, 1986.
12. Hahn KA, et al: Comparison of survey radiography with ultrasonography and x-ray computed tomography for clinical staging of subcutaneous neoplasms in dogs. *J Am Vet Med Assoc 196*:1795, 1990.
13. Hahn KH, et al: Single-phase methylene diphosphate bone scintigraphy in the diagnostic evaluation of dogs with osteosarcoma. *J Am Vet Med Assoc 196*:1483, 1990.
14. Hawkins EC, DeNicola DB: Tracheal wash and bronchoalveolar lavage fluid evaluation in the diagnosis of pulmonary mycosis in the dog. *J Am Vet Med Assoc 197*:79, 1990.
15. Hawkins EC, et al: Bronchoalveolar lavage fluid cytology in dogs with malignant lymphoma. Proceedings of the 8th Annual Veterinary Medical Forum, American College of Veterinary Internal Medicine, Washington, DC, May, 1990.
16. Herring DS, Bjornton G: Physics, facts and artifacts of diagnostic ultrasound. *Vet Clin North Am 15*:1107, 1985.
17. Jain NC: Cytochemistry of normal and leukemic lymphocytes. *In* Jain NC (ed): *Schalm's Veterinary Hematology*. Lea & Febiger, Philadelphia, 1986.
18. Karakousis CP, et al: Chromosomal changes in soft tissue sarcomas. *Arch Surg 122*:1257, 1987.
19. Kraft SL, et al: Canine brain anatomy on magnetic resonance images. *Vet Radiol 30*:147, 1989.
20. MacWilliams PS: Cytologic techniques in cancer diagnosis. *In* Withrow SJ, MacEwen EG (eds): *Clinical Veterinary Oncology*. J.B. Lippincott, Philadelphia, 1989.
21. Madewell BR, et al: Ras proteins detected and discriminated in canine

neoplasms by selective use of antisera. Proceedings of the 9th Annual Conference, Veterinary Cancer Society, Raleigh, NC, Oct, 1989.

22. Merkel DE, et al: Flow cytometry, cellular DNA content, and prognosis in human malignancy. *J Clin Oncol 5*:1690, 1987.
23. Mullins JI, et al: Viral transduction of c-myc gene in naturally occurring feline leukemias. *Nature 308*:856, 1984.
24. Nowell PC: Chromosomal approaches to oncogenes and oncogenesis. *Fed Am Soc Exper Biol 2*:3054, 1988.
25. Ordóñez NG: Application of immunocytochemistry in the diagnosis of poorly differentiated neoplasms and tumors of unknown origin. *Cancer Bull 41*:142, 1989.
26. Osborne CA: General principles of biopsy. *Vet Clin North Am 4*:213, 1974.
27. Patnaik AK, et al: Canine cutaneous mast cell tumor: Morphologic grading and survival time in 83 dogs. *Vet Pathol 21*:469, 1984.
28. Perman V, et al: Bone marrow biopsy. *Vet Clin North Am 4*:293, 1974.
29. Perman V, et al: Lymph node biopsy. *Vet Clin North Am 4*:281, 1974.
30. Remvikos Y, et al: DNA flow cytometry applied to fine needle sampling of human breast cancer. *Cancer 61*:1629, 1988.
31. Richardson RC, Rebar AH: Collection techniques in veterinary cytology. *In* Rebar AH (ed): *Handbook of Veterinary Cytology*. Ralston Purina Co., St. Louis, 1978, pp 2–14.
32. Rosenthal RC, MacEwen EG: Treatment of lymphoma in dogs. *J Am Vet Med Assoc 196*:774, 1990.
33. Rutteman GR, et al: Flow cytometric analysis of DNA ploidy in canine mammary tumors. *Cancer Res 48*:3411, 1988.
34. Sandusky GE, et al: Diagnostic immunohistochemistry of canine round cell tumors. *Vet Pathol 24*:495, 1987.
35. Shofer FS, et al: Histopathologic and dietary prognostic factors for canine mammary carcinoma. *Breast Cancer Res Treat 13*:49, 1989.
36. Sickel-Suntanello BJ, et al: Technical and statistical improvements for flow cytometric DNA analysis of paraffin-embedded tissue. *Cytometry 9*:598, 1988.
37. Spandidos DA: Cellular oncogenes, mutations and cancer. *Anticancer Res 3*:121, 1983.
38. Twardock AR, Hornof WJ: Nuclear medicine. *In* Theilen GH, Madewell BR (eds): *Veterinary Cancer Medicine*. 2nd ed. Lea & Febiger, Philadelphia, 1987, pp 85–92.
39. Withrow SJ, Lowes N: Biopsy techniques for use in small animal oncology. Proceedings of the Oncology Short Course, Colorado State University, Fort Collins, CO, Jan, 1981.
40. Yokota J, et al: Alterations of myc, myb, and ras^{Ha} proto-oncogenes in cancers are frequent and show clinical correlation. *Science 231*:261, 1986.
41. Young KM: Myeloproliferative disorders. *Vet Clin North Am 15*:769, 1985.

CHAPTER 150 Surgical Therapy

Stephen H. Levine

Cancer has been viewed as either a surgically curable or incurable disease. A cure was potentially possible if the neoplasm could be completely removed. If complete removal of the neoplasm was not feasible, it was considered inoperable and incurable.

As understanding of neoplasia has evolved, so have newer and more effective multidisciplinary treatment regimens. A neoplasm is no longer looked on as an entity separate from its host, requiring surgical excision before it spreads. A neoplasm is a struggle between the host's immune resistance and the intrinsic forces within the tumor promoting its growth. It is the balance between these opposing forces that determines whether a tumor survives or is destroyed by host responses.

ROLE OF SURGERY IN ONCOLOGICAL THERAPY

Conventionally, the role of surgery in oncological therapy involved sharp surgical excision of the neoplasm with a scalpel. Surgeons now use more modern techniques such as electrosurgery, cryosurgery, and laser surgery.

Although many tumors are amenable to surgical therapy alone, a surgeon is now a member of a much larger team that considers all aspects of patient/tumor relationships.

Undetectable metastasis is the major cause of failure of surgical treatment of neoplasia. In most instances, the neoplasm has metastasized by the time it is diagnosed.[4]

Surgery in the overall management of tumor patients includes definitive, palliative, and exploratory procedures, combination therapies, and surgery as immunotherapy.

Definitive Procedures

Surgery alone may be curative in the treatment of many neoplasms if the neoplasm is confined to a nonvital organ or region and amenable to complete removal. Common examples in dogs include tumors of the skin, mammary glands, and genitalia. Complete surgical cure of neoplasms in other sites is potentially possible but less likely because of metastatic disease. These sites include the endocrine and musculoskeletal systems, the gastrointestinal and urinary tracts, and the spleen.

A few surgical procedures have been shown to prevent the formation of certain neoplasms. For example, it has been shown that ovariohysterectomy performed on a bitch before 2 years of age decreases the frequency of mammary tumors later in life.[3, 16] Orchiectomy also inhibits development of canine perianal gland tumors.

Palliative Procedures

The goal of some surgical procedures is to locally reduce a tumor mass, despite local invasion or metastasis, to provide relief for a patient. For example, many fibrosarcomas grow slowly and recur locally.[1, 2, 7, 8, 15, 17] Repeated removal of such masses may reduce clinical signs and allow the animal to live a comfortable existence. Amputation of a limb with osteosarcoma may be included in this category. Although amputation does not increase survival time, removal of a limb may reduce the pain and problems associated with the local disease and make the patient more comfortable for several months.[5] Newer evidence now suggests that amputation in conjunction with chemotherapy may significantly increase survival time.

Exploratory Procedures

Surgical procedures are used to establish a diagnosis and prognosis for neoplastic conditions. Exploratory celiotomy or thoracotomy is used to confirm a suspicion of neoplasia based on history, physical examination, laboratory data, and radiography. Direct exposure with palpation sometimes is the only way to further define a mass observed radiographically or ultrasonographically. Observation of the tumor and metastases in other sites can aid as a prognostic tool or indicate other treatment. Biopsy specimens are often taken during exploratory procedures for microscopic examination.

Combination Therapy

Many neoplasms are now managed with a multidisciplinary approach that has provided veterinary surgeons with an expanding role in treatment. A surgeon may now be a member of a team that includes immunologists, radiologists, pathologists, oncologists, pharmacologists, and biochemists. Surgically reducing the tumor load is an important aspect of any multidisciplinary approach. The most effective treatments include maximum reduction of tumor cell mass by surgery or radiation. Surgical removal often results in improved immunocompetence.[4, 13] In addition, residual microfoci or tumor cells are more sensitive to chemotherapy than the primary tumor because metastases often have a richer blood supply and a more rapid rate of cell turnover.[13]

Surgery as Immunotherapy

Immunotherapy in the treatment of neoplasia involves the stimulation or moderation of a patient's immune system to damage or destroy neoplastic cells.

Cancer surgery is perhaps the most frequently used form of immunotherapy. Evidence suggests that a host's immune defenses can be limited by a growing neoplasm. Certain neoplasms are able to evade an immune attack by specific and nonspecific immunosuppression of the host. Growing neoplasms constantly shed soluble tumor-associated antigens in the blood, and these circulate alone or as antigen-antibody complexes. These serum antigens inhibit the lymphocyte-mediated destruction of tumor cells *in vitro* and may have a similar role *in vivo*.[13]

In addition to blocking tumor-specific antigens, a growing neoplasm often causes nonspecific immunosuppression. Humoral factors produced by the neoplasm or in response to it can be found in the sera of patients and may cause general immunosuppression.[11] The extent of immunosuppression correlates with the stage of disease and size of tumor burden. This immunosuppression is reversed by removing the growing neoplasms. Therefore, any therapeutic maneuver that reduces tumor mass may reverse both specific and nonspecific immunosuppression and alter the immune balance in favor of the patient. In this respect, surgery is immunotherapy because it effectively decreases neoplastic cell mass and increases patients' immunocompetence.

In veterinary medicine, immunotherapy has given inconsistent results.

COMPONENTS OF IMMUNOTHERAPY

Active Specific Immunotherapy

The basic assumption that tumor cells contain antigens that the host may recognize as foreign is the basis of active specific immunotherapy. It is still controversial. Production of effective tumor vaccines based on these antigens is theoretically possible. A significant problem is that experimentally produced tumors are often heterogeneous with respect to drug sensitivity, metastatic capacity, and immunogenicity. Although occasional encouraging results have been reported, much research still needs to be done to prove the clinical effectiveness of such an approach.

Passive Immunotherapy

Passive immunotherapy involves administration of immune mediators to the patient. These mediators include immune lymphocytes, specific antibodies, complement, transfer factor, and "immune" RNA preparations.

Successful results have been reported with the administration of immune lymphocytes and immune sera, but the technical problems associated with these procedures render them clinically unusable.[18]

Nonspecific Immunotherapy

Nonspecific immunotherapy uses various agents that nonspecifically stimulate the immune system to destroy tumors. How these agents work is not completely understood. These agents are broadly classified as biological modulators or chemical immunostimulators.

The biological modulators are bacteria including a mixed bacterial vaccine of *Streptococcus pyogenes* and *Serratia marcescens*; bacillus Calmette-Guérin, an attenuated strain of *Mycobacterium bovis*; and *Corynebacterium parvum*. Studies using these agents have produced inconsistent results.[18]

Freund adjuvant and vaccinia virus have been used as nonspecific immunotherapeutic agents.

Chemical immunostimulants were investigated because of the inconsistencies and problems in using biological modulators. Drugs of the imidothiazole class (levamisole and thiabendazole) are the most widely known of these agents. Originally developed as anthelmintics, they have immune-potentiating properties. Clinical results have been discouraging.[18]

Interferon is a group of glycoproteins produced by various animal cells. Originally investigated as antiviral agents, their potential for antitumor properties has been considered. Interferon may have some antitumor effects that are partly mediated by the immune system.

PREOPERATIVE CONSIDERATIONS

Many factors affect the selection of patients with neoplasms for surgical therapy. A neoplasm's biological behavior, location, and extent are considered, as well as a patient's overall health. Curability is not always feasible, yet surgery often improves the quality of life without eliminating the disease.

Individual patients must be completely and objectively evaluated before any treatment is considered or initiated. The majority of patients with neoplasms are older animals. In addition to their tumor, these patients are more likely to have other systemic or metabolic disorders. A thorough history and physical examination are essential, as well as a complete blood count, electrocardiogram, and laboratory assessment of renal and hepatic function.

Tumor boundaries are defined before therapy to determine whether the neoplasm is localized, invasive, or metastatic. Surrounding tissues and regional lymph nodes are carefully palpated for evidence of metastasis. Bone close to a neoplasm is radiographically evaluated for tumor invasion.

Thoracic radiographs are evaluated if the neoplasm has a tendency for pulmonary metastasis. Pulmonary metastases may be undetected on radiographic examination if their cross-sectional diameter is less than that of a major pulmonary vessel.[4] Therefore, a "negative" chest radiograph does not ensure the absence of metastasis. Thoracic radiographs are also a valuable aid in assessing a patient's cardiopulmonary status.

SURGICAL MANAGEMENT

Anesthesia

Newer anesthetic agents with minimal cardiopulmonary suppressive effects are ideal. Indwelling intravenous catheters and maintenance fluid therapy are used in most oncological procedures. These are often lengthy procedures with considerable potential for hemorrhage. Neoplasms in appropriate locations may be amenable to epidural or regional nerve blocks.

Local anesthetic agents may greatly distort the architecture of neoplasms, increase the difficulty of microscopic interpretation, and potentiate metastasis.[14] They should probably be avoided in tumor resections.

General anesthesia and surgery suppress immunocompetence.[6, 12] This may be significant if a patient is already immunosuppressed by a neoplasm.

Surgical Technique

Aseptic surgical technique is an important aspect in all forms of surgery and is particularly important in surgery of neoplasia. Patients with neoplasia are often debilitated and immunosuppressed and have an increased risk of infection. Strict aseptic techniques must be maintained to minimize the chances of surgically induced infection. Preoperative prophylactic antibiotics may also be considered.

A wide area round the lesion is prepared for surgery, should a larger incision be needed. Wide exposure is thus provided at the surgery site, aiding excision of the tumor with minimal manipulation and trauma.

Tissue Handling

Minimal, gentle handling of neoplastic tissues is imperative. Excessive surgical trauma may cause exfoliation of tumor cells into the wound and systemic circulation.[3, 4, 13, 19] This warning applies to the preoperative and operative periods. Excessive manipulation of a neoplasm or even a single injection of saline results in a tremendous increase in the shedding of cells and clumps of cells by neoplasms. These clumps of cells are most likely to survive and grow as metastatic foci.[13]

Margins

The best opportunity for surgical cure of neoplasia is at the first operation. A wide margin of normal tissue must be excised to ensure total removal of the neoplasm. The scalpel should pass only through normal tissues on all sides of the tumor. Normal tissue margins of at least 1 cm should suffice in all but the most highly malignant neoplasms. Fortunately, animals usually have enough loose skin to allow closure of surgical wounds. In certain sites it may be difficult to close the defect, but it is still imperative to include normal tissue margins. Rather than leaving tumor cells to regrow, it is preferable to leave the surgical wound open to heal by granulation or consider immediate or future reconstructive procedures.

Histological examination of specimen margins is recommended to determine the presence of microscopic invasion into normal tissues, which might suggest a second, wider surgical resection.

En Bloc Resections

An *en bloc* resection is removal of the primary tumor, intervening lymphatics, and regional lymph node in continuity. It is indicated only when a regional lymph node is in close proximity to a primary neoplasm. Removal of the primary tumor and lymph node through separate incisions could leave tumor cells behind in lymphatic channels.

An increasing understanding of the myriad functions that the lymph nodes perform has been accompanied by a decrease in the "radical" nature of surgical procedures. Routine lymph node removal with excisional biopsies is often contraindicated because lymph nodes are more than mechanical filters designed to remove foreign agents. The regional lymph nodes respond to tumor-specific antigens and are the body's first line of immune defense.[10] Random removal of the lymph nodes may actually impair defense mechanisms and shorten survival time.

Although controversial, it is generally recommended that only those lymph nodes that are clinically affected be removed. This determination is often difficult even for the most experienced surgeons. In addition to metastatic invasion by a tumor, a lymph node may be enlarged owing to hyperplasia secondary to tumor-antigen stimulation or to hemorrhage or infection within the tumor. If the lymph node is enlarged because it is producing stimulated lymphocytes, it should not be excised because it is one of the main defense mechanisms. However, if a lymph node is enlarged because of metastatic invasion, it should be removed. In the clinical situation, it is still probably wise to remove those lymph nodes that definitely appear involved, as well as those that are suspicious.

POSTOPERATIVE MANAGEMENT

Each surgically treated neoplasm is unique and may pose specific postoperative management problems that are as important as the surgical procedure itself. As an example, surgical resection of a functional pancreatic beta-cell adenocarcinoma may cause diabetes. A patient with surgically induced diabetes requires close monitoring of blood glucose and may ultimately require insulin therapy. Surgical management of thyroid neoplasms in both dogs and cats may also require prolonged treatment with thyroid hormone and calcium supplementation if the parathyroids were included in the resection.

Special diets and stool softeners may be indicated in various gastrointestinal-colonic resections. Some patients may require pharyngostomy tubes, gastrostomy tubes, nasogastric tubes, thoracic drains, and so on that require close supervision and postoperative maintenance. Depending on the surgical procedure used, administration of antibiotics during the postoperative period may be indicated.

Although adjuvant therapy may be started before surgery, other phases of combination therapies are often implemented in the immediate postoperative period. Many factors must be considered before initiating therapy: Will the neoplasm respond better to immediate postoperative radiation therapy or should it be delayed until some healing has occurred. If chemotherapy is used, should it be initiated before, during, or after the operation. A plan must be clearly laid out before any action is taken.

STAGING

Owners frequently request information on survival rates of animals affected with various neoplasms. This information is available for only a few neoplasms, but our knowledge in this area is constantly expanding.

To standardize classification and aggressiveness of various neoplasms, staging systems have been designed.[9] The objectives of a classification (staging) system are (1) to aid clinicians in planning treatment, (2) to establish prognosis, (3) to assist in evaluating results, (4) to facilitate the exchange of information between treatment centers, and (5) to assist in investigating neoplasia.

The most widely accepted staging system is the TNM designation (T, tumor; N, regional lymph node; M, distant metastasis). An example of the complete TNM system for mammary gland neoplasia is shown in Table 150–1. A tumor classified as $T_1N_0M_0$ is small and noninvasive. A $T_3N_2M_1$ is a large, locally invasive tumor with distant metastases.

TABLE 150–1. CLINICAL STAGING* OF CANINE MAMMARY TUMORS

T: Primary tumor	
T_0	No evidence of tumor (use for rechecks after surgical removal of 1° tumor)
T_1	Tumor less than 1 cm maximum diameter (a) not fixed, (b) fixed to skin, (c) fixed to muscle
T_2	Tumor 1 to 3 cm maximum diameter (a) not fixed, (b) fixed to skin, (c) fixed to muscle
T_3	Tumor greater than 3 cm maximum diameter
N: Regional lymph nodes (RLN)	
N_0	No RLN involved
N_1	Ipsilateral RLN involved (a) not fixed, (b) fixed
N_2	Bilateral RLN involved (a) not fixed, (b) fixed
M: Distant metastasis	
M_0	No evidence of distant metastasis
M_1	Distant metastasis (distant nodes included)

*Approved by World Health Organization, Geneva, April 1978.

POSTOPERATIVE FOLLOW-UP

The intensity of postoperative follow-up is dictated by the type of neoplasm being treated. Patients with highly aggressive malignancies are re-evaluated frequently. A thorough physical examination is performed at each visit, including palpation of the original surgical site for evidence of local recurrence and the regional lymph nodes for metastasis.

Follow-up examinations may include thoracic radiographs to assess pulmonary metastasis or abdominal radiographs to evaluate the mesenteric or sublumbar lymph nodes. Other patients may require laboratory evaluations of hepatic or renal function to detect metastases. Evaluation of such parameters as blood glucose, insulin, thyroid hormone, or calcium levels may be indicated.

Careful repeat examinations are important not only for care of individual patients but also for comparison and evaluation of various treatment regimens. Re-examinations allow development of rational clinical protocols and establishment of more accurate prognoses.

Finally, knowledge obtained from necropsies on patients dying of tumor recurrence, euthanasia, or totally unrelated circumstances provides information on a neoplasm's biological behavior and the efficacy of various surgical procedures.

CONCLUSIONS

The treatment of neoplasia is no longer totally within a surgeon's realm. While surgeons are constantly developing newer, more effective, and less traumatic techniques to deal with neoplasia, complete management demands a concerted, combined effort by clinicians of various specialties. Surgeons must have an understanding of the biological behavior of each neoplasm encountered to appreciate the newer and expanding indications for surgery in therapy. Proper execution of a diagnostic and therapeutic plan for each neoplasm must encompass a comprehensive presurgical, surgical, and postsurgical evaluation.

References

1. Abbas JS, et al: The surgical treatment and outcome of soft-tissue sarcoma. *Arch Surg 116*:765, 1981.
2. Bostock DE, Dye MT: Prognosis after surgical excision of fibrosarcomas in cats. *J Am Vet Med Assoc 175*:727, 1979.
3. Brodey RS: Surgical treatment of cancer in the dog. *J Am Vet Med Assoc 166*:494, 1975.
4. Brodey RS: Surgery. *In* Theilen GH, Madewell BR (eds): *Veterinary Cancer Medicine*. Lea & Febiger, Philadelphia, 1979, pp 67–79.
5. Brodey RS, Abt DA: Results of surgical treatment in 65 dogs with osteosarcoma. *J Am Vet Med Assoc 168*:1032, 1976.
6. Bruce DL, Wingard DW: Anesthesia and the immune response. *Anesthesiology 34*:271, 1971.
7. Castro EB, et al: Surgical therapy of fibrosarcomas of the extremeties. *Arch Surg 107*:284, 1973.
8. Devereux DF, et al: Surgical treatment of low grade soft tissue sarcomas. *Am J Surg 143*:490, 1982.
9. Engstrom PF: The impact of cancer staging on cancer management in the community hospital. *In* Sutnick AI, Engstrom PF (eds): *Oncologic Medicine*. University Park Press, Baltimore, 1976, pp 125–139.
10. Fisher B, Fisher ER: Studies concerning the regional lymph node in cancer. I. Initiation of immunity. *Cancer 27*:1001, 1971.
11. Harvey HJ: General principles of veterinary oncologic surgery. *J Am Anim Hosp Assoc 12*:335, 1976.
12. Lee YTN: Effect of anesthesia and surgery on immunity. *J Surg Oncol 9*:425, 1977.
13. Morton DL, Wells SA: Immunobiology of neoplastic disease. *In* Sabiston DC (ed): *Textbook of Surgery*. W.B. Saunders, Philadelphia, 1977, pp 583–622.
14. Peyton WT: Danger in the use of local infiltration anesthesia in operations upon malignant tumors. *Ann Surg 11*:453, 1940.
15. Rosenberg SA, et al: Prospective randomized evaluation of the role of limb sparing surgery, radiation therapy, and adjuvant chemoimmunotherapy in the treatment of adult soft tissue sarcomas. *Surgery 84*:62, 1978.
16. Schneider R, et al: Factors influencing canine mammary cancer development and postsurgical survival. *J Natl Cancer Inst 43*:1249, 1969.
17. Suit MD, et al: Management of patients with sarcoma of soft tissue in an extremity. *Cancer 31*:1247, 1973.
18. Susaneck SJ: Immunotherapy. *In* Slatter DH (ed): *Textbook of Small Animal Surgery*. W.B. Saunders, Philadelphia, 1985, pp 2400–2405.
19. Withrow SJ: Surgical management of cancer. *Vet Clin North Am 7*:13, 1977.

CHAPTER 151

Radiation Therapy

Gary R. Johnston, Marcia B. Whiteley, David B. Kestenman, and Daniel A. Feeney

Ionizing radiation alone or in combination is accepted as a treatment for neoplasia. Radiotherapeutic equipment is found in most veterinary teaching institutions. Increased interest by veterinary radiologists trained in radiation therapy has resulted in consistent radiotherapy protocols for many neoplasms. Demands by owners for an aggressive approach to tumor management have influenced interest in radiation therapy.

PRINCIPLES OF RADIATION THERAPY

Radiobiology

Radiobiology is the study of the interaction between ionizing radiation and living matter. Radiation therapy is the administration of ionizing radiation and its absorption by normal and neoplastic tissue. Therapeutic forms of ionizing radiation include x-ray, gamma-ray, electrons, neutrons, and other charged particles that randomly deposit their energy within matter in discrete clusters of ionization.[14, 27, 38, 63] This deposited energy is greater than the chemical binding energies of the molecules within the tissues. Ionization of the molecule results in ejection of orbital electrons that can lead to chemical changes within the vicinity of the ionization and eventually damage biologically important intracellular structures, particularly DNA. The density of local ionization depends on the absorber and the velocity and charge of the ionizating radiation.[27, 39] Charged particles (electrons and protons) have a lower velocity and a greater charge than electromagnetic radiation (x-rays and gamma-rays) and ionize more densely but dissipate their energy over a shorter tract for the equivalent energy.

Conversion of kinetic energy to biological damage by ionization within the cell can result from direct interaction between the ionizing photon or particle and the critical molecule or from indirect interaction of chemically reactive free radicals of water ionization and their subsequent interaction with regional molecules.[14, 27, 38, 63] Indirect mechanisms of biological damage predominate. Free radicals can fix radiation damage and result in irreversible chemical bonds. Nuclear DNA is the cellular target, damage to which is responsible for cell death.[14, 27, 38, 63] Ionizing radiation produces various reversible and irreversible lesions in the DNA molecule, including single- and double-strand breaks and alterations within the nucleic acid bases. Two mechanisms of radiation-induced cell death are recognized: mitotic cell death and interphase death.[38, 58, 63] Mitotic cell death occurs with moderate but lethal doses of radiation and results in the ultimate failure of cells to pass through mitosis after having completed one or more relatively normal mitoses. Alternatively, in more sensitive cells or cells receiving large doses of radiation, a cell may degenerate in interphase and fail to reach its first mitosis.

Radiosensitivity, Radioresponsiveness, and Radiocurability

The radiosensitivity of cells is related to their mitotic rate, further reproductive capabilities, and degree of differentiation and specialization. These criteria have

TABLE 151–1. CATEGORIES OF MAMMALIAN CELL RADIOSENSITIVITY

Cell Type	Example	Radiosensitivity
Vegetative intermitotic cells	Intestinal crypt cells, germinal layer of the epidermis	High
Differentiating intermitotic cells	Myelocytes, erythroblasts	Moderate to high
Multipurpose connective tissue cells	Fibroblasts, endothelial cells	Moderate to low
Reverting postmitotic cells	Hepatocytes, renal tubular cells, smooth-muscle cells	Moderate to low
Fixed postmitotic cells	Nerve cells, skeletal muscle, erythrocytes	Low

Modified from Rubin P, Casarett GW: *Clinical Radiation Pathology*. W.B. Saunders, Philadelphia, 1968, p.6.

been used to categorize mammalian cells on the basis of their relative radiosensitivity (Table 151–1).[14, 38, 65] Cells with a high mitotic rate and no differentiation between divisions, called *vegetative intermitotic cells* (intestinal crypt cells, basilar layer of the epidermis), are highly radiosensitive. Cells that do not divide and are highly differentiated and specialized are called *fixed postmitotic cells* and are radioresistant; examples include nervous tissue and skeletal muscle cells.

Radiosensitivity is also influenced by other factors unrelated to a cell's mitotic activity and degree of differentiation. Tumor size, cell type, a patient's condition, and the presence of infection influence radiosensitivity. Radiosensitivity is defined as the ability of radiation to biologically damage cells in normal or neoplastic tissue.[58]

Radioresponsiveness has frequently been equated with radiosensitivity. However, radioresponsiveness is the time required for visible structural or functional changes to occur and is measured by the rate at which the clinical manifestations of radiation injury take place.[58]

Radiocurability is the ability of ionizing radiation to reduce the number of malignant cells below a critical level so that no further clinical manifestations occur during a patient's remaining lifetime.[58] Radiocurability in humans is recognized if no tumor regrowth occurs within 5 years of radiotherapy treatment. In companion animals, radiocurability is accepted if no tumor regrowth occurs within 2 years of treatment. A tumor that shrinks rapidly after irradiation is radioresponsive. A tumor that shrinks very slowly is considered nonradioresponsive. Either tumor may be radiocurable. Failure to decrease the size of a tumor during or shortly after radiotherapy does not constitute a radiotherapy failure if neither continued tumor growth nor subsequent metastases ensue. Connective tissue tumors such as fibrosarcomas respond much more slowly (if at all) than epithelial tumors. The terminology is defined in Table 151–2.

Intracellular damage resulting from irradiation may cause cell death or recovery. The purpose of multiple external beam treatments is to use the varied characteristics of normal and neoplastic cells to enhance proliferation of normal cells and to promote mitotic cell death of tumor cells. Four factors, called the "four R's" of radiotherapy—repair, repopulation, redistribution, reoxygenation—are involved in designing radiotherapy protocols.[27, 100]

Repair of sublethal injury is possible to a greater degree in normal cells than in neoplastic cells. This advantage is increased by dividing the total dose into a number of smaller doses (fractionation), because the neoplastic cells, unlike normal cells, may have neither sufficient time nor the capability to repair sublethal injury before a subsequent dose is administered.

Repopulation by regeneration of stem cells may differ between normal and neoplastic cells. In normal tissues, restoration to preirradiation patterns of cell differentiation and rate of mitosis is a complex process under homeostatic control. The ability of neoplastic cells to regenerate and repopulate relative to normal tissues under external homeostatic control occurs at a slower rate. If normal tissues have a more rapid regrowth relative to tumor tissues after irradiation, these tissues would be less responsive to the effects of fractionated radiotherapy treatments. However, evidence suggests that tumor cells can respond to the stress of fractionated irradiation by increasing proliferation rates as well.[100]

Redistribution of cells within the cell cycle is another possible advantage of fractionated radiotherapy. Cells surviving a dose of radiation tend to synchronize in resistant phases of the cell cycle. Theoretically, it may be possible to develop treatment protocols to selectively disadvantage the tumor cells once synchronized. However, the rate at which individual cells progress through the cell cycle varies considerably, resulting in a phase difference between cells and decreasing the probability

TABLE 151–2. RADIOTHERAPY FOR COMPANION ANIMAL NEOPLASMS*

Tumor Type	Radiosensitivity	Responsiveness	Curability
Canine transmissible venereal tumors	High	Rapid	Excellent
Perianal adenomas	High	Rapid	Excellent
Squamous cell carcinoma	Variable†	Moderate to rapid	Fair to good
Fibrosarcoma	Low to moderate†	Slow	Poor to fair
Mast cell tumors	Moderate	Moderate to slow	Good to fair
Melanocarcinomas	Low	Slow	Poor to none
Osteosarcoma	Low	Slow	Poor to none

*Based on the authors' clinical experience in radiotherapy of companion animal neoplasms.
†Biological behavior after radiotherapy varies with location on the patient and species.[40, 76, 78]

that surviving cells will be in a resistant phase at the time of the next radiation fraction.

Reoxygenation of hypoxic cells is a result of several complex processes. Tumors larger than 150 to 200 μm are composed of a relatively radiosensitive, oxygenated population and a more radioresistant, hypoxic population.[38] The presence of hypoxic radioresistant cells is considered one of the major causes of postirradiation recurrence. Oxygenated cells are more sensitive to radiation than hypoxic cells and are selectively killed during fractionated treatment. A reduced population of oxygenated cells after radiation reduces the separation of hypoxic cells from blood vessels and results in more effective oxygen diffusion. Decreased tissue pressure within the tumor after radiation, because of a reduced number of tumor cells, reopens compressed blood vessels and increases vascular flow in areas of previous hypoxia. The net effect of reoxygenation is increased sensitivity of previously hypoxic cells to subsequent dose fractions.

RADIOBIOLOGICAL BASIS OF RADIATION THERAPY AND TISSUE TOLERANCE

The response of normal tissue in an irradiated field is the limiting factor in planning radiotherapy.[27, 30, 31, 33, 58, 70, 80] If only tumoricidal doses are considered, any tumor can be controlled by an appropriate dose of ionizing radiation. The goal is to cure without normal tissue complications. However, the risk must be evaluated for each patient. Although tumor control is the major objective, the risk of major, potentially life-threatening complications yet decreases the probability of tumor control. If the complications encountered can be managed medically or surgically, a protocol that uses a maximum dose of radiation to increase the probability of tumor control may be chosen. Tissue tolerance and acceptable level of complications vary between institutions and radiotherapists. Tolerance doses have been derived from clinical and experimental data for various tissues.[22, 64] In human radiotherapy, a minimum tissue tolerance dose (TD 5/5) results in no more than a 5 per cent severe complication rate within 5 years.[64, 66] The maximum tissue tolerance dose (TD 50/5) results in no more than a 50 per cent severe complication rate within 5 years of treatment.[64, 66] Definitions for companion animals have not been determined.

NORMAL TISSUE REACTION TO IONIZING RADIATION

Radiation injury depends on the relative radiosensitivity of the tissues receiving the radiation. Concurrent infection, trauma, or other diseases may influence the degree of tissue injury by radiation. Of primary consideration in radiation injury is turnover of parenchymal cells and its relationship to microcirculation.[64, 65] Also, the radiosensitivity of the parenchymal tissue relative to stromal tissues is important in determining acute and chronic effects of radiotherapy injury.[64] Rapidly renewing parenchymal tissues, such as the basilar layer of the epidermis, are vegetative intermitotic cells.[64] These cells are highly radiosensitive, compared with more radioresistant vascular and stromal tissues. Moderate radiation doses may destroy the more radiosensitive basilar layer of the epidermis with minimal damage to the more radioresistant vascular and stromal elements. However, the ability of vegetative intermitotic cells to regenerate and repopulate after irradiation depends on their survival and the integrity of supporting vascular and stromal structures. Large doses of radiation may cause necrosis of the more radiosensitive parenchymal tissues remaining in regeneration and repopulation, to be followed by chronic progressive injury mediated by vascular damage and interstitial fibrosis (increased histohematic connective tissue barrier).[64, 65] The end result of the vascular injury may be ischemia and necrosis even if more radiosensitive parenchymal tissues have repopulated to preirradiation levels.

A major problem is that acute radiotherapy changes do not predict later chronic changes. In slow, nonrenewing cell systems such as the brain and spinal cord, heart, liver, and kidneys, minimal or no acute functional change may be recognized after moderate to high doses of radiation. Later vascular changes may not be encountered for several months. Accurate prediction of late radiotherapy injury is tenuous even if the acute manifestations are well recognized.

METHODS OF RADIOTHERAPY

External Beam Radiotherapy (Teletherapy)

External beam radiotherapy uses a source of ionizing radiation separated at a distance from the patient. The primary beam of radiation is limited by collimation to expose only a specified area of the patient. The sources of external beam radiotherapy currently available in veterinary institutions include orthovoltage x-ray, cobalt 60 (^{60}Co), cesium 137 (^{137}Cs), and linear accelerators.

Orthovoltage Radiotherapy

Orthovoltage radiotherapy uses x-rays with a low to medium energy range of 150 to 400 kVp.[67] The quality of radiation produced by orthovoltage x-ray is further described by its half-value layer (HVL). The HVL is defined as the amount of absorber required to reduce the intensity of the primary beam by one-half. The HVL for orthovoltage x-ray beams ranges from 4 mm of aluminum to 4 mm of copper.

Orthovoltage x-ray therapy has many limitations compared with higher-energy x-rays and gamma-rays in the megavoltage range (in excess of 1 MeV). The ability to penetrate tissue and achieve adequate depth of dose is a major limitation. With orthovoltage radiotherapy, the dose at depth decreases exponentially with increasing depth beneath the skin surface. With megavoltage radiotherapy, the maximum dose is below the skin surface, thus achieving a degree of "skin sparing." Orthovoltage has a major limitation in this respect because the dose the skin can tolerate may be too small to allow tumoricidal doses for deep tumors. Another disadvantage of orthovoltage radiotherapy is the disparity of dose distribution between soft tissue and bone in the same field. A primary x-ray beam with a HVL of 2 mm of copper delivers a dose to bone that may be 1.5 times greater than the dose in soft tissue. Doses greater than the tolerated dose for bone can result if tumoricidal doses to soft tissue are in the range of 4,500 to 5,000 cGy.* With megavoltage radiotherapy, minimal differential absorption occurs between bone and soft tissue. Although orthovoltage radiotherapy has major limitations, it is the most commonly used method in veterinary institutions in North America. Its major advantages are its simplicity, low cost, and reduced requirements for environmental shielding compared with those for megavoltage equipment.

Supervoltage Radiotherapy

Supervoltage teletherapy uses x-rays, gamma-rays, or electrons in an energy range in excess of 500 KeV.[67] ^{60}Co, ^{137}Cs, x-rays, and electron teletherapy units are limited to a few veterinary institutions. Both gamma-rays and x-rays are forms of electromagnetic radiation; however, they differ in their origin. Gamma-rays originate from spontaneous nuclear decay of a radioactive isotope, and x-rays originate from an event outside the nucleus. ^{60}Co has an average gamma-ray energy of 1.25 MeV, a half-life of 5.3 years, and a HVL of 12 mm of lead. ^{137}Cs has a gamma-ray energy of 0.66 MeV, a half-life of 30 years, and a HVL of 6.6 mm of lead. ^{137}Cs gamma emissions are intermediate in energy between orthovoltage (400 KeV[0.400 MeV]) and megavoltage ^{60}Co emissions (1.25 MeV). The greater energy of ^{137}Cs radiation provides a higher percentage depth dose penetration in the tissues than orthovoltage radiation. Because of its lower energy, less shielding is required than that for ^{60}Co. However, ^{137}Cs has low specific activity (disintegrations per second) and therefore low radiation output; its percentage depth dose is only modestly better than orthovoltage; and it has minimal if any skin-sparing effect compared with ^{60}Co. Although ^{137}Cs has advantages over orthovoltage radiotherapy, the added advantages of depth dose penetration, skin sparing, and uniform dose distribution for soft tissue and bone, as well as ease of equipment maintenance (compared with linear accelerators), make ^{60}Co the most practical method for veterinary radiotherapy. High-energy x-ray and electron beam therapy from linear accelerators in the energy range of 4 to 35 MeV are standard in human radiotherapy centers. At present, only one veterinary institution has linear accelerator capability.

Interstitial Brachytherapy

With interstitial brachytherapy, a radioisotope sealed in a metallic container, usually a seed, needle, or applicator, is placed in or on the patient.[33, 39, 90, 97] Radiation is administered in one prolonged dose over minutes, hours, or days. The sources may subsequently be removed, depending on the physical half-life of the isotope. The primary advantage of brachytherapy is that the sources are placed in the tumor, providing maximum tumor dose while minimizing the dose to surrounding normal tissues. The disadvantages of brachytherapy include (1) exposure to the personnel involved in placing the sources, (2) the necessary isolation facilities required for hospitalization of a patient to prevent environmental contamination with lost sources, and (3) exposure to the animal's owner or trainer.

In interstitial brachytherapy, organ tolerance depends on the volume of tissue implanted, much like teletherapy tolerance depends on field size. The tolerance dose decreases as the size of the volume implant increases.[39] Implant volumes less than 10 cm^3 can tolerate higher doses than implant volumes in excess of 200 cm^3. Consequently, implant volumes less than 5 cm in diameter are more suitable for implant therapy. The radioactive isotopes currently available to veterinary radiotherapists include ^{60}Co, ^{137}Cs, gold 198 (^{198}Au), iridium-192 (^{192}Ir), and iodine 125 (^{125}I).[39, 90, 97] The most important factor in selecting a therapeutic radionuclide is its half-life. Radiation quality, radiation safety, availability, and economy are also considered when selecting a radionuclide.

Systemic Radiotherapy

The internal use of radionuclides resembles interstitial brachytherapy except that the radioactive source is submicroscopic. The radionuclides can be administered orally, intravenously, or into the peritoneal or pleural space. Their localization into normal or neoplastic tissue depends on the chemical characteristics of the radionuclide. The application of systemic radiotherapy is limited to selected neoplastic diseases that cannot be adequately treated by teletherapy, chemotherapy, surgery, or other treatment methods. ^{131}I has been used to treat feline hyperthyroidism, as well as metastatic thyroid carcinoma in people and animals.[12, 43, 56, 62, 87] Phosphorus 32 (^{32}P) is currently used for treatment of polycythemia vera and palliation of chronic leukemia and metastatic cancers to bone.[67, 72] ^{32}P and ^{198}Au are used for palliation of malignant pleural and peritoneal effusions.[67] The disadvantages of systemic radiotherapy are similar to those with brachytherapy: A patient becomes radioactive, and the environment may become contaminated. Urine and feces must be handled as radioactive waste. Animals receiving systemic radiotherapy must be monitored during confinement to ensure that the level of radioactivity is safe for the general human population before they can be released. Systemic radiotherapy is currently limited to institutions with confinement facilities.

SEQUENCE OF RADIOTHERAPY IN COMBINATION WITH SURGERY

Surgery and radiotherapy are the major potentially curative methods available for veterinary tumor treatment. Surgery and irradiation may be used in several combinations. Surgery may be used to salvage early radiotherapy failures but is considered less effective in

*1 Centigray (cGy) = 0.01 gray = 1 rad; 1 gray (Gy) = 100 rad.

late radiotherapy failure.[27, 58] Radiotherapy may be used in surgical failures but is considered less effective because gross recurrence and distant metastasis usually have already occurred.[27, 58] Surgery and radiotherapy may be used to treat different areas. For example, surgical resection of tonsillar carcinomas with regional irradiation of the lymph nodes has been reported in dogs.[50] Surgery and irradiation may be used in a combined treatment protocol to treat the same area. Surgical failures occur because microscopic disease is not removed, even with radical resection. Radiation failure occurs because of the inability of the exponential cell-killing characteristics of ionizing radiation to reduce the tumor cell burden below a level that can be managed by a patient's immune system. This is especially important in the treatment of large masses, because the probability of recurrence increases with increasing tumor size.[27, 58] Clinical data suggest that 5,000 cGy given over 5 weeks eliminates microscopic neoplastic disease in 90 per cent of human patients.[27] It is logical to assume that surgery and radiotherapy can be complementary, surgery removing the gross mass and irradiation eliminating microscopic foci. Irradiation may be preoperative, intraoperative, or postoperative.[27, 36, 58]

Preoperative Radiotherapy

The arguments in favor of preoperative radiotherapy include the following: rendering a locally diffuse tumor removable, decreasing the required extent of surgical resection of normal tissues, and rendering nonviable any malignant cells that may be inadvertently implanted surgically in the wound or circulatory system.[26] Radical surgical resection has been associated with distant metastasis in human clinical studies.[26, 27, 58] The argument against preoperative radiotherapy concerns impaired wound healing, which is directly proportional to the radiation dose.[26, 27, 58] Tumor shrinkage from preoperative radiotherapy may cause a client to refuse or delay curative resection or a surgeon to perform less radical resection.[26, 27, 58] Clinical and experimental data on increased cure rates for preoperative compared with those for postoperative radiotherapy are *inconclusive*. The optimum dose of preoperative radiotherapy varies with the tumor cell type and location. In humans, the total dose of preoperative radiotherapy is from 2,000 cGy in eight treatments to 5,000 cGy in 20 treatments.[58] The interval between preoperative radiotherapy and surgery is usually 3 to 6 weeks.[58] However, a 24- to 48-hour interval between the two procedures has been reported.[27] Preoperative radiotherapy may be of benefit in neoplasms with a high incidence of postoperative recurrence.

Intraoperative Radiotherapy

Radiotherapy during surgery has received increased recognition in human oncology. Accurate beam collimation to encompass the tumor and the ability to displace sensitive organs outside the radiation field are the major advantages of such therapy. The major disadvantage is the expense of combined radiotherapy and a surgical facility. When less than optimum facilities exist, anesthetized patients must be moved to a nonsterile area for radiation of the open surgical field. The risk of introducing pathogens under these circumstances is considerable. The trend in human radiotherapy centers is to design special operating rooms in the radiotherapy area. Single doses of 1,000 to 3,000 cGy of orthovoltage x-rays or electrons (from linear accelerators) are currently used.[36] Application to veterinary radiotherapy is limited because of the expense. It has been used in selective intra-abdominal tumors with some success.[86, 98, 101]

In general, radiotherapy during surgery is reserved for diffuse neoplasms that are not responsive to postoperative fractionated external beam megavoltage radiation or interstitial brachytherapy. Principles of radiotherapy and clinical experience of normal tissue tolerance suggest that the risk of long-term complications increases with a smaller number of higher-dose fractions for a specified total dose.[76] Large single doses of radiotherapy may result in fibrosis, stricture formation, loss of function, and necrosis. The decision to use this method of treatment must take into account the organs involved, the probability of long-term survival (long enough for complications to occur), the quality of life after treatment, and the therapeutic advantage over more conventional approaches.

Postoperative Radiotherapy

The primary indication for postoperative radiotherapy is a local neoplasm that cannot be completely removed. When the inaccuracies of assessing tumor involvement have been clarified by surgery, radiotherapy can be better adjusted.[26, 27] A higher total dose of irradiation can be given compared with preoperative or intraoperative radiotherapy.[26, 27] Surgical resection and healing are favored in the irradiated field compared with preoperative or intraoperative radiotherapy. Postoperative radiotherapy has several disadvantages: (1) Distant metastases may be produced by the surgical procedure, (2) surgery may decrease vascularity and predispose to tissue hypoxia, and (3) tumor proliferation may occur before irradiation is initiated if surgical healing is prolonged. Veterinary radiotherapists often elect to have the tumor border reduced by surgery, followed by radiotherapy immediately or 2 to 4 weeks postoperatively. It has been suggested that if irradiation is not begun immediately after surgery, it should be delayed about 3 weeks to permit tissue healing and decrease the likelihood of radiation-induced dehiscence.[77, 95] However, this philosophy is controversial. The decision to combine surgery and radiotherapy follows careful consideration of the cell type, extent of local invasion, and physical characteristics of the tumor.

RADIATION COMBINED WITH NONSURGICAL TREATMENT

The presence of hypoxic cells in a solid tumor is a major consideration in radiotherapy because of their relative radioresistance compared with normal and neoplastic oxygenated cells. Hyperthermia and administration of hypoxic cell sensitizers (i.e., misonidazole) and radioprotectants (WR 2721) have been investigated to overcome hypoxia and increase the therapeutic effect. Sequential or simultaneous use of chemotherapy in combination with surgery and radiation[56] has been used to improve the therapeutic ratio.

Hyperthermia

Temperatures of 104°F (40°C) or greater are used to treat tumors. Hyperthermia may be used as a primary treatment method or combined with radiotherapy or chemotherapy. The therapeutic effects of hyperthermia have been observed in cell cultures and in spontaneous tumors in companion animals.[10, 15, 32, 54, 81, 83] Cell death by heat alone begins at 107.6° to 109.4°F (42° to 43°C) (tissue temperature). The lethal intracellular effects of heat are the result of rupture of plasma membranes, disruption of mitochondria, clumping of nuclear chromatin, and focal cytoplasmic swelling.[54, 74] These effects depend on time and temperature. In mice with implanted tumors, the destructive effects of heat began at 107.6°F (42°C).[18] For each degree rise in temperature above 107.6°F, the time required to produce the same biological effects was halved.[18] Results using hyperthermia alone for squamous cell carcinomas with tissue temperatures from 109.4° to 112°F (43° to 44.5°C) for 30 minutes have been encouraging, with complete regression of the tumor in several patients.[32, 54] Clinical hyperthermia in combination with either interstitial brachytherapy or teletherapy has been used in human and veterinary radiotherapy. Encouraging results for squamous cell carcinomas and fibrosarcomas using combined hyperthermia and radiotherapy have been reported in dogs and cats.[10, 54] The results using hyperthermia and radiotherapy for canine osteosarcoma are less encouraging.[48]

Local or systemic hyperthermia may be used. Radiofrequency, microwave, ultrasound, and water immersion or whole-body chambers are currently used.

No definite evidence shows that tumor cells are more sensitive to heat than normal tissues. The local tumor environment that has an important role in hyperthermic killing of tumors cells is substantially different from normal tissue.[74] A tumor's microenvironment consists of areas of necrosis, hypoxia, and reduced pH. The primitive vascularity of tumors reduces their ability to dissipate heat. The net result is that the tumor tissue has a higher temperature than the normal surrounding tissues. The decreased pH in a tumor and the reduced nutrition of the tumor cells may also increase their sensitivity to high temperatures. Hypoxic cells found in a tumor are more resistant to radiation than oxygenated cells but are more sensitive to heat than oxygenated cells.[21]

The rationale for combining hyperthermia and radiotherapy is based on their synergistic effects. Results in clinical trials using hyperthermia either alone or in combination with other methods are encouraging. However, protocols for specific tumors are either incomplete or still under investigation. The use of hyperthermia and radiotherapy is limited to educational or research institutions. Heat alone by localized radiofrequency instruments has been used for localized tumors in animals.*

Hypoxic Cell Sensitizers

Chemical sensitizers selectively increase the sensitivity of hypoxic tumor cells to radiation without altering the response of oxygenated cells.[9] Nitroheterocyclic compounds with affinity for electrons sensitize hypoxic cells to radiation.[2, 60] Radiosensitizers may have a similar mechanism of action to oxygen on cells by promoting effects of radiation within cells.[1, 60] Hypoxia protects cells against the effects of radiation by a factor of 2.5 to 3.0 compared with well-oxygenated cells. With adequate concentrations of radiosensitizers *in vitro*, this level of hypoxic protection is reduced and may approach the level of sensitivity of oxygenated cells.[2, 68, 69]

Nitromidazoles have displayed encouraging radiosensitizing properties in investigations of animal tumors. Metronidazole and misonidazole are radiosensitizers that have been extensively investigated. Misonidazole has been used extensively in clinical trials in humans.[3] Nausea, vomiting, and neurotoxicity are complications of multiple-dose regimens with misonidazole.[3] To limit neurotoxicity to an acceptable clinical level in humans, the total dose of misonidazole recommended is 10.5 to 15.0 g/m^2.[96] This reduces the number of doses (of radiation and therapeutic cell sensitizers) that can be administered to between 4 and 10 (less than the 20 to 40 doses that would be administered with a conventional multifractionated radiotherapy protocol).

The use of misonidazole and irradiation for treatment of fibrosarcomas in dogs has been reported.[17] However, no statistical difference was found in survival rates between those dogs treated with radiation alone and those treated with radiation and misonidazole.

Agents that Protect Against Radiation

Oxidation of biological molecules by free radicals produced from irradiation of intracellular water is an accepted cause of radiation injury. These molecules may be DNA or associated proteins. Certain sulfhydryl compounds, such as cysteamine and cystine, have protective capacities during irradiation. Depletion of sulfhydryl compounds is reported to increase cellular radiosensitivity.[94, 102] The addition of exogenous sulfhydryl compounds protects aerated cells yet provides only minimal protection to hypoxic cells.[94, 102] It is likely that these compounds are scavengers of free radicals or competitors for the oxidative effects of the radiation-induced free radicals, thus permitting repair of sublethal diseases. If normal tissues can be protected, total radiation doses could be increased, resulting in greater tumor control without increased damage to normal tissue. Several sulfhydryl compounds that have been developed provide protection *in vitro* and *in vivo*. WR2721 protects normal aerated tissues without protecting the hypoxic tumor cells.[84, 93, 94, 102] WR2721 and radiation have been

*See references 10, 19, 20, 32, 34, 37, and 81.

used experimentally for the treatment of spontaneous tumors in dogs.[84] Dogs treated with WR2721 and radiation had milder dermatitis than dogs treated with radiation alone.[84] Longer tumor regression and reduced damage to normal tissues were obtained in dogs with spontaneous neoplasms treated with WR2721 and radiation.[74] More clinical trials are necessary to determine the therapeutic gain obtained with radioprotectants and radiation in spontaneous neoplasms of companion animals. Their use in combination with radiation, radiosensitizers, and hyperthermia requires further investigation.

Chemotherapy

The combination of chemotherapy and radiation has received little attention by veterinarians, although considerable attention has been given to combined chemotherapy and radiation for human adult and pediatric neoplasms.[27] Increased therapeutic ratios are obtained in large mediastinal masses of Hodgkin's disease when chemotherapy is used to shrink the tumor mass so the radiotherapist can reduce the field size and irradiate less lung tissue and a smaller tumor mass.

Therapeutic results are improved using combined chemotherapy for head and neck tumors in humans.[99] Combinations have been recommended in the treatment of pediatric Wilms' tumor, Hodgkin's disease, rhabdomyosarcoma, and leukemia of the central nervous system.[27] Radiation therapy, testosterone, and menadiol sodium diphosphate were used unsuccessfully to treat an undifferentiated mammary carcinoma in an 11-year-old female pointer.[72] Menadiol sodium diphosphate, a synthetic vitamin K preparation, has been used as an early radiosensitizer but is reported to have little activity. Its use with radiation for spontaneous tumors in dogs has been reported.[72] Surgery or radiotherapy followed by chemotherapy was recommended for the treatment of canine osteosarcoma.[8] Cisplatin and radiation have been used in combination for treatment of urinary bladder carcinoma in two dogs, with reduction in tumor size.[52] Chemotherapy and radiation have been recommended in the treatment of tonsillar squamous cell carcinoma and other tumors in dogs and cats.[11, 71, 96]

Chemotherapeutic agents such as antibiotics, alkylating agents, and antimetabolites may be used with radiation therapy to prevent metastasis during irradiation of the primary tumor.[27] These compounds act as apparent sensitizers and potentiate effects of radiation.[38] In reality, they do not increase the lethal effects of radiation but probably add to the effect of radiation.[38] The early and late effects of chemotherapeutic drugs are well known. The severity of complications encountered when radiation and chemotherapy are simultaneously combined may produce unacceptable complications that are more severe than if either had been used alone.[56] The toxicity of each compound and its potential effect if used in conjunction with radiation should be considered. The toxicity of commonly used chemotherapy agents combined with radiation is listed in Table 151–3. Additional investigations using radiation therapy and chemotherapy are needed to determine if survival rates are increased over those with treatment by either irradiation or chemotherapy alone (see Chapter 152).

APPLICATIONS

Evaluation Before Radiotherapy

Evaluation before radiotherapy is critical and directly influences the decision to accept a patient for radiotherapy. The minimum data base for each patient should include a physical examination, complete blood count, urinalysis, serum chemistry profile, thoracic radiographs, abdominal radiographs (and abdominal ultrasonography if the neoplasm is caudal to the diaphragm), radiographs of the primary tumor if near osseous structures, and a biopsy. If lymphadenopathy is identified, a biopsy should be performed to determine if inflammatory or metastatic disease is present. Thoracic radiographs may show if metastases are present, in addition to assessing the cardiopulmonary system. Abdominal radiographs are recommended with tumors of the perineum, anus, and hind legs to evaluate caudal retroperitoneal lymph nodes. With occult bone pain without radiographic lesions or in cases with radiographic evidence of osseous involvement, nuclear imaging with a radiopharmaceutical that localizes to bone (i.e., ^{99m}Tc-MDP) may be helpful in radiotherapy treat-

TABLE 151–3. MAJOR TOXIC EFFECTS OF DRUGS COMMONLY USED IN CONJUNCTION WITH RADIOTHERAPY

Complication	Vincristine	Actinomycin D	Cyclophosphamide	Adriamycin	High-Dose Methotrexate	Cisplatin[45]
Leukopenia	–	+	+ +	+ + +	+ + +	+ + +
Thrombocytopenia	–	+ + +	+	+	+ +	+ + +
Neurotoxicity	+ +	–	–	–	–	+
Cardiotoxicity	–	–	+	+ + +	–	+
Cystitis	–	–	+ + +	–	–	–
Mucositis	–	+ +	–	+ +	+ + +	–
Gastrointestinal toxicity	+ +	+ +	+ +	+ +	–	+ + +
Cellulitis	+ +	+ +	–	+ +	–	–
Erythema	–	+ +	–	–	+	–
Pulmonary	—	—	—	—	—	+ + +
Renal toxicity	–	—	—	—	—	+ + +
Hepatotoxicity	–	–	–	–	+ + +	—

Increased number of + signs denotes increasing severity and frequency of complications.

Complications represented by + are for combined protocols of chemotherapeutic agents and radiation.

From Suton WW, Chan RC: Irradiation and chemotherapy in pediatric tumors. *In* Fletcher GH (ed): *Textbook of Radiotherapy*. Lea & Febiger, Philadelphia, 1980, p. 639.

ment planning, but its availability is limited. In tumors of the nasal passages or central nervous system, computed tomography is beneficial and essential in radiotherapy treatment planning when multiportal protocols are used.[82, 88] A serum chemistry profile detects coexisting hepatic or renal insufficiency. Patients with these insufficiencies are considered poor anesthetic risks and may have a decreased life expectancy.

A biopsy is a prerequisite to radiotherapy by providing a cell-type diagnosis, thereby determining the overall prognosis. However, the biopsy technique may influence the accuracy of the diagnosis. Fine-needle biopsies should not be considered definitive except in mast cell tumors because of the hit-or-miss nature of the technique. In addition, cell distortion may preclude an accurate diagnosis. An excisional biopsy is recommended because it provides veterinary pathologists with an adequate nontraumatized sample. In abdominal neoplasia, ultrasonographically guided needle biopsy may be less invasive than excisional biopsy and yet provide the same degree of diagnostic accuracy as excisional biopsy. If excisional biopsy is not appropriate, a trephined core or wedge biopsy sample should be obtained. A qualified veterinary histopathologist should evaluate tissue samples for histological diagnosis, degree of malignancy, tumor staging, and completeness of an excisional biopsy.

Selection of Patients

Radiation therapy is not a panacea for all neoplasms, nor should it be considered a last-ditch effort when all other therapies have failed to control a tumor. A practitioner may be reluctant to refer a patient because of age and life expectancy. However, the physical examination should determine a patient's general health. An older patient in good physical condition is a potential candidate for radiotherapy. The data from the evaluation determine if concurrent disease exists and may preclude radiation therapy. Neoplasms such as lymphosarcoma, lymphoblastic leukemia, systemic mast cell sarcomas, and metastatic neoplasms should be treated with chemotherapy. In general, the physical characteristic of a tumor determines treatment. Superficial neoplasms that are not locally invasive are surgically resected. Superficial tumors that are localized but invasive may be effectively treated by radiation. Surgical resection followed by radiation frequently is appropriate for tumor therapy. Surgical resection is recommended even in invasive tumors to reduce the size of the tumor mass, because tumor volume adversely affects radiocurability. The greater the number of cells, the greater the total dose required to cure the tumor. Because normal tissue tolerance is the factor that limits dose in radiotherapy, adequate tumoricidal doses may not be obtained in large tumor masses if the normal tissues are treated to the tolerance level.

Selection of Radiotherapy

The selection of radiotherapy for an individual case depends on the location and physical characteristics of the tumor and the availability of radiotherapy facilities. ^{60}Co or ^{137}Cs needles, ^{125}I and ^{198}Au seeds, and ^{181}Ir ribbons or wire can be used for localized superficial tumors that cannot be surgically resected. However, brachytherapy requires special facilities for housing patients. Some older patients in good physical condition may not tolerate hospitalization and may be treated as outpatients with either orthovoltage or telecobalt therapy.

Brachytherapy using a ^{90}Sr applicator is suitable for the treatment of superficial inflammatory and neoplastic lesions of the cornea. ^{90}Sr is a beta emitter and produces particles that have a small range of penetration before attenuation by tissues. Fifty per cent of beta radiation is attenuated by 1 mm of soft tissue.[67]

Superficial lesions up to 5 mm in depth can be effectively treated using low-energy x-rays. An orthovoltage x-ray unit operated at 150 kVp and 15 mA may have an effective photon energy of 47 KeV and a HVL of approximately 6.5 mm of aluminum. Fifteen per cent of the x-ray photons are attenuated within the first 5 mm of tissue, and 50 per cent within the first 2 cm of tissue.[7] Low-energy x-ray photons can be used for superficial tumors over the abdomen when the underlying intestine can be protected. However, these low-energy x-rays should not be used to treat superficial lesions directly over bone. Low-energy x-rays are disproportionately absorbed by bone. Radiation doses in excess of bone tolerance may occur if therapeutic doses between 3,500 and 4,500 cGy are used to treat the soft tissues of the tumor.

For treating deep tumors, high-energy orthovoltage x-ray may be used. An orthovoltage x-ray unit operated at 250 kVp and 15 mA with appropriate added filtration has an effective photon energy of 100 to 140 KeV and a HVL between 1.5 and 4.0 mm of copper, providing a 50 per cent depth dose at 3 to 6 cm depth depending on the field size.[7] High-energy orthovoltage x-rays can be used for the treatment of tumors 3 to 4 cm in depth. The main limitation at these depths is the excessive surface dose, which can be avoided in some patients by using multiple treatment portals. High-energy orthovoltage x-ray also delivers a slightly higher dose to bone than to soft tissue.

High-energy gamma rays from ^{60}Co have an average energy of 1.25 MeV. Photon and electrons from linear accelerators may be in excess of 2 MeV. These megavoltage radiotherapy units have the advantage of delivering tumoricidal doses to deep-seated tumors yet sparing skin because the maximum dose is several millimeters below the skin surface. Bone and soft tissue attenuate radiation similarly with megavoltage radiation; consequently, a more even distribution of dose is obtained. Supervoltage and megavoltage radiation are currently limited by availability. With increasing interest in radiation therapy, it is anticipated that the availability of supervoltage radiation will increase in veterinary institutions.

Cure Versus Palliation

The ultimate goal in radiation therapy is to deliver a tumoricidal dose with an acceptable degree of complications. With large nonresectable tumors, radiotherapy may be used as a palliative treatment. Tumoricidal doses of 4,000 to 4,500 cGy may produce unacceptable complications in large fields or sensitive anatomical regions, and doses of 2,500 to 3,500 cGy may be necessary to reduce the size of the tumor. Single-fraction treatments during surgery for locally diffuse tumors are palliative. Clients may wish to treat the primary site of a metastatic tumor if the quality of life for a patient can be temporarily improved.

Specific Application to Selected Tumors

The tumors most frequently treated by radiotherapy are listed in the Appendix at the end of this chapter. The 1- and 2-year survivals were obtained from the veterinary literature and are referenced in the Appendix. Most veterinary radiotherapists treat malignant neoplasms by delivering a total dose of 4,000 to 5,000 cGy in ten fractions at a rate of three fractions per week.[85] These doses result in acceptable complication rates. Benign tumors and other benign lesions such as lick granulomas and rodent ulcers are treated with a total dose of 600 to 2,400 cGy given in one to four fractions.

FAILURE OF RADIOTHERAPY AND COMPLICATIONS

Failure of radiotherapy results from an inadequate field size to cover the primary tumor site and failure to detect regional or distant metastases. Careful evaluation before therapy may disclose regional lymph node involvement. Examination of an excisional biopsy specimen may determine if the tumor extends beyond the edge of the resected sample. Failure of radiotherapy may also result from the inherent resistance of the tumor because of hypoxic cells or because adequate lethal doses could not be delivered without exceeding regional normal tissue tolerance.

Complications of radiation therapy are primarily limited to the site of irradiation. Nausea and vomiting are not encountered unless the abdominal viscera are irradiated directly or unless during the course of treating periabdominal neoplasms sufficient doses are given to these organs. Complications of radiotherapy suggest that the radiation dose exceeded the tolerance of normal tissue in the field. Necrosis is the most common long-term sequel if tissue or organ tolerance is exceeded. Tissue or organ atrophy and fibrosis may be the end result of radiotherapy, depending on the dose and schedule (total and per fraction), specific tissue, and size of the field.

Because the surface dose is usually greater than the maximum tumor dose with orthovoltage radiotherapy, the most common sites for injury are the skin and mucous membranes. Epilation, depigmentation, and moist desquamation are the most frequently encountered complications.[44] It is important that these complications be explained to clients before radiotherapy. Epilation is encountered with surface skin doses in excess of 500 cGy. It is often a temporary complication of radiotherapy. The hair frequently grows back but may be a different color and less dense. Moist desquamation may be encountered with orthovoltage radiotherapy when surface doses range from 4,000 to 5,000 cGy, depending on the field size and treatment schedule. Moist desquamation is a result of injury to the germinal layer of the epidermis. Sloughing of the epidermis results in a thin desquamated epithelium, and hyperemia and vascular injury result in a serous exudate. Moist desquamation occurs around the seventh fraction of a ten-fraction protocol and reaches its peak intensity 10 to 14 days after therapy. This reaction usually subsides 2 to 3 weeks after therapy. Owners should be instructed to keep the area clean and free of encrusted debris and prevent the animal from mutilating the area. Inflammation of mucous membranes occurs in treatment of oral tumors, and its pathogenesis is similar to that of moist dermatitis. Because of the skin-sparing characteristics of megavoltage radiotherapy, serious skin injury is uncommon, but subcutaneous fibrosis and regional distortion can be seen.

Radiation-induced bone necrosis may occur after orthovoltage radiotherapy. The absorbed dose in both bone and soft tissues in an orthovoltage-treated field can be calculated to avoid overtreatment of bone.

References

1. Adams GE: Hypoxia-mediated drugs for radiation and chemotherapy. *Cancer 48*:696, 1981.
2. Adams GE, et al: Electron-affinic sensitizers VII: A correlation between structures. 1: Electron reduction potentials and efficiencies of some nitromidazoles as hypoxic cell radiosensitizers. *Radiat Res 67*:9, 1976.
3. Adams GE, et al: Hypoxic cell sensitizers in radiobiology and radiotherapy. *Br J Cancer 37*:(Suppl III):1, 1978.
4. Adams WM, et al: Radiotherapy of malignant nasal tumors in 67 dogs. *J Am Vet Med Assoc 191*:311, 1987.
5. Allan GS, Gillette EL: Response of canine mast cell tumors to radiation. *J Nat Cancer Inst 63*:691, 1979.
6. Banks WC, Morris E: Results of radiation treatment of naturally occurring animal tumors. *J Am Vet Med Assoc 166*:1063, 1975.
7. Bewley DK, et al: Central axis depth dose data for use in radiotherapy. *Br J Radiol 17*(Suppl)1, 1983.
8. Bostock DE, Owen LN: Chemotherapy of canine and feline neoplasms. *J Small Anim Pract 13*:359, 1972.
9. Brady LW: Radiation sensitizers: Their use in the clinical management of cancer. *In* Brady LW, DeVita VT (eds): *Cancer Management*. Vol 5. Masson, New York, 1980.
10. Brewer WG, Turrel JM: Radiotherapy and hyperthermia in the treatment of fibrosarcomas in the dog. *J Am Vet Med Assoc 181*:146, 1982.
11. Brooks MD, et al: Chemotherapy versus chemotherapy and radiotherapy in the treatment of tonsillar squamous cell carcinoma in the dog. *J Vet Intern Med 2*:206, 1988.
12. Broome MR, et al: Predictive value of tracer studies of ^{131}I treatment in hyperthyroid cats. *Am J Vet Res 49*:193, 1988.
13. Carllisle CH, Gould S: Response of squamous cell carcinoma of the nose of the cat to treatment with x-rays. *Vet Radiol 23*:186, 1982.
14. Casaret AP: *Radiation Biology*. Prentice-Hall, Englewood Cliffs, NJ, 1968, pp 7–30, 57–89, 159–170.
15. Connor WG, et al: Localized current field heating as an adjunct to radiation therapy. I. The use of LCF hyperthermia and irradiation in the treatment of spontaneous animal tumors. *Radiat Environ Biophys 17*:219, 1980.
16. Couto CG, et al. Central nervous system lymphosarcoma in the dog. *J Am Vet Med Assoc 184*:809, 1984.
17. Creasey WA, et al: Pharmacokinetic and antitumor studies with radiosensitizers misonidazole in dogs with spontaneous fibrosarcomas. *Am J Vet Res 43*:1015, 1982.
18. Crile G: The effects of heat and radiation on cancers implanted on the feet of mice. *Cancer Res 23*:372, 1963.
19. Dewhirst MW, et al: Local control and distant metastases in primary canine malignant melanomas treated with hyperthermia and/or radiotherapy. *Int J Hyperthermia 1*:219, 1985.
20. Dewhirst MW, et al: Correlation between initial and long-term responses of spontaneous pet animal tumors to heat and radiation or radiation alone. *Cancer Res 43*:5735, 1983.
21. Dritschilo A, Piro AJ: Therapeutic implications of heat as related to radiation therapy. *Semin Oncol 8*:83, 1981.
22. Ellis F: Tolerance of normal tissues and tumors to radiation. *Front Radiat Ther Oncol 12*:101, 1978.
23. Evans SM: Canine hemangiopericytoma. A retrospective analysis of response to surgery and orthovoltage radiation. *Vet Radiol* 28:13, 1987.
24. Evans SM, et al: Prognostic factors and survival after radiotherapy for

intranasal neoplasms in dogs: 70 cases (1974–1985). *J Am Vet Med Assoc 194*:1460, 1989.
25. Evans SM, Thrall DE: Postoperative orthovoltage radiation therapy of parotid salivary gland adenocarcinoma in three dogs. *J Am Vet Med Assoc 182*:993, 1983.
26. Fletcher GH: Combination of irradiation and surgery. *Int Adv Surg Oncol 2*:55, 1979.
27. Fletcher GH: *Textbook of Radiotherapy*. 3rd ed. Lea & Febiger, Philadelphia, 1980, pp 103–180, 219–224, 637–661.
28. Giger U, et al: Orthovoltage radiotherapy of primary lymphoma of bone in a dog. *J Am Vet Med Assoc 195*:627, 1989.
29. Gillette EL: Radiation therapy of canine and feline tumors. *J Am Anim Hosp Assoc 12*:359, 1976.
30. Gillette EL: Radiation therapy. *In* Kirk RW (ed): *Current Veterinary Therapy VII*. W.B. Saunders, Philadelphia, 1977, pp 479–482.
31. Gillette EL: Radiotherapy. *In* Theilen GH, Madewell BR (eds): *Veterinary Cancer Medicine*. Lea & Febiger, Philadelphia, 1979, pp 85–94.
32. Gillette EL: Large animal studies of hyperthermia and irradiation. *Cancer Res 39*:2242, 1979.
33. Gillette EL: Radiation therapy. *In* Carlson WD (ed): *Carlson's Veterinary Radiology*. 3rd ed. Lea & Febiger, Philadelphia, 1977, pp 477–489.
34. Gillette EL, et al: Response of oral carcinoma to heat and radiation. *Int J Radiat Oncol Biol Phys 13*:1861, 1987.
35. Goldson AL: Past, present and prospects of intraoperative radiotherapy (IOR). *Semin Oncol 8*:59, 1981.
36. Graves GM, et al: Canine hemangiopericytoma: 23 cases (1967–1984). *J Am Vet Med Assoc 192*:99, 1988.
37. Grier RL, et al: Hyperthermic treatment of superficial tumors in cats and dogs. *J Am Vet Med Assoc 177*:227, 1980.
38. Hall EJ: *Radiobiology for the Radiologist*. 2nd ed. Harper & Row, Hagerstown, MD, 1978, pp 27, 31–62, 81–92, 95–110, 113–128, 171–194, 195–202.
39. Hilaris BS: *Handbook of Interstitial Brachytherapy*. Publishing Sciences Group, Acton, Inc, 1975, pp 1–43, 61–85.
40. Hilmas DE, Gillette EL: Radiotherapy of spontaneous fibrous connective-tissue sarcomas in animals. *J Natl Cancer Inst 56*:365, 1976.
41. Hitt ME, et al: Radiation treatment for thymoma in a dog. *J Am Vet Med Assoc 190*:1187, 1987.
42. Hutson C, et al: Radiotherapy of squamous cell carcinoma of the mandible in 4 cats. Proceedings 8th meeting, International Veterinary Radiology Association, Sydney, Australia, Aug. 1988, p 75.
43. Johns HE, Cunningham JR: *The Physics of Radiology*. 3rd ed. Charles C Thomas, Springfield, IL, 1978, pp 532–579.
44. Johnston GR, Feeney DA: Radiotherapy of the extremities: Tissue tolerance and complications. *Vet Radiol 24*:130, 1983.
45. Knapp DW, et al: Cisplatin toxicity in cats. *J Vet Intern Med 1*:29, 1987.
46. Langham RF, et al: X-ray therapy of selected odontogenic neoplasms in the dog. *J Am Vet Med Assoc 170*:820, 1977.
47. LeCouteur RA, et al: X-ray computed tomography of brain tumors in cats. *J Am Vet Med Assoc 183*:301, 1983.
48. Lord PF, et al: Increased skeletal metastasis of spontaneous canine osteosarcoma after fractionated systemic hyperthermia and local X-irradiation. *Cancer Res 41*:4331, 1981.
49. Lord PF, et al: Osteogenic sarcoma of the nasal cavity in a cat: Postoperative control with high dose-per-fraction radiation therapy and metronidazole. *Vet Radiol 23*:23, 1982.
50. MacMillan R, et al: Surgery and regional irradiation for treatment of canine tonsillar squamous cell carcinomas: Retrospective review of eight cases. *J Am Anim Hosp Assoc 18*:311, 1982.
51. Marmor JB, et al: Treatment of spontaneous tumors in dogs and cats by hyperthermia induced by ultrasound. *Int J Radiat Oncol Biol Phys 4*:967, 1978.
52. McCaw DL, Lattimer JC: Radiation and cisplatin for treatment of canine urinary bladder carcinoma: A report of two case histories. *Vet Radiol 29*:264, 1988.
53. McChesney SL, et al: Radiotherapy of soft tissue sarcomas in dogs. *J Am Vet Med Assoc 194*:60, 1989.
54. Miller RC, et al: Prospects for hyperthermia in human cancer therapy. Part I: Hyperthermic effects in man and spontaneous animal tumors. *Radiology 123*:489, 1977.
55. Mitchell M, et al: Canine thyroid carcinomas: Clinical occurrence, staging by means of scintiscans and therapy of 15 cases. *Vet Surg 8*:112, 1979.
56. Moore JV: Timing and dose in experimental combinations of cytotoxic drugs and radiation. *Appl Radiol 11*:113, 1982.
57. Morgan JP, Carlson WD: X-irradiation of perianal gland neoplasms in the dog. *J Am Vet Med Assoc 143*:1227, 1963.
58. Moss WT, et al: *Radiation Oncology: Rationale, Technique, Results*. 5th ed. C.V. Mosby, St. Louis, 1979, pp 1–51.
59. Ogilvie GK, et al: Papillary squamous cell carcinoma in three dogs. *J Am Vet Med Assoc 192*:933, 1988.
60. Phillips TL: Sensitizers and protectors in clinical oncology. *Semin Oncol 8*:65, 1981.
61. Postorino NC, et al: Prognostic variables for canine hemangiopericytoma: 50 cases (1979–1984). *J Am Anim Hosp Assoc 24*:501, 1988.
62. Riknberk A: Hyperthyroidism in the dog and its treatment with radioactive iodine. *Tijdschr Diergeneeskd 91*:789, 1966.
63. Ritter MA: The radiobiology of mammalian cells. *Semin Oncol 8*:3, 1981.
64. Rubin P: The radiographic expression of radiotherapeutic injury: An overview. *Semin Roentgenol 9*:5, 1974.
65. Rubin P, Casarett GW: *Clinical Radiation Pathology*. W.B. Saunders, Philadelphia, 1968, pp 1–61.
66. Rubin P, Casarett GW: A direction for clinical radiation pathology. The tolerance dose. *Front Radiat Ther Oncol 6*:1, 1972.
67. Selmon J: *The Basic Physics of Radiation Therapy*. 2nd ed. Charles C Thomas, Springfield, IL, 1976, pp 120–172, 311–318, 472–533.
68. Sheldon PW, et al: Radiosensitization of C3H mouse mammary tumors by a 2-nitromedazole drug. *Br J Cancer 30*:560, 1975.
69. Sheldon PW, et al: Radiosensitization of C3H mouse mammary tumors using fractionated dose of x-rays with the drug Ro-07-0582. *Br J Radiol 49*:76, 1975.
70. Silver IA: Use of radiotherapy for the treatment of malignant neoplasms. *J Small Anim Pract 13*:351, 1972.
71. Silver IA, Carter DB: Radiotherapy and chemotherapy for domestic animals. II. Treatment of malignant tumors in dogs and cats. *Acta Radiol 2*:457, 1964.
72. Smith M, Turrel JM: Radiophosphorus (^{32}P) treatment of bone marrow disorders in dogs: 11 cases (1970–1987). *J Am Vet Med Assoc 184*:554, 1984.
73. Straw RC, et al: Use of radiotherapy for the treatment of intranasal tumors in cats: Six cases (1980–1985). *J Am Vet Med Assoc 189*:927, 1986.
74. Suit HD: Hyperthermic effects on animal tissues. *Radiology 123*:483, 1977.
75. Thrall DE: Orthovoltage radiotherapy of oral fibrosarcomas in dogs. *J Am Vet Med Assoc 179*:159, 1981.
76. Thrall DE: Orthovoltage radiotherapy of canine transmissible venereal tumor. *Vet Radiol 23*:21, 1982.
77. Thrall DE: Principles of radiation therapy in cancer. *In* Ettinger SJ (ed): *Textbook of Veterinary Internal Medicine*. 2nd ed. W.B. Saunders, Philadelphia, 1983, pp 393–405.
78. Thrall DE, Adams WM: Radiotherapy of squamous cell carcinomas of the canine nasal plane. *Vet Radiol 23*:193, 1982.
79. Thrall DE: Orthovoltage radiotherapy of acanthomatous epulides in 39 dogs. *J Am Vet Med Assoc 184*:826, 1984.
80. Thrall DE, Biery DN: Principles and application of radiation therapy. *Vet Clin North Am Small Anim Pract 7*:35, 1977.
81. Thrall DE, Dewhirst MW: Use of radiation and/or hyperthermia for treatment of mast cell tumors and lymphosarcoma in dogs. *Vet Clin North Am Small Anim Pract 15*:835, 1985.
82. Thrall DE, Harvey CE: Radiotherapy of malignant nasal tumors in 21 dogs. *J Am Vet Med Assoc 183*:663, 1983.
83. Thrall DE, et al: Response to cell *in vitro* and tissues *in vivo* to hyperthermia and x-irradiation. *Adv Radiat Biol 6*:211, 1976.
84. Thrall DE: Evaluation of radiation of WR-2721 in dogs with spontaneous tumors. *In* Brady LW (ed): *Cancer Management*. Vol 5. *Radiation Sensitizers: Their Use in the Management of Cancer*. Masson, New York, 1980, pp 343–347.
85. Thrall DE, et al: A review of treatment planning in veterinary radiation oncology. *Vet Radiol 30*:194, 1989.
86. Turrel JM: Intraoperative radiotherapy of carcinoma of the prostate gland in ten dogs. *J Am Vet Med Assoc 190*:48, 1987.
87. Turrel JM, et al: Thyroid carcinoma causing hyperthyroidism in cats: 14 cases (1981–1986). *J Am Vet Med Assoc 193*:359, 1988.
88. Turrel JM, et al: Radiotherapy of brain tumors in dogs. *J Am Vet Med Assoc 184*:82, 1984.
89. Turrel JM, et al: Prognostic factors for radiation treatment of mast cell tumors in 85 dogs. *J Am Vet Med Assoc 193*:936, 1988.
90. Turrel JM, Koblik PD: Techniques of afterloading iridium-192 interstitial brachytherapy in veterinary medicine. *Vet Radiol 24*:278, 1983.
91. Turrel JM, et al: Response to radiation therapy of recurrent lymphangioma in a dog. *J Am Vet Med Assoc 193*:1432, 1988.
92. Turrel JM, Theon AP: Single high-dose irradiation for selected canine rectal carcinomas. *Vet Radiol 27*:141, 1986.
93. Utley JF, et al: Protection of normal tissues by WR2721 during fractionated radiotherapy. *Int J Radiat Oncol Biol Phys 1*:699, 1976.
94. Utley JF, et al: Differential radioprotection of enoxic and hypoxic mouse mammary tumors by a thiophosphate compound. *Radiology 110*:213, 1980.
95. Vikram B: Importance of the time interval between surgery and postoperative radiation therapy in the combined management of head and neck cancer. *Int J Radiat Oncol Biol Phys 5*:1837, 1979.
96. Walker MA: A review of drugs that may be used in conjunction with radiotherapy. *Vet Radiol 23*:220, 1982.
97. Walker MA: A review of permanent interstitial implant radiotherapy using radon-22 and iodine-125. *Vet Radiol 23*:223, 1982.
98. Walker MA, Breider M: Intraoperative radiotherapy of canine bladder cancer. *Vet Radiol 28*:200, 1987.
99. Weaver A, et al: Combined modality therapy for advanced head and neck cancer. *Am J Surg 140*:549, 1980.
100. Withers HR: The four R's of radiotherapy. *In* Lett JT, Adler H (eds): *Advances in Radiation Biology*. Vol 5. Academic Press, New York, 1975, pp 241–271.
101. Withrow SJ, et al: Intraoperative irradiation of 16 spontaneously occurring canine neoplasms. *Vet Surg 18*:7, 1989.
102. Yuhas JM: Improvement of lung tumor radiotherapy through differential chemoprotection of normal and tumor tissue. *J Natl Cancer Inst 48*:1255, 1972.

APPENDIX:

Survival Data for Neoplasms with Multimodality Therapy Using Radiation Therapy*

Tumor Type/Location	Number of Tumors	Type of Radiation	Survival Data	Reference
Acanthomatous				
Epulis				
Oral	39	O	85% (33/39)—1 year survival 67% (26/39)—2 year survival Range = 1—102 months survival Mean = 38 months survival	Thrall[79]
Adenocarcinoma				
Anal gland	3	O	50% (1/2)—1 year survival NED	Silver and Carter[71]
Mammary	15	O, X (Sx, H)	For responses > 1 month duration (1 and 2 year survivals NG) XRT w/o H CR = 12.5% (1/8) PR = 62.5% (5/8) NR = 25% (2/8) XRT + H CR = 57.1% (4/7) PR = 42.8% (3/7) NR = 0% (0/7)	Dewhirst et al[19]
Nasal	38	O, C, CS, X (Sx)	1 and 2 year survivals NG 18.7 months mean survival 12.0 months mean survival	Adams et al[4]
Nasal (feline)	1	X	0% (0/1)—1 year survival	Straw et al[73]
Parotid	3	O (Sx)	100% (3/3)—1 year survival NED 100% (2/2)—2 year survival NED	Evans and Thrall[25]
Brain tumors				
Canine 2 Meningiomas 1 Astrocytoma 1 Undifferentiated sarcoma	4	C (Chx)	100% (2/2)—1 year survival 0% (0/2)—2 year survival Range = 176–497 days Mean survival = 329 days Median survival = 322 days	Turrel et al[88]
Canine lymphosarcoma	3	C (Chx)	0% (0/3)—1 year survival	Couto et al[16]
Feline lymphosarcoma	1	C	0% (0/1)—1 year survival	LeCouteur et al[47]
Urinary bladder				
11 Transitional cell carcinomas 1 Leiomyosarcoma 1 Rhabdomyosarcoma	13	Cs (IO)	61.5% (8/13)—1 year survival 5.4% (2/13)—2 year survival	Walter and Breider[98]
Transitional cell carcinoma	2	C (Chx)	0.0% (0/2)—1 year survival	McCaw and Lattimer[52]
Carcinomas				
Tonsillar carcinoma (mixed)	27	O	33% (9/27)—1 year survival	Silver[70]
Undifferentiated nasal carcinoma	7	O, C, Cs, X	1 and 2 year survivals NG 5.2 months mean survival	Adams et al[4]
Undifferentiated nasal carcinoma	7	O (Ch, Sx)	40% (2/5)—1 and 2 year survival	Thrall and Harvey[82]
Nasal carcinoma	49	O (Sx)	54%—1 year survival 43%—2 year survival 35%—3 year survival 13.5 months median survival	Evans et al[24]
Undifferentiated nasal carcinoma (feline)	1	X	100% (1/1)—1 and 2 year survival	Straw et al[73]
Chondrosarcoma				
Nasal	3	O (Sx)	33.3% (1/3)—1 and 2 year survival	Thrall and Harvey[82]
Nasal (feline)	1	X	0% (0/1)—1 year survival	Straw et al[73]

APPENDIX:

Survival Data for Neoplasms with Multimodality Therapy Using Radiation Therapy* *Continued*

Tumor Type/Location	Number of Tumors	Type of Radiation	Survival Data	Reference
Fibrosarcoma				
Oral	17	O (n = 14), O + Sx (n = 3)	13% (2/15)—1 year survival 7% (1/15)—2 year survival	Thrall[75]
Oral	9	O (Ch)	29% (2/7)—1 year survival 14% (1/7)—1.5 year survival	Creasey et al[17]
Oral	6	O (H)	60% (3/5)—1 year survival 40% (2/5)—2 year survival	Brewer and Turrel[10]
External nasomaxillary	4	O (H)	66% (2/3)—1 year survival (1 dog LTF at 70 days post-XRT) 2 year survival NG (2 dogs LTF)	Brewer and Turrel[10]
Location NG	268	O + other	53% (142/268)—1 year survival	Silver[70]
Location NG	13	O, C, FN	O or C (1 and 2 year survival NG) 23% (3/13)—S 15% (2/13)—TR 8% (1/13)—US FN (1 and 2 year survival NG) 23% (3/13)—TR 23% (3/13)—US 8% (1/13)—U	Banks and Morris[6]
Location NG	16	O, X (H, Sx)	XRT (for responses > 1 month; and 2 year survival NG) 33% (3/9)—CR 56% (5/9)—PR 11% (1/9)—NR XRT + H (for responses > 1 month; 1 and 2 year survival NG) 43% (3/7)—CR 29% (2/7)—PR 29% (2/7)—NR	Dewhirst et al[20]
Head and neck	26	O, C	27% (7/26)—1 year survival TC	Gillette[29]
Head, legs, thorax, digits, inguinal area	26	O (Sx)	16% (4/25)—1 year survival NED 5% (1/22)—2 year survival NED	Hilmas and Gillette[40]
Hemangiopericytoma				
Extremities, head, neck, trunk	22	O	68.4% (13/19)—1 year survival NED 50% (8/16)—2 year survival NED	Evans[23]
Extremities, lip, throracic wall	8	X (Sx)	66.6% (4/6)—1 year survival NED 40% (2/5)—2 year survival NED	Postorino et al[61]
Extremities, thorax, flank	5	O (Sx)	40% (2/5)—follow-up duration NG, NED	Graves et al[36]
Histiocytoma				
Location NG	3	O, C, FN	O or C 33.3% (1/3)—S 33.3% (1/3)—TR FN 33.3% (1/3)—S	Banks and Morris[6]
Lymphosarcoma				
Cutaneous	2	NG	100% (2/2)—1 and 2 year survival NED	Thrall and Dewhirst[81]
Nasal	3	X	100% (3/3)—1 year survival 100% (1/1)—2 year survival	Straw et al[73]
Skeletal	1	O	100% (1/1)—1 and 2 year survival	Giger et al[28]
Nasal (feline)	3	X	100% (3/3)—1 year survival 2 year survival unknown	Straw et al[73]
Lymphangioma	1	C	100% (1/1)—1 and 2 year survival NED	Turrel et al[91]
Mast cell sarcoma				
Extremities, trunk	95 (85 dogs)	O, C (Sx, Chx)	78.8% (68/85)—1 year survival NED 77%—2 year survival NED Mean = 62.7 months survival Median = 17 months survival	Turrel et al[89]

Appendix continued on following page

APPENDIX:

Survival Data for Neoplasms with Multimodality Therapy Using Radiation Therapy* *Continued*

Tumor Type/Location	Number of Tumors	Type of Radiation	Survival Data	Reference
Extremities, head, thoracic wall, scrotum	20	O (Sx)	XRT 66% (2/3)—1 and 2 year survival XRT + Sx 100% (13/13)—1 year survival 100% (6/6)—2 year survival	McChesney et al[53]
Extremities	2	O	100% (1/1)—1 year survival NED	Silver and Carter[71]
Inguinal, other?	52	O, C (Sx)	48% (25/52)—1 year survival TC	Gillette[29]
Location NG	93	O, other?	51% (47/93)—1 year survival	Silver[70]
Location NG	28	O, X (H, Sx)	XRT: For responses > 1 month duration CR = 33% (5/15) PR = 46% (6/13) NR = 31% (4/13) XRT + H CR = 77% (10/13) PR = 15% (2/13) NR = 0% (0/13)	Dewhirst et al[19]
Cutaneous, location NG	23	O, C	43.5% (19/23)—1 year survival NED	Allan and Gillette[5]
Location NG	16	O, C	O or C 13% (2/16)—S 32% (5/16)—TR 56 (9/16)—US	Banks and Morris[6]
Melanoma				
Oral, dermal	34	X (H)	XRT 7.7% (1/13)—1 year survival NED XRT + H 23.8% (5/21)—1 year survival NED	Dewhirst et al[19]
Oral	16	O, X (H, Sx)	XRT: For responses > 1 month duration CR = 12.5% (1/8) PR = 62.5% (5/8) NR = 25% (2/8) XRT+H CR = 100% (8/8) PR = 0% (0/8) NR = 0% (0/8)	Dewhirst et al[19]
Some oral, others location NG	9	O, C, FN	O or C 33.3% (3/9)-S 44.7% (4/9)—TR FN 11% (1/9)-TR 11% (1/9)-US	Banks and Morris[6]
Foot, inguinal region, thigh	1 dog (3 areas)	O	0% (0/1)—1 year; died 127 days post-XRT	Silver and Carter[71]
Location NG	26	O, other	45% (12/26)—1 year survival	Silver[70]
Odontogenic tumors				
Adamantinoma	14	O	91% (10/11)—1 year survival NED 75% (6/8)—2 year survival NED	Langham et al[46]
Ameloblastic odontoma	2	O	100% (2/2)—1 and 2 year survival	Langham et al[46]
Osteosarcoma				
Dorsum of nose	1	O (Sx, Chx)	100% (1/1)—1 and 2 year survival	Lord et al[49]
Extremities	7	O (H)	14% (1/7)—1 year survival NED	Lord et al[48]
Location NG	3	O (Chx)	0% (0/3)—1 year survival	Silver and Carter[71]
Location NG	31	O, other	0% (0/31)—1 year survival	Silver[70]

APPENDIX:

Survival Data for Neoplasms with Multimodality Therapy Using Radiation Therapy* *Continued*

Tumor Type/Location	Number of Tumors	Type of Radiation	Survival Data	Reference
Location NG	18	O, C, FN	O or C 22.2% (4/18)—TR 16.7% (3/18)—US FN 5.5% (1/18)—S 16.7% (3/18)—TR 38.9% (7/17)—US	Banks and Morris[6]
Parosteal osteosarcoma	3	O, C, FN	O or C 33.3% (1/3)—US FN 66.7%(2/3)—US	Banks and Morris[6]
Perianal glands				
Adenoma	23	O, C	O or C 87% (20/23)—S 9% (2/23)—TR 4% (1/23)—US	Banks and Morris[6]
Adenoma and carcinoma	101	O, C + castration	47% (47/101)—1 year survival	Gillette[29]
Adenoma and carcinoma	56 (44 dogs)	O + castration	55.7% (29/52)—1 year survival NED (4 dogs LTF by 1 year) 32.5% (13/40)—2 year survival NED (16 dogs LTF by 2 years)	Morgan and Carlson[57]
Prostatic carcinoma	10	O (intraoperative) + Chx	11% (1/9)—1 and 2 year survival Range = 41–750 days Mean survival = 196 days Median survival = 114 days	Turrel[86]
Rectal adenocarcinoma	6	O	50% (2/4)—1 year survival NED (2 dogs LTF by 1 year) 25% (1/4)—2 year survival NED Range = 5–31 months survival Mean = 11.3 months survival Median = 7 months survival	Turrel and Theon[92]
Rodent ulcer	2	O, C	100% (2/2)—S	Banks and Morris[6]
Sarcomas (misc)				
Oral, cell type NG	179	O, other	61% (109/179)—1 year survival	Silver[70]
Extremities, oral cavity, head, neck, trunk (includes fibrosarcoma, neurofibrosarcoma, and hemangiopericytoma)	43	X	30%—1 year TC-35 Gy 35%—1 year TC-40 Gy 48%—1 year TC-45 Gy 67%—1 year TC-50 Gy 12%—2 year TC-40 Gy 33%—2 year TC-50 Gy	McChesney et al[53]
Nasal chondrosarcoma, myxosarcoma, undifferentiated sarcoma, osteosarcoma	15	O, C, Cs, X (Sx)	Mean = 11.9 months survival Median = 8.1 months survival	Adams et al[4]
Leiomyosarcoma (location NG)	3	O, C	66.7% (2/3)—S 33.3% (1/3)—TR	Banks and Morris[6]
Nasal (unspecified cell type)	1	O (Sx)	100% (1/1)—1 year survival (died at 13 months post-XRT)	Thrall and Harvey[82]
Spindle cell sarcoma (gingiva)	1	O (Sx)	0% (0/1)—1 year survival (euthanized at 68 days post-XRT due to recurrence)	Silver and Carter[71]
Spindle cell sarcoma (ocular, conjunctival)	1	O, P	100% (1/1)—1 year survival (NED at 615 days post-XRT)	Silver and Carter[71]
Neurosarcoma (elbow)	1	O (Chx)	100% (1/1)—2 year survival (NED at 813 days post-XRT)	Silver and Carter[71]

Appendix continued on following page

APPENDIX:

Survival Data for Neoplasms with Multimodality Therapy Using Radiation Therapy* *Continued*

Tumor Type/Location	Number of Tumors	Type of Radiation	Survival Data	Reference
Squamous cell carcinoma				
Extremity, head, penis	11	O (Chx)	37.5% (3/8)—1 year survival Range = 52–458 days survival Mean = 267 days survival	Silver and Carter[71]
Gingiva	3	O (Sx)	100% (2/2)—1 and 2 year survival	Ogilvie et al[59]
Head, neck	52	O, C	34% (18/52)—1 year TC	Gillette[29]
Mandible	4	O, C (Sx)	NED Range = 1–14 months survival Mean = 5.5 months survival	Hutson et al[42]
Nasal	7	O, Cs, C, X (Sx)	Mean = 6.3 months survival Median = 6.1 months survival	Adams et al[4]
Nasal	1	O (Sx)	Survived 5 months post-XRT	Thrall and Harvey[82]
Nasal plane	Gp A = 62	O	Group A 37% (23/62)—2 year survival 26% (16/62)—3 year survival	Carllisle and Gould[13]
	Gp B = 26	O	Group B 57% (15/26)—2 year survival	
Nasal plane	8	O, B	Range = 3–14 months survival Mean = 6.6 months survival Median = 6 months survival	Thrall and Adams[78]
Oral, dermal	49	O, X (H, Sx)	XRT (for responses > 1 month) 44% (11/25) = CR 28% (7/25) = PR 28% (7/25) = NR XRT + H (for responses > 1 month) 62.5% (15/24) = CR 29.2% (7/24) = PR 8.3% (2/24) = NR	Dewhirst et al[19]
Oral	38	C, X (H)	XRT = 47.6% (10/21)—1 year survival XRT + H = 64.7% (11/17)—1 year survival	Gillette et al[34]
Tonsillar	8	C (Sx)	13% (1/8)—1 and 2 year survival	MacMillan et al[50]
Tonsillar	2	O	50% (1/2)—1 and 2 year survival	Silver and Carter[71]
Location NG	428	O and other	78% (334/428)—1 year survival	Silver[70]
Location NG	36	O, C, FN	O, C 25% (9/36)—S 22% (8/36)—TR 14% (5/36)—US 14% (5/36)—US FN 5.5% (2/36)—S 5.5% (2/36)—S 14% (5/36)—US	Banks and Morris[6]
Transmissible venereal tumor				
Genital area, flank, ear, chest wall	18	O	100% (18/18)—1 year survival 100% (13/13)—2 year survival	Thrall[76]
Location NG	28	O, C	100% (28/28)—2 year survival	Banks and Morris[6]
Thymoma	1	O (Chx)	0% (0/1)—1 year (partial remission for 6 months)	Hitt et al[41]
Thyroid carcinoma	4	C, ^{131}I	3/4 dogs tumor free > 2 months post-XRT	Mitchell et al[55]

APPENDIX:

Survival Data for Neoplasms with Multimodality Therapy Using Radiation Therapy* *Continued*

Tumor Type/Location	Number of Tumors	Type of Radiation	Survival Data	Reference
Tumor cell type CA, carcinoma SA, sarcoma Definition of follow-up NED, no evidence of disease SURV, survival LTF, lost to follow-up Other abbreviations NG, not given XRT, radiation therapy			Type of radiation O, orthovoltage B, brachytherapy P, plesiotherapy C, cobalt 60 Cs, cesium X, electrons or megavoltage x-rays FN, fast neutrons Gy (gray) = 100 rad Adjunct therapy Sx, surgery Chx, chemotherapy H, hyperthermia Tumor response Cr, complete regression of all clinical disease PR, at least 50% reduction in tumor volume NR, <50% reduction or continued growth U, unknown CR, complete regression of all disease PR, at least 50% reduction in tumor volume NR, <50% volume reduction or continued growth TC, no evidence of tumor growth beyond original tumor size	

CHAPTER 152

Chemotherapy

Robert C. Rosenthal

For at least 40 years, chemotherapy has had a role in cancer management in human and animal patients. More than 50 agents (including hormones) are useful in human medicine,[7] but the number of practical use in veterinary medicine is smaller. The biological and pharmacological principles underlying the rational use of these drugs provide an important basis for the chemotherapist. These principles have been thoroughly reviewed.[56, 58, 60, 66]

The goal of chemotherapy is to cure the disease, but how frequently a true chemotherapeutic cure is obtained in veterinary medicine is debatable.[66] Transmissible venereal tumor may be cured with various chemotherapeutic approaches alone,[2, 5, 52] but this tumor clearly represents the exception to the rule.[66]

Even if a total cure is unobtainable by chemotherapy alone, other benefits are accrued from its use. Chemotherapy may help control generalized rapidly progressive disease not amenable to surgery or radiotherapy or may help increase the disease-free interval after other initial treatment. It may help prevent spread of a neoplasm by controlling early metastases that are proliferating rapidly and have a relatively small likelihood of containing resistant cells. Chemotherapy may also benefit patients by providing symptomatic relief of related problems and temporary restoration of deteriorated function.[25, 66]

Surgery is the treatment of choice for most solid tumors. In some cases, radiotherapy is effective for localized disease. Neither is able to deal with systemic or undetected metastatic disease. Metastatic disease is the primary cause of death in patients with neoplasia regardless of mode of treatment.[16] Clearly, the more effective the chemotherapy in controlling the distant spread of the disease, the longer a patient's survival.

DRUG RESISTANCE

The emergence of resistance is related to the mutation rate of the genetically unstable neoplastic cells and to tumor mass. The larger the number of tumor cells (tumor mass), the greater the number and proportion of resistant clones. Once such clones emerge, clinical resistance develops relatively rapidly; approximately six doublings are required for a 95 per cent chance of no resistant cells to become a less than 5 per cent chance of no resistant cells. Thus, the probability of success in treating micrometastatic disease or a small mass is greater than in treating a large tumor burden.[17]

Resistance to a drug may develop by several means. Acquired resistance may occur with decreased activation or increased deactivation of the drug by neoplastic cells. Resistance may also be related to impermeability of the tumor cell to the drug, increased rates of removal of drugs from tumor cells, shifts in enzyme specificity, increased repair of cytological lesions, or bypassing of inhibited reactions with alternate biochemical pathways.[25, 49, 57]

TOXICOSES

Efficacy and toxicity of these drugs must be balanced. Chemotherapeutic protocols are most often limited by host toxicosis. Recalling one of the biological bases for chemotherapy—that proliferating neoplastic cells can be attacked most effectively as they pass around the cell cycle—helps explain some of the more commonly noted toxicoses related to rapidly renewing tissues. The most commonly encountered problems relate to gastrointestinal toxicity, bone marrow suppression, and immunosuppression.[9, 39] Vomiting and anorexia may be noted as the gastrointestinal epithelium is affected. Although this problem is usually not life threatening, it can be detrimental to patients. Antiemetics may be helpful.[3, 13, 15, 31, 69] Other gastrointestinal toxicoses seen less frequently include diarrhea, stomatitis, esophagitis, and peptic ulcer.[23]

Bone marrow damage leading to leukopenia and immune suppression affecting both humoral and cell-mediated immunity is a serious problem associated with chemotherapy. Bone marrow damage may affect all cellular components of blood. Anemia and thrombocytopenia may be life threatening, but leukopenia and the associated risk of infection are more common problems. Patterns of myelosuppression differ with the agent given; some are more profound and persistent than others. Chemotherapy may need to be postponed until white blood cell numbers in the peripheral blood are acceptable. Recommended leukocyte counts at which to postpone therapy vary.[25, 27, 28] One such guideline is 4,000 total white blood cells per microliter with at least 2,500 granulocytes per microliter. As veterinary chemotherapists use more intensive protocols, these guidelines may be amended to reflect acceptance of more myelosuppression (to gain an increased likelihood of cure) and improved methods of dealing with myelosuppression. The use of hematopoietic growth factors offers interesting potential.[20, 35, 38, 43] Generally, chemotherapy can be reinstituted in 1 to 2 weeks based on a return to normal white blood cell parameters. When resuming chemotherapy, it may be advisable to decrease the dosage of the offending drug by 25 per cent.

Immunosuppression relates closely to bone marrow toxicosis and myelosuppression. There is great variation in the amount of immunosuppression encountered with chemotherapy, and clinicians must be constantly aware of its dangers. The combination of reduced nonspecific immunity (myelosuppression) and impaired humoral and cell-mediated immunity can render patients prone to life-threatening infection with little or no means of defense. Fortunately, immunosuppression associated with chemotherapy usually does not last long beyond the time of drug administration. Nonetheless, chemotherapeutic protocols should include as few immunosuppressive drugs as feasible without compromising the treatment. Cyclophosphamide is the most immunosuppressive of the commonly used anticancer agents.[7, 24]

Less common problems involve other body systems. Hemorrhagic cystitis associated with cyclophosphamide is a well-known complication that limits prolonged use.[14] The bladder is not the only susceptible organ of the genitourinary system. The kidneys are subject to damage from methotrexate, streptozotocin, L-asparaginase, and other chemotherapeutic agents. Sterility in males and congenital malformations are also possible complications. Skin reactions and alopecia are less frequent in animals than humans but do occur.[10] Clipped hair may not regrow or may regrow a different color. Wire-haired and curly-coated breeds seem more likely than others to develop alopecia. Cats may be more likely to have problems with alopecia than dogs. The lungs, liver, heart, and central nervous system all are subject to damage from various chemotherapeutic agents, although manifestations are less common.

The list of possible complications of chemotherapy is long. It is ironic that anticancer drugs themselves may be mutagenic. Their increased use may reveal this to be a more serious problem than is currently appreciated.

SAFE HANDLING OF CHEMOTHERAPEUTIC AGENTS

Anticancer drugs are valuable, but because they are damaging to cells, actively cycling cells in particular, those who use them must be aware of the potential for problems to arise. A prudent handler of anticancer drugs takes a conservative but reasonable approach to all aspects of storing, preparing, administering, and disposing of these agents.[51, 64, 70] Risks stem from the inherent toxicity of the drugs and the extent of exposure by inhalation, ingestion, or absorption. There are no universally accepted or practiced techniques to limit exposure. Each individual should be constantly aware of potential exposures and means to decrease them.[51, 65, 70]

1. Unpack anticancer drugs carefully. Store them on a shelf away from busy areas, preferably in a locked cabinet.

2. Never eat, drink, smoke, or apply cosmetics where anticancer drugs are prepared or administered.

3. Reconstitute these materials in a well-ventilated area. A class II vertical containment hood is ideal. Place an absorbent pad under the working area.

4. Prepare and administer anticancer drugs with unpowdered surgical latex gloves. Gowns and goggles also decrease exposure.

5. Use syringes and intravenous sets with Luer-Lok fittings. Do not fill syringes more than three-quarters full. Large-bore needles require less pressure but are more likely to drip.

6. Consult package inserts for directions regarding spills.

7. Ensure that patients are well restrained during administration.

Ideal means of disposing of anticancer drugs or the excreta of treated canine and feline patients do not exist. Problems are compounded by the lack of knowledge about absolute limits of exposure and practical means of testing for exposure. In most settings, the risk of exposure is probably quite small and can be minimized by using proper work habits.

GUIDELINES FOR CHEMOTHERAPY

Although patients may benefit from a single chemotherapeutic drug, the use of drugs in combination has advantages. Chemotherapeutic drugs kill a constant fraction of tumor cells independently of the total number of cells, and the fraction killed by one drug is independent of that killed by another. Drugs can be used in combination to attack different specific portions of the cell cycle. Drugs that have different major toxicities are chosen, thus limiting toxicity of any other type and allowing each drug to be used in a full dose. Combination chemotherapy also helps limit the problems of inherent drug resistance and the emergence of resistant subpopulations due to acquired resistance.[9] Intermittent treatment schedules allow intensive attack on a neoplasm and a rest period for recovery of normal cells before the next treatment.[8] In theory, added benefit is accrued from intensifying the chemotherapeutic attack when small numbers of neoplastic cells remain. At the biochemical level, combinations may act by sequential, concurrent, or complementary inhibition,[25] and it may be possible to design protocols based on these drug interactions. To date the most successful combined regimens are empirical, using drugs individually active against a tumor.[8] There are many unanswered questions about not only the best combinations for any particular neoplasm but also how best to schedule chemotherapy in relation to surgery, radiotherapy, biological therapy, and hyperthermia. A few principles of combination chemotherapy follow:

1. Use drugs effective as single agents.
2. Use drugs with different mechanisms of action.
3. Use drugs with different toxicities.
4. Use an intermittent treatment schedule.

Several criteria must be met before undertaking chemotherapy.[9, 28] A thorough history and physical examination supported by an appropriate data base are necessary. In all cases, a histological diagnosis of malignancy is imperative. An understanding of the biological behavior of the tumor aids in prognostication and in selection of drugs with a known effect against the tumor. The clinician must also understand the drugs and their adverse effects. Toxic responses to drugs vary among species, and human dosages cannot be adopted without modification. Safe dosage schedules for the species being treated are used. Monitoring the toxicoses associated with the treatment and evaluating patients' responses follow. Both are important to the proper management of chemotherapy. Monitoring toxicosis to alter or limit treatment is needed for the well-being of patients. Patients are evaluated to judge the effect of treatment on the disease as well as recovery from toxic effects. No chemotherapy should be undertaken without the owner's full understanding and cooperation in terms of the goals of the therapy as well as the costs and the necessary commitment to regular follow-up. Not all owners elect chemotherapy; some opt for no therapy and some for euthanasia. Chemotherapy can help extend a patient's comfortable life in some instances. The quality of a patient's life is the primary consideration in offering chemotherapy as a realistic alternative in treatment of neoplasia.

DRUGS USED IN CHEMOTHERAPY

Chemotherapeutic agents are broadly classified to help make them more easily understood, yet each drug has its own characteristics and peculiarities. Comments on selected drugs (Table 152–1) aid in effective, rational chemotherapy. Note that doses are expressed as milligrams per square meter (body surface area) rather than milligrams per kilogram. This method is presumed to be physiologically more accurate in determining dosages of chemotherapeutic drugs[26]; however, for some drugs, a body weight method might be preferable.[44, 46, 48] Weight in grams is converted to body surface area (m^2) by a fractional exponential function:

$$m^2 = \frac{Km \times W^{2/3}}{10^4}$$

where m^2 is the body surface area in square meters, W is the body weight in grams, and Km is a species-specific constant (10.1 for dogs, 10.0 for cats). Table 152–2 is a conversion table for dogs. The table is also applicable to domestic cats but is not appropriate for larger nondomestic cats.

Alkylating Agents

Alkylating agents have an alkyl radical ($R\text{-}CH_2\text{-}CH_2+$) substituted for a hydrogen atom. Alkylation causes breaks in the DNA molecule and cross-linking of the twin strands of DNA. Cross-linking interferes with DNA replication and RNA transcription.[24, 66] Most of these compounds contain more than one alkylating group. The alkylating agents are not specific for the cell cycle phase.

TABLE 152–1. CHEMOTHERAPEUTIC AGENTS COMMONLY USED IN VETERINARY MEDICINE

	Brand Name (Manufacturer)	Possible Indications	Suggested Dosages	Toxicity
Alkylating agents				
Cyclophosphamide	Cytoxan (Mead Johnson)	Lymphoreticular neoplasms, mammary and lung carcinomas, miscellaneous sarcomas	50 mg/m^2 PO or IV 4 days/week, or 200 mg/m^2 IV weekly	Leukopenia, anemia, thrombocytopenia (less common), nausea, vomiting, sterile hemorrhagic cystitis
Chlorambucil	Leukeran (Burroughs Wellcome)	Lymphoreticular neoplasms, chronic lymphocytic leukemia	2 mg/m^2 PO 2 to 4 days/week	Mild leukopenia, thrombocytopenia, anemia, nausea, vomiting (not common)
Nitrogen mustard	Mustragen (Merck Sharp & Dohme)	Lymphoreticular neoplasms	5 mg/m^2 IV; cautious topical application (10 mg/50 ml water)	Leukopenia, thrombocytopenia, nausea, vomiting, anorexia; contact dermatitis
Melphalan	Alkeran (Burroughs Wellcome)	Multiple myeloma, monoclonal gammopathies, lymphoreticular neoplasms	1.5 mg/m^2 PO for 7 to 10 days, repeat cycle	Leukopenia, thrombocytopenia, anemia, anorexia, nausea, vomiting
Dacarbazine	DTIC (Dome Laboratories)	Malignant melanoma, various sarcomas	200 mg/m^2 IV for 5 days every 3 weeks	Leukopenia, thrombocytopenia, anemia, nausea, vomiting, diarrhea (often decreases with later cycles)
Antimetabolites				
Methotrexate	Methotrexate (Lederle)	Lymphoreticular neoplasms, myeloproliferative disorders, various carcinomas and sarcomas	2.5 mg/m^2 PO daily; 0.5–0.8 mg/kg IV as indicated by protocol	Leukopenia, thrombocytopenia, anemia, stomatitis, diarrhea, hepatopathy, renal tubular necrosis
6-Mercaptopurine	Purinethol (Burroughs Wellcome)	Lymphosarcoma, acute lymphocytic leukemia, granulocytic leukemia	50 mg/m^2 PO daily until response or toxicity	Leukopenia, nausea, vomiting, hepatopathy
5-Fluorouracil	Fluorouracil (Roche Laboratories)	Various carcinomas and sarcomas	150–200 mg/m^2 IV weekly	Leukopenia, thrombocytopenia, anemia, anorexia, nausea, vomiting, diarrhea, stomatitis
	Efudex Cream (Roche Laboratories)	Cutaneous tumors	Apply BID for 2 to 4 weeks	
Cytosine arabinoside	Cytosar-U (Upjohn)	Lymphosarcoma, myeloproliferative disorders	100 mg/m^2 SC or IV drip for 4 days	Leukopenia, thrombocytopenia, anemia, nausea, vomiting, anorexia
Plant Alkaloids				
Vincristine	Oncovin (Eli Lilly)	Transmissible venereal tumor, lymphosarcoma	0.5 mg/m^2 IV weekly	Peripheral neuropathy, paresthesia, constipation
Vinblastine	Velban (Eli Lilly)	Lymphosarcoma, various carcinomas	2.0 mg/m^2 IV weekly	Leukopenia, nausea, vomiting
Antibiotics				
Doxorubicin	Adriamycin (Adria Laboratories)	Lymphosarcoma, osteogenic sarcoma, various carcinomas and sarcomas	30 mg/m^2 IV every 3 weeks (do not exceed 240 mg/m^2 total)	Leukopenia, thrombocytopenia, nausea, vomiting, cardiac toxicity, reactions during administration
Bleomycin	Blenoxane (Bristol Laboratories)	Squamous cell carcinomas, other carcinomas	10 mg/m^2 IV or SC for 3 to 9 days, then 10 mg/m^2 IV weekly (do not exceed 200 mg/m^2 total)	Allergic reactions following administration, pulmonary fibrosis
Hormones				
Prednisolone		Lymphoreticular neoplasms, mast cell tumors, central nervous system tumors	Vary widely depending on indication: 60 mg/m^2 PO daily to 20 mg/m^2 PO every 48 hours	Hyperadrenocorticism, secondary adrenocortical insufficiency
Diethylstilbestrol		Perianal adenomas, prostatic neoplasms (adjunctive)	1.1 mg/kg IM once (do not administer more than 25 mg) or 1 mg PO every 72 hours	Bone marrow toxicity, feminization
Miscellaneous				
L-Asparaginase	Elspar (Merck Sharp & Dohme)	Lymphoreticular neoplasms	10,000 units per m^2 intraperitoneally	Anaphylaxis, leukopenia
o,p'-DDD	Lysodren (Calbiochem)	Adrenocortical tumors	50 mg/kg PO daily to effect, then 50 mg/kg PO every 7 to 14 days as needed	Adrenocortical insufficiency
Cisplatinum	Platinol (Bristol Laboratories)	Osteosarcoma, other sarcomas and carcinomas	50–70 mg/m^2 IV every 28 days with appropriate saline diuresis	Renal damage, gastrointestinal upset, myelosuppression

TABLE 152–2. CONVERSION TABLE OF WEIGHT IN KILOGRAMS TO BODY SURFACE AREA IN SQUARE METERS FOR DOGS

kg	m²	kg	m²
0.5	0.06	26.0	0.88
1.0	0.10	27.0	0.90
2.0	0.15	28.0	0.92
3.0	0.20	29.0	0.96
4.0	0.25	30.0	0.96
5.0	0.29	31.0	0.99
6.0	0.33	32.0	1.01
7.0	0.36	33.0	1.03
8.0	0.40	34.0	1.05
9.0	0.43	35.0	1.07
10.0	0.46	36.0	1.09
11.0	0.49	37.0	1.11
12.0	0.52	38.0	1.13
13.0	0.55	39.0	1.15
14.0	0.58	40.0	1.17
15.0	0.60	41.0	1.19
16.0	0.63	42.0	1.21
17.0	0.66	43.0	1.23
18.0	0.69	44.0	1.25
19.0	0.71	45.0	1.26
20.0	0.74	46.0	1.28
21.0	0.76	47.0	1.30
22.0	0.78	48.0	1.32
23.0	0.81	49.0	1.34
24.0	0.83	50.0	1.36
25.0	0.85		

Cyclophosphamide is the most widely used alkylating agent in veterinary medicine. It has been administered for lymphoreticular neoplasia, various sarcomas and carcinomas, mast cell tumors, and transmissible venereal tumors, as a single agent and with other drugs.[27, 66] Cyclophosphamide requires activation to its active metabolite 4-hydroxycyclophosphamide by the liver microsomal oxidase system and must be given orally or intravenously. Hematological and gastrointestinal toxicoses are dose limiting. Leukopenia is most severe within a week or two of administration, with recovery usually following within 10 days. Anemia and thrombocytopenia are less common.[7, 24]

A unique and important problem associated with cyclophosphamide is sterile hemorrhagic cystitis. Active metabolites of cyclophosphamide cause mucosal ulceration, necrosis of smooth muscle and small arteries, and hemorrhage and edema in the urinary bladder. The renal pelves may also be affected. Patients may show signs of hematuria, pollakiuria, and stranguria.[14] Early recognition of signs, diuresis, and cessation of cyclophosphamide administration help limit the problem. Some cases may persist and require more aggressive therapy, such as instillation of a 1 per cent formalin solution into the bladder.[67] Measures helpful in avoiding sterile hemorrhagic cystitis include (1) not administering cyclophosphamide to a patient with concurrent cystitis or hematuria; (2) administering the daily dose in the morning and providing free access to fresh water and ample opportunity to urinate at all times; and (3) being certain the patient urinates before the owners retire for the night. Gastrointestinal and skin toxicities may sometimes occur and require dosage adjustment.

Chlorambucil is often used in chemotherapy of canine lymphosarcoma as a replacement for cyclophosphamide, either in maintenance regimens or when myelosuppression or sterile hemorrhagic cystitis has been a problem. Although chlorambucil acts more slowly than cyclophosphamide and has less myelosuppressive effect, regular monitoring of white blood cell parameters is warranted. Melphalan is most useful in multiple myeloma but also in lymphoreticular neoplasia, mammary and lung carcinomas, and osteogenic sarcoma.[27, 66] Dacarbazine may be useful in lymphoma in dogs[18] but is not widely used. Nitrogen mustard is rarely used systemically, but topical application is helpful in cutaneous lymphoma.[1, 12]

Antimetabolites

Antimetabolites are structural analogues of normal metabolites required for cell function and replication. They damage cells by interacting with cell enzymes (1) by substituting for a metabolite needed in a key molecule, rendering it functionally abnormal; (2) by competing successfully with a normal metabolite for the catalytic site of a key enzyme; or (3) by competing with a normal metabolite that acts at an enzyme regulatory site to alter the catalytic rate of a key enzyme.[24]

The antimetabolites are S-phase–specific drugs. They are highly schedule dependent, and many questions regarding their best use remain unanswered.[7, 24]

Methotrexate acts in S phase to inhibit dihydrofolate reductase competitively and interferes with both DNA and RNA synthesis.[24, 66] This folic acid antagonist is used in the treatment of lymphoreticular neoplasms and myeloproliferative disorders as well as metastatic transitional cell tumor, transmissible venereal tumor, Sertoli cell tumor, and osteogenic sarcoma.[27, 66] Damage to the bone marrow and gastrointestinal tract can be severe; with high-dose regimens, appropriately timed "rescue" may be achieved by administering citrovorum factor (folinic acid), the specific antidote. More commonly in veterinary medicine, methotrexate is given in a low-dose regimen that is far less toxic.[66]

The purine analogue 6-mercaptopurine interferes with purine synthesis and interconversion and is used for lymphocytic and granulocytic leukemias.[66] Useful pyrimidine analogues include 5-fluorouracil and cytosine arabinoside. 5-Fluorouracil inhibits thimidylate synthetase and interferes with DNA synthesis. It also blocks uracil phosphatase and inhibits use of preformed uracil in RNA.[24] 5-Fluorouracil is used in the treatment of various carcinomas. Hematological and gastrointestinal toxicoses are important.[7, 66] It is not used in cats because of severe neurotoxicosis. Cytosine arabinoside blocks DNA synthesis by inhibiting DNA polymerase, blocking conversion of cytosine to dioxycytodine. In addition to S-phase action, cytosine arabinoside also blocks progression of cells from G_1 to S.[7] Administration by the subcutaneous route or by slow intravenous drip during a prolonged period may thus be beneficial in the recruitment and synchronization of neoplastic cells. Myelosuppression is the major dose-limiting toxicosis, although gastrointestinal signs ranging from anorexia to vomiting may be observed.[7]

Antibiotics

The antitumor antibiotics, like the plant alkaloids, are natural products, derived from strains of the soil fungus *Streptomyces*. They are cytotoxic, nonspecific for cell cycle phase, and damage DNA by binding DNA and inhibiting DNA or RNA synthesis.[24] Doxorubicin is the most frequently used in veterinary medicine. Hematological, gastrointestinal, and cardiac toxicoses are important.[13, 46, 62] Renal disease may be significant in cats.[11, 40] Although signs of gastrointestinal upset, vomiting, and diarrhea can usually be treated symptomatically, myelosuppression may be a dose-limiting problem in the short term.[7, 62] Cumulative cardiac toxicosis results in a dose-related cardiomyopathy. All patients receiving doxorubicin should have initial chest radiographs, an electrocardiogram, and an echocardiogram. Re-evaluation as feasible should precede each treatment, and therapy should be discontinued if serious abnormalities develop (decreased size of QRS complexes, premature ventricular contractions, arrhythmias, or echocardiographic changes denoting cardiomyopathy). Dosages are reduced if hepatic damage develops.

Doxorubicin is administered slowly through a free-flowing intravenous line. Extravasation causes serious sloughing and is treated promptly with saline dilution through the same (unremoved) needle used to administer the drug after attempts to aspirate extravasated drug. Cold packs are applied as often as possible for a week at least. Slough following extravasation may be noted in 7 to 10 days. Local palliative treatments may make patients more comfortable but probably do not markedly alter the course.[13, 29] Restlessness, facial swelling, or head shaking may signal excessively rapid administration. If these signs are seen, administration is stopped temporarily and started at a slower rate when signs abate. Pretreatment with antihistamines may help avoid some of these complications. Despite its apparently numerous drawbacks, doxorubicin has had wide application in the treatment of canine lymphosarcoma as both a first- and second-line drug[4, 6, 45, 50] and for various carcinomas and sarcomas with limited success.[27, 45, 66]

Bleomycin has had limited use in squamous cell carcinoma in animals. Although bleomycin is not a myelosuppressive drug, pulmonary fibrosis may be a lethal complication.[66]

Plant Alkaloids

Vincristine and vinblastine are alkaloids extracted from *Vinca rosea*.[54] They act specifically in M phase by binding with the microtubular protein tubulin and blocking mitosis by interfering with chromosomal separation in metaphase. Although vincristine and vinblastine have a common mechanism of action, resistance to one does not imply resistance to the other.[24] They also have different major toxicities. Vincristine affects the nervous system. Paresthesia, loss of deep tendon reflexes, and sensory neuropathy are more easily assessed in human patients than animals.

Lymphoid hypoplasia and constipation are more frequent veterinary complications.[54] Vinblastine toxicity is primarily hematological. Myelosuppression may be a severe problem.[7] Like doxorubicin, these drugs cause sloughing if injected perivascularly. The reaction is usually not as severe and may develop up to 7 days after injection. Treatment is similar to that described for doxorubicin except that hot packs, rather than cold, are used.[29]

Both vincristine and vinblastine are used to treat lymphoreticular neoplasms. Vincristine is the treatment of choice for transmissible venereal tumor and is used for sarcomas and carcinomas.[2, 5, 27, 52] Vinblastine is used to treat carcinomas and mast cell tumors.[27, 66]

Hormones

The potential for hormonal intervention in neoplasia is great. Unlike other chemotherapeutic agents, hormones are not primarily cytotoxic. Hormonal agents are more selective than cytotoxic drugs in their actions.[55] Peptide hormones interact with cell membrane-bound nucleotide cyclase systems such as those that convert adenosine triphosphate (ATP) to cyclic adenosine monophosphate (cyclic AMP). Cyclic AMP acts as a "second messenger" to deliver and amplify regulatory signals to intracellular sites. Steroid hormones enter cells and bind to a specific receptor protein. "Transformation" ("activation") of this newly formed complex allows it to pass the nuclear membranes, where it binds to DNA. This binding alters the transcription of the cell's messenger RNA, resulting in synthesis of new protein. Steroid-induced increases in free fatty acids may cause dissolution of the nuclear membrane, leading to cell death.[7, 28, 42] The lysis associated with corticosteroid-induced cell death may be initiated by activation of endonucleases.[68]

Adrenal corticosteroids have important uses in therapy of lymphosarcoma and mast cell tumors and may be of benefit in central nervous system neoplasms because of their ability to cross the blood-brain barrier. The major effects of these drugs in brain tumors relates to the reduction of peritumor inflammation and edema. Their beneficial actions in other solid tumors probably also relate more to anti-inflammatory effects than to direct antitumor effects.

Sex hormones have been used in the treatment of hormone-dependent tumors of mammary, prostatic, or perianal gland origin. Hormonal therapy may be supplemental or ablative. Antiestrogenic therapy currently remains experimental. Hormones also have a valuable role as replacement therapy after ablative surgery, in the management of some metastatic problems, and in paraneoplastic syndromes such as hypercalcemia and anemia.[55]

Miscellaneous Agents

A number of other drugs are also used to treat neoplasia in animals.

L-Asparaginase is an enzyme derived from bacteria. By hydrolyzing asparaginase to aspartic acid and ammonia, L-asparaginase deprives neoplastic cells that lack the ability to synthesize L-asparaginase of extracellular sources, thereby rapidly inhibiting protein synthesis. L-Asparaginase acts against cells in G_1.[7, 24] It is effective in canine lymphoreticular neoplasms.[53, 59, 66] Anaphylaxis has been the most dangerous side effect. Other toxicities include gastrointestinal disturbances, hepatotoxicity, hemorrhagic pancreatitis, and coagulation defects.[7, 22, 63]

The cell cycle–nonspecific drug *o,p'*-DDD directly suppresses both normal and neoplastic adrenocortical cells.[7] With proper management, *o,p'*-DDD may be beneficial in patients with inoperable adrenocortical carcinoma as well as with adrenocortical hyperplasia secondary to a pituitary neoplasm.[24] In addition to hypoadrenocorticism, toxic manifestations include vomiting, diarrhea, and depression.[7]

Streptozocin is a cell cycle phase–nonspecific antibiotic derived from *Streptomyces achromogenes*. It inhibits DNA synthesis, nicotinamide-adenine dinucleotide and its reduced form, and enzymes important in gluconeogenesis.[24] Streptozocin has been suggested to treat islet cell carcinoma but has generally been considered too toxic for use in dogs.[66]

Platinum complexes have tumoricidal activity; *cis*-dichlorodiammineplatinum (CDDP) is a cell cycle phase–nonspecific drug that inhibits DNA synthesis and has some alkylating activity.[47] It has been used in veterinary medicine for various tumors.[21, 30, 33, 34] CDDP toxicity is significant.[44, 47] CDDP causes nausea and vomiting, which may be severe and prolonged. Renal insufficiency is usually the dose-limiting toxicosis, but myelosuppression may also occur.[18] Brisk saline diuresis before and after administration and use of antiemetics help limit renal damage and gastrointestinal disturbances.[44, 47] CDDP should not be given to cats because of dose-related primary pulmonary toxicosis.[34] The most clearly defined indication for CDDP is adjunctive treatment of osteosarcoma in dogs.[41, 61]

Of the drugs available to treat neoplasia, it is not clear that the best use of any single drug—let alone the best drug combination or multimodality therapy—has been clearly established for any neoplasm. An understanding of the drugs available for use and their mechanisms, indications, and toxicities helps rational chemotherapy.

MULTIMODALITY THERAPY

As the treatment of neoplasia becomes more a part of everyday practice, most veterinarians will be concerned with questions about the best ways to use surgery and chemotherapy together and to a lesser extent, radiotherapy, hyperthermia, and biological response modification. Surgery and radiotherapy are local treatments; chemotherapy and biological response modification are systemic. Hyperthermia may be either local or systemic. Surgical excision remains the most widely recommended therapy for tumors in pets.

The classic approach to combining modalities has been to use local therapy, usually surgery but sometimes radiotherapy, first and alone. Patients were observed until the disease recurred. At the time of relapse, chemotherapy might have been attempted. This approach lessened the likelihood of a favorable response to drug therapy because of the late and recurrent nature of the disease. Now it is common practice to plan adjuvant chemotherapy as part of the initial treatment for diseases with a high metastatic rate, such as osteosarcoma and thyroid carcinoma in dogs.[32, 37, 41, 61] Although local therapy is important in reducing the total tumor burden by removing or reducing the bulk of the primary, the known biological behavior of many of the commonly encountered tumors suggests that cure is not attained by these means. It is here that chemotherapy, planned and conducted with other treatments, is likely to be most beneficial. When applied to the much smaller tumor burdens left after surgery, chemotherapy may have a better chance of working. Whether adjunctive chemotherapy brings about a cure seems to depend on the metastatic burden at the time of the primary therapy.[19]

Another means of combining modalities is neoadjuvant chemotherapy, the use of drugs before the definitive treatment, surgery or radiotherapy, for the primary. By using chemotherapy first, it may be possible to reduce the size of the surgical or radiation field even if the chemotherapy itself is not curative. Noncurative cytoreduction (by surgery or radiation) leads to increased proliferation, which in turn leads to increased resistance, increased shedding of tumor cells, and increased protection in sanctuaries. Neoadjuvant chemotherapy should help diminish these problems. In addition, early chemotherapy may have an effect on undetected micrometastatic disease. Some implications for surgery are obvious; any significant decrease in the size of the primary makes the surgical procedure easier and less deforming. Also, even if tumor cells are dislodged at surgery, they may have been sterilized by chemotherapy and therefore be less likely to cause spread by direct implantation. The smaller the tumor burden at surgery, the less the chance that disseminated intravascular coagulation will be a problem. Neoadjuvant chemotherapy is not without potential disadvantages. There is always the possibility that the tumor will be totally unresponsive to the chosen drugs and that the patient will suffer unwarranted toxicosis, immunosuppression, and delay in other more effective therapy.

The concepts of combined or multimodality therapy are still relatively new to veterinary medicine. Serious thought should be given to planning the entire course of treatment to present a client with a fully developed plan that includes whatever approaches might benefit the patient. It is worthwhile, then, to have in mind the indications for and problems with various combinations of surgery, radiotherapy, and chemotherapy. In general, in combined modality treatments, chemotherapy and biological therapy can be considered useful to combat micrometastatic disease, radiotherapy to sterilize local-regional disease, and surgery to remove the gross tumor. The true role of either local or systemic hyperthermia is unknown. The most commonly considered combination probably is surgery followed by chemotherapy. For diseases known not to be cured by surgery alone, the consideration of postoperative drugs is attractive but has not been fully evaluated. Tumors that might benefit from such therapy (but have not been proved to do so) include gastrointestinal tumors, malignant mammary tumors, some malignant melanomas, soft-tissue sarcomas, and squamous cell carcinomas. In any case, adjuvant chemotherapy should not be undertaken unless there is some evidence that the tumor being treated is responsive to the drug used.

A significant problem is evaluation of the efficacy of adjunctive treatment. If surgery were curative, unneeded adjunctive therapy would appear to have been beneficial, the owner would have assumed unwarranted expense, and the patient would have suffered unnecessary toxicoses. In addition, there has been much concern about the effects of chemotherapy on wound healing. Although in experimental situations some chemotherapeutic drugs can affect some phases of healing, the clinical effects are minimal.[36]

References

1. Ackerman L: Cutaneous T cell-like lymphoma in the dog. *Comp Cont Educ Pract Vet 6*:37, 1984.
2. Brown NO, et al: Follow-up on chemotherapy of venereal tumors. *J Am Vet Med Assoc 177*:676, 1980.
3. Burrows CF: Metoclopramide. *J Am Vet Med Assoc 183*:1341, 1983.
4. Calvert CA, Leifer CE: Doxorubicin for treatment of canine lymphosarcoma after development of resistance to combination chemotherapy. *J Am Vet Med Assoc 179*:1011, 1981.
5. Calvert CA, et al: Vincristine for treatment of transmissible venereal tumor in the dog. *J Am Vet Med Assoc 181*:163, 1982.
6. Carter RF, et al: Chemotherapy of canine lymphoma with histopathological correlation: Doxorubicin alone compared to COP as first treatment regimen. *J Am Anim Hosp Assoc 23*:587, 1987.
7. Carter SK, Livingston RB: Drugs available to treat cancer. *In* Carter SK, et al (eds): *Principles of Cancer Treatment*. McGraw-Hill, New York, 1981.
8. Carter SK, Livingston RB: Principles of cancer chemotherapy. *In* Carter SK, et al (eds): *Principles of Cancer Treatment*. McGraw-Hill, New York, 1981.
9. Chabner BA: The role of drugs in cancer treatment. *In* Chabner BA (ed): *Pharmacologic Principles of Cancer Treatment*. W.B. Saunders, Philadelphia, 1982.
10. Conroy JD: The etiology and pathogenesis of alopecia. *Comp Cont Educ Pract Vet 1*:806, 1979.
11. Cotter SM, et al: Renal disease in five tumor-bearing cats treated with Adriamycin. *J Am Anim Hosp Assoc 21*:405, 1985.
12. Couto CG: Cutaneous lymphomas. *Proc Kal Kan Symp 11*:71, 1988.
13. Couto CG: Toxicity of anticancer chemotherapy. *Proc Kal Kan Symp 10*:37, 1987.
14. Crow SE, et al: Cyclophosphamide induced cystitis in the dog and cat. *J Am Vet Med Assoc 171*:259, 1977.
15. Davis LE: Pharmacologic control of vomiting. *J Am Vet Med Assoc 176*:241, 1980.
16. Fidler IJ: General concepts of tumor metastasis in the dog and cat. *J Am Anim Hosp Assoc 12*:374, 1976.
17. Goldie JH, Coldman AJ: A mathematical model for relating the drug sensitivity of tumors to their spontaneous mutation rate. *Cancer Treat Rep 63*:1727, 1979.
18. Gray KN, et al: Histologic classification as an indication of therapeutic response in malignant lymphoma in dogs. *J Am Vet Med Assoc 184*:814, 1984.
19. Griswold DP: Body burden of cancer in relationship to the therapeutic outcome: consideration of preclinical evidence. *Cancer Treat Rep 70*:81, 1986.
20. Groopman JE, et al: Hematopoietic growth factors: Biology and clinical applications. *N Engl J Med 321*:1449, 1989.
21. Hahn KA, Richardson RC: Use of cisplatin for control of metastatic malignant mysenchymoma and hypertrophic osteopathy in a dog. *J Am Vet Med Assoc 195*:351, 1989.
22. Hansen JF, Carpenter RH: Fatal acute systemic anaphylaxis and hemorrhagic pancreatitis following asparaginase treatment in a dog. *J Am Anim Hosp Assoc 19*:977, 1983.
23. Harris JB: Nausea, vomiting and cancer treatment. *CA 28*:194, 1977.
24. Haskell CM: Drugs used in cancer chemotherapy. *In* Haskell CM (ed): *Cancer Treatment*. W.B. Saunders, Philadelphia, 1980.
25. Haskell CM: Principles of cancer chemotherapy. *In* Haskell CM (ed): *Cancer Treatment*. W.B. Saunders, Philadelphia, 1980.
26. Henness AM, et al: Use of drugs based on square meters of body surface area. *J Am Vet Med Assoc 171*:1076, 1977.
27. Hess PW: Principles of cancer chemotherapy. *Vet Clin North Am 7*:21, 1977.
28. Hess PW, et al: Chemotherapy of canine and feline tumors. *J Am Anim Hosp Assoc 12*:350, 1976.
29. Hessen JA: Protocol for treatment of vesicant antineoplastic extravasation. *Hosp Pharm 24*:705, 1989.
30. Himsel CA, et al: Cisplatin chemotherapy for metastatic squamous cell carcinoma in two dogs. *J Am Vet Med Assoc 189*:1575, 1986.
31. Hosgood G: Pharmacologic features of butorphanol in dogs and cats. *J Am Vet Med Assoc 196*:135, 1990.
32. Jeglum KA, Wherat A: Chemotherapy of canine thyroid carcinoma. *Comp Cont Educ Pract Vet 5*:96, 1983.
33. Knapp DW, et al: Cisplatin therapy in 41 dogs with malignant tumors. *J Vet Intern Med 2*:41, 1988.
34. Knapp DW, et al: Cisplatin toxicity in cats. *J Vet Intern Med 1*:29, 1987.
35. Kurzman ID, et al: Effect of colony-stimulating factors on monocyte function and number of circulating monocytes in normal dogs. *Proc Vet Cancer Soc 9*:80, 1989.
36. Laing EJ: The effect of antineoplastic agents on wound healing: guidelines for the combined use of surgery and chemotherapy. *Comp Cont Educ Pract Vet 11*:136, 1989.
37. LaRue SM, et al: Limb-sparing treatment for osteosarcoma in dogs. *J Am Vet Med Assoc 195*:1734, 1989.
38. Laver J, Moore MAS: Clinical use of recombinant human hematopoietic growth factors. *J Natl Cancer Inst 81*:1370, 1989.
39. MacEwen EG: Cancer chemotherapy. *In* Kirk RW (ed): *Current Veterinary Therapy VII*. W.B. Saunders, Philadelphia, 1980.
40. Mauldin GN, et al: Efficacy and toxicity of doxorubicin and cyclophosphamide used in the treatment of selected malignant tumors in 23 cats. *J Vet Intern Med 2*:60, 1988.
41. Mauldin GN, et al: Canine osteosarcoma treatment by amputation versus amputation and adjuvant chemotherapy using doxorubicin and cisplatin. *J Vet Intern Med 2*:177, 1988.
42. Meyers FH, et al: The adrenocortical steroids. *In* Meyers FH, et al (eds): *Review of Medical Pharmacology*. 6th ed. Lange Medical Publications, Los Altos, Cal., 1978.
43. Obradovich JE, et al: Evaluation of recombinant canine granulocyte colony-stimulating factor as an inducer of granulopoiesis in the dog: A pilot study. *Proc Vet Cancer Soc 9*:62, 1989.
44. Ogilvie GK, et al: Evaluation of cisplatin-induced emesis in dogs with malignant neoplasia: 115 cases (1984–1987). *J Am Vet Med Assoc 195*:1399, 1989.
45. Ogilvie GK, et al: Phase II evaluation of doxorubicin for treatment of various canine neoplasms. *J Am Vet Med Assoc 195*:1580, 1989.
46. Ogilvie GK, et al: Acute and short-term toxicoses associated with the administration of doxorubicin to dogs with malignant tumors. *J Am Vet Med Assoc 195*:1584, 1989.
47. Page R: Cisplatin, a new antineoplastic drug in veterinary medicine. *J Am Vet Med Assoc 186*:288, 1985.
48. Page RL, et al: Unexpected toxicity associated with use of body surface area for dosing melphalan in the dog. *Cancer Res 48*:288, 1988.
49. Perti P, Mini E: Drug resistance in cancer: An overview of the clinical aspects. *J Chemother 1*:5, 1989.
50. Posterino NC, et al: Single agent therapy with Adriamycin for canine lymphosarcoma. *J Am Anim Hosp Assoc 25*:221, 1989.
51. Power LA: ASHP technical assistance bulletin on handling cytotoxic drugs in hospitals. *Am J Hosp Pharm 42*:131, 1985.
52. Richardson RC: Canine transmissible venereal tumor. *Comp Cont Educ Pract Vet 3*:951, 1981.
53. Rogers KS: L-Asparaginase for treatment of lymphoid neoplasia in dogs. *J Am Vet Med Assoc 194*:1626, 1989.
54. Rosenthal RC: Clinical applications of *vinca* alkaloids. *J Am Vet Med Assoc 179*:1084, 1981.
55. Rosenthal RC: Hormones in cancer therapy. *Vet Clin North Am 12*:67, 1982.
56. Rosenthal RC: Chemotherapy. *In* Slatter DH (ed): *Textbook of Small Animal Surgery*. W.B. Saunders, Philadelphia, 1985.
57. Rosenthal RC: Drug resistance in cancer chemotherapy. *In* Kirk RW (ed): *Current Veterinary Therapy IX*. W.B. Saunders, Philadelphia, 1986, pp 471–472.
58. Rosenthal RC: Chemotherapy. *In* Withrow SJ, MacEwen EG (eds): *Clinical Veterinary Oncology*. J.B. Lippincott, Philadelphia, 1989.
59. Rosenthal RC, MacEwen EG: Treatment of lymphoma in dogs. *J Am Vet Med Assoc 196*:774, 1990.
60. Schabel FM: The use of tumor growth kinetics in planning "curative" chemotherapy of advanced solid tumors. *Cancer Res 29*:2384, 1969.
61. Shapiro W, et al: Use of cisplatin for treatment of appendicular osteosarcoma in dogs. *J Am Vet Med Assoc 192*:507, 1988.
62. Susaneck SJ: Doxorubicin therapy in the dog. *J Am Vet Med Assoc 182*:70, 1983.
63. Swanson JF, et al: Cerebral thrombosis and hemorrhage in association with L-asparaginase administration. *J Am Anim Hosp Assoc 22*:749, 1986.

64. Swanson LV: Potential hazards associated with low-dose exposure to antineoplastic agents: Part I. Evidence for concern. *Comp Cont Educ Pract Vet 10*:293, 1988.
65. Swanson LV: Potential hazards associated with low-dose exposure to antineoplastic agents: Part II. Recommendations for minimizing exposure. *Comp Cont Educ Pract Vet 10*:616, 1988.
66. Theilen GH, et al: Chemotherapy. *In* Theilen GH, Madewell BR (eds): *Veterinary Cancer Medicine*. 2nd ed. Lea & Febiger, Philadelphia, 1987.
67. Weller RE: Intravesical instillation of dilute formation for treatment of cyclophosphamide-induced hemorrhagic cystitis in two dogs. *J Am Vet Med Assoc 172*:1206, 1978.
68. Wielckens K, et al: Glucocorticoid-induced lymphoma cell death: The good and the evil. *J Steroid Biochem 27*:413, 1987.
69. Willard MD: Some newer approaches to the treatment of vomiting. *J Am Vet Med Assoc 184*:590, 1984.
70. Yodaiken RE, Bennett C: OSHA work-practice guidelines for personnel dealing with cytotoxic (antineoplastic) drugs. *Am J Hosp Pharm 43*:1193, 1986.

CHAPTER 153

Skin and Subcutis

Ralph A. Henderson and
William G. Brewer, Jr.

The skin is the origin of about one-third of canine neoplasms. Owner observations draw the attention of veterinarians to these masses, usually at a time that curative excision is possible. Likewise, the skin accounts for one-fourth of feline tumors, the second most common site, with lymphohematopoietic tumors being more common. Skin tumors in cats are more likely to be malignant than in dogs.[63, 76] The variety of cell types of cutaneous tumors results from cellular transformation of the different epithelial and mesenchymal skin components (Fig. 153–1).

Benign tumors are commonly denoted by the suffix *-oma.* Malignant neoplasms of ectodermal or neuroectodermal origin (epidermis and mucosa) are commonly denoted by the suffix *carcinoma,* which is also used as a generic name for these tumors. A prefix may be added to clarify the predominant differentiated tissue in the malignancy (e.g., *adenocarcinoma* signifies a carcinoma that appears histologically to be forming glands). Malignancies arising from the tissues of mesoderm or endoderm are most commonly denoted by the suffix *sarcoma,* also used as a common generic name. A prefix is added to clarify the dominant differentiated tissue (e.g., *hemangiosarcoma* denotes a malignant mesodermal tumor originating from blood vessels).

Important features of clinical management of skin tumors are covered in this chapter. The non-neoplastic tumefactions that must be included in a complete differential diagnosis of neoplasia are not discussed: hyperplasia/injury (epidermal callus, hygroma), cystic entrapment of cellular debris (epidermal inclusion cyst, dermoid cysts), mineral deposition (calcinosis circumscripta, heterotopic bone formation), infection (staphylococcal pyogranuloma, *Mycobacterium leptomurium* in cats, nocardiosis, actinomycosis, pheohyphomycosis, sporotrichosis, blastomycosis, histoplasmosis, cryptococcosis, coccidioidomycosis, zygomycosis), nonseptic inflammation (nodular panniculitis,[8] nodular fasciitis, eosinophilic granuloma, acral lick granuloma, deep sterile steriod-responsive pyogranuloma), and unknown causes (generalized nodular dermatofibrosis/renal cystadenocarcinomas of German shepherds).[28]

DERIVATION OF SKIN TUMORS

The basal lamina invests the entire body. The epidermis and mucous membranes, derivatives of embryonic *ectoderm,* rest on the basal lamina. The superficial epidermal layers are dying cells; they form the cornifying layers and do not undergo neoplastic change. The deep or basal layer of the epidermis, called the *stratum germinativum,* is composed of melanocytes and basal cells; the latter differentiate into prickle cells. Both benign and malignant *epidermal (skin) tumors* arise from these cells.

The basal lamina and epidermis deeply invaginate into the dermis and subcutis, forming the origin of each gland or hair follicle. Hair follicles and glands are called, corporately, the *adnexa.* The follicles, glands, and ducts are lined by epidermis, and in the hair follicle, the inner root sheath is a continuation of the basal layer. In addition to glands, each hair follicle may have an erector

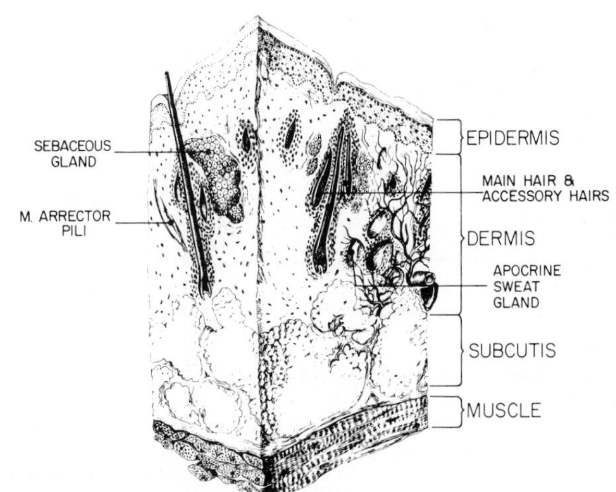

FIGURE 153–1. Cutaneous tumors may arise from the epidermis, hair, or glands (adnexa) or from cells of the dermis or hypodermis. (From Swaim SF: *Surgery of Traumatized Skin: Management and Reconstruction in the Dog and Cat.* W.B. Saunders, Philadelphia, 1980.)

pili (smooth) muscle. Benign and malignant tumors arise here and are referred to as *adnexal tumors.*

Cutaneous sebaceous, apocrine sweat, and merocrine glands, singly or in combination, form specialized glands, some of which have unique locations, such as the caudal tail gland (sebaceous and apocrine sweat), circumanal gland (sebaceous), and anal sac gland (sebaceous and apocrine sweat). Perianal glands are masses of large polygonal cells with no secretory activity located deep to the circumanal glands. Sebaceous glands are most numerous in the lips, anus, and dorsum of the body. The large coiled apocrine sweat glands are usually located with hair follicles and are especially numerous in the facial and interdigital skin. The smaller coiled merocrine sweat glands are found in the footpads, deep in the dermohypodermal junction. Malignant neoplasms of the adnexa are referred to as *adnexal carcinomas* and, though histologically distinct, possess similar behavior.

The *dermis* is directly beneath the basal lamina and is composed of blood vessels, lymphatics, nerves, adipose tissue, histiocytes, mast cells, connective tissue, and ground substance. The subcutis (hypodermis) is a network of connective tissue, nerves, blood vessels, and adipose tissue deep to the dermis. Females have a thicker subcutis than males.[2] Because of the deep invaginations of the hair follicles and glands, these glands appear in the dermis and subcutis in histological sections, and thus epidermal tumors may form "beneath" the epidermis.

REACHING A THERAPEUTIC DECISION

Staging

Clients often first notice cutaneous lumps or ulcers and request a professional opinion. If a veterinarian first notices the lesion, it is usually a secondary finding during a thorough examination for another complaint. The answers to two questions form the foundation of therapy. The answer to the first question, "What is the lesion?" establishes the *diagnosis.* The answer to the second, "What is the extent of the lesion?" establishes the *stage* (Fig. 153–2). In addition, the general health and reserve function of the vital organs (heart, liver, kidneys, and lungs), influence what therapy a patient can withstand. In some instances, the second question is answered first, and because the lesion is localized, the first question is answered after excisional biopsy.

Tumor staging establishes whether local therapy is likely to be sufficient or whether advanced extent of disease requires systemic therapy. *TNM staging* is based on physical characteristics of the tumor (T), palpation and clinical examination of the local and regional lymph nodes (N), and metastasis (M). Mast cell tumor and cutaneous lymphoma are exceptions to this TNM format because of their systemic involvement. When multiple tumors coexist, each is located and measured, but the one with the highest T value is used for prognostication. When coexisting tumors differ with regard to N and M stages, advanced N stage supersedes T values in prognosis and therapy. Advanced M stage takes precedence over both T and N.

Staging can be limited by the lack of sensitivity of some methods, such as the inability of radiography to reveal most pulmonary metastases smaller than 2 mm; and by lack of specificity, such as the inability of palpation to establish the degree of local infiltration of tumor. Adequate staging requires progressive inspection of T, N, and M using increasingly sophisticated methods to enhance detection and definition, especially selecting methods appropriate for the anticipated biological behavior of the lesion.

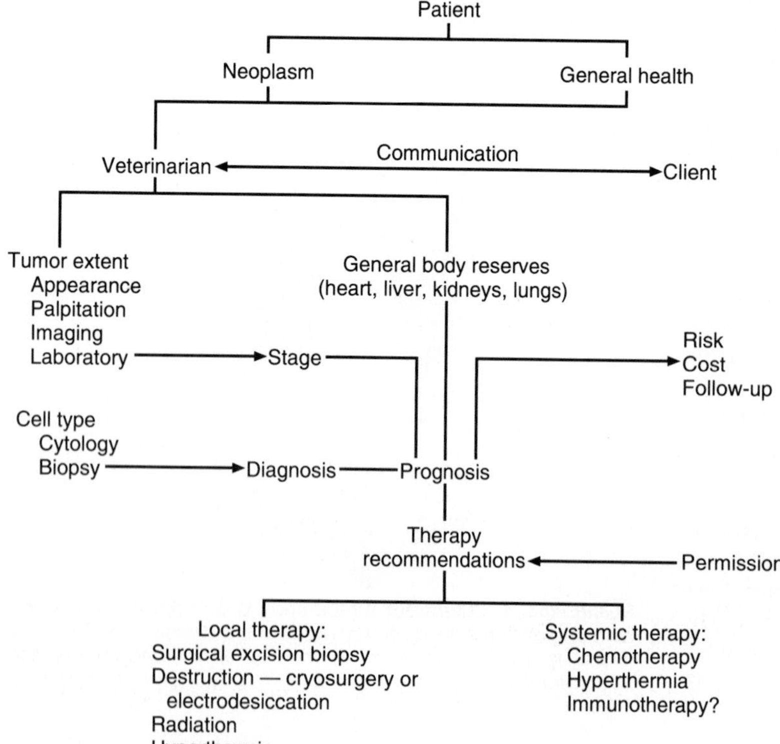

FIGURE 153–2. Algorithm of diagnostic data accumulation to establish specific therapeutic recommendations for skin tumors.

Cytology and Biopsy

Because prognosis and therapy are influenced by cell type and histological grade, early identification of the tumor by cytology and follow-up by histopathological evaluation are optimal. Cutaneous tumors such as malignant melanoma, mast cell tumor, and fibrosarcoma require wide primary excision. With experience, cytological evaluation is an invaluable aid in treatment planning.[1] Tumors frequently may be classified as carcinoma (epidermal, adnexal), round cell (melanoma, lymphoma, plasmacytoma, histiocytoma, mast cell tumor, transmissible venereal tumor), or supporting tissue (soft-tissue tumors). Identification of one of these tumors by fine-needle cytological study, tissue scrapings, or smears can lead to a complete excision biopsy as the initial therapeutic plan.

General Therapeutic Options

Whenever localization of a skin tumor allows, complete *surgical excision* is the treatment of choice because immediate cure is provided (Fig. 153–3). Complete excision must include the tumor and an adequate margin of normal tissue and must preclude accidental inoculation of the surgical wound with tumor cells. Localized skin tumors that are not resectable or that are incompletely resected may respond to *radiation* therapy with or without the combination of *hyperthermia.* These procedures may be followed by excision or systemic therapy. *Chemotherapy* with or without hyperthermia and *immunotherapy* are best suited for use with disseminated neoplasms or to enhance the efficacy of surgery or radiation.

A combination of modalities is used to manage large

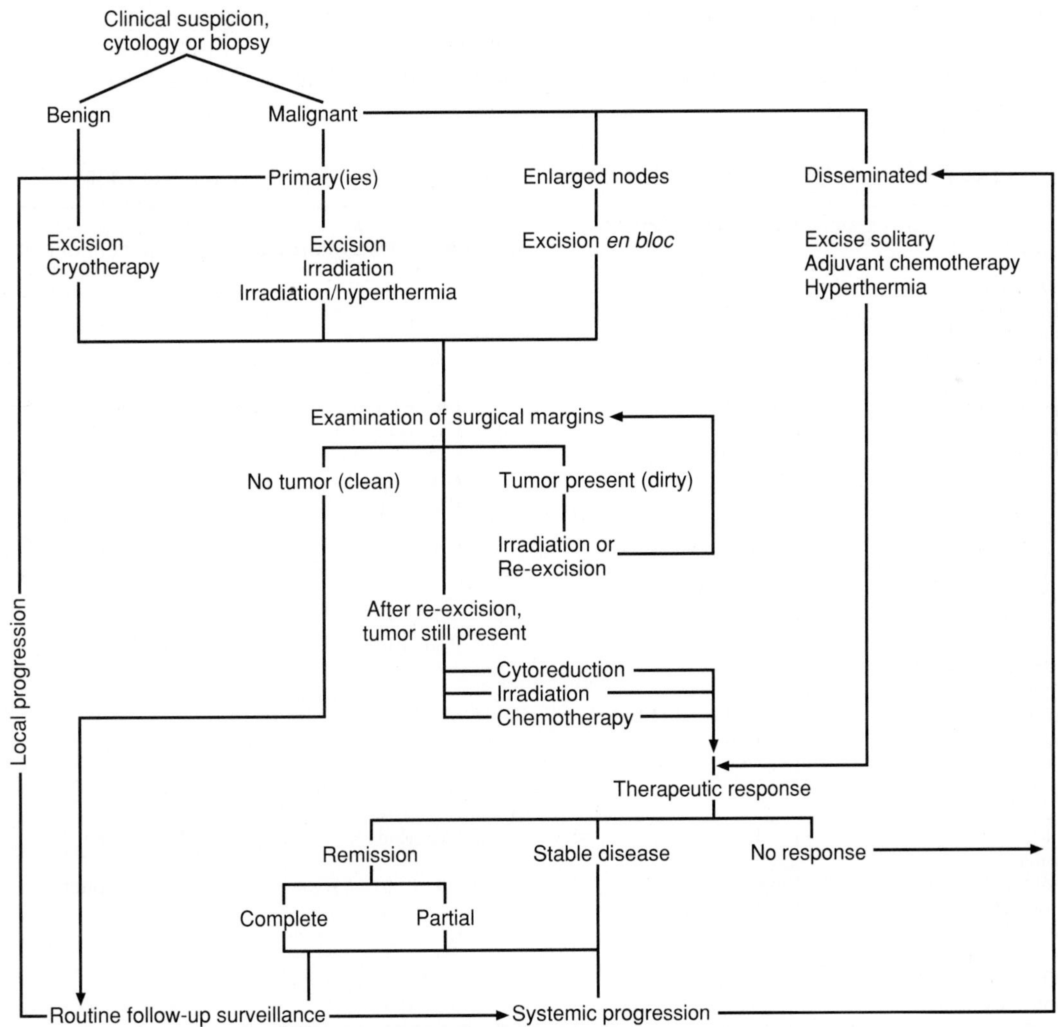

FIGURE 153–3. Algorithm of therapeutic selection, interpretation of response, and routine follow-up surveillance depending on the extent of involvement.

infiltrative or metastatic processes comprehensively by attempts to eradicate the primary tumor, treat or remove affected or potentially affected nodes, and manage sites of distant metastasis (Table 153–1). The goal is to reduce the tumor burden progressively to the point that a patient's own immune system is able to remove the final vestiges of a disseminated neoplasm.

EPIDERMAL AND ADNEXAL TUMORS

Epidemiology and Etiology

Epidermal tumors account for up to 28 per cent of canine tumors and include the basal cell tumors, melanocytic tumors (discussed with round-cell tumors), and prickle cell tumors. The incidence in cats is roughly half that in dogs. Although primarily a disease of older animals, these lesions also afflict young animals.[55, 76]

The causes of epidermal neoplasms (drawn from multiple species) are known and range from viral induction of papillomas to chemical (creosote) carcinogenesis of squamous cell carcinomas, but the cause of most canine and feline epidermal neoplasms is unknown.

Pathology

Typical epidermal neoplasms are derived from ectoderm and neuroectoderm. They are common on all surfaces of the body. The tumors take their names from their cells of origin, and in most instances, malignant cell types have a benign counterpart: squamous cell carcinoma and squamous papilloma from the prickle cell layer, malignant melanoma and benign melanomas/nevi from melanogenic neuroectodermal cells; sebaceous, ceruminous, sweat, and perianal gland adenocarcinomas and adenomas from those respective cell types. A benign counterpart to adenocarcinoma of the apocrine gland of the anal sac has not been reported. Some epithelial tumors are benign despite local invasion, rarely exhibit a malignant counterpart, and even more rarely metastasize: basal cell adenoma from the basal layer and tricoepithelioma, pilomatricoma, and tricholemmoma from hair follicles.[63]

The majority of epithelial tumors are composed of pleomorphic cells that are roundish to polyhedral rather than spindle shaped. Malignancy is characterized by increasing pleomorphism, heterochromia, and the presence of mitotic figures. Melanomas may exhibit a spin-

TABLE 153–1. SUGGESTED FIRST TREATMENT OPTIONS FOR PRIMARY AND METASTATIC SITES

Cell Type	Treatment(s)/Adjuvant or Primary	Treatment of Involved Node	Treatment of Metastases
Epidermal origin			
Basal cell tumor	Exc/Rad		
Squamous papilloma	Exc		
Squamous cell carcinoma	Exc/Rad, Rad.-Hth	Exc, Rad	Pl
Benign sebaceous	Exc		
Sebaceous adenoma	Exc/Rad	Exc, Rad	AC, Pl
Perianal adenoma	Exc, castration/rad	Exc, Rad-Hth	Estrogen ?
Perianal adenocarcinoma	Exc, castration/rad	Exc, Rad-Hth	Pl, AC
Adenocarcinoma, anal sac	Exc/rad, Rad-Hth	Exc, Rad-Hth	AC
Sweat gland carcinoma	Exc/Rad	Exc/Rad	Pl
Hair follicle tumors	Exc		
Adnexal carcinoma	Exc/Rad, Rad-Hth	Exc, Rad	5C, AC
Mesenchymal origin (spindle cells)			
Benign, soft-tissue	Exc		
Sarcoma, soft-tissue	Exc/Rad, Rad-Hth	Rad-Hth	AC, VAC, M
Lipoma, encapsulated	Exc		
Lipoma, infiltrative	Exc, amputation		
Hemangiopericytoma	Exc/Rad, Rad-Hth		
Lymphangioma	Exc/Rad		
Nerve sheath tumors	Exc		
Hemangiosarcoma	Exc		AC, VAC, M
(Round cells)			
Mast cell tumor	Exc/Rad	Exc, Rad	Prednisone, Hth
Histicytoma	Exc		
Lymphoma, cutaneous	Biopsy, Exc		See Lymphoma
Plasmacytoma	Exc/Rad		
Transmissible venereal tumor	Biopsy, Rad, O	O	O/A
Melanoma, benign	Exc		
Malignant, melanoma	Exc/Rad, Rad-Hth	Exc, Rad	Hth & Pl or Melphalan

Adjuvants (/ . . .) are listed for incomplete or ineffective primary therapy or as an alternate therapy. Excision (Exc) implies any primary ablative attempt (including cryosurgery or electrodesiccation) and added ablative attempts if earlier attempts were incomplete. Radiation (Rad) may be effective as a primary treatment for several neoplasms, but due to expense and relative lack of availability, it is primarily considered here for cases in which excision is not possible. Radiation may be an alternative to re-excision for some cell types when re-excision is not possible. The quantitative benefits of hyperthermia (Hth) have not been established but are suspected. The chemotherapy protocols are suggested first choices for surgical adjuvant or systemic disease. Individual toxicities and specific contraindications should be reviewed before administration. Chemotherapeutic regimens are represented by single or grouped letters. The letters used represent conventional protocols or the following agents: A, doxorubicin; C, cyclophosphamide; V or O, vincristine; M, Mitoxantrone; P, prednisone; Pl, cisplatin; 5, 5-fluorouracil.

dle, epithelial, or mixed collage of cell types. Some carcinomas can appear scirrhous, so the differential diagnosis of poorly differentiated carcinomas must also include poorly differentiated sarcomas. Some carcinomas exhibit typical paraneoplastic characteristics, presumably associated with their neuroectodermal association.

Carcinomas are locally invasive. Small carcinomas that have not invaded deeper than the basal lamina are referred to as carcinomas *in situ.* Once they have invaded through the basal lamina, carcinomas metastasize via blood and lymph. Carcinomas are more likely to spread via local and regional lymphatics than blood vessels. Distant metastases commonly affect the lungs, bones, kidneys, and central nervous system tissue.

Diagnosis

Epidermal tumors may be exophytic, sessile, or crateriform. The surface may be ulcerated. They frequently are very firm at their margin, hence the derivation of their latin prefix, *carcino-,* meaning "hard." A minimum data base includes local examination and determination of lymphatic and thoracic involvement. Carcinomas usually exfoliate easily, and cytological preparations like fine-needle aspiration reveal sheets or "rafts" of cells and individual cells with malignant characteristics. Local and regional lymph nodes are examined, and survey radiographs of the lungs obtained.

Basal Cell Tumors

Basal cell tumors, also known as *basal cell carcinoma, basal cell epithelioma,* and *basiloma,* increase in frequency near the mean ages of 6 years in dogs and 10 years in cats.[95] Neither sex is predisposed, but poodles, mixed breeds, and cocker spaniels are more commonly affected. The head and trunk of dogs are the most common sites. Grossly, the lesions are firm, round, raised, solitary, and hairless and may be ulcerated. They rarely infiltrate adjacent structures. Microscopically, they are aggressive, with varying cell morphology and numerous mitoses,[88] but their clinical course is usually benign. Cystic cavities are more common in cats than dogs.[103] Complete surgical excision or biopsy and cryodestruction are the treatments of choice. Radiation may be used for unresectable lesions. The recurrence rate is low, and the prognosis is favorable.

Squamous Cell Carcinoma

Squamous cell carcinoma arises from keratinocytes in the *stratum germanitivum/spinosum.*[77] Direct or reflected solar irradiation, radiation therapy, petroleum-based chemicals, and chronic trauma have been associated with their occurrence in humans and animals. Skin with little or no pigment is more commonly affected, but no particular sex or breed is predisposed. The peak occurrence in dogs is at 9 years.[98] Common locations on dogs include the toes, scrotum, nose, anus, and abdomen. The eyelids, ears, and nose are commonly affected in cats. Associated hypercalcemia has been reported in cats.[50]

The most characteristic lesion is that of a chronic nonhealing wound. Both proliferative cauliflower lesions and ulcerated craters covered with fibrinonecrotic debris are common. The surface is often pink with fine granular off-white nodules. The histopathological criterion necessary to diagnose squamous cell carcinoma is the presence of desmosomes. Depending on the degree of differentiation, deep rete pegs and keratin accumulations are seen. Squamous cell carcinoma may aggressively invade into adjacent tissue including bone. It usually metastasizes first via lymphatics and later by blood. Squamous cell carcinomas of the inguinal area and nail bed metastasize earlier and exhibit a more aggressive behavior.

The treatment of choice is complete excision or biopsy followed by cryodestruction or electrodesiccation. Depending on tumor size and location, surgical margins of 1 to 3 cm are included. Amputation of digits, ears, and nose are possible and cosmetically acceptable. Affected regional nodes are removed *en bloc.* Even with apparent complete excision, recurrence or distant metastasis occurs. In our experience, radiation therapy (45 to 50 Gy; x- or gamma rays) is unpredictable; some lesions regress quickly during therapy, others respond transiently, and others do not respond. Intravenous cisplatin (40 to 60 mg/m^2) has yielded partial to complete responses of primary and metastatic lesions for 2 to 15 weeks.[43, 90] The prognosis for tumors detected and adequately treated while localized is favorable; however, large and invasive lesions are difficult to treat effectively, and the prognosis is guarded. Application of sunscreens and the use of other protective measures should be considered mandatory for animals after treatment and are advised as prophylactic for lightly pigmented animals that receive chronic exposure to intense sunlight.

Sebaceous Gland Tumors

The sebaceous glands are located over the entire body, and other modified sebaceous glands include the perianal glands, tarsal glands of the eyelid, and ceruminous glands of the ears. Sebaceous lesions account for 7.9 per cent of canine skin tumors.[85] Four stages of hyperactive sebaceous development are reported: adenomatous or nodular (senile) hyperplasia (53 per cent), sebaceous epithelioma (37 per cent), sebaceous adenoma (7.5 per cent), and sebaceous adenocarcinoma (1.7 per cent).[85, 93] All are more common in older dogs, and certain breeds are over-represented.[85, 96]

Adenomatous hyperplasia occurs anywhere on the body, especially the limbs, trunk, and eyelids, and frequently at multiple sites. Individual foci are characterized as wartlike or nodular (half are ulcerated), up to 0.5 cm in diameter, melanotic or pale yellow on cross section, and containing aggregates of mature and immature sebaceous components. Sebaceous epitheliomas are indistinguishable from hyperplasia grossly but are usually larger (0.5 to 5.0 cm). Adenomas are firm, well circumscribed, freely movable, frequently hairless, warty, and occasionally ulcerated. These lesions are benign.[63] Larger adenomas may be excised, but biopsy and electrodesiccation or freezing under local anesthesia is the safest and most convenient therapy for smaller lesions. Large (0.5 to 2.0 cm) sebaceous epitheliomas of the eyelids have been associated with incomplete excision and recurrence.

Sebaceous gland carcinoma is a rare tumor of older dogs, especially cockers and poodles. Compared with adenomas and hyperplasia, carcinomas are frequently larger (though half are less than 2 cm), possess more ill-defined borders, and are often ulcerated. About half of carcinomas occur on the head.[97] Because metastasis is unlikely, complete excision including a border of normal tissue is usually curative. In one study, only 15 per cent recurred.[97] If complete excision is not possible, adjuvant radiation is considered.

Perianal Tumors

Perianal gland adenomas/carcinomas are the most common neoplasms of male dogs. The ratio of benign to malignant cell types is about 4:1.[76] Adenomas occur less frequently in females (10:1) and not at all in cats. Malignant perianal tumors are less common (1:10) and occur infrequently in female dogs and cats.[76] Cocker spaniels, beagles, German shepherds, dachshunds, English bulldogs, and fox terriers may be more frequently affected with adenomas. German shepherds and Arctic Circle breeds are more affected by adenocarcinomas.[107] Tumors of the perianal region of a bitch are more likely to be malignant, possibly of anal sac origin.

Perianal glands are modified sebaceous glands[25, 48] that are anatomically distributed with heaviest concentration around the anus, prepuce, and tail head and lighter patchy distribution on other areas of the trunk. In response to androgens, these cells grow throughout a male dog's lifetime and are normally characterized by the hyperplastic or prominent anus and caudal (tail head) glands of older male dogs. Benign tumors are solitary or multiple, slow growing, soft, and often ulcerated. Malignant tumors are indistinguishable from benign except by microscopic examination. Malignant tumors other than those of perianal origin also occur in this area, mandating histological diagnosis for every tumor.[60] Well-differentiated benign tumors with low numbers of mitoses can metastasize via lymphatics to the sacral, hypogastric, or medial iliac lymph nodes. Malignant tumors are locally invasive and metastatic. Cytologically, large polyhedral cells resembling hepatocytes characterize adenomas. Adenocarcinomas exhibit greater pleomorphism and altered staining characteristics. Rectal palpation, as well as thoracic and especially lateral radiographs of the abdomen, are used for staging. Enlarged sublumbar lymph nodes may cause ventral colonic deviation.

The treatment for adenomas is castration and tumor excision.[111] Although adenomas regress with castration, the 10 to 20 per cent occurrence of adenocarcinomas makes excisional biopsy prudent. Adenomas are sensitive to radiation and estrogen. We consider estrogen therapy unsafe and unwarranted as a treatment for benign tumors. Although the value of castration for adenocarcinomas has not been completely documented,[107, 111] castration is recommended in conjunction with excision of the tumor and a margin of normal tissue. We have measured temporary regression of both primary and metastatic sites after castration. In addition, excision of metastatic sublumbar nodes is associated with long-term remission, but involvement of the terminal aorta and vena cava arborization makes dissection difficult. Adjuvant radiation is recommended for adenocarcinoma that is not resectable or incompletely excised, as well as for sublumbar metastases. Dogs that stage at $T_2N_0M_0$ or greater have decreased survival time.[107] Mithramycin has induced remission experimentally.[65]

Adenocarcinoma of the Apocrine Glands of the Anal Sac

The second clinically important tumor associated with perianal tissues is the apocrine gland adenocarcinoma of the anal sac.[41, 62] Adenocarcinoma of the apocrine glands of the anal sac is reported only in bitches, and although bitches may also have other tumors of the perianal area, malignancy should be considered likely in all perianal tumors in bitches. The lesions are associated with the anal sacs. This tumor secretes a parathormone-like substance that raises serum calcium levels above normal in 85 per cent[80] and may cause dystrophic soft-tissue calcification and renal failure.[41, 62] Hypercalcemia is treated by saline diuresis and furosemide. Like the perianal adenomas, the sacral, hypogastric (intrapelvic), and medial iliac (caudal sublumbar) lymph nodes are the local and regional nodes that are inspected during staging for metastasis (67 per cent).[80] Pulmonary metastasis usually occurs later than lymphatic metastasis. Treatment is by aggressive excision and adjuvant radiation if excision is incomplete. Lymph node metastases usually respond at least transiently to radiation. Thirty to 50 per cent recurred after excision, with a mean survival of 9.5 months.[80] Chemotherapy with cyclophosphamide and melphalan was unsuccessful.[38] Serum calcium is useful for diagnosing recurrence because metastatic foci secrete the parathormone-like protein.

Sweat Gland Tumors

Sweat gland tumors are uncommon neoplasms of older dogs and cats.[108] No breed or sex predisposition has been confirmed. The head, neck, back, and flank are most commonly affected, but other sites are involved. Sweat gland tumors have no typical clinical presentation. The malignant tumors may be sharply or poorly demarcated and may be large.[64] They may be cystic to solid. Five major classes are distinguished, including cystadenoma of apocrine sweat glands, spiradenoma, papillary syringoadenoma, mixed variety, and carcinoma of the sweat glands.[108]

Excision of adenomas is curative. Few survival data are available for sweat gland adenocarcinoma. The tumor and involved nodes are excised. Irradiation may be effective for inducing remission or as an adjuvant to incomplete surgical excision. Adenocarcinomas are invasive and metastasize readily.[64]

Hair Follicle Tumors

Pilomatricomas, tricoepitheliomas, and tricolemmoma probably originate from hair matrix, primitive hair matrix or basal cells, and the outer root sheath, respectively. Hair follicle tumors are most common in older animals and are located on the dorsum of the head or trunk, especially in Kerry blue terriers, schnauzers, and poodles. These breeds may have more than one hair growing from each follicle. Hair follicle tumors are rare in cats.[76] The skin over the tumor is often hairless and thinned or ulcerated. Central calcification, melanin deposition, and an inflammatory capsule are common. Although neither invasion or metastasis is common, tricoepitheliomas may be locally invasive, and pilomatricomas invade and metastasize.[49] Complete excision of a localized neoplasm is curative.[63] If the tumor is compressed or keratin escapes into the subcutis, inflammation ensues.

Intracutaneous Cornifying Epithelioma

Intracutaneous cornifying epithelioma commonly occurs at an average age of 5 years, more commonly affects Norwegian elkhounds, and occurs three times more frequently in males.[93] The lesions are small, firm nodules characterized by a hard keratin plug protruding from a pore and are differentiated from inverted papillomas.[24] They are frequently multiple. When secondarily infected, they resemble a draining sinus tract. They are not invasive, do not metastasize, and do not recur after excision.

SOFT-TISSUE SARCOMAS AND MESENCHYMAL NEOPLASMS

Epidemiology and Etiology

Soft-tissue sarcomas account for 14 to 17 per cent of canine tumors and encompass more than 20 different tumors and subtypes. The incidence in cats is half that in dogs. Although the lesions occur late in life, they also afflict young animals.[55, 76] In most instances, the malignant cell type has a benign correlate. For instance, the malignant cell type leiomyosarcoma has, for a benign counterpart, the leiomyoma. The actual listing of the tumors classified as soft-tissue sarcomas varies between references. The World Health Organization Classification of animal tumors defines soft tissue as all nonepithelial extraskeletal tissue but excludes hematopoietic, lymphoid, glia, neuroectodermal portions of the peripheral and autonomic nervous system, paraganglionic structures, and mesothelial and synovial structures. The similarity of behavior of some of the malignant types of the latter excluded tissues to the accepted or classic soft-tissue sarcomas make their simultaneous discussion convenient. The cellular origins of some sarcomas are unclear. This chapter attempts to deal primarily with those soft-tissue sarcomas located in the dermis and subcutis, but the behavior of the same tumors deeper within the body is similar.

The cause of most soft-tissue sarcomas of the skin of dogs and cats is unknown. A cause-and-effect relationship has been established between feline sarcoma virus and multiple fibrosarcomas in young cats,[92] as distinguished from solitary fibrosarcoma in older cats. Chronic and single-event trauma and foreign implants have been implicated in subcutaneous and musculoskeletal sarcoma in both dogs and cats.[14, 91, 94] Ionizing radiation, chemicals, and parasite migration have been implicated in sarcoma development in various tissues.

Pathology

Soft-tissue sarcomas are mesodermal tumors usually arising in connective tissue. They are common on the limbs, trunk, head and neck, and retroperitoneum and internally may arise in virtually any parenchymatous organ. The tumors take their names from their cells of origin: fibrosarcomas from fibroblastic connective tissue, myxosarcoma from primitive cells that manufacture ground substance, liposarcoma from fat,[61, 99] leiomyosarcoma from smooth muscle, rhabdomyosarcoma from skeletal muscle, hemangiosarcoma from blood vessels (angiosarcoma if vascular spaces do not exist), lymphangiosarcoma from lymphatics, malignant hemangiopericytoma from pericytes, and malignant schwannoma from Schwann cells. The major primary bone tumors, osteosarcoma and chondrosarcoma, are found arising as extraskeletal variants.[83] Malignant fibrous histiocytoma[37, 52] may arise from a primitive mesenchymal cell capable of either fibroblastic or histiocytic differentiation. A number of sarcomas have unclear origins. Synovial cell sarcoma may derive from periosteum rather than synovium. Granular cell myoblastoma may originate from striated muscle. A number of sarcomas fail to show the characteristics necessary for classification or are so poorly differentiated that they are called *undifferentiated sarcomas.*[63]

The majority of sarcomas are composed of large, elongated malignant cells with a so-called spindle-cell pattern. Although most sarcomas are easily diagnosed, the differential diagnosis of poorly differentiated sarcomas also includes poorly differentiated carcinomas. To add further confusion, some carcinomas exhibit a sarcomatoid or scirrhous appearance, and the microscopically aggressive, but benign, condition nodular fasciitis must also be ruled out. In one study of human soft-tissue sarcomas, review of the primary pathologist's diagnosis by another pathologist resulted in corroboration of diagnosis in 66 per cent of cases, disagreement about sarcoma subtype in 27 per cent, and disagreement about whether the diagnosis was actually a sarcoma in 6 per cent.[74] Rebiopsy or pathological review may be of value if the clinical impression disagrees with the histopathological opinion.

Sarcomas form their own vascular capillary spaces as they grow. These spaces are usually lined by neoplastic cells, not endothelium, as seen in most carcinomas. Sarcomas do not contain lymphatics, and although they may invade lymphatics, their most typical route of metastasis is by blood.

Diagnosis

Soft-tissue sarcomas are likely to have no clinical sign other than a painless mass. They occassionally cause lameness or other dysfunction because of their location. Sarcomas usually feel fleshy when palpated, but their density may range from fluctuant to firm. Sarcomas must be distinguished from lipomas, the commonly occurring primary differential. Lipomas are recognized for their slow growth and their tendency to occur in obese dogs at multiple characteristic sites. Careful palpation and continued observation may be all that is necessary to manage such cases. Solitary masses found on thinner dogs or in uncharacteristic sites should be examined more thoroughly.

In some cases, fat may be radiographically distinguished from a sarcoma by differential density, but other causes of masses with the same radiographic tissue density of sarcomas cannot be distinguished. Likewise, fine-needle aspiration may not be reliable for diagnosis of sarcomas because of their poor exfoliation during aspiration, and they may be invested in fat that could be aspirated, giving the false impression of lipoma. Very large or rapidly growing tumors may have necrotic centers and be misdiagnosed as abscessation. The accuracy of aspiration may be enhanced by using a progressively larger needle; however, an aspirate that contains no sarcoma cells does not preclude the presence of a sarcoma. For these reasons, negative findings on fine-needle aspirates are verified by biopsy. The biopsy is planned with definitive treatment in mind and should provide the pathologist with enough tissue to determine both type and histopathological grade.

Staging

The TNM system, currently advocated for staging soft-tissue sarcomas, is not associated with prognosis, even in small tumors 2 to 5 cm maximum diameter (T_2) with no local nodal or distant metastases (N_0M_0). The reason for the inadequacy of clinical staging to provide prognostic support is that it appears that both anatomical site and histopathological grade influence survival. Anatomically, sarcomas become less curable the more proximal the location, and location determines the ease of resection, the most efficacious method of treatment. In humans, histopathological grade is the single most important prognostic factor, irrespective of histological type. For these reasons, a TNMG system has been recommended to stage soft-tissue sarcomas: *G* represents the histological grade, the light microscopic impression of the degree of malignancy, which is interpreted as low, medium, and high grades (malignancy).[109] In that system, the grade influences the stage more than T, N, or M. Low malignancy is grade 1 and is given the stage grouping of I. Grades 2 (medium) and 3 (high) are staged II and III. If the lymph node is involved, the tumor is always staged at least III, and if gross local invasion or distant metastasis is present, the stage is increased to IV. In the latter two instances, the anatomical grade is used irrespective of the histopathological grade. This staging system would have to be proved to be prognostically valuable in a large number of cases before being uniformly adopted.

General Therapy and Response

Surgery is the most important form of treatment for soft-tissue sarcomas, primarily in the form of "radical" excisions that include not only wide margins, but also deep margins including normal fascia and muscle up to full-thickness body wall and, as needed, amputation. The rationale for such surgery is high local recurrence. The primary surgical feature of these tumors is that they frequently appear encapsulated and are often "shelled" or enucleated. The apparent capsule is a pseudocapsule, and the shelling out leaves microscopic neoplastic infiltration within the tissue, a source of recurrence. If an excision with smaller conservative margins is used for diagnosis, the excision site and appropriate margins are re-excised as soon as a histopathological diagnosis is confirmed. Wide 3- to 4-cm margins are preferred.

Although sarcomas are frequently considered radiation resistant, the most common adjuvant for soft-tissue sarcomas is radiation therapy, and it is used as a primary therapy for unresectable and recurrent neoplasms. Most commonly, the postoperative surgical field is irradiated when resection is incomplete, but preoperative radiation is used to reduce the neoplasia to a resectable volume. Radiation is administered in doses ranging from 3,500 to more than 5,000 cGy in 10 to 18 fractions. Higher radiation doses seem able to overcome the relative resistance of these tumors. Tumors with greater cellularity (less connective tissue) and higher-grade malignancy may respond more rapidly than tumors with more connective tissue and low-grade malignancy. Local control for 1 year ranges up to 67 per cent at 5,000 cGy but declines to 33 per cent at 2 years.[59]

Likewise, the responsiveness of sarcomas to chemotherapy is variable. In humans, response rates range from 40 to 50 per cent in rhabdomyosarcomas, neurogenic sarcomas, and synovial sarcomas down to 15 to 20 per cent for osteosarcomas and mesotheliomas.[40] Some sarcomas such as childhood rhabdomyosarcomas and Kaposi and alveolar soft-part sarcomas respond exceptionally well to chemotherapy. In animals, single-agent chemotherapy with doxorubicin and mitoxantrone has shown overall response rates of 22 per cent[67, 84] and 17.7 per cent,[66] respectively. Other agents frequently used in humans and animals include dacarbazine, methotrexate, actinomycin D, cyclophosphamide, lomustine (CCNU), cisplatin, and vincristine. In both humans and pet animals, combination doxorubicin and cyclophosphamide or vincristine, doxorubicin, and cyclophosphamide are commonly used. Responses in animals vary from 2 to 6 months in our experience.

Hyperthermia is effective therapy for soft-tissue sarcoma.[53] The evidence in animals is not so profound, but the general consensus suggests that hyperthermia probably enhances the efficacy of radiation and chemotherapy in this group of tumors, especially those with low vascularity. Likewise, little is reported on immunotherapy of soft-tissue sarcomas in animals. Bacille Calmette-Guérin immunotherapy in cats with feline sarcoma virus–induced neoplasms was ineffective.[6] The combined use of surgery, chemotherapy (vincristine, cyclophosphamide, methotrexate), and immunotherapy (mixed bacterial vaccine) caused partial or complete responses in various feline tumors including sarcomas.[16]

Specific Tumor Idiosyncrasies and Prognosis

Fatty Tumors

Lipomas are benign, usually well circumscribed, and easily excised.[101] Injection with calcium chloride has been reported but may cause severe tissue necrosis.[3] A subclass of lipomas is infiltrative and possess a benign histological appearance but invade adjacent structures.[10, 36, 51, 58, 60] These infiltrative lipomas are indistinguishable from encapsulated lipomas until resection is attempted. Twelve of 17 cases have been in females. They may occur in any site but commonly afflict the limbs. Adequate excision includes the muscles that are being invaded. Recurrence is likely if excision is inadequate. Amputation may be required if function is impaired and excision is impossible. Attachment to bone or invasion of it may be accompanied by tumor mineralization and has been reported as a parosteal lipoma.[31]

Hemangiopericytoma

Hemangiopericytomas are characterized by infiltrative growth, high recurrence rate after incomplete excision, and low metastatic potential. They are most frequently seen on the limbs but occur anywhere. Early intervention and initial aggressive surgery are necessary for cure. Advanced tumors can be repeatedly excised because metastasis is uncommon. Although one report correlated a mitotic index of nine or lower with improved prognosis,[12] subsequent reports could not substantiate that finding.[39, 73] The reported recurrence rate with surgery alone is approximately 25 per cent. The reported recurrence rate of 50 per cent with the combination of surgery and radiation possibly reflects selection of radiation as an adjuvant in the more advanced cases. The duration of response ranges from 1 month to years.[33] In our experience, many inoperable hemangiopericytomas regress for 3 to 9 months when treated with gamma irradiation; not all respond, and one was reported to metastasize after x-radiation alone.[59]

Lymphangioma/Sarcoma

Lymphangioma/sarcomas are extremely rare tumors that, especially when malignant, possess unusual features, both aspects perhaps contributing to underdiagnosis. Sarcomas occur frequently on the trunk, are difficult to diagnose, and metastasize early. Cure is unlikely. Palliative attempts are directed as with other sarcomas.[81] Lymphangioma may respond to gamma irradiation even when recurrent after surgery.[106]

Nerve Sheath Tumors

Nerve sheath tumors are associated with tumefaction, slow progression, and paresis. Diagnosis is by clinical signs, neuroradiography, and surgical exploration and biopsy. They have a very high rate of recurrence.[13, 100]

Hemangiosarcoma

Although most commonly a malignancy of parenchymatous organs, hemangiosarcoma is one of the most common soft-tissue sarcomas in dogs, especially German shepherds. Metastasis is common, and death is almost assured; 100 of 104 dogs in one series died.[18] In cats, metastasis is rare when the primary tumor is not within the abdominal cavity (50 per cent).[82] Chemotherapy alone or as an adjuvant may prolong the mean survival time of 4 months by an additional 2 to 4 months.

ROUND-CELL TUMORS

With the exception of melanoma, round-cell tumors are also of mesenchymal origin. Because of their unique round cell shape and discrete cytoplasmic membranes, they are usually discussed separately. They exfoliate well on aspiration and are usually easier to identify than other mesenchymal or cutaneous neoplasms. Six tumor types are included in the round-cell classification: mast cell tumor, histiocytoma, lymphosarcoma, plasmacytoma, transmissible venereal tumor, and melanoma.

Mast Cell Tumor

Mast cell tumors account for 7 to 21 per cent of all skin tumors and 11 to 27 per cent of all malignant skin tumors in dogs.[26, 32, 75] In cats, they account for 2 to 15 per cent of all skin tumor types.[56, 77, 86] Mast cell tumors can occur in dogs or cats of any age but are most frequently encountered at mean ages of 8.5 years and 8.2 years, respectively.[34, 69] A breed predisposition is noted in boxers, Boston terriers, bulldogs, and related breeds,[72] but there is no sex predisposition. One study of mast cell tumors in cats reported that a spontaneously regressing multicentric histiocytic form of mast cell tumors predominately afflicted Siamese cats that were younger than 4 years.[110] Some reports state that male cats are at an increased risk for developing mast cell tumors,[34, 77] whereas other studies have shown no sex predisposition.[45, 86]

Canine mast cell tumors occur primarily in the dermis and subcutaneous tissues. In cats, mast cell tumors arise from the dermis, subcutaneous tissues, and viscera, with the visceral form usually involving the spleen or liver.

Mast cell cytoplasmic granules contain several different vasoactive substances, especially histamine and heparin, and are responsible for the metachromatic staining characteristics of the cells. With toluidine blue staining, heparin stains red and is found in highest concentrations in mature mast cells whereas histamine stains blue and is found in highest concentration in immature mast cells.[77] Poorly differentiated mast cell tumors may have few or no cytoplasmic granules. In cats, a histiocytic form of mast cell tumor has been described, primarily in young (less than 4 years old) Siamese cats, with cytoplasmic granules that stain poorly with toluidine blue but are readily apparent with electron microscopy.[110]

The function of normal mast cells and clinical signs of the neoplastic cells are related to the substances contained in the cytoplasmic granules. In addition to histamine and heparin, mast cell granules contain serotonin, leukotrienes, prostaglandins, and proteolytic enzymes. Most interest has centered on the effects of histamine and its effects on the gastrointestinal tract. Histamine stimulates H_2 receptors on gastric parietal cells, causing increased acid production, and also increases gastrointestinal motility, leading to gastroduodenal ulceration and vomiting. In addition, histamine causes increased venule permeability, which contributes to decreased blood flow to the stomach and further enhancement of ulcer formation. One necropsy study showed that 83 per cent of dogs with mast cell tumors had some degree of gastroduodenal ulceration.[47] The effects of histamine and other granule constituents contribute to poor wound healing and hemorrhage, which are frequently associated with mast cell tumors.

Histological grading systems have been developed for mast cell tumors. The grading system used in dogs is based on tumor cellularity and on nuclear and cytoplasmic features of the cells.[11, 46, 71] Tumors are divided into three grades: well differentiated, intermediate, and anaplastic. Unfortunately, the earlier studies[11, 46] used grade I to describe anaplastic tumors and grade III to describe well-differentiated tumors (directly opposite to most grading schemes). The grading system used by Patnaik and colleagues[71] is consistent with that used in other tumor types where grade I is well differentiated and grade III is anaplastic. Readers are cautioned to inquire about which grading system their pathologist uses, because the grades have prognostic significance.

Pathological grading of cutaneous mast cell tumors in cats is not as well defined as in dogs. One study that examined 23 cutaneous mast cell tumors in cats[19] failed to show any prognostic significance when the canine mast cell tumor grading system was applied to cats. Another study of 65 surgically excised feline cutaneous mast cell tumors divided the tumors into either a compact form (45 per cent) or a diffuse form (55 per cent).[45] Based on a follow-up questionnaire to referring veterinarians, 12 of 17 diffuse and only 6 of 15 compact tumors recurred or metastasized. This observation may represent a variability in behavior or imply that the diffuse form is more difficult to excise completely. Another study evaluating 23 cutaneous mast cell tumors in cats[19] described both the previously mentioned histocytic mast cell tumors of Siamese cats and a more traditional appearing mast cell tumor. Although the histiocytic form had a benign course and often spontaneously regressed, the latter type consisted of both benign solitary masses and a more anaplastic form that frequently recurs or metastasizes.

The most common sites of involvement of canine mast cell tumors are the trunk and perineum (50 per cent), extremities (40 per cent), and head and neck (10 per cent). Multiple sites are involved approximately 11 per cent of the time.[26, 64] Tumor size ranges from 1 to 10 cm in diameter, and masses are usually firm and raised. In another form, because of collagen breakdown caused by mast cell granule products, the tumor mass is ill defined, soft, and almost edematous. On palpation, this form is frequently confused with lipoma.

In cats, some reports list a predilection for the head and neck[77, 86] but others do not.[45] The occurrence of the histiocytic form in Siamese cats less than 4 years of age was discussed earlier. Reports suggest that cutaneous mast cell tumors in cats are more frequent than the visceral form and that solitary cutaneous tumors are more frequent than the multiple form.[45, 110] In cats, cutaneous tumors are firm, raised, and up to 1 cm in diameter.

Dogs have a broad range of clinical histories. Tumor growth rate is variable and ranges from slow-growing masses to those that grow and metastasize rapidly. The appearance ranges from small solitary dermal nodules with well-defined borders, to ill-defined alopecic erythematous, to an ulcerated mass. They may be firm or fluctuant, and palpation can cause degranulation to occur, leading to erythema and swelling in the area. Mast cell tumors can metastasize via lymphatics or hematogenously and infiltrate fascial planes locally. Because of the high content of vasoactive amines, coagulopathies including disseminated intravascular coagulopathy may occur secondarily. The effects of histamine on the gastrointestinal tract can lead to anorexia, vomiting, diarrhea, and gastroduodenal ulceration.

Inguinal and perineal canine mast cell tumors recur and metastasize more frequently than tumors located on other areas of the body.[22, 85, 103]

Cats are most likely to have a solitary tumor that is benign, although more aggressive forms do exist. Clinical signs are similar to those in dogs, although there is no evidence that tumors in one cutaneous site are more aggressive than those at another.

Diagnosis of mast cell tumors is based on clinical characteristics as well as cytological or histological evaluation. Mast cell tumors are usually easily diagnosed by cytological study, which aids in planning the surgical procedure, but histological assessment of canine tumors does allow grading of the tumor, which has shown prognostic significance in several studies.[11, 46, 71] In cats, histological evaluation may also afford prognostic information.[19, 45] It also allows evaluation of excision and the need for additional therapy.

A complete history and physical examination are important in the evaluation of patients with mast cell tumors. It is important to determine whether the animal has had previous mast cell tumors. The physical examination should include a careful search for the presence of other masses as well as lymphadenopathy, and the finding of either necessitates that they be aspirated.

Additional diagnostic tests include hematological studies, serum chemistry evaluation, and urinalysis. Anemia may suggest gastroduodenal ulceration (mild responsive anemia early, microcytic hypochromic in chronic stage), anemia of chronic disease, or even erythrophagocytosis by the tumor cells as has been reported in cats.[57] In addition, eosinophilia and basophilia have been reported in humans[29] and in a dog with systemic mastocytosis.[30] Buffy coat smears have been recommended to increase the chance of detecting circulating mast cells, but one small study[68] suggested that bone marrow aspirates may be more sensitive in detecting systemic mastocytosis.

Radiographs of the thorax are of limited value[56] because metastasis of cutaneous mast cell tumors to the lungs is rare and usually results in a diffuse pattern. In our experience, mast cell tumors that involve the axillary or superficial cervical lymph nodes frequently show involvement of intrathoracic lymph nodes on radiographs. Abdominal radiographs may demonstrate lymph node enlargement in cases that involve the rear limbs or especially the inguinal and perineal regions in dogs. Additionally, they may show splenic involvement in cats. Organomegaly can be further evaluated with ultrasonography and aspiration cytological study.

Occult blood tests of the stool can be used to evaluate animals for gastroduodenal ulceration; however, false positives may occur with gastrointestinal parasites or myoglobin from meat in the diet.

A clinical staging form has been proposed by the World Health Organization[70] (Table 153–2), although no studies have been carried out to show the prognostic significance of this form. The primary mode of therapy for mast cell tumors is wide surgical excision with at least 3-cm margins of normal tissue. All excised tissues are examined for completeness of excision, and the tumor is also graded. Studies of dogs[11, 71] have shown that survival time does correlate with histological grade (Table 153–3). If the tumor is incompletely excised, a second more radical operation is performed or the tumor bed is treated with radiation.

Radiation therapy is considered as postsurgical treatment for intermediate and poorly differentiated tumors. It is of benefit as the primary therapy for inoperable or recurrent tumors and involved lymph nodes that are not excised.[105]

Once the tumor is no longer localized, treatment becomes palliative and success rates quite variable. Most studies deal with the treatment of mast cell tumors in dogs, but similar treatment recommendations can be made for treatment of cats with multicentric cutaneous mast cell tumors. Our experience with a few cats is that treatment is palliative and provides comfort for up to 6 months. Bulky disease associated with disseminated tumors is treated the same as localized disease. Various chemotherapeutic protocols involving vinca alkaloids or cyclophosphamide have been proposed for mast cell tumors, but no studies show that such protocols are more efficacious than corticosteroids alone. Corticosteroid therapy usually involves the use of oral prednisolone or prednisone given at 40 mg/m^2 PO daily for 7 days, then 20 mg/m^2 PO every other day. Dosages may be adjusted depending on the response of the tumor and the animal. Triamcinolone is used less frequently but can be used intralesionally at 1 mg/cm^2 of tumor every 2 weeks.

TABLE 153–2. CLINICAL STAGING OF CANINE MAST CELL TUMORS

Stage	
I:	Solitary dermal tumor
II:	Solitary dermal tumor + lymph node involvement
III:	Multiple dermal tumors
IV:	Any tumor with distant metastasis
Each stage further divided into	
a:	Without signs of systemic disease
b:	With signs of systemic disease

Side effects caused by release of products from mast cell tumors are severe enough that they are treated directly. Animals with mast cell tumors are at risk for gastroduodenal ulceration secondary to histamine. This complication is treated with H_2 blockers (e.g., cimetidine, 5 mg/kg PO TID to QID; or ranitidine, 0.5 mg/kg PO BID). The most frequently used gastrointestinal protectant for treatment of ulceration is sucralfate (500 mg PO TID for animals $<$18 kg and 1 g PO TID for animals $>$18 kg). Sucralfate interferes with the absorption of cimetidine; therefore, cimetidine must be given either 45 minutes before or 2 hours after sucralfate. H_1 antagonists such as diphenhydramine (2 mg/kg PO TID) have been suggested to prevent the suppressive effects of histamine on fibroblast activity during wound healing.[56]

Hyperthermia enhances the efficacy of radiation therapy for localized mast cell tumors.[104] A small study of dogs suggests that whole-body hyperthermia is beneficial for the treatment of generalized mast cell tumors, especially when total tumor volume is less than 2 cm^3.[104]

Several studies of dogs suggest than mast cell tumors are unlikely to recur if they have not done so by 6 months after treatment.[11, 22, 35]

Histiocytoma

Histiocytomas are a common tumor in dogs; a few similar tumors have been reported in cats.[56, 56a] These benign tumors arise from the monocyte macrophage population of the skin and account for 10 to 20 per cent of all skin tumors. Purebred dogs, especially boxers and dachshunds, are at increased risk.[102] Approximately half the tumors occur in dogs younger than 3 years.

TABLE 153–3. SURVIVAL TIMES OF DOGS WITH CUTANEOUS MAST CELL TUMORS TREATED WITH SURGERY ALONE

	No. of Dogs	Per Cent Surviving	Days After Surgery
Bostock[11]			
Well differentiated	39	77	210
Intermediate differentiation	30	45	210
Anaplastic	45	13	210
Patnaik et al[71]			
Well differentiated	30	93	1,500
Intermediate differentiation	36	47	1,500
Anaplastic	17	6	1,500

Histiocytomas are usually solitary tumors, but multiple forms have been reported. The tumors frequently are rapidly growing, dome-shaped masses with the surface being alopecic and inflamed to ulcerated. They are most commonly located in the head and neck regions. Although histiocytomas may spontaneously regress in 2 to 3 months, they are frequently excised because of their clinical appearance. Recurrence is uncommon, and metastasis does not occur.[9] Malignant fibrous histiocytomas were discussed earlier with soft-tissue sarcomas.

Cutaneous Lymphosarcoma

Lymphosarcoma uncommonly involves the skin of dogs and cats. It may do so as an extension of multicentric lymphosarcoma or as a primary disease. It occurs in older dogs (mean age = 9.5 years)[17] and cats (mean age = 11 years).[21] Cats with the tumor are feline leukemia virus negative,[21] as are older cats with other forms of lymphosarcoma.

Clinically, the tumors may appear as simple erythema, crusting, ulcers, or nodules. These tumors frequently involve the dermis and subcutis and are derived from type B lymphocytes.[44] Mycosis fungoides is a tumor that begins as a superficial scaling lesion and is of T-cell lineage, affecting both dogs and cats.[20, 89]

Diagnosis for dogs and cats with lymphosarcoma is the same as for any animal with lymphosarcoma. It allows determination of whether the disease is primary or multicentric in nature and assists in appropriate planning of therapy.

Therapy of cutaneous lymphosarcoma includes surgery, radiation therapy, and chemotherapy. Unfortunately, the response of cutaneous lymphosarcoma to treatment is variable and frequently disappointing. The greatest success is in dogs with solitary lesions that can be completely excised or treated with radiation therapy.[17] Cats, even with solitary lesions, do poorly despite therapy, except in the case of one cat with mycoses fungoides that was treated with fibronectin.[20, 21] Dogs and cats with multiple lesions or disease that is part of multicentric lymphosarcoma are treated with standard chemotherapy protocols.

Plasmacytoma

Plasmacytomas[7, 78] are solitary broad-based, round, circumscribed, alopecic cutaneous or mucocutaneous lesions that occur in older dogs, especially cocker spaniels. Cats are also affected. The lips, feet, and ears are most commonly affected. Neither sex is more commonly affected. No special clinical or biochemical findings are documented. Local invasion including bone is noted. Surgical excision results in cure. The recurrence ranges from 3 to 30 per cent. Recurrent lesions respond to reexcision. In our experience, response to radiation is transitory.

Transmissible Venereal Tumor

Canine transmissible venereal tumor is a transmissible, usually nonmalignant tumor that becomes metastatic in only 5 per cent. The tumor is spread by the implantation of intact tumor cells. The tumor cells have a different chromosome number than the dog. As the name implies, it usually involves the genitalia but can affect the skin, usually by direct implantation of tumor cells into abraded skin or less frequently by metastasis from a primary site. The cutaneous form may present as solitary or multiple subcutaneous or dermal nodules. The overlying skin may be intact, alopecic, or ulcerated.

When the skin is afflicted, a careful search is made for other sites of involvement. Therapy consists of surgery, radiation therapy, or chemotherapy. Surgery may be effective for localized lesions, but recurrence ranges from 20 per cent for local lesions to 60 per cent for extragenital lesions.[4] More invasive or extensive localized lesions respond well to radiation therapy, with total dosage recommendations varying from 15 to 45 Gy given in divided doses.[42] Episiotomy may be required for exposure if orthovoltage is used. Localized or more extensive tumors also respond well to chemotherapy with vincristine (0.5 mg/m^2 IV[5, 15, 23] weekly) or doxorubicin (30 mg/m^2 IV every 3 weeks[54]). Treatment is continued until remission is complete.

Malignant Melanoma

Melanomas are of neuroectodermal origin and are frequently round or epithelioid, but they are also seen as spindle cells histologically, giving the impression of a mesodermal sarcoma—hence the old name *melanosarcoma.* They also are seen in mixed cellular populations. Likewise, the degree of pigmentation varies. These features are not associated with prognosis.

Cutaneous melanomas are common in dogs (approximately 6 per cent of all skin tumors)[27] and rare in cats.[56, 56a] These tumors occur most frequently in dogs 7 to 14 years of age, in males, and in breeds with dark skin pigmentation.[27] In dogs, most cutaneous melanomas are benign except for ones of the nail bed and mucocutaneous regions (see the earlier section on oral melanoma). An exception to the mucocutaneous rule, eyelid melanomas are usually benign. Benign tumors are frequently solitary, dome-shaped, well-circumscribed, pigmented nodules that vary from 0.5 to 2.0 cm in diameter. In cats, both benign and malignant forms occur in equal numbers.

The benign forms are usually of little consequence and respond to simple excision.[87] Suspected malignant lesions necessitate complete diagnosis, including thoracic radiographs for metastatic disease. Therapy for malignant masses includes wide surgical excision, which may include amputation for digital melanomas. Radiation therapy of the primary site may also be considered. The use of combined cisplatin and whole-body hyperthermia has demonstrated some therapeutic benefit. No matter what therapeutic modalities are used, the response of malignant melanomas to treatment is usually poor.

References

1. Akerman M, et al: Aspiration cytology of soft tissue tumors. *Acta Orthop Scand 56*:407, 1985.
2. Al-Bagdadi F, Lovell J: The integument. *In* Evans HE, Christensen GC (eds): *Miller's Anatomy of the Dog.* W.B. Saunders, Philadelphia, 1979, p 78.

3. Albers GW, Theilen GH: Calcium chloride for treatment of subcutaneous lipomas in dogs. *J Am Vet Med Assoc 186*:492, 1985.
4. Amber EI, Henderson RA: Canine transmissible venereal tumor: Evaluation of surgical excision of primary and metastatic lesions in Zaria-Nigeria. *J Am Anim Hosp Assoc 18*:350, 1982.
5. Amber EI, et al: Single-drug chemotherapy of canine transmissible venereal tumor with cyclophosphamide, methotrexate, or vincristine. *J Vet Intern Med 4*:144, 1990.
6. Bachman D, et al: Effect of bacille Calmett-Guérin immunotherapy on feline sarcoma virus-induced neoplasms in the cat. *Am J Vet Res 43*:475, 1982.
7. Baer KE, et al: Cutaneous plasmacytomas in dogs: A morphologic and immunohistochemical study. *Vet Pathol 26*:216, 1989.
8. Baker BB, Stannard AA: Nodular panniculitis in the dog. *J Am Vet Med Assoc 167*:752, 1975.
9. Bender WM, Mueller GH: Multiple, resolving, cutaneous histiocytoma in a dog. *J Am Vet Med Assoc 194*:535, 1989.
10. Berzon JL, Howard PE: Lipomatosis in dogs. *J Am Anim Hosp Assoc 16*:253, 1980.
11. Bostock DC: The prognosis following surgical removal of mastocytomas in dogs. *J Small Anim Pract 14*:27, 1973.
12. Bostock DE, Dye MT: Prognosis after surgical excision of canine fibrous connective tissue sarcomas. *Vet Pathol 17*:581, 1980.
13. Bradley RL, et al: Nerve sheath tumors in the dog. *J Am Anim Hosp Assoc 18*:915, 1982.
14. Braund KG: Foreign-body induced sarcomas. *In* Becker FF (ed): *Cancer.* Plenum, New York, 1975, p 485.
15. Brown NO, et al: Chemotherapeutic management of transmissible venereal tumors in 30 dogs. *J Am Vet Med Assoc 176*:983, 1980 (and follow-up letter *177*:676, 1980).
16. Brown NO, et al: Combined modality therapy in the treatment of solid tumors in cats. *J Am Anim Hosp Assoc 16*:719, 1980.
17. Brown NO, et al: Cutaneous lymphosarcoma in the dog: A disease with variable clinical and histologic manifestations. *J Am Anim Hosp Assoc 16*:565, 1980.
18. Brown NO, et al: Canine hemangiosarcoma: Retrospective analysis of 104 cases. *J Am Vet Med Assoc 186*:56, 1985.
19. Buerger RG, Scott DW: Cutaneous mast cell neoplasia in cats: 14 cases (1975–1985). *J Am Vet Med Assoc 190*:1440, 1987.
20. Caciolo PL, et al: A case of mycoses fungoides in a cat and literature review. *J Am Anim Hosp Assoc 19*:505, 1983.
21. Caciolo PL, et al: Cutaneous lymphosarcoma in the cat: A report of nine cases. *J Am Anim Hosp Assoc 20*:491, 1983.
22. Calvert CA: Canine viral and transmissible neoplasms. *In* Green CE (ed): *Clinical Microbiology and Infectious Diseases of the Dog and Cat.* W.B. Saunders, Philadelphia, 1984, pp 472–473.
23. Calvert CA, et al: Vincristine for treatment of transmissible venereal tumor in the dog. *J Am Vet Med Assoc 181*:163, 1982.
24. Campbell KL, et al: Cutaneous inverted papillomas in dogs. *Vet Pathol 25*:67, 1988.
25. Chaisiri N, Pierripoint CG: Steriod-receptor interaction in a canine anal adenoma. *J Small Anim Pract 20*:405, 1979.
26. Cohen D, et al: Epidemiological analysis of the most prevalent sites and types of canine neoplasia observed in a veterinary hospital. *Cancer Res 34*:2859, 1974.
27. Conroy J: Canine skin tumors. *J Am Anim Hosp Assoc 19*:91, 1983.
28. Cosenza SF, Seely JC: Generalized nodular dermatofibrosis and renal cystadenocarcinomas in a German shepherd dog. *J Am Vet Med Assoc 189*:1587, 1986.
29. Cryer PE, Kissane JM: Systemic mastocytosis. *Am J Med 61*:671, 1976.
30. Davies AP, et al: Noncutaneous systemic mastocytosis and mast cell leukemia in a dog: Case report and literature review. *17*:361, 1981.
31. Doige CE, et al: Parosteal lipoma in a dog. *J Am Anim Hosp Assoc 16*:87, 1980.
32. Dorn ER, et al: Survey of animals neoplasms in Alameda and Contra Costa counties, California. II. Cancer morbidity in dogs and cats from Alameda County. *J Natl Cancer Inst 40*:307, 1968.
33. Evans SM: Canine hemangiopericytoma: A retrospective analysis of response to surgery and orthovoltage radiation. *Vet Radiol 28*:13, 1987.
34. Garner FM, Lingeman CH: Mast cell neoplasms of the domestic cat. *Vet Pathol* 7:517, 1970.
35. Gilette EL: Radiation therapy of canine and feline tumors. *J Am Anim Hosp Assoc 12*:359, 1976.
36. Gleisler CA, et al: Infiltrating lipomas in the dog. *Vet Pathol 16*:623, 1979.
37. Gleisler CA, et al: Malignant fibrous histiocytoma in dogs and cats. *Vet Pathol 16*:199, 1979.
38. Goldschmidt MH, Zoltowski C: Anal sac adenocarcinoma in the dog: 14 cases. *J Small Anim Pract 22*:119, 1981.
39. Graves GM, et al: Canine hemangiocytoma: 23 cases (1967–1984). *J Am Vet Med Assoc 192*:99, 1988.
40. Greenall MJ, et al: Chemotherapy for soft tissue sarcoma. *Surg Gynecol Obstet 162*:193, 1986.
41. Hause WR, et al: Pseudohyperparathyroidism associated with adenocarcinomas of anal sac origin in four dogs. *J Am Anim Hosp Assoc 17*:373, 1981.
42. Herron MA: Tumors of the canine genital system. *J Am Anim Hosp Assoc 19*:981, 1983.
43. Himel CA, et al: Cisplatin chemotherapy for metastatic squamous cell carcinoma in two dogs. *J Am Vet Med Assoc 189*:1575, 1986.
44. Holmberg CA, et al: Canine malignant lymphomas: Comparison of morphologic and immunologic parameters. *J Natl Cancer Inst 56*:125, 1976.
45. Holzinger EA: Feline cutaneous mastocytomas. *Cornell Vet 63*:87, 1973.
46. Hottendorf GH, Nielson SW: Survey of 300 extirpated canine mastocytomas. *Zentralbl Veterinarmed [A] 14*:272, 1967.
47. Howard EB, et al: Mastocytoma and gastroduodenal ulceration. *Vet Pathol 6*:146, 1969.
48. Isitor GN: Comparative ultrastructural study of normal, adenomatous, carcinomatous, and hyperplastic cells of canine hepatoid circumanal glands. *Am J Vet Res 44*:463, 1983.
49. Johnson RP: Malignant pilomatrixoma in an old English sheepdog. *Can J Vet Med 24*:392, 1983.
50. Klausner JS, et al: Hypercalcemia in two cats with squamous cell carcinomas. *J Am Vet Med Assoc 196*:103, 1990.
51. Kramek BA, et al: Infiltrative lipomas in three dogs. *J Am Vet Med Assoc 186*:81, 1985.
52. Latimer CA, et al: Azathioprine in the management of fibrous histiocytoma in two dogs. *J Am Anim Hosp Assoc 19*:155, 1983.
53. Lehti PM, et al: Improved survival for soft tissue sarcoma of the extremities by regional hyperthermic perfusion, local excision and radiation therapy. *Surg Gynecol Obstet 162*:149, 1986.
54. MacEwen EG: Canine transmissible venereal tumor. *In* Withrow SJ, MacEwen EG (eds): *Clinical Veterinary Oncology.* J.B. Lippincott, Philadelphia, 1989, pp 421–425.
55. MacVean DW, et al: Frequency of canine and feline tumors in a defined population. *Vet Pathol 15*:700, 1978.
56. Macy DW, MacEwen EG: Mast cell tumors. *In* Withrow SJ, MacEwen EG (eds): *Clinical Veterinary Oncology.* J.B. Lippincott, Philadelphia, 1989, pp 156–166.
56a. Macy DW, Reynolds HA: The incidence, characteristics and clinical management of skin tumors of cats. *J Am Anim Hosp Assoc 17*:1026, 1981.
57. Madewell BR, et al: Mast cell phagocytosis of red blood cells in a cat. *Vet Pathol 20*:638, 1983.
58. McChesney AE, et al: Infiltrative lipoma in dogs. *Vet Pathol 17*:316, 1980.
59. McChesney SM, et al: Radiotherapy of soft-tissue sarcomas in dogs. *J Am Vet Med Assoc 194*:60, 1989.
60. McGavin MD, Fishburn F: Perianal adenoma of apocrine origin in a dog. *J Am Vet Med Assoc 166*:388, 1975.
61. Messick JB, Radin MJ: Cytologic, histologic and ultrastructural characteristics of a canine mixoid liposarcoma. *Vet Pathol 26*:520, 1989.
62. Meuten DJ, et al: Hypercalcemia in dogs with adenocarcinoma derived from apocrine glands of the anal sac: Biochemical and histomorphometric investigations. *Lab Invest 48*:428, 1983.
63. Nielsen SW: Classification of tumors in dogs and cats. *J Am Anim Hosp Assoc 19*:13, 1983.
64. Nielsen SW, Cole CR: Canine mastocytoma—a report of 100 cases. *Am J Vet Radiol 19*:417, 1958.
65. Nishikawa S, et al: Effects of mithramycin on transplantable canine perianal gland carcinoma (CAC-9) in nude mice: Biochemical, histomorphometric, and ultrastructural investigations. *Vet Pathol 23*:698, 1986.
66. Ogilvie GK, et al: Phase II evaluation of mitoxantrone against various canine neoplasms. *J Am Vet Med Assoc 198*:1618, 1991.
67. Ogilvie GK, et al: Acute and short-term toxicity associated with the administration of doxorubricin to dogs with malignant tumors. *J Am Vet Med Assoc 195*:1584, 1989.
68. O'Keefe DA, et al: Systemic mastocytosis in the dog. *J Vet Intern Med 1*:75, 1987.
69. Orkin M, Schwartzman RM: A comparative study of canine and human dermatology: Cutaneous tumors: The mast cell and human mastocytoma. *J Comp Dermatol 32*:451, 1959.
70. Owen LN: *TNM Classification of Tumors in Domestic Animals.* World Health Organization, Geneva, 1980.
71. Patnaik AK, et al: Canine cutaneous mast cell tumor: Morphologic grading and survival time in 83 dogs. *Vet Pathol 21*:469, 1984.
72. Peters JA: Canine mastocytoma excess risk as related to ancestry. *J Natl Cancer Inst 42*:435, 1969.
73. Postorino NC, et al: Prognostic variables for canine hemangiopericytoma: 50 cases (1979–1984). *J Am Anim Hosp Assoc 24*:501, 1988.
74. Presant CA, et al: Soft-tissue and bone sarcoma histopathology peer review: The frequency of disagreement in diagnosis and the need for second pathology opinions, the southeastern cancer study group experience. *J Clin Oncol 4*:1658, 1986.
75. Priester WA: Skin tumors in domestic animals. Data from 21 U.S. and Canadian colleges of veterinary medicine. *J Natl Cancer Inst 50*:457, 1973.
76. Priester WA, McKay FA: *The Occurrence of Tumors in Domestic Animals.* National Cancer Institute Monograph 54. US Department of Health and Human Services, Bethesda, 1980.
77. Pulley LT, Stannard AA: Tumors of the skin and soft tissues. Moulton JE (ed): *Tumors in Domestic Animals.* University of California Press, Berkeley, 1990, pp 23–87.

78. Rakich PM, et al: Mucocutaneous plasmacytomas in dogs: 75 cases (1980–1987). *J Am Vet Med Assoc 194*:803, 1989.
79. Richardson RC, et al: Metastatic canine hemangiopericytoma. *J Am Vet Med Assoc 182*:705, 1983.
80. Ross JT, et al: Abstract: Adenocarcinoma of the apocrine gland of the anal sac in the dog: A retrospective study of 31 dogs. Proceedings of the 25th Meeting of the American College of Veterinary Surgeons, New Orleans, Feb. 1990, p 71.
81. Rudd RG, et al: Lymphangiosarcoma in dogs. *J Am Anim Hosp Assoc 25*:695, 1989.
82. Scavelli TD, et al: Hemangiosarcoma in the cat: Retrospective evaluation of 31 surgical cases. *J Am Vet Med Assoc 187*:817, 1985.
83. Schema CJ, et al: Extraskeletal sarcomas in 2 dogs. *J Am Vet Med Assoc 194*:1452, 1989.
84. Schoster JV, Wyman M: Remission of orbital sarcoma in a dog, using doxorubicin therapy. *J Am Vet Med Assoc 172*:1101, 1978.
85. Scott DW, Anderson WI: Canine sebaceous gland tumors: A retrospective analysis of 172 cases. *Canine Pract 15*:19, 1990.
86. Scott DW: Feline dermatology 1900–1978: A monograph. *J Am Anim Hosp Assoc 16*:419, 1980.
87. Scott DW, et al: Nevi in the dog. *J Am Anim Hosp Assoc 20*:505, 1984.
88. Seiler RJ: Granular basal cell tumors in the skin of 3 dogs: A distinct clinical entity. *Vet Pathol 18*:23, 1983.
89. Shadduck JA, et al: A canine cutaneous lymphoproliferative disease resembling mycoses fungoides in man. *Vet Pathol 15*:716, 1978.
90. Shapiro W, et al: Cisplatin for treatment of transitional cell and squamous cell carcinomas in dogs. *J Am Vet Med Assoc 193*:1530, 1988.
91. Sinibaldi K, et al: Tumors associated with metalic implants in animals. *Clin Orthop 118*:257, 1976.
92. Snyder SP, Theilen GH: Transmissible feline fibrosarcoma. *Nature 221*:1074, 1969.
93. Stannard AA, Pulley LT: Intracutaneous cornifying epithelioma (keratoacanthoma) in the dog: A retrospective study of 25 cases. *J Am Vet Med Assoc 167*:385, 1975.
94. Stevenson S, et al: Fracture-associated sarcoma in the dog. *J Am Vet Med Assoc 180*:1189, 1982.
95. Strafuss AC: Basal cell tumors in dogs. *J Am Anim Hosp Assoc 9*:322, 1976.
96. Strafuss AC: Sebaceous gland adenomas in dogs. *J Am Vet Med Assoc 169*:640, 1976.
97. Strafuss AC: Sebaceous gland carcinoma in dogs. *J Am Vet Med Assoc 169*:325, 1976.
98. Strafuss AC: Squamous cell carcinoma in dogs. *J Am Vet Med Assoc 168*:425, 1976.
99. Strafuss AC, Bozarth AJ: Liposarcoma in dogs. *J Am Anim Hosp Assoc 9*:183, 1973.
100. Strafuss AC, et al: Schwannoma in a dog. *J Am Vet Med Assoc 163*:245, 1973.
101. Strafuss AC, et al: Lipomas in dogs. *J Am Anim Hosp Assoc 9*:555, 1973.
102. Taylor DON, et al: Morphologic and biologic characteristics of the canine histiocytoma. *Cancer Res 29*:83, 1969.
103. Theilen GH, Madewell B: Tumors of the skin and subcutaneous tissues. *In* Theilen GH, Madewell B (eds): *Veterinary Cancer Medicine.* 2nd ed. Lea & Febiger, Philadelphia, 1987, p 311.
104. Thrall DE, Dewhirst MW: Use of radiation and hyperthermia for treatment of mast cell tumors and lymphosarcoma in dogs. *Vet Clin North Am 15*:835, 1985.
105. Turrel JM, et al: Prognostic factors for radiation treatment of mast cell tumors in 85 dogs. *J Am Vet Med Assoc 193*:936, 1988.
106. Turrel JM, et al: Response to radiation therapy of recurrent lymphangioma in a dog. *J Am Vet Med Assoc 193*:1432, 1988.
107. Vail DM, et al: Perianal adenocarcinoma in the canine male: A retrospective study of 41 cases. *J Am Anim Hosp Assoc 26*:329, 1990.
108. Weiss E, Frese K: Tumors of the skin. *Bull WHO 50*:79, 1974.
109. White RAS: Clinical diagnosis and management of soft-tissue sarcomas. *In* Gorman NT (ed): *Contemporary Issues in Small Animal Practice: Oncology.* Churchill Livingstone, New York, 1986, p 243.
110. Wilock BP, et al: The morphology and behavior of feline cutaneous mastocytomas. *Vet Pathol 23*:320, 1986.
111. Wilson GP, Hayes HM: Castration for treatment of perianal gland neoplasms in the dog. *J Am Vet Med Assoc 1704*:1301, 1979.

CHAPTER 154 Alimentary Tract, Liver, and Pancreas

J. S. Klausner and R. M. Hardy

OROPHARYNGEAL NEOPLASIA

Neoplasia of the oral and pharyngeal cavities is the fifth most common canine and the seventh most common feline malignancy.[35] The incidence is 20/100,000/year in dogs and 11/100,000/year in cats.[35] Malignant and benign tumors arising from dental and nondental tissues have been described (Table 154–1).[14, 28, 36, 57, 138, 150] Squamous cell carcinoma and malignant melanoma are the most frequent malignant oral tumors in dogs, whereas squamous cell carcinoma and fibrosarcoma are most common in cats.

Most oral tumors arise from the gingiva in dogs and from the gingiva or tongue in cats. Canine tongue tumors are uncommon, with squamous cell carcinomas, granular cell myoblastomas, melanomas, mast cell tumors, and fibrosarcomas most frequent.[7] Sublingual squamous cell carcinoma is the most common tongue tumor in cats.

Although oral tumors may be encountered in dogs and cats of any age, older animals have an increased risk (Table 154–2). Exceptions include fibrosarcomas in large dogs, which occur more frequently in younger dogs; papillary squamous cell carcinomas, described in dogs less than 6 months of age; undifferentiated oral tumors, identified in dogs younger than 2 years; and virus-induced papillomatosis, which is typically identified in dogs younger than one year.[7, 105, 120, 150, 158]

TABLE 154–1. CANINE AND FELINE OROPHARYNGEAL TUMORS

Nonodontogenic neoplasia
Benign tumors
Papilloma, fibroma, lipoma, chondroma, osteoma, hemangioma, histiocytoma, fibromatous epulis, ossifying epulis
Malignant tumors
Malignant melanoma, squamous cell carcinoma, fibrosarcoma, acanthomatous epulis, adenocarcinoma, undifferentiated carcinoma, hemangiosarcoma, lymphosarcoma, osteosarcoma, transmissible venereal tumor, mast cell tumor, neuroendocrine cell tumor, granular cell myoblastoma
Odontogenic neoplasia
Odontoma
Ameloblastoma

TABLE 154–2. EPIDEMIOLOGICAL FEATURES AND BIOLOGICAL BEHAVIOR OF CANINE OROPHARYNGEAL NEOPLASMS

	Malignant Melanoma	Fibrosarcoma	Tonsillar Squamous Cell Carcinoma	Nontonsillar Squamous Cell Carcinoma
Mean age (years)	11	7.6	9.6	8.8
Male/female	4.2:1	1.8:1	1.5:1	1:1
Bone involvement (%)	57	68	ND*	77
Regional lymph node involvement (%)	15	11	35	45
Distant metastases (%)	66	23	41	36

*Not determined.

Data from Todoroff RJ, Brody RS: Oral and pharyngeal neoplasia in the dog: a retrospective survey of 361 cases. *J Am Vet Med Assoc 175*:567, 1979.

The risk of developing oral melanomas and fibrosarcomas is greater in male dogs.[34] Breeds with a high incidence of oral tumors include the cocker spaniel, weimaraner, German shepherd, German shorthaired pointer, golden retriever, and boxer. Small breeds have a higher incidence of malignant melanomas and tonsillar carcinomas, whereas fibrosarcomas and nontonsillar squamous cell carcinomas are more common in large dogs.

The incidence of tonsillar squamous cell carcinomas is higher in urban dogs than in rural dogs, prompting speculation of an environmental cause.[125] Dogs with heavily pigmented oral mucosa are predisposed to malignant melanomas.[34]

Biological Behavior

Epulides arise from the periodontal stroma, are typically located in the gingiva near the incisor teeth, and are more common in dogs than in cats.[8, 40] Three types have been described.[41] The fibromatous and ossifying epulides are benign tumors that form pedunculated nonulcerating, noninvasive masses. Acanthomatous epulides are locally invasive, causing bone destruction, but do not metastasize (Fig. 154–1).

Ameloblastomas, the most common tumors of dental laminar epithelium, are expansile, slow-growing tumors.[40] They are often cystic, producing large radiolucent areas within bone. Although they are locally invasive, ameloblastomas typically do not metastasize. Inductive fibroameloblastoma, a rare odontogenic tumor primarily affecting young cats, is locally invasive in bone but does not metastasize.[41]

Malignant melanomas grow rapidly and are characterized by early gingiva and bone invasion and metastases to regional lymph nodes and lungs (see Table 154–2). They usually arise on the gingiva, buccal mucosa, or lips. Melanomas are firm and black but may be nonpigmented. Surface ulceration and necrosis are common.

Nontonsillar squamous cell carcinomas are most fre-

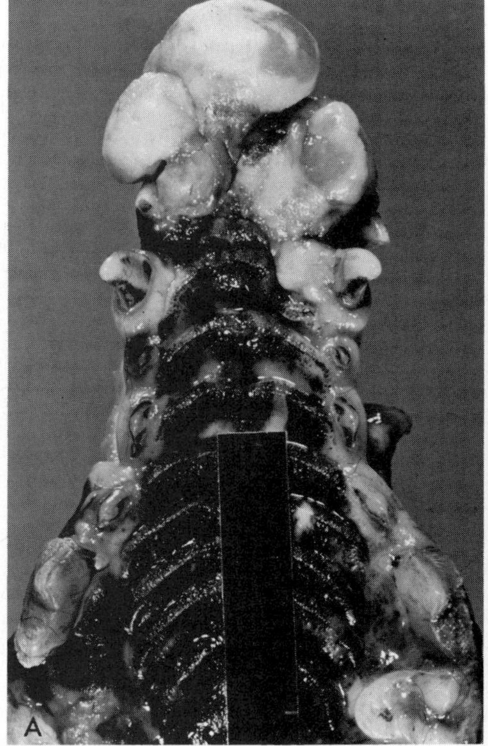

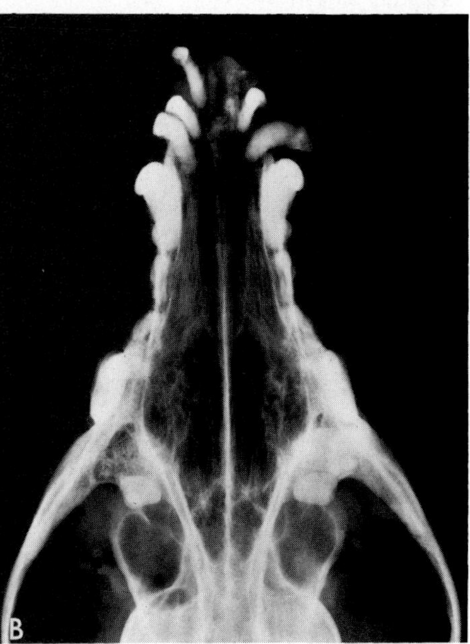

FIGURE 154–1. *A*, Upper jaw of a 16-month-old mixed-breed dog extensively infiltrated by an acanthomatous epulis. *B*, Ventrodorsal radiograph of the maxilla. Note the extensive bone lysis surrounding the incisor teeth.

quently identified arising from the gingiva rostral to the canine teeth in dogs and under the tongue in cats.[138, 150] They appear as irregular, ulcerated masses. Bone invasion is present in 77 per cent of canine tumors.[150] In both dogs and cats, regional lymph node involvement is uncommon. Distant metastasis has been reported in 3 to 36 per cent of dogs and is rare in cats.[98, 150] Papillary squamous cell carcinomas, identified in young dogs, are locally invasive into bone but do not metastasize.[105]

Tonsillar squamous cell carcinomas appear as plaque-like or cauliflower lesions affecting one tonsil. They are locally invasive and frequently spread to the cervical lymph nodes and to distant sites. In one series, 98 per cent of dogs had regional lymph node metastasis and 63 per cent had distant metastasis.[14]

Fibrosarcomas are typically firm, fleshy tumors that arise from the gingiva, hard palate, or buccal mucosa. Gingival fibrosarcomas are frequently identified in the maxillary arcade between the canine and carnassial teeth.[150] They are locally invasive in gingiva and bone. Metastasis to regional lymph nodes and distant sites is uncommon. Aggressive local tissue invasion has been noted in fibrosarcomas that are histologically well differentiated.

TABLE 154–3. CLINICAL STAGING SYSTEM FOR TUMORS OF THE ORAL CAVITY

T: Primary tumor
- T_0 No evidence of tumor
- T_1 Tumor < 2 cm maximum diameter
  - T_{1a} Without bone invasion
  - T_{1b} With bone invasion
- T_2 Tumor 2 to 4 cm maximum diameter
  - T_{2a} Without bone invasion
  - T_{2b} With bone invasion
- T_3 Tumor > 4 cm maximum diameter
  - T_{3a} Without bone invasion
  - T_{3b} With bone invasion

N: Regional lymph nodes (RLN)
- N_0 No evidence of RLN involvement
- N_1 Movable ipsilateral nodes
  - N_{1a} Nodes histologically negative
  - N_{1b} Movable histologically positive
- N_2 Movable contralateral or bilateral nodes
  - N_{2a} Nodes histologically negative
  - N_{2b} Nodes histologically positive
- N_3 Fixed nodes

M: Distant metastasis
- M_0 No evidence of distant metastasia
- M_1 Distant metastasis present

Stage Groupings

Stage	T	N	M
I	T_1	N_0, N_{1a}, or N_{2a}	M_0
II	T_2	N_0, N_{1a}, or N_{2a}	M_0
III*	T_3	N_0, N_{1a}, or N_{2a}	M_0
IV	Any T		
	Any T	Any N_{2b} or N_3	M_0
	Any T	Any N	M_1

*Any bone involvement.
From World Health Organization: *Report of the Second Consultation on the Biological Behavior and Therapy of Tumors of Domestic Animals.* WHO, Geneva, 1978.

Clinical Signs and Diagnosis

Clinically, oral tumors produce proliferative or occasionally ulcerative lesions. Associated signs may include decreased appetite, halitosis, tooth loss, and bloody salivation. Dyspnea is common with large tonsillar or posterior pharyngeal tumors. Histological examination of oral lesions is necessary to differentiate neoplastic from inflammatory lesions and to determine the cell of origin of neoplastic tissue.

Regional lymph nodes are carefully palpated for enlargement, and aspiration biopsy is performed on abnormal nodes. Metastasis to regional lymph nodes occurs in approximately 17 per cent of oral tumors and is most often identified in melanomas, mastocytomas, and tonsillar carcinomas.[161]

Radiographs of underlying bone are obtained in animals with tumors that adhere to bone to aid in determining clinical stage. Radiographically, involved bones usually appear lytic, but proliferative lesions are occasionally observed. Bone invasion occurs in 60 per cent of dogs with oral tumors.[161] A negative radiograph does not preclude bone involvement. Chest radiographs are obtained to rule out pulmonary metastasis.

Clinical staging for oral tumors is based on tumor size and the presence of bone invasion, regional lymph node involvement, and distant metastasis (Table 154–3). The clinical stage is determined after careful physical examination of the oral cavity, palpation and biopsy of regional lymph nodes, and thoracic radiology. Most dogs with oral tumors have stage III or stage IV disease at diagnosis.[161]

Treatment

Animals without evidence of pulmonary involvement should receive aggressive local therapy (surgery, radiation therapy, or cryosurgery). Survival times are short unless the local tumor is completely excised and tumor cells eliminated from underlying bone.

Surgical Therapy

Benign and malignant tumors that do not involve bone are surgically excised. A 2-cm margin of normal tissue is removed with the tumor. For tumors in which bone invasion is suspected or has been demonstrated radiographically, the tumor and underlying bone are removed. Various procedures for mandibulectomy and maxillectomy have been described, and the procedures are well tolerated by most patients.[9, 121, 130, 160, 163]

Epulides are cured by aggressive surgical treatment. In 25 dogs with various epulides (40 per cent acanthomatous, 32 per cent ossifying, 28 per cent fibromatous), local recurrence after surgical removal was noted in only two cases.[8]

In dogs and cats with malignant oral tumors, mandibulectomies and maxillectomies have increased survival times compared with surgical excision alone, but local recurrence and metastatic disease remain significant problems (Table 154–4).

TABLE 154–4. RESPONSE OF CANINE OROPHARYNGEAL NEOPLASMS TO SURGICAL EXCISION[150] OR PARTIAL MANDIBULECTOMY[129]

Neoplasm	Treatment	Median Survival (Months)	Local Recurrence (%)	Metastasis %
Malignant melanoma	Excision	3	ND	ND
	Mandibulectomy	7.3	9.5	52.4
Nontonsillar squamous cell carcinoma	Excision	2	ND	ND
	Mandibulectomy	15.8	0	7.1
Fibrosarcoma	Excision	1	ND	ND
	Mandibulectomy	7	44.4	22.2

ND, not determined.

Radiation Therapy

Local radiation therapy can produce long-term remissions and cures of radiosensitive tumors (squamous cell carcinoma, acanthomatous epulis, dental tumors). It can be used alone, as an adjuvant to surgical excision, or combined with hyperthermia.[62, 76, 147, 148, 149, 150]

In 39 dogs with acanthomatous epulides, only 3 dogs had recurrence after orthovoltage therapy, but other malignant tumors developed at the previously irradiated site in 7 dogs.[149]

In dogs with nontonsillar squamous cell carcinomas, mean survival times after radiation therapy were significantly longer in dogs having local tumor excisions before radiation therapy (34 months) than in dogs treated with radiation therapy alone (16 months).[68] Dogs younger than 6 years and those with tumors rostral to the second premolar have increased survival times.[45]

Short-term benefit has been documented in dogs with tonsillar squamous cell carcinomas treated with radiation and chemotherapy (cisplatin, doxorubicin) compared with those receiving chemotherapy alone.[15]

Survival times in cats with oral squamous cell carcinomas are shorter than in dogs.[154] Median survival time in nine cats treated with radiation without prior surgery was 4 months. Only one cat lived longer than 1 year.[68]

Long-term results of radiation therapy for oral fibrosarcomas and malignant melanomas in dogs are disappointing, although responses occur.[148]

Chemotherapy

Chemotherapy can be used to provide palliative relief in dogs and cats with disseminated oral tumors. Short-term benefits have been documented in dogs with oral squamous cell carcinomas treated with cisplatin[134] and in cats with fibrosarcomas and squamous cell carcinomas treated with doxorubicin and cyclophosphamide.[84]

Prognosis

Acanthomatous epulides can be cured by either surgical excision or radiation therapy. In a small percentage of dogs treated with radiation, secondary malignant tumors have developed at the previously irradiated site.

Long-term survival and cures have been achieved in dogs with nontonsillar squamous cell carcinomas with radical surgical excisions and radiation therapy, especially with rostrally located tumors. Neither surgery nor radiation therapy significantly affects survival time in cats with oral squamous cell carcinomas. Survival time in dogs with tonsillar carcinomas is short, although limited benefit occurs after combination radiation and chemotherapy.[15]

In dogs with oral melanomas, local control can often be achieved after partial maxillectomy or mandibulectomy, but most treated animals die of metastatic disease.[129] Oral fibrosarcomas often do not metastasize but frequently recur at the surgical site.

ESOPHAGEAL NEOPLASIA

Esophageal neoplasia is rare in dogs and cats except for osteosarcomas and fibrosarcomas associated with *Spirocerca lupi*.[20, 77, 98, 156] A study of 5,854 canine neoplasms at necropsy revealed only 19 esophageal tumors.[137] In another report, only two primary esophageal tumors were identified in 49,229 dogs in an 11-year period.[126] Feline esophageal tumors occur more frequently in Great Britain than in the United States; 5 esophageal carcinomas were found in a series of 200 feline neoplasms.[32] No esophageal tumors were identified in a series of 46 feline alimentary tract tumors in the United States.[12] Neoplasms that metastasize to the esophagus include thyroid carcinomas, pulmonary neoplasms, and gastric carcinomas.[77, 126]

Leiomyoma is the most frequently identified benign esophageal neoplasm.[13, 17, 33] Clinical signs result from obstruction of the esophageal lumen. Leiomyomas may be found incidentally at necropsy.

Carcinomas arise from squamous epithelium of the esophagus and infiltrate the lumen, muscularis, and serosa. Annular constriction of the esophagus may result. Metastases to trachea, lung, and mediastinal lymph nodes occur.[20, 85, 126]

Strong evidence suggests that *S. lupi* is an important etiological factor in the development of esophageal osteosarcomas and fibrosarcomas. Esophageal sarcomas are frequent in areas of the world where *S. lupi* is endemic; lesions associated with *S. lupi* (vertebral spondylosis, aortic scarring or aneurysm) are frequent in dogs with esophageal sarcomas; and sarcomatous changes have been described in fibroblasts in *S. lupi* granulomas.[6] Esophageal sarcomas frequently metastasize to the lungs, and a high incidence of hypertrophic pulmonary osteoarthropathy has been noted.

Clinical Signs

Clinical signs of esophageal neoplasia result from obstruction or altered esophageal motility. Regurgitation, dysphagia, and weight loss are common. Regurgitation may result in aspiration pneumonia and respiratory signs.

Diagnosis

Esophagoscopy, radiographic evaluation, and thoracotomy can be used to establish a diagnosis of esophageal neoplasia. Esophagoscopy may reveal the presence of nodules, ulcerations, mucosal irregularities, lack of distensibility, or stricture. Mucosal lesions can be sampled through the endoscope with a punch biopsy instrument.

Retention of gas in the esophageal lumen and displacement of mediastinal structures may be noted on survey radiographs.[126] Evaluation of contrast radiographs may reveal an irregular mucosal surface, luminal narrowing, retention of contrast medium within the esophagus, or thickening of the esophageal wall. Fluoroscopy may reveal decreased esophageal peristalsis.

Treatment and Prognosis

Neoplasia of the esophagus is associated with a poor prognosis. Small tumors can be surgically removed. Unfortunately, the diagnosis of esophageal neoplasia is often established late in the disease course, precluding surgical resection.

GASTRIC NEOPLASIA

Gastric neoplasms are uncommon in dogs and cats. Adenocarcinoma is the most common canine gastric tumor but accounts for less than 1 per cent of all canine malignancies.[13, 80]

The incidence of gastric tumor in cats is less than in dogs. Lymphosarcoma is the most frequent feline gastric neoplasm.[12]

Gastric tumors generally occur in older animals, with vomiting and weight loss the most frequent clinical signs. Signs are usually attributable to gastric outflow obstruction or mucosal ulceration.

Benign Gastric Tumors

Leiomyoma is the most common benign gastric tumor in dogs.[60, 111, 131] The average age of dogs with gastric leiomyomas is 16 years. Leiomyomas originate in the muscle layers of the stomach wall and usually grow into the gastric lumen. They may not cause clinical signs or may be associated with vomiting, especially if outflow obstruction is present. Treatment is by surgical removal.

Adenomatous polyps result from benign gastric mucosal proliferation. Both single and multiple polyps have been reported in the canine stomach.[30, 37, 59, 60, 101] Grossly, polyps are raised sessile or pedunculated lesions. They may be associated with vomiting, may cause pyloric outflow obstruction, or may be an incidental finding at necropsy.

Malignant Gastric Tumors

Malignant gastric tumors of dogs and cats include adenocarcinomas, lymphosarcomas, fibrosarcomas, leiomyosarcomas, and squamous cell carcinomas.[12, 13, 119] Gastric lymphosarcoma may result in nodular, diffusely infiltrative, or ulcerative lesions.[44] The stomach may be the only organ involved, or the disease may be generalized. Therapy includes surgical removal of nodular lesions and chemotherapy.

Adenocarcinomas account for 42 to 72 per cent of all malignant gastric tumors in dogs.[38, 65, 80, 87, 103, 122] Gastric adenocarcinomas occur in older dogs, usually between the ages of 7 and 13 years, with a peak incidence at 8 years. Males are more commonly affected. An increased prevalence has been noted in rough collies and Staffordshire bull terriers.[144] Geographical differences in occurrence similar to those described in humans have not been identified in dogs. Lymphosarcoma is the most frequent feline gastric tumor.

Environmental and hereditary factors increase the risk of gastric cancer in humans.[81, 127] Substances suspected of being carcinogenic include those associated with pickling or smoking of food for preservation; benzpyrene derived from cooking; and nitrosamines from high-nitrate-containing food.[96] In addition, blood type, atrophic gastritis, and pernicious anemia have been associated with gastric adenocarcinomas in humans. Canine gastric adenocarcinomas have been induced by intragastric administration of nitrosamine.[74] The lower frequency of gastric adenocarcinoma in dogs compared with humans may result from an inherent resistance of the canine stomach to carcinogens or to the shorter life span of dogs.[80]

Gastric adenocarcinomas are usually located in the pyloric antrum or along the lesser curvature of the stomach (Fig. 154–2). Three anatomical types have been described: (1) diffuse infiltration of tumor in the gastric wall, resulting in a thickened, nondistensible stomach (linitis plastica); (2) plaque-like mucosal lesions usually with large central ulcers; and (3) raised polypoid lesions.[101] The neoplasm originates in the mucosa and spreads laterally, frequently involving all layers of the gastric wall. Histologically, large pleomorphic tumor cells may be randomly arranged (diffuse type) or may have a distinct glandular structure (intestinal type).[112] Variable amounts of mucin and large central vacuoles

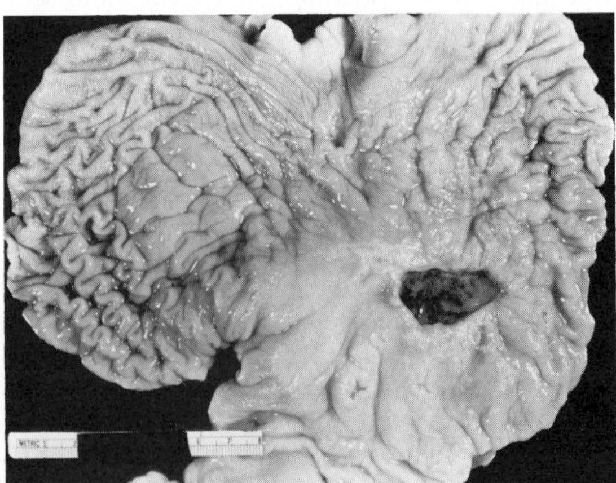

FIGURE 154–2. Large nonperforating ulcer on the lesser curvature of the stomach resulting from a gastric adenocarcinoma in an 11-year-old female basset hound.

may be present within the neoplastic cells. A marked fibrous connective reaction commonly accompanies gastric adenocarcinoma. Early metastasis to regional lymph nodes and liver is common. Other metastatic sites include the spleen, omentum, adrenal glands, myocardium, and lungs.[60]

Clinical Signs

Chronic vomiting, weight loss, and anorexia are usually noted. In addition, hematemesis, melena, and abdominal pain may be detected. Rarely, an abdominal mass may be palpated. Ascites, icterus, and dyspnea often denote metastatic spread. The duration of the illness is generally less than 3 months.

Diagnosis

Chronic vomiting and weight loss in an older dog suggest gastric adenocarcinoma. A microcytic hypochromic anemia may be present if mucosal ulceration results in gastric bleeding. Results of a fecal occult blood test may be positive.

Changes detected on abdominal radiographs are usually minimal. An anterior abdominal mass or gastric dilation may be apparent. Contrast radiography, either a barium series or double-contrast gastrogram, is usually required to detect gastric lesions (Fig. 154–3). Abnormalities associated with adenocarcinoma include (1) delayed gastric emptying; (2) pyloric or lesser curvature filling defects; (3) thickened gastric wall; (4) mucosal ulceration; and (5) loss of normal rugal pattern.[131] Significant abnormalities persist on multiple films. Fluoroscopy is useful to confirm suspicious lesions and to assess gastric motility. Diffuse infiltration of the gastric wall results in gastric hypomotility.

Gastric lesions can also be detected with a flexible gastroscope. Gastric neoplasms are raised masses that project into the stomach lumen or thickened rugal folds. Mucosal ulceration or inability to distend the stomach may be apparent.[144] Tumors that diffusely infiltrate the gastric wall are often difficult to see. Directed biopsy of lesions can be achieved with biopsy forceps passed through the gastroscope. It is sometimes difficult to obtain diagnostic biopsy samples from submucosal tumors.

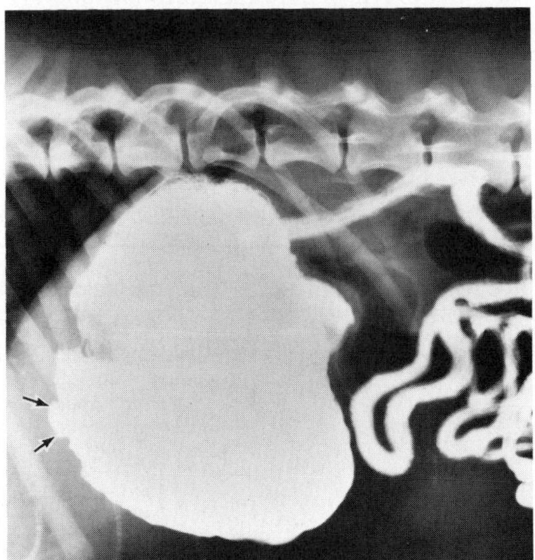

FIGURE 154–3. Lateral radiograph following stomach tube administration of barium demonstrating multiple filling defects and a large ulcer *(arrows)* in the anterior margin of the stomach of a 4-year-old male standard poodle. Laparotomy revealed extensive infiltration of the lesser curvature of the stomach by adenocarcinoma.

Surgical exploration is used to confirm a diagnosis of gastric neoplasia, to assess the extent of the tumor in the stomach, and to detect the presence of metastases in regional lymph nodes and the liver. Tissue can be obtained for histopathological evaluation from primary and metastatic lesions.

Treatment

Complete surgical excision is the treatment of choice for gastric adenocarcinomas. Depending on the size and location of the lesion, either segmental resection or partial gastrectomy is selected. Because the pyloric area of the stomach is often involved, a gastroduodenostomy or gastrojejunostomy may be required.[157] Enlarged regional lymph nodes are removed. Extensive gastric involvement may preclude complete excision of the primary tumor. Removal of a portion of the neoplasia may provide palliative relief and increased survival time.[106]

Chemotherapy has not been adequately evaluated in canine gastric adenocarcinoma patients. Chemotherapy has been used in humans with extensive metastatic disease and as an adjuvant after complete surgical excision of gastric adenocarcinomas.[29, 97] Objective responses in humans have been obtained with 5-fluorouracil, mitomycin-C, carmustine (BCNU), and doxorubicin (Adriamycin).[82] Duration of responses with single agents is generally brief, lasting approximately 4 months, but combination therapy can extend response time to 10 months. A beneficial effect of adjuvant chemotherapy has been demonstrated in humans.

In dogs and cats with gastric lymphosarcoma, multiple-drug chemotherapy is indicated if the tumor cannot be removed and is probably indicated after surgical resection of localized lesions.

Prognosis

Factors that influence prognosis of gastric adenocarcinoma in humans include depth of tumor involvement in the gastric wall, involvement of regional lymph nodes, and distant metastases.[81] Most dogs with gastric adenocarcinoma have extensive involvement at diagnosis. Survival time in untreated dogs is generally less than 3 months after the onset of clinical signs. Survival after tumor excision is less than 6 months,[34, 80, 87, 106] although 5-year survival in one dog has been reported.[37] Earlier gastroscopic diagnosis and adjuvant chemotherapy after surgery may improve the prognosis.

INTESTINAL NEOPLASIA

Intestinal neoplasms are uncommon in dogs and cats. Intestinal adenocarcinoma represents 0.33 per cent of canine malignancies and 0.4 to 2.9 per cent of feline malignancies.[111, 118] Intestinal tumors occur most frequently in the colon and rectum of dogs and small intestine of cats.

In dogs, adenocarcinomas are identified more frequently in the intestine than leiomyosarcomas, lymphosarcomas, fibrosarcomas, or carcinoids.[13, 55, 60, 61, 111] Adenomatous polyps are the most common canine rectal tumor.[63] In cats, intestinal lymphosarcoma is identified more frequently than adenocarcinoma or mast cell tumors.[61] Benign tumors of the feline intestine are rare.

Intestinal neoplasms usually occur in older animals (Table 154–5), and males are more frequently affected than females. German shepherds and Siamese cats are predisposed to adenocarcinomas,[111, 152] and boxers have a high incidence of intestinal lymphosarcoma.[13]

Benign Neoplasms

Leiomyomas occur infrequently in the small and large intestine of dogs and cats.[13, 16, 31, 32, 61] They arise from smooth muscle in the intestinal wall and are usually nonulcerated but may obstruct the intestinal lumen. Leiomyomas are occasionally an incidental finding at necropsy.

Adenomatous polyps occur most frequently in the canine rectum.[60, 61, 107] Male and female dogs are equally affected; the mean age of occurrence is 6.9 years; Collies are predisposed.[132] Grossly, rectal polyps vary from a few millimeters to several centimeters in diameter. They are raised, sessile, or pedunculated and may occur in grapelike clusters.[98] Single or multiple polyps may be present. Histologically, well-differentiated columnar cells cover the surface of the polyp and a fibrous stalk connects the base of the polyp to the mucosa. Polyps generally do not recur after surgical removal. Although carcinomatous change has been described in polyps,[132, 135] there is little clinical evidence that adenomatous polyps represent a premalignant lesion in dogs.

Malignant Neoplasms

Adenocarcinomas occur most frequently in the rectum, colon, and jejunum of dogs and in the ileum of cats (Table 154–5).[14, 32, 61, 72, 79, 132] Small-intestine adenocarcinomas appear as firm, annular, constrictive masses. Neoplastic proliferation begins in the mucosa and spreads throughout the intestinal wall. Extensive stromal fibrosis and muscle hypertrophy contribute to intestinal stenosis. Four histological types of adenocarcinomas have been described: solid, acinar, papillary, and mucinous.[113] The biological behavior of the four types is similar, but each has a predilection for different sites within the intestinal tract.

Intestinal adenocarcinomas frequently metastasize to regional lymph nodes, especially mesenteric and iliac nodes (see Table 154–5). Widespread abdominal lymph node involvement may occur. Diffuse metastasis to peritoneal surfaces (carcinomatosis) results in ascites. Metastasis to abdominal and thoracic viscera including the liver, spleen, kidneys, myocardium, and lungs has been reported.[13, 61, 118, 119]

Lymphosarcoma is most frequently identified in the jejunum of dogs and ileum of cats.[12, 32, 61] Rectal and colonic involvement occurs less commonly (Fig. 154–4). Multiple sites within the intestinal tract are frequently involved. Grossly, lesions may be fusiform or nodular. Large segments of the intestine may be diffusely thickened. Metastasis to regional lymph nodes, the kidneys, and liver is common. Affected cats are usually feline leukemia virus negative.

Leiomyosarcomas have been reported infrequently throughout the intestinal tract of dogs and cats.[19, 55, 61, 111] Cecal and jejunal involvement is most common. Leiomyosarcomas usually arise in the outer muscular layers, are nodular, and may result in intestinal perforation. Metastasis is to regional lymph nodes and the liver.[61]

Intestinal carcinoids occur in the duodenum, ileum, colon, and rectum of dogs[25, 56, 113] and ileum and duodenum of cats.[18, 75] Carcinoids are uncommon and arise from enterochromaffin cells (Kulchitsky cells) in the intestinal mucosa. Enterochromaffin cells contain high levels of 5-hydroxytryptamine (serotonin) and are characterized by intracytoplasmic argyrophilic granules. In humans, release of biologically active amines from carcinoid tumors can result in the carcinoid syndrome, which is characterized by cutaneous flushing, abdominal

TABLE 154–5. EPIDEMIOLOGICAL FEATURES AND BIOLOGICAL BEHAVIOR OF CANINE AND FELINE INTESTINAL NEOPLASMS

	Mean Age (years)	Male/Female	Breed Predisposition	Frequent Sites in Intestine	Frequent Metastatic Site
Canine					
Adenocarcinoma	9	1.8:1	German Shepherd	Rectum, colon jejunum	Regional lymph nodes, peritoneum, lung, liver
Leiomyosarcoma	11	1:2	None	Cecum, jejunum	Regional lymph nodes, liver
Lymphosarcoma	6.5	1.6:1	Boxer	Jejunum, ileum	Regional lymph nodes, liver, spleen
Feline					
Adenocarcinoma	11	2.5:1	Siamese	Ileum	Regional lymph nodes, peritoneum, omentum
Lymphosarcoma	10.5	1.4:1	None	Ileum, duodenum	Regional lymph nodes, omentum, liver

Data from Brody RC, Cohen D: An epizootiologic and clinicopathologic study of 95 cases of gastrointestinal neoplasm in the dog. Scientific Proceedings, 101st Annual Meeting, American Veterinarians Medical Association, 1964, pp 167–179; Patnaik AK, Hurvitz A, Johnson GF: Canine gastrointestinal neoplasms. *Vet Pathol* 14:547, 1977; and Turk MAM, Russell TS: Nonhematopoietic gastrointestinal neoplasia in cats: A retrospective study of 44 cases. *Vet Pathol* 18:614, 1981.

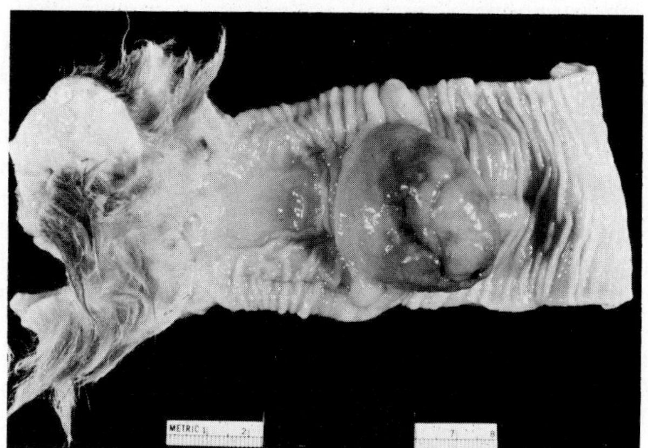

FIGURE 154–4. Ulcerated nodular rectal mass from a 5-year-old Shetland sheepdog diagnosed as lymphosarcoma. There was no evidence of lymphosarcoma in other organs.

pain, diarrhea, and dyspnea.[5] Canine carcinoid tumors usually metastasize to regional lymph nodes and the liver.[114]

Intestinal mast cell tumors are more frequently identified in cats[2] than in dogs.[110] Feline mast cell tumors produce firm, nonulcerated thickenings of the intestinal wall. Metastases to the mesenteric lymph node, liver, and spleen are frequently observed.

Clinical Signs

Clinical signs associated with intestinal neoplasia result from bleeding, intestinal obstruction, peritonitis, or malabsorption. Intermittent vomiting and diarrhea, weight loss, and inappetence characterize small-intestinal tumors. Tenesmus, bloody mucoid feces, constipation, rectal prolapse, and increased frequency of defecation are frequent signs with large-intestinal tumors.

Intestinal bleeding, which occurs with ulcerative lesions, may result in anemia, thrombocytopenia, and hypoproteinemia. Results of fecal occult blood tests are positive. Abdominal pain and fever occur with peritonitis resulting from intestinal perforation. Malabsorption occurs when intestinal villi become filled with neoplastic cells, lymphatics become blocked by neoplastic cells, or tumors cause complete or partial intestinal obstruction.

Diagnosis

Intestinal neoplasia is suspected when an older dog or cat is presented with progressive weight loss and clinical signs referable to the intestinal tract. Unexplained bleeding from the intestinal tract, anemia, ascites, abdominal mass, or peritonitis suggests possible intestinal neoplasia.

Intestinal tumors are often identified by abdominal palpation. A nodular mass or diffuse thickening of intestinal loops may be noted. Mesenteric lymph nodes may be enlarged. Diagnosis can sometimes be established by cytological examination of an aspiration biopsy of the abnormal mass.

Rectal examination may reveal a polypoid lesion or stricture. Proctoscopic evaluations may reveal a proliferative tumor, ulceration, mucosal irregularity, or stenosis. Lesions can be sampled with a punch biopsy instrument passed through the proctoscope.

Survey abdominal radiographs and contrast studies (upper gastrointestinal series, barium enema) often show abnormalities (Figs. 154–5 and 154–6). Radiographic abnormalities may include (1) an abdominal mass; (2) intestinal accumulation of fluid, gas, or ingesta; (3) delayed intestinal transit time; (4) mural lesions associated with luminal filling defects; (5) mucosal ulceration; and (6) thickening of the intestinal wall and displacement of adjacent bowel loops.[48, 55] Nodular, patchy, irregular abdominal densities may be noted if diffuse peritoneal metastasis has occurred.

Endoscopic biopsy is sometimes possible for proximal duodenal tumors. Excisional or incisional biopsy of distal intestinal tumors can be performed at laparotomy.

Treatment

Polyps in the rectum and distal colon can be surgically removed by pedicle ligation, electrocautery, or cryosurgery after digital exteriorization or rectal prolapse.[111, 141]

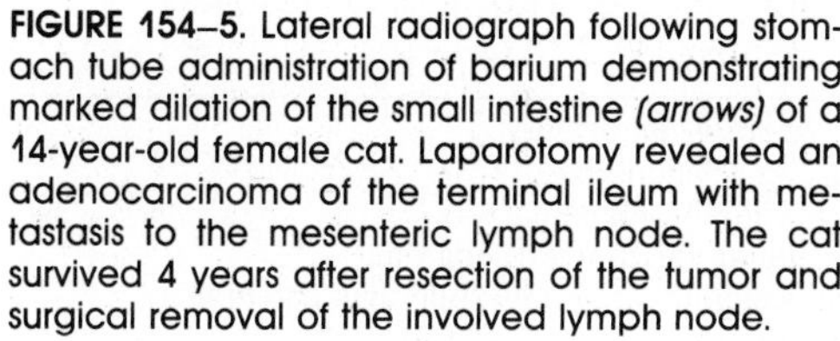

FIGURE 154–5. Lateral radiograph following stomach tube administration of barium demonstrating marked dilation of the small intestine *(arrows)* of a 14-year-old female cat. Laparotomy revealed an adenocarcinoma of the terminal ileum with metastasis to the mesenteric lymph node. The cat survived 4 years after resection of the tumor and surgical removal of the involved lymph node.

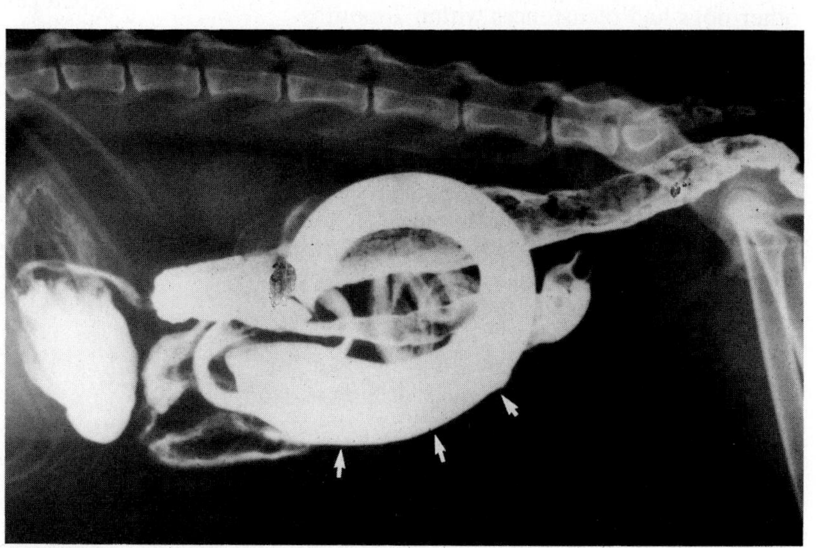

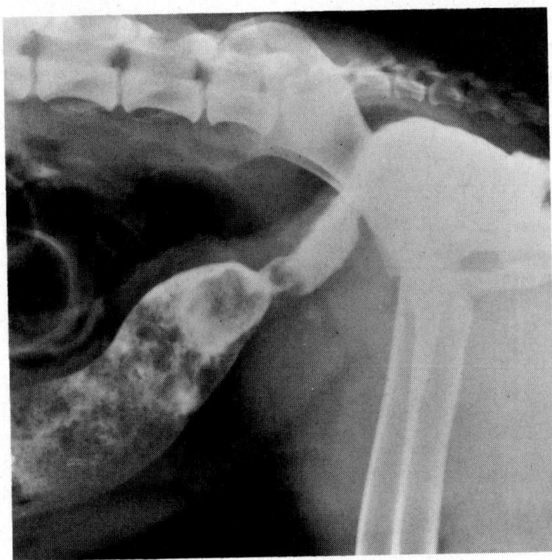

FIGURE 154–6. Lateral radiograph after administration of a barium enema revealed an annular constriction resulting from an infiltrating adenocarcinoma of the distal colon and rectum in a 7-year-old female German shepherd.

Wide surgical excision and intestinal anastomosis compose the treatment of choice for most malignant intestinal tumors. *En bloc* excision including the tumor, mesentery, and regional lymph nodes may offer the best chance of cure.[146] Tumor removal can provide palliative relief even in the presence of metastatic disease.

Pelvic osteotomy may be required to gain adequate exposure in animals with midrectal tumors. A rectal pull-through or a dorsal approach to the rectum can be used to expose distal rectal tumors.[3, 90] Complications of rectal surgery including wound dehiscence, stricture, fecal incontinence, and infection have limited the usefulness of these procedures.

Radiation therapy may provide an alternative to surgery in some dogs with rectal adenocarcinomas. Single high-dose radiation therapy has been used to treat dogs with tumors less than 3 cm in diameter.[155] Transient tenesmus was the only significant complication. Three dogs were disease free at 5, 6, and 31 months. Three other dogs had recurrences within 7 months.

Chemotherapy has little effect on intestinal adenocarcinomas. In humans, treatment of intestinal carcinomas with 5-fluorouracil produced objective responses in only 20 per cent of cases.[27] The effectiveness of adjuvant chemotherapy has not been well evaluated in dogs.

Isolated nodular lymphosarcoma lesions can be surgically excised. Follow-up combination chemotherapy is probably indicated. Multiple intestinal lesions or metastatic disease is best treated by chemotherapy alone.

Prognosis

The prognosis after removal of polyps and other benign tumors is usually favorable.[63] Recurrences are infrequent.

In general, intestinal adenocarcinomas are associated with a guarded to poor long-term prognosis. In one report, mean survival time in 23 dogs with colorectal adenocarcinomas treated with stool softeners was 15 months, whereas dogs treated with cryosurgery had a mean survival time of 24 months and dogs treated by radical surgical excision had a mean survival time of only 0.2 month.[26] Dogs with annular tumors had shorter survival times (1.6 months) than dogs with single, pedunculated, polypoid tumors (32 months) or dogs with nodular or cobblestone-like lesions (12 months). Mean survival time in 14 dogs with epithelial tumors of the rectum treated by local resection or rectal pull-through was 6.9 months.[159] Local recurrence was noted in most cases.

In cats with intestinal adenocarcinomas, survival times after surgical resection are short, although a small percentage of cats, even those with metastasis to mesenteric lymph nodes, have survived longer than 2 years.[71]

The prognosis for dogs with intestinal leiomyosarcomas is better than for dogs with adenocarcinomas. Three of five dogs treated with surgical resection were alive at 12, 17, and 20 months after surgery.[16]

Dogs and cats with intestinal lymphosarcoma generally respond poorly to therapy, although transient improvement may be noted after surgical resection of segmental lesions.

HEPATIC NEOPLASIA

Primary Hepatic Tumors

Primary hepatic tumors are uncommon in dogs and cats. They constitute from 0.6 to 1.3 per cent of all tumors.[114] Primary hepatic tumors are identified in 0.63 to 2.6 per cent of all necropsies.[114, 142, 151] A large veterinary tumor registry estimates the occurrence to be 1.6:100,000 patient years.[83]

Hepatic tumors arise from epithelial or mesenchymal tissues (Table 154–6). The two most common are hepatocellular carcinoma and cholangiocellular carcinoma. Hepatic neoplasia is nearly always a disease of aged dogs and cats. The mean age of occurrence is between 10 and 11 years of age, although affected animals as young as 2 years have been reported.[21, 83, 114, 142] No known breed predisposition is noted in dogs or cats. Hepatocellular carcinomas and various sarcomas of hepatic origin occur slightly more frequently in male dogs, whereas cholangiocellular carcinomas are slightly more common in female dogs.[114] One study of cats found that

TABLE 154–6. CLASSIFICATION OF PRIMARY HEPATIC NEOPLASIA

Tumors of epithelial origin
Hepatocellular adenoma
Cholangiocellular adenoma
Hepatocellular carcinoma (hepatoma)
Cholangiocellular carcinoma (bile duct carcinoma)
Hepatic carcinoids
Tumors of mesenchymal origin
Hemangiosarcoma
Fibrosarcoma
Extraskeletal osteosarcoma
Leiomyosarcoma

females were more likely than males to develop cholangiocellular carcinomas.[21]

Multiple etiological factors have been associated with development of primary hepatic tumors in humans and laboratory animals.[145] Causative factors include (1) chemicals such as azo-compounds, nitrosamines, aflatoxins, methylcholanthrene, acetylaminofluorene, *Senecio* alkaloids, chlorinated hydrocarbons, cycasin, and vinyl chloride, (2) Thorotrast, (3) androgens, (4) malnutrition, (5) cirrhosis, (6) hepatitis B virus, and (7) parasites (schistosomiasis, clonorchiasis).[145] Of this list, aflatoxins, polycyclic hydrocarbons, cycasin, and dimethylnitrosamine are well-documented carcinogens. Although the incidence of hepatic neoplasia associated with cirrhosis is high in humans, this association in dogs and cats is rare. Only 6 animals of 110 with primary liver tumors also had histological evidence of cirrhosis; 4 had hepatocellular carcinoma, and 2 had cholangiocellular carcinoma.[114]

The metastatic potential of primary hepatic tumors is high. The rate of metastasis ranges from 61 per cent for hepatocellular carcinomas to 93 per cent for hepatic carcinoids.[114] Metastasis occurs by direct extension to other parts of the liver or to adjacent organs and through blood and lymph to distant sites. The most common sites for metastases of epithelial tumors are regional lymph nodes and the lungs.[114] Metastatic hepatic mesenchymal tumors most often metastasize to the spleen.[114] Additional sites of metastases for primary hepatic tumors include the brain, kidneys, omentum, peritoneum, adrenals, pancreas, gastrointestinal tract, spine, and pituitary gland.[114, 145]

Hepatocellular Carcinomas

Hepatocellular carcinomas are the most common hepatic neoplasms. They accounted for 76 of 159 (47.7 per cent) primary hepatic tumors identified in two extensive necropsy studies.[116, 151] Clinical signs, although nonspecific, generally denote hepatic failure. Lethargy, weakness, anorexia, weight loss, a pendulous abdomen, and vomiting are common. Less frequently observed signs include ascites, diarrhea, jaundice, and dyspnea. The most significant finding on physical examination is a palpable abdominal mass in as many as 80 per cent of patients with hepatocellular carcinoma.[151] In most cases, the mass is readily localized to the liver.

The ultimate diagnosis of hepatocellular carcinoma requires histological confirmation. Hematological, biochemical, and radiological findings are useful for localizing the disease to the liver and supporting the need for a biopsy. Hematological abnormalities include mild to moderate anemia in approximately 50 per cent and neutrophilia in two-thirds of patients.[116] Biochemical abnormalities compatible with liver disease are also present in significant numbers of animals with primary liver tumors.[116, 142, 151] Hepatic enzyme abnormalities are not specific for neoplastic disease; rather, they resemble those in a large number of non-neoplastic inflammatory hepatic diseases. Moderate to marked increases in serum alanine transaminase and aspartate transaminase are common. Serum alkaline phosphatase concentrations are dramatically increased in most patients (82 per cent).[142] Biochemical evidence of functional hepatic failure is less frequently observed. Serum bilirubin concentrations are increased (usually mildly) in 26 per cent of patients, and albumin concentrations are often normal. Increases in serum albumin were reported in 18 per cent of these patients,[114] whereas hypoalbuminemia was found in 16 per cent.[114, 142, 151] Blood or serum glucose concentrations were evaluated in 65 animals with hepatocellular carcinoma. Only four (6 per cent) had evidence of hypoglycemia. Although infrequent, hypoglycemia may be so severe that it is the primary reason for a patient's being examined.[143]

Additional diagnostic tests that may be useful with hepatocellular carcinomas include radiography, cytological study of abdominal effusions, ultrasonography, and biopsy. Because an abdominal mass is generally palpable, survey radiographs localize the lesion to the liver and may determine if extrahepatic abdominal metastases exist. If ascites is present, survey radiographs may have limited usefulness. Abdominal ultrasonography may add significantly to diagnostic information.[43, 47, 104] Ultrasonography allows for characterization of the internal architecture of hepatic masses, confirms the site of origin, defines the extent of disease, allows for specific localization of palpable masses not easily seen when ascites exists, and identifies metastases presurgically.[47] It does not provide information about specific tumor type, and the sonographic findings are not pathognomonic. Additional diagnoses that must be ruled out when finding focal or multifocal infiltrative lesions ultrasonographically include abscesses, cysts, hematomas, and focal nodular hyperplasia.[47] Because these tumors frequently metastasize to the lungs, thoracic radiographs are included in the evaluation of these patients. Cytological evaluations of abdominal fluid in animals with hepatocellular carcinomas are most often unrewarding. Biopsy of abdominal masses of undetermined etiology is the diagnostic method of choice. Biopsy techniques include fine-needle aspiration, needle core, and incisional and excisional biopsy. Aspiration or needle core biopsies are rapid and technically simple and carry minimal risk. However, establishing a diagnosis of hepatocellular carcinoma from small biopsy samples is difficult. Hepatocellular carcinoma cells frequently retain a normal appearance, mitoses are uncommon, and reasonably normal architecture is maintained.[99]

Exploratory celiotomy is the diagnostic method of choice. Not only does surgery allow a visually guided biopsy, but surgical excision may be attempted if no metastases are seen. Hepatocellular carcinomas do not fulfill the usual criteria of malignancy.[99] They are most often found as large solitary masses with a predisposition for the left lateral hepatic lobe.[114] These lesions are generally well encapsulated and grow by expansion and compression of adjacent tissue. Their malignant potential is often based on size and degree of local invasion in the absence of detectable metastases.[99] Unfortunately, metastases are present at diagnosis in 61 per cent of hepatocellular carcinomas.[116]

Because many animals with hepatocellular carcinomas have single large masses (Fig. 154–7), surgical excision

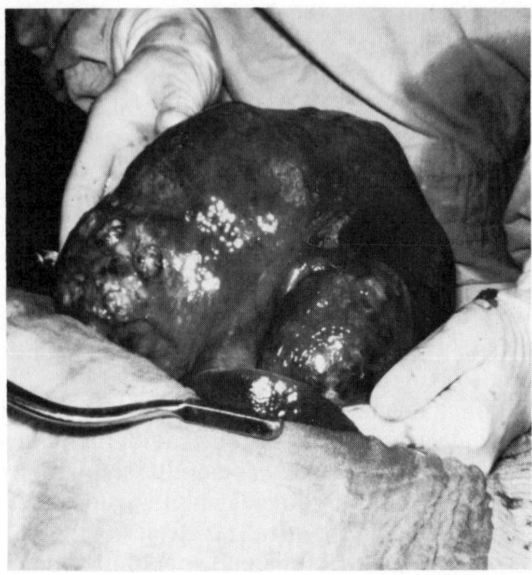

FIGURE 154–7. Typical large solitary hepatocellular carcinoma at surgery.

remains the therapy of choice. Unfortunately, the debilitated state, age, and degree of hepatic or other organ failure in such animals make major surgery a challenging task. Alternatives to surgical excision in humans include ligation of either the venous or arterial supply to the affected lobe and adjunctive chemotherapy. Significant improvement has been noted in human patients with surgically inoperable or metastatic hepatocellular carcinomas by segmental ligation of the portal vein.[64] Tumor vascularity significantly affects whether venous or arterial ligation is selected. Hypovascular neoplasms respond best to segmental portal venous ligation, whereas hypervascular tumors show greater regression if segmental hepatic artery ligation is performed. Estimations of tumor vascularity are made using presurgical hepatic radioisotopic scans. Chemotherapy in humans involves the use of systemic or intra-arterial 5-fluorouracil or methotrexate.[145] No controlled clinical studies in animals support the use of chemotherapy for nonresectable hepatic neoplasms or as adjunctive therapy.[123]

The prognosis for dogs and cats with hepatocellular carcinoma is usually poor. The high rate of metastasis, size, degree of invasion, and debilitated state of patients often preclude corrective surgery. Even when surgery is performed, survival for less than 80 days is reported for most malignant hepatocellular carcinomas.[123]

Cholangiocellular Carcinoma (Bile Duct Carcinoma)

Cholangiocellular carcinomas occur slightly less often than heptocellular carcinomas. Thirty-nine of 142 (27 per cent) of primary hepatic neoplasms were of this type.[114, 151] These tumors arise primarily from intrahepatic bile duct epithelium, although in rare instances tumors may arise from the extrahepatic bile ducts or gallbladder.[162] Causative factors for these tumors in dogs and cats include infestations with the Chinese liver fluke, *Clonorchis sinensis,* and exposure to either *o*-aminoazotoluene or the organic sulfite insecticide aramite.[99]

Clinical signs are quite similar to those described for animals with hepatocellular carcinomas. Weight loss, anorexia, depression, vomiting, and an enlarged abdomen are common. Jaundice occurs in 13 to 23 per cent.[115, 151] Hepatomegaly is usually detected during abdominal palpation.

The diagnosis of cholangiocellular carcinoma is made by microscopic evaluation. Hematological and biochemical data are similar to those for hepatocellular carcinoma. Increased serum concentrations of alanine transaminase, aspartate transaminase, and serum alkaline phosphatase are common.[21, 115, 151] Biochemical data do not differentiate these two primary hepatic neoplasms.

The most important diagnostic and therapeutic procedure is exploratory celiotomy. Cholangiocellular carcinomas are often of the massive type, involving primarily the left lateral lobe. Metastases are even more common than with hepatocellular carcinomas, occurring in roughly 87 per cent of cases in dogs and 78 per cent of cases in cats.[21, 115] Metastases occur most often in the regional lymph nodes, lungs, and peritoneum, although widespread metastases are frequent. The prognosis for animals with this tumor is poor because of widespread dissemination before diagnosis and their infiltrative nature.

Hepatic Carcinoids

Hepatic carcinoids are infrequently identified in dogs and cats.[1, 114, 117] Investigators identifying this neoplasm concluded that they had observed carcinoids because of the large number of necropsies they performed (12,245) and their awareness of the microscopic features of these tumors. Hepatic carcinoids originate from neuroectodermal tissue scattered throughout the liver. These cells are classified as enterochromaffin or APUD cells. *APUD* is an acronym for a biochemical characteristic of this group of cells (i.e., they are capable of *a*mine *p*recursor *u*ptake and *d*ecarboxylation). Embryologically similar cells are responsible for the development of insulinomas and gastrinomas discussed at the end of this section. Of 110 primary hepatic tumors identified, 15 were of this cell type.[114] Hepatic carcinoids occur at a slightly younger mean age (8 years) than other hepatic malignancies (10 years). Except for the absence of hepatomegaly, clinical signs, diagnostic criteria, and prognosis for carcinoids are similar to those of the other two primary carcinomas affecting the liver. At necropsy, all 15 were diffuse throughout all liver lobes. Severe hemorrhage and necrosis were present in the liver of all dogs. Extrahepatic metastases were identified in 14 of 15 cases.

Nonepithelial Hepatic Neoplasms

Both benign and malignant tumors of mesenchymal origin occur within the liver of dogs and cats. They are much less common than epithelial tumors. Tumors recognized include hemangiosarcoma,[151] fibrosarcoma,[151] leiomyosarcoma,[114] hepatic mixed sarcoma,[88, 99] and extraskeletal osteosarcoma.[66] Clinical features of hepatic sarcomas are similar to those of other primary tumors; therefore, biopsy is the sole method of differentiation. No effective therapy, short of early surgical excision, is known. The prognosis is poor.

Hepatocellular Adenoma, Nodular Hyperplasia

Nodular hyperplasia is a frequent finding in aged dogs, reportedly occurring in from 15 to 60 per cent.[100] Differentiation of nodular hyperplasia from hepatocellular adenomas is difficult.[46, 114] Nodular hyperplasia occurs most often in dogs over 11 years old and is not a "precancerous" lesion.[46] Lesions range from 0.1 to 5.0 cm in diameter, may be single or multiple, and are not associated with clinical signs. They are most often noted during exploratory surgery or at necropsy, and it is important to distinguish them from hepatocellular carcinomas histologically.

Tumors Metastatic to the Liver (Secondary Tumors)

The liver is a major site for metastasis of tumors. The liver, via its portal circulation, is a filter between abdominal organs and the systemic circulation. It is vulnerable to metastatic cells circulating in the portal system, originating primarily from the gastrointestinal tract. In two series of 3,258 necropsies, 224 metastases to the liver were identified (6.8 per cent of the total).[86, 151] This rate is 2.6 times that for primary hepatic neoplasms. The rate at which nonhepatic malignancies metastasized to the liver was from 30.6 per cent[151] to 36.8 per cent,[86] a rate that exceeds that for the lungs (24.2 per cent).[151] The mean age of occurrence for metastatic liver cancer was 7.8 years, whereas that for primary hepatic malignancies was 10 years.

Clinical signs associated with metastatic liver tumors are variable. Most often, signs relate to the type and location of the primary tumor. The degree of hepatic involvement must be significant before signs of hepatic failure develop. Hepatomegaly, which is common with primary hepatic neoplasms, is uncommon with metastatic tumors.[142, 151] Metastatic disease of the liver induces less dramatic changes in hepatic biochemical profiles than does primary hepatic neoplasia, and abnormalities are less predictable. When biochemical abnormalities are identified, they do not correlate with the extent of neoplastic infiltration.[86, 142, 151] Mild to moderate increases in alanine transaminase occur in 46 to 70 per cent.[86, 142, 151] The serum alkaline phosphatase rise may be mild to marked in approximately half the patients, reflecting the degree of major bile duct obstruction. Hyperbilirubinemia occurs in 30 to 46 per cent of cases.[86, 142, 151] Aspartate transaminase is the most sensitive liver enzyme in hepatic metastatic neoplasms, being elevated in 87 per cent of cases.[86] If patients in which creatine kinase values were also increased are excluded, this figure drops to 81 per cent. Unfortunately, this leaves from 19 to 30 per cent of dogs with metastatic hepatic neoplasia with normal biochemical profiles.

Tumors metastasizing to the liver arise from three major sources: hematopoietic cells, epithelium, and mesenchyme.[5] Hematopoietic neoplasms accounted for 81 of 129 secondary liver tumors (63 per cent), with lymphosarcoma being the most prevalent (67 cases).[151] Epithelial tumors were the next most common, 27 of 129 (21 per cent), with pancreatic adenocarcinomas being the most notable tumor type (9 of 27). Mesenchymal tumors were the least common type of secondary liver tumor, accounting for 21 of 129 cases (16 per cent).[151] Hemangiosarcoma was the primary tumor diagnosis in 15 of 21 sarcomas, and 19 originated in the spleen. Therapy for these tumors is directed at the primary neoplasm, if possible. Because signs and laboratory abnormalities of hepatic disease may dominate the clinical picture, a diagnosis of disseminated carcinoma may not be made until results of a liver biopsy have been obtained. The prognosis is poor.

PANCREATIC NEOPLASIA

Neoplasms of the pancreas arise primarily from epithelial tissue (Table 154–7). The two most important neoplasms are pancreatic adenocarcinoma and pancreatic islet cell adenocarcinoma. Neoplasms of the pancreas are uncommon in both dogs and cats. Estimates on their frequency are from 0.05 to 1.88 per cent of all tumors in dogs[145] and from 1.1 to 2.8 per cent in cats.[99, 124] Adenocarcinomas are strongly associated with increasing age. Mean age of occurrence is 10 years in dogs (range 5 to 16 years) and 12 years in cats. Cats older than 15 years have an especially high risk. The only canine breed at increased risk is the Airedale.

Pancreatic Adenocarcinomas

Pancreatic adenocarcinomas arise from both ductular and acinar tissue of the exocrine pancreas. Ductular carcinomas predominate.[69] These tumors metastasize readily, frequently before clinical diagnosis. Metastases occur most often in the liver, retroperitoneum, and mesenteric lymph nodes.[99] Less common metastatic sites

TABLE 154–7. CLASSIFICATION OF PANCREATIC TUMORS IDENTIFIED IN DOGS AND CATS

Epithelial tumors
Exocrine
Adenoma
Adenocarcinoma
Malignant foregut carcinoid
Undifferentiated carcinomas
Endocrine
Islet cell adenoma
Islet cell adenocarcinoma (insulinoma, gastrinoma)
Nonepithelial tumors
Unclassified
Metastatic tumors
Tumor-like lesions
Nodular hyperplasia
Hyperplasia of pancreatic ducts
Ectopic pancreatic tissue
Cysts

Data from Kircher D, Nielsen S: Tumors of the pancreas. *Bull WHO 53*:195, 1976.

include the lungs, duodenum, adrenals, kidneys, heart, and gallbladder.

Clinical signs are often nonspecific and frequently relate more to the primary metastatic site (liver) than the organ of origin. Weight loss, anorexia, depression, vomiting, and jaundice are common.[4] Pancreatic adenocarcinomas frequently compress the common bile duct, producing jaundice (Fig. 154–8). Signs of maldigestion occur in association with pancreatic adenocarcinomas, but this is rare.[89] These tumors are generally small and rarely palpable in dogs, but in cats, a cranial abdominal mass is often detected.[21]

A definitive antemortem diagnosis is rarely made except via exploratory celiotomy. These animals often die or are euthanized, with the diagnosis established at necropsy. Serum amylase and lipase concentrations are usually normal, except when rapidly invading tumors produce mild signs of pancreatitis. Biochemical profiles most often suggest that liver rather than pancreatic disease is present. Mild increases in alanine aminotransferase, with moderate to marked rises in serum alkaline phosphatase and serum bilirubin, are typical of metastatic pancreatic adenocarcinoma. Radiographs may detect evidence of mass lesions, peritoneal fluid accumulation, or carcinomatosis.[4] Abdominocentesis, with or without lavage, may help establish a diagnosis. Pancreatic adenocarcinomas exfoliate readily, and cytological study of peritoneal fluid suggests abdominal malignancy. Cytological evaluations rarely establish the site of origin for the exfoliated carcinoma cells, but the prognosis is not altered.

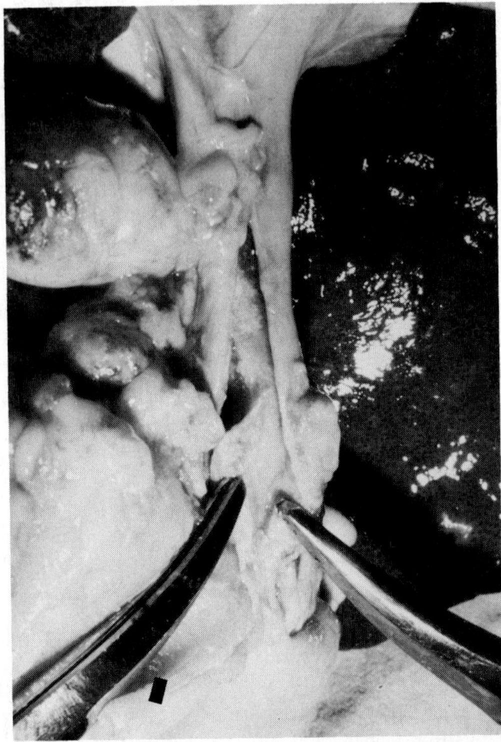

FIGURE 154–8. Pancreatic adenocarcinoma (at tip of scissors) invading the common bile duct in a 5-year-old Brittany spaniel. Clinical signs were those associated with extrahepatic bile duct obstruction.

The prognosis for animals with pancreatic adenocarcinoma is invariably poor owing to the tendency for early and widespread metastases. Occasional cases in humans have responded to 5-fluorouracil. Therapy for solitary lesions is surgical removal.

Pancreatic Adenoma/Hyperplasia

Pancreatic hyperplasia is a frequent finding in aged dogs and cats.[21, 99] Pancreatic adenoma is rare, although precise microscopic criteria for separation of these two entities are equivocal.[69, 99] These lesions are small white to tan nodules within the pancreas, rarely larger than 1 to 4 mm, and have no clinical significance.

Pancreatic Islet Cell Tumors

Two major pancreatic islet cell neoplasms have been recognized. The most common is insulinoma or functional tumor of the pancreatic beta cells. Gastrinoma is much less common. Gastrinomas are islet cell tumors arising from pancreatic G cells, which secrete gastrin. Neither of these neoplasms occurs with any frequency in cats.[69, 91]

Insulinomas

Insulinomas are less frequently recognized than pancreatic acinar cell carcinomas. Approximately 200 had been reported up until 1990, with few cases documented in cats.[21, 22, 69, 91, 92, 128] Between 60 and 70 per cent of these neoplasms are functional. Although the term *insulinoma* is commonly applied to these neoplasms, the vast majority are islet cell carcinomas.[69, 140] Even tumors that appear benign microscopically often develop recurrent signs of disease at variable intervals postoperatively because of the presence of metastases that were not identified at surgery. The mean age of occurrence is between 9 and 10 years, with a range between 4 and 15 years old.[22, 49, 78, 139] Large dogs at increased risk include Irish setters, golden retrievers, boxers, German shepherds, standard poodles, fox terriers, and mixed breeds.[73, 78, 92, 102, 124] Seventy-two per cent of affected dogs weigh more than 25 kg.[78] No sex predilection exists.

Clinical signs are variable, but all are related to hypoglycemia induced by excessive production of insulin by the tumor or to catecholamine release secondary to hypoglycemia. Hypoglycemic convulsions or collapse may occur in two-thirds of dogs with insulinomas. Weakness and ataxia (particularly of the rear limbs), muscle tremors, dullness, disorientation, and decreased exercise tolerance are also common.[22, 24, 73, 92, 139] The rate of decline in blood glucose concentration rather than the absolute value determines the type and severity of signs. A rapid reduction in blood glucose generally results in signs of catecholamine release (weakness, hunger, tachycardia), whereas a slower decline generally is associated with neurological manifestations.[102, 153] The duration of clinical signs before diagnosis ranges from 1 day to 3 years, with a mean of 3 months.[22, 73, 92] Nearly one-third have been treated nonspecifically for an idiopathic seizure disorder before diagnosis.[22, 92] Signs are nearly always intermittent, and long periods may elapse between episodes of clinically apparent hypoglycemia. Signs become more frequent as the disease progresses. Generally, a poor correlation exists between the time an animal is fed and the onset of clinical signs.

Confirming a diagnosis of insulinoma is uncomplicated. Routine hematological, biochemical, and urinalysis findings in these patients are usually normal except for fasting or nonfasting hypoglycemia. The majority have blood glucose values less than 70 mg/100 ml on initial evaluations.[22, 51, 73] Once hypoglycemia is confirmed, the next step is to validate that it is due to relative or absolute insulin excess and not some other cause. Multiple alternative diagnoses exist for hypoglycemia in dogs and cats, and they are simultaneously searched for in hypoglycemic animals (Table 154–8). Serum is analyzed for insulin concentration from any hypoglycemic sample in which another obvious cause of the hypoglycemia is not identified. Normal fasting serum immunoreactive insulin concentrations range from 5 to 26 microunits/ml from most veterinary laboratories.[52, 102] The mean fasting insulin concentration in one large series of cases was 71.4 microunits/ml.[22] Approximately 75 per cent have elevated serum insulin concentrations when initially evaluated, and a diagnosis of insulinoma is highly likely. In the remaining 25 per cent in which initial insulin values are in the normal range, support for a presumptive diagnosis of insulinoma may be made by comparing the ratio between blood glucose and insulin in a number of ways. When these ratios are abnormal, they support a relative excess of insulin to glucose in peripheral blood. Comparisons may be made between the ratio of insulin to glucose (I/G), between the ratio of glucose to insulin (G/I), or by calculating an amended insulin glucose ratio (AIGR). Values supporting relative insulin excess for I/G are >0.23 microunit/mg, for G/I are <3.31 microunits/mg, and for AIGR are >30 microunits/mg.[70] The AIGR is calculated as follows:

$$\text{AIGR (microunits/mg)} = \frac{\text{serum insulin (microunits/ml} \times 100}{\text{Plasma glucose (mg/100ml)} - 30}$$

In most studies, if the blood glucose level is less than or equal to 30 mg/100 ml, one has been substituted for the denominator. Using the latter calculation for determining the AIGR increases the sensitivity of this ratio but decreases its specificity.[42, 51, 70, 78] The result is that more false-positive diagnoses are made and potentially unnecessary surgery is performed. If hypoglycemia is not detected on random blood samples and insulinoma is still suspected, several provocative tests can be performed to stimulate neoplastic islet cells to release insulin and induce hypoglycemia. These include "prolonged" fasting, intravenous or oral glucose tolerance tests, L-leucine tolerance, and glucagon tolerance and tolbutamide tolerance tests. All the provocative tests, except fasting, are expensive, time-consuming, unreliable, or high risk (tolbutamide tolerance) and do not improve diagnostic accuracy. Most dogs with insulinoma can be made hypoglycemic by simple fasting for 8 to 12 hours or less.[49, 51, 73, 139] When fasting dogs to induce

TABLE 154–8. DIFFERENTIAL DIAGNOSIS FOR HYPOGLYCEMIA

Increased Utilization	Decreased Production/ Availability	Miscellaneous
Insulinoma	Hepatic failure (acquired/ congenital)	Insulin overdose
Extrapancreatic neoplasms	Hypoadrenocorticism (Addison's)	Laboratory artifact
Sepsis	Puppy hypoglycemia	
Hunting dog hypoglycemia	Uremia	
Polycythemia	Starvation	
Pregnancy	Malabsorption	
	Hypopituitarism	
	Hypothyroidism	
	Glycogen storage disease	

hypoglycemia, testing is started in the morning so they may be monitored throughout the day. Blood glucose measurements are made every 2 to 3 hours until hypoglycemia (< 60 mg/100 ml) is detected.[49] A serum insulin concentration is measured on the first hypoglycemic sample, and an AIGR, I/G, or G/I ratio calculated if necessary. Patients are monitored closely throughout the testing period, particularly if seizures are the primary presenting complaint. Once hypoglycemia associated with hyperinsulinism is confirmed, exploratory surgery is recommended. When serum insulin assays are not available, exploratory surgery is considered if other known causes of hypoglycemia have been ruled out (see Table 154–8). Routine survey radiographs of the abdomen are of no diagnostic value, because these neoplasms are too small to be detected.[49, 92] Ultrasonography may be able to identify primary tumors within the pancreas or metastases in adjacent organs.[49] Thoracic radiographs are consistently negative for pulmonary metastases, even if present, and do not aid in staging the disease.[49, 92]

Preoperative treatment of dogs with insulinomas varies depending on the severity of hypoglycemia and the presence or absence of other clinical signs (e.g., seizures, weakness, collapse). Feeding three to six small daily meals of a diet high in protein and complex carbohydrates often reduces or eliminates clinical signs. Semimoist diets high in simple sugars are avoided. The addition of prednisone or the oral hyperglycemic agent diazoxide may also help preoperatively to stabilize patients that fail to respond to frequent feedings alone. Hypoglycemia may be so severe that intravenous 5 or 10 per cent dextrose may be needed to maintain blood glucose concentrations in the normal range, even though the patient is eating.

Patients are given no food for 8 to 12 hours preoperatively, and blood glucose concentrations are maintained by intravenous 5 per cent dextrose. At exploratory surgery, the pancreas is gently but thoroughly palpated for evidence of tumor nodules. Nearly all have readily identifiable round 1- to 2.5-cm-diameter solitary (85 per cent) or multiple tumor nodules visible in the pancreas (Fig. 154–9).[22, 51] Unfortunately, approximately 45 per cent of patients also have metastases to regional lymph

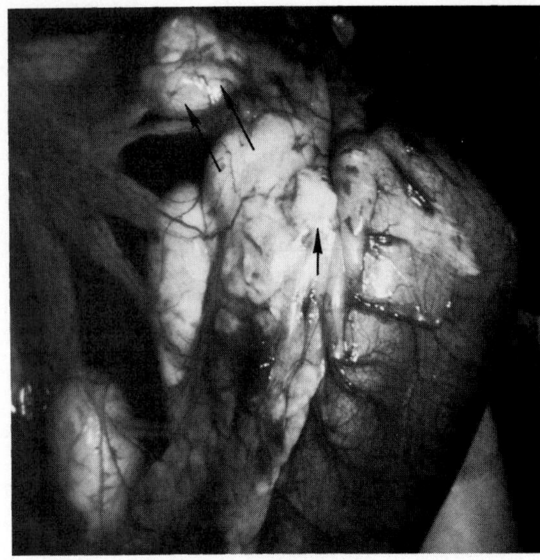

FIGURE 154–9. Insulinoma *(single arrow)* with metastasis to the regional lymph node *(double arrows)*.

nodes or the liver at surgery.[22, 92] Tumors are identified with equal frequency within the left (splenic) or right (duodenal) limb of the pancreas. Much less commonly identified sites are the body or angle of the pancreas, and rare diffuse nonpalpable tumors have been reported.[51, 73] An isolated case of a primary ectopic insulinoma localized to the duodenal wall was reported.[136]

Intravenous methylene blue (Methylene Blue Injection 1 per cent*) may aid in identifying primary and metastatic insulinomas in dogs.[53, 54, 136] Methylene blue intensely stains neoplastic islet cells, helping to differentiate them from surrounding normal tissue; 3 mg/kg is diluted in 250 ml of 0.9 per cent sterile saline and given over 30 to 40 minutes. Maximal staining of the tumor occurs approximately 30 minutes after the infusion is begun. Hemolytic anemia may develop if this dosage is exceeded, owing to Heinz body formation. If no primary tumor is identified and the diagnosis is likely, consider blind resection of 50 per cent of the pancreas in case diffuse islet cell neoplasia is present.[51]

The postoperative course for dogs with insulinomas is variable. Recognized complications include persistent hypoglycemia, surgically induced pancreatitis, diabetes mellitus, acquired epilepsy, and diffuse polyneuropathy.[22, 24, 49, 51, 92, 133] Persistent hypoglycemia develops in dogs in which the primary tumor is inoperable or metastases are present at surgery. This complication is reported in 20 to 27 per cent of cases.[22, 92] As much tumor as possible is removed surgically, because this modifies the severity of postoperative hypoglycemia even though there is no chance of a cure.

Pancreatitis is an infrequent complication in dogs. Patients with signs of pancreatitis are given no oral food and water for 36 to 48 hours. Intravenous 5 per cent dextrose is necessary only if hypoglycemia persists during the postoperative period. Otherwise, balanced fluid and electrolyte solutions and broad-spectrum antibiotics are administered.

Development of diabetes mellitus is a unique paradox of this disease. Prolonged increases in tumor insulin and subsequent hypoglycemia may lead to atrophy of normal islet tissue. Partial pancreatectomy to control the tumor may also decrease insulin reserves. Diabetes may develop in 15 to 29 per cent of dogs in the postoperative period.[22, 49, 50, 92] In many cases, the hyperglycemia is transient, lasting from a few days to 2 months. In others, the condition may last for years and require chronic insulin therapy. Gradual growth of metastases often results in correction of the diabetes. Signs of hypoglycemia eventually recur. These dogs need careful monitoring, because signs of insulin overdose and tumor recurrence are similar.

Rare complications of insulinomas are acquired epilepsy and chronic diffuse polyneuropathy.[10, 24, 49, 133] Recurrent severe hypoglycemia is hypothesized to result in organic brain damage that subsequently serves as a seizure focus, even though hypoglycemia is corrected. The seizures in some dogs respond to anticonvulsants.

Occasional dogs have persistent moderate to severe ataxia even though hypoglycemia has been corrected.[10, 24, 49, 133] A peripheral polyneuropathy recognized in dogs with insulinomas is characterized by decreased patellar reflexes, decreased conscious proprioception, and electromyography findings compatible with axonal degeneration.

Medical treatment of dogs with insulinomas is considered in the preoperative period to stabilize their disease before surgery. Medical therapy is also of value in dogs in which surgery is not performed. Medical management is helpful in controlling signs in dogs with metastatic disease. Methods to control hypoglycemia include frequent feeding, reduced exercise, glucocorticoids, oral hyperglycemic agents, somatostatin analogues, and islet cell cytotoxic drugs. Dogs with recurrent hypoglycemia are fed between four and six times per day, offering a high-protein diet that is low in simple sugars and high in complex carbohydrates.[102] Such diets may induce less stimulation of tumor-produced insulin or at least provide calories at frequent intervals. Prednisone or prednisolone is given twice daily to stimulate gluconeogenesis. Initial dosages are 1.0 to 4 mg/kg/day, BID. This dosage may be increased up to 2 mg/kg/day in refractory cases.

The oral hyperglycemic agent diazoxide (Proglycem) is helpful in controlling signs of hypoglycemia in as many as 70 per cent of dogs.[49, 109, 153] The duration of clinical response is 2 to 15 months, with a mean of 6.5 months.[92] This agent has no antineoplastic effects; rather, it controls hypoglycemia by inhibiting insulin release from tumor cells, by promoting hepatic gluconeogenesis and glycogenolysis through stimulation of the sympathetic nervous system, by decreasing peripheral glucose use, and by augmenting free fatty acid mobilization.[49, 102] Recommended dosages are 5 to 30 mg/kg BID. Anorexia, vomiting, and diarrhea are the main adverse reactions to diazoxide; decreasing the dose and giving the drug with meals reduce these reactions.[102] Combining diazoxide with another thiazide derivative, hydrochlor-

*Elkins-Sinn Co., Cherry Hill, NJ.

thiazide (Aldoril, 2 to 4 mg/kg BID) may potentiate the effects of diazoxide.[102, 153]

The somatostatin analogue SM 201–945 was given to five dogs with insulinomas, 10 to 20 μg BID to TID, and clinical signs resolved in two.[164] Somatostatin is a potent inhibitor of growth hormone, insulin, glucagon, and gastrin. This drug holds promise for future alternative methods of managing this disease.

Alloxan, a drug toxic to both islet cells and renal tubular epithelium, has been tried in a limited number of dogs with metastatic insulinomas.[51] When given as a single intravenous injection to five dogs at 65 mg/kg, four of five became hyperglycemic in 3 to 5 days. Hyperglycemia persisted for several months in two dogs, and in the other two, prolonged euglycemia developed. Renal failure is a significant complication and may develop in approximately 10 per cent of dogs given this drug. Further evaluation of this agent is warranted.

Streptozotocin, a drug with antineoplastic activity against islet cells, has been used in two cases of metastatic insulinomas in dogs.[93, 94] It was highly nephrotoxic in these two animals, and further investigations are needed before it can be recommended for clinical use in dogs.

The prognosis for dogs with functional islet cell tumors is highly variable but generally poor. Surgical cures of insulinomas are not expected. If patients are monitored postoperatively for evidence of recurrent hypoglycemia, it invariably develops. In some cases, a second or third operation to remove metastatic tumors after signs recur may allow further significant disease-free time for the animal. Prognostic factors associated with decreased survival are age at the time of diagnosis (younger dogs have shorter survival times), high preoperative serum insulin concentrations, and the presence of distant metastases at surgery.[22] If the tumor is confined to the pancreas (stage 1), survival is significantly longer than dogs in stage 2 (regional node involvement) or stage 3 (regional node and distant metastases). Mean survival times for dogs that are euglycemic after surgery varies from 11 to 17 months.* Although dogs in which hypoglycemia persists postoperatively generally survive only briefly, combinations of surgical and medical therapy have resulted in animals living as long as 3½ years postoperatively.[139]

Gastrinomas

Functional nonbeta islet cell pancreatic tumors have been documented for a number of years in humans. These tumors produce a syndrome that is characterized by excessive gastric acid production (hyperchlorhydria), peptic esophagitis, and gastric or duodenal ulceration. This complex of signs, when caused by a gastrin-secreting tumor of pancreatic islets, is known as the Zollinger-Ellison syndrome.

Nine cases were reported to document the existence of pancreatic islet cell tumors that secrete gastrin in dogs, and one case in a cat.† Clinical findings have been fairly consistent. Animals range in age from 3 to 9 years, and no breed or sex predisposition is identified. Presenting complaints usually include depression, anorexia, vomiting, diarrhea, and weight loss. Vomiting of blood or melena and abdominal pain were observed in 11 per cent of cases.[50] Laboratory abnormalities include regenerative anemia, neutrophilic leukocytosis, hypoproteinemia, hypoalbuminemia, hypochloremia, hypokalemia, and mild increases in alanine aminotransferase and alkaline phosphatase. Endoscopic abnormalities include erosive esophagitis; gastritis; ulcerations in the esophagus, stomach, and duodenum; and gastric mucosal hypertrophy.[11] A barium swallow identifies ulcerations and prominent gastric mucosal folds. Perforations of the ulcers and regional peritonitis have also been reported. Ultrasonography may be useful to identify primary tumors in the pancreas or hepatic metastases.

A definitive diagnosis is based on identifying a pancreatic islet cell neoplasm and documentation of elevated fasting serum gastrin concentrations. Normal fasting serum gastrin concentrations in dogs are between 20 and 190 pg/ml and in cats between 28 and 135 pg/ml.[11, 50] Serum gastrin concentrations in dogs with gastrinomas have been from 360 to 2,780 pg/ml and in one cat, 1,000 pg/ml.

Most dogs and cats with gastrinomas are treated by a combination of medical and surgical approaches. Most are extremely sick when initially evaluated. As such, surgical exploration is delayed until patients are stabilized by medical management, except when a perforated gastric or duodenal ulcer exists. Medical management includes supportive care for anemia; correction of fluid, electrolyte, and acid base abnormalities; and control of the ulcer. Ulcer care usually involves the use of H_2-receptor antagonists such as cimetidine (5 mg/kg four to six times daily), or ranitidine (2 mg/kg TID), and the ulcer protective agent sucralfate (0.25 g in cats and 0.5 to 1 g in dogs, given every 8 hours, 30 minutes before H_2-receptor antagonists).[108] Once patients are stabilized, exploratory surgery is recommended. Surgery has the benefits of being both a diagnostic and therapeutic technique and adding valuable prognostic information. Gastrinomas are generally small, similar to insulinomas, and surgical removal of primary and metastatic tumors is attempted. In addition, severe ulcers may be better managed surgically than medically.

The prognosis for animals with gastrinomas is poor. Most have had metastatic disease when the diagnosis was first made and survive briefly. In any animal with idiopathic gastric or duodenal ulcers, if serum gastrin concentrations cannot be obtained, abdominal exploration is warranted to examine the pancreas for tumors.

*See references 22–24, 49, 73, 78, 92, and 139.
†See references 11, 39, 50, 58, 67, 95, 140, and 164.

References

1. Alexander R, Kock R: Primary hepatic carcinoid (APUD cell carcinoma) in a cat. *J Small Animal Pract 23*:767, 1982.
2. Alroy J, et al: Distinctive intestinal mast cell neoplasms of domestic cats. *Lab Invest 33*:159, 1975.
3. Anderson G, et al: Rectal resection in the dog: A new surgical approach and evaluation of its effect on fecal continence. *Vet Surg 16*:119, 1987.
4. Anderson N, Johnson D: Pancreatic carcinoma in the dog. *J Am Vet Med Assoc 150*:286, 1967.
5. Anlyan W: Carcinoid tumors and the carcinoid syndrome. *In* Sabiston DC (ed): *Textbook of Surgery*. W.B. Saunders, Philadelphia, 1977, p 1045.
6. Bailey W: *Spirocerca lupi:* A continuing injury. *J Parasitol 58*:1, 1972.

7. Beck ER, et al: Canine tongue tumors: A retrospective review of 57 cases. *J Am Anim Hosp Assoc 33*:525, 1986.
8. Bjorling DE, et al: Surgical treatment of epulides in dogs: 25 cases (1974–1984). *J Am Vet Med Assoc 109*:1315, 1987.
9. Bradley RL, et al: Mandibular resection for removal of oral tumors in 30 dogs and 6 cats. *J Am Vet Med Assoc 184*:460, 1984.
10. Braund K, et al: Insulinoma and subclinical peripheral neuropathy in two dogs. *J Vet Intern Med 1*:86, 1987.
11. Breitschwerdt E, et al: Hypergastrinemia in canine gastrointestinal disease. *J Am Anim Hosp Assoc 22*:585, 1986.
12. Brody R: Alimentary tract neoplasia in the cat: A clinicopathologic survey of 46 cases. *Am J Vet Res 27*:74, 1966.
13. Brody R, Cohen D: An epizootiologic and clinicopathologic study of 95 cases of gastrointestinal neoplasm in the dog. Scientific Proceedings of the 101st Annual Meeting of the American Veterinary Medical Association, Chicago, July 1964, p 167.
14. Brody RS: Biologic behavior of canine oral and pharyngeal neoplasms. *J Small Anim Pract 11*:45, 1970.
15. Brooks MB, et al: Chemotherapy versus chemotherapy plus radiotherapy in the treatment of tonsillar squamous cell carcinoma in the dog. *J Vet Intern Med 2*:206, 1988.
16. Bruecker K, Withrow S: Intestinal leiomyosarcomas in six dogs. *J Am Anim Hosp Assoc 24*:281, 1987.
17. Campbell J, Pirie H: Leiomyoma of the oesophagus in a dog. *Vet Rec 77*:624, 1965.
18. Carakostas M, et al: Malignant foregut carcinoid in a domestic cat. *Vet Pathol 16*:607, 1979.
19. Carb A, Barrett R: Leiomyosarcoma of the cecum in the dog. *J Am Anim Hosp Assoc 14*:631, 1978.
20. Carb A, Goodman D: Oesophageal carcinoma in the dog. *J Small Anim Pract 14*:91, 1973.
21. Carpenter J, et al: Tumors and tumor-like lesions. *In* Holzworth J (ed): *Diseases of the Cat*. W.B. Saunders, Philadelphia, 1987, p 500.
22. Caywood D, et al: Pancreatic insulin-secreting neoplasms: Clinical, diagnostic, and prognostic features in 73 dogs. *J Am Anim Hosp Assoc 24*:577, 1988.
23. Caywood D, et al: Pancreatic islet cell adenocarcinoma: Clinical and diagnostic features of six cases. *J Am Vet Med Assoc 176*:714, 1979.
24. Chrisman C: Postoperative results and complications of insulinomas in dogs. *J Am Anim Hosp Assoc 16*:677, 1980.
25. Christie G, Jabara A: Two cases of malignant intestinal neoplasms in dogs. *J Comp Pathol 74*:90, 1964.
26. Church EM, et al: Colorectal adenocarcinoma in dogs: 78 cases (1973–1984). *J Am Vet Med Assoc 191*:727, 1987.
27. Cline M, Haskell C: *Cancer Chemotherapy*. W.B. Saunders, Philadelphia, 1980.
28. Cohen D, Brody RS: Epidemiologic aspects of oral and pharyngeal neoplasms of the dog. *J Am Vet Med Assoc 25*:1776, 1964.
29. Comis R: The therapy of stomach cancer. *In* Carter SK, Glatstein E, and Livingston RB (eds): *Principles of Cancer Treatment*. McGraw-Hill, New York, 1982, p 420.
30. Conroy J: Multiple gastric adenomatous polyps in a dog. *J Comp Pathol 79*:465, 1969.
31. Cotchin E: Neoplasms in cats. *Proc R Soc Med 45*:671, 1952.
32. Cotchin E: Further observations of neoplasms in dogs with particular reference to the site of origin and malignancy. *Br Vet J 110*:218, 1954.
33. Culbertston R, et al: Esophageal/gastric leiomyoma in the laboratory Beagle. *J Am Vet Med Assoc 183*:1168, 1983.
34. Dorn A, et al: Gastric carcinoma in a dog. *J Small Anim Pract 17*:109, 1976.
35. Dorn RC, Priester W: Epidemiology. *In* Theilen GK, Madewell BR (eds): *Veterinary Cancer Medicine*. Lea & Febiger, Philadelphia, 1987, p 27.
36. Dorn RC, Priester WA: Epidemiologic analysis of oral and pharyngeal cancer in dogs, cats, horses, and cattle. *J Am Vet Med Assoc 169*:1202, 1976.
37. Douglas S, et al: The surgical relief of gastric lesions in the dog; report on seven cases. *Vet Rec 86*:743, 1970.
38. Drake J, Hime J: Gastric carcinoma in the dog; two further cases. *J Small Anim Pract 6*:131, 1965.
39. Drazner F: Canine gastrinoma: A condition analogous to the Zollinger-Ellison syndrome in man. *Calif Vet 35*:6, 1981.
40. Dubielzig R: Proliferative dental and gingival diseases of dogs and cats. *J Am Anim Hosp Assoc 18*:577, 1982.
41. Dubielzig R, et al: The nomenclature of periodontal epulides in dogs. *Vet Pathol 16*:209, 1979.
42. Edwards D: It's time to unamend the insulin-glucose ratio. *J Am Vet Med Assoc 188*:951, 1986.
43. Evans S: The radiographic appearance of primary liver neoplasia in dogs. *Vet Radiol 28*:192, 1987.
44. Evans S, De Frate L: Gastric lymphosarcoma in a dog; a case report. *Am Coll Vet Radiol 21*:55, 1980.
45. Evans SM, Shofer F: Canine oral nontonsillar squamous cell carcinoma. Prognostic factors for recurrence and survival following orthovoltage radiation. *Vet Radiol 29*:129, 1988.
46. Fabry A, et al: Nodular hyperplasia of the liver in the beagle dog. *Vet Pathol 19*:109, 1982.
47. Feeney D, et al: Two-dimensional gray-scale ultrasonography for assessment of hepatic and splenic neoplasia in the dog and cat. *J Am Vet Med Assoc 184*:68, 1984.
48. Feeney D, et al: Chronic bowel obstruction caused by primary intestinal neoplasia. *J Am Anim Hosp Assoc 18*:67, 1982.
49. Feldman E: Hyperinsulinism in a dog. *Mod Vet Pract 60*:995, 1979.
50. Feldman E, Nelson R: Gastrointestinal endocrinology. *In* Feldman E, Nelson R (eds): *Canine and Feline Endocrinology and Reproduction*. W.B. Saunders, Philadelphia, 1987, p 375.
51. Feldman E, Nelson R: Hypoglycemia. *In* Feldman E, Nelson R (eds): *Canine and Feline Endocrinology and Reproduction*. W.B. Saunders, Philadelphia, 1987, p 304.
52. Feldman EC, et al: Amended insulin glucose ratio. *J Am Vet Med Assoc 188*:1277, 1986.
53. Fingeroth J, Smeak D: Intravenous methylene blue infusion for intraoperative identification of pancreatic islet cell tumors in dogs. Part II. Clinical trials and results in four dogs. *J Am Anim Hosp Assoc 24*:175, 1988.
54. Fingeroth JM, et al: Intravenous methylene blue infusion for intraoperative identification of parathyroid gland and pancreatic islet cell tumors in dogs. Part I. Experimental determination of dose-related staining efficacy and toxicity. *J Am Anim Hosp Assoc 24*:165, 1988.
55. Gibbs C, Pearson H: Localized tumours of the canine small intestine: A report of twenty cases. *J Small Anim Pract 27*:507, 1986.
56. Giles R, et al: Carcinoid tumors in the small intestine of a dog. *Vet Pathol 11*:340, 1974.
57. Gorlin RJ, et al: The oral and pharyngeal pathology of domestic animals: A study of 487 cases. *Am J Vet Res 20*:1032, 1959.
58. Happe R, et al: Zollinger-Ellison syndrome in three dogs. *Vet Pathol 17*:177, 1980.
59. Happe R, et al: Multiple polyps of the gastric mucosa in two dogs. *J Small Anim Pract 18*:179, 1977.
60. Hayden D, Nielsen S: Canine alimentary neoplasia. *Zentralbl Veterinaermed [A] 20*:1, 1973.
61. Head K, Else R: Neoplasia and allied conditions of the canine and feline intestine. *Vet Ann 21*:190, 1981.
62. Hilmes D, Gilette E: Radiotherapy of spontaneous fibrous connective-tissue sarcomas in animals. *J Natl Cancer Inst 56*:365, 1976.
63. Holt PE, Lucke VM: Rectal neoplasia in the dog: A clinicopathological review of 31 cases. *Vet Rec 116*:400, 1985.
64. Honjo I, et al: Ligation of a branch of the portal vein for carcinoma of the liver. *Am J Surg 30*:296, 1975.
65. Howell J: Two cases of mucin-secreting carcinoma of the stomach of the dog. *J Comp Pathol 74*:94, 1964.
66. Jeraj K, et al: Primary hepatic ostersarcoma in a dog. *J Am Vet Med Assoc 179*:1000, 1981.
67. Jones B, et al: Peptic ulceration in a dog associated with an islet cell carcinoma of the pancreas and an elevated plasma gastrin level. *J Small Anim Pract 17*:593, 1976.
68. Kestenman D, et al: Treatment experience of oropharyngeal squamous cell carcinoma in the dog and cat using orthovoltage and cobalt-60 radiation therapy: 1978–1988. *J Am Vet Med Assoc,* in press.
69. Kircher D, Nielsen S: Tumors of the pancreas. *Bull WHO 53*:195, 1976.
70. Knowlen G, Schall W: The amended insulin-glucose ratio: Is it really better? *J Am Vet Med Assoc 185*:397, 1984.
71. Kosovsky J, et al: Small intestinal adenocarcinoma in cats: 32 cases (1979–1985). *J Am Vet Med Assoc 192*:233, 1988.
72. Krook L: On gastrointestinal carcinoma in the dog. *Acta Pathol Microbiol Scand 38*:43, 1956.
73. Kruth SA, et al: Insulin secreting islet cell tumors: Establishing a diagnosis and the clinical course for 25 dogs. *J Am Vet Med Assoc 181*:54, 1982.
74. Kurihara M, et al: A new method for producing adenocarcinomas in the dog with *N*-ethyl-*N*-nitro-*N*-nitrosoguanidine. *Gann 65*:168, 1974.
75. Lahellec M, Joncourt A: Etude clinique et histologique d'une tumeur carcinoide du grele chez un chat. *Bull Acad Vet Fr 45*:363, 1972.
76. Langham R, et al: Oral adamantinomas in the dog. *J Am Vet Med Assoc 146*:474, 1965.
77. Lawson D, Pirie H: Conditions of the canine oesophagus—II. Vascular rings, achalasia, tumors and perioesophageal lesions. *J Small Anim Pract 7*:117, 1966.
78. Leifer C, et al: Insulin secreting tumors: Diagnosis and medical and surgical management in 55 dogs. *J Am Vet Med Assoc 188*:60, 1986.
79. Lingeman C, Garner F: Comparative study of intestinal adenocarcinomas of animals and man. *J Natl Cancer Inst 48*:325, 1972.
80. Lingeman C, et al: Spontaneous gastric adenocarcinomas of dogs: A review. *J Natl Cancer Inst 47*:137, 1971.
81. Longmire W: Carcinoma of the stomach. *In* Sabiston DC (ed): *Textbook of Surgery*. W.B. Saunders, Philadelphia, 1977, p 983.
82. MacDonald J, et al: 5-FU, mitomycin C and Adriamycin: A new combination program for advanced gastrointestinal cancer. *Proc Am Soc Clin Oncol 176*:264, 1976.
83. MacVean D, et al: Frequency of canine and feline tumors in a defined population. *Vet Pathol 15*:700, 1978.
84. Mauldin GN, et al: Efficacy and toxicity of doxorubicin and cyclophosphamide used in the treatment of selected malignant tumors in 23 cats. *J Vet Intern Med 2*:60, 1988.

85. McCaw D, et al: Squamous cell carcinoma of the esophagus in a dog. *J Am Anim Hosp Assoc 16*:561, 1980.
86. McConnell M, Lumsden J: Biochemical evaluation of metastatic liver disease in the dog. *J Am Anim Hosp Assoc 19*:173, 1983.
87. McDonald A: Primary gastric carcinoma of the dog: Review and case report. *Vet Surg 7*:70, 1978.
88. McDonald R, Helman G: Hepatic malignant mesenchymoma in a dog. *J Am Vet Med Assoc 188*:1052, 1986.
89. McIntosh-Bright J: Pancreatic adenocarcinoma in a dog with a maldigestion syndrome. *J Am Vet Med Assoc 187*:420, 1985.
90. McKeown D, et al: Over-the-top approach to the caudal pelvic canal and rectum in the dog and cat. *Vet Surg 13*:181, 1984.
91. McMillan F, et al: Functional pancreatic islet cell tumor in a cat. *J Am Anim Hosp Assoc 21*:741, 1985.
92. Melhaff C, et al: Insulin producing islet cell neoplasms: Surgical considerations and general management in 35 dogs. *J Am Anim Hosp Assoc 21*:607, 1985.
93. Meyer D: Pancreatic islet cell carcinoma in a dog treated with streptozotocin. *Am J Vet Res 37*:1221, 1976.
94. Meyer D: Temporary remission of hypoglycemia in a dog with an insulinoma after treatment with streptozotocin. *Am J Vet Res 38*:1201, 1977.
95. Middleton D, Watson A: Duodenal ulceration associated with gastrin secreting pancreatic tumor in a cat. *J Am Vet Med Assoc 183*:461, 1983.
96. Miller A: Epidemiology of gastrointestinal cancer. *In* Stroehlein JR, Romsdale MM (eds): *Gastrointestinal Cancer.* Raven Press, New York, 1981, p 31.
97. Moertel C: Carcinoma of the stomach: Prognostic factors and criteria of response to therapy. *In* Staquet MJ (ed): *Cancer Therapy: Prognostic Factors and Criteria of Response.* Raven Press, New York, 1975, p 229.
98. Moulton J: Tumors of the alimentary tract. *In* Moulton JE (ed): *Tumors in Domestic Animals.* University of California Press, Berkeley, 1978, p 240.
99. Moulton J: Tumors of the pancreas, liver, gallbladder and mesothelium. *In* Moulton JE (ed): *Tumors in Domestic Animals.* University of California Press, Berkeley, 1978.
100. Mulligan RM: *Neoplasms of the Dog.* Williams & Wilkins, Baltimore, 1949.
101. Murray M, et al: Primary gastric neoplasia in the dog. *Vet Rec 91*:474, 1972.
102. Nelson RW, Foodman MS: Medical management of canine hyperinsulinism. *J Am Vet Med Assoc 187*:78, 1985.
103. Nielsen S, Schroder J: Gastric carcinoma of dogs: Report of three cases. *North Am Vet 34*:640, 1953.
104. Nyland T: Ultrasonic patterns of canine hepatic lymphosarcoma. *Vet Radiol 25*:167, 1984.
105. Ogilvie GK, et al: Papillary squamous cell carcinoma in three young dogs. *J Am Vet Med Assoc 192*:933, 1988.
106. Olivieri M, et al: Gastric adenocarcinoma in a dog: Six-and-one-half month survival following partial gastrectomy and gastroduodenostomy. *J Am Anim Hosp Assoc 20*:78, 1984.
107. Palminteri A: The surgical management of polyps of the rectum and colon of the dog. *J Am Vet Med Assoc 148*:771, 1966.
108. Papich M: Medical therapy for gastrointestinal ulcers. *In* Kirk RW (ed): *Current Veterinary Therapy.* W.B. Saunders, Philadelphia, 1989, p 911.
109. Parker A, et al: Diazoxide treatment of metastatic insulinoma in a dog. *J Am Anim Hosp Assoc 18*:315, 1982.
110. Patnaik A, Twedt D: Intestinal mast cell tumor in a dog. *J Small Anim Pract 21*:207, 1980.
111. Patnaik A, et al: Canine gastrointestinal neoplasms. *Vet Pathol 14*:547, 1977.
112. Patnaik A, et al: Canine gastric adenocarcinoma. *Vet Pathol 15*:600, 1978.
113. Patnaik A, et al: Canine intestinal adenocarcinoma and carcinoid. *Vet Pathol 17*:149, 1980.
114. Patnaik A, et al: Canine hepatic neoplasms: A clinicopathologic study. *Vet Pathol 17*:553, 1980.
115. Patnaik A, et al: Canine bile duct carcinoma. *Vet Pathol 18*:439, 1981.
116. Patnaik A, et al: Canine hepatocellular carcinoma. *Vet Pathol 18*:427, 1981.
117. Patnaik A, et al: Canine hepatic carcinoids. *Vet Pathol 18*:445, 1981.
118. Patnaik A, et al: Feline intestinal adenocarcinoma. *Vet Pathol 13*:1, 1976.
119. Patnaik AK, Lieberman PH: Gastric squamous cell carcinoma in a dog. *Vet Pathol 17*:250, 1980.
120. Patnaik AK, et al: A clinicopathologic and ultrastructural study of undifferentiated malignant tumors of the oral cavity in dogs. *Vet Pathol 23*:170, 1986.
121. Penwick RC, Nunamaker DM: Rostral mandibulectomy: A treatment for oral neoplasia in the dog and cat. *J Am Anim Hosp Assoc 23*:19, 1987.
122. Pollock S, Wagner B: Gastric adenocarcinoma or linitis plastica in a dog. *Vet Med Small Anim Clin 68*:139, 1973.
123. Postorino N: Hepatic Tumors. *In* Withrow SJ, MacEwen EG (eds): *Veterinary Clinical Oncology.* J.B. Lippincott, Philadelphia, 1989, p 196.
124. Priester W: Data from eleven United States and Canadian colleges of veterinary medicine on pancreatic carcinoma in domestic animals. *Cancer Res 34*:1372, 1974.
125. Reif JS, Cohen D: The environmental distribution of canine respiratory tract neoplasms. *Arch Environ Health 22*:136, 1971.
126. Ridgway R, Suter P: Clinical and radiographic signs in primary and metastatic esophageal neoplasms of the dog. *J Am Vet Med Assoc 174*:700, 1979.
127. Robbins S: The stomach. *In* Robbins S (ed): *Pathologic Basis of Disease.* W.B. Saunders, Philadelphia, 1974, p 911.
128. Rogers K, Luttgen P: Hyperinsulinism. *Comp Cont Educ Pract Vet 7*:829, 1985.
129. Salisbury SK, Lantz GC: Long-term results of partial mandibulectomy for treatment of oral tumors in 30 dogs. *J Am Anim Hosp Assoc 24*:285, 1988.
130. Salisbury SK, et al: Partial maxillectomy and premaxillectomy in the treatment of oral neoplasia in the dog and cat. *Vet Surg 15*:16, 1986.
131. Sautter J, Hanlon G: Gastric neoplasia in the dog: A report of 20 cases. *J Am Vet Med Assoc 168*:691, 1976.
132. Seiler R: Colorectal polyps of the dog: A clinicopathologic study of 17 cases. *J Am Vet Med Assoc 174*:72, 1979.
133. Shahar R, et al: Peripheral polyneuropathy in a dog with functional islet B-cell tumor and widespread metastasis. *J Am Vet Med Assoc 187*:175, 1985.
134. Shapiro W, et al: Cisplatin for treatment of transitional cell and squamous cell carcinomas in dogs. *J Am Vet Med Assoc 193*:1530, 1988.
135. Silverman S: Carcinoma arising in adenomatous polyps. *Dis Colon Rectum 14*:191, 1971.
136. Smeak D, et al: Intravenous methylene blue as a specific stain for primary and metastatic insulinoma in a dog. *J Am Anim Hosp Assoc 24*:478, 1988.
137. Smith H, Jones T: *Veterinary Pathology.* Lea & Febiger, Philadelphia, 1966, p 266.
138. Stebbins KE, et al: Feline oral neoplasia: A ten-year survey. *Vet Pathol 26*:121, 1989.
139. Steinberg H: Insulin secreting pancreatic tumors in the dog. *J Am Anim Hosp Assoc 16*:695, 1980.
140. Straus E, et al: Canine Zollinger-Ellison syndrome. *Gastroenterology 72*:380, 1977.
141. Straw R: Tumors of the intestinal tract. *In* Withrow SJ, MacEwen EG (eds): *Clinical Veterinary Oncology.* J.B. Lippincott, Philadelphia, 1989, p 200.
142. Strombeck D: Clinicopathologic features of primary and metastatic neoplastic disease of the liver in dogs. *J Am Vet Med Assoc 173*:267, 1978.
143. Strombeck D, et al: Hypoglycemia and hypoinsulinemia associated with hepatoma in a dog. *J Am Vet Med Assoc 169*:811, 1976.
144. Sullivan M, et al: A study of 31 cases of gastric carcinoma in dogs. *Vet Rec 120*:79, 1987.
145. Theilen GH, Madewell BR: Tumors of the digestive tract. *In* Theilen GH, Madewell BR (eds): *Veterinary Cancer Medicine.* Lea & Febiger, Philadelphia, 1979.
146. Theilen GH, Madewell BR: Tumors of the digestive tract. *In* Theilen GJH, Madewell BR (ed): *Veterinary Cancer Medicine.* Lea & Febiger, Philadelphia, 1987, p 499.
147. Thompson JM, et al: Hyperthermia and radiation in the management of canine tumors. *J Small Anim Pract 28*:457, 1987.
148. Thrall D: Orthovoltage radiotherapy of oral fibrosarcomas in dogs. *J Am Vet Med Assoc 179*:159, 1981.
149. Thrall DE: Orthovoltage radiotherapy of acanthomatous epulides in 39 dogs. *J Am Vet Med Assoc 184*:826, 1984.
150. Todoroff R, Brody R: Oral and pharyngeal neoplasia in the dog: A retrospective survey of 361 cases. *J Am Vet Med Assoc 175*:567, 1979.
151. Trigo F, et al: The pathology of liver tumors in the dog. *J Comp Pathol 92*:21, 1982.
152. Turk M, et al: Nonhematopoietic gastrointestinal neoplasia in cats; a retrospective study of 44 cases. *Vet Pathol 18*:614, 1981.
153. Turnwald G, Troy G: Hypoglycemia, Part II—clinical aspects. *Comp Cont Educ Pract Vet 6*:115, 1984.
154. Turrel J: Principles of radiation therapy. *In* Theilen GR, Madewell BR (eds): *Veterinary Cancer Medicine.* Lea & Febiger, Philadelphia, 1987, p 144.
155. Turrel J, Theon A: Single high-dose irradiation for selected canine rectal adenocarcinomas. *Vet Radiol 27*:141, 1986.
156. Vernon F, Roudebush P: Primary esophageal carcinoma in a cat. *J Am Anim Hosp Assoc 16*:547, 1982.
157. Walter MC, et al: Pylorectomy and gastrodenostomy in the dog: Technique and clinical results in 28 cases. *J Am Vet Med Assoc 187*:909, 1985.
158. Watrach AM, et al: Canine papilloma: Progression of oral papilloma to carcinoma. *J Natl Cancer Inst 45*:915, 1970.
159. White R, Gorman N: The clinical diagnosis and management of rectal and pararectal tumours in the dog. *J Small Anim Pract 28*:87, 1987.
160. White RAS, et al: The surgical management of bone-involved oral tumors in the dog. *J Small Anim Pract 26*:693, 1985.
161. White RAS, et al: Clinical staging for oropharyngeal malignancies in the dog. *J Small Anim Pract 26*:581, 1985.
162. Willard M, et al: Neuroendocrine carcinoma of the gallbladder in a dog. *J Am Vet Med Assoc 192*:926, 1988.
163. Withrow SJ, Hommberg D: Mandibulectomy in the treatment of oral cancer. *J Am Anim Hosp Assoc 19*:273, 1983.
164. Zerbe C, et al: Pancreatic polypeptide and insulin secreting tumor in a dog with duodenal ulcers and hypertrophic gastritis. *J Vet Intern Med 3*:178, 1989.

CHAPTER

155 Cardiovascular System

Phillip N. Ogburn

Tumors may arise from numerous sites in the body and involve various tissues within the heart, pericardium, or peripheral vessels; benign and malignant tumors may develop (Table 155–1). Primary tumors of the heart are uncommon[15, 32] and most often arise from the right atrium.[27, 31] Reports of cardiac neoplasia in small animals have dealt mainly with two neoplasms, chemodectoma or aortic body tumors and hemangiosarcoma. Chemodectomas are common heart base tumors in dogs and are observed predominantly in males of brachycephalic breeds, boxers and Boston terriers.[57] Hemangiosarcoma, the most common primary malignant tumor of the heart, is found frequently in golden retrievers, Labrador retrievers, German shepherds, and poodles.[27, 40–42, 48]

Because of their slower growth patterns and singular nature, the rare benign tumors of the heart—myxoma, fibroma, and leiomyoma—often remain unrecognized until massive destruction of the myocardium or obstructive vascular changes occurs.

Metastatic tumors of the heart in dogs occur late in the course of a malignancy and are infrequently diagnosed antemortem. Metastatic tumors arise most commonly from mammary adenocarcinoma, peripheral hemangiosarcoma, squamous cell carcinoma, and undifferentiated malignant oral tumors.[30]

Primary cardiac tumors in cats are exceedingly rare.[29, 39] Isolated cases of pericardial mesothelioma,[54] fibrosarcoma,[45] and chemodectoma[8] and 18 cases of hemangiosarcoma with metastatic cardiac involvement have been documented.[39] Lymphosarcoma, which accounts for one-third of all feline tumors, is the most common metastatic tumor.[19]

Neoplasms of peripheral vascular origin are more common in dogs than cats. Hemangiosarcoma is the most prevalent neoplasm and may arise from the spleen, liver, right atrium, lungs, skin, bone, brain, and other organs in dogs.[27, 40–42, 48]

The antemortem diagnosis of cardiac tumors is challenging because they are rare and exhibit nonspecific clinical manifestations. Some neoplasms, like hemangiosarcoma of the heart, have certain clinical features (e.g., fragmentation anemia) that may provide valuable clues to their presence. The possibility of cardiac neoplasia should be considered in aged dogs with clinical signs of heart failure, especially in breeds with a high predisposition toward neoplasia.

Refinements in echocardiography, angiocardiography, fine-needle aspiration biopsy, cardiopulmonary bypass, and surgical techniques, as well as advances in radiation and chemotherapy, have made early diagnosis and treatment possible for some animals.

TABLE 155–1. COMMON CARDIOVASCULAR TUMORS

Cardiac	
Benign	Fibroma
	Myxoma
	Rhabdomyoma
Malignant	Chemodectoma (aortic body tumor)
	Fibrosarcoma
	Hemangiosarcoma
	Lymphosarcoma
	Mammary gland adenocarcinoma
	Melanosarcoma
	Mesothelioma
	Rhabdomyosarcoma
Vascular	
Benign	Hemangioma
Malignant	Hemangiosarcoma
	Chemodectoma (carotid body tumor)

PRIMARY CARDIAC NEOPLASMS

Hemangiosarcoma (angiosarcoma, hemangioendothelioma), a highly malignant tumor of endothelial origin, is more commonly found in dogs than cats. The incidence of hemangiosarcoma in dogs is 25 to 100 times greater than in the human population.[38] Hemangiosarcoma is reported in 0.3 to 2 per cent of canine necropsies and represents approximately 5 per cent of all nonskin primary malignant neoplasms in dogs.[35, 38, 40] A predilection is noted in middle-aged to aged male German shepherds, boxers, and golden retrievers.

In two postmortem studies, 40[40] to 50 per cent[27] of hemangiosarcomas arose from the heart as primary tumors. In a retrospective study of 104 dogs, only 3 per cent originated from the heart but 63 per cent arose from the spleen.[6] The difference in these observations may relate to different populations of dogs or to the difficulty in establishing a primary site when multiple tissues are affected.

Primary cardiac hemangiosarcoma frequently originates in the right atrium at the crista terminalis, a ridge of muscle at the juncture of the right atrium and right auricle (Fig. 155–1), or within the right auricle.[2] Hematogenous metastasis to the lungs, liver, spleen, kidneys, brain, and subcutaneous tissue is common. Signs of right-sided congestive heart failure, with hemorrhagic pericardial fluid, often develop in dogs. Examination of affected dogs may reveal anemia, tachycardia, arrhythmias, muffling of heart sounds, dyspnea, and enlargement of the liver and spleen. More than 50 per cent of affected dogs are borderline to severely anemic.[27] The anemia, often a microangiopathic hemolytic anemia, is characterized by moderate numbers of crenated erythrocytes, schistocytes, poikilocytes, and anisocytes, as well as polychromasia.[43] Patients with hemangiosarcoma may be predisposed to disseminated intravascular co-

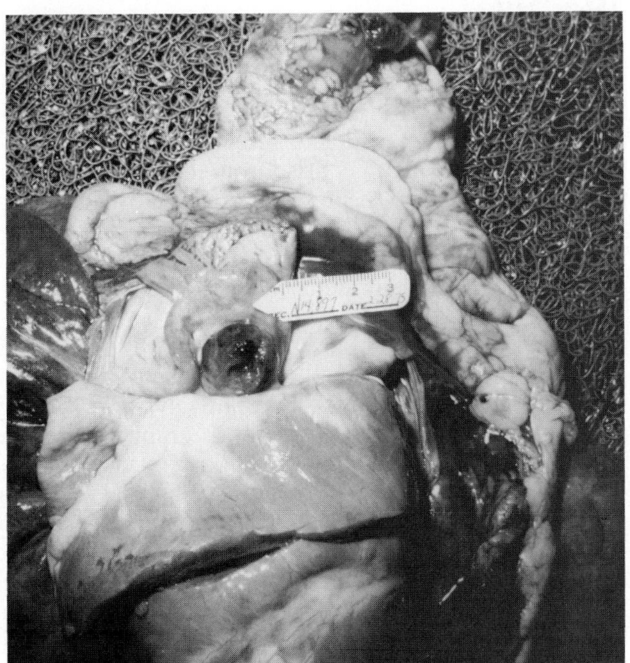

FIGURE 155–1. A circumscribed primary cardiac hemangiosarcoma, 2 cm in diameter, at the junction of the right auricle and atrium in a 9-year-old male Labrador retriever.

agulation. With disseminated intravascular coagulation, the depletion of clotting factors and excessive fibrinolysis cause clotting inadequacy leading to hemorrhage.[12, 28]

Chemodectomas arise from the nonchromaffin paraganglia of the aortic bodies (aortic body tumor, heart base tumor).[25] Although common in older male dogs,[10, 21] they are rare in cats.[8] Chemodectoma is not a hormone-secreting tumor like pheochromocytoma. Clinical signs relate to disease caused by local tissue alteration or metastasis. It has a smooth surface and varies in color and consistency from reddish-brown and fleshy to gray-white and hard. Aortic body tumors may infiltrate the wall of the pulmonary artery or aorta and frequently invade the atria or pericardium.[57] Associated tumors in dogs include interstitial cell testicular tumor, pheochromocytoma, seminoma, adenomatous thyroid neoplasm, and hemangiosarcoma.[21] Aortic body tumors are usually benign, grow slowly, and often become large. Malignant forms may aggressively invade veins, nerves, and lymphatics and metastasize to the lungs, lymph nodes, myocardium, kidneys, brain, and bone.[17, 26, 34, 36] In one study of 29 dogs, 13 per cent of dogs with this neoplasm had evidence of malignancy.[57]

Clinical signs are often those of congestive heart failure (e.g., dyspnea, cough, cyanosis, hepatomegaly, venous engorgement, and ascites). Subcutaneous edema of the head, neck, and forelimbs is sometimes observed. Chemodectoma and other tumors that are situated at the heart base, ectopic thyroid, and parathyroid tumors displace the great vessels, heart, and trachea. These tumors may be visible as diffuse radiodense masses extending from the dorsal cardiac silhouette or heart base. A bloody pericardial effusion is often encountered and may cause cardiac tamponade. Because chemodectomas do not exfoliate, cytological evaluation of the pericardial fluid usually is not diagnostic.

Myxomas account for 30 to 50 per cent of primary cardiac tumors in humans but are rare in dogs.[26, 44] Myxomas are benign neoplasms derived from mesenchymal cells of the subendocardial region. They form polypoid pedunculated masses that arise from the subendocardium of the atria or ventricles, often extending through and sometimes partly occluding the atrioventricular orifice. In humans, they are most often found in the left atrium, but most reports describe the location on the right side of the heart in dogs. Complete surgical excision along the base of the mass with a rim of unaffected endocardium and myocardium is the treatment of choice in dogs.[5]

Fibromas are benign connective tissue tumors that may be of congenital origin[33] and appear less frequently in the heart than elsewhere in the body. In the cardiac chambers, they may be amenable to surgical excision. Clinical signs of the neoplasm relate to mechanical interference of blood flow, and because they are found most frequently in the right heart, clinical signs may mimic tricuspid valve dysfunction or other causes of right-sided heart failure.[31]

Mesotheliomas are rare mesodermal neoplasms that can arise from the pleural, pericardial, or peritoneal cavities. When neoplastic cells arise within the pericardium, they can involve both the parietal and visceral layers, giving the pericardium a shaggy appearance. Mesothelioma may also be nodular and invade adjacent fat, myocardium, local lymphatics, and lymph nodes.[24] Reports of the tumor in dogs[7, 24] and cats[53] do not describe other organ involvement. Most mesotheliomas evolve spontaneously and are sometimes congenital.[1, 4, 18] Asbestosis is a precipitating cause of pleural mesothelioma in humans.[49] Clinical signs of right-sided congestive heart failure, muffling of heart sounds, weak femoral pulses, and exercise intolerance are caused by effusions within the pericardium.

Rhabdomyoma is a benign striated muscle tumor that seldom occurs in the heart.[23] This neoplasm may represent anomalous formation of myocardial fibers, discernible as one or more discrete gray nodules that project into the ventricular lumen.[26]

Sarcomas, other than hemangiosarcoma, occurring as primary cardiac tumors are infrequently reported in dogs[29] and cats, although melanosarcoma, fibrosarcoma, chondrosarcoma, and leiomyosarcoma all have been described in dogs.[56] The physical features of these tumors vary depending on their degree of malignancy.

METASTATIC CARDIAC NEOPLASMS

Although metastatic cardiac tumors occur 10 to 40 times more frequently in humans than do primary cardiac tumors, the opposite is true in dogs. Hemangiosarcoma, pulmonary adenocarcinoma, mammary gland adenocarcinoma, squamous cell carcinoma, and undifferentiated malignant oral tumors (Fig. 155–2) are the most commonly observed metastatic tumors in dogs but occur with low frequency.[29]

Hemangiosarcoma often arises from the right atrium,

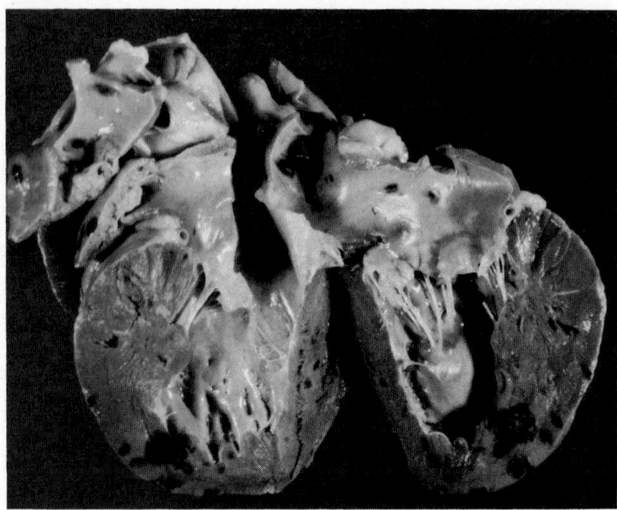

FIGURE 155–2. Metastasis to the left atrium and ventricle from an oral melanosarcoma in a 14-year-old male golden retriever.

but neoplasms may originate from peripheral organs or tissues such as the spleen, liver, or bone and metastasize to the heart and lungs because they have access to vascular channels. Metastatically affected animals exhibit signs similar to those with a primary neoplasm in the heart, except that they may have dominating clinical signs related to the organ from which the tumor arose (e.g., bone pain and abdominal discomfort).

Lymphosarcoma, the most common metastatic heart tumor in cats, rarely invades the hearts of dogs. Its cause in cats is an oncogenic RNA virus (oncornavirus) of the family *Retroviriidae.*[20] Cardiac involvement may exhibit two forms of distribution. In the nodular form, the neoplasm is smoothly nodular, with masses sometimes becoming very large. Neoplasms may resemble fatty accumulations, although they are prone to central necrosis. In the diffusely infiltrative form, the myocardium is irregularly thickened and gray-white, resembling myocardial degeneration and fibrosis. The pericardium, cardiac chambers, and great vessels may be involved.

The cranial mediastinal form of lymphosarcoma has the greatest tendency to afflict the myocardium.[54] Clinical signs of dyspnea, wheezing, coughing, and cyanosis occur with pleural effusion, and large cranial mediastinal masses may displace the heart and cause incompressibility of the cranial chest.

PERIPHERAL VASCULAR NEOPLASMS

Hemangioma, a benign tumor of endothelial cells, must be differentiated from vascular malformations, inflamed hematomas, and vascularized neoplasms. These neoplasms are more prevalent in older dogs (> 9 years) with pigmented skin, Scottish terriers, Airedales, Kerry blue terriers, and Labrador retrievers.[48]

These dark-red to reddish-black tumors may develop in any location but are usually found in the subcutis or dermis of the leg, flank, neck, face, eyelid, or scrotum.[52] They are ovoid to discoid, 0.5 to 3.0 cm in diameter, and firm. Histologically, they consist of endothelium-lined spaces that may contain blood, lymph, or thrombi.[48] If located in scrotal tissue or other sensitive, exposed areas of the body, excessive bleeding may result from trauma or self-mutilation.[52] Tumor recurrence is not a problem after complete resection of the mass.

Hemangiosarcoma may arise from many tissues; however, the most common sites of peripheral origin in dogs are the spleen, liver, bone, and skin. Hemangiosarcomas have a high metastatic potential, and survival rates are discouraging. Frequent metastatic sites include the liver, lungs, heart, and brain.

Clinical findings include various signs relating to the degree of organ involvement and metastatic spread. The course of clinical signs may be relatively short, usually 1 to 3 weeks, in which dogs begin to exhibit progressive lethargy, pallor, anorexia, weight loss, weakness, and dyspnea. Acute collapse related to internal bleeding within the thorax or abdomen is common. Dogs may recover only to have signs recur. Icterus may be noted with hemothorax or hemoperitoneum. Renal involvement may be suggested by periodic to persistent hematuria and proteinuria.[12] Cutaneous forms characteristically have soft, dark, fluctuant subcutaneous masses that are not often ulcerated. Bone involvement may produce pain in the affected area, lameness, and radiographic evidence of bone lysis.

Abdominal palpation is helpful in detecting masses involving the spleen, liver, and kidneys. Gentle palpation is recommended, because the tumors are fragile and affected dogs are uncomfortable.

Pulmonary metastases form small miliary nodules in the parenchyma; they may not be identifiable on routine thoracic radiographs. As pulmonary involvement progresses, the lesions may become more evident and pleural effusions may occur. A serosanguineous to hemorrhagic fluid that does not clot is often encountered by paracentesis.

Hematological evaluation of peripheral blood may help in diagnosis because a majority of dogs with hemangiosarcoma exhibit regenerative anemia. Erythrocyte regeneration is uncommon in dogs with other forms of neoplasia, when it is more common to note suppression of hematopoiesis.[27, 58] Disseminated intravascular coagulation may be encountered when large quantities of blood are sequestered in tumor sites. The diagnosis is established by the presence of hemorrhage at other locations, with decreasing numbers of platelets, increasing prothrombin time, and decreased fibrinogen.[37]

The treatment of choice for hemangiosarcoma is surgical removal, but because most tumors have metastasized by the time they are recognized, the prognosis is guarded. Chemotherapy has been tried but with limited success in bringing about temporary remission and increased survival time.[11, 12, 14] Various chemotherapeutic agents including cyclophosphamide, vincristine, methotrexate, and doxorubicin have been used, but reports describe no significant difference in survival time.[6, 16]

Chemodectomas originating from the carotid bodies (carotid body tumor) occur less frequently but are more often malignant than chemodectomas originating from the aortic body. The carotid body tumor is a unilateral mass near the angle of the jaw.[22] Clinical signs of dysphagia or dyspnea due to compression of the esophagus or trachea may be encountered as the mass enlarges and invades surrounding structures.

Multicentric neoplastic transformation of chemoreceptor tissue occurs frequently, as 65 per cent of carotid body tumors also have concurrent aortic body tumors. In 30 per cent of affected dogs, metastasis occurs to the lungs, bronchial and mediastinal lymph nodes, liver, pancreas, kidneys, and bone.[13]

Neoplasms of the carotid body are often rounded, red, and thinly encapsulated and surround the bifurcation of the common carotid artery.[47] Carotid body tumors involve the mastoid process and the vagus, accessory, and hypoglossal cranial nerves. The cranial sympathetic ganglion and trunk may be invaded.[13] Pulsation of the neoplasm may be seen in the neck. These neoplasms must be differentiated from ectopic thyroid and parathyroid tumors. They displace the trachea and surrounding structures.[26]

Carotid body tumors are difficult to remove surgically because of local extension into vessel walls and nerves. The high degree of malignancy, with metastatic involvement of other structures, dictates a guarded prognosis. Chemodectomas are radiosensitive, and some animals may respond.[55]

DIAGNOSIS OF CARDIAC NEOPLASIA

Cardiac neoplasia should be suspected as a potential cause of heart failure in dogs with a breed predisposition to certain tumor types. Clinical signs of heart failure—exercise intolerance, dyspnea, fluid retention, arrhythmias, weak arterial pulses, and abnormal heart sounds—are common to many neoplastic disorders as well as to the usual causes of failure, valvular endocardiosis and myocardial degeneration.

Radiography may be useful in determining the presence of cardiac neoplasms and in detecting metastasis. Radiographic changes include cardiomegaly, abnormal cardiac silhouette, tracheobronchial lymph node enlargement, vena cava distension, elevation of the trachea, pleural effusion, and pulmonary edema. The cardiac silhouette may increase in size and become circular if pericardial effusion occurs. Dorsal displacement of the trachea at the heart base, accompanied by tissue density ventral to the trachea and pericardial effusion, is often recognized with heart base tumors.

An electrocardiogram can provide supportive information relating to the presence of pericardial effusion because the QRS amplitude often becomes dampened or reduced. Low-voltage QRS complexes, accompanied by electrical alternans, suggest pericardial effusion. Arrhythmias, although nonspecific for tumor involvement, suggest serious myocardial disease, especially with other clinical features of failure.

Echocardiography helps define the presence, location, and size of cardiac masses and documents the presence of pericardial effusion.[50, 51] With echocardiography, a more accurate list of differential diagnoses may be made because certain tumors have a location and physical

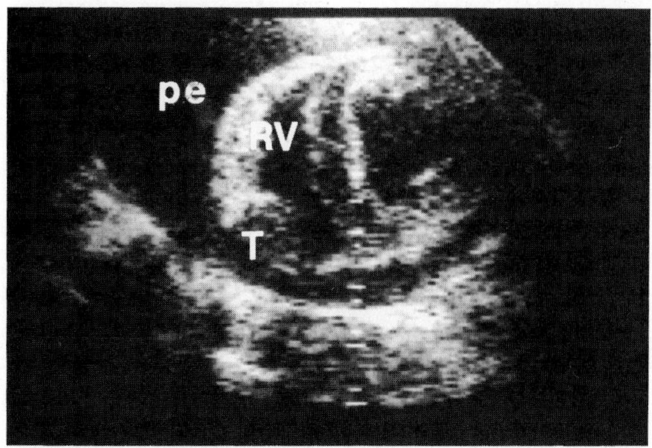

FIGURE 155–3. Two-dimensional echocardiogram. Eight-year-old male golden retriever with primary cardiac hemangiosarcoma. Short-axis view of the heart from a right parasternal position. Pericardial effusion (pe) is present, allowing excellent observation of the entire heart. The well-circumscribed neoplasm (T) is identifiable within the wall of the right ventricle (RV).

features that allow some differentiation (Fig. 155–3). Primary and metastatic hemangiosarcomas are often found in the right atrium. Aortic body tumors arise at the base of the aorta between the aorta and the pulmonary artery. Pericardial effusion is common to both of these conditions. Myxomas are exclusively found within the cardiac chambers, as are most fibromas and other forms of benign tumor, fibroma, chondroma, and rhabdomyoma. Metastatic tumors, various sarcomas, and adenocarcinomas may produce lesions within the walls of the right and left ventricle and interventricular septum. These tumors are more difficult to identify because the tissue density may be similar to cardiac muscle. Necrosis and modification of the morphology of the ventricular or atrial walls may allow detection by careful two-dimensional echocardiographic study. The more accurately tumors can be identified, the more likely a treatment plan can be developed and a prognosis established.

Biopsy of cardiac masses is difficult, often requiring exploratory thoracotomy. Tissue from intramural lesions can be obtained by guided transvenous myocardial biopsy catheters. Neoplastic involvement of the myocardium might be missed if the tumor is not distributed throughout the structure. Information about the nature of most cardiac tumors should await surgical exploration. A diagnosis can sometimes be established by identifying neoplastic cells in pericardial effusions. Mesotheliomas and other tumors that exfoliate may be identified by cytological evaluation of pericardial fluid.

Both angiocardiography and intracardiac pressure measurements can provide valuable complementary information to echocardiography by further defining the location and extent of cardiac luminal involvement and the neoplasm's effect on hemodynamic performance.[9, 50] Angiocardiograms (Fig. 155–4) help a surgeon determine if resection of the mass is surgically feasible.[3, 5] Surgical relief of right ventricular outflow tract obstruction by a large myxoma has been described.[5]

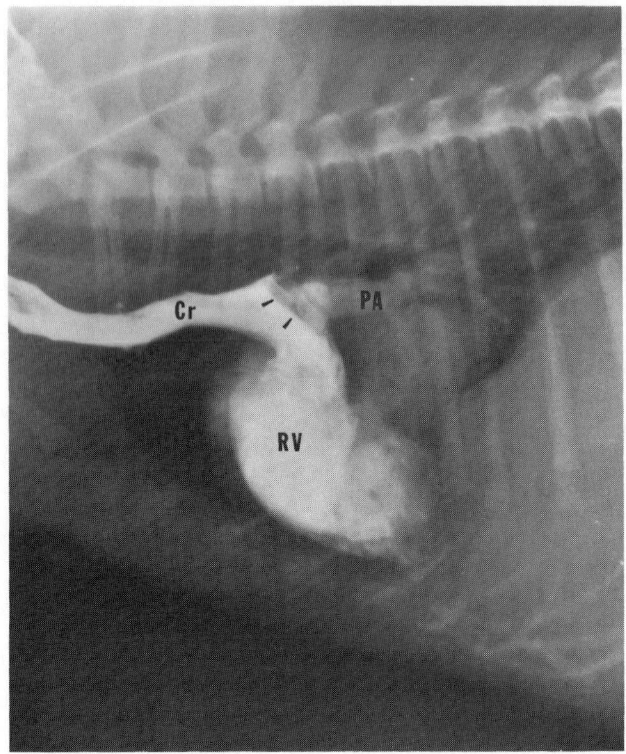

FIGURE 155–4. A nonselective angiocardiogram showing impaired caudal right atrial filling caused by an invasive aortic body tumor. Arrows show the cranial edge of the mass, which caused a redirection of blood flow in the right atrium. (RV, right ventricle; Cr, cranial vena cava; PA, pulmonary artery.)

TREATMENT OF CARDIAC NEOPLASIA

Solitary cardiac tumors that have not metastasized may be treated surgically if they are accessible and do not involve large portions of the myocardial wall. Careful preoperative screening of space-occupying lesions via echocardiography and angiocardiography can provide enough information to make surgery worthwhile. Exploratory thoracotomy is indicated as a diagnostic or a therapeutic procedure to treat certain neoplastic conditions of the heart and pericardium.[2] Solitary hemangiomas or hemangiosarcomas, which are isolated to the right atrial wall, and fibromas and myxomas located in the right heart are the most surgically approachable. Resection of right atrial hemangiosarcoma can be accomplished, but surgical and postoperative complications, coagulopathies, arrhythmias, and tumor recurrence are expected.[2, 46] Mean survival time in one group was 4 months.[2] Surgical removal of some intraluminal cardiac masses in the right heart is possible without cardiopulmonary bypass if the mass is pedunculated, as are some myxomas and fibromas.[5] Surgical success depends on finding small isolated tumors in approachable locations.

Aortic body tumors can be resected rarely, but removal of the pericardial sac when pericardial tamponade is a problem can relieve clinical signs and extend an animal's life. Irradiation of these tumors has resulted in remission in a few animals.[55]

There is little useful information about the chemotherapy of cardiac tumors, although some success is claimed in the therapy of hemangiosarcoma.[12, 16] Chemotherapy has the potential to extend survival in dogs or cats with cardiac lymphosarcoma, although there are no data to support this claim.

Recent developments in diagnostic methods and aggressive approaches in surgery have extended the hope for long-term survival in dogs with certain forms of cardiac neoplasia. Surgical removal of a right ventricular tumor allowed recovery and freedom of recurrence for more than 2 years.[5] I have observed complete long-term recovery of two dogs, one with a right atrial hemangioma and the other with right atrial hemangiosarcoma, after surgical removal. Unfortunately, many animals with cardiac neoplasia have metastatic or locally invasive disease at diagnosis, limiting our ability to improve survival time with surgery or chemotherapy. With widespread disease, the prognosis is grave.

References

1. Andrews EJ: Pleural mesothelioma in a cat. *J Comp Pathol 83*:259, 1973.
2. Aronsohn M: Cardiac hemangiosarcoma in the dog: A review of 38 cases. *J Am Vet Med Assoc 187*:922, 1985.
3. Atkins CE, et al: Diagnosis of an intracardiac fibrosarcoma using two-dimensional echocardiography. *J Am Anim Hosp Assoc 20*:131, 1984.
4. Baskerville A: Mesothelioma in the calf. *Vet Pathol 4*:149, 1967.
5. Bright JM, et al: Right ventricular outflow obstruction caused by primary cardiac neoplasia: Clinical features in two dogs. *J Vet Intern Med 4*:12, 1989.
6. Brown NO, et al: Canine hemangiosarcoma: Retrospective analysis of 104 cases. *J Am Vet Med Assoc 186*:56, 1985.
7. Brunner P: Papillary polypus mesothelioma of the pericardium of a dog. *Virchows Arch [A] 357*:257, 1972.
8. Buergelt CD, Das KM: Aortic body tumor in a cat: A case report. *Vet Pathol 5*:84, 1968.
9. Cantwell HD, et al: Angiographic diagnosis of heartbase tumor in the dog. *J Am Anim Hosp Assoc 18*:83, 1982.
10. Capen CC: Tumors of the endocrine glands. *In* Moulton JE (ed): *Tumors in Domestic Animals*. University of California Press, Berkeley, 1978, pp 372–429.
11. Couto CG, Helfand SC: VAC chemotherapy for metastatic and non-resectable soft tissue tumors in the dog. Proceedings of the Veterinary Cancer Society, 6th Annual Conference. *6*:28, 1986.
12. Crow SE: Hematuria associated with renal hemangiosarcoma in a dog. *J Am Vet Med Assoc 176*:531, 1980.
13. Dean MJ, Strafuss AC: Carotid body tumors in the dog: A review and report of four cases. *J Am Vet Med Assoc 166*:1003, 1975.
14. deMadron E, et al: Use of chemotherapy for treatment of cardiac hemangiosarcoma in a dog. *J Am Vet Med Assoc 190*:887, 1987.
15. Detweiler DK: Wesen und Haufigkeit von Herzkrankheiten bei Hunden. *Zentralbl Veterinarmed 9*:317, 1962.
16. Fees DL, Withrow SJ: Canine hemangiosarcoma. *Comp Cont Educ Pract Vet 3*:1047, 1981.
17. Gliatto JM: Multiple organ metastasis in an aortic body tumor in a boxer. *J Am Vet Med Assoc 191*:1110, 1987.
18. Grant CA: Congenital tumors of calves. Report of 2 cases of mesothelioma and a tumor apparently of reticuloendothelial origin. *Zentralbl Veterinarmed 5*:231, 1958.
19. Hardy WD: Hematopoietic tumors of cats. *J Am Anim Hosp Assoc 17*:921, 1981.
20. Hardy WD, McClelland AJ: Feline leukemia virus: Its related diseases and control. *Vet Clin North Am 7*:93, 1977.
21. Hayes HM, Fraumeni JF. Chemodectoma in dogs: Epidemiologic comparisons with men. *J Natl Cancer Inst 52*:1455, 1974.
22. Hubben K, et al: Carotid body tumor in the dog. *J Am Vet Med Assoc 137*:411, 1960.
23. Hulland TJ: Tumors of muscle. *In* Moulton JE (ed): *Tumors in Domestic Animals*. University of California Press, Berkeley, 1978, pp 75–88.
24. Ikede BO, et al: Pericardial mesothelioma with cardiac tamponade in a dog. *Vet Pathol 17*:496, 1980.
25. Jackson C: The incidence and pathology of tumors of domesticated animals in South Africa: A study of the Onderstepoort collection of neoplasms with special reference to their histopathology. *J Vet Sci Anim Ind 6*:1, 1936.
26. Jubb KVF, Kennedy PC: The circulatory system: Neoplasms of the heart.

In Jubb KVF, Kennedy PC (eds): *Pathology of Domestic Animals*. Academic Press, New York, 1970, pp 121–122.
27. Kleine LJ, et al: Primary cardiac hemangiosarcoma in dogs. *J Am Vet Med Assoc 157*:326, 1970.
28. Legendre AM, Krehbiel JD: Disseminated intravascular coagulation in a dog with hemothorax and hemangiosarcoma. *J Am Vet Med Assoc 171*:1070, 1977.
29. Liu SK: Pathology of feline heart diseases. *Vet Clin North Am 7*:323, 1977.
30. Liu SK, Hsu FS: Neoplasms of the heart and large vessels. *In* Liu SK, Hsu FS (eds): *An Atlas of Cardiovascular Pathology*. Wonder Enterprise and Shin Chaan Colar Printing, Tainan, Taiwan, ROC, 1989, pp 347–364.
31. Lombard CW, Goldschmidt MH: Primary fibroma in the right atrium of a dog. *J Small Anim Pract 21*:439, 1980.
32. Loppnow H von: Zur kasuistik primarer herztumoren beim hund (Zwei falle von hamangiom am rechten herzohr). *Berl Munch Tierarztl Wochenschr 74*:214, 1961.
33. McAllister HA Jr: Primary tumors of the heart and pericardium. *In* Sommers SC, Rosen PP (eds): *Pathology Annual:* Part 2. Appleton-Century-Crofts, New York, 1979, pp 325–355.
34. Montgomery DL, et al: Malignant aortic body tumor with metastasis to bone in a dog. *Vet Pathol 17*:241, 1980.
35. Moulton JE: Tumors of the skin and soft tissues. *In* Moulton JE (ed): *Tumors in Domestic Animals*. University of California Press, Berkeley, 1978, pp 35–36.
36. Nilsson T: Heart-base tumors in dogs. *Acta Pathol Microbiol Scand 37*:385, 1955.
37. O'Keefe DA, et al: Coagulation abnormalities associated with neoplasia. *Vet Clin North Am Small Anim Pract 18*:157, 1988.
38. Oksanen A: Haemangiosarcoma in dogs. *J Comp Pathol 88*:585, 1978.
39. Patnaik AJ, Liu SK: Angiosarcomas in cats. *J Small Anim Pract 18*:191, 1977.
40. Pearson GR, Head KW: Malignant haemangioendothelioma (angiosarcoma) in the dog. *J Small Anim Pract 17*:737, 1976.
41. Pirie HM: The pathology of heart diseases in the dog. *J Small Anim Pract 8*:175, 1967.
42. Priester WA, McKay FW: The occurrence of tumors in domestic animals. *Natl Cancer Inst Monogr 54*:1, 1980.
43. Rebar AH, et al: Microangiopathic hemolytic anemia associated with radiation induced hemangiosarcoma. *Vet Pathol 17*:443, 1980.
44. Roberts SR: Myxoma of the heart in a dog. *J Am Vet Med Assoc 134*:185, 1959.
45. Ryan CP, Walder EJ: Feline fibrosarcoma of the heart. *Calif Vet 8*:12, 1980.
46. Scavelli TD, et al: Hemangiosarcoma in the cat: Retrospective evaluation of 31 surgical cases. *J Am Vet Med Assoc 187*:817, 1985.
47. Scotti TM: The carotid body tumor in dogs. *J Am Vet Med Assoc 132*:413, 1958.
48. Stannard AA, Pulley LT: Tumors of the skin and soft tissues. *In* Moulton JE (ed): *Tumors in Domestic Animals*. University of California Press, Berkeley, 1978, pp 16–74.
49. Stanton MF, Wrench C: Mechanisms of mesothelioma induction with asbestos and fibrous glass. *J Natl Cancer Inst 48*:797, 1972.
50. Swartout MS, et al: Intracardiac tumors in two dogs. *J Am Anim Hosp Assoc 23*:533, 1987.
51. Thomas WP, et al: Detection of cardiac masses in dogs by two-dimensional echocardiography. *Vet Radiol 25*:65, 1984.
52. Thornburg LP, Breitschwert EB: Canine hemangioma of the scrotum with fatal bleeding: a case report. *J Am Anim Hosp Assoc 12*:797, 1976.
53. Tilley LR, et al: Pericardial mesothelioma with effusions in a cat. *J Am Anim Hosp Assoc 11*:60, 1975.
54. Tilley LR, et al: Cardiovascular tumors in the cat. *J Am Anim Hosp Assoc 17*:1009, 1981.
55. Turrel JM: Principles of radiation therapy. Part II—Clinical applications. *In* Theilen GH, Madewell BR (eds): *Veterinary Cancer Medicine*. Lea & Febiger, Philadelphia, 1987, pp 144–156.
56. Vicini DS, et al: Cardiac fibrosarcoma in a dog. *J Am Vet Med Assoc 189*:1486, 1986.
57. Yates WD, et al: Chemoreceptor tumors diagnosed at the Western College of Veterinary Medicine. 1967–1979. *Can Vet J 21*:124, 1980.
58. Zook BC: Some spontaneous cardiovascular lesions in dogs and cats. *Adv Cardiol 13*:148, 1974.

CHAPTER 156 Hematopoietic System

Stuart C. Helfand and David M. Vail

CANINE HEMATOPOIETIC SYSTEM

Lymphoma

Epidemiology

Lymphoma (lymphosarcoma) is defined as a lymphoid neoplasm primarily affecting lymph nodes or other solid visceral organs such as the liver or spleen.[27, 110] With an annual incidence of 24:100,000, lymphoma accounts for 5 per cent of all canine malignant neoplasia and 83 per cent of all canine hematopoietic malignancies.[36, 110, 192] Middle-aged to older (median age of 5.5 to 9.1 years) dogs are primarily affected, with no sex predilection.[89, 192] Although it can occur in any purebred or mixed-breed dog, it may be more prevalent in German shepherds, boxers, poodles, basset hounds, and Saint Bernards.[89, 192]

Etiology

The cause of canine lymphoma is unknown. A retroviral etiology for certain forms has been demonstrated in cats, chickens, cattle, and humans. Numerous reports describe C-type virus particles in canine lymphoma tissue and increased reverse transcriptase activity in some canine lymphoma and lymphoid leukemia samples.[19, 78, 98, 156, 212] A viral etiology is unconfirmed.

Diagnostics and Staging

Various classifications are used because of the varied presentations for canine lymphoma. Traditionally, canine lymphoma is classified according to anatomical site (Table 156–1); the majority are multicentric.[27, 36] Dogs with multicentric lymphoma usually are presented because of increased lymph node size, nonspecific signs of

TABLE 156–1. ANATOMICAL FORMS OF CANINE LYMPHOMA

Anatomical Form	Frequency (Percentage of Total Cases)
Multicentric	84
Alimentary	6.9
Cutaneous	6.3
Mediastinal	2.2
Miscellaneous	0.6

inappetence, weight loss, polyuria/polydypsia, and lethargy. Other presentations, related to anatomical site (e.g., diarrhea with gastrointestinal, dyspnea with cranial mediastinal lymphoma), are discussed later.

The differential diagnosis for lymphadenopathies includes infectious diseases (e.g., bacterial, viral, parasitic, and fungal), immune-mediated diseases (e.g., systemic lupus), and other neoplasms metastatic to lymph nodes. The diagnosis of lymphoma is best established after biopsy. Although fine-needle aspirates of lymph nodes, spleen, or liver can suggest neoplasia, conclusive histological diagnosis from lymph node biopsy is recommended. An entire accessible lymph node should be removed to preserve tissue architecture. It is best not to sample lymph nodes draining more reactive areas of the body (e.g., submandibular lymph nodes in the presence of periodontal disease) to decrease the likelihood of reactive lymphoid hyperplasia masking the neoplastic disease.

In addition to histological confirmation, diagnostic procedures may allow clinical staging according to the World Health Organization[233] (Table 156–2). Complete staging includes a complete blood count (CBC), platelet count, bone marrow aspirate/core, biochemistry profile, and thoracic and abdominal radiographs. CBC and platelet count values are especially important, because the presence of myelosuppression or cytopenia may necessitate modification of the chemotherapeutic protocols initiated. Morrison and colleagues have recommended bronchoalveolar lavage to further stage canine lymphoma, because 6 of 15 dogs with lymphoma that had the procedure required an upgrade of staging from III or IV to V.[150] The prognostic or clinical significance resulting from a change in clinical stage following bronchoalveolar lavage is unknown.

Up to 96 per cent of dogs with multicentric lymphoma have one or more hematological, biochemical, or bone marrow abnormalities.[131] Hematological disorders reported in decreasing order[131] include atypical circulating immature lymphocytes (65 per cent), thrombocytopenia (49 per cent), eosinopenia (48 per cent), altered bone marrow myeloid/erythroid ratio (44 per cent), anemia (38 per cent), bone marrow infiltration with neoplastic lymphocytes (36 per cent), and nucleated erythrocytes (18 per cent). The anemia is usually chronic (normocytic, normochromic, and nonregenerative); however, a small percentage have indices compatible with blood loss or hemolysis. Bone marrow involvement occurs in 23 to 83 per cent of lymphoma cases.[131, 178, 209, 220, 222] Bone marrow cores are more diagnostic of infiltration than aspirates; a 57 per cent incidence was found in 53 dogs studied. Only 27 per cent of dogs were diagnosed with leukemias based on peripheral smears alone; therefore, more than half of leukemic dogs are understaged without bone marrow analysis.

TABLE 156–2. WORLD HEALTH ORGANIZATION CLINICAL STAGING FOR LYMPHOMA*

Stage	Criteria
I	Involvement limited to single lymph node or lymphoid tissue in a single organ (excluding bone marrow)
II	Involvement of many lymph nodes in regional area (with or without tonsils)
III	Generalized lymph node involvement
IV	Liver and/or spleen involvement (with or without stage III)
V	Manifestations in blood and involvement of bone marrow and/or other organ systems (with or without stages I to IV)

*Each stage is subclassified into (a) without systemic signs and (b) with systemic signs.

From World Health Organization: *TNM Classification of Tumors in Domestic Animals*. World Health Organization, Geneva, 1980.)

Attempts have been made to subclassify canine lymphoma histologically into low-, moderate-, and high-grade subtypes[18, 91] (Table 156–3). The majority of multicentric canine lymphomas are moderate to high grade. Efforts to immunophenotype canine lymphoma for subclassification are not clinically applicable at present.[78, 102, 197]

Radiographically, 60 per cent of dogs with lymphoma have sternal lymph node enlargement, 55 per cent splenomegaly, 50 per cent sublumbar lymph node enlargement, and 47 per cent hepatomegaly.[2] Although none of these radiographic abnormalities are diagnostic, they can be useful in staging.

Ophthalmic abnormalities are common in dogs with lymphoma. Complete ophthalmic examinations per-

TABLE 156–3. NATIONAL CANCER INSTITUTE WORKING FORMULATION FOR CLASSIFICATION OF NON-HODGKIN'S LYMPHOMA; FREQUENCY IN 92 CANINE CASES IN PERCENTAGE OF CASES

Grade	Abbreviation	Cell Type	Percentage of Cases
Low	DSL	Diffuse small lymphocytic cell	6.5
	FSC	Follicular small cleaved cell	1.0
	FM	Follicular mixed small cleaved and large cell	0
Intermediate	FL	Follicular large cell	0
	DSC	Diffuse small cleaved cell	4.0
	DM	Diffuse mixed small cleaved and large cell	1.0
	DL	Diffuse large cell, noncleaved or cleaved	13.0
High	IB	Immunoblastic, secretory or nonsecretory	11.0
	LB	Lymphoblastic, nonconvoluted or convoluted	30.0
	SNC	Diffuse small noncleaved cells	26.0
Unclassified			6.5

Modified from Carter RF, et al: Chemotherapy of canine lymphoma with histopathological correlation: Doxorubicin alone compared to COP as first treatment regimen. *J Am Animal Hosp Assoc 23*:587, 1987.

formed on 98 dogs revealed that 37 per cent had one or more abnormalities.[100] These include uveitis, hemorrhage, and ocular infiltration. Dogs with ocular changes are more likely to have hematological abnormalities, and 75 per cent of those with ocular hemorrhage were thrombocytopenic.

Overall, 15 to 20 per cent of dogs with multicentric lymphoma and approximately half of those with mediastinal forms are hypercalcemic.[131, 230] The majority of dogs with bone marrow infiltration in one study were hypercalcemic, lending support to the presence of a hormone-like substance, likely an osteoclast-activating factor, elicited by the neoplastic cells in the bone marrow.[131] Hypercalcemia in dogs with lymphoma was reported to be due to a parathyroid hormone-like protein, and in dogs for which lymphocyte typing was investigated, the tumors were composed of T cells.[228, 229] A thorough investigation for lymphoma is carried out whenever hypercalcemia of unknown origin is encountered, including careful physical examination with special attention to lymph nodes, thoracic radiographs, and bone marrow aspirate. Abdominal ultrasonography and exploratory laparotomy may be necessary before a diagnosis can be made.

Prognostic Indicators

Age, body weight, and breed do not affect duration, remission, or overall survival. Most larger studies fail to reveal a relationship between clinical stage and response to therapy[122, 124]; however, bone marrow involvement (especially with associated CBC abnormalities) is associated with decreased long-term survival.[23, 123] Although not all reports agree, female dogs have significantly prolonged remission and survival times, median survival of 375 days for females compared with 214 for males.[124] Neutering was not a risk factor for either sex. Attempts to correlate survival with histopathological grade have failed.[18, 231] Dogs with low-grade histology based on the National Cancer Institute Working Formulation are significantly less likely to attain remission; however, their overall survivals are similar to high-grade lymphomas.[18] These data imply that if one could initially identify the small percentage of low-grade canine lymphomas, affected animals could be spared the side effects of systemic chemotherapy, thereby increasing quality of life without compromising length of survival. Dogs with high-grade lymphoma may indeed survive because of therapy, whereas those with low-grade disease survive despite therapy.

Therapy of Multicentric Lymphoma

Without treatment, most dogs with lymphoma die in 4 to 6 weeks.[11] Treatment of canine lymphoma can be quite gratifying because of the high percentage of complete remission and good quality of life throughout the length of remission. With few exceptions, canine lymphoma is a systemic disease and requires systemic therapy to achieve remission and lengthen survival. Systemic chemotherapy is the therapy of choice for canine lymphoma. Although single-agent chemotherapy may be less expensive and less toxic, with the notable exception of doxorubicin, it is not as effective as combination chemotherapy. All drugs used in combination protocols should have proven efficacy alone before they are incorporated into a protocol. There are nearly as many chemotherapeutic protocols published for canine lymphoma as there are veterinary oncologists. The ideal chemotherapeutic protocol remains in question. Inherent drawbacks in comparing survival and remission data in various published protocols include the small numbers involved; lack of randomization; different staging systems and staging criteria; various study endpoints, including the reasons for euthanasia or death; use of mean versus median; varied drug dosages, routes of administration, and duration; and the lack of histological grading. Published protocols with reported remission and survival data are presented (Table 156–4). Regardless of the protocol used, the majority of published reports have comparable remission rates and remission and survival durations. MacEwen and colleagues[128] reported median remission and survival times of 214 and 351 days, respectively, after induction chemotherapy with vincristine, cyclophosphamide, doxorubicin, and either native L-asparaginase or PEG-L-asparaginase (a conjugate of L-asparaginase with polyethylene glycol) followed by maintenance therapy with native or conjugated L-asparaginase. These remission and survival times are the longest yet recorded for canine lymphoma treatment protocols. PEG-L-asparaginase was as effective as native L-asparaginase but was better tolerated. Unlike humans, dogs with lymphoma are still rarely cured; all protocols apparently reach the same 6- to 8-month remission failure. Readers are referred to the chapters on chemotherapy and tumor biology for discussion of tumor drug resistance and treatment failures.

Drug therapy for multicentric lymphoma may have to be altered based on the presence of one or more cytopenias. Most importantly, thrombocytopenia ($<$ 75,000/μl) and neutropenia ($<$ 2,500/μl) are cause for concern. Common chemotherapeutics that spare bone marrow and are usually safe with low white blood cell and platelet counts include prednisone, L-asparaginase, and vincristine. If myelosuppression is due to concurrent chemotherapy, discontinuing the chemotherapy for 5 to 7 days, repeating the CBC/platelet count, and reinstituting therapy at a decreased dose or frequency may be necessary.

Lymphoma is a drug-sensitive tumor; rapid tumor cell death is the rule rather than the exception. Lymphoma cells are so exquisitely sensitive that a serious life-threatening sequel of therapy known as *tumor lysis syndrome* can develop. Breakdown of tumor cells releases nucleic acid purines, lactate, and uric acid, causing hyperuricemia, hyperphosphatemia, hyperkalemia, hypocalcemia, and lactic acidosis.[105] These by-products must be cleared by renal excretion, hepatic metabolism, or a combination of the two. Although tumor lysis syndrome is common in human patients with widespread lymphoma, it is rare in dogs. The rarity of this condition may be due to hepatic uricase, which converts uric acid to allantoin, an enzyme system not present in humans or Dalmatians.[105, 161] Two dogs with lymphoma devel-

TABLE 156–4. PUBLISHED CHEMOTHERAPEUTIC PROTOCOLS FOR CANINE LYMPHOMA

Drug Protocol	Case Numbers	Complete Remission Rate (%)	Median (Mean) Remission Time (Days)	Median (Mean) Survival Time (Days)	Reference
1. CTX, 50 mg/m² PO daily × 4 days/week × 8 Ara-C, 100 mg/m² IV daily × 4 days VCR, 0.5 mg/m²/week IV × 8 Prednisone, 40 mg/m² × 7 days, then 20 mg/m² every 2 days thereafter Maintenance: CTX, 50 mg/m²/day PO × 4 days/week Prednisone, 10 mg/m² BID every 48 hours or 6-MP, 50 mg/m²/day PO or MTX, 2.5 mg/m² PO BID weekly	20	65	66	186	Couto[27]
2. CTX, 300 mg/m² PO every 3 weeks VCR, 0.75 mg/m²/week IV × 4 weeks, then every 3 weeks Prednisone, 1 mg/kg/day PO × 21 day, then every 2 days	77	75	180	N/R	Cotter[23]
3. Protocol 2 above for 7 weeks, then doxorubicin, 30 mg/m² replaces every third CTX treatment. All therapy stopped at 78 weeks	46	83	210	N/R	Cotter and Goldstein[26]
4. VCR, 0.7 mg/m² IV day 1, 14 L-Asparaginase, 400 IU/kg IP or IM day 1 CTX, 200–250 mg/m² IV day 7 MTX, 0.6–0.8 mg/kg IV day 7 Repeat procedure above, except use L-asparaginase for rescue only; substitute chlorambucil (1.4 mg/kg) PO for CTX if dog is in remission	147	77	140	265	MacEwen et al[123, 124]
5. Doxorubicin, 30 mg/m² IV every 21 days × 5 courses	37	59	131	230	Pastorino et al[173]
6. Protocol 5 plus rescue with CTX, VCR, prednisone, L-asparaginase	21	76	206 (189)	270 (265)	Carter et al[18]

CTX, cyclophosphamide; Ara-C, cytosine arabinoside; VCR, vincristine; 6-mR, 6-mercaptopurine; MTX, methotrexate.
Modified from MacEwen EG, Young KM: Canine lymphoma and lymphoid leukemias. *In* Withrow SJ, MacEwen EG (eds): *Clinical Veterinary Oncology*. J.B. Lippincott, Philadelphia, 1989.

oped tumor lysis syndrome after staged whole-body radiotherapy.[105] It may be wise to consider the possibility of tumor lysis syndrome when treating dogs with large tumor burdens and to maintain hydration to decrease its development.

Therapy for hypercalcemia secondary to lymphoma is best accomplished by attaining disease remission. If necessary, diuresis with high-sodium crystalloids (0.9 per cent sodium chloride) delivered at twice maintenance volumes alone or in combination with furosemide is usually successful. The addition of prednisone decreases serum calcium levels; however, it should only be started after a diagnosis. Salmon calcitonin, mithramycin, and newer diphosphonates are not yet evaluated in animals.

Dogs with stage III and IV lymphoma have altered carbohydrate metabolism that parallels alterations in human cancer patients suffering from the paraneoplastic syndrome of cancer cachexia.[218, 219] They were hyperlactatemic and insulin resistant. Infusion of lactated Ringer solution or dextrose-containing solutions exacerbated elevated blood lactate levels. Although the clinical significance of these elevations in lactic acid is unknown, it may be prudent to avoid such fluid types when considering fluid replacement therapy.

Splenectomy in specific cases of canine lymphoma has been reported[13] but should receive limited use. Human lymphoma patients with increased survival after splenectomy are those with splenic rupture, autoimmune complications, massive splenomegaly, or lymphoma present solely in the spleen.[13]

Rescue therapy, defined as an attempt to re-establish remission once an animal's disease reasserts itself, has not been carefully studied in animals. If the disease returns while an animal is on chemotherapy, those drugs being used should be discontinued in favor of alternates. However, if a drug used in the past was not currently being used when the disease returned, it may still be an effective choice and can be reinstated if superior alternatives do not exist. Reports on the use of doxorubicin alone[16] or doxorubicin in combination with dacarbazine[223] in small groups of dogs revealed rates of reinduction of complete remission of 33 and 24 per cent, respectively. Although no prospective randomized studies on rescue chemotherapy exist, most investigators believe the likelihood of attaining a new remission and the length of the subsequent remission are usually half that of the previous success.

Immunotherapy

A growing number of studies have been devoted to combining immunotherapy (either specific or nonspecific stimulation of the immune system) with traditional chemotherapy to increase length and quality of remissions. MacEwen and colleagues[122] reported on 98 dogs with lymphoma that were randomized into either chemotherapy alone (vincristine, cyclophosphamide, methotrexate, and L-asparaginase) versus chemotherapy plus the nonspecific immunomodulator levamisole. No significant difference in response resulted between therapy groups. Early studies combining systemic chemotherapy with autogenous tumor vaccines prepared from the dog's own tumor did result in increased duration of remission and total survival time.[37] These tumor vaccines included the nonspecific immunostimulant Freund adjuvant, which subsequently was shown to enhance remission and survival as well on its own as when combined with tumor cells.[232]

Reports have combined chemotherapy with more specific forms of immunotherapy, including intralymphatic delivery of autochthonous tumor cell vaccines without Freund adjuvant.[94–96] Overall remission and survival duration are not significantly altered with autochthonous vaccines, although a trend toward increased survival is apparent with the addition of the vaccines. Comparison of data from the vaccine trials is potentially flawed because they were nonrandomized studies and results are compared with historical rather than concurrent controls. Percentage and duration of remissions reported with chemotherapy alone in these studies did not compare favorably with more commonly reported protocols, thereby potentially skewing the comparisons. Administration of specific monoclonal antibodies against canine lymphoma cell antigens is now being evaluated.[90, 92, 188]

Radiation Therapy With or Without Bone Marrow Transplantation

Radiation therapy alone for multicentric lymphoma, including staged total-body irradiation, shows limited promise.[106] Total-body irradiation with bone marrow transplant techniques is now being evaluated.[3, 41, 193, 227] In these studies, dogs are typically first placed in complete remission with combination chemotherapy. Then, after a short (usually 2 weeks) rest from chemotherapy, their bone marrow is harvested, processed, and preserved. Dogs then receive total-body irradiation followed immediately by reinfusion of autologous bone marrow. Long-term cures have been reported. With improved techniques, newer broad-spectrum antibiotics, and greater availability of bone marrow growth factors, the morbidity and mortality traditionally inherent in these procedures may diminish. The greatest limitation of total-body irradiation and autologous bone marrow transplant is ensuring that bone marrow is free of tumor cells at collection. This limitation can be overcome only after detection capabilities or cell separation techniques improve.

Extranodal Lymphoma

Extranodal lymphoma includes those forms that occur in nonlymphoid sites (gastrointestinal, cutaneous, peripheral and central nervous system, nasal, bone). Clinical staging is important in suspected extranodal lymphoma to ensure that the disease is not a sequel to the more common multicentric nodal forms of lymphoma and to determine whether the disease is indeed localized to the extranodal site. Extranodal lymphoma that is determined to be a local disease after thorough staging can be treated locally (i.e., surgery, radiotherapy) without systemic chemotherapy.

Alimentary Lymphoma

In a large compilation of alimentary lymphoma cases,[35] the majority arose in the gastrointestinal tract; they were rarely solitary and often metastasized to liver and local lymph nodes and were rarely amenable to surgical extirpation. Male dogs may be at greater risk for alimentary lymphoma. Clinical signs are nonspecific but involve vomiting and diarrhea, sometimes with blood. The majority of dogs are hypoalbuminemic; a third are anemic. Although upper gastrointestinal contrast radiography can be suggestive, exploratory laparotomy is necessary for diagnosis. Superficial biopsy samples derived endoscopically are rarely diagnostic because the disease begins in the submucosa and is often associated with extensive lymphocytic-plasmacytic mucosal infiltration that may be misdiagnosed as benign. The major differential diagnosis for alimentary lymphoma is lymphocytic-plasmacytic enteritis; immunohistochemical stains are the only reliable method to differentiate the two in humans. Lymphocytic-plasmacytic enteritis may be preneoplastic, as reported in three Basenjis.[10]

Therapy is usually unrewarding[35]; few cases of vigorous combination chemotherapy for alimentary lymphoma are reported. Clinical responses are noted, but remission usually lasts only a few weeks. For a small number, long-term remissions have been achieved with either combination chemotherapy[35] or combination surgery and chemotherapy.[109]

Cutaneous Lymphoma*

Cutaneous lymphoma usually begins primarily but occasionally is secondary to multicentric forms of the disease. Three histologically distinguishable subclasses of cutaneous lymphoma have been reported: the more common mycosis fungoides (cutaneous T-cell-like lymphoma), histiocytic lymphoma, and Woringer-Kolopp disease (epidermotropic T-cell lymphoma).[7, 97] Sezary's syndrome, a probable variant of cutaneous T-cell lymphoma accompanied by circulating lymphoma cells, also occurs.[214] Some believe the term *T-cell-like* should be used when definitive cell phenotyping is not performed, because the names are commonly applied on the basis of criteria established in human literature. Lymphomatoid papulosis (a continuous, self-healing, clinically benign variant of cutaneous lymphoma) may represent a preneoplastic condition.[31]

Clinical findings with cutaneous lymphoma are variable. Lesions can be solitary or multiple, with the majority eventually developing into systemic multicentric disease. Mycosis fungoides is referred to as "the great imitator" because it may clinically mimic other skin disorders including seborrhea, pemphigus, and pyoderma. It may begin as a mild eczematous pruritic plaque and progress to nodular tumors, from which its name is derived. Mycosis fungoides refers to its mushroom-like appearance (Fig. 156–1). Approximately half

*See references 1, 7, 14, 22, 29, 31, 39, 97, 142, and 214.

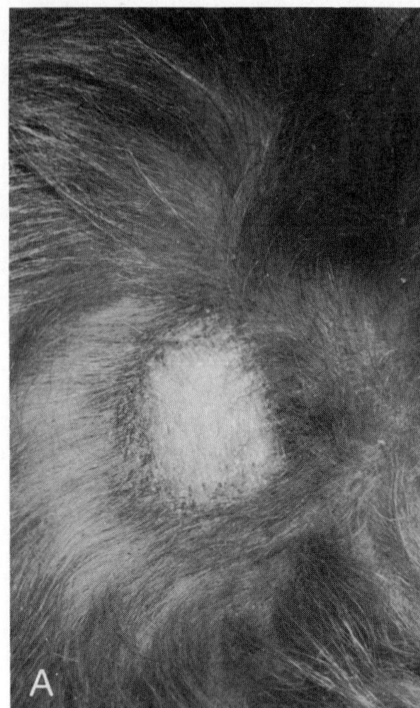

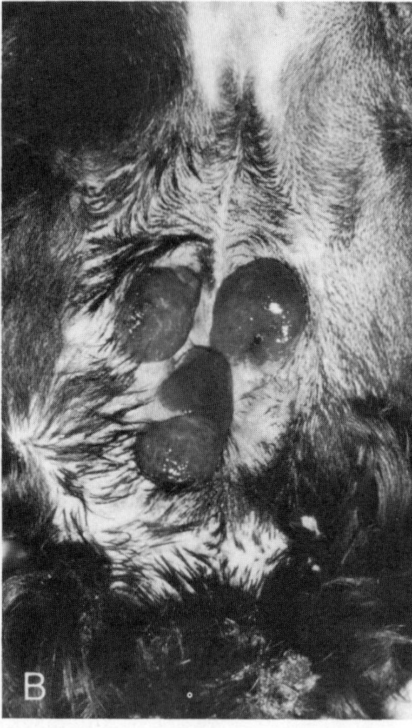

FIGURE 156–1. *A*, Mild pruritic plaque histologically determined to be mycosis fungoides in a 4-year-old golden retriever. *B*, More classic mushroom-like lesions of mycosis fungoides in the perineum of a 6-year-old springer spaniel.

of the reported cases of cutaneous lymphoma are pruritic.

Therapy depends on the extent of disease. If a solitary lesion is noted and thorough clinical staging, as previously discussed for multicentric lymphoma, fails to reveal systemic disease, local therapy including surgery or radiotherapy may produce a cure. Fractionated radiotherapy to a total dose of 30 to 45 Gy has been associated with long-term control[7, 22, 143] and is ideally delivered as superficial electron therapy. Topical nitrogen mustard (mechlorethamine) has some efficacy; however, thorough client education on handling of hazardous drugs and waste is necessary. Most published reports do not describe positive treatment responses, but we have found that the disease can be successfully controlled, with long-term survival. Couto reports that five of six dogs responded to combination chemotherapy with COAP (cyclophosphamide, vincristine, cytosine arabinoside, and prednisone); median remissions and survivals were 250 and 399 days, respectively.[29] Responses have been reported in human patients receiving oral vitamin A analogues known as *retinoids.*[99] A small number of dogs have been successfully treated with oral 13 *cis*-retinoic acid (Accutane), with prolonged complete remissions resulting after failure of more traditional therapy. Such therapy is preliminary.

Mediastinal Lymphoma

Dogs with mediastinal lymphoma are often presented with respiratory signs or precaval syndrome (i.e., facial and forelimb edema) secondary to the mass effect of the tumor. Forty to 50 per cent of thymic lymphomas are associated with hypercalcemia; therefore, polyuria/polydipsia, anorexia, and weakness may also be present. Hypercalcemia does not have a prognostic effect[190]; however, anterior mediastinal lymphoma itself is associated with decreased duration of remission. The differential diagnosis for mediastinal lymphoma includes ectopic thyroid tumors, heart base tumors, thymoma, and pulmonary lymphomatoid granulomatosis.

Lymphoma of the Nervous System

Lymphoma of the nervous system is an unusual finding in dogs, although not uncommon in humans.[12, 34, 38, 194] In human patients with multicentric lymphoma, the central nervous system (CNS) is often the site of eventual treatment failure, partly because of lack of blood-brain barrier penetration by many of the drugs used. The majority of CNS lymphomas reported in dogs are secondary to systemic disease, although primary CNS lymphoma does occur. Signs relative to intracranial disease including seizure activity, dementia, and coma occur if the lesions are intracranial, whereas signs referable to cord compression or peripheral nerve dysfunction accompany lymphoma in these locations. Diagnosis of nervous system lymphoma includes a complete lymphoma staging procedure as well as a cerebrospinal fluid (CSF) aspirate, computed tomographic (CT) scan, or myelogram if available. All dogs in one group of eight with CNS lymphoma had elevated abnormal lymphocytes in CSF fluid, and the majority had elevated CSF protein levels, both of which are rare in CNS lymphoma in humans.[34] Biopsy may be necessary for eventual diagnosis if neoplastic lymphocytes are not present in the CSF.

Therapy for nervous system lymphoma depends on tumor location, the capabilities of drugs to cross the blood-brain barrier, and the presence of disease outside the nervous system. Surgical intervention for diagnosis or removal of accessible tumors has been successfully performed. More commonly, surgery must be combined with adjuvant chemotherapy or radiotherapy. Of the agents commonly used in dogs, only prednisone and cytosine arabinoside (ara-C) consistently cross the blood-brain barrier in therapeutic concentrations.[199] Ara-C can be delivered intrathecaly (20 mg/m^2) after removing an equal volume of CSF, at a dosage of 100 mg/m^2 SC daily for 4 consecutive days every 3 weeks, or as a continuous 4-day infusion given at 100 mg/m^2/day diluted in saline or a balanced electrolyte solution. If the CNS lymphoma is accompanied by disease elsewhere in the body, the ara-C is incorporated into a more traditional combination therapy protocol. Radiotherapy has also been successfully used for treating CNS lymphoma because of exquisite sensitivity of lymphocytes to radiation. Various fractionation protocols up to a total dose of 30 Gy have been reported. However, we have safely used 45 Gy in 3 Gy fractions daily. Of six dogs treated with either systemic chemotherapy or chemotherapy and radiotherapy (30 Gy), all had improvement of disease of short duration (weeks to 3 months).[34]

Lymphoma of Bone

Few reports describe osseous involvement of lymphoma in dogs.[50, 154, 201, 217] These cases often occurred in younger animals with multiple osseous sites. As with other forms of extranodal involvement, thorough clinical staging to rule out systemic disease can be followed by local therapy including surgery or radiotherapy (Fig. 156–2). Most apparent primary cases eventually recur systemically, although often not for many months or years.

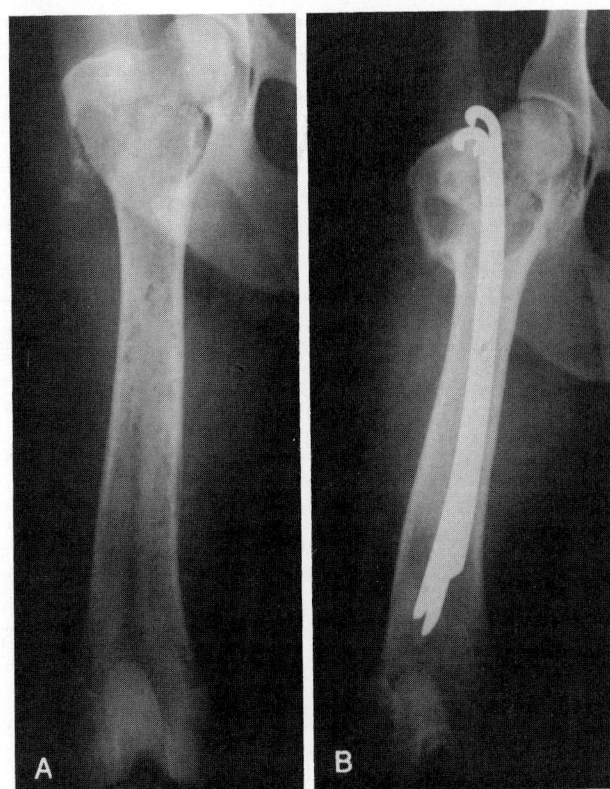

FIGURE 156–2. *A,* Osseous lymphoma resulting in a pathological fracture of the proximal femur of a 7-year-old Dalmatian. *B,* The same femur, now healed, after Rush pin fixation and local radiotherapy in combination with systemic doxorubicin chemotherapy.

Lymphoid Leukemia

Leukemia is defined as the proliferation of neoplastic hematopoietic cells in the bone marrow; such cells may not be circulating in the peripheral blood.[28] The two general categories of lymphoid leukemia are chronic lymphocytic leukemia and acute lymphoblastic leukemia.

Acute Lymphoblastic Leukemia

Acute lymphoblastic leukemia is uncommon.[28, 55, 137, 139] No sex, breed, or weight predilection exists, and most patients are of late middle age. The majority have absolute leukocytosis with circulating abnormal lymphocytes, and only 10 per cent are classified as having aleukemic leukemia (bone marrow involvement without peripheral blood involvement). Clinical signs can include fever, generalized and abdominal pain, anorexia, splenomegaly, and pale mucous membranes. Anemia was reported in 40 per cent of patients with acute lymphoblastic anemia, and 25 per cent are thrombocytopenic.[28]

Diagnosis depends on documentation of abnormal lymphocytes in the bone marrow or peripheral blood. Some forms of the disease are blastic and undifferentiated, making special stains necessary to differentiate myeloproliferative conditions (Table 156–5). Acute lymphoblastic leukemia may be clinically differentiated from late stages of lymphoma by the acute progression of disease, lesser likelihood of lymphadenopathy (<50 per cent), poor response to therapy, and shorter survival. Only 19 per cent of cases responded to vincristine and prednisone therapy, with a median survival of 19 days,[137] whereas 46 per cent (6/13) responded to vincristine, prednisone, and asparaginase in combination with blood replacement therapy. Those responding had a median survival of 150 days versus 15 days for unresponsive dogs.[139]

Chronic Lymphocytic Leukemia

Chronic lymphocytic leukemia, defined as an abnormal proliferation of morphologically normal mature lymphocytes in the bone marrow or peripheral blood, is rare in dogs.[33, 75, 111] These abnormal cells can infiltrate other hematopoietic tissue or solid organs. No breed predilection is noted. A male/female ratio of 1.8:1 is reported, and the disease mainly afflicts older dogs. Presenting complaints are nonspecific and include lethargy, inappetence, polyuria/polydipsia, bleeding diathesis, intermittent lameness, and episodes of collapse. Two-thirds have lymphadenopathy and splenomegaly. Pale mucous membranes and pyrexia are commonly found. One case of chronic lymphocytic leukemia with cutaneous lymphoma has been reported.[33] Twenty-one of 22 dogs in one report had leukocytosis, the majority were anemic (normocytic, normochromic, and nonregenerative), and approximately half were thrombocytopenic.[111] Thirty-six per cent were hyperglobulinemic, 50

TABLE 156–5. CYTOCHEMICAL REACTIONS IN BLAST CELLS OF ACUTE LEUKEMIAS

Leukemia	Sudan Black B	Peroxidase (Leukocyte)	PAS	CAE	NSE	Peroxidase (Platelet)
AML	+	+	+	+	−	
AMML	+	±	±	+	+	
AMoL	−	±	±	−	+*	
Erythroleu	−	−	+	−	−	
Meg L			+			+
ALL	−	−		+†	+‡	
Undiff	−	−	−	−	−	−

PAS, periodic acid-Schiff; CAE, chloroacetate esterase; NSE, nonspecific esterase; AML, acute myelogenous leukemia; AMML, acute myelomonocytic leukemia; AMoL, acute monocytic leukemia; Erythroleu, erythroleukemia; Meg L, acute megakaryocytic leukemia; ALL, acute lymphoblastic leukemia; Undiff, undifferentiated leukemia. +, positive; −, negative; ±, weakly or occasionally positive.
*Sodium fluoride sensitive.
†Coarse blocks of PAS-positive material in cytoplasm.
‡Focal positivity.
Modified from Young KM: Myeloproliferative disorders. *Vet Clin North Am 15*:776, 1985.

per cent had monoclonal gammopathies on serum electrophoresis, and 40 per cent had Bence Jones proteins in the urine, suggesting B-cell origin.

Therapy for chronic lymphocytic leukemia in humans and dogs is recommended only if a patient is symptomatic or if anemia, hyperglobulinemia, splenomegaly, or lymphadenopathy is present. The prognosis greatly exceeds that for acute lymphocytic leukemia. Leifer and colleagues[111] treated 22 dogs using vincristine, prednisone, and chlorambucil, with a resultant normalization of white blood cell counts in 70 per cent and median survival of 348 days. Splenectomy significantly increases survival in human patients with aggressive forms of chronic lymphocytic leukemia[169]; however, no studies of dogs support these findings.

Myeloproliferative Disorders

Myeloproliferative disorders are a group of nonlymphocytic bone marrow cell disorders in which proliferation of one, several, or all of the marrow cell lines is present.[65, 236] These disorders are considered neoplastic or preneoplastic and can be benign or malignant. Because bone marrow stem cells are pluripotent, one form of myeloproliferative disorders can evolve into another, and rarely is just one cell line involved.

Specifically, myeloproliferative disorders have two primary forms. One involves uncontrolled proliferation of a mature, well-differentiated bone marrow cell line and is referred to as *chronic* myeloproliferative disorder. The other involves proliferation of a poorly differentiated cell line incapable of maturation and is classified as acute myeloproliferative disorder. The various forms reported in dogs are listed in Table 156–6. Chronic myeloproliferative disorders can eventually terminate in a blast crisis, characterized by an acute shift from more differentiated cancer cells to a highly undifferentiated leukemic cell type. This switch is associated with poor survival.[112, 171, 236]

Diagnosis is based on documentation of neoplastic cells and the absence of those diseases associated with bone marrow hyperplasia or hypoplasia. Such conditions include ehrlichiosis, multicentric lymphoma, estrogen toxicity, or lead poisoning. Special stains are often necessary to differentiate undifferentiated forms of myeloproliferative disorders (see Table 156–5). Diagnosis of polycythemia vera, a chronic myeloproliferative disorder, is based on increased red blood cell mass, the absence of disease capable of causing secondary polycythemia (e.g., dehydration, hypoxia, erythropoietin-producing tumor), and normal erythropoietin levels. The prognosis is guarded at best for chronic myeloproliferative disorders and grave for acute myeloproliferative disorders.

Although many treatment protocols have been published for myeloproliferative disorders, readers are

TABLE 156–6. CLASSIFICATION OF MYELOPROLIFERATIVE DISORDERS (MPD) AND REPORTS IN THE VETERINARY LITERATURE

Name	Abnormal Cell or Tissue Type	References
Acute MPD		
Acute myelogenous leukemia	Myeloblasts	8, 17, 28, 55, 67, 189
Acute myelomonocytic leukemia	Myeloblasts, monoblasts	6, 28, 32, 51, 55, 85, 115, 176, 181
Acute monocytic leukemia	Monoblasts	28, 55, 107
Erythroleukemia	Erythroblasts, myeloblasts	116
Basophilic leukemia	Basophils and precursors	125
Acute megakaryocytic leukemia	Megakaryoblasts, collagen	15, 67
Eosinophilic leukemia	Eosinophils and precursors	
Undifferentiated leukemia	Blast cells	
Chronic MPD		
Polycythemia vera	Erythrocytes	141, 170, 204
Chronic myelogenous leukemia	Neutrophils, late precursors	112, 171
Primary thrombocythemia	Platelets	204
Myelofibrosis	Megakaryocytes, collagen	76

urged to check with a veterinary oncologist for the latest treatment alternatives as they become available. The radioactive nuclide ^{32}P, which is incorporated into bone $CaPO_4$ and emits beta particles, has been successfully used to treat chronic myeloproliferative disorders, polycythemia vera, and essential thrombocythemia.[204, 236] Phlebotomy can also be used successfully for polycythemia vera. Hydroxyurea has been used with more limited success in polycythemia vera and other chronic types of myeloproliferative disorders, but it does not alter or forestall the terminal blast crisis.

Low-dose cytosine arabinoside (10 mg/m^2 SC BID for 14 to 28 days) has produced favorable results in humans with acute myeloproliferative disorders, including acute myeloproliferative leukemia,[5, 144, 146, 226] and in one case of feline lymphoblastic leukemia.[72] The mechanism by which this low dose of ara-C works is not understood; there is *in vitro* evidence for induction of terminal differentiation in neoplastic cells (i.e., the immature tumor cell is compelled to grow up and die). Initial reports with low-dose ara-C revealed high remission rates with low drug toxicity. Reports now suggest that low-dose ara-C is associated with significant life-threatening myelosuppression and may not be superior to more aggressive traditional chemotherapy.[4, 101]

Plasma Cell Neoplasms

Of the three primary clinical forms of plasma cell neoplasms, the most common is multiple myeloma. The other two occur uncommonly and are solitary plasmacytoma of bone and extramedullary plasma cytoma.[126, 127, 138, 177]

Multiple Myeloma

Multiple myeloma, the neoplastic proliferation of a clone of plasma cells, occurs primarily in aged dogs, with no sex predilection.[138] German shepherds may be at greater risk. Seventy-five per cent of affected dogs have a monoclonal gammopathy, either of the IgG or IgA subtype. Primary macroglobulinemia (Waldenström's disease) a rare tumor intermediate between plasma cell and lymphocytic neoplasm, is accompanied by hyperglobulinemia due to elaboration of IgM. A small percentage of B-cell lymphomas may also elicit immunoglobulins. Differentials for monoclonal gammopathy include ehrlichiosis and benign hypergammaglobulinemia syndrome, which has been described in dogs.[77] Light-chain (Bence Jones) proteins may be detectable in the urine. These proteins are not detected by routine urine dipstick analysis and require phoretic techniques to be identified. Clinical signs attributable to multiple myeloma are nonspecific and include anorexia, listlessness, and polyuria/polydipsia. Most patients have lameness secondary to paresis or pain, and half possess a bleeding diathesis (epistaxis or gingival bleeding) secondary to hyperviscosity syndrome, or thrombocytopenia/thrombocytopathia.[138]

The majority of dogs with multiple myeloma have nonregenerative, normocytic/normochromic anemia, approximately one-third are thrombocytopenic, and 10 per cent have circulating abnormal plasmacytes. Fifteen to 20 per cent of patients with multiple myeloma are hypercalcemic secondary to bone resorption due to osteoclast-activating factors or other substances elicited by the tumor.

Diagnosis of multiple myeloma usually follows documentation of bone marrow plasmacytosis ($>$ 20 to 30 per cent plasma cells), osteolytic bone lesions, and serum or urine myeloma proteins. Histological confirmation may be necessary in cases that do not elicit all three abnormalities. The differential diagnosis for plasmacytosis is considered and includes carcinomas, connective tissue disorder, liver disease, hypersensitivity states, and infections.

The short-term prognosis for multiple myeloma is normally favorable, and long-term remissions are the rule. The long-term prognosis is grave because cures are rare. Extensive bone lesions, light-chain proteinuria, hypercalcemia, and anemia are negative prognostic signs. A clinical staging protocol has been proposed, but it does not have prognostic significance.[138] Combination chemotherapy using melphalan (0.1 mg/kg PO daily for 10 days, followed by 0.05 mg/kg daily) with prednisone (0.5 mg/kg daily for 10 days, then every other day) results in remission rates of 90 per cent and median survival times of 540 days.[138] Serum protein levels normalize within 2 to 3 months. Fractures accompanying multiple myeloma can be treated by surgical reduction in combination with chemotherapy or radiotherapy. Healing normally accompanies remission of the multiple myeloma. Rescue therapy is not well documented once remission is lost. Doxorubicin, vincristine, and dexamethasone combinations work well in humans and may be of benefit in dogs.[203]

Solitary Plasmacytoma of Bone

Solitary plasmacytoma of bone is rare in animals.[126] Two cases in dogs were not accompanied by a secretory protein, and both eventually developed systemic multiple myeloma, as is the case for 50 per cent of human cases.[52] Localized lesions can be treated with either surgery or radiotherapy. Careful clinical staging and a strict re-evaluation schedule should be established because of the propensity to develop systemic disease.

Extramedullary Plasmacytoma

Although extramedullary plasmacytoma is infrequent, one pathological study suggested it may be more common.[177] Seventy-five cases were reported equally between sexes and primarily in aged dogs (mean 9.7 years). It occurs primarily as a solitary mucocutaneous lesion of the mouth but also can affect the feet, trunk, and ears. Two of 75 cases had concurrent lymphoma, and 2 of 75 dogs had or developed multiple myeloma. Cure was by local surgical resection in 40 of 57 dogs treated, with a median disease-free interval of 11.8 months; this number continues to rise as most dogs under study are still alive and free of disease. The prognosis is very favorable for solitary extramedullary plasmacytoma in dogs. Radiation therapy is also effective for treatment in humans.[52]

FELINE HEMATOPOIETIC SYSTEM

A discussion of hematopoietic malignancy (lymphoma/leukemia complex) in cats is virtually synonymous with a review of neoplastic diseases induced by feline leukemia virus (FeLV). Approximately 25 per cent of FeLV-induced diseases are neoplastic, and the majority of these are lymphoid and hematopoietic malignancies. Lymphoid and hematopoietic malignancy account for 30 per cent of all feline tumors, and 90 per cent of these are malignant lymphomas.[42] FeLV-induced immunosuppressive (and other degenerative) syndromes are probably of greater relevance to veterinarians providing surgical care to FeLV-infected cats than are the overtly neoplastic illnesses. This section concentrates primarily on findings related to the natural history, diagnosis, therapy, and prevention of FeLV infection, as well as diagnosis, prognosis, and therapy in cats. Readers are referred to other sources for more comprehensive reviews of FeLV.[59, 183, 184, 211, 215] A discussion of the feline immunodeficiency virus (FIV) is also included.

Natural History of FeLV

Classification

FeLV is a single-stranded RNA virus of the subfamily Oncovirinae, a group belonging to the family Retrovirinae.[49] These viruses are unique because they contain the enzyme *reverse transcriptase,* enabling the viral RNA genome to be copied into a complementary strand of DNA that is ultimately integrated permanently into the genome of infected cells.[184] The integrated viral genome is called a *provirus.* The genome of the provirus can subsequently be transcribed by normal feline enzymes to produce viral structural proteins and new copies of viral RNA that combine to form new, infectious virus.[224] Alternatively, the provirus can remain quiescent within the feline genome in a latent or untranscribed state.

Viral Structure

FeLV is composed of an internal core containing RNA, reverse transcriptase, and several proteins, one of which has relevance to the clinical detection of FeLV infection.[184] The 27,000-dalton major core protein, also referred to as *p27,* forms the substrate for the widely used indirect fluorescent antibody (IFA) and enzyme-linked immunoassay (ELISA) tests for FeLV infection.[62, 71, 119, 121] The outer envelope, encoded for by the envelope (env) genes, consists of a 70,000-dalton glycoprotein (gp70) present as "knobs" that are attached to the outer end of the 15,000-dalton transmembrane "spikes" (p15E). Protein gp70 binds the virus to susceptible feline cells.[182] Protein p15E mediates many immunosuppressive effects characteristic of FeLV.[184] Although the core proteins and p15E are highly conserved between isolates of FeLV, gp70 is composed of (at least) three distinct subtypes that each evoke unique virus-neutralizing antibody responses in host cats. Various individual serological responses to gp70 define the three major subgroups (serotypes) of FeLV: FeLV-A, FeLV-B, FeLV-C.[196] From a clinical perspective, individual subgroups of FeLV influence the spectrum of disease in FeLV-infected cats.

Subgroups and Spectrum of Disease

FeLV-A is found in all FeLV-positive cats and is contagious between cats.[88] By itself, FeLV-A probably is responsible for general immunosuppression in infected cats (due to p15E) but not neoplastic disease. Cats infected with FeLV-A can remain disease free for several years, but the stress of elective operations (e.g., ovariohysterectomy, castration) or other disease processes (e.g., trauma, abscesses) can precipitate clinical illness.

A form of FeLV-A referred to as *variant A* induces a progressive and fatal immunodeficiency syndrome in affected cats.[88, 152, 151, 159] In contrast to FeLV-A, in which infected cells are not destroyed by the provirus, variant A infection causes progressive lysis of lymphoid and bone marrow stem cells, leaving the cat an immunological cripple. Affected cats are highly vulnerable to systemic bacterial infections and usually die within weeks of developing variant A infection. This specific FeLV-induced immunological disease has been called *feline acquired immunodeficiency syndrome* (FAIDS). Variant A is replication defective and requires association with FeLV-A for pathogenicity.[151]

FeLV-B is found in 49 per cent of FeLV-infected cats, and it is always associated with FeLV-A.[60] FeLV-B is formed when FeLV-A provirus recombines with sequences of the endogenous feline genome.[210] FeLV-B isolates (in association with FeLV-A) are implicated in a spectrum of neoplastic diseases including thymic lymphoma and myeloproliferative diseases.[60, 182]

FeLV-C is also a recombinant or mutated variety of FeLV-A. FeLV-C is replication defective and always induces erythroid hypoplasia within weeks to months of FeLV-C expression. A bone marrow aspirate from an FeLV-C–infected cat shows a decrease or absence of erythroid precursor cells that is nonreversible.[157] Veterinarians providing care to cats with FeLV-induced anemia are faced with a progressively fatal condition that is unresponsive to therapy. Feline oncornavirus-associated cell membrane antigen (FOCMA), previously thought to be a tumor-specific antigen expressed on the surface of cells transformed by FeLV, is related to gp70 of FeLV-C.[206, 225] Cats that develop antibodies to FOCMA are protected against development of lymphoma but not non-neoplastic FeLV-induced abnormalities.[61] FOCMA antibody lyses cells expressing FeLV-C gp70 on the surface and can directly neutralize some FeLV-C virus particles.[182] An important immunological response of cats infected with FeLV seems to be the ability to contain FeLV-C infected cells through FOCMA antibody development. Although the other subgroups (or combinations) induce fatal conditions, specific immunoprotective strategies other than virus-neutralizing antibodies (i.e., anti-gp70 antibody) have not been recognized in FeLV-infected cats to protect as completely as FOCMA antibodies.[59, 195]

Genetic Pathogenesis of FeLV-Induced Disease

FeLV-infected cat cells are destroyed quickly when large amounts of unintegrated FeLV DNA accumulate within the cytoplasm. This is the pathogenesis for FeLV variant A disease.[152] It is the association of the integrated provirus with host genomic sequences, called *proto-oncogenes,* that determines the phenotypic expression of malignancy. Loss of transcriptional regulatory control of a normal cellular proto-oncogene, following FeLV-provirus insertion into the genome, can derange normal expression of the growth-promoting gene and result in excessive cellular proliferation. This is the cause of many cases of feline lymphoma in which a cellular gene that is important for growth, *c-myc,* is "switched on" by elements of the provirus.[153] Alternatively, cellular proto-oncogenes can undergo rearrangement by combining with FeLV provirus sequences. The genetic recombination, when transcribed, results in a malignant phenotype. About 20 per cent of FeLV-induced thymic lymphomas and all fibrosarcomas induced by the feline sarcoma virus (FeSV) are the result of virus-host genetic recombinations.[9, 153] Because virus-host genetic recombination recurs *de novo* in FeLV-infected cats, those cats that develop fibrosarcomas do not pose a risk to other cats for development of fibrosarcomas. However, they are still contagious for the FeLV that gave rise to FeSV by genetic recombination.

Transmission and Pathogenesis of FeLV Infection

The sequence of events following exposure of a susceptible cat to FeLV has been described.[163, 185] A sound understanding of these events can form the basis for rational clinical decisions when dealing with cats that have been exposed to FeLV. FeLV is usually transmitted through the saliva of one infected cat to the oral or nasal mucous membranes of another cat via licking and grooming. FeLV infects lymphocytes and macrophages in the tonsils and oral pharynx after viral attachment to these cells by gp70.[185] Virus is replicated intracellularly for 2 to 4 days, and infected cells drain to the regional lymph nodes in the neck.[185] Most cats successfully neutralize the virus by this stage through production of virus-neutralizing antibody and are subsequently immune to FeLV infection.[61] In cats that do not eliminate virus, the infected cells leave the nodes and circulate hematogenously for 2 to 14 days. Infected cells seed numerous lymphoid tissues, in which many more cells become infected. By 7 to 21 days after exposure, infected cells enter the bone marrow in large numbers and the very sensitive, mitotically active blood cell precursors become infected.[185] By 4 to 6 weeks, a cat is persistently viremic and has greater than a 95 per cent chance of remaining infected for life.[59] After 4 weeks, virus is disseminated to numerous mucosal and glandular epithelial cells by infected neutrophils and platelets. Sites include the oronasal pharynx, salivary glands, and mucosa of the urinary bladder and gastrointestinal tract. Virus is shed into the environment in saliva and urine.[81] FeLV can also infect unborn fetuses *in utero* (through horizontal transmission), and infection of young kittens occurred on occassion by virus secretion into the milk of lactating queens.[60] Most persistently FeLV-infected cats die within 3.5 years of developing chronic infection.[140]

Latent Infection of FeLV

The past several years have yielded important information about the phase of FeLV infection known as *latency.*[132, 166, 186] Latently infected cats do not actively shed virus and are not viremic. However, FeLV can be isolated from the bone marrow of these cats after *in vitro* bone marrow culture.[166, 186] These cats have virus-neutralizing antibodies in their serum and are apparently recovered from FeLV infection.[160]

Latent FeLV infections probably represent a phase of recovery after exposure to FeLV in cats that develop immunity.[160, 166, 182] By 4 to 6 weeks after exposure, most cats restrict infection to the bone marrow and lymph nodes.[80, 185] Many of these cats neutralize whole virus, but if provirus is contained within the genome of bone marrow cells, these cells can survive from months to years with provirus inserted. These cells do not actively produce infective FeLV, or if they do, the cat's immune mechanisms quickly prevent systemic release of virus. Therefore, cats test negative for cell-associated viremia (by IFA methods), although small numbers are intermittently positive by ELISA testing. Over time, virus cannot be isolated from bone marrow of latently infected cats, suggesting that the infection has been completely extinguished. For most cats, latency lasts between 9 and 16 months after initial exposure.[160] Several factors contribute to the duration of latency, including the size of the viral burden, FeLV subgroup, and health of the cat when exposed to FeLV.[182] The larger the viral challenge, the greater the tendency for cats to develop latent infections. Cats with other viral illnesses or immune system stress at FeLV exposure are also more likely to develop latent infections.

Based on the nature of latency, it is obvious that there is no simple, widely available method to test for this phase of FeLV infection. From the clinical perspective, it is important to recognize the risk of these cats reverting to a FeLV-producing status. Should this occur, these cats are sources of infective virus to other cats and increase their own chance for a FeLV-associated illness. Latently infected cats are not usually predisposed to development of diseases associated with FeLV, even after prolonged follow-up.[160] One report described a higher than expected prevalence of FeLV-negative lymphoma, nonregenerative anemia, and neurological disease in latently infected cats from multiple-cat households.[166] Research has also demonstrated immunological defects of neutrophils in latently infected cats.[103] The dysfunction of neutrophils resulted in decreased phagocytic ability equivalent to that of FeLV-viremic cats. Such an abnormality might increase the risk for infection of latently infected cats and possibly the chance for virus-negative tumors owing to decreased surveillance of emerging tumor cells.

There is no evidence that latently infected cats routinely transmit FeLV to susceptible cats.[160] On rare occasions, queens with latent infection have shed infectious virus in the milk, but colostral antibodies usually protect the kittens from infection. It is probable that such cats have lower levels of virus-neutralizing antibodies and, once identified, probably should not be bred.[160] Maintenance of the latent state and its subsequent eradication depend on a cat's immunological responses. One experimental method of reactivating viral expression is to immunosuppress latently infected cats with prolonged treatment of high doses of glucocorticosteroids. It is important that cats with latent infection are not further immunocompromised either iatrogenically by administration of glucocorticosteroids, by infection with other viruses, or by superimposition of stressful situations including elective surgery. Most clinicians are not able to confirm latency for every cat presented for surgical (or medical) problems, so a complete history aimed at uncovering a cat's FeLV exposure history is essential. It is vital to decrease indiscriminate glucocorticosteroid therapy and to avoid subjecting animals to elective surgery (e.g., ovariohysterectomy, castration) shortly after FeLV exposure. Although not diagnostic, ELISA-positive, IFA-negative cats are suspect for latency and should be retested.

In summary, the key points of FeLV latency relative to clinical (surgical) care are as follows: (1) The cats are not viremic and thus not contagious. (2) Latency is probably a "normal" phase of recovery from FeLV exposure. (3) Minimized stress and immunosuppression probably aid a cat in permanently extinguishing FeLV infection.

Clinical Diagnostic Testing for FeLV

From the standpoint of providing surgical care to cats, it is recommended that a cat showing any of the myriad FeLV-associated clinical or laboratory abnormalities be tested for FeLV infection before surgery. FeLV-induced neoplasms, composed chiefly of lymphoma/leukemia, and fibrosarcoma (especially in cats younger than 5 years), constitute only about one-fourth of the FeLV-related disease spectrum. These conditions are often obvious, so it is unlikely that such cats will inadvertently have surgery. It is more likely that cats with non-neoplastic FeLV-associated immunosuppressive and degenerative conditions will have surgery without prior testing of their FeLV status. Cats can show many signs, including anemia, bacterial infections, respiratory (viral) infections, gingivitis, and reproductive problems.[59] FeLV testing consists of two basic types: IFA and ELISA. Clinicians engaged in surgery should be familiar with the principles of both tests and interpretation of results.

For rapid screening of FeLV status, ELISA has proved to be a reliable, simple, and quick method for testing cats in a clinical setting. ELISA has been subject to a great deal of scrutiny and discussion about its accuracy.[86, 87, 120] This test, like the IFA, determines the presence of the FeLV core protein p27. Because it is a highly sensitive test, cats can be positive by ELISA and negative by IFA. These "false" positive cats can actually reflect an early stage of FeLV infection when soluble p27 is detectable in serum but cell-associated viremia, a prerequisite for a positive IFA result, has not yet developed.[121] Since its introduction, ELISA testing for FeLV has improved markedly because of development of monoclonal antibodies that are highly specific for epitopes of p27. Therefore, the likelihood of obtaining a truly "false" positive result is far less today than previously. The main reason for a positive ELISA result in a cat that is not FeLV infected is improper sample preparation. Incomplete washing of test samples, especially when hemolyzed serum or whole blood is used, contributes to nonspecific binding of the monoclonal antibody reagents. False-positive ELISA results are sometimes a problem when saliva is tested for FeLV antigen. Cross-reactions with oral flora sometimes cause false-positive ELISA results when saliva is tested for FeLV antigen. Cats being screened for FeLV before a surgical procedure thus should have serum samples tested when ELISA methods are used. ELISA of tears has been useful although inconsistent because FeLV-infected cats do not always shed p27 in the tears.[71] False-positive reactions have been associated with antimouse antibodies in some uninfected cats.[117]

A positive ELISA result suggests FeLV antigenemia (and infection) but does not confirm persistent FeLV infection. It is possible that a cat with a positive ELISA result is in the early stages of a FeLV infection that it may subsequently eliminate. To maximize a cat's chances of extinguishing infection, it is essential to minimize stress, including postponing any elective surgical procedures. Concurrently, determination of persistent FeLV infection should be verified by the IFA test on a blood or bone marrow sample. Cats that are IFA positive only rarely clear viremia.[60] A cat that is ELISA positive and IFA negative should be retested at intervals for at least several months (e.g., 3 to 6). If a cat is consistently ELISA positive and IFA negative, it is possible that such an animal has a compartmentalized FeLV infection. Complete virus is confined to a specific anatomical site (e.g., bone marrow), but viral antigen (p27) circulates systemically. These cats are latently infected with FeLV and probably are at risk for development of persistent viremia if stressed. Younger cats are most susceptible to FeLV infection. It is this population that is presented more often for elective surgical procedures including ovariohysterectomy, castration, and onychectomy. Therefore, appropriate screening of young cats is warranted before surgical procedures, especially because of unknown prior FeLV exposure in this population of cats (e.g., strays, animals acquired from animal shelters).

Therapy of FeLV Infection

Although no effective therapies can reliably eliminate persistent FeLV infection, several experimental approaches have been investigated. Some of these include reverse transcriptase inhibitors,[21, 25] bone marrow transplantation,[25] whole-body hyperthermia,[130] and staphylococcal protein A.[45, 104, 205] This substance is a cell wall constituent of *Staphylococcus aureus* Cowan I that binds to the Fc region of IgG and has great affinity for circulating immune complexes.[45] Staphylococcal protein A is also mitogenic for T- and B-lymphocytes and stimulates production of immunologically active lymphokines such as interferon by effector cells.[45] Some FeLV-infected cats treated either by interperitoneal injections of staphylococcal protein A or by external perfusion of plasma over columns containing staphylococcal protein A have been reported to eliminate FeLV infections and showed improvement of FeLV-associated lymphoma and myeloproliferative disorders.[45, 205] Immunological responses in cats that eliminated FeLV infection and experienced tumor remissions included development of antibodies to FeLV subgroup C envelope glycoprotein, gp70, which likely mediated antibody-dependent cytotoxicity of lymphoma cells.[205] As mentioned earlier, FeLV-C gp70 is a major component of the novel lymphoma membrane protein referred to as *FOCMA*.[206] Antibody to gp70 can also neutralize FeLV *in vivo*.[195] Staphylococcal protein A enhances neutrophil function in cats with FeLV viremia.[104]

Because responses of FeLV-infected cats to staphylococcal protein A have been limited and variable, the future role for this substance in the therapy of FeLV is uncertain.

Vaccination Against FeLV

The first commercial vaccine against FeLV was marketed in 1985. Since that time, considerable controversy and confusion have ensued about the efficacy of this product regarding its ability to confer immunity to FeLV-vaccinated cats.* A randomized blind trial of the vaccine demonstrated that unvaccinated cats developed persistent viremia approximately three times more often than vaccinates when these animals cohabited with FeLV-infected cats for prolonged periods.[172] This study was one of the most convincing to date to demonstrate efficacy of the subunit vaccine. Another study did not confirm protective claims for the vaccine.[108] There were several differences between the two studies. In the trial that demonstrated efficacy, three doses of vaccine were administered before test cats were exposed to the FeLV viremic cats, 6 weeks after the final vaccination. In the trial that did not demonstrate efficacy, vaccinated cats were given only two doses of vaccine and were exposed to FeLV viremic cats after only 2 weeks. Other data by the vaccine's manufacturer, using a second-generation version of the subunit vaccine, suggested protection against FeLV infection, viral persistence, and tumor formation.[58] Other FeLV vaccines introduced after 1985 by additional manufacturers have not been subjected to as rigorous scrutiny as the first vaccine.

Several conclusions about FeLV vaccination can be stated. Strict adherence to the manufacturer's recommended vaccination procedure is essential. Despite the proper vaccination schedule, some cats are not protected. All cats should be FeLV negative before vaccination, but in the clinical situation, the possibility of prior FeLV exposure can never be ruled out. Cats at highest risk for FeLV infection, such as those in multicat households or cats younger than 1 year, are most likely to benefit from FeLV vaccination. FeLV vaccination should be considered for cats at risk before they undergo elective surgical procedures.

*See references 108, 135, 155, 158, 162, 165, and 200.

Lymphomas

Lymphomas (malignant lymphomas, lymphosarcomas) are the most common malignancies in cats and account for approximately one-third of all tumors in this species.[59] The majority of hemolymphatic tumors (i.e., 60 to 90 per cent) are lymphomas,[30] making them important and frequently encountered clinical entities. FeLV is causally associated with 70 per cent of lymphomas and has been implicated in development of FeLV-negative lymphomas as well.[63, 187]

Lymphomas are malignancies arising in solid lymphoid tissues such as lymph nodes, spleen, liver, thymus, or Peyer patches. In advanced cases, tumor cells can also infiltrate the bone marrow. By contrast, lymphoid malignancy that originates in the bone marrow is usually classified as lymphoid leukemia. Although these distinctions may appear academic, they are clinically relevant because as a group, cats with lymphoma have a better treatment prognosis than cats with leukemia.[24] Sometimes it is not possible to determine the primary site of disease because of its wide anatomical distribution. Such a distinction may not be clinically relevant because of the poor prognosis for cats with advanced lymphoma.[148] Lymphomas can also affect nonlymphoid tissues, resulting in a conglomerate of anatomical presentations. In advanced cases, nonlymphoid locations can develop as tumor cells spread from the primary lymphoid sites. Alternatively, lymphoma can arise exclusively in sites other than the primary lymphoreticular tissues, presenting as so-called extranodal lymphomas.[30] Frequently involved sites of extranodal lymphoma include the kidneys, skin, CNS, and eyes. Because of the assortment of clinical presentations, lymphoma can mimic various illnesses.

Lymphoma has been classified using several criteria, including histological features, immunophenotypic markers, cytochemical staining, and anatomical distribution.[79, 187, 202, 211, 220, 221] These diagnostic classification systems have in common the goal of gaining a better understanding of the biology and natural history of lymphoma, which can ultimately affect therapy. Feline lymphoma is a heterogeneous disease of lymphocytes, and identification of prognostic factors through the use of diagnostic classification schemes is an important strategy to gain these insights.

Histological Classification of Feline Lymphomas

Histological classification of lymphomas entails evaluation of individual cell morphology and the architectural arrangement of these cells within the tumor. It has been known for some time that as in humans, feline lymphomas are histopathologically heterogeneous.[208] Numerous schemes to classify lymphomas in humans have been published, and some have been applied to feline lymphomas.[79, 220] From a clinical standpoint, a histopathological classification system that implies biological behavior (and indirectly, prognosis) is obviously desirable. This approach has proved useful in humans, although numerous classifications using various nomenclatures for overlapping histological features have resulted in confusion.[191] In an effort to develop a unified clinical pathological approach for the classification of lymphomas in humans, the National Cancer Institute Working Formulation has emerged.[191]

The morphological criteria of the Working Formulation have been applied to more than 600 cases of feline lymphoproliferative disease.[221] Specimens were classified by nuclear and cytoplasmic features as well as nodal distribution of malignant cells (i.e., follicular malignant cells confined to lymph follicles or diffuse malignant cells widespread throughout the entire node). More than 600 cases of feline lymphoproliferative disease were reviewed: 8.6 per cent were low-grade, 35.1 per cent were intermediate-grade, and 55.2 per cent were high-grade tumors. The remaining 1.1 per cent were plasmacytomas. These figures include 1.6 per cent of chronic lymphocytic leukemias included within the low-grade group and 3.7 per cent of acute lymphocytic leukemias within the high-grade group. More than one-third of all feline lymphomas were of the immunoblastic type, and these tumors did not have a topographical predilection. Approximately 7 per cent of feline lymphomas were of the diffuse mixed type characterized by sclerosis and frequently by focal involvement of the intestinal mucosa. These tumors are highly "homed" to the lamina propria and the submucosa of the intestine and often form bulky tumors while relatively sparing the muscular wall. In a number of cases, these lesions had been excised surgically, with long-term survival of the animal. The recognition of this tumor subtype and its tendency to be localized has important implications for surgical management.

Less than 1 per cent of feline lymphomas had follicular architecture, and in this respect cats are like dogs and cows and unlike humans in which some 25 per cent of lymphomas have this architectural pattern. Lymphoblastic lymphomas, which are a subtype of the high-grade tumors, constituted less than 3 per cent of the population and occurred in cats at about the same level as in humans and at a much lower level than in dogs.

Mitotic rates were low in low-grade tumors and high in high-grade tumors. Mitotic rates were highly variable in the intermediate-grade lymphomas, being high in the follicular large and diffuse large cell variants and very low in the diffuse mixed and diffuse small cleaved cell types. It is anticipated that remission in response to chemotherapy would be most easily obtained in those lymphomas with a high proliferative rate, although this may be short-lived. Remission would likely be difficult to obtain in those tumors with a low mitotic rate, although these lesions would be much more slowly progressive.

Considerable variation in age of animals was noted within the various cell types, but low-grade tumors occured in animals 10 years of age or older whereas high-grade tumors occurred in animals 6 years old or younger. Clinical features for each biopsy sample were not provided.

A term that often produces confusion for clinicians is the diagnosis of *histiocytic* lymphoma. The cells of these tumors are not histiocytes and in the Working Formulation are referred to as *immunoblastic lymphoma.*[191] Morphologically, these are large cells containing large nuclei with prominent, often multiple, nucleoli. The cytoplasm is pale staining. The majority of feline lymphomas are composed of this cell type. Clinicians are encouraged to consult a pathologist about their biopsy samples if the nomenclature of a biopsy report is unfamiliar or confusing. It is hoped that a standardized effort to classify feline lymphomas histologically will be adopted by all veterinary pathologists in the future.[221]

Immunological and Cytochemical Characterization of Feline Lymphomas

The majority of lymphomas in cats are composed of T cells transformed by FeLV.[20, 64] Further immunological and cytochemical classification of feline lymphomas was reported by Rojko and others.[187] In this study, thymic lymphomas induced by the Rickard strain of FeLV were composed of immature thymic lymphocytes. Lymphomas associated with other strains of FeLV showed heterogeneity in the cells of origin and reflected markers or immunological behavior suggestive of helper T-lymphocytes, monocyte/macrophage lineage, and null cells (pre-T, pre-B lymphocytes). This heterogeneity may reflect origin of some lymphomas from hematopoietic progenitor cells infected with FeLV in the bone marrow.[187] Lymphomas arising in the the alimentary tract are usually of B-lymphocyte origin.[79] Most affected cats test negative for FeLV infection.

Anatomical Classification of Feline Lymphomas

Mediastinal Lymphoma

The majority of cats with lymphoma in the thoracic cavity are FeLV positive.[59] Structures involved can include lymph nodes in the mediastinum and remnants of the thymus, especially in kittens. Clinically, it is usually impossible to identify specific tissues affected when tumors are large (Fig. 156–3). This form of lymphoma is common in cats and most often affects young animals between 2 and 3 years of age. Mediastinal lymphoma has been extensively recognized worldwide although varying in prevalence geographically. It was reported as the most common form of lymphoma in England and the second most common form in California and New York.[56, 59, 211] A frequently cited study from Scotland described an 18 per cent prevalence rate for the mediastinal form of feline lymphomas.[129] Affected cats most often show respiratory signs compatible with extrapulmonary, intrathoracic lung compression owing to the large tumor and malignant pleural effusion it induces. A restrictive breathing pattern characterized by tachypneic shallow breaths and slightly forced expiration is typical. Cats often show nonspecific signs such as an-

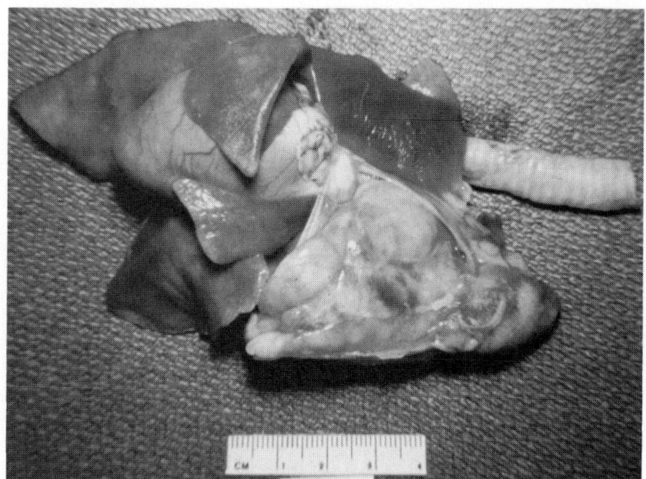

FIGURE 156–3. Mediastinal lymphoma involving the thymus and mediastinal lymph nodes in a young cat.

orexia, depression, listlessness, and vomiting before demonstrating overt respiratory signs. Affected cats cough rarely. Cats are commonly presented on an emergency basis for life-threatening respiratory signs. Physical examination confirms respiratory embarrassment, muffled heart sounds (which are often displaced caudally), and decreased thoracic compressibility. Horner's syndrome is occasionally present owing to compression of the vagosympathetic trunk by the mediastinal mass (Fig. 156–4).

Mediastinal lymphoma should always be high on the list of differential diagnoses when young cats are presented with restrictive breathing patterns. Additional causes of these signs include other causes of pleural effusion such as pyothorax, feline infectious peritonitis, congestive heart failure, or chylothorax (which sometimes accompanies lymphoma); space-occupying lesions such as thymoma, other tumors, or diaphragmatic hernia; and chest wall lesions such as rib fractures.

Radiographs of the thorax reveal a space-occupying mass in the mediastinum, elevation of the trachea, and usually pleural effusion (Fig. 156–5*A*). Given the advanced stage of chest disease evident on radiographs, it is easy to understand why these cats do not tolerate stress or restraint well. It is essential to minimize handling when radiographing dyspneic cats.

Definitive diagnosis of mediastinal lymphoma is made by microscopic examination of tumor tissue or pleural effusion. Fine-needle aspiration through the lateral chest wall using a small-gauge needle is a reliable method to sample the mass or fluid.[148] Diagnostic cytological samples are frequently obtained (Fig. 156–6). Cytological features of thymoma are distinct from lymphoma.[175]

A complete work-up is always recommended to stage lymphoma in the mediastinum (or any other site). Lymphoma in the chest is usually confined to that location, but some cats have a leukemic hemogram showing bone marrow infiltration by cancer cells. This represents a

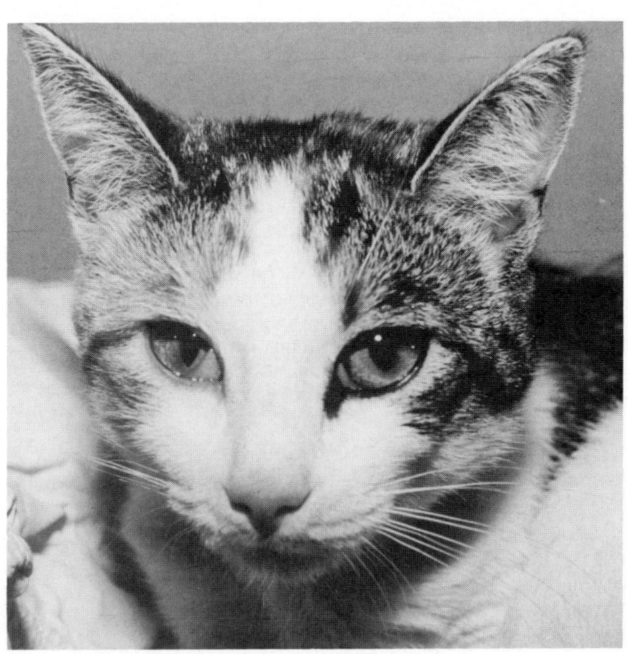

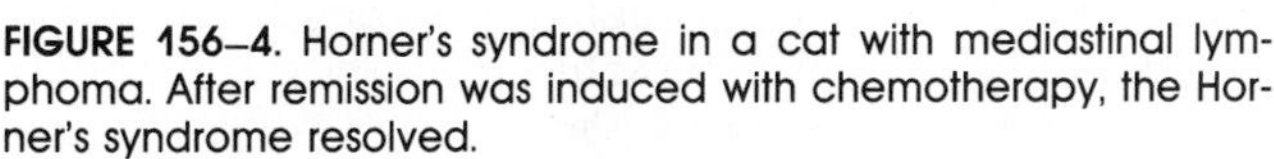

FIGURE 156–4. Horner's syndrome in a cat with mediastinal lymphoma. After remission was induced with chemotherapy, the Horner's syndrome resolved.

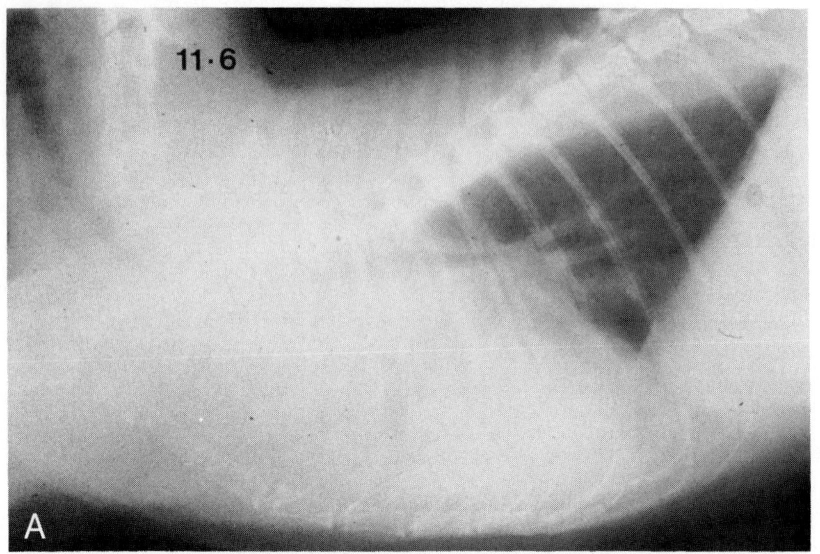

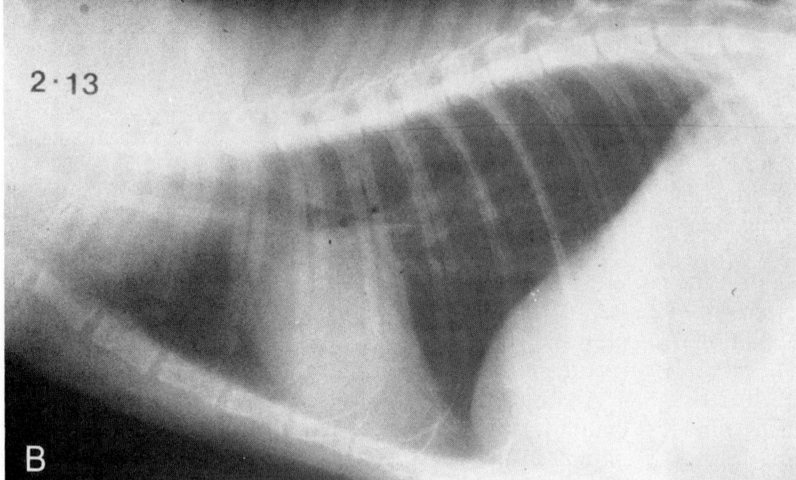

FIGURE 156–5. *A,* Lateral thoracic radiograph of a cat with mediastinal lymphoma. The trachea is elevated, and pleural effusion is present. *B,* After initiation of chemotherapy, remission of this tumor is complete.

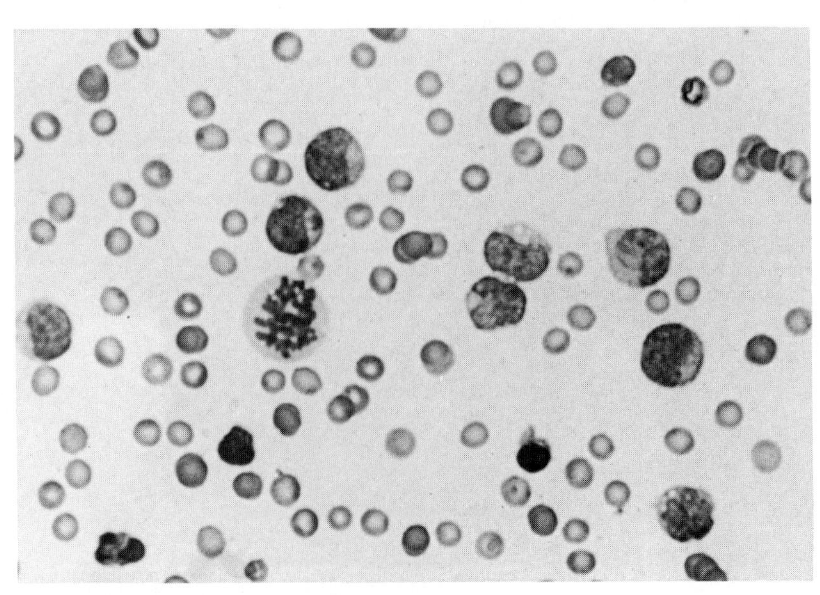

FIGURE 156–6. Photomicrograph of pleural fluid from a cat with mediastinal lymphoma. A mitotic figure and several large, immature lymphocytes are seen. The smallest cells in the background are red blood cells, and several small lymphocytes are also present. (× 100.)

more advanced stage of disease and carries a poorer prognosis (see the later section on prognosis).

Chemotherapy is used to treat lymphoma in the chest, and several protocols have been advocated (Table 156–7). Most cats with mediastinal lymphoma experience rapid shrinkage of tumor mass and improvement of malignant pleural effusion once chemotherapy is instituted (Fig. 156–5*B*).

Alimentary Lymphoma

The epizootiology of alimentary lymphoma differs from the mediastinal form in several respects. Affected cats are usually middle-aged (8 years old), and only a minority (30 per cent) are FeLV positive.[59] In a study of California cats, roughly one-third of animals with lymphoma had the alimentary form,[211] and almost half of the cats in the study from Scotland had lymphoma affecting the alimentary tract.[129]

Alimentary lymphoma involves the stomach, small intestine, or large intestine. It can be solitary or diffuse and result in thickened stomach and bowel walls (Fig. 156–7) or frank obstruction of the gastrointestinal tract by a tumor mass. A common site of obstruction is the ileocecocolic area. Alimentary lymphoma often progresses to involve mesenteric lymph nodes, the liver, and spleen, making this anatomical classification broader than the term *alimentary* implies. Kidney involvement is sometimes also included in this classification.

Cats with alimentary lymphoma demonstrate gastrointestinal signs that are usually chronic (weeks to months) but can be acute. These can include vomiting (not necessarily associated with eating), small-bowel diarrhea, large-bowel diarrhea (with blood and mucus),

TABLE 156–7. PUBLISHED CHEMOTHERAPEUTIC PROTOCOLS FOR FELINE LYMPHOMA

Drug Protocol	Number of Cases	Complete Remission Rate (%)	Median Remission Time (days)	Median Survival Time (days)	Reference
1. VCR, 0.75 mg/m² IV/week × 4 CTX, 300 mg/m² PO day 1, 22 Prednisone, 2 mg/kg/day PO After day 22, VCR and CTX given together every 3 weeks Treat for 1 year.	38	79	321	NS	Cotter[24]
2. VCR, 0.025 mg/kg IV day 1, 15 CTX, 10 mg/kg IV day 8	62	52	112	49	Jeglum et al[93]
MTX, 0.8 mg/kg IV or PO on day 22	With prednisone: 44	NS	NS	70	
Rescue drugs: Used if not in remission; frequency not stated Prednisone, 5 mg PO/day L-Asparaginase, 400 IU/kg	With L-asparaginase: 36	NS	NS	84	
3. VCR, 0.025 mg/kg IV day 1, 15 L-Asparaginase, 400 IU/kg IP on day 1 CTX, 10 mg/kg IV day 8 MTX, 0.8 mg/kg IV day 22 Prednisone, 2 mg/kg PO/day × 1 year *Repeat* × 8 weeks, L-asparaginase used only initially; then repeat every 10 days × 8; then every 2 weeks × 7 months. Year 2: treat every 3 weeks; year 3: every 4 weeks; Year 4: every 6 weeks; year 5: every 8 weeks	103	62	NS	210	Mooney et al[148]
4. *Induction* 50 mg/m² PO daily × 4 days VCR, 0.5 mg/m²/week IV Ara-C, 100 mg/m²/day IV infusion or SC × 2 days, week 1 only Prednisone, 40 mg/m² PO × 7 days, then 20 mg/m² PO every 2 days *Repeat* for 6 weeks *Intensification* (if not in remission after induction) L-Asparaginase, 10,00020,000 IU/m² SC one time *Maintenance* (if in remission) CLR, 2 mg/m² every other day or 20 mg/m² PO every 14 days MTX, 2.5 mg/m² PO 2–3 times/week Prednisone, 20 mg/m² every other day	NS	NS	NS	NS	Couto[30]

VCR, Vincristine; CTX, Cyclophosphamide; MTX, Methotrexate; Ara-C, Cytosine arabinoside; CLR, Chlorambucil; NS, Not stated.

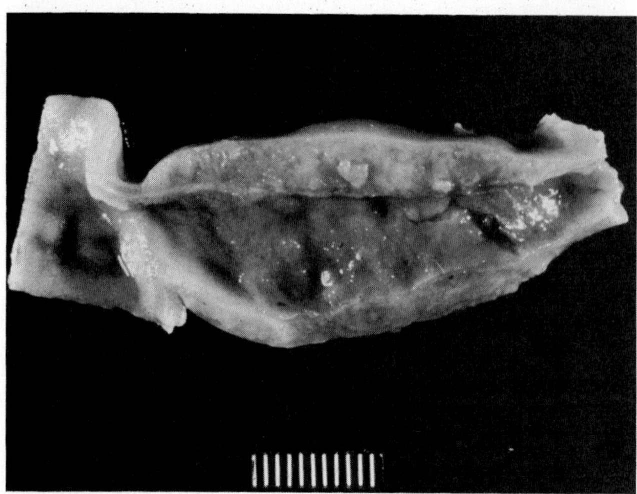

FIGURE 156–7. Lymphoma infiltrating a section of small intestine of a cat, causing mural thickening, lack of bowel pliability, and intestinal obstruction.

weight loss, and inappetence. When the disease has been chronic, physical examination often reveals that cats are underweight and sometimes cachectic. Abdominal palpation may reveal mass(es) associated with the bowel or mesenteric lymph nodes. Thickened loops of intestinal wall can occasionally be felt in a thin cat with diffuse intestinal disease, but this finding has been greatly exaggerated in veterinary literature. Hepatosplenomegaly can also be palpated when present. Although physical and historical signs might suggest alimentary or gastrointestinal lymphoma, this form of malignancy is not as readily diagnosed as the mediastinal form. Differential diagnoses include hyperthyroidism, diabetes mellitus, and in cats with mesenteric masses, feline infectious peritonitis.

The diagnosis is confirmed by microscopic examination of tumor cells obtained from a fine-needle aspirate of intestinal wall or mass or via laparotomy with incisional/excisional surgical biopsy. Laparotomy has the advantage of facilitating staging of the disease through the sampling of multiple sites of the alimentary tract. There is a risk, however, that incisions into the lymphomatous bowel might dehisce owing to poor healing at the tumor site. Biopsy specimens can also be obtained with the use of an endoscope inserted *per os* or *per rectum*. This technique allows multiple sampling in a noninvasive manner with rapid recovery and earlier institution of cytotoxic chemotherapy that could otherwise affect healing of a laparotomy incision. The small size of individual samples poses minimal risk of intestinal perforation. The major disadvantages of endoscopic biopsy include inability to obtain samples deep into the mucosa or superficial submucosa. Lymphoma has a tendency to "preferentially" affect the lamina propria and submucosa in cats.[221] Also, it is difficult to examine the entire intestine with the endoscope.

Radiographs of the gastrointestinal tract, especially contrast series using barium sulfate, sometimes demonstrate mucosal irregularities that suggest mural lymphoma or frank obstruction. For many, effective use of the endoscope has superseded radiological studies in diagnosis of alimentary lymphoma.

One report described chronic lymphocytic-plasmacytic enteritis progressing to overt lymphoma in several cats.[40] The gastrointestinal signs associated with lymphocytic-plasmacytic enteritis resolved with dietary management, and subsequent biopsy samples showed resolution of lesions. From 6 to 18 months later, gastrointestinal signs recurred and new specimens revealed lymphoma. A role for chronic inflammatory bowel disease in the natural history of alimentary lymphoma in cats is speculative.

The treatment of choice for alimentary lymphoma is chemotherapy (see Table 156–7). Surgery is used to palliate obstructions and may result in long-term remissions if lesions are focal.[221] Some cats experience long survivals (i.e., $>$ 1 year) when treated with multiagent chemotherapy.[24, 93]

Multicentric Lymphoma

Multicentric lymphoma usually includes lymphomas that are widely disseminated to many lymphoid tissues. The peripheral lymph nodes are most often involved, but additional lymphoid structures affected include the spleen, liver, and bone marrow. Although some investigators[59, 211] include cats with primary lymphoid neoplasia of the bone marrow and blood in the multicentric category, others[30, 93] suggest that primary involvement of the bone marrow constitutes a separate classification of lymphoid leukemia. From the viewpoint of survival of treated cats (see the later section on prognosis), it is most appropriate to exclude cats with lymphoid leukemia from the multicentric classification, given the uniformly worse prognosis for the leukemics.[24, 148] Additional confusion about classification arises when trying to group cats with lymphomas in nonlymphoid tissues. For example, cats with renal lymphoma are sometimes included with multicentric patients for the purpose of analyzing survival data by stage,[148] whereas others separate renal involvement entirely.[24, 93]

Most cats (80 per cent) with multicentric lymphoma are FeLV positive and are younger (mean age 4 years).[59] Cats with multicentric lymphoma are presented for various complaints depending on extent of disease. Enlarged, nonpainful peripheral lymph nodes often are incidental findings by conscientious cat owners. Hepatosplenomegaly is frequently present, and some cats also have enlarged tonsils. Extranodal involvement is frequently found with primary multicentric lymphoid disease, and sites include the kidneys (usually bilaterally), eyes, CNS, and less often the skin.

The high prevalence of FeLV infection in cats with multicentric lymphoma accounts for a large number of cats with anemia and other FeLV-associated problems concurrent with lymphoma.[30, 148] Affected cats should undergo complete staging before chemotherapy, the usual treatment of choice (see Table 156–7). The prognosis for affected cats varies based on clinical stage and FeLV status (see the later section on prognosis).[148]

Miscellaneous Lymphomas

A group of lymphomas arising in various extralymphoid sites are often referred to as *miscellaneous lymphomas.* Most commonly affected sites are the kidneys, eyes, CNS, and skin. A study of 28 cases of feline renal lymphoma reported a mean age of 7 years for these cats; 50 per cent were FeLV positive.[149] Various degrees of azotemia were present, but the magnitude of azotemia did not always correlate with survival time. Involvement of the CNS was a frequent sequel to renal lymphoma, causing death of 40 per cent of the cats studied. In all cats in this study, lymphoma involved tissues beyond the kidneys. All cats received chemotherapy (see Table 157–7), and the majority experienced clinical remissions. A summary of clinical aspects of other extranodal lymphomas in cats has been published.[30]

Treatment and Prognosis of Feline Lymphomas

Feline lymphomas are treated with systemic multiagent chemotherapy because the malignancy usually affects more than one body site and lymphoma cells are sensitive to various drugs. Surgery, radiotherapy, and immunotherapy have more limited use. Radiotherapy is useful for local control of lymphoma because of the extreme sensitivity of lymphoid cells. It is occasionally used with chemotherapy when rapid remissions are urgent, as in some cases of mediastinal lymphoma.[30] Immunotherapy, principally using staphylococcal protein A, has demonstrated efficacy and continues to be investigated.[45, 205]

Chemotherapeutic agents most used to treat feline lymphoma include vincristine, cyclophosphamide, L-asparaginase, methotrexate, cytosine arabinoside, and prednisone (see Table 156–7). Curiously, doxorubicin, an important agent in the long-term control of canine lymphoma, has not enjoyed similar popularity in the treatment of feline lymphoma. Several investigators have recommended the use of doxorubicin for cats with lymphoma,[30, 136] but there are no reports of treatment results. Chemotherapeutic protocols, as well as remission and survival times reported by several oncologists, are detailed in Table 156–7.

One of the most confusing aspects encountered when comparing results obtained with various protocols is the tendency of researchers to subdivide responses by anatomical form of lymphoma.[24, 93] The problem with this approach is that the natural behavior of feline lymphomas does not always lend itself to simplified anatomical classification schemes, and anatomical distribution does not necessarily imply total body tumor burden. In addition, anatomical groupings are subjective and vary among investigators. For this reason, some oncologists have favored classification of lymphoma by stage rather than location.[147] The staging system proposed differs from that of the World Health Organization. One report using this approach did not determine anatomical location to significantly affect therapeutic response.[148] Regardless of location, 62 per cent of all 103 treated cats experienced complete remission and had a median survival of 7 months. One-third of these cats survived at

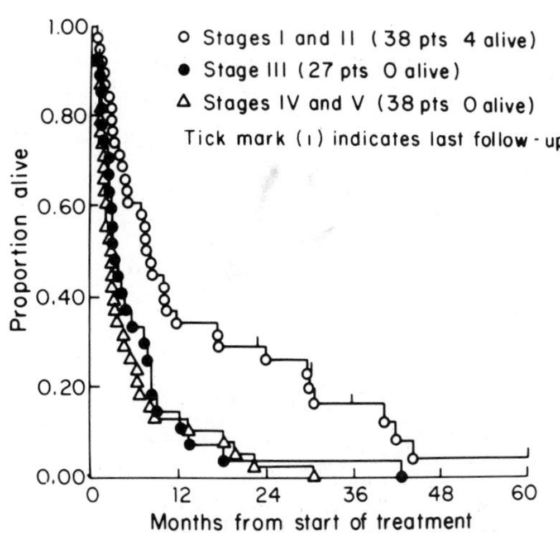

FIGURE 156–8. Correlation of survival time and stage of lymphoma in cats treated with chemotherapy. Cats with less advanced disease (stages I and II) had the longest median survival time (7.6 months), whereas cats with the most advanced stages (IV and V) had the shortest median survival time (2.6 months). Median survival time for cats with stage III lymphoma was 3.2 months. (From Mooney SC, et al: Treatment and prognostic factors in lymphoma in cats: 103 cases (1977–1981). *J Am Vet Med Assoc 194*:696, 1989.)

least 1 year. The study showed that two variables, namely clinical stage and FeLV status, significantly affected prognosis. Those cats with less advanced stages (stages I and II) lived significantly longer than cats with advanced disease (Fig. 156–8). Cats that were FeLV negative with lymphoma also survived longer than FeLV-positive cats (Fig. 156–9). A correlation of survival time, stage of disease, and FeLV status showed that advanced tumor stages or FeLV infection carried an equally poor prognosis (Fig. 156–10).

Lymphoid Leukemias

Lymphoid leukemias are characterized by the proliferation of malignant lymphoid cells primarily within the

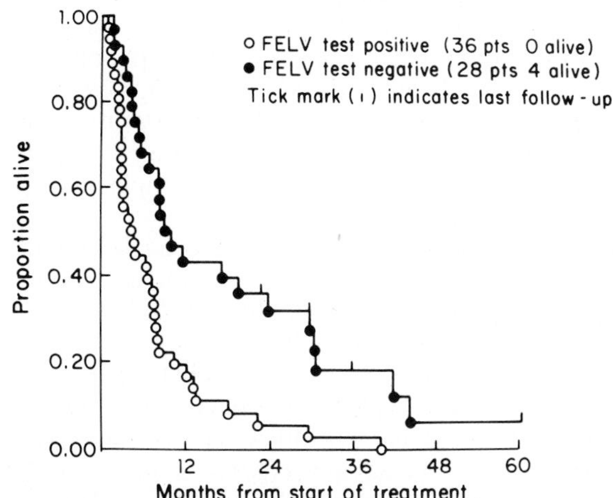

FIGURE 156–9. Correlation of survival time and FeLV status in cats with lymphoma that achieved complete remission with chemotherapy. The median survival time for FeLV-positive cats was 4.2 months versus 9 months for FeLV-negative cats. (From Mooney SC, et al: Treatment and prognostic factors in lymphoma in cats: 103 cases (1977–1981). *J Am Vet Med Assoc 194*:696, 1989.)

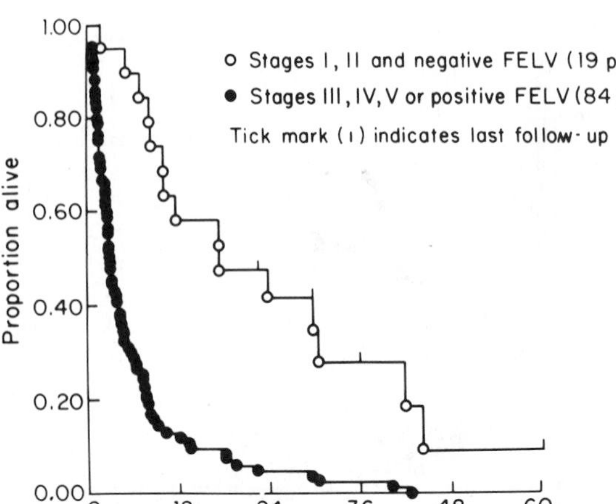

FIGURE 156–10. Correlation of survival time, stage of disease, and FeLV status in cats with lymphoma treated with chemotherapy. Cats that were FeLV negative with less advanced disease (stages I and II) had a long median survival time of 17.5 months compared with FeLV-positive cats with more advanced lymphoma (stages III, IV, and V) that had a median survival time of only 2.9 months. (From Mooney SC, et al: Treatment and prognostic factors in lymphoma in cats: 103 cases (1977–1981). *J Am Vet Med Assoc* *194*:696, 1989.)

bone marrow. Malignant cells usually but not always circulate in the blood and infiltrate organs of the reticuloendothelial system. Therefore, leukemia is a bone marrow disease that spreads peripherally whereas lymphoma is a disease that originates peripherally and progresses centrally. This distinction is of clinical relevance because the prognosis for lymphoma is usually more favorable than for true leukemia.

In cats, most lymphoid leukemias are an immature, blastic cell type. This form of leukemia, referred to as *acute lymphoblastic leukemia* is characterized by rapid onset, fulminant course, and relatively poor response to chemotherapy. The hallmark of the diagnosis is identification of large numbers ($\geq$ 30 per cent) of these cells in a bone marrow aspirate. The peripheral blood smear usually contains large numbers of lymphoblasts, and white blood cell counts often exceed 50,000/μl; pancytopenia can also be present.[30, 54, 213] Poorly differentiated blasts may require cytochemical staining to confirm a lymphoid lineage; negative staining reactions suggest the presence of lymphoid cells.[48]

Clinical signs of acute lymphoblastic leukemia are nonspecific and include lethargy, anorexia, vomiting, and diarrhea. Physical abnormalities include pallor, splenomegaly, hepatomegaly, mildly enlarged lymph nodes, and fever. Most animals are FeLV positive.

Although chemotherapy can effectively lower the cell counts, only a small percentage of treated cats attain complete remission. In one report, 27 per cent of cats with acute lymphoblastic leukemia attained complete remission, compared with 79 per cent of cats with lymphoma.[24] Unless cats attained complete remission, survival time was short. The median survival for the 27 per cent of responding cats was 7 months. The chemotherapeutic approach for treating acute lymphoblastic leukemia is usually the same as for lymphoma,[24] but one report described a short-term remission in a cat with lymphoid leukemia using a low dose (10 mg/m^2) of cytosine arabinoside injected subcutaneously twice daily.[72]

Chronic lymphocytic leukemia is rare in cats. The low occurrence of this form of lymphoid neoplasia suggests it is not an important consequence of FeLV infection. Two cases were described by Couto, and both cats tested negative for FeLV infection by ELISA, although in one cat, FeLV could be reactivated from the bone marrow.[30]

Chronic lymphocytic leukemia is characterized by excessive numbers of mature (well-differentiated) lymphocytes that are produced in the bone marrow. Affected cats have shown nonspecific signs including lethargy, inappetence, vomiting, and diarrhea. Physical examination revealed hepatosplenomegaly but not lymphadenopathy.

Based on limited experience, a less aggressive chemotherapeutic approach is warranted. Chlorambucil (2 mg/m^2 PO every other day) plus prednisone (20 mg/m^2 PO every other day) can improve clinical signs.

Plasma Cell Neoplasms

In contrast to dogs, malignancies affecting plasma cells are rarer in cats.[30, 70] Most reports of feline plasma cell disease are of multiple myeloma, a condition in which large numbers of malignant plasma cells replicate primarily in the bone marrow (Fig. 156–11).[43, 83, 145] As in other species, the abnormal plasma cells, all derived from the same malignant clone, secrete large quantities of an identical class of immunoglobulin referred to as a *paraprotein* or *M component.* Most reports of feline multiple myeloma have described the paraprotein as IgG. An unusual case of IgA myeloma was reported in a cat with a pleural effusion and *Salmonella typhimurium* infection.[70] The large amount of circulating immunoglobulin can cause serum hyperviscosity when the paraprotein is of high molecular weight, such as IgA. Impaired CNS blood flow and capillary hemorrhages result. The clinical signs referable to hyperviscosity include neurological abnormalities, retinal hemorrhages/degeneration, and cardiac failure, all of which have been reported in cats.[70, 83]

Other clinical signs associated with multiple myeloma in cats are nonspecific and have included vomiting, anorexia, listlessness, and neurological abnormalities such as circling.[43, 70, 83] High plasma protein concentration, neurological signs, and retinal lesions are also compatible with feline infectious peritonitis. The diagnosis of multiple myeloma is confirmed by finding bone marrow infiltration by plasma cells, hyperproteinemia with monoclonal gammopathy on serum protein electrophoresis, and Bence Jones proteins in the urine. Bence Jones proteins are light chains (i.e., incomplete immunoglobulin molecules) and are not detected by routine dipstick testing of the urine. Although osteolytic lesions are a common finding in canine multiple myeloma, they are uncommon in cats.[30]

There are limited reports of therapy for cats with

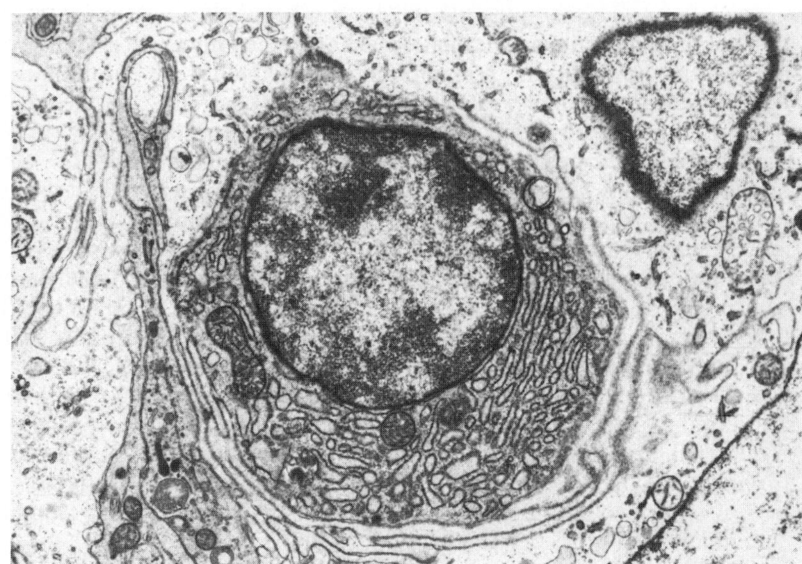

FIGURE 156–11. Ultrastructure of a plasma cell from the bone marrow of a cat with multiple myeloma. Within the cytoplasm is abundant rough endoplasmic reticulum typical of plasma cells. (×12,400.)

multiple myeloma.[43] Cats, like dogs, have been treated with a combination of the alkylating agent melphalan (0.5 mg PO once a day for 10 days; then 0.5 mg PO every other day) and prednisone. One report described improvement in three of five affected cats treated with this regimen, but their survival times were short (4 to 9 months) compared with dogs.[43] Multiple myeloma is a more aggressive disease in cats than in dogs.

Myeloproliferative Disorders

Acute

Any cell line in the bone marrow has the potential to undergo malignant transformation. The pluripotent nature of bone marrow cells often results in malignant cells that are poorly differentiated and morphologically difficult to classify. More than one cell line can be involved, sometimes simultaneously and occasionally sequentially.[68, 198] Collectively, primary bone marrow malignancies are classified as leukemia, but given the variety of cell lines that can be involved, the term *myeloproliferative disorder* is more accurate. These diseases can constitute as much as 30 per cent of hemolymphatic neoplasia in cats.[211] The majority (70 to 90 per cent) of affected cats test positive for FeLV infection.[211]

The clinical and pathological features of acute myeloproliferative disorders are ubiquitous regardless of the individual cell line(s) affected. Acute onset of signs is the norm, and cats are depressed, anorectic, and lethargic. Physical examination reveals pale mucous membranes, hepatomegaly, splenomegaly, and sometimes mildly enlarged lymph nodes and fever. The diagnosis of myeloproliferative disease is confirmed by examination of the peripheral blood and bone marrow, which demonstrate various abnormalities. The bone marrow contains large numbers of atypical immature blasts and decreased numbers of normal precursor cells. Other hemolymphatic organs are also infiltrated. These cells often circulate in the peripheral blood in high numbers and are present on the blood smear. White blood cell counts can be quite high (> 200,000/μl), but leukemic cells sometimes are primarily confined to the bone marrow, resulting in a low white blood cell count. Most cats are neutropenic, thrombocytopenic, and profoundly anemic. Based on morphological features, specific leukemic disorders described in cats include acute myelogenous leukemia, acute monocytic leukemia, acute myelomonocytic leukemia, undifferentiated leukemia (formerly reticuloendotheliosis), erythremic myelosis (a proliferation of erythroid precursors), erythroleukemia, and megakaryocytic leukemia.[65] Acute eosinophilic leukemia experimentally induced by FeLV is also described.[113] Because of the aggressive and rapid clinical course of most myeloproliferative diseases in cats, the majority are classed as acute leukemias. Most of these leukemias affect the white cell series; however, erythremic myelosis is characterized by large numbers of nucleated red blood cells in the peripheral blood despite a low packed cell volume and inadequate reticulocyte response.

In addition to morphology, efforts can be made to distinguish involved cell lines by using cytochemical stains in cats.[48] From a clinical perspective, the uniformly grave prognosis for cats with myeloproliferative diseases does not warrant this time-consuming procedure. Chemotherapy for cats with myeloproliferative diseases has not been successful and therefore is not routinely recommended.[54, 73, 74] For surgeons, the importance of these diseases lies in the knowledge of their poor prognosis, making surgical procedures in affected cats unwarranted.

Chronic

Cats, in contrast to dogs, have relatively few chronic myeloproliferative disorders. One group of chronic abnormalities recognized in cats are the myelodysplastic syndromes, also referred to as *hematopoietic dysplasias* and *preleukemic syndromes.*[134] The hallmark of these disorders is peripheral blood cytopenias, especially leukopenia, but any or all of the blood lines can be affected. Ineffective hematopoiesis by a defective clone of myeloid cells in the marrow is responsible for the abnormal blood findings.[114] Despite marked peripheral blood cytopenia, bone marrow aspiration reveals normal to increased cellularity due to the presence of large numbers of very immature granulocytic precursors and gives the picture of a maturation arrest.[66] These hematological abnormalities can persist for weeks to years, during which time affected cats can show anorexia, lethargy, weight loss, intermittent fever, and infections.[133, 134] Some animals die of these problems. Some cats eventually develop overt acute leukemia, usually characterized by large numbers of neoplastic blast cells in the blood and bone marrow.[133, 134] For this reason, myelodysplasia is sometimes referred to as *preleukemic syndrome.*

Most affected cats are young and are FeLV positive.[134] The importance of recognition of feline myelodysplastic syndromes lies in the poor long-term prognosis associated with these syndromes. Rarely, however, individual cats have spontaneously recovered.[66] Therapy for feline myelodysplastic syndromes has not been worthwhile,[134] although newer approaches are being aimed at reversing the arrested bone marrow maturation by inducing cellular differentiation.[180, 216] Low-dose injections of cytosine arabinoside (10 mg/m^2 BID SC) have most often been used for this purpose. One cat with acute leukemia showed short-term improvement with this therapy.[72]

Polycythemia rubra vera is another chronic myeloproliferative disease that has occasionally been reported in cats.[30, 179] The condition is characterized by autonomous proliferation of red blood cell precursors in the bone marrow, resulting in an excessive number of circulating red blood cells. A very high packed cell volume, usually greater than 70 per cent, is present despite low to normal serum erythropoietin activity.[30] Clinical signs, probably the result of hyperviscosity, hypervolemia, and vascular thrombosis, are chiefly neurological. Emergency treatment consists of phlebotomy, initially removing at least 20 ml of blood per kilogram, plus saline replacement. Because the blood is thick, a large-gauge needle works best. Hydroxyurea (15 mg/kg) can be used to suppress erythropoiesis. This drug is extremely myelosuppressive in cats, and close monitoring of the hemogram is essential.

Feline Immunodeficiency Virus

Feline immunodeficiency virus (FIV) was discovered in 1987.[164] Since that time, considerable information has been forthcoming about its biology, epizootiology, and clinical syndromes.[53, 82, 84, 118, 234, 235]

Like FeLV, FIV is a retrovirus (family Retrovirinae), but unlike FeLV, it is a lentivirus, endowing it with more similarities to other immunodeficiency viruses including those of humans and simians.[207] Infections by lentiviruses are characteristically asymptomatic for long periods before clinical signs are evidenced.[57] FIV preferentially infects T-lymphocytes, resulting in selective destruction of helper T cells.[46, 235] Helper T-lymphocytes are pivotal to the generation of the cell-mediated immune response. This is in contrast to FeLV, which not only infects lymphocytes but also replicates in all nucleated cells of the myeloid lineages. Infection with FIV is lifelong, whereas many cats initially infected by FeLV are able to eradicate this virus.[235]

FIV, like other lentiviruses, elicits an early antibody response in infected cats, with seroconversion detectable within 2 to 4 weeks of (experimental) infection.[235] Induction of antibodies to viral proteins does not eliminate viremia, because FIV routinely coexists with these antibodies. The presence of FIV antibody is therefore a highly reliable sign of FIV infection.[235] Both IFA and ELISA techniques have been used to detect FIV antibodies, and an ELISA test kit is commercially available.

Seroepidemiological studies have demonstrated a worldwide prevalence of FIV infection.[53, 84, 118, 174, 234] The majority of positive cats are sick. Of sick cats tested, 14 per cent in the United States and 44 per cent in Japan were positive for FIV infection.[84, 234] The high prevalence of infection in the Japanese cats was attributed to the larger number of free-roaming cats in that country.[84] A much lower prevalence was noted in healthy cats tested in these studies, suggesting that FIV is endemic rather than epidemic.[168] Viral transmission is probably most often accomplished through bite wounds.[234, 235] This is because infected cats shed virus in their saliva and likely explains the greater prevalence for free-roaming male cats to test positive owing to their aggressive territorial behavior.[234, 235] Although virus can be recovered from the blood, serum, plasma, CSF, and saliva of infected cats, close contact (other than biting) is a relatively inefficient method for horizontal transmission.[168] Other routes of transmission are uncommon to nonexistent, including venereal, *in utero,* and neonatal via colostrum, milk, and maternal grooming.[168] In nature, cats most often identified with FIV infections have been between 5 and 7 years old, reflecting the long prodromal period associated with lentivirus infection.[84, 234]

Once a cat is infected by FIV, three stages characterize the clinical course. Four to 6 weeks after infection, an initial acute stage is seen, typified by neutropenia and generalized lymphadenopathy in most cats with low-grade fever and malaise in some.[168] Histological examination of the lymph nodes shows follicular hyperplasia with dysplasia.[168] Peripheral lymphadenopathy lasts between 3 and 6 months, whereas neutropenia reportedly lasts between 2 and 9 weeks.[207] Less frequently, experimentally infected cats developed superficial bacterial skin infections.[207] A period of relative normalcy, which can last from months to years, follows the acute phase.[168]

The third and final stage is considered the terminal stage, when cats demonstrate the much publicized acquired immunodeficiency syndrome (AIDS).[168] Development of mild to moderate anemia (either regenerative or nonregenerative) and recrudescence of neutropenia signal the onset of the terminal stage.[168] Cats show various clinical syndromes that can be single or multiple in any one cat and wax and wane from months to years before death.[207] The most frequent (50 per cent) finding is chronic progressive oral infection affecting the gingiva, periodontal tissues, cheeks, or tongue.[168] Gingivitis and stomatitis can be purulent and necrotizing or show plasmacytic infiltration. Chronic upper respiratory tract infections affect about 25 per cent of cats and are sometimes associated with conjunctivitis and oral ulcers. Chronic bacterial skin infections (often due to *Staphylococcus*) and otitis externa are noted in about 50 per cent of FIV-AIDS cats.[168] Chronic diarrhea due to enteritis is present in 10 per cent.[82, 168] Histological findings include enterocyte necrosis; fused, atrophic villi; and dilated crypts.[207] Vague signs including weight loss, inappetence, recurrent fevers, generalized or localized lymphadenopathy, or neurological behavioral changes are encountered in about 30 per cent of FIV-positive cats.[82, 168] Neurological signs described include dementia, twitching of the face and tongue, and psychoses (e.g., hiding, aggression, pacing).[168] Cats develop various infections, some of which are unusual or opportunistic, such as toxoplasmosis, cryptococcosis, candidiasis, generalized demodectic and notoedric mange, and hemobartonellosis.[82, 84, 168] This list is probably incomplete. Ocular disease affecting the anterior uveal tract, anterior vitreous, and retina has also been reported.[47] Lymphoma and myeloproliferative diseases have also developed in FIV-positive cats that were FeLV negative.[234] Several solid tumors including squamous cell carcinoma, mammary carcinoma, and adnexal lung tumor have been recognized in FIV-infected cats.[82, 84] The role of FIV in the pathogenesis of neoplasia is unknown.

Although approximately 10 to 15 per cent of clinically sick cats with FIV infection are coinfected with FeLV, this finding does not appear to represent an increased risk of FeLV infection in cats infected by FIV.[84, 234] However, cats that are infected with both retroviruses reportedly died earlier and had more severe clinical disease than cats infected with FIV alone.[53, 84, 234] Preexistent FeLV infection greatly potentiates the expression and spread of FIV, thereby increasing the severity of the initial and chronic (terminal) stages of FIV infection.[167]

Treatment of FIV-infected cats is symptomatic and directed at control of secondary/opportunistic infections and providing general supportive care. Cats usually respond favorably to early treatments but become more refractory with time, most likely because of continued deterioration of the immune system.[168] With proper care, it is possible for some cats to enjoy years of comfortable life. Antiviral drugs that inhibit reverse transcriptase, such as azidothymidine, have shown hematological toxicity in cats.[69] Treatment of infected cats with the purine analogue 9-(2-phosphonomethoxyethyl) adenine suppressed replication of FIV, resulting in improvement of opportunistic infections and clinical signs of stomatitis, gingivitis, and diarrhea.[44] Immunological manipulations through administration of combinations of interferons and interleukin-2 represent another possible therapeutic approach.[207]

Spread of FIV is probably best controlled by segregating FIV-positive cats. Because the major mode of transmission is via bites, keeping cats indoors, restricting free roaming, neutering males to reduce their fighting, and avoiding introduction of stray or feral cats without prior FIV testing are strategies to break the cycle of infection.[168] Because FIV does not replicate in human cells, is labile in the environment, and slow to induce clinical disease, immediate euthanasia is probably not warranted.[168, 174]

Several key points about FIV are important to surgeons. Cats demonstrating neutropenia or anemia on a presurgical screen should be tested for FIV (as well as FeLV). Similarly, cats considered in high-risk groups for FIV should also be tested before surgery. After thorough client education, nonelective surgery could be performed on asymptomatic FIV-infected cats, but more frequent monitoring of surgical wounds and concurrent administration of antibiotics are prudent.

References

1. Ackerman L: Cutaneous T cell-like lymphoma in the dog. *Comp Cont Educ Pract Vet 6*:37, 1984.
2. Ackerman N, Madewell BR: Thoracic and abdominal radiographic abnormalities in the multicentric form of lymphosarcoma in dogs. *J Am Vet Med Assoc 176*:36, 1980.
3. Appelbaum FR, et al: Marrow transplant studies in dogs with malignant lymphoma. *Transplantation 39*:499, 1985.
4. Aul C, Schneider W: The role of low-dose cytosine arabinoside and aggresive chemotherapy in advanced myelodysplastic syndromes. *Cancer 64*:1812, 1989.
5. Baccarani M, et al: Low dose arabinosyl cytosine for treatment of myelodysplastic syndromes and subacute myeloid leukemia. *Leukemia Res 7*:539, 1983.
6. Barthel CH: Acute myelomonocytic leukemia in a dog. *Vet Pathol 11*:79, 1974.
7. Barton CL: Cytologic diagnosis of cutaneous neoplasia: An algorithmic approach. *Comp Cont Educ Pract Vet 9*:29, 1987.
8. Bennet JM, et al: Proposals for the classification of the acute leukemias. *Br J Haematol 33*:451, 1976.
9. Besmer P: Acute transforming feline retroviruses. *Curr Top Microbiol Immunol 107*:1, 1983.
10. Breitschwerdt EB, et al: Clinical and epidemiologic characterization of a diarrheal syndrome in Basenji dogs. *J Am Vet Med Assoc 180*:914, 1982.
11. Brick JO, et al: Chemotherapy of malignant lymphoma in dogs and cats. *J Am Vet Med Assoc 153*:47, 1968.
12. Britt JO, et al: Malignant lymphoma of the meninges in two dogs. *J Comp Pathol 94*:45, 1984.
13. Brooks MB, et al: Use of splenectomy in the management of lymphoma in dogs: 16 cases (1976–1985). *J Am Vet Med Assoc 191*:1008, 1987.
14. Brown NO, et al: Cutaneous lymphosarcoma in the dog: A disease with variable clinical and histologic manifestations. *J Am Anim Hosp Assoc 16*:565, 1980.
15. Cain R, et al: Platelet dysplasia associated with megakaryoblastic leukemia in a dog. *J Am Vet Med Assoc 188*:529, 1986.
16. Calvert CA, Leifer CE: Doxorubicin for the treatment of canine lymphosarcoma after development of resistance to combination chemotherapy. *J Am Vet Med Assoc 179*:1011, 1981.
17. Cameron TP, et al: Irradiation of a dog with myelogenous leukemia. *J Am Vet Med Assoc 154*:279, 1969.
18. Carter RF, et al: Chemotherapy of canine lymphoma with histopathological correlation: Doxorubicin alone compared to COP as first treatment regimen. *J Am Anim Hosp Assoc 23*:587, 1987.
19. Chapman NL, et al: A preliminary report on virus-like particles in canine leukemia and derived cell cultures. *Cancer Res 27*:18, 1967.
20. Cockerell GL, et al: Characterization of feline T- and B-lymphocytes and identification of an experimentally induced T-cell neoplasm in the cat. *J Natl Cancer Inst 57*:907, 1976.
21. Cogan DC, et al: Effect of suramin on serum viral replication in feline leukemia virus-infected pet cats. *Am J Vet Res 47*:2230, 1986.
22. Cotter GW, et al: Palliative radiation treatment of cutaneous mycosis fungoides—a dose response. *Int J Radiat Oncol Biol Phys 9*:1477, 1983.
23. Cotter SM: Treatment of lymphoma and leukemia with cyclophosphamide, vincristine, and prednisone: I. Treatment of dogs. *J Am Anim Hosp Assoc 19*:159, 1983.
24. Cotter SM: Treatment of lymphoma and leukemia with cyclophosphamide, vincristine, and prednisone: II. Treatment of cats. *J Am Anim Hosp Assoc 19*:166, 1983.
25. Cotter SM: Treatment of retroviral infections. Proceedings of the 7th American College of Veterinary Internal Medicine Forum. Vol 7. San Diego, May 1989, pp 909–912.
26. Cotter SM, Goldstein MA: Comparison of two protocols for maintenance of remission in dogs with lymphoma. *J Am Anim Hosp Assoc 23*:495, 1987.

27. Couto CG: Canine lymphomas: Something old, something new. *Comp Cont Educ Pract Vet 7*:291, 1985.
28. Couto CG: Clinicopathologic aspects of acute leukemias in the dog. *J Am Vet Med Assoc 186*:681, 1985.
29. Couto CG: Cutaneous lymphomas. Proceedings of the 11th Annual Kal Kan Symposium. Vol 11. Columbus, Ohio, Oct. 1987, pp 71–77.
30. Couto CG: Oncology. *In* Sherding RG (ed): *The Cat: Diseases and Clinical Management*. Churchill Livingstone, New York, 1989, pp 589–647.
31. Couto CG, Helfand SC: Chemotherapy for canine cutaneous lymphoma. Proceedings of the 5th Annual Conference of the Veterinary Cancer Society. Vol 5. West Lafayette, Ind., Oct. 1985, p 16.
32. Couto CG, Kallet AJ: Preleukemic syndrome in a dog. *J Am Vet Med Assoc 184*:1389, 1984.
33. Couto CG, Sousa C: Chronic lymphocytic leukemia with cutaneous involvement in a dog. *J Am Anim Hosp Assoc 22*:374, 1986.
34. Couto CG, et al: Central nervous system lymphosarcoma in the dog. *J Am Vet Med Assoc 184*:809, 1984.
35. Couto CG, et al: Gastrointestinal lymphoma in 20 dogs. *J Vet Intern Med 3*:73, 1989.
36. Crow SE: Lymphosarcoma (malignant lymphoma) in the dog: Diagnosis and treatment. *Comp Cont Educ Pract Vet 4*:283, 1982.
37. Crow SE, et al: Chemoimmunotherapy for canine lymphosarcoma. *Cancer 40*:2102, 1977.
38. Dallman MJ, Saunders GK: Primary spinal cord lymphosarcoma in a dog. *J Am Vet Med Assoc 189*:1348, 1986.
39. da Silva Curiel JMA, et al: Multiple mucocutaneous lymphosarcoma in a dog. *Can Vet J 29*:1001, 1988.
40. Davenport DJ, et al: Progression of lymphocytic-plasmacytic enteritis to gastrointestinal lymphosarcoma in three cats. Proceedings of the 7th Annual Conference of the Veterinary Cancer Society. Vol 7 (Suppl). Madison, Wis., Oct. 1987.
41. Deeg HJ, et al: Autologous marrow transplantation as consolidation therapy for canine lymphoma: Efficacy and toxicity of various regimens of total body irradiation. *Am J Vet Res 46*:2016, 1985.
42. Dorn CR, et al: Survey of animal neoplasms in Alameda and Contra Costa Counties, California. II. Cancer morbidity in dogs and cats from Alameda County. *J Natl Cancer Inst 40*:307, 1968.
43. Drazner FH: Multiple myeloma in the cat. *Comp Cont Educ Pract Vet 4*:206, 1982.
44. Egberink H, et al: Suppression of feline immunodeficiency virus infection *in vivo* by 9-(2-phosphonomethoxyethyl) adenine. *Proc Natl Acad Sci USA. 87*:3087, 1990.
45. Engelman RW, et al: Clinicopathologic responses in cats with feline leukemia virus-associated leukemia-lymphoma treated with staphylococcal protein A. *Am J Pathol 118*:367, 1985.
46. English RV: Update on feline immunodeficiency virus. *Vet Cancer Soc Newletter 14*:1, 1990.
47. English RV, et al: Intraocular disease associated with feline immunodeficiency virus infection in cats. *J Am Vet Med Assoc 196*:1116, 1990.
48. Facklam NR, Kociba GJ: Cytochemical characterization of feline leukemic cells. *Vet Pathol 23*:155, 1986.
49. Fenner F: The classification and nomenclature of viruses. Summary of results of meetings of the International Committee on Taxonomy of Viruses in Madrid. *Intervirology 6*:1, 1975.
50. Giger U, et al: Orthovoltage radiotherapy of primary lymphoma of bone in a dog. *J Am Vet Med Assoc 195*:627, 1989.
51. Green RA, Barton CL: Acute myelomonocytic leukemia in a dog. *J Am Anim Hosp Assoc 13*:708, 1977.
52. Greenberg P, et al: The treatment of solitary plasmacytoma of bone and extramedullary plasmacytoma. *Am J Clin Oncol 10*:199, 1987.
53. Grindem CB, et al: Seroepidemiologic survey of feline immunodeficiency virus infection in cats of Wake County, North Carolina. *J Am Vet Med Assoc 194*:226, 1989.
54. Grindem CB, et al: Morphological classification and clinical and pathological characteristics of spontaneous leukemia in 10 cats. *J Am Anim Hosp Assoc 21*:227, 1985.
55. Grindem CB, et al: Morphological classification and clinical and pathological characteristics of spontaneous leukemia in 17 dogs. *J Am Anim Hosp Assoc 21*:219, 1985.
56. Gruffydd-Jones TJ, et al: Clinical and radiological features of anterior mediastinal lymphosarcoma in the cat. *Vet Rec 104*:304, 1979.
57. Haase AT: Pathogenesis of lentivirus infections. *Nature 322*:130, 1986.
58. Haffner K: 1987–1989 efficacy studies of Leukocell and Leukocell 2. Proceedings of the 8th American College of Veterinary Internal Medicine Forum. Vol 8. 1990, pp 415–418.
59. Hardy WD, Jr: The feline leukemia virus. *J Am Anim Hosp Assoc 17*:951, 1981.
60. Hardy WD Jr, MacEwen EG: Feline retroviruses. *In* Withrow, MacEwen (eds): *Clinical Veterinary Oncology*. J.B. Lippincott, Philadelphia, 1989, pp 362–380.
61. Hardy WD Jr, et al: Biology of feline leukemia virus in the natural environment. *Cancer Res 36*:582, 1976.
62. Hardy WD Jr, et al: Detection of the feline leukemia virus and other mammalian oncornaviruses by immunofluorescence. *In* Dutcher RM, Chieco-Bianchi L, (eds): *Unifying Concepts of Leukemia*. Karger, Basel, 1973, pp 778–799.
63. Hardy WD Jr, et al: Development of virus nonproducer lymphosarcomas in pet cats exposed to FeLV. *Nature 288*:90, 1980.
64. Hardy WD Jr, et al: A feline leukemia and sarcoma virus-induced tumor specific antigen. *Nature 270*:249, 1977.
65. Harvey JW: Myeloproliferative disorders in dogs and cats. *Vet Clin North Am 11*:349, 1981.
66. Harvey JW: Myeloproliferative disorders in the cat. Proceedings of the 52nd Annual Meeting of the American Animal Hospital Association. Orlando, Fla., Mar. 1985, pp 442–447.
67. Harvey JW, et al: Myeloproliferative disease with megakaryocytic predominance in a dog with occult dirofilariasis. *Vet Clin Pathol 11*:5, 1982.
68. Harvey JW, et al: Feline myeloproliferative disease: Changing manifestations in the peripheral blood. *Vet Pathol 15*:437, 1978.
69. Haschek WM, et al: Zidovudine toxicity to cats infected with feline leukemia virus. *J Fundam Appl Toxicol 14*:764, 1990.
70. Hawkins EC, et al: Immunoglobulin A myeloma in a cat with pleural effusion and serum hyperviscosity. *J Am Vet Med Assoc 188*:876, 1986.
71. Hawkins EC, et al: Use of tears for diagnosis of feline leukemia virus infection. *J Am Vet Med Assoc 188*:1031, 1986.
72. Helfand SC: Low dose cytosine arabinoside-induced remission of lymphoblastic leukemia in a cat. *J Am Vet Med Assoc 191*:707, 1987.
73. Henness AM, Crow SE: Treatment of feline myelogenous leukemia: Four case reports. *J Am Vet Med Assoc 171*:263, 1977.
74. Henness AM, et al: Monocytic leukemia in three cats. *J Am Vet Med Assoc 170*:1325, 1977.
75. Hodgkins EM, et al: Chronic lymphocytic leukemia in the dog. *J Am Vet Med Assoc 177*:704, 1980.
76. Hoenig M: Six dogs with features compatible with myelonecrosis and myelofibrosis. *J Am Anim Hosp Assoc 25*:335, 1989.
77. Hoenig M, O'Brien JA: A benign hypergammaglobulinemia mimicking plasma cell myeloma. *J Am Anim Hosp Assoc 24*:688, 1988.
78. Hohenhaus AE, et al: Lymphocyte blastogenesis, immunophenotype and identification of reverse transcriptase activity in dogs with lymphoid neoplasia. Proceedings of the 9th Annual Conference of the Veterinary Cancer Society. Vol 9 (Suppl). Raleigh, N.C., Oct. 1989.
79. Holmberg CA, et al: Feline malignant lymphomas: Comparison of morphologic and immunologic characteristics. *Am J Vet Res 37*:1455, 1976.
80. Hoover EA, et al: Feline leukemia virus infection: Age-related variation in response of cats to experimental infection. *J Natl Cancer Inst 57*:365, 1976.
81. Hoover EA, et al: Host-virus interactions in progressive versus regressive feline leukemia virus infection in cats. Cold Spring Harbor Conference on Cell Proliferation. Vol 7. Cold Spring Harbor, Sept. 1980, pp 635–651.
82. Hopper CD, et al: Clinical and laboratory findings in cats infected with feline immunodeficiency virus. *Vet Rec 125*:341, 1989.
83. Hribernik TN, et al: Serum hyperviscosity associated with IgG myeloma in a cat. *J Am Vet Med Assoc 181*:169, 1982.
84. Ishida T, et al: Feline immunodeficiency virus infection in cats of Japan. *J Am Vet Med Assoc 194*:221, 1989.
85. Jain NC, et al: Clinical-pathological findings and cytochemical characterization of myelomonocytic leukaemia in 5 dogs. *J Comp Pathol 91*:17, 1981.
86. Jarrett O, et al: Detection of transient and persistent feline leukemia virus infections. *Vet Rec 110*:225, 1982.
87. Jarrett O, et al: A comparison of three methods of feline leukemia virus diagnosis. *Vet Rec 110*:325, 1982.
88. Jarrett O, et al: The frequency of feline leukemia virus subgroups in cats. *Int J Cancer 21*:334, 1978.
89. Jeglum KA: Malignant lymphoma in the dog. *Comp Cont Educ Pract Vet 1*:503, 1979.
90. Jeglum KA, Steplewski Z: A phase I clinical trial of murine anti-dog lymphoma monoclonal antibody. Proceedings of the 7th Annual Conference of the Veterinary Cancer Society. Vol 7. Madison, Wis., Oct. 1987, p 24.
91. Jeglum KA, et al: Prognostic value of the NCI working formulation in canine lymphoma treated with chemotherapy and chemoimmunotherapy. Proceedings of the 7th Annual Conference of the Veterinary Cancer Society. Vol 7. Madison, Wis., Oct. 1987, p 24.
92. Jeglum KA, et al: A phase II study of adjuvant cytotoxic monoclonal antibodies in canine lymphoma. Proceedings of the 8th Annual Conference of the Veterinary Cancer Society. Vol 8. Estes Park, Col., Oct. 1988, p 36.
93. Jeglum KA, et al: Chemotherapy of lymphoma in 75 cats. *J Am Vet Med Assoc 190*:174, 1987.
94. Jeglum KA, et al: *In vitro* immune monitoring of antibody response in dogs given chemoimmunotherapy for lymphoma. *Am J Vet Res 50*:488, 1989.
95. Jeglum KA, et al: Intralymphatic autochthonous tumor cell vaccine in canine lymphoma. *J Biol Response Mod 5*:168, 1986.
96. Jeglum KA, et al: Chemotherapy versus chemotherapy with intralymphatic tumor cell vaccine in canine lymphoma. *Cancer 61*:2042, 1988.
97. Johnson JA, Patterson JM: Canine epidermotropic lymphoproliferative disease resembling pagetoid reticulosis in man. *Vet Pathol 18*:487, 1981.
98. Kakuk TJ, et al: Experimental transmission of canine malignant lymphoma to a Beagle neonate. *Cancer Res 28*:716, 1968.

99. Kessler JF, et al: Isotretinoin and cutaneous helper T-cell lymphoma (mycosis fungoides). *Arch Dermatol 123*:201, 1987.
100. Krohne SDG, et al: Ocular involvement in canine lymphosarcoma, a retrospective study. Proceedings of the 7th Annual Conference of the Veterinary Cancer Society. Vol 7. Madison, Wis., Oct. 1987, p 27.
101. Kumar L, et al: Low-dose cytosine arabinoside in acute nonlymphoblastic leukemia. *Cancer 63*:415, 1989.
102. Ladiges WC, et al: Phenotypic characterization of canine lymphoma, using monoclonal antibodies and a microlymphocytotoxicity assay. *Am J Vet Res 49*:870, 1988.
103. Lafrado L, et al: Immunodeficiency in latent feline leukemia virus infections. *Vet Immunol Immunopathol 21*:39, 1989.
104. Lafrado LJ, et al: Biological effects of staphylococcal protein A immunotherapy in cats with induced feline leukemia virus infection. *Am J Vet Res 51*:482, 1990.
105. Laing EJ, Carter RF: Acute tumor lysis syndrome following treatment of canine lymphoma. *J Am Anim Hosp Assoc 24*:691, 1988.
106. Laing EJ, et al: Half-body radiotherapy in the treatment of canine lymphoma. *J Vet Intern Med 3*:102, 1989.
107. Latimer KS, Dykstra MJ: Acute monocytic leukemia in a dog. *J Am Vet Med Assoc 184*:852, 1984.
108. Legendre AM, et al: Efficacy of a feline leukemia virus vaccine in a natural exposure challenge. *J Vet Intern Med 4*:92, 1990.
109. Leib MS, Bradley RL: Alimentary lymphosarcoma in a dog. *Comp Cont Educ Pract Vet 9*:809, 1987.
110. Leifer CE, Matus RE: Canine lymphoma: Clinical considerations. *Semin Vet Med Surg 1*:43, 1986.
111. Leifer CE, Matus RE: Chronic lymphocytic leukemia in the dog: 22 cases (1974–1984). *J Am Vet Med Assoc 189*:214, 1986.
112. Leifer CE, et al: Chronic myelogenous leukemia in the dog. *J Am Vet Med Assoc 183*:686, 1983.
113. Lewis MG, et al: Retroviral-associated eosinophilic leukemia in a cat. *Am J Vet Res 46*:1066, 1985.
114. Linman JW, Bagby GC Jr: The preleukemic syndrome (hematopoietic dysplasia). *Cancer 42*:854, 1978.
115. Linnabary RD, et al: Acute myelomonocytic leukemia in a dog. *J Am Anim Hosp Assoc 14*:71, 1978.
116. Liu S, Carb AV: Erythroblastic leukemia in a dog. *J Am Vet Med Assoc 152*:1511, 1968.
117. Lopez NA, Jackson RH: False-positive reactions associated with anti-mouse activity in serotests for feline leukemia virus antigen. *J Am Vet Med Assoc 195*:741, 1989.
118. Lutz H, et al: Felines T-lymphotropes lentivirus (FTLV): Experimentelle infektion und vorkommen in einigen ländern Europas. [Feline T-lymphotropic lentivirus (FTLV): Experimental infection and occurrence in some European countries]. *Kleintierpraxis 33*:455, 1988.
119. Lutz H, et al: Monoclonal antibodies to three epitopic regions of feline leukemia virus p27 and their use in enzyme-linked immunosorbent assay of p27. *J Immunol Methods 56*:209, 1983.
120. Lutz H, et al: Detection of feline leukemia virus infection. *Feline Pract 10*:13, 1980.
121. Lutz H, et al: Course of feline leukemia virus infection and its detection by enzyme-linked immunosorbent assay and monoclonal antibodies. *Am J Vet Res 44*:2054, 1983.
122. MacEwen EG, et al: Levamisole as adjuvant to chemotherapy for canine lymphosarcoma. *J Biol Response Mod 4*:427, 1985.
123. MacEwen EG, et al: Cyclic combination chemotherapy of canine lymphosarcoma. *J Am Vet Med Assoc 178*:1178, 1981.
124. MacEwen EG, et al: Evaluation of some prognostic factors for advanced multicentric lymphosarcoma in the dog: 147 cases (1978–1981). *J Am Vet Med Assoc 190*:564, 1987.
125. MacEwen EG, et al: Treatment of basophilic leukemia in a dog. *J Am Vet Med Assoc 166*:376, 1975.
126. MacEwen EG, et al: Nonsecretory multiple myeloma in two dogs. *J Am Vet Med Assoc 184*:1283, 1984.
127. MacEwen EG, et al: Extramedullary plasmacytoma of the gastrointestinal tract in two dogs. *J Am Vet Med Assoc 184*:1396, 1984.
128. MacEwen EG, et al: A double-blind randomized study to evaluate PEG-L-asparaginase versus native L-asparaginase in canine lymphoma. Proceedings of the 9th Annual Conference of the Veterinary Cancer Society. Vol 9. Raleigh, N.C., Oct. 1989, pp 1–3.
129. Mackey LJ, Jarrett WFH: Pathogenesis of lymphoid neoplasia in cats and its relationship to immunologic cell pathways. I. Morphologic aspects. *J Natl Cancer Inst 49*:853, 1972.
130. Macy DW, et al: Dose response of whole body hyperthermia on cats infected with the feline leukemia virus. Proceedings of the 9th Annual Conference of the Veterinary Cancer Society. Vol 9. Raleigh, N.C., Oct. 1989, pp 87–88.
131. Madewell BR: Hematological and bone marrow cytological abnormalities in 75 dogs with malignant lymphoma. *J Am Anim Hosp Assoc 22*:235, 1986.
132. Madewell BR, Jarrett O: Recovery of feline leukaemia virus from non-viraemic cats. *Vet Rec 112*:339, 1983.
133. Madewell BR, et al: Hematologic abnormalities preceding myeloid leukemia in three cats. *Vet Pathol 16*:510, 1979.
134. Maggio L, et al: Feline preleukemia: An animal model of human disease. *Yale J Biol Med 51*:469, 1978.
135. Mastro JM, et al: Feline leukemia vaccine: Efficacy, contents, and probable mechanism. *Vet Immunol Immunopathol 11*:205, 1986.
136. Matus RE: Lymphoma in the cat: Prognosis and response to chemotherapy. Proceedings of the 7th American College of Veterinary Internal Medicine Forum. Vol 7. San Diego, May 1989, pp 888–891.
137. Matus RE, et al: Acute lymphoblastic leukemia in the dog: a review of 30 cases. *J Am Vet Med Assoc 183*:859, 1983.
138. Matus RE, et al: Prognostic factors for multiple myeloma in the dog. *J Am Vet Med Assoc 188*:1288, 1986.
139. Matus RE, et al: Acute lymphoblastic leukemia in 13 dogs: Pathologic and immunologic studies and response to chemotherapy. Proceedings of the 7th Annual Conference of the Veterinary Cancer Society. Vol 7. Madison, Wis., Oct. 1987, p 30.
140. McClelland AJ, et al: Prognosis of healthy feline leukemia virus infected cats. *In* Hardy WD Jr, et al (eds): *Feline Leukemia Virus*. Elsevier, New York, 1980, pp 121–126.
141. McGrath CJ: Polycythemia vera in dogs. *J Am Vet Med Assoc 164*:1117, 1974.
142. McKeever PJ, et al: Canine cutaneous lymphoma. *J Am Vet Med Assoc 180*:531, 1982.
143. Micaily B, et al: Total electron beam and total nodal irradiation for therapy of patients with cutaneous T-cell lymphoma. *Int J Radiat Oncol Biol Phys 11*:1111, 1985.
144. Michalewicz R, et al: Cell differentiation and therapeutic effect of low doses of cytosine arabinoside in human myeloid leukemia. *Leukemia Res 8*:783, 1984.
145. Mills JN, et al: A case of multiple myeloma in a cat. *J Am Anim Hosp Assoc 18*:79, 1982.
146. Moloney WC, Rosenthal DS: Treatment of early acute nonlymphatic leukemia with low dose cytosine arabinoside. *Haematol Blood Transf 26*:59, 1981.
147. Mooney SC, Hayes AA: Lymphoma in the cat: An approach to diagnosis and management. *Semin Vet Med Surg 1*:51, 1986.
148. Mooney SC, et al: Treatment and prognostic factors in lymphoma in cats: 103 cases (1977–1981). *J Am Vet Med Assoc 194*:696, 1989.
149. Mooney SC, et al: Renal lymphoma in cats: 28 cases (1977–1984). *J Am Vet Med Assoc 191*:1473, 1987.
150. Morrison WB, et al: Bronchoalveolar lavage fluid analysis assisted staging of canine lymphoma. Proceedings of the 9th Annual Conference of the Veterinary Cancer Society. Vol 9. Raleigh, N.C., Oct. 1989, pp 29–30.
151. Mullins JI, et al: FeLV-FAIDS-induced immunodeficiency syndrome in cats. *Vet Immunol Immunopathol 21*:25, 1989.
152. Mullins JI, et al: Disease-specific and tissue-specific production of unintegrated feline leukemia virus variant DNA in feline AIDS. *Nature 319*:333, 1986.
153. Neil JC, et al: Transduction and rearrangement of the myc gene by feline leukemia virus in naturally occurring T-cell leukemias. *Nature 308*:814, 1984.
154. Ogilvie GK, et al: Malignant lymphoma with cardiac and bone involvement in a dog. *J Am Vet Med Assoc 194*:793, 1989.
155. Olsen RG, Sharpee RL: Letter to the editor. *Feline Pract 16*:4, 1986.
156. Onions D: RNA dependent DNA polymerase activity in canine lymphosarcoma. *Eur J Cancer 116*:345, 1980.
157. Onions D, et al: Selective effect of feline leukemia virus on early erythroid precursors. *Nature 296*:156, 1982.
158. Ott RL: Letter to the editor. *Feline Pract 16*:9, 1986.
159. Overbaugh J, et al: Molecular cloning of a feline leukemia virus that induces fatal immunodeficiency disease in cats. *Science 239*:906, 1988.
160. Pacitti AM: Latent feline leukaemia virus infection: A review. *J Small Anim Pract 28*:1153, 1987.
161. Page RL, et al: Uric acid and phosphorous excretion in dogs with lymphosarcoma. *Am J Vet Res 47*:910, 1986.
162. Pedersen NC: Letter to the editor. *Feline Pract 16*:8, 1986.
163. Pedersen NC, et al: Studies of naturally transmitted feline leukemia virus infection. *Am J Vet Res 38*:1523, 1977.
164. Pedersen NC, et al: Isolation of a T-lymphotropic virus from domestic cats with an immunodeficiency-like syndrome. *Science 235*:790, 1987.
165. Pedersen NC, et al: Evaluation of a commercial feline leukemia virus vaccine for immunogenicity and efficacy. *Feline Pract 15*:7, 1985.
166. Pedersen NC, et al: Biological behavior of tumors and associated retroviruses in cats inoculated with Snyder-Theilen fibrosarcoma virus and the phenomenon of tumor recurrence after primary regression. *Infect Immun 143*:631, 1984.
167. Pedersen NC, et al: Feline leukemia virus infection as a potentiating cofactor for the primary and secondary stages of experimentally induced feline immunodeficiency virus infection. *J Virol 64*:598, 1990.
168. Pedersen NC, et al: Feline immunodeficiency virus infection. *Vet Immunol Immunopathol 21*:111, 1989.
169. Pegourie B, et al: Splenectomy during chronic lymphocytic leukemia. *Cancer 59*:1626, 1987.
170. Peterson ME, Randolph JF: Diagnosis of canine primary polycythemia and management with hydroxyurea. *J Am Vet Med Assoc 180*:415, 1982.

171. Pollet, L, et al: Blastic crisis in chronic myelogenous leukemia in a dog. *J Small Anim Pract 19*:469, 1978.
172. Pollock RVH, Scarlett JM: Randomized blind trial of a commercial FeLV vaccine. *J Am Vet Med Assoc 196*:611, 1990.
173. Postorino NC, et al: Single agent therapy with Adriamycin for canine lymphosarcoma. *J Am Anim Hosp Assoc 25*:221, 1989.
174. Povey RC, Hawkins GJ: Feline immunodeficiency virus: A commentary. *Can Vet J 30*:559, 1989.
175. Rae CA, et al: A comparison between the cytological and histological characteristics in thirteen canine and feline thymomas. *Can Vet J 30*:497, 1989.
176. Ragan HA, et al: Acute myelomonocytic leukemia manifested as myelophthisic anemia in a dog. *J Am Vet Med Assoc 169*:421, 1976.
177. Rakich PM, et al: Mucocutaneous plasmacytomas in dogs: 75 cases (1980–1987). *J Am Vet Med Assoc 194*:803, 1989.
178. Raskin RE, Krehbiel JD: Prevalence of leukemic blood and bone marrow in dogs with multicentric lymphoma. *J Am Vet Med Assoc 194*:1427, 1989.
179. Reed C, et al: Polycythemia vera in a cat. *J Am Vet Med Assoc 157*:85, 1970.
180. Roberts JD, et al: Low-dose cytosine arabinoside in the myelodysplastic syndromes and acute myelogenous leukemia. *Cancer 56*:1001, 1985.
181. Rohrig KE: Acute myelomonocytic leukemia in a dog. *J Am Vet Med Assoc 182*:137, 1983.
182. Rojko JL: Biology of the feline leukemia virus. Proceedings of the 10th Annual Kal Kan Symposium. Columbus, Ohio, Oct. 1986, pp 89–95.
183. Rojko JL, Hardy WD Jr: Feline leukemia virus and other retroviruses. *In* Sherding RG (ed): *The Cat: Diseases and Clinical Management.* Churchill Livingstone, New York, 1989, pp 229–332.
184. Rojko JL, Olsen RG: Immunobiology of the feline leukemia virus. *Vet Immunol Immunopathol 6*:107, 1984.
185. Rojko JL, et al: Pathogenesis of experimental feline leukemia virus infection. *J Natl Cancer Inst 63*:759, 1979.
186. Rojko JL, et al: Reactivation of latent feline leukemia virus infection. *Nature 298*:385, 1982.
187. Rojko JL, et al: Feline lymphomas: Immunological and cytochemical characterization. *Cancer Res 49*:345, 1989.
188. Rosales C, et al: Cytolytic activity of murine anti-dog lymphoma monoclonal antibodies with canine effector cells and complement. *Cell Immunol 115*:420, 1988.
189. Roscher AA, et al: Acute myelogenous leukemia. *J Am Vet Med Assoc 136*:491, 1960.
190. Rosenberg MP, et al: Prognostic factors in dogs with lymphoma and hypercalcemia. Proceedings of the 9th Annual Conference of the Veterinary Cancer Society. Vol 9. Raleigh, N.C., Oct. 1989, p 69.
191. Rosenberg SA (Chairman): Non Hodgkin's Lymphoma Classification Project. National Cancer Institute sponsored study of classifications of non-Hodgkin's lymphomas. *Cancer 49*:2112, 1982.
192. Rosenthal RC: Epidemiology of canine lymphosarcoma. *Comp Cont Educ Pract Vet 4*:855, 1982.
193. Rosenthal RC: Autologous bone marrow transplantation for lymphoma. Proceedings of the 6th American College of Veterinary Internal Medicine Forum. Vol 6. Washington, D.C., May 1988, pp 397–399.
194. Rosin A: Neurologic disease associated with lymphosarcoma in ten dogs. *J Am Vet Med Assoc 181*:50, 1982.
195. Russell PH, Jarrett O: The occurrence of feline leukemia virus neutralizing antibodies in cats. *Int J Cancer 22*:351, 1978.
196. Sarma PS, Log T: Subgroup classification of feline leukemia and sarcoma viruses by viral interference and neutralization tests. *Virology 54*:160, 1973.
197. Sarmiento UM, Valli VEO: A canine lymphocyte surface antigen detectable by a monoclonal antibody (DT200). *Can J Vet Res 51*:110, 1987.
198. Schalm OW: Myeloproliferative disorders in the cat. 3. Progression from erythroleukemia into granulocytic leukemia. *Feline Pract 5*:31, 1975.
199. Scott-Moncrieff C, et al: Plasma and CSF pharmacokinetics of intravenous cytosine arabinoside in dogs. Proceedings of the 8th Annual Conference of the Veterinary Cancer Society. Vol 8. Estes Park, Col., Oct. 1988, p 10.
200. Sharpee RL, et al: Feline leukemia virus vaccine: Evaluation of safety and efficacy against persistent viremia and tumor development. *Comp Cont Educ Pract Vet 8*:267, 1986.
201. Shell L, et al: Generalized skeletal involvement of a hematopoietic tumor in a dog. *J Am Vet Med Assoc 194*:1077, 1989.
202. Slayter MV, et al: Feline malignant lymphoma: Log-linear multiway frequency analysis of a population involving the factors of sex and age of animal and tumor cell type and location. *Am J Vet Res 45*:2178, 1984.
203. Smith L, Alexanian R: Treatment strategies for plasma cell myeloma. *CA 35*:214, 1985.
204. Smith M, Turrel JM: Radiophosphorus (32P) treatment of bone marrow disorders in dogs: 11 cases (1970–1987). *J Am Vet Med Assoc 194*:98, 1989.
205. Snyder HW Jr, et al: Remission of FeLV-associated lymphosarcoma and persistent viral infection after extracorporeal immunoadsorption of plasma using staphylococcal protein A columns: Details of immune response. *Semin Hematol 26* (Suppl): 25, 1989.
206. Snyder HW, et al: The feline oncornavirus-associated cell membrane antigen (FOCMA) is related to but distinguishable from FeLV-C gp70. *Virology 131*:315, 1983.
207. Sparger EE: Feline immunodeficiency virus. Proceedings of the 12th Annual Kal Kan Symposium. Columbus, Ohio, Oct. 1988, pp 35–41.
208. Squire RA: A cytologic study of malignant lymphoma in cattle, dogs, and cats. *Am J Vet Res 26*:97, 1965.
209. Squire RA, et al: Clinical and pathologic study of canine lymphoma: Clinical staging, cell classification, and therapy. *J Natl Cancer Inst 51*:565, 1973.
210. Stewart MA, et al: Nucleotide sequences of a feline leukemia virus subgroup A envelope gene and long terminal repeat and evidence for the recombinational origin of subgroup B viruses. *J Virol 58*:825, 1986.
211. Theilen GH, Madewell BR: Feline hematopoietic neoplasms, sarcomas, and related conditions. *In* Theilen GH, Madewell BR (eds): *Veterinary Cancer Medicine.* Philadelphia, Lea & Febiger, 1987, pp 354–381.
212. Thomley FM, et al: Reverse transcriptase activity and particles of retroviral density in cultured canine lymphosarcoma supernatants. *Br J Cancer 47*:277, 1983.
213. Thrall MA: Lymphoproliferative disorders. Lymphocytic leukemia and plasma cell myeloma. *Vet Clin North Am 11*:321, 1981.
214. Thrall MA, et al: Cutaneous lymphosarcoma and leukemia in a dog resembling sezary syndrome in man. *Vet Pathol 21*:182, 186, 1984.
215. Tompkins MB, et al: Immunopathogenesis of feline leukemia virus infections. *Companion Animal Practice 2*:15, 1988.
216. Tricot G, et al: Low dose cytosine arabinoside (Ara-C) in myelodysplastic syndromes. *Br J Haematol 58*:231, 1984.
217. Turnwald GH, et al: Lymphosarcoma with osseous involvement in a dog. *J Am Anim Hosp Assoc 24*:350, 1988.
218. Vail DM, et al: Exacerbation of hyperlactatemia by infusion of lactated Ringer's solution in dogs with lymphoma. *J Vet Intern Med. 4*:228, 1990.
219. Vail DM, et al: Alterations in carbohydrate metabolism in canine lymphoma. *J Vet Intern Med 4*:8, 1990.
220. Valli VE, et al: Histocytology of lymphoid tumors in the dog, cat, and cow. *Vet Pathol 18*:494, 1981.
221. Valli VE, et al: Anatomical and histological classification of feline lymphoma using the National Cancer Institute Working Formulation. Proceedings of the 9th Annual Conference of the Veterinary Cancer Society. Vol 9 (Suppl). Raleigh, N.C., Oct. 1989.
222. Van Pelt RW, Conner GH: Clinicopathologic survey of malignant lymphoma in the dog. *J Am Vet Med Assoc 152*:976, 1968.
223. Van Vechten M, et al: Treatment of relapsed canine lymphoma with doxorubicin and dacarbazine. *J Vet Intern Med 4*:187, 1990.
224. Varmus HE: Form and function of retroviral proviruses. *Science 216*:812, 1982.
225. Vedbrat SS, et al: Feline oncornavirus-associated cell membrane antigen: A viral and not a cellularly coded transformation-specific antigen of cat lymphomas. *Virology 124*:445, 1983.
226. Weh HJ, et al: Treatment of acute myeloid leukemia and myelodysplastic syndrome by low dose cytosine arabinoside. *Haematol Blood Transf 29*:60, 1985.
227. Weiden PL, et al: Prolonged disease-free survival in dogs with lymphoma after total-body irradiation and autologous marrow transplantation consolidation of combination-chemotherapy-induced remissions. *Blood 54*:1039, 1979.
228. Weir E, et al: Hypercalcemia in canine lymphosarcoma is associated with the T-cell subtype and with secretion of a PTH like factor. Proceedings of the 8th Annual Conference of the Veterinary Cancer Society. Vol 8. Estes Park, Col., Oct. 1988, p 16.
229. Weir EC, et al: Humoral hypercalcemia of malignancy in canine lymphosarcoma. *Endocrinology 122*:602, 1988.
230. Weller RE: Paraneoplastic disorders in dogs with hematopoietic tumors. *Vet Clin North Am 15*:805, 1986.
231. Weller RE, et al: Histologic classification as a prognostic criterion for canine lymphosarcoma. *Am J Vet Res 41*:1310, 1980.
232. Weller RE, et al: Chemoimmunotherapy for canine lymphosarcoma: A prospective evaluation of specific and nonspecific immunomodulation. *Am J Vet Res 41*:516, 1980.
233. World Health Organization: *Classification of Tumors in Domestic Animals.* Geneva, World Health Organization, 1980.
234. Yamamoto JK, et al: Epidemiologic and clinical aspects of feline immunodeficiency virus infection in cats from the continental United States and Canada and possible mode of transmission. *J Am Vet Med Assoc 194*:213, 1989.
235. Yamamoto JK, et al: Pathogenesis of experimentally induced feline immunodeficiency virus infection in cats. *Am J Vet Res 49*:1246, 1988.
236. Young KM: Myeloproliferative disorders. *Vet Clin North Am 15*:769, 1985.

CHAPTER

157

Central Nervous System

Rodney S. Bagley, Joe N. Kornegay, Rodney L. Page, and Donald E. Thrall

Central (CNS) and peripheral nervous system (PNS) neoplasia occurs commonly in dogs and cats. General considerations of nervous system neoplasia are addressed early in this chapter, followed by specific descriptions of common tumor types, metastatic disease, and systemic manifestations.

CLASSIFICATION

CNS tumors may be classified as either primary or secondary by their cells of origin (Table 157–1).[94, 95, 103, 178] Primary tumors include those arising from neuroepithelial, meningeal, vascular, germ cell, nerve sheath, lymphoid, and malformed tissue. The term *glioma* refers to all tumors originating from cells derived from the medullary (neural) plate. These include astrocytomas, oligodendrogliomas, glioblastomas, choroid plexus papillomas, ependymomas, medulloblastomas, and other tumors that are either rare or have not yet been reported in dogs and cats. Secondary tumors reach the brain by local extension or hematogenous metastasis.

Spinal tumors are often additionally classified according to their location relative to the dura as extradural, intradural-extramedullary, and intramedullary.

INCIDENCE

Brain tumors occur more commonly in dogs than other domestic species.[178] The incidence of nervous system tumors in dogs and cats is estimated to be 14.5 and 3.5, respectively, per 100,000 at risk.[178] Astrocytoma[62, 194] or meningioma[50] is the most common brain tumor of dogs. One large series of canine brain tumors included roughly similar numbers of each, 118 astrocytomas and 106 meningiomas.[103] Twenty-seven of 69 (39 per cent) histologically confirmed brain tumors were meningiomas.[65] Astrocytoma was the next most frequent tumor type, accounting for 10 per cent. These data suggest that meningiomas may be increasing in frequency or, alternatively, that astrocytomas now occur less commonly. Changes in breed popularity may be a factor (discussed later). Meningioma is the most common primary brain tumor of cats.[40, 89, 195]

Most spinal tumors in dogs occur extradurally.[97, 110, 192] These tumors generally arise from bone and include osteosarcoma, fibrosarcoma, hemangiosarcoma, multiple myeloma, and chondrosarcoma. Various tumors also metastasize to vertebrae, ultimately causing spinal cord compression.[19, 20, 172, 189] Lymphosarcoma is the most common soft-tissue extradural spinal tumor in dogs.[26, 139] Nerve sheath tumors (schwannoma, neurofibroma)[11] and meningiomas[46] account for most intradural-extramedullary tumors in dogs. Neuroepitheliomas occur less commonly.[6, 168] Meningiomas can arise in any location but concentrate near nerve roots,[53] originating from arachnoid rest cells.[132] Intramedullary tumors are rare. Astrocytoma and ependymoma are the most common primary tumor types,[63, 122, 131, 170] whereas hemangiosarcoma is the most common secondary tumor.[182] Lymphosarcoma is the predominant spinal tumor of cats[85, 195]; most occur extradurally. Primary vertebral tumors,[119, 134] meningiomas,[72, 140, 193] nerve sheath tumors,[186] and gliomas[2, 64] occur infrequently.

The age at onset of brain tumors varies, but most dogs are older than 5 years. The median age of 86 dogs with brain tumors was 9 years.[65] Younger animals can be affected. CNS tumors occurring in young animals include medulloblastoma (Fig. 157–1), epidermoid cyst, and teratoma. Certain breeds have a higher incidence of specific tumor types. Brachycephalic breeds are predisposed to astrocytomas, oligodendrogliomas, glioblastomas, and pituitary tumors, whereas meningiomas may be more common in dolichocephalic breeds.[132] Canine breeds that are over-represented include the boxer, golden retriever, Doberman pinscher, Scottish terrier, and Old English sheepdog.[65]

Gender predilection is not well established. Gliomas were more common in males and meningiomas in females.[103] A similar gender predilection is seen in humans with brain tumors.[150] No gender bias occurred in 28 dogs

TABLE 157–1. CLASSIFICATION OF CENTRAL NERVOUS SYSTEM NEOPLASIA OF DOGS AND CATS

Primary tumors	*Secondary tumors*
Neuroepithelial	Local extension
Astrocytoma	Osteoma
Oligodendroglioma	Pituitary adenoma
Glioblastoma multiforme	Olfactory carcinoma
Choroid plexus papilloma	Hematogenous metastases
Ependymoma	Hemangiosarcoma
Medulloblastoma	Melanoma
Spongioblastoma	Carcinoma
Ganglioglioma	Miscellaneous
Pinealoma	
Mixed; unclassified	
Meningeal	
Meningioma	
Meningeal sarcoma	
Lymphoid	
Lymphosarcoma	
Reticulosis (neoplastic forms)	
Malformed tissues	
Epidermoid-dermoid cyst	
Craniopharyngioma	
Vascular	
Hemangioblastoma	
Germ cell	
Teratoma	
Nerve sheath	
Neurinoma (schwannoma)	
Neurofibroma	

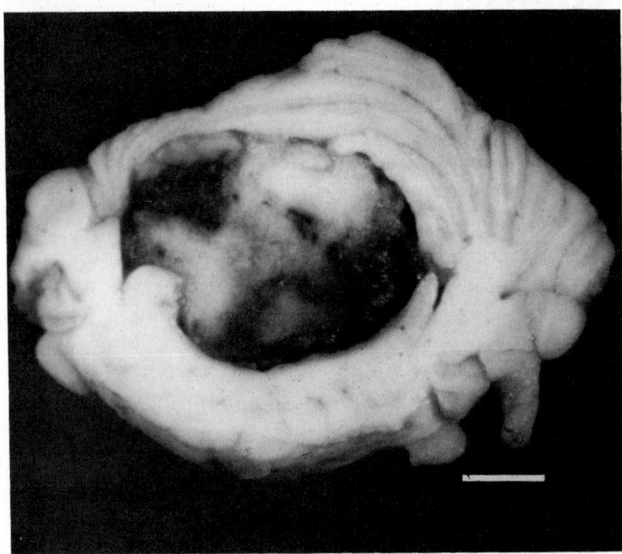

FIGURE 157–1. Transverse section of cerebellum and brain stem from an 8-month-old male Sharpei with a 2-week course of progressive ataxia and subsequent seizures and left-sided torticollis. A somewhat circular mass, shown on histopathological evaluation to be a medulloblastoma, is seen dorsal to the brain stem. Seizures were presumed to result from hydrocephalus that had occurred secondary to obstruction of the fourth ventricle. (Bar = 0.5 cm.)

with meningiomas in another series.[127] Meningiomas are recognized more commonly in male cats.[114] A male predilection for spinal tumors in dogs has been reported.[192]

CLINICAL FINDINGS

It is important to establish the anatomical level of lesions responsible for neurological disease in animals. Clinical signs associated with neoplasia depend on the location, rate of growth, and associated secondary effects of the tumor. Specific areas may be involved because of direct effects of the tumor or secondarily due to complications such as edema or brain herniation. If signs resulting from these secondary effects are more prominent than those associated with the tumor itself, absolute localization of the primary lesion by examination alone may be difficult.

Rapidly growing tumors usually cause acute neurological dysfunction, whereas slowly expanding tumors cause insidious disease, evolving over a year or more in some cases.[70] Hemorrhage within the tumor may lead to acute deterioration after a prolonged course in humans.[76] We have encountered similarly affected patients (Fig. 157–2). Underlying systemic abnormalities such as disseminated intravascular coagulopathy and thrombocytopenia, drug therapy (anticoagulants, chemotherapeutic agents), and hypertension increase the chance of intracranial hemorrhage.

A complete physical and neurological examination is imperative in any patient suspected of having CNS disease. Neurological signs may occur in association with extraneural disease owing to local extension or metabolic derangement. Papilledema has been noted in some animals with brain tumors.[123] Bilateral papilledema is essentially pathognomonic for raised intracranial pressure but not necessarily for brain neoplasia.

Several typical clinical patterns are characteristic of localized CNS disease (Fig. 157–3). Signs seen with forebrain lesions include circling (usually ipsilateral to the lesion); head pressing; behavioral abnormalities; sensorium changes; seizures; and contralateral vision, motor, and conscious proprioceptive deficits. Seizures occur in some animals for prolonged periods before diagnosis.[50]

Involvement of the floor of the calvarium (Fig. 157–4) can lead to a characteristic set of signs termed *cavernous sinus syndrome* in man. Similar signs occur in dogs.[93] As they course from the brain stem to the orbital fissure, cranial nerves III, IV, VI, and the ophthalmic division of V penetrate the dura in the cavernous sinuses. Sympathetic fibers from the cervical ganglia enter the cranial cavity with the internal carotid arteries and

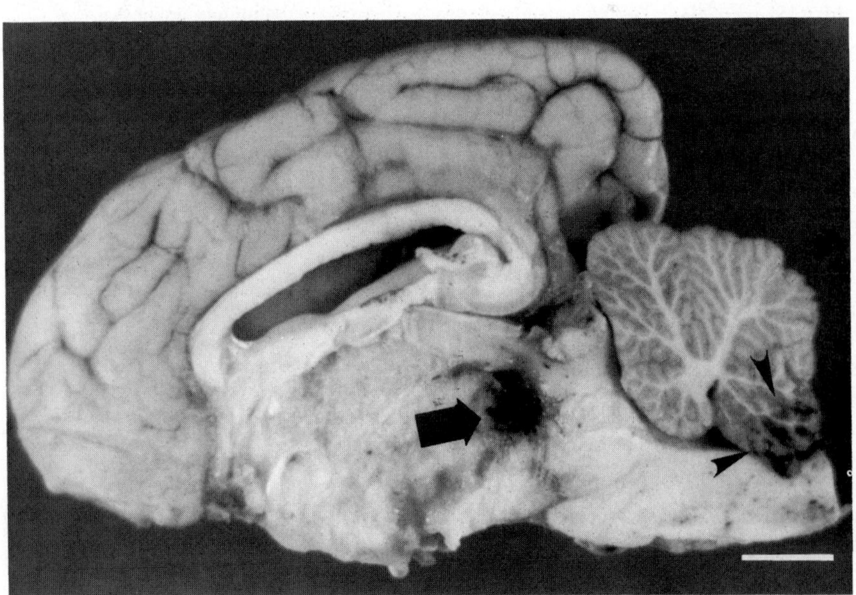

FIGURE 157–2. Sagittal section of brain from a 2-year-old male German shepherd with acutely progressive depression, circling, blindness, apnea, and death over an 11-hour period. Much of the thalamus is occupied by a poorly defined mass that had histological features of a pituitary carcinoma. A focus of black discoloration *(arrow)* that was shown to be hemorrhage microscopically is noted dorsally. The caudal cerebellar vermis *(arrowheads)* is discolored subsequent to foramen magnum brain herniation. There was also caudal transtentorial brain herniation. Tumor necrosis and hemorrhage were presumed to have contributed to the herniation and the dog's acute clinical deterioration. (Bar = 0.75 cm.)

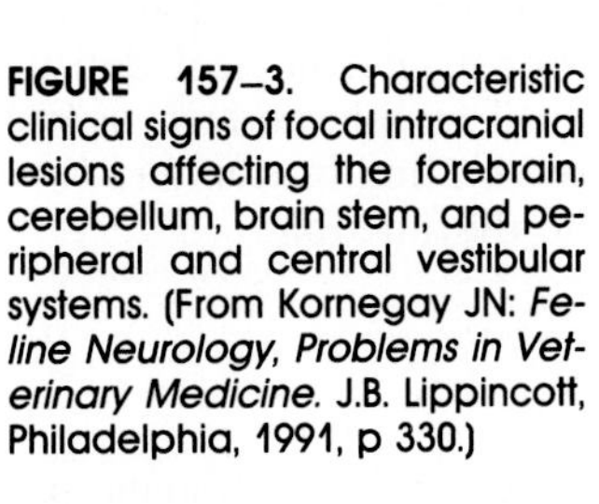

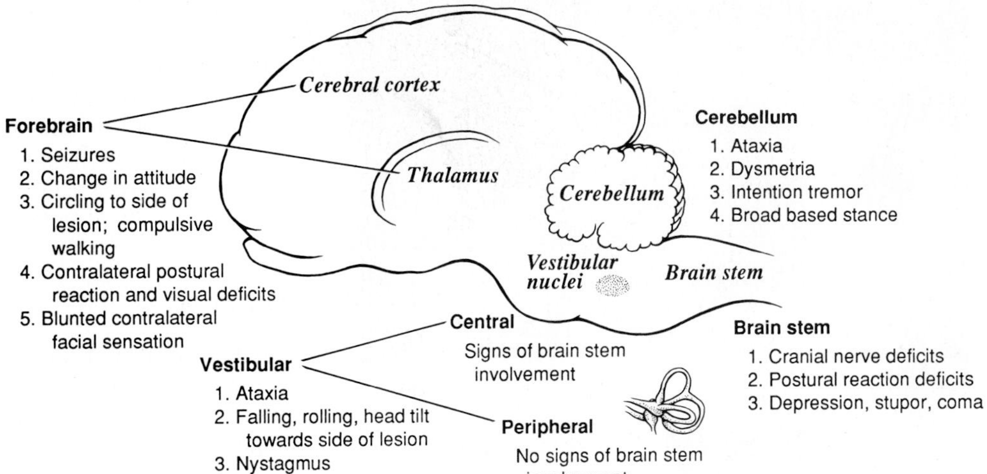

FIGURE 157–3. Characteristic clinical signs of focal intracranial lesions affecting the forebrain, cerebellum, brain stem, and peripheral and central vestibular systems. (From Kornegay JN: *Feline Neurology, Problems in Veterinary Medicine.* J.B. Lippincott, Philadelphia, 1991, p 330.)

also pass through the cavernous sinuses to innervate the eyes.[102] Dogs with tumors of the cavernous sinuses often have parasympathetic, sympathetic, sensory, and motor deficits in the ipsilateral eye.[93] Involvement of the optic nerves or chiasm can cause additional ipsilateral or bilateral blindness and loss of pupillary light reflexes.[28, 157]

When the brain stem is affected, cranial nerve and long tract signs occur. Lesions at the cerebellopontine angle often involve cranial nerves V, VII, and VIII, leading to atrophy of the temporal and masseter muscles (Fig. 157–5) and loss of facial and ocular sensation (V); inability to blink and sagging of the lip (VII); and head tilt, nystagmus, and ataxia (VIII). Tumors affecting the middle or inner ear can cause signs of cranial nerve VII and VIII dysfunction and Horner's syndrome.[69] Involvement of the reticular activating system and descending tracts leads to depression and tetraparesis, respectively. Animals with cerebellar tumors may have dysmetria and intention tremor.

Spinal cord tumors are localized by the presence of upper motor neuron or lower motor neuron signs in the pelvic and thoracic limbs (Fig. 157–6). Monoparesis and associated lower motor neuron signs (Fig. 157–7) suggest peripheral nerve, nerve root, or ventral horn cell involvement. Reviews of the principles of neurological lesion localization are available.[30] Neuroanatomical localization does not establish cause but is important in formulating a differential diagnosis. Some tumors affect specific spinal cord areas; neuroepitheliomas involve the area of the thoracolumbar junction,[6, 168] whereas meningiomas[46] and nerve sheath tumors[11] commonly occur in the cervical area.

In one study, acute onset of signs was noted in 40 per cent of extradural tumors, 60 per cent of intradural-extramedullary lesions, and 100 per cent of intramedullary tumors.[97] Clinical signs of intramedullary neoplasms may occur acutely owing to edema and hemorrhage.[53] Signs in animals with intramedullary tumors can also progress insidiously. Pain is often a feature of

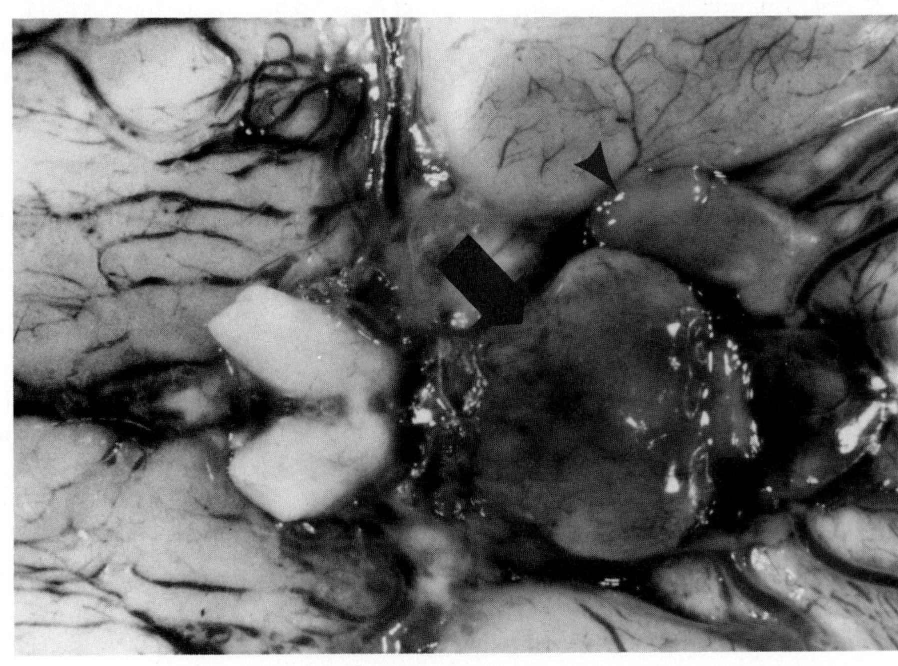

FIGURE 157–4. Ventral surface of the brain from a 7-year-old female mixed-breed dog with progressive dysfunction involving cranial nerves III, V, and VI. The dog's oculovestibular eye movements were absent bilaterally, and facial sensation was depressed. Euthanasia was performed at the owner's request. The pituitary gland *(arrow)* and the left oculomotor nerve *(arrowhead)* are coated by poorly defined gelatinous material that extended to the cavernous sinuses and involved other cranial nerves on further dissection. A diagnosis of lymphosarcoma was made on histological evaluation.

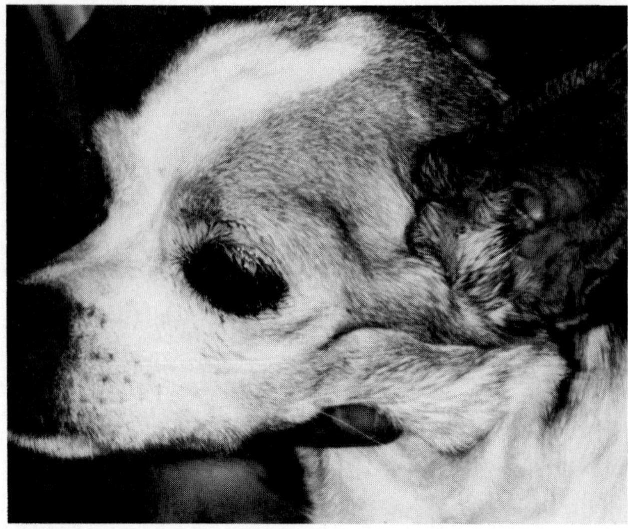

FIGURE 157–5. Photograph of a 16-year-old female Chihuahua with a 3-week history of left temporal and masseter muscle atrophy and more recent ataxia and left-sided head tilt. Because of the atrophy, the zygomatic arch on the left side is clearly delineated. A lesion involving the left trigeminal and vestibular nerves was suspected, and a meningioma was identified at this level (see Fig. 157–16). The tumor was grossly resected, but the dog became nonambulatory after surgery. Although the dog remained nonambulatory, it survived approximately 15 months after surgery, when seizures necessitated euthanasia. Necropsy was not performed. (Courtesy of Dr. L. Gainsburg.)

extradural and intradural-extramedullary lesions but not usually intramedullary tumors. Intramedullary tumors may cause pain on paraspinal palpation, possibly because of either encroachment or tension of tumor on the nerve rootlets or ischemia due to effects of the tumor on nerve root vasculature.

Peripheral nerve tumors usually cause monoparesis that may initially be mistaken for lameness arising from a musculoskeletal lesion. Definitive signs of neural involvement, such as knuckling and neurogenic muscle atrophy (see Fig. 157–7), suggest the actual cause. Pain may be noted on extension of the limb or manipulation of the involved region. Ipsilateral loss of the panniculus reflex and Horner's syndrome aid in localizing tumors affecting the brachial plexus. A mass can be identified on axillary palpation.[11, 187] General anesthesia may be needed to decrease pain and allow complete palpation.[187] These tumors often compress or invade the spinal cord.

Tumors affecting cranial nerves may initially cause signs of specific neural dysfunction. If the tumor is outside the cranial vault, the signs may remain localized. Enlargement of intracranial tumors can lead to brain stem compression and additional neurological deficits. Dissemination of hematological neoplasia such as myelomonocytic leukemia can lead to infiltration and compression of cranial nerves and dysfunction.[17]

DIAGNOSIS

After the lesion has been localized to a specific part of the nervous system, appropriate diagnostic tests discussed next can be performed to establish a definitive diagnosis.

Survey Radiography (see Chapter 70)

Survey radiographs of the skull are of limited value in evaluating intracranial neoplasia. Exceptions are tumors involving the skull (Fig. 157–8), nasal tumors invading the cribriform plate, and either bone atrophy or sclerosis adjacent to tumors such as meningiomas. Calcification occurring in psammomatous meningiomas may also be seen on survey radiographs. Various views have been used to identify these changes.[132]

Radiography can be useful in evaluating spinal neoplasia. Osteoproduction and osteolysis due to vertebral tumors may be seen on survey radiographs (Fig. 157–9). Expansion of the vertebral canal is seen with some intradural-extramedullary and intradural tumors (Fig. 157–10*A*). Intervertebral foramina may expand subsequent to proximally enlarging peripheral nerve neoplasms (see Fig. 157–10*A*).

Contrast Radiography

Contrast radiographs may be helpful in providing evidence of intracranial neoplasia. Several different contrast media have been used. Meglumine iothalamate and iohexol for intravascular and subarachnoid injection, respectively, are fairly safe, but adverse reactions occur.[181, 191]

Angiography. Cerebral angiography is an invasive procedure for viewing the cerebral vasculature. An iodinated contrast medium (0.38 ml/kg meglumine

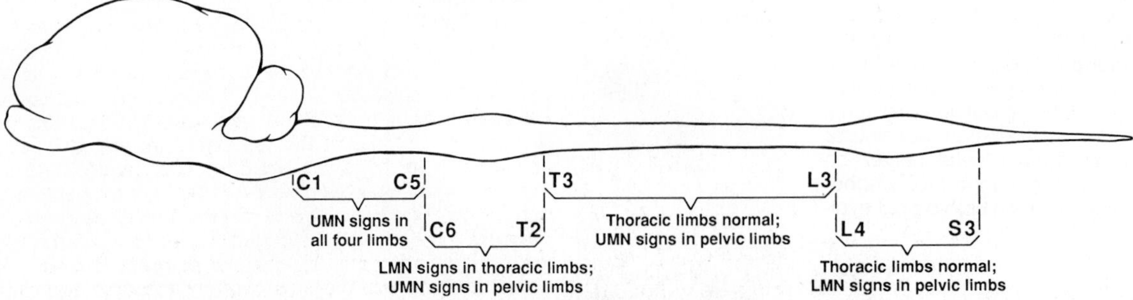

FIGURE 157–6. Neurological clinical signs in animals with lesions affecting the spinal cord at C1–C5, C6–T2, T3–L3, and L4–S3. (From Kornegay JN: *Feline Neurology, Problems in Veterinary Medicine.* J.B. Lippincott, Philadelphia, 1991, p 329.)

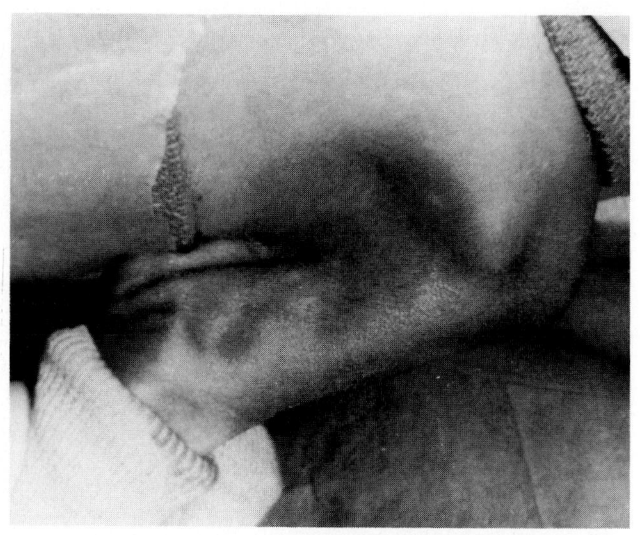

FIGURE 157–7. The right thoracic limb of a 6-year-old male mixed-breed dog with progressive thoracic limb lameness and subsequent paresis. Note the marked atrophy of the triceps muscle group. Pain was expressed on axillary palpation. Diffuse denervation was present in these and other muscles of this limb on electromyographic examination. Neoplasia involving nerves of, or roots contributing to, the brachial plexus on the right side was suspected. Results of myelography were normal. The right axillary area was explored, and peripheral nerves of the plexus were enlarged (see Fig. 157–39) and firm. Resected tissue had histological features of a malignant schwannoma. Deterioration of function in this limb followed surgery. Amputation was advised but declined.

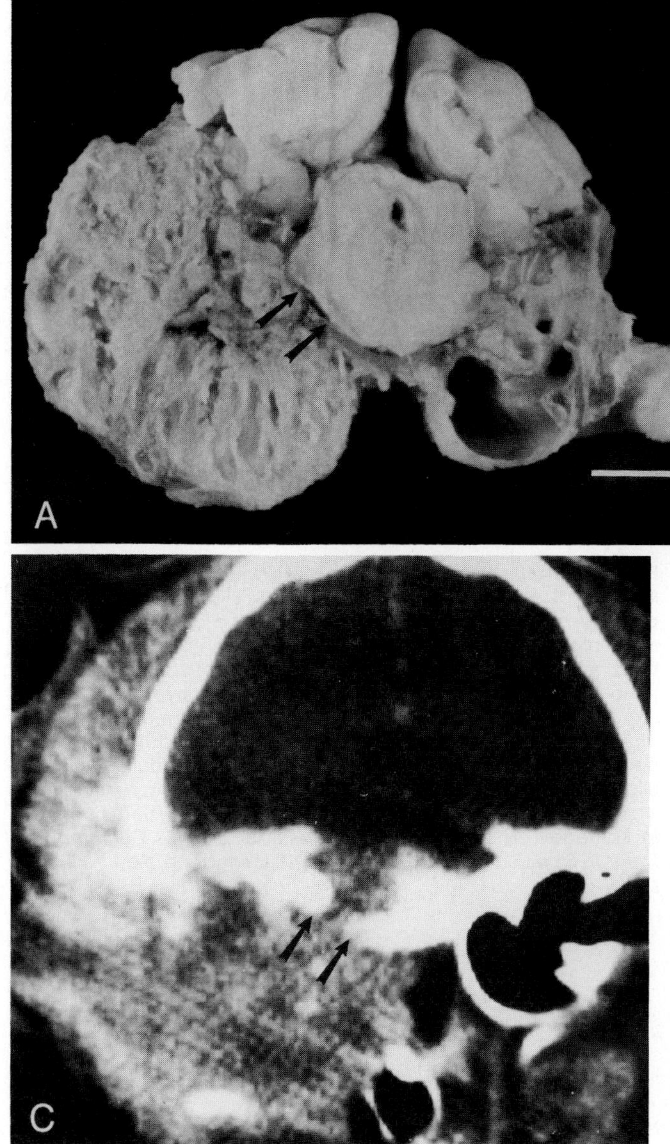

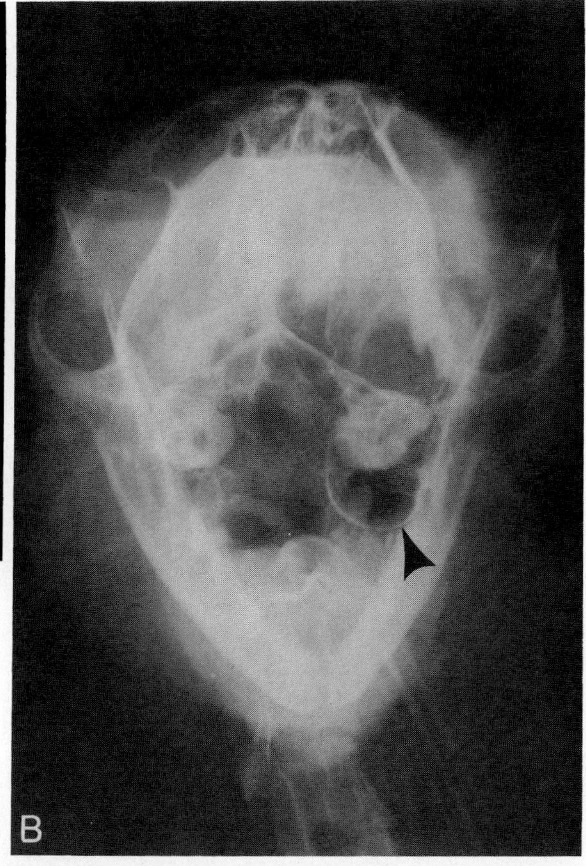

FIGURE 157–8. Transverse pathological section of brain and skull *(A)*, survey skull radiograph *(B)*, and computed tomography scan *(C)* from a 5-year-old female domestic cat with initial signs of otitis externa and peripheral vestibular disease and subsequent clinical evidence of brain stem involvement. Palpation revealed a mass at the base of the left ear. A proliferative lesion has obliterated the left tympanic bulla and invades the calvaria (*arrows* in *A* and *C*). Compared with the right tympanic bulla that can be seen clearly in *B (arrowhead)*, the left bulla is obscured. However, the nature of the underlying lesion is poorly defined in the survey radiograph. The cat was euthanized, and squamous cell carcinoma was diagnosed on microscopic examination of the lesion. (Bar = 0.75 cm in *A*.) (From Kornegay JN: *Feline Neurology, Problems in Veterinary Medicine.* J.B. Lippincott, Philadelphia, 1991, p 422.)

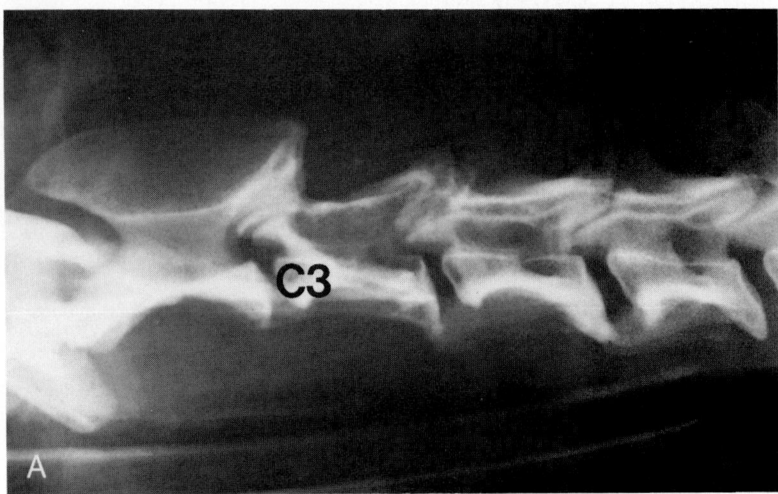

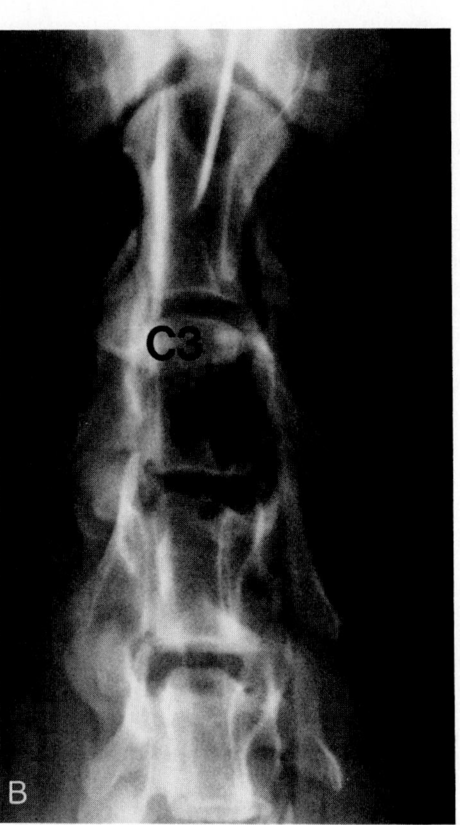

FIGURE 157–9. Lateral *(A)* and ventrodorsal *(B)* radiographs of the cervical vertebral column from an 8-year-old female Labrador retriever with progressive tetraparesis. A large lytic area involves the vertebral arch of C3. A diagnosis of osteosarcoma was made at necropsy. (From Kornegay JN: Vertebral diseases of large breed dogs. *In* Kornegay JN [ed]: *Neurologic Disorders.* Vol 5. *Contemporary Issues in Small Animal Practice.* Churchill Livingstone, New York, 1986, pp 197–215.)

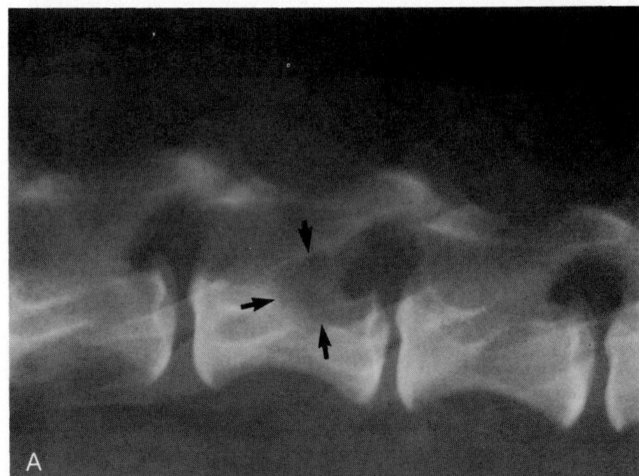

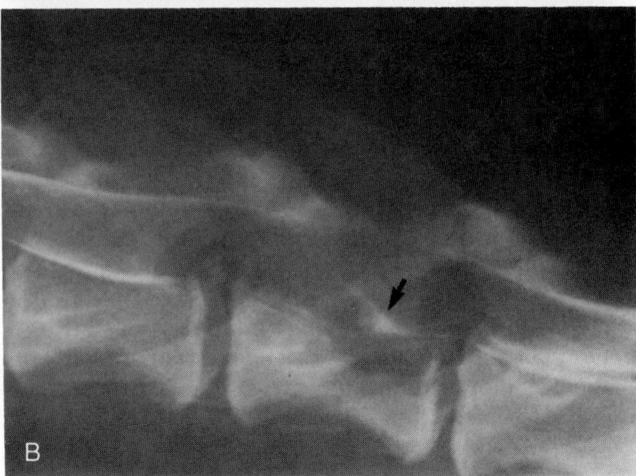

FIGURE 157–10. Lateral radiograph *(A)* and myelogram *(B)* of the lumbar spine of a 5-year-old male Welsh corgi with progressive paraparesis that was most pronounced in the right pelvic limb. The right intervertebral foramen at L5–L6 *(arrows)* is enlarged in *A*, presumably as a result of the compressive effects of a nerve root tumor involving the right L5 nerve root. Bone atrophy has also caused the dorsal lamina of L5 to be less distinct when compared with that of either L4 or L6. The ventral contrast column in *B* divides cranial to the intervertebral foramen at L5–L6 *(arrow)*. An intradural-extramedullary nerve root tumor with microscopic features of a neurofibroma was resected. (From Kornegay JN: Central nervous system neoplasia. *In* Kornegay JN [ed]: *Neurologic Disorders.* Vol 5. *Contemporary Issues in Small Animal Practice.* Churchill Livingstone, New York, 1986, pp 79–108.)

iothalamate [Conray-60]) is injected through a catheter in the internal carotid artery.[35] Arterial and venous phases can be studied. Distortion of the vascular architecture suggests a space-occupying lesion. Contrast medium may be retained in a tumor after clearing from the rest of the brain.[5]

Cavernous Sinus Venography. The venous vasculature on the floor of the skull can be observed by injecting contrast medium (5 to 10 ml) into one of the angularis oculi veins.[126] Lesions can be indirectly identified because of distortion of the normal vascular pattern.

Optic Thecography. With optic thecography, a contrast medium is injected intrathecally (0.2 ml/kg metrizamide at a concentration of 166 mg/ml) at the cerebellomedullary cistern.[90] Skull radiographs are taken after the head has been tilted ventrally at a 30° angle from the horizontal plane for 6 minutes. The extension of the subarachnoid space around the optic nerves can be observed to evaluate neoplastic disease involving the optic nerves.

Myelography. Subarachnoid injection of a contrast medium (iohexol or metrizamide, approximately 40 mg I/kg) outlines the spinal cord and allows definition of compressive lesions. Epidural injection defines the extradural space, helping to identify compressive lesions in the lumbosacral area. Three classic myelographic patterns are associated with extradural, intradural-extramedullary (Fig. 157–10*B*), and intramedullary lesions (Fig. 157–11).[53] Absolute distinction between intradural-extramedullary and intramedullary tumors is not always possible. Further studies including computed tomography (CT), magnetic resonance imaging (MRI), or surgery may be needed to accurately locate the cause and the extent of an intradural lesion.

Scintigraphy

Scintigraphy has been used to diagnose intracranial neoplasia in dogs and cats.[73, 125] A radionuclide such as technetium-99 is injected intravenously and accumulates in brain parenchyma, where the blood-brain barrier is disrupted. Radioactivity is detected by using a gamma camera. This appears to be most useful in detecting masses of at least 1 cm in diameter in the cerebrum or thalamus.[73]

Electrophysiology

Electroencephalography can be used to identify abnormalities and asymmetry in the brain. Tumors themselves are electrically silent. Deep lesions of the brain may not cause electroencephalographic abnormalities.[132] Neuronal damage by the tumor can result in abnormal electrical activity. Focal slowing of the recording to 0.5 to 3.0 potentials per second (delta waves) overlying the tumor occurs most commonly in humans.[47] Nonspecific patterns have also been identified in dogs and cats.[134, 147]

Brain stem auditory evoked response testing may support a diagnosis of a brain stem abnormality without identifying a cause. Electromyography can define spontaneous activity induced by peripheral nerve and spinal lesions.[22] These changes are not specific for nervous system neoplasia.

Cerebrospinal Fluid Analysis

Changes in cerebrospinal fluid (CSF) associated with intracranial neoplasia vary. Tumors are classically said to cause albuminocytological dissociation (elevated protein without a concurrent increase in white blood cells). However, changes reflecting inflammation can be en-

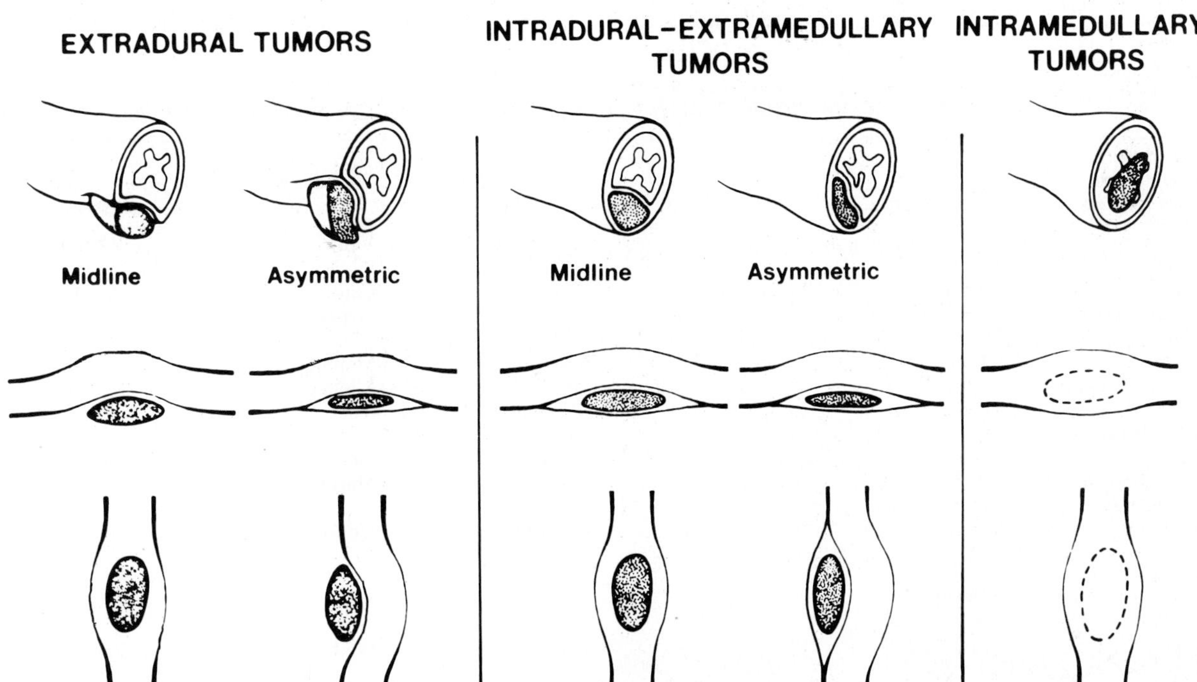

FIGURE 157–11. Myelographic patterns seen on lateral *(top)* and ventrodorsal *(bottom)* views with extradural, intradural-extramedullary, and intramedullary spinal neoplasms. (From Kornegay JN: Central nervous system neoplasia. *In* Kornegay JN [ed]: *Neurologic Disorders.* Vol. 5. *Contemporary Issues in Small Animal Practice.* Churchill Livingstone, New York, 1986, pp 79–108.)

countered with CNS neoplasia.[3, 8, 18] One study found that the pleocytosis associated with meningiomas was more severe than that associated with other tumor types.[3] In lymphosarcoma and diffuse meningeal tumor infiltration, CSF cytological analysis may be diagnostic.[26, 61] Pleocytosis may be associated with a poorer prognosis.[65]

Electrophoresis of CSF can help establish a diagnosis of CNS disease.[8, 161] Albumin typically increases because of blood-brain barrier disruption. Globulins also may increase, presumably because of increased endothelial cell permeability.[161] Tumors in the ventricular system of humans are more likely to produce blood-brain barrier dysfunction and transudation of serum proteins than are noninvasive parenchymal tumors.[49] An increase in the globulin fraction alone may be more consistent with a primary inflammatory process; however, increased gamma-globulin concentrations occur with some brain tumors and may denote intrathecal IgG production by tumor cells.[8, 161] Monoclonal gammopathy associated with multiple myeloma can also cause CNS dysfunction.[177]

Brain herniation subsequent to CSF collection is a risk in animals with increased intracranial pressure.[81] Computed tomography (CT) may be helpful in identifying mass lesions and should be performed, if possible, before CSF collection. If CSF collection is imperative in animals suspected of having increased intracranial pressure, the lumbar cistern is sampled, because the cerebellomedullary cistern may be obliterated by herniating tissue. Lumbar puncture does not decrease the risk of brain herniation.

Computed Tomography

Computed tomography, coupled with magnetic resonance imaging, has largely replaced other techniques for diagnosis of intracranial neoplasia in man and is being used more commonly in animals. The features of most brain tumors of dogs and cats have been well characterized.[79, 174] Features are defined before and after intravenous injection of an iodinated contrast medium (meglumine iothalamate, 600 to 900 mg I/kg) (Fig. 157–12; Table 157–2). Contrast medium is normally excluded by the blood-brain barrier but often leaks through the abnormal or damaged barrier in tumors. Secondary effects, such as vasogenic edema, mass effect, and hydrocephalus, can be detected (Fig. 157–13). Spinal lesions may be defined with CT as well (Fig. 157–14).

Magnetic Resonance Imaging

Magnetic resonance imaging (MRI) is superior to CT for viewing intracranial tumors in humans.[12] This is especially true of posterior fossa lesions. The techniques, physical principles, and normal anatomy of the canine brain, as observed on MRI, have been reviewed.[79, 83] Limited data on the features of individual brain tumors in dogs and cats also have been reported (Fig. 157–15).[78, 79, 124] Most brain tumors have low signal intensity on T1-weighted images (Fig. 157–15*A*) and high signal intensity on those that are T2 weighted. That brain edema has similar features creates problems in defining tumor margins, particularly with intra-axial lesions. Contrast media such as gadolinium-DTPA are beneficial in making this distinction (Fig. 157–15*B*).[43, 85]

Biopsy

Biopsy is required for definitive histological diagnosis of CNS neoplasia. By defining the tumor type, treatment can be planned and a more accurate prognosis given. Although this would be desirable with all CNS lesions, biopsy often is not practical, particularly when there is

TABLE 157–2. COMPUTED TOMOGRAPHY FEATURES OF 50 PRIMARY CANINE BRAIN TUMORS

Computed Tomographic Characteristics	Meningioma	Astrocytoma	Pituitary Gland Tumor	Choroid Plexus Tumor	Oligodendroglioma
Location	Rostral or caudal fossae	Rostral fossa	Sella turcica	Ventricular system	Rostral fossa
Orientation	Peripheral	Parenchymal	Ventral	Central	Parenchymal
Noncontrast tumor density	Iso- or hyperdense	Iso- or hyperdense	Iso- or hyperdense	Hyperdense	Hypodense
Mass effect	Moderate	Marked	Minimal	Minimal	Marked
Peritumoral edema	Minimal	Marked	Minimal	Minimal	Moderate
Presence of hydrocephalus	17% (3/18)	None	50% (4/8)	None	33% (1/3)
Relative size*	Medium	Large	Small	Small	Large
Degree of contrast enhancement	Marked	Marked	Moderate	Marked	Minimal
Uniformity of contrast enhancement	Uniform	Nonuniform	Uniform	Uniform	Nonuniform
Presence of ring effect	11% (2/18)	30% (3/10)	None	None	33% (1/3)
Margination	Well defined	Poorly to well defined	Well defined	Well defined	Poorly defined

*Large = greater than 2 cm in diameter; medium = 1 to 2 cm in diameter; small = less than 1 cm in diameter.
(From Turrel JM, et al: Computed tomographic characteristics of primary brain tumors in 50 dogs. *J Am Vet Med Assoc 188:*851, 1986.)

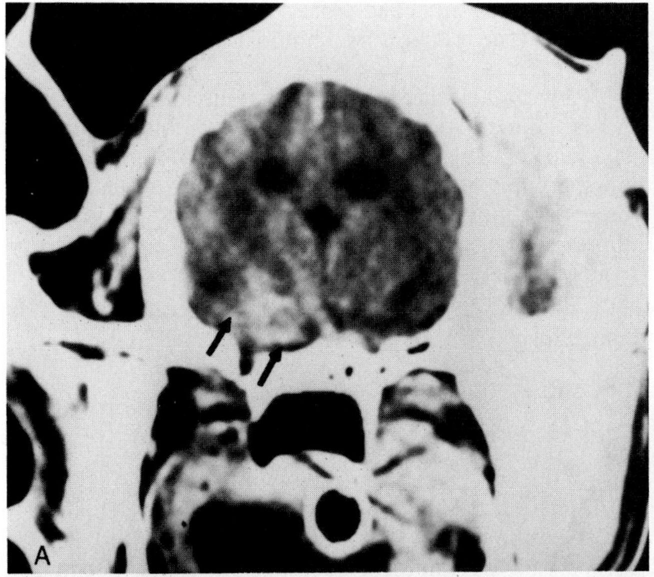

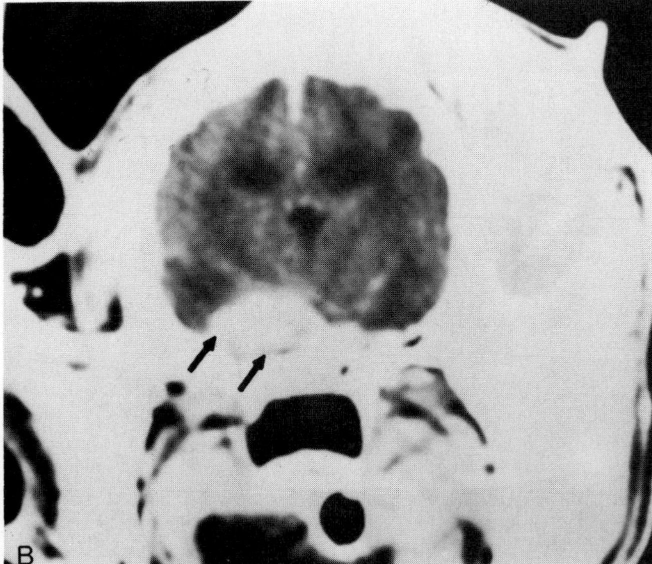

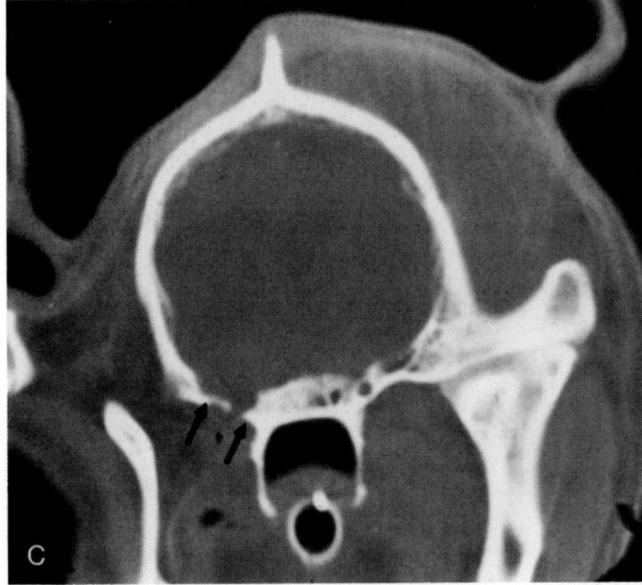

FIGURE 157–12. Transverse computed tomography images at the level of the thalamus from a 6-year-old male Doberman pinscher with chronic left temporal and masseter muscle atrophy and more recent ataxia and depression. *A* was obtained before contrast administration and *B* afterward. A somewhat irregular area of increased radiopacity *(arrows)*, presumably corresponding to a focus of either mineralization or hemorrhage, is seen in *A*. This area enhances homogeneously in *B (arrows)*. *C* was obtained using window settings that allow definition of bony detail. Bone lysis is seen ventrally *(arrows)*. The dog died, and a histopathological diagnosis of meningeal sarcoma, with bony extension, was made at necropsy. (Courtesy of Duke University Medical Center. From Kornegay JN: Imaging brain neoplasia. Computed tomography and magnetic resonance imaging. *Vet Med Rep 2*:372, 1990.)

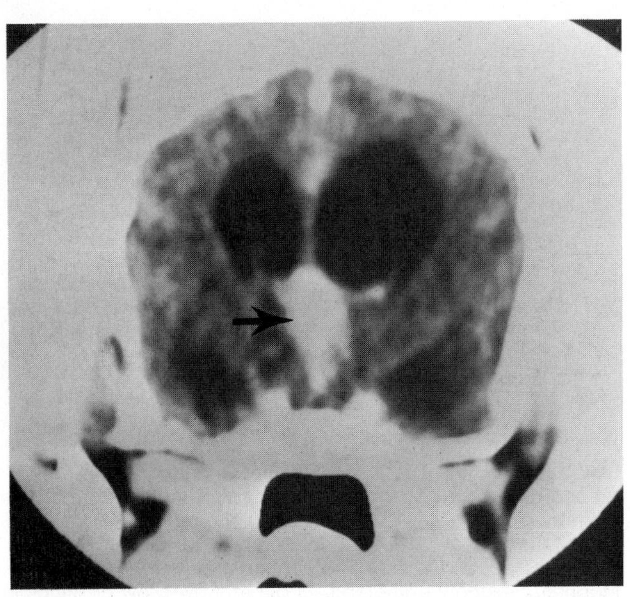

FIGURE 157–13. Iodine-enhanced transverse computed tomography image at the level of the thalamus from a 10-year-old male miniature pinscher with progressive neurological dysfunction. A homogeneously enhancing mass *(arrow)* is present in the third ventricle, and secondary obstructive hydrocephalus is seen. The mass had microscopic features of a choroid plexus papilloma. (Courtesy of Duke University Medical Center. From Kornegay JN: Central nervous system neoplasia. *In* Kornegay JN [ed]: *Neurologic Disorders.* Vol 5. *Contemporary Issues in Small Animal Practice.* Churchill Livingstone, New York, 1986, pp 79–108.)

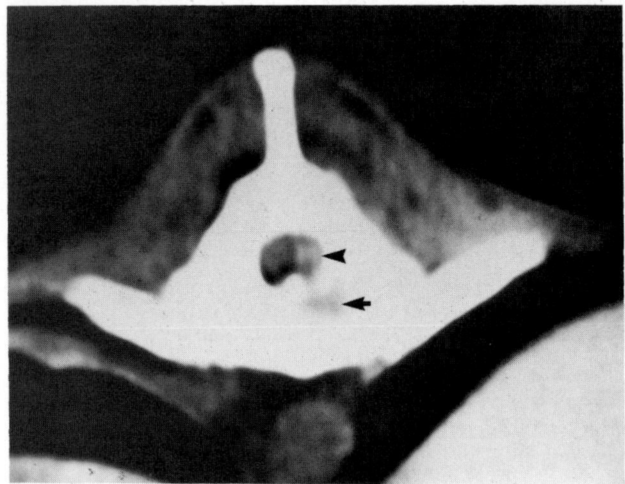

FIGURE 157–14. Iodine-enhanced transverse computed tomography image at the level of T12 of a 9-year-old male basset hound with progressive paraparesis. An area of lysis *(arrow)* within the vertebral body communicates with the vertebral canal. A mass within the canal *(arrowhead)* has displaced the spinal cord to the left. Tissue removed at surgery had microscopic features of an anaplastic adenocarcinoma. A primary tumor was not identified. (Courtesy of Duke University Medical Center. From Kornegay JN: Central nervous system neoplasia. *In* Kornegay JN [ed]: *Neurologic Disorders.* Vol 5. *Contemporary Issues in Small Animal Practice.* Churchill Livingstone, New York, 1986, pp 79–108.)

a high risk of subsequent neurological impairment. Intracranial biopsy in animals has generally been done by means of craniotomy. Stereotactic biopsy guided by CT has decreased the need for exploratory surgery in humans but has not been used commonly in animals. Peripheral nerve tumors should also be sampled by biopsy.[164]

Neoplasia has classically been subdivided on the basis of characteristic histological features. Immunocytochemical markers have been used to identify tumor types more definitively.[107, 179] Using immunohistological techniques and antisera against major canine immunoglobulin classes has allowed some cases of reticulosis to be reclassified as lymphosarcoma.[180]

TREATMENT

Medical Treatment

Glucocorticoids

Treatment of neoplasia involving the nervous system is directed at both the primary lesion and the secondary effects of the tumor. Glucocorticoids are commonly used to decrease peritumoral edema. The exact mechanism by which steroids decrease brain edema is not known. Fluid extravasation may be decreased because of decreased tumor capillary permeability, reduced oxygen free radical activity, and altered exchange of sodium and water across endothelial cells.[185] Alternatively, glucocorticoids may increase the rate of fluid reabsorption by decreasing CSF production at the choroid plexus. Clinical benefits from steroids in human patients with brain tumors have correlated with decreased cerebral white matter water content.[185]

From a diagnostic standpoint, steroid administration alters the CT appearance of brain tumors and decreases

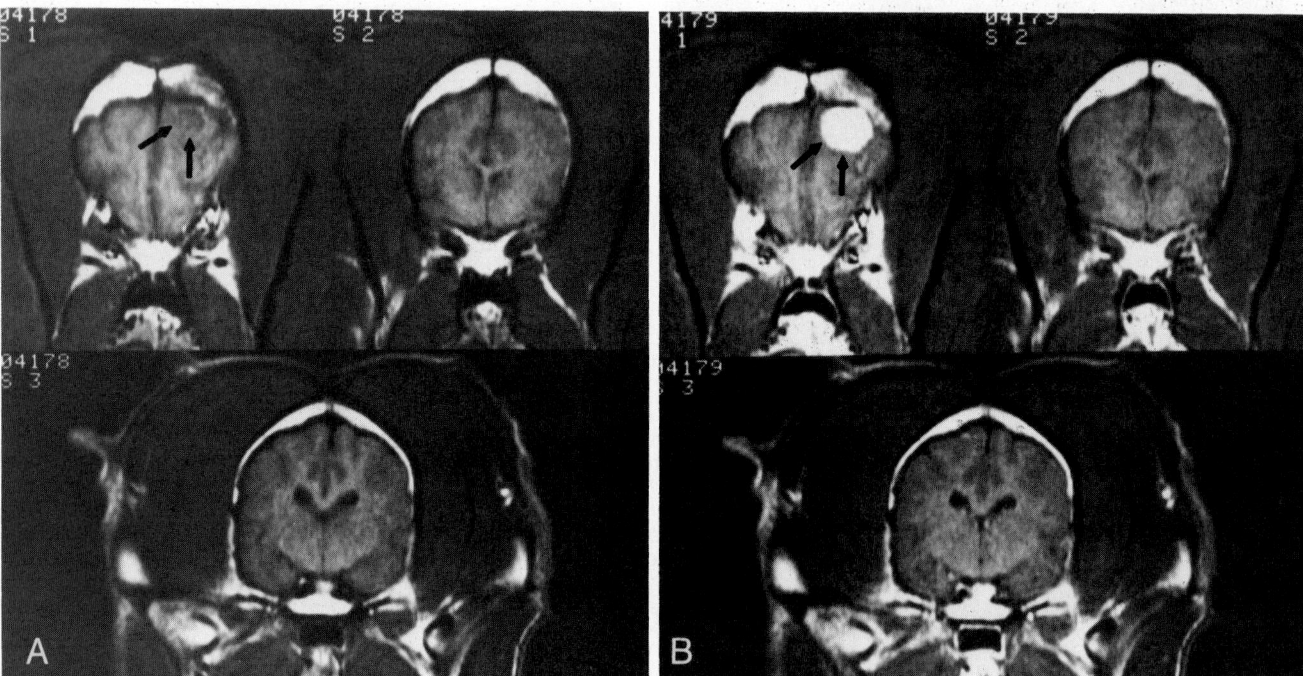

FIGURE 157–15. Transverse magnetic resonance images from a 9-year-old male boxer with seizures. The images were obtained before *(A)* and after *(B)* administration of the contrast medium gadolinium-DTPA. The three sections are at the level of the frontal cortex *(top left)*, basal nuclei *(top right)*, and thalamus *(bottom)* in each series. Before gadolinium-DTPA, a poorly defined area of decreased signal intensity is seen in the right frontal cortex dorsally *(arrows)*. This area enhances uniformly after gadolinium-DTPA *(arrows)*. A tumor with histopathological features of a meningioma was resected surgically. (Spin echo; TR, 500 msec; TE, 20 msec.) (From Thomson CE, et al: Magnetic resonance imaging—a general overview of principles and examples in veterinary neurodiagnosis. *Vet Radiol Ultrasound,* in press.)

the intensity of contrast enhancement in humans and presumably in animals.[59, 60, 99, 111, 145] Concomitant steroid therapy may also decrease the concentration of chemotherapeutic agents within brain tumors.[185] Glucocorticoids may have other deleterious effects, so monitoring of patients is imperative. The dosage required for clinical improvement is variable. Dogs and cats with rapidly progressive clinical signs receive a fast-acting glucocorticoid (prednisolone sodium succinate [15 to 30 mg/kg IV] or dexamethasone [2 mg/kg IV] repeated BID if needed; not to exceed two doses). Smaller doses are used for maintenance.

Hyperosmolar Agents

If cytotoxic edema is suspected, hyperosmolar agents such as mannitol (1 g/kg at 2 ml/minute as a bolus) can be administered. In some human studies, furosemide (0.7 mg/kg IV) administered 20 minutes after the mannitol seems to potentiate its antiedema effect.[137] If hemorrhage has occurred subsequent to the tumor, mannitol may leak from the vasculature, drawing water with it. This potentially can increase the overall mass effect and lead to acute neurological deterioration. The incidence of this phenomenon in animals with brain tumors is unknown. In human studies, gliomas are more often associated with hemorrhage than are meningiomas.[76]

Chemotherapy

The efficacy of certain chemotherapeutic regimens in management of brain tumors is limited because the blood-brain barrier impedes passage of some agents. This shortcoming is partially countered by the fact that some tumors disrupt the barrier. Furthermore, the blood-tumor barrier is not as effective in blocking delivery of certain drugs.[152]

Chemotherapeutic agents used for various brain tumors in human beings have included cytosine arabinoside, nitrosoureas, procarbazine, cisplatin, hydroxyurea, and 5-fluorouracil.[152] When given as a single bolus by intravenous injection, cytosine arabinoside achieves a CSF/serum ratio of 0.7, which is theoretically efficacious for brain neoplasia. Plasma and CSF cytosine arabinoside drug levels were monitored in normal dogs after intravenous bolus injection.[151] Delayed distribution of drug to the CSF compartment best fitted a one-compartment model. Plasma/CSF concentrations were 1.0. Cytosine arabinoside may be expected to distribute well into the CSF of dogs and be potentially useful for management of CNS neoplasia. This drug has been used with some success in combination with other systemic chemotherapeutic agents in treating lymphosarcoma involving the CNS in dogs.[26] In humans, longer infusion times of over 96 hours may increase the amount of cytosine arabinoside in the CSF.[112]

The nitrosoureas, carmustine and lomustine, are highly lipid soluble and cross the blood-brain barrier. Several dogs with histologically confirmed glial tumors improved after administration of these agents alone or in combination with other forms of treatment.[34, 165] Dosages of 50 to 80 mg/m^2 of body surface area have been given at intervals of 6 to 8 weeks.

Intrathecal therapy is used in certain CNS neoplasms in humans. The goal is to bypass the blood-brain barrier and achieve higher concentrations of drug in the CSF. Dogs with neural lymphosarcoma have been treated with intrathecal cytosine arabinoside.[26] This drug may remain at therapeutic levels after intrathecal injection for longer periods because less cytidine deaminase is available in the CSF to break down the drug.[26, 188] Methotrexate has also been used intrathecally in humans.[112]

Other mechanisms by which effects of the blood-brain barrier may be at least partially attenuated include increased drug dose, intra-arterial injection, and use of hyperosmolar agents to open the barrier.[152] Although hyperosmolar agents such as mannitol are effective in opening the normal blood-brain barrier, effects on the blood-tumor barrier have been inconsistent. Such therapy could conceivably have toxic effects on normal brain while the tumor itself remained unaffected.[152]

Chemotherapeutic agents used to treat extracranial neoplasia can cause neurological complications. These side effects may be inappropriately attributed to brain metastasis. Examples include the neurotoxic effects of 5-fluorouracil[57] and neural thrombosis and hemorrhage associated with L-asparaginase.[171] Clinical signs associated with 5-fluorouracil neurotoxicosis in dogs and cats include hyperexcitability, nervousness, muscle tremors, and ataxia.[57] In human patients, optic neuritis, euphoria, and signs of cerebellar dysfunction have been noted.[105, 184]

Anticonvulsants

Anticonvulsants may be necessary to control seizures secondary to intracranial neoplasia. Some animals develop seizures after intracranial surgery, so prophylactic administration of anticonvulsants is indicated. Potential drug interactions with chemotherapeutic agents should be evaluated before administration.

Surgery

Surgery should be contemplated in patients with brain tumors to aid in both diagnosis and therapy. In our hospital, affected dogs that had surgery had an increase in survival time as compared with dogs receiving only symptomatic care.[65] The mean survival time of dogs undergoing surgery was only 2 months. Others have reported longer survival times in dogs and cats with brain tumors managed by surgery alone. The average survival time in one series of 19 dogs and cats with assorted tumors was 236 days.[118] A number of factors, including those detailed at the conclusion of this section, clearly affect survival duration.

Most reports of surgical management of brain tumors in animals have concerned meningiomas (Fig. 157–16).[89, 155] Surgical considerations for this tumor type are discussed later in the section on meningioma. Principles discussed in that section pertain to other extra-axial tumors. Intra-axial lesions are much more difficult to treat by surgery alone. Although benign tumors conceivably can be completely resected, cytoreduction and biopsy generally are all that is practical. Adjunctive

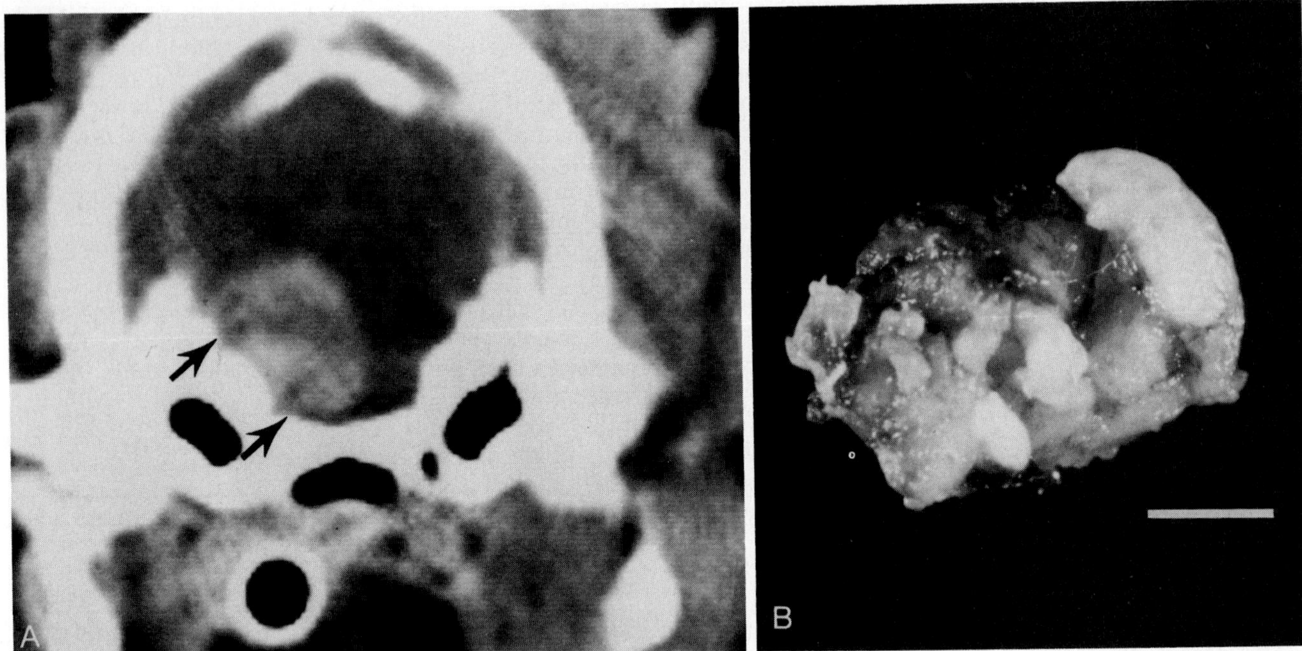

FIGURE 157–16. Iodine-enhanced transverse computed tomography image *(A)* and resected tumor *(B)* from the dog illustrated in Figure 157–5. A homogeneously enhancing mass is present in the caudal fossa on the left side *(arrows)*. The mass appears to have a broad point of origin from the area of the petrous temporal bone. Meningioma was suspected and confirmed on histological evaluation of the resected tumor. (Courtesy of Duke University Medical Center.) (Bar in *B* = 0.3 cm.)

therapies such as irradiation, chemotherapy, or both are then indicated.

Irradiation

Irradiation increases the survival time of humans with several types of primary brain tumors[154] and has been used to treat affected animals.[36, 65, 91, 92, 175] Dogs treated with irradiation alone or in combination with surgery had improved survival times over dogs treated symptomatically.[65] A total dose of 45.6 to 48.0 Gy has generally been administered to the whole brain, using 12 fractions of 3.8 to 4.0 Gy three times weekly. Smaller fractions have also been used daily. Somewhat similar protocols have been used by others.[36, 91, 92] Clinical improvement may occur within 2 weeks of irradiation; actual reduction in tumor size may not be noted on CT for several months.[91] In some dogs, clinical long-term improvement occurs despite persistence of significant tumor volume on CT examination (Fig. 157–17).

As with any form of therapy, the benefits of irradiation must be balanced against potential complications, such as necrosis of normal brain, damage to extracranial structures including the eyes and skin, and tumor necrosis with associated hemorrhage.[54] Brain necrosis due to irradiation occurs in some human patients within a few weeks to months after treatment (early delayed necrosis) and after months or even years in others (late delayed necrosis).[84] These late effects are more deleterious and are usually progressive and irreversible. The severity of irradiation-induced necrosis is related to the total dose administered and the volume of normal brain irradiated.[84] Necrosis has been encountered in human patients receiving total doses of 50 to 60 Gy or more. Injury may range from demyelination to coagulative necrosis of white matter.[1]

Several mechanisms probably contribute to the late effects of irradiation on the brain. Hydrocephalus, leukoencephalopathy, and cortical metabolic derangements have been documented.[29] Hydrocephalus may occur because of irradiation-induced fibrosis of the leptomeninges, with reduction in CSF absorption across the arachnoid villi. Leukoencephalopathy apparently occurs because of increased capillary permeability and subsequent transudation of fluid into the interstitial space. Low-density contrast-enhancing foci of irradiation-induced necrosis seen on CT may be confused with tumor; MRI may be more sensitive.[1] Although similar pathological effects of irradiation have been seen experimentally in dogs,[45] changes have not been well documented in animals with spontaneous brain tumors.[91] As longer survival times are achieved by more efficient control of intracranial neoplasms, these secondary effects of irradiation may become more apparent.

Methods used to augment effects of irradiation on tumor have included radiation sensitizers, heavy-particle radiotherapy, interstitial implants of radioisotopes (brachytherapy), hyperthermia, and unconventional fractionation schemes.[116] Implants of the radioisotope ^{125}I have been used in humans with brain tumors[55] and on a limited basis in affected animals.[78] Although brachytherapy theoretically allows selective dosing of the tumor while the remainder of the brain is spared, undertreatment of the tumor periphery may lead to recurrences.

Hypoxic cells are up to three times more resistant to

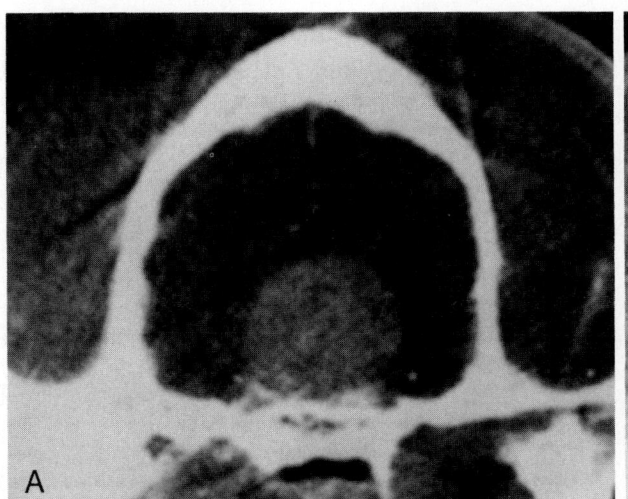

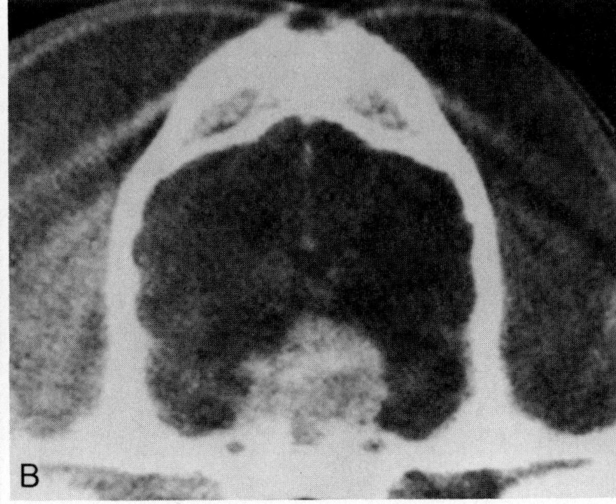

FIGURE 157–17. Iodine-enhanced transverse computed tomography images from a 6-year-old female bull terrier with a 3-month history of progressive signs of right forebrain dysfunction before *(A)* and 1 year after irradiation *(B)* for a suspected pituitary gland tumor. Studies of endocrine function were compatible with pituitary-dependent hyperadrenocorticism. In both images, a homogeneous, roughly circular mass is located on the midline on the floor of the middle fossa. The size of the mass is reduced after irradiation. Clinical signs in the dog resolved after irradiation despite persistent tumor. The dog was functional for 41 months, at which time recurrence of neurological dysfunction, again referable to the right forebrain, necessitated euthanasia. On re-evaluation by computed tomography at that time, the mass had enlarged to roughly its pretreatment size.

irradiation than those that are well oxygenated.[116] Drugs such as misonidazole may sensitize them to the effects of irradiation.[162] Hyperthermia also acts synergistically with radiation, particularly against hypoxic cells.[33, 121] Use of localized hyperthermia has a similar drawback to brachytherapy; the periphery of the tumor may be underheated, leading to recurrences.[98] Accordingly, whole-body hyperthermia has been used in some clinical trials of extracranial neoplasms in humans[136] and has been used in combination with either external beam irradiation or brachytherapy in several dogs with brain tumors.[65, 78] Radiation administered by boron neutron capture therapy may also be more effective in overcoming the effects of hypoxia than conventional radiotherapy. Several dogs with brain tumors have been treated using this modality, with apparent radiographic and clinical improvement.[108, 109]

Clearly, numerous factors affect prognosis in dogs with intracranial neoplasia. Factors associated with increased survival in a retrospective review of 86 dogs with brain tumors were mode of therapy (surgery and/or cobalt-radiation versus symptomatic), tumor type (meningiomas and primary tumors versus other tumor types and secondary tumors, respectively), CSF results (normal or albuminocytological dissociation versus other changes), degree of initial neurological dysfunction (mild versus moderate/severe), tumor volume (small versus medium/large), and multiplicity of brain involvement (solitary versus multiple).[65]

TUMOR TYPES

The following section describes more common CNS neoplasms. Specific details that may aid in the diagnosis and treatment of these tumors have been included.

Meningioma

Incidence and Classification

Meningiomas are tumors of mesenchymal origin. Intracranial, optic nerve, spinal, and paranasal meningiomas occur. Meningiomas have been divided on histological features into meningotheliomatous (endotheliomatous or syncytial), fibrous, transitional, psammomatous, or anaplastic types.[13] There is little difference in prognosis for these different types in humans. Solitary meningiomas are common in both dogs and cats. Cats, in particular, may have multiple tumors.[195] Dolichocephalic breeds of dogs may be at increased risk.[132] Golden retrievers may be affected disproportionately. An unexplained increased incidence of meningiomas has been noted in cats with mucopolysaccharidosis I.[58]

Meningiomas occur more commonly intracranially than in the vertebral canal in both dogs and cats. Optic nerve meningiomas are usually constricted by bone of the optic foramina but occasionally extend into the cranial cavity.[52, 86, 129] Paranasal meningiomas include many histological types; in one study, eight of ten tumors extended from the nasal area to the brain.[128] The frontal lobes, falx cerebri, and cerebellopontine angle are frequent intracranial sites for meningiomas in dogs (Fig. 157–18).[132] Most meningiomas in cats occur over the cerebral convexities.[114]

Spinal meningiomas are more common in the cervical area.[46] The mean age at diagnosis of 13 dogs with spinal meningiomas was 9.5 years; a 2:1 male/female distribution was noted.[46]

Clinical Features

Clinical signs encountered with these tumors vary depending on the part of the nervous system involved.

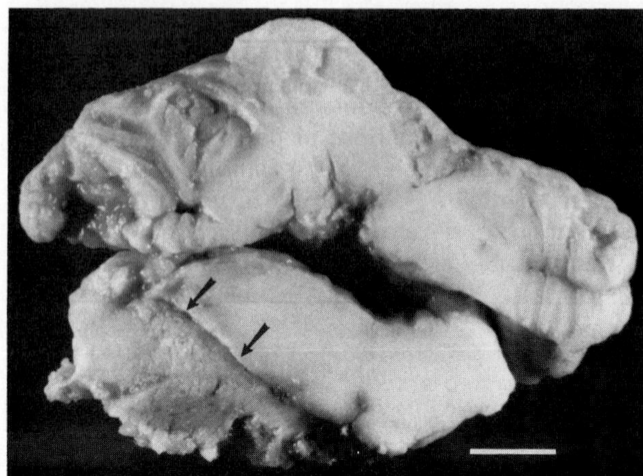

FIGURE 157–18. Transverse section of brain at the level of the medulla oblongata and cerebellum from an 11-year-old female coonhound with intermittent episodes of signs related to left-sided vestibular dysfunction. The dog was euthanized without treatment. The medulla oblongata is displaced dorsally by a ventrolaterally positioned, well-demarcated mass *(arrows)*. The mass had histological features of a meningioma at necropsy. (Bar = 0.5 cm.)

Interestingly, human patients with meningiomas more commonly have extraneural primary malignancies, compared with patients with non-neoplastic CNS lesions and patients with non-CNS disease.[7] This observation does not necessarily imply a direct cause-and-effect relationship between meningiomas and primary extraneural neoplasia. Patients with meningiomas may simply remain asymptomatic for long periods, thus allowing development of other spontaneous neoplasms.

A high incidence of seizures has been reported in dogs with paranasal tumors, presumably because of edema and various degrees of hemorrhage and necrosis frequently occurring in adjacent brain.[128] Only two of ten dogs in that study had clinical signs of nasal cavity disease. The *en plaque* meningioma can arise from the floor of the skull and adhere to it, frequently affecting cranial nerves II through VIII.[132] Plaque-like meningiomas also may extend over the brain dorsally (Fig. 157–19).

Spinal meningiomas frequently cause hyperesthesia and progressive paresis.[46]

Diagnosis

Hyperostosis of the skull may be seen on survey radiographs in patients with meningiomas. Modified views have been used in an attempt to better appreciate this effect.[132] On CT evaluation, the precontrast appearance of meningiomas varies from isodense to either hyperdense or hypodense.[79, 174] Uniform contrast enhancement is noted in most tumors (Fig. 157–20). Hyperostosis of the skull generally is not encountered in dogs but may occur in cats.

Changes usually are not noted on survey radiographs in animals with spinal meningiomas.[46] Thinning of the dorsal lamina may be noted. On myelographic evaluation, either an intradural-extramedullary or intramedullary pattern may be seen (Fig. 157–21). CT may also identify the tumor.

Treatment

Treatment for meningiomas includes surgical cytoreduction/resection (see Fig. 157–16) and irradiation, alone or combined.[65, 78, 82, 89, 91, 92] Resection of benign rostral fossa tumors carries a favorable prognosis, as long as the tumor is resected entirely and a wide rim of meninges is removed. Meningiomas over the cerebral convexities are most easily resected. Some tumors recur, even when complete gross resection has apparently been accomplished. Tumors on the floor of the skull are difficult to remove without associated clinical deterioration. *En plaque* meningiomas adjacent to the brain stem are particularly difficult to expose adequately. Standard lateral and suboccipital approaches to the brain[120] often allow observation of only the rostral and caudal portions of the tumor, respectively. Although both surgical approaches can be used concurrently, the tumor's midsection may still be inadequately exposed. A ventral approach, perhaps through the middle ear, might be more useful, but clinical experience in animals is lacking.

The cerebral cortex can be retracted with less risk of deterioration; accordingly, in contrast to caudal fossa lesions, tumors in the middle and rostral fossae can be exposed relatively well. Exposure of rostrally positioned tumors is further complicated by the frontal sinuses. Transfrontal approaches[32, 82] expedite exposure but also increase the risk of infection. Laterally and ventrally positioned tumors can be exposed by performing a limited craniotomy ventral to the frontal sinus.[92] Involvement of the dorsal sagittal sinus by tumors on the dorsal

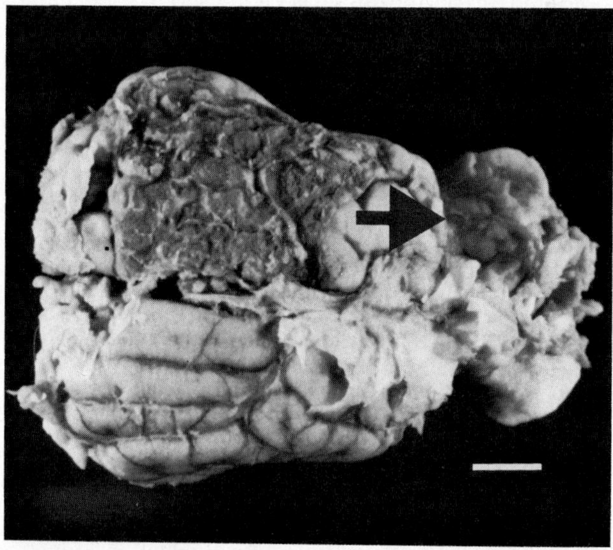

FIGURE 157–19. Gross overview of the dorsum of the cerebrum from a 13-year-old female collie with seizures of 3 weeks duration and mild, poorly localizing neurological deficits. Evaluation of computed tomography and magnetic resonance images identified a left frontal mass, most compatible with a meningioma, and additional diffuse changes over the dorsal cerebrum attributed potentially to local spread of tumor. The owner declined treatment, and the dog was eventually euthanized. Necropsy was performed. The left frontal mass is seen here *(arrow)*; in addition, the dorsal meninges are markedly thickened by neoplastic tissue (caudal to *arrow*). Meningioma with local extension (meningioma en plaque) was diagnosed histologically. (Bar = 1 cm.)

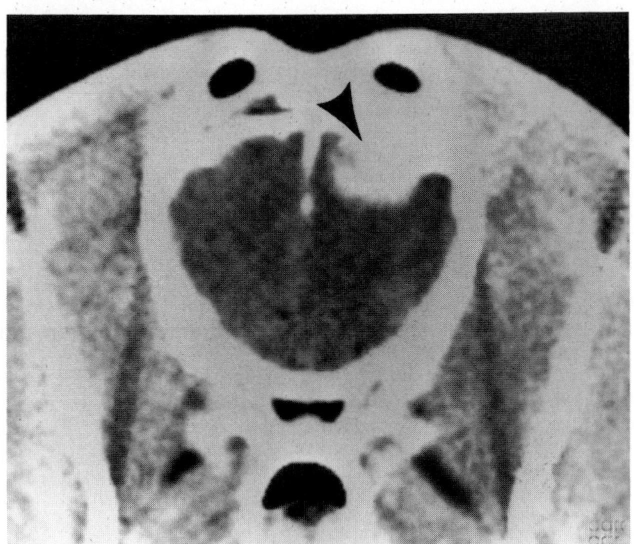

FIGURE 157–20. Iodine-enhanced transverse computed tomography image at the level of the frontal cortex from the dog illustrated in Figure 157–15. A homogeneously enhancing mass with a broad base and sharply defined margins is present at the periphery of the right frontal cerebral cortex *(arrowhead)*. A zone of decreased radiopacity, presumably corresponding to edema, is seen around the tumor. There is slight right-to-left mass effect. These features were believed to be most compatible with meningioma, which was confirmed on histopathological evaluation of the resected tumor. (Courtesy of Duke University Medical Center. From Kornegay JN: Central nervous system neoplasia. *In* Kornegay JN [ed]: *Neurologic Disorders.* Vol 5. *Contemporary Issues in Small Animal Practice.* Churchill Livingstone, New York, 1986, pp 79–108.)

midline creates additional difficulties. Although tumor and the sinus are generally grossly separable, wide excision is precluded, and poorly defined tumor foci can lead to recurrence.

Surgical cytoreduction may be beneficial when complete resection is impossible. A few dogs with paranasal meningiomas have remained free of clinical signs 1 year after surgery despite tumor recurrence.[128]

Although meningiomas have generally been thought to be radiation resistant, longer survivals have been achieved in humans with surgery and irradiation than with surgery alone.[4] General indications for radiation in affected human patients include incomplete resection, malignant histological features, and progressive or recurrent disease after curative surgery.[160] Irradiation seems to improve survival of dogs with meningiomas as well.[65, 91, 92] Some dogs with large frontal meningiomas treated by surgery and radiation have survived more than 1 year despite persistent tumor.[92] Radiation alone also may be beneficial; one dog survived for 791 days after radiation and had only a small residual focus of tumor.[91]

Six of nine dogs with spinal meningiomas that were operated on improved.[46] In each case, the only gross finding at surgery was enlargement of the dural tube before durotomy. Four of the nine dogs had indistinct or nonexistent margins between the spinal cord and tumor. Results of surgery were poor in dogs that had intumescence lesions, ventrally located tumors, iatrogenic spinal cord injury, or spinal cord invasion.[46]

Astrocytoma

Incidence and Classification

Intracranial astrocytomas (Fig. 157–22) afflict both dogs and cats. Various histological types occur in humans and dogs. Tumors may be graded based on their biological activity (low versus high grade; grade I to IV, denoting increasing malignancy) or the predominant cell type (fibrillary, protoplasmic, gemistocytic, or pilocytic). Astrocytoma is the most common glial tumor in dogs. Ninety-two of 341 gliomas were astrocytomas in one study;[178] another series of 215 gliomas included 118 astrocytomas.[103] Middle-aged boxers and Boston terriers are most often affected.[95, 132] Cerebral involvement is common.[103, 132] The spinal cord is also affected relatively often (Fig. 157–23). Astrocytoma is the most common glioma affecting cats but occurs infrequently.[40, 95, 147]

Diagnosis

The CT appearance of astrocytomas varies with the biological behavior of the tumor.[79, 174] Well-differentiated tumors have variable but uniform density on precontrast scans. Necrosis and hemorrhage in anaplastic tumors result in a mottled appearance. On contrast medium administration, most tumors enhance markedly, but some show minimal enhancement. Although enhancement is generally uniform (Fig. 157–24*A*), a ring pattern is seen in anaplastic tumors because of central necrosis. MRI may allow clearer tumor delineation (Fig. 157–24*B*).

The immunocytochemical marker for human astrocytic tumors is glial fibrillary acidic protein (GFAP) stain-

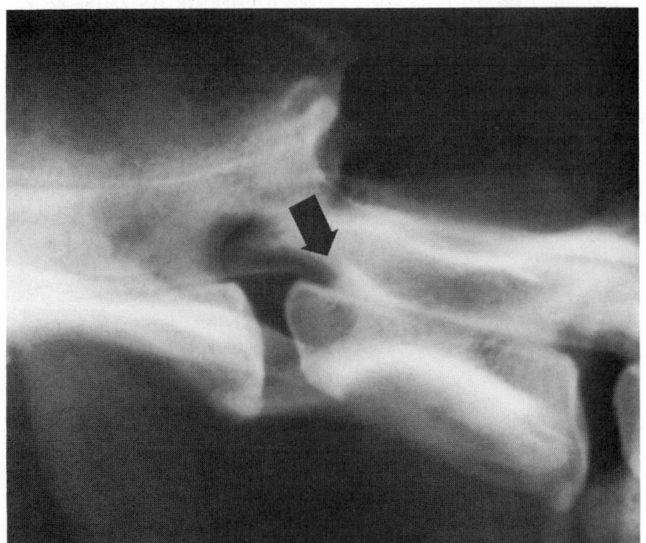

FIGURE 157–21. Lateral cervical myelogram from an 8-year-old male golden retriever with left thoracic limb monoparesis and eventual tetraparesis. Contrast medium has accumulated within the ventral subarachnoid space dorsal to the cranial aspect of the C3 vertebral body *(arrow)*. This golf tee pattern is characteristic of intradural-extramedullary lesions. The resected mass had histological features of a meningioma. External beam irradiation was done postoperatively, and the dog was clinically normal 1 year later.

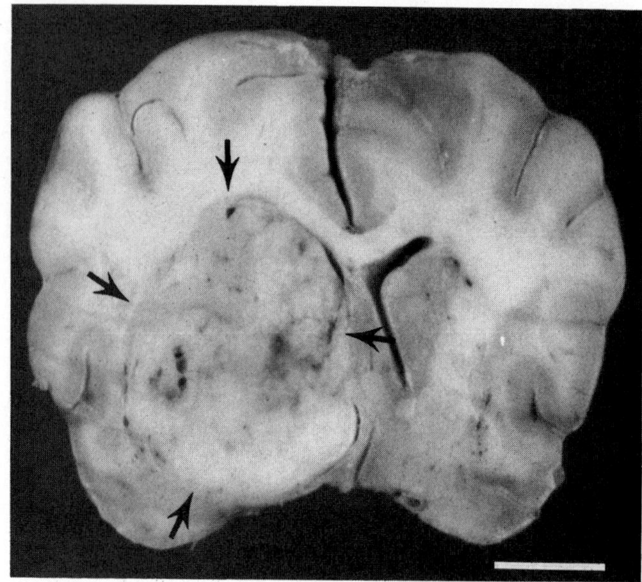

FIGURE 157–22. Transverse section of brain at the level of the basal nuclei from a 13-year-old male standard poodle that collapsed and died acutely. A large, relatively well demarcated mass *(arrows)* has obliterated the basal nuclei on the left side, resulting in moderate left-to-right mass effect. A histological diagnosis of astrocytoma was made. (Bar = 0.75 cm.)

ing. In one study, only 12 of 19 canine tumors classified histologically as astrocytomas were unequivocally positive for GFAP.[179] In humans with astrocytomas, GFAP is consistently demonstrated in both differentiated and anaplastic tumors. Canine astrocytomas may not be as well differentiated as their human counterparts; alternatively, some tumors originally classified as astrocytomas actually may have originated from other cell types.[178]

Treatment

There have been few reports on treatment of astrocytomas in animals.[34, 78, 165] Benign tumors can be resected. Variables that correlated with increasing survival in one large series of humans with surgically treated supratentorial low-grade astrocytomas were gross total surgical removal, lack of major preoperative deficit, long duration of symptoms before surgery, seizures as a presenting symptom, lack of major postoperative neurological deficit, and surgery performed in recent decades.[88] That there was a positive correlation with long duration of symptoms and seizures was attributed to the indolent nature of tumors in these patients. Not surprisingly, outcome was poorer when there were symptoms of increased intracranial pressure, befitting the more aggressive nature of these tumors. In this same study, postoperative radiation was most beneficial in older patients with incompletely removed tumors. Chemotherapy may also reduce tumor mass or at least delay growth in affected dogs.[34, 165]

Glioblastoma Multiforme

Glioblastoma multiforme is an aggressive tumor that shares many features with high-grade astrocytomas.[16, 141] Necrosis and hemorrhage are especially prominent. This tumor occurs relatively infrequently in dogs and is rare in cats. Twenty-five were included in one series of 215 canine gliomas affecting the brain.[103] Another series of 341 gliomas of the brain of dogs contained 40 glioblastomas.[178] Tumors classified as glioblastomas are undoubtedly called anaplastic astrocytomas or undifferentiated gliomas by others and vice versa.

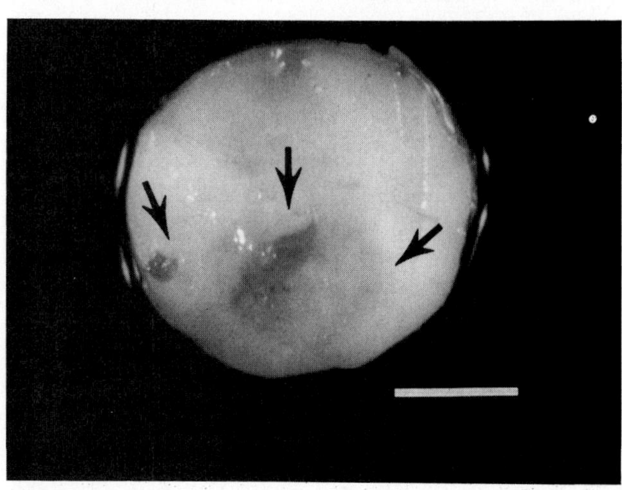

FIGURE 157–23. Transverse section of spinal cord from a 7-year-old female bulldog with progressive paraparesis over a period of 2 weeks. An intramedullary pattern was noted on myelography, and the dog was euthanized without treatment. The spinal cord contains a poorly defined mass *(arrows)* that had histological features of an astrocytoma. (Bar = 0.3 cm.)

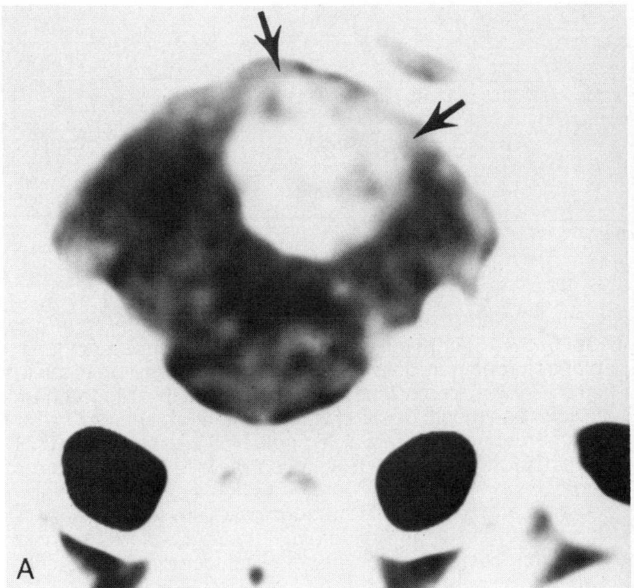

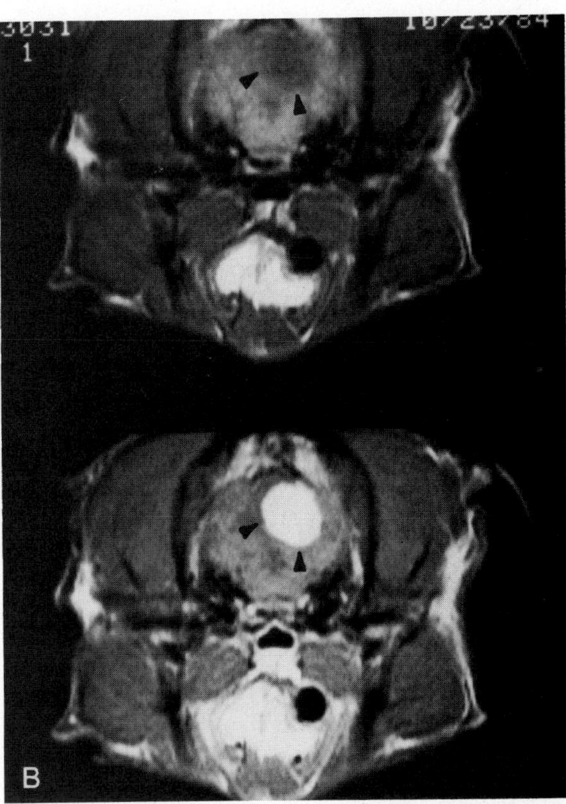

FIGURE 157–24. Transverse iodine-enhanced computed tomography *(A)* and magnetic resonance images before (*B*, top) and after (*B*, bottom) administration of gadolinium-DTPA from a 4-year-old male Pekingese with a 1-month history of ataxia and seizures. A somewhat heterogeneously enhancing mass is seen in the cerebellum in *A (arrows)*. In the magnetic resonance images, the mass has low signal intensity before contrast administration *(arrowheads)* and uniform high signal intensity after gadolinium-DTPA *(arrowheads)*. The resected mass had histological features of an astrocytoma. (Courtesy of Duke University Medical Center. *B*, from Kornegay JN: Imaging brain neoplasia. Computed tomography and magnetic resonance imaging. *Vet Med Rep* 2:372, 1990.)

Although these tumors classically are locally invasive, surprisingly well differentiated masses can be seen, particularly with the giant-cell form of the tumor in humans.[141] The same appears to be true of dogs (Fig. 157–25).

Middle-aged and older brachycephalic dogs are predisposed; most tumors affect the cerebrum or thalamus.[95] Multiple lesions may be noted. Principles of diagnosis and treatment are similar to those described for anaplastic astrocytomas but more extreme. More aggressive forms of treatment discussed earlier in the general sections on radiation and chemotherapy have been developed particularly for this tumor.

Ependymoma

Ependymomas arise from ependymal cells. They are more common in the spinal cord[96] (Fig. 157–26) in dogs but can also arise intracranially. Ependymomas are rare in both dogs and cats. Only 4 ependymomas were identified in 215 glial brain tumors in dogs; 3 of these were in the third ventricle, and 1 was in the cerebellum.[103] Another study of 341 gliomas in the brains of dogs contained 19 ependymomas, but their location was not stated.[178] A single ependymoma was included in 87 feline CNS tumors.[195] The CT appearance in the few reported canine cases has been variable.[174] Treatment of affected animals has not been described. Craniospinal radiation alone or combined with surgery improves duration of survival in human patients.[133, 146]

Choroid Plexus Tumors

Incidence and Classification

Choroid plexus tumors are derived from epithelial cells of the choroid plexus. The absence of both cilia and blepharoplasts distinguishes this tumor from ependymomas.[104, 141, 142] Choroid plexus tumors occur relatively frequently in dogs but rarely in cats. Twenty-five choroid plexus tumors were included in one series of 215 dogs with glial brain tumors.[103] Another study of 341 canine brain gliomas included 42 choroid plexus tumors.[178] Histologically benign papillomas and more malignant carcinomas are encountered. Any part of the ventricular system can be involved; however, the fourth ventricle is affected most frequently (Fig. 157–27).[95, 197] Most tumors occur at the level of the lateral apertures. The left side may be preferentially affected.[197] Intracranial and spinal metastasis may occur through the CSF (Fig. 157–28).[103, 126, 196]

Clinical Features

Middle-aged and older dogs are generally affected, but tumors can occur in young dogs.[70, 95] In one series, all affected dogs were males.[197] Brachycephalic dogs are not predisposed, as they are to most gliomas.[95] Signs of

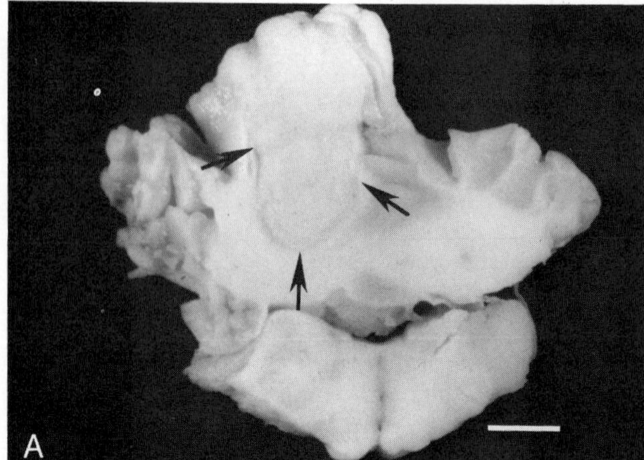

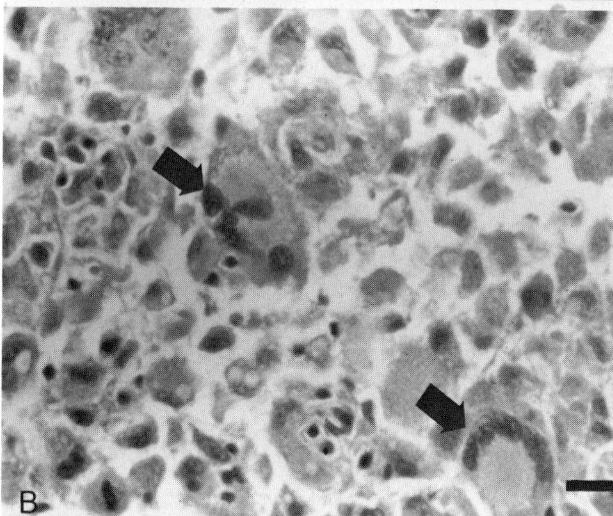

FIGURE 157–25. Transverse section of brain at the level of the medulla oblongata and cerebellum *(A)* and photomicrograph of this lesion *(B)* from a 3-year-old male mixed-breed dog with attitude change and ataxia of one month duration and more recent seizures. On evaluation of cerebrospinal fluid, nucleated cells (465/μl) and protein (373 mg/dl) were increased. A mixed population of cells, including rare multinucleates, was present. The dog died without treatment. A relatively well demarcated mass is seen in the cerebellum (*arrows* in *A*). A similar lesion was noted in the midbrain. Both tumors were composed of a heterogeneous population of cells, including multinucleates (*arrows* in *B*) and foci of necrosis. A diagnosis of giant cell glioblastoma multiforme was made. (Bar = 0.5 cm in *A* and 25 μm in *B;* H & E stain in *B.*)

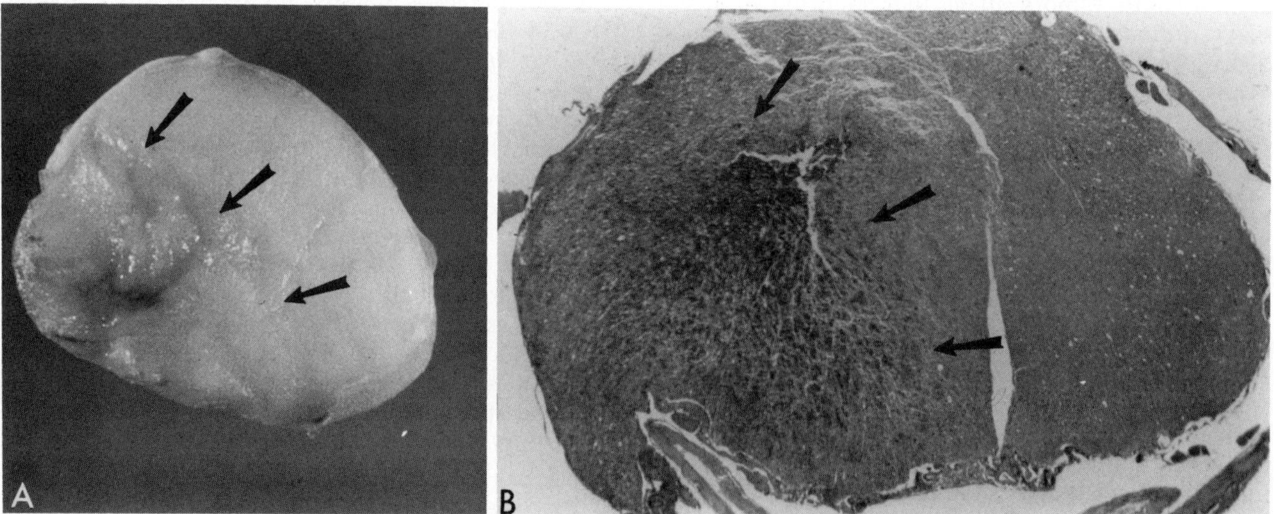

FIGURE 157–26. Transverse gross *(A)* and microscopic *(B)* sections of spinal cord from an 11-year-old female bichon frise with progressive paraparesis leading to paraplegia. An intramedullary lesion was identified within the spinal cord at T13–L1 at surgery. The dog was euthanized. The left lateral and ventral funiculi contain a poorly defined mass that had histological features of an ependymoma (*arrows* in both).

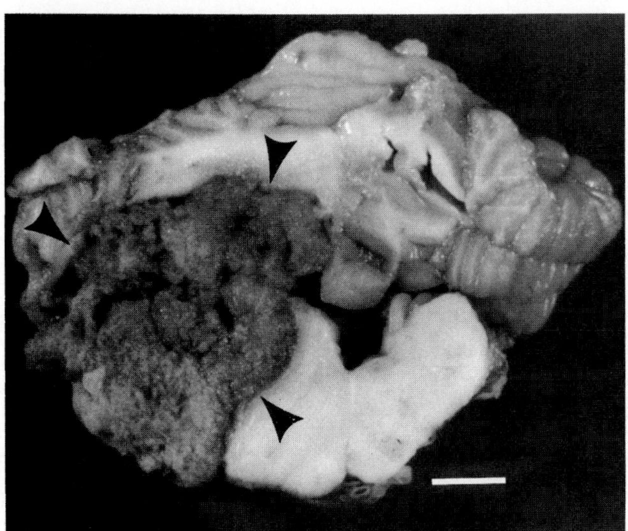

FIGURE 157–27. Transverse section of brain at the level of the medulla oblongata and cerebellum from a 7-year-old male Irish setter with progressive ataxia and left-sided head tilt. Further evaluation was declined by the owner, and the dog was euthanized. A large, well-demarcated mass *(arrowheads)* at the level of the left lateral aperture has markedly compressed and displaced the medulla oblongata and cerebellum. A histological diagnosis of choroid plexus papilloma was made at necropsy. (Bar = 0.5 cm.)

vestibular disease are frequently noted. On rare occasions, paraparesis due to spinal metastasis may precede intracranial signs.[103]

Diagnosis

Tumors are generally well delineated on CT evaluation. All five choroid plexus tumors in one report were associated with the ventricular system and were hyperdense on precontrast scans.[174] Some tumors may also be isodense.[79] Choroid plexus tumors usually show marked contrast enhancement and well-defined tumor margins with both CT and MRI (Fig. 157–29). Minimal peritumoral edema and no evidence of hydrocephalus were observed in one report;[174] hydrocephalus is commonly noted when the third ventricle is involved (Fig. 157–30). Large tumors in the fourth ventricle also may obstruct CSF outflow, leading to hydrocephalus. Excessive CSF production by functional choroid plexus tumors can also conceivably lead to hydrocephalus.[101]

Treatment

Treatment is reported rarely. We have unsuccessfully attempted to resect two tumors.[78] As with meningiomas, caudal fossa tumors are difficult to expose adequately. Tumors within the third or lateral ventricles must be approached by incising either the cerebrum or corpus callosum. Given the epithelial origin of this tumor, radiation could be beneficial.

Oligodendroglioma

Incidence and Classification

Oligodendrogliomas selectively affect brachycephalic dogs.[194] One series of 341 canine gliomas affecting the brain included 99 oligodendrogliomas.[178] Another series of 215 canine glial brain tumors contained 60 oligodendrogliomas.[103] Cats are rarely affected.[159] Most tumors are relatively well demarcated, but some are infiltrative. Ventricular invasion occurs, and hemorrhage is also noted.

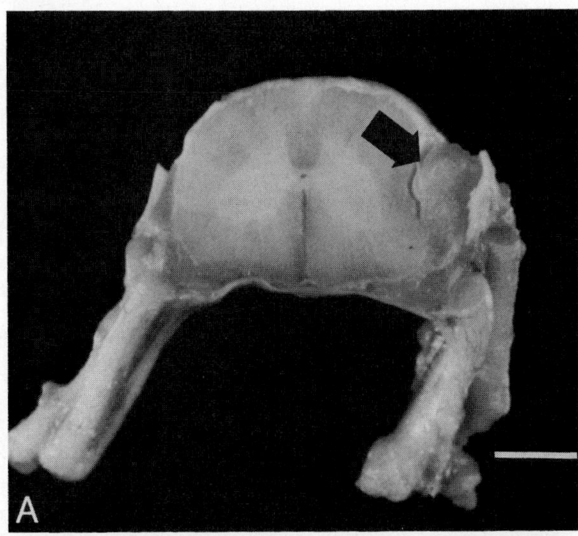

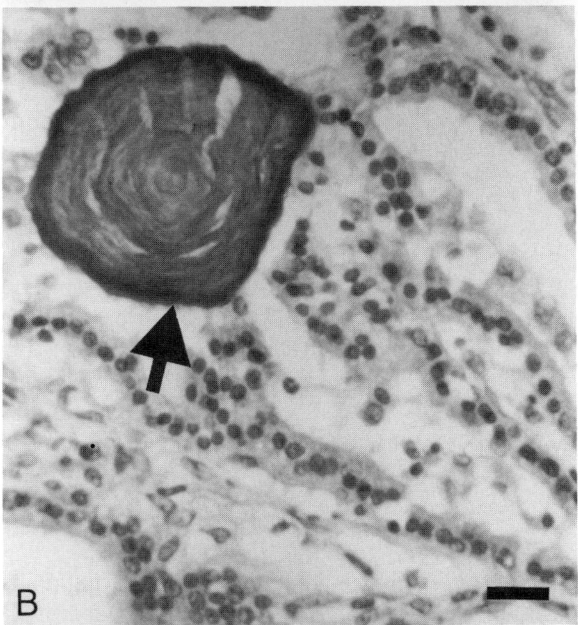

FIGURE 157–28. Transverse section of lumbar spinal cord and nerve roots *(A)* and photomicrograph of focus of tumor *(B)* from a 5-year-old male golden retriever with a history of seizures of 5 months duration and more recent progressive paraparesis. Computed tomography of the skull was normal. On myelography, a pattern consistent with an intramedullary lesion was noted in the caudal lumbar area. Laminectomy revealed several small, relatively poorly defined, subdural masses. One mass was sampled and had histological features of an epithelial tumor, as well as foci of mineralization (*arrow* in *B*). A primary tumor site was not identified elsewhere in the body. The owners declined further treatment, and the dog was euthanized. At necropsy, two small masses were noted in the brain, and several subdural spinal lesions were found (arrow in *A*). Histological evaluation was most compatible with a choroid plexus tumor. Tumors were not identified elsewhere in the body. A diagnosis of choroid plexus carcinoma, with spinal metastasis, was made. (Bar = 0.3 cm in *A* and 25 μm in *B;* H & E stain in *B*.)

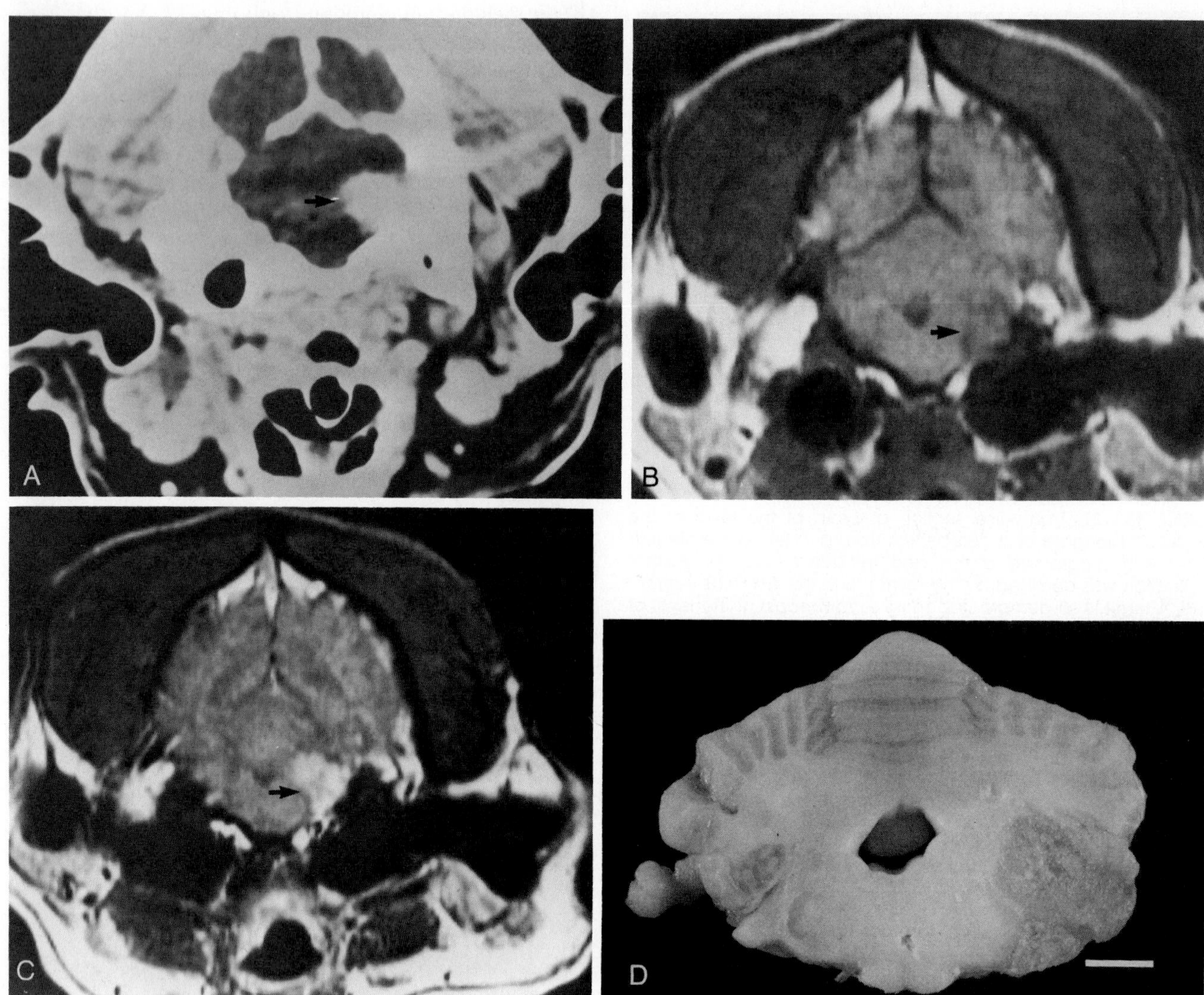

FIGURE 157–29. Iodine-enhanced transverse computed tomography image *(A)* and magnetic resonance images before *(B)* and after *(C)* gadolinium-DTPA administration in a 13-year-old male Old English sheepdog with head tilt to the right and ataxia. A mass, later shown to be a choroid plexus papilloma *(D)*, is seen to the right of the medulla oblongata in *A–D (arrows)*. Anatomical detail is better in the magnetic resonance images, with tumor differentiation being best after gadolinium-DTPA. (Bar in *D* = 0.5 cm.) (Courtesy of Duke University Medical Center. From Kornegay JN: Central nervous system neoplasia. *In* Kornegay JN [ed]: *Neurologic Disorders.* Vol 5. *Contemporary Issues in Small Animal Practice.* Churchill Livingstone, New York, 1986, pp 79–108.)

Diagnosis

On CT, oligodendrogliomas vary from hypodense to hyperdense on noncontrast scans and have minimal to marked contrast enhancement (Fig. 157–31*A*).[79, 174] On immunocytochemical staining, these tumors are typically GFAP and myelin basic protein (MBP) negative.[179] Initially, the negative MBP staining was surprising; however, the degree of cellular differentiation necessary for MBP expression may not be achieved by malignant oligodendrocytes. Similarly, although myelin-associated glycoprotein is a marker of undifferentiated oligodendrocytes in tissue culture, only 3 of 11 oligodendrogliomas expressed this marker in one study.[179]

Treatment

Treatment of oligodendrogliomas has not been described in dogs and cats. Benign cerebrocortical tumors conceivably can be resected. Radiation and chemotherapy may be beneficial.

Pituitary Gland Tumors

Incidence and Classification

Pituitary gland tumors occur relatively frequently in dogs but are rare in cats. Micro- and macroadenomas and adenocarcinomas occur (see Fig. 157–2).[36, 37, 148] Pituitary gland tumors in humans grow in an inferior direction because a complete dural adhesion encircling the pituitary stalk impedes superior growth.[39] The dural adhesion overlying the pars nervosa in dogs is also complete. Because most canine pituitary gland tumors involve the pars distalis of the adenohypophysis, dorsal growth is favored and diencephalic encroachment and hypothalamic dysfunction result.[36, 37, 39, 132, 148] These tumors can also extend dorsally and laterally along the

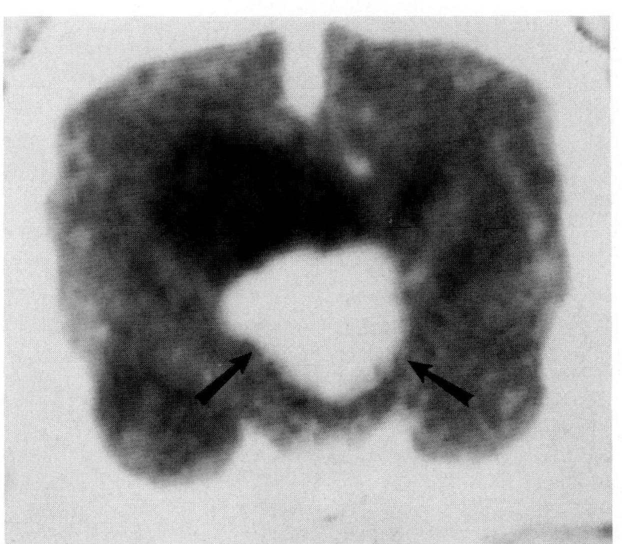

FIGURE 157–30. Iodine-enhanced transverse computed tomography image from a 14-year-old female mixed-breed dog with a 4-week history of altered attitude, left-sided circling, and right hemiparesis. A homogeneously enhancing mass *(arrows)* is seen in the area of the third ventricle. There is marked dilation of the left lateral ventricle, presumably due to obstruction of the interventricular foramen on that side. The tumor, shown histologically to be a choroid plexus papilloma, was partially resected by approaching through the dilated left lateral ventricle; however, the dog died the day after surgery. (Courtesy of Duke University Medical Center. From Kornegay JN: Imaging brain neoplasia. Computed tomography and magnetic resonance imaging. *Vet Med Rep* 2:372, 1990.)

base of the brain, leading to additional features of brain stem involvement.

Clinical Features

The mean time from diagnosis of pituitary-dependent hyperadrenocorticism to occurrence of neurological signs in eight dogs in one study was 12.8 months.[148] Affected dogs generally deteriorated rapidly once neurological signs were observed. Systemic signs of hyperadrenocorticism may also occur.

Diagnosis

On noncontrast CT scans, most pituitary gland tumors are isodense but some are hyperdense.[79, 174] Tumors usually enhance uniformly (Fig. 157–32). Occasional tumors cannot be seen on either noncontrast or contrast scans. Hydrocephalus was observed in half of the cases in one study[174] but is rare in our experience.[79]

Hyperadrenocorticism may result from excess adrenocorticotropic hormone (ACTH) production.[36, 37, 148] In five of eight cases of large pituitary tumors in dogs, high-dose dexamethasone did not decrease serum cortisol concentrations to a degree necessary to diagnose pituitary-dependent hyperadrenocorticism.[148] The pituitary origin of these tumors was confirmed by evaluating ACTH levels.

Treatment

Treatment of human patients has included surgical resection and radiation. There was no difference in survival rate in patients managed by concomitant surgery and radiation and those receiving radiation alone in one study.[54] Trans-sphenoidal surgical approaches to the pituitary gland have been described in dogs.[66, 87] Because many tumors affecting dogs are relatively large macroadenomas and carcinomas, this surgical approach is unlikely to allow exposure necessary for complete resection.[36] Irradiation is the most effective treatment for large pituitary gland tumors (see Fig. 157–17).[35, 36] The mean and median survival time after radiation in one study of six affected dogs was 740 and 743 days, respectively.[37] Secretion of ACTH by the tumor may not

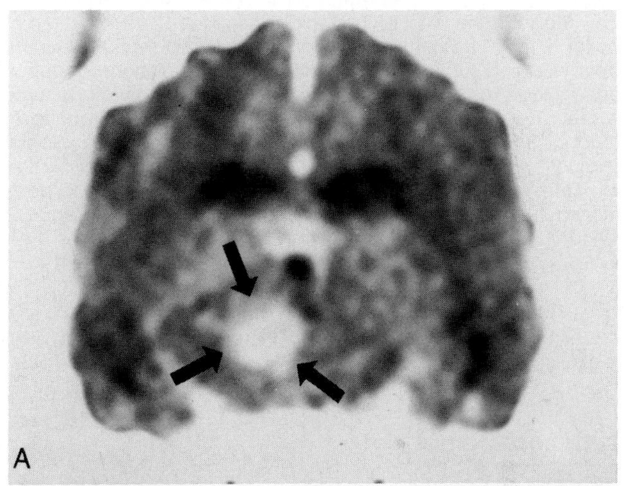

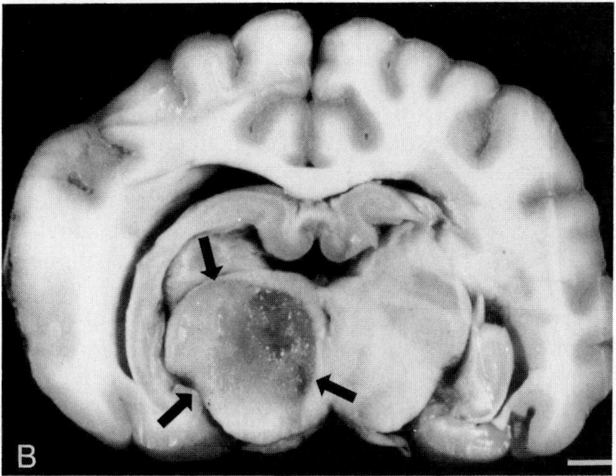

FIGURE 157–31. Iodine-enhanced transverse computed tomography image *(A)* and pathological specimen *(B)*, both at the level of the thalamus, from an 8-year-old male German shepherd with a 4-week history of progressive signs of left forebrain dysfunction. A homogeneously enhancing intra-axial mass *(arrows)* is seen in the left thalamus in *A*. A glioma was suspected; irradiation was offered but declined by the owner. The dog was euthanized. A somewhat gelatinous mass, corresponding to the lesion seen on computed tomography, is seen in *B (arrows)*. On histological evaluation, the tumor had features of an oligodendroglioma. (Bar = 0.5 cm in *B*.) (Computed tomography image courtesy of Duke University Medical Center.)

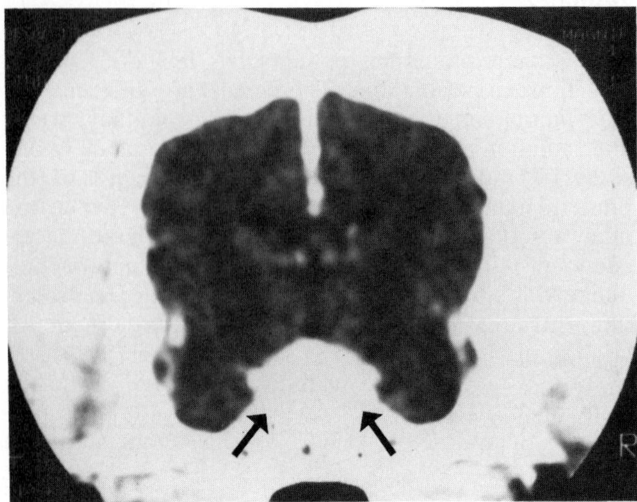

FIGURE 157–32. Iodine-enhanced transverse computed tomography image at the level of the thalamus from a 12-year-old female boxer with a 1-month course of polydipsia/polyuria, abnormal behavior, and subtle neurological dysfunction. A homogeneously enhancing mass *(arrows)*, suspected to be a pituitary gland tumor, is seen. Treatment was declined, and the dog was euthanized. A diagnosis of pituitary adenoma was made on histopathological evaluation at necropsy. (Courtesy of Duke University Medical Center. From Kornegay JN: Imaging brain neoplasia. Computed tomography and magnetic resonance imaging. *Vet Med Rep 2*:372, 1990.)

decrease for 6 to 12 months, so medication to normalize cortisol levels may be necessary initially.[37]

Lymphosarcoma

Incidence and Classification

Lymphosarcoma affects the nervous system in both dogs (Fig. 157–33) and cats (Fig. 157–34). Both primary and secondary involvement occur. In two series of dogs, spinal cord and peripheral and cranial nerve involvement were most common.[26, 139] Systemic disease generally is present; however, the nervous system may be affected exclusively.[27] Strict meningeal involvement may also occur.[15] Concomitant CNS and cutaneous lymphosarcoma have been noted.[31]

Neoplastic reticulosis of the CNS is a form of primary lymphoreticular disease (Fig. 157–35). Criteria have been established to define differences between inflammatory and neoplastic diseases in this group; mixed lesions exist.[41, 75] Some lesions previously classified as inflammatory have been reclassified as B-cell lymphomas after immunocytochemical evaluation.[180] Focal neoplastic lesions occur in some dogs; additional, at times subclinical, foci are frequently found elsewhere in the CNS.

Lymphosarcoma in cats most commonly affects the epidural space of the vertebral canal (see Fig. 157–34).[25, 85, 195] Most tumors are solitary, but multiple sites may be involved. Many cats with renal lymphosarcoma have CNS involvement.[106] Differences in CNS versus systemic immunity may increase CNS susceptibility to metastasis from extraneural sites.

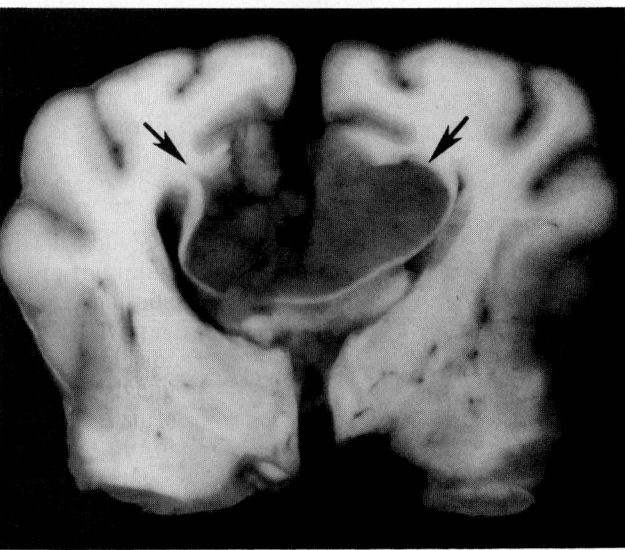

FIGURE 157–33. Transverse section of brain at the level of the thalamus from a 6-year-old male Scottish terrier with progressive neurological dysfunction, including seizures. The dog died acutely before it could be evaluated critically. A large, roughly round mass *(arrows)* involves the corpus callosum and cingulate gyri bilaterally. The tumor had histological features of lymphoma.

Clinical Features

Lymphosarcoma typically causes progressive neurological dysfunction. Acute deterioration, presumably associated with hemorrhage, occurs in some cases, particularly with cervical lesions in cats.[85] Most dogs with neural lymphosarcoma have additional systemic involvement. Although this may be true of affected cats, only 11 of 24 cats with spinal lymphosarcoma had extraneural organ involvement.[85]

Diagnosis

Leukemia may be evident on evaluation of peripheral blood in both dogs and cats. Cats without leukemia may still have bone marrow involvement, so examination of

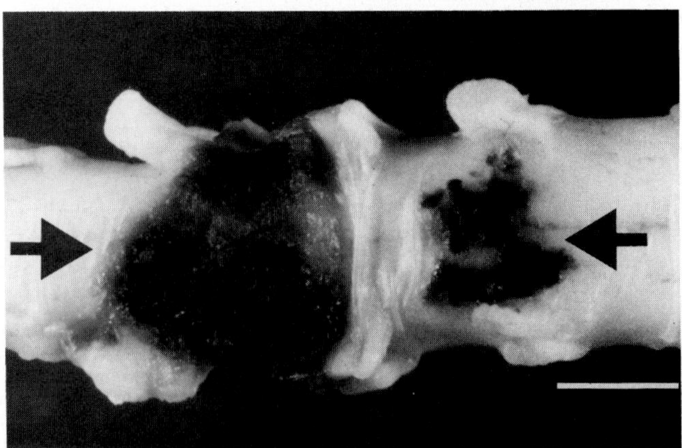

FIGURE 157–34. Ventral view of the spinal cord from a 1-year-old female domestic cat with progressive tetraparesis. The cat was euthanized without benefit of definitive diagnostic procedures. Neoplastic tissue identified as lymphosarcoma on microscopic examination is seen *(arrows)*. (Bar = 0.5 cm.)

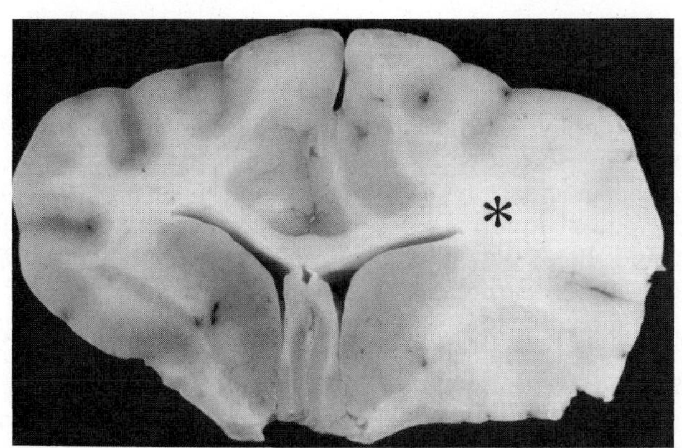

FIGURE 157–35. Transverse section of brain from a 3-year-old female pug with progressive signs of forebrain disease. The right corona radiata *(asterisk)* is expanded and poorly distinguished from the overlying cerebral cortex. On microscopic examination, a marked mixed population of mononuclear cells was seen. The lesion was believed to be most compatible with neoplastic reticulosis or granulomatous meningoencephalomyelitis. Because of the breed, consideration must also be given to the syndrome of "pug encephalitis."

an aspirate is indicated.[25] Survey radiographs generally are normal in animals with spinal cord lesions, because bone involvement is unusual. On myelographic evaluation, an extradural pattern is most common in dogs and cats (Fig. 157–36). Extension to the spinal cord can result in an intramedullary pattern. Most affected cats are positive for feline leukemia virus.[85] Neoplastic cells can be seen on CSF evaluation.[26, 85] Brain lesions are identified with CT. Biopsy may be necessary for diagnosis.

Treatment

Treatment of lymphosarcoma may include surgery, systemic and intrathecal chemotherapy, radiation, or combinations of these. Rapid reduction of tumor mass occurs within hours of delivering a single large dose of radiation (500 to 1000 cGy) in extraneural lymphosarcoma in cats.[100] Two dogs with spinal lymphosarcoma that improved after craniospinal radiation and chemotherapy subsequently died.[26] One dog had a seizure and died 84 days after onset of therapy; the other dog developed leukopenia/thrombocytopenia and disseminated intravascular coagulopathy within several days. Human patients with cerebral involvement routinely are irradiated, irrespective of surgical intervention[67]; surgery alone does not improve the prognosis in humans with neural lymphosarcoma.[113, 130] Laminectomy or craniotomy may be necessary to confirm the diagnosis in advance of chemotherapy and radiation.

Various chemotherapeutic protocols have been used to treat animals with lymphosarcoma. Few data are available on those with neural involvement. Some affected dogs have received concomitant irradiation and chemotherapy, as described earlier.[26] Neurological deficits in one dog in this same study resolved for at least 3 months after chemotherapy alone. A dog with spinal lymphosarcoma lived for 13 months after initial laminectomy and chemotherapy.[77] Cytosine arabinoside has been incorporated into some lymphosarcoma protocols to decrease the incidence of CNS metastasis.[26]

Glucocorticoid treatment may improve some animals with neoplastic reticulosis.[144] Subsequent deterioration is common. Radiation has led to improvement in a few patients.[156] Chemotherapy also may be beneficial.

Nerve Sheath Tumors

Incidence and Classification

The term *nerve sheath tumor* refers collectively to schwannoma, neurofibroma, neurilemmoma, neurinoma, and neurofibrosarcoma.[11] The Schwann cell is the predominant cell of origin for both neurofibroma and schwannoma.[48, 56] These tumors occur relatively commonly in dogs but are rare in cats. Cervical nerve roots are usually affected in dogs (Fig. 157–37).

Clinical Features

Clinical signs vary with the nerve roots affected but often include thoracic limb muscle atrophy (see Fig.

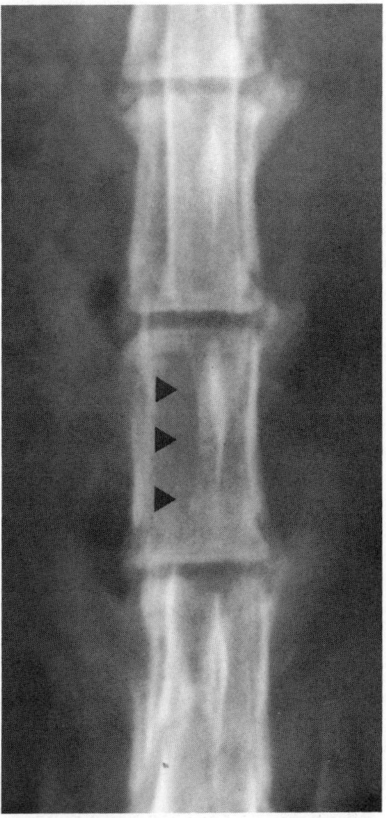

FIGURE 157–36. Ventrodorsal myelogram from a 6-month-old female domestic cat with progressive paraplegia and a cranial mediastinal mass. The contrast medium is displaced from right to left *(arrowheads)* over the bodies of L2–L4. The cat was positive for feline leukemia virus, and multifocal lymphosarcoma was suspected. Combined chemotherapy and radiation were administered, and clinical improvement was noted. The cat died 5 months later. A necropsy was not performed. (From Kornegay JN: *Feline Neurology, Problems in Veterinary Medicine.* J.B. Lippincott, Philadelphia, 1991, p 367.)

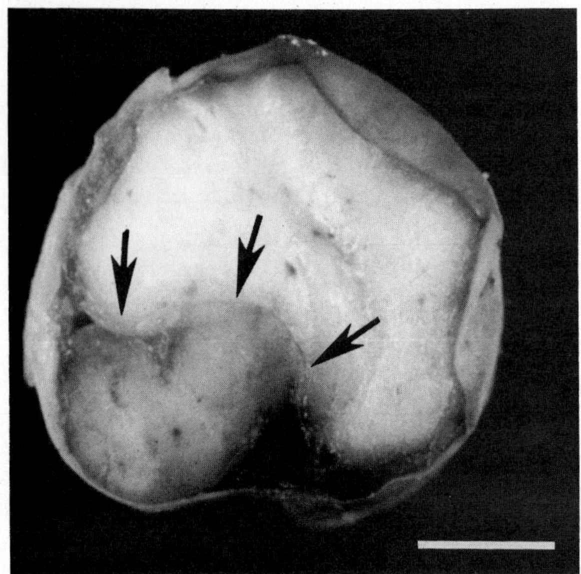

FIGURE 157–37. Transverse section of cervical spinal cord from a 9-year-old male Labrador retriever with progressive paraparesis and eventual cervical hyperesthesia. A compressive lesion was identified with myelography at C5–C6, and a laminectomy was performed. The dog was euthanized when tumor extending to the subarachnoid space was noted. A distinct, roughly round mass is seen within the subarachnoid space ventrolateral to the C6 spinal cord segment on the left side *(arrows)*. Schwannoma was diagnosed on histological evaluation. (Bar = 0.3 cm.)

157–7), lameness, ipsilateral Horner's syndrome, hyperesthesia, and licking or chewing at the foot or carpus. Extension to the spinal cord can lead to additional involvement of the other thoracic limb and paraparesis.[11] Tumors usually originate in the dorsal nerve root, causing pain initially and spinal cord compression later.[11] An axillary mass can be palpated in some animals.[11, 164, 188] Many of these animals have a long history of an undiagnosed lameness of the affected forelimb.

Diagnosis

Diagnosis of peripheral tumors may be difficult unless a palpable mass is present. Electromyographic evidence of denervation aids in defining the underlying neural nature of the lesion. Intervertebral foramina may be enlarged on survey radiographs because of expansion of the tumor or the pulsation of the tumor vasculature (see Fig. 157–10).[11] Regardless of whether clinical signs of spinal cord involvement are present, myelography should always be performed to identify potential intradural tumor extension. An intradural-extramedullary pattern is seen (see Fig. 157–10). Parenchymal extension is more common in the thoracolumbar area.[11] CT allows more precise characterization of lesions (Fig. 157–38).

Treatment

Treatment has centered on surgical resection or debulking of nerve root tumors. Both peripheral and spinal components must be removed. If an intradural-extramedullary tumor is diagnosed, laminectomy, durotomy, and tumor removal are indicated. Nerve roots are explored to the limits of the incision in these cases to determine if the tumor has originated or extended peripherally. Peripheral tumor generally cannot be completely resected with a laminectomy alone. Exploration of the brachial plexus allows definition of the extent of peripheral involvement.[74, 153] Surgical resection usually cannot be achieved without causing severe denervation; amputation is often necessary.

The sequence of operations is reversed in dogs that do not have clinical or myelographic evidence of spinal cord compression. Exploration of the brachial plexus is initially indicated. Affected nerves are firm and discolored on gross evaluation (Fig. 157–39).[11, 164] Some peripheral tumors can be resected; amputation is generally indicated. The proximal extent of the tumor is determined at amputation. Tumor extending proximally often cannot be resected using this surgical approach, and a laminectomy is required. Despite aggressive staged management, the prognosis is poor for most affected dogs. Tumor extends to the thoracic sympathetic chain in some cases, and the risk of spinal recurrence is great. Most dogs deteriorate again within 6 months of surgery. Limited experience with postoperative radiation has not been promising.

Germ Cell Tumors

Germ cell tumors are infrequent in animals.[24, 169, 176] Doberman pinschers are particularly susceptible.[176] Most tumors occur in the rostrosellar area, leading to visual and pupillary abnormalities. Similar tumors in humans are radiosensitive.[44]

Medulloblastoma

Medulloblastoma is a tumor that classically affects the cerebellum of children. Young dogs and cats also are occasionally affected by this tumor (see Fig. 157–1).[95] Of 341 glial canine brain tumors, 20 were medulloblastomas.[178] Only 2 medulloblastomas were included in another series of 215 canine gliomas.[103] This tumor is even more rare in cats. No medulloblastomas were reported in a series of 87 CNS tumors identified in 75 cats in one study.[195] Individual cases have been reported.[2, 42, 95, 166] The cerebellum is typically involved in both dogs and cats. In all domestic animal species thus far studied, these tumors grow rapidly and can metastasize to the meninges via the CSF.[95] Compression of the fourth ventricle can lead to hydrocephalus in affected animals, leading to additional signs of forebrain disease. Treatment of affected animals has not been described. Combinations of surgery, radiation, and chemotherapy are generally used in affected children, at times leading to decreased learning ability.[38]

Vascular Tumors and Malformations

Vascular tumors and malformations occur in both the spinal cord and brain in animals.[23, 167, 190] Cerebral angioendotheliomatosis is a rare form of lymphoma in humans.[67] Proliferating tumor cells enter arteries, cap-

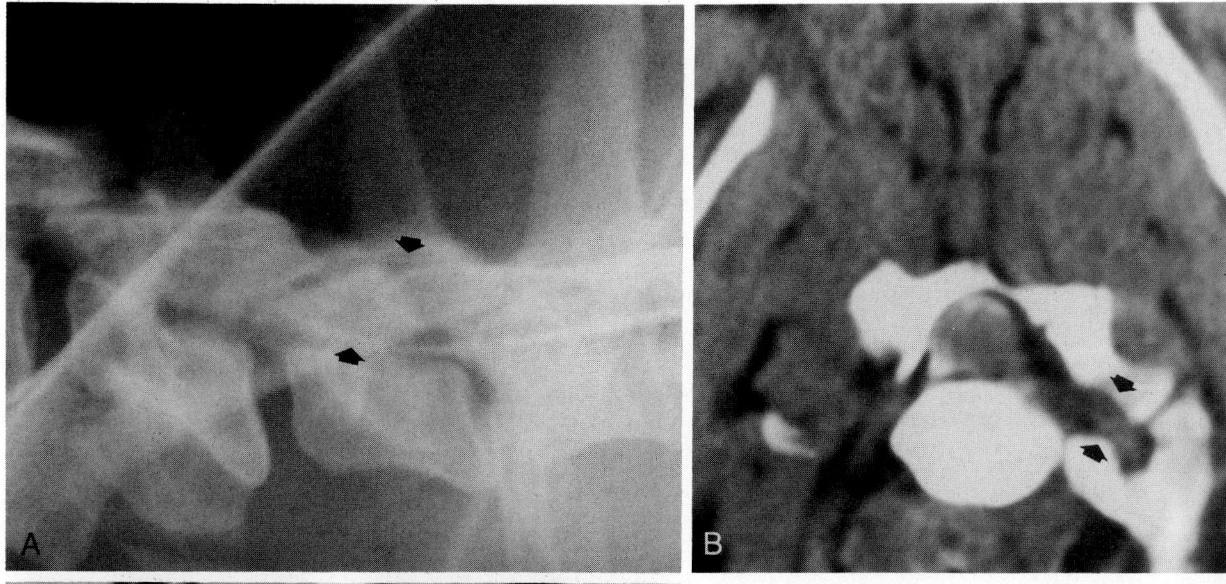

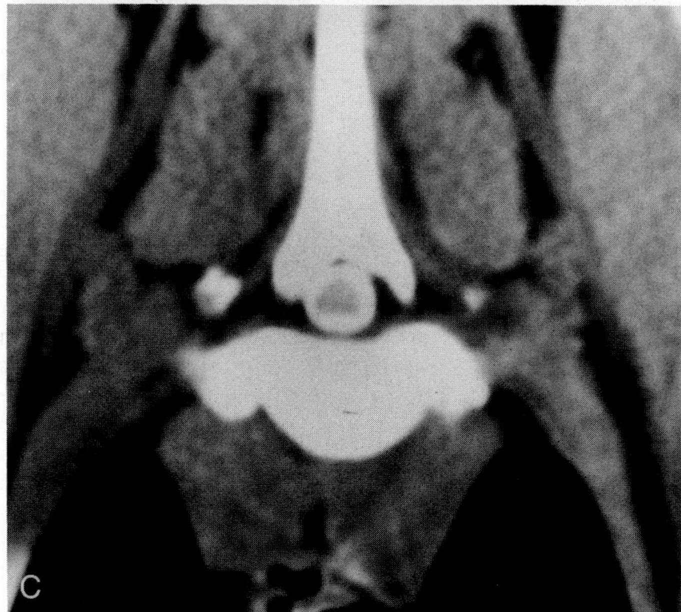

FIGURE 157–38. Lateral myelogram *(A)* and transverse computed tomography images *(B, C)* made approximately 12 hours after the myelogram from an 11-year-old male Labrador retriever with initial right thoracic limb lameness and subsequent tetraparesis. The myelogram was performed by lumbar injection. Both the ventral and dorsal contrast columns *(arrows)* are attenuated at the level of C7 in *A*. A similar but more poorly defined pattern was seen on the ventrodorsal view. The computed tomography image in *B* was obtained near the level of the C7–T1 interspace. The image is slightly tangential, with the first rib being seen only on the right side. However, when compared with the image obtained caudad to the point of compression at T3 in *C*, the contrast medium is attenuated and has been displaced and the intervertebral foramen on the right side *(arrows)* appears enlarged. A nerve sheath tumor involving the C8 nerve root on the right side was suspected and confirmed at surgery. The dog initially improved; however, recurrence of signs 4 months later necessitated euthanasia. Necropsy was not performed. (Computed tomography images courtesy of Duke University Medical Center.)

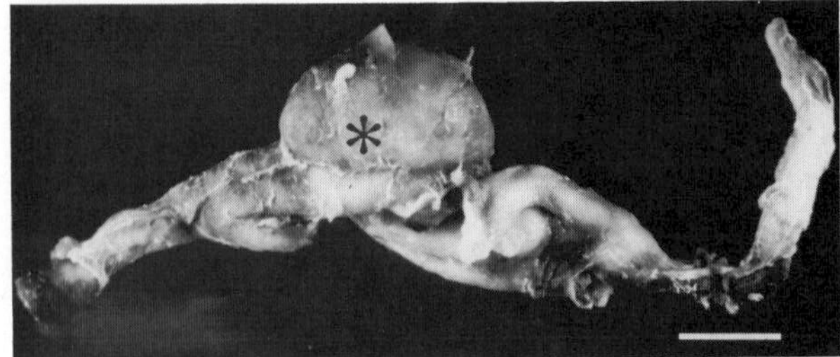

FIGURE 157–39. Resected neural tissue from the right thoracic limb of the dog illustrated in Figure 157–7. This dog had progressive monoparesis and neoplastic involvement of multiple nerves of the brachial plexus. The nerve shown here is enlarged and contains a bulbous expansion *(asterisk)*. A histological diagnosis of malignant schwannoma was made. (Bar = 1 cm.)

illaries, and venules in single or many organs.[167] A single case of cerebral angioendotheliomatosis was reported in a 6-year-old male Doberman pinscher.[167] The blood vessels of the brain were filled with small mononuclear tumor cells. No tumor invasion of the neuropil was noted. Clinical signs may relate, at least partially, to poor cerebrovascular perfusion.[167]

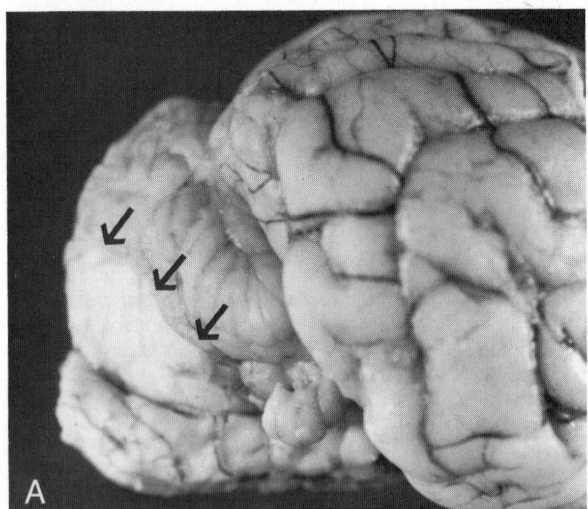

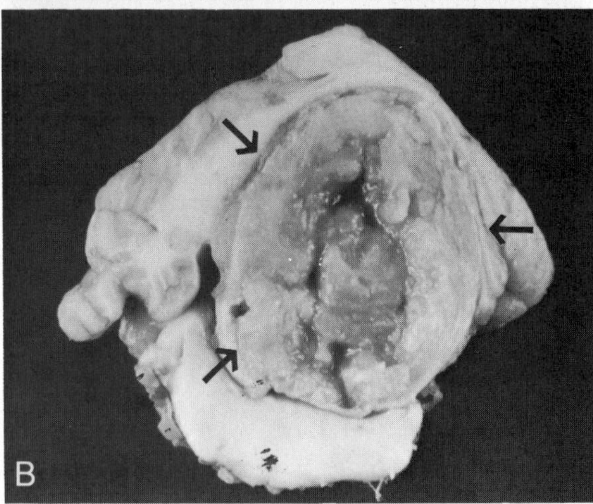

FIGURE 157–40. Lateral *(A)* and transverse *(B)* sections of brain from a 2-year-old male English setter with acute onset of signs of right-sided central vestibular disease. A well-circumscribed mass is seen at the caudoventral aspect of the cerebellum in *A* and dorsal to the brain stem in *B* (*arrows* in each). This mass contained keratin and was lined by squamous epithelium on microscopic examination. A diagnosis of intracranial epidermoid cyst was made. (From Kornegay JN, Gorgacz EJ: Intracranial epidermoid cysts in three dogs. *Vet Pathol 19*:646, 1982.)

Epidermoid Cysts

Epidermoid and dermoid cysts afflict the brain or spinal cord.[68, 80, 173] These cysts occur because of entrapment and subsequent growth of primordial epithelial cells during closure of the neural tube.[143] Most tumors in dogs have occurred in the fourth ventricle (Fig. 157–40).[80] Mechanical implantation of epidermal cells after trauma has resulted in morphologically similar cysts in humans.[10, 21, 158] Treatment of affected dogs has not been described.

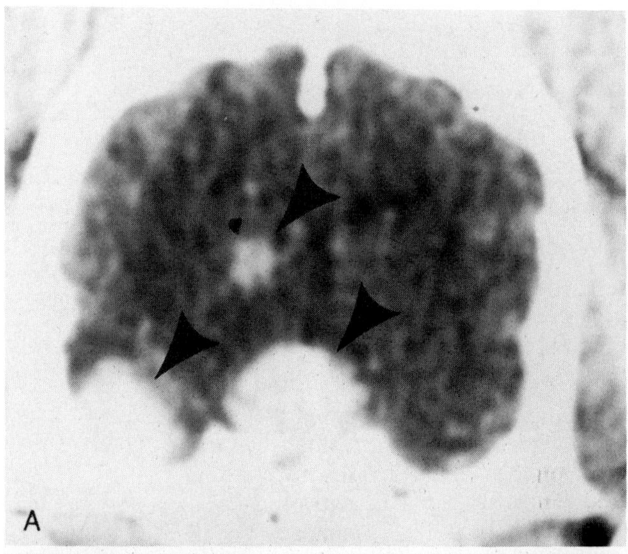

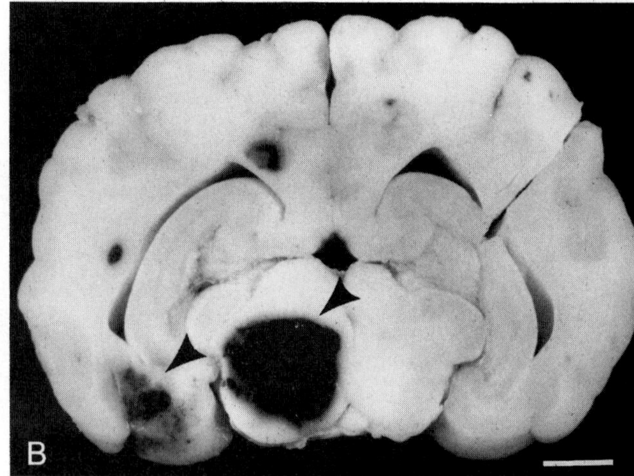

FIGURE 157–41. Iodine-enhanced transverse computed tomography image *(A)* and pathological section at a similar level *(B)* from a 9-year-old male Staffordshire terrier with progressive neurological dysfunction referable principally to the brain stem. Multiple enhancing lesions *(arrowheads)* thought to most likely represent metastatic neoplasia are noted in the computed tomography image. On evaluation of computed tomography of the abdomen, additional hepatic involvement was noted, and the dog was euthanized. Tumors corresponding to the principal two lesions seen in *A* are noted in the pathological section in *B (arrowheads)*. A histological diagnosis of widely metastatic hemangiosarcoma was made on evaluation at necropsy. (Computed tomography image courtesy of Duke University Medical Center.) (Bar in *B* = 0.7 cm.)

Neuroepithelioma

Neuroepitheliomas typically affect the spinal cord at T10–L2 in young dogs.[6, 30, 168] Some have referred to this tumor as *medulloepithelioma.*[97] Some spinal tumors previously classified as ependymomas may actually be neuroepitheliomas.[30, 168] German shepherds may be overrepresented. The origin of the tumor is unknown. Immunocytochemical studies do not support a neuroectodermal origin,[6, 168] and several investigators have suggested that this tumor is a form of nephroblastoma.[6, 14, 168] One tumor, referred to as a *teratomatous medulloepithelioma,* contained foci of hyaline cartilage and cysts lined by stratified squamous epithelium.[9] Surgery is helpful if performed early before irreversible damage to the spinal cord has occurred.[30] Metastasis has not been observed.[168]

Metastatic Disease

Many tumors metastasize to the CNS. In some cases, neurological signs may precede those associated with the primary tumor.[163] Hemangiosarcoma (Fig. 157–41), carcinomas, and melanoma metastasize most commonly. Twelve of 85 dogs with hemangiosarcoma had brain metastasis in one study.[183] A higher incidence of brain metastasis was associated with radiographic evidence of pulmonary involvement. The CNS is particularly susceptible to spread of systemic lymphosarcoma.[26, 106]

Hemangiosarcoma is the principal metastatic tumor affecting the spinal cord.[194] Most spinal cord metastases are extradural, but intramedullary lesions are encountered (Fig. 157–42). In a small series of human patients with spinal cord metastases, intramedullary tumors were associated neither with extradural foci nor with spread into the subarachnoid space.[71] This observation suggested that these tumors reached the cord hematogenously rather than by either direct extension or perineural spread.

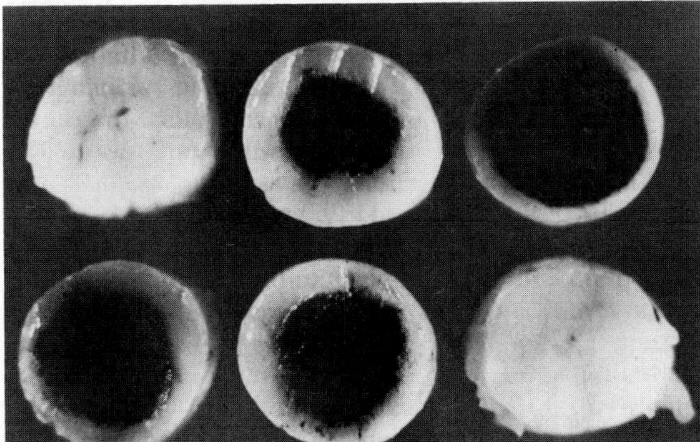

FIGURE 157–42. Transverse serial sections of thoracic spinal cord from a 10-year-old male mixed-breed dog with progressive paraparesis and eventual paraplegia. Findings on myelography were normal. A small dermal mass on the dorsum of the thorax was removed and interpreted as a malignant melanoma on microscopic examination. Spinal metastasis was considered possible, and the dog was euthanized. No obvious gross connection was found between the area of the resected dermal mass and the spinal cord. Spinal cord sections illustrated were taken from the caudal thoracic area and extend from cranial *(upper left)* to caudal *(lower right).* The spinal cord is largely effaced by a round black mass that had histological features of malignant melanoma.

Systemic Manifestations of Central Nervous System Neoplasia

The nervous system has an integral role in the control of many body functions. Neoplastic involvement thus can alter the normal homeostatic environment of the host and create systemic signs alone or in addition to neurological dysfunction. An astrocytoma involving the diencephalon in a dog resulted in weight loss and behavioral abnormalities similar to diencephalic syndrome in humans.[117] Weight loss and emaciation, despite a normal appetite, were related to abnormal concentrations of growth hormone or fat-mobilizing substance. Hypothalamic involvement can also decrease thirst, leading to hypernatremia. Bradycardia in one patient with meningioma may have occurred because of increased intracranial pressure and an associated Cushing effect or because of effects on sympathetic pathways.[51]

A craniopharyngioma was associated with hypothyroidism and diabetes insipidus in a dog.[115] These tumors commonly involve the pituitary/hypothalamic region, accounting for the constellation of associated metabolic defects. Adiposogenital syndrome due to hypothalamic involvement was reported in another dog with this tumor type.[149] Certain other derangements that occur secondary to human nervous system neoplasia have not been recognized in dogs and cats.[1, 138]

References

1. Adams RD, Victor M: Intracranial neoplasms. *In Principles of Neurology.* 4th ed. McGraw-Hill, New York, 1989, p 516.
2. Averill DR: Tumors of the nervous system. *In* Holzworth J (ed): *Diseases of the Cat.* W.B. Saunders, Philadelphia, 1987, p 554.
3. Bailey CS, Higgins RJ: Characteristics of cisternal cerebrospinal fluid associated with primary brain tumors in the dog: A retrospective study. *J Am Vet Med Assoc 188*:414, 1986.
4. Barbaro NM, et al: Radiation therapy in the treatment of partially resected meningiomas. *Neurosurgery 20*:525, 1987.
5. Bartels JE, et al: Neuroradiology. *In* Horlein BF (ed): *Canine Neurology.* 3rd ed. W.B. Saunders, Philadelphia, 1978, p 103.
6. Baumgartner W, Peixoto PV: Canine neuroepitheliomas, a rare spinal cord tumour in young dogs. Report of three cases. Proceedings of the European Society of Veterinary Neurology Meeting, Paris, Oct. 1987.
7. Bellur SN, et al: Association of meningiomas with extraneural primary malignancy. *Neurology 29*:1165, 1979.
8. Bichsel P, et al: Immunoelectrophoretic determination of albumin and IgG in serum and cerebrospinal fluid in dogs with neurological diseases. *Res Vet Sci 37*:101, 1984.
9. Blass CE, et al: Teratomatous medulloepithelioma in the spinal cord of a dog. *J Am Anim Hosp Assoc 24*:51, 1988.
10. Blockey NJ, Schorstein J: Intraspinal epidermoid tumors in the lumbar region of children. *J Bone Joint Surg [Am] 43*:556, 1961.
11. Bradley RL, et al: Nerve sheath tumors in the dog. *J Am Anim Hosp Assoc 18*:915, 1982.
12. Brant-Zawadzki M, et al: Primary intracranial tumor imaging: A comparison of magnetic resonance and CT. *Radiology 150*:435, 1984.
13. Braund KG: Central nervous system meningiomas. *Comp Cont Educ Vet Pract 8*:241, 1986.
14. Bridges CH, et al: Spinal cord nephroblastoma in a dog. *Proc Am Coll Vet Pathol 35*:97, 1984.
15. Britt JO, et al: Malignant lymphoma of the meninges in two dogs. *J Comp Pathol 94*:45, 1984.
16. Burger PC: Malignant astrocytic neoplasms: Classification, pathologic anatomy, and response to treatment. *Semin Oncol 13*:16, 1986.
17. Carpenter JL, et al: Bilateral trigeminal nerve paralysis and Horner's syndrome associated with myelomonocytic neoplasia in a dog. *J Am Vet Med Assoc 191*:1594, 1987.

18. Carrillo JM, et al: Intracranial neoplasm and associated inflammatory response from the central nervous system. *J Am Anim Hosp Assoc 22*:367, 1986.
19. Cello RM, Olander H: Cord compression and paraplegia in a dog secondary to pancreatic carcinoma. *J Am Vet Med Assoc 142*:1407, 1963.
20. Cho DY, et al: Adenocarcinoma in the duodenum and vertebrae in a dog. *J Am Vet Med Assoc 169*:317, 1976.
21. Choremis C, et al: Intraspinal epidermoid tumors (cholesteatomata) in patients treated for tuberculous meningitis. *Lancet 2*:437, 1956.
22. Chrisman CL: Electromyography in the localization of spinal cord and nerve root neoplasia in dogs and cats. *J Am Vet Med Assoc 166*:1074, 1975.
23. Cordy DR: Vascular malformations and hemangiomas of the canine spinal cord. *Vet Pathol 16*:275, 1979.
24. Cordy DR: Intracranial germinoma in a dog. *Vet Pathol 21*:357, 1984.
25. Cotter SM: Feline leukemia virus induced disorders in the cat. *Vet Clin North Am 6*:367, 1976.
26. Couto CG, et al: Central nervous system lymphosarcoma in the dog. *J Am Vet Med Assoc 184*:809, 1984.
27. Dallman MJ, Saunders GK: Primary spinal cord lymphosarcoma in a dog. *J Am Vet Med Assoc 189*:1348, 1986.
28. Davidson MG, et al: Acute blindness associated with intracranial tumors. *J Am Vet Med Assoc 199*:155, 1991.
29. DeAngelis LM, et al: Radiation-induced dementia in patients cured of brain metastases. *Neurology 39*:789, 1989.
30. de Lahunta A: *Veterinary Neuroanatomy and Clinical Neurology*. W.B. Saunders, Philadelphia, 1983.
31. Dennis JS, Schmidt DA: Cutaneous and central nervous system lymphoma in a dog. *J Am Anim Hosp Assoc 23*:31, 1987.
32. De Wet PD, et al: Surgical approach to the rostral cranial fossa by radical transfrontal craniotomy in the dog. *J South African Vet Assoc 53*:40, 1982.
33. Dewey WC, Freeman ML: Rationale for use of hyperthermia in cancer therapy. *Ann NY Acad Sci 335*:372, 1980.
34. Dimski DS, Cook JR: Carmustine-induced partial remission of an astrocytoma in a dog. *J Am Anim Hosp Assoc 26*:179, 1990.
35. Dorn AS: A standard technique for canine cerebral angiography. *J Am Vet Med Assoc 161*:1669, 1972.
36. Dow SW, LeCouteur RA: Radiation therapy for canine ACTH-secreting pituitary tumors. *In* Kirk RW (ed): *Current Veterinary Therapy X*. W.B. Saunders, Philadelphia, 1989, p 1031.
37. Dow SW, et al: Response of dogs with functional pituitary macroadenomas and macrocarcinomas to radiation. *J Small Anim Pract 31*:287, 1990.
38. Duffner PK, et al: Late effects of treatment on the intelligence of children with posterior fossa tumors. *Cancer 51*:233, 1983.
39. Eigenmann JE, Lubberink AAME: *In* Slatter DH (ed): *Textbook of Small Animal Surgery*. Vol II. W.B. Saunders, Philadelphia, 1985, p 1840.
40. Engle GC, Brodey RS: A retrospective study of 395 feline neoplasms. *J Am Anim Hosp Assoc 5*:21, 1969.
41. Fankhauser R, et al: Reticulosis of the central nervous system (CNS) in dogs. *In* Brandly CA, Cornelius CE (eds): *Advances in Veterinary Science and Comparative Medicine*. Vol 16. Academic Press, New York, 1972, p 35.
42. Fankhauser R, et al: Tumours of the nervous system. *Bull WHO 50*:53, 1974.
43. Felix R, et al: Brain tumors: MR imaging with gadolinium-DTPA. *Radiology 156*:681, 1985.
44. Fields JN, et al: Suprasellar germinomas: Radiation therapy. *Radiology 164*:247, 1987.
45. Fike JR, et al: Computed tomography analysis of the canine brain: Effects of hemibrain X irradiation. *Radiation Res 99*:294, 1984.
46. Fingeroth JM, et al: Spinal meningiomas in dogs: 13 cases (1972–1987). *J Am Vet Med Assoc 191*:720, 1987.
47. Fischer-Williams M: Brain tumors and other space occupying lesions (with a section on oncological CNS complications). *In* Niedermeyer E, da Silva FL (eds): *Electroencephalography*. Urban and Schwarzenberg, Baltimore, 1982, p 197.
48. Fisher ER, Vuzevski VD: Cytogenesis of schwannoma (neurilemmoma), neurofibroma, dermatofibroma, and dermatofibrosarcoma as revealed by electron microscopy. *Am J Clin Pathol 49*:2, 1968.
49. Fishman RA: Cerebrospinal fluid in diseases of the nervous system. W.B. Saunders, Philadelphia, 1980, p 288.
50. Foster ES, et al: Clinical signs of tumors affecting the rostral cerebrum in 43 dogs. *J Vet Intern Med 2*:71, 1988.
51. Freeman KP, et al: Bradycardia associated with meningioma in a dog. *J Am Vet Med Assoc 187*:838, 1985.
52. Geib LW: Ossifying meningioma with extracranial metastasis in a dog. *Pathol Vet 3*:247, 1966.
53. Gilmore DR: Intraspinal tumors in the dog. *Comp Cont Educ 5*:55, 1983.
54. Grigsby PW, et al: Results of surgery and irradiation or irradiation alone for pituitary adenomas. *J Neurooncol 6*:129, 1988.
55. Gutin PH, et al: Brachytherapy of recurrent malignant brain tumors with removable high-activity iodine-125 sources. *J Neurosurg 60*:61, 1984.
56. Harkin JC, Reed RJ: Tumors of the peripheral nervous system. *Atlas of Tumor Pathology*. 2nd Series, Fascicle 3, Armed Forces Institute of Pathology, Washington, D.C., 1968.
57. Harvey HJ,: Neurotoxicosis associated with the use of 5-fluorouracil in five dogs and one cat. *J Am Vet Med Assoc 177*:277, 1977.
58. Haskins ME, McGrath JT: Meningiomas in young cats with mucopolysaccharidosis I. *J Neuropathol Exp Neurol 42*:664, 1983.
59. Hatam A, et al: Effect of dexamethasone treatment on the volume and contrast enhancement of intracranial neoplasms. *J Comput Assist Tomogr 7*:295, 1983.
60. Hatam A, et al: Effect of dexamethasone treatment on peritumoral brain edema: evaluation by computed tomography. *J Comput Assist Tomogr 6*:586, 1982.
61. Hay WH, et al: Disseminated meningeal tumor in a dog. *J Am Vet Med Assoc 191*:692, 1987.
62. Hayes HM, et al: Occurrence of nervous-tissue tumors in cattle, horses, cats, and dogs. *Int J Cancer 15*:39, 1975.
63. Hayes KC, Schieffer B: Primary tumors in the CNS of carnivores. *Pathol Vet 6*:94, 1969.
64. Haynes JS, Leininger JR: A glioma in the spinal cord of a cat. *Vet Pathol 19*:713, 1982.
65. Heidner GL, et al: A retrospective study of 86 dogs with brain tumors; identification of prognostic variables and response to treatment. *J Vet Intern Med 19*:412, 1990.
66. Henry RW, et al: Transoral hypophysectomy with mandibular symphysiotomy in the dog. *Am J Vet Res 43*:1825, 1982.
67. Hochberg FH, Miller DC: Primary central nervous system lymphoma. *J Neurosurg 68*:835, 1988.
68. Howard-Martin M, Bowles MH: Intracranial dermoid cyst in a dog. *J Am Vet Med Assoc 192*:215, 1988.
69. Indrieri RJ, Taylor RF: Vestibular dysfunction caused by squamous cell carcinoma involving the middle and inner ear in two cats. *J Am Vet Med Assoc 4*:471, 1984.
70. Indrieri RJ, et al: Choroid plexus papilloma associated with prolonged signs of vestibular dysfunction in a young dog. *J Am Anim Hosp Assoc 16*:263, 1980.
71. Jellinger K, et al: Intramedullary spinal cord metastases. *J Neurol 220*:31, 1979.
72. Jones BR: Spinal meningioma in a cat. *Aust Vet J 50*:229, 1974.
73. Kallfelz FA, et al: Scintigraphic diagnosis of brain lesions in the dog and cat. *J Am Vet Med Assoc 172*:589, 1978.
74. Knecht CD: Surgical approach to the brachial plexus in small animals. *J Am Anim Hosp Assoc 13*:592, 1977.
75. Koestner A, Zeman W: Primary reticuloses of the central nervous system in dogs. *Am J Vet Res 23*:381, 1962.
76. Kondziolka D, et al: Significance of hemorrhage into brain tumors: Clinicopathological study. *J Neurosurg 67*:852, 1987.
77. Kornegay JN: Spinal cord/peripheral nerve tumors. Proceedings of the 14th Annual Veterinary Surgical Forum, Chicago, IL, October 1986, p 84.
78. Kornegay JN: Central nervous system neoplasia. *In* Kornegay JN (ed): *Neurologic Disorders: Contemporary Issues in Small Animal Practice*. Vol 5. Churchill-Livingstone, New York, 1986, p 78.
79. Kornegay JN: Imaging brain neoplasia. Computed tomography and magnetic resonance imaging. *Vet Med Rep 2*:372, 1990.
80. Kornegay JN, Gorgacz EJ: Intracranial epidermoid cysts in three dogs. *Vet Pathol 19*:646, 1982.
81. Kornegay JN, et al: Clinicopathologic features of brain herniation in animals. *J Am Vet Med Assoc 182*:1111, 1983.
82. Kostolich M, Dulisch ML: A surgical approach to the canine olfactory bulb for meningioma removal. *Vet Surg 16*:273, 1987.
83. Kraft SL, et al: Canine brain anatomy on magnetic resonance images. *Vet Radiol 30*:147, 1989.
84. Lampert PW, Davis RL: Delayed effects of radiation on the human central nervous system. "Early" and "late" delayed reactions. *Neurology 14*:912, 1964.
85. Lane SB, et al: Feline spinal lymphosarcoma: A retrospective evaluation of 24 cases. *J Vet Intern Med,* in press.
86. Langham RF: Primary retrobulbar meningioma of the optic nerve of a dog. *J Am Vet Med Assoc 159*:175, 1971.
87. Lantz GC, et al: Transsphenoidal hypophysectomy in the clinically normal dog. *Am J Vet Res 49*:1134, 1988.
88. Laws ER, et al: Neurosurgical management of low-grade astrocytoma of the cerebral hemispheres. *J Neurosurg 61*:665, 1984.
89. Lawson DC: Cerebral meningioma in the cat: Diagnosis and surgical treatment of ten cases. *J Am Anim Hosp Assoc 20*:333, 1984.
90. LeCouteur RA, et al: Indirect imaging of the canine optic nerve using metrizamide (optic thecography). *Am J Vet Res 43*:1424, 1982.
91. LeCouteur RA, et al: Radiation response of autochthonous canine brain tumors. *Int J Radiat Oncol Biol Phys 13*:166, 1987.
92. LeCouteur RA, et al: Combined surgical debulking and irradiation for the treatment of a large frontal meningioma in 8 dogs. Proceedings of the 7th Annual Conference of the Veterinary Cancer Society, Madison, Wis. Oct. 1987.
93. Lewis GT, et al: Ophthalmoplegia caused by thyroid adenocarcinoma invasion of the cavernous sinuses in the dog. *J Am Anim Hosp Assoc 20*:805, 1984.
94. Luginbuhl H: Comparative aspects of tumors of the nervous system. *Ann NY Acad Sci 108*:702, 1963.

95. Luginbuhl H, et al: Spontaneous neoplasms of the nervous system in animals. *Prog Neurol Surg 2*:85, 1968.
96. Luttgen PJ, Bratton GR: Spinal cord ependymoma: A case report. *J Am Anim Hosp Assoc 12*:788, 1976.
97. Luttgen PJ, et al: A retrospective study of twenty-nine spinal tumours in the dog and cat. *J Small Anim Pract 21*:213, 1980.
98. Lyons BE: Localized hyperthermia in the treatment of malignant brain tumors using an interstitial microwave antennae array. *IEEE Trans Biomed Eng 31*:53, 1984.
99. Macdonald DR, et al: Steroid-induced CT changes in patients with recurrent malignant gliomas. *Neurology 37* (Suppl 1):300, 1987.
100. MacEwen EG, et al: Management of feline neoplasms. *In* Holzworth J (ed): *Diseases of the Cat.* W.B. Saunders, Philadelphia, 1987, p 597.
101. Matson DD, Crofton FDL: Papilloma of the choroid plexus in childhood. *J Neurosurg 17*:1002, 1960.
102. McClure RC: The cranial nerves, *In* Evans HE, Christensen GC (eds): *Miller's Anatomy of the Dog.* 2nd ed. W.B. Saunders, Philadelphia, 1970, p 903.
103. McGrath JT: Morphology and classification of brain tumors in domestic animals. Abstracts for Conference on Brain Tumors in Man and Animals. Research Triangle Park, N.C., Sept. 1984.
104. Milds HJ, Olafsen P: Primary brain tumors in small animals. *Cornell Vet 26*:159, 1936.
105. Moertel GG: Cerebellar ataxia associated with fluorinated pyrimidine therapy. *Cancer Chemother Rep 41*:15, 1964.
106. Mooney SC, et al: Renal lymphoma in cats: 28 cases (1977–1984). *J Am Vet Med Assoc 191*:1473, 1987.
107. Moore AS, et al: Immunohistochemical evaluation of intermediate filament expression in canine and feline neoplasms. *Am J Vet Res 50*:88, 1989.
108. Moore MP, et al: Boron neutron capture therapy for the treatment of canine brain tumors. Proceedings of the 7th Annual American College of Veterinary Internal Medicine Forum, San Diego, CA, May 1989, p 623.
109. Moore MP, et al: Boron neutron capture therapy for treatment of brain tumors in dogs. *J Vet Intern Med 4*:128, 1990.
110. Morgan JP, et al: Vertebral tumors in the dog: A clinical, radiologic, and pathologic study of 61 primary and secondary lesions. *Vet Radiol 21*:197, 1980.
111. Muller W, et al: CT-analyses of cerebral tumors under steroid therapy. *Neuroradiology 26*:293, 1984.
112. Murphy SB, Donaldson SS: Pediatric lymphoma. *In* Carter SK, et al (eds): *Principles of Cancer Treatment.* McGraw Hill, New York, 1982, p 882.
113. Murray K, et al: Primary malignant lymphoma of the central nervous system: Results of treatment of 11 cases and review of the literature. *J Neurosurg 65*:600, 1986.
114. Nafe LA: Meningiomas in cats: A retrospective clinical study of 36 cases. *J Am Vet Med Assoc 174*:1224, 1979.
115. Neer TM, Reavis DU: Craniopharyngioma and associated central diabetes insipidus and hypothyroidism in a dog. *J Am Vet Med Assoc 182*:519, 1983.
116. Nelson DF, et al: Recent and current investigations of radiation treatment for malignant gliomas. *Semin Oncol 13*:46, 1986.
117. Nelson RW, et al: Diencephalic syndrome secondary to intracranial astrocytoma in a dog. *J Am Vet Med Assoc 179*;1104, 1981.
118. Niebauer GW, et al: Clinical results of intracranial surgeries performed in 30 dogs and cats during the past 5 years. Proceedings of the European Society for Veterinary Neurology Meeting, Berne, Oct. 1989, p 62.
119. O'Brien D, et al: Osteosarcoma of the vertebra causing compression of the thoracic spinal cord in a cat. *J Am Anim Hosp Assoc 16*:497, 1980.
120. Oliver JE Jr: Surgical approaches to the canine brain. *Am J Vet Res 29*:353, 1968.
121. Page RL, et al: Whole body hyperthermia. Rationale and potential use for cancer treatment. *J Vet Intern Med 1*:110, 1987.
122. Palmer AC: Clinical and pathological aspects of cervical disc protrusion and primary tumors in the dog. *J Small Anim Pract 11*:63, 1970.
123. Palmer AC: Clinical signs including papilloedema associated with brain tumors in twenty-one dogs. *J Small Anim Pract 15*:359, 1974.
124. Panciera DL, et al: Magnetic resonance imaging in two dogs with central nervous system disease. *J Small Anim Pract 28*:587, 1987.
125. Parker AJ, et al: Scintigraphic imaging of acute unilateral lesions in the brain parenchyma of three dogs. *J Am Anim Hosp Assoc 18*:926, 1982.
126. Patnaik AK, et al: Choroid plexus carcinoma with meningeal carcinomatosis in a dog. *Vet Pathol 17*:381, 1980.
127. Patnaik AK, et al: Intracranial meningioma: A comparative pathologic study of 28 dogs. *Vet Pathol 23*:369, 1986.
128. Patnaik AK, et al: Paranasal meningioma in the dog: A clinicopathologic study of ten cases. *Vet Pathol 23*:362, 1986.
129. Paulsen ME, et al: Primary optic nerve meningioma in a dog. *J Am Anim Hosp Assoc 25*:147, 1989.
130. Pollack IF, et al: Prognostic factors in the diagnosis and treatment of primary central nervous system lymphoma. *Cancer 63*:939, 1989.
131. Prata RG: Diagnosis of spinal cord tumors in the dog. *Vet Clin North Am 7*:165, 1977.
132. Prata RG, Carillo JM: Oncology—nervous system. *In* Slatter DH (ed): *Textbook of Small Animal Surgery.* W.B. Saunders, Philadelphia, 1985, p 2499.
133. Read G: The treatment of ependymoma of the brain or spinal canal by radiotherapy: A report of 79 cases. *Clin Radiol 35*:163, 1984.
134. Redding RW, Knecht CE: *Atlas of Electroencephalography in the Dog and Cat.* Praeger, New York, 1984.
135. Reidarson TH, et al: Thoracic vertebral osteosarcoma in a cat. *J Am Vet Med Assoc 192*:1102, 1988.
136. Robbins HI: Role of whole-body hyperthermia in the treatment of neoplastic disease: Its current status and future prospects. *Cancer Res 44*(Suppl):4878, 1984.
137. Roberts PA, et al: Effect on intracranial pressure of furosemide combined with varying doses and administration rates of mannitol. *J Neurosurg 66*:440, 1987.
138. Robertson GL, Berl T: Pathophysiology of water metabolism. *In* Brenner BM, Rector FC (eds): *The Kidney.* W.B. Saunders, Philadelphia, 1986, p 408.
139. Rosin A: Neurologic disease associated with lymphosarcoma in ten dogs. *J Am Vet Med Assoc 181*:50, 1982.
140. Ross J, Wyburn RS: A report on the clinical investigation of a paraplegic cat. *N Z Vet J 17*:251, 1969.
141. Rubinstein LJ: Tumors of the central nervous system. *Atlas of Tumor Pathology,* 2nd series, Fascicle 6, Armed Forces Institute of Pathology, Washington, DC, 1972.
142. Russell DS, Rubinstein LJ: *Pathology of Tumors of the Nervous System.* 3rd ed. Williams & Wilkins, Baltimore, 1971.
143. Russell DS, Rubinstein LJ: Congenital tumors of maldevelopmental origin. *In* Russell DS, Rubinstein LJ (eds): *Pathology of Tumors of the Nervous System.* Williams & Wilkins, Baltimore, 1977, p 30.
144. Russo ME: Primary reticulosis of the central nervous system in dogs. *J Am Vet Med Assoc 174*:492, 1979.
145. Sage MR: Blood-brain barrier: Phenomenon of increasing importance to the imaging clinician. *AJNR 138*:887, 1982.
146. Salazar OM, et al: Improved survival in cases of intracranial ependymoma after radiation therapy. *J Neurosurg 59*:652, 1983.
147. Sarfaty D, et al: Cerebral astrocytoma in four cats: Clinical and pathologic findings. *J Am Vet Med Assoc 191*:976, 1987.
148. Sarfaty D, et al: Neurologic, endocrinologic and pathologic findings associated with large pituitary tumors in dogs: Eight cases (1976–1984). *J Am Vet Med Assoc 193*:854, 1988.
149. Saunders LZ, Richard C: Craniopharyngioma in a dog with apparent adiposogenital syndrome and diabetes insipidus. *Cornell Vet 42*:490, 1952.
150. Schoenberg BS: The epidemiology of central nervous system tumors. *In* McGuire WL (ed): *Oncology of the Nervous System.* Martinus Nijhoff, Boston, 1983, p 1.
151. Scott-Moncrieff C, et al: Plasma and CSF pharmacokinetics of intravenous cytosine arabinoside (AraC) in dogs. Program and Abstracts, Veterinary Cancer Society, 8th Annual Conference. Estes Park, Col., Oct. 1988, p 10.
152. Shapiro WR, Shapiro JR: Principles of brain tumor chemotherapy. *Semin Oncol 13*:56, 1986.
153. Sharp NJH: Craniolateral approach to the canine brachial plexus. *Vet Surg 17*:18, 1988.
154. Sheline GE, Wara WM: Radiation therapy of brain tumors. *In* Youmans JR (ed): *Neurological Surgery.* 2nd ed. Vol 5. W.B. Saunders, Philadelphia, 1982, p 3096.
155. Shell L, et al: Surgical removal of a meningioma in a cat after detection by computerized axial tomography. *J Am Anim Hosp Assoc 21*:439, 1985.
156. Sisson AF, et al: Radiation therapy of granulomatous meningoencephalomyelitis of dogs. Proceedings of the 7th Annual Veterinary Medical Forum, San Diego, CA, May 1989, p 1031.
157. Skerritt GC, et al: Bilateral blindness in a dog due to invasion of the optic chiasma by a glioma. *J Small Anim Pract 27*:97, 1986.
158. Smith CML, Timperley WR: Multiple intraspinal and intracranial epidermoids and lipomata following gunshot injury. *Neuropathol Appl Neurobiol 10*:235, 1984.
159. Smith DA, Honhold N: Clinical and pathological features of a cerebellar oligodendroglioma in a cat. *J Small Anim Pract 29*:269, 1988.
160. Solan MJ, Dramer S: The role of radiation therapy in the management of intracranial meningiomas. *Int J Radiat Oncol Biol Phys 11*:675, 1985.
161. Sorjonen DC: Total protein, albumin quota, and electrophoretic patterns in cerebrospinal fluid of dogs with central nervous system disorders. *Am J Vet Res 48*:301, 1987.
162. Stadler B, et al: Misonidazole and irradiation in the treatment of high-grade astrocytomas: Further report of the Vienna study group. *Int J Radiat Oncol Biol Phys 10*:1713, 1984.
163. Stampley AR, et al: Meningeal carcinomatosis secondary to a colonic signet-ring carcinoma in a dog. *J Am Anim Hosp Assoc 23*:655, 1987.
164. Steinberg HS: Brachial plexus injuries and dysfunctions. *Vet Clin North Am 18*:565, 1988.
165. Steinberg HS: Treatment of intracranial neoplasms of dogs and cats. Proceedings of the 13th Annual Kal Kan Symposium for the Treatment of Small Animal Diseases, Neurology and Ophthalmology, Columbus, OH, Oct. 1989, p 43.
166. Sullivan ND: The nervous system. *In* Jubb KVF, et al (eds): *Pathology of Domestic Animals.* 3rd ed. Academic Press, New York, 1985, p 201.

167. Summers BA, de Lahunta A: Cerebral angioendotheliomatosis in a dog. *Acta Neuropathol (Berl) 68*:10, 1985.
168. Summers BA, et al: A novel intradural extramedullary spinal cord tumor in young dogs. *Acta Neuropathol (Berl) 75*:402, 1988.
169. Summers BA, et al: Intracranial germ cell tumors in two dogs. *J Small Animal Pract 30*:39, 1989.
170. Suter PF, et al: Myelography in the dog: Diagnosis of tumors of the spinal cord and vertebrae. *J Am Vet Radiol Soc 12*:29, 1972.
171. Swanson JF, et al: Cerebral thrombosis and hemorrhage in association with L-asparaginase administration. *J Am Anim Hosp Assoc 22*:749, 1986.
172. Szczech GM, et al: Chemodectoma with metastasis to bone in a dog. *J Am Vet Med Assoc 162*:376, 1973.
173. Tomlinson J, et al: Intraspinal epidermal cyst in a dog. *J Am Vet Med Assoc 193*:1435, 1988.
174. Turrel JM, et al: Computed tomographic characteristics of primary brain tumors in 50 dogs. *J Am Vet Med Assoc 188*:851, 1986.
175. Turrel JM, et al: Radiotherapy of brain tumors in dogs. *J Am Vet Med Assoc 184*:82, 1984.
176. Valentine BA, et al: Suprasellar germ cell tumors in the dog: A report of five cases and review of the literature. *Acta Neuropathol 76*:94, 1988.
177. van Bree H, et al: Cervical cord compression as a neurologic complication in an IgG multiple myeloma in a dog. *J Am Anim Hosp Assoc 19*:317, 1983.
178. Vandevelde M: Brain tumors in domestic animals: An overview. Abstracts for Conference on Brain Tumors in Man and Animals. Research Triangle Park, N.C., Sept. 1984.
179. Vandevelde M, et al: Immunocytochemical studies in canine neuroectodermal brain tumors. *Acta Neuropathol (Berl) 66*:111, 1985.
180. Vandevelde M, et al: Immunohistological studies on primary reticulosis of the canine brain. *Vet Pathol 18*:577, 1981.
181. Walter PA, et al: Diagnosis and treatments of adverse reactions to radiopaque contrast agents. *In* Kirk RW (ed): *Current Veterinary Therapy IX*. W.B. Saunders, Philadelphia, 1986, p 47.
182. Waters DJ, Hayden DW: Intramedullary spinal cord metastasis in the dog. *J Vet Intern Med 4*:207, 1990.
183. Waters DJ, et al: Intracranial lesions in dogs with hemangiosarcoma. *J Vet Intern Med 3*:222, 1989.
184. Weissm AJ, et al: An evaluation of 5-fluorouracil in malignant disease. *Ann Intern Med 55*:731, 1961.
185. Weissman DE: Glucocorticoid treatment for brain metastases and epidural spinal cord compression: A review. *J Clin Oncol 6*:543, 1988.
186. Wheeler SJ, et al: Myelography in the cat. *J Small Anim Pract 26*:143, 1985.
187. Wheeler SJ, et al: The diagnosis of brachial plexus disorders in dogs: A review of twenty-two cases. *J Small Anim Pract 27*:147, 1986.
188. Winkelman MD, Hines JD: Cerebellar degeneration caused by high dose cytosine arabinoside: A clinicopathologic study. *Ann Neurol 43*:520, 1983.
189. Wise DT, et al: Posterior paresis caused by extension of hemangiosarcoma from lungs to thoracic vertebrae of a dog. *J Am Vet Med Assoc 171*:544, 1977.
190. Withrow SJ, Doige CE: Subperiosteal vertebral hematoma as a cause of acute paraplegia in two dogs. *J Am Anim Hosp Assoc 15*:295, 1979.
191. Wood AK: Iohexol and iopamidol: New nonionic contrast media for myelography in dogs. *Comp Cont Educ Vet Pract 1*:32, 1988.
192. Wright JA: The pathological features associated with spinal tumors in 29 dogs. *J Comp Pathol 95*:549, 1985.
193. Yoshioka MM: Meningioma of the spinal cord in a cat. *Comp Cont Educ Pract Vet 9*:34, 1987.
194. Zaki FA: Spontaneous central nervous system tumors in the dog. *Vet Clin North Am Small Anim Pract 7*:153, 1977.
195. Zaki FA, Hurvitz AI: Spontaneous neoplasms of the CNS of the cat. *J Small Anim Pract 17*:773, 1976.
196. Zaki FA, Kay WJ: Carcinoma of the choroid plexus in a dog. *J Am Vet Med Assoc 164*:1195, 1974.
197. Zaki FA, Nafe LA: Choroid plexus tumors in the dog. *J Am Vet Med Assoc 176*:328, 1980.

CHAPTER 158 Eye and Orbit

Stephen I. Bistner

LID TUMORS

Tumors of the eyelids may occur at any age but are frequently encountered in middle-aged and older dogs (8 to 9 years). In dogs, epithelial lid tumors predominate six to one over mesenchymal tumors, and roughly 75 per cent of the tumors are histologically classified as benign.*

Canine Cutaneous Histiocytoma

Cutaneous histiocytoma is unique to canine skin. Tumor cells arise from the monocyte-macrophage cells of the skin. The incidence is 117:100,000 dogs, accounting for 10.7 per cent of all canine neoplasms reviewed in a 3-year period. The tumor is commonly noted in dogs younger than 2 years, with a decreasing incidence in older dogs. Cutaneous histiocytoma is more frequently found in boxers and possibly dachshunds and especially involves the skin of the head.[19, 35, 47, 53, 71, 77]

The tumors are pink, fleshy, circular, epilated lesions that may involve the lids (Fig. 158–1). The lesions appear erythematous, may become ulcerated, and may range in diameter from 0.5 to 4.0 cm and involve only the skin. If the tumor ulcerates, inflammation may spread to the underlying dermis.

The histological appearance and distribution of infiltrating lymphocytes have been described.[53] An immune response to the lesions may occur, and some lesions may spontaneously regress or completely disappear. Individual histiocytic cells may have a high mitotic index, but the tumors are benign. Pathologists may diagnose the tumors as malignant in humans because of the mitotic index.

Because the tumors involve only the skin, they can be removed in a number of ways. Cryosurgery can be performed on small lesions. On larger lesions, especially those involving the lid margin, a split-thickness lid resection can be performed, the skin and associated tumor removed, and the lid skin closed from side to side. Alternatively, a vertical or horizontal pedicle graft can be created if the lesion involves more than one-fourth of the lid margin.[16, 70] Histiocytomas do not recur if completely removed.

*See references 16, 17, 19, 48, 49, 58, 70, and 71.

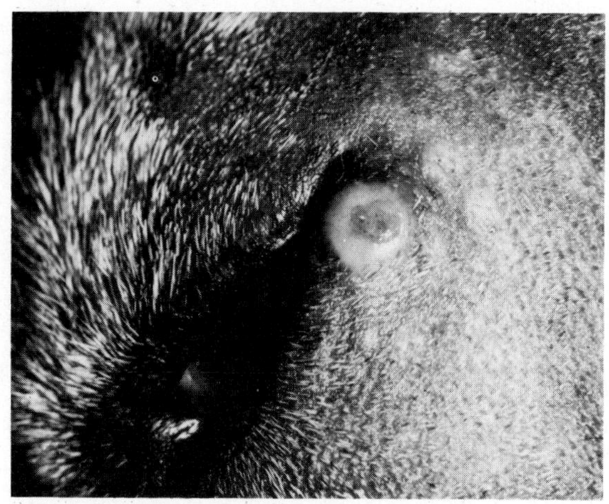

FIGURE 158–1. A canine histiocytoma of the skin at the lateral canthus. These benign tumors usually occur in young animals and involve the epidermis and underlying dermis.

Papillomas (Verrucas, Warts)

Papillomas are benign epithelial tumors that are common in dogs, accounting for 1 to 25 per cent of all skin neoplasms.[15, 16, 48, 70, 71]

Cutaneous papillomas involving the lids are most commonly encountered in dogs older than 8 years.[16] They may have a broad base or may be on a narrow, pedunculated stalk. The epidermis of the tumor becomes thickened and may appear cauliflower-like with numerous projections (Fig. 158–2). As the tumors grow larger, they are easily traumatized, their surface ulcerates, and they bleed. The tumors do not invade the underlying dermis. Papillomas are frequently found (17 to 20 per cent of lid tumors) in older dogs and may be multiple on one lid.[16, 70]

Because these tumors involve only the epidermis, surgical full-thickness wedge resection of the lid is not necessary. These growths can be treated by cryosurgery or split-thickness resection of the skin tumor from the lid. If the tumor is completely removed, regrowth does not occur. Cutting the pedunculated stalk of a papilloma may remove the mass of the tumor, but the small remaining stalk may regrow.

Basal Cell Tumors (Basal Cell Carcinoma, Basal Cell Epithelioma)

Basal cell tumors arise from the basal layers of the epidermis or embryonal stratum germinativum or within hair follicles or cells of sebaceous glands.

Basal cell tumors account for 10 to 12 per cent of canine skin tumors, with dogs in the 7- to 9-year-old group having the highest incidence. The incidence of basal cell tumors may be higher in cats than in dogs, as high as 26 per cent of all epithelial skin tumors.[19, 27, 71]

The tumors may be found on the lids. Size varies from 0.5 to 10 cm, and the skin is elevated, firm, erythematous, and frequently ulcerated. They do not invade locally but frequently extend into the dermis and are usually well encapsulated. Basal cell tumors are classified by histological appearance into solid, garland, medusoid, adenoid, cystic, and basosquamous types.[71, 72]

Basal cell tumors are benign and if entirely removed do not recur. If a tumor involves the lid margin and can be palpated over the dermis as well as epidermis, full-thickness wedge resection is indicated. Cryotherapy may be used.

Squamous Cell Carcinoma

Squamous cell carcinoma is the most malignant of the epithelial tumors. These lesions originate from the squamous epithelial cells of the epidermis, and the incidence in dogs and cats varies from 3 to 20 per cent of cutaneous tumors. The tumor is more frequently found in animals with lightly pigmented skin after chronic sunlight exposure or long periods of dermatosis. The head, tips of the ears, and eyelids in lightly pigmented or white animals (e.g., white cats) are most frequently affected.[15, 27, 55, 71, 73]

A lesion starts as an epitheliomatous plaque progressing through stages of carcinoma *in situ* and invasive carcinoma. The tumors frequently spread rapidly, in-

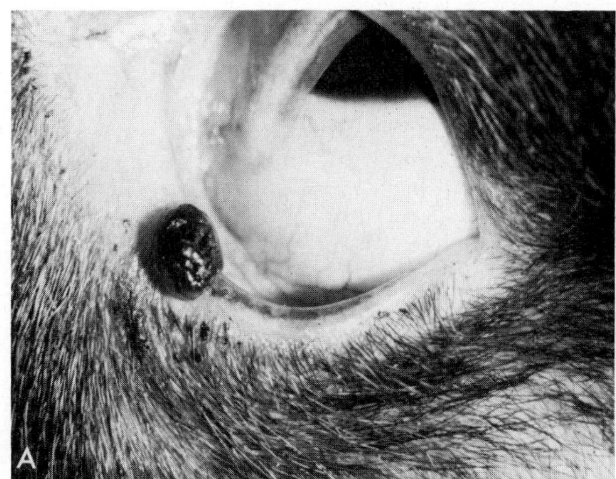

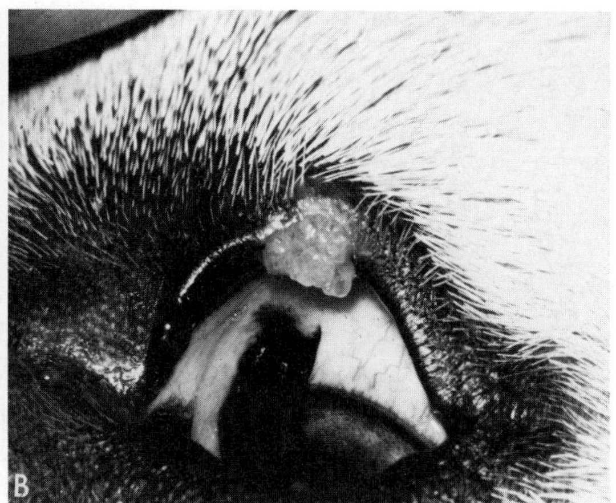

FIGURE 158–2. *A* and *B*, Fibropapillomas of the lid margin. These are commonly seen on the lids of older dogs and may be multiple, with more than one tumor on the lid. They are benign and epithelial in origin.

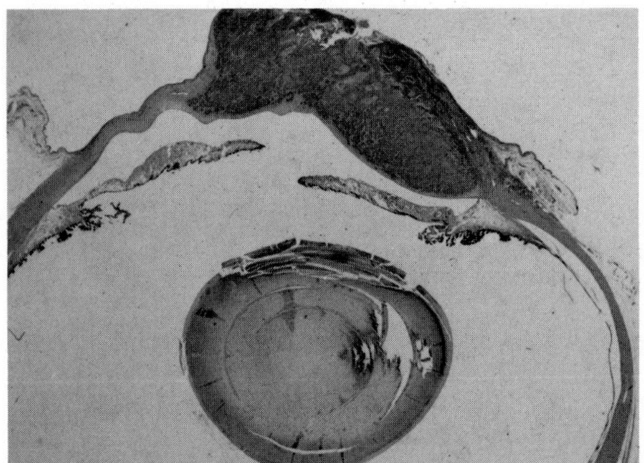

FIGURE 158–3. Squamous cell carcinoma of the cornea that has grown throughout the corneal stroma but has failed to penetrate the Descemet membrane and the anterior chamber.

vade, and are necrotic. They are easily traumatized and tend to bleed. Some tumors consist of cells that are very anaplastic, spread rapidly, and metastasize to regional lymph nodes and lungs. Diagnosis can usually be based on biopsy of the lesion and histological examination. The tumor should be staged (Figs. 158–3 through 158–7).[55]

ADNEXAL TUMORS

Tumors of the sebaceous glands of the lids are the most common adnexal tumors in older dogs (mean age 9.5 years).[16] They arise from the tarsal (meibomian) glands of the lids and are common in older dogs. Tumors arising from sebaceous glands can be subdivided into adenomas, adenocarcinomas, and adenomatous hyperplasia.[15, 21, 36, 50, 71]

Tarsal gland adenomas involve the lid margin. As the tumor enlarges, tumor tissue grows through the lid margin. The overlying skin may be pigmented, or the tumor may be easily traumatized and may ulcerate and bleed. Examination of the palpebral conjunctiva reveals that the conjunctiva is elevated because of the tumor growing within the substance of the lid (Figs. 158–8 and 158–9).

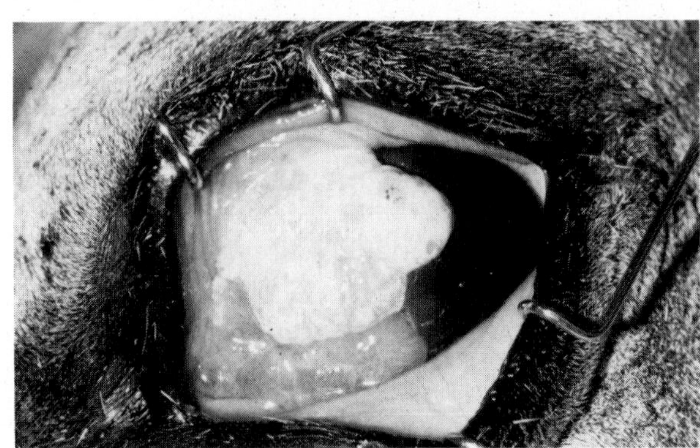

FIGURE 158–5. A squamous cell carcinoma of the third eyelid as well as the cornea.

These tumors are most easily removed when they are small. Full-thickness wedge resection of the lid is performed, and if all tumor tissue is removed, regrowth does not take place. If the tumor is an adenoma, it is benign and noninvasive. If the tumor mass penetrates the margin of the lid and only this extruding tumor tissue is removed, the tumor regrows until the core of the tumor tissue arising from the gland is surgically resected.[16]

Melanomas

Normal melanocytes are dendritic cells and are located within the epidermis at the epidermal-dermal junction between the cells of the basal layer. Melanoblasts, the precursors of melanocytes, are derived from neuroectodermal tissue.[24]

Melanomas involve the skin of older dogs, with an average age of 9 to 10 years. The incidence of dermal melanomas is approximately 5 to 7 per cent of skin tumors. Skin melanomas most frequently afflict Scottish terriers, Boston terriers, Airedale terriers, and springer spaniels. The increased incidence in these breeds may be associated with increased skin pigmentation. The

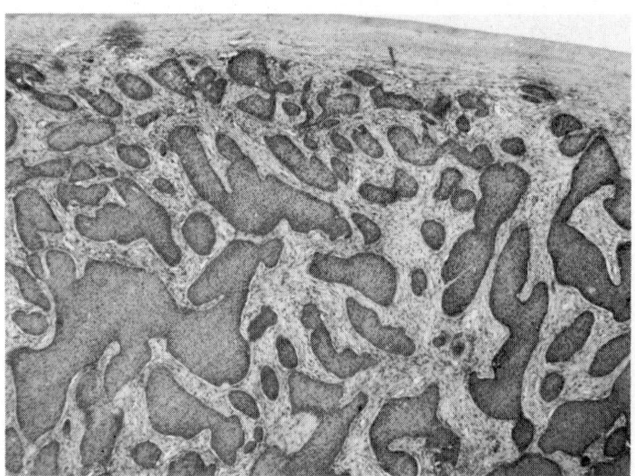

FIGURE 158–4. Histological section of the squamous cell carcinoma in Figure 158–3 (higher magnification). Nests of squamous tumor cells are present throughout the corneal stroma.

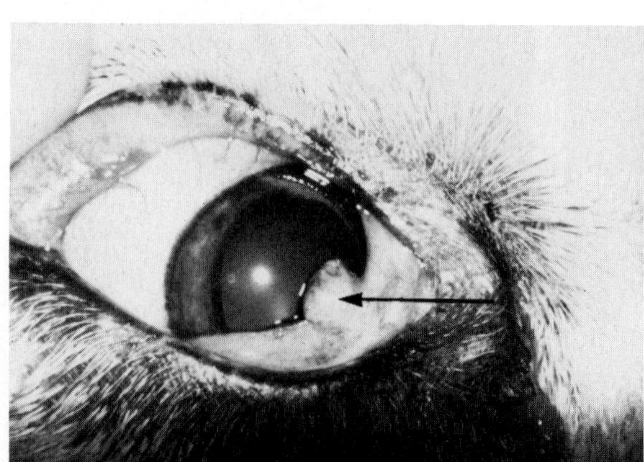

FIGURE 158–6. Early squamous cell carcinoma on the margin of the third eyelid in a dog. Early surgical removal or cryosurgery is indicated.

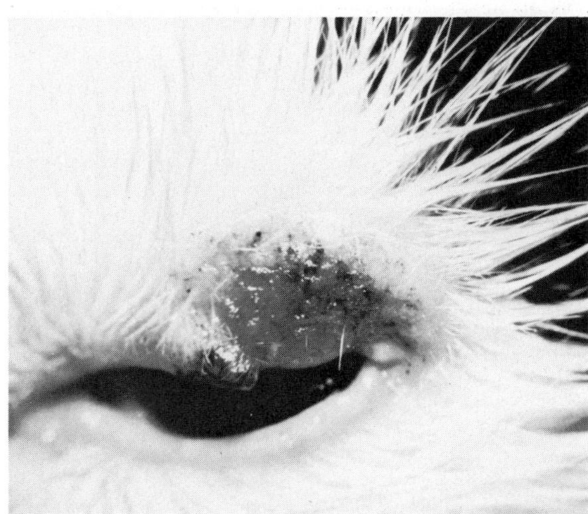

FIGURE 158–7. Squamous cell carcinoma of the lids of a white cat. Early recognition and wide surgical excision may be curative. Advanced lesions should be staged, and more radical therapy is required.

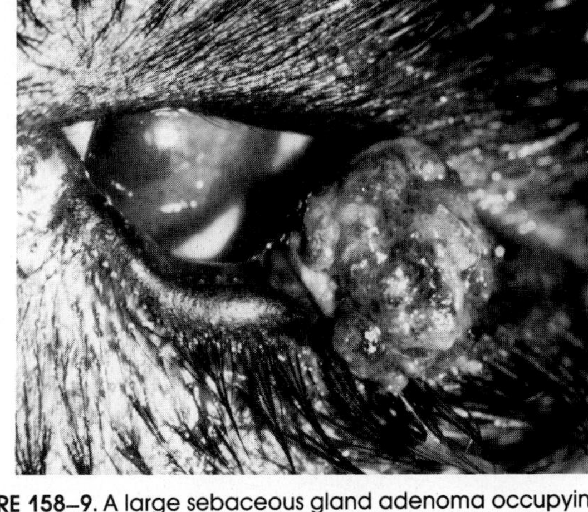

FIGURE 158–9. A large sebaceous gland adenoma occupying half of the lid margin. Although this tumor is benign, when this large the mass can be easily ulcerated and bleed.

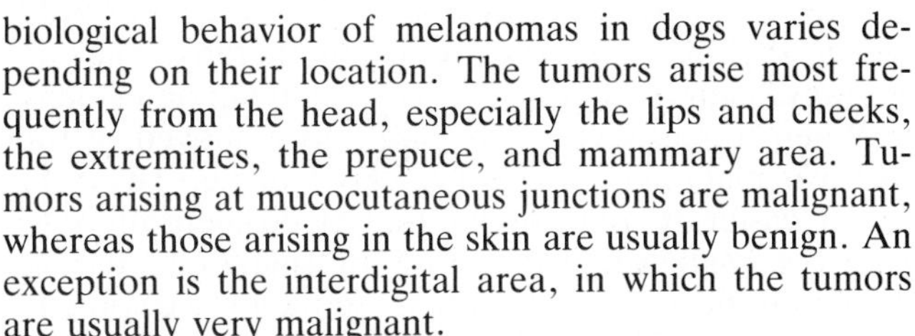

biological behavior of melanomas in dogs varies depending on their location. The tumors arise most frequently from the head, especially the lips and cheeks, the extremities, the prepuce, and mammary area. Tumors arising at mucocutaneous junctions are malignant, whereas those arising in the skin are usually benign. An exception is the interdigital area, in which the tumors are usually very malignant.

A classification of skin melanomas in dogs has been established.[24, 71] Benign growths are subdivided according to the presence of abnormal melanocytes at the epidermal-dermal junction. Benign melanocytic growths that show such junctional activity are called *junctional melanocytomas*. Dermal melanocytomas do not have junctional activity and are subdivided into fibrous and cellular tumors. Malignant melanomas invade the dermis and surrounding connective tissue and metastasize.

The more complicated system of dermal melanoma formation used in humans to refer to nevi formation and junctional and compound nevi cannot be easily applied to dogs.

Melanocytic tumors with junctional activity develop from flat black maculae into elevated, often pedunculated lesions that may be from 0.5 to 1.0 cm in diameter. Some junctional nevi regress spontaneously.[24, 71]

Benign dermal melanomas are well-circumscribed, elevated masses covered by thin, hairless skin. They usually measure 0.5 to 2.0 cm. Malignant melanomas are usually larger than benign dermal melanomas. These tumors usually are rapidly growing and locally invasive, and the overlying skin may be ulcerated. Fortunately, most melanomas of the lids of dogs are either benign junctional or benign dermal (Figs. 158–10 and 158–11).

Bostock has reviewed the prognosis after surgical removal of canine melanomas.[18] Ten per cent of dogs that were diagnosed as having benign dermal melanomas died of the disease. Dogs with malignant melanomas of the skin had a 70-week median survival time, and 45 per cent of the dogs died of the tumor in 2 years. The major histological type found in malignant dermal mel-

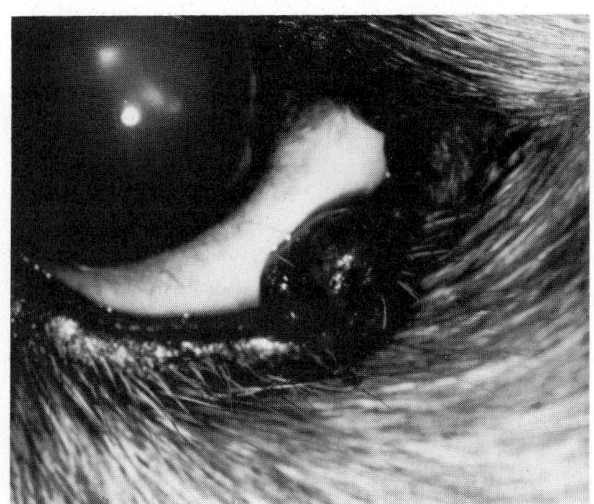

FIGURE 158–8. A sebaceous gland adenoma of the tarsal glands of the lower lid. This is the most common type of benign growth of the lids in older dogs.

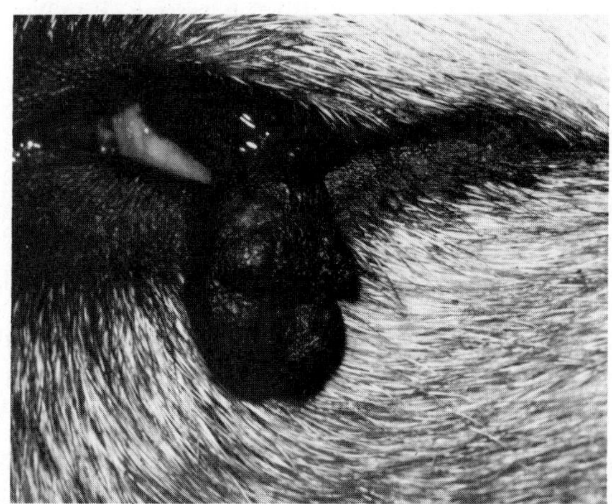

FIGURE 158–10. A melanoma of the lower lid in a dog. Melanomas of the lid are usually benign compared with those arising from mucous membrane surfaces.

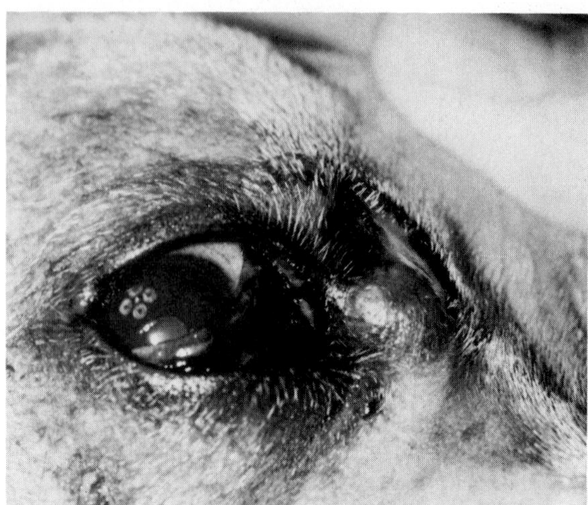

FIGURE 158–11. A malignant melanoma of the skin and subcutaneous tissue of the medial canthus of a 9-year-old Cairn terrier. The tumor had been surgically removed on three occasions. The time from first surgical removal to metastasis of the melanoma was 9 months.

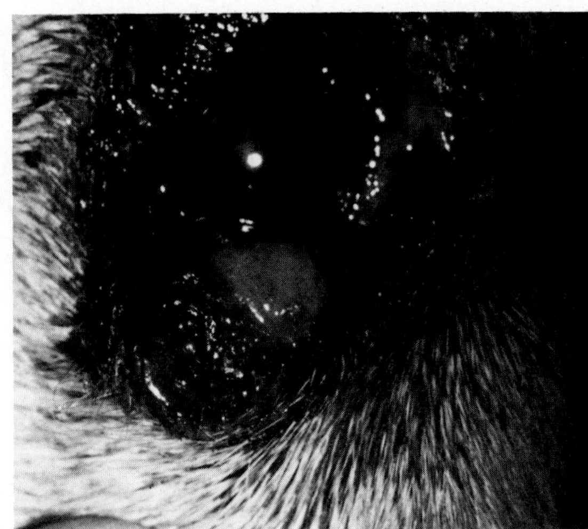

FIGURE 158–12. A canine mast cell tumor involving half of the lower lid.

anomas was epithelioid; the dogs had a mean survival time of 24 weeks, and 73 per cent died after 2 years.

Besides the histological type involved in tumor formation, the mitotic activity is also significant in determining prognosis. Dogs with melanomas with two or less mitotic figures per 10 high-power fields had a median survival time of 104 weeks and a 10 per cent mortality after 2 years. Dogs with tumors that had three or more mitotic figures per 10 high-power fields had a 30-week median survival time and a 73 per cent mortality after 2 years.

Mast Cell Tumors

Mast cells are a normal component of connective tissue. The terms *mast cell tumor, mastocytoma, mast cell sarcoma*, and *mastocytosis* may be used interchangeably. Mast cell tumors in dogs represent 7 to 21 per cent of all skin tumors and 11 to 27 per cent of all malignant skin tumors. These tumors are most frequently encountered in dogs 8 to 10 years of age. There is a breed predilection in the boxer, Boston terrier, English bulldog, and English bull terrier.[15, 32, 39, 50, 71]

The most common sites for those mastocytomas arising from the dermis and subcutaneous tissue are the trunk, perineal region, and head and neck.[16] Lid tumors are elevated, nodular, and firm. Hair is lost from the skin, and the tumors frequently ulcerate on the surface (Fig. 158–12).

Diagnosis of mast cell tumor can be made on impression smears or fine-needle aspirates of the tumor. The smears are stained with new methylene blue, a Romanowsky stain, or toluidine blue to demonstrate the metachromatically staining granules of heparin, histamine, serotonin, and eosinophilic chemotactic substance.

Mast cell tumors may be benign or malignant. A histological system to classify these tumors according to degree of malignancy and a clinical staging system have been developed.[76] Each patient's treatment is based on histological findings and clinical staging. Treatment of lid tumors is by full-thickness wedge resection. Additional therapy may involve chemotherapy, radiation therapy, immunotherapy, or any combination of these.

When a mastocytoma is surgically removed, a wide surgical margin of at least 2 cm is made. Thus, it is much easier to remove lid tumors cosmetically when they are small. Surgical removal of isolated lid mast cell tumors is most successful when the tumor is confined to stage 1, in which there is no lymph node, peripheral blood, or bone marrow involvement. Cryosurgery can be used for small mast cell tumors.

TUMORS OF THE CONJUNCTIVA, THIRD EYELID, AND CORNEA

Tumors of the conjunctiva may involve the third eyelid or the bulbar or palpebral conjunctiva. Conjunctival papillomas usually occur on the lid margins or the third eyelid (Fig. 158–13). They may be pigmented and tend to be pedunculated. Histological study usually reveals frond- or finger-like projections covered by acanthotic epithelium and lined by a core of connective tissue.

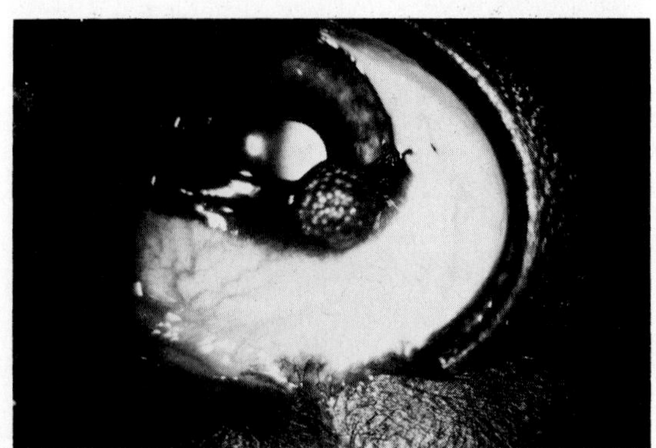

FIGURE 158–13. A fibropapilloma on the margin of the third eyelid. This fibropapilloma was on a sessile base and could have been removed either surgically or with cryosurgery.

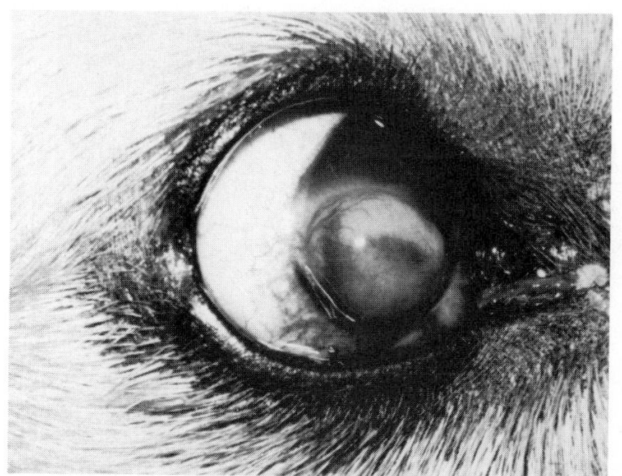

FIGURE 158–14. A benign fibrous histiocytoma that developed on the conjunctiva and grew to invade the corneal stroma.

Carcinoma of the conjunctiva often develops at the perilimbal area or on the third eyelid. The earliest lesion is a leukoplakia or slightly raised fleshy mass (see Figs. 158–5 and 158–6). In these early cases, the epithelium is replaced by atypical pleomorphic epithelial cells, and the epithelium is two to five times thicker than normal. The normal polarity of epithelial cells is lost, and mitotic figures are frequently observed in the abnormal cells. The basement membrane of the epithelium is intact, and the subepithelial tissue is not invaded.[45, 46, 82] Carcinomas of the conjunctiva spread through the epithelial basement membrane and into the stroma or across the limbus and into the cornea (Fig. 158–14; see also Fig. 158–11).

Dermoids are congenital tumors of the cornea and conjunctiva. A dermoid (dermolipoma) is a choristoma, a congenital tumor composed of elements normally not present in that location (Fig. 158–15). Dermoids often arise on the conjunctiva and cross the limbus to involve the cornea. The dermoid is usually composed of epidermis with epidermal appendages (hair follicles, sebaceous glands, keratin). Treatment is by superficial keratectomy. If all the tumor tissue is removed, it does not recur.[45, 82]

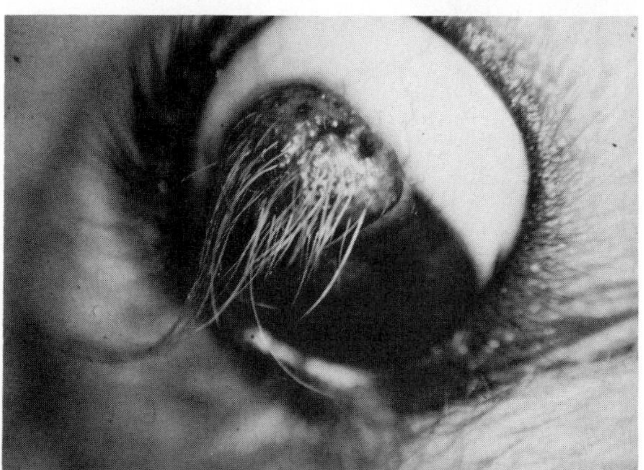

FIGURE 158–15. A corneal dermoid on the conjunctiva and cornea. Complete surgical removal of the dermoid by a superficial keratectomy will prevent any further growth or irritation.

INTRAOCULAR TUMORS

Intraocular tumors are not frequently recognized. Reports in the literature cover a total of 24 primary intraocular tumors and 11 secondary intraocular tumors. More intraocular tumors do undoubtedly occur, but the eye, especially the posterior pole, is seldom examined.*

A number of clinically significant signs may suggest the development of an intraocular tumor:

1. The iris may be altered in color, shape, thickness, or mobility. With melanomas, changes in pigmentation and thickness may be diffuse or focal.
2. Keratitis and corneal edema may be associated with neoplastic growth in the iris and invasion of the anterior chamber, damaging the corneal endothelium.
3. Uveitis commonly accompanies lymphosarcomatous infiltration of the anterior uveal tract.
4. Secondary glaucoma may develop when tumor tissue invades the anterior uveal tract.
5. Conjunctival and deep scleral vascularization may be noted over the area of the tumor cell infiltration in the anterior uveal tract.
6. Additional signs that may be observed with intraocular tumor metastasis include intraocular bleeding, lens luxation, and retinal detachments.

Intraocular tumors can be classified as primary or secondary. Primary tumors arise directly from the neuroepithelium of the retina, ciliary body, or iris; from cells of neural crest origin; from vascular endothelium; or from smooth muscle or neural mesenchymal elements. The most common primary intraocular tumor is melanoma, which occurs in two forms, localized and diffuse.†

Epibulbar Melanomas

Black masses that appear in the sclera, usually near or at the limbus, present a difficult differential diagnosis. The tissue mass may be an epibulbar melanoma arising in the scleral or episcleral tissues and not invading the sclera to involve deeper intraocular tissues. Epibulbar masses may, however, be extensions of intraocular melanomas arising from the ciliary body or iris and growing into the sclera and episcleral tissue. Careful ocular examination usually differentiates the two (Fig. 158–16).[8, 25, 40, 44, 57]

1. Extensions of intraocular melanomas usually have a well-developed vascular supply in the sclera.
2. Gonioscopic examination may show evidence of intraocular spread of melanoma into the sclera.
3. The iris may show evidence of intraocular involvement with melanoma.
4. Tumor involvement may be seen by dilating the pupil and, using indirect ophthalmoscopy, examining the peripheral retina and pars plana ciliary body area.

Based on a limited study of dogs, epibulbar melanomas may be more aggressive in their growth patterns in

*See references 1, 6, 7, 11, 17, 48, 56, 58, 69, and 70.
†See references 1–3, 14, 26, 29, 31, 63, 66, 74, 78, 80, and 81.

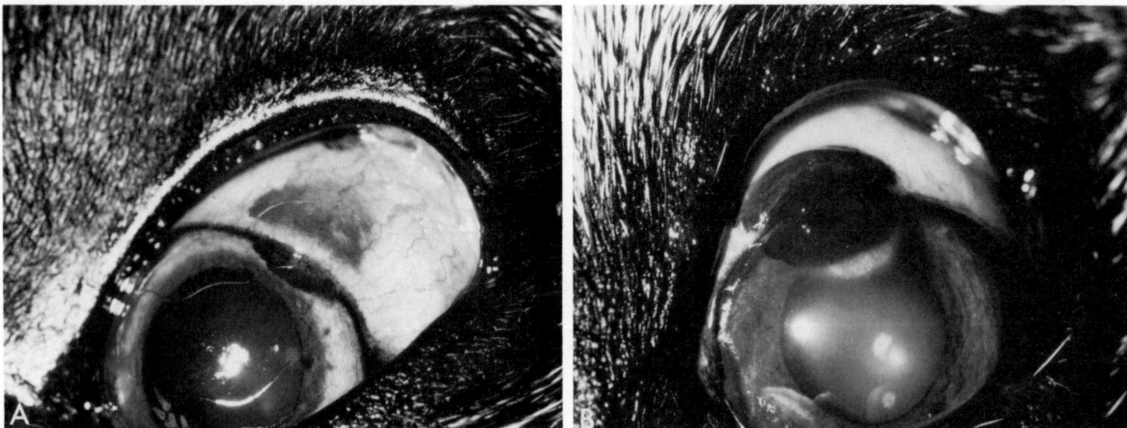

FIGURE 158–16. *A* and *B*, Episcleral melanomas in a dog. Note that the melanomas are arising on the episcleral tissue and involve the conjunctiva and that there is regrowth of melanoma into the cornea. Examination of the iris and anterior drainage angle using a gonioscopic lens failed to reveal any spread of the tumor into deeper ocular structures.

young dogs. In this series, tumor growth invaded the cornea from the sclera and grew into the corneal stroma. In older dogs (7 to 11 years), the epibulbar melanomas remained in the sclera and episcleral tissue.[57, 77]

If epibulbar melanomas do not invade and do not grow into the cornea or through the sclera, surgical removal is not recommended. If the tumors begin to grow, either complete enucleation or scleral wall resection with a scleral transplant is performed.

True melanomas of the posterior choroid are rare in domestic animals.[1, 3, 14, 31, 69, 80] Melanomas usually arise from the pigmented epithelial cells of the ciliary processes, ciliary body, or posterior iridal surface. The growths are not usually recognized until one of the following takes place: (1) A black, elevated mass becomes visible in the well-vascularized sclera adjacent to a thickening of the iris stroma; (2) the surface of the iris assumes a different shape, and iris pigmentation is altered; (3) the anterior chamber is partially filled with pigmented tissue, altering the pupillary space; or (4) hyphema and secondary glaucoma obliterate the anterior ocular segment.

Treatment of intraocular melanomas is being re-evaluated in humans as well as animals. In dogs, melanomas that involve only portions of the iris and small areas of the ciliary body may be treated by surgical sector iridectomy. If postoperative complications are not severe, results have been good, usually without recurrence or metastasis.[1, 22, 57]

More extensive intraocular melanoma in dogs presents a surgical dilemma. Should the diseased eye be enucleated? Unfortunately, we do not have extensive follow-up reports on intraocular melanomas in dogs. Evidence suggests that intraocular melanomas in dogs grow within the globe but rarely metastasize to regional lymph nodes and lungs.[1, 77] Combined data from reports in the veterinary literature on intraocular melanomas in small animals document confirmed tumor metastasis in 7 of 129 cases.[28, 75] My experience is that if the melanoma is surgically disturbed (i.e., cut during enucleation), rapid spread and dissemination are likely to follow. Another problem encountered with intraocular melanomas in dogs is that if left alone, the tumor may grow through the scleral wall or cribriform plate and enter the orbit (Figs. 158–17 and 158–18).

Canine choroidal melanomas are distinct entities compared with anterior uveal melanomas.[31] The tumors consist of polyhedral cells with no mitotic figures and minimal nuclear anaplasia and do not metastasize. The retina overlying the tumor tissue is usually detached. In two reported melanomas, the basement membrane of the retinal epithelium was disrupted and tumor infiltrated into the retina and subretinal space. Posterior choroidal melanoma in small animals is much more rarely encountered than anterior uveal melanoma.

Wilcock and Peiffer[81] reported the morphology and behavior of primary ocular melanomas in 91 dogs, and classified the tumors into two groups: benign and partially malignant melanomas. The most accurate classification scheme for separating tumors into these categories was the mitotic index of the tumor. Of the

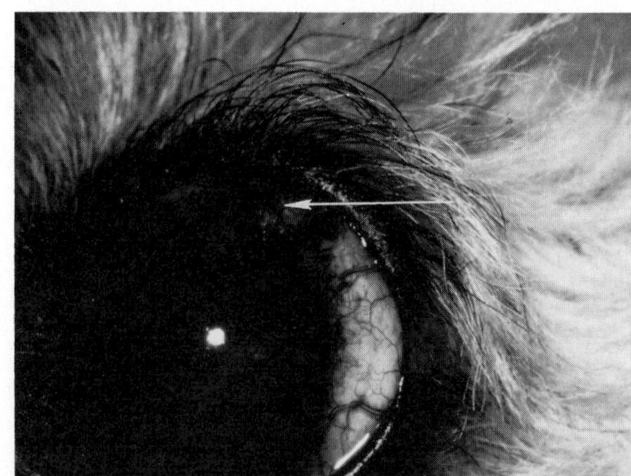

FIGURE 158–17. A pigmented mass in the superior aspect of the sclera of a dog. The pigmented mass is elevated, and examination of the iris and anterior drainage angle revealed that this melanoma arising from the ciliary body was not grossly visible until the tumor grew into the sclera. In this case, because of the rapid growth of the tumor, the eye was enucleated.

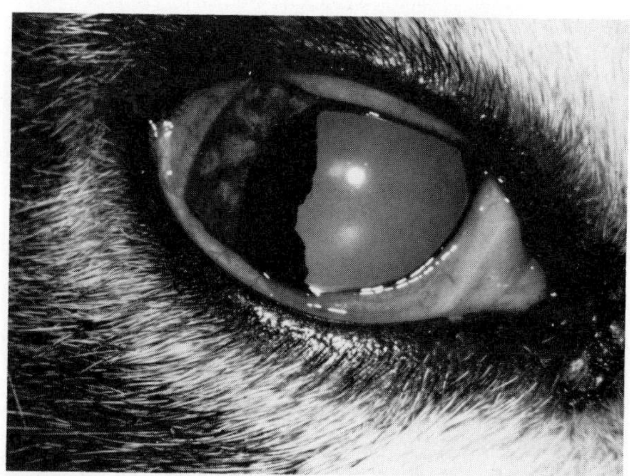

FIGURE 158–18. A melanoma arising from the ciliary body and involving the iris and penetrating the sclera in a dog. The tumor was not recognized until it grew through the sclera.

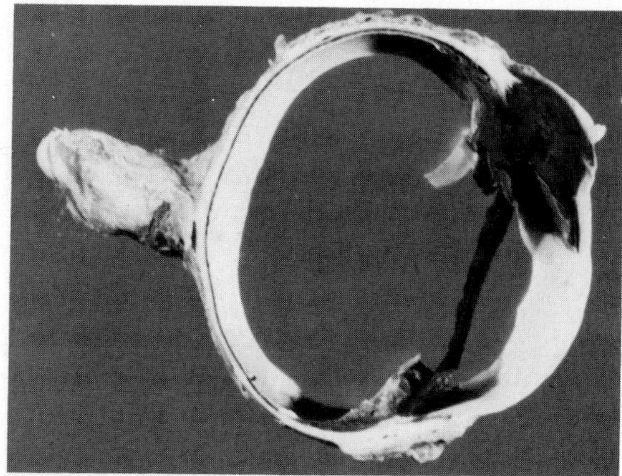

FIGURE 158–19. Diffuse malignant melanoma arising from the iris and ciliary body of a cat.

reported cases, 75 were benign and 16 were histologically malignant. Three had confirmed metastasis. Unlike the scheme for the Callender classification of human melanomas, cell type of growth within the tumor tissue did not predict metastatic potential. A scheme based on mitotic index was used to classify intraocular melanomas (Table 158–1).

Harling and colleagues[40] reported four cases of feline limbal melanomas that closely resemble canine epibulbar melanomas. All cats were at least 8 years old, and the tumors were slow growing and locally invasive but did not metastasize.

Diffuse Feline Melanomas

In cats, the melanoma is more diffuse, involves the iris stroma, and results in infiltration of the anterior drainage angle with development of secondary glaucoma (Fig. 158–19). Neoplastic cells may be seen in the anterior chamber as well as on the anterior lens capsule. The types of tumor cells seen are predominantly anaplastic epithelioid and balloon cells. These more diffuse tumor types may spread more rapidly throughout the anterior ocular segment. Their metastatic potential is controversial.[1–3, 26, 63] The treatment of choice is enucleation.

TUMORS OF NONPIGMENTED EPITHELIAL CELLS

Patnaik and Mooney described 29 cats with feline melanomas.[60] Nineteen involved the eye; 16 of these were intraocular, and 3 were palpebral. The ciliary body and iris were involved in 12, and the average age of affected cats was 11 years. Eight intraocular tumors were described as mixed melanoma cell types, six as epithelioid, and two as spindle cell. Metastasis occurred in cats with intraocular melanomas in 63 per cent and in all cats with palpebral melanomas.

The second most frequently observed intraocular tumors are growths arising from the nonpigmented epithelium of the ciliary body and ciliary processes. These neuroepithelial tumors can be classified morphologically on the basis of whether the tumor is derived from mature neuroepithelium or primitive medullary epithelium. Tumors arising from mature neuroepithelium include adenomas and adenocarcinomas. Tumors arising from more primitive neuroepithelial tissue include medulloepitheliomas and teratoid medulloepitheliomas.*

TABLE 158–1. CLASSIFICATION OF INTRAOCULAR MELANOMAS

Histological Class	Mitotic Index*	Behavior After Enucleation
Melanocytoma	<2	0/52
Melanoma	>4	3/9 Confirmed metastasis 1/9 Suspected metastasis

*Total mitosis in 10 high-power (approximately 430×) microscopic fields.

Neuroepithelial Tumors

Neuroepithelial tumors usually are not recognized until they become large enough to be seen through the pupil. More of the tumor mass can be seen if the pupil is dilated. The growth can be deceiving because only a small amount of tumor tissue may be visible in the pupillary space while much more extensive tumor may be present in the vitreous and posterior chamber (Fig. 158–20).

Peiffer[61] reported 11 canine and 2 feline ciliary body tumors. Six in dogs were adenomas, and five were adenocarcinomas. The two reported cases in cats were adenocarcinomas. Adenocarcinomas of the ciliary body arising from the nonpigmented epithelium grow within the eye and usually do not spread from the eye. Enlarging tumors frequently grow between the iris and the lens, pushing the lens into a posteriorly subluxated position. Increasing tumor size may partially obliterate the anterior chamber, leading to secondary glaucoma and necessitating enucleation.

Histologically, the more mature tumors of neuroepithelial tissue—adenomas and adenocarcinomas—are characterized by proliferation of nonpigmented ciliary

*See references 1, 9, 10, 12, 13, 34, 37, 51, 52, and 79.

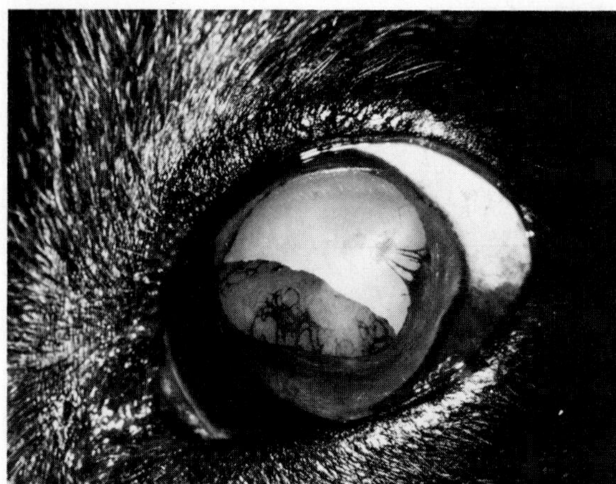

FIGURE 158–20. The second most common intraocular tumor found in dogs and cats arises from the nonpigmented epithelial tissue of the ciliary body and ciliary processes. These tumors are not usually noticed until the tumor mass is large enough to be seen through the pupil.

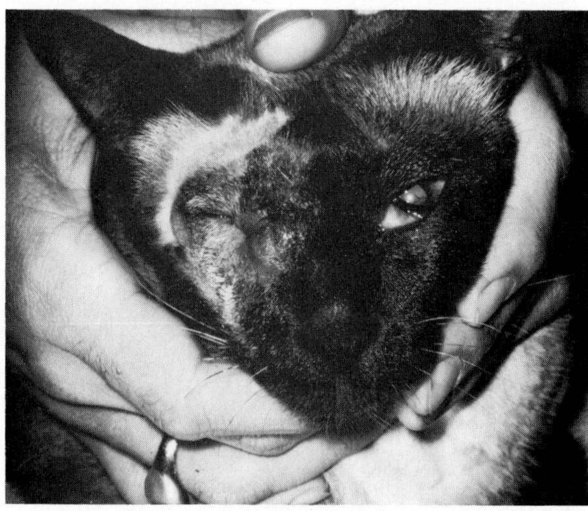

FIGURE 158–21. Lymphosarcoma involving the periorbital tissues of the right eye as well as infiltrating the uvea of the left eye in a Siamese cat. Deep biopsy of the tissue surrounding the right eye was necessary to confirm the diagnosis of lymphosarcoma.

epithelium. Cells are proliferated in the form of cords, convoluted strands, or pseudorosettes. An eosinophilic staining mucoid material within the center of the rosette may be a precursor of vitreous. Although these growths can be locally invasive, they are seldom malignant or metastatic. The more primitive neuroepithelial tumors contain multilayered sheets and tubular structures formed by elongated polarized neuroblastic cells that resemble primitive retina. The teratoid medulloepitheliomas contain structures not normally found as derivatives of the medullary epithelium of the optic cup. These include tissues containing neurons and glia resembling brain, islands of hyaline cartilage, embryonic mesenchyme, and skeletal muscle fibers. These tumors may be locally invasive, but metastasis to other areas is uncommon.[51, 52, 79] Tumors of the nonpigmented epithelium of the ciliary body are removed by enucleation.

Secondary Intraocular Tumors

The most common secondary intraocular tumor is lymphosarcoma.[23, 54, 62, 67] Immature lymphocytes commonly infiltrate the third eyelid and anterior uveal tract; infiltration may result in a greatly thickened iris and an irregular, usually miotic pupil. Hypopyon frequently develops, and a severe flare (increased protein) in the anterior chamber obscures the iris and lens from view. Deep scleral injection and conjunctival chemosis are noted. Thickening of the iris with infiltration of immature lymphocytes can lead to narrowing of the anterior drainage angle and secondary glaucoma.

Lymphocytic infiltration may also involve the posterior choroid, precipitating exudative retinal detachment and an outpouring of immature lymphocytes and protein into the vitreous cavity. Retinal hemorrhages and vitreal bleeding may also be observed. The ocular manifestations of lymphosarcoma in cats are often bilateral, although one eye may show more advanced changes (Figs. 158–21 and 158–22).[1, 23, 62, 69, 70]

Metastatic neoplasms from distant sites most commonly involve the anterior uveal tract. The most frequent tumor type is secondary adenocarcinoma, with metastasis most frequently from the kidney, thyroid, mammary gland, or nasal cavity. Diagnosis of metastatic intraocular tumor requires a careful evaluation of the animal to discover the primary tumor. Transmissible venereal tumors may also metastasize to the eye as well as orbital tissue.[1, 13] Hemangiosarcomas may metastasize to the uveal tract and result in intraocular hemorrhage and secondary glaucoma.

Cats may be afflicted with a unique form of intraocular sarcoma that may develop secondary to chronic uveitis or ocular trauma.[30] These tumors are usually spindle cell sarcomas with pluripotential cells. Tumor tissue may contain osteoid material. Peiffer and colleagues[64] reported 13 cats with intraocular sarcomas during an 8-

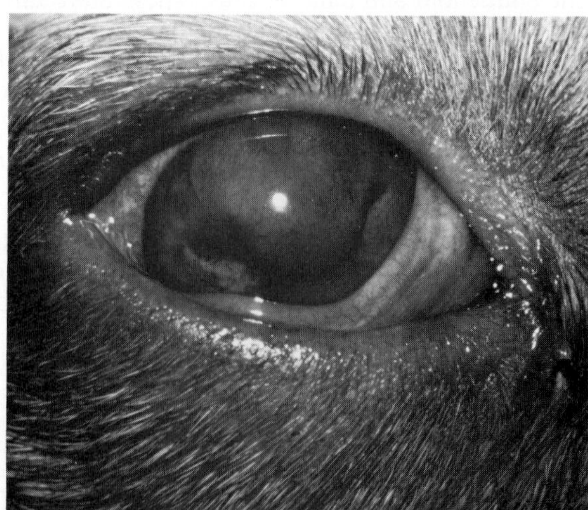

FIGURE 158–22. Anterior uveal lymphoid infiltration in a dog with lymphosarcoma. The entire uveal tract is filled with immature lymphocytes, and secondary glaucoma, uveitis, and exudative retinal detachments may be observed.

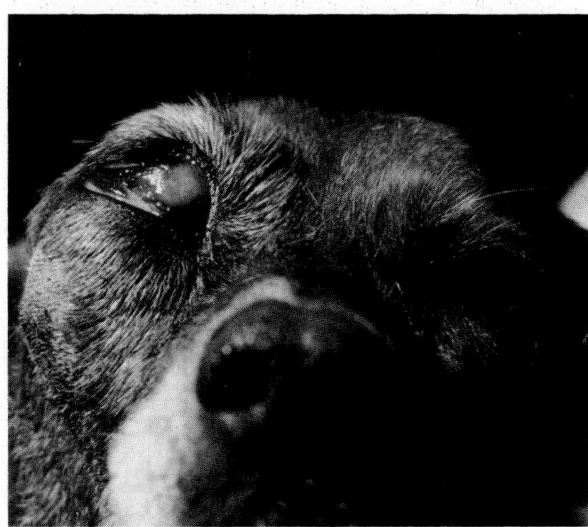

FIGURE 158–23. Severe exophthalmos caused by a rapidly growing meningioma of the optic nerve that filled the orbital cavity in a dog.

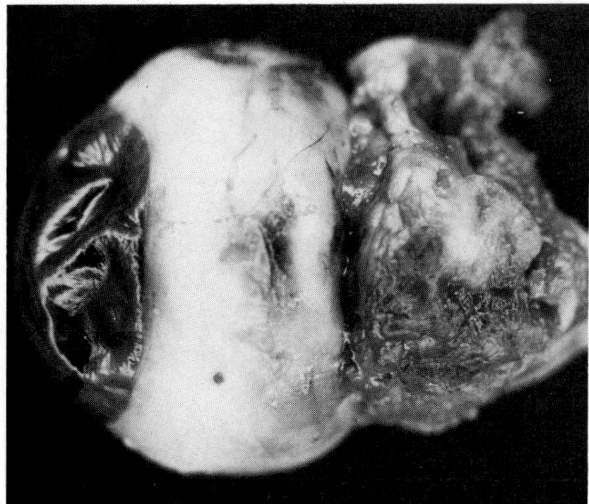

FIGURE 158–24. Meningioma of the optic nerve as shown in Figure 158–23.

year period. The mean age was 12 years. Five cats had previous trauma, and six cats had a history of chronic uveitis. These tumors are locally aggressive and frequently do metastasize to adjacent soft tissue and regional lymph nodes. Of the 12 cats in this study, 7 experienced tumor-related death. Early enucleation of globes suspected of having ocular sarcoma formation is indicated after careful evaluation for metastatic lesions.

ORBITAL TUMORS

Orbital tumors may be primary, arising from one of the many tissues within the orbit, or secondary, spreading by direct extension from the sinuses, nose, and lacrimal gland. Orbital tumors in animals are uncommon.*

Tumors arising primarily from the orbit are sarcomas and meningiomas. Sarcomas are usually anaplastic, spread diffusely, and many metastasize rapidly to regional lymph nodes and lungs. The tumors often destroy surrounding bone, producing lytic lesions visible on radiographs. These lesions often spread from the orbit into the mouth or nasal cavity.

Meningiomas are usually benign tumors originating from arachnoid cells.† They may be classified into (1) primary meningiomas that originate from intraorbital optic nerve sheath or (2) secondary meningiomas that arise within the cranium and extend into the orbit directly through bone or by extension through the optic foramen along sheaths of the optic nerve (Figs. 158–23 and 158–24).

Meningiomas have also been classified according to cell type. There is controversy about the naming of these cell types. Two types are identified: endotheliomatous and fibroblastic. Endotheliomatous meningioma is composed of polygonal epithelium-like cells with ill-defined cell borders. The cells are diffuse and arranged in elongated sheets or islands separated by scanty vascular connective tissue trabeculae. Cells are almost always present in whorls closely wrapped around one another. The whorls appear fairly frequently with a hyalinized and calcified center and are termed *psammoma bodies*. The word *psammoma* is derived from the Greek *psammos*, meaning "sand."

The tumor cells of fibroblastic meningiomas are composed of elongated fusiform cells arranged in wavy interlacing fascicles. A well-developed network of collagen and reticulin fibers is interposed between individual cells. Occasional whorls and psammoma bodies may be found.[65] Meningiomas are locally invasive but usually do not metastasize.[4, 5, 20, 43]

Secondary orbital neoplasms usually include nasal carcinoma, anaplastic sarcoma, fibrosarcoma, squamous cell carcinoma, chondrosarcoma, rhabdomyosarcoma,

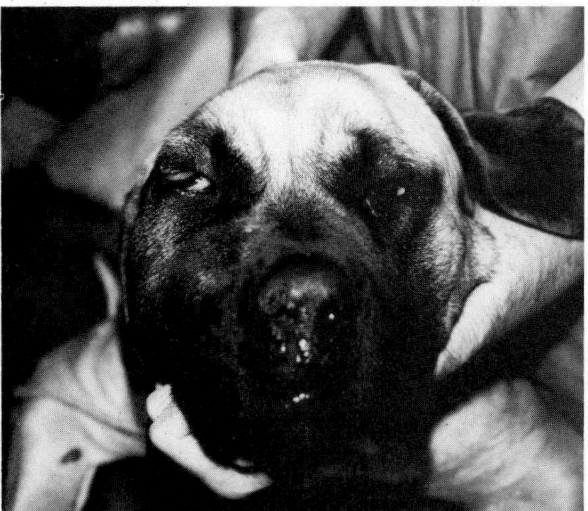

FIGURE 158–25. A 2-year-old dog with a rapidly growing periorbital and orbital mass deforming the right side of the face and compressing the right globe in the orbit. The tumor is typical of the anaplastic sarcomas that involve the periorbital area of young dogs.

---

*See references 1, 4, 5, 16, 20, 33, 38, 41–43, and 59.

†See references 4, 5, 20, 33, 38, 43, 46, and 65.

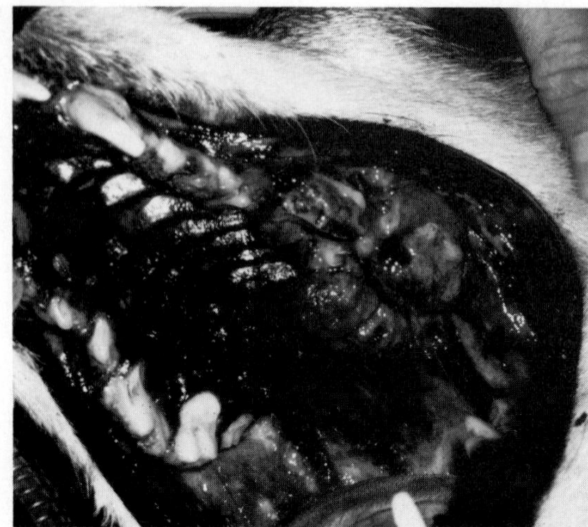

FIGURE 158–26. The anaplastic sarcoma in Figure 158–25 has grown through the mouth and destroyed large areas of the zygomatic and maxillary bones.

osteosarcoma, hemangiosarcoma, chondroma, liposarcoma, and malignant melanoma.

Primary anaplastic sarcomas of the periorbital area have been observed in a series of dogs 1 to 3 years of age. These tumors are small when first recognized but grow rapidly and metastasize early to regional lymph nodes. The cells are anaplastic, with large numbers of mitotic figures. Bone near these tumors usually undergoes lysis on radiographic examination (Figs. 158–25 and 158–26).

Orbital and retro-orbital tumors usually have the following clinical signs:

1. Slowly progressive exophthalmos. Positional deviation of the globe may develop if the tumor is outside the posterior orbital cone of muscles (e.g., tumor of zygomatic salivary gland that causes upward deviation of the globe).
2. Secondary exposure keratitis.
3. Loss of vision; dilated, unresponsive pupil.
4. Optic nerve edema, atrophy, retinal detachment.
5. Impaired mobility of the globe.
6. Protrusion of the third eyelid.

Orbital tumor can be diagnosed via a number of techniques:

1. Contrast orbital venography may demonstrate a retro-orbital vascular compressive lesion but cannot differentiate the type of mass present.
2. Ultrasonography demonstrates an abnormal mass and its extent but not its type.
3. Radiography of the orbit.
4. Retro-orbital aspiration and cytological examination.
5. Surgical exploration of the orbit. In many instances, the results of this technique allow a decision to be made about the extent of a retro-orbital mass (i.e., whether it can be surgically removed or if the orbit must be surgically exenterated).[16, 70]

Treatment of orbital neoplasms depends on the extent of the lesion, whether metastasis is present, and the tumor type.[41, 59, 68, 83]

References

1. Acland GM: Intraocular tumors in dogs and cats. *Comp Cont Educ 1*:558, 1979.
2. Acland GM, et al: Diffuse iris melanoma in cats. *J Am Vet Med Assoc 176*:52, 1980.
3. Aguirre GD, et al: Melanoma of the choroid in a dog. *J Am Anim Hosp Assoc 20*:471, 1984.
4. Andrews EJ: Clinicopathologic characteristics of meningiomas in dogs. *J Am Vet Med Assoc 163*:151, 1973.
5. Barnett KC, Kelly DF: Retrobulbar and chiasmal meningioma in a dog. *J Small Anim Pract 8*:391, 1967.
6. Barron CN, Saunders LZ: Intraocular tumors in animals. II. Primary nonpigmented intraocular tumors. *Cancer Res 19*:1171, 1959.
7. Barron CN, et al: Intraocular tumors in animals. III. Secondary intraocular tumors. *Am J Vet Res 24*:835, 1963.
8. Belkin PV: Malignant melanoma of the bulbar conjunctiva in a dog. *Vet Med Small Anim Clin 70*:957, 1975.
9. Bellhorn RW: Ciliary body adenocarcinoma in a dog. *J Am Vet Med Assoc 159*:1124, 1971.
10. Bellhorn RW: Secondary ocular adenocarcinoma in three dogs and a cat. *J Am Vet Med Assoc 160*:302, 1972.
11. Bellhorn RW: Ocular neoplasia. *In* Kirk RW (ed): *Current Veterinary Therapy VI*. W.B. Saunders, Philadelphia, 1977, pp 652–655.
12. Bellhorn RW, Henkind P: Adenocarcinoma of the ciliary body adenoma. *Pathol Vet 5*:122, 1968.
13. Bellhorn RW, Vainisis SJ: Successful removal of ciliary body adenoma. *Mod Vet Pract 50*:47, 1969.
14. Bessanich MM: Canine uveal melanomas: Series and literature review. *J Am Anim Hosp Assoc 23*:415, 1987.
15. Bevier D, Goldschmidt MH: Skin tumors in the dog: Part I. Epithelial tumors and tumorlike lesions. Part II. Tumors of soft (mesenchymal) tissues. Part III. Lymphohistiocytic and melanocytic tumors. *Comp Cont Educ 3*:389, 506, 588, 1981.
16. Bistner SI, et al: *Atlas of Veterinary Ophthalmic Surgery*. W. B. Saunders, Philadelphia, 1977.
17. Blodi FC, Ramsey FK: Ocular tumors in domestic animals. *Am J Ophthalmol 64*:627, 1967.
18. Bostock DE: Prognosis after surgical excision of canine melanomas. *Vet Pathol 16*:32, 1979.
19. Brodey RS: Canine and feline neoplasms. *Adv Vet Sci 14*:341, 1970.
20. Buyukmihci N: Oribital meningioma with intraocular invasion in a dog. Proceedings of the American College of Veterinary Ophthalmology, Las Vegas, Nev., Oct. 1976, pp 1–3.
21. Buyukmihci N, Karpinski LG: Cosmetic removal of a sebaceous adenocarcinoma of the eyelid. *Vet Med Small Anim Clin 70*:1091, 1975.
22. Carter JD: Extraocular extension of ocular melanoma. *Vet Med Small Anim Clin 70*:819, 1975.
23. Cello RM, Hutcherson B: Ocular changes in malignant lymphosarcoma of dogs. *Cornell Vet 52*:492, 1962.
24. Conroy JD: Melanocytic tumors of domestic animals. *Arch Dermatol 96*:372, 1967.
25. Cook CS, et al: Malignant melanoma of the conjunctiva in a cat. *J Am Vet Med Assoc 186*:505, 1985.
26. Cordy RH: Primary intraocular melanoma in a Siamese cat. *Vet Pathol 14*:648, 1977.
27. Cotchin E: Skin tumors of cats. *Res Vet Sci 2*:353, 1961.
28. Cottrill NB, et al: Bilateral orbital parosteal osteoma in a cat. *J Am Anim Hosp Assoc 23*:405, 1987.
29. Diters RW, et al: Primary ocular melanoma in dogs. *Vet Pathol 20*:379, 1983.
30. Dubielzig RR: Ocular sarcoma following trauma in three cats. *J Am Vet Med Assoc 184*:578, 1984.
31. Dubielzig RR: Choroidal melanomas in dogs. *Vet Pathol 22*:582, 1985.
32. Garner FM, Lingeman CH: Mast cell neoplasms of domestic cat. *Pathol Vet 7*:517, 1970.
33. Geib LW: Ossifying meningioma with extracranial metastasis in a dog. *Pathol Vet 3*:247, 1966.
34. Gelatt K: Excision of adenocarcinoma of iris and ciliary body. *J Am Anim Hosp Assoc 6*:59, 1970.
35. Gelatt KN: Histiocytoma of the eyelid of a dog. *Vet Med Small Anim Clin 70*:305, 1975.
36. Gelatt KN: Meibomian adenoma in a dog. *Vet Med Small Anim Clin 70*:962, 1975.
37. Glickstein JM, Allen HL: Malignant ciliary body adenocarcinoma in a dog. *J Am Vet Med Assoc 165*:455, 1974.
38. Gross S, et al: Tumors involving the orbit of the dog. Proceedings of the 10th Annual Meeting of the American College of Veterinary Ophthalmology, San Francisco, Nov. 1979, pp 229–240.

39. Hallstrom M: Mastocytoma of the third eyelid of a dog. *J Small Anim Pract 11*:769, 1970.
40. Harling DE, et al: Feline limbal melanoma: Four cases. *J Am Anim Hosp Assoc 22*:795, 1986.
41. Hause WR: Treatment of musculoskeletal tumors of the dog and cat, selected cases. Proceedings of the 4th Annual Kal-Kan Symposium, 1980, pp 45–51.
42. Hayden DW: Squamous cell carcinoma in a cat with intraocular and orbital metastasis. *Vet Pathol 13*:332, 1976.
43. Henderson JW: *Orbital Tumors*, 2nd ed. B. C. Decker, New York, 1980.
44. Hendy-Ibbs PM: Familial feline epibulbar dermoids. *Vet Rec 116*:13, 1985.
45. Hogan MJ, Zimmerman LE: *Ophthalmic Pathology*, 2nd ed. W. B. Saunders, Philadelphia, 1962, pp 344–466.
46. Jakobiec FA: *Ocular and Adnexal Tumors*. Aesculapius, Birmingham, 1978.
47. Kelly DF: Canine cutaneous histiocytoma: A light and electron microscopic study. *Pathol Vet 7*:12, 1970.
48. Kircher CH, et al: International histologic classification of tumors of domestic animals. Tumors of the eye and adnexa. *Bull WHO 50*:135, 1974.
49. Kircher CH, et al: Tumors of the eye and adnexia. *Bull Org Mond Sante 50*:135, 1974.
50. Krehbiel JD, Langham RF: Eyelid neoplasms of dogs. *Am J Vet Res 36*:115, 1975.
51. Lahav M, et al: Malignant teratoid medulloepithelioma in a dog. *Vet Pathol 13*:11, 1976.
52. Langloss JM, et al: Malignant intraocular teratoid medulloepithelioma in three dogs. *Vet Pathol 12*:343, 1976.
53. Lockerall GL, Slauson DO: Patterns of lymphoid infiltrate in canine histiocytoma. *J Comp Pathol 89*:193, 1979.
54. MacEwen EG, Hess PW: Canine lymphosarcoma and leukemia. *In* Kirk RW (ed): *Current Veterinary Therapy VI*. W. B. Saunders, Philadelphia, 1977, pp 473–479.
55. Madewell BR, et al: Sunlight-skin cancer association in the dog. *J Cutan Pathol 8*:434, 1981.
56. Magrane WG: Tumors of the eye and orbit in the dog. *J Small Anim Pract 6*:165, 1965.
57. Martin CL: Canine epibulbar melanomas and their management. Proceedings of the 10th Annual Meeting of the American College of Veterinary Ophthalmology, Nov. 1979, pp 113–139.
58. Morgan G: Ocular tumors in animals. *J Small Anim Pract 10*:563, 1969.
59. Owen LN: Biological behavior and therapy of osteosarcoma in the dog. Proceedings of the 4th Kal-Kan Symposium, 1980, pp 59–62.
60. Patnaik AK, Mooney S: Feline melanoma: A comparative study of ocular, oral, and dermal neoplasms. *Vet Pathol 25*:105, 1988.
61. Peiffer RL: Ciliary body epithelial tumors in the dog and cat; a review of thirteen cases. *J Small Animal Pract 24*:347, 1983.
62. Peiffer RL, et al: Lymphosarcoma, small lymphocyte type, with ocular manifestations in a dog. *J Canine Pract 3*:50, 1976.
63. Peiffer RL Jr, et al: Malignant melanoma of the iris and ciliary body in cat. *Mod Vet Pract 58*:854, 1977.
64. Peiffer RL, et al: Primary ocular sarcomas in the cat. *Small Anim Pract 29*:105, 1988.
65. Russell DS, Rubinstein LJ: Tumors of meninges and related tissues. *In Pathology of Tumors of the Nervous System*. 3rd ed. Williams & Wilkins, Baltimore, 1972, pp 50–52.
66. Ryan AM, Diters RW: Clinical and pathologic features of canine ocular melanomas. *J Am Vet Med Assoc 184*:60, 1984.
67. Saunders LZ, Barron CN: Intraocular tumours in animals. IV. Lymphosarcoma. *Br Vet J 120*:25, 1964.
68. Saunders LZ, Barron CN: Primary pigmented intraocular tumors in animals. *Cancer Res 18*:234, 1958.
69. Saunders LZ, Rubin LF: *Ophthalmic Pathology of Animals*. S. Karger, New York, 1975, pp 232–233.
70. Slatter DH: *Fundamentals of Veterinary Ophthalmology*. 2nd ed. W. B. Saunders, Philadelphia, 1990.
71. Stannard AA, Pulley TL: Tumors of the skin and soft tissues. *In* Moulton JE (ed): *Tumors in Domestic Animals*. 2nd ed. University of California Press, Berkeley, 1978, pp 16–74.
72. Strafuss AC: Basal cell tumors in dogs. *J Am Vet Med Assoc 169*:322, 1976.
73. Strafuss AC: Sebaceous gland carcinomas in dogs. *J Am Vet Med Assoc 169*:325, 1976.
74. Swanson JF, Dubelzig RR: Ocular tumors. *In* Withrow SJ, MacEwen EG (eds): *Clinical Veterinary Oncology*. J. B. Lippincott, Philadelphia, 1989.
75. Szymanski C: Multiple myeloma with hyperviscosity syndrome in a dog. Proceedings of the Annual Meeting of the American College of Veterinary Ophthalmology, Las Vegas, Nev., Oct. 1976, pp 143–145.
76. Tams TR, Macy DW: Canine mast cell tumors. *Comp Cont Educ 3*:869, 1981.
77. Taylor DON, et al: Morphologic and biologic characteristics of the canine cutaneous histiocytoma. *Cancer Res 29*:83, 1969.
78. Trucksa R, McLean I: Intraocular canine melanomas. Proceedings of the 12th Annual Meeting of the American College of Veterinary Ophthalmology, 1981, pp 103–114.
79. Verwer MAJ, Thije PA: Tumor of the epithelium of the ciliary body in a dog. *J Small Anim Pract 8*:627, 1967.
80. Weisse I, et al: Benign melanoma of the choroid in a beagle: Ophthalmological, light and electron microscopical investigations. *Vet Pathol 22*:586, 1985.
81. Wilcock BP, Peiffer RL Jr: Morphology and behavior of primary ocular melanomas in 91 dogs. *Vet Pathol 23*:418, 1986.
82. Yanoff M, Fine B: *Ocular Pathology*. Harper & Row, Hagerstown, MD, 1975, pp 619–685.
83. Ziegler JL (ed): *Sarcomas of Soft Tissue and Bone in Childhood*. National Cancer Institute Monograph, 56, NIH Publication 81–2162, Bethesda, MD, 1981.

CHAPTER 159 Reproductive Systems

Shirley D. Johnston

Tumors of the female and male reproductive organs of companion animals comprise those of the ovaries, uterus, vagina and vestibule, mammary glands, testes, prostate, and penis. Canine and feline mammary tumors and canine testicular tumors are among the most common neoplasms in these species and are ones in which knowledge of tumor type, behavior, treatment options, and prognosis is essential for optimal management of patients. Tumors of the canine ovaries and prostate are common and often pose both diagnostic and therapeutic challenges. The World Health Organization (WHO) clinical staging of animal tumors of the reproductive tract based on character of the primary tumor (T), lymph nodes (N), and presence of distant metastasis (M) (Tables 159–1 and 159–2) is recommended as a diagnostic guide for assessing these tumors in clinical patients and for trying to accumulate standardized data for future conclusions on optimal treatment and survival time.[210]

TABLE 159–1. WORLD HEALTH ORGANIZATION CLINICAL STAGES OF CANINE TUMORS OF THE FEMALE REPRODUCTIVE ORGANS

	Site of Primary Tumor		
	Ovary	*Uterus*	*Vulva and Vagina*
T: Primary tumor			
T_0	No evidence of T	No evidence of T	No evidence of T
T_1	T limited to one ovary	Small noninvasive T	T ≤ 1 cm in its main dimension, superficial
T_2	T limited to both ovaries	Large or invasive T	T > 1 cm and < 3 cm in main dimension, minimal infiltration
T_3	T extending into ovarian bursa	T invading neighboring structures	T > 3 cm or deep infiltration present
T_4			T infiltrating neighboring structures
N: Regional lymph nodes	[Sublumbar]	[Lumbar, iliac, sacral]	[Inguinal, iliac, sacral]
N_0	No regional LN involved	No regional LN involved	No regional LN involved
N_1	Regional LN involved	Regional LN involved	Movable unilateral nodes
N_2		Juxtaregional LN involved	Movable bilateral nodes
N_3			Fixed nodes
M: Distant metastasis			
M_0	No evidence of distant metastasis	No evidence of distant metastasis	No evidence of distant metastasis
M_1	Evidence of metastasis	Evidence of metastasis	Distant metastasis present
M_{1a}	In the peritoneal cavity	In the peritoneal cavity	
M_{1b}	Beyond the peritoneal cavity	Beyond the peritoneal cavity	
M_{1c}	Both peritoneal cavity and beyond	In and beyond the peritoneal cavity	

T, tumor; LN, lymph nodes.
From World Health Organization: Internal Report of the Second WHO Consultation on the Biological Behaviour and Therapy of Tumours of Domestic Animals, Geneva, 1979 (unpublished WHO document VPH/CMO/79.17).

TABLE 159–2. WORLD HEALTH ORGANIZATION CLINICAL STAGES OF CANINE MAMMARY TUMORS

T: Primary tumor	
T_0	No evidence of T
T_1	T < 5 cm maximum diameter
T_2	T 5 to 10 cm maximum diameter
T_3	T 11–15 cm maximum diameter; muscle fixation
T_4	T > 15 cm maximum diameter; whole gland involved; infiltration of underlying tissue
N: Regional lymph nodes (RLN) (axillary, superficial inguinal)	
N_0	No regional LN involved
N_1	Ipsilateral regional LN involved
N_2	Bilateral regional LN involved
N_3	Distant LN involved
NR	LN previously removed
M: Distant metastasis	
M_0	No evidence of lung metastasis
M_1	Solitary lung metastasis
M_2	Multiple lung metastasis
M_3	Other nonlung sites of metastasis
M_4	Solitary or multiple lung metastasis and other nonlung metastatic sites

T, tumor; LN, lymph nodes.
From World Health Organization: Internal Report of the Second WHO Consultation on the Biological Behaviour and Therapy of Tumours of Domestic Animals, Geneva, 1979 (unpublished WHO document VPH/CMO/79.17).

Female

OVARIAN NEOPLASIA

Incidence

The incidence of spontaneously occurring ovarian neoplasia is low; primary ovarian tumors were reported in 38 of 4,067 (0.9 per cent) canine patients with neoplasia and in 4 of 1,153 (0.3 per cent) feline patients with neoplasia.* In dogs, ovarian tumors occur with equal frequency in the right and left ovaries and occasionally in both.[48, 162] Although granulosa cell tumors occur in patients as young as one 14-month-old golden retriever and a 6-month-old domestic shorthair cat, risk increases with age, especially for epithelial tumors (Table 159–3).[37, 67, 82, 186] In 71 ovarian neoplasms, median ages of dogs with different tumor types were similar, and all were more than 10 years old, except for a mean age of 4 years in seven animals with teratomas. Mean age of 18 cats with ovarian neoplasia was 6.9 years (range 0.17 to 20 years).[67] A statistically significant increased risk was noted in pointers for epithelial ovarian tumors and in English bulldogs for granulosa-theca tumors in 94 cases, although each breed had only three animals with the tumor.[82] Mongrels have a decreased risk of malignant ovarian tumors and about the same risk as purebreds for benign tumors of the ovaries.

Ovarian tumors may arise from epithelial, gonadal-stromal, or germ cell tissue in the ovary (see Table 159–3); primary mesodermal tumors or metastatic tumors

*See references 28, 43, 45, 47, 83, 146, and 147.

TABLE 159–3. INCIDENCE OF OVARIAN TUMOR TYPE IN BITCHES AND QUEENS

Ovarian Tumors Reported in Companion Animals	Tumor Occurrence in Bitches							Tumor Occurrence in Queens			
	Dow [55]	Cotchin [48]	Norris, et al.[150]	Hayes and Young [83]	Patnaik and Greenlee[162]	Total, Canine		Nielsen[148]	Gelberg and McEntee [67]	Total, Feline	
Epithelial origin							(46%)				(9%)
Adenoma/cystadenoma	10	20	20	23	12	85		1	1	2	
Adenocarcinoma/ cystadenocarcinoma	1	7	3	32	21	64		1		1	
Undifferentiated			10			10					
Gonadal-stromal origin							(34%)				(59%)
Granulosa cell tumor	13	30	15	22	12	92		5	9	14	
Granulosa-theca cell tumor											
Thecoma				1		1					
Luteoma		1				1			5	5	
Sertoli cell tumor			6		12	18					
Unspecified			5			5					
Germ cell origin							(12%)				(28%)
Dysgerminoma		8	11	2	7	28		6		6	
Teratoma		1	2	4	1	8		2	1	3	
Teratocarcinoma				1	6	7					
Mesodermal origin							(4%)				
Mixed mesodermal			1			1					
Leiomyoma			1	1		2					
Fibroma	1			2		3					
Sarcoma, undifferentiated		2	4	2		8					
Metastatic origin							(4%)				(3%)
Lymphosarcoma	2					2					
Uterine adenocarcinoma			1			1		1		1	
Mammary adenocarcinoma	1		3			4					
Skin tumor, unspecified			1			1					
Transmissible venereal tumor			1			1					
Unclassified				4		4					
Totals:	28	69	84	94	71	346		10	22	32	

also occur.[10] Occurrence, pattern of metastasis, and ability of the tumor to secrete ovarian hormones are influenced by the tissue of origin. Tumors of epithelial cell origin are most common in bitches, and gonadal-stromal origin in queens. The granulosa cell tumor is the single most common ovarian tumor of both species.

Size of ovarian tumors in dogs ranges from less than 1 to 15,000 cm^3, and in cats from less than 1 to more than 1,000 cm^3 (Fig. 159–1).[67, 162] Twenty-nine per cent of 71 canine ovarian tumors metastasized, with highest rates (48 to 50 per cent) in adenocarcinomas and teratocarcinomas; distant metastasis was more common in the latter.[67] Six of 22 ovarian neoplasms in cats metastasized. Granulosa cell tumors may produce estrogen, progesterone, or both, leading to paraneoplastic syndromes of persistent estrus, estrogen-induced pancytopenia, cystic endometrial hyperplasia, or pyometra. Persistent estrus occurs in queens with dysgerminomas or granulosa cell tumors.[67]

Ovarian fibromas were observed in 12 of 92 bitches treated with mibolerone, a synthetic androgen used for estrus suppression, for more than 9 years in an experimental trial; tumors were not observed in 60 control bitches or in 55 bitches treated with three to five times the efficacious dose of mibolerone used for estrus suppression.[179] Thirteen of 13 bitches treated with injections of 15 to 60 mg of diethylstilbestrol in oil every 4 to 6 weeks (90 to 495 mg total dose) developed ovarian neoplasia, most of which were papillary carcinomas; 9 of these bitches developed metastases. Hormonal withdrawal from five affected dogs was followed, 10.5 to 14.5 months later, by regression of the tumors.[98, 99]

Diagnosis

Ovarian tumors may be diagnosed at ovariohysterectomy if small and benign or may be associated with signs of a palpable and sometimes painful abdominal mass, persistent estrus, aplastic anemia, or pyometra. Other signs may be referable to metastasis of malignant neoplasms, which may spread to abdominal, thoracic, and central nervous system locations. A complete physical and neurological examination, a hemogram, abdominal and thoracic radiography, and ovarian and uterine ultrasonography are indicated for patients suspected of having ovarian neoplasia. If functional neoplasia is suspected, vaginal cytological study to look for cornification (an indicator of estrogen secretion) and serum progesterone measurement for values exceeding 2 ng/ml are indicated.

Ovarian tumors are staged clinically (see Table 159–1).[210] Regional lymph nodes are the sublumbar nodes.

Adenoma/Cystadenoma

Ovarian adenomas are some of the most common primary ovarian tumors in bitches. They range in diameter from a few millimeters to more than 10 cm. A

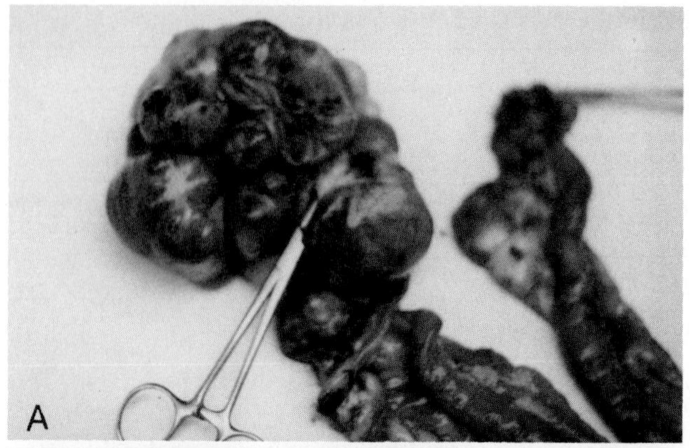

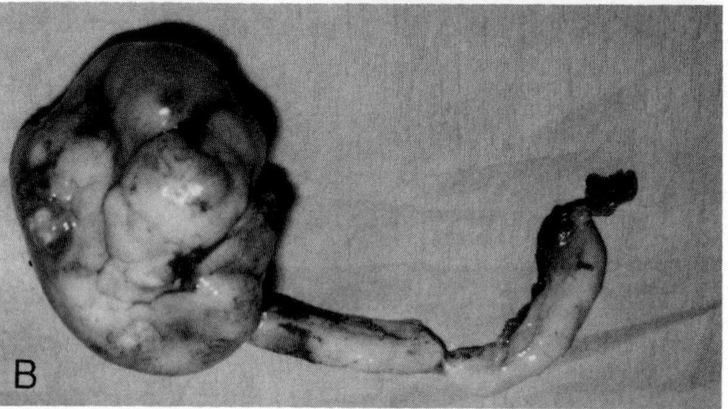

FIGURE 159–1. Gross appearance of ovarian neoplasia of the right ovaries of an 11-year-old female English setter with a cystadenocarcinoma *(A)* and a 4-year-old female domestic long-haired cat with a granulosa cell tumor *(B)*.

bilateral cystadenoma, with the tumor in the left ovary measuring 7.5 × 5.2 × 4.5 cm, has been described in queens.[67] Ovarian epithelial proliferation, neoplasia, and metastasis can be induced by prolonged estrogen administration in dogs, but the role of endogenous estrogen in spontaneously occurring tumors is unknown.[158] In 29 spontaneous ovarian adenomas in bitches, age at diagnosis ranged from 6 to 14 years, and 8 of 11 patients were nulliparous.[48, 55, 113, 162] Five of 12 bitches with unilateral adenoma of the ovary had a contralateral cystic ovary.[162] Of seven, six had abdominal distension, three vomited, and one had abdominal pain on palpation. Because four of these animals had pyometra and ten had cystic endometrial hyperplasia, hormonal function was attributed to the cystadenomas, although these changes are common in all old, intact female dogs.[48, 162] One cystadenoma described in a 9-year-old cat occurred with a lipoma in the presence of signs of persistent estrus, virilization, and cystic endometrial hyperplasia.[149] Diagnosis is by histopathological examination after excision.

Adenocarcinoma/Cystadenocarcinoma

Ovarian adenocarcinoma or cystadenocarcinoma usually occurs in bitches older than 9 years.[162] Metastases to omentum, sublumbar lymph nodes, liver, and lungs are described in approximately half the cases.[48, 55, 71, 162] Clinical signs include an enlarged abdomen, ascites, and hydrothorax when metastases are present in the liver and lungs. This tumor is rare in cats but has been described in a 5-year-old queen with an abdominal mass, ascites, and hair loss; metastases were present throughout the pelvis and in the peritoneum, liver, and lungs.[149]

Granulosa Cell Tumor

The granulosa cell tumor, which arises from ovarian sex cords, is the most common primary ovarian tumor in dogs and cats (see Fig. 159–1). Age at diagnosis ranges from 14 months to 16 years in dogs (median age 12 years in 12 cases) and 6 months to 20 years in cats (mean age 7.9 years in 8 cases).* Tumors are as large as 15 × 22 × 28 cm, may weigh 4.7 kg in dogs, and may reach 5 cm in diameter in cats.[11, 67] In one survey, 10 of 13 bitches with this tumor were nulliparous.[55] Common clinical signs include abdominal distension and the presence of a palpable abdominal mass. Functional tumors may produce estrogens (leading to vulvar enlargement, sanguineous vulvar discharge, persistent estrus, alopecia, or aplastic pancytopenia), progesterone (leading to cystic endometrial hyperplasia/pyometra complex), or both.[48, 82, 123, 149, 150] Metastases occurred in about 20 per cent of affected dogs and in 10 of 17 affected cats.† Metastasis occurs by direct extension to the liver, spleen, kidneys, pancreas, adrenals, gastrointestinal tract, and uterus and by lymphatic/hematogenous spread to mesenteric and bronchial lymph nodes, meninges, and cerebrum.‡ One bilateral and one extraovarian granulosa cell tumor have been reported in cats.[13, 149]

Thecoma

Thecomas originate from ovarian stromal tissue. An 8 × 10-cm thecoma was removed from the left ovary of

*See references 6, 37, 55, 67, 126, 150, and 162.
†See references 4, 13, 14, 67, 149, and 162.
‡See references 4, 6, 13, 14, 37, 57, and 67.

a 10-year-old toy poodle with a history of depression, vomiting, and anestrus for 18 months.[61]

Sertoli Cell Tumor

Ovarian tumors arising from sex cord stroma demonstrate a histological pattern similar to that of Sertoli cell tumors of the testes. Eighteen were described among 155 canine ovarian neoplasms, and one was found in a cat.[93, 150, 162] Tumors occurred in dogs 9 to 15 years of age, and metastasis was present in one. One anaplastic Sertoli-Leydig tumor was 15,000 cm^3.[162] In nine bitches in which the uterus was examined histologically, cystic endometrial hyperplasia was present, and two bitches had a contralateral cystic ovary. One bitch had signs of prolonged estrus, two had purulent vaginal discharge, one had alopecia, and two had mammary carcinomas. The feline ovarian Sertoli cell tumor occurred in the right ovary of a 6-year-old domestic shorthaired queen with cystic endometrial hyperplasia; there was no evidence of metastasis.[93]

Dysgerminoma

Dysgerminomas are malignant tumors arising from undifferentiated germ cells of the ovary; they are comparable to seminomas in males. They constitute about 8 per cent of canine and almost 20 per cent of feline ovarian tumors.* Tumor diameter may range from 2 to 30 cm in dogs and from 1 to 9 cm in cats. Dysgerminomas affected dogs from 5 to 20 years of age and cats from 1 to 17 years of age.[34, 50, 67, 96, 189, 198] Bilateral dysgerminomas have been reported in both dogs and cats, but most are unilateral; 20 to 30 per cent metastasize to adjacent peritoneum, adrenals, kidneys, mesenteric lymph nodes, pancreas, liver, or mediastinal nodes.†

Teratoma (Dermoid Cyst)

Teratomas are germ cell tumors that show somatic differentiation beyond the primordial germ cell stage into masses with three germ layers (ectoderm, mesoderm, entoderm). They have been called *dermoid cysts* because the masses typically include cysts lined by hair and keratinized squamous epithelium; they often contain sebaceous fluid, sweat glands, cartilage, fat, muscle fiber, bone, nervous tissue, connective tissue, teeth, and glandular epithelium. These tumors arise from the gonads of young animals and may originate in the embryonic or fetal stage of development.[65] Age range at diagnosis of dogs with this tumor is 1 to 11 years, and in cats 2 to 6 years.‡

Tumor diameter varies from 2 to 30 cm in dogs and to as much as 15 cm in cats.[38, 50, 72, 73, 173, 187] Clinical signs include abdominal enlargement with a palpable mass, weight loss, anorexia, and vomiting. Some patients are asymptomatic or are presented for pregnancy diagnosis after breeding when their abdomen appears enlarged.[208] Radiographically, these tumors are the most likely of all primary ovarian tumors to demonstrate calcific densities.

*See references 34, 48, 50, 67, 72, 150, 162, and 185.
†See references 12, 50, 67, 72, 101, 118, 162, 183, and 189.
‡See references 25, 38, 50, 51, 65, 72, 73, 103, 173, 187, and 208.

Teratocarcinoma

Teratocarcinomas are undifferentiated teratomas containing both mature and embryonal elements; they frequently show radiographic calcific densities and may weigh as much as 5 kg.[163] They are much less common than teratomas but have been reported in 11 bitches ranging from 2 to 10 years of age.[49, 73, 162, 163] Metastases occurred to the adjacent omentum, regional lymph nodes, pancreas, lung, mediastinum, peripheral lymph nodes, ulna, olecranon, and tibial crest. Clinical signs included abdominal enlargement, depression, anorexia, weight loss, and lameness with bone metastases.

Treatment and Prognosis

Ovariohysterectomy is the treatment of choice for patients with ovarian neoplasia, because some ovarian tumors are bilateral, tumor extension to the uterus can occur, and cystic endometrial hyperplasia leading to pyometra is common in aging females in which primary ovarian tumors occur. Excision of the tumor and affected ovary alone may be indicated in young, valuable purebred patients with an ovarian mass strongly suggestive of a teratoma (large tumor with calcific densities, no evidence of metastasis or sex steroid secretion by the tumor); one such dog was able to reproduce successfully after tumor excision.[208] Care is taken not to rupture fluid-filled cysts during surgery, because peritoneal implantation of tumor cells from such fluid may occur. The prognosis is favorable with benign tumors without aplastic anemia but poor with metastasis or bone marrow suppression.

Chemotherapy of dogs with metastatic adenocarcinomas or granulosa cell tumors has been reported, although little information is available on its short- or long-term effectiveness. Cyclophosphamide (2.2 mg/kg PO once daily while the white blood cell count exceeds 2,000/cm^3) has been recommended for metastatic ovarian tumors.[27] One dog with metastatic ovarian papillary cystadenocarcinoma in the thorax and peritoneal cavity was treated with oral cyclophosphamide (50 mg/m^2) on days 1, 3, and 5 of each week and oral chlorambucil (8 mg/m^2) on days 2 and 4 for 3.5 months until the onset of hemorrhagic cystitis. The dog was then treated with chlorambucil and 1-(2-chloroethyl)-3-cyclohexyl-1-nitrosourea (CCNU), 130 mg/m^2 PO at 6-week intervals, decreasing to a dose of 90 mg/m^2 over 4.5 months. This second regimen was discontinued 8 months after the original diagnosis because of repeated neutropenia and septicemia. The dog was asymptomatic for 2 months thereafter. Intraperitoneal administration of triethylenethiophosphoramide (0.4 to 0.8 mg/kg) has been recommended after paracentesis to control malignant intraperitoneal effusions.[82] Immunotherapy of metastatic canine ovarian cancer with mixed bacterial toxins also has been advocated.[82]

UTERINE TUBE (OVIDUCT) NEOPLASIA

Tumors of the uterine tube reported in pathological surveys of bitches include a papillary cystadenoma of the mesovarium, a cauliflower-like adenoma, an adenocarcinoma with implantation to the peritoneal cavity, and a lipoma of the ovarian bursa.[43, 124] Tumors of this organ are rare (2 in a survey of 4,187 canine neoplasms), and no information is available on signalment, history, tumor behavior, or suggested treatment. Tumors of the uterine tube have not been reported in cats.

UTERINE NEOPLASIA

Incidence

Uterine tumors accounted for 11 of 3,073 (0.36 per cent) and 9 of 2,361 (0.31 per cent) canine tumors from all organs, and 9 of 776 (1.2 per cent) and 11 of 1,086 (1.0 per cent) canine tumors of the reproductive organs in surveys in the United States and Great Britain.[29, 44, 47] Single cases of feline uterine neoplasia have been reported in surveys of 464, 372, and 256 tumor cases (0.2 to 0.4 per cent) and in 1 of 68 cases (1.5 per cent) of tumors of the feline reproductive organs.[45, 47, 57, 176] Uterine tumors occurred in dogs and cats from 5 to 12 years of age.

Uterine tumor types in companion animals include those of epithelial (adenoma, adenocarcinoma) and mesenchymal (fibroma, fibrosarcoma, leiomyoma, leiomyosarcoma, lipoma, and lymphosarcoma) origin.* The most common of these in bitches is leiomyoma, which accounted for 10 of 11 and 7 of 9 primary uterine tumors in two surveys.[29, 142] German shepherd bitches with hereditary dermatofibrosis show a high incidence of uterine leiomyomas and multifocal renal cystadenocarcinomas.[138] Although rare, other primary uterine tumor types, such as adenocarcinomas, may occur and metastasize in bitches.[199] Endometrial adenocarcinoma is the most common feline uterine tumor, and uterine leiomyomas, leiomyosarcomas, and fibromas have also been described.[182] Endometrial adenocarcinoma in cats may metastasize to the peritoneum, mesentery, ovaries, regional lymph nodes, adrenal glands, liver, diaphragm, lungs, brain, and eyes.[17, 18, 128, 157, 166]

Diagnosis

Clinical signs in animals with uterine neoplasia depend on tumor type, size, and pattern of metastasis, if any. In dogs, signs of illness are rare and are referable to site of metastasis, if present, as in one case with hemorrhage into the pericardial sac after tumor metastasis to the myocardium.[199] Cats may have an intermittent cough after spread of a uterine tumor to the thorax and may suffer blindness with motor incoordination after metastasis to the central nervous system.[17, 157, 166]

Because uterine tumors are rare and often benign, diagnosis is generally made at ovariohysterectomy or necropsy. Some uterine masses are detected by abdominal palpation or radiographic/ultrasonographic examination of the uterus in patients suspected of having pyometra (Fig. 159–2).[164] The uterus of cats and dogs generally cannot be identified ultrasonographically unless it contains fluid, a fetus, or a neoplastic mass. Pyometra is common in aged intact bitches and queens

*See references 29, 43, 47, 59, 60, 70, 107, 124, 142, and 151.

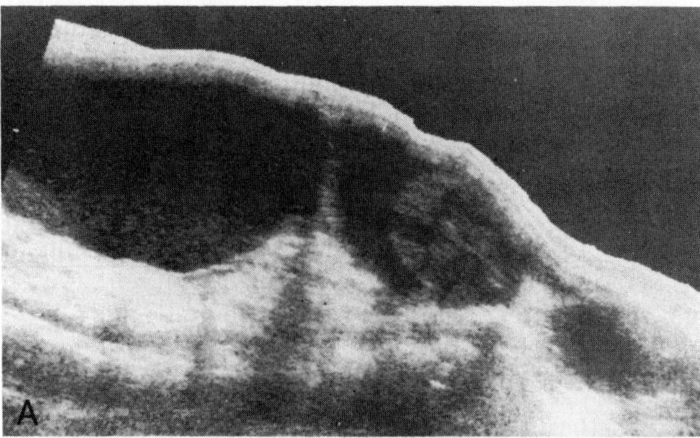

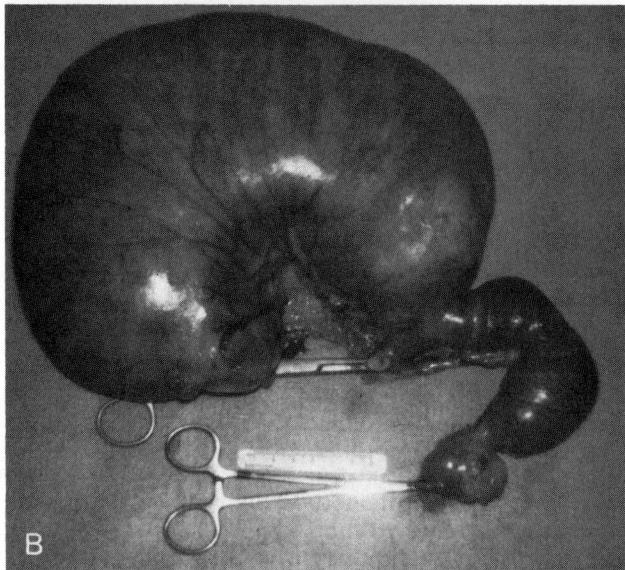

FIGURE 159–2. Ultrasonographic *(A)* and gross *(B)* appearance of a uterine leiomyoma in the left uterine horn of an 11-year-old female miniature poodle. (*A*, from Feeney DA, Johnston GR: *Textbook of Veterinary Diagnostic Radiology.* W. B. Saunders, Philadelphia, 1986, p 462.)

and may be a concurrent finding unrelated to the presence of a primary uterine tumor.[54]

Uterine tumors in bitches and queens may be staged according to the protocol shown in Table 159–1, which is based on behavior of the primary tumor (T), regional lymph node involvement (N), and the presence of metastasis (M).[210] The regional lymph nodes draining the uterus are the lumbar, internal and external iliac, and sacral nodes.

Treatment and Prognosis

Ovariohysterectomy with routine aftercare is the treatment of choice for canine and feline patients with primary uterine neoplasia, following abdominal and thoracic radiography to seek evidence of metastatic disease. These tumors generally occur in older animals, and malignant tumors consist of multifocal nodules, suggesting complete hysterectomy. Chemotherapy may be considered after surgery for patients with metastasis and should be chosen on the basis of tumor type. The prognosis is excellent for patients with leiomyomas or other benign tumors and poor for those with metastatic disease.

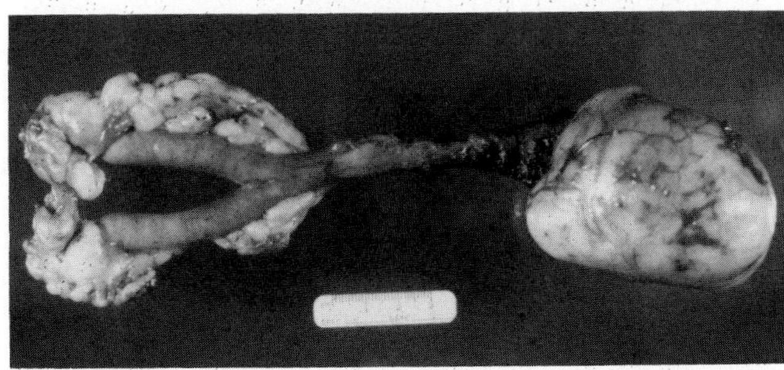

FIGURE 159–3. Leiomyoma of the vagina of a 13-year-old female miniature poodle.

VAGINAL NEOPLASIA

Incidence

Vaginal and vestibular tumors are the most common female reproductive neoplasms in bitches, excluding those of the mammary gland; 123 were reported in a survey of 191 genital tumors from 4,187 tumors from all sites. No feline vaginal tumors were reported in three studies comprising 1,115 tumors from all sites,[45, 57, 176] although single cases of vaginal neoplasia have been reported.[108, 207, 209]

Most canine vaginal tumors are leiomyomas (Fig. 159–3) and transmissible venereal tumors (Fig. 159–4). Of 205 cases of vaginal neoplasia in three reports, 146 (71 per cent) were leiomyomas.[29, 112, 191] In 99 cases of vaginal neoplasia, vaginal leiomyomas, fibromas, and polyps were classified together because they are derived from the smooth muscle of the vulva or vagina and differ only in amount of fibrous connective tissue.[191] Transmissible venereal tumors account for 19 of the remaining 59 cases, followed by leiomyosarcomas (13), lipomas (9), squamous cell carcinomas (4), nerve sheath tumors (3), fibrous histiocytomas (2), and single cases of benign melanoma, myxoma, myxofibroma, hemangiosarcoma, osteosarcoma, adenocarcinoma, mast cell sarcoma, transitional cell carcinoma, and epidermoid carcinoma. Vaginal fibrosarcoma, reticulum cell sarcoma, and lymphosarcoma also occur in dogs,[43, 94, 124, 142] vaginal leiomyoma (and fibroma) in cats.[108, 194, 207, 209]

Age of animals with vaginal tumors ranges from 2 to 18 years and depends on tumor type.[191] Transmissible venereal tumors, which are transmitted at copulation and by close contact, occur in younger bitches than other vaginal tumor types. In 185 cases of canine vaginal neoplasia, average ages of dogs with transmissible venereal tumors and leiomyomas were 4.2 and 10.8 years,

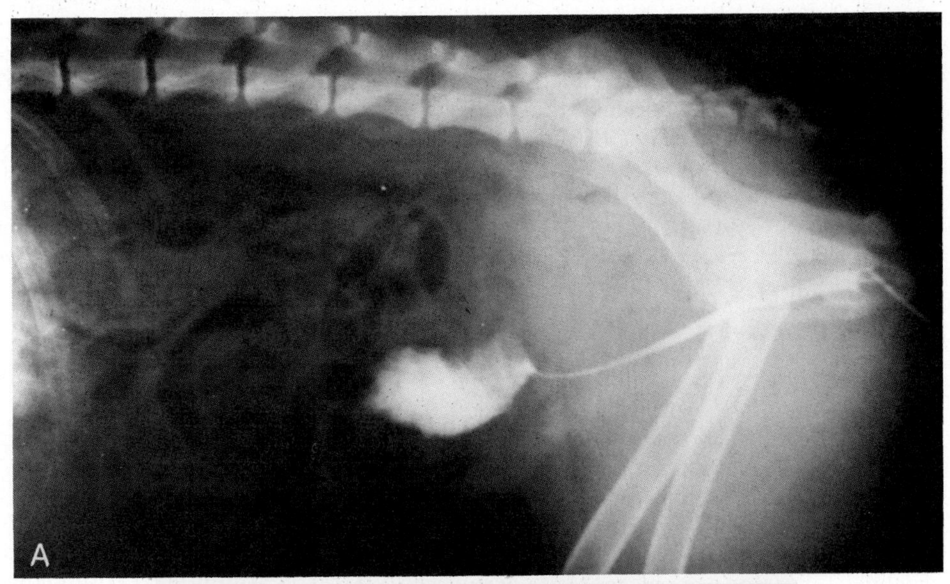

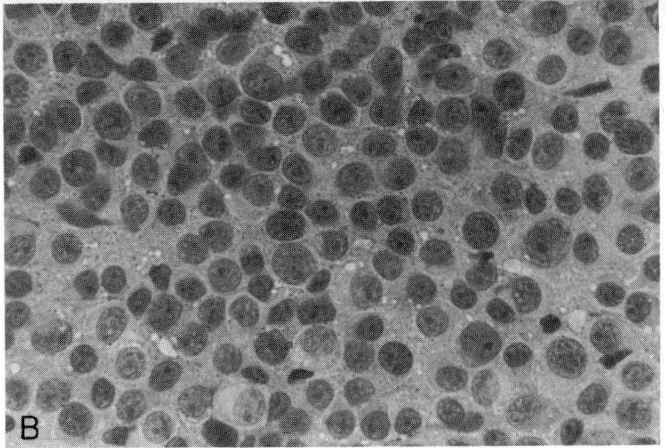

FIGURE 159–4. Radiographic *(A)* and histological *(B)* appearance of a transmissible venereal tumor encircling the cranial vagina and impinging on the urinary bladder of a 4-year-old mixed-breed dog.

respectively.[112, 191] The boxer, poodle, and German shepherd had the highest incidence; proportions of animals of these breeds in the populations were not provided. Vaginal leiomyomas have been reported in two female cats, ages 8 and 14 years.[209]

Vaginal tumors may occur in sexually intact and spayed bitches. Because leiomyomas have been reported in guinea pigs given exogenous estrogen and because the vagina is a target tissue for sex steroids during the normal reproductive cycle, some investigators have suggested that vaginal leiomyomas in bitches are hormonally induced.[112, 191, 205] Occurrence of this tumor in both spayed and intact bitches argues against this hypothesis, as does the observation that this tumor is not associated significantly with estrous irregularity.[29] There is no evidence that ovariohysterectomy prevents development of malignant vaginal neoplasia or improves prognosis. Intact bitches may be at greater risk for vaginal transmissible venereal tumor via copulation than spayed bitches, but both groups can acquire the tumor by implantation to the skin or nasopharynx.[9]

Metastases from vaginal tumors are rare, because most are benign. Leiomyosarcomas spread to the regional lymph nodes, spleen, lungs, and spinal cord[29, 86] and may recur after surgical excision without metastasizing.[29] Transmissible venereal tumors metastasized in 5 of 385 (1.3 per cent) animals in an experimental transplantation study;[110] the frequency of metastasis in spontaneous disease is unknown. Cells from transmissible venereal tumors may spread by transplantation to the skin, lip, nasal passages, tongue, pharynx, and tonsils; by direct extension to the cervix, uterus, and uterine tubes; or by hematogenous/lymphatic spread to regional lymph nodes, intestine, spleen, liver, lungs, and central nervous system.*

Diagnosis

Vaginal tumors range in diameter from 2 to 20 cm in bitches and 2 to 8 cm in queens.[29, 86, 209] The location of tumors within the vestibule and vagina in 49 dogs[191] included the vulvar lips or vestibule (16), vulvar/vaginal roof (15), vulvar/vaginal floor (9), perineal/perivulvar region (7), and cervix (2). No correlation is noted between location of vaginal masses and histological type in dogs.

Clinical signs of vaginal neoplasia include bulging of the perineum, prolapse of tissue from the vulva, dysuria, pollakiuria, tenesmus, and obstruction to copulation in intact females. If the tumor becomes irritated, infected, or necrotic, it may be associated with a sanguineous or purulent vaginal discharge. Urinary incontinence occurs secondary to the presence of a benign vaginal tumor.[174]

Digital palpation of the vestibule and vagina and vaginal cytological study are performed in patients with any of these signs, followed by vaginoscopic examination and, if indicated, contrast vaginography to determine the site of origin and extent of the mass. Rectal palpation may permit localization and characterization of vaginal masses in toy-breed bitches and queens when vaginal palpation is not possible. Differential diagnoses for vaginal masses include vaginal prolapse, primary vaginal neoplasia, and metastatic neoplasia from another site. Primary vaginal tumors are tentatively distinguished from vaginal prolapses based on the age of the bitch (prolapses occur in young animals, tumors in older ones), the origin of the mass (prolapses usually arise from the floor of the vagina cranial to the urethral orifice, tumors may arise elsewhere), and time of occurrence of the mass in relation to the estrous cycle (prolapses occur during proestrus and estrus and regress, tumors do not). Vaginal metastases from primary tumors originating in the urinary tract and mammary gland have been reported, and metastasis may occur from other primary sites as well. Diagnosis of vaginal neoplasia in bitches is based on detection of a vaginal mass by inspection, palpation, vaginoscopy, or retrograde vaginography and by histological confirmation of tumor type.

*See references 1–3, 16, 41, 120, 127, 145, 152, 167, 170, 175, 184, and 204.

Leiomyoma

Vaginal and vestibular leiomyomas occur in bitches 5 to 16 years of age and frequently afflict boxers and multiparous bitches.[29, 109] Duration of clinical signs before diagnosis is 1 day to 2 years (mean 7 weeks) for intraluminal and 2 months to 2 years (mean 24 weeks) for extraluminal tumors.[29] Both types of tumors are slow growing and are associated with tenesmus and dysuria. Constipation due to rectal compression may occur in cats.[209]

Leiomyosarcoma

Vaginal and vestibular leiomyosarcomas occur in bitches older than 9 years and have not been described in cats.[29, 88] Clinical signs include perineal swelling, weakness, and dysuria. These tumors may recur after excision and metastasize to the regional lymph nodes, lungs, and cervical spinal cord.

Transmissible Venereal Tumor

Transmissible venereal tumors are transplantable tumors that usually contain 58 to 59 chromosomes, of which 17 to 19 are metacentric, in contrast to normal canine cell complements of 78 acrocentric chromosomes.[3, 143, 171, 201] Surface antigen and histocompatability studies suggest that the tumor resulted from chromosomal translocations (the joining of two chromosomes into one) in one single tumor, with subsequent maintenance and spread in canine populations worldwide.* Transmissible venereal tumor was the first tumor to be transmitted by contact of tumor cells, but not cell-free extracts, to mucous membrane or scarified skin surfaces.

Tumor transmission, growth, and metastasis depend on the immunological status of the animal to which it is transplanted. It grows rapidly and metastasizes in pups and immunosuppressed adults and grows slowly or regresses in normal adult dogs.[19, 20, 40] Regression of trans-

*See references 39, 41, 58, 89, 91, 97, 117, 143, 172, and 197.

missible venereal tumor was reported in dogs that were infected with canine parvovirus or inoculated with modified live parvovirus vaccine, perhaps as a result of a direct oncolytic effect of the virus or of a host immunological mechanism.[211]

Treatment and Prognosis

Because most vaginal neoplasms are benign, surgical excision is the treatment of choice, with a guarded to favorable prognosis. Extent of the mass is determined before surgery, and exfoliative cytological study is used to determine tumor type. Thoracic and abdominal radiographs are obtained to search for metastases. Most vaginal tumors in bitches are round, well circumscribed, and easy to remove surgically via an episiotomy. Complete vulvovaginectomy and perineal urethrostomy have been described in three dogs with malignant, infiltrative vaginal neoplasia. Urine scalding and urinary tract infection were postoperative complications; survival times were 9 weeks to 10 months.[21]

Transmissible venereal tumors may regress spontaneously in patients with normal immune systems. They respond well to surgical excision, chemotherapy, and orthovoltage radiotherapy.* Treatment is recommended in most cases because of the small risk of metastasis, the difficulty in detecting spread to abdominal organs, and the complexity of evaluating the immune system. Choice of surgical excision, chemotherapy, or radiation therapy is influenced by tumor location, the presence or absence of metastases, and available treatment methods.

Wide surgical excision of the vaginal tumor via episiotomy is usually recommended when the tumor is a single one that is easily accessible. Tumor cell transplantation at the incision site may cause recurrence; electrosurgery may minimize this risk.[192] A disadvantage of surgical treatment is the high rate of tumor recurrence (17 to 58 per cent).[9, 35, 193] Surgical excision of a large primary tumor may be used with later chemotherapy or radiotherapy with good success.[32, 35, 193]

Chemotherapy with vincristine (0.025 mg/kg IV, not to exceed 1 mg), administered once weekly after a hemogram to search for leukopenia, is effective. Of 41 dogs of both sexes with primary or recurrent (but not metastatic) transmissible venereal tumor, 39 experienced complete tumor regression after 2 to 7 weeks of vincristine therapy.[35] One dog that did not respond to vincristine alone showed tumor regression after subsequent doxorubicin therapy; a second dog did not respond to either drug. Advantages of chemotherapy are the high cure rate, ease of administration, and usefulness with metastatic or multifocal disease. A disadvantage is the presence of side effects, which include vomiting and transient leukopenia; these occurred in 5 of the 41 cases (13 per cent) cited earlier.[35] Effectiveness of chemotherapy in the presence of metastatic disease is not well documented.

Orthovoltage radiotherapy in a single dose of 1,000 rad cured seven of eight dogs.[193] Ten others were treated up to six times at 2- to 21-day intervals, with total radiation doses up to 3,000 rad. All had tumor-free periods of 1 year after therapy, despite recurrence of tumors following previous surgical or chemotherapy. None of the dogs had metastatic disease, but one had multicentric tumors, which were treated with 1,000 rad per site. Disadvantages of radiotherapy are lack of availability and the need for an accessible tumor.

Immunotherapy of transmissible venereal tumors has been effective in experimental studies but has not been widely evaluated clinically.[90] Tumors regress when serum from patients in remission is administered to dogs with active tumor growth.[165]

Choice of therapy for patients with transmissible venereal tumor depends on tumor location, the presence or absence of metastasis, and the availability of radiotherapy. Wide electrosurgical excision is recommended for accessible tumors, followed by chemotherapy for recurrent or metastatic disease. Alternatively, some clients might choose radiotherapy over surgery for a primary tumor, or even chemotherapy alone. The prognosis is favorable for all patients except those with metastasis to the central nervous system.

*See references 9, 15, 32, 33, 35, 95, and 172.

MAMMARY NEOPLASIA

Incidence

Patient Signalment

Dogs. The mammary glands are the most common site of neoplasia in female dogs; tumors of these glands accounted for 42 per cent of 2,917 tumors in all sites and 82 per cent of 1,086 tumors of the female reproductive organs.[29, 47, 52] Bitches have a greater incidence of mammary neoplasia than other female domestic animals or women.[31] Mammary neoplasia is rare in bitches younger than 2 years; its frequency increases dramatically after 6 years and peaks at 10 to 11 years, thereafter declining.[42, 53, 140, 141] Median ages in four surveys totaling 991 animals ranged from 9 to 11 years.[46, 64, 177] Age at peak incidence is the same for neutered and intact females.[31]

Intact bitches have a three- to sevenfold greater risk of developing mammary cancer than neutered females.[66, 141, 168] Ovariectomy has a detectable sparing effect on the incidence of mammary tumors when it is performed before the first estrus (0.5 per cent), after one but before the second estrus (8 per cent), or after two but less than four estrous cycles (26 per cent). After 2.5 years of age or four estrous cycles, ovariectomy has slight or no sparing effect.[130, 178] Irregular estrous cycles, parity, fecundity, and false pregnancy do not influence the incidence of mammary tumors.[30, 76, 177, 178, 200]

Increased risk of mammary neoplasia has been reported in the Airedale terrier, Brittany spaniel, Boston terrier, cocker spaniel, English setter, English springer spaniel, fox terrier, German shorthaired pointer, Great Pyrenees, Irish setter, keeshond, Labrador retriever, pointer, poodle, and Samoyed.[42, 52, 136] Reduced risk for mammary neoplasia has been reported for mixed-breed bitches, Chihuahuas, and boxers.[42, 52, 136] Mammary tumors may occur in any of the five pairs of mammary glands and are most common in the two caudal

TABLE 159–4. INCIDENCE OF MAMMARY TUMOR TYPES IN BITCHES AND QUEENS

Tumor Type	Canine				Feline			
	Cotchin[46]	Moulton et al[140]	Bostock[23]	Total	Cotchin[45]	Hayden[80]	Hayes et al	Total
Carcinomas								
Adenocarcinoma, unspecified	14	239			38	27	94	
Adenocarcinoma, tubular	19	56	251					
Adenocarcinoma, papillary		91	141			19		
Adenocarcinoma, papillary-cystic							1	
Solid carcinoma	39	116	276			2		
Spindle cell carcinoma					1			
Anaplastic carcinoma	10		66			2	16	
Squamous cell carcinoma	5	39					2	
Mucinous carcinoma								
Solid adenocarcinoma								
				1,362 (40%)				202 (86%)
Sarcomas								
Osteosarcomas	23							
Fibrosarcomas		2					1	
Osteochondrosarcomas								
Unspecified	50	7	50				1	
				132 (4%)				2 (0.8%)
Carcinosarcomas (malignant mixed tumors)	27	115	10				4	
				152 (4%)				4 (1.7%)
Benign tumors								
Adenomas	8	70	82		6	2	11	
Papillomas						1		
Fibromas	2							
Fibroadenomas (benign mixed tumors)	230	616	740			2	4	
Lipomas	9						2	
Myoepithelioma		15						
Benign mesenchymal tumors			9					
				1781 (52%)				28 (12%)
Total	436	1366	1625	3427	45	55	136	236

pairs.[28, 46, 131, 140, 141, 200] Multiple mammary tumors of the same or different histological type are common, occurring in up to 66 per cent of affected bitches.[31, 140, 178]

Cats. Mammary tumors are the third most common neoplasm in cats, following skin and lymphoid tumors, and may account for up to 76 per cent of reproductive tumors.[28, 45, 52] Age incidence increases most dramatically after 6 years and peaks at 10 to 11 years in intact females, thereafter declining.[53, 203] Intact female cats have seven times greater risk of mammary neoplasia than neutered females.[53] Siamese were over-represented in one survey of 132 cats with mammary neoplasia.[84] All four pairs of feline mammary glands are at equal risk.[27, 45, 203]

Incidence of Tumor Type and Patterns of Metastasis

Dogs. About half of all canine mammary tumors are benign; most benign tumors are fibroadenomas, and most malignant tumors are adenocarcinomas (Table 159–4).* Metastasis of malignant mammary cancer to many different organs occurs; in surveys of 100 and 223 dogs with malignant tumors, 93 and 77 per cent, respectively, had metastatic lesions, with most animals showing metastasis to the lungs and lymph nodes.[63, 139] Mammary carcinomas in dogs metastasize most commonly to regional lymph nodes and then lungs. Mammary sarcomas in dogs metastasize most often to the lungs, suggesting spread of tumor emboli by venous rather than lymphatic drainage.[31, 63, 140, 181, 192] Common metastatic sites of malignant mammary tumors include the liver, kidneys, adrenals, spleen, pancreas, diaphragm, ovaries, heart, bone, urethral and vestibular submucosa, skeletal muscle, eyes, and brain.[31, 63, 131, 135, 140, 192] Bony metastases may not be obvious on routine necropsy examination unless careful radiological or pathological searches are made.[31]

In women, inflammatory mammary carcinoma is a mammary tumor characterized by mammary erythema, edema, firmness, and warmth, with or without a discrete mammary mass. It is highly metastatic, and tumor cell obstruction of subepidermal lymphatics is usually present. Ten cases of inflammatory mammary carcinoma in dogs, found in a review of 225 mammary tumor cases, were reported; all dogs had rapidly enlarging, diffusely enlarged mammary glands, some with distinct nodules.[188] The dogs were presented for mammary neoplasia, mas-

*See references 23, 31, 46, 52, 53, 63, 66, 77, 140, and 168.

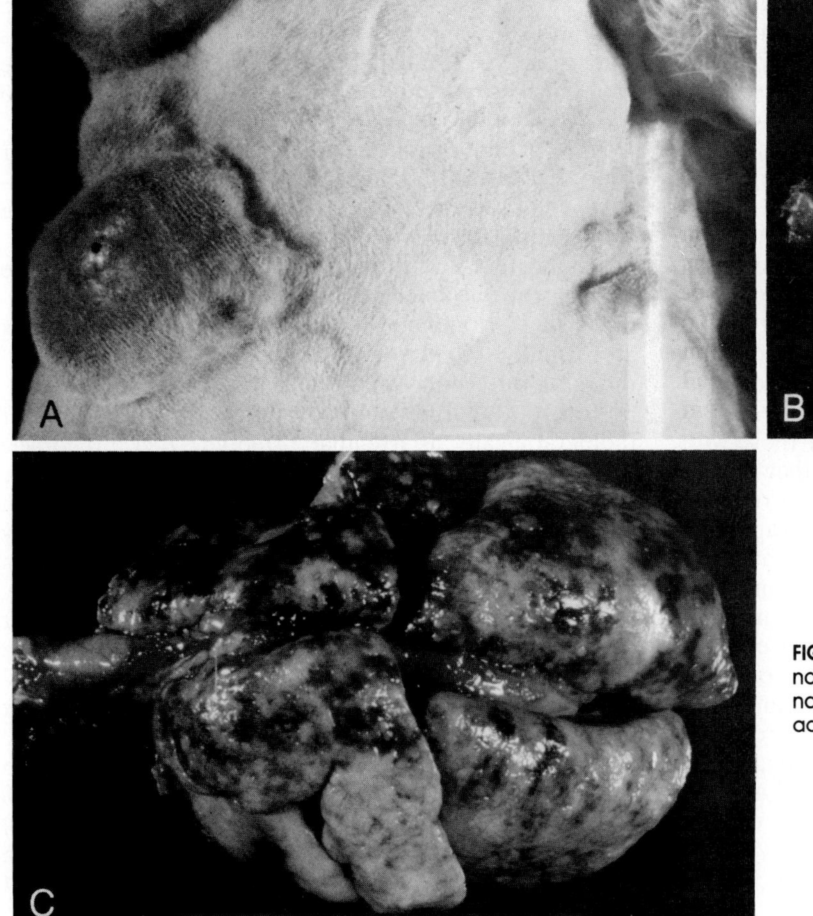

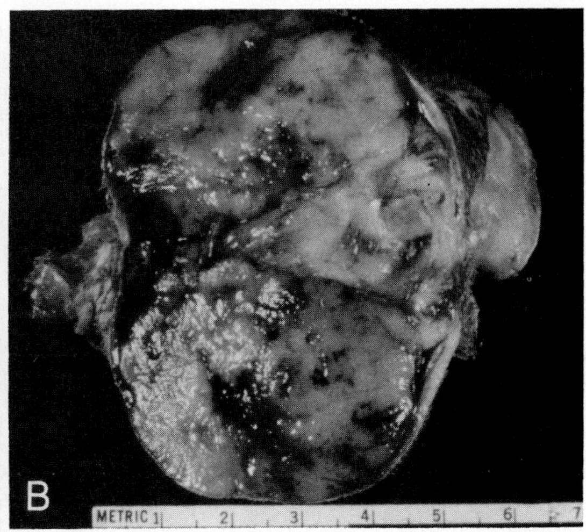

FIGURE 159–5. Gross appearance of the mammary nodule *(A)*, excised mammary tumor *(B)*, and pulmonary infiltrate with metastases *(C)* of a feline mammary adenocarcinoma.

titis, allergy, rash, or lameness secondary to hindlimb edema. The most common tumor type was adenocarcinoma, with squamous cell carcinoma, scirrhous carcinoma, solid carcinoma, and malignant mixed mammary tumor represented. Metastases were widespread, and pulmonary and nodal metastases were present in seven and nine dogs, respectively.

Regional lymph nodes for the three cranial pairs of mammary glands are the axillary nodes, and for the two caudal pairs the superficial inguinal nodes. Anastomosis of lymphatics occurs infrequently between the third and fourth pairs; lymphatics may cross the midline.[181] Mammary tumors of the third glands most commonly spread to the axillary nodes rather than the inguinal.[63]

Cats. Nearly 90 per cent of feline mammary tumors are malignant, and most are adenocarcinomas (see Table 159–4; Fig. 159–5).[45, 80, 129, 153] Metastases are present in more than 90 per cent of cats with malignant mammary tumors and may occur in the lungs (84 per cent), regional lymph nodes (83 per cent), pleura, liver, spleen, omental fat, pancreas, adrenals, kidneys, ovaries, heart, brain, and vertebral column.[36, 45, 80, 129, 148, 203] Lymphatic drainage of the two cranial mammary glands is to the axillary node, and of the two caudal glands to the superficial inguinal lymph node. Lymphatics do not connect anterior and posterior glands or cross the midline, but small veins may serve as a metastatic route.[80, 148] Mammary tumors of different histological type have occurred in the same cat, and cats with mammary tumors have been reported to have radiographic lesions suggesting metastasis although they were a pulmonary abscess or primary lung tumor.[26, 84, 144]

Influence of Reproductive Hormones on Occurrence

The ovarian steroids, estrogen and progesterone, are regarded as having a role in the etiology of mammary tumors in companion animals because (1) nearly all of these tumors occur in females, (2) early ovariectomy greatly decreases the risk of these tumors in cats and dogs, and (3) administration of exogenous progestogens may cause tumor development and growth in these species.*

Estrogen and progesterone bind protein receptors in the cytosol of target tissue cells, after which the steroid-receptor complex moves into the nucleus, binds to chromatin material, and causes synthesis of proteins that influence the cell's function. Receptor assays of mammary tumor tissue in humans, dogs, and cats have demonstrated that some tumor cytosols are rich in

*See references 45, 47, 53, 66, 69, 80, 84, 88, 100, 136, 148, 190, 196, and 203.

estrogen and progesterone receptors.* In humans, tumors rich in estrogen receptors alone or estrogen and progesterone receptors regress after additive (antiestrogen) or ablative (ovariectomy, adrenalectomy, hypophysectomy) endocrine therapy; tumors rich in progesterone receptors only and tumors lacking receptors do not respond to endocrine therapy, and affected patients have a poorer prognosis than those with receptor-rich tumors.[125]

Of canine mammary adenocarcinomas, 50 to 53 per cent are estrogen receptor rich, and 44 per cent are rich in both estrogen receptors and progesterone receptors.[75, 116, 160, 161, 169] In 87 malignant canine mammary tumors, no relationship was found between signalment, parity, false pregnancies, or progestogen administration and receptor status, but survival of patients with receptor-rich tumors was significantly greater than for those with receptor-poor tumors. These data suggest that the 44 per cent of dogs with receptor-rich tumors may respond favorably to ovariectomy or antiestrogen therapy. Although reports in the veterinary literature state that ovariectomy at time of mammary tumor excision is not associated with increased survival time, that may be because patients with receptor-rich tumors were not evaluated separately.[8] Most of the small number of feline mammary tumors examined for receptor content were estrogen receptor negative and progesterone receptor positive or negative, which in humans is a diagnostic profile associated with poor prognosis.[105, 106, 161] A small number of cats with metastatic mammary cancer did not respond to antiestrogen (tamoxifen) therapy.[104]

Diagnosis

Initial diagnosis of mammary neoplasia is based on signalment (age, age at ovariectomy if performed), history (of reproductive cycles, lactation, or progestogen therapy), and physical examination (presence of one or more mammary masses, enlargement of regional lymph nodes, evidence of dyspnea, cough, lymphedema, lameness). Mammary tumors in both dogs and cats are firm, well-demarcated nodules that vary in diameter from several millimeters to 10 to 20 cm. Mixed mammary tumors often contain regions of bone formation and may be hard. Large tumors may be traumatized and ulcerated.[206] Because mammary tumor metastases may occur in nearly every organ of the body, signs referable to a compromised organ are variable and may include lameness, dyspnea, anterior uveitis, and central nervous system deficits.[31, 111, 114, 131, 135] Hypercalcemia, which disappeared after excision of a canine mammary tumor, has been reported.[31] Differential diagnosis in cats includes nodular mammary hypertrophy.[5, 81, 92, 180]

Cytological examination of fine-needle aspiration biopsy samples, nipple secretions, or scrapings of ulcerated surfaces of mammary masses are obtained in all cases because of the ease and low cost of these procedures, but results are interpreted with caution. When cytological findings of 75 canine mammary masses, of which 36 were malignant, were examined and compared with later histological diagnosis, false-positive diagnoses were made in 3 and 0 per cent of the cases by two cytologists, respectively, and false-negative diagnoses were made in 22 and 36 per cent; the positive predictive value of the procedure thus was 90 to 100 per cent, and the negative predictive value was 59 to 75 per cent.[7] Cytological criteria such as variable nuclear size, nuclear giant forms, high nucleus/cytoplasm ratio, variable nucleolar number, and abnormal nucleolar shape and size were significant predictors of malignancy.[7]

Diagnostic tests for evidence of metastasis include thoracic and abdominal radiographs and ultrasonography of the abdomen. Metastatic lesions in the thorax are usually circular, well-defined radiodensities, although a diffuse interstitial pattern with lymphatic infiltration by tumor cells may occur; bony lesions appear radiographically as irregular osteolytic foci.[31] Thoracic radiographs of 55 female dogs with mammary tumors (31 malignant and 24 benign) suggested the presence of metastasis in 11 of the 17 dogs in which pulmonary metastasis was detected at necropsy and in one dog in which the lungs were normal at necropsy, corresponding to a sensitivity of 65 per cent, a specificity of 97 per cent, and a diagnostic accuracy of 87 per cent. Six false negatives and one false positive occurred.[195] The metastases were less than 4 mm in diameter in four of the six false negatives. Radionuclide imaging of the skeletal system of dogs with mammary neoplasia has also been advocated, although 16 abnormal scans observed in 30 affected dogs were associated with non-neoplastic (14) or other concurrent neoplasia (1) lesions in most; in only 1 of the 30 dogs did such scanning reveal occult bone metastases.[154, 155]

Definitive diagnosis is based on histopathological examination of an excision biopsy specimen. Several histological grading systems have been proposed to provide prognostic information. In general, the more highly differentiated tumors (with tubule or acinar formation) and those with fewer mitotic figures and more regular nuclear size and shape have a more favorable prognosis.[68, 78, 79, 132, 134] Commercially available steroid receptor assays for human mammary tumors may be performed on canine tumors, but the cost of these assays may be more than performing ovariohysterectomy to confer protection in the 44 per cent of dogs with receptor-rich malignant tumors. Neither receptor assay nor ovariohysterectomy is advocated for cats. Flow cytometric DNA analysis and microspectrophotometric DNA measurements have been used to investigate canine mammary tumors because nuclear DNA content in some human tumors predicts tumor behavior, but results are equivocal.[85, 137]

Mammary tumors in dogs and cats are staged according to the behavior of the primary tumor (T), regional lymph node involvement (N), and the presence of distant metastasis (M), if any (see Table 159–2).[210]

Treatment and Prognosis

Surgical Excision

Surgical excision of all canine and feline mammary tumors is recommended for patients undergoing treat-

*See references 74, 75, 105, 106, 116, 121, 160, 169, and 202.

ment for this tumor, with the possible exception of dogs with inflammatory mammary carcinoma, which in humans adversely influences the risk of rapid spread.[188] Six categories of surgical excision of canine mammary tumors have been reported:

1. Removal of the tumor alone (lumpectomy)
2. Removal of the affected gland only (simple mastectomy)
3. Removal of the affected and ipsilateral glands (regional mastectomy)
4. Removal of the affected gland, the regional lymph nodes, and all intervening glands and lymphatics (*en bloc* dissection)
5. Removal of all glands on the affected side (unilateral mastectomy)
6. Bilateral mastectomy (simultaneous or staged)

The type of surgery does not influence survival time or cancer-free survival time.[8, 115, 133] In one study of dogs treated by simple mastectomy (211) or *en bloc* dissection (42), both groups had similar postsurgical survival rates.[133] The type of surgical excision (categories 1, 2, 3, 5, or 6 above) had no effect on cancer-free interval in 63 dogs with malignant mammary neoplasia.[8] No significant difference in survival time or cancer-free survival time was noted between dogs treated by simple (35) or unilateral mastectomy (33).[116] These results suggest that lumpectomy or simple mastectomy of affected glands, with excision of regional lymph nodes for staging, may be the surgical treatment of choice. Concurrent ovariectomy or ovariohysterectomy of an affected intact bitch should be considered, because such treatment increases survival time in dogs (approximately 44 per cent) with receptor-rich tumors.[161] Most reports in the veterinary literature describe no beneficial effect of ovariectomy at mastectomy (all malignant mammary tumors); in one study of 59 bitches, mean survival time was 18.5 months in bitches treated with both operations, compared with 6.1 months in bitches treated with mastectomy alone.[8, 62, 64, 159, 178] If performed at the same time, ovariectomy precedes mastectomy to avoid seeding the abdomen with exfoliated tumor cells.

En bloc dissection or unilateral mastectomy has been advocated for surgical management of feline malignant mammary neoplasia, in which frequent lymphatic penetration occurs.[115, 203] In one survey of 91 cats with mammary adenocarcinoma, cats receiving unilateral mastectomies had significantly longer disease-free intervals but no different survival times when compared with cats that received simple mastectomies.[115] Ovariectomy is not indicated for intact affected patients of this species, because most feline tumors are receptor poor.

Chemotherapy

Results of mammary cancer treatment in humans suggest that antiestrogen therapy or chemotherapy may be of therapeutic value in some bitches with mammary cancer following surgical excision if metastasis to regional lymph nodes or other parts of the body is demonstrated; however, there are no conclusive reports documenting effectiveness or safety of such treatment in dogs. Antiestrogen treatment (tamoxifen citrate [Nolvadex], 10 to 20 mg PO BID) may be indicated for receptor-rich mammary adenocarcinomas after ovariectomy.[119] Fifteen bitches with advanced malignant mammary cancer did not respond to combination cytoxin, vincristine, and methotrexate chemotherapy, but bitches with evidence of early metastatic disease and lymph node excision for staging have not been studied critically in chemotherapeutic trials.[23] A chemotherapeutic protocol using doxorubicin (30 mg/m^2 IV on day 1) and cyclophosphamide (100 mg/m^2 on days 3 through 6) repeated at 21-day intervals until remission or death has been advocated for dogs, without documentation of its effectiveness.[119]

Fourteen cats with advanced mammary adenocarcinoma treated with doxorubicin and cyclophosphamide on a 6-day regimen repeated at 21-day intervals until death or withdrawal from the study tolerated the chemotherapy, except for anorexia.[102] Three of 11 cats available for long-term follow-up had complete response to chemotherapy (regression of all signs of tumor for at least 4 weeks), 2 had partial response (more than 50 per cent reduction in tumor mass), and 4 had no response; survival time in those with complete or partial response was 45 to 344 days and in those with no response was 4 to 106 days. The treatment protocol was doxorubicin (Adriamycin, 30 mg/m^2 IV) on day 1 and cyclophosphamide (Cytoxan, 100 mg/m^2 PO) on days 3 through 6. In a later report, the same protocol but with a lower dose of doxorubicin (25 mg/m^2 IV) and cyclophosphamide (50 mg/m^2 PO) was associated with a partial response in 7 of 14 affected cats, although survival was not prolonged.[122] Transient anorexia occurred in 78 per cent of cats.

Radiation Therapy

Radiation therapy has not been well evaluated in canine mammary neoplasia. It is suggested as the treatment of choice for inflammatory mammary carcinoma in dogs, based on results of this treatment in women.[188]

Immunotherapy

In two reports, immunotherapy of dogs with malignant mammary tumors was associated with increased survival time or regression of pulmonary metastases.[24, 31] Intravenous BCG (bacillus Calmette-Guérin) at 1-, 2-, and 4-week intervals and then every 8 weeks until 1 year after mastectomy was associated with a median survival time of more than 100 weeks, compared with 24 weeks for the control groups, suggesting a BCG-induced delay in pulmonary metastasis.[24] Therapy of 76 dogs with the nonspecific immune modulator levamisole (5 mg/kg PO three times weekly until death or withdrawal from the study) after simple or unilateral mastectomy did not show a significant difference in either cancer-free interval or survival pattern compared with untreated dogs.[156]

Prognosis

Prognosis for cats and dogs with mammary cancer is influenced by tumor size, histological type of the tumor, mode of growth, and clinical stage.[22, 56]

In 34 dogs with malignant mammary tumor size less than 5 cm (maximum diameter) and no local invasion or distant metastasis, survival times were not different from 34 dogs with benign mammary tumors.[8] Eleven of 14 dogs that died of mammary cancer showed distant metastasis or gross local invasion. Seventy-five per cent of 253 dogs with malignant mammary tumors did not survive more than 2 years after simple mastectomy or *en bloc* dissection.[132, 134] The type of surgical excision in 253 and 97 dogs with mammary neoplasia did not influence cancer-free interval and was not a prognostic indicator. In a histological survey of 232 dogs that underwent mastectomy for mammary neoplasia, the frequency of tumor recurrence after surgery was significantly less in patients with tumors exhibiting noninvasive proliferation, greater nuclear differentiation, and diffuse lymphoid cellular reactions. Inflammatory mammary carcinomas have an extremely poor prognosis, with estimated survival times of less than a few months.[188]

In cats, average survival time after mammary tumor detection was reported as 12.3 months in 56 cats, and 1-year survival rates were significantly higher in cats with well-differentiated tumors with low or medium grades of pleomorphism and a low number of mitotic figures.[203] Maximum survival (50 per cent) was reported in cats with tumor volumes less than 8 cm^3.[23] Median survival times for 91 cats with mammary adenocarcinomas were 4.5 years for cats with tumors less than 8 cm^3, 2.0 years for cats with tumors of 9 to 27 cm^3, and 6 months for cats with tumors larger than 28 cm^3; nine cats with carcinoma *in situ* were cured by surgical excision.[115]

For both dogs and cats, lymphatic infiltration (with peripheral lymphedema or satellite nodules between the tumor and regional nodes), metastatic lesions, infiltration of the body wall, rapid tumor growth, or recurrence augurs a poor prognosis.

References

1. Abbott PK: Venereal transmissible tumor on eyelid of dog. *Aust Vet J 42*:29, 1966.
2. Adams EW, Slaughter LJ: A canine venereal tumor with metastasis to the brain. *Pathol Vet 7*:498, 1970.
3. Adams EW, et al: Cytogenic observations on the canine venereal tumor in long-term culture. *Cornell Vet 71*:336, 1981.
4. Aliakbrai S, Ivoghli B: Granulosa cell tumor in a cat. *J Am Vet Med Assoc 174*:1306, 1979.
5. Allen HL: Feline mammary hypertrophy. *Vet Pathol 10*:501, 1973.
6. Allen HL, Franklin GA: Malignant granulosa cell tumor in a bitch. *J Am Vet Med Assoc 166*:447, 1975.
7. Allen SK, et al: Cytologic differentiation of benign from malignant canine mammary tumors. *Vet Pathol 23*:649, 1986.
8. Allen SW, Mahaffey EA: Canine mammary neoplasia: Prognostic indicators and response to surgical therapy. *J Am Anim Hosp Assoc 25*:540, 1989.
9. Amber EI, Henderson RA: Canine transmissible venereal tumor: Evaluation of surgical excision of primary and metastatic lesions in Zaria-Nigeria. *J Am Anim Hosp Assoc 18*:350, 1982.
10. Andersen AC, Simpson ME: *The Ovary and Reproductive Cycle of the Dog (Beagle)*. Geron-X, Los Altos, CA, 1973.
11. Andersen GL: Granulosa cell tumor in a dog. *Comp Cont Educ 8*:158, 1986.
12. Andrews EJ, et al: A histopathological study of canine and feline ovarian dysgerminomas. *Can J Comp Med 38*:85, 1974.
13. Arnbjerg J: Extra-ovarian granulosa cell tumor in a cat. *Feline Pract 10*:26, 1980.
14. Baker E: Malignant granulosa cell tumor in a cat. *J Am Vet Med Assoc 129*:322, 1956.
15. Banks WC: Results of radiation treatment of naturally occurring animal tumours. *J Am Vet Med Assoc 166*:1063, 1975.
16. Barron CN, et al: Intraocular tumors in animals. V. Transmissible venereal tumor of dogs. *Am J Vet Res 24*:1263, 1963.
17. Bellhorn R: Secondary ocular adenocarcinoma in three dogs and a cat. *J Am Vet Med Assoc 160*:302, 1972.
18. Belter LF, et al: Endometrial adenocarcinoma in a cat. *Pathol Vet 5*:429, 1968.
19. Bennett BT: Tumor-blocking and -inhibitory serum factors in the clinical course of canine transmissible venereal tumor. *Cancer Res 35*:2942, 1975.
20. Beschomer WE, et al: Isolation and characterization of canine venereal tumor-associated inhibitory and blocking factors. *Cancer Res 39*:3920, 1979.
21. Bilbrey SA, et al: Vulvovaginectomy and perineal urethrostomy for neoplasms of the vulva and vagina. *Vet Surg 18*:450, 1989.
22. Bostock DE: The prognosis following surgical excision of canine mammary neoplasms. *Eur J Cancer 11*:389, 1975.
23. Bostock DE: Neoplasia of the skin and mammary glands in dogs and cats. *In* Kirk RW (ed): *Current Veterinary Therapy VI*. W. B. Saunders, Philadelphia, 1977, pp 493–496.
24. Bostock DE, Gorman NT: Intravenous BCG therapy of mammary carcinoma in bitches after surgical excision of the primary tumor. *Eur J Cancer 14*:879, 1978.
25. Britt JO, Howard EB: An ovarian teratoma in a dog. *Canine Pract 8*:41, 1981.
26. Britt JO, et al: Simultaneous mixed mammary tumor and adenocarcinoma in a cat. *Feline Pract 9*:41, 1979.
27. Broadhurst JJ: Neoplasms of the reproductive system. *In* Kirk RW (ed): *Current Veterinary Therapy V*. W. B. Saunders, Philadelphia, 1974, pp 928–937.
28. Brodey RS: Canine and feline neoplasia. *Adv Vet Sci Comp Med 14*:309, 1970.
29. Brodey RS, Roszel JF: Neoplasms of the canine uterus, vagina and vulva. A clinicopathologic survey of 90 cases. *J Am Vet Med Assoc 151*:1294, 1967.
30. Brodey RS, et al: The relationship of estrous irregularity, pseudopregnancy, and pregnancy and the development of K9 mammary neoplasms. *J Am Vet Med Assoc 149*:1047, 1966.
31. Brodey RS, et al: Canine mammary gland neoplasms. *J Am Anim Hosp Assoc 19*:61, 1983.
32. Brown NO, et al: Chemotherapeutic management of transmissible venereal tumor in 30 dogs. *J Am Vet Med Assoc 176*:983, 1980.
33. Brown NO, et al: Follow-up on chemotherapy of venereal tumors. *J Am Vet Med Assoc 177*:676, 1980.
34. Buergelt CD: Dysgerminomas in two dogs. *J Am Vet Med Assoc 153*:553, 1968.
35. Calvert CA, et al: Vincristine for treatment of transmissible veneral tumors in the dog. *J Am Vet Med Assoc 181*:163, 1982.
36. Chen HC: A case of feline papilliferous mammary adenocarcinoma with widespread metastases. *Can J Comp Med 32*:465, 1968.
37. Chestnutt RK: Granulosa cell tumor in a Golden Retriever. *Vet Med Small Anim Clin 75*:444, 1980.
38. Clayton HM: A canine ovarian teratoma. *Vet Rec 96*:567, 1975.
39. Cohen D: Detection of humoral antibody to the transmissible venereal tumor of the dog. *Int J Cancer 10*:207, 1972.
40. Cohen D: The biological behavior of the transmissible venereal tumour in immunosuppressed dogs. *Eur J Cancer 9*:253, 1973.
41. Cohen D: The transmissible venereal tumor of the dog—a naturally occurring autograft? *Isr J Med Sci 14*:14, 1978.
42. Cohen D, et al: Epidemiological analysis of the most prevalent sites and types of canine neoplasia observed in a veterinary hospital. *Cancer Res 34*:2859, 1974.
43. Cotchin E: Further observations on neoplasms in dogs with particular reference to site of origin and malignancy. *Br Vet J 110*:218, 1954.
44. Cotchin E: Neoplasia in the dog. *Vet Rec 66*:879, 1954.
45. Cotchin E: Neoplasia in the cat. *Vet Rec 69*:425, 1957.
46. Cotchin E: Mammary neoplasms of the bitch. *J Comp Pathol 68*:1, 1958.
47. Cotchin E: Some tumors of dogs and cats of comparative veterinary and human interest. *Vet Rec 71*:1040, 1959.
48. Cotchin E: Canine ovarian neoplasms. *Res Vet Sci 2*:133, 1961.
49. Crane SW, et al: Malignant ovarian teratoma in a bitch. *J Am Vet Med Assoc 167*:72, 1975.
50. Dehner LP, et al: Comparative pathology of ovarian neoplasms. 3. Germ cell tumors of canine, bovine, feline, rodent and human species. *J Comp Pathol 80*:299, 1970.
51. Dillberger JE, Altman NH: A canine ovarian germ cell tumor with extraembryonic differentiation. *Vet Pathol 24*:96, 1987.
52. Dorn CR, et al: Survey of animal neoplasms in Alameda and Contra Costa counties, California. I. Methodology and description of cases. *J Natl Cancer Inst 40*:295, 1968.
53. Dorn CR, et al: Survey of animal neoplasms in Alameda and Contra Costa counties, California. II. Cancer morbidity in dogs and cats from Alameda County. *J Natl Cancer Inst 40*:307, 1968.

54. Dow C: Experimental production of the cystic-hyperplasia-pyometra complex in the bitch. *J Pathol Bacteriol 78*:267, 1959.
55. Dow C: Ovarian abnormalities in the bitch. *J Comp Pathol 70*:59, 1960.
56. Else RW, Hannant D: Some ultrastructural findings on spontaneous and cultured canine and feline mammary carcinomas. Proceedings of the 6th World Congress of the World Small Animal Veterinary Association, Amsterdam, Oct. 1977, pp 91–92.
57. Engle CG, Brodey RS. A retrospective study of 395 feline neoplasms. *J Am Anim Hosp Assoc 5*:21, 1969.
58. Epstein RB, Bennett BT: Histocompatibility typing and course of canine venereal tumors transplanted into unmodified random dogs. *Cancer Res 34*:788, 1974.
59. Esplin DG, Wardrip SJ: Uterine carcinoma with metastasis to the myocardium. *J Am Anim Hosp Assoc 20*:261, 1984.
60. Evans JG, Grant DI: A mixed mesodermal tumour in the uterus of a cat. *J Comp Pathol 87*:635, 1977.
61. Faulkner RT: Removal of a thecoma in a poodle. *Vet Med Small Anim Clin 73*:451, 1978.
62. Fidler IJ, et al: Biological behavior of canine mammary neoplasms. *J Am Vet Med Assoc 151*:1311, 1967.
63. Fidler IJ, Brodey RS: A necropsy study of canine malignant mammary neoplasms. *J Am Anim Hosp Assoc 151*:710, 1967.
64. Fowler EH, et al: Biologic behavior of canine mammary neoplasms based on a histogenetic classification. *Vet Pathol 3*:197, 1974.
65. Frye FL: Canine ovarian teratoma. *Vet Med Small Anim Clin 78*:1863, 1983.
66. Frye FL, et al: Characteristics of canine mammary gland tumor cases. *Anim Hosp 3*:1, 1967.
67. Gelberg HB, McEntee K: Feline ovarian neoplasms. *Vet Pathol 22*:572, 1985.
68. Gilbertson SR, et al: Canine mammary epithelial neoplasms: Biologic implications of morphologic characteristics assessed in 232 dogs. *Vet Pathol 20*:127, 1983.
69. Giles RC, et al: Mammary nodules in beagle dogs administered investigational oral contraceptive steroids. *J Natl Cancer Inst 60*:1351, 1978.
70. Gilmore CE: Tumors of the female reproductive tract. *Mod Vet Pract 45*:38, 1964.
71. Greene JA, et al: Ovarian papillary cystadenocarcinoma in a bitch: Case report and literature review. *J Am Anim Hosp Assoc 15*:351, 1979.
72. Greenlee PG, Patnaik AK: Canine ovarian tumors of germ cell origin. *Vet Pathol 22*:117, 1985.
73. Gruys E, et al: Four canine ovarian teratomas and a nonovarian feline teratoma. *Vet Pathol 13*:455, 1976.
74. Hamilton JM, et al: Oestrogen receptors in feline mammary carcinomas. *Vet Rec 99*:477, 1976.
75. Hamilton JM, et al: Oestrogen receptors in canine mammary tumors. *Vet Rec 101*:258, 1977.
76. Hamilton JM, et al: Serum prolactin concentrations in canine mammary cancer. *Vet Rec 102*:127, 1978.
77. Hampe JF, Misdorp W: Tumors and dysplasias of the mammary gland. *Bull WHO 50*:111, 1974.
78. Harvey HJ: General principles of veterinary oncologic surgery. *J Am Anim Hosp Assoc 12*:335, 1976.
79. Harvey HJ, Gilbertson SR: Canine mammary gland tumors. *Vet Clin North Am 7*:213, 1977.
80. Hayden DW: Feline mammary tumors. *J Small Anim Pract 12*:687, 1971.
81. Hayden DW, et al: Feline mammary hypertrophy/fibroadenoma complex: Clinical and hormonal aspects. *Am J Vet Res 42*:1699, 1981.
82. Hayes A, Harvey HJ: Treatment of metastatic granulosa cell tumor in a dog. *J Am Vet Med Assoc 174*:1304, 1979.
83. Hayes HM, Young JL: Epidemiologic features of canine ovarian neoplasms. *Gynecol Oncol 6*:348, 1978.
84. Hayes HM, et al: Epidemiologic features of feline mammary carcinoma. *Vet Rec 108*:476, 1981.
85. Hellmen E, et al: Comparison of histology and clinical variables to DNA ploidy in canine mammary tumors. *Vet Pathol 25*:219, 1988.
86. Helphrey ML: Vulvar leiomyosarcoma metastatic to the spinal cord in a dog. *J Am Vet Med Assoc 172*:583, 1978.
87. Helphrey ML: Vulvar leiomyosarcoma metastatic to the spinal cord in a dog. *J Am Vet Med Assoc 172*:583, 1978.
88. Hernandez FJ, et al: Feline mammary carcinoma and progestagens. *Feline Pract 5*:45, 1975.
89. Hess A, Cunningham B: *In vitro* correlates of the *in vivo* course of the canine transmissible venereal tumor studied by mixed lymphocyte-tumor cultures. *Transplant Proc 7*:507, 1975.
90. Hess AD, et al: *In vitro* and *in vivo* response of canine venereal tumors to intralesional BCG therapy. *Proc Am Soc Clin Oncol 17*:29, 1976.
91. Higgins DA: Observations on the canine transmissible venereal tumor as seen in the Bahamas. *Vet Rec 79*:67, 1966.
92. Hinton M, Gaskell CJ: Non-neoplastic mammary hypertrophy in the cat associated either with pregnancy or with oral progestagen therapy. *Vet Rec 100*:277, 1977.
93. Hofmann W, et al: Sex cord stromal tumor of the cat: So-called androblastoma with Sertoli-Leydig cell pattern. *Vet Pathol 17*:508, 1980.
94. Howell JMC, et al: A 6 year survey of tumours of dogs and cats removed surgically in private practice. *J Small Anim Pract 11*:793, 1970.
95. Idowu AL: A retrospective evaluation of four surgical methods of treating canine transmissible venereal tumour. *J Small Anim Pract 25*:193, 1984.
96. Ishmael J: Dysgerminoma of the ovary in a bitch. *J Small Anim Pract 11*:697, 1970.
97. Ivoghli B: Canine transmissible venereal tumor in Iran. *Vet Pathol 14*:289, 1977.
98. Jabara AG: Canine ovarian tumours following stilboestrol administration. *Aust J Exp Biol 37*:549, 1959.
99. Jabara AG: Induction of canine ovarian tumours by diethylstilboestrol and progesterone. *Aust J Exp Biol 40*:139, 1962.
100. Jabara AG: Two cases of mammary neoplasms arising in male dogs. *Aust Vet J 45*:476, 1969.
101. Jackson ML, et al: Ovarian dysgerminoma in a bitch. *Can Vet J 26*:285, 1985.
102. Jeglum KA, et al: Chemotherapy of advanced mammary adenocarcinoma in 14 cats. *J Am Vet Med Assoc 187*:157, 1985.
103. Jergens A, et al: Ovarian teratoma in a bitch. *J Am Vet Med Assoc 191*:81, 1987.
104. Johnston SD: Personal observation, 1982.
105. Johnston SD, et al: Progesterone receptors in spontaneously occurring feline mammary adenocarcinomas. Proceedings of the 73rd Annual Meeting of the American Association for Cancer Research, St. Louis, July 1982, p 238.
106. Johnston SD, et al: Progesterone receptors in feline mammary adenocarcinomas. *Am J Vet Res 45*:379, 1984.
107. Joshi KV, et al: A case of uterine adenocarcinoma in a dog. *Indian Vet J 44*:114, 1967.
108. Joshua JO: *The Clinical Aspects of Some Diseases of Cats*. J. B. Lippincott, Philadelphia, 1965, pp 119–140.
109. Kang TB, Holmberg DL: Vaginal leiomyoma in a dog. *Can Vet J 24*:258, 1983.
110. Karlson AG, Mann FC: The transmissible venereal tumor of dogs: Observations on forty generations of experimental transfers. *Ann NY Acad Sci 54*:1197, 1952.
111. Knight D, Hamilton JM: An unusual case of metastatic mammary carcinoma in a bitch. *Vet Rec 90*:570, 1972.
112. Kydd DM, Burnie AG: Vaginal neoplasia in the bitch: A review of forty clinical cases. *J Small Anim Pract 27*:255, 1986.
113. Ladds PW: Ovarian serous cystadenoma in a dog. *Cornell Vet 61*:482, 1971.
114. Ladds PW, et al: Canine ocular adenocarcinoma of mammary origin. *J Am Vet Med Assoc 156*:6369, 1970.
115. MacEwen EG, et al: Prognostic factors for feline mammary tumors. *J Am Vet Med Assoc 185*:201, 1984.
116. MacEwen EG, et al: Estrogen receptors in canine mammary tumors. *Cancer Res 42*:2255, 1982.
117. Magne ML, et al: Urinary tract carcinomas involving the canine vagina and vestibule. *J Am Anim Hosp Assoc 21*:767, 1985.
118. Manderino D: Dysgerminoma in a dog. *Mod Vet Pract 68*:241, 1987.
119. Mann FA: Canine mammary gland neoplasia. *Canine Pract 11*:22, 1984.
120. Manning PJ, Martin PD: Metastasis of canine transmissible venereal tumor to the adenohypophysis. *Pathol Vet 7*:148, 1970.
121. Martin PM, et al: Multiple steroid receptors in human breast cancer. *Cancer Chemother Pharmacol 2*:107, 1979.
122. Mauldin GN, et al: Efficacy and toxicity of doxorubicin and cyclophosphamide used in the treatment of selected malignant tumors in 23 cats. *J Vet Intern Med 2*:60, 1988.
123. McCandlish IAP, et al: Hormone producing ovarian tumors in the dog. *Vet Rec 105*:9, 1979.
124. McEntee K, Nielsen SW: Tumors of the female genital tract. *Bull WHO 53*:217, 1976.
125. McGuire WL: An update on estrogen and progesterone receptors for primary and advanced breast cancer. *In* Iacobelli S, et al (eds): *Hormones and Cancer*. Raven Press, New York, 1980, pp 337–344.
126. McKee WM: Granulosa cell tumour and attempted chemotherapy in a 17-month-old bitch. *Vet Rec 117*:501, 1985.
127. McLeod CG, Lewis JE: Transmissible venereal tumor with metastasis in 3 dogs. *J Am Vet Med Assoc 161*:199, 1972.
128. Meier H: Carcinoma of the uterus of the cat. Two cases. *Cornell Vet 46*:188, 1956.
129. Misdorp W: Malignant mammary tumors in the dog and cat compared with the same in women. Inaugural Dissertation, Utrecht, 1964.
130. Misdorp W: Canine mammary tumours: Protective effect of late ovariectomy and stimulating effect of progestins. *Vet Q 10*:26, 1988.
131. Misdorp W, den Herder BA: Bone metastasis in mammary cancer. A report of 10 cases in the female dog and some comparisons with human cases. *Br J Cancer 20*:496, 1966.
132. Misdorp W, Hart AAM: Canine mammary carcinoma. I. Prognosis. *J Small Anim Pract 20*:385, 1979.
133. Misdorp W, Hart AAM: Canine mammary cancer. II. Therapy and causes of death. *J Small Anim Pract 20*:395, 1979.
134. Misdorp W, Hart AAM: Prognostic factors in canine mammary cancers. *J Natl Cancer Inst 56*:779, 1976.
135. Misdorp W, et al: Canine malignant mammary tumors. I. Sarcomas. *Vet Pathol 8*:99, 1971.

136. Mitchell L, et al: Mammary tumors in dogs: Survey of clinical and pathological characteristics. *Can Vet J 15*:131, 1974.
137. Mollermark G, et al: Distribution of nuclear DNA-content in canine mammary tumours. *J Small Anim Pract 29*:309, 1988.
138. Moriello KA: Dermatology update: Applying recent advances to practice. *Vet Med 85*:160, 1990.
139. Moulton JE, et al: Mammary tumors in a colony of beagle dogs. *Vet Pathol 23*:741, 1986.
140. Moulton JE, et al: Canine mammary tumors. *Pathol Vet 7*:189, 1970.
141. Mulligan RM: Mammary cancer in the dog: A study of 120 cases. *Am J Vet Res 36*:1391, 1975.
142. Mulligan RM: Mesenchymal and neurilemmal tumors in the dog. *Arch Pathol 71*:512, 1961.
143. Murray M, et al: A study of the cytology and karyotype of the canine transmissible venereal tumor. *Res Vet Sci 10*:565, 1969.
144. Nafe LA, et al: Mammary tumors and unassociated pulmonary masses in two cats. *J Am Vet Med Assoc 175*:1194, 1979.
145. Ndiritu CG, et al: Extragenitally located TVT in dogs. *Mod Vet Pract 11*:940, 1977.
146. Nielsen SW: Classification of tumors in dogs and cats. *J Am Anim Hosp Assoc 19*:13, 1983.
147. Nielsen SW: Tumors of the genital tract. *In* Catcott EJ (ed): *Feline Medicine and Surgery*, American Veterinary Publications, Wheaton, IL, 1964, pp 165–168.
148. Nielsen SW: The malignancy of mammary tumors in cats. *North Am Vet 33*:245, 1952.
149. Norris HJ, et al: Pathology of feline ovarian neoplasms. *J Pathol 97*:138, 1969.
150. Norris HJ, et al: Comparative pathology of ovarian neoplasms. IV. Gonadal stromal tumors of canine species. *J Comp Pathol 80*:399, 1970.
151. Novinsky MA: Zur frage uber die impfung der krebsigen geschwulste. *Zentralbl Med Wiss 14*:790, 1876.
152. Oduye OO, et al: Metastatic transmissible venereal tumor in dogs. *J Small Anim Pract 14*:625, 1973.
153. Ogilvie GK: Feline mammary neoplasia. *Comp Cont Educ 5*:384, 1983.
154. Ogilvie GK, et al: Use of radionuclide imaging to identify malignant mammary tumor bone metastasis in dogs. *J Am Vet Med Assoc 195*:220, 1989.
155. Ogilvie GK, et al: Malignant lymphoma with cardiac and bone involvement in a dog. *J Am Vet Med Assoc 194*:793, 1989.
156. Ogilvie GK, et al: Evaluation of effects of levamisole and surgery on canine mammary cancer. *J Biol Response Mod 4*:418, 1985.
157. O'Rourke MD, Geib LW: Endometrial adenocarcinoma in a cat. *Cornell Vet 60*:598, 1970.
158. O'Shea JD, Jabara AG: The histogenesis of canine ovarian tumors induced by stilbestrol administration. *Pathol Vet 4*:137, 1967.
159. Osipov NE, et al: Spontaneous mammary gland tumors of dogs as a model for experimental tumor therapy. *Bull Exp Biol Med 74*:948, 1972.
160. Panko WB, et al: Canine mammary adenocarcinoma: Biochemical and endocrinologic similarities to human breast cancer. *Cancer Treat Rep 63*:1169, 1979.
161. Parodi AL, et al: Canine and feline mammary cancers as animal models for hormone dependent human breast tumors. *Prog Cancer Res Ther 31*:357, 1984.
162. Patnaik AK, Greenlee PG: Canine ovarian neoplasms: A clinicopathologic study of 71 cases including histology of 12 granulosa cell tumors. *Vet Pathol 24*:509, 1987.
163. Patnaik AK, et al: Metastasizing ovarian teratocarcinoma in dogs. A report of 2 cases and review of the literature. *J Small Anim Pract 17*:235, 1976.
164. Poffenbarger EM, Feeney DA: Use of gray-scale ultrasonography in the diagnosis of reproductive disease in the bitch: 18 cases. *J Am Vet Med Assoc 189*:90, 1986.
165. Powers RD: Immunologic properties of canine transmissible venereal sarcoma. *Am J Vet Res 29*:1637, 1968.
166. Preiser H: Endometrial adenocarcinoma in a cat. *Pathol Vet 1*:485, 1964.
167. Prier JE, Johnson JH: Malignancy in a canine transmissible venereal tumor. *J Am Vet Med Assoc 145*:1092, 1964.
168. Priester WA: Occurrence of mammary neoplasms in bitches in relation to breed, age, tumor type, and geographical region from which reported. *J Small Anim Pract 20*:1, 1979.
169. Raynaud JP, et al: Spontaneous canine mammary tumors: A model for human endocrine therapy? *J Steroid Biochem 15*:201, 1981.
170. Rensburg IB: Extragenital malignant transmissible venereal tumor in a bitch. *J South Afr Vet Assoc 51*:199, 1980.
171. Richards DA, Pencis RE: Transmissible venereal tumors. *Canine Pract 3*:23, 1976.
172. Richardson RC: Canine transmissible venereal tumor. *Comp Cont Educ 3*:951, 1981.
173. Riser WH, et al: Dermoid cyst of the canine ovary. *J Am Vet Med Assoc 134*:27, 1959.
174. Sahay PN, et al: Urinary incontinence in a bitch caused by vaginal fibroma. *Vet Rec 116*:76, 1985.
175. Sastry GA: A case of metastatic venereal tumor in a bitch. *Indian Vet J 42*:658, 1965.
176. Schmidt RE, Langham RF: A survey of feline neoplasms. *J Am Vet Med Assoc 151*:1325, 1967.
177. Schneider R: Comparison of age, sex and incidence rates in human and canine breast cancer. *Cancer 26*:419, 1970.
178. Schneider R, et al: Factors influencing canine mammary cancer developments and post surgical survival. *J Natl Cancer Inst 43*:1249, 1969.
179. Seaman WJ: Canine ovarian fibroma associated with prolonged exposure to mibolerone. *Toxicol Pathol 13*:177, 1985.
180. Seiler RJ, et al: Total fibroadenomatous change of the mammary glands of two spayed cats. *Feline Pract 9*:25, 1979.
181. Silver IA: Symposium on mammary neoplasia in the dog and cat. I. The anatomy of the mammary gland of the dog and cat. *J Small Anim Pract 7*:689, 1966.
182. Sorribas CA: Submucous uterine fibroma in a cat. *Mod Vet Pract 68*:493, 1987.
183. Smith CW: Dysgerminoma in a dog: A case report. *J Am Anim Hosp Assoc 9*:585, 1973.
184. Spence JA, et al: Metastasis of a transmissible venereal tumor to the pituitary. *J Small Anim Pract 19*:175, 1978.
185. Stein BS: Tumors of the feline genital tract. *J Am Anim Hosp Assoc 17*:1022, 1981.
186. Stein BS, Velders RW: What is your diagnosis? *J Am Vet Med Assoc 165*:749, 1974.
187. Storm RE: Dermoid cyst of the ovary. *North Am Vet 28*:30, 1947.
188. Susaneck SJ, et al: Inflammatory mammary carcinoma in the dog. *J Am Anim Hosp Assoc 19*:971, 1983.
189. Taylor DON, Dorn CR: Dysgerminoma in a 20-year-old female German shepherd dog. *Am J Vet Res 28*:587, 1967.
190. Taylor GN, et al: Mammary neoplasia in a closed beagle colony. *Cancer Res 36*:2740, 1976.
191. Thacher C, Bradley RL: Vulvar and vaginal tumors in the dog: A retrospective study. *J Am Vet Med Assoc 183*:690, 1983.
192. Theilen GH, Madewell BR: *Veterinary Cancer Medicine*. Lea & Febiger, Philadelphia, 1979.
193. Thrall DE: Orthovoltage radiotherapy of canine transmissible venereal tumors. *Vet Radiol 23*:217, 1982.
194. Thrasher JP: Neoplasms of dogs. *J Am Vet Med Assoc 138*:27, 1961.
195. Tiemessen I: Thoracic metastases of canine mammary gland tumors—a radiographic study. *Vet Radiol 30*:249, 1989.
196. Tomlinson MJ, et al: Feline mammary carcinoma: A retrospective evaluation of 17 cases. *Can Vet J 25*:435, 1984.
197. Tutt JB: Transmissible venereal tumor in a boxer bitch. *Vet Rec 84*:13, 1969.
198. Vardija VG, Ajinkya SM: A case of dysgerminoma in a dog. *Indian Vet J 46*:475, 1969.
199. Wardrip SJ, Esplin DG: Uterine carcinoma with metastasis to the myocardium. *J Am Anim Hosp Assoc 20*:261, 1984.
200. Warner MR: Age incidence and distribution of mammary dysplasias in young beagle bitches. *J Natl Cancer Inst 57*:57, 1976.
201. Weber WT, et al: Chromosome studies of a transplanted and a primary canine venereal sarcoma. *J Natl Cancer Inst 35*:537, 1965.
202. Weijer K: Feline malignant mammary tumors. IV. Oestrogen receptors. *In* Weijer K (ed): *Feline Mammary Tumor and Dysplasias*. Drukkerij Van der Molen, Oosthuizen, Netherlands, 1979, pp 51–54.
203. Weijer K, et al: Feline malignant mammary tumors. I. Morphology and biology: Some comparisons with human and canine mammary carcinomas. *J Natl Cancer Inst 49*:1697, 1972.
204. Weir EC, Pond MJ: Extragenital occurrence of transmissible venereal tumor in the dog. Literature review and case reports. *J Am Anim Hosp Assoc 14*:532, 1978.
205. Weller RE, Park JF: Vaginal leiomyoma and polyps in a beagle dog. *Calif Vet 37*:6, 1983.
206. White SD, et al: Cutaneous metastases of a mammary adenocarcinoma resembling eosinophilic plaques in a cat. *Feline Pract 15*:27, 1985.
207. Whitehead JE: Neoplasia in the cat. *Vet Med Small Anim Clin 62*:357, 1967.
208. Wilson RB, et al: Ovarian teratoma in two dogs. *J Am Anim Hosp Assoc 21*:249, 1985.
209. Wolke RE: Vaginal leiomyoma as a cause of chronic constipation in the cat. *J Am Vet Med Assoc 143*:1103, 1963.
210. World Health Organization: Report of the second consultation on the biological behaviour and therapy of tumours of domestic animals. Geneva, Switzerland, 1979, pp 18–20.
211. Yang TJ, Jones JB: Canine transmissible venereal sarcoma: Transplantation studies in neonatal and adult dogs. *J Natl Cancer Inst 51*:1915, 1973.

Male

TESTICULAR NEOPLASIA

Incidence

Testicular neoplasia is the second most common tumor of male dogs (following skin) and is more common than in any other domestic mammal or humans.[22, 27, 28, 42, 48] Testicular tumors constitute 4 to 7 per cent of all canine neoplasms, and 90 per cent of tumors of the male genitalia.[15, 21, 22, 79]

The three major tumors of the canine testicle are the Sertoli cell tumor, seminoma, and interstitial cell tumor, which occur with approximately equal frequency.[19, 22, 48, 74, 86] Tumor size, secretion of testicular hormones, and incidence of metastasis vary with histological type. Testicular tumors cause noticeable testicular enlargement, have a low incidence of metastasis, and are cured by castration; Sertoli cell tumors may secrete estrogen, causing feminizing signs or aplastic pancytopenia (Fig. 159–6). More than one testicular tumor of the same or different type per dog or per testis is fairly common.[29, 68, 110] In four reports comprising 788 dogs with testicular neoplasia, the incidence of bilateral neoplasia ranged from 21 to 45 per cent and of multiple testicular neoplasia from 11 to 55 per cent.[29, 48, 68, 110] Individual cases of testicular fibrosarcoma, gonadoblastoma, granulosa cell tumor, hemangioma, leiomyoma of the tunica vaginalis, schwannoma, and undifferentiated sarcoma/carcinoma also occur in dogs.[19, 48, 94, 105, 110, 122]

Cryptorchidism increases the risk of testicular neoplasia in dogs by as much as 13.6 times; risk factors reported by tumor type are 23 times for Sertoli cell tumors, 16 times for seminomas, and 1.6 times for interstitial cell tumors.[22, 48, 68, 97, 102, 110] Cryptorchidism also predisposes to testicular neoplasia in humans; such risk does not decrease with early surgical orchiopexy into the scrotum, suggesting that a dysgenetic gonad rather than abdominal environment may cause tumor development.[6, 48] Testicular tumors occur with equal frequency in right and left scrotal testes and more frequently in the right testis (R/L = 1.8:1) in cryptorchid dogs, matching the 1.9:1 right-to-left ratio of cryptorchid testes in dogs without neoplasia.[6, 7, 22, 102]

Age incidence is influenced by tumor type and location of the affected testis. Tumors occur in dogs from 2 to 17 years old.[111, 126] Risk increases for all intact male dogs until 10 to 14 years of age and then declines.[22, 48, 103] Mean age of incidence for each of the tumor types decreases in cryptorchid testes. Mean age of occurrence for Sertoli cell tumors was 11 years for scrotal testes (n=50), 8.8 years for inguinal testes (n=24), and 7.8 years for abdominal testes (n=34).[102] Mean age for seminomas was 10.5 years for scrotal testes (n=45), 9.1 years for inguinal testes (n=15), and 7.5 years for abdominal testes (n=8).[102] Mean age for interstitial cell tumors was 11.5 years in all dogs (n=45).[22]

Breed predisposition to testicular neoplasia occurs in the border collie, boxer, Cairn terrier, Chihuahua, Pekingese, Pomeranian, poodle, miniature schnauzer, Shetland sheepdog, Siberian husky, and Yorkshire terrier.[51, 119, 126] Breed predisposition to Sertoli cell tumors has been reported in the boxer, Cairn terrier, border collie, Shetland sheepdog, Pekingese, and Weimaraner, and to seminomas in German shepherds.[48, 126] Low risk of testicular neoplasia is reported in mixed-breed dogs, dachshunds, beagles, and Labrador retrievers.[48, 119] Miniature schnauzers have a syndrome of cryptorchidism, Sertoli cell tumor in the abdominal testis, and persistence of the müllerian duct in individuals that are phenotypically and chromosomally male.[9, 10, 59, 84, 87] A seminoma occurred in the gonad of a lateral hermaphrodite collie.[120]

Testicular tumors are rarely reported in cats. None were present in 1,576 feline tumors (from both sexes).[20, 21, 27, 70] Single case reports have documented Sertoli cell tumors, undifferentiated carcinomas, an adenoma, and a testicular teratoma.[75, 115]

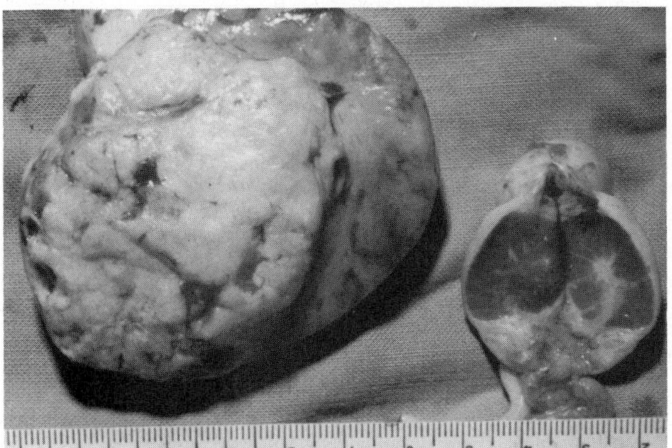

FIGURE 159–6. Sertoli cell tumor of the right testis and contralateral testicular atrophy of the left testis in an 8-year-old male bulldog with feminizing signs.

Diagnosis

Testicular neoplasia in dogs or cats is diagnosed by palpation of a testicular mass in a scrotal or ectopic testis, followed by excision biopsy and histopathological evaluation. Interstitial cell tumors are the smallest of the canine testicular tumors and may be an incidental finding at necropsy or may be detected by testicular ultrasonography in a patient with abnormal testicular texture on palpation or abnormal semen quality (Fig. 159–7).[34]

Paraneoplastic syndromes such as feminization (gynecomastia, attraction of males), alopecia, or blood dyscrasia (pancytopenia) may cause clinical signs in addition to testicular enlargement, for which dogs with testicular neoplasia are admitted.* These are attributed

*See references 3, 7, 32, 66–68, 74, 76, 79, and 111.

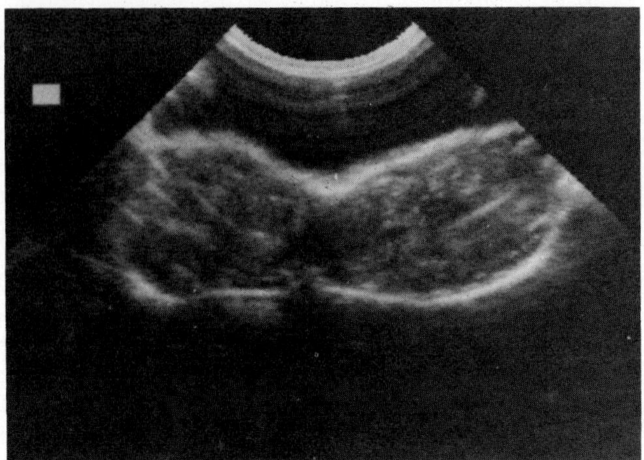

FIGURE 159–7. Ultrasonographic appearance of bilateral Sertoli cell neoplasia in scrotal testes of a 15-year-old male cocker spaniel. Hypoechoic regions represent areas of necrosis.

to sex steroid secretion by tumor cells and usually to estradiol secretion by Sertoli cell tumors, which account for the majority of testicular tumors associated with these syndromes. Circulating estradiol concentrations may not be elevated in affected dogs, but elevation in urinary estrogens, *in vitro* production of estrogens by tumor explants, and increased concentrations of estradiol in spermatic vein blood from the affected compared with the nonaffected testis support such production.* Feminization and pancytopenia are similar to those in dogs treated with exogenous estrogen, and these signs subside after successful removal of the tumor. Slight elevation of serum progesterone level was reported in a dog with a Sertoli cell tumor, although the assay was performed after administration of an adrenocorticotropic hormone stimulation test, which may have influenced the result.[36]

*See references 7, 9, 17, 22, 68, 79, 98, 111, and 112.

Other abnormalities that are androgen dependent and associated with testicular neoplasia in older male dogs include prostatic disease, perineal hernia, perianal gland adenoma, and perianal gland adenocarcinoma.[7, 68] Secretion of elevated plasma concentrations of testosterone by an interstitial cell tumor in a dog has been reported, although most dogs with these tumors have normal peripheral serum testosterone concentrations.[109] These concurrent disorders also afflict older intact male dogs without testicular neoplasia. Torsion of a neoplastic scrotal or cryptorchid testis occurs occasionally, leading to signs of anorexia, vomiting, marked testicular swelling and pain, and a painful abdomen; torsion most often occurs in an abdominal testis containing a Sertoli cell tumor.[61, 81, 96] Paraneoplastic syndromes have not been associated with testicular neoplasia in cats.

Metastasis is uncommon in canine testicular neoplasia and varies with tumor type. It has not been reported in cats nor in dogs with more than one testicular tumor type.[68] Clinical staging of canine testicular tumors is by behavior of the primary tumor (T), regional lymph node involvement (N), and the presence of metastasis (M) (Table 159–5).[130] Regional lymph nodes are the sublumbar and inguinal nodes.

Sertoli Cell Tumors

Sertoli cell tumors are the most easily recognized canine testicular tumors because they are the largest of the three types, are most likely to occur in ectopic testes, and are most likely to secrete estrogens and be

TABLE 159–5. WORLD HEALTH ORGANIZATION CLINICAL STAGES OF CANINE TUMORS OF THE MALE REPRODUCTIVE ORGANS

	Site of Primary Tumor		
	Testis	***Prostate***	***Penis and Prepuce***
T: Primary tumor			
T_0	No evidence of T	No evidence of T	No evidence of T
T_1	T restricted to testes	Intracapsular T, surrounded by normal gland	T ≤ 1 cm in main dimension, superficial
T_2	T invading tunica albuginea		T > 1 cm and < 3 cm in main dimension
T_3	T invading rete testis and/or epididymis		T > 3 cm or deep infiltration present
T_4	T invading spermatic cord and/or scrotum		T infiltrating neighboring structures
N: Regional lymph nodes	[Sublumbar, inguinal]	[Internal and external iliac]	[Superficial inguinal]
N_0	No regional LN involved	No regional LN involved	No regional LN involved
N_1	Ipsilateral regional LN involved	Regional LN involved	Movable unilateral nodes
N_2	Contralateral or bilateral regional LN involved	Regional and juxtaregional LN involved	Movable bilateral nodes
N_3			Fixed nodes
M: Distant metastasis			
M_0	No evidence of metastasis	No evidence of metastasis	No evidence of metastasis
M_1	Distant metastasis present Specify sites	Distant metastasis present Specify sites	Distant metastasis present Specify sites

T, tumor; LN, lymph nodes.
From World Health Organization: Internal Reports of the First and Second WHO Consultations on the Biological Behaviour and Therapy of Tumours of Domestic Animals, Geneva, 1978 and 1979 (unpublished WHO documents VPH/CMO/78.15 and 79.17).

associated with paraneoplastic syndromes.[7, 22, 68, 79] They range in diameter from 1 mm to more than 10 cm; on cut section they are homogeneous and pale yellow–gray or cream colored.[22, 29, 110] Feminizing signs in dogs with Sertoli cell tumors include gynecomastia with or without mammary gland secretion, a pendulous prepuce, attraction of males, and loss of libido. Bilaterally symmetrical alopecia in these dogs has been attributed to estrogen-induced atrophy of hair follicles and sebaceous glands.[7, 110]

Blood dyscrasias in dogs with Sertoli cell tumors are similar to those caused by exogenous estrogen administration and include early anemia, thrombocytopenia, and leukocytosis, followed by later decline in leukocyte count and pancytopenia.[12] Bone marrow aplasia may persist for months after estrogen administration and may be more life threatening than any other aspect of testicular tumors.[80] Blood dyscrasias were described in 8 of 76 (11 per cent), 8 of 60 (13 per cent), and 4 of 17 (23 per cent) dogs with Sertoli cell tumors.[79, 99, 111] Signs of the blood dyscrasia included anorexia, weakness, acute collapse, and hematuria. Three of 16 dogs with blood dyscrasias survived after castration, antibiotic and fluid therapy, and administration of hematinics, androgenic steroids, and blood or platelet-rich plasma; the others died or were euthanized.[79, 111]

Metastasis occurred in 18 of 197 (9 per cent) dogs with Sertoli cell tumors.* Metastases occur most frequently to the inguinal and sublumbar lymph nodes; metastasis to the lungs, mediastinal lymph nodes, liver, spleen, kidneys, pancreas, mesenteric lymph nodes, and nipple also has been described.

Sertoli cell tumors in cats may be unilateral or bilateral and may cause gross gonadal enlargement; they are not associated with paraneoplastic syndromes.[75]

Seminoma

Canine seminomas are round, 1 mm to 10 cm in diameter, and pale cream color or gray.[29, 110] Paraneoplastic syndromes attributable to hormone secretion by seminomas are less common than with Sertoli cell tumors, but a few cases of feminization, alopecia, or blood dyscrasia have been described.[3, 22, 68, 79] Testicular torsion was reported in an abdominal testicle with a seminoma.[96]

Metastases of seminomas were present in 8 of 204 (4 per cent) dogs.[22, 29, 68, 110] The most common sites of metastasis are the sublumbar lymph nodes, followed by the mesenteric lymph nodes, spleen, lungs, meninges, and eyes.†

Seminoma has not been reported in cats.

Interstitial Cell Tumor

Canine interstitial cell tumors are smaller than other canine testicular tumors, 1 mm to 9 cm in diameter, with 88 per cent less than 2 cm in diameter.[29, 110] They may be incidental findings at necropsy in testes that were not enlarged antemortem. On cut surface, they are ochre to yellow, soft friable masses that are sharply demarcated from adjacent seminiferous tubules.

A few dogs with interstitial cell tumors have shown feminization, alopecia, or blood dyscrasia, which are most characteristic of dogs with Sertoli cell tumors.[22, 68, 79] Intra-abdominal testicular torsion has been described in a 9-year-old unilateral cryptorchid Labrador retriever with a 30 × 10 × 10-cm interstitial cell tumor in the retained right testis; the dog recovered uneventfully after castration.[81]

Prostatic disease (20 of 67 cases) and perianal gland neoplasia (31 of 67 cases) have been described in dogs with interstitial cell tumors; most tumors do not secrete elevated concentrations of androgens, which might explain these findings.[68]

Metastasis is rare in interstitial cell tumors and was reported in only 2 of 332 (0.6 per cent) cases.[22, 29, 68, 110] The two had tumor cells in the sublumbar lymph nodes and lungs; one dog also had inguinal lymph node lesions, and the other had a neoplastic nodule in the spleen.[22, 29]

Interstitial cell tumors have not been reported in cats.

Treatment and Prognosis

Treatment of canine and feline testicular neoplasia is bilateral castration. Hemicastration may be considered in valuable breeding animals if ultrasonography of the contralateral testicle shows no evidence of bilateral neoplasia and if semen evaluation reveals viable sperm. Atrophy of the contralateral testicle due to elevated intrascrotal temperature caused by the tumor may reduce fertility.

Radiotherapy of caudal abdominal metastatic seminoma in four dogs after castration has been described.[71] Cesium 137 was administered at total doses ranging from 17 to 40 Gy in eight to ten fractions administered three times weekly. The tumor regressed in all four dogs, and the dogs survived for 6 to 57 months. Three of the four died of unrelated causes and showed no evidence of tumor at necropsy. The fourth was euthanized for undetermined pulmonary disease 43 months after therapy.

The prognosis for patients with testicular neoplasia is favorable in the absence of metastasis and blood dyscrasia. Signs of feminization disappear 2 to 6 weeks after castration unless metastases are present.[14, 73, 126] Pancytopenia at surgery or as late as 2 months afterward is associated with a poor to grave prognosis, even with aggressive supportive therapy.

PROSTATIC NEOPLASIA

Incidence

The incidence of prostatic neoplasia is based on a necropsy study of 4,500 dogs, in which 15 (0.33 per cent) had prostatic adenocarcinoma.[125] Other reported estimates are that prostatic adenocarcinoma occurs in 0.29 to 0.6 per cent of all male dogs and 1.4 to 5.8 per cent of those with carcinomas.[19, 60, 106] Prostatic neoplasia occurs more often in dogs than in other domestic species.[62]

*See references 7, 22, 29, 68, 99, 110, 116, and 126.

†See references 22, 29, 49, 68, 110, 113, and 128.

TABLE 159–6. TUMOR TYPE, SIGNALMENT, CLINICAL SIGNS AND PATTERNS OF METASTASIS IN DOGS WITH PROSTATIC NEOPLASIA

	O'Shea[93]	Leav and Ling[62]	Taylor[118]	Weaver[125]	Durham and Dietze[31]	Bell et al[5]	Total
Tumor type							
Adenocarcinoma	6	20	9	15	12	31	93
Carcinoma			2				2
Transitional cell carcinoma	1						1
Signalment							
Number of dogs	7	20	11	15	12	31	96
Number intact	6	16		15		21	58/73
Number male/castrated	1	4		0		10	15/73
Age range, years	9–12	6–15	6–12	6–14	5–12	6–18	5–18
Age mean, years	11.3	10.1	8.5	8.8	9.3	9.9	
Number of breeds	5	13	9	9	8	18	
Clinical signs							
Emaciation	2	14	2	4	8	11	41
Tenesmus	1	9	1	8	8	14	41
Dysuria	1	6	5	11		8	31
Urethral bleeding/hematuria	1	5	3	2	9	7	27
Lameness		10	1	4	6	2	23
Polydipsia/polyuria		6		3		4	13
Lumbar pain		6	1		3		10
Dyspnea	2					4	6
Metastasis present (number)	5/5	20/20	6/7	13/13	11/12	24/31	79/88
Iliac lymph nodes	2	15	2	13	11	9	52
Lungs	2	13	3	5	6	16	45
Urinary bladder	2	10	2	9	6	7	36
Rectum	1	6		9	3	6	25
Pelvic muscle	3	5	1	12			21
Bone		7		3	5	3	18
Kidneys		2	3	4		5	14
Liver		1	1	1		9	12
Mesentery	1	7			3		11
Heart		3				5	8
Adrenals		2		1		5	8
Spleen		2				6	8
Ureter				4			4
Mediastinal lymph node	1						1

Most canine prostatic tumors are adenocarcinomas (Table 159–6). Poorly differentiated carcinoma, fibromyoma, leiomyoma, sarcoma, squamous cell carcinoma, transitional cell carcinoma, and secondary metastatic neoplasia to the prostate also have been described.[40, 42, 45, 65]

Prostatic adenocarcinoma generally is diagnosed in older dogs (see Table 159–6); mean age of 96 affected dogs in 6 studies ranged from 8.5 to 11.3 years.[5, 31, 62, 93, 125] This tumor occurs in both neutered and intact males. Results of early surveys suggested that intact males were at greater risk of developing this tumor, but two reports of 43 and 31 cases noted that 44 per cent and 32 per cent, respectively, were castrated; the risk of developing prostatic cancer was calculated at 2.39 times greater for neutered than intact dogs.[5, 35, 45, 62, 89, 93] Although prostatic adenocarcinoma in humans may respond to antiandrogen therapy, there is no evidence that the canine tumor is hormonally dependent. Castration does not prevent development of prostatic neoplasia in dogs, nor does it alter behavior of the tumor in affected dogs.* There is no known breed predisposition.

Prostatic adenocarcinoma has been reported in older cats (10 to 17 years).[46, 50, 92, 129]

*See references 26, 30, 33, 52, 62, 69, and 125.

Diagnosis

The major clinical signs in dogs with prostatic neoplasia are emaciation, tenesmus, dysuria, and urethral bleeding/hematuria (see Table 159–6). Clinical signs in cats include hematuria, dysuria, pollakiuria, and outflow obstruction of the urinary tract.[46, 92, 129] On physical examination, the prostate usually is palpably enlarged and firm and may be asymmetrical, cystic, or irregularly nodular; enlarged sublumbar lymph nodes may be palpable per rectum.[62, 125] The size of the neoplastic gland varies greatly; the largest prostate in 15 cases was 8 × 6 × 5 cm.[125]

Survey radiography of affected dogs generally reveals prostate enlargement, although the size of the affected gland varies greatly and may not differ from that of dogs with benign prostatic hypertrophy.[38, 62, 125] Multifocal, irregularly shaped parenchymal mineral densities were observed on radiographs of 4 of 7 dogs with prostate cancer and in a dog with chronic prostatitis in 30 dogs with prostate disease.[38] Irregularity and filling defects of the prostatic urethra have been detected in both dogs and cats by retrograde urethrography.[46] Narrowing of the prostatic urethra and asymmetrical distribution of the prostatic parenchyma may occur but are not specific for prostatic neoplasia.[38] Prostatic ultrasonography of ten dogs with prostatic adenocarcinoma revealed increased echogenicity in six, decreased echogenicity in two, and a mixed, mottled appearance in one (Fig. 159–8).[5] Thoracic metastases appear as diffuse structured or nonstructured interstitial lung disease. Eight of ten cases with locomotor disturbance had radiographic evidence of osteolytic or proliferative metastasis to vertebrae, pelvis, or long bones.[46] Hypertrophic osteopathy has been described in a dog with prostatic adenocarcinoma without thoracic metastasis.[104]

Diagnostic methods to evaluate dogs with suspected prostatic adenocarcinoma include cytological examination of ejaculate, prostatic massage, and biopsy by urethral brush, aspiration, punch, incision, or excision of the prostate gland.[5, 58, 63, 91] An iliac lymph node is aspirated at biopsy if possible.[13, 62, 100, 125] Ejaculation and prostatic massage are noninvasive and are attempted initially, although dogs in pain may not achieve erection and ejaculation, and even when samples are obtained, they may not be diagnostic. Needle aspiration of the prostate may be performed using a perirectal or transabdominal approach and a long spinal needle. Punch biopsy is performed perirectally, transrectally, or transabdominally after sedation and local anesthesia and may be followed by transient hematuria. Needle and punch biopsy are contraindicated if an abscess is present, because localized peritonitis may follow. Because prostatic adenocarcinoma commonly occurs in glands that are also hypertrophic and may have cysts or infection, biopsy specimens are interpreted with caution.[14] Of 15 canine prostatic adenocarcinomas, 6 were diagnosed as cysts or infection after initial biopsy.[125] In 25 dogs with prostatic disease, 5 of which had prostatic cancer confirmed by histological evaluation, 22 of 23 dogs (96 per cent) were correctly predicted using cytological differentiation, as were 4 of the 5 neoplasia cases.[91]

Normal canine prostatic tissue contains three glycoproteins: human prostate-specific antigen (PSA), prostate-specific acid phosphatase (PSAP), and canine prostatic secretory protease (CPSP).[72] Immunohistochemical staining of 31 canine prostatic adenocarcinomas revealed the presence of CPSP in 8, PSAP in 3, and PSA in 2. Investigations of these antigens may permit future serological detection of these proteins as tumor markers in malignant and metastatic disease.

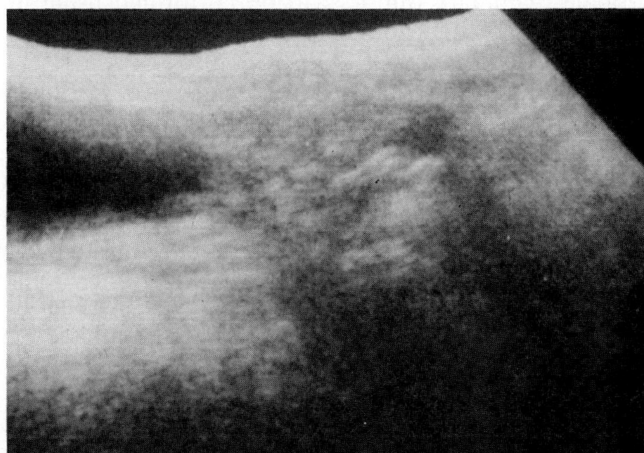

FIGURE 159–8. Ultrasonographic appearance of prostatic adenocarcinoma in an 11-year-old male castrated mixed-breed dog. The region to the right of the dark trigone of the urinary bladder is characterized by hyper- and hypoechoic mottled areas.

Metastatic lesions are common with canine prostatic adenocarcinoma and were detected in 79 of 88 dogs listed in Table 159–6. Metastases were found most often in the iliac lymph nodes, the lungs, the urinary bladder, and the rectum and may occur in other tissues, including bone.[64] Metastasis has also been described in the cerebrum in a patient with facial paralysis and loss of balance.[41] Pulmonary metastases were present in a 10-year-old neutered male cat with prostatic adenocarcinoma; survey radiographs taken before euthanasia did not reveal thoracic disease.[46]

Clinical staging of prostatic tumors is by behavior of the primary tumor (T), regional lymph node involvement (N), and the presence of metastasis (M) (see Table 159–5).[130] Regional lymph nodes are the internal and external iliac nodes.

Treatment and Prognosis

The only treatments available for prostate neoplasia in dogs are surgical excision and radiotherapy during surgery. Neither procedure is associated with a favorable prognosis, because metastasis usually has occurred before diagnosis. Prostatectomy is associated with a high incidence of urinary incontinence as a result of decreased urethral pressures, particularly of the skeletal muscle external urethral sphincter, and detrusor instability.[4, 43, 44] There are no published data documenting increased survival time after prostatectomy of affected dogs.

Intraoperative orthovoltage radiotherapy of ten dogs with prostatic carcinoma using 20 to 30 Gy per dog resulted in survival times of 41 to 750 days after treatment.[123] Five of these dogs with localized carcinoma had uneventful recuperative periods, improvement of clinical signs within a week, and complete response within 3 months after treatment. Four of the dogs were euthanized because of progression of clinical signs. Doxorubicin, 5-fluorouracil, and cyclophosphamide were administered to two dogs after irradiation. Results suggest that intraoperative radiotherapy may effectively treat some patients without metastasis.

Survival after diagnosis of prostatic neoplasia in dogs depends on pathological grade and the presence of metastasis. Fourteen dogs with signs lasting 1 to 6 months had postadmission survival times of 1 to 29 (mean 2.75) months.[125]

NEOPLASIA OF THE PENIS AND PREPUCE

Incidence

Tumors of the canine penis and prepuce include epithelial tumors (papilloma, squamous cell carcinoma), fibropapillomas (fibroma), transmissible venereal tumor, and other mesenchymal tumors (fibrosarcoma, lymphosarcoma, hemangiosarcoma, mast cell sarcoma), including a chondrosarcoma of the os penis.[2, 23, 42, 95] They constitute 0.24 per cent of tumors in male dogs, with an age-standardized incidence of 2 cases per 100,000 male dogs per year.[108] Age incidence for these tumors is unknown except for transmissible venereal tumors, which occur in young, free-roaming dogs. In one report, 45 of 78 cases of penile transmissible venereal tumor were present in dogs less than 4 years of age, and 19 were present between 5 and 7½ years.[82] The incidence of penile neoplasia is not influenced by neutering, except for decreased risk of acquiring transmissible venereal tumor venereally after castration.

Tumors of the penis and prepuce have not been reported in cats.

Diagnosis

Patients with penile or preputial neoplasia may be presented for a preputial mass, preputial hemorrhage, lack of libido, phimosis, or stranguria secondary to urethral obstruction.[2, 82, 95, 124] Occasional patients with transmissible venereal tumors may also have tumor in the nasal passages, causing epistaxis.[83] Papillomas and transmissible venereal tumors often appear as pedunculated masses that ulcerate and bleed, whereas squamous cell carcinomas may appear wartlike and progress to masses greater than 5 cm in diameter.[56]

Transmissible venereal tumors were first identified in 1876.[88] They behave similarly in males and females, with rapid growth, invasion, and metastasis in immune-compromised individuals and spontaneous regression in some normal individuals. Tumor spread may occur by transplantation to the skin, the nasal or pharyngeal mucosa, or the orbit or by hematogenous/lymphogenous spread to the regional lymph nodes, liver, spleen, intestine, lungs, or brain.[1, 16, 25, 37, 90, 131] The incidence of metastasis is unknown in spontaneous disease but was 1.3 per cent experimentally.[57]

Diagnosis of penile or preputial neoplasia is based on observation of a preputial or intrapreputial mass followed by histological examination of a fine-needle aspirate or excision biopsy of the mass. These tumors are staged by the TNM scheme in Table 159–5.[130] Regional lymph nodes are the superficial inguinal nodes.

Treatment and Prognosis

Tumors of the penis and prepuce are removed by wide surgical excision, using electrocautery to minimize bleeding.[119] Male dogs are kept away from females in estrus to minimize penile bleeding associated with erection. With recurrent, invasive, or metastatic transmissible venereal tumors, chemotherapy with vincristine (0.025 mg/kg IV, not to exceed 1 mg) once weekly after a hemogram to look for leukopenia may be administered until there is no longer evidence of disease.[8, 11] Orthovoltage radiotherapy using a single dose of 1,000 rad is effective.[121] Radiotherapy with 4,000 to 6,000 rad in 500-rad fractions three times weekly has been recommended following surgical excision of a squamous cell carcinoma.[24] Penile amputation and urethrostomy are indicated when tumor involvement is extensive or when urethral patency cannot be maintained.[24, 56] The prognosis for benign tumors of the penis and for transmissible venereal tumors is favorable in the absence of central nervous system metastasis; the prognosis is guarded to poor with carcinomas and sarcomas.

MAMMARY NEOPLASIA IN MALES

Incidence

The incidence of mammary tumors in male dogs and cats is low. In five reports including 1,705 dogs with mammary neoplasms, only 15 affected animals were males.[18, 39, 55, 78, 117] In six reports of 311 cats with malignant mammary tumors, 4 were neutered males, and none were intact males.[18, 47, 77, 85, 107, 127]

Mammary tumor types reported in 25 cases in male dogs consisted of 20 malignant and 5 benign tumors.[53–55, 101] These included adenocarcinoma (seven), malignant mixed mammary tumor (five), carcinoma (four), benign mixed mammary tumor (fibroadenoma) (two), adenoma (two), osteosarcoma (two), cystadenochondroma (one), spindle cell carcinoma (one), and undifferentiated sarcoma/carcinoma (one). Average age at diagnosis was 10.9 years (n = 18), and castration status was not reported. Affected mammary glands were equally represented on right and left sides. The fourth and fifth glands were most commonly involved, and one dog had bilateral adenocarcinomas. Metastases to lymph nodes and lungs have been reported.

In four cases of mammary neoplasia in male cats, all occurred in castrated males. Information on patients' age, survival, tumor type, or length of survival was not given.[18, 77, 127]

Diagnosis

Diagnosis is based on inspection and palpation of a mammary mass followed by excision biopsy and tumor histological assessment. Because the reported male canine mammary tumors are predominantly malignant and some metastasized to lymph nodes and lungs,[53, 54] radiographs of the chest and abdomen are advised to search for metastasis before surgical excision. Clinical staging of male mammary tumors can be performed using the TNM scheme (see Table 159–2).[130]

Treatment and Prognosis

Without clinical evidence of metastasis, excision biopsy of mammary tumors in male dogs and cats is recommended. Until more information is available on these rare tumors, the prognosis is based on histological study of the tumor type and its expected behavior in females.

References

1. Amber EI, Adeyanju JB: Oronasal transmissible venereal tumor in a dog. *Mod Vet Prac 67*:154, 1986.
2. Ball V, Rossi P: Cancer of the prepuce and glans (round celled sarcoma) with ganglial metastasis in a dog. *Vet J 84*:530, 1928.
3. Barsanti JA, et al: Alopecia associated with a seminoma. *J Anim Hosp Assoc 15*:33, 1979.

4. Basinger RR, et al: Urodynamic alterations associated with clinical prostatic diseases and prostatic surgery in 23 dogs. *J Am Anim Hosp Assoc 25*:385, 1989.
5. Bell FW, et al: Prostatic adenocarcinoma in 31 dogs—clinical and pathologic features. *J Am Vet Med Assoc 199*:1623, 1991.
6. Brodey RS: Canine and feline neoplasia. *Adv Vet Sci Comp Med 14*:309, 1970.
7. Brodey RS, Martin JE: Sertoli cell neoplasms in the dog. The clinicopathologic and endocrinological findings in 37 dogs. *J Am Vet Med Assoc 133*:249, 1958.
8. Brown NO, et al: Chemotherapeutic management of transmissible venereal tumor in 30 days. *J Am Vet Med Assoc 176*:983, 1958.
9. Brown TT, et al: Male pseudohermaphroditism, cryptorchidism and Sertoli cell neoplasia in three miniature schnauzers. *J Am Vet Med Assoc 169*:821, 1976.
10. Bruinsma DL, Ackerman LA: Male pseudohermaphroditism in a miniature schnauzer. *Vet Med/Small Anim Clin 78*:1568, 1983.
11. Calvert CA, et al: Vincristine for treatment of transmissible venereal tumor in the dog. *J Am Vet Med Assoc 181*:163, 1982.
12. Chiu T: Studies of estrogen-induced proliferative disorders of hemopoietic tissues in dogs. PhD Thesis, University of Minnesota, 1974.
13. Clark L, English PB: Carcinoma of the prostate gland in a dog. *Aust Vet J 42*:214, 1966.
14. Coffin DL, et al: Functional Sertoli cell tumor with metastases in a dog. *J Am Vet Med Assoc 121*:352, 1952.
15. Cohen D: Epidemiological analysis of the most prevalent sites and types of canine neoplasia observed in a veterinary hospital. *Cancer Res 34*:2859, 1974.
16. Cohen D: The transmissible venereal tumor of the dog—a naturally occurring allograft? *Isr J Med Sci 14*:14, 1978.
17. Comhaire F, et al: Testosterone and oestradiol in dogs with testicular tumours. *Acta Endocrinol 77*:408, 1974.
18. Cotchin E: Neoplasms in small animals. *Vet Rec 63*:67, 1951.
19. Cotchin E: Further observations on neoplasms in dogs with particular reference to site of origin and malignancy. Part I: Male genital, skeletal, lymphatic and other systems. *Br Vet J 110*:274, 1954.
20. Cotchin E: Neoplasia in the cat. *Vet Rec 69*:425, 1957.
21. Cotchin E: Some tumours in dogs and cats of comparative veterinary and human interest. *Vet Rec 71*:1040, 1959.
22. Cotchin E: Testicular neoplasms in dogs. *J Comp Pathol 70*:232, 1960.
23. Crocker WJ: Three thousand autopsies. *Cornell Vet 9*:142, 1919.
24. Crow SE: Neoplasms of the reproductive organs and mammary glands of the dog. *In* Morrow DA (ed): *Current Therapy in Theriogenology*. W. B: Saunders, Philadelphia, 1980, pp 640–646.
25. Dass LL, et al: Malignant transmissible venereal tumor. *Canine Pract 13*:15, 1986.
26. Deklerk DP, et al: Comparison of spontaneous and experimentally induced canine prostatic hyperplasia. *J Clin Invest 64*:842, 1979.
27. Dorn CR, et al: Survey of animal neoplasms in Alameda and Contra Costa counties, California. I. Methodology and description of cases. *J Natl Cancer Inst 40*:295, 1968.
28. Dorn CR, et al: Survey of animal neoplasms in Alameda and Contra Costa counties, California. II. Cancer morbidity in dogs and cats from Alameda county. *J Natl Cancer Inst 40*:307, 1968.
29. Dow C: Testicular tumours in the dog *J Comp Pathol 72*:247, 1962.
30. Dube JY, et al: Effect of endocrine manipulations on the levels of cytosolic and nuclear receptors for androgens in dog prostate. *Invest Urol 18*:418, 1981.
31. Durham SK, Dietze AE: Prostatic adenocarcinoma with and without metastasis to bone in dogs. *J Am Vet Med Assoc 188*:1432, 1986.
32. Edwards DF: Bone marrow hypoplasia in a feminized dog with a Sertoli cell tumor. *J Am Vet Med Assoc 178*:494, 1981.
33. Ehrlichman RJ, et al: Differences in the effects of estradiol on dihydrotestosterone-induced prostatic growth of the castrate dog and rat. *Invest Urol 18*:466, 1981.
34. Eilts BE, et al: Use of ultrasonography to diagnose Sertoli cell neoplasia and cryptorchidism in a dog. *J Am Vet Med Assoc 192*:533, 1988.
35. Evans JE Jr, et al: Prostatic adenocarcinoma in a castrated dog. *J Am Vet Med Assoc 186*:78, 1985.
36. Fadok VA, et al: Hyperprogesteronemia associated with Sertoli cell tumor and alopecia in a dog. *J Am Vet Med Assoc 188*:1058, 1986.
37. Fallon RK, Swayne DE: Canine transmissible venereal tumor: A diagnostic dilemma. *Comp Cont Educ 6*:415, 1984.
38. Feeney DA, et al: Canine prostatic disease—comparison of radiographic appearance with morphologic and microbiologic findings: 30 cases (1981–1985). *J Am Vet Med Assoc 190*:1018, 1987.
39. Frye FL, et al: Characteristics of canine mammary gland tumor cases. *Anim Hosp 3*:1, 1967.
40. Gorman NT, et al: A case of transitional cell carcinoma of the canine urethra. *J Am Anim Hosp Assoc 20*:817, 1984.
41. Grant CA: Carcinoma of the canine prostrate. *Acta Pathol Microbiol Scand 40*:197, 1957.
42. Hall WC, et al: Tumours of the prostate and penis. *Bull WHO 53*:247, 1976.
43. Hardie EM, et al: Complications of prostatic surgeons. *J Am Anim Hosp Assoc 20*:50, 1984.
44. Hardie EM, et al: Prostatectomy vs drainage for treatment of prostatic disease in the dog. *Vet Surg 1*:69, 1989.
45. Hargis AM, Miller LM: Prostatic carcinoma in dogs. *Comp Cont Educ 5*:647, 1983.
46. Hawe RS: What is your diagnosis? *J Am Vet Med Assoc 182*:1257, 1983.
47. Hayden DW: Feline mammary tumors. *J Small Anim Pract 12*:687, 1971.
48. Hayes HM, Pendergrass TW: Canine testicular tumors: Epidemiologic features of 410 dogs. *Int J Cancer 18*:482, 1976.
49. HogenEsch H, et al: Seminoma with metastases in the eyes and the brain in a dog. *Vet Pathol 24*:278, 1987.
50. Hornbuckle WE, Kleine LJ: Medical management of prostatic disease. In Kirk RW (ed): *Current Veterinary Therapy VII*. W. B. Saunders, Philadelphia, 1980, pp 1146–1150.
51. Howard EB, Nielsen SW: Neoplasia of the boxer dog. *Am J Vet Res 26*:1121, 1965.
52. Isaacs JT, Coffey DS: Changes in dihydrotestosterone metabolism associated with the development of canine benign prostatic hyperplasia. *Endocrinology 108*:445, 1981.
53. Jabara AG: Canine mixed tumours. *Aust Vet J 36*:212, 1960.
54. Jabara AG: Canine mammary carcinomata. *Aust Vet J 36*:389, 1960.
55. Jabara AG: Two cases of mammary neoplasms arising in male dogs. *Aust Vet J 45*:476, 1969.
56. Johnston DE: Tumors of the prepuce and penis. *In* Catcott EJ (ed): *Canine Surgery*. American Veterinary Publications, Wheaton, IL, 1965, pp 622–626.
57. Karlson AG, Mann FC: The transmissible venereal tumor of dogs: Observations on forty generations of experimental transfers. *Ann NY Acad Sci 54*:1197, 1952.
58. Kay ND, et al: Cytological diagnosis of canine prostatic disease using a urethral brush technique. *J Am Anim Hosp Assoc 25*:517, 1989.
59. Kedzieski M: Sertoli-cell tumor in a cryptorchid dog. *Mod Vet Pract 65*:865, 1984.
60. Krook L: A statistical investigation of carcinoma in the dog. *Acta Pathol Microbiol Scand 35*:407, 1954.
61. Laing EJ, et al: Spermatic cord torsion and Sertoli cell tumor in a dog. *J Am Vet Med Assoc 183*:879, 1983.
62. Leav I, Ling GV: Adenocarcinoma of the canine prostate gland. *Cancer 22*:1329, 1968.
63. Leeds EB, Leav I: Perineal punch biopsy of the canine prostate gland. *J Am Vet Med Assoc 154*:925, 1969.
64. Lee-Parritz DE, Lamb CR: Prostatic adenocarcinoma with osseous metastases in a dog. *J Am Vet Med Assoc 192*:1569, 1988.
65. Leibs MS, et al: Squamous cell carcinoma of the prostate gland in a dog. *J Am Anim Hosp Assoc 22*:509, 1986.
66. Lindberg R, et al: Sertoli cell tumors associated with feminization, prostatitis, and squamous metaplasia of the renal tubular epithelium in a dog. *J Small Anim Pract 17*:451, 1976.
67. Lindo DE, Glenn HH: Bilateral Sertoli cell tumor in a canine cryptorchid with accompanying pathologic lesions. *Can Vet J 10*:145, 1969.
68. Lipowitz AJ, et al: Testicular neoplasms and concomitant clinical changes in the dog. *J Am Vet Med Assoc 143*:1364, 1973.
69. Lloyd JW, et al: Androgens and estrogens in the plasma and prostatic tissue of normal dogs and dogs with benign prostatic hypertrophy. *Invest Urol 13*:220, 1975.
70. MacVean DW, et al: Frequency of canine and feline tumors in a defined population. *Vet Pathol 15*:700, 1978.
71. McDonald RK, et al: Radiotherapy of metastatic seminoma in the dog: Case reports. *J Vet Intern Med 2*:103, 1988.
72. McEntee M, et al: Adenocarcinoma of the canine prostate: Immunohistochemical examination for secretory antigens. *Prostate 11*:163, 1987.
73. McNeil PE, Weaver AD: Massive scrotal swelling in two unusual cases of canine Sertoli cell tumour. *Vet Rec 106*:144, 1980.
74. McQueen SD, et al: An unusual case of Sertoli cell neoplasia in a dog. *Vet Med Small Anim Clin 69*:1449, 1974.
75. Meier H: Sertoli-cell tumor in the cat. Report of two cases. *North Am Vet 37*:979, 1956.
76. Michaels J: Sertoli cell tumor in a collie dog. *Vet Med Small Anim Clin 69*:192, 1974.
77. Misdorp W: Malignant mammary tumors in the dog and cat compared with the same in women. Inaugural Dissertation, Utrecht, 1964.
78. Mitchell L, et al: Mammary tumors in dogs: Survey of clinical and pathologic characteristics. *Can Vet J 15*:131, 1974.
79. Morgan RV: Blood dyscrasias associated with testicular tumors in the dog. *J Am Anim Hosp Assoc 18*:970, 1982.
80. Morris BJ: Fatal bone marrow depression as a result of Sertoli cell tumor. *Vet Med Small Anim Clin 78*:1070, 1983.
81. Naylor RW, Thompson SMR: Intraabdominal testicular torsion. A report of two cases. *J Am Anim Hosp Assoc 15*:763, 1979.
82. Ndiritu CG: Lesions of the canine penis and prepuce. *Mod Vet Pract 60*:712, 1979.
83. Ndiritu CG, et al: Extragenitally located transmissible venereal tumor in dogs. *Mod Vet Pract 11*:940, 1977.
84. Neuman RH: Pyometra and a Sertoli cell tumor in a hermaphroditic dog. *Vet Med Small Anim Clin 74*:1757, 1979.
85. Nielsen SW: The malignancy of mammary tumors in cats. *North Am Vet 33*:245, 1952.

86. Nielsen SW, Lein DH: Tumours of the testis. *Bull WHO 50*:71, 1974.
87. Norrdin RW: A male pseudohermaphrodite dog with a Sertoli cell tumor, mucometra and vaginal glands. *J Am Vet Med Assoc 156*:204, 1970.
88. Novinsky MA: Zur frage uber die impfung der krebsigen geschwulste. *Zentral Med Wiss 14*:790, 1876.
89. Obradovich J, et al: The influence of castration on the development of prostatic carcinoma in the dog. *J Vet Intern Med 1*:183, 1987.
90. Oduye OO, et al: Metastatic transmissible venereal tumor in dogs. *J Small Anim Pract 14*:625, 1973.
91. Olson PN, et al: Disorders of the canine prostate gland: Pathogenesis, diagnosis and medical therapy. *Comp Cont Educ 9*:613, 1987.
92. Osborne CA: Personal communication, 1983.
93. O'Shea JP: Studies on the canine prostate gland. II. Prostatic neoplasms. *J Comp Pathol 73*:244, 1963.
94. Patnaik AK, Liu SK: Leiomyoma of the tunica vaginalis in a dog. *Cornell Vet 65*:228, 1975.
95. Patnaik AK, et al: Two cases of canine penile neoplasm: Squamous cell carcinoma and mesenchymal chondrosarcoma. *J Am Anim Hosp Assoc 24*:403, 1988.
96. Pearson H, Kelly DF: Testicular torsion in the dog: A review of 13 cases. *Vet Rec 97*:200, 1975.
97. Pendergrass TW, Hayes HM: Cryptorchidism and related defects in dogs: Epidemiologic comparisons with man. *Teratology 12*:51, 1975.
98. Pierrepoint CG, et al: Steroid metabolism of a Sertoli cell tumor of the testis of a dog with feminization and alopecia and of the normal canine testis. *J Endocrinol 38*:61, 1967.
99. Post K, Kilborn SH: Canine Sertoli cell tumor: A medical records search and literature review. *Can Vet J 28*:427, 1987.
100. Rabaut SM, Kelch WJ: Undifferentiated carcinoma in the canine prostate. *Mod Vet Pract 60*:401, 1979.
101. Raflo CP, Diamond SS: Neoplasm of the mammary papilla in a male dog. *Am J Vet Res 41*:953, 1980.
102. Reif JS, Brodey RS: The relationship between cryptorchidism and canine testicular neoplasia. *J Am Vet Med Assoc 155*:2005, 1969.
103. Reif JS, et al: A short study of canine testicular neoplasia. *J Am Vet Med Assoc 175*:719, 1979.
104. Rendano VT, Slauson DO: Hypertrophic osteopathy in a dog with prostatic adenocarcinoma and without thoracic metastasis. *J Am Anim Hosp Assoc 18*:719, 1979.
105. Rothwell TLW, et al: Schwannoma in the testis of a dog. *Vet Pathol 23*:629, 1986.
106. Schlotthauer CF, Millar JAS: Carcinoma of the prostate gland in dogs—a report of three cases. *J Am Vet Med Assoc 99*:239, 1941.
107. Schmidt RE, Langham RF: A survey of feline neoplasms. *J Am Vet Med Assoc 151*:1325, 1967.
108. Schneider R: Epidemiological aspects of mammary and genital neoplasia. *In* Morrow DA (ed): *Current Therapy in Theriogenology*. W. B. Saunders, Philadelphia, 1980, pp 636–639.
109. Scott DW, Reimers TJ: Gland and perianal gland hyperplasia associated with testicular neoplasia and hypertestosteronemia in a dog. *Canine Pract 13*:15, 1986.
110. Scully RE, Coffin DL: Canine testicular tumors. *Cancer 5*:592, 1952.
111. Sherding RG, et al: Bone marrow hypoplasia in eight dogs with Sertoli cell tumor. *J Am Vet Med Assoc 178*:497, 1981.
112. Siegel ET, et al: An estrogen study in the feminized dog with testicular neoplasia. *Endocrinology 80*:272, 1967.
113. Simon J, Rubin SB: Metastatic seminoma in a dog. *Vet Med Small Anim Clin 74*:941, 1979.
114. Spackman CJA, Roth L: Prostatic cyst and concurrent Sertoli cell tumor in a dog. *J Am Vet Med Assoc 192*:1096, 1988.
115. Stein BS: Tumors of the feline genital tract. *J Am Anim Hosp Assoc 17*:1022, 1981.
116. Strutt CS: Sertoli cell carcinoma and multiple metastasis in a dog. *Cornell Vet 57*:597, 1967.
117. Taylor GN, et al: Mammary neoplasia in a closed beagle colony. *Cancer Res 36*:2740, 1976.
118. Taylor PA: Prostatic adenocarcinoma in a dog and a summary of 10 cases. *Can Vet J 14*:162, 1973.
119. Theilen GH, Madewell BR: *Veterinary Cancer Medicine*. Lea & Febiger, Philadelphia, 1979.
120. Thomas TN, et al: Lateral hermaphroditism and seminoma in a dog. *J Am Vet Med Assoc 189*:1596, 1986.
121. Thrall DE: Orthovoltage radiotherapy of canine transmissible venereal tumors. *Vet Radiol 23*:217, 1982.
122. Turk JR, et al: A canine testicular tumor resembling gonadoblastoma. *Vet Pathol 18*:201, 1981.
123. Turrel JM: Intraoperative radiotherapy of carcinoma of the prostate gland in ten dogs. *J Am Vet Med Assoc 190*:48, 1987.
124. Wasman SC: Cancer of the penis. *Vet Med 50*:31, 1955.
125. Weaver AD: Fifteen cases of prostatic carcinoma in the dog. *Vet Rec 109*:71, 1981.
126. Weaver AD: Survey with follow-up of 67 dogs with testicular Sertoli cell tumours. *Vet Rec 113*:105, 1983.
127. Weijer K, et al: Feline malignant mammary tumors. I. Morphology and biology: Some comparisons with human and canine mammary carcinomas. *J Natl Cancer Inst 49*:1697, 1972.
128. Weller RE, Palmer B: Metastatic seminoma in a dog. *Mod Vet Pract 64*:275, 1983.
129. Whitehead JE: Diseases of the male reproductive system. *In* Catcott EJ (ed): *Feline Medicine and Surgery*. American Veterinary Publications, Wheaton, IL, 1964, pp 292–294.
130. World Health Organization: Report of the second consultation on the biological behaviour and therapy of tumours of domestic animals. Geneva, Switzerland, 1979.
131. Yang TJ: Metastatic transmissible venereal sarcoma in a dog. *J Am Vet Med Assoc 190*:555, 1987.

CHAPTER 160 Urinary System

Dennis D. Caywood, Jeffrey S. Klausner, and Patricia A. Walters

NEOPLASMS OF THE KIDNEY

Incidence

Benign renal neoplasms are less common than malignant renal tumors in dogs and cats and are primarily observed in older animals.* Renal adenoma is one of the more commonly encountered benign neoplasms of the kidneys (Table 160–1). Kidney adenomas have no breed or sex predilection. Renal interstitial cell tumors, arising from the fibroblast-like cell of the renal stroma, are common in humans, are noted in 26 to 42 per cent of human autopsies, and have also been recognized in dogs.[26] The tumors are multiple and generally bilateral, located near the corticomedullary junction. Most renal interstitial cell tumors are incidental necropsy findings in dogs older than 10 years. There is no breed or sex predilection. Other benign renal neoplasms include hemangioma, papilloma, lipoma, and fibroma.

Tubular cell carcinomas are the most common primary malignant neoplasms of the kidneys.* As in humans, the incidence is higher in males (Tables 160–1 and 160–2). The tumor may be hormonally induced, and originate

*See references 4, 15, 17, 41, 48, 62, and 67.

*See references 4, 17, 20, 28, 41, 48, 62, 67, and 70.

TABLE 160–1. TYPE, AGE, AND SEX OF 523 DOGS WITH PRIMARY RENAL NEOPLASMS

Tumor Type	Sex				Age (Years)		
	Number of Cases	*Male*	*Female*	*Not Determined*	*Mean*	*Range*	*Not Determined*
Epithelial tissue							
Adenoma	16	9	6	1	10.2	3–15	1
Renal carcinoma	280	148	103	29	7.7	1–15	37
Transitional cell carcinoma	18	7	11	0	8.2	5–13	0
Squamous cell carcinoma	11	8	3	0	8.6	4–14	0
Connective tissue							
Fibroma	4	3	1	0	9.5	5–13	0
Fibrosarcoma	40	25	15	0	9.35	1–15	0
Lipoma	7	0	7	0	7.7	1–13	0
Liposarcoma	1	0	1	0	—	5	0
Chondroma	1	1	0	0	13	13	0
Osteoma	2	2	0	0	4	3–5	0
Myxoma	1	1	0	0	—	8	0
Reticulum cell sarcoma	1	1	0	0	—	3	0
Unclassified sarcoma	17	8	9	0	9.1	6 months–15 years	0
Muscle tissue							
Rhabdomyosarcoma	1	1	1	0	—	12	0
Leiomyoma	1	1	0	0	—	—	1
Leiomyosarcoma	3	2	0	1	9	5–13	1
Vascular tissue							
Hemangioma	7	4	3	0	11.3	8–15	0
Hemangiosarcoma	67	35	32	0	10.8	5–15	3
Mixed tissue							
Nephroblastoma	40	19	16	5	5.6	6 months–13 years	0
Teratoma	4	2	2	0	2.8	1–5	0
Hamartoma	1	1	0	0	—	5	0

*Data from the Veterinary Medical Data Program and Caywood DD, Osborne CA: Urinary system. *In* Slatter DH (ed): *Textbook of Small Animal Surgery*. W.B. Saunders, Philadelphia, 1985, pp 2561–2574.

from the renal tubular epithelial cells.[73] The incidence increases with age in cats and dogs. It has not been determined whether carcinomas arise directly from renal tubular cells, by evolution through adenomatous hyperplasia, or from renal cortical adenomas.[73] Bilateral and multiple renal cystadenocarcinomas have been associated with a syndrome of generalized nodular dermatofibrosis in German shepherds.[19, 54, 83] The disease is hereditary, with an autosomal dominant pattern.

Nephroblastoma is a congenital neoplasm derived from the pluripotential metanephrogenic blastema, which allows production of epithelial and connective tissue elements.[3, 62, 74] It is part of the developing kidney and is associated with continued growth but abnormal

TABLE 160–2. TYPE, AGE, AND SEX OF 71 CATS WITH PRIMARY RENAL NEOPLASMS

Tumor Type	Sex				Age (Years)		
	Number of Cases	*Male*	*Female*	*Not Determined*	*Mean*	*Range*	*Not Determined*
Epithelial tissue							
Adenoma	3	1	2	0	—	13	2
Renal carcinoma	31	15	6	10	9.2	1–13	6
Transitional cell carcinoma	6	5	1	0	10.8	6–15	1
Squamous cell carcinoma	3	2	1	0	—	13	2
Connective tissue							
Lipoma	2	1	1	0	4	3–5	0
Fibrosarcoma	2	2	2	0	9	5–13	0
Unclassified sarcoma	10	1	2	7	6.8	6 months–13 years	8
Muscle tissue							
Leiomyosarcoma	2	0	1	1	—	22	1
Vascular tissue							
Hemangiosarcoma	1	1	1	0	—	3	0
Mixed tissue							
Nephroblastoma	11	3	1	7	4.3	1–8	5

*Data from the Veterinary Medical Data Program and Caywood DD, Osborne CA: Urinary system. *In* Slatter DH (ed): *Textbook of Small Animal Surgery*. W.B. Saunders, Philadelphia, 1985, pp 2561–2574.

differentiation.[3, 62, 74] The neoplasm occurs more often in young dogs and cats, although many cases have been observed in dogs and cats 4 years of age and older (see Tables 160–1 and 160–2). No breed or sex predilection is apparent.

Transitional cell and squamous cell carcinomas of the canine renal pelvis are much less common than the same types of tumors in the urinary bladder and are rare in cats (see Tables 160–1 and 160–2). The fact that urothelium maintains the embryonic potential to produce mucus-secreting glandular epithelium and squamous epithelium in addition to transitional epithelium accounts for different morphological urothelial carcinomas, including transitional cell carcinomas and squamous cell carcinomas.[73] The sequence of events leading to development of transitional cell and squamous cell neoplasms is similar in all species.[17, 61, 73] Studies of humans, dogs, and laboratory animals have revealed that urothelial cellular hyperplasia precedes formation of many malignant transitional cell neoplasms.[73]

Renal fibrosarcomas, hemangiosarcomas, and undifferentiated sarcomas are frequently encountered neoplasms of the kidneys of dogs (see Table 160–1). Other sarcomas are less common than epithelial neoplasms or nephroblastomas (Tables 160–1 and 160–2).

Metastatic neoplasms are commonly found in the kidneys, possibly because of the large blood volume that the kidneys receive and their abundant supply of capillaries.[22, 62, 73, 90] Renal lymphomas are generally considered metastatic neoplasms associated with the alimentary form of the disease.[17, 60, 66, 90] Malignant lymphoma is the most common renal neoplasm of cats but is less frequent in dogs. Approximately 40 per cent of feline renal lymphomas are confined to the kidneys.[60]

Clinical Signs and Laboratory Findings

Clinical signs vary with location, size, and duration of neoplasia. Neoplasms of the renal pelvis are usually associated with local signs (hematuria, hydronephrosis, and others) that precede polysystemic signs (Fig. 160–1).[4, 17, 48, 67] This pattern is often opposite to that in patients with renal parenchymal neoplasms.[4, 17, 48, 67]

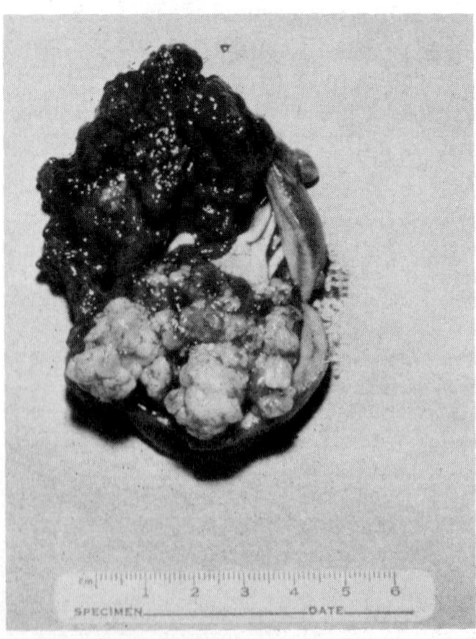

FIGURE 160–1. Transitional epithelial polyps of the renal pelvis in a 9-year-old male schnauzer.

Benign renal neoplasms are rarely significant and are usually incidental necropsy findings. An exception is canine renal hemangioma.[17, 67] This neoplasm is frequently associated with constant or intermittent gross hematuria and various degrees of enlargement of the affected kidney.[24, 27, 42, 50, 51, 65]

Clinical signs of renal tubular cell carcinomas are nonspecific and may not suggest involvement of the urinary system initially.* Local signs include persistent or intermittent gross or microscopic hematuria and abdominal distension with an associated palpable mass.[17, 48, 53, 63, 67] Enlarged kidneys caused by neoplasia must be differentiated from enlarged kidneys caused by hydronephrosis or polycystic disease.[17, 67] In addition, neoplastic enlargement of the kidneys must be differentiated from neoplastic enlargement of one or both adrenal glands and the ovaries, spleen, liver, pancreas, and intestine.[17, 67] Even though both kidneys are involved, a sufficient quantity of functional renal parenchyma may persist to prevent signs of renal failure.[17, 67] Extensive bilateral involvement of the kidneys that destroys 70 to 75 per cent or more of the nephrons is associated with signs of progressive renal insufficiency.[17, 67]

Polysystemic signs unrelated to the urinary tract are common and may be the first clinical manifestation of renal carcinomas.[17, 67] In 54 dogs with primary renal neoplasms, the most common clinical complaints were anorexia, depression, and weight loss. In the same study, an abdominal mass was palpated in 43 per cent with renal neoplasms.[48] Anemia and pyrexia are common.† Proteinuria is the most consistent nonspecific laboratory finding.[48] Polysystemic clinical signs may be related to production of excessive quantities of erythrocyte-stimulating factor, renin, parathormone, prostaglandins, and other hormones by these neoplasms.[11, 32, 88] Polycythemia has been observed in dogs and cats with renal adenomas and renal tubular cell carcinomas that elaborated excessive quantities of erythrocyte-stimulating factor.[11, 32, 88] Clinical signs may be caused by metastatic lesions and may be the first evidence of their presence.

Renal tubular cell carcinomas spread by direct extension through the renal capsule or renal pelvis and by invasion of intrarenal veins and lymphatics.[17, 62, 67, 73] Invasion and growth of renal tubular cell carcinomas into renal veins can occur and may account for the high incidence of lung metastases.[17, 62, 67, 73] One study revealed that 48 per cent of dogs with renal tubular cell carcinomas had pulmonary metastasis on initial radiographic examination.[48] In the same study, renal transitional cell carcinomas did not show initial radiographic evidence of pulmonary metastasis.[48] This may reflect a tendency for transitional cell carcinomas to metastasize later, metastasize less frequently, or manifest clinical signs earlier. Invasion of the renal vein is less common in dogs than in humans.[48] The most common sites of

*See references 13, 36, 44, 48, 53, 63, 93, and 96.

†See references 13, 17, 36, 48, 63, 67, and 97.

metastases in dogs and cats are the lungs, lymph nodes, liver, brain, and bone.[48] Any tissue may be affected, and metastases to unusual sites are common. Many dogs have metastatic lesions when renal tubular cell carcinoma is diagnosed.[48] Metastasis may occur before the onset of urinary signs.[48]

Clinical signs associated with nephroblastomas are similar to those associated with renal tubular cell carcinomas. Hypertrophic osteopathy has been observed in dogs with renal tumors.[9, 10, 16] In one case, characteristic bony lesions of this syndrome developed in the absence of detectable pulmonary metastases.[16]

Nephroblastomas are usually unilateral; bilateral involvement has been reported.[17] If the tumor penetrates the renal capsule, local invasion of perinephric fat, posterior abdominal muscles, diaphragm, and neighboring organs may occur.[3, 48, 49] Distant metastases occur via the lymphatics into pararenal and para-aortic lymph nodes or, more commonly, by venous metastasis from the renal vein into the vena cava. The most common site of metastasis is the lung, followed by the liver, mesentery, and lymph nodes.*

In cats, alimentary lymphoma may be associated with extensive renal involvement. Both kidneys are usually affected and may be palpated as enlarged asymmetrical structures in the abdominal cavity.[17, 60, 66, 90] Renal failure caused by bilateral renal lymphoma occurs more commonly in cats than dogs.[66] Clinical signs include progressive weight loss, depression, anorexia, vomiting, and diarrhea. Cachexia, fever, anemia, and secondary infections occur during terminal phases.[17, 60, 66, 90]

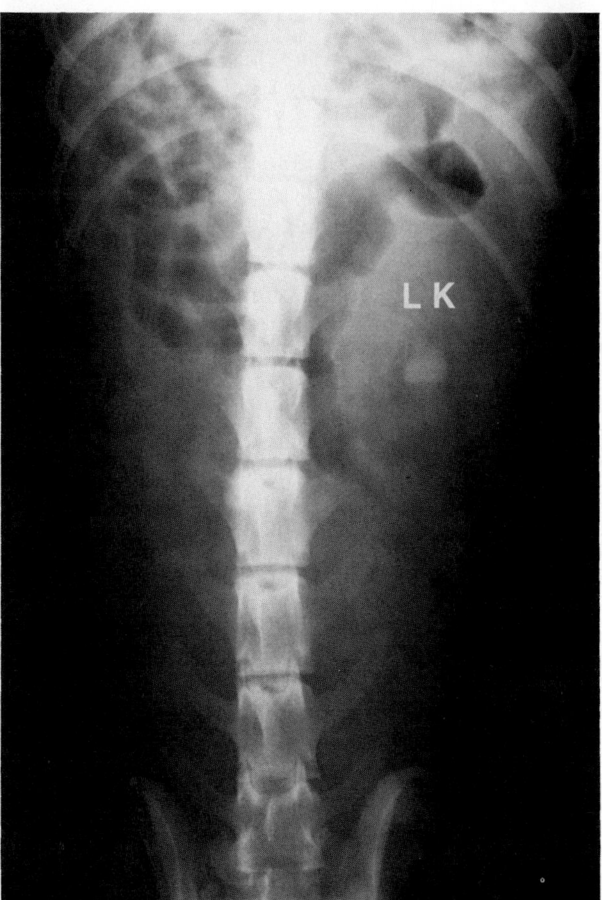

FIGURE 160–2. Ventrodorsal abdominal radiograph of a 6-year-old female Irish water spaniel with renal tubular cell carcinoma of the left kidney. Note the diffuse enlargement of the left kidney (LK). The round radiopaque density is a superimposed nipple.

Diagnosis

Plain abdominal radiographs often reveal an abdominal mass (Figs. 160–2 and 160–3). In one study evaluating abdominal radiographs of 43 dogs with renal neoplasms, abdominal masses were detected in 81.4 per cent and correctly identified as kidney in 53.5 per cent.[48] In the same study, abdominal mass was identified by ultrasonography in 100 per cent of the dogs evaluated with renal neoplasms and correctly identified as kidney in 84.6 per cent (Fig. 160–4).[48] Intravenous urography allowed observation of a renal mass in 96.2 per cent of the dogs evaluated.[48] Intravenous urography not only allows localization of the neoplasm but may permit estimation of the extent of renal parenchymal involvement. Distortion in the shape of the renal pelvis and diverticula and retention of contrast medium are generally seen in the neoplastic kidney (Figs. 160–1 and 160–5). Lack of excretion of detectable quantities of radiopaque contrast material suggests severe hydronephrosis. Selective angiography may also be performed to delineate the precise location and extent of renal destruction (Fig. 160–6). Renal neoplasms associated with enlargement of the kidneys must be differentiated from hydronephrosis and polycystic disease.[17, 67] Thoracic radiographs are taken when renal neoplasm is suspected, to aid in clinical staging for therapy.

A definitive antemortem diagnosis may be established by microscopic identification of neoplastic cells from biopsy specimens of the kidney or detection of neoplastic cells in urine sediment. Needle biopsy of a unilateral renal neoplasm may be inadvisable if treatment by

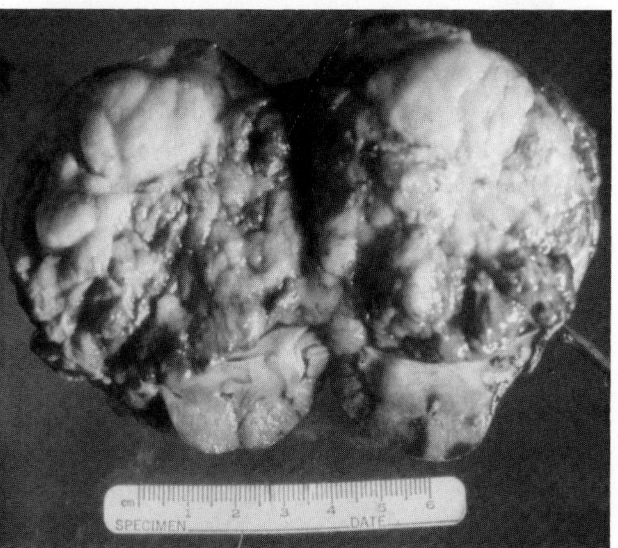

FIGURE 160–3. Renal tubular cell carcinoma of the left kidney of the dog in Figure 160–2.

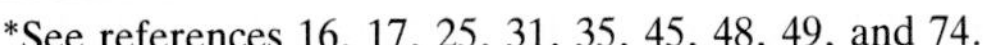

*See references 16, 17, 25, 31, 35, 45, 48, 49, and 74.

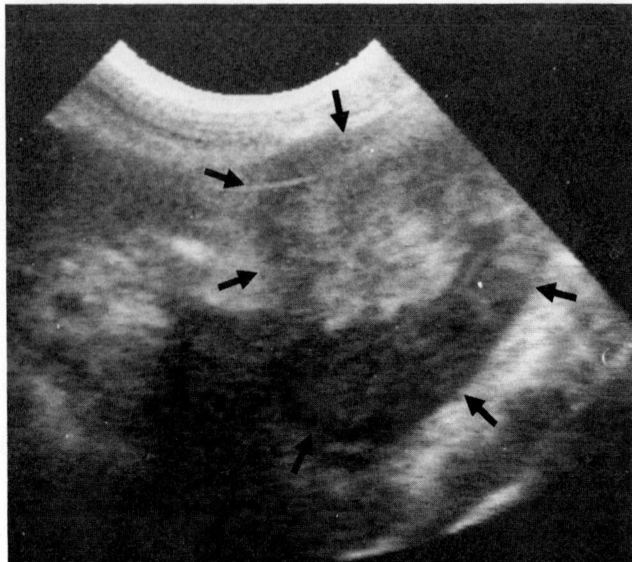

FIGURE 160–4. Sagittal real-time sector sonogram of the left kidney of the dog in Figure 160–2. Note the diffusely invasive mixed-echoic left renal mass *(arrows)*. Severe architectural disruption and loss of recognizable renal anatomy are common with this tumor type.

surgical extirpation is contemplated, because the potential for iatrogenic metastasis exists.[17, 67] Exploratory laparotomy is advised because a biopsy sample may be obtained with less risk of metastasis, the abdomen may be explored for metastases, and nephrectomy can be performed for treatment.

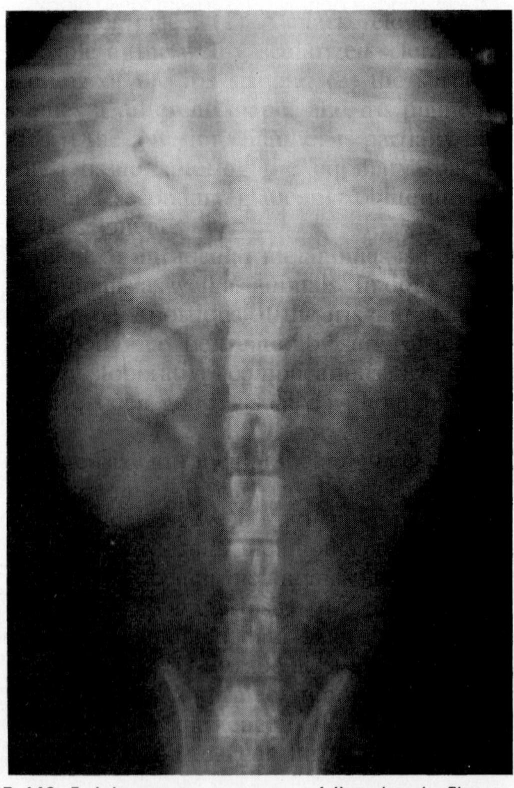

FIGURE 160–5. Intravenous urogram of the dog in Figure 160–1. Note the thin rim of cortical tissue opacified on the left kidney.

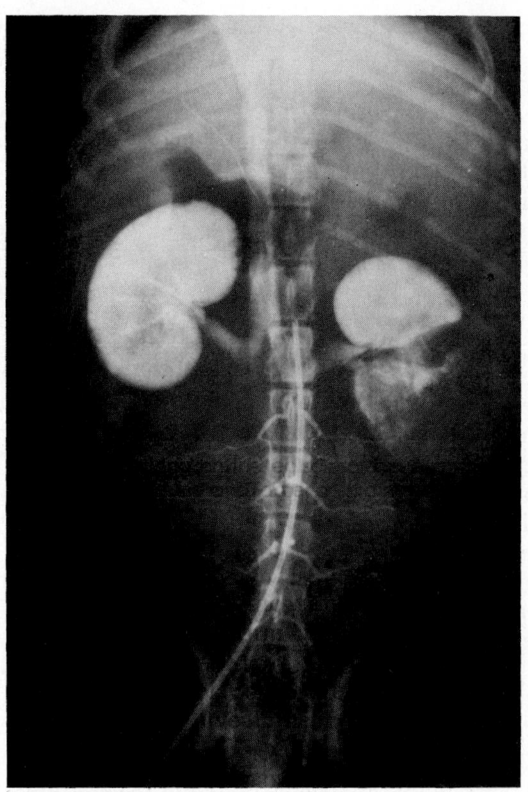

FIGURE 160–6. Selective angiogram of the left kidney of a 10-year-old female miniature poodle with a primary renal hemangioma. Note the lack of filling of the distal pole in the left kidney.

Treatment

Therapy is based on clinical staging (Table 160–3).[95] If the tumor has not metastasized and if the opposite kidney is not neoplastic and has adequate function, nephrectomy and partial ureterectomy are indicated. Preoperative abdominal palpation is restricted to pre-

TABLE 160–3. WORLD HEALTH ORGANIZATION CLINICAL STAGES OF CANINE TUMORS OF THE KIDNEYS

T: Primary tumor	
T_0	No evidence of tumor
T_1	Small tumor without deformation of the kidney
T_2	Solitary tumor with deformation and/or enlargement of the kidney
T_3	Tumor invading perinephric structures (peritoneum) and/or pelvis, ureter, and/or renal blood vessels (renal vein)
T_4	Tumor invading neighboring structures
N: Regional lymph nodes (RLN) (lumbar LN)	
N_0	No RLN involved
N_1	Ipsilateral RLN involved
N_2	Bilateral RLN involved
N_3	Other LN involved (abdominal and pelvic LN)
M: Distant metastasis	
M_0	No evidence of metastasis
M_1	Distant metastasis—specify sites
M_{1a}	Single metastasis
M_{1b}	Multiple metastases in one organ
M_{1c}	Multiple metastases in various organs

Data from World Health Organization: Internal report of the Second Consultation of the Biological Behaviour and Therapy of Tumours of Domestic Animals, Geneva, 1979 (unpublished WHO document VPH/CMO/79.17).

vent rupture of the tumor and seeding of the abdomen with neoplastic cells.[17, 49, 73, 74] Adequate surgical exposure, careful manipulation of the affected kidney, and ligation of the renal vein are advised before mobilizing the tumor to prevent release of neoplastic cells into the blood stream. In addition to complete removal of the tumor, the associated ureter is removed, because metastasis may occur anywhere along its length. If the lymph nodes are enlarged and abnormal, systematic dissection and excision of regional lymph nodes are advised to prevent incomplete removal of tumor cells within lymphatics.[17, 49, 73, 74] Little information in the veterinary literature describes the use of x-ray or chemotherapeutic agents in the treatment of renal tubular cell carcinomas. Clinical and experimental studies in humans suggest limited success.[22] In humans, aggressive or invasive renal tubular cell carcinomas receive adjuvant cytotoxic chemotherapy. Combinations of 5-fluorouracil, doxorubicin, and cyclophosphamide have been used in dogs, but evidence of an objective response is lacking.[22] Medroxyprogesterone has been used in humans with some success in causing partial regression or arresting the growth of renal tubular cell carcinomas.[22]

Chemotherapy is effective against nephroblastomas in humans. Actinomycin D has prevented metastasis.[30, 31, 34, 43, 78] In addition to showing laboratory evidence of direct tumoricidal effect, this drug is also a radiosensitizer that augments the effect of radiation on nephroblastomas.[43, 45, 74] Vincristine has also been used with success in the treatment of nephroblastomas in humans. It is much less toxic than actinomycin D and has a synergistic effect when combined with it.[34, 45, 73, 74] Its use in combined therapy may greatly decrease the risks of toxic side effects of actinomycin D.

The use of radiotherapy for nephroblastoma is limited in veterinary medicine but has significantly improved survival times in humans.[25, 73, 74] It is probable that cells dislodged during surgery or left behind because of incomplete excision are destroyed by x-rays.[25, 73, 74] Radiotherapy is initiated shortly after surgery or administered during surgery by single-dose external beam megavoltage or brachytherapy.

A unilateral nephroblastoma with metastases was successfully controlled in a 1-year-old female mixed-breed dog by surgical extirpation of the right kidney, local irradiation of tissue adjacent to the right kidney, and periodic administration of actinomycin D (0.015 mg/kg daily for 5 days).[16] Combination therapy, incorporating principles of surgical management, radiotherapy, and chemotherapy, is extremely effective in management of nephroblastomas in humans. Cure rates of 70 to 80 per cent have been reported, even in patients with metastatic disease.[34, 45, 73, 74]

In one study, feline renal lymphoma was treated with combination chemotherapy consisting of vincristine, L-asparaginase, cyclophosphamide, methotrexate, cytosine arabinoside, and prednisone.[60] Response was related to clinical stage and the presence or absence of a positive result on a test for feline leukemia virus (Tables 160–4 and 160–5).[60]

Prognosis

The prognosis depends on the type, location, and extent of neoplastic involvement, the presence or absence of metastasis, and the biological behavior of the neoplasm. Long-term survival has been reported after complete surgical extirpation of a unilateral malignant neoplasm. Unfortunately, early diagnosis is not the rule and metastasis is often present, particularly with parenchymal tumors. With bilateral renal involvement or metastases or when treatment is not provided, the prognosis is guarded to poor. Limited survival data reflect the grave prognosis associated with primary renal neoplasms, particularly those with advanced disease at diagnosis. In a study of dogs that had primary renal neoplasms, underwent nephrectomy, and were alive 21 days after surgery, those with renal tubular cell carcinomas had a mean survival of 6.8 months (range 1 to 18 months), those with renal transitional cell carcinomas had a mean survival of 11 months (range 1 to 25 months), and two dogs with nephroblastomas survived 4 and 21 months, respectively.[48]

In a study in which renal lymphoma was diagnosed, staged, and treated in 28 cats, cats that had stage 2

TABLE 160–4. CLINICAL STAGING SYSTEM FOR FELINE LYMPHOMA

Stage 1:	Single tumor (extranodal) or single anatomic area (nodal)
	Includes primary intrathoracic tumors
Stage 2:	Single tumor (extranodal) with regional lymph node involvement
	Two or more nodal areas on the same side of the diaphragm
	Two (extranodal) tumors with or without regional lymph node involvement on the same side of the diaphragm
	A primary, resectable, gastrointestinal tract tumor, usually in the ileocecal area, with or without involvement of associated mesenteric lymph nodes only
Stage 3:	Two tumors (extranodal) on opposite sides of the diaphragm
	Two or more nodal areas cranial and caudal to the diaphragm
	All extensive primary unresectable intra-abdominal disease
	All paraspinal or epidural tumors, regardless of other tumor site(s)
Stage 4:	Stages 1 to 3 with liver and/or spleen involvement
Stage 5:	Stages 1 to 4 with initial involvement of CNS and/or bone marrow

From Mooney SC, et al: Renal lymphoma in cats: 28 cases (1977–1984). *J Am Vet Med Assoc 191:*1473, 1987.

TABLE 160–5. SURVIVAL TIMES OF 28 CATS WITH RENAL LYMPHOMA ACCORDING TO STAGE OF DISEASE

Stage	Number of Cats	Mean Survival Time (Days)	Number of FeLV-Positive Cats/Mean Survival Time (Days)	Number of FeLV-Negative Cats/Mean Survival Time (Days)
2	11	396+	4/168	7/526+
3	5	30	4/27	3/31
4	6	213+	2/105	4/267+
5	6	321+	6/321+	267+

FeLV, feline leukemia virus.

From Mooney SC, et al: Renal lymphoma in cats: 28 cases (1977–1984). *J Am Vet Med Assoc 191:*1473, 1987.

TABLE 160–6. TYPE, AGE, AND SEX OF 21 DOGS WITH PRIMARY NEOPLASMS OF THE URETER

	Sex				Age (Years)		
Tumor Type	Number of Cases	Male	Female	Not Determined	Mean	Range	Not Determined
Epithelial tissue							
Papilloma	1	1	0	0	—	2	0
Transitional cell carcinoma	18	6	12	0	9	5–15	0
Muscle tissue							
Leiomyoma	2	0	2	0	13	11–15	0

Data from the Veterinary Medical Data Program and Caywood DD, Osborne CA: Urinary system. *In* Slatter DH (ed): *Textbook of Small Animal Surgery.* W.B. Saunders, Philadelphia, 1985, pp 2561–2574.

lymphomas (see Table 160–4) and had negative results on testing for feline leukemia virus had the best prognosis compared with other stages, with a mean survival time of greater than 526 days (see Table 160–5).[60]

NEOPLASMS OF THE URETER

Primary neoplasms of the canine ureter are rare. Ureteral neoplasms are more common in females with transitional cell carcinoma being the most common type. (Table 160–6).[5, 17, 38, 52, 67] A favorable prognosis is associated with nephroureterectomy of benign and malignant neoplasms confined to the ureter. Clinical signs are usually associated with hydronephrosis.[5, 17, 38, 52, 67] Neoplasms originating from abdominal organs or tissues may encroach on ureters, occlude their lumina, and cause hydronephrosis. Occlusion of the distal ends of ureters by bladder neoplasia invading the trigone is the most common cause of neoplastic involvement of the ureters.[17, 67] Primary neoplasms of the ureter have not been reported in cats.

NEOPLASMS OF THE URINARY BLADDER

Epidemiology

Bladder tumors are more frequent than tumors in other sites in the urinary tract but account for less than 1 per cent of all canine and feline neoplasms.[21, 40, 44, 92] Bladder tumors are more common in dogs than cats, possibly because of a difference in the metabolism of potentially carcinogenic agents, including tryptophan (Tables 160–7 and 160–8).[12] They are more frequent in female dogs and male cats.[40, 68, 77, 92] In both dogs and cats, bladder tumors are more common in older animals, except for rhabdomyosarcomas, which are frequently identified in young dogs.[14, 68, 75, 77, 82, 92] The average ages of dogs and cats with bladder tumors are 8.3 years and 9.1 years, respectively. Breeds with an increased risk include the Scottish terrier, Shetland sheepdog, beagle, and collie.[40] Dogs from countries with a high level of industrial activity are at risk for bladder cancer.[39]

TABLE 160–7. TYPE, AGE, AND SEX OF 1164 DOGS WITH PRIMARY NEOPLASMS OF THE URINARY BLADDER

	Sex				Age (Years)		
Tumor Type	Number of Cases	Male	Female	Not Determined	Mean	Range	Not Determined
Epithelial tissue							
Papilloma	36	9	23	4	10.6	3–15	3
Adenoma	3	1	1	1	10.3	8–13	1
Adenocarcinoma	78	43	35	0	8.9	2–15	0
Squamous cell carcinoma	50	11	38	1	9.9	5–15	1
Transitional cell carconoma	797	287	507	3	10.9	6 months–15 years	7
Unclassified carcinoma	42	8	13	21	8.9	4–13	15
Muscle tissue							
Leiomyoma	12	1	2	9	12.7	12–13	7
Leiomyosarcoma	50	26	24	0	9.4	1–15	0
Botryoid rhabdomyosarcoma	20	7	10	3	1.3	6 months–5 years	4
Connective tissue							
Myxoma	1	1	0	0	13	—	0
Fibroma	12	1	2	10	7	4–11	7
Neurofibroma	6	0	6	0	10.5	3–13	0
Fibrosarcoma	21	7	13	1	8.6	1–15	1
Unclassified sarcoma	16	7	7	2	3.5	1–8	1
Vascular tissue							
Hemangioma	2	1	0	1	10	—	1
Hemangiosarcoma	18	11	7	0	9.7	2–15	0

Data from the Veterinary Medical Data Program and Caywood DD, Osborne CA: Urinary system. *In* Slatter DH (ed): *Textbook of Small Animal Surgery.* W.B. Saunders, Philadelphia, 1985, pp 2561–2574.

TABLE 160–8. TYPE, AGE, AND SEX OF 69 CATS WITH PRIMARY NEOPLASMS OF THE URINARY BLADDER

Tumor Type	Sex				Age (Years)		
	Number of Cases	*Male*	*Female*	*Not Determined*	*Mean*	*Range*	*Not Determined*
Epithelial tissue							
Papilloma	5	3	1	1	6.7	4 months–15 years	0
Cystadenoma	1	0	1	0	—	12	0
Adenocarcinoma	6	1	4	1	9.2	5–15	1
Squamous cell carcinoma	2	1	0	1	—	8	1
Transitional cell carcinoma	41	17	21	3	10.4	3–15	1
Unclassified carcinoma	5	3	0	2	13.3	13–14	2
Connective tissue							
Myxosarcoma	1	1	0	0	—	6	0
Fibrosarcoma	2	0	2	0	6.5	5–8	0
Muscle tissue							
Leiomyoma	4	1	3	0	6	1–12	0
Leiomyosarcoma	2	0	2	0	9.8	8.5–11	0

Data from the Veterinary Medical Data Program and Caywood DP, Osborne CA: Urinary system. *In* Slatter DH (ed): *Textbook of Small Animal Surgery*. W.B. Saunders, Philadelphia, 1985, pp 2561–2574.

Etiology, Pathology, and Biological Behavior

Although the cause of spontaneously occurring bladder neoplasms in animals has not been established, prolonged mucosal contact with carcinogenic substances in urine is suspected to be important. Experimentally, bladder tumors in dogs have resulted after oral administration of chemical carcinogens, many of which were aromatic hydrocarbons.[64] Two reports have documented an association between chronic administration of cyclophosphamide and transitional cell carcinomas in the bladder of dogs.[55, 89]

In both dogs and cats, malignant tumors are identified more frequently than benign tumors, and malignant epithelial tumors are more common than malignant connective tissue tumors (see Tables 160–7 and 160–8). Secondary tumors of the urinary bladder are infrequent.

Papillomas typically occur in older dogs and may be single or multiple.[68] Ulceration, which frequently is aggravated by bacterial infection, is commonly associated with persistent hematuria. Clinically, papillomas may be difficult to distinguish from polyps associated with polypoid cystitis.[46]

Fibromas are most common in older dogs, may be single or multiple, and are usually associated with bacterial urinary tract infection.[29] Cystic uroliths have been identified in approximately one-third of animals. Prognosis after surgical removal is favorable.

Transitional cell carcinomas are the most common primary malignant tumors of the urinary bladder in dogs and cats.[14, 40, 68, 69] They typically occur as nonpapillary solitary projections into the bladder lumen, often arising from the trigone region. Invasion of the bladder wall is common, and the mucosa and underlying muscle layers may be completely replaced by neoplastic tissue. Tumors may occlude the urethra or ureters. Most grow slowly and metastasize relatively late in their course.[22] Metastasis has been identified in 50 per cent of dogs and 40 per cent of cats.[68, 69] Frequent metastatic sites include the lungs, regional lymph nodes, kidneys, liver, and prostate.[68]

Sarcomas are much less common than carcinomas but when present are usually characterized by diffuse invasive growth into the bladder wall and metastases.[68] Rhabdomyosarcomas, identified most frequently in young large dogs, probably originate from a pluripotential mesodermal stem cell arising from the urogenital ridge.[37, 47, 71, 75, 80] They are typically located at the neck of the bladder, are locally invasive, often do not metastasize, and frequently result in hypertrophic osteopathy.

Secondary bladder tumors account for only 5 per cent of urinary tract neoplasms.[68] Most secondary bladder tumors arise from the urethra and prostate.[14]

Clinical Findings and Diagnosis

Clinical signs commonly associated with bladder tumors include persistent or intermittent hematuria, increased frequency of urination, dysuria, and urinary incontinence.[68, 77] No sign is pathognomonic for neoplasia; animals with bacterial urinary tract infection, urolithiasis, and other lower urinary tract disorders demonstrate similar signs. Partial or complete obstruction of the urethra or ureters may result in signs referable to renal failure. Polydipsia, noted in 33 per cent of dogs with bladder tumors,[14] may be psychogenic because concentrated urine is usually produced after water deprivation.[24] Signs may be present from a few days to months before a diagnosis is established.[14]

Early and potentially curable neoplasms do not produce abnormalities that can be detected by physical examination alone. Later, thickening of the bladder wall or a firm mass within the bladder can be palpated. Cystic calculi may be associated with bladder tumors and may be detected by abdominal palpation. Sublumbar lymph nodes are occasionally enlarged. Swollen and painful extremities resulting from hypertrophic osteopathy are noted in dogs with transitional cell carcinomas, rhabdomyosarcomas, and neurofibrosarcomas.[10, 56, 71, 75] Hypertrophic osteopathy is most often identified in dogs with rhabdomyosarcomas and is typically not associated with pulmonary lesions (Fig. 160–7).

Hematological and biochemical findings are usually

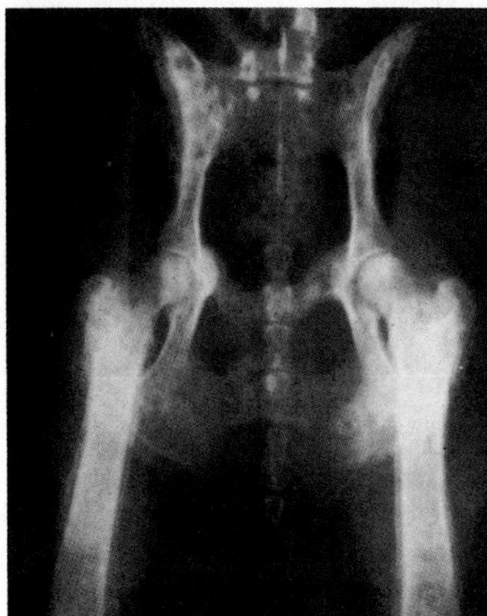

FIGURE 160–7. Hypertrophic osteopathy of the pelvis and femurs of a 2-year-old Doberman pinscher with a rhabdomyosarcoma of the urinary bladder.

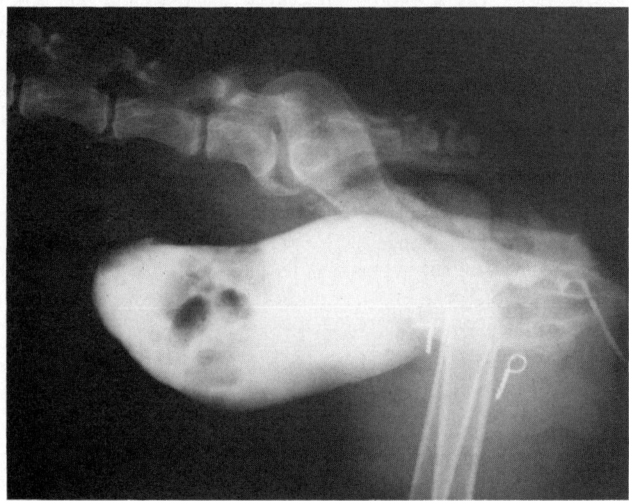

FIGURE 160–8. Positive contrast cystogram of a 14-year-old female spayed mixed-breed dog with transitional cell carcinoma of the urinary bladder. Note the irregularly marginated lobular radiolucent filling defects (masses) in the apical region of the bladder.

normal unless urinary obstruction has resulted in azotemia. Hematuria and mild proteinuria are consistently noted in urinalyses. Pyuria may be observed, especially if urinary tract infection is present. Cats are typically feline leukemia virus negative.[69]

Cytological examination of the urine sediment is useful in establishing a diagnosis, especially in patients with transitional cell carcinomas.[14, 76, 77] Clusters of large anaplastic epithelial cells with prominent nuclear membranes and nucleoli, high nucleus/cytoplasm ratio, and variability in nuclear size are seen. Similar cells are occasionally observed in urine samples from animals with severe inflammatory cystitis, and results are always interpreted with other clinical and laboratory findings.[16] Evaluation of urine sediments from dogs with rhabdomyosarcomas typically reveals large numbers of inflammatory cells and small numbers of small tumor cells with an eccentric nucleus and one or two prominent nucleoli.[75] Evaluation of the urine sediment is performed before contrast radiography because hypertonic contrast solutions can distort normal epithelial cells.

Radiography usually provides presumptive evidence of bladder cancer, is useful for determining clinical stage, and can demonstrate ureteral obstruction and hypertrophic osteopathy. Survey abdominal radiographs may appear normal or may reveal calcification of the bladder wall, urolithiasis, bladder distension, bladder displacement, or increased size of the sublumbar lymph nodes.[14, 77] Tumors are readily demonstrated by contrast cystography (pneumocystography, positive-contrast cystography, or double-contrast cystography). Carcinomas typically appear as space-occupying masses arising from the bladder trigone and protruding into the bladder lumen (Fig. 160–8). Diffuse thickening of the bladder wall is occasionally noted. Polypoid lesions, not at the trigone, are more likely to be benign.[94] Infrequently, severe inflammatory cystitis is associated with radiographic lesions that are similar to those in carcinoma. This is especially true with polypoid cystitis.[46] Ureteral obstruction, if present, can be demonstrated by intravenous urography.

Thoracic radiographs are obtained to determine the presence or absence of metastatic disease. In a study of 11 dogs with pulmonary metastases from transitional cell carcinomas of the bladder or urethra, four radiographic patterns were noted: (1) diffuse unstructured increase in interstitial density, (2) localized interstitial or alveolar infiltrates, (3) multiple interstitial nodules, and (4) normal pulmonary opacity.[87] The diffuse unstructured interstitial pattern, which can be confused with pulmonary aging changes, was most frequent. Hilar lymphadenopathy was noted in one dog. Findings on pulmonary radiographs are frequently negative at initial diagnosis.

Ultrasonography can be used to demonstrate bladder tumors, to determine the extent of disease, and to document ureteral obstruction (Figs. 160–9 and 160–10).[1] Compared with cystography, ultrasonography has the advantage of being noninvasive and usually does not require sedation.

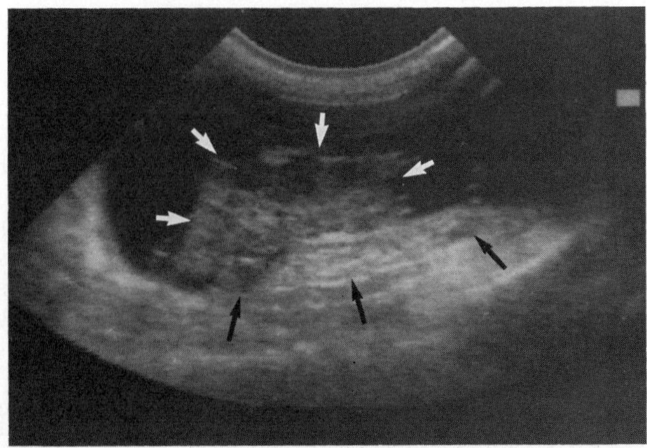

FIGURE 160–9. Sagittal real-time sector sonogram of the urinary bladder of the dog in Figure 160–9. Note the solid mixed-echoic mass *(arrows)*, which originates from the bladder wall and projects into the bladder lumen.

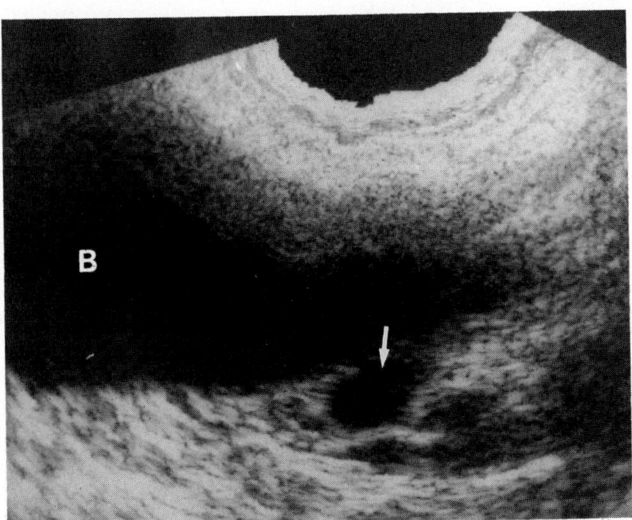

FIGURE 160–10. Sagittal real-time sector sonogram of the urinary bladder of an 8-year-old male German shepherd with a previously surgically removed squamous cell carcinoma of the urinary bladder (B). Note the dilated anechoic ureter *(arrow)* entering the bladder trigone.

History, physical findings, urine sediment examination, and radiographic and ultrasonographic evaluations are useful in establishing a presumptive diagnosis of bladder neoplasia. Biopsy is required to establish a definitive diagnosis and to determine histological type. Material for histopathological examination can be obtained by catheter biopsy of the tumor,[58] cystoscopy,[18] or exploratory celiotomy. If a celiotomy is performed, the iliac lymph nodes are carefully examined for evidence of metastatic disease. Evaluation of the depth of bladder wall invasion, the presence or absence of regional lymph node involvement, and the presence or absence of distant metastases is required to determine the clinical stage of disease (Table 160–9).

Treatment

Considerations in the choice of therapy for animals with bladder tumors include the tumor type, the extent and location of the tumor within the bladder, the presence or absence of metastatic disease, and the presence of concurrent problems such as renal failure, ureteral or urethral obstruction, bacterial urinary tract infection, or urolithiasis.

Animals with benign bladder tumors can often be successfully treated by surgical removal of the tumor if the tumor does not involve the bladder trigone or neck. Ninety-five per cent of dogs with urinary bladder fibromas were symptom free at least 3 months after tumor excision.[29] Seven dogs with papillomas, two with hemangiomas, and two with leiomyomas were alive 6 months to 5 years after partial cystectomy.[14] Long-term survival has also been reported in cats after surgical excision of leiomyomas and fibromas.[77]

The optimum therapy for animals with malignant bladder tumors has not been determined. Treatment measures that have been attempted include surgery (partial cystectomy or total cystectomy with urinary diversion), radiation therapy, chemotherapy, immunotherapy, and combinations of these. Extensive disease at diagnosis and a high prevalence of metastatic disease have resulted in only short-term benefits in most animals using these approaches. Use of the World Health Organization clinical staging system for bladder tumors (see Table 160–9) aids in defining appropriate therapy.

Partial cystectomy can be used to remove tumors without extensive trigonal involvement. A full-thickness cystectomy is performed, leaving a wide margin of normal-appearing tissue. More than 80 per cent of the bladder can be removed without significant loss in capacity.[94] Ureteral transplantation to the body of the bladder may be necessary. Tumors are handled as little as possible to prevent seeding of neoplastic cells in the abdominal cavity or incision line.[2] Survival times after partial cystectomy are short because of tumor recurrence or metastatic disease.[77]

Techniques for total cystectomy and urinary diversion have been described, but complications from the diversion procedure or the presence of metastatic disease have resulted in short-term benefit.[6, 8, 59, 81] Five months was the longest survival time in 10 dogs with bladder or urethral transitional cell carcinomas after complete removal of the bladder and proximal urethra and ureterocolonic anastomosis.[81] Six dogs had metastatic disease at death. Complications from the diversion procedure include intermittent vomiting, anorexia, neurological abnormalities, hyperchloremic metabolic acidosis, and pyelonephritis.

Radiation therapy (external beam or during surgery) has been attempted with bladder tumors. Tumor control has been short, and complication rates are high. Thirteen dogs with bladder tumors were treated with radiation after partial excision of their tumors.[86] Sixty-one per cent were alive at 1 year, 46 per cent at 18 months, and 23 per cent at 2 years. One dog survived longer than 70 months. Persistence or recurrence of tumor was noted in 46 per cent and metastasis in 30 per cent. Postradiotherapy complications, which were severe in some cases, included increased frequency of urination

TABLE 160–9. WORLD HEALTH ORGANIZATION CLINICAL STAGES OF CANINE TUMORS OF THE URINARY BLADDER

T: Primary tumor	
T_{is}	Carcinoma *in situ*
T_0	No evidence of primary tumor
T_1	Superficial papillary tumor
T_2	Tumor invading the bladder wall, with induration
T_3	Tumor invading neighboring organs (prostate, uterus, vagina, anal canal)
The letter *m* added to the appropriate T category denotes multiple tumors	
N: Regional lymph nodes (RLN) (internal and external iliac LN)	
N_0	No RLN involved
N_1	RLN involved
N_2	RLN and juxtaregional nodes involved
M: Distant metastasis	
M_0	No evidence of metastasis
M_1	Distant metastasis present–specify sites

Data from World Health Organization: Internal Report of the Second Consultation on the Biological Behaviour and Therapy of Tumours of Domestic Animals, Geneva, 1979 (unpublished WHO document VPH/CMO/79.17).

(46 per cent), urinary incontinence (46 per cent), cystitis (38 per cent), and stranguria (15 per cent). Increased frequency of urination probably resulted from bladder wall fibrosis. Seven dogs with bladder tumors received radiation during surgery, followed by fractionated external beam radiation (five dogs) after partial tumor excision.[94] Mean survival time of the dogs completing treatment was 5 months, and no dog lived longer than 13 months. Five of six dogs undergoing necropsy had evidence of viable tumor. Urinary incontinence and hydroureter were frequent complications. Two dogs with bladder carcinomas received fractionated external beam radiation and cisplatin.[57] Clinical improvement and a decrease in tumor size were noted in both dogs, but survival times were less than 7 months.

In humans with superficial bladder tumors, intravesical chemotherapy with agents such as doxorubicin, triethylene thiophosphoramide, and mitomycin-C has been useful in reducing recurrence rates.[72] With invasive disease, systemic combination chemotherapy has resulted in complete and partial remission rates of 45 to 70 per cent. The most effective chemotherapeutic protocols have included combinations of cisplatin, methotrexate, cyclophosphamide, 5-fluorouracil, or cyclophosphamide.

Few reports are available on the use of systemic or local chemotherapy in animals with bladder cancer, and only palliative benefits have been documented. Cisplatin was used to treat eight dogs with bladder or urethral transitional cell carcinomas.[79] One partial response was noted, and four dogs had stable disease from 7.5 to 8.5 months. In seven dogs, subjective improvements consisting of apparent growth arrest and partial relief of symptoms were noted after therapy with combinations of intravesicular instillations of triethylene thiophosphoramide or 5-fluorouracil or both and systemic administration of 5-fluorouracil, doxorubicin, or cyclophosphamide.[23]

Immunotherapy with bacillus Calmette-Gúerin (BCG) has been beneficial in humans with superficial bladder tumors.[72] Injection of BCG into bladders of previously sensitized dogs resulted in cystitis.[7] Two of seven dogs with bladder tumors treated with BCG at the time of partial tumor excision benefited from the therapy.[93]

Palliation of signs is possible with currently available treatment methods and attentive symptomatic and supportive care. Because of urothelial damage and urinary retention, animals with bladder tumors are susceptible to bacterial urinary tract infection. Invasive procedures, such as catheterization, are kept to a minimum. Urine is cultured frequently, and urinary tract infections are treated vigorously with antibiotics chosen on the basis of sensitivity tests. Diagnostic methods that facilitate earlier diagnosis and new approaches to surgery, chemotherapy, and radiation therapy need to be evaluated if survival times in animals with bladder cancer are to be significantly improved.

Prognosis

The prognosis for benign tumors that can be completely resected surgically is favorable. The long-term prognosis for most malignant bladder tumors is poor because of extensive bladder wall invasion at diagnosis and a high incidence of metastasis. Surgery, chemotherapy, or radiation therapy may reduce the tumor burden enough to induce short-term improvement in clinical signs. Treatment of urinary tract infection or urolithiasis also alleviates clinical signs.

NEOPLASMS OF THE URETHRA

Epidemiology

Primary tumors of the urethra are uncommon. More females are affected than males, and tumors usually occur in older animals (Table 160–10), with a mean age of 10.4 yrs.[84, 91] Urethral neoplasms are usually located in the prostatic urethra in males and the distal urethra or throughout the urethra in females. Beagles may have an increased risk.[91]

TABLE 160–10. TYPE, AGE, AND SEX OF 340 DOGS WITH PRIMARY NEOPLASMS OF THE URETHRA

	Sex				Age (Years)		
Tumor Type	*Number of Cases*	*Male*	*Female*	*Not Determined*	*Mean*	*Range*	*Not Determined*
Epithelial tissue							
Adenoma	5	1	0	4	—	5	4
Adenocarcinoma	17	5	11	1	11.3	5–15	1
Squamous cell carcinoma	35	5	30	0	10.5	5–13	0
Transitional cell carcinoma	275	36	239	0	7	6 months–15 years	5
Unclassified carcinoma	1	0	1	0	—	15	0
Connective tissue							
Fibroma	1	1	0	0	—	5	0
Myxoma	1	1	0	0	—	13	0
Myxosarcoma	1	0	1	1	—	9	0
Muscle tissue							
Leiomyoma	1	0	1	0	—	8	0
Rhabdomyosarcoma	1	1	0	0	—	3	0
Vascular tissue							
Hemangiosarcoma	2	0	2	0	9.5	9–10	0

Data from the Veterinary Medical Data Program and Caywood DD, Osborne CA: Urinary system. *In* Slatter DH (ed): *Textbook of Small Animal Surgery*. W.B. Saunders, Philadelphia, 1985, pp 2561–2574.

Etiology, Pathology, and Biological Behavior

The cause of urethral neoplasia has not been established. In humans, chronic urethral irritation has been suggested as a predisposing factor.[33] Transitional cell carcinoma is the most common urethral tumor (see Table 160–10). Local invasion into the bladder occurs in one-third of cases.[91] Urethral neoplasms grow slowly and metastasize late. Metastasis to local lymph nodes or the lung occurs in approximately 30 per cent of dogs with urethral tumors.[84]

Clinical Findings and Diagnosis

Chronic dysuria is a frequent clinical sign. Hematuria, urinary incontinence, and urethral discharge may also be noted. If urethral obstruction is present, postrenal azotemia may develop. A posterior abdominal mass and bladder distension may be noted on abdominal palpation. A urethral mass can often be palpated *per rectum*. Vaginoscopy may reveal a mass protruding from the urethral orifice. Urethral catheterization is often difficult or impossible. Neoplastic cells may be seen in urine sediment.

Survey abdominal radiographs may reveal a posterior abdominal mass, bladder distension, sublumbar lymphadenopathy, or vertebral lysis. Urethral tumors are readily demonstrated by contrast radiography. A positive-contrast urethrogram is the technique of choice if the urethra can be catheterized. If catheterization is impossible, a positive-contrast vaginogram or intravenous urogram may enhance observation of the urethra. Typical lesions include multiple poorly marginated intraluminal masses that result in a generalized moth-eaten appearance of the urethra (Fig. 160–11).[85] Extension of contrast medium into periurethral tissues may be noted. Chest radiographs are obtained to rule out pulmonary involvement.

History, physical findings, and radiography usually localize the disease to the urethra. Urethral tumors are definitively diagnosed by biopsy. Material for histopathological examination can be obtained by catheter biopsy of the urethra or surgical exploration of the pelvic urethra.[58] A pelvic osteotomy is usually required to expose the tumor adequately and to evaluate its extent.

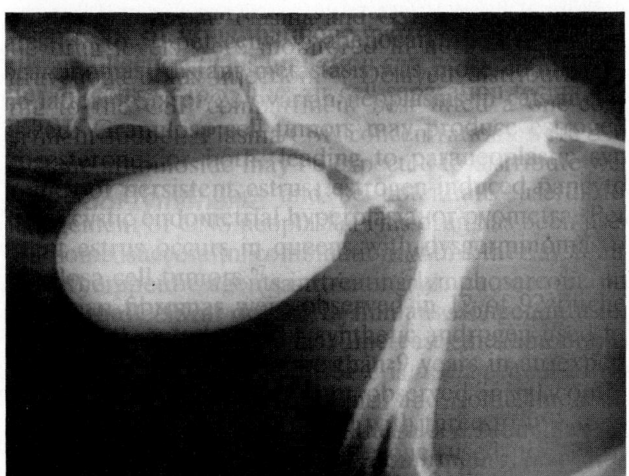

FIGURE 160–11. Lateral positive contrast retrograde urethrocystogram from an 8-year-old female spayed Shih Tzu with transitional cell carcinoma of the urethra. Note the irregular margination of the proximal urethral lumen.

Treatment

As with bladder tumors, urethral neoplasms are diagnosed late in their course, and optimum therapy has not been determined. Therapeutic options include surgical excision, radiation therapy, or chemotherapy. The usefulness of partial urethrectomy followed by trigonal colonic anastomosis or antepubic urethrostomy is limited by frequent trigonal involvement.[93] Complete urethrectomy, cystectomy, and urinary diversion are associated with the same problems described for bladder neoplasia. Tumor progression may be delayed in some cases by radiation therapy or chemotherapy. Survival times of 1 and 4 months were reported in two dogs treated with radiation therapy.[94] Cisplatin chemotherapy produced stabilization of disease in two dogs for 4 and 8 months.[79] Cyclophosphamide and doxorubicin may also be valuable for palliation.

Prognosis

The long-term prognosis for dogs with urethral tumors is poor because of extensive local disease at diagnosis and a high rate of metastasis. Radiation therapy or chemotherapy may result in reduction of clinical signs and increased survival time by several months.

References

1. Abu-Yousef MM: Ultrasound of bladder tumors. *Semin Ultrasound CT MR* 7:275, 1986.
2. Anderson WI, et al: Presumptive subcutaneous surgical transplantation of urinary bladder transitional cell carcinoma in a dog. *Cornell Vet 79*:263, 1989.
3. Balsaver AM, et al: Ultrastructural studies in Wilms' tumors. *Cancer 22*:417, 1968.
4. Baskin GB, DePaoli A: Primary renal neoplasms of the dog. *Vet Pathol 14*:591, 1977.
5. Berzon JL: Primary leiomyosarcoma of the ureter of a dog. *J Am Vet Med Assoc 175*:374, 1979.
6. Bjorling DE, et al: Bilateral ureteroileostomy and perineal urinary diversion in dogs. *Vet Surg 14*:204, 1985.
7. Bloomberg SD, et al: The effects of BCG on the dog bladder. *Invest Urol 12*:423, 1975.
8. Bovee KC, et al: Trigonal-colonic anastomosis: A urinary diversion procedure in dogs. *J Am Vet Med Assoc 174*:184, 1979.
9. Brody RS, Craig PH: Hypertrophic osteoarthropathy in a dog with pulmonary metastasis arising from a renal adenocarcinoma. *J Am Vet Med Assoc 132*:231, 1958.
10. Brody RS, et al: Hypertrophic pulmonary osteoarthropathy in a dog with carcinoma of the urinary bladder. *J Am Vet Med Assoc 162*:474, 1973.
11. Brown NO: Paraneoplastic syndromes of humans, dogs and cats. *J Am Anim Hosp Assoc 17*:911, 1981.
12. Brown RR, Price JM: Quantitative studies on metabolites of tryptophan in the urine of the dog, cat, rat and man. *J Biol Chem 219*:985, 1956.
13. Burger GT, et al: Renal carcinoma in a dog. *J Am Vet Med Assoc 171*:282, 1977.
14. Burnie AG, Weaver AD: Urinary bladder neoplasia in the dog: A review of seventy cases. *J Small Anim Pract 24*:129, 1983.
15. Caywood DD, Osborne CA: Urinary system, oncology. *In* Slatter DH (ed): *Textbook of Small Animal Surgery*. W. B. Saunders, Philadelphia. 1985, pp 2561–2574.
16. Caywood DD, et al: Hypertrophic osteoarthropathy associated with an atypical nephroblastoma in a dog. *J Am Anim Hosp Assoc 16*:855, 1980.
17. Caywood DD, et al: Neoplasms of the canine and feline urinary tract. *In*

Kirk RW (ed): *Current Veterinary Therapy VII*. W. B. Saunders, Philadelphia, 1980, pp 1203–1212.
18. Cooper JE, et al: Cystoscopic examination of male and female dogs. *Vet Rec 115*:571, 1984.
19. Cosenza SF, Seely JC: Generalized nodular dermatofibrosis and renal cystadenocarcinomas in a German shepherd dog. *J Am Vet Med Assoc 189*:1587, 1986.
20. Cotchin E: Neoplasia in the cat. *Vet Rec 60*:425, 1957.
21. Cotchin E: Spontaneous carcinoma of the urinary bladder of the dog. *Br Vet J 115*:431, 1959.
22. Crow SE: Urinary tract neoplasms in dogs and cats. *Comp Cont Educ 7*:607, 1985.
23. Crow SE, Klausner JS: Management of transitional cell carcinomas of the urinary bladder. *In* Kirk RW (ed): *Current Veterinary Therapy VIII*. W. B. Saunders, Philadelphia, 1983, pp 1119–1121.
24. Crow SE, et al: Hematuria associated with renal hemangiosarcoma in a dog. *J Am Vet Med Assoc 176*:531, 1980.
25. D'Angio GJ: Radiation therapy in Wilms' tumor. *JAMA 204*:124, 1968.
26. Diters RW, Wells M: Renal interstitial cell tumors in the dog. *Vet Pathol 23*:74, 1986.
27. Dunn WH: Renal neoplasms of dogs. *J Am Vet Med Assoc 84*:119, 1934.
28. Engle GC: A retrospective study of 395 feline neoplasms. *J Am Anim Hosp Assoc 5*:21, 1969.
29. Esplin DG: Urinary bladder fibromas in dogs: 51 cases (1981–1985). *J Am Vet Med Assoc 190*:440, 1987.
30. Farber S, et al: Clinical studies of actinomycin D with special reference to Wilms' tumor in children. *Ann NY Acad Sci 89*:421, 1960.
31. Garrett RA, et al: Metastatic renal nephroma: Survival following therapy. *J Urol 98*:444, 1967.
32. Gorse MJ: Polycythemia associated with renal fibrosarcoma in a dog. *J Am Vet Med Assoc 192*:793, 1988.
33. Grabstald H: Tumors of the urethra in men and women. *Cancer 32*:1236, 1973.
34. Greene FL, Donaldson MH: Chemotherapy of Wilms' tumor. *New Physician 19*:598, 1970.
35. Gross RE, Neuhauser EBP: Treatment of mixed tumors of the kidney in childhood. Pediatrics *6*:843, 1950.
36. Habermann RT, Williams FP: Papillary cystic adenocarcinoma of a kidney in a dog. *J Am Vet Med Assoc 142*:1011, 1963.
37. Halliwell WH, Ackerman N: Botryoid rhabdomyosarcoma of the urinary bladder and hypertrophic osteoarthropathy in a young dog. *J Am Vet Med Assoc 165*:911, 1974.
38. Hanika C, Rebar AH: Ureteral transitional cell carcinoma in the dog. *Vet Pathol 17*:643, 1980.
39. Hayes H, et al: Bladder cancer in pet dogs: A sentinel for environmental cancer? *Am J Epidemiol 114*:229, 1981.
40. Hayes HM: Canine bladder cancer: Epidemiologic features. *Am J Epidemiol 104*:673, 1976.
41. Hayes HM, Fraumeni JF: Canine renal neoplasm: Epidemiologic features. *Cancer Res 37*:2553, 1977.
42. Hitt ME: Hematuria of renal origin. *Comp Cont Educ 8*:14, 1986.
43. Howard R: Actinomycin D in Wilms' tumor: Treatment of lung metastasis. *Arch Dis Child 40*:200, 1965.
44. Jabara AG: Three cases of primary malignant neoplasms arising in the canine urinary system. *J Comp Pathol 78*:335, 1968.
45. James DH, et al: Childhood malignant tumors—concurrent chemotherapy with dactinomycin and vincristine sulfate. *JAMA 197*:1043, 1966.
46. Johnston SJ, et al: "Canine polypoid cystitis." *In* Kirk RW (ed): *Current Veterinary Therapy VII*. W. B. Saunders, Philadelphia. 1980, pp 1137–1138.
47. Kelly DF: Rhabdomyosarcoma in the urinary bladder of a dog. *Vet Pathol 18*:375, 1973.
48. Klein MK, et al: Canine primary renal neoplasms: A retrospective review of 54 cases. *J Am Anim Hosp Assoc 24*4431, 1988.
49. Ladd WE: Embryoma of the kidney (Wilms' tumor). *Ann Surg 108*:885, 1938.
50. Lappin MR: Hematuria and extreme neutrophilic leukocytosis in a dog with renal tubular carcinoma. *J Am Vet Med Assoc 192*:793, 1988.
51. Lee R, et al: Persistent hematuria in a dog due to a discrete renal hemangioma. *J Small Anim Pract 15*:621, 1974.
52. Liska WD, Patnaik AK: Leiomyoma of the ureter of a dog. *J Am Anim Hosp Assoc 13*:83, 1977.
53. Lucke VM, Kelley DF: Renal carcinoma in the dog. *Vet Pathol 13*:264, 1976.
54. Luim B, Moe L: Hereditary multifocal renal cystadenocarcinomas and nodular dermatofibrosis in the German shepherd dog: Macroscopic and histopathologic changes. *Vet Pathol 22*:447, 1985.
55. Macy DW, et al: Transitional cell carcinoma of the bladder associated with cyclophosphamide administration. *J Am Anim Hosp Assoc 19*:965, 1983.
56. Mandel M: Hypertrophic osteoarthropathy secondary to neurofibrosarcoma of the urinary bladder in a cocker spaniel. *Vet Med Small Anim Clin 7*:1307, 1975.
57. McCaw DL, Lattimer JC: Radiation and cisplatin for treatment of canine urinary bladder carcinoma—a report of two case histories. *Vet Radiol 29*:264, 1988.
58. Melhoff T, Osborne CA: Catheter biopsy of the urethra, urinary bladder and prostate gland. *In* Kirk RW (ed): *Current Veterinary Therapy VI*. W. B. Saunders, Philadelphia, 1977, pp 1173–1184.
59. Montgomery RD, Hankes GH: Ureterocolonic anastomosis in a dog with transitional cell carcinoma of the urinary bladder. *J Am Vet Med Assoc 190*:1427, 1987.
60. Mooney SC, et al: Renal lymphoma in cats: 28 cases (1977–1984). *J Am Vet Med Assoc 191*:1473, 1987.
61. Mulligan RM: Comparative pathology in human and canine cancer. *Ann NY Acad Sci 108*:642, 1963.
62. Nielsen S, Moulton JR: Tumors of the urinary system. *In* Moulton JR (ed): *Tumors in Domestic Animals*. 3rd ed. University of California Press, Berkeley, 1990, pp 458–478.
63. Nielson SW, Archibald J: Canine renal disorders. III. Renal carcinoma in 3 dogs. *North Am Vet 36*:36, 1955.
64. Okajima E, et al: Urinary bladder tumors induced by *N*-butyl-*N*-(4-hydroxybutyl)nitrosamine in dogs. *Cancer Res 41*:1958, 1981.
65. Osborne CA, et al: Feline renal pelvic carcinoma. *J Am Vet Med Assoc 159*:1238, 1971.
66. Osborne CA, et al: Renal lymphoma in the dog and cat. *J Am Vet Med Assoc 158*:2058, 1971.
67. Osborne CA, et al: Neoplasms of the kidney. *In Canine and Feline Urology*. W. B. Saunders, Philadelphia, 1972, pp 255–260.
68. Osborne CA, et al: Neoplasms of the canine and feline urinary bladder: Incidence, etiologic factors, occurrence and pathologic features. *Am J Vet Res 29*:2041, 1968.
69. Patnaik AK, et al: A histopathologic study of twenty urinary bladder neoplasms in the cat. *J Small Anim Pract 27*:433, 1986.
70. Peterson ME: Inappropriate erythropoietin production from a renal carcinoma in a dog with polycythemia. *J Am Vet Med Assoc 179*:995, 1981.
71. Pletchner JM, Dalton L: Botryoid rhabdomyosarcoma in the urinary bladder of a dog. *Vet Pathol 18*:695, 1981.
72. Richie JP, et al: Cancer of the urinary bladder. *In* DeVita VT, et al (eds): *Cancer: Principles and Practice of Oncology*. J. B. Lippincott, Philadelphia, 1989, pp 1008–1022.
73. Rickham PP: Malignant tumors involving the genitourinary system. *In* Johnson JH, Scholtmeyer RJ (eds): *Problems in Pediatric Urology*. Excerpta Medica, Amsterdam, 1972, pp 180–236.
74. Rickham PP: Wilms' tumor. *In* Rob C, Smith R (eds): *Operative Surgery*. Butterworth, London, 1970, pp 65–66.
75. Rozel JF: Cytology of urine from dogs with botryoid sarcoma of the bladder. *Acta Cytol 16*:443, 1972.
76. Rozengurt N, et al: Urinary cytology of a canine bladder carcinoma. *J Comp Pathol 96*:581, 1986.
77. Schwarz PD, et al: Urinary bladder tumors in the cat: A review of 27 cases. *J Am Anim Hosp Assoc 21*:237, 1985.
78. Schweisquth O, Schleinger MJ: Actinomycin D associated with irradiation in the treatment of Wilms' tumor. *Ann Radiol 10*:657, 1967.
79. Shapiro W, et al: Cisplatin for treatment of transitional cell and squamous cell carcinomas in the dog. *J Am Vet Med Assoc 193*:1530, 1988.
80. Stamps P, Harris DL: Botryoid rhabdomyosarcoma of the urinary bladder of a dog. *J Am Vet Med Assoc 153*:1064, 1968.
81. Stone EA, et al: Ureterocolonic anastomosis in ten dogs with transitional cell carcinoma. *Vet Surg 17*:147, 1988.
82. Strafuss AC, Dean MJ: Neoplasms of the canine urinary bladder. *J Am Vet Med Assoc 166*:1161, 1975.
83. Suter M, et al: Generalized nodular dermatofibrosis in six alsatians. *Vet Pathol 20*:632, 1983.
84. Tarvin G, et al: Primary urethral tumors in dogs. *J Am Vet Med Assoc 172*:931, 1978.
85. Ticer G, et al: Transitional cell carcinoma of the urethra in four female dogs: Its urethrographic appearance. *Vet Radiol 21*:12, 1980.
86. Walker M, Breider M: Intraoperative radiotherapy of canine bladder cancer. *Vet Radiol 28*:200, 1987.
87. Walter PA, et al: Radiographic appearance of pulmonary metastases from transitional cell carcinoma of the bladder and urethra of the dog. *J Am Vet Med Assoc 185*:411, 1984.
88. Waters DJ, Prueter JC: Secondary polycythemia associated with renal disease in the dog: Two case reports and review of the literature. *J Am Anim Hosp Assoc 24*:109, 1988.
89. Weller RE, et al: Transitional cell carcinoma of the bladder associated with cyclophosphamide therapy in a dog. *J Am Anim Hosp Assoc 15*:733, 1979.
90. Willson JE, Gillmore CE: Malignant lymphoma in a cat with involvement of the kidneys demonstrated radiographically. *J Am Vet Med Assoc 140*:1068, 1962.
91. Wilson GP, et al: Canine urethral cancer. *J Am Anim Hosp Assoc 15*:741, 1979.
92. Wimberly HC, Lewis RM: Transitional cell carcinoma in the domestic cat. *Vet Pathol 16*:223, 1979.
93. Withrow SJ: Tumors of the urinary system. *In* Withrow SJ, MacEwen EG (eds): *Clinical Veterinary Oncology*. J. B. Lippincott, Philadelphia, 1989, pp 312–324.
94. Withrow SJ, et al: Intraoperative irradiation of 16 spontaneously occurring canine neoplasms. *Vet Surg 18*:7, 1989.
95. World Health Organization: Internal report of the Second Consultation of the Biological Behaviour and Therapy of Tumours of Domestic Animals, Geneva, 1979 (unpublished WHO document VPH/CMO/79.17).
96. Yang YH: The multicentric renal adenocarcinomas *in situ* of a dog. *Pathol Microbiol 29*:181, 1966.
97. Zontine WJ: Renal neoplasia and hematuria. *Pulse 8*:8, 1966.

CHAPTER

161

Musculoskeletal System

David J. Waters

Neoplasms of bone may arise from tissue elements within bone (primary bone tumors) or may secondarily invade bone either by local extension or distant metastasis (secondary bone tumors). In dogs and cats, primary bone tumors far outnumber secondary bone tumors, although precise data on the relative prevalence of each are lacking. The majority of canine and feline primary bone tumors are malignant. Neoplasms of joints are less common than bone neoplasms. Neoplasms of skeletal muscle are rare.

CLINICAL SIGNS OF BONE NEOPLASMS

The most frequent clinical signs in dogs and cats with appendicular bone tumors are pain or lameness referable to the primary tumor. A palpable swelling or mass may not be evident at presentation. Careful evaluation for pain in response to deep palpation of bone is critical to distinguish bone tumors from more common disease entities associated with lameness, such as anterior cruciate ligament rupture or degenerative joint disease. Pain and lameness may be gradual in onset and may persist for several weeks or months. Clinical signs are relentless, and lameness is progressive; worsening of lameness after exercise or "warming out of lameness" is not a typical observation. Pathological fracture associated with bone neoplasms may cause sudden onset of nonweightbearing lameness.

Clinical signs in dogs and cats with axial skeletal neoplasms reflect tumor location. Neoplasms of the skull or nasal cavity may be associated with seizures, exophthalmos, pain on opening the mouth, facial deformity, nasal discharge, or sneezing. Neoplasms of ribs are usually externally palpable and may be associated with dyspnea secondary to intrathoracic extension of the tumor or associated pleural effusion. Spinal neoplasms may produce paresis or pain with extradural compression or nerve root compromise. Pathological fracture of vertebrae may result in sudden onset of myelopathic signs. Neoplasms of the pelvis may be associated with lameness but more frequently result in tenesmus or stranguria due to pelvic canal compromise.

DIAGNOSIS OF BONE NEOPLASMS

Radiographs are useful in assessing the extent of bone involvement and distinguishing bone neoplasms from other non-neoplastic conditions such as fractures, osteomyelitis, and metabolic bone disease. Radiographic changes such as cortical destruction and periosteal new bone formation may support a diagnosis of bone neoplasia but are seldom pathognomonic for a histological type.[58, 59, 73, 102, 147] The formation of reactive bone between the periosteum and cortex at the transition zone of the neoplasm (the so-called Codman triangle) is not pathognomonic for osteosarcoma and may be seen with neoplastic or non-neoplastic processes.[73, 147] Definitive diagnosis is based on histopathological evaluation.[153]

BONE BIOPSY

Bone biopsy is important in the diagnosis and management of bone tumors in dogs and cats. Two techniques of closed biopsy have received the most attention: Michele trephine and Jamshidi needle biopsy. Biopsy of 32 bone tumors in 28 dogs using a Michele trephine was reported.[214] After a stab skin incision and retraction of underlying soft tissue, core biopsy samples of the near cortex and medullary cavity were collected. With the help of radiographs, core samples were obtained from both the center zone and transition zone of the lesion. Radiographs after biopsy were used to confirm the biopsy site. Postbiopsy splintage was used in some dogs to decrease the risk of pathological fracture associated with biopsy. Center zone biopsy yielded positive tumor in a significantly greater number of samples than transition zone biopsies.[214] Tumor was identified in 83.9 per cent of center zone biopsy samples but only 54.5 per cent of transition zone samples. Two samples per lesion (i.e., concurrent center and transition zone biopsy) improved diagnostic accuracy. Postbiopsy fracture rate was 3 per cent.

In another study, biopsy of 62 bone lesions in 59 small animals was performed using a Jamshidi needle.[155] Two or three samples were obtained from the center zone of the lesion. Fifty-one of 62 (82.3 per cent) lesions were accurately identified as a specific tumor type or a non-neoplastic process.[155] Postbiopsy complications were not reported. Jamshidi needle biopsy was performed easily and safely, and its high accuracy rate made it valuable in diagnosis of bone lesions.

Definitive statements about the value and reliability of bone biopsy in diagnosis of bone lesions are based on the following criteria: (1) the probability of attaining a biopsy diagnosis of "neoplasia" from neoplastic lesions, (2) the probability of attaining a correct biopsy diagnosis of "non-neoplastic" from non-neoplastic lesions, (3) the probability of attaining a correct biopsy diagnosis of "osteosarcoma" from osteosarcoma lesions. (4) the probability that a biopsy diagnosis of "osteosarcoma" is accurate, and (5) the ability to accurately identify the particular histological type of neoplastic lesions. Data from two biopsy series[155, 214] are summarized in Table 161–1. Bone biopsy using the Michele trephine or Jamshidi needle techniques yielded a diagnosis of tumor in more than 90 per cent of neoplastic lesions. The probability of attaining a bone biopsy diagnosis of "non-neoplastic" from non-neoplastic le-

TABLE 161–1. SUMMARY OF TWO CANINE BONE BIOPSY SERIES

	Michele Trephine[214]	Jamshidi Needle†[155]
Probability of biopsy diagnosis "neoplasm" from neoplastic lesions	30/32 (94%)	54/59 (92%)
Probability of biopsy diagnosis "non-neoplastic" from non-neoplastic lesions	N/A*	3/3 (100%)
Probability of biopsy diagnosis "osteosarcoma" from osteosarcoma lesions	25/30 (83%)	40/48 (83%)
Probability that biopsy diagnosis "osteosarcoma" is accurate	25/25 (100%)	41/41 (100%)
Ability of biopsy to accurately identify a particular histological type of neoplastic lesion		
All biopsies	27/32 (84%)	48/59 (81%)
Nonosteosarcoma biopsy diagnosis	2/7 (29%)	7/18 (39%)

*All lesions in this series were neoplastic.
†Sixty-two bone lesions from 57 dogs, one cat, and one ferret were sampled in this series.

sions remains unknown, because only 3 of 94 lesions were non-neoplastic. The likelihood of an erroneous diagnosis of tumor following biopsy of a non-neoplastic tumor-like lesion of bone has not been established. The probability of a biopsy diagnosis of "osteosarcoma" from osteosarcoma lesions was 83 per cent. All 66 lesions with a biopsy diagnosis of osteosarcoma were ultimately confirmed as osteosarcoma. The diagnostic accuracy of biopsy in identification of histological type was 81 to 84 per cent. This accuracy rate decreased to 29 to 39 per cent for lesions in which the biopsy diagnosis was not osteosarcoma. Because osteosarcoma represented 83 per cent of the lesions in these two series, an 83 per cent accuracy rate for histological type could have been achieved *without* performing biopsy but instead guessing that all tumors were osteosarcoma.

Thus, it is important that the potential usefulness as well as limitations of bone biopsy be kept in perspective. A biopsy diagnosis of osteosarcoma may be accepted with great confidence, and biopsy accurately identifies tumor in more than 90 per cent of neoplastic lesions. A biopsy diagnosis of reactive bone or a histological type of bone tumor other than osteosarcoma is interpreted with caution, because more than 50 per cent of these lesions are ultimately identified as osteosarcoma on further histological evaluation. Careful planning, proper biopsy technique, and close cooperation between surgeon and pathologist are recommended.

CLINICAL STAGING AND PATHOLOGICAL FEATURES OF BONE NEOPLASMS

The World Health Organization TNM Classification of canine and feline bone tumors[142] is presented in Table 161–2. Because regional lymph node metastases occur infrequently in patients with primary sarcomas of bone, clinical staging is usually limited to the primary tumor and the presence or absence of metastatic disease (i.e., a TM system). Use of a standardized system of clinical staging is critical so that results of treatment protocols may be compared between patients with equivalent stage of disease and interpreted appropriately. Unfortunately, clinical staging data for dogs with primary bone tumors are infrequently reported.[79]

The majority of primary bone tumors arise from within the medullary cavity or cortical bone, so-called central or medullary bone neoplasms. A subset of primary bone tumors distinct from these classic tumors arises from outside the cortex (presumably from the periosteum), so-called juxtacortical, parosteal, or periosteal bone neoplasms. Although the criteria and nomenclature used to describe these nonclassic bone neoplasms are inconsistent,[169] biological behavior and clinicopathological features of certain nonclassic tumors in humans are well characterized (e.g., parosteal [juxtacortical] osteosarcoma is recognized as a low-grade malignancy with a 10-year survival rate approaching 90 per cent).[133] Because the prognosis for humans with parosteal osteosarcoma is much better than with central osteosarcoma, a favorable prognosis for parosteal bone neoplasms in dogs and cats might also be expected. Although parosteal osteosarcoma and fibrosarcoma have been reported in dogs and cats,* insufficient data are available to confirm this hypothesis. In small animals, parosteal osteosarcoma has most frequently been reported in cats and is discussed separately from classic osteosarcoma in the later section on feline bone tumors.

Central osteosarcoma is classified by the nature of the predominant mesenchymal component (e.g., osteoblastic, chondroblastic, fibroblastic, telangiectatic).[34, 155, 169] In 600 human patients, differences in classification were not associated with differences in 5-year survival.[43] The prognostic utility of subclassification data in dogs and cats with osteosarcoma is unproven.[153] The prognosis for telangiectatic osteosarcoma in humans and animals is controversial.[61, 83, 118, 169] The concept of heterogeneity within different regions of these tumors is important because it provides insight into a potential shortcoming of bone biopsy in distinguishing osteosarcoma from nonosteogenic sarcomas of bone.

Invasion of the joint space by primary sarcomas of bone occurs infrequently. This characteristic has been useful in distinguishing primary sarcomas of bone from conditions such as rheumatoid arthritis, septic arthritis,

*See references 7, 16, 29, 34, 40, 52, 66, 85, 104, 153, 159, and 196.

TABLE 161–2. WORLD HEALTH ORGANIZATION TNM CLASSIFICATION OF CANINE AND FELINE TUMORS OF BONE

T: Primary tumor
- T_0 No evidence of tumor
- T_1 Tumor confined within the medulla and cortex
- T_2 Tumor extends beyond the periosteum
- Multiple tumors should be classified independently.

M: Distant metastasis
- M_0 No evidence of distant metastasis
- M_1 Distant metastasis detected (specify sites)

From Owen LN: *TNM Classification of Tumors in Domestic Animals.* World Health Organization, Geneva, 1980.

and synovial sarcoma. The "barrier" capability of cartilage has been attributed to collagenase inhibitors, which may directly inhibit tumor cell invasion or inhibit neoangiogenesis.[20, 91] The impact of bone tumors on nearby joints is unknown, because the cytological characteristics of synovial fluid from joints adjacent to metaphyseal lesions are poorly characterized.[93]

TREATMENT OF BONE NEOPLASMS

Surgery is the most important therapeutic modality in treatment of musculoskeletal neoplasms. Adjunctive therapy using cytotoxic chemotherapy, radiation therapy, or immunotherapy has been reported and is discussed later.

After thorough evaluation of patients, amputation with or without adjunctive therapy is the standard treatment for tumors of the appendicular skeleton. Radiographs of the primary lesion are important in characterizing the extent of bone involvement. Radiographs may underestimate the diaphyseal extent of bone tumors, and scintigraphic evaluation of the primary tumor has been recommended in candidates for tumor resection and limb salvage.[95] Because of the risk of intramedullary spread of tumor cells, neoplasms of the humerus and femur are treated by forequarter amputation or scapulohumeral/coxofemoral disarticulation techniques. Thoracic radiographs are performed so that pulmonary metastases may be detected, although negative radiographs do not rule out metastatic disease. Ventrodorsal and right and left lateral thoracic radiographic views are recommended.[96, 97, 143] Survey skeletal radiography[98] or bone scintigraphy[11, 69, 94, 209] may assess involvement of other parts of the skeleton. A thorough orthopedic examination is critical so that concurrent non-neoplastic orthopedic abnormalities, such as severe degenerative joint disease, may be identified in the other limbs. Concurrent musculoskeletal abnormalities, particularly in large and giant breeds, may make a patient unsuitable for amputation. Application of a nonweightbearing sling to the tumor-bearing appendage may also be useful in predicting postamputation mobility. When these aspects of case selection are considered, clients are usually satisfied after limb amputation regardless of postoperative survival time. Biopsy of the lesion is indicated if results of histopathological examination would affect treatment. The need for biopsy evaluation of bone neoplasms before amputation is controversial. Jamshidi needle biopsy[155] performed before amputation has been recommended. If radiographs are definitive for a primary bone neoplasm and limb salvage is not an option, amputation *without* biopsy is a legitimate approach. Amputation is a pain-relieving procedure with a potential for cure and provides the pathologist with an opportunity to evaluate the neoplasm *in toto*.

In patients with axial skeletal neoplasms, local tumor control after surgical excision may be difficult. Normal surgical margins may be impossible to achieve, particularly with neoplasms of the skull or vertebrae. The role of chemotherapy or radiation therapy in the management of primary bone sarcomas of the axial skeleton is unclear.[77, 78, 121, 176]

PRIMARY BONE TUMORS IN DOGS

Osteosarcoma of the Canine Appendicular Skeleton

Incidence and Biological Behavior

Osteosarcoma is the most common canine bone neoplasm, accounting for approximately 80 per cent of primary bone tumors.[24] It is more common in the appendicular than axial skeleton.[24, 210] Appendicular osteosarcoma exhibits a "close to the knee, away from the elbow" site predilection, and the distal radius is the most common primary site.[24, 58, 102] Most tumors are metaphyseal, although diaphyseal osteosarcoma occurs.[56, 161, 184] Body size is an important risk factor; large and giant breeds may have up to 150 times greater risk than dogs weighing less than 10 kg.[194] As with most neoplasms, the etiology of osteosarcoma is largely unknown, although osteosarcoma may arise in abnormal bone (e.g., bone infarcts), at the site of previous fractures (see the later section on fracture-associated sarcoma), or after exposure to radioisotopes or radiation therapy.[126, 191] Histologically, the presence of tumor osteoid distinguishes osteosarcoma from nonosteogenic malignant bone neoplasms (e.g., chondrosarcoma, fibrosarcoma).

Older dogs are most frequently affected, although a biphasic peak incidence (2 and 9 years) has been reported.[24] Although monostotic disease (one bone lesion) is most frequently encountered, multiple bone involvement has been reported.[43, 85, 98, 141] Four of 42 (9.1 per cent) dogs with osteosarcoma had multiple bone lesions detected on survey skeletal radiography[98]; survey skeletal radiography was more useful than thoracic radiography in detecting disease isolated from the primary lesion. It remains undetermined whether multiple skeletal lesions in dogs represent multiple primary neoplasms or metastatic lesions.

Appendicular osteosarcoma in dogs has a high metastatic rate, with micrometastatic disease or detectable metastases present in most individuals at initial presentation.[22] The lungs are the most frequent site of metastases, although more intensive adjuvant chemotherapy protocols have been associated with an apparent change in metastatic pattern. Dogs receiving chemotherapy after amputation or as part of a limb salvage protocol have a lower incidence of pulmonary metastases and more frequent bone involvement.[39, 99, 124] Whether this phenomenon represents a true change in metastatic pattern or merely a prolongation of survival allowing expression of a more advanced stage of the disease process is unknown.

Treatment and Prognosis

Data from 62 dogs with appendicular osteosarcoma[22] are frequently cited as the historical standard against which subsequent studies have been compared. Median survival for these dogs with appendicular osteosarcoma after amputation and for three dogs with rib osteosarcoma following excision was 18 weeks, with a 6-month survival rate of 26 per cent and 1-year survival rate of

10.7 per cent.[22] Although thoracic radiographs reveal pulmonary metastases in only 5 to 10 per cent of dogs with appendicular osteosarcoma at initial presentation,[98, 102] tumor metastasis has often taken place, as evidenced by the poor prognosis for cure after amputation.

Because micrometastatic disease is likely to be present in most dogs with appendicular osteosarcoma at amputation, investigations have focused on agents and modalities with the potential to control or prevent metastatic disease. Antiplatelet therapy[72, 163] and "prophylactic" lung irradiation[144] failed to alter metastatic rate or influence survival in dogs with appendicular osteosarcoma. In some instances, prolonged survival has been reported in dogs receiving cytotoxic chemotherapy or immunotherapy after surgical control of the primary tumor,[113, 124, 145, 175, 188] whereas other studies have shown no benefit.[39, 68, 114, 128, 202]

Prolonged survival has been reported in dogs after amputation and postoperative chemotherapy. In one study,[175] 19 dogs with appendicular osteosarcoma underwent nonrandomized treatment with amputation (n=8 dogs) or amputation followed by cisplatin (40 to 50 mg/m^2 IV every 28 days for two to six treatments) (n=11 dogs). Dogs treated with amputation and adjuvant cisplatin had significantly longer median survival time (43 weeks) than dogs treated with amputation alone (14.5 weeks). Acute renal failure attributable to cisplatin renal toxicity was not observed, and transient vomiting, which occurred in 9 of 11 dogs during or shortly after cisplatin infusion, was self-limiting. Cisplatin administration before amputation also prolonged survival but offered no advantage over postoperative cisplatin therapy.[188]

Thirty-six dogs with appendicular osteosarcoma underwent nonrandomized treatment with amputation (n=19) or amputation followed by adjuvant chemotherapy (n=17).[124] Adjuvant chemotherapy was initiated 2 weeks postoperatively as follows: doxorubicin (30 mg/m^2 IV) on day one, cisplatin (60 mg/m^2 IV) on day 21, followed by a second cycle repeated 3 weeks later. Median survival of 19 dogs treated with amputation alone was 25 weeks. One-year survival rate was 21 per cent; all dogs were dead at 16 months. Necropsy data were not available for dogs that underwent amputation alone. Median survival of 19 dogs (17 appendicular, 2 axial) that underwent amputation and adjuvant chemotherapy was 43 weeks. One-year survival rate was 37 per cent. Four of five dogs that survived 2 years or more eventually died of osteosarcoma-related disease; one dog was still alive at 25 months. Although necropsy data were limited to 5 of 18 nonsurvivors in the adjuvant chemotherapy group, follow-up radiographs revealed that metastatic disease had developed in all nonsurvivors. Bone lesions were identified in 8 of 18 (44 per cent) nonsurvivors. Clinical signs of drug toxicity were not observed.

Limb salvage, consisting of *en bloc* tumor excision, cortical allografting, and bone plate application, combined with preoperative radiation therapy and intravenous or intra-arterial cisplatin, has also prolonged survival in dogs with osteosarcoma.[99] Median survival in 20 dogs was 32 weeks; tumor necrosis greater than 80 per cent on histological examination was correlated with effective local tumor control.[99] There is no evidence that dogs with osteosarcoma treated with limb salvage survive longer than dogs treated with amputation and adjuvant chemotherapy.[206]

Amputation followed by adjuvant immunotherapy using liposome-encapsulated muramyl tripeptide (MTP-PE) prolongs metastasis-free interval and survival in dogs with appendicular osteosarcoma.[113] In a randomized double-blind trial, 14 dogs underwent amputation and received intravenous MTP-PE treatment twice weekly for 8 weeks. Thirteen dogs that underwent amputation and received empty liposomes served as controls. At amputation, all dogs were free of radiographically evident pulmonary metastases. Metastasis-free interval was determined using thoracic radiography and was defined as the time from amputation to appearance of pulmonary metastases. Median metastasis-free interval in dogs treated with amputation and MTP-PE was 24 weeks, versus only 8 weeks in dogs treated with amputation alone. Median survival in MTP-PE–treated dogs was 32 weeks, with 4 of 14 (29 per cent) dogs still alive 17 to 32 months after amputation.[111, 113] Median survival in 13 dogs treated with amputation alone was 11 weeks, and all dogs died with metastatic disease. Significant adverse side effects attributable to MTP-PE treatment were not reported. Prolongation of metastasis-free interval and survival was attributed to the ability of MTP-PE–activated macrophages to destroy tumor cells.[113] Preliminary data suggest that dogs with appendicular osteosarcoma treated with amputation and adjuvant cisplatin, followed by MTP-PE treatment, have longer survival than amputation-adjuvant cisplatin–treated dogs that did not receive immunotherapy.[111]

Surgical resection of pulmonary metastases has been reported in humans[10, 65, 129, 158] and dogs[208] with osteosarcoma. The rationale for surgical management of pulmonary metastases is that measurable metastatic disease (i.e., nonmicrometastatic disease) in the lungs responds poorly to chemotherapy and immunotherapy.[10] Criteria for selection of patients for pulmonary metastectomy are evolving and include (1) health status sufficient to survive thoracotomy, (2) sustained primary tumor control, (3) absence of detectable extrathoracic neoplastic disease, and (4) likelihood of resectability of pulmonary metastases.[10, 65, 129, 158, 208] Resectability of metastatic disease is most likely in patients without mediastinal or thoracic wall involvement and in patients with relatively few pulmonary metastases. Pulmonary metastases may be quantified using thoracic radiography or computed tomography. Involvement of both right and left lung lobes should not be considered a contraindication to metastectomy, because median sternotomy enables the surgeon to resect bilateral disease. Survival data from humans with osteosarcoma after pulmonary metastectomy are encouraging, with 40 per cent of patients alive and disease free after 5 years.[158] The presence of three or fewer pulmonary nodules on computed tomography was the most important favorable prognostic factor in human patients.[158]

Pulmonary metastectomy has been reported in 16

dogs with appendicular osteosarcoma.[208] Primary tumor control had been achieved in all dogs via limb salvage or amputation. Detectable disease was confined to the thoracic cavity, and fewer than 6 pulmonary nodules were present on thoracic radiographs. Approximately 50 per cent of dogs developed new pulmonary lesions within 3 months of metastectomy. Seven of 16 (44 per cent) dogs were alive and disease free at a median of 18 weeks after thoracotomy. None of the dogs received postthoracotomy chemotherapy. This study demonstrated that pulmonary metastectomy can be performed with acceptable morbidity in a select group of dogs with osteosarcoma. Additional follow-up data are needed to quantitate the extended survival time afforded by these procedures and further clarify criteria for case selection.

Osteosarcoma of the Canine Axial Skeleton

Axial skeletal involvement is present in approximately 25 per cent of dogs with osteosarcoma.[24] Because of the location of axial skeletal neoplasms, tumor-free surgical margins may be difficult to achieve. Tumor-related death has usually been a consequence of inadequate local tumor control rather than metastatic disease. Although the biological behavior of axial skeletal osteosarcoma is less aggressive than appendicular skeletal osteosarcoma,[63] this statement is difficult to substantiate. Much of the information about these tumors is from dogs in which conservative surgery was performed or treatment was not attempted. A low metastatic rate might be expected in these patients, because many underwent early euthanasia owing to poor local tumor control. More radical surgical techniques such as mandibulectomy,[168, 207] rib resection and thoracic wall reconstruction,[21, 49] and hemipelvectomy[187] have shown acceptable morbidity. Follow-up data from dogs treated with these more aggressive surgical techniques are needed to better assess the metastatic potential of these tumors.

Osteosarcoma of the Skull

Osteosarcoma of the skull is most common in boxers; giant breeds are under-represented.[75] Because calvarial osteosarcomas tend to be purely osteoproductive, lytic lesions of the calvarium are more likely to represent nonosteogenic tumors or inflammatory disease.[75] A metastatic rate of 30 per cent was reported in 13 dogs that underwent necropsy.[75] Complete surgical excision of these tumors may be difficult or impossible.

Osteosarcoma of the Mandible

Osteosarcoma is one of the five most common tumors of the canine mandible, along with melanoma, squamous cell carcinoma, fibrosarcoma, and acanthomatous epulis. Although previous reports suggest that axial skeletal osteosarcoma has a lower metastatic rate and longer clinical course than appendicular osteosarcoma,[63, 75] this statement is largely unsubstantiated with regard to mandibular osteosarcoma. Necropsy data on dogs with mandibular osteosarcoma are limited to fewer than ten cases.[25, 75, 151, 207] In a review of dogs that underwent mandibulectomy, osteosarcoma was the histological type of mandibular neoplasm with the least favorable prognosis.[168] Median survival for six dogs after mandibulectomy was 1.5 months.[168]

Osteosarcoma of the Rib

Osteosarcoma is the most common rib tumor in dogs[55]; 11 of 15 (73 per cent) primary rib tumors were osteosarcoma.[55] Distant metastases were identified in 5 of 11 (45 per cent) cases; all dogs with metastatic disease had pulmonary metastases. Intrathoracic expansion of these tumors may result in a "tip of the iceberg" phenomenon in which only a scarcely discernible mass may be externally palpable. Treatment consists of *en bloc* excision of the tumor followed by thoracic wall reconstruction using polypropylene mesh or alternative materials.[21, 49] The prognosis for dogs with untreated rib osteosarcoma is poor, with less than 10 per cent of dogs surviving more than 4 months after diagnosis.[55] Expected survival after surgical excision of these tumors is unknown. Two dogs with rib osteosarcoma survived 1 and 4 months after tumor excision.[28]

Osteosarcoma of the Vertebrae

Osteosarcoma is the most common canine extradural spinal neoplasm,[156] representing 12 of 26 (46 per cent) primary vertebral tumors in one series; multiple vertebral involvement was reported in 25 per cent.[135] The radiographic appearance of vertebral osteosarcoma is inconsistent and nonspecific.[135] The metastatic rate of vertebral osteosarcoma is poorly characterized, probably because of early and often catastrophic consequences of the primary lesion. Surgical excision of these tumors is often impossible.

Extraskeletal Osteosarcoma in Dogs

Incidence and Biological Behavior

Osteosarcoma arising in nonosseous tissues is termed *extraskeletal osteosarcoma*; it is rare in dogs, accounting for less than 2 per cent of all canine osteosarcomas.[148] Osteoid-producing malignant mixed neoplasms (carcinosarcomas) of mammary gland and thyroid and osteosarcomas of the esophagus associated with *Spirocerca lupi* infection are generally excluded from this classification.[148, 170] The cause of extraskeletal osteosarcoma in dogs is unknown, although trauma has been implicated in the formation of ocular osteosarcoma in cats.[131, 211] Jejunal osteosarcoma associated with a retained surgical sponge was reported in one dog.[146] Previous radiation therapy has been implicated in extraskeletal osteosarcoma development in humans,[181] and extraskeletal osteosarcoma of the liver has been produced experimentally with aflatoxin in nonhuman primates.[177]

Although 80 per cent of extraskeletal osteosarcoma in humans involves soft tissues of the extremities, more than 80 per cent of canine extraskeletal osteosarcomas involve visceral organs including the eyes, spleen, liver, adrenal glands, kidneys, small intestine, testes, and vagina.[148, 170] No breed predilection has been reported; older dogs (mean age 11 years) are most often affected.[148] Extraskeletal osteosarcoma exhibits aggressive biological behavior in dogs and humans.[148, 181] Distant metastases were reported in 7 of 11 (64 per cent) dogs with extraskeletal osteosarcoma.[148] Regional lymph nodes were the most frequent site of metastatic disease.[148]

Treatment and Prognosis

Extraskeletal osteosarcoma must be differentiated from myositis ossificans or dystrophic calcification associated with neoplastic or inflammatory lesions.[4, 105, 160] Diagnosis of extraskeletal osteosarcoma relies on the demonstration of primitive osteoid with a relatively uniform pattern of sarcomatous cells.[170] Survey skeletal radiography[98] or bone scintigraphy[94] is recommended to distinguish extraskeletal osteosarcoma from a primary bone neoplasm with soft-tissue extension or metastasis. Treatment is surgical excision. The prognosis depends on the operability of the primary lesion and the presence or absence of metastases. The prognosis is guarded owing to local invasiveness and metastatic disease.[148]

NONOSTEOGENIC PRIMARY MALIGNANT NEOPLASMS OF THE CANINE APPENDICULAR SKELETON

Nonosteogenic primary malignant neoplasms account for 10 to 15 per cent of tumors in the canine appendicular skeleton.[87] Fibrosarcoma, chondrosarcoma, and hemangiosarcoma are the most prevalent nonosteogenic primary appendicular skeletal neoplasms. Other histological types are less common or rare and include liposarcoma,[23, 28, 44, 59, 63] lymphosarcoma,[28, 60, 139, 195] myeloma,[63, 108] giant-cell tumor,[42, 85, 100] and malignant fibrous histiocytoma.[105]

Fibrosarcoma of the Appendicular Skeleton

Incidence and Biological Behavior

Fibrosarcoma is the third most common primary bone neoplasm in dogs, accounting for up to 9 per cent of all canine bone tumors.[87] Appendicular skeletal involvement is present in 30 to 40 per cent.[87, 105] Radiographically, fibrosarcoma is predominantly lytic but in some instances may mimic osteosarcoma.[59]

Disagreement exists about the origin of fibrosarcoma of bone, because some pathologists believe all fibrosarcomas of bone have an extramedullary origin.[182] Distinguishing between central fibrosarcoma and tumors of parosteal or soft-tissue origin may be difficult histologically, and this distinction is best made with clinical information. Parosteal and soft-tissue fibrosarcoma are typically associated with a palpable mass; radiographically, tumor predominance is extracortical. Central fibrosarcoma may not be associated with a palpable mass and radiographically may have considerable osseous involvement in the absence of a large soft-tissue component. Histological evaluation of multiple tissue sections is critical to distinguish fibrosarcoma from osteosarcoma forming scant quantities of osteoid. The absence of osteoid in a single tissue section may erroneously lead to a diagnosis of fibrosarcoma.

Appendicular fibrosarcoma is less malignant than oronasal fibrosarcoma[150] and slower to metastasize than appendicular osteosarcoma.[2, 87, 150] Although a metastatic rate of 6 per cent was reported in 17 dogs with fibrosarcoma, the specific characteristics of these neoplasms (i.e., axial versus appendicular, central versus soft tissue) were not reported.[108] Additional necropsy data are limited to fewer than five cases, and patient outcome following amputation limited to three dogs.[25, 28, 33, 59, 150, 164] Statements about the biological behavior or "prognosis for cure" in dogs with appendicular fibrosarcoma are difficult to substantiate.

Review of case records from the University of Minnesota and Colorado State University Veterinary Teaching Hospitals of dogs with central fibrosarcoma of the appendicular skeleton revealed nine cases. Criteria for inclusion were (1) physical examination and radiographic findings supportive of a primary bone tumor of central origin and (2) histological diagnosis of fibrosarcoma based on evaluation of tissue specimens obtained after surgical excision (limb salvage), amputation, or necropsy. Animals with biopsy diagnosis alone were excluded from study. Tumors of suspected soft-tissue origin with secondary bone invasion were excluded. Most dogs with appendicular fibrosarcoma were large; six of nine dogs weighed more than 30 kg. Mean age was 7.8 years, and the distal radius was more frequently affected. Clinical signs in all dogs were referable to the primary lesion, and pathological fracture was present in more than 50 per cent. One of nine had evidence of pulmonary metastases on thoracic radiographs at initial presentation. No dogs had confirmed multiple bone involvement.

Treatment and Prognosis

Seven of nine dogs in the same series underwent amputation or limb salvage. Two of seven (29 per cent) dogs were alive 1 year postoperatively; two of three were alive 1 year after amputation.[25, 28, 59] Although the number of reported cases is small, the prognosis for cure after surgical treatment of central fibrosarcoma of the appendicular skeleton is poor.

Chondrosarcoma of the Appendicular Skeleton

Incidence and Biological Behavior

Chondrosarcoma is a malignant cartilage-producing neoplasm that usually arises *de novo* within bone. It occasionally occurs at the site of a previous bone lesion (e.g., secondary chondrosarcoma associated with an osteochondroma).[45, 153] Although chondrosarcoma represents 10 per cent of all canine bone tumors,[26, 28, 102] it represents a much lower percentage of appendicular neoplasms. In one study, chondrosarcoma represented 2 of 34 (6 per cent) nonosteogenic neoplasms of the appendicular skeleton.[59] In the largest retrospective study of canine chondrosarcoma, only 4 of 35 (11 per cent) tumors were appendicular[26]; all 4 dogs were euthanized at diagnosis, and none had detectable metastatic disease.[26]

Treatment and Prognosis

Appendicular chondrosarcoma may be the canine primary malignant bone neoplasm with the best prognosis for cure after amputation. Two cases of long-term survival after limb salvage have been reported.[90, 198]

Hemangiosarcoma of the Appendicular Skeleton

Incidence and Biological Behavior

Hemangiosarcoma is a malignant neoplasm arising from endothelial cells, with highest frequency in male German shepherds.[31] The spleen and right atrium are the most frequently reported primary sites; less than 5 per cent of dogs with hemangiosarcoma have bone involvement.[31] In one series, hemangiosarcoma accounted for 4 per cent of all canine primary bone tumors.[87] The proximal humerus, femur, ribs, and vertebrae are the most frequently affected skeletal sites.[15] Distribution between the appendicular and axial skeleton is approximately equal.[15, 87] The proximal humerus is the most frequently involved site in dogs with appendicular skeletal hemangiosarcoma, accounting for 7 of 11 (64 per cent) dogs.[15] Radiographically, hemangiosarcoma is predominantly lytic and may demonstrate considerable intramedullary extension without dramatic cortical or periosteal changes. A sizable soft-tissue mass may accompany limb lesions in more than 50 per cent.[15] Because of the lytic nature of this neoplasm, pathological fracture may be a sequel[8, 15, 36] (Fig. 161–1).

It may be difficult to determine whether hemangiosarcoma bone lesions represent primary bone tumors or metastatic lesions. Thus, the use of the term *metastatic rate* may be inappropriate for hemangiosarcoma of bone. In 11 dogs with appendicular hemangiosarcoma, the primary lesion was bone in 3 dogs, spleen in 3, subcutis in 1, and uncertain in 4.[15] Nonosseous organ involvement was present in 15 of 17 (88 per cent) dogs with appendicular hemangiosarcoma at necropsy.[8, 15, 41, 47]

Treatment and Prognosis

If hemangiosarcoma of bone is suspected, a thorough search for other osseous and extraosseous lesions is indicated; ultrasonographic evaluation of the liver, spleen, and heart is recommended. Pulmonary metastases in dogs with hemangiosarcoma may be difficult to confirm on thoracic radiographs, because these lesions may assume a diffuse interstitial pattern that mimics pulmonary aging changes.[201] Because of the aggressive nature of this neoplasm and the frequent presence of extraosseous disease, the prognosis for dogs with appen-

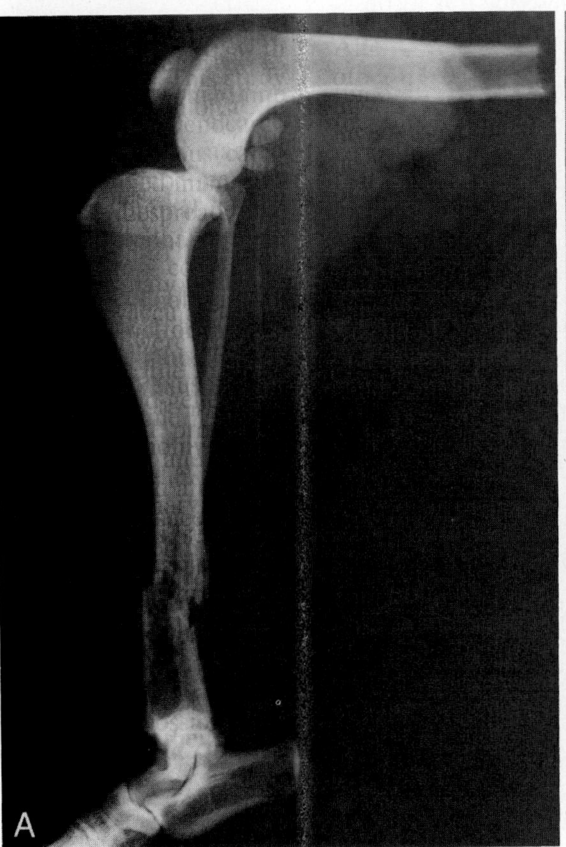

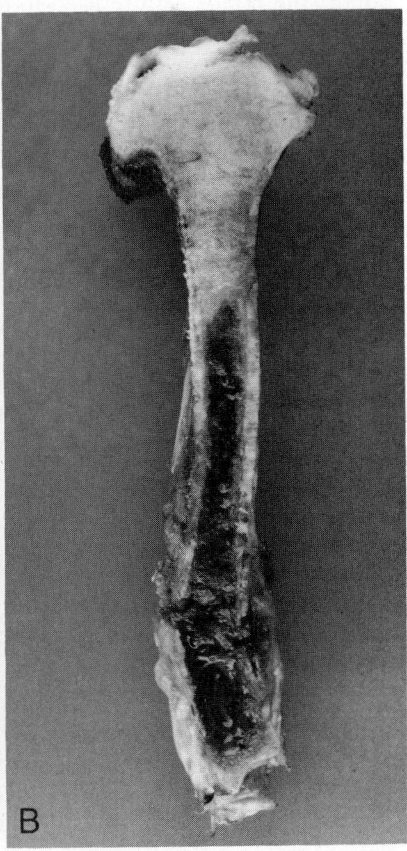

FIGURE 161–1. *A*, Lateral radiograph of the right tibia of an 11-year-old terrier with sudden onset of hindlimb lameness. *B*, Longitudinal section of the tibia after amputation, showing intramedullary tumor and hemorrhage. Diagnosis was hemangiosarcoma of the distal tibia with pathological fracture.

dicular hemangiosarcoma is guarded. Mean survival time in five dogs after amputation was less than 5 months.[15, 47] These data are similar to postsplenectomy survival data for dogs with splenic hemangiosarcoma.[31, 86] A dog with hemangiosarcoma of the femur survived for 13 months after coxofemoral disarticulation and adjuvant chemotherapy with doxorubicin and cyclophosphamide.[41]

NONOSTEOGENIC MALIGNANT NEOPLASMS OF THE CANINE AXIAL SKELETON

Nonosteogenic malignant neoplasms of the axial skeleton reported with reasonable frequency in dogs include vertebral neoplasms, sinonasal chondrosarcoma, multilobular osteochondrosarcoma of the skull, and chondrosarcoma of the rib. Surgical excision is important in treatment of at least two of these conditions, multilobular osteochondrosarcoma and chondrosarcoma of the rib.

Multilobular Osteochondrosarcoma

Incidence and Biological Behavior

Multilobular osteochondrosarcoma is an osteocartilaginous tumor in dogs. It arises from the mandible, maxilla, or cranium. Histologically, the tumor consists of islands of partially or completely calcified cartilage or osseous tissue surrounded by a neoplastic mesenchymal cell stroma.[153] Radiographically, it displays a lobulated appearance with well-defined borders. Despite the characteristic histological and radiographic features of this tumor, the nomenclature used to describe it is inconsistent. Previous descriptions include *chondroma rodens, calcifying aponeurotic fibroma*, and *multilobular osteoma/chondroma*.[127, 174, 186, 215] Although it was once considered benign,[153] evidence now suggests this tumor to be a low-grade malignancy.[186]

Treatment and Prognosis

Because the prognosis for dogs with multilobular osteochondrosarcoma depends on local tumor control, treatment focuses on complete surgical excision. However, despite radical surgical excision, tumor location may make tumor-free margins impossible to achieve. Seven of 12 (58 per cent) dogs treated with surgical excision had local recurrence; 4 with complete excision had no local recurrence.[186] Only one of four with complete excision developed metastases, whereas metastatic disease developed in six of eight dogs with incomplete surgical excision. The lungs were the most frequent site of metastases.

Because this tumor grows slowly, the disease-free interval may be prolonged despite incomplete surgical excision. The median interval from surgery to local recurrence was 14 months[186]; signs referable to metastatic disease were seen in two of seven dogs with metastases, and mean interval from detection of pulmonary metastases to death was 11 months. Thus, prolonged survival in dogs with multilobular osteochondrosarcoma is possible despite metastatic disease.

Chondrosarcoma of the Rib

Incidence and Biological Behavior

Chondrosarcoma has a predilection for the axial skeleton and is the second most common canine primary rib neoplasm.[55] Boxers may be at increased risk for rib chondrosarcoma, but not chondrosarcoma of the skull or nasal cavity.[26] Clinically, this neoplasm is often indistinguishable from rib osteosarcoma. Both neoplasms usually occur at the costochondral junction, frequently exhibit an intrathoracic component that exceeds the extrathoracic portion, and may possess similar radiographic features[26] (Fig. 161–2). Metastatic rate was 50 per cent in six dogs that had rib chondrosarcoma and underwent necropsy.[26, 55]

Treatment and Prognosis

Treatment consisting of surgical excision and thoracic wall reconstruction may result in long-term survival.

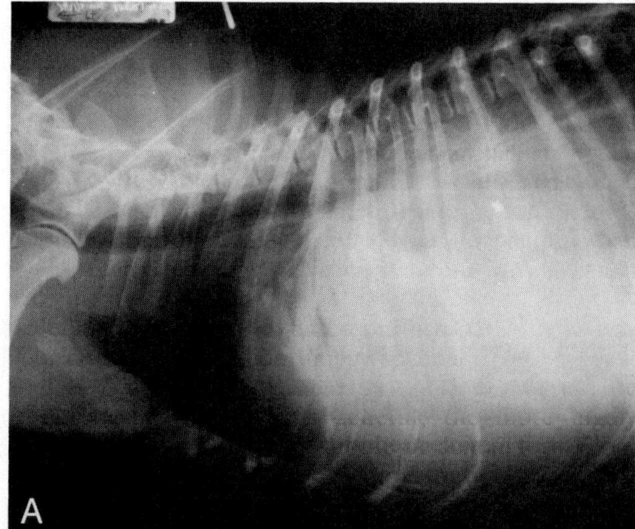

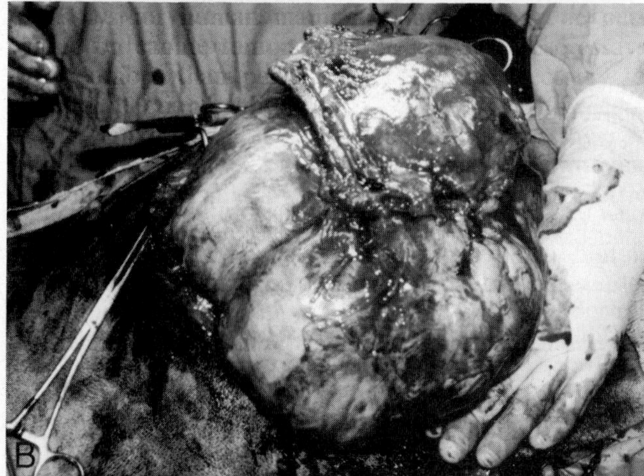

FIGURE 161–2. *A*, Lateral thoracic radiograph of a 9-year-old German shepherd with mild dyspnea. *B*, Intraoperative photograph of large intrathoracic neoplasm originating from the left ninth rib. Diagnosis was chondrosarcoma. After rib resection and thoracoplasty with polypropylene mesh, the dog has remained disease free for 27 months.

Data on the surgical treatment of ten dogs with rib chondrosarcoma demonstrate an 86 per cent 1-year survival rate in dogs surviving beyond the perioperative period.[26, 55] Local recurrence 4 to 5.5 years after surgical excision has been reported and may respond to a second surgical excision.[26]

Nonosteogenic Vertebral Neoplasms

Approximately 50 per cent of vertebral neoplasms are metastatic lesions, 25 per cent are osteosarcomas, 15 per cent are chondrosarcomas, and the remaining 10 per cent are other nonosteogenic primary malignant bone neoplasms, including fibrosarcoma, hemangiosarcoma, and myeloma.[110, 135, 189, 212, 213] The radiographic features of primary and secondary vertebral neoplasms are similar, because both groups are osteodestructive and may involve multiple vertebrae.[135] Information on the management of vertebral neoplasms in dogs is limited. Complete surgical excision of vertebral neoplasms is often impossible. Nonosteogenic sarcomas of bone are generally radioresistant, and radiation-induced spinal cord damage may be a sequel to irradiation of vertebral lesions. Responsiveness of chondrosarcoma to radiation therapy is controversial[77] and cytotoxic chemotherapy is ineffective.[176] Although retinoic acid inhibits growth of chondrosarcoma in cell culture, its therapeutic efficacy is unproven.[176, 190] Chemotherapy and radiotherapy are unproven in treatment of fibrosarcoma of bone.[121] Cytotoxic chemotherapy using doxorubicin has been used in dogs with hemangiosarcoma of soft tissues.[78] Myeloma is usually a nonsurgical disease, and early cases may respond to melphalan and prednisone.[112]

Sinonasal Chondrosarcoma

In 285 dogs with sinonasal neoplasms, chondrosarcoma was the most common nonepithelial tumor reported,[149] accounting for 34 of 285 (12 per cent) sinonasal tumors, and was the only histological type noted more frequently in younger (age 1 to 8 years) than older dogs. Osteosarcoma was 6 per cent of the neoplasms in that series. Metastatic rate for both sinonasal chondrosarcoma and osteosarcoma was approximately 10 per cent.[149] Cytoreductive surgery or radiation therapy has been used in the treatment of dogs with sinonasal chondrosarcoma.[1, 53]

SECONDARY BONE TUMORS IN DOGS AND CATS

Secondary bone tumors may involve bone either via local invasion or distant metastasis. Local invasion of bone is most frequently encountered in dogs and cats with squamous cell carcinoma of the oral cavity or digits, fibrosarcoma of the oral cavity or extremities, and synovial sarcoma (see the sections in this chapter on neoplasms of digits, feline bone tumors, and neoplasms of joints).

Bone Metastases

Bone metastases represent tumor cell foci that have become established within bone after hematogenous dissemination from a remote primary neoplasm. The prevalence of bone metastases in dogs is generally low.[27, 106, 108] In a prospective necropsy study, 24 of 141 (17 per cent) dogs with malignant neoplasms and visceral metastases also had macroscopic bone metastases.[62] During the same period, 26 dogs with primary bone tumors were identified. Thus, 12.4 per cent of dogs with malignant neoplasms had primary bone tumors, and 11.5 per cent had skeletal metastases.[62]

There is convincing evidence that bone destruction associated with bone metastases is mediated by local factors and that direct bone lysis by tumor cells is generally a late event.[12, 57] Prostaglandin E may have a major role in bone resorption associated with human breast carcinoma metastases.[12, 57] Estrogens increase bone-resorbing activity and prostaglandin E production of human breast carcinoma cells *in vitro*.[197] This observation is consistent with the observation that estrogen receptor–positive breast cancer has a greater propensity for bone metastasis.[197]

It is well recognized that the distribution of metastases cannot be explained solely by mechanical factors such as anatomical proximity and organ vascularity.[12, 80, 205] The observation that certain histological types of neoplasms exhibit an apparent propensity for establishing metastases in particular organs has fostered the concept of differential organ susceptibility to metastases ("seed and soil" hypothesis).[205] Adhesive factors that facilitate arrest, chemotactic factors that facilitate escape from the vascular space into tissue, and growth factors that stimulate tumor growth within tissue have been implicated in the pathogenesis of bone metastases.[12, 117, 120, 137] Skeletal metastases have a predilection for red bone marrow, where the marrow sinusoids are vulnerable to penetration and escape by tumor cells.[12] The release of chemotactic substances during normal bone remodeling has been proposed as a possible explanation for the propensity of some tumors to metastasize to bone.[117, 120] Type I collagen and collagen fragments are chemotactic for certain tumor cells *in vitro*.[137] Products of bone resorption may also serve as growth factors that promote tumor cell proliferation.[120]

The pathogenesis of bone metastases with prostatic carcinoma, a tumor with a propensity for skeletal metastases in dogs and humans, is interesting. Two observations are that (1) prostatic carcinoma metastases are consistently osteoproductive and osteolysis is rare[84] and (2) in humans, the growth rate of bone metastases of prostatic carcinoma is often more rapid than the growth rate of the primary tumor.[35] Because of the osteoproductive nature of these metastases, it is unlikely that bone resorption–associated chemotactic or growth factors could account for this neoplasm's propensity for skeletal metastases or rapid growth in bone. Human prostatic carcinoma cells are stimulated by mammalian bone marrow–derived mitogenic factors *in vitro*, whereas nonprostatic tumor cell lines show little response.[35]

Neoplasms of the mammary glands, lungs, liver, thyroid, and prostate are the most frequent primary tumors in dogs with bone metastases.[27, 62, 88] In one study, 21 of 24 (88 per cent) skeletal metastases were of epithelial origin.[62] Twenty-one per cent of dogs with epithelial malignancy and visceral metastases had bone metastases, whereas bone metastases were present in only 6 per cent of dogs with metastatic mesenchymal tumors.[62] Ribs, vertebrae, femur, and humerus were the most frequent sites of metastatic lesions.[27, 62, 88, 106] In one study, 14 of 24 (58 per cent) of dogs had two or more bones affected; approximately two-thirds of dogs with lesions of the humerus or femur were affected bilaterally.[62] Lesions of the femur and humerus were most frequent in the proximal metaphysis or diaphysis.[62] Dogs with skeletal metastases almost invariably had visceral metastases.[62] Not infrequently, the primary tumor is never identified.[167]

Bone lesions in dogs with prostatic adenocarcinoma are most frequent in caudal lumbar vertebrae.[48, 135] Periosteal new bone formation is characteristically present, particularly on the ventral surface; one or more vertebrae may be affected.[48, 135] Bone metastases were identified in 5 of 12 (42 per cent) dogs with prostatic adenocarcinoma.[48] In that study, weight loss and lumbar pain were more common in dogs with bone metastases. No specific histological features predicted the presence or absence of bone metastases.[48]

Although many of the radiographic features of bone metastases are nonspecific, certain considerations such as signalment, history, and anatomical site may distinguish these lesions from primary bone tumors or other tumor-like lesions of bone. For example, metaphyseal bone lesions of the distal radius in giant breeds of dogs are more likely to be osteosarcomas than metastatic lesions. However, a metastatic lesion should be suspected in a dog with a diaphyseal long-bone lesion and a previous history of mammary gland adenocarcinoma. Metastatic bone tumors may be osteolytic or osteoproductive. Multiple skeletal metastases must be distinguished from osteosarcoma involving multiple bones or polyostotic non-neoplastic conditions of bone such as bacterial or fungal osteomyelitis,[5, 17, 132, 165] bone cysts,[13, 70, 173] or panosteitis.

Serum calcium concentrations in most dogs with metastatic bone neoplasms are normal. Hypercalcemia in dogs with malignancy (e.g., lymphosarcoma, apocrine gland adenocarcinoma of the anal sac) is secondary to the elaboration of tumor-derived humoral factors that possess parathyroid hormone-like activity—humoral hypercalcemia of malignancy.[203, 204] Local osteolysis by bone metastases is seldom implicated. Local osteolysis by bone metastases is responsible for hypercalcemia in the majority of hypercalcemic humans with breast cancer.[136]

Definitive diagnosis of bone metastases relies on histopathological evaluation of appropriate tissue specimens. Management of patients focuses on primary tumor control and assessment of the extent of metastatic disease. Although extensive literature on the management of human cancer patients with bone metastases is available,[67, 185] similar data for dogs are lacking. Fewer than 40 per cent of dogs with bone metastases have clinical signs referable to bone lesions.[62] It is plausible that euthanasia of dogs early in the course of the metastatic process may account for the relatively high percentage of clinically occult bone metastases and overall low reported prevalence of bone metastases. Prolonged survival of tumor-bearing dogs receiving aggressive multimodality therapy is likely to increase the clinical importance of bone metastases in small animals.

FELINE BONE TUMORS

Primary bone tumors are uncommon in cats, representing only 20 of 395 (5.1 per cent) feline neoplasms.[50] Although osteosarcoma is the most frequently reported primary bone tumor in cats,[34, 196] squamous cell carcinoma is the most common feline neoplasm involving bone.[159] Bone metastases are infrequent in cats.[34, 167]

As in dogs, most feline bone tumors are malignant. Feline bone neoplasms are characterized by a lower metastatic rate.[196] Wide surgical excision or amputation is likely to result in a more favorable prognosis in cats than in dogs with malignant bone neoplasms. Statements about the biological behavior and prognosis of feline bone neoplasms must be interpreted in light of the paucity of data. Only the most common bone tumors of cats are discussed here. A more complete discussion may be found elsewhere.[34]

Feline Osteosarcoma

Incidence and Biological Behavior

Osteosarcoma is the most common primary bone tumor of cats, representing 70 per cent of primary bone tumors.[196] Older cats are most frequently affected (mean age 10 years).[196] Appendicular skeletal neoplasms are more prevalent than axial skeletal neoplasms, and a predilection for the metaphyses of long bones of the hindlimbs has been suggested.[34, 196] Unlike in dogs, lesions of the distal radius are uncommon. Although the radiographic features of feline osteosarcoma are variable, long-bone lesions are predominatly lytic whereas skull lesions are osteoproductive.[172] Solitary osteolytic metaphyseal long-bone lesions in older cats are considered osteosarcoma until proven otherwise (Fig. 161–3). Osteosarcoma in cats behaves less aggressively than canine osteosarcoma. A metastatic rate of 16 per cent was reported in 32 cats that had osteosarcoma and underwent necropsy.[50, 159, 196]

Treatment and Prognosis

Wide surgical excision or amputation is the treatment of choice for feline osteosarcoma; the prognosis depends on location. Because amputation maximizes the likelihood of tumor-free margins, cats with appendicular osteosarcoma have a better prognosis for long-term survival than cats with axial osteosarcoma.[16] In one study, 6 of 12 (50 per cent) cats that had appendicular osteosarcoma and underwent amputation were alive at 13 to 64 months postoperatively; median survival of cats that died was 49 months.[16] In that same study, six of seven cats with axial skeletal osteosarcoma were treated with surgery, radiation, or chemotherapy; median survival was 5.5 months.[16] Remission for longer than 2 years has been reported in a cat with osteosarcoma of the nasal cavity after cytoreductive surgery, orthovoltage radiotherapy, and metronidazole.[109]

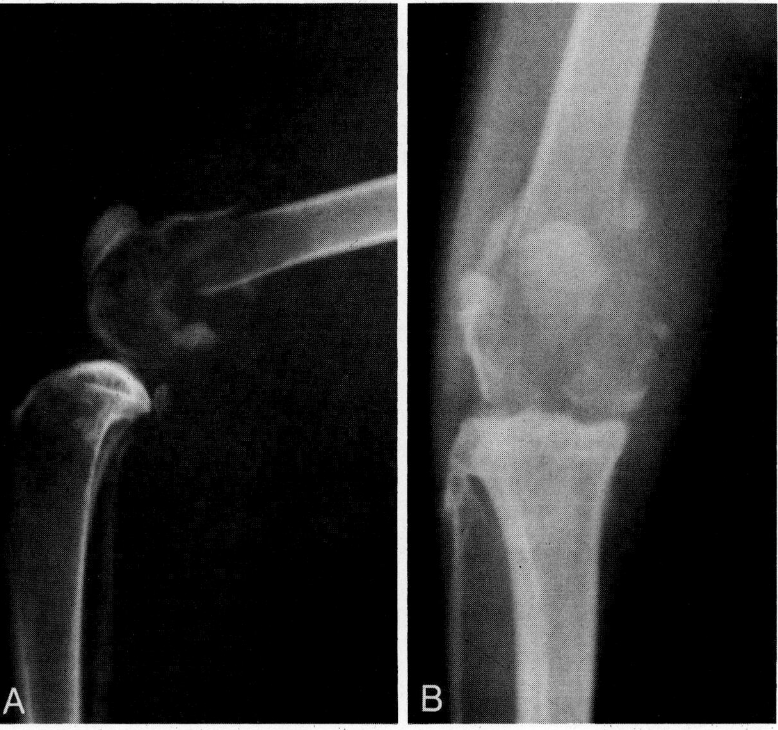

FIGURE 161–3. Lateral *(A)* and craniocaudal *(B)* radiographs of the right distal femur of an 11-year-old domestic shorthaired cat with osteosarcoma and pathological fracture. Osteolysis is frequently the predominant feature of appendicular osteosarcoma in cats.

Feline Parosteal (Juxtacortical) Osteosarcoma

Parosteal osteosarcoma is distinct from central osteosarcoma because it arises from tissue (presumably periosteum) outside the cortex or medullary cavity. Parosteal osteosarcoma represented 8 of 55 (14 per cent) tumors in four series of feline bone tumors.[16, 104, 159, 196] This neoplasm may be distinguished from central osteosarcoma by its gross, radiographic, and histological appearance. In cats, parosteal osteosarcoma is a painless growth on the surface of the skull or long bones. Radiographs reveal a well-circumscribed osteoproductive lesion. A radiolucent line of demarcation between the tumor and underlying cortical bone may be present. Histologically, the neoplasm is composed of fibrous, osseous, and cartilaginous tissue elements. Metastases have been reported[66] but are uncommon. Amputation or wide surgical excision is recommended. The prognosis for humans with parosteal osteosarcoma is much better than for central osteosarcoma.[51, 133] The situation in cats in unknown.

Feline Chondrosarcoma

Chondrosarcoma is rare in cats, representing only 4 of 103 (3.9 per cent) bone tumors.[50, 104, 159] The scapula is the most frequently reported site.[30, 50, 104, 172] Amputation has been reported in the treatment of three cats with chondrosarcoma.[30, 104] Two cats died of tumor-related causes at 7 and 52 weeks, and one cat remained disease free at 18 weeks.

Feline Fibrosarcoma

Primary fibrosarcoma of bone is rare in cats.[101, 104, 159, 193, 196] More commonly, secondary bone invasion by fibrosarcoma originating in soft tissue is reported.[30, 104] In one series in which all fibrosarcomas of bone were considered secondary bone tumors, solitary fibrosarcoma was noted in 11 of 28 (39 per cent) cats with soft-tissue tumors involving bone.[104] This solitary form of fibrosarcoma in older cats must be distinguished from feline sarcoma virus–associated multicentric fibrosarcoma in young cats.[74] After amputation, disease-free intervals greater than 10 months occurred in three cats with appendicular fibrosarcoma.[101, 104, 193]

Feline Squamous Cell Carcinoma

Local bone invasion by squamous cell carcinoma in cats occurs most frequently with tumors of the oral cavity and less frequently the digits (see the later section on neoplasia of the digits). Radiographs reveal destructive lesions, but variable osteoproduction may be present.[159] Histologically, squamous cell carcinoma is characterized by keratin-producing malignant epithelial cells. Keratin "pearls" should not be mistaken for osteosarcoma-associated tumor osteoid.

Feline Solitary Osteochondroma and Osteochondromatosis

An osteochondroma is a trabecular bone exostosis covered by a cartilaginous cap.[34, 154] Solitary osteochondromas in cats involve the axial skeleton or the physeal regions of long bones.[172, 196] These are well circumscribed and often amenable to local excision. Although local recurrence or malignant transformation is possible, the prognosis for cats with solitary osteochondroma is favorable after surgical excision.[172]

Osteochondromatosis, or multiple cartilaginous exostoses, is distinct from solitary osteochondroma.[154] Feline osteochondromatosis is characterized by multiple exostotic lesions involving the cranium, scapula, ribs, vertebrae, or pelvis; appendicular skeletal lesions are rare. Relentless growth distinguishes feline osteochondromatosis from canine multiple cartilaginous exostoses, a condition that is nonprogressive after skeletal maturity.[154] As the disease progresses in cats, lesions acquire increasingly more sarcoma-like characteristics. The role of retrovirus infection in cats with osteochondromatosis remains unclear, although type C virus particles have been identified in tumors.[154] Affected cats frequently test positive for feline leukemia virus, and survival beyond 1 year after diagnosis has not been reported.[172] The clinicopathological features of osteochondromatosis/multiple cartilaginous exostoses in dogs and cats have been extensively reviewed.[154]

FRACTURE-ASSOCIATED SARCOMA IN DOGS AND CATS

Incidence and Clinicopathological Features

Fracture-associated sarcomas are primary bone tumors that develop at the site of previous fractures (Fig. 161–4). This name is more accurate than *implant-associated sarcoma* because cases have occurred when no fracture fixation was used.[184] Fracture-associated sarcoma should not be confused with pathological fractures, which are fractures occurring in abnormal bone.[18] Fracture-associated sarcoma is most frequently reported with fractures that have undergone a complicated or disturbed healing process (e.g., comminuted fractures, osteomyelitis, delayed union or nonunion).[183] Osteosarcoma arising in a cortical allograft used to repair a comminuted femoral fracture has been reported.[199] Persistent heightened local bone activity associated with allograft incorporation may have had a role in the pathogenesis of malignant transformation.[199]

Both internal and external fixation devices have been incriminated in the pathogenesis of fracture-associated sarcoma.[178, 184] The fixation device or metallic implant may serve as an innocent bystander, or corrosion of implants with subsequent metallic ion-induced carcinogenesis may be important (e.g., Jonas, intramedullary splint).[179] The increased frequency with which bone plates are implicated most likely reflects the increased use of these implants in comminuted and complicated fractures.

In 62 dogs, the mean age at fracture was 1.9 years, and the mean interval from fracture to appearance of neoplasm was 6.3 years.[183] Osteosarcoma is the most common histological type, representing more than 90 per cent of reported fracture-associated sarcomas.[178, 184] Distribution differs from the classic canine osteo-

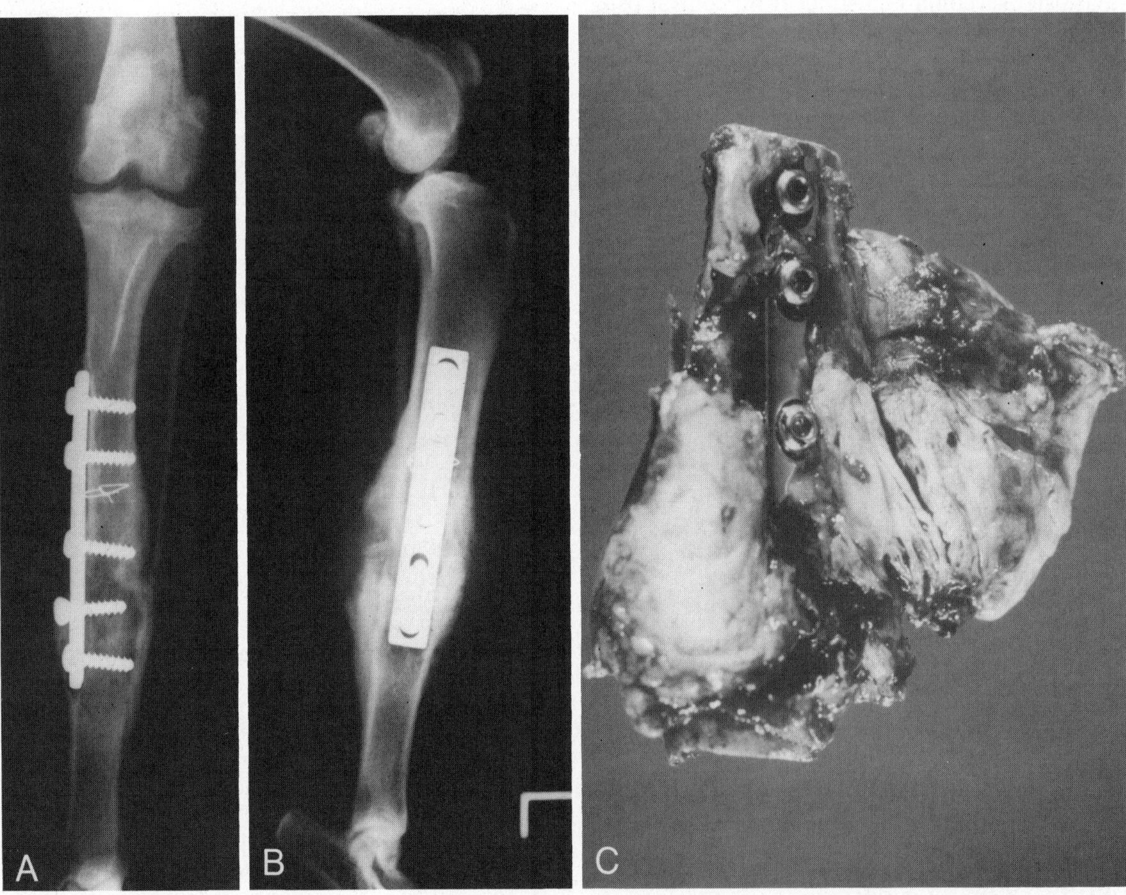

FIGURE 161–4. Fracture-associated sarcoma in an 8-year-old Labrador retriever with hindlimb lameness and cutaneous draining tracts that developed 7 years after plate fixation of a left tibial fracture. Craniocaudal *(A)* and lateral *(B)* radiographs of the tibia reveal osteolysis and osteoproduction in association with the plate. Gross specimen *(C)* shows neoplastic tissue in close proximity to the plate.

sarcoma.[24, 58, 102] More than 80 per cent of fracture-associated sarcomas are diaphyseal, and the femur is the most frequent bone affected in dogs, consistent with the high prevalence of femoral diaphyseal fractures. Fracture-associated sarcoma represents approximately 5 per cent of canine osteosarcomas.[28, 58, 89] In humans, fewer than 20 cases of bone sarcomas associated with prostheses or metallic implants have been reported.[122]

Biological Behavior, Treatment, and Prognosis

Metastases were reported in 6 of 42 (14 per cent) dogs with fracture-associated sarcoma.[184] Biological behavior is not well characterized, and it is unclear whether dogs with fracture-associated osteosarcoma have a more favorable prognosis than dogs with classic osteosarcoma. Diaphyseal location of these neoplasms may facilitate limb salvage techniques that might otherwise be abandoned in dogs with metaphyseal lesions.

Implications for Treating Fractures

The surgeon should select a means of fracture fixation that maximizes the likelihood of uncomplicated repair, particularly in dogs with comminuted long-bone fractures. In dogs with disturbed fracture healing, particularly chronic osteomyelitis, implant removal is recommended after healing is complete. Tumor development is predicted in only 5 to 10:10,000 total fractures or 10 to 30:10,000 fractures repaired with internal fixation.[76, 178] An attempt to prevent fracture-associated sarcoma is *not* the rationale for plate removal after repair of uncomplicated fractures. Positive bacterial cultures have been reported in 40 per cent of dogs at plate removal after uncomplicated fractures.[180] The clinical significance of these occult infections is unknown.

NEOPLASMS OF THE DIGITS

Squamous cell carcinoma, melanoma, and mast cell sarcoma are the most common neoplasms involving the digits. Squamous cell carcinoma is most frequently associated with bone involvement. Reports of osteosarcoma and other primary bone neoplasms involving the phalanges are infrequent.[87]

Digital squamous cell carcinoma may be solitary[107] or involve multiple digits.[54, 116, 140] Physical examination reveals lameness associated with one or more painful, swollen digits. Radiographs typically reveal a destructive process with soft-tissue swelling. Clinically and radiographically, this condition may mimic osteomyelitis.

Squamous cell carcinoma involving several digits has been reported.[54, 116, 140] All dogs were large (> 20 kg), and had black skin and black haircoat (e.g., Labrador retriever, standard poodle, giant schnauzer). All tumors arose from nail bed epithelium, with invasion and destruction of the second or third phalangeal bones. As many as six digits were amputated during a 4-year period.[54, 116, 140] Metastases to local lymph nodes were identified in two dogs.[116] Six dogs remained disease free 6 to 24 months postoperatively.[54, 116, 140] Feline squamous cell carcinoma of several digits also occurs.[32, 152]

Lameness attributable to digital metastases may be the initial manifestation of pulmonary carcinoma in cats.[34, 125, 134] Swelling of several digits is accompanied by radiographic evidence of phalangeal osteolysis and new bone formation. Fixed exsheathment of the claws is consistent.[125] Thoracic radiographs reveal the pulmonary neoplasm(s). Metastatic disease is frequently present in the kidneys and in hindlimb muscles.[125, 134]

BENIGN BONE TUMORS

Benign tumors are a small percentage of primary bone tumors.[87, 153] Osteoma,[3, 59, 87, 102] osteoid osteoma,[105] ossifying fibroma,[108, 153] enchondroma,[153] chondroma,[64, 73, 108] and osteochondroma[154] are reported. Few data on the prevalence and clinicopathological features of these neoplasms are available. They are generally slow growing and do not metastasize. Complete surgical excision is curative, although tumor location may make this impossible.

NON-NEOPLASTIC BONE TUMORS

Radiographic features and biological behavior of non-neoplastic lesions are important because these lesions may mimic bone neoplasms and may be difficult to distinguish. Biopsy and histopathological examination may be necessary. Alternatively, sequential radiographic evaluation may be used. The disease conditions that are discussed in this section represent an incomplete list of the non-neoplastic tumor-like lesions of bone reported in dogs and cats. Other lesions including panosteitis, craniomandibular osteopathy, hypertrophic osteopathy, and hypervitaminosis A are discussed elsewhere.

Osteomyelitis

Radiographic features of osteomyelitis may mimic bone neoplasms.[73, 102, 147] Fungal osteomyelitis lesions associated with *Coccidioides immitis*[5, 132] or *Blastomyces dermatitidis*[17, 165] infection may be particularly difficult to distinguish from neoplasia (Fig. 161–5).

A syndrome of septic arthritis and osteomyelitis of the coxofemoral joint occurs in mature dogs.[171] Five of six dogs had unilateral coxofemoral joint involvement, and one dog was affected bilaterally.[171] Anorexia, lethargy, and unilateral coxofemoral pain were the most common signs. Initial radiographic changes were subtle. In advanced cases, radiographs revealed an osteolytic lesion involving the proximal femur, with periacetabular new bone formation extending along the ilium and ischium. The presence of radiographic changes on both sides of the coxofemoral joint is helpful in distinguishing this syndrome from primary bone tumors or ischemic necrosis of the femoral head. *Staphylococcus aureus* (n = 3), *Streptococcus* (n = 1), and *Clostridium* (n = 1) were isolated from five of five coxofemoral joints that were cultured. Blood-borne infection was suspected because affected joints had not been subjected to previous surgical or nonsurgical trauma. Positive bacterial cultures from synovial fluid or adjacent bone are useful in distinguishing this syndrome from villonodular

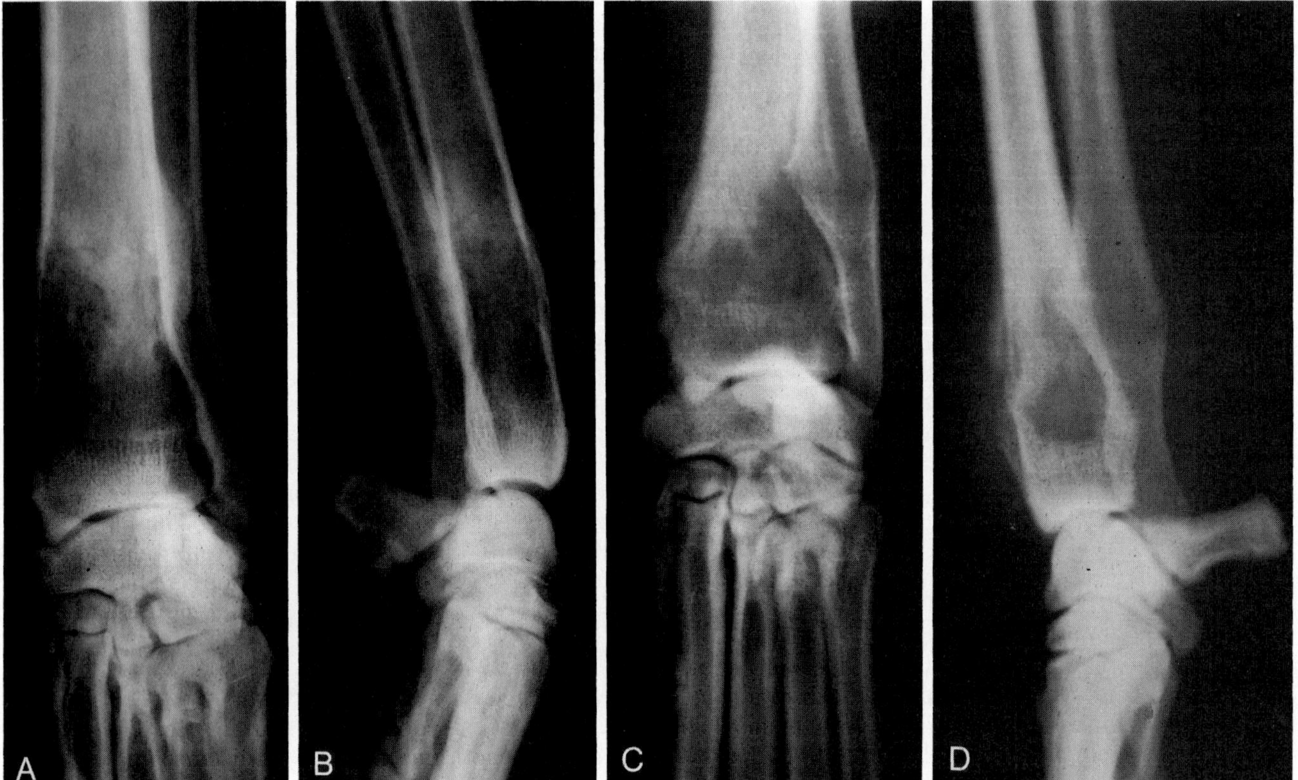

FIGURE 161–5. Craniocaudal *(A)* and lateral *(B)* radiographs of the distal radius and ulna of a dog with osteosarcoma. Craniocaudal *(C)* and lateral *(D)* radiographs of the distal radius and ulna of a dog with blastomycosis. The radiographic features of mycotic osteomyelitis often mimic those of bone neoplasms.

synovitis[92] or synovial sarcoma. Surgical drainage and débridement of the affected joint, with femoral head and neck excision and systemic antibiotic therapy, were successful in maintaining or restoring acceptable limb function.[171]

Simple or Benign Bone Cyst

Simple bone cysts have been reported in dogs.[13, 70, 173] The distal radius and ulna of young (< 18 months) large dogs are most frequently affected.[173] The characteristic radiographic features of simple bone cysts (lytic, expansile metaphyseal lesions with little or no periosteal new bone formation) often distinguish these lesions from osteosarcoma, which may also occur in young dogs. Most lesions are fluid filled, unicameral (single compartment), and lined by a thin membrane. Multiple bone cysts are found in approximately 40 per cent of affected dogs, particularly Doberman pinschers.[173] The prognosis after drainage and curettage is favorable. Local recurrence or malignant transformation has not been reported. The cause of simple bone cysts remains unknown.

Aneurysmal Bone Cyst

Although frequently reported in humans,[133, 138, 166] aneurysmal bone cysts are rare in dogs[19, 162] and cats.[14, 34, 104, 105, 200] This lesion is not a true cyst because it has no epithelial lining. Aneurysmal bone cysts are distinguished from simple bone cysts by the presence of multiple blood-filled spaces separated by fibrous tissue and fine bone trabeculae.[166] Histologically, the absence of spindle-shaped malignant cells distinguishes aneurysmal bone cysts from hemangiosarcoma of bone and telangiectatic osteosarcoma. Although aneurysmal bone cysts may occur with pre-existing lesions of bone,[123] the cause remains unknown.

Human patients with aneurysmal bone cysts have been treated with surgical curettage,[166] radiation,[138] or embolization.[38] A recurrence rate of 30 per cent after curettage was reported.[166] Reports of spontaneous healing as well as regression after simple biopsy may suggest a conservative approach.[119] The ideal therapy for dogs and cats with aneurysmal bone cysts has not been established.

Bone Infarction

Multifocal medullary infarctions are reported in dogs with bone neoplasms.[46, 98, 157, 164] Radiographically, bone infarctions are medullary radiopacities that represent bone proliferation secondary to hypoxia.[46] All dogs reported with bone infarctions had or eventually developed primary bone sarcomas.[46, 98, 157, 164] Because infarction-associated necrosis alone may not cause pain or lameness, the true prevalence of bone infarction is unknown.[46] Miniature schnauzers are over-represented, accounting for 38 per cent of dogs with infarction-associated osteosarcoma.[46, 164] A relationship between bone infarction, fibrocartilaginous embolic myelopathy,[37] and hyperlipidemia[6] is possible in miniature schnauzers.

NEOPLASMS OF JOINTS (SYNOVIAL SARCOMA)

Incidence and Biological Behavior

"Synovial sarcoma" or malignant synovioma most frequently involves the joints of dogs and cats.[103, 115] These neoplasms do not arise within the joint, because marked differences in immunohistochemical staining of human synovial sarcoma cells and normal synovial cells suggest a periarticular origin.[130] In humans, synovial sarcomas remote from joints have been reported; neoplasms involving tendon sheaths occur in dogs and cats.[34, 115]

Synovial sarcoma is uncommon in dogs, representing only 9 of 394 (2.3 per cent) canine bone neoplasms or tumor-like lesions of bones.[108] Synovial sarcoma is rare in cats.[34, 50, 115, 159] These neoplasms consist of two cell types: synovium-like (epithelioid) cells and a sarcomatous (spindle cell) element. Tumors with a predominance of the sarcomatous cell type may be difficult to distinguish from fibrosarcoma.

Lameness is the most common presenting sign in dogs with synovial sarcoma. The mean age of affected dogs is 7 to 8 years (range 1 to 14 years).[103, 115] Examination of the affected joint may reveal swelling, pain, and decreased range of motion. A palpable mass may not be identifiable.[103] Radiographic lesions may be limited to soft-tissue swelling but frequently include cortical destruction and periosteal reaction. Radiographic evidence of a destructive lesion involving bones on both sides of a joint suggests synovial sarcoma (Fig. 161–6). The stifle and elbow are sites of predilection, representing 23 of 31 (74 per cent) synovial sarcomas reported.[103, 115] Tumors are usually adherent to the external surface of the fibrous joint capsule; extension through the joint capsule occurred in only 3 of 13 (23 per cent) cases.[103] Metastases were detected radiographically or microscopically in 8 of 31 (26 per cent) dogs with synovial sarcoma.[103, 115]

Treatment and Prognosis

Duration of clinical signs referable to synovial sarcoma varies, with a mean of 7.9 months (range 1 week to 60 months).[103] These neoplasms apparently exhibit an entire spectrum of biological behavior (i.e., low to high-grade malignancy); the prognosis after surgical excision is somewhat unpredictable. Although amputation is the recommended treatment, data regarding prognosis after amputation are limited. A long (2 years) disease-free interval after amputation is possible.[115] Local recurrence 6 to 24 weeks after amputation has been reported and may not be accompanied by metastases.[103] Three-year survival after excisional biopsy and combination chemotherapy (doxorubicin, cyclophosphamide) has been reported.[192]

NEOPLASMS OF SKELETAL MUSCLE

Neoplasms of skeletal muscle are extremely rare.[34, 81] Primary malignant tumors (rhabdomyosarcoma) predominate; malignant melanoma, hemangiosarcoma, and lymphosarcoma are most frequently associated with skeletal muscle metastases.[82] The two most frequently reported tumors of striated muscle in dogs do not involve skeletal muscle. Botryoid rhabdomyosarcoma, a urinary bladder neoplasm of young dogs, is known for its association with hypertrophic osteopathy.[71] Granular cell myoblastoma, a tumor of myoblast origin, is the second most frequently reported tongue neoplasm in dogs.[9]

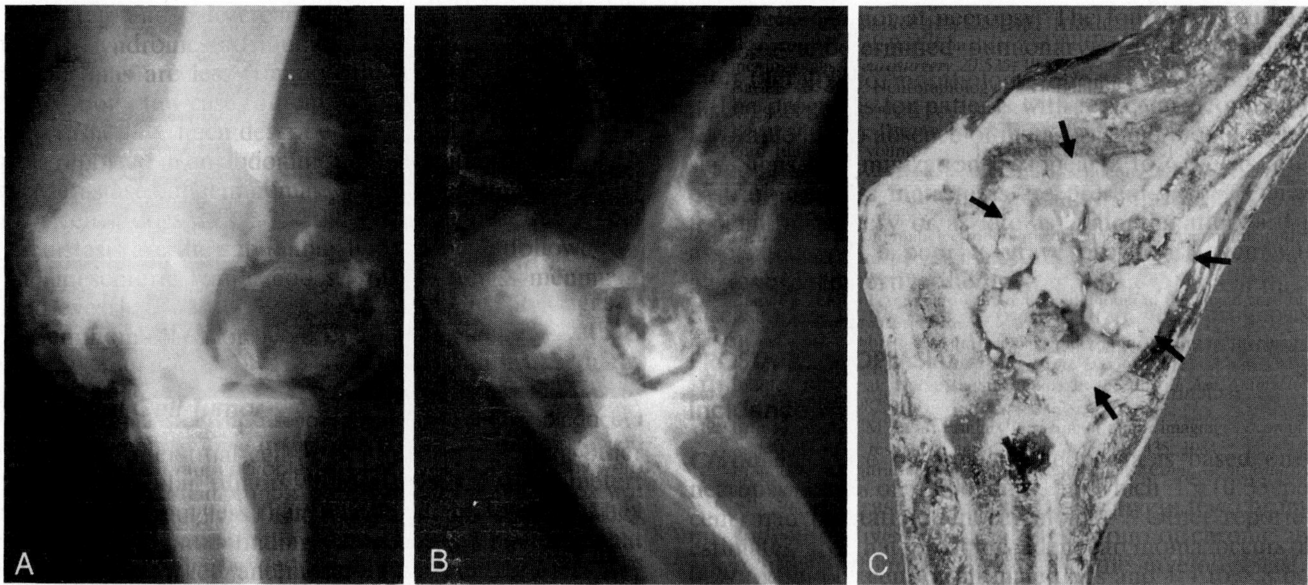

FIGURE 161–6. Craniocaudal *(A)* and lateral *(B)* radiographs of the right elbow of a 12-year-old golden retriever with extensive osteolysis of the distal humerus and proximal radius and ulna. Gross specimen *(C)* shows tumor *(arrows)* surrounding the joint. Diagnosis was synovial sarcoma.

Definitive statements about the biological behavior, treatment, and prognosis of skeletal muscle neoplasms in dogs and cats cannot be made.

References

1. Adams WM, et al: Radiotherapy for malignant nasal tumors in 67 dogs. *J Am Vet Med Assoc 191*:311, 1987.
2. Alexander JW, Patton CS: Primary tumors of the skeletal system. *Vet Clin North Am Small Anim Pract 13*:181, 1983.
3. Alexander JW, Patton CS: Musculoskeletal system. *In* Slatter DH (ed): *Textbook of Small Animal Surgery*. W.B. Saunders, Philadelphia, 1985, pp 2575–2583.
4. Allan CJ, Soule EH: Osteogenic sarcoma of the somatic soft tissues: Clinicopathologic study of 26 cases and review of literature. *Cancer 27*:1121, 1971.
5. Armstrong PJ, DiBartola SP: Canine coccidioidomycosis: A literature review and report of eight cases. *J Am Anim Hosp Assoc 19*:937, 1983.
6. Armstrong PJ, Ford RB: Hyperlipidemia. *In* Kirk RW (ed): *Current Veterinary Therapy X*. W.B. Saunders, Philadelphia, 1989, pp 1046–1050.
7. Banks WC: Parosteal osteosarcoma in a dog and a cat. *J Am Vet Med Assoc 158*:1412, 1971.
8. Barber DL, et al: Primary osseous hemangiosarcoma in a dog. *J Am Vet Radiol Soc 14*:17, 1973.
9. Beck ER, et al: Canine tongue tumors: A retrospective review of 57 cases. *J Am Anim Hosp Assoc 22*:525, 1986.
10. Belli L, et al: Resection of pulmonary metastases in osteosarcoma: A retrospective analysis of 44 patients. *Cancer 63*:2546, 1989.
11. Berg J, et al: Bone scintigraphy in the initial evaluation of dogs with primary bone tumors. *J Am Vet Med Assoc 196*:917, 1990.
12. Berrettoni BA, Carter JR: Mechanisms of cancer metastasis to bone. *J Bone Joint Surg [Am] 68*:308, 1986.
13. Biery DN, et al: Bone cysts in the dog. *J Am Vet Radiol Soc 17*:202, 1976.
14. Biller DS, et al: Aneurysmal bone cyst in a rib of a cat. *J Am Vet Med Assoc 190*:1193, 1987.
15. Bingel SA, et al: Haemangiosarcoma of bone in the dog. *J Small Anim Pract 15*:303, 1974.
16. Bitetto WV, et al: Osteosarcoma in cats: 22 cases (1974–84). *J Am Vet Med Assoc 190*:91, 1987.
17. Bone DL: Osteomyelitis due to canine blastomycosis. *J Vet Orthopedics 3*:15, 1984.
18. Boulay JP, et al: Pathological fracture of long bones in the dog. *J Am Anim Hosp Assoc 23*:297, 1987.
19. Bowles MHY, Freeman K: Aneurysmal bone cyst in the ischia and pubes of a dog: A case report and literature review. *J Am Anim Hosp Assoc 23*:423, 1987.
20. Brem H, Folkman J: Inhibition of tumor angiogenesis mediated by cartilage. *J Exp Med 141*:427, 1975.
21. Bright RM: Reconstruction of thoracic wall defects using Marlex mesh. *J Am Anim Hosp Assoc 17*:415, 1981.
22. Brodey RS, Abt DA: Results of surgical treatment in 65 dogs with osteosarcoma. *J Am Vet Med Assoc 168*:1032, 1976.
23. Brodey RS, Riser WH: Liposarcoma of bone in a dog: A case report. *J Am Vet Radiol Soc 7*:27, 1966.
24. Brodey RS, Riser WH: Canine osteosarcoma: A clinicopathologic study of 194 cases. *Clin Orthop 62*:54, 1969.
25. Brodey RS, et al: A clinical and radiological study of canine bone neoplasms. Part I. *J Am Vet Med Assoc 134*:53, 1959.
26. Brodey RS, et al: Canine skeletal chondrosarcoma: A clinicopathologic study of 35 cases. *J Am Vet Med Assoc 165*:68, 1974.
27. Brodey RS, et al: Metastatic bone neoplasms in the dog. *J Am Vet Med Assoc 148*:29, 1966.
28. Brodey RS, et al: Canine bone neoplasms. *J Am Vet Med Assoc 143*:471, 1963.
29. Brogdon JD, et al: Parosteal osteosarcoma of the mandible in a dog. *J Am Vet Med Assoc 194*:1079, 1989.
30. Brown NO, et al: Soft tissue sarcomas in the cat. *J Am Vet Med Assoc 173*:744, 1978.
31. Brown NO, et al: Canine hemangiosarcoma: Retrospective analysis of 104 cases. *J Am Vet Med Assoc 186*:56, 1985.
32. Brown PJ, et al: Multiple squamous cell carcinoma of the digits in two cats. *J Small Anim Pract 26*:323, 1985.
33. Brunnberg VL, et al: Knochentumoren beim hund nach trauma und osteosynthese. *Kleintierpraxis 25*:143, 1980.
34. Carpenter JL, et al: Tumors and tumor-like lesions. *In* Holzworth J (ed): *Diseases of the Cat: Medicine and Surgery*. W.B. Saunders, Philadelphia, 1987, pp 406–596.
35. Chackal-Roy M, et al: Stimulation of human prostatic carcinoma cell growth by factors present in human bone marrow. *J Clin Invest 84*:43, 1989.
36. Childers HE: Radiologic diagnosis of a hemangiosarcoma in a dog. *J Am Vet Med Assoc 157*:1379, 1970.
37. Cook JR: Fibrocartilaginous embolism. *Vet Clin North Am Small Anim Pract 18*:581, 1988.
38. Cory DA, et al: Aneurysmal bone cysts: Imaging findings and embolotherapy. *Am J Roentgenol 153*:369, 1989.
39. Cotter SM, Parker LM: High-dose methotrexate and leucovorin rescue in dogs with osteogenic sarcoma. *Am J Vet Res 39*:1943, 1978.
40. Cottrill NB, et al: Bilateral orbital parosteal osteoma in a cat. *J Am Anim Hosp Assoc 23*:405, 1987.
41. Crow SE: Primary hemangiosarcoma of the femur in a dog. *Mod Vet Pract 58*:343, 1977.
42. Crow SE, et al: Giant cell tumor (osteoclastoma) in a dog. *J Am Anim Hosp Assoc 15*:473, 1979.
43. Dahlin DC, Coventry MB: Osteogenic sarcoma: A study of six hundred cases. *J Bone Joint Surg [Am] 49*:101, 1967.
44. Davis PE, et al: Multiple liposarcoma of bone marrow origin in a greyhound. *J Small Anim Pract 15*:445, 1974.
45. Doige CE, et al: Chondrosarcoma arising in multiple cartilaginous exostoses in a dog. *J Am Anim Hosp Assoc 14*:605, 1978.
46. Dubielzig RR, et al: Bone sarcomas associated with multifocal medullary bone infarction in dogs. *J Am Vet Med Assoc 179*:64, 1981.
47. Dueland R, Dahlin DC: Hemangioendothelioma of canine bone. *J Am Anim Hosp Assoc 8*:81, 1972.
48. Durham SK, Dietze AE: Prostatic adenocarcinoma with and without metastasis to bone in dogs. *J Am Vet Med Assoc 188*:1432, 1986.
49. Ellison GW, et al: Reconstructive thoracoplasty using spinal fixation plates and polypropylene mesh. *J Am Anim Hosp Assoc 17*:613, 1981.
50. Engle GC, Brodey RS: A retrospective study of 395 feline neoplasms. *J Am Anim Hosp Assoc 5*:21, 1969.
51. Enneking WF, et al: The surgical treatment of parosteal osteosarcoma in long bones. *J Bone Joint Surg [Am] 67*:125, 1985.
52. Evans JE, et al: Parosteal osteosarcoma in a dog. *J Am Anim Hosp Assoc 20*:813, 1984.
53. Evans SM, et al: Prognostic factors and survival after radiotherapy for intranasal neoplasms in dogs: 70 cases (1974–85). *J Am Vet Med Assoc 194*:1460, 1989.
54. Ewing GP, et al: Multiple squamous cell carcinoma of the nail bed in the canine. *Calif Vet 22*:16, 1968.
55. Feeney DA, et al: Malignant neoplasia of canine ribs: Clinical, radiographic, and pathologic findings. *J Am Vet Med Assoc 180*:927, 1982.
56. Feeney DA, et al: A mid-diaphyseal osteosarcoma of the humerus in a dog: A case report. *J Am Anim Hosp Assoc 18*:910, 1982.
57. Galasko CSB: Mechanisms of lytic and blastic metastatic disease of bone. *Clin Orthop 169*:20, 1982.
58. Gibbs C, et al: The radiological features of osteosarcoma of the appendicular skeleton in dogs: A review of 74 cases. *J Small Anim Pract 25*:177, 1984.
59. Gibbs C, et al: The radiological features of nonosteogenic malignant tumours of bone in the appendicular skeleton of the dog: A review of thirty-four cases. *J Small Anim Pract 26*:537, 1985.
60. Giger U, et al: Orthovoltage radiotherapy of primary lymphoma of bone in a dog. *J Am Vet Med Assoc 195*:627, 1989.
61. Gleiser CA, et al: Telangiectatic osteosarcoma in the dog. *Vet Pathol 18*:396, 1981.
62. Goedegebuure SA: Secondary bone tumours in the dog. *Vet Pathol 16*:520, 1979.
63. Goldschmidt MH, Thrall DE: Malignant bone tumors in the dog. *In* Newton CD, Nunamaker DM (eds): *Textbook of Small Animal Orthopedics*. J.B. Lippincott, Philadelphia, 1985, pp 887–898.
64. Goldschmidt MH, Thrall DE: Benign bone tumors in the dog. *In* Newton CD, Nunamaker DM (eds): *Textbook of Small Animal Orthopedics*. J.B. Lippincott, Philadelphia, 1985, pp 899–902.
65. Goorin AM, et al: Prognostic significance of complete surgical resection of pulmonary metastases in patients with osteogenic sarcoma: Analysis of 32 patients. *J Clin Oncol 2*:425, 1984.
66. Griffith JW, et al: Parosteal osteosarcoma with pulmonary metastases in a cat. *Vet Pathol 21*:123, 1984.
67. Habermann ET, Lopez RA: Metastatic disease of bone and treatment of pathological fractures. *Orthop Clin North Am 20*:469, 1989.
68. Hahn KA, et al: Remission and survival length observed in dogs receiving amputation and adjunctive cisplatin chemotherapy for osteogenic sarcoma. Abstracts of the 8th Annual Conference of the Veterinary Cancer Society, Estes Park, Col., Oct. 1988, p 11.
69. Hahn KA, et al: Single-phase methylene diphosphate bone scintigraphy in the diagnostic evaluation of dogs with osteosarcoma. *J Am Vet Med Assoc 196*:1483, 1990.
70. Halliwell WH: Tumor-like lesions of bone. *In* Bojrab MJ (ed): *Pathophysiology in Small Animal Surgery*. Lea & Febiger, Philadelphia, 1981, pp 716–728.
71. Halliwell WH, Ackerman N: Botryoid rhabdomyosarcoma of the urinary bladder and hypertrophic osteoarthropathy in a young dog. *J Am Vet Med Assoc 165*:911, 1974.
72. Hamilton HB, et al: Effect of RA 233 on metastasis in dogs with osteosarcomas. *Am J Vet Res 48*:1380, 1987.
73. Hanlon GF: A radiologic approach to bone neoplasms. *Vet Clin North Am Small Anim Pract 12*:329, 1982.

74. Hardy WD: The feline sarcoma viruses. *J Am Anim Hosp Assoc 17*:981, 1981.
75. Hardy WD, et al: Osteosarcoma of the canine skull. *J Am Vet Radiol Soc 8*:5, 1967.
76. Harrison JW, et al: Osteosarcoma associated with metallic implants: Report of two cases in dogs. *Clin Orthop 116*:253, 1976.
77. Harwood AR, et al: Radiotherapy of chondrosarcoma of bone. *Cancer 45*:2769, 1980.
78. Helfand SC: Chemotherapy for nonresectable and metastatic soft tissue tumors. Proceedings of the 10th Kal Kan Symposium, Columbus, Ohio, Oct. 1986, pp 133–142.
79. Henness AM, et al: Combination therapy for canine osteosarcoma. *J Am Vet Med Assoc 170*:1076, 1977.
80. Horak E, et al: Analysis of organ-specific effects on metastatic tumor formation by studies *in vitro*. *J Natl Cancer Inst 76*:913, 1986.
81. Hulland TJ: Muscles and tendons. *In* Jubb KVF, et al (eds): *Pathology of Domestic Animals*. 3rd ed. Academic Press, Orlando, FL, 1985, pp 193–194.
82. Hulland TJ: Tumors of muscle. *In* Moulton JE (ed): *Tumors in Domestic Animals*. 2nd ed. University of California Press, Berkeley, 1978, pp 75–88.
83. Huvos AG, et al: Telangiectatic osteogenic sarcoma: A clinicopathologic study of 124 patients. *Cancer 49*:1679, 1982.
84. Jacobs SC: Spread of prostatic cancer to bone. *Urology 21*:337, 1983.
85. Jacobson SA: *The Comparative Pathology of the Tumors of Bone*. Charles C Thomas, Springfield, IL, 1971.
86. Johnson KA, et al: Splenomegaly in dogs: Predictors of neoplasia and survival after splenectomy. *J Vet Intern Med 3*:167, 1989.
87. Jongeward SJ: Primary bone tumors. *Vet Clin North Am Small Anim Pract 15*:609, 1985.
88. Kas NP, et al: Metastatic bone neoplasms in dogs, cats and a lion. *Zentralbl Veterinarmed [A] 17*:909, 1970.
89. Knecht CD, Priester WA: Osteosarcoma in dogs: A study of previous trauma, fracture, and fracture fixation. *J Am Anim Hosp Assoc 14*:82, 1978.
90. Kramek BA, et al: Surgical repair of a pathological fracture due to chondrosarcoma: A case report. *J Am Anim Hosp Assoc 21*:643, 1985.
91. Kuettner KE, et al: Morphological studies on the resistance of cartilage to invasion by osteosarcoma cells *in vitro* and *in vivo*. *Cancer Res 38*:277, 1978.
92. Kusba JK, et al: Suspected villonodular synovitis in a dog. *J Am Vet Med Assoc 182*:390, 1983.
93. Lagier R: Synovial reaction caused by adjacent malignant tumors: anatomicopathological study of three cases. *J Rheumatol 4*:65, 1977.
94. Lamb CR: Bone scintigraphy in small animals. *J Am Vet Med Assoc 191*:1616, 1987.
95. Lamb CR, et al: Preoperative measurement of canine primary bone tumors, using radiography and bone scintigraphy. *J Am Vet Med Assoc 196*:1474, 1990.
96. Lang J, et al: Sensitivity of radiographic detection of lung metastases in the dog. *Vet Radiol 27*:74, 1986.
97. La Rue SM, Withrow SJ: Tumors of the skeletal system. *In* Withrow SJ, MacEwen EG (eds): *Clinical Veterinary Oncology*. J.B. Lippincott, Philadelphia, 1989, pp 234–252.
98. LaRue SM, et al: Radiographic bone surveys in the evaluation of primary bone tumors in dogs. *J Am Vet Med Assoc 188*:514, 1986.
99. LaRue SM, et al: Limb-sparing treatment for osteosarcoma in dogs. *J Am Vet Med Assoc 195*:1734, 1989.
100. LeCouteur RA, et al: A case of giant cell tumor of bone (osteoclastoma) in a dog. *J Am Anim Hosp Assoc 14*:356, 1978.
101. Levitt L, Doige CE: Primary intraosseous fibrosarcoma in a cat. *J Am Vet Med Assoc 194*:1601, 1989.
102. Ling GV, et al: Primary bone tumors in the dog: A combined clinical, radiographic, and histologic approach to early diagnosis. *J Am Vet Med Assoc 165*:55, 1974.
103. Lipowitz AJ, et al: Synovial sarcoma of the dog. *J Am Vet Med Assoc 174*:76, 1979.
104. Liu SK, et al: Primary and secondary bone tumours in the cat. *J Small Anim Pract 15*:141, 1974.
105. Liu SK: Tumors of bone and cartilage. *In* Bojrab MJ (ed): *Pathophysiology in Small Animal Surgery*. Lea & Febiger, Philadelphia, 1981, pp 690–711.
106. Liu SK, Harvey HJ: Metastatic bone neoplasms in the dog. *In* Bojrab MJ (ed): *Pathophysiology in Small Animal Surgery*. Lea & Febiger, Philadelphia, 1981, pp 712–715.
107. Liu SK, Hohn RB: Squamous cell carcinoma of the digit of the dog. *J Am Vet Med Assoc 153*:411, 1968.
108. Liu SK, et al: Primary and secondary bone tumors in the dog. *J Small Anim Pract 18*:313, 1977.
109. Lord PF, et al: Osteogenic sarcoma of the nasal cavity in a cat: Postoperative control with high dose-per-fraction radiation therapy and metronidazole. *Vet Radiol 23*:23, 1982.
110. Luttgen PJ, et al: A retrospective study of twenty-nine spinal tumors in the dog and cat. *J Small Anim Pract 21*:213, 1980.
111. MacEwen EG: Adjuvant chemotherapy and immunotherapy for canine osteosarcoma. Proceedings of the 8th American College of Veterinary Internal Medicine Forum, Washington, D.C., May 1990, pp 949–952.
112. MacEwen EG, Hurvitz AI: Diagnosis and management of monoclonal gammopathies. *Vet Clin North Am Small Anim Pract 7*:119, 1977.
113. MacEwen EG, et al: Therapy for osteosarcoma in dogs with intravenous injection of liposome-encapsulated muramyl tripeptide. *J Natl Cancer Inst 81*:935, 1989.
114. Madewell BR, et al: Amputation and doxorubicin for treatment of canine and feline osteogenic sarcoma. *Eur J Cancer 14*:287, 1978.
115. Madewell BR, Pool R: Neoplasms of joints and related structures. *Vet Clin North Am Small Anim Pract 8*:511, 1978.
116. Madewell BR, et al: Multiple subungual squamous cell carcinomas in five dogs. *J Am Vet Med Assoc 180*:731, 1982.
117. Magro C, et al: Adhesion, chemotaxis, and aggregation of Walker carcinosarcoma cells in response to products of resorbing bone. *J Natl Cancer Inst 74*:829, 1985.
118. Mahaffey EA, Greene CE: Hemothorax associated with telangiectatic osteosarcoma in a dog. *J Am Vet Med Assoc 187*:270, 1985.
119. Malghem J, et al: Spontaneous healing of aneurysmal bone cysts: A report of three cases. *J Bone Joint Surg [Br] 71*:645, 1989.
120. Manishen WJ, et al: Resorbing bone stimulates tumor cell growth: A role for the host microenvironment in bone metastasis. *Am J Pathol 123*:39, 1986.
121. Marks KE, Bauer TW: Fibrous tumors of bone. *Orthop Clin North Am 20*:377, 1989.
122. Martin A, et al: Osteosarcoma at the site of total hip replacement. *J Bone Joint Surg [Am] 70*:1561, 1988.
123. Martinez V, Sissons HA: Aneurysmal bone cyst: A review of 123 cases including primary lesions and those secondary to other bone pathology. *Cancer 61*:2291, 1988.
124. Mauldin GN, et al: Canine osteosarcoma: Treatment by amputation versus amputation and adjuvant chemotherapy using doxorubicin and cisplatin. *J Vet Intern Med 2*:177, 1988.
125. May C, Newsholme SJ: Metastasis of feline pulmonary carcinoma presenting as multiple digital swelling. *J Small Anim Pract 30*:302, 1989.
126. McChesney SL, et al: Radiotherapy of soft tissue sarcomas in dogs. *J Am Vet Med Assoc 194*:60, 1989.
127. McLain DL, et al: Multilobular osteoma and chondroma (chondroma rodens) with pulmonary metastasis in a dog. *J Am Anim Hosp Assoc 19*:359, 1983.
128. Meyer JA, et al: Canine osteogenic sarcoma treated by amputation and MER: An adverse effect of splenectomy on survival. *Cancer 49*:1613, 1982.
129. Meyer WH, et al: Thoracotomy for pulmonary metastatic osteosarcoma: An analysis of prognostic indicators of survival. *Cancer 59*:374, 1987.
130. Miettinen M, Virtanen I: Synovial sarcoma—a misnomer. *Am J Pathol 117*:18, 1984.
131. Miller WW, Boosinger TR: Intraocular osteosarcoma in a cat. *J Am Anim Hosp Assoc 23*:317, 1987.
132. Millman TM, et al: Coccidioidomycosis in the dog: Its radiographic diagnosis. *J Am Vet Radiol Soc 20*:50, 1979.
133. Mirra JM, et al: *Bone Tumors: Diagnosis and Treatment*. J.B. Lippincott, Philadelphia, 1980.
134. Moore AS, Middleton DJ: Pulmonary adenocarcinoma in three cats with non-respiratory signs only. *J Small Anim Pract 23*:501, 1982.
135. Morgan JP, et al: Vertebral tumors in the dog: A clinical, radiologic, and pathologic study of 61 primary and secondary lesions. *Vet Radiol 21*:197, 1980.
136. Mundy GR: Hypercalcemia of malignancy revisited. *J Clin Invest 82*:1, 1988.
137. Mundy GR, et al: Collagen and collagen-derived fragments are chemotactic for tumor cells. *J Clin Invest 68*:1102, 1981.
138. Nobler MP, et al: The cure of aneurysmal bone cyst: Irradiation superior to surgery in an analysis of 33 cases. *Radiology 90*:1185, 1968.
139. Ogilvie GK, et al: Malignant lymphoma with cardiac and bone involvement in a dog. *J Am Vet Med Assoc 194*:793, 1989.
140. O'Rourke M: Multiple digital squamous-cell carcinomas in 2 dogs. *Mod Vet Pract 66*:644, 1985.
141. Owen LN: An account of multiple osteosarcomata of bone in dogs having multicentric or metastatic origin. *Br J Radiol 38*:520, 1965.
142. Owen LN: *TNM Classification of Tumors in Domestic Animals*. World Health Organization, Geneva, 1980.
143. Owen LN: Clinical diagnosis and management of bone neoplasia. In Gorman NT (ed): *Oncology*. Churchill Livingstone, New York, 1986, pp 271–293.
144. Owen LN, Bostock DE: Prophylactic x-irradiation of the lung in canine tumors with particular reference to osteosarcoma. *Eur J Cancer 9*:747, 1973.
145. Owen LN, et al: Studies on therapy of osteosarcoma in dogs using BCG vaccine. *J Am Vet Radiol Soc 18*:27, 1977.
146. Pardo AD, et al: Primary jejunal osteosarcoma associated with a surgical sponge in a dog. *J Am Vet Med Assoc 196*:935, 1990.
147. Park RD: Radiographic diagnosis of long bone neoplasms in the dog. *Comp Cont Educ Pract Vet 3*:922, 1981.
148. Patnaik AK: Canine extraskeletal osteosarcoma and chondrosarcoma: A clinicopathologic study of 14 cases. *Vet Pathol 27*:46, 1990.

149. Patnaik AK, et al: Canine sinonasal skeletal neoplasms: Chondrosarcomas and osteosarcomas. *Vet Pathol 21*:475, 1984.
150. Peiffer RL, et al: Fibrosarcoma involving the skeleton of the dog. *Vet Med Small Anim Clin 69*:1143, 1974.
151. Penwick RC, Nunamaker DM: Rostral mandibulectomy: A treatment for oral neoplasia in the dog and cat. *J Am Anim Hosp Assoc 23*:19, 1987.
152. Pollack M, et al: Metastatic squamous cell carcinoma in multiple digits of a cat: Case report. *J Am Anim Hosp Assoc 20*:835, 1984.
153. Pool RR: Tumors of bone and cartilage. *In* Moulton JE (ed) *Tumors in Domestic Animals*. 2nd ed. University of California Press, Berkeley, 1978, pp 89–149.
154. Pool RR: Osteochondromatosis. *In* Bojrab MJ (ed): *Pathophysiology in Small Animal Surgery*. Lea & Febiger, Philadelphia, 1981, pp 641–649.
155. Powers BE, et al: Jamshidi needle biopsy for diagnosis of bone lesions in small animals. *J Am Vet Med Assoc 193*:205, 1988.
156. Prata RG, Carillo JM. Nervous system. *In* Slatter DH (ed): *Textbook of Small Animal Surgery*. W.B. Saunders, Philadelphia, 1985, pp 2499–2522.
157. Prior C, et al: Radial diaphyseal osteosarcoma with associated bone infarctions in a dog. *J Am Anim Hosp Assoc 22*:43, 1986.
158. Putnam JB, et al: Survival following aggressive resection of pulmonary metastases from osteogenic sarcoma: Analysis of prognostic factors. *Ann Thorac Surg 36*:516, 1983.
159. Quigley PJ, Leedale AH: Tumors involving bone in the domestic cat: A review of fifty-eight cases. *Vet Pathol 20*:670, 1983.
160. Rao U, et al: Extraosseous osteogenic sarcoma: Clinicopathological study of eight cases and review of literature. *Cancer 41*:1488, 1978.
161. Rendano VT, et al: Osteosarcoma in the middiaphysis of the radius in the dog: A neoplastic process that initially mimicked a benign process. *Vet Radiol 28*:127, 1987.
162. Renegar WR, et al: Aneurysmal bone cyst in the dog: A case report. *J Am Anim Hosp Assoc 15*:191, 1979.
163. Richardson RC, et al: An adjuvant study of nafazatrom in resected canine osteogenic sarcomas. Abstracts of the 7th Annual Conference of the Veterinary Cancer Society, Madison, Wis., Oct. 1987, pp 39–40.
164. Riser WH, et al: Bone infarctions associated with malignant bone tumors in dogs. *J Am Vet Med Assoc 160*:411, 1972.
165. Roberts RE: Osteomyelitis associated with disseminated blastomycosis in nine dogs. *Vet Radiol 20*:124, 1979.
166. Ruiter DJ, et al: Aneurysmal bone cysts: A clinicopathological study of 105 cases. *Cancer 39*:2231, 1977.
167. Russell RG, Walker M: Metastatic and invasive tumors of bone in dogs and cats. *Vet Clin North Am Small Anim Pract 13*:163, 1983.
168. Salisbury SK, Lantz GC: Long-term results of partial mandibulectomy for treatment of oral tumors in 30 dogs. *J Am Anim Hosp Assoc 24*:285, 1988.
169. Schajowicz F, McGuire MH: Diagnostic difficulties in skeletal pathology. *Clin Orthop 240*:281, 1989.
170. Schena CJ, et al: Extraskeletal osteosarcoma in two dogs. *J Am Vet Med Assoc 194*:1452, 1989.
171. Schrader SC: Septic arthritis and osteomyelitis of the hip in six mature dogs. *J Am Vet Med Assoc 181*:894, 1982.
172. Schrader SC, Sherding RG: Disorders of the skeletal system. *In* Sherding RG (ed): *The Cat: Diseases and Clinical Management*. Churchill Livingstone, New York, 1989, pp 1264–1292.
173. Schrader SC, et al: Bone cysts in two dogs and a review of similar cystic bone lesions in the dog. *J Am Vet Med Assoc 182*:490, 1983.
174. Selcer BA, McCracken MD: Chondroma rodens in dogs: A report of two case histories and a review of the veterinary literature. *J Vet Orthopedics 2*:7, 1981.
175. Shapiro W, et al: Use of cisplatin for treatment of appendicular osteosarcoma in dogs. *J Am Vet Med Assoc 192*:507, 1988.
176. Shives TC, et al: Chondrosarcoma of the spine. *J Bone Joint Surg [Am] 71*:1158, 1989.
177. Sieber SM, et al: Induction of osteogenic sarcomas and tumors of the hepatobiliary system in nonhuman primates with aflatoxin B1. *Cancer Res 39*:4545, 1979.
178. Sinibaldi K, et al: Tumors associated with metallic implants in animals. *Clin Orthop 118*:257, 1976.
179. Sinibaldi KR, et al: Osteomyelitis and neoplasia associated with use of the Jonas intramedullary splint in small animals. *J Am Vet Med Assoc 181*:885, 1982.
180. Smith MM, et al: Bacterial growth associated with metallic implants in dogs. *J Am Vet Med Assoc 195*:765, 1989.
181. Sordillo PP, et al: Extraosseous osteogenic sarcoma: A review of 48 patients. *Cancer 51*:727, 1983.
182. Spjut HJ, et al: *Atlas of Tumor Pathology: Tumors of Bone and Cartilage*. Armed Forces Institute of Pathology, Washington, DC, 1971, pp 280–292.
183. Stevenson S: Fracture-associated sarcomas. Paper presented at the 10th Annual Canine Advanced Course, Internal Fixation of Fractures and NonUnions. Columbus, OH, March 1987.
184. Stevenson S, et al: Fracture-associated sarcoma in the dog. *J Am Vet Med Assoc 180*:1189, 1982.
185. Stoll BA, Parbhoo S: *Bone Metastasis: Monitoring and Treatment*. Raven Press, New York, 1983, pp 201–406.
186. Straw RC, et al: Multilobular osteochondrosarcoma of the canine skull: 16 cases (1978–1988). *J Am Vet Med Assoc 195*:1764, 1989.
187. Straw RC, et al: Partial or complete hemipelvectomy in the management of sarcomas in six dogs and two cats. Abstracts of the 9th Annual Conference Veterinary Cancer Society, Raleigh, N.C., Oct. 1989, pp 47–48.
188. Straw RC, et al: Amputation and cisplatin for treatment of canine osteosarcoma. *J Vet Intern Med 5*:205, 1991.
189. Suter PF, et al: Myelography in the dog: Diagnosis of tumors of the spinal cord and vertebrae. *J Am Vet Radiol Soc 12*:29, 1971.
190. Thein R, Lotan R: Sensitivity of cultured human osteosarcoma and chondrosarcoma cells to retinoic acid. *Cancer Res 42*:4771, 1982.
191. Thrall DE, et al: Bone sarcoma following orthovoltage radiotherapy in two dogs. *Vet Radiol 24*:169, 1983.
192. Tilmant LT, et al: Chemotherapy of synovial cell sarcoma in a dog. *J Am Vet Med Assoc 188*:530, 1986.
193. Tischler SA, Owens JM: Ulnar fibrosarcoma in a cat. *Mod Vet Pract 67*:39, 1986.
194. Tjalma RA: Canine bone sarcoma: Estimation of relative risk as a function of body size. *J Natl Cancer Inst 36*:1137, 1966.
195. Turnwald GH, et al: Lymphosarcoma with osseous involvement in a dog. *J Am Anim Hosp Assoc 24*:350, 1988.
196. Turrel JM, Pool RR: Primary bone tumors in the cat: A retrospective study of 15 cats and a literature review. *Vet Radiol 23*:152, 1982.
197. Valentin-Opran A, et al: Estrogens and antiestrogens stimulate release of bone resorbing activity by cultured human breast cancer cells. *J Clin Invest 75*:726, 1985.
198. Vasseur PB: Limb salvage in a dog with chondrosarcoma of the tibia. *J Am Vet Med Assoc 187*:620, 1985.
199. Vasseur PB, Stevenson S: Osteosarcoma at the site of a cortical bone allograft in a dog. *Vet Surg 16*:70, 1987.
200. Walker MA, et al: Aneurysmal bone cyst in a cat. *J Am Vet Med Assoc 167*:933, 1975.
201. Waters DJ, et al: Intracranial lesions in dogs with hemangiosarcoma. *J Vet Intern Med 3*:222, 1989.
202. Weiden PL, et al: Canine osteosarcoma: Failure of intravenous or intralesional BCG as adjuvant immunotherapy. *Cancer Immunol Immunother 11*:69, 1981.
203. Weir EC, et al: Adenylate cyclase-stimulating, bone resorbing and B TGF-like activities in canine apocrine cell adenocarcinoma of the anal sac. *Calcif Tissue Int 43*:359, 1988.
204. Weir EC, et al: Humoral hypercalcemia of malignancy in canine lymphosarcoma. *Endocrinology 122*:602, 1988.
205. Weiss L, et al: Organ vascularity and metastatic frequency. *Am J Pathol 101*:101, 1980.
206. Withrow SJ: Limb-sparing for canine osteosarcoma: Current status and future prospects. Paper presented at the 9th Annual Conference of the Veterinary Cancer Society, Raleigh, NC, October 1989.
207. Withrow SJ, Holmberg DL: Mandibulectomy in the treatment of oral cancer. *J Am Anim Hosp Assoc 19*:273, 1983.
208. Withrow SJ, et al: Pulmonary metastectomy for canine osteosarcoma. Abstracts of the 8th Annual Conference of the Veterinary Cancer Society, Estes Park, CO, Oct. 1988, p 2.
209. Wolff RK, et al: Comparison of bone scans and radiography for detecting bone neoplasms in dogs exposed to 238 PuO2. *Am J Vet Res 41*:1804, 1980.
210. Wolke RE, Nielsen SW: Site incidence of canine osteosarcoma. *J Small Anim Pract 7*:489, 1966.
211. Woog J, et al: Osteosarcoma in a phthisical feline eye. *Vet Pathol 20*:209, 1983.
212. Wright JA: The pathological features associated with spinal tumours in 29 dogs. *J Comp Pathol 95*:549, 1985.
213. Wright JA, et al: The clinical and radiological features associated with spinal tumours in thirty dogs. *J Small Anim Pract 20*:461, 1979.
214. Wykes PM, et al: Closed biopsy for diagnosis of long bone tumors: Accuracy and results. *J Am Anim Hosp Assoc 21*:489, 1985.
215. Zaki FA, et al: Calcifying aponeurotic fibroma in a dog. *J Am Vet Med Assoc 166*:384, 1975.

CHAPTER

162

Respiratory System

Theresa W. Fossum and Kenita S. Rogers

Primary tumors of the respiratory system are rare in dogs and cats, especially compared with humans, in whom lung cancer has become the leading cause of cancer death in men and is fast becoming the leading cause in women. With improved medical care, animals are living longer and owners are more frequently seeking veterinary care for their geriatric pets. Clinicians thus are increasingly called on to both recognize and treat neoplasia in the pet population.

NEOPLASMS OF THE NASAL AND PARANASAL SINUSES

Epidemiology and Pathology

Neoplasms of the nasal cavity and paranasal sinuses are rare in most domestic species. These tumors apparently occur almost twice as frequently in dogs as in cats, with reported prevalences varying from 0.3 to 2.4 per cent of canine tumors surveyed.[16, 59, 113] Prevalence of sinonasal tumors in one survey was 81:100,000 cases[59]; in a more recent study, 120 cases were identified in 15,644 necropsies.[82]

Intranasal tumors generally occur in older animals, with a median reported age of 10 years in dogs and 12 years in cats.[58, 113] Mean age varies according to histological diagnosis; the mean age of dogs with chondrosarcomas is less than that of dogs with other tumor types (7 years versus 9 years).[82] In dogs 1 to 4 years of age, chondrosarcomas are more commonly diagnosed than all other tumor types.[82] Soft-tissue tumors involving the nasal cavity have been reported in dogs as young as 1 year.[82]

Male dogs and cats have a higher incidence of sinonasal neoplasms than females, irrespective of histological diagnosis.[59, 82] A similar trend has been reported in human beings, possibly related to occupational exposure to carcinogens and hormonal influences.[27, 96] Castration before administration of a carcinogen that affects primarily the nasal and paranasal cavities, thyroid, liver, urinary tract, and prostate of rats prevents induction of nasal tumors, suggesting androgenic dependency of these neoplasms.[85] Genetic influences and environmental factors probably also have a role in humans; however, no significant differences have been found in the incidence of sinonasal neoplasia between dogs from urban areas and those from rural settings.[87] In several studies, mixed-breed dogs have been well represented, leading one investigator to suggest that environmental factors might be more important than genetic factors in the epidemiology of these tumors.[58]

Breeds reported to be at increased risk for sinonasal tumors include the Airedale terrier, basset hound, Old English sheepdog, Scottish terrier, collie, Shetland sheepdog, and German shorthair pointer.[58] Dolichocephalic breeds may have a higher incidence of nasal tumors than brachycephalic dogs, but dolichocephalic and mesencephalic breeds appear to be equally affected.[9]

Sinonasal tumors may be classified histologically as epithelial, nonepithelial, or miscellaneous (Table 162–1).[82] Neoplasms of epithelial origin are the most common, with adenocarcinomas being the single most frequent histological diagnosis in dogs. In cats, some investigations have reported epithelial tumors to be the most common[16, 59]; others have found nonepithelial tumors, particularly those of lymphoreticular origin, to be most prevalent.[102] Nonepithelial tumors of skeletal origin (i.e., chondrosarcoma and osteosarcoma) account for approximately one-fifth of the canine tumors. In humans, carcinomas are more common than adenocarcinomas, and soft-tissue sarcomas, particularly lymphosarcoma, are more common than tumors of skeletal origin.[82]

The metastatic rate of nasal tumors is low,[102, 113] with metastasis occurring late in the natural course. In one survey, 49 of 120 dogs that had sinonasal tumors and underwent necropsy had metastasis.[82] The most common site of metastasis was the brain (28.3 per cent), followed in decreasing order of frequency by the lymph nodes,

TABLE 162–1. HISTOLOGICAL CLASSIFICATION OF CANINE SINONASAL NEOPLASMS

	Number of Neoplasms	% of Total Neoplasms
Epithelial		
Squamous cell carcinoma		
Nonkeratinizing	54	18.9
Keratinizing	27	9.5
Adenocarcinoma	90	31.6
Nonepithelial		
Skeletal		
Chondrosarcoma	34	11.9
Osteosarcoma	17	6.0
Soft tissue		
Lymphosarcoma	14	4.9
Fibrosarcoma	10	3.5
Hemangiosarcoma	7	2.5
Muscular origin	6	2.0
Fibrous histiocytoma	5	1.8
Malignant nerve sheath	3	1.0
Miscellaneous		
Adenocarcinoid	7	2.5
Esthesioneuroblastoma	5	1.8
Carcinoid	4	1.4
Melanoma	2	0.7
Total	285	100

From Patnaik AK: Canine sinonasal neoplasms: Clinicopathological study of 285 cases. *J Am Anim Hosp Assoc 25*:103, 1989.

lungs, and liver.[82] The rate of metastasis varied with different histological types. Esthesioneuroblastomas had the highest rate (100 per cent), followed by neuroendocrine tumors (80 per cent); both usually metastasized to the brain. Approximately half of the epithelial tumors had evidence of metastasis, usually to the regional lymph nodes and lungs.[82] None of the dogs with keratinizing squamous cell carcinomas had metastasis to the lungs, but 9 per cent had regional lymph node metastasis. In accordance with previous reports, skeletal tumors of this region had a low incidence of metastasis, with the lungs being the most common site.[82] In one study of six cats with nasal tumors, none had evidence of metastasis at the onset of treatment, and prolonged survival (more than 1 year) in those with lymphoreticular tumors following radiotherapy suggested that metastasis was very slow or did not occur.[102]

Clinical Presentation

Duration of clinical signs varies, but most animals have clinical signs for more than 1 month before definitive diagnosis and many have signs for longer than 6 months.[59, 102, 113] Initial clinical signs are often intermittent, but they tend to become more persistent as the tumor develops. Nasal tumors often respond to conservative therapy, such as antibiotics, leading to delayed definitive diagnosis.

Clinical signs in dogs with tumors involving the nasal cavity include epistaxis, swelling of the facial region (including exophthalmos), nasal discharge, sneezing or snuffling, dyspnea, ocular discharge, bleeding from the oral cavity, and seizures (Fig. 162–1).[58, 113] Epistaxis or nasal discharge is usually unilateral, although bilateral discharge may occasionally be noted depending on the location and extent of the tumor. In bacterial and fungal infections, by comparison, the nasal discharge is usually bilateral and purulent. Foreign bodies and bleeding diatheses may also cause unilateral nasal discharge. Sneezing may be paroxysmal in dogs with nasal tumors and may be violent enough to lead to epistaxis. Clinical signs in cats are similar, with most evaluated for sneezing and nasal discharge and occasionally epistaxis.[102]

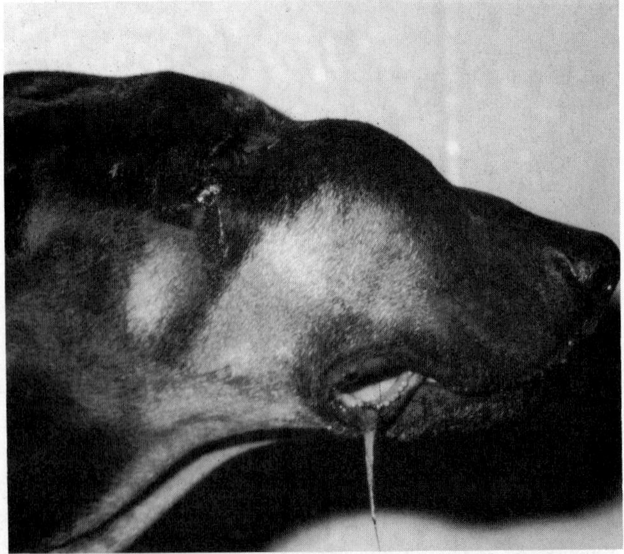

FIGURE 162–1. Marked nasal deformity in an 8-year-old Doberman pinscher with a nasal tumor histologically diagnosed as an osteosarcoma.

Neurological signs may be the predominant clinical finding in dogs and cats with nasal tumors. In one study of five dogs and two cats with nasal tumors, abnormalities noted included seizures, behavior changes, obtundation, paresis, ataxia, circling, visual deficits, and proprioceptive deficits.[98] These animals had no clinical signs related to the respiratory tract and no evidence of metastasis. Neurological signs were related to erosion of the cribriform plate by the tumor and invasion and compression of the olfactory and frontal regions of the brain.

Clinical signs may vary according to histological type. Seizures are more common in dogs with carcinoids and esthesioneuroblastomas than with tumors of epithelial origin, presumably because of differences in metastatic patterns. Dyspnea may be more common with epithelial neoplasms, and sneezing has been reported to occur most commonly in dogs with chondrosarcomas.[82]

Diagnostic Evaluation

Laboratory examination of dogs and cats with nasal tumors should be performed to assess anesthetic risk in geriatric patients and to rule out underlying disease secondary to coagulopathies, but abnormalities are uncommon. If epistaxis has been severe or chronic, anemia may be noted. Rarely is the white blood cell count abnormal even in the presence of a secondary bacterial infection. Affected animals are carefully evaluated for clotting abnormalities by assessing platelet numbers, bleeding from venipuncture sites, or the presence of ecchymoses, petechiae, melena, hematuria, or retinal hemorrhages. If appropriate tests are available, coagulation is assessed by activated clotting time, prothrombin time, or partial thromboplastin time. Diseases or syndromes such as ehrlichiosis, immune-mediated thrombocytopenia, multiple myeloma, systemic hypertension, polycythemia vera, and hyperviscosity syndrome may cause epistaxis and must be ruled out.[9] Cats are evaluated for feline leukemia virus and feline immunodeficiency virus infections.

Before general anesthesia in a patient suspected of having a nasal tumor, thoracic radiography and aspiration of regional lymph nodes are performed and evaluated for the presence of metastasis. Radiographs of the skull usually require general anesthesia to obtain satisfactory positioning. High-quality nasal radiographs help define the extent and location of disease and are recommended before performing rhinoscopy, nasal flushes, or surgical biopsies. Recumbent lateral, dorsoventral, open-mouth ventrodorsal, and frontal sinus views are generally performed. Oblique views may occasionally be necessary to outline lesions that are masked by bony structures or superimposed over them. Of these various views, the open-mouth ventrodorsal view consistently provides the most information by allowing examination of the entire turbinate region and reducing superimposition of the mandibles.[52]

Radiographs are evaluated for the presence of increased soft-tissue density of the nasal cavity or frontal sinuses, bone lysis, destruction of the normal turbinate pattern, new bone formation, and the presence of foreign bodies (Figs. 162–2 and 162–3).[90] Early nasal tumors are often difficult to recognize radiographically because at this stage they resemble inflammatory changes; in fact, it is important to remember that neoplastic and inflammatory lesions cannot be accurately differentiated on the basis of radiographic appearance.[52] Lesions resulting in considerable bone destruction are usually neoplastic, although severe fungal or bacterial infections may also cause bone lysis. Increased soft-tissue density may be seen in both neoplastic and inflammatory diseases.[90] Extension into the frontal sinus or the contralateral nasal cavity and destruction of the hard palate suggest an aggressive process. An increased soft-tissue density in the frontal sinus, without bony erosion, should not be interpreted as evidence of neoplastic extension into the frontal sinus because obstruction of outflow secondary to a nasal tumor often results in accumulation of fluid in this cavity (Fig. 162–4). Destruction of the cribriform plate may signal extension into the brain and a poor prognosis.

Computed tomography (CT) may be helpful in defining the extent of disease in animals with nasal tumors, both for prognosis and for planning of radiation therapy. It may also be helpful in patients with minimal or no neurological signs but with evidence of destruction of the rostral portion of the calvarium radiographically. Both plain and contrast-enhanced CT studies may be useful. In one report, CT provided specific evidence of invasion of tumor into the frontal and olfactory lobes, compression of the right lateral ventricle, dilation of the

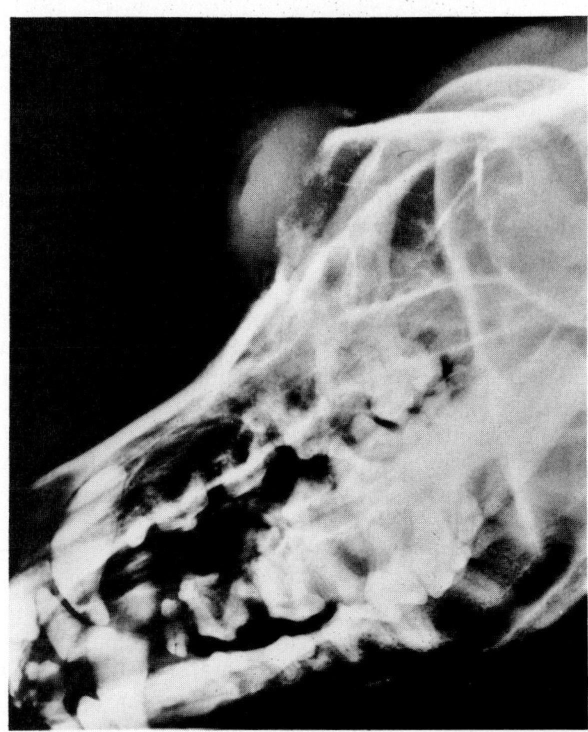

FIGURE 162–3. Lateral skull radiograph of a 5-year-old male collie presented for evaluation of an aggressive sinonasal neoplasm. Note the lysis of the frontal bone and the associated soft-tissue swelling. The tumor was histologically diagnosed as a squamous cell carcinoma.

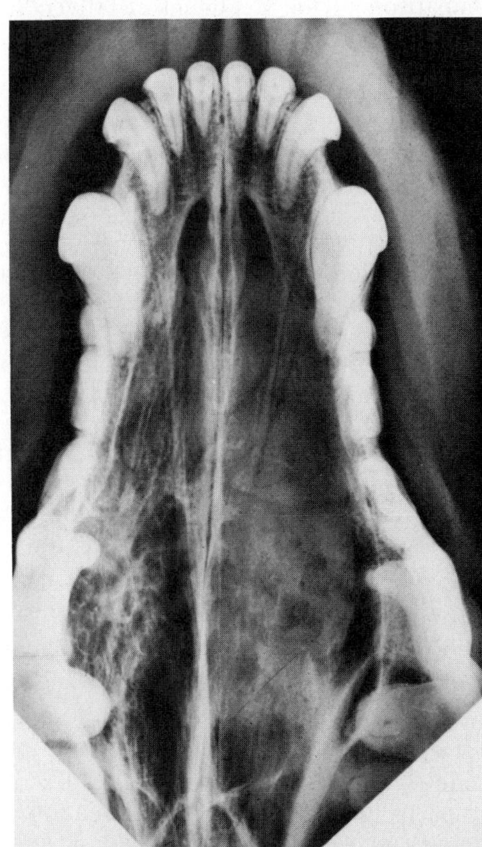

FIGURE 162–2. Ventrodorsal open-mouth radiograph of a 6-year-old mixed-breed dog presented for evaluation of stertorous respiration and a right-sided nasal discharge. Note the increased soft-tissue density in the right nasal cavity with destruction of nasal turbinates. The tumor was diagnosed histologically as a chondrosarcoma.

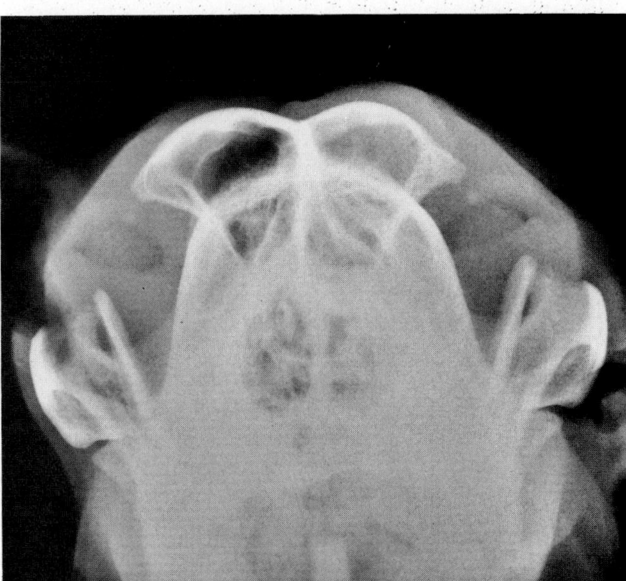

FIGURE 162–4. Frontal sinus view of a 6-year-old mixed-breed dog presented for evaluation of a nasal fibrosarcoma. Note the opacity in the left frontal sinus caused by fluid accumulation. The neoplasm did not invade the frontal sinus.

left lateral ventricle, and deviation of the falx cerebri.[93] Contrast-enhanced CT showed disruption of the blood-brain barrier in the same patient, suggesting invasion of the mass into the right olfactory lobe.

Visual examination of the palate and nasal area is performed under general anesthesia. Rhinoscopy, using dental mirrors or fiber-optic endoscopes to evaluate the caudal nasopharynx and otoscopic cones or endoscopes to evaluate the ventral nasal meatus, may be performed.[90] Unfortunately, the presence of nasal discharge and blood makes meticulous examination of the nasal cavity difficult. Using a small arthroscope that allows fluid to be flushed simultaneously into the nose facilitates inspection.

Definitive diagnosis is made by cytological or histopathological evaluation of specimens obtained by nasal flushing techniques or by biopsy. Both of these procedures require that the animal be anesthetized with an endotracheal tube inserted. The cuff of the endotracheal tube should be inflated to prevent aspiration of blood or other materials during the procedure.

Although a number of techniques have been described to flush the nasal cavity, we prefer to use a rigid polypropylene male urinary catheter or the outer protective shield of a Sovereign catheter* that has been attached to a plastic syringe connecter (with the metal stylet removed). The end of the catheter is cut off at a sharp angle. To prevent inadvertent entry into the calvarium in patients with lysis of the cribriform plate, the distance from the medial canthus of the eye to the external nares is measured and the catheter marked to correspond to this length. Gauze sponges are placed above the soft palate and below the external nares to collect fluid and tissues dislodged during flushing. A 35-ml syringe is attached to the catheter, and 15 to 30 ml of saline flushed into the nasal cavity. The gauze sponges are evaluated for the presence of tissue and debris. Cytological examination of the tissues is performed, and separate samples saved for microbiological examination, including fungal and bacterial cultures. If sufficient quantities are obtained, samples are also submitted for histopathological examination. Neoplasia was identified in 50 per cent of all tumor cases in one study using similar techniques.[57] Hemorrhage may occur after this procedure but is generally mild and of short duration.

If sufficient quantities of tissue are not obtained for diagnostic purposes, the same catheter, attached to a 12-ml syringe, can be used to obtain a transnostril core biopsy sample of the involved area. The location of the lesion is discerned from the radiographs, and the catheter is advanced through the tumor several times while negative pressure is applied to the syringe. On withdrawal of the catheter from the nares, the barrel of the syringe is removed and a small amount of air added to the syringe. This air is then used to propel the tissue sample forcefully from the syringe hub onto a microscope slide or into a formalin-filled container. Repeated sampling at various angles may be necessary to obtain sufficient tissue. The use of a biopsy needle* has also been described; however; tube aspiration was preferable to needle biopsies, particularly with mucoid tumors.[115] These techniques are more helpful with epithelial tumors than connective tissue tumors. Nasal biopsies are more likely than nasal flushes to yield samples that lead to a definitive diagnosis.

When the previously described techniques do not result in a diagnosis, surgical exploration and biopsy may be necessary. Generally, in such cases the diagnostic procedure is combined with the therapeutic procedure (rhinotomy and debulking). Cytological study or frozen section examination of tissues is helpful in such cases.

*Sovereign Indwelling Catheter Feline Needle Gauge; Monoject, Division of Sherwood Medical, St. Louis, MO.

*Tru-Cut Disposable Biopsy Needle, Travenol Laboratories Inc., Morton Grove, IL.

Therapy

Most therapeutic modalities for nasal tumors in dogs are directed at control of local disease. Because of the location of tumor and the advanced stage at which it is typically diagnosed, palliation measures are often unsuccessful and fraught with complications. A number of treatment options have been reported, including surgical debulking, surgical debulking combined with radiation therapy, radiation therapy alone, chemotherapy, immunotherapy, and cryosurgery. However, because of inconsistent surgical techniques, inadequate or deficient staging of the tumors, and inconsistent reporting methods, comparison of the treatment effectiveness within or between studies is difficult.

Rhinotomy

Surgery as the sole treatment of dogs with nasal tumors has not resulted in prolonged survival times. Median survival times in three separate studies were 3, 4, and 5 months.[57, 59, 75] The poor response to surgery in dogs with nasal tumors is due to the advanced nature of most tumors at the time of diagnosis, a propensity for these tumors to invade bones that are inaccessible or that cannot be surgically removed, and lack of appreciable encapsulation, all of which make it impossible in most cases to remove the tumor. Surgery may palliate clinical signs in some dogs by removing tissues that are obstructing respiration and by decreasing epistaxis. Permanent tracheostomy may benefit some dogs that have severe respiratory difficulties and in which other treatment options are not feasible.

Radiation Therapy

Radiotherapy appears to be the most effective treatment for nasal tumors.[1, 9, 52, 57, 75, 105] Most studies have investigated orthovoltage (125 to 400 KeV) irradiation,[1, 57, 59, 75] although occasional reports have described the use of megavoltage (>1 KeV) x-irradiation.[1, 88] The optimum dosage and method of delivery have not been determined. The dosage delivered to the tumor in most reports has approximated 4,000 rad in ten fractions given on alternate days,[9, 57, 102] although lower total doses, particularly after surgical debulking when tumor burden is low and the remaining cells are well oxygenated, should be investigated.[105] Adams compared megavoltage irradiation (cobalt or linear accelerator) with softer deep radiation (cesium or orthovoltage) and found that the dogs with the longest median survival (15.2 months) were those that had adenocarcinomas and were treated with cytoreductive surgery and softer deep radiation.[1] Radiotherapy of nasal tumors in cats reportedly results in as good an outcome or better than in dogs with similar disease. In one study of six cats with nasal tumors (three lymphoreticular origin, one chondrosarcoma, one undifferentiated carcinoma, and one adenocarcinoma), the median survival time from initiation of radiotherapy was 19 months.[102]

Whether radiation therapy should be combined with surgical debulking is controversial.[91, 105] One reason for doing so is to improve a dog's clinical status before radiation therapy. One investigator found that after surgery, dyspnea due to nasal cavity obstruction, nasal discharge, and epistaxis were decreased considerably.[105] Second, uniform penetration of large tumor masses with orthovoltage radiation is difficult. Finally, if debulking is not performed before surgery, clinical signs of obstruction may increase as the tumor mass dies. One study found that survival times of dogs that were treated with softer radiation alone (without surgery) were shorter than those that were treated with the two modalities combined.[1] However, cytoreductive surgery did not improve survival times of dogs that were treated with megavoltage irradiation.[1]

Complications associated with megavoltage irradiation of the nasal and paranasal cavities are frequent in dogs. In one study, 17 of 29 (58.6 per cent) dogs treated with this form of radiotherapy developed severe ocular complications consisting of keratitis, conjunctivitis, cataracts, and keratoconjunctivitis sicca.[88] Additional potential complications include alopecia, changes in skin texture, and bone necrosis.

Other Therapeutic Modalities

Cryosurgery as the principal therapy has not appreciably prolonged the survival times of dogs with nasal tumors.[112] A complication associated with this form of therapy is necrosis of the hard palate secondary to excessive freezing and destruction of the palatine blood supply. Local recurrence is common, particularly near the cribriform plate or caudal nasal area around the orbit.[112]

Immunotherapy using two adjuvants, MBV (a heat-killed mixture of *Streptococcus pyogenes* and *Serratia marcescens*) and levamisole, was reported in six dogs. Dogs treated with immunotherapy alone lived a median of 3 months, those treated with immunotherapy and surgery lived 7 months, and untreated dogs lived 5 months.[57]

Course of Disease and Prognosis

The prognosis for dogs with nasal tumors is generally poor. In patients not treated and those treated with surgery, chemotherapy, immunotherapy, and cryosurgery, the mean survival time is generally 3 to 5 months.[113] Improvement in this survival period has been accomplished with radiation therapy combined with surgical debulking (discussed earlier), with mean reported survival times of 8 to 25 months. The prognosis for carcinomas is better than for sarcomas, and adenocarcinomas appear to have the best overall prognosis.[113] It is unlikely that therapy will result in cure in most dogs, and more successful local control may lead to increased detection of metastasis.[113] Conversely, the prognosis for cats with lymphoid neoplasia of the nasal cavity is favorable. In one study of six cats with intranasal neoplasia, the clinical improvement appeared to be complete, rapid, and long lasting, particularly in those with lymphoreticular neoplasms.[102]

One unusual neoplasm associated with a much more favorable long-term prognosis than those previously mentioned is intranasal transmissible venereal tumor. Clinical signs associated with intranasal transmissible venereal tumor are similar to those of other tumors of this location (epistaxis, sneezing), and the tumor may appear as a space-occupying mass within the nasal cavity. Bone lysis may occasionally be noted. If the tumor is localized, radiation therapy may be curative. Chemotherapy with vincristine is also effective in treating localized or metastatic transmissible venereal tumor.

NEOPLASMS OF THE LARYNX AND TRACHEA

Epidemiology and Pathology

Tumors of the larynx and trachea are extremely rare in dogs and cats, and most reports in these species are individual case reports. In a 10-year retrospective survey of 56,413 surgical pathology accessions and 7,444 necropsy case reports, laryngeal tumors were identified in 13 dogs and 11 cats.[94] In another study of 11,774 malignancies, only 11 canine and 2 feline laryngeal tumors were identified.[86] Of 289 hematopoietic tumors in cats, 2 tracheal tumors and no laryngeal tumors were identified.[83] Laryngeal tumors occur much more frequently in humans, accounting for 2 per cent of all malignancies, and development of these tumors has been associated with smoking and alcohol consumption.[111, 113] Tracheal tumors, independent of lung tumors, are also exceedingly rare in human beings.

Laryngeal tumors generally occur in older animals, with most affected dogs being between the ages of 7 and 12 years and cats between 8 and 17 years.[94] As with nasal tumors, a male predilection has been reported in dogs, cats, and humans.[94, 111] No breed predilection has been determined in either species.[94] Tracheal tumors, on the other hand, often occur in adolescent dogs.[30, 36, 43]

Many different tumor types affect the canine larynx, including adenocarcinoma, myxochondroma, fibrosarcoma, fibropapilloma, chondroma, chondrosarcoma, osteosarcoma, melanoma, rhabdomyoma, rhabdomyosarcoma, mast cell tumor, oncocytoma, lipoma, squamous cell carcinoma, and undifferentiated carcinoma.* In cats, lymphosarcoma is most commonly identified; squa-

*See references 8, 15, 19, 33, 47, 62, 65, 80, 94, and 111.

mous cell carcinoma and adenocarcinoma have also been reported.[94, 100, 107] More than 95 per cent of laryngeal tumors in humans are squamous cell carcinomas. These tumors occur secondary to chronic irritation, which initially results in dysplastic changes of the laryngeal mucosa with chronic inflammation, squamous metaplasia, and polypoid proliferation.[56, 111, 113] Rhabdomyomas and oncocytomas are laryngeal tumors that appear histologically similar with light microscopy; electron microscopy and immunocytochemistry are necessary to discern the striated muscle origin of the former tumor and thus differentiate it from the latter (which derives its name from the cell of origin, the oncocyte).[65] Oncocytes are epithelial cells that are found in small quantities in a number of organs including the larynx, thyroid, pituitary, and trachea. These tumors occur in young dogs[65, 80] and warrant special consideration because long-term survival without evidence of metastasis, following surgical resection, has been reported.[15, 65] Tracheal osteochondromas may occur in dogs younger than 1 year.[30, 36, 43, 114] These masses probably reflect a malfunction of osteogenesis and are benign.[113] Other tracheal tumor types that have been found in dogs include chondrosarcoma, osteosarcoma, mast cell tumor, squamous cell carcinoma, and leiomyoma.[3, 13, 19, 22, 41] In cats, squamous cell carcinoma, adenocarcinoma, and lymphosarcoma have been reported.[8, 23, 95, 108]

Filaroides osleri (Oslerus osleri) is a nematode that forms nodules in the trachea and mainstem bronchi of dogs. These lesions must be differentiated from neoplastic lesions.[50] Definitive diagnosis of this parasite may be difficult because larva are shed only intermittently in the feces. The diagnosis is based on identifying eggs, larvae, or adult worms in bronchoscopically obtained biopsy specimens or by identifying the larvae in feces. Treatment consisting of anthelmintic therapy and surgical resection has met with varying degrees of success.[26]

Reports of the incidence of metastasis of laryngeal and tracheal tumors in dogs and cats are not available; in humans, 60 per cent of the patients with carcinoma present with local disease only, 30 per cent have regional node metastasis, and 10 per cent have local metastasis.[113]

Clinical Presentation and Physical Examination Findings

As with nasal tumors, laryngeal and tracheal tumors are often well advanced at diagnosis. In humans, these tumors are usually diagnosed at an earlier stage, when subtle changes in voice are noticed. Clinical signs associated with laryngeal tumors in dogs and cats include dyspnea, voice change, coughing, loud tracheal sounds, nasal discharge, neck swelling, cyanosis, stertorous respiration while sleeping, choking episodes, tachypnea, and exercise intolerance. The most common signs in dogs are a hoarse bark or loss of voice, with subsequent onset of exertional dyspnea and cough.[111] Patients with tracheal tumor generally have respiratory distress, coughing, and exercise intolerance.[113]

Laryngeal and tracheal tumors are usually not palpable externally,[113] and oral pain with laryngeal tumors may make examination difficult. With laryngeal tumors, radiography usually reveals a reduction in diameter of the laryngeal air space by an intraluminal mass; however, there may be no correlation between the severity of the respiratory distress and the obstruction. Radiographic involvement of tissues outside the immediate vicinity of the larynx is unusual.[111] Radiography, combined with physical examination, should differentiate laryngeal tumors from other causes of upper respiratory dyspnea including collapsing larynx, elongated soft palate, laryngeal paralysis, and tracheal collapse. Under general anesthesia, these tumors can be sampled by biopsy.

Tracheal tumors usually appear radiographically as a mass that is narrowing or obstructing the tracheal lumen. Osteochondromas are often radiodense and easily identified on plain radiographs (Fig. 162–5). Contrast esophagograms or esophagoscopy may occasionally be indicated to rule out esophageal involvement. Biopsy of tracheal tumors is more difficult than that of laryngeal tumors but can usually be performed using either a fiberoptic endoscope or a rigid bronchoscope. Size, consistency, and nature of attachment of the tumor to the tracheal wall are noted. Histopathological identification of tumor type before therapy helps determine the extent of surgical resection indicated.

Therapy

Because of the advanced stage of most laryngeal tumors at diagnosis, therapy is difficult; however, oncocytomas and rhabdomyomas warrant a favorable prognosis after partial laryngectomy.[15, 65] Successful total laryngectomy and permanent tracheoscopy have also been reported in a dog with an extensive laryngeal mast cell tumor,[29] and laryngotomy and surgical resection of

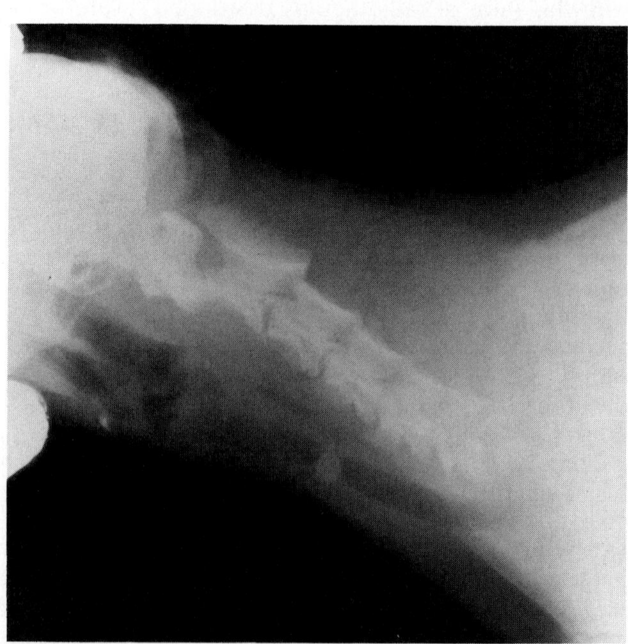

FIGURE 162–5. Lateral cervical radiograph of a 6-month-old Doberman puppy presented for evaluation of dyspnea and exercise intolerance. Note the radiopaque density in the trachea. The tumor was diagnosed histologically as an osteochondroma.

an undifferentiated carcinoma resulted in resolution of clinical signs in an 11-year-old dog.[15] This dog was free of respiratory signs 10 months after surgery. Radiation therapy may be beneficial in treating laryngeal lymphosarcoma.[113] Although the primary laryngeal tumor in many human patients can be treated successfully, a high percentage of these patients (20 per cent) develop secondary tumors.

Although prognosis is related to histological type, the prognosis for many tracheal tumors is excellent,* primarily because the trachea can be readily resected and anastomosed. One study has demonstrated that in adult dogs, 12 per cent of the total tracheal length (approximately four rings) may be resected and anastomosed without generating undue tension at the anastomosis.[46, 104] In puppies, as much as 25 per cent of the total trachea length may be removed.[46] Successful treatment of tracheal osteochondromas and leiomyoma has been reported in dogs without resection of tracheal rings[13, 106]; however, with most tracheal tumors, resection and anastomosis of the affected rings are indicated (Figs. 162–6 and 162–7).[3, 22, 41, 114] Successful treatment of tracheal tumors in cats with tracheal resection and anastomosis has also been reported.[7, 23, 95]

PRIMARY PULMONARY NEOPLASIA

Epidemiology and Pathology

The development of spontaneous primary pulmonary neoplasia is uncommon in dogs and cats. The average incidence has been estimated to be 1.24 per cent for dogs and 0.38 per cent for cats.[70] This low incidence contrasts with the occurrence of lung tumors in humans, in whom this form of neoplasia is the leading cause of cancer death in men 35 years of age and older and the second leading cause of cancer death in women ages 35 to 74 years. If current trends continue, lung cancer will overtake breast cancer as the leading cause of cancer death in women in the near future.[67] Although the incidence of primary lung cancer is low in dogs and cats, knowledge of its existence is important for two reasons. First, a rational basis for the diagnosis and treatment of individual cases in companion animals must be founded on clinical manifestations, biological behavior, and response to therapy. Second, dogs have made valuable contributions as experimental models for the development of pulmonary neoplasia in the presence of carcinogens.[5, 25, 37]

*See references 3, 22, 23, 41, 95, 106, and 114.

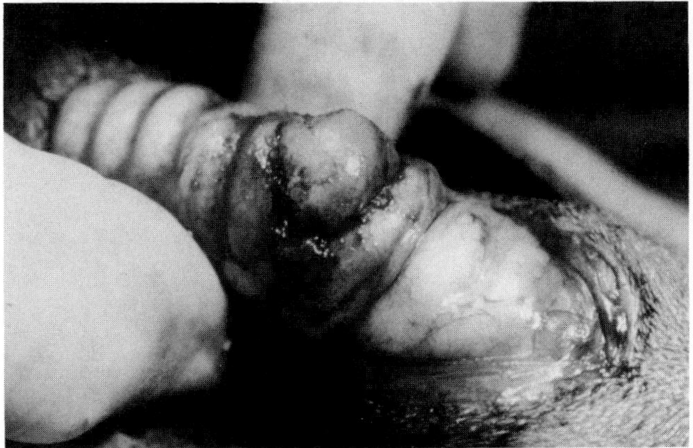

FIGURE 162–6. Intraoperative photograph showing appearance of the tumor in Figure 162–5 after incision of the annular ligament. (Photograph courtesy of H. Phil Hobson, Texas A&M University)

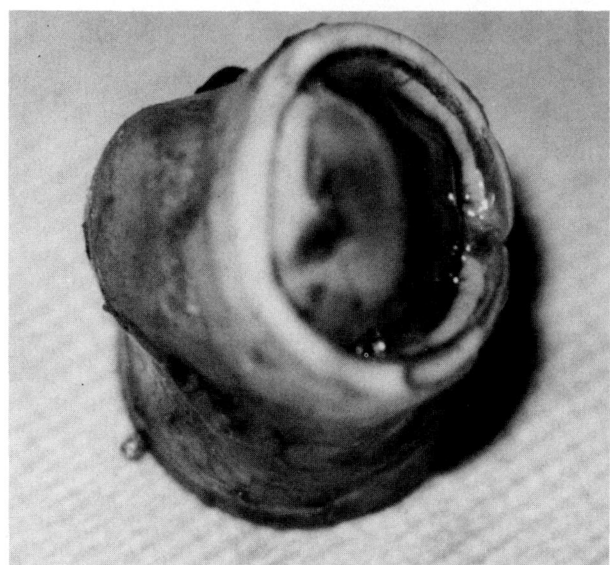

FIGURE 162–7. Section of the trachea incorporating the tumor in Figure 162–6 after tracheal resection and anastomosis. (Photograph courtesy of H. Phil Hobson, Texas A&M University)

The average age of dogs with primary lung tumors is 10 to 11 years; these tumors seldom occur in animals younger than 7 years. Anaplastic carcinomas occur at a slightly younger age (8 to 9 years) than adenocarcinomas. Cats are often slightly older when primary lung tumors are diagnosed (12 years). There is no sex or breed predilection, although boxers were over-represented in two studies.[18, 87]

The classification of primary lung tumors is usually based on the prevailing histological pattern.[66, 70, 71] This method is preferred because the advanced nature of these tumors often precludes more specific anatomical localization of tumor origin. Adenocarcinomas are the most common histological type found in dogs and cats, with squamous cell carcinoma and anaplastic carcinomas being identified more rarely.[18, 24, 71]

Squamous cell carcinomas are more commonly diagnosed than adenocarcinomas in humans, although the pattern is changing as more women develop lung cancer.[67] Adenocarcinoma and bronchoalveolar carcinomas are usually found peripherally, in the subpleural space, and most arise from terminal bronchi, bronchioles, or alveoli. Anaplastic carcinomas are found in any location in the lungs and often develop from alveoli or terminal bronchioles. Squamous cell carcinomas usually arise from larger bronchi and are most commonly found in the hilar region of the lung. Pulmonary carcinomas tend to be expansive or infiltrative, with poorly defined margins that may blend in with surrounding fibrous stroma.[70]

The diaphragmatic lobes are most frequently involved, with the right lung lobes more often affected than the left. Cavitation may be a feature due to tumor necrosis. Although it is uncommon for pulmonary carcinomas to adhere to the thoracic wall, direct extension of the tumor to surrounding structures may occur, with invasion of the hilar region and mediastinum.

Primary pulmonary tumors of connective tissue origin are rare. Those reported include osteosarcoma, fibrosarcoma, and hemangiosarcoma.[70, 101] Even more rare are benign pulmonary tumors,[70] including papillary adenoma, bronchial adenoma, fibroma, myxochondroma, and plasmacytoma. Other neoplastic diseases that may affect the lungs as a primary event are lymphomatoid granulomatosis, carcinoids, and malignant histiocytosis.[70, 81, 89, 113] Most lung tumors are advanced in their course at the time of diagnosis in animals; consequently, determination of the precise origin is difficult. Further confounding the recognition of histological tumor type is the frequent presence of more than one tissue type within a single tumor.

Although the risk factors for the development of pulmonary neoplasia have been largely defined in humans, the controversy about the role of environment and pollutants in lung cancer in dogs and cats is unsettled. Studies on the role of living in rural and urban environments have produced conflicting results,[77, 87] and evidence regarding natural risk factors is inconclusive. Exogenous factors associated with lung cancer in experimental animals and humans include ionizing radiation and atmospheric pollutants such as nickel carbonyl, asbestos, benzopyrene, and aromatic amines.[70]

Primary lung tumors metastasize early and aggressively. A necropsy study showed that 100 per cent of squamous cell carcinomas and 90 per cent of anaplastic carcinomas had metastasized by the time of primary lesion detection, whereas approximately 50 per cent of adenocarcinomas had metastasized.[18] One of the most common sites of metastasis is the lungs themselves, where spread can occur via lymphatics, pulmonary blood vessels, or airway transmigration. In addition, direct invasion into the mediastinum, pleura, pericardium, and diaphragm may occur. Regional lymph nodes are common metastatic sites, and their involvement is an important prognostic factor.[76] Extrathoracic sites in dogs may include bone, kidneys, liver, spleen, heart, pleura, skeletal muscle, and occasionally brain.[68] Feline tumors metastasize most commonly to long bones, vertebrae, and skeletal muscle.[63] Other sites include the lymph nodes, brain, eyes, spleen, diaphragm, and heart. The TNM system is recommended for clinical staging of primary pulmonary tumors.[76, 78]

Clinical Presentation

Pulmonary neoplasia sometimes is an incidental finding when thoracic radiographs are evaluated for an unrelated problem. In one study, approximately 25 per cent of dogs with lung tumors presented with no clinical signs related to the respiratory system.[77] Most lung tumors cause no clinical signs in their early stages[70]; however, the owner may report clinical signs apparent for weeks to months. These clinical signs may be a direct result of the primary tumor or may be a consequence of metastatic lesions or paraneoplastic syndromes.

The presenting signs depend on tumor location, growth rate, structures invaded, cell type, the presence of previous pulmonary disease, attentiveness of the owner, the presence of metastatic disease, and associated paraneoplastic syndromes. The most commonly reported sign is a nonproductive cough. Other signs include hemoptysis, fever, lethargy, exercise intolerance, weight loss, dysphagia, and anorexia. Signs referable to the respiratory tract are noted in only one-third of cats, and coughing is only occasionally encountered in cats.[63]

Respiratory distress may be associated with significant lung replacement with neoplastic tissue or the development of hemothorax, pneumothorax, or malignant pleural effusion. Lameness or swollen legs may be associated with metastasis to bone or skeletal muscles or with the development of hypertrophic osteopathy (Figs. 162–8 and 162–9). Signs related to regional spread and metastasis may include dysphagia, pleural or pericardial effusion, ascites, or cranial vena cava syndrome.[11] Ocular metastasis in a cat led to anisocoria, subretinal hemorrhage, retinal detachment, and optic neuropathy.[39]

Paraneoplastic syndromes are well documented in humans with lung cancer but are rare in animals, with the most commonly associated change being hypertrophic osteopathy. This condition is nonspecific and may be associated with primary or metastatic pulmonary neoplasia, neoplastic conditions involving the kidneys or bladder, and non-neoplastic conditions such as hypertension, bacterial endocarditis, and infection with *Dirofilaria immitis* and *Spirocerca lupi*.[17, 38, 74, 103, 109] Hypertrophic osteopathy usually affects all four limbs and has a characteristic radiographic pattern of periosteal

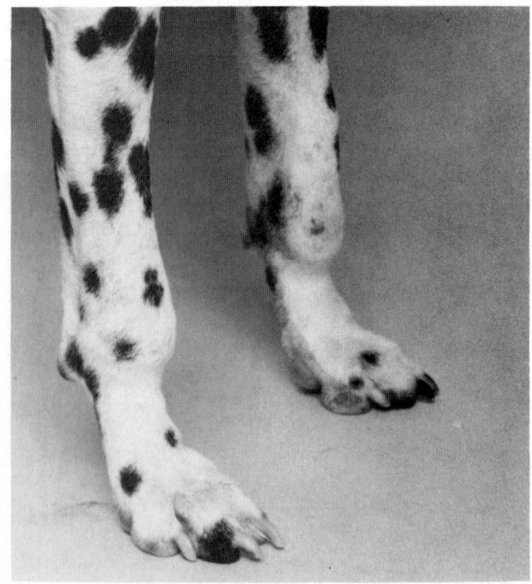

FIGURE 162–8. Marked bilateral limb swelling in a 9-year-old Dalmatian with hypertrophic osteopathy and primary lung neoplasia.

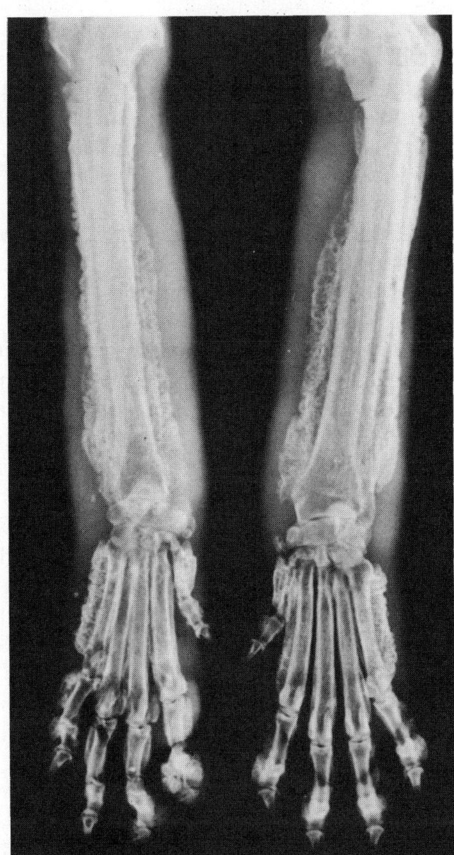

FIGURE 162–9. Anterior-posterior radiograph of forelimbs in an aged German shepherd with primary pulmonary neoplasia. Characteristic radiographic findings in hypertrophic osteopathy include soft-tissue swelling and extensive periosteal proliferation of bones of the extremities.

new bone formation and soft-tissue swelling. Swelling of the limbs or lameness may be noted by the owner. Hypertrophic osteopathy may regress in 2 weeks to 7 months after surgical excision of the primary lung mass. It may also recur with development of further metastases.[17, 77] The cause of hypertrophic osteopathy is unknown, but growth hormone, estrogens, neurogenic factors, and circulatory factors may have a role.[67, 103] Other paraneoplastic syndromes include hypercalcemia, paraplegia and neuromyopathy, and secretion of adrenocorticotropic hormone.[73, 77, 99]

Diagnostic Evaluation

Clinical suspicions may be pursued with several diagnostic procedures after a complete history and physical examination. Surgical biopsy remains the most definitive method of diagnosis, with only 38.6 per cent of cases being definitively diagnosed before surgery or necropsy in one study.[77] Thoracic radiography is a valuable noninvasive diagnostic tool. The most common presentation is a solitary nodular density in a dorsal caudal lung lobe; peripheral lesions are more commonly observed than perihilar disease in animals (Fig. 162–10).[66] Neoplasia is more commonly found in the larger, right lung lobes of dogs but is more evenly distributed between the right and left caudal lobes in cats.[45] Vessels and adjacent bronchi tend to bend around the neoplasm as it expands.[75] Multiple miliary lesions are less commonly seen. The radiographic pattern may be classified as solitary nodular, multiple nodular, or disseminated infiltrative. Occasionally, there are multiple discrete lesions within a single lobe or multiple lobes; these may represent metastatic disease or perhaps multicentric primary neoplasia. No typical radiographic pattern characterizes feline lung neoplasia; the appearance is more variable than in dogs and humans.[45, 63] Pleural effusion is more common in cats but is usually due to concurrent decompensated cardiomyopathy rather than extension of neoplasm into the pleural space.[63]

The views recommended to maximize radiographic resolution of pulmonary nodules include a ventrodorsal and both right and left lateral recumbency. Lung lesions may remain undetected in recumbent lateral radiographs when the affected lung is dependent because of increased opacity of surrounding lung tissue.[84] For accurate interpretation, it is extremely important that patients be properly positioned and the films be of high quality. Despite their diagnostic value, thoracic radiographs are insensitive in detecting primary or metastatic lung tumors. The nodules must be at least 1 cm in diameter to be reliably recognized with conventional radiography. This represents approximately 30 doublings of the tumor cells, implying that the lesion is far advanced in its natural course at initial recognition.

Large mass lesions may appear less well demarcated than smaller nodular lesions owing to compression of adjacent pulmonary parenchyma.[58] Cavitating lesions are usually thick-walled structures with a roughened inner surface surrounded by abnormal lung tissue. They may contain one large or several small central lucencies. Linear shadows that are 2 mm or more in width and

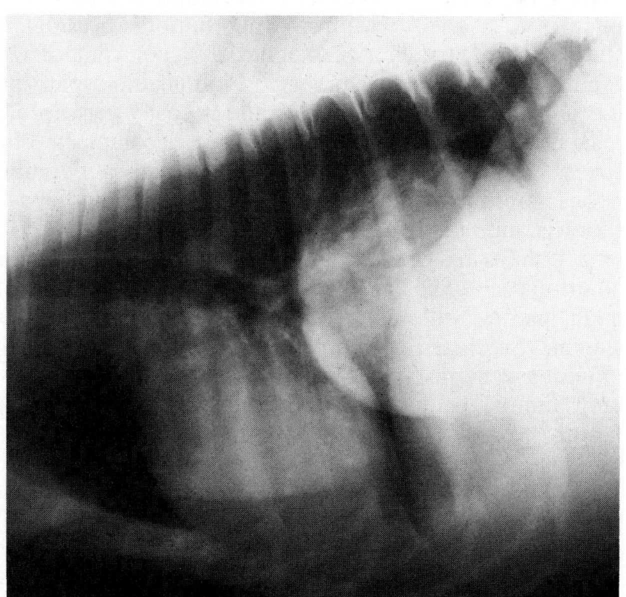

FIGURE 162–10. Lateral thoracic radiograph of an 8-year-old coonhound. A large solitary mass in the left caudal lung lobe was histologically diagnosed as a primary pulmonary adenocarcinoma.

nonbranching may be neoplasm that is spreading via intrapulmonary lymphatics. Intrathoracic calcification of lesions can occur with inflammatory as well as neoplastic masses. Although calcification suggests a benign lesion in humans, this may not be the case in veterinary medicine.[45] Other important factors to note radiographically are intrathoracic lymphadenopathy and pleural effusion, but the absence of enlarged hilar lymph nodes does not rule out metastatic disease. Enlarged intrathoracic lymph nodes or pleural effusion suggests advanced disease and warrants a guarded prognosis. Pleural fluid or atelectasis complicates radiographic detection of a neoplastic mass. The differential diagnosis of nodular pulmonary disease includes granulomatous conditions, metastatic neoplasia, pneumonia, abscesses, and infarcts.

An additional noninvasive technique that can be performed at many referral centers is a pulmonary perfusion scan. Most scans are performed by venous administration of ^{99m}Tc-labeled macroaggregated albumin. This technique is quite sensitive but relatively nonspecific. Perfusion scans allow detection of small (subsegmental) defects that are peripherally located and distributed more or less evenly throughout the lungs.[6, 58] A scan may detect lesions at the diaphragmatic border of the lungs; these are not readily seen on thoracic radiographs owing to superimposition of the hepatic shadow.

Collection of specimens for cytological evaluation and culture and sensitivity testing can be accomplished by several methods, including transtracheal lavage, percutaneous fine-needle aspirates, and bronchoscopy. Collection and evaluation of sputum are helpful in 40 to 80 per cent of cases in humans, but sputum is difficult to collect in animals. The value of transtracheal lavage depends on communication of the neoplastic mass with an airway and ability of the mass to exfoliate. Fine-needle aspiration cytology may be helpful in approximately 50 per cent of cases.[63] Although not used frequently to diagnose primary lung tumors, cytological study yielded a definitive diagnosis 79 per cent of the time when used before surgery.[77] Fine-needle aspiration has a low risk of complications and is easily performed.

Biopsy of a pulmonary mass may be accomplished by several methods, including bronchoscopy, a percutaneous approach, and exploratory thoracotomy.[6, 100] A thoracotomy is often necessary for definitive diagnosis of a pulmonary mass. Each lung lobe is palpated for additional nodules and secondary lesions, and biopsy of hilar lymph nodes is performed for accurate clinical staging. Surgical resection is not indicated with intrapulmonary metastasis, distant metastasis of a primary lung tumor, or lung metastasis of a distant primary tumor.[11]

Therapy

Wide surgical resection is the treatment of choice for solitary nodules confined to one lobe or one lung after the anesthetic risk to the patient has been assessed. Patients are selected for surgery if they have a solitary mass or multiple masses involving a single lobe with no evidence of distant metastasis or extrapleural involvement.[58] An intercostal approach to the thoracotomy is preferred over median sternotomy because it provides adequate exposure for lobectomy and lymph node biopsy.[75] Partial lobectomy is recommended only for very peripherally located tumors; total lobectomy is the technique of choice. An automatic stapling device allows a safe, fast, and efficient method for lung removal.[51, 64]

Chemotherapy is routinely used for particular histological types of neoplasia in humans, but its use in animals with pulmonary neoplasia has been limited. Chemotherapy may be considered when lesions are inoperable, surgery is contraindicated for other reasons, or lesions recur after surgical resection.[63] Cisplatin and vincristine have been used on a limited basis and have resulted in a measurable response.[64] Although radiation is used in humans as adjunctive therapy, it is largely untried in veterinary medicine. Normal lung tissue may not accept a radiation dose required to kill tumor without complications such as fibrosis. The use of chemotherapy and radiation therapy for treatment of primary pulmonary neoplasia warrants further investigation in veterinary medicine.

Course of Disease and Prognosis

Although the prognosis for patients with primary pulmonary neoplasia remains guarded, it is not as uniformly dismal as discussed in several early reports.[18] This fact can probably be attributed to earlier detection of lesions with more routine use of thoracic radiographs as a screening procedure.[63, 64] The best prognosis is for patients with solitary lesions of small diameter (<5 cm), negative lymph nodes, no malignant pleural effusion, and diagnosis before the development of respiratory symptoms. Under these circumstances, more than 50 per cent of dogs can live at least 1 year postoperatively. Dogs with tumors in the lung periphery or near the base of a lung have longer survival times than those with involvement of an entire lobe, just as those with small tumors have better survival than those with large tumors.[113] Survival in humans is linked to the presence or absence of respiratory signs at the time of diagnosis. Dogs with respiratory signs at the time of diagnosis and surgery have shorter survival times than dogs without signs.[75] Survival times are greater with differentiated adenocarcinomas; undifferentiated adenocarcinomas are more invasive and metastasize more frequently. One study found that the most important prognostic factor related to tumor remission and survival in dogs after surgery was lymph node involvement at the time of surgery.[76] Other valuable parameters in predicting survival time were failure to find distant metastatic disease or large lymph nodes in the presurgical evaluation and finding a localized primary tumor that was not invasive into surrounding tissue.

The prognosis for most cats with primary lung tumor is poor owing to the advanced nature of disease at the time of diagnosis and aggressive metastatic behavior. Most patients eventually die or are destroyed because of recurrence of the primary tumor or metastatic disease.

METASTATIC PULMONARY NEOPLASIA

Epidemiology and Pathology

Metastasis is a major cause of treatment failure in cancer patients. The lung is second only to regional lymph nodes in incidence of metastatic disease. Metastatic pulmonary neoplasia is encountered far more commonly than primary lung tumors in dogs and cats and represents an important differential diagnosis for nodular lung disease. Because pulmonary metastatic disease represents an advanced stage of neoplasia, its recognition is also vital in formulating a rational therapeutic plan and an accurate prognosis.

Development of metastatic disease is the culmination of a complicated series of events requiring tumor and host interaction. The process of metastasis is not random, and the tumor cells must accomplish a cascade of linked sequential steps if a metastatic lesion is to develop. A metastatic tumor cell must leave the primary tumor and invade local host tissue. It must then enter the circulation, survive in circulation, arrest at the distant vascular bed, extravasate into the organ interstitium and parenchyma, and multiply to initiate a metastatic colony.[54] The development of metastasis for most neoplasms implies that the disease is advanced in its course, and a poor prognosis is warranted. Tumors with a high likelihood of resulting in pulmonary metastasis include mammary carcinoma, thyroid carcinoma, hemangiosarcoma, osteosarcoma, transitional cell carcinoma, squamous cell carcinoma, and oral and digital melanoma.

Clinical Presentation

The history and physical examination of patients with metastatic pulmonary neoplasia may be nonspecific, but several important factors should be considered. First, a complete history and thorough physical examination may reveal the site of the primary neoplastic lesion. This site is particularly important because definitive diagnosis of the primary lesion may be more easily accomplished than discovering the histological origin of the metastases noninvasively. Second, clinical signs relative to the respiratory disease may include cough, exercise intolerance, or dyspnea. Nonspecific clinical signs that may be associated with metastatic neoplasia include weight loss, anorexia, and lethargy. If metastatic lesions are present in other organs, clinical signs may be associated with these lesions (i.e., bone pain and lameness with bone metastasis). Additionally, certain paraneoplastic syndromes, particularly hypertrophic osteopathy, can be associated with metastatic pulmonary nodules as well as primary lung neoplasia.[103]

Diagnostic Evaluation

Clinical findings supporting metastatic disease rather than primary pulmonary neoplasia are multiple pulmonary masses, the presence of a nonpulmonary mass, and the previous excision of a malignant mass.[63] If pulmonary metastasis is the only detectable sign of neoplasia, the diagnostic evaluation is directed at identifying the primary tumor.[100] When evaluating thoracic radiographs, it may be difficult to differentiate metastatic pulmonary neoplasia from a distant primary site and pulmonary metastasis from a primary pulmonary tumor. Compared with primary lesions, metastatic tumors are generally smaller and more circumscribed (Fig. 162–11). Metastatic nodules are usually located in the peripheral or middle portions of the lung and do not cause noticeable displacement or obstruction of bronchi. Cavitation is usually not encountered with pulmonary metastatic disease. Multiple nodules associated with primary lung tumors often consist of one large mass and smaller secondary nodules. When multiple nodules are metastases, several large masses and various smaller lesions are usually present. The most accurate view for detecting pulmonary metastasis is the right lateral recumbent view, and it is recommended that this view always be included in the diagnostic evaluation.[49] Because of the varied patterns of metastatic spread to the pulmonary parenchyma, not all metastatic lesions appear as distinct nodular densities. The radiographs may show only an increased unstructured interstitial opacity, which could be interpreted as changes compatible with age.[110]

Additional methods of diagnostic evaluation that may be helpful in determining the presence or extent of pulmonary metastatic neoplasia are pulmonary perfusion scans and fine-needle aspiration cytology. Obviously, careful evaluation of the primary neoplastic lesion can be invaluable in determining further diagnostic and therapeutic courses. The presence of other metastatic lesions may be determined by survey radiographs, nuclear imaging, ultrasonography, or cytological or histopathological evaluation.

Therapy

The presence of metastasis implies that a primary neoplasm can no longer be treated as a local entity but

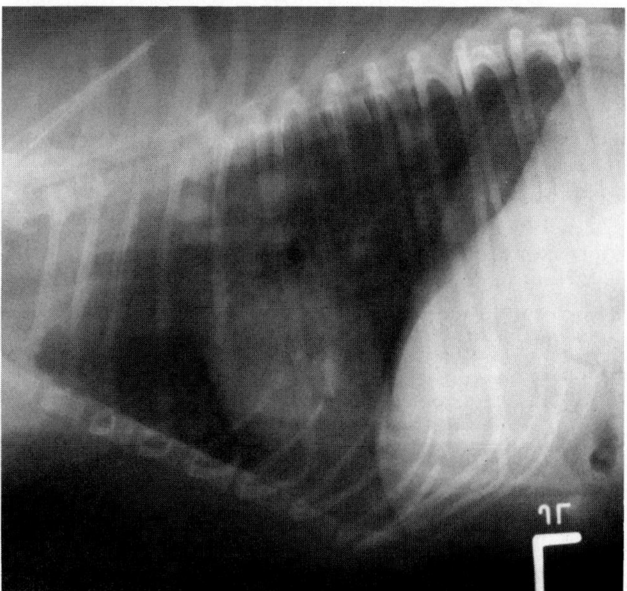

FIGURE 162–11. Lateral thoracic radiograph of a 14-year-old mixed-breed dog. Multiple discrete pulmonary masses of different sizes represent metastatic foci from mammary adenocarcinoma.

must be considered a systemic disease. Chemotherapy has been the standard for treating metastatic disease because of its ability to be distributed throughout the body. The response of each patient depends on the tissue type of the primary tumor and its inherent ability to respond to chemotherapy. Chemotherapy directed at the primary tumor may also have a role in altering the expected metastatic pattern.[28]

Surgical management of solitary or slow-growing metastases has been attempted with some success in veterinary patients.[116] As an increased understanding of the mechanisms of tumor cell invasion is developed, progress may be made in developing pharmacological strategies to block or prevent various steps in the cascade of events leading to metastasis.

MALIGNANT PLEURAL EFFUSION

Pleural effusion may be associated with either primary thoracic neoplasia, such as pleural mesothelioma, or metastatic pulmonary tumors. The clinical signs in these patients often result from fluid, which reaccumulates rapidly after thoracentesis, rather than from growth of the tumor itself in the pleura or lungs or on the chest wall. Few reports in the veterinary literature have described the treatment of pleural effusion of malignant origin.[97] Malignant effusions are apparently much more common in humans, accounting for between 25 and 53 per cent of pleural effusion encountered in general hospitals.[60] The most common cause of exudative effusions in humans is malignancies. The tumors most commonly associated with pleural effusion in humans are those arising from the lungs, breasts, and ovaries, as well as the lymphomas.[60]

Although malignant cells are identified in 25 to 87 per cent of pleural effusion occurring in humans with cancer,[60] in our experience, identification of neoplastic cells in pleural effusion of cats and dogs is less common. Additionally, malignant cells are difficult to differentiate from reactive mesothelial cells, which exfoliate in response to the pleural effusion. Techniques being evaluated to increase the sensitivity and specificity of malignant fluid evaluation include flow cytometry, pleural fluid cytogenetics, immunohistochemistry, and analysis of biochemical parameters such as carcinoembryonic antigen. There are few reports of the efficacy of these techniques.

Treatment of malignant pleural effusion is directed at controlling the primary tumor. When there is no effective systemic treatment and clinical signs related to the effusion predominate, treatment of the effusion may be indicated to prolong an animal's life. Intracavitary instillation of chemotherapeutic agents or radioactive isotopes has been effective in the treatment of malignant pleural effusions in humans[32, 42, 44]; the latter was reported in a dog.[97] Although the mechanism of action of most intracavitary agents in humans is unknown, their effectiveness appears to be due to their ability to cause pleurodesis, rather than their antineoplastic effects. Pleurodesis has been used in dogs to treat pleural effusion[12, 48]; however, its effectiveness is unproven. Such details as proper agent, dose, and instillation method have been adapted primarily from human clinical trials or from experimental studies in other species and need to be more closely evaluated in dogs.

Mesotheliomas are rare tumors in dogs. They arise from mesodermal cells of the pleural, pericardial, and peritoneal surfaces.[40, 69] A documented association between mesothelioma and exposure to asbestos has been noted in humans, and in one study, three of five dogs with mesotheliomas had asbestos particles in their lungs at necropsy; asbestos particles were not found in the lungs of control dogs in the same study.[10] These tumors are highly effusive, and clinical signs are usually related to the presence of large amounts of serosanguineous fluid, which inhibits normal respiration. Diagnosis of mesothelioma is generally made by open biopsy; examination of pleural fluid is rarely helpful because reactive mesothelial cells and neoplastic mesothelial cells are difficult to differentiate cytologically.[69]

Metastasis of mesotheliomas to intrathoracic organs is common in dogs, and therapy is generally restricted to controlling pleural effusion. Intracavitary administration of chemotherapeutic agents and pleurectomy have resulted in significant clinical improvement in some human patients.[14, 61] However, median survival in patients treated with intrapleural therapy was only 8 months in one study.[61] The prognosis in dogs for long-term survival is similarly poor.[69]

TUMORS OF THE THORACIC WALL AND STERNUM

Primary tumors of the ribs are uncommon in dogs; however, these tumors are usually malignant, have a high metastatic rate, and generally develop in young dogs, with a mean reported age in one study of 4 years.[31] Osteosarcomas are the most common neoplasm of the canine rib, followed by chondrosarcoma; the costochondral junction is the usual site of origin.[20, 31, 55] Most rib tumors cause a localized swelling of the thoracic wall; however, pleural effusion without evidence of a thoracic mass has been reported in two dogs with primary rib

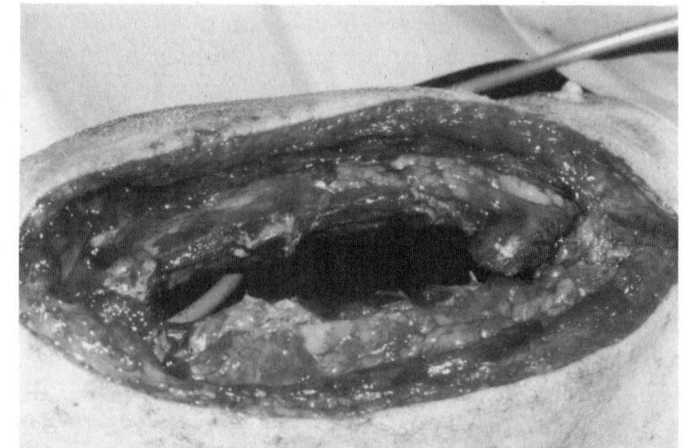

FIGURE 162–12. A dog with sternal osteomyelitis showing the defect created after removal of the caudal three-quarters of the fifth and the entire sixth, seventh, and eighth sternebrae. A portion of the xiphoid cartilage was left intact. (From Fossum TW, et al: Partial sternectomy for sternal osteomyelitis in the dog. *J Am Anim Hosp Assoc 25*:435, 1989.)

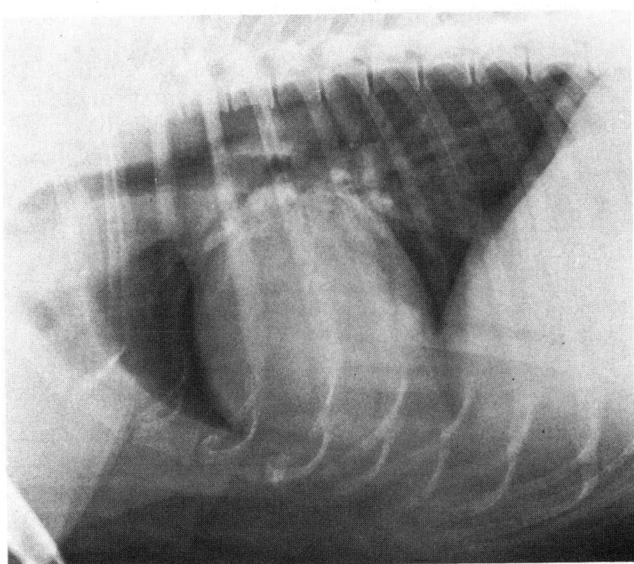

FIGURE 162–13. Lateral thoracic radiograph of the same dog as in Figure 162–12 after partial sternectomy had been performed. (From Fossum TW, et al: Partial sternectomy for sternal osteomyelitis in the dog. *J Am Anim Hosp Assoc 25*:435, 1989.)

tumors and metastatic pulmonary lesions.[31] Other clinical signs of rib tumors are weight loss and dyspnea.

A tentative diagnosis of the cell type can usually be made by fine-needle aspiration of the mass, but definitive diagnosis usually requires histological examination of a biopsy specimen. Although pleural effusion is common in dogs with rib tumors, identification of neoplastic cells in the fluid is uncommon.[31] Because of the high rate of pulmonary metastasis, the prognosis for dogs with rib tumors is poor. In one study of 15 dogs with primary rib tumors, more than 90 per cent of the dogs died or were euthanized within 4 months of the diagnosis.[31]

Although also rare, both metastatic and primary tumors of the sternum have been reported in dogs.[4, 55, 91] In humans, metastatic tumors involving the sternum are more frequently recognized than primary tumors.[53] The distant primary site is most commonly the thyroid, kidney, breast, testicle, lung, stomach, or rectum.[53] Primary neoplasms of the bony chest account for 7 to 8 per cent of all bone tumors in humans, and although primary rib tumors are frequently benign, tumors of the sternum are typically malignant.[92] Similar generalizations are difficult to make in dogs because of the infrequency with which sternal tumors have been reported. However, chondrosarcomas and osteosarcomas involving the sternebrae have been reported in dogs.[4, 55]

When a diagnosis of sternal neoplasia is made, the diseased bone as well as normal surrounding tissue should be removed (Fig. 162–12). Unlike most bones in the body, the sternebrae can be removed with little decrease in function.[35] Successful treatment of sternal osteomyelitis after resection of large portions of the sternebrae has been reported in dogs and humans; and the procedure would likely benefit dogs with primary sternal neoplasia (Fig. 162–13).[2, 21, 35, 72, 79]

References

1. Adams WM, et al: Radiotherapy of malignant nasal tumors of 67 dogs. *J Am Vet Med Assoc 191*:311, 1987.
2. Arnold PG, Pairolero PC: Chondrosarcoma of the manubrium. *Mayo Clin Proc 53*:54, 1978.
3. Aron DN, et al: Primary tracheal chondrosarcoma in a dog: A case report with description of surgical and anesthetic techniques. *J Am Anim Hosp Assoc 16*:31, 1985.
4. Atwell RB, Seiler R: Primary osteosarcoma of the sternum of a dog. *Aust Vet J 54*:585, 1978.
5. Auerbach O, et al: Effects of cigarette smoking in dogs. II. Pulmonary neoplasms. *Arch Environ Health 21*:754, 1970.
6. Bauer T, Thomas WP: Pulmonary diagnostic techniques. *Vet Clin North Am 13*:273, 1983.
7. Beaumont PR: Intratracheal neoplasia in two cats. *J Small Anim Pract 23*:29, 1982.
8. Beaumont PR, et al: Mast cell sarcoma of the larynx in a dog: A case report. *J Small Anim Pract 20*:19, 1979.
9. Beck ER, Withrow SJ: Tumors of the canine nasal cavity. *Vet Clin North Am 15*:521, 1985.
10. Becklake MR: Asbestos-related diseases of the lung and other organs: Their epidemiology and implications for clinical practice. *Am Rev Respir Dis 114*:11, 1976.
11. Bell FW: Neoplastic diseases of the thorax. *Vet Clin North Am 17*:31, 1987.
12. Birchard SJ, Gallagher L: Use of pleurodesis in treating selected pleural diseases. *Comp Cont Educ Pract Vet 10*:826, 1988.
13. Black AP, et al: Primary tracheal leiomyoma in a dog. *J Am Vet Assoc 179*:905, 1981.
14. Brenner J, et al: Malignant mesothelioma of the pleura. *Cancer 49*:2431, 1982.
15. Bright RM, et al: Laryngeal neoplasia in two dogs. *J Am Vet Med Assoc 184*:738, 1984.
16. Brodey RS: Canine and feline neoplasia. *Adv Vet Sci Comp Med 14*:309, 1970.
17. Brodey RS: Hypertrophic osteoarthropathy in the dog: A clinico-pathologic survey of 60 cases. *J Am Vet Med Assoc 159*:1242, 1971.
18. Brodey RS, Craig PH: Primary pulmonary neoplasia in the dog: A review of 29 cases. *J Am Vet Med Assoc 147*:1628, 1965.
19. Brodey RS, et al: Osteosarcoma of the upper airway in the dog. *J Am Vet Med Assoc 155*:1460, 1969.
20. Brodey RS, et al: Canine skeletal chondrosarcoma: A clinicopathological study of 35 cases. *J Am Vet Med Assoc 165*:55, 1974.
21. Brodin H, Linden K: Resection of the walls of the sternum and the cartilaginous parts of costae I-IV. *Acta Chir Scand 1315*:118, 1959.
22. Bryan RD, et al: Tracheal leiomyoma in a dog. *J Am Vet Med Assoc 178*:1069, 1981.
23. Cain GR, Manley P: Tracheal adenocarcinoma in a cat. *J Am Vet Med Assoc 182*:614, 1983.
24. Carpenter JL, et al: Tumors and tumor-like lesions. *In* Holzworth J (ed): *Diseases of the Cat: Medicine and Surgery*. W.B. Saunders, Philadelphia, 1987, pp 406–596.
25. Clarke WJ, et al: Bronchiolo-alveolar tumors of the canine lung following inhalation of plutonium particles. *Am Rev Respir Dis 90*:963, 1964.
26. Clayton HM: The management and treatment of respiratory nematode infections in small animals. *Vet Ann 23*:254, 1983.
27. Clifford P: On the epidemiology of nasopharyngeal carcinoma. *Invest J Cancer 5*:21, 1970.
28. Cotter SM, Parker LM: High-dose methotrexate and leucovorin rescue in dogs with osteogenic sarcoma. *Am J Vet Res 39*:1943, 1978.
29. Crowe DT, et al: Total laryngectomy for laryngeal mast cell tumor in a dog. *J Am Anim Hosp Assoc 22*:809, 1986.
30. Dubielzig RR, Dickey DL: Tracheal osteochondroma in a young dog. *Vet Med Small Anim Clin 73*:1288, 1978.
31. Feeney DA, et al: Malignant neoplasia of the canine ribs: Clinical, radiographic, and pathologic findings. *J Am Vet Med Assoc 180*:927, 1982.
32. Fentiman IS, et al: Control of pleural effusions in patients with breast cancer. *Cancer 52*:737, 1983.
33. Flanders JA, et al: Laryngeal chondrosarcoma in a dog. *J Am Vet Med Assoc 190*:68, 1987.
34. Fossum TW, et al: Partial sternectomy for sternal osteomyelitis in the dog. *J Am Anim Hosp Assoc 25*:435, 1989.
35. Gibbs C, et al: Radiological features of intra-nasal lesions in the dog: a review of 100 cases. *J Small Anim Pract 20*:515, 1979.
36. Gourley RM, et al: Tracheal osteochondroma in a dog: A case report. *J Small Anim Pract 11*:327, 1970.
37. Hahn FF, et al: Primary pulmonary neoplasms in beagle dogs exposed to aerosols of 144 CE in fused-clay particles. *J Natl Cancer Inst 50*:675, 1973.
38. Halliwell WH, Ackerman P: Botryoid rhabdomyosarcoma of the urinary bladder and hypertrophic osteoarthropathy in a young dog. *J Am Vet Med Assoc 165*:911, 1974.
39. Hamilton HB, et al: Pulmonary squamous cell carcinoma with intraocular metastasis in a cat. *J Am Vet Med Assoc 185*:307, 1984.

40. Harbison ML, Godleski JJ. Malignant mesothelioma in urban dogs. *Vet Pathol 20*:531, 1983.
41. Harvey HJ, Sykes G: Tracheal mast cell tumor in a dog. *J Am Vet Med Assoc 180*:1097, 1982.
42. Hausheer FH, Yarbro JW: Diagnosis and treatment of malignant pleural effusion. *Cancer Metastasis Rev 6*:23, 1987.
43. Hough JD, et al: Tracheal osteochondroma in a dog. *J Am Vet Med Assoc 170*:1416, 1977.
44. Jones GR: Treatment of recurrent malignant pleural effusion by iodized talc pleurodesis. *Thorax 24*:69, 1969.
45. Koblik PD: Radiographic appearance of primary lung tumors in cats. *Vet Radiol 27*:66, 1986.
46. Kotake Y, Grillo HG: Reduction of tension at the anastomosis following tracheal resection in puppies. *J Thorac Cardiovasc Surg 71*:600, 1976.
47. Ladds PW, Webster DR: Pharyngeal rhabdomyosarcoma in a dog. *Vet Pathol 8*:256, 1971.
48. Laing EJ, Norris AM: Pleurodesis as a treatment for pleural effusion in the dog. *J Am Anim Hosp Assoc 22*:193, 1986.
49. Lang J, et al: Sensitivity of radiographic detection of lung metastases in the dog. *Vet Radiol 27*:74, 1986.
50. Lappin MR, Prestwood AK. *Oslerus osleri*: Clinical case, attempted transmission, and epidemiology. *J Am Anim Hosp Assoc 24*:153, 1988.
51. LaRue SM, et al: Lung resection using surgical staples in dogs and cats. *Vet Surg 16*:238, 1987.
52. Legendre AM, et al: Canine nasal and paranasal sinus tumors. *J Am Anim Hosp Assoc 19*:115, 1983.
53. le Roux BT, Shama DM: Resection of tumors of the chest wall. *Curr Probl Surg 20*:345, 1983.
54. Liotta LA, Stetler-Stevenson WG: Principles of molecular cell biology of cancer: Cancer metastasis. *In* DeVita VT, et al (eds): *Cancer—Principles and Practice of Oncology*. 3rd ed. J.B. Lippincott, Philadelphia, 1989, pp 98–115.
55. Lui SK, et al: Primary and secondary bone tumors in the dog. *J Small Anim Pract 18*:313, 1977.
56. MacComb WS, Fletcher GH: *Cancer of the Head and Neck*. Williams & Wilkins, Baltimore, 1967, pp 192–213.
57. MacEwen EG, et al: Nasal tumors in the dog: Retrospective evaluation of diagnosis, prognosis, and treatment. *J Am Vet Med Assoc 170*:45, 1976.
58. Madewell BR, Theilen GH: Tumors of the respiratory tract and thorax. *In* Theilen GH, Madewell BR (eds): *Veterinary Cancer Medicine*. 2nd ed. Lea & Febiger, Philadelphia, 1987, pp 535–565.
59. Madewell BR, et al: Neoplasms of the nasal passages and paranasal sinuses in domesticated animals as reported by 13 veterinary colleges. *Am J Vet Res 37*:851, 1976.
60. Malden LT, Tattersall MHN: Malignant effusions. *Q J Med 58*:221, 1986.
61. Markman M, et al: Cisplatin administered by the intracavitary route as a treatment for malignant mesothelioma. *Cancer 58*:18, 1986.
62. McConnell EE, et al: Melanoma in the larynx of a dog. *J South Afr Vet Med Assoc 42*:189, 1971.
63. Mehlhaff CJ, Mooney S: Primary pulmonary neoplasia in the dog and cat. *Vet Clin North Am 14*:1061, 1985.
64. Mehlhaff CJ, et al: Surgical treatment of primary pulmonary neoplasia in 15 dogs. *J Am Anim Hosp Assoc 20*:799, 1984.
65. Meuten DJ, et al: Canine laryngeal rhabdomyoma. *Vet Pathol 22*:533, 1985.
66. Miles KG: A review of primary lung tumors in the dog and cat. *Vet Radiol 29*:122, 1988.
67. Minna JD, et al: Cancer of the lung. *In* DeVita VT, et al (eds): *Cancer—Principles and Practice of Oncology*. 3rd ed. J.B. Lippincott, Philadelphia, 1989, pp 591–705.
68. Moore JA, Taylor HW: Primary pulmonary adenocarcinoma with brain stem metastasis in a dog. *J Am Vet Med Assoc 192*:219, 1988.
69. Morrison WB, Trigo FJ: Clinical characterization of pleural mesothelioma in seven dogs. *Comp Cont Educ Pract Vet 6*:342, 1984.
70. Moulton JE: Tumors of the respiratory system. *In* Moulton JE (ed): *Tumors in Domestic Animals*. 2nd ed. University of California Press, Los Angeles, 1978, pp 216–239.
71. Moulton JE, et al: Classification of lung carcinomas in the dog and cat. *Vet Pathol 18*:513, 1981.
72. Myre TT, Kirklin JW: Resection of tumors of the sternum *Ann Surg 144*:1023, 1956.
73. Nafe LA, et al: Hypercalcemia associated with epidermoid carcinoma in a dog. *J Am Vet Med Assoc 176*:1253, 1980.
74. Nafe LA, et al: Hypertrophic osteopathy in a cat associated with renal papillary adenoma. *J Am Anim Hosp Assoc 17*:659, 1981.
75. Norris AM, et al: Oncology of the respiratory system. *In* Slatter DH (ed): *Textbook of Small Animal Surgery*. W.B. Saunders, Philadelphia, 1985, pp 2583–2592.
76. Ogilvie GK, et al: Prognostic factors for tumor remission and survival in dogs after surgery for primary lung tumor: 76 cases (1975–1985). *J Am Vet Med Assoc 195*:109, 1989.
77. Ogilvie GK, et al: Classification of primary lung tumors in dogs: 210 cases (1975–1985). *J Am Vet Med Assoc 195*:106, 1989.
78. Owen LN: *TNM Classification of Tumors of Domestic Animals*. World Health Organization, Geneva, 1981.
79. Paris F, et al: Total sternectomy for malignant disease. *J Thorac Cardiovasc Surg 80*:459, 1980.
80. Pass DA, et al: Canine laryngeal oncocytomas. *Vet Pathol 17*:672, 1980.
81. Pastorino NC, et al: Canine pulmonary lymphomatoid granulomatosis: 8 cases (1981–1986). *J Vet Intern Med 3*:15, 1989.
82. Patnaik AK: Canine sinonasal neoplasms: Clinicopathological study of 285 cases. *J Am Anim Hosp Assoc 25*:103, 1989.
83. Patnaik AK, et al: Nonhematopoietic neoplasms in cats. *J Natl Cancer Inst 54*:855, 1975.
84. Pechman RD: Effect of dependency versus nondependency on lung lesion visualization. *Vet Radiol 28*:185, 1987.
85. Pour PM, Sepan KR: The role of testosterone in the nasal cavity tumors induced by *N*-nitrosobis(2-oxypropyl)amine in rats. *Carcinogenesis 9*:1417, 1988.
86. Priester WA, McKay FW: The occurrence of tumors in domestic animals. National Cancer Institute, Bethesda, 1980.
87. Reif JS, Cohen D: The environmental distribution of canine respiratory tract neoplasms. *Arch Environ Health 22*:136, 1971.
88. Roberts SM, et al: Ophthalmic complications following megavoltage irradiation of the nasal and paranasal cavities in dogs. *J Am Vet Med Assoc 190*:43, 1987.
89. Rosin A, et al: Malignant histiocytosis in Bernese mountain dogs. *J Am Vet Med Assoc 188*:1041, 1986.
90. Rudd RG, Richardson DC: A diagnostic and therapeutic approach to nasal disease in dogs. *Comp Cont Educ Pract Vet 7*:103, 1985.
91. Russell RG, Walker M: Metastatic and invasive tumors of bone in dogs and cats. *Vet Clin North Am 13*:163, 1983.
92. Sabanthan S, et al: Primary chest wall tumors. *Ann Thorac Surg 39*:4, 1985.
93. Sackman JE, et al: X-ray computed tomography-aided diagnosis of nasal adenocarcinoma, with extension to the skull and central nervous system, in a dog. *J Am Vet Med Assoc 194*:1073, 1989.
94. Saik JE, et al: Canine and feline laryngeal neoplasia: A 10-year survey. *J Am Anim Hosp Assoc 22*:359, 1986.
95. Schneider PR, et al: Histiocytic lymphosarcoma of the trachea in a cat. *J Am Anim Hosp Assoc 15*:485, 1979.
96. Shanmugaratnam K, et al: Histopathology of nasopharyngeal carcinoma: Correlations with epidemiology, survival rates and other biological characteristics. *Cancer 44*:1029, 1979.
97. Shapiro W, Turrell J: Management of pleural effusion secondary to metastatic adenocarcinoma in a dog. *J Am Vet Med Assoc 192*:530, 1988.
98. Smith MO, et al: Neurologic abnormalities as the predominant signs of neoplasia of the nasal cavity in dogs and cats: Seven cases (1973–1986). *J Am Vet Med Assoc 195*:242, 1989.
99. Sorjonen DC, et al: Paraplegia and subclinical neuromyopathy associated with a primary lung tumor in a dog. *J Am Vet Med Assoc 180*:1209, 1982.
100. Stann SE, Bauer TG: Respiratory tract tumors. *Vet Clin North Am 15*:535, 1985.
101. Stephens LC, et al: Primary pulmonary fibrosarcoma associated with *Spirocerca lupi* infection in a dog with hypertrophic pulmonary osteoarthropathy. *J Am Vet Med Assoc 182*:496, 1983.
102. Straw RC, et al: Use of radiotherapy for the treatment of intranasal neoplasia in cats: six cases (1980–1985). *J Am Vet Med Assoc 189*:927, 1986.
103. Susaneck SJ, Macy DW: Hypertrophic osteopathy. *Comp Cont Educ Pract Vet 4*:689, 1982.
104. Tangner CH, Hedlund CS: Tracheal surgery in the dog—Part 1. *Comp Cont Educ Pract Vet 5*:599, 1983.
105. Thrall DE, Harvey CE: Radiotherapy of malignant nasal tumors in 21 dogs. *J Am Vet Med Assoc 183*:663, 1983.
106. Troy GC: Surgical removal of a tracheal osteochondroma. *Canine Pract 5*:47, 1978.
107. Vasseur PB, Patnaik AK: Laryngeal adenocarcinoma in a cat. *J Am Anim Hosp Assoc 17*:639, 1981.
108. Veith LA: Squamous cell carcinoma of the trachea in a cat. *Feline Pract 4*:30, 1974.
109. Vulgamott JC, Clark RG: Atrial hypertension and hypertrophic pulmonary osteopathy associated with aortic valvular endocarditis in a dog. *J Am Vet Med Assoc 177*:243, 1980.
110. Walter PA, et al: Radiographic appearance of pulmonary metastases from transitional cell carcinoma of the bladder and urethra of the dog. *J Am Vet Med Assoc 185*:411, 1984.
111. Wheeldon EB, et al: Neoplasia of the larynx in the dog. *J Am Vet Med Assoc 180*:642, 1982.
112. Withrow SJ: Cryosurgical therapy for nasal tumors in the dog. *J Am Anim Hosp Assoc 18*:585, 1982.
113. Withrow SJ: Tumors of the respiratory system. *In* Withrow SJ, MacEwen EG (eds): *Clinical Veterinary Oncology*. J.B. Lippincott, Philadelphia, 1989, pp 215–233.
114. Withrow SJ, et al: Treatment of tracheal osteochondroma with an overlapping end-to-end anastomosis. *J Am Anim Hosp Assoc 14*:469, 1978.
115. Withrow SJ, et al: Aspiration and punch biopsy techniques for nasal tumors. *J Am Anim Hosp Assoc 21*:551, 1985.
116. Withrow SJ, et al: Pulmonary metastasectomy for canine osteosarcoma. The 8th Annual Conference of the Veterinary Cancer Society, Estes Park, CO, Oct, 1988, p 2.

SECTION 17

Anesthetic Considerations in Surgery

Richard M. Bednarski
William W. Muir III ■ *Section Editors*

CHAPTER 163 Anesthetics and Techniques

William W. Muir III

Veterinary surgeons are frequently presented with an apparently normal healthy dog or cat requiring an elective surgical procedure; however, on many occasions, a patient may not be normal or healthy. Frightened patients may attempt to hide or escape or may become aggressive. In either situation, the sympathetic nervous system is activated, producing effects that often mask clinical problems. Some patients are very young or very old, necessitating special medical and laboratory tests to evaluate cardiac, hepatic, and renal function. Others may have an undiagnosed or diagnosed illness, may have suffered extensive trauma, or may be severely debilitated. Many patients may be receiving drugs to control or prevent allergies, eliminate parasites, combat infections, or treat specific organ system failure (heart, kidneys, endocrine). All of these situations raise important questions about decisions regarding the choice and amount of drugs to produce chemical restraint, immobilization, and anesthesia. The knowledge and skill of the veterinary surgeon, the training and skill of technical assistants, and the type of anesthetic and monitoring equipment available must be considered to identify the best approach. This chapter discusses the many drugs and drug combinations used to produce chemical restraint and anesthesia.[1–18]

DEFINITIONS (Table 163–1)

Chemical restraint refers to a drug-induced state that produces favorable behavior modification, sedation, analgesia, or muscle relaxation. Anesthesia includes two of these qualities, analgesia and muscle relaxation, but also incorporates hypnosis or unconsciousness. No currently available chemical restraining or anesthetic drugs can produce the ideal degree of each of these properties in every patient. Thorough familiarity with a select few allows a surgeon to produce safe and effective anesthesia in almost all clinical situations.

DRUGS USED AS PREANESTHETIC MEDICATION OR FOR SHORT SURGICAL PROCEDURES

Drugs currently approved for chemical restraint in dogs and cats are used (1) as preanesthetic medication, (2) to produce short-term immobilization, (3) intraoperatively as adjuncts to intravenous or inhalation anesthesia, and (4) postoperatively to provide analgesia and calm recovery. These drugs can be placed into one of three broad categories: sedatives, nonopioid analgesics, and opioid analgesics. The term *sedative* is used interchangeably with *tranquilizer* in veterinary medicine because both are used to calm patients. The combination of a sedative or an alpha$_2$-adrenoceptor agonist (xylazine or another nonopioid analgesic) with an opioid analgesic

TABLE 163–1. DEFINITION OF USEFUL TERMS IN ANESTHESIA

Term	Definition
Premed	Preanesthetic medication
Neuroleptanalgesic	The combination of a sedative and opioid analgesic
Bolus	Rapid intravenous injection of a drug or drugs
Crash induce	Rapid induction of anesthesia
Tube	To place an endotracheal tube in a patient's trachea by way of the oral cavity
Bag	Squeeze the rebreathing bag on an anesthetic machine to ventilate the patient
Mask induce	Induction of anesthesia by breathing an inhalation anesthetic from a mask
Deep	Unconsciousness characterized by marked central nervous system depression
Light	Almost conscious
Stabilized	Cardiopulmonary systems are being supported and are normal
General anesthesia	Hypnosis (unconsciousness) analgesia and muscle relaxation produced by injectable or inhalation drugs
Balanced anesthesia	Production of general anesthesia by two or more drugs
Dissociative anesthesia	Production of general anesthesia by ketamine or tiletamine/zolazepam

TABLE 163–2. DRUGS COMMONLY USED TO PRODUCE CHEMICAL RESTRAINT

Drug Group	Examples	Dose Range (mg/kg)	Primary Effect
Sedatives			
Phenothiazines	Acepromazine	0.02–0.4 (maximum 4 mg total)	Calming, muscle relaxation
Butyrophenones	Droperidol	Not applicable	Antiemetic, calming?
Benzodiazepines	Diazepam, midazolam, others	0.2–0.4; 0.2–0.4	Muscle relaxation, anticonvulsant
Nonopioid analgesics			
$Alpha_2$ agonists	Xylazine, medetomidine	0.5–1.1; 0.01–0.02	Sedation, muscle relaxation, analgesia
$Alpha_2$ antagonists	Yohimbine, tolazoline	0.2; 3.0–5.0	Antagonizes $alpha_2$ agonists
Opioid analgesics			
Opioid agonists	Morphine, meperidine, oxymorphone	0.1–0.3; 2.0–6.0; 0.05–0.1	Analgesia, sedation
Opioid agonists/antagonists	Butorphanol, pentazocine, nalbuphine, buprenorphine	0.2–1.0; 2.0–4.0; 0.15–0.2; 0.005–0.01	Analgesia, sedation?, antagonize opioid agonists
Opioid antagonists	Naloxone	0.005–0.01	Antagonize opioid agonists
Neuroleptanalgesics	Acepromazine-meperidine	0.2/2.0	Sedation, analgesia, neuroleptanesthesia
	Acepromazine-oxymorphone	0.2/0.1	
	Diazepam-oxymorphone	0.2/0.1	
	Diazepam-morphine	0.2/0.2	
	Xylazine-oxymorphone	0.5/0.05–0.1	
	Droperidol-fentanyl (Innovar-Vet)	1 ml/10–25 kg	
	Midazolam/butorphanol	0.2/0.2	
Anticholinergics	Atropine, glycopyrrolate	0.01–0.02; 0.005–0.01	Prevent salivation, bradycardia; produce mydriasis, ileus

*Used as adjuncts to preanesthetic medication or anesthesia.

(e.g., morphine, meperidine) makes up a fourth drug combination group referred to as *neuroleptanalgesics* (Table 163–2). An advantage of several of these drug categories is their potential for antagonism or reversibility (see Table 163–2). The $alpha_2$-adrenoceptor agonist xylazine can be antagonized by either yohimbine or tolazoline. Similarly, the opioid agonists morphine, meperidine, and oxymorphone can be antagonized by either an opioid agonist/antagonist (butorphanol and others) or the opioid antagonist naloxone. Naloxone, a specific opioid antagonist, antagonizes opioid-induced central nervous system depression, respiratory depression, and analgesia. This has important clinical implications because it permits an opioid agonist like morphine to be antagonized by an opioid agonist/antagonist (butorphanol), thereby maintaining some degree of analgesia. The antagonists for diazepam, midazolam, and flumazenil are effective in speeding recovery after diazepam/ketamine or tiletamine/zolazepam combinations.

Tranquilizers and Sedatives

Acepromazine is the only phenothiazine sedative (tranquilizer) in common use in small animal practice. Acepromazine is the most predictable and effective phenothiazine available and is the least likely to produce side effects (see Table 163–2). All phenothiazine tranquilizers produce calmness and indifference, reduce aggressive behavior, and bring about muscle relaxation by depressing the reticular activating system and brain stem and inhibiting effects of the central neurotransmitters norepinephrine and dopamine. Most animals can be aroused given sufficient stimulus. Phenothiazines are also noted for their $alpha_1$-adrenoceptor blocking effect, which is important systemically in producing hypotension. The severity of hypotension is dose related, presenting important clinical implications for the use of other potentially hypotensive drugs. Other pharmacological activities of phenothiazine tranquilizers include antiadrenergic, antiarrhythmic (they abolish halothane sensitization to catecholamines), antifibrillatory, antihistaminic, antiemetic, antipyretic, antishock, and anticonvulsant effects. This anticonvulsant property makes phenothiazines effective in inhibiting ketamine and tiletamine/zolazepam-induced seizures even though they are also known to lower seizure threshold by a separate mechanism. The ability of phenothiazines to lower seizure threshold is important in patients with organic brain disease (neoplasia), inherited or familial epilepsy, or encephalitis. Other potential side effects include hypotension, hypothermia, and occasionally profound bradycardia. Bradycardia is atypical because heart rate usually increases as a reflex response to reduction in arterial blood pressure or decreases slightly in excited animals because of sedation. Increases in central nervous system cholinergic activity are responsible for profound bradycardia, which is treatable with atropine or glycopyrrolate. Packed cell volume and platelets may decrease after phenothiazine administration because of erythrocyte sequestration in the spleen and hemodilution caused by fluid movement into the vascular compartment from the interstitial fluid. Dogs and cats have accidentally received massive overdoses (10 to 20 times the recommended dose) of acepromazine without ill effect other than pronounced and prolonged depression and hypotension. Fluid therapy, occasional administration of an alpha$_1$-adrenoceptor agonist (phenylephrine), and supportive therapy are generally all that is needed to ensure complete recovery. Acepromazine is compatible and additive with all drugs used as preanesthetic medication or for general anesthesia, but a fatal drug interaction has been reported when diathal, thiamylal, and acepromazine were administered to dogs. The muscle relaxant and respiratory depressant effects of general anesthetics are also potentiated when acepromazine is administered to dogs or cats receiving organophosphate medications.

The butyrophenone tranquilizers are typified by droperidol, the tranquilizing portion of the neuroleptanalgesic Innovar-Vet, and offer few if any real practical advantages over acepromazine (see Table 163–2). They are almost identical to the phenothiazines pharmacologically and toxicologically, although they are much better antiemetics, do not lower seizure threshold, and are not as likely to produce hypotension. They are poor sedatives when used alone. Most dogs and cats show no signs of sedation when recommended dosages are administered, and many become disoriented and unresponsive to commands.

Benzodiazepines

Recommended doses of diazepam and midazolam produce no better sedative or calming effects than the butyrophenones, although calming is observed in aged, sick, or debilitated patients (see Table 163–2). All the benzodiazepines are appetite stimulants. The major advantages of these drugs are their lack of significant cardiopulmonary depressant effects, their muscle relaxant properties, and their ability to inhibit seizures. They possess antiarrhythmic properties and are synergistic with thiobarbiturates, opioids, and possibly, alpha$_2$ agonists. One potential problem associated with the use of diazepam is its diluent, propylene glycol. Rapid intravenous administration of diazepam to dogs and cats may produce bradycardia, hypotension, and transient periods of cardiac arrest. Although rarely fatal, this effect deserves consideration. Midazolam is a water-soluble benzodiazepine and should not cause this problem. Midazolam is slightly more potent than diazepam but has a shorter duration of action. Clinical trials using midazolam in dogs and cats suggest that it can be used interchangeably with diazepam. All benzodiazepines are potentially reversible with a benzodiazepine antagonist, flumazenil. This effect could be of significant clinical benefit to dogs or cats that have received tiletamine/zolazepam (Telazol), because zolazepam has a prolonged duration of action in some animals.

Nonopioid Analgesics

The nonopioid analgesics xylazine and medetomidine produce analgesic, sedative, and muscle relaxant effects by combining with central nervous system alpha$_2$ adrenoceptors. Central nervous system sympathetic outflow is substantially reduced. These drugs also stimulate peripheral alpha$_1$ and alpha$_2$ adrenoceptors, potentially producing marked cardiopulmonary depression. Respiratory rate and tidal volume, heart rate, and cardiac output decrease after administration of xylazine. Arterial blood pressure first increases and then decreases. Intravenous xylazine administration can produce first-, second-, and third-degree heart block in dogs and cats and has on occasion caused cardiac arrest. Xylazine-induced bradycardia is partially responsive (atropine or glycopyrrolate) but may require more specific therapy by administering an alpha$_2$-adrenoceptor antagonist. Xylazine induces vomiting in approximately 25 per cent of dogs and 50 to 75 per cent of cats and enhances cardiac sensitization to catecholamines produced by halothane and augmented by thiobarbiturates. These side effects have limited the use of xylazine in small animal practice, although xylazine is an excellent adjunct (sedative, analgesic, muscle relaxant) when used at reduced doses or in combination with ketamine for short surgical procedures. Xylazine markedly decreases the amount of intravenous and inhalation anesthetic required to produce and maintain anesthesia (see Table 163–2). Yohimbine and tolazoline are alpha$_2$-adrenoceptor antagonists that specifically antagonize xylazine's effects by competitively blocking and displacing it from alpha$_2$ adrenoceptors. Sedation, analgesia, and muscle relaxation are abolished within 1 to 2 minutes of intravenous administration of either drug. Some dogs and cats may become excited or cry in pain once xylazine has been antagonized. Doxapram, a central nervous system and specifically a respiratory center stimulant, also speeds recovery in dogs and particularly in cats recovering from xylazine sedation. Doxapram is not as effective as yohimbine or tolazoline in reversing xylazine, but its use may be more practical because it returns patients to a higher level of consciousness without eliminating analgesia.

Opioid Analgesics and Neuroleptanalgesia

The opioid analgesics are a large family of drugs that are used as preanesthetic medication, for sedation and analgesia during surgery, to reduce the amount of general anesthetic required, and postoperatively to provide analgesia and potentially reverse opioid agonists (see Table 163–2). Many new opioid analgesics have been developed because of improved understanding of their receptor pharmacology. Opioid analgesics produce their diverse effects, including analgesia, by interacting with one or more opioid receptors (Table 163–3). Depending on the receptor(s) stimulated, sedation and analgesia or excitement and analgesia can be produced. Respiratory depression is common once a dog or cat is made unconscious, and bradycardia and occasional hypotension can be produced in dogs administered opioid agonists or agonist/antagonists. Most dogs and cats vomit after intramuscular or intravenous administration of some opioid agonists. These drugs not only affect multiple receptors but produce both opioid agonistic and antagonistic effects. Butorphanol can be used as an analgesic or to antagonize the opioid agonist morphine (see Table 163–2). Most currently available opioid agonists/antagonists are not effective sedatives compared with opioid agonists. Fentanyl, the opioid agonist com-

TABLE 163–3. OPIOID RECEPTOR CLASSIFICATION AND EFFECTS

Receptor*	Effects	Agonists†	Dose Range (mg/kg)
Mu (μ)	Analgesia	Morphone	0.1–0.3
	Respiratory depression	Meperidine	2–6
	Bradycardia	Oxymorphone	0.05–0.1
	Miosis	Fentanyl	0.005–0.01
Kappa (κ)	Sedation	Morphine	
	Analgesia	Meperidine	
	Minimal respiratory depression	Oxymorphone	
		Butorphanol	0.2–1.0
		Buprenorphine	0.005–0.01
		Nalbuphine	0.15–0.2
Sigma (σ)	Excitement	Nalbuphine	
	Tachycardia		
	Tachypnea	Butorphanol	
	Mania		
Delta (δ)	Analgesia	Butorphanol	
	Hypotension		

*The opioid receptor subtypes, locations, and number have not been completely determined in dogs and cats.
†Large doses of any opioid may affect all opioid receptors.

ponent of Innovar-Vet, is an extremely effective analgesic (100 times more potent than morphine) but a poor sedative, hence its combination with droperidol. The combination of excellent analgesic properties and poor sedative effects has led veterinarians to become adept at combining opioids with sedatives (see Table 163–2). For example, administration of oxymorphone to a dog or cat produces good analgesia but poor sedation and may result in excitement, hyperexcitability, and mania. The addition of acepromazine, diazepam, midazolam, or xylazine to oxymorphone, however, produces excellent analgesia and mild (diazepam) to moderate (acepromazine) sedation to neuroleptanesthesia (acepromazine, xylazine), depending on the dose. One advantage of drug combinations using xylazine and an opioid analgesic is the ability to reverse their effects totally with an alpha$_2$ antagonist (tolazoline) and an opioid antagonist (naloxone) or opioid agonist/antagonist (butorphanol).

Anticholinergics

The anticholinergic drugs atropine and glycopyrrolate are frequently administered as preanesthetics. They reduce salivary and tracheal secretions, dilate airways, prevent or reverse parasympathetically induced bradycardias, and cause mydriasis. Glycopyrrolate has a longer duration of action than atropine and does not cross the blood-brain or placental barriers, thereby avoiding unwanted central nervous system or fetal effects. Potential deleterious effects of these drugs are tachycardia, cardiac arrhythmias, and ileus—important considerations in dogs with cardiac or gastrointestinal disease. Routine use of anticholinergics in dogs and cats is controversial because the majority of anesthetic techniques in current use do not produce excessive salivation or bradycardia. Bradycardia, when it does occur, is more often a sign of anesthetic overdose or a deep plane of anesthesia than increased parasympathetic tone. Anticholinergics are useful in preventing or reversing bradycardia caused by xylazine and opioid analgesics. Specific types of surgical procedures such as correction of patent ductus arteriosus, cervical disc removal, and excision of bladder neoplasia may benefit from prior anticholinergic administration by preventing vagally induced bradycardias.

DRUGS USED TO PRODUCE GENERAL ANESTHESIA

Drugs commonly used to produce general anesthesia in dogs and cats include hypnotics, dissociative anesthetics, and inhalation anesthetics (Table 163–4). Nitrous oxide is used to provide analgesia but has lost popularity in recent years because of the development of new inhalation anesthetics and the administration of potent opioid agonists (fentanyl, oxymorphone) during surgery.

Barbiturates and Other Hypnotics

Thiamylal and thiopental are ultrashort-acting thiobarbiturates that are popular for producing short-term intravenous anesthesia, inducing general anesthesia before inhalation anesthesia, and reinducing anesthesia in animals that have become light during inhalation anesthesia (Table 163–4). When used at appropriate dosages, thiobarbiturates are among the safest and most cost-effective drugs available. They produce hypnosis and muscle relaxation by depressing all areas of the central nervous system and inhibiting polysynaptic reflexes. Dogs and cats that are made unconscious do not respond to painful stimuli but may feel pain during recovery. Nonopioid and opioid drugs should be used as preanesthetic medication or for postanesthetic analgesia, depending on the surgical procedure. All barbiturates produce dose-dependent depression of respiration. Hypotension is possible after large or bolus doses. Thiobarbiturates can produce ventricular arrhythmias, particularly bigeminy, and augment cardiac sensitization to catecholamines produced by halothane. Thiobarbiturate arrhythmias are generally inconsequential, and most disappear shortly after induction of anesthesia. Prean-

TABLE 163–4. GENERAL ANESTHETICS

Anesthetic Drug	Drug	Intravenous Dose Range (mg/kg)
Hypnotics		
Barbiturates	Thiamylal	4–8
	Thiopental	5–10
	Methohexital	5–10
	Pentobarbital	20–30
Imidazoles	Etomidate	0.5–1.5
Alkylphenols	Proprofol	4.0–8.0
Dissociative Anesthetics		
Cyclohexylamines	Ketamine	2–5
	Tiletamine/zolazepam	0.5–3.0
*Inhalation Anesthetics**	Methoxyflurane	0.25–1.0%
	Halothane	0.5–1.5%
	Isoflurane	1.0–2.5%
Gases	Nitrous oxide	40–70%

*Assume semiclosed system at an oxygen flow rate equal to 20 ml/kg/minute.

esthetic medication with acepromazine usually prevents them. If cardiac arrhythmias persist or cause hemodynamic complications (weak pulse, prolonged capillary refill time, poor mucous membrane color), they are treated with lidocaine (0.5 to 1.0 mg/kg). One of the most disturbing properties of the thiobarbiturates is that they are cumulative. The anesthetic duration of thiamylal and thiopental is related to reduction of their plasma drug concentration due to redistribution into muscle and then fat, not metabolism and excretion. More than 95 per cent of the original dose is still present after recovery from a bolus dose of either thiamylal or thiopental. The clinical significance is that multiple readministrations of either drug eventually produce plasma concentrations that depend on metabolism by the liver and excretion by the kidneys to terminate drug effects. Because the biological half-life for these drugs is between 5 and 7 hours in dogs and cats, the total time for recovery may exceed 24 hours (five half-lives). Dogs and cats that are extremely excited or frightened before induction of anesthesia may require much higher doses of thiobarbiturate. Increases in muscle blood flow caused by fear or excitement hasten their redistribution and lower plasma concentrations and therefore brain concentrations, resulting in rapid recovery. The opposite is true in depressed and dehydrated patients and patients in shock. Small doses of thiobarbiturates may produce immediate and prolonged unconsciousness owing to a centralization of blood volume and poor muscle blood flow. Acidosis and hypoproteinemia prolong and increase the intensity of thiobarbiturate anesthesia by slowing elimination and increasing the amount of free (active) drug in the plasma, respectively. Diuresis and administration of sodium bicarbonate speed thiobarbiturate elimination. Recovery is prolonged in sight hounds (greyhounds, whippets, borzois, Afghans) after thiobarbiturate administration. The reason for this is unclear but is partially related to the slow liver metabolism of both drugs. Dogs and cats showing signs of stress during recovery, paddling, or vocalizing should be given diazepam.

Alternatives to thiobarbiturate induction include methohexital (an ultrashort-acting barbiturate), etomidate, and propofol. These drugs are rapidly metabolized in both the plasma and liver, are not cumulative, and can be used in sight hounds without prolonging recovery. Etomidate is not as likely to produce cardiopulmonary depression as methohexital, but both drugs are noted for their side effects (excitement, paddling, regurgitation), including seizures during induction, unless proper preanesthetic medication has been used (see Table 163–4). Preanesthetic medication using any sedative, nonopioid, or opioid analgesic greatly reduces or eliminates side effects without markedly prolonging recovery from anesthesia. One noteworthy disadvantage of etomidate is its cost; because of its safety, it is an excellent alternative to thiobarbiturates and methohexital in high-risk patients and emergency situations. Pentobarbital, a short-acting (45 to 60 minutes) barbiturate, is no longer recommended as a general anesthetic because of its comparatively pronounced cardiopulmonary depressant effects. When administered in low doses (2 to 6 mg/kg IV), it is an excellent adjunct to anesthesia, producing hypnosis and muscle relaxation without noticeably prolonging recovery.

Cyclohexylamines

The dissociative anesthetics ketamine and tiletamine/zolazepam are used as preanesthetic medication for restraint, as general anesthetics, and intraoperatively as adjuncts to anesthesia (see Table 163–4). They provide excellent superficial analgesia by depressing various areas of the brain. Cardiovascular function is usually maintained or improved and respiration is only transiently depressed after intravenous administration and unchanged following intramuscular administration. Anesthesia is characterized by salivation; an apneustic breathing pattern (breath holding); active corneal, palpebral, swallowing, and laryngeal reflexes; and waxy rigidity of the neck and extremities. The pupils dilate, intraocular pressure increases, and skeletal muscle relaxation is poor. Inadequate muscle relaxation, the potential for seizures during induction and recovery from anesthesia, and the development of emergence delirium during recovery from anesthesia have caused ketamine to be used in combination with acepromazine, xylazine, diazepam (see Table 163–2), or thiobarbiturates. These drug combinations are safe and effective when appropriate dosages are used and markedly improve skeletal muscle relaxation, visceral analgesia, and recovery from anesthesia. Ketamine and tiletamine are relatively safe drugs but almost always produce significant increases in arterial blood pressure and tachycardia, an important consideration in patients with congenital or acquired heart disease. Excessive rises in arterial blood pressure increase myocardial work, which, when combined with tachycardia, markedly increases myocardial oxygen consumption, predisposing to cardiac arrhythmias, myocardial ischemia, and heart failure. Administration of intravenous or intramuscular doses of ketamine to aged patients or patients with undiagnosed heart disease has resulted in pulmonary edema and acute

TABLE 163–5. CLINICALLY RELEVANT PROPERTIES OF INHALATION ANESTHETICS

Drug	Analgesia	Muscle Relaxation	Respiration	Circulation	Quality of Induction/Recovery	Other
Methoxyflurane	Good	Good	Depressed	Generally acceptable	Good/fair	Prolonged recovery, toxic metabolite and environmental pollutants
Halothane	Fair	Fair	Generally acceptable	Hypotension	Good/good	Sensitization of the myocardium to catecholamines
Isoflurane	Good	Good	Depressed	Hypotension	Good/fair	Rapid recovery producing emergence delirium

heart failure. Ketamine and tiletamine/zolazepam are contraindicated with severe liver or renal disease because of their extended action due to prolonged drug elimination. Furthermore, ketamine and tiletamine are not used in patients with head trauma or brain hemorrhage because of increases in arterial blood pressure and cerebrospinal fluid pressure. Their use in dogs or cats with urethral obstruction is not contraindicated provided renal function is normal.

Inhalation Anesthetics

Methoxyflurane, halothane, and isoflurane are inhalation anesthetics used to produce and maintain general anesthesia for all types of surgical procedures (Table 163–5). Inhalation anesthetics offer increased controlability compared with injectable drugs. Problems associated with environmental pollution and drug toxicity, the paucity of antagonists for injectable drugs, and the availability of new short-acting intravenous drugs are worth considering before investing in expensive and often cumbersome inhalation anesthetic equipment. Inhalation anesthetics provide safe and effective long-term general anesthesia. Methoxyflurane is an excellent muscle relaxant and analgesic but is noted for its prolonged recovery periods *if dosage is not controlled correctly.** A large percentage of the methoxyflurane inhaled (approximately 50 per cent) is metabolized to trifluoroacetic acid and fluoride ions, which are toxic to the kidneys. Dogs and cats administered methoxyflurane and other potentially nephrotoxic drugs (tetracycline, gentamicin) have died of acute renal failure. More importantly, pollution of the environment by methoxyflurane could lead to toxicity in operating room personnel.

Halothane is a fair analgesic and muscle relaxant but generally provides excellent anesthesia when preanesthetic medications are used. Induction and recovery from anesthesia are rapid. Halothane produces hypotension more rapidly than methoxyflurane but is not as potent a respiratory depressant at anesthetic concentrations. Halothane sensitizes the myocardium to catecholamine-induced arrhythmias; this is made worse by the use of xylazine as preanesthetic medication and induction with thiobarbiturates. This problem is easily prevented by avoiding xylazine as preanesthetic medication when using halothane and using low doses (4 to 8 mg/kg) of thiobarbiturates for induction of anesthesia (see Table 163–4). Halothane is metabolized to a significant extent (25 per cent), although it seldom causes organ system toxicity (specifically liver toxicity). Halothane can induce malignant hyperthermia in susceptible dogs and cats, but this is very rare. Environmental pollution is a potential risk to operating room personnel.

Isoflurane, a relatively new inhalation anesthetic, is rapidly increasing in popularity because of its purported safety for patients and minimal metabolism (little or no toxic metabolites), and because it produces relatively rapid induction and recovery from anesthesia. Isoflurane produces excellent short- or long-term anesthesia in birds and reptiles. It does not sensitize the myocardium to catecholamines like halothane but can produce marked hypotension and respiratory depression (see Table 163–5). Recovery from anesthesia can be so rapid in some dogs and cats that excitement and delirium may occur, requiring resedation. Despite these problems, when isoflurane is appropriately used, its advantages outweigh its disadvantages. One practical consideration is cost. Isoflurane is less potent and more volatile than methoxyflurane or halothane, requiring higher concentrations to maintain anesthesia.

Nitrous oxide can be used to add analgesia and muscle relaxation. It must be administered as at least 40 to 70 per cent of the inspired gas concentration in normal dogs and cats if any real beneficial effect is to be derived, and it should not exceed 70 per cent of the inspired gas concentration if hypoxia is to be avoided (see Table 163–4). Nitrous oxide hastens induction of anesthesia (second gas effect) and can produce hypoxia during recovery, owing to its rapid elimination from the blood, if oxygen is discontinued before nitrous oxide. Despite potential hypoxia, nitrous oxide is a safe drug when used appropriately and does not produce

TABLE 163–6. NONDEPOLARIZING NEUROMUSCULAR BLOCKING DRUGS (NNBD) AND THEIR ANTAGONISTS

NNBDs	IV Dose (μg/kg)	Duration of Action (Minutes)
Pancuronium	15–20	10–90
Vecuronium	10–20 (dog)	20–40 (dog)
	20–40 (cat)	10–15 (cat)
Atracurium	100–250	20–30
NNBD Antagonists*		**IV Dose (mg/kg)**
Neostigmine		0.02–0.04
Pyridostigmine		0.1–0.2
Edrophonium		1.0–1.2

*Should be preceded by an anticholinergic (0.01 mg/kg IM or IV glycopyrrolate).

*Editor's note.

cardiopulmonary depression. It produces no known toxic metabolites and decreases the concentration of inhalation anesthetic (methoxyflurane, halothane, isoflurane) required.

NEUROMUSCULAR BLOCKING DRUGS

The peripheral neuromuscular blocking drugs can be used as adjuncts to anesthesia and surgery but are infrequently used in veterinary surgery (Table 163–6). As a group, they are known for their inability to produce hypnosis, their tendency to cause respiratory depression, their lack of analgesia, and their propensity to cause hypothermia secondary to skeletal muscle relaxation. Depolarizing (succinylcholine) and nondepolarizing drugs are available, although nondepolarizing (pancuronium, vecuronium, atracurium) drugs are currently preferred because of their predictable duration of action and reversibility with acetylcholinesterase inhibitors (see Table 163–6). When used at recommended dosages with adequate analgesia and controlled ventilation, nondepolarizing neuromuscular blocking drugs are excellent adjuncts to surgery and provide unparalleled muscle relaxation. Muscle paralysis may greatly facilitate fracture repair and exploration of the abdominal cavity or permit uninterrupted delicate surgery of the eye. Their use is unlikely to increase, given the previous potential complications and the necessity of close nursing care during recovery to ensure adequate return of ventilation.

References

1. Booth NH: Hypnotics, sedatives, and anticonvulsants. *In* Booth NH, McDonald LE (eds): *Veterinary Pharmacology and Therapeutics*. 6th ed. Iowa State University Press, Ames, 1988, pp 275–289.
2. Booth NH: Inhalant anesthetics. *In* Booth NH, McDonald LE (eds): *Veterinary Pharmacology and Therapeutics*. 6th ed. Iowa State University Press, Ames, 1988, pp 181–211.
3. Booth NH: Intravenous and other parenteral anesthetics. *In* Booth NH, McDonald LE (eds): *Veterinary Pharmacology and Therapeutics*. 6th ed. Iowa State University Press, Ames, 1988, pp 212–274.
4. Booth NH: Neuroleptanalgesics, narcotic analgesics, and analgesic antagonists. *In* Booth NH, McDonald LE (eds): *Veterinary Pharmacology and Therapeutics*. 6th ed. Iowa State University Press, Ames, 1988, pp 290–328.
5. Booth NH: Nonnarcotic analgesics. *In* Booth NH, McDonald LE (eds): *Veterinary Pharmacology and Therapeutics*. 6th ed. Iowa State University Press, Ames, 1988, pp 329–362.
6. Gleed RD: Tranquilizers and sedatives. *In* Short CE (ed): *Principles and Practice of Veterinary Anesthesia*. Williams & Wilkins, Baltimore, 1987, pp 16–27.
7. Lumb WV, Jones EW: The barbiturates. *In* Lumb WV, Jones EW (eds): *Veterinary Anesthesia*. 2nd ed. Lea & Febiger, Philadelphia, 1984, pp 279–306.
8. Lumb WV, Jones EW: General anesthesia. *In* Lumb WV, Jones EW (eds): *Veterinary Anesthesia*. 2nd ed. Lea & Febiger, Philadelphia, 1984, pp 199–212.
9. Lumb WV, Jones EW: The inhalation anesthetics. *In* Lumb WV, Jones EW (eds): *Veterinary Anesthesia*. 2nd ed. Lea & Febiger, Philadelphia, 1984, pp 213–240.
10. Lumb WV, Jones EW: Methods and equipment for administration of inhalation anesthetics. *In* Lumb WV, Jones EW (eds): *Veterinary Anesthesia*. 2nd ed. Lea & Febiger, Philadelphia, 1984, pp 241–278.
11. Lumb WV, Jones EW: The muscle relaxants and other adjuvants to anesthesia. *In* Lumb WV, Jones EW (eds): *Veterinary Anesthesia*. 2nd ed. Lea & Febiger, Philadelphia, 1984, pp 333–356.
12. Lumb WV, Jones EW: Preanesthetic agents. *In* Lumb WV, Jones EW (eds): *Veterinary Anesthesia*. 2nd ed. Lea & Febiger, Philadelphia, 1984, pp 165–198.
13. Short CE: Anticholinergics. *In* Short CE (ed): *Principles and Practice of Veterinary Anesthesia*. Williams & Wilkins, Baltimore, 1987, pp 8–15.
14. Short CE: Barbiturate anesthesia. *In* Short CE (ed): *Principles and Practice of Veterinary Anesthesia*. Williams & Wilkins, Baltimore, 1987, pp 58–69.
15. Short CE: Dissociative anesthesia. *In* Short CE (ed): *Principles and Practice of Veterinary Anesthesia*. Williams & Wilkins, Baltimore, 1987, pp 158–172.
16. Short CE: Inhalant anesthetics. *In* Short CE (ed): *Principles and Practice of Veterinary Anesthesia*. Williams & Wilkins, Baltimore, 1987, pp 70–90.
17. Short CE: Neuroleptanalgesia and alpha-adrenergic receptor analgesia. *In* Short CE (ed): *Principles and Practice of Veterinary Anesthesia*. Williams & Wilkins, Baltimore, 1987, pp 47–57.
18. Short CE: Pain, analgesics, and related medications. *In* Short CE (ed): *Principles and Practice of Veterinary Anesthesia*. Williams & Wilkins, Baltimore, 1987, pp 28–46.

CHAPTER 164 Equipment and Techniques for Inhalation Anesthesia

Richard M. Bednarski

Nitrous oxide and the four commonly used volatile inhalation anesthetics—methoxyflurane, halothane, enflurane, and isoflurane—are administered using many types of equipment. Various breathing circuits and vaporizers are used to produce the same result, delivery of oxygen and anesthetic to the patient and removal of carbon dioxide (CO_2). A particular breathing circuit can be used with diverse fresh gas (oxygen and nitrous oxide) flow rates. This chapter reviews the components of the anesthetic machine and the various breathing circuits available for administration of inhalation anesthetics. Emphasis is on rational selection and use of a breathing circuit. A more complete discussion of use and function of the anesthetic machine can be found elsewhere.[2, 10, 11]

THE ANESTHETIC MACHINE

A generic anesthetic machine consists of (1) a source of oxygen and anesthetic and (2) a breathing circuit through which the mixture of anesthetic and oxygen is delivered to a patient's airway in exchange for exhaled CO_2 (Fig. 164–1).

Oxygen and nitrous oxide are usually supplied to the anesthetic machine from high-pressure cylinders. Alternatively, oxygen can be supplied from an oxygen-gen-

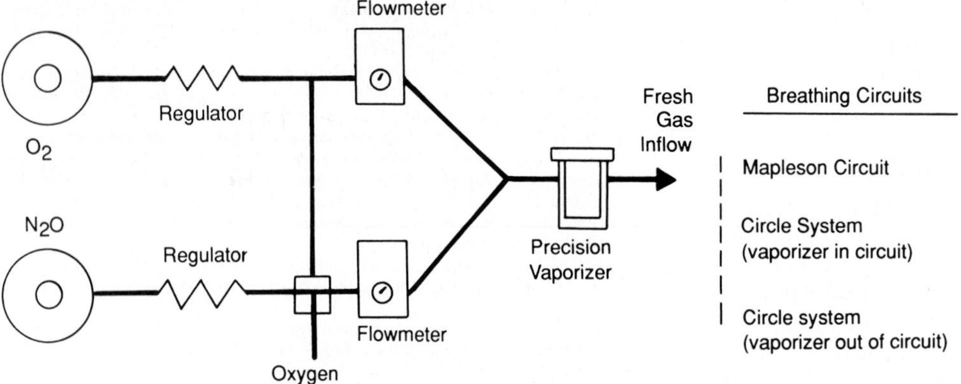

FIGURE 164–1. Schematic diagram of an anesthetic machine and its connection to various breathing circuits.

erating device, or in extremely high-use situations, oxygen can be supplied from insulated containers of liquid oxygen. A full high-pressure cylinder of oxygen is pressurized to approximately 2,000 psi, whereas the pressure within a nitrous oxide cylinder is 750 psi. A pressure regulator reduces incoming cylinder pressure to approximately 50 psi. The regulator delivers a constant pressure to the flowmeters from fluctuating cylinder pressures. Most machines are equipped with an oxygen regulator that connects to a portable E-sized cylinder. An additional regulator for nitrous oxide may be present. A separate regulator is required when large nonportable cylinders are used for the gas supply.

Many newer machines are equipped with an oxygen fail-safe device downstream from the pressure regulators to stop the flow of nitrous oxide in the event that the oxygen supply is disconnected or the oxygen supply pressure drops by 50 per cent. Some of these fail-safe devices have an audible alarm.

The flowmeter assemblies receive gas from the regulators at a pressure of 50 psi. Individual flowmeters for oxygen and nitrous oxide may be preset. The flowmeters control and indicate the flow of gas passing through. The flowmeters consist of smoothly tapered hollow glass tubes. A variable flow of gas, determined by rotation of the flowmeter control knob, enters the bottom of the tube and causes an indicator float to rise within the tube. The greater the flow rate, the higher the float rises, and the flow rate is read from a scale printed along the float. Some machines are equipped with two oxygen flowmeters. One indicates flow rates from 0 to 1 L/minute, and the other indicates flows greater than 1 L/minute. This flowmeter configuration is preferable when using low-flow systems.

Volatile liquid anesthetic is transformed into a vapor within the anesthetic vaporizer. Two types of vaporizers are in use. Most recently manufactured anesthetic vaporizers are agent-specific devices that deliver a constant known output despite changes in ambient temperature or the flow rate of gas passing through the vaporizer (Fig. 164–2). These "precision" vaporizers can be used with any type of breathing circuit. A disadvantage of this vaporizer is that it is expensive to purchase and should only be used for one anesthetic. The other type of vaporizer, referred to as a "draw-over" type, is limited to a location within a circle breathing circuit. Examples of this type of vaporizer include the Ohio Number 8 Vaporizer (Fig. 164–3) and the Stephans Universal Vaporizer (Fig. 164–4). The output of these vaporizers varies with the flow of gas passing through the vaporizer, the ambient temperature, the length of time the vaporizer is in use, and the type of anesthetic used.[4] These vaporizers are not readily adaptable for use with Mapleson breathing circuits.

ANESTHETIC BREATHING CIRCUITS

Breathing circuits have been classified according to numerous confusing schemes.[2] Words such as *open, semiopen, semiclosed*, and *closed* mean different things to different people, and a more useful classification is based on a functional description of the components present and the fresh gas flow rates used.[4] Many breathing circuit configurations exist. Two types are commonly used in small animal anesthesia, Mapleson circuits and circle rebreathing systems.

Mapleson Circuits

Mapleson circuits depend on the fresh gas flow to remove exhaled CO_2 (Fig. 164–5). If relatively high fresh gas flow rates are used, these circuits are nonrebreathing circuits. They are mechanically simple, consisting of a fresh gas delivery line, corrugated tubing, a breathing bag, and pressure relief valve or opening. Relative simplicity and low cost are major advantages. Another advantage is that these systems are relatively easy to clean. The Mapleson A, D, and F are in common use (see Fig. 164–5).

The Mapleson A system, also called a *Magill system*, was the first modern anesthetic breathing system developed and is still popular in Great Britain. Fresh gas enters the system near the breathing bag, and excess gas is discharged through a pressure relief valve located near the attachment of the endotracheal tube. Fresh gas flow rates during spontaneous ventilation should be equal to the patient's minute ventilation (tidal volume × frequency) to prevent rebreathing of exhaled CO_2. The disadvantage of this system is that it cannot be used reliably during controlled ventilation because high fresh

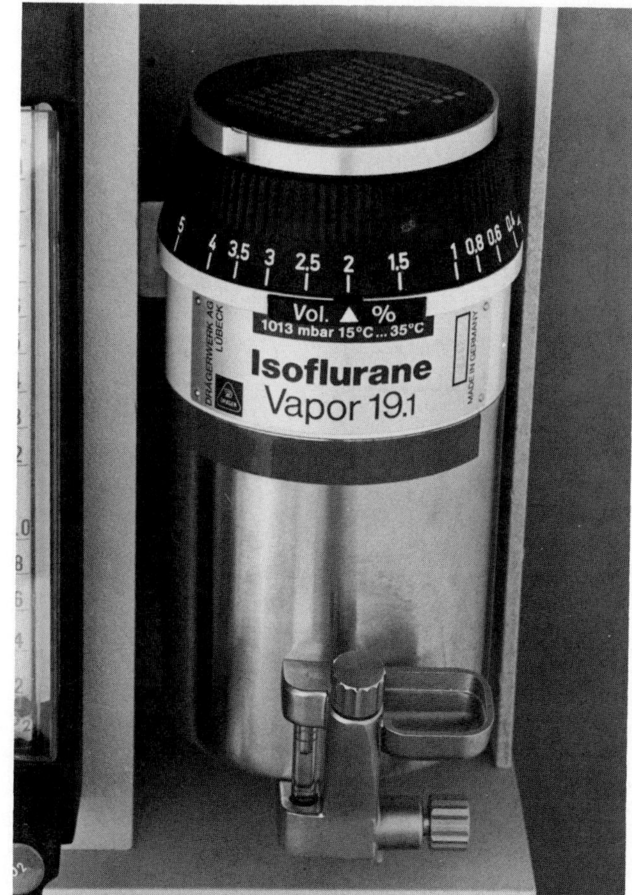

FIGURE 164–2. Precision vaporizer for delivery of isoflurane. (N. A. Dragar, Telford, PA.)

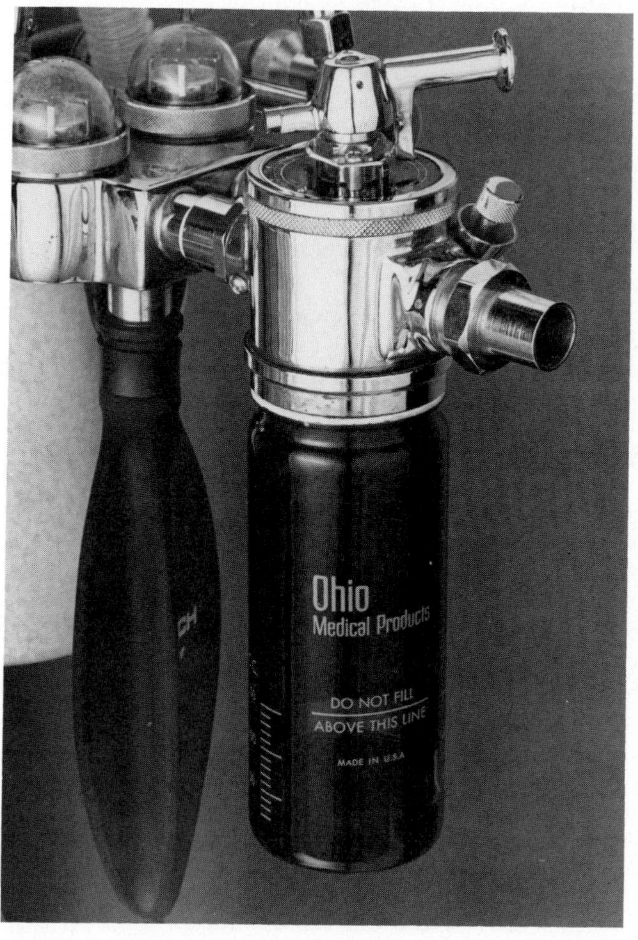

FIGURE 164–3. Draw-over vaporizer. This vaporizer is located within the circle. (Anaquest, Madison, WI.)

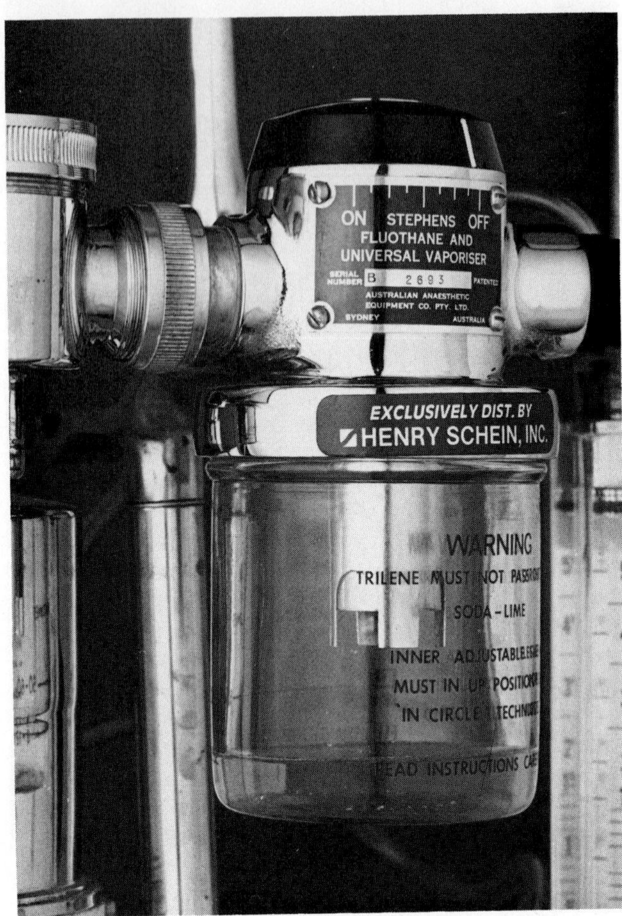

FIGURE 164–4. Draw-over vaporizer. This vaporizer is located within the circle. (Henry-Schein Inc., Port Washington, NY.)

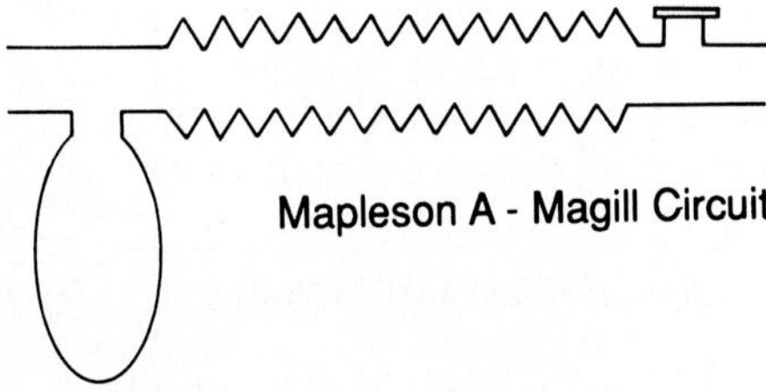

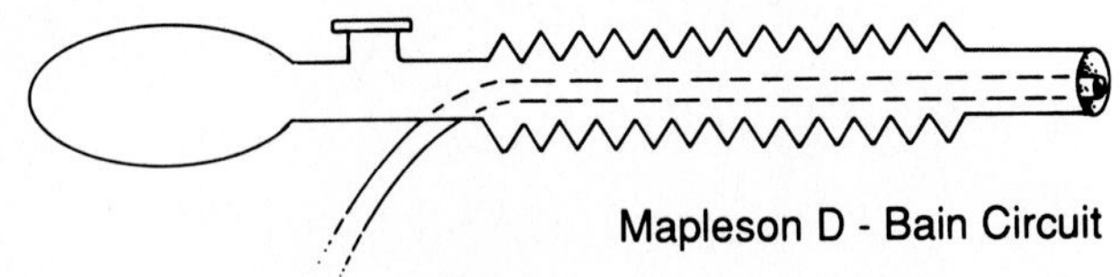

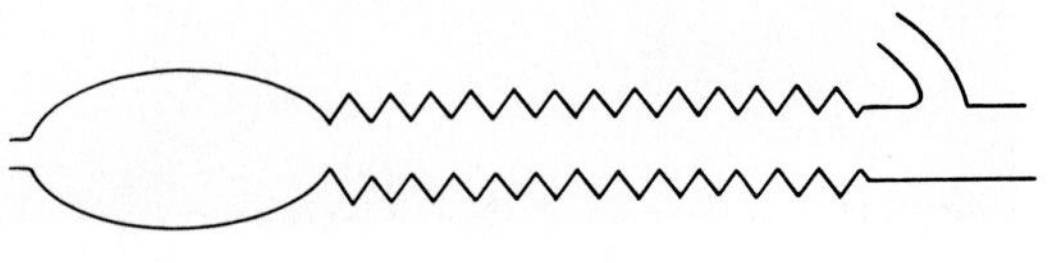

FIGURE 164–5. Schematic of Mapleson breathing circuits. All circuits consist of a breathing bag, fresh gas delivery hose, and a corrugated hose for removal of exhaled gas. In addition, the Magill circuit uses a pressure relief valve.

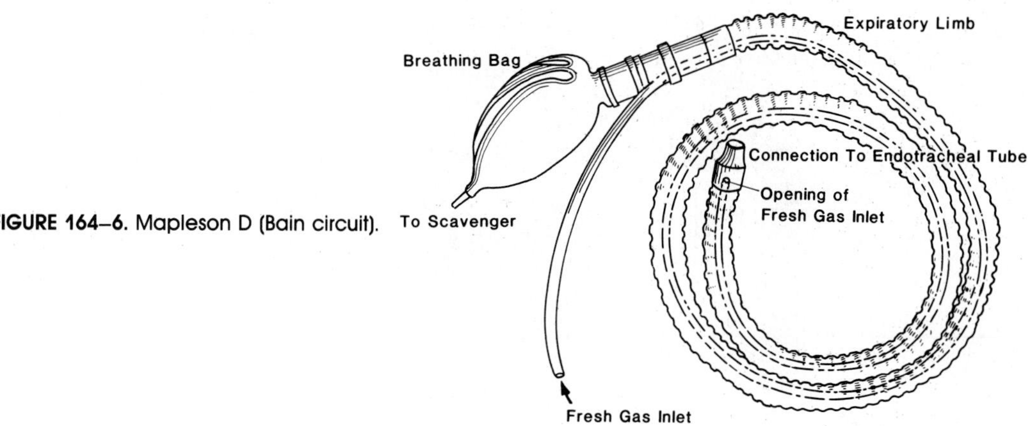

FIGURE 164–6. Mapleson D (Bain circuit).

gas flow rates are necessary to prevent rebreathing of CO_2.[8] This is because of the location of the pressure relief valve relative to the fresh gas inflow.

The Mapleson D and F circuits are functionally similar. An example of the Mapleson D circuit in common use is the coaxial or Bain circuit (Fig. 164–6). Fresh gas flows through the inner hose of the coaxial tube and passes to the patient near the endotracheal tube connection. Exhaled gas flows around the inner tube, through the corrugated tube, toward the reservoir bag. The Jackson-Rees modification of the Ayres T piece (Fig. 164–7) is an example of the Mapleson F system. Fresh gas is delivered to the patient near the endotracheal tube connection, and exhaled gas flows through the corrugated tube to exit through the tail of the reservoir bag. The D and F systems can be used with spontaneous or controlled ventilation. Fresh gas flow rates are adjusted to at least 1.5 to 3 times minute ventilation to eliminate rebreathing of exhaled gases.[1,5] Fresh gas flow rates as low as 100 to 150 ml/kg can be used.[1,7] These relatively low fresh gas flow rates permit partial rebreathing of exhaled gas but do not result in hypercarbia.[7] The advantage of these lower flow rates is maintenance of a warmer, more humid airway.

Circle Rebreathing Systems

The circle rebreathing anesthetic system was first introduced by Sword in 1929.[13] The advantage of the circle system is that relatively low fresh gas flow rates are used. Fresh gas flow can be low because of the presence of CO_2-absorbent material within the circuit.

Components of the Circle System

(Figs. 164–8 and 164–9)

Exhaled CO_2 is removed from the circle breathing circuit via a chemical reaction, whereas with the Mapleson systems CO_2 is removed by the flushing action of high fresh gas flow rates. Exhaled CO_2 reacts with water and a hydroxide of the alkaline earth metals to form carbonate and water. The chemical reaction is exothermic. The reaction also lowers the pH of the absorbent material, and a pH-sensitive indicator changes color to signal exhaustion of absorbent material. Unidirectional valves direct gas flow away from the patient through one breathing hose and to the patient through the other hose. These valves prevent the patient from rebreathing exhaled gas before it passes through the CO_2-absorbent canister.

The paired breathing hoses conduct inhaled gas to and exhaled gas away from the patient. The tubes are corrugated to prevent kinking. Standard 22-mm-diameter hoses are suitable for use with medium to large (heavier than 5 kg) animals. Smaller-diameter hoses are more suitable for patients weighing less than 5 kg. These smaller hoses decrease the overall volume and response time of the circle system.

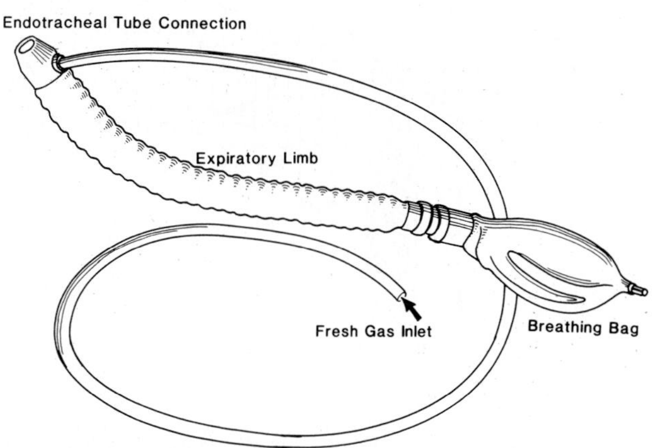

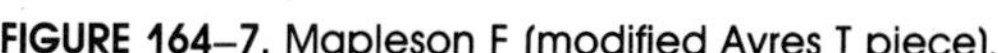

FIGURE 164–7. Mapleson F (modified Ayres T piece).

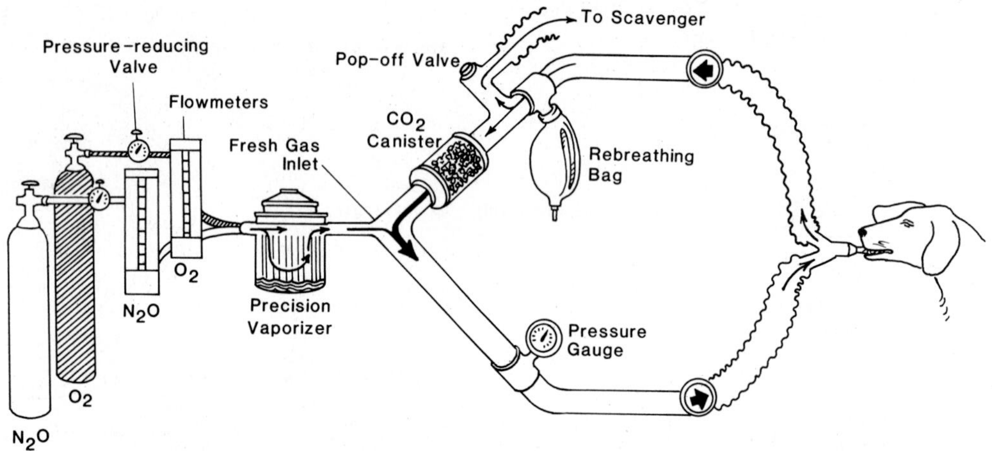

FIGURE 164–8. Circle rebreathing system with the vaporizer located out of the circle.

The pressure relief valve vents gas to the atmosphere via the waste gas scavenging system. The valve in the fully open position allows gas to escape when pressure within the breathing circuit reaches 0.5 to 1.5 cm H_2O. The valve is closed to ventilate the patient manually.

The breathing bag provides visual assessment of ventilation. It is a compliant structure and expands and contracts with each exhalation and inhalation. The bag, depending on its compliance, remains inflated to some degree throughout the respiratory cycle. The bag can be compressed to deliver a breath manually. Too large a bag makes visual assessment of ventilation difficult and also adds unnecessary volume to the circuit; too small a bag provides an inadequate reservoir for large tidal volumes. A 1-L bag is suitable for cats and small dogs, a 2-L bag for medium-sized dogs, and a 3-L bag for large dogs.

The fresh gas inlet delivers oxygen and anesthetic gas to the breathing circuit. This inflow of gas replenishes the oxygen and anesthetic gas removed from the circuit by the patient. If fresh gas flow rate is in excess of that removed by the patient, the excess gas fills the breathing system and exits through the pressure relief valve (semiclosed system). If the fresh gas inflow matches uptake by the patient, no gas flows out of the pressure relief valve (closed system).

An anesthetic vaporizer can be located within the anesthetic circle (see Fig. 164–9). These vaporizers are simply constructed. They are suitable for use with all the commonly used volatile agents and are particularly useful during closed-system anesthesia because their output does not directly depend on the fresh gas flow rate.[12] The wick is left in the vaporizer only when methoxyflurone is used.

Fresh Gas Flow Rates

The increasing use of relatively expensive isoflurane and the heightened awareness of the dangers of exposure to trace anesthetic gas concentrations have sparked interest in using economical anesthetic techniques. A way to minimize anesthetic cost is to minimize the fresh gas flow rate. The lower the fresh gas flow rate, the less anesthetic used. The minimum flow rate of oxygen that

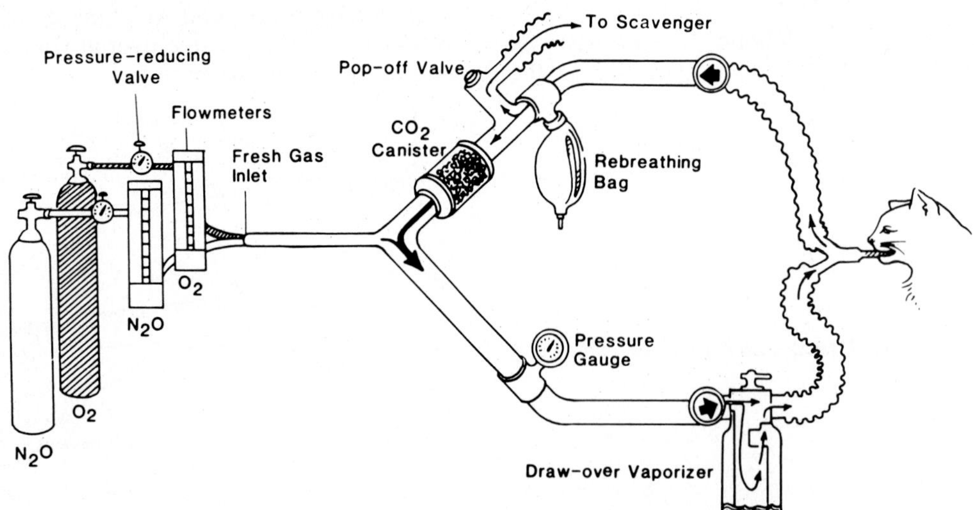

FIGURE 164–9. Circle rebreathing system with the vaporizer located within the circle.

TABLE 164–1. MAINTENANCE VAPORIZER SETTINGS FOR PRECISION VAPORIZERS

Anesthetic	Mapleson System*	Semiclosed Circle†	Closed Circle‡
Halothane	1.0–2.0	1.0–2.0	2.0–4.0
Isoflurane	1.25–2.5	1.5–2.75	3.0–5.0
Methoxyflurane	0.2–1.0	0.25–2.0	2.0–3.0
Enflurane	2.0–3.5	2.5–4.0	4.0–6.0

Vaporizer dial settings are for temperature- and flow-compensated (precision) vaporizers.
*Fresh gas flow rates ≥ 100–150 ml/kg/minute.
†Fresh gas flow rates = 20 ml/kg/minute.
‡Fresh gas flow rates = 3–6 ml/kg/minute.

can be used with the circle system just equals a patient's minute oxygen consumption: $10 \times$ body weight $(kg)^{3/4}$, or approximately 3 to 6 ml/kg.[9] For example, a 15-kg dog requires an oxygen flow rate of approximately 80 ml/minute. This low flow rate can be used immediately after anesthetic induction and intubation and continued throughout the anesthetic period when an in-circle vaporizer is used. This is possible because vaporization of the anesthetic within the vaporizer depends on the minute ventilation and not the fresh gas flow.[12] When an out-of-circle vaporizer is used, relatively high oxygen flow rates (1 to 3 L/minute) are initially needed to rapidly deliver the anesthetic vapor leaving the vaporizer into the circle. Oxygen flow rate can be decreased within 20 minutes of induction to closed-system flow rates. Maintenance vaporizer settings for out-of-circle vaporizers during closed-system anesthesia are high (Table 164–1) because the low fresh gas flow carrying anesthetic into the circle carries only small volumes of volatile anesthetic with it. A disadvantage of a closed-system flow rate with an out-of-circle vaporizer arrangement is that anesthetic concentration cannot be changed rapidly without increasing the oxygen flow rate. The pressure relief valve is opened, and the fresh gas flow is increased to between 1 and 3 L/minute. The fresh gas flow is returned to a closed-system flow rate when a patient reaches the desired anesthetic plane. This difficulty in rapidly increasing anesthetic depth is not a problem with an in-circle arrangement because low fresh gas flow rates do not impede the anesthetic rate of rise.

The disadvantage of the relatively slow rate of change in anesthetic concentration, when using closed-system flow rates with an out-of-circle vaporizer, can be eliminated by using flow rates that are greater than the minute oxygen consumption. The higher flow rate more rapidly delivers anesthetic into the circle system and facilitates the rate of change of anesthetic concentration. A maintenance oxygen flow rate of 20 ml/kg/minute allows a rapid rate of change and is also economical. This oxygen flow rate of 20 ml/kg/minute is high enough to avoid hypoxia if nitrous oxide is used. Nitrous oxide should not be used with closed-system flow rates unless an oxygen analyzer is inserted into the circle. This is because the concentration of nitrous oxide can gradually increase relative to the oxygen concentration, resulting in a hypoxic gas mixture.

CHOICE OF ANESTHETIC BREATHING CIRCUITS

The choice of anesthetic breathing circuit is primarily determined by a patient's size. Resistance to breathing is greater in a circle system than a Mapleson system. The relatively small tidal volume of a small patient does not adequately mix the gas within the circle. Studies confirm that patients as small as 2.5 kg can be safely anesthetized using a circle system.[3, 6] Debilitated dogs or cats or those that have pulmonary disease and weigh between 2.5 and 5 kg retain better cardiopulmonary function when anesthetized with Mapleson systems.

References

1. Conway CM, et al: Spontaneous ventilation with the Bain system. *Br J Anaesth 49*:1245, 1977.
2. Dorsch JA, Dorsch SE: *Understanding Anesthesia Equipment*. 2nd ed. Williams & Wilkins, Baltimore, 1984.
3. Graff TD, et al: Acid-base balance in infants during halothane anesthesia with the use of an adult circle-absorption system. *Anesth Analg 43*:583, 1964.
4. Hamilton WK: Nomenclature of inhalation anesthetic systems. *Anesthesiology 25*:3, 1964.
5. Harrison GA: The effect of the respiratory flow pattern on rebreathing in a T-piece system. *Br J Anaesth 36*:206, 1964.
6. Hartsfield SM, Sawyer DC: Cardiopulmonary effects of rebreathing and nonrebreathing systems during halothane anesthesia in the cat. *Am J Vet Res 37*:1461, 1976.
7. Manley SV, McDonell WN: Clinical evaluation of the Bain breathing circuit in small animal anesthesia. *J Am Anim Hosp Assoc 15*:67, 1979.
8. Mapleson WW: Theoretical considerations of the effect of rebreathing in two semi-closed anaesthetic systems. *Br Med Bull 14*:64, 1958.
9. Moens Y: Introduction to the quantitative technique of closed circuit anesthesia in dogs. *Vet Surg 17*:98, 1988.
10. Muir WW, et al: *Handbook of Veterinary Anesthesia*. CV Mosby, St Louis, 1989.
11. Short CE (ed): *Principles and Practice of Veterinary Anesthesia*. Williams & Wilkins, Baltimore, 1987.
12. Soma LR, Klide AM: Techniques and equipment for inhalation anesthesia in small animals. *J Am Vet Med Assoc 152*:957, 1968.
13. Sword BC: Closed circle method of administration of gas anesthesia. *Anesth Analg 9*:198, 1930.

CHAPTER

165 Anesthesia for Elective Soft-Tissue and Orthopedic Procedures

James S. Gaynor and Thomas K. Day

Elective soft-tissue operations are the most widely performed procedures in veterinary medicine, including elective ovariohysterectomy and castration. Dogs and cats presented for these procedures are usually young and healthy and have no systemic diseases. Other commonly performed elective procedures include ear cropping and cosmetic removal of benign masses of the integument. Animals in the latter group vary in age and physical condition. Orthopedic procedures are also commonly performed, including fracture repair, metabolic bone defect repair, amputations, and corrective long-bone surgery.

A systematic review of history, physical examination findings, and laboratory data is essential for safe and effective anesthesia.

PREANESTHETIC PREPARATION

Medications that the animal is currently receiving are noted so that potential drug interactions can be avoided (Table 165–1). Past physical health and vaccination status are ascertained. Sexually mature females should have a thorough reproductive history focusing on the most recent estrus or pregnancy. Any history of an abnormal estrous cycle or possible pregnancy is investigated further during the physical and laboratory examination.

Elective operations other than sterilization require a more detailed history because older dogs and cats may show signs of systemic disorders. Questions concerning tolerance to exercise, eating habits, and water consumption assist in identifying problems with the cardiovascular, renal, and endocrine systems.

A recent history detailing respiratory pattern, urination, defecation, and temperament can provide valuable information about systemic disorders, particularly those resulting from trauma. Physical examination and laboratory findings become more important in these patients.

Accurate measurement of body weight is essential because it assists in proper dosing of potentially dangerous anesthetic drugs. Mental state and temperament are observed. Excitable or vicious animals require more intense preoperative sedation than those that are quiet and depressed. Mucous membrane color and capillary refill time are evaluated. Pale mucous membranes suggest anemia, and slow capillary refill (>1 to 2 seconds) suggests cardiovascular dysfunction.

Thoracic auscultation and palpation of peripheral pulses assist evaluation of cardiopulmonary function. Any abnormal findings such as heart murmurs, pulse deficits, or abnormal lung sounds are pursued with electrocardiography, radiography, and more specific testing.

The abdomen is palpated to determine the presence of organomegaly, which is important in female patients presented for ovariohysterectomy with a history suggesting pregnancy.

Close evaluation of the cardiopulmonary system in trauma patients may reveal arrhythmias due to myocardial contusion, labored breathing due to pneumothorax or pulmonary contusions, or severe anemia from trauma-associated blood loss. Thoracic radiography can be performed to assist in the diagnosis of fractured ribs, pulmonary contusions, pneumothorax, and diaphragmatic hernia. Electrocardiogram tracings are important to evaluate possible cardiac arrhythmias or ST-T segment depression suggesting traumatic myocarditis. Serial packed cell volume (PCV) and total protein (TP) are determined if internal hemorrhage is suspected.

PHYSICAL STATUS

A classification system for veterinary patients based on that established by the American Society of Anesthesiologists can be used to classify the risk of anesthesia (Table 165–2).

TABLE 165–1. POTENTIAL DRUG INTERACTIONS

Drug 1	Drug 2	Interaction
Acepromazine	Organophosphates (anthelmintics, insecticides)	Acepromazine enhances anticholinesterase inhibitory effects of organophosphates
Nondepolarizing muscle relaxants	Aminoglycoside antibiotics	Potentiation of neuromuscular blockade
Barbiturates, hypnotics	Chloramphenicol, H_2 blockers (cimetidine and ranitidine)	Enhanced duration of action of barbiturates and hypnotics due to inhibition of hepatic microsomal enzyme activity
Barbiturates, hypnotics	Phenobarbital	Decreased duration of action of barbiturates and hypnotics due to hepatic microsomal enzyme induction
Halothane, methoxyflurane	Beta blockers	Potentiation of negative inotropy

TABLE 165–2. CLASSIFICATION OF PATIENT'S PHYSICAL STATUS

Category	Description	Example
I	Normal, healthy patient	Six-month-old patient presented for elective sterilization with no discernible systemic disease
II	Patient with mild systemic disease	Uncomplicated fracture, compensated heart disease (mitral regurgitation)
III	Patient with severe systemic disease, limiting activity but not incapacitating	Anemia, fever, cachexia, compensated renal disease
IV	Patient with severe, incapacitating systemic disease that is a constant threat to life	Trauma (pneumothorax, uroabdomen), noncompensated heart disease or uremia
V	Moribund patient not expected to live 24 hours with or without surgery	Terminal malignancy, severe trauma

Most young, healthy patients admitted for elective sterilization are excellent risks for anesthesia (class I). Healthy geriatric animals and those animals with simple fractures not resulting from major trauma, as well as obese patients, are placed in class II. Class III includes patients with a history of major trauma and those with compensated chronic heart disease or anemia. Anesthetic management of class IV and V patients is discussed in subsequent chapters.

LABORATORY DATA

The laboratory data required to perform anesthesia safely are based on physical status and age (Table 165–3). A minimum laboratory data base for class I and II patients includes PCV and TP determinations. These can be performed simultaneously with a small amount of blood, microhematocrit capillary tubes, and centrifuge.

The laboratory data for patients in classes II and III may vary depending on history and physical examination. More laboratory tests may be needed in older patients to assess systemic function properly. The tests include a complete blood count (CBC), chemistry profile, and urinalysis. A CBC and chemistry profile are ideal in an animal 5 to 10 years of age, but alternative, less expensive tests include blood dipstick tests for BUN and glucose and manual blood smear examination. A CBC and profile are evaluated in animals older than 10 years. Ancillary tests or procedures such as radiography, electrocardiography, or ultrasonography are considered if any abnormalities are found on physical examination or laboratory data.

ANESTHETIC TECHNIQUES

A safe anesthetic plan is formulated after considering the animal's temperament, physical status, previous medical history, current medication, and the type of procedure to be performed. The anesthetic plan encompasses choice of anesthetic drugs, their route of administration, fluid support, temperature regulation, monitoring, and postanesthetic care.

Food but not water is withheld for 8 to 12 hours before anesthesia, except in dogs less than 3 kg or neonates, to help ensure an empty stomach and minimize vomiting and aspiration of gastric contents. Blood glucose should be evaluated preoperatively and supplemented if necessary in neonates and dogs weighing less than 3 kg.

INTRAVENOUS CATHETERIZATION

A peripheral vein is catheterized before administering intravenous anesthetic drugs. A patent intravenous line allows administration of fluids during the perianesthetic period and, if necessary, rapid administration of emergency medications. Over-the-needle catheters, through-the-needle catheters, and butterfly needles can be used.

Over-the-needle catheters have an inner stylet with a beveled edge for venipuncture. The catheter, which can consist of various materials such as Teflon or polyethylene, is advanced, and the stylet withdrawn once in the vein. These catheters are inexpensive. Over-the-needle catheters are technically easy to insert and maintain patent. A 20-gauge 5-cm catheter is suitable for use in dogs or cats weighing more than 3 kg. A 22-gauge 3.8-cm catheter is suitable for use in dogs or cats weighing less than 3 kg.

Through-the-needle catheters are expensive. The catheter size is smaller than the needle through which it passes. It is difficult with this type of catheter to administer large volumes of fluids rapidly. These catheters also predispose to hematoma formation at the venipuncture site. Through-the-needle catheters initially require slightly more technical skill to insert. They may be more difficult to insert in small peripheral veins because of the relatively large needle diameter. They are generally easier to maintain for long periods because of their length and are advantageous in the intensive care unit. A 17-gauge 11-cm catheter is usually suitable

TABLE 165–3. MINIMUM LABORATORY DATA BASED ON PATIENT'S PHYSICAL STATUS

Physical Status Category	Minimum Laboratory Data
I	Packed cell volume, total protein
II	Packed cell volume, total protein, Azostick
III*	Complete blood count, blood urea nitrogen, creatinine
IV*	Complete blood count, chemistry profile, urinalysis
V*	Complete blood count, chemistry profile, urinalysis, blood gas

*Laboratory data obtained are determined by the signalment, physical examination, and history.

for use in animals weighing more than 7 kg. A 19-gauge 11-cm catheter is suitable for use in animals weighing less than 7 kg.

A butterfly catheter consists of a short needle with two plastic wings attached distally. It is very easy to lacerate the vessel inadvertently because the needle portion of the catheter remains in the vein. Butterfly catheters are potentially adequate for short-term use. Their insertion is simple in healthy, calm dogs and cats.

The most common location for catheter insertion is the cephalic vein in both dogs and cats. The lateral saphenous vein in dogs and the medial saphenous vein in cats may be cannulated if the cephalics are not accessible or appropriate. The jugular vein can also be cannulated and is preferred for long-term catheterization or when large volumes of fluids or hyperosmotic drugs are to be administered.

FLUID ADMINISTRATION

Fluid administration is a useful adjunct to general anesthesia. Intravenous fluids expand the effective vascular volume, which may be reduced by anesthetic drugs. A balanced electrolyte or isotonic solution is recommended for routine fluid replacement in normal, healthy animals. Examples include 0.9 per cent saline, Ringer solution, lactated Ringer solution, and various dextrose (2.5, 5 per cent) combinations. Fluids are administered at 5 to 10 ml/kg/hour in normal, healthy patients. The PCV and TP are determined during prolonged procedures or if significant blood loss is encountered. Blood or plasma is administered if PCV decreases to 20 or TP decreases to 3.5 g/100 ml.

ROUTES OF DRUG ADMINISTRATION

The onset of drug action and duration of effect are longer after the intramuscular and subcutaneous routes than after the intravenous route. The intramuscular and subcutaneous routes are most useful for fractious or excitable animals and are the most commonly used routes of premedication. The intravenous route produces greater peak effect and has a shorter onset and duration of action than the intramuscular and subcutaneous routes and requires a cooperative patient. The advantage of the intravenous route is that the onset of the desired effect is more rapid. Further, some useful preanesthetic drugs like diazepam have a more predictable action after intravenous administration. The intramuscular and subcutaneous routes may also be less predictable than the intravenous.

ANESTHETIC TECHNIQUES

The following examples represent anesthetic plans for routine elective operations. An understanding of the pharmacology of the anesthetic drugs (Chapter 163) is necessary for safe anesthetic administration.

Aggressive Dog

Signalment

A 4-year-old 50-kg intact male rottweiller was presented for prophylactic dental cleaning and polishing.

History, Physical Examination, and Laboratory Data

Current vaccinations; no current problems; unable to handle; PCV = 39, TP = 7.4, heartworm negative.

Premedication

Innovar-Vet, 3 ml IM (60 mg droperidol + 1.2 mg fentanyl).

Induction

Thiamylal sodium, 200 to 400 mg IV.

Maintenance

Halothane; semiclosed circle rebreathing system; 1 L/minute oxygen flow; lactated Ringer solution, 500 ml/hour.

Routine Soft-Tissue Surgery—Dog

Signalment

A 6-month-old 12-kg alert female mixed-breed was presented for ovariohysterectomy.

History, Physical Examination, and Laboratory Data

Current vaccinations, normal on examination; no previous estrus; PCV = 44; TP = 7.9; heartworm and fecal negative.

Premedication

Acepromazine, 1.5 mg IM.

Induction

Thiamylal sodium, 50 to 100 mg IV.

Maintenance

Halothane; semiclosed circle rebreathing system; 250 to 500 ml/minute oxygen flow and lactated Ringer's solution.

Routine Orthopedic Surgery—Dog

Signalment

An 8-year-old 4-kg neutered male poodle was presented for repair of ruptured anterior cruciate ligament.

History, Physical Examination, and Laboratory Data

Three-day duration of lameness; positive anterior drawer in right rear limb; otherwise normal on physical examination; PCV = 38; TP = 7.1; blood urea nitrogen = 15; creatinine = 0.7; heartworm and fecal negative.

Premedication

Midazolam, 0.8 mg IM + butorphanol, 0.8 mg IM, or oxymorphone, 0.4 mg IM.

Induction

Thiamylal sodium, 16 to 32 mg IV.

Maintenance

Methoxyflurane; Bain circuit nonrebreathing system; 600 to 800 ml/minute oxygen flow; lactated Ringer solution, 40 ml/hour; fentanyl, 0.009 mg IV when dog shows signs of inadequate analgesia.

Soft-Tissue Surgery—Sight Hound

Signalment

A 6-month-old 32-kg intact male greyhound was presented for castration.

History, Physical Examination, and Laboratory Data

Normal on examination, PCV = 44; TP = 7.5.

Premedication

Acepromazine, 2 mg IM.

Induction

Combination of diazepam, 9 mg, + ketamine, 175 mg IV.

Maintenance

Halothane; semiclosed circle rebreathing system; 650 to 1,000 ml/minute oxygen flow.

Routine Soft-Tissue Surgery—Cat

Signalment

Eight-month-old 4.4-kg Siamese cat was presented for elective ovariohysterectomy and front onychectomy.

History, Physical Examination, and Laboratory Data

Normal on examination, PCV = 41; TP = 7.3.

Premedication

Ketamine, 24 mg, oxymorphone, 0.3 mg, + acepromazine, 0.2 mg IM.

Induction

Thiamylal, 25 mg IV; cat unable to be intubated—additional thiamylal 5 mg IV.

Maintenance

Halothane; Bain nonrebreathing system; 750 to 900 ml/minute oxygen flow.

Aggressive Cat

Signalment

A 4-year-old 7-kg intact male cat was presented for abscess drainage; extremely aggressive.

History, Physical Examination, and Laboratory Data

Current vaccinations including feline leukemia virus; normal on examination; unable to sample blood.

Premedication

Combination of ketamine, 50 mg, + acepromazine, 0.35 mg IM; still unable to restrain for catheterization.

Induction

Induction chamber with 4 per cent halothane delivered with 100 per cent oxygen (6 L/minute).

Maintenance

Halothane; Bain nonrebreathing system; 1.0 to 1.5 L/minute oxygen flow.

Routine Orthopedic Surgery—Cat

Signalment

A 10-year-old 6-kg castrated male cat was presented for a fractured femur.

History, Physical Examination, and Laboratory Data

Cat was hit by a car hours earlier and is lame on rear leg; radiographs confirm pneumothorax and a femur fracture; all else normal; PCV = 32; TP = 6.4. Forty-eight hours later, the pneumothorax has resolved; the electrocardiogram is normal.

Premedication

Combination of butorphanol, 1.2 mg, + midazolam, 1.2 mg IM.

Induction

Thiamylal, 40 mg IV.

Maintenance

Isoflurane; Bain nonrebreathing system; 1.0 to 1.5 L/minute oxygen flow; lactated Ringer solution, 60 ml/hour.

Postoperative Analgesia

Butorphanol, 24 mg IM.

CHAPTER 166 Anesthesia for the Trauma or Shock Patient

William J. Tranquilli

PREOPERATIVE EVALUATION

Proper care of trauma victims requires advance planning, an ordered protocol, and efficient use of time and resources. Rapid evaluation and treatment are possible when a team approach is taken in the emergency room with each member of the team taking responsibility for preassigned duties. Airway, breathing, circulation, and neurological status are quickly assessed after the patient's arrival. Periodic assessment of circulation and ventilatory and neurological function are made during the initial treatment period. A trauma score has been developed,[32] and a modified version of this scoring method is included (Table 166–1). A low score signifies severe trauma and a poor prognosis.

Traumatized patients are often presented close to cardiopulmonary collapse or cardiac arrest, which may result from many factors including severe myocardial ischemia, malignant dysrhythmias, hypoxemia associated with severe lung damage, hemorrhagic shock or cardiomyopathy, acid-base or electrolyte abnormalities, drug toxicosis, profound vagal tone such as is associated with the oculocardiac reflex, and electrocution.[30] Because many anesthetic drugs depress cardiopulmonary function, anesthesia enhances the likelihood of cardiovascular collapse or cardiac arrest. As a general rule, anesthesia is not undertaken until the patient's condition has been assessed and stabilized. Patients with a history of severe trauma should always be considered likely candidates for developing shock.

Providing anesthesia for burned and crushed patients presents unique problems. Opioids should be considered with any technique to enhance pre- and postoperative analgesia. Ventilation may be necessary if lung damage has occurred. These patients may not respond normally to muscle relaxants.[26] Within 24 hours of injury, succinylcholine administration is associated with a rapid increase in serum potassium concentration, which can cause cardiac arrest. In contrast, these patients are often refractory to nondepolarizing muscle relaxants (e.g., pancuronium and vecuronium). The principles of treatment for patients with electric burns are similar to those for patients with thermal burns. If the burn is located in the oral cavity, severe swelling of pharyngeal tissues may complicate efforts to intubate. The extent of burn is often misleading. Small cutaneous lesions may overlie extensive areas of devitalized tissue and muscle. Accordingly, these patients are carefully observed for myoglobinemia and renal failure as well as neurological deficits.[32]

ANESTHETIC MANAGEMENT OF TRAUMA PATIENTS

Premedication

Preoperatively, vagal influences on cardiopulmonary function and excess secretions can be controlled by atropine or glycopyrrolate. Anticholinergics are not recommended for routine use in trauma patients because they often increase heart rate and oxygen consumption while predisposing to cardiac dysrhythmias.[2] A full stomach should be assumed, and measures to prevent aspiration before anesthesia induction need to be considered. Aspiration of acid gastric contents (pH < 2.5) can result in pneumonitis. Several steps can be taken to minimize vomiting and aspiration. These include glycopyrrolate administration to increase pH of gastric contents,[36] positioning an animal to reduce gastric pressure, immediate intubation of unconscious patients, and availability of suction to clear the pharynx of gastric reflux.[8]

Analgesics or sedatives can be given to help allay pain, fear, and apprehension during the preoperative period. Sedative doses of barbiturates are contraindicated in patients that are excited, delirious, or in pain because small doses can enhance these actions.[8] Butorphanol (0.1 mg/kg IV) or oxymorphone (0.05 mg/kg IV) may be administered in small incremental doses if analgesia is needed. Diazepam (0.2 mg/kg IV) or midazolam (0.2 mg/kg IV or IM) can be combined with the opioid if greater central nervous system depression is desirable. Benzodiazepines are not usually administered alone in alert animals because they can induce unpredictable behavior in both dogs and cats. Low doses can induce profound central nervous system depression in depressed dogs.[17] Acepromazine (0.05 mg/kg) can be combined with butorphanol or oxymorphone to induce neuroleptanalgesia if shock or severe blood loss is unlikely. Acepromazine increases vascular capacity and can reduce cardiac filling and reduce blood pressure. Hypovolemic patients with compensatory vasoconstriction can rapidly vasodilate and decompensate after acepromazine administration. If volume replacement has been adequate before acepromazine administration, decreasing arterial resistance (alpha blockade) may improve perfusion to some vital organs (e.g., kidneys and intestines). Intramuscular meperidine (1 to 2 mg/kg) provides a moderate degree of sedation and analgesia in cats. Ketamine (1 to 3 mg/kg IV or IM) can also be given preoperatively (cats) or in combination with diazepam or midazolam (dogs or cats). A 1:1 combination of tiletamine and zolazepam (Telazol) also produces dose-dependent central nervous system depression and muscle relaxation. Cardiopulmonary function is fairly well maintained in both dogs and cats.

TABLE 166—1. PROGNOSTIC TRAUMA SCORE

Trauma	Value	Points	Score
A. Respiratory rate/minute:	10 to 20	4	
Number of respirations in 15	20 to 30	3	
seconds, multiply by 4	>30	2	
	<5	1	A___
B. Respiratory effort: shallow or	Normal	1	
labored		0	B___
C. Systolic blood pressure: systolic cuff pressure, by either	>90	4	
	70 to 90	3	
auscultation or palpation	50 to 69	2	
	<50	1	C___
D. Capillary refill: normal/			
refill in 2 seconds		2	
Delayed more than 2 seconds		1	
None/no refill		0	D___
E. CNS function scale			
1. Mentation:			
Alert		4___	
Stuporous		3___	
Comatose		2___	
2. Eye opening:			
Spontaneously		4___	
To voice		3___	
To pain		2___	
Will not open		1___	
3. Motor responses:			
Responds to voice		5___	
Purposeful movement		4___	
(pain)		3___	
Withdraw (pain)		2___	
Flexion (pain)		1___	E___
No response			

A low score denotes severe trauma and a poor prognosis.

Total score___

Anesthetic Induction

The most commonly used induction drugs are the ultrashort-acting barbiturates thiopental and thiamylal. Barbiturates depress myocardial function and baroreceptor reflexes.[4] They are respiratory depressants and poor analgesics. Intravenous thiobarbiturate administration can cause venodilation and decreases in venous return, cardiac output, and blood pressure. Thiopental increases renal blood flow in the presence of moderate blood loss.[31] The degree of barbiturate-induced myocardial depression correlates with the peak blood concentration and is a function of dose and rate of injection.[34] Barbiturates are highly protein bound, and normal pharmacokinetics are influenced by a patient's acid-base status, albumin content, and concurrent drug administration. Trauma victims are often acidotic and hypoproteinemic, so a reduced induction dose should be anticipated. Thiobarbiturates are used cautiously in patients with pre-existing cardiac arrhythmias because they are arrhythmogenic when given rapidly or in large doses. Alternatives to thiobarbiturates should be used in severely hypovolemic, hypotensive patients or when severe cardiac disease or pre-existing dysrhythmias are present. Simultaneous administration of diazepam (0.2 mg/kg) or lidocaine (2.0 mg/kg) decreases barbiturate requirement and the incidence of cardiac arrhythmias.[33]

Inhalation anesthetics, unlike injectable agents, are retrievable should an adverse response result.[16] Inhalation anesthetics are as hypotensive as barbiturates and are only safer as induction agents because they are more controllable and homeostatic mechanisms have longer to compensate for the depressant effects of inhalants during induction. Halothane, enflurane, isoflurane, and methoxyflurane all induce dose-dependent cardiopulmonary depression. Isoflurane is least depressant at equipotent (e.g., 1.5 minimum alveolar concentration) concentrations. Induction with an inhalation anesthetic alone is not recommended if the dog or cat is alert and likely to struggle.

Ketamine is one of the few anesthetics with cardiovascular stimulant properties. It increases blood pressure secondary to increased sympathetic activity, heart rate, and cardiac output in healthy patients.[18] Ketamine also induces a direct myocardial depressant effect in patients whose sympathetic system is maximally stressed by hemorrhagic shock.[40] This is often the case in traumatized patients. Ketamine is contraindicated in patients with hypertrophic or restrictive cardiomyopathy (e.g., cats with idiopathic cardiomyopathy and normal left ventricular contractility), because it may induce tachycardia and further decrease preload.[2] Ketamine may be a good choice for inducing anesthesia in large or giant-breed dogs suffering from cardiogenic shock and myocardial failure as defined by poor contractility (dilated cardiomyopathy). It does not provide good muscle relaxation, and spontaneous movement is common when it is given alone. Ketamine is not recommended for anesthetic induction of trauma patients with severe closed head injury because it can increase intracranial pressure.

Muscle relaxation and sedation are enhanced when benzodiazepines are combined with ketamine, barbiturates, or opioids. Diazepam (0.2 mg/kg IV) and ketamine (2 to 3 mg/kg IV) can be given in rapid sequence to induce anesthesia in traumatized dogs or cats.[16] Delivery of low concentrations of halothane or isoflurane (0.5 to 1.0 per cent) by face mask completes the induction if the patient is not sufficiently depressed after diazepam-ketamine administration. Isoflurane is less arrhythmogenic than halothane and is preferred for mask induction of any trauma victim exhibiting dysrhythmias or suspected of having severe myocardial contusions.[15, 20] Dysrhythmias occurring during halothane anesthesia have been abolished after halothane discontinuation and the administration of isoflurane at similar concentrations.[20]

Opioid induction usually necessitates concomitant use of an adjunctive tranquilizer-sedative (neuroleptanalgesia) or inhalation anesthetic. Intravenous opioid administration is preceded by preoxygenation and atropine to prevent bradycardia. Meperidine and morphine intravenously administered to dogs induce a dose-dependent histamine release that can cause hypotension. Intravenous oxymorphone has not been associated with histamine release. Oxymorphone is commonly given intravenously to depressed trauma victims, in small increments (0.05 mg/kg) along with diazepam (0.2 mg/kg) until intubation is possible.[16] Alternatively, midazolam (0.2 mg/kg) and oxymorphone (0.1 to 0.2 mg/kg) can be administered intramuscularly to induce neuroleptanalgesia.[2] Opioids and benzodiazepines are a useful induction combination in patients with hypovolemia, cardiogenic shock, septic shock, or dehydration because they do not cause myocardial depression or severe vasodilation. Opioid inductions are slower than those achieved with barbiturates or dissociatives and are *not* recommended if rapid intubation of the airway is necessary for a patient's survival.

Etomidate is useful for induction in patients in shock or with severe chronic cardiac disease. Etomidate produces minimal hemodynamic alterations and cardiac depression at 0.5 to 2.0 mg/kg IV.[13] Adrenocortical suppression may follow induction of anesthesia, but this is of limited concern when etomidate is given as a single bolus to a hemodynamically unstable patient for whom anesthesia may be lifesaving.[32] Etomidate is useful for patients in compensated or decompensated (congestive) heart failure whether caused by acquired chronic atrioventricular valvular disease or myocardial failure (dilated cardiomyopathy).

Anesthetic Maintenance

The first priority during maintenance of anesthesia is adequate ventilation. Mechanical ventilation may be necessary for normal gas exchange. Second, preservation of hemodynamic stability is essential. This is achieved by providing adequate intravascular volume, administering positive inotropes if necessary, and using anesthetic drugs judiciously. The natural tendency is to choose an anesthetic for trauma patients that is an adrenergic stimulant or is associated with little hypotensive affect when given to a healthy animal. However, there are limited data to suggest the superiority of stimulant drugs for maintenance of anesthesia during severe hypovolemic shock or in patients with severe central nervous system injury.[32] Ketamine's overall cardiovascular effects in hypovolemic pigs were similar to those of thiopental.[40]

Dissociatives

Ketamine given with diazepam or midazolam can be used to maintain anesthesia for short periods in cardiovascularly unstable patients. Ketamine is repeated at an approximate dosage of 1 to 2 mg/kg/IV every 20 to 30 minutes or as necessary to keep the patient anesthetized.[16] Diazepam or midazolam can also be repeated (0.2 mg/kg/IV) every 30 to 60 minutes or as necessary to provide adequate muscle relaxation.[16] Recovery can be prolonged with repeated injections. Duration of anesthesia should be limited to less than 2 hours. Long recoveries may be problematic in cats because they metabolize benzodiazepines more slowly than dogs. Similarly, tiletamine plus zolazepam (Telazol) may be useful when given in low doses for minimal restraint. These injectable regimens are often supplemented with low concentrations of halothane or isoflurane (0.5 to 1.0 per cent) if anesthesia is extended.

Inhalation Agents

Nitrous oxide does not offer any hemodynamic advantage over halothane when administered to hypovolemic animals.[39] The use of high concentrations of nitrous oxide (70 per cent) cannot be routinely recommended because trauma patients frequently have pulmonary contusions with increased venous admixture, and large arterial-alveolar oxygen gradients. Nitrous oxide is contraindicated if pneumo- or hemothorax is present. Similarly, in patients with a distended abdomen or diaphragmatic hernia resulting in respiratory compromise, nitrous oxide is avoided. Nitrous oxide stimulates cerebral metabolism and causes increased cerebral blood flow and intracranial pressure.[35] Accordingly, nitrous oxide is not advocated for trauma patients with severe head or open eye injury.

Isoflurane, like halothane and methoxyflurane, is hypotensive but does not sensitize the myocardium to the arrhythmogenic effects of catecholamines as does halothane.[21] Isoflurane depresses the myocardium less and is a more potent vasodilator. Consequently, isoflurane is the preferred inhalation agent in patients with congestive heart failure or those with severe dysrhythmias. Like halothane, isoflurane should not be used in hypovolemic shock before volume replacement.[16] Myocardial depression coupled with peripheral vasodilation can result in decreased coronary perfusion and an increased likelihood of myocardial ischemia in severely volume-depleted patients. Myocardial depression and hypotension can be minimized by using as low a concentration of inhalation anesthetic as possible. Ventricular dysrhythmias occurring during light halothane anesthesia can often be converted to sinus rhythm by simply increasing halothane concentration.[28] Attempting to abolish arrhythmias may be unwise because cardiopulmonary collapse could result in patients with questionable cardiopulmonary reserve.[28] It is common practice to administer a muscle relaxant to humans to help prevent their movement when using low inhalant concentrations. Unfortunately, human patients have recalled surgical events under these conditions.[32] Preanesthetic or operative administration of an opioid or benzodiazepine tranquilizer can ensure adequate central nervous system depression during low-dose inhalation anesthesia. Fentanyl (0.002 mg/kg) or oxymorphone (0.02 mg/kg) is preferred for supplemental surgical analgesia in hypovolemic patients.

Regional and Local Anesthesia

Epidural or spinal blocks are contraindicated in trauma patients with severe hemorrhage. Sympathetic blockade induced by local anesthetics can cause acute hypotension. Epidural or intrathecal administration of opioids or $alpha_2$ agonists may prove effective alternatives to local anesthetics in providing analgesia without sympathetic blockade.[37, 38] Morphine (0.1 mg/kg in 0.25 ml/kg of saline) administered in the caudal epidural space has provided analgesia for up to 10 hours without motor impairment. The degree and duration of analgesia can be enhanced by the simultaneous administration of an opioid and $alpha_2$ agonist.[7] Superficial lacerations and wounds of the extremities can be managed with infiltration of local anesthetic (e.g., lidocaine) in severely depressed, calm, and stoic patients. Local blocks commonly used include the intercostal nerve block,[3] intrapleural infusion, and peripheral nerve blocks of the extremities. Intravenous infusions of local anesthetic distal to tourniquet placement can also provide effective analgesia for digit amputation, laceration repair, and nail removal.[24]

Anesthetic Support

Several choices of fluids are available for use in hypovolemic patients undergoing anesthesia and surgery. Contraction of extracellular volume occurs with hemorrhage as the intravascular compartment is autotransfused with interstitial fluid. Intravenous administration of a crystalloid solution such as lactated Ringer restores this depletion and expands intravascular volume to help maintain cardiac output. Patients generally should be given 20 to 40 ml/kg IV before anesthetic induction. Fluids can be given rapidly into the intraosseous space of the tibia and femur if necessary.[10] Patients in hypovolemic shock can be given one blood volume (80 ml/kg dog; 60 ml/kg cat) of isotonic electrolyte solution in the first hour. Animals can rapidly decompensate after anesthetic drug injection, when underlying hypovolemia is unmasked as severe hypotension.[16] Not all isotonic solutions are optimal. Although 5 per cent dextrose in water and lactated Ringer with 2.5 per cent dextrose are isotonic, once glucose is metabolized, the remaining fluid is hypotonic and contains either all (5 per cent dextrose) or half (2.5 per cent dextrose) free water, which rapidly leaves the vascular compartment.[22] Even nonglucose isotonic crystalloid solutions remain intravascular for only 30 to 60 minutes before redistributing throughout the entire extracellular space.[6]

Colloid solutions probably have little advantage in resuscitating hypovolemic patients, although this opinion is controversial.[9] Colloid solutions maintain intravascular volume for 2 to 5 hours but have associated complications. Dextran solutions can cause bleeding disorders and allergic reactions.[11, 12] Protein solutions can impair pulmonary function if they extravasate into damaged lung.[19] Hydroxyethyl starch (6 per cent solution in normal saline) is a glucose polymer that has proved useful as a volume expander when the dose is limited to less than 20 ml/kg.[29] This solution is hypertonic and must be administered slowly to avoid rapid fluid shifts and volume overload.[10]

Increasing evidence suggests that hypertonic saline may be beneficial in the early treatment of hypovolemic and hemorrhagic shock.[23] Intravenous administration of small volumes (4 to 6 ml/kg) of 7.5 per cent hypertonic saline results in beneficial cardiovascular effects in dogs and cats.[5, 25, 27] Increases in blood pressure and cardiac output appear to be mediated by pulmonary-vagal reflexes and increased plasma volume coupled with a venoconstrictor effect.[25]

Red blood cells are administered when extreme blood loss ($>$40 per cent of blood volume) occurs. Fresh whole blood ($<$6 hours old) is preferable. Only 12 per cent of the original platelets remain viable in human whole blood after 1 day of storage. Similar reductions may occur in stored blood of domestic animals. Regardless of age, whole blood is preferred to packed red blood cells.[32] Fresh-frozen plasma is reserved for specific coagulation disorders.[1] Most clotting disorders are secondary to large-volume fluid replacement in acute trauma, resulting in dilutional thrombocytopenia. Surgery and anesthesia are delayed until the packed cell volume can be increased to above 20 per cent. The best method of assessing adequate fluid and blood replacement is to assess vital signs, urine output (1 to 2 ml/kg /hour is optimal), serial hematocrit, and total protein values when ongoing losses and replacement are occurring simultaneously.

Traumatized dogs and cats often have metabolic acidosis due to shock, hypothermia, and generalized stress. Ventilation of the lungs to induce a mild respiratory alkalosis helps normalize blood pH. Improved tissue perfusion (fluids) and renal and hepatic function should resolve the problem. Treatment with sodium bicarbonate is reserved for severe metabolic acidosis. Rapid, vigorous sodium bicarbonate therapy may be detrimental for the treatment of lactic acidosis because bicarbonate depresses both arterial pressure and cardiac output.[14] More important measures in treating metabolic acidosis are fluid administration, adequate ventilation, and rewarming. Patients with normal liver function can often develop metabolic alkalosis 6 to 24 hours after large-volume replacement with lactated Ringer solution.

Hypothermia is treated. Hypothermia is frequently

associated with reduced kidney function, poor platelet activity, low glucose utilization, shivering and increased oxygen consumption by nonvital tissues, metabolic acidosis, and decreased metabolism of anesthetics.[32] Warming fluids and blood before administration helps maintain body temperature, reduces blood viscosity, and improves tissue blood flow. Warm water blankets and heat lamps may help prevent further heat loss, but the patient is not rewarmed rapidly. The operating room should not be cold.

Normal urine output is maintained to prevent acute oliguric renal failure. Unfortunately, there is no formula to predict the degree of hypoperfusion that results in renal failure. Maintenance of renal function and diuresis is necessary to reduce intracranial pressure if head injury has occurred. Myoglobinemia must be treated by vigorous diuresis following skeletal muscle crush or electrocution. Mannitol can be administered (0.5 g/kg IV bolus) once fluid volume and blood pressure are normal. Furosemide (1 mg/kg) and dopamine (2 to 5 μg/kg/minute) can be used to increase renal blood flow and water and solute excretion. Maintaining a functional renal system is essential for a favorable outcome after massive tissue damage.[32]

In summary, diagnosis and therapeutic management of trauma patients are difficult because several organ systems may be injured simultaneously, each with its own vital function and therapeutic priority. For example, a dog that has been hit by a car may have head injuries of unknown severity, a ruptured spleen, lung contusions, arrhythmias suggesting cardiac contusion and ischemia, a broken leg with massive muscle damage, and myoglobinuria. Head and lung injuries suggest fluid restriction, whereas rapid fluid administration is necessary for treatment of shock and prevention of renal damage.

References

1. Baldini M, et al: The viability of stored human platelets. *Blood 16*:1669, 1960.
2. Bednarski RM: Anesthesia and pain control. *In* Kirby R, Stamp GL (eds): *Veterinary Clinics of North America: Critical Care.* W.B. Saunders, Philadelphia, 1989, p 1223.
3. Berg RJ, Orton EC: Pulmonary function in dogs after intercostal thoracotomy: Comparison of morphine, oxymorphone, and selective intercostal nerve block. *Am J Vet Res 47*:471, 1986.
4. Bernards C, et al: Effect of anesthetic induction agents on baroreceptor function. *Anesthesiology 63*:A31, 1985.
5. Bitterman H, et al: Use of hypertonic saline in the treatment of hemorrhagic shock. *Circ Shock 21*:271, 1987.
6. Cervera LA, Moss G: Crystalloid distribution following hemorrhage and hemodilution. *J Trauma 14*:506, 1974.
7. Cousins MJ, Mather LE: Intrathecal and epidural administration of opioids. *Anesthesiology 61*:276, 1989.
8. Evans T: Anesthesia and monitoring for trauma and critical care patients. *In* Slatter DH (ed): *Textbook of Small Animal Surgery.* W.B. Saunders, Philadelphia, 1985, pp 2702–2711.
9. Gallagher TJ, et al: Large volume crystalloid resuscitation does not increase extravascular lung water. *Anesth Analg 64*:323, 1985.
10. Garvey MS: Fluid and electrolyte balance in critical patients. *In* Kirby R, Stamp GL (eds): *Veterinary Clinics of North America: Critical Care.* W.B. Saunders, Philadelphia, 1989, pp 1021–1058.
11. Giesecke AH Jr: Anesthesia for trauma surgery. *In* Miller RD (ed): *Anesthesia.* Churchill Livingstone, New York, 1981, pp 1247–1264.
12. Giesecke AH, Jenkins MT: Fluid therapy. *Clinical Anesthesia 11*:57, 1976.
13. Gooding JM, Corssen G: Effect of etomidate on the cardiovascular system. *Anesth Analg 56*:717, 1977.
14. Graf H, et al: Evidence for the detrimental effect of bicarbonate therapy on hypoxic lactic acidosis. *Science 227*:754, 1985.
15. Harvey RC, Short CE: The use of isoflurane for safe anesthesia in animals with traumatic myocarditis or other myocardial sensitivity. *Canine Pract 10*:18, 1983.
16. Haskins SC: Anesthetic considerations in patients with cardiovascular debilitation. Proceedings of the 7th American College of Veterinary Internal Medicine Forum, San Diego, May 1989.
17. Haskins SC, et al: Cardiovascular changes in dogs given diazepam and diazepam-ketamine. *Am J Vet Res 47*:795, 1986.
18. Haskins SC, et al: Ketamine in dogs. *Am J Vet Res 46*:1855, 1985.
19. Holcraft JW, et al: Sepsis in the baboon: Factors affecting resuscitation and pulmonary edema in animals resuscitated with Ringer's lactate versus plasmanate. *J Trauma 17*:600, 1977.
20. Hubbell JAE, et al: Change of inhalation anesthetic agents for management of ventricular premature depolarizations in anesthetized cats and dogs. *J Am Vet Med Assoc 185*:643, 1984.
21. Joas TA, Stevens WC: Comparison of the arrhythmic doses of epinephrine during forane, halothane, and fluroxene anesthesia in dogs. *Anesthesiology 35*:48, 1971.
22. Layon AJ, Kirby RR: Fluids and electrolytes in the critically ill. *In* Civetta JM, et al (eds): *Critical Care.* J.B. Lippincott, Philadelphia, 1988, pp 451–474.
23. Layon J, et al: Hypertonic saline as a resuscitation solution in hemorrhagic shock. *Anesth Analg 66*:154, 1987.
24. LeBlanc PH: The practical use of local anesthesia for the small animal veterinarian. Proceedings of the Eastern States Veterinary Conference, Anesthesia Section, Orlando, Jan, 1990, pp 8–9.
25. Lopes OU, et al: Hypertonic sodium restores mean circulatory filling pressure in severely hypovolemic dogs. *Hypertension 8*(Suppl 1):1195, 1986.
26. Martyn J: Clinical pharmacology and drug therapy in the burned patient. *Anesthesiology 65*:67, 1986.
27. Muir WW, Sally J: Small volume resuscitation with hypertonic saline solution in hypovolemic cats. *Am J Vet Res 50*:1883, 1989.
28. Muir WW, et al: Increasing halothane concentration abolishes anesthesia-associated arrhythmias in cats and dogs. *J Am Vet Med Assoc* 192:1730, 1988.
29. Munoz E, et al: Effect of hydroxyethyl starch versus albumin on hemodynamic and respiratory function in patients in shock. *Crit Care Med 8*:255, 1980.
30. Pascoe PJ: Emergency care medicine. *In* Short CE (ed): *Principles and Practice of Veterinary Anesthesia.* Williams & Wilkins, Baltimore, 1987, pp 558–598.
31. Priano LL: Renal hemodynamic alterations following administration of thiopental, diazepam, or ketamine in conscious hypovolemic dogs. *Adv Shock Res 9*:173, 1983.
32. Priano LL: Trauma. *In* Barash PG, et al: *Clinical Anesthesia.* J.B. Lippincott, Philadelphia, 1989, pp 1365–1377.
33. Rawlings CA, Kolata RJ: Cardiopulmonary effects of thiopental/lidocaine combination during anesthetic induction in the dog. *Am J Vet Res 44*:144, 1983.
34. Roberts JG: Intravenous anesthetic agents. *In* Prys-Roberts C (ed): *The Circulation in Anesthesia. Applied Physiology and Pharmacology.* Blackwell Scientific Publications, Oxford, England, 1980, pp 311–327.
35. Sakabe T, et al: Cerebral effects of nitrous oxide in the dog. *Anesthesiology 48*:195, 1978.
36. Salem MR, et al: Premedicant drugs and gastric juice pH and volume in pediatric patients. *Anesthesiology 44*:216, 1976.
37. Tung AS, Yaksh TL: The antinociceptive effects of epidural opiates in the cat: Studies on the pharmacology and the effects of lipophilicity in spinal analgesia. *Pain 12*:343, 1982.
38. Valverde A, et al: Epidural morphine reduces halothane MAC in the dog. *Can J Anaesth 36*:629, 1989.
39. Weiskopf RB, Bogetz MS: Cardiovascular actions of nitrous oxide and halothane in hypovolemic swine. *Anesthesiology 63*:509, 1985.
40. Weiskopf RB, et al: Cardiovascular and metabolic sequelae of inducing anesthesia with ketamine or thiopental in hypovolemic swine. *Anesthesiology 60*:214, 1984.

CHAPTER

167 Anesthesia and the Urinary System

Diane E. Mason

Veterinary surgeons often encounter situations in which it is necessary to anesthetize an animal that has disease involving the urinary system. The surgical procedure may be directly related to the urinary system, as in repair of a traumatic bladder rupture in a dog. It is also common for an animal to need surgery that does not involve the urinary tract, although the animal's condition is complicated by renal disease. This chapter reviews important functions of the urinary system, highlights interactions between anesthesia and the kidneys, and suggests techniques to minimize risk of anesthesia with urinary system dysfunction.

Two primary functions of the urinary system are to excrete end products of cellular metabolism and to control the concentrations of various constituents in body fluids. These functions allow the kidneys to maintain a normal extracellular environment for all cells so that tissues can function unimpeded by biochemical disturbances. The kidneys also secrete hormones that regulate systemic and renal hemodynamics, promote red blood cell production, and regulate calcium, phosphorus, and bone metabolism. This chapter addresses urinary system disorders that result in an inability of the kidneys to carry out their normal physiological processes, as evidenced by the presence of azotemia.

Azotemia is the accumulation of nitrogenous products of cellular metabolism (urea and creatinine) that are eliminated by glomerular filtration in the kidneys[2]; at least 75 per cent of the glomeruli in the kidneys are not filtering. Azotemia has various causes and may be temporary or permanent. Any process that disrupts normal function of the urinary system may also cause fluid, electrolyte, and acid-base imbalances. When azotemia is accompanied by metabolic derangement, the condition is described as renal failure.[2] Table 167–1 compares the three types of azotemia and lists characteristic metabolic changes expected if these conditions progressed to renal failure.

EFFECTS OF ABNORMAL RENAL FUNCTION ON ANESTHESIA

Some functional and metabolic changes that result from disease in the urinary system can have a significant impact on an animal's ability to tolerate anesthesia. One concern is the impact that the diseased kidney will have on the pharmacokinetics of anesthetic drugs. Most anesthetics are weakly ionized and have high lipid solubility, allowing the drug to penetrate the blood-brain barrier into the central nervous system, the site of action of most anesthetics. The kidneys are an important pathway in the elimination of highly ionized, relatively lipid insoluble drugs or the polar metabolites of drugs that have been transformed by the liver. Few anesthetic drugs rely on the kidneys for primary elimination. There are a few exceptions to this rule (Table 167–2). A number of anesthetic drugs undergo hepatic biotransformation, and their metabolites, which retain some pharmacological activity, are eliminated by the kidneys (see Table 167–2). These metabolites usually have a lower degree of activity than the parent compound, and reduced clearance at the kidneys does not markedly affect the duration of response of an animal with short-term anesthetic use. With chronic administration of drugs in this category, accumulation of active metabolites may have a significant impact on an animal's recovery on discontinuation of the drug.

The most important effect of renal disease on the pharmacokinetics of anesthetic drugs results from changes in body fluid composition. Azotemia can have marked effects on drug pharmacokinetics. It causes increased sensitivity to thiobarbiturates, and a decreased thiobarbiturate dose is recommended for patients with renal disease.[4] Azotemia influences the plasma protein binding of these drugs. Less protein binding results in a higher concentration of unbound (active) thiopental, making more drug available to cross the blood-brain barrier and produce an anesthetic effect. Other drugs that are highly protein bound, such as diazepam and midazolam, may also be affected in this way, and reduced doses are usually indicated.

EFFECTS OF ANESTHESIA ON RENAL FUNCTION

The effects of anesthetic drugs on renal function in animals with impaired kidneys are of concern because the potential exists to inadvertently exacerbate the renal disease with anesthesia. This can occur through direct effects of certain anesthetic drugs that are nephrotoxic or it can occur with relatively nontoxic drugs by indirect effects on hemodynamics, neuroendocrine responses, and urine production.

Among anesthetic drugs, only the inhalation agent methoxyflurane directly causes nephrotoxicity. Methoxyflurane undergoes biotransformation to fluoride ion, which is a potent inhibitor of renal metabolic processes.[3] In normal dogs, the renal dysfunction produced by methoxyflurane is transient, and normal function returns in a few days.[10] The right combination of pre-existing renal damage, duration of exposure, and compromised renal perfusion may potentiate irreversible renal tubular disease in a dog or cat with a urinary tract disorder. Methoxyflurane is to be avoided in animals with renal disease or those with the potential to develop acute nephrotoxicity from other causes. Methoxyflurane can be especially deleterious when used in combination with other nephrotoxic drugs (Table 167–3).

TABLE 167–1. AZOTEMIA: DIFFERENTIATION AND ANTICIPATED METABOLIC CHANGES

	Prerenal	Primary Renal	Postrenal
Blood urea nitrogen	Increased	Increased	Increased
Creatinine	Increased	Increased	Increased
Urine specific gravity	>1.040	<1.030	Variable
Urinalysis	Normal	Abnormal	Abnormal
Urine volume	Decreased	Variable	None/decreased
PCV/Total protein	Increased	Anemic (CRF)	Increased
Potassium	Normal	Increased (ARF)	Increased
Phosphorus	Normal	Increased	Increased
Metabolic acidosis	Slight	Compensated	Uncompensated

ARF, acute renal failure; CRF, chronic renal failure; PCV, packed cell volume.

Anesthetic drugs that are not nephrotoxic may have profound effects on renal function. The functional unit of the kidneys is the glomerulus, and filtration within the glomeruli is a function of capillary hydrostatic pressure, which depends on renal blood flow. Renal blood flow is a product of systemic arterial blood pressure and compliance of the renal vasculature. Therefore, renal blood flow and glomerular function may be depressed as a consequence of systemic hypotension, renal vasoconstriction, or a combination of the two. Decreased renal blood flow during the anesthetic period is a problem for patients with renal disease for two reasons. First, regulation of extracellular fluid composition is arrested during the period of circulatory compromise. Second, significant further damage to diseased renal tissue could result, either from a prolonged period of poor renal perfusion (ischemia) or from the concentration of toxic metabolites in urine secondary to inadequate urine volume. Without sufficient washout of these toxic substances from the renal tubules as urine is produced, postanesthetic acute tubular necrosis can result, and irreparable kidney damage can occur in an animal that suffered from only mild renal compromise preoperatively.[6]

In the absence of extrinsic neural or hormonal influences, renal blood flow is maintained fairly constant within a mean arterial pressure range of 80 to 180 mm Hg.[3] Renal blood flow diminishes markedly if the mean arterial blood pressure drops below 80 mm Hg. A goal of anesthesia in animals with renal disease is to maintain renal perfusion through use of anesthetic drugs that are less likely to produce hypotension, appropriate fluid therapy, and inotropic support when fluid therapy is not adequate to maintain blood pressure within the acceptable range.

Even with adequate mean blood pressure, renal perfusion can be inadequate if renal vascular resistance is too high. The blood vessels of the kidneys are richly innervated by sympathetic nerve fibers that mediate vasoconstriction through alpha-adrenergic receptors. To minimize renal vasoconstriction in an animal with renal disease, one should prevent sympathetic nervous system stimulation and increases in circulating catecholamines. Stress, excitement, pain, and light anesthetic planes all can result in sympathetic stimulation. Animals with renal disease respond most favorably if given adequate sedation, analgesia, and stress-free handling. Drugs such as ketamine or tiletamine can cause an increase in systemic catecholamine levels, and though they support systemic blood pressure, they may cause an increase in renal vascular resistance and can depress renal function. Potent alpha-agonist drugs like xylazine cause marked elevations in both peripheral and renal vascular resistance and are contraindicated in patients with renal disease. Alpha-adrenergic blocking agents such as acepromazine or droperidol (the tranquilizer portion of Innovar-Vet) may protect against the reduction in renal cortical perfusion that occurs as a result of sympathetic stimulation or endogenous catecholamine release. Care must be taken with these drugs because systemic vasodilatation can result in significant hypotension if adequate fluid therapy is not provided.

All general anesthetic drugs in animals with or without renal disease temporarily depress renal function as a result of diminished cardiac output. Renal blood flow in the operative period is influenced by endocrine activity, as well. Antidiuretic hormone (vasopressin) is the most important hormonal regulator of urine volume. Many general anesthetic agents, opioids, hemorrhage, and positive-pressure ventilation induce release of antidiuretic hormone, thus decreasing urine production and increasing urine concentration during and after anesthesia. Fortunately, the effects of antidiuretic hormone can be over-ridden by adequate fluid therapy and diuretics.[8]

Epidural anesthesia may produce minimal alterations in renal function. Epidural anesthesia blocks sympa-

TABLE 167–2. RELATIVE IMPORTANCE OF RENAL ELIMINATION FOR VARIOUS ANESTHETIC DRUGS

Primary Elimination	Partial Elimination	Renal Elimination of Active Metabolites	Decreased Protein-Bound Fraction
Ketamine (cats)	Atropine	Diazepam	Thiobarbiturates
Gallamine	Glycopyrrolate	Lidocaine	Methohexital
Neostigmine	Pancuronium	Ketamine	Diazepam
	Phenobarbital	Meperidine	Midazolam

TABLE 167–3. DRUGS WITH POTENTIAL FOR NEPHROTOXICITY

Aminoglycosides
Amphotericin B
Arsenical anthelmintics
Cephalosporins
Methoxyflurane
Nonsteroidal anti-inflammatory drugs
Penicillins
Sulfonamides
Tetracyclines

thetic fibers in the thoracolumbar spine and prevents renal vasoconstriction. Provided blood pressure is well maintained with intravenous infusion of balanced electrolyte solutions, epidural anesthesia can be a safe alternative to general anesthesia in compromised animals.

It is important to remember that the renal effects of anesthetics are dose related and are favorably influenced by adequate repletion of extracellular fluid with intravenous fluid therapy. Operative management of patients has a much larger role in successful anesthesia of animals with renal disease than does the choice of anesthetic drugs.

FLUID THERAPY FOR PATIENTS WITH RENAL DISEASE

One of the keys to successful anesthetic management of animals with renal disease is maintaining proper intravascular volume throughout the anesthetic and operative period. The aims are to optimize renal perfusion, maintain urine production, and reduce ischemic or toxic insult to kidneys that are already compromised. Many patients with acute renal diseases, such as acute renal failure or acute obstructive disease of the urinary tract, present with significant dehydration and oliguria. Preoperative administration of intravenous fluids is a necessity in these animals. A balanced electrolyte solution such as lactated Ringer is usually appropriate to restore circulating blood volume. Depending on preoperative electrolyte concentrations, 0.9 per cent sodium chloride may be suitable to stimulate urine production. Improved urine production can often be used as a means of monitoring the adequacy of fluid administration and determining the need for other pharmacological stimulants of renal function. Adequate urine production is 1 to 2 ml/kg/hour. If less than 0.5 ml/kg/hour of urine is produced despite efforts at rehydration, diuretics should be considered before anesthesia. Mannitol (0.25 to 0.5 g/kg) is a good choice for operative diuresis. Its peak effect occurs within 30 minutes, and it can be diluted in the fluids that an animal is receiving for hydration. It is compatible with the use of other drugs, like furosemide or dopamine infusion. Mannitol protects against toxic or ischemic damage to kidneys over and above its effects as a diuretic. Pretreatment with mannitol before aortic cross-clamping and total renal ischemia results in reduced postanesthetic renal failure in humans undergoing aortic aneurysm repair.[9] There are contraindications to the use of mannitol. Mannitol should not be used in an animal that is already overhydrated, has renal hypertension, or suffers from congestive cardiac disease because it causes plasma volume expansion, which may result in peripheral edema or congestive heart failure.

Fluid therapy is maintained at an initial rate of 10 ml/kg/hour during anesthesia. The rate of fluid therapy may need to be adjusted during anesthesia, depending on hemodynamic status and urine production. Useful indices for determining the adequacy of operative fluid therapy include systemic blood pressure (mean blood pressure >80 mm Hg), central venous pressure (<10 cm H_2O), or urine output (>0.5 ml/kg/hour). These monitoring techniques are not difficult or expensive to institute, though they require the placement of an arterial catheter, a jugular venous catheter, or a urinary catheter.

There are other factors to consider in animals with chronic renal disease, in addition to adequate operative fluid therapy. Patients with chronic renal damage may be deficient in erythropoietin, a hormone that is produced by the kidneys and stimulates red blood cell production. In addition, azotemia shortens red blood cell life span, and gastrointestinal bleeding from uremic ulcers may occur. A nonregenerative anemia is not unusual in animals with chronic renal disease. With a hematocrit between 25 and 30 per cent, the animal compensates for the anemia owing to an increase in 2,3-diphosphoglyceric acid in the red blood cells and a shifting of the oxyhemoglobin dissociation curve to the right, allowing more oxygen to be delivered to the tissues. With the risk of further blood loss during a surgical procedure, an animal may benefit from blood transfusion before or during anesthesia. If the hematocrit falls to 15 per cent or less, blood transfusion is recommended.

Azotemia can also be associated with prolonged bleeding time despite normal platelet numbers. Azotemia interferes with platelet function and markedly increases the risk of surgical bleeding. Pretreatment with desmopressin acetate (DDAVP, 1 μg/kg SC) may be beneficial in minimizing the risk of prolonged bleeding. It has been useful in treatment of platelet dysfunction due to von Willebrand's disease in Doberman pinschers and for uremic coagulopathy in humans.[5, 7]

ACID-BASE AND ELECTROLYTE DISORDERS OF RENAL DISEASE

Depending on the etiology and chronicity of an animal's renal disease, various electrolyte and acid-base disorders may be present, and some pose great risk with respect to anesthesia (see Table 167–1). Table 167–4 represents both the minimum and supplemental laboratory data that may be beneficial to assess renal disease patients adequately. Metabolic acidosis is a common finding with most types of renal disease. An increase in the anion gap occurs in these patients because of the accumulation of organic acids such as sulfates and phosphates, normally excreted by the kidneys. The pH of the animal may reflect varying degrees of compensatory response for this acidosis. If an animal has a metabolic

TABLE 167–4. PREANESTHETIC LABORATORY DATA FOR ANIMAL WITH URINARY DYSFUNCTION

Minimum Data	Supplemental Data
Blood urea and creatinine levels	Coagulation profile
Urinalysis (specific gravity, sediment)	Electrocardiogram
Hematocrit	Complete blood count, calcium
Total protein	Thoracic/abdominal radiographs
Electrolytes (Na, K, Cl)	Systemic blood pressure
	Blood gas analysis
	Urine output

TABLE 167–5. DRUGS CONSIDERED SAFEST FOR ANIMALS WITH RENAL DISEASE

Benzodiazepines
Phenothiazines
Anticholinergics
Opioids
Thiobarbiturates
Neuroleptanalgesics
Isoflurane
Epidural anesthesia

acidosis with a pH greater than 7.25, the appropriate preanesthetic treatment is fluid therapy to improve both tissue perfusion and urine production, reducing the base deficit. If an animal's pH is less than 7.20, fluid therapy is warranted, followed by sodium bicarbonate therapy if the response to fluid therapy is inadequate. It is important to treat conservatively when determining the amount of sodium bicarbonate to administer. Several complications might result from sodium bicarbonate administration in a patient with renal disease: volume overload, hyperosmolality, overshoot alkalosis, and tetany if a uremic patient is hypocalcemic. To minimize the likelihood of these complications, treat with only half of the calculated extracellular fluid bicarbonate deficit: $\frac{\text{body weight (kg)} \times 0.3 \times \text{base deficit}}{2}$. A relatively safe dose of sodium bicarbonate to use if the base deficit is unknown is 0.5 mEq/kg.

Hyperkalemia is sometimes found in patients with renal disease. Hyperkalemia can be extreme and immediately life threatening in acute obstructive renal disorders. Even moderate elevations in serum potassium can impart significant increase in risk of anesthesia, potentiating the cardiovascular depressant effects of anesthetic drugs and predisposing to arrhythmias. If an animal has a serum potassium level greater than 6 mEq/L, preoperative fluid therapy with a balanced electrolyte solution reduces the potassium to normal levels through improved urine production and dilutional effects. If the serum potassium is greater than 6.5 mEq/L and cardiac effects such as bradycardia or spiked T waves are evident on an electrocardiogram, then more aggressive treatment is warranted. This treatment might include one or more of the following: intravenous 5 per cent dextrose and regular insulin, sodium bicarbonate administration, administration of calcium gluconate, or the use of ion-exchange resins. The aim is to lower the serum potassium into the normal range to make the animal a safer candidate for anesthesia.[1]

SUGGESTED ANESTHETIC TECHNIQUES FOR RENAL DISEASE

Specific anesthetic drug choices are less important in these animals than overall management practices.

Premedication

Stress and excitement should be minimized in animals with compromised renal function. Premedication is a wise idea, unless the animal is extremely depressed as a result of its disease. Central nervous system depression markedly enhances an animal's sensitivity to sedative drugs, and when central nervous system signs are evident, the fewer drugs that can be used in the animal, the better the animal will respond and recover. Tranquilization is indicated if the animal appears nervous or objects to handling, as during catheter placement. Sedation with opioids is considered for an animal that is in pain, because the systemic response to pain is accompanied by renal vasoconstriction. Fluid therapy and diuresis are important in conjunction with the use of opioids to overcome the effects of antidiuretic hormone release. No matter what premedicant is chosen, reductions in dose are usually indicated if an animal is azotemic. Anticholinergics can be used for premedication. Vomiting can be a significant preanesthetic and postanesthetic problem in azotemic animals. Glycopyrrolate may be preferable to atropine because of its minimal central nervous system effects and its efficacy in diminishing gastric volume and acidity.

Induction and Anesthesia

All intravenous induction drugs used in veterinary medicine are acceptable for use in patients with urinary

TABLE 167–6. GUIDELINES FOR ANESTHETIC MANAGEMENT FOR RENAL DISEASE

Consider preoperative fluid therapy.
Consider diuretics (mannitol, 0.5 g/kg IV) along with fluid therapy before anesthesia to maintain urine production. Furosemide can also be used for this purpose if normovolemia is ensured.
Minimize elevations in catecholamines due to excitement, pain, light anesthetic planes (provide adequate sedation, analgesia).
Maintain adequate circulating blood volume and cardiac output during anesthesia.
Use inotropic drugs when necessary to maintain cardiac output. Dopamine is the drug of choice. At doses of 0.5 to 2 μg/kg/minute, it has a renal vasodilatory effect and increases urine flow and sodium and creatinine clearance. At >10 μg/kg/minute, the alpha-adrenergic effects of dopamine will predominate, causing renal vasoconstriction and decreased renal perfusion despite an increase in systemic blood pressure.
Avoid drugs that may trigger high levels of circulating catecholamines or act as alpha-adrenergic receptor agonists. Ketamine and tiletamine should also be avoided if an animal has renal hypertension.
Catheterize the bladder and measure urine production and urine specific gravity in response to drug and fluid therapy during anesthesia and in the postoperative period. Urine production should be > 0.5 ml/kg/hour.

tract disease. Thiobarbiturates are safe provided that a reduced dose is used and adequate volume replacement is carried out to prevent significant hypotension. Preoxygenation in an anemic animal before induction enhances blood oxygen content and increases the margin of safety in the initial few minutes of anesthesia, especially if the animal has a period of apnea immediately after induction. Mask inductions with inhalation anesthetics can also be used and may be the technique of choice in an animal that is depressed or well sedated. Methoxyflurane should not be used because of its potential to cause nephrotoxicity. Both halothane and isoflurane are effective inhalation agents; however, isoflurane offers the advantage of minimal biotransformation and little likelihood for tissue toxicity. Table 167–5 lists drugs considered safe for use in animals with urinary system disorders. Not all of these drugs are appropriate choices in every animal. One must take into consideration concurrent problems, medical history, and other factors when making up an anesthetic regimen. Table 167–6 is a summary of anesthetic management in cases of renal disease. With preparation, monitoring, and postoperative care, animals with urinary tract dysfunction can be safely and adequately anesthetized.

References

1. Chew DJ: Electrolytes and osmolality. *In* Fenner WR (ed): *Quick Reference to Veterinary Medicine*. J.B. Lippincott, Philadelphia, 1982, pp 489–511.
2. Chew DJ, DiBartola SP: *Manual of Small Animal Nephrology*. Churchill Livingstone, New York, 1986, pp 55–77.
3. Cousins MJ, et al: Anaesthesia and the kidney. *Anaesth Intensive Care 11*:292–320, 1983.
4. Ghoneim MM, Pandya H: Plasma protein binding of thiopental in patients with impaired renal or hepatic function. *Anesthesiology 42*:545, 1975.
5. Kraus KH, et al: Effect of desmopressin acetate (DDAVP) on bleeding times and plasma von Willebrand factor in Doberman pinscher dogs with von Willebrand's disease. *Vet Surg 18*:59, 1989.
6. Maddern PJ: Anaesthesia for the patient with impaired renal function. *Anaesth Intensive Care 11*:321, 1983.
7. Manucci PM, et al: Deamino-8-D-arginine vasopressin shortens the bleeding time in uremia. *N Engl J Med 308*:8, 1983.
8. Mazze RI: Renal physiology and the effects of anesthesia. *In* Miller RD (ed): *Anesthesia*. Vol 2. 2nd ed. Churchill Livingstone, New York, 1986, pp 1223–1248.
9. Mazze RI, Barry KG: Prevention of functional renal failure during anesthesia and surgery by sustained hydration and mannitol infusion. *Anesth Analg 46*:61, 1967.
10. Pedersoli WM: Serum fluoride concentration, renal and hepatic function results in dogs with methoxyflurane anesthesia. *Am J Vet Res 38*:949, 1977.

CHAPTER 168

Anesthesia for the Central Nervous System and Ophthalmic Surgery

Central Nervous System

Ralph C. Harvey
Robert R. Paddleford

Anesthesia alters central nervous system (CNS) physiology. The alteration of neurological function by anesthesia can have deleterious effects on patients with pre-existing CNS disorders. With optimal anesthetic management, some neurological disorders (e.g., seizures and altered intracranial pressure) can be improved.

Many patients require anesthesia for diagnostic evaluation of neurological disorders. Increasingly used diagnostic neurological procedures that require either general anesthesia or heavy sedation include electroencephalography (EEG), myelography, alternate imaging techniques, and electrodiagnostic testing.

Veterinary neurosurgical anesthesia more often concerns patients with spinal cord than intracranial disorders. Surgery for intervertebral disc disease is the most frequently performed. Increased use of advanced imaging techniques, such as computed tomography and magnetic resonance imaging, has led to more intracranial surgery. Consideration of the dynamics of intracranial pressure, cerebral blood flow, and cerebrospinal fluid production and flow are important in neurosurgical patients.

PHYSIOLOGICAL CONCERNS

Blood supply to the CNS is tightly controlled by autoregulatory mechanisms in normal awake animals. Alteration in cerebral blood flow can result from changes in arterial oxygen and carbon dioxide concentrations and in mean arterial pressure and venous outflow (Fig. 168–1). Because these are dramatically influenced by the effects of general anesthesia, considerable fluctuations can occur in cerebral blood flow during anesthesia.[10, 19, 24–26]

The brain and spinal cord are protected within the bony skull and vertebral column. Increases in blood flow within the noncompliant cranial vault cause an increase in intracranial volume and pressure.[24–26] Once increases in cerebral blood flow cause the intracranial volume to exceed the limits of effective compliance

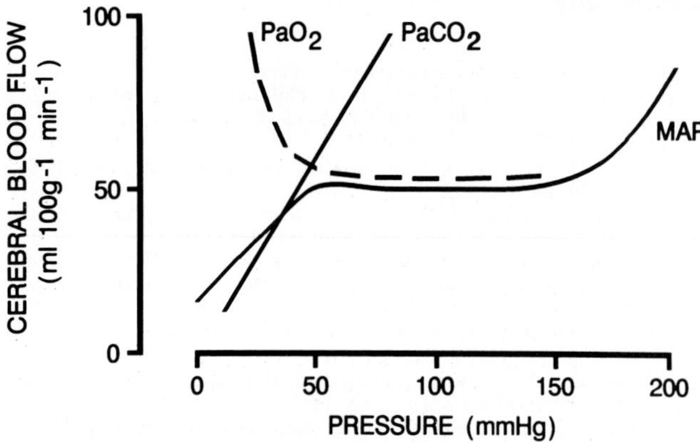

FIGURE 168–1. Cerebral blood flow is influenced by arterial oxygenation (PaO_2), alveolar ventilation ($PaCO_2$), and arterial pressure (MAP). (From Stoelting RK: *Pharmacology and Physiology in Anesthetic Practice.* J.B. Lippincott, Philadelphia, 1987.)

(represented by position A in Fig. 168–2), intracranial pressure sharply increases. When intracranial pressure is already increased by intracranial masses, trauma, or derangement of autoregulation, slight changes in intracranial volume greatly increase intracranial pressure.[25] The results of substantial increases in intracranial pressure include life-threatening systemic manifestations, worsening of cerebral ischemia, and eventually brain herniation.[24]

Autoregulation of Cerebral Blood Flow

Autoregulation of brain blood flow is usually effective in the range of mean arterial pressures from approximately 60 to 140 mm Hg. Within this range of blood pressures, many factors including intracranial tumors, hypercapnea, severe hypoxia, and many anesthetics interfere with autoregulation[15, 19, 24] and alter intracranial pressure.

Blood vessels supplying tumors or diseased tissue in the brain may be fully dilated at all times. There is no autoregulation of blood flow in these tissues. When such areas are present, increases in flow to normal brain tissues may effectively "steal" blood flow from abnormal tissues that lack autoregulation. This diversion of blood away from diseased areas can occur if hypercapnea develops as a result of anesthetic depression of ventilation.

Cerebral Metabolic Rate

Anesthetic-induced depression of the CNS is usually accompanied by decreased cerebral metabolic rate or cerebral metabolic oxygen requirement. This decrease in oxygen requirement can be protective in possible relative ischemia during anesthesia and neurosurgery. There are conflicting reports on the efficacy of various anesthetics in reducing cerebral metabolic oxygen requirement, as with the relative effects of anesthetics on cerebral blood flow and intracranial pressure. Isoflurane and barbiturates contribute substantially to reduced cerebral metabolic oxygen requirement and afford some cerebral protection.[19]

Blood Gases and Cerebral Blood Flow/Intracranial Pressure Dynamics

Cerebral blood flow increases when arterial oxygenation decreases below 50 mm Hg. The relationship between $Pa{CO_2}$ and cerebral blood flow is linear for $Pa{CO_2}$ between 20 and 80 mm Hg.[14] (see Fig. 168–1). Cerebral blood flow increases by about 2 ml/minute/100 g of brain tissue for every 1 mm Hg increase in $Pa{CO_2}$. Hyperventilation electively reduces cerebral blood flow, resulting in cerebral vasoconstriction and reduced tissue bulk. Hyperventilation can divert blood flow preferentially to diseased tissues lacking autoregulation at the expense of normal brain.[2] Deliberate hyperventilation to reduce intracranial pressure can be risky as an adjunct to deliberate hypotension when mean arterial blood pressures are less than 50 mm Hg. The ensuing ischemia could be deleterious to normal brain tissues if a diversion of cerebral blood flow takes remaining blood flow.[2, 16] The rapid and substantial reduction in cerebral blood flow and intracranial pressure by hyperventilation makes hyperventilation valuable for immediately reducing brain bulk to facilitate intracranial surgery and reduce acute brain swelling.

Fluid Therapy

Restriction of intravenous fluids to only that volume necessary to maintain adequate circulating volume is recommended in neurosurgical patients with increased intracranial pressure.[9, 17] Excessive fluid volume is associated with decreased venous outflow and increased risk of compounding cerebral edema. Diuretic therapy is frequently indicated in medical management of patients with intracranial masses and elevated intracranial pressure or cerebral edema.[4]

Dextrose administration should be adjusted to the situation. Hyperglycemia is contraindicated in animals with cerebral ischemia, and cerebral edema can be exacerbated by administration of isotonic dextrose. Its

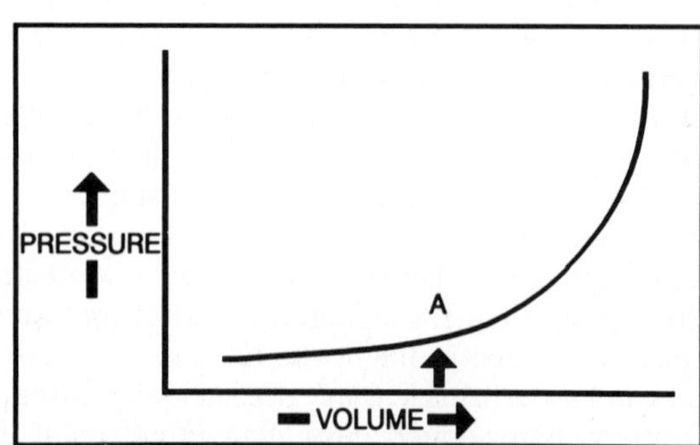

FIGURE 168–2. Increasing volume within the intracranial compartment causes little increase in pressure until a critical volume is reached. Beyond the limits of compliance, increases in volume greatly increase intracranial pressure. (From Shapiro HM: *In* Miller RM [ed]: *Anesthesia.* 2nd ed. Churchill Livingstone, New York, 1986, p 1566.)

use decreases seizures after metrizamide myelography and is indicated in hypoglycemic seizures or hypoglycemic coma.[10, 13, 24]

Glucocorticosteroid Therapy

Glucocorticoids are effective in treating some forms of cerebral edema.[8] Corticosteroids reduce the increased intracranial pressure resulting from brain tumors and hydrocephalus. Glucocorticoid therapy should be considered in the management of patients with cerebral edema associated with primary or metastatic brain neoplasia, trauma, some types of hemorrhage, and contusion. Steroid therapy is probably of little value once cerebral ischemia has occurred. Glucocorticosteroid therapy should optimally begin the day before neurosurgery when possible. Dexamethasone is recommended at 0.25 mg/kg every 8 hours, with a dose of 0.25 to 1 mg/kg IV after induction of anesthesia.[4] Because dexamethasone administration reduces the rate of CSF formation in dogs,[8, 22] there may be some value to steroid administration in the preanesthetic management of hydrocephalic patients considered at risk of further increases in intracranial pressure. Corticosteroids are contraindicated in infectious CNS diseases.

Positional Effects

Further increases in intracranial pressure can result from gravitational, procedural, or positional interference with drainage of venous blood from the head. Jugular venous occlusion from surgical positioning of the head, from the use of a neck leash, or from obtaining jugular venous blood samples or placement of jugular vein catheters can rapidly result in dangerously increased intracranial pressure in patients with pre-existing increases.[4] Slight elevation of the head above the level of the heart with the neck in a neutral position facilitates venous drainage and reduces intracranial pressure. Extreme elevation of the head during neurosurgery is avoided to minimize the risk of venous air embolization.[26]

DELIBERATE HYPOTENSION

Deliberate hypotension is occasionally indicated during neurosurgery. Controlled and deliberate reduction of arterial pressure, primarily with sodium nitroprusside or isoflurane, reduces operative blood loss in general surgery and is an adjunct to neurosurgery to reduce intracranial volume.[2, 4, 18, 24, 26]

Reduction of arterial blood pressure is rarely necessary in anesthetized animals, particularly if volatile anesthetics are used. Reduction in blood pressure is achieved by titrated administration of increased concentrations of volatile anesthetics (preferably isoflurane).[26] Isoflurane anesthesia is the favored method for producing deliberate hypotension because it has a rapid onset of action, produces no toxic metabolites, is easy to titrate to the desired effect, probably does not cause deleterious derangements of blood flow to critical tissues, and is rapidly reversed.

Among many techniques effective in producing deliberate and controlled hypotension, intravenous infusion of sodium nitroprusside (3 to 20 μg/kg/minute) is effective and can be safer than techniques based on other injectable drugs. Nitroprusside is metabolized to cyanide, and both its rate of infusion and total dose delivered are minimized. A maximum rate of 0.5 mg/kg/hour has been recommended.[4] Nitroprusside as well as other antihypertensive agents with vasodilatory properties (e.g., hydralazine and calcium antagonists) can cause cerebral vasodilatation, thereby actually increasing cerebral blood flow and intracranial pressure.[27]

Continuous monitoring of arterial blood pressure by arterial catheterization is required for safe management of deliberate hypotension regardless of the technique used. Mean arterial pressures should not be reduced below 50 mm Hg in controlled hypotension.[24, 26] Reduction in arterial pressure can be precipitous, and further physiological support must be immediately available. Deliberate hypotension may increase the likelihood of vasospasm, may contribute to ischemia, and may impair autoregulation.

ANESTHETIC CONCERNS

Volatile Anesthetics

Volatile anesthetics increase cerebral blood flow and alter cerebral metabolic oxygen requirement to various degrees (Figs. 168–3 and 168–4).[7, 10, 24–26] Because increased cerebral blood flow and intracranial pressure are also influenced by carbon dioxide retention, respiratory depression associated with volatile anesthesia can be responsible for clinically significant increases in intracranial pressure. Regional changes in distribution of cerebral blood flow result from administration of volatile anesthetics such that our understanding of cerebrovascular effects based on global estimates of cerebral blood flow in animals may be inaccurate.[15]

Halothane blocks autoregulation, increasing cerebral blood flow and intracranial pressure.[5, 6] Methoxyflurane, enflurane, and isoflurane all interfere with autoregulation less than halothane.[26] At 1.1 times the minimum alveolar concentration (MAC) levels of anesthesia, cerebral blood flow increases almost 200 per cent with

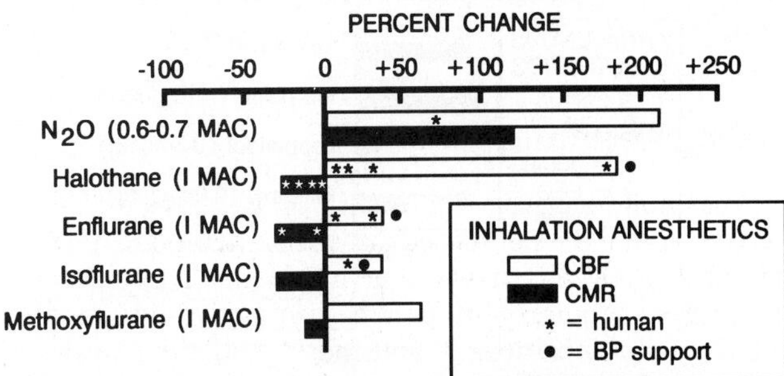

FIGURE 168–3. Alteration in cerebral blood flow (CBF) and cerebral metabolic rate (CMR) by volatile anesthetics. (From Shapiro HM: *Neuroanesthesia: Physiologic and Pharmacologic Principles. ASA Annual Refresher Course Lectures.* American Society of Anesthesiologists, Park Ridge, IL, 1980.)

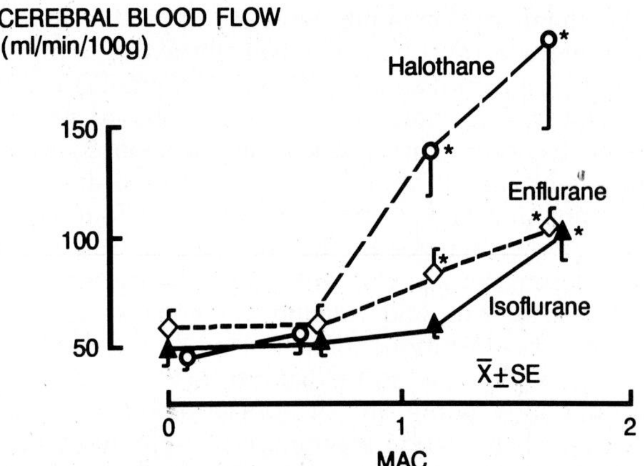

FIGURE 168–4. Cerebral blood flow increases with increasing concentration of volatile anesthetics (expressed as multiples of minimum alveolar concentration). (From Eger EI: *Isoflurane [Forane]. A Compendium and Reference.* Ohio Medical Products, Madison, WI, 1984.)

halothane but only about 40 per cent with enflurane and is unchanged with isoflurane.[7, 25] The alteration of cerebral blood flow by volatile anesthetics depends on dose (see Fig. 168–4).

Modest hyperventilation to reduce arterial carbon dioxide to about 30 mm Hg eliminates the volatile anesthetic-induced increase in cerebral blood flow.[5] Hyperventilation is rapidly effective in reducing cerebral blood flow and intracranial pressure or in preventing their rise in patients at risk. Hyperventilation is easy and cost free and is the safest method available to decrease intracranial pressure. Modest hyperventilation should be incorporated into the anesthetic technique for animals with intracranial masses or other disorders of autoregulation because of the respiratory depression of general anesthesia and the potential rise in cerebral blood flow and intracranial pressure. Nitrous oxide has substantial cerebrovascular effects, profoundly increasing in cerebral blood flow and intracranial pressure.

Injectable Anesthetics

Most injectable anesthetics cause significant reductions in cerebral metabolic oxygen requirement, cerebral blood flow, and intracranial pressure (Fig. 168–5).[4, 10, 19, 24–26] The value of barbiturates as therapy for cerebral ischemia/hypoxia is controversial. It is likely that barbiturates are protective if administered before the insult but of little value if administered after signs have developed. As with glucocorticoids, barbiturates may be of value in avoiding postoperative sequelae to surgical trauma. Barbiturate anesthesia can prolong anesthetic recovery. CNS depression associated with residual barbiturates can seriously obscure postoperative evaluation and prevent meaningful neurological evaluation.

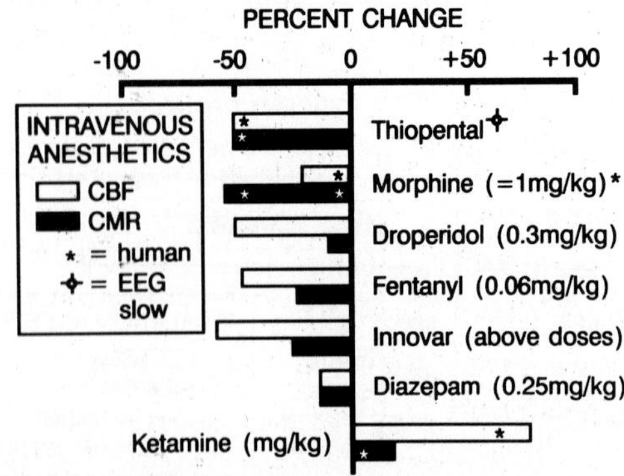

FIGURE 168–5. Alteration in cerebral blood flow (CBF) and cerebral metabolic rate (CMR) by injectable anesthetics. (From Shapiro HM: *Neuroanesthesia: Physiologic and Pharmacologic Principles. ASA Annual Refresher Course Lectures.* American Society of Anesthesiologists, Park Ridge, IL, 1980.)

The dissociative anesthetics represent a notable exception to the reduction in cerebral blood flow, intracranial pressure, and cerebral metabolic oxygen requirement characteristic of most injectable anesthetics (see Fig. 168–5).[4, 10, 24–26] EEG activity also increases with dissociative anesthesia. Convulsant activity ranging from muscle twitching to seizures is an infrequent adverse effect. Patients with a history of seizure-related disorders, intracranial masses, craniocerebral trauma, and other conditions potentially increasing intracranial pressure should not receive dissociative anesthetics.

SPECIFIC ANESTHETIC MANAGEMENT

Electroencephalography and Seizure Disorders

Dose-dependent CNS depression of EEG activity by most anesthetics is characteristic and has led to the development of EEG-based anesthetic monitoring techniques.[12] Notable exceptions include the dissociatives and enflurane. Enflurane anesthesia can be accompanied by increased EEG activity extending to seizures, particularly if a patient is hyperventilated and hypocarbic.[10, 26]

Seizure disorders can be exacerbated or improved by anesthetic management. Increased seizure activity associated with administration of the phenothiazine (e.g., acepromazine) and butyrophenone (e.g., droperidol) tranquilizers[11] contraindicates their use in seizure-prone patients and in patients undergoing diagnostic EEG. Control of seizures by administration of diazepam and midazolam can be desirable for other procedures in seizure-prone patients but obscures characteristic activity in diagnostic EEGs.

Isoflurane anesthesia frequently causes a characteristic intermittent suppression of EEG "burst activity"[20, 23] and may interfere with diagnostic information. Recommended anesthetic technique for diagnostic EEG evaluation and for procedures other than EEGs in seizure-prone patients is summarized (Table 168–1).

Myelography and Intervertebral Disc Disease

Anesthetic management for surgical decompression of cervical or thoracolumbar intervertebral disc herniation includes (1) protection from seizures and complications associated with administration of myelographic contrast agents, (2) pain relief, (3) maintenance of spontaneous ventilation, and (4) management of concurrent disorders such as urinary incontinence or other factors predisposing to adverse recovery. Recom-

TABLE 168–1. ANESTHETIC MANAGEMENT FOR SEIZURE-PRONE PATIENTS AND FOR DIAGNOSTIC ELECTROENCEPHALOGRAPHY

Control of seizures
Treatment or avoidance of hypoglycemia.
Avoid phenothiazine (e.g., acepromazine) and butyrophenone (e.g., droperidol) tranquilizers.
Benzodiazepine (diazepam, 0.4 mg/kg IM or IV) tranquilization or barbiturate (phenobarbital, 2 to 5 mg/kg IM) sedation.
Intravenous induction with thiobarbiturate (thiamylal or thiopental) but not methohexital.
Inhalational induction with isoflurane or halothane but not with enflurane.
Avoidance of increases in cerebral blood flow and intracranial pressure.

Diagnostic electroencephalography
Avoid preanesthetic tranquilizers and sedatives.
Intravenous induction with thiobarbiturate.
Maintain light plane of anesthesia with halothane or incremental thiobarbiturate if necessary to prolong duration.
Infiltration of temporal muscles with lidocaine as an alternative to general anesthesia.

mended anesthetic technique is summarized in Table 168–2.

Radiographic contrast myelography is frequently performed in the immediate preoperative period to localize the lesion(s) and identify the site for decompression. Patient management is designed to optimize conditions for both diagnostic (radiographic) and therapeutic procedures, because they are often performed during the same anesthetic period. Dural puncture for sampling of CSF or for administration of myelographic contrast agent requires a depth of anesthesia less than a surgical plane but adequate to prevent patients' movement and subsequent trauma.

Avoidance of potent respiratory depressants and a light surgical plane of anesthesia will maintain spontaneous ventilation during myelography. Among the less frequent complications associated with myelography are respiratory depression, respiratory arrest, and cardiac arrhythmias.[21] Respiratory depression is probably referable to effects of the contrast agent or the brain stem and medullary respiratory centers. As such, respiratory effects are most likely to be associated with "high" myelograms, typically those in which contrast agent ascends to the brain and brain stem. Seizure activity and the other potential adverse side effects of myelography are reduced with either iopamidol or iohexol rather than metrizamide.[3, 28]

Maintenance of spontaneous ventilation not only allows rapid recognition of respiratory depression as an adverse drug effect but also facilitates recognition of airway obstruction. Hyperflexion of the cervical spine for cisternal collection of cerebrospinal fluid and for cervical administration of myeolographic contrast can easily kink endotracheal tubes, resulting in airway obstruction. Armored or spiral wire endotracheal tubes are resistant to kinking; however, these tubes are radiopaque and are unsuitable for use in cervical and cranial radiographic studies. Close attention to adequacy of the airway and spontaneous ventilation is important.

Cervical disc disease can be associated with increased

TABLE 168–2. ANESTHETIC MANAGEMENT FOR MYELOGRAPHY AND INTERVERTEBRAL DISC DISEASE

Myelography and surgical decompression
Benzodiazepine tranquilization (e.g., diazepam, 0.4 mg/kg IV).
Low-dose opioid agonist-antagonists (e.g., butorphanol, 0.4 mg/kg IM).
Anticholinergics if indicated.
Intravenous induction with thiobarbiturate or inhalational induction with isoflurane or halothane by mask.
Avoid hyperflexion/extension of neck in patients with cervical trauma, instability, and disc disease.
Maintenance of protected airway and spontaneous ventilation (for recognition of side effects of myelography and to minimize vertebral sinus blood flow during surgery).
Fluid therapy with dextrose for metrizamide myelography.
Positioning to avoid venous occlusion.
Postoperative analgesics as needed.

risk of cardiac arrhythmias.[26] Increased vagal stimulation during ventral surgical approaches to the cervical spine can occur from retraction of the carotid sheath during ventral approach to the cervical spine. Postoperative pain frequently is more intense with cervical than thoracolumbar surgical repair.

Patients having lost deep-pain perception are surgical emergencies. Rapid-sequence induction using intravenous general anesthetics rather than inhalational induction of anesthesia is indicated if the animal has, or may have, a full stomach. The fact that these animals do not feel painful stimuli in the rear limbs suggests that these areas can preferentially be used for placement of injections and intravenous catheters without contributing additional stress to the patients.

Intracranial Masses and Elevated Intracranial Pressure

Animals with intracranial masses, dysfunctional cerebral blood flow autoregulation, or increased intracranial pressure are at risk of rapid deterioration during anesthesia. Anesthetic monitoring should address the physiologic variables associated with altered intracranial pressure. Venous and arterial pressures and airway or arterial sampling for carbon dioxide analysis are included if possible. Management of anesthesia for these patients is summarized in Table 168–3. Optimal anes-

TABLE 168–3. ANESTHETIC MANAGEMENT FOR PATIENTS WITH ELEVATED CBF/ICP AND FOR INTRACRANIAL SURGERY

Preanesthetic critical care management and stabilization (including glucocorticosteroid and diuretic therapy as indicated)
Fluid therapy limited to minimize cerebral edema but adequate to support circulation
Avoid potent respiratory depression, jugular venous occlusion, and coughing at induction of anesthesia and during recovery
Avoid dissociatives, halothane, enflurane, and nitrous oxide
Intravenous barbiturate induction of anesthesia
Minimal concentrations of isoflurane, supplemented with opioids or barbiturates for maintenance of anesthesia
Modest hyperventilation (30 mm Hg) to reduce CBF/ICP
Postoperative critical care with support of ventilation and circulation as indicated

thetic management can substantially improve a patient's status and the outcome of intracranial procedures.

Advance Imaging and Electrodiagnostic Techniques

Computed tomography, magnetic resonance imaging, and positron emission tomography are increasingly used in veterinary referral centers. Application of these techniques can greatly facilitate identification and definition of many intracranial and spinal cord lesions. Unique and sometimes exotic requirements for anesthetic equipment and monitoring are associated with facilities that house these imaging units.[1, 25]

Advanced eletrodiagnostic procedures including electroretinography, visual evoked potential, auditory evoked response, brain stem auditory evoked response, and somatosensory evoked response similarly have become valuable diagnostic tools in referral centers. In many cases, significant limitations are placed on the choice of anesthetic drugs to maximize the diagnostic value of these procedures.[12]

References

1. Burk NS: Anesthesia for magnetic resonance imaging. *Anesth Clin North Am 7*:707, 1989.
2. Cottrell JE: Deliberate hypotension. Annual Refresher Course Lectures, American Society of Anesthesiologists, Section 245, pp 1–7.
3. Cox FH: The use of iopamidol for myelography in dogs: A study of twenty-seven cases. *J Small Anim Pract 27*:159, 1986.
4. Dayrell-Hart B, Klide AM: Intracranial dysfunctions: Stupor and coma. *Vet Clin North Am Small Anim Pract 19*:1209, 1989.
5. Drummond JC, Todd MM: The response of the feline cerebral circulation to Pa_{CO_2} during anesthesia with isoflurane and halothane and during sedation with nitrous oxide. *Anesthesiology 62*:268, 1985.
6. Drummond JC, et al: CO_2 responsiveness of the cerebral circulation during isoflurane anesthesia and nitrous oxide sedation in cats. *Anesthesiology 57*:A333, 1982.
7. Eger EI: *Isoflurane (Forane). A Compendium and Reference.* Ohio Medical Products, Madison, WI, 1984.
8. Franklin RT: The use of glucocorticoids in treating cerebral edema. *Comp Cont Educ 6*:422, 1984.
9. Frost EAM: Central nervous system trauma. *Anesth Clin North Am 5*:565, 1987.
10. Gilroy BA: Neuroanesthesiology. *In* Slatter D (ed): *Textbook of Small Animal Surgery*. W. B. Saunders, Philadelphia, 1985.
11. Gleed RD: Tranquilizers and sedatives. *In* Short CE (ed): *Principles and Practice of Veterinary Anesthesia.* Williams & Wilkins, Baltimore, 1987.
12. Goodrich JT: Electrophysiologic measurements: Intraoperative evoked potential monitoring. *Anesth Clin North Am 5*:477, 1987.
13. Gray PR, et al: Effect of intravenous administration of dextrose or lactated Ringer's solution on seizure development in dogs after cervical myelography with metrizamide. *Am J Vet Res 48*:1600, 1987.
14. Grubb RL, et al: The effects of changes in Pa_{CO_2} on cerebral blood volume, blood flow, and vascular mean transit time. *Stroke 5*:530, 1974.
15. Hansen TD, et al: Regional distribution of cerebral blood flow with halothane and isoflurane. *Anesthesiology 69*: 332, 1988.
16. Harp JR, Wollman H: Cerebral metabolic effects of hyperventilation and deliberate hypotension. *Br J Anaesth 45*:256, 1973.
17. Hirshfeld A: Fluid and electrolyte management in neurosurgical patients. *Anesth Clin North Am 5*:491, 1987.
18. Osborn I: Choice of neuroanesthetic technique. *Anesth Clin North Am 5*:531, 1987.
19. Rampil IJ, et al: I653 and isoflurane produce similar dose-related changes in the electroencephalogram of pigs. *Anesthesiology 69*:298, 1988.
20. Riedesel DH: Diagnostic or experimental surgical procedures. *In* Short CE (ed): *Principles and Practice of Veterinary Anesthesia.* Williams & Wilkins, Baltimore, 1987.
21. Sato O, et al: The effect of dexamethasone phosphate on the production rate of cerebrospinal fluid in the spinal subarachnoid space of dogs. *J Neurosurg 39*:480, 1973.
22. Schwartz AE, et al: Electroencephalographic burst suppression in elderly and young patients anesthetized with isoflurane. *Anesth Analg 68*:9, 1989.
23. Shapiro HH: Neurosurgical anesthesia and intracranial hypertension. *In* Miller RD (ed): *Anesthesia*. 2nd ed. Churchill Livingstone, New York, 1986, pp 1563–1620.
24. Stoelting RK: *Pharmacology and Physiology in Anesthetic Practice*. J.B. Lippincott, Philadelphia, 1987.
25. VanPoznak A: Special considerations for veterinary neuroanesthesia. *In* Short CE (ed): *Principles and Practice of Veterinary Anesthesia.* Williams & Wilkins, Baltimore, 1987.
26. Warner DS: [Report of scientific meeting]. *Anesthesiology 68*:663 1988.
27. Wheeler SJ, Davies JV: Iohexol myelography in the dog and cat: A series of one hundred cases and a comparison with metrizamide and iopamidol. *J Small Anim Pract 26*:247, 1985.
28. Yamada S, et al: Safety limits of controlled hypotension in humans. *Acta Neurochir 42*:14, 1988.

Anesthesia for Ophthalmic Surgery

John W. Ludders

No single medical or surgical condition or type of patient characterizes patients presenting for ophthalmic surgery. To anesthetize animals for ophthalmic surgery, one must be able to safely manage young and old, healthy and sick, minor elective and severe emergencies. No single anesthetic technique exists for all animals for ophthalmic procedures. This section focuses on a few key considerations for safer anesthetic management of patients presenting for ophthalmic surgery, with particular attention given to patients with increased intraocular pressure.

The two goals for anesthetic management of patients undergoing ophthalmic surgery are (1) to avoid increases in intraocular pressure and (2) to support cardiopulmonary function.

INTRAOCULAR PRESSURE

Intraocular pressure is influenced by several major physiological factors, including aqueous humor fluid dynamics, choroidal blood volume, central venous pressure, vitreous humor volume, and extraocular muscle tone.[3] Aqueous humor fluid dynamics are determined by aqueous production and drainage; anything that influences either production or drainage will cause changes in aqueous humor fluid volume and will affect intraocular pressure. Choroidal blood volume is affected by a number of factors including local autoregulatory mechanisms, systolic blood pressure, central venous pressure, and Pa_{CO_2}.[3] Coughing, vomiting, straining, and positive-pressure ventilation can cause sudden increases in central venous pressure, thus increasing intraocular pressure. Increases in Pa_{CO_2} can increase choroidal blood volume. All of these factors can be affected by both anesthetic drugs and anesthetic techniques.

Most anesthetic medications used in veterinary medicine decrease intraocular pressure by reducing cardiac output or systemic blood pressure or both, relaxing extraocular muscles, or increasing aqueous outflow. Barbiturates reduce intraocular pressure primarily by relaxation of the extraocular muscles and by facilitating aqueous humor outflow. Narcotics are acceptable induction agents, especially for patients with cardiac disease, but some (morphine, fentanyl) may need to be preceded by an anticholinergic because they increase vagal tone and cause bradyarrhythmias.

Early studies demonstrated that ketamine caused an increase in intraocular pressure. Studies now suggest that intraocular pressure actually decreased by 25 per cent in patients receiving ketamine and premedicated with diazepam and meperidine.[3] Intraocular pressure decreased by 12% in monkeys anesthetized with ketamine.[5] The disadvantages of ketamine are the loss of the blink reflex, precipitation of nystagmus, and prolonged and atactic recovery. Ketamine has proved safe and useful for induction when combined with sedatives such as diazepam.

PREANESTHETIC ASSESSMENT AND MEDICATION

Anesthetic management always begins with a review of a patient's medical history, which familiarizes the clinician with past problems, medications, and circumstances surrounding physical conditions or current ocular problems. Inquiries about current medications identify potential adverse drug interactions between ophthalmic and anesthetic drugs. A complete physical examination is essential for developing an anesthetic plan tailored to each patient.

Although adequate ventilation is important for any anesthetized patient, it can have greater importance for patients with eye disease. Patients with ophthalmic disease are frequently medicated with a carbonic anhydrase inhibitor such as acetazolamide (Diamox) or dichlorphenamide (Daranide) for control of intraocular pressure. These drugs can produce a significant metabolic acidemia,[6] and hyperventilation is a normal compensatory mechanism. It is not unusual to observe these patients breathing deeply and rapidly before anesthesia while resting quietly in their cages. Anesthetic-induced hypoventilation worsens a patient's acidosis and complicates anesthetic management. Acidosis lowers the threshold for cardiac arrhythmias and reduces cardiac contractility. It is preferable to correct metabolic acidosis with bicarbonate before anesthesia and surgery. During anesthesia, fluids may be administered to maintain intravascular volume and adequate perfusion of vital tissues and organs. A light plane of anesthesia and support of ventilation help overcome anesthetic-induced ventilatory depression.

Severe bradyarrhythmias and cardiac arrest due to stimulation of the oculocardiac reflex have been documented and occur infrequently.[1, 8] The oculocardiac reflex is due to direct pressure or traction on extraocular muscles. This reflex is more likely to occur in dogs with both inadequate relaxation of the extraocular muscles and hypoventilation.[2] As a protective measure against the oculocardiac reflex and other vagally mediated cardiac arrhythmias, patients are premedicated with an anticholinergic such as atropine (0.02 mg/kg IM or SC) or glycopyrrolate (0.01 mg/kg IM or SC). The surgeon should stop manipulating the eye and administer either atropine or glycopyrrolate intravenously to block the parasympathetic nervous system if heart block or bradyarrhythmias occur during anesthesia. Glycopyrrolate is associated with a lower incidence of tachycardia and dysrhythmias than atropine.[4] To avoid atropine- or glycopyrrolate-induced tachycardia, one-half of the intramuscular dose is given intravenously, and 3 minutes is allowed to elapse before another injection is administered. Atropine's CNS effects may become obvious before its peripheral effects when administered intravenously at doses of less than 0.015 mg/kg.[7] Thus, heart rate can further decrease before it increases.

ANESTHETIC MANAGEMENT

The combined effects of a tranquilizer and narcotic (neuroleptanalgesia) may be used to both calm and provide pain relief, facilitating management of patients with increased intraocular pressures or corneal lacerations (see Chapter 163).

Induction to anesthesia should be stress free. Gentle, patient restraint and a quiet environment sustain the effects of preanesthetic sedatives and tranquilizers, thus limiting patients' excitement. This in turn helps to minimize increases in intraocular pressure and reduce unnecessary challenges to the cardiopulmonary system.

Extra care should be taken to protect patients' eyes. Direct pressure around or on the eyes should be avoided during induction. The edges of an anesthetic mask should not rub against the eyes. Jugular venous blood flow must not be impeded because impediment to flow can cause a marked increase in intraocular pressure due to high venous pressure and reduced aqueous drainage. Tight collars are removed before induction, and strangleholds are avoided.

Anesthesia can be induced with any standard anesthetic induction technique. Selection of an induction technique is determined by the general health of the patient, as well as the availability of drugs and equipment.

Intubation is always recommended for animals under general anesthesia. Intubation is not performed if anesthesia is too light and the animal is resistant. Marked increases in intraocular pressure have been recorded during and after difficult intubation, and these increased pressures have persisted well into the surgical period.[3] Gentle intubation with the animal at an appropriate level of anesthesia minimizes laryngeal stimulation and reduces the chance for increases in IOP.

All inhalant anesthetics—methoxyflurane, halothane, isoflurane, and nitrous oxide—reduce intraocular pressure as much as 35 to 50 per cent of awake values.[3] During general anesthesia with inhalant anesthetics, the

TABLE 168–4. GENERAL EFFECTS OF SOME MUSCLE PARALYTICS

Drug	Histamine Release	Sympathetic Stimulation	Vagal Stimulation	Duration of Effect	Effect on Intraocular Pressure
Succinylcholine	+	–	+	Short	Increase
Atracurium	+	–	–	Intermediate	No effect
Vecuronium	–	–	–	Intermediate	No effect
Pancuronium	–	+ +	–	Long	No effect

plane of anesthesia is often deepened to eliminate undesirable ocular responses such as nystagmus and palpebral reflexes. This practice is potentially dangerous. Anesthetic depression of cardiopulmonary function depends on dose. A patient's head is frequently covered with surgical drapes, making it difficult to monitor traditional signs of anesthetic depth such as jaw tone, mucous membrane color, capillary refill time, lingual pulse, and ocular reflexes. Reduced monitoring and a deepening plane of anesthesia place anesthetized patients at increased risk for anesthetic-induced cardiopulmonary failure. A blood pressure monitor, such as a Doppler flow probe monitor or oscillometric device, coupled with an electrocardiogram may help to overcome difficulties of monitoring.

Central or peripheral muscle relaxants may be used to ensure a quiet eye and as an alternative to deep general anesthesia. Routine use of such newer peripheral muscle relaxants such as atracurium and vecuronium offers specific advantages such as an intermediate duration of action (10 to 20 minutes), minimal cardiovascular effects, minimal if any histamine release, and no effect on intraocular pressure (Table 168–4).[9] Peripheral muscle relaxants are not anesthetics, do not produce unconsciousness or provide analgesia, and are not used alone. Once paralyzed, a patient must be mechanically ventilated. Adequate ventilation can be achieved with airway pressures of 10 to 15 cm H_2O and ventilatory frequencies of 8 to 12 breaths per minute. Obesity or pulmonary disease may require increased airway pressures or respiratory frequencies. Every effort is made not to redose a peripheral muscle relaxant near the end of a surgical procedure because this prolongs recovery. Recovery from anesthesia and muscle paralysis is faster when a patient is normothermic; metabolism and excretion are slowed by hypothermia. The combination of atropine (0.02 mg/kg IV) followed by neostigmine (0.02 mg/kg IV) is used to reverse the effects of peripheral muscle relaxants. Administration of more than three doses of reversal drugs without effect signals residual effects of other anesthetic drugs or hypothermia. Cardiopulmonary support (fluids, ventilation) while warming the patient facilitates recovery.

Recovery is as important as anesthesia induction and maintenance. A quiet, struggle-free recovery is important to avoid trauma to the eyes.

References

1. Blanc VF, et al: The oculocardiac reflex: A graphic and statistical analysis in infants and children. *Can Anaesth Soc J 30*: 360, 1983.
2. Clutton RE, et al: Significance of the oculocardiac reflex during ophthalmic surgery in the dog. *J Small Anim Pract 29*: 573, 1988.
3. Cunningham AJ: Intraocular pressure—physiology and implications for anesthetic management. *Can Anesth Soc J 32*:195, 1986.
4. Greenan J: Cardiac dysrhythmias and heart rate changes at induction of anaesthesia: A comparison of two intravenous anticholinergics. *Acta Anaesthesial Scand 28*: 182, 1984.
5. Hahnenberger RW: Influence of cataleptoid anesthetic agents on the intraocular pressure in monkeys (*Macaca fascicularis*). *Acta Ophthalmol 54*: 491, 1976.
6. Haskins SC, et al: Effect of acetazolamide on blood acid-base and electrolyte values in dogs. *J Am Vet Med Assoc 179*: 792, 1981.
7. Muir WW: Effects of atropine on cardiac rate and rhythm in dogs. *J Am Vet Med Assoc 172*: 917, 1978.
8. Smith RB, et al: The oculocardiac reflex and sino-atrial arrest. *Can Anaesth Soc J 19*: 138, 1972.
9. Torda TA: The new relaxants. A review of the clinical pharmacology of atracurium and vecuronium. *Anaesth Intensive Care 15*:72, 1987.

CHAPTER 169 Anesthesia for Upper Airway and Thoracic Surgery

Jane E. Quandt and Marc R. Raffe

Management of respiratory disease during anesthesia is important in surgical practice. The overall goal is to maintain or support normal respiratory tract function. This chapter presents general patient management principles that are important to the respiratory disease patient and applies these principles to specific disease conditions that are encountered in companion animal practice.

Normal pulmonary function is disrupted during general anesthesia, and knowledge of the effects of anesthetic drugs on respiratory function and on control of breathing is important. The respiratory patient is fragile and must be managed in a calm, efficient manner until anesthetic induction and airway patency can be secured. Preoperative assessment is critical in evaluating the location, extent, and severity of respiratory disease. Obvious injury or disease to the chest wall, diaphragm, pulmonary tree, or trachea is stabilized prior to anesthetic induction so that pulmonary gas exchange can remain unrestricted. The degree of dysfunction associated with the disease must be understood so that surgical preparation of the patient can occur with minimal additional stress. The patient is supported with oxygen and handled gently. Emergency supplies and drugs should be accessible during induction and maintenance of anesthesia.

MANAGEMENT OF RESPIRATORY PATIENT DURING ANESTHESIA

Airway Management Techniques

Several techniques are available for ensuring a patent airway. The most common is orotracheal intubation using a cuffed endotracheal tube. A high-volume, low-pressure cuff is preferred to seal the airway should ventilatory support be necessary. A laryngoscope is valuable for rapid, accurate intubation because it facilitates laryngeal observation. Alternate techniques of airway management may be necessary if orotracheal intubation cannot be performed because of the surgical procedure or pre-existing disease. Tracheostomy or pharyngostomy intubation is performed in these cases. The animal is initially intubated after anesthetic induction, and tracheostomy or pharyngostomy is performed aseptically. Oxygen and an anesthetic gas can be adminstered by face mask until the airway is supported by one of these techniques if intubation is not possible during the initial period. The surgical approach for tracheostomy is performed, and if the patient was previously intubated orotracheally the tracheostomy tube is introduced as the orotracheal tube is withdrawn. A cuffed tracheostomy tube is preferred to allow the airway to be sealed. Pharyngostomy intubation is performed using an endotracheal tube, which is introduced through the aseptically prepared pharyngostomy incision. The tube is guided into position through the larynx after withdrawal of the orotracheal tube.[2, 4, 10, 14]

Ventilatory Support

The respiratory patient may require ventilatory support during anesthesia because of the combined effects of the presenting disease and the anesthetic drugs. The goal of ventilatory support is to mimic normal ventilation. Tidal volume is approximately 15 ml/kg. Normal respiratory rate is 6 to 12 breaths per minute. The maximum airway pressure during ventilation is 15 to 18 cm H_2O in the dog and 12 to 15 cm H_2O in the cat. Increased airway pressure of 20 to 30 cm H_2O may be required to maintain adequate volume in open chest procedures. The ratio of inspiration to expiration is 1:2 or 1:3.[3, 13, 17] At least twice as much time should be spent in the expiratory as in the inspiratory phase.

Ventilation can be provided by manual compression of the reservoir bag or by mechanical ventilation. Two types of mechanical ventilators are available: pressure-cycled ventilators, such as the Bird ventilator, and volume-cycled ventilators, such as the Ohio and Metomatic* ventilators. A volume-cycled ventilator has a preset tidal volume delivered regardless of airway pressure generated in delivering the breath. A pressure-limited ventilator delivers the gas volume until a preset pressure value is reached. The tidal volume varies, depending on changes in respiratory compliance and resistance.[13, 17]

Ventilatory support is usually administered as intermittent positive-pressure ventilation, which mimics normal breathing. Gas volume is delivered during the respiratory cycle with return to baseline airway pressure between breaths. Additional techniques may be used with intermittent positive-pressure ventilation to improve gas exchange in compromised patients. Positive end-expiratory pressure can be used with intermittent positive-pressure ventilation to help keep small airways open. Gas exchange following lung trauma or during pulmonary edema is improved by the increase in functional residual capacity. Typically, a baseline airway pressure of 5 to 10 cm H_2O is maintained between breaths. A similar technique, continuous positive airway pressure can be used in patients who are ventilating spontaneously. Continuous positive airway pressure allows the animal to take spontaneous breaths while maintaining a basal positive airway pressure. This technique is useful at the beginning or end of a surgical procedure that induces significant lung atelectasis.[3, 13, 17] A commercially available positive end-expiratory pressure valve† can be inserted into the expiratory limb of the breathing circuit. Alternatively, the scavenging hose of the pressure-relief (pop-off) valve can be mechanically restricted to produce the desired degree of positive end-expiratory pressure.

Resistance to ventilation may be encountered during ventilatory support. Inadequate anesthetic depth may be the cause; however, increased anesthetic depth may be undesirable because of additional cardiorespiratory depression. Supplemental analgesia can be provided by using incremental doses of fentanyl or oxymorphone. These drugs produce effective analgesia with minimal cardiorespiratory depression. Doses during or after surgery are generally one-fourth the induction dosages. Muscle relaxants may be indicated to overcome patient resistance and allow surgery to proceed. Atracurium besylate or pancuronium bromide are the drugs of choice. Both drugs are given by a slow intravenous injection. Atracurium and pancuronium produce minimal cardiovascular effects. Tachycardia following administration of pancuronium is the major side effect. Concentration of inhalant anesthetic can be decreased following administration of a muscle relaxant, or following supplemental analgesia, unless inadequate anesthesia is the initial cause of patient resistance.

---

*Bird Products Corp., Palm Springs, CA; Ohio Medical Products, Madison, WI.

†Vital Signs, Inc., Tutore, NJ.

Reversal of muscle relaxation may be necessary after surgery to re-establish spontaneous breathing. Neostigmine or edrophonium chloride is used for this reversal, but each can be dangerous because of its muscarinic effects which can cause bradycardia. An anticholinergic is administered with the reversal drug. The endpoint of reversal is the animal's ability to ventilate adequately to maintain relative normocarbia.[9, 11, 17]

Monitoring

The parameters to monitor in the respiratory patient are similar to those monitored in other patients. Evaluation of cardiorespiratory parameters, tissue perfusion, and anesthetic depth are critical issues. The extent of monitoring varies with patient age and severity of the pre-existing disease.[3, 6, 12]

Monitoring parameters in cases of minimal respiratory disease include respiratory rate and chest excursions, mucous membrane color and blood color at the surgery site, and pulse. Visual observation of the animal and reservoir bag, and use of an esophageal stethoscope, accomplish this. Patients with pre-existing cardiorespiratory disease are monitored for tidal volume and oxygen status by noninvasive methods or by arterial blood gas analysis. Additional emphasis is placed on the assessment of oxygenation and tissue perfusion in patients with special considerations regarding their pre-existing cardiorespiratory disease.

Qualitative evaluation of respiratory function includes respiratory rate and pattern in the spontaneously breathing animal. Color and refill of mucous membranes provide information regarding oxygen delivery to tissues. Quantitative methods of respiratory gas analysis require expensive and specialized equipment. Arterial blood gas evaluation provides information regarding adequacy of ventilation and gas exchange. Pulse oximetry is a technique that works by noninvasive placement of a sensor on the skin or mucous membranes. Common probe sites in companion animals are the tongue and tail base. Normal hemoglobin saturation value, as measured by pulse oximetry, is 98 to 100 per cent, moderate desaturation occurs at less than 90 per cent, and severe hypoxemia occurs at or below 85 per cent. Capnometry measurement of carbon dioxide (in expired gas) can be used to evaluate overall integrity of the respiratory tract.[18, 19]

Monitoring cardiovascular parameters provides corollary information about gas exchange. Tachycardia may be a sign of inadequate anesthetic depth, hypoxemia, or hypercapnia. Bradycardia may reflect anesthetic overdose, terminal hypoxemia, or extreme hypercapnia. Diminished heart sounds may indicate reduced mechanical activity of the heart resulting from the factors listed previously. Mucous membrane color is a qualitative indicator of gas exchange and peripheral perfusion.[1, 3, 6, 12]

An electrocardiographic monitor is used to detect dysrhythmias associated with impaired gas exchange. Dysrhythmia of atrial or ventricular origin can occur as a condition secondary to respiratory disease and associated hypoxemia or hypercapnia.[1, 3, 6, 12]

Blood pressure can be influenced by hypoxemia or hypercapnia. Normal blood pressure values are 100 to 160 mm Hg systolic pressure, 60 to 100 mm Hg diastolic pressure, and 80 to 120 mm Hg mean arterial pressure. Hypoxemia and hypercapnia are associated with an initial increase in blood pressure followed by a secondary reduction as the magnitude of the hypoxemia and hypercapnia increases.[1, 3, 6, 12]

MANAGEMENT OF RESPIRATORY PATIENT DURING RECOVERY

The recovery period is critical for the respiratory patient. Continued evaluation of the patient's gas exchange is imperative. Maintaining a clear, unobstructed airway through proper positioning of the patient is important. Until the patient demonstrates the ability to maintain a clear, unobstructed airway, airway support is essential. Adequacy of ventilation can be assessed with a respirometer. The respirometer can be attached to the end of the endotracheal tube or tight-fitting face mask that is placed over the nose and mouth. A minimum tidal volume of 10 ml/kg should be present. Assisted ventilation should continue if the animal has a tidal volume less than this value. Availability of equipment to provide supplemental airway support and oxygenation following extubation is important to prevent hypoxemia and hypoventilation in the immediate postoperative period. Evaluation of the patient following extubation should continue for 15 minutes. Assessment of mucous membrane color and refill, respiratory rate and effort, and heart rate and pulse quality provides information regarding patient stability.[3]

Patients undergoing thoracotomy require additional consideration. Pulmonary reinflation after surgery is ensured by direct observation of lung inflation prior to closure. Evacuation of the pleural cavity to restore the normal relationship between the lungs and chest wall must occur. In most cases, a chest drain is inserted through the thoracic wall prior to closure. The tube is used to remove air and fluid from the pleural cavity. Following closure, the animal is rolled in several positions during tube aspiration to remove any residual air or fluid. The tube is clamped to prevent reintroduction of air into the pleural space, and a loose wrap is placed on the thorax. A radiograph is obtained to confirm intrapleural location if the tube is inserted after the chest is closed.[3, 10]

Pain relief following thoracic surgery may be necessary to ensure adequate gas exchange. The risk of respiratory depression associated with analgesic drugs is usually outweighed by improved tidal volume and reduced respiratory effort, which result from analgesia. Pain relief can be provided by several methods. Intercostal nerve block after lateral thoracotomy is useful for providing analgesia. Bupivacaine hydrochloride (Marcaine 0.5%) is recommended for analgesia because it provides 6 to 8 hours of analgesia per administration. Intercostal nerve block requires an injection at individual nerve locations. Two nerve segments on either side of the incision are blocked. An injection of 0.5 ml per nerve is used. Blocking the intercostal nerves decreases the amount of systemic analgesic required. Intercostal nerve blocks can be used in the dog and the cat. Bupivacaine may also be infused through the chest drain to provide analgesia by intrapleural analgesia. Bupivacaine is combined with saline (1:1 v/v) prior to injection into the thoracic chest tube. The patient is positioned so that the surgical site is down, permitting greatest contact between bupivacaine and surgical site. The duration of analgesia ranges from 4 to 12 hours with this technique.

Opioids can also be used for pain relief in the postthoracotomy patient. Opioid agonists such as morphine (0.1 to 0.3 mg/kg) and oxymorphone (0.05 to 0.1 mg/kg) and buprenorphine hydrochloride (Buprenex) (0.005 to 0.01 mg/kg) can also be used to provide analgesia. Butorphanol's analgesic duration is shorter than that of oxymorphone; buprenorphine is longer in duration than butorphanol. Oxymorphone or butorphanol in combination with a tranquilizer works well in the cat for postsurgical pain management. Buprenorphine does not produce central nervous system depression.[3, 6, 7, 8, 10]

SPECIFIC CONDITIONS

Upper-Airway Corrective Procedures. Laryngeal procedures such as partial laryngectomy for laryngeal paralysis and removal of everted laryngeal saccules are usually performed through an oral approach. These procedures may require an unguarded airway or alternate airway management. Fortunately, surgical correction is usually quick. The anesthetic goal during these procedures is to maintain spontaneous ventilation and provide an uninhibited airway. Oxygen insufflation (3 to 10 L/min) via sterile rubber or silicone tubing introduced into the airway maintains adequate oxygenation during this period. Preoperatively, airway management equipment such as a laryngoscope, endotracheal tubes and an Ambu bag* or anesthetic machine should be readily available. The availability of suction equipment for evacuation of blood is important. A low dose of acepromazine or a neuroleptanalgesic such as droperidol-fentanyl (Innovar-Vet) can be used to calm the animal if it shows signs of respiratory distress. Innovar-Vet or a thiobarbiturate is intravenously titrated to provide anesthesia for the procedure. A new sedative-hypnotic drug, propofol (Diprivan) also works well for these procedures. The anesthetic depth is adjusted to minimize laryngeal reflexes during surgical resection. The animal is given corticosteroids at the completion of the procedure to decrease inflammation. Oral intubation, airway suctioning, and recovery with oxygen support are performed. The endotracheal tube cuff is inflated to help minimize introduction of blood into the trachea. The cuff is kept partially inflated during extubation to remove blood clots. Ventilation is closely observed during recovery. Postoperative tranquilization or sedation may be indicated during recovery to minimize struggling and excitement, which increase oxygen demand.[3–5, 15]

*Mercury Medical, Clearwater, FL.

Tracheal Procedures. Tracheal lacerations, tracheal collapse, and tracheal neoplasia are the most common diseases encountered that require anesthetic support. Surgical procedures on the trachea require airway support. Preoperative management includes patient stabilization, premedication to reduce increased respiratory effort associated with excitement, and preoxygenation. Anesthetic induction is rapid and airway control is achieved (Tables 169–1 and 169–2). Sedative-hypnotics such as thiobarbiturates or propofol can be safely used in cases without concurrent cardiovascular disease. Orotracheal intubation is accomplished as quickly as possible. Premeasurement of tube length ensures correct positioning of the tube beyond the lesion. A small-diameter tube may be necessary to bypass the lesion. Following intubation and cuff inflation, ventilatory support is provided as required. Insufflation of oxygen through a bronchoscopic side port, or airway support through an endotracheal tube adapter with a side port for bronchoscope insertion, is preferred to prevent hypoxemia during bronchoscopic examination.

Continuation of airway maintenance for as long as possible is desirable during emergence from anesthesia. Elective tracheostomy and tracheostomy tube placement are performed at this time if long-term ventilatory support is anticipated. Supplemental oxygen administered by nasal catheter or face mask can prevent hypoxemia in the immediate postanesthetic period.

Chest Wall Injuries. Chest wall injuries are often associated with trauma and require special consideration

TABLE 169–1. SUGGESTED AGENTS FOR DOGS WITH RESPIRATORY DISEASE

Agent	Advantages	Disadvantages
Premedication		
Acepromazine	Minimal respiratory depression	Hypotension
Opioids	Analgesia Minimal cardiovascular effects	Respiratory depression
Midazolam	Minimal cardiovascular effects	Respiratory depression
Atropine or glycopyrrolate	Decreases salivation	Increases heart rate
Induction		
Thiobarbiturate	Rapid onset with short duration	May cause arrhythmias and apnea
Methohexital sodium	Rapid onset with short duration	May cause arrhythmias and apnea
Propofol	Rapid onset with very short duration	May cause apnea
Ketamine or tranquilizer	Cardiorespiratory stability	Slow onset Laryngeal tone Tachycardia
Opioid or tranquilizer	Cardiorespiratory stability	Slow onset Laryngeal tone
Maintenance		
Methoxyflurane	Analgesia	Slow induction and recovery
Halothane	Rapid induction and recovery	Hypotension Catecholamine-induced arrhythmias
Isoflurane	Rapid induction and recovery	Respiratory depression

TABLE 169–2. SUGGESTED AGENTS FOR CATS WITH RESPIRATORY DISEASE

Agent	Advantages	Disadvantages
Premedication		
Acepromazine	Minimal respiratory depression	Hypotension
Midazolam	Minimal cardiovascular effects	Respiratory depression
Atropine or glycopyrrolate	Decreases salivation	Increases heart rate
Ketamine	Rapid onset	Salivation Tachycardia Irregular respiratory pattern
Induction		
Thiobarbiturate	Rapid onset with short duration	May cause arrhythmias
Methohexital sodium	Rapid onset with short duration	May cause arrhythmias
Propofol	Rapid onset with very short duration	May cause apnea
Ketamine or tranquilizer	Cardiorespiratory stability	Slow onset Laryngeal tone Tachycardia
Maintenance		
Methoxyflurane	Analgesia	Slow induction and recovery
Halothane	Rapid induction and recovery	Hypotension Catecholamine-induced arrhythmias
Isoflurane	Rapid induction and recovery	Respiratory depression

because of their effects on respiratory mechanics and gas exchange. Traumatic myocarditis is often associated with chest wall injury. Myocardial contusion is suspected in all cases of blunt chest trauma. It is usually manifested by cardiac arrhythmias not attributed to other causes, such as pre-existing disease or shock. Attempts are made to stabilize cardiac rhythm prior to anesthesia. Arrhythmogenic anesthetics such as xylazine hydrochloride, thiobarbiturates, and halothane are avoided if traumatic myocarditis is present.

Flail chest, if present, must be presumed to cause inadequate respiration. Preoperative patient management includes stabilization of the flail segment of the chest prior to anesthesia. The patient can be placed in lateral recumbency with the flail side down to improve ventilation when emergency stabilization cannot be performed. Pulmonary parenchymal injury is assumed. Preoxygenation is provided during the preparation and induction periods to facilitate oxygen transport. Anesthetic techniques that provide rapid induction are selected (see Tables 169–1 and 169–2); orotracheal intubation is immediately initiated. Because intermittent positive-pressure ventilation reverses the phasic changes in transthoracic pressures associated with normal ventilation, it provides a pneumatic splint to a flail segment. Anesthetic maintenance is usually provided by inhalational agents. Monitoring techniques associated with the high-risk patient include analysis of arterial blood gases and electrocardiography. Airway maintenance following surgical correction is continued for as long as possible. Supplemental oxygenation maintains systemic oxygenation during postoperative hypoventilation and ventilation/perfusion mismatching. Pain management by local nerve blocks and by parenteral analgesics facilitates normal breathing in the postsurgical period. External bandages are not tightly wrapped around the thorax. The clinician should be able to introduce one hand comfortably between the underside of the bandage and the chest wall.[3, 15]

Penetrating chest wall trauma requires aggressive management. Pneumothorax and hemothorax must be assumed to be present in all cases until proved otherwise. Preoperative stabilization including supplemental oxygen, thoracentesis, or thoracostomy tube placement is performed prior to anesthetic induction. Anesthetic management is similar to that described previously.[3, 15]

Pleural Space Disease. Space-occupying lesions such as hemothorax, pyothorax, pneumothorax, chylothorax, and intrapleural masses create abnormal pulmonary compliance and dynamics. Animals with one or more of these conditions are at high risk, because anesthesia, respiratory depression, and ventilation/perfusion mismatching further compromise the patient's ability to maintain normal gas exchange and oxygenation.

Preoperative stabilization is critical. Drainage of fluid or air from the pleural space by thoracentesis or placement of a thoracostomy tube re-establishes cardiorespiratory stability prior to anesthesia. Supplemental oxygen administration by nasal catheter or face mask is important in the preoperative period. Continued monitoring of cardiorespiratory parameters during anesthetic preparation and induction is needed to verify stabilization and to evaluate continued fluid or air accumulation within the pleural cavity. Induction techniques that permit rapid control and management of the airway are preferred in cases with no or minimal cardiovascular dysfunction (see Tables 169–1 and 169–2). Anesthetic maintenance with inhalation anesthesia is acceptable. Because of potential entrapment and volume expansion in the pleural space, nitrous oxide is not used unless continued chest drainage is provided.[3, 14, 15]

Postoperative management includes continued drainage of the pleural cavity until air or fluid cannot be withdrawn. Supplemental oxygenation is critical to offset poor tidal volume and gas exchange associated with the underlying disease and the residual anesthetic effects.

Diaphragmatic Hernia. A patient with traumatic hernia is stabilized before surgical repair is attempted. Supplemental oxygenation by nasal catheter or face mask is beneficial. Positional changes can transiently improve ventilation. A vertical head-up posture can produce partial repositioning of visceral structures and improve ventilation. If gastric entrapment and dilation have occurred, percutaneous gastrocentesis can be performed to reduce intragastric volume prior to surgical correction.[3, 15, 16]

Like other space-occupying masses, a diaphragmatic hernia produces pulmonary compression with hypoxemia when the patient is stressed. Visceral displacement into the thoracic cavity causes a reduced venous return to the heart as a result of compression of the heart and great vessels. Ventilation is supported immediately following induction and orotracheal intubation. Positive-pressure ventilation should not exceed 15 to 20 cm H_2O pressure at which level too rapid re-expansion of atelectatic lung regions and subsequent pulmonary edma may occur. The risk of these complications is greater following re-expansion of a chronically atelectatic lung. Blood pressure is monitored to ensure adequate venous return and cardiac output. Hypotension may continue or become progressively worse. Inotropic support with dopamine or dobutamine infusion improves myocardial contractility and cardiac output. Infusion is necessary to maintain plasma levels, as both drugs have a short (1- to 2-minute) half-life. The dose range is 2 to 10 μg/kg per minute. Dopamine is diluted in a 250-ml bag of normal saline or 5 per cent dextrose and delivered to effect using a 60 drops/ml drip set. Improved pulse quality, heart rate, blood pressure, and capillary perfusion are positive endpoints of these drugs. Tachycardia or arrhythmias can develop if the infusion rate is too rapid.[3, 15, 16]

Peritoneopericardial hernia is usually diagnosed in young puppies and kittens shortly after birth. Reduced cardiac output may occur because of cardiac compression associated with visceral displacement into the pericardial sac. Premedication reduces stress of handling and of intravenous catheter placement. A neuroleptanalgesic or ketamine-tranquilizer combination can be used for anesthetic induction. Mask induction using isoflurane works well in most pediatric patients (see Chapter 172). Management is similar to that described for other thoracotomy procedures.[3, 6, 15]

Primary Pulmonary Disease. The lung may undergo several disease processes that require surgical correction. Foreign bodies, abscesses, neoplasia, and lung lobe torsion may require partial or total lobectomy as part of the treatment. Preoperative assessment of cardiorespiratory function is critical. Physical examination, thoracic radiography, and if possible, evaluation of arterial blood gases are indicated in reduced gas exchange associated with primary pulmonary disease.[3, 15]

These patients are considered at risk for anesthetic complications. Preoxygenation is provided during the preparation and induction period to facilitate oxygen transport. Anesthetic techniques that provide rapid induction are selected (see Tables 169–1 and 169–2). Orotracheal intubation and initiation of ventilatory support by intermittent positive-pressure ventilation are immediately performed. Low levels of positive end-expiratory pressure (5 cm H_2O) may be added during surgery to maintain alveolar inflation.

Monitoring techniques associated with the high-risk patient, including assessment of arterial blood gases, are helpful. Airway maintenance following surgical correction is provided for as long as possible. Supplemental oxygenation is usually required in these patients. Thoracostomy tube placement is indicated if ongoing pleural effusion is anticipated. The tube is maintained until no evidence of air or fluid accumulation is noted. Pain management by local nerve blocks and parenteral analgesics facilitates normal breathing in the postoperative period.

Patent Ductus Arteriosus. The young animal that has minimal cardiovascular changes can tolerate surgery quite well. Dogs can be premedicated with an opioid and atropine or with a low dose of acepromazine intramuscularly. Induction is with ultrashort-acting barbiturates, a ketamine-tranquilizer combination, neuroleptanalgesic agents, or gas. Cats can be premedicated with ketamine, a ketamine-tranquilizer combination, or a neuroleptanalgesic. Induction techniques are the same as those described for the dog. Anesthesia is maintained with inhalation anesthesia. Once the animal is intubated, intermittent positive-pressure ventilation is begun. The actual ligation of the patent ductus arteriosus is done in stages. Trial ligation of the patent ductus arteriosus indicates the potential of reflex bradycardia because of an increase in blood volume going to the left side of the circulation. Administration of anticholinergic drugs to inhibit vagal reflexes usually reverses reflex bradycardia.[3, 15]

Pericardial Disease. Cardiac tamponade can cause significant hemodynamic changes that can be aggravated during anesthesia. Patients with this condition are considered cardiac cripples because the heart cannot effectively pump, thus causing decreased cardiac output. Bradycardia, if present, increases the severity of cardiac dysfunction. The strategy for anesthetic management is to select agents that minimally depress myocardial contractility and cardiac rate. An opioid-atropine combination administered intramuscularly is used for premedication. Induction by mask or a narcotic-tranquilizer combination or diazepam-ketamine combination administered intravenously, is recommended. Barbiturates are best avoided. Premedication in the cat with a low dose of a ketamine-midazolam or opioid-tranquilizer combination is preferred. Mask induction or intravenous administration of ketamine in a low dose facilitates intubation for induction. Topical anesthesia of the larynx with lidocaine facilitates intubation. Intermittent positive-pressure ventilation decreases cardiac output. Drugs providing inotropic support are commonly used during surgery and postoperatively.[3, 15]

References

1. Benumof JL, Alfery DD: Anesthesia for thoracic surgery. *In* Miller RD (ed): *Anesthesia*. Vol 2. 2nd ed. Churchill Livingstone, New York, 1986, p 1380.
2. Dulisch ML: Skull and mandibular fractures. *In* Slatter D (ed): *Textbook of Small Animal Surgery*, Vols I and II. W. B. Saunders, Philadelphia, 1985, p 2286.
3. Faggella AM, Raffe, MR: Non-cardiac surgical diseases of the thorax. *Vet Clin North Am Small Anim Pract 17*:469, 1987.
4. Grandage J: The oral cavity and pharynx. *In* Slatter D (ed): *Textbook of Small Animal Surgery*. W. B. Saunders, Philadelphia, 1985, p 638.
5. Grandy JL, Steffy EP: Anesthesia and the respiratory system. *In* Slatter D (ed): *Textbook of Small Animal Surgery*. W. B. Saunders, Philadelphia, 1985, p 2621.
6. Haskins SC: Monitoring the anesthetized patient. *In* Short CE (ed): *Principles and Practice of Veterinary Anesthesia*. Williams & Wilkins, Baltimore, 1987, p 455.
7. Heel RC, et al: Butorphanol: A Review of Its Pharmacological Properties and Therapeutic Efficacy. ADIS Press, Australia Pty Ltd., Auckland, 1978, p 474.
8. Heel RC, et al: *Buprenorphine: A Review of Its Pharmacological Properties and Therapeutic Efficacy*. ADIS Press, Australia Pty Ltd., Auckland, 1979, p 82.
9. Klein LV: Neuromuscular Blocking Agents. *In* Short CE (ed): *Principles and Practice of Veterinary Anesthesia*. Williams & Wilkins, Baltimore, 1987, p 134.
10. Muir WW, Hubbell JAE: Anesthetic procedures and techniques in small

animals. *In* Muir WW (ed): *Handbook of Veterinary Anesthesia.* C. V. Mosby, St. Louis, 1989, p 202.
11. Muir WW, Hubbell JAE: Neuromuscular blocking drugs. *In: Handbook of Veterinary Anesthesia* C. V. Mosby, St. Louis, 1989, p 108.
12. Muir WW, Hubbell JAE: Patient monitoring during anesthesia. *In: Handbook of Veterinary Anesthesia.* C. V. Mosby, St. Louis, 1989, p 165.
13. Muir WW, Hubbell JAE: Ventilation and Mechanical Assist Devices. *In: Handbook of Veterinary Anesthesia.* C. V. Mosby, St. Louis, 1989, p 153.
14. Nelson AW: Lower respiratory system. *In* Slatter DH (ed): *Textbook of Small Animal Surgery* W. B. Saunders, Philadelphia, 1985, p 1014.
15. Paddleford RR: Anesthetic considerations in patients with preexisting problems or conditions. *In* Paddleford RR: *Manual of Small Animal Anesthesia.* Churchill Livingstone, New York, 1988, p 270.
16. Punch PI, Slatter D: Diaphragmatic hernias. *In* Slatter D (ed): *Textbook of Small Animal Surgery.* W. B. Saunders, Philadelphia, 1985, p 869.
17. Shawley RV: Controlled ventilation and pulmonary function. *In* Short CE (ed): *Principles and Practice of Veterinary Anesthesia.* Williams & Wilkins, Baltimore, 1987, p 419.
18. Swedlow DB: Capnometry and capnography: The anesthesia disaster early warning system. *Seminars on Anesthesia* Vol V. 3:194, 1986.
19. Tremper KK, Barker, SJ: Pulse oximetry. *Anesthesiology 70*:98, 1989.

CHAPTER 170 Anesthesia for Gastrointestinal Surgery

Michael B. Curtis

GASTROINTESTINAL PHYSIOLOGY AND EFFECTS OF ANESTHESIA

Hepatic Blood Flow. To function properly, the liver depends on a dual blood supply from the portal vein and the hepatic artery. This hepatic circulation responds to autoregulation, sympathetic stimulation, hypoxia, and hypercapnia. Anesthetics change hepatic blood flow by decreasing cardiac output, arterial blood pressure, and vascular tone, thus inhibiting the normal autoregulation of hepatic blood flow. Anesthetics can also alter hepatic blood flow by changing sympathetic tone. As cardiac output falls in response to an anesthetic, there is a proportional drop in hepatic blood flow. Isoflurane produces the least reduction in portal blood flow, and increases hepatic artery blood flow.[5] Halothane decreases blood flow from both sources in proportion to the dose-related decrease in cardiac output. Methoxyflurane also causes a marked reduction in hepatic blood flow.[13]

Among the opioids, morphine at a low dose (1 mg/kg) increases cranial mesenteric blood flow, an effect that is consistent with its stimulation of the release of catecholamines from the adrenal medulla. Other opioids, based on their ability to maintain or decrease cardiac output, have a minimal effect or decrease hepatic blood flow.

Biliary System. The biliary system is essential to the elimination of several metabolic by-products, particularly with regard to the metabolism and elimination of certain anesthetic drugs. Certain opioids increase intrabiliary pressure and can be potentially harmful in patients with confirmed or suspected obstructive biliary disease. Inhalant anesthetics have little effect on intrabiliary pressure but a possible effect on the formation of bilirubin.[3]

Drug Metabolism. Virtually all anesthetics undergo a certain degree of hepatic biotransformation, and several agents are capable of stimulating hepatic microsomal enzymes of the mixed-function oxidase system. Both halothane and methoxyflurane induce hepatic microsomal enzymes, particularly with prolonged or multiple exposures. Under conditions in which the enzymes are induced, the level of potentially harmful metabolites generated from the biotransformation of the inhalant anesthetics may be increased, leading to organ toxicity.

Another factor that contributes to hepatic damage during exposure to halothane and methoxyflurane is hypoxia. If hypoxia exists, metabolism of halothane can lead to the production of free radicals, rather than to the nontoxic trifluoracetic acid produced under aerobic conditions. The free radicals can in turn lead to lipid peroxidation of the hepatocyte. Both enzyme induction and hypoxia are required to produce halothane-associated hepatitis in the rat; however, there may be species variability in susceptibility, as other experimental models have shown greater sensitivity.[2] As much as 50 per cent of methoxyflurane is metabolized in the liver, compared with 20 per cent for halothane. Unlike halothane, methoxyflurane produces free fluoride ions in its normal metabolic degradation. As a result, the risk of liver damage is increased in patients exposed to methoxyflurane, particularly in patients with pre-existing hepatocellular disease, or with enzymes induced by phenobarbital or prior exposure to anesthetic agents.

Isoflurane is an inhalant anesthetic that undergoes no measurable hepatic metabolism. As such, it does not produce hepatic toxicity, even under conditions of hypoxia and enzyme induction. Nitrous oxide undergoes no hepatic metabolism and is useful in the management of patients with liver disease. In the presence of hypoxia, however, hepatic cellular damage can occur with this agent.

Acepromazine is a phenothiazine tranquilizer that undergoes extensive and prolonged hepatic metabolism. Hepatic microsomal enzymes may be induced with multiple exposures. Acepromazine in patients with severe liver disease may have a prolonged duration of action and increases the metabolic demand placed on the already compromised liver. The phenothiazines also reduce the central nervous system threshold for seizures, and their effects could be potentiated in patients with seizure activity associated with hepatic encephalopathy. The opioids also require a significant amount of hepatic biotransformation. The duration of activity for most opioids is less than for acepromazine, suggesting more rapid metabolism. The primary advantage of the opioids in patients with liver disease is the ability to reverse the effects of the drug with a specific antagonist. The benzodiazepines, despite fairly extensive biotransformation in the liver, and some active intermediates, are safe for patients with compensated liver disease, as they produce only mild depression of the central nervous system and have few side effects.

Both the thiobarbiturates and the cyclohexylamines (ketamine and tiletamine) undergo redistribution after administration, causing plasma levels to drop rapidly. Despite redistribution, the rate of thiobarbiturate metabolism is still a significant factor in their duration of action. Without prior induction of microsomal enzymes, recovery from a sleep dose of thiopental sodium is much longer in greyhounds than in mixed-breed dogs receiving the same dose.[11] Methohexital is more rapidly metabolized than thiobarbiturates, and allows more rapid recovery. Methohexital has been used with good results in the sight hounds. Hepatic disease prolongs the duration of action of thiobarbiturates and can also prolong the recovery of dogs from large doses of cyclohexylamines.

The half-life of thiamylal elimination in cats is 14.5 hours.[14] This half-life would probably be even longer in cats with hepatic dysfunction. In dogs, cyclohexylamines undergo a significant degree of liver metabolism. In cats, however, the major portion of ketamine is eliminated via the kidneys, and the anesthetic duration of ketamine in liver disease is more predictable.[7]

Certain neuromuscular blockers require at least partial metabolism in the liver to terminate their activity. Vecuronium depends almost entirely on the liver for clearance and should be avoided in patients with liver disease. Pancuronium bromide has a prolonged duration in patients with liver disease, despite minimal liver metabolism. Succinylcholine is metabolized by plasma cholinesterase, an enzyme produced mainly by the liver. Succinylcholine's duration of action can be prolonged in patients with liver disease. Preferred muscle relaxants for patients with liver disease include atracurium besylate, metabolized in the plasma, and gallamine triethiodide, which is primarily excreted in the urine.

Carbohydrate Metabolism. Glucose homeostasis depends on normal hepatic function. In cases of severe liver disease, hypoglycemia is possible and dextrose supplementation should be considered. Probably the only anesthetic drug with a clinically significant effect on glucose levels is xylazine, which is capable of producing marked hyperglycemia.[4] This response is probably blunted in the patient with liver disease because of inadequate glucose reserves, but significant hyperglycemia may result if dextrose is administered supplementally.

Coagulation. Most of the coagulation factors are produced in the liver. It is possible to reduce these factors in severe liver disease to the point at which coagulation abnormalities are seen. Tests for adequate coagulation are performed prior to surgery, and replacement therapy is initiated if coagulation is impaired. Treatment with vitamin K can be attempted if a vitamin K deficiency is suspected to increase the production of coagulation factors. Twenty-four to 48 hours are required after vitamin K administration for coagulation factors to be restored.

Protein. The liver is also responsible for production of albumin. Hypoalbuminemia can result from hepatic dysfunction. Significant hypoalbuminemia usually occurs late in the course of hepatic disease after 80 per cent or more of the liver is involved. Replacement therapy is appropriate for severe reductions in albumin (<1.5 g/dl). Albumin replacement alone may not reduce peripheral edema and is not considered potentially harmful to the kidney. Replacement therapy has been required with mild to moderate reductions in protein, but the dose of anesthetic drugs that are highly protein bound should be reduced (thiobarbiturates, benzodiazepines). This measure prevents major elevations in the active unbound fraction of these drugs, which would lead to more pronounced effects and prolonged durations of action. The thiobarbiturate dose for a healthy patient (relative to cardiovascular function) should be reduced by one-third to one-half, depending on the degree of hypoalbuminemia.

Cerebral Sensitivity. Sensitivity to certain anesthetic agents is increased in many patients with liver disease, even after a decrease in dose consistent with the severity of the disease. The number of neuroinhibitory receptors (α-aminobutyric acid) is increased during chronic liver failure. Drugs that act via the α-aminobutyric acid receptors (barbiturates and benzodiazepines) may therefore have a greater effect under these conditions.

Alimentary Tract

Salivary Glands. The salivary glands are controlled by the autonomic nervous system, and anesthetic agents that affect this system can also affect the volume and viscosity of saliva. Indications for the use of anticholinergics include oral surgery, mask induction in brachycephalic breeds when airway security could be compromised, animals that salivate excessively prior to anesthesia, and animals that have laryngeal disease and have previously undergone or are considered at high risk for pathologic aspiration. Use of atropine can lead to dysrhythmias. Glycopyrrolate is less likely to produce dysrhythmias, and its antisialagogue effect is two to three times that of atropine.[6, 10]

Gastrointestinal Motility. A number of anesthetics alter gastrointestinal motility. How motility is affected must be considered in relation to the surgical procedure being performed and to the condition of the animal. Decreased motility is desirable in any animal with a full stomach that must be anesthetized quickly, as it reduces the risk of vomiting and aspiration. In contrast, the patient with pre-existing ileus (often with accompanying anorexia) might benefit by the use of drugs that stimulate gastrointestinal motility. The anticholinergics decrease gastrointestinal motility and pressure across the lower esophageal sphincter, potentially making regurgitation easier for the patient.[1] Acepromazine, diazepam, and oxymorphone decrease pressure across the lower esophageal sphincter, and fentanyl-droperidol, xylazine, pentobarbital sodium, halothane, and methoxyflurane produce marked reductions in gastrointestinal motility. Acepromazine and ketamine have little effect on motility, and thiopental increases motility of certain portions of the gastrointestinal tract.[15]

Morphine, oxymorphone, and meperidine have a spasmogenic effect on the gastrointestinal system. They increase sphincter smooth-muscle tone and nonpropulsive contractions. Morphine, oxymorphone, and fentanyl can also frequently cause transient vomiting shortly after administration, secondary to stimulation of the central nervous system. Xylazine is also associated with emesis and, when administered as a premedicant, consistently produces vomiting in cats, and to a lesser degree in dogs.[7] Butorphanol and pentazocine also decrease motility of the small intestine. Adjunctive agents used in anesthesia that can affect motility include neostigmine and metoclopramide hydrochloride, both of which increase gastrointestinal motility significantly.

Gastrointestinal Secretions. Both atropine and glycopyrrolate decrease gastric acidity and volume in patients in which vomiting and aspiration, or gastric reflux, is probable. The pH of gastric contents is important in determining the degree of damage to the respiratory or esophageal mucosa should aspiration or reflux occur; greater damage is associated with lower pH. Glycopyrrolate is more effective than atropine in increasing pH. Cimetidine and ranitidine are more consistent than the anticholinergics in decreasing gastric acidity. Cimetidine inhibits hepatic microsomal enzymes. Metoclopramide has also been used to decrease gastric volume by increasing gastric motility.

Gas Distension. Distension of the gastrointestinal tract can be increased by the addition of nitrous oxide. Nitrous oxide is avoided when significant amounts of gas are known or suspected to be present in the gastrointestinal tract (or other closed space). If severe enough, gas distension of the stomach, and occasionally the intestines, can lead to reduced ventilation and venous return. These patients can usually be stabilized by passage of a stomach tube for decompression and use of controlled ventilation, but severe cases may require rapid percutaneous decompression.

The effects of other anesthetics on a distended portion of the gastrointestinal tract are relative to their effects[3] on motility and blood flow. Agents that dramatically decrease cardiac output also decrease blood flow to the gastrointestinal tract. Isoflurane maintains better intestinal blood flow than does halothane. Drugs that increase gastrointestinal motility are used cautiously in a patient with an obstructive lesion and severe gas distension, as the increased intraluminal pressure caused by these agents could lead to rupture of the distended segment. Opioids are considered carefully in this type of patient.

PREANESTHETIC CONSIDERATIONS

Fasting. The most effective approach to managing many of the potential anesthetic problems associated with the gastrointestinal system consists of withholding food from the patient if possible, for 8 to 12 hours prior to anesthesia. This recommendation is modified in neonates, aged patients, and animals weighing less than 3 kg. Often, water is also withheld for up to 2 hours prior to anesthesia; however, this precaution should be omitted if there is any indication of volume depletion. Prolonged fasting may be inappropriate in many emergency situations or in very small patients with high metabolic rates. Rapid-sequence induction, in which the airway is quickly intubated, is indicated to help prevent aspiration. Emetics are never indicated except in cases of ingested toxins. These agents do not reliably empty the stomach and are stressful to the patient.

Clinical Data Base

Liver. In most cases, animals with advanced hepatic disease do not require emergency anesthesia unless another unrelated problem exists. Thus, adequate time is allowed to evaluate hepatic dysfunction with appropriate laboratory tests. Assessment of hepatic function usually involves the evaluation of liver enzymes, direct and indirect bilirubin, and albumin (total protein or solids). Blood urea nitrogen is often decreased in patients with portosystemic shunts. More elaborate tests of hepatic function can be pursued if liver disease is suspected, but not confirmed, from these screening tests. These tests include the analysis of bile acids, urinary bile pigments, and clearance of organic anion dyes removed from the circulation by the liver (sulfobromophthalein sodium and indocyanine green). Evaluation of a patient with a portosystemic shunt often includes a determination of baseline ammonia level and an ammonia tolerance test.

Increased levels of the commonly measured liver enzymes reflect cellular necrosis and loss of cell membrane integrity; however, these elevated levels of enzymes have several other possible explanations. Enzyme elevations that are considered specific for hepatocellular disease include alanine aminotransferase and sorbitol dehydrogenase; γ-glutamyltransferase is more specific for biliary tissue and is elevated with cholestasis.

The specificity of the test can be increased by using the ratio of direct to total bilirubin. Decreases in this ratio indicate increased bilirubin production. Increases are due to hepatic dysfunction, with marked increases suggesting obstructive biliary disease.

Hypoproteinemia is a supportive finding in suspected liver disease, because albumin is produced in the liver. It cannot be used as a primary diagnostic tool, as there are multiple non–liver-related reasons for hypoproteinemia, which must also be considered. Coagulation is evaluated if any or all of these tests suggest liver disease. Evaluation of activated clotting time constitutes minimal testing, and if possible, prothrombin time, partial thromboplastin time, and fibrin degradation products are tested.

Gastrointestinal Tract. Laboratory data that might be useful in the evaluation of these patients depend on the specific disease process. Patients that have chronic vomiting or diarrhea, gastric dilatation–volvulus, or an obstructive lesion can all be expected to have some degree of acid-base and electrolyte disorder. Hydration status and electrolyte levels are always part of the minimum data base for this type of patient. Analysis of blood gases, when possible, is useful in the evaluation of these patients, and when considered with the electrolyte values, it helps determine the appropriate type of fluid therapy. Electrocardiography is performed prior to anesthesia if significant electrolyte imbalances are present, and in all cases of gastric dilatation–volvulus. The electrocardiogram is monitored regularly, as dysrhythmias may develop later with these disorders.[8]

Stabilization

Liver. Patients with liver disease may require replacement therapy for low levels of albumin, or for inadequate coagulation factors. Vomiting, associated renal disease, anorexia, and hypoglycemia may require various types of crystalloid fluid therapy to correct hypovolemia and acid-base, electrolyte, and glucose disorders.

Gastrointestinal Tract. Often the patient with an acute abdomen is presented in shock. Initial stabilization consists of establishing at least one large-bore intravenous catheter and administering crystalloid fluid therapy and shock doses of steroids. In the case of gastric dilatation–volvulus, decompression is attempted with a stomach tube.

Acid-base and electrolyte disorders are usually present with gastric dilatation–volvulus, obstructions of the gastrointestinal tract, vomiting, and diarrhea. Patients with gastric dilatation–volvulus often develop metabolic acidosis because of volume depletion and lactic acidosis; this is not consistent, and with frequent vomiting, metabolic alkalosis may be present. Metabolic acidosis is a common sequela to diarrhea. Acid-base and electrolyte status is evaluated rapidly, and fluid replacement can be tailored to the patient's individual needs. Hypovolemia, acidosis, and hyperkalemia or hypokalemia all precipitate cardiac dysrhythmias, and can be life threatening if not corrected rapidly, particularly if ischemic necrosis of the stomach or intestines is suspected.

ANESTHETIC MANAGEMENT CONSIDERATIONS

Liver

There are several potential complications when anesthesia is administered to a patient with hepatic dysfunction. Most of these are related to alterations in the normal liver processes (Table 170–1).

Anesthesia for the patient with a portosystemic shunt can be complicated by any or all of the problems listed in Table 170–1 as well as by hepatic encephalopathy. This problem is secondary to impaired hepatic metabolism of protein, accumulation of ammonia, and production of false neurotransmitters. Efforts are made to stabilize the patient neurologically by decreasing ammonia levels prior to anesthesia. This change is accomplished by altering the diet to decrease protein intake. These patients usually have normal or mildly increased hepatic enzyme levels and normal bilirubin levels. The severity of the shunt determines how functional the liver is, and this dictates the type and dose of anesthetic agents. The benzodiazepines work well for light sedation;[6] however, in depressed shunt patients, the initial dose is low (0.05 to 0.2 mg/kg). Opioids can be used for greater sedation (oxymorphone, 0.05 to 0.2 mg/kg; meperidine, 2 to 4 mg/kg). The dose is reduced in more depressed patients, and it is probable that their duration of action is prolonged. The advantage of opioids is that they can be reversed with specific antagonists.

TABLE 170–1. ANESTHETIC COMPLICATIONS ASSOCIATED WITH HEPATIC DISEASE

Anticipated Problems	Anesthetic Considerations
Decreased hepatic blood flow	Administer adequate fluid therapy. Use isoflurane, nitrous oxide, opioids, and diazepam to maintain blood flow.
Decreased drug metabolism	Minimize doses of anesthetic agents. Use drugs not dependent on hepatic metabolism (isoflurane, nitrous oxide). Use reversible drugs (opioids).
Hypoglycemia	Supplement dextrose-containing fluids (5% or 2.5%, 10 ml/kg/hr). Avoid xylazine.
Coagulation defects	Administer vitamin K therapy. Administer fresh plasma or cryoprecipitate.
Hypoproteinemia	Administer fresh or stored plasma. Administer dextran 40 or 70, or hetastarch.
Biliary spasm	Avoid certain opioid agonists (oxymorphone).
Anesthetic-induced hepatitis	Avoid repeated, prolonged exposure to halothane and methoxyflurane.

The commonly employed induction agents can often be used at a reduced dose in minimally affected patients. Reducing the thiobarbiturate dosage compensates for decreased albumin and protein binding, decreased metabolism, potentially decreased volume of distribution, and a postulated increase in central nervous system sensitivity. It is preferable to induce patients with more severe manifestations of disease using a mask with isoflurane. Isoflurane is preferable for maintenance of anesthesia, as it undergoes minimal hepatic metabolism. Isoflurane and nitrous oxide should be the only agents used in the most severely compromised and critical shunt patients. Small doses of fentanyl (0.001 to 0.002 mg/kg) can be titrated intravenously if isoflurane alone is inadequate for surgery. Atracurium (0.1 to 0.2 mg/kg is the safest and most predictable of the neuromuscular blockers in portosystemic shunt patients.

Oral Cavity

Lesions of the oropharyngeal region rarely have systemic effects that influence the choice of anesthetic agents. Selection of drugs is based primarily on the overall health of the patient, with consideration given to decreasing salivary secretions, inhibiting vagal stimulation during manipulation of the airway, and rapidly securing an airway. The major anesthetic problems associated with oropharyngeal surgery are related to mechanical difficulties that may be encountered during the procedure. These include the possibility of aspiration of blood or debris with an unsecured airway, space-occupying masses that either make intubation difficult or are difficult to work on with an endotracheal tube in place, and an inability to expose the airway via an oral approach because of craniomandibular osteopathy or extensive trauma.

Several techniques are used to secure an airway under difficult conditions. If the larynx and trachea can be exposed with a laryngoscope, a small feeding tube or urinary catheter can be passed into the trachea and used as a guide to introduce a larger endotracheal tube. A small piece of tubing can be introduced percutaneously into the trachea in the cervical region if the larynx cannot be exposed, and then can be passed in a retrograde manner out the oral cavity. The tubing can be used to guide the endotracheal tube into the airway. If a fiber-optic bronchoscope is available, the endotracheal tube can be positioned over it and inserted into the airway, using it as a guide.

The endotracheal tube can be introduced into the pharynx through the site used for a pharyngotomy tube. This procedure is most easily accomplished by intubating the animal orally, removing the Y-piece adapter from the endotracheal tube (while maintaining the position securely), inserting hemostats through the skin at the entry site for a pharyngotomy tube, grasping the proximal end of the endotracheal tube with the hemostats, and pulling it through the skin. If all of these measures are insufficient, a tracheostomy can be performed, and the airway secured with a tracheostomy or endotracheal tube.

Cuffed endotracheal tubes should be securely in position whenever feasible. The oral and pharyngeal regions are thoroughly flushed of blood and debris and the cuffed endotracheal tube is maintained in the airway until the patient has regained airway reflexes. The patient is extubated with the cuff partially inflated, and the head positioned lower than the body. Steroids or furosemide are often used if edema or inflammation is expected.

Esophagus

Animals with obstructive lesions of the esophagus are evaluated for aspiration pneumonia, volume depletion, electrolyte imbalance, and poor nutritional status due to a prolonged period of decreased intake. Esophageal masses in some patients may partially obstruct the trachea, resulting in variable amounts of dyspnea and difficult intubation. Animals with an obstructive esophageal lesion or megaesophagus are at high risk for regurgitation and aspiration. To reduce this possibility, induction and intubation are performed rapidly to secure the airway. The agents best suited to this type of induction are thiobarbiturates and cyclohexylamines. The endotracheal tube is cuffed, long, and relatively stiff to prevent collapse of the trachea during esophageal manipulation. The tube is positioned well below the site of esophageal injury (beyond the thoracic inlet). If the esophageal damage is within the thorax, the anesthetist should be alert for the development of pneumothorax and pneumomediastinum. Other useful techniques are preoxygenation of patients with aspiration pneumonia, and evaluation of megaesophagus patients for myasthenia gravis, as this condition can affect the time needed for the animal to regain muscle strength in recovery.

Stomach and Intestines

The choice of anesthetics is based on many of the previously addressed considerations and is discussed using the patient with gastric dilatation–volvulus as an example. Dogs with this disorder are often in the most critical condition of the gastrointestinal patients, and the concerns in other disorders are similar and usually less complicated by multiple-system involvement. The pancreas may be damaged by increased venous back pressure, and myocardial depressant factor is released and contributes to myocardial depression. The acid-base and electrolyte imbalances that develop increase cardiac irritability, as do increased catecholamine levels from autonomic imbalance. Gastric decompression of the patient is performed as soon as possible after presentation to minimize damage done by gastric distension. Treatment of the dysrhythmias consists of lidocaine (1 to 2 mg/kg IV bolus) followed by infusion at 40 to 80 μg/kg/min procainamide (0.5 mg/kg) in refractory animals.[9]

Premedication is tailored to physical status. Premedication may not be needed in very depressed patients, or a low dose of diazepam can be given intravenously (0.1 mg/kg) to maintain a more consistent plane of anesthesia than could be accomplished with gas alone. Patients with only mild depression may require heavier premedication to maintain cardiovascular stability. Butorphanol (0.2 mg/kg) or oxymorphone (0.1 mg/kg) is effective, and each can be combined with low doses of acepromazine (0.03 mg/kg), for its antiarrhythmic effect, if the patient is adequately hydrated.

The severely depressed patient can often be induced by mask, using maintenance concentrations of inhalant anesthetic if vomiting has not been a factor. Other acceptable techniques for induction include slow intravenous titration of oxymorphone (up to 0.2 mg/kg) or fentanyl (up to 0.005 mg/kg), or a combination of diazepam (0.2 mg/kg) and ketamine (2 to 4 mg/kg) administered intravenously. Maintenance is accomplished with isoflurane, as it maintains cardiac contractility better than halothane and does not sensitize the myocardium to catecholamines. Supplemental fentanyl can be used safely during surgery. Nitrous oxide is avoided with distended abdominal organs, as it enlarges gas pockets.

Controlled ventilation may be necessary if the abdominal distension impairs the animal's ability to ventilate. Airway pressure is kept to a minimum (15 to 20 cm H_2O) to prevent excessive intrathoracic pressure and subsequent decreased venous return. Arterial blood gases are monitored if possible. Operative use of a positive inotropic agent (dopamine or dobutamine, 2 to 5 μg/kg per minute) may be needed to support patients with severely depressed myocardial contractility and cardiac output. Intensive monitoring continues in recovery, as dysrhythmias frequently develop postoperatively.[8] Supplemental oxygen therapy or controlled ventilation may be needed if severe ventilation/perfusion mismatches have developed. Oxygen levels are maintained below 50 per cent during long-term ventilatory support, and a tracheostomy tube may be required. If vomiting has occurred, the airway is protected until recovery of airway reflexes is complete.

Peritonitis and Ascites

Animals with peritonitis may be severely ill, exhibiting varying degrees of shock, abdominal fluid accumulation, and endotoxemia. Large accumulations of fluid can distend the abdomen, displace the diaphragm cranially, and compromise ventilation. Positioning the patient in dorsal recumbency further inhibits the patient's ventilation. These patients require control of ventilation and higher than normal airway pressures (20 to 30 cm H_2O) to compensate for decreased compliance. Abdominal effusion (modified transudate) is considered a "third-space fluid" and is in equilibrium with the circulating blood volume. This fluid may also contain a substantial amount of protein. Rapid withdrawal of this fluid during surgery can result in dramatic falls in blood pressure and in hypoproteinemia. Intravenous replacement with a crystalloid solution dilutes the remaining plasma protein. When medically appropriate, fluid from an abdominal effusion should be reduced gradually over the course of several days through the use of restricted salt diets and diuretics or through repeated abdominocentesis in the awake patient.

Crystalloids are rapidly administered intravenously with a replacement ratio of 3 L to every 1 L lost if a hypotensive crisis develops during rapid fluid withdrawal in surgery. Protein must be replaced by the administration of plasma if hypotension and rapid crystalloid therapy results in dilutional hypoproteinemia. Hypertonic saline has been suggested for the treatment of hypovolemic shock.[12] This therapy requires intravenous administration of 7 per cent sodium chloride, increases the cardiac output via increased contractility, and helps re-establish adequate blood pressure. Dilutional hypoproteinemia is not a significant factor, because large volumes of the intravenous solution are not required.

Respiratory depressants are avoided in patients with depressed ventilation. Large doses of xylazine, acepromazine, barbiturates, and inhalant anesthetics are avoided, because these all potentiate cardiovascular depression associated with shock. The patient is placed in lateral recumbency for as long as possible, and two intravenous catheters are placed. Administration of antibiotics, flunixin meglumine, and steroids may be appropriate prior to anesthesia. Ventilation is monitored in recovery to ensure that it is adequate.

Perianal Surgery

The major problems associated with surgery in this area usually result from a head-down surgical position. This positioning results in cranial displacement of the diaphragm, decreased lung volumes, and respiratory depression. The problem becomes more significant in large or obese patients, or in those with pre-existing respiratory disease. Controlled ventilation may be required in many of these patients. Elevated intracranial pressure, decreased cardiac output, and decreased arterial blood pressure are also consequences of this positioning.

References

1. Cotton BR, Smith G: Comparison of the effects of atropine and glycopyrrolate on lower esophageal sphincter pressure. *Br J Anaesth 53*:875, 1981.
2. Cousins MK: Mechanisms and evaluation of hepatotoxicity. *1984 ASA Annual Refresher Course Lectures, 204*:1, 1984.
3. Engelking LR, et al: Effects of isoflurane anesthesia on equine liver function. *Am J Vet Res 45*:616, 1984.
4. Feldberg W, Symonds HW: Hyperglycemic effect of xylazine. *J Vet Pharmacol Ther 3*:197, 1980.
5. Gelman S, et al: Liver circulation and function during isoflurane and halothane anesthesia. *Anesthesiology 61*:726, 1984.
6. Greenan J: Cardiac dysrhythmias and heart rate changes at induction of anaesthesia: A comparison of two intravenous anticholinergics. *Acta Anaesthesiol Scand 28*:182, 1984.
7. Lumb WV, Jones EW: *Veterinary Anesthesia*. 2nd ed. Lea & Febiger, Philadelphia, 1984.
8. Muir WW: Gastric dilatation-volvulus in the dog, with emphasis on cardiac arrhythmias. *J Am Vet Med Assoc 180*:739, 1982.
9. Muir WW, Bonagura JD: Treatment of cardiac arrhythmias in dogs with gastric distension-volvulus. *J Am Vet Med Assoc 184*:1366, 1984.
10. Rammamurthy S, et al: Glycopyrrolate as a substitute for atropine: A preliminary report. *Anesth Analg 50*:732, 1971.
11. Robinson EP, et al: Barbiturate anesthesia in Greyhound and mixed-breed dogs: Comparative cardiopulmonary effects, anesthetic effects, and recovery rates. *Am J Vet Res 47*:2105, 1986.
12. Schertel ER, Muir WW: Shock: Pathophysiology, monitoring, and therapy. *In* Kirk RW (ed): *Current Veterinary Therapy X, Small Animal Practice*. W. B. Saunders, Philadelphia, 1989, p 316.
13. Tranquilli WJ, et al: Systemic and regional blood flow distribution in unanesthetized swine and swine anesthetized with halothane and nitrous oxide, halothane, or enflurane. *Anesthesiology 56*:369, 1982.
14. Wertz EM, et al: Pharmacokinetics of thiamylal in cats. *Am J Vet Res 49*:1079, 1988.
15. Zontine WJ: Effects of chemical restraint drugs on the passage of barium sulfate through the stomach and duodenum of dogs. *J Am Vet Med Assoc 162*:878, 1973.

CHAPTER 171 Anesthesia and the Endocrine System

Cynthia M. Trim

Considerable endocrine and metabolic changes occur during and after anesthesia and surgery. Anesthetic agents can influence the endocrine response to anesthesia and surgery, but surgical stress has a greater influence. During surgery, cortisol, growth hormone, prolactin, luteinizing hormone, antidiuretic hormone, and catecholamine concentrations increase variably, whereas thyrotropin and testosterone decrease. Renin may be released, and aldosterone synthesized. Metabolic changes after surgery include a negative nitrogen balance, sodium retention and potassium loss, reduced water and glucose tolerance, and increased plasma concentration of free fatty acids. Various factors initiate these changes: fear and apprehension, pain, surgery, some anesthetic agents, and consequences of anesthetic technique such as blood pH changes, hypercapnia, hypoxia, fluid loss, handling of tissues, and sepsis. The responses may be modified by the nutritional and medical state of the patient. Goals of anesthetic management include minimizing the stress response to surgery by alleviating fear, apprehension, and pain and maintaining adequate respiratory and cardiovascular function. Patients with pre-existing endocrine malfunction may require specific medical therapy and selective use of anesthetic drugs.

THE PANCREAS

Diabetes Mellitus

The most important goal in the anesthetic management of the diabetic animal is to prevent hypoglycemia, which can result in brain damage. A practical approach is to produce moderate hyperglycemia (100 to 250 mg/100 ml) for a short time and to anticipate and avoid serious abnormalities of fluid and electrolyte balance. Prolonged hyperglycemia is avoided, because it is associated with decreased resistance to infection and increased morbidity.

The diabetic patient is investigated for evidence of hyperadrenocorticism or decreased renal function in addition to undergoing routine examination before anesthesia. Peripheral neuropathy may exist without clinical signs of nervous system malfunction. Postural hypotension may develop because of impaired vascular reflexes when the autonomic nervous system is involved.

If possible, anesthesia is scheduled for the morning so that the patient can be monitored for the rest of the day while laboratory facilities are available. A simple successful technique for managing the controlled diabetic is as follows. The patient is fed and treated normally on the day before surgery. On the morning of surgery, food is withheld, and only half the usual dose of insulin is administered. Blood glucose is measured before anesthesia, and if the value is less than 80 mg/100ml, syrup or dextrose solution is administered before proceeding. Infusion of 5 per cent dextrose in water at 5 ml/kg per hour during anesthesia should maintain adequate blood glucose concentration. A non–dextrose-containing solution, such as lactated Ringer solution, is also given at 5 ml/kg per hour to maintain blood volume. Adequate surveillance can be provided for short procedures by measuring blood glucose at the end of anesthesia and again several hours after anesthesia, when the effect of the morning insulin administration is increasing. Blood glucose is measured at least every 2 hours during long procedures. Uneven absorption of insulin may occur in the anesthetized patient because of alterations in regional blood flow produced by anesthetic drugs, or increased absorption may occur from vasodilation caused by placing the animal on a heating pad. The peak effect of most insulin preparations occurs several hours after surgery has been completed. Thus, one must ensure that the patient eats its evening meal, if it is able to do so, or receives additional dextrose and has its blood glucose monitored. Most diabetic patients return to their usual routine of insulin and feeding by the day after anesthesia.

Insulin requirement increases during pregnancy, but this requirement is reduced by one-half when the placenta separates, necessitating more frequent monitoring of blood glucose. Consequently, a patient who has already received a regular dose of insulin and is undergoing cesarean section is at greater risk for hypoglycemia.

Preoperative anxiety and the surgical procedure may cause hyperglycemia through sympathetic stimulation and release of glucocorticoids. Most anesthetic drugs, with the exception of xylazine, cause only a minor change in blood glucose. Administration of xylazine causes a decrease in serum insulin and an increase in plasma glucose (200 to 500 per cent increase in cats and 69 per cent increase in dogs) for 3 to 4 hours. Choice of anesthetic drugs depends on physical status of the patient and requirements of the procedure to be performed. Satisfactory drug combinations include induction of anesthesia with a neuroleptanalgesic combination or a thiobarbiturate, and maintenance of anesthesia with an inhalant. The anesthetic technique chosen should allow the patient to recover quickly so that the normal routine of feeding and insulin treatment can be instituted as soon as possible.

A poorly regulated diabetic patient should be hospitalized and stabilized for 2 to 3 days before anesthesia. Anesthesia for uncontrolled diabetics is more complicated. The patient's fluid, electrolyte, acid-base, and blood glucose status are evaluated and treated. Blood glucose may need to be measured every 30 minutes during anesthesia. Insertion of a urinary catheter to monitor urine production and glucose is not done routinely in diabetics because of the risk of infection, but it is valuable in the uncontrolled diabetic. The urine is allowed to drain continuously through the catheter to evaluate glucose accurately.

Insulinoma

Avoidance of hypoglycemia is the main concern in the management of anesthetic patients with a beta-cell tumor of the pancreas. Fasting the patient before anesthesia is necessary but can result in dangerously low blood glucose levels. Hypoglycemia occurs within 4 to 6 hours of beginning a fast in some dogs with insulinoma. Therefore, monitoring of blood glucose levels and infusion of 5 per cent dextrose solution begin during the preanesthetic preparation.

A convenient access site for blood sampling is established before anesthesia, as is placement of the venous catheter used for fluid infusion. The lingual veins are large enough in most dogs to be used for direct puncture during anesthesia. A theoretical argument can be made for choosing anesthetic drugs that decrease cerebral metabolic rate and therefore presumably decrease cerebral metabolism of glucose. Barbiturates, neuroleptic techniques, and inhalant anesthetics decrease cerebral metabolism. Nitrous oxide has variable effects but increases cerebral metabolic rate in dogs. The increase can be partially counteracted by the prior administration of a thiobarbiturate. Ketamine produces a marked increase in cerebral metabolic rate. Various anesthetic drug combinations have been used successfully for this surgery.[9] Prior treatment with diazoxide may increase the percentage of active thiobarbiturate by altering protein binding. Slower administration of a decreased amount of thiobarbiturate may be advisable in these patients.

Obese dogs with insulinoma benefit from controlled ventilation during anesthesia. Excessive hyperventilation is avoided, because lowered carbon dioxide levels decrease cerebral blood flow and thus decrease glucose delivery to the brain. Infusion of 5 per cent dextrose, in addition to balanced electrolyte solution, continues during anesthesia. Blood glucose is measured hourly. Hypoglycemia is difficult to recognize during anesthesia. Signs attributable to the sympathetic nervous system, such as sweating, tachycardia, hypertension, or hypotension, may occur, but seizures may be masked by anesthetic drugs. Severe hypoglycemia may occur during manipulation of the tumor, whereas a marked increase in blood glucose may occur after its removal. The latter change does not always occur, because several tumors may be present, but not apparent, during surgery. The patient may even exhibit transient diabetes mellitus. Consequently, blood glucose is measured frequently during and after surgery, and treatment is adjusted accordingly.

Pancreatitis

Patients with pancreatitis are often dehydrated and azotemic, and they may be in hypovolemic or endotoxic shock. In one group of dogs with pancreatitis, 88 per cent were hyperglycemic and 52 per cent were hypocalcemic.[8] Treatment before anesthesia should ensure replacement of blood volume, restoration of urine production, and correction of hypocalcemia. The patient is also evaluated for cardiac dysrhythmias or respiratory distress syndrome, which may alter the management of anesthesia.

Anticholinergic drugs decrease gastrointestinal motility, can result in accumulation of fluid, distension of the antrum of the stomach, and increased pancreatic enzyme secretion. Usually, however, anesthetic agents decrease gastric fluid volume, regardless of whether anticholinergic drugs such as atropine and glycopyrrolate are used. Consequently, use of an anticholinergic agent during anesthesia to counteract anesthetic drug–induced, or surgically induced, bradycardia is not contraindicated. Anesthetic drugs are chosen for an individual patient, and dose rates are decreased according to the degree of pre-existing central nervous system depression. The combination of tiletamine and zolazepam (Telazol) is contraindicated in patients with pancreatic disease.

Arterial blood pressure is monitored constantly throughout surgery, because manipulation of the inflamed pancreas may cause release of vasoactive substances, resulting in vasodilation and hypotension. The decrease in blood pressure may be so severe that aggressive treatment with fluids, vasoconstrictive drugs, or cardiac stimulants may be indicated.

THE THYROID GLAND

Hypothyroidism

Hypothyroidism increases the sensitivity of the central nervous system to anesthetic drugs. Patients may also be slow to recover from anesthesia and be sedated for longer than usual because of decreased hepatic metabolic rate. Normal response to pancuronium and reversal with neostigmine have been reported.

Hypothyroidism may be accompanied by hypotension and a decrease in cardiac output as much as 40 per cent because of reductions in heart rate and stroke volume. Structural degeneration of the myocardium and impaired cellular metabolism of the myocardium from decreased thyroid hormone are suggested causes. Hypothyroid patients are usually hypothermic and vasoconstricted and may have a low blood volume. Therefore, anesthetic drugs that cause vasodilation may precipitate hypotension. The combination of anesthesia and decreased cardiovascular function may explain why hypotension readily develops in these patients.

Preanesthetic considerations include evaluation for diabetes mellitus. Preferably, elective procedures should be postponed until the patient is rendered euthyroid. Most patients with mild hypothyroidism tolerate anesthesia and surgery well, but severe hypothyroidism increases the risks associated with anesthesia and surgery. A single intravenous injection of L-thyroxine (20 to 40 μg/kg), given several hours before anesthesia, has been suggested for patients that have severe untreated hypothyroidism and require emergency anesthesia and surgery.[5] Anesthetic drugs are chosen and administered with the knowledge of decreased anesthetic requirement and decreased cardiovascular function. Tranquilizers, sedatives, or narcotics are used in extremely small doses. Thiobarbiturates are titrated in small increments rather than administered as a bolus. Anesthesia can be maintained with low concentrations of an inhalation agent. Controlled ventilation may be necessary during anesthesia because hypothyroidism decreases respiratory function and hypoxic ventilatory drive. The patient is observed during recovery to ensure adequate ventilation. Balanced electrolyte solution is infused intravenously during anesthesia to promote adequate flow of urine.

Patients with overt hypothyroidism may have a 40 per cent decrease in metabolic rate, which results in a subnormal body temperature and an inability to increase core temperature in response to low-temperature stress. During anesthesia and the early postoperative period, the hypothyroid patient is particularly susceptible to hypothermia. Hypothermia further decreases the patient's requirement for anesthetic drugs. Shivering during recovery increases oxygen demand and stresses the cardiovascular and respiratory systems at a time when they may not be able to respond. Hypoxemia and secondary cardiac dysrhythmias may result.

Hyperthyroidism

Cardiovascular abnormalities are common in hyperthyroid patients. In a survey of 131 cats with hyperthyroidism, the mean resting heart rate exceeded 240 beats/min, 16 cats had congestive heart failure, and 40 cats had electrocardiographic changes indicating left ventricular enlargement.[7] Atrial and ventricular dysrhythmias and intraventricular conduction disturbances were also described. Treatment with antithyroid drugs, given to render the patient euthyroid before surgery, should decrease the risk of cardiac failure during anesthesia, because ventricular hypertrophy is reversible, disappearing when the patient becomes euthyroid. Heart rates exceeding 240 beat/min can be decreased by administration of propranolol, a beta-adrenergic blocking agent. Propranolol reduces cardiac contractility and heart rate, prolongs atrioventricular conduction, and decreases blood pressure. The recommended dosage for cats is 2.5 to 5.0 mg every 8 hours as required to decrease the resting heart rate to within the normal range.[6] Propranolol is not given to patients in congestive heart failure. The disadvantages of propranolol treatment in relation to general anesthesia are increased myocardial depression and imbalance of the sympathetic nervous system that may contribute to cardiovascular collapse in circumstances such as blood loss. Because of the cardiovascular effects of preoperative administration of propranolol, anesthetic drug delivery is decreased. Intraoperative administration of propranolol may cause significant myocardial depression and hypotension. The required dose of propranolol during anesthesia is extremely small (0.1 mg).

Atropine and glycopyrrolate potentiate tachycardia in hyperthyroid patients and are avoided. Thiobarbiturates have an antithyroid activity and may be the induction agent of choice. Ketamine causes sympathetic stimulation and catecholamine release, which may have a deleterious effect on cardiovascular function. Avoidance of the use of ketamine in unstabilized hyperthyroid animals has been recommended.[1] Acepromazine (0.1 mg/kg) and ketamine (5 mg/kg), given intramuscularly, provide satisfactory sedation before induction of anesthesia with halothane or isoflurane.[3] Low doses of diazepam and ketamine have been used to immobilize cats for thyroid scanning without producing obvious complications. Xylazine is used cautiously, as it may increase the incidence of dysrhythmias. Narcotic drugs may be used as part of the anesthetic technique. Halothane decreases plasma thyroxine concentrations and has been used successfully to maintain anesthesia for thyroidectomy.

The electrocardiogram is monitored for dysrhythmias, and balanced electrolyte solution (5 ml/kg per hour) is infused during anesthesia. Despite polyuria, signs of renal malfunction are usually absent. Large thyroid tumors may have a well-developed blood supply, resulting in excessive blood loss during surgery. Damage to the recurrent laryngeal nerve during surgery can result in laryngeal collapse and airway obstruction after extubation, requiring tracheotomy.

Hypocalcemia can occur 24 to 72 hours after surgery, even when an effort is made to preserve the parathyroid glands; this condition requires treatment with calcium and vitamin D.

THE ADRENAL GLANDS

Hyperadrenocorticism

Excessive production of cortisol from the adrenal cortex (hyperadrenocorticism) may be suspected in a patient that has polyuria, polydipsia, polyphagia, pendulous abdomen, alopecia and thin skin, and hyperpigmentation. Hyperadrenocorticism results either from a cortisol-producing adrenocortical adenoma or carcinoma (Cushing's syndrome) or from excessive stimulation of the adrenal glands by hypersecretion of adrenocorticotropic hormone from the pituitary gland (Cushing's disease).

The metabolic and biochemical changes characteristic of hyperadrenocorticism present specific anesthetic problems. Approximately 10 per cent of dogs with hyperadrenocorticism, and a higher proportion of cats with hyperadrenocorticism, also have diabetes mellitus, requiring additional management. Hypokalemia can complicate anesthesia by causing muscle weakness, bradycardia, ventricular dysrhythmias, and hypotension. The potassium deficit is determined and corrected before anesthesia. A small number of dogs develop dystrophic calcification of the skin, abdominal organs, and bronchi. Bronchial calcification and fibrosis may contribute to pulmonary insufficiency and are identified preoperatively using radiography. Osteoporosis may also be present, and care must be taken when handling the patient to avoid fractures. Obesity and muscle weakness result in hypoventilation during anesthesia, and controlled ventilation may be necessary. There is no reason for choosing one anesthetic agent over another on the basis of adrenal disease.

Surgery for adrenalectomy may be associated with acute massive blood loss; therefore, two venous catheters are placed in preparation for rapid fluid infusion. Surgically created pneumothorax is also a possible complication because of the proximity of the adrenal glands to the diaphragm. The intensity of monitoring of the cardiovascular and respiratory systems during anesthesia depends on the physical status of the patient. Heart rate and blood pressure, blood loss, and rate and depth of breathing are assessed frequently. Once the tumor has been identified, dexamethasone is added to the intravenous fluids and administered at 0.02 to 0.04 mg/kg over approximately 6 hours, as adrenalectomy may result in an acute decrease in circulating cortisol level.[2] Mineralocorticoid and glucocorticoid replacement therapy is instituted postoperatively.

Hypoadrenocorticism

Adrenocortical insufficiency may be caused by adrenal failure (Addison's disease) or may be secondary to a pituitary or hypothalamic lesion, long-term administration of glucocorticoids, treatment with mitotane, or bilateral adrenalectomy. Patients with hypoadrenocorticism may be depressed, weak, anorexic, and vomiting. Hyponatremia and hyperkalemia are frequently present, although some patients may have normal electrolyte values. Decreased aldosterone production by the adrenal cortex results in excessive sodium and water loss by the kidney and in potassium retention. Severe hyponatremia affects the central nervous system and may cause seizures or coma. Astrocytes swell, and neurotransmitter release is impaired. The actions of local and inhalant anesthetics are potentiated, and smaller doses than usual are adequate for anesthesia in these patients. Hypovolemia and decreased cardiac output result from sodium and water depletion. Microcardia may be observed in thoracic radiographs. Blood volume must be restored before anesthesia, and anesthetic agents must be administered carefully to minimize cardiovascular depression. Thiopental and thiamylal must be used with caution. Hyperkalemia decreases resting membrane potentials in the heart, slows heart rate and conduction velocity, and may result in atrioventricular block. Bradycardia may progress to sinus arrest or ventricular fibrillation. Hypoventilation is also more likely to occur. Fluid therapy should precede anesthesia to decrease the serum potassium concentration to less than 6.5 mEq/L.

One of four dogs with hypoadrenocorticism may have hypercalcemia, the magnitude of which is related to the severity of adrenocortical insufficiency but is usually mild. Hypercalcemia may cause bradycardia, and atrioventricular block, vasoconstriction, and hypertension with a reduction in blood volume. Anesthetic drugs that cause vasodilation can cause hypotension. Before anesthesia, serum calcium is restored to near normal by treatment with 0.9 per cent saline infusion and glucocorticoid therapy.

Prerenal azotemia is present in some dogs and cats with hypoadrenocorticism. Increased intensity of action of anesthetic drugs or prolonged duration of action may occur in these patients because of altered protein binding from azotemia and acidosis, and slowed elimination of the drugs and their metabolites.

Action potentials generated from the neuromuscular junction have had decreased amplitude in experimental animals with adrenal insufficiency. Prolonged neuromuscular blockade with pancuronium has been reported in a human patient suspected of having inadequate replacement of adrenocortical hormones.

Thus, the preoperative assessment of the patient with hypoadrenocorticism includes measurement of serum electrolytes. Surgery is delayed, if possible, so that treatment to correct abnormal electrolyte values and to expand blood volume can be provided. An additional dose of corticosteroid is usually administered before anesthesia to patients that have been on long-term steroid therapy. Although sudden hypotension may occur during surgery as a result of acute adrenal insufficiency, other causes such as hypoxemia, interruption of venous return by the surgeon, decreased blood volume, or endotoxemia must be considered. A venous catheter is inserted before anesthesia, and an infusion of saline is started.

A solution of 5 per cent dextrose in water is given if hypoglycemia is present. Etomidate, an ultrashort-acting intravenous anesthetic for use in high-risk patients suppresses adrenal function and is avoided. Smaller amounts of anesthetic drugs than are usually administered are needed for induction of anesthesia. Controlled ventilation may be necessary during anesthesia. The dosage of neuromuscular blocking agents is reduced. Stress from surgery is minimized by providing a quiet induction of anesthesia, adequate depth of anesthesia, sufficient fluid therapy during surgery, and prevention of pain postoperatively.

Pheochromocytoma

Pheochromocytoma is an adrenal medullary tumor that secretes norepinephrine, both norepinephrine and epinephrine, or, in a few cases, dopamine. Periodic release of catecholamines produces tachycardia, hypertension, restlessness, panting, collapse, and sudden death. Large tumors may constantly secrete catecholamines, resulting in persistent hypertension that leads to venous congestion, cardiomyopathy, and congestive heart failure. Particular emphasis is placed on preoperative evaluation of the cardiovascular system, including examination of the electrocardiogram for cardiac dysrhythmias. Contracted blood volume may be suspected from changes in thoracic radiographs or from elevated packed cell volume. The patient is examined for evidence of neoplastic invasion of adjacent structures and for involvement of other endocrine organs.

Treatment for several days before surgery with phenoxybenzamine, a long-acting, alpha-adrenergic blocking agent, is recommended. The drug decreases hypertension by preventing vasoconstriction. The recommended dosage for oral-administration phenoxybenzamine is initially 0.2 to 0.4 mg/kg twice daily, with a gradual increase in dose rate until blood pressure is within the normal range.[5] Propranolol may be required to treat tachycardia, but must only be administered after adequate alpha-adrenergic blockade has been produced.[4]

Atropine is not used because it potentiates the chronotropic effects of epinephrine. Low doses of phenothiazine tranquilizers may be useful for patients with cardiac arrhythmias. Xylazine increases the sensitivity of the myocardium to catecholamine effects and to cardiac arrhythmias. The use of droperidol-fentanyl (Innovar-Vet) is controversial. Droperidol-fentanyl (Innovar) has been used successfully as an induction agent in humans and has been recommended because droperidol reduces the pressor response to epinephrine. Other case reports have suggested that droperidol has been associated with the release of catecholamines from the tumors. Morphine and meperidine are not used because they cause histamine release. Low doses of acepromazine, diazepam, midazolam, fentanyl, or oxymorphone are not contraindicated. Thiopental and thiamylal have been used satisfactorily for induction of anesthesia in dogs with pheochromocytoma. Ketamine is a less desirable induction agent because it increases circulating catecholamine levels, heart rate, and blood pressure when used alone or with xylazine or diazepam. Halothane may be used to maintain anesthesia; however, isoflurane causes less myocardial sensitization to catecholamines and decreases the potential for cardiac arrhythmia development. A greater arrhythmogenicity has been demonstrated with halothane–nitrous oxide anesthesia than with halothane alone.

Endotracheal intubation causes tachycardia and increased blood pressure. The intravenous administration of lidocaine before intubation in dogs reduces this response. One specific induction technique for dogs involves administration of thiopental and lidocaine in alternate small doses, flushing the catheter with saline between injections to prevent precipitation, until anesthesia is sufficient for tracheal intubation or until the total dose for thiopental (11 mg/kg) and lidocaine (8.8 mg/kg) is reached.

Heart rate, arterial blood pressure, electrocardiogram, and body temperature are monitored closely during induction and maintenance of anesthesia. Excitement, hypoxia, and hypercapnia are avoided. Measurement of arterial blood pressure using a catheter inserted into a peripheral artery is advisable (if possible), as measurement using indirect methods may be difficult because of intense vasoconstriction. Dysrhythmias may be of various types and may require appropriate treatment. Sinus tachycardia should disappear after the tumor is removed, and treatment may not be needed provided that the arterial pressure and capillary refill time are adequate. Low doses of propranolol (0.05 to 0.01 mg/kg IV) are useful for limiting sinus tachycardia and preventing ventricular arrhythmias. Balanced electrolyte solution, such as lactated Ringer Solution, is infused to maintain blood volume. Phentolamine has been used to treat hypertension resulting from catecholamine release during manipulation of the tumor, either as an intravenous bolus (0.02 to 1.0 mg/kg) or by infusion (10 mg in 100 ml of 5 per cent dextrose in water), until the desired effect is achieved. Sodium nitroprusside has been advocated as better for this purpose; however, treatment of hypotension between catecholamine surges can be difficult.[4] Hypotension may develop after the tumor is removed or in the postoperative period as a result of withdrawal of catecholamine influence. Increased fluid administration or blood transfusion is the best treatment for this hypotension.

References

1. Court MH, et al: Anesthetic management of small animal patients with endocrine disease. *Br Vet J 144*:323, 1988.
2. Feldman EC, et al: Therapy for spontaneous canine hyperadrenocorticism. *In* Kirk RW (ed): *Current Veterinary Therapy X: Small Animal Practice*. W. B. Saunders, Philadelphia, 1989.
3. Flanders JA, et al: Feline thyroidectomy: A comparison of postoperative hypocalcemia associated with three different surgical techniques. *Vet Surg 16*:362, 1987.
4. Hull CJ: Phaeochromocytoma: Diagnosis, preoperative preparation, and anaesthetic management. *Br J Anaesth 58*:1453, 1986.
5. Peterson ME: Pathophysiological changes in the endocrine system. *In* Short CE (ed): *Principles and Practice of Veterinary Anesthesia*. Williams & Wilkins, Baltimore, 1987.
6. Peterson ME: Treatment of feline hyperthyroidism. *In* Kirk RW (ed): *Current Veterinary Therapy X: Small Animal Practice*. W. B. Saunders, Philadelphia, 1989.
7. Peterson ME, et al: Feline hyperthyroidism: Pretreatment clinical and laboratory evaluation of 131 cases. *J Am Vet Med Assoc 183*:103, 1983.
8. Schaer M: A clinicopathologic survey of acute pancreatitis in 30 dogs and 5 cats. *J Am Anim Hosp Assoc 15*:681, 1979.
9. Trim CM: Anesthesia and the endocrine system. *In* Slatter D (ed): *Textbook of Small Animal Surgery*. W. B. Saunders, Philadelphia, 1985.

CHAPTER

172 Pediatric and Geriatric Anesthetic Techniques

Elaine P. Robinson

The term *pediatric* is applied to the first 12 weeks of postnatal life in puppies and kittens. Using similar terms to those used for human babies, *neonate* (newborn) describes puppies and kittens in the first 2 weeks of life, and *infant* describes those between 2 and 6 weeks of age.[15] Defining the term *geriatric* is more difficult because aging is a gradual process with much species and individual variation. One suggestion is that dogs and cats can be considered aged when they have completed 75 to 80 per cent of their expected life spans.[3] This definition implies 6 years of age for Great Danes and other giant dogs, 8 to 10 years for medium and large breeds of dogs, and 12 to 15 years for cats, toy dogs, and smaller terrier breeds.[4]

PHYSIOLOGICAL, PATHOPHYSIOLOGICAL, AND PSYCHOLOGICAL DIFFERENCES BETWEEN AGE GROUPS

Puppies and kittens are immature at birth and have long neonatal periods compared with domestic ungulates. Reflexes and responses develop slowly in the first 4 weeks of life but are similar to those of adults by 6 to 8 weeks.[2, 7, 15] Physiological changes of pediatric animals are summarized in Table 172–1.

Psychologically, pediatric puppies and kittens are distressed easily and resist handling, even for simple procedures. They vocalize loudly but normally do not bite or scratch. Exceptions to this may be wild animals, those unsocialized to humans, and those with highly developed protective instincts. Painful manipulations must be minimized, and handling must be performed gently and sympathetically. This requirement applies particularly to the 7- to 8-week ("fear-imprint") stage when stressful experiences with strange people may negatively affect the bonding process for the rest of the animal's life.

Some pathophysiological changes are expected in older animals because of the aging process. These changes have been reviewed extensively elsewhere,[3, 4, 8, 9, 11, 12] and they are summarized in Table 172–2. Age-related decline in function of the central nervous, cardiovascular, respiratory, hepatic, renal, and endocrine systems is progressive and often well tolerated. The degree of degeneration and the impact of intercurrent diseases, however, influence the ability of the older animal to tolerate the stress of anesthesia. Thorough preanesthetic assessment of each animal by the clinician is vital. Even then, there may be a narrow margin between what is normal and what is abnormal for an older animal. Often, older dogs and cats are calm and tolerant of handling; however, some animals may be blind or senile and disoriented.

Injectable drugs are usually given intramuscularly to young and old dogs and cats. Usually, uptake from muscle is reliable. Subcutaneous absorption of drugs may be delayed or incomplete in old animals because of loss of elasticity, increases in fat deposits, and reduced blood flow to skin and subcutaneous tissues. In general, pediatric and geriatric animals are more sensitive than young healthy animals to anesthetic drugs; changes in

TABLE 172–1. PHYSIOLOGICAL DIFFERENCES IN YOUNG COMPARED WITH YOUNG ADULT ANIMALS

Pediatric Differences	Effects
Immature hepatic microsomal enzyme system until 6–12 weeks of age.	May delay metabolism of drugs.
Immature renal function until 4–8 weeks of age.	Slow clearance of fluids; increased Na^+ loss; inability to conserve fluids.
Poor vasomotor control.	Greater susceptibility to hypotension and hypothermia.
Large body surface area; lack of subcutaneous fat; inability to shiver.	Greater susceptibility to hypothermia.
Neonatal heart has immature innervation, is less able to increase force of contraction, and is more rate dependent.	Greater susceptibility to hypotension in response to bradycardia.
Respiratory system has less alveoli, less surfactant, higher gas-flow resistance, greater chest-wall expansion, and increased alveolar ventilation.	More rapid inhalation anesthetic induction; less oxygen reserve; greater fluctuations of anesthetic depth during spontaneous ventiliation.
Reduced response to high $Paco_2$ or low Pao_2.	Newborn may respond to hypoxia by depressing ventilation.
Low blood glucose and low blood calcium levels.	Routine preanesthetic blood glucose determination advisable.
Newborn hemoglobin contains 70% to 80% fetal hemoglobin.	Hemoglobin has greater affinity for oxygen, and it gives oxygen less readily to tissues ("shift to left").
Total body water is 75% of body weight (60% in adult); extracellular fluid is 40% of body weight in the newborn (20% in adult); less intracellular fluid reserves; higher water turnover; very low fat content (2%–3% of body weight).	Drugs confined to extracellular fluid relatively less potent (e.g., atropine); perianesthetic fluid supplementation is important.
Greater percentage of cardiac output to brain; increased permeability of blood-brain barrier.	More rapid, profound anesthetic effects.

Modified from Robinson EP: Anesthesia of pediatric patients. *Comp Cont Educ Prac Vet* 5:1004, 1983.

TABLE 172–2. PHYSIOLOGICAL DIFFERENCES IN GERIATRIC COMPARED WITH YOUNG ADULT ANIMALS

Geriatric Differences	Effects
Liver function may be decreased by lipidosis, neoplasia, cirrhosis, or decreased hepatic blood flow.	Metabolism of injectable drugs is reduced, and duration of action increased.
Chronic renal failure and loss of nephrons.	Slow clearance of drugs.
Decreased blood volume, blood pressure, and cardiac output. A significant number have cardiac disease, especially chronic valvular disease.	Reduced ability to compensate for hemodynamic changes such as hypovolemia.
Poor thermoregulation.	Hypothermia is common during and following surgery.
Physiologic vagotonia is common.	Heart rates are often slower; tachycardia may indicate first-stage heart failure.
Decreased lung elasticity; chronic bronchitis; fibrotic vasculature; stiffened chest wall; less active protective reflexes; neoplasia; emphysema; reduced ventilatory function.	Slower induction and recovery to inhalation anesthesia.
V/Q mismatch in lungs—low resting Pa_{O_2}.	Reduced ability to respond to hypercapnia and hypoxia.
Low resting thyroid hormone (T_3 and T_4) levels.	Obesity, decreased drug metabolism, hypothermia, poor cardiac function.
Inappropriate adrenal response more common.	Although basal cortisol levels may be normal, "adrenal exhaustion" can occur with stress of anesthesia; Cushing's disease also common.
Diabetes mellitus more common.	Ketoacidosis, diuresis, liver disease.
Decline in central nervous system activity and increased percentage of CO to brain; increased permeability of blood-brain barrier; deterioration of neuromuscular function.	Reduced doses of anesthetic drugs needed; blindness and deafness can disorientate animal; more rapid profound anesthetic effects.
Total body water decreases from 60%–50% of body weight; intracellular fluid decreases to 30%, and extracellular fluid remains constant at 20%; fat often increases up to 25%–40% of body weight.	Lipid-soluble drugs (thiobarbiturates, ketamine) have larger volume distribution (are less potent); water-soluble drugs (midazolam), are more potent.

CO, cardiac output; T_3, triiodothyronine; T_4, thyroxin; V/Q ventilation/perfusion.

distribution and metabolism account for most of the differences. Major factors affecting distribution of drugs include differences in body composition, fluid compartments, fat stores, plasma binding, blood-brain barrier permeability, and cardiac output (see Tables 172–1 and 172–2).

PREANESTHETIC ASSESSMENT

Elective procedures on puppies and kittens require a minimum preoperative data base that includes history, physical examination including an accurate body weight, and packed cell volume and plasma protein; expected values are listed in (Table 172–3). Vaccination status, anthelmintic therapy, and overall condition of the puppy or kitten are assessed. Signs of nasal discharge, diarrhea, dehydration, or pyrexia (greater than 103.5°F [39.7°C] in a calm animal) indicate concurrent disease and are investigated before anesthesia.

Preoperative assessment of all geriatric animals should be thorough and directed to evaluation of cardiac, renal, and hepatic systems. Careful taking of history and examination of the animal help indicate major organ systems at risk. Minimum data base includes complete blood count, serum enzymes and chemistries (at least alanine aminotransferase, alkaline phosphatase, blood urea nitrogen, and creatinine), urinalysis, preoperative electrocardiogram, and microfilarial evaluation in heartworm areas.[5] The owner of the animal should be informed of the value of these tests, which warn of potential organ failure during anesthesia and surgery. Other tests pertinent to the specific disease present are indicated preoperatively. If cardiac disease, renal dis-

TABLE 172–3. AGE-RELATED PHYSIOLOGICAL VALUES

Value	Newborn	2 Weeks	6 Weeks	Adult	Geriatric
Heart rate	160–200	180–210	180–200	80–130	80–150
Respiratory rate	40	40	20–30	10–20	10–20
Tidal volume (ml/kg)	2–3	2–3	2–3	2–3	2–3
Arterial blood pressure (torr)	60/40	80/50	90/60	120/70	110/60
Pa_{CO_2} (torr)	33	—	—	38	40
Pa_{O_2} (torr)	60–80	—	—	80–100	70–80
pH	7.45	—	—	7.4	7.4
Plasma bicarbonate (mEq/L)	14–20	—	—	18–24	18–24
Blood volume (% body weight)	—	8.5	—	8	7
Hemoglobin (g/dl)	17	10	10	15	15
Packed cell volume (%)	55	27–32	28–35	46	46
Erythrocytes (10^6/cu mm)	6	3.2	4.9	8	8

Modified from Robinson EP: Anesthesia of pediatric patients. *Comp Cont Educ Pract Vet 5*:1004, 1983.

ease, or diabetes mellitus is diagnosed, the animal is treated and stabilized before anesthesia, if possible.

CHOICE AND MANAGEMENT OF ANESTHETIC DRUGS

The basic principles of anesthetic management are similar for pediatric and geriatric animals: Large or multiple doses of injectable drugs, undue handling, stress and alarm, and overhydration with excess intravenous fluids are avoided. Excitable pediatric and geriatric animals benefit from properly dosed preanesthetic sedation and tranquilization. Oxygenation, ventilation, heart rate and rhythm, blood pressure, fluid balance, and body temperature are monitored and maintained.

EARLY NEUTERING AND EAR-CROPPING

Early neutering is gaining widespread acceptance, especially in animal shelters. Extensive experience has been gained in one shelter in which more than 3,000 surgical procedures have been performed on puppies and kittens.[16] The usual age at which the procedure is performed is 6 to 8 weeks, although on occasion, 3- to 4-week-old puppies and kittens have been neutered. Various anesthetic techniques have been tried, but the combination of acepromazine, xylazine, and ketamine has proved to be the most effective and efficient method. The combination is 10 ml (1000 mg) ketamine, 2 ml (200 mg) xylazine, and 1 ml (10 mg) acepromazine. The intramuscular dose is 0.22 ml/kg of body weight. Atropine is not used as a routine preanesthetic agent. The procedure lasts approximately 3 minutes, and puppies are awake and active within 30 minutes. Kittens recover more slowly, in 1 to 2 hours. When tiletamine-zolazepam (Telazol) is used, recovery is slower.[16]

Vaccination and worming are performed at least 72 hours before surgery. Puppies and kittens are given no food overnight, and water is withdrawn 3 hours before surgery. To allow ease of breathing, the legs are left free and not tied down during surgery. A considerable volume of free fluid escapes when the abdomen is opened in females, which is normal—absence of fluid implies dehydration, which may require fluid therapy. Doxapram and sodium prednisolone succinate (Solu-delta Cortef) are given to all puppies and kittens (Solu-delta Cortef, 1.0 mg/kg, intraperitoneally) postoperatively to improve breathing and arousal and to combat "shock".[17] Anesthesia-related deaths have included two 3- to 4-week-old kittens that became apneic and one puppy that had a slow recovery and was extremely hypothermic.[16]

A previous recommendation for ear-cropping was to inject atropine and fentanyl-droperidol (Innovar-Vet) intramuscularly and then a low dose of pentobarbital intravenously.[15] Alternatively, tiletamine-zolazepam (6 to 13 mg/kg IM) can be used. Potential complications with this drug include apnea and excitable recovery in dogs and prolonged 24-hour recovery in cats. Several adjunctive drugs have been used with tiletamine-zolazepam, including xylazine and butorphanol in dogs,[1] and acepromazine. Another alternative is a combination of acepromazine, diazepam, and ketamine, injected intravenously.[17] Acepromazine (0.9 ml [9 mg]) is combined in the bottle with ketamine (10 ml [1000 mg]). For procedures lasting less than 15 minutes (e.g., cropping of an 8-week-old miniature Schnauzer), the combination is given intravenously (0.5 ml/4.5 kg of body weight), along with diazepam (0.25 ml [1.25 mg] per 4.5 kg of body weight). Recovery usually occurs within 10 minutes of surgery. In larger puppies (e.g., in ear cropping of a Doberman pinscher) or in procedures of longer duration, anesthesia is induced with one-half to one-third the recommended dose rate of the acepromazine, ketamine, and diazepam combination. The puppy is intubated, and anesthesia is continued with either halothane or isoflurane.

HIGH-RISK PEDIATRIC PATIENTS AND COMPLEX PEDIATRIC PROCEDURES

Simple inhalation anesthesia using either a chamber or mask for induction of anesthesia is often preferred in depressed or sick puppies and kittens.[10, 15] Preoxygenation for approximately 5 minutes with a face mask is desirable if the puppy or kitten can tolerate the procedure without struggling. Isoflurane is now the inhalant of choice because of rapid induction and recovery from anestheia, relative stability of the cardiovascular system, and freedom from toxic effects. Halothane, with or without nitrous oxide, is still used. The main complications with halothane are related to intraoperative arterial hypotension and the possibility of cardiac arrhythmias.

The use of preanesthetic tranquilizers or sedatives depends on the temperament of the young animal and its physical condition. Xylazine and high doses of acepromazine are not used in high-risk pediatric animals because they are associated with cardiovascular depression and prolonged sedation. Sedative-analgesics are useful in puppies. Oxymorphone (Numorphan) in a dose of 0.1 to 0.2 mg/kg IM, and atropine, in a dose of 0.04 mg/kg IM, are suitable. This combination helps prevent bradycardia, which is particularly important for young animals, in which cardiac output is directly related to heart rate. Emesis and hypotension are minimal after oxymorphone administration. Restraint and immobilization can be produced in kittens or puppies by combinations of ketamine (6 to 11 mg/kg IM) and midazolam (0.1 mg/kg IM) with or without butorphanol (0.4 mg/kg IM) or oxymorphone (0.05 to 0.1 mg/kg IM) for analgesia. Atropine can also be given to small kittens and puppies to prevent excessive salivation and possible airway obstruction. Atropine should probably be avoided in puppies and kittens of less than 2 weeks of age because of the immaturity of vagal innervation and the limited cardiac effects of the drug.[3] Furthermore, atropine may increase viscosity of secretions and lead to plugging of airways with thick mucus.

THORACOTOMY FOR CONGENITAL CARDIAC ANOMALY

Preoperative status and intraoperative status dictate anesthetic management. Otherwise healthy puppies with patent ductus arteriosus can be treated like healthy animals undergoing elective procedures with certain exceptions, noted later. Acid-base and electrolyte abnormalities are corrected preoperatively if possible. For intracardiac surgery, the patient is crossmatched, and compatible whole blood is prepared, before surgery. Fresh whole blood is preferred because of its maximum oxygen-carrying ability. Electrolyte solutions are a poor substitute for blood lost in pediatric patients, as the hemoglobin levels of these animals are already low (see Table 172–3). Blood infusion is started immediately prior to the incision into the heart. For a 3-kg puppy or kitten, a 75-ml blood loss would constitute a severe hemorrhage (greater than 25 per cent of total blood volume), and a loss of 150 ml (50 per cent of total blood volume) would probably be fatal.

Hypotensive drugs such as acepromazine, meperidine, and halothane are best avoided. Anesthetic drugs that are arrhythmogenic should be avoided. These include xylazine, halothane, thiobarbiturates, and ketamine. If ketamine is used in kittens, only small preanesthetic doses (4 to 10 mg/kg IM) are used, to avoid prolonged or severe tachycardia. Isoflurane is used as the primary anesthetic. Oxymorphone or fentanyl can be used intravenously as an adjunctive analgesic drug. Muscle-relaxant drugs are usually not necessary in these small patients. Intraoperatively, I prefer atracurium at 0.1 mg/kg IV. This nondepolarizing muscle blocker has a short duration of action, rarely needs to be reversed postoperatively, and does not rely on hepatic or renal function for degradation and excretion.

Because the chest is so compliant in pediatric patients, overinflation of the lungs by positive-pressure ventilation should be avoided. Airway pressures of 15 to 18 cm H_2O are sufficient when the chest is closed. The pressure can be increased to 20 to 25 cm H_2O when the chest is opened after visible inspection of the lungs. Although pediatric ventilators are available (e.g., Veterinary Anesthesia Ventilator Model 2000* with 300 ml bellows), most surgeons prefer to ventilate these young animals manually. Blood gases during surgery are difficult to obtain, so pulse oximetry and end-expired respiratory gas monitoring (Datex Capnomac and Cardiocap†) are helpful in monitoring adequacy of ventilation. Blood gas values measured from lingual veins correlate well with arterial values.[19] Collection and measurement of microcapillary samples in dogs have been described.[13]

Fluid therapy at 4 ml/kg per hour may consist of lactated Ringer solution, Plasmolyte-148, which contains no lactate, or a mixture of dextrose and electrolytes (e.g., one-half strength lactated Ringer solution plus 2.5 per cent dextrose, or 0.45 per cent saline plus 2.5 per cent dextrose). Dextrose is particularly valuable in preventing hypoglycemia. Oxygen therapy can be continued postoperatively using a mask or oxygen chamber. Puppies and kittens, unless severely depressed, do not tolerate nasal catheters for oxygen administration.[6]

Postoperative pain relief is vital, as young animals respond violently to pain. Incisional pain can be relieved with intercostal nerve blocks of three to four nerves, using the local anesthetic bupivacaine (Marcaine) (0.5 per cent, 0.5 ml per nerve). The nerve blocks are performed by the surgeon before closure. Opioids can be used for analgesia; butorphanol, morphine, or oxymorphone can be used in puppies and kittens.[18] Sometimes tranquilizers such as diazepam, or even acepromazine, are added to a narcotic to enhance sedation. Unless immediate reversal of opioids used during anesthesia is desired to revive the animal, the use of a partial reversal antagonist such as nalbuphine (Nubain) is preferable, so that some analgesia remains. Nalbuphine is administered intravenously or intramuscularly in a dose of 0.1 mg/kg.

*Hallowell, Pittsfield, MA.
†Datex, Tewksbury, MA.

ELECTIVE GERIATRIC PROCEDURES

All older patients should be considered "high-risk," even those undergoing dental work or other short procedures. Rarely can satisfactory dental work be performed using only sedation, and few veterinarians contemplate local anesthetic dental blocks. General anesthesia has the advantage of providing oxygenation, airway protection from blood, water, and tartar, and the ability to ventilate the patient.

If preoperative sedation is needed in dogs for tooth extractions and other painful procedures, one of the opioid analgesic drugs (oxymorphone, 0.1 mg/kg IM, or morphine, 1 mg/kg IM) can be administered. Opioids can be antagonized or partially antagonized at the end of the procedure, if necessary. Naloxone is an opioid antagonist, and nalbuphine is a partial opioid antagonist (see previous section). Diazepam (Valium) (0.2 mg/kg IV) or midazolam (Versed) (0.1 mg/kg IV or IM) provides good preoperative sedation with minimal side effects.

Rapid anesthetic induction without premedication can be accomplished using thiobarbiturates in healthy dogs and cats. These drugs are given slowly to effect. Ketamine (4 to 6 mg/kg IV) and diazepam (0.2 mg/kg IV), or ketamine and midazolam (0.1 mg/kg IV), can be used. Oxymorphone (0.1 mg/kg IV) and diazepam (0.2 mg/kg IV), or oxymorphone and midazolam (0.1 mg/kg IV), are also effective. Oxymorphone is injected slowly and followed immediately with diazepam or midazolam to prevent excitement. Another opioid-based induction regimen is fentanyl (Sublimaze) (0.1 mg/kg IV) and intravenously administered diazepam or midazolam. Fentanyl is injected slowly and followed immediately with diazepam. Propofol (Diprivan) (6 to 8 mg/kg IV without premedication, 1 to 4 mg/kg IV after premedication) is a relatively new drug that is approved for use in humans and produces smooth induction and recovery from anesthesia. Cardiac arrhythmias are uncommon, and recovery is rapid and complete. The drug provides little analgesia, and as with the barbiturates, respiratory depression is common.

For geriatric patients, isoflurane is the drug of choice for maintenance of anesthesia for any procedure longer than 5 minutes. Intravenous fluid therapy is advisable, even during routine dental procedures, to maintain blood volume and urine production. A balanced electrolyte solution at a low rate of replacement (1 ml/3 kg per hour) is recommended. If the patient has heart disease, a non–sodium-containing solution such as 5 per cent dextrose can be used.

HIGH-RISK GERIATRIC PATIENTS AND COMPLEX GERIATRIC PROCEDURES

Many anesthetic approaches and complications outlined previously apply equally well to high-risk geriatric animals. Simple anesthesia using mask induction with isoflurane and continuing with isoflurane for anesthetic maintenance may be satisfactory for many depressed older patients; however, if inhalation anesthesia alone is insufficient, then a more balanced anesthetic regimen is desirable. Neuroleptanalgesia with the combinations of benzodiazepines (diazepam, midazolam) with opioids (oxymorphone, fentanyl, butorphanol) can produce sedation, analgesia, and sleep, the effects depending on route of administration and dose.[12] Because of the hypotensive and prolonged effects of droperidol, fentanyl-droperidol is now rarely used in older dogs, except in those that are vicious. It is still used as an immobilizing, restraining combination in that situation. Inhalation anesthesia with isoflurane, analgesia with an opioid, and muscle relaxation with atracurium produce a balanced anesthesia in which each drug contributes its specific effects and therefore can be used in smaller doses. Preoxygenation with a face mask and 100 per cent oxygen administered for 5 minutes before anesthetic induction greatly benefits geriatric animals. Thiobarbiturates are best avoided in these animals, but any of the other injectable induction techniques listed in the previous section can be used. Ketamine may produce tachycardia, which is undesirable in animals with heart failure. I prefer the fentanyl-diazepam combination or propofol for high-risk geriatric dogs, and propofol for cats.

All animals should have an intravenous catheter in place throughout administration of the anesthetic, both for fluid and drug administration. An unexpected emergency can then be handled more effectively and successfully. Continuous monitoring of the electrocardiogram should start before induction of anesthesia. Blood pressure and body temperature are monitored in all patients. Dinamap* and Doppler† blood pressure monitors can be used for indirect measurements. In medium-size or larger dogs, more accurate blood pressure readings can be obtained by arterial catheterization of the cranial tibial artery. Heart rate and heart sounds can be monitored continuously via an esophageal stethoscope. Pulse oximetry (if available) is performed; sensors can be placed on the tongue, ear or vulva. Decreases in oxygen saturation below 90 per cent indicate hypoxemia ($Pa_{O_2} < 80$ mm Hg) and are treated by ventilating the patient with oxygen. Respiratory gas monitoring is used, if available, in high-risk geriatric animals. Inspired and expired carbon dioxide, oxygen, and anesthetic gas monitoring provides continual measurements during anesthesia and can be valuable in assessing the condition of the patient. Blood component therapy is indicated if packed cell volume is less than 20 per cent, total plasmaproteins is less than 4.0 g/dl, or platelet count is less than 2×10^5 per μl. Urine production is monitored in uremic animals and in those undergoing prolonged or radical procedures. A catheter introduced into the bladder can be attached to a closed tubing-bag system for urine collection during anesthesia. A minimum of 1 ml/kg of body weight of urine should be produced each hour. Decreased urine production warrants more rigorous fluid therapy, dopamine infusions, or even diuretics, such as furosemide or mannitol.[14]

Old anesthetized animals are handled gently, as they can easily suffer bruising and skeletal injuries. Skeletal osteoporosis in geriatric animals can make bones susceptible to fractures. Animals with skull or spinal injuries snould be carefully supported during transportation. Older animals tolerate nasal catheters postoperatively for supplementary oxygen administration.[6] Postoperative analgesic drugs may be necessary as described for pediatric animals. Local anesthesia should be considered as an alternative. Useful techniques include epidural blocks (perineal surgery, postoperative pain relief), local infiltrations (superficial tumor removal), retrograde intravenous block (peripheral limb surgery).

*Critikon, Tampa, FL.
†Parks Labs, Beaverton, OR.

ANESTHETIC EQUIPMENT

Endotracheal tube intubation, laryngoscope blades, and choice of anesthetic circuits for pediatric dogs and cats have been reviewed elsewhere.[15] The same equipment is suitable for geriatric toy dogs and cats.

References

1. Benson GJ, et al: Abstract: Clinical evaluation of Telazol-xylazine-butorphanol anesthesia for ovariohysterectomy in dogs. *Vet Surg 18*:405, 1989.
2. Breazile JE: Neurologic and behavioral development in the puppy. *Vet Clin North Am Small Anim Pract 8*:31, 1978.
3. Dodman NH, et al: Aging changes in the geriatric dog and their impact on anesthesia. *Comp Cont Educ Pract Vet 6*:1106, 1984.
4. Evans T: Anesthesia for the geriatric patient. *Vet Clin North Am Small Anim Pract 11*:653, 1981.
5. Faulkner RT: Preoperative consideration of the surgical patient. *In* Slatter DH (ed): *Textbook of Veterinary Surgery*. W. B. Saunders, Philadelphia, 1985, pp 242–248.
6. Fitzpatrick RK, Crowe DT: Nasal oxygen administration in dogs and cats: Experimental and clinical investigations. *J Am Anim Hosp Assoc 22*:293, 1986.
7. Fox MW: *Canine Pediatrics*. Charles C Thomas, Springfield, IL, 1966.
8. Kaufman GM: Renal function in the geriatric dog. *Comp Cont Educ Pract Vet 6*:1087, 1984.
9. MacDougall DF, Barker J: An approach to canine geriatrics. *Br Vet J 140*:115, 1984.
10. Meyer RE: Anesthesia for neonatal and geriatric patients. *In* Short CE (ed): *Principles and Practice of Veterinary Anesthesia*. Williams & Wilkins, Baltimore, 1987, pp 330–337.
11. Mosier JE: Effect of aging on body systems of the dog. *Vet Clin North Am Small Anim Pract 19*:1, 1989.
12. Paddleford RR: Anesthetic considerations for the geriatric patient. *Vet Clin North Am Small Anim Pract 19*:13, 1989.
13. Quandt JE, et al: Evaluation of toenail blood samples for blood-gas analysis (abstract). *Vet Surg 18*:407, 1989.
14. Robinson EP: Anaesthesia and renal disease. *Aust Vet Pract* 7:137, 1977.
15. Robinson EP: Anesthesia of pediatric patients. *Comp Cont Educ Pract Vet* 5:1004, 1983.

16. Shepler CJ: Report from Memphis Animal Shelter. Personal communication, 1990.
17. Smith FO: Personal communication, 1990.
18. Tranquilli WJ, et al: Selecting the right analgesics: Indications and dosage requirements. *Vet Med 84*:692, 1989.
19. Wagner AE, et al: Abstract: A comparison of arterial and lingual venous blood gases in anesthetized dogs. *Vet Surg 18*:408, 1989.

CHAPTER 173

Anesthesia for Cesarean Section

Peter W. Hellyer

Anesthetic techniques for cesarean section must be tailored to provide adequate surgical anesthesia for the dam while minimizing maternal and fetal depression. Maternal physiological changes increase the risk of anesthetic-related complications for the dam. Anesthetics and anesthetic adjuncts affect the fetus either directly by crossing the placenta or indirectly by altering maternal cardiopulmonary function. Selection of the most appropriate anesthetic technique depends on the status of the dam, viability of the fetuses, expected advantages and disadvantages of the technique, and experience of the veterinarian.

MATERNAL PHYSIOLOGICAL CHANGES

Cardiovascular Changes. The maternal cardiovascular system is markedly changed during pregnancy to meet increased metabolic demands during gestation and parturition.[1, 2, 4, 6] In the normal dam, increased blood volume provides an adequate reserve to compensate for large quantities of blood and fluid lost at delivery. The contracting uterus acts as an additional reservoir of blood, providing autotransfusion for the dam. Partial vena caval occlusion and aortic compression, resulting in hypotension, may occur in animals placed in dorsal recumbency. Dogs, and presumably cats, are resistant to supine hypotension at term.[9, 10] Dehydration, bleeding, and inhibition of maternal compensatory mechanisms by anesthetic drugs increase the potential for supine hypotension. Changes in position (tilting to left or laterally to right), reduction of the time spent in dorsal recumbency, and additional cardiovascular support (intravenous fluids and inotropic agents) may be necessary in animals that show signs of hypotension. Decreases in maternal cardiac output and arterial blood pressure during anesthesia reduce uterine and placental blood flow and threaten fetal viability. Reflex increases in endogenous catecholamines can induce intense vasoconstriction of the uterine artery. Similarly, exogenously administered alpha-adrenergic agonists cause vasoconstriction of the uterine artery and decreased uterine blood flow. Inotropic agents with predominately beta-adrenergic activity are chosen when augmentation of cardiac output and arterial blood pressure is required.

Respiratory Changes. Physiological changes that occur during pregnancy significantly alter respiratory function and decrease respiratory reserves.[1, 3, 12] Cranial displacement of the diaphragm by the enlarging uterus is primarily responsible for the mechanical changes in respiratory function. Resting lung volume, particularly functional residual capacity, is decreased. Reductions in functional residual capacity are significant for several reasons. Maternal oxygen reserves are diminished because the amount of air in the lungs at the end of an expiration is reduced. Closing capacity, the lung volume at which dependent airways begin to close, is normally less than functional residual capacity in young healthy adults. Closing capacity does not change during pregnancy; however, reductions in lung volume move functional residual capacity and closing capacity closer together.[11] The resulting ventilation/perfusion inequalities and intrapulmonary shunting increase the tendency for maternal hypoxemia. Increases in maternal oxygen demand increase the tendency toward hypoxemia during periods of hypoventilation. Limiting the time spent in dorsal recumbency and increasing the inspired concentration of oxygen minimize the effects of reduced functional residual capacity.

Acid-Base Changes. Hyperventilation during pregnancy results in decreased Pa_{CO_2}. Maternal pH remains normal, representing compensated respiratory alkalosis.[1] Maternal pH in the normal, unmedicated animal may rise during the early stage of labor. Increased minute ventilation, secondary to pain and anxiety, is responsible for the early rise in maternal pH. As labor progresses, metabolic acidosis occurs; subsequently, maternal pH returns to normal or becomes acidotic. Lactic acid is the main metabolite responsible for the metabolic acidosis.[1] The acid-base status of animals presented for emergency cesarean section varies widely from respiratory alkalosis to metabolic acidosis. Respiratory depression from tranquilizers, sedatives, and narcotics may increase Pa_{CO_2}, exacerbating concomitant metabolic acidosis. Maternal acidosis prior to delivery is preferably treated with hyperventilation. Sodium bicarbonate is used only if necessary, because it may aggravate fetal acidosis. Sodium bicarbonate transiently increases maternal and fetal Pa_{CO_2}. Placental transfer of carbon dioxide is rapid, whereas bicarbonate may require 1 to 3 hours to cross the placenta.[1] Consequently, if delivery is expected within 30 to 60 minutes, sodium bicarbonate is avoided.

Gastrointestinal Changes. Gastrointestinal changes that occur during pregnancy place the dam at an increased risk of regurgitation and aspiration.[2, 7, 9] Dams for elective cesarean section are denied food overnight to decrease the risk of regurgitation and aspiration. All dams, particularly those presented for emergency section, are considered to have a full stomach and be at high risk of regurgitation and aspiration. Fasting reduces the likelihood of regurgitation; however, it does not ensure an empty stomach. Following induction of general anesthesia, tracheal intubation is performed rapidly with a cuffed endotracheal tube. Maintenance of anesthesia with a face mask is not recommended, because aspiration can occur. The risk of regurgitation and aspiration continues into the postoperative period; therefore, extubation should be performed only after return of swallowing reflexes.

SPECIFIC ANESTHETIC DRUGS

As stated previously, anesthetics and anesthetic adjuncts affect the fetus either directly by crossing the placental barrier or indirectly by altering maternal cardiopulmonary function. Drug-induced cardiopulmonary depression (both maternal and fetal) is dose dependent, necessitating the use of low doses of anesthetic drugs. Drugs with different spectrums of activity are combined to obtain satisfactory surgical analgesia while minimizing fetal and maternal depression.

Anesthetic Premedications. Anticholinergics, atropine or glycopyrrolate, are given to decrease salivary secretions and provide vagal blockade during anesthesia. Glycopyrrolate does not cross the placental barrier and therefore does not alter fetal heart rate. Anticholinergics may be administered intravenously as needed. Anticholinergics are administered only to those patients in which excessive salivary secretions (interfering with airway patency) or bradycardia is likely.

Phenothiazines (acepromazine, promazine) decrease anxiety and motor activity and produce calming. Phenothiazines cross the placenta rapidly and can be found in fetal blood within 2 minutes of intravenous administration. Clinically useful dosages do not affect the neonate.[7] Phenothiazines induce peripheral alpha-adrenergic blockade and vasodilation, which may result in maternal hypotension. The hypotensive effects of the phenothiazines are aggravated by the large amount of fluid and blood lost by the dam during cesarean section. Phenothiazines are not administered to a dam that is already compromised by dehydration, hypovolemia, or shock. Acepromazine administered in low doses (0.025 to 0.05 mg/kg IM) in combination with an opioid usually sedates a nervous dam adequately for epidural analgesia. During anesthesia, volume replacement with an intravenous crystalloid solution (10 to 20 ml/kg/per hour) is essential, especially when a phenothiazine is used for premedication. Phenothiazine tranquilizers are used only in low dosages, and when absolutely necessary, to manage an apprehensive or nervous dam.

Xylazine produces calming, muscle relaxation, and analgesia, and it induces severe respiratory depression in both the dam and the fetus.[2] Cardiac output falls because of a decrease in heart rate and transient increase in peripheral vascular resistance. Uterine and placental blood flow may decrease, leading to fetal depression. Although xylazine is used in small animals for routine surgical procedures, its use in the dam is contraindicated.[2]

Diazepam and midazolam may produce mild calming and muscle relaxation. They produce minimal cardiopulmonary depression (maternal and fetal), making them useful premedications. They are most beneficial when administered intravenously prior to induction of anesthesia. Dams that are already relatively calm, depressed, or compromised respond most favorably to the calming and sedative effects of benzodiazepines. Nervous or anxious dogs may respond favorably to diazepam or midazolam administered intramuscularly with an opioid analgesic.

Narcotic agonists are frequently used alone or in combination with sedatives and tranquilizers to produce analgesia and sedation. Opioids readily cross the placenta and concentrate in the fetus as a result of maternal-fetal pH differences (ion trapping).[2] Central nervous system depression and respiratory depression are common in neonates. Opioids may induce maternal respiratory depression and bradycardia. The cardiopulmonary depressant effects of these drugs are mild, however. Opioid-induced bradycardia is treated with atropine or glycopyrrolate. Maternal and fetal hypoxemia can be avoided by administering oxygen to the dam if respiratory depression becomes significant. Opioids by themselves do not provide surgical anesthesia; however, their potent analgesic properties greatly reduce the amount of other anesthetic drugs required. Naloxone, an opioid antagonist, completely reverses all opioid-induced effects, including respiratory and central nervous system depression and analgesia.

Ketamine is frequently administered intramuscularly to cats as an anesthetic premedication. Ketamine rapidly crosses the placental barrier, causing dose-dependent fetal depression. Low doses of ketamine (1 mg/kg IV, 5 mg/kg intramuscularly) administered to cats cause minimal neonatal depression.[8] Ketamine's sympathomimetic effects may increase uterine tone and decrease uterine and placental blood flow. Alternatively, its stimulatory effects on the cardiovascular system may help to maintain uterine blood flow in a hypovolemic or depressed animal. Concurrent administration of diazepam is beneficial in decreasing ketamine-induced muscle rigidity.

Induction Drugs. Anesthetic induction drugs rapidly cross the blood-brain barrier and, therefore, rapidly cross the placental barrier. Varying degrees of fetal and neonatal depression occur after induction of anesthesia, depending on the specific anesthetic induction drug used, the dose, and the time from induction of anesthesia to delivery. Ultrashort-acting barbiturates affect the fetus minimally if administered in low doses (less than 8 mg/kg) as a single bolus.[8, 11] The duration of action of the ultrashort-acting barbiturates is due primarily to redistribution. Subsequent boluses maintain maternal plasma concentrations, preventing redistribution of drug away from the fetus. Maternal recovery from anesthesia is faster with methohexital than with thiopental because of the former's shorter elimination half-life. Neonatal viability following thiopental anesthesia is similar to that following methohexital anesthesia; therefore, methohexital does not offer any advantage over thiopental. Pentobarbital is contraindicated because of its association with prolonged anesthetic recovery, neonatal respiratory depression, and a high incidence of neonatal mortality.

Ketamine, administered intravenously in low doses, is a useful induction anesthetic in dogs and cats. Dogs should be given diazepam intravenously, prior to or concurrently with ketamine to prevent convulsions and muscle rigidity. Ketamine's stimulatory effects on the cardiovascular system may be particularly beneficial in dams that are depressed, dehydrated, or hypovolemic. Dams in shock are given ketamine with caution, as they may respond with marked cardiovascular depression instead of cardiovascular stimulation.

Propofol, a new alkyl phenol anesthetic, may be useful for cesarean section. Propofol's cardiopulmonary effects are similar to those of thiopental. Propofol's main advantage is a short duration of action following an intravenous bolus or continuous infusion. Preliminary studies in women, anesthetized for cesarean section with propofol, suggest that neonatal depression is minimal and well tolerated.[5]

Inhalant Anesthetics. All inhalant anesthetics rapidly cross the blood-brain barrier and placental barrier.[2, 7, 8] Neonatal depression is related to the duration and depth of anesthesia. Deep anesthesia depresses maternal cardiovascular function, further depressing the fetus. The choice of agent depends on the dam's physical status, the availability of agents, and the experience of the anesthetist. Inhalant anesthetics are administered for as short a time as possible prior to delivery, to minimize fetal depression. Alveolar concentrations of inhaled anesthetics rise more rapidly in pregnant than in nonpregnant patients as a result of pregnancy-induced increases in minute ventilation and decreases in lung volume. The dosage requirements for inhalants to induce anesthesia are decreased in pregnant patients. Consequently, induction of anesthesia with inhalant anesthetics may occur rapidly, and care must be taken to prevent overanesthetizing the animal. Halothane, isoflurane, and methoxyflurane are commonly used inhalant anesthetics for cesarean section. Halothane and isoflurane are preferred over methoxyflurane, because they are more controllable and because recovery from anesthesia, both maternal and fetal, is more rapid with these agents. Isoflurane has a greater margin of cardiovascular safety than halothane, making it useful for the compromised dam. Both halothane and isoflurane cause profound uterine relaxation, which may increase uterine hemorrhage and prolong surgery. The addition of 50 per cent nitrous oxide may be beneficial by decreasing the dose required of the more potent inhalant anesthetic. Maternal oxygenation is monitored closely, and the nitrous oxide is discontinued if hypoxemia develops.[8]

Local Anesthetics. Local and regional anesthetic techniques are frequently used for cesarean section to minimize maternal and fetal depression.[2, 7, 8] Significant fetal depression may occur as a result of excessive doses or inadvertent intravenous administration of local anesthetics. Neonatal toxicity is manifested as severe central nervous system depression, convulsions, bradycardia, and hypotension. Maternal hypotension from sympathetic blockade may reduce uteroplacental perfusion, leading to fetal hypoxemia and acidosis.[2] Cranial migration of epidurally administered local anesthetics may cause respiratory depression or paralysis. Elevation of the dam's head and careful attention to proper epidural technique, as well as avoidance of excessive doses of local anesthetic, minimize maternal and fetal complications. Maternal hypotension is usually avoided by appropriate intravenous fluid therapy.

Neuromuscular Blockers. Neuromuscular blocking drugs are not commonly used in veterinary anesthesia for cesarean section; however, these drugs may be useful to improve skeletal muscle relaxation during light anesthesia.[2] Maternal ventilation and analgesia must be provided. Fetal depression is unlikely because these drugs cross the placental barrier minimally. Neuromuscular blocking agents used in veterinary medicine include succinylcholine, pancuronium, vecuronium, and atracurium. Vecuronium and atracurium are preferred because of their short duration of action, lack of cumulative effects, and minimal cardiovascular effects.

ANESTHETIC TECHNIQUES

The physical status of animals presented for cesarean section varies widely. The specific anesthetic technique chosen should require drugs and equipment familiar to the practitioner, provide adequate surgical anesthesia for the dam, avoid maternal and fetal cardiopulmonary depression, and minimize deleterious effects in the neonate. Minimal effective doses of anesthetic drugs are given, and the anesthetic period is kept as short as possible. If the dam is tractable, the surgery site is clipped and scrubbed prior to induction of anesthesia to minimize the interval between induction and delivery. Dams are given a crystalloid solution (e.g., lactated Ringer solution) intravenously at 10 to 20 ml/kg/hour throughout the anesthesia. Preoxygenation for 3 to 5 minutes prior to induction of anesthesia is recommended if the dam tolerates a face mask. Adequate personnel should be available to monitor the dam and provide supportive care for the neonates. Representative examples of acceptable anesthetic protocols are presented in Table 173–1.

Dams presenting for emergency cesarean section usually exhibit varying degrees of dehydration, hypovolemia, hypotension, metabolic acidosis, and shock. Hypovolemia may be treated with an intravenous crystalloid solution administered at 50 to 100 ml/kg/hour. The dam is monitored closely for hypervolemia, pulmonary edema, and hypoproteinemia. Catecholamines

TABLE 173–1. REPRESENTATIVE ANESTHETIC REGIMENS FOR CESAREAN SECTION

Species	Drug or Technique	Dosage	Comment
Elective cesarean section			
Dogs	1. Lidocaine (2%)		Assistant required for restraint. Oxygen administered by face mask. Additional tranquilizers may be required. Glycopyrrolate given as needed.
	a. Epidural	1 ml/3–5 kg	
	b. Line block	8 mg/kg max. dose	
	Oxymorphone	0.05–0.2 mg/kg	
	2. Droperidol-fentanyl (Innovar-Vet)	1 ml/20–30 kg IV	Supplemental dose of droperidol-fentanyl or fentanyl may be needed. Inhalant given in low dosage until delivery.
	Glycopyrrolate	0.01 mg/kg, as needed to effect	
	Isoflurane		
	Halothane*		
	N_2O	50% N_2O/50% O_2	
Cats	Ketamine	5 mg/kg IM	Fetal depression occurs with excessive doses. Lidocaine (0.25 ml) applied to arytenoid cartilages facilitates intubation.
	Ketamine	1–3 mg/kg IV to effect	
	Isoflurane*		
	Halothane		
	N_2O		
Emergency cesarean section			
Dogs	1. Diazepam	0.2 mg/kg IV	Narcotics used to keep dose of inhalant low. Patient may decompensate with excessive dose of inhalant.
	Ketamine	5.5 mg/kg IV	
	Isoflurane*	0.5–1.0 %	
	Oxymorphone	0.05–0.1 mg/kg IV	
	2. Diazepam	0.2 mg/kg IV	Supplemental doses of oxymorphone may be needed.
	Oxymorphone	0.05–0.1 mg/kg IV	
	Line block	Lidocaine 2%	
Cats	Diazepam	0.2 mg/kg IV	Topical lidocaine facilitates intubation.
	Ketamine	1–2 mg/kg IV	
	Oxymorphone	0.05 mg/kg IV	
	Isoflurane*	0.05–1.0%	

Techniques listed for emergencies are also suitable for elective cesarean sections.
*Inhalant anesthetics are used in low concentrations, and only if necessary, until the fetuses are delivered.

are used to treat hypotension unresponsive to fluid therapy. Alpha-adrenergic agonists cause vasoconstriction of the uterine artery, thereby decreasing uterine and placental blood flow. Catecholamines with predominantly beta-adrenergic activity, such as dobutamine or ephedrine, are preferred for inotropic support. Dobutamine is my drug of choice and is administered as a continuous intravenous infusion at 1 to 10 μg/kg per minute. Ephedrine can be administered at a dosage of 0.3 mg/kg IV.[2] Maternal acidosis is treated with hyperventilation following endotracheal intubation. Sodium bicarbonate may be administered as needed once the fetuses have been delivered.

CARE OF THE NEWBORN

Immediately on delivery, each neonate's head and airway is cleared of membranes and fluids. The respiratory tract may be cleared of fluid by cradling the neonate in the hands and gently swinging it in a head-down position. The head and neck must be supported to prevent injury. Alternatively, a bulb syringe may be used to aspirate fluids from the oral pharynx. The neonate is gently rubbed with a towel; this action dries the neonate and stimulates its breathing. Because it is susceptible to chilling,[2] the neonate is kept in a warm environment, preferably 85° to 90°F (30° to 32°C), and it is placed with the dam as soon as she has recovered from anesthesia.

Neonates that are cyanotic are given oxygen by face mask. Endotracheal intubation and assisted ventilation may be necessary in the presence of severe respiratory depression or apnea. Respiratory depression may be treated with doxapram or naloxone administered sublingually, intramuscularly, or intravenously. Breathing may be stimulated with sublingual doxapram at 1 to 2 drops in kittens and 1 to 5 drops in puppies.[2] Naloxone (a few drops to effect, sublingually) is used to reverse neonatal respiratory depression if the dam was given opioids prior to delivery. Neonates administered naloxone to reverse opioid-induced respiratory depression must be observed closely over the next few hours for signs of a recurrence of the opioid effects.

References

1. Albright GA, et al: Physiology of pregnancy. *In* Albright GA, et al (eds): *Anesthesia in Obstetrics: Maternal, Fetal, and Neonatal Aspects*. 2nd ed. Butterworths, Boston, 1986, pp 41–79.
2. Benson GJ, Thurmon JC: Anesthesia for cesarean section. *In* Burke TJ (ed): *Small Animal Reproduction and Infertility: A Clinical Approach to Diagnosis and Treatment*. Lea & Febiger, Philadelphia, 1986, pp 353–371.
3. Cheek TG, Gutsche BB: Maternal physiologic alterations during pregnancy. *In* Shnider SM, Levinson G (eds): *Anesthesia for Obstetrics*. 2nd ed. Williams & Wilkins, Baltimore, 1987, p 3.
4. Concannon PW, et al: Pregnancy and parturition in the bitch. *Biol Reprod* *16*:517, 1977.
5. Dailland P, et al: Intravenous propofol during cesarean section: Placental transfer, concentrations in breast milk, and neonatal effects. A preliminary study. *Anesthesiology 71*:827, 1989.
6. Gibbs CP: Maternal physiology. *Clin Obstet Gynecol 24*:525, 1981.
7. Goodger WJ, Levy W: Anesthetic management of the cesarean section. *Vet Clin North Am 3*:85, 1973.
8. Marcella KL, Short CE: Anesthetic management of the pregnant animal. *Comp Cont Educ Pract Vet 6*:942, 1984.
9. Probst CW, Webb AI: Postural influence on systemic blood pressure, gas exchange, and acid/base status in the term-pregnant bitch during general anesthesia. *Am J Vet Res 44*:1963, 1983.

10. Probst CW, et al: Postural influence on systemic blood pressure in large full-term pregnant bitches during general anesthesia. *Vet Surg 16*:471, 1987.
11. Shnider SM, Levinson G: Obstetric anesthesia. *In* Miller RD (ed) *Anesthesia*. 2nd ed. Churchill Livingstone, New York, 1986, p 1681.
12. Weinberger SE, et al: Pregnancy and the lung. *Am Rev Resp Dis 121*:559, 1980.

CHAPTER 174 Common Complications and Anesthetic Emergencies

A. Thomas Evans

SLOW INDUCTION

Absorption of drugs from intramuscular sites is often unpredictable and depends on the blood flow in relation to local tissue. For example, an anesthetic dose of ketamine injected into the epaxial muscles may accidentally be deposited subcutaneously or in fat. The subcutaneous and fat tissues have a poor blood supply, and the drug is poorly absorbed. Induction of anesthesia is slow, and a surgical plane of anesthesia may not be reached. Slow induction and recovery from intravenous injection are seen with certain breeds and body conformations. The recommended intravenous dose of thiobarbiturates in sight hounds or other lean dogs or cats often results in slow induction with long anesthetic times and recovery periods.[10] One explanation for this phenomenon is that the injected dose of thiobarbiturates is redistributed quickly, prolonging the onset of anesthesia. Additional drugs must be administered, resulting in high plasma concentrations and prolonged anesthesia.

There are several reasons for slow induction of anesthesia with inhalation agents. Speed of induction depends on factors that determine the anesthetic alveolar partial pressure. The alveolar partial pressure is in equilibrium with arterial partial pressure, which is in turn in equilibrium with brain partial pressure, which is related to anesthetic depth. The alveolar partial pressure is affected by the concentration of the inspired anesthetic. Common causes for a low inspired anesthetic concentration include an empty vaporizer and patient disconnection from the anesthetic system. Excessively high fresh gas flow rates (oxygen, nitrous oxide) delay the rate of anesthetic rise in a breathing system using an in-the-circle vaporizer, and low fresh gas flow rates delay rate of anesthetic rise in a breathing system using an out-of-the-circle vaporizer.

Apnea or hypoventilation can slow anesthetic induction. Apnea or hypoventilation can be due to a relative overdose of induction drugs. The resulting respiratory depression limits the anesthetic concentration in the alveolus. The type of anesthetic breathing system is also important when slow induction occurs. A system with a large volume has a long time constant (volume of system divided by the gas flow into the system), resulting in a relatively slow rate of anesthetic induction. Finally, the high solubility of inhaled anesthetics in rubber or plastic components of the system may contribute to slowing of induction and delayed recovery.

The transfer of inhaled anesthetic from the alveoli to arterial blood is influenced by the blood:gas solubility and cardiac output. Slow induction of inhalation anesthesia may be due in part to the use of a relatively soluble anesthetic (methoxyflurane). Anesthetics of intermediate solubility (halothane, isoflurane) provide faster induction. A high blood solubility means that a large amount of inhaled anesthetic must be dissolved in the blood before equilibrium is reached with the gas phase.

Sometimes, slow induction is observed even though anesthetics with intermediate blood:gas partition coefficients are used. One explanation is that the patient has developed a large intrapulmonary shunt, reducing the number of alveoli participating in gas exchange. The use of methoxyflurane in this situation may speed induction.

An increase in cardiac output slows anesthetic induction. Increased blood flow through the lungs removes anesthetic and carries it to highly perfused tissue beds. This explains why induction is slower in an excited dog or cat. If the animal is also hyperventilating, the low Pa_{CO_2} causes cerebral vasoconstriction, limiting anesthetic delivery to the brain, and further slowing induction.

SLOW RECOVERY

Many of the same factors influence recovery and induction (e.g., ventilation, anesthetic solubility, and cardiac output). One important difference is that metabolism of the inhaled anesthetic can influence the rate of decline of alveolar partial pressure, which is an important factor for methoxyflurane. Metabolism is a principal determinant in the rate of decline of methoxyflurane. Metabolism with halothane is as important as ventilation, whereas the isoflurane alveolar partial pressure decline is due to ventilation.[2] A decrease in cardiac output due to excessive anesthetic depth, hypothermia, or hypovolemia slows removal of anesthetic gas from tissues.

A slow recovery from thiobarbiturates or ketamine anesthesia may reflect acidosis, low plasma protein concentration, or compromised kidney and liver function.[11] Ketamine is approximately 50 per cent protein bound in the cat and is at least partially excreted in the urine.

Anesthesia recovery is longer in greyhounds than in non-greyhound mixed breeds given thiopental, thiamylal, and methohexital.[10] Long recovery from thiobarbiturate anesthesia in greyhounds is probably due to a decrease in tissue distribution and metabolic clearance. Slow recovery from anesthesia could also be due to accidental hypothermia that results in slow metabolism of anesthetic drugs. If severe enough, hypothermia produces anesthesia.

INADEQUATE ANESTHETIC DEPTH

Several of the reasons for a patient's premature recovery from inhalation anesthesia have been discussed in the section on slow induction. When a patient awakens prematurely from inhalation anesthesia, the anesthetist should first evaluate the anesthetic equipment. Problems would result from an empty vaporizer, disconnected oxygen lines, large leaks within the anesthetic circuit, inappropriate fresh gas flow rates, or too strong a vacuum from the waste gas scavenger system, which could evacuate the anesthetic circuit. The endotracheal tube is inspected for proper insertion or for leaks in the endotracheal tube cuff. A relatively short endotracheal tube can dislodge from the trachea.

Surgical stimulation is one of the primary reasons for a patient's awakening during surgery. Premature awakening sometimes occurs after peritoneal incision, opening of a joint capsule, or traction on the ovarian ligament or spermatic cord. Administration of supplemental anesthetic drugs may be necessary to maintain adequate anesthetic depth. Hyperthermia, accidental or as a by-product of disease (fever), increases anesthetic requirements.

EXCESSIVE ANESTHETIC DEPTH

Many factors decrease the need for anesthesia. Hypothermia decreases the need for anesthesia because of its generalized depressant effects on metabolic rate and central nervous system function. Requirements for halothane and methoxyflurane in dogs fall 5 per cent with each degree centigrade from 37°C. Other factors that increase potency of inhalant anesthetics are hyponatremia, pregnancy, anemia, other anesthetic drugs, severe hypoxemia, shock, and increasing age. Increased potency during pregnancy is related to increased steroid concentration. Pregnancy may be associated with reductions in minimum alveolar concentration (MAC) of 20 to 30 per cent with halothane and methoxyflurane and 40 per cent for isoflurane. Anemia also reduces the requirement for anesthetic. With halothane, potency was increased when the arterial oxygen content decreased below 4.3 ml of oxygen per 100 ml blood.[3] This finding may explain why anemic animals are easily induced.

Acepromazine, opioids, and xylazine decrease anesthetic requirement. Anesthetic requirement is less in older animals than in neonates or younger animals.

Accidental or relative anesthetic overdose can occur. Inappropriate use of a vaporizer or failure to monitor the patient adequately can result in deep anesthesia. Treatment of overdose of inhalant anesthetic involves turning off the vaporizer, flushing the breathing system with oxygen, and ventilating the patient to remove anesthetic. Assisted ventilation continues at 8 to 12 breaths per minute, at an inspired pressure of 15 to 20 cm of H_2O, until the patient recovers.

BREATHING PROBLEMS DURING ANESTHESIA

Hypoventilation

Hypoventilation or apnea may occur in anesthetized animals as a result of an overdose of anesthetics, obstruction of the airway, a space-occupying lesion in the thorax (diaphragmatic hernia or chylothorax), or the peculiar effects of certain drugs. An anesthetic overdose results in a slow respiratory rate and small tidal volumes. Carbon dioxide accumulation and respiratory acidosis result from anesthetic-induced insensitivity to carbon dioxide. Apnea may occur for several minutes before breathing is stimulated. Occasionally, when cats anesthetized with a ketamine-diazepam mixture or tiletamine-zolazepam (Telazol) are intubated and are maintained with isoflurane and oxygen, they are apneic until the Pa_{CO_2} is greater than 80 mm Hg. This severe hypoventilation is in part due to a ketamine- or tiletamine-induced apneustic breathing pattern and the respiratory depressant activity of isoflurane. Premedicants such as xylazine and the opioids can induce significant hypoventilation during inhalation anesthesia.

Airway obstruction can occur from aspiration of regurgitated stomach contents, kinking of the endotracheal tube, or small larynx, elongated soft palate, and redundant pharyngeal tissue in brachycephalic breeds. Periodically, an animal demonstrates a pharyngeal, tracheal, or cervical mass that apparently causes no airway obstruction. The tumor may obstruct the airway, however, after induction of anesthesia and subsequent relaxation of pharyngeal tissue. This airway obstruction is manifested as exaggerated breathing efforts and no gas flow. Intubation must be immediate. Hypoventilation during surgery can also result from physical pressure on the thorax. If the surgical procedure is long, the surgeon may rest an arm on the thorax, thereby limiting respiratory excursion.

Several abnormal breathing patterns that occur during anesthesia result in hypoventilation.[8] Cheyne-Stokes respiration is characterized by periods of apnea of 15 to 20 seconds separated by approximately equal periods of hyperventilation with tidal volumes that wax and wane. Cheyne-Stokes breathing is caused by an abnormally functioning respiratory control mechanism, which may be due to reduced brain blood flow as occurs in cardiac failure. Damage to the respiratory center may also increase feedback gain of the respiratory center in response to changes in P_{CO_2} and blood pH. Biot's breathing is an abnormal respiratory pattern in which respirations are faster and deeper than normal with interspersed pauses. Each breath has the same tidal volume and does not wax and wane. Kussmaul's breathing is characterized by deep regular breaths that resemble sighs; it sometimes accompanies severe metabolic acidosis. Apneustic breathing, a deep inhalation followed by breath holding and then an exhalation followed immediately by another inhalation, usually occurs after administration of ketamine or tiletamine-zolazepam.[7] Short inefficient breathing movements may occur at the end of inhalation anesthesia.

Hyperventilation

Hyperventilation can occur at the beginning of anesthesia when the patient is lightly anesthetized. The stimulation of intubation coupled with light anesthesia may cause the animal to take several deep breaths, which are followed by apnea. During this time, $PaCO_2$ slowly increases to a point that stimulates the patient to breathe. Surgical stimulation may also cause a period of hyperventilation during maintenance of anesthesia. Increasing anesthetic depth prevents hyperventilation. Hyperventilation can also occur in response to hypoxemia or as a compensatory response to severe metabolic acidosis.

Tachypnea

Inhalant anesthetics generally produce dose-dependent decreases in breathing. Like other inhalant anesthetics, isoflurane decreases the rate of breathing. The effect of inhalant anesthetics on frequency of breathing probably reflects central nervous system depression. Halothane and isoflurane occasionally increase respiratory rate, which is characterized as rapid, shallow, and regular. This type of breathing is commonly seen in dogs of small breeds, particularly if they are overweight.

HYPOTENSION

Preanesthetic drugs such as phenothiazine tranquilizers and intravenous opioids can cause hypotension. Acepromazine can cause hypotension if administered intravenously in a dose greater than 0.4 mg/kg. The hypotension caused by acepromazine is due to $alpha_1$-adrenoceptor antagonism. Induction drugs, including the barbiturates, can cause hypotension, especially if a relative overdose has been administered. Severity of hypotension depends on the barbiturate dose, rate of injection, and physical status of the patient. As with phenothiazine tranquilizers, pre-existing hypotension, hypovolemia, or cardiac disease may predispose the patient to hypotension regardless of the dose following administration of thiopental.[11] Inhalant anesthetics cause dose-related hypotension.

When administered intraoperatively as anesthetic adjuncts, ketamine and butorphanol induce hypotension. Surgical maneuvers leading to hypotension include obstruction of venous return and hemorrhage, either acutely or over long periods. Hypotension can result from cardiac dysrhythmias (see later). Excessively fast or slow heart rates, or asynchronous myocardial activity from multiple premature beats, can reduce cardiac output. Treatment of hypotension involves eliminating its cause, for example, lightening anesthesia, restoring venous return, increasing intravascular volume, inducing vasoconstriction with alpha-adrenergic agonists, stimulating cardiac output with positive inotropic agents (dopamine, dobutamine), reversing drug effects if an antagonist is available, and re-establishing normal cardiac rhythm (Table 174–1).

DYSRHYTHMIAS

Cardiac dysrhythmias can result from traumatic myocarditis, gastric dilatation–volvulus, electrolyte disturbances, or congestive heart failure. Dysrhythmias can also result from anesthetic drugs or surgical conditions such as hypoxemia, inadequate anesthetic depth, or electrolyte imbalance.

Bradycardia

During general anesthesia, bradycardia is more ominous than tachycardia and may require treatment. Bradycardia can result from drug effects, hypothermia, and autonomic reflexes. Xylazine, phenothiazine tranquilizers (acepromazine), opioids, and inhalant anesthetics can cause bradycardia. A declining heart rate of less than 60 beats/min is treated with intravenous atropine or glycopyrrolate. Decreasing the depth of anesthesia and treatment of hypothermia may also be required.

Ventricular dysrhythmias during halothane anesthesia can be associated with halothane-induced myocardial sensitivity to circulating catecholamine concentrations. Certain drugs such as ketamine and xylazine and the thiobarbiturates predispose patients to halothane-induced ventricular dysrhythmias. Acepromazine and diazepam inhibit dysrhythmias. Halothane-catecholamine dysrhythmias are associated with light planes of anesthesia and can be abolished by deepening anesthesia or changing inhalant anesthetics.[5, 9] Other pharmacological treatments for dysrhythmias include atropine, acepromazine, and lidocaine. Atropine works by increasing the sinus rate and overriding the abnormal focus. Acepromazine blocks alpha receptors and reduces afterload on the heart, and lidocaine decreases spontaneous automatic depolarization and has a variable effect on atrioventricular nodal conduction.

Tachycardia

Tachycardia occurs during anesthesia as a result of surgical stimulation, administration of atropine or glycopyrrolate, hyperthermia, or anesthetic effects. Meperidine causes tachycardia, probably because of its structural similarity to atropine. Ketamine causes tachycardia because it stimulates the sympathetic nervous system. Treatment of tachycardia is not required in the healthy patient, because anesthetic-induced effects gradually decrease and surgical stimulation decreases as anesthetic

TABLE 174–1. MANAGEMENT OF COMPLICATIONS ASSOCIATED WITH ANESTHESIA

Complication	Treatment	Trade Name	Dosage	Side Effects
Excitement, delirium	Acepromazine	PromAce	0.2 mg/kg IM	Prolonged recovery
	Diazepam	Valium	0.5 mg/kg IV, IM	Hypothermia
Hypoventilation	Oxygen	—	—	Excitement from mask
	Ventilation	—	—	Respiratory depression
	Doxapram	Dopram V	1–2 mg/kg IV	Excitement
Laryngospasm	Lidocaine spray	Xylocaine 2%		
	Lidocaine jelly	—	—	—
Dyspnea	Oxygen	—		
	Tracheostomy	Portex*	—	Hyperventilation
	Ventilation (14 mg/kg)	—		
Pneumothorax	Oxygen	—		
	Chest tubes	—	—	Hyperventilation
	Ventilation (14 mg/kg)	—		Infection
Cardiac arrhythmias:				
Tachycardia	Fluids (lactated Ringer solution)	—	10–20 ml/kg IV per hour	Bradycardia
	Propranolol	Inderal	0.05–0.1 mg/kg IV	Hypotension
Bradycardia	Glycopyrrolate	Robinul V	0.005 mg/kg IV	Tachycardia
Ventricular arrhythmia	Lidocaine	Xylocaine	Dogs: 0.5 mg/kg IV Cats: 0.2 mg/kg IV	Bradycardia
	Procainamide	Pronestyl	10–20 mg/kg IM	Hypotension
Hypotension	Fluids (lactated Ringer solution)	—	10–20 ml/kg IV per hour	—
	Dopamine	Intropin	3–5 μg/kg IV per minute	Arrhythmias
	Dobutamine	Dobutrex	3–5 μg/kg IV per minute	Hypertension, central nervous system toxicity
Blood or fluid loss	Fluids (lactated Ringer solution)	—	40–90 ml/kg IV per minute	Overhydration, edema
	Blood	—	10–40 ml/kg IV	Allergic reaction
Hypothermia	Warmed fluids (lactated Ringer solution)	—	5–10 ml/kg IV per hour	Overhydration, edema
	H_2O heating pad	Goymer†	—	
	Heating lamp	—	—	
Hypoglycemia	Dextrose 50%	—	1–2 ml/kg IV	Hyperosmolality
Metabolic acidosis	Sodium bicarbonate	—	0.5–1.0 mEq/kg IV every 10 minutes	Metabolic alkalosis, hypokalemia, hyperosmolality
Hyperkalemia	Sodium bicarbonate	—	0.5–1.0 mEq/kg IV	As above
	0.9% sodium chloride	—	10–40 ml/kg IV per hour	
	Calcium chloride	—	0.5 ml/kg IV	Tachycardia
Hyperpyrexia	Oxygen			
	Fluids (lactated Ringer solution)		5–10 mg/kg IV per hour	Hypothermia
	Tranquilizers	PromAce	0.4 mg/kg IM	
	Dantrolene sodium		2–4 mg/kg IV	
Prolonged recovery	Doxapram	Dopram V	1–2 mg/kg IV	Central nervous system excitement
	Yohimbine	—	0.25 mg/kg IV	
	Yobine	—	0.6 mg/kg IV	
Postoperative pain	Morphine sulfate		0.02–0.5 mg/kg IM	Respiratory depression
	Pentazocine	Talwin-V	0.2–0.5 mg/kg IM	

*Shiley Inc., Irvine, CA.
†Goymer, Orchard Park, NY.

levels stabilize. Tachycardia must be avoided if myocardial disease is present.

VISUAL DISTURBANCE

Ketamine may cause transient blindness. A similar response has been noticed in cats after administration of a tiletamine-zolazepam combination.

CARDIOPULMONARY ARREST

Cardiopulmonary arrest is the most dreaded of the anesthetic complications. Probably less than 25 per cent of arrest victims return to normal. Treatment requires fast action by a team of personnel knowledgeable in the physiology and pharmacology of cardiac arrest.

The mechanism of blood flow during cardiopulmonary resuscitation (CPR) is still the cause of some debate. One theory holds that blood flow during CPR is due to direct pressure on the heart from movement of the thoracic wall pressing on the heart during external thoracic massage (cardiac pump theory). Another proposal explains forward movement of blood during CPR as a result of an increase in intrathoracic pressure with each compression of the chest wall (thoracic pump theory). This theory has recently gained support from evidence in arrested human patients that coughing generates arterial pressure and cardiac output. The mechanism of blood flow during CPR in dogs and cats is probably a combination of the cardiac pump and thoracic pump theories. Small dogs, puppies, and cats, which have compliant chest walls, probably generate most of their cardiac output during CPR from the cardiac pump. But larger dogs and animals with noncompliant chest walls generate forward blood flow via the thoracic pump. Neither mechanism of blood flow protects the brain from ischemic or hypoxic injury during external chest massage. This lack of success with external thoracic massage requires an early decision to switch to internal thoracic massage.

Diagnosis of cardiac arrest involves recognition of the obvious symptoms (Table 174–2). After confirmation of a diagnosis of cardiac arrest, the guidelines *A* through *D* for CPR are followed: *A*irway, *B*reathing, *C*ardiac massage, and *D*efinitive or *D*rug therapy. A patent airway is always obtained or confirmed through intubation. The patient is ventilated at a rate of 4 to 5 breaths per minute at an inspiratory pressure of 15 to 20 cm H_2O. If the patient has been anesthetized with inhalant anesthetics, a faster respiratory rate is used initially to help clear residual anesthetic effects. The anesthetic circuit is repeatedly flushed to remove the inhalation anesthetic. Excessive ventilation causes respiratory alkalosis and is avoided. External thoracic massage is initiated with the patient in right lateral recumbency and with the patient's back toward the resuscitator. This position facilitates intracardiac injections and prevents the animal from sliding across the table during thoracic compressions. An early decision must be made to switch to internal thoracic massage if external efforts are ineffective because of poor brain perfusion during external thoracic massage. Internal thoracic massage may be initiated after no more than 2 to 3 minutes of external thoracic massage, by making an incision through the left fifth intercostal space. A quick clip and scrub are completed prior to the thoracic incision. The pericardial sac does not need to be opened before internal massage is started. The massage rate for either external or internal massage is approximately 100 compessions per minute. The main drawback with this method is its requirement of an early decision for internal thoracic massage. This decision may seem like a bold move, but it is the only way to ensure optimum early perfusion of the brain. Figure 174–1 shows a simplified protocol for administering CPR.

TABLE 174–2. SIGNS OF CARDIAC ARREST

No palpable heartbeat. Heartbeat may be present but is not strong enough to be palpated (i.e., electrical-mechanical dissociation).
No palpable pulse
Apnea
Lack of jaw tone/no muscle tone
Lack of surgical hemorrhage
Cyanosis in the surgical field
Cyanosis or paleness of the mucous membranes
Dilated pupils (after 3 to 4 minutes of arrest)

The most important drug to administer during CPR is epinephrine (adrenalin). A high dose of epinephrine decreases the number of countershocks needed to reverse ventricular fibrillation in dogs. A study evaluating this dose demonstrated that 10 of 10 dogs survived a 10-minute period of ventricular fibrillation when administered the high dose compared with a greater number of countershocks and a longer time required for resuscitation when they were given a lower dose of epinephrine (0.14 mg/10 kg).[1] Epinephrine is given early and in high doses (1 mg/10 kg).

A central injection of epinephrine is recommended, even though a vena caval catheter is not usually present. Circulation times during closed-chest CPR were 62.7 seconds after central injection and 93.6 seconds after peripheral injection. Circulation times were shorter during open-chest CPR, with times shortest after central injection.[4] One or two doses should be given intravenously during external massage, with additional doses given during internal massage. Alternate routes to intravenous injection are intratracheal or intracardiac injection. Intratracheal administration is accomplished by diluting the dose of epinephrine with 4 or 5 ml of saline and squirting the solution down the endotracheal tube while the animal's head is held toward the ceiling. Ventilation is performed two or three times to push the solution further into the lungs. Intracardiac injection of epinephrine is the third option. It can result in accidental drug deposition into the myocardium. The dose of epinephrine for intracardiac injection is one-fourth of the intravenous dose.

This method improves the chances of resuscitation during classic cardiac arrest (asystole), electrical-mechanical dissociation, and ventricular fibrillation. Conversion of ventricular fibrillation to normal sinus rhythm is best accomplished by direct current countershock. For internal defibrillation, 20 to 40 joules are used, and for external defibrillation, 200 to 400 joules are used.

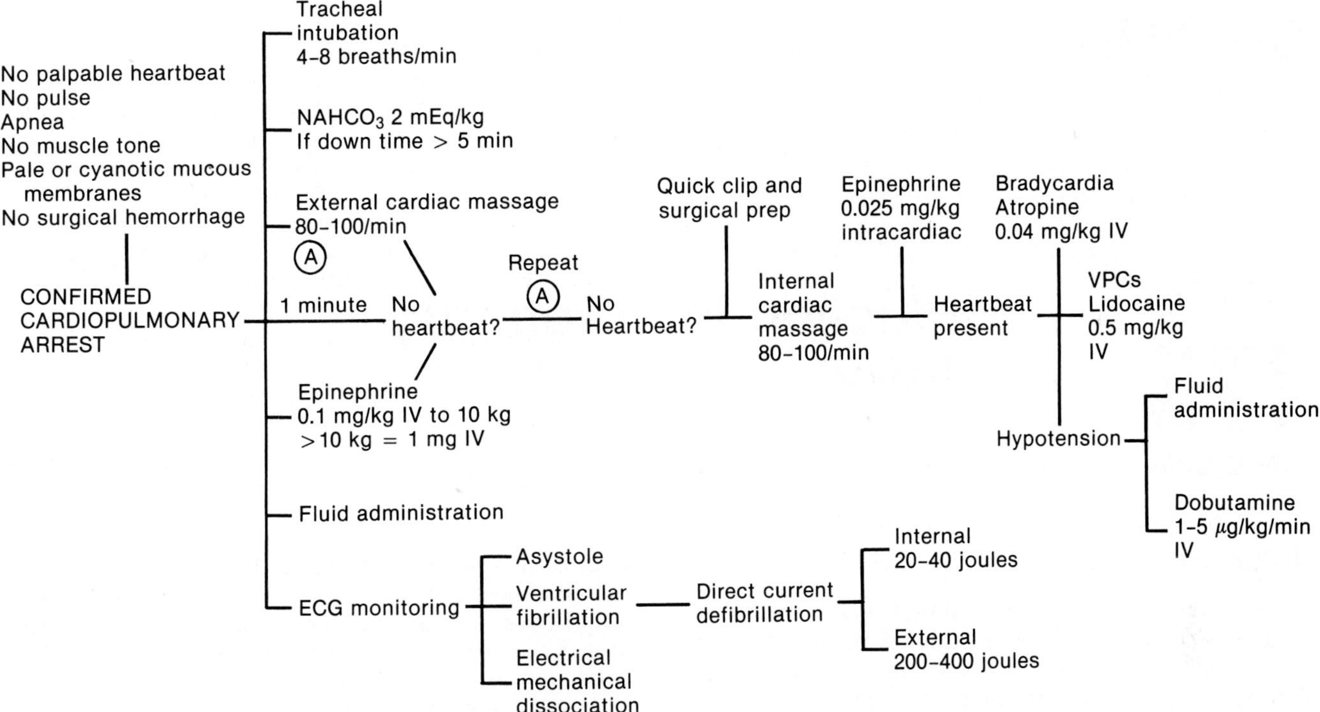

FIGURE 174–1. An algorithm for CPR. This simplified protocol for CPR is used to resuscitate animals that have the potential for surviving cardiac arrest. Because early restoration of brain perfusion is the most important goal to be achieved, a quick decision for internal cardiac massage is required. (ECG, electrocardiogram; $NAHCO_3$, sodium bicarbonate; VPCs, ventricular premature contractions).

A second drug to consider during treatment of cardiac arrest is sodium bicarbonate. Acidosis in arterial blood is not as common or severe as originally thought. Bicarbonate is given if the arrest has been present for longer than 5 minutes. Sodium bicarbonate is probably not required if resuscitation begins immediately after the cardiac arrest. Paradoxical acidosis of the cerebrospinal fluid is not a problem if sodium bicarbonate is administered during administration of CPR. Sodium bicarbonate administration improves both arterial and venous pH and increases the blood Pco_2. Approximately 1.0 mEq/kg of sodium bicarbonate is administered every 10 minutes during resuscitation. Rapid manual chest compressions (120 compressions per minute) along with bicarbonate therapy and fluid loading can increase survival time. Rapid manual compression by itself does not improve recovery. Adversely, sodium bicarbonate can induce hyperosmolarity and hypernatremia. Sodium bicarbonate overdose also induces transient alkalosis with arrhythmias. Acidosis does not affect defibrillation threshold.[6]

Lidocaine and atropine can be helpful during cardiac arrest. They are used to treat ventricular dysrhythmias and bradycardias respectively. These drugs are not included in the primary treatment protocol (see Fig. 174–1).

Aftercare requires good nursing with attention to adequacy of ventilation, fluid load, blood pressure, and arterial pH. Animals with the best prognosis show fast and steady recovery from the hypoxic insult, though some may make a complete neurologic recovery after 12 to 24 hours of postresuscitation delirium. Various protocols to improve neurologic survival, involving calcium antagonists, free radical scavengers, and iron chelators, have been proposed and have met with some success in certain studies. None of the new treatment regimens have resulted in satisfactory long-term neurologic recovery.

References

1. Burnette DD, Jameson SJ: Comparison of standard versus high dose epinephrine in the resuscitation of cardiac arrest in dogs. *Ann Emerg Med 19*:8, 1990.
2. Carpenter RL, et al: The extent of metabolism of inhaled anesthetics in humans. *Anesthesiology 65*:201, 1986.
3. Cullen DJ, Eger EI: The effects of hypoxia and isovolemic anemia on the halothane requirement (MAC) of dogs. III. The effects of acute isovolemic anemia. *Anesthesiology 32*:46, 1970.
4. Emerman CL, et al: Effect of injection site on circulation times during cardiac arrest. *Crit Care Med 16*:1138, 1988.
5. Hubbell JAE, et al: Changes of inhalation anesthetic agents for management of ventricular premature depolarizations in anesthetized cats and dogs. *J Am Vet Med Assoc 185*:643, 1984.
6. Kerber RE, et al: Effect of ischemia, hypertrophy, hypoxia, acidosis and alkalosis on canine defibrillation. *Am J Physiol 244*:4825, 1983.
7. Muir WW, Hubbell JAE: Blood pressure response to acetylpromazine and lenperone in halothane anesthetized dogs. *J Am Anim Hosp Assoc 21*:285, 1985.
8. Muir WW, Hubbell JAE: Respiratory emergency. *In* Muir WW (ed): *Handbook of Veterinary Anesthesia.* C. V. Mosby, St. Louis, 1989, pp 272–284.
9. Muir WW, et al: Increasing halothane concentration abolishes anesthesia-associated dysrhythmias in dogs and cats. *J Am Vet Med Assoc 192*:1730, 1988.
10. Robinson EP, et al: Barbiturate anesthesia in greyhound and mixed-breed dogs: Comparative cardiopulmonary effects, anesthetic effects, and recovery rates. *Am J Vet Res 47*:2105, 1986.
11. Soma LR: Intravenous anesthetic agents. *In Textbook of Veterinary Anesthesia.* William & Wilkins, Baltimore, 1971, pp 265–268.

SECTION 18

Dentistry

Albert S. Dorn ■ *Section Editor*

CHAPTER 175 Introduction to Veterinary Dentistry

Albert S. Dorn

HISTORICAL PERSPECTIVES

The evolution of dentistry and oral surgery as subspecialties of veterinary practice parallels the development of veterinary medicine. Many of the procedures and concepts used in current veterinary practice are based on ideas and techniques developed over the centuries.

For hundreds of years, little information on canine dentistry appeared in the veterinary literature, because treatment of abnormal and diseased teeth consisted of extraction, usually by a barber-surgeon.[14] In 1832, Delabere Blaine published his veterinary outlines and his third edition of *Canine Pathology*, which contains occasional references to dentistry and oral surgery.[2]

In 1908, Dr. Louis A. Merillat published *Animal Dentistry and Diseases of the Mouth*, the first text completely devoted to the practice of veterinary and animal dentistry.[11]

Merillat hypothesized on the future of dentistry and veterinary medicine:

> *When dentistry in animals is more generally recognized as an important if not essential feature of animal therapeutics, and when dental operations by reason of greater skill are made easier, the veterinary [sic] will then treat the art of dentistry with the same dignity as the other branches of surgery. . . . The limited number of patients will probably always prevent evolution of animal dentistry into a special profession. The veterinarian, will therefore, be required to perfect himself in the practice of this art.*[11]

Anatomically, Merillat divided the tooth into the crown, neck, fang, and roots. The terminology has been updated since this early observation.[11]

Merillat also described the eruption of the deciduous or temporary teeth of the dog. Not all the observations regarding the eruption and loss of deciduous teeth were correct: however, this early contribution was important in promoting awareness of the importance of canine dental disease.

In 1925, Hobday published the third edition of the book, *Surgical Diseases of the Dog and Cat*. This text described a variety of conditions of the canine mouth, oral cavity, and teeth, including one condition called "pus in the antrum," now known as carnassial tooth abscess or abscess of the upper fourth premolar tooth. Dental deposits on the teeth were described as a disease of old dogs, usually manifested by malodorous breath, pain on eating and drinking, and secondary pyorrhea. Hobday wrote, "Treatment includes scaling and removal of dental deposits from the enamel surfaces of the teeth. Usually the patient is awake with the mouth muzzled shut and the instrument is applied close to or under the gum and drawn towards the crown of the tooth. Occasionally teeth must be extracted as part of the treatment of this disease."[10]

In 1938, Garbutt described a variety of conditions of the teeth and the oral cavity and speculated on the importance of a regular program of cleaning the teeth and dental prophylaxis in veterinary practice. He suggested prevention of dental deposits by brushing the teeth with a solution of table salt and pumice. When a large quantity of tartar was present on the teeth, the teeth were cleaned with the patient placed under general anesthesia. Garbutt recommended that owners bring the animals to the veterinarian twice a year for dental prophylaxis and treatment. This recommendation was the first suggestion that dental prophylaxis prevents tartar accumulation and loss of teeth, and the recommended program of brushing teeth on a regular basis accompanied by scaling and polishing at a veterinary clinic still holds merit.[7]

Garbutt also discussed dental eruption in dogs, stating that 42 permanent teeth are arranged like the temporary teeth with the exception of the large molar teeth. The problem of permanent tooth eruption before the deciduous teeth fall out was described. If deciduous teeth are removed before the permanent teeth erupt, the permanent teeth are given a chance of aligning properly, whereas they may erupt improperly if the deciduous teeth remain in the mouth.[7] This suggestion of early removal of deciduous teeth is one of the first reports of treatment of malocclusion. This practice has grown in popularity with dog breeders in recent years and is known as intraceptive orthodontics.

CURRENT STATUS AND IMPORTANCE

In the 1960s various specialties developed in veterinary medicine and were given recognition by the American Veterinary Medical Association as board certified specialties. Most of these specialties were clinical disciplines and included medicine, surgery, radiology, ophthalmology, and anesthesiology.

The American Veterinary Medical Association was aware of the growing interest in dentistry and published an editorial in *Journal of the American Veterinary Medical Association* in 1967 entitled "Veterinary Dentistry."[4] Interestingly, this report stated that dentistry would never be employed in animals to the same extent it is employed in humans. Increased awareness of veterinarians on this subject would direct efforts toward preserving teeth and put less emphasis on extraction as the "first resort."

As specialties were developing, practicing veterinarians formed interest groups and societies for the exchange of ideas in clinical disciplines. One of these groups was the American Society of Veterinary Dentistry, which was organized in 1978. Within 5 years, seminars lasting 1 to 2 days on small animal dentistry and oral surgery were offered at major national meetings. Practitioners became more aware of the importance of dental treatment in the overall health care of their patients.

New textbooks devoted exclusively to veterinary dentistry were soon available to practicing veterinarians. These new texts and their authors included *Concepts in Veterinary Dentistry* by Tholen (1983),[15] *Veterinary Dentistry* by Harvey (1985),[9] *Veterinary Dentistry* by Eisenmenger and Zetner (1985),[5] and an issue of *Veterinary Clinics of North America* devoted to dentistry, edited by Frost (1986).[6] General texts on small animal medicine and surgery now include topics on dental diseases and dental restorative procedures.

In 1986, the Academy of Veterinary Dentistry was established to promote continuing education in dentistry. Academy membership is based on credentials and test results, and nearly 40 veterinarians, most in private practice, have qualified and joined the academy. In 1989, the American Veterinary Medical Association College was founded as a clinical specialty recognized by the American Veterinary Medical Association. Membership to this college is based on formalized residency training, credentials evaluation, and successful completion of an examination. In a period of about 10 years, veterinary dentistry has evolved from being an area of passing clinical interest to being recognized as a clinical specialty by the American Veterinary Medical Association.

Dental and oral surgical cases now make up a significant portion of small animal surgical practice. The authors of one report examined the surgical logs of 78 small animal practices in California in which 10,088 operative procedures were performed on 9,520 patients.[16] As expected, soft-tissue procedures, including elective ovariohysterectomy and orchidectomy, constituted 74% of the cases. Next in importance were dental procedures, which were 12% of the total. When these rankings were compared with the Veterinary Medical Teaching Hospital at the University of California-Davis over a 6-month period, soft-tissue procedures were 70% and dental procedures were 7% of the operations performed. In both situations, the importance of dentistry and oral surgery was clearly documented, suggesting significant demand for veterinary dental services.

In another report, 63 anesthetized dogs were surveyed at a veterinary teaching hospital for the incidence of dental disease.[8] Most dogs had some dental abnormalities such as wear facets, missing teeth, increased mobility, fractures, and pulp exposure. Other data, including location of dental abnormalities, diet, and periodontal indices, are included in this report. The most important conclusion is the high incidence of dental diseases in the canine population.

DENTAL CLASSIFICATION

Teeth are classified into simple or complex types based on the interrelationships of dental anatomic structures including enamel, cementum, dentin, and pulp. Simple teeth and complex teeth are also known as brachydont (short crown) and hypsodont (high crown), perspectively. All the teeth of the dog, cat, and human are simple, or brachydont, teeth.[1] This concept is important, because many of the details and techniques for dental therapy described in human dental textbooks and literature are applicable through modification to veterinary dentistry. Because complex teeth are found in other species, readers are referred to appropriate texts for additional information.[5, 9, 11]

DENTAL STRUCTURES AND FUNCTION

The teeth are derived from ectodermal and mesodermal tissues that are firmly attached in the mandible and maxilla and serve as aids in prehension and mastication.[13] The basic histologic structures of the simple tooth are enamel, dentin, pulp, and cementum, which are arranged in a definite pattern (Fig. 175–1).[3]

Enamel, the outer covering of the tooth, is the hardest substance in the body. Enamel is found only on the crown and completely covers and protects the dentin

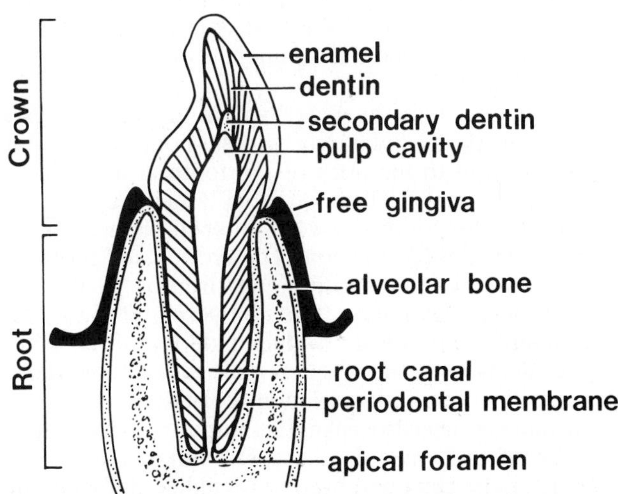

FIGURE 175–1. The anatomy of a normal tooth is illustrated with the relationship of tissues, including enamel, dentin, pulp chamber, root canal, and the periodontal membrane and ligaments.

from external exposure. Enamel is about 96 per cent inorganic material, and the remaining 4 per cent is organic matrix and water. The mineral content of enamel is greater than that of dentin, cementum, or bone.

Dentin, which forms the bulk of the tooth, is just deep to the enamel and separates this structure from the pulp cavity. In an intact normal tooth, dentin is not visible because it is covered by enamel and cementum. Dentin is a calcified tissue similar to bone and composed of 70 per cent minerals and 30 per cent organic material and water. Dentin is perforated by numerous canals called dentinal tubules, which contain dentinal fibers. These fibers form the cytoplasm of the cells located within the pulp chamber. These special cells of the pulp cavity, which are shared by both the dentin and pulp chamber, are called odontoblasts. The nucleus of the odontoblast is located in the pulp cavity and is surrounded by cytoplasm, but part of the odontoblast extends into the dentinal tubules, ensuring the vitality of the dentin. A modified type of dentin, or irregular dentin, is found in older teeth along the pulp chamber wall or near areas of attrition or tooth wear.[13]

The central structure of the tooth is the pulp cavity or chamber. The pulp contains blood vessels and nerves that enter the tooth through an apical foramen located at the apex of the root. Pulp is the only noncalcified tissue of a tooth and contains soft connective tissue, odontoblasts, and other intracellular substances. In young animals, the cells of the pulp tissue are more numerous, including fibroblasts, histiocytes, undifferentiated mesenchymal cells, and additional odontoblasts.

Cementum is a hard bony tissue that covers the dentin of the tooth root and contains crystallized minerals. Cementum has cells irregularly scattered throughout, but blood vessels and nerves are absent. Cementum is not as hard as dentin because it is about 50 per cent mineral and 50 per cent organic material and water. Cementum attaches the tooth to the alveolus with the periodontal ligaments and to the surrounding alveolar bones. This attachment to these two different tissues literally suspends the tooth in the alveolar socket. Cementum is a dynamic tissue that is produced intermittently by the periodontal ligament throughout the life of the tooth.

The gingiva may be described as the oral mucosa attached to the alveolar process (the bone surrounding the tooth) and to the neck of the tooth at a crevice or crevicular groove. This epithelial attachment of the gingiva to the tooth must be intact and healthy for normal periodontal function. The crevice and tooth are constantly exposed to saliva and bacteria in the oral cavity, which may damage the epithelium of the sulcus. This damage progresses to the underlying connective tissue, deepening the gingival sulcus, forming dental deposits, and initiating periodontal disease.

Advancing age also changes the pulp cavity. Secondary dentin is formed continuously with increasing age, and the pulp chamber becomes smaller and the root canal narrower. These changes are universal and normal, not pathological.

The teeth are surrounded by the mandible and maxilla, and the specific bone that surrounds and supports the teeth is called the alveolar process. The alveolar process is composed of the lamellated bone and the supporting bone. The lamellated bone is the bone of the wall of the tooth socket or dental alveolus, whereas the supporting bone is composed of the cortical plate and trabecular bone. In some areas, the alveolar process is thin and contains little or no trabecular bone, resulting in fusion of the lamellated bone and cortical plate. The alveolar process supports the tooth roots on the facial, lingual, and palatal sides, extending between the teeth, and into the furcations of multirooted teeth. The alveolar process also separates teeth on the mesial and distal sides of the roots.[13]

DENTAL ANATOMY

The teeth are divided into four types, based on gross appearance, anatomical location in the mouth, and function. These four types of teeth are incisors, canine teeth, premolars, and molars.[12]

Incisor teeth are located in the rostral part of the mouth, embedded in the incisive bones of the maxilla or mandible. These teeth are long, slender, arched slightly forward, and laterally compressed. All incisors have single roots.

The four canine teeth are of considerable importance to carnivorous animals. These teeth are the longest in the mouth, with large roots that are nearly twice as long as the crowns. Each canine tooth has a single root, which is intimately attached into the mandible or maxilla.

The cheek teeth just posterior to the canines are the premolars. In the permanent dentition, there are four premolar teeth on each side of the jaw, numbered from rostral to caudal. The first premolar may have one or two roots, whereas the remainder of the premolar teeth have two roots. The only exception is the upper fourth premolar or carnassial tooth, which has three roots. The crowns of the premolars usually have two pointed cusps, which mesh with the premolar crowns of the opposite arch, resulting in a shearing action during chewing (Fig. 175–2).

The large variation in the shapes of canine skulls results in considerable variation in the space between, and the location of, the premolar teeth. Occasionally, premolar teeth are absent, a condition called anodontia. This trait varies with different breeds of dogs, and purebred associations have established standards for their specific breeds.

Molar teeth are located caudal to the premolar teeth and have no deciduous predecessors. There are two molars on each side of the upper jaw and three molars on each side of the lower jaw. Each upper molar tooth has three diverging roots. The lower two molars are unique in that the first molar tooth is much larger than the other two more caudal molars. All the mandibular molars have two roots (Table 175–1).

Along with the canine teeth, the carnassial teeth (those relating to eating flesh) are the largest teeth in the mouth. The upper fourth premolar tooth is the carnassial tooth in the maxillary arcade, whereas the

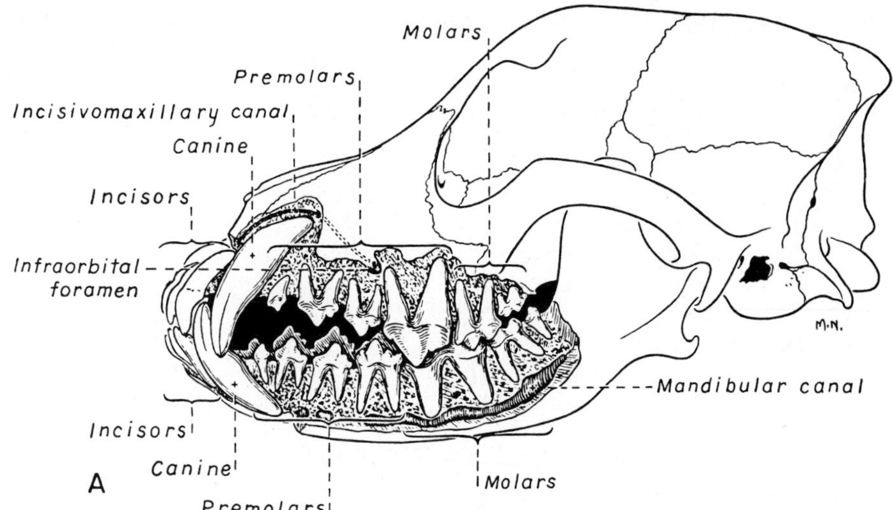

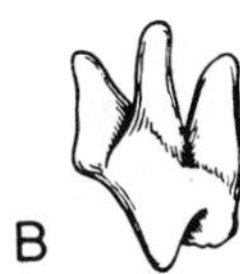

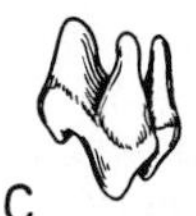

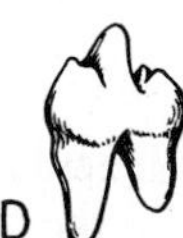

FIGURE 175–2. Jaws and teeth of an adult dog. *A*, Lateral view of jaws, sculptured to show tooth roots. *B*, Left upper fourth premolar (carnassial tooth), anterolateral aspect. *C*, Left upper first molar, anterolateral aspect. *D*, Left lower first molar (carnassial tooth), anterolateral aspect. (From Evans HE, Christensen GC: *Miller's Anatomy of the Dog.* 2nd ed. W. B. Saunders, Philadelphia, 1979, p 415.)

lower first molar tooth is the carnassial tooth in the mandibular arcade. These teeth are also called sectional or shearing teeth. The upper and lower carnassial teeth are in close proximity when the bite is closed, creating the strong shearing mechanism that is important in carnivorous alimentation.[12]

DENTAL FORMULAS AND NOTATION

Because teeth are classified by anatomic location and form (incisors, canine teeth, premolars, molars), the arrangement can be expressed in a dental formula. The types of teeth are indicated as follows: incisors (I), canine teeth (C), premolars (P), molars (M), with the maxillary teeth written above the mandibular teeth. The permanent teeth are always represented by upper-case letters (I, C, P, M), and the deciduous teeth are written with lower-case letters (i, c, p, m).

The phylogenetically complete dental formula for mammals, found only in the wild boar and mole, is:[9]

$$\frac{3I \quad 1C \quad 4P \quad 3M}{3I \quad 1C \quad 4P \quad 3M} = 44 \text{ teeth}$$

All domestic species have variations of this dental formula, and the formula for the permanent dentition of the dog is (Fig. 175–3):

$$\frac{3I \quad 1C \quad 4P \quad 2M}{3I \quad 1C \quad 4P \quad 3M} = 42 \text{ teeth}$$

The formula for the permanent dentition of the cat is (Fig. 175–4):

$$\frac{3I \quad 1C \quad 3P \quad 1M}{3I \quad 1C \quad 2P \quad 1M} = 30 \text{ teeth}$$

Since the formula for deciduous teeth can be expressed in a similar manner using lower-case letters, the deciduous dental formula for the dog is:

$$\frac{3i \quad 1c \quad 3p}{3i \quad 1c \quad 3p} = 28 \text{ teeth}$$

The deciduous dental formula for the domestic cat is:

TABLE 175–1. THE NUMBER OF ROOTS FOR THE TEETH

Basic Tooth Group	Number of Roots
Incisors	
Central incisor	1
Intermediate incisor	1
Lateral incisor	1
Canine Teeth	1
Premolars	
First premolar	1
Second premolar	2
Third premolar	2
Fourth premolar*	3
Fourth premolar (lower arcade)	2
Molars	
First molar (upper arcade)	3
First molar (lower arcade)*	2
Second molar (upper arcade)	2
Third molar (lower arcade)	1

*The fourth upper premolar and the first lower molar are termed carnassial teeth, because they are capable of shearing.

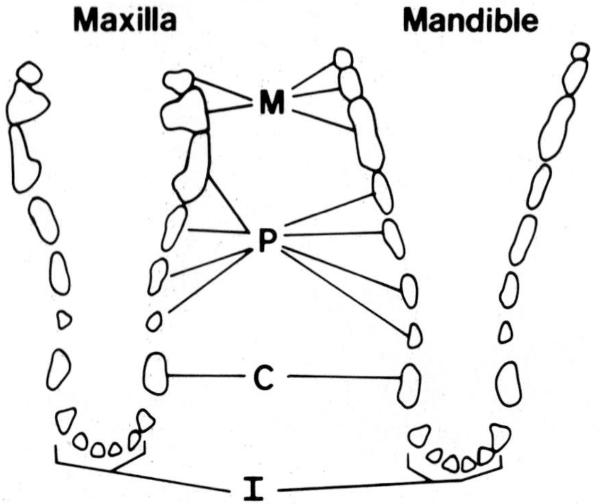

FIGURE 175–3. The various teeth of the dog are identified in this diagram of the maxilla and mandible. (I, incisor; C, canine; P, premolar; M, molar.)

TABLE 175–2. ERUPTION SCHEDULE FOR PERMANENT TEETH IN THE DOG

Basic Tooth Group	Eruption Time
Incisors	
Central incisor	2 to 5 months
Intermediate incisor	2 to 5 months
Lateral incisor	4 to 5 months
Canine Teeth	5 to 6 months
Premolars	
First premolar	4 to 5 months
Second premolar	6 months
Third premolar	6 months
Fourth premolar	4 to 5 months
Molars	
First molar	5 to 6 months
Second molar	6 to 7 months
Third molar	6 to 7 months

In general, permanent teeth erupt earlier in large-breed dogs.

$$\frac{3i \quad 1c \quad 3p}{3i \quad 1c \quad 2p} = 26 \text{ teeth}$$

Deciduous teeth are also known as primary teeth, and in the dog, these teeth erupt early in life.[12] The sequence for eruption of primary teeth is:

1. Dog is born edentulous (without teeth).
2. Central incisors, intermediate incisors, and canine teeth erupt during first 4 weeks.
3. Lateral incisors erupt at 5 to 6 weeks of age.
4. Premolars erupt at 4 to 8 weeks of age.

In general, the gross appearance of the deciduous teeth of the dog is similar to that of the permanent teeth. The incisors and canine teeth appear similar to the secondary or permanent teeth of the same location. There are three deciduous premolar teeth. The first appears similar to P1, the second appears similar to P3, and the third deciduous tooth appears similar to the carnassial tooth of the upper or lower dental arcade. The permanent teeth erupt at different times, and the eruption dates are given in Table 175–2. Permanent teeth erupt earlier in larger breeds of dogs and later in smaller breeds of dogs.

A common clinical problem in some breeds of dogs is retention of deciduous teeth, especially the canine teeth. The deciduous teeth do not fall from the mouth when the associated permanent teeth erupt, resulting in malocclusion and crowding of permanent teeth. This problem is discussed in a later chapter.

Different systems have been described for recording dental lesions on medical records.[5, 6, 9] The usual and most widely accepted system uses upper-case letters for describing permanent teeth (I, C, P, M) and lower-case letters for describing deciduous teeth (i, c, p, m). The teeth are also numbered in a rostral-to-caudal direction for each major type of tooth. If the tooth is in the upper or maxillary arcade, the number is written as a superscript, and if the tooth is located in the mandibular or lower arcade, a subscript number is used. If the tooth is located on the left side of the mouth, the number precedes the letter, whereas if the tooth is located on the right side, the tooth number follows the letter. Some examples of this notation are:

Permanent upper left canine tooth	$= {}^{1}C$
Permanent lower right second premolar	$= P_2$
Permanent upper left carnassial tooth	$= {}^{4}P$
Permanent lower left carnassial tooth	$= {}_{1}M$
Deciduous lower right intermediate incisor	$= i_2$
Deciduous upper left canine tooth	$= {}^{1}c$
Deciduous lower left carnassial tooth	$= {}_{3}p$

Another system of notation adapted from human dentistry uses continuous numbering for all the permanent teeth (Fig. 175–5). The numbering system starts with the upper right second molar as number 1, and continues around the maxillary arcade to the left second molar, which is number 20. The numbering continues onto the mandibular arcade, where the lower left third molar is number 21 and the lower right third molar is number 42. The numbers of the upper canine teeth are

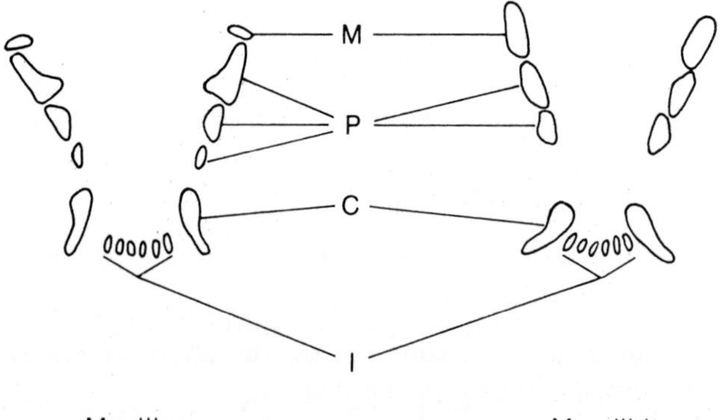

FIGURE 175–4. The various teeth of the cat are identified in this diagram of the maxilla and mandible. (I, incisor; C, canine; P, premolar; M, molar.) (From Frost P, Williams, CA: Feline Dental Disease. *Vet. Clin. North Am 16*:851, 1986.)

7 and 14 and of the lower canine teeth are 28 and 35 (all multiples of 7). This method has not gained wide acceptance in veterinary practice.[5]

A third method of dental notation uses (+) and (−) signs, and numbers teeth from the median plane of the oral cavity. The canine tooth on either side of the maxillary arcade would be +4. The canine teeth on the mandibular arcade would be −4. The upper carnassial teeth would be +8. Obviously, one must indicate right or left before the numerical notation to indicate the affected side.[5]

DENTAL TERMINOLOGY

Dental anatomical terminology can be confusing to veterinarians not accustomed to reading dental literature. Occasionally, terms are used that are not anatomically correct. Newer textbooks and reports have now described these terms, which have been accepted by veterinary anatomists.[15, 17, 18] Some of the common veterinary dental terms are pictured on Figure 175–6. Common veterinary dental terms are:

Rostral —toward the nose (cranial)
Caudal —toward the tail
Labial —toward the lips
Lingual —toward the tongue
Buccal —toward the cheek
Facial —toward the face or lips
Mesial —toward the center line of the dental arch
Distal —away from the center line of the dental arch
Contact —where a tooth touches an adjacent tooth
Occlusal—biting surface
Coronal —toward the crown
Apical —toward the root

All of these terms are used to describe the relationships between teeth, oral structures, and locations within the oral cavity. These terms are also used to describe the location of pathological lesions on the teeth or adjacent oral structures.

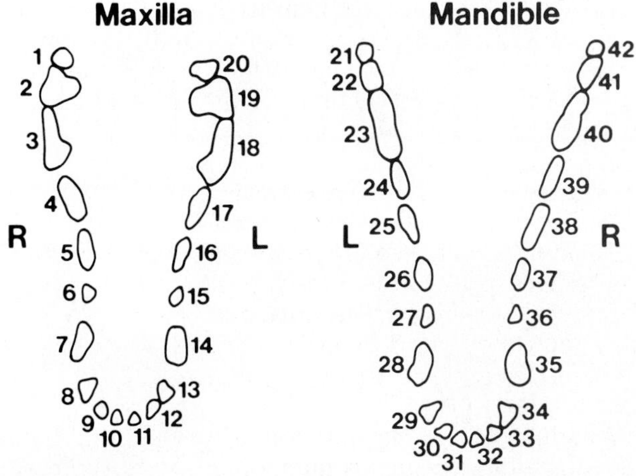

FIGURE 175–5. A numerical system for tooth identification in the dog. The numbering begins at the upper right side and ends at the lower right side. (Modified from Eisenmenger E, Zetner K: *Veterinary Dentistry.* Lea & Febiger, Philadelphia, 1985.)

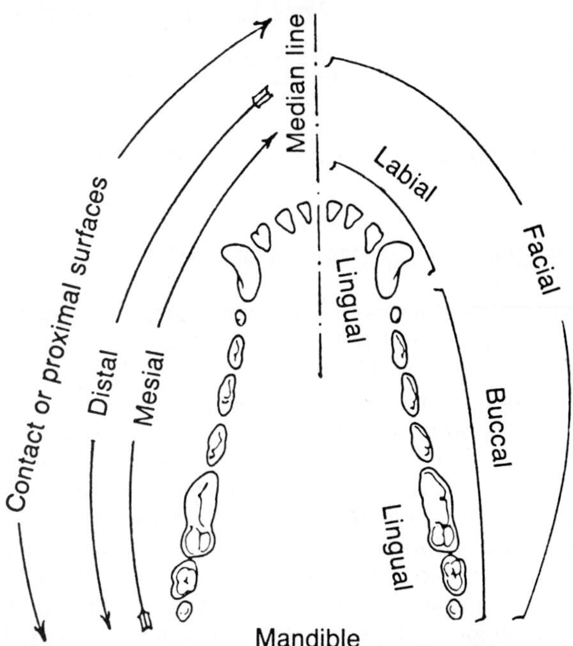

FIGURE 175–6. The common dental anatomical terms are illustrated on this diagram of the canine mandible. (From Wiggs RB: Canine oral anatomy and physiology. *Comp Cont Educ Pract Vet 11*:1476, 1989.)

References

1. Anderson NV: *Veterinary Gastroenterology.* Lea & Febiger, Philadelphia, 1980.
2. Barbee-Lomax JW: Delabere Pritchett Blaine: A biographical note. *J Small Anim Pract 2*:135, 1961.
3. Dorn AS: Dentistry in the Geriatric Dog. *Vet Clin North Am 11*:689, 1981.
4. Editorial: Veterinary dentistry. *J Am Vet Med Assoc 150*:634, 1967.
5. Eisenmenger E, Zetner K: *Veterinary Dentistry.* Lea & Febiger, Philadelphia, 1985.
6. Frost P, Williams CA: Feline dental disease. *Vet Clin North Am 16*:851, 1986.
7. Garbutt RJ: *Diseases and Surgery of the Dog.* Orange Judd Publishing Co., New York, 1938.
8. Golden AL, et al: A survey of oral and dental diseases in dogs anesthetized at a veterinary hospital. *J Am Anim Hosp Assoc 18*:891, 1982.
9. Harvey CE: *Veterinary Dentistry.* W. B. Saunders, Philadelphia, 1985.
10. Hobday FTG: *Surgical Diseases of the Dog and Cat.* 3rd ed. Chicago Medical Book Co., Chicago, 1925.
11. Merillat LA: *Animal Dentistry and Diseases of the Mouth.* Daniels Co. Press, Chicago, 1908.
12. Miller ME: *Anatomy of the Dog.* W. B. Saunders. Philadelphia, 1964.
13. Permar D: *Oral Embryology and Microscopic Anatomy.* 5th ed. Lea & Febiger, Philadelphia, 1972.
14. Smithcors JF: *Evolution of the Veterinary Art.* Veterinary Medicine, Kansas City, MO, 1957.
15. Tholen MA: *Concepts in Veterinary Dentistry.* Veterinary Medicine, Edwardsville, KS, 1983.
16. Vasseur PB, et al: The volume and distribution of surgical cases in 78 small animal practices in California. *J Am Anim Hosp Assoc 17*:161, 1981.
17. Wiggs RB: Canine oral anatomy and physiology. *Comp Cont Educ Pract Vet 11*:1475, 1989.
18. Zontine WJ: Canine dental radiology: Radiographic technique, development, and anatomy of the teeth. *J Am Vet Rad Soc 16*:75, 1975.

CHAPTER 176

Dental Pathology and Microbiology

Frank J. M. Verstraete

DEVELOPMENTAL ANOMALIES OF TEETH

Many disturbances of the development and growth of oral structures and the teeth have been recognized in the dog and cat. These dental disturbances may be manifested as abnormalities of shape, number, eruption and exfoliation, or structure. In addition, a number of occlusal problems may occur. These dental anomalies may have a genetic background or may be caused by a variety of environmental factors interfering with fetal or neonatal development.[40, 103] In humans, hereditary factors and pathological environmental conditions account for about 10 per cent of developmental anomalies, and the remaining 80 per cent are idiopathic.[85] Whether these figures also apply to the dog and cat is unknown.

Abnormal Shape

Gemination, Fusion, and Concrescence

Gemination, fusion, and concrescence are developmental disturbances in the shape of teeth.[56, 85] Gemination (or dichotomy) refers to an attempt at division of a single tooth bud. This attempt results in the incomplete formation of two teeth. The clinical appearance is usually that of a tooth with a longitudinal coronal groove and a single root (Fig. 176–1). Fusion and concrescence of teeth denote a joining of two tooth buds to form a single structure. Fusion may be complete or incomplete, but the dentin is always confluent. In concrescence, the teeth involved have completely separated dentin, but the cementum of the roots is confluent. Fusion can affect two normally present teeth but can also occur between a normal tooth and a supernumerary tooth. It may be difficult or impossible to differentiate between fused and dichotomous teeth.[56, 85]

These anomalies are rare in animals. Colyer, in his monumental work on the dental disorders of wild and domestic animals, found gemination in the dog and in 12 wild animal species.[20] Most epidemiological studies on the dental disorders of the dog and the cat do not mention fusion or gemination of teeth.[61, 66, 69, 80] Kuiper and colleagues described two cases of incisor gemination, and one case of suspected fusion, in the dog.[52]

Most documented dichotomous teeth in the dog involve incisor teeth,[4, 21, 52] although gemination or fusion involving the upper third premolar in a dog and in a cat has been recorded.[96] In animals, geminated or fused teeth are usually of only academic interest, especially when the incisors are affected.[78] They may give rise to periodontitis as a result of the altered gingival contour and occlusal trauma, and malocclusion may be present.[96] Extraction may be indicated.

Dilaceration and Supernumerary Roots

Dilaceration is a sharp curve in the root, which is probably caused by trauma to the dental follicle.[85] Supernumerary roots are anatomical variations that are occasionally seen in the dog and cat and that mainly affect the upper premolars, and the third premolar in particular (see Fig. 176–1). Dilaceration and supernumerary roots may be clinically important if extraction of the involved teeth is indicated.

Other Abnormalities

The term *dens in dente* refers to a well-recognized developmental abnormality in humans, characterized by an invagination of the enamel and dentin from the surface of the tooth crown.[85] Food impaction and caries may arise. This condition has been mentioned in the veterinary literature.[40, 41] Enamel pearls have been described in the dog.[83] An enamel pearl is a small, focal, excessive mass of enamel on the surface of the tooth, most frequently found near the cementoenamel junction or in the bifurcation of dental roots.

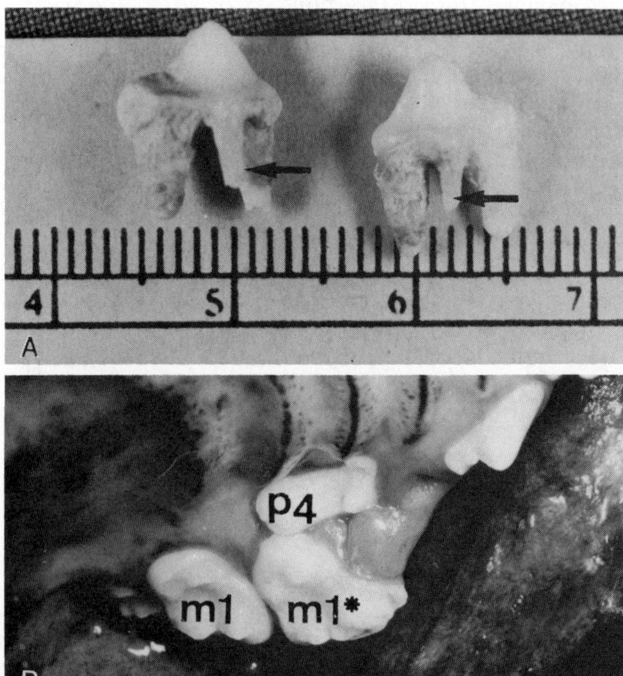

FIGURE 176–1. Abnormal shape and number of teeth: *A,* Upper third premolars with a supernumerary root *(arrows)* in a dog. *B,* Supernumerary upper first molar (m1*) in a dog, causing incomplete eruption of the fourth premolar (p4). (m1, upper first molar.)

Abnormal Number

Anodontia and Oligodontia

Anodontia is the complete congenital absence of teeth, which may involve both the deciduous and the permanent dentition. This condition is extremely rare in the dog and cat.[4, 95] Oligodontia, or partial anodontia, is the congenital absence of one or more teeth. This condition is common.[4, 20] Both anodontia and oligodontia are differentiated from false anodontia and oligodontia, or pseudoanodontia and pseudo-oligodontia, which involve absence of teeth as a result of extraction, trauma, periodontitis, or failure to erupt.

Oligodontia is much more common in the permanent dentition than in the deciduous dentition.[40] If deciduous teeth are missing, the corresponding permanent teeth are likely to be absent.[40] The first premolar and the third molar are most often affected in the dog.[29, 69] The upper second premolar in the cat has been the subject of considerable investigation, and absence of this small tooth is common in certain populations.[61, 62]

Oligodontia is usually considered serious, and radiographic techniques have been described for the early diagnosis of missing teeth in the dog.[30] Oligodontia is not a recent development—it occurred in prehistoric dogs.[15] The genetic implications of oligodontia are complex.[86, 103]

Polyodontia

Polyodontia, or supernumerary teeth, are less common than missing teeth.[4, 69] A 13 per cent prevalence in the dog was noted by Kuiper and associates.[51] Certain breed variations have been recognized.[20] In both humans and dogs, supernumerary teeth are more common on the upper jaw.[4] A supernumerary premolar mesial to the first premolar and a supernumerary molar distal to the last molar are most common in the dog and are of minimal clinical importance.[52, 69, 86] A well-recognized entity is the mesiodens, which is a supernumerary upper incisor found between the two first incisors. The prevalence of the mesiodens has been found to be 39 per cent and 26 per cent in the bulldog and boxer, respectively.[2] Supernumerary teeth in the middle of the premolar and molar row are extremely rare. These teeth may cause malocclusion and crowding as well as incomplete eruption or impaction of adjacent teeth (see Fig. 176–1). Although a genetic cause has been suggested, the pathogenesis of polyodontia remains unclear.[52, 86, 103]

Abnormal Eruption and Exfoliation

Retained Deciduous Teeth

Delayed exfoliation of deciduous incisors and canine teeth is common in the dog, especially in toy breeds, and its occurrence in the cat has been recorded.[17, 109] In the extreme form, deciduous teeth may persist after the eruption of the permanent teeth. A strong genetic basis for this condition has been suggested, although the exact pattern has not been determined.[29, 79, 103] A multifactorial pathogenesis, as found in humans, should be considered.[85]

A deciduous tooth may persist because of the absence of the corresponding permanent tooth and the resulting incomplete root resorption.[4, 16] In most cases, the permanent tooth develops normally, although the time and direction of eruption are influenced by the retained deciduous tooth. Permanent incisors erupt at a site immediately caudal to the retained deciduous incisors. Retained deciduous canine teeth cause a lingual deviation of the erupting lower canine teeth and a facial deviation of the upper canine teeth. Furthermore, retained deciduous teeth alter the gingival contour, with plaque and debris accumulating between the deciduous and permanent teeth.[17, 29]

Embedded and Impacted Teeth

Embedded teeth are individual teeth that are unerupted, usually because of a lack of eruptive force.[85] Embedded canine teeth are seen in the dog and are usually of traumatic origin, although embedded teeth are a possible sequel to distemper.[14, 50] An impacted tooth is prevented from erupting by some mechanical barrier in the eruption path.[40, 85] A dentigerous cyst may develop around the crown of the impacted tooth.[33, 64, 85] Partially embedded or impacted teeth that communicate with the oral cavity may develop periodontitis.[85]

Abnormal Structure

Enamel Hypoplasia

Enamel hypoplasia is the incomplete or defective formation of organic enamel matrix of teeth.[85] Hereditary and environmental forms occur in humans,[85] but only the environmental form is recognized in dogs. Enamel hypoplasia occurs as a result of damage to the ameloblasts while the teeth are developing.[22, 28] This damage can be caused by a variety of infectious and noninfectious conditions.[85] Epitheliotropic virus infections, particularly distemper, are the most important causes.[6, 28, 50, 51]

Mild enamel hypoplasia is characterized by irregular enamel, the areas of which initially appear as opaque but soon become brown-stained. Small irregular pits may be present. In the more severe form, a band-shaped absence or extreme thinning of the enamel is visible (Fig. 176–2).[22, 29, 50] The location of the lesions on the tooth is related to the developmental stage in which the ameloblasts were damaged.[6, 28] Teeth with enamel hypoplasia are predisposed to staining and calculus accumulation because of the rough surface.[6, 29]

Enamel hypoplasia affects the entire dentition as a result of distemper and other systemic causes. Arnbjerg noted a high incidence of generalized root hypoplasia with distemper-induced enamel hypoplasia.[6] Trauma to the developing dental follicles may result in enamel hypoplasia of one or more teeth.

Enamel hypoplasia occurring in the dog and resulting from excessive fluoride intake during tooth formation has been recorded.[37, 58] The pathophysiological factors are similar to those of distemper enamel hypoplasia. Damage to ameloblasts occurs, but interference with the calcification process of the matrix may take place.[85]

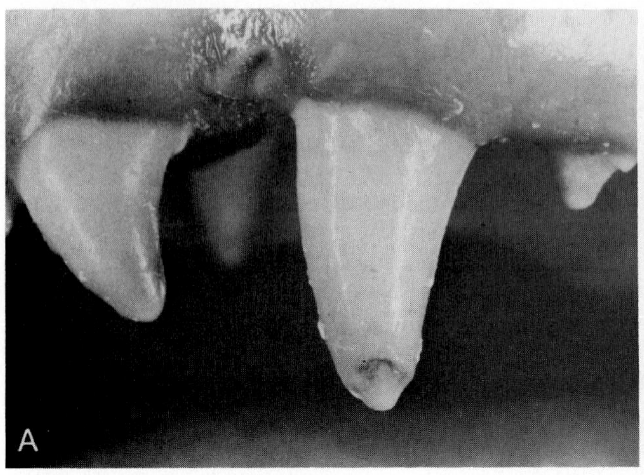

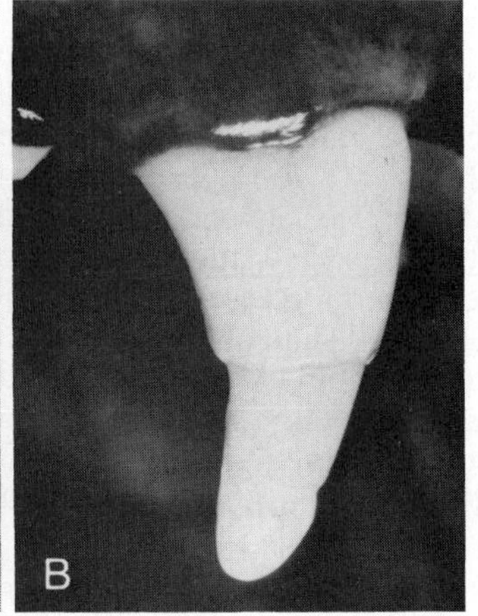

FIGURE 176–2. Enamel hypoplasia in the dog. *A,* Mild form showing opaque and stained areas as well as irregular pits. *B,* More severe form characterized by a band-shaped absence of enamel.

Odontogenesis Imperfecta

Odontogenesis imperfecta, or odontodysplasia, is a rare condition in humans and in dogs.[7, 67, 85] The shape of an affected tooth is markedly altered and irregular, often with radiological evidence of defective mineralization. One or several teeth in a localized area may be affected. The etiology is uncertain, although local factors such as trauma and osteomyelitis have been implicated.[67] Generalized odontodysplasia was found in two young dogs with severe renal disease.[25]

Tetracycline Staining

Tetracycline administered during tooth development becomes incorporated in the enamel and dentin and causes a permanent brown-yellow-orange discoloration.[10, 29] This drug should not be administered to dogs and cats before the age of 5 months or to pregnant female animals.[41] Treatment of this condition by bleaching has been used on an experimental and limited clinical basis in the dog.[100, 101, 107, 108]

INJURIES TO TEETH

Attrition

Attrition is the wearing away of dental substance due to occlusal contact and mastication. Attrition is usually a normal and physiological process, associated with aging. Attrition may be abnormal and enhanced because of malocclusion, with one or more teeth wearing abnormally against others.[40] This abnormality is initially manifested by wear facets, a common finding in the dog.[36] As wear continues, dentin is exposed, and sclerosis of the exposed dentinal tubules takes place. The rougher surface of the dentin stains easily, with the slightly yellowish dentin contrasting with the surrounding white enamel. As attrition proceeds, a brown spot may become visible in the center of the occlusal table, because of the exposure of secondary or tertiary dentin. Loss of dental substance by attrition is usually minimal in carnivores that have a normal diet.[29, 40]

Abrasion

Abrasion refers to the pathological wearing away of dental substance through an abnormal mechanical process.[85] Abnormal chewing habits such as biting stones, pathological gnawing,[40] and cage-biting are common causes of abrasion. Chewing on metal cage bars results in typical lesions, characterized by a considerable loss of dental substance on the distal aspect of the teeth, particularly the upper canine teeth and third incisors.[29] Traces of metal can be seen on the affected dental surfaces (Fig. 176–3).[41] This condition predisposes the animal to fractures of the affected teeth.[29] Pulp exposure may occur if the rate of formation of tertiary dentin cannot keep pace with the abrasion.[40]

Dental Fractures

Types

Dental fractures are common in the dog and cat, with an incidence of 14 per cent in the cat[80] and 27 per cent in the dog.[36] Fahrenkrug reported a higher incidence in young dogs.[32] In the cat, fractures mainly involve the canine teeth.[80] Reported figures regarding the location of dental fractures in the dog differ.[29, 36] Dental fractures in the dog and the cat have not been systematically classified. The World Health Organization classification of dental fractures in humans[3] can be modified for use in the dog and cat (Table 176–1 and Fig. 176–4).

Pathophysiology

Enamel fractures and uncomplicated crown fractures are of little clinical importance in small animals. The dog is largely resistant to caries. The exposed dentin is initially sensitive, and this sensitivity disappears because of sclerosis of the dentinal tubules and formation of tertiary dentin in the pulp chamber. Dentin is rougher than enamel and facilitates plaque and calculus accumulation. Sharp fracture edges may cause soft tissue trauma and can be rounded off if necessary.[40]

Crown-root fractures involve the periodontal ligament and may lead to periodontitis because of the altered gingival contour. A small fracture fragment and the

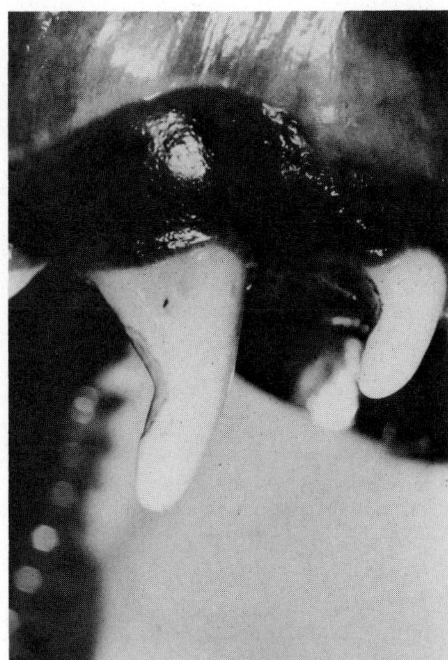

FIGURE 176–3. Abrasion of the distal aspect of the upper third incisor and canine tooth due to cage-biting in a dog.

TABLE 176–1. CLASSIFICATION OF DENTAL FRACTURES

Category	Definition
Enamel infraction or fracture	A chip fracture or crack of the enamel only
Uncomplicated crown fracture	A fracture involving enamel and dentin, but not exposing the pulp
Complicated crown fracture	A fracture involving enamel and dentin and exposing the pulp
Uncomplicated crown-root fracture	A fracture involving enamel, dentin, and cementum, but not exposing the pulp
Complicated crown-root fracture	A fracture involving enamel, dentin, and cementum and exposing the pulp
Root fracture	A fracture involving dentin, cementum, and the pulp

From Andreasen JD: *Traumatic Injuries of the Teeth.* 2nd ed. Munksgaard, Copenhagen, 1981.

overlying unsupported gingiva can be removed to restore physiological contour. Many crown-root fractures lead to irreversible periodontitis and indicate extraction. Complicated crown fractures cause pulp exposure and ensuing endodontic disease.[29, 40]

Root fractures of traumatic origin are infrequently seen; iatrogenic fractures are common. A root tip left behind may become covered by bone and gingiva in the absence of infection.[74] Alternatively, pulp necrosis may take place and lead to sequestration. An existing periapical granuloma does not resolve in the presence of a retained root fragment. Pathological root fractures are common in the cat because of external odontoclastic resorption lesions associated with periodontitis.[75]

Other Injuries to Dental Tissues

Injuries to periodontal tissues are rarely diagnosed, with the exception of lateral luxation, extrusive luxation, and exarticulation. Lateral luxation is characterized by displacement of the tooth and comminution or fracture of the alveolar socket.[3] Extrusive luxation and exarticulation are the partial and complete displacement of the tooth from its socket, respectively.[3] Immediate repositioning or reimplantation of the tooth, followed by splinting, is indicated.[40] No data are available regarding the success rate in veterinary medicine, but in humans,

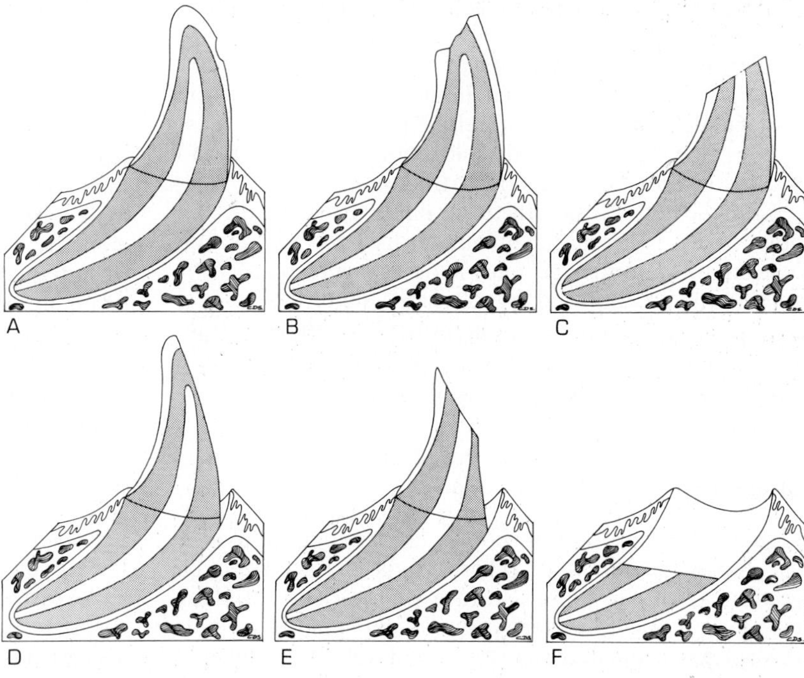

FIGURE 176–4. Classification of dental fractures. *A,* Enamel fracture. *B,* Uncomplicated crown fracture. *C,* Complicated crown fracture. *D,* Uncomplicated crown-root fracture. *E,* Complicated crown-root fracture. *F,* Root fracture.

the rate of long-term failure due to root resorption is high.[3]

Response to Trauma

Dentin-Pulp Complex

Secondary dentin is formed by the odontoblasts after root formation has been completed.[91] The continuous deposition of dentin results in a progressive reduction in the size of the pulp chamber. The formation of secondary dentin occurs as a response of the tooth to stimuli of the normal aging process. Tertiary dentin (also referred to as irregular secondary dentin or reparative dentin) results from the irritation of odontoblastic processes within the dentinal tubules.[85, 91] Tertiary dentin is produced by the odontoblasts that are directly affected by the irritation. Irritation of the odontoblastic processes may occur in a variety of conditions during which dentin is exposed.

In attrition, abrasion, and uncomplicated dental fractures, the formation of tertiary dentin usually seals off the pulp cavity effectively. With progressive wear, the tertiary dentin may become clinically evident as a brown spot in the center of the occlusal surface. This condition can be differentiated from an exposed root canal through use of a dental explorer.[41] The brown color results from the irregular tertiary dentin, which stains easily. With severe abrasion, pulp exposure may occur if tertiary dentin formation cannot keep pace with rapid wear. Severe irritation of the odontoblastic process may lead to pulp necrosis, even in the absence of direct pulp exposure. This irritation may occur in active carious lesions or when irritating restorative materials are applied directly onto dentin.

Exposed dentin is painful, because of the presence of intradental nerve fibers and fluid movement through the tubules.[44, 91] Pain is manifested by sensitivity to heat, cold, and pressure, and it eventually disappears as the calcification of the primary dentinal tubules is followed by sclerosis.[85]

Occasionally, the integrity of the hard tissues of the tooth are not distorted, but hemorrhage occurs in the root canal, with subsequent pulpal necrosis. This process may be demonstrated by discoloration of the crown and is an indication for endodontic treatment.[40]

Complicated dental fractures imply exposure of the pulp cavity. The initial inflammatory response is evidenced by hemorrhage and signs of acute pain. This stage may be followed by transient superficial pulpal hyperplasia, known as "pulp polyp" in humans (Fig. 176–5).[3] Invariably, migration of bacteria into the pulp occurs rapidly, ultimately leading to pulpal necrosis.[46, 87, 102]

Resorption

Internal resorption is poorly understood and may accompany endodontic disease. It is characterized by resorption of the pulpal surface of the dentin and by filling of the dental defect with vascular pulp tissue.[85] If resorption occurs in the crown, discoloration and enamel perforation may take place.[40] Internal resorption indicates endodontic treatment.

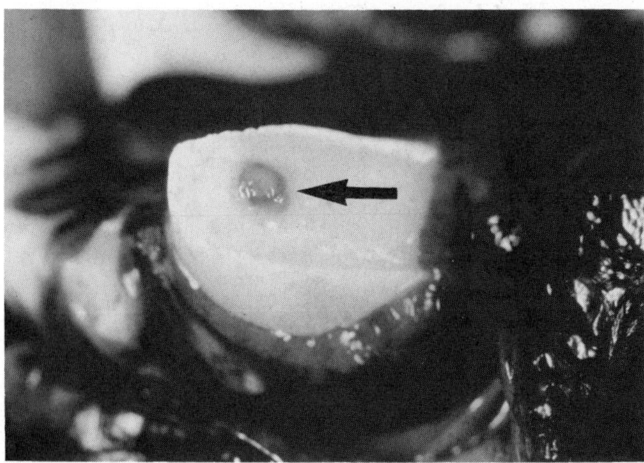

FIGURE 176–5. Recent complicated crown-root fracture of a mandibular canine tooth in a dog, with evidence of superficial pulpal hyperplasia ("pulp polyp") *(arrow).*

External resorption refers to resorption that begins on the root surface. The role of osteoclasts in this condition is unclear.[85] External resorption may be associated with periapical disease, periodontal trauma (including reimplantation of exarticulated teeth), tumors, cysts, and excessive orthodontic forces. Localized resorption at the cementoenamel junction is a well-recognized condition in cats and is known as external odontoclastic resorption. This type of resorption is characteristic of periodontal disease in cats.[75, 81, 84]

CARIES

Caries is a microbial disease of the calcified tissues of the tooth, characterized by demineralization of the inorganic portion and destruction of the organic substance of the tooth.[85] The etiology is complex, and no consensus is found regarding the relative importance of acid-producing bacteria, proteolytic bacteria, and the role of chelation.[85]

The reported prevalence of caries in the dog varies from 0.5 to 35 per cent.[9, 34, 51, 66, 69] Most authors agree that the prevalence is low.[29, 36, 40, 51, 69, 82] A possible explanation for the discrepancies in the reported prevalence rates of caries in the dog is that most authors fail to define detailed criteria for diagnosing caries.[34] This problem emphasizes the need for thorough and repeatable surveys based on accepted principles of epidemiology. Data regarding the prevalence of caries in the cat are unavailable (external odontoclastic resorption does not fulfill the criteria for caries).[75, 81, 84]

Caries in the dog may occur as pit or fissure caries (class I cavities) on the occlusal surface, or as smooth-surface caries (class V cavities) around the tooth neck.[31] Fissure caries are the most common and usually affect the upper and lower first molars (Fig. 176–6).[9, 66] Cervical caries should be differentiated from external resorption as previously described. The extent of carious lesions has been classified as superficial, intermediate,

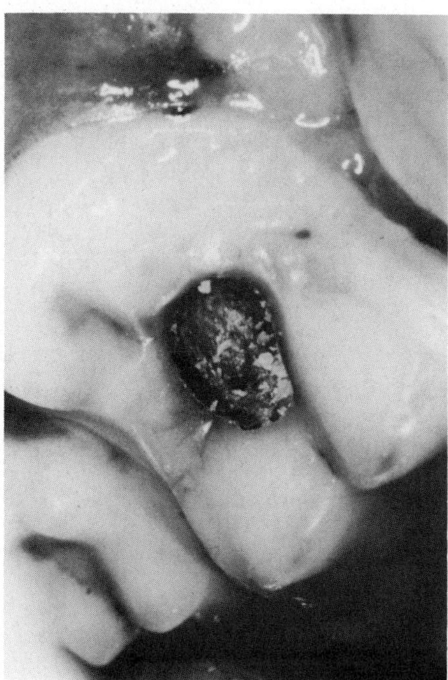

FIGURE 176–6. Carious lesion of the occlusal surface of an upper first molar in a dog.

or deep, depending on whether it involves enamel only, enamel and dentin, or enamel, dentin, and pulp, respectively.[51] An early carious lesion usually appears brown or black and feels slightly soft or sticky when probed with a fine dental explorer.[85] A carious cavity involving the dentin is filled with disintegrated dental substance and debris. The walls of the cavity are lined with contaminated decalcified dentin, in contrast with resorption defects, which are lined by healthy, hard dental substance.[85]

Clinical signs associated with intermediate carious lesions are difficulty in eating and jaw chattering,[40] which can be attributed to the irritation of intradental nerve fibers and odontoblastic processes in the dentinal tubules.[44, 91] Pulpitis may ensue; it is invariably present with deep carious lesions.[40]

Reasons for low prevalence of caries in the dog have been proposed.[34, 51] The morphology of the teeth is not conducive to caries. The conical shape and the absence of deep, narrow occlusal fissures and pits promote natural cleaning. The only teeth with large occlusal surfaces are the first molars, which are most commonly affected by caries. The salivary pH and urea concentration are higher in dogs than in humans, and these factors cause neutralization of the acids formed by bacteria.[34] *Streptococcus mutans* and *Lactobacillus* spp. have been isolated, rarely, from the mouths of normal dogs and from dogs with periodontal disease.[21, 79] Experimental attempts to induce carious lesions in the dog have proved difficult.[57]

ODONTOGENIC TUMORS

Epulides

The term *epulis* is derived from the Greek *epi-oulon,* meaning "on the gum." It is a descriptive clinical term applied to a variety of neoplastic and non-neoplastic tumors that appear on the gingiva as circumscribed elevated lesions. The nature of these lesions should be determined histologically (Fig. 176–7).

The epulis has been described as the most common benign oral tumor in the dog. In other reports, this tumor is not even mentioned, making it difficult to compare relative incidence.[40, 53, 94, 97] This discrepancy can be attributed to continuing confusion regarding the origin and nomenclature of the epulis. Dubielzig and associates recognized three types, namely, fibromatous, ossifying, and acanthomatous.[27] The common origin of these tumors is the periodontal ligament. In a later publication, Dubielzig and Thrall clearly differentiate between the acanthomatous epulis and the ameloblastoma.[24] A number of authors subsequently challenged the Dubielzig classification. Bostock and White questioned the common origin of these tumors.[18] These authors recognize the ameloblastoma, but reclassify the fibromatous and ossifying epulides as peripheral odontogenic fibromas, and the acanthomatous epulis as a basal cell carcinoma. Conversely, Reichart and coworkers found inflammatory fibrous hyperplasia with and without metaplastic bone formation and plexiform epithelial hyperplasia, and they regarded the acanthomatous epulis as an ameloblastoma.[76]

Most recently, these classifications and well-described histological criteria for similar tumors in humans were used in classifying a large series of epulides.[96b] It was found that the majority of epulides could be classified as focal fibrous hyperplasia. This non-neoplastic localized gingival hyperplasia coincides with what has been referred to as fibrous epulis.[39] Chronic gingivitis may lead to nodular proliferation and granulation tissue. These lesions may be associated with underlying periodontal disease.[23] The rest of the lesions that were previously diagnosed as fibromatous and ossifying epulides, were reclassified as peripheral odontogenic fibroma (WHO type), in agreement with current criteria in human oral pathology.[19, 35] Most so-called acanthomatous epulides were found to be peripheral ameloblastoma. The peripheral ameloblastoma is a tumor believed to originate either in the connective tissue of the gingiva from remnants of the dental lamina (rests of Serres) or from the basal cell layer of the oral mucosa.[96a] This tumor should not be called a basal cell carcinoma, which is a primary tumor of skin originating from the primordium of dermal appendages.[55] If a basal cell carcinoma were to occur in the mouth, it would be extremely rare and would originate from ectopic germ cells of skin appendages. The peripheral ameloblastoma should not be confused with the central ameloblastoma, which is a well recognized entity that is distinct from the acanthomatous epulis.[24, 27]

Generalized gingival hyperplasia has been called an epulis, but the term is a misnomer. Generalized gingival hyperplasia is occasionally seen in the boxer and collie.[23] Gingival hyperplasia has been noted to occur in the dog and cat after the experimental administration of certain drugs.[43, 47] Fibrous epulis, or non-neoplastic localized gingival hyperplasia, also occurs but is a separate entity.[39] Chronic gingivitis may lead to nodular proliferative lesions characterized by inflammatory infiltration

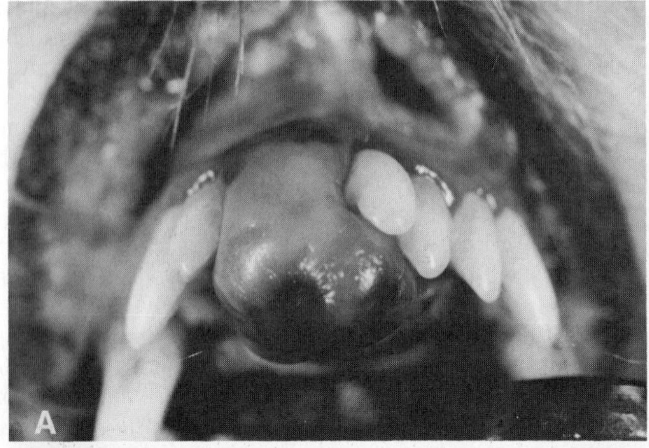

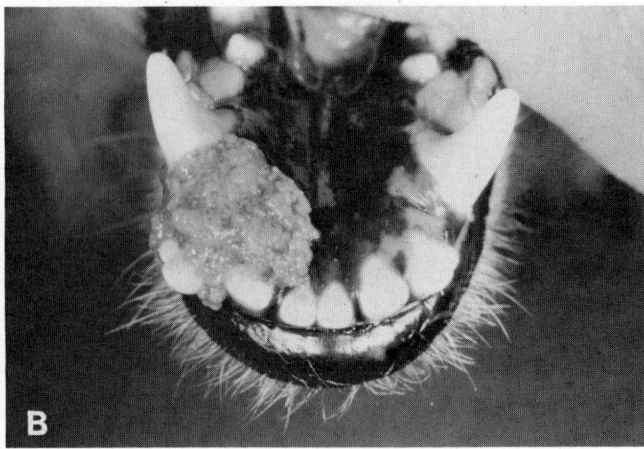

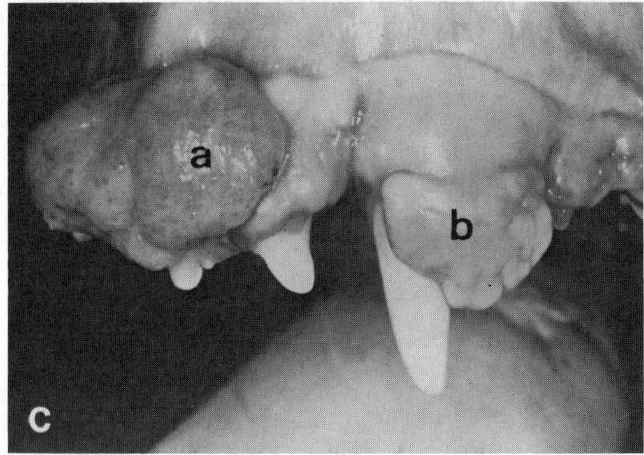

FIGURE 176–7. A wide variety of tumors may appear clinically as epulides in the dog. *A*, Peripheral odontogenic fibroma (WHO type). *B*, Peripheral ameloblastoma (acanthomatous epulis). *C*, Squamous cell carcinoma (a) and focal fibrous hyperplasia (b) in the same oral cavity, illustrating the need for multiple biopsies.

and granulation tissue. These lesions may be associated with underlying periodontal disease.[23]

Odontogenesis and Induction

Odontogenic tumors are rare in the dog and cat.[17, 22, 25, 95] To understand the classification of odontogenic tumors, it is important to consider the reciprocal interactions of mesenchymal and epithelial tissues during odontogenesis.[95] The epithelial dental lamina invaginates to form the enamel organ. The inner enamel organ epithelium consists of the preameloblasts. The mesenchymal odontoblast precursors migrate to the basement membrane and eventually make contact with the preameloblasts. The preameloblasts then induce the odontoblasts to form the dentin. In turn, the odontoblasts influence the ameloblasts and these cells start secreting the enamel matrix. The mesenchymal stroma enclosed in the developing dental follicle is induced to take on the characteristics of dental pulp. As tooth formation is completed, the odontogenic epithelium disappears leaving the epithelial rests of Malassez behind in the periodontal ligament.[10] These clusters of epithelial cells retain their odontogenic potential, which may subsequently be expressed in neoplasia.[22]

Classification

A variety of odontogenic tumors have been described, and their classification is based on the type of cell differentiation, on cell interaction, and on the presence of induction.[42, 73, 99] Three tumor types are classified as noninductive, indicating that the neoplastic epithelial cells do not influence the surrounding mesenchymal cells. They are ameloblastoma, adenomatoid odontogenic tumor, and calcifying epithelial odontogenic tumor. Tumor types in which induction of mesenchymal tissue does occur are ameloblastic fibroma, dentinoma, and ameloblastic odontoma. In addition to these categories are the complex and compound odontomas. These various tumors are grouped under the heading "benign tumors" in the human World Health Organization classification.[42, 73] Apart from the inductive and noninductive tumors, a group of primary connective-tissue tumors exists. This group includes the odontogenic fibroma, myxoma, and cementoma. Most of these tumor types have been recognized in the dog and cat.*

Central Ameloblastoma

The most common odontogenic tumor, except for the peripheral odontogenic fibroma (WHO type) and the peripheral ameloblastoma is the central ameloblastoma, which is occasionally referred to incorrectly as adamantinoma.[23, 53] This tumor usually appears as a locally invasive neoplasm with osteolysis around the tooth roots and with cystic changes.[18, 23, 24, 55] The classic

*See references 1, 23, 24, 26, 70, 88, 98, and 99.

histological appearance of a central ameloblastoma is a follicular arrangement of ameloblasts and stellate reticulum cells, resembling the basic structure of the enamel organ.[24, 60] Central ameloblastoma in the dog is often characterized by focal keratinization.[24] Metastasis has not been described.

Odontoma

An odontoma is a tumor in which both the epithelial and the mesenchymal cells are well differentiated, resulting in the formation of all types of dental tissue. An odontoma is probably a hamartoma rather than a neoplasm.[60] The dental tissues may exhibit normal relationships to one another.[85] An odontoma in which toothlike structures are present indicates advanced cellular differentiation and is referred to as a compound odontoma. An odontoma in which the conglomerate of dental tissues bears no resemblance to a tooth is called a complex odontoma.[85] Odontomas have been diagnosed in young dogs and in cats.[99] An odontoma may be associated with unerupted teeth or a dentigerous cyst, or it may be attached to an otherwise normal tooth (Fig. 176–8).[49]

Ameloblastic Fibroma

Ameloblastic fibroma in young cats has been described as inductive fibroameloblastoma.[23, 26, 88] This tumor is characterized by ameloblastic epithelial cells arranged around dental pulp–like stroma. The rostral maxilla is the most common site. This tumor may be locally invasive; however, metastasis has not been recorded (see Fig. 176–8).[26, 40]

Diagnosis and Clinical Staging

The principles of clinical staging and diagnosis of oropharyngeal tumors are well established,[40, 45, 77, 105] and they would apply also to epulides and odontogenic tumors. Because epulides may be a variety of pathological entities, the diagnosis and therapeutic plan are not based on gross appearance.[45] A biopsy submitted for histopathological examination by a pathologist experienced in oral pathology is essential. An incisional biopsy is performed, using a biopsy punch or a scalpel. If more than one tumor is present, multiple biopsies are taken (see Fig. 176–7). Atraumatic technique and minimal manipulation of the tumor are important. General anesthesia is recommended. Radiographs are obtained to determine the presence and extent of bone infiltration.

Therapy

The therapeutic plan is based on the clinical and radiographic findings and, most important, the result of the histopathological examination (Fig. 176–9).[45] Benign or hyperplastic lesions confined to the gingiva may be

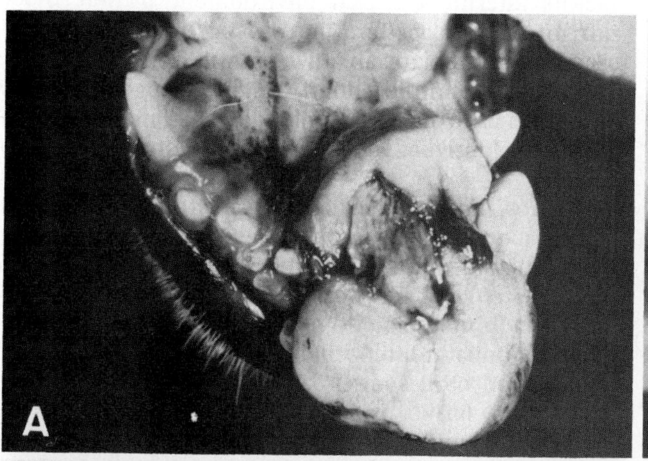

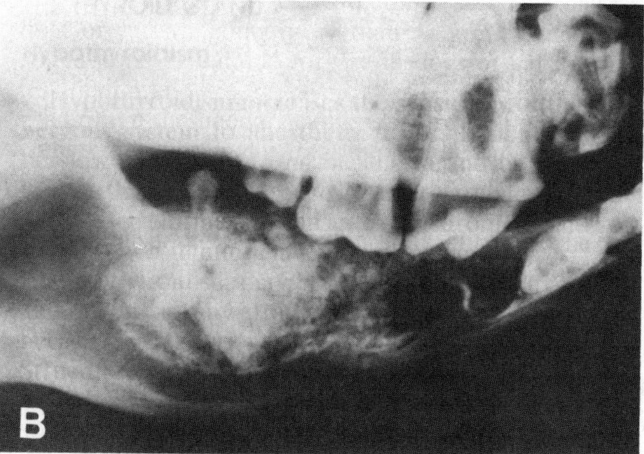

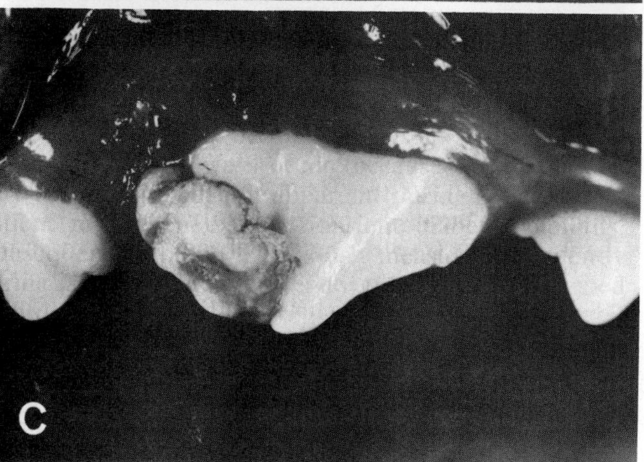

FIGURE 176–8. Odontogenic tumors in the dog. *A*, Central ameloblastoma of the rostral part of the mandible. *B*, Radiograph of a complex odontoma of the caudal part of the body of the mandible. *C*, Compound odontoma associated with the crown of an upper fourth premolar.

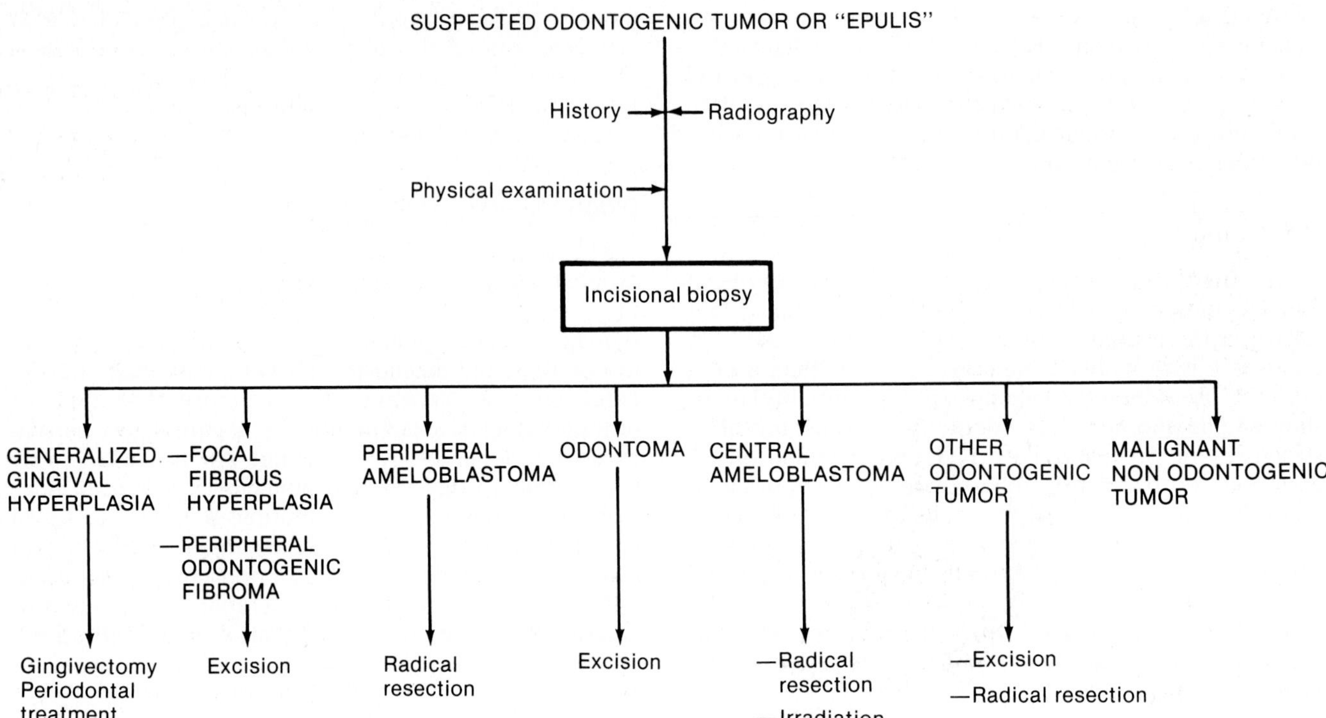

FIGURE 176–9. Management of suspected odontogenic tumors and epulides.

removed by local excision. Regrowth has been noted with a benign tumor such as peripheral odontogenic fibroma.[18] If possible, a wide margin of normal tissue is excised. One should strive for a physiological gingival contour and should treat associated periodontal disease.

Local excision is not indicated if bone infiltration is evident or if the tumor is malignant. Rather, such lesions are candidates for radical resection techniques.[40, 77] Radical resection is the method of choice for treating the peripheral ameloblastoma (acanthomatous epulis).[12, 18, 40, 77, 104] Most odontogenic tumors are locally invasive and potentially malignant, and radical resection is presumably indicated.[77] An exception is the odontoma, which is well circumscribed and can be removed by conservative excision, based on human experience.[49] Specimens are submitted for histopathological examination of the wound edges to confirm complete removal.

Irradiation of peripheral (acanthomatous epulis) and central ameloblastoma in the dog is well documented, and good results are reported.[53, 54, 92] Malignant tumor formation at the sites of previously irradiated epulides has been recorded.[93, 106] Osteoradionecrosis is a serious complication.[93]

DENTAL MICROBIOLOGY

Oral Ecology

A variety of bacteria are normally present in the oral cavities of humans and animals.[65] The bacterial composition of the oral cavity varies, however, according to the animal species.[21] A delicate balance exists between the resident flora and the oral environment.[65] The qualitative and quantitative composition of the bacterial flora is influenced by local environmental factors as well as by interactions between microorganisms.[38, 65] Important factors altering the oral environment include dietary changes, dental treatment, restorations and orthodontic appliances, and antibiotic therapy. Bacteriological examination of samples taken from patients is of little value because of the diversity of bacteria present and the lack of a quantitative method.[38]

Canine Oral Bacteriology

Diverse aerobic, facultative, and anaerobic bacteria are present in the canine oral cavity.[8] These bacteria have been studied mainly with specific reference to their association with bite wounds[8, 79] and periodontitis.[47, 89, 90] The frequency with which individual bacterial species are isolated depends on culture methods, sampling site, canine breed, and oral health status.[38, 48]

Comparing data on this subject is difficult. In normal dogs, *Streptococcus* spp., *Staphylococcus aureus* and *Staphylococcus epidermidis, Pasteurella multocida, Simonsiella* spp., the Enterobacteriaceae, and many other bacterial organisms have consistently been found.[8, 48, 71, 79] Interestingly, *Streptococcus mutans* is rare in the dog.[21, 79]

The high incidence of *P. multocida* is important in the pathophysiology of bite wounds.[5, 8] Anaerobic bacteria are also important and outnumber aerobic bacteria. Those isolated include *Bacteroides* spp., *Fusobacterium spp., Veillonella* spp., and *Lactobacillus* spp.[48] The subgingival and supragingival plaque flora associated with periodontitis has also been studied extensively. Although the bacterial population in periodontitis is the same as is found in the normal mouth, the proportions differ largely. The flora associated with periodontitis is predominantly anaerobic.[48, 65, 72, 90] The subgingival flora mainly includes gram-negative bacteria such as *Fusobacterium nucleatum* and *Bacteroides asaccharolyticus,* whereas the supragingival flora comprises a greater proportion of gram-positive bacteria.[90] Spirochetes are present in great numbers.[72] A *Spirillum* organism was isolated from beagles with necrotizing ulcerative gingivitis.[68]

Bacteremia may occur during and following periodontal treatment and dental extraction, and a variety of bacteria have been isolated from the blood of these patients.[13, 38, 110] This bacteremia may lead to heart valve colonization or hematogenous infection of surgical wounds created at the same time of the dental treatment.[13, 38] Dental procedures should not be performed at the same time as other surgical procedures.[13, 38]

Feline Oral Bacteriology

The normal oral flora of the cat has not been well documented. *P. multocida* was found in 80 per cent of cats.[5] The bacteria associated with periodontitis in the cat have received attention.[63] Anaerobic gram-negative rods such as black-pigmented *Bacteroides* spp. similar to *B. gingivalis* were isolated in increasing numbers with severe periodontitis. Love and associates[59] found *B. tectum* as the most common *Bacteroides* species and associated this organism with fight wound abscesses and pyothorax.

References

1. Abbott DP, et al: Calcifying epithelial odontogenic tumours in three cats and a dog. *J Comp Pathol 96*:131, 1986.
2. Aitchison J: Incisor dentitions of short-muzzled dogs. *Vet Rec 76*:165, 1964.
3. Andreasen JD: *Traumatic Injuries of the Teeth.* 2nd ed. Munksgaard, Copenhagen, 1981.
4. Arnall L: Some aspects of dental development in the dog—III. Some common variations in the dentitions. *J Small Anim Pract 2*:195, 1962.
5. Arnbjerg J: *Pasteurella multocida* from canine and feline teeth, with a case report of glossitis calcinosa in a dog caused by *P. multocida. Nord Vet Med 30*:324, 1978.
6. Arnbjerg J: Schmelz- und Wurzelhypoplasien nach Staupe. *Kleintierpraxis 31*:313, 1986.
7. Arnjberg J, Reibel J: Dentinogenesis imperfecta bei zwei Hunde. *Kleintierpraxis 33*:463, 1988.
8. Baillie WE, et al: Aerobic bacterial flora of oral and nasal fluids of canines with reference to bacteria associated with bites. *J Clin Microbiol 7*:223, 1978.
9. Bell AF: Dental disease in the dog. *J Small Anim Pract 6*:421, 1965.
10. Bennett IC, Law DB: Incorporation of tetracycline in developing enamel and dentin in dogs. *J Dent Child 34*:93, 1967.
11. Bhaskar SN: *Orban's Oral Histology and Embryology.* 9th ed. C. V. Mosby, St Louis, 1980.
12. Bjorling DE, et al: Surgical treatment of epulides in dogs: 25 cases (1974–1984). *J Am Vet Med Assoc 190*:1315, 1987.
13. Black AP, et al: Bacteremia during ultrasonic teeth cleaning and extraction in the dog. *J Am Anim Hosp Assoc 16*:611, 1980.
14. Bodingbauer J: Retention of teeth in dogs as a sequel to distemper infection. *Vet Rec 72*:636, 1960.
15. Bodingbauer J: Oligodontia and polyodontia in prehistoric dogs. *Vet Rec 75*:668, 1963.
16. Bodingbauer J: Korrelation zwischen Oligodontie und Milchzahnpersistenz als Fehlerquelle bei der Beurteilung des Hundegebisses. *Kleintierpraxis 21*:12, 1976.
17. Bodingbauer J: Milchzahnpersistenz beim Hund. *Kleintierpraxis 23*:339, 1978.
18. Bostock DE, White RAS: Classification and behaviour after surgery of canine "epulides." *J Comp Pathol 97*:197, 1987.
19. Buchner A, et al: Peripheral odontogenic fibroma. *Oral Surg Oral Med Oral Pathol 64*:432, 1987.
20. Colyer F: *Variations and Diseases of the Teeth of Animals.* John Bale, Sons and Danielsson, London, 1936.
21. Dent VE, Marsch PD: Evidence for a basic plaque microbial community on the tooth surface in animals. *Arch Oral Biol 26*:171, 1981.
22. Dubielzig RR: The effect of canine distemper virus on the ameloblastic layer of the developing tooth. *Vet Pathol 16*:268, 1979.
23. Dubielzig RR: Proliferative dental and gingival diseases of dogs and cats. *J Am Anim Hosp Assoc 18*:577, 1982.
24. Dubielzig RR, Thrall DE: Ameloblastoma and keratinizing ameloblastoma in dogs. *Vet Pathol 19*:596, 1982.
25. Dubielzig RR, et al: Dental dysplasia in two young uremic dogs. *Vet Pathol 23*:333, 1986.
26. Dubielzig RR, et al: Inductive fibroameloblastoma, an unusual dental tumor of young cats. *J Am Vet Med Assoc 174*:720, 1979.
27. Dubielzig RR, et al: The nomenclature of periodontal epulides in dogs. *Vet Pathol 16*:209, 1979.
28. Dubielzig RR, et al: Lesions of the enamel organ of developing dog teeth following experimental inoculation of gnotobiotic puppies with canine distemper virus. *Vet Pathol 18*:684, 1981.
29. Eisenmenger E, Zetner K: *Tierärztliche Zahnheilkunde.* Verlag Paul Parey, Berlin, 1982.
30. Emily P: Intraoral radiology. *Vet Clin North Am Small Anim Pract 16*:801, 1986.
31. Emily P: Restorative dentistry. *Vet Clin North Am Small Anim Pract 16*:895, 1986.
32. Fahrenkrug P: *Handbuch der Zahnbehandlung in der Kleintierpraxis.* 4th ed. A. Albrecht G.m.b.H., Aulendorf, 1988.
33. Field EA, et al: The removal of an impacted maxillary canine and associated dentigerous cyst in a Chow: A case report. *J Small Anim Pract 23*:159, 1982.
34. Gardner AF, et al: Dental caries in domesticated dogs. *J Am Vet Med Assoc 140*:433, 1962.
35. Gardner DG: The peripheral odontogenic fibroma: An attempt at clarification. *Oral Surg Oral Med Oral Pathol 54*:40, 1982.
36. Golden AL, et al: A survey of oral and dental diseases in dogs anesthetized at a veterinary hospital. *J Am Anim Hosp Assoc 18*:891, 1982.
37. Grancher D, et al: Fluorose beim Hund. *Kleintierpraxis 33*:203, 1988.
38. Greene CE: *Clinical Microbiology and Infectious Diseases of the Dog and Cat.* W. B. Saunders, Philadelphia, 1984.
39. Greenwood AM, O'Brien FV: The fibrous epulis in the dog. *J Oral Pathol 4*:67, 1975.
40. Harvey CE: *Veterinary Dentistry.* W. B. Saunders, Philadelphia, 1985.
41. Harvey CE: Oral, dental pharyngeal, and salivary gland disorders. *In* Ettinger SA (ed): *Textbook of Veterinary Internal Medicine.* 3rd ed. W. B. Saunders, Philadelphia, 1989.
42. Head KW: Tumors of the upper alimentary tract. *Bull World Health Organ 53*:145, 1976.
43. Heijl L, Sundin Y: Nitrendipine-induced gingival overgrowth in dogs. *J Periodontol 60*:104, 1988.
44. Hirvonen TJ, et al: The excitability of dog pulp nerves in relation to the condition of dentine surfaces. J Endod *10*:294, 1984.
45. Hoyt RF, Withrow SJ: Oral malignancy in the dog. *J Am Anim Hosp Assoc 20*:83, 1984.
46. Isermann GT, Kaminski EJ: Pulpal response to bacteria in the dog. *Oral Surg Oral Med Oral Pathol 48*:353, 1979.
47. Ishikawa J, Glickman I: Gingival response to the systematic administration of sodium diphenyl hydantoin (Dilantin) in cats. *J Periodontol 32*:149, 1961.
48. Isogai E, et al: Oral flora of mongrel and beagle dogs with periodontal disease. *Jpn J Vet Sci 51*:110, 1989.
49. Kaugars GE, et al: Odontomas. *Oral Surg Oral Med Oral Pathol 67*:172, 1989.
50. Köstlin R, et al: Zur Oligodontie und Schmelzhypoplasie beim Hund. *Kleintierpraxis 27*:11, 1982.
51. Kuiper JD, Van der Gaag I: Cariës, emailhypoplasie en tandverkleuringen bij de hond. *Tijdschr Diergeneeskd 107*:457, 1982.
52. Kuiper JD, et al: Polydontie en afwijkende tandvormen bij de hond. *Tijdschr Diergeneeskd 107*:451, 1982.
53. Langham RF, et al: Oral adamantinomas in the dog. *J Am Vet Med Assoc 146*:474, 1965.
54. Langham RF, et al: X-ray therapy of selected odontogenic neoplasms in the dog. *J Am Vet Med Assoc 170*:820, 1977.
55. Lever WF, Schaumburg-Lever G: *Histopathology of the Skin.* 7th ed. J. B. Lippincott, Philadelphia, 1990.
56. Levitas TC: Gemination, fusion, twinning and concrescence. *J Dent Child 32*:93, 1965.
57. Lewis TM: Resistance of dogs to dental caries: A two-year study. *J Dent Res 44*:1354, 1965.
58. Loeffler K, et al: Fluorose beim Hund. *Kleintierpraxis 24*:167, 1979.
59. Love DN, et al: *Bacteroides* species from the oral cavity and oral-associated diseases of cats. *Vet Microbiol 19*:275, 1989.

60. Lucas RB: *Pathology of Tumours of the Oral Tissues.* 4th ed. Churchill Livingstone, Edinburgh, 1984.
61. Lüps P: Gebiss- und Zahnvariation an einer Serie von 257 Hauskatzen (Felis silvestris f. catus L., 1758). *Zool Abh Staatl Mus Tierk Dresden 34*:155, 1977.
62. Lüps P: Vergleichende Untersuchung am zweiten oberen Vorbackenzahn P2 der Hauskatze Felis silvestris f. catus. *Z Säugetierkunde 45*:245, 1980.
63. Mallonee DH, et al: Bacteriology of periodontal disease in the cat. *Arch Oral Biol 33*:677, 1988.
64. Manfra Marretta S, et al: An iatrogenic dentigerous cyst in a dog. *J Vet Dent 6*:11, 1989.
65. McGhee JR, et al: *Dental Microbiology.* Harper & Row, Philadelphia, 1982.
66. Meyer R, Suter G: Epidemiologische und morphologische Untersuchungen am Hundegebiss—I. Mitteilung: Epidemiologische Untersuchungen. *Schweiz Arch Tierheilkd 118*:307, 1976.
67. Meyer R, et al: Epidemiologische und Morphologische Untersuchungen am Hundegebiss—II. Mitteilung: Morphologische Untersuchungen. *Schweiz Arch Tierheilkd 122*:503, 1980.
68. Mikx FHM, Van Campen GJ: Microscopical evaluation of the microflora in relation to necrotizing ulcerative gingivitis in the beagle dog. *J Periodont Res 17*:576, 1982.
69. Mooser M: Zahnärztlich-vergleichende Untersuchungen am 425 Hundeschädeln. *Schweiz Arch Tierheilkd 100*:209, 1958.
70. Nold JB, et al: Ameloblastic odontoma in a dog. *J Am Vet Med Assoc 185*:996, 1984.
71. Nyby MD, et al: Incidence of *Simonsiella* in the oral cavity of dogs. *J Clin Microbiol 6*:87, 1977.
72. Page RC, Schroeder HE: *Periodontitis in Man and Other Animals.* Karger, Basel, 1982.
73. Pindborg JJ, Kramer IRH: *International Histological Classification of Tumours No. 5—Histological Typing of Odontogenic Tumours, Jaw Cysts and Allied Lesions.* World Health Organization, Geneva, 1971.
74. Plata RL, Kelln EE: Intentional retention of vital submerged roots in dogs. *Oral Surg Oral Med Oral Pathol 42*:100, 1976.
75. Reichart PA, et al: Periodontal disease in the domestic cat. *J Periodont Res 19*:67, 1984.
76. Reichart PA, et al: Epulides in dogs. *J Oral Pathol Med 18*:92, 1989.
77. Richardson RC, et al: Oral neoplasms in the dog: A diagnostic and therapeutic dilemma. *Comp Cont Educ Pract Vet 5*:441, 1983.
78. Ross DL: Veterinary dentistry. *In* Ettinger SJ (ed): *Textbook of Veterinary Internal Medicine—Diseases of the Dog and Cat.* Vol 2. W. B. Saunders, Philadelphia, 1975.
79. Saphir DA, Carter GR: Gingival flora of the dog with special reference to bacteria associated with bites. *J Clin Microbiol 3*:344, 1976.
80. Schlup D: Epidemiologische und morphologische Untersuchungen am Katzengebiss—I. Mitteilung: Epidemiologische Untersuchungen. *Kleintierpraxis 27*:87, 1982.
81. Schlup D, Stich H: Epidemiologische und morphologische Untersuchungen am Katzengebiss—II. Mitteilung: Morphologische Untersuchungen der "neck lesions." *Kleintierpraxis 27*:179, 1982.
82. Schneck GW: Caries in the dog. *J Am Vet Med Assoc 150*:1142, 1967.
83. Schneck GW: A case of enamel pearls in a dog. *Vet Rec 92*:115, 1973.
84. Schneck GW: Neck lesions in the teeth of cats. *Vet Rec 99*:100, 1976.
85. Shafer WG, et al: *A Textbook of Oral Pathology.* 4th ed. W. B. Saunders, Philadelphia, 1983.
86. Skrentny TT: Preliminary study of the inheritance of missing teeth in the dog. *Wien Tierarzt Mschr 51*:231, 1964.
87. Stabholz A, Sela MN: The role of oral microorganisms in the pathogenesis of periapical pathosis. I. Effect of *Streptococcus mutans* and its cellular constituents on the dental pulp and periapical tissue of cats. *J Endod 9*:171, 1983.
88. Stebbins KE, et al: Feline oral neoplasia: A ten-year survey. *Vet Pathol 26*:121, 1989.
89. Syed SA, et al: The predominant cultivable dental plaque flora of beagle dogs with gingivitis. *J Periodont Res 15*:123, 1980.
90. Syed SA, et al: The predominant cultivable dental plaque flora of beagle dogs with periodontitis. *J Clin Periodontol 8*:45, 1981.
91. Ten Cate AR: *Oral Histology: Development, Structure, and Function.* 2nd ed. C. V. Mosby, St. Louis, 1985.
92. Thrall DE: Orthovoltage radiotherapy of acanthomatous epulides in 39 dogs. *J Am Vet Med Assoc 184*:826, 1984.
93. Thrall DE, et al: Malignant tumor formation at the site of previously irradiated acanthomatous epulides in four dogs. *J Am Vet Med Assoc 178*:127, 1981.
94. Todoroff RJ, Brodey RS: Oral and pharyngeal neoplasia in the dog: A retrospective study of 361 cases. *J Am Vet Med Assoc 175*:567, 1979.
95. Ueberberg H: Beobachtungen einer sogenannten Anodontie bei einer Hauskatze. *Zentralbl Veterinar med [A] 12*:193, 1965.
96. Verstraete FJM: Anomalous development of the upper third premolar in a dog and a cat. *J South Afr Vet Assoc 56*:131, 1985.
96a. Verstraete FJM, et al: The histological nature of epulides in dogs. *J Comp Pathol 106*:169, 1992.
97. Vos JH, Van der Gaag I: Canine and feline oral-pharyngeal tumours. *J Vet Med A 34*:420, 1987.
98. Vos JH, et al: A feline dental tumor resembling calcifying epithelial odontogenic tumor in man. *Vet Pathol 22*:508, 1985.
99. Walsh KM, et al: Epithelial odontogenic tumours in domestic animals. *J Comp Pathol 97*:503, 1987.
100. Walton RE, et al: External bleaching of tetracycline stained teeth in dogs. *J Endod 8*:536, 1982.
101. Walton RE, et al: Internal bleaching of tetracycline-stained teeth in dogs. *J Endod 9*:416, 1983.
102. Watts A, Paterson RC: Migration of materials and microorganisms in the dental pulp of dogs and rats. *J Endod 8*:53, 1982.
103. Wegner W: Genetisch bedingte Zahnanomalien. *Prakt Tierarzt 5*:19, 1987.
104. White RAS, Gorman NT: Wide local excision of acanthomatous epulides in the dog. *Vet Surg 18*:12, 1989.
105. White RAS, et al: Clinical staging for oropharyngeal malignancies in the dog. *J Small Anim Pract 26*:581, 1985.
106. White RAS, et al: Sarcoma development following irradiation of acanthomatous epulis in two dogs. *Vet Rec 118*:668, 1986.
107. Wiggs RB: Bleaching vital teeth in canines. *J Vet Dent 5*:15, 1988.
108. Wiggs RB: Bleaching nonvital teeth in canines. *J Vet Dent 6*:9, 1989.
109. Wissdorf H, Hermanns W: Persistierende Milchhakenzähne (Cd) im Oberkiefer einer Hauskatze. *Kleintierpraxis 19*:14, 1974.
110. Withrow SJ: Dental extraction as a probable cause of septicemia in a dog. *J Am Anim Hosp Assoc 15*:345, 1979.

CHAPTER 177

Dental Extractions and Complications

Albert S. Dorn

The brand of dentistry specializing in the extraction of teeth is called exodontics, and tooth extraction, or exodontia, was a common procedure in veterinary medicine for many years. Teeth were extracted when the alveolar attachments were destroyed by chronic periodontal disease, at which stage the affected teeth could be removed without effort or special instruments. Improvements in veterinary dentistry, such as periodontal therapy, endodontic repair, and crown restoration, permit the preservation of teeth, and extraction has become the treatment of last resort.

Some indications for extraction still exist, but improvements in techniques and instrumentation have made this task much easier for the veterinary practitioner. New elevators, dental engines, and the use of mucoperiosteal flaps have improved techniques, resulting in less trauma to the patient.

INDICATIONS FOR DENTAL EXTRACTIONS

A variety of indications for the extraction of teeth in veterinary practice have been described.[3] These indications include the following:

1. Gross decay or caries
2. Fractured crown or root with the fracture extending into the pulp
3. Advanced periodontal disease
4. Supernumerary teeth
5. Malocclusion
6. Retained deciduous teeth
7. Teeth in the fracture line (mandible or maxilla)
8. Periapical abscess

Significant caries (decay) is rare in the dog, but various lesions occur frequently in the cat. Carious lesions are often too advanced to undergo restoration, because the lesions often occur subgingivally and are not observed. If decay is too aggressive and invades the pulp chamber, extraction is the only possible treatment.

A fractured crown or root with exposure of the pulp chamber may require extraction, depending on the extent and location of the injury. The tooth may be partially restored or endodontically treated if the root is undamaged. If injury involves only the original crown, a cast crown restoration can be cemented to a healthy root. Failure to treat or extract the tooth leads to chronic inflammation, pulpitis, necrotic pulp, and periapical abscess.

Advanced periodontal disease is one of the most common indications for extraction of teeth. Usually, teeth are loose because of destruction of the periodontal ligaments and supporting structures of the teeth. If two-thirds of the supporting structure has been destroyed, restoration is impossible and extraction is necessary. These teeth are usually quite movable and may be extracted without effort or special instruments.

Supernumerary teeth are defined as extra teeth in the dental arcade. The most frequent cause is retained deciduous teeth, but occasionally, extra incisors or premolars are present. These extra teeth are extracted to allow appropriate occlusion and interdigitation of cheek teeth.

Malocclusion can result from a variety of causes, including congenital defects such as wry jaw, supernumerary teeth, retained deciduous teeth, or trauma. Whenever possible, the primary cause of the problem is addressed. Selected extractions may resolve the problem.

Retained deciduous teeth act similarly to supernumerary teeth. When a deciduous tooth is retained, it is extracted immediately, because failure to remove a primary tooth often results in malocclusion of the secondary tooth at that location. Retained deciduous teeth predispose the surrounding permanent teeth to premature periodontal disease by allowing accumulation of dental plaque and calculus.

Teeth located in the fracture line of a traumatized maxilla and mandible are extracted. These teeth may have disrupted blood supply from trauma, and damage to pulp can occur, with secondary pain and inflammation. Removal of teeth from the fracture site prevents interference with the normal healing process. The veterinary surgeon must exercise care not to cause additional trauma during extraction.

Periapical abscess formation may be another indication for dental extraction when endodontic restoration is inappropriate. Periapical abscess occurs after chronic exposure or infection of the pulp and often causes localized pain and swelling. In advanced cases, a fistula from the abscess to the lip, face, or surrounding gingiva occurs. The tooth must be endodontically treated by apicoectomy and retrograde sealing, or by extraction.

A variety of other indications for dental extractions have been described in the human literature and may apply to animals.[1] These additional indications include the following:

1. Teeth interfering with intraoral appliances such as splints or orthodontic devices
2. Teeth not restorable by operative dentistry
3. Impacted or unerupted teeth
4. Malposed teeth not amenable to orthodontic correction
5. Retained roots and parts of teeth from previous extractions
6. Teeth traumatizing surrounding soft tissue
7. Teeth surrounding oral neoplasia that would interfere with treatment
8. Teeth directly involved with or affected by oral neoplasia

Intraoral appliances have been used frequently for the treatment of fractures and for orthodontic corrections.[3, 8] These appliances are secured to existing oral structures such as teeth, mandible, or maxilla, by cement, wires, brackets, or composites. Proper fit may require the extraction of selected teeth that interfere with the placement of appliances, and careful evaluation of occlusion must be performed before extracting teeth for this purpose.

Advanced caries, trauma to the crown, or enamel hypoplasia may result in a tooth that is unsuitable for restoration. When teeth cannot be repaired by restorative dental techniques, extraction may be the only acceptable alternative.

Removal of impacted or unerupted teeth is controversial, and in veterinary practice, these teeth are usually not removed. If the impacted tooth interferes with normal occlusion or eruption of adjacent teeth, extraction is indicated. Surgical incision of the superficial gingival tissue may facilitate eruption and is considered before extraction.

Malposed or malaligned teeth not amenable to orthodontic correction may be extracted. Occasionally, orthodontic appliances are unsuitable for particular animals, or owners may be unwilling to comply with the requirements of orthodontic care.

During a previous extraction attempt, or because of previous trauma or injury, root fragments may be retained in the dental arcade. Broken roots from deciduous-tooth extractions usually resorb and cause little difficulty, but the effects of root remnants from permanent teeth vary. Clinical signs such as pain, salivation, gingival hyperplasia, and local irritation may necessitate extraction of the affected root fragment. Care is used to extract the entire root remnant so that the wound heals rapidly and without complication.

Cats and dogs have a high incidence of oral neoplasia. Teeth may be surrounded by the neoplastic tissue or, in rare instances, may be the neoplastic tissue of origin. The presence of teeth in the dental arcade may affect aspects of the treatment plan such as radical surgery or radiation therapy. If teeth interfere with the treatment protocol for an oral tumor, or if treatment can be enhanced by the removal of teeth, extraction is indicated. Loss of teeth is acceptable in successful oral neoplasia therapy.

TECHNIQUES FOR DENTAL EXTRACTION—MUCOPERIOSTEAL FLAPS

An important consideration in dental extraction is whether the entire crown and parts of the root of the tooth are exposed. This situation necessitates exposure of the labial or buccal cortical plate of bone surrounding the affected tooth.[3, 8] The first step is to remove the overlying soft tissue away from the bone, and because the periosteum is reflected with the gingiva and mucous membrane, the exposure is called a mucoperiosteal flap (Fig. 177–1).

Mucoperiosteal flaps are designed to provide access to the surgical site, maintain tissue integrity, anticipate anatomical and pathological variations, and reposition the soft tissue properly.[11] When creating a mucoperiosteal flap, the following principles are observed:

1. Maintain adequate blood supply.
2. Extend the incision beyond the affected area.
3. Design flap for maximum visibility.
4. Make incision through periosteum and mucosa.
5. Use sharp blades and tissue elevators.
6. Elevate the root from a distal direction.
7. Avoid sharp angles in the incisions.
8. Undermine attached mucosa for suturing.
9. Remove residual blood from site.
10. Suture for primary closure.

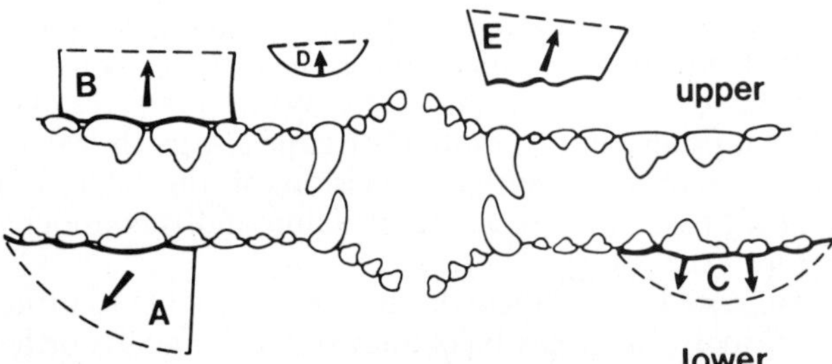

FIGURE 177–1. Various types of mucoperiosteal flaps are illustrated. The arrows indicate the direction of reflection. (A, triangular flap; B, rectangular flap; C, envelope flap; D, semilunar flap; E, Leubke-Oschenbein flap.) (Modified from Levine N [ed]: *Current Treatment in Dental Practice.* W. B. Saunders, Philadelphia, 1986.)

Various mucoperiosteal flaps have been described. They are generally divided into two types: full mucoperiosteal flaps and limited mucoperiosteal flaps.[11] Full mucoperiosteal flaps include the triangular flap, the rectangular flap, and the envelope flap. Limited mucoperiosteal flaps include the semilunar flap and the Leubke-Oschenbein flap.

Full mucoperiosteal flaps are used for extractions and periodontal surgery. Limited mucoperiosteal flaps have specific applications such as retrieval of a retained root fragment or exposure of the apical delta for an endodontic procedure.

PRINCIPLES OF DENTAL EXTRACTIONS

Infection, restriction of mouth opening, caries, fracture, tooth mobility, and tooth alignment in the dental arch all affect extraction techniques. Radiography of the dental arch is performed, especially if the teeth are thought to be primary and if the surgeon is uncertain whether secondary teeth will erupt at the same site.

The surgical site is properly prepared. Ultrasonic scaling or cleaning of the adjacent teeth may be necessary if advanced periodontal disease is present. Topical antiseptics are applied to the surgical site to reduce the number of local bacteria. Chlorhexidine can be sprayed on the extraction site or applied topically.

In multirooted teeth, consideration must be given to division of the crown to facilitate extraction (Fig. 177–2). Crown division is especially important if the periodontal ligaments are intact and the tooth is well supported and attached within the bony alveolus.

Crown division can be performed with dental engines and handpieces, power drills and burs, or manual saws. The preferred method requires a high-speed dental handpiece with a round bur, or a low-speed handpiece with a diamond disc.[5] After the crown is divided, a dental elevator can be inserted to apply leverage using the other cusps or crown fragments of the same tooth. This technique prevents damage to the crowns of adjacent teeth.

EQUIPMENT FOR DENTAL EXTRACTIONS

Dental Elevators

The most important instrument for the extraction of teeth is the dental elevator. Elevators are available in different sizes with a variety of tips, which are used to free the tooth from the alveolar attachment. Extraction of large teeth in large breeds requires a large elevator, whereas extraction of feline teeth necessitates a small elevator or an apical root tip elevator. If a large elevator is used on a small dental arcade, the result may be fracture of the adjacent bone, the alveolus, or the entire mandible or maxilla.

The goal is to stretch, break, or cut peridontal fibers

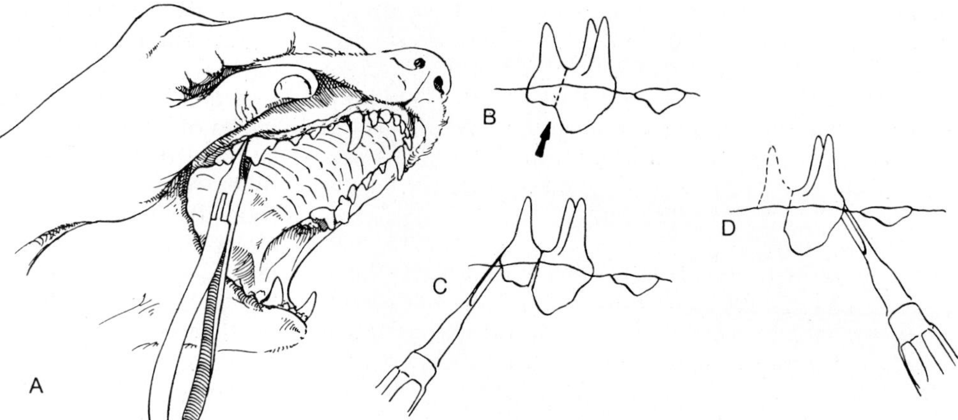

FIGURE 177–2. Carnassial tooth extraction. *A* and *B*, The tooth is cut into one- and two-root sections (see dotted line). *C* and *D*, The separated sections are removed in turn. (From Harvey CE: *Veterinary Dentistry.* W. B. Saunders, Philadelphia, 1985, p 102.)

or ligaments, a small number at a time, until the tooth is loose enough to extract. Most extraction techniques begin with use of the elevator tip to cut the periodontal fibers down to the crest of the alevolar bone. The tips of the dental elevators must be sharpened, as with other precision surgical instruments. Exposure of the neck of the tooth can be facilitated by the use of a mucoperiosteal envelope flap.

One method involves pushing the tip of the elevator down into the alveolar socket.[2, 10] As the elevator moves into the periodontal ligament space, the fibers are cut around the circumference of the root, and the tooth is displaced out of the alveolus. Application of rotational pressure while the elevator tip is deep in the alveolus, parallel to the long axis of the root, is also useful in breaking the periodontal ligaments. When the root is moving freely, extraction forceps are applied to grasp the tooth, break down the remaining small fibers, and remove the tooth.

In another technique for elevator application, the elevator is placed perpendicular to the long axis of the root at the level of the alveolar crest.[6] The elevator is rotated, and the cutting edge is forced toward the tooth, producing elevation in small increments. Pressure is gradually increased and rapidly repeated. This manner of elevator application is used around the entire circumference of the tooth, elevating and lifting against the periodontal ligaments. As this technique continues, the tooth gradually loosens, and extraction forceps are applied to finish the procedure.

A third method of elevator application is indicated only for multirooted teeth.[2, 8] An elevator is inserted into the furcation, the space between the roots, so that it is perpendicular to the long axis of the root (Fig. 177–3). The elevator acts as a wedge, and when rotated as previously described, it forces the intact tooth from the alveolus.

The choice of elevators for extraction varies for each surgeon, depending on the type of patients treated, the preferred shape of the elevator tip, and the hand size of the surgeon.[15] An assortment of elevators is needed, including both pointed and flat elevator tips to cut periodontal fibers.

The apical root tip or number 78S elevator has a delicate, sharp, pointed tip on a small handle and is designed to remove apical root fragments that remain in the alveolus after root breakage (Fig. 177–4).[9] The elevator is also used to loosen and elevate small deciduous teeth prior to extraction. The sharp point permits cutting of the periodontal fibers during insertion, but because of the delicate shape of the tip, only limited rotational force can be exerted.

Extraction Forceps

Extraction forceps are also used in exodontia, to grasp the tooth after elevation and withdraw it from the alveolus. If excessive force is exerted with the extraction forceps, the tooth may break, resulting in root fragment retention.

Certain principles for the application and use of forceps have been described:[1]

1. Select the correct forceps.
2. Grasp the forceps near the ends of the handle.
3. Apply the long axis of the forceps beak parallel to the long axis of the tooth.
4. Place the forceps on the root structure.
5. Grasp the root firmly to prevent slippage.
6. Place the forcep beak so that impingement on adjacent teeth does not occur.

Extraction forceps can be used to loosen teeth in the dental alveolus before insertion of an elevator.[1] The forceps are applied to the neck of the tooth, and lingual and labial pressure is alternately applied, enlarging the alveolus. The tooth is rotated mesially and lifted from the alveolus. Some surgeons have recommended a pause

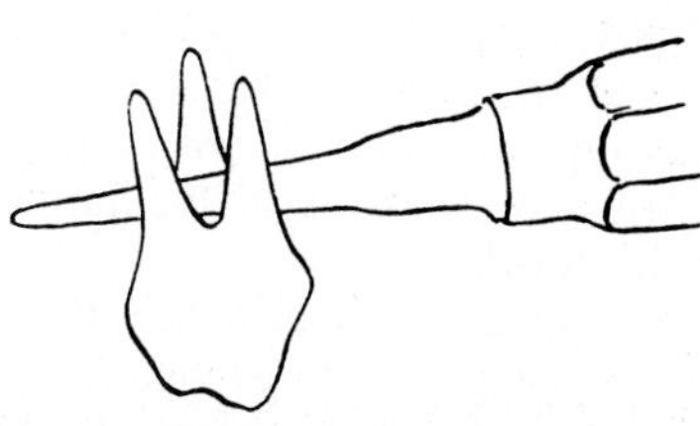

FIGURE 177–3. Tooth extraction. The neck of the root elevator is used as a wedge between roots (furcation area) of a multirooted tooth. (From Harvey CE: *Veterinary Dentistry.* W. B. Saunders, Philadelphia, 1985, p 101.)

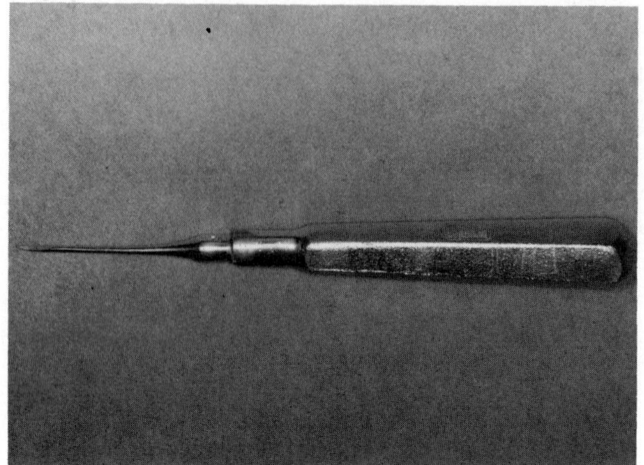

FIGURE 177–4. The apical root (number 78S) elevator is useful for extracting deciduous teeth as well for removing retained root tips. (Premier Dental Products Co., Norristown, PA.)

after the initial movement of the tooth, to allow hemorrhage into the alveolus, which places pressure on the periodontal ligaments from the apical direction.[10] The significance of this maneuver is controversial, but there is no apparent contraindication. If the initial forceps application is unsuccessful in loosening the tooth, a dental elevator used in combination with a mucoperiosteal flap facilitates exposure and loosening of the tooth.

Extraction forceps are available in a variety of shapes and sizes and are standardized by a numerical identification.[15] Common sizes include number 150 (universal upper incisor forceps) and number 151 (universal lower incisor forceps). Variations include numbers 150A and 151A, similar to numbers 150 and 151 but with beaks that do not close, and pediatric sizes 150S and 151S. Other extraction forceps with application to veterinary surgery are number 62 (universal upper and lower deciduous forceps with a straight handle) and number 101 (universal upper and lower deciduous forceps with short beaks). Because the numbers are standardized between manufacturers and suppliers, the source of the instruments is not as important as the specific instrument indicated for a certain task or operation.

Dental Drills and Burs

Dental drills, burs, and discs are used as aids in extractions. Drills and burs can aid in exposure of a tooth, especially if the tooth is firmly attached to the alveolar bone at the neck. After creating a mucoperiosteal flap, a bur on a high-speed or low-speed handpiece can be used to remove the alveolar crest and allow elevation of the tooth.

When an adequate mucoperiosteal flap is created, a bur can detach the periodontal ligaments around the alveolus. After the tooth is removed, the dental bur may be used to reduce the alveolar crest and the bone located at the furcation, the space between the roots of a multirooted tooth. This bone, called intraradicular bone, may protrude through the healed gingiva after extraction, and removal of the intraradicular bone facilitates wound closure.

A dental drill, bur, or disc can be used to divide the crown of a tooth to be extracted. A tooth crown should be divided into the same number of pieces as there are roots. Most cheek teeth in the dog and cat have two roots, the exceptions being the upper carnassial and first molar teeth of the dog, which have three roots. Different techniques for root division have been proposed, including a high-speed handpiece with burs, a low-speed handpiece with burs, and a low-speed handpiece with a diamond disc.

A dental drill and burs are used to remove root fragments retained in the alveolus after extraction.[3, 6] Roots may break off during elevation or during improper forceps application. Some teeth are more brittle, such as endodontically treated teeth or nonvital teeth, and root breakage is difficult to avoid.

An alternative to previously described extraction techniques is the use of a dental drill and burs to obliterate teeth completely. In small animals such as cats and some breeds of dogs, manipulation and leverage of teeth with elevators and extraction forceps may result in fracture of the mandible or maxilla. In crown and root pulverization, the dental bur is applied to the root remnant after the crown is removed, and the root, periodontal ligaments, and intraradicular bone are completely pulverized, leaving only the bony alveolus.[3]

Another mechanical technique that may have applications to tooth extraction is the use of high-frequency oscillation. In one report, teeth were extracted nine times faster by this method, which left no remnants of periodontal ligaments, crown fragments, or root fractures.[12]

COMPLICATIONS OF EXTRACTIONS

A variety of complications of dental extractions in the dog and cat have been described. The following six complications are the most common:[8]

1. Hemorrhage
2. Fracture of the mandible
3. Root retention
4. Necrosis of bone around extraction site
5. Oronasal fistula
6. Functional abnormalities

Hemorrhage may occur in animals with clotting abnormalities or chronic renal disease. If an animal is suspected of having a blood clotting problem, appropriate laboratory tests are performed before the extraction. Serosanguineous drainage is expected after extractions, but excessive hemorrhage is abnormal.

The problem of maxillary and mandibular fracture was noted earlier in the section on root pulverization as an alternate extraction technique. Small dogs, cats, and animals with chronic periodontal disease are at greatest risk. Fractures may be avoided by careful surgical technique and by manual support of the maxilla and mandible during the dental manipulations.

Root retention and breakage of teeth during extraction may occur because of improper elevation, underlying dental disease, caries, necrotic pulp, or previous endodontic therapy. Radiography may be advisable before extraction to detect retained roots or broken deciduous teeth. Isolated normal vital roots located below the level of surrounding bone may be covered by bone and gingiva following healing and may be difficult to identify.[14] During extraction, attempts are made to remove root remnants using an apical root tip elevator or root pulverization.

Necrosis of bone occasionally follows extraction. If the remaining alveolar socket does not form a clot, it may become a source of infection and irritation, and in extreme cases, osteomyelitis may occur. Advanced cases are called alveolar osteitis or "dry socket," and this complication is discussed later.

Oronasal fistula may occur after extraction and is usually associated with upper canine teeth or lateral incisors with advanced periodontal disease. Small, narrow-nosed dogs are at highest risk. Before extraction of these teeth is considered, a complete periodontal examination, including probing, is performed, at which time the surgeon can determine whether oronasal fistula will be a postoperative complication.

If an oronasal fistula occurs, it is best corrected using a buccal flap or a double reposition flap.[4] With either procedure, the closure should not be attempted until the surrounding tissue is sufficiently healed; this may require a period of 20 to 60 days after extraction.

Functional abnormalities are rare but can include difficult chewing or abnormal position of the lips or tongue. Most animals learn to accommodate to these changes, although occasionally reconstructive surgery of the lips may be necessary to make the animal more comfortable. Reconstructive procedures are usually performed after satisfactory recovery from the extractions.

Various other complications of extractions have been described and include the following:[1, 11]

1. Gingival abrasions, tears, and lacerations
2. Fractures of the alveolus
3. Temporomandibular joint dislocation
4. Broken instruments
5. Bacteremia and systemic infection
6. Alveolar osteitis (dry socket)

Gingival abrasions, lacerations, and tears occur when dental elevators and extraction forceps are used improperly. When an elevator is placed into the gingival sulcus, the gingiva may be torn. If this problem is anticipated, a mucoperiosteal flap should be made at the extraction site before beginning the elevation. After the tooth is extracted and the intraradicular bone is removed, the flap can be sutured across the site.

Fractures of the alveolus may be desirable if they facilitate removal of intraradicular bone. Conversely, alveolar fractures may weaken the supporting bone and lead to a complete fracture, especially of the mandible. If a fracture results from extraction, radiographs are obtained to evaluate the extent of the trauma. Conservative treatment and support are usually adequate.

Temporomandibular joint dislocation occurs in small breeds of dogs and cats when excessive force is used to elevate or extract teeth. To prevent this complication, the mandible is supported carefully with manual pressure during elevation and extraction. Temporomandibular joint dislocations are usually managed by manual reduction and support with a muzzle.

During the extraction, instruments can break within the alveolus. This problem occurs particularly with delicate instruments such as the apical root tip elevator. Leverage must not be applied with delicate instruments, as retrieval of a broken instrument from the alveolus is difficult. If an instrument is broken, the piece is retrieved by root pulverization or by preparation of a mucoperiosteal flap with an apical approach.

Bacteremia and septicemia have been reported as probable complications to dental extraction.[16] In one case, this problem occurred when general dental prophylaxis and associated extractions were performed in conjunction with an exploratory laparotomy. This dog had not received an antibiotic and died 8 hours after the operation. At necropsy, diffuse fibrinous peritonitis, chronic glomerulonephritis, and endocarditis were identified. Given this case and other unpublished reports, surgical procedures should probably not be performed in conjunction with dental prophylaxis and extraction. If the two procedures must be performed concurrently, appropriate administration of an antibiotic is indicated.

Alveolar osteitis is an extension of one of the previous complications, necrosis of bone at the extraction site. This condition is also known as fibrinolytic alveolitis, alveolitis sicca dolorosa, or dry socket, and it is commonly reported after human oral surgery. It usually starts about 48 hours after extraction of a mandibular tooth (usually a molar) and is characterized by excruciating pain, absence of normal blood clot in the wound, and a foul odor in the mouth. The usual causes in humans are as follows:

1. Insufficient blood supply
2. Excess trauma to the site
3. Dense bone
4. Local infiltration with vasoconstrictors
5. Abnormal blood clotting
6. Clot disruption by irrigation, sucking, or chewing
7. Smoking

Specific reports of this condition in animals are not found, although necrosis of bone at the surgical site has been suggested as a complication.[8] The actual incidence of this complication in veterinary surgery is difficult to establish because of the lack of careful observation of the oral cavity following extractions. One reason for the lower incidence in veterinary dentistry is that oral wounds heal more rapidly in the dog because of canine saliva.[9]

Recent reports have placed greater emphasis on increased fibrinolytic activity of blood as a primary cause of this problem in humans, hence the name *fibrinolytic alveolitis.*[11] In one report, fibrinolytic activity of blood in patients undergoing oral surgery was compared preoperatively and postoperatively, and patients developing alveolitis sicca showed a significant increase in fibrinolytic activity after extractions, suggesting one predisposing factor.[7] The significance of this report for animals is unknown; however, the increase in the number of dogs identified with blood clotting problems should alert the surgeon to the possibility of this complication.

Various techniques have been recommended to reduce the incidence of infections and alveolar osteitis following extraction. One report recommends soluble tetracycline powder applied topically to the extraction sites during surgery.[15] Other materials including soluble gelatin sponge (Gelfoam) and oxidized regenerated cellulose (Surgicel) have been advocated as biological dressings, and polylactic acid shows promise in preventing alveolar osteitis.[13]

References

1. Archer WH: *Oral and Maxillofacial Surgery*. 5th ed. W. B. Saunders, Philadelphia, 1975.
2. Blogg R: Exodontia in the dog. *Aust Vet J 39*:57, 1963.
3. Bojrab MJ, Tholen M: *Small Animal Oral Medicine and Surgery*. Lea & Febiger, Philadelphia, 1990.
4. Ellison GW, et al: A double reposition flap technique for repair of recurrent oronasal fistulas in dogs. *J Am Anim Hosp Assoc 22*:803, 1986.
5. Fisfis NH, et al: Use of a dental drill in extracting the fourth premolar tooth in dogs. *Vet Med Small Anim Clin 67*:879, 1972.
6. Frost P (ed): Dentistry. *Vet Clin North Am 16*:967, 1986.
7. Gersel-Pedersen N: Blood fibrinolytic activity before and after oral surgery. *Int J Oral Surg 6*:42, 1977.
8. Harvey CE: *Veterinary Dentistry*. W. B. Saunders, Philadelphia, 1985.
9. Huebasch RF, Hansen LS: A histopathologic study of extraction wounds in dogs. *Oral Surg Oral Med Oral Pathol 28*:187, 1969.
10. Kaplan ML, Jeffcoat MK: A tooth extraction procedure: Exodontia for veterinarians. *Canine Pract 7*:33, May-June 1980.
11. Levine N (ed): *Current Treatment in Dental Practice*. W. B. Saunders, Philadelphia, 1975.
12. Muman ED, Miller AS: The application of a frequency oscillation method for tooth extraction in dogs. *Lab Anim Sci 25*:228, 1975.
13. Olsen RAJ, et al: A comparative study of polylactic acid, Gelfoam, and Surgicel in healing extraction sites. *Oral Surg Oral Med Oral Path 53*:441, 1982.
14. Plata RL, Pellon EE: Intentional retention of vital submerged roots in dogs. *Oral Surg Oral Med Oral Path 42*:100, 1976.
15. Preisch SD: The effect of tetracycline on the incidence of postextraction alveolar osteitis. *J Oral Maxillofac Surg 45*:1029, 1987.
16. Withrow SJ: Dental extraction as a probable cause of septicemia in the dog. *J Am Anim Hosp Assoc 15*:345, 1979.

CHAPTER 178 Periodontal Disease

T. Keith Grove

Periodontal disease is an oral infection that results from the chronic retention of bacteria at the junction of the tooth and the gingiva.[12, 15] When bacteria are present for about 1 week, the soft tissue surrounding the teeth (the gingiva) becomes acutely inflamed. The term *gingivitis* refers to swelling, redness, tenderness, and bleeding in the soft tissue around the tooth. It can be resolved by removing accumulated bacteria from the neck of the tooth. Gingivitis alone does not cause loss of support around the teeth. Gingivitis often becomes chronic in dogs and cats because periodic tooth cleaning is not practiced. It may remain without progressing into more severe disease, or periodontitis may follow.

Periodontitis may develop around teeth with gingivitis because of the chronic presence of bacterial products around the teeth. Periodontitis involves deep inflammation, loss of supporting alveolar bone, and destruction of fibrous connective tissue attachment at the neck of the tooth. It is usually a slowly progressive asymptomatic infection that causes tooth loss by destruction of tooth supporting tissue rather than the tooth itself.

Treatment of periodontal disease is primarily surgical. Medical treatment to counter bacterial infection and eliminate destructive inflammation shows promise but requires root débridement to be effective. Further surgical treatment improves access to the roots, removes offending roots that cannot be treated, or regenerates support that was lost because of periodontitis.

EXAMINATION

Changes in color and contour of the gingiva suggest periodontal disease. Nonpigmented gingiva is a uniform coral pink. Red and purple areas signify inflammation and arouse suspicion that gingivitis, and perhaps periodontitis, are present.

Swelling of the gingival margin is another early indicator of periodontal disease. The healthy gingival margin is sharp and tight against the neck of the tooth. Swelling of a fluid or fibrotic nature in the attached gingiva is a sign of more extensive inflammation around the teeth and suggests periodontitis (Fig. 178–1).

With gingivitis, there is an increase in the flow of fluid from the gingival crevice as well as a tendency to bleed when the gingival margin is touched lightly with an instrument. Teeth with periodontitis show a similar tendency to bleed when probed underneath the gingival margin and may exhibit a purulent exudate from the gingival space.

Periodontitis that has destroyed support for the teeth can be seen on dental radiographs as resorption of bone around the neck of the tooth (Fig. 178–2). Normally, the interdental bone is within 1 to 2 mm of the cementoenamel junction, and the inter-radicular bone completely fills the space between roots. Epithelium attaches at the cementoenamel junction for at least 1 mm, and at least 1 mm of connective tissue exists between alveolar

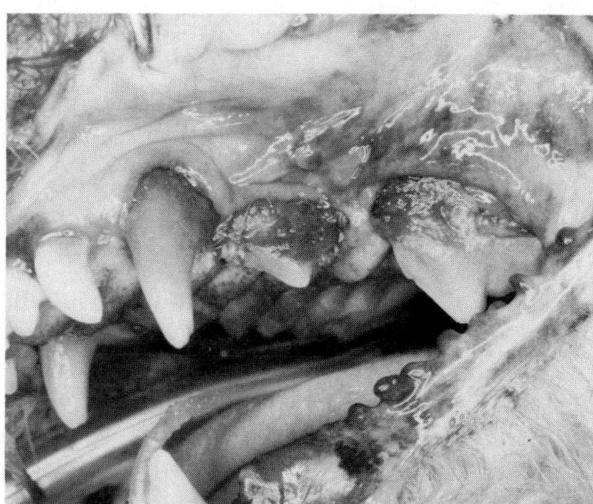

FIGURE 178–1. Photograph of dog with advanced periodontitis shows accumulation of debris, recession, and soft-tissue inflammation.

bone and epithelium (Fig. 178–3). Radiographs showing that bone support has receded more than 2 mm from the cementoenamel junction usually indicate periodontitis.

The periodontal probe is the cornerstone for examination and diagnosis of periodontal disease. This thin probe is calibrated in millimeters at the tip. This instrument measures the depth of the gingival crevice when it is inserted between the gingiva and tooth (Fig. 178–4). It can measure the distance between the gingival margin and the cementoenamel junction, assess the firmness of the gingiva, and evaluate the flow and character of fluid from the gingival space. A periodontal chart can be created to indicate anatomical changes associated with disease and to describe the severity of inflammation.

Commonly, periodontal charting begins with drawing the relationship of the free gingival margin to the cementoenamel junction on a diagram of the teeth. The depth of the gingival crevice is measured, and a second line is drawn that is apical to the free gingival margin. The second line is the attachment level, the anatomical point at which the periodontium and the tooth are attached. When this distance is greater than 2 mm below the cementoenamel junction, loss of periodontal attachment has occurred.

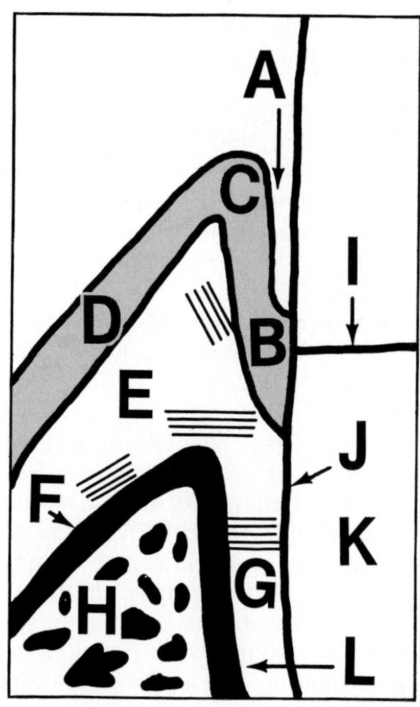

FIGURE 178–3. Diagram demonstrating cervical relationships of normal dental and periodontal anatomy. (A, gingival space (crevice); B, epithelial attachment; C, free gingival margin; D, attached gingiva; E, gingival connective tissue; F, outer cortical plate of alveolar process; G, periodontal ligament; H, medullary bone; I, cementoenamel junction; J, cementum; K, radicular dentin; L, alveolar bone.)

When bleeding or purulent exudate is observed on probing, a mark is placed on the chart to indicate active periodontal disease. Serial periodontal chartings demonstrate progress or resolution of inflammation and are useful in determining prognosis.

DIAGNOSIS

When the gingiva is inflamed but no loss of tissue attachment to the root has occurred, the diagnosis is gingivitis. Gingivitis can be described as subclinical (histological changes and increased fluid production only), marginal (affecting the gingival margin only),

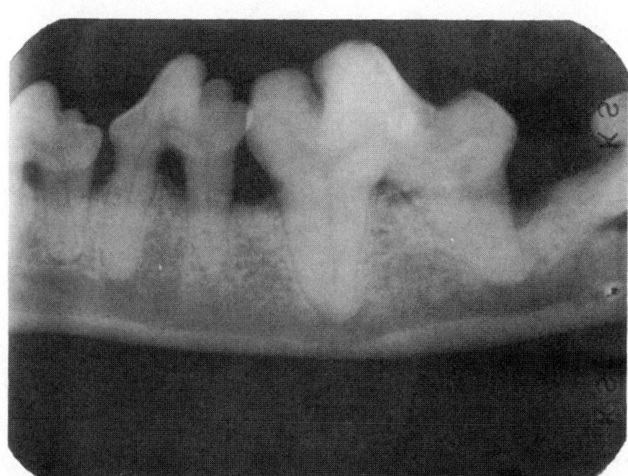

FIGURE 178–2. Radiograph of a dog with periodontitis shows loss of bone around teeth due to periodontitis.

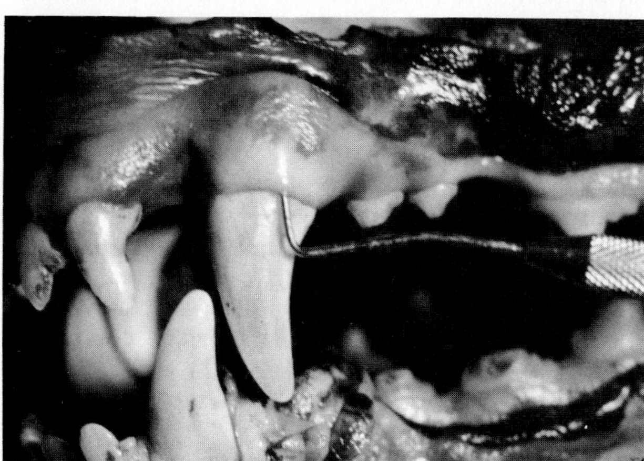

FIGURE 178–4. Probe inserted into the gingival space to measure and evaluate it for inflammation.

acute (short duration and acute inflammation), or chronic (long duration with chronic inflammatory infiltrate).

Periodontitis involves loss of attachment (loss of tooth-supporting tissue) and inflammation in supporting tissue deeper than the gingiva. To diagnose periodontitis, loss of attachment and inflammation must be demonstrated. Periodontitis is incipient (beginning loss of attachment), mild (< 25 per cent support loss), moderate (> 25 per cent < 50 per cent support loss), or severe (> 50 per cent support loss). Thus, gingivitis may be diagnosed on visual examination based on change in tissue color, but a diagnosis of periodontitis requires measurement.

The overall diagnosis of gingivitis or periodontitis may be further modified to provide a better description of the pathogenesis or behavior of the periodontal disease process in that patient. Thus, the term *rapidly progressive periodontitis* may describe severe lesions in young patients, *hormonal gingivitis* may describe increased inflammation in pregnant patients, and so forth. In human patients, subgroups of the population have been identified as exhibiting varying presentations of periodontal disease.

TREATMENT

Preventive Therapy

Periodontal disease is preventable if the teeth can be kept clean. Hygiene is important for all patients. Initiation of hygiene control in patients at sexual maturity represents good preventive medicine. Toothbrushing, antiseptic mouth rinses, and regular professional prophylaxis are recommended to keep the teeth clean to prevent disease.

Systemic Phase

Systemic problems that predispose patients to periodontal disease must be identified. Diabetes mellitus due to defects in neutrophil function decreases the patient's resistance to periodontal infection. All animals should have a physical examination and appropriate laboratory testing to ensure that systemic problems do not affect the successful surgical treatment of periodontal disease. When identified, systemic diseases that require treatment are resolved before surgery.

Hygiene Phase

Initial periodontal treatment involves removing plaque and calculus from the teeth above and below the gingival margin. This treatment allows some resolution of inflammation and, depending on the degree of damage, may be sufficient to control periodontal disease.[9]

Ultrasonic scaling along with copious water irrigation is the fastest method of removing gross accretions from the teeth. A universal tip can be used to reach most areas. The instrument is held with a pen grasp and moved lightly up and down the surface of the tooth to avoid overheating or gouging the surface. Because the root surface is softer than the crown, it is important not to use the point of the instrument against the root. After all visible calculus, plaque, and stain are removed, the instrument is inserted to the depth of the gingival space. It is withdrawn at each stroke to remove dislodged debris. When the surface of the tooth feels smooth and clean, ultrasonic débridement is complete.

After ultrasonic scaling, the root is probed with a number 17 explorer to identify residual roughness or calculus that was missed. These areas are smoothed with a number 13 or number 14 Columbia curette until they feel hard and even (Fig. 178–5). Particular attention is paid to feeling for calculus in the furcations, at the cementoenamel junction, at the depth of the gingival space, and at the line angles (e.g., rostral-buccal or caudal-lingual surface) of the teeth, as these are the areas where most operators miss calculus.[5]

After being thoroughly cleaned and smoothed by scaling and root planing, the teeth are polished. Smooth surfaces accumulate less debris and are easier to clean in the future because the calculus cannot interlock mechanically with the tooth. The prophylaxis angle attached to a slow-speed handpiece polishes efficiently. Polishing occurs slightly under the gingival margin if a rubber cup is loaded with polishing paste and pressed gently against the tooth as it rotates in the handpiece. The teeth remain moist during polishing to minimize overheating.

After the cleaning, the mouth is irrigated, and the patient is discharged with a 2-week supply of 0.1 to 0.2 per cent chlorhexidine solution. Owners are instructed to rinse the mouth twice daily for 30 seconds with this solution to allow healing with minimal bacterial

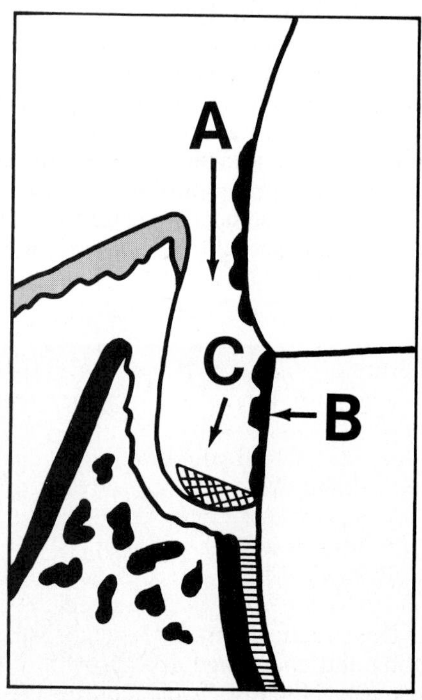

FIGURE 178–5. Curette engaging the root surface at the bottom of a periodontal pocket to begin planing the root smooth and clean after gross scaling with an ultrasonic cleaner. (A, periodontal pocket; B, calculus and debris; C, curette in cross section.)

contamination.[16, 21] Toothbrushing can begin the day after cleaning. A hard diet is offered because it decreases plaque mass on teeth.

About 1 month after cleaning, re-evaluation should occur, and any periodontal surgery necessary can take place. The healing that occurs during the month after thorough cleaning may be enough to resolve the gingival inflammation and the bleeding on probing. Even when pocket depth is greater than 5 mm at re-evaluation, surgery is not necessary if bleeding on probing and inflammation have resolved. Gums that are no longer inflamed are cleaned in 3 to 6 months. Many animals respond to this therapy.

Surgical Phase

Surgery is indicated when pocket depth is 5 mm or greater and bleeding on probing does not resolve after thorough tooth cleaning.[13] It may also be indicated for soft-tissue and bone grafts. Most surgical patients have deep pockets with inflammation after tooth cleaning and re-examination in 1 month. In general, opening the area by surgery provides better access to the root surface so that hidden calculus can be exposed to view and removed.[5] If residual inflammation is present after scaling and if the initiating calculus can be identified and removed without surgery, surgery is unnecessary. The initiating factors for periodontal disease are on the root surface, not in the soft tissue; therefore, soft-tissue surgery in itself is not corrective.

Inverse-Bevel Repositioned Flaps for Root Débridement

The goal of inverse-bevel repositioned flaps is to reflect the soft tissue away from the teeth, remove granulation tissue around the roots, and thoroughly clean the roots down to the periodontal attachment. This procedure eliminates etiological factors associated with inflammation.[3]

The procedure starts with an incision in the gingival crevice, beginning at the free gingival margin and extending to the alveolar crest (Fig. 178–6). The incision is extended around all affected teeth in that area and connected interdentally so that buccal and lingual flaps can be raised (Fig. 178–7). A sharp periosteal elevator is used to reflect the soft tissue past the mucogingival junction. Granulation tissue is removed from the underside of the flap with curettes, scissors, or tissue nippers. The roots are irrigated, surrounding granulation tissue is removed, and all calculus and root roughness are eliminated with curettes. Simple interrupted 3-0 sutures are used to oppose flap edges between the teeth, and the flaps are returned to their former level (hence the term *repositioned*). Moist gauze is compressed against the gingiva, which adapts the underside of the flap to the teeth. This practice eliminates dead space that could delay healing and encourage downgrowth of epithelium into the space. Nonabsorbable sutures, if used, are removed in 7 days.

During the first 2 weeks after surgery, the dentogingival junction is irrigated with 0.1 to 0.2 per cent chlorhexidine twice daily for 30 seconds. Although resolution of inflammation ordinarily occurs after periodontal surgery, the accumulation of bacteria on the teeth eventually re-establishes inflammation in the area. Surgical patients should undergo tooth cleaning every 3 to 12 months, depending on inflammatory level, to prevent recurrence. Owners are encouraged to brush the patient's teeth daily and provide a hard diet or chew toys to aid debris removal. All periodontal surgery patients are treated the same postoperatively, despite differences in the surgical procedure. When compliance with home care and recall for scaling are not expected, surgery is not performed. Rather, thorough cleanings are scheduled on a regular basis.

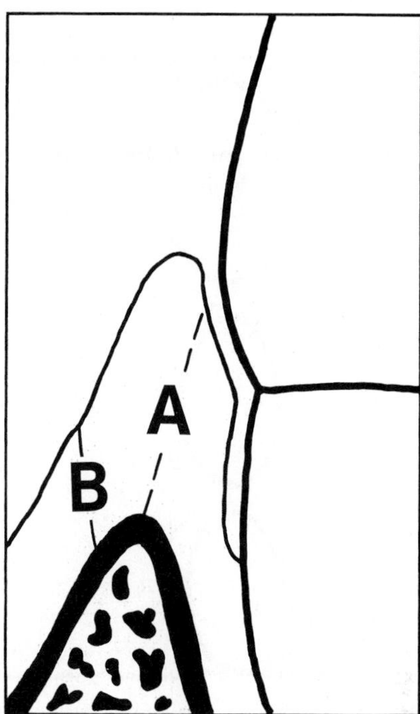

FIGURE 178–6. Incisions used in flap surgery. (A, inverse-bevel intrasulcular incision; B, inverse-bevel incision for apically positioned flap.)

Inverse-Bevel Apically Positioned Flaps for Pocket Reduction

Inverse-bevel apically positioned flaps are indicated to expose the root surface, decrease pocket depth, and increase the amount of attached gingiva. They are produced by making an incision around the neck of the teeth 1 to 3 mm away from the free gingival margin (see Fig. 178–6). This incision is directed toward the alveolar process so that it undermines the gingiva adjacent to the tooth. Other operations are similar to inverse-bevel repositioned flaps for root débridement except that the edges of the flap are returned to just above the alveolar crest, rather than repositioned to the former location. This apical placement of the free gingival margin eliminates soft-tissue pockets and reduces the depth of intrabony pockets that have a pronounced soft-tissue component above them. Also, the mucogingival junction is

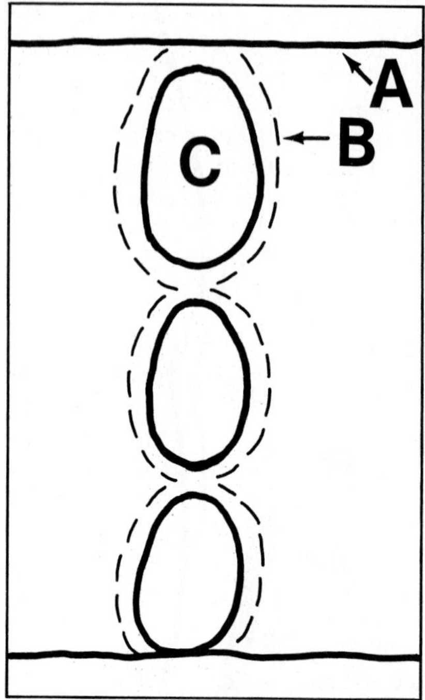

FIGURE 178–7. Occlusal view of three caudal teeth and incision outline for flap surgery (incision line is drawn at the level of the alveolar crest—not the free gingiva). (A, vertical releasing incisions [if necessary for exposure]; B, incision around the teeth; C, occlusal view of teeth.)

apically positioned, increasing the amount of attached gingiva around the teeth. Postoperative care is the same as for other periodontal surgery.

Osseous Flap Surgery

Osseous flap surgery is similar to inverse-bevel flap surgery except that it is intended as an approach for bone surgery. The goal is to eliminate pockets that have a bony margin by resecting the alveolar bone or the alveolar process that is irregular in contour. Thus, the primary difference between this operation and other flap operations is that it involves bone removal. No better prognosis has been reported with pocket elimination.[10] This operation is seldom used except for treating deep pockets with intractable inflammation below the bony crest that borders them. Osseous flap surgery is performed primarily for access, and ledges of bone are removed with chisels, rongeurs, or carbide burs (Fig. 178–8). When supporting bone is removed, the operation is called ostectomy. When nonsupporting bone is removed to eliminate pockets by improving flap adaptation, the procedure is called osteoplasty. Postoperative care is the same as for other periodontal surgery.

Crown Lengthening

When teeth are fractured below the gingival margin, normal tooth structure must be exposed to allow an accurate restoration. This operation involves removing bone and soft tissue to reposition the margins of a flap below the fracture line. It is also used on resorptive lesions in cats ("neck lesions") to restore teeth damaged by root resorption. Flap elevation is the same as reverse-bevel flap surgery, but bone is removed so that apical positioning of the flap allows supragingival exposure of the fracture line. The flap may need to be thinned at the margins to avoid excessive bone removal. The fracture line is at least 5 mm above the bone crest to allow connective-tissue attachment and epithelial adhesion over bone. Failure to leave enough space between bone and restorative margins predisposes the patient to poor healing. Postoperative care is the same as for other periodontal surgery.

Gingivectomy

Gingivectomy eliminates periodontal pockets through excision of excessive tissue above the alveolar crest. It is indicated when excessive tissue can be removed without creating abnormal gingival tissue contour. Pockets extending below the alveolar crest contraindicate gingivectomy when tissue removal would result in abnormal "reverse" architecture that would accumulate debris. The operation is begun by marking the depth of the pocket on the attached gingiva by applying pressure with a periodontal probe. The incision is started below the marks and is directed toward the depth of the pocket on the tooth. The resected tissue is removed with tissue nippers and curettes, the area is irrigated, and the roots are cleaned. Postoperative care is the same as for flap surgery.

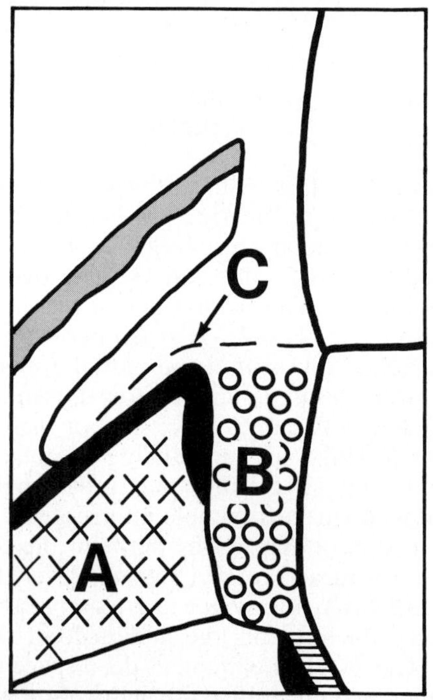

FIGURE 178–8. Alternatives for management of intrabony periodontal pockets after flap exposure. (A, osteoplasty to remove bony wall of pocket [X]; B, implanting bone or alloplastic material [O]; C, membrane placement [---] to exclude gingival tissue during healing.)

Gingivoplasty

Gingivoplasty reshapes the gingiva. The operation is the same as for gingivectomy except that the intent is to create normal tissue contour rather than to resect soft-tissue pockets. It is useful in treating gingival hyperplasia in which the gingiva needs to be recontoured (Fig. 178–9). Postoperative care is the same as for other periodontal surgery.

Recurrence of gingival hyperplasia indicates repetition of the operation at a later date. Patients that accumulate plaque and calculus postoperatively frequently have regrowth of excessive tissue.

Mucogingival Surgery

Mucogingival surgery increases the amount of attached gingiva or repositions the attached gingiva and alveolar mucosa. It is indicated when periodontal inflammation persists after cleaning because of an inadequate barrier of attached gingiva between alveolar mucosa and the periodontal attachment to the tooth. Dehiscences over roots caused by chewing hard objects and irritating restorations may create a need for mucogingival treatment. Pedicle flap surgery and soft-tissue grafts are types of mucogingival surgery.

Pedicle Flap Surgery. Gingival recession over prominent roots may be treated by rotating a pedicle of adjacent attached gingiva to the denuded area.[14] First, the margins of the defect are removed to expose gingival connective tissue. Next, a pedicle is created, allowing a full-thickness mucoperiosteal flap to be placed over the defect. Occasionally, a frenulum must be cut to keep lip movement from displacing a pedicle. The risk of displacement can be evaluated by tugging on the lip and looking for evidence of tension on the pedicle. When necessary, the frenulum is incised down to bone to relieve the tension. The margins are sutured, and the postoperative management is the same as for other types of periodontal surgery.

Soft-Tissue Grafts. Soft tissue may be harvested from one area of the mouth and transferred to bone or connective tissue in another area to increase tissue at the new site. The recipient area is denuded by sharp dissection and periosteal removal. Next, a donor site is chosen. The mucoperiosteum removed from the recipient site and aluminum foil are used as a template to harvest a partial-thickness (at least 2 mm thick) graft of connective tissue. The graft is sutured to the recipient site with simple interrupted sutures (4-0 or less). Wet gauze is used to apply pressure adapting the graft to the recipient bone for 1 minute to eliminate dead space. These grafts survive by plasmatic circulation the first week and must be sutured to intimate contact with the bed. When epithelium is transferred, it sloughs during the first 10 days. The lamina propria confers keratinizing potential on the graft. The keratinizing nature of the lamina propria is genetically determined and survives in its new location to influence the character of epithelium that migrates over it. As with pedicle grafts, interfering frenums may be resected to eliminate motion between the graft and the bed. Postoperative care is the same as for other periodontal surgery except that care is taken to ensure that the graft is not dislodged from the recipient site by vigorous irrigation or by chewing hard objects.

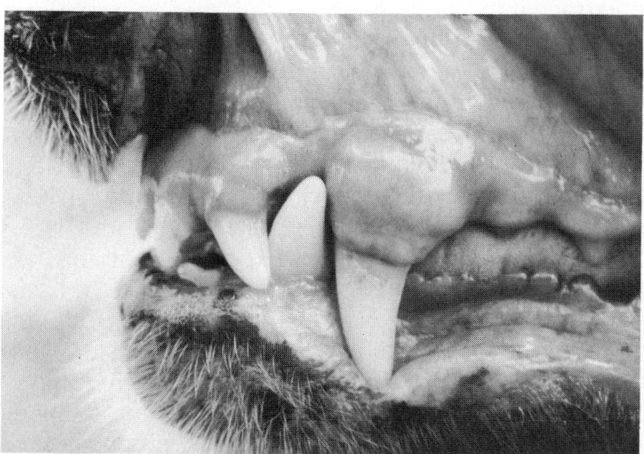

FIGURE 178–9. Fibrotic gingiva without pocket formation. This condition may indicate gingivoplasty if the area is becoming inflamed because of debris retention caused by poor contour.

Reconstructive Surgery for Intrabony and Furcation Defects

Bone and Alloplastic Implants. Bone may be harvested from the patient (autograft), another member of the same species (allograft), or a different species (xenograft) and used as a framework for defect closure in the host periodontium.[17] Crushed oral cancellous bone or frozen red marrow from the same individual is most effective in stimulating regeneration of new support. Bone morphogenic protein theoretically induces bone growth and occurs in its largest usable concentration in bone grafts. Freeze-dried bone grafts from other individuals of the same species have been successful and provide a source for graft material that does not require a second surgical operation. Concern over the transfer of disease and immunological intolerance may make this method of acquiring graft material less desirable.

Alloplastic (synthetic) materials can also form a scaffold for bone growth. Processed coral, nonresorbable synthetic hydroxyapatite, resorbable hydroxyapatite, and beta tricalcium phosphate are used for bone implants.

Placing of a bone graft or implant is initiated by inverse-bevel flap exposure. The soft tissue in the bone defect is removed, the roots are cleaned, and the defect is filled with the chosen material (see Fig. 178–8). The flaps are carefully adapted to the teeth, and the patient is administered tetracycline for 3 weeks, because complete wound closure and use of antibiotics enhance graft success.[20] Chlorhexidine solution is used to irrigate the mouth for the first 2 weeks postoperatively, to decrease bacterial contamination of the graft site. Evaluation of results requires about 1 year, with many cases not exhibiting maximum radiographic bone growth until that time.

Guided Tissue Regeneration. When gingival connective tissue and epithelium can be excluded from healing defects in the bone or furcation, progenitor cells from bone or periodontal tissues are used to repopulate the defect.[7] This process results in greater regeneration of the defect with return to normal structure.[6, 8, 18, 19] When these tissues are not excluded from the healing defect, such as occurs in conventional flap surgery, defects rarely fill with bone and periodontal ligament.

The operation begins with elevation of a mucoperiosteal flap. The bone defect or defect in the furcation area is débrided and the exposed roots are cleaned. Decalcifying the root surface with citric acid for 3 minutes has been effective in dogs to promote new attachment between healing periodontal tissue and the tooth. Decalcification cleans and detoxifies the root surface, exposing collagen in the dentin.[2, 22] All cementum must be removed for the dentin collagen to be exposed by citric acid; this removal is usually accomplished by thorough root planing. Tetracycline can be used as an acid to decalcify the root surface.[11] One 250-mg capsule of tetracycline hydrochloride is dissolved in 5 ml of water, and this solution (with pH of 1) is applied for 3 minutes to the root surface with a paintbrush. Tetracycline may also have some local antibiotic effect when used in this manner.[1] After the root surface is prepared, the defect may be implanted with bone or alloplastic material. Implants added to defects before membrane placement improve the amount of defect filling compared with placement of a membrane only.

Gore-Tex* may be used for this purpose and is highly inert. This membrane has been developed for use in human teeth and is commercially available. The membrane is trimmed to cover the defect plus 2 mm of surrounding bone, and it is then sutured tightly around the root surface (see Fig. 178–8).

The flaps are replaced and sutured interdentally. Oral chlorhexidine rinses are used for 2 weeks, and systemic tetracycline is administered for 3 weeks. The membrane is removed with a gentle tug in 4 to 6 weeks. Daily home care and professional supragingival cleaning every 3 months for the first year are suggested. This operation is suggested for regenerating deep intrabony defects on the palatal surface of maxillary canine teeth, where defects may extend to the nasal mucosa.

Maintenance Therapy

Although most surgical therapy for periodontal disease is initially successful in decreasing inflammation, and perhaps in regenerating lost tooth support, active involvement in an appropriate maintenance program is required for continued success. Each patient has different requirements for how often the dentition must be professionally cleaned. Variations are due to differences in disease severity at the beginning of therapy, disparity in owner compliance with daily home hygiene, and dissimilarities in host resistance to infection.

One way to establish an appropriate recall interval is to re-examine treated patients at 3-month intervals. If the clinician recognizes established gingivitis and bleeding on subgingival probing, the dentition is cleaned, and a new appointment is made for 1 month. If the gingiva is healthy 1 month after cleaning, the recall interval is appropriate for maintenance therapy to resolve recurrent gingivitis. If the gingiva is unhealthy or if loss of attachment has occurred since the last cleaning, the recall interval must be shortened. Most animals with severe periodontitis require cleaning approximately every 6 months. Animals that have not lost much attachment often do well with annual cleaning.

Maintenance cleaning differs from initial therapy in that subgingival scaling and root planing are not necessary in noninflamed gingival units; however, supragingival scaling with inspection of the subgingival environment for bleeding is required. Only those areas that bleed are scaled and root-planed subgingivally, because repeated root planing may initiate slight loss of gingival attachment. All teeth are polished, and for 2 weeks, 0.1 to 0.2 per cent chlorhexidine rinses are used twice daily for 30 seconds.

Periodontal charting to determine areas of increased disease activity is helpful in following patients after treatment. Measurements taken during recall scaling are compared with initial status; loss of more than 2 mm of attachment, as evaluated by clinical probing, is significant and indicates deteriorating status. Radiographs can be used in chronologically evaluating the attachment level on the rostral and caudal surfaces of teeth. Maintenance-phase radiographs can be compared with initial radiographs. Where additional loss of bone support can be appreciated, the disease has progressed.

Management of Combined Periodontal and Endodontic Lesions

Therapy becomes more complicated when the roots are not uniformly affected by periodontal disease and certain ones have advanced disease, or when endodontic lesions are present on teeth that require periodontal therapy (see Chapter 179).

Roots so severely affected by periodontal disease that they are painful or cause periodic abscess should be removed. Often, bone loss on multirooted teeth is similar on all roots. When little periodontal attachment remains, the offending tooth is extracted. When a multirooted tooth has one or more roots that are solid with little bone loss, the decision is more difficult. The choice of whether to retain a tooth because it has a good root or extract it because it has a bad root is a dilemma. When the tooth is not valuable, extraction is best, because comfortable retention of a bad root is probably not possible without special attention.

When a tooth is considered valuable (e.g., the maxillary fourth premolar in dogs) but has a hopelessly affected root, the surgeon can amputate the involved root and allow the tooth to survive. The tooth is first treated endodontically to prevent pain, contamination of the remaining canals with bacteria, and retarded periodontal healing, which might occur if the root were amputated first.[23] In general, the division of the roots must be exposed with a flap unless severe gingival recession has occurred in that area. The root is severed with a high-speed fissured bur at the point where it extends from the tooth. The surrounding area is smoothed into the general contour of the tooth so that no irregularities of the previous root remain. The tooth

*WL Gore & Assoc., Inc. Flagstaff, AZ.

must be treated by conventional endodontic techniques in all the remaining roots, and a filling, similar to that used for apical surgery in endodontics, is used to close the root canal space over the amputated root. The flap is replaced, and postoperative care is the same as for other periodontal surgery.

Periodontal Prosthesis

When attachment loss has been extensive and mobility of teeth prevents mastication without pain, the surgeon can join teeth together and use their combined support to avoid discomfort. Teeth selected for this procedure should have noninflamed periodontal status, increased mobility, and radiographic signs of secondary occlusal trauma. Individual crowns are constructed for the involved teeth, and these are joined together by soldered or cast joints. The splint is cemented as a unit to the involved teeth. Although this procedure does not change the mobility of individual teeth permanently, it does decrease mobility of the splinted section to a lesser degree.

Another indication for splinting teeth together with a prosthesis is food impaction. Food may become impacted between loose-touching teeth (teeth without proper tight interdental contact) by the opposing dentition. The impacted material can tear the periodontal attachment and initiate chronic periodontitis, which may lead to tooth loss. These teeth can be joined together with cast crowns, which prevent food impaction.

References

1. Al-Ali W, et al: The effect of local doxycycline with and without tricalcium phosphate on the regenerative healing potential of periodontal osseous defects in dogs. *J Periodontol 60*:582, 1989.
2. Albair WB, et al: Connective tissue attachment to periodontally diseased roots after citric acid demineralization. *J Periodontol 53*:515, 1982.
3. Ammons WF, Smith DH: Flap curettage: Rationale, technique, and expectations. *Dent Clin North Am 20*:215, 1976.
4. Becker W, et al: Periodontal treatment without maintenance: A retrospective study in 44 patients. *J Periodontol 55*:505, 1984.
5. Brayer WK, et al: Scaling and root planing effectiveness: The effect of root surface access and operator experience. *J Periodontol 60*:67, 1989.
6. Card SJ, et al: New attachment following the use of a resorbable membrane in the treatment of periodontitis in dogs. *Int J Periodont Restor Dent 9*:58, 1989.
7. Caton JG, et al: Periodontal regeneration via selective cell repopulation. *J Periodontol 58*:546, 1987.
8. Claffey N, et al: Placement of a porous membrane underneath the mucoperiosteal flap and its effect on periodontal wound healing in dogs. *J Clin Periodontol 16*:12, 1989.
9. *Consensus Report Discussion, Section II. World Workshop in Periodontics.* American Academy of Periodontology, Chicago, 1989, p II-15.
10. *Consensus Report Discussion, Section IV. World Workshop in Periodontics.* American Academy of Periodontology, Chicago, 1989, p IV-24.
11. Frantz B, Polson A: Tissue interactions with dentin specimens after demineralization using tetracycline. *J Periodontol 59*:714, 1988.
12. Grove TK: Periodontal disease. *Comp Cont Educ Pract Vet 4*:564, 1982.
13. Grove T: Periodontal therapy. *J Cont Educ Pract Vet 5*:660, 1983.
14. Hoag PM: Isolate areas of gingival recession: Etiology and treatment. *Calif Dent Soc Rev 72*:27, 1979.
15. Loe H, et al: Experimental gingivitis in man. *J Periodont 36*:177, 1965.
16. Killoy WJ: Quantity, nature, and time required for reccurrence of the microbial mass irrigated from the periodontal pocket. *J Am Soc Prev Dent 6*:17, 1976.
17. Mellonig JT: Bone grafts in periodontal therapy. *N Y State Dent J 52*:27, 1986.
18. Niederman R, et al: Regeneration of furca bone using Gore-Tex periodontal material. *Int J Periodont Restor Dent 9*:469, 1989.
19. Pfeifer J, et al: Epithelial exclusion and tissue regeneration using a collagen membrane barrier in chronic periodontal defects: A histological study. *Int J Periodont Restor Dent 9*:263, 1989.
20. Sanders JJ, et al: Clinical evaluation of freeze-dried bone allografts in periodontal osseous defects. Part II. Composite freeze-dried bone allografts with and without autogenous bone grafts. *J Periodontol 54*:1–8, 1983.
21. Southard SR, et al: The effect of 2% chlorhexidine digluconate irrigation on clinical parameters and the level of *Bacteroides gingivalis* in periodontal pockets. *J Periodontol 60*:302, 1989.
22. Tanaka K, et al: The effect of citric acid on retained plaque and calculus. *J Periodontol 60*:81, 1989.
23. Weine FS, et al: Endodontic emergency treatment following root amputation in periodontally involved teeth. *J Periodontol 41*:391, 1970.

CHAPTER 179 Endodontics and Root Canal Therapy

T. Keith Grove

Endodontic therapy is needed to retain a tooth with a necrotic pulp. The term *endodontics* refers to treatment inside the tooth. Therapy deals with the dental pulp—a specialized connective tissue containing unmyelinated nerves that sense only pain, blood vessels that nurture the odontoblasts lining the pulp cavity, and lymphatic vessels. The structures of the pulp have their primary role during tooth development. After the tooth is formed, the pulp is not essential to the function of the tooth, although teeth without vital pulp tissue may be less resilient and more prone to fracture. Thus, endodontic therapy is treatment of diseased pulp to allow preservation of affected teeth.

Fracture into the pulp is the most common indication for endodontic therapy in dogs (Figs. 179–1 and 179–2). Dental resorption is the most common indication in cats. Unlike in humans, dental caries is rarely an indication for endodontics in either dogs or cats.

Although no immediate loss of function usually occurs when the dental pulp is exposed to the oral cavity, many teeth with endodontic lesions, in time, are lost prematurely, affect adjacent structures adversely, or become painful. Early endodontic therapy on teeth with pulp disease can be used to retain these teeth in comfort as functional units. The sooner treatment is delivered after the initial endodontic insult, the more likely it will be

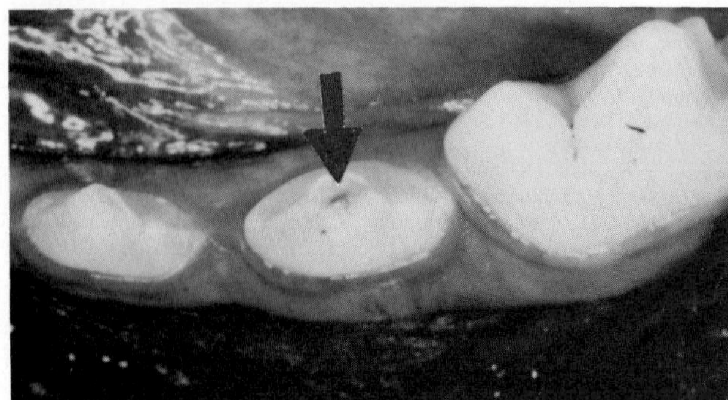

FIGURE 179–1. Fracture into the pulp horn on a mandibular fourth premolar, creating the need for endodontic therapy.

effective. As teeth with acute endodontic lesions are usually painful, early treatment avoids needless suffering. Because of the improved prognosis for teeth treated soon after pulp injury, and for humane reasons, endodontic treatment is a high-priority branch of dental therapy.

PATHOGENESIS OF THE ENDODONTIC LESION

The term *pulpal hyperemia* refers to reversible inflammation of the pulp due to trauma, and the term *pulpitis* refers to irreversible damage of the pulp due to trauma. Teeth with pulpal hyperemia are engorged with blood and inflammatory cells. Commonly, these teeth are hyperesthetic in humans and cause sharp pain of less than 1 minute in duration when stimulated by temperature changes or percussion. Resolution can occur if pressure from swelling does not result in cellular death within the pulp. Therapy in pulpal hyperemia is directed at preventing additional insult during healing and might take the form of adjusting the tooth out of occlusion, providing a soft diet at body temperature, or placing sedative dressings over the pulp after coronal tooth structure has been removed to allow for swelling. Unfortunately, early pulpal hyperemia is rarely diagnosed in veterinary patients because of their stoic nature and inability to communicate. It is much more common to diagnose pulpitis, because clinical signs of the disease become evident.

Pulpitis involves an irreversible lesion that leads to pulpal death. The pulp cannot regenerate, and when it dies, the odontoblasts that line the pulp cavity are cut off from their vascular supply so that they also die. This process devitalizes the dentin. The only part of the tooth that remains vital after pulpal death is the cellular cementum that covers the exterior surface of the root. (The ameloblasts that form enamel die after crown formation.)

Death of the pulp does not affect tooth function. The extension of the pulpal inflammatory process into the periodontium causes functional problems. Two common causes of pulpitis in the dog and cat are pulpitis caused by periodontal disease and pulpitis caused by dental disease. When pulpitis occurs as a result of periodontal disease (Fig. 179–3), the pulp is usually devitalized by extension of periodontal infection and inflammation into the apical nutrient canals or, less commonly, into accessory pulp canals along the side of the tooth. Thus, the pulp is secondarily affected as a result of periodontitis, and the process is given the term *periodontal-endodontic involvement.*

When pulpitis is caused by dental disease, the pulp is affected first, and the process extends secondarily out of the tooth into the periodontal tissues, usually near the tooth apex. This process is given the term *endodontic-periodontal involvement,* signifying that the endodontic lesion caused the periapical periodontitis.

When periodontal-endodontic involvement is present, drainage is established before the endodontic lesion is created. Therefore, although these lesions seriously shorten the life span of the tooth, they rarely result in extensive infiltration of the process into adjacent structures. Also, because relief of abscess pressure occurs readily, these lesions are less likely to be symptomatic than are primary endodontic lesions.

Primary endodontic lesions result in toxic tissue and products of bacterial breakdown that can cause necrosis,

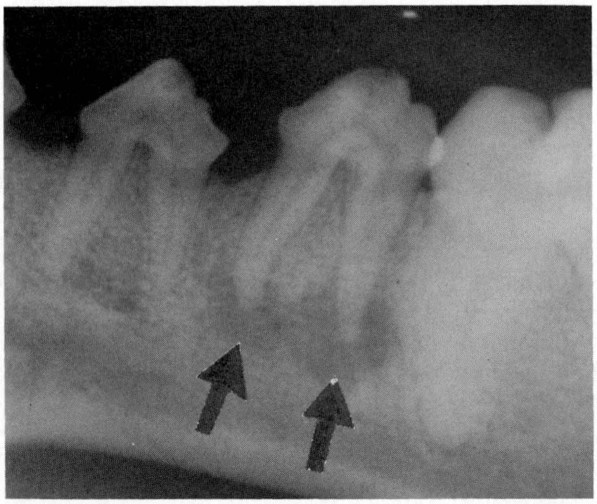

FIGURE 179–2. Radiograph of Figure 179–1, demonstrating periapical radiolucency from endodontic disease.

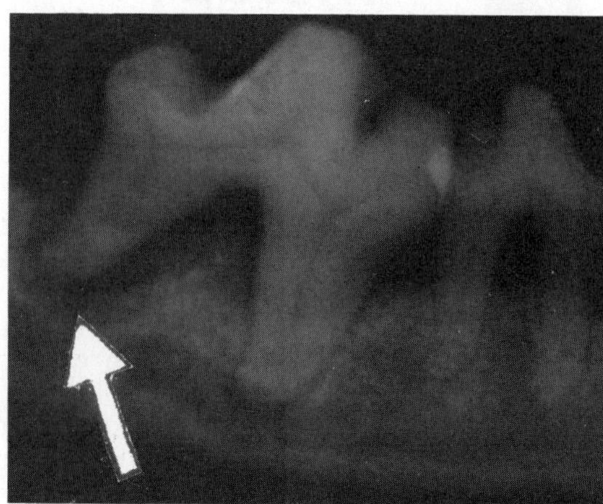

FIGURE 179–3. Radiograph showing periodontal disease on the caudal root of a mandibular first molar, which has caused devitalization of the pulp.

infection, and inflammation as they leave the tooth. The path of the abscess, cyst, or granuloma produced by these products may extend through bone or soft tissue and may drain locally. Occasionally, distant extension of the endodontic lesion may drain to the nose, orbit, intermandibular space, skin, or pharynx. Also, the process may become localized in bone or soft tissue as a large cyst, abscess, or area of cellulitis.

The two most common drainage patterns for primary endodontic lesions are (1) through the bone and exiting through the mucosa into the mouth and (2) along the periodontal ligament and exiting into the mouth by creation of a periodontal pocket between the gingiva and tooth. The first pattern creates a parulis or gum boil, which represents the end of a fistulous tract from the tooth. The second pattern creates a periodontal pocket that leads to the apex of the root.

The results of the endodontic lesion tend to persist until the tooth is lost. Without treatment, the pathological processes associated with endodontic disease rarely resolve. Most lesions have periods of quiescence and activity that are unpredictable. During periods of activity, the lesion usually causes progressive disease in surrounding tissues, which partially resolves during periods of quiescence. The lesion becomes more extensive as it becomes more chronic.

EXAMINATION

Endodontic lesions are usually diagnosed by a combination of visual, tactile, and radiographic signs. Many teeth are devitalized by fractures into the pulp. New fractures show obvious hemorrhage; older fractures produce necrotic tissue and debris in the pulp chamber. Familiarity with the anatomy of the tooth allows a diagnosis of endodontic involvement.

Teeth with pinpoint exposures of the pulp, as often occur with slab fractures of the maxillary fourth premolar in dogs, require tactile confirmation that exposure of the pulp has occurred. A fine, sharp probe is used to explore the suspected area while the patient is under general anesthesia or is sedated and the tooth is locally anesthetized. When the probe is successfully passed into the pulp chamber or canal, a diagnosis of endodontic involvement is made. Smooth, hard, discolored spots of dentin that occur on teeth with attrition and secondary dentin formation do not admit the probe (Fig. 179–3). These teeth need not be treated.

Radiography is useful in confirming endodontic disease in chronic lesions. Usually, about 2 weeks are required for an endodontic lesion to become visible in the apical area of a tooth with pulpal necrosis. Most cases are chronic when presented to the veterinarian, so that radiography of suspect teeth is appropriate.

The most anatomically correct view possible is used, and proper contrast is required for diagnosis. Early lesions simply appear as an interruption of the lamina dura, usually at the apex but occasionally along the side of the root. Later, lesions have some periapical radiolucency, usually in a circular or ovoid pattern.

The combination of radiographic and clinical evidence is highly predictive of endodontic disease. Such teeth are treated even without signs of pain or infection, because of the high probability of later problems developing and going unrecognized while pathological progression occurs. The best chance to retain normal anatomical structure occurs with the earliest intervention.

CONVENTIONAL ENDODONTIC TREATMENT

Once a diagnosis of pulpitis has been made, the most commonly used and predictable therapy is conventional endodontics. Conventional endodontics entails removal of contaminated debris from the root canal by a coronal approach and subsequent filling of the canal with biocompatible material so that the area around the tooth heals.[1] The purpose of conventional endodontics is to seal the nutrient foramen in the root so that no further seepage of necrotic debris or bacteria comes from the root. Because most teeth do not have accessory canals along the root, the focus of treatment is usually sealing of the apex of the root.

Access

Endodontic treatment is begun by gaining access to the root canals in a straight line. This step involves making an "access preparation" over each canal. A radiograph is used in estimating the proper position and angle for entering the pulp. Surgical-length 1557 carbide burs can be used in a high-speed handpiece to make an opening into the pulp above each root canal. This preparation is approximately 1.5 to 2.0 mm wide and enters the tooth surface at a 90° angle so that enamel rods are not undermined. The access opening is smooth so that files do not become caught on irregular edges when inserted into the tooth. Furthermore, the preparation should allow placement of the file to the apex of the tooth without the need to bend the file.

Cleaning

Once the access preparation has been cut, a number 10 or number 15 file is inserted to ensure that the operator can reach the apex without further modification. If necessary, the operator enlarges the access preparation while considering the fact that the more tooth structure is removed, the more likely the tooth is to fracture under stress. When access to the apex is assured, a barbed broach or file is used to remove as much of the pulp as possible. The canal is flushed with a 10 per cent solution of household bleach mixed with water. It is delivered to the apex by a fine hypodermic needle. Care must be taken not to irrigate the area under pressure and inadvertently drive hypochlorite solution into the periodontal area.

As each successively larger file is used, the operator ensures that the working length of the original file is maintained by obtaining an initial radiograph with the thinnest file in place and using a rubber stopper on the shank of the file as a marker. With a push-pull motion, the files are used in gentle débridement of the apex and walls of the pulp canal to loosen adherent debris (Fig. 179–4). As successively larger-diameter files are used,

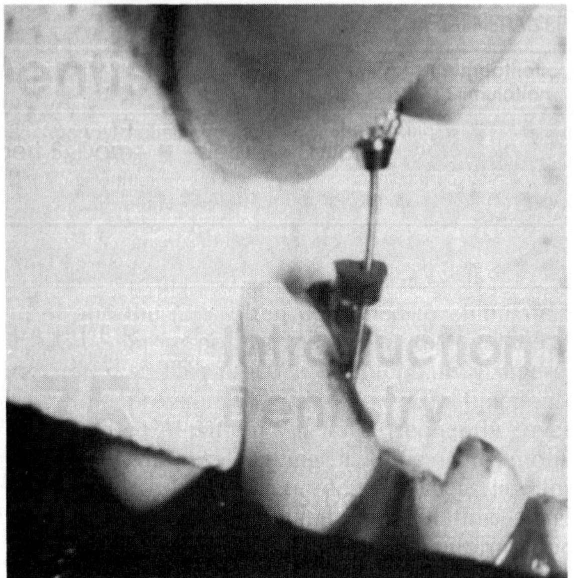

FIGURE 179–4. Debris exuding from canal as filing is done to clean the inside of the tooth.

they are preset with rubber stoppers at the same length, and the operator ensures that each file stopper relates exactly to the same point on the tooth. If a file does not reach the apex, further instrumentation of the tooth is needed so that working length is maintained. Carefully débriding the walls of the root canal, using a lubricant and chelating agent (e.g., urea peroxide and ethylenediamine tetra acetic acid [RC Prep]), and irrigating the area with hypochlorite solution after use of each file are helpful in maintaining working length.

Files can also be turned clockwise one-eighth to one-quarter turn and pulled out to enlarge canal size by boring out dentin with the flutes of the cutting end. This procedure may cause fracture of the file or of the root, especially with Hedstrom pattern files. The problem of wedging and root fracture persists with every file design.

Excessive instrumentation of the root canal is avoided to prevent mechanical weakening of the root, perforation of the apex with instruments, and breakage of instruments within the canal. The operator should cease instrumentation when the canal is clean and the apex has been prepared to a uniform size. This endpoint can be seen when clean dentin filings and irrigation fluid emerge after a file is used. Also, the tactile sensation of a snug fit between the file and end of the root should be appreciated. At this time, the canal is irrigated a final time with hypochlorite solution and dried with paper points. The paper points should emerge clean and dry (Fig. 179–5). If they do not, further filing and drying are necessary.

This process of cleaning and preparing the apex is completed on every root of multirooted teeth. Notation should be made of the width and length of each file that completes instrumentation of each clean, prepared root. At this stage, the root canal is ready to be filled.

Filling

The most traditionally acceptable, and usually the easiest, technique to perform confidently is the gutta-percha fill technique. In this technique, the operator selects a preformed gutta-percha point of the exact width and shape of the last file used in instrumentation of the apex. This point is seated to the end of the canal. It should fit snugly. It is withdrawn and dipped momentarily in chloroform to soften the outside of the point. After immediate insertion of this "master point" into the canal to the apex, it is quickly withdrawn and allowed to dry for 1 minute. This technique fits the point to the apical preparation exactly. Root canal sealer is mixed and spun into the canal to the apex with a spiral filler. The master point is coated with this sealer, and the point is seated to the apex. The point should fit snugly and resist removal slightly when fully seated. The excess gutta-percha is removed above the root canal with a warmed excavator. A root canal spreader is used to condense the master point against the root canal, and "accessory points" (thinner gutta-percha cones) are inserted into the space created to produce dense filling of the root canal. This process continues until the canal does not admit further cones and radiography demonstrates complete filling.

Alternate Method

One problem that occurs with longer teeth with large root canals, such as the canine teeth in dogs, is the difficulty of completely filling irregular wide areas of the canal with gutta-percha cones. Ultrafil,* a thermally softened injectable gutta-percha system, may be used to fill large volume irregular canals. This is especially helpful when the apex has been successfully filled with gutta-percha points driven into place with a plugger. More coronal aspects of the canal cannot be filled by preformed points because the canal is wider in the middle than in the coronal part. In this technique, very soft gutta-percha in injection cartridges can be extruded into the canal, and irregularities can be filled by con-

*The Hygienic Corp., Akron, OH.

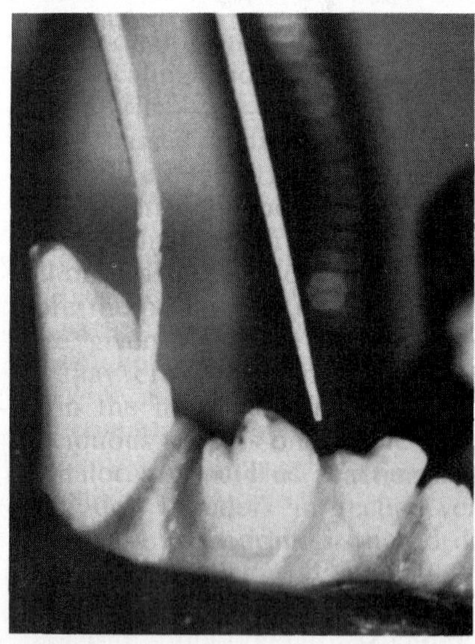

FIGURE 179–5. Paper points being used to dry the canal and give visual assurance that the canal is clean.

densing the soft gutta-percha with root canal pluggers dipped in alcohol.

The routine use of gutta-percha is encouraged because it compresses the root canal and drives the cement laterally into voids and accessory canals during seating of the points. When only root canal sealer is injected by syringe and hypodermic needle, it may not flow into all areas. Incomplete filling predisposes the patient to leakage of material between the inside of the tooth and the periodontium, which can perpetuate or aggravate periapical periodontitis.

Restoration

Conventional endodontic treatment is completed by filling the pulp canal with condensed gutta-percha and high compressive-strength cement (e.g., zinc phosphate) and placing a permanent filling (e.g., silver amalgam) in the access preparation. All endodontically treated teeth are covered with a cast metal crown to prevent breakage. Although not every endodontically treated tooth breaks, a significant number do, because they become more brittle after devitalization or because stress lines are set up during endodontic instrumentation. Maximum protection against breakage requires holding the coronal aspects of the tooth together with a cast metal crown.

SURGICAL ENDODONTICS

Surgical endodontics is an alternative to conventional endodontic technique. It is indicated when the standard coronal access cannot be performed, when previous treatment has failed, when sclerotic canals do not admit the file to the apex (Fig. 179–6), when prosthetic replacements interfere, or when filling at the apex remains incomplete after several attempts.

The term *surgical endodontics* connotes an approach to the endodontic system through the apex—a "reverse fill." The goal is to approach the apical area laterally or apically, to cut off a section of the apex, and to fill the root canal at the apex with an inert biocompatible material. It can be done coincidentally with coronal-approach endodontics to assure a dense, complete filling at the apex while directly treating or performing biopsy of diseased tissue in the apical area.[2] Because this approach enhances exposure and access, it can improve the outcome of endodontic therapy in difficult cases. Use of the surgical approach should be restricted, however, to situations in which the operator has some reason to doubt that conventional endodontics would produce an adequate result. Severe infection or anatomical abnormalities in the tooth may indicate a surgical approach. Indiscriminate use of the surgical approach is not advised, because increased morbidity may result from damage to normal anatomical structures during the surgical approach to the apex. Also, because surgical endodontics does not fill or clean the entire root canal, it does not prevent leakage of contaminated material out of accessory canals. For this reason, the operator should fill as much of the root canal as possible by the conventional approach at the same time at which surgical endodontics is performed.

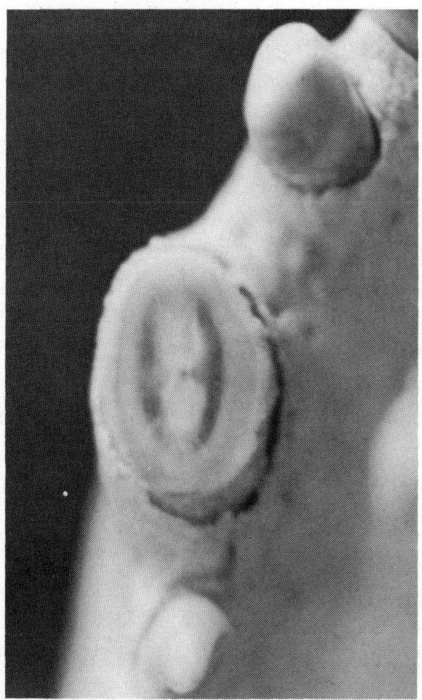

FIGURE 179–6. Sclerotic pulp chamber totally filled with dentin in an older dog.

Conventional endodontics and surgical endodontics can be performed at the same time, but on different roots of multirooted teeth. This situation occurs most frequently in treatment of the maxillary fourth premolar in older dogs, when the rostral buccal root is often sclerotic and must be treated by reverse filling.

Technique

The starting point for surgical endodontics is creation of a mucoperiosteal flap to expose the alveolar process over the apex of the tooth. Access to the apex can also start with an incision in the alveolar mucosa directly over the apex or with an extraoral approach through the skin of the face. These approaches are less commonly used because they increase the difficulty in locating the apex.

Usually, the incision is begun in the attached gingiva at a site just coronal to the mucogingival junction. It is made in full thickness through the periosteum and extended rostrally and caudally to the involved tooth, far enough to expose the apical region. A periosteal elevator is used to lift the flap off the bone, and when additional exposure is needed, a vertical releasing incision may be made at either end or at both ends of the incision. A sharp periosteal elevator must be used, and pressure must be applied directly on bone, to avoid tearing the flap. Partial-thickness flaps that preserve the periosteum on the bone are not recommended. They are technically difficult and may result in interruption of the blood supply.

Once the flap is elevated, it is kept moist with physiological saline while it is pushed out of the way or sutured to adjacent mucosa. This action prevents drying and preserves vitality. The flap acts as a bandage over the surgical site postoperatively, and if it undergoes necrosis, permanent dehiscence or fenestration may occur over that area.

After the flap approach is performed, the apex is located. Location of the apex is most simply accomplished by palpation if the root is prominent. Also, some patients with extensive periapical inflammation demonstrate obvious changes in the bone, such as cavitation through the cortical plate or discoloration signifying underlying disease. These clues can be used to find a site where a sharp explorer can be pushed through the bone and the apex of the tooth located in this manner.

When the apex cannot be located by sight or touch radiography is best used to estimate its position. Either a file, a triangular piece of radiopaque material (e.g., trimmed foil from a dental film packet), or an endodontic point laid over the root may be used to locate the apex. A surgical bur is used to mark the approximate location of the apex on the cortical bone.

Beginning above the apex (i.e., away from the occlusal surface), the operator gradually removes bone with a surgical-length 1557 bur, under irrigation, until the apex is located. At least 3 mm of vertical length at the apex must be exposed to cut back the apex sufficiently to find the end of the root canal. The approach is constructed so that the operator has room for access to the apex both laterally and above the apex. This room for access is necessary for exposure, for preparation of the apex to receive a filling, and for instrumentation to place the filling in the preparation.

After the apex and surrounding area are sufficiently exposed, the apex is amputated at an angle so that the end of the root canal can be seen and is accessible. This procedure creates an ovoid face at the end of the root, which is positioned toward the operator. This face should be smooth and even with the periodontal ligament. The cells of the periodontal ligament contribute substantially to filling of the defect created by surgery.

The root tip is cut back until all anatomical irregularities and diseased tissue that can interfere with healing are removed. Also, the root tip must be cut back until a definite root canal space can be seen (Fig. 179–7), because the terminal part of a normal canine or feline root usually has an apical delta rather than a patent single canal. Failure to cut back to the confluence of these apical arborizations results in a filling that does not seal the end of the root from the inside of the tooth. When severe sclerosis of the root canal has occurred, differences in color usually indicate where the root canal space was located. An oversize filling is put in this location to seal the root when the operator cannot exactly locate the remaining pulp space.

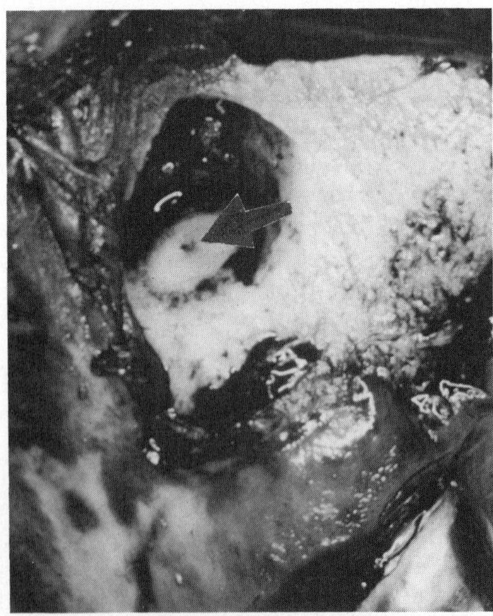

FIGURE 179–7. Apex exposed and amputated to the level of the terminal root canal (black spot indicated by *arrow*).

The apical preparation can be made with an inverted cone–shaped or pear–shaped carbide bur. This preparation must be undercut so that pressure that may build up in the root does not force the filling out of the tooth. Extensive or deep preparation is not needed if the apex has been cut back to the level of healthy root structure and patent root canal. Preparation that is 1 to 2 mm deep is sufficient.

The area is rinsed with physiological saline to flush away chips of bone and tooth. Excess fluid is removed from the area, and the apical preparation is dried with a cotton pellet. Total drying of the surface of the cut bone or periodontal area is not attempted, as this leads to more cellular damage.

Although several restorative materials have been used to fill the apical preparation, non-zinc silver amalgam is usually the best choice, because it is biocompatible, radiopaque, and easy to handle under slightly moist conditions. One disadvantage of this material is that small particles left in the surgical area can make postoperative radiographs look untidy.

A reverse-fill amalgam carrier can be used to deliver small increments of amalgam to the apex (Fig. 179–8). The amalgam is condensed with small pluggers, and the excess is removed with a fine amalgam carver. The area is flushed with normal saline, and a radiograph is obtained (Fig. 179–9).

The flap is replaced in the original position and secured by simple interrupted sutures for primary-intention healing. Dead space does not need to be closed in most areas where bone was removed over the root. Especially large areas of dead space can be filled with absorbable gelatin sponge, hydroxyapatite alloplastic material, or autogenous pulverized bone. If material is implanted in the surgical site, administration of antibiotics for 5 to 7 days is prudent. Grafting in an area of active infection is not recommended, although the use of gelatin sponge impregnated with antibiotics may be helpful. Reliance on proper débridement of infected tissues is preferable to local antibiotic treatment. Except in cases involving systemic predisposition to infection (e.g., diabetes mellitus), evidence of bacterial septicemia, fulminating local infection in the area of vital structures (e.g., eye, airway, or brain), or surgical implantation of material into the surgical site, postoperative antibiotic coverage is unnecessary.

Postoperative Care

After conventional and surgical endodontic therapy, patients are rechecked clinically and radiographically to assure success. The first re-examination is performed at 7 to 14 days, at which time the area is inspected for

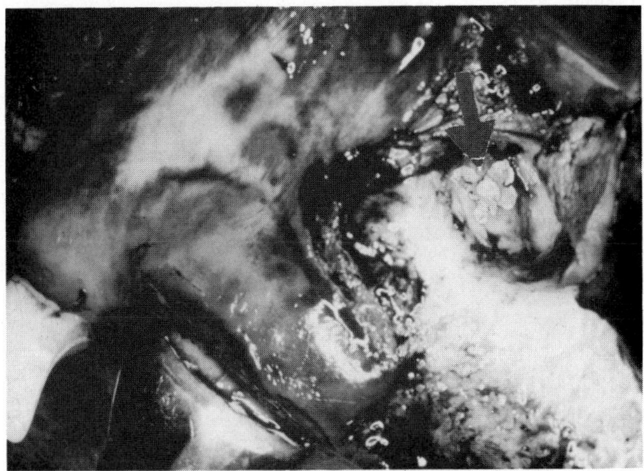

FIGURE 179–8. Amalgam placed in apical preparation *(arrow)*.

proper healing and sutures are removed. The area is evaluated for inflammation and the tooth is evaluated by palpation for increased mobility or pain. Poor healing indicates radiographic evaluation. Severe infection indicates extraction. Slightly increased mobility with inflammation indicates systemic antibiotic treatment and local antiseptic rinses twice daily with 0.1 to 0.2 per cent chlorhexidine acetate or chlorhexidine gluconate.

Radiographic evaluation is performed at 6 months, and yearly thereafter, for apparently successful cases. Clinical examination is also indicated at that time to check for increasing mobility, periodontal disease, and signs of periapical inflammation. When evaluating postoperative radiographs, the operator must compare the size of the periapical radiolucency with that on the original radiographs. Teeth with increasing radiolucency are usually failing and require retreatment, re-evaluation, or extraction, depending on the apparent progress of the lesion. Teeth with radiolucency that is the same or decreased are successful and require only continued monitoring.

Crowning of all endodontically treated teeth is prudent, as structural failure is more likely when endodontically treated teeth are stressed. Prosthetic crowns can be constructed immediately after conventional or surgical endodontics, without requiring time for further healing. Care is taken to ensure that the crown is not placed in hyperocclusion (too high), as such crown placement puts considerable pressure on the periapical area and perpetuates inflammation.

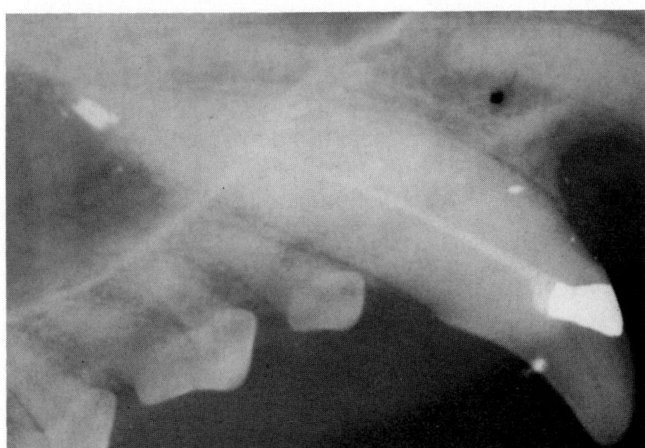

FIGURE 179–9. Maxillary canine tooth immediately after surgical endodontic treatment and incomplete conventional endodontic treatment. (Sclerosis prevented completion of the latter treatment.)

COMBINED ENDODONTIC–PERIODONTIC LESIONS

Management

Endodontic lesions often create periodontal problems. When both types of lesions are present, the question of which to treat first arises. In practice, both lesions often need to be treated concurrently. Theoretically, the best strategy is to treat the endodontic lesion first, wait for periodontal healing to determine the extent of the persistent periodontal lesion, and complete therapy with periodontal treatment. This plan for treatment is best because instrumentation of the root surface may remove attachment of periodontal ligament that would ordinarily heal after endodontics.

With a combined lesion, the operator should attempt to determine which lesion is primary. Obvious trauma to the crown (fracture, caries, resorption, and so forth) may indicate an initial endodontic lesion. Therefore, minimal instrumentation of the root surface is carried out, and the periodontal lesion is treated more aggressively after the 6-week postoperative evaluation of the endodontic result.

If the adjacent teeth have severely damaged periodontal support and primary endodontic damage to the tooth is not evident, the periodontal lesion is probably responsible for endodontic disease. In this situation, the periodontal lesion is treated surgically at the time of endodontic treatment.

Prognosis

The presence of chronic periodontal lesions communicating with and responsible for devitalized pulpal tissue indicates a poor prognosis for extensive periodontal repair after endodontic treatment. Elimination of the endodontic lesion, however, allows periodontal therapy to resolve inflammation. With periodic maintenance care, the prognosis is good, as with other treated cases of periodontitis.[3, 4]

Treatment of endodontic lesions may allow regeneration of normal periodontal anatomy around the tooth without specialized periodontal surgery. Acute endodontic/periodontal lesions draining through the periodontal area have an excellent prognosis for regeneration of normal periodontal tissue if endodontics are promptly initiated.[5]

References

1. Bolds DK, Grove TK: Ten tested tips for canine teeth. *Vet Forum* June 1988, p 18.
2. Grove TK: Apicoectomy and retrograde endodontics. *Vet Forum* October 1988, p 14.
3. Hirschfeld L, Wasserman B: A long-term survey of tooth loss in 600 treated periodontal patients. *J Periodontol 49*:225, 1978.
4. Ross I, Thompson R: A long-term study of root retention in the treatment of maxillary molars with furcation involvement. *J Periodontol 49*:238, 1978.
5. Weine FS, et al: Endodontic emergency treatment following root amputation in periodontally involved teeth. *J Periodontol 41*:391, 1970.

CHAPTER 180 Restorative Dentistry

B. Jean Hawkins

Dental restorations have been used for more than 2,000 years, and a wide variety of materials have been used to replace or restore teeth. Modern dentistry began in the 19th century when Greenwood invented the foot-powered dental drill. Shortly thereafter silver amalgam was introduced as a dental restorative material, initiating restorative dentistry.[6]

RESTORATIVE MATERIALS

Amalgam

Silver amalgam, the first dental restorative material in general use, was described first by Bell in 1819, and then by Travean in 1826. Later, in 1861, John Towes tested the physical properties of amalgam and discovered that marginal leakage resulted in further decay.[6]

In the past, amalgam had a composition within specified limits: silver 65 per cent (minimum), tin 29 per cent (maximum), copper 6 per cent (maximum), zinc 2 per cent (maximum), and mercury 3 per cent (maximum).[6] In 1963, Canadian researchers reported that increased levels of copper improved the characteristics of silver amalgam, and copper is now added as a blended alloy, or as a single silver-copper particle alloy. The amount of copper in amalgam ranges from 12 to 30 per cent, depending on the manufacturer.[6]

The advantage of higher copper content is that mercury has a chemical preference for bonding to copper instead of to tin. The mercury-tin bond, or gamma-2 phase of the traditional amalgam reaction, was the "weakest, softest, and most corrodible phase in the set metallurgical structure."[6] The preferable copper-tin reaction significantly reduces the weakness of silver amalgam.

Silver amalgams are constantly being improved. Different types of amalgam are available. They are type 1, "blended" amalgam (spheres with lathe-cut silver particles); type 2, consisting of spheres only; and type 3, consisting of spheroids (irregularly shaped particles that have a smooth surface). The blended alloys require more mercury to coat the increased surface area of the lathe-cut particles, producing a satisfactory plasticity. The blended alloys (type 1) are called "positive-pack" amalgams because they resist the condenser point during placement in a prepared cavity. This resistance results in tight marginal adaptation, which helps decrease marginal leakage and restoration failure.[5]

Spheroidal alloys (type 3) are described as intermediate in packing quality. These alloys offer some resistance to condensation but do not pack as tightly against the cavity wall as do the blended alloys. Spherical alloys (type 2) offer the least resistance to packing and are described as "plashy." The spheres slip past each other during condensation and make a tight marginal seal more difficult to achieve. The spherical and spheroidal alloys (types 2 and 3) require less mercury to achieve plasticity and are more carvable and polishable.[5]

A major disadvantage of amalgam in dentistry is the lack of any chemical bond with either enamel or dentin. Amalgam must be held in place by mechanical undercutting of the tooth with an inverted cone–shaped or pear–shaped bur, which weakens the tooth.

In spite of this disadvantage, silver amalgam alloys are the material of choice for posterior restorations on the occlusal surfaces of molars in the dog. They are the least sensitive to technique and strongest of the materials available. They are also quite suitable for the closure of access openings following endodontic procedures, because silver amalgam is unaffected by the eugenol component of zinc oxide–eugenol, the most common endodontic sealer.

When amalgam is used for restorations, cavity varnish liner is applied to all cavity preparations in vital teeth. The layer of varnish seals the open dentinal tubules and fills in the microscopic space between the amalgam and the cavity wall, until the corrosion reaction that seals the restoration to the margin has occurred (6 to 12 months). Cavity varnish minimizes marginal leakage. The setting time for the various alloys varies: 5 to 9 minutes for type 1, 5 to 7 minutes for type 2, and 4 to 5 minutes for type 3.[5]

Deeper carious lesions, which extend within 1 mm of the pulp chamber, require a rigid base to protect the pulp tissues. Satisfactory bases include various cements such as zinc phosphate, polycarboxylate, glass ionomer, or reinforced zinc oxide–eugenol.[5] Zinc phosphate is the least desirable because of the potential of pulpal irritation.

Most veterinary dentists use precapsulated silver amalgam instead of pellets and liquid mercury dispensers. A more uniform mix is obtained using a high-speed triturator based on directions of the manufacturer for length of mix.[5]

Unfortunately, amalgam restorative materials require 24 hours to set sufficiently to allow a high polish. If the veterinary patient is cooperative, the owner can polish an amalgam restorative on a buccal or lingual tooth surface with a pencil eraser the day after the restoration.

Composite Resins

Composite resins were developed in 1962 from synthetic materials to decrease the shrinkage experienced with polymethacrylate restorative resins. Since their initial development, composite resins have undergone changes and are based on the size of the filler particles. The first composites contained particles as large as 100 micrometers (μm), were not durable (the surface particles came out of the resin easily), stained easily, and could not be highly polished.

Newer microfilled composite resins (with particle sizes of 0.04 to 0.00004 μm) are highly polishable and are more durable than the earlier macrofilled counterparts, but they contain 20 per cent less filler. Hybrid composite resins have a mixture of large and small filler particles. Hybrid resins are not as shiny as the microfilled composite resins, but they do produce a smooth surface, which retards plaque accumulation.[1] Initially, the fillers were radiolucent quartz, but this material did not allow the detection of carious lesions under the restoration. At present, fillers are radiopaque and include barium, strontium, and zinc glass components.

Composite resins are of two types, based on curing method: chemical-cured resins and light-cured resins. Chemical-cured resins rely on benzoyl peroxide–tertiary amine mechanisms and are self-curing. Two paste systems polymerize when mixed and must be placed quickly into the prepared site. Problems include air voids and inconsistency of the mix. The light-cured composite resins eliminate some of these problems. At first, ultraviolet light was used to initiate the diketone polymerization reaction, but visible light (400 to 500 μm blue range) is now preferred. Light-cured restorative materials allow the operator more time for accurate placement and result in decreased porosity of the restoration. (The operator and other personnel should not look at the light unless a filter is used.) Composite restorative materials can be finished with polishing discs or special fine finishing diamond burs.[1]

Composite resins have many applications in veterinary dentistry, including cosmetic restorations, correction of enamel hypoplasia, and restoration of slab fractures of the upper fourth premolar teeth. Threaded pins should be placed in the dentin to increase retention of the restoration in these cases. Composite resins can also be used to close access openings after endodontic procedures. If zinc oxide–eugenol has been used in the endodontic procedure, the area is cleaned with alcohol and interfaced with zinc phosphate cement, light-cured calcium hydroxide or glass ionomer cement, because eugenol can interfere with polymerization of the composite resin. Glass ionomer cement placed on the dentin interface enhances the restoration by preventing microscopic leakage. The greatest disadvantage of composite restorative materials is their lack of durability, especially on occlusal surfaces.

Glass Ionomer Cements

Glass ionomer cements are the newest restorative material and are unique in that they form a chemical bond to the dentin and, to a lesser degree, the enamel.[7]

Glass ionomer cements are powder-liquid materials containing a glass portion, aluminosilicate, which has a high fluoride content. The fluoride is of benefit because the leaching of fluoride into the dental tissues prevents decay. The liquid portion is a type of polyacrylic acid.[7]

The glass ionomer bond occurs in two phases. Calcium polycarboxylate gel is formed initially, followed by aluminum polycarboxylate gel during the next 24 hours. The dentin and enamel of the affected tooth must be clean for proper bonding to occur. A slurry of pumice and water in a rubber polishing cup is used to clean the site if no caries are present. If the lesions are extensive, caries must be removed with a bur before restoration.

After the tooth is prepared, a "smear layer" of dentin remains, consisting of dentinal tubule that is clean, bent, or broken. The open tubules may allow odontoblastic material to migrate into the cleaned surface, resulting in contamination and a decreased chemical bond.[7] Accordingly, serious debate has arisen concerning the treatment of this smear layer. Pumice and water irrigation may be adequate; however, acid cleaning may be appropriate. The surface of the area to be bonded should be clean and slightly moistened with water.

Glass ionomer cements may be hand-mixed or premixed. The premixed products require special equipment and instruments, but the perfect powder/liquid ratio results in the strongest restoration.

After the cement is placed, a matrix is positioned and left in place during the first several minutes. A special waterproof glass ionomer varnish or cocoa butter is then placed over the restoration to prevent rapid dehydration. If the cement dries too rapidly, it cracks, and if it is contaminated with excess moisture, it becomes chalky and crumbles.[7]

Major advantages of glass ionomer cements include hard surface translucency, bonding to dentin, release of fluoride, and little accumulation of plaque. These cements are preferred for restoration of cervical line lesions (neck lesions) in feline teeth.[4] All involved teeth are radiographed before treatment, as many have undetected root resorption and should not be restored.[4] Glass ionomer cements are also excellent choices for filling access openings after endodontic procedures.

Glass ionomer cements with silver particles incorporated into the powder have been developed to provide extra strength. These mixtures are called cermets.[6] In veterinary treatment of feline cervical line lesions, this product has little advantage, because an occlusal surface is not involved in the procedure.

ACCESSORY MATERIALS

Cements

Cements have a variety of uses in veterinary dentistry. They are used as luting agents to hold restorations in place, and they are used as restorative materials if heavy filling is required. Cements can also be used as interfaces between restorative materials and normal dental tissues. The first cements were zinc phosphate and zinc oxide–eugenol, and these serve as a basis for comparison of other cements.[6] The four basic types of cements are based on the type of bonding to teeth: phosphate-bonded, phenolate-bonded, polycarboxylate-bonded, and polymer-bonded.[6]

Zinc phosphate is a phosphate-bonded cement. It is used as a luting agent, in temporary restorations, and for protection of vital dental tissues against thermal changes.[6] Zinc phosphate can be used as an interface between zinc oxide–eugenol and composite restorative materials, so that the eugenol does not interfere with the setting properties of the resin. Zinc phosphate is extremely sticky, and handling can be improved by coating the instruments or fingers with the zinc phosphate powder and forming a small ball.

Zinc oxide–eugenol is a phenolate-bonded cement. It is used as a root canal filling material, as a temporary filling material, and as a base for thermal insulation. The almost neutral pH produces minimal pulpal irritation. Unless it is reinforced (or light-cured), it fractures when placed under large occlusal restorations. Cavitec* is one commercially available brand of zinc oxide–eugenol.

Duralon† is a polycarboxylate cement usually used for luting of restorations. This cement has fluoride-releasing properties because it contains stannous fluoride. The liquid portion of this cement can be used to remove the smear layer prior to restoring cervical line lesions.[6]

Glass ionomer cements are polymer bonded and have undergone considerable changes since they were first developed. Most manufacturers of glass ionomer filling cements also produce a similar luting cement. The chemical bond produced with dentin and enamel plus the continual release of fluoride makes glass ionomer cements desirable for restorations as well as for luting agents in crown placement.[6] Glass ionomer cements may be used over a light-cured calcium hydroxide base for restorations or for pulpotomy of vital teeth of dogs and cats.

Liners

A cavity liner is a material used to protect vital pulp tissue and over which a restoration is to be placed. Two thin layers of a cavity varnish are often used to seal dentinal tubules and occupy the microscopic space between the cavity wall and a silver amalgam restoration until a sealing corrosion layer forms between the restoration and the tooth.[5] Examples of cavity varnishes used as liners are Copanol and Copanol-F‡.

Glass ionomer restorative materials usually do not require liners because they bond to dentin and are usually not irritating to the pulp when used properly.

Composite restorative materials bond only with etched enamel, which limits their usefulness (e.g., for cervical line lesions in cats). However, with a light-cured adhesive liner such as Scotchbond II,§ which bonds to dentin, a composite material can be used effectively. The composite material does bond with the adhesive, and then the etched enamel, to produce a strong, color-compatible restoration. Two such light-cured composites are Silux§ and Silar§.

Chemical-cured adhesives and chemical-cured composite restorative materials can also be used, but light-cured materials of all types are increasingly preferred because they allow longer placement time and a short curing time.

RESTORATION OF CARIES AND CERVICAL LINE LESIONS

Caries are the organic breakdown of tooth enamel from the by-products of certain microorganisms in the mouth. Normally, enamel protects the tooth from decay,[2] and exposed roots and dentin in dogs should be more susceptible to decay because of the lack of enamel covering. When they do occur in dogs, carious lesions are usually found in the occlusal surfaces of the molar teeth, where food can become trapped in the enamel pits and fissures, rather than on exposed root surfaces.

In the cat, cervical line lesions (also called cervical line erosions, neck lesions, or caries) are manifested differently in comparison with similar lesions in the dog. Cervical line lesions are characterized by "progressive, subgingival, osteoclastic resorption."[3] The usual location of these lesions is the gingival margin or neck of the tooth. Sixty-four per cent of the cats examined had some cervical line lesions present.[3]

These lesions are often covered by heavy plaque, calculus, and hyperplastic gingiva,[2] and they may not be detected unless an explorer is used. The buccal surfaces of the teeth are most often affected.[2] In my experience, the cervical line lesion of the lower molar seems to have a characteristic caudal-to-rostral (distal-to-medial) progression and has no significant calculus or gingival hyperplasia. This particular cervical line lesion is usually detected by exploring from the caudal aspect rostrally at the gingival margin of the lower first molar. Often, only a fragment of the rostral root holds the crown in place.

Cervical line lesions are either shallow (not into the pulp chamber) or deep (invading the pulp chamber). Affected teeth seldom die from pulpal exposure, as does a fractured tooth, but rather they form a pulpal polyp (viable pulp protruding from the pulp chamber) or granulation tissue. A recent study has shown that a significant number of teeth have subgingival lesions, alone or in combination with visible cervical line lesions.[2]

A variety of techniques have been proposed for the restoration of cervical line lesions. Radiographic examination of the affected teeth is necessary, as shallow cervical line lesions should not be restored unless radiographs indicate solid root structure.[4] Radiographs may also reveal retained root fragments, which are removed.

Teeth with cervical line lesions that extend into the pulp tissue are usually removed by extraction or pulverization with a high-speed drill and round bur. Retained roots, which may be identified by localized inflamed gingival areas, may also be removed by root pulverization. If a canine tooth is affected and has sufficient root structure, an endodontic procedure may be performed.

Glass ionomer cements are extremely useful for the restoration of certain cervical line lesions. The earlier section on glass ionomer cements contains a description of the procedure for the application of these cements into cervical line lesions after the dentin is prepared.

Shallow cervical line lesions may be treated conser-

*Kerr Manufacturing Co, Romulus, MI.
†Premier Dental Products, Norristown, PA.
‡Teledyne Dental Products, Saratoga, CA.
§3M, St. Paul, MN.

vatively (not given full restoration) with an application of ScotchBond II,* a light-cured material that seals the dentinal tubules. This treatment immediately relieves the sensitivity, and the release of fluoride from the adhesive protects the dentinal tissue from further erosion.

Patients with cervical line lesions are rechecked every 6 months. New lesions may have developed, restorations may have been lost, or the lesion may have progressed through the pulp chamber, in which case the tooth is extracted or treated endodontically after radiographic examination.

*3M, St. Paul, MN.

References

1. Bowen RL: Dental filling material comprising vinyl selane treated fused silica and a binder consisting of a reaction product of bisphenol and glycidyl acrylate. U.S. Patent 3,066,112, 1962.
2. Emily P: Restorative dentistry. *Vet Clin North Am 16*:895, 1986.
3. Frost P, Williams C: Feline dental disease. *Vet Clin North Am 16*:851, 1986.
4. Harvey C: Cervical line lesions in cats. American College of Veterinary Surgeons Meeting, October 1989.
5. Jordan RE, et al: Oral rehabilitation: Current therapy with silver amalgam. *In* Levine N, et al (eds): *Current Treatment in Dental Practice.* W. B. Saunders, Philadelphia, 1986, pp 83–101.
6. Smith D, Desjardin RP: Oral rehabilitation: Dental materials: Current status and future prospects. *In* Levine N, et al. (eds): *Current Treatment in Dental Practice.* W. B. Saunders, Philadelphia, 1986, pp 57–73.
7. Watson PA, McComb D: Operative dentistry: Recent advances in aesthetic restorative materials. *In* Levine N, et al (eds): *Current Treatment in Dental Practice.* W. B. Saunders, Philadelphia, 1986, pp 74–83.

CHAPTER 181 Occlusion and Orthodontics

Gary B. Beard

Orthodontics is the specialty involving the prevention and correction of dental and oral anomalies. It is subdivided into preventive, interceptive, and corrective orthodontics.

1. Preventive orthodontics is action taken to preserve and protect occlusion.[1, 11] With companion animals, this action usually involves counseling the owner to provide proper chew toys and exercises and to prevent the young animal from pulling or tugging on hard objects, such as metal or concrete. Behavior training and modification may be necessary in the young pet.
2. Interceptive orthodontics is action taken to intercept a potential or existing early malocclusion in the mixed dentition of developing and permanent teeth.[1, 11]
3. Corrective orthodontics is the treatment or manipulation of a definitive malocclusion in the permanent dentition.[1, 11]

NORMAL OCCLUSION

To determine malocclusion, one must first know and understand normal occlusion. Normal occlusion is based on the mesaticephalic skull and is characterized by a scissors bite (Fig. 181–1). The scissors bite is a shear mouth, that is, the mandibular incisors are in minimal contact with the lingual surfaces of the maxillary incisors.[15]

For more than half of the 148 breeds recognized by the American Kennel Club, a scissors bite is not mandatory. Breed standards describe only the correct canine occlusion. They do not state the relationship of the incisors and the number of teeth that should be present.[8]

TOOTH ERUPTION AND RETAINED DECIDUOUS TEETH

The retention of deciduous teeth past the normal eruption of permanent teeth is common in many breeds. The retention of these teeth for as short a period as 2 weeks can produce occlusal defects in the permanent dentition.[13] Malocclusions produce early wearing of the teeth (attrition); rotation and crowding of the teeth, resulting in periodontal disease; and in many instances,

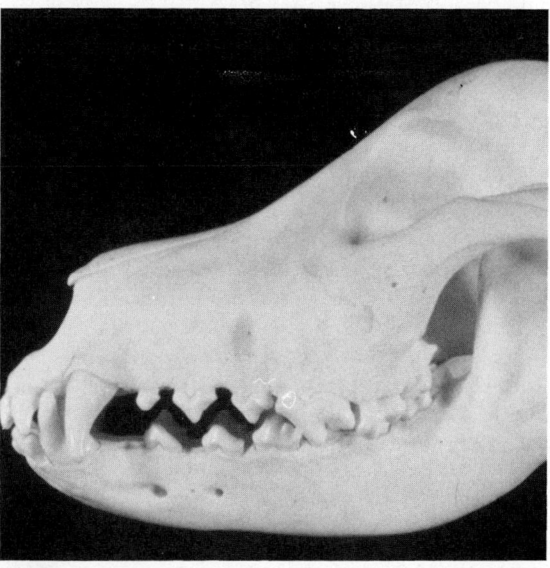

FIGURE 181–1. Normal occlusion appearing as a scissors bite in a canine skull.

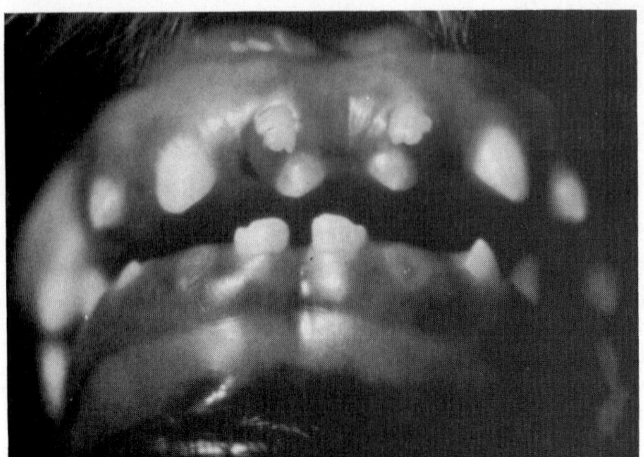

FIGURE 181–2. Periodontal lesions caused by the retention of maxillary central incisors. These lesions will persist if not treated promptly.

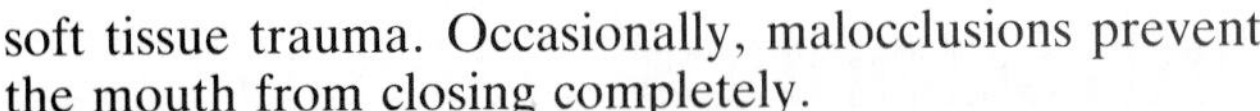

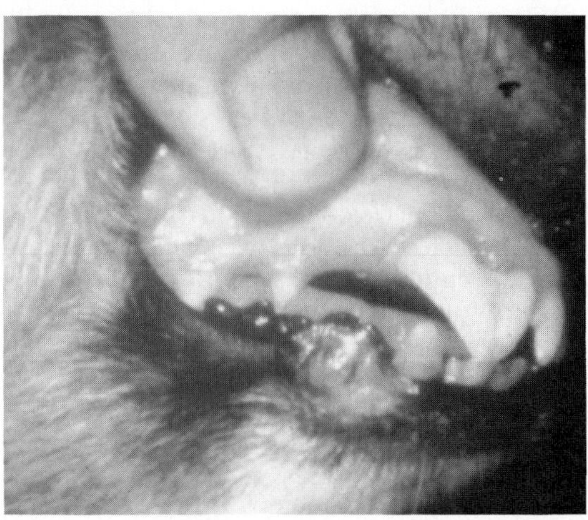

FIGURE 181–4. A rostrally displaced maxillary canine tooth caused by retention of the deciduous canine tooth. This condition is found frequently in shelties and other miniature breeds of dogs.

soft tissue trauma. Occasionally, malocclusions prevent the mouth from closing completely.

Changes are produced in the soft tissue when the permanent tooth erupts alongside the deciduous tooth. The permanent tooth surface in contact with the deciduous tooth is often deprived of normal periodontal tissues, and a slight periodontal defect can persist even after the loss or extraction of the deciduous tooth. Once a periodontal lesion is established, gradual progression is likely (Fig. 181–2).

The permanent teeth have a characteristic eruption pathway when the deciduous teeth are retained.[2] The incisors, lower canine teeth, and premolars erupt at positions lingual or palatal to the deciduous teeth. The lower canine teeth are "base narrow" and tend to damage the tissues of the hard palate as they erupt (Fig. 181–3). Frequently, the mandibular canine teeth do not fully erupt upon striking the palate. If the condition is not rectified before apexification, the full expression of length of the crown does not occur.[7, 8] Eruption of the maxillary canine teeth is rostral to the deciduous canine teeth, so that the interdental space between the lateral incisors and the canine teeth is closed (Fig. 181–4). The resulting occlusal defect is seen in the lower dentition. The lower canine teeth are forced in a forward (rostral) and lingual dissection to maintain their position anterior to the maxillary canine teeth. The resultant crowding of the anterior arch tends to move the lower incisors forward to produce an abnormal occlusion resembling prognathism. Anterior crossbite is also produced as the lower incisors rotate and are displaced in their eruptive efforts. Frequently, the mandibular lateral incisors are impacted and fail to erupt at all. In addition, the attrition produced as a result of striking of the maxillary lateral incisors by the mandibular canine teeth leads to complete destruction of both teeth (Fig. 181–5).

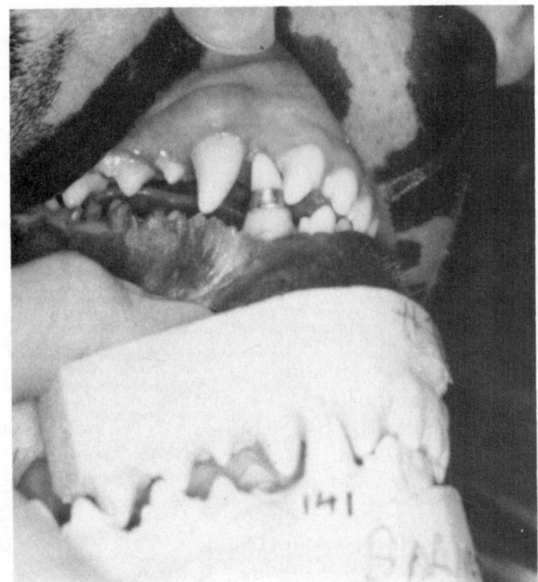

FIGURE 181–3. A model and appliance have been fashioned to correct this "base-narrow" mandibular canine tooth in a dog.

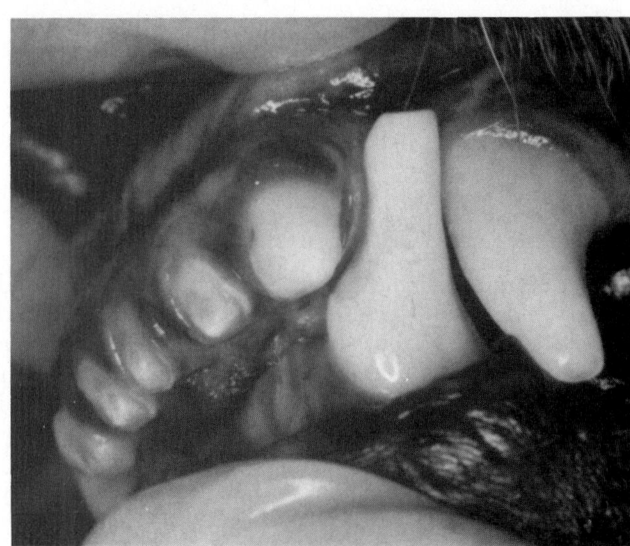

FIGURE 181–5. Attrition produced when the mandibular canine tooth strikes the maxillary lateral incisor can completely destroy both teeth.

Retained deciduous teeth should be extracted *immediately*. One should follow this rule: "Never allow two teeth of the same type to remain in the mouth at the same time."[7] The practitioner cannot wait for the deciduous teeth to fall out, even though the crowns may be loose. The root of the tooth directs the eruption path of the permanent tooth.[2]

INTERCEPTIVE ORTHODONTICS

The term *interceptive orthodontics* refers to instances in which a manifest malocclusion is developing because of hereditary patterns or extrinsic or intrinsic factors. A plan for serial extractions is developed to lessen the severity of the malformation and, in some instances, to eliminate its cause. Properly timed removal of deciduous teeth can allow considerable autonomous adjustment of space available in the dental arches.

In minor differences of jaw length in the young puppy, extraction of the deciduous incisors or canine teeth is often beneficial. This extraction allows the full genetic potential for growth of the mandible and maxilla to be expressed.[7, 10, 13, 18] In selecting teeth for extraction, the guiding principle is to remove those teeth that would interfere with the forward growth of the short jaw and, if possible, to leave those that tend to stop growth when the desired length has been achieved. This problem is referred to as "adverse dental interlock" and can be seen when a growth spurt allows the mandible or maxilla temporary acceleration of its normal growth pattern (Fig. 181–6).[3, 7] If the mandibular canine teeth are positioned caudal to the maxillary canine teeth, the growth pattern of lengthening the jaw proceeds, but the mandible bows ventrally. If the lower canine teeth are not released by extraction, phenotypical "overshoot" results.[19]

Similarly, if an adverse interlock of the maxillary incisors is caudal to the mandibular ones, extraction of the upper deciduous incisors hastens eruption of the permanent incisors and allows them to assume their correct position, rostral to the lower incisors. If the lower incisors are left, the permanent teeth lingual to the upper incisors are forced to assume a normal position. This technique usually results in improvement, if not complete correction, of minor differences in jaw length. All animals are entitled to healthy occlusions, but not all are entitled to perfect occlusions.[19]

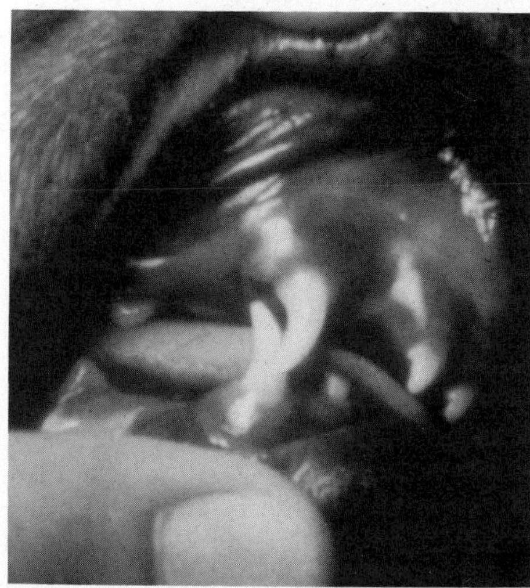

FIGURE 181–6. Adverse dental interlock resulting from accelerated growth of the maxilla. If not corrected by interceptive orthodontics, this condition will interfere with the pet's genetic potential for normal occlusion.

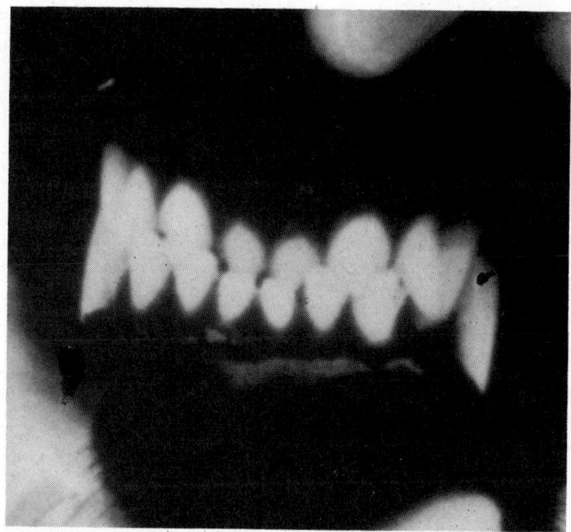

FIGURE 181–7. Class I malocclusion, anterior crossbite, caused by abnormal retention of deciduous incisors.

Shedding of the deciduous dentition is not left to chance but is kept on schedule through extraction of the tooth or teeth that have not been shed on time via normal processes.

MALOCCLUSION

Class I Malocclusion (Neutroclusion)

Class I malocclusion, or neutroclusion, is characterized by irregularities of individual teeth, but with a normal mesiodistal or rostral-caudal relationship of the mandibular and maxillary dental arches. Normal occlusion and class I malocclusion share the same premolar and molar relationship, but differ in the arrangement of the teeth in relation to the line of occlusion. This malocclusion essentially represents dental dysplasia. Rotations, individual tooth malpositions, missing teeth, and tooth size discrepancies fall under this classification (Fig. 181–7).[11, 17] Class I malocclusion is the largest single group of malocclusions.

In class I malocclusions, there is not enough space to accommodate all teeth. This situation may be due to prolonged retention of deciduous teeth, retained root tips of deciduous teeth, micrognathia, and extreme variations in tooth size, as in toy breeds of dogs. Incisors may be rotated or missing, and canine teeth may have insufficient room to erupt into their normal place in the dental arch. Premolars may be rotated or erupted buccally or lingually to the normal positions in the dental arch. For instance, if sufficient bone is not present in the mandibular symphysis, the central incisors start a downward and rostral shift that continues as the dog

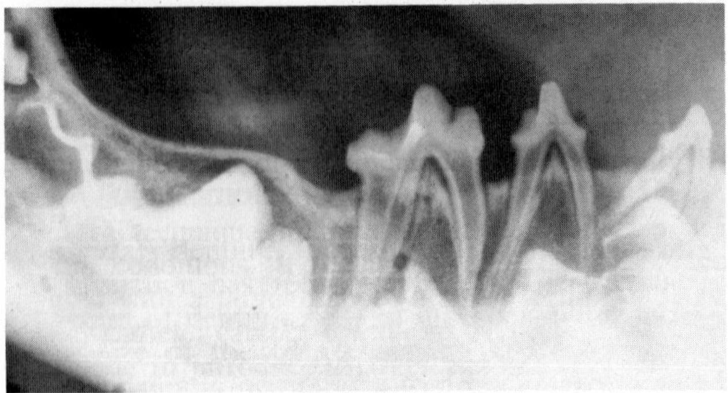

FIGURE 181–8. Permanent teeth in place as early as 6 to 8 weeks of age. This procedure is helpful in those breeds that require a full set of permanent teeth to be eligible for shows.

ages.[18] Not all malocclusions are "surface evident." A large percentage of class I malocclusions occur because of events of the critical developmental weeks, with most of the activity below the surface of the bone and gingiva.

The veterinarian should perform a thorough examination that should include consideration of breed predisposition, size of the dental arch, proper chewing exercises, and radiographic examination to determine the relative position of the permanent teeth as well as the proper number in those breeds that require a full set of teeth. These radiographs can be clinically evaluated in the very young animal well before eruption of the permanent teeth—as early as 6 weeks of age (Fig. 181–8).[8] Interceptive orthodontics including serial extractions can prevent a substantial number of these malocclusions if performed at the proper time.*

Class II Malocclusion (Distoclusion/Brachygnathia)

In class II malocclusion, the upper dental arch is in a rostral or anterior relationship to the lower dental arch, as reflected by the permanent premolars and the permanent canine teeth in the permanent dental arch. The maxillary canine teeth move forward into contact with the caudal edge of the mandibular canine teeth. The upper premolars drift over the top of their mandibular counterparts, and the angle of the mandible increases and moves in front of the condyle. This drift is also referred to as "overshoot" and occurs frequently in dolichocephalic breeds, such as the dachshund, collie, Italian greyhound, and Russian wolfhound (Fig. 181–9).

Brachygnathia, or the lack of growth of the mandible compared with the growth of the maxilla, results in an increase in space between the upper and lower incisors. The mandibular incisors may cause painful pressure necrosis in the maxillary gingiva. In some instances, the mandibular canine teeth are completely caudal and palatal to the maxillary canine teeth. When the mandibular canine teeth change their positions in relation to the upper canine teeth, a severe genetic abnormality is overriding the jaw and allowing the animal to maintain a dental relationship at the expense of the muscles of mastication.[18]

*See references 3, 4, 7, 9, 13, 18, and 19.

Class III Malocclusion (Mesioclusion/Prognathism)

The upper dental arch is caudal or posterior to the lower dental arch in class III malocclusion, as reflected by the molars, premolars, and canine teeth in their permanent dentition.

In describing growth patterns, Ross has presented the following analogy:

> "Consider the bone to be somewhat elastic in response to the interlock of the upper and lower teeth and the forces exerted by elongation growth. If mandibular growth is considered to come from the condylar region and elongation forces the mandibular development down and forward, it is easier to correlate the changes in mandibular form with the genetic abnormalities that produce growth deviations. Therefore, when extra jaw length is inherited, the first change noted is the forward shift of the premolars, canines, and incisors to the extent the interlocking action of the two arches will allow. Beyond that, the following changes begin to occur. The body of the mandible begins to curve ventrally, and there is visible increase in space between the cusp tips of the premolars. The angle of the mandible begins a posterior shift in response to the limitation of forward movement by the lower canine striking the maxillary lateral incisor. The lower incisors shift forward to come to a "cusp to cusp" relationship, referred to as a "level bite" by breeders and show enthusiasts. A strong growth push is required to entirely overcome the resulting dental interlock. When the mandibular canines move either lingual or labial to the maxillary lateral incisors, the genetic problem is a very serious one. The complete extent of the genetic problem is determined by the addition of the degree of anterior displacement, the degree of mandibular curvature, and the amount of distal shift present in the angle of the mandible. To evaluate only a single area (the incisors) leads to erroneous determinations of the genetic potential of individual animals."[18]

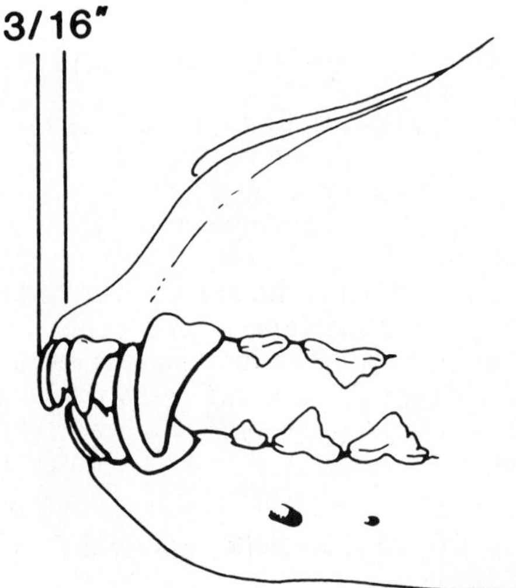

FIGURE 181–9. Class II malocclusion, or "overshoot," is any maxillary protrusion greater than three-sixteenths of an inch. This condition is common in dolichocephalic breeds.

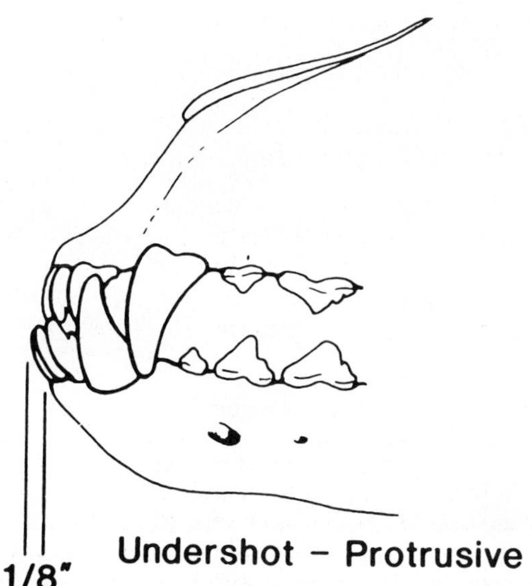

FIGURE 181–10. Class III malocclusion, or "undershoot," is any mandibular protrusion greater than one-eighth of an inch. This condition is normal for most brachycephalic breeds such as boxers and English bulldogs.

Prognathism is normal for brachycephalic breeds of dogs such as boxers and bulldogs, but it is an aberration in mesocephalic and dolichocephalic breeds (Fig. 181–10).

CORRECTIVE ORTHODONTICS—ETHICAL CONSIDERATIONS

The American Kennel Club and most veterinarians consider orthodontic therapy unethical when efforts are made to camouflage genetic malocclusions. At least 50 per cent of all malocclusions are acquired and have no genetic basis.[7, 8, 18] These problems can evolve from something as simple as a puppy's playing "tug-of-war," or a traumatic incident occurring while teeth are still deciduous. A large number of orthodontic problems occur because of retained deciduous teeth or untimely eruption of deciduous teeth.

Because the majority of requests for orthodontics in "show dogs" deal with anterior crossbite of the incisors, particular attention must be paid to the total occlusal relationships of all teeth. Any deviation from normal of the canine, premolar, or molar occlusion in these dogs suggests a genetic cause and precludes orthodontic therapy from ethical practitioners.* If only the incisors are involved and if all other occlusal parameters are normal, trauma, nutrition, disease, and retention of deciduous teeth are potential causes, and orthodontic therapy can be instituted.

PRINCIPLES OF ORTHODONTIC MOVEMENT

Malaligned teeth are moved into a more normal configuration to reduce the abnormal wear from one tooth's striking another, to allow the patient to close its mouth and chew more comfortably, and to reduce the high incidence of periodontal disease in animals with malocclusion. Malocclusions can be corrected at any age.[6] As a rule, the younger the patient, the faster the alterations are completed. Ideally, the 6-month-old to 1-year-old animal is preferred, and most movements can be accomplished in as little as 2 to 16 weeks.[4]

The movement of teeth has three basic prerequisites: sufficient space, adequate pressure, and the necessary anchorage.[11, 17] When constant pressure is applied to a tooth surface, bone is resorbed ahead of the drifting tooth and deposited behind it. This process results from the action of osteoclastic cells that are apparently phagocytic and from the action of osteoblasts. As the alveolus or tooth socket moves, maintaining space for tooth and periodontal membrane, bony reorganization occurs outside the alveolus. Ahead of the moving tooth, trabeculae show resorption on the side nearest the moving tooth, with deposition of bone on the side farthest away. Behind the moving tooth, bone is deposited on the side of the trabeculae nearest the tooth, while bone is resolved on the side away from the tooth to maintain a constant length of the trabecular structure. Constant pressure must be maintained to reposition the tooth properly. Retention of the tooth in its proper position is sometimes necessary for about 4 weeks.

ORTHODONTIC APPLIANCES

Intraoral Appliances

Intraoral appliances can be used successfully to treat malocclusions. Orthodontic acrylic (polymethyl methacrylate) may be used to form an active appliance or may be used as a retainer. It is supplied as a polymer (a powder in various colors) and as a monomer (a liquid). The two materials are mixed in gradual proportions and harden within minutes to form the acrylic appliance. Powder or liquid is added as needed to give the proper consistency. Acrylic appliances are almost always formed on an oral model to prevent thermal damage to the oral tissues during the curing phase, which produces an exothermic reaction. Forming the appliance on a model also allows for a more accurate and easier design of the appliance. Thickness can be altered by adding more liquid or powder, or by removing portions that are too thick with an acrylic bur. Holes can be drilled, wires can be embedded for attachment, and various pressure-producing units, such as expansion or retraction screws or memory finger wires, can be attached or embedded.

Certain acrylics with little exothermic reaction are safe for direct application in the mouth.[7–10]

The most common use of the acrylic appliance is for an inclined bite plane indicated for lingually displaced mandibular canine teeth. After the patient is anesthetized, a thorough dental prophylaxis is performed using a slurry mixture of flour pumice and water as the final polishing material. Fluorides added to pumice interfere with adhesion and are not used when adhesion of an orthodontic appliance is anticipated. Utility wax strips

*See references 3, 7–10, 12, 14, 18, 19, and 20.

are used to make a dam or to outline the area of application of acrylic. The acrylic should encompass the lingual aspect of the incisors, extending just beyond the distal margin of the maxillary canine teeth. A figure-of-eight wire snugly fitting around the canine teeth helps hold the acrylic to the teeth. This wire (20 to 24 gauge) is embedded in the acrylic as it is formed. The acrylic powder and liquid are added slowly and carefully to cover the entire area encompassed by the wax dam. Initially, it is very soft, and overspills are removed with a plastic spatula or a gauze sponge. A buildup of acrylic at the contact points of the lower canine teeth allows the force of mastication to move the teeth along an inclined plane into proper apposition.

Articulation with the acrylic plate must be checked. The patient must be extubated, the tongue retracted, and the mouth closed in a normal, tensionless fashion. This determination is performed before the acrylic sets, when it is still soft. The teeth make an impression into the acrylic, and a groove or inclined plane can be impressed into the soft material to guide the teeth into proper position (Fig. 181–11). After the acrylic has set and is very hard, the material can be further finished or angled with an acrylic bur after the utility wax dam has been removed. Some forward or rostral movement of the displaced canine teeth can be accommodated by grooving the acrylic in a rostral-labial direction to curve around the mesial margin of the maxillary canine teeth.

Direct Bonding

Improved cements and composite bonding techniques allow orthodontic movement through direct application of brackets or bands. The most common orthodontic problem for which this type of therapy is appropriate is

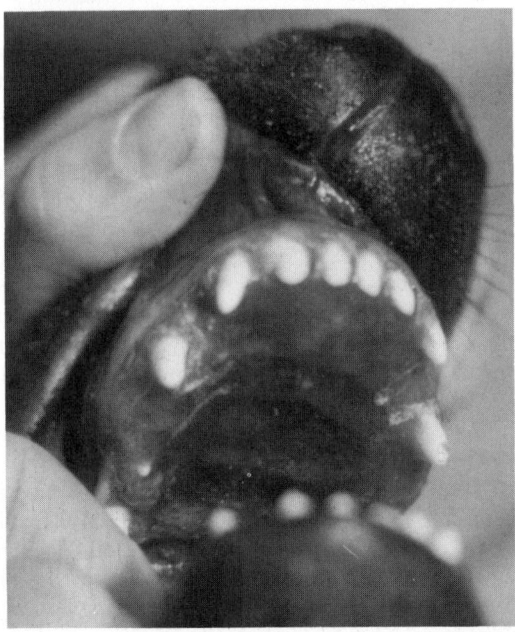

FIGURE 181–11. An inclined acrylic bite plane, in place in the patient's mouth, is used to correct base-narrow mandibular canine teeth.

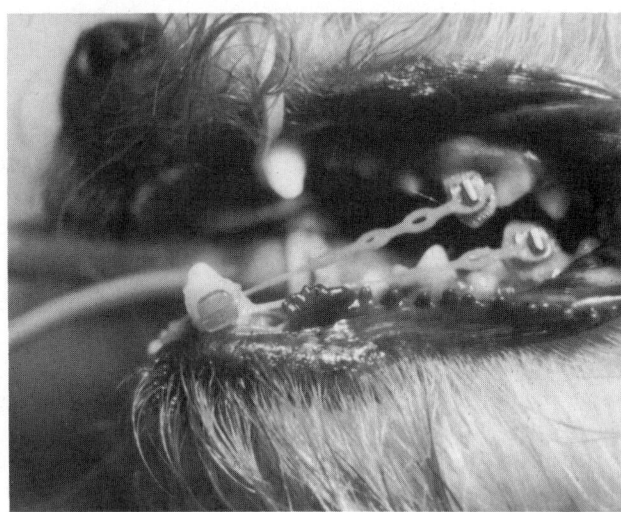

FIGURE 181–12. Brackets have been bonded to the mandibular canine tooth, the upper fourth premolar, and the lower first molar to retrude a protruded canine tooth with a "power chain." The double anchorage is necessary in toy breeds of dogs.

rostral protrusion of the maxillary canine teeth. Occasionally, the rostral protrusion of the mandibular canine teeth can be treated by this approach, and small movements and some rotation of incisors can be accomplished.

The procedures required before adhesion of any appliance, bracket, or band are as follows:

1. Clean the teeth thoroughly, and polish with a slurry of flour pumice and water.
2. Rinse copiously with water, and then dry the tooth with air.
3. Etch the tooth or teeth to be used with unbuffered phosphoric acid (30 to 50 per cent concentration), for 30 to 60 seconds. When properly etched, the tooth has a chalky white appearance.
4. Thoroughly rinse the acid from the teeth, being careful to remove any residue from oral tissues.
5. Dry the teeth with warm air.

A grooved orthodontic bracket or button can be attached to the labial and lingual surfaces of the canine tooth. A similar bracket is attached to the upper fourth premolar and the lower first molar, which are used as the anchor teeth. Attachment of the elastics to each side of the canine tooth produces even retraction without rotation (Fig. 181–12). If there is not enough open contact on the lower first molar to prevent striking by the upper fourth premolar when the mouth is closed, the bracket can be placed on the lingual surface of the molar.

Various elastics can be used in this situation, but most orthodontists prefer the energy chain. This elastic chain, or series of loops, is especially amenable to this procedure. With the chain under no tension, the loops from bracket to bracket are counted. About 75 per cent of this length is stretched and attached to the brackets. With the greater distance being from the maxillary canine tooth to the lower first molar, that length of chain will be greater. It should also be attached with the mouth moderately or halfway open to allow for stretching upon full opening of the mouth.

These elastics are changed at intervals of about 2 weeks because the elasticity is usually lost by then. In addition, the teeth and oral tissues are checked at regular intervals. The owner must adhere to a rigid program of daily oral hygiene and examination of the appliance. Successful outcome depends on full cooperation and compliance by the owner.

Depending on the size and age of the dog, a period of 8 to 12 weeks is required to move a tooth to the new position. Once the tooth is in place, it is retained with ligature wires or an acrylic splint for at least 4 weeks to allow the bone and tissue to reorganize. The same procedure can be used to retrude a rostrally displaced mandibular canine tooth, but results are accomplished much more slowly because of the dense mandibular bone.[3, 8, 12, 18]

Dental Impressions

Indirect applications of orthodontic appliances must be preceded by the development of a working model to enable the veterinarian or the dental laboratory technicians to fabricate the appliance. A good impression of the teeth that can be transformed into a stone model must be obtained and used by the dental technicians to produce a custom appliance for the individual patient. Good, clean, accurate impressions are the first step toward successful therapy.[7]

Impression trays are used to carry the putty-like alginate mixture to the mouth and hold it in position until it sets (Fig. 181–13). A number of prefabricated impression trays that are commercially available are designed especially for the dog and cat.

The most common impression material is dental alginate, which is supplied in fast and regular set. The fast set allows much time for mixing and obtaining an impression. The appropriate-size tray is selected and placed in the mouth to check whether a proper, inclusive impression can be obtained. The patient *must* be totally immobile during the taking of the impression. Any movement results in an altered impression and, subsequently, in an appliance that does not fit properly.[7] A general anesthetic must be used.[5] The alginate is measured exactly according to the manufacturer's instructions and mixed in a rubber mixing bowl. After being mixed to a creamy-smooth consistency, the alginate is placed in the tray, and the tray is placed in the patient's mouth. Once the teeth are set in the impression material, the tray must be held firmly and steadily until the material sets—approximately 2 minutes. The alginate assumes a latex-like consistency and rebounds when pressed. The tray is removed in one brisk movement away from the teeth. Close examination reveals whether a proper impression has been obtained; if not, the process is repeated. If stone models are not poured immediately, a water soaked paper towel is placed in the impression, and the impression put into a resealable plastic bag, to prevent drying and distortion.

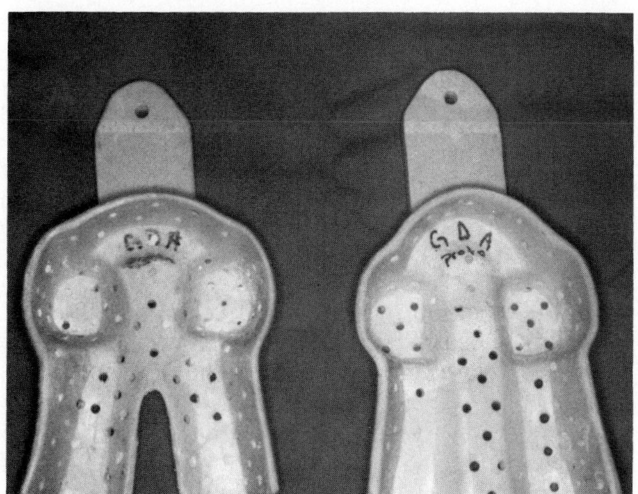

FIGURE 181–13. Custom-made impression trays are needed to fully cover the long canine teeth and irregularly shaped mouths of canine patients.

Stone Model Production

The various stone powders that are available differ in strength, setting time, and ability to reproduce detail. These different types are represented by different colors; pink stone is most often used in animals. Water is added to the stone and mixed in a rubber mixing bowl to produce a smooth, workable consistency. The mixture should flow but not run. The alginate impression, while still in the tray, is placed on an investment vibrator, and small amounts of the stone mixture are flowed into the impression with the vibrator running. The vibration allows more even filling with no trapped air bubbles to distort the model. Additional stone is used to thicken the base of the model, which adds strength and body. Several hours are necessary for the stone to harden, after which the alginate can be carefully removed or cut away (Fig. 181–14). For cases that require a faster setting time, the fast-setting stone is ready to use within approximately 15 minutes. This type of store powder is indicated for construction of an acrylic splint to use for fracture repair.[7]

Fixed Appliances

Once a study model is produced, designing the appliance to address the orthodontic problem is usually a simple task. If consultation is necessary, the model can be sent to a veterinary dental specialist or to a dental laboratory for confirmation of the appropriate therapy. The various types of appliances are as follows:

1. Acrylic splints
2. Expansion or jackscrews
3. Bands with hooks or buttons
4. Memory wires
5. Maryland bridge

The expansion screw is more substantial than the microscrew device and can be used to move one tooth or the entire arch segment.[3, 4] An acrylic plate is fash-

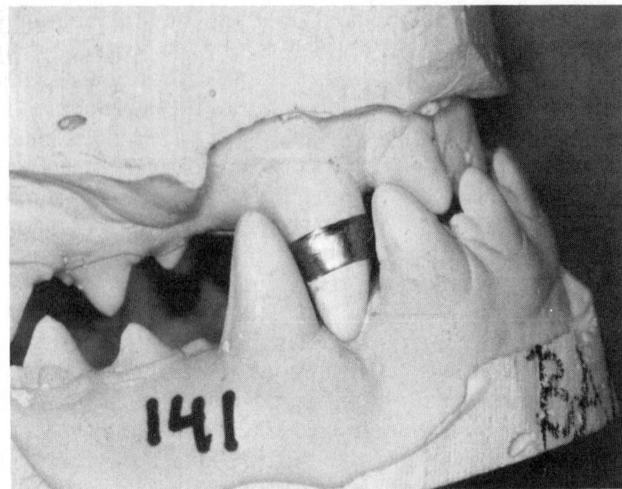

FIGURE 181–14. A stone model fashioned from an alginate impression of the mouth. Note the orthodontic band (a "W" wire appliance) around the lower canine tooth.

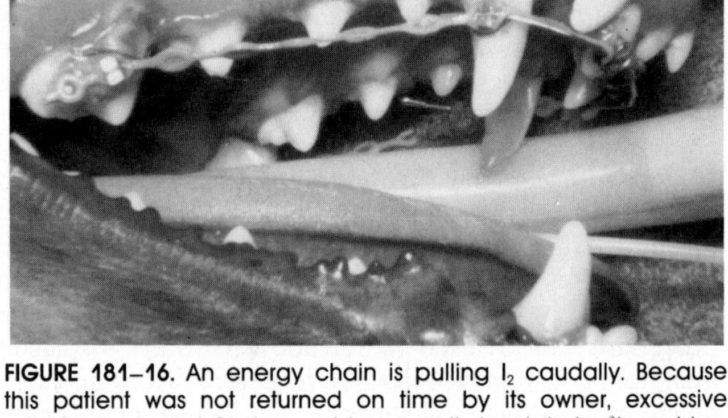

FIGURE 181–16. An energy chain is pulling I_2 caudally. Because this patient was not returned on time by its owner, excessive retrusion occurred. Such a problem usually leads to tooth avulsion. The use of direct bonding techniques with no stops is dangerous for this reason.

ioned to fit around and adhere to the maxillary canine teeth. The rostral segment is in contact with the teeth to be moved. The acrylic plate is sectioned with a diamond disc, and an expansion screw is positioned between the segments and embedded into the acrylic. The screw is positioned so that when the screw is turned once clockwise, it opens the plate by one-quarter of a millimeter. The teeth should move 1 mm in a 2-week period if the appliance screw is given one turn twice weekly. Few anterior crossbite problems need to be corrected more than 2 to 4 mm (Fig. 181–15).

Acrylic can also be used to embed elastic ligature thread (power thread), or to retract a tooth and also act as a stop to prevent the tooth from moving too far caudally. Grooves can be cut into the acrylic to guide the movement of a tooth into a proper position.

Orthodontic bands with hooks or buttons can be constructed on the model to attach the power chain or elastic ligature thread (Fig. 181–16). The advantages of brackets and buttons over direct bonding is that the bands are much more stable and withstand more pressure. They are useful in rotational movements and in retracting rostrally protruded canine teeth.[3, 7]

Memory wires were developed to return to the original shape no matter how much distortion occurred. This wire can be shaped into a "W" configuration and soldered to bands connected to the mandibular canine teeth on the prepared model. When placed and cemented in the patient's mouth, the "W" wire returns to its original shape. The force produced gives an even, steady pressure to move the lingually displaced canine teeth to their normal position. This movement takes place within 2 to 4 weeks in most patients. It does not constrict growth, is easy to construct, and is inexpensive. It is the preferred method of correcting this common malocclusion (Fig. 181–17).[3, 7]

Maryland bridge techniques involve a combination of cast-metal and resin-bonded restorative materials that

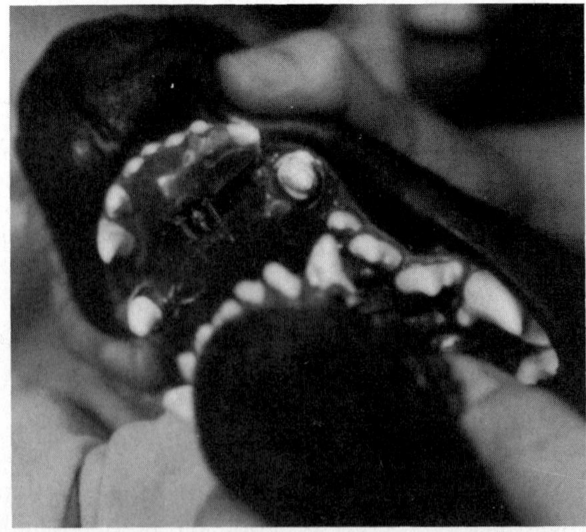

FIGURE 181–15. An acrylic maxillary expansion device, shown in place in the patient's mouth, is used to protrude the incisors in an anterior crossbite malocclusion.

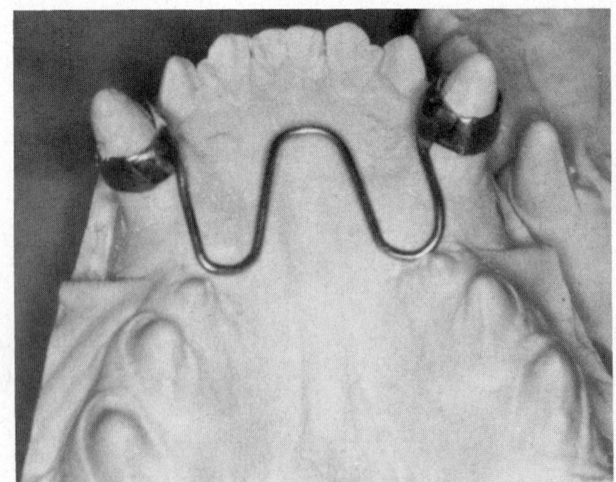

FIGURE 181–17. A "W" wire fashioned on the model of the patient's mouth to correct malocclusion from base-narrow mandibular canine teeth.

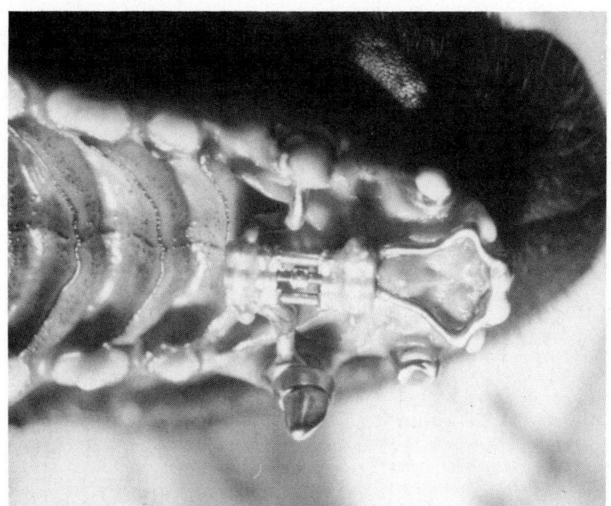

FIGURE 181–18. Maryland bridge technique for expansion of the maxillary incisors. Since the procedure was instituted, the device has been opened approximately 4 mm.

have been used in human dentistry for more than 15 years. Numerous refinements and improvements have been reported.[16] The development of improved composite resins and the substantiation that resin-bonded retainers withstand normal occlusal forces have contributed to the success of these procedures.

The Maryland "wings" are used to clasp or anchor the canine teeth and the appliance. A custom-cast framework of a polished base metal is attached to the wings, and an expansion screw can be fitted on a series of bars to protrude some or all of the maxillary incisors (Fig. 181–18). The Maryland wings are bonded to the canine teeth, and the anterior bands fit over the central incisors.

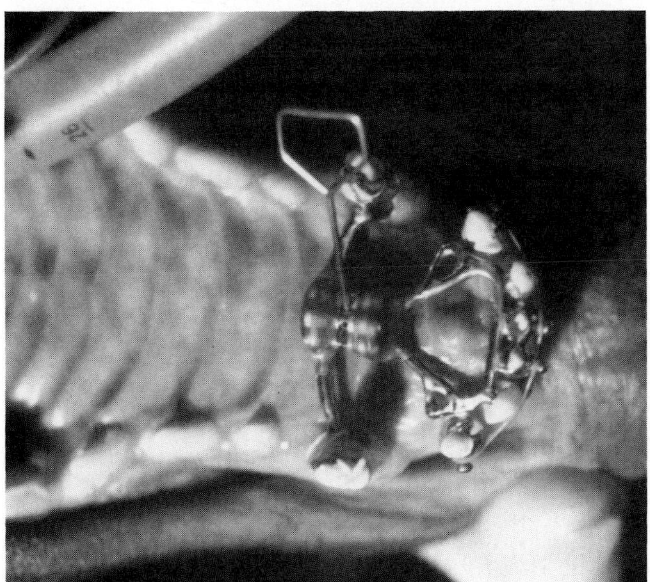

FIGURE 181–19. This Maryland bridge appliance shows the "key" in place to open the expansion screw device. The owner turns the appliance twice a week until the teeth are in place.

A curve in the bar involves the middle incisors. A series of custom-cast bands, with hooks or buttons attached, fit over individual or pairs of incisors, which further enhances the flexibility of the appliance. A retaining bar on the lingual surface of the maxillary incisors can be fitted with hooks or buttons to allow elastics to cause retrusion of lower incisors and prevent their further caudal movement once the incisors come in contact with the bar. The incisors can be retained to ensure proper positioning when the appliance is removed (Fig. 181–19).[4]

The same technique can be applied to moving rostrally displaced canine teeth caudally, by casting the appliance over the first three premolars and connecting them with a series of crossbars. Lingual and buccal hooks or buttons on the appliance are connected to cast bands on the canine teeth, with similar hooks or buttons attached to the lingual and labial surfaces by the energy chain. A guide plane and stop, built into the appliance, assure that the canine teeth move caudally into proper position and no farther. Retention of these teeth for at least 4 to 6 weeks is necessary. For this period of retention, the energy chain can be replaced by retentive wires from the teeth to the appliance.[4]

The appliance is made of light, polished metal that offers little area for food, hair, or other debris to accumulate, and is easily cleaned by brushing and flushing. Proper application to the teeth is essential, and the greatest success in securing these orthodontic appliances is with a composite luting cement or a resin-based cement for resin-bonded retainers.

Factors controlling the successful completion of an orthodontic procedure using the Maryland Bridge technique include the following:

1. A clean and *accurate* impression and model.
2. An accurate, well-made appliance that fits *exactly*.
3. *Strict adherence to technique* in applying cement and seating the appliance.
4. *Full client cooperation* in keeping the appliance clean, adjusting it if necessary, and keeping appointments needed for evaluation and monitoring of the progress of the procedure.

References

1. Angle E: *Treatment of Malocclusion of the Teeth, Angle System.* 1st ed. SS White Dental Manufacturing Company, Philadelphia, 1907.
2. Banks WJ: *Applied Veterinary Histology.* Williams & Wilkins, Baltimore, 1985.
3. Beard GB: Veterinary Dental Orthodontics. Scientific Proceedings, Western Veterinary Conference, Las Vegas, 1988.
4. Beard GB: Anterior Crossbite—Interceptive Orthodontics for Prevention; Maryland Bridge Technique for Correction. Proceedings, Academy of Veterinary Dentistry, New Orleans, 1988.
5. Beard GB: Veterinary dental anesthesiology. *J Vet Dent 7*:1, 1990.
6. Beard GB, Beard DM: Geriatric dentistry. *Vet Clin North Am 19*:1, 1989.
7. Beard GB, et al: Veterinary Dental Seminar, Course IV: Orthodontics. American Animal Hospital Association, 1990.
8. Emily P: Vetodontics notes. School of Veterinary Medicine, Colorado State University, Fort Collins, 1988.
9. Emily P: Veterinary Orthodontics. Scientific Proceedings, Western Veterinary Conference, Las Vegas, 1990.

10. Emily P: Veterinary orthodontics. Scientific proceedings, American Animal Hospital Association, San Francisco, 1990.
11. Graber TM: *Orthodontics: Principles and Practice.* W. B. Saunders, Philadelphia, 1967.
12. Grove JK: Straight facts on crooked teeth. *Vet Forum*, pp 30–31, August 1988.
13. Grove JK: Interceptive orthodontics. *Vet Forum*, p 15, April 1986.
14. Harvey CE: Diseases of the oral cavity. *In* Slatter D (ed): *Textbook of Small Animal Surgery*. W. B. Saunders, Philadelphia, 1985.
15. Hillmann DJ, Littlefield MA: Anatomy notes. Louisiana State University School of Veterinary Medicine, Baton Rouge, 1988.
16. Levine N: *Current Treatment in Dental Practice.* W. B. Saunders, Philadelphia, 1986.
17. Proffit WR: *Contemporary Orthodontics.* C. V. Mosby, St. Louis, 1986.
18. Ross DL: Orthodontics for the dog. *Vet Clin North Am 16*:5, 1986.
19. Ross DL: The oral cavity. *In* Kirk RW (ed): *Current Veterinary Therapy VI.* W. B. Saunders, Philadelphia, 1977.
20. Zetner K, Eisenmenger E: *Veterinary Dentistry*. Lea & Febiger, Philadelphia, 1985.

APPENDIX

Normal Laboratory Values for the Dog and Cat

By
George M. Peavy, DVM
Diplomate, American Board of Veterinary Practitioners,

Lon J. Rich, DVM, PhD
Diplomate, American College of Veterinary Pathology, and

Embert H. Coles, DVM, PhD
Professor Emeritus, Kansas State University

HEMATOLOGICAL VALUES

	Units	Dog	Cat
Erythrocytes (RBC)	$\times 10^6/\mu l$	5.5–8.5	7.5–10.5
Hemoglobin (Hb)	g/dl	12–18	10–15
Hematocrit (PCV)*	%	37–55	30–45
Mean corpuscular volume (MCV)	fL	60–77	39–55
Mean corpuscular Hb (MCH)	pg	19–25	13–17
Mean corpuscular Hb concentration (MCHC)	g/dl	32–36	32–36
Reticulocyte	%	0–1	0–2
RBC life span	days	120	70
RBC diameter	μ	6.7–7.2	5.5–6.3
Platelet count	$\times 10^3/\mu l$	200–500	200–500
Leukocytes (WBC)	$\times 10^3/\mu l$	6.0–17.0	5.5–19.5
Band/Neutrophils	%	0–3	0–3
	$\times 10^3/\mu l$	0–0.3	0–0.3
Segmented/Neutrophils	%	60–77	35–75
	$10^3/\mu l$	3.0–11.5	2.5–12.5
Lymphocytes	%	12–30	20–55
	$\times 10^3/\mu l$	1.0–4.8	1.5–7.0
Monocytes	%	3–10	1–4
	$\times 10^3/\mu l$	0.15–1.5	0–0.85
Eosinophils	%	2–10	2–12
	$\times 10^3/\mu l$	0.1–1.0	0–1.0
Basophils	%	rare	rare
	$\times 10^3/\mu l$	rare	rare
Total Blood Volume	ml/kg	80—90	60–66

From Jain NC: Schalm's Veterinary Hematology. 4th ed. Lea & Febiger, Philadelphia, 1986.
*Lower in young animals; higher range in greyhounds. Manual (centrifuge) method will be slightly higher than automated methods.

BLOOD CHEMISTRIES AND ELECTROLYTES

	Dog		Cat	
Test	***Traditional Units***	***S.I. Units***	***Traditional Units***	***S.I. Units***
ACTH	20–100 pg/dl	4.4–22 pmol/L*	20.0–61 pg/dl	4.4–13.4 pmol/l†
Alkaline phosphatase	20–200 IU/L	20–200 U/L	20–220 IU/L	20–220 U/L
ALT (SGPT)	10–90 IU/L	10–90 U/L	10–80 IU/L	10–80 U/L
Ammonia	19–120 μg/dl	11–70.5 μmol/l		
Amylase	250–3000 IU/L	250–3000 U/L	100–2000 IU/L	100–2000 U/L
APTT	14–18 seconds		18–22 seconds	
AST (SGOT)	10–90 IU/L	10–90 U/L	10–80 IU/L	10–80 U/L
Bicarbonate (HCO_3)‡	18–24 mEq/L	18–24 μmol/L	17–21 mEq/L	17–21 μmol/L
Bile acids				
Fasting	0.78–1.1 μg/ml	1.9–2.7 μmol/L	0.6–0.8 μg/ml	1.5–2.0 μmol/L
2 hours postprandial	2.4–4.3 μg/ml	6.0–10.6 μmol/L	3.1–3.7 μg/ml	7.5–9.1 μmol/L

Table continued on following page

BLOOD CHEMISTRIES AND ELECTROLYTES *Continued*

Test	Dog		Cat	
	Traditional Units	*S.I. Units*	*Traditional Units*	*S.I. Units*
Bilirubin				
Direct	0.0–0.3 mg/dl	0.0–5.1 μmol/L	0.0–0.3 mg/dl	0.0–5.1 μmol/L
Indirect	0.1–0.3 mg/dl	1.7–5.1 μmol/L	0.0–0.3 mg/dl	0.1–5.1 μmol/L
Total	0.1–0.6 mg/dl	1.7–10.2 μmol/L	0.1–0.6 mg/dl	1.7–10.2 μmol/L
BUN	10–25 mg/dl	3.6–8.9 mmol/L	10–30 mg/dl	3.6–10.7 mmol/L
Calcium	8.5–11.0 mg/dl	2.2–2.8 mmol/L	8.2–10.5 mg/dl	2.0–2.6 mmol/L
Chloride	105–116 mEq/L	105–116 mmol/L	115–125 mEq/L	115–125 mEq/L
Cobalamin (Vitamin B_{12})§	300–800 ng/L		200–1680 ng/L	
Cholesterol (Total)	120–255 mg/dl	3.1–6.6 mmol/L	90–200 mg/dl	2.3–5.2 mmol/L
Cholinesterase	2000–4000 IU/L	2000–4000 U/L	2000–4000 IU/L	2000–4000 U/L
CO_2 (Total)	18–24 mEq/L	18–24 mmol/L	8–24 mEq/L	18–24 mmol/L
Pco_2 (Partial pressure) ‖	38 mmHg	5.1 kPa	36 mm Hg	4.8 kPa
Cortisol (RIA)	1.0–5.0 μg/dl	0.03–0.14 μmol/L	0.1–3.5 μg/dl	0.0–0.1 μmol/L
CK (CPK)	20–120 IU/L	20–120 U/L	20–120 IU/L	20–120 U/L
Creatinine	1.0–2.2 mg/dl	88.4–194.5 μmol/L	0.8–2.0 mg/dl	70.7–176.8 μmol/L
Folate§	7.5–17.5 μ/L		13.4–38 μg/L	
Fibrinogen	100–400 mg/dl	1–4 g/L	100–400 mg/dl	1–4 g/L
Glucose	60–120 mg/dL	3.3–6.6 mmol/L	75–160 mg/dl	4.1–8.8 mmol/L
GGT (γ-glutamyltransferase)	1–10 IU/L	1–10 IU/L	1–10 U/L	1–10 IU/L
Immunoglobulins				
IgA	20–150 mg/dl	0.2–1.5 G/L	60–350 mg/dl	0.6–3.5 G/L
IgM	70–270 mg/dl	0.7–2.7 G/L	100–200 mg/dl	1.0–2.0 G/L
IgG	1000–2000 mg/dl	10–20 G/L	1000–2000 mg/dl	10–20 G/L
Insulin	<20 μU/ml	<145 pmol/L		
Iron ‖	30–180 μg/dl	5.37–32.2 μmol/L	68–215 μg/dl	12.2–38.5 μmol/L
Iron binding				
Capacity (Total)§	165–418 μg/dl	29.5–74.9 μmol/L		
Capacity (Unbound)§	170–222 μg/dl	30.4–39.7 μmol/L		
LDH ‖	45–233 IU/L	45–233 U/L	63–273 IU/L	63–273 U/L
Lipase	25–800 IU/L	25–800 U/L	25–250 IU/L	25–250 U/L
O_2 pressure ‖	85–100 mm Hg	11–13 kPa	78–100 mm Hg	10–13 kPa
Parathormone (PTH)	10–33 pg/dl			
Ph ‖	7.31–7.42		7.24–7.40	
Phosphorus	2.2–5.6 mg/dl	0.7–1.8 mmol/l	2.0–6.5 mg/dl	0.6–2.1 mmol/L
Potassium	3.6–5.8 mEq/L	3.6–5.8 mmol/L	3.7–4.6 mEq/L	3.7–4.6 mmol/L
Protein (Total) ‖	5.4–7.1 g/dl	54–71 g/L	5.4–7.8 g/dl	54–78 g/L
Albumin ‖	2.6–3.3 g/dl	26–33 g/L	2.1–3.3 g/dl	21–33 g/L
Globulins ‖	2.7–4.4 g/dl	27–44 g/L	2.6–5.1 g/dl	26–51 g/L
α_1	0.2–0.5 g/dl	2.0–5.0 g/L	0.2–1.1 g/dl	2–11 g/L
α_2	0.3–1.1 g/dl	3.0–11 g/L	0.4–0.9 g/dl	4.0–9.0 g/L
β_1	0.7–1.3 g/dl	7.0–13.0 g/L	0.3–0.9 g/dl	3.0–9.0 g/L
β_2	0.6–1.4 g/dl	6.0–14.0 g/L	0.6–1.0 g/dl	6.0–10.0 g/L
γ_1	0.5–1.3 g/dl	5.0–13.0 g/L	0.3–2.5 g/dl	3.0–25.0 g/L
γ_2	0.4–0.9 g/dl	4.0–9.0 g/L	1.4–1.9 g/dl	14–19.0 g/L
A/G ratio	0.4–1.6		0.9–2.6	
Prothrombin time	8–11 seconds		9–12 seconds	
SGOT (AST)	10–90 IU/L	10–90 U/L	10–80 IU/L	10–80 U/L
SGPT (ALT)	10–90 IU/L	10–90 U/L	10–80 IU/L	10–80 IU/L
Thrombin time	5–8 seconds		5–9 seconds	
Thyroid				
T_3 (RIA)	100–200 ng/dl	1.5–3.1 nmol/L	75–150 ng/dl	1.2–2.3 nmol/L
T_4 (RIA)	1.5–4.5 μg/dl	19.3–57.9 nmol/L	1.0–3.0 μg/dl	12.9–38.6 nmol/L
Free T_4 (RIA)	0.9–3.5 ng/dl	71.1–276–5 pmol/L	0.9–2.5 ng/dl	71.1–197.5 pmol/L
TLI (trypsin-like-immunoreactivity)¶	3.2–3.5 μg/L			
Urea nitrogen	10–25 mg/dl	3.6–8.9 mmol/L	10–30 mg/dl	3.6–10.7 mmol/L
Uric acid	0–2.0 mg/L	0–0.12 mmol/L	0–1.0 mg/L	0–0.06 mmol/L

Normal blood chemistry values vary between laboratories, depending on instrumentation and biochemical procedures. Standardized values are established by each individual laboratory.

*Data from Feldman EC, et al: Plasma adrenocorticotropin levels in normal dogs. *Am J Vet Res 38*:1643, 1977.

†Data from Smith MC, Feldman EC: Plasma endogenous ACTH concentrations and plasma cortisol responses to synthetic ACTH and dexamethasone sodium phosphate in healthy cats. *Am J Vet Res 48*:1719, 1987.

‡Data from Coles EH: *Veterinary Clinical Pathology*. 4th ed. W. B. Saunders, Philadelphia, 1986.

§Data from Meyer DJ, et al: *Veterinary Laboratory Medicine—Interpretation and Diagnosis*. W. B. Saunders, Philadelphia, 1991.

‖ Data from Kaneko JJ: *Clinical Biochemistry of Domestic Animals*. 4th ed. Academic Press, San Diego, 1989.

¶Data from Williams DA, Batt RM: Sensitivity and specificity of radioimmunoassay of serum trypsin-like immunoreactivity for the diagnosis of canine exocrine pancreatic insufficiency. *J Am Vet Med Assoc 192*:195, 1988.

CEREBROSPINAL FLUID

Test	Dog	Cat
Appearance	Clear, colorless	Clear, colorless
Specific gravity	1.0003–1.0006	1.003–1.006
Total protein	<25 mg/dl	<25 mg/dl
Globulin tests		
Pandy's test	Negative	Negative
Nonne-Apelt (Ross Jones)	Negative	Negative
Glucose	40–80 mg/dl 2.2–4.4 mmol/L 60% to 70% of blood glucose level	40–80 mg/dL 2.2–4.4 mmol/L 60% to 70% of blood glucose level
Cell count		
WBC	0–5/μl	0–5/μl
RBC	0–5/μl	0–5/μl
Cell type	Predominantly small lymphocytes, rare large mononuclear cells	Predominantly small lymphocytes, rare large mononuclear cells

Data from Coles EH: *Veterinary Clinical Pathology*. 4th ed. W. B. Saunders, Philadelphia, 1986.

SYNOVIAL FLUID

Test	Canine
Amount (ml)	0.01–1.00
pH	7–7.8
Erythrocytes ($\times 10^3/\mu l$)	0–320.0
Total leukocytes ($\times 10^3/\mu l$)	0–2.9
Neutrophils/μl	0–32
Monocytes/μl	0–838
Lymphocytes/μl	0–2436
Clasmatocytes/μl	0–166
Mucin clot	Tight, ropy clump Clear supernatant

From Sawyer DC: Synovial fluid of canine joints. *J Am Vet Med Assoc 143*:609, 1963.

URINE

	Dog	Cat
Specific gravity		
Minimum	1.001	1.001
Maximum	1.060	1.080
Usual limits	1.015–1.045	1.015–1.045
pH	6.0–7.0	6.0–7.0
Protein	0–Trace	0–Trace
Glucose	0	0
Ketones	0	0
Occult blood	0	0
Bilirubin	0–1	0–1
Urobilinogen		
Emlich Unit	1	1
Wallace and Diamond	<1:32	<1:32
Protein-creatinine ratio	<1*†	<0.7‡
Cortisol-creatinine ratio§	6–20	
Fractional clearance ‖		
Sodium	0–0.7%	0.24–0.96%
Potassium	0–20%	6.7–23.9%
Chloride	0–0.8%	0.41–1.33%
Calcium	0–0.4%	0.01–0.13%‡
Phosphorus	3–39%	17–73%

Data from Coles EH: *Veterinary Clinical Pathology*. 4th ed. W. B. Saunders, Philadelphia, 1986; and Osborne CA, et al: *Canine and Feline Urology*. W. B. Saunders, Philadelphia, 1972.

*Data from Grauer GF, et al: Estimation of quantitative proteinuria in the dog, using the protein-to-creatinine ratio from a random, voided sample. *Am J Vet Res 46*:2116, 1985.

†Data from White JV, et al: Use of protein to creatinine ratio in a single urine specimen for quantitative estimation of canine proteinuria. *J Am Vet Med Assoc 185*:88, 1984.

‡Data from Meyer DJ, et al: *Veterinary Laboratory Medicine—Interpretation and Diagnosis*. W. B. Saunders, Philadelphia, 1991.

§Data from Smiley LE, Peterson ME: Urinary corticosteroid/creatinine ratio as a screening test for canine hyperadrenocorticism. *Vet Int Med 4*:113, 1990.

‖ Data from Chew PJ, DiBartola SP: Diagnosis and pathophysiology of renal disease. *In* Ettinger SJ (ed): *Textbook of Veterinary Internal Medicine*. 3rd ed. W. B. Saunders, Philadelphia, 1989.

References

1. Chew PJ, DiBartola SP: Diagnosis and pathophysiology of renal disease. *In* Ettinger SJ (ed): *Textbook of Veterinary Internal Medicine.* 3rd ed. W. B. Saunders, Philadelphia, 1989.
2. Coles EH: *Veterinary Clinical Pathology.* 4th ed. W. B. Saunders, Philadelphia, 1986.
3. Feldman EC, et al: Plasma adrenocorticotropin levels in normal dogs. *Am J Vet Res 38*:1643, 1977.
4. Grauer GF, et al: Estimation of quantitative proteinuria in the dog, using the protein-to-creatinine ratio from a random, voided sample. *Am J Vet Res 46*:2116, 1985.
5. Jain NC: *Schalm's Veterinary Hematology.* 4th ed. Lea & Febiger, Philadelphia, 1986.
6. Kaneko JJ: *Clinical Biochemistry of Domestic Animals.* 4th ed. Academic Press, San Diego, 1989.
7. Meyer, DJ, et al: *Veterinary Laboratory Medicine—Interpretation and Diagnosis.* W. B. Saunders, Philadelpha, 1991.
8. Osborne CA, et al: *Canine and Feline Urology.* W. B. Saunders, Philadelphia, 1972.
9. Sawyer DC: Synovial fluid of canine joints, *J Am Vet Med Assoc 143*:609, 1963.
10. Smiley LE, Peterson ME: Urinary corticosteroid/creatinine ratio as a screening test for canine hyperadrenocorticism. *J Vet Int Med 4*:113, 1990.
11. Smith MC, Feldman EC: Plasma endogenous ACTH concentrations and plasma cortisol responses to synthetic ACTH and dexamethasone sodium phosphate in healthy cats. *Am J Vet Res 48*:1719, 1987.
12. White JV, et al: Use of protein to creatinine ratio in a single urine specimen for quantitative estimation of canine proteinuria. *J Am Vet Med Assoc 185*:88, 1984.
13. Williams DA, Batt RM: Sensitivity and specificity of radioimmunoassay of serum trypsin-like immunoreactivity for the diagnosis of canine exocrine pancreatic insufficiency. *Am Vet Med Assoc 192*:195, 1988.

Index

Note: Page numbers in *italics* refer to illustrations. Page numbers followed by t indicate tables.